COLOR ATLAS
AND TEXTBOOK OF
Diagnostic Microbiology

COLOR ATLAS AND TEXTBOOK OF
Diagnostic Microbiology

FIFTH EDITION

Elmer W. Koneman, M.D.
Section Chief, Microbiology Laboratory
Department of Pathology
Veterans Affairs Medical Center
Professor of Pathology
University of Colorado School of Medicine
Denver, Colorado

Stephen D. Allen, M.D.
Professor of Pathology
Indiana University School of Medicine
Director, Division of Clinical Microbiology
Indiana University Hospitals
Clinical Microbiologist
Wishard Memorial Hospital and
Roudebush Veterans Affairs Hospital
Indianapolis, Indiana

William M. Janda, Ph.D.
Associate Professor of Pathology
Associate Director, Clinical Microbiology Laboratory
The University of Illinois
College of Medicine at Chicago
Chicago, Illinois

Paul C. Schreckenberger, Ph.D., M.S.
Associate Professor of Pathology
Director, Clinical Microbiology Laboratory
The University of Illinois
College of Medicine at Chicago
Chicago, Illinois

Washington C. Winn, Jr., M.D., M.B.A.
Professor of Pathology
University of Vermont College of Medicine
Director, Clinical Microbiology Laboratory
Fletcher Allen Health Care
Burlington, Vermont

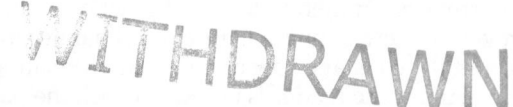

LIPPINCOTT WILLIAMS & WILKINS
A **Wolters Kluwer** Company

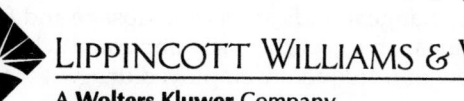

Philadelphia · Baltimore · New York · London
Buenos Aires · Hong Kong · Sydney · Tokyo

Acquisitions Editor: Andrew Allen
Editorial Assistant: Holly Collins
Project Editor: Susan Deitch
Production Manager: Helen Ewan
Production Coordinator: Kathryn Rule
Design Coordinator: Kathy Kelley-Luedtke

Fifth Edition

9   8   7   6   5

Library of Congress Cataloging-in-Publication Data

Color atlas and textbook of diagnostic microbiology / Elmer W. Koneman
    . . . [et al.]. — 5th ed.
      p.   cm.
    Includes bibliographical references and index.
    ISBN 0-397-51529-4
    1. Diagnostic microbiology—Atlases.   I. Koneman, Elmer W., 1932–

QR67.C64   1997
616'.01—dc21   96–37818
                                                                  CIP

Care has been taken to confirm the accuracy of the information presented
and to describe generally accepted practices. However, the authors,
editors, and publisher are not responsible for errors or omissions or for
any consequences from application of the information in this book and
make no warranty, express or implied, with respect to the contents of the
publication.

The authors, editors and publisher have exerted every effort to ensure
that drug selection and dosage set forth in this text are in accordance
with current recommendations and practice at the time of publication.
However, in view of ongoing research, changes in government regulations, and the constant flow of information relating to drug therapy and
drug reactions, the reader is urged to check the package insert for each
drug for any change in indications and dosage and for added warnings
and precautions. This is particularly important when the recommended
agent is a new or infrequently employed drug.

Some drugs and medical devices presented in this publication have Food
and Drug Administration (FDA) clearance for limited use in restricted
research settings. It is the responsibility of the health care provider to
ascertain the FDA status of each drug or device planned for use in their
clinical practice.

PREFACE

Users of previous editions of the *Color Atlas and Textbook of Diagnostic Microbiology* will immediately recognize that this fifth edition is larger. The increase in physical dimensions is consistent with that of other major textbooks, providing the advantage that illustrations and tables can be more effectively displayed in a larger page format. The increase in page number reflects a conservative culling of new information from a database that has continued to expand exponentially since the last edition.

The information in each of the 21 chapters in this text has been painstakingly revised. Numerous developments have taken place in the taxonomic classification and nomenclature of the clinically significant microbes since the publication of the fourth edition. In response to these changes, the hundreds of time-honored and new methods required for the isolation and identification of an ever-expanding array of microbes have been carefully evaluated, extensively revised, and updated. Of primary importance, a keen focus on the biochemical and physiological properties unique to each family, genus, and species of clinically relevant microorganisms has been retained in this text—fundamentals that nevertheless have been interwoven with recent applications of genetic principles and molecular techniques that offer a broader understanding of microbial life. The practical approaches to aid students and experienced laboratorians in the recognition of microorganisms and the diseases they cause are basic to this text.

A brief inventory of several chapters is in order. Chapter 1 is new, combining some of the information relative to new technologies presented in Chapter 21 of the fourth edition but adding sections on basic bacterial morphology and physiology. At the other end of the spectrum are expanded sections on the fundamentals and practical applications of molecular amplification techniques, including polymerase chain reaction, branched DNA assays, ribotyping, and nucleic acid sequencing. Chapters 2 and 3 provide an expanded view of current practices in the collection, transport, and laboratory work-up of clinical specimens and the array of infectious diseases by organ systems as related to the bacterial species identified in the clinical laboratory.

Chapter 4, The *Enterobacteriaceae*, includes information on 121 species and groups belonging to this family, including the presentation of eight new *Citrobacter* species and four new unnamed species formerly considered to be *Proteus vulgaris*. Three new color plates have been designed, and the most recent CDC tables of biochemical reactions are included. Chapter 5 includes an all new guide for the identification of glucose nonfermenting gram-negative rods and the most recent nomenclature changes and new species of this diverse group of bacteria. A new table in Chapter 6 lists the differential characteristics for 30 *Campylobacter*, *Arcobacter*, and *Helicobacter* species, including seven new *Campylobacter* species.

Chapter 7 on *Haemophilus* species includes descriptions of the *H. influenzae* type b vaccines and expanded discussions relative to emerging organisms and diseases, such as Brazilian purpuric fever and the recently described "cryptic genospecies" of haemophili found in the genital tract. Chapter 8 encompasses the miscellaneous, fastidious gram-negative bacilli, including an expanded discussion of organisms belonging to the genus *Bartonella* and its role in cat scratch disease and infections in immunocompromised hosts. Chapter 9 is an expanded discussion on the genus *Legionella* and related organisms. Chapter 10, on the family *Neisseriaceae*, includes complete discussions of the traditional pathogenic species and new *Neisseria* species that have been recently described, such as *N. weaveri* and *N. elongata* subspecies. Staphylococci and related organisms are presented in Chapter 11, with updates on newly described species and new methods for identifying and characterizing these organisms. Chapter 12 presents an expanded discussion of the streptococci and an update on clinically important vancomycin-resistant enterococci and "*Streptococcus*-like" bacteria, such as leuconostocs and pediococci. This chapter also includes a complete update on several newly described viridans streptococci and "streptococcus-like" genera, including *Vagococcus, Globicatella, Lactococcus,* and *Tetragenococcus*.

Chapter 15, Antimicrobial Susceptibility Testing, provides an expanded discussion of the mechanisms of antimicrobial resistance and the implications that expanding resistance has for laboratory testing and

v

treatment of patients. Computer-generated figures are used to explain these resistance mechanisms with utmost clarity.

In Chapter 16, several new AIDS-associated *Mycoplasma* species are presented in some detail. Chapter 17 includes much new information on mycobacteria species, particularly on the new molecular techniques being applied to the direct detection of antigen in clinical specimens, the culture confirmation of clinically significant species, and genetic approaches to antimycobacterial susceptibility testing. Clinical information relevant to each species is separated out in color-shaded correlation boxes for easy access.

Significant format changes have been made to the chapters on Mycology and Parasitology. Line drawings have been added to accompany the scores of photomicrographs to better depict the microscopic morphology of clinically significant fungi. These photomicrographs and accompanying illustrations are now interwoven within the text, making it easier for the reader to cross-check essential information. Illustrated and color-shaded life cycles of the clinically significant parasites have brought new life and expanded information to this chapter. The clinical information relevant to these parasites has been set off in separate color-highlighted correlation boxes to facilitate learning. An expanded presentation on the free-living amoeba and a new section on ectoparasites bring the Parasitology chapter to full completeness.

In Chapter 21, coverage of newly recognized or emphasized infectious agents (including prions, Ebola virus, and other filoviruses, arenaviruses, and hantaviruses) has been added to the wealth of information revised from the fourth edition. A discussion of the newly recognized *Ehrlichia* species also brings this chapter to completeness.

Thus, the fifth edition of the *Color Atlas and Textbook of Diagnostic Microbiology* is more colorful than ever. The modern, new cover design, liberal use of color illustrations throughout, and the many color-shaded boxes containing essential information are in keeping with the up-to-date status of the text. The larger physical size of the book not only allowed larger magnification of the color images but also made it necessary to replace almost all the photographs. The procedure charts have been collated alphabetically in the back of the text for easy access, regardless of which chapter the technique is cited in. The references cited at the end of each chapter are extensive and up-to-date, with a high percentage being published since the previous edition. The index is designed in great detail, with the use of extensive subtopics so that point pieces of information can be immediately cross-referenced to the appropriate pages on which they appear.

Repeating the last two paragraphs from the Preface to the fourth edition, we again pause to acknowledge the major contributions made by our retired or departed coauthors of previous editions. The spirit of the late V.R. Dowell, Jr. continues in this text. All who use this text will be enriched by the insight he provided in guiding us through the maze of nonfermenters and fastidious gram-negative bacilli, as presented in the first and second editions, at a time when meaningful algorithms and identification schema were first evolving. And, of course, we acknowledge his vast knowledge of anaerobic bacteria, which continues to lend such vibrancy to the revised Chapter 14 in this edition.

Our continued best wishes to our emeritus author, Herbert M. Sommers, M.D., whose general support and encouragement were instrumental in bringing the first three editions to fruition. His vast practical experience continues to shine through the chapters on gram-positive cocci, mycobacteria, and antimicrobial susceptibility testing, for which he made major contributions in the past. The spirits of Drs. Dowell and Sommers will never disappear as long as this *Color Atlas and Textbook of Diagnostic Microbiology* remains a viable entity and as long as the current authors, who knew them so well, have the privilege of transmitting their spirit of inquiry and clarity of scientific thought to those, present and future, who have a great thirst for learning.

With this, we leave the fascinating study of microbiology to the users of this text. Microbiology is no longer a simple discipline, and the emergence of AIDS, organ transplant programs, and the longevity of patients with various debilitating diseases make virtually every bacterial species presented in this text a potential pathogen. We have opted to tell the story as it is in all of its array rather than attempting to select what we feel may be important or what may meet the needs of every potential user of this text. We pass the challenge to the hundreds of teachers and faculty of taking this material and presenting it to each contingent of students as best fits their needs. We invite your feedback and appreciate the counsel and encouragement received from many of you in the past to make this text beyond what has been accomplished before.

ACKNOWLEDGMENTS

Special acknowledgments are given to Jean A. Siders for outstanding contributions to the chapter on Anaerobic Bacteriology, to the extent that she should be considered a coauthor of that chapter; to Fred Westenfield, MT(ASCP)SM, who contributed the significant Ectoparasite section to the Parasitology chapter; and to Debra Reardon, MT(ASCP) for major contributions to the revisions in the chapter on Antimicrobial Susceptibility Testing.

Recognition is also given to Jean A. Siders, MT (ASCP), MS, Ed Harris, MT (ASCP), MS, and Linda Marler, MT (ASCP), MS, for their assistance with the Gram-Positive Bacillus chapter and to Robin Martin, Kaye Pinkston, and Linda Wolters, MT(ASCP) for clerical assistance. Special recognition is also given to George Buckley (now deceased), who provided several illustrations included in Chapter 3.

We also express appreciation to the medical technologists and microbiologists who staff the microbiology laboratories at the Denver Veterans Affairs Hospital, the University of Colorado Hospital, the Indiana University Medical Center Hospitals, the University of Illinois/Chicago Hospital, and Fletcher Allen Health Care and also to the clinical pathology residents who rotate through these services. They collectively have provided both direct support and encouragement in countless ways to the authors, and indirect support by covering the day-to-day activities of laboratory practice during the innumerable hours when their chiefs were preoccupied with computer screens, library searches, and the review of galley proofs. Their input is reflected in much of the current information included in this text. We also appreciate the curbstone and written suggestions from medical technologists, pathologists and others for bringing improvements in materials presented in previous chapters.

CONTENTS

* With a contribution by Fred W. Westenfeld.

LIST OF COLOR PLATES

BASIC BACTERIOLOGY, CONCEPTS OF VIRULENCE, AND TECHNOLOGIC ADVANCES IN CLINICAL MICROBIOLOGY:
AN OVERVIEW

INTRODUCTION

Over the three centuries that have passed since Leeuwenhoek first observed bacteria and protozoa with his primitive microscope, a vast amount of knowledge has been accumulated about the small "animalcules" now collectively known as microorganisms. Microorganisms are found in all environments, including the soil, water, and air. They participate in all the vital life functions that are observed in higher, more complex life forms. These organisms are found in association with the nonliving environment and with other living things, including plants, animals, and humans. By their activities in these environments, microorganisms contribute immeasurably to the balance that allows all life to flourish. By studying microorganisms, the mechanisms of many life processes that occur in all forms of life have been elucidated. The role of microorganisms in nature and their contributions to the biologic and ecologic cycles that maintain the delicate balances within our environment are only now beginning to be fully appreciated. By necessity, the subsequent chapters in this text deal with the relatively small number of microorganisms that are capable of causing pathology and disease in humans. The story of pathogenic microorganisms—their morphology, physiology, biochemistry, and interactions as agents of infectious diseases in humans—is unfolded in the following chapters. This text captures only a small portion of an exponentially exploding data base regarding the numbers and kinds of organisms and the properties that enable them to cause disease. The material presented here is only a "snapshot" of clinical microbiology at the present time, with a respectful nod to the scientific advances in years past, and with a realization that the new technologies described in this and forthcoming chapters have already revolutionized laboratory practices and will continue to affect current and future approaches to the art and science of clinical microbiology.

By the close of the 19th century, Pasteur had experimentally dispelled the myth of spontaneous generation, and Koch, among others, had shown that microorganisms were able to cause infectious diseases. Although current techniques allow a more direct assessment of microbial virulence and pathogenicity, to some extent making Koch's postulates obsolete, the fundamental assumptions of those postulates still serve as a basis to unequivocally link microorganisms with the diseases they cause. The tenets of **Koch's postulates** are outlined in Box 1-1.

From a little over 100 years ago until the present, systems have evolved to put microorganisms into a logical classification scheme—into taxa based on morphology, phylogeny, physiology, biochemistry, and, most recently, genetic relatedness.

With the advent of solid culture media that enabled pathogenic organisms to be isolated in pure culture, it became necessary to develop a standardized "system"

by which newly isolated organisms could be accurately identified, named, and associated with a given disease state. The first step in becoming acquainted with these organisms is the same step that one must take when introduced to new people; you have to learn their names. So, as our survey of microorganisms as agents of human disease begins, it is important to first address how bacteria and other organisms are "named," that is, the science of taxonomy.

TAXONOMY: CLASSIFICATION, NOMENCLATURE, AND IDENTIFICATION OF BACTERIA

The taxonomy of bacteria specifically refers to three basic concepts: classification, nomenclature, and identification. **Classification** refers to the systematic division of organisms into related groups based on similar characteristics and includes species as the smallest and most definitive level of division. Although phylum or division, subphylum, class, subclass, order, suborder, and superfamily, are progressively more inclusive taxonomic groups (taxa) within the higher plant and animal kingdoms, the taxa comprising the family, genus, and species are the levels of classification most commonly used for the pathogenic bacteria, protozoa, and fungi. **Speciation** of microorganisms occurs at the time an organism is classified and named, although reclassification of individual microorganisms may occur from time to time.

Nomenclature refers to the naming of microorganisms. Nomenclature of microorganisms is governed by international rules developed and applied by scientists involved in taxonomy, so that an organism with a given name (*ie*, a species) is internationally recognized to be the same. These rules are published in the *International Code of Nomenclature of Bacteria*; the most recent revision of this document was published in 1992.[240] These rules are outlined in Box 1-2.

Both taxonomy and classification depend on the use of techniques for **identification**, which is essen-

> ## Box 1-1. Koch's postulates
>
> 1. A given organism must be present in every case of a given infectious disease.
> 2. The microorganism can be isolated from specimens associated with that disease state.
> 3. Inoculation of the isolate into susceptible animals produces a similar disease.
> 4. The same organism that is associated with the disease state can be recovered from representative specimens from the experimentally infected animal.

BOX 1-2. RULES OF THE NOMENCLATURE OF MICROORGANISMS

1. There is only one correct name for an organism. When more than one name exists for the same species, the oldest legitimate name for that organism has precedence. Occasionally proposed and accepted names may be changed to reflect proper latinized endings (*eg*, the name *Alloiococcus otitis* being changed to *Alloiococcus otitidis*).[3,271]

2. Names that cause error or confusion should be rejected.

3. All names are in Latin or are latinized (ie, given endings that agree in terms of proper usage and gender [masculine, feminine, neuter]) regardless of origin.
   a. The first word (**genus**) is always capitalized.
   b. The second word (**species** or specific epithet) is not capitalized.
   c. Both the genus and species name, together referred to as the **species**, are either <u>underlined</u> or *italicized* when appearing in print.
   d. The correct name of a species or higher taxonomic designations is determined by valid publication, legitimacy of the name with regard to the rules of nomenclature, and priority of publication.

tially the process of characterizing a given microorganism to determine its classification, its relatedness to other similar or dissimilar microorganisms, and, by these processes, assigning a name to the organism.

A bacterial species is a collection of strains that share many common characteristics. Strains are descendents of a pure culture isolate; the type strain represents the permanent example of the species and carries the reference name. The species name often reflects a morphologic feature or a biochemical characteristic of the microorganism or may commemorate a famous person (usually a microbiologist) or a place. All species are assigned to a genus, which is usually morphologically and biochemically well defined; however there is often subjectivity among microbiologists as to exactly what constitutes a genus and species. Genera are, in turn, assigned to tribes and families, each of which have general but distinctive morphologic, physiologic, and biochemical features. By accepted taxonomic convention, order names have the ending *-ales* (ie, the order *Eubacteriales*), family names have the latinized ending *-aceae* (*eg*, the family *Enterobacteriaceae*, the family *Neisseriaceae*), and tribe names end in *-eae* (*eg*, the tribe *Proteae*). Taxonomic groupings have been historically based on phenotypic characteristics.

Because phenotypes may change or additional biochemical characteristics may be discovered that preclude an organism from retaining a previous designation, name changes occur from time to time, much to the consternation of microbiologists and physicians alike. The current focus of taxonomy and nomenclature on genetic determinants reflecting relatedness (*eg*,

DNA homologies, DNA sequence analysis, 16S ribosomal RNA analysis) may finally enable microbiologists to establish more stable taxonomic systems where future name changes may occur less frequently.

As pointed out by Staley and Krieg (*Bergey's Manual of Systematic Bacteriology*, volume 1, 1984), "there is no 'official' classification of bacteria."[242a] New or revised species designations can be made by any investigator on publication of a legitimate name, following the rules of nomenclature cited previously. Once an organism name is published in the *International Journal of Systematic Bacteriology* (*IJSB*), it is considered to be validly published and is assumed to be correct unless challenged by subsequent publications. Challenges to the validity of a new species name are made by publishing a "request for an opinion" from the Judicial Commission of the International Union of Microbiological Societies. This commission usually refers the request to smaller bodies that deal with specific groups of organisms (*eg*, the International Committee on Systematic Bacteriology Subcommittee on the Taxonomy of *Pasteurellaceae* and Related Organisms). Criteria for valid publication of a new species proposal include:

1. The naming of the new species
2. Provision of a detailed description of the morphologic, biochemical, and genetic characteristics of the proposed new species
3. The designation and characterization of a living strain or "type strain" of the species. This type strain is sent to and deposited in reference-type culture collections (*eg*, the American Type Culture Collection [ATCC] and the National Type Culture Collection [NTCC])

Priorities for bacterial names were established between May 1, 1953 and January 1, 1980. At that time the first "Approved List of Bacterial Names" was published in *IJSB*.[238] This list was subsequently amended, updated, and republished in 1989.[239] Quarterly issues of *IJSB* routinely include lists of new species names. The descriptions of these new species are either published in *IJSB* or in a variety of other American and foreign journals; however, publication of the organism name in *IJSB* is required for validation of a species name, regardless of where the original species description is published. Before approval, new species names are commonly set off by quotation marks. Genus and species names appearing in *IJSB* can be changed according to the following rules:

1. In transferring a species from one genus to another, the species epithet is retained (*eg*, *Campylobacter pylori* became *Helicobacter pylori*).
2. If a type strain is found to actually belong to another genus, the type strain genus is considered invalid.
3. If an organism is included in two or more genera or has two or more species designations, the name of the genus/species containing the correct type strain is considered the valid name.

The optimal scheme for classification of bacteria would be one that is phylogenetic, that is, a scheme that reflects the evolutionary relatedness of microorganisms to one another. This type of classification system has only recently become truly feasible with the application of molecular and genetic techniques to bacterial systematics. Taxonomic groupings or **taxa** that were originally based on phenotypic characteristics are now being reassessed with molecular methods. These methods include **nucleic acid hybridization** and **ribosomal RNA (rRNA) sequence analysis** (discussed later). With the advent and expansion of these techniques into bacterial systematics, significant taxonomic changes have occurred and will continue to occur as more organisms are **genotypically** characterized by these techniques. Over the many years of clinical microbiology laboratory practice, methods for exhaustive **phenotypic characterization** of clinically significant microorganisms have been recognized, published, and codified to enable laboratories to determine if an organism belongs to a given species. The incorporation of such information into computerized data bases for use with bacterial identification kit systems has, in many cases, provided much needed organization to the vast amount of phenotypic data that has accumulated. Reference texts that serve as compendia for phenotypic descriptions of microorganisms include *Bergey's Manual of Systematic Bacteriology*, a four-volume set containing exhaustive information on phenotypic characteristics, and *Bergey's Manual of Systematic Bacteriology*, a single-volume work that essentially abstracts phenotypic information from the four-volume work. The phenotypic data found in these and other references and texts include information contained in points 1 through 8 in Box 1-3. Information on the genetic and molecular characterizations of microorganisms (point 9 in Box 1-3) await inclusion in the next editions of these manuals.

By analyzing organisms and applying the identification criteria listed above, microorganisms can be classified within the taxonomic framework described earlier and a final genus and species name can be determined. The primary role of the clinical microbiology laboratory is to provide physicians with accurate and timely identifications of microorganisms recovered from clinical specimens and to determine and provide information on the susceptibility of these microorganisms to antimicrobial agents. Physicians, in turn, use this information to guide their selection of appropriate therapeutic interventions, to monitor the clinical response of the patient, and to evaluate the patient's clinical course.

To provide the reader with sufficient background information for understanding subsequent chapters regarding specific bacterial pathogens and the diseases that they cause, the next section of this chapter deals with the general morphology, physiology, and virulence mechanisms of bacteria. This material provides the basic information necessary for understanding the nuances of morphology, staining properties, growth, metabolic features, and biochemical characteristics of the bacterial organisms discussed in the chapters to follow. Following this, a discussion of rapid biochemical, metabolic, immunologic, and serologic methods used in clinical microbiology is presented. The last sec-

---

BOX 1-3. METHODS FOR CHARACTERIZATIONS OF MICROORGANISMS

1. Cellular morphology (*eg*, cell shape, cell size, cellular arrangements)

2. Staining characteristics (*eg*, Gram stain, acid-fast stain)

3. Motility

4. Presence or absence of spores

5. Growth characteristics
   a. Rapidity of growth
   b. Morphology of colonies on growth media
   c. Optimal atmospheric conditions for growth (*eg*, requirements for oxygen, carbon dioxide, microaerophilic environments, etc)
   d. Optimal temperature for growth
   e. Colonial morphology on selective, nonselective, and differential media

6. Biochemical characteristics (*eg*, formation of distinct biochemical end-products, production of acid from various carbohydrates, presence of certain bacterial enzymes)

7. Serologic tests, including direct detection of antigens, as well as serologic detection of antibodies formed in response to infection

8. Analysis of metabolic end-products or structural components of organisms by various methods (spectroscopy, gas-liquid chromatography, high-pressure liquid chromatography)

9. Genetic analysis using nucleic acid probes and other molecular techniques (*eg*, polymerase chain reaction)

---

tion of this chapter addresses the new molecular genetic approaches to the detection and identification of microorganisms, including nucleic acid probe technology and gene amplification (*eg*, polymerase chain reaction). Subsequent chapters on specific bacterial, fungal, viral, and protozoal microorganisms address not only the classical laboratory approach to the isolation and identification of these organisms, but also newer technologies that are either in use at the present time or that are on the horizon for detection and characterization of these organisms and their pathogenic properties. The basic morphology and physiology of fungi, parasites, and viruses are presented in Chapters 19, 20, and 21, respectively.

Bacteria are **prokaryotic**, while fungi, protozoa, and other organisms are **eukaryotic**. Eukaryotic cells contain a nucleus with a nuclear membrane enclosing multiple chromosomes, whereas prokaryotic cells have a single chromosome that is not enclosed in a nuclear membrane. Eukaryotic cells also possess a variety of subcellular **organelles** having specialized functions, such as mitochondria (sites of aerobic respiration) and chloroplasts (sites of of photosynthesis in green plants). In fact, these subcellular organelles probably evolved from prokaryotic organisms that entered the eukaryotic cells and developed symbiotic relationships with them over time by losing metabolic functions associated with a free-living existence and developing features or attributes that benefited the "host" organism. Prokaryotic and eukaryotic cells differ substantially in many other characteristics, as briefly described in Table 1-1.

BASIC BACTERIAL ANATOMY AND PHYSIOLOGY

BACTERIAL SIZE AND SHAPE

Bacterial cells have a wide variety of sizes and shapes. They are generally 0.2 to 2 μm in diameter and 1 to 6 μm in length. Bacteria exist in four basic morphologies: spherical cells or **cocci**, rod-shaped cells or **bacilli**, spiral-shaped cells or **spirilla**, and comma-shaped cells or **vibrios**. Arrangements of coccal cells in pairs, chains, or clusters define groups of organisms called **diplococci**, **streptococci**, and **staphylococci**, respectively (Fig. 1-1). Rod-shaped organisms may be regular in morphology, may be somewhat shorter (ie, "coc-

cobacillary"), or may appear club or dumbbell shaped ("**coryneform**"). Comma-shaped cells generally define a basic characteristic of certain species (eg, *Vibrio* species). The same is true for certain other spiral-shaped bacteria (eg, *Campylobacter* species, *Borrelia* species, and *Treponema* species), where spiral formation may be loose (about 4 coils per organism) or tight (14 to 20 coils per organism). In addition to their size, shape, and cellular arrangement, bacteria can be further differentiated on the basis of their staining characteristics with **Gram stain**. Using this staining technique, most bacteria can be classified as gram-positive or gram-negative organisms. The Gram stain differentiates bacteria based on their cell wall structure and is discussed later in this chapter and again in Chapter 2. The structure of a generalized bacterial cell (both gram-positive and gram-negative) is depicted in Figure 1-2.

NUCLEAR STRUCTURE, DNA REPLICATION, TRANSCRIPTION, AND TRANSLATION

The inheritable characteristics of all living organisms are determined by the structure of the genetic material. The genetic material of an individual cell is composed

TABLE 1-1
PROPERTIES OF PROKARYOTIC AND EUKARYOTIC CELLS

CHARACTERISTIC	PROKARYOTIC CELLS	EUKARYOTIC CELLS
Major groups	Bacteria, blue-green algae	Algae, fungi, protozoa, plants, animals
Cell wall	Contains peptidoglycan, lipids, proteins	Absent; when present, contains chitin or cellulose (green plants)
Nuclear structure		
Nuclear membrane	Absent	Present
Chromosomes	Single, closed, circular, double-stranded DNA	Multiple, linear, chromosomes
Ploidy	Haploid	Diploid, haploid (fungi)
Transcription/translation	Continuous, with short-lived mRNA and polyribosome (polysome) formation	Discontinuous; long-lived mRNA transcribed in nucleus and translated in cytoplasm
Histones	Absent	Present
Cytoplasm		
Ribosomes	Present; 70S (50S + 30S)	Present; 80S (60S + 40S)
Mitochondria	Absent	Present
Golgi complex	Absent	Present
Endoplasmic reticulum	Absent	Present
Cytoplasmic membrane	Present; phospholipids, no sterols (except for *Mycoplasma* species)	Present; phospholipids and sterols (cholesterol, ergosterol)
Triglyceride fats	Absent	Present
Motility	Flagella (simple)	Flagella (complex); pseudopodia; other complex locomotor organs
Energy generation	Cytoplasmic membrane-associated	Mitochondria
Sexual reproduction	Absent (unnecessary)	Present (may alternate with asexual reproductive cycles)
Recombination/gene exchange	Chromosomal or plasmid gene exchange via transformation, transduction, or conjugation	Diploid zygote formed from haploid germ cells; meiosis results in genetic recombination

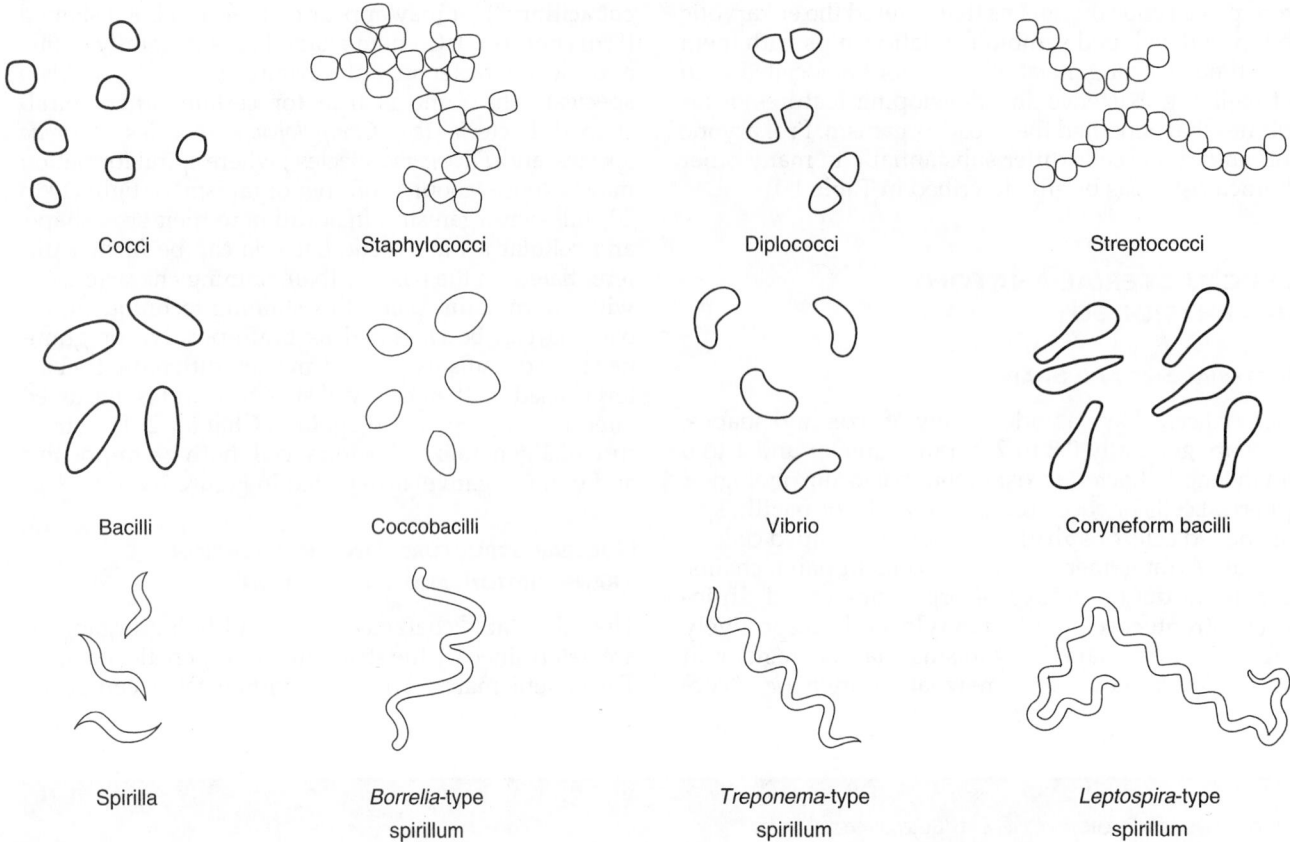

Cocci   Staphylococci   Diplococci   Streptococci

Bacilli   Coccobacilli   Vibrio   Coryneform bacilli

Spirilla   *Borrelia*-type spirillum   *Treponema*-type spirillum   *Leptospira*-type spirillum

Figure 1-1
Basic morphologies of various bacteria.

of **deoxyribonucleic acid (DNA)** organized into single or multiple chromosomes. Collectively, the genetic material is referred to as the organism's **genome**. In prokaryotic organisms, the genome is composed of a single, covalently closed, circular chromosome of double-stranded DNA (dsDNA). This circular chromosome, termed the **nucleoid**, is not bounded by a membrane, but is free in the cytoplasm in a discrete central portion of the bacterial cell. Bacterial cellular DNA measures 300 to 1400 μm in length and is present in the cell in a **supercoiled** state (*ie*, the double-stranded molecule is twisted up on itself like a "twisted" rubberband). Individual genes are arranged linearly on the chromosome. The nucleoid represents about 10% of the cell volume, although DNA is only 2% to 3% of the cell's dry weight. In *Escherichia coli*, the chromosome contains about 5×10^6 base pairs, and its length is about 1000 times the length of the bacterial cell in which it is contained. Unlike similar processes in eukaryotic cells, DNA replication and transcription of the DNA into messenger ribonucleic acid (mRNA) occur continually. The chromosome also appears to be attached to the inner aspect of the cell membrane at certain points. In eukaryotic organisms, the genetic material is organized into several chromosomes within the nucleus. The chromosomes are, in turn, associated with several basic proteins called **histones**, which help to stabilize chromosomal structure. The chromosomes

of eukaryotic organisms are separated from the rest of the cellular material by a **nuclear membrane**, which is composed of a lipid bilayer that is similar in composition to the cell membrane. The nuclear membrane also contains pores, which allow passage of small molecules into and out of the nucleus.

Nucleic acids of all bacteria, like other organisms, are composed of **polynucleotides** (a polymer consisting of nucleotides) that are comprised of the following three components (Fig. 1-3): (1) a cyclic, 5-carbon sugar (ribose in RNA, deoxyribose in DNA), (2) a purine (adenine, guanine) or pyrimidine (cytosine, thymine, uracil) base attached to the 1' carbon atom of the pentose by an *N*-glycosidic bond, and (3) a phosphate group (PO_3) attached to the 5' carbon of the pentose by a phosphodiester linkage. Deoxyribose moieties are linked together via alternating phosphate groups to form a chain that has a characteristic helical coil, and the bases are directed toward the central axis of the coil. Such a structure composes a single strand of nucleic acid (ssDNA).

The double helix structure of DNA, specifically, results from the interaction between two complementary single strands of nucleic acid. Complementarity is associated with the sequence of bases on a single strand and the hydrogen bonding that occurs between specific bases on the complementary strand (Fig. 1-4). The purine bases are adenine (A) and guanine (G), and the

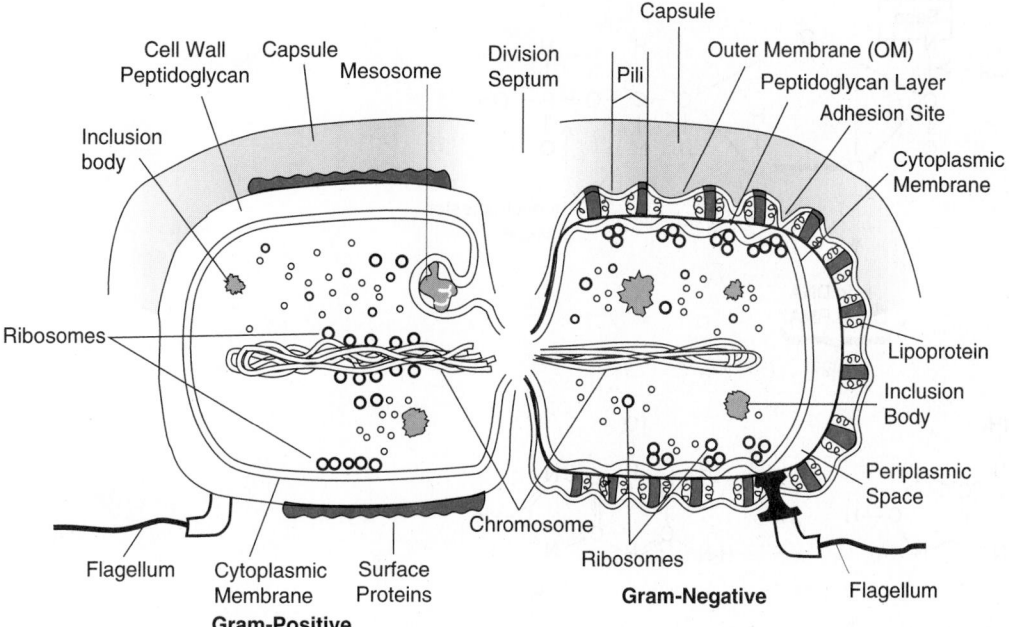

Figure 1-2
Cross-section through a generalized bacterial cell. The left half of this figure depicts the structure of a gram-positive bacterium; the right half shows the structure of a gram-negative bacterium.

pyrimidine bases are cytosine (C), thymine (T), and uracil (U). The purine adenine will specifically base-pair only with the pyrimidine thymine; the purine guanosine will specifically base-pair only with the pyrimidine cytosine. Antiparallel strains of ssDNA are held together by three hydrogen bonds between C and G and two hydrogen bonds between A and T (see Fig. 1-4). Native DNA exists as a double-stranded helix, whereas RNA exists primarily in a single-stranded form as **messenger RNA** (mRNA), and in partially double-stranded forms in **ribosomal RNA** (rRNA) and **transfer RNA** (tRNA) molecules. In all RNA species, uracil is present in place of thymine (see Fig. 1-3).

The sequence of purine and pyrimidine bases in DNA constitutes the genetic code, with specific codons (three base-pair sequences) coding for specific amino acids. Single-stranded mRNA is synthesized from dsDNA during the process of **transcription** by DNA-dependent RNA polymerase, in which a complementary strand of mRNA is synthesized with the "sense" strand of dsDNA as the template. The mRNA is "decoded" in association with several ribosomes in a **polysome-mRNA complex**, where the codon-anticodon base pairing occurs through molecules of **transfer RNA (tRNA)** during the process of **translation**. Transfer RNA molecules bear the specific anticodons corresponding to the codons of the mRNA and also carry the corresponding, covalently linked amino acid. Thus, the genetic code present in the DNA is translated into protein molecule "building blocks" and enzymes that, in turn, catalyze the synthesis and degradation of all the other cellular components. The synthesis of new DNA molecules, called **replication**, occurs by the uncoiling and "unzipping" of the dsDNA molecule by a

DNA gyrase enzyme, and the synthesis of complementary strands of DNA by a **DNA-dependent DNA polymerase**. Each new dsDNA molecule contains a single strand of the parent DNA. The relationship among DNA replication, RNA transcription, and translation of the genetic code into proteins is summarized in Figure 1-5.

Because the nucleotide sequence of DNA is unique to individual species of microorganisms, analysis of nucleic acid relatedness between and among microbes has become a powerful tool for taxonomists. Double-stranded DNA can be separated into its two component strands by heat or high salt concentrations. On cooling or on lowering the salt concentration, the two single strands will **reanneal** or **hybridize** into the double-stranded form by specific base pairing. The extent to which two single strands of DNA reanneal with one another is an indirect assessment of their relatedness and can be used to help determine whether two organisms are members of the same species. At the genetic level, species can be defined as strains of bacteria that exhibit 70% or more DNA relatedness and 5% or less divergence in related nucleotide sequences.[275] Even though this criterion holds for most microorganisms, some bacterial species have more than 70% DNA relatedness, yet are still considered distinct species because of their clinical significance. For example, *Neisseria gonorrhoeae* and *Neisseria meningitidis* are virtually identical when analyzed by nucleic acid hybridization, but the two species cause distinct clinical entities, the sexually transmitted disease gonorrhea and epidemic/endemic cerebrospinal meningitis, respectively.

Another application of nucleic acid technology to microbial taxonomy is **ribosomal RNA (rRNA) se-**

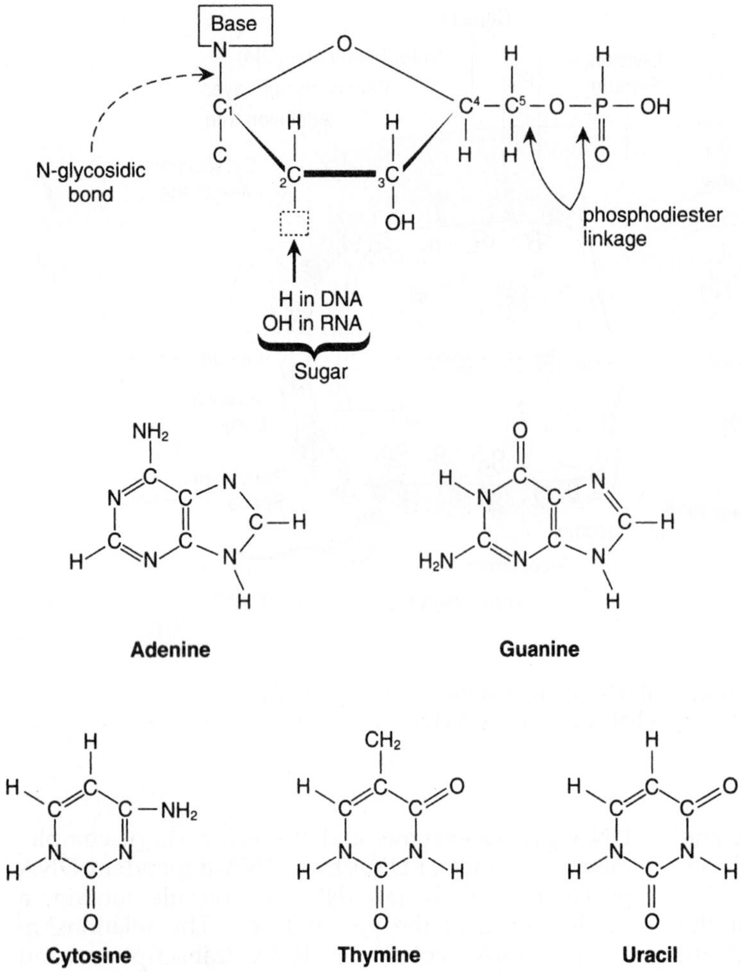

Figure 1-3
Molecular structure of polynucleotides and nucleic acid bases. Polynucleotides consist of a cyclic, 5-carbon sugar (ribose or deoxyribose), a purine or pyrimidine base attached to the 1' carbon atom of the sugar by an *N*-glycosidic bond, and a phosphate group linked to the 5' carbon of the sugar by a phosphodiester linkage. The structures of the two purine (adenine and guanine) and the three pyrimidine (cytosine, thymine, and uracil) bases also are shown.

quence analysis. The nucleotide sequences of the single-stranded RNA species that are incorporated into the subunits of the bacterial ribosome can be used to ascertain the relatedness of organisms because in individual species these sequences have remained highly conserved (*ie*, have not been altered by mutations) during evolution. Mutations in these highly conserved base sequences are usually lethal and organisms having such mutations do not usually survive and propagate. By examining the nucleotide sequences of the 16S rRNA, the phylogenetic relationships and evolution of organisms from common ancestral types can be ascertained. Ribosomal RNA sequence analysis is most useful for determining the relatedness of microorganisms above the genus level, although this technique has been used to validate existing phenotypic differences between closely related genera and species. Sequencing studies of ribosomal RNA molecules have also revealed nucleotide sequences that are unique to individual species. Because these unique RNA sequences are also highly conserved and exist in multiple copies within the ribosomes of a bacterial cell, synthetic oligonucleotides that can hybridize with these unique sequences can be used to detect and identify bacteria. Such an approach forms the basis for nucleic acid probe technology for direct detection of organisms in clinical specimens. These probes can also be applied to organisms recovered on culture media as a method of organism identification or can be used to detect these unique sequences directly in clinical specimens. Nucleic acid probe technology and its applications in clinical microbiology are discussed later in this chapter.

CYTOPLASM

The cytoplasm is an amorphous gel containing enzymes, ions, subcellular organelles serving various functions, and a variety of granules, many of which represent food and energy reserves. The cytoplasmic enzymes of prokaryotic cells function in both anabolic and catabolic processes; many of these enzymes are associated with the inner aspect of the cell membrane (see below). Prokaryotic cells lack separate, membrane-bounded subcellular organelles, whereas eukaryotic cells contain a variety of subcellular structures (eg, mitochondria, endoplasmic reticula, etc) composed of or bounded by phospholipid bilayer membranes. Intracellular cytoplasmic inclusions or granules represent accumulations of food reserves (polysaccharides, lipids, or polyphosphates). The numbers and types of storage granules vary with the medium and the functional state of the cells. Glycogen is the major storage

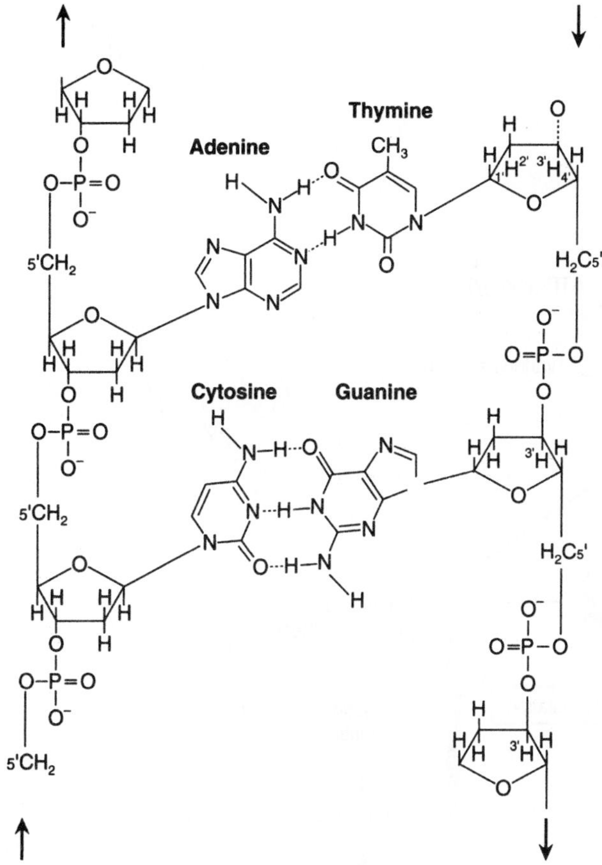

Figure 1-4
In the DNA molecule, the two polynucleotide strands of the DNA double helix are "anti-parallel," ie, the 3'-OH terminus of one strand is adjacent to the 5'-P terminus of the complementary strand. The bases, which are directed toward the central axis of the helix, hold the two polynucleotide strands together by relatively weak hydrogen bonds. Adenine pairs with thymine via two hydrogen bonds, while cytosine pairs with guanine via three hydrogen bonds. These interactive forces between the polynucleotide strands can be overcome by thermal energy (heat) or by strong alkali in the process of denaturation.

material of enteric bacteria, whereas some *Bacillus* and *Pseudomonas* species accumulate 30% or more of their dry weight as poly-β-hydroxybutyrate. High molecular weight polymers of polyhexametaphosphate known as **metachromatic granules** or **volutin** occur in *Corynebacterium* species, *Yersina pestis*, and *Mycobacteria* species. These volutin granules appear reddish pink when stained with methylene blue.

Both prokaryotic and eukaryotic organisms harbor large numbers of **ribosomes**, which are the sites of protein synthesis. In prokaryotic organisms, the ribosomes are 70S; in eukaryotic organisms, the ribosomes are 80S. The "S" refers to a Svedburg unit, which is an indirect measure of the size of the ribosome as determined by its rate of sedimentation when subjected to ultracentrifugal force. Ribosomal ribonucleic acid (rRNA) comprises 80% of the total cellular RNA. The 70S bacterial ribosome has a molecular weight of about 800,000 daltons and exists in a dissociated state as two subunits termed the 30S and the 50S subunits. The 30S subunit contains 16S RNA, whereas the 50S subunit contains both 23S and 5S RNA; both subunits also contain several specific ribosomal proteins. The remaining 20% of the cellular RNA is found as **transfer ribonucleic acid (tRNA)** and **messenger ribonucleic acid (mRNA)**. When complexed with an mRNA transcript from the DNA, the 50S and 30S ribosomal subunits form the intact 70S ribosome found in bacterial cells. Ribosome-mRNA aggregates termed **polyribosomes** or **polysomes** contain all components of the protein-synthesizing system; **polysomes** are essentially chains of 70S ribosomes (monomers) attached to messenger RNA (mRNA). Histone or histone-like proteins that stabilize the nascent polypeptides synthesized by the polysomes have only recently been found in small amounts in association with *Escherichia coli* DNA, whereas the occurrence of polyamine proteins (*eg*, putrescine and spermidine) associated with bacterial DNA is well known.

Extrachromosomal DNA is frequently present in the cytoplasm of prokaryotic organisms in the form of **plasmids**. Plasmids exist as covalently closed circles of dsDNA. They are generally not found in eukaryotic organisms, although some subcellular organelles in eukaryotic organisms (*eg*, mitochondria) do contain DNA molecules that resemble bacterial plasmids. Plasmids are capable of autonomous replication and are inherited by progeny bacterial cells. Plasmids may contain the genetic information for a variety of structures or functions related to bacterial virulence, including genes for antimicrobial resistance, virulence-related adhesins, toxin production, and resistance to heavy metal ions. Some bacteria may also possess **transposons**, which are sequences of DNA that are able to "jump" from one location to another in the bacterial genome.[161] Transposable sequences may be chromosomal or derived from plasmids.

CYTOPLASMIC MEMBRANE

The cytoplasm of all bacterial cells is surrounded by a cytoplasmic membrane. The bacterial cytoplasmic membrane lies immediately within the cell wall peptidoglycan layer in gram-positive bacteria and adjacent to the periplasmic space in gram-negative bacteria (discussed below). The basic structure of the cytoplasmic membrane is a phospholipid bilayer in which various constituent proteins are embedded. The membrane is comprised of 30% to 60% phospholipid and 50% to 70% protein by weight. Most bacterial cell membranes contain phosphatidyl glycerol, phosphatidyl ethanolamine, and diphosphatidyl glycerol; they do not contain sterols (*eg*, cholesterol or ergosterol). The only prokaryotic exceptions to this are the mycoplasmas and ureaplasmas, which incorporate sterols from the growth medium into their cell membranes. The fatty acids that compose the lipid portion of the phospholipid bilayer generally contain 15 to 18 carbon backbones and are usually saturated or mono-unsaturated.

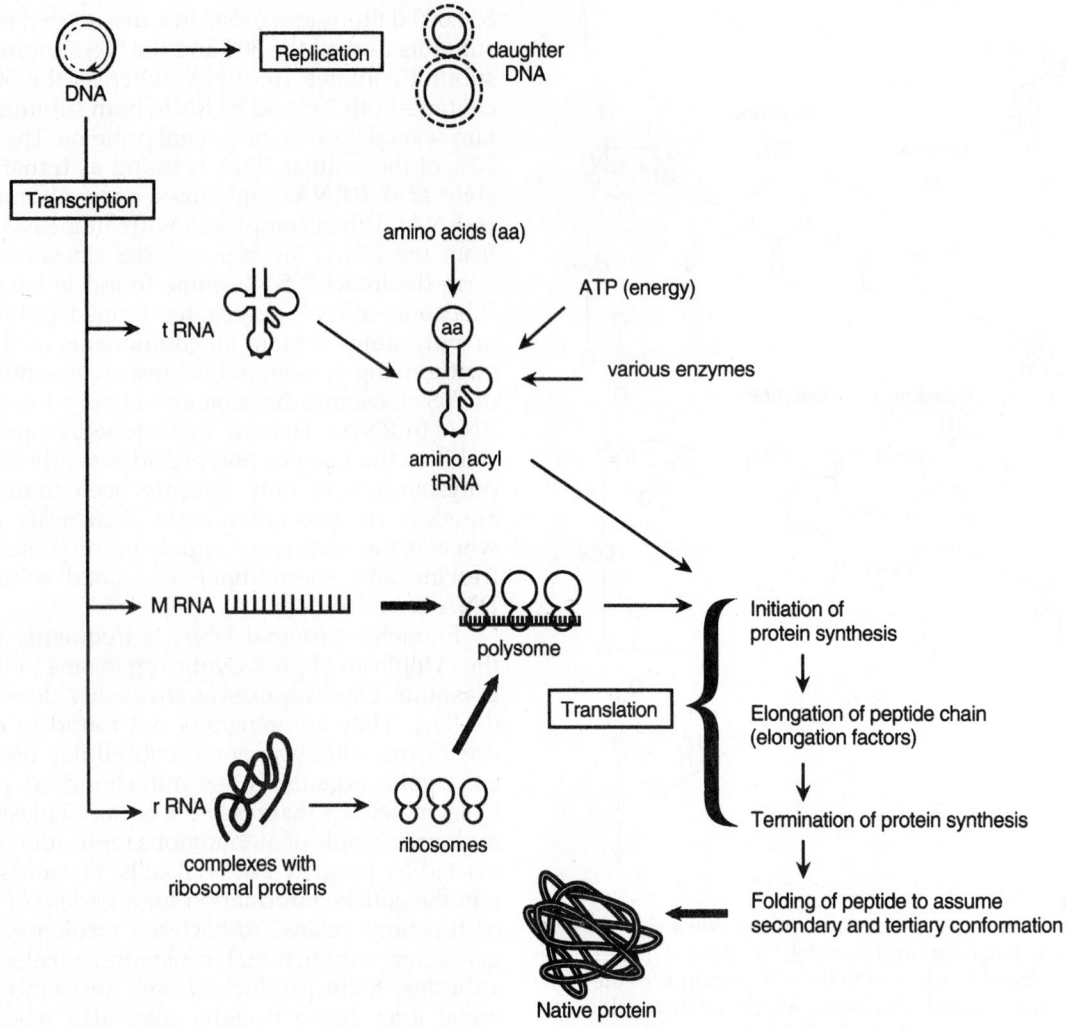

Figure 1-5

Replication, transcription, and translation of the genetic code in prokaryotic organisms. DNA is replicated by DNA-dependent DNA polymerase to produce two double-stranded DNA (dsDNA) molecules. The genetic code in the dsDNA is copied to produce a single-stranded RNA called messenger RNA (mRNA) during the process of transcription. Transfer RNA (tRNA) and ribosomal RNA (rRNA) are also transcribed. rRNA becomes complexed with specific proteins to form part of the structure of the ribosome. The mRNA becomes complexed with ribosomes to form polysomes, which are the site of protein sunthesis. On the polysome, codons specific for individual amino acids are recognized by anticodons on tRNA molecules by specific base pairing. Specific codons correspond to different amino acids attached to aminoacyl tRNA molecules. During the stages of translation, protein synthesis is initiated, polypeptide chains are elongated, and synthesis is eventually terminated with the release of a protein molecule.

The cell membrane of prokaryotes possesses several functions that are relegated to specialized subcellular organelles in eukaryotic organisms. The bacterial cell membrane contains enzymes that are active in cellular respiration and oxidative phosphorylation, peptidoglycan biosynthesis, and outer membrane biosynthesis in gram-negative bacteria. The cell membrane also functions in the synthesis and secretion of enzymes and bacterial toxins. The cytoplasmic membrane provides an insulating barrier across which energy can be built up in the form of a gradient or membrane potential; such energy may be used for flagellar movement, chromosomal mobilization, and so forth. The membrane also functions to retain metabolites and

exclude external compounds. Proteins in the cytoplasmic membrane are primarily involved in electron transport and oxidative phosphorylation, complex lipid biosynthesis, synthesis of cell wall constituents, and DNA replication. They are also involved in the active transport of materials into the cytoplasm. Such specific membrane-associated carrier proteins are termed **permeases. Mesosomes**, which are invaginations of the cytoplasmic membrane that extend into the cytoplasm, may function to increase the available membrane surface area for catabolic and anabolic cellular enzymes. The may also function in DNA replication and DNA duplex separation in actively growing cells.

BACTERIAL CELL WALLS

The bacterial cell wall provides structural rigidity, confers shape to the cell, and forms a physical barrier against the outside environment. The rigid component of the cell wall of all bacteria is composed of **peptidoglycan**. Peptidoglycan is found in all bacterial species except for the cell wall-less mycoplasmas and ureaplasmas. This structure is composed of a backbone of alternating carbohydrate moieties of **N-acetylglucosamine** and **N-acetylmuramic acid** in β-1,4 linkage (Fig. 1-6). Short tetrapeptides, generally composed of identical short chains of D- and L-amino acids, are attached to the N-acetyl muramic acid residues via a peptide bond to the lactyl group on C3. These short chains contain unusual amino acids not generally found in proteins, including D-isomers of glutamic acid and alanine (gram-positive bacteria) and *meso*-diaminopimelic acid (gram-negative bacteria). Some of these tetrapeptides are, in turn, linked to one another by short peptides forming cross-bridges between adjacent peptidoglycan strands (Fig. 1-7A). The types of amino acids found and the degrees of cross-linkage are variable components of the peptidoglycan structure. For example, in *Staphylo-coccus aureus*, most of the N-acetylmuramic acid residues are cross-linked to adjacent peptidoglycan strands by five glycine residues, therby providing a rather tight, rigid cell wall structure (see Fig. 1-7A). In gram-negative bacteria (*eg Escherichia coli*), the cross-linkage is directly between the *meso*-diaminopimelic acid of one peptidoglycan "chain" and the terminal D-alanyl residue on an adjacent strand (see Fig. 1-7B). Such cross-linking determines whether a cell wall structure is termed "tight" (highly cross-linked) or "loose."

GRAM-POSITIVE BACTERIAL CELL WALLS

The gram-positive bacterial cell wall (Fig. 1-8A) is almost 80 nm thick and is composed mostly of several layers of peptidoglycan; in fact, anywhere from 40% to greater than 80% of the dry weight of some gram-positive cell walls may be peptidoglycan. Trapped within this peptidoglycan matrix are a variety of proteins, polysaccharides, and unique molecules called **teichoic acids**. Teichoic acids are polymers of either **ribitol** (5-carbon) or **glycerol** (3-carbon) units joined together by **phosphodiester linkages** (Fig. 1-9). **Ribitol teichoic acids** are associated with the cell wall, whereas **glycerol teichoic acids** are associated with the inner aspect of the bacterial cell membrane. Ribitol teichoic acids are covalently linked to the peptidoglycan via the C6 hydroxyl group of N-acetylmuramic acid; the glycerol teichoic acids are linked to glycolipids of the cytoplasmic membrane. The latter molecules are termed **lipoteichoic acids**. They are linked to the outer lipid layer of the cell membrane and extend into the cell wall. Teichoic acids of different bacteria are further modified by addition of "R" groups including ester-linked D-alanine or D-lysine residues or O-glycoside-linked glucose, galactose, or N-acetylglucosamine. Teichoic acids stabilize the cell wall, maintain the association of the wall with the cell membrane, chelate small ions necessary for cell function and cell wall integrity, and participate in cellular interaction and adherence to mucosal or other surfaces. Teichoic acids may also function in peptidoglycan synthesis and septum formation during growth and reproduction and may also play a role in the competence of some gram-positive bacteria to undergo transformation (*eg*, pneumococci). In some organisms, the teichoic acids are antigenic and form the basis for antigenic grouping (*eg*, the group D antigen in group D streptococci and members of the genus *Enterococcus*). The C polysaccharide found in the cell walls of *Streptococcus pneumoniae* is a complex lipoteichoic acid composed of ribitol and phosphate substituted at various points with N-acetyl-D-galactosamine, D-glucose, N-acetyl-2,4-diamino-2,4,6-trideoxyhexose in O-glycosidic linkage and choline in diester linkage.

In the various groups of pathogenic gram-positive bacteria, other cell wall structures that are important virulence determinants may also be present. For example, M protein, a recognized virulence factor of group A β-hemolytic streptococci, is associated with lipoteichoic acids in the streptococcal cell wall and extends out of the wall as a fimbrial protein (see Chap. 12). The structure of the gram-positive cell wall is graphically represented in Figure 1-8A.

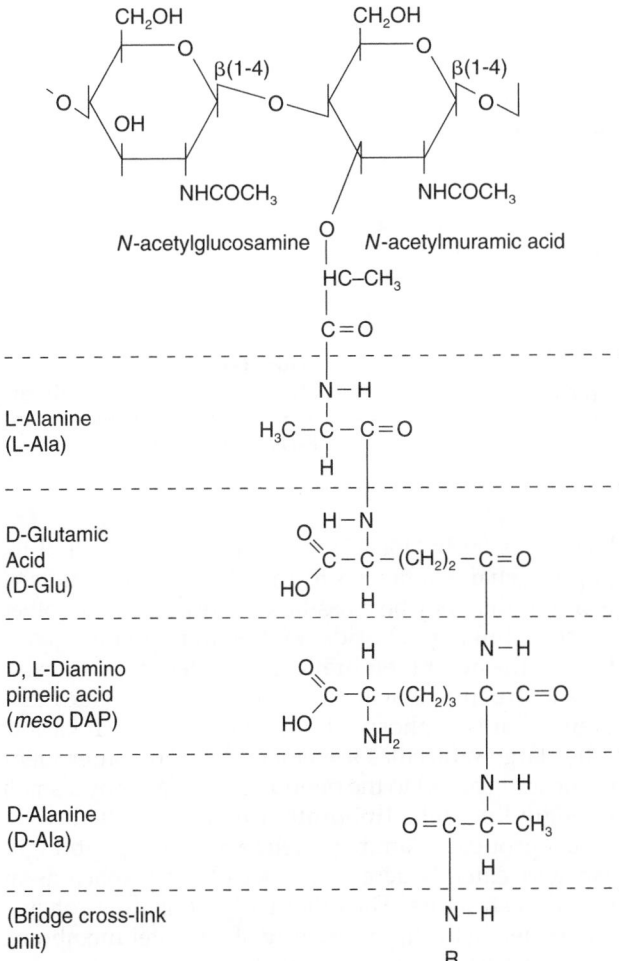

Figure 1-6
Structure of the repeating peptidoglycan unit of *Escherichia coli*.

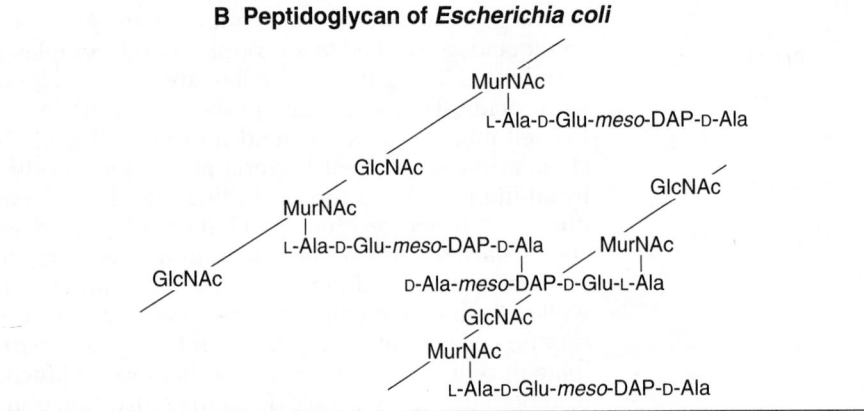

A Peptidoglycan of *Staphylococcus aureus*

Abbreviations: GlcNAc, *N*-acetyl-glucosamine; MurNAc, *N*-acetyl-muramic acid; Ala, alanine; Glu-NH$_2$, iso-glutamine; Lys, lysine; and Gly, glycine.

B Peptidoglycan of *Escherichia coli*

Abbreviations: See above; also Glu, glutamate; and DAP; diaminopimelate.

Figure 1-7
Structure of the peptidoglycan in *Staphylococcus aureus* (**A**) and *Escherichia coli* (**B**).

GRAM-NEGATIVE BACTERIAL CELL WALLS

The cell walls of gram-negative bacteria (see Fig. 1-8*B*) are thinner than those of gram-positive bacteria but are structurally more complex. Outside of the cytoplasmic membrane is a **periplasmic space**, an enzyme-containing compartment between the cytoplasmic membrane and the outer portions of the cell wall. A **single-unit thick peptidoglycan layer** forms the outer border of the periplasmic space. Because the peptidoglycan layer is only one layer thick, cross-linking occurs only to adjacent peptidoglycan strands rather than to layers of peptidoglycan either deeper in or more external to the individual cell surface. Cross-links are formed from the carboxyl group of the terminal D-alanine residue on one chain to the free amino group of a diaminopimelic acid residue on an adjacent chain (see Fig. 1-7*B*). The peptidoglycan layer of gram-negative

bacteria is fairly "loose"; that is, only about half of the peptide chains attached to the *N*-acetylmuramic acid residues that may be cross-linked are actually involved in cross-linking. Outside of the thin peptidoglycan layer is the **outer membrane**. This outer membrane has a basic structure that is similar to the cytoplasmic membrane, that is, a phospholipid bilayer in which various other large molecules are embedded. The outer membrane is anchored to the peptidoglycan layer by a small, strongly lipophilic **lipoprotein** that is attached to the amino group of diaminopimelic acid in the peptidoglycan and extends across the periplasmic space as an α-helical structure. The other end of this lipoprotein is embedded in the lipid structure of the outer membrane.

A structural component that is unique to the gram-negative outer membrane is **lipopolysaccharide (LPS)** (Fig. 1-10*A*). LPS molecules are the major surface anti-

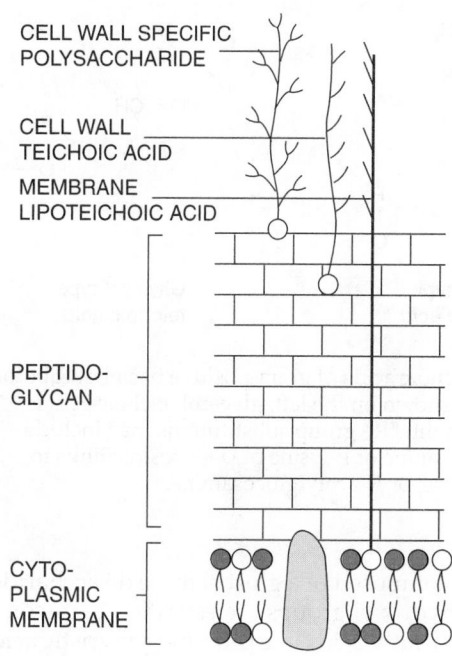

CELL WALL SPECIFIC POLYSACCHARIDE

CELL WALL TEICHOIC ACID

MEMBRANE LIPOTEICHOIC ACID

PEPTIDO-GLYCAN

CYTO-PLASMIC MEMBRANE

A. GRAM - POSITIVE

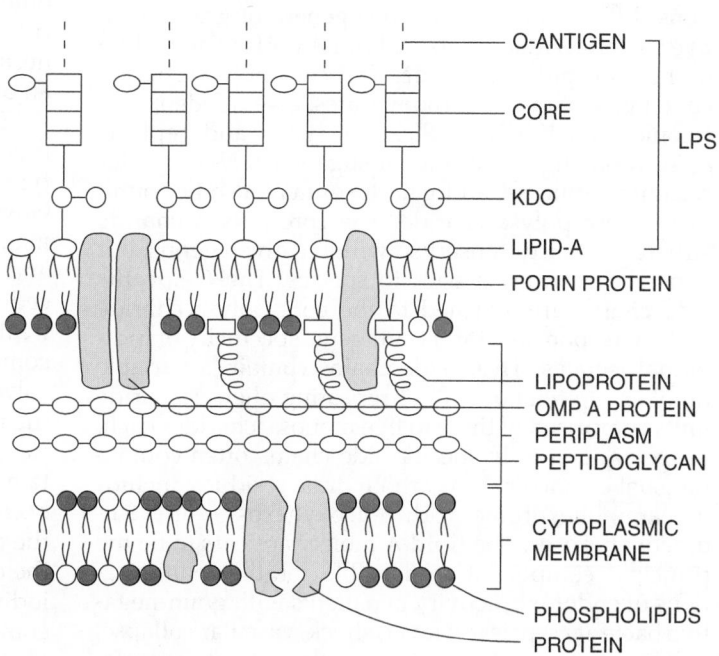

O-ANTIGEN

CORE

LPS

KDO

LIPID-A

PORIN PROTEIN

LIPOPROTEIN
OMP A PROTEIN
PERIPLASM
PEPTIDOGLYCAN

CYTOPLASMIC MEMBRANE

PHOSPHOLIPIDS
PROTEIN

B. GRAM - NEGATIVE

Figure 1-8
Structure of the cell wall of gram-positive (**A**) and gram-negative (**B**) bacteria. KDO, keto-deoxy-octulonate; LPS, lipopolysaccharide.

genic determinants (called **somatic** or **O antigens**) in gram-negative bacteria and are responsible for the **endotoxin** activity of gram-negative cells. LPS molecules are complex glycolipids composed of a complex lipid portion called **lipid A**, a **core polysaccharide** region that is generally similar in structure within a given bacterial genus or species, and **O-specific side chains**, which are regions of variable biochemical structure that impart unique serologic identity to gram-negative

species. The lipid A moiety of the LPS is embedded in the outer leaflet of the outer membrane, with the core polysaccharide and the O-specific side chains projecting from the outer membrane surface like whiskers. Each *Salmonella* species, for example, has characteristic O-specific side chains that provide valuable criteria for identification of the organism in the clinical laboratory. The structure of LPS has been studied most extensively in *Salmonella* species and *Escherichia coli*.

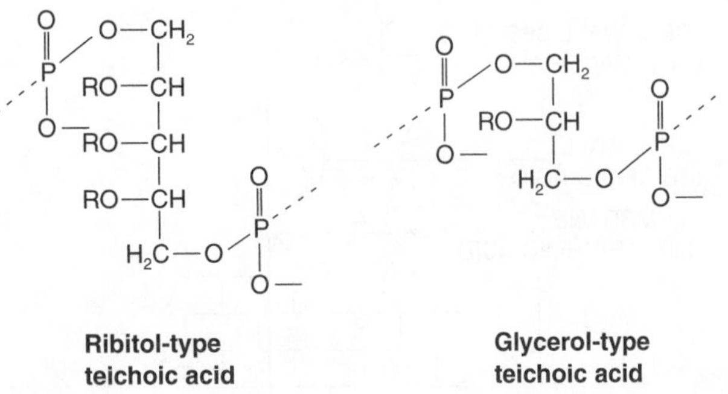

Ribitol-type teichoic acid   **Glycerol-type teichoic acid**

Figure 1-9
Structure of teichoic acids of gram-positive bacteria. Ribotol teichoic acid is shown on the left; glycerol teichoic acid is shown on the right. "R" group substitutions may include ester-linked D-alanine or D-lysine or O-glycosidic links to glucose, galactose, or N-acetylglucosamine.

Lipid A is composed of a glucosamine disaccharide in which the hydroxyl groups are esterified to uncommon β-hydroxy fatty acids like β-hydroxymyristic acid (C_{14}), myristomyristic acid, and lauromyristic acid (see Fig. 1-10B). Additional fatty acids may be attached via hydroxyl groups to other unsubstituted locations on the myristic acid molecule; these additional substitutions differ among the various genera of gram-negative bacteria. Attached to the lipid A portion of the LPS is the **core polysaccharide**. The core polysaccharide contains two unique carbohydrates: 2-keto-3-deoxyoctulonic acid (KDO), an 8-carbon sugar, and heptose, a 7-carbon sugar. Additional sugars (eg, N-acetylglucosamine, glucose, and galactose) may also be found in the core polysaccharide. The core polysaccharide structure is fairly conserved within a given genus, but it may vary from species to species. The **O-specific side chains** are attached to the core polysaccharide and are responsible for the antigenic specificity of individual isolates. These side chains contain a variable number (up to about 40) of repeating oligosaccharide units comprised of three to five monosaccharides each. These antigenically specific side chains often contain unusual or uncommon carbohydrate residues, including aminohexuronic acid, 6-deoxyhexoses, and 2,6-dideoxyhexoses. The **lipid A** moiety appears to be the principal component responsible for the manifestations of endotoxin activity in patients with gram-negative bacterial sepsis (eg, fever, shock, vascular collapse, and hemorrhage). Endotoxin can also activate complement and can cause disseminated intravascular coagulation. The generalized structure of the LPS of *Salmonella* species is shown in Figure 1-10A; the structure of lipid A, the core polysaccharides, and somatic antigens are shown in Figure 1-10B, C, and D, respectively.

Dissociation of the outer membrane LPS can be partially accomplished by treatment of cell suspensions with ethylenediamine tetraacetic acid (EDTA), which chelates the divalent cations of the outer membrane. Subsequent treatment with lysozyme hydrolyzes the peptidoglycan layer of gram-negative bacteria, and the cells may be lysed. The dependence of the integrity of the outer membrane on calcium and magnesium ions is one of the principal reasons for the in-

clusion of these ions in media used for antimicrobial susceptibility testing.

The gram-negative outer membrane also contains phospholipids and proteins. The phospholipids are similar to those found in the cytoplasmic membrane and include phosphatidyl ethanolamine and phosphatidyl glycerol. The outer membrane also contains proteins; some of these are present in greater concentrations than others, and these are called **principal** or **major membrane proteins**. These proteins fall into three major groups. **Porin proteins** are proteins that form trans-outer membrane channels through which low molecular weight materials are allowed into the periplasmic space. Many of these porin proteins have a "trimer" structure (ie, three identical proteins that form a "doughnut-shaped" pore). **Non-porin proteins** are transmembrane proteins that are associated with the peptidoglycan layer of the cell wall. They may function in exoenzyme production and secretion, binding to surfaces, or in binding of antimicrobial agents to their cell surface targets (eg, penicillin binding proteins). **Lipoproteins** are the smallest of the outer membrane proteins and stabilize the cell wall by covalent linkage with the peptidoglycan. Among the *Enterobacteriaceae*, an enterobacterial common antigen is also found in the outer membrane. This antigen is a linear polysaccharide composed of N-acetylglucosamine, N-acetylmannosaminuronic acid, and N-acetylfucosamine linked to an outer membrane phospholipid.

The structure of the bacterial cell wall has direct, practical importance to the microbiologist because the type of cell wall structure is largely responsible for the Gram stain reaction. This differential stain divides the majority of bacteria into two groups–the gram-positive and the gram-negative bacteria. In the Gram stain procedure, cells are (1) stained with **crystal violet;** (2) treated with **iodine** to form a crystal violet/iodine complex within the cell; (3) washed with an organic solvent (**acetone-alcohol**); and (4) stained again with the red counterstain **safranin**. In **gram-positive** bacteria, the purple crystal violet/iodine complex is retained within the cell after washing with acid-alcohol because the thick peptidoglycan layer does not allow the crystal violet-iodine complex to be washed out of the cell. In **gram-negative bacteria**, the crystal violet/iodine complex is leached from the cell (ie, the cells become colorless) due to disruption of the lipid-rich outer membrane by the acetone-alcohol organic solvent. These colorless cells must be counterstained to be seen under the light microscope; this counterstain is provided by safranin. Gram-positive bacteria appear blue-purple under the microscope; gram-negative bacteria are stained red by the safranin counterstain.

"ACID-FAST" BACTERIAL CELL WALLS

A modification of the gram-positive cell wall is seen in organisms belonging to the genera *Mycobacterium*, *Nocardia*, and *Corynebacterium*. In these organisms, lipids account for as much as 60% of the dry weight of the cell wall. These organisms contain molecules called **mycolic acids** in their cell walls. Mycolic

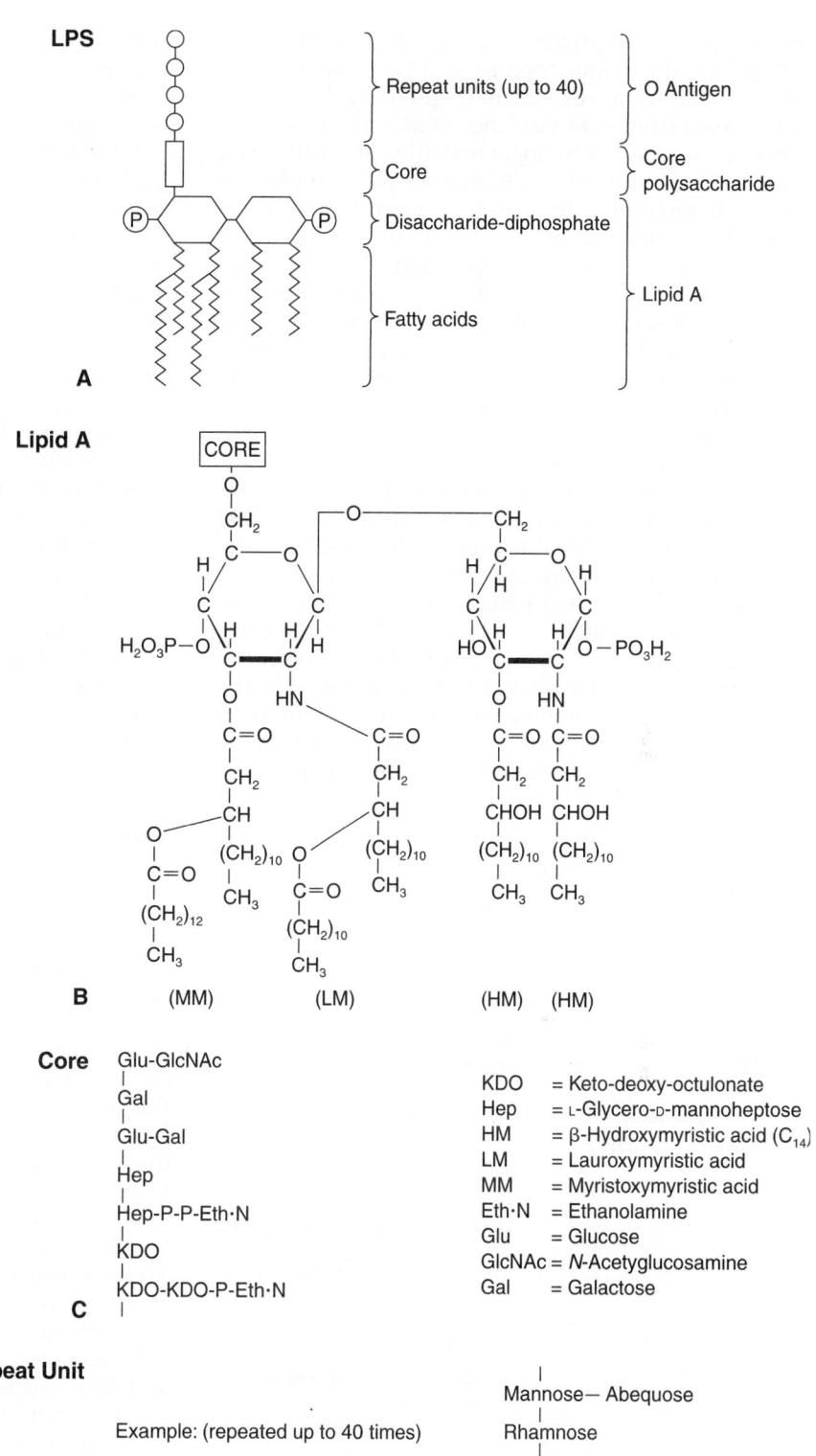

Figure 1-10
The lipopolysaccharide (LPS) of the gram-negative cell envelope. (**A**) Segment of the polymer showing the arrangements of the major constituents. (**B**) Structure of lipid A of *Salmonella typhimurium*. (**C**) Polysaccharide core. (**D**) Typical repeat unit (*Salmonella typhrimurium*). (Redrawn from Brooks GF et al: Jawetz, Melnick and Adelberg's Medical Microbiology, 19E. Norwalk, Connecticut, Appleton & Lange, 1991.)

acids are large, α-substituted, β-hydroxy fatty acids that occur as esters attached to cell wall polysaccharides. Mycolic acids vary in the number of carbon atoms; those with 30 carbons (C30) are found among the corynebacteria (corynemycolenic acids), those with C50 are found in *Nocardia* species (nocardic acids), and those with C90 or more constitute the mycolic acids found in the genus *Mycobacterium*.

The cell wall of mycobacteria contains a peptidoglycan layer, the structure of which is similar to that found in gram-negative bacteria. The peptidoglycan is attached to a branched-chain polysaccharide called **arabinogalactan** by phosphodiester bonds. The distal ends of the arabinogalactan are esterified to the high molecular weight mycolic acids just described. These high molecular weight glycolipids have carbon skeletons ranging in length from C_{78} to C_{90}. In *Mycobacterium tuberculosis*, the unique mycolic acid 6,6'-dimycolyltrehalose, is known as **cord factor** (Fig. 1-11A). This molecule is associated with virulence of *M. tuberculosis* and has a wide range of biologic activities, including cell membrane cytotoxicity, inhibition of polymorphonuclear cell migration, induction of granuloma formation, adjuvanticity, antitumour activity, and ability to activate the alternative complement pathway. The peptidoglycan-arabinogalactan-mycolic acid complex forms the skeleton of the mycobacterial cell wall. The hydrocarbon chains of the mycolic acids are intercalated with those of numerous wall-associated lipids and glycolipids. The wall-associated lipids include those with medium-length (C_{24} to C_{36}) and short (C_{12} to C_{20}) fatty acyl groups. These wall-associated lipids include trehalose sulfolipids (see Fig. 1-11B). The trehalose sulfolipids, typified by the principal sulfolipid of *M. tuberculosis* 2,3,6,6'-tetraacyltrehalose-2'-sulfate, are associated with mycobacterial virulence in that these molecules prevent phagosome-lysozyme fusion following phagocytosis of the mycobacterial cells, thereby allowing the organisms to survive as facultative intracellular parasites. Protruding through the peptidoglycan, the arabinogalactan, and the mycolic acid layers of the wall are substituted phospholipids (phosphatidylinositol mannosides) and lipopolysaccharides (lipoarabinomannans) that are attached to the outer leaflet of the mycobacterial cell membrane. These molecules provide a noncovalent link between the cell membrane and the cell wall. Proteins that are embedded in the mycobacterial cell wall are involved in biosynthesis and construction of the cell wall polymers and some apparently also function as porins.

Organisms that are acid-fast are stained red with the basic dye carbolfuchsin and are resistant to decolorization with acid-alcohol. Because of the hydrophobicity of the mycobacterial cell wall, penetration of the dye into the cell is enhanced by heat treatment (*ie*, the Ziehl-Neelsen method) or incorporation of detergent into the dye (*ie*, the Kinyoun method). Resistance to decolorization by acid-alcohol (*ie*, "acid-fastness") is associated with the mycolic acid-arabinogalactan moieties that constitute the bulk of wall materials external to the peptidoglycan layer. The soluble lipids contribute to but do not determine the acid-fast properties of mycobacterial cells because extraction of these lipids diminishes but does not destroy acid-fastness. Mechanical disruption of the cell wall and extraction of the cell wall lipids with ethanolic alkalis that remove both free and esterified lipids destroy the acid-fast properties of these organisms, indicating that the total lipid content of the cell wall is responsible for the acid-fast staining property.

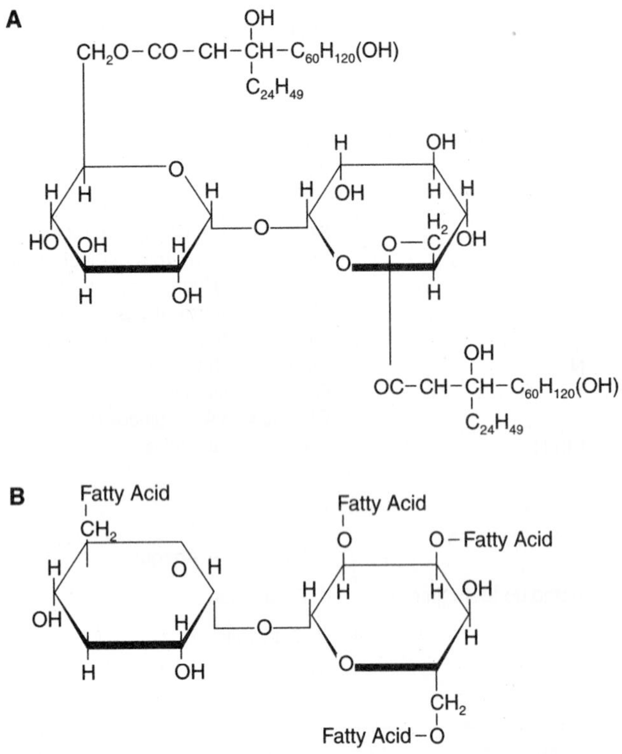

ENDOSPORES

Endospores are spherical or oval structures formed within certain bacterial species that represent a dormant or "resting" stage in the growth cycle of the organism. Among clinically significant bacteria, endospores are formed by only two bacterial genera; aerobic endospore-forming gram-positive bacilli belong to the genus *Bacillus*, and obligately anaerobic, endospore-forming gram-positive bacilli are members of the genus *Clostridium*. In these genera, endospores are formed in response to nutritional deprivation within the vegetative bacterial cell. They are highly resistant to the injurious effects of heat, drying, pressure, and many chemical disinfectants. Sterilization procedures (*ie*, 120°C for 15–20 minutes) are required to kill spores. The heat resistance of bacterial endospores is believed to be due to reduced amounts of water in the core of the spore itself. The size, shape, and location of incipient endospores in stationary phase cells of *Clostridium* and *Bacillus* species is helpful for characterization and identification of certain species within these two genera. The endospores may be spherical, subspherical, or oval in shape; they may differ in their location within the cell (*ie*, central, terminal, or subterminal); and they may or may not swell the cell. Endospores generally do not stain with routine staining methods like the Gram stain and appear as refractile, nonstaining bodies in smears.

Under the stimulus of certain environmental conditions such as the exhaustion of nutrients (*ie*, glucose, nitrogen, or phosphate) or exposure to suboptimal temperatures or redox potentials, the nuclear material divides into two nucleoids, and one becomes sepa-

Figure 1-11
Molecular structure of specialized lipids found in the cell wall of *Mycobacterium tuberculosis*. (**A**) Molecular structure of cord factor (6,6'-dimycolyltrehalose) produced by *Mycobacterium tuberculosis*. (**B**) Molecular structure of the principal sulfolipid (2,3,6,6'-tetraacyltrehalose-2'-sulfate) of *M. tuberculosis*.

rated from the other by a membranous septum. The septum then grows together and the spore core becomes engulfed in a double membrane. Between the two membranes, a cortex layer is deposited by the membranes. This cortex consists primarily of peptidoglycan material. The cortex layer thickens and accumulates calcium ions due to the chelating activity of a unique molecule called **dipicolinic acid**. The core becomes protected by the high concentration of calcium ions tightly cross-linking the peptidoglycan material and all available water in the spore is expelled. Several layers of the **spore coat** (a keratin-like substance that is rich in disulfide bonds) are laid down, and the endospore is liberated on the death and lysis of the mother vegetative cell. Endospores may remain viable for prolonged periods. When the spore is placed in a favorable environment in the presence of particular stimuli (*eg*, the presence of particular amino acids or carbohydrates and water), spore outgrowth occurs. On this stimulus, enzymes are activated, which degrade the spore cortex and release the peptidoglycan material, calcium ions, and dipicolinic acid. RNA synthesis begins, followed by protein synthesis and, eventually, DNA synthesis. A new vegetative cell results.

BACTERIAL SURFACE STRUCTURES

CAPSULES

Some bacteria possess a **capsule** external to the outer layer of the cell wall. The capsule may be thick or thin and may be closely or loosely associated with the external aspect of the cell wall. Loosely associated capsular material may also be referred to as a **slime layer**. Capsular material is usually **polysaccharide** in nature; they may be polymers of single monosaccharides (glucans, dextrans, levans) or **heteropolysaccharides** containing both hexose and pentose sugars, plus ribitol, glycerol, or other sugar alcohols. Phosphates are also frequently present. In some bacterial species, such as *Bacillus* species, the bacterial capsule is polypeptide in nature. The capsule is synthesized at the level of the cell membrane; components are synthesized and exported out of the cell by an isoprenoid lipid "carrier" system, where the components become attached to "primer" capsular material already present on the surface of the cell. In some cases, such as the glucan capsule of *Streptococcus mutans*, the capsule is synthesized by extracellular enzymes called **glucosyltransferases** that are secreted out of the cell. The action of these enzymes on dietary sucrose creates a branched, insoluble glucan matrix that then specifically interacts with receptors on the cell surface to create the glucan capsule. The glucan capsule has practical importance as a virulence factor because this material forms the matrix of dental plaque. Adherence of bacteria to this matrix, and the subsequent formation of acids from dietary sucrose, leads to the initiation of dental caries.

The bacterial capsule has several functions. It protects the cell from desiccation and from toxic materials in the environment (*eg*, heavy metal ions, free radicals) and promotes the concentration of nutrients at the bacterial cell surface because of its polyanionic nature. The capsule also plays a role in the adherence of bacteria to cells and mucosal surfaces. This adherence is necessary for many organisms to establish infections in appropriate hosts (discussed later). In addition, the capsule also offers resistance to the bactericidal action of complement and serum antibodies. Capsular material is usually antigenic and the serologic detection of the capsule forms the basis of the Quellung test, which can be used to identify or subtype several important human pathogenic bacteria, including *Streptococcus pneumoniae*, *Haemophilus influenzae* type b, *Klebsiella pneumoniae*, and *Neisseria meningitidis* serogroups. The capsular material of many microorganisms is synthesized in abundance and is shed into the surrounding fluid both in vivo and in vitro. This material can be detected in various body fluids (*eg*, serum, spinal fluid, and urine) during infection by certain encapsulated bacteria (*eg*, pneumococci, meningococci, and *H. influenzae* type b) and can be specifically detected and identified by electrophoresis or agglutination tests to provide a rapid diagnosis.

FLAGELLA

Bacterial flagella are long, filamentous appendages that arise at the level of the cytoplasmic membrane and extend through the cell wall into the surrounding medium. They are responsible for cellular motility. Flagella are usually found in rod-shaped, gram-negative bacteria, although motile, gram-positive rods (*eg*, *Listeria* species) and cocci (some *Enterococcus* species, *Vagococcus* species) are also found. Flagella differ in their numbers and their arrangements on cells. Bacteria with a single polar flagellum are termed **monotrichous**; those with two or more flagella originating at one pole or point are **lophotrichous**; those with a single flagellum located at two different points or poles are called **amphitrichous**; and those with two or more (a tuft) flagella at two points or poles of the cell are called **amphilophotrichous**. Organisms that have flagella arising over the entire cell surface are termed **peritrichous**.

In gram-negative bacteria, flagella have a complex structure consisting of three parts: the **filament**, the **hook**, and the **basal body** (Fig. 1-12). The flagellar filament is 13 to 17 nm in diameter and is variable in length. The filament is composed of parallel subfibrils of the protein flagellin (MW = 30,000–40,000 daltons), which interact to form a hollow cylinder. The filament is semirigid and forms a left-handed helix as it exits the cell. Flagellin has the capacity to self-assemble. Monomers of the protein are synthesized and passed through the lumen of the cylinder. At the growing tip of the flagellum helix, the monomer undergoes a conformational change and becomes added to the distal end of the flagellum. The hook is composed of another distinct protein and acts as a "sleeve" from which the flagellar filament emerges. The hook permits the transmission of a rotary motion from the basal body to the filament. The **basal body** is composed of complex rings connected by a rod-shaped structure. The **M, S, P**, and **L rings** are anchored in the membrane, the periplasmic space, the peptidoglycan, and the lipopoly-

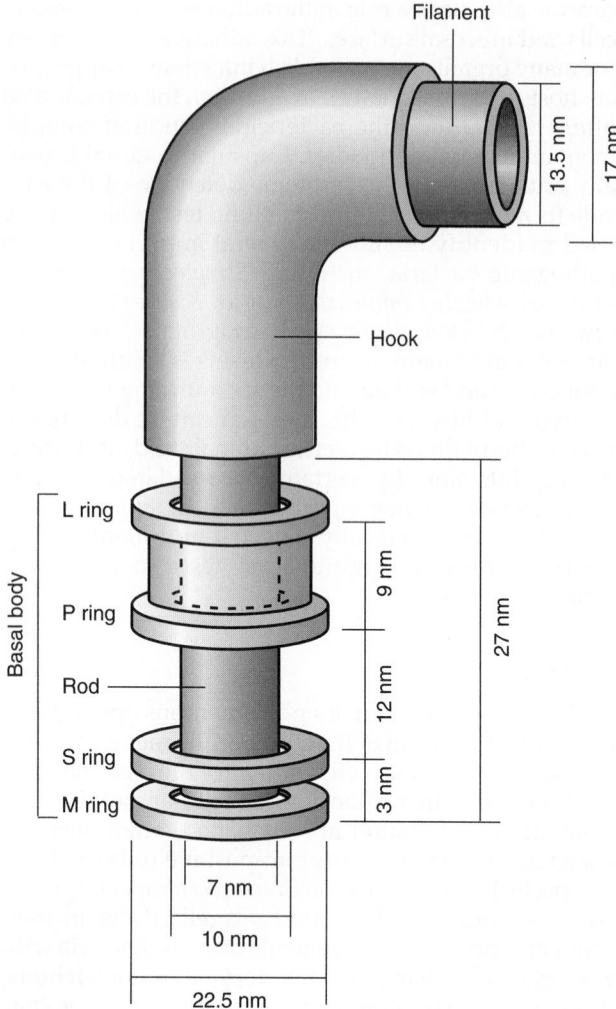

Figure 1-12
Ultrastructure of a flagellum from a gram-negative bacterium.

species, but also occurs in several other species. Flagellar antigens in gram-negative bacilli are referred to as H antigens, from the German word "hauch," meaning "breath." Complete serologic typing of salmonellae involves the identification of S (somatic antigen), H (flagellar antigens), and K (capsular) antigens.

FIMBRIAE (PILI)

Fimbriae or pili are smaller appendages found on the surface of many gram-negative bacteria. Although the terms "pili" and "fimbriae" have been used interchangeably, fimbriae is now used to describe any nonflagellar hairlike appendages, whereas pili is used to denote the fimbriae of gram-negative bacteria that function specifically in the transfer of DNA from one cell to another during the process of conjugation (ie, sex pili). Fimbriae are composed of a protein called **fimbrillin**, are 3 to 10 nm in diameter, and are 15 to 20 μm in length. The proteins form hollow tubes that appear to originate in the cell membrane but that lack the basal body and hook structures of flagella. These appendages are involved in specific pair formation for exchange of genetic material during conjugation and also serve as attachment sites for bacteriophages. Fimbriae also function as cellular organelles for attachment to cells or mucosal surfaces; fimbriae that serve this attachment function are often referred to as **adhesins**. Most adhesins display lectin-like binding to terminal carbohydrate residues like mannose moieties. For example, the adherence of enteric bacteria to mucosal surfaces that is mediated by type 1 or common pili can be inhibited by preincubation of the bacteria with mannose. Mannose attaches to the terminal portion of the adhesin and blocks adherence; therefore, type 1 pili are termed mannose-sensitive. Adhesins that are not affected by mannose are termed mannose-resistant. Differing lectin-like specificities are partly responsible for the tissue tropisms observed with a variety of bacterial species.

The role of fimbriae as virulence factors has been studied most extensively in *Neisseria gonorrhoeae*. Virulent strains of *N. gonorrhoeae* possess surface fimbriae and are able to avidly adhere to mucosal cells in the genital tract. The loss of fimbriae on repeated subculture in vitro renders these organisms unable to initiate urogenital infection due to lack of mucosal adherence. In addition, gonococci possess a large number of genes that code for structurally and antigenically distinct fimbrial proteins. When antibodies to one type of fimbrial protein are present, the organism is able to "switch off" production of the old protein and "switch on" production of a new fimbrial protein. Because of the ability of a single gonococcal strain to produce multiple, antigenically distinct fimbrial antigens, the use of fimbriae as candidate antigens for antigonococcal vaccines has been largely unsuccessful.

GENETIC EXCHANGE IN BACTERIA

Bacterial replication occurs by the process of binary fission, an asexual process that does not involve recombinational events and results in the generation of

saccharide outer membrane, respectively. At least 10 proteins comprise the outer ring structure in gram-negative bacteria. The ring structure attached to the cell membrane rotates as a part of an energy-dependent reaction, causing the rigid flagellar helix to turn like a propeller. The energy for this reaction is derived by the passage of protons from the outside into the cytoplasm via the basal body. The outer rings (L and P rings) evidently function as bearings, minimizing friction and leakage of materials from the cell at the points of flagellar insertion. In gram-positive bacteria, the flagellar structure is less complex and is composed of two rings. One ring structure anchors the flagellum to the plasma membrane; the second ring structure is embedded in the thick peptidoglycan layer.

Several species of flagellated organisms are also able to alter the expressed antigenic type of flagella that they produce; this process is known as **phase variation**. Phase variation occurs by the differential expression of genes coding for variously structured flagellin proteins. This phenomenon was first recognized in enteric gram-negative bacteria like *Salmonella*

two daughter cells that are identical to the parent cell. Several groups of bacteria, however, do have the ability to undergo genetic exchange and recombination with other organisms. Genetic exchange between bacteria occurs by one of three mechanisms: transformation, transduction, and conjugation (Fig. 1-13).

Transformation involves the uptake of free DNA from the surrounding environment. Cells that are physiologically capable of taking up and incorporating free DNA into their genomes are termed **competent**. Competence is usually a transient state that occurs toward the late exponential phase of growth. In competent gram-positive cells, small pieces of double-stranded DNA become bound to the cell by a cell surface receptor that is expressed during the competent period. As the DNA enters the cell, one strand is hydrolyzed by a surface-bound nuclease. Recombinational events between the single-stranded DNA and the homologous region of the bacterial chromosome result in integration of the transformed DNA into the bacterial genome. If homologous regions for the transforming DNA are lacking, the DNA strand does not integrate, genes on the particular DNA strand are not expressed, and the single-stranded DNA is degraded by endogenous restriction endonucleases. Competent gram-negative bacteria also possess receptors for DNA on the cell surface, but the process of DNA binding occurs simultaneously with the recognition of a nu-

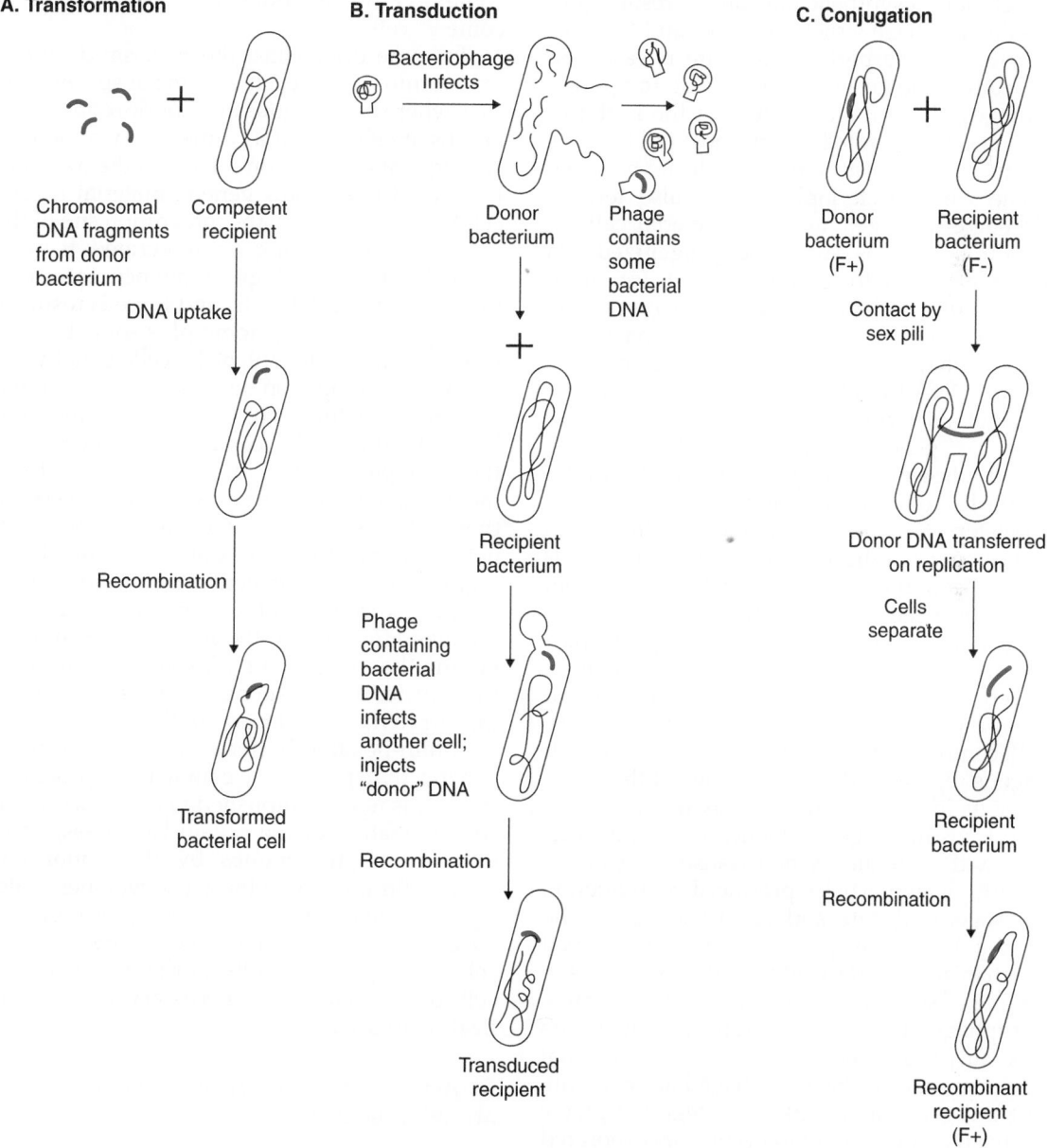

Figure 1-13
Mechanisms of gene transfer in bacteria. Microorganisms may exchange genetic material by any of three processes: transformation (**A**), transduction via bacteriophage (**B**), and conjugation (**C**).

cleotide sequence of 10 to 14 base-pairs that only allows DNA from closely related species to bind and enter the competent cell. Double-stranded DNA then enters the cell, but only one strand participates in the recombinational events that incorporate the transforming DNA into the genome of the recipient. Cells that normally do not express competence for genetic transformation can be made permeable to extracellular DNA by treatment with $CaCl_2$ or other salt solutions. Uptake of naked DNA by "artificially competent" bacteria is called **transfection**.

Transduction refers to the exchange of genetic information via bacteriophages. Bacteriophages (or simply "phages") are viruses that infect bacteria. Some bacteriophages are lytic; that is, after infecting the bacterial cell, the bacteriophage regulatory genes "take over" the cellular biosynthetic machinery, resulting in the expression of phage structural genes and the production of new phage particles that are released on lysis and death of the host bacterium. With **temperate bacteriophages**, the genetic material of the bacteriophage becomes incorporated into the host cell DNA as a "prophage" and replicates along with the bacterial chromosome. Such bacteriophages are also termed **lysogenic bacteriophages**, and the bacterial cell infected with this phage is said to be **lysogenized**. On **induction** by exposure to certain chemicals (eg, mitomycin C) or to ultraviolet irradiation, a lysogenic bacteriophage may be induced to begin production of new phages (ie, the phage becomes "lytic"). Excision of the bacteriophage DNA from the bacterial cell genome results in some bacteriophages containing not only "phage-specific" genes, but also host cell genes that were located adjacent to the site of phage DNA integration in the bacterial chromosome.

The transfer of genetic information during transduction may be generalized or specialized. **Generalized transduction** refers to the accidental, random packaging of host cell DNA into the capsid or "head" of the phage particle. Release of the mature phage particle on cell lysis and subsequent infection of another bacterial cell results in the introduction of "donor DNA" from the original host bacterium into the "recipient." Recombination of the transduced DNA with a homologous region on the chromosome of the recipient cell results in integration and subsequent expression of the transduced genes. Generalized transduction occurs with a frequency of 1 transducing phage per 10^5 to 10^8 phage particles produced on induction from the lysogenized state, and about 1% to 2% of the total length of the host cell genome may be transferred by this mechanism. **Specialized transduction** refers to the packaging of specific host cell genes into the transducing prophage. This type of transduction occurs with temperate phages that have specific chromosomal integration sites, such as bacteriophage **lambda**. Only those host cell genes that flank the integrated phage genome have the opportunity to become incorporated into the bacteriophage genome on induction from the lysogenic state. One specialized transducing phage is produced out of 10^5 to 10^6 new phage particles following induction.

Conjugation is the only mechanism of genetic exchange between bacteria that requires cell-to-cell contact. Gram-negative bacteria that are able to participate in conjugation possess a plasmid called the F plasmid that codes for a **sex pilus**. This specialized pilus functions as a vehicle for establishing contact with another bacterial cell and as a "tube" through which the DNA is passed during the conjugative process. Cells that possess F plasmids are termed F^+; cells that lack this plasmid are termed F^-. Once contact of an F^+ cell with an F^- cell is established by the sex pilus, the circular F plasmid begins to be replicated. During this process, one of the single strands of the plasmid DNA is passed through the pilus into the recipient cell. The single strand that is passed begins to be replicated as it enters the recipient cell, and the end result is two cells that contain complete conjugative plasmids (ie, both become F^+ cells).

In some organisms, the F plasmid becomes integrated into the host cell genome at specific integration sites where homologous nucleotide sequences are present. Establishment of a connection via the F pilus and subsequent conjugation results in the transfer of some F plasmid genes plus genetic material from the host cell that is adjacent to the integration site of the F plasmid. Cells possessing an integrated F plasmid are termed **Hfr cells** (high frequency recombinations). Mating between Hfr cells and F^- cells results in transfer of part of the F genome plus some host cell genes from the donor. Recipient F^- cells usually remain F^- following conjugation because only part of the F plasmid from the donor Hfr cell is transferred to the recipient cell during the conjugative process. Therefore, these recipient cells will not possess the full complement of genes that are subsequently necessary to synthesize the sex pilus. Recombination between the genetic material from the donor cell and homologous regions in the F^- recipient enables the donor DNA to become expressed in the recipient cell. The donor cell remains Hfr because the host cell chromosome (containing the integrated F plasmid) is replicated during the transfer of the genomic single-stranded DNA from the Hfr to the F^- cell through the sex pilus.

Gram-positive bacteria are also able to exchange genetic material via a conjugative process, but the transfer is not accomplished via a pilus, but rather by a co-aggregation of the organisms in response to production of **pheromones** by the donor bacterium. Under stimulation by these pheromones, potential recipient bacteria synthesize a receptor molecule that is specific for a conjugative adhesin present on the donor cell. Aggregation results in the establishment of the cell-to-cell connections necessary for plasmid mobilization to occur.

REQUIREMENTS FOR BACTERIAL GROWTH AND METABOLISM

CARBON

Bacteria can be divided into two large groups on the basis of their carbon requirement—the **lithotrophic** or **autotrophic** bacteria and the **organotrophic** or **heterotrophic** bacteria. The **lithotrophic bacteria** can use carbon dioxide as the sole source of carbon and synthesize from it the carbon "skeletons" for all their organic metabolites. They require only water, inorganic salts, and CO_2 for growth and their energy is derived either from light (**photolithotrophic bacteria**) or from the oxidation of one or more inorganic substances (**chemolithotrophic bacteria**). **Organotrophic bacteria** are unable to use CO_2 as their sole source of carbon but require it in an organic form, such as glucose. For these heterotrophic bacteria, a portion of the organic compound that serves as an energy source is also used for the synthesis of organic compounds required by the organism. A wide variety of other substances can also be used as exclusive or partial sources of carbon by different bacterial species. Among the most versatile bacteria are *Pseudomonas* species, some of which can use more than 100 different organic compounds as their sole source of carbon and energy. The relationships among energy sources, carbon sources, and electron donors for generation of energy are summarized in Table 1-2.

CARBON DIOXIDE

Some bacteria are able to use atmospheric CO_2 as a principal source of carbon for biosynthetic reactions. The energy for catalyzing this utilization may come from light energy (photolithotrophic bacteria) or from oxidation of inorganic molecules (chemolithotrophic bacteria). Organisms that require an organic source of carbon also require some CO_2 for certain macromolecular synthetic pathways, such as fatty acid biosynthesis. Carbon dioxide for these reactions is usually obtained from the breakdown of organic substrates occurring at the same time as the biosynthetic reactions.

OXYGEN

The oxygen requirement of a particular bacterium reflects the mechanism used for satisfying its energy needs. On the basis of their oxygen requirements, bacteria may be divided into five groups. **Obligate anaerobes** grow only under conditions of high reducing intensity and for which oxygen is toxic. **Aerotolerant anaerobes** are anaerobic bacteria that are not killed by exposure to oxygen. **Facultative anaerobes** are capable of growth under both aerobic and anaerobic conditions. **Obligate aerobes** have an absolute requirement for oxygen to be able to grow. **Microaerophilic organisms** grow the best under lower oxygen tension; higher oxygen tensions may be inhibitory. In obligate and facultative aerobes, the assimilation of glucose results in the terminal generation of the free radical superoxide (O_2^-). The superoxide is reduced by the enzyme superoxide dismutase to oxygen gas (O_2) and hydrogen peroxide (H_2O_2). Subsequently, the toxic H_2O_2 generated in this reaction is converted to water and O_2 by the enzyme **catalase**, which is found in aerobic and facultative bacteria, or by various **peroxidases**, which are found in several aerotolerant anaerobes.

NITROGEN

The nitrogen atoms of important biomolecules (*ie*, amino acids, purines, pyrimidines) come from ammonium ions (NH_4^+). The generation of ammonium ions starts with the reduction of atmospheric N_2 to NH_4^+ (ammonium ion or ammonia, NH_3). NH_4^+ is then assimilated into more complex macromolecules by way of the key compounds **glutamate** and **glutamine**. Certain species of bacteria (*Rhizobium* species, *Azotobacter* species) and blue-green algae are able to "fix" atmospheric N_2 into a more readily useable organic form. Because of the strength of the triple bonds in N_2, nitrogen fixation requires cellular energy in the form of adenosine triphosphate (ATP) and a powerful reductant. The process is catalyzed by a complex multienzyme system called the **nitrogenase complex**. In most nitrogen-fixing organisms, reduced ferredoxin is the source of electrons:

$$N_2 + 6e^- + 12\,ATP + 12\,H_2O \rightarrow 2\,NH_4^+ + 12\,ADP + 12\,P_i + 4H^+$$

The ability to fix nitrogen is primarily accomplished by the soil-dwelling bacteria mentioned above. However,

---

TABLE 1-2

ENERGY AND CARBON SOURCES OF BACTERIA

TYPE/EXAMPLES	ENERGY SOURCE(S)	CARBON SOURCE(S)	ELECTRON DONORS
Photolithotrophs Green sulfur bacteria Purple sulfur bacteria	Light	CO_2	Inorganic compounds (H_2S, S)
Photoorganotrophs Purple nonsulfur bacteria	Light	Organic compounds (and CO_2)	Organic compounds
Chemolithotrophs Hydrogen, sulfur, and denitrifying bacteria	Oxidation-reduction reactions	CO_2	Inorganic compounds (H_2, S, H_2S, Fe, NH_3)
Chemoorganotrophs	Oxidation-reduction reactions	Organic compounds	Organic compounds (glucose, and other carbohydrates)

some bacterial species that are involved in human disease, such as *Klebsiella pneumoniae* and certain *Clostridium* species are also able to fix atmospheric nitrogen.

Ammonium ions may also be generated by nitrate reduction. This is accomplished by two distinct physiologic mechanisms. **Assimilatory nitrate reduction** is a process in which nitrate is reduced to nitrite and hydroxylamine, which are then converted to ammonia for assimilation. **Dissimilatory nitrate reduction** is when nitrate serves as an alternative electron acceptor to oxygen (anaerobic respiration), with NO_2 or N_2 being the usual products. Nitrate assimilation is widespread in microorganisms and requires both nitrate and nitrite reductases, whereas dissimilatory nitrate reduction is seen only in anaerobic bacteria and facultative anaerobic bacteria growing at low oxygen tension (*ie*, in a broth). Ammonia generated by these mechanisms becomes incorporated into organic molecules by the action of the enzymes **glutamate dehydrogensase**, **glutamine synthetase**, and **glutamic acid synthase** (Fig. 1-14). The final products of these reactions are glutamine and glutamic acid, which then become the building blocks used in other biosynthetic reactions for the synthesis of several amino acids,

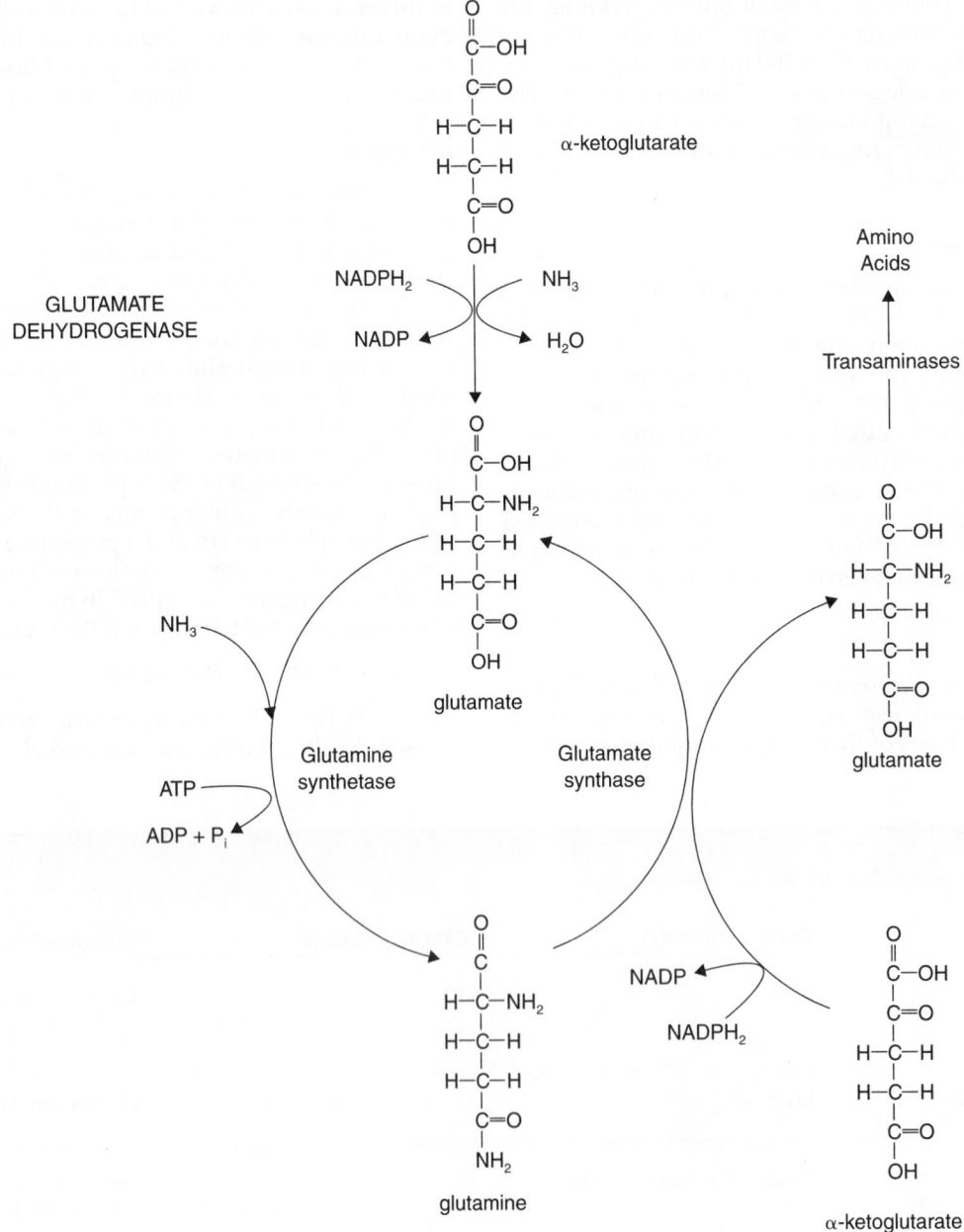

Figure 1-14
Nitrogen assimilation and metabolism via the enzymes glutamine synthetase, glutamate dehydrogenase, and glutamate synthase. This enzymatic system results in the formation of amino acids and other compounds.

purines, pyrimidines, and other necessary nitrogenous compounds (see Fig. 1-14).

GROWTH FACTORS

These substances promote growth of the organism and are provided by various body fluids and tissues in vivo and in the form of yeast extract and blood or blood products in vitro. These factors include B-complex vitamins, minerals, certain amino acids, purines, and pyrimidines. The B-complex vitamins play a catalytic role within the cell, acting either as components of coenzymes or as prosthetic groups of enzymes. Organisms that do not require an exogenous source of a given growth factor because they are capable of synthesizing their own are referred to as **prototrophic**. **Auxotrophic** organisms require the addition of the growth factor to culture media before growth can occur. Small amounts of a number of inorganic ions also are required by all bacteria. In addition to nitrogen, sulfur, and phosphorus, which are present as constituents of important biologic compounds, potassium, magnesium, and calcium are often functionally associated with certain anionic polymers. Magnesium divalent cations stabilize ribosomes, cell membranes, the cell wall, and nucleic acids and are also required for the activity of many enzymes. Potassium is also required for the activity of a number of enzymes, and in gram-positive bacteria its concentration in the cell is influenced by the teichoic acid content of the cell wall. Most organisms also require zinc, iron, manganese, copper, and cobalt. Certain physical requirements for growth include optimal growth temperature, pH, and oxidation/reduction potential.

KINETICS OF BACTERIAL GROWTH

During growth in fluid culture medium, bacteria display a uniform growth curve, as expressed in logarithmic numbers of bacteria over time. A typical bacterial growth curve is shown in Figure 1-15. The **lag phase** is a period of physiologic adjustment and "gearing up," when the cell synthesizes new enzymes, cofactors, and essential metabolic intermediates, and the intracellular

pools of nutrients are established. During the **increasing growth phase**, cell growth begins as enzymatic reaction rates begin to approach their steady-state rates. During the **logarithmic growth phase**, cell growth and cell division are occurring at their maximal rates. This rate is influenced by temperature, the type of carbon source being used, the rate-limiting concentrations of various essential nutrients, the types of nutrients available, and the oxygen tension or redox potential. During the **declining growth phase**, growth eventually ceases due to exhaustion of various nutrients from the medium. During the **stationary phase**, the number of viable cells has plateaued and the numbers of new organisms produced is equal to the numbers of cells that die due to lack of nutrients. During the **death phase**, cells begin to lyse and die.

GENERAL BACTERIAL METABOLISM AND ENERGY GENERATION

FERMENTATION

Bacterial metabolism is a dynamic balance between biosynthesis (anabolic reactions) and degradation (catabolic reactions). Catabolic reactions, in addition to providing smaller building blocks for subsequent biosynthetic processes, provide the energy to "drive" the biosynthetic reactions. In these processes, energy from the hydrolysis of chemical bonds is captured in the high energy phosphate bonds of **adenosine triphosphate (ATP)**. These bonds provide for the activation and continuation of other biochemical events. Using this energy, the bacterial cell wall, proteins, nucleic acids, and other structural and regulatory macromolecules are synthesized. Utilization of carbohydrates by bacteria and the conditions under which this utilization occurs are key characteristics for broadly characterizing bacteria. In general, many tests performed in the clinical microbiology laboratory involve the detection of the end-products of bacterial metabolism in spent culture fluids, either by pH indicators in the medium or by gas-liquid chromatogra-

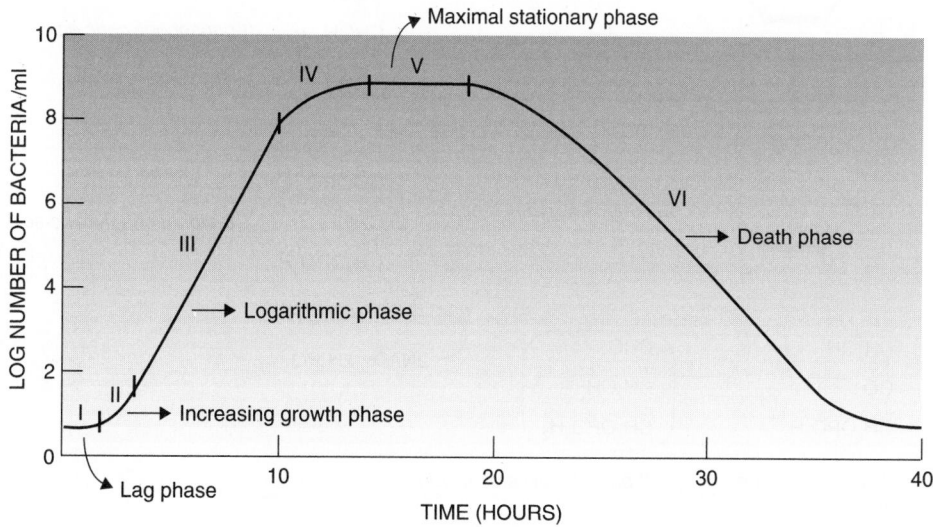

Figure 1-15
Kinetics of bacterial growth.

phy. The ability of a given microorganism to produce acid from a variety of carbohydrates (*eg*, maltose, sucrose, mannitol, mannose, etc) reflects the enzymatic capabilities of these organisms to initially convert such carbohydrates to **glucose**, which is the starting point for both aerobic and anaerobic carbohydrate catabolism.

Utilization of glucose under anaerobic conditions is termed **fermentation**. Fermentation occurs via glycolysis, with the end-product being **pyruvic acid** or **pyruvate**. The glycolytic pathway from glucose to pyruvate is shown in Figure 1-16. This pathway requires two ATP molecules for initial phosphorylation of glucose to glucose-6-phosphate and subsequent phosphorylation of fructose-6-phosphate to fructose-1,6-diphosphate. During glycolysis, ATP is generated at two points in the pathway. As a result of the conversion of 1,3-diphosphoglyceric acid to 3-phosphoglyceric acid, the energy derived from the oxidation of an aldehyde group is conserved as a high-energy phosphate bond in ATP. The conversion of phosphoenolpyruvate to

pyruvate results in the generation of another ATP molecule. Therefore, four ATP molecules are produced from every molecule of glucose during glycolysis by a process called **substrate level phosphorylation**, resulting in a net gain of two molecules of ATP. In addition to ATP, reducing power is also produced by the generation of $NADH_2$ from the cofactor NAD (nicotinamide adenine dinucleotide).

Glycolysis is not the sole pathway for carbohydrate metabolism in most organisms. Other pathways, such as the pentose phosphate and Entner-Doudoroff pathways, begin with glucose being converted to 6-phosphogluconic acid. In the pentose phosphate pathway, this hexose (6-carbon) is converted to ribulose-5-phosphate (5-carbon) and CO_2. From this point, enzymes known as **transketolases** and **transaldolases** convert this precursor to various 3-, 4-, and 5-carbon sugars. These carbohydrates, in turn, are used as building blocks for the biosynthesis of nucleic acid precursors. The Entner-Doudoroff pathway is used by aerobic bacteria that lack the enzymatic ability to convert fructose-

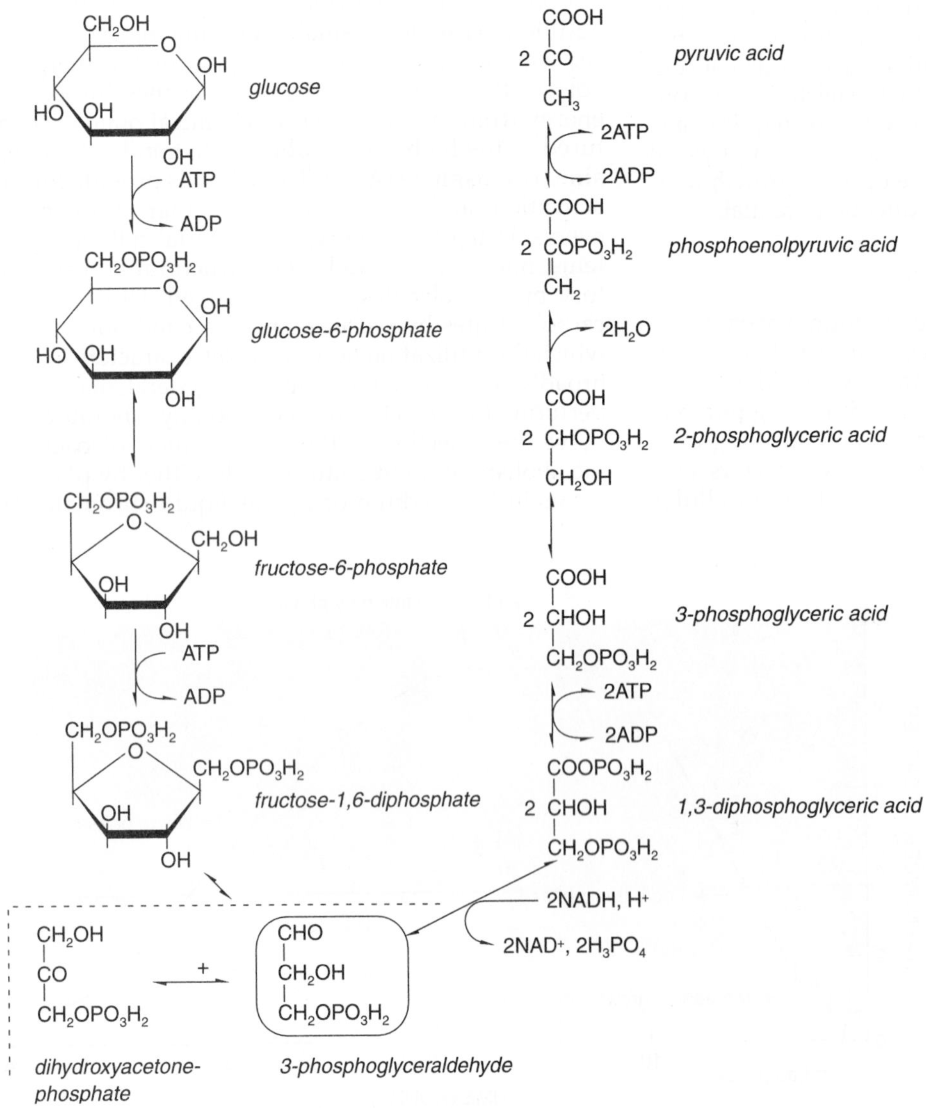

Figure 1-16
Glycolytic pathway.

6-phosphate to fructose-1,6-diphosphate in the glycolytic pathway. In this pathway, 6-phosphogluconic acid is dehydrated to generate 2-keto-3-deoxy-6-phosphogluconic acid, which is then cleaved to form glyceraldehyde-3-phosphate and pyruvate. In *Neisseria* and *Pseudomonas* species, the pyruvate is then converted to enthanol and CO_2 (see Chaps. 4 and 5).

UTILIZATION OF PYRUVATE

Pyruvate may enter a variety of pathways, resulting in several different end-products. It is these end-products that are often useful in categorizing the organisms isolated in the clinical microbiology laboratory. The metabolic pathways shown in Figures 1-17 and 1-18 include:

Pathway #1—Homolactic fermentation (homofermentative). In this pathway, the simplest of fermentations, the sole product of glucose fermentation is lactic acid. No gas is formed. Homolactic fermentation of glucose is characteristic of the streptococci, enterococci, pediococci, and lactobacilli.

Pathway #2—Heterolactic fermentation. Pyruvate is metabolized to acetaldehyde and ethanol, with the release of CO_2. This type of pathway is seen in *Leuconostoc* species, some lactobacilli, and yeasts.

Pathway #3—Mixed acid fermentation. In this metabolic pathway, pyruvate is metabolized to a number of different products (acetic acid, ethanol, succinic acid, formic acid). The nature and amounts of the various acids depend on the nature of the organism. All of the *Enterobacteriaceae* produce formic acid, which is converted to H_2 and CO_2.

Pathway #4—Butanediol fermentation. In this pathway, pyruvate is the precursor to **acetoin** (acetylmethylcarbinol), which, in the presence of hydrogen, is reduced to **2,3-butanediol**. This reduction reaction is slowly reversible in air under alkaline conditions; the acetoin that is synthesized can be detected by the additon of α-naphthol. This is the basis of the Voges-Proskauer test, which uses α-naphthol in the presence of alkali to detect acetoin (VP test). This pathway is seen in the *Klebsiella-Enterobacter-Serratia-Hafnia* group of the family *Enterobacteriaceae*. The conversion of some of the pyruvate to 2,3-butanediol reduces the amount of acid relative to the mixed acid pathway described above and is responsible for the methyl-red (MR) reaction used to separate *E. coli* and related organisms (MR+/VP−) from the *Klebsiella-Enterobacter-Serratia-Hafnia* group (MR−/VP+).

Pathway #5—Butyric acid fermentation. Butyric acid formation is characteristic of the clostridia. Two molecules of pyruvate condense to form **acetoacetic acid**, which is subsequently reduced to **butyric acid**. In some *Clostridium* species, variable quantities of butyric acid may be reduced further to **butanol**, **acetone**, **isopropanol**, and

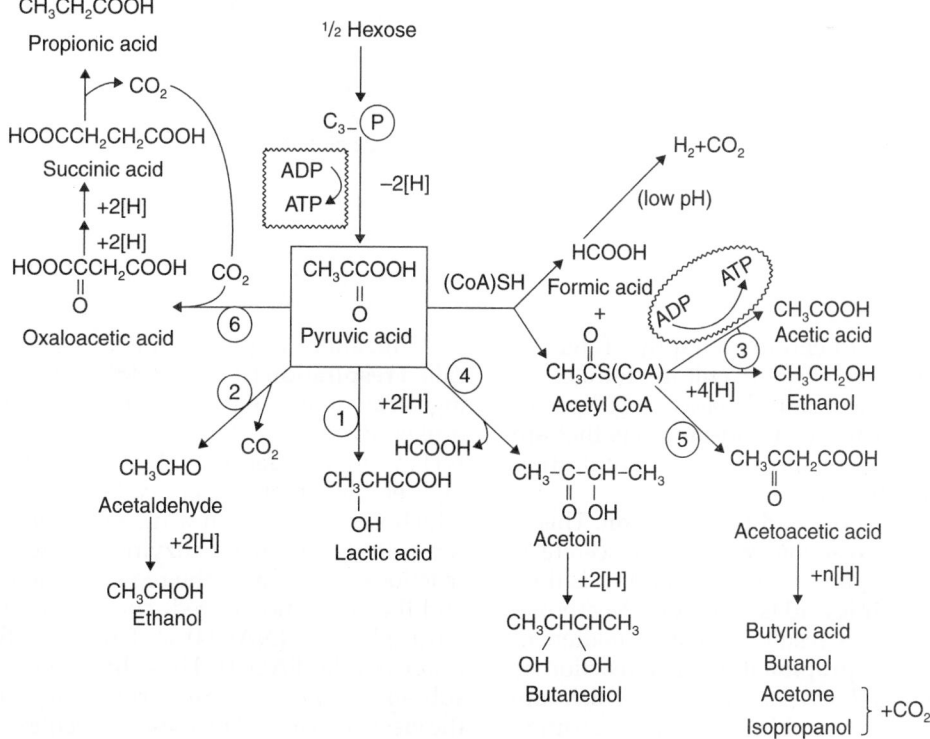

Figure I-17
Fate of pyruvate formed during anaerobic fermentation.

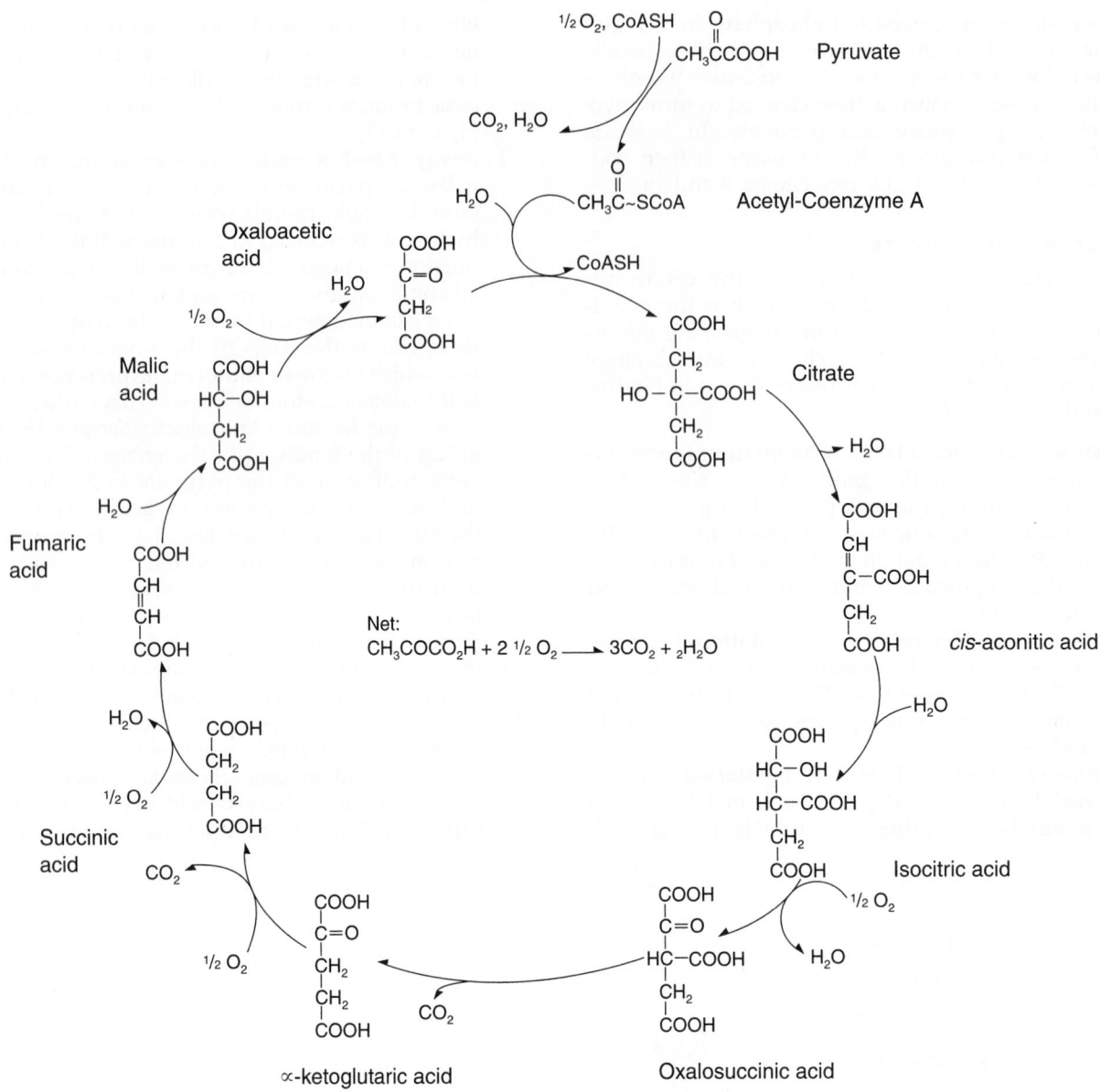

Figure 1-18
Krebs' tricarboxylic acid cycle.

ethanol. Gas-liquid chromatography of derivatives prepared from spent culture filtrates of *Clostridium* species and *Fusobacterium* species may contain a variety of end-products that are helpful for genus- or species-level identification of these anaerobic bacteria.

Pathway #6—Propionic acid fermentation. This is a cyclic-type of reaction where oxaloacetate is formed from CO_2 and pyruvate, and this is then reduced to **succinic acid (succinate)**. Decarboxylation of succinate results in the formation of **propionic acid (propionate)**. This reaction is seen in *Propionibacterium* species, which are gram-positive, anaerobic, non–spore-forming bacilli.

Utilization of glucose under aerobic conditions is called **respiration** (see Fig. 1-18). Pyruvate formed during fermentation enters the Krebs' cycle, where it is broken down to CO_2 and H_2O with the generation of ATP. Oxidative decarboxylation of pyruvate yields the high-energy intermediate called acetyl-coenzyme A, which condenses with a molecule of oxaloacetate to form citrate and free coenzyme A. A series of oxidative reactions ensues with the regeneration of oxaloacetate and the generation of reducing power in the forms of reduced NAD (NADH) and reduced flavin adenine dinucleotide (FADH). These high-energy compounds subsequently enter the electron transport chain, where the electrons carried by these molecules are transferred through a series of cytochrome enzymes. Energy created by the transfer of electrons in the chain generates ATP. The final electron acceptor in the electron transport chain is oxygen, with the final product being water. Complete oxidation of glucose via anaerobic glycolysis and the aerobic Krebs' cycle results in a net gain of 38 ATP molecules per mole of glucose as compared with the net generation of only 2 ATP molecules per mole of glucose via the glycolytic (fermentative) pathway alone. In addition to the generation of ATP during aerobic metabolism, the Krebs' cycle also provides the cell with precursors or intermediate compounds used in the biosynthesis of several other cellular components, such as purines, pyrimidines, amino acids, and lipids. The cycle also serves a catabolic function by providing a venue for the oxidative breakdown of these same macromolecules.

BACTERIAL VIRULENCE AND PATHOGENICITY

DEFINITIONS AND CONCEPTS

Pathogenicity refers to the ability of an organism to cause disease. Organisms that are capable of causing disease under the appropriate circumstances are called **pathogens**. **Virulence** refers to the degree of pathogenicity within a group or species of microorganisms. Virulence is not generally attributable to single discrete factors but depends on several parameters related to the organism, the host, and their interaction. In general, virulence encompasses two features of a pathogenic microorganism: its **infectivity** (*ie*, the ability to initiate an infection) and the **severity** of the condition produced. Highly virulent, moderately virulent, or avirulent strains may occur within a species or group of organisms that are generally considered to be pathogenic.

Infection of the host by an organism is a necessary step in the production of disease. However, infection does not always cause disease. **Colonization** of a host with normal flora organisms is, in a broad sense, infection. The normal flora organisms become established in and on the host early in life and persist throughout the life of the host. When host defense mechanisms are abrogated, these endogenous organisms may cause pathology and disease. Although certain organisms are always associated with pathology when present (*eg, Neisseria gonorrhoeae*), other organisms (*eg, Neisseria meningitidis*) appear to cause disease only under certain circumstances.

REQUIREMENTS FOR PATHOGENICITY

The first step in the establishment of an infectious process resides in the ability of a microorganism to enter the host and to initiate infection. The initial contact depends on the ability of the organism to attach to and survive on the host's mucous membrane surfaces. Some organisms will attach to epithelial cells without invasion of the deeper tissues. In such cases, toxin(s) elaborated by the organisms are usually responsible for the pathology. Examples of such organisms include *Bordetella pertussis* and *Vibrio cholerae*. Certain organisms attach to the mucosal epithelial cells and subsequently penetrate this barrier. Further multiplication of the organisms in the subepithelial tissues results in tissue destruction. More invasive organisms may attach, penetrate the epithelial cell surfaces, begin to multiply, and extend into the deeper tissues; such organisms may eventually gain access to the bloodstream, causing widespread or disseminated infection. Some bacteria species, such as mycobacteria and brucellae, attach, invade, multiply, and subsequently adapt themselves to a continued existence within the host, usually by taking up residence within cells of the reticuloendothelial system.

Many organisms are highly specific in the types of tissues that they may infect. For example, *Neisseria meningitidis* may be found as a normal inhabitant of the throat but may invade the meninges and the bloodstream. *Streptococcus pneumoniae* may also inhabit the throat and nasopharynx, yet it preferentially invades the lower respiratory tract when causing disease. Tissue specificity may be related to the presence of specific receptors for bacterial attachment or the presence of nutrients (*eg*, certain amino acids, ions, or carbohydrates). A classic example of this nutritional dependence is seen with *Brucella abortus*, the cause of contagious abortion in cattle. This organism has a specific growth requirement for the sugar alcohol **erythritol**, which is present in high concentrations in the bovine uterus and placental tissue. Hence, this organism may actually "home in" on the bovine genital tract due to this nutritional prediliction.

VIRULENCE FACTORS OF MICROORGANISMS

ADHESINS

To infect a host, microorganisms must first adhere to the mucosal surface. Bacterial adherence is usually a specific process involving bacterial cell surface structures that are generally known as **adhesins** and complementary **receptors** on the surface of susceptible cells. Bacterial adhesins may include fimbriae, components of the bacterial capsule, lipoteichoic acids that project outside of the peptidoglycan of the cell wall of gram-positive bacteria, or other cell surface antigens. Specific examples of well-characterized adhesins in pathogenic microorganisms include the adherence fimbriae of *Neisseria gonorrhoeae*, mannose-sensitive and mannose-resistant fimbriae of uropathogenic and enteropathogenic *E. coli*, and lipoteichoic acids of group A β-hemolytic streptococci.

AGGRESSINS

To survive and multiply within the host, many organisms produce a variety of substances that allow them to avoid or circumvent host defense mechanisms. These substances, termed **aggressins**, include capsules and extracellular slime substances, surface proteins and carbohydrates, enzymes, toxins, and other small molecules. The capsular structures of some bacteria enable the organisms to avoid phagocytosis by preventing interaction between the bacterial cell surface and phagocytic cells or by concealing bacterial cell surface components that would otherwise interact with phagocytic cells and lead to their ingestion. Specific antibodies directed against capsular material leads to **opsonization** of the microorganisms. Following opsonization, encapsulated bacteria are readily and rapidly ingested and killed by phagocytic cells. Organisms that possess polysaccharide capsules that behave as aggressins include *Streptococcus pneumoniae, Neisseria meningitidis, Haemophilus influenzae* type b, *Klebsiella pneumoniae,* and group B β-hemolytic streptococci.

Some bacteria possess surface proteins or enzymes that play a role in adherence and also contribute to microbial virulence in other ways. For example, the **M protein of group A β-hemolytic streptococci** has multiple effects on the the immune system of the host, including impairment of complement function and lytic effects on polymorphonuclear leukocytes. **Protein A**, a cell wall protein of *Staphylococcus aureus,* is able to bind immunoglobulin (IgG) molecules by their Fc region. Because antibody-mediated phagocytosis (*ie,* opsonization) is Fc receptor dependent, protein A may interfere with this process. The presence of protein A may also inhibit the activation of complement by the staphylococcal cell wall by masking the peptidoglycan moieties that are known to have complement-activating activity. Some bacteria can produce a protease that is able to hydrolyze and inactivate secretory immunoglobulins (IgA). This immunoglobulin acts locally to prevent bacterial adherence; hydrolysis of IgA by bacterial protease, therefore, fosters mucosal colonization.

Some aggressins act after phagocytosis has occurred by interfering with phagosome/lysosome fusion and with the activity of the myeloperoxidase system. The mycobacteria and brucellae are able to adapt to an intracellular existence within host cells by elaborating substances that prevent intracellular destruction of organisms. In the mycobacteria, this is due to the presence of cell wall-associated sulfolipids that become incorporated into the inner aspect of the phagosome and prevent lysosome/phagosome fusion. Other organisms like *Listeria monocytogenes* and *Staphylococcus aureus* secrete enzymes such as **catalase** and **superoxide dismutase** that inhibit organism destruction by the myeloperoxidase system of phagocytic cells. Taking up residence within phagocytic cells by these mechanisms also contributes to virulence by protecting the organisms from destruction by specific antibodies and complement. An intracellular existence also has a significant influence on therapy. Infections with organisms such as *Brucella* species and *Francisella tularensis* must be treated with antibiotics that are able to act intracellularly (*eg,* tetracyclines, aminoglycosides) to affect these "protected" organisms.

Many bacteria produce enzymes or toxins or possess cellular constituents that have direct toxic or necrotizing effects on host inflammatory cells and other components of the immune system. The leukocidins produced by *Staphylococcus aureus* cause degranulation, swelling, and lysis of polymorphonuclear

cells. The lipopolysaccharide of gram-negative bacteria may delay or blunt the acute inflammatory response, allowing the organism to establish itself within the host with relative ease. Some organisms have cell surface properties that render them resistant to the bactericidal effects of normal human serum. This property may facilitate dissemination of the bacteria via the bloodstream and lymphatics, leading to overwhelming systemic infection or to the establishment of infected foci at sites distant from the site of the initial infection. Some of these components confer resistance to the effects of antibacterial lysosomal proteins such as lysozyme, lactoferrin, and cationic proteins.

The invasive properties of some bacteria are attributed to the elaboration of enzymes that act extracellularly. Many gram-positive pathogenic bacteria, such as *Staphylococcus aureus* and group A β-hemolytic streptococci, produce **hyaluronidase**, an enzyme that promotes the spread of the organism through the connective tissues by depolymerizing hyaluronic acid, the ground substance responsible for cell-to-cell adhesion. Group A streptococci and staphylococci also elaborate enzymes that hydrolyze fibrin clots (streptokinase and staphylokinase) and facilitate the spread of organisms in the tissues. *Clostridium histolyticum, Clostridium perfringens,* and *Clostridium septicum* produce **collagenases,** which break down the collagen matrix of muscle and connective tissue and facilitate the extension of the organisms into these tissues to cause necrotizing fasciitis and gas gangrene.

Most pathogenic bacteria produce **siderophores,** which are small molecules that are secreted by the organism and that scavenge iron from the host during infection. Iron is a requirement for virulence in several bacteria. The production of siderophores is considered a virulence factor because some of them apparently protect microorganisms from the killing effects of normal human serum. They are produced by a wide variety of organisms including the *Enterobacteriaceae* (**enterobactins**), *Neisseria* species (**gonobactins** and **meningobactins**), *Mycobacterium* species (**mycobactins**), and *Pseudomonas* species (**pyochelins**). In addition, the production of many extracellular microbial products, including toxins, is partially regulated by the concentrations of iron in the surrounding medium. For example, the expression of the β-phage structural gene for diphtheria toxin in lysogenized *Corynebacterium diphtheriae* cells depends on iron levels.

Although plasmids themselves are not virulence factors, the genes that code for many of the bacterial cell products responsible for virulence frequently reside on bacterial plasmids. **R factors** (plasmids that contain genes coding for resistance to antimicrobial agents) may be considered as virulence factors because the acquisition of resistance to antimicrobial agents fosters continued growth and spread of bacterial infections despite therapeutic intervention. Some bacteria also contain plasmids that code for **sex pili** and **chromosomal mobilization**. These two factors enable a microorganism to transfer genetic material (either plasmid-borne, chromosomal, or both) to other organisms. Plasmids may also bear the genes that code for colonization antigens, serum resistance, iron chelation and transport, toxin and hemolysin production, and undefined intracellular survival functions. *Shigella, Salmonella, Yersinia,* and *"Shigella"*-like *E. coli* strains contain plasmids that are known to contribute to their virulence.

EXOTOXINS AND ENDOTOXINS

Toxins of microbial origin fall into two groups: **exotoxins** and **endotoxins**. Bacterial exotoxins are the most potent biologic toxins known. Exotoxins are produced mostly by gram-positive bacteria, although some gram-negative bacteria elaborate them as well. Exotoxins are usually protein in nature and are heat labile. Because they are proteins, many can be inactivated or destroyed by proteolytic enzymes. Some exotoxins only become activated after partial hydrolysis ("nicking") by proteolytic enzymes (see below). The toxic activity of many exotoxins can be destroyed by formaldehyde treatment (toxoid development) and neutralized by specific antibodies. Exploitation of these properties led to the development of the diphtheria and tetanus toxoids that are used for active immunization against diphtheria and tetanus, respectively. In the case of tetanus, botulism, diphtheria, and cholera, the signs and symptoms of these diseases are due entirely to the effects of the toxins elaborated by these bacteria.

Tetanus is due to the systemic effects of **tetanospasmin**, the toxin produced by *Clostridium tetani*. Tetanospasmin is released on cell lysis after bacterial growth under anaerobic conditions (*eg*, in deep puncture wounds). The toxin is produced initially as a single peptide (MW = 160,000 daltons). On release from the bacterial cell, the toxin peptide is "nicked" by proteolytic enzymes to form two polypeptide chains connected by a disulfide bond. Under reducing conditions, the two peptides are split into a heavy (β) chain (MW = 107,000 daltons) and a light (α) chain (MW = 53,000 daltons). The receptor-binding site of the intact toxin molecule resides in the β chain. The α chain is internalized and moves from the peripheral nerves to the central nervous system (CNS) by retrograde axonal transport. This toxin acts by blocking presynaptic inhibition of the CNS, causing spastic paralysis, "lockjaw," and generalized convulsions. Toxin is elaborated in puncture wounds during anaerobic growth of *C. tetani*. When tetanus toxin reaches the CNS (spinal cord and cerebellum), it becomes rapidly fixed to its receptor, a ganglioside containing stearic acid, sphingosine, glucose, galactose, *N*-acetylglucosamine, and *N*-acetyl neuraminic acid (sialic acid). The spasmogenic effect of the toxin is due to its action on presynaptic reflexes involving interneurons in the spinal cord. The toxin blocks the normal postsynaptic inhibition of spinal motor neurons following afferent impulses by preventing the release of inhibitory neurotransmitters (*ie*, γ-aminobutyric acid, glycine). Resulting sensitivity to excitatory impulses, unchecked by inhibitory mechanisms, produces the generalized spastic paralysis characteristic of tetanus.

Botulism results from the ingestion of toxins formed by *Clostridium botulinum* growing in food, the principal vehicles being improperly canned fruits and vegetables (generally home canned), condiments, and fish products. Wound contamination with the organism has been associated with noninvasive infection and toxin formation (wound botulism). *Clostridium botulinum* can also colonize the intestinal tract of infants and produce toxin at that site (infant botulism). Toxin accumulates in cells of *C. botulinum* during spore germination and active vegetative cell growth, but it is only released on cell lysis. The seven serologic types of *C. botulinum* are types A, B, C-α, D, E, F, and G, and each produces an immunologically type-specific toxin. Toxin types A, B, E, and F affect humans. These toxins are aggregates of two or three kinds of proteins. Botulinal toxin is produced as a progenitor protein with a molecular weight of about 150,000 daltons. These toxins are produced as inert molecules that become activated after proteolysis, but proteolytic cleavage is internal to the peptide molecules and the toxins do not change in molecular weight following activation. After absorption from the gastrointestinal tract, the toxin reaches susceptible neurons (at neuromuscular junctions and peripheral autonomic synapses) via the bloodstream. There it becomes bound to presynaptic terminals, where it blocks the release of acetylcholine from cholinergic motor nerve endings. Symptoms include weakness, dizziness, nausea, blurring of vision, slurring of speech, dilatation of pupils, urinary retention, general flaccid paralysis of skeletal muscles, and respiratory paralysis.

Diphtheria is another example of an illness caused primarily by the action of a toxin. Interestingly, only those strains of *Corynebacterium diphtheriae* that contain a lysogenic bacteriophage (the β corynephage) are able to produce diphtheria toxin. The structural genes for the toxin (called the *tox* gene) is part of the bacteriophage's genome. The toxin molecule is formed by *C. diphtheriae* in association with the cell membrane and is secreted from the cell as a single peptide with a molecular weight of about 63,000 daltons. On gentle proteolysis, the single peptide is cleaved into two major chains, designated as A and B, that are connected by disulfide bonds. Peptide A contains the the enzymatic activity of the molecule that inhibits protein synthesis; peptide B is responsible for binding of the toxin molecule to its target receptor. On binding to the target cell, the disulfide bonds are reduced and peptide A (MW = 24,000 daltons) enters the cell. Peptide A inhibits protein synthesis by the adenoribosylation of **elongation factor 2** (EF-2), an enzyme that is required for translocation of the polypeptidyl-tRNA from the acceptor site to the donor site on the eukaryotic ribosome. The adenoribosyl group (ADPR) is transferred from **nicotinamide adenine dinucleotide (NAD)** to EF-2 by the peptide A toxin subunit, rendering EF-2 inactive:

$$NAD^+ + EF\text{--}2 \xrightarrow[A]{\text{toxin peptide}} ADPR{:}EF\text{--}2 \text{ complex} + \text{nicotinamide} + H^+$$

Treatment of the intact toxin with formalin renders a **toxoid** that cannot be split into A and B subunits.

Therefore, the toxoid lacks the ability to catalyze its toxic intracellular effects, yet it retains its antigenicity. Immunity to diphtheria is generally mediated by the presence of antibodies against the toxin.

All the signs and symptoms of cholera caused by *Vibrio cholerae* result from the rapid loss of fluid from the gut. Increased electrolyte secretion is caused by a protein enterotoxin. The enterotoxin (MW = 84,000 daltons) consists of a binding subunit (subunite B) that consists of five identical monomers (MW = 11,500 daltons for each subunit) and an active subunit, subunit A (MW = 27,000 daltons). The mode of action of cholera toxin is described in Chapter 6.

Endotoxins are produced only by gram-negative bacteria and consist primarily of lipopolysaccharide (LPS). LPS, as described earlier, is a structural component of the gram-negative outer membrane, representing the somatic (O) antigenic determinants. Endotoxins are heat stable, are not detoxified by formaldehyde treatment, and are only partially neutralized by specific antibodies. Compared with many of the exotoxins, endotoxins are of relatively low toxicity. Although endotoxin may escape into the surrounding fluids (as "blebs" on the surface of gram-negative bacteria), the whole cell generally retains the major portion of the toxic activity. The biologic and toxic activities of endotoxin are broad. Nanogram amounts of endotoxin cause fever in humans and the release of endogenous pyrogen. Larger doses cause hypotension, lowered polymorphonuclear leukocyte and platelet counts from increased margination of these cells toward the walls of small blood vessels, hemorrhage, and sometimes disseminated intravsacular coagulation due to the activation of clotting mechanisms. Endotoxin is also mitogenic for B lymphocytes and stimulates the release of several cytokines from macrophages.

TECHNOLOGIC ADVANCES IN CLINICAL MICROBIOLOGY

Most of this text deals with pathogenic organisms and methods for their identification. Although conventional approaches to identification (*eg*, sugar fermentations, chemical detection of metabolic by-products, etc) are still valid and useful, several others are now available. With the introduction of "modified conventional" and rapid chromogenic enzyme substrate tests in the late 1960s, the development of kit systems using these tests for identification of the *Enterobacteriaceae* (*eg*, the original API strip), and the introduction of antimicrobial susceptibility instrumentation (the old Pfizer "AutoBac" system), "rapid methods" and "rapid reporting" truly became a feasible goal for clinical microbiology laboratories. These methods have not only decreased the turn-around time for patient results, but have increased the clinical relevance of the information provided by the laboratory. A gram-negative bacillus recovered from a blood culture at 9 o'clock in the morning could now be identified, along with antibiotic susceptibility results, by 1 o'clock that afternoon, rather than the 24 to 48 hours necessary with conventional methods. Following this significant departure from past practices, new technologies for use in clinical microbiology laboratories have literally exploded. The next section of this chapter addresses these technologic advances in general terms. Specific rapid methods and applications of new technologies are addressed in those chapters dealing with specific microorganisms and the diseases associated with them.

RAPID BACTERIAL IDENTIFICATION/DETECTION METHODS

In contrast to the use of conventional, growth-dependent procedures for bacterial identification, the use of chromogenic enzyme substrate tests and chromatographic procedures allows the laboratory to accurately and rapidly identify many species of microorganisms. Chromogenic enzyme substrates detect preformed enzymes in bacteria and may allow specific organism identifications when considered along with growth on selective or differential media, colonial characteristics, and cell morphology on a gram-stained smear. These new tests could be used, along with traditional "spot tests" such as catalase and oxidase tests, to provide accurate presumptive identifications of clinically significant microorganisms. Gas chromatography and various modifications of this technique can be used to detect specific bacterial products directly in clinical specimens or to provide ancillary information for genus- or species-level bacterial identification.

CHROMOGENIC ENZYME SUBSTRATE TESTS

Enzyme substrate analogs for bacterial identification are not a new concept in bacterial identification systems. The "classical" test using this technology is the ONPG test for detection of β-galactosidase, where the colorless compound *o*-nitrophenyl-β-D-galactopyranoside is hydrolyzed and the yellow colored *o*-nitrophenol moiety is released. The synthesis of several other colorless compounds that yield a colored hydrolysis product, either directly or after addition of a developing reagent, has revolutionized the rapid identification of bacterial species by detection of phenotypic enzymatic characteristics. Other chromogenic substrates may yield colored end-products when they are either reduced or oxidized by bacterial enzymes. "Classical tests" in this category include the cytochrome oxidase test and the nitrate reduction test. Table 1-3 lists the general categories of bacterial enzymes, the substrates used for their detection, and the enzymatic reactions that result in an observable end point.

The most commonly used enzymatic substrates for bacterial identification are those for glycosidase and aminopeptidase enzymes. Substrates for glycosidases are usually various types of mono- and disaccharides that are linked to *ortho*- or *para*-nitrophenol. On hydrolysis by glycosidases that are specific for individual carbohydrates or classes of carbohydrates, the yellow nitrophenol moiety is released. Aminopeptidase substrates are generally *p*-nitroanilide or β-naphthylamide derivatives of amino acids. Hydrolysis of *p*-nitroanilide

TABLE 1-3
BACTERIAL ENZYMES AND MODES OF ACTION ON VARIOUS CHROMOGENIC SUBSTRATES

ENZYME CLASS	SPECIFIC ENZYMES	MODE OF ACTION
Oxidoreductases	Cytochrome oxidase	Tetra methyl-p-phenylenediamine reacts directly with cytochrome c to produce a blue-colored compound (see Chart 16).
	Nitrate reductase	Nitrate is first reduced to nitrite. Two reagents are then used: sulfanilic acid reacts with nitrite to form a diazonium salt; α-naphthylamine functions as a diazo dye coupler to form a red color (see Chart 53).
Dehydrogenases	Reasuzurin Tetrazolium	Many dyes are colorless when in the reduced stage; however, with the loss of hydrogen ions (oxidation) they develop pigmented complexes. These compounds are reduced by flavin-linked enzymes of bacterial transport systems.
Amino acid hydrolases	Tryptophanase	Hydrolysis of tryptophane yields indole, which can be detected by observing the red color that develops on addition of p-dimethylaminobenzaldehyde.
Glycosidases	Chromogenic carbohydrate analogues: orthonitrophenyl-β-D-galactopyranosidase (ONPG)	Orthonitrophenyl moieties are linked to various carbohydrates through an ester linkage—hydrolysis leads to release of yellow-colored orthonitrophenol.
Aminopeptidases	Chromogenic amino acid analogues: amino acid linked to p-nitroaniline or β-naphthylamine	Hydrolysis of the amino acid p-nitroanilide releases a free amino acid and the yellow p-nitroaniline chromophore; a diazo dye coupler is required to detect free β-naphthylamide.

substrates releases p-nitroaniline, a yellow compound that is detected directly. The β-naphthylamine that is released by enzymatic hydrolysis of the naphthylamide amino acid analogs is detected by the addition of a colorless diazo-dye coupler such as p-dimethylaminocinnamaldehyde, which results in the formation of a pink or red-colored end product.

Using such substrates, rapid tests for specific bacterial identifications have been developed and are in use in many laboratories. One such test is the **pyrrolidonyl arylamidase (PYR) test**. Once the hemolytic character of a streptococcal isolate has been determined, this test can be used to identify both group A streptococci and *Enterococcus* species (see Chap. 12). β-Hemolytic streptococci that are PYR positive are group A streptococci; nonhemolytic or α-hemolytic streptococci that are PYR positive are enterococci.[288,292] Specific identification of pathogenic *Neisseria* species may also be accomplished with chromogenic substrate tests. If an oxidase-positive, gram-negative diplococcal isolate is recovered on modified Thayer-Martin (MTM) agar and produces only prolylaminopeptidase, the organism may be identified as *Neisseria gonorrhoeae*. Similarly, the demonstration of β-galactosidase activity in an organism with the same morphology and also growing on MTM medium specifically rules out the gonococcus and allows an identification of *Neisseria lactamica* to be made (see Chap. 10).[109,116]

Chromogenic substrate tests and modified "conventional" tests have been combined into kit systems that are able to identify a variety of bacterial species.

These systems are in common use in clinical laboratories the world over. This state of the art technology is directed toward providing bacterial identifications that are rapid, standardized, and reproducible. For example, the RapID NH system (Innovative Diagnostic Systems, Atlanta, GA), the Vitek NHI card (bio Merieux-Vitek, Inc, Hazelwood, MO), and the HNID panel (Dade/Microscan, West Sacramento, CA) provide 4-hour identifications for *Neisseria* species, *Haemophilus* species, and a variety of other fastidious gram-negative bacilli (see Chaps. 7, 8, and 10).[114,115] Reliable identification of the clinically significant anaerobic bacteria can be achieved with the RapID ANA II (Innovative Diagnostic Systems), the An-IDENT system (bio Merieux-Vitek, Inc., Hazelwood, MO), and the Vitek Anaerobe Identification (ANI) card.[41,208,227] This technology has also been applied to the identification of clinically significant yeasts and yeastlike fungi.[134,199] All of these systems use an expanded battery of glycosidase and aminopeptidase enzyme substrates to obtain a characteristic enzyme "profile." Comparison of the profile of an individual isolate to reactions for a large number of strains in a computerized data base allows specific identifications to be made within 4 hours. Some kit systems, such as the Rapid Strep (bio Merieux-Vitek, Hazelwood, MO) and the ID32 Strep systems (bio Merieux, La Balme les Grottes, France) also include modified conventional tests (eg, esculin hydrolysis, acid production from carbohydrates) in the panel of substrates used for identification.[77,83] Additional discussions of kit systems for bacterial identification are included in subsequent chapters. Evaluations of these rapid chromogenic substrate tests and kits have shown them to be reliable and accurate methods for identifying the organisms for which they are intended.

FLUOROGENIC ENZYME SUBSTRATE TESTS

A related application of rapid chromogenic substrate tests is the use of fluorogenic enzyme substrates for detection of bacterial enzymes and identification of microorganisms. Such substrates are used in the semi-automated MicroScan autoSCAN "Walkaway" (W/A) Rapid Bacterial Identification System (Dade/Baxter, West Sacramento, CA), which provides 2-hour bacterial identifications based on the release of fluorescent products of hydrolysis from a variety of fluorogenic substrates.[200,252] These substrates are composed of carbohydrate or amino acid moieties linked through glycoside or peptide linkages to compounds such as 4-methylumbelliferone (eg, 4-methylumbelliferyl- β-D-galactopyranoside, 4-methylumbelliferyl-β-D-glucuronide, etc) and 4-methylcoumarin (eg, L-alanine-4-methylcoumarin, L-glutamic acid-4-methylcoumarin, etc) that produce fluorescent end-products on hydrolysis by bacterial enzymes. Because the enzymes are preformed in the bacterial inoculum and the test instrument's detection systems are highly sensitive to low levels of fluorescence, prolonged incubation of the unknown bacteria to produce a detectible end point is not required and readings as soon as 2 hours after inoculation are possible.

CHROMATOGRAPHIC IDENTIFICATION METHODS

Chromatography is based on the premise that compounds have differing solubilities when exposed to different immiscible materials or phases. The principle of chromatography is to achieve an absorption equilibrium between two phases, one mobile and the other stationary. Mobile and stationary phases obtain for virtually all types of chromatography. Thin-layer chromatography uses a moving liquid phase and a stationary solid phase; differing solubilities of materials in mixtures between the two phases achieves a separation of the components of the mixture. In gas-liquid chromatography (GLC), an inert carrier gas (eg, nitrogen, helium, or argon) is the mobile phase, into which the sample for analysis is injected. The stationary phase consists of a solid matrix (eg, silica or celite) coated with an inert, easily volatilized liquid, such as carbowax or methyl silicone. These materials are coated onto the inner surface of a coiled, capillary glass tube ("column") that is enclosed in a heating unit. The sample to be analyzed is volatilized by heat at the port of injection into the column, where it immediately mixes with the stream of carrier gas. Compounds present in the sample become distributed between the inert and mobile phases of the column by their relative affinities for the phase coated onto the column. Compounds with low affinity pass through the column most rapidly and are detected first; those with higher affinity move through the column more slowly and emerge last. The time between injection of a given ma-

terial into the column and its appearance in the detection system is called the **retention time**. This retention time, under defined conditions of temperature, type of carrier gas, and type of column packing, is constant; therefore, unknown compounds can be identified by comparison with known, similarly prepared specimens run through the same column.

The basic components of a GLC system include an oven containing the packed column through which a regulated flow of carrier gas is passed, a heated port where the sample to be analyzed is injected and immediately volatilized, and a detector system to measure the unknown components as they emerge from the distal end of the column. The detector may be either a thermal conductivity (hot wire) detector, a flame ionization detector, or an electron-capture detector. Thermal conductivity detectors can be used for analysis of most end-products of bacterial metabolism. Flame ionization detectors are more sensitive and versatile but require the presence of hydrogen and air in the system to feed the flame source. Electron-capture detectors are extremely sensitive and are most often used in research settings or reference laboratories, where, in one application, body fluids are examined directly for the presence of trace quantities of bacterial metabolites. The detection signals are amplified and translated to a pen-scroll recorder, where tracings are made on moving calibrated paper. The retention times of materials in the analyte are compared with retention times of similarly prepared controls, allowing the identification of unknown metabolites. The heights of "peaks" on the tracing are directly proportional to the amount of a given metabolite in a specimen.

Gas-liquid chromatography has found its greatest application in anaerobic bacteriology.[107,137] These bacteria produce a variety of short-chain fatty acids, alcohols, and amines that can be extract from broth media by aqueous or organic solvents. For example, volatile, short-chain fatty acids such as acetic, propionic, isobutyric, and butyric acid can be extracted from culture medium using an acid-ether mixture. Nonvolatile acids such as succinate and fumarate must first be converted to methyl esters by treatment with methanol before they can be extracted. This last step is accomplished by raising the pH to around 11.0 and extracting the broth with chloroform. Based on the Gram stain reaction and the types of volatile and nonvolatile fatty acids produced during growth in broth, genus-level identifications of most obligately anaerobic bacteria can be achieved.[107]

Chromatographic methods like GLC can also be used to assist in the identification of a wide variety of other bacterial species and yeasts species as well.[36,80,89,102,118,119,120,123,140,146,148,163,174–177,248,267,274] When organisms are grown under rigidly standardized conditions, the chemical compositions of their various components remain constant. High-performance liquid chromatography (HPLC) can be used to analyze the long-chain fatty acid components of bacterial cell walls and membranes. Organisms grown under standard conditions are harvested and saponified with hydroxide to release the long-chain fatty acids from the intact cells. These fatty acids are methylated to render them volatile, extracted with an organic solvent (hexane:methyl *tert*-butyl ether [1:1]), and injected into a column containing a cross-linked phenylmethyl silicone liquid phase adsorbed onto fused silica with hydrogen as the carrier gas. Detection of the derivated fatty acid methyl esters is accomplished with a flame ionization detector. The detector uses a mixture of burning oxygen and hydrogen to ignite the organic compounds; ionized particles in the sample then pass between two oppositely charged wires, causing a fluctuation in the current that is measured and translated into a permanent record.

Abel and colleagues[1] first suggested that microorganisms may be classified by gas chromatographic analysis of the components of the bacterial cell walls and membranes. These early concepts have found current application in the Microbial Identification System (MIS or MIDI) (Microbial ID Inc., Newark, DE), a sophisticated, automated cellular fatty acid bacterial identification system that is commercially available. With this system, extracted bacterial cell wall fatty acid methyl esters are analyzed on a Hewlett-Packard 3890A gas chromatograph (Avondale, PA) equipped with a flame ionization detector, automatic sampler, integrator, and computer. Organism identifications are based solely on computer comparison of the unknown organism's fatty acid methyl ester profile with the profiles of a predetermined library of known isolates using covariance matrix-pattern recognition software. Osterhout and associates[188] found that the Microbial ID system correctly identified 478 of 532 clinical isolates (90%) and reference strains of gram-negative nonfermentative bacteria. Of those strains where GLC identifications did not agree with biochemical criteria, the majority belonged to the genera *Acinetobacter*, *Moraxella*, and *Alcaligenes*, or were *Pseudomonas pickettii*. Other discrepancies were encountered when reference strains were not adequately characterized or when it was not possible to differentiate between chemotaxonomically closely related strains. Stoakes and coworkers compared the MIS with conventional methods for identifying staphylococci and found complete agreement with reference identifications for 87.8% of 470 isolates tested.[244]

Various chromatographic procedures, particularly thin-layer chromatography, HPLC, and capillary gas chromatography, have been extremely useful for identification of *Mycobacterium* species and related genera.[26,34,35,53,89,147,254,257] With these particular organisms, chromatographic techniques primarily detect mycolic acid esters that comprise part of the cell wall of these organisms. These methods are in use in various reference and state laboratories throughout the country and an analysis/computerized data base system (the MIS discussed above) is commercially available for this purpose. GLC has also proven to be useful for the identification of fastidious organisms that are biochemically inert in conventional identification systems, such as *Bartonella* species, *Brucella* species, *Streptobacillus moniliformis*, *Francisella tularensis*, and other fastidious gram-negative bacilli.[21,48,118,221,276,277] Future improvements in the system will undoubtedly increase the accuracy of identifications and will expand the utility of the GLC approach to the identification of other bacterial genera.

Gas-liquid chromatographic approaches have also been used to detect bacterial and fungal agents and their products directly in clinical specimens. Brooks and his associates, using frequency-pulsed electron capture GLC, have detected various organism-specific products (*eg*, acid, alcohol, amine, and hydroxy acid moieties) in extracts of several types of biologic fluids.[27–30] In diarrheal stool specimens, *Clostridium difficile* could be detected by the presence of isocaproic acid and *Shigella* species demonstrated species-specific fatty acid profiles. Stool containing rotavirus was characterized by decreased quantities of isobutyric, isovaleric, and valeric acids. Brooks and coworkers also demonstrated that major causative agents of bacterial meningitis (*Haemophilus influenzae* type b, *Neisseria meningitidis* serogroups B and C, *Klebsiella pneumoniae*, and *Streptococcus pneumoniae*) could be detected and differentiated by performing GLC on extracts of cerebrospinal fluid (CSF).[29] DeRepentigny and colleagues also used GLC methods to detect arabinitol and mannans in serum in the diagnosis of invasive *Candida* infections in cancer patients.[57,58] Although these techniques require sophisticated equipment and are currently largely limited to research laboratories, the application of GLC and mass spectrometry nevertheless represent almost unlimited potential for future applications in clinical microbiology laboratories.

IMMUNOLOGIC METHODS IN CLINICAL MICROBIOLOGY

Applications of chromogenic substrates and GLC have been generally limited to the rapid identification of microorganisms growing on agar media and in broth media, respectively. However, the development of methods to directly detect microbial antigens using antibodies as diagnostic reagents is a relatively new technology that is couched in basic, classical immunology and has gained widespread acceptance as a method for the rapid diagnosis of certain infectious diseases. Newer immunologic procedures have also changed the methods currently used for detection of antibodies in the serologic diagnosis of infections or the determination of immune status. After a brief review of basic immunologic concepts, the application of these concepts to direct detection of antigens and antibodies will be discussed.

ANTIGENS AND ANTIBODIES: BASIC DEFINITIONS

An **antigen** is a substance that evokes the formation of antibodies in an animal that is immunized or infected with that antigen. An antigen is generally "immunogenic," that is, it has the capability to stimulate antibody formation and is also able to specifically combine with the antibodies that are formed against it. Not all parts of an antigen may be equally immunogenic, and those parts of the molecule that interact with and are most often recognized by antibodies are called **immunodominant antigenic determinants** or **epitopes**. The unique characteristics of each antigen depend on the types and sequences of amino acids in proteins and their secondary, tertiary, and quaternary structures, and on the chemical and structural composition of polysaccharides, glycoproteins, and nucleic acids. The structures of all these biomolecules are genetically determined.

Some types of molecules have common antigenic determinants and will be recognized by antibodies directed against them. For example, the C1 portions of the light chains from the various immunoglobulin classes contain common antigenic determinants that allow them to be recognized by the same antibodies. These antigen-antibody combinations are termed "cross-reactive." Cross-reactions of antibodies with common or closely related antigens may be clinically important in some disease states. For example, it is believed that the cardiac damage that occurs during the development of rheumatic heart disease may be related to the cross-reactivity of cell surface antigens of group A β-hemolytic streptococci and antigens found in the sarcolemma of heart muscle (see Chap. 12).[22] Following streptococcal pharyngitis, these antibodies are formed and subsequently bind to heart tissue. This activates the complement cascade, resulting in damage to the heart muscle. Similar reactions occurring in the glomerular basement membrane of the kidney and in the synovial tissue lining the joint spaces may also be responsible for poststreptococcal glomerulonephritis and arthritis, respectively.[22]

Antibodies or immunoglobulins (Ig) can be divided into five classes based on their structure: IgG, IgM, IgA, IgD, and IgE (Fig. 1-19). IgG molecules are composed of two light and two heavy chains and have two sites for the binding of specific antigens. IgM molecules are composed of five monomers that resemble an IgG molecule; that is, each monomer is composed of two heavy and two light polypeptide chains and has two antigen-combining sites (Fab sites). IgM molecules are formed very early in the immune response and at very low levels, followed by the appearance of much larger amounts of IgG to the same antigen. IgA occurs in multimeric forms (*ie*, from one to four monomers) and accounts for less than 10% of the serum Ig. It is, however, the principal antibody form found on mucosal surfaces and in extracellular secretions, such as colostrum, respiratory and genital tract mucin, tears, and saliva. IgD is similar in structure to IgG but is found in extremely low quantities in serum. IgE is present only in trace amounts in serum, but these antibodies play a major role in allergic reactions, including severe anaphylactic shock. The genesis of the cellular and humoral immune response and their interactions that result in the production of specific antibodies are beyond the scope of this text; this material is found on other textbooks devoted to immunology and immunogenetics.

In clinical microbiology, molecules of IgG, in particular, can be used to detect specific bacterial antigens. These IgG molecules may be **polyclonal** or **monoclonal**. Polyclonal antibodies are generally purified from animals that are immunized with the antigen of interest. Consequently the antibodies produced against a complex antigen are reactive with a variety of differ-

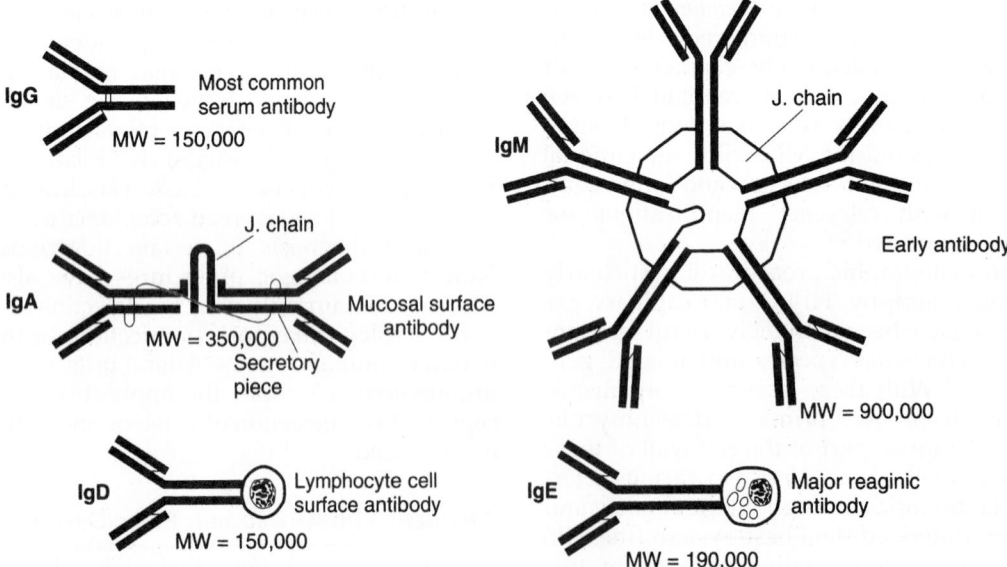

Figure 1-19
Classes of human immunoglobulins. Antibodies belong to five structural and functional classes designated IgG, IgM, IgA, IgD, and IgE. The basic structural unit of members in each class consists of two pairs of polypeptides (two heavy chains and two light chains) joined by disulfide bonds and each unit has two antigen combining sites. Some Ig types have other structural components (J chain in IgM, secretory piece in IgA).

ent immunogenic determinants or epitopes. Monoclonal antibodies are antibodies that are produced against specific epitopes of an antigen; these antibodies, therefore, are highly specific. Because monoclonal antibodies have revolutionized antigen detection methods so profoundly, the manufacture and production of these molecules will be briefly discussed. First, however, the types of reactions in which these antibodies are used in the clinical laboratory will be addressed.

TYPES OF ANTIGEN-ANTIBODY REACTIONS

PRECIPITIN REACTIONS

The basic type of antigen-antibody reaction is the precipitin reaction. This reaction is found in test systems that allow the free diffusion of antigen and antibody fronts toward one another. At a critical point of interface, where the concentrations are optimal, a visible precipitate composed of combined antigens and antibodies forms. In a single-diffusion system, antibody is incorporated into an agar gel into which antigen is allowed to diffuse. In the tube method, antigen is overlaid onto agar containing antisera, and one or more precipitin lines form at zones of equivalence. In radial immunodiffusion, antibody is contained in agar that is coated onto a glass slide. Material containing antigen is then placed into circular wells cut into the agar. During incubation, the antigen diffuses into the agar and a ring of precipitate forms. The diameter of the ring is directly proportional to the amount of antigen present in the material, and semiquantitative results on the concentration of the antigen can be obtained by comparing the diameter of the precipitin reaction with those of material containing known quantities of antigen. The most commonly used conventional immunodiffusion procedure is **double diffusion**. In this technique, both antigen and antibody are placed in wells adjacent to one another, and the materials diffuse out and toward one another. A line of precipitate then forms between the lines when concentrations of equivalence are reached. Double diffusion may take up to 48 hours to reach an interpretable result. Countercurrent immunoelectrophoresis (CIE) uses double-diffusion technology, but it uses an electric current running through the agarose support matrix to speed up the migration of the antigen and antibody toward one another. These methods may be used for the detection of both antibody or antigen in body fluids.

One precaution in performing precipitin procedures is to recognize the possibility of false-negative reactions caused by prozone or postzone phenomena. If antibody is in excess (ie, in concentrations far in excess of available antigen), a false-negative (prozone) reaction occurs because molecular lattices, which make up the visible precipitate, do not form. In contrast, postzone reactions occur when antigen is in excess and antibodies become saturated with antigens such that lattice formation characteristic of precipitin reactions does not occur. In cases in which high concentrations of antigen or antibody are anticipated, false-negative prozone or postzone phenomena, respectively, can be avoided by performing repeat tests on serial dilutions of the specimen.

Although all of the methods described above (ie, tube diffusion, radial diffusion, double diffusion) have been used for detection of bacterial antigens in body fluids (eg, CSF, pleural fluid, etc), CIE was the only method that gained acceptance in clinical practice because of the relative rapidity of the test (30–60 minutes as compared with 24–48 hours for double diffusion). However, even this method has been largely supplanted by the more rapid latex particle agglutination and staphylococcal coagglutination procedures described below. Conventional double-diffusion methods are still used for the serologic diagnosis of fungal infections such as aspergillosis, blastomycosis, histoplasmosis, and coccidioidomycosis (ie, fungal immunodiffusion testing). In these tests, antigens from these organisms are reacted with patient sera and with control sera containing antibodies in double-diffusion tests. The development of precipitin lines of identity with the positive control sera and with the patient's serum indicates the presence of these antifungal antibodies. The presence or absence of certain bands in fungal immunodiffusion has diagnostic and prognostic significance (see Chap. 19).

AGGLUTINATION REACTIONS

Agglutination reactions can be defined as the specific immunochemical aggregation of particles (bacteria, erythrocytes, synthetic latex particles) coated with antigen or antibody that can be used to detect either soluble antibodies or antigens, respectively. Antigens or antibodies are attached to the particulate surfaces either by intramolecular electrical forces or by covalent bonds. Clumping of the carrier particles occurs as an indicator of the antigen-antibody interactions occurring on the surface of the carriers.

Either antigens or antibodies can be detected by agglutination reactions, depending on the reactant that is bound to the carrier. For example, detection of rubella antibodies by latex agglutination is accomplished by mixing latex particles to which immunodominant antigens of the rubella virus are attached with serum specimens and looking for agglutination (ie, rubella-specific antibodies).[243] Direct detection of group A streptococcal antigen in throat swabs is accomplished by extracting the swab with either low pH (nitrous acid) or with enzymes and reacting the fluid extract with latex beads coated with anti-group A streptococcal antibodies.[210] In either case, interconnecting lattices are formed between the carriers and the analyte to cause easily visible secondary agglutination.

Agglutination reactions are more sensitive than precipitin reactions because of the direct nature of the antigen/carrier/antibody interaction. The sensitivity and the ability of these reactions to occur at high dilutions allows semiquantitative measurements of antigens or antibodies to be made in many cases. In the case of antibodies, semiquantitative results can be derived by determining the highest dilution of serum that produces a visible agglutination reaction. In this context, such reactions may be likened to end point determinations for the macroscopic flocculation procedure used in the quantitative rapid plasma reagin (RPR) card test (see Chap. 18). Changes in agglutination titer in acute and convalescent specimens may provide retrospective serologic diagnoses in a manner similar to a complement fixation or hemagglutination inhibition test. In the semiquantitative determination of antigen concentrations, an end point titer of a patient specimen (eg, CSF) may be compared to end point agglutination titers obtained with a serially diluted preparation of a known concentration of antigen.

Comparisons of titers in sequential specimens may have direct applications to patient care. For example, a decrease in the CSF titer of capsular polysaccharide antigen is directly related to therapeutic response in patients with *Cryptococcus neoformans* meningitis.[63] Conversely, a rising titer or a persistently elevated titer in a patient who has been treated for this infection is an excellent indicator of posttreatment relapse.

Latex is the most common of several inert particles (bentonite, collodion, tanned erythrocytes, and charcoal are others) that can be used to absorb different groups of antigens, including proteins, carbohydrates, and DNA. Covalent bonding of proteins to latex is possible and provides a stable linkage that encourages maximum reaction with antigens or antibodies, depending on the system being used. The particle serves as a polystyrene core that is coated with a shell of another polymer that can bind to protein.

Coagglutination is also widely used, particularly in the detection of antigens of various streptococcal groups, *Neisseria meningitidis* and *Neisseria gonorrhoeae*, *Haemophilus influenzae*, *Streptococcus pneumoniae*, and others (reagents available from Karo- Bio Diagnostics AB, Huddinge Sweden). Certain strains of *Staphylococcus aureus* (the Cowan strain, ATCC 12498) have a high content of surface protein A. Protein A on the *S. aureus* cell wall binds the Fc portion of the immunoglobulin molecule, leaving the Fab portion free to bind antigen. Visible agglutination of the staphylococcal cells serves as a positive test to indicate antigen-antibody binding.

Antibody-coated latex particles or staphylococci serve as the basis for several commercially available systems for direct detection of bacterial and other microbial antigens in body fluids. One important application has been the detection of soluble capsular antigens of several agents of acute and chronic meningitis, namely, *Haemophilus influenzae*, *Streptococcus pneumoniae*, *Neisseria meningitidis*, group B streptococci, *Escherichia coli*, and *Cryptococcus neoformans*. Commercial tests for bacterial antigen detection include the Directigen (Becton Dickinson Microbiology Systems, Cockeysville, MD), Bactigen (Wampole Laboratories, Cranbury, NJ), and Wellcogen (Wellcome Diagnostics, Dartford, England) systems (all latex particle agglutination tests) and the Phadebact coagglutination test (KaroBio Diagnostics, Huddinge, Sweden). Tests can be completed within 15 minutes and perform with sensitivities approaching 90% or greater and with specificities in the range of 97% to 99%. Tilton and colleagues examined the CSF from 157 patients suspected

of having meningitis (34 had a positive diagnosis).[256] Of these, CIE detected 76%, the Phadebact coagglutination test detected 76%, Directigen latex test detected 82%, and the Bactigen latex test detected 93%. It was concluded from this study that latex agglutination was more sensitive than either coagglutination or CIE. Sippel and coworkers examined specimens from 162 patients with bacterial meningitis.[237] They found that the Directigen test detected *H. influenzae* type b antigen in 83% of 83 patients with meningitis caused by this agent, detected *Streptococcus pneumoniae* capsular antigen in 77% of 39 patients with pneumococcal meningitis, and found *Neisseria meningitidis* capsular antigen in 93% of 40 patients with meningococcal meningitis. Ingram and associates found that the Wellcogen test provided a specific diagnosis of meningitis in 92% of those with *H. influenzae* type b, 100% of those with meningitis due to *N. meningitidis* serogroups A and Y, 36% of those with *N. meningitidis* serogroup C, and 69% of patients with meningitis due to *S. pneumoniae*.[112]

Latex agglutination assays may also be applied to other specimen types to provide a rapid diagnosis. Ajello and colleagues found commercial latex agglutination tests valuable for the direct detection of antigens in serum and urine specimens in patients with bacterial pneumonia.[4] In a study of 44 patients with bacterial pneumonia (23 with *Streptococcus pneumoniae*, 13 with *Haemophilus influenzae* type b, and 11 with other species), antigen was detected in over 90% of cases of hemophilus pneumonia with both the Directigen and the Bactigen latex agglutination test systems. However, the sensitivities for detecting cases of pneumococcal pneumonia were only 27% for Directigen and 38% for Bactigen.

SOLID PHASE IMMUNOASSAYS

Solid phase immunoassay, an extension of the basic principles discussed above, refers to the binding of either antigen or antibody to a variety of solid materials, such as polystyrene microtube wells or plastic beads. For example, solid phase systems designed for the detection of antibody in an unknown sample have antigen bound to the solid phase (Fig. 1-20). The initial reaction occurs when the specimen to be tested is incubated for a prescribed time with the solid phase. Specific antibody binds to the immobilized antigen. After the reaction mixture is washed to remove any extraneous materials, an antiglobulin conjugated with a "tag" is added and incubated in the reaction vessel. In radioimmunoassay (RIA) procedures, the tag is a radioactive isotope (eg, ^{32}P or ^{125}I); in enzyme immunoassay (EIA) methods, the tag is an enzyme. In commercially available EIA systems for detecting human antibodies, the conjugate is frequently alkaline phosphatase- or horseradish peroxidase-labeled antihuman immunoglobulin raised in goats. If the initial antigen-antibody reaction has occurred, the antiglobulin (with its radioactive or enzyme tag) binds to the antibody. The final step in these assays is the detection of radioactive or enzymatic activity. This is done with a scintillation counter, which detects either β or γ emis-

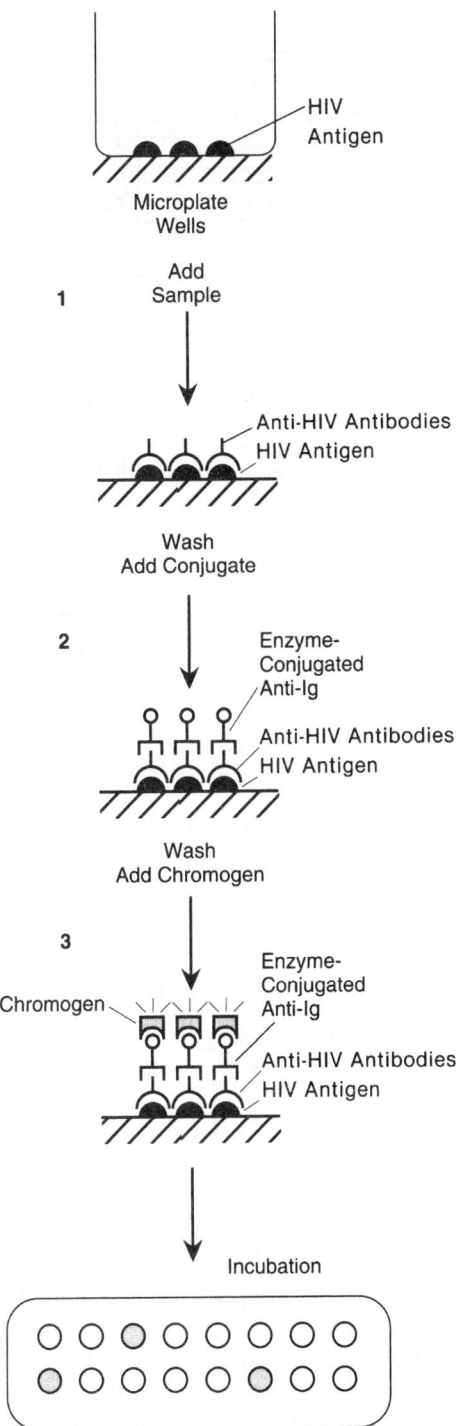

Figure I-20

Principles of enzyme immunoassay (EIA). This figure shows the EIA procedure for the detection of antibodies against HIV-1. Partially purified HIV-1 antigens are absorbed onto microplate wells. In *step 1*, serum is added and incubated. Anti-HIV-1 antibodies, if present, bind to the antigen. Following a wash step, anti-human immunoglobulin that is conjugated with an enzyme is added (*step 2*). After a second wash step, a chromogenic enzyme substrate is added. Absorbances for individual wells are read spectrophotometrically, and test results are interpreted by comparison with positive and negative controls performed in the same test.

sions, or by the addition of an enzyme substrate that generally yields a colored end-product that is detected visually or with a spectrophotometer. A positive reaction indicates that antibody was present in the original sample, and the intensity of the reaction is proportional to the concentration of antibody in the specimen. A diagrammatic representation of an EIA for detection of anti-human immunodeficiency virus type 1 antibodies is shown in Figure 1-20.

Most RIAs use a competitive-type assay system. In the quantitative test for antibodies, the solid phase system is first standardized using an unlabeled bound antigen and a standard concentration of antibody that is labeled with a radioactive tag. The unknown sample containing the antibody to be tested (which is unlabeled) is added to the assay system. The amount of labeled antibody displaced from the antigen is proportional to the amount of unlabeled antibody present in the test sample. The antibody concentration in the unknown sample is determined by comparing readings to those on a standard curve. The curves are derived by determining the degree of inhibition of binding of labeled antibody mixed with serial dilutions of known amounts of unlabeled antibody. The approach is similar when antigens are being detected by this method, except that a labeled antigen is used to quantitate free antigen in the specimen.

Radioimmunoassay has achieved wide use in clinical chemistry, clinical endocrinology, and toxicology, but it has not found significant routine applications in clinical microbiology. RIA procedures in current use include tests for steroid hormones (*eg*, aldosterone, cortisone, progesterone) and peptide hormones (corticotropin, follicle-stimulating hormone, vasopressin). Testing for markers for hepatitis B infection (HBsAg, HBsAb, HBcAb, HBeAg, HBeAb) is still done by RIA in some laboratories but has largely been replaced by EIA technology. Although RIA has great sensitivity and specificity, the problems associated with radioactive waste disposal and the instability of certain radionuclides has limited the expansion of RIA techniques.

Enzyme immunoassays grew out of the need to circumvent the disadvantages of using radioisotopes in clinical laboratories. EIA techniques were initially developed in Europe, where the use of radioactive compounds is limited and strictly controlled. EIA techniques not only overcome the precautions required for handling radioactive substances, but they also avoid certain technical problems inherent in the rapid decay of the radionuclide or outdating of reagents. Commercially available EIA test kits for the detection of antibodies in serum have become more widely available over the past 5 years, and have supplanted, in many cases, the more time-consuming and laborious procedures such as complement fixation and hemagglutination inhibition assays for viral serology.[55,167,168,206,269] In fact, EIA methods are the recommended format for the newer serologic tests, such as the screening tests for detection of antibodies to human immunodeficiency virus (HIV)-1 and HIV-2.[49,88]

Serologic procedures that have EIA technology as their basis have also been modified to increase their utility as specific diagnostic or confirmatory test methods. The Western blot procedure for HIV-1 antibodies is an example of such a modification (Fig. 1-21).[49,88] In the HIV-1 Western blot procedure, HIV-1 that is grown in tissue culture is partially purified from cell cultures and solubilized by detergent treatment. Using polyacrylamide gel electrophoresis, the HIV-1 proteins are fractionated on the basis of molecular weight, with the low molecular weight proteins migrating farther than the high molecular weight proteins and glycoproteins. A sheet of nitrocellulose paper is placed on the gel and the HIV-1 proteins are electrophoretically "transblotted" or transferred onto the nitrocellulose sheet. This sheet is then cut into strips for use as the "solid phase" in the assay. Serum that is repeatedly reactive in the HIV-1 EIA screening test is diluted and incubated with the nitrocellulose strip. If present, HIV-1 antibodies will bind to specific viral antigens on the strip. After washing, the strips are incubated with goat anti-human antibodies that are conjugated with horseradish peroxidase or alkaline phosphatase. After another wash step, enzyme substrate is added to the strip. At this time, colored bands will appear on the strip in areas where an initial antibody-antigen reaction has occurred. The position of these bands and comparison of the patterns with positive control samples enables reactivity of a given sample with specific viral antigens to be assessed and an interpretation to be made.[49,88]

Enzyme immunoassay techniques have also been adapted to the detection of bacterial, fungal, and parasite antigens in various types of clinical specimens. Bacterial antigens that can be detected by EIA methods include the capsular antigens of *S. pneumoniae*, *H. influenzae* type b, and *N. meningitidis*, and the cell wall antigen of group A streptococci.[162,290] The recent availability of enzyme-linked immunosorbent assays (ELISA) for the detection of *Giardia lamblia* and *Cryptosporidium*-specific antigen directly in stool has brought ELISA technology into a diagnostic area that has seen relatively little innovation since the introduction of specimen preservation and staining techniques.[2,128,295] Although fungal serology is still performed primarily by complement fixation and immunodiffusion, research in this area shows promise for the development of EIA methods as adjunctive tests in the diagnosis of systemic fungal infections such as *Coccidioides immitis*.[126]

Direct detection of chlamydial and viral antigens in patient specimens is currently an exciting area in virology. To date, EIA antigen detection methods have found their most widespread applications in the detection of hepatitis B surface antigen in serum, rotavirus in stool specimens, and respiratory syncytial virus in respiratory tract secretions.[99] In these cases, large amounts of antigen are generally present during the acute phases of the illnesses. The sensitivity of these assays may be compromised, however, by the trapping of antigen in the specimen (*eg*, mucoid stool or tenacious respiratory tract secretions) and the affinity of antigens produced "in vivo" (*ie*, in the patient) for antibodies produced "in vitro" (*ie*, monoclonal antibodies or polyclonal antibodies raised in animals and bound to a solid phase). A diagram of an antigen capture assay for detection of *Chlamydia trachomatis* is presented in Figure 1-22.

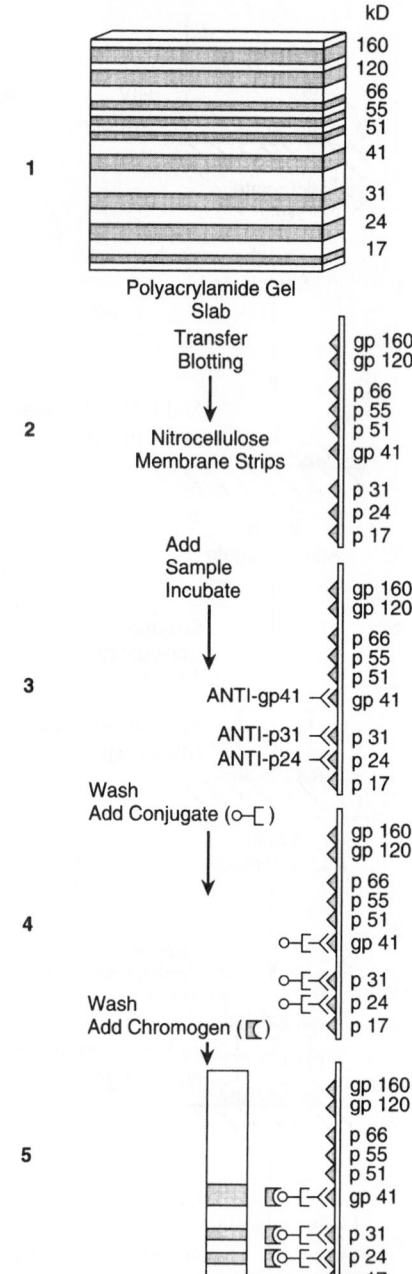

Figure 1-21

Western blot technique for detection of anti-HIV-1 antibodies. In *step 1*, virus that is grown in tissue culture is solubilized, partially purified, and subjected to electrophoresis in a polyacrylamide slab gel. This separates the viral proteins and glycoproteins by their molecular weights. In *step 2*, the antigens in the gel are electrophoretically "transblotted" onto a nitrocellulose sheet, which is then cut into strips. The strips are then incubated (*step 3*) with the test sample (serum). After washing away unbound material, an enzyme-labeled conjugate is added (*step 4*). This material binds to antibodies from the serum sample that have bound to the strip. After another wash step, the enzyme's chromogen substrate is added, and colored bands appear on the strip at the sites of initial antibody reactivity. In this diagram, reactivity is shown with gp41, p24, and p31, confirming that the serum sample contains anti-HIV-1 antibodies. (Figure courtesy Sandler SG, in DeVita VI Jr, Hellman S, Rosenberg SA [eds]: AIDS Etiology, Diagnosis, Treatment, and Prevention, 2nd ed., p 128. Philadelphia: JB Lippincott Co., 1988.)

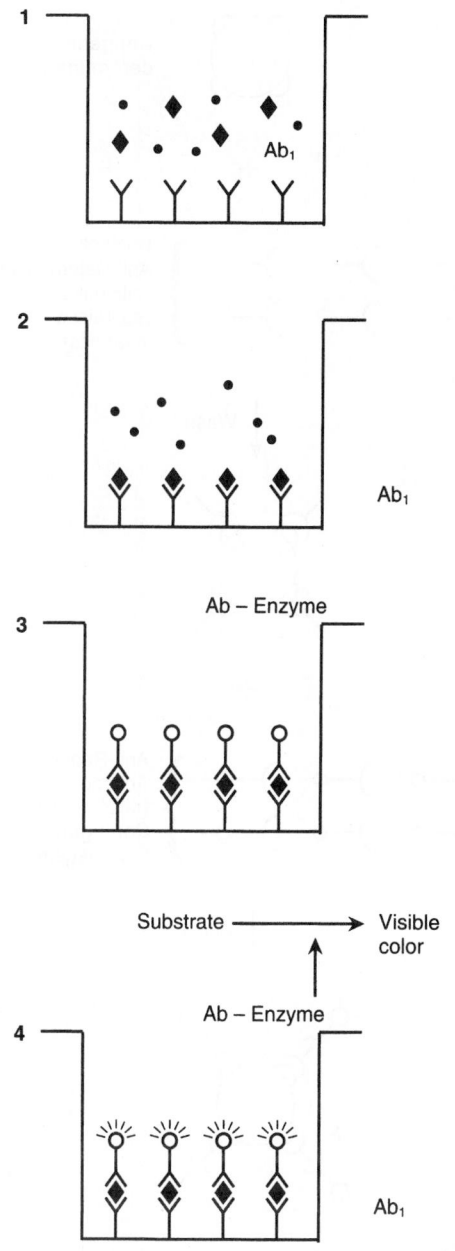

Figure 1-22
Enzyme immunoassay antigen capture technique for *Chlamydia trachomatis*. In this technique, antibody directed against the antigen to be detected is bound to the solid phase. Endocervical swab specimen washings are added to the well (*step 1*). Chlamydiae present in the urogenital sample are "captured" by the solid phase antibody. After a wash step, anti-chlamydia antibody that is conjugated to an enzyme is added (*step 2*) and reacts with the solid phase antibody-bound antigen. After another wash step, enzyme substrate is added (*step 3*), and a visible color is detected.

In addition to EIAs for detection of HIV-1 antibodies, capture EIAs for HIV-1 p24 antigen have also been licensed for diagnostic testing purposes and are now required (along with anti-HIV-1 antibodies) for testing of units of blood before transfusion.[129] Detection of HIV-1 p24 antigen in serum may be clinically useful in certain situations.[5] HIV-1 p24 antigen may be detected

in early infection before the production of antibodies and disappears with seroconversion.[149,272,273] The antigen reappears in the serum with the progression of clinical disease. The p24 antigen test has clinical and research utility in monitoring the response of antigenemic patients to antiviral chemotherapy and may be of diagnostic importance in the detection of infected neonates, who will be positive for antibodies to HIV-1 due to transplacental acquisition. In the latter instance, viral antigens that are complexed with antibody in neonatal serum specimens may not be free to react in competitive antigen capture assays. New generations of the serum p24 HIV-1 antigen assay that are being used in current research protocols include a pretreatment step that dissociates antigen-antibody complexes, releasing the p24 antigen so that it may react with the capture antibody on the assay's solid phase.[103]

IMMUNOFLUORESCENCE METHODS

Immunofluorescence provides an alternative to EIA as a means for detecting and localizing antigens in making the diagnosis of bacterial, fungal, parasitic, and viral diseases. This technique may also be used to detect antibodies for retrospective diagnosis of infectious diseases. For detection of antigens, specific antibody is conjugated to a fluorescent compound (usually fluorescein isothiocyanate), resulting in a sensitive tracer with unaltered immunologic reactivity. The conjugated antiserum is added to cells or tissues on a slide and becomes fixed to antigens, forming a stable immune complex. Nonreacting materials are removed by washing, and the preparation is then dried and observed with a fluorescence microscope. Antigens bound specifically to fluorescent antibody can be detected as bright apple green or orange yellow objects against a dark background depending on the fluorochrome and filters being used. Immunofluorescence techniques may be direct or indirect. Direct immunofluorescence tests are usually used for antigen detection, whereas the indirect method can be used for both antigen and antibody detection (*ie,* serology).

Direct immunofluorescence techniques (Fig. 1-23) involve direct application of the labeled conjugate to the material being examined, followed by a 15- to 30-minute period of incubation in a humid environment at 35° to 37°C to allow the antigen-antibody reaction to occur. After a wash step to remove unbound conjugate, the preparation is air dried and mounted for observation under a microscope fitted with an appropriate fluorescent light source and barrier filters. In the indirect procedure (Fig. 1-24), the material to be examined is first overlaid with an excess of unlabeled immune serum directed at the antigen and allowed to react for 30 to 45 minutes at 35° to 37°C. The specimen is washed with phosphate-buffered saline solution and then reacted with fluorescein-tagged antiserum against the species of immunoglobulin used in the initial reaction (*eg,* fluorescein-conjugated anti-human antibody raised in goats). After washing the background free of extraneous materials, the presence of

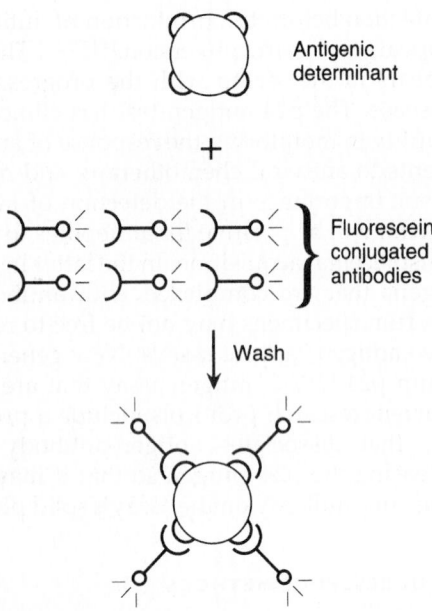

Figure 1-23
Schematic diagram of a direct immunofluorescence assay (DFA). In the DFA method, the antigen (*eg*, respiratory specimens for respiratory syncytial virus, urogenital specimen for chlamydia) is placed in the well of an FA slide and reacted directly with a fluorescein-conjugated monoclonal antibody directed against the antigen. After incubation and washing, the slide is examined for characteristic fluorescence.

microscopic fluorescence indicates the presence of antigen. The direct method is simple and rapid to perform with fewer nonspecific reactions; however, it is less sensitive. The indirect method is more sensitive and gives brighter fluorescence; however, it is less specific and subject to increased cross-reactivity.[31]

Direct immunofluorescence assays (DFA) are limited to the detection of antigen, whereas indirect immunofluorescence assays (IFA) can be used to detect both antigens or antibodies (Fig. 1-25). The latter is the basis for IFA tests for detection of antibodies to primarily against viral agents (*eg*, cytomegalovirus [CMV], measles, etc). In the IFA procedure, slides with virus-infected tissue culture cells fixed in discrete FA test slide wells are overlaid with serial dilutions of patient serum. After incubation and washing, a fluorescein-labeled goat or rabbit antibody directed against human immunoglobulin (conjugate) is added to each of the slide areas containing the viral antigens. After washing, the slides are inspected with a fluorescence microscope and an end point (*ie*, the highest dilution of serum producing positive immunofluorescence) can be detected. Changes in titer may be determined by inspection of slides reacted with serial dilutions of acute- and convalescent-phase sera that are performed together at the same time. Indirect assays can also be performed using enzyme-labeled conjugates (*eg*, horseradish peroxidase) instead of fluorochrome-tagged reagents. These enzyme conjugate tests can be read with a light rather than a fluorescence microscope.

Immunofluorescence and enzyme immunoassay approaches each have their own advantages and dis-

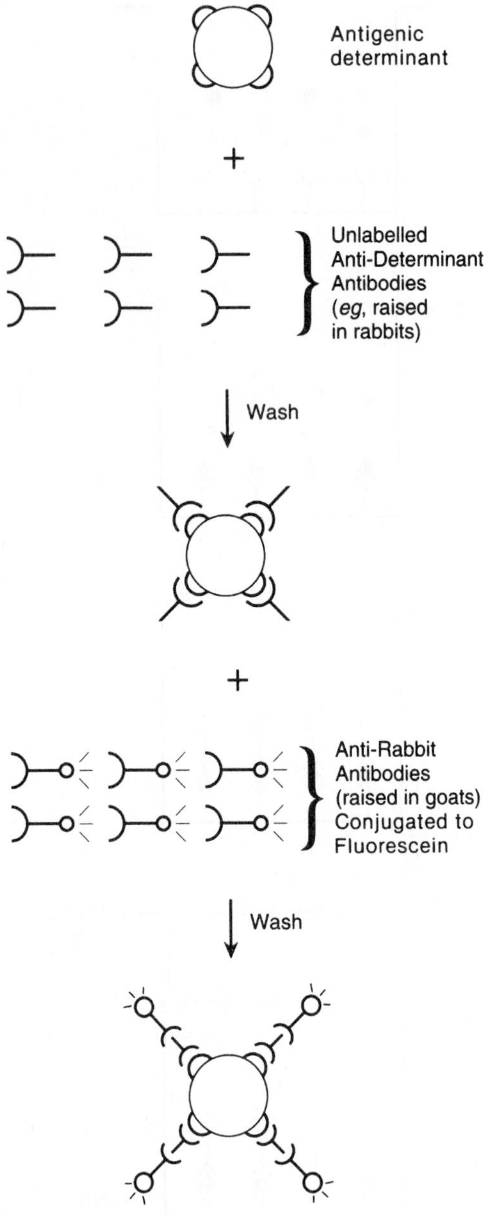

Figure 1-24
Schematic diagram of an indirect immunofluorescence assay (IFA) for antigen detection. In this method, the specimen (eg, sputum for *Legionella*) is reacted with an excess of unlabeled antibodies directed against the antigen. After a wash step, fluorescein-conjugated antibodies directed against the species of antibody used in the initial reaction (eg, fluorescein-labeled anti-rabbit Igs raised in goats) are overlaid on the FA slide. After washing, the slide is examined for specific fluorescence. With *Legionella*, for example, unlabeled rabbit antibodies against a large number of serotypes can be used for the first step in the procedure, while only a single fluorescein-conjugated goat anti-rabbit Ig is required for the second step. If *Legionella* organisms were to be detected by a DFA method, separate fluorescein-labeled conjugates for each serotype would be required.

advantages. The use of EIA methods for antigen detection is advantageous in high-volume laboratories where many samples are examined daily for a single determinant (*eg*, *Chlamydia trachomatis* or respiratory syncytial virus).[124,247] Although immunofluorescence

Step 1

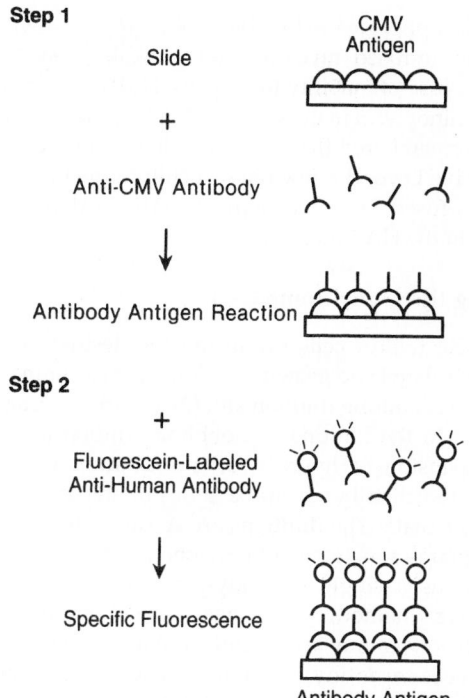

Figure 1-25
Indirect fluorescent antibody (IFA) method for antibody detection. In this method, antigen (*eg,* cytomegalovirus [CMV]-infected tissue culture cells) is fixed onto an FA slide and reacted with patient serum. If anti-CMV antibodies are present, they bind to the antigens on the slide. After a washing step, a fluorescein-conjugated goat anti-human antibody is overlaid on the slide. This results in labeling of the CMV-infected cells on the slide and indicates the presence of anti-CMV antibodies in the initial serum specimen. Titers can be determined by performing the assay with twofold dilutions of serum and reading for the highest serum dilution resulting in a proscribed degree of fluorescence.

techniques are considerably more labor intensive, the ability to directly observe the background cellular elements in certain direct antigen test procedures to determine the adequacy of the specimen is a distinct advantage of DFAs over antigen-capture EIA methods. For example, because *Chlamydia trachomatis* preferentially infects cervical columnar epithelial cells, the presence of squamous epithelial cells and a preponderance of segmented neutrophils, erythrocytes, or excess mucus indicates that the specimen is inadequate for diagnostic purposes. Adequate specimens show a preponderance of intact cuboidal and columnar epithelial cells. This assessment can be made with the direct fluorescent antibody test and incorporated into the laboratory report, allowing the physician to weigh clinical evidence of chlamydial infection along with the possibility that a negative report may actually reflect an inadequately collected cervical specimen. Such determinations cannot be made with the antigen-capture EIAs for *C. trachomatis*. In addition to *C. trachomatis*, direct fluorescent antibody reagents are available for the detection of several organisms, including *Giardia lamblia*, *Cryptosporidium parvum*, and *Pneumocystis carinii*.[128,283,295]

MONOCLONAL ANTIBODIES

A natural outgrowth of the serologic principles and techniques described previously has been the attempts to purify antigens to reduce the heterogeneity of antisera. Antigen molecules with only a single epitope are rarely encountered; rather, hundreds or even thousands of potential antigenic determinants may exist on a cell surface or within the mix of other substances. When these mixed antigens are injected into an animal, an equal number of lymphocyte clones are stimulated. Even though each clone produces a specific antibody, the final result is a highly heterogeneous mixture of antibody molecules, the specificity and affinity of which are often unknown and difficult to control from batch to batch. When these polyclonal antisera are used in bacterial test systems, cross-reactivity may occur, either because antigenic determinants are shared by different species or because mutations may result in the evolution of epitopes sufficiently close in specificity to produce detectable reactions. Attempts to produce pure antigens through adsorption techniques have only been partially successful.

As the science of serologic testing evolved, the view was held that the availability of an antibody that possesses a high degree of molecular homogeneity with a narrow specificity for a single, antigenic epitope without cross-reactivity would solve many of the problems encountered in the use of polyclonal antibodies. Highly specific monoclonal antibodies, the product of a single clone of lymphoid cells, gradually emerged as a by-product of the investigations in cell fusion and hybridoma technology conducted by Kohler and Milstein.[138] Because of their discovery, it is now possible to isolate cloned lines of single lymphocytes that produce unique antibody molecules. The main breakthrough was not that a single line of monoclonal antibody-producing cells could be isolated, but rather that these mouse lymphocytes could be fused with mouse myeloma cells to produce hybrid cells with two important inherent properties: (1) the capability of producing monospecific antibodies (acquired from the parent lymphocytes) and (2) the ability to grow permanently in culture, a gift of immortality passed on from the myeloma cells. Thus, individual monoclonal antibodies can now be produced in a continuous and almost endless supply.

MONOCLONAL ANTIBODY PRODUCTION

The production of monoclonal antibodies follows seven distinct steps.

1. Selection of antigen (need not be pure);
2. Immunization of the animal;
3. Fusion of animal spleen lymphocytes and myeloma cells;
4. Formation of antibody-producing hybridomas;
5. Cloning of desired isolated hybridomas;
6. Screening for antibodies—use of selection techniques;
7. Mass production of desired monoclonal antibodies.

Details of these procedures are included in Box 1-4.

BOX 1-4. PROCEDURE FOR PRODUCTION OF MONOCLONAL ANTIBODIES

Selection of Antigen

Monoclonal antibodies can be produced against any substance recognized as an antigen by the immune system of the animal being injected. Using a pure antigen is ideal. In fact, certain antigens, such as chemically purified drugs used for assays (eg, digoxin), may be homogeneous. Even so, one can never guarantee that an antigenic determinant will consist of only one epitope. The fact that impure antigens can be used in monoclonal antibody production is a chief advantage over conventional methods used to proudce polyclonal antibodies.

Animal Immunization

The chief objectives in the immunization procedure are to prime the immune system of the animal to avidly recognize all antigens injected, to maximally stimulate B-lymphocyte clones, and to have the spleen cells divide at a high rate. In the production of monoclonal antibodies, the BALB/cj mouse strain is most commonly used. The antigen is injected subcutaneously or intraperitoneally, with the simultaneous injection of Freund's adjuvant. Injections are repeated at weekly intervals and a final "booster" injection is given intravenously approximately 3 days before spleen cells are harvested. At the end of the injection schedule, the animal is killed and the spleen is aseptically removed.

Fusion of Splenic Lymphocytes and Myeloma Cells

The animal spleen is placed in sterile culture medium containing antibiotics. The splenic tissue is teased to release cells and to form a slurry. This material is passed through a mesh to obtain single cells. Ficoll is added and the slurry is centrifuged to remove red blood cells. Polyethylene glycol (PEG) is added to the slurry to reduce intercell surface tension; this brings the cells into close proximity to one another and allows their membranes to fuse. Dimethylsulfoxide (DMSO) is added to the fusion mixture to maximize cell-to-cell contact. Finally, the cells are packed into a pellet by gently centrifuging the mixture for 5 minutes. Thus, at the end of these steps, the preparation consists of unfused myeloma cells, unfused lymphocytes, and a few fused hybrid lymphocyte-myeloma cells (it should be recognized that splenic lymphocytes and myeloma cells fuse with a frequency of only about $1/10^5$ or 10^6 cells).

Selection of Hybrid Lymphocyte-Myeloma Cells

Unfused myeloma cells rapidly outgrow the hybrids and must be removed in some manner. The myeloma cells used for fusion are grown in the presence of 8-azoguanine, a drug that causes the cells to permanently switch off the production of hypoxanthine phosphoribosyl transferase (HRPT), an enzyme that is needed to continue growth. If these HRPT-negative cells are suspended in a medium containing hypoxanthine, aminopterin, and thymidine (HAT medium), only the hybridoma cells will grow successfully. The hybridoma cells inherit HRPT from the splenic lymphocytes with which they fused and will survive. The unfused myeloma cells, unable to synthesize DNA because of inability to produce HRPT, will be killed by the aminopterin in the selective HAT medium. It should also be remembered that unfused splenic lymphocytes do not survive beyond a few days in culture medium; therefore, the fused lymphocyte-myeloma hybrid cells alone survive in the HAT medium.

Cloning the Hybridoma Cells

The single hybrid cells producing the desired antibody must be isolated and grown as a clone. Two techniques can be used: (1) limiting dilution and (2) growth in an agar gel medium. In the limiting or doubling dilution technique, the suspension of hybrids (after maximum growth) is diluted and distributed into a series of sterile wells in a microtiter plate. The dilutions are so calculated that each well contains an average of only one cell that can then be replaced as a single antibody-producing clone. In the alternative method, using agarose gel supplemented with serum, amino acids, and antibiotics, the dividing hybrid cells form tiny, spherelike clusters. These spheres can be selected with a Pasteur pipette and transferred to microtube wells for further culture and ultimately for assay to determine whether the desired antibody is being produced.

Screening for Desired Antibodies

In the fusion step of the procedure of producing monoclonal antibodies, many lymphocytes other than those producing the desired monoclonal antibodies may have fused. In fact, less than 5% of the hybrid cells out of those selected actually produce the desired specific antibodies. Thus, assays of the selected cell lines are required to determine if the desired antibody is being produced. RIAs, EIAs, precipitin techniques, and blotting techniques can be used for this phase of the procedure.

Mass Production of Monoclonal Antibodies

Once the desired clone of hybrid cells has been selected, the next step is the production of large quantities of monoclonal antibodies. The peritoneal cavity of mice, preferably the same strain that was used for the initial immunization step, can be used to grow the selected hybrid cell clone. First, the peritoneal cavity is injected with an organic irritant, such as pristeane, to produce a chemical peritonitis. Next, the selected hybrid cell line is injected into the peritoneal cavity. Within days, a tumor known as a hybridoma develops. This tumor produces large quantities of monoclonal antibodies that can be harvested by aspirating the ascitic fluid from the mouse's peritoneal cavity. A tumor-bearing mouse will survive for 4 to 6 weeks, during which time large quantities of antibody can be harvested. Hybridomas can also be grown in tissue cultures where highly purified antibodies are produced without the potential of contamination from serum, nonspecific interference from ascites proteins, or cross-reactivity of histoincompatibility antibodies derived from the mouse tissues.

APPLICATIONS OF MONOCLONAL ANTIBODIES

Monoclonal antibodies have been produced against many clinically relevant antigens.[186] The applications are far too numerous to cite in detail, and microbiologists must remain in touch with current publications to determine which new development may be of use in their laboratories. Monoclonal antibodies produced for specific epitopes of a wide variety of viruses, bacteria, parasites, and fungi have been reported in the medical literature.[2,139,204] Monoclonal antibody conjugates are now used in many commercial systems in both immunofluorescence and EIA formats.[124,247] In addition to the direct detection of microbial structural antigens, monoclonal antibodies are also being used with increased frequency for the identification of enteric toxins, including those produced by *Shigella* species, *Campylobacter* species, uropathogenic and toxigenic strains of *Escherichia coli*, and *Vibrio* species, among others.[56,67] This approach introduces a totally new way of looking at the relationship of microorganisms and infectious diseases. Instead of the conventional focus on detection and identification of the organisms themselves, these reagents allow the specific detection of microbial virulence factors that may be shared by several bacterial species that cause a given symptom complex. For example, it may be more important to know that an enteric toxin is the cause of hyperosmotic diarrhea, rather than receiving the information that the patient is infected with *Shigella* species, *Escherichia coli*, *Vibrio* species, and so forth.

MOLECULAR METHODS IN CLINICAL MICROBIOLOGY

NUCLEIC ACID PROBES

In broad terms, a nucleic acid probe is a sequence of single-stranded nucleic acid that can hybridize specifically with its complementary strand via nucleic acid base pairing. A probe may be constructed to detect either DNA or RNA. Probes may be small (as few as 20 nucleotides in length) or large (several thousand nucleotides in length). The basic principle behind DNA probe technology is **hybridization**, which involves denaturation of dsDNA into single strands and detection of ssDNA with a labeled, complementary ssDNA probe (Fig. 1-26). Probe hybridization can be used to demonstrate genetic relatedness (*eg*, sequences of homologous base sequences) in the DNA of different organisms, and, in this way, has been used extensively in efforts to construct phylogenetic taxonomic schemes, usually by probe analysis of highly conserved 16S rRNA sequences. In the diagnostic laboratory, DNA probes are being used for culture confirmation as an alternative to conventional, time-consuming, or labor-intensive methods. DNA probes are also being used for detection of fastidious organisms directly in clinical specimens; these direct probe methods are much less sensitive when used without DNA amplification procedures (discussed later) because the numbers of a specific organisms present in a clinical specimen may fall below the sensitivity of the probe assay. In the absence of amplification procedures prior to probe testing, commercially available probes may detect as few as 10^4 to 10^6 copies of a specific nucleic acid sequence, while amplification used along with probe detection may detect 10 or fewer copies of a specific nucleotide sequence. When probes are used to confirm the identity of a cultured organism, the number of target copies far exceeds the threshold of test sensitivity. However, in testing clinical specimens directly, this threshold may or may not be met.

Probes were initially developed in research settings and involved the use of sophisticated recombinant DNA technology, including the use of restriction endonucleases and plasmid or viral cloning vehicles, and entailed procedures for sequence detection, probe labeling, and probe production.[258] As a result of basic research in this area, unique nucleotide sequences of bacterial, viral, fungal, or parasitic organisms can now be determined using automated biochemical sequencers. Computerized analysis of these nucleotide sequences allows recognition of oligonucleotide sequences (*ie*, sequences of 50–70 base-pairs) that are unique to a given microorganism. A "synthetic sequence" of nucleotides can then be "manufactured" (again using automated nucleic acid synthesizers), labeled, and used as hybridization probes for detection of the unique sequence in an organism grown in culture or directly in a clinical specimen. The details for the "old method" of nucleic acid probe construction (*ie*, insertional inactivation, nick translation, etc) may be found in Chapter 21 of the previous edition of this textbook.

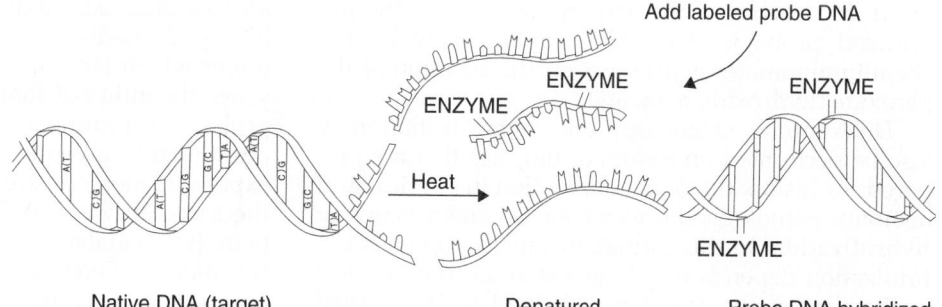

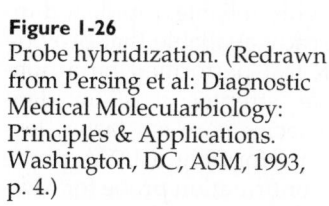

Figure 1-26
Probe hybridization. (Redrawn from Persing et al: Diagnostic Medical Molecularbiology: Principles & Applications. Washington, DC, ASM, 1993, p. 4.)

Native DNA (target)

Heat

Add labeled probe DNA

ENZYME   ENZYME   ENZYME

ENZYME

Denatured (single stranded) DNA

Probe DNA hybridized to target DNA

Detection of probe reactivity with unknown organisms or specimens can be accomplished by a variety of techniques. Nitrocellulose paper filters are able to bind denatured ssDNA very tightly but will not bind native dsDNA. A heat- or alkali-denatured sample can be passed through a nitrocellulose filter, and the ssDNA will bind tightly to the filter along the deoxyribose-phosphate-deoxyribose "backbone" of the strand. This filter is then incubated with the labeled probe under optimal hybridization conditions, followed by thorough washing and exposure to a single strand-specific nuclease to "chew up" any labeled, unbound probe. The filter can then be assayed in a scintillation counter or can be overlayed with X-ray film for autoradiographic detection. If an enzyme-labeled probe is used, the filter is exposed to the enzyme substrate. If the hybridization reaction has occurred, a colored "spot" will appear in that area of the filter. This type of hybridization-detection format is known as a "dot blot" hybridization assay.

Early probe work involved labeling of the probe with radioactive compounds such as ^{32}P and detecting positive probe reactions by autoradiography or scintillation counting. Non-radiolabeled probes were then developed that used enzymes (horseradish peroxidase, alkaline phosphatase) or affinity labels such as biotin as labels for detection of hybridized probes. Commercially available nucleic acid probes use chemiluminescence for detection. The probes are synthesized and then linked to an acridinium ester. After the hybridization step, nonhybridized probe is chemically removed from the reaction mixture, leaving only the acridinium ester-labeled probe that has become hybridized to the target molecule. Detection is accomplished by the addition of hydrogen peroxide and hydroxide. This results in hydrolysis of the ester linkage and the generation of light energy, which is detected by a chemiluminometer. This reporter molecule-detection format was developed by GenProbe (San Diego, CA) and is used in their AccuProbe™ product line for culture confirmation and in the PACE 2 systems for direct detection of *Chlamydia trachomatis* and *Neisseria gonorrhoeae* in clinical specimens. Chemiluminescent probe assays are performed in a liquid phase from start to finish and do not require the use of filters, radioactivity, or enzyme substrates. Removal of unhybridized, labeled probe is accomplished by a differential hydrolysis step rather than repeated wash steps. Because the reaction occurs in a single phase, the kinetics of the hybridization reaction are much more rapid. Hydrolysis of the acridinium ester on the hybridized probe is detected instantaneously by the chemiluminometer instrument on the addition of the peroxide/hydroxide reagents.

DNA probe technology and hybridization may also be performed on tissues or biopsies that are prepared for histopathologic examination in surgical and anatomic pathology; this technique is known as **in situ hybridization**. In this format, the ability to detect hybridization depends to a large extent on the physical availability of the target nucleic acid to the labeled probe. Different tissue fixation methods may affect this availability and, conversely, the size of the probe may limit its ability to reach target nucleotide sequences in the fixed specimen. When initially developed, in situ hybridization procedures also used radioactively labeled probes and autoradiography detection methods. Biotinylated probes are now the most commonly used reagents for in situ hybridization. Detection is accomplished by reacting the tissues with avidin-horseradish peroxidase (avidin-HRP). The avidin moiety of avidin-HRP stoichiometrically binds to the biotin attached to the probe. Exposure to the HRP enzyme substrate results in a colorimetric reaction that can be detected with a light microscope. With in situ hybridization, the pathologist can appreciate the presence of specific probe reactivity in the context of cellular architecture and the presence of other hallmarks of infection (ie, presence of organisms within granulomas, microabscesses, etc). In situ hybridization has its greatest applications in the detection of organisms that are difficult to grow in culture, such as human papillomaviruses, Epstein-Barr virus, hepatitis B virus, and HIV-1.[86,98,262,280]

APPLICATIONS OF NUCLEIC ACID PROBES

Although nucleic acid probe technology is more expensive than conventional approaches, the decrease in turn-around time afforded by some applications of this technology may significantly affect patient outcome by providing a more rapid diagnosis, thereby decreasing ancillary costs and length of stay in the hospital. Probes for direct detection of pathogenic organisms in clinical specimens may be advantageous, particularly for organisms for which reliable culture systems are not available or practical. This is true of bacterial organisms like *Bartonella* species and viruses such as the human papillomaviruses, parvovirus B-19, and HIV. Direct detection probes may also be advantageous for fastidious pathogens like *Neisseria gonorrhoeae* and *Chlamydia trachomatis*, particularly if specimens are collected at remote clinic sites and sent to reference laboratories for organism detection.[157] Direct detection probes, however, lack an amplification step and are usually more sensitive than conventional culture methods, but less sensitive than probe tests performed after some sort of target amplification technique. At the present time, however, only a few probes are approved by the Food and Drug Administration and commercially available for use in clinical microbiology laboratories in the United States (Table 1-4). Most of these are culture confirmation probes that are used to identify organisms that have already grown on solid or in liquid media.[52] Given the economic constraints under which laboratories have been placed in recent years, the utility of some of these culture confirmation probes for routine use in the clinical laboratory is questionable, given that highly reliable, rapid, and inexpensive methods are already available that provide the same answers. A PYR test performed on a non-hemolytic, catalase-negative "streptococcus" for identification of *Enterococcus* species is much faster, less costly, and as accurate as performing a DNA probe test. A test like the culture confirmation probe for *Neis-*

TABLE 1-4

COMMERCIALLY AVAILABLE PROBE TESTS FOR USE IN CLINICAL LABORATORIES

APPROVED APPLICATION	ORGANISMS DETECTED

Culture confirmation only	Bacteria
	   Campylobacter species *(C. jejuni, C. coli, C. lari)**
	   Enterococcus species*
	   *Haemophilus influenzae**
	   *Listeria monocytogenes**
	   *Mycobacterium avium**
	   Mycobacterium avium complex*
	   *Mycobacterium gordonae**
	   *Mycobacterium intracellulare**
	   Mycobacterium kansasii
	   Mycobacterium tuberculosis complex*
	   *Neisseria gonorrhoeae**
	   Streptococcus agalactiae (Group B β-hemolytic streptococci)*
	Fungi
	   *Blastomyces dermatiditis**
	   *Coccidioides immitis**
	   *Cryptococcus neoformans**
	   *Histoplasma capsulatum**

Direct detection in clinical specimens	Bacteria
	   *Chlamydia trachomatis**
	   Gardnerella vaginalis†
	   *Legionella pneumophila**
	   *Neisseria gonorrhoeae**
	   Streptococcus pyogenes (Group A β-hemolytic streptococci)*
	Fungi
	   Candida species†
	Protozoa
	   Trichomonas vaginalis†
	Viruses
	   Human papillomavirus‡

* Gen-Probe, Inc., San Diego, CA
† MicroProbe Corp., Bothell, WA
‡ Digene Diagnostics, Inc., Silver Spring, MD

seria gonorrhoeae, which has been demonstrated to be 100% sensitive and specific, may have utility as a reliable confirmatory test in certain instances, such as confirmation of presumptive gonococcal isolates recovered from children as indicators of sexual abuse.[117,155] The culture confirmation probes for *Histoplasma capsulatum*, *Blastomyces dermatiditis*, *Coccidioides immitis*, and *Cryptococcus neoformans* clearly present distinct advantages over conventional procedures for identification due to their high sensitivity and specificity and their "user friendliness."[245]

Probe tests that are already being used in many clinical laboratories include those for the identification of *Mycobacteria* species.[91,180] As indicated in Table 1-4, culture confirmation probes are available for several clinically important mycobacteria. In contrast to conventional confirmatory test procedures for these organisms, probe tests are rapid, highly sensitive and specific, and require only small inocula for test performance.[91] Most laboratories use these probes in conjunction with the BACTEC radiometric system for detection of mycobacteria, thereby providing an amplified specimen for probe testing.[50,51,197] Growth of *Myobac-*

terium tuberculosis and other clinically significant isolates occurs more rapidly in the BACTEC system than on conventional solid media. Once the BACTEC system signals a positive growth index, the contents of the bottle can be reacted directly with the mycobacterial probes to identify the organisms on the same day as their detection by the BACTEC system. This is in contrast with subculture of the positive BACTEC bottle to solid growth media, incubation for several days, and inoculation of conventional identification tests. Mixed mycobacterial infections have also been detected using these probe tests.[50]

Probe technology has literally exploded in recent years; perusal of the clinical microbiology literature over the last 5 to 10 years reveals that probes have been developed for a wide variety of organisms. DNA probes have been developed for the detection of several viruses; most of these probes have been used in clinical research studies and with and without prior target amplification procedures. DNA probes have been described for CMV, rotavirus, herpes simplex viruses, enteric adenoviruses, hepatitis B virus, and Epstein-Barr virus, to name a few.[7,46,66,76,79,101,150,181,229,242]

Probes have also been developed for the identification of organisms that are difficult to detect or identify, including *Mobiluncus* species, *Campylobacter* species, *Legionella* species, *Haemophilus ducreyi*, *Chlamydia trachomatis*, *Mycobacterium kansasii*, *Mycobacterium avium*, *Mycobacterium intracellulare*, and *Mycobacterium paratuberculosis*.[71,72,95,110,156,192,193,198,217,250,265,279] Probes have also been applied to epidemiologic studies to pinpoint bacterial strains involved in outbreaks. For example, using a DNA fingerprint technique, Kristiansen and coworkers pinpointed the source of a strain of *Neisseria meningitidis* to family contacts in an outbreak of group B meningococcal disease among school children in northern Norway.[141] Probes have also been used for the direct detection of important, genetically encoded virulence factors in culture isolates or in clinical specimens, including the enterotoxin genes of *Escherichia coli* and *Clostridium perfringens* (the latter to confirm outbreaks of food poisoning), the detection of shiga-like toxins I and II, and the detection and differentiation of *Staphylococcus aureus* strains encoding enterotoxins A, B, C and toxic shock syndrome toxin 1.[9,173,182,184,263,268] Probes also have been developed for the direct detection of genes encoding resistance to antimicrobial agents.[92,251] Daly and associates identified 325 of 327 isolates of *Streptococcus agalactiae*, *Haemophilus influenzae*, and *Enterococcus* species from pediatric patients using the Accuprobe culture confirmation probes described above.[52]

Advances in probe technology have overcome many of the disadvantages of the earlier DNA probes; namely, the shelf life of nonisotopic probes has been extended, the sensitivity and specificity have been improved, and the number of base-pair sequences required for hybridization to produce a positive "signal" have been markedly reduced. However, the ultimate goal of detecting small quantities of DNA in clinical specimens, providing virtually immediate diagnoses, is now on the immediate horizon through the marriage of probe technology and the newly emerging DNA amplification technology.

Gene Amplification: Polymerase Chain Reaction and Other Amplification Techniques

Polymerase chain reaction (PCR) refers to a highly sensitive technique by which minute quantities of specific DNA or RNA sequences can be enzymatically amplified to the extent that a sufficient quantity of material is available to reach a threshold "signal" for detection.[195] The impetus for development of this new technology grew from basic research performed by Mullis and other scientists working at the Cetus Corporation and the Department of Human Genetics, Emerysville, CA.[74,178,179,222] The technique can be used to detect very small amounts of specific nucleic acid material in clinical specimens where bacterial, viral, or fungal agents are thought to play a causative role. The fundamental basis of this technology is that each infectious disease agent possesses a unique "signature sequence" in its DNA or RNA composition by which it can be identified. PCR is a method by which repeated cycles of oligonucleotide-directed DNA synthesis of these target "signature sequences" is carried out in vitro.

METHODOLOGY OF PCR

Polymerase chain reaction is a "target amplification" technique. This means that a target sequence of DNA is identified and amplified to such an extent that it can be detected. PCR is performed using an automated, computerized "hot block" called a thermal cycler (Perkin-Elmer Corp, Norwalk, CT). The "ingredients" necessary for the reaction—dsDNA of interest, single-stranded oligonucleotide "primers," deoxynucleotide triphosphates (usually labeled with ^{32}P), and "*Taq* DNA polymerase"—are placed together in a small vial, which, in turn, is placed in the block. The thermal cycler is able to elevate, hold, and cool the temperature of the vials in a manner that allows initial DNA denaturation and then repeated cycles of DNA synthesis and denaturation to occur. The initial denaturation step "melts" the dsDNA at 95° to 100°C. Single-stranded, oligonucleotide "primers" that flank the DNA sequence of interest (*ie*, that which needs to be amplified) are allowed to anneal to the denatured DNA strands during a cooling step. Extension of the primers by DNA synthesis is done by a thermostable *Taq* polymerase (purified from *Thermus aquaticus*, a thermophilic bacterium that lives in hot springs at temperatures of 70–75°C). Repetition of the heat denaturing-primer annealing-primer extension reaction sequence results in the amplification of the DNA sequence that is located between the primers. A typical PCR protocol for amplification of a target sequence consists of 30 to 50 thermal cycles, with a doubling of the number of target sequences occurring with each cycle. A diagrammatic representation of PCR and gene amplification is shown in Figure 1-27.

Detection of the PCR end-products may be accomplished by electrophoretically separating the components of the final amplified sample in agarose or acrylamide gels, followed by staining of the gel for 15 minutes in the running buffer containing a couple of drops of 2 mg/mL ethidium bromide. The gel separation can then be visualized on a shortwave ultraviolet radiation transilluminator, comparing the separated bands with those of a standard run in parallel. The amplified target DNA or RNA sequences can also be detected more specifically by hybridization of the amplified DNA to a synthetic, labeled probe that is complementary to all or part of the amplified DNA sequence. Using PCR technology, DNA can be amplified exponentially, by an average of a factor of 10^7, until a desired concentration of nucleic acid products is reached to attain a threshold level for the detection system being used.

Several modifications of the basic PCR technique have also been described. One such modification is **mutliplex PCR**. With this modification, multiple primer pairs for different target molecules are included in the same amplification mixture. Such a preparation can theoretically be used to simultaneously amplify target sequences for several pathogenic microorganisms in a

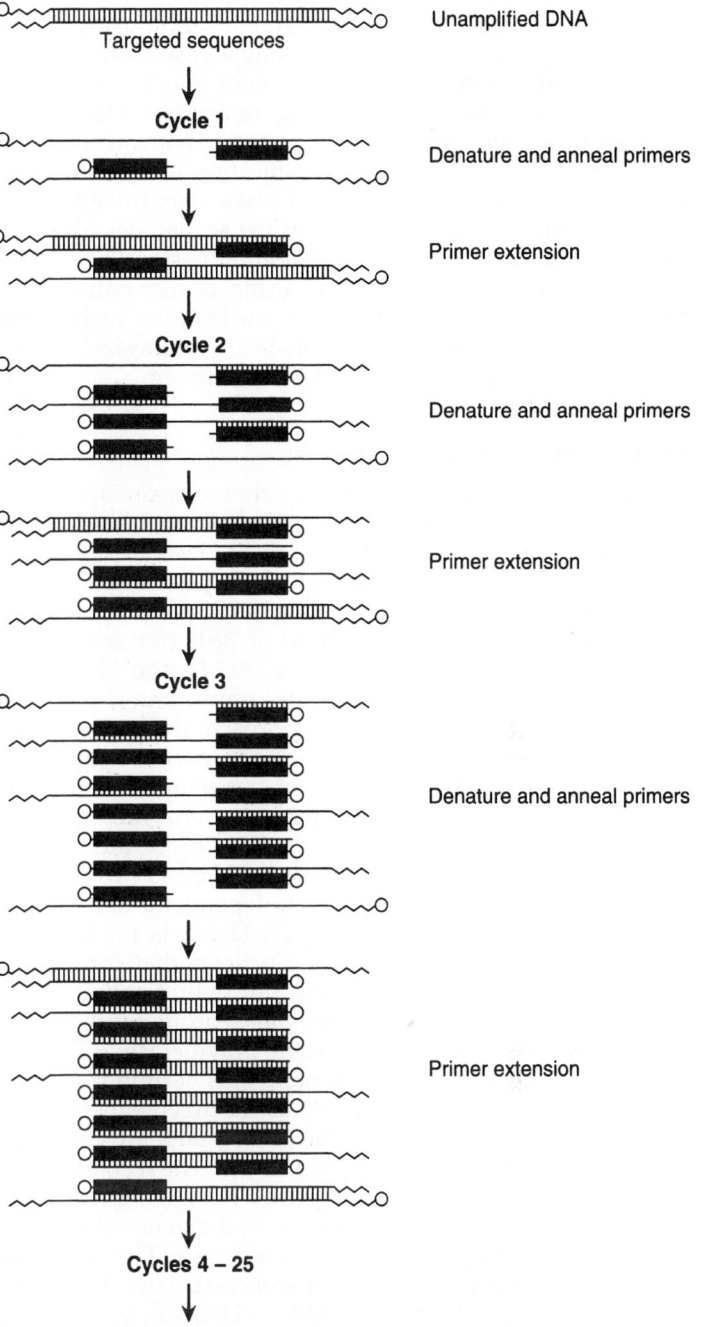

Figure 1-27
Polymerase chain reaction (PCR). The first step in the PCR sequence is the denaturation of the unamplifed dsDNA. As denaturation occurs, oligonucleotide primers that flank the nucleic acid region of interest anneal to the denatured, unamplified DNA. The primers are extended by a heat-stable DNA polymerase (*Taq* polymerase) that synthesizes complementary strands of the denatured DNA (*cycle 1*). The resulting dsDNA molecules are then denatured by heat again, the primers anneal to these ssDNA molecules, and the *Taq* polymerase, in turn, synthesizes complementary strands (*cycle 2*). This cycle is repeated many times, and with each cycle, the number of copies of the DNA sequence located between the opposing primers is doubled. This results in at least a 10^5-fold increase in the copy number of the DNA sequence. This sequence can then be detected by sequence-specific nucleic acid probes.

single reaction vial. In some applications of this technique, one set of primers is used to amplify an internal "control" sequence while the other set is used to prime the amplification of the DNA sequence of interest. Such an approach verifies that the amplification of the desired target has occurred. Multiplex PCR has been used to detect the structural genes for toxins A and B in *Clostridium difficile* and the structural gene *mec*A, which codes for the low-affinity penicillin-binding protein in oxacillin-resistant strains of staphylococci.[87,169] Multiplex PCR would be a desirable approach for clinical laboratory use because one could theoretically use a "cocktail" of primer pairs targeted to amplify the "sig-

nature sequences" (*eg*, 16S rRNA) of several pathogenic microorganisms in a single PCR reaction. Detection of the various amplicons could then be accomplished with "species-specific" hybridization probes.

Nested PCR is a technique in which several rounds of amplification are performed with one set of primers, and the product of this amplification is subsequently amplified using another set of primers that lie within the internal sequence amplified by the first primer set (*ie*, the second set of primers is "nested" within the sequence amplified with the first primer set). Nested PCR is extremely sensitive, but it does have some disadvantages, including the need to transfer reaction products synthesized with the first set of primers to another reaction vial for subsequent amplification using the "nested" set of primers, thus risking aerosolization of the amplified DNA. This requirement may be circumvented by physically separating the reaction mixtures for the the first and second primer sets with an oil phase in the same vial. After amplification using the first pair of primers, the separated phases are mixed and the contents reamplified using the second set of primers. Another method for performing nested PCR in the same reaction vial involves using primer pairs that are enriched with appropriate nucleotides such that the melting temperatures of the DNA synthesized during the two amplification cycles are different.

OTHER AMPLIFICATION TECHNIQUES

Since the description of PCR, other elegant approaches to amplification of target nucleic acid have been described. Kwoh and coworkers described a method called **transcription-based amplification**, which has subsequently been called **NASBA** (nucleic acid sequence-based amplification) or **3SR** (for self-sustaining sequence replication) (Fig. 1-28).[144] The 3SR technique has its greatest utility in amplification of ssRNA rather than DNA. In this approach, DNA that is complementary to the target RNA sequence is synthesized first; this DNA is then used as a template for transcription. The 3SR technique uses three enzymes in the reaction mixture: a reverse-transcriptase (RT, purified from avian myeloblastosis virus), RNase H (from E. coli), and bacteriophage T7 DNA-dependent RNA polymerase. Initially, a DNA copy (cDNA) is made from a target RNA sequence using primers that contain some target-specific sequences (for hybridization of the primers to part of the target) plus a promoter region for binding the phage T7 RNA polymerase. RT makes a cDNA copy of the target, thus forming a cDNA/target RNA hybrid. The RNase H enzyme then degrades the strand of RNA in the cDNA/target RNA hybrid, leaving the single-stranded cDNA. The second primer binds to the newly synthesized cDNA, the RT enzyme binds to the second primer, and extends the primer using the cDNA strand as a template. The result is a dsDNA copy of the target sequence. After this sequence of events, both strands of the DNA copy are flanked by T7 RNA polymerase promoter regions and both strands can serve as templates for this enzyme. Consequently, several antisense RNA copies of the target sequence are produced from this dsDNA molecule by the action of the T7 enzyme. These RNAs can then act as templates for RT, once again resulting in a dsDNA molecule, both strands of which can then by transcribed by the T7 RNA polymerase to produce several copies of the RNA target (see Fig. 1-28). 3SR does not require a thermal cycler and is best suited for detection of ssRNA targets. 3SR techniques have been described for detection of point mutations resulting in zidovudine resistance in strains of HIV-1.[90]

The **strand displacement amplification (SDA) technique** (Fig. 1-29) exploits the fact that, following "nicking" of a single strand of dsDNA by a site-specific restriction endonuclease, DNA polymerase can bind and synthesize a complementary copy of the ssDNA; the nicked strand becomes displaced from the strand being copied during the process of DNA synthesis. Incorporation of α-thio substituted nucleotides (eg, deoxyadenoside 5'-[α-thio]-triphosphate) into the reaction mixture renders the newly synthesized strands resistant to nicking by the endonuclease enzyme. Double-stranded DNA molecules having a single strand with incorporated α-thio substitutions can only be cut by the restriction enzymes in the "native strand," so the ssDNA that is displaced during the copying process can subsequently act as a template for binding of the primer and extension of the nucleotide strands. Single-strand nicking and subsequent polymerization and strand displacement continue to occur because of the continual regeneration of unaltered, single-strand "nick-able" sites in duplex molecules. SDA techniques have been reported for the detection of *Mycobacterium tuberculosis* in sputum specimens.[61]

Polymerase chain reaction, 3SR, and SDA deal with amplification of a target sequence that is subsequently detected with some type of probe. Other amplification methods do not amplify the number of target molecules, but amplify the "probe" used to detect the genetic sequence of interest. Two types of assays use the probe amplification approach: Qbeta replicase amplification and the ligase chain reaction (LCR).[159,287]

The Qbeta replicase method makes use of a "replicase" enzyme that is able to synthesize the genomic RNA of bacteriophage Qbeta (Fig. 1-30). The RNA genome of phage Qbeta has several ssRNA "loops" and partially double-stranded regions (like a molecule of tRNA). In the amplification test, a naturally occurring variant of the phage particle called MDV-1 is used; this variant behaves as a substrate for the Qbeta replicase enzyme and can be manipulated such that an oligonucleotide "probe" sequence can be inserted into one of the "loops." The MDV-1-"probe" is added to the reaction mixture and binds to its target sequence (if the target is in dsDNA, heat is used to denature the DNA, enabling the probe to hybridize). Once the probe region in the loop of the molecule anneals to its recognition sequence, it becomes resistant to hydrolysis by RNase; RNase treatment hydrolyzes the unbound probe and a wash step removes these molecules from the reaction mixture. Addition of Qbeta replicase enzyme to the probe-target complex and subsequent incubation results in specific amplification of the probe. The Qbeta replicase amplification method can be used to detect either DNA or RNA targets.

Ligase chain reaction, or **LCR**, is another probe amplification technique (Fig. 1-31). Single-stranded target DNA is incubated with oligonucleotide probes that bind to the target in an end-to-end fashion. A thermostable DNA ligase then "ligates" or joins the two probes together.[14] The resulting duplex is heated, causing denaturation and separation of the target ssDNA and the ligated probes. The ligated probes and the target again bind probe sequences in an end-to-end fashion, followed by ligation to form another duplex. These steps are repeated several times. Geometric accumula-

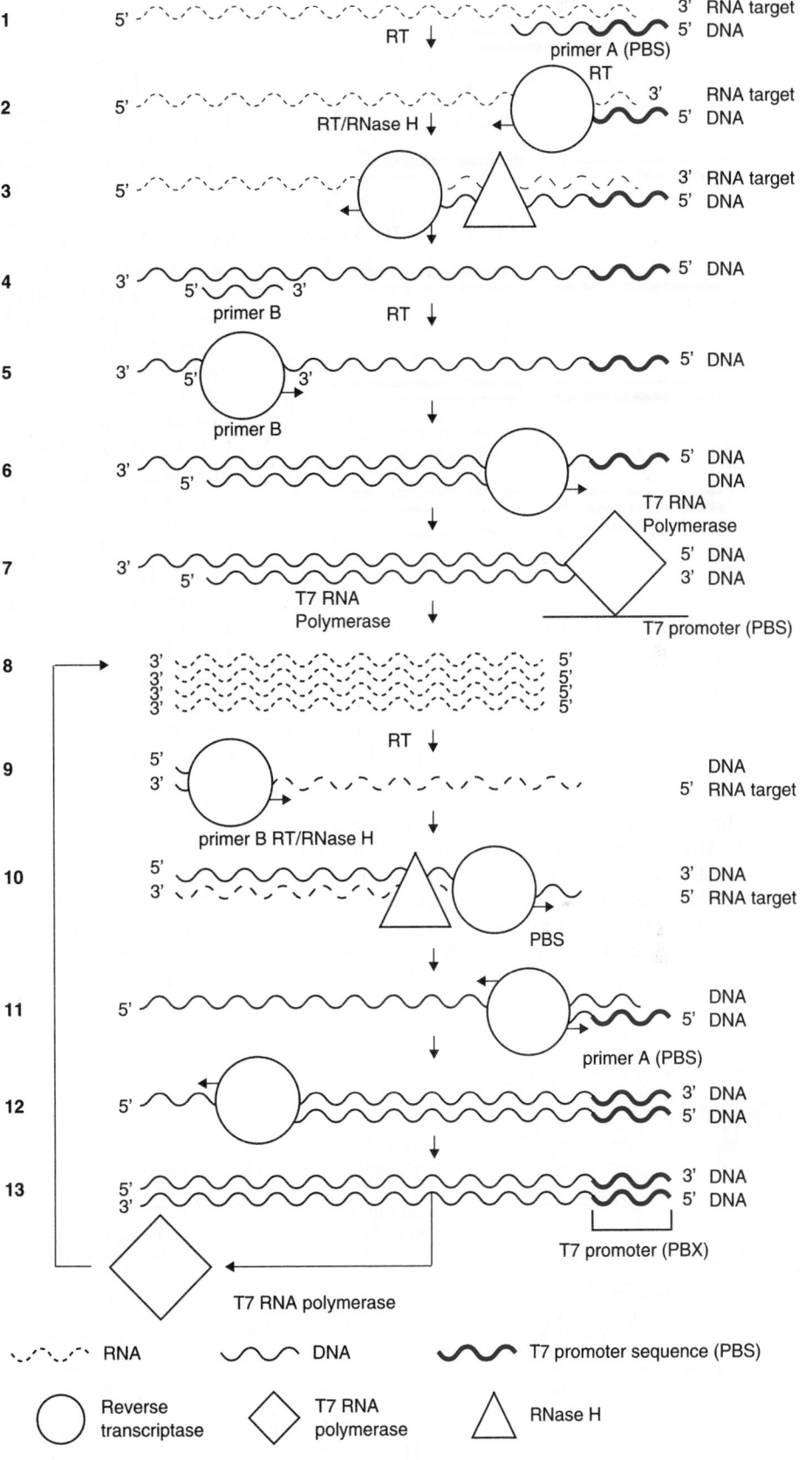

Figure 1-28
3SR (self-sustaining sequence replication). (Redrawn from Persing et al: Diagnostic Medical Molecularbiology: Principles & Applications. Washington, DC, ASM, 1993, p. 67.)

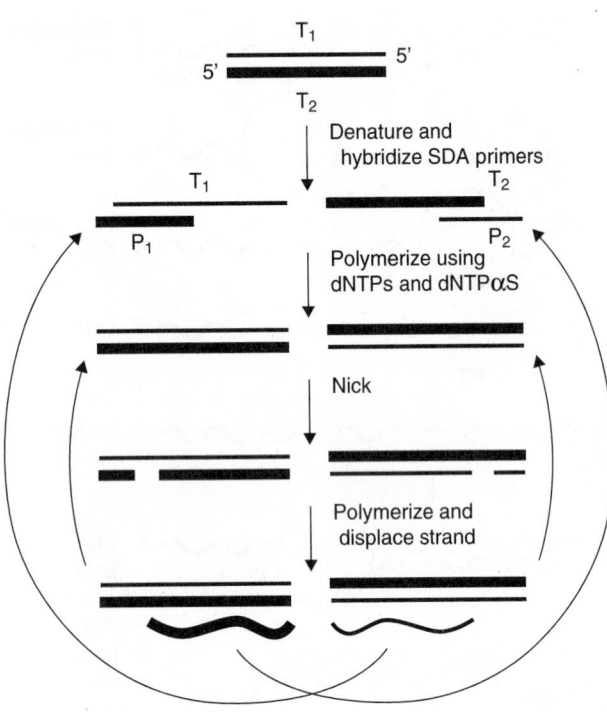

Figure 1-29
Strand displacement amplification (SDA). T, and T₂ are target sequences; P, and P₂ are primers. (Redrawn from Persing et al: Diagnostic Medical Molecularbiology; Principles & Applications. Washington, DC, ASM, 1993, p. 69.)

tion of the the ligation products results in probe amplification. Attachment of functional groups (biotin, enzymes) to the probes results in labeling of the ligated probe products, enabling them to be detected.

Another approach to amplification is one where the signal generated by the probe is amplified rather than the number of target molecules (as in PCR, 3SR, and SDA) or the number of probes (as in LCR and *Qbeta* replicase approaches). Signal amplification techniques work by either attaching additional functional "reporter" groups onto a probe or by increasing the intensity of the signal generated by a probe. Unlike PCR, based methods, these types of assays are not subject to the contamination problems described later for PCR, but some workers have found the method to be less sensitive, so specimens that contain very few target molecules may not be detected with signal amplification methods. An example of signal amplification is the **branched-chain DNA method** (developed by Chiron Corporation) (Fig. 1-32). In this method, target DNA is released from a specimen, and the DNA is denatured to single strands. The single-stranded target DNA binds to small oligonucleotide "capture probes" that anneal to contiguous "runs" of nucleotides. "Extender probes" also anneal to the "captured" target oligonucleotide at sequences adjacent to the capture probes. These extender probes also contain sequences that anneal to single-stranded oligonucleotides that form the "tail" of a large branched amplification "multimer." Enzyme-labeled oligonucleotides (the reporter molecules) then hybridize to the ssDNA branches of the large multimer via homologous base pairing, forming a dsDNA "tree" (see Fig. 1-32). Addition of the enzyme substrate generates an amplified signal. Branched-chain DNA assays have been described for detection of several viruses, including HIV-1, hepatitis C, and CMV, and have been used to assess viral load and the response of patients to therapy with various antiviral agents, including zidovudine, ganciclovir, and α-interferon.[59,190,215,235]

TECHNICAL PROBLEMS WITH PCR

Although the basic theory of PCR and gene amplification is relatively simple, a number of technical problems currently prevent this technology from becoming

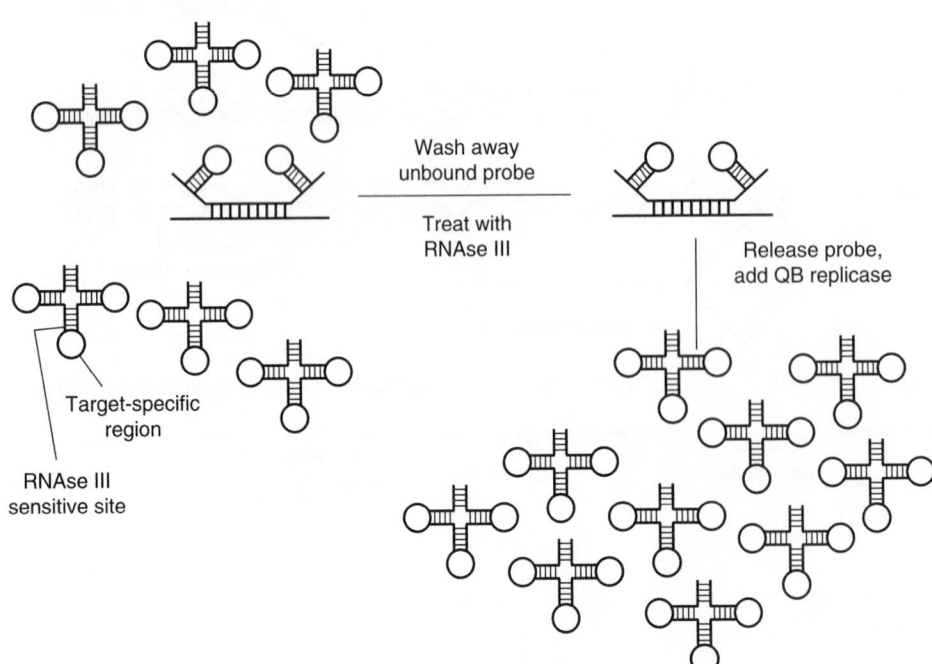

Figure 1-30
Qbeta replicase-based probe amplification. (Redrawn from Persing et al: Diagnostic Medical Molecularbiology: Principles & Applications. Washington, DC, ASM, 1993, p. 73.)

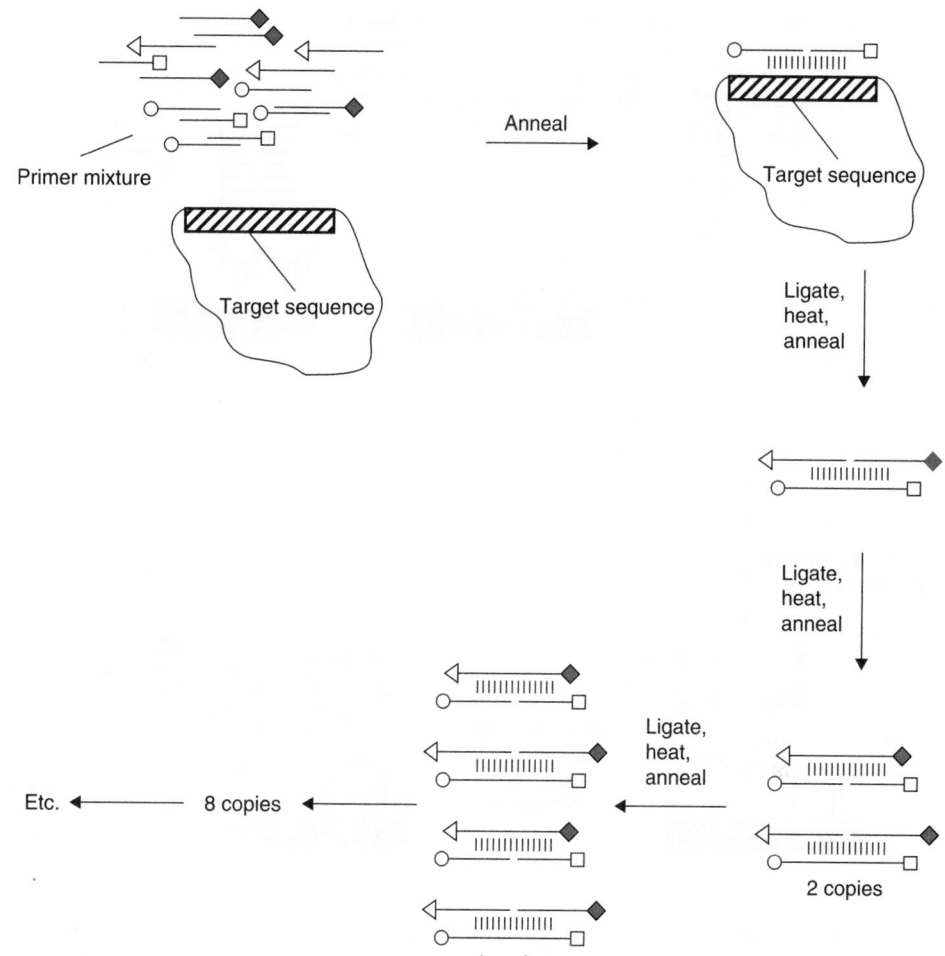

Figure 1-31
Ligase chain reaction. (Redrawn from Persing et al: Diagnostic Medical Molecularbiology: Principles & Applications. Washington, DC, ASM, 1993, p. 74.)

a staple of clinical laboratory testing.[73,195,286] One major problem is false-positive reactions caused by the introduction of contaminating nucleic acids into the reaction mixtures. Nucleic acid contamination may originate from cross-contamination due to a single specimen containing large numbers of target molecules, contamination of reagents by DNA derived from previously analyzed samples, and accumulation of PCR products (amplicons) in the laboratory by repeated amplification of the same target. In PCR, LCR, and SDA amplification systems, DNA amplicons are the main source of contamination, whereas with 3SR and Q*beta* replicase approaches, RNA products are responsible for contamination. "Amplicon buildup" in laboratory reagents, glassware, autoclaves, and ventilation systems may be a serious problem. Each PCR vessel, after amplification, may contain as many as 10^{12} copies of an amplicon; thus, even a tiny aerosol droplet can contain a significant number of contaminating targets. However, various methodologic modifications are now available to circumvent the contamination problem.[196]

Despite these problems, PCR techniques are being successfully used in several research centers where variables can be carefully controlled. These variables include not only the physical space, but also the functions of the laboratory workers within that space.

Ehrlich[73] outlined specific provisions that must be afforded in any laboratory desiring to engage in PCR analyses (Box 1-5).

Space and staffing requirements for performance of PCR analyses currently preclude all but select research laboratories from using this technology in a diagnostic sense. The lack of efficient ways to detect the amplicons after amplification by PCR is also a deterrent to the implementation of this technology in most clinical laboratories. The use of gel electrophoresis, filter membrane hybridization, and radioactive probes is a time-consuming and labor-intensive activity requiring highly trained and dedicated personnel. The introduction of nonisotopic detection formats coupled with automation may represent a partial solution for this problem in the future. PCR will not reach universal applications similar to other current technologies in clinical microbiology laboratories until formal instruction in molecular techniques are introduced into clinical training programs for medical technologists, pathology residency training programs, and clinical microbiology fellowships. National standards for test performance, proficiency testing, and quality control and quality assurance will need to be written, adopted, and in place before PCR technology can truly be implemented in clinical laboratories to any great extent. Fi-

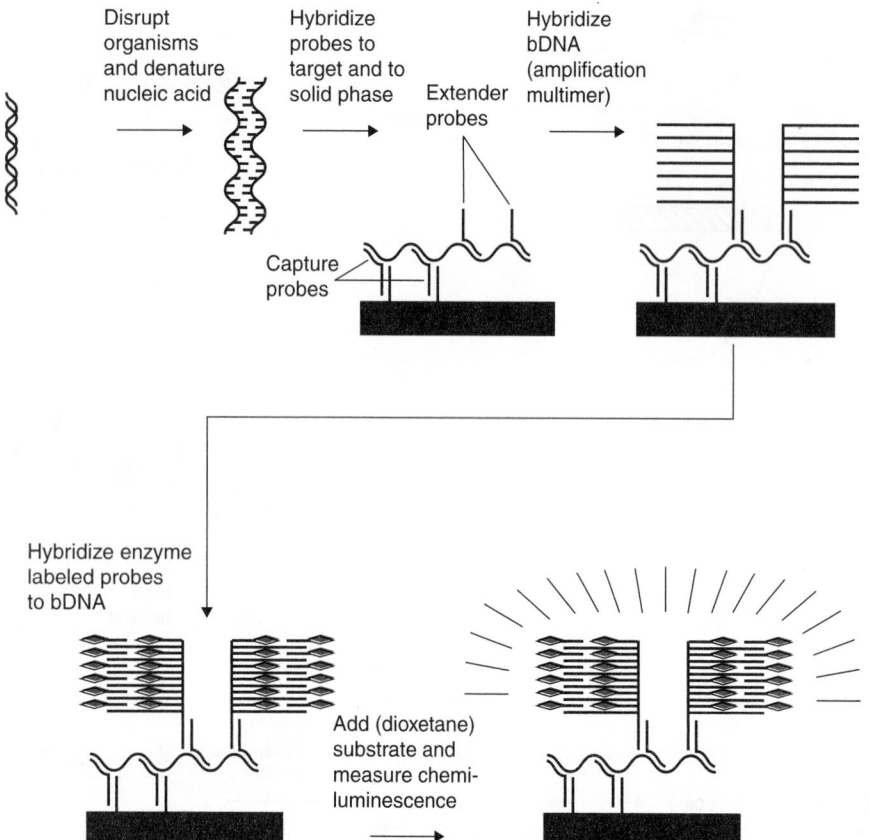

Disrupt organisms and denature nucleic acid

Hybridize probes to target and to solid phase

Extender probes

Hybridize bDNA (amplification multimer)

Capture probes

Hybridize enzyme labeled probes to bDNA

Add (dioxetane) substrate and measure chemi-luminescence

Figure 1-32
Branched DNA (bDNA)-based signal amplification.

nancial considerations are also important because it may be many years before the costs for amplification and nucleic acid probe approaches to infectious disease diagnosis can be justified as compared to the conventional bench methods currently being used.

APPLICATIONS OF PCR TECHNOLOGY IN CLINICAL MICROBIOLOGY

Polymerase chain reaction and other amplification and detection techniques have a variety of applications in the clinical microbiology laboratory (Tables 1-5 through 1-8). In clinical bacteriology, PCR may be used for direct detection/identification of microorganisms, detection of genes coding for virulence factors, determining the presence of genes responsible for antimicrobial resistance, and typing of bacterial isolates in epidemiologic investigations. Detection and identification of organisms by PCR is probably most valuable for those bacteria that grow slowly, that are difficult to grow on conventional media, or that lack sensitive culture systems. PCR detection and identification protocols have been described for several bacteria; among these are *Mycobacterium tuberculosis*, other mycobacteria, *Chlamydia trachomatis*, *Bartonella* species, *Bordetella pertussis*, *Brucella* species, *Francisella tularensis*, and *Mycoplasma* species.[18,24,32,43,69,121,209,259] Although nucleic acid probes have been successful in the culture confirmation of *Mycobacterium* species, as mentioned before, probes lack the sensitivity to directly detect mycobacterial DNA or rRNA in sputum and other clinical spec-

imens without amplification. Both basic and applied research is currently underway to develop PCR methods for amplification of repetitive DNA or rRNA sequences specific for *Mycobacterium tuberculosis*, with the vision that the diagnosis of tuberculosis may be reduced to a 1- or 2-day procedure instead of the several days to weeks required by conventional methods.[24,75,100] Processing of the specimens, extraction of nucleic acids specific for *Mycobacterium* species, and amplification could be performed on the first day, with analyses of products being done on the second day. The AMPLICOR PCR *Mycobacterium tuberculosis* test (Roche Molecular Systems, Branchburg, NJ), a commercial adaptation of PCR methodology, shows promise for the direct detection of *M. tuberculosis* in clinical specimens.[20]

Polymerase chain reaction and other methods have been used to detect and characterize genes coding for various bacterial virulence factors such as enterotoxins and antimicrobial resistance factors. Kato and colleagues reported that toxigenic and nontoxigenic strains of *Clostridium difficile* could be differentiated by using oligonucleotide primers from nonrepeating sequences of the toxin A gene to amplify a 1,266-bp DNA product.[125] The extracted DNA from nontoxigenic *C. difficile* strains did not hybridize, indicating that they lacked the toxin A gene. Victor and coworkers used PCR to amplify a highly conserved region of the A subunit of the heat-labile enterotoxin gene of *Escherichia coli*. These heat labile toxin-producing strains were responsible for about 9% of nondiagnosed

---

BOX 1-5. REQUIREMENTS FOR FACILITIES PERFORMING PCR

1. The facility should provide for at least three separate functions to accommodate specimen receiving, reaction setup, and amplification/analysis, with each of the three conducted in separate rooms with individual air supply and egress with 100% air exchange with the outside and no air exchange among the rooms. Each of the laboratory rooms should also have an airlock.

2. The specimen-receiving laboratory should be staffed by individuals who have no contact with DNA or amplification products. This laboratory may also serve as the sample processing, aliquoting, and storage facility and should be located as far as possible from the amplification laboratory, with negative pressure into the hallways.

3. The setup laboratory should have positive pressure to the hall and to the amplification laboratory so that the movement of uncontrolled air flow is from the clean laboratory to the amplification (dirty) laboratory. The amplification/analysis laboratory, conversely, should have a negative pressure to the hall and setup laboratory so that when people pass through the airlock the net flow of air is into the laboratory and out of the hall.

4. These laboratories should not directly interconnect and the laboratory personnel should be segregated by task.

5. Each laboratory should be completely equipped with its own reagent preparation area. There should be absolutely no trafficking of any materials between the laboratories, particularly from the dirty laboratory to the clean laboratory. The use of disposable laboratory materials, prealiquoted reagents, and positive-displacement pipettes is also recommended.

---

diarrhea in their study series.[268] The genes that code for resistance to methicillin in staphylococci have also been amplified and detected by PCR.[127]

Polymerase chain reaction technology has also been evaluated for the diagnosis of syphilis and other spirochetal diseases. Grimprel and colleagues found that PCR was a useful adjunct in the diagnosis of congenital syphilis for detecting *Treponema pallidum* in amniotic fluid from pregnant women with untreated syphilis.[96] Several studies have demonstrated the value of PCR in the diagnosis of Lyme disease. Rosa and Schwan were the first to apply PCR to the detection of *Borrelia burgdorferi*, with 17 of 18 strains examined being successfully detected.[219] The outer surface protein A gene, located on a linear plasmid within the spirochete, has been used as a PCR target for the detection of *B. burgdorferi*. Wise and Weaver, in contrast, used a 419–base-pair region of the flagellin gene sequence of *B. burgdorferi* as the target sequence for PCR.[281] Using a nonradioactive, gene-specific probe, sensitivity at a level of 1 to 10 spirochetes was achieved. Kron and colleagues used PCR in epidemiologic studies to detect *B. burgdorferi* in tissue obtained

from infected ticks, providing an alternative to tick dissection and indirect fluorescent antibody analysis.[142]

This technology has also had research applications in diagnostic parasitology. Tachibana and associates differentiated between pathogenic and nonpathogenic isolates of *Entamoeba histolytica* by using the PCR technique to amplify a nucleotide sequence coding for a 30,000-megadalton virulence-associated antigen.[246] Kirchhoff and colleagues used PCR for *Trypanosoma cruzi* to monitor infection in experimentally infected mice.[133,172] During the acute illness, PCR detected organisms in the bloodstream 4 days earlier than microscopic examination. PCR was also positive throughout the chronic phase of the illness, whereas microscopic positivity was intermittent. PCR methods have also been published for the direct detection of *Toxoplasma gondii*. In one report, the nucleic acid of as few as 10 individual organisms could be detected in the presence of DNA from 100,000 leukocytes.[33] A PCR-based method for diagnosis of microsporidial infection, specifically *Enterocytozoon bieneusi*, has been reported that uses primer pairs adjacent to a unique sequence in the small subunit rRNA.[54]

Polymerase chain reaction and other amplification techniques are particularly useful and highly sensitive for the detection of viral agents, many of which cannot be cultivated in routinely used tissue culture systems. In a study by Puchhammer-Stockl and colleagues, varicella-zoster virus DNA was detected in the CSF of symptomatic patients with varicella-zoster virus infection after PCR amplification.[207] Arthur and coworkers detected the DNAs of human polyomaviruses BK and JC in brain tissue and urine following PCR amplification using a single pair of 20-base oligonucleotide primers complementary to shared sequences in the same region of both viruses.[11] Cao and associates applied PCR to rapid detection of cutaneous herpes simplex virus infections.[37] Cassol and associates have amplified CMV DNA in clinical specimens obtained from bone marrow transplant patients.[40] PCR technology has also been successfully applied to the detection of human papillomavirus in normal and abnormal cervical tissue.[236,293] These techniques have also been used for the detection of various hepatitis viruses (eg, hepatitis E in stool, hepatitis C in serum).[17,59,260]

Polymerase chain reaction and other molecular biologic techniques have become powerful tools for the diagnosis and management of HIV-1 infections.[211,284] Use of PCR and HIV-1-specific probes has determined that HIV-1 may be detectable in peripheral blood lymphocytes of infected persons for 3 to 6 months before seroconversion occurs.[111,130,160,189] PCR techniques may also help in diagnosing HIV-1 infection in the newborn, where serologic diagnostic methods are stymied by the presence of transplacental antibodies.[42,153,218] Gene amplification methods have also been used to assess the meaning of transiently or persistently indeterminate Western immunoblots for HIV-1. These studies indicate that persons who are at low risk for HIV-1 infection and who have indeterminate Western blot patterns are rarely, if ever, infected with HIV-1.[113] With the approval of antiviral drugs for treatment of HIV

TABLE 1-5
Selected Applications of Amplification Techniques in Clinical Bacteriology

Agent	Amplification Method	Application	References
Aureobacterium species	PCR	Identification of clinical isolate	224
Bordetella pertussis	PCR, nested PCR	Detection	32, 214
Borrelia burgdorferi	Nested PCR	Detection before, during, and after therapy	226
Brucella species		Detection/identification	164
Burkholderia pseudomallei	PCR	Identification/detection in buffy coats and pus	62
Campylobacter species	PCR	Identification by analysis of 16S rRNA	38
CDC group IV-c-2	PCR	Typing of outbreak-associated isolates	171
Chlamydia trachomatis	PCR	Diagnosis in asymptomatic patients	259
	AMPLICOR PCR	Evaluation of commercial diagnostic kit	194, 209
Coagulase-negative staphylococci	Multiplex PCR	*mecA* detection for methicillin resistance	264, 291
Corynebacterium diphtheriae	PCR	Detection of toxigenic strains	170
Escherichia coli O157:H7	Multiplex PCR	Detection of toxigenic strains	82
Haemophilus ducreyi	Multiplex PCR	Direct detection in genital ulcer specimens	187
Helicobacter pylori	PCR	Detection of organism in gastric biopsies	145
Legionella pneumophila	PCR	Molecular typing of outbreak-associated strains	94
Leptospira interrogans	PCR	Identification of leptospiral serovars	296
Mycobacterium avium complex	PCR	Differentiation of *M. avium* and *M. intracellulare*	43
Mycobacterium tuberculosi	PCR	Diagnosis of pulmonary tuberculosis	18, 105
	AMPLICOR PCR	Evaluation of commercial diagnostic kit	20, 39, 60, 282
	SDA	Detection in respiratory tract specimens	68
	PCR	Diagnosis of mycobacteremia	78
	Qbeta	Direct detection in clinical specimens	234
Neisseria gonorrhoeae	LCR	Direct detection in urogenital swab specimens	45
Salmonella typhi	PCR	Typing and detection of resistance plasmids	104
Staphyloccoccus aureus	Multiplex PCR	Detection of methicillin resistance	264
Streptococcus pneumoniae	PCR	Detection of autolysin and penicillin binding proteins	261
Streptococcus pyogenes	PCR	Strain typing by analysis of M protein genes	16
Treponema pallidum	Multiplex PCR	Direct detection in genital ulcer specimens	187
Yersinia enterocolitica	PCR	Strain typing	278

infection (*ie*, reverse transcriptase inhibitors, protease inhibitors, etc), PCR and other amplification techniques have been developed to monitor mutations in the *pol* region of the viral genome for analyses of zidovudine-resistant HIV-1 strains.[151,152] Relationships between HIV-1 RNA levels in plasma and clinical dis-

ease progression have been delineated using amplification studies.[108,191,201,215,233] As a result, both PCR and branched-chain DNA approaches are now considered state of the art for monitoring viral load, assessing levels of HIV-1 replication in infected individuals, and quantitating responses to various therapeutic interven-

TABLE 1-6

SELECTED APPLICATIONS OF AMPLIFICATION TECHNIQUES IN CLINICAL MYCOLOGY

AGENT	AMPLIFICATION METHOD	APPLICATION	REFERENCES
Aspergillus species	PCR	Detection in bronchoalveolar lavage specimens	266
Candida species	PCR	Identification and characterization by DNA "fingerprints"	253
Pneumocystis carinii	PCR	Detection in respiratory tract specimens	154

tions. Last of all, PCR and probe methods have been developed to differentiate HIV-1 from HIV-2 and have been used to demonstrate the presence of both viruses in a few patients.[212,213,216]

EPIDEMIOLOGIC TYPING METHODS

In the past, subtyping and characterization of bacterial isolates implicated in nosocomial infections or outbreaks were performed by phenotypic methods, such as biotyping, serotyping, phage typing, and susceptibility to bacteriocins. Biotyping is based on metabolic activities of the organism such as utilization of carbohydrates or production of certain metabolic end-products. Biotyping methods, however, generally lack reproducibility and discriminatory ability. For example, strains of *Haemophilus influenzae* may have identical biotyping reactions (based on production of indole, urease, and ornithine decarboxylase production, see Chap. 7) but may show different patterns on analysis

TABLE 1-7

SELECTED APPLICATIONS OF AMPLIFICATION TECHNIQUES IN CLINICAL VIROLOGY

AGENT	AMPLIFICATION METHOD	APPLICATION	REFERENCES
Adenovirus	PCR	Subgenus identification of human isolates	131
Cytomegalovirus	PCR	Detection of virus in blood, cerebrospinal fluid	97, 183, 270
Enteroviruses	PCR	Detection in clinical specimens; strain typing	10, 289
Hepatitis C	PCR bDNA	Detection in serum Quantitation of virus in serum and plasma	17 59
Hepatitis E	PCR	Detection in stool and serum	260
Herpes simplex virus 2	PCR	Evaluation of treatment outcomes	64
Herpes simplex viruses 1 and 2	Multiplex PCR	Direct detection in genital ulcer specimens	187
Human herpesviruses 6 and 7	PCR	Development and direct detection in lymph node specimens	230
Human immunodeficiency virus	NASBA, PCR, bDNA PCR	Quantitation of HIV-1 in serum (viral load) Quantitation of HIV-1 RNA and proviral DNA	215 158
Human papillomavirus	in situ PCR	Detection of virus in cervical carcinomas	13
Human parvovirus B19	PCR	Direct detection of virus in serum	106
Measles virus	PCR	Detection of virus in urine	220
Respiratory syncytial virus	PCR	Differentiation of vaccine- and wild-type RSV strains; subtyping of isolates	93, 294
Rubella virus	PCR	Diagnosis of congenital rubella in utero and during infancy	25

TABLE 1-8
SELECTED APPLICATIONS OF AMPLIFICATION TECHNIQUES IN CLINICAL PARASITOLOGY

AGENT	AMPLIFICATION METHOD	APPLICATION	REFERENCES
Enterocytozoon bieneusi	PCR	Development of primers and probes; detection in intestinal biopsies	54, 81
Encephalitozoon hellem	PCR	Diagnosis/follow-up of disseminated infection	65
Plasmodium species	PCR	Detection of malaria parasites in blood specimens	132
Toxoplasma gondii	PCR	Diagnosis/follow-up of disseminated toxoplasmosis	12, 70
Trypanosoma cruzi	PCR	Detection compared with microscopic methods	133

of cell wall proteins, indicating that the two strains are really different. Antimicrobial susceptibility patterns have also been used for strain characterization, especially when organisms associated with clusters of infections had unique or uncommon susceptibility profiles. However, the ability of organisms to rapidly acquire plasmids or transposable elements coding for antimicrobial resistance somewhat limits this approach.[8,161] Bacteriophage typing (usually used for staphylococci) and susceptibility to bacteriocins (*eg*, pyocin typing of *Pseudomonas aeruginosa*) are largely limited by the lack of availability of high-quality reagents and standardization.[23,202] Although serotyping has been the reference method for strain characterization of certain organisms (*eg*, somatic and flagellar typing of *Salmonella* species), this technique is also limited by reagent availability. The ability of serotyping to differentiate among strains may also be limited by the overrepresentation of certain serotypes among clinically significant isolates and the presence of serologically nontypeable strains. Monoclonal antibodies for strain typing have demonstrated significant utility for some organisms, such as *Neisseria gonorrhoeae*, but overrepresentation of certain gonococcal serovars may require the use of additional typing methods (*eg*, auxotyping for nutritional requirements, see Chap. 10) to achieve adequate discrimination among strains.[135,136] Molecular analyses of bacterial ultrastructural molecules such as lipopolysaccharides, principle outer membrane proteins, and nucleic acids are now the methods of choice for characterization of microorganism strains. This has come about largely due to the development of highly discriminatory molecular separation techniques (*eg*, polyacrylamide gel electrophoresis [PAGE]), the availability of computerized analytical programs, and the virtual explosion of nucleic acid technology—the development of probes and amplification techniques.

Typing of bacteria by analysis of whole cell proteins can be accomplished by a technique called **multilocus enzyme electrophoresis**. This method characterizes cellular proteins by electrophoretically separating them in a starch gel matrix and then exposing the gels to chromogenic substrates for the detection of enzymatic activities.[232] Differing mobilities of enzyme proteins in the starch gel matrix translates to differences in polypeptide sequences that are actually encoded in the DNA of the bacterium. Therefore, organisms with different enzymatic mobilities can be said to be different strains.

Nucleic acid-based typing methods include plasmid analysis, restriction endonuclease analysis, DNA probe fingerprinting, and PCR fingerpinting. Analysis of plasmid content was among the first of the nucleic acid-based methods used for characterizing organisms.[166] These autonomous transmissible extrachromosomal DNA molecules can be relatively easily extracted from cells and separated by agarose gel electrophoresis based on their size. Plasmid analysis is an appropriate analytical method for investigating outbreaks that are somewhat restricted as to time and place.[122,225] The discriminatory ability of simple plasmid analysis is not adequate for long-term epidemiologic investigations because the organisms may gain or lose plasmids and transposons when exposed to selective pressures (*eg*, changes in antibiotic usage) over time. Plasmid extraction and treatment with restriction endonucleases before electrophoresis significantly increases the utility of plasmid analysis.

Restriction endonuclease analysis relies on the use of enzymes produced by various bacteria called **restriction endonucleases**. These are enzymes that cut DNA at specific recognition sequences composed of four to six base-pairs. Commonly used restriction endonucleases include *Eco*RI (from *E. coli*), *Hind*III (from *H. influenzae*), and *Bam*HI (from *Bacillus amyloliquefaciens*). To perform the fingerprinting assay, chromosomal or plasmid DNA is isolated and treated with the restriction endonuclease. This treatment results in the generation of several fragments, the sizes of which are determined by the content of recognition sequences in the molecule. Separation of the fragments is achieved by electrophoresis in an agarose gel and visualization is accomplished by staining the gel with ethidium bromide. The differences (polymorphism) in the size of DNA fragments generated by restriction endonuclease treatment is termed **restriction fragment length polymorphism**, or **RFLP** (Fig. 1-33). Using this method, iso-

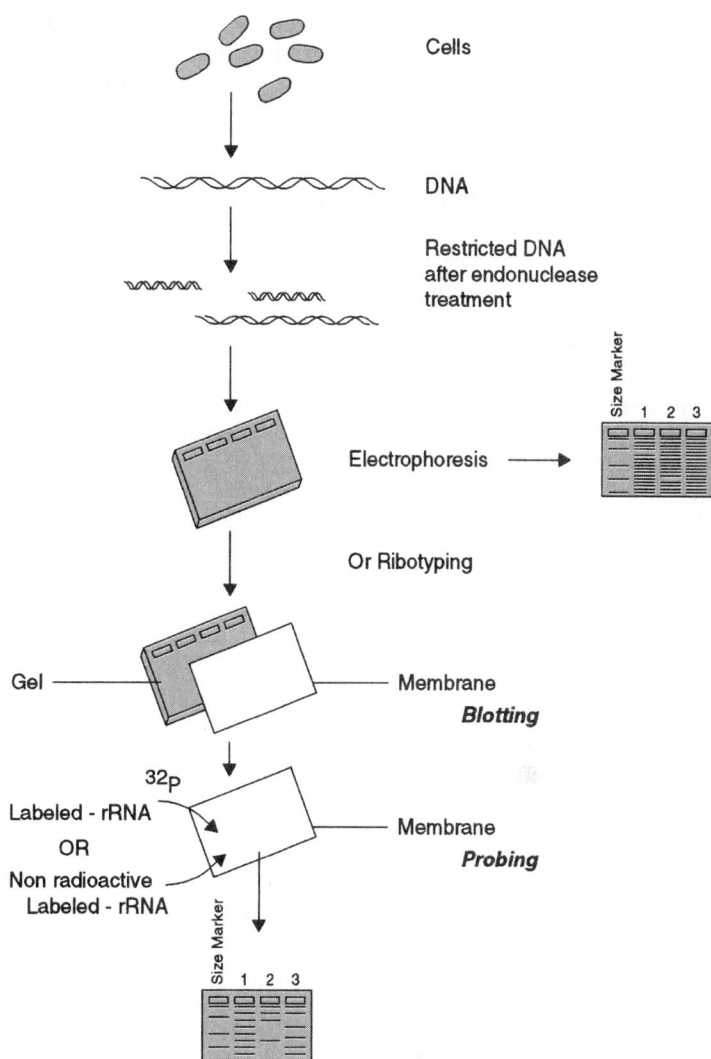

Figure 1-33
Procedure for restriction fragment length polymorphism analysis and ribotyping. (Redrawn from Persing et al: Diagnostic Medical Molecularbiology: Principles & Applications. Washington, DC, ASM, 1993, p. 35.)

lates from nosocomial outbreaks or clusters can be analyzed to see if they have the same or different RFLPs. **Pulsed-field gel electrophoresis (PFGE)** is a specialized type of RFLP analysis.[228] In PFGE, suspensions of whole bacterial cells are placed in agarose plugs, lysed in situ, and treated with restriction enzymes that generate a small number of relatively large restriction fragments. The fragments are then electrophoresed in an electric field where the polarities of the electric field are periodically reversed rather than being kept constant. This method produces fewer, larger DNA fragments that are cleanly separated into resolved bands on electrophoresis. PFGE analysis has been applied to epidemiologic studies of a wide variety of organisms.[15,85,143,185,203,205,231,255,285]

Analysis by RFLP can also be coupled with DNA probe analysis. This is accomplished by transblotting the electrophoresed DNA onto nitrocellulose paper (called a Southern blot) and exposing the paper with the separated adherent restriction fragments to a labeled probe or probes. Autoradiography is used to detect hybridization if the probes are labeled with a radionuclide. Biotinylated probes can be reacted with

avidin-horseradish peroxidase and then exposed to the enzyme substrate to generate a colored "band" where the probe has hybridized. The probes used for these analyses may be hybridizable to chromosomal DNA fragments, specific DNA sequences (*eg*, those that code for virulence factors like toxin production), or rRNA. Analysis of restriction fragments with probes that detect rRNA is called **ribotyping**. Ribotyping has been widely used for epidemiologic characterization and subtyping of many species of bacteria.[19,44,143,203,205,231,255]

Polymerase chain reaction methods used in combination with the techniques outlined above also show great potential for typing or subtyping bacterial isolates for epidemiologic purposes. Following PCR amplification of a specific DNA sequence or sequences, the amplicons may be treated with restriction endonucleases to generate polymorphic restriction fragments. These fragments are then analyzed electrophoretically (PCR-RFLP analysis). Large amounts of homogeneous DNA fragments can be generated for analysis with modification of the PCR procedures (*eg*, use of "nested" PCR). PCR-RFLP analysis of 16S rRNA can actually be used to identify new species of microorganisms or verify the relatedness of organisms because these genes are highly conserved within species. PCR-based sequence characterization has been used to identify newly described or noncultivable organisms and to subtype a wide variety of bacterial and fungal pathogens, including mycobacteria, *Legionella pneumophila*, *Clostridium difficile*, *Helicobacter pylori*, *Bartonella* species, *Mycoplasma pneumoniae*, *Aspergillus* species, and *Cryptococcus* species.[6,16,37,47,84,94,165,223,241,249] PCR and other amplification techniques may also be used to generate discrete segments of DNA that can be directly sequenced by automated DNA sequencing procedures. Using this approach, the actual sequence of nucleotides in a fragment of DNA can be determined.

The PCR and other amplification techniques may have profound effects in shortening the time and increasing the accuracy of diagnosing a variety of microbial infections. Ehrlich[74] makes the plea that initial priorities in the applications of the PCR technology be directed toward the detection of those infectious agents for which alternative testing is costly and cumbersome, or in which delays in diagnosis are caused by the slow growth of organisms in conventional culture systems. He suggests the possible development of panels of tests, in which discreet amplification of signature DNA sequences of several organisms simultaneously be designed for use by specific medical specialties. For example, Ehrlich poses the possibility of offering a "liver panel," consisting of tests for hepatitis viruses (types A, B, C, D, E, and F), CMV, and Epstein-Barr virus. Through a multidisciplinary approach combining the efforts of research scientists working in our academic institutions, the resources available from industry, the astute diagnostic acumen of dedicated clinicians, and the laboratory know-how of technologists and technicians in diagnostic laboratories, the ease and accuracy with which infectious disease syndromes can be diagnosed in the future is virtually boundless.

REFERENCES

1. Abel K, de Schmertzing H, Peterson JI: Classification of microorganisms by analysis of chemical composition. I. Feasibility of utilizing gas chromatography. J Bacteriol 85:1039–1044, 1963
2. Addiss DG, Mathews HM, Stewart JM et al: Evaluation of a commercially available enzyme-linked immunosorbent assay for *Giardia lamblia* antigen in stool. J Clin Microbiol 29:1137–1142, 1991
3. Aguirre M, Collins MD: Phylogenetic analysis of *Alloiococcus otitis* gen. nov., sp. nov., an organism from human middle ear fluid. Int J Syst Bacteriol 42:79–83, 1992
4. Ajello GW, Bolan GA, Hayes PS: Commercial latex agglutination tests for detection of *Haemophilus influenzae* type b and *Streptococcus pneumoniae* antigens in patients with bacteremic pneumonia. J Clin Microbiol 25:1388–1391, 1987
5. Allain J, Laurian Y, Paul DA et al: Serological markers in early stages of human immunodeficiency virus infection in hemophiliacs. Lancet ii:1233–1236, 1986
6. Anderson MJ, Gull K, Denning DW: Molecular typing by random amplification of polymorphic DNA and M13 Southern hybridization of related paired isolates of *Aspergillus fumigatus*. J Clin Microbiol 34:87–93, 1996
7. Andiman W, Gradoville L, Heston R, et al: Use of cloned probes to detect Epstein-Barr viral DNA in tissues of patients with neoplastic and lymphoproliferative diseases. J Infect Dis 248:976–977, 1983
8. Archer GL, Dietrick DR, Johnston JL: Molecular epidemiology of transmissible gentamicin resistance among coagulase-negative staphylococci in a cardiac surgery unit. J Infect Dis 151:243–251, 1985
9. Archer GL, Karchmer AW, Vishniavsky N et al: Plasmid pattern analysis for the differentiation of infecting from noninfecting *Staphylococcus epidermidis*. J Infect Dis 149: 913–920, 1984
10. Arola A, Santti J, Ruuskanen O et al: Identification of enteroviruses in clinical specimens by competitive PCR followed by genetic typing using sequence analysis. J Clin Microbiol 34:313–318, 1996
11. Arthur RR, Dagostin S, Shah KV: Detection of BK virus and JC virus in urine and brain tissue by polymerase chain reaction. J Clin Microbiol 27:1174–1179, 1989
12. Aubert D, Foudrinier F, Villena I et al: PCR for diagnosis and follow-up of two cases of disseminated toxoplasmosis after kidney grafting. J Clin Microbiol 34: 1347, 1996
13. Baay MFD, Quint WHV, Koudstaal J et al: Comprehensive study of several general and type-specific primer pairs for detection of human papillomavirus DNA by PCR in paraffin-embedded cervical carcinomas. J Clin Microbiol 34:745–747, 1996
14. Barany F: Genetic disease detection and DNA amplification using cloned thermostable ligase. Proc Natl Acad Sci USA 88:189–193, 1991
15. Barbier N, Saulnier P, Chachaty E et al: Random amplified polymorphic DNA typing versus pulsed-field gel electrophoresis for epidemiological typing of vancomycin-resistant enterococci. J Clin Microbiol 34: 1096–1099, 1996
16. Beall B, Facklam RR, Thompson T: Sequencing *emm*-specific PCR products for routine and accurate typing of group A streptococci. J Clin Microbiol 34:953–958, 1996
17. Beardsley AM, Gowans EJ, Burrell CJ et al: Enhanced amplification of hepatitis C virus (HCV) cDNA by PCR: Detection of HCV RNA in archival sera. J Clin Microbiol 34:1581–1582, 1996
18. Bennedsen J, Thomsen VO, Pfyffer GE et al: Utility of PCR in diagnosing pulmonary tuberculosis. J Clin Microbiol 34:1407–1411, 1996
19. Bennekov T, Colding H, Ojeniyi B et al: Comparison of ribotyping with genome fingerprinting of *Pseudomonas aeruginosa* isolates from cystic fibrosis patients. J Clin Microbiol 34: 202–204, 1996

20. BERGMANN JS, WOODS GL: Clinical evaluation of the Roche AMPLICOR PCR *Mycobacterium tuberculosis* test for detection of *M. tuberculosis* in respiratory specimens. J Clin Microbiol 34:1083–1085 1996

21. BERNARD K, COOPER C, TESSIER S ET AL: Use of chemotaxonomy as an aid to differentiate among *Capnocytophaga* species, CDC group DF-3, and aerotolerant strains of *Leptotrichia buccalis*. J Clin Microbiol 29:2263–2265, 1991

22. BISNO AL: Chapter 176 *Streptococcus pyogenes*. In Mandell GL, Douglas RG, Dolin R (eds): *Mandell, Douglas, and Bennett's Principles and Practice of Infectious Diseases*, 4th ed, pp 1768–1799. New York, Churchill Livingstone, 1995

23. BLAIR JE, WILLIAMS REO: Phage typing of staphylococci. Bull WHO 24:771–784, 1961

24. BODDINGHAUS B, ROGALL T, FLOHR T ET AL: Detection and identification of mycobacteria by amplification of rRNA. J Clin Microbiol 28:1751–1759, 1990

25. BOSMA TJ, CORBETT KM, ECKSTEIN MB ET AL: Use of PCR for prenatal and postnatal diagnosis of congenital rubella. J Clin Microbiol 33:2881–2887, 1995

26. BRENNAN PJ, HEIFETS M, ULLOM BP: Thin-layer chromatography of lipid antigens as a means of identifying nontuberculous mycobacteria. J Clin Microbiol 15:447–455, 1982

27. BROOKS JB: Gas-liquid chromatography as an aid in rapid diagnosis by selective detection of chemical changes in body fluids. In Coonrod JD, Kunz LJ, Ferrano MJ (eds): The Direct Detection of Microorganisms in Clinical Samples, pp 313–334. New York, Academic Press, 1983

28. BROOKS JB, DANESHVAR MI, HABERBERGER RL, MIKHAIL IA: Rapid diagnosis of tuberculous meningitis by frequency-pulsed electron-capture gas-liquid chromatography detection of carboxylic acids in cerebrospinal fluid. J Clin Microbiol 28:989–997, 1990

29. BROOKS JB, KELLOGG DS JR, SHEPHERD ME, ALLEY CC: Rapid differentiation of the major causative agents of bacterial meningitis by use of frequency-pulsed electron capture gas-liquid chromatography: Analysis of amines. J Clin Microbiol 11:52–58, 1980

30. BROOKS JB, NUNEX-MONTIEL OL, BASTA MT ET AL: Studies of stools from pseudomembranous colitis, rotaviral and other diarrheal syndromes by frequency-pulsed electron capture gas-liquid chromatography. J Clin Microbiol 20:549–560, 1984

31. BROWN SL, BIBB WF, MCKINNEY RM: Retrospective examination of lung tissue specimens for the presence of *Legionella* organisms: Comparison of an indirect fluorescent antibody system with direct fluorescent antibody testing. J Clin Microbiol 19:468–472, 1984

32. BUCK GE: Detection of *Bordetella pertussis* by rapid-cycle PCR and colorimetric microwell identification. J Clin Microbiol 34:1355–1358, 1996

33. BURG JL, GROVER CM, POULETTY P, BOOTHROYD JC: Direct and sensitive detection of a pathogenic protozoan, *Toxoplasma gondii*, by polymerase chain reaction. J Clin Microbiol 27:1787–1792, 1989

34. BUTLER WR, AHEARN DG, KILBURN JO: High-performance liquid chromatography of mycolic acids as a tool in the identification of *Corynebacterium*, *Nocardia*, *Rhodococcus*, and *Mycobacterium* species. J Clin Microbiol 23:182–185, 1986

35. BUTLER WR, JOST KC, KILBURN JO: Identification of mycobacteria by high-performance liquid chromatography. J Clin Microbiol 29:2468–2472, 1991

36. CANONICA FP, PISANO MA: Identification of hydroxy fatty acids in *Aeromonas hydrophila*, *Aeromonas sobria* and *Aeromonas caviae*. J Clin Microbiol 22:1061–1062, 1985

37. CAO M, XIAO X, EGBERT B ET AL: Rapid detection of cutaneous herpes simplex virus infection with the polymerase chain reaction. J Invest Dermatol 92:391–392, 1989

38. CARDARELLA-LEITE P, BLOM K, PATTON CM ET AL: Rapid identification of *Campylobacter* species by restriction fragment length polymorphism analysis of a PCR-amplified fragment of a gene coding for 16S rRNA. J Clin Microbiol 34:62–67, 1996

39. CARPENTIER E, DROUILLARD B, DAILLOUX M ET AL: Diagnosis of tuberculosis by AMPLICOR *Mycobacterium tuberculosis* test: A multicenter study. J Clin Microbiol 33:3106–3110, 1996

40. CASSOL SA, POON MC, PAL R, ET AL: Primer-mediated enzymatic amplification of cytomegalovirus (CMV) DNA. Application to the early diagnosis of CMV infection in marrow transplant recipients. J Clin Invest 83:1109–1115, 1989

41. CELIG DM, SCHRECKENBERGER PC: Clinical evaluation of the RapID-ANA II panel for identification of anaerobic bacteria. J Clin Microbiol 29:457–462, 1991

42. CHADWICK EG, YOGEV R, KWOK S ET AL: Enzymatic amplification of the human immunodeficiency virus in peripheral blood mononuclear cells from pediatric patients. J Infect Dis 160:954–959, 1989

43. CHEN Z-H, BUTLER WR, BAUMSTARK BR ET AL: Identification and differentiation of *Mycobacterium avium* and *Mycobacterium intracellulare* by PCR. J Clin Microbiol 34:1267–1269

44. CHETOUI H, DELHALLE E, OSTERRIETH P ET AL: Ribotyping for use in studying molecular epidemiology of *Serratia marcescens*: Comparison with biotyping. J Clin Microbiol 33:2637–2642, 1995

45. CHING S, LEE H, HOOK III EW ET AL: Ligase chain reaction for detection of *Neisseria gonorrhoeae* in urogenital swabs. J Clin Microbiol 33:3111–3114, 1995

46. CHOU S, MERIGAN TC: Rapid detection and quantitation of human cytomegalovirus in urine through DNA hybridization. N Engl J Med 308:921–925, 1983

47. COLLIER MC, STOCK F, DEGIROLAMI PC ET AL: Comparison of PCR-based approaches to molecular epidemiologic analysis of *Clostridium difficile*. J Clin Microbiol 34:1153–1157, 1996

48. COLOE PJ, SINCLAIR AJ, SLATTERY JF ET AL: Differentiation of *Brucella ovis* from *Brucella abortus* by gas-liquid chromatographic analysis of cellular fatty acids. J Clin Microbiol 19:896–898, 1984

49. CONSTANTINE NT, CALLAHAN JD, WATTS DM: Supplemental tests for HIV-1 infection. In Constantine NT, Callahan JD, Watts DM (eds): *Retroviral Testing: Essentials for Quality Control and Laboratory Diagnosis*, pp 59–87. Boca Raton, FL, CRC Press, 1992

50. CONVILLE PS, KEISER JF, WITEBSKY FG: Mycobacteremia caused by simultaneous infection with *Mycobacterium avium* and *Mycobacterium intracellulare* detected by analysis of a BACTEC 13A bottle with the Gen-Probe kit. Diagn Microbiol Infect Dis 12:217–219, 1989

51. CONVILLE PS, KEISER JF, WITEBSKY FG: Comparison of three techniques for concentrating positive BACTEC 13A bottles for mycobacterial DNA probe analysis. Diagn Microbiol Infect Dis 12:309–313, 1989

52. DALY JA, CLIFTON NL, SESKIN KC, GOOCH WM III: Use of rapid, nonradioactive DNA probes in culture confirmation tests to detect *Streptococcus agalactiae*, *Haemophilus influenzae* and *Enterococcus* spp. from pediatric patients with significant infections. J Clin Microbiol 29:80–82, 1991

53. D'AMATO JJ, KNISLEY C, COLLINS MT: Characterization of *Mycobacterium paratuberculosis* by gas-liquid and thin-layer chromatography and rapid demonstration of mycobactin dependence using radiometric methods. J Clin Microbiol 25:2380–2383, 1987

54. DA SILVA AJ, SCHWARTZ DA, VISVESVARA GS ET AL: Sensitive PCR diagnosis of infections by *Enterocytozoon bieneusi* (microsporidia) using primers based on the region coding for small-subunit rRNA. J Clin Microbiol 34:986–987, 1996

55. DEMMLER G, STEINBERG S, BLUM G ET AL: Rapid enzyme linked immunosorbent assay for detecting antibody to varicella-zoster virus. J Infect Dis 157:211–212, 1988

56. DEREE JM, SCHWILLENS P, VAN DEN BORCH JF: Monoclonal antibodies for serotyping of the P fimbriae of uropathogenic *Escherichia coli*. J Clin Microbiol 24:121–125, 1986

57. DEREPENTIGNY L, KUYKENDALL RJ, REISS E: Simultaneous determination of arabinitol and mannose by gas-liquid chromatography for the rapid diagnosis of invasive candidiasis in cancer patients. J Clin Microbiol 17:1166–1169, 1983

58. DEREPENTIGNY L, MARR LD, KELLER JW, ET AL: Comparison of enzyme immunoassay and gas-liquid chromatography for the rapid diagnosis of invasive candidiasis in cancer patients. J Clin Microbiol 21:972–979, 1985

59. DETMER J, LAGIER R, FLYNN J ET AL: Accurate quantification of of hepatitis C virus (HCV) RNA from all HCV genotypes by using branched-chain DNA technology. J Clin Microbiol 34:901–907, 1996

60. DEVALLOIS A, LEGRAND E, RASTOGI N: Evaluation of AMPLICOR MTB test as an adjunct to smears and culture for direct detection of *Mycobacterium tuberculosis* in the French Caribbean. J Clin Microbiol 34:1065–1068, 1996

61. DEY M, DOWN J, HOWARD A ET AL: Strand displacement amplification (SDA) of *M. tuberculosis* DNA from clinical isolates. Abstracts of the 93rd General Meeting of the American Society for Microbiology. Abstract U-41, p 176, 1993

62. DHARAKUL T, SONGSIVILAI S, VIRIYACHITRA S ET AL: Detection of *Burkholderia pseudomallei* DNA in patients with septicemic melioidosis. J Clin Microbiol 34:609–614, 1996

63. DIAMOND RD, BENNETT JE: Prognostic factors in cryptococcal meningitis: A study of 111 cases. Ann Intern Med 80:175–177, 1981

64. DIAZ-MITOMA F, RUBEN M, SACKS S ET AL: Detection of viral DNA to evaluate outcome of antiviral treatment of patients with recurrent genital herpes. J Clin Microbiol 34:657–663, 1996

65. DIDIER ES, ROGERS LB, BRUSH AD ET AL: Diagnosis of disseminated microsporidian *Encephalitozoon hellem* infection by PCR-Southern analysis and successful treatment with albendazole and fumagillin. J Clin Microbiol 34:947–952, 1996

66. DIMETROV DH, GRAHAM DY, ESTES MK: Detection of rotaviruses by nucleic acid hybridization with cloned DNA of simian rotavirus SA11 genes. J Infect Dis 152:293–300, 1985

67. DONOHUE-ROLFE A, KELLEY MA, BENNISH M ET AL: Enzyme-linked immunosorbent assay for shigella toxin. J Clin Microbiol 24:65–58, 1986

68. DOWN JA, O'CONNELL MA, DEY MS ET AL: Detection of *Mycobacterium tuberculosis* in respiratory tract specimens by strand displacement amplification of DNA. J Clin Microbiol 34:860–865, 1996

69. DRANCOURT M, MOAL V, BRUNET P ET AL: *Bartonella (Rochalimaea) quintana* infection in a seronegative hemodialyzed patient. J Clin Microbiol 34:1158–1160, 1996

70. DUPON M, CAZENAVE J, PELLEGRIN J-L ET AL: Detection of *Toxoplasma gondii* by PCR and tissue culture in cerebrospinal fluid and blood of human immunodeficiency virus-seropositive patients. J Clin Microbiol 33:2421–2426, 1995

71. EDELSTEIN PH: Evaluation of the Gen-Probe DNA probe for the detection of *Legionellae* in culture. J Clin Microbiol 23:481–484, 1986

72. EDELSTEIN PH, BRYAN RN, ENNS RK ET AL: Retrospective study of Gen-Probe rapid diagnostic system for detection of *Legionellae* in frozen clinical respiratory tract samples. J Clin Microbiol 25:1022–1026, 1987

73. EHRLICH HA: Caveats of PCR. Clin Microbiol Newsletter 13:149–151, 1991

74. EHRLICH HA, GELFAND DH, SAIKI RK: Specific DNA amplification. Nature 331:461–472, 1988

75. EISENACH KD, CAVE MD, BATES, JH, CRAWFORD ST: Polymerase chain reaction amplification of a repetitive DNA sequence specific for *Mycobacterium tuberculosis*. J Infect Dis 161:977–981, 1990

76. ESPY MJ, SMITH TF: Detection of herpes simplex virus in conventional tube cell cultures and in shell vials with a DNA probe kit and monoclonal antibodies. J Clin Microbiol 26:22–24, 1988

77. FACKLAM RR, RHODEN DL, SMITH PB: Evaluation of the Rapid Strep system for identification of clinical isolates of *Streptococcus* species. J Clin Microbiol 20:894–898, 1984

78. FOLGUEIRA L, DELGADO R, PALENQUE E ET AL: Rapid diagnosis of *Mycobacterium tuberculosis* bacteremia by PCR. J Clin Microbiol 34:512–515, 1996

79. FORGHANI B, DURPIS KW, SCHMIDT NJ: Rapid detection of herpes simplex virus DNA in human brain tissue by in-situ hybridization. J Clin Microbiol 22:656–658, 1985

80. FOX A, ROGERS JC, FOX KF ET AL: Chemotaxonomic differentiation of *Legionellae* by detection and characterization of aminodideoxyhexoses and other unique sugars using gas chromatography-mass spectrometry. J Clin Microbiol 28:546–552, 1990

81. FRANZEN C, MOLLER A, HEGENER P ET AL: Detection of microsporidia (*Enterocytozoon bieneusi*) in intestinal biopsy specimens from human immunodeficiency virus-infected patients by PCR. J Clin Microbiol 33:2294–2296, 1996

82. FRATAMICO PM, SACKITEY SK, WIEDMANN M ET AL: Detection of *Escherichia coli* O157:H7 by multiplex PCR. J Clin Microbiol 33:2188–2191, 1995

83. FRENEY J, BLAND S, ETIENNE J ET AL: Description and evaluation of the semiautomated 4-hour rapid ID32 Strep method for identification of streptococci and members of related genera. J Clin Microbiol 30: 2657–2661, 1992

84. FUJIMOTO S, MARSHALL SB, BLASER MJ: PCR-based restriction fragment length polymorphism typing of *Helicobacter pylori*. J Clin Microbiol 32:331–334, 1994

85. FUJITA M, FUJIMOTO S, MOROOKA T ET AL: Analysis of strains of *Campylobacter fetus* by pulsed-field gel electrophoresis. J Clin Microbiol 33:1676–1678, 1995

86. GAL AA, UNGER ER, KOSS MN ET AL: Detection of Epstein-Barr virus in lymphoepithelioma-like carcinoma of the lung. Mod Pathol 4:264–268, 2991

87. GEHA DJ, UHL JR, GUSTAFERRO CA ET AL: Multiplex PCR for identification of methicillin-resistant staphylococci in the clinical laboratory. J Clin Microbiol 32:1768–1772, 1994

88. GEORGE JR, SCHOCHETMAN G: Serologic tests for the detection of human immunodeficiency virus infection. In Schochetman G, George JR (eds.): *AIDS Testing: Methodology and Management Issues*, pp 48–78. New York, Springer-Verlag, 1992

89. GEURRANT GO, LAMBERT MA, MOSS CW: Gas-chromatographic analysis of mycolic acid cleavage products in mycobacteria. J Clin Microbiol 13:899–907, 1987

90. GINGERAS TR, PRODANOVICH P, LATIMER T ET AL: Use of self-sustained sequence replication amplification reaction to analyze and detect mutations in zidovudine-resistant human immunodeficiency virus. J Infect Dis 164:1066–1074, 1991

91. GONZALEZ R, HANNA BA: Evaluation of Gen-Probe DNA hybridization systems for the identification of *Mycobacterium tuberculosis* and *Mycobacterium avium-intracellulare*. Diagn Microbiol Infect Dis 8:69–77, 1987

92. GOOTZ TD, TENOVER FC, YOUNG SA ET AL: Comparison of three DNA hybridization methods for detection of the aminoglycoside 2'-O-adenyl-transferase gene in clinical bacterial isolates. Antimicrob Agent Chemother 28:69–73, 1985

93. GOTTSCHALK J, ZBINDEN R, KAEMPF L ET AL: Discrimination of respiratory syncytial virus subgroups A and B by reverse transcription-PCR. J Clin Microbiol 34:41–43, 1996

94. GRATTARD F, BERTHELOT P, REYROLLE M ET AL: Molecular typing of nosocomial strains of *Legionella pneumophila* by arbitrarily primed PCR. J Clin Microbiol 34: 1595–1598, 1996

95. GRIMONT PA, GRIMONT F, DESPLACES N ET AL: DNA probe specific for *Legionella pneumophila*. J Clin Microbiol 21:431–437, 1985

96. GRIMPREL E, SANCHEZ PJ, WENDEL GD: Use of polymerase chain reaction and rabbit infectivity testing to detect *Treponema pallidum* in amniotic fluid, fetal and neonatal sera and cerebrospinal fluid. J Clin Microbiol 29:1711–1718, 1991

97. GRUNDY JE, EHRNST A, EINSELE H ET AL: A three-center European external quality control study of PCR for detection of cytomegalovirus DNA in blood. J Clin Microbiol 34:1166–1170, 1996

98. GUARNER J, DEL RIO C, CARR D ET AL: Non-Hodgkin's lymphoma in patients with human immunodeficiency virus infection: Presence of Epstein-Barr virus by in situ hybridization, clinical presentation, and follow-up. Cancer 68:2460–2465, 1991

99. HALSTEAD DC: Noncultural methods for diagnosing respiratory syncytial virus infections. Clin Microbiol Newsletter 9:181–185, 1987

100. HANCE AJ, GRANDCHAMP B, LE'VY-FRE'HAULT ET AL: Detection and identification of mycobacteria by amplification of mycobacterial DNA. Mol Microbiol 3:843–849, 1989

101. HAMMOND G, HANNAN C, YEH T ET AL: DNA hybridization for diagnosis of enteric adenovirus infection from directly spotted human fecal specimens. J Clin Microbiol 25:1881–1885, 1987

102. HAYWARD NJ, JEAVONS TH, NICHOLSON AJC ET AL: Methyl mercaptan and dimethyl disulfide production from methionine by *Proteus* species detected by headspace gas liquid chromatography. J Clin Microbiol 6:187–194, 1977

103. HENRARD DR, WU S, PHILLIPS J ET AL: Detection of p24 antigen with and without immune complex dissociation for longitudinal monitoring of human immunodeficiency virus type 1 infection. J Clin Microbiol 33:72–75, 1995

104. HERMANS PWM, SAHA SK, VAN LEEUWEN WJ ET AL: Molecular typing of *Salmonella typhi* from Dhaka (Bangladesh) and development of DNA probes identifying plasmid-encoded drug-resistant isolates. J Clin Microbiol 34:1373–1379, 1996

105. HERRERA EA, SEGOVIA M: Evaluation of *mtp-40* genomic fragment amplification for specific detection of *Mycobacterium tuberculosis* in clinical specimens. J Clin Microbiol 34:1108–1113, 1996

106. HICKS KE, BEARD S, COHEN BJ ET AL: A simple and sensitive DNA hybridization assay used for the routine diagnosis of human parvovirus B19 infection. J Clin Microbiol 33:2473–2475, 1995

107. HOLDEMAN LV, CATO EP, MOORE WEC (EDS): Anaerobe Laboratory Manual, 4th ed. Blacksburg, VA, Virginia Polytechnic Institute and State University, 1977

108. HOLODNIY M, KATZENSTEIN DA, SENGUPTA S ET AL: Detection and quantification of human immunodeficiency virus RNA in serum by use of the polymerase chain reaction. J Infect Dis 163:862–866, 1991

109. HOSMER ME, COHENFORD MA, ELLNER PD: Preliminary evaluation of a rapid colorimetric method for identification of pathogenic *Neisseria*. J Clin Microbiol 24:141–142, 1986

110. HUANG ZH, ROSS BC, DWYER B: Identification of *Mycobacterium kansasii* by DNA hybridization. J Clin Microbiol 29:2125–2129, 1991

111. IMAGAWA DT, LEE MH, WOLINSKY SM ET AL: Human immunodeficiency virus type 1 infection in homosexual men who remain seronegative for prolonged periods. N Engl J Med 320:1458–1462, 1989

112. INGRAM DL, PEARSON AW, OCCHIUTI AR: Detection of bacterial antigens in body fluids with the Wellcogen *Haemophilus influenzae* b, *Streptococcus pneumoniae* and *Neisseria meningitidis* (ACYW135) latex agglutination tests. J Clin Microbiol 18:1119–1121, 1983

113. JACKSON JB, MACDONALD KL, CADWELL J ET AL: Absence of HIV infection in blood donors with indeterminate Western blot tests for antibody to HIV-1. N Engl J Med 322:217–220, 1990

114. JANDA WM, BRADNA JJ, RUTHER P: Identification of *Neisseria* spp., *Haemophilus* spp., and other fastidious gram-negative bacteria with the MicroScan *Haemophilus-Neisseria* identification panel. J Clin Microbiol 27:869–873, 1989

115. JANDA WM, MALLOY PJ, SCHRECKENBERGER PC: Clinical evaluation of the Vitek *Haemophilus-Neisseria* identification card. J Clin Microbiol 25:37–41, 1987

116. JANDA WM, MONTERO M: Premarket evaluation of the BactiCard *Neisseria*. Abstracts of the 95th General Meeting of the American Society for Microbiology. Abstract C-303, p 53, 1995

117. JANDA WM, WILCOSKI LM, MANDEL KL ET AL: Comparison of monoclonal antibody-based methods and a ribosomal ribonucleic acid probe test for *Neisseria gonorrhoeae* culture confirmation. Eur J Clin Microbiol Infect Dis 12:177–184, 1993

118. JANTZEN E, BERDAL BP, OMLAND T: Cellular fatty acid composition of *Francisella tularensis*. J Clin Microbiol 10:928–930, 1979

119. JANTZEN E, BRYN K, BERGAN T, BOVRE K: Gas chromatography of bacterial whole cell methanolysates. V. Fatty acid composition of neisseriae and moraxellae. Acta Pathol Microbiol Scand Sect B 82:767–779, 1974

120. JANTZEN E, BRYN K, BERGAN T, BOVRE K: Gas chromatography of bacterial whole cell methanolysates. VII. Fatty acid composition of *Acinetobacter* in relation to the taxonomy of *Neisseriaceae*. Acta Pathol Microbiol Scand Sect B 83:569–580, 1975

121. JENSEN JS, ULDUM SA, SONDERGAARD-ANDERSON J ET AL: Polymerase chain reaction for detection of *Mycoplasma genitalium* in clinical samples. J Clin Microbiol 29:46–50, 1991

122. JOHN JF JR, TWITTY JA: Plasmids as epidemiologic markers in nosocomial gram-negative bacilli: Experience at a university and review of the literature. Rev Infect Dis 8:693–704, 1886

123. KANEDA T: Fatty acids in the genus *Bacillus*. I. Iso and anteiso-fatty acids as characteristic constituents of lipids in 10 species. J Bacteriol 29:894–903, 1967

124. KAO C-L, MCINTOSH K, FERNIE B ET AL: Monoclonal antibodies for the rapid diagnosis of respiratory syncytial virus infection by immunofluorescence. Diagn Microbiol Infect Dis 2:199–206, 1984

125. KATO N, OU C, KATO H ET AL: Identification of toxigenic *Clostridium difficile* by the polymerase chain reaction. J Clin Microbiol 29:33–37, 1991

126. KAUFMAN L, SEKHON AS, MOLEDINA N ET AL: Comparative evaluation of commercial Premier EIA and microimmunodiffusion and complement fixation for *Coccidioides immitis* antibodies. J Clin Microbiol 33:618–619, 1995

127. KAZUHISA M, MINAMIDE W, WADA K ET AL: Identification of methicillin-resistant strains of staphylococcus by polymerase chain reaction. J Clin Microbiol 29:2240–2244, 1991

128. KEHL KSC, CICIRELLO H, HAVENS PL: Comparison of four different methods for detection of *Cryptosporidium* species. J Clin Microbiol 33:416–418, 1995

129. KENNY C, PARKIN J, UNDERSHILL G ET AL: HIV antigen testing. Lancet i:565–566, 1987

130. KESSLER H, BLAAUW B, SPEAR J ET AL: Diagnosis of human immunodeficiency virus infection in seronegative homosexuals presenting with an acute viral syndrome. JAMA 258:1196–1199, 1987

131. KIDD AH, JONSSON M, GARWICZ D ET AL: Rapid subgenus identification of human adenovirus isolates by a general PCR. J Clin Microbiol 34:622–627, 1996

132. KIMURA M, MIYAKE H, KIM H-S ET AL: Species-specific PCR detection of malaria parasites by microtiter plate hybridization: clinical study witrh malaria patients. J Clin Microbiol 33:2342–2346, 1995

133. KIRCHHOFF LV, VOTAVA JR, OCHS DE ET AL: Comparison of PCR and microscopic methods for detecting *Trypanosoma cruzi*. J Clin Microbiology 34:1171–1175, 1996

134. KITCH TT, JACOBS MR, MCGINNIS MR ET AL: Ability of RapID Yeast Plus system to identify 304 clinically significant yeasts within 5 hours. J Clin Microbiol 34:1069–1071, 1996

135. KNAPP JS, SANDSTROM EG, HOLMES KK: Overview of epidemiologic and clinical applications of auxotype/serovar classification of *Neisseria gonorrhoeae*. In Schoolnik GK (ed): *The Pathogenic Neisseriae*, pp 6–12. Washington, DC, American Society for Microbiology, 1985

136. KNAPP JS, TAM MR, NOWINSKI RC ET AL: Serological classification of *Neisseria gonorrhoeae* with use of monoclonal antibodies to gonococcal outer membrane protein I. J Infect Dis 150:44–48, 1984

137. KODAKA H, LOMBARD GL, DOWELL VR JR: Gas-liquid chromatography technique for detection of hippurate hydrolysis and conversion of fumarate to succinate by microorganisms. J Clin Microbiol 16:962–964, 1982

138. KOHLER G, MILSTEIN C: Continuous culture of fused cells secreting antibodies of predefined specificity. Nature 256:495–497, 1975

139. KOLK AHJ, HO ML, KLASTER PR ET AL: Production and characterization of monoclonal antibodies to *Mycobacterium tuberculosis*, *M. bovis* (BCG) and *M. leprae*. Clin Exp Immunol 58:511–521, 1984

140. KOTILAINEN P, HUOVINEN P, EEROLA E: Application of gas-liquid chromatographic analysis of cellular fatty acids for species identification and typing of coagulase-negative staphylococci. J Clin Microbiol 29:3125–322, 1991

141. KRISTIANSEN B, SORENSEN B, BJORVATN B ET AL: An outbreak of group B meningococcal disease. Tracing the causative strain of *Neisseria meningitidis* by DNA fingerprinting. J Clin Microbiol 23:764–767, 1986

142. KRON MA, GUPTA A, MACKENZIE CD: Identification of related DNA sequences in *Borrelia burgdorferi* and two strains of *Leptospira interrogans* by using polymerase chain reaction. J Clin Microbiol 29:2338–2340, 1991

143. KUHN I, BURMAN LG, HAEGGMAN S ET AL: Biochemical fingerprinting compared with ribotyping and pulsed-field gel electrophoresis of DNA for epidemiological typing of enterococci. J Clin Microbiol 33:2812–2817, 1995

144. KWOH DY, DAVIS GR, WHITFIELD KM ET AL: Transcription-based amplification system and detection of amplified human immunodeficiency virus type 1 with a bead-based sandwich hybridization format. Proc Natl Acad Sci USA 86:1173–1177, 1989

145. LAGE AP, FAUCONNIER A, BURETTE A ET AL: Rapid colorimetric hybridization assay for detecting amplified *Helicobacter pylori* DNA in gastric biopsy specimens. J Clin Microbiol 34:530–533, 1996

146. LAMBERT MA, MOSS CW: Cellular fatty acid compositions and isoprenoid quinone contents of 23 *Legionella* species. J Clin Microbiol 465–473, 1989

147. LAMBERT MA, MOSS CW, SILCOX VA ET AL: Analysis of mycolic acid cleavage products and cellular fatty acids of *Mycobacterium* species by capillary gas chromatography. J Clin Microbiol 23:731–736, 1986

148. LAMBERT MA, PATTON, CM, BARRETT TJ, MOSS CW: Differentiation of *Campylobacter* and *Campylobacter*-like organisms by cellular fatty acid composition. J Clin Microbiol 25:706–713, 1987

149. LANGE J, GOUDSMIT J: Decline of antibody reactivity to HIV core proteins secondary to increased production of HIV antigen. Lancet i:448, 1987

150. LANGENBERG A, SMITH D, BRAKEL CL ET AL: Detection of herpes simplex virus DNA from genital lesions by in situ hybridization. J Clin Microbiol 26:933–937, 1988

151. LARDER BA, DARBY G, RICHMAN DD: HIV with reduced sensitivity to zidovudine (AZT) isolated during prolonged therapy. Science 246:1731–1732, 1989

152. LARDER BA, KEMP SD: Multiple mutations in HIV-1 reverse transcriptase confer high-level resistance to zidovudine (AZT). Science 246:1155–1158, 1989

153. LAURE F, COURGNAUD V, ROUZIOUX C ET AL: Detection of HIV DNA in infants and children by means of polymerase chain reaction. Lancet 2:538–541, 1988

154. LEIBOVITZ E, POLLACK H, MOORE T ET AL: Comparison of PCR and standard cytological staining for detection of *Pneumocystis carinii* from respiratory tract specimens from patients with or at high risk for infection by human immunodeficiency virus. J Clin Microbiol 33:3004–3007, 1996

155. LEWIS JS, KRANIG-BROWN D, TRAINOR DA: DNA probe confirmatory test for *Neisseria gonorrhoeae*. J Clin Microbiol 28:2349–2350, 1990

156. LIM SD, TODD J, LOPEZ J ET AL: Genotypic identification of pathogenic *Mycobacterium* species by using a nonradioactive oligonucleotide probe. J Clin Microbiol 29:1276–1278, 1991

157. LIMBERGER RJ, BIEGA R, EVANCOE A ET AL: Evaluation of culture and the Gen-Probe PACE 2 assay for detection of *Neisseria gonorrhoeae* and *Chlamydia trachomatis* in endocervical specimens transported to a state health laboratory. J Clin Microbiol 30:1162–1166, 1992

158. LIN HJ, HAYWOOD M, HOLLINGER FB: Application of a commercial kit for detection of PCR products to quantification of human immunodeficiency virus type 1 RNA and proviral DNA. J Clin Microbiol 34:329–333, 1996

159. LIZARDI P, GUERRA C, LOMELI H ET AL: Exponential amplification of recombinant-RNA hybridization probes. Biotechnology 6:1197–1202, 1988

160. LOCHE M, MACH B: Identification of HIV-infected seronegative individuals by a direct diagnostic test based on hybridization to amplified viral DNA. Lancet ii:418–421, 1988

161. LUPSKI JR: Molecular mechanisms for transposition of drug-resistance genes and other movable genetic elements. Rev Infect Dis 9:357–368, 1987

162. MACONE AB, ARAKERE G, LETOURNEAU JM ET AL: Comparison of a new rapid enzyme-linked immunosorbent assay with latex particle agglutination for the detection of *Haemophilus influenzae* type b infections. J Clin Microbiol 21:711–714, 1985

163. MARUMO K, AOKI Y: Discriminant analysis of cellular fatty acids of *Candida* species, *Torulopsis glabrata*, and *Cryptococcus neoformans* determined by gas-liquid chromatography. J Clin Microbiol 28:1509–1513, 1990

164. MATAR GM, KHNEISSER IA, ABDELNOOR AM: Rapid laboratory confirmation of human brucellosis by PCR analysis of a target sequence on the 31-kilodalton *Brucella* antigen DNA. J Clin Microbiol 34:477–478, 1996

165. MATAR GM, SWAMINATHAN B, HUNTER SB ET AL: Polymerase chain reaction-based restriction fragment length polymorphism analysis of a fragment of the ribosomal operon from *Rochalimaea* species for subtyping. J Clin Microbiol 31:1730–1734, 1993

166. MAYER LW: Use of plasmid profiles in epidemiologic surveillance of disease outbreaks and in tracing the transmission of antibiotic resistance. Clin Microbiol Rev 1:228–243, 1988

167. MAYO DR, BRENNAN T, SIRPENSKI SP ET AL: Cytomegalovirus antibody detection by three commercially available assays and complement fixation. Diagn Microbiol Infect Dis 3:455–459, 1985

168. MCHUGH TM, CASAVANT CH, WILBER JC ET AL: Comparison of six methods for the detection of antibody to cytomegalovirus. J Clin Microbiol 22:1014–1019, 1985

169. MCMILLIN DE, MULDROW LL, LAGGETTE SJ: Simultaneous detection of toxin A and toxin B genetic determinants of *Clostridium difficile* using the multiplex polymerase chain reaction. Can J Microbiol 38:81–83, 1992

170. MIKHAILOVICH VM, MELNIKOV VG, MAZUROVA IK ET AL: Application of PCR for detection of toxigenic *Corynebacterium diphtheriae* strains isolated during the Russion diphtheria epidemic, 1990 through 1994. J Clin Microbiol 33:3061–3063, 1995

171. MOISSENET D, TABONE M-D, GIRARDET J-P ET AL: Nosocomial CDC group IVc-2 bacteremia: Epidemiological investigation by randomly amplified polymorphic DNA analysis. J Clin Microbiol 34:1264–1266, 1996

172. MOSER DR, KIRCHHOFF LV, DONELSON JE: Detection of *Trypanosoma cruzi* by DNA amplification using the polymerase chain reaction. J Clin Microbiol 27:1477–1482, 1989

173. MOSLEY SL, ECHEVERRIA P, SERIWATANA J ET AL: Identification of enterotoxigenic *Escherichia coli* by colony hybridization using three enterotoxigenic gene probes. J Infect Dis 145:863–869, 1983

174. MOSS CW: Gas-liquid chromatography as an analytical tool in microbiology. J. Chromatogr 203:337–347, 1981

175. MOSS CW, DEES SB, GUERRANT GO: Gas-liquid chromatography of bacterial fatty acids with a fused-silica capillary column. J Clin Microbiol 12:127–130, 1980

176. MOSS CW, KAI A, LAMBERT MA, PATTON CM: Isoprenoid quinone content and cellular fatty acid composition of *Campylobacter* species. J Clin Microbiol 19:772–776, 1984

177. MOSS CW, SHINODA T, SAMUELS JW: Determination of cellular fatty acid compositions of various yeasts by gas-liquid chromatography. J Clin Microbiol 16:1073–1079, 1982

178. Mullis KB: The unusual origin of the polymerase chain reaction. Sci Am 262:56–65, 1990

179. Mullis KB, Faloona FA: Specific synthesis of DNA in vitro via a polymerase-catalyzed chain reaction. Methods Enzymol 155:335–350, 1987

180. Musial CE, Tice LS, Stockman L et al: Identification of mycobacteria from culture by using the Gen-Probe rapid diagnostic system for *Mycobacterium avium* complex and *Mycobacterium tuberculosis* complex. J Clin Microbiol 26:2120–2123, 1988

181. Myerson D, Hackman RC, Meyers JD: Diagnosis of cytomegaloviral pneumonia by in-situ hybridization. J Infect Dis 150:272–277, 1984

182. Neill RJ, Fanning GR, Delahoz F et al: Oligonucleotide probes for detection and differentiation of *Staphylococcus aureus* strains containing genes for enterotoxins A, B and C and toxic shock syndrome toxin 1. J Clin Microbiol 28:1514–1518, 1990

183. Nelson CT, Istas AS, Wilkerson MK et al: PCR detection of cytomegalovirus DNA in serum as a diagnostic test for congenital cytomegalovirus infection. J Clin Microbiol 33:3317–3318, 1995

184. Newland JW, Heill RJ: DNA probes for shiga-like toxins I and II and for toxin-converting bacteriophages. J Clin Microbiol 26:1292–1297, 1988

185. Ng L-K, Carballo M, Dillon JR: Differentiation of *Neisseria gonorrhoeae* isolates requiring proline, citrulline, and uracil by plasmid content, serotyping, and pulsed-field gel electrophoresis. J Clin Microbiol 33:1039–1041, 1995

186. Nowinski RC, Tam MR, Goldstein LC et al: Monoclonal antibodies for diagnosis of infectious diseases in humans. Science 219:637–644, 1983

187. Orle KA, Gates CA, Martin DH et al: Simultaneous PCR detection of *Haemophilus ducreyi, Treponema pallidum*, and herpes simplex virus types 1 and 2 from genital ulcers. J Clin Microbiol 34:49–54, 1996

188. Osterhout GJ, Shull VH, Dick JD: Identification of clinical isolates of gram-negative nonfermentative bacteria by an automated cellular fatty acid identification system. J Clin Microbiol 29:1822–1830, 1991

189. Ou CK, Kwok J, Mitchell SW et al: DNA amplification for direct detection of HIV-1 in DNA of peripheral blood mononuclear cells. Science 239:295–297, 1988

190. Pachi CA, Kern DG, Sheridan PJ et al: Quantitative detection of HIV RNA in plasma using a signal amplification probe assay. Program Abstracts of the 32nd Interscience Conference on Antimicrobial Agents and Chemotherapy. Antimicrob Agents Chemother, abstract 1247, American Society for Microbiology, Washington, DC, 1992

191. Pan L-Z, Werner A, Levy JA: Detection of plasma viremia in human immunodeficiency virus-infected individuals at all clinical stages. J Clin Microbiol 31:283–288, 1993

192. Parsons LM, Shayegani M, Waring AL, Bopp LH: DNA probes for identification of *Haemophilus ducreyi*. J Clin Microbiol 27:1441–1445, 1989

193. Pasculle AW, Veto GE, Krystofiak S et al: Laboratory and clinical evaluation of a commercial DNA probe for the detection of *Legionella* species.

194. Pasternak R, Vuorinen P, Kuukankorpi A et al: Detection of *Chlamydia trachomatis* infections in women by AMPLICOR PCR: Comparison of diagnostic performance with urine and cervical specimens. J Clin Microbiol 34:995–998, 1996

195. Persing DH: Polymerase chain reaction: Trenches to benches. J Clin Microbiol 29:1281–1285, 1991

196. Persing DH, Cimino GD: Amplification product inactivation methods. In Persing DH, Smith TF, Tenover FC, White TJ (eds): *Diagnostic Molecular Biology: Principles and Applications*, pp 105–121. Washington, DC, American Society for Microbiology, 1993

197. Peterson EM, Lu R, Floyd C et al: Direct identification of *Mycobacterium tuberculosis, Mycobacterium avium*, and *Mycobacterium intracellulare* from amplified primary cultures in BACTEC media using DNA probes. J Clin Microbiol 27:1543–1547, 1989

198. Peterson EM, Oda R, Alexander R, et al: Molecular techniques for the detection of *Chlamydia trachomatis*. J Clin Microbiol 27:2359–2363, 1989

199. Pfaller MA, Preston T, Bale M et al: Comparison of the Quantum II, API Yeast-Ident, and AutoMicrobic systems for identification of clinical yeast isolates. J Clin Microbiol 26:2054–2058, 1988

200. Pfaller MA, Sahm D, O'Hara CO, et al: Comparison of the AutoSCAN-W/A rapid bacterial identification system and the Vitek AutoMicrobic System for identification of gram-negative bacilli. J Clin Microbiol 29:1422–1428, 1991

201. Piatek M, Saag MS, Yang LC et al: High levels of HIV-1 in plasma during all stages of infection determined by competitive PCR. Science 259:1749–1754, 1993

202. Pitt TL: Epidemiological typing of *Pseudomonas aeruginosa*. Eur J Clin Microbiol Infect Dis. 14:209–217, 1988

203. Poh CL, Yeo CC, Tay L: Genome fingerprinting by pulsed-field gel electrophoresis and ribotyping to differentiate *Pseudomonas aeruginosa* serotype 011 strains. Eur J Clin Microbiol Infect Dis 11:817–822, 1992

204. Polonelli L, Castagnola M, Morace G: Identification and serotyping of *Microsporum canis* isolates by monoclonal antibodies. J Clin Microbiol 23:609–615, 1986

205. Prevost G, Jaulhac B, Piemont Y: DNA fingerprinting by pulsed-field gel electrophoresis is more effective than ribotyping in distinguishing among methicillin-resistant *Staphylococcus aureus* isolates. J Clin Microbiol 30:967–973, 1992

206. Pruneda RC, Dover JC: A comparison of two passive agglutination procedures with enzyme-linked immunosorbent assay for rubella antibody status. Am J Clin Pathol 86:768–770, 1986

207. Puchhammer-Stockl A, Popow-Kraupp T, Heinz FX et al: Detection of varicella-zoster virus DNA by polymerase chain reaction in the cerebrospinal fluid of patients suffering from neurological complications associated with chicken pox or herpes zoster. J Clin Microbiol 29:1513–1516, 1991

208. Quentin C, Desailly-Chanson M-E, Bebear C: Evaluation of AN-Ident. J Clin Microbiol 29:231–235, 1991

209. Quinn TC, Welsh L, Lentz A et al: Diagnosis by AMPLICOR PCR of *Chlamydia trachomatis* infection in urine samples from women and men attending sexually transmitted disease clinics. J Clin Microbiol 34:1401–1406, 1996

210. RADESTSKY M, WHEELER RC, ROE MH ET AL: Comparative evaluation of kits for rapid diagnosis of group A streptococcal disease. Pediatr Infect Dis 4:274–281, 1985

211. RANKI A, VALLE S, KROHN M: Long latency precedes overt seroconversion in sexually transmitted human immunodeficiency virus infection. Lancet ii:589–593, 1987

212. RAY F, SALUUN D, LESBORDES JL ET AL: HIV-1 and HIV-2 double infection in Central African Republic. Lancet i:1391–1392, 1986

213. RAYFIELD M, DECOCK K, HEYWARD WL ET AL: Mixed human immunodeficiency virus (HIV) infection of an individual: Demonstration of both HIV-1 and HIV-2 proviral sequences by polymerase chain reaction. J Infect Dis 158:170–176, 1988

214. REIZENSTEIN E, LINDBERG L, MOLLBY R ET AL: Validation of a nested *Bordetella* PCR in pertussis vaccine trial. J Clin Microbiol 34:810–815, 1996

215. REVETS H, MARISSENS D, DE WIT S ET AL: Comparative evaluation of NASBA HIV-1 RNA QT, AMPLICOR HIV Monitor, and QUANTIPLEX HIV RNA assay, three methods for quantification of human immunodeficiency virus type 1 RNA in plasma. J Clin Microbiol 34:1058–1064, 1996

216. REY MA, GIRARD PM, HARZIC M ET AL: HIV-1 and HIV-2 double infection in French homosexual male with AIDS-related complex. Lancet i:388–389, 1987

217. ROBERTS MC, HILLIER SL, SCHOENKNECHT FD ET AL: Comparison of gram stain, DNA probe and culture for the identification of *Mobiluncus* in female genital specimens. J Infect Dis 152:74–77, 1985

218. ROGERS MF, OU C-Y, RAYFIELD M ET AL: Use of the polymerase chain reaction for early detection of the proviral sequence of human immunodeficiency virus in infants born to seropositive mothers. N Engl J Med 320:1649–1654, 1989

219. ROSA PA, SCHWAN TG: A specific and sensitive assay for the Lyme disease spirochete *Borrelia burgdorferi* using the polymerase chain reaction. J Infect Dis 160:1018–1029, 1989

220. ROTA PA, KHAN AS, DURIGON E ET AL: Detection of measles virus RNA in urine specimens from vaccine recipients. J Clin Microbiol 33:2485–2488, 1996

221. ROWBOTHAM TJ: Rapid identification of *Streptobacillus moniliformis*. Lancet 2:567, 1983

222. SAIKI PK, GELFAND DH, STOFFEL S ET AL: Primer-directed enzymatic amplification of DNA with a thermostable DNA polymerase. Science 239:487–491, 1988

223. SASAKI T, KENRI T, OKAZAKI N ET AL: Epidemiological study of *Mycoplasma pneumoniae* infections in Japan based on PCR-restriction fragment length polymorphism of the P1 cytadhesion gene. J Clin Microbiol 34:447–449, 1996

224. SAWELJEW P, KUNKEL J, FEDDERSEN A ET AL: Case of fatal systemic infection with an *Aureobacterium* sp: Identification of isolate by 16S rRNA gene analysis. J Clin Microbiol 34:1540–1541, 1996

225. SCHABERG DR, ZERVOS M: Plasmid analysis in the study of the epidemiology of nosocomial gram-positive cocci. Rev Infect Dis 8:705–712, 1986

226. SCHMIDT B, MUELLEGGER RR, STOCKENHUBER C ET AL: Detection of *Borrelia burgdorferi*-specific DNA in urine specimens from patients with erythema migrans before

and after antibiotic therapy. J Clin Microbiol 34:1359–1363, 1996

227. SCHRECKENBERGER PC, CELIG DM, JANDA WM: Clinical evaluation of the Vitek ANI card for identification of anaerobic bacteria. J Clin Microbiol 26:225–230, 1988

228. SCHWARTZ DC, CANTOR CR: Separation of yeast chromosome-sized DNAs by pulsed field gradient gel electrophoresis. Cell 37:67–75, 1984

229. SCOTTO J, HADCHOUEL M, HERY C ET AL: Detection of hepatitis B virus DNA in serum by simple spot hybridization technique: Comparison with results for other viral markers. Hepatology 3:279–284, 1983

230. SECCHIERO P, ZELLA D, CROWLEY RW ET AL: Quantitative PCR for human herpesviruses 6 and 7. J Clin Microbiol 33:2124–2130, 1995

231. SEIFERT H, GERNER-SMIDT P: Comparison of ribotyping and pulsed-field gel electrophoresis for molecular typing of *Acinetobacter* isolates. J Clin Microbiol 33, 1402–1407, 1995

232. SELENDER RK, CAUGANT DA, OCHMAN H ET AL: Methods for multilocus enzyme electrophoresis for bacterial population genetics and systematics. Appl Environ Microbiol 51:873–884, 1986

233. SEMPLE MN, LOVEDAY C, WELLER I ET AL: Direct measurement of viraemia in patients infected with HIV-1 and its relationship to disease progression and zidovudine therapy. J Med Virol 35:38–45, 1991

234. SHAH JS, LIU J, BUXTON D ET AL: *Q-beta* replicase-amplified assay for detection of *Mycobacterium tuberculosis* directly from clinical specimens. J Clin Microbiol 33:1435–1441, 1995

235. SHEN LP, KOLBERG JA, SPAETE RR ET AL: A quantitative method for detection of human cytomegalovirus DNA using a branched DNA enhanced label amplification assay. Abstract 92nd General Meeting of the American Society for Microbiology, abstract S54, p 408, American Society for Microbiology, Washington, DC, 1992

236. SHIBATA D, FU YS, GUPTA JW ET AL: Detection of human papillomavirus in normal and dysplastic tissue by the polymerase chain reaction. Lab Invest 59:555–559, 1988

237. SIPPEL JE, HIDER PA, CONTRONI G: Use of Directigen latex agglutination test for detection of *Haemophilus influenzae*, *Streptococcus pneumoniae*, and *Neisseria meningitidis* antigens in cerebrospinal fluid from meningitis patients. J Clin Microbiol 20:884–886, 1984

238. SKERMAN VBD, MCGOWAN V, SNEATH PHA: Approved list of bacterial names. Int J Syst Bacteriol 30:225–420, 1980

239. SKERMAN VBD, MCGOWAN V, SNEATH PHA (EDS): Approved list of bacterial names, amended edition. American Society for Microbiology, Washington, DC, 1989

240. SNEATH PHA (ED): International code of nomenclature of bacteria. Bacteriologic code, 1992 revision. American Society for Microbiology, Washington, DC, 1992

241. SORRELL TC, CHEN SCA, RUMA P ET AL: Concordance of clinical and environmental isolates of *Cryptococcus neoformans* var. *gattii* by random amplification of polymorphic DNA analysis and PCR fingerprinting. J Clin Microbiol 34:1253–1260, 1996

242. SPECTOR SA, RUA JA, SPECTOR DH ET AL: Detection of human cytomegalovirus in clinical specimens by DNA-DNA hybridization. J Infect Dis 150: 121–126, 1984

242a. STALEY JT, KRIEG NR: Classification of procaryotic organisms: an overview. In Krieg NR, Holt JG (eds): *Bergley's Manual of Systematic Bacteriology*, vol 1. pp 1–4. Baltimore, Williams & Wilkins

243. STEECE RS, TALLEY MS, SKEELS MR ET AL: Comparison of enzyme-linked immunosorbent assay, hemagglutination inhibition, and passive latex agglutination for determination of rubella immune status. J Clin Microbiol 21:140–142, 1985

244. STOAKES L, JOHN MA, LANNIGAN R ET AL: Gas-liquid chromatography of cellular fatty acids for identification of staphylococci. J Clin Microbiol 32:1908–1910, 1994

245. STOCKMAN L, CLARK KA, HUNT JM ET AL: Evaluation of commercially available acridinium ester-labeled chemiluminescent DNA probes for culture identification of *Blastomyces dermatiditis*, *Coccidioides immitis*, *Cryptococcus neoformans*, and *Histoplasma capsulatum*. J Clin Microbiol 31:845–850, 1993

246. TACHIBANA H, IHARA S, KOBAYASHI S ET AL: Differences in genomic DNA sequences between pathogenic and nonpathogenic isolates of *Entamoeba histolytica* identified by polymerase chain reaction. J Clin Microbiol 29:2234–2239, 1991

247. TAM MR, STAMM WE, HANDSFIELD HH ET AL: Culture independent diagnosis of *Chlamydia trachomatis* using monoclonal antibodies. N Engl J Med 310:1146–1150, 1984

248. TAYLOR AJ, SKINNER PR: Gas liquid chromatography in medical microbiology. Med Lab Sci 40:375–385, 1983

249. TELENTI A, MARCHESI F, BALZ M ET AL: Rapid identification of mycobacteria to the species level by polymerase chain reaction and restriction enzyme analysis. J Clin Microbiol 31:175–178, 1993

250. TENOVER FC, CARLSON LC, BARBAGALLO S, NACHAMKIN I: DNA probe culture confirmation assay for identification of thermophilic *Campylobacter* species. J Clin Microbiol 28:1284–1287, 1990

251. TENOVER FC, GOOTZ TD, GORDON KP ET AL: Development of a DNA probe for the structural gene of the 2'-O-adenyl-transferase aminoglycoside-modifying enzyme. J Infect Dis 150:678–687, 1984

252. TENOVER FC, MIZUKI TS, CARLSON LG: Evaluation of autoSCAN-W/A automated microbiology system for the identification of non-glucose-fermenting gram-negative bacilli. J Clin Microbiol 28:1628–1634, 1990

253. THANOS M, SCHONIAN G, MEYER W ET AL: Rapid identification of *Candida* species by DNA fingerprinting with PCR. J Clin Microbiol 34:615–621, 1996

254. THIBERT L, LAPIERRE S: Routine application of high-performance liquid chromatography for identification of mycobacteria. J Clin Microbiol 31:1759–1763, 1993

255. THONG K-L, NGEOW Y-F, ALTWEGG M ET AL: Molecular analysis of *Salmonella enteriditis* by pulsed-field gel electrophoresis and ribotyping. J Clin Microbiol 33:1070–1074, 1995

256. TILTON RC, DIAS F, RYAN RW: Comparative evaluation of three commercial products and counterimmunoelectrophoresis for the detection of antigens in cerebrospinal fluid. J Clin Microbiol 20231–234, 1984

257. TISDALL PA, DEJOUNG DR, ROBERTS GD, ANHALT JP: Identification of clinical isolates of mycobacteria with gas-liquid chromatography alone. J Clin Microbiol 10:506–514, 1979

258. TOTTEN PK, HOLMES KK, HANDSFIELD HH ET AL: DNA hybridization technique for the detection of *Neisseria gonorrhoeae* in men with urethritis. J Infect Dis 148:462–471, 1983

259. TOYE B, PEELING RW, JESSAMINE P ET AL: Diagnosis of *Chlamydia trachomatis* in asymptomatic men and women by PCR assay. J Clin Microbiol 34:1396–1400, 1996

260. TURKOGLU S, LAZIZI Y, MENG J ET AL: Detection of hepatitis E virus RNA in stools and serum by reverse transcription-PCR. J Clin Microbiol 34:1568–1571, 1996

261. UBUKATA K, ASAHI Y, YAMANE A ET AL: Combinational detection of autolysin and penicillin-binding protein 2B genes of *Streptococcus pneumoniae* by PCR. J Clin Microbiol 34:592–596, 1996

262. UNGER ER, CHANDLER FW, CHENGGIS ML ET AL: Demonstration of human immunodeficiency virus by colorimetric in situ hybridization: A rapid technique for formalin-fixed paraffin-embedded material. Mod Pathol 2:200–204, 1989

263. VAN DAMME-JONGSTEN M, RODHOUSE J, GILBERT RJ, NOTERMANS S: Synthetic DNA probes for detection of enterotoxigenic *Clostridium perfringens* strains isolated from outbreaks of food poisoning. J Clin Microbiol 28:131–133, 1990

264. VANDENBROUCKE-GRAULS CMJE, KUSTERS JG: Specific detection of methicillin-resistant *Staphylococcus* species by multiplex PCR. J Clin Microbiol 34:1599, 1996

265. VARY PH, ANDERSEN PR, GREEN E ET AL: Use of highly specific DNA probes and the polymerase chain reaction to detect *Mycobacterium paratuberculosis* in Johne's disease. J Clin Microbiol 28:933–937, 1990

266. VERWEIJ PE, LATGE J-P, RIJS AJMM ET AL: Comparison of antigen detection and PCR assay using bronchoalveolar lavage fluid for diagnosing invasive pulmonary aspergillosis in patients receiving treatment for hematological malignancies. J Clin Microbiol 33:3150–3153, 1996

267. VEYS A, CALLEWAERT W, WALKENS E, VAN DEN ABBEELE K: Application of gas-liquid chromatography to the routine identification of nonfermenting gram-negative bacteria in clinical specimens. J Clin Microbiol 27:1538–1542, 1989

268. VICTOR T, DUTOIT R, VAN ZYL J ET AL: Improved method for the routine identification of toxigenic *Escherichia coli* by DNA amplification of a conserved region of the heat-labile toxin A subunit. J Clin Microbiol 29:158–161, 1991

269. VIKERFORS T, LINDEGREN G, GRANDIEN M ET AL: Diagnosis of influenza A virus infections by detection of specific immunoglobulins M, A and G in serum. J Clin Microbiol 27:453–458, 1989

270. VOGEL J-U, CINATL J, LUX A ET AL: New PCR assay for rapid and quantitative detection of human cytomegalovirus in cerebrospinal fluid. J Clin Microbiol 34:482–483, 1996

271. VON GRAEVENITZ A: Revised nomenclature of *Alloiococcus otitis*. J Clin Microbiol 31:472, 1993

272. VON SYDOW M, GAINES H, SONNERBORG A ET AL: Antigen detection in primary HIV infection. Br Med J 295:238–240, 1988

273. WALL R, DENNING D, AMOS A: HIV antigenaemia in acute HIV infection. Lancet i:566, 1987

274. WALLACE PL, HOLLIS DG, WEAVER RE, MOSS CW: Characterization of CDC group DF-3 by cellular fatty acid analysis. J Clin Microbiol 27:735–737, 1989

275. WAYNE LG, BRENNER DJ, COLWELL RR ET AL: Report of the ad hoc committee on reconciliation of approaches to bacterial systematics. Int J Syst Bacteriol 37:463–464, 1987

276. WELCH DF, HENSEL DM, PICKETT DA ET AL: Bacteremia due to *Rochalimaea henselae* in a child: Practical identification of isolates in the clinical laboratory. J Clin Microbiol 31:2381–2386, 1993

277. WELCH DF, PICKETT DA, SLATER LN ET AL: *Rochalimaea henselae* sp. nov., a cause of septicemia, bacillary angiomatosis, and parenchymal bacillary peliosis. J Clin Microbiol 30:275–280, 1992

278. WEYNANTS V, JADOT V, DENOEL PA ET AL: Detection of *Yersinia enterocolitica* serogroup O:3 by a PCR method. J Clin Microbiol 34:1224–1227, 1996

279. WILKINSON HW, SAMPSON JS, PLIKAYTIS BB: Evaluation of a commercial gene probe for identification of *Legionella* cultures. J Clin Microbiol 23:217–220, 1986

280. WILSON RW, CHENGGIS ML, UNGER ER: Longitudinal study of human papillomavirus infection of the female urogenital tract by in situ hybridization. Arch Pathol Lab Med 114:155–159, 1990

281. WISE DJ, WEAVER TL: Detection of Lyme disease bacterium, *Borrelia burgdorferi*, by using the polymerase chain reaction and a nonradioisotopic gene probe. J Clin Microbiol 29:1523–1526, 1991

282. WOBESER WL, KRAJDEN M, CONLY J ET AL: Evaluation of Roche AMPLICOR PCR assay for *Mycobacterium tuberculosis*. J Clin Microbiol 34:134–139, 1996

283. WOLFSON JS, WALDRON MA, SIERRA LS: Blinded comparison of a direct immunofluorescent monoclonal antibody staining method for identification of *Pneumocystis carinii* in induced sputum and bronchoalveolar lavage specimens of patients infected with human immunodeficiency virus. J Clin Microbiol 28:2136–2138, 1990

284. WOLINSKY SM, RINALDO CR, KWOK S ET AL: Human immunodeficiency virus type 1 (HIV-1) infection a median of 18 months before a diagnostic Western blot: Evidence from a cohort of homosexual men. Ann Intern Med 111:961–972, 1989

285. WONG H-C, LU K-T, PAN T-M ET AL: Subspecies typing of *Vibrio parahaemolyticus* by pulsed-field gel electrophoresis. J Clin Microbiol 34:1535–1539, 1996

286. WRIGHT PA, WYNFORD-THOMAS W: The polymerase chain reaction: Miracle or mirage? A critical review of its uses and limitations in diagnosis and research. J Pathol 162:99–117, 1990

287. WU DY, WALLACE RB: The ligation amplification reaction (LAR)—amplification of specific DNA sequences using sequential rounds of template-dependent ligation. Genomics 4:560–569, 1989

288. YAJKO DM, LAWRENCE J, NASSOS P ET AL: Clinical trial comparing bacitracin with Strep-A-Chek for accuracy and turnaround time in the presumptive identification of *Streptococcus pyogenes*. J Clin Microbiol 24:431–434, 1986

289. YERLY S, GERVAIX A, SIMONET V ET AL: Rapid and sensitive detection of enteroviruses in specimens from patients with aseptic meningitis. J Clin Microbiol 34:199–201, 1996

290. YOLKEN RH, DAVIS D, WINKELSTEIN J ET AL: Enzyme immunoassay for detection of pneumococcal antigen in cerebrospinal fluid. J Clin Microbiol 20:802–805, 1984

291. YORK MA, GIBBS L, CHEHAB F ET AL: Comparison of PCR detection of *mecA* with standard susceptibility testing methods to determine methicillin resistance in coagulase-negative staphylococci. J Clin Microbiol 34:249–253, 1996

292. YOU MS, FACKLAM RR: New test system for identification of *Aerococcus*, *Enterococcus*, and *Streptococcus*. J Clin Microbiol 24:607–611, 1986

293. YOUNG LS, BEVAN IS, JOHNSON MA ET AL: The polymerase chain reaction: A new epidemiological tool for investigating cervical human papillomavirus. Br Med J 298:14–18, 1989

294. ZHENG H, PERET TCT, RANDOLPH VB ET AL: Strain-specific reverse transcriptase PCR assay: Means to distinguish candidate vaccine from wild-type strains of respiratory syncytial virus. J Clin Microbiol 34:334–337, 1996

295. ZIMMERMAN SK, NEEDHAM CA: Comparison of conventional stool concentration and preserved-smear methods with Merifluor *Cryptosporidium*/*Giardia* direct immunofluorescence assay and ProSpecT *Giardia* EZ microplate assay for detection of *Giardia lamblia*. J Clin Microbiol 33:1942–1943, 1995

296. ZUERNER RL, ALT D, BOLIN CA: IS*I533*-based PCR assay for identification of *Leptospira interrogans* sensu lato serovars. J Clin Microbiol 33:3284–3289, 1995

INTRODUCTION TO MICROBIOLOGY
PART I: THE ROLE OF THE MICROBIOLOGY LABORATORY IN THE DIAGNOSIS OF INFECTIOUS DISEASES: GUIDELINES TO PRACTICE AND MANAGEMENT

INTRODUCTION

THE CLINICAL MICROBIOLOGY LABORATORY: AN EXPANDING ROLE

The chief functions of the clinical medical microbiology laboratory are to examine and culture specimens for microorganisms, to make accurate species identification of important isolates and to perform antibiotic susceptibility tests when indicated. These tasks will assist physicians in the diagnosis and treatment of infectious diseases. Microbiology data are also valuable in monitoring the course of antibiotic therapy and in providing epidemiologic information for defining common sources of infection. Whereas in the past two or three decades the major focus of clinical laboratory activity has been directed toward internal quality control and maintaining accuracy and precision of test results, the emphasis currently and in the decades ahead will be on how discriminating clinicians will be in utilizing laboratory services and how effectively they apply laboratory test results to the care and management of patients. A new vocabulary is evolving—"quality assurance" (QA), "laboratory utilization," "outcome indicators," "assessment monitors," "standards of care," and the like, terms that are now becoming as familiar in laboratory circles as the well-known quality control expressions "accuracy," "precision," "sensitivity," and "predictive values."

Under the impetus of the Joint Commission on Accreditation of Healthcare Organizations (JCAHO) and other local and state commissions and peer review organizations, hospitals are now required to have active quality assurance and laboratory utilization committees, with the charge 1) to evaluate all aspects of patient care within each institution, 2) to establish criteria and standards of care, 3) to institute monitors to assess the degree of accordance with these standards, and 4) to make recommendations to correct any practices found to be out of compliance. As mentioned later in this chapter, the implementation of the JCAHO program, as outlined here, has been tempered in many laboratories as a clear working definition of "quality of care" has proved difficult to derive. Therefore, initial enthusiasm for establishing a complex hospital-wide quality assurance program has taken more the form of implementing a few monitors in areas for which problems have been defined and improvement is possible. In whatever form it may take in a given institution, the overall concept of quality assurance is sound and laboratory personnel should continue to take an active role in establishing the criteria and standards of medical care related to laboratory utilization. An entire section later in this chapter is devoted to a formal presentation of what is now called "quality assurance," including guidelines for the practical implementation of procedures and practices in microbiology laboratories.

Color Plates for Chapter 2 are found between pages 80 and 81.

THE DIAGNOSTIC CYCLE

The diagnostic cycle shown in Figure 2-1 provides a useful model to understand the role the microbiology laboratory plays in the practice of quality assurance. Shown are the sequence of steps involved in collecting, processing, and analyzing clinical specimens submitted for culture, leading to information that can be used to establish the clinical and laboratory diagnosis of infectious diseases.

The diagnostic cycle begins with the patient who consults a physician because of signs or symptoms suggesting an infectious disease. Cultures from one or more anatomic sites may be indicated, depending on the findings of medical history and physical examination. An appropriate specimen for culture must be collected and a transport container(s) selected that will maintain the viability of any pathogenic organisms during transit. The specimen container must be properly labeled with the patient's name, location, date and time of collection, and type of specimen. This information along with the physician's orders must be transcribed to a laboratory request form, entered into a computer data file, or both. Ideally the request form should include essential clinical findings, a working diagnosis, and any information that may require laboratory personnel to apply other than routine procedures to recover uncommon or particularly fastidious microorganisms. Physicians should either call the laboratory or indicate on the laboratory request slip if an infectious disease, caused by less commonly encountered or fastidious microorganisms, is suspected.

Certain culture media required for the optimum recovery of certain fastidious or slow-growing microorganisms may not be available or used in many laboratories. For example, the recovery of bacterial species belonging to the genera *Brucella*, *Pasteurella*, *Moraxella*, *Haemophilus*, *Neisseria*, *Leptospira*, *Vibrio*, *Campylobacter*, and *Legionella*, among others, may require special culture media or alternative techniques. Physicians should be apprised of the specific organisms that will be missed by the routine culture techniques being used in any given laboratory, so that special requests can be made when appropriate. Within the subspecialized areas of mycobacteriology, mycology, and virology, it is particularly helpful for laboratory personnel to know more exactly which fungal or viral disease is clinically suspected, because special culture media, adjusted incubation temperatures, or alternative analytical techniques may be necessary.

Once the specimen is received in the laboratory, the information on the request form is entered into a computer file or log book. The specimens are examined visually and, depending on the physician's order and the nature of the specimen, wet mounts and smears may be prepared and stained for microscopic examination. Observations may or may not be immediately

THE DIAGNOSTIC CYCLE

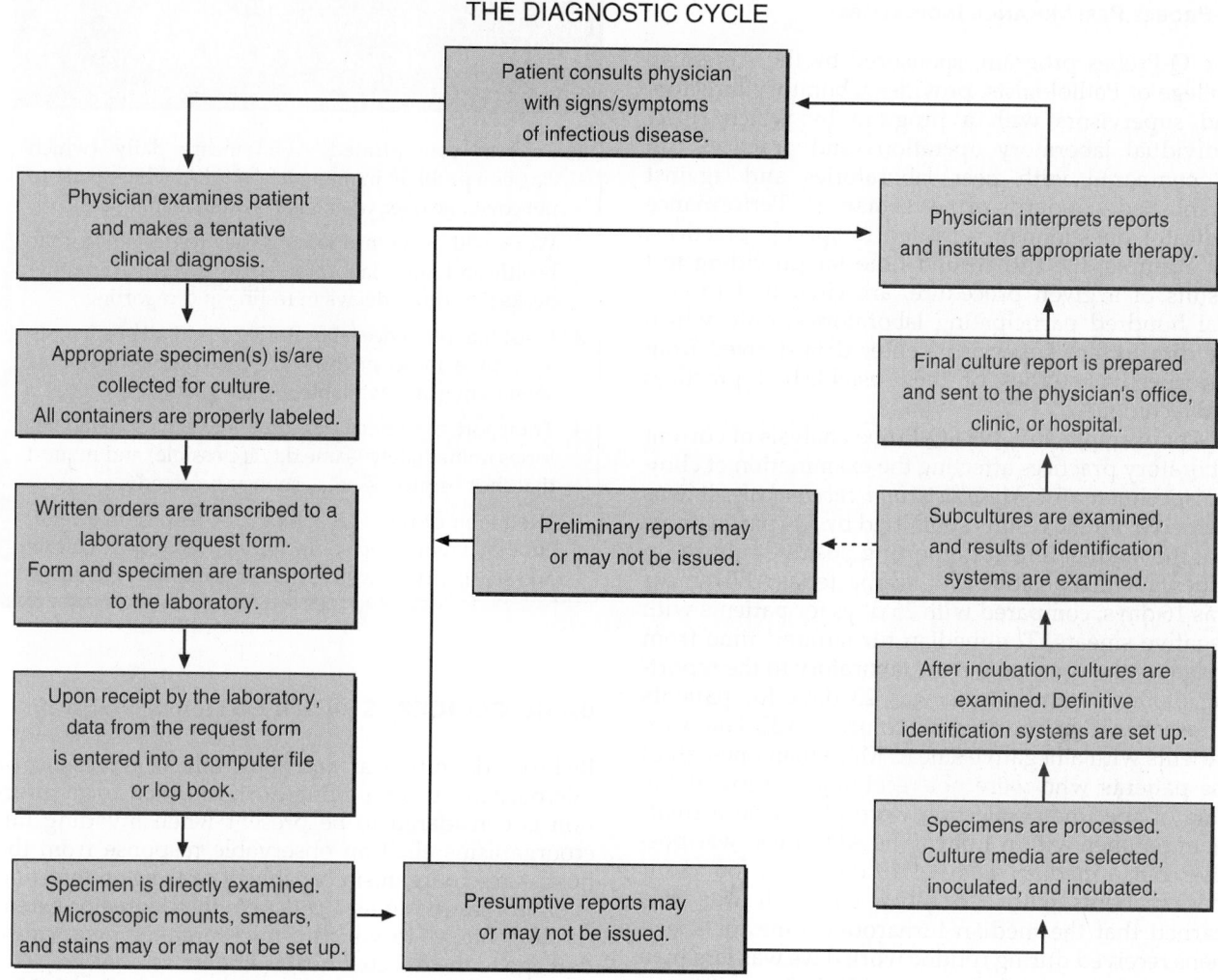

Figure 2-1.
The clinical and laboratory diagnosis of infectious disease: A schematic overview of the diagnostic cycle.

reported to the physician depending on the definitiveness of the results. Timely information may often be used to establish a presumptive diagnosis and to institute a specific course of therapy.

Specimens that require definitive identification of potentially pathogenic microbes are processed further. One or more culture media are selected, or if viral diseases are suspected, appropriate cell lines are chosen that will be inoculated with a portion of the specimen. All agar plates are streaked for colony isolation; then plates, broths, and cell cultures are placed in an incubator with appropriate temperature and environmental conditions to maximize the growth and replication of microbes. After a specified incubation period, the cultures are examined both visually and microscopically. Often presumptive microbial identifications can be made. A final report is issued if a definitive answer can be given; if not, the report should be delayed while subcultures and additional test procedures are performed to identify the organisms definitively.

Each step in this cycle must be monitored to assure accuracy and precision of performance. Although di-

rectly involved in only a portion of the cycle, microbiologists must assume responsibility for seeing that policies and practices are in place by which all specimens are properly collected and transported to the laboratory and that timely and accurate reports are issued to maximize the quality of patient care.[38] Laboratory directors and supervisors must also pay ongoing attention to the evolution of new technologies that may provide more rapid results, with equal or greater accuracy, at less cost.[6] An open line of two-way communication must be maintained between physicians and their support personnel in offices, clinics, and hospitals as taxonomy changes, direct-detection systems become available, and the interpretation of laboratory reports changes. Ten areas of emphasis in nurturing communications between infectious disease physicians and microbiology personnel have been outlined by Matsen.[40]

The reader is also directed to a publication by D'Amato and Isenberg,[15] in which the broad aspects of microbiologic laboratory utilization and several deficiencies in operations and corrective actions are reviewed that may lead to more cost-effective practice.

Q-PROBES PERFORMANCE INDICATORS

The Q-Probes program, sponsored by the American College of Pathologists, provides laboratory directors and supervisors with a program by which select individual laboratory operations and practices can be compared with peer laboratories and against established standards of performance.[59] Performance indicator questionnaires related to specific practices, for example, the turnaround time for providing test results of a given procedure, are circulated to several hundred participating laboratories, onto which the directors or supervisors enter data derived from retrospective studies of their established practices and techniques.

For example, in a 1994 Q-Probe analysis of current laboratory practices affecting the examination of clinical specimens for *Mycobacterium tuberculosis*, it was learned from the results submitted by 534 participants that the median time for reporting positive cultures in patients with a positive acid-fast bacteria (AFB) smear was 16 days, compared with 25 days for patients with negative smears. The median turnaround time from arrival of the specimen in the laboratory to the reporting of final identification was 23 days for patients whose smear was positive, in contrast to 32.9 days for patients with a negative smear. More than one-half of the patients who were not receiving therapy at the time of specimen collection were placed on a treatment regimen within 1 day if the AFB smear was positive, but a median delay of 13 days was found for those patients with a negative smear. It was also learned that the median turnaround time for specimens received during routine work days was less than 24 hours; however, this increased to 41 hours if specimens were received on Saturday, presumably because many institutions do not process specimens submitted for mycobacterial culture on weekends. Final reports were also significantly delayed for specimens sent to a reference laboratory, by as long as 1 week in some instances.

In light of these Q-Probe results and based on the Centers for Disease Control and Prevention (CDC) performance standards, the CDC has recommended guidelines for ensuring faster turnaround times (Box 2-1).

The CDC further recommends that clinical laboratories provide rapid results of testing of clinical specimens, to help control the spread of tuberculosis (Box 2-2).

The information derived from the Q-Probe responses and the guidelines and recommendations derived therefrom provide each laboratory director or supervisor with a valuable benchmark for implementing specific changes in procedures and practices in his or her individual laboratory. The underlying focus is not only to improve the quality of patient care, but also to establish an early diagnosis of an infectious disease so that the possibility of spread in the community can be minimized.

BOX 2-1. CDC RECOMMENDATIONS REGARDING LABORATORY TURNAROUND TIMES

1. Perform concentrated AFB smears daily (which causes a problem in many laboratories where personnel coverage over weekends is often inadequate).

2. Work with reference laboratories (especially public health and state laboratories) to investigate bottlenecks that cause delays in testing and reporting.

3. Insist that reference laboratories report all positive results by a rapid method (e.g., telephone or fax) as soon as they are available.

4. Transport specimens or cultures to reference laboratories immediately (same day if possible) and request that they be processed as soon as received.

5. Use the most rapid technology, or request that reference laboratories do so (including radiometric culture and sensitivity, as well as nucleic acid probe identifica-

---

BASIC CONCEPTS OF INFECTIOUS DISEASE

By broad definition, an *infection* implies the presence of microorganisms in a living host. In practice, an infection is considered to be present when invading microorganisms elicit an observable response from the host. A microorganism capable of causing an infection is often referred to as a *pathogen*; the degree or extent (pathogenicity) to which a microorganism can cause damage to the infected host is known as *virulence*.

This response may be localized at the site of infection or may be generalized or systemic. The local

---

BOX 2-2. CDC RECOMMENDATIONS REGARDING CONTROL OF TUBERCULOSIS

1. Clinical specimens should reach the laboratory within 24 hours of collection.

2. Smear results should reach the physician within 24 hours after specimen receipt in the laboratory.

3. Isolates should be definitively identified to species level within 17 to 21 days of specimen receipt.

4. Antibiotic susceptibility results should reach physicians within 28 days of specimen receipt. Susceptibility results for *M. tuberculosis* can be assessed most rapidly using the BACTEC or equivalent rapid method.

5. Inoculation of liquid medium as primary culture.

6. Identify growth in liquid medium as acid–fast and use molecular probes, inhibition of growth in NAP, or mycologic aid procedures for rapid identification.

reaction to infection takes the form of inflammation. *Inflammation* is a general term referring to that abnormal alteration of tissues or organs caused by injury or tissue destruction. The local inflammatory response caused by infectious agents can be divided into acute suppurative (or purulent), chronic, and granulomatous infections.

ACUTE SUPPURATIVE (OR PURULENT) INFECTION

An acute suppurative infection elicits an inflammatory response in which pus is formed. Pus is a liquid material with a specific gravity exceeding 1.013, containing large numbers of segmented neutrophils, the hallmarks of acute inflammation. *Cellulitis* is often used to describe involvement of loose subcutaneous connective tissue in which the purulent exudate spreads between layers of the involved tissues. *Abscess* is the term used when segmented neutrophils become localized in a walled-off area of suppurative inflammation. *Necrosis* refers to cell death or destruction of tissue at the site of pus formation.

CHRONIC INFECTION

A chronic infection is a long-standing infection in which the cellular inflammatory response includes predominantly mononuclear inflammatory cells—lymphocytes, plasma cells, and monocytes.

GRANULOMATOUS INFECTION

Granulomatous infection is a subtype of chronic infection in which granulomas are formed. A *granuloma* can be most simply defined as focal collections of large activated macrophages or histiocytes that have an increased capacity for phagocytosis and digestion of foreign particles. These cells are also called "epithelioid" cells because they have some resemblance to squamous epithelial cells. Several macrophages often aggregate to form multinucleated giant cells. In certain granulomas a particular type of necrosis, called caseous necrosis, may be found in which the tissue has a cheeselike consistency. The presence of multinucleated giant cells and caseous necrosis are characteristic of tuberculosis but they may also be seen in certain other infections.

THE INFECTED HOST

An infection is referred to as *opportunistic* when a microbial agent not commonly causing disease causes inflammation in an immunocompromised or debilitated host. Other terms commonly used to describe the interaction of microbes and the infected host are commensalism, symbiosis, and parasitism. *Commensalism* (also referred to as *colonization*) is a relation in which a microorganism lives on or within a host in such a way that neither one derives benefit or harm; examples of commensal organisms are the α-hemolytic streptococci that colonize the upper respiratory tract and a variety of *Staphylococcus* species and yeasts that inhabit the skin. *Symbiosis* is a relation in which a microorganism lives on or within a host such that both derive mutual advantage or benefit. A symbiotic bacterium is *Escherichia coli* that colonizes the bowel, deriving nutrients and energy from the host; and, for the host, it synthesizes the vitamin K required to prevent bleeding disorders. *Parasitism* is a relation in which one microorganism lives on or within a host and gains benefit at the expense of the host. *Salmonella typhi, Corynebacteria diphtheriae,* and *Bordetella pertussis* are examples of parasites; that is, bacteria that live within host tissue but in return cause typhoid fever, diphtheria, and whooping cough, respectively, to the detriment, morbidity, and on occasion mortality of the host. A *saprophyte* is a microorganism that lives on dead organic matter. *Saprophytes* are generally not pathogenic to humans except in cases of immunosuppression or chronic debilitating disease, when superinfections may occur.

Whether an infectious disease occurs in the presence of an organism depends on the relation between the host's resistance, the organism's virulence, and sometimes, the effects of prophylactic therapy. To establish an infectious disease, an organism must:

1. Reach the host and find a portal of entry
2. Overcome the host defenses
3. Invade and proliferate in the host tissues and produce toxins or other virulence factors
4. Be capable of resisting host defenses

Organisms may reach the host by exogenous routes (inhalation, ingestion, direct contact, or inoculation) or endogenous routes (following breaks in natural barriers, change in virulence of "normal flora," or changes in host defense mechanisms).

ORGANISM VIRULENCE

Bacteria have a variety of virulence mechanisms, or they produce factors that allow their persistence in the tissues or result in toxic effects on the host. Bacteria must find a portal of entry into the host, usually a result of barrier breaks in the skin or mucous membranes, caused either by mechanical injury or by a variety of underlying conditions compromising the integrity of epithelial linings, including metabolic disorders, other infections, invading neoplasms, and effects of chemotherapy, to mention a few. Microbes that invade the bloodstream may resist secondary host defenses, such as developing capsules that prevent phagocytosis and producing factors that protect against the oxidative burst of neutrophil lysosomal granules once phagocytosis occurs, thereby allowing a protective intracellular existence. A variety of enzymes may be produced, including proteases (the leukocidens of staphylococci, for example) that destroy immunoglobulins or leukocytes, β-lactamases that inactivate antibiotics, lecithinases that interrupt cell membranes, leading to tissue necrosis and gas gangrene, and hemolysins that can destroy red blood cells.

Catalase, coagulase, hyaluronidase, streptokinase, and elastase are among other destructive enzymes that may be produced by several virulent species of bacteria. *Helicobacter pylori* has a unique mechanism by which it is protected from the extremely low acidic environment of the gastric mucosa. Through strong urease activity, a cloud of ammonia surrounds each bacterial cell, neutralizing the low pH of the gastric acid and producing a microenvironment conducive to survival and proliferation.

Factors that facilitate attachment of bacterial cells to cutaneous or mucous membrane surfaces are important virulence mechanisms that prevent bacteria from being swept away, allowing them to penetrate and proliferate in the underlying tissues. Gram-negative bacteria possess specialized appendages called fimbriae, or pili, and outer membrane proteins that effect attachment to host cell surfaces. Siegfried and coworkers,[62] in a study of 168 strains of *E. coli* isolated from cases of pyelonephritis and lower urinary tract infections in children, found expression of P fimbriae and cell-surface hydrophobicity among several important virulence factors, particularly for those strains causing pyelonephritis. Similarly, Foxman and coworkers,[20] found that the *E. coli* strains expressing fimbrial adhesions I–IV, F1845 pili, Pap and Prs pili, S fimbriae, and type 1 pili were important virulence factors of isolates recovered from women aged 18 to 40 years with first-time urinary tract infections.

Juskova and Ciznar,[32] using a biotinylated ^{32}P probe for the detection of P fimbriae in urinary isolates of *E. coli*, were able to separate probe-positive pathogenic strains from nonpathogenic strains that were probe-negative. Tarkkanen and associates[63] also demonstrated type 1 fimbriae as an important virulence factor in pathogenic urinary tract strains of *Klebsiella pneumoniae*, particularly in binding to urinary slime. Adherence factors may also play an important role in nosocomial, catheter-related urinary tract infections. Roberts and coworkers[57] found that bacterial strains causing catheter-related urinary tract infections adhered to silicone and red rubber catheters; no adherence was noted with catheters having a hydrophilic surface, which was related to a delay in the onset of significant bacteriuria. Adherence mechanisms may also play a role in catheter-associated infections related to bacterial biofilm formation on infected catheters.[49]

Surface components of gram-positive organisms, such as lipoteichoic acids (streptococci) and M-proteins (staphylococci), may serve as adherence factors in causing infections. Certain strains of streptococci, notably *S. mutans*, are rich in surface dextrans that effect preferential adherence to dental surfaces, prerequisite to formation of dental plaque and caries.[69] Surface dextrans are also important in effecting the adherence of *S. mutans* and *S. sanguis* to fibrin–platelet clots on the surfaces of damaged heart valves, making these two species particularly prone to cause bacterial endocarditis.[14]

Toxin production also serves as an important virulence mechanism for many bacterial species. Exotoxins, secreted from the bacterial cell, are produced primarily by gram-positive bacteria. The exotoxins of *Corynebacterium diphtheriae*, *Clostridium tetani*, *Clostridium botulinum*, and *Shigella dysenteriae* are among the most powerful poisons known. These are all neurotoxins that have their target activity distant from the primary sites of infection. *Clostridium difficile* produces a powerful exotoxin that causes a severe, necrotizing, pseudomembranous infection of the colon; *Staphylococcus aureus* produces a variety of toxins related to hemolytic and necrotizing pyogenic infection, exfoliative dermatitis, toxic shock syndrome, and food poisoning. An erythrogenic toxin produced by *Streptococcus pyogenes* manifests as scarlet fever. Cholera toxin, composed of five "B" subunits responsible for binding to the GM1 ganglioside receptors on epithelial surfaces, and an active A2 subunit that activates cyclic-AMP leading to accumulation of water and electrolytes in the bowel and severe hypertonic, watery diarrhea.[23]

Endotoxins, integral to the bacterial cell wall, are associated with gram-negative bacteria. Endotoxins consist of a highly conserved lipid A core firmly anchored to the cell membrane and a highly variable, surface-accessible carbohydrate segment that determines the "O" (somatic) antigenic specificity of the bacteria. Clinically, endotoxins mediate the septic shock syndromes associated with overwhelming gram-negative sepsis. The biologic effects of endotoxin can be detected by measurement of the gelling of an amebocyte lysate from the horseshoe crab (*Limulus*) or by immunologic methods.[69]

MECHANISMS OF HOST RESISTANCE

Primary host defenses include anatomic barriers, such as the intact epithelium, nasal hairs, cilia in the respiratory tract, the mucous layer lining the gut, and the flow of liquids in the respiratory and intestinal tracts, aided by coughing or swallowing and peristalsis, respectively. Physiologic factors that inhibit bacterial growth and minimize the chance for infections include high or low pH or oxygen tensions in many tissues and organs that render them unsuitable for the proliferation of microorganisms; chemical inhibitors to bacterial growth, such as the production of proteases in the gastrointestinal tract; the presence of bile acids; activation of lysozymes in saliva and tears; and the accumulation of fatty acids on the surface of the skin. Any barrier breaks in the skin and mucous membrane, such as the presence of an indwelling venous catheter, temporary dysfunction of the ciliary action of the respiratory tract that occurs in smokers, ileus for whatever reason in the bowel, and obstruction to the flow of secretions, such as in the bile and pancreatic ducts or in the urinary tract, can lead to the local proliferation of bacteria and potential onset of infection.

Structural differences in organs and tissues and differences in activities are often responsible for the susceptibility to infections between genders and at various ages. Urinary tract infections are one example, being more common in males at young and advanced ages, the former results from a high prevalence of urinary tract anomalies and the latter from urinary obstruction secondary to chronic prostatism. Because of the short urethra and trauma from sexual activity, middle-aged females are more prone to acquiring cystitis and lower urinary tract infections.

The normal flora on mucous membranes and in the bowel also tend to inhibit the proliferation of pathogens by competing for nutrients or cell membrane binding sites, and by producing inhibitors called bacteriocins. For example, fungal infections, particularly with yeasts, commonly occur in patients whose normal flora has been reduced or eliminated by long-term antibiotic therapy.

Secondary or internal host defenses include the presence of naturally occurring humoral substances (complement, lysozyme, and opsonins) in plasma and other body secretions, phagocytosis by circulating segmented neutrophils and fixed macrophages in the reticuloendothelial system, and the production of humoral (IgM, IgG, and IgA) antibodies and cell-mediated immune responses. The activation of complement by bacteria in the early stages of infection, usually by the alternate pathway in the absence of immunoglobulins, particularly C3b, serves to link the bacteria to receptors on the cell membrane, enhancing attachment, phagocytosis, and subsequent killing. Nonimmune-derived compounds such as the opsonic glycoprotein, fibronectin, and surfactant also facilitate phagocytosis before immunoglobulins are produced in response to any given acute infection.[70] Immunologically specific cellular immunity is mediated through thymus-derived T lymphocytes, particularly the CD4 lymphocytes, which possess immunologic memory, helper function for other T lymphocytes and regulate the response of B cells to many antigens.[50,51]

Obviously, any defects in humoral and cellular defenses will increase the susceptibility of a host to infection. Hypogammaglobulinemia, with deficiencies in both IgA and IgG globulins, deficiency in plasma complement, leukopenia, functional defects of neutrophils and monocytes, and a variety of neoplastic and metabolic debilitating diseases, predispose humans to recurrent infections. Individuals infected with the human immunodeficiency virus (HIV), with its particular tropism for, and destruction of, CD4 lymphocytes, are particularly prone to infections with a variety of bacterial, fungal, parasitic, and viral infectious disease agents. These often are resistant to most antimicrobial drugs, resulting in relentless recurrent and progressive infections.

Other factors that affect host resistance include 1) age (the very young and the very old are more susceptible to infections) and nutritional status of the host; 2) presence of chronic or debilitating diseases such as diabetes, cardiovascular diseases, and malignancies; 3) use of certain short- and long-term modes or agents of therapy, including radiation, chemotherapy, corticosteroids, immunodepressants and antibiotics; 4) toxic ingestion of alcohol and drugs; and 5) factors such as trauma, undue physical or emotional stress, and the presence of foreign material at the site of infection.

CLINICAL MANIFESTATIONS OF INFECTION: SIGNS AND SYMPTOMS

Signs and symptoms of infection may be generalized or systemic, or they may be focal or localized to a given organ or organ system. Early Greek and Roman physicians recognized four cardinal signs of inflammation:

1. Dolor (pain)
2. Calor (heat)
3. Rubor (redness)
4. Tumor (swelling)

The underlying mechanisms predisposing to these signs are not well known. The initiating pathophysiologic mechanism is the dilation of blood vessels caused by a complex cascade of vasoactive amines and other chemical mediators.[13] The local release of chemical mediators results in increased blood flow, with venous and capillary congestion (calor and rubor), and increased permeability of vessels, with fluid, blood, and proteins escaping into the extracellular spaces (dolor and tumor). Segmented neutrophils are attracted to the area of irritation by chemotactic substances and escape through the permeable vasculature into the extracellular spaces (pus formation).

GENERAL OR SYSTEMIC SIGNS AND SYMPTOMS OF INFECTION

In the acute phase of infection, the patient may experience fever (often high-grade and spiking), chills, flushing (vasodilation), and an increase in pulse rate. Patients with subacute or chronic infections may present with minimal or vague symptoms—intermittent low-grade fever, weight loss or fatigability, and lassitude. Toxic reactions to bacterial products may produce eczematous or hemorrhagic skin reactions or a variety of neuromuscular, cardiorespiratory, or gastrointestinal signs and symptoms, initial indicators of an underlying infectious disease.

Radiographic manifestations of infectious disease include pulmonary infiltrates, fibrous thickening of cavity linings, the presence of gas and swelling in soft tissues or of radiopaque masses, or accumulation of fluid within body cavities and organs.

Laboratory values suggesting an infectious disease in patients with minimal or early symptoms include an elevation in the erythrocyte sedimentation rate (ESR), peripheral blood leukocytosis or monocytosis and alterations in plasma proteins. Elevations in gammaglobulins or the presence of certain reactants, such as C-reactive protein, or the production of type-specific antibodies may also indicate infection.

LOCAL SIGNS OF INFECTION

The cardinal signs of infection are the unmistakable manifestations of local infection. Localized redness and heat and the production of a swelling or tumorous mass generally can be observed, either visually if present on the external surfaces, or from radiographs or other noninvasive techniques (echograms, computed tomography scans, nucleomagnetic resonance, and such). If nerve endings are irritated or stretched by the expanding mass, pain may be experienced either in the immediate area or in adjacent or distant sites through complementary efferent pathways (known as "referred" pain). The presence of a draining sinus and the excretion of a purulent exudate are also indications of a local inflammatory or infectious process. Any of these signs and symptoms should direct the physician to collect material for direct microscopic examination and culture.

The specific signs and symptoms of infection manifest in the several organ systems (respiratory, gastrointestinal, urinary tract, genital, or other) will be presented in detail in Chapter 3 where these individual sites of infection are discussed.

SPECIMEN COLLECTION

Once an infectious disease is suspected, appropriate cultures must be ordered or techniques directed toward the serologic detection of antigens or antibodies should be requested. As discussed in Chapter 1, new techniques are evolving that use monoclonal antibodies, DNA probes, and other nonculture procedures for the rapid and direct detection of antigens in body fluids. Pathologists, microbiologists, and medical technologists are available in most institutions and communities to assist physicians in selecting the proper specimens for culture and in ordering the appropriate tests to achieve the maximum recovery or detection of microorganisms.

The proper collection of a specimen for culture is possibly the most important step in the ultimate confirmation that a microorganism is responsible for the infectious disease process. A poorly collected specimen not only may result in failure to recover important microorganisms, but may also lead to incorrect or even harmful therapy if treatment is directed toward a commensal or contaminant. For example, assume that *Klebsiella pneumoniae*, a legitimate cause of human pneumonia, as the species name would indicate, has been recovered from the sputum of a patient with clinical pneumonia. *Klebsiella pneumoniae* is also known to colonize the nasopharynx. If the sputum in this theoretical case has been improperly collected and consisted primarily of saliva, the recovery of *K. pneumoniae* may not reflect the true cause of the pneumonia, but merely nasopharyngeal colonization. Treatment for *K. pneumoniae* could be improper and may, by chance, be effective only if the bacterial species causing the pneumonia had an antibiotic susceptibility pattern similar to that of *K. pneumoniae*. If *Pseudomonas aeruginosa* had actually been the causal agent, the therapy selected may have been in error.

The following are fundamental considerations in the collection of specimens:

1. The specimen must be material from the actual infection site and must be collected with a minimum of contamination from adjacent tissues, organs, or secretions. For example, throat swabs for strepto-

coccal screening should be taken from the peritonsillar fossae, while avoiding contact of the swab with other areas in the oropharynx. Contamination of sputum or lower respiratory specimens with oropharyngeal secretions must also be minimized. Failure to culture the depths of a wound or draining sinus without touching the adjacent skin, inadequate cleansing of the periurethral tissue and perineum before collecting a clean-catch urine sample from a woman, contamination of an endometrial sample with vaginal secretions, and failure to reach deep abscesses with aspirating needles or cannulas are other examples for which laboratory results may be misleading. Swabs, by and large, are inferior in the collection of most specimens and the use of aspiration needles and catheters should be encouraged.

2. Optimal times for specimen collection must be established for the best chance of recovery of causative microorganisms. Knowledge of the natural history and pathophysiology of the infectious disease process is important in determining the optimal time for specimen collection. Although classic typhoid fever is currently a relatively rare disease in the United States, the progression of the infectious process in this disease is a prime example of the importance of proper timing in specimen collection (Fig. 2-2). The causative microorganism can be recovered optimally from the blood during the first week of illness. Culture of the feces or urine is usually positive during the second and third weeks of illness. Serum agglutinins begin to rise during the second week of illness, reaching a peak during the 5th week, and remain detectable for many weeks after clinical remission of the disease.

Monitors should be established in clinical microbiology laboratories to limit the frequency with which repeat specimens are obtained from the same

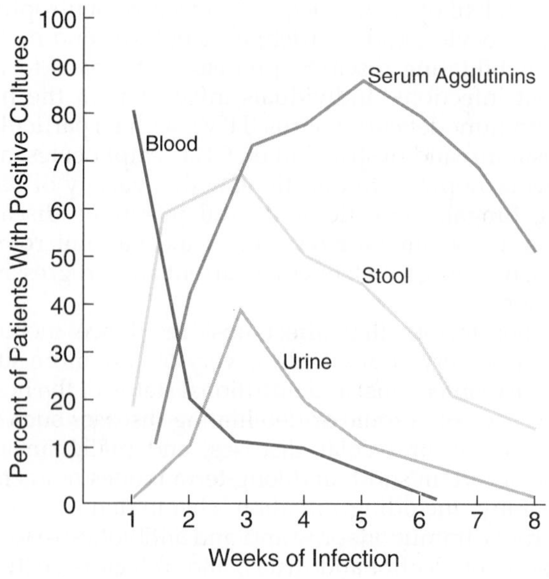

Figure 2-2.
Culture and serologic diagnosis of typhoid fever.

anatomic sites. Obtaining daily sputum cultures to diagnose bacterial pneumonia or obtaining more than one stool specimen in 24 hours for the detection and recovery of animal parasites is an unnecessary duplication of effort. Three blood culture sets in 24 hours and repeat draws of two or three sets on the second day for a septicemic episode are generally sufficient to establish a diagnosis. At least two sets of blood cultures should be drawn for each bacteremic episode to maximize the recovery of microorganisms. The drawing of blood samples for determination of antimicrobial drug levels must be carefully correlated with the times of administration of antibiotics to establish accurate peak and valley concentrations.

Routine throat, sputum, urine, and wound cultures should be limited to one in each 24-hour period. The first-morning, deep-cough sputum specimens should be obtained on 3 successive days to confirm the diagnosis of pulmonary tuberculosis. Once the diagnosis of pulmonary tuberculosis is established, repeat sputum collections should be no more frequent than once a week, primarily to monitor the efficacy of therapy.

For the recovery of intestinal ova and parasites, obtaining one stool specimen daily or every other day for a total of three samples is usually adequate. When routine stool cultures continue to be negative in the face of strong clinical evidence of intestinal parasitic disease, collection immediately following a purge may be rewarding. Siegel and coworkers[61] present strong evidence that stool specimens for the recovery of enteric pathogens or for the detection of ova and parasites should not be accepted from patients who have been in the hospital for 3 days or longer. They found during a 3-year period that only 1 of 191 stools for enteric pathogens and none of 90 ova and parasite examinations were positive in a group of patients in whom collections were made after 3 days of hospitalization. Similar results obtained from an unpublished study at the University of Colorado Health Sciences Center Microbiology Laboratory led to implementation of this "no examination for stool parasites after 3-day" policy. These authors estimate that eliminating stool cultures and ova and parasite examinations on hospitalized patients could realize a nationwide savings of as much as 20 to 30 million dollars per year. Fan, et al.[18a] have suggested a similar policy for rejection of stool specimens for bacterial pathogens. The yield is so low that stool examination for bacterial pathogens should be performed only if there is plausible clinical or epidemiologic evidence to do so.

Because of the high risk of contamination or overgrowth with more rapidly growing commensal bacteria, 24-hour collections of clinical materials for culture, particularly of sputum and urine, should be discouraged. On the other hand, Kaye[34] has shown that urine from normal persons may be inhibitory or bactericidal for some microorganisms, particularly if the urine pH is 5.5 or lower (acidic), if the osmolality is high, or if the urea concentration is in-

creased. The ability of bacteria to grow in urine may represent a failure in a host defense mechanism.

3. A sufficient quantity of specimen must be obtained to perform the culture techniques requested. Guidelines should be established outlining what constitutes a sufficient volume of material for culture. In most cases of active bacterial infections, sufficient quantities of pus or purulent secretions are produced; thus, volume is not a problem. Mermel and Maki[46] advise that clinical laboratory personnel should routinely monitor the volume of blood in blood culture bottles as a quality assurance measure. They discovered that 15% of blood culture specimens from adults in their hospital were being collected in 3.5-mL pediatric tubes; another 5% that were drawn in 10-mL adult tubes contained less than 5-mL of blood. Standard-volume cultures had a substantially higher detection rate for septicemia (92%) than did low-volume cultures (69%). They calculated that the yield of organism recovery from adult blood cultures increased by 3%/mL of blood collected.

In chronic or milder forms of infection, it may be difficult to procure sufficient material; the submission of a dry swab or scant secretions to the laboratory with the hope that something will grow is frequently an exercise in futility and, possibly, of considerable cost to the patient. Swab cultures are easy to obtain, but often lead to spurious results. Inadequate samples should be held until the physician or ward nurse can be reached to determine if a repeat collection can be conveniently made. If not and if the culture is still clinically indicated, the specimen can be processed; however, the laboratory report should include a statement on the condition of the specimen when received.[5] Obviously, exceptions may be necessary for neonates and young children.

All too frequently, 0.5 mL or less of material labeled "sputum" or "bronchial washings" is delivered to the laboratory with a request for routine, AFB and fungal cultures. Such specimens may not represent pulmonary secretions from the site of infection, and the low volume may be insufficient to enable performance of all the procedures requested. Tubes containing holding broth such as phosphate yeast glucose (PYG) can be provided into which the physician can directly inoculate whatever amount of material that can be collected. In this way, the specimen can be divided in the laboratory for inoculation to a variety of primary isolation media. In some institutions, several tubes are provided, each containing culture media optimal for the recovery of mycobacteria, fungi, and viruses. If the secretions obtained are minimal, the physician must choose which tube to inoculate based on the clinical information available.

4. Appropriate collection devices, specimen containers, and culture media must be used to ensure optimal recovery of microorganisms.

Sterile containers should be used for collection of most specimens. It is also important that containers be constructed for ease of collection, particularly if the patients are required to obtain their own specimens. Narrow-mouthed bottles are poorly designed for collection of sputum or urine samples. The containers should also be provided with tightly fitted caps or lids to prevent leakage or contamination during transport.

Swabs are commonly used for obtaining many types of cultures; however, they are generally inferior to other methods for collecting specimens, and their use should be discouraged as much as possible. If swabs are used, certain precautions should be taken. Cotton swabs may contain residual fatty acids, and calcium alginate may emit toxic products that may inhibit certain fastidious bacteria: thus, use of swabs tipped with Dacron or polyester may be indicated. Specimens should not be allowed to remain in contact with the swab any longer than necessary. Except for throat swabs, for which drying does not seem to affect the recovery of streptococci, swabs should be placed in a transport medium or moist container to prevent drying and death of bacteria. Good recovery of most bacterial species from these tubes has been demonstrated for up to 48 hours or longer. The use of culture tubes containing semisolid Stuart's or Amies' transport medium, with or without charcoal, also serves as an adequate means for holding swab cultures during transport. Organism recovery from swabs may be enhanced by placing the swab in 0.5 to 1.0 mL of saline or tryptic soy broth and vortexing for 20 seconds before inoculation.[19]

In general the use of swabs for collection of specimens for recovery of anaerobic bacteria in particular is discouraged; rather, aspiration with a needle and syringe is recommended. In either event, specimens once collected must be protected from exposure to ambient oxygen and kept from drying until they can be processed in the laboratory. A number of transport containers suitable for anaerobic specimens are listed in Table 2-1, some of which are commercially available.

Regardless of the transport system used, the major task is to reduce the time delay between collection of specimens and inoculation of media to a minimum. For example, if rectal swabs are used for the recovery of *Shigella* species from patients with bacillary dysentery, the material collected should be inoculated directly onto the surface of MacConkey medium or into gram-negative (GN) enrichment broth. Even the use of a holding or transport medium may jeopardize the recovery of certain strains. Urethral or cervical secretions obtained for the recovery of *Neisseria gonorrhoeae* also should be inoculated directly onto the surface of chocolate agar or one of several selective culture media. Likewise, upper respiratory specimens intended for isolation of *Bordetella pertussis* should be inoculated for fresh Bordet-Gengou agar or equivalent at the bedside or in the clinic, unless an appropriate transport agar is used (see Chapter 8).

5. Whenever possible, obtain cultures before the administration of antibiotics.

Obtaining cultures before the use of antibiotics is particularly recommended for recovery of organisms that are usually highly susceptible to antibiotics, such as β-hemolytic streptococci from throat specimens, *N. gonorrhoeae* from genitourinary samples, or *Haemophilus influenzae* or *N. meningitidis* from cerebrospinal fluid (CSF). However, administration of antibiotics does not necessarily preclude recovery of other microorganisms from clinical specimens.

The action of many antibiotics may be bacteriostatic, not bactericidal; thus, microorganisms may be recovered when transferred to an environment devoid of antibiotic (a fresh culture medium). Also, the concentration of antibiotic at the site of infection may be lower than the minimal inhibitory concentration for the organism in question, and recovery in culture is not a problem. Therefore, one should always make an attempt to culture these sites, although the results must be interpreted accordingly or qualified in the written report.

6. The culture container must be properly labeled.

Each culture container must have a legible label, with the following minimum information:

Name _____

ID _____

Source _____

Doctor _____

Date/hour _____

Figure 2-3 (page 80) illustrates a culture tube with a label that has been properly filled out. Use the patient's full name and avoid initials. The identification number may be the hospital number, clinic or office number, home address, or social security number, depending on the circumstances. The physician's name or office title is necessary should consultation or early reporting be required. The specimen source should be noted so that special culture media can be selected if required. The date and time of collection should appear on the label to ensure that the specimen is processed within an acceptable length of time. Other potentially useful information includes the clinical diagnosis and the antibiotic treatment history of the patient.

SPECIMEN TRANSPORT

The primary objectives in the transport of diagnostic specimens, whether within the hospital or clinic, or externally by mail to a distant reference laboratory, is to maintain the sample as near its original state as possible with minimum deterioration and to minimize hazards to specimen handlers by using tightly fitting collection devices that are confined within proper protective containers. Adverse environmental conditions, such as exposure to extremes of heat and cold, rapid changes in pressure (during air transport), or excessive drying should be avoided. If prolonged delay is expected before the specimen can be processed (e.g.,

TABLE 2-1

TRANSPORT CONTAINERS FOR ANAEROBIC SPECIMENS

CONTAINER	RATIONALE OR DESCRIPTION	PRODUCT
Syringe and needle for aspiration	Fresh exudate or liquid specimens can be transported to the laboratory after bubbles are carefully expelled from the syringe and the tip of the needle is inserted into a sterile stopper. This procedure is valid only if the specimen can be transported to the laboratory without delay. This practice is under question because of the chance of HIV transmission from needlestick injury.	Standard equipment from several commercial laboratory supply companies
Tube or vial	Tube or vial contains semisolid holding medium, an atmosphere of 5% CO_2, a reducing agent, and reazurin indicator to give visual indication of anaerobiosis. The tube is used primarily for insertion of swab specimens; the vials are used for inoculation of liquid specimens.	Port-A-Cul System, Becton Dickinson Microbiology Systems, Cockeysville MD Anaerobic Transport Medium, Anaerobe Systems, San Jose CA Anaport and Anatube, Scott Laboratories, Fiskeville RI
Swab/plastic jacket system	Plastic tube or jacket is fitted with a swab and contains either Cary–Blair, Amies transport, or prereduced (PRAS) medium. The culturette system also includes a vial or chamber separated by a membrane that contains chemicals resulting in generation of CO_2 catalysts, and desiccants to "scavenger" any residual O_2 that may get into the system.	Anaerobic Culturette System, Becton Dickinson Microbiology Systems, Cockeysville MD PRAS Anaerobic Transport System, Remel Inc., Lenexa KS
Bio-bag or plastic pouch	Transparent plastic bag containing a CO_2-generating system, palladium catalyst cups, and an anaerobic indicator. The bag is sufficiently large to enclose an inoculated petri dish containing prereduced media, or a biochemical identification microtube tray such as for performing Minitek tests. Bag or pouch is sealed after inoculated plates have been inserted and the CO_2-generating system is activated. The advantage of these systems is that the plates can be directly observed through the thin, clear plastic of the bag for visualization of early growth of colonies.	Pouch System, Difco Laboratories, Detroit MI Bio-bag, Becton Dickinson Microbiology Systems, Cockeysville MD

more than 4 days), it is generally preferable to freeze the specimen at −70°. A −20° freezer may be used (it must be nondefrosting) if the periods of storage are brief.

Sputum samples that have been collected primarily for recovery of mycobacteria and fungi may be shipped without further treatment if collected in sterile propylene or polyethylene containers. To avoid breakage during transport, do not use glass containers.

Most fluid specimens, particularly urine samples, should be transported to the laboratory as quickly as possible. In a hospital setting, a maximum 2-hour time limit between collection and delivery of specimens to the laboratory is recommended.[4,29] This time limit poses a problem for specimens collected in physicians' offices. Urine transport containers containing a small amount of boric acid may be used if rapid transport is not possible. A holding or transport medium can be used for most other specimens, following the manufac-

turer's instructions. Stuart, Amies, and Carey-Blair transport media are most frequently used (Box 2-3).

This medium is essentially a solution of buffers with carbohydrates, peptones and other nutrients and growth factors excluded, designed to preserve the viability of bacteria during transport without allowing their multiplication. Sodium thioglycolate is added as a reducing agent to improve recovery of anaerobic bacteria, and the small amount of agar provides a semisolid consistency to prevent oxygenation and spillage during transport. Sodium borate solution can be recommended as a preservative for shipping specimens suspected of containing mycobacteria to distant laboratories.[56] Sucrose-phosphate-glutamate is a good transport buffer medium for recovery of certain viruses, such as herpesvirus. Warford and associates[67] report that a viral transport system, the Transporter (Bartels Immunodiagnostics, Bellevue WA) has also been successfully used in the recovery of viruses.

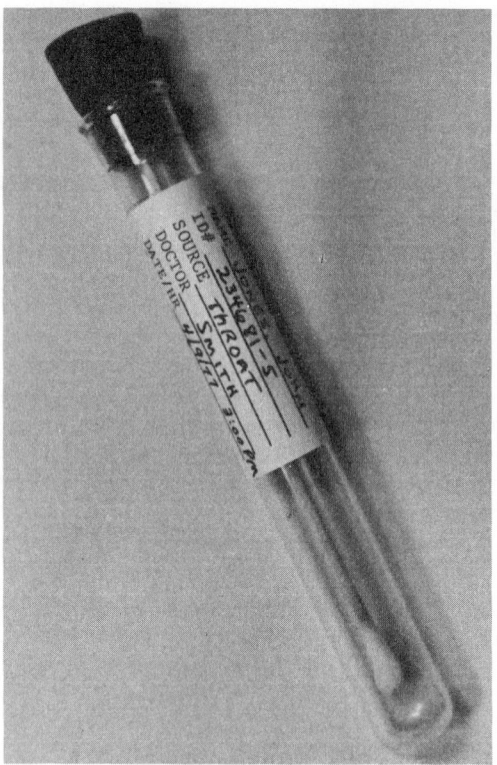

Figure 2-3.
A culture transport tube with a properly written identification label.

All microbiology specimens to be transported through the United States mail must be packaged under strict regulations specified by the Public Health Service. A complete list of etiologic agents that are included under these regulations is available on request from the CDC and is accompanied by a presentation of several recommended standard procedures published by the National Committee for Clinical Laboratory Standards.[48]

Specimens must be packaged to withstand shocks or pressure changes that may occur during handling

and cause the contents to leak. A leaking container not only predisposes the specimen to potential contamination, but may also expose mail handlers or personnel at the receiving site to pathogenic microorganisms. Figure 2-4 illustrates the proper technique for packaging and labeling etiologic agents. The primary container (test tube, vial) must be fitted with a watertight cap and surrounded by sufficient packing material to absorb the fluid contents should a leak occur. In turn, this container is placed in an secondary container, preferably constructed of metal, fitted with a screw-cap lid. The primary and secondary containers are then enclosed in an outer shipping carton constructed of corrugated fiberboard, cardboard, or Styrofoam.

Dry ice is considered a hazardous material. A shipping carton containing dry ice as a refrigerant for a specimen must be marked **"DRY ICE FROZEN MEDICAL SPECIMEN."** The packaging should be such that carbon dioxide gas can escape, preventing a buildup of pressure that could rupture the container. The dry ice should be placed outside the secondary container along with shock-absorbent material in such a manner that the secondary container does not become loose inside the outer container as the dry ice sublimates.

In addition to the address label, the outer container must also have the etiologic agents/biomedical material label (with its red logo against a white background) affixed as well as a notice to the carrier, as illustrated in Figure 2-5 (page 82).

SPECIMEN RECEIPT AND PRELIMINARY OBSERVATIONS

In most clinical laboratories, a special area is designated for the receipt of culture specimens. Because of the increasing possibility that laboratory personnel may incur a laboratory-acquired infection from specimens potentially contaminated with pathogenic bacteria or viruses, initial observations and handling should be performed under a laminar-flow hood. Personnel should wear protective clothing as appropriate—laboratory coats, rubber gloves and, in some instances, surgical masks. Previously, these precautions were taken only for specimens carrying hazard labels; however, because it is not possible to determine if a patient may be harboring a transmittable disease, or if a given sample may contain a highly contagious pathogen, it is prudent to practice special care when handling all specimens.

The processing of specimens includes the following: 1) the entry of essential data into a log book or computer terminal; 2) visual examination and determination of whether all criteria for acceptance are met (see section on criteria for specimen rejection immediately below); and 3) for certain specimens, the microscopic examination of direct mounts or stained smears to establish a presumptive diagnosis.

BOX 2-3. STUART'S TRANSPORT MEDIUM	
Sodium chloride	3 g
Potassium chloride	0.2 g
Disodium phosphate	1.25 g
Monopotassium phosphate	0.2 g
Sodium thioglycollate	1.0 g
Calcium chloride, 1% aqueous	10.0 g
Magnesium chloride, 1% aqueous	10.0 g
Agar	4.0 g
Distilled water to equal	1.0 L
pH = 7.3	

COLOR PLATES

CHAPTERS 2–6

GRAM STAIN EVALUATION OF SPUTUM SMEARS

The quality of sputum samples can be evaluated by counting the relative numbers of squamous epithelial cells and segmented neutrophils per low-power field in a gram-stained smear. The presence of squamous epithelial cells indicates contamination with oropharyngeal secretions. In contrast, bacterial pneumonia will produce large numbers of segmented neutrophils that can be detected in sputum samples. The following are photomicrographs of Gram-stained smears of sputum samples illustrating the relative presence of the various cellular components.

A. Low-power view of Gram-stained sputum smear revealing full field of squamous epithelial cells and absence of segmented neutrophils. This specimen represents saliva, would give a low quality score, and is not acceptable for culture.

B. The squamous epithelial cell shown here is heavily colonized with gram-positive bacteria. The overgrowth of bacterial cells in sputum specimens generally indicates that the specimen has been delayed in transit to the laboratory and any semiquantitative results will be of little value.

C. This Gram-stained sputum smear shows a mixture of squamous cells and segmented neutrophils. The presence of segmented neutrophils indicates that a nidus of infection exists somewhere in the respiratory tract; however, the squamous epithelial cells indicate contamination with upper respiratory tract secretions. This type of sputum smear is difficult to interpret because upper respiratory tract infections cannot be distinguished from lower respiratory tract infections.

D. Full field of neutrophils and virtual absence of squamous epithelial cells. This is a high-quality sputum sample that provides a good chance for producing relevant results.

E. Higher-power view of sample in **D** revealing scattered segmented neutrophils against a background of pink-staining mucous threads.

F. Smear of an induced sputum sample stained with Diff Quick, illustrating several ciliated, columnar epithelial cells. These cells have origin in the lower respiratory tract and, when present in a sputum smear such as seen here, indicate a high-quality specimen from which relevant results can be potentially obtained.

G. High-power view of a Gram-stained sputum specimen illustrates the morphology of a ciliated columnar epithelial cell. Note the distinct cilia atop the flared terminal end of this eosinophilic-staining columnar epithelial cell.

H. Toluidine blue stain of an induced sputum specimen revealing mononuclear inflammatory cells consistent with alveolar macrophages. As in columnar epithelial cells, alveolar macrophages have origin deep within the lower respiratory tract and their presence in sputum samples increases the significance of any bacterial species recovered.

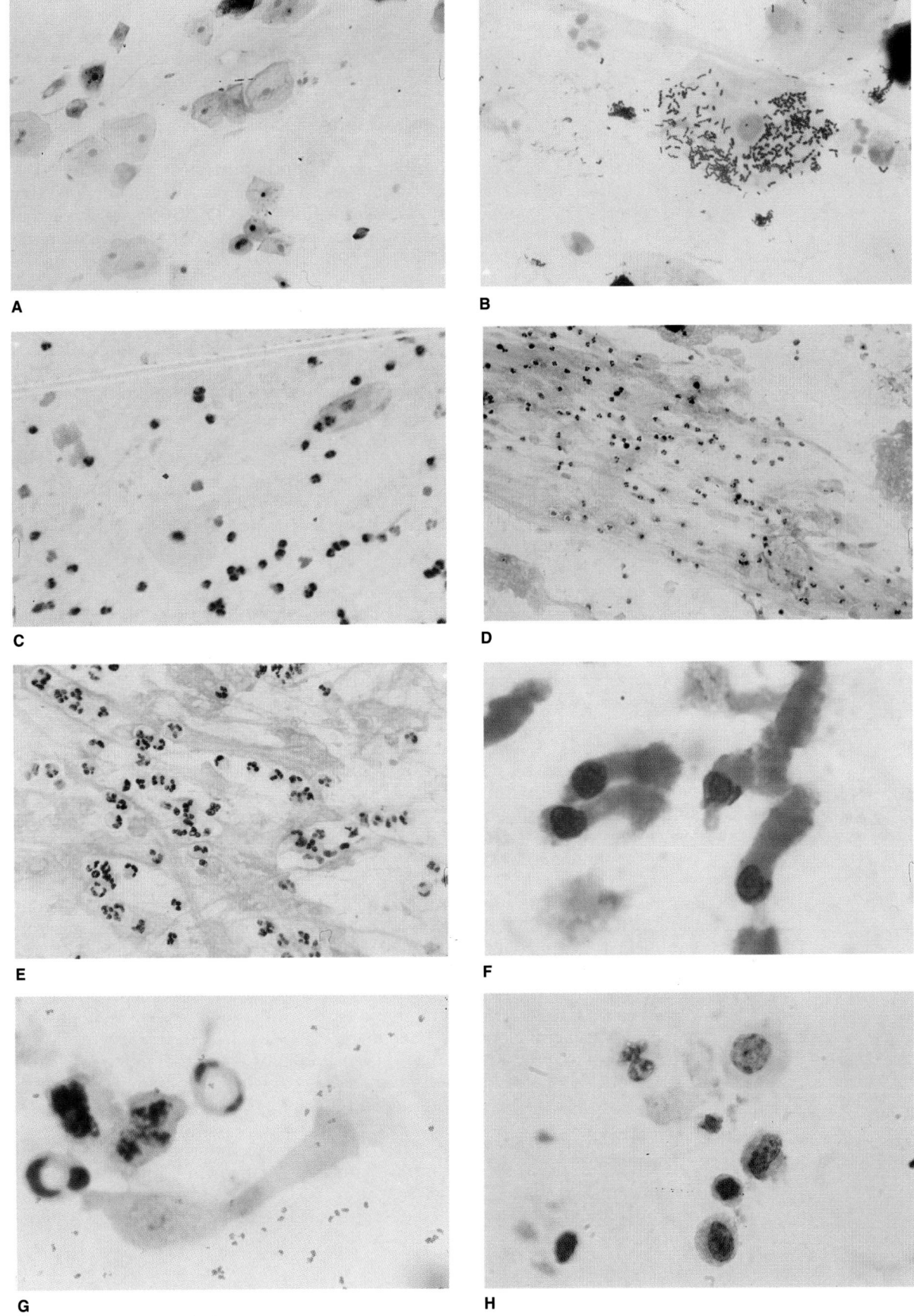

A

B

C

D

E

F

G

H

MISCELLANEOUS STAINS USED IN MICROBIOLOGY

Because many of the microbes of medical importance have refractive indices near that of water, stains are needed to make possible their detection and study. A variety of stains have been developed over the years, each designed to highlight internal organelles or specific components of the cell wall. The following are illustrations of selected stains and some of their applications.

A. *Gram's stain.* The most common stain used in the microbiology laboratory is designed to differentiate between those bacteria that can retain crystal violet dye and appear deep blue-black after decolorization (gram-positive) from those that cannot and stain red (gram-negative). Illustrated here is a Gram-stained preparation revealing red-staining, gram-negative bacilli.

B. *Acid-fast.* This stain is commonly used to demonstrate a variety of acid-fast organisms, including *Nocardia* species in sputum specimens and *Cryptosporidium* oocysts in fecal samples. Shown here are clusters of red-staining, acid-fast bacilli in a liver biopsy specimen of a patient with AIDS. The organisms stain red with the acid-fast stain, and those shown here were identified as belonging to the *Mycobacterium avium-intracellulare* complex.

C. *Direct fluorescence.* Fluorescent dyes (rhodamine and auramine) react directly with the cell wall of mycobacteria. Fluorescein-conjugated antibodies are also available to demonstrate a variety of microbial agents using the direct fluorescent antibody test. Shown here are yellow-green, fluorescing mycobacteria in a sputum concentrate from a patient with pulmonary tuberculosis.

D. *Acridine orange.* This rapid fluorescent stain is used to demonstrate bacterial forms in direct smears and mounts of biologic fluids. It is particularly useful in detecting gram-negative bacteria in positive blood culture broths, which may be missed in Gram stains because of the deep red-staining debris in the background. Shown here is a long, rod-shaped bacterium, with a characteristic orange glow, when microscopically observed with a fluorescence microscope.

E. *Methylene blue.* This nonspecific, rapid stain is used to demonstrate bacteria and other microbes in direct smears. Illustrated here are bacilli that have taken the blue stain. One important application is in the detection of bacteria in direct smears of cerebrospinal fluid in cases of suspected acute meningitis, particularly gram-negative species, that may be obscured by the red background staining of the proteinaceous material.

F. *Calcofluor white.* This autofluorescent whitening agent has the property of coupling with carbohydrate moieties in the cell walls of fungi. Shown here are brilliant yellow-green staining hyphae in a direct calcofluor white-stained mount as observed with a fluorescent microscope.

G. *Wright-Giemsa.* This stain is commonly used to demonstrate the cellular elements in peripheral blood and bone marrow smears. In microbiology, the stain is most commonly used to detect intraerythrocytic (plasmodia, babesiae) and exoerythrocytic (trypanosomes, microfilaria) parasites, chlamydial inclusions, and, as shown here, the intracellular yeast forms of *Histoplasma capsulatum*.

H. *Periodic acid–Schiff (PAS).* This general stain is used to demonstrate polysaccharide-rich cell walls. It has specific applications in detecting fungi in tissue sections and smears. Recognized here is the fruiting body of *Aspergillus* species in an aspirate of a fungus ball lesion of the lung surrounded by red-staining *Aspergillus* spores.

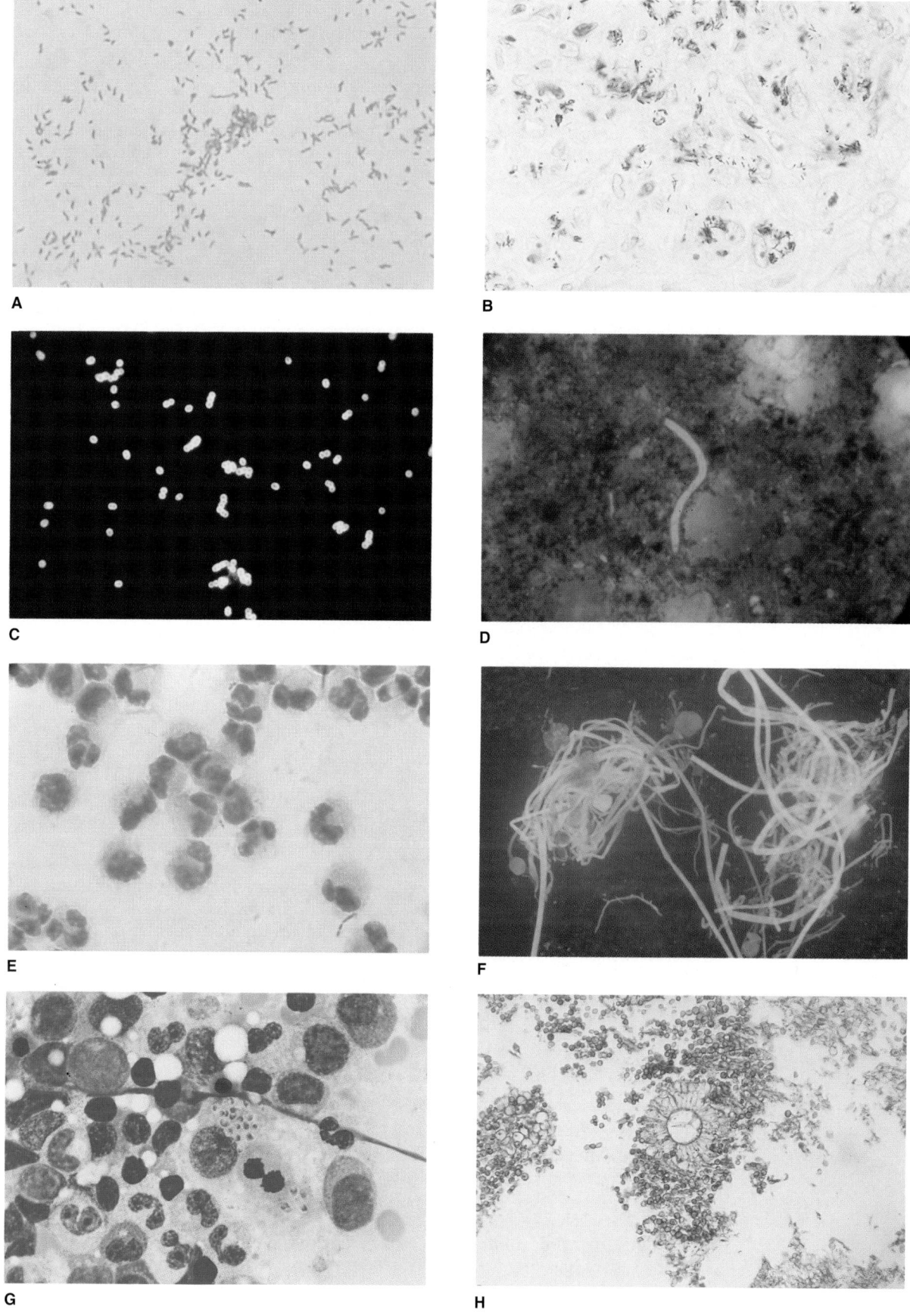

A

B

C

D

E

F

G

H

PRESUMPTIVE BACTERIAL IDENTIFICATION BASED ON OBSERVING COLONIAL
MORPHOLOGY

Microbiologists use various characteristics of bacterial colonies that grow on the
surface of agar culture media to make a presumptive identification of the group
or genus and as a guide in selecting differential tests to determine the final
species identification. Size, shape, consistency, color, and pigment production
by the colonies, as well as the presence of hemolytic reactions on blood agar, are
the criteria commonly used.

A. Blood agar plate on which are growing round, yellow-white, entire, convex,
nonhemolytic colonies of *Staphylococcus* species.

B. Colonies growing on blood agar illustrating distinct zones of β-hemolysis
around the colonies. The relation between the size of the colonies and the zones
of hemolysis is used to differentiate between certain species. Shown here are
Streptococcus species, which commonly have a lower ratio of colony size to hemolytic zones, in contrast with *Staphylococcus* species, in which the relative size
of the colonies is generally larger.

C. Blood agar plate demonstrates the greenish discoloration of the agar, characteristic of α-hemolysis. Growing on this plate are tiny, clear colonies of viridans
streptococci, with larger zones of α-hemolysis.

D. Opaque, dull gray, somewhat moist colonies growing on blood agar (*left*) and
MacConkey agar (*right*), suggestive of one of the members of the family *Enterobacteriaceae*. The growth on MacConkey agar shows no red pigmentation, indicating that the organism is a non-lactose fermenter. The bacteria shown here are
Salmonella species.

E. Dry, wrinkled colonies of a *Bacillus* species. Similar-appearing, wrinkled
colonies are also seen with *Pseudomonas stutzeri*.

F. Yellow-pigmented colonies on blood agar. Pigment production is an important
feature in the differential identification of many bacterial species, particularly
those belonging to several groups of nonfermentative bacilli. The colonies
shown here are those of *Flavobacterium* species after 48 hours of incubation, with
the last 24 hours of incubation being at room temperature. The intensity of pigment is often accentuated after additional incubation at room temperature.

G. Distinctly mucoid colonies growing on blood agar. The mucoid consistency of
colonies is generally secondary to the production of capsules, a protective
mechanism used by several bacterial species in defense against phagocytosis.
Pseudomonas species, *Klebsiella pneumoniae*, *Streptococcus pneumoniae*, and *Cryptococcus neoformans* are among the more commonly recovered microbial species
producing mucoid colonies. The colony shown here is *Streptococcus pneumoniae*.

H. Grey semitranslucent colonies of *Eikenella corrodens* growing on blood agar.
Note the halo appearance around the colonies illustrating the "pitting" characteristic of the species.

I. Grey, smooth, semitransparent colonies of *Capnocytophaga ochracea*. Note the
mistlike extension of the colonies illustrating the gliding motility characteristic
of *Capnocytophaga* species.

J. White, dry, chalky colony of *Nocardia* species. *Streptomyces* species produce
similar-appearing colonies. These presumptive identifications can be confirmed
if the musty basement odor characteristic of these species can be detected.

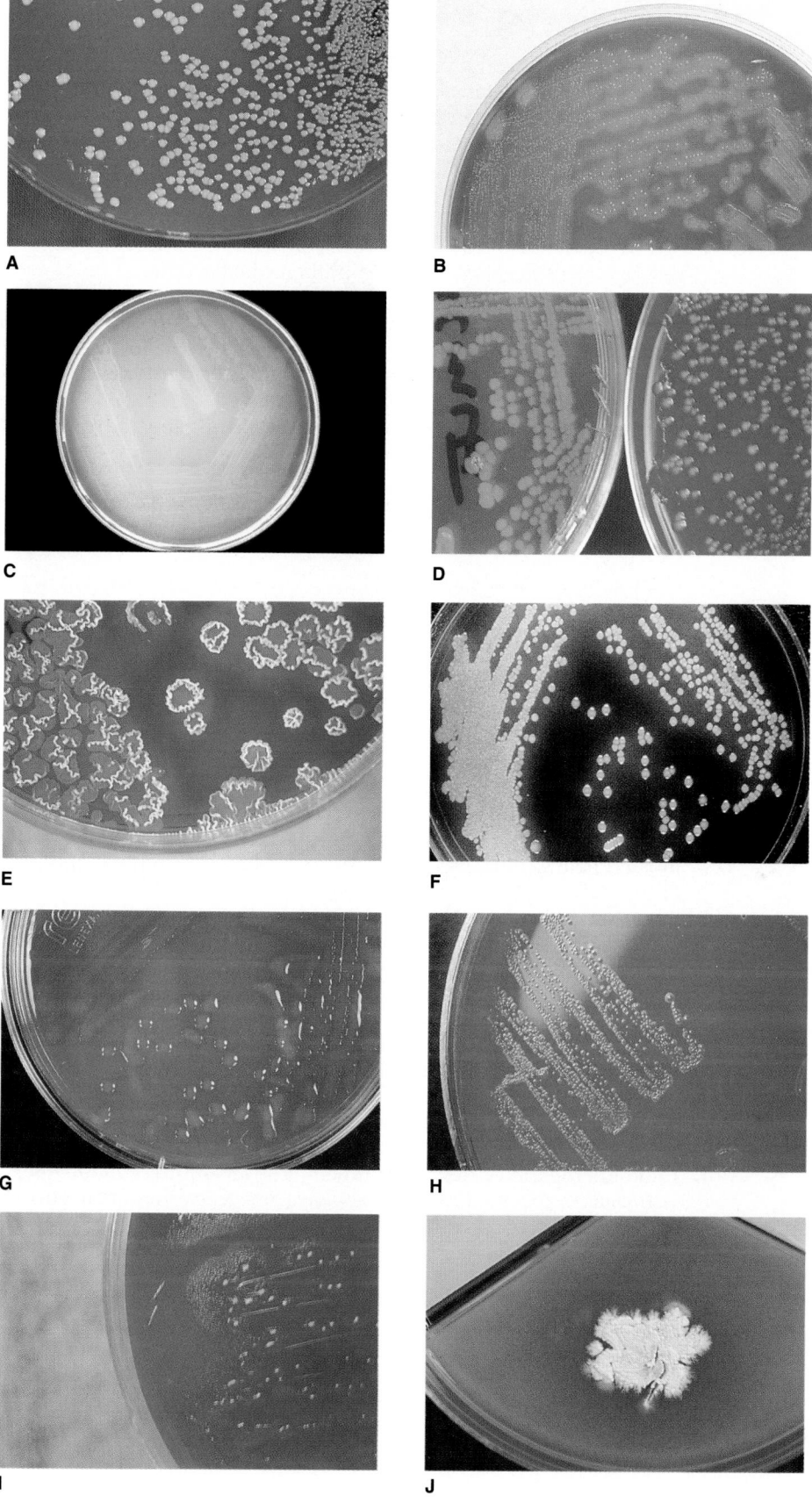

A

B

C

D

E

F

G

H

I

J

PRESUMPTIVE BACTERIAL IDENTIFICATION BASED ON OBSERVING MICROSCOPIC
CELLULAR MORPHOLOGY IN STAINED SMEAR PREPARATIONS

Gram stain of bacteria, in addition to other staining techniques, is one of the
more important determinations in the presumptive identification of microorganisms. The morphology of the bacterial cells, their arrangement, and their
staining characteristics are often distinctive enough to allow a presumptive
identification in a Gram-stained smear. The microscopic characteristics suggestive of several groups of bacteria are included in this plate.

A. Relatively slender, gram-positive bacilli arranged in Chinese letter pattern suggesting one of the coryneform (diphtheroids) bacteria.

B. Gram-positive, spore-forming bacilli. The aerobic spore formers belong to the
genus *Bacillus*; the anaerobic spore formers belong to the genus *Clostridium*.
Illustrated here are spore-forming cells of *Bacillus sphaericus*.

C. Direct Gram's stain of a purulent exudate illustrating gram-positive cocci
arranged in small clusters, characteristic of *Staphylococcus* species.

D. Direct smear of a necrotic exudate from a case of myonecrosis. The tiny, gram-
positive cocci seen in this photomicrograph are streptococci.

E. Direct Gram's stain of a smear of purulent sputum demonstrating gram-positive
diplococci, characteristic of *Streptococcus pneumoniae*.

F. Purulent exudate form the chest wall of a patient with acute, suppurative
empyema. Against the background of segmented neutrophils are numerous
gram-positive, branching bacilli. *Actinomyces* species and *Nocardia* species can
produce a picture similar to this; however, in this case, a pure culture of *Bifidobacterium* species was recovered in anaerobic culture.

G. Gram-stained preparation of a direct smear of urine sediment from a case of
acute cystitis. Note the several gram-negative bacilli amid the background segmented neutrophils. *Escherichia coli* was recovered in pure culture.

H. Gram-stained preparation of a direct smear prepared from a purulent urethral
exudate of a sexually active male, illustrating the intracellular, gram-negative,
diplococci characteristic of *Neisseria gonorrhoeae*. The bacterial cells are paler staining in this photograph than normally seen by direct microscopic examination.

I. Photomicrograph of a sputum smear illustrating a few segmented neutrophils
in the background, and a diffuse infiltration with many short, gram-negative
bacilli some of which appear to be surrounded by a halo. *Klebsiella pneumoniae*
grew out in culture.

J. Photomicrogaph of delicate, branching gram-positive filaments suggestive of
Actinomyces species. *Propionibacterium acnes* grew out in culture.

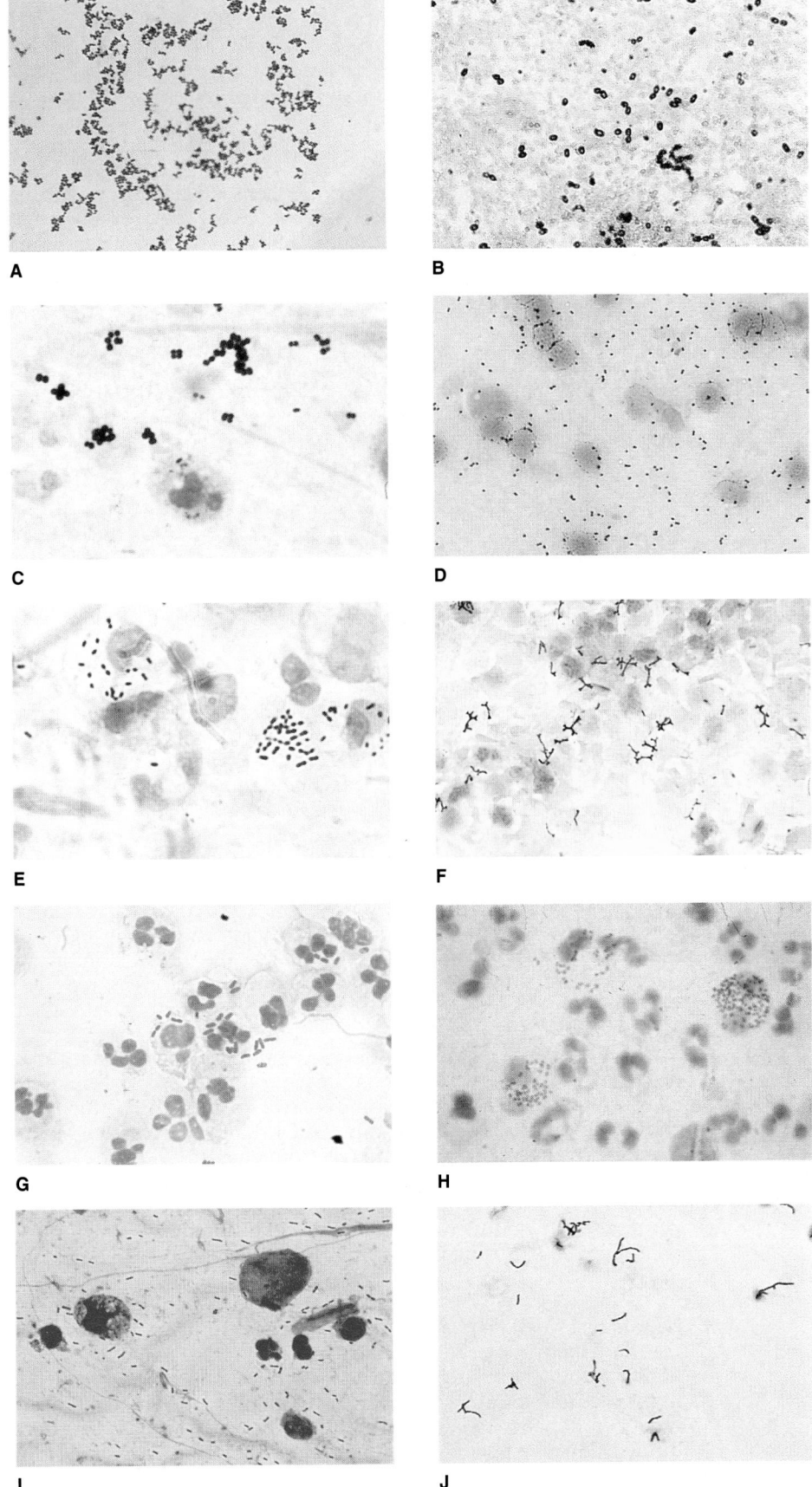

A

B

C

D

E

F

G

H

I

J

PRESUMPTIVE IDENTIFICATION OF THE *ENTEROBACTERIACEAE*

Presumptive identification of the *Enterobacteriaceae* is based on the appearance of colonies growing on primary isolation media and on an assessment of certain biochemical reactions. By definition, for an organism to be classified within the *Enterobacteriaceae*, it must ferment glucose, producing acid or acid and gas; reduce nitrates to nitrites; and exhibit no cytochrome oxidase activity.

A. A Gram stain of a sputum smear showing characteristic short, plump, gram-negative rods that are typical for members of the *Enterobacteriaceae*. Also depicted are two polymorphonuclear leukocytes, suggesting an on-going infectious process in this patient. In this case the culture confirmed the organism to be *K. pneumoniae*.

B. Mixed culture showing 24-hour growth on blood agar of two morphotypes of large gram-negative rods and a third morphotype of a smaller organism that can be suspected to be a gram-positive species. One morphotype can be seen as large, shiny, white colonies while the other morphotype appears as large, grey colonies with irregular edges. Both these colony types can be suspected to be gram-negative rods typical for members of the *Enterobacteriaceae*. Also present are many small, white, entire colonies typical of one of the gram-positive cocci.

C. Large, mucoid, glistening, pink colonies on MacConkey agar typical of many *Klebsiella* and *Enterobacter* species. By their appearance alone, these colonies can be suspected to be one of the species of *Enterobacteriaceae*.

D. Swarming pattern of a motile strain of *Proteus* species on chocolate agar plate.

E. Series of Kligler iron agar (KIA) slants illustrating several reaction patterns. Tube on the far left illustrates an acid (yellow) slant and acid (yellow) butt, indicating both glucose and lactose fermentation. Also note the space at the bottom of the tube and the split in the agar in the middle of the tube which indicates gas (CO_2) production by the organism. Copious amounts of CO_2, such as seen here, are usually produced only by organisms belonging to Tribe V (*Klebsielleae*). The second tube from the left shows an acid/acid reaction but without the presence of gas, typical of the type of reaction seen with *E. coli*. The third tube from the left illustrates an alkaline (red) slant/acid butt characteristic of a nonlactose fermenter. The fourth tube illustrates a red slant/black butt indicating hydrogen sulfide (H_2S) production. When this type of reaction is seen with an oxidase-negative organism, the assumption is made that the butt portion of the tube is acid (yellow), indicating glucose fermentation even though the yellow color is masked due to the H_2S production. The reaction in the fifth tube (*far right*) red/red is typical of nonfermenting gram-negative bacilli that ferment neither lactose nor glucose.

F. Three tubes of purple broth media containing Durham tubes to demonstrate gas formation. The two tubes on the right illustrate acid from glucose (yellow color) compared with the negative control on the left. The tube on the far right shows the collection of gas within the Durham tube characteristic of an organism that produces both acid and gas from glucose.

G. Cytochrome oxidase test revealing a positive purple color reaction (*left*) compared with a negative reaction on the right (no blue color within 10 seconds—see Chart 16). Any organism giving a positive reaction can be excluded from the family *Enterobacteriaceae*.

H. Nitrate test media containing Durham tubes to demonstrate nitrogen gas formation. The tube on the left shows a positive (red) reaction after addition of α-naphthylamine and sulfanilic acid. The test organism had reduced the nitrates in the medium to nitrites, which reacted with the reagents to form the red pigment p-sulfobenzene-azo-α-naphthylamine (see Chart 53). The tube in the middle also depicts a positive nitrate reaction, but in this case all the nitrate was first reduced to nitrite and then further reduced to nitrogen gas indicated by the collection of gas within the Durham tube. Since there is no nitrite in the tube, there is no red color when the reagents are added. The tube on the far right shows no red color and no gas and depicts a negative test for nitrate reduction.

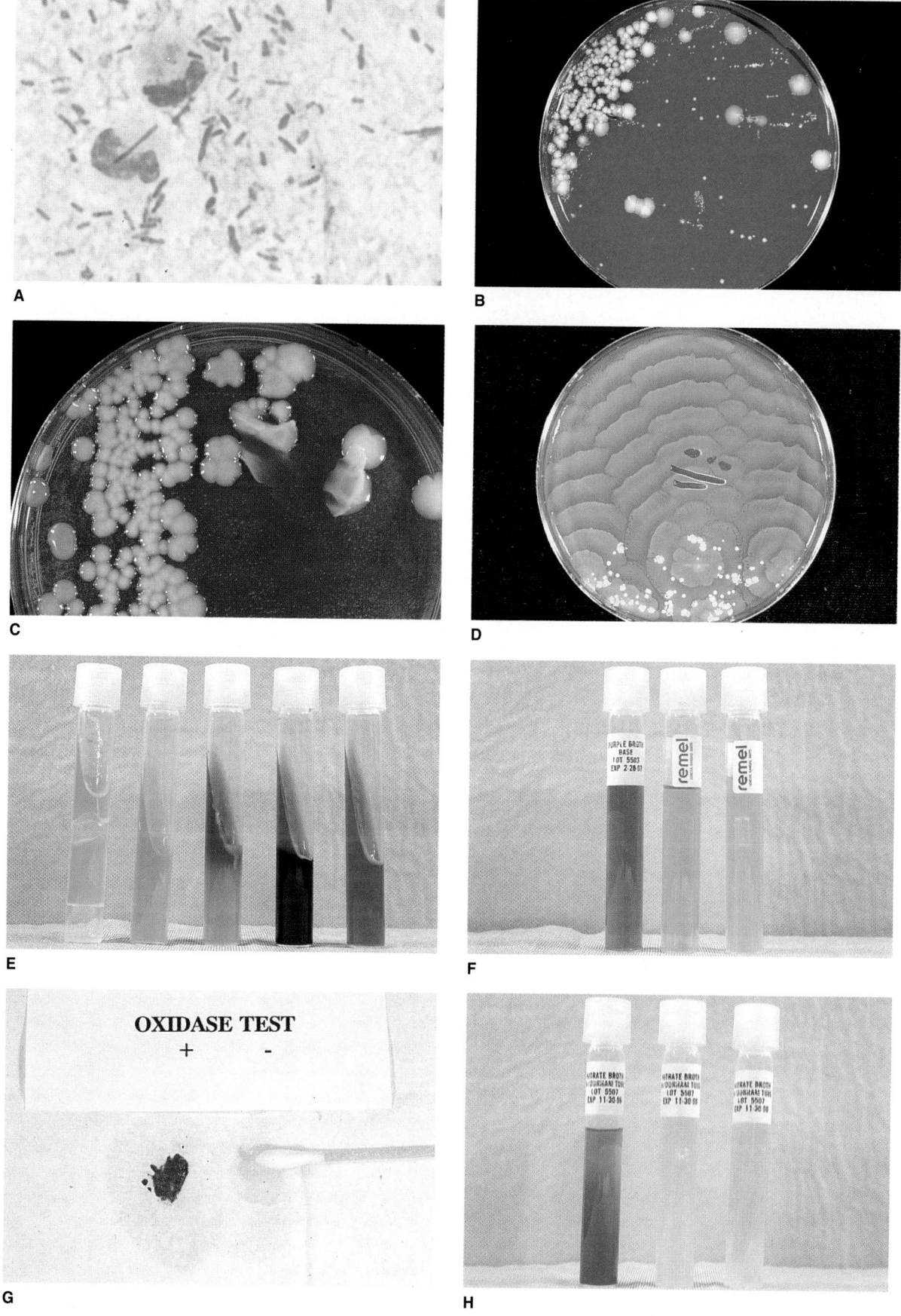

A

B

C

D

E

F

G

OXIDASE TEST

+   −

H

APPEARANCE OF THE *ENTEROBACTERIACEAE* COLONIES ON MACCONKEY AND EMB AGARS

MacConkey and eosin methylene blue (EMB) agars are two commonly used selective primary isolation media for presumptive differentiation of lactose-fermenting from non-lactose-fermenting members of the *Enterobacteriaceae*. On MacConkey agar, lactose-fermenting colonies appear red because of the acid conversion of the indicator, neutral red. On EMB, a green metallic sheen is produced by avid lactose fermenters when production of acid is sufficient to lower the pH to approximately 4.5 or below.

A. Surface of MacConkey agar with 24-hour growth of red, lactose-fermenting colonies. The diffuse red color in the agar surrounding the colonies is produced by organisms that avidly ferment lactose, producing large quantities of mixed acids, and cause precipitation of the bile salts in the medium surrounding the colonies (*eg, Escherichia coli*).

B. Surface of MacConkey agar illustrating both red, lactose-fermenting colonies and smaller, clear non-lactose-fermenting colonies.

C. and D. Surface of EMB agar plates illustrating the green sheen produced by avid lactose- (or sucrose) fermenting members of the *Enterobacteriaceae*. Most strains of *E. coli* produce colonies with this appearance on EMB agar, and since *E. coli* is among the most frequent isolates from clinical specimens, the appearance of such colonies can often serve as presumptive identification of *E. coli*. However, characteristics other than the production of a green sheen on EMB must be assessed before an organism can be definitively identified as *E. coli*, since other lactose-fermenting *Enterobacteriaceae* can have a similar appearance.

E. and F. Surface of EMB agar plates illustrating a mixed culture of *E. coli* (green sheen colonies) and *Shigella* species. Most *Shigella* species do not ferment lactose and, thus produce nonpigmented, semitranslucent colonies on EMB agar. Other species incapable of fermenting lactose produce colonies that appear similar to those illustrated in these photographs.

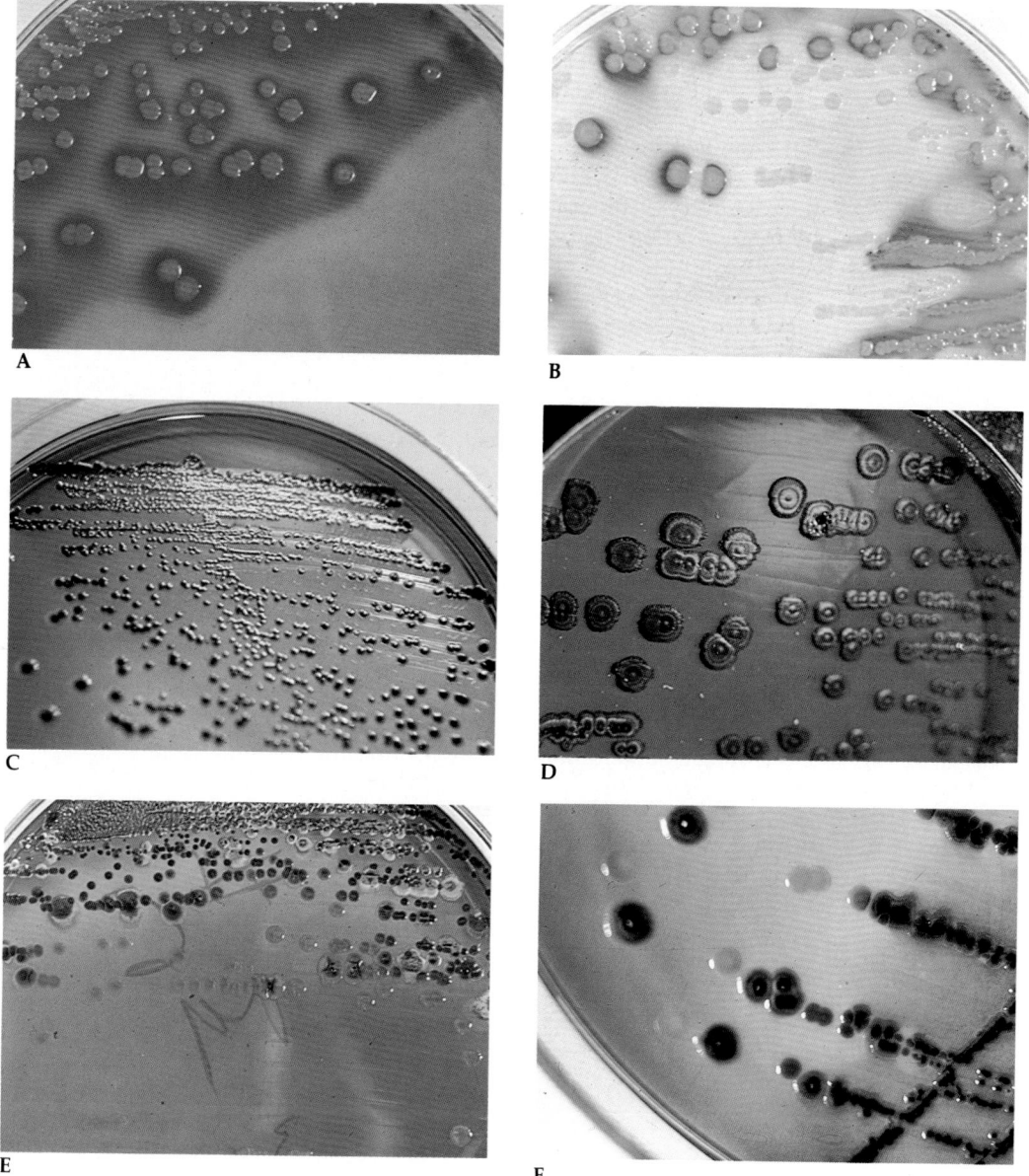

A

B

C

D

E

F

APPEARANCE OF THE *ENTEROBACTERIACEAE* ON XLD AND HE AGAR PLATES

Several types of media more selective than MacConkey or EMB agars are commonly used in clinical microbiology laboratories for recovering select members of the *Enterobacteriaceae*. Xylose-lysine-deoxycholate (XLD) and Hektoen enteric (HE) agars are most commonly used; highly selective media such as bismuth sulfate agar are used only for special applications. These media not only have the capability of separating lactose from non-lactose fermenters but can detect hydrogen sulfide (H_2S)-producing microorganisms as well.

A. Surface of XLD agar illustrating yellow conversion of the medium from acid-producing colonies of *E. coli*.

B. Non-lactose-fermenting colonies (no acid conversion of the medium) of *Salmonella* species growing on the surface of XLD agar. Note the black pigmentation of some of the colonies, indicating H_2S production.

C. Photograph illustrating an XLD agar plate inoculated with a 50/50 mixture of *E. coli* and *Salmonella* species. Note the preponderant growth of the *Salmonella* species (red colonies) compared with the few yellow, lactose-fermenting colonies of *E. coli* that have been effectively inhibited. The distinct pink halo around the *Salmonella* colonies indicates the decarboxylation of lysine, a helpful feature in differentiating *Salmonella* species (positive) from H_2S-producing colonies of *Proteus* species.

D. XLD agar plate inoculated with an H_2S-producing strain of a *Proteus* species. Note the lack of a light pink halo around the colonies, indicating the lack of lysine decarboxylation (compare with the colonies shown in **C**).

E. Surface of HE agar illustrating yellow acid production by colonies of *E. coli*.

F. Surface of HE agar illustrating the faint green (colorless) colonies of non-lactose-fermenting members of the *Enterobacteriaceae*.

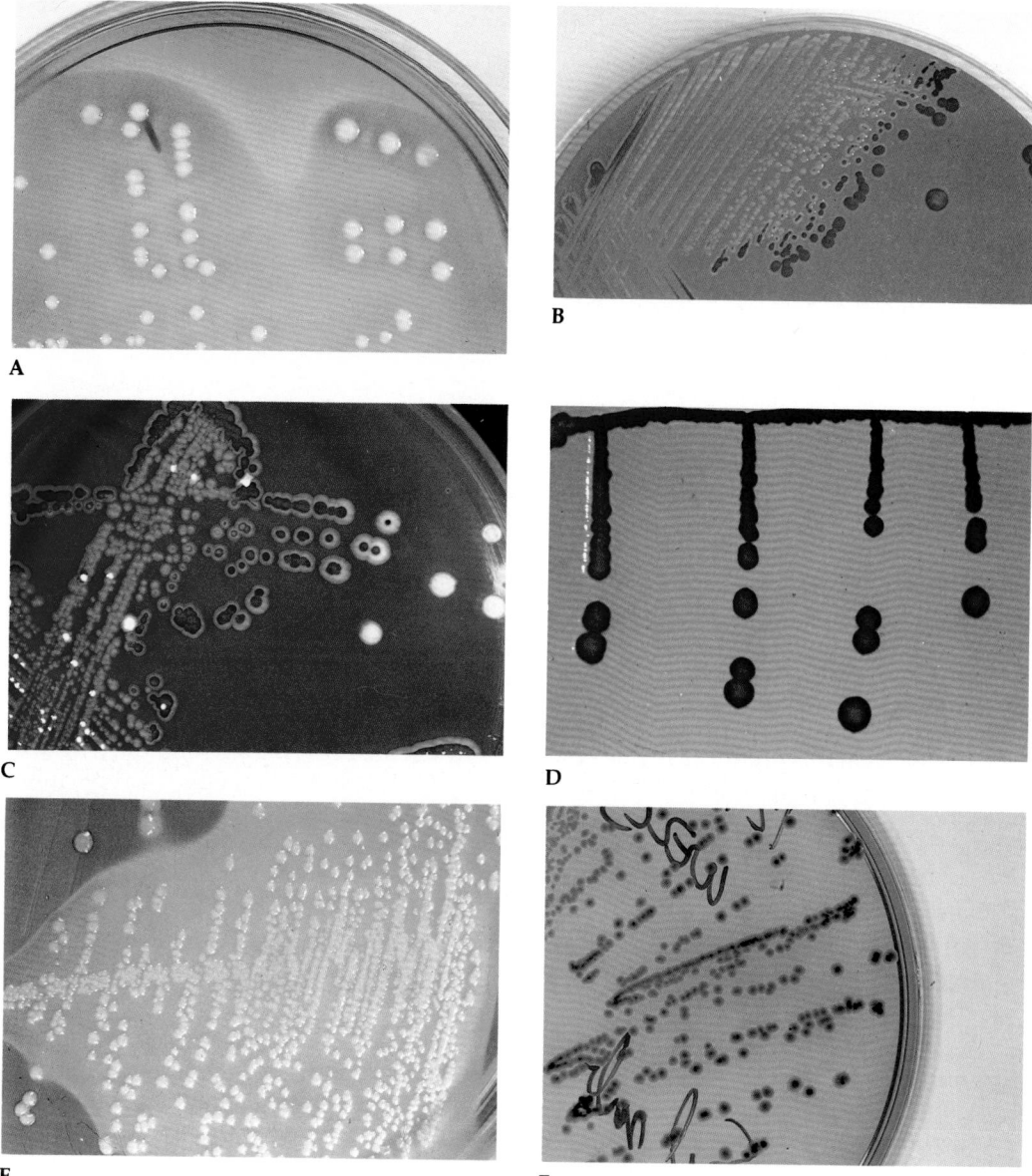

A

B

C

D

E

F

DIFFERENTIAL CHARACTERISTICS OF THE *ENTEROBACTERIACEAE*

A. *Ortho*-nitrophenyl-β-D-galactopyranoside (ONPG) test showing a positive (yellow) reaction (*left*) compared with the negative control (*right*). A positive reaction indicates that the organism is capable of producing β-galactosidase, an enzyme required for the initial degradation of lactose, releasing the yellow colored *ortho*-nitrophenol.

B. Sulfide indole motility (SIM) semisolid agar tube (*right*) and Kligler iron agar (KIA) slant (*left*), illustrating the differences in sensitivity in detecting hydrogen sulfide (H_2S) by different media. The diffuse delicate blackening in the SIM tube is produced by a motile, weak H_2S-producing organism (in this case *S. typhi*). Note that the H_2S produced in the less sensitive KIA tube appears only in the middle of the tube at the interface of the slant and butt and is the typical appearance of *S. typhi* in this medium.

C. and D. Four tubes demonstrating the indole (I), methyl red (MR), Voges-Proskauer (VP), and citrate (C) tests. These four tests when performed together constitute the classic IMViC reactions. The formation of indole from tryptophan is indicated by a red color upon the addition of Kovac's reagent (*far left tube*, **C**). The development of a red color in the MR tube indicates a drop in pH to 4.4 or below, indicative of strong mixed acid fermenters (*second tube from left*, **C**). A red color in the VP tube indicates the presence of acetoin (acetylmethylcarbinol) formed from pyruvate in the butylene glycol metabolic pathway (*third tube from left*, **D**). Growth on the slant of Simmon's citrate agar and conversion of the bromthymol blue indicator to an alkaline blue color indicates that the organism can utilize sodium citrate as the sole source of carbon (*last tube on right*, **D**). **C** shows the reactions for *E. coli* ($++--$). **D** shows the reactions for *Klebsiella/Enterobacter* ($--++$).

E. Two tubes on left show negative (light yellow) and positive (dark green) phenylalanine deaminase reactions. The green color is produced by the reaction between the $FeCl_3$ reagent and phenylpyruvic acid in the medium, resulting from the deamination of phenylalanine (see Chart 60). The three tubes on the right are Christensen's urea agar slants. The third in from the right shows a strong positive (red color throughout the medium indicating an alkaline reaction from degradation of urea), compared with the negative control on the far right (yellow color throughout). The reaction in the second tube from the right (red color in slant only) is produced by organisms such as *Klebsiella* species and certain *Enterobacter* species that are weak urease producers.

F. Four tubes containing Moeller decarboxylase medium covered with a layer of mineral oil to effect an anaerobic environment (see Chart 18). Reading from left to right: a growth control tube devoid of amino acid (growth is indicated by conversion to a yellow color due to the fermentation of glucose in the medium), arginine, lysine, ornithine. The bromcresol purple indicator is yellow at an acid pH and purple at an alkaline pH. Thus, any tube that appears purple indicates an alkaline pH, the reaction produced by organisms that can decarboxylate the amino acid contained in the medium. The organism pictured here is arginine negative and lysine and ornithine positive and is the typical reaction seen with *E. aerogenes*.

G. Lysine iron agar (LIA) is used to differentiate enteric organisms based on their ability to decarboxylate or deaminate lysine and to form H_2S. Organisms that decarboxylate lysine produce an alkaline (purple) reaction in the butt of the tube (*middle tube*). Organisms that deaminate lysine produce a red slant over an acid (yellow) butt (*tube on far left*). Bacteria that produce H_2S cause blackening of the medium mainly in the middle and the butt of the tube (*also seen in tube on far left*). The tube on the far left is lysine deaminase positive and lysine decarboxylase negative. The middle tube is lysine deaminase negative and lysine decarboxylase positive. The tube on the far right is negative for both lysine deaminase and lysine decarboxylase.

H. Tubes of motility medium. Motile organisms will show diffuse growth away from the line of inoculation (*left tube*); nonmotile organisms show growth only along the stab line (*right tube*). Also available is motility medium to which 2,3,5-triphenyltetrazolium chloride (TTC) is added. Growth of organisms capable of reducing TTC will appear red along the stab line as well as in the area into which the cells have migrated, making it easier to differentiate between motile and nonmotile bacteria. (Photo courtesy of Health and Education Resources, Inc., Bethesda, MD)

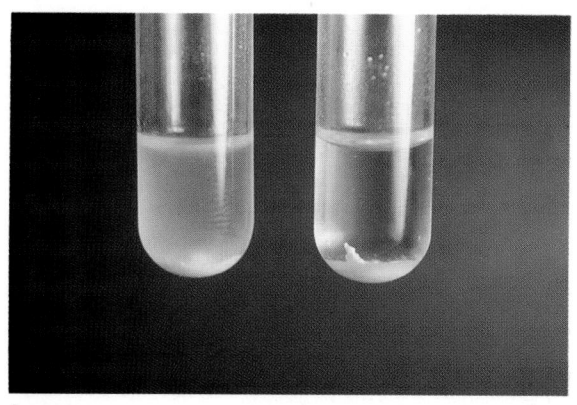

A

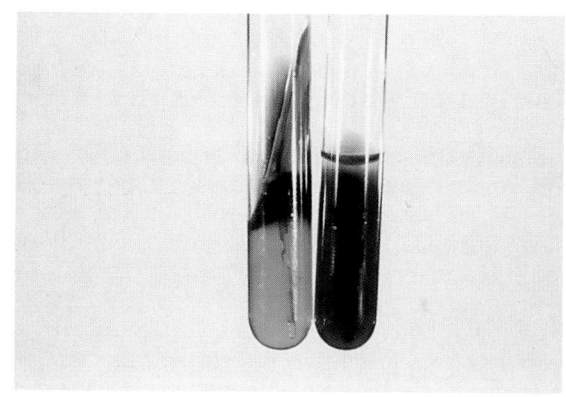

B

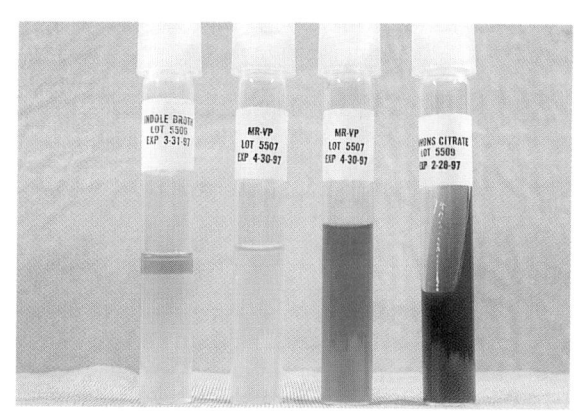

C

D

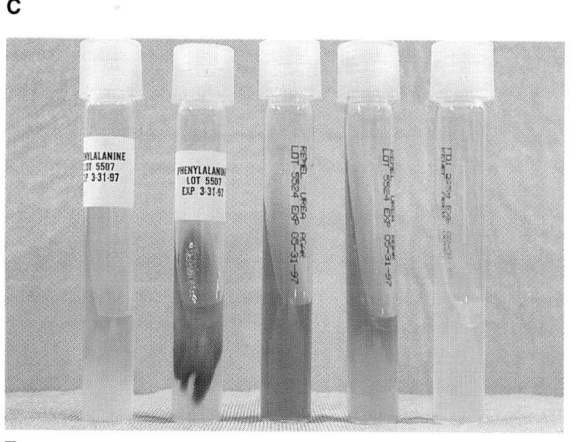

E

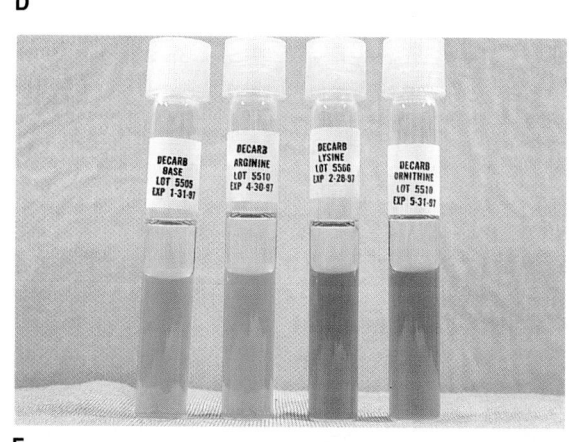

F

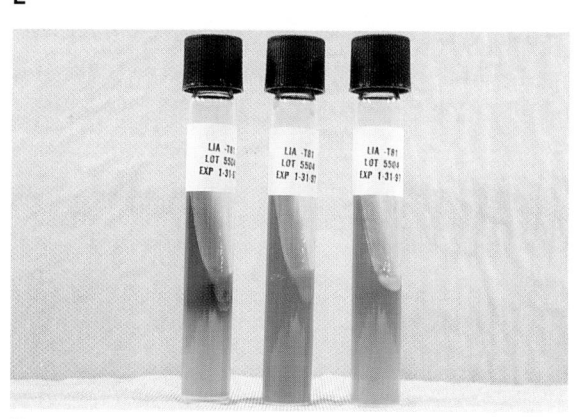

G

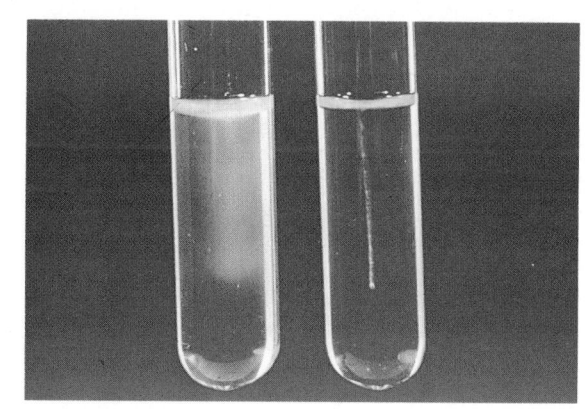

H

PACKAGED MICROBIAL IDENTIFICATION SYSTEMS

A number of packaged microbial identification systems are currently available that contain stable reagents and media designed for determining biochemical characteristics.

A. API 20-E strips illustrating method of inoculation and the appearance of strip following inoculation and incubation. A suspension of the organism to be tested is transferred with a pipette into each of the 20 media compartments. Color reactions are read after 18 to 24 hours of incubation at 35°C. The manufacturer supplies worksheets for recording the visual interpretation of the color reactions, which are then converted into a seven-digit biotype number.

B. The BBL Crystal Enteric/Nonfermenter identification system contains a lid with 30 dehydrated substrates on the tips of the plastic prongs. A test suspension is prepared and added to all 30 wells in the base unit. The lid is then aligned with the base and snapped in place whereby the test inoculum rehydrates the dried substrates and initiates test reactions. After incubation, panels are read upside-down using the BBL Crystal light box. The wells are examined for color changes and a 10-digit profile number is generated and entered on a PC in which the BBL Crystal Electronic codebook has been installed, to obtain the identification.

C. The IDS Rapid onE system consists of a plastic tray with 18 reaction cavities. Reaction cavities contain dehydrated reactants, and the tray allows the simultaneous inoculation of each cavity with a predetermined amount of inoculum. Test 18 is bifunctional, containing two separate tests in the same cavity. Each test is interpreted visually for color changes after 4 hours of incubation at 35°C. The 19 test results plus oxidase are scored in the appropriate boxes of the report form and a seven-digit profile code is generated similar to that shown in **A**.

D. Enterotube II tubes after 18 to 24 hours of incubation at 35°C. The color reactions can be interpreted visually and converted to a biotype number using a worksheet similar to that shown in **A**. The Enterotube II is easily inoculated by removing the plastic cap from one end and touching the tip of the self-contained inoculating needle to the top of an isolated colony to be identified. The needle is then pulled through the entire length of the tube, thus transferring colonies from the tip of the needle into each of the media compartments.

E. Micro-ID system illustrating color reactions within the reagent tablets in the first five centrally located chambers (*reading from left to right*) and within the lower portions of the remaining chambers. A bacterial suspension is delivered with a pipette into each of the reaction chambers followed by incubation for 4 hours at 35°C. Interpretations are made visually and the results converted into a five-digit biotype number using worksheets supplied by the manufacturer.

F. Biolog GN Microplate system consisting of a 96-well microtiter plate containing 95 carbon substrates and a redox indicator-tetrazolium dye. If a carbon substrate is utilized by the inoculated bacteria, the colorless dye is irreversibly reduced and forms a purple color. With the use of a computer screen, purple wells are coded as positive and colorless wells are coded as negative. The computer then matches the "metabolic fingerprint" of the inoculated organism with those in the database and generates the most likely identification.

G. MicroScan gram-negative ID panel. The microtubes are inoculated with a heavy suspension of the organism to be identified and incubated at 35°C for 15 to 18 hours. The panels can be interpreted visually, after which the biochemical results are converted into a seven- or eight-digit biotype number that is looked up in a codebook supplied by the manufacturer. An automated tray reader can also be used that is combined with a computer identification system. Some trays also include antibiotics for performing broth microdilution susceptibility testing. The panels can also be used with the MicroScan Walkaway automated instrument system. (Photographed by Leon J. LeBeau, University of Illinois at Chicago).

H. Vitek system consisting of (*from left to right*) vacuum-sealer module, reader-incubator, computer-printer, and computer monitor. This system is used with the Vitek test cards for fully automated bacterial identification and antibiotic susceptibility testing.

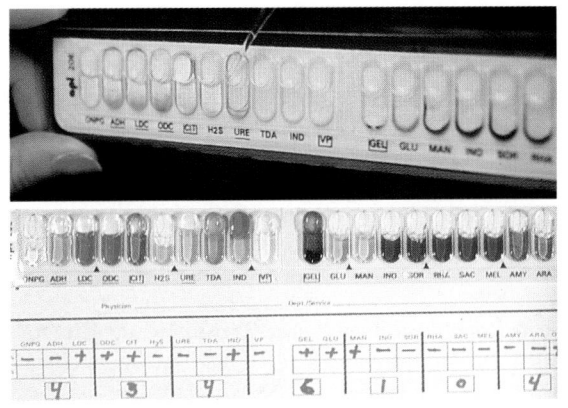

A

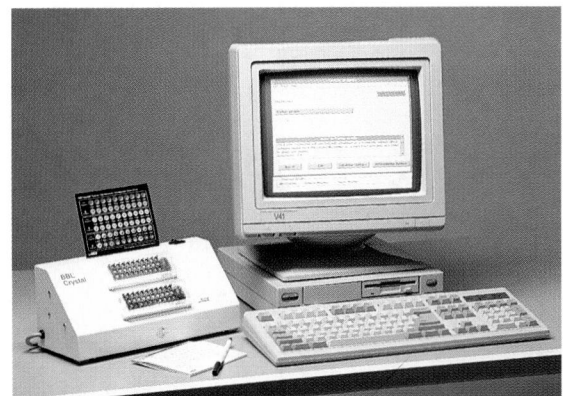

B

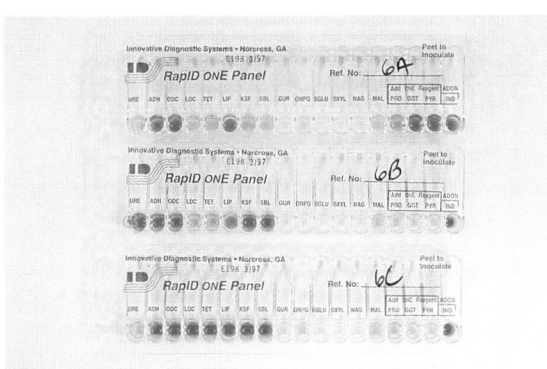

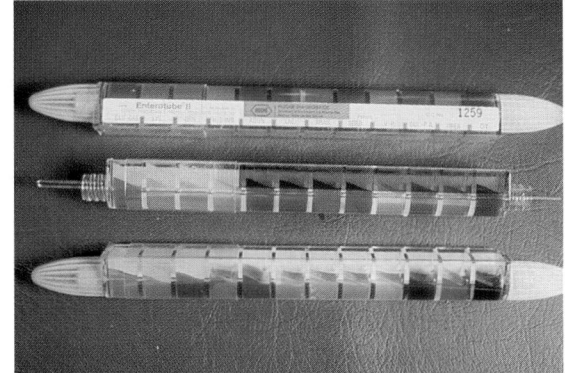

C

D

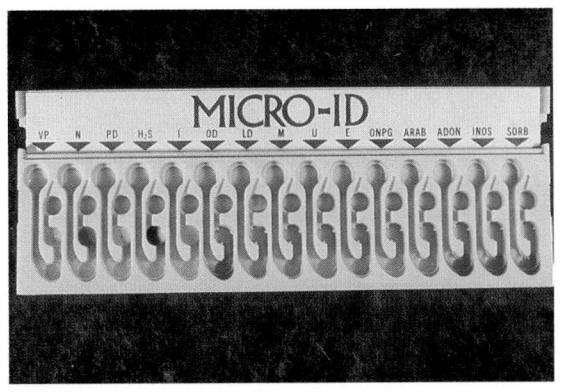

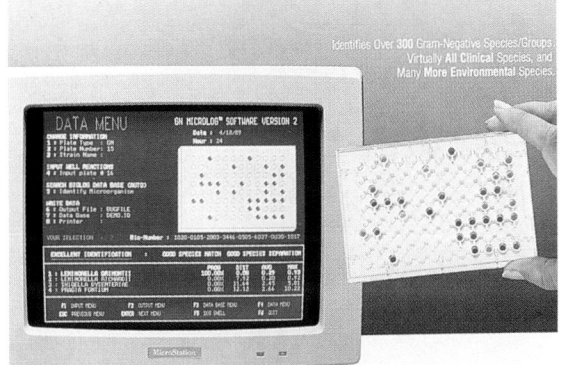

E

F

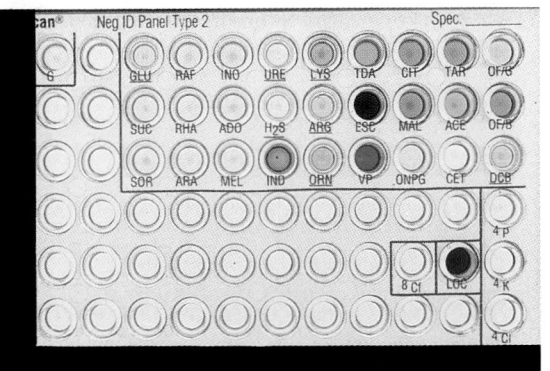

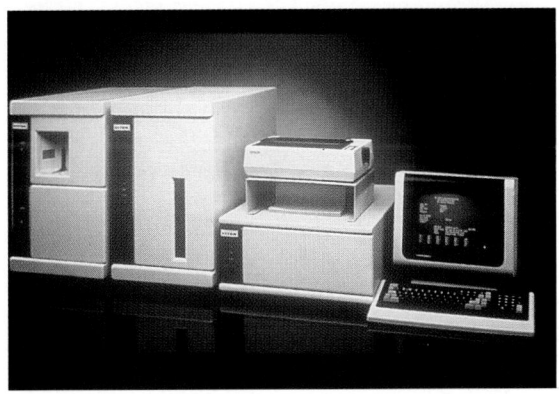

G

H

IMPORTANT CHARACTERISTICS FOR DISTINGUISHING NONFERMENTATIVE
GRAM-NEGATIVE BACILLI

A. The KIA tube on the right shows an alkaline slant/alkaline butt reaction characteristic of a nonfermenting organism; the tube on the left shows an acid slant/acid deep reaction indicating fermentation of dextrose and lactose (characteristic of many species of the *Enterobacteriaceae*). No acid production in Kliger iron agar (KIA) or in triple sugar iron (TSI) agar indicates the inability of nonfermenting bacteria to utilize the lactose or the dextrose in KIA (or the sucrose in TSI).

B. Cytochrome oxidase test. The formation of a blue color within 10 seconds after smearing a test colony on filter paper saturated with the oxidase reagent (tetramethyl-*p*-phenylenediamine dihydrochloride) indicates cytochrome oxidase activity, a characteristic helpful in identifying many species of nonfermenters. All members of the *Enterobacteriaceae* are cytochrome oxidase negative.

C. Failure to grow on MacConkey agar or inhibited growth on MacConkey agar is a clue that a gram-negative rod may be a nonfermenter. Although many species of nonfermenters are capable of growing on MacConkey agar, the lack of growth on this medium, as illustrated on the right side of this split frame, excludes the *Enterobacteriaceae*, all members of which grow well on MacConkey (*left side*).

D. Oxidative utilization of glucose. Illustrated here are two tubes of Hugh-Leifson oxidative-fermentative (OF) medium. The tube on the right is open to the atmosphere, whereas the tube on the left is covered with mineral oil to exclude exposure to atmospheric oxygen. Acid (yellow color) is seen only in the top portion of the open tube, indicating that the organism is capable of oxidizing glucose but incapable of fermenting glucose.

E. Tubes of Motility B medium containing 2,3,5-triphenyltetrazolium chloride (TTC). Motility is often difficult to observe with nonfermentative bacteria since the organisms tend to grow only in the upper (most aerobic) portion of the tube. The addition of tetrazolium aids in detecting motility because organisms capable of reducing TTC will appear red along the stab line as well as in the area into which the cells have migrated, making it easier to differentiate between motile and nonmotile bacteria.

F. Plate of trypticase soy agar inoculated with a yellow, pigment-producing bacterium. Pigment production is an important differential characteristic in identifying nonfermentative gram-negative bacilli. The organism depicted here is *Brevundimonas vesicularis*.

G. Tubes of Flo and Tech agar inoculated with *Pseudomonas aeruginosa* viewed under visible light. These media are used to enhance the production of two pigments: pyoverdin (fluorescein), which appears as a yellow diffusible pigment on Flo agar, and pyocyanin, which appears as a turquoise-blue pigment of Tech agar. Although three species on nonfermentative bacilli produce pyoverdin (*P. aeruginosa*, *P. fluorescens*, and *P. putida*), only one species (*P. aeruginosa*) produces pyocyanin.

H. Tubes of Flo and Tech agar inoculated with *Pseudomonas aeruginosa* viewed under ultraviolet (UV) light using a Wood's lamp. Note that the Flo agar tube (*on the left*) fluoresces, while the Tech agar tube (*on the right*) does not fluoresce under UV light. Only pyoverdin pigment, which is enhanced by growing the organism on Flo agar, fluoresces under UV light.

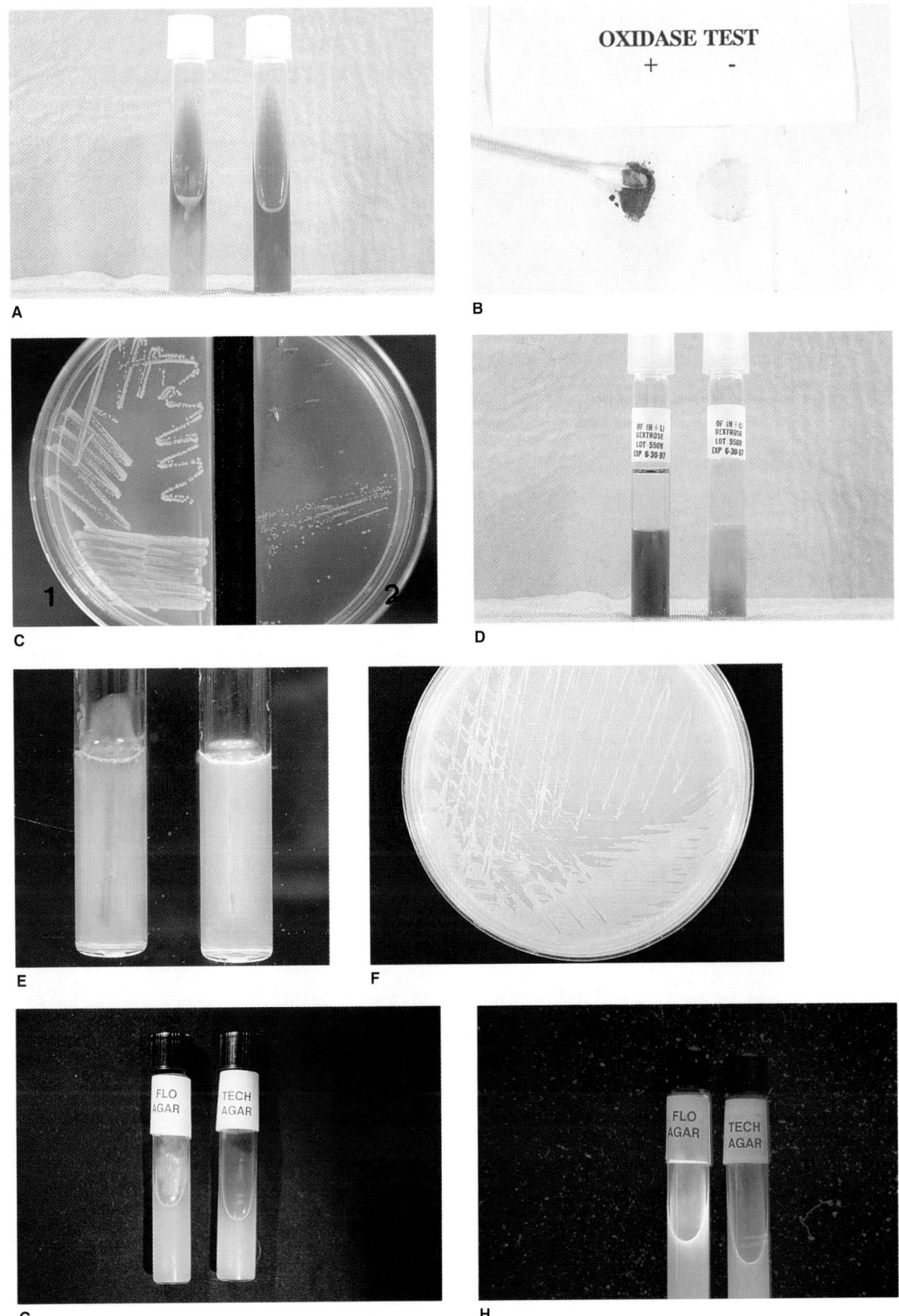

A

B

C

D

E

F

G

H

TESTS USED IN THE IDENTIFICATION OF NONFERMENTATIVE GRAM-NEGATIVE BACILLI

A. Two tubes of Christensen's urea illustrating the fuchsia red color of a positive test (*right*) compared with a negative control (*left*). A rapid positive urease reaction (<4 hr) is seen with the following species of nonfermentative bacilli: *Bordetella bronchiseptica*, CDC Group IVc-2, *Oligella ureolytica*, and *Bergeyella zoohelcum*.

B. Two tubes demonstrating nitrate reduction (*on the left*) and nitrite reduction (*on the right*). Both tubes contain a Durham tube to demonstrate nitrogen gas formation. The tube on the left depicts the reduction of nitrate to nitrogen gas, and the tube on the right demonstrates the reduction of nitrite to nitrogen gas. Note that there is more gas formed in the tube on the right indicating that quantitatively more nitrogen gas is formed from nitrite than nitrate during the same incubation period. Production of gas from both nitrate and nitrite is typical of the Stutzeri group as well as *Alcaligenes xylosoxidans* subsp. *xylosoxidans*.

C. Three tubes of tryptophan broth showing a negative indole reaction (*left*), a positive indole reaction (*center*), and an orange indole reaction (*right*). The two tubes on the left illustrate the type of positive and negative indole reactions obtained using the xylene extraction method followed by the addition of Ehrlich's reagent (see Chart 40). A positive indole reaction is noted by the appearance of a red band at the interface of the tryptophane broth and the xylene layer. The indole positive nonfermentative bacilli include *Balneatrix*, *Bergeyella*, *Chryseobacterium*, *Empedobacter*, *Weeksella* and some unnamed CDC groups. A peculiar orange indole reaction (*tube on far right*) is observed when Kovac's reagent is added to tryptophane broth that has been inoculated with *Comamonas acidovorans*. This reaction is observed only with Kovac's reagent and is due to the formation of anthranilic acid from tryptophane. The reaction may take over 1 hour to develop following the addition of Kovac's reagent.

D. Four tubes of Moeller decarboxylase medium covered with a layer of mineral oil. *Reading from left to right:* lysine, arginine, ornithine, control tube devoid of amino acid. With the nonfermentative bacilli, negative tests remain the same color as the original uninoculated tubes, while positive decarboxylation reactions appear darker purple owing to the formation of alkaline amines causing a more alkaline pH in the tube. The positive lysine decarboxylase reaction illustrated here occurs with only two species of nonfermentative bacilli: *Stenotrophomonas maltophilia* and *Burkholderia cepacia*. (Photographed by Leon J. LeBeau, University of Illinois at Chicago)

E. Split frame showing two tubes of esculin agar viewed under visible light (*on the left*), and the same two tubes viewed under ultraviolet light from a Wood's lamp (*on the right*). When esculin is hydrolyzed by a microorganism the glycoside esculin is converted to esculetin and glucose. The esculetin reacts with an iron salt (ferric citrate) in the medium to form a dark brown or black complex (*second tube from left*). The production of a dark brown or black pigment may be difficult to discern if the organism itself produces a brown or deep-colored pigment. Since esculin is a fluorescent compound, true esculin hydrolysis can be determined by observing for the absence of fluorescence. The brightly fluorescing tube in the right frame (*second tube from far right*) depicts the reaction observed with a negative esculin reaction. The tube on the far right shows marked squelching of fluorescence, particularly in the slant, indicating that the test organism is capable of hydrolyzing esculin.

F. API NFT strips illustrating the 24-hour (*top*) and 48-hour (*bottom*) reactions. Note that the first eight tests (*reading left to right*) are conventional colorimetric reactions, while the remaining 12 tests are carbon assimilation reactions that are read as positive if turbid growth appears or is negative in the absence of turbidity. Users of this system should note that the strip is incubated at 30°C rather than the usual 35°C. (Photographed by Leon J. LeBeau, University of Illinois at Chicago)

G. Remel Uni-N/F system illustrating the circular plate containing 11 independently sealed peripheral wells and a center well containing medium for detecting indole and hydrogen sulfide production. The constricted GNF tube (*second from the right*) is used for detection of glucose fermentation and nitrogen gas (*below the constriction*) and fluorescein production on the slant. The nonconstricted 42P tube (*far right*) is used to test for growth at 42°C and pyocyanin pigment production. (Photographed by Leon J. LeBeau, University of Illinois at Chicago)

H. The Rapid NF Plus system demonstrating the typical reactions seen with *P. aeruginosa*. The system consists of a plastic tray containing 10 reaction cavities. Seven of the reaction cavities (4 through 10) are bifunctional, containing two separate tests in the same cavity. The system is inoculated with a heavy suspension of the test organism and incubated for 4 hours at 35°C. Following incubation, bifunctional tests are first scored before the addition of reagent providing the first test result (*top row*). The same cavity is scored again after the addition of reagent to provide the second test result (*bottom row*). The reactions obtained with these 17 tests plus oxidase provide 18 test scores.

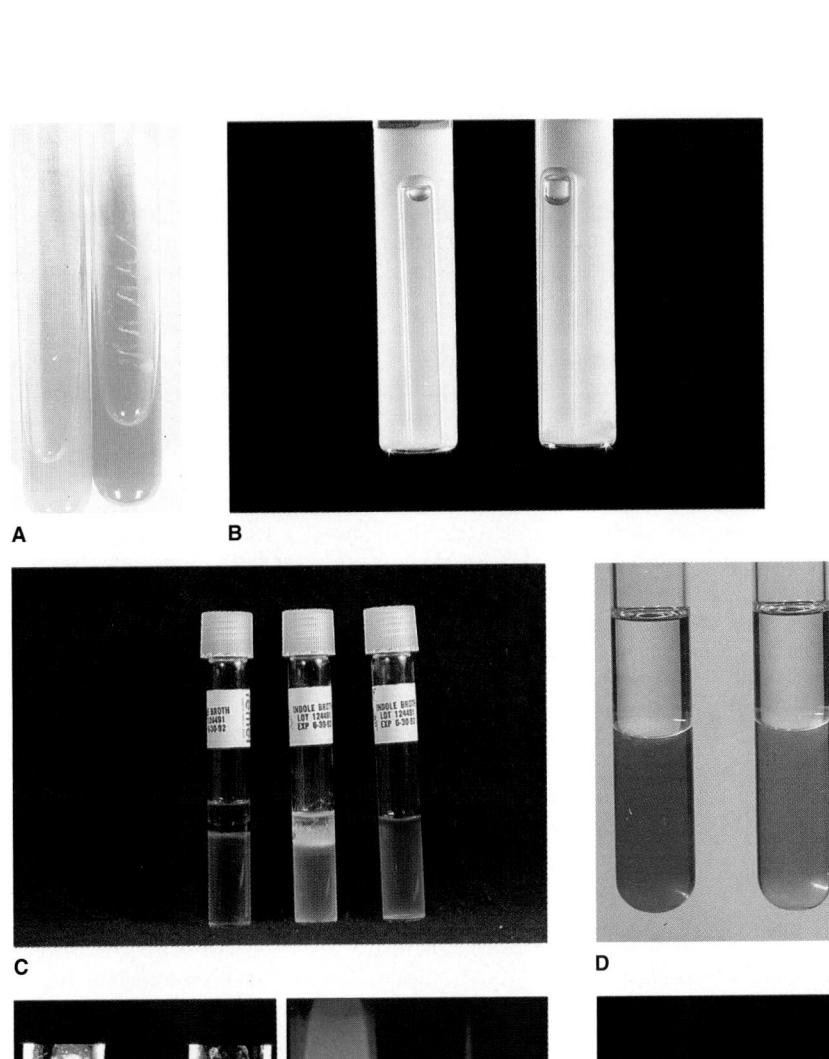

A

B

C

D

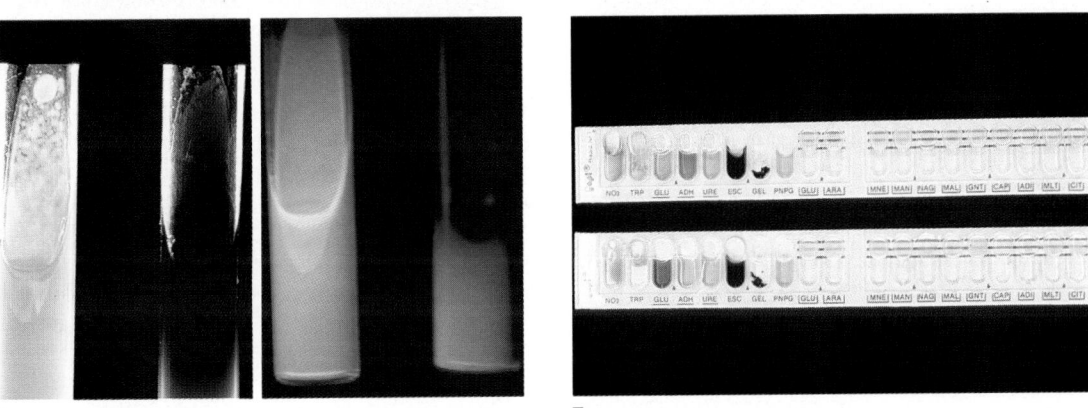

E

F

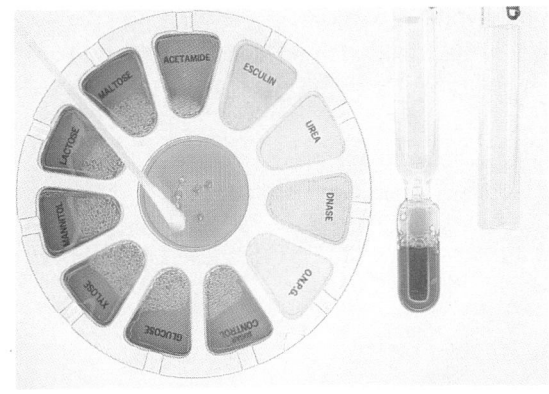

G

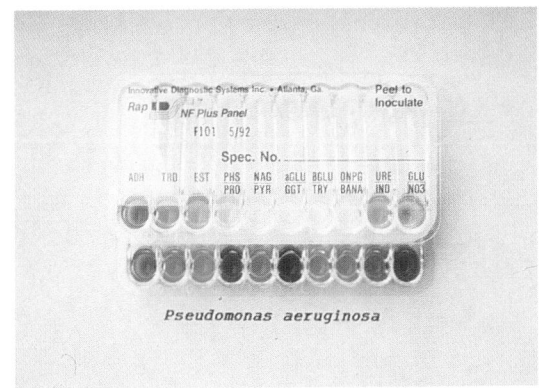

H

Pseudomonas aeruginosa

COLONIAL AND MICROSCOPIC MORPHOLOGY OF CERTAIN NONFERMENTATIVE
BACILLI

Some species of nonfermentative gram-negative bacilli have characteristic features that can be observed on growth media or in gram-stained preparations. An awareness of these features can be an aid in making a correct species identification.

A. Blood agar plate demonstrating growth of *Alcaligenes faecalis* after 48 hours incubation at 35°C. Colonies are white and glistening; in older cultures colonies tend to spread at the outer border of the colonies. This species typically gives off a fruity odor sometimes described as smelling like green apples.

B. Mucoid strain of *Pseudomonas aeruginosa* on MacConkey agar. Colonies can be extremely mucoid and runny. This is the typical appearance of *P. aeruginosa* strains that are isolated from the sputum of patients with cystic fibrosis. (Photographed by Leon J. LeBeau, University of Illinois at Chicago)

C. *Pseudomonas stutzeri* on blood agar medium. Note the characteristic dry, wrinkled colonies that are typical of this species. One should immediately think of *P. stutzeri* when a nonfermentative bacillus produces this type of colony on blood agar. (Photographed by Leon J. LeBeau, University of Illinois at Chicago)

D. Blood agar plate illustrating growth of *Stenotrophomonas maltophilia* on blood agar. The dull yellow pigment is distinctive for this species but at times may be difficult to visualize. Colonies may also appear dark tan to lavender upon continued incubation, particularly if left at room temperature.

E. Gram stain preparation illustrating gram-negative coccobacilli. *Acinetobacter* and *Moraxella* species are the nonfermentative bacilli that characteristically have this staining morphology. The smear depicted here was made from a broth culture of *A. baumannii*.

F. *Acinetobacter baumannii* on MacConkey agar showing a pink to light lavender appearance that is typical for this species. Often a bluish pigmentation may be observed, particularly striking in colonies grown on EMB agar, where it is described as a "cornflower" blue.

G. and H. A useful test for distinguishing between *Neisseria* species and *Moraxella* species is to grow the organisms on blood agar around a penicillin disk. Both organisms are susceptible to penicillin and will demonstrate a zone of inhibition around the penicillin disk **(G)**. After overnight incubation, a Gram stain can be performed on colonies taken from the edge of the zone of inhibition. *Neisseria* species are true cocci and in the presence of subinhibitory concentrations of penicillin will continue to stain as gram-negative diplococci (*right side,* **H**). *Moraxella* species are coccobacilli and in the presence of subinhibitory concentrations of penicillin will form bizarre rod-shaped cells (*left side,* **H**). (Photographed by Leon J. LeBeau, University of Illinois at Chicago)

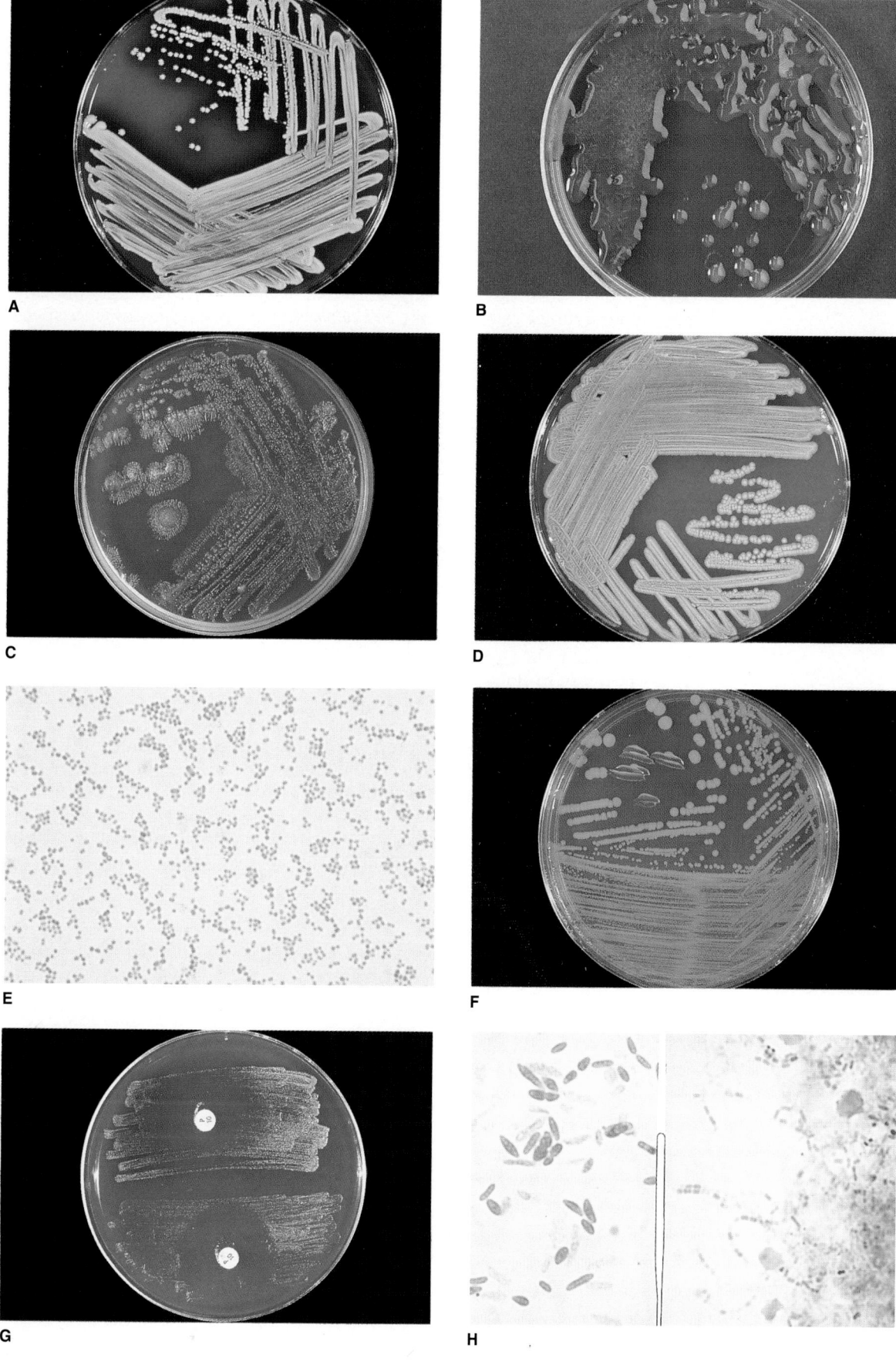

A

B

C

D

E

F

G

H

COLONIAL AND MICROSCOPIC MORPHOLOGY OF CERTAIN NONFERMENTATIVE
BACILLI (CONTINUED)

A. Three plates showing growth of *Methylobacterium* species. Poorest growth is observed on blood agar medium (*bottom*), slightly better growth is seen on buffered charcoal yeast extract agar (BCYE, *upper left*), while the best growth is observed on Sabouraud dextrose agar (*upper right*). Colonies appear dry and exhibit a deep pink or coral pigmentation. These colonies absorb ultraviolet light and appear dark when held under a Wood's lamp.

B. Gram stain of *Methylobacterium* species showing characteristic gram-negative bacilli containing vacuoles.

C. Sabouraud dextrose agar growing *Roseomonas* species. These are light pink, mucoid, almost runny colonies. Like *Methylobacterium* species, *Roseomonas* species also grow best on Sabouraud's agar, however, they do not absorb UV light and do not appear dark when held under a Wood's lamp.

D. Gram stain of *Roseomonas* species showing characteristic gram-negative coccoid forms. These bacteria were previously referred to as the "pink coccoid group" of nonfermenting bacilli.

E. MacConkey agar plate showing growth of *Agrobacterium radiobacter*. Even though these bacteria are nonfermenters, they rapidly oxidize lactose and consequently appear as pink colored, extremely mucoid colonies on MacConkey agar. These organisms can be easily confused with a lactose-positive fermenter, however, they are oxidase positive, which automatically excludes any members of the *Enterobacteriaceae*.

F. Gram stain of CDC Group EO-2 prepared from broth culture. Two characteristic gram-negative staining, "O-shaped" colonies can be observed in the center of this frame.

G. Gram stain of *Neisseria weaveri* prepared from broth culture. Unlike the typical diplococcal appearance of most *Neisseria* species, this species is characterized by cells exhibiting a rod-shaped morphology.

H. Gram stain of *Neisseria elongota* prepared from broth culture. This is another atypical *Neisseria* species that exhibits rod-shaped rather than diplococcal morphology.

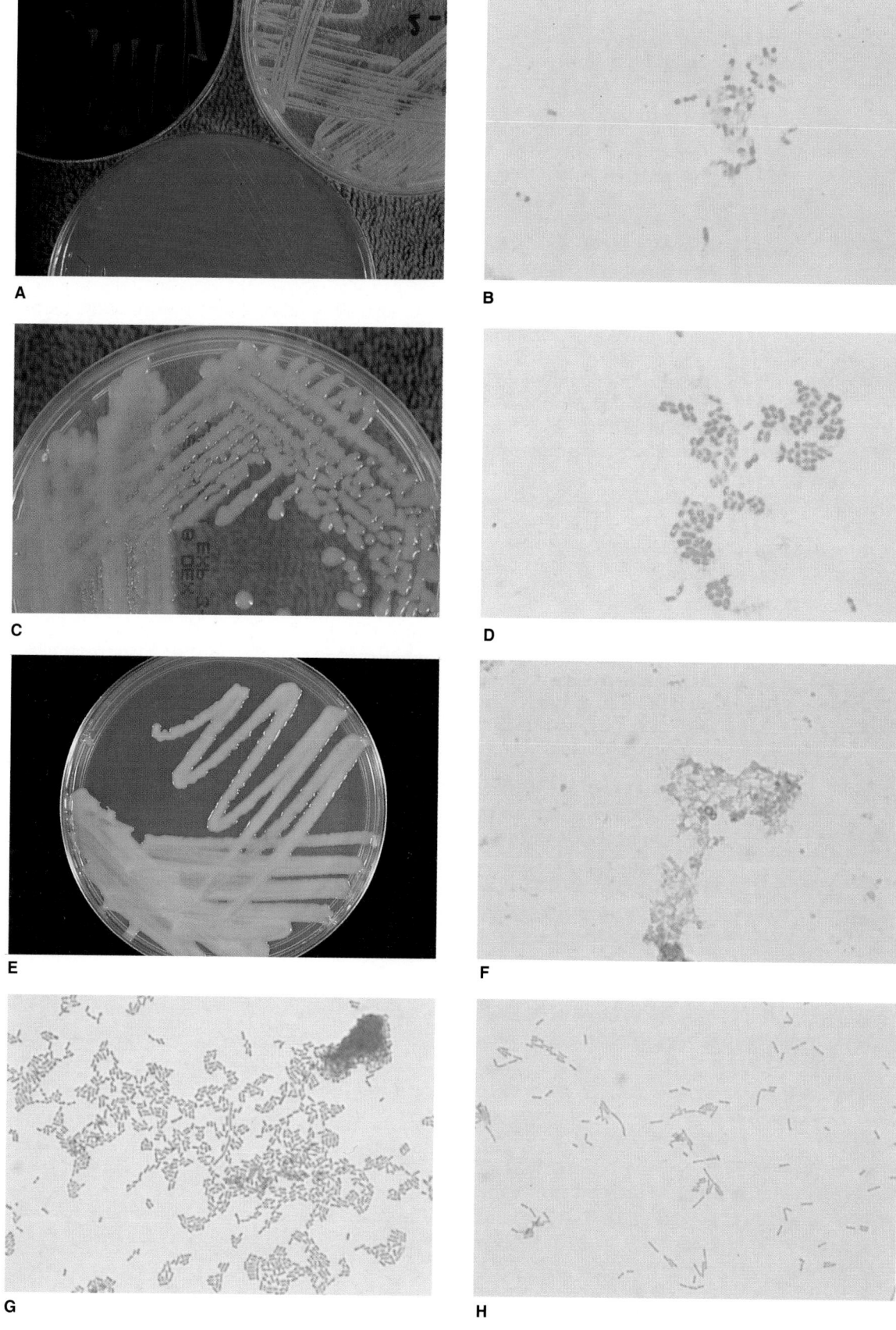

A

B

C

D

E

F

G

H

LABORATORY IDENTIFICATION OF *CAMPYLOBACTER* SPECIES

A. Gram stain of *Campylobacter jejuni* illustrating pleomorphic gram-negative bacilli, with short, curved, and spiral forms. Note that some cells connect to form gull-winged and "S" shapes.

B. *C. jejuni* growing on nonselective *Brucella* agar plate following isolation from stool using the membrane filter technique (described in text). Note that growth has occurred only in the area of the plate underneath where the filter had been placed.

C. Close-up view of *C. jejuni* on blood agar illustrating raised, gray-white, and somewhat mucoid colonies.

D. Growth of *C. jejuni* on Campy BAP agar illustrating the tendency of the organism to grow along the streak lines.

E. Tubes showing the rapid hippurate reaction. Purple color develops with the addition of ninhydrin when hippurate has been hydrolyzed to form glycine and benzoic acid (*positive tube on left compared with negative control on right*). Of the *Campylobacter* species, only *C. jejuni* gives a positive hippurate reaction.

F. *Brucella* blood agar plate showing growth of *C. jejuni* around cephalothin and nalidixic acid disks. Note that with *C. jejuni* a zone of inhibition forms around the nalidixic acid disk (*right*), indicating that this species is susceptible to nalidixic acid but resistant to cephalothin. This test is easy to perform and allows presumptive identification of *C. jejuni*.

G. Triple sugar iron (TSI) agar slant reactions illustrating the hydrogen sulfide (H$_2$S) reactions of several species. The tube to the extreme left illustrates the lack of H$_2$S, characteristic of *C. jejuni*, *C. fetus* subsp. *fetus*, and *C. fetus* subsp. *venerealis*. Tubes 2, 4, and 5 (*reading from left*) illustrate a strong butt reaction, characteristic of *C. sputorum* biovar *bubulus*, *C. sputorum* biovar *fecalis*, or *C. sputorum* biovar *sputorum*. Tube 3 illustrates a strong slant reaction characteristic of *C. mucosalis*.

H. Silver-stained tissue section of superficial gastric mucosa demonstrating clusters of blue-black staining bacilli along the epithelial lining, consistent with the bacillary forms of *Helicobacter pylori*. When observed in a Gram-stained preparation, the individual cells are long, thick, and curved.

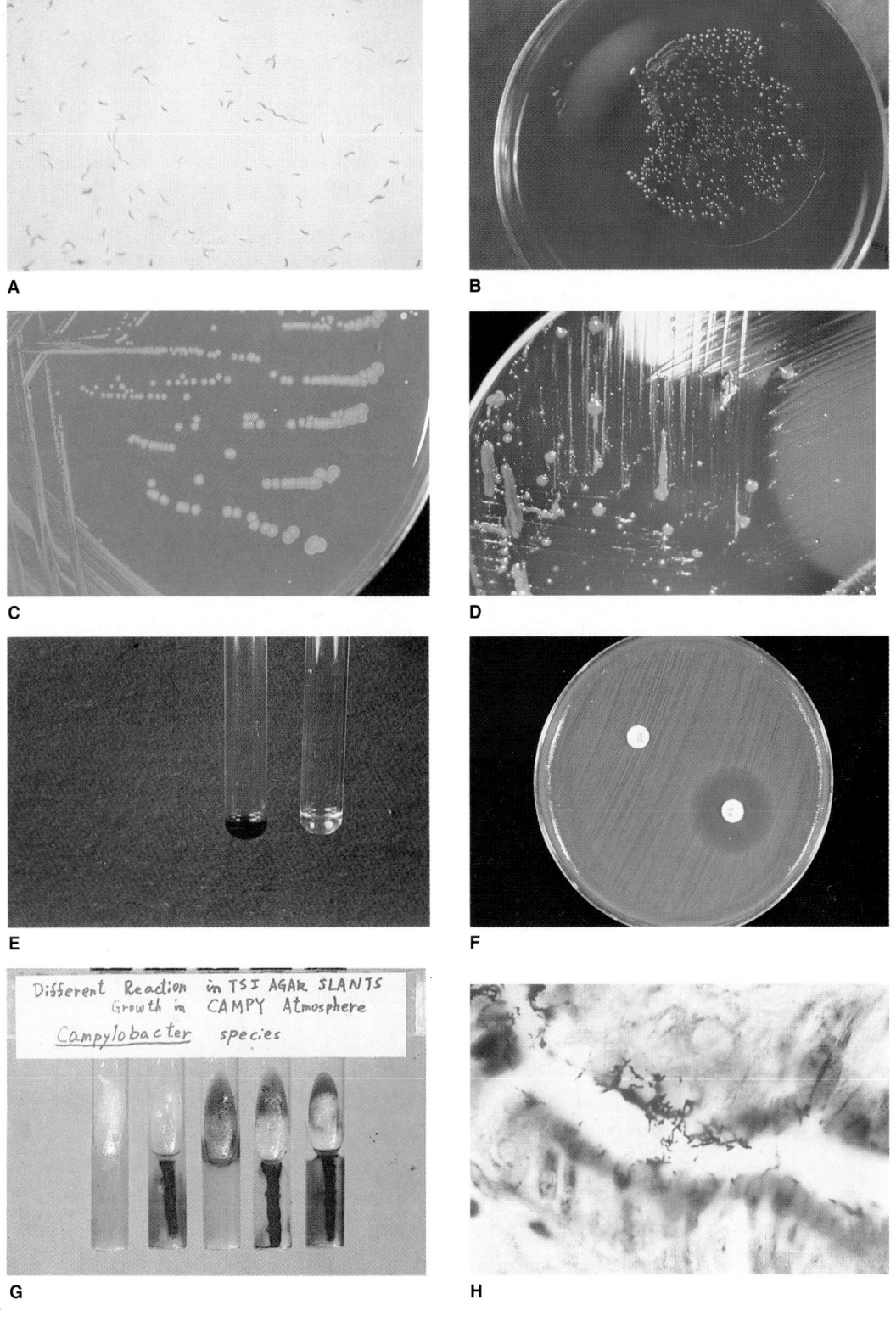

A

B

C

D

E

F

G

Different Reaction in TSI AGAR SLANTS
Growth in CAMPY Atmosphere
Campylobacter species

H

LABORATORY IDENTIFICATION OF *VIBRIO CHOLERAE* AND OTHER *VIBRIO* SPECIES

A. Appearance of *Vibrio cholerae* on thiosulfate citrate bile sucrose (TCBS) agar. The yellow colonies result from citrate utilization and the formation of acid from utilization of the sucrose in the medium. The appearance of yellow colonies on this medium is virtually diagnostic of *V. cholerae.*

B. Colonies of *V. parahaemolyticus* growing on TCBS agar illustrating the characteristic semitranslucent, green-gray appearance.

C. Gelatin agar with white, opaque colonies of *V. cholerae.* Note the opalescence of the agar adjacent to the colonies, indicating hydrolysis and denaturation of the gelatin.

D. Gram stain of *V. vulnificus* illustrating gram-negative bacterial cells with the curved, rod-shaped morphology typical of *Vibrio* species.

E. Positive string test with *V. cholerae.* When colonies of *V. cholerae* are mixed in a drop of 0.5% sodium deoxycholate, they produce a viscous suspension that can be drawn into a string when the inoculating loop is slowly raised from the side.

F. Positive slide agglutination test for *V. cholerae* using polyvalent O antiserum.

G. Blood agar plate illustrating the relatively large, intensely β-hemolytic colonies of the El Tor biotype of *V. cholerae.*

H. Chicken erythrocyte agglutination test. Classic strains of *V. cholerae* do not agglutinate chicken erythrocytes (*top*), in contrast to the El Tor biotype (*bottom*), which is capable of agglutinating the erythrocytes.

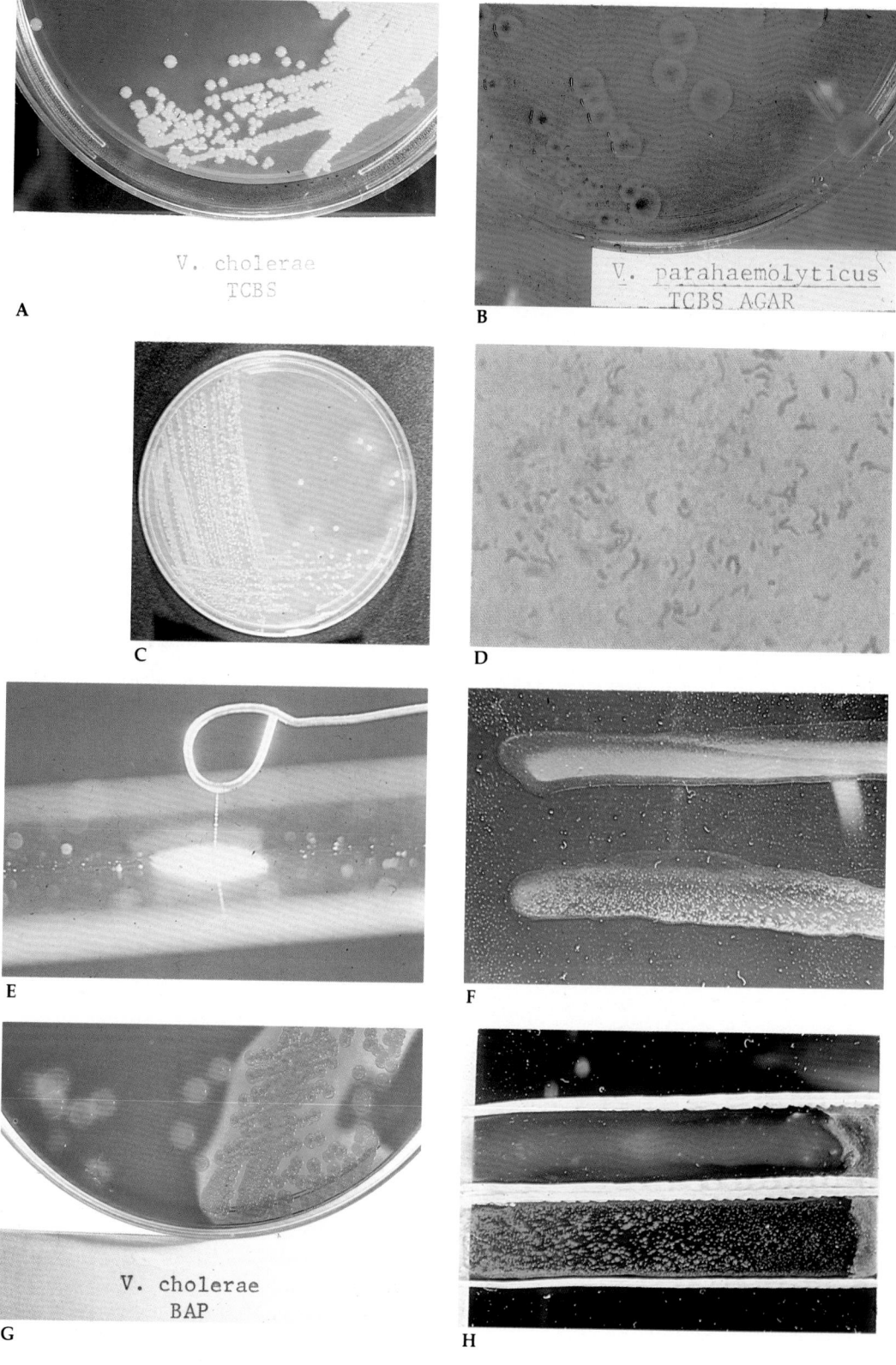

A V. cholerae TCBS

B V. parahaemolyticus TCBS AGAR

C

D

E

F

G V. cholerae BAP

H

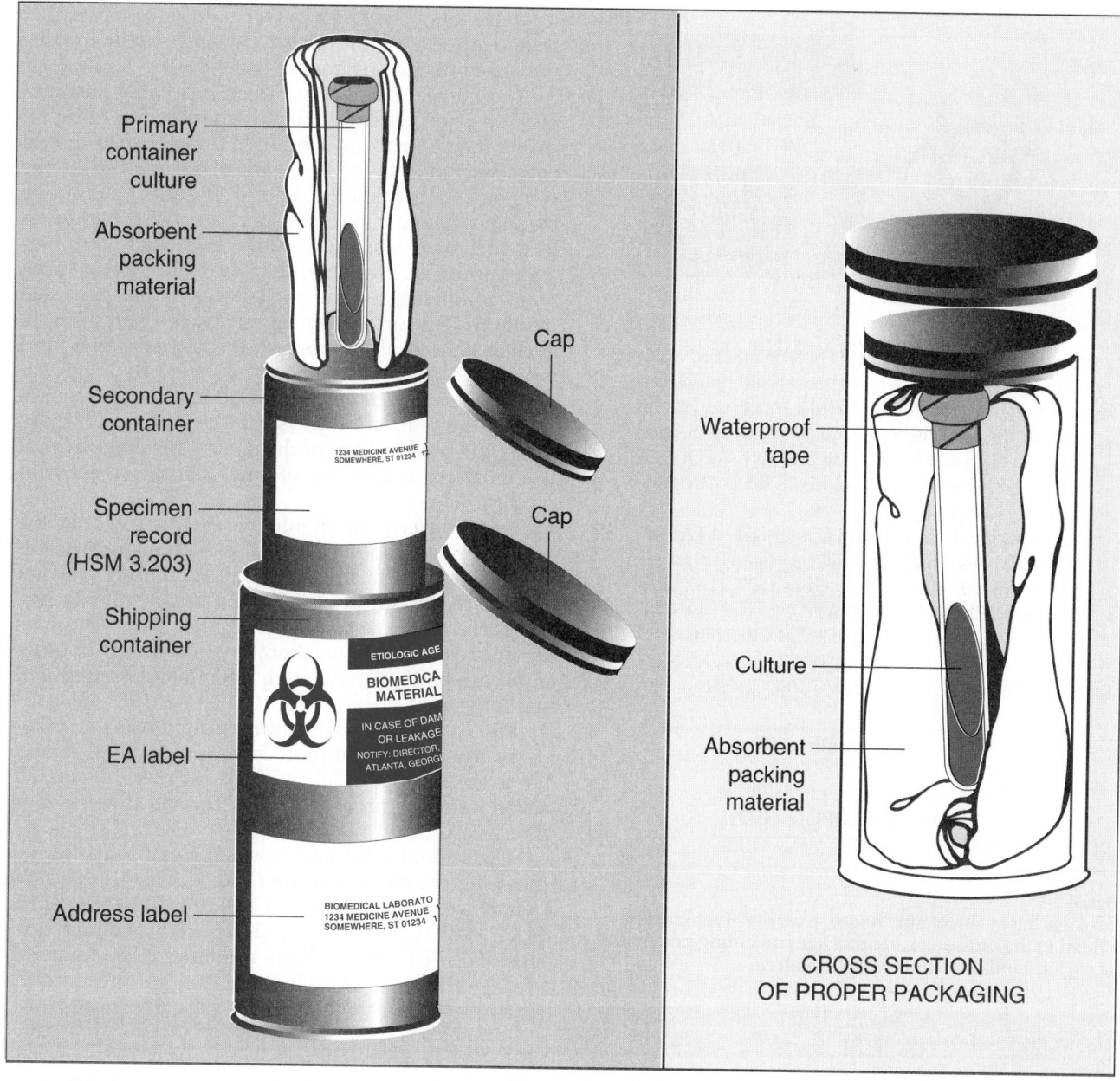

Primary container culture

Absorbent packing material

Secondary container

Specimen record (HSM 3.203)

Shipping container

EA label

Address label

Cap

Cap

1234 MEDICINE AVENUE
SOMEWHERE, ST 01234

ETIOLOGIC AGE
BIOMEDICA
MATERIAL
IN CASE OF DAM
OR LEAKAGE
NOTIFY: DIRECTOR,
ATLANTA, GEORG

BIOMEDICAL LABORATO
1234 MEDICINE AVENUE
SOMEWHERE, ST 01234

Waterproof tape

Culture

Absorbent packing material

CROSS SECTION
OF PROPER PACKAGING

Figure 2-4.
Proper technique for packaging of biologically hazardous materials. (CDC Laboratory
Manual. DHEW publication No. [CDC] 74-8272, Atlanta, Centers for Disease Control, 1974)

CRITERIA FOR SPECIMEN REJECTION

Criteria for rejection of unsuitable specimens for culture must be established in all laboratories.[19] Each request slip and specimen label must be checked to see that all essential information is included: patient's name, hospital or outpatient number, age, gender, location or address, name of physician, source of specimen, date of collection, and procedures requested. A short clinical history and presumptive diagnosis are other pieces of information that are often helpful. Improper or incomplete information is not sufficient, per se, to refuse a specimen. Recollection should be en-

couraged, but if the specimen cannot be recollected, a responsible person should be contacted to make corrections. A comment should be entered on the final report that the specimen was received improperly labeled, and the person's name or initials verifying the specimen identity should also appear. If the type of specimen can be ascertained, it may be acceptable in certain cases to issue a report: "specimen appears to be _____." If not, the specimen should be rejected. Whenever discrepancies occur, a written record of how the situation was handled and names of the individual contacted should be entered on the back of the requisition.

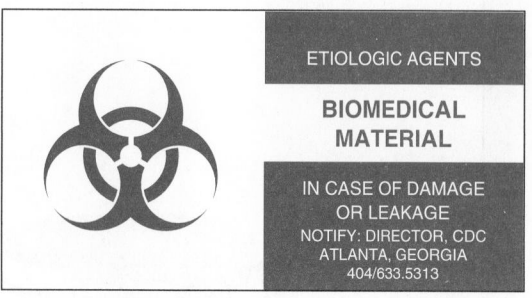

NOTICE TO CARRIER

This package contains LESS THAN 50 ml of AN ETI-OLOGIC AGENT, N. O. S., is packaged and labeled in accordance with the U.S. public Health Service Interstate Quarantine Regulations (42 CFR, Section 72.25(c), (1) and (4), and MEETS ALL REQUIREMENTS FOR SHIPMENT BY MAIL AND ON PASSENGER AIRCRAFT.

This shipment is EXEMPTED FROM ATA RESTRICTED ARTICLES TARIFF 6-D (see General Requirements 386 ([d] [1]) and from DOT HAZARDOUS MATERIALS REGULATIONS (see 49 CRF, Section 173, 386 [d] [3]). SHIPPERS CERTIFICATES, SHIPPING PAPERS, AND OTHER DOCUMENTATION OR LABELING ARE NOT REQUIRED.

_____   _____
Date   Signature of Shipper

CENTERS FOR DISEASE CONTROL
ATLANTA, GEORGIA 30333

Figure 2-5.
Etiologic agents logo and "notice to carrier" that must be affixed to the outside of any package containing potentially hazardous and infectious biologic materials.

A list of specimen types or culture requests that should appear on the reject list and should not be processed further appears in Box 2-4.

The names of other specimen types may also appear on rejection lists. When a specimen is to be rejected, the person who submitted the specimen should be contacted and made aware of the nature of the problem. As a rule of thumb, every effort should be made not to reject specimens that are difficult to recollect, such as cerebrospinal fluid, bronchial washings, and so on. Cultures should be set up on these specimens following routine procedures or using special media to recover a particular suspected pathogen. In such instances, the decision can be made afterward whether to report the results; and, if reported, the condition of the specimen should be indicated, transferring to the requesting physician the responsibility to apply the data in light of the clinical history, physical examination, and results of other laboratory determinations.

Rejection criteria should be clearly listed in the ward manual, and in-service classes to instruct hospital personnel in the importance of submitting relevant specimens for culture should be conducted on a regular basis. Recurring problems and their solutions should be published in laboratory newsletters or other publications that may reach hospital personnel and staff physicians.

The cost savings by instituting rigid rejection criteria in any given institution can be substantial, as outlined by Morris, et al.[46a] These workers evaluated seven tests and procedures for cost and time savings (Box 2-5).

The annual laboratory cost savings for instituting these seven practices at the Duke University Medical Center were calculated as: $999, $1,662, $2,991, $525, $4,447, $4,931, and $12,293, respectively, or a total savings of $27,848. In addition, a total of 1,082 hours of

---

BOX 2-4. SPECIMEN TYPES OR CULTURE REQUESTS THAT SHOULD BE REJECTED

1. Any specimen received in formalin. The only exception might be large specimens in which the time of exposure to formalin is short (less than 1 hour). In these instances, the tissue should be bisected with a sterile knife or scissors and an innermost portion sampled for culture.

2. Twenty-four-hour sputum collections. It is difficult to prevent contamination, and individual collections containing a high concentration of microorganisms will be diluted out by subsequent, less-concentrated samples.

3. Smears of secretions from uterine cervix, vaginal canal, or anus for Gram's stain detection of *Neisseria gonorrhoeae.*

4. A single swab submitted for multiple requests; for example, "aerobes, anaerobes, fungus, and tuberculosis."

5. Submission in an improper, nonsterile, or obviously contaminated container in which portions of the specimen have leaked out. Any leaking container having a biohazard label should be handled with extreme care.

6. Culture plates that are overgrown or dried out. One exception might be a culture plate obtained for the recovery of one of the pathogenic fungi (see Chapter 19). At times, one of the slower-growing pathogenic fungi will still grow on top of bacteria or another mold. Consultation with the physician may be in order.

7. Specimens that are obviously contaminated, as evidenced by the presence of foreign materials, such as barium, colored dyes, or oily chemicals.

8. The following specimens are not acceptable for anaerobic culture: gastric washings, midstream urine, prostatic secretions collected transurethrally, feces (except for the recovery of *Clostridium* species associated with gastrointestinal disease—*C. difficile, C. perfringens, C. septicum*), ileostomy or colostomy swabs, throat, nose, or other oropharyngeal specimens (except specimens obtained from deep tissue during oral surgery), superficial skin, and environmental cultures.

BOX 2-5. REJECTION CRITERIA OF SPECIMENS EFFECTIVE COST SAVINGS

REJECTED SPECIMENS	CRITERIA FOR REJECTION
CSF culture for fungi	Not performed for nonimmunocompromised patients if chemistry values and cell counts performed on CSF are normal.
CSF culture for mycobacteria	Not performed for nonimmunocompromised patients if chemistry values and cell counts performed on CSF are normal.
Stool culture for bacterial enteric pathogens	Not performed if cultures were ordered after patient was in the hospital more than 3 days.
Stool examination for ova and parasites	Not performed if cultures were ordered after patient was in the hospital more than 3 days.
Culture of endotracheal suction aspirates	Not performed if more than 10 squamous epithelial cells/lower power field or no organisms are observed on Gram stain.
Broth backup of bacterial cultures	Used only for tissue biopsies or certain fluids: continuous ambulatory peritoneal dialysis fluid or CSF from patients with shunts.
Bacterial antigens on CSF	Tests not performed because true-positives do not alter therapy and false-positives may lead to additional costs, prolonged hospitalization, and complications.

From Morris AJ, Smith LK, Mirrett S, Reller LB: Cost and time savings following introduction of rejection criteria for clinical specimens. *J Clin Microbiol* 34:355–357, 1996

personnel time were saved to perform other tasks. Schreckenberger and Janda (personal communication) recorded even greater laboratory cost savings at the University of Illinois/Chicago by instituting three other practices:

1. Decreasing the rejection criteria for sputum from more than 25 squamous epithelial cells (SEC) to more than 10 SEC: rejection rate increased from 8% to 35% at an annual savings of $77,832.
2. Rejecting endotracheal suction specimens if no bacteria are seen on Gram stain: $9,588 savings per year.
3. Eliminating routine urine cultures on asymptomatic prenatal screens: 2928 specimens per year eliminated, equaling $105,408 annual savings.

These figures are quite impressive, and each laboratory director must evaluate what cost-saving practices may be applicable for implementation in individual laboratories.

MICROSCOPIC EXAMINATION

The reasons for microscopic examination of clinical materials have been emphasized by several authors.[4,7,21,29,30] First, the number and percentage of segmented neutrophils that are present usually indicate the magnitude and type of inflammatory response. Second, the quality of the specimens can be validated and the observation of bacteria, mycelial elements, yeast forms, parasitic structures, or viral inclusions may provide sufficient information to render an immediate presumptive diagnosis, leading to specific therapy. Third, direct microscopic examination may also give immediate presumptive evidence that species of anaerobic bacteria are present.

The examination of wet mounts of unstained materials by phase contrast or darkfield microscopy is useful for demonstrating motility, spirochetes and endospores. Giemsa, Wright's, or acridine orange stains may be helpful in observing bacterial forms that stain poorly or that have little contrast from background material.

Direct Gram's stains of clinical material may also be used to determine whether a specimen is representative of the site of infection. This technique has been applied to the evaluation of sputum samples. From the relative numbers of squamous epithelial cells and segmented neutrophils in direct Gram stains of sputum samples, Bartlett[5] has devised a grading system for evaluating sputum samples (Box 2-6).

Using this system, negative numbers are assigned to a smear when squamous epithelial cells are observed, indicating contamination with oropharyngeal secretions (saliva). Positive numbers are assigned for the presence of segmented neutrophils, indicating the

BOX 2-6. BARTLETT'S GRADING SYSTEM FOR ASSESSING THE QUALITY OF SPUTUM SAMPLES

NO. OF NEUTROPHILS PER 10 × LOW-POWER FIELD	GRADE
<10	0
10–25	+1
>25	+2
Presence of mucus	+1

NO. OF EPITHELIAL CELLS PER 10 × LOW-POWER FIELD	
10–25	−1
>25	−2
Total*	

*Average the number of epithelial cells and neutrophils in about 20 or 30 separate 10× microscopic fields and then calculate the total. A final score of 0 or less indicates lack of active inflammation or contamination with saliva. Repeat sputum specimens should be requested.

presence of active infection. The magnitude of these negative and positive designations depends on the relative numbers of epithelial cells and segmented neutrophils as shown in the outline of Bartlett's grading system. A final score of 0 or less indicates either lack of inflammatory response or presence of significant salivary contamination, thus invalidating the specimen. Representative photomicrographs of gram-stained sputum preparations illustrating this grading system are shown in Color Plate 2-1.

A similar grading system has been proposed by Murray and Washington[47] (Box 2-7).

The large number of epithelial cells in groups 1 to 4 of this system indicates contamination with oropharyngeal secretions and invalidates the samples. Only group 5 specimens are considered clinically relevant. In a clinical study, Van Scoy[66] recommends that sputum samples containing more than 25 neutrophils be accepted for culture even if more than 10 epithelial cells are present (group 4). Conversely, the absence of neutrophils in the absence of squamous epithelial cells does not discount the possibility of an infection, particularly if the patient is neutropenic. Also, the sputum grading system cannot be employed if pulmonary infections caused by mycobacteria, most fungi, and viruses are suspected.

For further information of the collection, transport and processing of specimens, refer to Isenberg and associates.[29]

MICROSCOPIC TECHNIQUES

A number of techniques may be used in the direct microscopic examination of clinical specimens, either to demonstrate the presence of microorganisms or to observe certain biochemical, physiologic, or serologic characteristics. The techniques more commonly used in clinical microbiology laboratories are outlined in Table 2-2. Because the refractive index of bacteria and other microorganisms is similar to that of the mounting medium, they are not visible when examined by bright-field illumination. Therefore, certain manipulations of the light source may be necessary. Often it is helpful to reduce the amount of light entering the field by closing the iris diaphragm, reducing the contrast between the object being observed and the background. The common practice of lowering the condenser to achieve this effect is discouraged.

DIRECT STAINS

Biologic stains are generally required to visualize bacteria adequately and demonstrate the fine detail of internal structures. The introduction of stains in the mid-19th century was, in large part, responsible for the major advances that have occurred in clinical microbiology and in other fields of diagnostic microscopy during the past 100 years. Today, we are so dependent on biologic stains that it is difficult to realize how the study of bacteria could have progressed before their introduction. The chemical formulas, components and purposes of the stains commonly used in the microbiology laboratory are shown in Table 2-3 (pages 87 and 88).

Stains consist of aqueous or organic preparations of dyes or groups of dyes that impart a variety of colors to microorganisms, plant and animal tissues, or other substances of biologic importance. Dyes may be used as direct stains of biologic materials, as indicators of pH shifts in culture media, as oxidation–reduction indicators to demonstrate the presence or lack of anaerobic conditions and to demonstrate physiologic functions of microorganisms using so-called supravital techniques.

Almost all biologically useful dyes are derivatives of coal tar. The fundamental chemical structure of most dyes is the benzene ring. Dyes are generally composed of two or more benzene rings connected by well-defined chemical bonds (chromophores) that are associated with color production. Although the underlying mechanism of the color development is not totally understood, it is theorized that certain chemical radicals have the property of absorbing light of different wavelengths, acting as chemical prisms. Some of the more common chromophore groupings found in dyes are: $C = C$, $C = O$, $C = S$, $C = N$, $N = N$, $N = O$, and NO_2. (Note the presence of these groups in the chemical formulas of the stains shown in Table 2-3.) The depth of color of a dye is proportional to the number of chromophore radicals in the compound.

Dyes differ from one another in the number and arrangement of these rings and in the substitution of hydrogen atoms with other molecules. For example, there are three key single substitutions for one hydrogen atom of benzene that constitute the basic structure of most dyes: 1) substitution of a methyl group to form toluene (methylbenzene), 2) substitution of a hydroxyl group to form phenol (carbolic acid), and 3) the substitution of an amine group to form aniline (phenylamine). Most stains used in microbiology are derived from aniline and are called aniline dyes.

CH₂	OH	NH₂
Toluene (Methylbenzene)	Phenol (Carbolic acid)	Aniline (Phenylamine)

BOX 2-7. MURRAY AND WASHINGTON'S GRADING SYSTEM FOR ASSESSING THE QUALITY OF SPUTUM SAMPLES

	EPITHELIAL CELLS PER LOW-POWER FIELD	LEUKOCYTES PER LOW-POWER FIELD
Group 1	25	10
Group 2	25	10–25
Group 3	25	25
Group 4	10–25	25
Group 5	<10	25

TABLE 2-2
TECHNIQUES FOR DIRECT EXAMINATION OF UNSTAINED SPECIMENS

METHODS AND MATERIALS	PURPOSE	TECHNIQUES
Saline Mount Sodium chloride, 0.85% (aqueous) Glass microscope slides, 3 × 1-inch Coverslips Paraffin–petrolatum mixture (Vaspar)	To determine biologic activity of microorganisms, including motility or reactions to certain chemicals, or serologic reactivity in specific antisera. The latter includes the quellung (capsular swelling) reaction used to identify different capsular types of *Streptococcus pneumoniae* and *Haemophilus influenzae*.	Disperse a small quantity of the specimen to be examined into a drop of saline on a microscope slide. Overlay a coverslip and examine directly with a 40 × or 100 × (oil immersion) objective of the microscope, closing the iris diaphragm to reduce the amount of transmitted light. To prevent drying, ring the coverslip with a small amount of paraffin–petrolatum before overlaying the specimen drop on the slide.
Hanging-drop Procedure Hanging-drop glass slide (This is a thick glass slide with a central concave well.) Coverslip Physiologic saline or water Paraffin–petrolatum mixture	The hanging-drop mount serves the same purpose as the saline mount, except there is less distortion from the weight of the coverslip and a deeper field of focus into the drop can be achieved. This technique is generally used for studying the motility of bacteria.	A small amount of paraffin–petrolatum mixture is placed around the lip of the well on the undersurface of the hanging-drop slide. Cells from a bacterial colony to be examined are placed in the center of the coverslip, into a small drop of saline or water. The slide is inverted and pressed over the coverslip, guiding the drop of bacterial suspension into the center of the well. The slide is carefully brought to an upright position for direct examination under the microscope.
Iodine Mount Lugol's iodine solution: Iodine crystals, 5 g Potassium iodide, 10 g Distilled water, 100 mL Dissolve KI in water and add iodine crystals slowly until dissolved. Filter and store in tightly stoppered bottle. Dilute 1:5 with water before use. Microscope slides, 3 × 1-inch Coverslips	Iodine mounts are usually used in parallel with saline mounts when examining feces or other materials for intestinal protozoa or helminth ova. The iodine stains the nuclei and intracytoplasmic organelles so that they are more easily seen. Iodine mounts cannot be used to the exclusion of saline mounts because iodine paralyzes the motility of bacteria and protozoan trophozoites.	A small amount of fecal matter or other material is mixed in a drop of the iodine solution on a microscope slide. This is mixed to form an even suspension, and a coverslip is placed over the drop. The mount is then examined directly under a microscope. If this is to be delayed or if a semipermanent preparation for future study is desired, the edges of the coverslip can be sealed with the paraffin–petrolatum mixture.
Potassium Hydroxide (KOH) Mount Potassium hydroxide, 10% (aqueous) Microscope slides, 3 × 1-inch Coverslips	The KOH mount is used to aid in detecting fungus elements in thick mucoid material or in specimens containing keratinous material, such as skin scales, nails, or hair. The KOH dissolves the background keratin, unmasking the fungus elements to make them more apparent.	Suspend fragments of skin scales, nails, or hair in a drop of 10% KOH. Add coverslip over the drop and let sit at room temperature for about a half hour. The mount may be gently heated in the flame of a Bunsen burner to accelerate the clearing process. Do not boil. Examine under a microscope for fungal hyphae or spores.
India Ink Preparation India Ink (Pelikan brand) or Nigrosin (granular)* Microscope slides, 3 × 1-inch Coverslips	India ink or nigrosin preparations are used for the direct microscopic examination of the capsules of many microorganisms. The fine granules of the india ink or nigrosin give a semiopaque background against which the clear capsules can easily be seen. This technique is particularly useful in visualizing the large capsules of *Cryptococcus neoformans* in cerebrospinal fluid, sputum, and other secretions.	Centrifuge the cerebrospinal fluid or other fluid specimens lightly to concentrate any microorganisms in the sediment. Emulsify a small quantity of the sediment into a drop of india ink or nigrosin on a microscope slide and overlay with a coverslip. Do not make the contrast emulsion too thick, or the transmitted light may be completely blocked. Examine the mount directly under a microscope, using the 10 × objective for screening and the 40 × objective for confirmation of suspicious encapsulated microorganisms.

(Continued)

TABLE 2-2 (Continued)
Techniques for Direct Examination of Unstained Specimens

Methods and Materials	Purpose	Techniques
Darkfield Examination Compound microscope equipped with a darkfield condenser Microscope slides, 3 × 1-inch Coverslips Physiologic saline Applicator sticks or curet Paraffin–petrolatum mixture	Darkfield examinations are used to visualize certain delicate microorganisms that are invisible by brightfield optics and stain only with great difficulty. This method is particularly useful in demonstrating spirochetes from suspicious syphilitic chancres for *Treponema pallidum*.	The secretion to be examined is obtained from the patient. In the case of a chancre, the top crust is scraped away with a scalpel blade and a small quantity of serous material is placed on a microscope slide. Ring a coverslip with paraffin–petrolatum mixture and place over the drop of material. Examine the mount directly under a microscope fitted with a darkfield condenser with a 40 × or 100 × objective. Spirochetes will appear as motile, bright "corkscrews" against a black background.
Neufeld's Quellung Reaction Homologous anticapsular serum Physiologic saline Microscope slides, 3 × 1-inch Coverslips	When species of encapsulated bacteria are brought into contact with serum containing homologous anticapsular antibody, their capsules undergo a change in refractive index to produce "swelling" that is visible by microscopic examination. This serologic procedure is useful in identifying the various types of *Streptococcus pneumoniae* and *Haemophilus influenzae* in biologic fluids or in cultures.	A loopful of material, such as emulsified sputum, body fluid, or broth culture, is spread over a 1-cm area in two places on opposite ends of a microscope slide. A loopful of specific anticapsular typing serum is spread over the area of one of the dried preparations; the opposite area is overlaid with a loopful of saline to serve as a control. Each area is overlaid with a coverslip and examined under the 100 × (oil immersion) objective of the microscope. Organisms showing a positive reaction appear surrounded with a ground-glass, refractile halo owing to capsular swelling. Compare the test preparation with the saline control where no capsular swelling occurs.

*Available from Harleco Co., Philadelphia, PA

All biologic dyes have a high affinity for hydrogen. When all the molecular sites that can bind hydrogen are filled, the dye is in its reduced state and is generally colorless. In the colorless state, the dye is called a leuko compound. Looking at this concept from the opposite view, a dye retains its color only as long as its affinities for hydrogen are not completely satisfied. Because oxygen generally has a higher affinity for hydrogen than many dyes, color is retained in the presence of air. This allows certain dyes, such as methylene blue, to be used as an oxidation–reduction indicator in an anaerobic environment, such as a GasPak jar (BBL, Division of Becton-Dickinson and Co., Cockeysville MD) because the indicator becomes colorless in the absence of oxygen.

In broad terms, dyes are referred to as acidic or basic, designations not necessarily indicating their pH reactions in solution, but rather, whether a significant part of the molecule is anionic or cationic. From a practical standpoint, basic dyes stain structures that are acidic, such as the nuclear chromatin in cells; acidic dyes react with basic substances, such as cytoplasmic structures. If both nuclear and cytoplasmic structures are to be stained in a given preparation, combinations of acidic and basic dyes may be used. A common example is the hematoxylin (basic) and eosin (acidic), or H & E, stain used in the examination of tissue sections.

THE USE OF STAINS IN MICROBIOLOGY

Microbiologists are encouraged to perform direct microscopic examination on specimens submitted for culture. Not only may it be possible to provide the physician with a rapid presumptive diagnosis, but also the detection of specific microorganisms may serve as a guide for selecting appropriate culture media and to provide a valuable quality control comparison with isolates recovered. The positive findings for various staining procedures and diseases that can be suspected for the various specimen types that are submitted to microbiology laboratories are listed in Table 2-4. The following is a brief description of the stains most commonly used.

Gram's Stain. Gram's stain, discovered a little over 100 years ago by Hans Christian Gram, is most commonly used for direct microscopic examination of specimens and subcultures (the formula can be found in Table 2-3). The staining procedure is explained in Box 2-8.

TABLE 2-3

COMMON BIOLOGIC STAINS USED IN BACTERIOLOGY

STAIN	CHEMICAL FORMULA	INGREDIENTS		PURPOSE
Loeffler's methylene blue	Tetramethyl thionin	Methylene blue Ethyl alcohol, 95% Distilled water	0.3 g 30 mL 100 mL	This is a simple direct stain used to stain a variety of microorganisms, specifically used to detect bacteria in cerebrospinal fluid smears in suspected cases of bacterial meningitis.
Gram's stain	Crystal Violet (Hexamethylpararosanilin) Dimethyl Phenosafranin	Crystal violet 　Crystal violet 　Ethyl alcohol, 95% 　NH₄ oxalate 　Distilled water Gram's iodine 　Potassium iodide 　Iodine crystals 　Distilled water Decolorizer 　Acetone 　Ethyl alcohol, 95% Counterstain 　Safranin 0 　Ethyl alcohol, 95% 　Add 10 mL to distilled water	2g 20 mL 0.8 g 100 mL 2 g 1 g 100 mL 50 mL 50 mL 2.5 g 100 mL 100 mL	This is a differential stain used to demonstrate the staining properties of bacteria of all types. Gram-positive bacteria retain the crystal violet dye after decolorization and appear deep blue. Gram-negative bacteria are not capable of retaining the crystal violet dye after decolorization and are counterstained red by the safranin dye. Gram-staining characteristics may be atypical in very young, old, dead, or degenerating cultures. Staining of cyst forms of *Pneumocystis carinii* (Gram–Weigert modification—see Plate 20-7*H*).
Ziehl-Neelsen acid-fast stain	Carbolfuchsin (Triaminotriphenylmethane)	Carbolfuchsin 　Phenol crystals 　Alcohol, 95% 　Basic fuchsin 　Distilled water Acid alcohol, 3% 　HCl, concentrated 　Alcohol, 70% Methylene blue 　Methylene blue 　Glacial acetic 　Distilled water	2.5 mL 5 mL 0.5 g 100 mL 3 mL 100 mL 0.5 g 0.5 mL 100 mL	Acid-fast bacilli are so called because they are surrounded by a waxy envelope that is resistant to staining. Either heat or a detergent (Tergitol) is required to allow the stain to penetrate the capsule. Once stained, acid-fast bacteria resist decolorization, whereas other bacteria are destained with the acid alcohol.
Fluorochrome	Auramine O Rhodamine B Acridine orange	Auramine O Rhodamine B Glycerol Phenol Distilled water	1.5 g 0.75 g 75 mL 10 mL 50 mL	This fluorochrome dye stains mycobacteria selectively by binding to the mycolic acid in the cell wall. This stain demonstrates mycobacteria better than conventional acid-fast stains and permits screening of smears at lower magnification because organisms are more easily seen.
		AO powder Sodium acetate buffer (pH 3.5) (Add about 90 mL 1 M HCl to 100 mL 1 M Na acetate)	20 mg 190 mL	Acridine orange is a stain particularly well adapted for the demonstration of bacteria in blood culture broth, cerebrospinal fluid, urethral smears, or other exudates where they may be present in relatively small numbers, as low as 10^4 CFU mL, or when they are obscured by a heavy background of polymorphonuclear leukocytes or other debris. At pH below 4.0, bacteria and yeast cells stain brilliant orange against a black, light green, or yellow background.

TABLE 2-3 *(Continued)*
COMMON BIOLOGIC STAINS USED IN BACTERIOLOGY

STAIN	CHEMICAL FORMULA	INGREDIENTS		PURPOSE

Wright's–Giemsa	Polychrome methylene blue
	Methylene blue
	Methylene azure
	Eosin
	
	Methylene azure B
		Powdered Wright's
		  stain
		Powdered Giemsa
		  stain
		Glycerin
		Absolute methyl
		  alcohol
		Mix in brown
		  bottle and let
		  stand 1 month
		  before using.
			9 g
			
			1 g
			90 mL
			
			2910 mL
				Wright's–Giemsa is commonly used for staining the cellular elements of the peripheral blood smear. It is useful in micriobiology for the demonstration of intracellular organisms such as *Histoplasma capsulatum* and *Leishmania* species (see Color Plate 20-6H). The stain is also useful in demonstrating intracellular inclusions in direct smears of skin or mucous membranes, such as corneal scrapings for trachoma.

Lactophenol aniline blue	Aniline blue	Phenol crystals Lactic acid Glycerol Distilled water Dissolve ingredients, then add: Aniline blue	20 g 20 g 40 mL 20 mL 0.05 g	Because of the sulfonic groups, the dye is strongly acidic and has been used as a counterstain for unfixed tissues, bacteria, and protozoa, in combination with other dyes. Currently it is most commonly used for the direct staining of fungal mycelium and fruiting structures, which take on a delicate light blue color.

Crystal violet (gentian violet) serves as the primary stain, binding to the bacterial cell wall after treatment with a weak solution of iodine, which serves as the mordant to bind the dye. Some bacterial species, because of the chemical nature of their cell walls, have the ability to retain the crystal violet even after treatment with an organic decolorizer, such as a mixture of equal parts of 95% ethyl alcohol and acetone. Dye-retaining bacteria appear blue-black when observed under the microscope and are called gram-positive. Certain bacteria lose the crystal violet primary stain when treated with the decolorizer, presumably because of the high lipid content of their cell wall. These decolorized bacteria then pick up the safranin counterstain and appear red when observed under the microscope and are called gram-negative (Color Plate 2-2A). The visualization of certain fastidious gram-negative bacilli can be improved by adding carbolfuchsin to the sapronin counterstain. These gram-stained reactions, when observed in conjunction with the types (cocci and bacilli) and arrangements of bacterial cells, can be used to make presumptive identifications (see Table 2-4).

The more common Gram's stain applications have been reviewed by Friedly.[21] Gram-positive cocci in clusters suggest staphylococci; in chains, they suggest streptococci. Gram-positive, lancet-shaped diplococci, particularly when seen in smears made from sputum samples, are characteristic of *Streptococcus pneumoniae*; gram-negative, kidney-shaped diplococci are characteristic of *Neisseria* species. Large, gram-positive bacilli suggest *Bacillus* or *Clostridium* species; small gram-positive bacilli suggest *Listeria* species or one of the coryneforms (diphtheroids) if "Chinese-letter" arrangements are observed. Curved, gram-negative rods in diarrheal stool specimens suggest *Vibrio* species or, if corkscrew forms are also seen, *Campylobacter* species. Gram-negative bacilli are the bacteria most commonly encountered in clinical laboratories and include the *Enterobacteriaceae*, the nonfermentative bacilli, *Haemophilus* species, and a variety of fastidious species. A variety of gram-stained images are included in Color Plate 2-4, which is discussed in more detail in a later section of this chapter.

Gram's stain can also be used to identify nonbacterial forms such as trichomonads, strongyloides larvae, *Pneumocystis carinii* cysts, and *Toxoplasma gondii* trophozoites, although not as sensitive as other special stains used for visualizing these parasites. These various applications demonstrate the versatility of the Gram's stain.

Acid-Fast Stains. Mycobacteria are coated with a thick, waxy material that resists staining; however,

TABLE 2-4

DIAGNOSIS OF INFECTIOUS DISEASE BY DIRECT EXAMINATION OF CULTURE SPECIMENS

SPECIMEN	SUSPECTED DISEASE	LABORATORY PROCEDURE	POSITIVE FINDINGS
Throat culture	Diphtheria	Gram's stain	Delicate pleomorphic gram-positive bacilli in Chinese letter arrangement
		Methylene blue stain	Light–blue-staining bacilli; with prominent metachromatic granules
	Acute streptococcal pharyngitis	Direct fluorescent antibody technique (after 4–6 hours incubation in Todd-Hewitt broth)	Fluorescent cocci in chains; use positive and negative controls with each stain
Oropharyngeal ulcers	Vincent's disease	Gram's stain	Presence of gram-negative bacilli and thin, spiral-shaped bacilli
Sputum Transtracheal aspirates Bronchial washings	Bacterial pneumonia	Gram's stain	Variety of bacterial types; *Streptococcus pneumoniae* with capsules particularly diagnostic
	Tuberculosis Pulmonary mycosis	Acid-fast stain Gram's stain, Wright-Giemsa's stain or Calcofluor white Gram-Weigert stain	Acid-fast bacilli Budding yeasts, pseudohyphae, true hyphae, or fruiting bodies
Cutaneous wounds or purulent drainage from subcutaneous sinuses	Bacterial cellulitis	Gram's stain	Variety of bacterial types; suspect anaerobic species
	Gas gangrene (myonecrosis)	Gram's stain	Gram-positive bacilli suggesting *Clostridium perfringens;* spores usually not seen
	Actinomycotic mycetoma	Direct saline mount Gram's stain or modified acid–fast stain	"Sulfur granules" Delicate, branching gram-positive filaments; *Nocardia* species may be weakly acid-fast
	Eumycotic mycetoma	Direct saline mount Gram's stain or lactophenol cotton blue mount	White, grayish, or black grains True hyphae with focal swellings or chlamydospores
Cerebrospinal fluid	Bacterial meningitis	Gram's stain	Small gram-negative pleomorphic bacillic (*Haemophilus* species) Gram-negative diplococci (*Neisseria meningitidis*) Gram-positive diplococci (*Streptococcus pneumoniae*)
		Methylene blue stain	Bacterial forms that stain blue-black
		Acridine orange stain	Bacterial forms that glow brilliant orange under ultraviolet illumination
	Pneumococcal meningitis	Quellung reaction (type-specific antisera)	Swelling and ground-glass appearance of bacterial capsules
	Cryptococcal meningitis	India ink or nigrosin mount	Encapsulated yeast cells with buds attached by thin thread
	Listeriosis	Gram's stain Hanging-drop mount	Delicate gram-positive bacilli Bacteria with tumbling motility

(Continued)

TABLE 2-4   *(Continued)*
DIAGNOSIS OF INFECTIOUS DISEASE BY DIRECT EXAMINATION OF CULTURE SPECIMENS

SPECIMEN	SUSPECTED DISEASE	LABORATORY PROCEDURE	POSITIVE FINDINGS
Urine	Yeast infection	Gram's stain or Wright-Giemsa stain	Pseudohyphae or budding yeasts
	Bacterial infection	Gram's stain	Variety of bacterial types
	Leptospirosis	Darkfield examination	Loosely coiled motile spirochetes
Purulent urethral or cervical discharge	Gonorrhea	Gram's stain	Intracellular gram-negative diplococci
	Chlamydial infection	Direct fluorescent antibody stain of smear	Elementary bodies
Purulent vaginal discharge	Yeast infection	Direct mount or Gram's stain	Pseudohyphae or budding yeasts
	Trichomonas infection	Direct mount	Flagellates with darting motility
	Gardnerella vaginalis	Pap stain or Gram's stain Measure pH of vaginal secretions	"Clue cells" or pH of vaginal secretions > 5.5
Penile or vulvar ulcer (chancre)	Primary syphilis	Darkfield mount of chancre secretion	Tightly coiled motile spirochetes
	Chancroid	Gram's stain of ulcer secretion or aspirate of inguinal bubo	Intracellular and extracellular small gram-negative bacilli
Eye	Purulent conjunctivitis	Gram's stain	Variety of bacterial species
	Trachoma	Giemsa stain of corneal scrapings	Intracellular perinuclear inclusion clusters
Feces	Purulent enterocolitis	Gram's stain	Neutrophils and aggregates of staphylococci
	Cholera	Direct mount of alkaline peptone water enrichment	Bacilli with characteristic darting motility; no neutrophils
	Parasitic disease	Direct saline or iodine mounts. Examine purged specimens.	Adult parasites or parasite fragments; protozoa or ova
Skin scrapings, nail fragments, or plucked hairs	Dermatophytosis	10% KOH mount	Delicate hyphae or clusters of spores
	Tinea versicolor	10% KOH mount or lactophenol cotton blue mount	Hyphae and spores resembling spaghetti and meatballs
Blood	Relapsing fever *(Borrelia)*	Wright's or Giemsa stain Darkfield examination	Spirochetes with typical morphology
	Blood parasites: malaria, trypanosomiasis, filariasis	Wright's or Giemsa stain Direct examination of anticoagulated blood for the presence of microfilaria	Intracellular parasites (malaria, babesia) Extracellular forms: trypanosomes or microfilaria

once stained the bacterial cells resist decolorization by strong organic solvents such as acid alcohol. Consequently, these bacteria are known as acid-fast, a phenomenon first discovered in 1881 by Ziehl and Neelsen.

Special treatment is required for the primary stain, carbolfuchsin, to penetrate the waxy material of the acid-fast bacilli. Heat is used in the conventional Ziehl-Neelsen technique. After the carbolfuchsin is overlaid on the surface of the smear to be stained, the flame of a

1. Make a thin smear of the material for study and allow to air dry.

2. Fix the material to the slide by passing the slide three or four times through the flame of a Bunsen burner so that the material does not wash off during the staining procedure. Some workers now recommend the use of alcohol for the fixation of material to be gram-stained (flood the smear with methanol or ethanol for a few minutes).

3. Place the smear on a staining rack and overlay the surface with crystal violet solution.

4. After 1 minute (less time may be used with some solutions) of exposure to the crystal violet stain, wash thoroughly with distilled water or buffer.

5. Overlay the smear with Gram's iodine solution for 1 minute. Wash again with water.

6. Hold the smear between the thumb and forefinger and flood the surface with a few drops of the acetone–alcohol decolorizer, until no violet color washes off. This usually takes 10 seconds or less.

7. Wash with running water and again place the smear on the staining rack. Overlay the surface with safranin counterstain for 1 minute. Wash with running water.

8. Place the smear in an upright position in a staining rack, allowing the excess water to drain off and the smear to dry.

9. Examine the stained smear under the 100× (oil) immersion objective of the microscope. Gram-positive bacteria stain dark blue; gram-negative bacteria appear pink-red.

which immunologic reactions can be visualized in direct smears of biological fluids or secretions and in tissue sections. Fluorochrome/protein ratios vary with different reagents to produce optimal staining of the desired objects, with a minimum of nonspecific background interference. The current development of monoclonal antibodies, which are monospecific to their respective antigens, has led to the preparation of fluorescent reagents for direct and indirect detection of several antigens of causal agents in human and animal specimens: *Chlamydia trachomatis*, *Legionella* species, *Treponema pallidum*, *Toxoplasma gondii*, and several viruses, including varicella-zoster, HSV-1 and 2, influenza A and B, cytomegalovirus, and respiratory syncytial virus among others.

Fluorescence microscopy is an exacting technique that requires a microscope of high quality, with the proper combination of microscope objectives, bright and darkfield condensers, a mercury arc or halogen ultraviolet light source, and appropriate combinations of exciter and barrier or suppression filters. Achromatic objectives are satisfactory for most applications, except in research applications in which expensive apochromatic lenses may be needed to achieve maximum illumination and resolution. The selection of microscope slides and coverslips of proper thickness, and the use of low-fluorescing immersion oils and mounting fluids that have figuration of the system being used, are critical for optimal performance.

The choice of filters in fluorescence microscopy is also critical to successful work. Four filters are required in sequence: 1) one to absorb heat, to prevent damage to the exciter filter; 2) an exciter filter with a wave bandwidth appropriate for the wavelength of light produced by the excited fluorochrome; 3) a red-absorbing filter to block out any red light emitted by the blue excitation filters; and 4) a barrier filter to absorb any of the residual short-wavelength incident excitation light, allowing only the longer-wavelength visible light to pass. Suboptimal performance of a fluorescence microscope system is often due to poor selection of filter combinations. Manufacturers of fluorescence equipment provide information and consultation so that users can achieve optimal performance of their systems. Fluorescence systems, using epi-illumination, blue light halogen lamps that do not require expensive transformers, and interference filters with maximum absorption peaks at the longer visible wavelengths, are now available within a price range acceptable to most clinical laboratories. McKinney and Cherry[43] provide a succinct review of immunofluorescence microscopy for those wishing to study the subject in more detail.

Bunsen burner is passed back and forth beneath the slide. The smear is heated to steaming, stopping short of boiling. The Kinyoun modification of the acid-fast stain is called the "cold method" because a surface-active detergent, such as Tergitol is used rather than heat treatment.

With either of these stains, the acid-fast bacilli appear red against either a green or blue background depending on the counter-stain used (Color Plate 2-2*B*). Although this method is satisfactory for most mycobacteria, certain weakly acid-fast strains of rapidly growing species (*Mycobacterium fortuitum/chelonae* complex) may stain better with the Ziehl-Neelsen method (further discussion can be found in Chapter 17).

Fluorescent Stains. Fluorescein isothiocyanate (FITC) and tetramethylrhodamine isothionate (TMRI) are two commonly used fluorochromes that, on excitation with ultraviolet or short-wavelength, visible light, emit light waves in the visible range, with absorption maxima of 490 nm and 555 nm, respectively. These fluorochromes bind chemically with a variety of proteins, including antigens and antibodies, providing a label or tag by

Fluorochrome Stains for Mycobacteria. The fluorochrome dyes auramine and rhodamine can also be used to demonstrate acid-fast bacilli. Viewed by fluorescence microscopy, the bacterial cells appear yellow against a dark background when potassium permanganate is used as a counterstain (Color Plate 2-2C). Use of the fluorescence procedure facilitates the screening of smears, particularly when a 25× objective is being used. This objective provides magnification low enough to scan wide microscopic fields, yet sufficiently high to see the yellow light points emanating from the fluorescing bacterial cells (Color Plate 2-2C). Higher magnification can be used to confirm suspicious objects observed with 25× lens.

The acid-fast stains can also be used to identify other nonbacterial microorganisms. The oocysts of *Cryptosporidium* species and *Isospora belli*, two coccidian organisms that have been incriminated as important etiologic agents in "gay bowel syndrome," are acid-fast and can be easily detected in acid-fast–stained preparations of stool specimens (Color Plate 20-2J).

Acridine Orange. The acridine orange (AO) stain is being used more frequently in microbiology laboratories to detect bacteria in smears prepared from fluids and exudates in which bacteria are expected to be in low concentration (10^3 to 10^4 colony-forming units [CFU]/mL) or are trapped within a heavy aggregate of background debris, making them difficult to visualize by conventional-staining procedures. The stain was originally used by microbiologists to demonstrate bacteria in soil samples. As in the application of fluorochrome dyes in studying acid-fast bacilli, smears stained with AO and examined under ultraviolet light can be more rapidly and efficiently screened at low-power magnifications (100×), reserving study at magnifications of 450× or higher when suspicious forms are visualized. The stain detects both living and dead bacteria, but does not indicate whether they are gram-negative or gram-positive. Once bacteria have been detected using the AO stain, a Gram's stain must be used to determine their differential-staining characteristics (Color Plate 2-2D).

The use of AO stains has been recommended in routine examination of blood culture broth, because the technique is sensitive enough to eliminate the need for 24-hour blind subcultures.[35,42] Lauer and associates[36] have found the AO stain to be more sensitive than the Gram's stain in detecting bacteria in CSF sediments, particularly when gram-negative organisms are present. The AO stain has also been useful in screening urine specimens for significant bacteriuria.[27] Box 2-9 outlines how to prepare an AO stain.

Toluidine Blue and Methylene Blue. Toluidine blue, a stain closely related to azure A and methylene blue, is being used more frequently in the staining of lung biopsy imprints and respiratory secretions for the rapid detection of *Pneumocystis carinii*. Methylene blue stains should be performed on spinal fluid sediments along with Gram's stains. The gram-negative–staining bacterial cells of *H. influenzae* and *N. meningitidis* often do not stand out against the red-staining background in Gram's stains; using methylene blue, polymorphonuclear leukocytes stain blue, and the bacterial cells are also deep blue and easier to detect against the light gray-staining background (Color Plate 2-2E). Methyl-

---

BOX 2-9. PREPARATION OF AN AO STAIN

Ingredients: AO powder 20 mg, sodium acetate buffer 290 mL, HCl 1M

Reagent preparation: Add 20 mg AO powder (JT Baker Chemical Co., Phillipsburg NJ) to 290 mL of sodium acetate buffer (stock solution of 100 mL of 2 molar [M]$CH_2COONa.3H_2O$ and 90 mL of 1 M HCl); 1 M HCl should be added as necessary to maintain the differential staining of the bacteria against the background debris.[36] The staining solution should be stored in a brown bottle at room temperature.

Procedure: The stain is performed by flooding air-dried and methanol-fixed smears of the material to be examined with the AO stain for 2 minutes, followed by a washing with tap water. The stained slides are dried and examined with a microscope equipped with an ultraviolet light source.

---

ene blue stains can be advocated as an adjunct to Gram's stains in laboratories where the inaccessibility to a fluorescence microscope precludes the use of the AO procedure.

A variety of procedures can be used to identify microorganisms in direct examinations. A summary of specimen types, various suspected infectious diseases, and direct examination procedures are summarized in Table 2-4.

Calcofluor White. Calcofluor white, a colorless dye used in industry to whiten textiles and paper, has two properties that make it useful in microbiology: 1) binding to β1-3, β1-4-polysaccharides (specifically cellulose and chitin); and 2) fluorescence when exposed to long-wavelength ultraviolet and short-wavelength visible light. Because the cell walls of fungi and plants are rich in chitin, calcofluor white is a valuable fluorochrome stain for the rapid detection of fungi in wet mounts, smears, and tissue sections. The stain has been most useful in detecting yeast cells, hyphae, and pseudohyphae in skin and mucous membrane scrapings. In particular, when mixed with 10% potassium hydroxide, mounts of skin scrapings can be rapidly screened for dermatophytes. When viewed microscopically under ultraviolet light, fungal structures display a brilliant apple-green or a ghostly blue-white (Color Plate 2-2F), depending on the wavelength of the exciter light. These structures are readily differentiated from background debris, cells, and tissue fragments. Calcofluor white has the added advantage that tissue sections can be subsequently stained with periodic acid–Schiff stain (PAS), Gomori methenamine silver (GMS), or other special stains without interference, should confirmation of findings or the availability of permanent slides be desired. The calcofluor white-staining technique is rapid and provides good definition of fungal fine structures and better contrast from the background than the widely used lactophenol analine blue stain.[25]

Silver Stains.   Certain bacteria, namely the spirochetes (including the recently recognized agent of Lyme disease, *Borrelia burgdorferi*) and the small bacillary organisms associated with cat scratch disease, are not readily stained by conventional methods. Presumably these organisms are either too slender to be visualized by brightfield microscopy, or they are in sufficiently low concentrations that they are not detected. Darkfield microscopy has been used to identify *T. pallidum*, the etiologic agent of syphilis, and other nontreponemal spirochetes, such as *Leptospira* species. One limitation of the darkfield procedure is the necessity to quickly examine wet, moist specimens containing living organisms. The silver stain has been used to observe these organisms in tissue sections.

The Warthin-Starry and Steiner-Steiner silver impregnation stains have been used for years to demonstrate spirochetes in formalin-fixed tissue sections. Kantoff and associates[33] propose that the histologic stain may be more effective in demonstrating the Lyme-associated spirochetes than darkfield examination and that skin biopsies may provide a reliable means for establishing the diagnosis. Recently, Duray and associates[17] have suggested use of a modified Dieterle stain to demonstrate the spirochetes of *B. burgdorferi* in tissue sections from patients with Lyme disease. This modification can be rapidly performed and is less susceptible to strict temperature control and instability of reagents than other silver-staining methods. *Borrelia burgdorferi* spirochetes stain black or brown-black against a tan-yellow background and vary in length from 4 μm to 39 μm. They can be distinguished from the spirochetes of *T. pallidum*, which are generally shorter in length (less than 256 μm) and more tightly coiled (see Color Plate 18-1*A*). Because spirochetes usually are not seen in large numbers in infected human tissues and often occur singly, screening of numerous oil immersion fields is usually required.

Wright's-Giemsa Stain.   The Wright's-Giemsa stain is commonly used for staining the cellular elements of the peripheral blood smear. This stain has little use in the staining of bacteria, but is used primarily to detect the intracellular yeast forms of *Histoplasma capsulatum* or the intracellular amastigotes of *Leishmania* species or *Trypanosoma cruzi* (Color Plate 2-2*G*). The stain is also helpful in demonstrating certain intracellular viral inclusions, such as may be observed in corneal scrapings in patients with trachoma (see Table 2-3).

Periodic Acid–Schiff.   The periodic acid–Schiff stain is based on the oxidation of hexoses and hexosamines by periodic acid, which breaks their pyranose rings, producing dialdehydes that react with Schiff reagent. Schiff reagent is a triphenylmethane dye prepared from basic fuchsin or *p*-rosanaline by reduction with sulfuric acid. Most substances that contain hexoses or hexosamines are PAS-positive, staining red against a green or blue background depending on the counterstain used. The stain is most frequently used in the staining of tissue sections to demonstrate fungal elements (Color Plate 2-2*H*).

PROCESSING OF CULTURES

After a specimen for culture has been received in the microbiology laboratory, the following key decisions must be made to recover and identify microorganisms that may be present:

1. Select primary culture media appropriate for the particular specimen type.
2. Determine the temperature and atmosphere of incubation to recover all organisms of potential significance.
3. Determine which of the isolates recovered on primary media require further characterization.
4. Determine whether antimicrobial susceptibility tests are required once the identification of the organism is known.

No single approach can be expected to serve the needs of all laboratories and clinical practice settings. The approach toward clinical microbiology in a 50-bed rural community hospital will differ from that used in a large, multidepartment medical center. Common to all is the recognition of the difficulties involved in maintaining quality services in the face of more and more stringent cost-containment policies. Laboratory directors and supervisors must work toward weeding out much of the clinically irrelevant work that was performed in the past. One hopes that the day of the "pan-culture" is over; that is, the indiscriminate ordering of cultures from all accessible body sites, in the hope of recovering a pathogenic organism, from patients with vague or ill-defined symptoms, such as fever of unknown origin, without localizing signs.

McCabe and Stottmeier[41] have noted this dilemma by pointing out that various "special interests" have adversely affected functions within hospitals and laboratories. Frequently, an extensive microbiology workup of a cadre of organisms known to be commensal or normal flora, often with orders to perform susceptibility tests, is carried out solely because a chief of service wants it done routinely. The decision of how far to process the individual specimen cultures must be based on a thorough knowledge of the host–parasite relations that apply in any given case. For the past two decades, many microbiologists have been attempting to practice what Bartlett calls "processing control";[4] that is, "restricting the processing and reporting of culture specimens to the production of predictably useful information."

SELECTION OF PRIMARY CULTURE MEDIA

From among the several hundred culture media commercially available, in addition to numerous "private" formulations that have been reported in the medical literature, only a few are required for daily use. Agar plates are commonly used. Inoculation of broth media for primary recovery of organisms should be limited only to those specimens, such as body fluids, needle biopsies, or deep tissue aspirations, in which recovery of even a few organisms in low concentration may be significant, or for which the chance for recovery of an anaerobe is reasonable. The past practice of routinely inoculating thioglycolate broth to recover hidden anaerobes has been abandoned in most laboratories. Except in special instances, the recovery of an organism in broth culture only after 4 or 5 days of incubation will have little clinical relevance. This practice also leads to the recovery of large numbers of contaminants.[46b] Bacterial isolates in very low concentrations are rarely significant, and the prolonged time for recovery will usually be too late for effective management. There are exceptions, such as the prolonged incubation time required for the recovery of *Brucella* species from blood and other specimens, or the recovery of *Cardiobacterium hominis* in patients with suspected bacterial endocarditis. In these situations, clinicians must be informed that the routine procedures used in a given laboratory may not recover certain organisms, and that the clinical suspicion of a rare or clinically confusing clinical condition must be clearly indicated on the request slip so that appropriate special media can be included in the workup.

It is currently recommended that only enriched, prereduced CDC or other suitable anaerobe blood agar plates be used for the recovery of anaerobes from most clinical specimens. If thioglycolate broth is used, the presence of growth after several days of incubation, in the face of no growth or the appearance of only an isolated colony on agar media, should probably be interpreted as minimal or rare growth and costly subcultures for biochemical characterization should not be performed. A Gram's stain of a drop of the broth isolate usually serves as a reliable guide for correlation with culture findings and determination of whether further analysis of the organism is necessary.

Media may be selective or nonselective. Nonselective media are free of inhibitors and support the growth of most microorganisms encountered in clinical laboratories. Five percent sheep blood agar is the most commonly used nonselective medium and is included in the battery of primary isolation media for virtually every clinical specimen. Horse blood, or sheep blood, agar supplemented with additives such as IsoVitalex, which includes various heme products, is preferred for the recovery of *H. influenzae* because it has no inhibitory effects on bacterial growth and is a rich source of factor X. Human blood is recommended for the recovery of *Gardnerella vaginalis*, for which, in addition to promoting good growth, hemolysis not seen on sheep blood agar can be observed, providing one clue to the presumptive identification.

Blood agar can be made selective by adding one or more antibiotics or certain chemicals. Kanamycin and vancomycin are added to blood agar (KV agar) used to recover anaerobic gram-negative bacilli (e.g., *Bacteroides* species); a combination of four or five antibiotics (bacitracin, novobiocin, colistin, cephalothin, polymyxin B, or others) are added to Campy-BAP to permit the recovery of *Campylobacter jejuni* from the heavy concentration of mixed flora in stool specimens. Colistin and nalidixic acid or phenylethyl alcohol can be added to blood agar to inhibit the growth of gram-negative bacteria in contaminated specimens, thereby

enhancing the recovery of gram-positive organisms. Fung and associates[22] have cautioned that CNA agar inhibits most strains of *Staphylococcus saprophyticus*. They recommend that blood agar should be used in addition to CNA for urine specimens obtained from female outpatients.

MacConkey agar is the selective culture medium most commonly used to inhibit gram-positive organisms. Bile salts and crystal violet are the active inhibitors, eosin Y and methylene blue are the inhibitors used in eosin methylene blue (EMB) agar. The formulas for these selective media are included in Chapter 4, the *Enterobacteriaceae*.

Enrichment broth is used to recover pathogenic organisms from specimens, such as feces, in which there is a heavy concentration of commensal organisms. For example, *Escherichia coli* and other "enteric" commensals are held in a prolonged lag phase of growth by the inhibitors in the enrichment broth, allowing the relatively few bacterial cells of *Salmonella* and *Shigella* species, in specific, to enter an uninhibited log phase of growth, during which they can better compete for survival.

The routine media used in a microbiology laboratory and a list of organisms that will not be recovered unless specifically requested should be published in a laboratory newsletter or manual. Physicians will then know for which infectious disease syndromes they will need to inform the laboratory that the anticipated causative organism is not covered by the culture media routinely used.

Techniques for Transfer and Culturing of Clinical Specimens

Once a specimen has "passed" the various criteria for rejection and has been accepted for culture, appropriate portions must be transferred to the various culture media described in the foregoing. This activity is also usually carried out in a designated part of the laboratory known as the "streak-out" area. The transfer of all specimens to culture media should be carried out under a biologic safety cabinet or laminar air hood where a glass or plastic shield is protecting the neck and face of the user. Although it is the policy in most hospitals to tag all potentially infectious specimens with a special biohazard label, it is not possible to completely screen all such samples. Therefore, the best policy is to handle all specimens as if they were highly infectious. Personnel should be required to wear rubber gloves when handling most specimens; the wearing of a surgical mask is optional, but is usually unnecessary.

The streak-out bench should be equipped with all of the implements and have the appropriate culture media readily available that will be needed for transferring specimens. Because most culture media must be refrigerated, a portable cart that extends the surface work area is often used. These carts can be stocked each morning with plates and tubes; any unused items can be returned to the refrigerator at the end of the day. When not in use, the media carts can be wheeled into a walk-in refrigerator.

Although full-time personnel working in the setup area may have memorized the culture media required for each specimen type, it is advisable to have appropriate charts and instructions posted on a bulletin board or included in a bench manual for use by those who are required to provide coverage during off hours. Every attempt should be made to use well-trained personnel, under close supervision, for the processing of specimens. Errors or misjudgments made during this link in the diagnostic cycle can negate all the expertise one may apply in the reading and interpretation of cultures. Expert microbiologists and technologists are often caught short in making a definitive diagnosis because inadequate or incorrect media were selected for a specimen. Options for the selection of specific culture media for the processing of specimens from various body sites (depending on the microorganisms to be recovered) will be presented in later sections of this chapter.

TECHNIQUES FOR THE CULTURING OF SPECIMENS

The equipment required for the primary inoculation of specimens is relatively simple. A Nichrome or platinum inoculating wire or loop is recommended (Fig. 2-6), with one end inserted into a cylindrical handle for easy use. The surface of agar media in petri plates may be inoculated with the specimen by several methods, one of which is shown in Figure 2-7. The primary inoculation can be made with a loop, swab, or other suitable device. Once the primary inoculum is made, a loop or straight wire can be used to spread the material into the four quadrants of the plate, as illustrated in Figure 2-8. The inoculum is successively streaked with a back-and-forth motion into each quadrant by turning the plate at 90-degree angles. The loop or wire should be sterilized between each successive quadrant streak. The purpose of this technique is to dilute the inoculum sufficiently on the surface of the agar medium so that well-isolated colonies of bacteria, known as colony-forming units (CFU) can be obtained. The isolated colonies can then be subcultured individually to other media to obtain pure culture isolates that can be studied on differential media. When streaking out blood agar plates with throat swabs submitted for

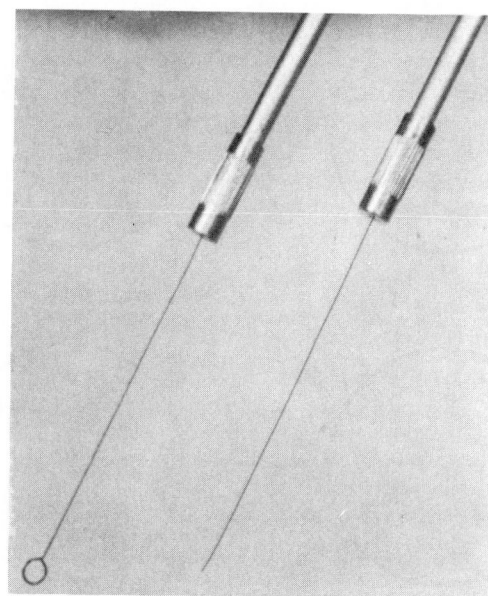

Figure 2-6.
Loop and straight wires commonly used for transfer and inoculation of specimens and cultures.

streptococcal screens, multiple stabs should be made in the areas of inoculation to unmask the oxygen-labile hemolysins, enhancing the detection of β-hemolytic streptococci. Also, bits of tissue that have been submitted for the recovery of fungi should be submerged beneath the surface of the agar. The initial growth of many species of fungi is enhanced in the microaerophilic atmosphere just beneath the agar surface.

The streaking technique used for inoculation of agar media for semiquantitative colony counts is illustrated in Figure 2-9. Nonferrous (Nichrome or platinum) inoculating loops, calibrated to contain either 0.01 or 0.001 mL of fluid, are immersed into an uncentrifuged urine sample. The loop is then carefully removed and the entire volume delivered to the surface of an agar plate by making a single streak across the center. The inoculum is spread evenly at right angles to the primary streak; then the plate is turned 90 de-

Figure 2-7.
The surface of an agar plate being inoculated with a specimen contained within an inoculating loop. Inoculation is accomplished by first touching the surface of the agar in one small area, then streaking the surface with a back and forth motion in a pattern shown in Figure 2-8, to obtain isolated colonies.

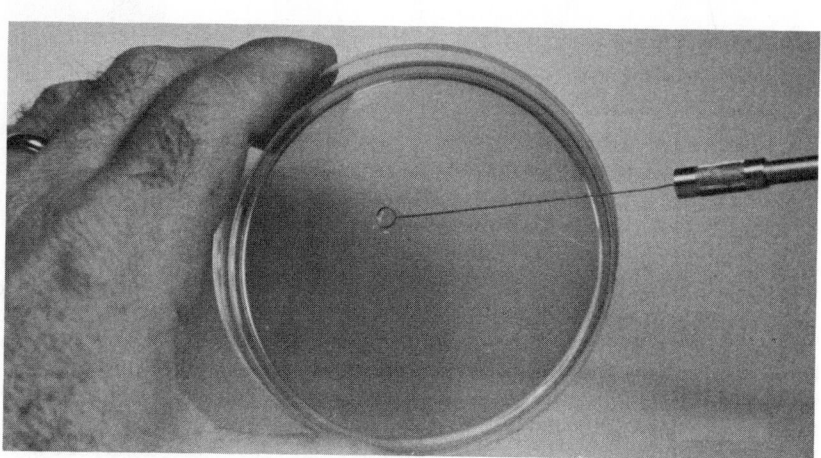

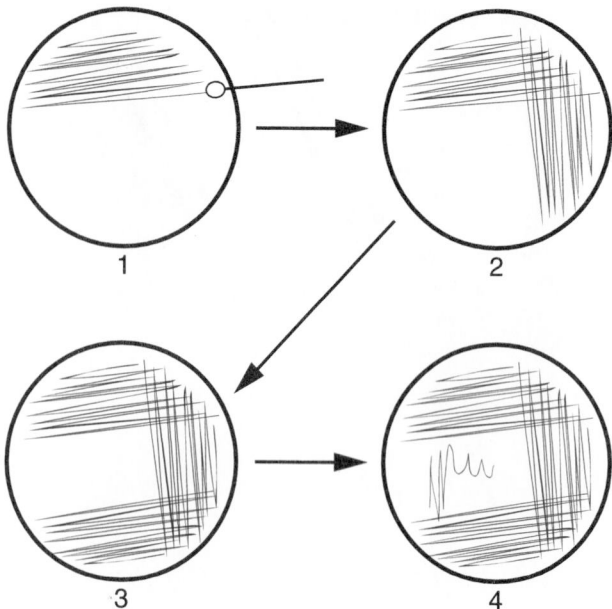

Figure 2-8.
Streaking patterns for the inoculation of specimens onto culture plates to obtain isolated bacterial colonies.

grees and the inoculum is spread to cover the entire surface. In some laboratories, two plates are inoculated, one with the 0.01- and the other with the 0.001-mL loop, serving as a quality control check. Although the inoculating loops are calibrated to deliver the volume of urine prescribed, accuracy can vary with an error rate of ±50%, particularly when using the 0.001-mL loop.[1] Vertical sampling from a small container may deliver only 50% of the prescribed volume; horizontal sampling at a 45-degree angle from a large container may deliver 150% of volume. Microbiologists should be aware of these potential errors and derive a standard angle for sampling in their laboratory, based on the volume of containers being used.

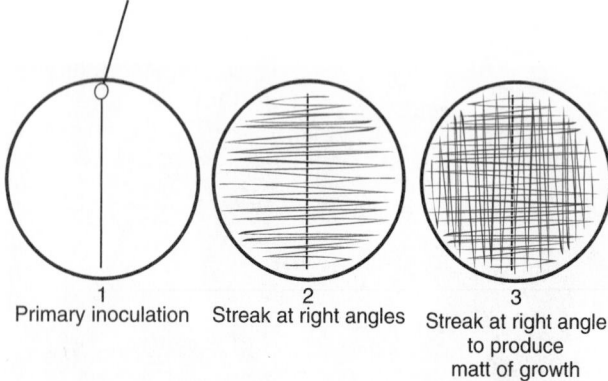

1	2	3
Primary inoculation	Streak at right angles	Streak at right angle to produce matt of growth

Figure 2-9.
Culture plates demonstrating streaking patterns of specimen for which a semiquantitative bacterial count is to be performed.

Accuracy and precision studies on the volume of inoculum can be done photometrically, by adding a loopful of gentian violet sampled from a 60-mL reservoir of dye in a 100 × 20-mm petri dish to 2 mL of water in a cuvette and reading it in a spectrophotometer set at 590 nm, or manometrically, by noting the change in weight when a loopful of water is delivered to a filter paper disk placed in the pan of a highly sensitive analytical balance (Gram-atic, Mettler Instrument Corp., Hightstown NJ). Devices are available to deliver a standard inoculum from fluid samples.[39]

After 18 to 24 hours of incubation, the number of bacteria in urine samples is estimated by counting the number of colonies that appear on the surface of the media. As illustrated in Figure 2-10, approximately 50 colonies can be counted. If a 0.001-mL loop had been used to inoculate the medium, the number of colonies would be multiplied by 1000. Therefore, the count in this illustration is 50,000 CFU/mL.

Media in tubes may be liquid, semisolid (0.3% to 0.5% agar) or solid (1% to 2% agar). Semisolid agar is suitable for motility testing. Broth medium in a tube can be inoculated by the method shown in Figure 2-11. The tube should be tipped at an angle of approximately 30 degrees and an inoculating loop touched to the inner surface of the glass, just above the point where the surface of the agar makes an acute angle. When the culture tube is returned to its upright position, the area of inoculation is submerged beneath the surface. Laboratory directors and microbiology supervisors must determine which specimens should be

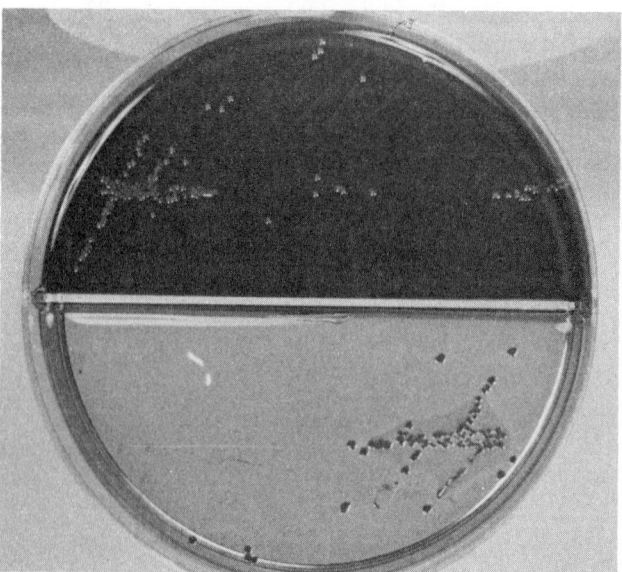

Figure 2-10.
Blood agar–MacConkey agar biplate previously streaked for semiquantitative colony count, as illustrated in Figure 2-9. Approximately 50 colonies appear on each side of this plate. If a 0.001-calibrated semiquantitative urine inoculating loop had been used for streaking each medium, the colony count would be 20 × 1,000–50,000 colony-forming units (CFU).

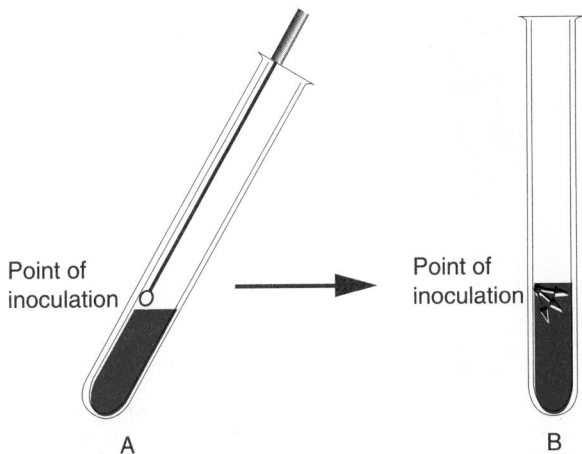

Figure 2-11.
Technique for inoculating a tube of broth medium. (**A**) Slant the tube and inoculate the tube by touching the moist inner surface of the glass tube at the acute angle of the meniscus. (**B**) Return the tube to an upright position, which has the effect of submerging the point of inoculation under the surface.

routinely transferred to broth cultures. Often considerable time can be wasted in tracking down the identity of a clinically insignificant organism that grows in broth culture in low concentration after only 4 or 5 days of incubation. In most instances, organisms causing infections are in sufficient concentration to be recovered on appropriate agar plates. Thus, broth cultures can be eliminated for most specimens, including those submitted for anaerobic culture. Whether to set up broth cultures on body fluids is a matter of personal preference based on experiences within a given practice setting.

Slants of agar medium are inoculated by first stabbing the depth of the agar, followed by streaking the slant from bottom to top with an S-motion as the inoculating wire is removed (Figs. 2-12 and 2-13). When inoculating semisolid tubed agar for motility testing, it is important that the inoculating wire be removed along the exact same track used to stab the medium. A fanning motion can result in a growth pattern along the stab line that may be falsely interpreted as bacterial motility.

Certain specimens may require centrifugation or filtering to concentrate any microbes that may be present. Tenacious, mucoid sputum samples may be liquefied with *N*-acetylcystine (Mucomist) to facilitate even streaking of the agar surface. Sputum samples to be processed for the recovery of *Mycobacterium* species must also be treated with sodium hydroxide to minimize the overgrowth of bacterial contaminants. Other specimens, such as urine and stool suspensions submitted for the recovery of mycobacteria, can also be briefly treated with NaOH to eliminate colonizing bacteria. Similarly, antibiotics can be added to control bacterial overgrowth in culture media and cell line suspensions used for the recovery of viruses. Specific applications can be found in Chapters 17 and 21.

Body fluids, such as those obtained from thoracentesis and paracentesis, should first be allowed to settle and then aliquots of the sediment centrifuged to further concentrate any bacteria that are present. Requests may be made to provide blood culture bottles for the direct inoculation of peritoneal fluid in suspected cases of an entity called spontaneous bacterial peritonitis. The use of blood culture bottles inoculated with peritoneal fluid at the bedside, rather than submitting the specimen to the laboratory for later processing, has been reported to increase the yield of organisms by as much as 50%, particularly in making the diagnosis of spontaneous bacterial peritonitis.[24,28,58] The negative features of this practice are that it does not provide a means for making semiquantitative estimates of the concentration of bacteria present in the original specimen, and it may not allow the detection of more than one bacterial species if a rapidly growing strain is present. The practice of using blood culture bottles for fluid specimens is currently limited to peritoneal fluid in cases of suspected spontaneous bacterial peritonitis; it does not apply to the recovery of organisms from other specimens, such as thoracentesis fluid, joint fluid, cerebrospinal fluid, and such.

Cerebrospinal fluid specimens, particularly for the recovery of *Cryptococcus neoformans*, should be centrifuged and portions of the sediment transferred to appropriate culture media; or preferably, the fluid should be passed through a 0.45-μm microbiological filter to trap any of the larger yeast cells that may be present.

Microorganisms differ in their optimal temperatures of incubation. In small laboratories, in which resources may be limited, it may not be possible to provide all of the incubation temperatures optimal for growth of all clinical isolates. Most microorganisms

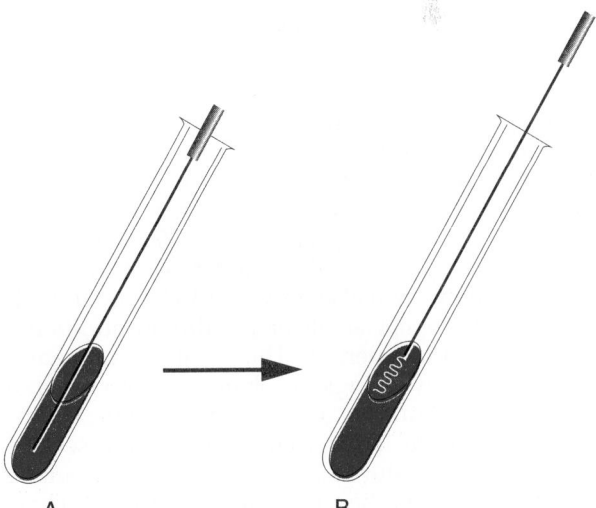

Figure 2-12.
The technique for inoculating an agar slant with a straight inoculating wire: (**A**) Stab the deep of the agar slant to within 2–3 mm of the bottom of the glass. If the bottom of the glass is touched, atmospheric air may enter, negating the anaerobic conditions. (**B**) Slowly remove the wire and streak the agar surface with a back and forth "S" motion.

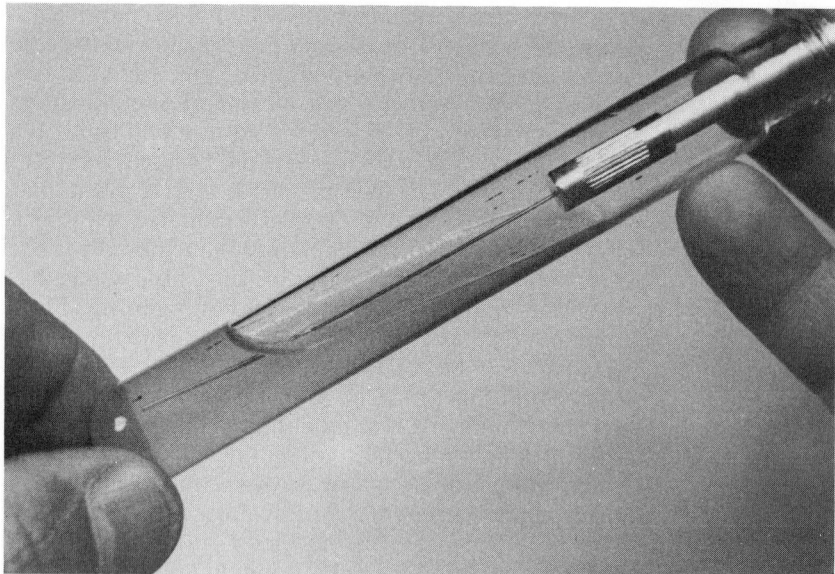

Figure 2-13.
The technique for inoculating an agar deep with a straight wire, as illustrated in Figure 2-12A. The deep of the medium is stabbed with the wire to within 2–3 mm of the bottom of the tube; then, after slowly removing the needle, the agar surface is streaked with a back and forth "S" motion, as illustrated in Figure 2-12B.

grow at 35°C; thus, if only one incubator is provided, it should be set at 35°C. Even organisms such as *Campylobacter jejuni*, which grows optimally at 42°C, will grow at 35°C if an additional 24 or 48 hours of incubation are allowed. The growth of most organisms is enhanced by an atmosphere of 5% to 10% CO_2. If only an ambient air, non-CO_2 incubator is available, the culture tubes and plates can be placed in a candle extinction jar and the entire assembly placed in the incubator. Conversely, an ambient air environment can be maintained in a CO_2 incubator by placing the cultures into a holding jar with a tightly fitted lid (an anaerobic jar or chamber is suitable). It should be realized, however, that organisms such as *C. jejuni*, which requires a reduced oxygen tension of 5% or below, will have difficulty growing in a candle jar in which the oxygen concentration is in the range of 10%.

Many microorganisms grow optimally within a narrow temperature range; others have a relatively wide range within which they can be recovered. The optimum temperature for growth of *C. jejuni* at 42°C was just mentioned. Most fungi grow optimally at 30°C; however, most can be recovered at room temperature or 35°C on appropriate media. *Yersinia enterocolitica* grows optimally at room temperature; however, most strains will also grow at 35°C, even though colonies may appear small or require an additional 24-hour incubation period. Thus, only infrequently will access to only a single incubator compromise the capability of a laboratory to recover most clinically important bacteria. In large laboratories where several incubation temperatures can be provided, organism recoveries will often be more rapid, and the appearance of colonies more true to form. Occasionally, incubation at room temperature for an extended time may be necessary to demonstrate certain biochemical or physical characteristics, such as pigment production and motility. These various adjustments will be learned through experience and by trial and error.

Probably more important than the mode of incubation is prevention of wide fluctuations in temperature. Even if cultures are incubated at room temperature, care should be taken to see that the tubes and plates are protected from air-conditioning drafts or heat vents through which convection currents can produce considerable fluctuations in temperature during on–off cycles. Incubators should be carefully controlled for temperature, with no more than ±1° to 2° fluctuations from day to day. Incubators should be located or protected so that control dials cannot be easily disturbed by cleaning personnel during off hours.

Humidity control within the incubator is also important. Most organisms grow maximally when the humidity is 70% or higher, and culture media tends to deteriorate more rapidly when undue drying or desiccation is allowed. The recovery of *H. pylori*, in particular, and to a lesser extent, *N. gonorrhoeae* require an atmosphere with high humidity. Most incubators purchased during the past several years have built-in water reservoirs by which chamber humidity can be regulated; if not, open pans of water can be placed on shelves to provide moisture through evaporation. Incubators must also be periodically checked for inadvertent spills that can cause contamination or a buildup of chemicals from reagents that may be inhibitory to bacterial growth.

INTERPRETATION OF CULTURES

Interpretation of primary cultures after 24 to 48 hours of incubation requires considerable skill. From initial observations, the microbiologist must assess the colonial growth and decide whether additional procedures are required. This assessment is made by noting the characteristics and relative number of each type of colony recovered on agar media; by determining the purity, Gram reaction and morphology of the bacteria in each type of colony; and by observing changes in the media surrounding the colonies, which reflect specific metabolic activities of the bacteria recovered.

GROSS COLONY CHARACTERISTICS

Assessment of gross colony characteristics is usually performed by visually inspecting growth on the surface of agar plates. Inspection of cultures is carried out by holding the plate in one hand and observing the surface of the agar for the presence of bacterial growth (Fig. 2-14). Standard culture plates are 100 mm in diameter and are convenient to hold in one hand. Each plate must be studied carefully, because the bacteria initially recovered from specimens are often in mixed culture and a variety of colonial types may be present. Pinpoint colonies of slow-growing bacteria may be overlooked among larger colonies, particularly if there is any tendency for growth to spread over the surface of the plate.

During examination, plates should be tilted in various directions, under bright, direct illumination, so that light is reflected from various angles. We highly recommend use of a hand lens or a dissecting microscope to assist in the detection of tiny or immature colonies and to better observe their characteristics (Fig. 2-15). Blood agar plates should also be examined when transilluminated by bright light from behind the plate to detect hemolytic reactions in the agar (Fig. 2-16).

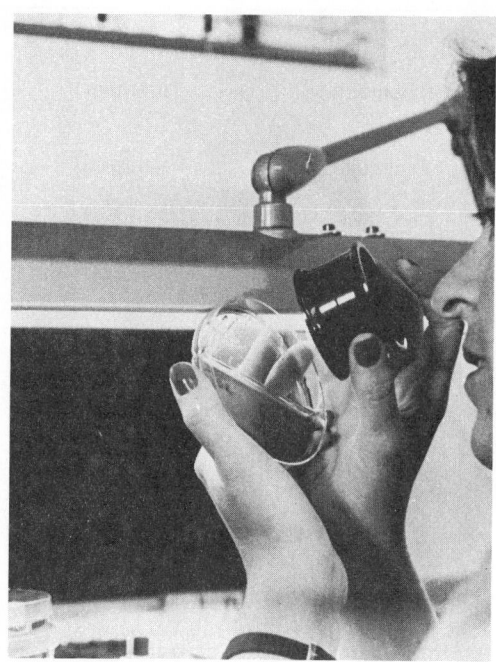

Figure 2-15.
The technique, using a hand lens, for examining colonies growing on the surface of an agar plate.

Figure 2-17 provides terms and illustrations helpful when describing bacterial colonies. Additional guidelines are outlined in Boxes 2-10 through 2-12.

Although difficult to describe specifically, odors produced by the action of certain bacteria in plating media and in liquid media can be very helpful in the tentative identification of the microorganisms involved. Examples of microorganisms exhibiting distinctive odors include *Pseudomonas* species: grape juice; *Proteus* species: burned chocolate; *Eikenella corrodens*: bleach; *Alkaligenes faecalis* (*odorans*): freshly cut

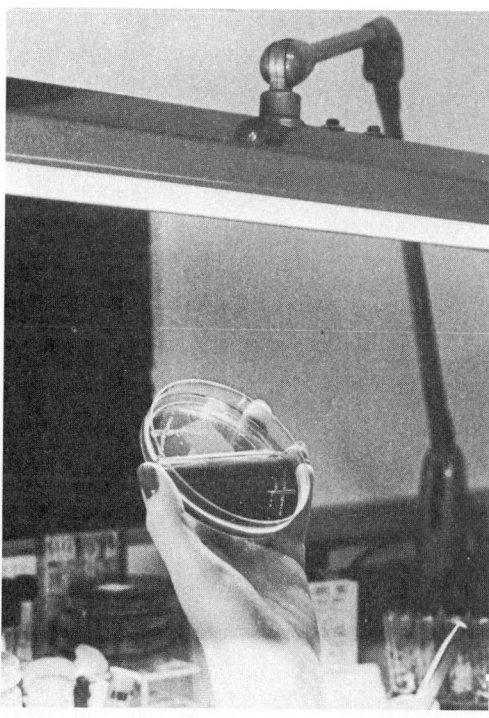

Figure 2-14.
The technique for examining the surface of an agar plate by direct, oblique-reflected light.

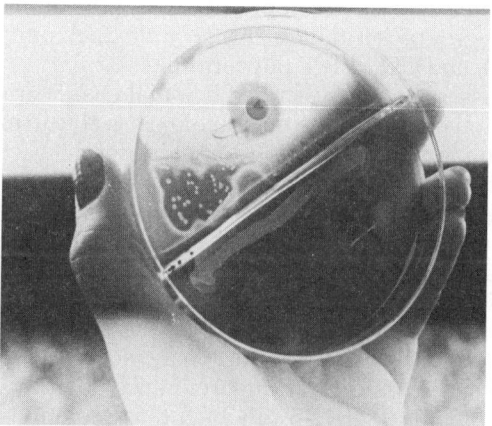

Figure 2-16.
The technique for examining colonies growing on the surface of an agar plate, using transmitted light. This technique is helpful in assessing the hemolytic properties of colonies growing on blood agar.

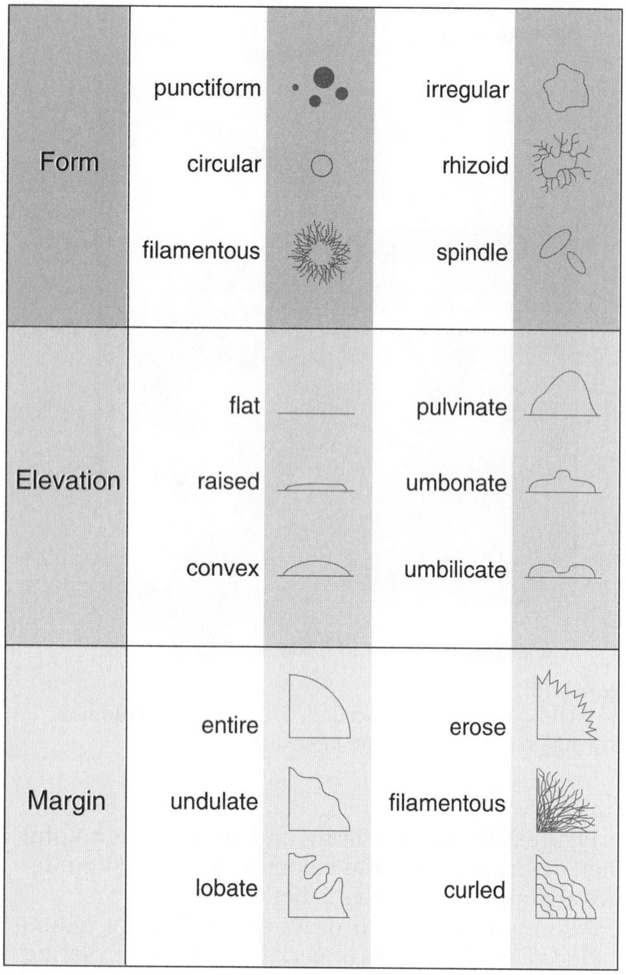

Figure 2-17.
Illustrations of a variety of morphologic colony forms, with labels of terms for each.

BOX 2-10. CHARACTERISTICS OF COLONIES USED IN THE IDENTIFICATION OF BACTERIA

Size: diameter in millimeters

Form: punctiform, circular, filamentous, irregular, rhizoid, spindlelike

Elevation: flat, raised, convex, pulvinate, umbonate, umbilicate

Margin (edge of colony): entire, undulant, lobate, erose, filamentous, curled

Color: white, yellow, black, buff, orange, other

Surface: glistening, dull, other

Density: opaque, translucent, transparent, other

Consistency: butyrous, viscid, membranous, brittle, other

See also fig. 2-17 and Color Plate 2-3

GRAM'S STAIN EXAMINATION

Preliminary impressions, based on observation of colony characteristics, can be further confirmed by studying gram-stained smears, a technique that is relatively simple to perform. The top and center of the colony to be studied is first touched with the end of a straight inoculating wire, taking care not to touch the adjacent agar (Fig. 2-18, page 102). The portion of the colony to

---

apples; *Corynebacterium* species, DF-3: "fruity"; *Nocardia* and *Streptomyces* species: musty basement; *Clostridium* species: fecal, putrid; *Bacteroides melaninogenicus* group: acrid; *Pasteurella multocida*: pungent (indole); and CDC EF-4: popcorn-like.

By assessing the described colonial characteristics and action on media, the microbiologist is able to make a preliminary identification of the different bacteria isolated by primary culture. These characteristics are helpful in selecting other appropriate differential media and tests to complete the identification of the isolates. To better illustrate this approach to bacterial identification, Table 2-5 lists some of the more commonly encountered colonial types, the group of bacteria to suspect for each, additional tests required for definitive identification, and reference to the exact frame in Color Plate 2-3 in which these colony types are illustrated.

The initial inspection of colonies for preliminary identification of bacteria is one of the cornerstones of diagnostic microbiology and is discussed in detail in later chapters devoted to specific groups of pathogenic bacteria and other microorganisms.

BOX 2-11. REACTIONS IN AGAR MEDIA USED IN THE IDENTIFICATION OF BACTERIA

Hemolysis on blood agar
  Alpha: partial clearing of blood around colonies with green discoloration of the medium; outline of red blood cells intact
  Beta: zone of complete clearing of blood around colonies owing to lysis of the red blood cells
  Gamma: no change in the medium around the colony; no lysis or discoloration of the red blood cells
  Alpha prime: halo of incomplete lysis immediately surrounding colonies, with a second zone of complete hemolysis at the periphery
Pigment production in agar medium
  Water-soluble pigments discoloring the medium
  Pyocyanin
  Fluorescent pigments
  Nondiffusable pigments confined to the colonies
Reaction in egg yolk agar
  Lecithinase: zone of precipitate in medium surrounding colonies
  Lipase: "pearly layer," an iridescent film in and immediately surrounding colonies, visible by reflected light
  Proteolysis: clear zone surrounding colonies

be sampled is emulsified in a small drop of water or physiologic saline on a microscope slide to disperse the individual bacterial cells (Fig. 2-19). After the slide has air dried, the bacterial film is fixed to the glass surface either by using heat, quickly passing the slide four or five times through the flame of a Bunsen burner, or by flooding with methanol or ethanol for a few minutes. The fixed smear is then placed on a staining rack and the Gram's stain is performed as described in Box 2-8.

The stained smear should be examined microscopically using an oil immersion objective. In addition to the Gram's stain reaction of the bacterial cells (gram-positive bacteria appear blue; gram-negative bacteria appear red or pink), three other characteristics are helpful in making a preliminary identification of isolates: 1) size and shape of the bacterial cells, 2) arrangement of the bacterial cells, and 3) presence or lack of specific structures or organelles (spores, metachromatic granules, swollen bodies, or other features).

In making a preliminary identification of bacterial isolates, the microbiologist should evaluate each of

TABLE 2-5
PRELIMINARY BACTERIAL IDENTIFICATION BY COLONIAL TYPES

COLONIAL TYPE	BACTERIAL GROUP	ADDITIONAL TESTS	FRAME OF PLATES ILLUSTRATING TYPE
Convex, entire edge, 2–3 mm, creamy, yellowish, zone of β-hemolysis	*Staphylococcus*	Catalase Coagulase DNase Mannitol utilization Tellurite reduction Novobiocin resistance Furazolidone resistance	2–3A
Convex or pulvinate, translucent, pinpoint in size, butyrous, wide zone of β-hemolysis	*Streptococcus*	Catalase A disk 6.5% NaCl tolerance Bile-esculin CAMP test Hippurate hydrolysis L-Pyrrolidonyl-β-naphthylamide (PyR)	2–3B, C
Umbilicate or flat, translucent, butyrous or mucoid, broad zone of α-hemolysis	*Pneumococcus*	P disk Bile solubility	2–3G

Pulvinate, semiopaque, gray, moist to somewhat dry, β-hemolysis may or may not be present	*Escherichia coli* and other Enterobacteriaceae	Multiple tests
		  Indole
		  Methyl red
		  Voges-Proskauer reaction
		  Citrate
		  Decarboxylases
		  Urease
		  Phenylalanine
		  Carbohydrate fermentations
			2–3D

Flat, gray; spreading as thin film over agar surface; burned chocolate odor	*Proteus*	Phenylalanine deaminase Urease Lysine deaminase	
Flat, opaque, gray to greenish, margins erose or spreading, green-blue pigment, grapelike odor	*Pseudomonas*	Cytochrome oxidase Fluorescence of carbohydrate assimilations Denitrification DNase Hydrolysis of acetamide Growth at 42°C	

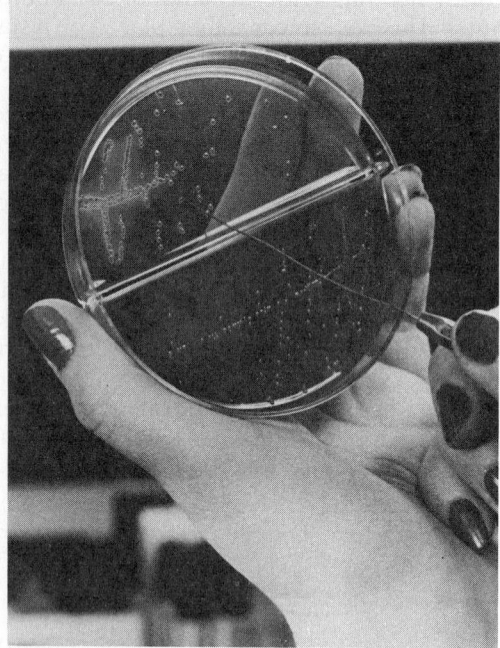

Figure 2-18.
The technique for picking an isolated bacterial colony with a straight wire for subculture to another medium.

these characteristics. Although other approaches to screening for bacteria, such as acridine orange stains, the Automicrobic System (AMS, Vitek, Hazelwood, MO) and the Bac-T-Screen device (Vitek) have been advocated, none is more sensitive than the Gram's stain in detecting significant bacterial concentrations in urine samples.[37,52] A series of photomicrographs of several stains illustrating a number of the morphologic

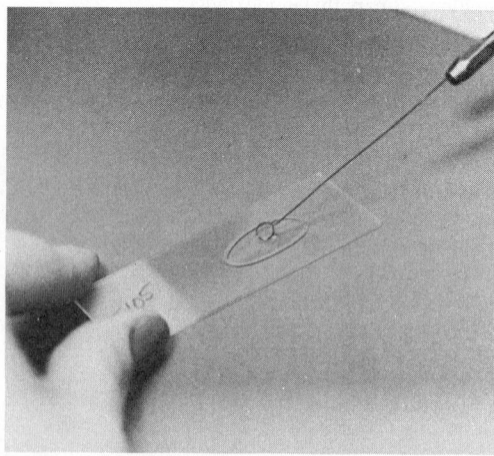

Figure 2-19.
The technique for preparing a smear for a Gram stain. The top portion of an isolated bacterial colony, as illustrated in Figure 2-18, is touched with an inoculating wire or loop, then the tip of the loop is submerged in a drop of water, or physiologic saline, on a glass slide, the inoculum emulsified, and the preparation left to air-dry before heat fixation and staining.

cells types and spatial arrangements of bacteria commonly encountered in clinical laboratories are shown in Color Plate 2-4.

With the information derived from the examination of bacterial colonies and gram-stained smears of cells, the microbiologist is able to proceed toward identifying isolates without performing differential tests. For example, a raised, creamy, yellow hemolytic colony on blood agar that shows gram-positive cocci in clusters in a gram-stained preparation suggests staphylococcus (see Color Plate 2-4C). A pinpoint translucent beta-hemolytic colony with blood agar showing gram-positive cocci in chains is most probably a streptococcus (see Color Plate 2-4D).

The microbiologist soon learns, however, not to rely solely on the examination of gram-stained smears because the staining reactions may be variable, particularly with very young or older colonies. Gram's stain morphology of most bacteria is most characteristic when smears are prepared from an 18- to 24-hour broth subculture, a time when the bacterial cells are in log phase of growth. Often, the Gram's stain morphology is less characteristic when smears are prepared from colonies growing on agar surfaces.

Microbiologists should provide as much preliminary information to the physician as possible. In selected cases, such as when observing bacteria in a blood culture broth or directly in infected CSF, this type of preliminary information can be quite useful in directing specific antibiotic therapy before final species identification or antimicrobial susceptibility test results are available.

PRELIMINARY IDENTIFICATION BASED ON METABOLIC CHARACTERISTICS

Most tests used to assess the biochemical or metabolic activity of bacteria, by which a final species identification can be made, are performed by subculturing the primary isolate to a series of differential test media, the results of which can then be interpreted after 1 or more days of additional incubation.

The initial observations and interpretations of culture plates should be used to determine whether the microorganism(s) recovered should be further identified and whether antibiotic susceptibility tests should be performed. Although to some extent these determinations must be based on observations of individual cultures, certain guidelines can be used to reduce the amount of unnecessary and costly work required. A major decision must be made as to how to handle cultures with mixed bacterial colonies. Although polymicrobic infections do occur, particularly when mixed aerobic and anaerobic bacterial species are recovered from deep wounds or visceral organs, this same mixture of organisms from cultures of urine, the respiratory tract, or superficial skin wounds or ulcers must be interpreted differently. Thus, the decision on how far to process the culture must be based on a fundamental understanding of how bacteria cause infections in different anatomic sites.

Bartlett[4] has recommended that routine cultures that grow three or more organism types should not be further processed. He suggests that reports be issued on the basis of gross plate morphology without complete identification and that no antibiograms be performed. We agree with this analysis that, except in unusual circumstances, the recovery of three or more organisms from specimens obtained from nonsterile sites most commonly represent colonization or contamination. Repeat cultures may be indicated if there is clinical evidence of infection. Our experience is similar to that reported by Bartlett—repeat cultures rarely confirm isolation of the same bacterial pathogens, particularly if clean-catch or closed catheter urine specimens are obtained.

Another problem is the receipt of specimens from the same source on successive days. If organisms with the same gross colony characteristics are observed in repeat cultures, the report can indicate that no significant change has been observed and detailed biochemical characterization and antibiograms are not necessary. However, if second cultures are received after an arbitrary interval of time, perhaps 5 days or 1 week, repeat complete identifications and antibiograms are indicated because a change in flora or antibiotic susceptibility patterns may be the cause for persistent infection. One must be careful in referring the susceptibility patterns of current isolates of *P. aeruginosa* to previous cultures, because induced resistance, manifesting only after exposure to certain antibiotics, particularly select cephalosporins, will result in the delayed production of specific cephalosporinases inactivating antibiotics used to treat infections. The mechanisms of antibiotic-induced resistance are discussed in Chapter 15.

The decision on how far to proceed in making final species identifications and in performing antibiotic susceptibility tests may depend on what is observed in gram-stained smears or the original specimen. Because Gram's stains are not always performed on all specimens, it may be wise to prepare unstained smears of certain specimens (e.g., wounds and body fluids) to reserve for Gram's staining if the decision is made to further process certain isolates. If the bacterial colonies are consistent with what is seen in gram-stained smears, there is more impetus to complete the identification and perform antibiograms.

DIRECT BIOCHEMICAL PROCEDURES FOR MAKING PRELIMINARY BACTERIAL IDENTIFICATIONS

Certain preliminary observations or a direct rapid test can be performed on select colonies. Frequently, an isolate can be identified to a level that is clinically useful based on these assessments alone. For example, the lactose-utilizing properties of gram-negative bacilli can be directly evaluated from MacConkey agar by observing the red pigmentation of the colonies; H_2S production may be detected on Hektoen and XLD agars by observing colonies with black centers. The decarboxylation of lysine can also be suspected when observing colonies growing on XLD agar. A red halo around the colony, indicating an alkaline pH shift, indicates the decarboxylation of lysine.

The following are direct tests that can be performed on isolated colonies recovered on primary culture plates.

THE CATALASE TEST

A few drops of 3% hydrogen peroxide are placed directly on a colony. Rapid effervescence indicates production of molecular oxygen and a positive test (see Chart 10). Accurate results may be difficult to obtain if the test is performed on colonies growing on blood agar because of the presence of peroxidase in erythrocytes. The peroxidase reaction produced by erythrocytes is delayed and weak, however, and can usually be readily differentiated from the immediate and highly active reactions produced by catalase-positive bacteria. The catalase test is frequently used to differentiate staphylococci (positive) from streptococci (negative).

THE BILE SOLUBILITY TEST

Two methods for determining bile solubility are commonly used. As an initial screen, a few drops of a 10% solution of sodium deoxycholate solution are placed on colonies suspected of being *Streptococcus pneumoniae*. Pneumococcal colonies completely lyse and disappear after about 30 minutes (see Chart 5). Because this test is sometimes difficult to interpret, the tube test is easier to read. An inoculum from the unknown bacterial colony can be suspended in a 10% solution of deoxycholate (bile salts) until turbidity is achieved. The clearing of the turbidity within 30 to 60 minutes after incubation at 35°C indicates bile solubility (see Chart 5).

THE SLIDE COAGULASE TEST

A colony suspected of being *Staphylococcus* species is emulsified in a drop of rabbit plasma on a glass slide. Bacterial clumping within 2 minutes indicates the presence of bound coagulase and constitutes a positive test result (see Chart 13). Several commercial systems are available for performing the coagulase test.[2,8] The one advantage is standardization of the method and interpretation of results. Sero STAT Staphtm (Scott Laboratories, Fiskville RI), AccuStaph (Carr-Scarborough Microbiologicals, Stone Mountain GA), Staphylatex (American Scientific Products, McGaw Park IL), and Staphyloslide (BBL Microbiology Systems, Cockeysville MD) are all based on the detection of protein A or clumping factor, characteristic of coagulase-positive strains. Aldridge and associates[2] found good correlation between these products and conventional plasma-based tests. The only exception was occasional false-negative results with methicillin-resistant strains of *S. aureus*. It is recommended that negative-reacting, methicillin-resistant strains be confirmed with a tube coagulase or the thermonuclease test.

THE DIRECT SPOT INDOLE TEST

A small portion of the colony to be tested is transferred from a nonselective medium, such as blood or chocolate agar, to a strip of filter paper that has been saturated with Kovac's reagent or *p*-dimethylamino-cinnamaldehyde (PACA) solution. The immediate development of a red color with Kovac's reagent indicates the presence of indole and a positive test (see Chart 40). PACA is more sensitive than Kovac's reagent, and a positive test reaction is indicated by the rapid development of a blue color. In many laboratories, dry-appearing, lactose-positive, spot indole-positive colonies appearing after 24 hours of incubation on MacConkey's agar, particularly on isolates from the urinary tract are presumptively identified as *E. coli*, and further tests are usually not performed. In these cases, the spot indole must be performed on colonies growing on parallel blood agar plates, because the pigmentation of the lactose-positive colonies on MacConkey's agar will make interpretation of the color reaction difficult.

CYTOCHROME OXIDASE TEST

A portion of the colony to be tested is smeared on the reagent-impregnated area of an oxidase test strip. The immediate development of a blue color indicates cytochrome oxidase activity and a positive test result (see Chart 16). Cytochrome oxidase tests are useful for the initial categorization of many bacterial species that have distinctive colonial morphology. Oxidase-positive colonies can be discounted as belonging to the *Enterobacteriaceae* and often help identify certain bacterial species that produce cytochrome oxidase, such as *Aeromonas* species, *Plesiomonas* species, *Pseudomonas* species and *Pasteurella* species.

MUG TEST

Other direct tests can be used to screen for certain organisms from primary isolation plates, offering potent savings on time-consuming and costly differentiation procedures. One is the MUG (4-methylumbelliferyl-β-D-glucuronidase) test, based on detecting the capability of the unknown organism to produce β-glucuronidase (can be used as a screen for *E. coli* instead of the spot indole test discussed earlier). The MUG reagent, in tubes or impregnated in dehydrated disks, after inoculation with a heavy suspension of the unknown organism, will fluoresce from release of 4-methylumbelliferone if glucuronidase is present. We have found the Remel MUG test (Remel Inc., Lenexa KA) to be accurate and easy to interpret. Indole can also be detected by adding Kovac's indole reagent to the MUG tube, making this combination test a valuable method for screening lactose-fermenting enteric bacilli.

PYR SUBSTRATE

Bosley and associates[9] have described the use of L-pyrrolidonyl-β-naphthylamide (PyR) substrate for the rapid identification of enterococci. After 4 hours of incubation following heavy inoculation of the substrate with a liquid suspension of the unknown organism prepared from a primary isolation plate, the production of a red color after adding *N,N*-methyl-aminocinnamaldehyde reagent is indicative of group D enterococci (group A streptococci are also PyR-positive, but can usually be differentiated by morphologic criteria; see Chart 61). The techniques and interpretations of the foregoing procedures are discussed in greater detail in subsequent chapters. In an era of stringent cost containment, it is imperative that microbiologists apply their skills of observation and use of a few select characteristics to presumptively identify bacterial species whenever possible. Developing this microbiologic "sixth sense" can also be helpful in verifying the results obtained from packaged kit systems or from automated instruments. On occasion, the biotype numbers issued by these systems may be in conflict with colonial, Gram stain, and biochemical "spot tests," and continued study may be in order to prevent issuing an erroneous report.

BACTERIAL SPECIES IDENTIFICATION AND SELECTION OF DIFFERENTIAL CHARACTERISTICS

Preliminary bacterial identification can be made by observing colonial characteristics and gram-stained morphology, as discussed in the foregoing. However, the final characterization of an unknown bacterial isolate to identify it to the genus and species levels is usually accomplished by testing for certain enzyme systems that are unique to each species and serve as identification markers. In the laboratory, these enzyme systems are detected by inoculating a small portion of a well-isolated bacterial colony into a series of culture media containing specific substrates and chemical indicators that detect pH changes, or by the presence of specific by-products. The clinical microbiologist must select appropriate sets of differential characteristics that will permit the identification of each group of bacteria.

For the final identification of bacteria within any given group, several dozen characteristics are available from which to choose. In Table 2-6 are listed several groups of bacteria commonly encountered in the clinical laboratory and the characteristics often selected for identifying species within these groups. The various schema in which these characteristics are used in the identification of the several bacterial groups listed are discussed in detail in subsequent chapters.

Species identifications, the determination of biotype numbers, and antibiotic profiles may be helpful in determining if an isolate from one site, such as in blood cultures, is identical with a similar organism from another site which may be the source of the septicemia. Recovery of *Streptococcus pneumoniae* from sputum or *E. coli* from a urine specimen has more significance if the same strain is concomitantly recovered from a blood culture. Recovery of the same yeast species from two or more sites may indicate disseminated infection; whereas, if the strains are different, simple colonization or contamination is more likely. Biotype numbers and antibiograms may also be helpful in determining

TABLE 2-6
DIFFERENTIAL CHARACTERISTICS COMMONLY USED FOR IDENTIFYING BACTERIA WITHIN VARIOUS GROUPS

BACTERIAL GROUP SUGGESTED BY GROSS COLONY AND MICROSCOPIC FEATURES	DIFFERENTIAL CHARACTERISTICS COMMONLY MEASURED	BACTERIAL GROUP SUGGESTED BY GROSS COLONY AND MICROSCOPIC FEATURES	DIFFERENTIAL CHARACTERISTICS COMMONLY MEASURED
Staphylococci	Catalase production Cytochrome oxidase activity Oxidative or fermentative (OF) glucose utilization Mannitol fermentation Coagulase production DNase activity Novobiocin resistance Furazolidone resistance	Nonfermentative gram-negative bacilli	Oxidative or fermentative (OF) glucose utilization Growth on MacConkey agar Cytochrome oxidase activity Motility Nitrate reduction Denitrification of nitrates and nitrites Gluconate reduction Fluorescein pigment production Pigment production Lysine decarboxylase activity Utilization of 10% lactose and glucose Penicillin sensitivity Catalase production Urease production Indole production Hydrolysis of acetamide Hydrolysis of esculin
Streptococci including S. pneumoniae	Catalase production Bacitracin susceptibility (A disk) 6.5% NaCl tolerance Reaction on bile–esculin agar Sodium hippurase production Bile solubility Optochin sensitivity (P disk) L-Pyrrolidonyl-β-naphthylamide (PyR)		
Enterobacteriaceae	Lactose fermentation Nitrate reduction Cytochrome oxidase activity Decarboxylase or dihydrolase activity (lysine, ornithine, and arginine) Hydrogen sulfide production Indole production Citrate utilization Methyl red reaction Motility o-Nitrophenyl galactosidase activity (ONPG test) Production of acetylmethyl carbinol (Voges-Proskauer reaction) Urease production	Neisseria Branhamella Moraxella	Growth on modified Thayer-Martin medium Cytochrome oxidase activity Nitrate reduction Carbohydrate utilization: glucose, maltose, sucrose, lactose Penicillin sensitivity
		Haemophilus	Catalase production Cytochrome oxidase activity Growth on sheep blood agar Nitrate reduction Requirements for CO_2 for growth Indole production Utilization of sucrose Requirement for growth factors X (hemin), V (NAD) Porphyrin formulation

if an isolate recovered at some time in the past is the same as a similar isolate currently recovered from the same source. If the species is identical, a treatment failure is probable if the biotypes and antibiograms are different, and a new unrelated infection is more likely.

ANTIBIOTIC SUSCEPTIBILITY TESTING

Decisions must be made whether to perform antibiotic susceptibility tests on organisms recovered from clinical specimens. Not all isolates should be tested, even if physicians have made the usual request for "culture and sensitivities." Antibiograms should not be performed on bacterial species with known patterns of susceptibility and resistance. For example, antibiotic susceptibility tests on β-hemolytic streptococci are not indicated because all strains are susceptible to penicillin. In Bartlett's experience, only 1.43% of hospitalized patients who developed bacteremia from urinary tract infections were infected with bacteria resistant to either amikacin or ampicillin, or both.[7] Extra costs can extend into many thousands of dollars per year if susceptibility tests are routinely performed on urinary tract isolates just to prevent the use of ineffective antibiotics empirically selected. Susceptibility testing should not be done on organisms considered to be contaminants, or when three or more species are recovered. Most microbiologists also refrain from performing susceptibility tests on fungi and mycobacteria; rather, when indicated, specimens are sent to reference laboratories.

β-Lactamase tests should be performed for all clinically significant isolates of *H. influenzae* and *N. gonorrhoeae*. Penicillin-resistant, β-lactamase-producing strains are being encountered with increasing frequency and must be detected before antibiotic therapy is begun.

In most laboratories, the number of antibiotics on which susceptibility testing can be performed is usually 15 or fewer; this group of select antibiotics is called a panel. The selection process should be done in consultation with hospital pharmacists and medical service committees so that the panel of antibiotics chosen for susceptibility testing conforms to local patterns of practice. A cascade for the selective reporting of antimicrobial susceptibility test results has been instituted in many laboratories to help prevent the emergence of resistant bacterial strains. The programmed cascade reports (displays) to the physicians and ward personnel only select drugs for any given bacterial isolate. A broader panel of antibiotics is tested, and the profiles of restricted drugs are available upon request. Each laboratory director, in consultation with the infectious disease and pharmacy services must decide on the cascade appropriate to the formulary and local patterns of practice. Box 2-13 provides examples of programmed cascades (if the first drug listed in a given group is resistant, the next drug in the group is reported, and so on). Thus, less than a half dozen antibiotics are reported for any given organism group. Although physicians may initially feel too restricted by the availability of results on such a select group of antibiotics, the programmed cascade is usually accepted after a period of usage.

Panels for other groups of organisms have also been suggested.[65] It is common practice to reserve certain antibiotics for use only against multiple-resistant organisms. See Chapter 15 for a listing of antibiotics that are often included on such panels.

USE OF SUSCEPTIBILITY TEST RESULTS FOR ORGANISM IDENTIFICATION

Susceptibility test results can also be used to validate bacterial identifications, particularly those that may be derived from data from one of the automated or semiautomated instruments. Certain common susceptibility patterns are well-established through common usage; therefore, if an instrument suggests an organism identification that is inconsistent with an anticipated susceptibility pattern, repeat testing may be in order. Table 2-7 shows the expected susceptibility patterns of several commonly encountered bacterial species.

Thus, *E. coli* and *Salmonella* species are usually susceptible to most antibiotics. Patterns of resistance are

---

BOX 2-13. CASCADE OF ANTIBIOTIC USAGE

Enterobacteriaceae

1. Ampicillin → ampicillin/sulbactam → mezlocillin → timentin
2. Gentamicin → tobramycin → amikacin → } ceftazidime ciprofloxacin imipenem aztreonam
3. Cefazolin → cefuroxime → ceftriaxone →
4. Trimethoprim/sulfamethoxazole
5. Nitrofurantoin (for urine isolates only)

Pseudomonas aeruginosa

1. Aminoglycosides:
   Gentamicin → tobramycin → amikacin
2. Cefotaxime-ceftriaxone → ceftazidime
3. Piperacillin → piperacillin/tazobactam → imipenem timentin → mezlocillin → aztreonam
4. Ofloxacin → ciprofloxacin

Enterococcus species

1. Ampicillin → Ampicillin/sulbactam → pipericillin → imipenem
2. Vancomycin → ofloxacin → chloramphenicol → doxycycline
3. Gentamicin synergy (high level)
4. Streptomycin synergy (high level)
5. Nitrofurantoin (urine isolates only)

---

ampicillin and carbenicillin for *K. pneumoniae*; ampicillin and cephalothin for *Enterobacter* species; tetracycline and nitrofurantoin for *P. mirabilis*; and ampicillin, cephalothin, and tetracycline for *Serratia marcescens*. In addition to these bacterial species, *Enterococcus* species tend to be resistant to penicillin and cephalothin, and *S. aureus* is often resistant to penicillin and ampicillin. Methicillin-resistant strains of *S. aureus* are also frequently encountered. Knowledge of the in-house susceptibility test results can be used not only to guide antibiotic therapy before susceptibility test results are known, but also to validate organism identifications made by automated instruments.

THE REPORTING OF RESULTS

Reports of microbiology culture results should be issued as soon as useful information becomes available. Gram-positive results on smears prepared from clinical materials or the observations made from direct antigen detection procedures should be telephoned immediately to the physician or ward. Such information may be urgently needed to initiate the next steps in the management of a patient with an infection. The

TABLE 2-7

ANTIBIOTIC SUSCEPTIBILITY PATTERNS OF GRAM-NEGATIVE BACILLI: DENVER VETERANS AFFAIRS HOSPITAL, 1994–1995

DRUG	ACINETOBACTER SPECIES (26)*	CITROBACTER FREUNDII (28)	ESCHERICHIA COLI (605)	ENTEROBACTER AEROGENES (49)	ENTEROBACTER CLOACAE (133)	KLEBSIELLA OXYTOCA (66)	KLEBSIELLA PNEUMONIAE (236)	PROTEUS MIRABILIS (97)	PROTEUS VULGARIS (8)	PSEUDOMONAS AERUGINOSA (392)	SERRATIA MARCESCENS (38)
Amikacin	100%†	100%	100%	100%	100%	100%	100%	100%	100%	94%	100%
Ampicillin	19	21	68	0	2	3	2	94	0	0	18
Ampicillin/sulbactam	64	73	87	43	50	90	92	97	100	2	52
Cefazolin	0	21	98	17	17	95	99	100	0	0	0
Cefotetan	23	79	100	63	63	100	100	100	100	0	100
Ceftazidime	100	93	100	70	81	100	100	100	100	99	100
Ceftriaxone	73	89	100	100	85	100	100	100	100	80	100
Cephalothin	0	37	89	6	11	94	89	100	0	0	0
Ciprofloxacin	50	96	100	96	95	100	100	100	100	83	100
Gentamicin	50	100	97	98	96	97	97	99	100	88	100
Imipenem	82	100	100	100	100	100	100	90	80	92	100
Mezlocillin	59	93	90	97	90	90	87	97	100	91	100
Ofloxacin	59	100	100	90	92	100	93	100	100	86	96
Piperacillin	64	100	80	93	90	95	95	97	100	97	100
Tobramycin	92	100	100	100	96	97	97	100	100	93	100
Trimethoprim/ sulfamethoxazole	58	79	84	98	91	96	90	85	100	4	92

*Total number of strains tested
†Percent of strains sensitive

results of blood cultures should be reported as soon as they become positive. Also, the recovery of enteric pathogens from stool specimens or detection of mycobacteria and fungi in any specimen should be made known to the physician without delay.

Timely preliminary and interim reports should be issued as a matter of policy. For example, preliminary reports on negative blood cultures should be issued within 48 hours; if the patient is still febrile, additional cultures should be obtained. An interim report of "negative culture" may be helpful, because the physician may wish to reevaluate the case pending the final report. Final reports should be issued within 48 hours if possible.

Microbiologists must be familiar with a state's statutes governing their responsibility for handling reportable diseases. For example, in the state of Illinois, a new regulation has recently been issued making it mandatory to report positive gonococcal cultures in patients younger than 11 years of age. Most state public health laboratories have a "Report of a Communicable Disease" card available on request, along with a list of reportable diseases. Such information may be helpful in curbing a local outbreak of an infectious disease and should be made available as soon as possible.

QUALITY ASSURANCE: DEFINITION AND APPLICATIONS

Medical care facilities should have in effect an ongoing system to evaluate the quality of medical care being provided, designated by the term "quality assurance" (QA). The quality of care may be difficult to define, and for that reason, many institutions have either altered their standards or changed the focus of attention. Thompson[64] has defined *quality* in reference to patient care as the "optimal achievable result for each patient, the avoidance of physician-induced (iatrogenic) complications and the attention to patient and family needs in a manner that is both cost-effective and reasonably documented." Donabedian[16] has further stated, "the quality of care is proportional to the extent to which possible improvements in the quality of life are attained as a result of that care, with the assumption that cost is no object."

The definitions of "high" and "acceptable" patient care have been vague in practice; thus, standards of performance have been difficult to delineate, and quality assurance is no longer practiced with as much enthusiasm in many institutions. Nevertheless, assessments of quality must still be addressed by medical audit and peer review committees, who still must make judgments based on established criteria and standards. Individuals assigned to these committees continue to struggle with assessing outcomes, either based on hard data related to morbidity, mortality, and disability statistics; or, more subjectively, based on judgments of whether adverse reactions or progression of disease could have been averted. It is unfortunate that formal quality assurance programs are on the wane, as this practice potentially provided an approach to measuring the level of care being provided as an institution, with failures to meet established standards directed to collective practices and not necessarily to the failure of given individuals.

The JCAHO 10-step model for quality assurance monitoring and evaluation was published in the fourth edition of this textbook. Readers are referred to that text if the formal program spelled out in this model is still being practiced in the institution being served. The model is not reproduced here.

Nevertheless, it may be prudent for directors and supervisors of microbiology laboratories to continue certain quality assurance monitoring of what practices are in effect, particularly those that are substandard and may potentially compromise patient care. The following monitors may be prudent to continue depending, on the local situation:

1. Blood culture utilization: With what frequency are single-set blood cultures being received?
2. With what frequency are blood cultures contaminated with skin flora?
3. How often are clean-voided urine cultures contaminated?
4. Culture utilization: How frequently are more than three blood cultures during 24 hours, more than three fecal specimens for parasites, or duplicate cultures of all types, from a single patient, being received in the laboratory?
5. How frequently do blood culture vials contain less than the recommended volume of blood?

Threshold performance levels for each of these monitors must be established by the microbiology staff, in conjunction with the infectious disease service and, perhaps, with the approval of the quality assurance committee. For example, the following threshold levels have been set for the foregoing listed monitors: 1) 5% or less of blood cultures should be single sets; 2) 3% or less of blood cultures should contain contaminating skin flora; 3) 10% or less of urine samples should have colony counts in the range of 10^1 to 10^4 (an indicator of contamination); 4) more than three blood cultures in a 24-hour period, more than three stool specimens for parasite examination, or duplicate cultures should occur no more than 2% of the time; and 5) the frequency for receipt of less than the recommended volume of blood should be found in 5% or fewer blood culture vials.

The director and supervisor for each microbiology laboratory should determine what practices are to be monitored and the threshold levels. It has been suggested that no more than two or three monitors be in effect at any given time, focusing on those practices for which casual observations indicate that a problem may exist. If a given monitor indicates that the threshold has been exceeded, specific corrective actions must be taken, documented, and follow-up assessment for the effectiveness of the corrective action should be made. It should be emphasized that quality assurance monitors may be formulated to correct problems in microbiology practice that go beyond the immediate confines of laboratory operations. For example, Bartlett[7] describes the microbiology practices that have been monitored at the Hartford Hospital: 1) the appropriate ordering of urine cultures, 2) the frequency with which collection times are not recorded on the request slip, 3) the frequency and sources of poor quality specimens, 4) the frequency with which culture specimens are delayed in transit beyond 2 hours, and 5) the frequency with which patients are treated with drugs to which in vitro resistance has been shown. Additional in-laboratory monitors that may be optionally implemented include the predictive value of direct smear and culture results; testing deficiencies (classic quality control); personnel errors versus equipment or material errors; frequency with which reports must be revised; turnaround times for gram-stained smears, urinalysis, or other tests; the frequency with which preliminary reports are delayed beyond 2 days; and the frequency with which final reports are delayed beyond 5 days.

In those laboratories electing to continue one or more monitors, quality assurance will continue to be used to detect potential problems that can be corrected. Thresholds for evaluation must be identified, which when exceeded based on the cumulative data collected, will trigger a more intensive evaluation.

RISK MANAGEMENT

Most health care facilities are currently involved in risk management. In fact, many hospitals and clinics have established formal risk management offices, fully funded and staffed, to help reduce to a minimum the chances for accidents or high-risk practices that potentially may cause harm to employees and patients alike. Although the major impetus for this practice may be directed toward reducing costly workman compensation claims and malpractice suits, in a larger sense risk management efforts are to help ensure a safe working environment and an atmosphere in which patients can receive the latest that medical technology has to offer, without fear of being harmed.[55]

Working in conjunction with the quality assurance committee, a risk manager is assigned to investigate cases in which quality management falls below the established thresholds, or situations in which employees or patients may be at undue risk. After reviewing the details of the situation with the appropriate representatives of the department involved, and after gathering the necessary data, the risk manager submits a condensed report to the quality assurance committee, with recommendations for corrective actions. A dialogue continues between the risk manager and the committee chairman until an appropriate plan of action is agreed upon. The department's compliance with the corrective action plans is then monitored.

Although the major focus of risk management is directed toward patient care, the clinical laboratory participates in seeing that all operations are in compliance with the overall practices and policies. If equipment or instruments are damaged because of fire or electrical accidents, or if personnel are injured, or they contract serious laboratory-acquired infections, work flow may be disrupted with a delay in producing laboratory results. Thus, for the most part, laboratory risk management is related to implementing and monitoring laboratory safety practices, directed more to employees than to patients. Liability for injury clearly rests with the employer, even though the negligence leading to the injury is that of a fellow worker.[31] This is why risk managers of the future will be so insistent on conducting safety-oriented education courses and seeing that all rules and regulations of laboratory safety are implemented.

LABORATORY SAFETY

Although it is the legal responsibility of hospital and laboratory managers to provide for a safe working environment, employees must also bear the responsibilities for adhering to safety standards outlined in the *Laboratory Safety Manual,* to bring to the attention of the supervisor any hazards or potential hazards that may be encountered during work activities, and to seek immediate medical attention for any potentially job-related injury.[31]

One person in the laboratory should be designated the safety officer, whose duties are to see that safety standards and guidelines are written and published, that employees are informed of these standards through regularly scheduled laboratory safety courses and in-service briefings, and that a system is in place to monitor compliance. The safety officer will work closely with the hospital risk manager to reconcile and correct any breaches of conduct or any irregularities discovered.

UNIVERSAL PRECAUTIONS

Since the advent of the acquired immunodeficiency syndrome (AIDS) epidemic, extraordinary efforts have been made to prevent laboratory-acquired infections with HIV. The practices and procedures follow closely those that have been in place to prevent the laboratory spread of hepatitis B virus (HBV). The following are recent statistics published by the CDC relative to transmission risks for HIV and HBV:[10] the risk for acquiring HIV following needlestick from a source patient with HIV is 0.5%; in contrast, acquiring HBV infection following needlestick from an HBV carrier ranges from 6% to 30%. It is estimated that each year a total of 12,000 health care workers become accidentally infected with HBV, with some 250 dying from complications of the disease and 700 to 1200 will become carriers. As of July 31, 1988, CDC surveillance studies of 860 health care workers exposed, by needlestick or splashes to skin or mucous membrane, to blood from patients known to be HIV-infected revealed that only four seroconverted (prevalence rate of 0.45%). Three of these patients experienced an acute retroviral syndrome and had no known nonoccupational risk factors. Thus, the CDC, jointly with OSHA, have established the following universal precautions:[11]

1. Blood and body fluids from all patients must be handled as infectious material. All patients should be assumed to be infectious for HIV and other blood-borne pathogens.
2. All specimens of blood and body fluids should be put in a well-constructed container, with a secure lid, to prevent leaking during transport.
3. All persons processing blood and body fluid specimens (e.g., removing tops from vacuum tubes) should wear gloves—plus a face shield (or a mask with glasses or goggles)—if blood or body fluids are expected to splatter.
4. Workers must change gloves and wash hands when finished processing specimens.
5. Workers should never pipette by mouth; use mechanical devices.
6. Use of needles and syringes should be limited to situations in which there is no alternative.
7. Laboratory work surfaces should be decontaminated with an appropriate chemical germicide after a spill of blood or other body fluids and when work activities are completed.
8. Contaminated materials used in laboratory tests should be decontaminated before reprocessing or be placed in bags and disposed of in accordance with institutional policies.
9. All persons should wash their hands after completing laboratory activities and should remove protective clothing before leaving the laboratory.

The CDC–OSHA recommendations[12] for postexposure follow-up are: Once an exposure has occurred, a blood sample should be drawn after consent is obtained from the individual from whom exposure occurred and tested for hepatitis B surface antigen (HBsAg) and HIV antibody. For exposure to a source individual found to be positive for HBsAg, the worker who has not previously been exposed should receive the vaccine series and a single dose of hepatitis B immune globulin (HBIG) within 7 days of exposure. If previously exposed, the worker should be tested for antibody to HBsAg and given one dose of vaccine and one dose of HBIG if the antibody level in the worker's blood sample is inadequate (less than 10 SRU by RIA or negative by EIA). If the source individual is negative for HBsAg and the worker has not been vaccinated, opportunity should be taken to provide hepatitis B vaccination. Thus, provisions must be made to see that hepatitis testing is done with a rapid turnaround time to provide timely results.

For any blood exposure to a source individual who has AIDS, who is positive for HIV infection, the worker should be counseled concerning the risk of infection and evaluated clinically and serologically for evidence of HIV infection as soon as possible after exposure.[12] The worker should be advised to report and seek medical evaluation for any acute febrile illness (particularly one that includes fever, rash, or lymphadenopathy) that occurs within 12 weeks after exposure. Seronegative workers should be retested at 6 weeks, 12 weeks, and 6 months after exposure to determine whether transmission has occurred. During the follow-up period, workers should refrain from activities (blood donation, unprotected sexual intercourse) that may lead to transmission of the virus.

In the extremely rare chance that seroconversion may occur, the worker must be further counseled by an HIV specialist concerning future management and the possibility of zidovudine (ZDV) prophylaxis.[12]

Laboratory workers are also subject to exposure to infectious disease agents other than HIV and HBV. Miller and associates[44] report on a 25-year experience of laboratory-acquired human infections at the National Animal Disease Center (NADC) in Ames, Iowa, an institution conducting research on domestic diseases of livestock and poultry. Because several zoonotic diseases are under investigation, the level of risk among workers is somewhat greater than in the average clinical laboratory. From 1960 to 1985, 128 laboratory exposures to zoonotic organisms were reported at NADC. Of these, 34 resulted in laboratory-associated infections. *Brucella*, *Mycobacterium*, and *Leptospira* species represented 74% of the laboratory-acquired infections. Brucellosis accounted for 47% of the cases, leptospirosis 27%, and mycobacteriosis for 9% of cases. *Salmonella* and *Chlamydia* species, Newcastle virus, and *Trichophyton* species accounted for the other laboratory-acquired infections at NADC.

The authors also summarize the previous reported surveys of laboratory-acquired infections by Pike,[53,54] Wedam,[68] and by the National Institutes of Health. The ten most frequent laboratory-acquired infections from these cumulated studies were 1) brucellosis, 2) Q-fever, 3) typhoid fever, 4) tularemia, 5) tuberculosis, 6) typhus, 7) infectious hepatitis, 8) Venezuelan equine encephalitis, 9) coccidioidomycosis, and 10) psittacosis. Mecoli-Kamp and Fletcher-Gutowski[45] report an outbreak of brucellosis (*B. melitensis* biotype 3) among eight microbiology laboratory employees at William Beaumont Hospital in Royal Oak, Michigan. The mode of transmission was assumed to be airborne, following subculture of a frozen stock culture of *B. melitensis* biotype 3 to fresh medium, without the use of a biohazard hood. Hoerl and coworkers[26] report a case of acquired typhoid fever with postinfection complications in a 22-year-old medical technology student after participating in a laboratory exercise in which *S. typhi* was studied as an unknown isolate. All of these case studies emphasize the importance for the practice of universal precautions as cited in the foregoing.

GENERAL SAFETY RULES AND REGULATIONS

Laboratory workers are advised not to take unnecessary risks. Carelessness, negligence, and unsafe practices may result in serious injuries, not only to the individual, but to coworkers and patients as well. The following are general considerations that will make working in microbiology laboratories less of a risk:

1. Each employee should be instructed on the location and operation of each of all safety equipment and facilities, such as fire blankets, fire extinguishers,

showers, and eye wash fountains. Each of these must be readily accessible in the laboratory.

2. Personal protective equipment (surgical gloves, lab coats, and such) should be worn when indicated. Laboratory coats should be worn (with buttons closed) at all times while in the laboratory, and removed when leaving the laboratory.

3. Personal habits and grooming must be put in perspective. Long hair must be tied such that it will not interfere with equipment or reagents. Application of cosmetics in the work area is prohibited. Sandals and open style shoes do not afford proper foot protection and are not acceptable. Smoking is prohibited in the laboratory. As much as possible, keep fingers, pencils, and other implements out of the mouth. Horseplay and practical jokes must be contained.

4. Contact lenses, especially the soft ones, absorb certain solvents and may be a hazard from splashes and spills. Employees are strongly advised not to wear contact lenses in the laboratory, or to wear safety glasses when working with caustic or infective materials.

5. Eating or storing food and beverages in the laboratory or in the laboratory refrigerators is not permitted. A refrigerator should be designated specifically to store employee lunches.

6. Mouth pipetting of any material is absolutely prohibited. A variety of suitable pipetting aids are available.

7. Laboratory personnel with current skin infections, acute respiratory infections, or other contagious diseases should avoid patient contact.

ROUTINE SAFETY PRECAUTIONS

CENTRIFUGATION

1. Before centrifuging any item, check tubes, vials, or bottles for cracks. Periodically replace the rubber cushions in the bottoms of the trunions and remove any broken glass that may have accumulated.

2. Make sure that the centrifuge is properly balanced before use. Check the trunion rings and tube carriers to be sure the weights match.

3. Wait for the centrifuge to come to a complete stop before opening the lid to remove samples. Use only the braking device to bring the rotation to a more rapid and complete stop.

4. Should breakage of a tube occur in the centrifuge, first turn off the instrument, wait at least 20 minutes before opening the lid, and, after donning mask and gloves, thoroughly clean and disinfect the inside of the centrifuge.

5. As part of the routine maintenance program, each centrifuge should be thoroughly cleaned with a suitable disinfectant on each day of use. Preventive maintenance of all working parts should be on a regular schedule—quarterly or semiannually as appropriate.

NEEDLES AND GLASSWARE

1. Discard all chipped or cracked glassware in appropriate containers.

2. Pick up broken glass with a brush and pan; do not use hands.

3. Glass articles should not be discarded in the sink or loosely in a wastebasket where paper articles are being discarded. They can cut the fingers and hands of individuals removing the refuge.

4. Used needles and lancets must be placed into appropriate used-needle containers to be disposed of in a safe manner.

5. Avoid removing needles or exchanging needles on syringes as much as possible. The practice of changing needles before discharging venipuncture blood into blood culture bottles has been abandoned in most hospitals.

ELECTRICAL SAFETY

1. All personnel must know the location of master switches and circuit breaker boards. Do not attempt to repair any instrument while it is still plugged in.

2. Plugs or cords that are broken, frayed, or worn should not be used.

3. Outlets must not be overloaded. Never use gang-type plugs.

4. All cord and plug-type electrical equipment should have grounded power cords and plugs. Equipment that is double insulated or provided with a nonconductive enclosure may have undergrounded power cords and plugs. All shocks, including small tingles, must be immediately investigated.

5. Extension cords should be used only in compliance with the overall hospital policies and procedures.

CORRIDOR CAUTIONS

1. Open doors into corridors with caution. Watch out for swinging doors. If there is a window in the door, look out to be certain the way is clear before opening the doors.

2. Keep to the right when approaching corridor intersections and when using stairways. Walk, never run, in halls, rooms, and stairwells.

3. Watch for hall hazards such as beds, carts, or tables. Watch out for articles on the floor, such as paper clips, electrical cords, loose tiles, and spilled liquids. Only one side of the corridor should be used for the temporary storage of movable equipment.

LIFTING

1. Back injuries are among the most frequent causes of debilitating illness among personnel. Avoid lifting heavy objects when possible. Always get help.

2. If objects must be lifted alone, exercise the following precautions:
   a. Have a good footing. Keep feet about 10 inches apart.
   b. Bend at the knees to grasp the object.

c. Keep the object close to you and get a firm hold.
d. Keep the arms and back as straight as possible and lift gradually upward by straightening the legs.

HANDLING SPECIMENS AND SPILLS

1. Specimens should be collected in sturdy containers with adequate closure to prevent spillage or leakage. All specimens must be considered a potential hazard.
2. Cuts on hands should be adequately covered with adhesive bandages. Wear disposable gloves if the work activity involves contact with blood, serum, plasma, or other specimens.
3. If a sample shows evidence of breakage, leakage, or soiling inside a specimen container, put on gloves and transfer as much of the specimen as possible to a second sterile container. Also rewrite any pertinent information from the old to the new container.
4. Blood-contaminated specimen requisitions should be rejected. Handle such a requisition only with gloves if processing is necessary in an emergency. Notify the requestor that such contaminated materials present a health hazard.
5. Wash hands thoroughly with soap and water several times a day and, particularly, after handling specimens before leaving for a coffee or lunch break.
6. Flood any area, where blood and serum spills have occurred, with disinfectant solution. Wearing gloves, use paper towels or gauze sponges to absorb the liquid, followed by a thorough wash with water. Bag all contaminated materials for disposal as infectious waste.

HANDLING OF WASTES

1. Set aside certain sinks in the laboratory to dispose of blood or urine specimens. Hand washing should not be allowed in these sinks.
2. Biohazard bags (so labeled) must be used to dispose of all potentially contaminated samples—blood tubes, specimen containers, pipettes, pipette tips, reaction vessels, stoppers, and such. Leave sufficient room at the top so that the bag can be easily closed and secured with an elastic band.
3. Dispose of glassware and sharps in appropriate hard-walled containers. When filled, such containers should be sealed with tape and placed in appropriate labeled waste boxes for proper disposal.
4. Remove filled biohazard bags to designated waste areas as frequently during the day as necessary to avoid buildup.
5. Immerse contaminated reusable glassware into disinfectant solution. Thoroughly rinse with water and autoclave before reusing.

CHEMICALS

1. Flash point: volatile combustible substances give off vapors along the surface of the liquid. The *flash point* is the lowest possible temperature at which a sufficient concentration of vapors is produced for a flame to occur. The classification of chemicals based on flash points and boiling points is:
   a. Flammables
      1) Class IA: Flash point, 40°F; boiling point, 65°F (e.g., ethers, acetaldehyde)
      2) Class IB: Flash point, 73°F; boiling point, 100°F (e.g., ethanol, acetone, gasoline)
      3) Class IC: Flash point, 73°F to 99°F (e.g., isopropyl alcohol, xylene)
   b. Combustibles:
      1) Class II: Flash point, 100°F to 139°F (e.g., ethylene glycol, glacial acetic acid)
      2) Class III: Flash point, 140°F (e.g., aniline, glycerol, mineral oil)
2. Storage safety cans and cabinets must be located away from sources of heat, flame, sparks, and exits. Storage areas should be adequately ventilated and of limited access to personnel.
3. All containers should be clearly labeled with 1) content, 2) hazard warnings, 3) special precautions, 4) date received/prepared, 5) date opened/put in use, 6) expiration date, and 7) manufacturer.
4. In case of a liquid chemical spill:
   a. Confine the spill to as small an area as possible
   b. Neutralize acids with disodium carbonate
   c. Neutralize alkalis with 1% boric acid
   d. For larger amounts of acids or bases, flush with large amounts of water after neutralization
   e. Clean any areas that have been splashed by the spill
   f. For flammable and toxic liquid spills, use an absorbent to reduce the vapor pressure and prevent possible ignition of the liquid.
5. Disposal of chemicals
   a. Wear rubber gloves, a rubber apron, and goggles
   b. Remove all items from the sink designated for disposal. Start a nonsplashing stream of cold water into the sink
   c. Slowly pour the liquid as close to the drain as possible without splashing. Only quantities less than 500 mL can be disposed of in the sink drain
   d. Continue to run cold water for several minutes after completion
   e. Dispose of water-soluble organic solvents (methanol, acetone) as described in the foregoing. For water-insoluble organic liquids, only quantities less than 100 mL can be disposed of as just described. For quantities over 100 mL, consult with the hospital safety officer or the local Environmental Health and Safety Office.

FIRE

1. Every hospital employee is responsible for preventing fires and assisting in minimizing losses should fire occur.
2. Keep work areas free of trash accumulation and excess flammable materials. Corridors, passageways, aisles, and stairs must be kept free of obstructions that may inhibit exit or add fuel to a fire.
3. Be aware of ignition sources, open flames, heating elements, and sparks gaps (motors, light switches, friction, and static). More than 22% of hospital

fires are caused by faulty wiring; 33% are due to smoking.

4. Personnel should be instructed in the differences in, and use of, fire extinguishers for the four classes of fire:
   a. Class A: Fires involving ordinary combustible materials such as wood, paper, cloth, and plastics; use a pressurized water extinguisher (type A).
   b. Class B: Fires involving flammable liquids, such as alcohol, gasoline, kerosene, and grease; use a carbon dioxide extinguisher (type B)
   c. Class C: Fires involving energized electrical equipment in which a resulting shock hazard owing to electrical conductivity may exist. Never use a water extinguisher; use a dry chemical type extinguisher (type C)
   d. Class D: Fires involving combustible metals, such as magnesium and potassium. Special techniques are required. Immediately call the local fire station.
5. Fire blankets are used to smother clothing by wrapping the victim in the blanket. If clothing should catch fire, drop to the ground and roll to smother the flame against the floor. **Do not run for the blanket**—airflow will only fan the flames and result in more serious injury.
6. Comply with all local fire regulations. Participate in periodic fire drills as conducted by the hospital. Each employee should know the fire drill procedure and the evacuation route for their area of the laboratory

QUALITY CONTROL

Historically, laboratory involvement in what is now risk management has been in the form of quality control. Quality control in the narrow sense has consisted of an on-going, systematic assessment of work to ensure that the final product conforms—to an acceptable degree—to previously established tolerance limits of precision and accuracy. The quality of work performed must continue as before; however, laboratory directors and supervisors must now realize that quality control is only one facet in the larger arenas of quality assurance and risk management, as defined earlier. Moreover, supervisors of low-volume laboratories may decide to limit the types of procedures or services offered; however, the procedures selected must be controlled within the same tolerance limits as similar procedures performed in large laboratories.

For further information on quality control of laboratory items not covered in this text, a number of pamphlets are available from the College of American Pathologists, and August and coworkers[3] have recently published an ASM CumiTech providing an update of current guidelines.

In a broad sense, quality control in microbiology is more an art than a science. It involves intangible items such as common sense, good judgment, and constant attention to detail. Programs should be organized with well-defined objectives in mind. In the end, high-level laboratory performance requires an alert, interested, and well-motivated laboratory staff. Emphasis is shifting to some extent away from rigorous point-by-point details of in-laboratory quality control to a broader assessment of quality assurance in patient care. It may be more important to ensure that timely reports are made available to physicians and are maximally used to direct patient care, rather than worrying whether, for example, a daily indole reaction is in control.

A basic microbiology quality control program lists several specific items that must be considered when implementing the various phases of the program. Bartlett[4] developed a quality control program and discusses different levels of activity ranging from basic to most advanced. Using his outline, a supervisor can select the level of activity that is appropriate for the personnel and volume of work in any given laboratory.

The Commission on Laboratory Inspection and Accreditation of the College of American Pathologists (CAP) has established standards for accreditation of medical laboratories, including an inspection checklist for microbiology laboratories. This checklist provides microbiology supervisors with valuable guidelines for making a point-by-point assessment of the quality control needs in their laboratories. The Q-Probes program described earlier in this chapter should also be considered as an aid in establishing quality control standards in light of the results derived from quality assurance monitors.

At the onset, a quality control coordinator must be selected. The duties of the coordinator must be clearly established and appropriate authority conferred to the extent that problems can be efficiently handled when they arise. It is the coordinator's responsibility to establish the minimal standards for quality control that are to be met by the laboratory and to outline the several steps to be taken for daily monitoring and surveillance of all facets of the program.

The coordinator should see that all activities are clearly described in a quality control manual, in which should also be outlined clearly the details of all quality control practices, such as the procedures and schedules for monitoring equipment function; the monitoring of all media and reagents for reactivity, expiration dates, reaction patterns of the various challenge organisms, and all proficiency testing results. Appropriate forms must be designed to collect data in the form of columns of numbers, graphs, or diagrams by which any item out of control can be quickly observed. The coordinator also must review all control records and verify that all incidences out of control and the corrective actions taken are clearly notated. A brief review of the several components of a quality control program follows.

COMPONENTS OF A QUALITY CONTROL PROGRAM

Any previous discussion of quality control must now be superseded with the impending provisions of the new Clinical Laboratory Improvement Act (CLIA), the preliminary provisions of which were spelled out by the Health Care Financing Administration (HCFA) in the March 14, 1990 *Federal Register*. To paraphrase from this document, "we (HCFA) are revising the regulations to remove outdated, obsolete and redundant requirements, are making provisions for new technologies and are placing increased reliance on outcome measures of performance . . . We intend to revise personnel standards so that personnel requirements are not focused principally on qualifications but on the accurate performance of laboratory tests."

Also, HCFA has gone on record with the intent to update current internal quality control requirements for each specialty and subspecialty, taking into consideration current and future technological advances. The punitive thrust of the new HCFA approach is apparent in their intent to disapprove licensure of any specialty or subspecialty that does not meet quality control performance standards. Every laboratory (including both independent and hospital-based laboratories) seeking Medicare approval or CLIA licensure must enroll and participate successfully in an approved proficiency testing (PT) program. The requirements for successful performance in proficiency testing as specifically related to the microbiology laboratory include the following.

1. Each laboratory can participate in only one proficiency testing program that meets the criteria established by HCFA. The proficiency testing agency must provide HCFA with a description of samples that it plans to include in its annual program.
2. There shall be a minimum of four testing events annually in each area of activity (bacteriology, mycology, parasitology, and virology), each providing a minimum of five samples per testing event (mycobacteriology has only two events a year). In the bacteriology subgroup, samples representative of the six major groups of bacteria must be included: *Enterobacteriaceae*, gram-positive bacilli, gram-positive cocci, gram-negative cocci, and miscellaneous gram-negative bacteria.
3. The laboratory must examine or test, as applicable, the PT samples it receives from the PT program in the same manner it tests patient specimens. The samples must be examined or tested with the regular patient workload by personnel who routinely perform the test.
4. The laboratory may not test the samples with a greater frequency of testing than it routinely tests patient samples.
5. A laboratory that performs tests on PT samples may not engage in any interlaboratory communications pertaining to the results of the proficiency testing sample. The laboratory may not send the samples or portions of samples to another laboratory for analysis.
6. Failure to attain an overall testing event score of at least 80% is unsatisfactory performance. Failure to achieve an overall testing event score of satisfactory for two consecutive testing events or two of three consecutive testing events is unsuccessful performance. A laboratory failing the PT requirements for

a testing event would have to enroll in an enhanced PT program or demonstrate successful performance for three successive testing events before receiving reinstatement as a Medicare approved or CLIA licensed laboratory for the specialty or subspecialty.

Those wishing to implement a quality control program or to revise a program already in effect should follow the guidelines established by the accrediting agencies' inspection and accreditation checklists. The following are the essential components of the guidelines established by the College of American Pathologists (Box 2-14).

MONITORING LABORATORY EQUIPMENT

A preventive maintenance program to ensure proper functioning of all electrical and mechanical equipment should be established in all microbiology laboratories. Equipment should be checked at prescribed time intervals; certain working parts should be replaced after a specified period of use, even though they may not appear worn. A brief list of some of the equipment, the monitoring procedures to be carried out, and the frequency and tolerance limits is shown in Table 2-8. Assignments should be made among laboratory personnel to ensure that all inspections are carried out and all data are recorded accurately onto charts or in maintenance manuals; this permits detection of upward or downward trends immediately and appropriate corrective action can be taken before serious errors result. The temperature of incubators, refrigerators, freezers, water baths, and heating blocks must be determined and recorded daily with thermometers calibrated by the Bureau of Standards. The concentration of CO_2 in all CO_2 incubators must also be determined daily. For any reading that falls outside of the established quality control range, the cause must be determined and the defect quickly corrected.

MONITORING CULTURE MEDIA, REAGENTS, AND SUPPLIES

To meet cost-containment policies, most inspection checklists for quality control of culture media permit acceptance of the documented records of the manufacturers and suppliers of commercial products, without the necessity of a second in-house evaluation. However, it is recommended that manufacturers' claims of quality control on all prepared lots of culture media should not be blindly accepted without periodic direct or indirect surveillance. In fact, the National Committee for Clinical Laboratory Standards (NCCLS), in the Performance Standard, "Quality Assurance for Commercially Prepared Microbiological Culture Media" (M22-T, Vol 7[5], 1988), recommends that in-house quality control monitoring of the selective agar used for recovery of *Campylobacter* species (Campy-BAP, for example), chocolate agar, and the selective media used for the recovery of pathogenic *Neisseria* species (Modi-

BOX 2-14. DEVELOPING A PROCEDURE MANUAL

One of the most important documents for directing day-to-day activities in the microbiology laboratory is an up-to-date procedure manual. All of the various activities of the laboratory should be clearly outlined, bound into one or more volumes, and placed in an accessible part of the laboratory, for ready reference by all employees at all times.

The exact order in which the material is to appear in the manual to best meet the needs of the laboratory must be determined by the microbiology supervisor. The following are items that should appear in all procedure manuals:

1. Names, addresses, and telephone numbers of the laboratory director, staff pathologists, doctoral scientists, supervisors, and all employees.

2. List of all general policies and regulations of the microbiology laboratory.

3. List of the exact locations of equipment, media, reagents, and supplies, particularly if the laboratory is covered by part-time personnel on evenings and weekends.

4. Complete description of all forms, reports, and files used in the microbiology laboratory.

5. Detailed description of all techniques and procedures that are performed in the laboratory.

6. List of all media and reagents used, including full descriptions of their formulations and instructions for preparation.

7. List of all identification schemes used in identifying and classifying microorganisms.

8. Names, addresses, telephone numbers, and the procedures and policies of other reference laboratories pertaining to shipment of reference samples.

Inclusion of all quality control procedures, with specific details on the frequency and manner in which each item is to be carried out.

Current laboratory inspection guidelines require that the procedure manual be revised and updated at least once a year and that the initials of the laboratory director or supervisor appear for each procedure, indicating that the update has been accomplished.

fied Thayer Martin, or equivalent) continue to be in effect. This requirement is currently under investigation because the number of failures in most laboratories is sufficiently small that the cost/benefit ratio is questionable. However, until the issue is settled, the present practice must remain in effect. Some laboratories also monitor in-house any media containing antibiotics, such as blood agar containing SXT (for inoculation of strep-screen throat cultures), anaerobic kanamycin–vancomycin blood agar, and the like.

A list of suggested organisms and acceptable results for the culture media most commonly used in clinical laboratories is found in Table 2-9. Quality control stock organisms may be maintained in the laboratory by subculturing bacterial isolates recovered as part of the routine work, or dried stock organisms, such as ATCC (American Type Culture Collection, 12301 Parklawn Dr. Rockville MD), Bactrol disks (Difco Laboratories, Detroit MI), or Bac-Check disks (Roche Diagnostics, Division of Hoffmann-LaRoche, Inc., Nutley NJ). Ideally, each batch of media should be checked with the most fastidious requirements to grow or produce biochemical activity. The availability of in-house bacterial stains may be required to supplement those commercially available.

Each culture tube, plate of medium, and reagent must bear a label that clearly indicates the content and dates of preparation and expiration. "Coded" culture tubes, plated media, and reagents should be referenced in such a way that even nonlaboratory personnel would be able to interpret the code. All antimicrobial susceptibility disks must be tested at least weekly with standard control organisms of known susceptibil-

ity, such as *Escherichia coli* (ATCC 25922), *Staphylococcus aureus* (ATCC 25923), *Streptococcus fecalis* (ATCC 29212), and *Pseudomonas aeruginosa* (ATCC 27853). The acceptable zone diameter ranges of these organisms for the more commonly used antibiotics is presented in Chapter 15.

Each batch of tubed or plated media must also undergo sterility testing, particularly media in which components are added after sterilization. Sterility checks must be done both visually and by subculture. Certain selective media, for example, may sufficiently suppress the visible growth of bacteria; however, viable organisms may appear on subculture. Prepared media should also be visually observed for other signs of deterioration, such as discoloration, turbidity, color changes, and status of hydration.

The frequency with which quality control testing of media and reagents (including serologic reagents) is performed must be determined by each laboratory director, in keeping with local practices and according to manufacturers' instructions for all commercial products used.

PERSONNEL

An accredited laboratory must be directed by a pathologist, other physician, or a person with a doctoral degree in a specific area of laboratory science. This requirement is being challenged and may be relaxed by the time this text is published. The laboratory must be staffed at all times with a qualified supervisor who has at least 4 years of laboratory experience.

TABLE 2-8

QUALITY CONTROL SURVEILLANCE PROCEDURES OF COMMONLY USED MICROBIOLOGY EQUIPMENT

EQUIPMENT	PROCEDURE	SCHEDULE	TOLERANCE LIMITS
Refrigerators	Recording of temperature*	Daily or continuous	2°C–8°C
Freezers	Recording of temperature*	Daily or continuous	−8°C to −20°C −60°C to −75°C
Incubators	Recording of temperature*	Daily or continuous	35.5°C ± 1°C
Incubators (CO_2)	Measuring of CO_2 content Use blood gas analyzer or Fyrite† device	Daily or twice daily	5%–10%
Water baths	Recording of temperature*	Daily	36°C–38°C 55°C–57°C
Heating blocks	Recording of temperature*	Daily	±1°C of setting
Autoclaves	Test with spore strip (*Bacillus stearothermophilus*)	At least weekly	No growth of spores in subculture indicates sterile run
pH meter	Test with pH-calibrating solutions	With each use	±0.1 pH units of standard being used
Anaerobic jars	Methylene blue indicator strip	With each use	Conversion of strip from blue to white indicates low O_2 tension
Anaerobic glove box	*Clostridium novyi* type B culture	Run periodically	Growth indicates very low O_2 tension. It is used only where extremely low O_2 tension is required.
	Methylene blue indicator solution	Continuously or daily	Solution remains colorless if O_2 tension is low.
Serology rotator	Count revolutions per minute	With each use	180 RPM ± 10 RPM
Centrifuges	Check revolutions with tachometer	Monthly	Within 5% of dial indicator setting
Safety hoods	Measure air velocity‡ across face opening	Semiannually or quarterly	50 ft of airflow per minute ± 5 ft/min

*Each monitoring thermometer must be calibrated against a standard thermometer.
†Bacharach Instrument Co., Pittsburgh, PA
‡Velometer Jr., Alnor Instrument Co., Chicago, IL

Quality control of personnel requires an effective continuing education program. In-service training must be an ongoing activity. Personnel should be encouraged to participate as often as possible in local, regional, and national seminars and workshops. All laboratories should participate in one or more of the available proficiency test services and these should be used as teaching exercises. Proficiency testing programs should be made available to personnel, particularly those who work evenings or weekends; to ensure that errors are not being made, provisions must be made for test results to be reviewed by a person on the regular shift.

Blind unknown samples for laboratory testing should also be circulated periodically with test runs, and any discrepancies in the results should be discussed openly, and the sources of errors should be pinpointed and corrected. Supervisory personnel should check all results for accuracy, reproducibility, and compliance with quality control standards. Laboratory techniques should be carefully evaluated for safety, to prevent both laboratory-acquired infections and the transmission of infectious agents by laboratory personnel to members of their families in the home environment.

SPACE

One remaining issue that is related to both quality control and safety is the problem of laboratory space. A minimum of 100 ft² of working space per full-time equivalent employee (FTE) is recommended; however, many laboratories fall short of this minimum requirement. Lack of sufficient space to perform adequately the tasks necessary for high-quality work is about the most frequent deficiencies cited by CAP laboratory inspectors. Elin and associates[18] have surveyed several laboratories in teaching hospitals to determine workload, space, and personnel allocations—information that may be of interest to microbiologists who wish to compare their recommendations with the actual in-laboratory situations.

MEDIUM	CONTROL ORGANISMS	EXPECTED REACTIONS
Blood agar	Group A *Streptococcus* *S. pneumoniae*	Good growth, β-hemolysis Good growth, α-hemolysis
Bile–esculin agar	*Enterococcus* species α-Hemolytic *Streptococcus*, not group D	Good growth, black No growth; no discoloration of media
Chocolate agar	*Haemophilus influenzae* *Neisseria gonorrhoeae*	Good growth Good growth
Christensen urea agar	*Proteus mirabilis* *Klebsiella pneumoniae* *Escherichia coli*	Pink throughout (positive) Pink slant (partial positive) Yellow (negative)
Simmons citrate agar	*K. pneumoniae* *E. coli*	Growth or blue color (positive) No growth, remains green (negative)
Cystine trypticase (CTA) agar Dextrose	*N. gonorrhoeae* *Branhamella catarrhalis*	Yellow (positive) No color change (negative)
Sucrose	*Escherichia coli* *N. gonorrhoeae*	Yellow (positive) No color change (negative)
Maltose	*Salmonella* species, or *N. meningitidis* *N. gonorrhoeae*	Yellow (positive) No color change (negative)
Lactose	*N. lactamicus* *N. gonorrhoeae*	Yellow (positive) No color change (negative)
Decarboxylases Lysine	*K. pneumoniae* *Enterobacter sakasakii*	Bluish (positive) Yellow (negative)
Arginine (dihydrolase)	*E. cloacae* *Proteus mirabilis*	Bluish (positive) Yellow (negative)
Ornithine	*P. mirabilis* *K. pneumoniae*	Bluish (positive) Yellow (negative)
Deoxyribonuclease (DNase)	*Serratia marcescens* *E. cloacae*	Zone of clearing (add 1 N HCl) No zone of clearing
Eosin–methylene blue agar	*E. coli* *K. pneumoniae* *Shigella flexneri*	Good growth, green metallic sheen Good growth, purple colonies, no sheen Good growth, transparent colonies (lactose negative)
Hektoen enteric agar	*Salmonella typhimurium* *S. flexneri* *E. coli*	Green colonies with black centers Green transparent colonies Growth slightly inhibited, orange colonies
Indole (Kovac's)	*E. coli* *K. pneumoniae*	Red (positive) No red color (negative)
Kligler iron agar	*E. coli* *Shigella flexneri* *Pseudomonas aeruginosa* *Salmonella typhimurium*	Acid slant/acid deep Alkaline slant/acid deep Alkaline slant/alkaline deep Alkaline slant/black deep
Lysine iron agar	*S. typhimurium* *Shigella flexneri* *P. mirabilis*	Purple deep and slant, + H$_2$S Purple slant, yellow deep Red slant, yellow deep

(Continued)

TABLE 2-9 *(Continued)*
QUALITY CONTROL OF COMMONLY USED MEDIA: SUGGESTED CONTROL ORGANISMS AND EXPECTED REACTIONS

MEDIUM	CONTROL ORGANISMS	EXPECTED REACTIONS
MacConkey agar	*E. coli* *P. mirabilis* *Enterococcus* species	Pink colonies (lactose positive) Colorless colonies, no spreading No growth
Malonate	*E. coli* *K. pneumoniae*	No growth Good growth, blue (positive)
Motility (semisolid agar)	*P. mirabilis* *K. pneumoniae*	Media cloudy (positive) No feather edge on streak line (negative)
Nitrate broth or agar	*E. coli* *Acinetobacter lwoffi*	Red on adding reagents No red (negative)
Phenylethyl alcohol blood agar	*Streptococcus* species *E. coli*	Good growth No growth
o-Nitrophenol-β-D-galactopyranoside (ONPG)	*Serratia marcescens* *Salmonella typhimurium*	Yellow (positive) Colorless (negative)
Phenylalanine deaminase	*P. mirabilis* *E. coli*	Green (add 10% $FeCl_3$) No green (negative)
Salmonella–Shigella (SS) agar	*S. typhimurium* *E. coli*	Colorless colonies, black centers No growth
Voges–Proskauer	*K. pneumoniae* *E. coli*	Red (add reagents) No development (negative)
Xylose–lysine–dextrose (XLD) agar	*Salmonella* species *E. coli* *Shigella* species	Red colonies (positive lysine) Yellow colonies (positive sugars) Transparent colonies (negative)

REFERENCES

1. ALBAERS AC, FLETCHER RD: Accuracy of calibrated-loop transfer. J Clin Microbiol 18:40–42, 1983
2. ALDRIDGE KE, KOCOS C, SANDERS CV, ET AL: Comparison of rapid identification assays for *Staphylococcus aureus*. J Clin Microbiol 19:703–704, 1984
3. AUGUST MJ, HINDLER JA, HUBER TW, SEWELL DL: Quality control and quality assurance practices in clinical microbiology. Washington, DC, the American Society for Microbiology, Cumitech 3A, May, 1990
4. BARTLETT RC: A plea for clinical relevance in microbiology. Am J Clin Pathol 61:867–872, 1974
5. BARTLETT RC: Medical Microbiology: Quality Cost and Clinical Relevance. New York, John Wiley & Sons, 1974
6. BARTLETT RC: Cost containment in microbiology. Clin Lab Med 5:761–791, 1985
7. BARTLETT RC: Leadership for quality. ASM News 57:15–21, 1991
8. BERKE A, TILTON RC: Evaluation of rapid coagulase methods for the identification of *Staphylococcus aureus*. J Clin Microbiol 23:916–919, 1985
9. BOSLEY GS, FACKLAM RR, GROSSMAN D: Rapid identification of enterococci. J Clin Microbiol 18:1275–1277, 1983
10. CENTERS FOR DISEASE CONTROL: Recommendations for prevention of HIV transmission in health care settings. Lab Med 19:88–95, 1988
11. CENTERS FOR DISEASE CONTROL: Guidelines for prevention of transmission of human immunodeficiency virus and hepatitis B virus to heath-care and public-safety workers. MMWR 38:1–37, 1989
12. CENTERS FOR DISEASE CONTROL: Public health service statement on management of occupational exposure to human immunodeficiency virus, including considerations regarding ziduvudine postexposure use. MMWR 39:#RR1, Jan 26, 1990
13. COTRAN RS, KUMER V, ROBBINS SL: Robbin's Pathologic Basis of Disease, 4th ed, pp 39–86. Philadelphia, WB Saunders, 1989
14. CRAWFORD I, RUSSELL C: Comparative adhesion of seven species of streptococci isolated from the blood of patients with subacute bacterial endocarditis to fibrin–platelet clots in vitro. J Appl Bacteriol 60:127–133, 1986
15. D'AMATO RF, ISENBERG HD: Practical and fiscally responsible application of clinical microbiology to patient care. ASM News 57:22–26, Jan 1991

16. DONABEDIAN D: Needed research in the assessment of and monitoring of the quality of medical care. National Center for Health Services Research Report Series. DHEW Pub (PHYS) 78-3219 (Hyattsville MD), July, 1978

17. DURAY PH, KUSNITZ A, RYAN J: Demonstration of the Lyme disease spirochete by a modified Dieterle stain method. Lab Med 16:685–687, 1985

18. ELIN RJ, ROBERTSON EA, SEVER GA: Workload, space and personnel of microbiology laboratories in teaching hospitals. Am J Clin Pathol 82:78–84, 1984

18a. FAN K, MORRIS, AJ, RELLER LB: Application of rejection criteria for stool cultures for bacterial enteric pathogens. J Clin Microbiol 31:2233–2235, 1993

19. FORBES BA, GRANATO PA: Processing specimens for bacteria. In Murray P (ed): Manual of Clinical Microbiology, 6th ed, Chap 21, p 266. Washington DC, American Society for Microbiology, 1995

20. FOXMAN B, ZHANG L, PALIN K, ET AL: Bacterial virulence characteristics of Escherichia coli isolates from first-time urinary tract infection. J Infect Dis 171:1514–1521, 1995

21. FRIEDLY G: Importance of bacterial stains in the diagnosis of infectious disease. J Med Technol 1:823–833, 1985

22. FUNG JC, McKINLEY G, TYBURSKI, MB, ET AL: Growth of coagulase-negative staphylococci on colistin–nalidixic acid agar and susceptibility to polymyxins. J Clin Microbiol 19:714–716, 1984

23. GUERRANT RL: Lessons from diarrheal diseases: demography to molecular pharmacology. J Infect Dis 169:1206, 1994

24. HALLAK A: Spontaneous bacterial peritonitis. Am J Gastroenterol 84:345–350, 1989

25. HAGEAGE CJ JR, HARRINGTON BJ: Use of calcofluor white in clinical mycology. Lab Med 15:109–115, 1984

26. HOERL D, ROSTKOWSKI C, ROSS, SL WALSH TJ: Typhoid fever acquired in a medical technology teaching laboratory. Lab Med 19:166–168, 1988

27. HOFF RG, NEWMANN E, STANECK JL: Bacteriuria screening by use of acridine orange-stained smears. J Clin Microbiol 21:513–516, 1984

28. HOLLEY JL, MOSS AH: A prospective evaluation of blood culture versus standard plate techniques for diagnosing peritonitis in continuous ambulatory peritoneal dialysis. Am J Kidney Dis 13:184–188, 1989

29. ISENBERG HD, WASHINGTON JA, DOERN G, AMSTERDAM D: Collection, handling and processing of specimens. In Balows A (ed): Manual of Clinical Microbiology, 5th ed, Chap 3, pp 15–28. Washington DC, American Society for Microbiology, 1991

30. JACOBSON JT, BURKE JP, JACOBSON JA: Ordering patterns, collection, transport and screening of sputum cultures in a community hospital. Infect Control 2:307–311, 1981

31. JAMES AN: Legal realities and practical applications in laboratory safety management. Lab Med 19:84–87, 1988

32. JUSKOVA E, CIZNAR I: Application of biotinylated and ^{32}P probes for detection of P-fimbriae in urinary E. coli. Folia Microbiol 38:259–263, 1993

33. KANTOFF PW, SHUPACK JL, GREENE JB: Histologic demonstration of intradermal spirochetes in a patient with Lyme disease. Am J Med Sci 287:40–42, 1984

34. KAYE E: Antibacterial activity of human urine. J Clin Invest 42:2374–2390, 1968.

35. KLEIMAN MB, REYNOLDS JK, SCHRIBER RL, ET AL: Rapid diagnosis of neonatal bacteremia with acridine orange-stained buffy coat smears. J Pediatr 105:419–421, 1984

36. LAUER BA, RELLER LB, MIRRETT S: Comparisons of acridine orange and Gram stains for detection of microorganisms in cerebrospinal fluid and other clinical specimens. J Clin Microbiol 14:201–205, 1981

37. LIPSKY BA, PLORDE JJ, TENOVER FC, ET AL: Comparison of the AutoMicrobic system, acridine orange-stained smears and gram-stained smears in detecting bacteriuria. J Clin Microbiol 22:176–181, 1985

38. LORIAN V (ED): Medical Microbiology in the Care of Patients, 2nd ed. Baltimore, Williams & Wilkins, 1983

39. LUND ME, HAWKINSON RW: Evaluation of the Prompt inoculation system for preparation of standardized bacteria inocula. J Clin Microbiol 18:84–91, 1985

40. MATSEN JM: The role of the infectious disease physician in hospital clinical microbiology laboratories. Bull NY Acad Med 63:605–611, 1988

41. McCABE WR, STOTTMEIER KD: Clinical Significance of aerobic gram-negative bacilli. In Lorian V (ed): Significance of Medical Microbiology in the Care of Patients. Baltimore, Williams & Wilkins, 1982

42. McCARTHY LR, SENNE JE: Evaluation of acridine orange stain for detection of microorganisms in blood cultures. J Clin Microbiol 11:281–285, 1980

43. McKINNEY RM, CHERRY SB: Immunofluorescence microscopy. In Lennette EH (ed): Manual of Clinical Microbiology, pp 891–897. Washington DC, American Society for Microbiology, 1985

44. MILLER CD, SONGER JR, SULLIVAN JF: A twenty-five year review of laboratory-acquired human infections at the National Animal Disease Center. Am Ind Hyg Assoc 48:271–275, 1987

45. MECOLY-KAMP C, FLETCHER-GUTOWSKI SM: Laboratory Acquired Brucellosis. Chicago, American Society of Clinical Pathologists, Check Sample MB-4, 1990

46. MERMEL LA, MAKI DG: Detection of bacteremia in adults; consequences of culturing an inadequate volume of blood. Ann Intern Med 119:270–272, 1993

46a. MORRIS AJ, SMITH LK, MIRRETT S, RELLER LB: Cost and time savings following introduction of rejection criteria for clinical specimens. J Clin Microbiol 34:355–357, 1996

46b. MORRIS AJ, WILSON SJ, MARX CE, ET AL: Clinical impact of bacteria and fungi recovered only from broth cultures. J Clin Microbiol 33: 161–165, 1995

47. MURRAY PR, WASHINGTON JA II: Microscopic and bacteriologic analysis of expectorated sputum. Mayo Clin Proc 50:339–344, 1975

48. NATIONAL COMMITTEE FOR CLINICAL LABORATORY STANDARDS (NCCLS): Standard Procedures for the Handling and Transport of Diagnostic Specimens and Etiologic Agents. Villanova PA, 1980

49. NICKEL JC, COSTERTON JW, McLEAN RJ, OLSON M: Bacterial biofilms: influence on the pathogenesis, diagnosis and treatment of urinary tract infections. J Antimicrob Chemother 33 (suppl A):31–41, 1994

50. NOELLE RJ, SNOW EC: Cognate interactions between helper T cells and B cells. Immunol Today 11:361, 1990

51. NOELLE RJ, SNOW EC: T helper cell-dependent B cell activation. FASEB J 5:2770, 1991

52. PFALLER MA, BAUM CA, NILES AC, ET AL: Clinical laboratory evaluation of a urine screening device. J Clin Microbiol 18:674–679, 1983

53. PIKE RM: Laboratory associated infections: summary and analysis of 3,921 cases. Health Lab Sci 13:105–114, 1976.

54. PIKE RM: Laboratory-associated infections: incidence, fatalities, causes and prevention. Annu Rev Microbiol 33:41–66, 1979

55. RICHARDS P, RATHBURN K: Medical Risk Management: Preventive Strategies for Heath Care Providers. Rockville MD, Aspen Press, 1983

56. RICHARDS WD, WRIGHT HS: Preservation of tissue specimens during transport to mycobacteriology laboratories. J Clin Microbiol 17:393–395, 1983

57. ROBERTS JA, KAACK MB, FUSSELL EN: Adherence to urethral catheters by bacteria causing nosocomial infections. Urology 41:338–342, 1993

58. RUNYON BA, UMLAND ET, MERLIN TR: Inoculation of blood culture bottles with ascitic fluid: improved detection of spontaneous bacterial peritonitis. Arch Intern Med 147:73–75, 1987

59. SCHIFMAN RB, VALENSTEIN PN: Q-Probes: Laboratory Diagnosis of Tuberculosis Data Analysis and Critique. Chicago IL, College of American Pathologists, 1994

60. SEWELL CM, CLARRIDGE JE, HOUNG EJ, ET AL: Clinical significance of coagulase-negative staphylococci. J Clin Microbiol 16:236–239, 1984

61. SIEGEL DL, EDELSTEIN PH, NACHAMKIN I: Inappropriate testing for diarrheal disease in the hospital. JAMA 263:979–982, 1990

62. SIEGFRIED L, KMETOVA M, PUZOVA H, ET AL: Virulence-associated factors in *Escherichia coli* strains isolated from children with urinary tract infections. J Med Microbiol 41:127–132, 1994

63. TARKKANEN AM, ALLEN BL, WILLIAMS PH, ET AL: Fimbriation, capsulation, and iron-scavenging systems of *Klebsiella* strains associated with human urinary tract infection. Infect Immun 60:1187–1192, 1992

64. THOMPSON R, CITED IN GRAHAM NO: Quality Assurance in Hospitals, p 9. Rockville MD, Aspen Publication, 1982

65. THORNSBERRY C: Susceptibility testing: General considerations. In Balows A (ed): Manual of Clinical Microbiology, 5th ed, pp 1059–1064. Washington DC, American Society for Microbiology, 1991

66. VAN SCOY RE: Bacterial sputum cultures: A clinician's viewpoint. Mayo Clin Proc 52:39–41, 1977

67. WARFARD AL, EVELAND WB, STRONG CA, ET AL: Enhanced virus isolation by use of the transporter for a regional laboratory. J Clin Microbiol 19:561–562, 1984

68. WEDAM AG, BARKLEY WE, HILLMAN A: Handling of infectious agents. J Am Vet Med Assoc 161:1557–1565, 1972

69. WINN WC JR: Bacterial diseases. In Damjanou I, Linder J (eds): Anderson's Pathology. CV Mosby, St. Louis MO, 1996

70. YANG KD, BOHNSACK JF, HILL HR: Fibronectin in host defenses: implications in the diagnosis, prophylaxis, and therapy of infectious diseases. Pediatr Infect Dis J 12:234, 1993

INTRODUCTION TO MICROBIOLOGY
PART II: GUIDELINES FOR THE COLLECTION, TRANSPORT, PROCESSING, ANALYSIS, AND REPORTING OF CULTURES FROM SPECIFIC SPECIMEN SOURCES

INTRODUCTION

In keeping with the model of the diagnostic cycle presented in Chapter 2, the focus of this chapter will be on the several steps necessary to establish the diagnosis of infections involving specific organ systems. In each of the sections that follow, the more common signs and symptoms of infections involving the specific organ systems will be presented, followed by a description of the unique procedures involved in the proper collection, transport, and processing of clinical specimens to ensure the recovery of pathogenic organisms (Table 3-1). The exact methods by which the common pathogenic bacteria found in each organ system are identified will be reviewed only briefly here, as details can be found in the individual chapters devoted to an in-depth presentation of the various groups of microbes. Emerging over the past 5 years has been the increasing implementation of the direct identification of microorganisms in clinical specimens using a variety of molecular techniques. Select procedures that have found their way into clinical laboratories are briefly introduced here. More information is available in Chapter 1 and in the chapters that follow that are devoted to presentations of the various organism groups. It may well be that many of the classic culture techniques as described here will be replaced by the time this edition becomes available; however, during this transition period these fundamentals of microbiology remain essential learning.

INFECTIONS OF THE RESPIRATORY TRACT

The respiratory tract is broadly divided into the upper tract (the oropharynx and nasopharynx) and the lower tract (the larynx, trachea, bronchi, and the alveolar air sacks of the lungs). For purposes of this discussion, the middle ear is also considered part of the upper respiratory tract because it is connected to the posterior pharynx through the eustachian tube.

INFECTIONS OF THE UPPER RESPIRATORY TRACT

Acute pharyngitis is the most common infection of the upper respiratory tract. Three important causes must be considered: streptococcal, viral, and diphtheritic. Diphtheria is primarily an infection of children, occurring in sporadic outbreaks, although adults may become infected, particularly in lower socioeconomic groups. The thick blue-white or gray membrane that covers the posterior pharynx, with marked edema of the underlying and surrounding tissues, can usually be differentiated from the fire-red throat of acute streptococcal pharyngitis. Viral infection, probably the most common cause of acute pharyngitis, is more difficult to differentiate from streptococcal infection. Adenoviruses, Epstein-Barr virus, and Coxsackie A viruses are the more common causes of viral pharyngitis; however, attempts to recover these agents are uncommonly attempted in most

clinical laboratories. The relatively high cost for viral cultures and the unavailability of a viruses reference laboratory in many locales are deterring factors. Rather, the diagnosis of viral pharyngitis is usually made by exclusion or empirically by knowing "what is going around" in the community.

Laboratory microbiologists should attempt to help the physician make a diagnosis by clearly distinguishing between "strep screens" and "routine throat cultures" for determining the etiology of acute upper respiratory tract infections. Confusion arises when the physician orders routine throat cultures for acute pharyngitis, and the laboratory reports the presence of *Staphylococcus aureus*, various gram-negative bacilli, *Haemophilus influenzae*, or other organisms that do not cause primary pharyngitis. In many laboratories, routine throat cultures are not included in test menus, offering a strep screen only.

Interpretation of throat culture results also must take into account the presence of the "normal" or "indigenous" bacterial flora of the oropharynx. α-Hemolytic streptococci (*Streptococcus mutans* and *S. salivarius*, and such), *Neisseria* species other than *N. gonorrhoeae*, coagulase-negative staphylococci (occasionally *S. aureus*), *Haemophilus hemolyticus*, *Streptococcus pneumoniae*, certain members of the family *Enterobacteriaceae* (particularly in hospitalized patients), yeasts including *Candida albicans* and, on occasion, β-hemolytic streptococci other than group A are normally present in varying combinations and concentrations. If the recovery of other organisms, such as *N. gonorrhoeae*, *B. pertussis*, or *C. diphtheriae*, or in rare instances, viral agents, is clinically indicated, the physician must so inform the laboratory so that special culture procedures will be used.

STREPTOCOCCAL PHARYNGITIS

Streptococcal pharyngitis may be clinically suggested by observing an inflamed and edematous pharyngeal mucosa in a patient who complains of throat pain, difficulty on swallowing, and secondary symptoms such as fever, headache, and occasionally a scarlatiniform rash.[68] Purulent exudates over the posterior pharynx and tonsillar area may also be observed. The presence of a tough, fibrinous, gray membrane ("pseudomembrane"), collections of pus, either within abscesses or exuding from draining sinuses, or the presence of mucosal ulcerations may indicate an infectious disease other than acute pharyngitis, and cultures other than throat swabs may be necessary.

Collection of Throat Cultures. The proper method for obtaining a throat swab specimen is shown in Figure 3-1 (page 125). A bright light from over the shoulder of the specimen collector should be focused into the oral cavity so that the swab can be guided to the posterior pharynx. The patient is instructed to tilt his or her head back and breathe deeply. The tongue is gently de-

TABLE 3-1

THE DIAGNOSIS OF BACTERIAL INFECTIONS AT DIFFERENT BODY SITES

SITE OF INFECTION	PRESENTING SIGNS AND SYMPTOMS	SPECIMENS TO CULTURE	BACTERIAL SPECIES POTENTIALLY ASSOCIATED WITH INFECTIONS
Respiratory tract	Upper tract—nose and sinuses 　Headache 　Pain and redness over malar area 　Rhinitis 　Radiograph: sinus consolidation, fluid levels, or membrane thickening Upper tract—throat and pharynx 　Redness and edema of mucosa 　Exudation of tonsils 　Pseudomembrane formation 　Edema of uvula 　Gray coating of tongue: "strawberry tongue" 　Enlargement of cervical nodes	Acute 　Nasopharyngeal swab 　Sinus washings Chronic 　Sinus washings 　Surgical biopsy specimen 　Swab of posterior pharynx 　Swab of tonsils (abscess) 　Nasopharyngeal swab	*Streptococcus pneumoniae* *Streptococcus*, β-hemolytic group A *Staphylococcus aureus* *Haemophilus influenzae* *Klebsiella* spp. and other *Enterobacteriaceae* *Bacteroides* spp. and other anaerobes (sinus) *Streptococcus*, β-hemolytic group A *Corynebacterium diphtheriae* *Neisseria gonorrhoeae* *Bordetella pertussis*
	Lower tract—lungs and bronchi 　Cough: bloody or profuse 　Chest pain 　Dyspnea 　Consolidation of lungs 　　Rales and rhonchi 　　Diminished breath sounds 　　Dullness to percussion 　　Radiographic infiltrates 　　Cavity lesions 　　Empyema	Sputum (poor return) Blood Bronchoscopy secretions Transtracheal aspirate Lung aspirate or biopsy	*Streptococcus pneumoniae* *Haemophilus influenzae* *Staphylococcus aureus* *Klebsiella pneumoniae* and other *Enterobacteriaceae* *Moraxella catarrhalis* *Legionella* spp. *Mycobacterium* spp. *Fusobacterium nucleatum, Prevotella melaninogenicus*, and other anaerobes *Bordetella* species
Middle ear	Serous or purulent drainage Deep pain in ear and jaw Throbbing headache Red bulging tympanic membrane	Acute 　No culture 　Nasopharyngeal swab 　Tympanic membrane aspirate Chronic: drainage of external meatus	Acute 　*Streptococcus pneumoniae* and other streptococci 　*Haemophilus influenzae* Chronic 　*Pseudomonas aeruginosa* 　*Proteus* spp. 　Anaerobic bacteria
Gastrointestinal tract	Upper—stomach and duodenum 　Gastritis and peptic ulcer disease Lower—small and large intestine 　Diarrhea 　Dysentery 　　Purulent 　　Mucous 　　Bloody 　Cramping abdominal pain	Gastric or duodenal biopsy Stool specimen Rectal swab or rectal mucus Blood culture (typhoid fever)	*Helicobacter pylori* *Campylobacter jejuni* and other *Campylobacter* spp. *Salmonella* spp. *Shigella* spp. *Escherichia coli* (toxigenic strains) *Vibrio cholerae* and other *Vibrio* spp. *Yersinia* species *Clostridium difficile* (demonstration of toxin)
Urinary tract	Urinary bladder infection 　Pyuria 　Dysuria 　Hematuria 　Pain and tenderness; suprapubic or lower abdomen Kidney infection 　Back pain 　Tenderness: costovertebral angle (CVA)	Clean-catch midstream urine Catheterized urine Suprapubic aspiration of urine	*Enterobacteriaeceae* 　*Escherichia coli* 　*Klebsiella* spp. 　*Proteus* spp. *Enterococcus* spp. *Pseudomonas aeruginosa* *Staphylococcus aureus, S. epidermidis*, and *S. saprophyticus*

(Continued)

SITE OF INFECTION	PRESENTING SIGNS AND SYMPTOMS	SPECIMENS TO CULTURE	BACTERIAL SPECIES POTENTIALLY ASSOCIATED WITH INFECTIONS

Genital tract	Males
	  Urethral discharge: serous or purulent
	  Burning on urination
	  Terminal hematuria
	Females
	  Purulent vaginal discharge
	  Burning on urination
	  Lower abdominal pain, spasm, and tenderness
	  Mucous membrane chancre or chancroid
		Urethral discharge
		Prostatic secretions
		
		Uterine cervix
		Rectum (anal sphincter swab)
		Urethral swab
		
		Darkfield examination
			Neisseria gonorrhoeae (*N. meningitidis*)
			Haemophilus ducreyi
			Treponema pallidum (syphilis)
			Mobiluncus spp. and other anaerobes
			Gardnerella vaginalis
			Nonbacterial:
			  Trichomonas vaginalis
			  Candida albicans
			  Mycoplasma spp.
			  Chlamydia trachomatis
			  Herpes simplex virus

Central nervous system	Headache Pain in neck and back Stiff neck Straight-leg raising: positive Kernig's sign Nausea and vomiting Stupor to coma Petechial rash	Spinal fluid Subdural aspirate Blood culture Throat or sputum culture	*Neisseria meningitidis* *Haemophilus influenzae* *Streptococcus pneumoniae* *Streptococcus*, β-hemolytic groups A and B (group B in infants) *Enterobacteriaceae*: debilitated patients, infants, and postcraniotomy *Listeria monocytogenes*
Eye	Conjunctival discharge: serous or purulent Conjunctival redness (hyperemia): pink eye Ocular pain and tenderness	Purulent discharge Lower cul-de-sac Inner canthus	*Haemophilus* spp. *Moraxella* spp. *Neisseria gonorrhoeae* *Staphylococcus aureus* *Streptococcus pneumoniae* *Streptococcus pyogenes* *Pseudomonas aeruginosa* (report stat)

Blood	Spiking fever
	Chills
	Cardiac murmur (endocarditis)
	Petechiae: skin and mucous membranes
	"Splinter hemorrhages" of nails
	Malaise
		Blood: three or four cultures per day at 1-h intervals or longer
		Any suspected primary site of infection:
		  Cerebrospinal fluid
		  Respiratory tract
		  Skin—umbilicus
		  Skin—ear
		  Wounds
		  Urinary tract
			Streptococcus spp.
			  Group A—all ages
			  S. viridans (endocarditis)
			  Groups A, B, D—neonates
			  S. pneumoniae
			Staphylococcus aureus
			Listeria monocytogenes
			Corynebacterium jekeium
			Haemophilus influenzae
			HACEK group (see Chap. 8)
			Echerichia coli and other "coliforms"
			Salmonella typhi
			Pseudomonas aeruginosa
			Bacteroides fragilis and other anaerobic bacteria

Wounds	Discharge: serous or purulent Abscess: subcutaneous or submucosal Redness and edema Crepitation (gas formation) Pain Ulceration or sinus formation	Aspirate of drainage Deep swab of purulent drainage Tissue biopsy	*Staphylococcus aureus* *Streptococcus pyogenes* *Clostridium* spp., *Bacteroides* spp., and other anaerobic bacteria *Enterobacteriaceae* *Pseudomonas aeruginosa* *Enterococcus* species
Bones and joints	Joint swelling Redness and heat Pain on motion Tenderness on palpation Radiograph: synovitis or osteomyelitis	Joint aspirate Synovial biopsy Bone spicules or bone marrow aspirate	*Staphylococcus aureus* *Haemophilus influenzae* *Streptococcus pyogenes* *Neisseria gonorrhoeae* *Streptococcus pneumoniae* *Enterobacteriaceae* *Mycobacterium* species

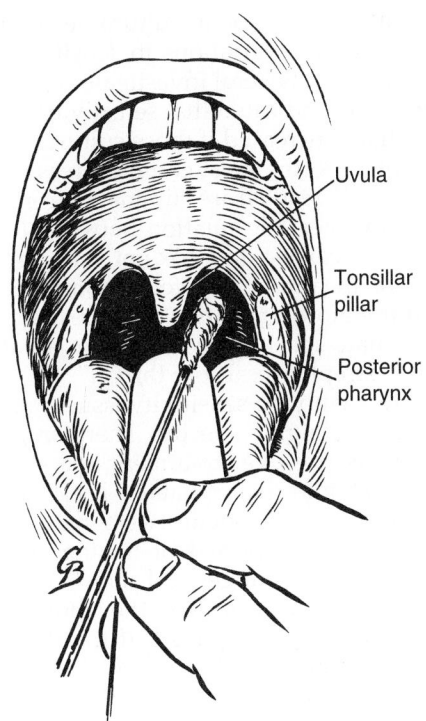

Uvula

Tonsillar pillar

Posterior pharynx

Figure 3-1.
Throat culture technique: The patient is asked to open the mouth widely and phonate an "ah." The tongue is gently depressed with a tongue blade and a swab is guided over the tongue into the posterior pharynx. The mucosa behind the uvula and between the tonsillar pillars is swabbed with a gentle back-and-forth sweeping motion.

pressed with a tongue blade to visualize the tonsillar fossae and posterior pharynx. The swab is extended between the tonsillar pillars and behind the uvula. Care should be taken not to touch the lateral walls of the buccal cavity or the tongue to minimize contamination with commensal bacteria. Having the patient phonate a long "ah" serves to lift the uvula and helps prevent gagging. The tonsillar areas and the posterior pharynx should be firmly rubbed with the swab. Any purulent exudate should also be sampled.

For the recovery of viruses from the upper respiratory tract, nasopharyngeal specimens are usually considered superior to throat swabs or washings. Frayha and coworkers[56] found no differences between nasopharyngeal swabs and nasopharyngeal aspirates in the overall recovery of viruses from the nasal passages in 125 patients studied; however, Isenberg and associates[91] report that nasopharyngeal washings are superior for the recovery of respiratory syncytial and possibly parainfluenza viruses. They also caution that calcium alginate swabs may inactivate and compromise the recovery of herpesvirus.

After collection, the swab should be placed immediately into a sterile tube or other suitable container for transport to the laboratory. If the recovery of only group A β-hemolytic streptococci is desired (i.e., a strep screen), swabs may be allowed to dry during transport without compromising the recovery of vi-

able organisms. Some reference laboratories recommend that swab tips be placed in a desiccant, such as silica gel, to suppress survival of commensal organisms and improve the recovery of group A streptococci. Swabs for the recovery of viral agents should be placed in a special transport medium (see Chap. 21).

Culture for Group A β-Hemolytic Streptococci. Organisms other than group A β-hemolytic streptococci, including β-streptococcal groups B, C, F, and G, on occasion may cause acute pharyngitis. When symptoms are associated with recovery of these organisms, the cardiac and renal sequelae seen following group A streptococcal pharyngitis generally do not occur, and the pharyngitis tends to be mild and self-limited. For the vast majority of throat cultures, culture medium for the sole recovery of group A β-hemolytic streptococci should be inoculated.

Recovery and identification of group A streptococci in throat swabs is accomplished by inoculating a 5% sheep blood agar plate for organism isolation and making two or three stabs into the agar in inoculated and uninoculated areas of the plate. Stabbing the agar forces some of the inoculum into a subsurface, partially anaerobic environment, and allows detection of both oxygen-labile and oxygen-stable streptococcal hemolysins (see Chap. 12). After 18 to 24 hours of incubation, the plate is examined for the presence of β-hemolytic colonies. Negative cultures should be incubated for an additional 24 hours before discarding as negative.

β-Hemolytic colonies that are determined to be streptococci by gram-staining and catalase testing can then be confirmed by either presumptive or definitive methods (see Chap. 12). Presumptive methods include testing for susceptibility to bacitracin and sulfamethoxazole–trimethoprim, whereas definitive methods include serologic grouping by latex or coagglutination methods. Direct application of bacitracin differential disks to the surface of nonselective primary blood agar plates for more rapid presumptive identification of group A streptococci in culture is not recommended.[122] The normal flora may partially inhibit the growth of group A streptococci, especially in areas of more confluent growth. However, if an inhibitory blood agar is used, in which antibiotics such as sulfamethoxazole–trimethoprim (SXT) have been added, the recovery of group A streptococci within 18 to 24 hours is markedly improved. Kurzynski and associates[121] also found that the direct placement of a bacitracin differential disk on SXT blood agar plates is acceptable for the recovery of group A streptococci. Anaerobic incubation increases the detection of group A streptococcal strains that produce only oxygen-labile streptolysin O and inhibits much of the normal flora.[127] The optimal conditions for the recovery of group A β-hemolytic streptococci from throat cultures has been reviewed by Kellogg.[101]

Direct Detection of Group A Streptococci on Throat Swabs. Direct detection of streptococcal antigen on throat swabs has become accepted practice in many clinic and laboratory settings.[101] All direct detection methods require extraction of the group A streptococcal antigen from the swab after collection and before detection. The original method for extraction of group-specific polysaccharide antigens of β-hemolytic streptococci was the use of nitrous acid.[47] Acid-extraction techniques and subsequent detection methods provide results within 10 to 15 minutes.[143,165] Antigen extraction can also be accomplished with cell–wall-active enzymes; however, these methods usually take an hour or more to perform.

Several methods for antigen detection in extracts have been described and are currently used.[26,59,60,88,216] Detection of antigen in nitrous acid extracts by coagglutination was the first procedure employed, and subsequently several kits using latex beads coated with antibody as the detection reagent were marketed.[217] More recently, enzyme immunoassay (EIA) detection methods have been successfully applied.[234] The EIA-based detection methods may have several advantages over latex methods, including increased sensitivity and specificity, ease of interpretation, and built-in quality control standards. Stranjord and coworkers[234] evaluated the EIA-based ICON Strep A test kit (Hybritech, Inc., San Diego CA) in a pediatric emergency room and an acute care clinic and concluded that the system had better specificity and positive predictive values than the latex particle test. An EIA-based test using anti–group A streptococcal antibodies conjugated to liposomes (Q Test Strep, Becton Dickinson, Franklin Lakes NJ) has also been successful in detecting antigen in extracts of throat swab specimens.[59]

A chemiluminescent nucleic acid probe assay for the direct detection of group A streptococci in pharyngeal specimens is commercially available (Group A Streptococcus Direct Test [GP-ST], Gen Probe, San Diego CA). In a study of 1103 pharyngeal swab specimens, Heiter and Bourbeau[73] found that the GP-ST assay was 93.5% sensitive and 99.7% specific for the detection of group A streptococci when compared with culture. The sensitivity, specificity, and positive and negative predictive values for the DNA probe were 89%, 96%, 86%, and 97%, respectively, in a study by Steed and associates[229] of the direct detection of group A streptococci from 277 throat swabs collected from pediatric patients. The false-negative DNA probe results occurred in specimens containing fewer than five colony-forming units (CFU) on culture. The authors reiterate the American Heart Association statement that a small number of S. pyogenes in throat isolates do not differentiate a carrier from an acutely infected individual. The researchers for both of these studies found the DNA probe assay to be highly sensitive, specific, and easy to use. Because of the need for specialized equipment and high costs for controls required for each run, the GP-ST assay is not suitable for point of care testing in the physician office or clinic setting nor in most clinical laboratories. In large-volume reference laboratories, the rapid turnaround time compared with culture and the potential labor savings from batching makes this procedure worth considering.

Facklam[51] reviewed the performance of 18 commercial direct streptococcal antigen detection kits in comparison with conventional culture techniques. The studies reveal wide variations in sensitivity, ranging from 62% to 100%. Several investigators (and kit manufacturers) have indicated that sensitivity rates would be substantially increased if those cultures growing 30 or fewer colonies (the most common reason for false-negative "rapid" results) are eliminated from statistical analysis. However, the relation between low colony counts and the carrier state has not yet been resolved. Furthermore, the presence of few colonies on a culture plate, and therefore a negative direct test, may also reflect inadequate specimen collection in a patient who indeed has "streptococcal sore throat."

In contrast with the sensitivity issues, all of the direct systems are highly specific. Therefore, if a direct antigen test is positive, treatment for streptococcal pharyngitis should be initiated. Facklam[51] recommends that physicians obtain two throat swabs from patients clinically suspected of having streptococcal pharyngitis. A direct antigen test should be performed on one of the swabs; if positive, the laboratory testing for that specimen is completed. If the direct antigen test is negative, the second swab should be used to set up a standard culture.

A theoretical advantage of direct antigen detection methods is that the results are more rapidly available than conventional culture results, making it possible to diagnose and prescribe immediate specific therapy in a physicians's office setting at the time the patient presents. However, directors and supervisors of hospital laboratories have frequently opted against using direct testing methods, for quick turnaround of results is less of a factor, and all negative antigen tests must be followed up with culture, requiring the somewhat cumbersome need for obtaining two swabs. Also, because no one test brand has emerged as superior, it may also be difficult to decide which to choose if an affirmative decision is made. Radestsky and associates[180] also cautioned against overuse of direct antigen test systems. They pointed out that the total technologist time involved in the processing, test performance, and interpretation of a rapid test procedure on a single specimen (and, therefore, several specimens) can be surprisingly long, thereby negating the value of rapid turnaround time. In addition, owing to current staffing constraints in many laboratories, the rapid tests are not done immediately but are run in batches. This further erodes the concept of rapid results and rapid reporting. Other parameters, such as relative costs per kit per test, shelf life, storage temperatures, performance times, and customer training requirements must be figured in the decision to employ a particular rapid streptococcal detection method.

With the extensive literature on this subject that has accumulated over the past decade reflecting both good and bad experiences with these methods, it may be difficult for users to decide whether to introduce a direct antigen detection method in their laboratory. Radetsky and coworkers[181] counsel that laboratories should do parallel studies comparing whatever direct antigen kit system they select with the conventional methods being used before a test procedure is adopted. In their view, the antigen detection system should be implemented only if a correlation of 95% or greater is achieved.

Recovery of Miscellaneous Pathogens From Throat Cultures. Laboratories must be prepared to handle requests to recover and identify bacterial species from throat cultures for less commonly encountered diseases. Diphtheria is an acute infectious disease, caused by toxigenic *Corynebacterium diphtheriae*, in which the presence of a gray pseudomembrane covering the mucous membrane of the oropharynx is an initial clue to diagnosis. In suspected cases, nasopharyngeal cultures should be obtained in addition to throat cultures. The specimen should be inoculated onto a slant of Loeffler's serum glucose medium (or modified Pai medium), a cystine-tellurite agar plate (e.g., Tinsdale agar), and 5% sheep blood agar. The interpretation of growth on these media, leading to the identification of *C. diphtheriae*, is discussed in Chapter 13.

Bordet-Gengou potato infusion agar has been the time-honored medium for the recovery of *Bordetella pertussis* from patients with suspected whooping cough. However, Regan and Lowe[185] found that charcoal agar with horse blood and cephalexin was superior as an isolation medium (see Chap. 8). This medium is also available as a combination transport and enrichment medium. At one time, the use of cough plates was advocated; however, collection of specimens from the nares with a nasopharyngeal swab is currently recommended. Gilligan and Fisher[58] reiterate the importance of collecting appropriate specimens for culture in establishing the laboratory diagnosis of pertussis, a procedure they found to be more sensitive than the direct fluorescent antibody test. For optimum results, a Bordet-Gengou or Regan-Lowe agar plate should be inoculated at the bedside by streaking the surface of the agar plate, and streaking the plate for isolation with a sterile loop.[85] Plates are then immediately placed into a CO_2-enriched environment at 35°C. The identification of *B. pertussis* is further discussed in Chapter 8.

Because culture is slow and insensitive, several methods for the direct detection of *B. pertussis* in nasopharyngeal swabs or aspirates have been used. A direct fluorescent assay (DFA) using a fluorescein-conjugated antibody offered some promise. However, investigators found an unacceptably high rate of false-positive reactions, particularly for commercially available reagents using polyclonal antibodies, primarily caused by extensive cross-reaction with normal nasopharyngeal and oral microbial flora.[50,141] In a study of 5683 cases of pertussis in a northern Alberta, Canada epidemic in 1989 to 1991, Ewanowich and associates[50] found that 84.6% of DFA-positive, culture-negative assays were also polymerase chain reaction (PCR)-negative, again demonstrating the insensitivity of this method. Several current studies indicate that PCR assays are the most sensitive method for diagnosing pertussis. In an outbreak of pertussis in Finland,[71] the PCR assay was 100% sensitive compared with culture, and it was also positive in 65 of 157 culture-negative specimens obtained from symptomatic patients; the PCR assay was sensitive to 25 bacteria per reaction tube. In addition to use as a diagnostic tool, it was suggested that PCR for detection of *B. pertussis* organisms may be helpful as a tool for the evaluation of vaccine efficacy and for tracing the transmission and spread to asymptomatic persons. In laboratories with assay capabilities, the PCR assay can provide accurate results within 24 hours.

When the clinical history or physical examination indicates that *Neisseria gonorrhoeae* may be the cause of pharyngitis, a selective medium for the pathogenic *Neisseria* species should be inoculated in addition to a 5% sheep blood agar plate (see Chap. 10). *N. meningitidis* may also be present in throat cultures and must be differentiated biochemically from *N. gonorrhoeae* when required.

Whether to culture for *Haemophilus influenzae* in throat cultures is problematic. In many laboratories, selective media for recovery of *H. influenzae* are used only for infants and children up to 2 years of age; recovery in older children and adults is done only on request. Acute obstructive epiglottitis is one potentially serious infection known to be caused by *H. influenzae*, and this infection may be seen in both adults and children. In these patients, blood cultures are usually positive, and throat culture for *H. influenzae* is noncontributory or may even be dangerous to collect in these severely ill patients. *H. influenzae* probably does not cause acute pharyngitis, although clinicians often relate that symptomatic patients who have this organism predominating in throat cultures improve with antibiotic therapy.

H. influenzae and other *Haemophilus* species will not grow on sheep blood agar because X factor (hemin) and V factor (NAD) are not readily available in sheep blood. In some laboratories, agar medium containing horse blood is used for recovery of *Haemophilus* species. Horse blood is rich in both X and V factors, and the hemolytic quality of the organisms can also be determined. A 10-μg bacitracin disk can also be placed in the streak area to inhibit organisms other than *Haemophilus* species, or the medium can be made selective by the addition of bacitracin. If a selective medium is not used, inoculated sheep blood agar plates can be cross-streaked with a β-hemolytic strain of *Staphylococcus aureus*. The latter organism lyses red cells in the medium, providing X factor, and secretes V factor during growth. The growth of small satellite colonies of pale-staining, gram-negative coccobacilli around the staphylococcal streak after 24 hours of incubation provides a presumptive identification of *Haemophilus* species. Additional tests (discussed in Chap. 7) may be performed for confirmation.

In summary, a single 5% sheep blood agar plate (or a selective blood agar plate containing sulfamethoxazole–trimethoprim) streaked for isolation with two or three stab marks and incubated aerobically is sufficient for most throat cultures when streptococcal sore throat is suspected. By special request, selective media for the recovery of *C. diphtheriae*, *B. pertussis*, *N. gonorrhoeae* (or *N. meningitidis*), *H. influenzae*, or other unusual pathogens may be required in certain cases.

INFECTIONS OF THE ORAL CAVITY

Bacteria, fungi, and viruses commonly cause a variety of infections of the oral cavity. In fact, a specimen labeled "buccal mucosa," "tongue," "gums," or "inner lip" should alert microbiologists that the cause may be a microorganism other than bacteria. Various bacterial species cause periodontal disease and mucosal ulcerative infections often related to immunosuppression. Necrotizing, ulcerative gingivostomatitis (Vincent's infection or "trench mouth") is a synergistic infection involving multiple oral anaerobic bacteria, and culture is not indicated. However, because the condition at times may accompanied by sepsis and metastatic infection, blood cultures should always be obtained in suspected cases. Observing gram-negative, fusiform-shaped bacilli and spirochetes in gram-stained smears prepared from an ulcerative buccal or gingival ulcer is helpful for presumptive diagnosis of these conditions. Cultures of the mouth and oral cavity are rarely helpful because of the presence of many species of commensal anaerobes. Gingivostomatitis may also be caused by herpes simplex virus (HSV-1), presenting as painful vesicular lesions of the oral mucosa. High fever and submandibular lymphadenopathy are also usually present. Infection with HSV-1 is more commonly seen as vesicular fever blisters or cold sores on the orolabial mucosa.

Capnocytophaga species, fusiform bacteria that are normally present in the oropharynx, have also been associated with the presence of oral mucosal ulcerations and positive blood cultures, particularly in patients with severe neutropenia.[249] These organisms may frequently be recovered on selective media for pathogenic *Neisseria* because of their resistance to vancomycin, colistin, and trimethoprim. By using a selective medium similar in formulation to selective neisseria medium, Rummens and associates[195] recovered *Capnocytophaga* species from 96% of oropharyngeal cultures compared with only a 6% recovery on chocolate agar plates inoculated in parallel.

If the clinical history reveals a long-standing, non-healing mucosal ulcer in the oral cavity, the possibility of the cutaneous extension of a systemic fungal disease must be considered. Bacteria rarely cause nonhealing ulcers in the oral cavity, and recovery of what may be considered a potential pathogen should be discounted until other conditions can be ruled out. An immediate diagnosis of histoplasmosis or blastomycosis may be possible by observing typical yeast forms in direct saline or potassium hydroxide mounts of material scraped from the base or margins of the ulcer. A tissue biopsy for histologic study and direct examination of exudative material may be required. White patches on the oral mucosa or the more extensive involvement of the oral cavity with production of a thick, curdlike exudate may be caused by *Candida albicans*, a diagnosis that can be made by observing the pseudohyphae and budding blastoconidia in a gram-stained smear of the exudate.

NASOPHARYNGEAL CULTURES

Obtaining nasopharyngeal specimens is of little practical value. In epidemiologic studies, nasopharyngeal cultures may be helpful in detecting carriers of *Streptococcus pyogenes*, *Corynebacterium diphtheriae*, or *Neisseria meningitidis*. Nasopharyngeal swab cultures are of limited value in helping establish the diagnosis of acute otitis media[206] or bacterial sinusitis[49] but are the specimen of choice for the isolation of *Bordetella pertussis*.[85] Nasopharyngeal swabs and aspirates are equally effective for the diagnosis of viral respiratory infections.[56]

Nasopharyngeal specimens are obtained under direct vision using over-the-shoulder illumination. With the thumb of one hand, gently elevate the tip of the nose. Moisten the tip of a small flexible wire nasopharyngeal swab with sterile water or saline and gently insert it into one of the nares. Guide the swab backward and upward along the nasal septum until a distinct give of resistance indicates that the posterior pharynx has been reached. Gently remove the swab. If while guiding the swab undue resistance is met, attempt the procedure through the opposite nares.

INFECTIONS OF THE LOWER RESPIRATORY TRACT

CLINICAL SYMPTOMS

Infections of the lower respiratory tract may involve the trachea and bronchial tree (tracheitis, bronchitis, and bronchiolitis) or the lung tissue (alveolitis and pneumonia), or both. Presenting symptoms usually include cough and varying degrees of sputum production. In cases of allergic bronchopulmonary infections caused by *Aspergillus* species and other fungi, tenacious mucin plugs containing eosinophils, Charcot-Leyden crystals, and hyphal fragments may be microscopically observed in sputum. Fever may or may not be present. Chest pain may be diffuse, vague and constant, or localized and intermittent, accentuated by deep respiration, if pleuritis is present. Shortness of breath and dyspnea usually indicate involvement of the terminal bronchioles and alveoli in a more diffuse pneumonitic process. Physical signs pointing to the lower respiratory tract include rales and rhonchi, diminished breath sounds, and localized dullness to percussion in cases of lobar pneumonia.[40]

Certain bacterial pneumonias exhibit distinctive pathologic and radiologic patterns of disease. Consolidation of a single lobe of the lung (lobar pneumonia) is primarily caused by *Streptococcus pneumoniae*, *Klebsiella pneumoniae*, or *Legionella pneumophila*. *K. pneumoniae* also has a tendency to produce "currant jelly" sputum because the invading organisms cause tissue damage and hemorrhage into the alveoli. Each of these organisms can also produce multifocal bronchopneumonia, although *Escherichia coli* is the more common cause, often complicated by empyema and septicemia. *Pseudomonas aeruginosa* and *Serratia marcescens* are associated with a severe necrotizing pneumonia in immunosuppressed patients.

Lung abscesses, often evolving into cavitary lesions, are seen with several species of anaerobes and *Staphylococcus aureus*. Cavitary lesions, principally of the upper lobes, are classically produced by *Mycobacterium tuberculosis*, although the pulmonary lesions caused by certain pathogenic fungi, such as *Histoplasma capsulatum* and *Coccidioides immitis*, can also cavitate. *Mycoplasma pneumoniae* commonly produces peribronchial, interstitial infiltrates but may also cause multifocal consolidation. Diffuse pneumonia in immunosuppressed or immunocompromised patients may indicate infections by *Pneumocysits carinii* or *Mycobacterium avium-intracellulare* complex, or by cytomegalovirus.

SPECIMEN COLLECTION TECHNIQUES

Sputum Specimens.   Our inability to adequately prevent contamination by oral secretions and difficulty in obtaining secretions representative of the lower respiratory tract significantly compromise the diagnostic utility of coughed and expectorated sputum samples for culture. Having the patient brush his or her teeth and gargle with water immediately before obtaining the sputum specimen reduces the number of contaminating oropharyngeal bacteria. Spada and colleagues[222] showed a 1-log decrease in the mean concentration of contaminating bacteria from $3.6 \pm 7.5 \times 10^8$ to $3.7 \pm 7.2 \times 10^7$ in sputum samples obtained from patients immediately following a simple mouth wash. They suggest that comparing the organisms recovered from "spit" and post-mouthwash sputum samples may provide a guideline for determining which bacterial species may be potentially important in causing pneumonia. Avoid using proprietary mouthwashes or gargles that may contain antibacterial substances.

Early-morning sputum samples should be obtained because they contain pooled overnight secretions in which pathogenic bacteria are more likely to be concentrated. Twenty-four-hour collections should be discouraged because there is not only a greater likelihood of contamination, but bacterial pathogens that may be in high concentration in one sample potentially become diluted with the addition of subsequent, more watery specimens. When sputum production is scant, induction with nebulized saline may be effective in producing a sample more representative of the lower respiratory tract (avoid the use of "saline for injection," many preparations of which may contain antibacterial substances).[187]

Special sputum collection devices are commercially available through laboratory supply companies, or a sterile wide-mouth jar with a tightly fitted screw-cap lid can be used. To prevent contamination of the outside of the container, the patient should be instructed to press the rim of the container under the lower lip to catch all of the expectorated cough sample.[4]

Translaryngeal (Transtracheal) Aspiration.   Translaryngeal aspirations may be indicated when

1. The patient is debilitated and cannot spontaneously expectorate a sputum sample.
2. Routine sputum samples have failed to recover a causative organism in the face of clinical bacterial pneumonia.
3. An anaerobic pulmonary infection is suspected.

The translaryngeal aspiration technique is illustrated in Figure 3-2. After the skin is locally anesthetized, the cricothyroid membrane is pierced with a 14-gauge needle through which a 16-gauge polyethylene catheter is threaded into the lower trachea. Secretions are aspirated with a 20-mL syringe. If secretions are scant, the physician may inject a small amount of sterile water or saline, thereby inducing a paroxysm of coughing. Translaryngeal aspiration is a traumatic procedure and should be done only after careful consideration of the patient's clinical condition, the potential value of the information to be derived, and whether an alternative, less risky procedure may be more efficient. Detection of microorganisms in gram-

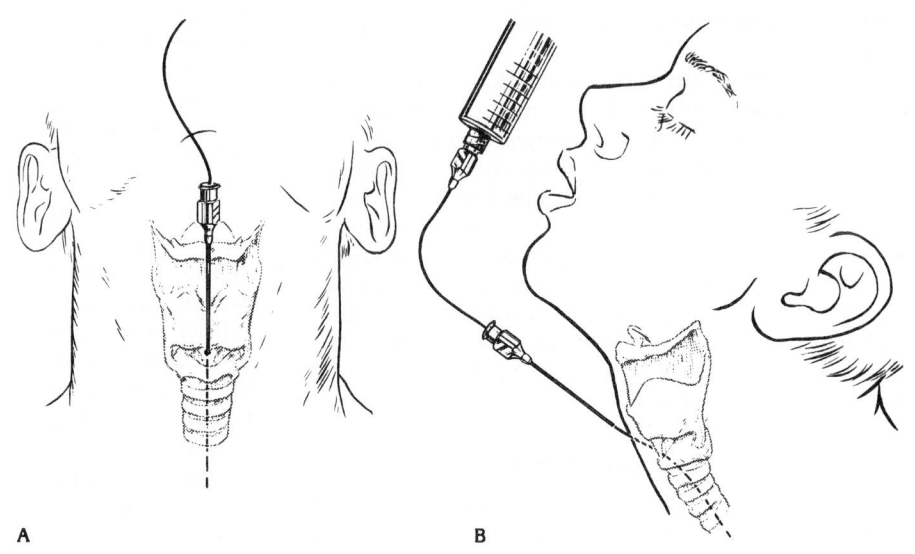

Figure 3-2.
(**A**) Front and (**B**) side views of translaryngeal (transtracheal) aspiration techniques: A 14-gauge needle is passed percutaneously through the cricothyroid membrane. A polyethylene catheter is threaded through the needle and extended into the trachea. A syringe is attached to the catheter, and material is aspirated by pulling on the plunger.

A   B

stained smears of tracheal secretions often predicts bacteremia in newborns.[212]

Bronchoscopy. Fiberoptic bronchoscopy is a technique being employed more frequently for obtaining transbronchial biopsies and brushings, particularly in patients with lung abscesses or other suspected deep pulmonary infections. The bronchial brush technique uses a telescoping double catheter plugged with polyethylene glycol at the distal end to protect a small bronchial brush. This technique is recommended for the optimal recovery of aerobic and obligate anaerobic bacteria from deep-seated pulmonary lesions.[8] Discrete sampling of focal lesions may be accomplished after fluoroscopic localization of the tip of the bronchoscope. Specimens that cannot be cultured immediately should be placed into a holding–transport medium for delivery to the laboratory. The success of this procedure depends on the following: 1) obtaining ample brush material from the distal bronchioles and alveoli to make several slides, 2) preparing a full set of special stains and multiple cultures, and 3) searching for more than one type of microorganism.

Bronchoalveolar Lavage. Bronchoalveolar lavage involves the injection of 30 to 50 mL of physiologic saline through a fiberoptic bronchoscope that has been threaded into the peripheral bronchiolar ramifications. The saline is then aspirated and submitted for smear preparation and culture. The semiquantitative cultures of respiratory secretions obtained by protected bronchial brush and alveolar lavage techniques have been useful in diagnosing pneumonia in intubated patients undergoing ventilation.[31] Organism colony counts higher than 10^3/mL that demonstrate intracellular bacteria in more than 25% of the inflammatory cells are indicators of pneumonia that requires specific treatment.

Additional procedures may be helpful in determining the etiology of respiratory infections when cultures are negative or nonrevealing. Blood cultures should always be obtained during the acute phases of pneumonia. *Streptococcus pneumoniae* may be recovered from the blood in 25% to 30% of patients with pneumococcal pneumonia, often when sputum cultures are negative.[152]

As with the group A streptococci and pharyngitis, rapid direct detection tests are being used with increasing frequency to diagnose lower respiratory tract infections. Direct fluorescent antibody tests are available to detect a variety of antigens in direct smears, touch preparations, and tissue sections. Touch preparations should always be prepared from transbronchial and open-lung biopsy tissues. *Pneumocystis carinii*, the tissue forms of various fungi, mycobacteria, viral inclusions, and other bacteria can often be observed by using one of several stains described in the next section of this chapter.

LABORATORY DIAGNOSIS OF BACTERIAL PNEUMONIA

Although distinctive patterns of pulmonary infection can occasionally be recognized, the isolation of the causative microorganisms is almost always required to make a definitive diagnosis. Sputum samples should be processed as soon after collection as possible. A significant decrease in recoverable organisms from sputum samples after 20 hours of refrigeration has been found,[169] although there was no compromise in the number or quality of epithelial cells and segmented neutrophils. A decline in the number of viable tubercle bacilli that could be recovered from sputum after storage at room temperature for several days has also been found,[167] although the concentration of acid-fast bacilli seen in acid-fast stains was not reduced after 20 days.

The quality of sputum samples should also be assessed using one of the grading systems described in Chapter 2. Literature reviews are mixed on how valuable the assessment of the concentration and morphotype of bacteria in Gram stains of sputum might be. Bartlett and coworkers[9] first suggested that the identification of organism categories in gram-stained smears of sputum may be accurately performed. For example, the Gram stain identification of staphylococci, "bacteroides–haemophilus," and bacteria of mixed morphology were made in their hands, with 75% accuracy in high-quality sputum specimens. It has been demonstrated[244] that semiquantitative enumeration of the bacteria in gram-stained sputum cannot be reproduced from one technologist to another (or even with the same technologist examining smears on repeated occasions) and that such estimations should not be reported. On the other hand, a more optimistic report[62] suggests that sputum Gram stains on quality specimens, in a select population of adults with community-acquired pneumonia, may provide clinicians with enough information to initiate empiric antibiotic therapy. In either event, considerable experience and correlation of laboratory results with clinical indicators would be necessary before Gram stain interpretations of sputum samples would be of value. These grading systems for sputum samples do not apply in lower respiratory infections caused by mycobacteria, fungi, and viruses, for which purulent cell responses are not typically elicited.

The semiquantitation of stainable tubercle bacilli in sequential examinations of acid-fast smears of sputum may be of value in determining the efficacy of antituberculous drug therapy. A decrease from 4+ to 1+, to rare, or even to an absence of bacilli over a 4- to 6-week course of therapy indicates good drug response and may be used to determine when it may be safe to discharge a patient to home care.

The importance of the microorganisms recovered from respiratory samples must always be evaluated in light of clinical information. Interpretation of sputum cultures is particularly difficult because they are neither specific nor sensitive to evaluations of lower respiratory infections. Lentino and Lucks[130] have succinctly stated the problem based on their experience in a study of 249 patients with suspected pneumonia (Box 3-1).

This experience is not a unique observation limited to their laboratory and should discourage the use of sputum cultures to diagnose bacterial pneumonia. However, the practice will continue because sputum is easy to collect, requires no sophisticated equipment, and is low-cost compared with other invasive pulmonary procedures. In about 10% to 15% of cases, valuable clinical and prognostic information may be obtained.[62]

Because so many species of bacteria can be found as normal flora or commensals in the respiratory tract, establishing the bacterial etiology of acute and chronic bronchitis can also be difficult (Table 3-2). The recovery of *Streptococcus pneumoniae*, *Klebsiella pneumoniae*, *Haemophilus influenzae*, and *Moraxella* (*Branhamella*) *catarrhalis* as the predominant microorganism from respiratory secretions, particularly when these organisms are also recovered from concomitant blood cultures, supports their role in the development of acute pneumonia.[40,267] Induced sputum samples, collected after inhalation of nebulized saline, may be required to increase the yield of detection of certain organisms, particularly *Pneumocystis carinii* (see Chap. 20).

If pulmonary infections caused by mycobacteria, fungi, human parasites, or viruses are suspected, special techniques must be used to recover the etiologic agents, as outlined in the chapters devoted to each of these groups of microorganisms. Although the recovery of certain fungi, such as the dimorphic pathogens, usually indicates disease, other fungi, such as *Aspergillus* species, must be recovered repeatedly from successive samples before the diagnosis can be confirmed. The production of scanty sputum devoid of bacteria and often of segmented neutrophils in a patient with clinical signs of bronchitis or pneumonia may point to a viral etiology. Viral cultures are not as commonly obtained, either because the course of the disease is already too far along at the time patients initially present for examination or because of the prolonged length of time required to establish a diagnosis. The latter problem has been corrected to some degree by the application of new techniques such as immunofluorescence staining, enzyme-linked immunoassays (EIA), and nucleic acid probes with which viral particles or antigen determinants can be detected. For example, respiratory syncytial virus can be detected by directly examining respiratory secretions using these techniques, or as for influenza virus, rapid diagnosis may be accomplished by demonstrating positive FA or EIA tests performed on 24- or 48-hour cell cultures. Various kit systems are currently commercially available for use in diagnostic laboratories. Similarly, nucleic acid probes are commercially available for culture confirmation of several *Mycobacterium* species. (These techniques are discussed in detail in Chap. 17.)

INFECTIONS OF THE GASTROINTESTINAL TRACT

LOWER INTESTINAL INFECTIONS

CLINICAL SYMPTOMS

The most common presenting symptom pointing to an infection of the lower intestinal tract is diarrhea. Although diarrhea, which is largely host-specific, may be difficult to define in absolute terms, patients usually know when they have bowel movements in excess of normal and when the stool takes on a form that is softer or more liquid than usual. The diarrhea may be accompanied by cramping abdominal pain of varying degrees of severity. Dysentery is a term used to describe the condition in which diarrhea is accompanied by cramping abdominal pain and tenesmus (a term referring to painful straining when passing the stool). Dysentery results from "enteroinvasive" microorganisms that penetrate through the mucosa and cause inflammation of the intestinal wall. At the opposite end of the spectrum are the nonpainful, profusely watery diarrheal syndromes caused by *Vibrio cholerae* and other noninvasive "enterotoxigenic" bacteria that produce vibrio-like toxins (see Chap. 6 for full discussion of the action of these toxins).

COLLECTION OF FECAL SPECIMENS

The collection of diarrheal stools is not difficult. In cases of diarrhea, stool specimens should be collected in clean (not necessarily sterile), wide-mouthed containers that can be covered with a tight-fitting lid. These containers are also suitable for the collection of stool specimens for the direct detection of various enteric viruses (Norwalk, rotoviruses, adenoviruses, and such). These containers should be free of preservatives, detergents, or metal ions. Contamination with urine should also be avoided. If an intestinal parasite such as *Entamoeba histolytica*, *Giardia lamblia*, or *Cryptosporidium* species is suspected, a small portion of stool sample should be placed in preservatives, such as polyvinyl alcohol and 10% formalin. Stool specimens for detection of viruses should not be added to viral transport medium because the viral particles may be diluted out beyond the sensitivity of detection of the system being used.

TABLE 3-2
COMMENSAL FLORA AND PATHOGENIC BACTERIA IN THE RESPIRATORY TRACT

COMMENSAL FLORA	POTENTIAL PATHOGENS	RECOMMENDED ISOLATION MEDIA

α-Streptococci
 	
    S. mutans
    S. salivarius
    S. pneumoniae
	Group A, β-hemolytic streptococci
	
	Streptococcus pneumoniae
	Klebsiella pneumoniae and other Enterobacteriaceae
		5% sheep blood agar, with or without trimethoprim–sulfamethoxazole
		
		5% sheep blood agar and MacConkey (or eosin methylene blue) agar

β-Streptococci other than group A	Pseudomonas aeruginosa	5% sheep blood agar

Staphylococci:
    S. aureus
    S. epidermidis
	Neisseria gonorrhoeae and N. meningitidis	Modified Thayer-Martin (MTM)

Haemophilus spp.	S. aureus	Horse blood with colistin and nalidixic acid (CNA)
Neisseria spp.	Haemophilus influenzae type b and nontypeable H. influenzae	Chocolate agar
Corynebacterium spp. ("diphtheroids")	Corynebacterium diphtheriae	Loeffler's or Pai slant and serum–tellurite agar
Escherichia coli and other Enterobacteriaceae	Moraxella catarrhalis Capnocytophaga spp.	5% sheep blood or chocolate agar
Anaerobes	Bordetella pertussis Mycobacterium spp. Legionella pneumophilia and other legionellae	Bordet-Gengou potato agar or Regan and Lowe medium Löwenstein-Jensen (LJ) egg medium and/or Middlebrook 7H11 agar Charcoal yeast extract (CYE) agar

In some instances, the collection of a rectal swab rather than feces may be necessary, particularly in newborns or in severely debilitated adults. Because certain strains of *Shigella* species are susceptible to cooling and drying, rectal swabs may be more effective in recovering these organisms. Rectal swabs may be more effective than stool specimens[140] in recovering *Clostridium difficile* in hospitalized patients, presumably because delays in transport or specimen processing are circumvented. To perform the procedure, the rectal swab should be inserted just beyond the anal sphincter, avoiding direct contact with fecal material in the rectum. These swabs should immediately be inoculated onto culture media or placed in a suitable transport system to prevent drying. The VACUTAINER anaerobic specimen collector was also superior to Amies Transport Medium in the recovery of *C. difficile* from rectal swabs.[140] Rectal swabs are also necessary for diagnosis of rectal gonococcal infection.

UPPER INTESTINAL INFECTIONS

CLINICAL SYMPTOMS

Upper gastrointestinal symptoms of infection include anorexia, a feeling of nausea, occasionally overt vomiting, and upper abdominal pain. The pain may be generalized if the stomach and upper duodenum are diffusely inflamed (as may occur in cases of viral gastritis), localized to specific areas in the upper abdomen, or referred to regions of the back if the stomach wall is affected. Because of the very low pH of the gastric acid, 99.9% of ingested bacteria are killed within 30 minutes of exposure; therefore, gastritis from direct invasion of the stomach wall is rare. Two corollaries follow: 1) antacid therapy, which neutralizes the low gastric pH and 2) gastrectomy, in which most of the acid-forming mucosa is removed, predispose individuals to enteric infections from a variety of bacterial species. Guerrant[67] reports that the dose of *V. cholerae* required to cause infection in normal people (10^8 organisms per milliliter) was reduced to only 10^4/mL in volunteers who were given bicarbonate to neutralize gastric acidity.

Candida albicans (and less commonly other fungi such as *Aspergillus* species and *Zygomyces* species), which grow optimally in an acidic environment, may directly invade and produce localized inflammation of the gastroesophageal junction, particularly in debilitated or immunosuppressed patients. Difficulty in swallowing and pain radiating to the back may be experienced. The bacterium *Helicobacter pylori* (formerly *Campylobacter pylori*) has been associated with gastritis and peptic ulcer disease.[129,138,236] The organism has the unique biochemical property of rapidly and avidly hydrolyzing urea and releasing ammonium ions. The bacterial cells can presumably surround themselves with an alkaline cloud, thereby making it possible to survive the highly acid environment of the gastric mucosa.

The acute and often fulminant gastritis accompanied by generalized weakness and vomiting, experienced after ingesting food heavily contaminated with organisms such as *Staphylococcus aureus*, *Salmonella* species, *Clostridium perfringens*, and *Bacillus cereus*, does not result from direct bacterial invasion of the stomach wall; rather, it results from the direct emetic action of preformed neurotoxins on the central autonomic nervous system. The more protracted and vague symptoms of upper abdominal bloating, belching, or increased flatulence may be caused by infections of the duodenum and upper ileum by parasitic organisms such as *Giardia lamblia* and *Strongyloides stercoralis*.

OBTAINING SPECIMENS FROM THE UPPER GASTROINTESTINAL TRACT

Gastric specimens for culture are only rarely obtained and are limited to those few situations for which a diagnosis may not be possible by other means. For example, the diagnosis of pulmonary tuberculosis (particularly in infants and young children) may be made on gastric washings when repeated sputum samples have been negative. The bacterial agents of acute toxic food poisoning may be recovered from vomitus material.

Gastric biopsies are being performed with increasing frequency to detect *Helicobacter* (*Campylobacter*) *pylori*.[236] Biopsy specimens may be cultured for the recovery of *H. pylori*, a procedure rarely performed in clinical laboratories, in lieu of better techniques, examined histologically in stained sections for the presence of the characteristic slender, spiral-shaped organisms or tested for the presence of in vitro urease activity. In the latter test, biopsy material can be inoculated into Christensen's urea agar and observed for the characteristic pink-red color change. A commercial product, the CLOtest (Tri-med Specialties, Overland Park KS), has been successfully used, particularly in outpatient clinic settings. The urease produced by organisms contained within the biopsy material acts on the urea in the substrate producing NH_4^+ and a red color change. Polymerase chain reaction (PCR) has also been used successfully to directly detect *H. pylori* in gastric biopsy specimens. Lage and coworkers[125] report that PCR assays in which the *ureC* gene was amplified were at least as sensitive as culture for detecting *H. pylori*; detection of the *cagA* gene (cytotoxin-associated antigen) was particularly useful in the study of gastric biopsies.

The detection of *H. pylori*–specific serum immunoglobulin G (IgG) antibodies has been strongly associated with gastrointestinal infections with this organism in a number of recently reported studies.[78,118] Several commercial kit assays currently on the market have been evaluated[200] for the detection of *H. pylori*–

specific serum immunoglobulins, finding sensitivities ranging between 56% and 92%, indicating that each laboratory director must conduct in-house studies to determine which of the systems is most applicable. A 94% sensitivity and 99% specificity were found[179] between serum *H. pylori* antibody titers and endoscopic results in a study of 256 patients with active gastritis. However, serologic results must always be directly correlated with clinical findings, for *H. pylori* IgG antibodies may be found in patients without disease, indicating prior infection. The incidence of *H. pylori* antibody conversion also increases with age in the population as exposure increases.[94]

Aspirations of duodenal contents may be helpful in making the diagnosis of giardiasis and strongyloidiasis for which repeated stool examinations have failed to uncover the causative organisms. The use of the commercial "string test" (Enterotest, HEDECO, Palo Alto CA) is an alternative to passing a gastric tube. The Enterotest is a capsule containing a tightly wound string. Before the capsule is swallowed, the string is unravelled for a short distance and the end taped to the cheek. In about 30 to 60 minutes, when the capsule has reached the upper duodenum, the string is carefully removed and any mucus adhering to the strand is milked onto the surface of a glass slide for direct microscopic examination.

PROCESSING AND DIRECT MICROSCOPIC EXAMINATION OF FECAL SPECIMENS

Stool specimens should be examined and cultured as soon as possible after collection. Warm stools are examined from patients with suspected amebiasis to offer the best chance of detecting motile trophozoites. As the stool specimen cools, the drop in pH soon becomes sufficient to inhibit the growth of many *Shigella* and some *Salmonella* species.

Direct microscopic examination of a fecal emulsion or stained smear to evaluate the presence of fecal leukocytes, yeasts, or parasitic forms may be valuable as part of the workup of certain enteric infections. Flecks of blood or mucin should be selected if present. An emulsion of feces can be prepared in culture broth, physiologic saline, or water; 1 or 2 drops placed on the surface of a glass slide under a cover slip; and the mount directly examined microscopically. Microscopic examination of fecal smears for the detection of leukocytes may be unreliable for specimens that have been transported, refrigerated, frozen, or collected by swab.[145] An antilactoferrin latex bead agglutination test (LFLA) was more sensitive for the detection of fecal leukocytes in these compromised specimens. Also, the stool specimens obtained from patients with *Vibrio cholerae* consistently gave LFLA titers lower than 1:50, in contrast to patients with inflammatory bowel diarrhea caused by *Shigella* species and *C. difficile*, who had high titers.[145]

If a delay in processing is anticipated or if the specimen is to be sent to a distant reference laboratory, an appropriate preservative should be used. Equal quantities of a 0.033-M sodium or potassium phosphate buffer and glycerol can be used to recover pathogenic bacteria; polyvinyl alcohol (PVA) fixative is recommended for the preservation of ova and parasites. Stool specimens are not suitable for the detection of ova and parasites for 10 days following a barium enema; however, recovery of enteric bacterial pathogens is usually not compromised. The practice of adding a small amount of fecal specimen to GN or selenite enrichment broth for the recovery of *Shigella* and *Salmonella* species has been discontinued in many laboratories.

The direct detection of rotavirus antigen in stools may be useful because this agent is difficult to recover in culture. Several enzyme-linked immunosorbent assays are now available including Rotazyme (Abbott Laboratories, North Chicago, IL), IDL Rotavirus EIA (International Diagnostic Laboratories, Chesterfield MO), Rotaclone (Cambridge Bioscience, Hopkinton MA), and also latex procedures—Rotalex (Orion Diagnostica, Espoo, Finland) and Rotatest (Wampole laboratories, Cranbury NJ). The latex agglutination procedure is most applicable for the majority of clinical microbiology laboratories. Reagents that use monoclonal antibodies have been reported by Herman and associates[77] to have a higher correlation than those using polyclonal antibodies, reaching a sensitivity of 100% and a specificity of 97% in these investigators hands. They found an unacceptably high rate of false-positive reactions in neonates, an observation also supported by the work of others.[119,266] Viruses, other than rotavirus—such as Norwalk virus, adenovirus, calicivirus, astrovirus, and coronavirus—in stool specimens, most of which cannot be propagated using cell culture techniques, may be detected using EIA techniques; or, if commercial EIA or LA kits are not available, may require techniques of electron microscopy (EM) or immunoelectron microscopy (IEM). These approaches are discussed in Chapter 1.

Enzyme-linked immunosorbent assays (ELISA) are also available for the detection of *Giardia lamblia* antigen in feces. Nash and coworkers[157] report detection of giardia antigen in 92% of persons with microscopically verified giardiasis; three of 125 individuals without microscopically detectable *G. lamblia* were also antigen-positive. In a study of diaper specimens from 426 children attending 20 day care centers, 99 samples were microscopically positive for *G. lamblia*.[1] Of these, 93 (94%) were also ELISA-positive, using the commercially available ProSpecT/Giardia kit (Alexon, Inc., Mountain View CA), which detects *G. lamblia*–specific GSA-65 antigen. Of 534 tests negative for *G. lamblia*, 32 (6%) were ELISA-positive; however, on repeat examination, one or more additional stool specimens were microscopically positive. These authors found that any optical density reading higher than 0.040 was 98.0% sensitive and 100% specific for *G. lamblia*. Enzyme-linked procedures, although highly sensitive (with a range of 95% to 98%), require special equipment and are cost-effective only if a high volume of samples is assayed.[150]

Alles and coworkers,[5] in a study of 2696 consecutive fresh stool specimens collected over a 1-year period, found that a combination of direct immuno-fluorescent–monoclonal antibody assay for detection of both *G. lamblia* and *Cryptosporidium parvum* in stool specimens increased the detection rate by 49.4% and 69.6%, respectively, compared with conventional-staining techniques. The Merifluor monoclonal antibody reagent (Meridian Diagnostics, Inc., Cincinnati OH) was highly sensitive for the detection of *G. lamblia* cysts and *Cryptosporidium* oocysts in known positive stool specimens.[57] The *G. lamblia* cysts appeared as 11- to 15-μm diameter oval bodies, the *Cryptosporidium* oocysts as 4- to 6-μm diameter spherules, both appearing apple green and easily distinguishable. Eight specimens previously interpreted as negative by routine microscopic ova and parasite examinations (four *G. lamblia* and four *Cryptosporidium* spp.) were positive by the direct fluorescence method; these positive results were later confirmed after repeat examination of additional trichrome and modified acid-fast smears. Grigoriew and associates[66] also found that the Merifluor reagent detected *G. lamblia* cysts or *Cryptosporidium* oocysts either alone or in combination in 100 positive formalin–ether concentrated specimens; the direct fluorescent method detected one additional false-negative specimen for each parasite. These authors found the method to be rapid, accurate and simple to perform.

Mahbubani and coworkers[134] detected *G. lamblia* cysts by DNA amplification by PCR, using giardin gene as the target. Not only were they able to detect the giardin gene in the presence of low concentrations of organisms, but they were able to differentiate live from dead cysts. They found the amount of giardin mRNA and total RNA was significantly increased in live cysts following the induction of encystation. The application of these research techniques to the clinical laboratory will require extensive field studies using fresh patient specimens before the clinical relevance can be established. Perhaps of more immediate utility, Chaudhuri and colleagues[32] found that the detection of circulating IgM antibodies correlated with 96% sensitivity and specificity in an evaluation of a large number of sera collected from patients with known giardiasis and negative controls.

SELECTION OF CULTURE MEDIA FOR ENTERIC BACTERIAL PATHOGENS

The normal flora in the bowel, the recognized pathogens, and suggested culture media are shown in Table 3-3. The classic diarrheal agents *Salmonella* species and *Shigella* species are no less important today than previously, even though other recently described enteric pathogens have gained the limelight. Laboratory directors and microbiology supervisors must choose from a variety of culture media containing inhibitors to the growth of normal bowel flora to allow *Salmonella* and *Shigella* spp. to be selected out. Box 3-2 lists commonly used selective culture media for the recovery of enteric pathogens.

The use of a highly selective medium, such as Wilson-Blair bismuth sulfite agar, is limited to epidemics when it may be important to specifically recover *Sal-*

TABLE 3-3
COMMENSAL FLORA AND PATHOGENIC BACTERIA IN THE GASTROINTESTINAL TRACT

COMMENSAL FLORA	POTENTIAL PATHOGENS	RECOMMENDED ISOLATION MEDIA
None	**Upper tract**	
	Helicobacter pylori (stomach and duodenum)	Skirrow *Campylobacter* medium, chocolate agar, or Marshall brain–heart infusion medium with horse blood (fresh medium and high humidity during incubation required)
	Lower tract	
Escherichia coli and other nonpathogenic "enterics"	*Salmonella* spp. *Shigella* species	MacConkey (or EMB) agar Hektoen enteric (or XLD) agar SS agar (optional)
Pseudomonas spp. and most other nonfermenters	*E. coli* (enteropathogenic, enterotoxigenic)	GN or selenite enrichment broths (no longer recommended as a routine)
Coagulase-negative staphylococci	*Staphylococcus aureus*	Phenylethyl alcohol (PEA) or CNA blood agar
Enterococcus spp.	*Campylobacter* spp. *Vibrio cholerae* and halophilic *Vibrio* spp. *Yersinia enterocolitica*	Selective "campy" blood agar Thiosulfate citrate bile sucrose (TCBS) agar CIN (cefsulodin–irgasan–novobiocin) agar
Most anaerobes	*Clostridium difficile*	Cycloserine–cefoxitin–egg yolk–fructose agar (must do cytotoxin assay on stool specimens)

monella typhi from stool specimens. The formulations and interpretation of the various reactions of these media are described in detail in Chapter 4. Note that certain media are duplications and only one of the pair need be selected. The combination of MacConkey and HE agars and GN enrichment broth compose a commonly selected battery. Both GN and selenite enrichment broths must be subcultured to selective media within the first 4 to 8 hours of incubation because normal bowel flora will begin to break through after that time. Additionally, a selective culture medium (phenylethyl alcohol [PEA] or colistin–naladixic acid [CNA]) agars may be used to recover staphylococci or yeasts from stool specimens of newborns or individuals receiving prolonged antibiotic therapy. *Campylobacter jejuni*, a recognized cause of acute diarrheal syn-

drome,[18] is now recovered with greater frequency in many laboratories than either *Salmonella* or *Shigella* species or both. Thus, campylobacter-selective culture media should be used.[81] Because certain strains of *Campylobacter* species may be inhibited by the antibiotics contained within the campy-selective media, Steele and McDermott[230] have devised a filter paper technique by which the growth of *Campylobacter* species can be selected out of mixed culture by using a filter paper membrane placed on conventional antibiotic-free blood agar plates. The recovery of *Campylobacter* species, the specific formulations of selective culture media, a description of the filter paper technique, and conditions of incubation will be discussed in detail in Chapter 6.

Other bacterial species also are known to cause diarrheal syndromes; however, in most locales their prevalence is sufficiently low to preclude the routine use of selective media. *Vibrio* species (particularly *V. parahemolyticus*) cause diarrheal diseases in certain parts of the world. In the United States, vibrio enteritis has both geographic (southeastern Gulf Coast regions) and occupational (fish and animal handlers) predispositions; laboratories serving communities where these syndromes are prevalent may decide to routinely screen diarrheal stool specimens. The routine use of special culture media to recover *Vibrio* species from stool specimens is not recommended in geographic regions of low prevalence. A simple but effective screen for *Vibrio* species may be accomplished by adding oxidase reagent to an uninoculated blood agar plate and sampling positive colonies for confirmatory testing.

The decision of whether to routinely set up special media for *Yersinia enterocolitica* is somewhat more com-

---

BOX 3-2. CULTURE MEDIA FOR THE RECOVERY OF ENTERIC PATHOGENS

MacConkey agar or EMB agar (select one)

Xylose–lysine–deoxycholate (XLD) agar or Hektoen Enteric (HE) agar (select one)

GN enrichment plated to MacConkey and XLD or HE agar within 4 to 8 hours; or selenite enrichment to MacConkey and XLD or HE agar 8 to 12 hours after inoculation (a practice discontinued in many laboratories because the yield over solid media is low)

Campy-BAP (or equivalent) for recovery of *Campylobacter* species

plex. Kachoris and coworkers[98] conclude from their experience in the Boston area (only seven isolates of *Y. enterocolitica* from 3622 [0.2%] stool examinations) that it is not cost-effective to routinely culture all stool specimens for *Y. enterocolitica*. Their experience is probably mirrored in most other locales, and selective media (cefsulodin–Irgasan–novobiocin [CIN]) are used only in instances for which the routine battery of media has failed to disclose a pathogen in patients with protracted diarrhea. On the other hand, Barteluk and Noble[11] argue that in certain regions of the world, the prevalence of yersiniosis is sufficiently high to warrant laboratories to routinely use selective media. In their practice setting in Vancouver, British Columbia, 7% of stool samples and 10% of symptomatic patients yield *Y. enterocolitica* on CIN agar. They recommend that each laboratory director decide whether to routinely screen for *Yersinia* species based on local needs.

Aeromonas species and *Plesiomonas* species have also been incriminated in certain cases of diarrheal disease.[82] Enteric organisms, such as enterotoxigenic strains of *Escherichia coli*, *Arizona* species (now included in the genus *Salmonella*), and *Edwardsiella tarda*, are also putative etiologic agents in diarrheal syndromes. These organisms can be recovered without difficulty on enteric isolation media and require no special provisions other than being alert to the possibility of their recovery. Sorbitol MacConkey agar has been used in many laboratories for the recovery and presumptive identification of enterohemorrhagic strains of *E. coli* 0157:H7 (sorbitol-negative and, therefore, appearing as nonpigmented colonies). Park and associates[168] were able to detect *E. coli* O157 isolates by direct immunofluorescence antibody staining of fecal smears prepared from bleach-treated stools, detecting all culture-positive isolates from 336 abnormal fecal samples with no false-negative results. Nonmotile strains, strains possessing the H7 flagellar antigen, and one strain with a flagellar antigen other than H7 were detected without difficulty. Orenstein and Kotler[164] found both light and electron microscopic abnormalities (disarray, degeneration, and necrosis of surface epithelium) in biopsies of 52 patients with acquired immunodeficiency syndrome (AIDS), with coliform bacilli, primarily *E. coli*, linked to the histopathologic changes. They suggest that further precise characterization of *E. coli* strains causing these abnormalities be defined so that diarrheogenic bacterial infections can be diagnosed in patients with AIDS using stool specimens rather than endoscopic biopsies.

Other diarrhea-producing organisms of concern include *Clostridium perfringens*, *C. septicum*, and *C. difficile*. These organisms are discussed in detail in Chapter 14. *C. perfringens* is a common cause of food-borne disease, and *C. septicum* has recently been associated with neutropenic hemorrhagic enterocolitis. *C. difficile* can be recovered on cycloserine cefoxitin egg yolk fructose agar (CCFA); however, the advent of monoclonal antibody tests to detect the disease-producing toxin promises to replace culture and isolation procedures in the near future.

EPIDEMIOLOGIC CONSIDERATIONS IN EVALUATING PATIENTS WITH DIARRHEAL SYNDROMES

A detailed medical history from all subjects involved in outbreaks of enteritis is important for both diagnostic and epidemiologic studies. It is important to know if the immediate family members or those in close contact with the patient have also recently experienced acute diarrhea. Most cases of infectious diarrhea occur in clusters within families, groups sharing a common meal, or travelers. Information should always be elicited concerning travel to countries outside of the United States where certain diarrheal diseases may be endemic. Many cases of "traveler's diarrhea," "Montezuma's revenge," "Delhi belly," and other such descriptive designations are caused by enterotoxigenic strains of *E. coli*. Poor-quality water and food supplies, marginal cold-storage facilities, and contamination from people preparing foods in countries outside the United States put travelers more at risk. Travel to the East and Gulf Coast regions in the United States can expose one to infections with halophilic vibrios from ingestion of vibrio-contaminated shellfish. Drinking water taken directly from remote streams or headwaters places backpackers at risk for infections with *G. lamblia*. There is evidence that beavers, dogs, and other animals may be infected with *Giardia* species pathogenic for humans, explaining the cause of waterborne outbreaks.[1]

The recovery of mycobacteria from stool specimens may be accomplished in patients with AIDS. Kiehn and Cammarata[111] have suggested that acid-fast smears should first be made directly from unprocessed fecal material and not processed further if organisms are not seen. If acid-fast bacteria are detected, a suspension of 1 g of fecal material in 5 mL of Middlebrook 7H9 broth should be prepared, and the suspension processed by the NaOH decontamination procedure used for sputum specimens. Acid-fast stains of smears prepared from diarrheal stool specimens from patients with AIDS are also being effectively used in the detection of *Cryptosporidium* species and *Isospora belli* (for details, see Chap. 20).

URINARY TRACT INFECTIONS

The urinary tract is divided into two major divisions, upper (the kidneys, renal pelves, and ureters) and lower (urinary bladder and urethra). Upper urinary tract infections are most commonly ascending; that is, they originate in the urinary bladder and ascend through the ureters to the kidneys. Normally the vesicourethral valve prevents reflux of urine from the urinary bladder into the ureters. Individuals with urogenital anomalies, overdistention of the urinary bladder from outflow obstruction, or neurogenic malfunctions, or women with overdistention of the uterus during pregnancy are particularly susceptible to ascending urinary tract infections. Infections of the renal pelvis (pyelitis) and chronic pyelonephritis are the most common complications.

Upper urinary tract infections may result from hematogenous spread of bacteria into the glomeruli and renal cortex in patients with septicemia. Microfocal abscesses or acute suppurative pyelonephritis are common manifestations. Upper urinary tract infections resulting from hematogenous spread of bacteria are less common than those caused by ascending spread of bacteria.

CLINICAL SIGNS AND SYMPTOMS

The cardinal clinical manifestations of upper urinary tract infections are fever (often with chills) and flank pain. Frequency, urgency, and dysuria are more suggestive of infections of the urinary bladder and urethra. However, some patients with pyelonephritis or other upper urinary tract infections first develop symptoms consistent with lower tract infections. This lack of clear clinical differentiation between the two levels of infection underlies past attempts to develop a laboratory approach to the differential diagnosis.

Most lower urinary tract infections involve the urinary bladder, with potential spread to the prostate gland in males and to the urethra (acute urethral syndrome) in females. Frequent and painful urination of small amounts of turbid urine and suprapubic heaviness or pain are the usual clinical manifestations. Elderly persons may harbor asymptomatic urinary tract infections that are recognized only because the urine may appear cloudy or because segmented neutrophils and an increased concentration of bacteria are observed microscopically.

Bacteriuria and pyuria, either with or without overt symptoms, most commonly serve as the initial clues that a patient may be harboring a urinary tract infection. A urine culture is usually necessary to establish the etiology of disease because inflammatory conditions other than infections can also cause similar symptoms or pyuria.

HOST FACTORS

The prevalence of urinary tract infections varies with the gender and age of the patient. In neonates and infants, urinary tract infections are more common in boys, with an overall prevalence of about 1%. Most of these infections are associated with congenital anomalies. By the time children attend school, there is a higher prevalence in girls (1.2%) compared with boys (0.03%). This ratio remains consistent into adulthood. High rates of incidence occur in certain conditions, such as diabetes or pregnancy. In the elderly, higher rates of occurrence can be expected for both women (20%) and men (10%) in which predisposing conditions exist, such as obstructive uropathy from the prostate in men, poor emptying of the bladder from uterine prolapse in women, and the more frequent procedures requiring instrumentation in both men and women.

Compromised urine flow, whether mechanical or functional, is the most common underlying condition that predisposes patients to urinary tract infections. Mechanical obstruction can be caused by renal calculi, vesicourethral reflux, bladder neck obstruction, urethral strictures, and prostatic hypertrophy. Catheterization and other mechanical manipulations of the urinary tract put patients at high risk. The expansion of the uterus during pregnancy causes reduced urinary bladder capacity and external pressure on the ureters. External pressure on the ureters with compromised urine outflow can also result from large pelvic neoplasms, some of which actually invade the musculature or the lumen for the ureter and cause obstruction. Diabetic neuropathy, tabes dorsalis, and poliomyelitis are less common functional causes of compromised urine outflow. Spinal cord injuries account for neurogenic malfunctions of the lower urinary tract.

Organisms are rapidly removed by the flushing action of the urine flow. The intact mucosa is an effective barrier to bacterial invasion. The extremes of osmolality, high urea content, and low pH of the urine inhibit the growth of many species of bacteria. However, when mucosal rents or ulcers (caused by the insertion of instruments or catheters) are present, the pH and osmolality of the urine are altered (as in pregnancy), or if a high concentration of glucose is present in patients with diabetes mellitus, a greater chance exists that bacteria introduced into the bladder will multiply and cause infection. Foreign bodies, including renal calculi and indwelling catheters, serve as a nidus for bacterial growth and are a source for chronic and recurrent urinary tract infections.

COLLECTION OF URINE SAMPLES FOR CULTURE

Except for the urethral mucosa, which supports the growth of a microflora, the normal urinary tract is usually devoid of bacteria.[100] Because male and female urethras and the female periurethral area harbor microorganisms, urine can easily become contaminated with bacteria from the vaginal canal or perineum. Table 3-4 lists microorganisms that are considered contaminants and pathogens along with suggested isolation media.

MIDSTREAM COLLECTION TECHNIQUE

Urine samples are most commonly collected by obtaining the midstream flow by the clean-catch technique. Urine collection from women by the clean-catch technique requires personal supervision for best results.[123] The periurethral area and perineum are first cleansed with two or three gauze pads saturated with soapy water, using a forward to back motion, followed by a rinse with sterile saline or water. Bradbury[21] offers evidence that failure to clean the periurethral area and perineum in females may not adversely affect the quality of midstream urine samples for culture. Despite this counsel, we still recommend that the cleaning procedure of Kunin described in the following be carried out when collecting urine specimens for culture from females for most accurate results.

TABLE 3-4
COMMENSAL FLORA AND PATHOGENIC BACTERIA IN THE URINARY TRACT

COMMENSAL FLORA (CONTAMINANTS)	POTENTIAL PATHOGENS	RECOMMENDED ISOLATION MEDIA
Staphylococci coagulase-negative	*Escherichia coli*	5% sheep blood agar
Diphtheroid bacilli	*Klebsiella–Enterobacter–Serratia* spp.	MacConkey or eosin methylene blue agar
Escherichia coli and other "coliforms"	*Proteus mirabilis* and other *Proteus* spp.	Use of selective enterococcal medium (strep fecalis or "SF") is no longer recommended
Lactobacillus spp.	*Enterococcus* spp.	5% sheep blood agar
α-Hemolytic streptococci	*Staphylococcus aureus* and *S. saprophyticus* *Corynebacterium jeikeium* *Acinetobacter* spp.	5% sheep blood agar
Bacillus spp.	*Pseudomonas aeruginosa* and other pseudomonads *Neisseria gonorrhoeae*	Recovery of *Neisseria gonorrhoeae* may require chocolate or modified Thayer-Martin agar

The labia should be held apart during voiding, and the first few milliliters of urine passed into a bedpan or toilet bowl to flush out bacteria from the urethra (Figure 3-3). The midstream portion of urine is then collected in a sterile, wide-mouthed container that can be covered with a tightly fitted lid. The soapy water preparation is usually not required for men; rather, simple cleansing of the urethral meatus immediately before voiding and then collection of the midstream sample is usually sufficient.

Patients seen in a physician's office or in a clinic are frequently asked to obtain their own urine sample. This practice is acceptable if the patients are given precise instructions for properly collecting the specimen. It is recommended that these instructions be printed on a card that the patient can retain after receiving the verbal description. When the patients do not seem to comprehend or when language is a barrier, the nurse or office assistant should read through the instructions point by point or provide direct assistance in collecting the sample. An example of an instruction card, as outlined by Kunin,[113] is given in Box 3-3.

The accuracy of the urine collection procedure can be monitored over time by noting the frequency with which urine colony counts range between 10,000 and 100,000 CFU/mL. Most patients will have colony counts that fall outside of this range. Those free of infection will have no bacteria or fewer than 10^2 CFU/mL. Most with infection will have 100,000 CFU/mL or more. The frequency of intermediate counts should not exceed 5% to 10% if the urine collection procedures have been performed properly. Speci-

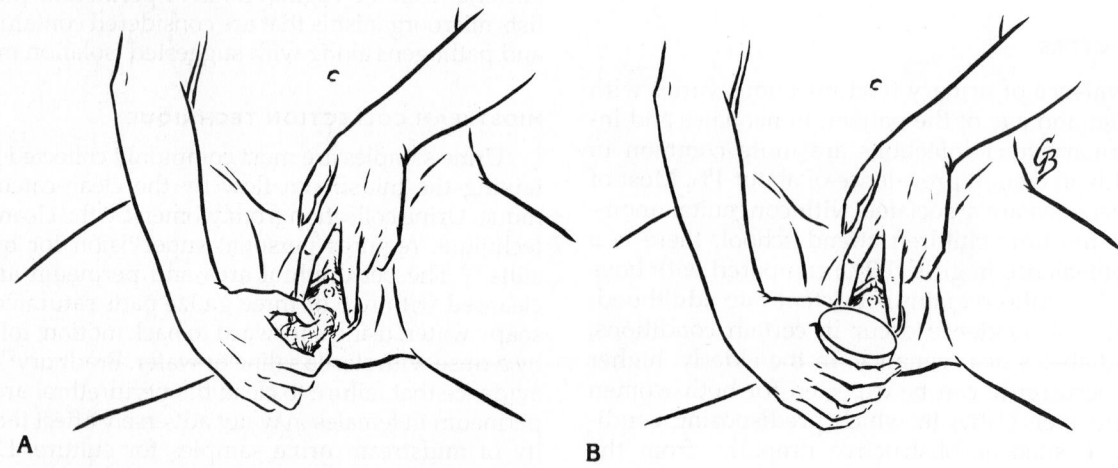

Figure 3-3.
Midstream clean-catch urine collection: (**A**) The labia are separated with the fingers and cleansed with a 4 × 4-inch gauze pad saturated with green soap. (**B**) The midstream portion of the urine is collected into a sterile container.

Box 3-3. Instructions for Obtaining Clean-Catch Urine Specimens (Females)

1. Remove underclothing completely and sit comfortably on the seat, swinging one knee to the side as far as you can.

2. Spread yourself with one hand, and continue to hold yourself spread while you clean yourself and collect the specimen.

3. Wash. Be sure to wash well and rinse well before you collect the urine sample. Using each of four separate 4″ × 4″ sterile sponges soaked in 10% green soap, wipe from the front of your body toward the back. Wash between the folds of the skin as carefully as you can.

4. Rinse. After you have washed with each soap pad, rinse with a moistened pad with the same front-to-back motion. Do not use any pad more than once.

5. Hold yourself apart and allow the first few drops of urine to pass into the toilet bowl. Hold the cup on the outside and pass the remaining urine into the cup.

6. Place the lid on the container or ask the nurse to do so for you.

mens should be processed within 2 hours after collection to achieve accurate colony counts.

The B-D Urine Collection Kit (Becton-Dickinson & Co., Cockeysville MD), designed to maintain the bacterial population in urine at room temperature for 24 hours, has been equally as effective as overnight refrigeration of specimens.[87] Although some decrease in colony count may be noted after prolonged storage, the system is recommended for transport of urine samples for which processing will be delayed up to 24 hours. Transport systems using boric acid may offer an alternative method for home or remote collection of urine samples. Jewkes and associates[93] conclude from a study of 84 children that urine collection in boric acid minimizes contamination, although growth of potential bacterial pathogens may also be inhibited in a small number of cases.

In a study of 1469 urine specimens obtained from children,[63] the Sage Products Urine Culture Tube (Sage Products Inc., Cary IL), which uses boric acid in a final concentration of 1.1%, was easy to use and was as effective as refrigeration in maintaining bacterial counts.

Collection of valid clean-catch urine specimens for culture from incontinent elderly men residing in nursing homes also poses a problem. Nicolle and colleagues[160] report success in diagnosing urinary tract infections in this population of patients by using an external collection device consisting of a sterile condom and leg bag. Before applying the condom, the glans penis was cleaned with soap and water and rinsed with sterile saline. The leg bag was examined every 10 to 15 minutes until a specimen was obtained.

Because contamination with low counts of bacteria occurred in almost 50% of the patients, rapid transport of the specimens to the laboratory and immediate transfer to culture media were required. Bacterial counts higher than 10^5 CFU/mL, particularly if obtained on two successive collections, had a high correlation with other indicators of urinary tract infection.

CATHETER COLLECTIONS

Catheterization for the expressed purpose of obtaining a urine specimen should be avoided if possible because of the high risk of introducing nosocomial infections. In fact, in a study of 105 women with suspected urinary tract infection,[248] the culture results obtained from midstream, clean-catch urine samples did not differ in sensitivity, specificity, or positive or negative predictive values from parallel in–out catheter specimens collected immediately after the midstream samples. Thus, catheterization should be restricted to those patients who are unable to produce a midstream sample, and it should be performed with meticulous attention to aseptic technique. The first several milliliters of urine from the catheter should be discarded to wash out any organisms that may have lodged in the catheter tip during transit through the urethra.

Urine samples can be obtained from an indwelling catheter using a number 28 needle and syringe. Be sure to disinfect the area where the needle puncture is to be made. Urine can be aspirated through the soft rubber connector between the catheter and the collecting tubing. Urine samples should not be obtained from catheter bags except from neonates or young infants when special precautions have been taken. Foley catheter tips are unsuitable for culture because they are invariably contaminated with urethral organisms.

SUPRAPUBIC ASPIRATION

Suprapubic aspirations are reserved almost exclusively for neonates, small children, and occasionally for adults with clinically suspected urinary tract infection in whom clean-catch samples have failed to establish a diagnosis. This technique is illustrated in Figure 3-4. The procedure is best performed when the bladder is full. The suprapubic skin overlying the urinary bladder is disinfected and sterile drapes or a towel used for spinal taps is put in place. In the immediate site where the tap is to be made, about 1 mL of anesthetic solution, such as 1% lidocaine HCl (Xylocaine), is injected subcutaneously. With the point of a sharply tapered surgical blade, make a small lance wound incision through the epidermidis. Through this wound, gently extend an 18-gauge, short-bevel spinal needle into the urinary bladder and aspirate 10 mL of urine into the syringe.

CULTURE OF URINE SPECIMENS

Both selective and nonselective media are required. A combination of 5% sheep blood agar and MacConkey agar is usually sufficient for the recovery of the organisms listed in Table 3-4, although some laboratories

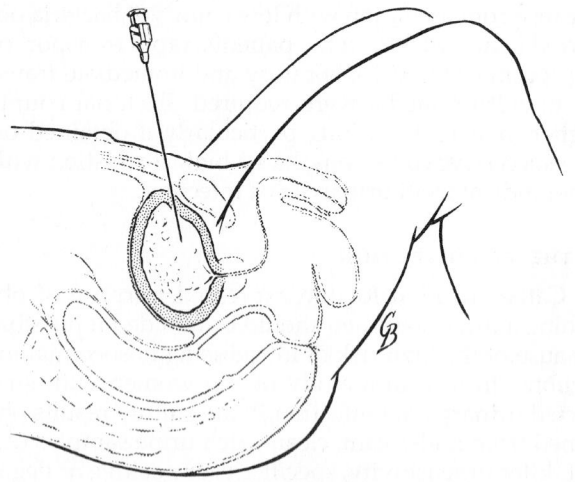

Figure 3-4.
Suprapubic urinary bladder aspiration. A needle is directed percutaneously into the urinary bladder just above the symphysis pubis. Urine can be removed with a syringe.

incorporate a medium selective for gram-positive bacteria as well (e.g., colistin–naladixic acid blood agar). In many laboratories, inoculation of duplicate plates with both the 0.01-mL and the 0.001-mL–calibrated loops is performed for comparison of counts as a quality control check. Only in rare instances, when a more fastidious organism such as *Neisseria gonorrhoeae* is suspected, is an enriched medium, such as chocolate agar, required to determine the cause of infection.

After delivering the inoculum from the calibrated loop, the surface of each agar plate should be completely streaked over all quadrants as demonstrated in Chapter 2 so that semiquantitative colony counts can be performed after incubation. A colony count of 10^5 CFU/mL or higher is the criterion used to determine if organism identification and susceptibility testing are to be performed. When the colony count is between 10^4 and 10^5 CFU/mL, or when two or more species are recovered, the decision to make identifications and perform susceptibility tests must be made on an individual, case by case basis. Cultures of catheterized or suprapubic urine specimens are usually analyzed in detail, even with low colony counts or with the recovery of multiple organism types. Colony counts as low as 10^2 CFU/mL of enteric gram-negative bacilli may be significant in female patients with the acute urethral syndrome;[226,227] however, the physician must alert the laboratory in suspected cases, because semiquantitative urine culture techniques are not designed to detect such low colony counts.

SCREENING TESTS

Because most urine specimens submitted to clinical laboratories for culture are negative or have bacterial colony counts below levels considered to be clinically significant, several nonculture-screening tests have been devised for the rapid detection of bacteriuria. The Gram stain is one inexpensive method for estimating

bacteriuria. In one study, the presence of (equal to or greater than) one organism per oil immersion field in uncentrifuged urine had a sensitivity of 94% and a specificity of 90% in reflecting colony counts of (greater than) 10^5 CFU/mL.[252] Yet the Gram stain is not used in most clinical laboratories as a urine-screening test because methodically reviewing the smears is too labor intensive.

COMMERCIAL SCREENING SYSTEMS

Several commercial screening test systems for the detection of bacteriuria or pyuria have been introduced, as reviewed by Needham.[158] One common approach is the use of a reagent-impregnated dipstick, designed to detect the presence of urine nitrite (Griess test) and to indirectly estimate the number of segmented neutrophils through the detection of leukocyte esterase activity (Ames Co., Elkhard IN; Biodynamics/Behringer-Manheim Co, Indianapolis IN).[175,197,258] The rationale for the nitrite test is that most urinary tract infections are caused by nitrate-reducing members of the family *Enterobacteriaceae* (particularly, *Escherichia coli*). This test lacks accuracy when used alone.[95,147] False-positive findings may result if the specimen has been delayed in transit and overgrown with nitrate-reducing bacteria or from drug interference; false-negative results are encountered if the organism causing the infection does not reduce nitrates (e.g., group D enterococci), the patient was on a vegetable-free diet (loss of an important source of nitrate), or the urine was collected too soon after previous voiding (within 4 to 6 hours), not providing sufficient time for nitrite concentrations to reach the lower chemical sensitivity of the test.

Leukocyte esterase (LE) is produced by segmented neutrophils. A reagent strip, impregnated with buffered indoxyl carboxylic acid ester and a diazonium salt, can be used to detect leukocyte esterase activity in the urine. One advantage of this test is that leukocytes need not be viable for LE activity to be detected. This test when performed alone correlated with ten or more white blood cells per high-power field (WBC/HPF) in the urine, with a sensitivity in the range of 88% and a specificity of 94%.[124] False-positive LE test findings may result from high urinary levels of ascorbic acid or albumin (300+ mg/dL) or from the effects of preservatives and detergents. Most false-negative results occur when urine WBC counts are in the marginal range of 5 to 10/HPF. Kierkegaard and associates[112] report that 35% of urine samples in their study turned from positive (30 WBC/HPF) to negative (10 WBC/HPF or fewer) when the urine was delayed in transit for 3 or more hours. Thus, the LE test may better reflect pyuria than does microscopic enumeration of neutrophils in settings where times of collection and delivery cannot be controlled.

The correlation of the combination nitrite–leukocyte esterase strip with bacteriuria at a breakpoint of 10^5 CFU/HPF is in the range of 79% to 93%, with a specificity of about 82% to 98%.[95,175,219,258] If a specificity as high as 98% can be reached using the combination strip, as found in the study by Smalley and Dittman,[219] urine specimens could be eliminated as negative without the need for culture. This high negative predictive value would be particularly useful in populations of patients anticipated to be free of urinary tract infections (those visiting postpartum clinics, for example). However, Murray and coworkers[155] found that the LN strip is too insensitive to recommend when attempting to detect urinary tract infections with bacterial concentrations less than 10^5 CFU/mL. In a multicenter study of 298 urine specimens with colony counts of fewer than 10^5 CFU/mL,[171] the LN strip detected 81% of cases. However, in a subset of 204 specimens with a combination of colony counts fewer than 10^5 CFU/mL and pyuria, the detection rate was increased to 95%.

The Bac-T-Screen (Marion Scientific, Div. Marion Laboratories, Inc., Kansas City MO), a bacterial detection device using vacuum suction in which the organisms in a diluted urine sample are trapped on a filter paper before staining, correctly detected 88.2% of urine samples containing concentrations of bacteria of 10^5 CFU/mL or higher.[174] The negative predictive value in this same study was 98.4%, comparing favorably with the predictive value of a negative urine Gram stain. One disadvantage of this system is the large number of samples (14% in their series) that could not be analyzed because of interfering chromogens in the urine or clogging of the filter.

One report[155] found that the Bac-T-Screen system (Vitek Systems Inc., Hazelwood MO) was the most sensitive screening test in detecting bacteriuria, predicting probable urinary tract infections with 98% accuracy. The authors cited the one major problem with the device of giving false-positive readings, most of which were for urine samples with numerous leukocytes or with colony counts of 10^4 CFU/mL or fewer. Pezzlo and coworkers[170] have previously pointed out the problem with false-positive results secondary to leukocytosis. On the other hand, detection of bacteriuria in symptomatic patients with fewer than 10^5 CFU/mL does not represent a false-positive result.

Colombrita and associates[35] report on the use of the BACTEC urine-screening system (Johnston Laboratories, Inc., Towson Md), which uses blood culture vials containing trypticase soy broth into which an aliquot of the urine sample to be tested is inoculated. The sensitivity of this system in their study of 852 urine samples was 97.6% at a breakpoint of 10^5 CFU/mL and 87% at a breakpoint of 10^4 CFU/mL. The specificity was 100%. In a multicenter study of 1500 urine samples with varying levels of bacteriuria and pyuria,[171] the Uriscreen system (Analytab Products, Plainview NY), a 2-minute catalase tube test to detect bacteriuria and pyuria, detected 93% of urine samples with bacteriuria with colony counts of 10^5 CFU/mL or higher, and 95% of specimens with CFUs of 10^2 or higher and pyuria. In a subset of 545 urines with probable pathogens and CFUs of 10^2 or higher, the rate of detection dropped to 85%. Most of the false-negative results were in urine samples without pyuria; false-positive results were caused by the detection of enzymes produced by somatic cells. The authors indicate that

Uriscreen is a rapid, manual, easy to perform enzymatic test with levels of performance similar to or greater (in specimens with pyuria) than the Chemstrip LN strip discussed earlier.

Urine-screening systems employing bioluminescence are also available. The Lumac System (3M Company, St. Paul MN) had a sensitivity of 92.4% and a specificity of 79.4% in a study of 986 urine samples, compared with culture.[42] The Monolight system had a sensitivity of 89.1% and a specificity of 81.8%. The authors conclude that either of these systems is sufficiently accurate to recommend for routine use, although costs are somewhat higher than for routine cultures. The UTIscreen (Los Alamos Diagnostics, Los Alamos NM), a system based on bioluminescence, was compared with the Bac-T-Screen (Vitek Systems Inc., Hazelwood MO), the Chemstrip LN strip (Boehringer Mannheim Diagnostics, BioDynamics, Indianapolis IN), and the Gram stain.[172,173] Of 276 urine samples with colony counts of 10^5 CFU/mL or more, the UTI screen detected 96%, the Bac-T-Screen 96%, the Chemstrip LN 90%, and the Gram stain 96%. At a breakpoint of 10^3 CFU/mL, the sensitivities were 91%, 95%, 89%, and 93%, and specificities were 79%, 55%, 57% and, 78%, respectively. Berger and associates[14] found that the catalase test may be helpful in screening for urinary tract infections, as their reagent correctly screened 83% of all urine samples and 97.6% of specimens containing significant numbers of leukocytes and bacteria. In contrast, other workers[70] determined that urine pH is of no value in detecting asymptomatic bacteriuria.

The use of the FlashTrack DNA Probe assay (Gen-Probe, San Diego CA) was reported in a study of 500 urine samples selected at random and screened for bacteriuria.[116] The target for the probe is not mentioned in the published paper. Of the 500 samples tested, 148 had colony counts of 10^5 CFU/mL or higher, 182 had 50,000 CFU/mL, and 234 had 10^4 CFU/mL or higher, as determined by semiquantitative culture. The sensitivity of the probe assay for these three urine categories was 96%, 97%, and 97%, respectively; the specificity was 78%, 67%, and 79%, respectively. The false-positive results were from urine samples that contained a significant number of bacteria after prolonged incubation or culture on chocolate agar, indicating that semiquantitative plate culture techniques, as routinely performed, may not be accurate in detecting fastidious bacteria. Although the FlashTrack assay was sensitive and performed better than the UTI-screen tests run in parallel, the major drawbacks, as cited by the authors, were the high cost and the complex protocol. Two centrifugation and three incubation steps were required in addition to the manual addition of reagents, requiring 2.5 hours before results were available. The performance was also less than acceptable for specimens with low bacterial counts.

Microbiologists are urged to carefully study the literature and to perform comparative studies in their own laboratories before deciding whether to implement one of the foregoing urine-screening methods.

This decision partly rests on the level of bacteriuria that must be detected.

INFECTIONS OF THE GENITAL TRACT

CLINICAL PRESENTATIONS AND APPROACHES TO ESTABLISHING A DIAGNOSIS

A purulent urethral discharge, appearing several days after sexual exposure to an infected partner, is the classic presenting symptom of acute genital gonorrhea in the male. The traditional approach to diagnosis is to examine a gram-stained preparation of the smear for the presence of intracellular gram-negative, biscuit-shaped diplococci. Although the presenting symptom in females may also be a urethral discharge, clinical manifestations are usually more complex, and varying degrees of exudative cervicitis, vaginitis, salpingitis, and pelvic inflammatory disease may be present. Examination of a gram-stained smear of cervical or urethral exudate alone is not sufficient to establish the diagnosis in the female because the cell morphology and staining characteristics of other bacterial species mimic the gonococcus; rather, the recovery of *Neisseria gonorrhoeae* in culture is necessary. Following traditional practice, selective gonococcal culture media incubated under increased CO_2 are inoculated with samples of cervical or urethral exudate, or both; or, the exudate is placed in an appropriate transport medium and delivered to a reference laboratory.

Currently, this traditional gonorrhea-oriented approach to the diagnosis of acute suppurative genital infections is changing for several reasons: 1) new and emerging clinical syndromes are being discovered, 2) *Chlamydia trachomatis* and herpes simplex (HSV-2) are more frequently recovered as significant pathogens,[20] and 3) new procedures based on the direct detection of pathogenic microorganisms or antigens in genital secretions are being implemented.

The incidence of *C. trachomatis* equals, or even exceeds, that of *N. gonorrhoeae* as a cause of acute suppurative genital infections.[83,198] The signs and symptoms of the two diseases are often indistinguishable from one another. *C. trachomatis* tends to produce less exudate and a lower concentration of segmented neutrophils than *N. gonorrhoeae*; however, these criteria are not always sufficient to separate the two diseases.[20] Furthermore, 20% of males and 40% of females with gonorrhea are coinfected with *C. trachomatis*; therefore, culture procedures to recover both organisms may be required in many cases, particularly when treatment fails.[235]

Asymptomatic infections are usually present in both males and females, particularly when *C. trachomatis* is the infecting agent. In certain cases of asymptomatic chlamydial infection, it may also be necessary to culture the sexual partner to establish a diagnosis. If both partners are infected, treatment of each will be required before cures can be effected. In cases of asymptomatic gonorrhea, other sites, such as the anal canal or the throat, may have to be cultured to establish the di-

agnosis, depending on the sexual practices of the patient as indicated by the medical history.

COLLECTION OF GENITAL SPECIMENS FROM MALES

A diagnosis of gonorrhea can be established in males who present with an acute suppurative urethritis in which gram-negative intracellular diplococci can be identified. Varying degrees of epididymitis and prostatitis may also be present. When urethral discharge is scant and intracellular diplococci are not seen in a random sample, collecting the first early morning specimen before urination may be helpful. Exudate may be expressed from the urethral orifice by gently "milking" the penis; if material is not readily obtained, the tip of a narrow-diameter cotton, rayon, or Dacron swab on a plastic or aluminum shaft may be inserted 3 to 4 cm into the anterior urethra. The swab should be left in place for a few seconds to allow the fibers to become saturated with the exudate. If a culture for chlamydia is being obtained, the swab should be rotated 360 degrees to dislodge some of the epithelial cells. In contrast with the organisms of *N. gonorrhoeae* that inhabit the exudate, *C. trachomatis* is strictly intracellular within the urethral epithelial cells.

A 12-hour water fast and the collection of mucin threads from the first early morning urine sample for a Gram stain may establish the diagnosis in occasional asymptomatic males who have negative urethral smears and cultures.[61] If intracellular gram-negative diplococci are still not seen, the possibility of nongonococcal urethritis secondary to *C. trachomatis* must be considered. Thus, cultures or direct detection tests for both *N. gonorrhoeae* and *C. trachomatis* may be necessary. Because both *N. gonorrhoeae* and *C. trachomatis* are susceptible to desiccation and cooling, the use of appropriate transport media is necessary if the causative organism is to be recovered in culture (see Chaps. 10 and 21).

COLLECTION OF GENITAL SPECIMENS FROM FEMALES

In females with signs and symptoms of acute genital infection, samples are most commonly obtained from the uterine cervix and the urethra. Cervical specimens are obtained with the aid of a speculum after clearing off the cervical mucus with a large swab. A smaller swab with a plastic shaft and a Dacron or polyester tip is recommended for obtaining the specimen.[135] The tip of the swab is inserted a few millimeters past the cervical os, rotated firmly to obtain both exudate and cervical cells, and removed, taking care not to touch the lateral walls of the vaginal canal. Urethral samples may be obtained by milking the urethra and collecting the discharge or, if no discharge is observed, by inserting a small urogenital swab into the urethra and leaving it in place for a few seconds to saturate the fibers with exudate.

In cases of deep pelvic inflammatory disease, cultures of the endometrium or aspirations of secretions by laparoscopy or culdoscopy may be necessary. Endometrial specimens are best obtained by inserting the swab through a narrow-bore catheter that has been introduced into the cervical canal, as illustrated in Figure 3-5. By using this technique, there is less chance of contaminating the specimen from secretions of the cervical os or the vaginal canal.

Direct smears of the obtained material should be made immediately to prepare a Gram stain, slide preparation, or both for direct antigen detection. The remaining material must be quickly inoculated to selective culture media or into a transport system. In a comparative study,[223] Culturette transport tube (Marion Scientific), which contains modified Stuart's transport medium, and the direct plating technique produced an almost identical 85% recovery of *N. gonorrhoeae* from culture-positive specimens. Swab transport systems containing charcoal are probably superior to the Culturette swabs because the charcoal helps neutralize toxic materials in the specimen.

RECOVERY OF ORGANISM TYPES FROM THE GENITAL TRACT

The majority of genital tract cultures are submitted to clinical microbiology laboratories for the recovery and identification of the two predominant pathogens— *Neisseria gonorrhoeae* and *Chlamydia trachomatis*. The recovery of the latter requires tissue culture procedures and will be discussed in further detail in Chapter 21.

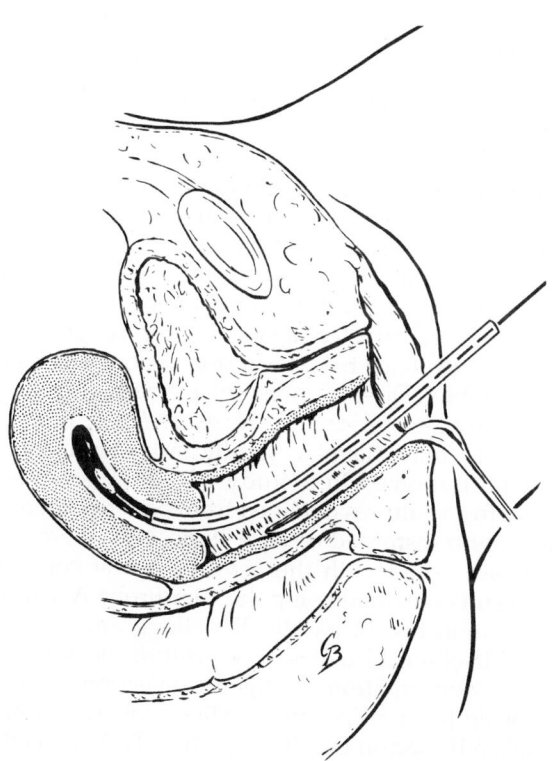

Figure 3-5.
Endometrial culture technique: Through a speculum, a catheter is introduced into the cervical os and a swab extended through the catheter into the endometrial cavity. This helps prevent contamination of the swab by contact with the vaginal wall or the cervical os.

Table 3-5 lists the commensal organisms in the genital tract, the pathogens, and suggested isolation media.

SPECIMEN COLLECTION KITS FOR SUSPECTED SEXUALLY TRANSMITTED DISEASES

To overcome some of the problems involved in obtaining adequate samples for the recovery of organisms in suspected cases of sexually transmitted diseases,[126] kits containing swabs, slides, and transport vials can be prepared in laboratories for use in clinics or physicians' office laboratories (Box 3-4). Such a kit helps ensure that the correct implements and transport media will be used. One such kit has been prepared for use at the University of Illinois Hospital in Chicago.

Each laboratory director can decide the appropriate items to include in the kit. Several commercial products are now available for the direct detection of chlamydial or viral antigens using enzyme-linked immunoassay procedures, latex agglutination, or fluorescein or enzyme-tagged monoclonal antibodies. These products can be included in the sample collection kit if direct antigen detection is currently being performed. In many instances, both swab cultures and the bedside smear preparations are required. With these techniques, definitive answers are often available within a few hours, at levels of sensitivity and specificity approaching 95% to 97% (see Chap. 21).

RECOVERY OF *NEISSERIA GONORRHOEAE*

N. gonorrhoeae is a fastidious bacterium that does not tolerate drying, sudden changes in temperature (particularly cooling), or an atmosphere low in CO_2. It requires an enriched medium and does not grow well in the presence of other commensal organisms that may be recovered from culture sites. The culture media and transport systems, therefore, have been designed to accommodate these somewhat stringent requirements.

Selective chocolate agar–based media containing various antibiotics are commonly used for recovery of *N. gonorrhoeae* from clinical specimens.[193] Users should be aware, however, that some strains of *N. gonorrhoeae* are inhibited by the concentrations of vancomycin contained in certain of the selective media.[146] Modified Thayer-Martin medium (MTM) is chocolate agar incorporating four antibiotics: vancomycin, colistin, nystatin, and trimethoprim lactate. Other selective media may contain varying concentrations of the antibacterial agents or different antifungal agents (e.g., Martin-Lewis medium, GC-Lect medium). Non–chocolate agar-based selective media, such as New York City medium,[52] are also available but are not as widely used. These media are discussed in more detail in Chapter 10.

In cases of urogenital gonococcal infection, the recovery of oxidase-positive, gram-negative diplococci on selective medium is usually sufficient to establish a presumptive diagnosis. Carbohydrate utilization or other confirmatory methods should always be performed to confirm the diagnosis and identify atypical strains and isolates from nongenital sources.

TABLE 3-5
COMMENSAL FLORA AND PATHOGENIC BACTERIA IN THE GENITAL TRACT

COMMENSAL FLORA (CONTAMINANTS)	POTENTIAL PATHOGENS	RECOMMENDED ISOLATION MEDIA
Escherichia coli and other "coliforms"	*Neisseria gonorrhoeae*	Modified Thayer-Martin medium or equivalent
Group D Streptococci	Group B streptococci	5% sheep blood agar
Lactobacillus spp.	*Enterococcus* spp.	5% sheep blood agar
Coagulase-negative staphylococci	*Gardnerella vaginalis*	V agar with protease peptone no. 3 and human blood
Many species of anaerobes	Certain anaerobes including *Actinonyces* spp. (associated with intrauterine devices) Virtually any organism in high concentration and in pure culture	Prereduced anaerobic blood agar plates, with and without selective agents 5% sheep blood agar, MacConkey agar or other special medium, depending on clinical diagnosis

Most microbiologists prefer the use of nutritive agar plate transport systems such as JEMBEC (Ames Co.), Bio-Bag (Marion Laboratories, Kansas City MO), or Gono-Pak (BBL Microbiology Systems, Cockeysville MD) for the transport of gonorrhea specimens. These systems consist of an individual agar plate of gonococcal-selective medium in a plastic, zip-locked bag containing a CO_2-generating tablet (see Chap. 2). Because proper preparation of the transport system before shipping cannot be guaranteed, with the chance that the appropriate concentration of CO_2 has not been maintained, reincubation of the specimen for an additional 24 to 48 hours at 35°C in a 5% CO_2 incubator in the reference laboratory is obligatory. These systems may have lost sufficient CO_2 to curtail growth, even though the organisms may still be viable.

Ebright and associates[45] found that the recovery rate of *N. gonorrhoeae* from modified Stuart's medium drops to 60% after 24 hours and to 27% after 48 hours.[45] If a transport container of Stuart's medium is used, transfer of the specimen to gonococcal-selective culture medium should occur as soon as possible (optimally within 6 hours).

Direct Detection of Gonococcal Antigen. Primarily for medicolegal reasons in the investigation of suspected sexual abuse cases, it is becoming increasingly necessary to confirm an isolate as *N. gonorrhoeae* by a second method employing a different principle. Monoclonal antibody tests directed against outer *N. gonorrhoeae* membrane proteins have been used as one such alternative method. Direct fluorescent antibody (DFA) tests have been used to identify *N. gonorrhoeae*; however, DFA tests may have a significantly high rate of misidentifications.[13] In a study of 395 *N. gonorrhoeae* isolates from cultures obtained from patients attending a sexually transmitted disease clinic, 4.5% were negative when tested with the Syva DFA test compared with results obtained using the Gen-Probe Accuprobe confirmation test in parallel.[13] Kellogg and Orwig,[104] tested 248 clinical isolates of *N. gonorrhoeae* with three culture confirmation antigen detection systems (GonoGen [Becton Dickinson Microbiology Systems], GonoGen II [Becton Dickinson], MicroTrak direct fluorescent-antibody test [Syva]), and with Rapid Fermentation Agar carbohydrates (Remel). The sensitivity for these four methods was 100%, 99.6%, 97.2%, and 97.6%, respectively. Of 62 isolates of other *Neisseria* species, none were misidentified as *N. gonorrhoeae* by GonoGen, MicroTrak, or the carbohydrate tests; how-

BOX 3-4. KIT FOR COLLECTION OF ORGANISMS IN SUSPECTED CASES OF SEXUALLY TRANSMITTED DISEASES

1. Two rayon-tipped, plastic-shaft swabs for collection of cervical, vaginal, or vesicle cultures.

2. One smaller Dacron-tipped, plastic-shaft swab for collection of chlamydial or gonococcal cultures from female urethra, with a tube of Amies charcoal transport medium.

3. One small-caliber, Dacron-tipped swab, with stainless steel shaft, for collection of cultures from male urethra.

4. One vial of 2SP viral transport fluid (0.2-M sucrose in 0.02-M phosphate buffer at pH 7.0 with 5% fetal calf serum and 50 μg/mL gentamicin) for the recovery of *Chlamydia trachomatis* and herpesvirus.

5. One vial of mycoplasma/ureaplasma transport medium (beef–heart/peptone base + yeast extract + horse serum +penicillin [100,000 μg/mL], polymyxin [5000 μg/mL], and amphotericin [5000 μg/mL]) for the recovery of *Mycoplasma* and *Ureaplasma* spp.

ever, seven of 22 (31.8%) *N. meningitidis* gave strong false-positive results with GonoGen II. The authors counsel that all GonoGen II-positive assays for *N. gonorrhoeae* should be confirmed by a second method.

Nucleic acid probe assays are also commercially available for the direct detection of *N. gonorrhoeae* from clinical specimens. In a study of 1750 specimens (496 females and 623 males) obtained from patients visiting the outpatient clinic of the Sexually Transmitted Diseases Department of the Westeinde Hospital, The Hague,[246] the Gen-Probe PACE 2 system performed with a sensitivity, specificity, and positive and negative predictive values of 97.2%, 99.1%, 90.6%, and 99.8%, respectively. Of a subset of 13 patients with positive probe results but negative cultures, 12 were thought to have gonococcal infection based on clinical and other laboratory parameters. The authors cite as one advantage of this system the ability to test for *C. trachomatis* on the same specimen; one disadvantage is the inability to determine β-lactamase production by the strains detected. In populations with a high percentage of β-lactamase–producing strains of *N. gonorrhoeae* (50% of isolates in the Hague study), antibiotic susceptibility studies may be necessary before the empiric use of ceftriaxone. In an unrelated study,[92] similar sensitivity, specificity, and predictive values were found for the direct diagnosis of gonorrhea using the PACE-2 system on endocervical specimens; the disadvantages were cited as the inability to determine specimen adequacy, the requirement for expensive instrumentation, and the inability to perform susceptibility studies. In a study of 7429 urethral swabs from men attending sexually transmitted disease clinics operated by the Houston Department of Health and Human Services, the Gen-Probe test correlated with gram-stained smear results 99.5% of the time for positive specimens, and 98.8% for negative specimens.[97]

DNA amplification techniques are also being applied to the direct diagnosis of gonorrhea in clinical specimens. Birkenmeyer and Armstrong[17] used a ligase chain reaction (LCR) directed against the multicopy *Opa* genes (*Omp*-II) and against multicopy pilin genes. Of 100 urogenital specimens assayed by LCR, 100% correlated with positive cultures and 97.8% correlated with negative cultures. Mahony and associates[136] developed a multiplex PCR assay for the simultaneous detection of *C. trachomatis* and *N. gonorrhoeae*, employing specific primers KL1-KL2 and HO2-HO3, respectively. The sensitivity of the M-PCR assay for detecting *C. trachomatis* was 100% and for *N. gonorrhoeae* was 92.3%; the specificities were 100% for both organisms. Although these assays are still being used primarily in research settings, clinical applications are sure to follow as PCR technology is introduced into more and more diagnostic laboratories.

CHLAMYDIA TRACHOMATIS

Specimens obtained for culture of *Chlamydia trachomatis* must immediately be placed in special transport medium (0.2-M sucrose in 0.02-M phosphate buffer [pH 7.0 to 7.2] with 5% fetal calf serum and 50 µg/mL final concentration of gentamicin). Maass and Dalhoff[133a] were able to recover 81% of stock strains after 12 hours that were stored at 22°C; 74% of strains were still recovered after 48 hours if refrigerated at 4°C. However, the stability of wild strains was less—primary isolates were not satisfactorily retrievable beyond 4 hours at 22°C or beyond 24 hours at 4°C. Thus, samples to be held longer than 24 hours require −75°C freezing.

Many laboratories use direct antigen detection procedures for the rapid diagnosis of chlamydial infections.[235] The MicroTrak system (Syva Co., Palo Alto CA) uses a fluorescent-tagged monoclonal antibody directed against chlamydial elementary bodies that can be detected by fluorescence microscopy.[55,239] Special slides that can be prepared by transferring a portion of the inoculum to the slide by rolling the tip of a secretion-saturated Dacron swab over the exposed surface are furnished by the manufacturer. The specimen is allowed to air dry and is forwarded to the laboratory for analysis. Recent evaluations of this system indicate that, in high-risk populations, when the presence of three or more elementary bodies are observed under oil immersion lenses, the sensitivity of the direct fluorescent method compared with tissue culture is 90%.[132,228,235,239] Well-trained personnel and a good microscope are required to achieve this level of accuracy.

Enzyme-linked assay (Chlamydiazyme—Abbott Laboratories) is another nonculture technique used for the detection of chlamydial antigens in clinical specimens.[96] In one study,[86] the sensitivity of the procedure compared with tissue culture averaged 78.8% for detecting urethral infections in males and 89.5% for detecting cervical infections in females. The specificity was 97% for both males and females in this same study. The use of enzyme-linked assays for diagnosing chlamydial infections is most appropriate for large-volume screening of high-risk populations. One disadvantage of enzymatic procedures compared with microscopic examinations is the inability to determine the quality of the specimen by evaluating cell morphology. The diagnosis of chlamydial infections is discussed in greater detail in Chapter 21.

Kellogg[102] advises that, in the wake of rapid and direct tests for the detection of *C. trachomatis* in endocervical specimens and the need to have adequate specimens to achieve acceptable levels of accuracy, periodic microscopic analysis for specimen quality should be implemented to help motivate personnel obtaining specimens. It is also advised[54] that EIA-reactive specimens with low positive readout quotients be confirmed by DFA. In this study,[54] of a subset of 236 genital swabs obtained from a medium-risk group for *C. trachomatis* infection and tested by EIA, 5.9% of patients would have been missed if the manufacturer's kit criteria alone were followed. Samples with an EIA quotient lower than 4.0, in particular, were subject to false-negative results and should be confirmed by DFA. Similarly, from data obtained from 6022 male and female urogenital specimens tested for *C. trachomatis* by the MicroTrak (Syva Company, San Jose CA) EIA assay,[28] only those samples giving optical densities within 0.499 AU above and 30% below the cutoff value required confirmation by DFA. In a study of 550 women from whom duplicate endocervical swabs were obtained and tested by the Syva Microtrak assay and Chlamydiazyme for the presence of *C. trachomatis*,[163] the former was found to be more sensitive (95% versus 79%).

Nucleic acid amplification techniques are being implemented in many laboratories for the diagnosis of *C. trachomatis* genitourinary infections. With an LCR assay, in which target sequences within the chlamydial cryptic plasmid were amplified, Schacter and associates[199] were able to detect *C. trachomatis* in 94% of 234 proved-positive endocervical specimens. Of these positive specimens, only 65% were detected in cell culture, indicating that LCR provides a sensitive nonculture method for diagnosing endocervical chlamydial infection. In a study of 234 endocervical specimens obtained from women in a high-risk female population,[144] the PACE 2 (Gen-Probe, San Diego CA) and the Amplicor (Hoffmann-LaRoche) PCR assays were though to offer an improvement in sensitivity (90% and 88% versus 81%, respectively) over the MicroTrak (Syva) EIA assay. With a PCR assay directed against the *C. trachomatis* 16S rRNA gene,[6] five elementary bodies was the lower level of detection. These investigators conclude that nucleic acid amplification techniques may facilitate investigations of persistent infection in culture-negative genitourinary infections.

Several recent studies indicate that PCR-based assays are also highly sensitive in detecting *C. trachomatis* DNA in urine specimens. A sensitivity of 93.8% and specificity of 99.9% were found[128] in the detection of *C. trachomatis* plasmid DNA in first-voided urine samples of 1932 women with suspected chlamydial genitourinary infections. Other investigators[39] found a 100% sensitivity and specificity of the Amplicor (Roche) PCR assay in detecting *C. trachomatis* in the urine specimens of 184 asymptomatic men attending a venereal disease clinic. An LCR-based assay with plasmid primers was able to detect *C. trachomatis* in urine samples of 12 and five culture-negative women and men, respectively, suspected of having genitourinary chlamydial infection.[245] In all cases, the presence of *C. trachomatis* was confirmed by a second LCR assay with primers based on chromosomal DNA. Both the LCx *Chlamydia trachomatis* LCR assay (Abbott) and the Amplicor *Chlamydia trachomatis* test (Roche) were much more sensitive than culture in the diagnosis of genitourinary tract infections in other studies.[30,31] Therefore, nucleic acid amplification assays performed on first-voided urine samples offer a rapid, noninvasive and highly sensitive approach to the diagnosis of chlamydial genitourinary infections in both men and women.

MISCELLANEOUS INFECTIONS

Herpes Simplex Virus Infections. Herpes infections most frequently manifest as vesicular lesions with an erythematous base on the glans penis, vulva, perineum, buttocks, or cervix. The vesicles are painful and may ulcerate. The genital lesions may be accompanied by systemic symptoms—fever, malaise, anorexia, and tender bilateral inguinal adenopathy. The vesicle fluid is rich in desquamated cells containing herpes virus and can be best obtained with a 27-gauge needle on a tuberculin syringe. If fluid is scant, the vesicle should be unroofed and the base of the ulcer firmly scraped with a Dacron (polyester) swab to remove some of the cells. Because herpes virus is also extremely sensitive to drying, immediate transfer of the specimen to viral transport medium is essential. The same 2SP transport medium used for *C. trachomatis* is also appropriate for herpes cultures.

Other Genital Ulcer Syndromes. In addition to herpes simplex-2, other genital ulcer syndromes include syphilis, chancroid (caused by *Haemophilus ducreyi*), lymphogranuloma venereum (caused by certain *C. trachomatis* serotypes), granuloma inguinale (caused by the difficult to isolate bacterium *Calymmatobacterium granulomatis*), and trauma. The chancres of syphilis differ from those of herpes in that they are painless and have indurated margins and a clean base. A darkfield examination of material, obtained from the base of the ulcer to detect the presence of spirochetes, is required to make the diagnosis of syphilis. Chancroid ulcers, in contrast to syphilitic chancres, are painful and do not have indurated margins. The primary pustule of lymphogranuloma venereum may resemble herpes simplex; however, this condition is usually recognizable by the massive bilateral necrotizing inguinal adenopathy. The primary lesion of granuloma inguinale is a subcutaneous nodule that erodes the surface, from which a beefy red, painless, elevated granulomatous lesion develops. The diagnosis is made by demonstrating the intracellular microorganisms known as "Donovan bodies" within histiocytes or monocytes on Wright's-stained impression smears. The human papillomavirus produces a variety of infections in the genital tract, including condyloma acuminata and flat warts. Some viral types may integrate into host cell DNA and cause epithelial neoplasia (see Chap. 21).

Vaginal Infections. Cultures of vaginal exudates for the recovery of pathogenic bacteria usually do not produce meaningful results. In cases of suppurative vaginal discharge, direct mounts or stained smears will often disclose the etiology. *Trichomonas vaginalis* classically produces a copious, frothy yellow or yellow-green discharge that collects in the posterior vaginal fornix. The discharge in candidiasis is typically more thick and curdlike, and the vaginal mucosa tends to be erythematous. Both of these infections can be diagnosed by observing the characteristic microscopic forms—the motile trophozoites of *T. vaginalis* and the budding yeast and pseudohyphal forms of *Candida* species—in direct wet mount preparations.

Bacterial Vaginosis. *Gardnerella vaginalis*, thought to be associated with bacterial vaginosis, most likely works synergistically with anaerobic bacteria belonging to the *Bacteroides* and *Peptococcus* genera in producing the characteristic malodorous discharge.[225] The recovery of *G. vaginalis* in the absence of mixed anaerobic flora and symptoms of bacterial vaginosis probably constitutes normal vaginal flora. It has been reported[46] that bacterial vaginosis (defined by clinical criteria) was not present in 55% of women from whom *G. vaginalis* was isolated. Observing dense aggregates of gram-negative bacilli on desquamated epithelial cells ("clue" cells) in stained smears of the vaginal secretion or the production of alkaline vaginal secretions (pH 4.5) should lead the clinician to suspect bacterial vaginosis.[137] False-positive rates as high as 18.5% have been reported because other bacteria can also attach to epithelial cells. A 10% false-negative rate has been reported owing to inhibition of bacterial attachment by IgA. However, when the clue cell test is combined with the amine production or "whiff" test (in which equal volumes of genital fluid and 10% KOH are mixed; perception of a fishy odor is a positive result), the predictive negative value of 99% provides a good screen for the absence of bacterial vaginosis.

Several media formulations have been used for the recovery of *G. vaginalis*, namely, chocolate agar, peptone–starch dextrose agar, sheep-blood beef infusion agar, V agar, Columbia–colistin–nalidixic acid (CNA) agar and others.[243] It has been suggested[65] that the essential ingredients include human blood (*G. vaginalis* hemolyzes human, but not sheep, rabbit, or horse bloods) and proteose peptone 3. However, in most practices the diagnosis of bacterial vaginosis is primarily based on correlating the clinical signs and symptoms with observations of a Gram stain of vaginal secretions.[162].

Mobiluncus curtisii and *M. mulieris* are also associated with bacterial vaginosis.[224] These are anaerobic, motile, curved gram-negative bacilli that require prolonged incubation periods of 7 days to several weeks for recovery. Thomason and coworkers[240] have described a selective and differential medium for the recovery of *Mobiluncus* species from mixed cultures. The medium consists of Columbia CNA agar with 5% packed red blood cells. Fetal calf serum (7%) was added to the rabbit blood supplement. For this reason, cultures are not routinely performed in most clinical laboratories. The importance of recognizing bacterial vaginosis clinically and establishing a laboratory diagnosis is emphasized.[84] In a study of 49 women with preterm labor, out of a subset of 12 who had concomitant bacterial vaginosis, eight (67%) had a 2.1-fold increase risk for preterm birth before 37 weeks of gestation. Bacterial vaginosis was also associated with low birth weight. The bacterial species commonly associated with bacterial vaginosis, specifically *Mobiluncus* species and high numbers of *Gardnerella vaginalis*, along with a variety of anaerobes, including *Prevotella* species, *Porphyromonas asaccharolytica*, *Fusobacterium nucleatum*, and *Peptostreptococcus* species, were associated with preterm delivery.

Elevated levels of vaginal fluid sialidase activity, probably derived from enzymatic activity of *Bacte-roides* species and *Prevotella* species,[24] and an elevation of vaginal fluid pH above 4.5 in conjunction with high levels of *G. vaginalis* (as determined by a specific DNA probe)[211] were other markers useful in confirming the diagnosis of bacterial vaginosis. Cook and associates[36] found that a persistent elevated pH and high polyamine and fatty acid levels in vaginal secretions along with clue cells in small numbers were valuable residual abnormalities predicting recurrence of bacterial vaginosis.

Acute Urethral Syndrome.   *N. gonorrhoeae* and *C. trachomitis* can also cause an acute urethral syndrome in females, in which patients may present with symptoms of urinary tract infections, such as frequency and dysuria; however, urine cultures are either negative or have colony counts of 10^2 CFU/mL or fewer.[226,227] Clinicians should inform the microbiology laboratory if the acute urethral syndrome is clinically suspected because routine urine culture techniques may not detect bacteria in such low concentrations. Urethral and cervical cultures for *N. gonorrhoeae* and *C. trachomatis* should be obtained from these patients.

Mycoplasma and Ureaplasma Infections.   The role of *Mycoplasma hominis* and *Ureaplasma urealyticum* as causes of genital tract infections is still unsettled. Twenty percent of healthy females are vaginal carriers of *M. hominis*; 60% carry *U. urealyticum*.[107] *U. urealyticum* may be one cause of nongonococcal urethritis; both *M. hominis* and *U. urealyticum* are thought to cause pelvic inflammatory disease in females and may be involved in premature labor, infertility, and septic abortion.[237] Specimens for culture must be immediately placed into a transport medium (trypticase soy broth with 0.5% bovine albumin and penicillin, 10,000 U/mL, the latter to suppress bacterial overgrowth). Transport media must be frozen at −70°C if cultures cannot be inoculated immediately. This group of organisms is discussed in detail in Chapter 16.

Endometritis.   Other bacterial species, notably members of the family *Enterobacteriaceae*, various anaerobes (*Bacteroides* species, *Peptostreptococcus* species, *Clostridium* species, the anaerobic actinomycetes and *Eubacterium nodatum*), β-hemolytic streptococci (particularly group B), are occasionally incriminated in genital tract infections. Endometritis can be caused by certain anaerobic bacteria, and a specific association has been reported between *Actinomyces israelii* and endometritis in women wearing plastic intrauterine devices.[43] The etiology is thought to involve the formation of a calcium carbonate nidus on the plastic in which the *Actinomyces* species grow. Women wearing copper devices are rarely infected, presumably because the metal is mildly bacteriostatic. Examination of gram-stained direct smears of genital secretions may be helpful to guide the selection of appropriate media in those instances when recovery of selected organisms is important.

INFECTIONS OF THE CENTRAL NERVOUS SYSTEM

CLINICAL SIGNS AND SYMPTOMS OF MENINGITIS

Patients with early acute meningitis may experience an influenzalike syndrome—sore and stiff neck, headache, low-grade fever, and lethargy. In elderly, debilitated, or immunosuppressed patients, unexpected alteration in mental status may be the only clue. Various degrees of confusion, agitation, disorientation, or coma may be observed. A positive Brudzinski's sign (resistance to passive neck flexion) and Kernig's sign (inability to extend the leg when the thigh is flexed at a 90° angle with the trunk) are signs of meningeal irritation. Subacute or chronic meningitis caused by tuberculosis or fungal infections may present with signs of increased intracranial pressure (papilledema, nausea, vomiting) and mental changes, such as disorientation, confusion, personality change and stupor.[139]

The CSF is normally water-clear, has no more than five lymphocytes per milliliter, has a glucose concentration between 45 and 100 mg/dL depending on the level of blood sugar, a protein concentration between 14 and 45 mg/dL, and is sterile. In cases of acute bacterial meningitis, cell counts may range between 500 and 20,000 segmented neutrophils per milliliter. In tuberculous or viral meningitis, lymphocyte counts between 200 and 2000/mL may be seen. In bacterial meningitis, the CSF glucose level is decreased (relative to blood glucose levels), and the CSF protein level is elevated. In acute viral meningitis, the WBC count is generally fewer than 500 cells per microliter. Mononuclear cells predominate, but substantial numbers of neutrophils may be present or even predominate at the onset. The glucose value is normal, and that of the protein is only slightly elevated. In subacute and chronic meningitis, a low-grade mononuclear pleocytosis is observed, the protein level is elevated, and the glucose level may or may not be decreased.

Meningitis is most prevalent in certain age groups or in patients with various underlying diseases. Meningitis in the neonate most commonly involves direct invasion of flora from the mother during vaginal delivery. Group B streptococci and *Escherichia coli* are the organisms most often recovered; *Listeria monocytogenes*, *Klebsiella pneumoniae*, *Serratia* species, *Pseudomonas* species, *Staphylococcus aureus*, and miscellaneous anaerobic bacteria are recovered less frequently.

Haemophilus influenzae is the most common cause of acute bacterial meningitis in the 6-month to 5-year age group; *Neisseria meningitidis* and *Streptococcus pneumoniae* are the next most common causes. These cases are frequently associated with bacteremia and extension of infection from adjacent sinuses or the middle ear following penetrating trauma, neurosurgery, or spinal anesthesia.

In adults, *S. pneumoniae* is the most common cause of bacterial meningitis. In young adults, *N. meningitidis* is also common. In the elderly, *E. coli* and other gram-negative bacilli are high in prevalence.[139] *Cryptococcus neoformans*, *Listeria monocytogenes*, and *Mycobacterium tuberculosis* cause indolent or chronic forms of meningitis in hosts with altered defenses; *E. coli*, *K. pneumoniae*, and staphylococci are most commonly recovered from patients with posttraumatic or postsurgical meningitis. Approximately 50% of acute meningitis associated with ventricular shunts is caused by coagulase-negative staphylococci.[139]

Viral meningitis has a seasonal association: enteroviruses and arboviruses are the agents most commonly recovered in summer and early fall; mumps and lymphocytic choriomeningitis virus (LCM) in winter and spring. Herpes simplex infections have no seasonal patterns.

Anaerobic bacteria are most frequently recovered from brain abscesses; anaerobic streptococci, *Porphyromonas* (*Bacteroides*) *melaninogenica* and other *Bacteroides* species, *Fusobacterium nucleatum*, *Eubacterium* species, and *Propionibacterium acnes* are the most commonly encountered species. The aerobic bacteria most commonly recovered include α-hemolytic streptococci, *S. aureus*, *S. pneumoniae*, gram-negative bacilli, and *Nocardia* species. The dematiaceous fungus *Xylohypha bantiana* (formerly *Cladosporium trichoides*) may also produce brain abscesses.[207]

COLLECTION OF SPECIMENS

Central nervous system (CNS) specimens for culture include CSF (obtained either by subdural tap, ventricular aspiration, or lumbar puncture), brain abscess aspirate, and brain biopsy. These samples are obtained by the physician under sterile operative conditions (the spinal tap technique is illustrated in Fig. 3-6).

The CSF obtained from lumbar spinal puncture is the most common CNS specimen received by the laboratory. Usually, three separate tubes of CSF fluid are submitted—tube 1 for cell counts and differential stains, tube 2 for Gram stains and culture, and tube 3 to test for protein and glucose, or for special studies such as VDRL, cryptococcal antigen, or cytology, depending on the clinical situation.

PROCESSING SPECIMENS

An orderly approach to the processing and culture of CSF specimens should be implemented. Too often, a small quantity of CSF is received with the order to perform bacterial, tuberculosis, and fungal cultures. A priority selection may be necessary based on the most probable etiologic agent in view of the patient's clinical presentation. It is questionable whether setting up tuberculosis or fungal cultures of crystal-clear spinal fluid specimens with no cellular or chemical abnormalities is useful. These cultures are virtually always negative, and it is tedious to make repeated examinations for the 4 to 6 weeks that they must be held. If there are sufficient organisms to recover in culture, active disease is virtually always present, and chemical or cellular changes will be present. Eliminating these extremely low-yield cultures may be suggested as a cost-saving measure. At the University of Vermont, approval of a pathologist is required for the processing

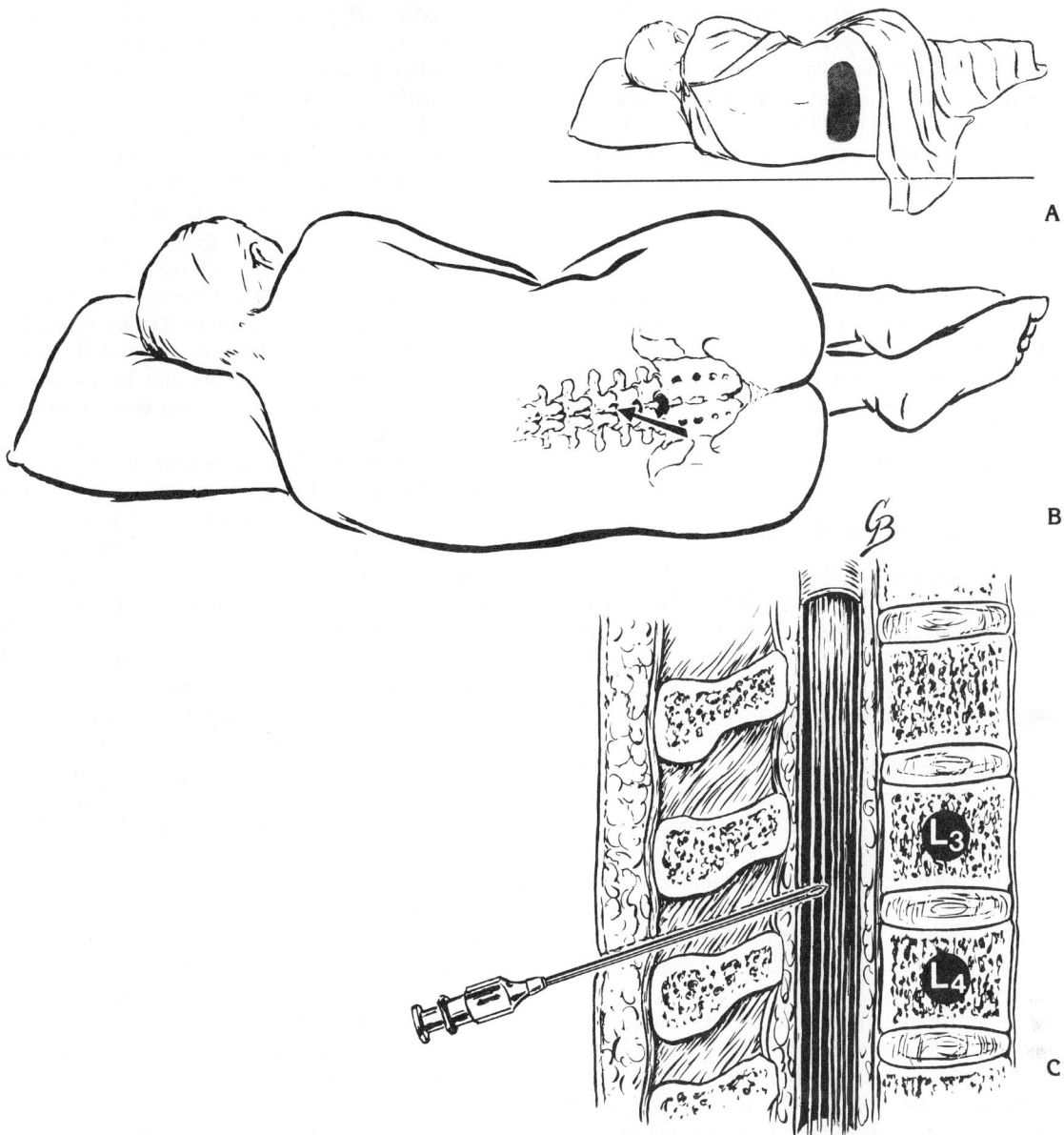

Figure 3-6.
Spinal tap technique: The patient lies on his or her side, with knees flexed and back arched
to separate the lumbar vertabrae. (**A**) The patient is surgically draped, and an area overlying the lumbar spine is disinfected. (**B**) The space between lumber vertabrae L-3 and L-4 is
palpated with the sterilely gloved forefinger, and (**C**) the spinal needle is carefully directed
between the spinous processes, through the intraspinous ligaments into the spinal canal.

of CSF for mycobacterial culture in the absence of features suggestive of past or current tuberculosis.

Examining stained smears of CSF sediment and
performing direct antigen detection tests may be helpful both in establishing a presumptive diagnosis and in
providing guidelines for the selection of culture media.
Microorganisms can often be detected in gram-stained
or methylene blue-stained CSF smears if they are present in concentrations of 10,000/mL (10^4) or more. It is
recommended that both a gram-stained and a methylene blue-stained smear be prepared in parallel. Gram-
negative organisms are often better observed in the
methylene blue-stained smear because the deep blue-

staining cells are easier to differentiate from the background debris. Safranin stains the background red in
the Gram stain, tending to obscure any pink-staining
bacteria. Smalley and Bradley[218] suggest that the leukocyte esterase (LE) test may substitute for the performance of cell counts on body fluids suspected of harboring bacteria. In a study of 63 culture-positive
peritoneal fluids, 85.7% also had positive LE reactions.
Six of the nine culture-positive and LE-negative fluids
grew only a few colonies of coagulase-negative
staphylococci isolates of questionable significance. De-
Lozier and Auerbach[38] report an overall sensitivity of
84.4% and a specificity of 98.1% using the dipstick

leukocyte esterase test (LET) on spinal fluids collected from 800 patients with suspected meningitis. The sensitivity of LET in culture-proved cases of bacterial meningitis was only 73%. They conclude that the LET is an adjunct to, but not a substitute for, CSF cell count and chemistry determination in the initial laboratory assessment of bacterial meningitis. For use in developing countries where laboratory tests for the examination of CSF may be limited, Moosa and coworkers[148] found that multireagent strips that estimate CSF glucose, protein, and leukocytosis may be of value. By using a Combur9 reagent strip (Boeringer Mannheim), they found that all but four of 234 (sensitivity of 97%) CSF samples obtained from children with suspected bacterial meningitis were not correctly identified. The strip gave a false-positive reaction in only two of 60 (2.9%) cases of viral meningitis.

DIRECT ANTIGEN DETECTION SYSTEMS

Several antigen detection systems are available for the direct detection of the polysaccharide capsular antigens of *H. influenzae*, *N. meningitidis*, *S. pneumoniae*, and group B streptococci in CSF. These detection systems have shown specificity and sensitivity in the 90% to 97% range and, when used in conjunction with the direct-staining techniques discussed later in this chapter, often provide rapid presumptive diagnoses on which specific antibiotic therapy can be based. Cuevas and associates[37] report the following levels of specificity and sensitivity, respectively, in using the latex particle agglutination test for the detection of bacterial antigens in the CSF of 91 patients with meningitis: *S. pneumoniae* 88% and 100%; *H. influenzae*, B 87% and 96%; *N. meningitidis* A, C, Y, W-135, 100% and 100%; and *N. meningitidis* B, 100% and 98%.

The initial enthusiasm for the rapid diagnosis of meningitis by antigen detection has been tempered by more recent experiences.[189] When performing latex particle agglutination tests for *H. influenzae* type b, group B streptococci, *N. meningitidis*, and *S. pneumoniae* on 1540 CSF specimens, obtained from patients with suspected acute bacterial meningitis, antigen was detected in only 27 samples.[182] The positive antigen results were helpful only in the management of neonates with group B streptococcal infections. These authors considered the latex text to be cost-ineffective. Feuerborn and coworkers[53] performed latex agglutination tests on spinal fluid samples for the detection of bacterial antigens in 176 patients with suspected meningitis. Antigen was detected in only five. They found that the CSF white blood cell count and differential were the best predictors of meningitis, and that latex agglutination tests should be limited to only patients with elevated CSF white counts. From the results of two other studies,[23,190] it may be concluded that the latex agglutination test is more sensitive than culture in the diagnosis of bacterial meningitis in patients who had received previous antibiotic therapy, presumably because bacterial growth was impaired. In a study of 1151 specimens from 791 children with suspected bacterial meningitis,[80] the sensitivity for detection of one of the

five classic CSF pathogens was 83.3% in CSF and 60% in urine. However, in the detection of all pathogens, the sensitivity was only 50% in CSF and 37.5% in urine. These authors emphasize that tests for the detection of bacterial antigen in CSF must be interpreted only in the light of clinical history and other CSF findings.

For future considerations, another study,[183] which used a seminested PCR assay and primers specific to conserved and variable regions in the 16S rRNA sequences of *N. meningitidis*, *H. influenzae*, *S. pneumoniae*, and *S. galactiae*, a sensitivity of 94% and specificity of 96% were found in the detection of these bacterial antigens. PCR inhibitors were considered the major cause of the few false results; this can be be improved as methods for separating bacteria from these inhibitors are perfected.

Direct tests for the detection of cryptococcal antigen in the spinal fluid, blood, or urine are also available, which have replaced the India ink test in many laboratories. In a study of 218 CSF specimens, which included 16 retrospective and six prospective cases of known cryptococcosis,[265] the IBL (International Biological Laboratories, Cranbury NJ) and the Myco-Immune (American Scientific Products, McGraw Park IL) cryptococcal latex antigen kits performed with 100% sensitivity in detecting cryptococcal antigen in the spinal fluid. In other studies,[238] the newly introduced monoclonal antibody-based latex agglutination test, Pastorex Cryptococcus (Sanofi-Diagnostics Pasteur, Marnes-La-Coquette, France), performed with equal sensitivity (97%) and specificity (100%) to the CALAS (Meridian Diagnostics, Inc., Cincinnati OH) and the Crypto-LA (International Biological Labs Inc., Cranbury NJ). The addition of pronase increased the sensitivity and specificity of the Pastorex and the CALAS assays. The Pastorex assay was also useful in detecting cryptococcal antigen in bronchoalveolar lavage and urine specimens, particularly in patients with AIDS. Positive antigen test results in these specimens serve to reinforce the presumptive diagnosis of cryptococcosis in these patients; for negative results, repeat cultures and antigen testing are indicated when clinical evidence of infection is strong.

False-positive reactions in serum caused by rheumatoid factor can be minimized by treating positive serum samples with pronase (Calbiochem-Behring Corp., LaJolla CA)[233]. Boom and associates[19] reported another case of false-positive cryptococcal latex agglutination reactions from contamination of spinal fluid samples with minute quantities of syneresis (agar condensation) fluid from agar plates. This source of contamination can be eliminated by taking care not to reintroduce the same inoculating needle back into the spinal fluid sample after streaking the surface of the agar plate. It was discovered[72] that immersing a platinum inoculating wire loop into the sample of CSF before performing the cryptococcal antigen latex test introduced interfering substances, leading to nonspecific agglutination; therefore it is recommended that the latex test be performed before subculturing.

A variety of nucleic acid techniques that provide DNA fingerprints, restriction fragment length polymorphism profiles, random primer amplified, and targeted primer PCR products and allow strain analyses of *C. neoformans* isolates from various sources have been reported in a plethora of papers appearing in the medical literature over the past 5 years. (See Chap. 1 for more information on these applications.)

Isolation of viral agents from CNS specimens requires special media and techniques that are discussed in more detail in Chapter 21. The direct detection of viral antigens in biopsy specimens using fluorescent-tagged monoclonal antibodies is now possible in making rapid diagnoses of viral encephalitides. Schlesinger and coworkers,[202] using a PCR-based amplification assay, detected HSV DNA in the CSF of three young women with signs and symptoms of meningitis, who had no history of genital herpetic lesions. They conclude that PCR can improve the recognition of HSV meningitis in patients presenting with aseptic meningitis.

CULTURE SETUP OF CSF SPECIMENS AND SELECTION OF CULTURE MEDIA

A list of pathogenic organisms that may be encountered in CSF and suggested media for their recovery are listed in Table 3-6. Many of the organisms listed tend to be fastidious and may be difficult to recover in culture; therefore, use of an enriched medium such as chocolate agar should always be included. Because *Haemophilus influenzae* is a common cause of meningitis, inoculation of the CSF specimen to chocolate agar and blood agar is essential. The blood agar plate after inoculation should be streaked across one quadrant with a β-hemolytic staphylococcus (staph streak technique) to provide factor V (NAD), which may be deficient in the medium. The chocolate agar will also recover another common pathogen, *N. meningitidis*. Because CSF is normally not contaminated, the use of a selective medium such as modified Thayer-Martin

(MTM) is not required to recover *N. meningitidis*. Inoculation of thioglycolate broth or an enriched eugonic broth may be helpful to recover fastidious organisms in low numbers.

Other pathogens, including *Listeria monocytogenes* and *Flavobacterium meningosepticum*, will grow on both the chocolate and blood agar plates. The colonies of *L. monocytogenes* may appear β-hemolytic and can be confused with β-hemolytic streptococci. The differential identification can be made by observing a gram-stained smear and performing a catalase test. *Listeria* species are gram-positive bacilli and are catalase-positive. *F. meningosepticum*, a somewhat fastidious gram-negative bacillus, is one of the etiologic agents of neonatal sepsis and can be suspected if yellow-pigmented colonies are observed on sheep blood or chocolate agars in the absence of growth on MacConkey agar.

Although *Cryptococcus neoformans* grows well on blood and chocolate agars and does not require the use of special media, CSF should be inoculated to a nutritious medium, such as brain–heart infusion agar with blood, if an infection caused by slower-growing fungi is suspected. Media containing antibiotics is not required. The processing of cultures for the recovery of mycobacteria and viruses are discussed in Chapters 17 and 21, respectively.

In preparing CSF specimens for culture, the fluid should be centrifuged to concentrate any bacteria that may be present. Centrifugation is also recommended for the recovery of *M. tuberculosis* in cases of suspected tubercular meningitis. A volume of at least 5 mL must be processed to have any chance to recover mycobacteria. The sediment can then be plated directly to Lowenstein-Jensen (LJ) egg infusion medium and Middlebrook 7H11 agar. As an alternative to centrifugation for the recovery of cryptococci, the CSF can be passed through a 0.45-μm bacterial filter (Millipore Corporation, Bradford MA) to concentrate the yeast

---

TABLE 3-6

COMMENSAL FLORA AND PATHOGENIC BACTERIA IN THE CEREBROSPINAL FLUID

COMMENSAL FLORA (CONTAMINANTS)	POTENTIAL PATHOGENS	RECOMMENDED ISOLATION MEDIA
Coagulase-negative staphylococci	*Neisseria meningitidis*	Chocolate agar (or modified Thayer-Martin)
Most streptococci		
Diphtheroids	*Haemophilus influenzae* group b	Chocolate agar with staph streak or colistin and nalidixic acid (CNA) agar
Lactobacilli	*Streptococcus pneumoniae*	5% sheep blood agar
Propionibacterium spp.	*Listeria monocytogenes* (rare enterics)	MacConkey (or eosin methylene blue) agar for "enterics"
Escherichia coli and other *Enterobacteriaceae*	*E. coli* *Flavobacterium meningosepticum* *Mycobacterium tuberculosis* and other *Mycobacterium* spp. (particularly in patients with the acquired immunodeficiency syndrome)	5% sheep blood agar Löwenstein-Jensen or Middlebrook 7H11 media

cells. The filters should be placed face down on the surface of the agar and moved to a new location every 3 or 4 days to permit the detection of colonial growth.

An excellent review of the approach to the laboratory diagnosis of meningitis has been published by Gran and Fedorko.[64]

WOUNDS AND ABSCESSES

CLINICAL PRESENTATIONS

The accumulation of pus, either within an abscess or exuding from a sinus tract or from a mucocutaneous surface, is one of the cardinal indicators of local sepsis. Varying degrees of redness, pain, and swelling may also be present. Exogenous wound infections include those associated with traumatic injury wounds or decubitus ulcers, animal or human bites, burns, or foreign bodies in the skin or mucous membranes.

Endogenous wounds and abscesses may be associated with appendicitis, cholecystitis, cellulitis, dental infections, osteomyelitis, empyema, septic arthritis, sinusitis, or many other internal infections. Many of these infections are nosocomial derived, secondary to invasive procedures, surgical manipulations, or placement of prostheses. Others derive from hematogenous spread from other primary sites of infection or by direct extension of bacterial contaminants from ruptured viscera, particularly the large intestine.

COLLECTION OF SPECIMENS

Surface wounds are often colonized with environmental bacteria, and swab samples often do not reflect the true cause of the infectious process. Aspiration of the loculated fluid or pus from the depths of pustular or vesicular wounds and abscesses with a sterile needle and syringe are the most desirable methods for collecting material for culture. The site from which the culture is to be obtained should first be decontaminated with surgical soap and 70% ethyl or isopropyl alcohol. In the past, it was permissible to use the aspirating syringe as the transport container provided the needle was capped. This practice has come under scrutiny because of the chance of transmitting the HIV virus by a needlestick. In any event, if a delay in processing of more than 30 minutes is anticipated, the specimen should be transferred to an anaerobic transport container, several of which are commercially available.

If material cannot be obtained with a needle and syringe, and a swab must be used, it may be necessary either to separate the wound margins with the thumb and forefinger of one hand (wearing a sterile glove) or make a small opening in a closed abscess with a scalpel blade before extending the tip of the swab deeply into the depths of the lesion with the other hand. Care should be taken not to touch the adjacent skin margins. The swab should then be either placed immediately into an appropriate anaerobic transport container or inoculated directly to culture media for anaerobes depending on circumstances.

CULTURE OF SPECIMENS

Because wounds may be contaminated with commensal flora commonly inhabiting the skin and mucous membranes, both selective and enriched nonselective media should be used to recover both eugonic and fastidious bacterial species. The suggested media for recovery of the pathogenic bacterial species recovered from wounds and abscesses are listed in Table 3-7. Specimens should be inoculated to plates of a 5%

TABLE 3-7
COMMENSAL FLORA AND PATHOGENIC BACTERIA FROM WOUND SPECIMENS

COMMENSAL FLORA (CONTAMINANTS)	POTENTIAL PATHOGENS	RECOMMENDED ISOLATION MEDIA
Corynebacterium spp.	*Staphylococcus aureus*	5% sheep blood agar
α-Hemolytic streptococci	β-Hemolytic streptococci	5% sheep blood agar and MacConkey (or eosin methylene blue) agar
Coagulase-negative staphylococci	Coryneform JK bacillus	5% sheep blood agar
Propionibacterium spp.	Enterococcus spp.	5% sheep blood agar

Bacillus spp.	*Escherichia coli*
	 Proteus spp.
	 Pseudomonas aeruginosa and other pseudomonads
	 Mycobacterium marinum
	 Nocardia species
	 Anaerobes:
	   Peptostreptococci
	   Bacteroides spp.
	   Clostridium perfringens
	   Actinomyces israelii
		5% sheep blood agar
		
		 Löwenstein-Jensen egg medium at 25°–30°C
		
		 Prereduced and vitamin K_1-supplemented anaerobic blood agar plates.

sheep blood agar, MacConkey agar, and chocolate agar as a minimum. Other selective media, such as CNA and PEA may be used if heavy contamination with gram-negative organisms is suspected.

Review of a gram-stained smear prepared from the specimen may serve as a helpful guide to the selection of appropriate culture media. Inoculation of thioglycolate broth is generally discouraged because clinically significant anaerobes will be recovered on prereduced anaerobic blood agar. If thioglycolate broth is used for the recovery of anaerobes, the medium should contain hemin and vitamin K₁ supplements. A selective prereduced blood agar medium supplemented with hemin, vitamin K_1 (3-phytylmenadione), and L1-cystine, as described in Chapter 14, is the isolation medium of choice. Use of a second enriched, prereduced blood agar plate containing kanamycin and vancomycin is optional.

All other pathogenic organisms listed in Table 3-7 will grow on one or more of the culture media suggested. The exceptions are *Sporothrix schenckii* and other dimorphic, pathogenic molds. Several fungal isolation media are available; the use of inhibitory mold agar is highly recommended (see Chap. 19).

EYE, EAR, AND SINUS INFECTIONS

Suppurative material from the conjunctiva of an infected eye should be collected from the cul-de-sac or from the inner canthus. A direct Gram stain of the material obtained should be prepared to determine the type of bacteria present. If trachoma is suspected, conjunctival scrapings should be smeared onto a glass microscope slide, air-dried, and fixed in absolute methanol. Chlamydial antigen detection systems are now available that use fluorescent-tagged monoclonal antibodies. The presence of the characteristic elementary bodies of *C. trachomatis* indicates a positive test. The sensitivity of these techniques is approximately 95%, and the answers can be available within 1 hour.

Because *Haemophilus influenzae* and other *Haemophilus* species commonly cause conjunctivitis, either chocolate agar or hemophilus isolation media should be used (see Chap. 7). Chocolate agar will also recover other relatively fastidious organisms, such as *Moraxella* species and *N. gonorrhoeae*, that occasionally cause infections, particularly in newborns and young children. Particular attention should be paid to the recovery and immediate identification of *Pseudomonas aeruginosa* from eye cultures, because this organism can be highly virulent and lead to rapidly progressive blindness. *Bacillus subtilis* may also cause eye infections following traumatic injury. The recovery of saprobic molds, particularly *Aspergillus niger* and *Fusarium* species from the ear and eye, respectively, may indicate cases of mycotic otitis media and mycotic keratitis. A selective fungal isolation medium (inhibitory mold agar or SABHI, for example) should be set up in suspected cases.

The possibility of keratitis caused by free-living amoeba belonging to the genus *Acanthamoeba* must be kept in mind, particularly in people wearing soft contact lenses.[231] The organisms may be seen either by microscopically examining a mount of superficial material from the lesion suspended in water; or by inoculating the surface of a blood agar plate with a mixed suspension of the specimen presumed to contain amoeba with a subculture of *E. coli*. The amoeba will feed on the *E. coli* and can be detected by observing the plate through a dissecting microscope for small blotches in the lawn of bacterial growth, or for the telltale tracks as the amoeba push aside the bacterial colonies as they migrate (see Chap. 20 for a more detailed discussion).

Cultures of the external auditory canal generally do not reflect the bacterial cause of otitis media unless the tympanic membrane has recently ruptured. Tympanic membrane aspiration is rarely performed for obtaining material for culture. On occasion, cultures of the posterior pharynx may reveal the organisms causing otitis media.

Cultures from the maxillary, frontal, or other sinuses should be collected by the syringe aspiration technique and cultures set up for recovery of both aerobic and anaerobic bacteria. Polymicrobial infection, usually including several species of anaerobic bacteria, is often found in cases of chronic sinusitis.

INFECTIONS OF THE BLOOD

CLINICAL PRESENTATIONS

Septicemia is a clinical syndrome characterized by fever, chills, malaise, tachycardia, hyperventilation, and toxicity or prostration, which results when circulating bacteria multiply at a rate that exceeds removal by phagocytes. "Failure to thrive" may indicate chronic septicemia in infants.

Bacteremia may be transient, intermittent, or continuous, reflecting several basic entry mechanisms of bacteria into the bloodstream. Transient bacteremia may occur when organisms, often comprising the normal flora, are introduced into the blood (e.g., following brushing of teeth, straining during bowel movements, or after a manipulative procedure). Intermittent bacteremia often occurs when bacteria from an infected site are spasmodically released into the blood from extravascular abscesses, empyemic cavities, or diffuse infections (cellulitis, peritonitis, septic arthritis). Continuous bacteremia usually occurs in cases where organisms have direct access to the bloodstream, such as subacute bacterial endocarditis, infected arteriovenous fistulas, intra-arterial catheters, or indwelling cannulae. However, the source of organisms may not be determined in up to one-third of bacteremias.

Several mechanisms play a role in the removal of microorganisms from the bloodstream. In healthy and immunocompetent hosts, a sudden influx of bacteria is usually cleared from the blood within 30 to 45 minutes. The liver and spleen play the primary role in clearing bacteria; intravascular neutrophils play only a minor role. Encapsulated bacteria are more difficult to clear; however, the presence of specific antibodies promotes clearance. Patients with debilitating or immunodeficiency diseases are at higher risk because circulating bacteria may not be cleared from the blood for hours.

Several other risk factors have been investigated by Weinstein and associates.[253] In their study of 500 episodes of bacteremia and fungemia, the overall mortality rate was 42%, with approximately half of these deaths attributed directly to septicemia. Risk factors and the relative mortality rates for each are shown in Table 3-8. Bryan[25] also emphasizes how positive blood cultures identify a population of patients at high risk of death. In studies cited, the author states that patients with positive blood cultures were 12 times more likely to die during hospitalization than those with negative blood cultures. From these experiences, it is imperative that the laboratory perform blood cultures correctly and report accurate results as soon as possible.

The critical factors that must be decided by laboratory directors include the type of collection, number and timing of blood cultures, the volume of blood to be cultured, the amount and composition of the culture medium, when and how frequently to subculture, and the interpretation of results. The following is a brief summary of these factors; reviews by Bartlett and associates,[10] Reller and coworkers,[188] and Washington[250] can be consulted for details.

BLOOD CULTURE COLLECTION

Because the mortality rate from septicemia may be 40% or higher in certain populations of hospitalized patients,[253] the timely recovery of bacteria from the patient's blood (bacteremia) can have great diagnostic and prognostic importance.

Every precaution should be taken to minimize the percentage of contaminated blood cultures. A quality assurance monitor tracing the incidence of contaminated samples should be performed at least once in all microbiology laboratories. Less than 3% of blood cultures should be contaminated. Bates and associates[12] estimate that a contaminant blood culture can lead to an increase of as much as 20% to 39% in a patient's hospital bill from an extended stay for intravenous antibiotic therapy and additional tests. They also emphasize the need to always have paired blood culture samples to indicate likely contamination if only one of the sets turns positive.

To reduce the chance of contaminating organisms from the skin, the venipuncture site should ideally be prepared as follows: 1) wash with soap, 2) rinse with sterile water, 3) apply 1% to 2% tincture of iodine or povidone-iodine and allow to dry for 1 or 2 minutes, and 4) remove the iodine with a 70% alcohol wash. In practice, the soap wash is usually omitted; however, the combined use of iodine compound and alcohol to disinfect the venipuncture site is essential. If the site must again be palpated after the iodine–alcohol preparation, the finger must be disinfected or a sterile glove worn. If povidone-iodine is used, step 4 must be omitted. However, be sure the povidone-alcohol solution is dry before making the venipuncture.

Blood cultures may be obtained either by using a needle and syringe (Fig. 3-7) or by the closed system, consisting of a vacuum bottle and double-needle collection tube. Obtaining blood for culture from indwelling intravenous or intra-arterial catheters has generally been discouraged. However, in a study of 200 catheter blood cultures compared with an equal number of peripheral blood cultures drawn at the same time,[263] there was a 96% correlation in positive cultures and a 98% correlation with negative cultures. Collignon and Munro[34] discuss the clinical significance of positive blood cultures from catheter lines, concluding that the recovery of fewer organisms than 15 CFU by a semiquantitative technique they describe, is less likely to reflect true septicemia. Shulman and associates[214] have discovered that only the first 0.3 mL of blood in infants and 1.0 mL from children need be discarded from central venous catheters when obtaining blood cultures from this source, a volume of blood considerably less than previously thought.

TABLE 3-8
MORTALITY RATES AND RISK FACTORS ASSOCIATED WITH BACTEREMIA[253]

CONDITION	MORTALITY (%)	RELATIVE RISK OF DEATH
Age of Patient		
<20	13.8	1.00
21–40	32.8	2.33
41–50	42.9	3.06
>50	49.8	3.55
Type of Organism		
Nonfermenters	27.7	6.84
(Pseudomonas aeruginosa)		
Enterobacteriaceae		
Escherichia coli	35.5	3.36
Klebsiella pneumoniae	48.0	4.52
Gram-positive cocci		
Staphylococcus aureus	32.7	3.08
Streptococcus pneumoniae	22.0	2.08
Enterococci	45.5	4.28
Unimicrobial bacteremia	37.7	
Polymicrobial bacteremia	63.0	5.96
Fungi	67.7	
Source of Infection		
IV catheter	1.1	1.00
Genitourinary	14.9	1.35
Foley catheter	37.8	3.38
Surgical wound (and burns)	42.9	3.88
Abscess	51.2	4.65
Respiratory infection	52.3	4.73
Predisposing Conditions		
Surgery	16.3	0.78
Trauma	27.3	1.30
Diabetes mellitus	30.0	1.43
Corticosteroids	33.3	1.59
Renal failure	37.5	1.79
Neoplasm	42.1	2.01
Cirrhosis	71.5	3.40

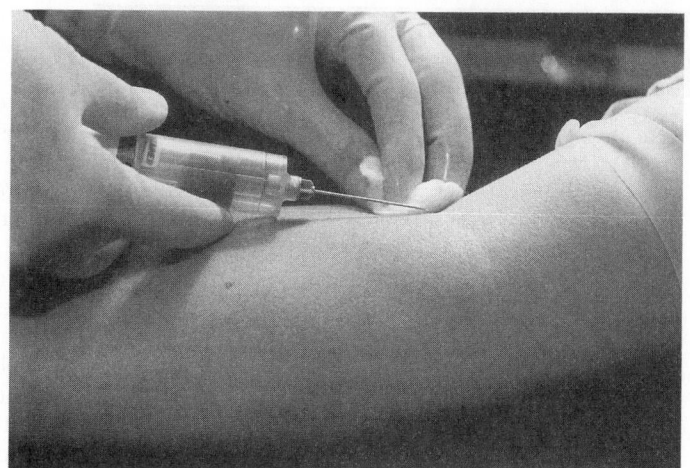

Figure 3-7.
Venipuncture technique for blood culture using a sterile needle and syringe: A tourniquet is applied to the upper arm above the venipuncture site to distend the antecubital veins. The site has previously been prepared with tincture of iodine and alcohol. The blood is removed with the syringe and needle and injected into an appropriate blood culture bottle. Rubber gloves must be worn during this procedure.

Because of the risk for acquiring hepatitis or HIV infections from accidental self-imposed needlesticks, the practice of switching to a sterile needle to inject blood culture bottles has been replaced by direct injection with the original phlebotomy needle. Krumholz and coworkers[120] found no significant difference in blood culture contamination rates between one group of patients for whom needles were switched between phlebotomy and injection of the bottles and the other group for whom needles were not switched. The validity of this study has been challenged.[48] On the other hand,[90] no significant difference was found in contamination rate in blood cultures from 303 children divided into three groups: no needle change (2.2% contamination rate), one needle change (0% contamination rate), and two needle changes (1.9% contamination rate). It was concluded that careful skin preparation is a more important than changing needles in reducing contamination of blood cultures. Independent studies,[29,220] also conclude that the changing of needles has no significant difference in contamination rates compared with direct injection.

NUMBER AND TIMING

Most investigators agree that routinely obtaining more than three blood cultures within 24 hours does not result in a significant increase in positive results.[10,188] Of cases ultimately proved to have positive blood cultures, 80% are positive within the first set, 90% by the second, and 99% by the third. Thus, a minimum of two blood culture sets per episode should be drawn.[251] One exception may be the situation described by Paisley and Lauer,[166] who suggest that in suspected community-acquired bacteremia in otherwise normal children, a single aerobic blood culture of adequate volume may be sufficient. In a study of hospital blood culture practices, Schifman and associates[201] discovered that the incidence of solitary blood cultures ranged from 1% to 99%, with a median of 26%. They estimate that as many as 18,000 episodes of bacteremia may be missed annually because of this practice. Between 20% and 30% of the solitary blood cultures they reviewed were not clinically indicated;

most of the others were ordered by physicians who were unaware that one culture is not sufficient. Focused intervention and global education have reduced solitary blood cultures from 40% to 24% in one hospital, and unnecessary draws were reduced from 38% to 12.5% in another hospital. They conclude that solitary blood cultures should be monitored in all hospitals and corrective actions be taken as appropriate.

Blood cultures should be drawn before the use of systemic antimicrobials if possible. However, just because a patient has been receiving antibiotics does not necessarily preclude obtaining samples, although this needs to be taken into consideration when culture results are interpreted.

Obtaining the blood culture one-half hour before a temperature spike is ideal because the highest concentration of organisms are circulating at that time. However, because the temperature spike is usually unpredictable, an educated guess must suffice in most cases when timing blood cultures. Box 3-5 lists guidelines for obtaining blood cultures in various conditions and situations.

It is general practice to draw sufficient blood for at least two bottles at each venipuncture; one is to be incubated anaerobically, the other vented through a cotton-plugged needle to allow atmospheric air to enter. This practice, however, is currently under challenge. A decline in the incidence of true anaerobic bacteremias has been documented.[41,44,210] In fact, Sharp[210] has recommended the use of two aerobic, rather than an aerobic and an anaerobic set, to increase the rate of yield, reserving the use of an anaerobic culture when clinically indicated. Most aerobic blood culture broths are in vacuum bottles that have a 5% to 10% concentration of CO_2 in the head gas to permit maximal yield of fastidious and CO_2-requiring (capnophilic) organisms to survive.

Murray and associates have further documented a significant change in the incidence of recovery of fungi (mostly yeasts) from blood cultures over the past decade, reaching a 3:1 ratio at Barnes Hospital in St. Louis.[156] These authors suggest that in institutions with a patient population who are at high risk for fungal infections, the advantage of replacing the anaero-

BOX 3-5. GUIDELINES FOR OBTAINING BLOOD CULTURES

In acute febrile illnesses (meningitis, bacterial pneumonia) when immediate empiric antibiotic therapy may be necessary, or for patients with infectious diseases (osteomyelitis, suppurative arthritis) who are to undergo emergency surgery, two separate samples should be drawn immediately in tandem, from opposite arms.

If the origin of a fever syndrome is unknown, two blood cultures can initially be drawn with an interval of 45 to 60 minutes. The reason for the time interval between draws is to determine if a continuous- or intermittent-seeding of the bloodstream exists. Two successive positive bottles drawn within a few minutes of each other may reflect the same bacteremic episode and are potentially less significant than two or more bottles drawn an hour or more apart in which recurrent bacteremia from an infective site is more probable. Two more sets of cultures can then be drawn 24 to 48 hours later, if necessary.

For patients with acute infective endocarditis, three blood cultures from three separate venipuncture should be drawn during the first 1 to 2 hours of evaluation and then therapy begun. In cases of suspected subacute bacterial endocarditis, obtain three blood cultures on the first day, spacing venipuncture at least 30 minutes apart. If these are negative, obtain two more sets on subsequent days. If cultures are persistently negative, despite positive clinical signs and symptoms (suspected culture-negative endocarditis with nutritionally dependent streptococci), the use of vitamin B_6 (pyridoxal)-supplemented culture media may be required (see Chap. 2).

bic bottle with a second aerobic bottle should be weighed. In fact, an increase in yield of microorganisms has been documented[151] when two aerobic bottles are used. In this study conducted at Duke University Medical Center, recovery rates from three different paired bottle systems were compared: 1) one aerobic and one anaerobic bottle (5 mL blood each); 2) two aerobic bottles (5 mL each); and 3) two aerobic bottles plus an extra anaerobic bottle when anaerobic infection was clinically suspected. The third approach had the largest yield of isolates. From their data, these investigators conclude that the use of two aerobic bottles with selective culturing for anaerobes will potentially increase the number of clinically important isolates by at least 6%.

VOLUME

Between 10 and 30 mL of blood should be drawn from adults during each venipuncture. The percentage yield of positive cultures drops significantly if less than 10 mL/bottle is obtained.[188] The need for a minimum of 10 mL up to a maximum 30 mL of blood per draw is also confirmed,[209] particularly for febrile immunocompromised patients and patients with infective endocarditis. There is a 17% increase in yield of positive blood cultures in patients from whom a 13- to 16-mL aliquot of blood has been drawn immediately after drawing a 6.5- to 8-mL aliquot.[7] The maximum average extra yield was as follows: S. aureus (26%), E. coli (16%), and S. pneumoniae (12%). In a study of over 13,000 blood cultures,[255] it was determined that the increase in yield of 10-mL draws over 5-mL draws was 7.2%, most marked for E. coli and other organisms belonging to the family Enterobacteriaceae. In infants and children who have a lower total blood volume, 1 to 5 mL of blood usually suffices for each culture. Blood for culture should be added to culture broth in a ratio of about 1:5 or 1:10 to dilute any inherent antibiotics, or other antibacterial substances.

In a hospital survey, Mermel and Maki[142] discovered that 15% of the blood culture specimens from adults had been drawn in 3.5-mL pediatric tubes, and another 5%, which was drawn in adult tubes, contained less than 5 mL of blood. In a matched pair study of 829 blood cultures with both standard volume (mean = 8.7 mL), and low-volume (mean = 2.7 mL), they found the detection rate of bloodstream infections were substantially reduced in the latter (92% compared with 69%). They estimated that the yield of blood cultures in adults increases approximately 3%/mL of blood cultured. Similarly, in a hospital audit,[178] only 17.5% of bottles examined contained the optimal amount of blood. Alfa and coworkers[3] warn that false-positive results will occur if bottles are overfilled. The vacuum in bottles may draw more than 10 mL; therefore, if phlebotomists are in the habit of drawing more than 10 mL of blood per draw and dividing the sample between more than one bottle, the first bottle may be overfilled. From these experiences, microbiology laboratory directors should consider implementing a blood culture volume quality assurance monitor and take remedial corrective actions as may be appropriate.

CULTURE MEDIUM

The medium used in blood culture bottles is multipurpose and nutritionally enriched: tryptic or trypticase soy, supplemented peptone broth, brain–heart infusion, Columbia broth, and brucella broth are commonly used. All are commercially available; however, variations in the composition of the same type of medium by different manufacturers makes comparisons and conclusions on the comparative yields of bacteria from each difficult to assess.

Most commercially available blood culture media contain the anticoagulant sodium polyanetholsulfonate (SPS) in concentrations varying from 0.025% to 0.05%. In addition to its anticoagulant properties (anticoagulation is a desired effect because certain bacteria do not survive well within the clot where phagocytosis by neutrophils and macrophages remains active), SPS also inactivates neutrophils and certain antibiotics, including streptomycin, kanamycin, gentamicin, and polymyxin, and precipitates fibrinogen, β-lipoproteins, B1C globulin, and other components of serum complement. SPS may also inhibit the growth of certain bacteria—*Peptostreptococcus anaerobius*, *N. gonorrhoeae*, *N. meningitidis*, and *Gardnerella vaginalis*. An anticoagulant culture broth may be required when one of these organisms is suspected of causing the septicemia. The inhibitory effect of SPS can be neutralized by adding gelatin to a final concentration of 1% to the medium.

Blood culture bottles with special broth formulations may be used in specific circumstances. Hypertonic sucrose (10%) has been advocated to improve the recovery of certain bacteria from patients receiving penicillin or cephalosporin analogues.[259] The use of these bottles has been largely discontinued in current practice.

Blood culture bottles incorporating synthetic antibiotic-removing resins (Antibiotic Removal Device [ARD]; Marion Laboratories, Inc. Kansas City MO, and the BACTEC 16 and 17 aerobic and anaerobic resin media, Johnston Laboratories, Townsend MD) into the broth has been advocated for use in patients who are receiving antibiotics. Significant improvement in the yield of some bacterial species from septicemic patients has been reported[131,247] through the use of resin bottles; Wright and associates,[264] on the other hand, could not corroborate these findings and suggest that any recommendations on the use of ARD await further studies. One such study has been conducted.[108] Of 1185 sets of blood cultures, aerobic BACTEC resin bottles (NR 16A and NR 17A) were more often positive (90 times versus 78) than standard BACTEC (NR 6A and NR 7A aerobic bottles); they yielded more organisms per culture and were more often positive after 1-day incubation. Also, in a study of 6839 paired blood cultures,[106] the use of resin media significantly improved the recovery of members of the family *Enterobacteriaceae*, *Enterococcus* species, *S. pneumoniae*, and viridans streptococci.

Blood cultures positive for *Mycobacterium* species, particularly in patients with AIDS, is on a marked increase. Shafer and coworkers[208] report that 15% of consecutive patients, in a study group in whom tuberculosis was newly diagnosed, had positive blood cultures for *M. tuberculosis*. Several mycobacterial blood culture media are currently available (BACTEC 13A bottles, Isolator/BACTEC 12B system, M7H11/BHI biphasic medium) to enhance recovery of mycobacteria from the blood, as recently reviewed.[2] This topic is covered in greater detail in Chapter 17.

LYSIS–CENTRIFUGATION BLOOD CULTURE SYSTEM

The Isolator system (formerly the DuPont Isolator, currently marketed by Wampole Laboratories, Cranbury NJ) is widely accepted as a blood culture method for improving the recovery of many microorganisms in suspected cases of septicemia, particularly fungemia. The Isolator is a special tube that contains saponin, a chemical that lyses both the red and the white blood cells. Approximately 7.5 to 10 mL of blood are added to the tube, which is then thoroughly mixed by inverting the tube several times, so that the lysis reaction can go to completion. The tube is then placed into an angle centrifuge and spun at 3000 rpm for 15 minutes to concentrate any microorganisms that may be present. After centrifugation, the sediment is aspirated and subcultured to appropriate media.

Several studies have shown that the collection and processing of blood cultures samples in Isolator tubes increases the percentage yield and decreases the time of recovery of certain microorganisms.[16,22,75,103,105,106,259] Bille and coworkers[16] showed a reduction of mean recovery time for yeasts from blood cultures from 4.90 days for conventional methods to 2.12 days for the Isolator (mean recovery rate of 8.0 days from 24.14 days in cases of *Histoplasma capsulatum* fungemia). They also found an overall 36.6% increase in the recovery rate of fungi from blood cultures through use of the Isolator system.

A two- to eightfold increase in contamination rates over conventional systems is the one significant problem in the use of the Isolator. The suggestion was made[111] that contamination can be reduced by using dry agar plates, disinfecting the work area, and processing samples in a vertical laminar air hood.

BLOOD CULTURE EXAMINATION

Blood culture bottles should be incubated at 35°C and examined visually for evidence of growth (hemolysis, gas production, or turbidity) during the first 6 to 18 hours after collection. For those using conventional broth media, bottles should be examined against bright fluorescent bulbs or with incandescent transmitted light. The surface of the sedimented blood layer should be examined because discrete colonies may be detected. Blind subcultures to chocolate agar plates should be made from all blood culture bottles (radiometric and agar–broth systems excluded) within 12 to 24 hours after collection and incubated aerobically in 5% to 10% CO_2 at 35°C. Blind anaerobic subcultures are usually not done in most laboratories. It is generally agreed, however, that both aerobic and anaerobic subcultures of all visually positive blood culture bottles should be set up.

Bottles should be visually examined daily for signs of growth. In a study of 20,155 blood culture bottles (trypticase soy broth and thiol broth),[153] only 32 trypticase soy bottles and 10 thiol bottles turned positive after 7 days of incubation. Fifteen of the 32 trypticase isolates and all of the thiol isolates were either recovered in other systems or were not considered clinically significant, indicating that holding blood cultures beyond 7 days is unnecessary. It has been confirmed[261] that 5 days of incubation are adequate when using the BacT/Alert blood culture system; however, certain fastidious organisms, including certain strains of *Brucella* and *Haemophilus* species, and relatively rare isolates of *Eikenella corrodens*, *Cardiobacterim hominis*, and *Actinobacillus* species may require longer incubation.

The routine microscopic examination of macroscopically negative blood culture bottles after 24 hours of incubation is probably not indicated because the number of organisms that can be detected by Gram stain (about 10^5 CFU) varies little from the 10^6 to 10^7 CFUs required to produce a visible turbidity of the broth.[188] Acridine orange stains are more sensitive, detecting 10^3 to 10^4 CFU/mL. Tierney and associates[242] report a 16.8% increase in the early detection of septicemia by examining macroscopically negative blood culture broths with the acridine orange stain.

AUTOMATED AND COMPUTERIZED BLOOD CULTURE SYSTEMS

The introduction of continuous-reading, automated and computed blood culture systems represents one of the significant advances in clinical microbiology practice over the past 5 years. Three such systems, the BacT/Alert (Organon Teknika, Durham NC), the BACTEC 9240/9120, and the Extra Sensing Power (ESP)(Difco Laboratories, Detroit MI), have found widespread use in the United States. The bioMerieux Vital blood culture system (bioMerieux Vitek, Hazelwood MO) has not received FDA clearance, although successful field trials have been conducted in Europe.

The BacT/Alert Blood Culture System. As the first continuous-monitoring blood culture system developed and marketed in the United States, the BacT/Alert system has found widespread implementation in clinical laboratories. Each blood culture bottle has a capacity to receive 10 mL of blood. As microorganisms grow in the blood–broth mixture, CO_2 is liberated. Bonded to the bottom of each bottle is a CO_2-sensitive chemical sensor that is separated from the blood–broth mixture by a unidirectional CO_2-permeable membrane. In the presence of CO_2, the sensor visibly turns from green to yellow, although the light-sensitive detector built into the instrument reacts before a color change is apparent.

Each bottle is placed bottom down into a receiving well in the data unit, directed by a bar code on the bottle label, which is integrated in the computer to match the patient identification data for each. Each data unit is a cabinet about the size of a small refrigerator which serves as a self-contained incubator, shaker, and detection device, with a capacity to hold either 240 or 120 bottles, depending on the model. Up to five modules can be linked through the same computer controls, reaching a total of 1440 bottles that can be monitored. The wells are arranged in two rows within a horizontal rack that gently rocks back and forth when the door to the data unit is closed. As each rack holds 20 bottles, 12 racks are contained in the 240 bottle data unit. At 10-minute intervals, a light beam from emitting diodes (one for each well) is projected through an excitation filter to reflect off the CO_2-sensitive sensor in the bottom of each bottle. The reflecting light is directed through an emission filter to a photosensitive detector that, in turn, is connected to a computer compiler. As soon as the accumulation of CO_2 is sufficient in the bottle to alter the sensor, an audible or visible "alert" is generated, and the position of the positive bottle is immediately flagged by the computer. Positive bottles can be immediately removed and further processed. A graph can be brought on the computer screen at any time to monitor the progress of CO_2 production.

The BACTEC 9440/9120 Blood Culture System. The BACTEC system consists of a self-contained incubator, agitator, and detection device, similar in appearance to the BacT/Alert system. There are two sizes, the 9240 model holds 240 bottles, the 9120 model holds 120 bottles; up to five modules can be linked to the same computer control unit. Similar to the BacT/Alert, each bottle has a sensor disk bonded to the inner bottom surface. The one operational difference between the BacT/Alert and the BACTEC systems is that the latter uses fluorescent, rather than spectral, light to detect changes in the CO_2 concentration in the broth–blood mixture. As CO_2 is produced in each bottle, its sensor emits a fluorescent light that passes an emission filter on the way to a light-sensitive diode. Bottles are also placed bottom down into receiving wells that are monitored once every 10 minutes. The voltage of the current reading of the diode is compared with the previous reading. If the voltage change exceeds a preset delta value, the microcomputer flags the bottle as positive. The position of the positive bottle is indicated on the computer screen, and that bottle can be pulled for further processing. A graph illustrating the progress of CO_2 production can be brought up on the computer screen at any time.

The whisky bottle shape of the blood culture bottle, with its long neck and excess headspace, does not require venting with atmospheric air after the blood culture is drawn, an advantage claimed by the manufacturer over the BacT/Alert bottle, which must be vented. The shape of the bottle also allows the blood to be drawn from the patient through a Vacutainer blood collection system, although this is not recommended by the manufacturer because of the danger of "back-flushing" of blood into the vein.

The Difco Extra Sensing Power (ESP) Blood Culture System. The Difco ESP blood culture system differs from the BacT/Alert and the BACTEC 9240/9120 system, described in the foregoing, as follows: 1) the production of CO_2 is monitored manometrically, 2) both gas consumption and production are monitored, and 3) changes in the concentrations of H_2 and O_2 in addition to CO_2 are detected.

The data unit is also a cabinet that serves as a self-contained incubator, agitator, and detector. Units with a capacity of 128 or 384 bottles are currently available, although more than one module can be linked to a central computer system. After inoculation of up to 10 mL of venous blood, each bottle is fitted with a disposable connector, which includes a recessed needle that penetrates the septum of the blood culture bottle. Each bottle is then placed in a defined position on a carrying rack that is aligned such that the connector attaches directly to a sensing probe located at the top of each position. Once the bottle is properly aligned, the pressure of the head gas is continuously monitored. A reading is taken every 12 minutes. When the change in reading exceeds a delta value, lights are illuminated that indicate the position of any positive bottle.

A reading may occur during a phase of consumption of H_2 and O_2. Oxygen consumption is accelerated at the time replicating organisms enter the log phase of growth. Therefore, a reading may be possible early in the incubation period before a detectable amount of CO_2 is produced. This is a distinct advantage for the ESP system, not only because readings usually occur 1 to 8 hours earlier than systems dependent only on CO_2 production; but also for the detection of asaccharolytic microorganisms that may never produce sufficient CO_2 to trip the indicator.

Vital Blood Culture System. The bioMerieux Vital blood culture system (bioMerieux Vitek, Hazelwood MO) is mechanically and electronically similar to the BacT/Alert and BACTEC 9240 systems. As yet, it has not received FDA approval and is not available in the United States, although it is in use in Europe. Each data unit consists of a cabinet containing four drawers within which are slots into which the blood culture bottles can be placed. The unique feature of this system is the incorporation of a soluble fluorescent molecule directly in the blood culture broth. As CO_2 accumulates in the broth–blood mixture, the detector molecules fluoresce, which is detected by a light ray directed through the center of each bottle. The position of the positive bottle is indicated through the computer database, and it can be easily removed and further processed.

O.A.S.I.S. Blood Culture System. The O.A.S.I.S. blood culture system (Unipath Ltd., Basingstoke, United Kingdom) is functionally similar to the Difco ESP system in that the production of CO_2 in the blood culture bottle is monitored manometrically by measuring changes in the headspace pressure. In contrast to the ESP system, the monitoring of pressure changes is noninvasive, achieved by monitoring the position of a flexible sealing septum with a scanning laser sensor. As with the ESP system, both the consumption and production of gas can be detected. In a field trial designed to evaluate the media, detection system, and associated detection algorithm,[232] the times to positivity were shorter with the O.A.S.I.S. system than with the BACTEC 460 system on samples run in parallel. The implementation of this system into clinical laboratories awaits the results of comparative clinical trials with other blood culture systems.

Manual Blood Culture Systems

THE OXOID SIGNAL SYSTEM. The Oxoid Signal System (Oxoid USA, Inc., Columbia MD) is a single-bottle blood culture system that also uses the production of CO_2 to determine early bacterial growth. The main blood culture bottle is similar to those used in other broth systems; however, the system uses a second plastic chamber, known as the signal chamber, which

is fitted at the bottom with a long needle. After the blood sample to be cultured has been inoculated into the main bottle, the signal chamber is connected by inserting the needle thorough the rubber stopper and positioning it below the surface of the culture medium. Growing and metabolizing bacteria produce CO_2. The resulting increase in pressure forces liquid into the signal chamber, which can be directly visualized and used for preparing Gram stains and subcultures. This system has been evaluated favorably.[154,204] A higher than normal number of false-positive results and a lower than normal yield of anaerobes remain problematical. Weinstein and coworkers[256] found an improved yield of organisms with the newly designed bottles that have an increased head-gas space and are subjected to agitation.

SEPTI-CHEK BLOOD CULTURE SYSTEM. The Septi-Chek (Roche Diagnostic Systems, Nutley NJ) biphasic agar slide blood culture system is also widely used. The Vacutainer agar–slant system (Becton Dickinson Vacutainer Systems, Rutherford NJ) is comparable in design with the Septi-Chek. These systems use a standard TSB broth blood culture bottle, designed for connection to a second plastic chamber that contains a paddle with agar surfaces. After the primary bottle is inoculated with the blood sample to be cultured, the plastic contained "slide" is screwed on. This slide contains a trisurface paddle faced with chocolate, MacConkey, and malt agar strips. The first "subculture" is made after 4 to 6 hours of incubation at 35°C by inverting the bottle and allowing broth to enter the slide's chamber, thereby flooding the agar surfaces. The bottle is then again placed upright for continuing incubation. The bottle can be inverted again at regular intervals to reinoculate the agar media on the paddle. The yield of certain bacterial species from the agar-slide systems is greater than obtained from conventional broth bottle methods.[49] Reimer and associates[186] found no statistical difference between the Septicheck and the Vacutainer agar–slant system in the overall recovery of clinically important microorganisms.

COMPARATIVE STUDIES

The comparative performance of these blood culture systems has been extensively studied over the past 5 years. Depending on the design of the study, the spectrum of microorganisms being recovered from clinical specimens, the volume of blood being cultured, and the exact types of bottles and media formulations being compared, one system may emerge as superior or inferior to another. Improvements in media formulations, the sensitivity of detectors, and the design of instruments continue to be made, and the results of a given study performed some months ago may not necessarily reflect the current technology. Therefore, each laboratory director and supervisor must weigh the previous results of other workers with the operation and needs of his or her individual laboratory when determining which if any new system should be implemented. Box 3-6 provides a selected and not inclusive

BOX 3-6. COMPARATIVE STUDIES

The BacT/Alert standard bottles are equivalent or superior to BACTEC radiometric and nonradiometric bottles.[254, 268]

The Pedi/BacT bottles are equivalent to the Isolator system for recovery of microorganisms in pediatric patients.[176]

The BactT/Alert standard bottles are inferior to the Isolator system for recovery of staphylococci and yeasts.[74, 133]

The BacT/Alert standard bottles are superior to the Isolator system in the speed of recovery and in the detection of aerobic and facultatively anaerobic gram-negative bacilli.[74]

The BacT/Alert FAN bottles are superior to BacT/Alert standard bottles in the recovery of both aerobic and anaerobic microorganisms.[254, 262]

The BacT/Alert Fan bottles are superior to the BACTEC Plus Aerobic/F bottles in the recovery of certain *Enterobacteriaceae* and *Pseudomonas aeruginosa* isolates and in the speed of detection of microbial *Staphylococcus aureus*.[177]

The BACTEC standard F bottles are equivalent or superior to BACTEC nonradiometric bottles in the recovery of microorganisms from blood cultures.[161]

The BACTEC Plus/Aerobic bottles are equivalent or superior to the oxoid signal system in the detection of microbial growth.[204]

The BACTEC Plus/F bottles are superior to BacT/Alert standard bottles in the detection of microbial growth.[221]

The BACTEC Aerobic Plus/F system detected microbial growth earlier than the Septi-Check Release system, although the latter showed an overall greater rate of recovery.[192]

The ESP system detected blood culture isolates in far less time than the Septi-Check system.[257]

The ESP system detected more organisms than did the BacT/Alert standard bottles, particularly *Staphylococcus aureus* and most anaerobic bacteria.[268]

The ESP system detected more organisms in a shorter time than the BACTEC NR660 system, particularly more yeasts, pneumococci, and episodes of bacteremia caused by *Staphylococcus epidermidis* and anaerobic bacteria.[149]

The ESP 80A and 80N bottles are inferior to the Isolator system in the overall detection of microorganisms in blood cultures.[33, 114]

---

list of recent comparative studies with cross-references that may be consulted for further information on how given systems have performed in research and clinical laboratories.

In summary, the advantages of continuous-monitoring blood culture systems include a decrease in laboratory work load, a decrease in the number of false-positive results and pseudobacteremia, a significant increase in the speed of detection and in the rate of microbial recovery. Disadvantages include a limited database for some systems, a limited selection of media selection, and the large size of the instruments for laboratories in which space is an issue. The decrease in laboratory work load is primarily because a technologist's time can be dedicated to processing only the positive cultures instead of loading and unloading instruments or subculturing and observing mostly negative specimens. However, because positive cultures may be "alerted" at any time requires an adjustment in staffing during off hours, depending on the requirements for reporting positive results to the clinical staff.

CLINICAL CONSIDERATIONS

To what extent the introduction of continuous-read blood culture systems has impinged on clinical practice is an important consideration. It can be argued by laboratory directors in whose laboratory manual or batch-read systems are in place, that to evaluate blood cultures on more than a 12- or 24-hour schedule is usually clinically irrelevant, in that most patients with clinical septicemia are covered empirically with antibiotics. The delay in obtaining a Gram stain evaluation or species identification of the organism(s) recovered does not usually affect clinical outcome, for the antibiotic regimen can then be changed if needed.

The counterargument holds that in institutions where continuous-read blood culture systems are in place, Gram stain information and species identifications occur on an average of 12 hours earlier than with manual systems. How access to early results may or may not affect the decision process of a given physician taking care of a patient with septicemia can only be anecdotal. To address this issue, the experience of implementing a continuous-read blood culture system in two Denver area hospitals can be cited.

The time to alert for positive blood cultures was analyzed for specimens submitted to the microbiology laboratories at the Denver Veterans Affairs Hospital between the period May 1993 through February 1994 ($n = 241$); and for the Provenant Health Care Partners (Denver Saint Anthony Central, Saint Anthony North, and Mercy Hospitals), for the period September through December 1993 ($n = 466$).[117] A BacT/Alert (Organon Teknika) continuous-read blood culture system was installed at the Denver VA Hospital and at St. Anthony Central Hospitals in April 1993 and April 1992, respectively. The data listed in Table 3-9 discloses that 24% of positive blood cultures were detected by 12 hours, 47% by 18 hours, and 63% by 24 hours at the Denver VA Hospital. At St. Anthony Central, percentage recovery rates for the same time periods were 44.8%, 61.5%, and 77.6%, respectively.

TABLE 3-9
BacT/Alert Blood Culture Study:
Relative Percentage Frequency of Positive Isolates

Veterans Affairs Hospital (n = 241)			Provenant Health Partners (n = 466)		
0–4 h	5	(2%)	0–4 h	16	(3.4%)
4–12 h	53	(22%)	4–12 h	183	(41.4%)
12–18 h	55	(23%)	12–18 h	78	(16.7%)
18–24 h	38	(16%)	18–24 h	75	(16.1%)
>24 h	90	(37%)	>24 h	104	(22.3%)

In Table 3-10 are listed the relative percentage frequency of bacterial species comprising 90% of the isolates recovered at the two hospitals. Although there is some insignificant difference in the order of the percentage recovery of bacterial species between the two institutions, some of this is artifactual in that there is less tendency at St. Anthony Central Hospital to definitively make species identifications, particularly for the coagulase-negative staphylococci. The only significant difference between the two institutions was the higher rate of recovery of S. pneumoniae from blood cultures submitted from the Provenant Partner Hospitals. Because almost all S. pneumoniae isolates were detected within 12 hours, it was felt that many cases may have been missed before the installation of the instrument because self-lysis of the bacterial cells may have occurred before the delayed reading of bottles inherent in the previous manual system.

The time to detection and the slope of the "growth curve" may have clinical meaning in some cases. Figure 3-8 illustrates the patterns of four basic curves within which the great majority of blood culture isolates fall. The rapid time to detection and steep slope of curve A most commonly is clinically significant, reflecting a relatively high concentration of circulating organisms at the time the blood cultures were drawn. For example, at the Denver VA Hospital, approximately 20% of Staphylococcus epidermidis blood culture isolates are re-

covered within 12 hours, usually from patients with indwelling line catheter infections. In contrast, 38% of S. epidermidis blood culture isolates are recovered after 24 hours (curve B or C). These most likely represent skin contaminants, usually of little clinical significance. E. coli and other members of the family Enterobacteriaceae become positive within 12 hours, reflecting the rapid doubling time of these isolates; most isolates of S. pneumoniae also follow this curve.

Many of the isolates following curve B are also clinically significant, representing a low inoculum of a pathogen at the time the blood is drawn, a slower-metabolizing organism, or an asaccharolytic species with low CO_2 output. Most of the bacterial species following curve C are clinically insignificant. One exception are yeast isolates, the alert for which is often delayed to 3 days or more. Curve D demonstrates a gradual production of CO_2, so slow that the delta change needed for an alert is not present. This curve is often seen in bottles that are overfilled, that have high white blood cell counts; or, on occasion, is produced by a slowly growing microorganism. It is not uncommon for Propionibacterium acnes to produce an alert between 4 and 5 days, almost always representing skin contamination.

Although these experiences do not solve the clinical relevance issue, nonetheless, conversations with several infectious disease specialists result in an almost unanimous affirmation that "sooner is better." In particular, many house officers at the Denver VA Hospital find it extremely valuable to know at 10:00 p.m. that a blood culture is positive with "gram-positive cocci in clusters" (or in chains), or with "short, fat gram-negative bacilli most likely one of the Enterobacteriaceae" rather than having to wait until the following morning for results. Several cases were specifically mentioned for whom being able to administer specific antibiotics was thought to significantly alter the course of a septicemia for the better. Although the BacT/Alert system was used in the studies presented in the foregoing, the results can be extrapolated to institutions using other continuous reading systems. One hopes that with ongoing experiences in many institutions, objective data

TABLE 3-10
BacT/Alert Blood Culture Study: Relative Percentage Frequency of Isolates by Species

Veterans Affairs Hospital (n = 202)			Provenant Health Partners (n = 209)		
Staphylococcus epidermidis, 44	(21.7%)		Staphylococcus spp., 48	(22.9%)	
Staphylococcus aureus, 36	(17.8%)		Escherichia coli, 33	(15.7%)	
Enterobacteriaceae spp., 24	(11.9%)		Streptococcus spp., 25	(12.0%)	
Streptococcus spp., 22	(10.9%)		Staphylococcus aureus, 25	(12.0%)	
Escherichia coli, 21	(10.4%)		Streptococcus pneumoniae, 22	(10.5%)	
Staphylococcus spp., 21	(10.4%)		Propionibacterium acnes, 12	(5.7%)	
Streptococcus pneumoniae, 7	(3.5%)		Staphylococcus epidermidis, 11	(5.3%)	
Propionibacterium acnes, 4	(2.0%)		Enterobacteriaceae spp., 10	(4.9%)	
Miscellaneous, 23	(11.4%)		Miscellaneous, 23	(11.0%)	

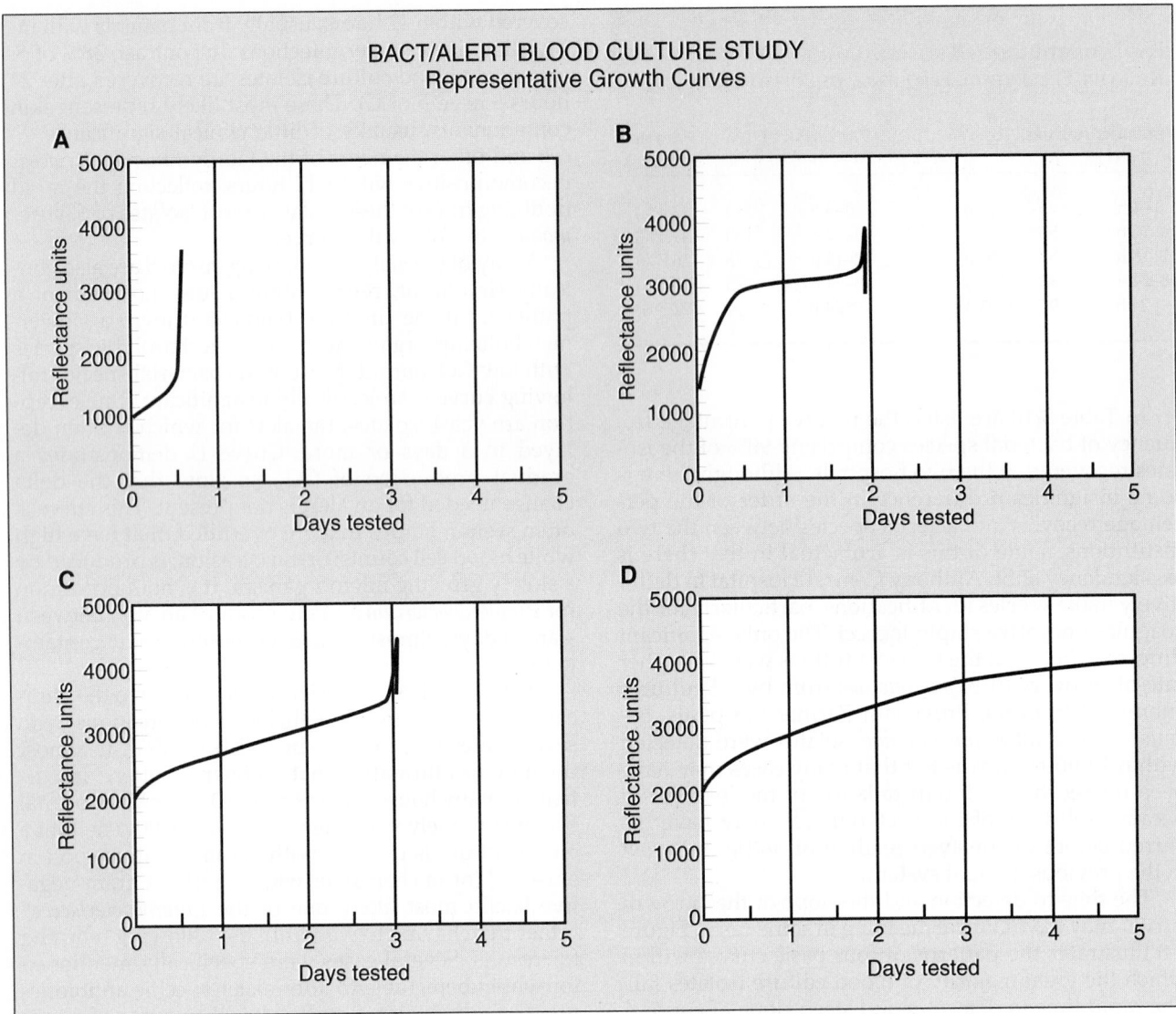

Figure 3-8.
Four prototype "growth curves" generated by the BacT/Alert Blood Culture system:
Curve *A* illustrates a short time to "alert" and a steep slope of the curve, most commonly
reflecting significant septicemia. Curve *B* demonstrates a time to alert within 2 days, representing either a slow-growing pathogen or one that produces CO_2 slowly. Curve *C* usually represents a skin contaminant in which a few bacterial cells were introduced into the
blood culture bottle during venipuncture. This curve, however, is often seen with certain
species of yeasts that tend to be slower growing or are weakly saccharolytic. Curve *4* represents an artifact caused by overfilling the bottle or a high white cell count in which low
levels of CO_2 are continuously being produced. *Propioniobacterium acnes* often produces an
alert between 4 and 5 days, usually representing a skin contaminant. Clinical correlation is
required to rule out a very slow-growing pathogen (such as *Brucella* spp., for example).

will be forthcoming in the near future to better resolve
this issue.

TISSUES AND BIOPSIES

Tissue samples for culture should be delivered
promptly to the laboratory in sterile gauze or in a
suitably capped, sterile container. Formalinized specimens are not suitable for culture unless the exposure

time has been short and the culture can be obtained
from a central portion of the tissue not exposed to
formalin.

Bone marrow cultures may be helpful in establishing the diagnosis of infectious granulomatous diseases
such as brucellosis, histoplasmosis, and tuberculosis.
Using the Isolator system to process the bone marrow
samples may be helpful in improving the recovery of
bacteria, particularly if the infections are caused by intracellular organisms.

REFERENCES

1. ADDISS DG, MATHEWS HM, STEWART JM, ET AL: Evaluation of a commercially available enzyme-linked immunosorbent assay for *Giardia lamblia* antigen in stool. J Clin Microbiol 29:1137–1142, 1991

2. AGY MB, WALLIS CK, PLORDE JJ, ET AL: Evaluation of four mycobacterial blood culture media. Diagn Microbiol Infect Dis 12:303–308, 1989

3. ALFA M, SANCHE S, ROMAN S, ET AL: Continuous quality improvement for introduction of automated blood culture instruments. J Clin Microbiol 33:1185–1191, 1995

4. ALLEN BW, DARRELL JH: Contamination of specimen container surfaces during sputum collection. J Clin Pathol 36:479–481, 1983

5. ALLES AJ, WALDRON MA, SIERRA LS, MATTIA AR: Prospective comparison of direct immunofluorescence and conventional staining methods for detection of *Giardia* and *Cryptosporidium* spp. in human fecal specimens. J Clin Microbiol 33:1632–1634, 1995

6. AN Q, LIU J, O'BRIEN W, ET AL: Comparison of characteristics of Q beta replicase-amplified assay with competitive PCR assay for *Chlamydia trachomatis*. J Clin Microbiol 33:58–63, 1995

7. APRI M, BENTZON MW, JENSEN J, FREDERIKSEN W: Importance of blood volume cultured in the detection of bacteremia. Eur J Clin Microbiol Infect Dis 8:838–842, 1989

8. BARTLETT JG, ET AL: Should fiberoptic bronchoscopy aspirates be cultured? Am Rev Respir Dis 114:73–78, 1976

9. BARTLETT RC, TETREAULT CJ, EVERS J, ET AL: Quality assurance of gram-stained direct smears. Am J Clin Pathol 72:984–990, 1979

10. BARTLETT RC, ELLNER PD, WASHINGTON JA II: Cumitech 1: Blood Cultures. Coordinating ed., JC Sherris. Washington DC, American Society for Microbiology, 1974

11. BARTELUK RL, NOBLE MA: Routine culturing of stool specimens for *Yersinia enterocolitica*. J Clin Microbiol 1616, 1988

12. BATES DW, GOLDMAN L, LEE TH: Contaminant blood cultures and resource utilization: The true consequences of false-positive results. JAMA 265:365–369, 1991

13. BEEBE JL, RAU MP, FLAGEOLLE S, ET AL: Incidence of *Neisseria gonorrhoeae* isolates negative by Syva direct fluorescent-antibody test but positive by Gen-Probe Accuprobe test in a sexually transmitted disease clinic population. J Clin Microbiol 31:2535–2537, 1993

14. BERGER SA, BOGOKOWSKY B, BLOCK C: Rapid screening of urine for bacteria and cells by using a catalase reagent. J Clin Microbiol 28:1066–1077, 1990

15. BHISITKUL DM, HOGAN AE, TANZ RR: The role of bacterial antigen detection tests in the diagnosis of bacterial meningitis. Pediatr Emerg Care 10:67–71, 1994

16. BILLE J. EDSON RS, ROBERTS GD: Clinical evaluation of the lysis–centrifugation blood culture system for the detection of fungemia and comparison with a conventional biphasic broth blood culture system J Clin Microbiol 19:126–128, 1984

17. BIRKENMEYER L, ARMSTRONG AS: Preliminary evaluation of the ligase chain reaction for specific detection of *Neisseria gonorrhoeae*. J Clin Microbiol 30:3089–3094, 1992

18. BLASER MJ, BERKOWITZ ID, LAFORCE FM, ET AL: *Campylobacter* enteritis: clinical and epidemiological features. Ann Intern Med 91:179–185, 1979

19. BOOM WH, PIPER DJ, RUOFF KL, ET AL: New cause for false-positive results with the cryptococcal antigen test by latex agglutination. J Clin Microbiol 22:856–857, 1985

20. BOWIE WR, HOMES KK: *Chlamydia trachomatis*. In Mandell GL, Douglas RG Jr, Bennett JE (eds): Principles and Practice of Infectious Diseases, 3rd ed, pp 1426–1437. New York, Churchill Livingstone, 1990

21. BRADBURY SM: Collection of urine specimens in general practice—to clean or not to clean? J R Coll Gen Pract 38:363–365, 1988

22. BRANNON P, KIEHN TE: Large scale clinical comparison of the lysis centrifugation and radiometer systems for blood culture. J Clin Microbiol 22:951–954, 1985

23. BRISITKUL DM, HOGAN AE, TANZ RR: The role of bacterial antigen detection tests in the diagnosis of bacterial meningitis. Pediatr Emerg Care 10:67–71, 1994

24. BRISELDEN AM, MONCLA BJ, STEVENS CE, HILLIER SL: Sialidases (neuraminidases) in bacterial vaginosis and bacterial vaginosis-associated microflora. J Clin Microbiol 30:663–666, 1992

25. BRYAN CS: Clinical implications of positive blood cultures. Clin Microbiol Rev 2:329–353, 1989

26. CAMPOS JM, CHARILAOU CC: Evaluation of Detect-A-Strep and the Culturette ten-minute strep ID kits for detection of group A streptococcal antigen in oropharyngeal swabs from children. J Clin Microbiol 22:145–148, 1985

27. CATRY MA, BORREGO MJ, CARDOSO J, ET AL: Comparison of the Amplicor *Chlamydia trachomatis* test and cell culture for the detection of urogenital chlamydial infections. Genitourin Med 71:247–250, 1995

28. CHAN EL, BRANDT K, HORSMAN GB: A 1-year evaluation of Syva MicroTrak *Chlamydia* enzyme immunoassay with selective confirmation by direct fluorescent-antibody assay in a high volume laboratory. J Clin Microbiol 32:2208–2211, 1994

29. CHAPNICK EK, SCHAFFER BC, GRADON JD, ET AL: Technique for drawing blood for cultures: is changing needles truly necessary? South Med J 84:1197–1198, 1991

30. CHARENSKY MA, JANG D, LEE H, ET AL: Diagnosis of *Chlamydia trachomatis* infections in men and women by testing first-void urine by ligase chain reaction. J Clin Microbiol 32:2682–2685, 1994

31. CHASTRE J, FAGON JY, SOLER P, ET AL: Diagnosis of nosocomial bacterial pneumonia in intubated patients undergoing ventilation: Comparison of the usefulness of bronchoalveolar lavage and the protected specimen brush. Am J Med 85:499–506, 1988

32. CHAUDHURI PP, SENGUPTA K, MANNA B, ET AL: Detection of specific anti-*Giardia* antibodies in the serodiagnosis of symptomatic giardiasis. J Diarrh Dis Res 10:151–155, 1992

33. COCKERILL FR, TORGERSON CA, REED GS, ET AL: Clinical comparison of Difco ESP, Wampole Isolator, and Becton Dickinson Septi-Check aerobic blood culturing systems. J Clin Microbiol 34:20–24, 1996

34. COLLIGNON PJ, MUNRO R: Laboratory diagnosis of intravascular catheter associated sepsis. Eur J Clin Microbiol Infect Dis 8:807–814, 1989

35. COLOMBRITA D, RAVIZZOLA G, PIRALI F, ET AL: Evaluation of BACTEC system for urine culture screening. J Clin Microbiol 27:118–119, 1989

36. COOK RL, RENDONDO-LOPEZ V, SCHMITT C, ET AL: Clinical, microbiological and biochemical factors in recurrent bacterial vaginosis. J Clin Microbiol 30:870–877, 1992

37. CUEVAS LE, HART CA, MUGHOGHO: Latex particle agglutination tests as an adjunct to the diagnosis of bacterial meningitis: a study from Malawi. Ann Trop Med Parasitol 83:375–379, 1989

38. DELOZIER JS, AUERBACH PS: The leukocyte esterase test for detection of cerebrospinal fluid leukocytosis and bacterial meningitis. Ann Emer Med 18:1191–1198, 1989

39. DOMEIKA M, BASSIRI M, MARDH PA: Diagnosis of genital *Chlamydia trachomatis* infections in asymptomatic males by testing urine by PCR. J Clin Microbiol 32:2350–2352, 1994

40. DONOWITZ GR, MANDELL GL: Acute pneumonia. In Mandell GL, Douglas RG Jr, Bennett JE (eds): Principles and Practice of Infectious Diseases, 3rd ed, pp 540–555. New York, Churchill Livingstone, 1990

41. DORSHER CW, ROSENBLATT JE, WILSON WR, ET AL: Anaerobic bacteremia: decreasing rate over a 15 year period. Rev Infect Dis 13:633–636, 1991.

42. DROW DL, BAUM CH, HIRSCHFIELD G: Comparison of the Lumac and Monolight systems for detection of bacteriuria by bioluminescence. J Clin Microbiol 20:797–801, 1984

43. DUGUID H, DUNCAN J. PARATT D, ET AL: *Actinomyces* and intrauterine devices. JAMA 248:1579–1580, 1982

44. DUNNE WM JR, TILLMAN J, HAVENS PL: Assessing the need for anaerobic medium for the recovery of clinically significant blood culture isolates in children. Pediatr Infect Dis J 13:203–106, 1994

45. EBRIGHT JR, SMITH KE, DREXLER L, ET AL: Evaluation of modified Stuart's medium in Culturettes for transport of *Neisseria gonorrhoeae*. Sex Transm Dis 9:45–47, 1983

46. ECHENBACH DA, HILLIER S. CRITCHLOW C, ET AL: Diagnosis and clinical manifestations of bacterial vaginosis. Am J Obstet Gynecol 158:819–828, 1988

47. EL KHOLY A, WANNAMAKER LW. KRAUSE RM. Simplified extraction procedure for serological grouping of beta-hemolytic streptococci. Appl Microbiol 28:836–839, 1974

48. ELLIOTT WO: Switching phlebotomy needles (letter). Ann Intern Med 114:94, 1991

49. EVANS FO, SYNDOR JB, MOORE WEC, ET AL: Sinusitis of the maxillary antrum. N Engl J Med 293:735–739, 1975

50. EWANOWICH CA, CHUI LW, PARANCHYCH MG, ET AL: Major outbreak of pertussis in Northern Alberta, Canada: analysis of discrepant direct fluorescent-antibody and culture results by using polymerase chain reaction methodology. J Clin Microbiol 311715–1725, 1993

51. FACKLAM RR: Specificity study of kits for detection of group A streptococci directly from throat swabs. J Clin Microbiol 25:504–508, 1987

52. FAUR YC, WEISBURD MH, WILSON ME: The selectivity of vancomycin and lincomycin in NYC medium for the recovery of *N. gonorrhoeae* from clinical specimens. Health Lab Sci 15:22–27, 1978

53. FEUERBORN SA, CAPPS WI, JONES JC: Use of latex agglutination testing in diagnosing pediatric meningitis. J Fam Pract 34:276–179, 1992

54. FONSECA K, MEGRAN DW, ANAND CM: Detection of *Chlamydia trachomatis* antigen by enzyme immunoassay: importance of confirmatory testing. J Clin Pathol 48:214–217, 1995

55. FORBES BA, BARTHOLOMA N, MCMILLAN J, ET AL: Evaluation of a monoclonal antibody test to detect chlamydia in cervical and urethral specimens. J Clin Microbiol 23:1136–1127, 1986

56. FRAYHA H, CASTRICIANO S, MAHONY J, CHERNESKY M: Nasopharyngeal swabs and nasopharyngeal aspirates equally effective for the diagnosis of viral respiratory diseases in hospitalized children. J Clin Microbiol 27:1387–1389, 1989

57. GARCIA LS, SHUM AC, BRUCKNER DA: Evaluation of a new monoclonal antibody combination reagent for direct fluorescence detection of *Giardia* cysts and *Cryptosporidium* oocysts in human fecal specimens. J Clin Microbiol 30:3255–3257, 1992

58. GILLIGAN PH, FISHER MC: Importance of culture in the laboratory diagnosis of *Bordetella pertussis* infections. J Clin Microbiol 20:891–893, 1984

59. GERBER MA, RANDOLPH MF, DEMEO KK: Liposome immunoassay for rapid identification of group A streptococci directly from throat swabs. J Clin Microbiol 28:1463–1464, 1990

60. GERBER MA, RANDOLPH MF, TILTON RC: Enzyme fluorescence procedure for rapid diagnosis of streptococcal pharyngitis. J Pediatr 108:421–423, 1985

61. GERSH I, KARSH H, KONEMAN EW: Asymptomatic chronic gonorrhoea in a male patient. Rocky Mt Med J 73:36–40, 1976

62. GLECKMAN R, DEVITA J, HIBERT D, ET AL: Sputum Gram stain assessment in community-acquired bacteremic pneumonia. J Clin Microbiol 26:846–849, 1988

63. GOODMAN LJ, KAPLAN RL, LANDOU W, ET AL: A urine preservative system to maintain bacterial counts. A laboratory and clinical evaluation. Clin Pediatr 24:383–386, 1985

64. GRAY LD, FEDORKO DP: Laboratory diagnosis of bacterial meningitis. Clin Microbiol Rev 5:130–145, 1992

65. GREENWOOD JR, PICKETT MJ, MARTIN WJ, ET AL: *Haemophilus vaginalis* (*Corynebacterium vaginale*): method for isolation and rapid biochemical identification. Health Lab Sci 14:102–106, 1977

66. GRIGORIEW GA, WALMSLEY S, LAW L, ET AL: Evaluation of the Merifluor immunofluorescent assay for the detection of *Cryptosporidium* and *Giardia* in sodium acetate formalin-fixed stools. Diagn Microbiol Infect Dis 19:89–91, 1994

67. GUERRANT RL: Gastrointestinal infections and food poisoning. Principles and definition of syndromes. In Mandell GL, Douglas RG Jr, Bennett JE (eds): Principles and Practice of Infectious Diseases, 3rd ed, p 839. New York, Churchill Livingstone, 1990

68. GWALTNEY JM JR: Pharyngitis. In Mandell GL, Douglas RG Jr, Bennett JE: Principles and Practice of Infect Disease, 3rd ed, Chap 43. New York, Churchill Livingstone, 1990

69. HARDY DJ, HULBERT BB, MIGNEAULT PC: Time to detection of positive BacT/Alert blood cultures and lack of need for routine subculture of 5- to 7-day negative cultures. J Clin Microbiol 30:2743–2745, 1992

70. HARLASS FF, DUFF P, HERD M: The evaluation of urine pH in screening for asymptomatic bacteriuria in pregnancy. Milit Med 155:49–51, 1990

71. HE Q, MERTSOLA J, SOINI H, ET AL: Comparison of polymerase chain reaction with culture and enzyme immunoassay for diagnosis of pertussis. J Clin Microbiol 31:642–645, 1993

72. HEELAN JS, CORPUS L, KESSIMIAN, N: False-positive reactions in the latex agglutination test for *Cryptococcus neoformans* antigen. J Clin Microbiol 29:1260–1261, 1991

73. HEITER BJ, BOURBVEAU PP: Comparison of the Gen-Probe Group A Streptococcus Direct Test with culture and a rapid streptococcal antigen detection assay for diagnosis of streptococcal pharyngitis. J Clin Microbiol 31:2070–2073, 1993

74. HELLINGER WC, CAWLEY JJ, ALVAREZ S, ET AL: Clinical comparison of the Isolator and BacT/Alert aerobic blood culture systems. J Clin Microbiol 33:1787–1790, 1995

75. HENRY NK, GREWELL CM, VAN GREVENHOF PE, ET AL: Comparison of lysis–centrifugation with a biphasic blood culture medium for the recovery of aerobic and facultatively anaerobic bacteria. J Clin Microbiol 20:413–416, 1984

76. HENRY NK, GREWELL CM, MCLIMANS CA, ET AL: Comparison of the Roche Septi-Check blood culture bottle with a brain heart infusion biphasic medium bottle and with a tryptic soy broth bottle. J Clin Microbiol 19:314–317, 1984

77. HERRMANN JE, BLACKLOW NR, PERRON DM, ET AL: Monoclonal antibody enzyme immunoassays for the detection of rotavirus in stool specimens. J Infect Dis 152:830–832, 1985

78. HERSCHL AM, BRANDSTATTER G, DRAGOSICS B, ET AL: Kinetics of specific IgG antibodies for monitoring the effect of anti-*Helicobacter pylori* chemotherapy. J Infect Dis 168:763–766, 1993

79. HILL DR: *Giardia lamblia*. In Mandell GL, Douglas RG Jr, Bennett JE (eds): Principles and Practice of Infectious Diseases, 3rd ed, pp 2110–2115. New York, John Wiley & Sons, 1990

80. HILL RB, ADAMS S, GUNN BA, EBERLY BJ: The effects of nonclassic pediatric bacterial pathogens on the usefulness of the Directigen latex agglutination test. Am J Clin Pathol 101:729–732, 1994

81. HODGE DS, TERRO R: Comparative efficacy of liquid enrichment medium for isolation of *Campylobacter jejuni*. J Clin Microbiol 19:434, 1984

82. HOLMBERG SP, SHELL WL, FANNING GR, ET AL: *Aeromonas* intestinal infections in the United States. Ann Interm Med 105:683–689, 1986

83. HOLMES KK: The chlamydia epidemic. JAMA 245:1718–1723, 1981

84. HOLST E, GOFFENG AR, ANDERISCH B: Bacterial vaginosis and vaginal microorganisms in idiopathic premature labor and association with pregnancy outcomes. J Clin Microbiol 32:176–186, 1994

85. HOPPE JE: Methods for isolation of *Bordetella pertussis* from patients with whooping cough. Eur J Clin Microbiol Infect Dis 7:616–620, 1988

86. HOWARD LV, COLEMAN PF, ENGLAND BJ, ET AL: Evaluation of Chlamydiazyme for the detection of genital infections caused by *Chlamydia trachomatis*. J Clin Microbiol 23:319–332, 1986

87. HUBBARD WA, SHALES PJ, MCCLATCHEY KD: Comparison of the B-D urine culture kit with a standard culture method and with MS-2. J Clin Microbiol 17:327–331, 1983

88. HUCK W, REED, BD, FRENCH T, MITCHELL RS: Comparison of the Directigen 1-2-3 group A strep test with culture for detection of group A beta-hemolytic streptococci. J Clin Microbiol 27:1715–1718, 1989

89. HUTCHINSON NA, THOMAS FD, SHANSON DC: The clinical comparison of Oxoid Signal with Bactec blood culture systems for the detection of streptococcal and anaerobic bacteraemias. J Med Microbiol 3l7:410–412, 1992

90. ISAACMAN DJ, KARASIC RB: Lack of effect of changing needles on contamination of blood cultures. Pediatr Infect Dis J 9:274–278, 1990

91. ISENBERG HD, WASHINGTON JA II, DOERN GV, AMSTERDAM D: Specimen collection and handling. In Balows A (ed), Manual of Clinical Microbiology, 5th ed. Washington DC, American Society for Microbiology, 1991

92. IWEN PC, WALKER RA, WARREN KI, ET AL: Evaluation of nucleic acid-based test (PACE 2C) for simultaneous detection of *Chlamydia trachomatis* and *Neisseria gonorrhoeae* in endocervical specimens. J Clin Microbiol 33:2587–2591, 1995

93. JEWKES FE, MCMASTER DJ, NAPIER WA, ET AL: Home collection of urine specimens—boric acid bottles or Dipslides? Arch Dis Child 65:286–289, 1990

94. JONES DM, ELDRIDGE J, FOX AJ, ET AL: Antibody to the gastric campylobacter-like organism (*Campylobacter pyloridis*): clinical correlation and distribution in the normal population. J Med Microbiol 22:57–62, 1986

95. JONES C, MACPHERSON DW, STEVENS DL: Inability of the Chemstrip LN compared with quantitative urine culture to predict significant bacteriuria. J Clin Microbiol 23:160–162, 1986

96. JONES MF, SMITH TF, HOUGLUM AJ, ET AL: Detection of *Chlamydia trachomatis* in genital specimens by the Chlamydiazyme test. J Clin Microbiol 20:465–467, 1984

97. JUCHAU SV, NACKMAN R, RUPPART D: Comparison of Gram stain with DNA probe for detection of *Neisseria gonorrhoeae* in urethras of symptomatic males. J Clin Microbiol 33:3068–3069, 1995

98. KACHORIS M, ROUFF KL, WELCH K, ET AL: Routine culture of stool specimens for *Yersinia enterocolitica* is not a cost-effective procedure. J Clin Microbiol 26:582–583, 1988

99. KELLOG JA, BANKERT DA, MANZELLA JP, ET AL: Clinical comparison of Isolator and thiol broth with ESP aerobic and anaerobic bottles for recovery of pathogens from blood. J Clin Microbiol 32:2050–2055, 1994

100. KAYE E: Antibacterial activity of human urine. J Clin Invest 42:2374–2390

101. KELLOGG JA.: Suitability of throat culture procedures for detection of group A streptococci and as reference standards for evaluation of streptococcal antigen detection kits. J Clin Microbiol 28:165–169, 1990

102. KELLOGG JA: Impact of variation in endocervical specimen collection and testing techniques on frequency of false-positive and false-negative Chlamydia detection results. Am J Clin Pathol 104:554–559, 1995

103. KELLOGG JA, MANZELLA JP, MCCONVILLE JH: Clinical laboratory comparison of the 10-mL Isolator blood culture system with BACTEC radiometric blood culture media. J Clin Microbiol 20:618–623, 1984

104. KELLOGG JA, ORWIG LK: Comparison of GonoGen, GonoGen II, and MicroTrak Direct Fluorescent-Antibody test with carbohydrate fermentation for confirmation of culture isolates of Neisseria gonorrhoeae. J Clin Microbiol 33:474–476, 1995

105. KELLY MT, BUCK GE, FOJTASEK MF: Evaluation of a lysis–centrifugation and biphasic bottle blood culture system during routine use. J Clin Microbiol 18:554–557, 1983

106. KELLY MT, ROBERTS, FJ, HENRY D, ET AL: Clinical comparison of Isolator and BACTEC 660 resin media for blood culture. J Clin Microbiol 28:1925–1927, 1990

107. KENNEY GE: Mycoplasmas. In Lennette EH (ed): Manual of Clinical Microbiology, pp 407–411. Washington DC, American Society for Microbiology, 1985

108. KERN W, KIRCHNER S, VANEK E: Resin versus standard blood culture media used with the new BACTEC automated infrared system: an evaluation in febrile granulocytopenic patients. Int J Med Microbiol 273:156–163, 1990

109. KHALIFA MA, ABDOH AA, SILVA FG, FLOURNOY DJ: Interpretation of multiple isolate urine cultures in adult male patients. J Natl Med Assoc 87:141–147, 1995

110. KIEHN TE, WONG B, EDWARDS FF, ET AL: Comparative recovery of bacteria and yeasts from lysis centrifugation and a conventional blood culture system. J Clin Microbiol 18:300–304, 1983

111. KIEHN TE, CAMARATA R: Comparative recoveries of Mycobacterium avium/Mycobacterium intracellulare from isolator lysis-centrifugation and BACTEC 13A blood culture systems. J Clin Microbiol 26:760–761, 1988

112. KIERKEGAARD H, RASMUSSEN UF, HORDER M, ET AL: Falsely negative urinary leucocyte counts due to delayed examination. Scand J Clin Lab Invest 40:259–261, 1980

113. KIRKLEY BA, EASLEY KA, BASILLE BA, WASHINGTON JA: Controlled clinical comparison of two lysis-based blood culture systems, Isolator and Septi-Check release, for detection of blood stream infections. J Clin Microbiol 31:2114–2117, 1993

114. KIRKLEY BA, EASLEY KA, WASHINGTON JA: Controlled clinical evaluation of Isolator and ESP aerobic blood culture systems for detection of blood stream infections. J Clin Microbiol 32:1547–1549, 1994

115. KLEIN RS, RECCO RA, CATALANO MT, ET AL: Association of Streptococcus bovis with carcinoma of the colon. N Engl J Med 297:800, 1977.

116. KOENIG C, TICK LJ, HANNA BA: Analyses of the Flas-Track DNA probe and UTIscreen bioluminescence tests for bacteriuria. J Clin Microbiol 30:342–345, 1992

117. KONEMAN, EW: Continuous-read blood culture systems. CAP Today, May, 1994

118. KOSUNEN TU, SEPPALA K, SARNA S. SIPPONEN P: Diagnostic value of decreasing IgG, IgA and IgM antibody titers after eradication of Helicobacter pylori. Lancet 339:393–395, 1992

119. KRAUSE PJ, HYANIS JS, MIDDLETON PJ: Unreliability of the Rotazyme ELISA test in neonates. J Pediatr 103:259–262, 1983

120. KRUMHOLZ HM, CUMMINGS S, YORK M: Blood culture phlebotomy: switching needles does not prevent contamination. Ann Intern Med 113:290–292, 1990

121. KURZYNSKI T, MEISE C, DAGGS R, ET AL: Improved reliability of the primary plate bacitracin test on throat cultures with sulfamethoxazole–trimethoprim blood agar plates. J Clin Microbiol 9:144–146, 1979

122. KURZYNSKI TA, MEISE C, VAN HOLTEN C: Evaluation of techniques for isolation of group A streptococci from throat cultures. J Clin Microbiol 13:891–894, 1981

123. KUNIN CM: Detection, Prevention and Management of Urinary Tract Infections: A Manual for the Physician, Nurse and Allied Health Worker, 2nd ed. Philadelphia, Lea & Febiger, 1974

124. KUSUMI RK, GROVER PJ, KUNIN CM: Rapid detection of pyuria by leukocyte esterase activity. JAMA 245:1653–1655, 1981

125. LAGE AP, GODRFOID E, FAUCONNIER A, ET AL: Diagnosis of Helicobacter pylori infection by PCR: comparison with other invasive techniques and detection of cagA gene in gastric biopsy specimens. J Clin Microbiol 33:2752–2756, 1995

126. LARSEN B: Problems in specimen collection for sexually transmitted diseases. J Reprod Med 30(supp):290–294, 1985

127. LAUER BA, RELLER LB, MIRRETT S: Effect of atmosphere and duration of incubation on primary isolation of group A streptococci from throat cultures. J Clin Microbiol 17:338–340, 1983

128. LEE HH, CHERNESKY MA, SCHACTER J, ET AL: Diagnosis of Chlamydia trachomatis genitourinary infection in women by ligase chain reaction assay of urine. Lancet 345:213–216, 1995

129. LEE A, HAZELL SL: Campylobacter pylori in health and disease: an ecological perspective. Microbial Ecol Health Dis 1:1–16, 1988

130. LENTINO JR, LUCKS DA: Nonvalue of sputum culture in the management of lower respiratory tract infections. J Clin Microbiol 25:759–762, 1988

131. LINDSEY JF, RILEY PE: In vitro antibiotic removal and bacterial recovery from blood with an antibiotic removal device. J Clin Microbiol 13:503–507, 1981

132. LIPKIN ES, MONCADA JV, SHAFER MA ET AL: Comparison of monoclonal antibody staining and culture in diagnosing cervical chlamydia infection. J Clin Microbiol 23:114–117, 1986

133. LYON R, WOODS G: Comparison of the BacT/Alert and Isolator blood culture systems for recovery of fungi. Am J Clin Pathol 103:660–662, 1995

133a. MAASS M, DALHOFF K: Transport and storage conditions for culture recovery of Chlamydia pneumoniae. J Clin Microbiol 33:1773–1776, 1995

134. MAHBUBANI MH, BEJ AK, PERLIN M, ET AL: Detection of *Giardia* cysts by using the polymerase chain reaction and distinguishing live from dead cysts. Appl Environ Microbiol 57:3456–3461, 1991

135. MAHONY JB, PHERNESKY MA: Effect of swab type and storage temperature in the isolation of *Chlamydia trachomatis* from clinical specimens. J Clin Microbiol 22:865–867, 1985

136. MAHONY JB, LUINSTRA KE, TYNDALL M, ET AL: Multiplex PCR for detection of *Chlamydia trachomatis* and *Neisseria gonorrhoeae* in genitourinary specimens. J Clin Microbiol 33:3049–3053, 1995

137. MARQUEZ-DAVILA G, MARTINEZ-BARREDA CE: Predictive value of the "clue cells" investigation and the amine volatilization test in vaginal infections caused by *Gardnerella vaginalis*. J Clin Microbiol 22:686–687, 1985

138. MARSHALL BJ, WARREN JR: Unidentified curved bacilli in the stomach of patients with gastritis and peptic ulceration. Lancet 1:1311–1315, 1984

139. McGEE ZA, BARINGER AB: Acute meningitis. In Mandell GL, Douglas RG Jr, Bennett JE (eds): Principles and Practice of Infectious Diseases, 3rd ed, pp 741–754. New York, Churchill Livingstone, 1990

140. McFARLAND LV, COYLE, MB, KREMER WH, STAFF WE: Rectal swab cultures for *Clostridium difficile* surveillance studies. J Clin Microbiol 25:2241–2242, 1987

141. McNICOL P, GIOERCKE SM, GRAY M, ET AL: Evaluation and validation of a monoclonal immunofluorescence reagent for direct detection of *Bordetella pertussis*. J Clin Microbiol 33:2868–2871, 1995

142. MERMEL LA, MAKI DG: Detection of bacteremia in adults: consequences of culturing an inadequate volume of blood. Ann Intern Med 119:270–272, 1993

143. MICEIKA BG, VITOUS AS, THOMPSON KD: Detection of group A streptococcal antigen directly from throat swabs with a ten-minute latex agglutination test. J Clin Microbiol 21:467–469, 1985

144. MIETTINÉN A, VUORINEN P, VARIS T, HALLSTROM O: Comparison of enzyme immunoassay antigen detection, nucleic acid hybridization and PCR assay in the diagnosis of *Chlamydia trachomatis* infection. Eur J Clin Microbiol Infect Dis 14:546–549, 1995

145. MILLER JR, BARRETT LJ, KOTLOFF K, GUERRANT RL: A rapid test for infectious and inflammatory enteritis. Arch Intern Med 154:2660–2664, 1994

146. MIRRETT S. RELLER LB, KNAPP JS: *Neisseria gonorrhoeae* strains inhibited by vancomycin in selective media and correlation with auxotype. J Clin Microbiol 14:94–99, 1981

147. MONTE-VERDE D, NOSANCHUK JS: The sensitivity and specificity of nitrite testing for bacteriuria. Lab Med 12:755–757, 1981

148. MOOSA AA, QUORTUM HA, IBRAHIM MD: Rapid diagnosis of bacterial meningitis with reagent strips. Lancet 345:1290–1291, 1995

149. MORELLO JA, LEITCH C, NITZ S, ET AL: Detection of bacteremia by Difco ESP blood culture system. J Clin Microbiol 32:811–818, 1994

150. MORINET F, FERCHAL F, COLIMON R, ET AL: Comparison of six methods for detecting human rotavirus in stools, Eur J Clin Microbiol 3:136–140, 1984

151. MORRIS AJ, WILSON ML, MIRRETT S, RELLER LB: Rationale for selective use of anaerobic blood cultures. J Clin Microbiol 31:2110–2113, 1993

152. MUFSON MA: *Streptococcus pneumoniae*. In Mandell GL, Douglas RG Jr, Bennett JE: Principles and Practice of Infect Disease, 4th ed, Chap 178. New York, Churchill Livingstone, 1990

153. MURRAY PR: Determination of the optimum incubation period of blood culture broths for the detection of clinically significant septicemia. J Clin Microbiol 85:481–485, 1985

154. MURRAY PR, NILES AC, HEEREN RL, ET AL: Comparative evaluation of the Oxoid Signal and Roche Septi-Chek Blood Culture Systems. J Clin Microbiol 26:2526–2530, 1988

155. MURRAY PR, SMITH FB, McKINNEY TC: Clinical evaluation of three urine screening tests. J Clin Microbiol 25:467–470, 1987

156. MURRAY PR, TRAYNOR P, HOPSON D: Critical assessment of blood culture techniques: analysis of recovery of obligate and facultative anaerobes, strict aerobic bacteria, and fungi in aerobic and anaerobic blood culture bottles. J Clin Microbiol 30:1462–1468, 1992

157. NASH TE, HERRINGTON DA, LEVINE MM: Usefulness of an enzyme-linked immunosorbent assay for detection of *Giardia* antigen in feces. J Clin Microbiol 25:1169–1171, 1987

158. NEEDHAM CA: Rapid detection methods in microbiology. Med Clin North Am 71:591–605, 1987

159. NG TM, FOCK KM, HO AL ET AL: Clotest (rapid urease test) in the diagnosis of *Helicobacter pylori* infection. Singapore Med J 33:568–569, 1992

160. NICOLLE LE, HARDING GKM, KENNEDY J ET AL: Urine specimen collection with external devices for diagnosis of bacteriuria in elderly incontinent men. J Clin Microbiol 26:1115–1119, 1988

161. NOLTE FS, WILLIAMS JM, JERRIS RC ET AL: Multicenter clinical evaluation of a continuous monitoring blood culture system using fluorescent-sensor technology (BACTEC 9240). J Clin Microbiol 31:552–557, 1993

162. NUGENT RP, KROHN MA, HILLIER SL: Reliability of diagnosing bacterial vaginosis is improved by a standardized method of Gram stain interpretation. J Clin Microbiol 29:297–301, 1991

163. OLSEN MA, SAMBOL AR, BOHNERT VA: Comparison of the Syva Microtrak enzyme immunoassay and Abbott Chlamydiazyme in the detection of chlamydial infections in women. Arch Pathol Lab Med 119:153–156, 1995

164. ORENSTEIN JM, KOTLER DP: Diarrhoegenic bacterial enteritis in acquired immune deficiency syndrome: a light and electron microscopy study of 52 cases. Hum Pathol 26:481–492, 1995

165. OTERO JR, REYES S, NORIEGA AR: Rapid diagnosis of group A streptococcal antigen extracted directly from swabs by an enzymatic procedure and used to detect pharyngitis. J Clin Microbiol 18:318–326, 1983

166. PAISLEY JW, LAUER BA: Pediatric blood cultures. Clin Lab Med 14:17–30, 1994

167. PARAMASIVAN CN, NARAYANA ASL, PRABHAKAR R ET AL: Effect of storage of sputum specimens at room temperature on smear and culture results. Tubercle 64:119–121, 1983

168. PARK CH, HIXON DL, MORRISON WL, COOK CB: Rapid diagnosis of enterohemorrhagic *Escherichia coli* 0157:H7 directly from fecal specimens using immunofluorescence stain. Am J Clin Pathol 101:91–94, 1994

169. PENN RL, SILBERMAN R: Effects of overnight refrigeration on microscopic evaluation of sputum. J Clin Microbiol 19:161–165, 1984

170. PEZZLO MT: Automated methods for detection of bacteriuria. Am J Med 75:71–78, 1983 (Infectious Disease Symposium)

171. PEZZLO MT, AMSTERDAM D, ANHALT JP ET AL: Detection of bacteriuria and pyuria by Uriscreen, a rapid enzymatic screening test. J Clin Microbiol 30:680–684, 1992

172. PEZZLO MT, IGE V, WOOLARD AP ET AL: Rapid bioluminescence method for bacteriuria screening. J Clin Microbiol 27:716–720, 1989

173. PEZZLO MT, WETKOWSKI MA, PETERSON EM ET AL: Detection of bacteriuria and pyuria within two minutes. J Clin Microbiol 21:578–581, 1985

174. PFALLER MA, BAUM CA, NILES AC ET AL: Clinical laboratory evaluation of a urine screening device. J Clin Microbiol 18:674–679, 1983

175. PFALLER MA, KOONTZ FP: Laboratory evaluation of leukocyte esterase and nitrite tests for the detection of bacteriuria. J Clin Microbiol 21:840–842, 1985

176. PICKETT DA, WELCH DF: Evaluation of the automated Bact-Alert system for pediatric blood culturing. J Clin Microbiol 103:320–323, 1995

177. POHLMAN JK, KIRKLEY BA, BASILLE BA, WASHINGTON JA: Controlled evaluation of BACTEC Plus Aerobic/F and BacT/Alert aerobic FAN bottles for detection of bloodstream infections. J Clin Microbiol 33:2856–2858, 1995

178. PORTER RC, LO P, LOW DE, ET AL: Utilization review of the use of BACTEC PLUS high-volume blood culture bottles. J Clin Microlbiol 31:2794–2795, 1993

179. PRONDVOST AD, ROSE SL, PAWLAK JW, ET AL: Evaluation of a new immunodiagnostic assay for *Helicobacter pylori* antibody detection: correlation with histopathological and microbiological results. J Clin Microbiol 32:46–50, 1994

180. RADETSKY MDCM, WHEELER RC, ROE MH, ET AL: Comparative evaluation of kits for rapid diagnosis of group A streptococcal disease. Pediatr Infect Dis 4:274–281, 1985

181. RADETSKY M, SOLOMON JA, TODD JK: Identification of streptococcal pharyngitis in the office laboratory: reassessment of new technology. Pediatr Infect Dis J 6:556–563, 1987

182. RATHORE MH, RATHORE S, EASLEY MA, AYUOUB EM: Latex particle agglutination tests on the cerebrospinal fluid. A reappraisal. J Fla Med Assoc 82:21–23, 1995

183. RADSTROM P, BACKMAN A, QIAN N, ET AL: Detection of bacterial DNA in cerebrospinal fluid by an assay for simultaneous detection of *Neisseria meningitidis*, *Haemophilus influenzae*, and streptocococci using a seminested PCR strategy. J Clin Microbiol 32:2738–2744, 1994

184. RATHORE MH, RATHORE S, EASLEY MA, AYOUB EM: Latex particle agglutination tests on the cerebrospinal fluid. A reappraisal. J Fla Med Assoc 82:21–23, 1995

185. REGAN J, LOWE F: Enrichment medium for the isolation of *Bordetella*. J Clin Microbiol 6:303–309, 1977

186. REIMER LG, RELLER LB, MIRRETT S: Controlled comparison of a new Becton Dickinson agar slant blood culture system with Roche Septi-Chek for the detection of bacteremia and fungemia. J Clin Microbiol 27:2637–2639, 1989

187. REIN MF, MANDELL GL: Bacterial killing by bacteriostatic saline solutions: potential for diagnostic error. N Engl J Med 289:794–795, 1973

188. RELLER LB, MURRAY PR, MacLOWRY JD: Cumitech 1A. Blood Cultures II. Washington DC, American Society for Microbiology, 1982

189. RINGELMANN R, HEYM B, KNIEHL E: Role of immunological tests in diagnosis of bacterial meningitis. Antibiot Chemother 45:68–78, 1992

190. RODRIQUEZ G, BOEHME C, SOTO L, ET AL: Diagnosis of bacterial meningitis by latex agglutination tests. Rev Med Chile 121:41–45, 1993

191. ROHNER P, PEPEY B, AUCKENTHALER R: Comparison of BACTEC aerobic Plus/F and Septi-check release blood culture media. J Clin Microbiol 34:126–129, 1996

192. ROHNER P, PEPEY B, AUCKENTHALER R: Comparison of BacT/Alert with Signal blood culture system. J Clin Microbiol 33:313–317, 1995

193. RONIN P, TANINO TT, HANDSFIELD HH: Isolation of *Neisseria gonorrhoeae* on selective and nonselective media in a sexually transmitted disease clinic. J Clin Microbiol 19:218–220, 1984

194. ROSTOFF JD, STIBBS HH: Isolation and identification of a *Giardia lamblia* specific stool antigen (GSA 65) useful in coprodiagnosis of giardiasis. J Clin Microbiol 23:905–910, 1986

195. RUMMENS J, FOSSEPRE J, DEGRUYTER M, ET AL: Isolation of *Capnocytophaga* species with a new selective medium. J Clin Microbiol 22:375–378, 1985

196. SALLUZZO R, REILLY K: The rational ordering of blood cultures in the emergency department. Qual Assur Util Rev 6:28–31, 1991

197. SAWYER KP, STONE LL: Evaluation of a leukocyte dipstick test used for screening urine cultures. J Clin Microbiol 20:820–821, 1984

198. SCHACHTER J, GROSSMAN M: Chlamydia infections. Annu Rev Med 32:45–61, 1981

199. SCHACHTER J, STAMM WE, QUINN TC, ET AL: Ligase chain reaction to detect *Chlamydia trachomatis* infection of the cervix. J Clin Microbiol 32:2540–2543, 1994

200. SCHEMBRI MA, LIN SK, LAMBERT JR: Comparison of commercial diagnostic tests for *Helicobacter pylori* antibodies. J Clin Microbiol 31:2621–2624, 1993

201. SCHIFMAN RB, STRAND CL, BRAUN E, ET AL: Solitary blood cultures as a quality assurance indicator. Qual Assur Util Rev 6:132–137, 1991

202. SCHLISINGER Y, TEBAS P, GAUDREAULT-KEENER, ET AL: Herpes simplex virus type 2 meningitis in the absence of genital lesions: improved recognition with use of the polymerase chain reaction. Clin Infect Dis 20:842–848, 1995

203. SCHULMAN RJ, PHILLIPS S. LAINE L, ET AL: Volume of blood required to obtain central venous catheter blood cultures in infants and children. Jpn J Parent Enteral Nutr 17:177–179, 1993

204. SCHWABE LD, RANDALL EL, MILLER-CATCHPOLE R, ET AL: A comparison of Oxoid Signal with nonradiometric

BACTEC NR-660 for detection of bacteremia. Diagn Microbiol Infect Dis 13:3–8, 1990

205. SCHWABE LD, THOMSON RB, FLINT KK, KOONTZ FP: Evaluation of BACTEC 9240 blood culture system using high-volume aerobic resin media. J Clin Microbiol 33:2451–2453, 1995

206. SCHWARTZ R, RODRIQUEZ WJ, MANN R, ET AL.: The nasopharyngeal culture in acute otitis media: a reappraisal of its usefulness. JAMA 241:2170–2173, 1979

207. SEAWORTH JB, KWON-CHUNG KJ, HAMILTON JD, ET AL: Brain abscess caused by a variety of *Cladosporium trichoides.* Am J Clin Pathol 79:747–752, 1983

208. SHAFER RW, GOLDBERG R, SIERRA M, GLATT AE: Frequency of *Mycobacterium tuberculosis* bacteremia in patients with tuberculosis in an area endemic for AIDS. Am Rev Respir Dis 140:1611–1613, 1989

209. SHANSON DC: Blood culture technique: current controversies. J Antimicrob Chemother 25(suppl C):17–29, 1990

210. SHARP S: Routine anaerobic blood cultures: still appropriate today? Clin Microbiol Newslett 13:179–181, 1991

211. SHEINESS D, DIX K, WATANABE S, HILLIER SL: High levels of *Gardnerella vaginalis* detected with an oligonucleotide probe combined with elevated pH as a diagnostic indicator of bacterial vaginosis. J Clin Microbiol 30:642–648, 1992

212. SHERMAN MP, CHANCE KH, GOLTZMAN BW: Gram's stain of tracheal secretions predict neonatal bacteremia. Am J Dis Child 138:848–850, 1984

213. SHIGEI JT, SHIMABUKURO JA, PEZZLO MT, ET AL: Value of terminal subcultures for blood cultures monitored by BACTEC 9240. J Clin Microbiol 33:1385–1388, 1995

214. SHULMAN RJ, PHILLIPS S, LAINE L, ET AL: Volume of blood required to obtain central venous catheter blood cultures in infants and children. Jpn J Parent Enteral Nutr 17:177–179, 1993

215. SIEGMAN-IGRA Y, KULKA T, SCHWARTZ D, KONFORTI N: Polymicrobial and monomicrobial bacteraemic urinary tract infection. J Hosp Infect 28:49–56, 1994

216. SLIFKIN M, GIL GM: Evaluation of the Culturette brand ten-minute group A strep ID technique. J Clin Microbiol 20:12–14, 1984

217. SLIFKIN M, GIL GM: Serogrouping of beta-hemolytic streptococci from throat swabs with nitrous acid extraction and the Phadebact streptococcus test. J Clin Microbiol 15:187–189, 1982

218. SMALLEY DL, BRADLEY ME: Correlation of leukocyte esterase activity and bacterial isolation from body fluids. J Clin Microbiol 20:1186, 1984

219. SMALLEY DL, DITTMANN AN: Use of leukocyte esterase-nitrate activity as predictive assays of significant bacteriuria. J Clin Microbiol 18:1256–1257, 1983

220. SMART D, BAGGOLEY C. HEAD J, ET AL: Effect of needle changing and intravenous cannula collection on blood culture contamination rates. Ann Emerg Med 22:1164–1168, 1993

221. SMITH JA, BRYCE EA, NGUI-YEN, ROBERTS FJ: Comparison of BACTEC 9240 and BacT/Alert blood culture systems in an adult hospital. J Clin Microbiol 33:1905–1908, 1995

222. SPADA EL, TINIVELLA A, CARLI S, ET AL: Proposal of an easy method to improve routine sputum bacteriology. Respiration 56:137–146, 1989

223. SPENCE MR, GUZIK DS, KATTA LR: The isolation of *Neisseria gonorrhoeae*—a comparison of three culture transport systems. Sex Transm Dis 10:138–140, 1983

224. SPIEGEL CA, ROBERTS M: *Mobiluncus* gen nov., *Mobiluncus curtisii* subsp., *curtisii* sp. nov., *Mobiluncus mulieris* sp nov., curved rods from the human vagina. Int J System Bacteriol 34:177–184, 1984

225. SPIEGEL CA: *Gardnerella vaginalis.* In Mandell GL, Douglas RG Jr., Bennett JE (eds): Principles and Practice of Infectious Diseases, 3rd ed, pp 1733–1735. New York, Churchill Livingston, 1990

226. STAMM WE, WAGNER KF, AMSEL R, ET AL: Causes of the acute urethral syndrome in women. N Engl J Med 303:409–415, 1980

227. STAMM WE, RUNNING K, MCKUVITT M, ET AL: Treatment of the acute urethral syndrome. N Engl J Med 304:956–958, 1981

228. STAMM WE, HARRISON HR, ALEXANDER ER, ET AL: Diagnosis of *Chlamydia trachomatis* infections by direct immunofluorescence staining of genital secretions—a multicenter trial. Ann Intern Med 101:638–641, 1984

229. STEED LL, KORGENSKI EK, DALY JA: Rapid detection of *Streptococcus pyogenes* in pediatric patient specimens by DNA probe. J Clin Microbiol 31:2996–3000, 1993

230. STEELE TW, MCDERMOTT SN: The use of membrane filters applied directly to the surface of agar plates for the isolation of *C. jejuni* from feces. Pathology 16:263–265, 1984

231. STEHR-GREEN JK, BAILEY TM, BRANDT FH, ET AL.: *Acanthamoeba* keratitis in soft contact lens wearers: a case control study. JAMA 258:57–60, 1987

232. STEVENS CM, SWAINE D, BUTLER C, ET AL: Development of O.A.S.I.S., a new automated blood culture system in which detection is based on measurement of bottle headspace pressure changes. J Clin Microbiol 32:1750–1756, 1994

233. STOCKMAN L, ROBERTS GD: Specificity of the latex test for cryptococcal antigen: a rapid, simple method for eliminating interference factors. J Clin Microbiol 16:965–967, 1982

234. STRANJORD TP, RICH EJ, QUAN L: Comparison of two antigen detection techniques for group A streptococcal pharyngitis in a pediatric emergency department. Pediatr Infect Dis J 11:1071–1072, 1987

235. TAM MR. STAMM WE, HANDSFIELD HH, ET AL: Culture-independent diagnosis of *Chlamydia trachomatis* using monoclonal antibodies. N Engl J Med 310:1146–1150, 1984

236. TAYLOR DE, HARGREAVES JA, LAI-KING NG, ET AL: Isolation and characterization of *Campylobacter pyloridis* from gastric biopsies. Am J Clin Pathol 87:49–54, 1987

237. TAYLOR-ROBINSON D: *Ureaplasma urealyticum* (T-strain mycoplasma) and *Mycoplasma hominis.* In Mandell GL, Douglas RG Jr, Bennett JE (eds): Principles and Practice of Infectious Diseases, 3rd ed, pp 1458–1462. New York, Churchill Livingston, 1990

238. TEMSTET A, ROUX P, POIROT JL, ET AL: Evaluation of a monoclonal antibody-based latex agglutination test for diagnosis of cryptococcosis: comparison with two tests using polyclonal antibodies. J Clin Microbiol 30:2544–2550, 1992

239. THOMAS B, EVANS RT, HAWKINS DA, ET AL: Sensitivity of detecting *Chlamydia trachomatis* elementary bodies in smears by use of fluorescein labeled monoclonal antibody—comparison with conventional chlamydia isolation. J Clin Pathol 37:812–816, 1984

240. THOMASON JL, SCHRECKENBERGER PC, LEBEAU LJ, ET AL: A selective and differential agar for anaerobic comma-shaped bacteria recovered from patients having motile rods and non-specific vaginosis. Scand J Urol Nephrol Suppl 86:125–128, 1984

241. THORPE TC, WILSON ML, TURNER JE, ET AL: BacT/Alert: an automated colorimetric microbial detection system. J Clin Microbiol 28:1608–1612, 1990

242. TIERNEY BM, HENRY NK, WASHINGTON JA II: Early detection of positive blood cultures by the acridine orange staining technique. J Clin Microbiol 18:830–833, 1983

243. TOTTEN PA, AMSEL R, HALE J, ET AL: Selective differential human blood bilayer media for isolation of *Gardnerella* (*Haemophilus vaginalis*). J Clin Microbiol 15:141–147, 1982

244. VALENSTEIN PN: Semiquantitation of bacteria in sputum Gram stains. J Clin Microbiol 26:1791–1794, 1988

245. VAN DOORNUM GJ, BUIMER M, PRINS M, ET AL: Detection of *Chlamydia trachomatis* infection in urine samples from men and women by ligase chain reaction. J Clin Microbiol 33:2042–2047, 1995

246. VLASPOLDER F, MUTSAERS JAEM, BLOG F, NOTOWICZ A: Value of a DNA probe assay (Gen-Probe) compared with that of culture for diagnosis of gonococcal infection. J Clin Microbiol 31:107–110, 1993

247. WALLIS C, MELNICK JL, WENDE RE, ET AL: Rapid isolation of bacteria from septicemic patients by use of an antimicrobial agent removal device. J Clin Microbiol 11:462–464, 1980

248. WALTER FG, KNOPP RK: Urine sampling in ambulatory women: midstream clean-catch versus catheterization. Ann Emerg Med 18:166–172, 1989

249. WARREN SS, ALLEN SD: Clinical, pathogenic and laboratory features of *Capnocytophaga* infections. Am J Clin Pathol 86:513–518, 1986

250. WASHINGTON JA II: Conventional approaches to blood culture. In Washington JA II (ed): The Detection of Septicemia, pp 48–86. CRC Press, West Palm Beach, FL, 1978

251. WASHINGTON JA: Collection, transport, and processing of blood cultures. Clin Lab Med 14:59–68, 1994

252. WASHINGTON JA II, WHITE CM, LAGANIERE M, ET AL: Detection of significant bacteriuria by microscopic examination of urine. Lab Med 12:294–296, 1981

253. WEINSTEIN MP, RELLER LB, MURPHY JR. LICHTENSTEIN KA: The clinical significance of positive blood cultures: a comprehensive analysis of 500 episodes of bacteremia and fungemia in adults. I. Laboratory and epidemiologic observations. Rev Infect Dis 5:54–70, 1983

254. WEINSTEIN MP, MIRRETT S, REIMER LG, ET AL: Controlled evaluation of BacT/Alert standard aerobic and FAN aerobic blood culture bottles for detection of bacteremia and fungemia. J Clin Microbiol 33:978–981, 1995

255. WEINSTEIN MP, MIRRETT S, WILSON ML, ET AL: Controlled evaluation of five versus ten milliliters of blood cultured in aerobic BacT/Alert blood culture bottles. J Clin Microbiol 32:2103–2106, 1994

256. WEINSTEIN MP, MIRRETT S, REIMER LG, RELLER LB: The effect of altered headspace atmosphere on yield and speed of detection of the Oxoid Signal blood culture system versus the BACTEC radiometric system. J Clin Microbiol 28:795–797, 1990

257. WELBY PL, KELLER DS, STORCH GA: Comparison of automated Difco ESP blood culture system with biphasic BBL Septi-Check system for detection of bloodstream infections in pediatric patients. J Clin Microbiol 33: 1084–1088, 1995

258. WENK RE, DUTTA D, RUDERT J, ET AL: Sediment microscopy, nitrituria and leukocyte esterasuria as predictors of significant bacteriuria. J Clin Lab Automation 2:117–121, 1982

259. WICHER K, KOSCINSKI D: Laboratory experience with radiometric detection of bacteremia with three culture media. J Clin Microbiol 20:668–671, 1982

260. WILSON ML, DAVIS TE, MIRRETT S, ET AL: Controlled comparison of the BACTEC high-blood–volume fungal medium, BACTEC plus 26 aerobic blood culture bottles, and 10-milliliter isolator blood culture system for detection of fungemia and bacteremia. J Clin Microbiol 31:865–871, 1993

261. WILSON ML, MIRRETT S, RELLER LB, ET AL: Recovery of clinically important microorganisms from the BacT/Alert blood culture system does not require 7 day testing. Diagn Microbiol Infect Dis 16:31–34, 1993

262. WILSON ML, WEINSTEIN MP, MERRITT S, ET AL: Controlled evaluation of BacT/Alert standard anaerobic and FAN anaerobic blood culture bottles for the detection of bacteremia and fungemia. J Clin Microbiol 33:2265–2270, 1995

263. WORMSER GP, ONORATO IM, PREMINGER TJ, ET AL: Sensitivity and specificity of blood culture obtained through intravascular catheters. Crit Care Med 18:152–156, 1990)

264. WRIGHT AJ, THOMPSON RL, MCLIMANS CA, ET AL: The antimicrobial removal device: a microbiological and clinical evaluation. Am J Clin Pathol 78:173–177, 1982

265. WU TC, KOO SY: Comparison of three commercial cryptococcal latex kits for detection of cryptococcal antigen. J Clin Microbiol 18:1127–1120, 1983

266. YOLKEN RH: Enzyme immunoassays for the detection of infectious antigens in body fluids: current limitations and future prospects. Rev Infect Dis 4:35–68, 1982

267. YUEN KY, SETO WH, ONG SG: The significance of *Branhamella catarrhalis* in bronchopulmonary infection—a case–control study. J Infect 19:2511–2516, 1989

268. ZWADYK P JR, PIERSON CL, YOUNG C: Comparison of Difco ESP and Organon Teknika BacT/Alert continuous-monitoring blood culture systems. J Clin Microbiol 32:11273–1279, 1994

THE *ENTEROBACTERIACEAE*

Gram-negative bacilli belonging to the *Enterobacteriaceae* are the most frequently encountered bacterial isolates recovered from clinical specimens. Widely dispersed in nature, these organisms are found in soil and water, on plants, and, as the family name indicates, within the intestinal tracts of humans and animals. Before the advent of antibiotics, chemotherapy, and immunosuppressive measures, the infectious diseases caused by the *Enterobacteriaceae* were relatively well defined. Diarrheal and dysenteric syndromes, accompanied by fever and septicemia in classic cases of typhoid fever, were known to be caused by *Salmonella* and *Shigella* species. Classic cases of pneumonia, characterized by production of brick-red or "currant jelly" sputum, were known to be caused by Friedlander's bacillus (*Klebsiella pneumoniae*). *Escherichia coli*, *Proteus* species, and various members of the *Klebsiella–Enterobacter* group were commonly recovered from traumatic wounds contaminated with soil or vegetative matter or from abdominal wound incisions following gastrointestinal surgery.

Thus, members of the *Enterobacteriaceae* may be incriminated in virtually any type of infectious disease and recovered from any specimen received in the laboratory. Immunocompromised or debilitated patients are highly susceptible to hospital-acquired infections, either after colonization with environmental strains or following invasive procedures, such as catheterization, bronchoscopy, colposcopy, or surgical biopsies, in which mucous membranes are traumatized or transected.

Endotoxic shock is one potentially lethal manifestation of infection with gram-negative bacteria, including the *Enterobacteriaceae*. Endotoxin is a complex pharmacologically active lipopolysaccharide that is contained within the cell wall of gram-negative species. This lipopolysaccharide is structured in three layers: 1) an outer variable carbohydrate portion that determines O-antigenic specificity (e.g., various *Salmonella* serotypes), 2) a middle core polysaccharide that is structurally similar among species, and 3) a central, highly conserved lipid moiety called lipid-A. The biologic effects of endotoxin have been demonstrated experimentally: small quantities injected intravenously into animals produce fever, leukopenia, capillary hemorrhage, hypotension, and circulatory collapse—symptoms that are, to a large extent, the same as those seen in humans with gram-negative sepsis.

The limulus lysate assay, which uses a reagent prepared from the amoebocytes of the horseshoe crab (*Limulus polyphemus*), has been employed with varying success in the diagnosis of endotoxic shock.[96] The lysate undergoes gelation when in contact with even trace amounts of endotoxin. More promising in the diagnosis of gram-negative sepsis is the development of monoclonal antibodies that can be used in enzyme-linked immunoassay or other techniques for the detection of lipid-A. The pharmacologic effects of endotoxin can be attributed primarily to lipid-A. It is highly antigenic and has determinants common to all strains of gram-negative bacilli. Thus, the detection of circulating lipid-A in patients with gram-negative sepsis, using a monoclonal antibody, could establish a diagnosis so that presumptive therapy could be started before the causative organism is recovered and identified.

Microbiologists must be alert to the emergence of any *Enterobacteriaceae* that are resistant to multiple antibiotics. The mechanisms by which resistance may develop are discussed in more detail in Chapter 15. Antibiotic resistance may evolve in formerly susceptible clinical isolates through the transfer of plasmids known as R factors or R plasmids. The gram-negative enteric bacteria commonly possess a single, large R plasmid that encodes for resistance to several antibiotics. An increasing percentage of strains within the genera *Enterobacter*, *Serratia*, *Klebsiella*, and *Providencia*, in addition to some indole-positive strains of *Proteus* and cephalothin-resistant strains of *Escherichia coli*, possess inducible β-lactamases that impart cross-resistance to many β-lactam antibiotics.[276,277] Inactivating enzymes are often chromosomally mediated and may be responsible for "breakthrough" resistance in patients who are being treated for septicemia. Disk diffusion susceptibility tests may not always detect resistant strains, particularly when testing the cephalosporins; thus, a broth dilution procedure may be indicated. Detecting these resistant strains is not only important in managing the patient from whom the isolate is recovered but also has important implications for surveillance of nosocomial infections. Specific clinical syndromes of individual genera and species are discussed in later sections of this chapter.

CHARACTERISTICS FOR PRESUMPTIVE IDENTIFICATION

What are the initial clues that an unknown isolate recovered from a clinical specimen may belong to the *Enterobacteriaceae*? In specimens other than feces, a gram-stained preparation may reveal short, plump, gram-negative bacillary or coccobacillary cells, ranging from 0.5 to 2 μm wide to 2 to 4 μm long (see Color Plate 4-1*A*). However, species differentiation cannot be made on the basis of only Gram stain morphology.

Characteristic colonial morphology of an organism growing on a solid medium may provide a second clue. Typically, members of the *Enterobacteriaceae* produce relatively large, dull gray, dry, or mucoid colonies on sheep blood agar, the latter suggesting encapsulated strains of *Klebsiella pneumoniae* (see Color Plate 4-1*B* and C). Hemolysis on blood agar is variable and indistinctive. Colonies appearing as a thin film or as waves (a phenomenon known as **swarming**) suggest that the organism is motile and probably a *Proteus* species (see Color Plate 4-1*D*). Colonies that appear red

Color Plates for Chapter 4 are found between pages 80 and 81.

on MacConkey agar or have a green sheen on eosin methylene blue (EMB) agar (see Color Plate 4-2) indicate that the organism is capable of forming acid from lactose in the medium.

Differentiation of the *Enterobacteriaceae*, however, is based primarily on the presence or absence of different enzymes coded by the genetic material of the bacterial chromosome. These enzymes direct the metabolism of bacteria along one of several pathways that can be detected by special media used in in vitro culture techniques. Substrates on which these enzymes can react are incorporated into the culture medium, together with an indicator that can detect either the utilization of the substrate or the presence of specific metabolic products. By selecting a series of media that measure different metabolic characteristics of the microorganisms to be tested, a biochemical profile can be determined for making a species identification.

SCREENING CHARACTERISTICS

Definitive identification of the members of the *Enterobacteriaceae* may require a battery of biochemical tests. Considerable time and possible misidentification can be avoided if a few preliminary observations are made to ensure that the organism being tested belongs to this group. If the organism is a gram-negative organism of another group, it may be necessary to use a different set of characteristics than that commonly used for the identification of the *Enterobacteriaceae*. With few exceptions, all members of the *Enterobacteriaceae* demonstrate the following characteristics:

- Glucose is fermented (see Color Plate 4-1*E* and *F*)
- Cytochrome oxidase is negative (see Color Plate 4-1*G*)
- Nitrate is reduced to nitrite (see Color Plate 4-1*H*).

CARBOHYDRATE UTILIZATION

It is common for laboratory microbiologists to refer to all carbohydrates as **sugars**. This is convenient in an operational sense, although it is understood that polyhedral alcohols, such as dulcitol and mannitol, or cationic salts of acetate or tartrate are not carbohydrates and thus are not truly sugars in a chemical sense.

The term **fermentation** is also used somewhat loosely in reference to the utilization of carbohydrates by bacteria, with terms such as **lactose fermenters** and **non-lactose fermenters**. By definition, fermentation is an oxidation–reduction metabolic process that takes place in an anaerobic environment, and instead of oxygen, an organic substrate serves as the final hydrogen (electron) acceptor. In bacteriologic test systems, this process is detected by observing color changes in pH indicators as acid products are formed. Acidification of a test medium may occur through the degradation of carbohydrates by pathways other than fermentation, or there may be ingredients other than carbohydrates in some media that result in acid end products. Although most bacteria that metabolize carbohydrates are facultative anaerobes, the utilization may not always be under strictly anaerobic conditions, as is observed in the production of acid products by bacterial colonies growing on the surface of agar media. Even though all tests used to measure an organism's ability to enzymatically degrade a "sugar" into acid products may not be "fermentative," these terms will be used in this text for convenience.

Basic Principles of Fermentation.   Pasteur's mid-19th century studies of the action of yeasts on wine provide the basis for our present understanding of carbohydrate fermentation. Pasteur observed that certain contaminating bacterial species produced a drop in the pH of wine (a carbohydrate substrate) from the production of a variety of acids. Full descriptions of the fermentative pathways by which a monosaccharide such as glucose is degraded evolved soon thereafter. Through a series of enzymatic glycolytic cleavages and transformations, the glucose molecule is split into a series of three carbon compounds, the most important of which is pyruvic acid. The chemical sequence by which glucose is converted to pyruvic acid is known as the **Embden–Meyerhof pathway** (EMP; Fig. 4-1). Many bacteria, including all *Enterobacteriaceae*, ferment glucose through the EMP to form pyruvic acid; the manner in which pyruvic acid is further used, however, varies among bacterial species. The alternative fates of pyruvic acid are the result of a variety of fermentation pathways, yielding quite different products (see Fig. 4-1).

Bacteria are differentiated by the carbohydrates they metabolize and the types and quantities of acids produced. These differences in enzymatic activity serve as one of the important characteristics by which the different species are recognized. It is important for students of microbiology to understand that in the glycolytic formation of pyruvic acid, adenosine triphosphate (ATP) is generated at the expense of the reduction of nicotinamide adenine dinucleotide (NAD) to $NADH_2$. For each glucose molecule that is fermented to form pyruvic acid, four hydrogen ions are consumed through the reduction of two NAD to two $NADH_2$. Since the total NAD in the cell is very limited, fermentation would cease very rapidly if the $NADH_2$ were not reoxidized in the further metabolism of pyruvic acid. Figure 4-2 depicts the fermentation of three molecules of glucose by means of two alternative pathways. For example, glucose fermentation by *Escherichia coli* occurs by means of the mixed acid fermentation pathway and results in the production of large quantities of acetic, lactic, and formic acids, with a marked drop in the pH of the test medium. This is detected by a positive methyl red test (see Fig. 4-2). On the other hand, the *Klebsiella–Enterobacter–Hafnia–Serratia* group metabolize pyruvic acid primarily through the butylene glycol pathway, producing acetyl methyl carbinol (acetoin) and a positive Voges-Proskauer (VP) test (see Fig. 4-2). Note that the principal end products in this latter pathway are alcohols, with only a small amount of acid produced, thus the methyl red test is usually negative for this group of organisms.

The gas resulting from fermenting bacteria is primarily a mixture of hydrogen and carbon dioxide

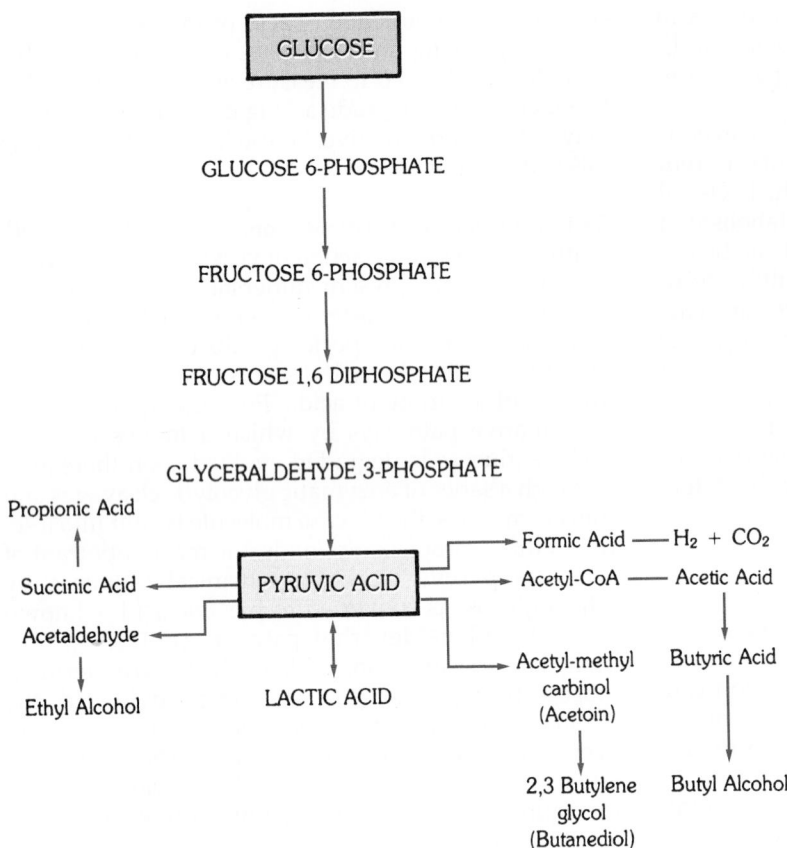

Figure 4-1
Fermentation of glucose to form pyruvate (Embden–Meyerhof pathway) and the alternative fates of pyruvic acid.

formed through the cleavage of formic acid. It is an accepted rule of thumb that any bacterium that forms gas in carbohydrate test medium must first form acid, which is self-evident from the EMP scheme in Figure 4-1. Gas is best detected by using a broth carbohydrate-fermentation medium into which small inverted Durham tubes have been placed (see Color Plate 4-1F). Even trace amounts of gas, which collect as bubbles under the Durham tubes, can be detected. Some species of *Enterobacteriaceae* lack the enzyme formic dehydrogenase and cannot cleave formic acid and, as a result, do not form even trace amounts of CO_2 (e.g., most species of *Shigella*). Conversely, organisms that use the butylene glycol pathway (i.e., VP positive) produce copious amounts of CO_2 (see Fig. 4-2). Therefore, when a large amount of gas is observed, one should consider members of the *Klebsiella–Enterobacter–Hafnia–Serratia* group as the likely identification.

The formation of ethyl alcohol by microorganisms is of utmost commercial importance in the manufacture of alcoholic beverages and organic reagents; however, it is of limited usefulness in the laboratory identification of bacteria.

The bacterial fermentation of lactose is more complex than that of glucose. Lactose is a disaccharide composed of glucose and galactose, connected through an oxygen linkage known as a **galactoside bond**. On hydrolysis, this bond is severed, releasing glucose and galactose. For a bacterium to metabolize lactose, two enzymes must be present: 1) β-galactoside permease,

permitting the transport of a β-galactoside, such as lactose, through the bacterial cell wall; and 2) β-galactosidase, the enzyme required to hydrolyze the β-galactoside bond once the disaccharide has entered the cell. The final acid reaction results from the degradation of glucose as shown in Figure 4-3.

Because lactose fermentation ultimately proceeds by way of glucose degradation through the EMP, it follows that any organism incapable of metabolizing glucose cannot form acid from lactose. This explains why glucose is omitted from the formulas of primary isolation media such as MacConkey agar and EMB agar: if it is not omitted, the ability to detect the lactose-fermenting capability of the test bacteria would be lost. In the test medium, the endpoint of lactose fermentation is the detection of acid production. A non–lactose-fermenting organism is one that lacks either one or both of the two enzymes required for lactose metabolism or lacks the ability to attack glucose. So-called late lactose-fermenters are believed to be organisms that exhibit β-galactosidase activity but show sluggish β-galactoside permease activity.

β-Galactosidase and the ONPG Test. *o*-Nitrophenyl-β-D-galactopyranoside (ONPG) is a compound structurally similar to lactose except that the glucose has been replaced by an *o*-nitrophenyl group. This rather ingenious manipulation of the molecule forms the basis for the ONPG test, which is outlined in Chart 57. This test detects the enzyme β-galactosidase far more

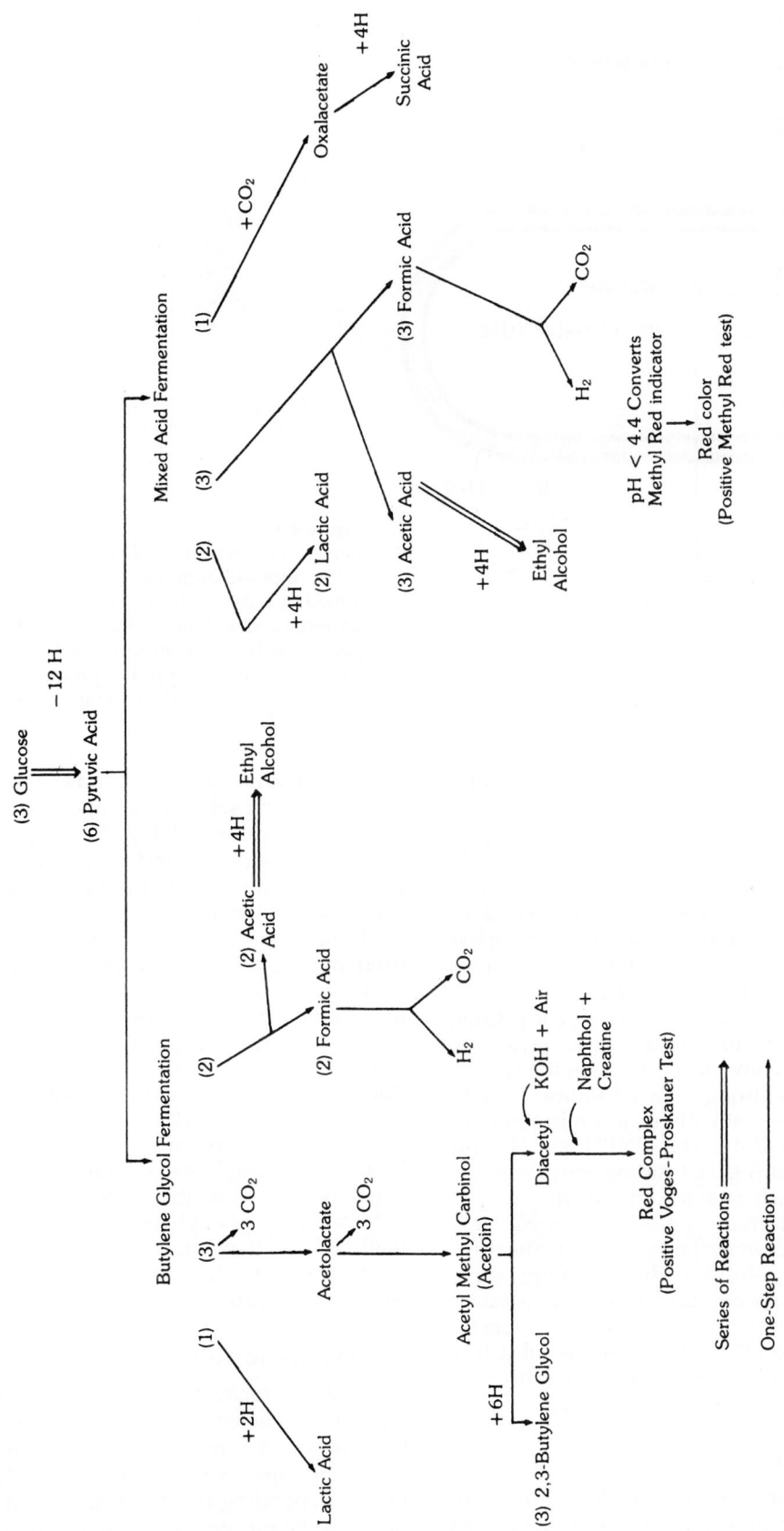

Figure 4-2
Mixed acid and butylene glycol pathways of glucose fermentation.

175

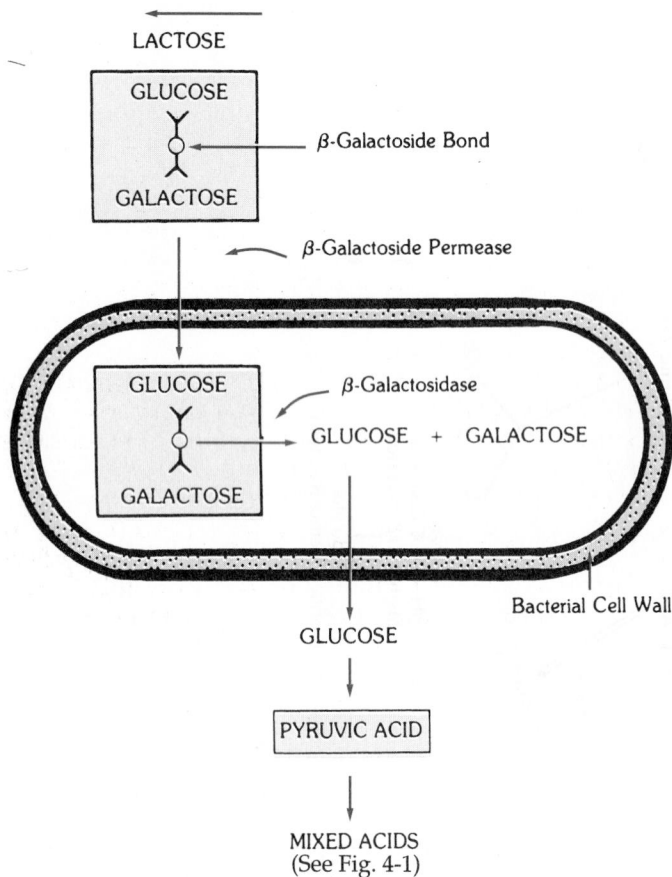

LACTOSE

GLUCOSE
Y
GALACTOSE

β-Galactoside Bond

β-Galactoside Permease

GLUCOSE — β-Galactosidase
Y
GALACTOSE → GLUCOSE + GALACTOSE

Bacterial Cell Wall

GLUCOSE

PYRUVIC ACID

MIXED ACIDS
(See Fig. 4-1)

Figure 4-3
Bacterial fermentation of lactose: Lactose, a disaccharide composed of molecules of glucose and galactose joined by a β-galactoside bond, diffuses through the bacterial cell wall under the action of β-galactoside permease. If the bacterium produces β-galactosidase, the lactose is hydrolyzed to produce glucose and galactose. The glucose is then metabolized as illustrated in Figure 4-1.

quickly than does the test for lactose fermentation previously described. This is helpful in identifying late lactose fermenters that are deficient in β-galactoside permease. ONPG permeates the bacterial cell more readily than lactose and, under the action of β-galactosidase, is hydrolyzed into galactose and *o*-nitrophenol (see Chart 57). *o*-Nitrophenol is a chromophore that is colorless when bound to D-galactopyranoside but is yellow in its free (unbound) form (see Color Plate 4-4A).

ONPG test tablets that can be easily reconstituted by adding a small amount of water are available commercially and are convenient for use in the laboratory. Organisms with strong β-galactosidase activity may produce a positive test within a few minutes after inoculation of the medium. The ONPG test is most helpful for detection of β-galactosidase activity in late lactose fermenters, such as some strains of *E. coli*, in which differentiation from species of *Shigella* (except certain strains of *S. sonnei*) may otherwise be difficult. The test is also helpful in distinguishing some strains of *Citrobacter* species and *Salmonella arizonae* (ONPG-positive) from most *Salmonella* species (ONPG-negative). The ONPG test is not a substitute for the determination of lactose fermentation because only the enzyme β-galactosidase is measured.

CYTOCHROME OXIDASE ACTIVITY

Any organism that displays cytochrome oxidase activity following the procedure and test conditions outlined in Chart 16 is excluded from the *Enterobacteriaceae*. The developing color reaction must be in-

terpreted within 10 to 20 seconds because many organisms, including selected members of the *Enterobacteriaceae*, may produce delayed false-positive reactions. Both oxidase-positive and oxidase-negative control organisms should be tested if there is difficulty in interpreting the cytochrome oxidase reaction.

The commercial cytochrome oxidase droppers are used most often because of their convenience. The color reactions are clearly visible within 10 seconds. If metal inoculating loops or wires are used in the laboratory for transferring bacteria to the oxidase reagent, those made from stainless steel or Nichrome may produce false-positive reactions, owing to trace amounts of iron oxide on the flamed surface of the metal. This problem can be circumvented by using plastic or platinum inoculating loops or by using wooden applicator sticks or cotton swabs to perform the oxidase test. Tetramethyl-*p*-phenylenediamine, rather than the dimethyl derivative, is most commonly used because the reagent is more stable, more sensitive, and less toxic (see Chart 16 and Color Plate 4-1G).

NITRATE REDUCTION

All *Enterobacteriaceae*, with the exception of certain biotypes of *Pantoea* (*Enterobacter*) *agglomerans* and certain species of *Serratia* and *Yersinia*, reduce nitrate to nitrite. Because a variable period of incubation (3 to 24 hours, depending on the system used) is required to perform the nitrate reduction test, it is not commonly used to prescreen unknown bacterial isolates. Rather, the test is used in most laboratories either to confirm the correct classification of an unknown microorganism or as an aid in determining the identification of bacterial species. Details of the nitrate reduction test are presented in Chart 53.

Any basal medium that supports the growth of the organism and contains a 0.1% concentration of potassium nitrate (KNO_3) is suitable for performing this test. Nitrate broth and nitrate agar in a slant are the media forms most commonly used in clinical laboratories. Because the enzyme nitrate reductase is maximally active under anaerobic conditions, ZoBell has recommended the use of semisolid agar.[329] Semisolid media also enhance the growth of many bacterial species and provide the anaerobic environment needed for enzyme activation. The addition of zinc dust to all negative reactions, as shown in Chart 53, should be a routine procedure. Most organisms capable of reducing nitrates will do so within 24 hours; some may produce detectable quantities within 2 hours. A rapid nitrate test has been described by Schreckenberger and Blazevic.[283] Both α-naphthylamine and sulfanilic acid are relatively unstable, so their reactivity should be determined at frequent intervals by testing with positive- and negative-control organisms. The diazonium compound that forms from the reaction of the reduced nitrate and reagents is also relatively unstable, and the color tends to fade; accordingly, readings should be made soon after the reagents are added (see Color Plate 4-1*H*).

CULTURE MEDIA USED FOR DETECTION OF CARBOHYDRATE FERMENTATION

A variety of different liquid or agar media can be used to measure the ability of a test organism to fermentatively utilize carbohydrates. The principle of carbohydrate fermentation is based on Pasteur's studies of bacteria and yeasts, written more than 100 years ago, which state that the action of many species of microorganisms on a carbohydrate substrate results in acidification of the medium. The formula of a typical basal fermentation medium contains trypticase (BBL), 10 g; sodium chloride, 5 g; phenol red, 0.018 g; and distilled water to equal 1 L.

The carbohydrate to be tested, such as glucose, is filter sterilized and added aseptically to the basal medium to a final concentration of 0.5% to 1.0%. Trypticase is a hydrolysate of casein that serves as a source for carbon and nitrogen; sodium chloride is an osmotic stabilizer; and phenol red is a pH indicator that turns yellow when the pH of the medium drops below 6.8. Color Plate 4-1*F* illustrates acid fermentation reactions in purple broth medium. All of the *Enterobacteriaceae* grow well in this type of medium, and the base formula used is a matter of personal preference. In addition to producing a pH color shift in fermentation culture media, the production of mixed acids, notably butyric acid, often results in a pungent, foul odor from the culture medium. When such an odor is detected, one should immediately be suspicious of the presence of one of the *Enterobacteriaceae* (in addition, the anaero-

bic bacteria produce characteristic metabolic products with distinctive odors).

USE OF KLIGLER IRON AGAR AND TRIPLE SUGAR IRON AGAR

In practice, microorganisms that are capable of fermenting glucose are commonly detected by observing the reactions they produce when grown on Kligler iron agar (KIA) or triple sugar iron (TSI) agar (Fig. 4-4; see Color Plate 4-1*E*). If an organism cannot ferment glucose, then an alkaline-slant–alkaline-butt (no change) reaction is observed (see Fig. 4-4*A*), indicating a lack of acid production and failure of the test organism to ferment any of the sugars present. This reaction alone is sufficient to exclude an organism from the *Enterobacteriaceae*. The formula for KIA is listed in Box 4-1 (the formula for TSI is identical except that 10 g of sucrose is added).

Several observations are important in studying the formulas of KIA and TSI. The incorporation of four protein derivatives—beef extract, yeast extract, peptone, and proteose peptone—makes KIA and TSI nutritionally very rich. The lack of inhibitors permits the growth of all but the most fastidious bacterial species (excluding the obligate anaerobes). For this reason, KIA and TSI agar can be used only when testing a bacterial species selected from a single colony recovered on primary or selective agar plates. Glucose and lactose (and sucrose in TSI medium) are evenly distributed throughout both the slant and deep portion of the tube. However, lactose is present in a concentration ten times that of glucose (similarly, the ratio of sucrose to glucose is 10:1 in TSI medium). This 10:1 ratio is important to the understanding of the biochemical principles discussed later. Ferrous sulfate as a hydrogen sulfide detector is somewhat less sensitive than other ferric or ferrous salts; therefore, there may be discrepancies in the hydrogen sulfide readings between KIA and TSI and other test media (see Color Plate 4-4*B*). The phenol red indicator is yellow below a pH of 6.8. Because the pH of the uninoculated medium is buffered at 7.4, relatively small quantities of acid production result in a visible color change.

BIOCHEMICAL PRINCIPLES

The biochemical principles underlying the reactions observed in KIA or TSI agar are illustrated in Figure 4-4. Note that the molten agar is allowed to solidify in a slant. This configuration results in essentially two reaction chambers within the same tube. The **slant** portion, exposed throughout its surface to atmospheric oxygen, is aerobic; the lower portion, called the **butt** or the **deep**, is protected from the air and is relatively anaerobic. It is important, when preparing the media, that the slant and the deep be kept equal in length, approximately 3 cm (1.5 in.) each, so that this two-chamber effect is preserved.

KIA and TSI tubes are inoculated with a long, straight wire. The well-isolated test colony recovered from an agar plate is touched with the end of the inoc-

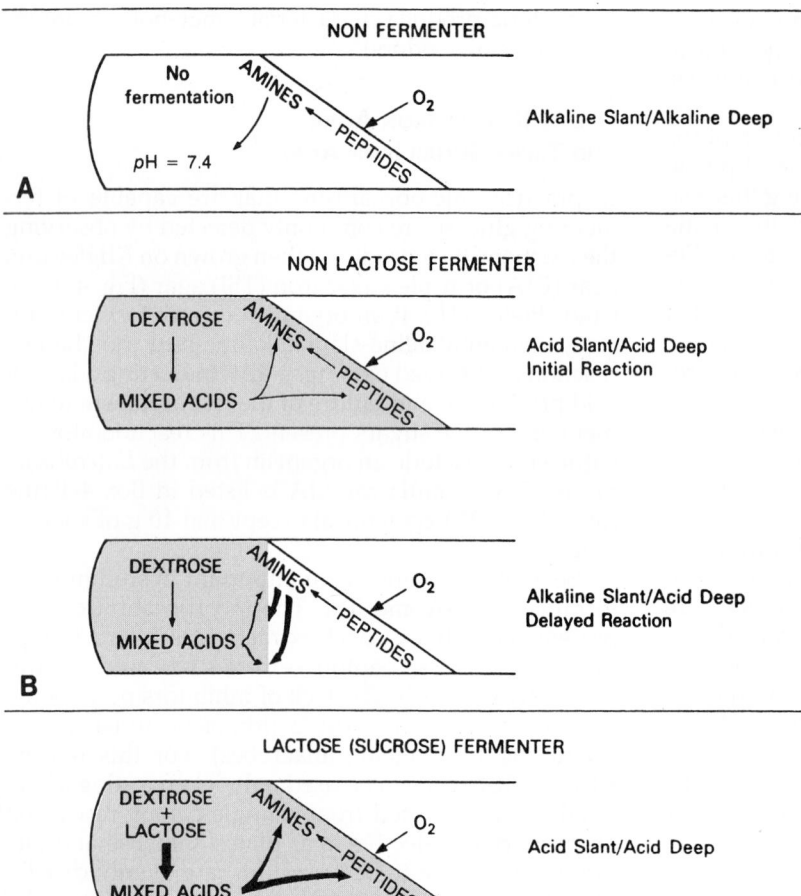

Figure 4-4
Three general types of reactions produced by bacteria growing on Kligler iron agar: (**A**) Nonfermentative bacilli that are unable to produce acids from the fermentation of glucose or lactose; there is no change in the medium (represented by *white*). (**B**) Initial acidification of both the deep and the slant of the medium (*shaded area*) by bacteria that ferment glucose, but the slant reverts back to alkaline pH as alkline amines are formed from the oxidative decarboxylation of peptides (derived from protein in the medium) near the surface. (**C**) Complete permanent acidification of both the deep and the slant of the tube by lactose-fermenting bacteria.

ulating needle, which is then stabbed into the deep of the tube, extending to within 3 to 5 mm of the bottom of the tube. When the inoculating wire is removed from the deep of the tube, the slant surface is streaked with a back-and-forth motion. Inoculated tubes are placed into an incubator at 35°C for 18 to 24 hours. The color photographs shown in Color Plates 4-1*E* and 5-1*A* reveal the reactions that are described in Box 4-2.

Thus, as shown in Figure 4-4*A* and in Plate 5-1*A*, without carbohydrate fermentation, no acids are formed, and the amine production in the slant together with the alkaline buffers produce a red color throughout the medium. The bacteria that produce this type of reaction are known as **nonfermenters** (see Chap. 5).

If the KIA tube is inoculated with a glucose-fermenting organism that cannot utilize lactose, only a relatively small quantity of acid can be obtained from the 0.1% concentration of glucose in the medium. Initially, during the first 8 to 12 hours of incubation, even this amount of acid may be sufficient to convert both the deep and the slant color to yellow. Within the next few hours, however, the glucose supply is completely exhausted and the bacteria begin oxidative degradation of the amino acids within the slant portion of the tube where oxygen is present. This results in the release of amines that soon counteract the small quantities of acid present in the slant; and by 18 to 24 hours, the entire slant reverts to an alkaline pH and the color returns to red. In the deep (anaerobic portion) of the tube, however, amino acid degradation is insufficient to counteract the acid formed, and the medium remains yellow. Thus, the alkaline-slant–acid-deep reaction on KIA (or TSI) is an important initial indicator that the test organism is a non–lactose-fermenter (see Fig. 4-4*B* and Color Plate 4-1*E*).

If the KIA tube is inoculated with a lactose-fermenting organism, then, even though the glucose is completely used up after the first 8 to 12 hours, fermentation continues as the organism is able to use lactose (present in ten times the concentration of glucose). Consequently, when the tube is examined at the end of 18 to 24 hours, acid production from fermentation of lactose is still occurring and both the slant and the

BOX 4-1. KLIGLER IRON AGAR

Beef extract, 3 g	Sodium chloride, 5 g
Yeast extract, 3 g	Sodium thiosulfate, 0.3 g
Peptone, 15 g	Agar, 12 g
Proteose peptone, 5 g	Phenol red, 0.024 g
Lactose, 10 g	Distilled water to equal 1 L
Glucose, 1 g	Final pH, 7.4
Ferrous sulfate, 0.2 g	

BOX 4-2. REACTIONS ON KIA

Alkaline Slant/Alkaline Deep (K/K)

No carbohydrate fermentation. This is characteristic of nonfermentative bacteria, such as *Pseudomonas aeruginosa.*

Alkaline Slant/Acid Deep (K/A)

Glucose fermented; lactose (or sucrose for TSI medium) not fermented. This is characteristic of non–lactose-fermenting bacteria, such as *Shigella* species.

Alkaline Slant/Acid (Black) Deep (K/A/H₂S)

Glucose fermented; lactose not fermented, hydrogen sulfide produced. This is characteristic of non–lactose-fermenting, hydrogen sulfide-producing bacteria, such as *Salmonella* species, *Citrobacter* species, and *Proteus* species.

Acid Slant/Acid Deep (A/A)

Glucose and lactose (or sucrose with TSI) fermented. This is characteristic of lactose-fermenting coliforms, such as *Escherichia coli* and the *Klebsiella–Enterobacter* species.

---

deep appear yellow, resulting in an acid-slant–acid-deep reaction (see Fig. 4-4*C* and Color Plate 4-1*E*).

Many microbiologists prefer TSI over KIA because the addition of sucrose to the formula helps screen for *Salmonella* and *Shigella* species, because neither of these (except rare strains) metabolizes either lactose or sucrose. Therefore, any acid–acid reaction of TSI indicates that either lactose, sucrose, or both have been fermented, excluding *Salmonella* and *Shigella.* It should also be remembered that *Yersinia enterocolitica* ferments sucrose, but not lactose; thus, on TSI the reaction will be acid–acid (similar to coliforms such as *E. coli*), but on KIA, the reaction will be alkaline–acid (similar to a non–lactose-fermenter). Consequently, when screening stool specimens for *Salmonella*, *Shigella*, and *Yersinia*, some might argue that KIA is preferable to TSI.

For the detection of hydrogen sulfide, which is colorless, the medium must include an indicator. Sodium thiosulfate is the source of sulfur atoms in most media used for hydrogen sulfide production. Iron salts (ferrous sulfate and ferric ammonium citrate) incorporated in the culture media then react with hydrogen sulfide to produce an insoluble black precipitate (ferrous sulfide). An acid environment is required for an organism to produce hydrogen sulfide and, therefore, a source of hydrogen ions must be provided. Because the deep of the KIA and TSI tubes becomes acidic with glucose fermentation (hydrogen ions increase), the blackening is often first seen or confined there, particularly with non–lactose-fermenting bacteria (see Color Plate 4-1*E*). Thus, it follows that a black deep should be

read as acid even if the usual yellow color is obscured by the black precipitate. KIA and TSI are less sensitive in the detection of hydrogen sulfide than other iron-containing media, such as sulfide indole motility (SIM) medium (see Color Plate 4-4*B*).

If an organism can be excluded from the *Enterobacteriaceae* before an extended battery of biochemical tests is set up, considerable time and labor will be saved. It is recommended that either a KIA or a TSI slant be set up on all isolates suspected of being one of the *Enterobacteriaceae* at the same time that differential test media of kit systems are set up. Even if an organism is a fermenter and is suspected of being one of the *Enterobacteriaceae*, a cytochrome oxidase test should be performed to exclude organisms belonging to other genera of fermenting bacteria, such as *Aeromonas, Plesiomonas, Vibrio,* and *Pasteurella* species, that are oxidase positive.

SELECTION OF PRIMARY ISOLATION MEDIA

Selective culture media must be used to recover the significant species of bacteria from specimens that may harbor a mixture of microorganisms. To make rational selections, microbiologists must know the composition of each formula and the purpose and relative concentration of each chemical or compound that is included. For example, it is not sufficient to know that bile salts are included in the formulas of a number of selective media to inhibit the growth of gram-positive and some of the more fastidious gram-negative bacterial species. For example, SS agar contains about five times the concentration of bile salts compared with MacConkey agar and is more inhibitory to *E. coli* and more selective for the recovery of *Salmonella* species from stool cultures.

For the recovery of the *Enterobacteriaceae* from clinical specimens that potentially harbor mixed bacteria, three general types of media are available: 1) nonselective media for primary isolation (e.g., blood agar); 2) selective or differential agars (e.g., MacConkey and Hektoen enteric agars); and 3) enrichment broths. Tables 4-1 and 4-2 compare different media commonly used in clinical practice. The formulas are complex and include ingredients that not only inhibit the growth of certain bacterial species (selective), but also detect several biochemical characteristics that are important in making a preliminary identification of the microorganisms present in the specimen (differential).

CHEMICALS AND COMPOUNDS USED IN SELECTIVE MEDIA

Box 4-3 lists the general types of chemicals and compounds used in selective media, including brief comments on the function of each.

SELECTIVE ISOLATION MEDIA

In 1905 MacConkey[194] first described a selective differential medium (neutral red–bile salt agar) that he used to isolate gram-negative enteric bacilli from specimens

TABLE 4-1
SELECTIVE DIFFERENTIAL MEDIA FOR RECOVERY OF ENTEROBACTERIACEAE

MEDIUM	FORMULATION		PURPOSE AND DIFFERENTIAL INGREDIENTS	REACTIONS AND INTERPRETATION
MacConkey agar (see Plate 4-2A and B)	Peptone	17 g	MacConkey agar is a differential-plating medium for the selection and recovery of the Enterobacteriaceae and related enteric gram-negative bacilli	Typical strong lactose fermenters, such as species of Escherichia, Klebsiella, and Enterobacter, produce red colonies surrounded by a zone of precipitated bile.
	Polypeptone	3 g		
	Lactose	10 g	The bile salts and crystal violet inhibit the growth of gram-positive bacteria and some fastidious gram-negative bacteria.	Slow or weak lactose fermenters, such as Citrobacter, Providencia, Serratia, and Hafnia, may appear colorless after 24 h or slightly pink in 24–48 h.
	Bile salts	1.5 g		
	Sodium chloride	5 g		
	Agar	13.5 g	Lactose is the sole carbohydrate. Lactose-fermenting bacteria produce colonies that are varying shades of red, owing to the conversion of the neutral red indicator dye (red below pH 6.8) from the production of mixed acids. Colonies of non–lactose-fermenting bacteria appear colorless or transparent.	Species of Proteus, Edwardsiella, Salmonella, and Shigella, with rare exceptions, produce colorless or transparent colonies.
	Neutral red	0.03 g		
	Crystal violet	0.001 g		Representative colonies, showing these various reactions, are shown in Color Plate 4-2.
	Distilled water to	1 L		
	Final pH = 7.1			
Eosin methylene blue (EMB) agar (see Color Plate 4-2C through F)	Peptone	10 g	EMB agar is a differential-plating medium that can be used in place of MacConkey agar in the isolation and detection of the Enterobacteriaceae or related coliform bacilli from specimens with mixed bacteria.	Typical strong lactose-fermenting colonies, notably Escherichia coli, produce colonies that are green-black with a metallic sheen.
	Lactose	5 g		
	Sucrose*	5 g		Weak fermenters, including Klebsiella, Enterobacter, Serratia, and Hafnia, produce purple colonies within 24–48 h.
	Dipotassium, PO₄	2 g	The aniline dyes (eosin and methylene blue) inhibit gram-positive and fastidious gram-negative bacteria. They combine to form a precipitate at acid pH, thus also serving as indicators of acid production.	
	Agar	13.5 g		Non–lactose-fermenters, including Proteus, Salmonella, and Shigella, produce transparent colonies.
	Eosin y	0.4 g		
	Methylene blue	0.065 g	Levine EMB, with only lactose, gives reactions more in parallel with MacConkey agar; the modified formula also detects sucrose fermenters.	Yersinia enterocolitica, a non–lactose, sucrose fermenter, produces transparent colonies on Levine EMB and purple to black colonies on the modified formula.
	Distilled water to	1 L		
	Final pH = 7.2			See Color Plate 4-2.

* Modified Holt-Harris Teague formula. Sucrose is not contained in Levine EMB agar.

containing mixtures of bacterial species. He incorporated lactose and the indicator neutral red into this medium to provide a visual means for detecting lactose utilization by the test organism. At that time, all non–spore-forming, gram-negative bacilli were still referred to as enteric organisms; however, microbiologists had recognized that certain species were more pathogenic to humans than others. The carbohydrate utilization patterns of several species of bacteria were already known by the turn of the century, and the fermentation of lactose, in particular, was recognized as an important marker for differentiating certain enteric pathogens. Holt-Harris and Teague[151] in 1916 described a medium with eosin and methylene blue as indicators for differentiating between lactose-fermenting and non–lactose-fermenting colonies. Sucrose was included in the medium to detect those members of the coliform group that ferment sucrose more readily than lactose.

MacConkey and EMB agars are only moderately inhibitory and are designed primarily to prevent growth of gram-positive bacteria from mixed cultures. Many species of fastidious gram-negative organisms are inhibited as well; however, all Enterobacteriaceae grow well. Table 4-1 compares the formulas, inhibitory ingredients, and key differential characteristics for MacConkey and EMB agars.

Deciding whether to use MacConkey or EMB agar is largely a matter of personal preference, because bacterial species that use lactose can be differentiated on both. MacConkey agar contains neutral red as the pH indicator and, as a result, lactose-metabolizing colonies appear pink from the production of mixed acids (see Color Plate 4-2A and B). Strong acid-producing bacteria, such as E. coli, form deep red colonies. Weaker acid-producing bacteria form light pink colonies or colonies that are clear at the periphery and have pink centers. On EMB agar, strong acid-producing bacteria form colonies that have a metallic sheen (see Color Plate 4-2C and D). The appearance of the sheen, caused by precipitation of dye in the colonies, is

TABLE 4-2

HIGHLY SELECTIVE MEDIA FOR RECOVERY OF *ENTEROBACTERIACEAE* FROM GASTROINTESTINAL SPECIMENS

MEDIUM	FORMULATION		PURPOSE AND DIFFERENTIAL INGREDIENTS	REACTIONS AND INTERPRETATION
Salmonella–Shigella (SS) agar	Beef extract	5 g	SS agar is a highly selective medium formulated to inhibit the growth of most coliform organisms and permit the growth of species of *Salmonella* and *Shigella* from environmental and clinical specimens. The high bile salts concentration and sodium citrate inhibit all gram-positive bacteria and many gram-negative organisms, including coliforms. Lactose is the sole carbohydrate and neutral red is the indicator for acid detection. Sodium thiosulfate is a source of sulfur. Any bacteria that produce hydrogen sulfide gas are detected by the black precipitate formed with ferric citrate (relatively insensitive). High selectivity of SS agar permits use of heavy inoculum.	Any lactose-fermenting colonies that appear are colored red by the neutral red. Rare strains of *Salmonella arizonae* are lactose fermenting, and colonies may simulate *Escherichia coli*. Growth of species of *Salmonella* is uninhibited, and colonies appear colorless with black centers, owing to hydrogen sulfide gas production. Species of *Shigella* show varying inhibition and colorless colonies with no blackening. Motile strains of *Proteus* that appear on SS agar do not swarm.
	Peptone	5 g		
	Lactose	10 g		
	Bile salts	8.5 g		
	Sodium citrate	8.5 g		
	Sodium thiosulfate	8.5 g		
	Ferric citrate	1 g		
	Agar	12.5 g		
	Neutral red	0.025 g		
	Brilliant green	0.033 g		
	Distilled water to	1 L		
	Final pH, 7.4			
Hektoen enteric (HE) agar (see Color Plate 4-3*E* and *F*)	Peptone	12 g	HE agar is a recent formulation devised as a direct-plating medium for fecal specimens to increase the yield of species of *Salmonella* and *Shigella* from the heavy numbers of normal flora. The high bile salt concentration inhibits growth of all gram-positive bacteria and retards the growth of many strains of coliforms. Acids may be produced from the carbohydrates, and acid fuchsin reacting with thymol blue produces a yellow color when the pH is lowered. Sodium thiosulfate is a sulfur source, and hydrogen sulfide gas is detected by ferric ammonium citrate (relatively sensitive).	Rapid lactose fermenters (such as *E. coli*) are moderately inhibited and produce bright orange to salmon pink colonies. *Salmonella* colonies are blue-green, typically with black centers from hydrogen sulfide gas. *Shigella* appear more green than *Salmonella,* with the color fading to the periphery of the colony. *Proteus* strains are somewhat inhibited; colonies that develop are small transparent, and more glistening or watery in appearance than species of *Salmonella* or *Shigella.* See Color Plate 4-3.
	Yeast extract	3 g		
	Bile salts	9 g		
	Lactose	12 g		
	Sucrose	12 g		
	Salicin	2 g		
	Sodium chloride	5 g		
	Sodium thiosulfate	5 g		
	Ferric ammonium citrate	1.5 g		
	Acid fuchsin	0.1 g		
	Thymol blue	0.04 g		
	Agar	14 g		
	Distilled water to	1 L		
	Final pH, 7.6			
Xylose lysine deoxycholate (XLD) agar (see Color Plate 4-3*A* through *D*)	Xylose	3.5 g	XLD agar is less inhibitory to growth of coliform bacilli than HE agar and was designed to detect shigellae in feces after enrichment in gram-negative broth. Bile salts in relatively low concentration make this medium less selective than the other two included in this table. Three carbohydrates are available for acid production, and phenol red is the pH indicator. Lysine-positive organisms, such as most *Salmonella* species, produce initial yellow colonies from xylose utilization and delayed red colonies from lysine decarboxylation. Hydrogen sulfide detection system is similar to that of HE agar.	Organisms such as *E. coli* and *Klebsiella–Enterobacter* species may use more than one carbohydrate and produce bright yellow colonies. Colonies of many species of *Proteus* are also yellow. Most species of *Salmonella* produce red colonies, most with black centers from hydrogen sulfide gas. *Shigella, Providencia,* and many *Proteus* species use none of the carbohydrates and produce translucent colonies. *Citrobacter* colonies are yellow with black centers; many *Proteus* species are yellow or translucent with black centers; salmonellae are red with black centers. See Color Plate 4-3.
	Lysine	5 g		
	Lactose	7.5 g		
	Sucrose	7.5 g		
	Sodium chloride	5 g		
	Yeast extract	3 g		
	Phenol red	0.08 g		
	Agar	13.5 g		
	Sodium deoxycholate	2.5 g		
	Sodium thiosulfate	6.8 g		
	Ferric ammonium citrate	0.8 g		
	Distilled water to	1 L		
	Final pH, 7.4			

BOX 4-3. CHEMICALS AND COMPOUNDS USED IN SELECTIVE MEDIA

Protein hydrolysates (e.g., peptones, meat infusion, tryptones, and casein): Proteins are cleaved by acids or enzymes into amino acids and peptides that can be used by bacteria to provide the carbon and nitrogen needed for bacterial metabolism.

Carbohydrates: A variety of disaccharides (e.g., lactose, sucrose, and maltose), hexoses (dextrose), and pentoses (xylose) are included in selective media for two purposes: 1) to provide a ready source of carbon for energy and 2) to serve as substrates in biochemical reactions for identification of unknown organisms.

Buffers: Balanced monosodium and disodium or potassium phosphates are most commonly used. Buffers provide 1) a stable pH for optimal growth of microorganisms, and 2) a standard reference pH for those media in which acid or alkaline reactions are used to identify microorganisms.

Enrichments (e.g., blood, serum, vitamin supplements, and yeast extracts): Growth supplements are added to media to recover fastidious organisms. Enrichments are less commonly used for the recovery of the *Enterobacteriaceae* because most members of this group grow without them.

Inhibitors: Various different compounds may serve to inhibit the growth of certain undesired bacterial species,

thus making the medium selective: 1) aniline dyes (e.g., brilliant green and eosin), 2) heavy metals (e.g., bismuth), 3) chemicals (e.g., azide, citrate, deoxycholate, selenite, and phenylethyl alcohol), and 4) antimicrobial agents (e.g., neomycin, colistin, vancomycin, and chloramphenicol). Their relative concentrations are important in determining the selectivity of the medium in which they are contained.

pH indicators: Fuchsin, methylene blue, neutral red, phenol red, and bromcresol purple are commonly used indicators in test media to measure pH shifts resulting from bacterial metabolism of given substrates.

Miscellaneous indicators: Other indicators may be included to detect specific bacterial products (e.g., ferric and ferrous ions for the detection of hydrogen sulfide).

Miscellaneous compounds and chemicals: Agar, a gelatinous extract of red seaweed, is commonly added to a medium, in varying concentrations, as a solidifying agent. Concentrations of 1% to 2% are used for plating media; concentrations of 0.05% to 0.3% are used for semisolid motility media; and trace amounts are added to anaerobic broth media to prevent convection currents and oxygen penetration. Sodium thiosulfate is commonly added to provide a source of sulfur.

---

highly suggestive of *E. coli*, although other strong acid producers, such as *Yersinia enterocolitica*, may have a similar appearance.

HIGHLY SELECTIVE ISOLATION MEDIA USED PRIMARILY FOR GASTROINTESTINAL SPECIMENS

Media are made highly selective by the addition of a variety of inhibitors to their formulas, generally in higher concentrations than in MacConkey and EMB agars. These media are used primarily to inhibit the growth of *E. coli* and other "coliforms," but they allow *Salmonella* and *Shigella* species to grow out from stool specimens.

Several selective media formulated for use in clinical laboratories are discussed here. The most commonly used are *Salmonella–Shigella* (SS) agar, xylose lysine deoxycholate (XLD) agar, and Hektoen enteric (HE) agar. These are described in Table 4-2.

Deciding which of these selective media to use for the recovery of enteric pathogens from fecal specimens depends both on personal preference and on the species to be selected. In general, these media are used in the clinical laboratory for the recovery of *Salmonella* and *Shigella* species from diarrheal stool specimens, or in public health laboratories to investigate possible fecal contamination of food and water supplies. Virtually all species of *Salmonella* grow well in the presence of bile salts, which explains why the gallbladder often

serves as one reservoir for human carriers. Bile salts are added to selective media because other species of enteric bacilli, including some of the more fastidious strains of *Shigella,* grow poorly or not at all. SS and HE agars contain relatively high concentrations of bile salts and are well adapted for recovering *Salmonella* species from specimens heavily contaminated with other coliform bacilli. However, because of its inhibitory effect on the recovery of certain strains of *Shigella* species, the routine use of SS agar as a single selective medium for isolation of enteric pathogens from stool specimens is not recommended.

XLD agar contains lactose, sucrose, and xylose;[295] thus, microorganisms that ferment these carbohydrates form yellow colonies (see Color Plate 4-3A). Bacteria incapable of fermenting these carbohydrates do not produce acids and form colorless colonies (see Color Plate 4-3B). Organisms that produce hydrogen sulfide form black pigment beginning in the center of the colonies (see Color Plate 4-3C). XLD agar also contains lysine. This is important because many species of *Salmonella* will ferment xylose and, therefore, will initially produce yellow colonies on XLD, but because these same species also decarboxylate lysine, the colonies will revert to pink after the small amount of xylose in the medium is used up. Lactose and sucrose, added in excess, prevent lysine-positive coliforms from similarly reverting. Because the decarboxylation of lysine results in the formation of strongly alkaline amines, a light pink halo may appear around the colonies on XLD agar (see Color Plate 4-3C). Black colonies without a pink halo are more suggestive of a hydrogen sulfide-producing strain of *Proteus* species (see Color Plate 4-3D).

The carbohydrates in HE agar are lactose, sucrose, and salicin.[176] Microorganisms capable of fermenting these carbohydrates also form yellow colonies (see Color Plate 4-3E); asaccharolytic strains produce colonies that are translucent or light green (see Color Plate 4-3F). Lactose- and sucrose-negative bacteria that acidify salicin may produce orange colonies. HE agar also contains ferric salts; thus hydrogen sulfide-producing colonies appear black. Bismuth sulfite and brilliant green agars are highly selective media that are not commonly used in clinical laboratories. They are difficult to prepare, and their shelf life is very short (48 to 72 hours). These media are specifically designed to recover *Salmonella typhi* from fecal specimens and are particularly useful when screening numerous patients in endemic areas or during an epidemic. *Salmonella* species (*S. typhi* in particular) can be suspected on these media because of the propensity to produce colonies with a black sheen.

ENRICHMENT MEDIA

As the name indicates, an enrichment medium is used to enhance the growth of certain bacterial species while inhibiting the development of unwanted microorganisms. Enrichment media are most commonly used in clinical laboratories for the recovery of *Salmonella* and *Shigella* species from fecal specimens. Enrichment broths are particularly helpful in the recovery of organisms from the stools of *Salmonella* carriers or from patients with light *Shigella* infections in whom the number of organisms may be as low as 200/g of feces. (*E. coli* and other enteric bacilli may reach massive concentrations, as high as 10^9/g of feces.)

Enrichment media work on the principle that *E. coli* and other gram-negative organisms, which constitute the normal fecal flora, are maintained in a prolonged **lag** phase by the inhibitory chemicals in the broth. *Salmonella* and *Shigella* species are far less inhibited, enter into a log phase of growth, and are more readily recovered from fecal samples. However, after several hours, the enrichment media no longer suppress the growth of *E. coli* and other enteric organisms, which will ultimately overgrow the culture. Thus, for maximal recovery of *Salmonella* and *Shigella* species from fecal samples, it is recommended that the enrichment broth be subcultured within 8 hours.

The two most commonly used enrichment media are selenite broth and gram-negative (GN) broth. Selenite broth is more inhibitory to the growth of *E. coli* and other enteric gram-negative bacilli than is GN broth. Thus, selenite broth is best adapted for the recovery of *Salmonella* or *Shigella* species from heavily contaminated specimens, such as feces or sewage. However, GN broth is used with greater frequency in clinical laboratories because it is less inhibitory to the growth of many of the more fastidious strains of

Shigella species. Enrichment of fecal specimens in GN broth for 4 to 6 hours and then subculturing to HE or XLD agar is the optimal technique for the recovery of *Shigella* species in suspected cases of bacillary dysentery. The formulas and salient characteristics of these two enrichment media are summarized in Table 4-3.

GUIDELINES FOR CHOOSING SELECTIVE ISOLATION MEDIA

The media listed in Tables 4-1 through 4-3 and the several combinations in which they can be used may be somewhat confusing. The following is a guide for selecting media that may be optimal in the recovery of the *Enterobacteriaceae* from clinical specimens.

For specimens other than feces or rectal swabs, a combination of MacConkey or EMB agar and a blood agar is usually sufficient. Media with greater inhibitory properties are not routinely required because the concentration of commensal flora or contaminating organisms is relatively low in most nonenteric specimens. Subculturing to a more inhibitory medium can be done in instances in which it appears necessary.

For fecal specimens or rectal swabs, it is necessary to select only one medium from each of the groups listed in Tables 4-1 and 4-2. The approach outlined in Box 4-4 is suggested.

DIFFERENTIAL IDENTIFICATION CHARACTERISTICS

Although a preliminary identification of the *Enterobacteriaceae* is possible based on colonial characteristics and biochemical reactions on primary isolation media, further species identification requires the determination of additional phenotypic characteristics that reflect the genetic code and unique identity of the organism being tested. It is the purpose of this discussion to review the salient features of the tests that measure these phenotypic characteristics and are commonly used in clinical laboratories. This orientation is necessary so that laboratory personnel can develop a fundamental understanding of the principles behind these procedures in order to recognize and correct any biochemical inconsistencies, problems with mixed cultures, or faulty techniques. It is not possible to discuss the variety of differential tests and numerous schemes available for the final species identification of the *Enterobacteriaceae*. However, several of the tests widely used in clinical laboratories to measure those metabolic characteristics by which all but a few rare or atypical species of the *Enterobacteriaceae* can be identified are listed in Box 4-5. Carbohydrate utilization and ONPG activity have been discussed previously.

INDOLE PRODUCTION

Indole is one of the degradation products from the metabolism of the amino acid tryptophan. Bacteria that possess the enzyme tryptophanase are capable of cleaving tryptophan, thereby producing indole, pyru-

TABLE 4-3

ENRICHMENT BROTHS FOR RECOVERY OF *ENTEROBACTERIACEAE*

BROTH	FORMULATION		PURPOSE AND DIFFERENTIAL INGREDIENTS	REACTIONS AND INTERPRETATION
Selenite broth	Peptone	5 g	Selenite F broth is recommended for the isolation of salmonellae from specimens, such as feces, urine, or sewage, that have heavy concentrations of mixed bacteria.	Within a few hours after inoculation with the specimen, the broth becomes cloudy.
	Lactose	4 g		Because coliforms or other intestinal flora may overgrow the pathogens within a few hours, subculture to *Salmonella–Shigella* (SS) agar or bismuth sulfite is recommended within 8–12 h.
	Sodium selenite	4 g	Sodium selenite is inhibitory to *Escherichia coli* and other coliform bacilli, including many strains of *Shigella*.	
	Sodium phosphate	10 g		
	Distilled water to	1 L	The medium functions best under anaerobic conditions, and a pour depth of at least 5 cm (2 in.) is recommended.	Overheating of the broth during preparation may produce a visible precipitate, making it unsatisfactory for use.
	Final pH = 7.0			
Gram-negative (GN) broth	Polypeptone peptone	20 g	Because of the relatively low concentration of deoxycholate, GN broth is less inhibitory to *E. coli* and other coliforms. Most strains of *Shigella* grow well. The deoxycholate and citrate are inhibitory to gram-positive bacteria.	GN broth is designed for the recovery of *Salmonella* and *Shigella* species when they are in small numbers in fecal specimens.
	Glucose	1 g		
	D-mannitol	2 g		The broth may become cloudy within 4–6 h of inoculation, and subculture to HE agar or XLD agar within that time is recommended.
	Sodium citrate	5 g		
	Sodium deoxycholate	0.5 g		
	Dipotassium phosphate	4 g	The increased concentration of mannitol over glucose limits the growth of *Proteus* species, nonetheless encouraging growth of *Salmonella* and *Shigella* species, both of which are capable of fermenting mannitol.	
	Monopotassium phosphate	1.5 g		
	Sodium chloride	5 g		
	Distilled water to	1 L		
	Final pH = 7.0			

vic acid, and ammonia. Indole can be detected in tryptophan test medium by observing the development of a red color after adding a solution containing *p*-dimethylaminobenzaldehyde (e.g., Ehrlich's or Kovac's reagent). The biochemistry and details of the indole test are schematically illustrated in Figure 4-5 and

Chart 40, respectively. A color reproduction is shown in Color Plate 4-4C.

The choice between Ehrlich's and Kovac's reagents is one of personal preference. Ehrlich's reagent is more sensitive and is preferred when testing nonfermentative bacilli or anaerobes in which indole production is

---

BOX 4-4. SELECTING A MEDIUM FOR FECAL SPECIMEN OR RECTAL SWAB

1. Inoculate the specimen directly to a MacConkey or EMB agar plate for primary isolation of all species of enteric gram-negative bacilli.

2. Directly inoculate either an XLD or an HE agar plate for the selective screening of *Salmonella* or *Shigella* species.

3. Enrich a small portion of the specimen by heavily inoculating either selenite or GN broth. If selenite is used, subculture to HE agar within 8 to 12 hours; if GN is used, subculture within 4 hours. **Note:** In the author's laboratory this step is not routinely performed unless screening asymptomatic patients for presence of a carrier state.

4. Incubate all plate cultures at 35°C for 24 to 48 hours. Select suspicious colonies for definitive biochemical or serologic testing.

BOX 4-5. TESTS USED TO MEASURE METABOLIC CHARACTERISTICS OF *ENTEROBACTERIACEAE*

Carbohydrate utilization

o-Nitrophenyl-β-D-galactopyranoside (ONPG) activity

Indole production

Methyl red

Voges-Proskauer test (production of acetyl methyl carbinol [acetoin])

Citrate utilization

Urease production

Decarboxylation of lysine, ornithine, and arginine

Phenylalanine deaminase production

Hydrogen sulfide production

Motility

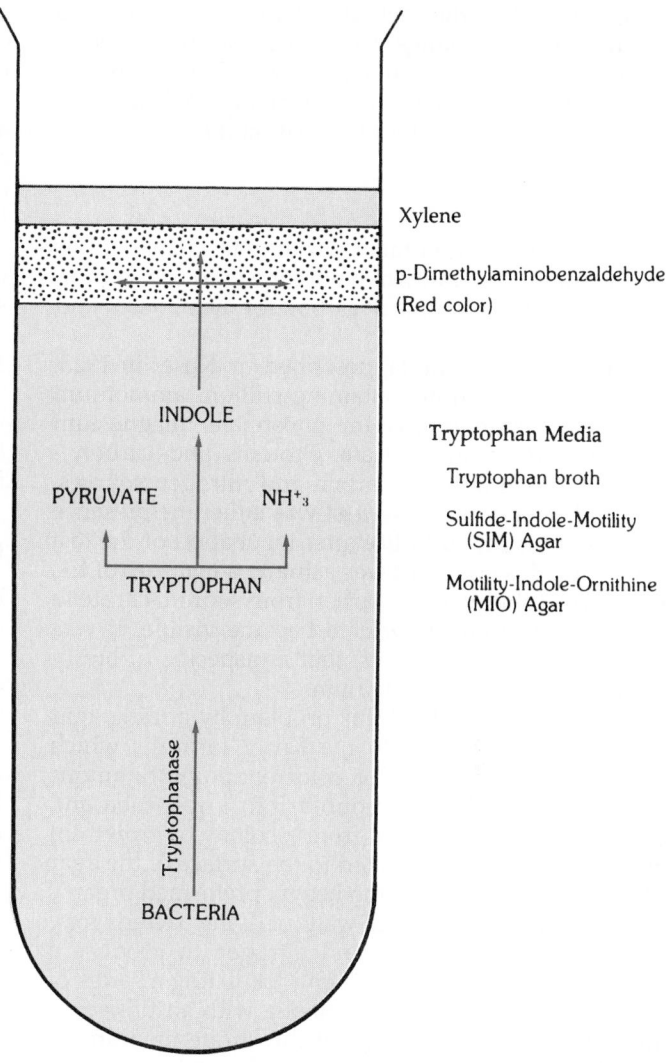

Figure 4-5
Formation of indole by tryptophanase-producing bacteria growing on a culture medium containing tryptophan. Indole is one of the immediate degradation products (in addition to pyruvic acid and ammonia) resulting from the deamination of tryptophan. Indole can be extracted from the aqueous phase of the medium by chloroform and detected by the addition of Ehrlich's reagent (dimethylaminobenzaldehyde).

minimal. Because indole is soluble in organic compounds, xylene or chloroform should be added to the test medium before adding Ehrlich's reagent. This extraction step is less critical for Kovac's reagent because amyl alcohol is used for the diluent (ethyl alcohol is used with Ehrlich's reagent).

METHYL RED TEST

A simplified schema showing only two alternative pathways (mixed acid and butylene glycol) for the metabolism of the pyruvate formed from the fermentation of glucose is shown in Figure 4-2. Bacteria that follow primarily the mixed acid fermentation route often produce sufficient acid to maintain a pH below 4.4 (the acid color breakpoint of the methyl red indicator). The methyl red test provides a valuable characteristic for identifying bacterial species that produce strong acids from glucose.

The details of the methyl red test are shown in Chart 48. The test, as originally described, requires 48 to 72 hours of incubation before a valid result can be obtained, an amount of time unacceptable to most clinical microbiology laboratories. Barry and coworkers[22]

have described a modification that can be read in 18 to 24 hours. A 0.5-mL aliquot of broth is used with a relatively heavy inoculum of the test organism. One or 2 drops of methyl red reagent are added after 18 to 24 hours of incubation at 35°C, and the development of red color indicates a positive test (see Color Plate 4-4C). The Barry modification is as accurate as the test originally described and saves a significant amount of time.

VOGES-PROSKAUER TEST

The details of the Voges-Proskauer test, shown in Chart 75, are based on the conversion of acetyl methyl carbinol (acetoin) to diacetyl through the action of potassium hydroxide and atmospheric oxygen. Diacetyl is converted into a red complex under the catalytic action of α-naphthol and creatine (see Color Plate 4-4D).

Note, in Figure 4-2, that the formation of acetoin and butylene glycol is an alternative pathway for the metabolism of pyruvic acid. Bacteria that use this pathway, such as certain strains within the *Klebsiella–Enterobacter–Serratia–Hafnia* group, produce only small quantities of mixed acids that may be insufficient to lower the pH of the methyl red medium enough to produce a color change. Consequently, most species of the *Enterobacteriaceae* that are Voges-Proskauer-positive, with rare exceptions, are methyl red-negative and vice versa (see Color Plate 4-4C and *D*).

CITRATE UTILIZATION

The principle of the citrate utilization test (Chart 12) is to determine the ability of an organism to use sodium citrate as the sole source of carbon for metabolism and growth.

The original formula, described by Koser in 1923, was a broth medium containing sodium ammonium phosphate, monopotassium phosphate, magnesium sulfate, and sodium citrate. Proteins and carbohydrates were omitted as carbon and nitrogen sources. The endpoint of the Koser test was either the presence or lack of visible turbidity after incubation of the test organism: this endpoint was actually a measure of the organism's ability to use carbon from sodium citrate to produce sufficient growth to become visible. It was soon recognized, however, that nonspecific turbidity could occur in Koser's medium.

Simmons[287] resolved this problem by adding agar and bromthymol blue to the Koser formula, which provided a more sensitive color endpoint. Simmons citrate agar medium is poured into a test tube and slanted. A light inoculum from a colony of growth of the test organism is streaked to the surface of the agar slant. If the inoculum is too heavy, preformed organic compounds within the cell walls of dying bacteria may release sufficient carbon and nitrogen to produce a false-positive test result. When inoculating a series of tubes of differential culture media with an unknown organism, it is important that the citrate medium be streaked first to prevent carryover of proteins or carbohydrates from the other media.

The production of a blue color in the test medium after 24 hours of incubation at 35°C indicates the presence of alkaline products and a positive citrate utilization test result (see Color Plate 4-4D). If carbon is used from sodium citrate, nitrogen is also extracted from the ammonium phosphate contained in the medium, releasing ammonia. Occasionally, visible growth is detected along the streak line before conversion of the medium to a blue color. This visible growth also indicates a positive test result. Malonate, acetate, and mucate are other anionic radicals commonly used to determine the ability of bacteria to use these simple compounds as a sole source of carbon.

The acronym IMViC (indole, methyl red, Voges-Proskauer, and citrate) was once used by sanitarians and epidemiologists to refer to those tests needed to detect fecal contamination of food and water. *Escherichia coli* has been used by public health officials for many years to indicate fecal contamination. *Enterobacter aerogenes* produces colonies on primary isolation media that often cannot be distinguished from *E. coli*. However, the recovery of *E. aerogenes* from food and potable water does not necessarily signify fecal contamination because the organism is widespread in soil, grasses, and vegetative matter. Therefore, a set of biochemical characteristics was needed to differentiate the two organisms. The IMViC tests were adopted to serve this purpose. Most strains of *E. coli* are indole- and methyl red-positive, with Voges-Proskauer and citrate being negative. *E. aerogenes* typically produces exactly opposite reactions (see Color Plates 4-4C and *D*). Although the individual characteristics included in the IMViC battery are still used in bacterial identification systems, they are used only infrequently as a specific test set.

In view of the complexity of differentiating over 100 species of *Enterobacteriaceae* presented in the next section of this text, it is interesting that there was a time when the major decisions in microbiology were relatively simple and could be made on the basis of only four easy-to-perform biochemical tests.

UREASE PRODUCTION

Microorganisms that possess the enzyme urease hydrolyze urea, releasing ammonia and producing a pink-red color change in the medium (see Color Plate 4-4E). The details of the urease test are shown in Chart 72.

Important differences between Stuart's urea broth and Christensen's urea agar should be noted. Stuart's broth is heavily buffered with phosphate salts at a pH of 6.8. Relatively large quantities of ammonia must be formed by the test organism before the buffer system is overcome and the medium's pH is elevated above 8.0 to produce a color change in the indicator. Stuart's broth, therefore, is virtually selective for *Proteus* species.

Christensen's urea agar[72] is less buffered than Stuart's urea broth and contains peptones and glucose. This enriched medium supports the growth of many species of bacteria that cannot grow in Stuart's broth, and the decreased buffer capacity permits the detection of smaller amounts of ammonia. Those organisms that produce less urease, such as certain species of *Klebsiella*, *Enterobacter*, *Brucella*, and *Bordetella bronchiseptica*, can be tested with Christensen's urea agar. For many of these species, a positive urease reaction is first detected by a pink-to-red color change in the slant portion of the agar (see Color Plate 4-4E). The slant initially turns red because the alkaline reaction, resulting from the splitting of small quantities of urea, is augmented by the amines formed from the oxidative decarboxylation of the amino acids in the air-exposed portion of the medium.

DECARBOXYLATION OF LYSINE, ORNITHINE, AND ARGININE

Many species of bacteria possess enzymes capable of decarboxylating specific amino acids in the test medium. The decarboxylase enzymes remove a molecule of CO_2 from an amino acid to form alkaline-reacting amines. The following are the amino acids most commonly tested and their amine degradation products:

Lysine → cadaverine
Ornithine → putrescine
Arginine → citrulline

A number of test systems have been described to measure this property, based on either detection of an alkaline pH shift in the test medium or direct measurement of the reaction products. For example, the amines resulting from the decarboxylation reaction can be detected with Ninhydrin reagent after extraction from the broth culture with chloroform. This is the relatively sensitive Carlquist reaction,[46] most commonly used for detecting the weak decarboxylase activity of many of the nonfermentative gram-negative bacilli and certain species of anaerobic bacteria.

The decarboxylase activity of the *Enterobacteriaceae* is most commonly measured in clinical microbiology laboratories with Moeller decarboxylase broth.[213] The details of this test are shown in Chart 18. The endpoint of the reaction is the production of an alkaline pH shift in the medium and the development of a blue-purple color after incubation with the test organism (see Color Plate 4-4F). Note, in the Moeller formula, included in Chart 18, that the medium is buffered at pH 6.0. This is more acidic than most culture media. This low pH is necessary because the decarboxylase enzymes are not optimally active until the pH of the medium drops below 5.5. The drop from 6.0 to 5.5 results from the growing bacteria that metabolize the small amount of glucose in the medium to produce mixed acids. A control tube, devoid of amino acid, must always be included when performing the decarboxylase test to ensure that this initial drop in pH has occurred. A yellow color change in the bromcresol purple indicator of the control tube shows acidification. Pyridoxal phosphate is included in the medium and acts as a coenzyme to further enhance the decarboxylase activity.

Many microbiologists prefer Falkow lysine broth[103] over the Moeller medium because the Falkow test depends on only an alkaline shift in pH indicator, and neither an anaerobic nor an acid environment is required. However, this medium cannot be used to detect lysine decarboxylase activity in certain members of the *Klebsiella–Enterobacter–Serratia–Hafnia* group. They produce acetyl methyl carbinol, which interferes with the final alkaline pH shift, leading to false-negative interpretations. Modifications in this medium form the basis of the motility indole ornithine (MIO)[92] semisolid agar used in clinical microbiology laboratories. Rapid methods for detecting ornithine[111] and lysine[45] decarboxylase activity in members of the *Enterobacteriaceae* have also been described.

Edwards and Fife[94] described a solid lysine decarboxylase medium based on the Falkow formula, which includes ferric ammonium citrate and thiosulfate for the detection of hydrogen sulfide. This medium is lysine iron agar (LIA), used in many laboratories as an aid in the identification of *Salmonella* species, most of which are both hydrogen sulfide-positive and lysine decarboxylase-positive. A black deep and a purple slant with LIA are virtually indicative of *Salmonella* species. Another advantage of LIA is that *Proteus* and *Providencia* species, both of which deaminate, rather

than decarboxylate, amino acids, can be detected by the development of a red color in the slant of the tube (see Color Plate 4-4G).

The lysine decarboxylase test is useful in differentiating lactose-negative *Citrobacter* species (0% positive) from *Salmonella* species (98% positive). Almost all strains of *Shigella sonnei* (more than 98%) possess ornithine decarboxylase activity, whereas only a few strains of *S. boydii* (2.5%) show such activity; *S. dysenteriae* and *S. flexneri* are ornithine-negative. The ornithine decarboxylase test is perhaps most useful in differentiating *Klebsiella* species (most species are negative) from *Enterobacter* species (most strains are positive).

PHENYLALANINE DEAMINASE PRODUCTION

The phenylalanine deaminase determination is useful in the initial differentiation of *Proteus*, *Morganella*, and *Providencia* species from other gram-negative bacilli. Only members of these genera, and a few relatively rare isolates of the *Enterobacter* group, possess the enzyme responsible for the oxidative deamination of phenylalanine. The test is easily performed, as outlined in Chart 60. Phenylpyruvic acid may be detected in as little as 4 hours if a heavy inoculum is used; however, 18 to 24 hours of incubation are generally recommended. The phenylalanine test medium employs yeast extract as the source for carbon and nitrogen. Meat extracts or protein hydrolysates contain varying amounts of naturally occurring phenylalanine that can lead to inconsistent results. The development of a green color after addition of the ferric chloride reagent is immediate and easy to visualize (see Color Plate 4-4E).

HYDROGEN SULFIDE PRODUCTION

The ability of certain bacterial species to liberate sulfur from sulfur-containing amino acids or other compounds in the form of H_2S is an important characteristic for their identification. The media most commonly used for the detection of H_2S and the sources for sulfur and the sulfide indicators are listed in Table 4-4.

The sequence of steps leading to the production and detection of H_2S in a test system is outlined in Box 4-6.

The differences in detecting H_2S production in the different media result from alteration in one or more of these conditions. H_2S detected in one medium may not be detected in another, and it is necessary to know the test system used when interpreting identification charts. SIM medium is more sensitive for the detection of H_2S than KIA, presumably because of its semisolid consistency, lack of carbohydrates to suppress H_2S formation, and use of peptonized iron as the indicator (see Color Plate 4-4B). KIA, on the other hand, is more sensitive than TSI agar because sucrose is believed to suppress the enzyme mechanisms responsible for H_2S production. Lead acetate is the most sensitive indicator and should be used whenever bacteria that produce only trace amounts of H_2S are tested. Unfortunately, lead acetate, when incorporated in culture media, also inhibits the growth of many fastidious bacteria, specif-

TABLE 4-4
MEDIA FOR THE DETECTION OF HYDROGEN SULFIDE (H₂S)

MEDIA	SULFUR SOURCE	H₂S INDICATOR
Bismuth sulfite	Peptones plus sulfite	Ferrous sulfate
Citrate sulfide agar	Sodium thiosulfate	Ferric ammonium citrate
Deoxycholate citrate agar	Peptones	Ferric citrate
Lysine iron agar	Sodium thiosulfate	Ferric ammonium citrate
Kligler iron agar	Sodium thiosulfate	Ferrous sulfate
Triple sugar iron agar	Sodium thiosulfate	Ferrous sulfate
Lead acetate agar	Sodium thiosulfate	Lead acetate
Salmonella–Shigella agar	Sodium thiosulfate	Ferric citrate
Sulfide–indole–motility medium	Sodium thiosulfate	Peptonized iron
Xylose–lysine–deoxycholate or Hektoen enteric	Sodium thiosulfate	Ferric ammonium citrate

ically the ones that may require a sensitive detector system. These organisms can be tested for production of H₂S by draping a lead acetate-impregnated filter paper strip under the cap of a culture tube of KIA medium. In this way, the extreme sensitivity of the lead acetate indicator can be used without incorporating it directly into the medium.

With all H₂S detection systems, the endpoint is an insoluble, heavy metal sulfide, which produces a black precipitate in the medium or on the filter paper strip. Because hydrogen ions must be available for H₂S formation, the blackening is first seen in test media in which acid formation is maximum, that is, along the inoculation line, within the deeps of slanted agar media, or in the centers of colonies growing on agar surfaces.

MOTILITY

Bacterial motility is another important determinant in making a final species identification. Bacteria move by means of flagella, the number and location of which vary among the different species. Flagellar stains are available for this determination (see Chap. 5).

Bacterial motility can be observed directly by placing a drop of culture broth medium on a microscope slide and viewing it under a microscope. Hanging-drop chambers are available so that the preparation can be viewed under higher magnification without danger of lowering the objectives onto the contaminated drop. This technique is used primarily for detecting the motility of bacterial species that do not grow well in semisolid agar media. However, *Enterobacteriaceae* do grow well, and tubes containing semisolid agar are most commonly employed.

Motility media have agar concentrations of 0.4% or less. At higher concentrations, the gel is too firm to allow the organisms to spread freely. Combination media, such as SIM medium[195] or MIO agar[92] have found wide use in clinical microbiology laboratories because more than one characteristic can be measured in the same tube. The motility test must be interpreted first because the addition of an indole reagent may obscure the results. Because SIM medium and MIO agar have a slightly turbid background, interpretations may be somewhat difficult with bacterial species that grow slowly in these media. In these cases, a motility test medium (Box 4-7) is recommended because it supports the growth of most fastidious bacteria and has a crystal-clear appearance.

The motility test is interpreted by making a macroscopic examination of the medium for a diffuse zone of growth flaring out from the line of inoculation (see Color Plate 4-4H). The use of tetrazolium salts in motility medium has been advocated as an aid in the visual detection of bacterial growth. Tetrazolium salts are colorless but are converted into insoluble red formazan complexes by the reducing properties of growing bacteria. In a motility test medium containing tetrazolium, the development of this red color helps trace the

BOX 4-6. HOW H₂S IS PRODUCED

1. Release of sulfide from cysteine or thiosulfate by bacterial enzymatic action
2. Coupling of sulfide (S²⁻) with a hydrogen ion (H⁺) to form H₂S
3. Detection of H₂S by iron, bismuth, or lead to produce insoluble, heavy metal sulfides that appear as a black precipitate

BOX 4-7. MOTILITY TEST MEDIUM (EDWARDS AND EWING)

Beef extract, 3 g	Agar, 4 g
Peptone, 10 g	Distilled water to equal 1 L
Sodium chloride, 5 g	Final pH, 7.3

spread of bacteria from the inoculation line. However, these salts may inhibit certain fastidious bacteria and cannot be used in all cases.

Of the *Enterobacteriaceae*, species of *Shigella* and *Klebsiella* are uniformly nonmotile. Most motile species of the *Enterobacteriaceae* can be detected at 35°C; however, *Yersinia enterocolitica*, in which flagellar proteins develop more rapidly at lower temperatures, is motile at 22°C (room temperature) but not at 35°C. *Listeria monocytogenes* is another bacterial species that requires room-temperature incubation before motility develops. *Pseudomonas aeruginosa*, an organism that grows well only in the presence of oxygen, produces a spreading film on the surface of motility agar and does not show the characteristic fanning out from the inoculation line because it does not grow in the deeper oxygen-deficient portions of the tube.

TAXONOMY OF THE *ENTEROBACTERIACEAE*

The application of new technologies to study the taxonomy of microorganisms has led to a rapid increase in the number of genera and species of bacteria that fit the general criteria for *Enterobacteriaceae*. In 1972, Edwards and Ewing[93] described 11 genera and 26 species belonging to the *Enterobacteriaceae*. In 1985, Farmer and associates[106] described 22 genera comprising 69 species and 29 enteric groups. In this chapter, 31 genera and 139 species, biogroups, and unnamed enteric groups of *Enterobacteriaceae* are described.

CLASSIFICATION OF *ENTEROBACTERIACEAE* BY TRIBES

The division of the *Enterobacteriaceae* into tribes is not used in the current edition of *Bergey's Manual* or in the Centers for Disease Control (CDC) classification because the authors believe that the use of tribes is of no diagnostic significance and of questionable taxonomic significance. This argument has validity from the perspective of pure classification. Yet, for those users of this text who are new to the field of microbiology and who must orient themselves to the complex and confusing *Enterobacteriaceae*, the tribe concept proposed by Ewing[98] has certain teaching and learning advantages. We agree with Ewing that his scheme, although imperfect, represents a good compromise between practical and ideal taxonomies.

The tribe concept provides both students and practitioners with a convenient method of grouping together the major genera within the family that share similar biochemical reactions and are of similar diagnostic importance. We believe it is important that practicing microbiologists maintain a base of knowledge that is firmly grounded in the morphology, physiology, and biochemistry of medically important bacteria. Furthermore, certain phenotypic patterns that allow easy subgrouping and clustering of related species must be committed to memory. This orientation is especially important if microbiologists use semiautomated and automated commercial systems with computer-assisted identification, because it serves as a quality control check to validate instrument-generated information. The use of the tribe concept as an approach to learning the *Enterobacteriaceae* serves these goals well and is the approach chosen for use in this text for teaching the key features of the established genera of the *Enterobacteriaceae*. The current species included in the established genera, sorted by tribes, are listed in Table 4-5.

KEY IDENTIFICATION CHARACTERISTICS FOR THE MOST COMMON SPECIES

Table 4-6 shows the key identification characteristics used in separating the established genera of the *Enterobacteriaceae* into seven tribes. Students should study this table and learn to categorize an unknown isolate into one of these tribes on the basis of reactions seen with these key tests. The following observations are made to assist students in identifying the most common species.

The members of the *Escherichieae* have the following key reactions: indole-positive, methyl red-positive, Voges-Proskauer-negative, citrate-negative (the classic example of mixed acid fermenters). They are negative for all the other key biochemical tests: hydrogen sulfide, phenylalanine deaminase, and urea. Note from Table 4-6 that *Shigella* species are similar to *Escherichia* species except they are negative for CO_2 gas and motility.

The *Edwardsielleae* are similar to *Escherichieae* except for the property of being hydrogen sulfide-positive. Students may wish to think of *Edwardsiella tarda* as hydrogen sulfide-positive *E. coli*. *Salmonelleae* resemble *Edwardsielleae* except that they are indole-negative and citrate-positive. *Citrobacter freundii* is similar to *Salmonella* except for being lysine-negative. *C. koseri* differs from *C. freundii* by being hydrogen sulfide-negative and indole-positive.

The *Klebsielleae* are composed of the Voges-Proskauer-positive members of the *Enterobacteriaceae*. As shown in Table 4-6 and illustrated in Figure 4-2, most members of this tribe produced copious amounts of CO_2, so much so that the deep portion of KIA and TSI slants is often pushed halfway up the tube. Notice that the *Klebsiella* species are nonmotile and that *Pantoea* is triple decarboxylase-negative (lysine-negative, arginine-negative, and ornithine-negative).

The *Proteeae* are separated from all others by virtue of being phenylalanine deaminase-positive, a feature unique to this tribe. The urea reaction for the species in the genus *Proteus* and *Morganella* as well as one of the

(text continues on page 196)

TABLE 4-5
IMPORTANT RECENT CHANGES IN THE ESTABLISHED GENERA OF THE *ENTEROBACTERIACEAE*

NEW DESIGNATION	PREVIOUS DESIGNATION	COMMENTS
Tribe I: *Escherichieae*		
Escherichia coli		Sorbitol (+) except for serotype 0157:H7. All other species are sorbitol (−).
E. coli inactive	Alkalescens-Dispar	Anaerogenic, lactose-negative (or delayed) and nonmotile.
E. blattae		Not found in human specimens. Isolated from cockroach feces.
E. fergusonii	Enteric group 10	Found in blood, urine, and feces: indole (+), sorbitol (−), LAO (+, −, +), lactose (−), but ONPG (+).
E. hermannii	Enteric group 11	Wounds and feces most common sources. Yellow pigmented, indole (+), sorbitol (−), LAO (−, −, +).
E. vulneris	Enteric group 1 API group 2 Alma group 1	Most strains from human wounds. Over half the strains are yellow-pigmented.
Shigella		The four species of *Shigella* and *E. coli* form a single species on the basis of DNA hybridization. *S. dysenteriae* (group A), *S. flexneri* (group B), and *S. boydii* (group C) are biochemically similar and must be separated by serologic methods. *S. sonnei* is ornithine (+).
Tribe II: *Edwardsielleae*		
Edwardsiella tarda	*Edwardsiella anguillimortifera* Asakusa group	Produce indole and abundant H_2S, ferment glucose and maltose, but not mannitol, lactose, sucrose, or arabinose. Found in cold-blooded animals. Opportunistic human pathogen. May cause wound infections and diarrhea.
E. tarda biogroup 1		Indole (+), H_2S (−), mannitol, sucrose, and arabinose-positive. Found in snakes, not a human clinical isolate.
E. hoshinae		Indole (−), H_2S (−), isolated from birds, reptiles, and water. Several isolates from human feces.
E. ictaluri		No human isolates, causes enteric septicemia in catfish.
Tribe III: *Salmonelleae*		
Salmonella	*S. choleraesuis* *S. typhi* *S. enteritidis*	All subgroups (subgenera) of *Salmonella* and *Arizona* are considered to belong to the same species. Organisms are now reported by genus and serotype, omitting reference to species.
Tribe IV: *Citrobactereae*		
Citrobacter amalonaticus	*Levinea amalonaticus*	H_2S (−), indole (+), adonitol (−), malonate (−). Primarily found in human feces, very rarely isolated from blood.
C. braakii	*Citrobacter* genomospecies 6	H_2S and indole are variable, adonitol (−), malonate (−). Isolated from human stools, urine, wounds and from animals and food.
C. farmeri	*C. amalonaticus* biogroup 1	Found primarily in human feces. Strains of biogroup 1 ferment sucrose, raffinose, α-methyl-D-glucoside, and melibiose and are citrate (−). *C. amalonaticus* usually have the opposite reactions.
C. freundii		H_2S (+), indole (−), adonitol (−), malonate (−). Found in urine, throat, sputum, blood, and wounds.

(Continued)

TABLE 4-5 *(Continued)*

IMPORTANT RECENT CHANGES IN THE ESTABLISHED GENERA OF THE *ENTEROBACTERIACEAE*

NEW DESIGNATION	PREVIOUS DESIGNATION	COMMENTS
Tribe IV: *Citrobactereae* (cont'd)		
C. gillenii	*Citrobacter* genomospecies 10	H_2S is variable, indole (−), adonitol (−), malonate (+). Found in human stool and food.
C. koseri	*Levinea malonatica* *C. diversus*	H_2S (−), indole (+), adonitol (+), malonate (+). Found in urine, throat, nose, sputum, and wounds. Rare cause of neonatal meningitis.
C. murliniae	*Citrobacter* genomospecies 11	H_2S is variable, indole (+), adonitol (−), malonate (−). Found in human stools and blood.
C. rodentium	*Citrobacter* genomospecies 9	H_2S (−), indole (−), adonitol (−), malonate (+). This organism has been isolated only from rodents.
C. sedlakii	*Citrobacter* genomospecies 8	H_2S (−), indole (+), adonitol (−), malonate (+). Found in human stools, blood, and wounds.
C. werkmanii	*Citrobacter* genomospecies 7	H_2S (+), indole (−), adonitol (−), malonate (+). Found in human stools and urine and from food.
C. youngae	*Citrobacter* genomospecies 5	H_2S and indole are variable, adonitol (−), malonate (−). Isolated from human stools and blood and from animals and food.
Tribe V: *Klebsielleae*		
Klebsiella oxytoca	Indole (+) *K. pneumoniae*	MIO (−, +, −). Common clinical isolate.
K. ornithinolytica	*Klebsiella* group 47	MIO (−, +, +). Isolated from blood, urine, sputum, and wounds.
K. planticola	*Klebsiella* species 2 *K. trevisanii*	Water and plant isolates; rare human clinical isolates.
K. pneumoniae subsp. *pneumoniae*		MIO (−, −, −). Common clinical isolate.
K. pneumoniae subsp. *ozaenae*	*K. ozaenae*	Biochemically inactive strain of *K. pneumoniae*. Causes atrophic rhinitis, a condition called ozena.
K. pneumoniae subsp. *rhinoscleromatis*	*K. rhinoscleromatis*	Biochemically inactive strain of *K. pneumoniae*. Causes a granulomatous disease known as rhinoscleroma.
K. terrigena		Soil and water isolates.
Enterobacter aerogenes		LAO (+, −, +). Common clinical isolate.
"*E. agglomerans* complex"	*Erwinia herbicola* *Erwinia milletiae*	Heterogeneous group of organisms representing over 13 DNA hybridization groups (HG). HG XIII has been transferred to the new genus *Pantoea* as *P. agglomerans*. Organisms that are LAO-negative (referred to as "triple decarboxylase negative") and are yellow pigmented were usually identified as *E. agglomerans* in the past.
E. amnigenus biogroup 1 *E. amnigenus* biogroup 2	Group H3	Two biogroups. Biogroup 1 ferment sucrose and raffinose, but not D-sorbitol. Biogroup 2 ferment D-sorbitol, but not sucrose or raffinose. Primarily water organisms. Have been isolated from human specimens, but no evidence that *E. amnigenus* can cause human infection.
E. asburiae	Enteric group 17 Atypical *Citrobacter*	Biochemically similar to *E. cloacae*. Nonmotile, VP (−), (79% + after 2 days), urea (+) (delayed). Isolated from variety of human sources: blood, urine, wounds, respiratory tract, feces.

(Continued)

NEW DESIGNATION	PREVIOUS DESIGNATION	COMMENTS
E. cancerogenus	*Erwinia cancerogena* Enterobacter taylorae Enteric group 19	Includes organisms formerly classified as *E. taylorae*. LAO (−, +, +), adonitol, inositol, sorbitol, raffinose, and melibiose all negative. Isolated from a variety of clinical sources including blood and spinal fluid.
E. cloacae		LAO (−, +, +). Common clinical isolate.
E. cloacae-like unnamed species 1		
E. cloacae-like unnamed species 2		
E. cloacae-like unnamed species 3		
E. dissolvens	*Erwinia dissolvens*	Closely related to *E. cloacae*. Not found in human clinical specimens.
E. gergoviae	Atypical *E. aerogenes*	LAO (+, −, +). Strong urease (+). Found in environment and urine and respiratory tract of humans. Rare isolates have been recovered from blood.
E. hormaechei	Enteric group 75	LAO (−, +, +). Biochemically closest to *E. taylorae* except is urea (+), sucrose (+), and esculin (−). Isolates reported from blood, wounds, and sputum.
E. intermedius	Group H1 *E. intermedium*	Water and soil isolates. No human isolates reported.
E. nimipressuralis	*Erwinia nimipressuralis*	Closely related to *E. cloacae*. Not found in human clinical specimens.
E. pyrinus	*Erwinia pirina*	Urease (+), most closely resembles *E. gergoviae*, is differentiated by its growth in KCN broth, acid production from myoinositol, and lack of acid production from raffinose. Causes brown leaf spot disease of pear trees.
E. sakazakii	Yellow-pigmented *E. cloacae*	LAO (−, +, +). Bright yellow pigment at 35°C. May cause meningitis, brain abscesses, and bacteremia in neonates.
Hafnia alvei	*Enterobacter hafniae*	Lactose (−), LAO (+, −, +), grows at 35°C, but biochemically more active at 25°C. Found in clinical specimens especially feces, occasionally from blood, sputum, urine, and wounds.
H. alvei biogroup 1	"*Hafnia protea*" *Obesumbacterium proteus* biogroup 1	Not a human clinical isolate. Occurs in breweries, where it grows in beer wort.
Pantoea agglomerans	*Enterobacter agglomerans* HG XIII *Erwinia herbicola* *Erwinia milletiae*	LAO (−, −, −) some may be yellow pigmented. Isolated from plant surfaces, seeds, and water, as well as from humans (wound, blood, urine, internal organs) and animals.
P. ananas	*E. agglomerans* HG VI *Erwinia ananas* *Erwinia uredovora*	Plant pathogen, causes pineapple rot.
P. citrea	New species	Isolated from Mandarin oranges in Japan.
P. dispersa	*E. agglomerans* HG III	Isolated from plant surfaces, seeds, humans, and the environment. Separated from *P. agglomerans* by negative salicin reaction.
P. punctata	New species	Isolated from Mandarin oranges in Japan.
P. stewartii subsp. *indologenes*	*Erwinia stewartii*	Cause of leaf spot on foxtail millet and pearl millet.

(Continued)

NEW DESIGNATION	PREVIOUS DESIGNATION	COMMENTS
P. stewartii subsp. *stewartii*	*Erwinia stewartii*	Causative agent of Stewart's bacterial wilt of corn.
P. terrea	New species	Isolated from soil in Japan.
Serratia entomophila		Resembles *S. marcescens* (arabinose −). Insect pathogen, no human isolates reported.
S. ficaria		Natural habitat is figs and fig wasps. Has been very rarely reported from human clinical specimens.
"*S.*" *fonticola*		Not really a species of *Serratia*. A water organism, rarely isolated from human specimens, mostly wounds.
S. grimesii	See *S. liquefaciens* group	Isolated from environment and human clinical specimens. Cannot be differentiated from other members of "*S. liquefaciens* group" by commonly used tests.
"*S. liquefaciens* group"	*Enterobacter liquefaciens* Different biogroups within the species *S. liquefaciens*	Consists of several DNA hybridization groups including species now named *S. proteamaculans*, and *S. grimesii*. Cannot be separated by currently used biochemical tests. Differ from *S. marcescens* by being L-arabinose (+). Report as "*S. liquefaciens* group."
S. marcescens		DNase (+), gelatin (+), L-arabinose (−) (other species are positive). Common clinical isolate. Red pigment produced by some strains.
S. odorifera biogroup 1 *S. odorifera* biogroup 2		Dirty, musty odor similar to potatoes. Two biogroups. Biogroup 1 is ornithine, sucrose, and raffinose positive and is predominantly isolated from sputum. Biogroup 2 is negative for these three reactions and has been recovered from blood and CSF.
S. plymuthica	*Bacterium plymuthica*	May have red pigment. Isolated from soil, water, sputum. Extremely rare in clinical specimens.
S. proteamaculans subsp. *proteamaculans*	See *S. liquefaciens* group	Cannot be separated from other members of "*S. liquefaciens* group" by currently utilized biochemical tests. Differs from *S. marcescens* by being L-arabinose (+).
S. proteamaculans subsp. *quinovora*	See *S. liquefaciens* group	Isolated from plants, wild rodents, insects, and water, but not yet from human clinical specimens.
S. rubidaea		Red pigment produced. Rarely isolated in humans.
Tribe VI: *Proteeae* *Proteus mirabilis*		H_2S (+), indole (−), ornithine (+). Common clinical isolate.
P. myxofaciens		No human isolates reported. Isolated only from living and dead gypsy moths.
P. penneri	*P. vulgaris* biogroup 1	Closely related to *P. vulgaris*, except that indole (−), salicin (−), esculin (−), and chloramphenicol-resistant.
P. vulgaris	*P. vulgaris* biogroup 2	H_2S (+), indole (+), ornithine (−). Common clinical isolate. Indole, salicin and esculin are positive.
P. vulgaris biogroup 3		Consists of four separate genetic species and are designated DNA groups 3, 4, 5, and 6. Indole (+), but salicin and esculin are (−).

(Continued)

NEW DESIGNATION	PREVIOUS DESIGNATION	COMMENTS
Tribe VI: *Proteeae* (cont'd)		
Morganella morganii subsp. *morganii*	*Proteus morganii*	H$_2$S (−), lysine, ornithine, and motility all variable; trehalose (−). Causes urinary tract infections and is cultured from many other body sites. Contains four biogroups designated A through D.
M. morganii subsp. *sibonii*	*M. morganii* biogroup 1	H$_2$S (−), lysine, ornithine variable; trehalose and motility (+). Contains three biogroups designated E through G.
M. morganii subsp. 3		
Providencia alcalifaciens	*P. alcalifaciens* biogroup 1, 2	Urea (−), adonitol (+), inositol (−). Generally isolated from diarrheic stools, particularly children.
P. heimbachae		Not a human clinical isolate. Found in penguin feces and an aborted cow fetus.
P. rettgeri	*Proteus rettgeri*	Urea (+), adonitol (+), inositol (+). Mostly isolated from urine of hospitalized and catheterized patients.
P. rustigianii	*P. alcalifaciens* biogroup 3 *P. friedericiana*	Urea (−), adonitol (−), inositol (−). Rarely found in clinical specimens, mostly from human feces.
P. stuartii	*P. alcalifaciens* biogroup 4	Urea (v), adonitol (−), inositol (+). Isolated most often from urine, less often from wounds, burns, and bacteremias. May cause nosocomial outbreaks.
Tribe VII: *Yersinieae*		
Yersinia aldovae	*Y. enterocolitica*-like group X2	Biochemically similar to *Y. enterocolitica*. Isolated from surface water, drinking water, and fish.
Y. bercovieri	*Y. enterocolitica* biogroup 3B	Biochemically similar to *Y. enterocolitica*. Isolated from human feces, water, soil, and raw vegetables.
Y. enterocolitica		May cause diarrhea, terminal ileitis, mesenteric lymphadenitis, arthritis, and septicemia in humans.
Y. frederiksenii	Biogroup of *Y. enterocolitica*	Mainly found in water, sewage, and fish. Occasionally found in human feces, blood, and sputum. Rarely associated with gastrointestinal illness.
Y. intermedia	Biogroup of *Y. enterocolitica*	Found in fresh water, sewage, and aquatic animals. Human isolates have been from stool, blood, wounds, and urine. Probably not a cause of gastrointestinal illness.
Y. kristensenii	Biogroup of *Y. enterocolitica*	Found in water, soil, and animals. Human isolates have been from stool, blood, and urine. No evidence that it can cause gastrointestinal illness.
Y. mollaretii	*Y. enterocolitica* biogroup 3A	Biochemically similar to *Y. enterocolitica*. Isolated from human feces, drinking water, meat, and raw vegetables.
Y. pestis	*Pasteurella pestis* *Y. pseudotuberculosis* subsp. *pestis*	Causative agent of plague.
Y. pseudotuberculosis		May cause mesenteric lymphadenitis, diarrhea, and septicemia in humans.
Y. rohdei		Biochemically similar to *Y. enterocolitica*. Isolated from dog feces, water, and human feces.
"*Y.*" *ruckeri*	"Red mouth bacterium"	Will probably be moved to a new genus. Fish pathogen. Human isolates are extremely rare.

IMViC, indole, methyl red, Voges-Proskauer, citrate; LAO, lysine–arginine–ornithine; MIO, motility–indole–ornithine; PAD, phenylalanine deaminase; HG, hybridization group; (+), ≥90% of strains positive; (−), ≥90% of strains negative; (v), variable.

TABLE 4-6
Key Identification Characteristics for the Most Common Enterobacteriaceae

	KIA	GAS	H₂S	MR	VP	IND	CIT	PAD	URE	MOT	LYS	ARG	ORN	ONPG
Tribe I: Escherichieae														
Genus: Escherichia														
E. coli	A/A	+	−	+	−	+	−	−	−	+	+	−/+	+/−	+
Genus: Shigella														
Groups A, B, C	Alk/A	−	−	+	−	−/+	−	−	−	−	−	−	−	−
S. sonnei	Alk/A	−	−	+	−	−	−	−	−	−	−	−	+	+
Tribe II: Edwardsielleae														
Genus: Edwardsiella														
E. tarda	Alk/A	+	+	+	−	+	−	−	−	+	+	−	+	−
Tribe III: Salmonelleae														
Genus: Salmonella	Alk/A	+	+	+	−	−	+	−	−	+	+	+/−	+	−
Tribe IV: Citrobactereae														
Genus: Citrobacter														
C. freundii	A/A; Alk/A	+	+	+	−	−	+	−	+/−	+	−	+/−	−/+	+
C. koseri	Alk/A	+	−	+	−	+	+	−	+/−	+	−	+/−	+	+
Tribe V: Klebsielleae														
Genus: Klebsiella														
K. pneumoniae	A/A	++	−	−	+	−	+	−	+	−	+	−	−	+
K. oxytoca	A/A	++	−	−	+	+	+	−	+	−	+	−	−	+
Genus: Enterobacter														
E. aerogenes	A/A	++	−	−	+	−	+	−	−	+	+	+	+	+
E. cloacae	A/A	++	−	−	+	−	+	−	+/−	+	−	+	+	+
Genus: Hafnia														
H. alvei	Alk/A	+	−	−/+	+	−	−	−	−	+	+	−	+	+
Genus: Pantoea														
P. agglomerans	A/A; Alk/A	−/+	−	−/+	+/−	−/+	+/−	−/+	−/+	+	−	−	−	+
Genus: Serratia														
S. marcescens	Alk/A	+	−	−/+	+	−	+	−	−	+	+	+	+	+
Tribe VI: Proteeae														
Genus: Proteus														
P. vulgaris	Alk/A	+/−	+	+	−	+	−/+	+	++	+*	−	−	−	−
P. mirabilis	Alk/A	+	+	+	+/−	−	+/−	+	++	+*	−	−	+	−
Genus: Morganella														
M. morganii	Alk/A	+	−	+	−	+	−	+	++	+	−	−	+	−
Genus: Providencia														
P. rettgeri	Alk/A	−	−	+	−	+	+	+	++	+	−	−	−	−
P. stuartii	Alk/A	−	−	+	−	+	+	+	−/+	+/−	−	−	−	−
P. alcalifaciens	Alk/A	+/−	−	+	−	+	+	+	−	+	−	−	−	−
Tribe VII: Yersinieae														
Genus: Yersinia														
Y. enterocolitica	Alk/A	−	−	+	−	+/−	−	−	+/−	−†	−	−	+	+

KIA, Kligler's iron agar; H₂S, hydrogen sulfide; MR, methyl red; VP, Voges-Proskauer; IND, indole; CIT, citrate; PAD, phenylalanine deaminase; URE, urease; MOT, motility; LYS, lysine; ARG, arginine; ORN, ornithine; ONPG, o-nitrophenyl-β-D-galactopyranoside; ++, strong positive reaction; +, 90% or more strains positive; −, 90% or more strains negative; +/−, 50%–90% of strains positive; −/+, 50%–90% of strains negative; shaded areas indicate key reactions.
* Swarming motility demonstrated on noninhibitory media.
† Nonmotile at 36°C, motile at 22°C.

Providencia species (*P. rettgeri*) is strongly positive. Both species of *Proteus* listed in Table 4-6 are hydrogen sulfide-positive and exhibit swarming motility.

The *Yersinieae* represented here by the most commonly isolated species, *Y. enterocolitica*, are very similar to members of the *Escherichieae*, except that *Y. enterocolitica* is usually urea-positive. Students may wish to think of *Y. enterocolitica* as urea-positive *E. coli*. Note that the motility for *Y. enterocolitica* is negative at 36°C but positive at 22°C.

Key reactions for students to remember are found in Box 4-8.

TRIBE *ESCHERICHIEAE*

The two genera within this tribe are *Escherichia* and *Shigella*. On first reflection these two groups of bacteria would not appear to be related because of differences in growth characteristics and appearance on the enteric isolation media (*E. coli* characteristically ferments lactose, *Shigella* species do not). *E. coli* is generally biochemically active compared with *Shigella* species, which tend to be inert. However, *E. coli* and *Shigella* species are closely related genetically; in fact, all four species of *Shigella* and *E. coli* form a single species on the basis of DNA hybridization studies.[36] However, because *Shigella* species are associated with a specific disease spectrum (bacillary dysentery) and because specific typing antisera for separating *E. coli* from *Shigella* are commercially available, *Shigella* species will continue to be classified in a separate genus, at least for now. Students should note, however, that certain late lactose-fermenting, nonmotile, and biochemically inactive strains of *E. coli* can be difficult to differentiate from *Shigella* species, and rare strains of *Shigella* species

(*S. flexneri*) also can produce gas from the fermentation of glucose. The pathogenic spectrum of *E. coli* is much broader than that of *Shigella* species, and toxigenic strains of *E. coli* can produce dysentery-like diarrheal syndromes indistinguishable from shigellosis. Serologic testing may be required in some instances to differentiate certain closely related strains. The key characteristics of the *Escherichieae* are given in Table 4-6.

Genus *Escherichia*. *E. coli* is the bacterial species most commonly recovered in the clinical laboratories and has been incriminated in infectious diseases involving virtually every human tissue and organ system. *E. coli* is one of the common organisms involved in gram-negative sepsis and endotoxin-induced shock. Urinary tract and wound infections, pneumonia in immunosuppressed hospitalized patients, and meningitis in neonates are other common infections caused by *E. coli*.

E. COLI THAT CAUSE GASTROENTERITIS. Certain strains of *E. coli* can cause enteritis or gastroenteritis by five distinct mechanisms, resulting in five different clinical syndromes.[188] See Table 4-7 and Clinical Correlation Boxes 4-1 through 4-5.[188]

DETECTION OF *E. COLI* 0157. The currently accepted methods for the detection or isolation of 0157 strains of *E. coli* are 1) assays for the detection of the 0157 serotype or Shiga-like toxins (SLTs) directly from stool; 2) direct plating on sorbitol MacConkey agar (SMAC),[199] cefixime-SMAC,[68] SMAC supplemented with cefixime and tellurite (CT-SMAC),[327] or media containing either 5-bromo-5-chloro-3-indoxyl-β-D-glucuronide[228] or 4-methylumbelliferyl-β-D-glucuronide;[299] and 3) immunomagnetic separation (IMS) using 0157-specific, antibody-coated beads, followed by bacteriologic culture.[69,168]

SPECIES OTHER THAN *E. COLI*. Strains designated in the CDC classification as *E. coli* inactive are anaerogenic (non–gas-producing), lactose-negative (or delayed), and nonmotile. These strains were previously known as the Alkalescens–Dispar serotype.

E. fergusonii (formerly CDC Enteric Group 10) has been recovered from blood, gallbladder, urine, and feces; however, its clinical significance has not been established.[106,107,118,120] It is differentiated from *E. coli* by being sorbitol- and lactose-negative, but adonitol- and cellobiose-positive. *E. hermannii* (formerly CDC Enteric Group 11) has been most commonly found in human wounds, sputum, and feces and is not believed to cause infection.[245] Of six strains recovered at the University of Illinois, four have been from leg wounds of patients with cellulitis, and one strain each has been recovered from urine and blood. The isolates recovered from wounds were mixed with other pathogenic species; however, the blood and urine isolates were present as the only isolates. *E. hermannii* strains are yellow-pigmented, indole-positive, and sorbitol-negative.[38] Because *E. hermannii* are sorbitol-negative, they appear biochemically similar to the 0157 serotype of *E. coli*. *E. vulneris* (formerly CDC Enteric Group 1) has a

---

BOX 4-8. KEY FACTS TO REMEMBER FOR IDENTIFYING *ENTEROBACTERIACEAE*

Hydrogen Sulfide–Positive

Edwardsiella tarda	*Proteus vulgaris*
Salmonella species	*Proteus mirabilis*
Citrobacter freundii	

Voges-Proskauer–Positive

Klebsiella species	*Pantoea* species
Enterobacter species	*Serratia* species
Hafnia species	

Phenylalanine Deaminase–Positive

Proteus species	*Providencia* species
Morganella species	

Nonmotile at 36°C

Shigella species	*Klebsiella* species
Yersinia species (motile at 22°C)	

TABLE 4-7
KEY FEATURES OF DIARRHEAGENIC *E. COLI*

TERM	ABBREVIATION	PATHOGENIC PHENOTYPE	SIGNS AND SYMPTOMS
Enterotoxigenic *E. coli*	ETEC	Elaboration of secretory toxins (LT, ST) that do not damage the mucosal epithelium	"Traveler's diarrhea." Profuse watery diarrhea is predominant symptom. Often accompanied by mild abdominal cramps. Dehydration and vomiting occur in some cases.
Enteropathogenic *E. coli*	EPEC	Adhere to epithelial cells in localized microcolonies and cause attaching and effacing lesions	Usually occurs in infants. Characterized by low-grade fever, malaise, vomiting, and diarrhea, with a prominent amount of mucus, but with no gross blood.
Enteroinvasive *E. coli*	EIEC	Invade epithelial cells	Dysentery; hallmarks are fever and colitis. Symptoms are urgency and tenesmus; blood, mucus, and many leukocytes in stool.
Enterohemorrhagic *E. coli*	EHEC	Elaboratorion of cytotoxins (SLT)	Bloody diarrhea without WBCs. Often no fever. Abdominal pain is common. May progress to HUS.
Enteroaggregative *E. coli*	EaggEC	Adhere to epithelial cells in a pattern resembling a pile of stacked bricks	Watery diarrhea, vomiting, dehydration and less commonly, abdominal pain.

CLINICAL CORRELATION BOX 4-1: ENTEROTOXIGENIC *E. COLI*

Enterotoxigenic strains (ETEC) form heat-labile (LT) or heat-stable (ST) enterotoxins that produce a secretory diarrhea ("traveler's diarrhea") similar to that of *Vibrio cholerae*.[130, 274] Surface attachment of the bacterial cells to the intestinal epithelial cells is prerequisite to toxin production. Toxin production is plasmid mediated and most commonly involves *E. coli* serogroups 06, 08, 015, 020, 025, 027, 063, 078, 080, 085, 092, 0115, 0128ac, 0139, 0148, 0153, 0159, and 0167.[252] ETEC infection usually follows ingestion of contaminated water or food, producing watery diarrhea, nausea, abdominal cramps, and low-grade fever. In infants, ETEC sometimes causes a disease known as "cholera infantum."[252]

Genus *Shigella*. *Shigella* species can be suspected in cultures because they are non–lactose-fermenters and tend to be biochemically inert. They typically do not produce gas from carbohydrates, with the exception of certain biogroups of *S. flexneri* that are aerogenic. Rare strains of *S. sonnei* can slowly ferment lactose (2%) and sucrose (1%), and most strains can decarboxylate ornithine—characteristics not shared by other *Shigella* species.

The CDC classification combines *S. dysenteriae* (group A), *S. flexneri* (group B), and *S. boydii* (group C) as "*Shigella*-serogroups A, B, C" because of their biochemical similarities. The presence of ornithine decarboxylase activity and β-galactosidase make most

CLINICAL CORRELATION BOX 4-2: ENTEROPATHOGENIC *E. COLI*

Enteropathogenic strains (EPEC) cause diarrheal syndromes primarily in infants.[122, 303] The pathogenesis is unclear; however, the inflammatory reactions and epithelial degenerative changes that are observed in tissue sections may be secondary to adhesive properties of the bacterium, believed to be plasmid related.[185] Serogroups 055, 086, 0111, 0119, 0126, 0127, 0128ab, and 0142 are most commonly involved.[252] EPEC illness is characterized by fever, malaise, vomiting, and diarrhea, with a prominent amount of mucus, but with no gross blood.[252]

high propensity for causing human wound infections, particularly of the arms and legs.[42,245] A single case of urosepsis caused by *E. vulneris* has been reported.[13] Over half of the strains are yellow-pigmented, and they are both indole- and sorbitol-negative. *E. blattae*, recovered from the intestinal tract of cockroaches, is indole-negative and does not ferment lactose. It has not been associated with human infections. *E. adecarboxylata* has been assigned to a new genus as *Leclercia adecarboxylata*.[292] The different biochemical reactions for the recognized species of *Escherichia* are shown in Table 4-8.

CLINICAL CORRELATION BOX 4-3: ENTEROINVASIVE *E. COLI*

Enteroinvasive strains (EIEC) are capable of penetrating the intestinal epithelial cells and producing an inflammatory diarrhea, similar to that caused by *Shigella* species.[303] As with *Shigella*, most strains are nonmotile, late- or non–lactose-fermenters, and anaerogenic. EIEC strains are suspected when blood, mucus, and segmented neutrophils are observed in fecal smears. The most commonly involved serogroups are 028ac, 029, 0112ac, 0124, 0136, 0143, 0144, 0152, and 0164.[252] The pathogenic mechanisms include invasion of the colonic mucosa, similar to *Shigella*, and proliferation within the epithelial cells, resulting in the cell death.

CLINICAL CORRELATION BOX 4-4: ENTEROADHERENT *E. COLI*

Enteroadherent *E. coli* (EAEC) is the term used to describe *E. coli* strains that are adherent to HEp-2 or HeLa cells; do not produce LT, ST, or VT; and are noninvasive, irrespective of the serogroups. EAEC strains produce different patterns of adherence to tissue cells. One pattern is characterized by formation of a "stacked brick" pattern of bacteria that are observed on both HEp-2 cells and glass coverslips.[252] Strains producing this pattern of adherence are referred to as enteroaggregative *E. coli* (EAggEC). To date, these strains have been recovered principally from children with chronic diarrhea.

strains of *S. sonnei* biochemically distinct from the other *Shigella* species. The inability to ferment mannitol distinguishes *S. dysenteriae*. The differential characteristics for the four species of *Shigella* are included in Table 4-9. Isolates recovered from stool specimens from patients with diarrheal disease, which are suspected of being *Shigella* species, should be biochemically categorized and the species confirmed by serologic testing. In the

near future, it may be possible to detect *Shigella* species and enteroinvasive strains of *E. coli* using DNA probes selected to detect the virulence plasmids responsible for coding the gene products that initiate intracellular penetration and bowel wall invasion.[32]

INCIDENCE AND SOURCES OF *SHIGELLA* INFECTIONS. Shigellosis is the most communicable of the bacterial di-

CLINICAL CORRELATION BOX 4-5: ENTEROHEMORRHAGIC *E. COLI*

Enterohemorrhagic *E. coli* (EHEC) strains produce bloody diarrhea in humans, probably secondary to toxin damage of vascular endothelial cells.[267] These strains also produce cytotoxic effects on Vero and HeLa cells, similar to those produced by the toxin of *Shigella dysenteriae* type 1. Because these strains are cytotoxic to Vero cells, the toxin is referred to by some as Verotoxin (VT) and the strains that produce the toxin as **Verotoxin**-producing *E. coli* or VTEC. Other researchers refer to this toxin as Shiga-like toxin (SLT) because it is biochemically very similar to the Shiga toxin produced by strains of *S. dysenteriae* serotype 1, and thus the term **Shiga-like toxin**-producing *E. coli* or SLTEC is also commonly used. The clinical significance of EHEC was not known until 1982, when these organisms were associated with two conditions of previously unknown etiology: hemorrhagic colitis[267] and hemolytic–uremic syndrome.[170] Patients with hemorrhagic colitis (also known as ischemic colitis) typically present with abdominal cramps and watery diarrhea, followed by a hemorrhagic discharge resembling lower gastrointestinal tract bleeding. There is no significant fever and an absence of inflammatory cells in the stool. Hemolytic–uremic syndrome is defined by a triad of features (acute renal failure, thrombocytopenia, and microangiopathic hemolytic anemia) and is the leading cause of acute renal failure in children. In its most common form, this syndrome is preceded by diarrheal illness that subsequently becomes bloody and resembles hemorrhagic colitis. A large portion of EHEC isolates belong to serotype 0157:H7. In early 1993, the largest *E. coli* food-poisoning outbreak to date caused by *E. coli* 0157:H7, occurred in the states of Washington, Idaho, California, and Nevada. Altogether, 582 culture-confirmed cases were re-

ported, causing 171 hospitalizations, 41 cases of HUS, and 4 deaths. Hamburgers from a single fast-food restaurant chain were implicated. The source of most cases of *E. coli*-related illnesses in the United States is considered to be ground beef. According to recent market-basket surveys, *E. coli* 0157:H7 is present in 1.0% to 2.5% of meat and poultry samples. It also turns up less frequently in supermarket samples of lamb and pork, although such isolates could arise from secondary contamination in the butchering area.[181] In the United States, cases have tended to occur in the last two-thirds of the year and in states bordering Canada. Isolation of *E. coli* 0157:H7 is possible only during the acute phase of illness, and the organisms may not be detectable 5 to 7 days after onset. The recovery of this serotype from stool is made simple because serotype 0157:H7 is sorbitol-negative. This property is the basis for a selective MacConkey agar that contains 1% D-sorbitol, rather than lactose to differentiate sorbitol-negative *E. coli* strains (colonies appear colorless, similar to lactose-negative colonies on regular MacConkey agar). Suspected isolates should be confirmed with specific 0157:H7 antisera. Although 0157:H7 is the prototypic serotype of EHEC in the United States, several other EHEC serotypes, such as 026:H11,[188] 048:H21,[128] 0103:H2,[200] 0111:NM (nonmotile),[66, 236] and 0145:NM,[188] have been recognized in other countries. Although non-0157 serotypes of EHEC are rare in the United States, one outbreak of hemorrhagic colitis caused by EHEC serotype 0104:H21 was reported among 11 patients in Helena, Montana in 1994.[65] To learn more about infections caused by EHEC, the review articles of Griffin and Tauxe,[133a] Karmali,[169] O'Brien and Holmes, [222] and Tarr, [293] may be consulted.

TABLE 4-8

DIFFERENTIATION OF SPECIES WITHIN THE GENUS ESCHERICHIA

BIOCHEMICAL TEST	E. COLI	E. HERMANNII	E. FERGUSONII	E. BLATTAE	E. VULNERIS
Indole	+	+	+	−	−
Methyl red	+	+	+	+	+
Voges-Proskauer	−	−	−	−	−
Citrate	−	−	V (17)	V (50)	−
Lysine decarboxylase	+	−	+	+	V (85)
Arginine dihydrolase	V (17)	−	−	−	V (30)
Ornithine decarboxylase	V (65)	+	+	+	−
ONPG	+	+	V (83)	−	+
Fermentation of					
Lactose	+	V (45)	−	−	V (15)
Sorbitol	+†	−	−	−	−
Mannitol	+	+	+	−	+
Adonitol	−	−	+	−	−
Cellobiose	−	+	+	−	+
Yellow pigment	−	+	−	−	V (50)

+, 90% or more strains are positive; −, 90% or more strains are negative; V, 11%–89% of strains are positive.
† Strains of E. coli belonging to serotype 0157:H7 are sorbitol negative.

arrheas. Humans serve as the natural host, and disease is transmitted by the fecal–oral route, with as few as 200 viable organisms being able to cause disease. Between 25,000 and 30,000 cases of shigellosis are reported annually in the United States. In 1993, 32,198 cases of shigellosis were reported to CDC, the highest number of cases reported in the United States in 42 years.[63]

S. sonnei is the serotype most commonly associated with diarrheal disease in the United States; however, symptoms tend to be mild and some patients may be asymptomatic.[137] It was the most common bacterial agent associated with water-borne disease outbreaks in the United States for the period 1986 to 1988.[54] S. dysenteriae is the least commonly recovered species in

TABLE 4-9

DIFFERENTIATION OF SPECIES WITHIN THE GENUS SHIGELLA

BIOCHEMICAL TEST	S. DYSENTERIAE	S. FLEXNERI	S. BOYDII	S. SONNEI
Serogroup	A	B	C	D
ONPG	−	−	−	+
Ornithine decarboxylase	−	−	−	+
Fermentation of				
Lactose	−	−	−	−
Mannitol	−	+	+	+
Raffinose	−	D	−	−
Sucrose	−	−	−	−
Xylose	−	−	D	−
Indole production	D	D	D	−

+, 90% or more strains are positive; −, 90% or more strains are negative; D, different strains are positive/negative.

CLINICAL CORRELATION BOX 4-6:
***SHIGELLA* INFECTION**

Fever, watery diarrhea with cramping abdominal pain, and generalized myalgias are the most common early symptoms suggesting shigellosis.[47] Fluid and electrolyte losses may also be noted early in the illness, owing to the action of enterotoxin on the intestinal epithelial cells. After 2 or 3 days, bowel movements become less frequent and the quantity of stool decreases, but the presence of bright red blood and mucus in the feces and the onset of tenesmus (straining at stool) indicate the dysenteric phase of illness, suggesting that bacterial penetration of the bowel has probably occurred. *Shigella* infections should be suspected in community-wide outbreaks of diarrheal illness that disproportionately affect young children. Outbreaks can occur at any time of the year, but are most common in the summer.

the United States, but is the most virulent serotype and the most common serotype isolated in third world countries. The belief that *Shigella* species remain confined to the bowel and neither invade the bowel lymphatics nor extend to other organs may no longer pertain. Drow and associates[88] reported the recovery of *S. flexneri* from a splenic abscess in a diabetic patient, indicating that extraintestinal sites of infection may be encountered.

TRIBE *EDWARDSIELLEAE*

Among the *Enterobacteriaceae*, the *Edwardsielleae* are the most recently described and were initially called the Asakusa group by Sakazaki and Murata[275] in 1962 and the Bartholomew group by King and Adler in 1964.[175] Ewing and associates suggested the name *Edwardsielleae* in 1965,[99] in honor of the prominent American microbiologist, P. R. Edwards. The *Edwardsielleae* consists of one genus, *Edwardsiella*, which has three species; however, only one species, *E. tarda*, is of medical importance. The chief reservoirs in nature are reptiles (especially snakes, toads, and turtles) and freshwater fish. The key characteristics that suggest *E. tarda* are given in Table 4-6.

A key feature of *E. tarda* is the production of abundant amounts of hydrogen sulfide. Except for this feature, the bacterium has biochemical properties similar to those of *Escherichia coli*. The organism also resembles some *Citrobacter* and *Salmonella* species by its production of hydrogen sulfide in TSI agar and its failure to use lactose. This failure to ferment lactose and many other carbohydrates is the basis for the species name *tarda*. A species similar to *E. tarda*, which is hydrogen sulfide-negative, but mannitol-, sucrose-, and arabinose-positive, has been designated "*E. tarda* biogroup 1."[109] This biotype is rarely encountered in laboratory practice and does not yet appear to have clinical significance.

In a series of studies by Clarridge and associates,[76] *E. tarda* has been cited as the cause of a variety of extraintestinal infections. Wound infections resulting

from trauma, often related to aquatic accidents, were frequent occurrences in their series; they also cite four cases of liver abscesses in which *E. tarda* was the predominant organism. Seven patients had typhoidal illnesses, an important differential consideration because *E. tarda* can simulate *Salmonella typhi* in culture. Wilson and colleagues[319] have reported a case of *E. tarda* bacteremia in a patient with sickle cell disease. Most reports of enteric illness describe a mild gastroenteritis that improves without therapy in 2 to 3 days. However, Vandepitte and associates[307] have reported one case of protracted diarrhea in a 2-month-old infant in whom *E. tarda* (of the same biogroup isolated from tropical aquarium fish in the home of the patient) was the only potential pathogen recovered. Marsh and Gorbach[201] reported the isolation of *E. tarda* from the stool of a patient with bloody diarrhea and sigmoidoscopic findings of multiple colonic ulcers and mucosal thickening consistent with Crohn's disease. The patient became asymptomatic after 2 days of antibiotic therapy. Iron availability has been thought to regulate the seriousness of *E. tarda* infection.[161,162] Iron overload, caused by such conditions as red cell sickling, leukemia, and cirrhosis, is associated with *E. tarda* septicemia.[161,319,324] Clusters of asymptomatic *E. tarda* infections are believed to occur in humans, and at least one such cluster has been reported among seven children and a teacher in a Florida day care center.[202]

Two other species in the genus *Edwardsiella* have been described. Grimont and associates[136] described *E. hoshinae*, initially recovered from birds, reptiles, and water. This species has also been recovered from human feces; however, it is not known to cause diarrhea. Hawke and coworkers[140] described *E. ictaluri*, an organism that has been recovered only from fish and, at present, has no clinical significance. The biochemical characterization of *Edwardsiella* species is shown in Table 4-10.

TRIBE *SALMONELLEAE*

The *Salmonelleae* contain a single genus, *Salmonella*, and are named after the American microbiologist, D. E. Salmon. Salmonellae have somatic (O) antigens that are lipopolysaccharide, and flagellar (H) antigens that are proteins. *S. typhi* also has a capsular or virulence (Vi) antigen. Biochemically, they are usually both lactose- and sucrose-negative. The key characteristics by which the genus *Salmonella* can be suspected are given in Table 4-6.

Classification of Salmonellae. The salmonellae are the most complex of all the *Enterobacteriaceae*, with more than 2200 serotypes described in the Kauffman-White schema. In this schema, the salmonellae are grouped (A, B, C, and so on) on the basis of somatic O antigens and are subdivided into serotypes (1, 2, and so on) by their flagellar H antigens (i.e., A1, A2, B1, B2). Prior to July 1, 1983, three species of *Salmonella* were used to report positive results: *S. choleraesuis*, *S. typhi*, and *S. enteritidis*, with most of the 2200 serotypes belonging to the last species, *S. enteritidis*. Presently, all former species and subgroups of *Salmonella* and *Arizona* are

TABLE 4-10
DIFFERENTIATION OF SPECIES WITHIN THE GENUS *EDWARDSIELLA*

BIOCHEMICAL TEST	E. TARDA	E. TARDA BIOGROUP I	E. HOSHINAE	E. ICTALURI
Indole	+	+	V (50)	–
Hydrogen sulfide	+	–	–	–
Motility	+	+	+	–
Fermentation of				
Mannitol	–	+	+	–
Sucrose	–	+	+	–
Arabinose	–	+	V (13)	–
Trehalose	–	–	+	–

+, 90% or more strains are positive; –, 90% or more strains are negative; V, 11%–89% of strains are positive.

considered to be the same species, but can be separated into six distinct subgroups, as listed in Box 4-9.

Beginning July 1, 1983, the CDC changed the method for reporting serotyping results so that all organisms identified as *Salmonella* were reported by genus and serotype, omitting reference to species (Box 4-10).

In day-to-day practice, unknown isolates from clinical specimens that are biochemically suggestive of *Salmonella* species are confirmed using polyclonal antisera containing antibodies to all the major subgroups. Subcultures of confirmed isolates are forwarded to public health laboratories, where serotype designations (e.g., *S.* serotype *typhimurium*) are made based on serologic reactions to O and H determinants.

IDENTIFICATION OF *SALMONELLA TYPHI*. Although most *Salmonella* serotypes cannot be distinguished by biochemical reactions, one serotype, namely *S. typhi*, does possess some unique biochemical characteristics that will allow it to be differentiated from other serotypes. First and foremost is the observation that strains of *S. typhi* produce only a trace amount of hydrogen sulfide, which is usually observed as a crescent-shaped wedge of black precipitate forming at the interface of the slant and butt in KIA or TSI media (Color Plate 4-4*B*). Additionally, *S. typhi* strains are noted to be less active biochemically than the more common serotypes and specifically are negative in the following reactions: Simmon's citrate; ornithine decarboxylase; gas from glucose; fermentation of dulcitol, arabinose, and rhamnose; and mucate and acetate utilization. Consequently, the authors believe that it is within the capabilities of most clinical laboratories to make a preliminary report of *S. typhi* or *Salmonella*

BOX 4-9. CLASSIFICATION OF *SALMONELLA*

Salmonella Subgroup 1: Includes Most Serotypes

S. typhi

S. choleraesuis

S. paratyphi

S. gallinarum

S. pullorum

Salmonella Subgroup 2

S. salamae

Salmonella Subgroup 3a

S. arizonae

Salmonella Subgroup 3b

S. diarizonae

Salmonella Subgroup 4

S. houtenae

Salmonella Subgroup 5

S. bongori

Salmonella Subgroup 6

S. choleraesuis subsp. *indica*

BOX 4-10. *SALMONELLA* NOMENCLATURE

PREVIOUS NOMENCLATURE	CURRENT NOMENCLATURE
Salmonella enteritidis serotype Enteritidis	*Salmonella* serotype enteritidis
S. enteritidis serotype Typhimurium	*Salmonella* serotype typhimurium
S. enteritidis serotype Heidelberg	*Salmonella* serotype heidelberg

species not *S. typhi* while the laboratory awaits specific serotype confirmation from their local public health laboratory.

INCIDENCE AND SOURCES OF SALMONELLOSES. Human infections with salmonellae are most commonly caused by ingestion of food, water, or milk contaminated by human or animal excreta. Salmonellae are primary pathogens of lower animals (e.g., poultry, cows, pigs, pets, birds, sheep, seals, donkeys, lizards, snakes), which are the principal source of nontyphoidal salmonellosis in humans. Interestingly, humans are the only known reservoir for *S. typhi*. Although the incidence of typhoid fever has declined in developed countries, sporadic outbreaks continue to occur. About 400 cases are reported annually in the United States. In contrast, about 50,000 cases of nontyphoid salmonellosis occur each year in the United States. About half of the salmonellosis epidemics are the result of contaminated poultry and poultry products. Salmonellae in the feces of hens contaminate the surface of eggs or penetrates internally through hairline cracks. In hens with ovarian infection, the organisms may gain access to the yolk. The Egg Products Inspection Act of 1970 requires pasteurization of all bulk egg products and federally supervised inspection of shell eggs for cracks.

Historically *S. typhimurium* has been the most frequently reported serotype, accounting for slightly more than 20% of isolates reported to the CDC.[55] However, from 1976 through 1991, the proportion of reported isolates of *S. enteritidis* in the United States increased from 5% to 20% and in 1989 and 1990 exceeded the isolation rate of *S. typhimurium*.[59] The largest single source outbreak of salmonellosis in U.S. history (16,000 culture-confirmed cases with epidemiologic data indicating 150,000 to 200,000 persons were actually infected) occurred in 1985 in Illinois and surrounding states and was traced to a faulty valve in a major commercial milk supply firm.[53] Several *S. enteritidis* outbreaks have occurred in the United States since 1990 that were associated with shell eggs.[55,57,59] An estimated 0.01% of all shell eggs contain *S. enteritidis*. Consequently, foods containing raw or undercooked eggs (e.g., homemade eggnog or ice cream, hollandaise sauce, Caesar salad dressing, homemade mayonnaise, and runny omelettes) pose a slight risk of infection with *S. enteritidis*.[57,59] In 1994, an outbreak of *S. enteritidis* infection was linked to a nationally distributed ice cream brand. Illnesses were documented in 41 states, and more than 200,000 persons were estimated to have been ill.[62] These outbreak serve as a constant reminder that modern technology is not immune to the ravages of infectious diseases that may occur in explosive and widespread epidemics.

Salmonellosis has also been associated with direct or indirect contact with reptiles (i.e., lizards, snakes, turtles). During the early 1970s, small pet turtles were an important source of salmonella infection in the United States. In 1975, The Food and Drug Administration prohibited the distribution and sale of small turtles, resulting in the prevention of 100,000 cases of

CLINICAL CORRELATION BOX 4-7: *SALMONELLA* INFECTION

Four clinical types of *Salmonella* infection may be distinguished:[137,286] 1) gastroenteritis, the most frequent manifestation, ranging from mild to fulminant diarrhea, accompanied by low-grade fever and varying degrees of nausea and vomiting; 2) bacteremia or septicemia without major gastrointestinal symptoms (*S. choleraesuis* is particularly invasive) characterized by high, spiking fever and positive blood cultures; 3) enteric fever, potentially caused by any strain of *Salmonella* species, usually manifested as mild fever and diarrhea, except for classic cases of typhoid fever (*S. typhi*), in which the disease progresses through a bimodal course, characterized by an early period (lasting 1 to 2 weeks) of fever and constipation, during which blood cultures are positive and stool cultures remain negative, followed by a second (diarrheic) phase during which blood cultures become negative and stool cultures will be positive; and 4) a carrier state in which persons with previous infection, especially with *S. typhi*, may continue to excrete the organism in their feces for up to 1 year following remission of symptoms. Of some concern is a recent report of lactose-positive strains of *S. virchow* causing bacteremia and meningitis.[271] Although detection of lactose-positive strains in the blood or cerebrospinal fluid would not be difficult, finding such strains in stool would pose a problem for most laboratories owing to the similarity in appearance to other lactose-positive coliforms present in stool specimens.

salmonellosis annually.[78] However, since 1986, the popularity of iguanas and other reptiles that can transmit infection to humans has given rise to an increased incidence of salmonella infections caused by reptile-associated serotypes.[64] Because young children are at increased risk for reptile-associated salmonellosis and severe complications (e.g., septicemia and meningitis), reducing exposure of infants or children younger than 5 years of age to reptiles is particularly important.

INFECTIONS DUE TO *SALMONELLA ARIZONAE*. Formerly classified as *Arizona hinshawii*, this species resembles salmonellae antigenically, clinically, and epidemiologically. It was first recovered in 1939 from diseased reptiles in Arizona and was initially called "S. dar-es-saalam type variety from Arizona." It was later distinguished from *Salmonella* but as of July 1, 1983 was reclassified as a serotype of the genus *Salmonella*. Although most *Salmonella* serotypes cannot be distinguished by biochemical reactions, *Salmonella* serotype *arizonae* can be easily differentiated on the basis of having positive malonate and negative dulcitol reactions. In addition, some strains ferment lactose, and all strains are ONPG positive. As a result of these unique biochemical reactions, a correct serotype designation can be easily made by most of the commercially available identification systems.

New Methods for Recovery and Characterization of Salmonellae. In addition to the classic media discussed previously (see Tables 4-1 through 4-3), new media have been described that are intended to improve the isolation of *Salmonella* species from stool samples. These include novobiocin–brilliant green–glucose agar (NGB),[85] novobiocin–brilliant green–glycerol–lactose agar (NBGL),[248] Rambach agar,[253] SM-ID medium (bioMerieux SA, France),[89,249] xylose–lysine–tergitol 4 (XLT4) medium,[212] and modified semisolid Rappaport Vassiliadis medium (MSRV).[12,84,129] The formulations and differential properties of these media are given in Table 4-11. In a study by Ruiz and associates comparing five plating media for isolation of *Salmonella*, NBGL media had the highest sensitivity (78.4%) and positive predictive value (61%) for direct recovery of *Salmonella* from stool.[270] These authors recommend the use of SM-ID for recovery of *S. typhi*, which is not detected on NBGL agar. Monnery and colleagues found SMID and Rambach agars to be considerably more specific than salmonella–shigella agar and Hektoen agar.[214] Dusch and Altwegg compared six media (Hektoen enteric agar [HE], Rambach agar, SM-ID medium, XLT4 agar, NBGL agar, and MSRV medium) and concluded that MSRV was the most sensitive medium tested for the isolation of nontyphoid salmonellae from stool; however, these authors noted that the semisolid nature of the medium was a disadvantage and requires careful handling in the laboratory. They noted that XLT4 had a sensitivity comparable with HE and nearly 100% specificity and can be considered an alternative for the isolation of salmonellae from stools.[90]

The 4-methylumbelliferyl caprilate test (MUCAP test; Biolife, Milano, Italy) is a fluorescence test for rapid identification of *Salmonella* strains directly from agar plates. The test consists of an eight-carbon-atom ester conjugated with methylumbelliferone. This substrate interacts with the salmonella C_8–esterase, leading to release of umbelliferone, which is strongly fluorescent at 365 nm. The test is performed by applying a drop of the reagent directly to suspect colonies on the agar surface and then observing for the appearance of blue fluorescence of the colony under a Wood's lamp within 5 minutes. Several studies have shown this test to provide nearly 100% sensitivity and specificity in detecting *Salmonella* strains and offers a useful and rapid adjunct to routine biochemical characterization of *Salmonella* strains.[4,229,272,273]

Other new techniques are being introduced that may significantly alter the future identification of *Salmonella* species, both in the clinical laboratory and in epidemiologic field studies. As an example of new applications, Olsvik and associates[230] traced the transmission of *S. typhimurium* strains from diseased cattle in four separate herds in Norway to human farm workers, by demonstrating identical cryptic plasmid profiles for the various isolates by using restriction endonuclease digestion techniques. As these authors point out, conventional serotyping and biotyping techniques are often not sufficiently specific to determine definitively that two or more isolates from different sources are, in fact, identical. Techniques, such as restriction endonuclease analysis or genetic probes, that detect nucleotide sequences in plasmids or in chromosomal DNA and RNA will make epidemiologic and diagnostic work in microbiology much more exacting in the future. These techniques are discussed in more detail in Chapter 1.

TRIBE *CITROBACTEREAE*

Included in the *Citrobactereae* are 1 genus—*Citrobacter*—and 11 species. The genus *Citrobacter* and the species *C. freundii* were designated in 1932 by Werkman and Gillen. In 1970 Frederiksen described a new species that he named *C. koseri*. In 1971, Young and coworkers proposed the name *Levinea malonatica* for a similar group of organisms, and in 1972 Ewing and Davis described *C. diversus*. Frederiksen examined all three strains and determined that they were phenotypically alike and proposed that the name *C. koseri* be restored as the valid name for this taxon.[115] In 1993, Brenner and colleagues, using DNA relatedness studies, showed that organisms identified as *C. freundii* consisted of a heterogeneous group representing several genetic species.[39] This work lead to the establishment of 11 genomospecies within the genus *Citrobacter*, as shown in Table 4-12.

The characteristics that suggest an isolate may belong to the genus *Citrobacter* are given in Table 4-6. The key characteristics that differentiate *C. freundii* and other H_2S-positive citrobacters from salmonellae are growth in KCN (*Salmonella* species are negative), absence of lysine decarboxylase activity (*Salmonella* species are positive), and the hydrolysis of ONPG (*Salmonella* species are negative). The biochemical differentiation among the *Citrobacter* species is shown in

TABLE 4-11

NEW MEDIA FOR RECOVERY OF SALMONELLA SPECIES FROM STOOL

MEDIUM	FORMULATION		PRINCIPLE AND INTERPRETATION
Novobiocin–brilliant green–glucose agar (NBG)	Tryptic soy agar	40 g	*Salmonella* colonies appear smooth and entire with medium- to large-sized, dark black, nucleated centers owing to H_2S production. In addition, reddening and a visible zone of clearing occurs in the medium around each colony. Coliforms are either inhibited or fail to produce black-centered colonies. Some *Citrobacter freundii* strains produce colonies indistinguishable from *Salmonella* species.
	Ferric ammonium citrate	1.5 g	
	Sodium thiosulfate pentahydrate	5 g	
	Phenol red (sodium salt)	80 mg	
	Glucose	1 g	
	Brilliant green	7 mg	
	Novobiocin	10 mg	
	Distilled water to	1 L	
	Final pH 7.3		
Novobiocin–brilliant green–glycerol–lactose agar (NBGL)	Trypticase soy agar	40 g	The detection of *Salmonella* spp. is based on the production of H_2S resulting in black colonies. Sufficient H_2S formation is achieved only by colonies that do not produce acid from glycerol or lactose, because a low pH interferes with H_2S formation. This results in colorless colonies for most *Proteus* and *Citrobacter* species.
	Ferric ammonium citrate	1.5 g	
	Sodium thiosulfate	5 g	
	Lactose	10 g	
	Glycerol	10 mL	
	Brilliant green	7 mg	
	Novobiocin	10 mg	
	Distilled water to	1 L	
Rambach agar	Propylene glycol	10 g	Detects ability of *Salmonella* spp. to metabolize propylene glycol. Suspect colonies on this medium are usually bright red. Contains moderate amount of bile salts to inhibit coliforms.
	Peptone	5 g	
	Yeast extract	2 g	
	Sodium desoxycholate	1 g	
	Neutral red	0.03 g	
	5-Bromo-4-chloro-3-indolyl-β-D-Galactopyranoside	0.1 g	
	Agar	15 g	
	Distilled water to	1 L	
SM-ID agar	Beef extract	3 g	Detection of *Salmonella* spp. is based on the formation of acid from the glucuronate and on the absence of β-galactosidase. *Salmonella* serotypes produce pinkish red colonies (sometimes with a colorless rim), whereas coliforms form other colors (green, blue, or violet) if they are positive for β-galactosidase, or remain colorless. Contains moderate amount of bile salts to inhibit coliforms.
	Bio-Polytone	6 g	
	Yeast extract	2 g	
	Bile salts	4 g	
	Neutral red	0.025 g	
	Tris buffer	0.65 g	
	Brilliant green	0.3 mg	
	Chromogen substrate 1 (galactopyranoside)	0.17 g	
	Sodium glucuronate	12 g	
	Chromogen substrate 2 (glucopyranoside)	0.026 g	
	Sorbitol	8 g	
	Agar	13.5 g	
	Distilled water to	1 L	
	Final pH 7.6 ± 0.2		
Modified Semisolid Rappaport–Vassiliadis Medium (MSRV)	Tryptose	4.59 g	Based on the swarming phenomenon of motile bacteria (*Salmonella* spp. and others) at reduced agar concentrations. After incubation the plates are checked for motile bacteria which appear as a halo of growth spreading out from the original inoculation point. Subcultures are taken from the edge of migration to check for purity and for further biochemical and serological tests. Coliforms are inhibited by a combination of increased osmotic pressure, malachite green, and incubation at 41° to 43°C
	Caesin hydrolysate acid	4.59 g	
	Sodium chloride	7.34 g	
	Potassium dihydrogen phosphate	1.47 g	
	Magnesium chloride (anhydrous)	10.93 g	
	Malachite green oxalate	0.037 g	
	Agar	2.7 g	
	Distilled water to	1 L	
	Novobiocin (2% solution) added after sterilization	1 mL	
	Final pH 5.2 ± 0.2		
Xylose–Lysine–Tergitol 4 (XLT4)	Bacto proteose peptone No. 3	1.6 g	This is a highly selective medium that substitutes the anionic surfactant Tergitol 4 for sodium desoxycholate found in XLD agar. The XLT4 agar completely inhibits the growth of all gram-positive bacteria and
	Bacto yeast extract	3.0 g	
	L-lysine	5.0 g	
	Bacto xylose	3.75 g	
	Bacto lactose	7.5 g	

(Continued)

TABLE 4-11 *(Continued)*

NEW MEDIA FOR RECOVERY OF *SALMONELLA* SPECIES FROM STOOL

MEDIUM	FORMULATION		PRINCIPLE AND INTERPRETATION
	Bacto saccharose	7.5 g	fungi, and either completely or strongly inhibits the growth of numerous gram-negative bacteria including *Proteus, Providence,* and *Pseudomonas.* In addition, *Citrobacter* species are somewhat inhibited and very rarely produce colonies with black centers after overnight incubation. *Salmonella* colonies (H_2S-positive) appear black or black-centered with a yellow periphery after 18–24 hours incubation. After continued incubation, the colonies become entirely black or pink to red with black centers. Rare strains of *Salmonella* that produce no H_2S display pink to pinkish yellow colonies that can be differentiated from bright yellow nonsalmonellae colonies.
	Ferric ammonium citrate	0.8 g	
	Sodium thiosulfate	6.8 g	
	Sodium chloride	5 g	
	Bacto agar	18 g	
	Bacto phenol red	0.08 g	
	Distilled water to	1 L	
	Final pH 7.4 ± 0.2		

Note: Rambach, XLT4, MSRV, NBG, and NBGL are not suitable for use in the isolation of typhoid *Salmonella* serotypes; only SM-ID detects salmonellae of such serotypes.

Table 4-13. Human isolates of all genomospecies except *C. koseri* have been obtained predominantly from stools.[39] Farmer and coworkers,[106] who reviewed strains referred to the CDC, cited *C. freundii* as a possible cause of diarrhea (although most fecal isolates do not appear to be associated with disease) and as a cause of isolated cases of extraintestinal infections. He also cites a possible association between *C. koseri* and outbreaks of meningitis and brain abscesses in neonates and reports the recovery of *C. amalonaticus* from a few blood cultures. Janda and colleagues at the Microbial Diseases Laboratory in California reported that *C. freundii* was the most common species identified from all body cites except feces. In gastrointestinal specimens, *C. freundii* ranked fourth behind *C. youngae, C. braakii,* and *C. werkmanii.*[163] *C. freundii* (complex) has been reported as a cause of gastrointestinal illness associated with imported Brie cheese,[52] and isolation of a

C. freundii strain that carries the *E. coli* 0157 antigen has been reported.[26] *C. koseri* has been most often isolated from urine and respiratory tract specimens.[148,192] *C. koseri* has also been reported with increasing frequency as a cause of sporadic and epidemic meningitis in neonates and young infants.[132,179,180,234,309] Brain abscesses are found in 75% of infants with *C. koseri* meningitis, a prevalence far higher than that reported for other bacteria that cause meningitis.[133,179] One-third of infants with *C. koseri* meningitis die, and at least 75% of survivors have severe neurologic impairment.[133] Other reports corroborate the tendency for *C. koseri* to cause meningitis and brain abscesses, particularly in association with the anaerobic gram-negative bacillus *Prevotella (Bacteroides) melaninogenica.*[11,81,189] *C. sedlakii* has been isolated from a catheterized urine specimen from a patient at the University of Illinois Hospital with a diagnosis of bacteremia. Genomospecies 9, recently named *C. rodentium,* has been isolated only from rodents and causes a disease in laboratory mice known as transmissible murine colonic hyperplasia.[279]

Identification of *Citrobacter* species is hampered because the new species are not yet included in the databases of most commercial identification systems. To assist laboratories in speciating the new *Citrobacter* species, O'Hara and colleagues have published a dichotomous key using conventional biochemical tests.[225] The susceptibility pattern of isolates also offers an aid to identification. *C. koseri* has an antibiotic susceptibility pattern similar to *Klebsiella* (i.e., resistant to ampicillin and ticarcillin), whereas *C. freundii* has a pattern more typical of *Enterobacter* species (i.e., resistant to ampicillin and first-generation cephalosporins).

TRIBE *KLEBSIELLEAE*

The tribe *Klebsielleae* includes four major genera—*Klebsiella, Enterobacter, Hafnia,* and *Serratia*—each of which includes several species that are overt and op-

TABLE 4-12

FORMER AND CURRENT SPECIES WITHIN THE GENUS *CITROBACTER*

FORMER SPECIES DESIGNATION	GENOMOSPECIES	CURRENT SPECIES
C. freundii complex	1	*C. freundii*
	5	*C. youngae*
	6	*C. braakii*
	7	*C. werkmanii*
	8	*C. sedlakii*
	9	*C. rodentium*
	10	*C. gillenii*
	11	*C. murliniae*
C. diversus	2	*C. koseri*
C. amalonaticus	3	*C. amalonaticus*
C. amalonaticus biogroup 1	4	*C. farmeri*

TABLE 4-13
Differentiation of Species Within the Genus *Citrobacter*

Biochemical Test	C. Koseri	C. Werkmanii	C. Sedlakii	C. Rodentium	C. Gillenii	C. Amalonaticus	C. Farmeri	C. Braakii	C. Freundii	C. Murliniae	C. Youngae
Adonitol	+	–	–	–	–	–	–	–	–	–	–
Malonate	+	+	+	+	+	–	–	–	–	–	–
Ornithine	+	–	+	+	–	+	+	+	–	–	–
Melibiose	–	–	+	–	V (67)	–	+	V (78)	+	V (33)	V (19)
Sucrose	V (44)	–	–	–	V (33)	V (13)	+	–	+	V (33)	V (14)
Indole	+	–	+	–	–	+	+	V (33)	V (38)	+	–
Dulcitol	V (38)	–	+	–	–	–	–	V (33)	V (13)	+	V (86)
H₂S	–	+	–	–	V (67)	V (13)	–	V (60)	V (75)	V (67)	V (67)

+, 90% or more strains positive; –, 90% or more strains negative; V, 11%–89% of strains positive; numbers in parentheses are percentage of strains giving positive reaction.
Data obtained from Brenner DJ et al. Int J Syst Bacteriol 43:645–658, 1993.

portunistic pathogens in humans. A new, fifth genus, *Pantoea*, has been added to accommodate the reclassification of the organism formerly named *Enterobacter agglomerans* biotype XIII and now called *Pantoea agglomerans*.[124] The key characteristics suggesting that an unknown isolate belongs to the *Klebsielleae* are given in Table 4-6. The biochemical differences between the major genera and species within the tribe are presented in Table 4-14.

Genus *Klebsiella*. The genus *Klebsiella* was named after Edwin Klebs, a late-19th century German microbiologist. The bacillus now known as *Klebsiella* was also described by Carl Friedlander, and for many years the "Friedlander bacillus" was well known as a cause of severe, often fatal, pneumonia. *K. pneumoniae* is the type species of this genus.

Klebsiella species are widely distributed in nature and in the gastrointestinal tracts of humans and animals. A *Klebsiella* species should be suspected when large colonies with a mucoid consistency are recovered on primary isolation plates. On MacConkey agar, the colonies typically appear large, mucoid, and red, with red pigment usually diffusing into the surrounding agar, indicating fermentation of lactose and acid production. Not all strains, however, are mucoid, and certain species of *Enterobacter* can closely simulate the *Klebsiella* species in screening tests. All *Klebsiella* species are nonmotile and most do not decarboxylate ornithine (*K. ornithinolytica* is ornithine-positive)—characteristics that are positive for most *Enterobacter* species. Many strains of *Klebsiella* hydrolyze urea slowly, producing a light pink color in the slant of

Christensen's urea agar. Production of indole from tryptophan can be used to separate the two principal species. *K. pneumoniae* is indole-negative, and *K. oxytoca* is indole-positive. Certain strains do not produce these classic reactions, which led to the naming of several additional species (Table 4-15).

K. pneumoniae is most frequently recovered from clinical specimens and can cause a classic form of primary pneumonia. It is infrequently found in the oropharynx of normal persons (1% to 6% carrier rate);[261] however, a prevalence as high as 20% may occur in hospitalized patients. This colonization may prove to be the source of lung infections that generally occur in patients with debilitating conditions such as alcoholism, diabetes mellitus, and chronic obstructive pulmonary disease.[261] The pneumonia tends to be destructive, with extensive necrosis and hemorrhage, resulting in the production of sputum that may be thick, mucoid, and brick red, or thin and "currant jellylike" in appearance. Lung abscesses, chronic cavitary disease, internal hemorrhage, and hemoptysis may be seen in severe cases. Pleuritis is commonly present, which explains why pleuritic pain is found in about 80% of patients. *K. pneumoniae* can also cause a variety of extrapulmonary infections, including enteritis and meningitis (in infants), urinary tract infections (in children and adults), and septicemia.

K. ozaenae and *K. rhinoscleromatis* are infrequent isolates that are now considered to be subspecies of *K. pneumoniae*; however, each is associated with a unique spectrum of disease. *K. ozaenae* is associated with atrophic rhinitis, a condition called ozena, and purulent infections of the nasal mucous membranes. Janda and

---

TABLE 4-14

DIFFERENTIATION OF THE MAJOR GENERA AND SPECIES WITHIN THE TRIBE *KLEBSIELLEAE*

	KLEBSIELLA		*ENTEROBACTER*		*PANTOEA*	*HAFNIA*	*SERRATIA*	
BIOCHEMICAL TEST	*PNEUMONIAE*	*OXYTOCA*	*AEROGENES*	*CLOACAE*	*AGGLOMERANS*	*ALVEI*	*MARCESCENS*	*LIQUEFACIENS*
Indole	−	+	−	−	V (20)	−	−	−
Motility	−	−	+	+	V (85)	V (85)	+	+
Lysine	+	+	+	−	−	+	+	+
Arginine	−	−	−	+	−	−	−	−
Ornithine	−	−	+	+	−	+	+	+
DNase (25°C)	−	−	−	−	−	−	+	V (85)
Gelatinase (22°C)	−	−	−	−	−	−	+	+
Fermentation of								
Lactose	+	+	+	+	V (40)	−	−	−
Sucrose	+	+	+	+	V (75)	−	+	+
Sorbitol	+	+	+	+	V (30)	−	+	+
Adonitol	+	+	+	V (25)	−	−	V (40)	−
Arabinose	+	+	+	+	+	+	−	+

+, 90% or more strains are positive; −, 90% or more strains are negative; V, 11%–89% of strains are positive.

TABLE 4-15

DIFFERENTIATION OF SPECIES WITHIN THE GENUS *KLEBSIELLA*

BIOCHEMICAL TEST	K. PNEUMONIAE	K. OZAENAE	K. RHINOSCLEROMATIS	K. ORNITHINOLYTICA	K. OXYTOCA	K. TERRIGENA	K PLANTICOLA
Indole	−	−	−	+	+	−	V (20)
Methyl red	−	+	+	+	V (20)	V (60)	+
Voges-Proskauer	+	−	−	V (70)	+	+	+
Urease	+	−	−	+	+	−	+
Lysine	+	V (40)	−	+	+	+	+
Ornithine	−	−	−	+	−	V (20)	−
ONPG	+	V (80)	−	+	+	+	+
Malonate	+	−	+	+	+	+	+
Growth at*							
5°C	−	−	−	+	−	+	+
10°C	−	−	−	+	+	+	+
41°C	+	NA	NA	+	+	−	+

+, 90% or more strains are positive; −, 90% or more strains are negative; V, 11%–89% of strains are positive; NA, results not available.
* Data from Farmer JJ III, Davis BR, Hickman-Brenner FW et al: Biochemical identification of new species and biogroups of *Enterobacteriaceae* isolated from clinical specimens. J Clin Microbiol 21:46–76, 1985.

colleagues[164] have also reported a case of corneal abscess caused by *K. ozaenae*. Reports of the isolation of *K. ozaenae* from blood, urine, and soft tissue suggests that the spectrum of disease caused by this organism is more extensive than has been previously thought.[127] *K. rhinoscleromatis* causes the granulomatous disease rhinoscleroma, an infection of the respiratory mucosa, oropharynx, nose, and paranasal sinuses. Clinical correlations should be made, when these species are recovered in cultures, to determine their medical significance in individual cases. Even though these two species are no longer considered to be true species but, rather, biochemically inactive strains of *K. pneumoniae*,[36] we believe that there is medical relevance in reporting the names *K. ozaenae* and *K. rhinoscleromatis* because of the specific disease association of these two strains.

Nearly half of the isolates of *K. oxytoca* submitted to the CDC have been from feces, with the next most common source being blood.[106] The newly named species, *K. terrigena*[156] and *K. planticola*,[17] reflect their sources in nature. *K. terrigena* closely resembles *K. pneumoniae* and has been isolated mainly from soil and water. Human isolates have been recovered from the feces of healthy humans[247] and the respiratory tract;[246] however, their capacity to cause human infection has not been shown. *K. planticola* (synonym *K. trevisanii*[112,123]) has been isolated primarily from botanical and aquatic environments. Human isolates have been recovered from the respiratory tract, urine, cerebrospinal fluid, and blood,[116,117] with the majority of

isolates representing colonization, rather than infection. See Table 4-15 for a listing of the characteristics by which these various species can be differentiated.

The higher incidence of infections due to *Klebsiella* species during the past decade probably reflects both an increase in nosocomial infections in debilitated or immunosuppressed patients and a trend toward greater antibiotic resistance. Klebsiellae have a tendency to harbor antibiotic-resistant plasmids; thus, infections with multiply antibiotic-resistant strains can be anticipated. Virtually all clinical strains are resistant to ampicillin, carbenicillin, and ticarcillin.[137] Of particular concern is the recent appearance of *Klebsiella* strains that posses plasmids that mediate resistance to extended-spectrum β-lactam drugs. This form of resistance is due to the production of unique β-lactamase enzymes, referred to as extended-spectrum β-lactamases, or ESBLs.[165,190] These enzymes have been seen mostly in strains of *K. pneumoniae* and *E. coli* and cause them to be resistant to most β-lactam drugs, including the third-generation cephalosporins. A unique feature of ESBLs is their ability to escape detection with most of the commonly used susceptibility test methods and the resultant concern that organisms possessing ESBLs are reported to be susceptible to antibiotics that, in fact, they are resistant to.[160,209] This subject is discussed in more detail in Chapter 15.

Genus *Enterobacter*. Because large amounts of gas are produced by many strains of the genus *Enterobacter*, for many years the type species was called *Aerobacter* *aerogenes.* The genus designation was changed to *Enterobacter* by Edwards and Ewing in 1962.

There are 16 species included in the genus *Enterobacter.* A recent development has been the removal of one of the biotypes of *E. agglomerans* and its placement in the genus *Pantoea.*[124] As a genus, *Enterobacter* has the general characteristics of the *Klebsielleae,* but can be differentiated from most *Klebsiella* species because they are motile and ornithine-positive. The biochemical characteristics by which the medically important species can be differentiated are included in Table 4-16. Four additional species (*E. intermedius, E. dissolvens, E. nimipressuralis,* and *E. pyrinus*) are found in the environment or as plant pathogens and have not been found in human clinical specimens.

E. aerogenes and *E. cloacae* are the species most commonly encountered in clinical specimens. They are widely distributed in water, in sewage, in soil, and on vegetables. They are part of the commensal enteric flora and are not believed to cause diarrhea, although a Shiga-like toxin-producing strain of *E. cloacae* has been isolated from the feces of an infant with hemolytic–uremic syndrome.[235] They are also associated with a variety of opportunistic infections involving the urinary tract, respiratory tract, and cutaneous wounds; and, on occasion, cause septicemia and meningitis.

E. sakazakii, known as yellow-pigmented *E. cloacae,*[104] has been found in several cases of neonatal meningitis and sepsis.[27,74,167,178,220,304] Fatality rates as high as 75% have been reported, indicating that this organism can be highly virulent and must be recognized in clinical laboratories. The bright yellow pigment (particularly intense if cultures are incubated at 25°C) and "tough" nature of the colonies are the initial clues that this organism is present (*Pantoea agglomerans* also produces a yellow pigment, usually less intense, and often only after delayed incubation at room temperature). The decarboxylase pattern of *E. sakazakii* (lysine-negative, arginine-positive, and ornithine-positive) helps to differentiate it from *E. aerogenes* (lysine-positive, arginine-negative, and ornithine-positive) and *P. agglomerans* (lysine-, arginine-, and ornithine-negative); and *E. sakazakii* does not ferment sorbitol, in contrast to *E. cloacae,* which does.

E. gergoviae causes urinary tract infections, and additional isolates have also been recovered from the respiratory tract and blood.[43] Biochemically it is closest to *E. aerogenes* (lysine-positive, arginine-negative, ornithine-positive), but is strongly urease-positive. It can be further differentiated by negative reactions in adonitol, inositol, and sorbitol, whereas *E. aerogenes* is positive for all three reactions.

TABLE 4-16

DIFFERENTIATION OF SPECIES WITHIN THE GENUS *ENTEROBACTER**

BIOCHEMICAL TEST	E. AEROGENES	E. CLOACAE	E. GERGOVIAE	E. SAKAZAKII	E. HORMAECHEI	E. CANCEROGENUS	E. AMNIGENUS BIOGROUP 1	E. AMNIGENUS BIOGROUP 2	E. ASBURIAE
Methyl red	−	−	−	−	V (57)	−	−	V (65)	+
Voges-Proskauer	+	+	+	+	+	+	+	+	−
Lysine	+	−	+	−	−	−	−	−	−
Arginine	−	+	−	+	V (78)	+	−	V (35)	V (21)
Ornithine	+	+	+	+	+	+	V (55)	+	+
Urease	−	V (65)	+	−	V (87)	−	−	−	V (60)
Motility	+	+	+	+	V (52)	+	+	+	−
Fermentation of									
Lactose	+	+	V (55)	+	−	−	V (70)	V (35)	V (75)
Sucrose	+	+	+	+	+	−	+	−	+
Adonitol	+	V (25)	−	−	−	−	−	−	−
Sorbitol	+	+	−	−	−	−	−	+	+
Raffinose	+	+	+	+	−	−	+	−	V (70)
Rhamnose	+	+	+	+	+	+	+	+	−
Melibiose	+	+	+	+	−	−	+	+	−
Yellow pigment	−	−	−	+	−	−	−	−	−

+, 90% or more strains are positive; −, 90% or more strains are negative; V, 11%–89% of strains are positive.
* Table includes only those *Enterobacter* species that have been isolated from human clinical specimens. Isolates that are triple decarboxylase negative may be *Pantoea* species, and isolates that are both lactose- and sucrose-negative but are lysine-positive may be *Hafnia alvei* (see Table 4-14).

E. cancerogenus (formerly called *Erwinia cancerogena, Enterobacter taylorae,* and CDC Enteric Group 19)[107,282] has been reported to cause a variety of clinical infections, including osteomyelitis after an open fracture,[317] wound infection,[257] urinary tract infection,[260,269] and bacteremia and pneumonia.[269] The key biochemical features are its lysine-negative, arginine-positive, and ornithine-positive reactions and its negative reactions in adonitol, inositol, sorbitol, raffinose, and melibiose. They are lactose-negative, but ONPG-positive, and we have noted that colonies growing on Mac-Conkey agar will develop purple centers after extended incubation.

E. asburiae (formerly called CDC Enteric Group 17, or atypical *Citrobacter*) is biochemically similar to *E. cloacae*; however, it is unique among the *Enterobacter* species by being nonmotile and Voges-Proskauer-negative. It has been reported from a variety of human sources, including blood, urine, wounds, respiratory tract, and feces.[41] We have found considerable variation in the ability of commercial identification systems to correctly identify this species.

E. amnigenus is primarily a water organism that has been isolated from human specimens; however, there is no evidence so far that *E. amnigenus* can cause human infection.[158]

E. hormaechei is a new species of *Enterobacter* named in 1989 after Estenio Hormaeche, a Uruguayan microbiologist who (with P. R. Edwards) proposed and defined the genus *Enterobacter*.[226] Formerly known as Enteric Group 75, it is biochemically closest to *E. taylorae* (now *E. cancerogenus*) except it is urea-positive, sucrose-positive, and esculin-negative. Isolates have been reported from blood, sputum, wounds, ear, gallbladder, and stool. In March 1993, CDC investigators identified a nosocomial outbreak of *E. hormaechei* septicemia in a neonatal intensive care unit. Five infants had positive blood cultures with *E. hormaechei*, and another infant had *E. hormaechei* tracheitis. Four additional infants were identified with *E. hormaechei* colonization. No deaths were reported. Environmental cultures showed the organism to be present on three isolettes and one doorknob.[50] A case of recurrent bacteremia caused by *E. hormaechei* has been seen at the University of Illinois Hospital in a 2-year-old patient with a neuroblastoma involving a left supraclavicular lymph node, an adrenal gland, and a perinaval lymph node.

Enterobacter species together with certain other members of the family *Enterobacteriaceae* (namely *C. freundii, Serratia* species, *Morganella morganii,* and *Providence* species) carry a gene for chromosomally encoded β-lactamase which can be induced by certain antibiotics, amino acids, or body fluids.[190] Unlike plasmid-mediated β-lactamases, these enzymes are not normally expressed. Only under the influence of an inducer or following mutation does the gene become activated and the enzyme expressed. It is a concern, therefore, that organisms harboring genes for inducible β-lactamases may show false susceptibility if tested in the unidued state. Recently, methods for the detection of resistance owing to inducible β-lactamases have been described.[154] This topic is discussed further in Chapter 15.

Genus Pantoea. In the early 1970s, *P. agglomerans* (then called *Enterobacter agglomerans*) was responsible for a nationwide outbreak of septicemia caused by contaminated intravenous fluids.[196] The new genus *Pantoea* was created in 1989 with the type species being *P. agglomerans*.[124] This taxon includes the former type strains of *Enterobacter agglomerans, Erwinia herbicola,* and *Erwinia milletiae*. *Pantoea* is derived from a Greek word meaning "of all sorts and sources," thus describing these bacteria that come from diverse geographic and ecologic sources. A second species, *P. dispersa,* has been isolated from plant surfaces, seeds, humans, and the environment. Both species are triple-decarboxylase-negative (lysine-negative, arginine-negative, and ornithine-negative), but can be separated by salicin, which is positive for *P. agglomerans* and negative for *P. dispersa*.[124] Five additional species found in soil and plants have been described (see Table 4-5)

Genus Hafnia. *H. alvei,* formerly *Enterobacter hafnia,* is the only species in the genus *Hafnia*. The biochemical characteristics are similar to those of *Enterobacter* species except that *H. alvei* does not produce acids from the following carbohydrates: lactose, sucrose, melibiose, raffinose, adonitol, sorbitol, dulcitol, and inositol (see Table 4-14). *H. alvei* can be distinguished from *Serratia* species because it does not produce lipase or deoxyribonuclease. We have also noted that, unlike other species of *Enterobacteriaceae,* this organism gives off a strong scent of human feces. The clinical significance of *H. alvei* is not well defined. The organism has been recovered from human feces in the absence of symptoms. Isolated cases of infection have been reported from persons in whom *H. alvei* has been recovered from wounds, abscesses, sputum, urine, blood, and other sites. In one of our laboratories (University of Illinois) *H. alvei* was isolated in pure culture from a chest wound of a patient following thoracic surgery. There is recent evidence to suggest that *H. alvei* may be an emerging cause of acute bacterial gastroenteritis.[6,254,255,259,266,318] Some strains of *H. alvei* posses the virulence-associated gene *eaeA* that is responsible for the adherence of the organism to epithelial cells and for formation of the characteristic attaching–effacing lesions in the intestinal brush border seen also with enterohemorrhagic and enteropathogenic *E. coli*.[7,185,265]

Genus Serratia. *Serratia* species are unique among the *Enterobacteriaceae* in producing three hydrolytic enzymes: lipase, gelatinase, and DNase. Resistance to colistin and cephalothin are additional distinguishing features. The biochemical differentiation of *Serratia* species is shown in Table 4-17.

S. marcescens is the most important member of the genus *Serratia* and is often associated with a variety of human infections, particularly pneumonia and septicemia in patients with reticuloendothelial malignancies who are receiving chemotherapeutic agents. At one time, the organism was used as a harmless commensal to trace environmental contamination, primarily because the characteristic red pigmentation of some strains was easy to spot in culture media. However, the organism is now recognized as an important pathogen with invasive properties and a tendency to resist many commonly used antibiotics. *S. marcescens* can be a significant nosocomial opportunist, as evidenced by a recent case of childhood meningitis following the use of contaminated benzalkonium chloride disinfectant solution.[278] The species referred to as *S. liquefaciens* is now known to be not a single species but a collection of several DNA hybridization groups, including species named *S. proteamaculans* and *S. grimesii*. Because the species that make up this hybridization group cannot be separated by currently used biochemical tests, it is suggested that members of this species be reported as "*Serratia liquefaciens* group." This group is differentiated from *S. marcescens* by virtue of its ability to ferment L-arabinose.

S. rubidaea, as its name would imply, produces colonies that are red-pigmented but is rarely isolated from human clinical specimens. Ursua and associates reported a case of *S. rubidaea* isolated from the bile and blood of a patient with a bile tract carcinoma who underwent invasive procedures.[306] *S. odorifera* produces a dirty, musty odor, similar to unpeeled potatoes. Two biogroups are described. Biogroup 1 is ornithine-, sucrose-, and raffinose-positive and is predominantly isolated from sputum; however, it has been reported to cause severe sepsis in elderly, compromised patients,[71,207] and catheter-associated sepsis in an adoles-

cent patient with thalassemia major who had been splenectomized.[126] Biogroup 2 is negative for these three reactions and has been recovered from blood and cerebrospinal fluid.[106] Strains of *S. plymuthica* may be red-pigmented and have been isolated from soil, water, and human sputum specimens. Although *S. plymuthica* is generally not considered to be a cause of serious human infections, recent reports have shown that it can be a significant pathogen causing chronic osteomyelitis,[328] wound infections,[48,75] community-acquired[258] and nosocomial bacteremia,[48,87,153] and has been isolated from the peritoneal fluid of a patient with cholecystitis.[48] *S. ficaria* has a natural habitat in figs and the fig wasp.[125] Isolation of this species from human specimens is extremely rare and usually is accompanied by a history of ingestion of figs.[82] *S. entomophila* is an insect pathogen, and no human isolates have been reported. "*S.*" *fonticola* is not really a species of *Serratia* and is likely to be reclassified. It is a water organism that has been rarely isolated from human clinical specimens, mostly wounds.[33,106,242]

TRIBE *PROTEEAE*

The *Proteeae* comprise three genera: *Proteus*, *Morganella*, and *Providencia*. The characteristics suggesting that an organism belongs to this tribe are given in Table 4-6.

TABLE 4-17
DIFFERENTIATION OF SPECIES WITHIN THE GENUS *SERRATIA**

BIOCHEMICAL TEST	S. MARCESCENS	S. LIQUEFACIENS	S. RUBIDAEA	S. PLYMUTHICA	S. FICARIA	S. FONTICOLA	S. ODORIFERA BIOGROUP 1	2
DNase (25°C)	+	V (85)	+	+	+	−	+	+
Lipase (corn oil)	+	V (85)	+	V (70)	V (77)	−	V (35)	V (65)
Gelatinase at 22°C	+	+	+	V (60)	+	−	+	+
Lysine (Moeller's)	+	+	V (55)	−	−	+	+	+
Ornithine (Moeller's)	+	+	−	−	−	+	+	−
Odor of potatoes	−	−	V	−	+	−	+	+
Red, pink, or orange pigment	V	−	V	V	−	−	−	−
Fermentation of								
L-Arabinose	−	+	+	+	+	+	+	+
D-Arabitol	−	−	V (85)	−	+	+	−	−
D-Sorbitol	+	+	−	V (65)	+	+	+	+
Sucrose	+	+	+	+	+	V (21)	+	−
Raffinose	−	V (85)	+	+	V (70)	+	+	−
Malonate utilization	−	−	+	−	−	+	−	−

+, 90% or more strains are positive; −, 90% or more strains are negative; V, 11%–89% of strains are positive.
* Data obtained from Table 4-24 and reference 125. Table includes only those *Serratia* species that have been isolated from human clinical specimens.

Genus Proteus. DNA relatedness studies have clarified the classification of organisms within the *Proteeae*. The genus *Proteus* now includes four named species: *P. vulgaris*, *P. mirabilis*, *P. myxofaciens*, and *P. penneri*, and four unnamed genomospecies that were formerly identified as biogroup 3 of *P. vulgaris*.[40] Strains of *P. vulgaris* have traditionally been placed into three biogroups as follows:

> *Proteus* biogroup 1: indole-, salicin-, esculin-negative; chloramphenicol-resistant
> *Proteus* biogroup 2: indole-, salicin-, esculin-positive
> *Proteus* biogroup 3: indole-positive, salicin- and esculin-negative

Proteus biogroup 1 is a single genetic species and is now known as *P. penneri*.[143] *Proteus* biogroup 2 is a single genetic species and will retain the name *P. vulgaris*. *Proteus* biogroup 3 consists of four separate genetic species that are designated DNA groups 3, 4, 5, and 6. Biochemical separation of the *Proteus* species and DNA groups is given in Table 4-18.

The genus *Proteus* is found in soil, water, and fecally contaminated materials. *Proteus* species exhibit the characteristic feature of swarming motility, which is observed on noninhibitory agar (e.g., BAP) as a wavelike spreading of the organism across the entire surface of the agar (see Color Plate 4-1D). Whenever swarming is observed, *Proteus* species should be suspected. *P. mirabilis* is the species most frequently recovered from humans, particularly as the causative agent of both urinary tract and wound infections. *P. vulgaris* is more commonly recovered from infected sites in immunosuppressed hosts, particularly those receiving prolonged regimens of antibiotics. As noted in Table 4-18, *P. vulgaris* is indole-positive, whereas *P. mirabilis* is indole-negative. Thus, by performing a rapid spot indole test on a characteristic swarming colony, a rapid presumptive identification of *P. mirabilis* or *P. vulgaris* can be made. The new species *P. penneri*[143] and *P. myxofaciens* are also indole-negative but are rarely encountered in clinical laboratories (the latter is a pathogen of gypsy moth larvae and has not been recovered from human specimens). Therefore, for practical purposes, the recovery of an indole-negative *Proteus* species can be presumptively identified as *P. mirabilis*. Virtually all strains of *P. mirabilis* are sensitive to ampicillin and cephalosporins, whereas *P. vulgaris* is resistant; therefore, most patients with clinical infection, from whom an indole-negative *Proteus* species is recovered, can be treated with one of the broad-spectrum penicillins or cephalosporins.

P. penneri closely resembles *P. vulgaris* but differs from *P. vulgaris* by being indole-, salicin-, and esculin-negative and failing to produce hydrogen sulfide in TSI. When *P. penneri* is suspected, a chloramphenicol susceptibility test should be performed for identification purposes. *P. penneri* is chloramphenicol-resistant, whereas other indole-negative *Proteus* species are chloramphenicol-susceptible (see Table 4-18).[143] Documented human infections with *P. penneri* have been limited mainly to the urinary tract and wounds of the abdomen, groin, neck, and ankle.[143,184] In one report a patient with leukemia was described who developed a *P. penneri* bacteremia with a concomitant subcutaneous thigh abscess, demonstrating the invasive potential of this bacterium.[97] Microbiologists are advised to be suspicious of any *P. vulgaris* isolates that are indole-negative and hydrogen sulfide-negative because these may possibly be isolates of *P. penneri*.

TABLE 4-18

DIFFERENTIATION OF SPECIES WITHIN MEMBERS OF THE GENUS *PROTEUS*

TEST	P. MIRABILIS	P. MYXOFACIENS	P. PENNERI	P. VULGARIS	DNA GROUP 3	4	5	6
Ornithine	+	−	−	−	−	−	−	−
Indole	−	−	−	+	+	+	+	+
Esculin	−	−	−	+	−	−	−	−
Salicin	−	−	−	+	−	−	−	−
Lipase	+	+	V (35)	V (56)	−	+	+	+
Tartrate	V (87)	+	V (89)	V (89)	−	+	+	+
Rhamnose	−	−	−	−	−	+	−	−
DNase	V (50)	V (50)	V (12)	V (86)	−	+	+	V (55)
Acetate	V (20)	−	V (12)	V (33)	−	−	V (11)	V (18)

+, 90% or more strains positive; −, 90% or more strains negative; V, 11%–89% of strains positive; numbers in parentheses are percentage of strains giving positive reaction.
Data obtained from: O'Hara C et al. Poster Session C-253, Am Soc Microbiol, Las Vegas, 1994.

Genus *Morganella*. On the basis of genetic studies performed by Brenner and colleagues in 1978, the organism previously designated *Proteus morganii* was reassigned to the new genus *Morganella* as *M. morganii*.[36] Studies by Jensen and colleagues have shown that *M. morganii* can be further separated into three DNA relatedness groups and seven biogroups. DNA relatedness group 1 contains biogroups A through D. DNA relatedness group 2 contains biogroups E and F and two-thirds of biogroup G (termed biogroup G-2). DNA relatedness group 3 contains the remaining one-third of biogroup G (termed biogroup G-1). Because G-1 and G-2 are phenotypically indistinguishable, Jensen and associates have proposed dividing *M. morganii* into just two subspecies based on trehalose fermentation.[166] *M. morganii* that are unable to ferment trehalose are designated *M. morganii* subsp. *morganii*, and those that are able to utilize trehalose are designated *M. morganii* subsp. *sibonii*.

M. morganii is a cause of both urinary tract and wound infections and has been implicated as a cause of diarrhea. Serious infections reportedly caused by *M. morganii* include a case of meningitis in a patient with AIDS[203] and a case of meningitis and brain abscess in an 8-day-old infant.[308] As shown in Table 4-6, the pattern of Simmons citrate-negative, hydrogen sulfide-negative, and ornithine decarboxylase-positive is characteristic of this genus. The biochemical differentiation of the subspecies and biogroups is given in Table 4-19.

Genus *Providencia*. Five species of *Providencia* are now recognized: *P. alcalifaciens*, *P. stuartii*, *P. rettgeri*, and the newly described species *P. rustigianii*[144] and *P. heimbachae*.[219]

All species of the genus *Providencia* deaminate phenylalanine, but only *P. rettgeri* consistently hydrolyzes urea. The biochemical differences of the species are shown in Table 4-20.

Except for causing urinary tract infections, for which Penner has cited several nosocomial outbreaks,[238] infections with *Providencia* species are uncommon and are limited to isolated case reports. All species may be recovered from feces; however, only *P. alcalifaciens* may be associated with diarrheal illness, usually in children. Hickman-Brenner and associates[144] designated *P. rustigianii* to what was previously known as *P. alcalifaciens* biogroup 3. This organism has also been recovered from feces; however, its role in diarrheal disease is still questionable. A new species, *P. heimbachae*, has been reported from penguin feces and an aborted cow fetus but as yet has not been isolated from humans.[219]

TRIBE *YERSINIEAE*

Three species of *Pasteurella*, including the causative agent of human plague, *P. pestis*, were formally assigned to a new genus, *Yersinia*, in the eighth edition of *Bergey's Manual* and placed in the *Enterobacteriaceae*. The name for the genus *Yersinia* was derived from the French bacteriologist Alexander Yersin, who in 1894, first identified the organism now called *Y. pestis*. The key characteristics of the *Yersinieae* are given in Table 4-6.

Although *Yersinia* species qualify biochemically for inclusion in the *Enterobacteriaceae*, the cells appear small and coccobacillary in gram-stained smears and may be small and pinpoint on MacConkey agar, particularly for certain strains of *Y. pestis* and *Y. pseudotuberculosis*. Colonies tend to be pinpoint in size after 24 hours of incubation on sheep blood agar. Optimal growth occurs from 25° to 32°C. Gray-white, convex colonies measuring 1 to 2 mm in diameter may be observed after 48 hours, if incubation is continued at room temperature.

Genus *Yersinia*. *Yersinia* is the only genus in the *Yersinieae*. Three species, *Y. pestis*, *Y. pseudotuberculosis*,

---

TABLE 4-19

DIFFERENTIATION OF SPECIES WITHIN THE GENUS *MORGANELLA*

BIOCHEMICAL TEST	*M. MORGANII* SUBSP. *MORGANII* BIOGROUPS				*M. MORGANII* SUBSP. *SIBONII* BIOGROUPS		
	A	B	C	D	E	F	G
Trehalose	−	−	−	−	+	+	+
Lysine	−	+	−	+	+	d+	−
Ornithine	+	+	−	−	+	−	+
Tetracycline (% susceptible)	100*	100	14	100	0	0	21
Motility	+	−	d+	−	+	+	+

+, 90% or more strains positive; −, 90% or more strains negative; V, 11%–89% of strains positive; d+, 50%–89% positive within 48 h.
* Strains with a zone of ≥28 mm around tetracycline were considered susceptible (MIC correlate, ≤2 µg/mL), and those with a zone diameter ≤15 mm were considered tetracycline resistant (MIC correlate, ≥32 µg/mL).
Data obtained from: Jensen KT et al. Int J Syst Bacteriol 42:613–620, 1992.

TABLE 4-20

DIFFERENTIATION OF SPECIES WITHIN THE GENUS *PROVIDENCIA*

BIOCHEMICAL TEST	*P. ALCALIFACIENS*	*P. RUSTIGIANII*	*P. HEINBACHAE*	*P. STUARTII*	*P. RETTGERI*
Urea hydrolysis	−	−	−	V (30)	+
Citrate utilization	+	−	−	+	+
Fermentation of					
Inositol	−	−	V (46)	+	+
Adonitol	+	−	+	−	+
Arabitol	−	−	+	−	+
Trehalose	−	−	−	+	−
Galactose	−	+	+	+	+

+, 90% or more strains are positive; −, 90% or more strains are negative.
Data obtained from Table 4-24 and reference 219.

and *Y. enterocolitica*, were included when the genus was transferred to the *Enterobacteriaceae*. In 1980, three new species were proposed for strains that were former subgroups of *Y. enterocolitica*:[25,37,44,305] *Y. frederiksenii* is the name given to the rhamnose-positive biogroup;[305] *Y. intermedia* is the designation for those atypical strains that ferment rhamnose, raffinose, and melibiose;[37] and *Y. kristensenii* is the name for the previous sucrose-negative, trehalose-positive biogroup of *Y. enterocolitica*.[25] Presently, 11 species are included in the genus *Yersinia*; however, only three (*Y. pestis, Y. pseudotuerculosis*, and *Y. enterocolitica*) have been unquestionably shown to be human pathogens. One species, *Y. ruckeri*, a fish pathogen and not known to cause human infection, will probably be moved to a new genus.[100] The differential characteristics for these various species are included in Table 4-21.

INCIDENCE AND SOURCE OF *Y. PESTIS* INFECTION. *Y. pestis* is endemic in various rodents, including rats, ground squirrels, prairie dogs, mice, and rabbits. Two epidemic forms of disease occur: **urban plague**, which is maintained in the urban rat population, and **sylvatic plague**, which is endemic in the western United States and is carried by prairie dogs, mice, rabbits, and rats. The organism is transferred from rodent to rodent or from rodent to human by the rat flea. From 1944 through 1993, 362 cases of human plague were reported in the United States, with most cases occurring in the Southwest.[256] During each successive decade of this period, the number of states reporting cases increased from three during 1944 to 1953, to 13 during 1984 to 1993, indicating the spread of human plague eastward to areas where cases previously had not been reported.[60] Human cases have been concentrated in two principal regions: 1) a southwestern area that includes New Mexico, northeastern Arizona, southern Colorado, and southern Utah; and 2) a Pacific Coast region located in California, Oregon, and western Nevada.[58] For the 10-year period 1984 through 1994 an average of 11 cases per year of human plague have been reported in the United States.[63] Between August

and October 1994 a large outbreak of human plague occurred in India where a total of 5150 suspected pneumonic or bubonic plague cases and 53 deaths were reported.[61]

Our colleagues at the Colorado Department of Health have noted that blood cultures are positive in approximately 80% of patients with bubonic plague and 100% of patients with septicemic plague. Gram stains of bubo aspirates show gram-negative rods in about two-thirds of cases, and Wright-Giemsa staining of peripheral blood smears often reveals the characteristic bipolar staining typical of yersinia. The colonies are slow growing on ordinary media and are said to have the appearance of beaten cooper when viewed under the stereoscope. The reaction observed on TSI agar in 24 hours is similar to that seen with *Pasteurella* species (i.e., weak acid production on the slant with little or no change in the butt).

Streptomycin is the treatment of choice for persons suspected to have plague: alternatives include tetracycline, chloramphenicol, and sulfonamides.[20]

INFECTIONS CAUSED BY *Y. PSEUDOTUBERCULOSIS*. *Y. pseudotuberculosis* is also endemic in a wide variety of animals, including fowl, and is responsible for mesenteric lymphadenitis, particularly in children who manifest a clinical disease simulating appendicitis. A septicemic form of *Y. pseudotuberculosis* infection occurs rarely and has been described mainly in patients with an underlying disorder, such as hepatic cirrhosis, hemochromatosis, or diabetes, with mortality rates as high as 75% despite antibiotic treatment.[191] The major biochemical tests that differentiate *Y. pseudotuberculosis* from *Y. enterocolitica* are ornithine decarboxylase, sucrose, and sorbitol. *Y. pseudotuberculosis* is negative for all three, whereas *Y. enterocolitica* is positive.

INFECTIONS CAUSED BY *Y. ENTEROCOLITICA*. *Y. enterocolitica* is widely distributed in lakes and reservoirs, and epizootic outbreaks of diarrhea, lymphadenopathy, pneumonia, and spontaneous abortions occur in various animals.[35] It is the most common species of *Yersinia* recovered from clinical specimens. The portal

TABLE 4-21
DIFFERENTIATION OF SPECIES WITHIN THE GENUS *YERSINIA*

BIOCHEMICAL TEST	Y. PESTIS	Y. PSEUDOTUBERCULOSIS	Y. ENTEROCOLITICA	Y. FREDERIKSENII	Y. INTERMEDIA	Y. KRISTENSENII	Y. ALDOVAE	Y. BERCOVIERI	Y. MOLLARETII	Y. ROHDEI
Indole	−	−	V (50)	+	+	V (30)	−	−	−	−
Ornithine	−	−	+	+	+	+	V (40)	V (80)	V (80)	V (25)
Motility 25°–28°C	−	+	+	+	+	+	+	+	+	NA
Fermentation of										
Sucrose	−	−	+	+	+	−	V (20)	+	+	+
Rhamnose	−	V (70)	−	+	+	−	−	−	−	−
Cellobiose	−	−	V (75)	+	+	+	−	+	+	V (25)
Sorbitol	V (50)	−	+	+	+	+	V (60)	+	+	+
Melibiose	V (20)	V (70)	−	−	V (80)	−	−	−	−	V (50)

+, 90% or more strains are positive; −, 90% or more strains are negative; V, 11%–89% of strains are positive;
NA, results not available.
Data obtained from Table 4-24 and references 24 and 314. All tests were done at 25°C to 28°C.

CLINICAL CORRELATION BOX 4-9: HUMAN PLAGUE

Three clinical forms of human plague may occur:

1. *Bubonic:* Incubation period of 7 days or less after a bite from an infected flea. Patients have high fever and painful bubo (inflammatory swelling of lymph node) in the groin (most common), axilla, or neck. It is the mildest form of plague; however, the fatality rate in untreated cases is approximately 75%.

2. *Pneumonic:* Shorter incubation (2 to 3 days); patients initially have fever and malaise, then develop pulmonary signs within 1 day. The pneumonic form is usually secondary to the bubonic process, although it may also result from direct exposure to respiratory droplets from another pneumonic patient or from infected cats.[95,316] The fatality rate exceeds 90% if untreated. Persons suspected of having pneumonic plague should be placed in respiratory isolation and reported immediately to public health authorities so that rapid diagnosis, environmental assessments, and control measures can be initiated.

3. *Septicemic:* In this form, 100% of patients become septic with positive blood cultures. Patients develop a hemorrhagic rash and intravascular clotting caused by the presence of endotoxin.

of entry in humans is the oral digestive route, with infection occurring in the terminal ileum that anatomically is adjacent to the appendix. The organism adheres to and penetrates the ileum, causing terminal ileitis, lymphadenitis, and acute enterocolitis, with secondary manifestations of erythema nodosum, polyarthritis, and less commonly, septicemia,[80,114] and endocarditis.[124a] There are over 50 serogroups of *Y. enterocolitica*; however, only five, designated 0:1,2a,3; 0:3; 0:5,27; 0:8; and 0:9, are generally considered pathogenic for humans.[28]

ASSOCIATION OF *Y. ENTEROCOLITICA* WITH TRANSFUSION REACTIONS. *Y. enterocolitica* was recovered from a unit of donor blood submitted to the University of Illinois Hospital Microbiology Laboratory for culture following a transfusion reaction. The recipient of the blood developed shaking chills and a shocklike syndrome after transfusion of about 50 mL of the contaminated unit. Similar cases have also been reported elsewhere, illustrating this organism's ability to grow at cold temperatures.[29,56,159,291,300] Investigation of these cases has led to the conclusion that blood contamination resulted from asymptomatic *Y. enterocolitica* bacteremia in the blood donors at the time of donation. Arduino and colleagues[10] have demonstrated that *Y. enterocolitica*, when inoculated into units of packed erythrocytes and stored at 4°C, can proliferate and produce endotoxin after a lag phase of 2 to 3 weeks. It is clear from these reports that *Y. enterocolitica* should be looked for whenever transfusion-associated bacteremia or endotoxemia is suspected. To learn more, the reader is referred to the review article by Wagner and coauthors.[310]

ASSOCIATION OF *Y. ENTEROCOLITICA* WITH HOUSEHOLD PREPARATION OF CHITTERLINGS. In countries where *Y. enterocolitica* has become an important cause of diarrhea, 0:3 is the predominant serotype, and pigs appear to be the major reservoir for infection.[294] A review of clinical isolates of *Y. enterocolitica* submitted to the Yersinia Reference Laboratory of the CDC from 1970 to 1980 and from 1986 to 1988, showed a shift in the preponderant serotype of *Y. enterocolitica* in the United States from 0:8 to 0:3. This shift coincides with an outbreak of gastroenteritis caused by *Y. enterocolitica* serotype 0:3 in Atlanta from November 1988 to January 1989. The outbreak involved 15 patients (all black), of which 14 were infants (median age, 3 months). All developed a febrile, diarrheal illness that was strongly associated with the household preparation of chitterlings, which are the large intestines of pigs. Although none of the infants had direct contact with the raw chitterlings, in nearly all cases the persons caring for the infants gave a history of cleaning chitterlings.[186] *Y. enterocolitica* was cultured from unopened containers of chitterlings, from the case households as well as from containers of chitterlings purchased from local supermarkets. In 10 of the 12 exposed households, the chitterlings were prepared for a Thanksgiving, Christmas, or New Year's meal. A survey of a grocery store chain in Atlanta revealed that the sale of chitterlings are largely restricted to the period from October through January, and peak in November. Data from other surveys support the association between chitterling preparation during the Thanksgiving to Christmas holiday period and cases of *Y. enterocolitica* infection and suggest that routine screening for *Y. enterocolitica* is warranted at certain hospitals, especially for children younger than 1 year of age.[187,208]

IDENTIFICATION OF *Y. ENTEROCOLITICA*. *Y. enterocolitica* is more biochemically reactive at room temperature than at 37°C. It has been our experience at the University of Illinois Hospital that isolates of *Y. enterocolitica* generally do not give an acceptable identification when set up on the Vitek system or the API 20E at an incubation temperature of 37°C. However, API 20E strips incubated at room temperature do provide an acceptable identification. This finding has been confirmed in recent published reports.[9,284]

Although antisera that can actually be used to serotype strains of *Y. enterocolitica* are not readily available, Farmer and colleagues have described four simple tests that can be used to screen for pathogenic serotypes. These tests include the pyrazinamidase test, salicin fermentation–esculin hydrolysis, D-xylose fermentation, and Congo red–magnesium oxalate (CR-MOX) agar used to determine Congo red dye uptake and calcium-dependent growth at 36°C.[105]

OTHER *YERSINIA* SPECIES. *Y. frederiksenii* is most commonly recovered from fresh water, foods, and nonirrigated soil and has only infrequently been recovered from human specimens. This organism can be recovered from stool specimens using MacConkey or SS agars incubated at 25°C for 48 hours, and cold enrichment techniques are rarely required. *Y. frederiksenii* is believed to be part of the commensal flora and does not cause diarrhea. Farmer and coworkers[106] cite a few human isolates, referred to the CDC, that were obtained from wound and respiratory samples.

Y. intermedia may also be recovered by cold enrichment from human fecal specimens, but it is probably not related to intestinal disease. Bottone[34] reviewed the medical literature to 1976, noting 21 case histories of extraintestinal infections with these atypical rhamnose-positive species. Of these cases, eight were from conjunctivitis and three were from urinary tract infections. Bottone added three more cases, representing urinary tract, conjunctival, and auxiliary abscess infections.

Farmer and coworkers[106] cite six specimens received at the CDC from which *Y. kristensenii* was recovered: four from stools, one from blood, and one from urine. Its pathogenic role has not yet been determined.

Four additional new species of *Yersinia* have been described that are all biochemically similar to *Y. enterocolitica*. All are very rare human isolates. *Y. rohdei* has been isolated from dog feces, water, and human feces.[8] *Y. aldovae* (formerly *Y. enterocolitica*-like group X2) has been found in surface water, drinking water, and fish.[24] *Y. mollaretii* (formerly *Y. enterocolitica* biogroup 3A) has been isolated from human feces, drinking water, meat, and raw vegetables.[314] *Y. bercovieri* (formerly *Y. enterocolitica* biogroup 3B) has been reported from human feces, water, soil, and vegetables.[314]

Recovery of *Yersinia* From Clinical Specimens. The recovery of *Yersinia* species is low in most clinical laboratories. Most strains of *Y. enterocolitica* will grow on selective enteric agars and will appear as small, lactose-negative colonies on MacConkey and SS agars in 48 hours. In some laboratories, plates of MacConkey agar inoculated with stool specimens suspected of harboring *Yersinia* species are routinely incubated at room temperature. *Y. enterocolitica*, in particular, can best be recovered from stool specimens that are incubated at 25°C. Cold enrichment of highly contaminated specimens, such as feces, by incubating cultures at 4°C for 1 to 3 weeks in phosphate-buffered saline before subculture onto enteric media, also enhances the recovery of *Y. enterocolitica*.[233] Weissfeld and Sonnenwirth[315] reported that pretreatment of stool with 0.5% potassium hydroxide at a ratio of 1:2 for 2 minutes, followed by plating onto enteric agar, resulted in the recovery of the highest number of *Yersinia* isolates. The superiority of cefsulodin–irgasan–novobiocin (CIN) agar for recovery of *Y. enterocolitica* from stool suspensions containing 10² colony-forming units or fewer has been reported by Head and colleagues.[141] The use of cold enrichment methods and specialized culture media, such as CIN agar, for the recovery of *Yersinia* is usually not required because, in cases of enterocolitis, the organisms are usually found in relatively high concentrations. The use of EMB agar is not recommended because *Y. enterocolitica* is sucrose-positive and will appear as a coliform on this medium. A similar problem

may also be encountered with the use of TSI, which also contains sucrose.

TRIBE *ERWINIEAE*

The *Erwinieae* are primarily pathogens in plants and only saprophytic in humans. Farmer believes that the concept of *Erwinia* as a separate genus is not useful in clinical microbiology because "true *Erwinia* species" represented by *E. amylovora*, do not grow at 35° to 37°C and are inactive biochemically in the tests used to identify *Enterobacteriaceae*. "*Enterobacter agglomerans* group" is the name used by the CDC for a heterogeneous group of bacteria that have been reported as various species of *Erwinia* in the literature.[106]

MISCELLANEOUS NEW GENERA OF *ENTEROBACTERIACEAE*

Table 4-22 is a listing of the more recently described and less common species of *Enterobacteriaceae*. New genus and species designations have evolved from DNA hybridization studies and biochemical characterizations performed on atypical strains referred to the CDC and other reference laboratories for identification and classification. Many of these new genus names have been applied to bacterial strains that, at one time, were designated atypical enteric groups at the CDC. Several enteric groups remain unnamed but will probably achieve genus status in the future when a sufficient number of strains are gathered.

IDENTIFICATION CHARACTERISTICS OF NEWER *ENTEROBACTERIACEAE*

The key identifying characteristics of several of the new genera are listed in Table 4-23. Learning the new genera need not be overly difficult if one remembers that most of these bacteria represent atypical strains closely related to well-established groups. For example, the closely related genera *Buttiauxella*[113] and *Kluyvera*[108] will phenotypically present as "citrate-positive *E. coli*"; the specific characteristics by which they can be differentiated are included in Table 4-23. Bacteria belonging to *Cedecea*[110,135] resemble *Serratia* because they are lipase-positive and are resistant to cephalothin and colistin; however, unlike *Serratia*, they do not hydrolyze gelatin or DNA. *Ewingella*,[134] *Rahnella*,[157] and *Tatumella*[149] will initially be grouped with *Pantoea agglomerans* because they are lysine-, ornithine-, and arginine decarboxylase-negative. The genera *Yokenella*[183] and *Obesumbacterium*[250] are similar to *Hafnia alvei*; *Moellerella*[146] can be considered phenylalanine-negative, lactose-positive *Providencia*; and *Leminorella*[147] can be thought of as phenylalanine- and urease-negative *Proteus* species. By using this orientation, identification is made somewhat easier.

The reaction patterns of these new genera and species have been incorporated into the numerical code files of most computer-assisted identification systems. Thus, the names of these genera and species may appear in the computer-generated reports of many commercial systems. In these instances, it may be nec-
(text continues on page 221)

TABLE 4-22
New Genera and Species in the Family *Enterobacteriaceae*

New Designation	Previous Designation	Comments
Arsenophonus nasoniae	New species	Not isolated from humans. Cause of the sun-killer trait in the parasitic wasp, *Nasonia vitripennis*.
Budvidia aquatica	"HG group"	H_2S (+). Frequently found in drinking and surface water. Has been isolated from human feces.
Buttiauxella agrestis	"Group F"	Biochemically closest to *Kluyvera*. Key reactions are IMViC (−, +, −, +), LAO (−, −, +), sucrose (−). Isolated from water. No human isolates reported.
B. brennerae	New species	
B. ferragutiae	"Group F" Enteric group 63	
B. gaviniae	"Group F" Enteric group 64	
B. izardii		
B. noackiae		
B. warmboldiae		
Cedecea davisae	"Enteric group 15—Davis subgroup"	*Cedecea* resemble *Serratia* because they are lipase (+), and resistant to colistin and cephalothin, but unlike *Serratia* are gelatin and DNase (−). *C. davisae* is most common species. Sputum is the most common source.
C. lapagei		Isolated from human respiratory tract specimens.
C. neteri	"*Cedecea* sp. 4" "*Cedecea* sp. strain 002"	Isolated from blood cultures of patient with valvular heart disease.
Cedecea sp. 3	"*Cedecea* sp. strain 001"	Isolated from sputum and heart blood at autopsy.
Cedecea sp. 5	"*Cedecea* sp. strain 012"	Toe wound.
Cedecea sp. 6		
Ewingella americana	Enteric group 40	IMViC (−, +, +, +), LAO (−, −, −). Strains may formerly have been classified as *Enterobacter agglomerans*, but differ by being arabinose (−). Have been recovered from sputa, wounds, and blood cultures.
Kluyvera ascorbata	Enteric group 8	Looks like *E. coli* except malonate, esculin, and citrate (+). Dark purple pigment on non–blood-containing media. Most common source is sputum, followed by urine, stool, and blood.
K. cochleae		
K. cryocrescens	Enteric group 8	Similar to *K. ascorbata* except grows and ferments glucose at 5°C.
K. georgiana	Enteric group 8 *Kluyvera* sp. group 3	
Leclercia adecarboxylata	Enteric group 41 *Escherichia adecarboxylata* *Enterobacter agglomerans* HG XI	IMViC (+, +, −, −), LAO (−, −, −). Yellow pigmented. Resembles *E. coli* on MacConkey and EMB agars. Isolated from a variety of clinical specimens, food, water, and the environment.
Leminorella grimontii	Enteric group 57	H_2S (+), TDA (−), LAO (−, −, −), IMViC (−, +, −, +). Isolated from human feces and urine.
L. richardii	Enteric group 57	Same as *L. grimontii* except for IMViC (−, −, −, −).
Leminorella species 3	Enteric group 57	

(Continued)

TABLE 4-22 *(Continued)*
NEW GENERA AND SPECIES IN THE FAMILY *ENTEROBACTERIACEAE*

NEW DESIGNATION	PREVIOUS DESIGNATION	COMMENTS
Moellerella wisconsensis	Enteric group 46	Looks like *E. coli* on enteric media. IMViC ($-$, $+$, $-$, $+$), LAO ($-$, $-$, $-$), lactose and sucrose ($+$). Originally isolated from stool cultures in Wisconsin.
Obesumbacterium proteus biogroup 2	*Flavobacterium proteus*	No human isolates reported. Common brewery contaminant. Grows slowly and is fastidious when incubated at 36°C, making it difficult to identify.
Photorhabdus luminescens	*Xenorhabdus luminescens* DNA group 5	Bioluminescent and biochemically inactive. Optimum growth at 25°C. Consists of five DNA hybridization groups. All human clinical isolates belong to DNA group 5. Colonies are yellow pigmented, produce an unusual hemolytic reaction, and are negative for nitrate reduction. Isolates have been from human wounds and blood.
Pragia fontium		H$_2$S ($+$), biochemically similar to *Budvicia*. Most strains from drinking water in Czechoslovakia.
Rahnella aquatilis *Rahnella* species 2	Group H2	LAO ($-$, $-$, $-$), nonmotile at 36°C, but motile at 25°C, PAD (wk $+$), no yellow pigment. May have been identified as *E. agglomerans* in past. All isolates have been from water except one strain from human burn wound.
Tatumella ptyseos	Group EF-9	Pinpoint colonies, slow growing, relatively inert. Motile at 25°C, but nonmotile at 35°C. Flagella are polar, lateral, or subpolar, rather than peritrichous. Large zones of inhibition are formed around disks containing penicillin (10 U). PAD very slow (wk $+$). Isolated from human clinical specimens particularly sputum.
Trabulsiella guamensis	Enteric group 90	H$_2$S ($+$) and biochemically similar to *Salmonella*. IMViC ($-$, $+$, $-$, $+$), lysine ($+$), arginine (50% $+$), ornithine ($+$). Isolates have been from soil and human feces. No evidence that it causes diarrhea.
Xenorhabdus beddingii	*Xenorhabdus nematophilus* subsp. *beddingii*	
X. bovienii	*Xenorhabdus nematophilus* subsp. *bovienii*	
X. japonicus		
X. nematophilus	*Achromobacter nematophilus*	Has been isolated only from nematodes.
X. poinarii	*Xenorhabdus nematophilus* subsp. *poinarii*	
Yokenella regensburgei	*Koserella trabulsii* Enteric group 45 Atypical *Hafnia*	Biochemically similar to *Hafnia alvei*. Differs by being colistin-resistant and VP ($-$). Isolated from wounds, throat, sputum, feces, and water.
Enteric group 58		Clinical isolates have been from wounds and feces.
Enteric group 59		Like *Enterobacter agglomerans* except arginine-positive. Recovered from sputum, wounds, and food.
Enteric group 60		Biochemically inactive. Recovered from urine and sputum.
Enteric group 68		DNase ($+$), but otherwise biochemically different from *Serratia*. Clinical isolates have been from urines.
Enteric group 69		Yellow pigmented and biochemically similar to *Enterobacter sakazakii*. Strains have been recovered from a slaughterhouse. No human isolates have been reported.

IMViC, indole, methyl red, Voges-Proskauer–citrate; LAO, lysine–arginine–ornithine; MIO, motility–indole–ornithine; PAD, phenylalanine deaminase; HG, hybridization group; ($+$), ≥90% of strains positive; ($-$), ≥90% of strains negative; (v), variable.

TABLE 4-23

New Genera of *Enterobacteriacea*

GENUS	GENUS CHARACTERISTICS	SPECIES AND DIFFERENTIATING CHARACTERISTICS				
			B. AGRESTIS	*KLUYVERA ASCORBATA*	*KLUYVERA CRYOCRESCENS*	
Buttiauxella	Indole −	Indole	−	+	+	
	MR/VP +/−	Lysine	−	+	V (23)	
Ferragut 1981[113]	Citrate +	Ascorbate	−	+	−	
	Lysine −	Glucose (5°C)	+	−	+	
(Group F, Gavini 1976)	Arginine −	Sucrose	−	+	+	
	Ornithine +					
	Sucrose −					
			C. DAVISAE	*C. LAPAGEI*	*C. NETERI*	SPEC 3	SPEC 5
Cedecea	ONPG +					
	MRVP + V (50–80)					
Grimont 1981[135]	Citrate +	Ornithine	+	−	−	−	V (50)
	Esculin +	Sucrose	+	−	+	V (50)	+
(Enteric group 15)	Lipase (corn oil) +	Sorbitol	−	−	+		+
	DNAse −	Raffinose	−	−	−	+	+
	Gelatin −	Xylose	+	−	+	+	+
	Colistin R	Melibiose	−	−	−	+	+
	Cephalothin R	Malonate	+	+	+	−	−
			E. AMERICANA	*P. AGGLOMERANS*		
Ewingella	Indole −	Arabinose	−	+		
Grimont 1983[134]	MR/VP +/+	Xylose	V (15)	+		
	Citrate +	Yellow pigment	−	V (75)		
(Enteric group 40)	Lysine −					
	Arginine −					
	Ornithine −					
			K. ASCORBATA	*K. CRYOCRESCENS*		
Kluyvera	Indole +	Ascorbate	+	−		
	MR/VP +/−	Glucose (5°C)	−	+		
Farmer 1981[108]	Citrate +	Lysine	+	V (23)		
	Malonate +					
(Enteric group 8)	Esculin +					
			L. ADECARBOXYLATA	*E. COLI*	*P. AGGLOMERANS*	
Leclercia	Indole +	Lysine	−	+	−	
Tamura et al, 1986[292]	MR/VP +/−	Adonitol	+	−	−	
(*Escherichia adecarboxylata*	Citrate −	Malonate	+	−	V	
Enteric group 41)	Lysine −	Yellow pigment	+	−	+	
	Arginine −					
	Ornithine −					
			L. GRIMONTII	*L. RICHARDII*	*PROTEUS SPECIES*	
Leminorella	H₂S+	Methyl red	+	−	+	
Hickman-Brenner 1985[147]	Phenylalanine −	Citrate	+	−	−/V (15–65)	
(Enteric group 57)	Mannose −	Dulcitol	V (83)	−	−	
	Arabinose +	Phenylalanine	−	−	+	
	Xylose +	Urease	−	−	+	
	L/A/O −/−/−	Arabinose	+	+	−	
			M. WISCONSENSIS	*PROVIDENCIA SPECIES*		
Moellerella	Indole −	Phenylalanine	−	+		
Hickman-Brenner 1984[146]	MR/VP +/−	Lactose	+	−		
(Enteric group 46)	Citrate +	Sucrose	+	V (15–50)		
	Lysine −	ONPG	+			
	Arginine −	Tyrosine	−	+		
	Ornithine −					
	Phenylalanine −					
	Colistin R					

(Continued)

TABLE 4-23 *(Continued)*
NEW GENERA OF *ENTEROBACTERIACEA*

GENUS	GENUS CHARACTERISTICS	SPECIES AND DIFFERENTIATING CHARACTERISTICS		
			O. PROTEUS 2	*HAFNIA ALVEI*	*H. ALVEI 1*

GENUS	GENUS CHARACTERISTICS		*O. PROTEUS 2*	*HAFNIA ALVEI*	*H. ALVEI 1*
Obesumbacterium Priest 1973[250]	Indole − MR/VP V (15)/− Citrate − Lysine + Ornithine + Motility −	Mannitol Salicin Arabinose	− − −	+ V (13) +	V (55) V (55) −

GENUS	GENUS CHARACTERISTICS		*R. AQUATILIS*	*P. AGGLOMERANS*
Rahnella Izard et al., 1979[157] ("Group H2")	Indole − MR/VP +/+ Citrate + Urea − Phenylalanine + wk L/A/O −/−/− Motility − (36°C)/ + (25°C)	Motility (36°C) Phenylalanine Yellow pigment	− + −	+ V (20) V (75)

GENUS	GENUS CHARACTERISTICS		*T. PTYSEOS*	*P. AGGLOMERANS*
Tatumella Hollis, 1981[149] (Biogroup EF-9)	Indole − MR/VP −/−/ (+ Coblentz) L/A/O −/−/− Phenylalanine + wk Sucrose + Gelatin −	Mannitol Phenylalanine Motility (36°C) Penicillin	− + − S	+ V (20) + R

GENUS	GENUS CHARACTERISTICS		*T. GUAMENSIS*	*SALMONELLA SUBGROUP 4*	*SALMONELLA SUBGROUP 5*
Trabulsiella McWhorter et al., 1991[206] Enteric group 90	H₂S + Indole V (40) MR/VP +/− Citrate + Lysine + Arginine V (50) Ornithine + KCN +	Dulcitol Lactose ONPG Malonate Growth KCN Mucate Ferm. D-Sorbitol	− − + − + + +	− − − − + − +	+ − + − + V (85) +

GENUS	GENUS CHARACTERISTICS		*Y. REGENSBURGEI*	*H. ALVEI*
Yokenella Kosako et al., 1984[183] *Koserella trabulsii* Enteric group 45	Indole − MR/VP +/− Citrate + Lysine + Ornithine + Cellobiose + Melibiose +	VP Citrate Melibiose Colistin R	− + + +	+ − − −

essary to visually check the individual reactions for accuracy and assess additional characteristics using Table 4-23 or the expanded tables published by the CDC and reproduced here in Table 4-24. Careful correlation of the biochemical activity with the growth patterns and appearance of colonies on agar media is usually enough to make accurate identifications. It cannot be overemphasized that students and microbiologists must retain a fundamental orientation to the morphology, physiology, and biochemistry of bacteria if accurate identifications are to be made.

CLINICAL SIGNIFICANCE OF NEWER *ENTEROBACTERIACEAE*

The seemingly endless reclassification and changes in bacterial taxonomy and the frequent addition of new genera and species might be discouraging for microbiology students and instructors alike. However, Farmer and associates conducted a study of scores of unclassified biogroups submitted for identification at the CDC and have brought order out of disarray in a landmark report that summarizes all of the old and *(text continues on page 228)*

TABLE 4-24

BIOCHEMICAL REACTIONS OF THE NAMED SPECIES, BIOGROUPS, AND ENTERIC GROUPS OF THE FAMILY ENTEROBACTERIACEAE*

Organism	Indole Production	Methyl Red	Voges-Proskauer	Citrate (Simmons')	Hydrogen Sulfide (TSI)	Urea Hydrolysis	Phenylalanine Deaminase	Lysine Decarboxylase	Arginine Dihydrolase	Ornithine Decarboxylase	Motility (36°C)	Gelatin Hydrolysis (22°C)	Growth in KCN	Malonate Utilization	D-Glucose, Acid	D-Glucose, Gas	Lactose Fermentation	Sucrose Fermentation	D-Mannitol Fermentation	Dulcitol Fermentation	Salicin Fermentation
Budvicia																					
B. aquatica†	0	93	0	0	80	33	0	0	0	0	27	0	0	0	100	53	87	0	60	0	0
Buttiauxella																					
B. agrestis	0	100	0	100	0	0	0	0	0	100	100	0	80	60	100	100	100	0	100	0	100
Cedecea																					
C. davisae†	0	100	50	95	0	0	0	0	50	95	95	0	86	91	100	70	19	100	100	0	99
C. lapagei†	0	40	80	99	0	0	0	0	80	0	80	0	100	99	100	100	60	0	100	0	100
C. neteri†	0	100	50	100	0	0	0	0	100	0	100	0	65	100	100	100	35	100	100	0	100
Cedecea sp. 3†	0	100	50	100	0	0	0	0	100	0	100	0	100	0	100	100	0	50	100	0	100
Cedecea sp. 5†	0	100	50	100	0	0	0	0	50	50	100	0	100	0	100	100	0	100	100	0	100
Citrobacter																					
C. freundii†	33	100	0	78	78	44	0	0	67	0	89	0	89	11	100	89	78	89	100	11	0
C. diversus (koseri)†	99	100	0	99	0	75	0	0	80	99	95	0	0	95	100	98	50	40	99	40	15
C. amalonaticus†	100	100	0	95	5	85	0	0	85	95	95	0	99	1	100	97	35	9	100	1	30
C. farmeri†	100	100	0	10	0	59	0	0	85	100	97	0	93	0	100	96	15	100	100	2	9
C. youngae†	15	100	0	75	65	80	0	0	50	5	95	0	95	5	100	75	25	20	100	85	10
C. braakii†	33	100	0	87	60	47	0	0	67	93	87	0	100	0	100	93	80	7	100	33	0
C. werkmanii†	0	100	0	100	100	100	0	0	100	0	100	0	100	100	100	100	17	0	100	0	0
C. sedlakii†	83	100	0	83	0	100	0	0	100	100	100	0	100	100	100	100	100	0	100	100	17
Citrobacter sp. 9†	0	100	0	0	0	100	0	0	0	100	0	0	0	100	100	100	100	0	100	0	0
Citrobacter sp. 10†	0	100	0	33	67	0	0	0	33	0	67	0	100	100	100	100	67	33	100	0	0
Citrobacter sp. 11†	100	100	0	100	67	67	0	0	67	0	100	0	100	0	100	100	67	33	100	100	33
Edwardsiella																					
E. tarda†	99	100	0	1	100	0	0	100	0	100	98	0	0	0	100	100	0	0	0	0	0
E. tarda biogroup 1†	100	100	0	0	0	0	0	100	0	100	100	0	0	0	100	50	0	100	100	0	0
E. hoshinae†	50	100	0	0	0	0	0	100	0	95	100	0	0	100	100	35	0	100	100	0	50
E. ictaluri	0	0	0	0	0	0	0	100	0	65	0	0	0	0	100	50	0	0	0	0	0
Enterobacter																					
E. aerogenes†	0	5	98	95	0	2	0	98	0	98	97	0	98	95	100	100	95	100	100	5	100
E. cloacae†	0	5	100	100	0	65	0	0	97	96	95	0	98	75	100	100	93	97	100	15	75
E. agglomerans group†	20	50	70	50	0	20	20	0	0	0	85	2	35	65	100	20	40	75	100	15	65
E. gergoviae†	0	5	100	99	0	93	0	90	0	100	90	0	0	96	100	98	55	98	99	0	99
E. sakazakii†	11	5	100	99	0	1	50	0	99	91	96	0	99	18	100	98	99	100	100	5	99
E. taylorae†	0	5	100	100	0	1	0	0	94	99	99	0	98	100	100	100	10	0	100	0	92
E. amnigenus biogroup 1†	0	7	100	70	0	0	0	0	9	55	92	0	100	91	100	100	70	100	100	0	91
E. amnigenus biogroup 2†	0	65	100	100	0	0	0	0	35	100	100	0	100	100	100	100	35	0	100	0	100
E. asburiae†	0	100	2	100	0	60	0	0	21	95	0	0	97	3	100	95	75	100	100	0	100
E. hormaechei†	0	57	100	96	0	87	4	0	78	91	52	0	100	100	100	83	9	100	100	87	44
E. intermedium	0	100	100	65	0	0	0	0	0	89	89	0	65	100	100	100	100	65	100	100	100
E. cancerogenus	0	0	100	100	0	0	0	0	100	100	100	0	100	100	100	100	0	0	100	0	100
E. dissolvens	0	0	100	100	0	100	0	0	100	100	100	0	100	100	100	100	0	100	100	0	100
E. nimipressuralis	0	100	100	0	0	0	0	0	0	100	0	0	100	100	100	100	0	0	100	0	100
Escherichia-Shigella																					
E. coli†	98	99	0	1	1	1	0	90	17	65	95	0	3	0	100	95	95	50	98	60	40
E. coli, inactive†	80	95	0	1	1	1	0	40	3	20	5	0	1	0	100	5	25	15	93	40	10
Shigella, O groups A, B, C†	50	100	0	0	0	0	0	0	5	1	0	0	0	0	100	2	0	0	93	2	0

Adonitol Fermentation	myo-Inositol Fermentation	d-Sorbitol Fermentation	l-Arabinose Fermentation	Raffinose Fermentation	l-Rhamnose Fermentation	Maltose Fermentation	d-Xylose Fermentation	Trehalose Fermentation	Cellobiose Fermentation	α-Methyl-d-Glucoside Fermentation	Erythritol Fermentation	Esculin Hydrolysis	Melibiose Fermentation	d-Arabitol Fermentation	Glycerol Fermentation	Mucate Fermentation	Tartrate, Jordan's	Acetate Utilization	Lipase (Corn Oil)	DNase at 25°C	Nitrate → Nitrite	Oxidase, Kovacs	ONPG‡ Test	Yellow Pigment	d-Mannose Fermentation
0	0	0	80	0	100	0	93	0	0	0	0	0	0	27	0	20	27	0	0	0	100	0	93	0	0
0	0	0	100	100	100	100	100	100	100	0	0	100	100	0	60	100	60	0	0	0	100	0	100	0	100
0	0	0	0	10	0	100	100	100	100	5	0	45	0	100	0	0	0	91	0	0	100	0	90	0	100
0	0	0	0	0	0	100	0	100	100	0	0	100	0	100	0	0	60	100	0	0	100	0	99	0	100
0	0	100	0	0	0	100	100	100	100	0	0	100	0	100	0	0	0	100	0	0	100	0	100	0	100
0	0	0	0	100	0	100	100	100	100	50	0	100	100	100	0	0	50	100	0	0	100	0	100	0	100
0	0	100	0	100	0	100	100	100	100	0	0	100	100	100	0	0	50	50	0	0	100	0	100	0	100
0	0	100	100	44	100	100	89	100	44	11	0	0	100	0	100	100	100	44	0	0	100	0	89	0	100
99	0	99	99	0	99	100	100	100	99	40	0	1	0	98	99	95	90	75	0	0	100	0	99	0	100
0	0	99	99	5	100	99	99	100	100	2	0	5	0	0	60	96	96	86	0	0	99	0	97	0	100
0	0	98	100	100	100	100	100	100	100	75	0	0	100	0	65	100	93	80	0	0	100	0	100	0	100
0	5	100	100	10	100	95	100	100	100	45	0	5	10	5	90	100	100	65	0	0	85	0	90	0	100
0	0	100	100	7	100	100	100	100	100	73	0	0	80	0	87	100	93	53	0	0	100	0	80	0	100
0	0	100	100	0	100	100	100	100	100	0	0	0	0	0	100	100	100	100	0	0	100	0	100	0	100
0	0	100	100	0	100	100	100	100	100	0	0	17	100	0	83	100	100	83	0	0	100	0	100	0	100
0	0	100	100	0	100	100	100	100	100	0	0	0	0	0	0	100	100	0	0	0	100	0	100	0	100
0	0	100	100	0	100	100	100	100	100	67	0	0	67	0	67	67	100	0	0	0	100	0	67	0	100
0	0	100	100	33	100	100	100	100	100	0	0	0	33	0	100	100	100	33	0	0	100	0	100	0	100
0	0	0	9	0	0	100	0	0	0	0	0	0	0	0	30	0	25	0	0	0	100	0	0	0	100
0	0	0	100	0	0	100	0	0	0	0	0	0	0	0	0	0	0	0	0	0	100	0	0	0	100
0	0	0	13	0	0	100	0	100	0	0	0	0	0	0	65	0	0	0	0	0	100	0	0	0	100
0	0	0	0	0	0	100	0	0	0	0	0	0	0	0	0	0	0	0	0	0	100	0	0	0	100
98	95	100	100	96	99	99	100	100	100	95	0	98	99	100	98	90	95	50	0	0	100	0	100	0	95
25	15	95	100	97	92	100	99	100	99	85	0	30	90	15	40	75	30	75	0	0	99	0	99	0	100
7	15	30	95	30	85	89	93	97	55	7	0	60	50	50	30	40	25	30	0	0	85	0	90	75	98
0	0	0	99	97	99	100	99	100	99	2	0	97	97	97	100	2	97	93	0	0	99	0	97	0	100
0	75	0	100	99	100	100	100	100	96	0	0	100	100	0	15	1	1	96	0	0	99	0	100	98	100
0	0	1	100	0	100	99	100	100	100	1	0	90	0	0	1	75	0	35	0	0	100	0	100	0	100
0	0	9	100	100	100	100	100	100	100	55	0	91	100	0	0	35	9	0	0	0	100	0	91	0	100
0	0	100	100	0	100	100	100	100	100	100	0	95	0	0	100	0	0	0	0	0	100	0	100	0	100
0	0	100	100	70	5	100	97	100	100	95	0	95	0	0	11	21	30	87	0	0	100	0	100	0	100
0	0	0	100	0	100	100	96	100	100	83	0	0	0	0	4	96	13	74	0	0	100	0	95	0	100
0	0	100	100	100	100	100	100	100	100	100	0	100	100	0	100	100	100	0	0	0	100	0	100	0	100
0	0	0	100	0	100	100	100	100	100	0	0	100	0	0	100	0	33	0	0	0	100	0	100	0	100
0	0	100	100	0	100	100	100	100	100	100	0	100	100	0	0	100	0	0	0	0	100	0	100	0	100
5	1	94	99	50	80	95	95	98	2	0	0	35	75	5	75	95	95	90	0	0	100	0	95	0	98
3	1	75	85	15	65	80	70	90	2	0	0	5	40	5	65	30	85	40	0	0	98	0	45	0	97
0	0	30	60	50	5	30	2	80	0	0	0	0	50	0	10	0	30	2	0	0	100	0	2	0	100

TABLE 4-24 *(Continued)*

BIOCHEMICAL REACTIONS OF THE NAMED SPECIES, BIOGROUPS, AND ENTERIC GROUPS OF THE FAMILY *ENTEROBACTERIACEAE**

Organism	Indole Production	Methyl Red	Voges-Proskauer	Citrate (Simmons')	Hydrogen Sulfide (TSI)	Urea Hydrolysis	Phenylalanine Deaminase	Lysine Decarboxylase	Arginine Dihydrolase	Ornithine Decarboxylase	Motility (36°C)	Gelatin Hydrolysis (22°C)	Growth in KCN	Malonate Utilization	D-Glucose, Acid	D-Glucose, Gas	Lactose Fermentation	Sucrose Fermentation	D-Mannitol Fermentation	Dulcitol Fermentation	Salicin Fermentation
S. sonnei†	0	100	0	0	0	0	0	0	2	98	0	0	0	0	100	0	2	1	99	0	0
E. fergusonii†	98	100	0	17	0	0	0	95	5	100	93	0	0	35	100	95	0	0	98	60	65
E. hermannii†	99	100	0	1	0	0	0	6	0	100	99	0	94	0	100	97	45	45	100	19	40
E. vulneris†	0	100	0	0	0	0	0	85	30	0	100	0	15	85	100	97	15	8	100	0	30
E. blattae	0	100	0	50	0	0	0	100	0	100	0	0	0	100	100	100	0	0	0	0	0
Ewingella																					
E. americana†	0	84	95	95	0	0	0	0	0	0	60	0	5	0	100	0	70	0	100	0	80
Hafnia																					
H. alvei†	0	40	85	10	0	4	0	100	6	98	85	0	95	50	100	98	5	10	99	0	13
H. alvei biogroup 1	0	85	70	0	0	0	0	100	0	45	0	0	0	45	100	0	0	0	55	0	55
Klebsiella																					
K. pneumoniae†	0	10	98	98	0	95	0	98	0	0	0	0	98	93	100	97	98	99	99	30	99
K. oxytoca†	99	20	95	95	0	90	1	99	0	0	0	0	97	98	100	97	100	100	99	55	100
K. ornithinolytica†	100	96	70	100	0	100	0	100	0	100	0	0	100	100	100	100	100	100	100	10	100
K. planticola†	20	100	98	100	0	98	0	100	0	0	0	0	100	100	100	100	100	100	100	15	100
K. ozaenae†	0	98	0	30	0	10	0	40	6	3	0	0	88	3	100	50	30	20	100	2	97
K. rhinoscleromatis†	0	100	0	0	0	0	0	0	0	0	0	0	80	95	100	0	0	75	100	0	98
K. terrigena	0	60	100	40	0	0	0	100	0	20	0	0	100	100	100	80	100	100	100	20	100
Kluyvera																					
K. ascorbata	92	100	0	96	0	0	0	97	0	100	98	0	92	96	100	93	98	98	100	25	100
K. cryocrescens†	90	100	0	80	0	0	0	23	0	100	90	0	86	86	100	95	95	81	95	0	100
Leclercia																					
L. adecarboxylata†	100	100	0	0	0	48	0	0	0	0	79	0	97	93	100	97	93	66	100	86	100
Leminorella																					
L. grimontii†	0	100	0	100	100	0	0	0	0	0	0	0	0	0	100	33	0	0	0	83	0
L. richardii†	0	0	0	0	100	0	0	0	0	0	0	0	0	0	100	0	0	0	0	0	0
Moellerella																					
M. wisconsensis†	0	100	0	80	0	0	0	0	0	0	0	0	70	0	100	0	100	100	60	0	0
Morganella																					
M. morganii ss morganii†	95	95	0	0	20	95	95	1	0	95	95	0	98	1	99	90	1	0	0	0	0
M. morganii biogroup 1†	100	95	0	0	15	100	100	100	0	80	0	0	90	5	100	93	0	0	0	0	0
M. morganii ss Sibonii 1†	50	86	0	0	7	100	93	29	0	64	79	0	79	0	100	86	0	7	0	0	0
Obesumbacterium																					
O. proteus biogroup 2	0	15	0	0	0	0	0	100	0	100	0	0	0	0	100	0	0	0	0	0	0
Pragia																					
P. fontium	0	100	0	89	89	0	22	0	0	0	100	0	0	0	100	0	0	0	0	0	78
Proteus																					
P. mirabilis†	2	97	50	65	98	98	98	0	0	99	95	90	98	2	100	96	2	15	0	0	0
P. vulgaris†	98	95	0	15	95	95	99	0	0	0	95	91	99	0	100	85	2	97	0	0	50
P. penneri†	0	100	0	0	30	100	99	0	0	0	85	50	99	0	100	45	1	100	0	0	0
P. myxofaciens	0	100	100	50	0	100	100	0	0	0	100	100	100	0	100	100	0	100	0	0	0

Adonitol Fermentation	myo-Inositol Fermentation	D-Sorbitol Fermentation	L-Arabinose Fermentation	Raffinose Fermentation	L-Rhamnose Fermentation	Maltose Fermentation	D-Xylose Fermentation	Trehalose Fermentation	Cellobiose Fermentation	α-Methyl-D-Glucoside Fermentation	Erythritol Fermentation	Esculin Hydrolysis	Melibiose Fermentation	D-Arabitol Fermentation	Glycerol Fermentation	Mucate Fermentation	Tartrate, Jordan's	Acetate Utilization	Lipase (Corn Oil)	DNase at 25°C	Nitrate → Nitrite	Oxidase, Kovacs	ONPG Test	Yellow Pigment	D-Mannose Fermentation
0	0	2	95	3	75	90	2	100	5	0	0	0	25	0	15	10	90	0	0	0	100	0	90	0	100
98	0	0	98	0	92	96	96	96	96	0	0	46	0	100	20	0	96	96	0	0	100	0	83	0	100
0	0	0	100	40	97	100	100	100	97	0	0	40	0	8	3	97	35	78	0	0	100	0	98	98	100
0	0	1	100	99	93	100	100	100	100	25	0	20	100	0	25	78	2	30	0	0	100	0	100	50	100
0	0	0	100	0	100	100	100	75	0	0	0	0	0	0	100	50	50	0	0	0	100	0	0	0	100
0	0	0	0	0	23	16	13	99	10	0	0	50	0	99	24	0	35	10	0	0	97	0	85	0	99
0	0	0	95	2	97	100	98	95	15	0	0	7	0	0	95	0	70	15	0	0	100	0	90	0	100
0	0	0	0	0	0	0	0	70	0	0	0	0	0	0	0	0	30	0	0	0	100	0	30	0	100
90	95	99	99	99	99	98	99	99	98	90	0	99	99	98	97	90	95	75	0	0	99	0	99	0	99
99	98	99	98	100	100	100	100	100	100	98	2	100	99	98	99	93	98	90	0	0	100	0	100	1	100
100	95	100	100	100	100	100	100	100	100	100	0	100	100	100	100	96	100	95	0	0	100	0	100	0	100
100	100	92	100	100	100	100	100	100	100	100	0	100	100	100	100	100	100	62	0	0	100	0	100	1	100
97	55	65	98	90	55	95	95	98	92	70	0	80	97	95	65	25	50	2	0	0	80	0	80	0	100
100	95	100	100	90	96	100	100	100	100	0	0	30	100	100	50	0	50	0	0	0	100	0	0	0	100
100	80	100	100	100	100	100	100	100	100	100	0	100	100	100	100	100	100	20	0	0	100	0	100	0	100
0	0	40	100	98	100	100	99	100	100	98	0	99	99	0	40	90	35	50	0	0	100	0	100	0	100
0	0	45	100	100	100	100	91	100	100	95	0	100	100	0	5	81	19	86	0	0	100	0	100	0	100
93	0	0	100	66	100	100	100	100	100	0	0	100	100	96	3	93	83	28	0	0	100	0	100	37	100
0	0	0	100	0	0	0	83	0	0	0	0	0	0	0	17	100	100	0	0	0	100	0	0	0	0
0	0	0	100	0	0	0	100	0	0	0	0	0	0	0	0	50	100	0	0	0	100	0	0	0	0
100	0	0	0	100	0	30	0	0	0	0	0	0	100	75	10	0	30	10	0	0	90	0	90	0	100
0	0	0	0	0	0	0	0	0	0	0	0	0	0	0	5	0	95	0	0	0	90	0	10	0	98
0	0	0	0	0	0	0	0	0	0	0	0	0	0	0	100	0	100	0	0	0	90	0	20	0	100
0	0	0	0	0	0	0	0	100	0	0	0	0	0	0	7	7	100	0	0	0	100	0	0	0	100
0	0	0	0	0	15	50	15	85	0	0	0	0	0	0	0	0	15	0	0	0	100	0	0	0	85
0	0	0	0	0	0	0	0	0	0	0	0	78	0	0	0	0	0	0	0	0	100	0	0	0	0
0	0	0	0	1	1	0	98	98	1	0	0	0	0	0	70	0	87	20	92	50	95	0	0	0	0
0	0	0	0	1	5	97	95	30	0	60	1	50	0	0	60	0	80	25	80	80	98	0	1	0	0
0	0	0	0	1	0	100	100	55	0	80	0	0	0	0	55	0	85	5	45	40	90	0	1	0	0
0	0	0	0	0	0	100	0	100	0	100	0	0	0	0	100	0	100	0	100	50	100	0	0	0	0

(Continued)

TABLE 4-24   *(Continued)*
BIOCHEMICAL REACTIONS OF THE NAMED SPECIES, BIOGROUPS, AND ENTERIC GROUPS OF THE FAMILY *ENTEROBACTERIACEAE**

Organism	Indole Production	Methyl Red	Voges-Proskauer	Citrate (Simmons')	Hydrogen Sulfide (TSI)	Urea Hydrolysis	Phenylalanine Deaminase	Lysine Decarboxylase	Arginine Dihydrolase	Ornithine Decarboxylase	Motility (36°C)	Gelatin Hydrolysis (22°C)	Growth in KCN	Malonate Utilization	D-Glucose, Acid	D-Glucose, Gas	Lactose Fermentation	Sucrose Fermentation	D-Mannitol Fermentation	Dulcitol Fermentation	Salicin Fermentation
Providencia																					
P. rettgeri[†]	99	93	0	95	0	98	98	0	0	0	94	0	97	0	100	10	5	15	100	0	50
P. stuartii[†]	98	100	0	93	0	30	95	0	0	0	85	0	100	0	100	0	2	50	10	0	2
P. alcalifaciens[†]	99	99	0	98	0	0	98	0	0	1	96	0	100	0	100	85	0	15	2	0	1
P. rustigianii[†]	98	65	0	15	0	0	100	0	0	0	30	0	100	0	100	35	0	35	0	0	0
P. heimbachae	0	85	0	0	0	0	100	0	0	0	46	0	8	0	100	0	0	0	0	0	0
Rahnella																					
R. aquatilis[†]	0	88	100	94	0	0	95	0	0	0	6	0	0	100	100	98	100	100	100	88	100
Salmonella																					
DNA group 1 strains[†]																					
Most serotypes[†]	1	100	0	95	95	1	0	98	70	97	95	0	0	0	100	96	1	1	100	96	0
S. typhi[†]	0	100	0	0	97	0	0	98	3	0	97	0	0	0	100	0	1	0	100	0	0
S. choleraesuis[†]	0	100	0	25	50	0	0	95	55	100	95	0	0	0	100	95	0	0	98	0	0
S. paratyphi A[†]	0	100	0	0	10	0	0	0	15	95	95	0	0	0	100	99	0	0	100	90	0
S. gallinarum[†]	0	100	0	0	100	0	0	90	10	1	0	0	0	0	100	0	0	0	100	90	0
S. pullorum[†]	0	90	0	0	90	0	0	100	10	95	0	0	0	0	100	90	0	0	100	0	0
DNA group 2 strains[†]	2	100	0	100	100	0	0	100	90	100	98	2	0	95	100	100	1	1	100	90	5
DNA group 3a strains[†]	1	100	0	99	99	0	0	99	70	99	99	0	1	95	100	99	15	1	100	0	0
DNA group 3b strains[†]	2	100	0	98	99	0	0	99	70	99	99	0	1	95	100	99	85	5	100	1	0
DNA group 4 strains[†]	0	100	0	98	99	0	2	100	70	100	98	0	95	0	100	100	0	0	98	0	60
DNA group 5 strains[†]	0	100	0	94	100	0	0	100	94	100	100	0	100	0	100	94	0	0	100	94	0
DNA group 6 strains[†]	0	100	0	89	100	0	0	100	67	100	100	0	0	0	100	100	22	0	100	67	0
Serratia																					
S. marcescens[†]	1	20	98	98	0	15	0	99	0	99	97	90	95	3	100	55	2	99	99	0	95
S. marcescens biogroup 1[†]	0	100	60	30	0	0	0	55	4	65	17	30	70	0	100	0	4	100	96	0	92
S. liquefaciens group[†]	1	93	93	90	0	3	0	95	0	95	95	90	90	2	100	75	10	98	100	0	97
S. rubidaea[†]	0	20	100	95	0	2	0	55	0	0	85	90	25	94	100	30	100	99	100	0	99
S. odorifera biogroup 1[†]	60	100	50	100	0	5	0	100	0	100	100	95	60	0	100	0	70	100	100	0	98
S. odorifera biogroup 2[†]	50	60	100	97	0	0	0	94	0	100	100	94	19	0	100	13	97	0	97	0	45
S. plymuthica[†]	0	94	80	75	0	0	0	0	0	0	50	60	30	0	100	40	80	100	100	0	94
S. ficaria[†]	0	75	75	100	0	0	0	0	0	0	100	100	55	0	100	0	15	100	100	0	100
S. entomophila	0	20	100	100	0	0	0	0	0	0	100	100	100	0	100	0	0	100	100	0	100
"Serratia" fonticola[†]	0	100	9	91	0	13	0	100	0	97	91	0	70	88	100	79	97	21	100	91	100
Tatumella																					
T. ptyseos[†]	0	0	5	2	0	0	90	0	0	0	0	0	0	0	100	0	0	98	0	0	55
Trabulsiella																					
T. guamensis	40	100	0	88	100	0	0	100	50	100	100	0	100	0	100	100	0	0	100	0	13
Xenorhabdus																					
X. luminescens (25°C)	50	0	0	50	0	25	0	0	0	0	100	50	0	0	75	0	0	0	0	0	0
X. luminescens DNA group 5[†]	0	0	0	20	0	60	0	0	0	0	100	80	20	0	100	0	0	0	0	0	0
X. nematophilus (25°C)	40	0	0	0	0	0	0	0	0	0	100	80	0	0	80	0	0	0	0	0	0
Yersinia																					
Y. enterocolitica[†]	50	97	2	0	0	75	0	0	0	95	2	0	2	0	100	5	5	95	98	0	20
Y. frederikensii[†]	100	100	0	15	0	70	0	0	0	95	5	0	0	0	100	40	40	100	100	0	92
Y. intermedia[†]	100	100	5	5	0	80	0	0	0	100	5	0	10	5	100	18	35	100	100	0	100

Adonitol Fermentation	myo-Inositol Fermentation	D-Sorbitol Fermentation	L-Arabinose Fermentation	Raffinose Fermentation	L-Rhamnose Fermentation	Maltose Fermentation	D-Xylose Fermentation	Trehalose Fermentation	Cellobiose Fermentation	α-Methyl-D-Glucoside Fermentation	Erythritol Fermentation	Esculin Hydrolysis	Melibiose Fermentation	D-Arabitol Fermentation	Glycerol Fermentation	Mucate Fermentation	Tartrate, Jordan's	Acetate Utilization	Lipase (Corn Oil)	DNase at 25°C	Nitrate → Nitrite	Oxidase, Kovacs	ONPG Test	Yellow Pigment	D-Mannose Fermentation
100	90	1	0	5	70	2	10	0	3	2	75	35	5	100	60	0	95	60	0	0	100	0	5	0	100
5	95	1	1	7	0	1	7	98	5	0	0	0	0	0	50	0	90	75	0	10	100	0	10	0	100
98	1	1	1	1	0	1	1	2	0	0	0	0	0	0	15	0	90	40	0	0	100	0	1	0	100
0	0	0	0	0	0	0	0	0	0	0	0	0	0	0	5	0	50	25	0	0	100	0	0	0	100
92	46	0	0	0	100	54	8	0	0	0	0	0	0	92	0	0	69	0	0	0	100	0	0	0	100
0	0	94	100	94	94	94	94	100	100	0	0	100	100	0	13	30	6	6	0	0	100	0	100	0	100
0	35	95	99	2	95	97	97	99	5	2	0	5	95	0	5	90	90	90	0	2	100	0	2	0	100
0	0	99	2	0	0	97	82	100	0	0	0	0	100	0	20	0	100	0	0	0	100	0	0	0	100
0	0	90	0	1	100	95	98	0	0	0	1	0	45	1	0	0	85	1	0	0	98	0	0	0	95
0	0	95	100	0	100	95	0	100	5	0	0	0	95	0	10	0	0	0	0	0	100	0	0	0	100
0	0	1	80	10	10	90	70	50	10	0	1	0	0	0	0	50	100	0	0	10	100	0	0	0	100
0	0	10	100	1	100	5	90	90	5	0	0	0	0	0	0	0	0	0	0	0	100	0	0	0	100
0	5	100	100	0	100	100	100	100	0	8	0	15	8	0	25	96	50	95	0	0	100	0	15	0	95
0	0	99	99	1	99	98	100	99	1	1	0	1	95	1	10	90	5	90	0	2	100	0	100	0	100
0	0	99	99	1	99	98	100	99	1	1	0	1	95	1	10	30	20	75	0	2	100	0	92	0	100
5	0	100	100	0	98	100	100	100	50	0	0	0	100	5	0	0	65	70	0	0	100	0	0	0	100
0	0	100	94	0	88	100	100	100	0	0	0	0	94	0	0	88	0	100	0	0	100	0	94	0	100
0	0	0	100	0	100	100	100	100	0	0	0	0	89	0	33	89	100	89	0	0	100	0	44	0	100
40	75	99	0	2	0	96	7	99	5	0	1	95	0	0	95	0	75	50	98	98	98	0	95	0	99
30	30	92	0	0	0	70	0	100	4	0	0	96	0	0	92	0	50	4	75	82	83	0	75	0	100
5	60	95	98	85	15	98	100	100	5	5	0	97	75	0	95	0	75	40	85	85	100	0	93	0	100
99	20	1	100	99	1	99	99	100	94	1	0	94	99	85	20	0	70	80	99	99	100	0	100	0	100
50	100	100	100	100	95	100	100	100	100	0	0	95	100	0	40	5	100	60	35	100	100	0	100	0	100
55	100	100	100	7	94	100	100	100	100	0	7	40	96	0	50	0	100	65	65	100	100	0	100	0	100
0	50	65	100	94	0	94	94	100	88	70	0	81	93	0	50	0	100	55	70	100	100	0	70	0	100
0	55	100	100	70	35	100	100	100	100	8	0	100	40	100	0	0	17	40	77	100	92	8	100	0	100
0	0	0	0	0	0	100	40	100	0	0	0	100	0	60	0	0	100	80	20	100	100	0	100	0	100
100	30	100	100	100	76	97	85	100	6	91	0	100	98	100	88	0	58	15	0	0	100	0	100	0	100
0	0	0	0	11	0	0	9	93	0	0	0	0	25	0	7	0	0	0	0	0	0	98	0	0	100
0	0	100	100	0	100	100	100	100	100	0	0	40	0	0	0	100	50	88	0	0	100	0	100	0	100
0	0	0	0	0	0	25	0	0	0	0	0	0	0	0	0	0	0	50	0	0	0	0	0	50	100
0	0	0	0	0	0	0	0	0	0	0	0	0	0	0	0	0	0	60	20	0	0	0	0	60	100
0	0	0	0	0	0	0	0	0	0	0	0	0	0	0	0	0	0	60	0	0	20	20	0	60	80
0	30	99	98	5	1	75	70	98	75	0	0	25	1	40	90	0	85	15	55	5	98	0	95	0	100
0	20	100	100	30	99	100	100	100	100	0	0	85	0	100	85	5	55	15	55	0	100	0	100	0	100
0	15	100	100	45	100	100	100	100	96	77	0	100	80	45	60	6	88	15	12	0	94	0	90	0	100

(Continued)

TABLE 4-24 *(Continued)*
BIOCHEMICAL REACTIONS OF THE NAMED SPECIES, BIOGROUPS, AND ENTERIC GROUPS OF THE FAMILY ENTEROBACTERIACEAE*

ORGANISM	Indole Production	Methyl Red	Voges-Proskauer	Citrate (Simmons')	Hydrogen Sulfide (TSI)	Urea Hydrolysis	Phenylalanine Deaminase	Lysine Decarboxylase	Arginine Dihydrolase	Ornithine Decarboxylase	Motility (36°C)‖	Gelatin Hydrolysis (22°C)	Growth in KCN	Malonate Utilization	D-Glucose, Acid	D-Glucose, Gas	Lactose Fermentation	Sucrose Fermentation	D-Mannitol Fermentation	Dulcitol Fermentation	Salicin Fermentation
Y. kristensenii[†]	30	92	0	0	0	77	0	0	0	92	5	0	0	0	100	23	8	0	100	0	15
Y. rohdei[†]	0	62	0	0	0	62	0	0	0	25	0	0	0	0	100	0	0	100	100	0	0
Y. aldovae	0	80	0	0	0	60	0	0	0	40	0	0	0	0	100	0	0	20	80	0	0
Y. bercovieri[†]	0	100	0	0	0	60	0	0	0	80	0	0	0	0	100	0	20	100	100	0	20
Y. mollaretii[†]	0	100	0	0	0	20	0	0	0	80	0	0	0	0	100	0	40	100	100	0	20
Y. pestis[†]	0	80	0	0	0	5	0	0	0	0	0	0	0	0	100	0	0	0	97	0	70
Y. pseudotuberculosis[†]	0	100	0	0	0	95	0	0	0	0	0	0	0	0	100	0	0	0	100	0	25
"Yersinia" ruckeri[†]	0	97	10	0	0	0	0	50	5	100	0	30	15	0	100	5	0	0	100	0	0
Yokenella (Koserella)																					
Y. regensburgei[†]	0	100	0	92	0	0	0	100	8	100	100	0	92	0	100	100	0	0	100	0	8
Enteric group 58[†]	0	100	0	85	0	70	0	100	0	85	100	0	100	85	100	85	30	0	100	85	100
Enteric group 59[†]	10	100	0	100	0	0	30	0	60	0	100	0	80	90	100	100	80	0	100	0	100
Enteric group 60[†]	0	100	0	0	0	50	0	0	0	100	75	0	0	100	100	100	0	0	50	0	0
Enteric group 63[†]	0	100	0	0	0	0	0	100	0	100	65	0	0	0	100	100	0	0	100	0	100
Enteric group 64[†]	0	100	0	50	0	0	0	0	50	0	100	0	100	100	100	50	100	0	100	0	100
Enteric group 68[†]	0	100	50	0	0	0	0	0	0	0	0	0	100	0	100	0	0	100	100	0	50
Enteric group 69[†]	0	0	100	100	0	0	0	0	100	100	100	0	100	100	100	100	100	25	100	100	100

* Each number gives the percentage of positive reactions after 2 days of incubation at 36°C (unless a different temperature is indicated).
† Known to occur in clinical specimens.

new genera of *Enterobacteriaceae* known as of January 1985.[106] As these investigators point out, up to 95% of all *Enterobacteriaceae* recovered in clinical laboratories are *Escherichia coli*, *Klebsiella pneumoniae*, and *Proteus mirabilis*; over 99% of the isolates belong to only 23 species, leaving less than 1% as the incidence of recovery for the several newly designated species. Thus, the bacteria listed in Table 4-22 are rarely encountered in most clinical laboratories; however, as Dr. Farmer has also stated, there are at least three reasons why these new species of *Enterobacteriaceae* are important to clinical microbiologists: 1) Some species cause serious human infections; 2) others occur in clinical specimens, but their causative role in disease is uncertain; and 3) many are biochemically similar to well-established species and thus can cause problems in identification. The clinical significance of the newer species that have been recovered from human clinical specimens is summarized as follows:

The genus *Buttiauxella* now contains seven species (see Table 4-22) that occur frequently and abundantly in the intestines of snails, slugs, and other mollusks.[218] A few strain have been isolated from unpolluted soil and drinking water, surface water, sewage, soil, and

fecal samples, but have not been isolated from primary sterile clinical specimens.[218]

Cedecea has been isolated from respiratory specimens,[16] blood,[110,197,239] a scrotal abscess,[15] cutaneous ulcer,[138] and lung tissue.[79] In most cases, however, an etiologic role for *Cedecea* in these infections was not proved.

Ewingella americana was described in 1983 and named in honor of the American bacteriologist, William Ewing.[134] The original strains were from human clinical specimens, including sputum, blood, throat, toe and thumb wounds, urine, and stool.[106,134] *E. americana* has been implicated in bacteremia,[86,244] an outbreak of bacteremia,[243] and an outbreak of pseudobacteremia.[205] It has also been associated with wound colonization[23] and conjunctivitis.[142]

The genus *Kluyvera* presently contains four species (see Table 4-22).[218] The original isolates of *Kluyvera* species were from human clinical specimens and the environment. The most common human sources have been sputum, followed by urine, stool, throat, and blood.[108] Environmental sources noted have been sewage, soil, kitchen food, water, milk, and a hospital sink.[108] There are only a few reports of serious infec-

Adonitol Fermentation	myo-Inositol Fermentation	D-Sorbitol Fermentation	L-Arabinose Fermentation	Raffinose Fermentation	L-Rhamnose Fermentation	Maltose Fermentation	D-Xylose Fermentation	Trehalose Fermentation	Cellobiose Fermentation	α-Methyl-D-Glucoside Fermentation	Erythritol Fermentation	Esculin Hydrolysis	Melibiose Fermentation	D-Arabitol Fermentation	Glycerol Fermentation	Mucate Fermentation	Tartrate, Jordan's	Acetate Utilization	Lipase (Corn Oil)	DNase at 25°C	Nitrate → Nitrite	Oxidase, Kovacs	ONPG‡ Test	Yellow Pigment	D-Mannose Fermentation
0	15	100	77	0	0	100	85	100	100	0	0	0	0	45	70	0	40	18	0	0	100	0	70	0	100
0	0	100	100	62	0	0	38	100	25	0	0	0	50	0	38	0	100	8	0	0	88	0	50	0	100
0	0	60	60	0	0	0	40	80	0	0	0	0	0	0	0	0	100	0	0	0	100	0	0	0	100
0	0	100	100	0	0	100	100	100	100	0	0	20	0	0	0	0	100	0	0	0	100	0	80	0	100
0	0	100	100	0	0	60	60	100	100	0	0	0	0	0	20	0	100	0	0	0	100	0	20	0	100
0	0	50	100	0	1	80	90	100	0	0	0	50	20	0	50	0	0	0	0	0	85	0	50	0	100
0	0	0	50	15	70	95	100	100	0	0	0	95	70	0	50	0	50	0	0	0	95	0	70	0	100
0	0	50	5	5	0	95	0	95	5	0	0	0	0	0	30	0	30	0	30	0	75	0	50	0	100
0	0	0	100	25	100	100	100	100	100	0	0	67	92	0	0	0	0	25	0	0	100	0	100	0	100
0	0	100	100	0	100	100	100	100	100	55	0	0	0	0	30	0	60	45	0	0	100	0	100	0	100
0	0	0	100	0	100	100	100	100	100	10	0	100	0	10	10	60	50	50	0	0	100	0	100	25	100
0	0	0	25	0	75	0	0	100	0	0	0	0	0	0	75	0	75	0	0	0	100	0	100	0	100
0	0	100	100	0	100	100	100	100	100	65	0	100	0	0	65	0	0	0	0	0	100	0	100	0	100
100	0	0	100	0	100	100	100	100	0	0	0	100	0	100	0	100	50	0	0	0	100	0	100	0	100
0	0	0	0	0	0	50	0	100	0	0	0	100	0	0	0	50	0	0	0	100	100	0	0	0	100
0	0	100	100	100	100	100	100	100	100	0	100	100	0	0	100	0	25	0	0	0	100	0	100	0	100

tions with *Kluyvera* species that involved the urinary tract,[302] the gallbladder,[297] the gastrointestinal tract,[3,101] and soft tissue of the forearm following a cut from a garbage can.[193] In addition, cases of catheter-related bacteremia[321] and mediastinitis and bacteremia following open-heart surgery[285] have been reported.

The clinical significance of *Leclercia adecarboxylata* is uncertain, but human isolates from blood, sputum, urine, stool, and wounds have been reported.[231,264,292] At the University of Illinois Hospital, *L. adecarboxylata* was found colonizing the endotrachea of a neonate and in a cystoscopic urine specimen from a patient in renal failure. In both cases, the organism was isolated along with other pathogen species; therefore, an etiologic role could not be established.

Leminorella has been isolated primarily from stool and urine.[147] It appears as lactose-negative colonies on primary plating media and gives an alkaline slant and a weak acid reaction with H₂S in the butt of TSI after 48 hours. Similar to *Proteus*, *Leminorella* species are H₂S-positive, D-mannose-negative, and tyrosine-positive, but unlike *Proteus*, they are urea- and phenylalanine-negative and L-arabinose-positive. So far, *Leminorella* has not been shown to cause human disease.

Moellerella wisconsensis was originally found in human stool samples, mainly from the state of Wisconsin.[146] It has also been isolated from water and animals and from clinical specimens other than stool, such as the gallbladder[223,320] and a bronchial aspirate.[311] On MacConkey agar, colonies appear bright red with precipitated bile around them; thus, they are indistinguishable from *E. coli* colonies.[146] Its pathogenic role in humans remains uncertain.

The natural habitat of *Rahnella aquatilis*, as its name implies, is water, and most isolates in the original CDC collection were from water, except two isolates from humans (one from a burn wound and the other from the bronchial washing of a HIV patient).[139] Of the few case reports of *R. aquatilis* in the literature, most describe infections in immunocompromised patients. In addition to the CDC isolates, others have reported the isolation of this organism from sputum (in a patient with chronic lymphocytic leukemia and emphysema),[73] the urinary tract (in a renal transplant patient),[5] and from a surgical wound possibly due to a nosocomial source.[198] Three cases of septicemia have been reported: one in a patient with acute lymphocytic leukemia,[131] a second in a pediatric patient after bone marrow transplantation,[152] and a third in an HIV-infected intravenous drug abuser.[121]

Of the original strains of *Tatumella ptyseos* studied at the CDC, 30 were from sputum, six from throat cultures, three from blood, and one each from a tracheal aspirate, a feeding tube, a pharynx, a stool, and urine.[149] There are three striking differences between *T. ptyseos* and other members of the *Enterobacteriaceae*: 1) strains produce a large zone of inhibition around penicillin; 2) it has a tendency to die on some laboratory media, such as blood agar, within 7 days; and 3) usually only one flagellum (either polar, subpolar, or lateral) is observed per cell.[149] The clinical importance of this organism is unknown.

Trabulsiella guamensis, which was formerly known as enteric group 90, is H₂S-positive and biochemically resembles *Salmonella* subgroups 4 and 5.[206] Strains have been isolated from vacuum cleaner dust, soil, and human feces; however, there is no evidence that it causes diarrhea. Its main interest to clinical microbiologist may be its possible misidentification as a strain of *Salmonella* (see Table 4-23).

Yokenella regensburgei was originally identified as NIH biogroup 9 by the National Institutes of Health in Japan[183] and later found to be identical to "*Koserella trabulsii*" (enteric group 45) named by workers from the Centers for Disease Control.[145,182] Since the name *Y. regensburgei* has priority over "*K trabulsii*" by virtue of prior publication, the use of the later name has been discontinued. In the original reports, *Y. regensburgei* had been recovered from the intestinal tracts of insects and well water, as well as human clinical specimens, including wounds of the limbs, the upper respiratory tract, urine, feces, and knee fluid.[145,183] More recently, Abbott and Janda have reported the recovery of *Y. regensburgei* from the blood of a patient with a transient bacteremia and from a knee wound of a patient with a diagnosis of septic knee.[1] The organism most closely resembles *H. alvei* from which it must be differentiated (see Table 4-23).

QUICK SCREENING METHODS FOR RAPID IDENTIFICATION

Escherichia coli, the bacterial isolate most frequently recovered in clinical laboratories, is often presumptively identified if an oxidase-negative, lactose-fermenting, dry colony on MacConkey agar gives a positive spot indole reaction (when tested on a colony growing on noninhibitory media, such as blood agar), particularly if the organism has been recovered in pure culture.[18] The spot indole test is also used in many laboratories for rapid speciation of swarming *Proteus* from primary isolation plates.[19] A rapid (2-minute) spot urease test has been described by Qadri and colleagues.[251] This test might be used to separate possible stool pathogens that require further biochemical testing from the nonpathogenic *Proteus–Providencia–Morganella* group. Taylor and Achanzar have reported using the catalase test (with 3% H₂O₂) as an aid in the identification of *Enter-obacteriaceae*.[296] They observed vigorous catalase reactions with *Serratia, Proteus,* and *Providencia*; moderate reactions with *Salmonella, Enterobacter, Klebsiella,* and rare *Escherichia*; and weak reactions with *Shigella* and most *Escherichia*. They report using the rapid catalase test for screening suspicious colonies on enteric media that mimic stool pathogens. Colonies of *Serratia, Proteus, Providencia,* or *Pseudomonas* are quickly eliminated by vigorous catalase reactions, in contrast with salmonellae, which give weak to moderate reactions, or shigellae, which are negative and, therefore, are flagged for further workup. Chester and Moskowitz[70] have reported on the catalase activity of many of the newer members of the *Enterobacteriaceae* and further advocate the use of catalase activity as a rapid supplemental test. Mulczyk and Szewczuk[217] suggested that the test for L-pyrrolidonyl peptidase (PYR) is of great value in differentiating between *Salmonella* and *Citrobacter freundii* complex strains. Other authors have also noted the value of using the PYR test for separating *Salmonella* and *E. coli* strains (both negative from *Citrobacter* spp. (PYR +).[67,155] Clearly, any of these approaches has validity in an era of cost-containment and the desire to receive test results quickly.

Yong and associates[325] have published a series of flow charts for the rapid (within 4 hours) screening of isolates of pathogenic members of the *Enterobacteriaceae*, based on the reactions derived from a series of rapid microbiochemical substrates to which is added a heavy inoculum of the bacterial unknown. In an evaluation of 7984 individual tests, a 99.8% agreement between conventional results and those derived from their system was demonstrated. They were able to identify accurately *Salmonella, Shigella, Edwardsiella, Aeromonas, Plesiomonas, Vibrio,* and *Yersinia* isolates from stool specimens. This method can be used in conjunction with the single-tube screening medium advocated by Thompson and Borczyk,[298] in which the detection of motility, β-galactosidase, and phenylalanine deaminase and the production of hydrogen sulfide and indole permit the accurate screening of enteric organisms recovered from stool specimens.

COMMERCIAL SCREENING KITS

Several commercial companies have marketed rapid detection kits for the identification of *E. coli*: E.COLI SCREEN (Carr-Scarborough, Stone Mountain GA); Lyfo-Kwik OMI (MicroBioLogics, St. Cloud MN); MUG Disk (Remel Inc., Lenexa KS); MUG Plus (Difco Laboratories, Detroit MI); and BactiCard *E. coli* (Remel, Lenexa KS).

These test systems are based on the finding that the majority of strains of *E. coli* are rapidly indole, ONPG (*o*-nitrophenyl-β-D-galactopyranoside), and MUG (4-methylumbelliferyl-β-D-glucuronide) positive.[91,174,301] The hydrolysis of MUG releases 4-methylumbelliferone, which is highly fluorescent when viewed under long-wave ultraviolet light. An interesting use of the MUG test is to screen isolates of *E. coli* for the detection of serotype 0157:H7 strains, which are the Shiga-like, toxin-producing strains associated with hemorrhagic colitis. This specific serotype is both sorbitol- and MUG-negative.

Also available is the RapID SS/u System (Innovative Diagnostic Systems, Inc., Atlanta GA), consisting of a set of 12 single-substrate chromogenic tests selected to identify rapidly the bacteria most commonly encountered in urinary tract infections (*E. coli, Proteus* species, *Klebsiella* species, *Serratia* species, *Enterobacter* species, *Pseudomonas* species, coagulase-negative staphylococci, enterococci, and others). Answers are available in 30 minutes to 2 hours, depending on the system used and the biochemical activity of the strain being tested. Another system called OMP and NGP Wee-Tabs (KEY Scientific Products, Round Rock TX) consists of two substrate tablets that together provide eight enzymatic tests, which, combined with urease, will identify approximately 95% of the *Enterobacteriaceae*. The tablets are rehydrated in a bacterial suspension, with results available in 2 to 4 hours.

COMMERCIAL SCREENING AGAR MEDIA

A new development in rapid screening methods is the coupled use of chromogenic agars and rapid spot tests for identification of bacteria directly from the surface of agar media. In 1984, Trepeta and Edberg demonstrated that the incorporation of an enzyme substrate into an agar media could facilitate organism identification.[301] Using *p*-nitrophenyl-β-D-glucuronide as a substrate, they were able to detect β-glucuronidase-producing bacteria using a fluorescent detection method. When used in combination with an indole spot test, they were able to demonstrate a rapid and presumptive identification of clinical isolates of *E. coli* with very high specificity.[301]

CPS ID2 (bioMerieux Vitek, Inc., Hazelwood MO) is a ready-to-use plated medium that contains chromogenic substrates for β-glucuronidase and β-glucosidase for use in the enumeration and presumptive identification of microorganisms from the urinary tract. The medium also permits direct testing for indole, tryptophane-deaminase, oxidase, and catalase activity. β-D-Glucuronidase activity (red colonies) and a positive indole reaction are used to identify *E.coli*. β-D-Glucosidase activity (blue colonies) is used to identify enterococci and enterobacteria belonging to the genera *Klebsiella, Enterobacter*, and *Serratia*. Colorless colonies that turn brown after the addition the R2 reagent (iron perchloride) are identified as *Proteus* species. An evaluation of this medium performed by Mazoyer and associates showed that CPS ID2 medium enables the presumptive identification of *E. coli*, enterococci, *Proteus* species, and bacteria belonging to the *Klebsiella, Enterobacter, Serratia* group with a specificity ranging from 98% to 100%. Sensitivity varied from 70% to 97% for polymicrobial cultures, and from 97% to 100% for monomicrobial cultures.[204]

The Rainbow UTI System (Biolog, Inc., Hayward CA) consists of Rainbow Agar CP-8 and a series of easy-to-use confirmatory spot tests that can be performed in seconds either on paper strips or directly on the agar medium. The Rainbow CP-8 agar is an opaque, chalky white agar containing nonfat milk, which provides an excellent background contrast for the various chromogenic reactions. Eight common pathogens form distinctive colored colonies on the agar: namely, *E. coli* (red), *K. pneumoniae* (blue), *P. mirabilis* (orange), *P. aeruginosa* (green), *E. faecalis* (white), *S. aureus* (gold), *K. oxytoca* (yellow), and *S. choleraesuis* (brown). Preliminary evaluations have shown that this medium provides a rapid, reliable identification of the most common urinary tract pathogens.[31,280]

The use of these screening systems is consistent with the current trend toward issuing results as soon as possible at lower cost. More expensive definitive test sets need not be set up if identifications can be made with the screening procedure.

CLASSIC IDENTIFICATION SYSTEMS

Systems for the identification and naming of microorganisms are either computer-assisted or manual. Before discussing the derivation and applications of numeric coding systems, two manual bacterial identification schemes that are still in use will be reviewed: 1) the cross-hatch or checkerboard matrix, and 2) the branching or dichotomous flow charts.

CHECKERBOARD MATRIX

Table 4-24 is a reproduction of the comprehensive identification table formulated by Farmer and colleagues for use at the CDC to identify all named species, biogroups, and unnamed enteric groups of the *Enterobacteriaceae*. This table is a classic example of the checkerboard matrix and demonstrates its advantages and disadvantages. The matrix is large, with 47 biochemical characteristics for 28 genera, 121 species, biogroups, and unnamed enteric groups. The numbers in the intersecting squares represent the percentage of strains that are positive or reactive against the various biochemical tests (listed in the vertical columns). A reaction is generally considered positive if 90% or more of the strains are reactive, negative if 10% or fewer of the strains fail to produce a result, and variable if 11% to 89% of reactions are positive. The ability to determine both the positive and negative reactions for the various characteristics being measured in this type of identification system results in a high degree of diagnostic accuracy. The major disadvantage of the checkerboard matrix is the tedium involved in matching point-by-point the various reactions against those derived from the test media and constructing the patterns that best match with a specific genus, species, or biogroup.

BRANCHING FLOW DIAGRAMS

During the 1960s, flow diagrams were designed to reduce the tedium of reading the checkerboard matrices and to facilitate the likely bacterial identification by tracing a series of positive and negative branch points in a dichotomous algorithm (Fig. 4-6). With the advent of automated instruments and packaged identification systems that rely on computer-assisted analyses of the various reactions of the characteristics being measured, flow diagrams are now used less frequently in clinical laboratories. One problem with flow diagrams has been the potential for inaccuracy if the reaction at a given branch point is either aberrant (i.e., not typical for the species), misinterpreted, or the result of the reactions of a mixed culture. Many flow diagrams are constructed to repeat some species names at several junctures to accommodate reactions that may be less than 100% or in the variable category. However, this built-in protection does not always apply for reactions that are misinterpreted, either by an automated instrument's detection system or by the human eye.

A modification of this approach is being used in many microbiology laboratories for the preliminary screening of commonly encountered bacterial species that are associated with specific infectious disease syndromes. Perry and colleagues[240] have presented a simple scheme for the rapid identification of multiple antibiotic-resistant members of the Enterobacteriaceae isolated from urine samples. Their scheme is based on only six conventional tests: lysine and ornithine decarboxylases, glucose and cellobiose fermentation, and indole and urease production, for which they have coined the acronym LOGIC identification system (see Fig. 4-6). In their initial report, the LOGIC system correctly identified 93% of the 300 strains tested.[240] Pattyn and associates[237] have published a modification of this system by adding two additional tests: oxidase and lactose fermentation. They report that the use of their system reduces the price of testing bacterial isolates by a factor of at least 20 and limits the frequency of use of more extensive identification systems to about 3%. They further note that an advantage of such a system, in contrast with automated or semiautomated systems, is that it requires thought, reasoning, and knowledge on the part of the student or microbiologist, who are not reduced to passive observers—a point well taken.

A system using a KIA and LIA tube (supplemented with tryptophan for detection of indole) is used in the microbiology laboratory at the University of Illinois Hospital for the screening of enteric pathogens from stool (Fig. 4-7). Definitive biochemical and serologic procedures are performed only on those isolates with presumptive positive reactions.

COMPUTER-AIDED SCHEMES

BioBASE (BioBASE, Inc, Boston MA) is a computer-enhanced numeric identification software package for use on personal computers (PC) that allows the user to create, update, and manipulate unlimited numbers of microbial databases. Conventional biochemical reactions on an unknown isolate are entered into the appropriate database whereby the program compares the unknown profile with that of any taxon in the database. To reach an identification verdict, BioBASE calculates identification scores, modal scores, and similarity indices of each taxon and compares them with the unknown's input data. The top-scoring microorganisms are then analyzed and weighted for a decision on identification, ranging from unacceptable to excellent. Miller and Alachi evaluated this program and report it to be user friendly, rapid and accurate, and state that it would be of value to any laboratory that uses conventional biochemicals.[210]

NUMERIC CODING SYSTEMS

The identification of the Enterobacteriaceae and many other families and groups of bacteria has been facilitated by the use of automated and packaged kit systems, by which organisms are identified with computer-assisted numeric codes. A numeric code is a system by which the several identifying characteristics of bacteria are translated into a sequence of numbers that represent one or more bacterial species. The fact that the identification of microorganisms is based on a series of positive and negative biochemical reactions makes computer programming easy because computer logic is also constructed on a sequence of positive and negative entries, using a binary numeric system. In binary logic there are only two numbers: "0" (or off) and "1" (or on). As can quickly be surmised, the identification characteristics of microorganisms can be easily translated into binary numbers by assigning a "1" to all positive reactions and a "0" to all negative reactions. This approach can be illustrated using the sequence of characteristics in the API 20E strip (bioMerieux Vitek, St. Louis) as a point of reference and converting the positive and negative reactions into binary numbers (Table 4-25).

If the binary numbers shown in Table 4-25 are read from top to bottom and rearranged horizontally, the following 21-digit binary number is derived:

101010000011111011100

Although computers are constructed to receive 1/0 bits of data from which to calculate meaningful results, the human mind cannot efficiently manipulate binary logic; therefore, binary codes must be converted into simpler mathematic systems to become usable. Conversion of the two-digit (binary) system into an eight-digit (octal) system serves this purpose. To understand the conversion of binary into octal numbers, visualize a series of three light bulbs. By turning different lights on and off, a total of eight combinations is possible, each of which can be represented by one of eight numbers ranging from 0 to 7. If all lights are off (−), the combination − − − is equivalent to octal 0. If only the left bulb is turned on (+), the combination + − − is equivalent to octal 1. Octal 2 is represented by the binary pattern − + −, and octal 3 by the pattern + + −. The octal equivalents of the eight combinations of a three-digit binary number are shown in Table 4-26.

To illustrate how binary numbers longer than three digits can be converted into their octal equivalents, use

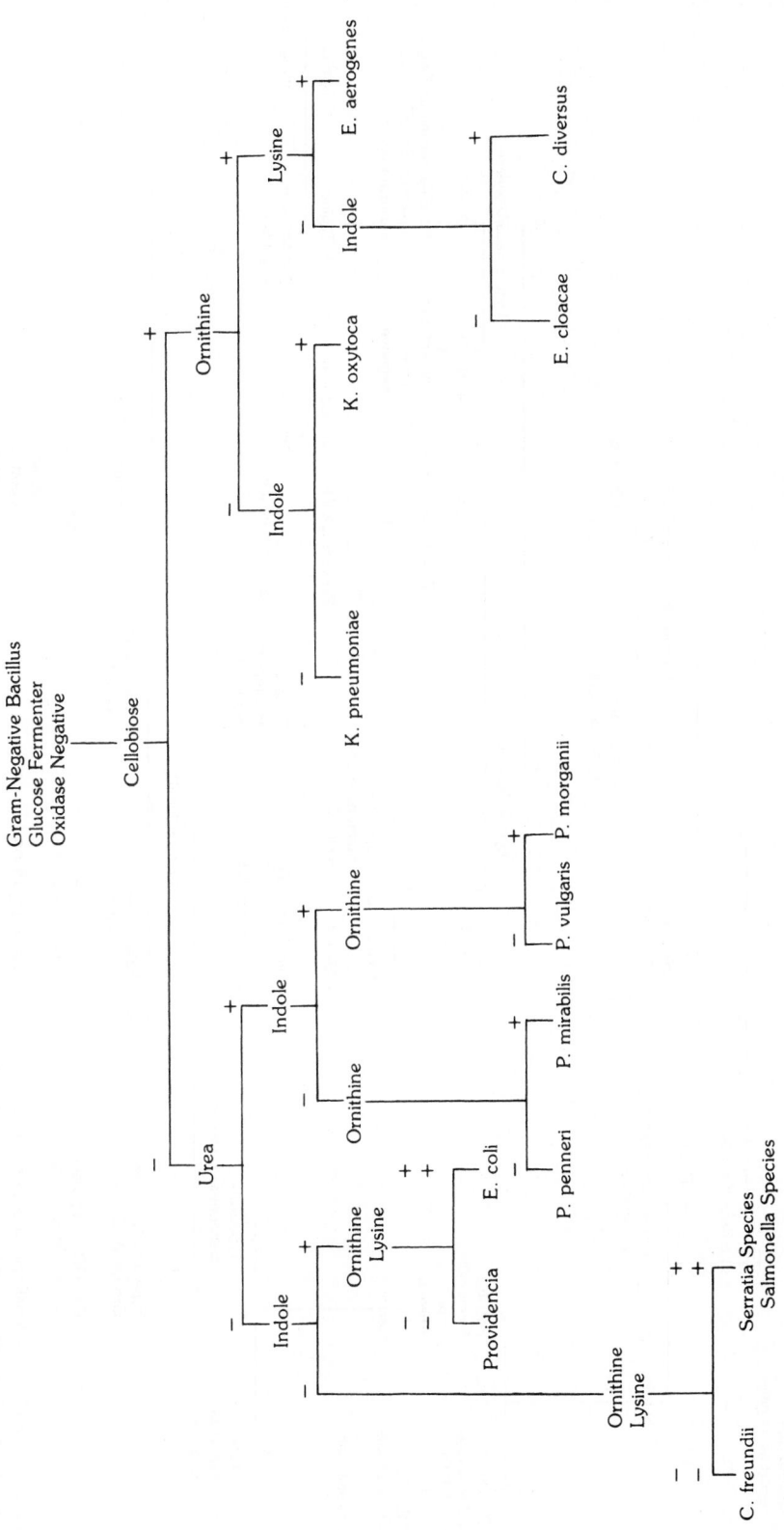

Figure 4-6

Flow diagram depicting the LOGIC system for biochemical identification of antibiotic-resistant *Enterobacteriaceae* isolates from urine. (Modified from Perry JD, Ford M, Hjersing N, Gloud FK: Rapid conventional scheme for biochemical identification of antibiotic-resistant *Enterobacteriaceae* isolates from urine. J Clin Pathol 41:1010–1012, 1988)

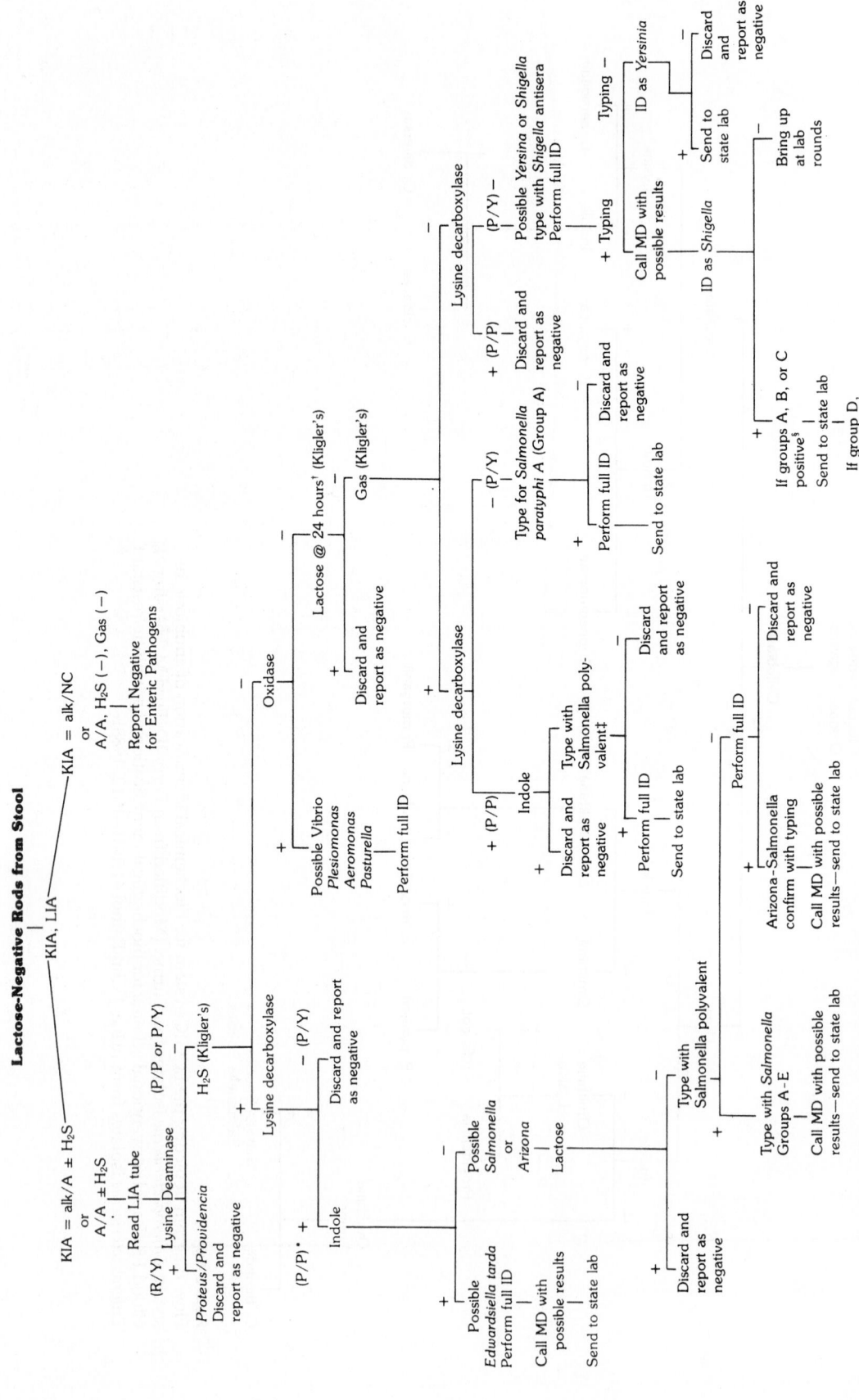

Figure 4-7
Schematic for screening of enteric pathogens from stool using KIA and modified LIA.

*Some strains of *C. freundii* will give a false-positive lysing decarboxylase (P/P) on LIA.
†Cultures of *Shigella sonnei* ferment lactose and sucrose slowly.
‡Some strains of *Salmonella* are H₂S negative.
§Certain biotypes of *Shigella flexneri* produce gas.

TABLE 4-25
BINARY CONVERSION OF REACTIONS OF UNKNOWN ORGANISM ON API 20-E STRIP

CHARACTERISTIC	REACTION	BINARY CONVERSION
ONPG	+	1
Arginine	−	0
Lysine	+	1
Ornithine	−	0
Citrate	+	1
Hydrogen sulfide	−	0
Urease	−	0
Triptophan deaminase	−	0
Indole	−	0
Voges-Proskauer	+	1
Gelatin	+	1
Glucose	+	1
Mannitol	+	1
Inositol	+	1
Sorbitol	+	1
Rhamnose	−	0
Sucrose	+	1
Melibiose	+	1
Amygdalin	+	1
Arabinose	−	0
Oxidase	−	0

the binary number that was derived from the API 20E reactions:

101010000111111011100

Beginning to the right, because binary numbers are read from right to left, divide the binary numbers into subsets of three:

101 010 000 111 111 011 100

Now convert each three-digit subset into its octal equivalent using the formula given in Table 4-26.

101 010 000 111 111 011 100
 5   2   0   7   7   6   1

The number 5207761 is far easier to remember and simpler to enter into a computer than the binary number 101010000111111011100.

A simpler way of remembering how to convert each binary triplet into its corresponding octal equivalent is to assign the following values (again reading from right to left): A value of 4 to a positive reaction for the first test in each triplet, a value of 2 to a positive reaction for the second test in each triplet, a value of 1 to a positive reaction for the third test in each triplet, and a value of 0 to any negative reactions (see Table 4-26).

These octal derivatives are known as **biotype numbers**, that is, a numeric representative of a series of phenotypic characteristics expressed by and unique to a particular bacterial species. It is important that everyone using biotype numbers, particularly those who are teaching students, understand that each number in the octal system is representative of three biochemical characteristics and that the number itself represents a pattern of positive and negative reactions. There is great danger that modern microbiologists consider biotype numbers as magic figures that can be read from charts or put into computers to derive automatic organism identification, thus losing sight not only of the biochemical reactions that they represent, but also of the biochemical principles on which the discipline of microbiology is based.

READING THE OCTAL NUMBER IN NUMERICAL CODE REGISTERS

All manufacturers who have packaged identification kits on the market, and the designers of many manual systems as well, publish numeric code registers in which hundreds of biotype numbers are matched with one or more bacterial species that are unique for that number. For example, for the biotype number 5207761, derived from the API 20E set of reactions used in the previous example, the following species are listed in the API 20E Profile Index: *Serratia marcescens*: acceptable identification; *S. marcescens*: 1/243; and *S. rubidaea*: 1/2,859.

The message in the API Profile Index for biotype number 5207761 for *S. marcescens* "Acceptable Identification" indicates that *S. marcescens* can be reported. This assessment is based on a computer-derived calculation of the percentage likelihood that *S. marcescens* is the correct identification compared with all the other organisms entered into the database.

THE ESTIMATED FREQUENCY OF OCCURRENCE

The frequency figures listed with each individual species name (in the previous example, 1/243 for *S. marcescens*) indicate the number of strains selected at random that would have a biotype number similar to the strain being studied. In other words, if one were to randomly test 243 *S. marcescens*, there is a chance of 1 in 243 that you will encounter this exact biochemical pattern. Whereas, if you tested 2859 randomly selected *S. rubidaea*, you would have a 1 in 2859 chance of finding a strain of this exact biotype. This figure does not directly indicate the percentage likelihood that one of these species is the correct name, so the user cannot determine from this statistic how viable one of the choices might be.

TABLE 4-26
OCTAL CONVERSION OF BINARY CODE

BINARY	CONVERSION FORMULA	OCTAL
− − −	0 + 0 + 0 =	0
+ − −	1 + 0 + 0 =	1
− + −	0 + 2 + 0 =	2
+ + −	1 + 2 + 0 =	3
− − +	0 + 0 + 4 =	4
+ − +	1 + 0 + 4 =	5
− + +	0 + 2 + 4 =	6
+ + +	1 + 2 + 4 =	7

THE CALCULATION OF LIKELIHOOD

The identification of an unknown organism with a given biotype number is based on the calculation of percentage likelihood between the unknown biotype number and each taxon stored in the memory of the computer. Code registers that list percentage likelihood figures are more useful for everyday decision making in the laboratory. Any identification that has a likelihood of 90% or greater can be reported, those that are near 90% may be easily identified with one or two additional tests, and those with very low likelihood percentages can probably be discounted. The use of messages such as "excellent identification," "acceptable identification," and "very good identification" in the API system implies that there is a percentage likelihood of 90% or greater. However, when the message describes an identification as "questionable" or "doubtful" and the percentage likelihood is not given, the user is unable to make any assessments concerning the likelihood that an unknown represents a certain species. For students and microbiologists who may be trying to understand this concept for the first time, an example for calculating percentage likelihood and frequency of occurrence is given in Table 4-27.

RESOLVING DISCREPANCIES

It must be pointed out that all answers derived from computer-based identification systems, whether or not they represent 90% or more confidence, must be interpreted in conjunction with other information available on the unknown organism—the colonial morphology, reactions on various isolation media, cellular morphology on Gram stain, results of presumptive biochemical reactions, antibiotic susceptibility patterns, and clinical setting.

When discrepancies occur, visualization of the tubes, reaction chambers, or microcupules, in which the reactions have taken place, may be necessary. In many instances, the visual interpretation of certain reactions may differ from that detected by instruments. When recalculated, the new biotype number may indicate an alternative bacterial identification that is much more in keeping with preliminary and supplemental observations.

Also, any given species may have several biotype numbers because one or more individual reactions may be variable. Consequently, designating bacterial species by biotype numbers may have epidemiologic value in recognizing the emergence of clusters of similar isolates in a given practice setting. For example, recovery of many *E. coli* from a given environment or series of cultures may be of limited value; however, knowing that all of the organisms have the same biotype number may be invaluable. In this way, it may be possible to trace the agents causing hospital nosocomial outbreaks or community-wide epidemics to a common source. Biotype analysis may also lead to a better understanding of the relation between virulence of bacterial variants and the presence or absence of certain biochemical characteristics.

PACKAGED KIT IDENTIFICATION SYSTEMS

The concept of combining a series of differential media or substrates in a single package, selected to aid in identifying members of a group of bacteria, is a logical development. In fact, the availability of packaged identification systems evolved naturally, almost as a practical necessity. The microorganisms currently known to cause infectious diseases are not only legion, but also are often fastidious and require a large battery of biochemical tests for identification. It is beyond the capability of many laboratories to maintain the diversity of conventional media required. The compact construction (requiring little storage space), easily visible chemical reactions, long shelf life, and standardized quality control provided by the manufacturers of these kits make them very convenient for use in microbiology laboratories. They are especially useful in low-volume laboratories, where there may not be the time nor technical expertise to make many of these identifications and where quality control is more difficult to maintain.

OVERVIEW OF PACKAGED SYSTEMS

It has now become almost standard practice in many clinical laboratories to use one or more available packaged systems for the identification of certain groups of microorganisms. Many of the systems have been in use for a decade or more, a sufficient time for most microbiologists to overcome the initial reluctance to give up the time-honored conventional methods. Improvements in kit design, the inclusion of alternative or additional substrates, and changes in reagents to improve the specificity and sensitivity of biochemical reactions, all have served to correct inaccuracies in the initial systems. Extensive testing in diagnostic and research laboratories has demonstrated a 95% or greater agreement between most packaged identification systems and conventional methods in the identification of microorganisms. Thus, packaged systems have found wide acceptance in clinical laboratories for the following reasons:

1. Their accuracy has proved to be comparable with that of conventional identification systems. Evaluations of several systems have been made at the CDC by Smith and associates.[288] In all evaluations, two criteria were used for measuring the performance of a product: 1) a comparison of each test in the product with its conventional counterpart and 2) the accuracy of identification made using the product.
2. Several of the systems have a long shelf life—6 months to 1 year—so that outdating of media, a problem particularly with conventional systems, is minimized.
3. The systems require only a minimum of space for storage and incubation.
4. Some of the systems are as easy or easier to use than conventional methods. Inoculation is simple, reactions are generally clear-cut within 24 hours, and

TABLE 4-27
CALCULATION OF FREQUENCY OF OCCURRENCE AND PERCENTAGE LIKELIHOOD

The identification of an unknown profile is based on the calculation of likelihood between the unknown profile and each species of organism stored in the memory of the computer. To test your understanding of frequency of occurrence and percentage likelihood, work through the following example. For ease in explaining the calculations, this example is based on only four biochemical tests and three species.

Step 1. An unknown organism gives the following profile:

	IND	MR	VP	CIT
Unknown	+	−	+	−

Step 2. Known biochemical reactions of three species of *Enterobacteriaceae* for the four tests (shown as percentage of positive reactions).

	IND	MR	VP	CIT
Serratia marcescens	1	20	98	98
Enterobacter agglomerans	20	50	70	50
Klebsiella oxytoca	99	20	95	95

Step 3. Frequencies of occurrence of observed reactions (+ − + −) for each species. *Note:* When a test result of the unknown is positive (IND and VP in this example), the probability of the positive reaction of the test listed in the database is used for the calculation. When the test result of the unknown is negative (MR and CIT), the probability of the negative reaction is 1 minus the probability of positive reactions.

	IND	MR	VP	CIT
Serratia marcescens	.01	.80	.98	.02
Enterobacter agglomerans	.20	.50	.70	.50
Klebsiella oxytoca	.99	.80	.95	.05

Step 4. Calculation of frequencies of occurrence of observed profile (+ − + −) for each species. The frequency of occurrence is calculated by multiplying together all the frequencies of occurrence of the reactions.

> *Serratia marcescens*
> $= .01 \times .80 \times .98 \times .02 = .0001568$
> *Enterobacter agglomerans*
> $= .20 \times .50 \times .70 \times .50 = .0350000$
> *Klebsiella oxytoca*
> $= .99 \times .80 \times .95 \times .05 = \underline{.0376200}$
> $.0727768$

Step 5. Identification percentages. Each frequency is divided by the sum of all the frequencies, then multiplied by 100 to give the %ID. The sum of the percentages of identification is equal to 100.

> *Serratia marcescens*
> $\%ID = (.001568/.0727768) \times 100 = 0.21\%$
> *Enterobacter agglomerans*
> $\%ID = (.0350000/.0727768) \times 100 = 48.1\%$
> *Klebsiella oxytoca*
> $\%ID = (.0376200/.0727768) \times 100 = 51.7\%$

Step 6. Order of likelihood

1.	*Klebsiella oxytoca*	%ID = 51.7
2.	*Enterobacter agglomerans*	%ID = 48.1
3.	*Serratia marcescens*	%ID = 0.21

What is the likelihood that *Klebsiella oxytoca* is the correct answer among the three species in the database?
(*Answer:* From step 5, the answer is 51.7%; however, there is a 48.1% likelihood that the unknown organism is *Enterobacter agglomerans*; therefore, additional tests would have to be set up to correctly identify this unknown organism.)
How frequently will *Klebsiella oxytoca* give this particular reaction profile?
(*Answer:* From step 4, 3.8% of the time; in other words, not very often.)

---

the availability of computer-assisted file registers makes final identification easy and accurate.

Whether to use one of the packaged identification systems and which one to select is largely a matter of personal preference. The ease of inoculation, the ability to select only the characteristics to be measured, the manipulation required in adding reagents after incubation, and the availability of interpretive charts or computed databases are the main items that potential users should consider before selecting a system. If strict attention is paid to the instructions provided by the manufacturer, essentially the same degree of accuracy and reliability of performance can be attained, with only minor differences in the sensitivity of individual tests.

SPECIFIC IDENTIFICATION SYSTEMS

API 20E

The API 20E identification system (bioMerieux Vitek, Inc., Hazelwood MO) has become the reference method against which the accuracy of other systems is compared. The 21 characteristics that can be determined by the API 20E system make it among the largest test sets of the packaged kits. The system identifies a high percentage of bacterial species within 24 hours, without the need to determine additional physiologic characteristics (Color Plate 4-5A). This system is among the most frequently used in clinical laboratories and has a large database that includes common and atypical strains. The API Profile Index, which can be used manually or with computer assistance, provides the frequency probability of several strains that must be considered for each biotype number. Thus, the accuracy of identification of the members of the *Enterobacteriaceae* is maximized. Castillo and Bruckner found that the API 20E system correctly identified 97.7% of 339 clinical and stock isolates.[49] The system is somewhat cumbersome to inoculate—a problem, however, that is overcome quickly with practice. After inoculation, the strips must be handled carefully so that the bacterial suspensions do not spill and contaminate the surrounding environment. Practice is required to interpret occasional borderline reactions, which can affect the biotype number and the final identification. Occasionally, biotype numbers may not appear in the profile register; however, the manufacturer maintains a telephone number for consultation. The design of the system, the operating procedures, substrates included, and evaluation studies are shown in Table 4-28.

API RAPID 20E SYSTEM

The API Rapid 20E (RE) 4-hour system is similar to the API 20E strip, with a few important modifications.[173] The RE cupules are smaller, and the substrates are not buffered, resulting in more rapid reactions. Because the cupule volumes are small and the inoculum is prepared to the density of only a 0.5 McFarland barium sulfate standard, only one or two well-isolated colonies are required to set up the strip.

In a comparative study of 441 clinical isolates of the *Enterobacteriaceae*, Overman and associates[232] found that the RE strip gave identifications identical with those derived from the 20E system 94% of the time, with only 3% misidentifications (correct but low-sensitivity an-

swers were given for the remaining 3%). Thus, these authors conclude that the RE strip, having the advantage of providing definitive answers within 4 hours, is an acceptable alternative for the identification of the commonly encountered members of the *Enterobacteriaceae*.

BBL CRYSTAL ENTERIC/NONFERMENTER ID SYSTEM

The BBL Crystal E/NF identification system (Becton Dickinson Microbiology Systems, Cockeysville MD) is a miniaturized identification method employing modified conventional and chromogenic substrates. It is intended for the identification of clinically significant aerobic gram-negative bacteria that belong to the family *Enterobacteriaceae*, as well as some of the more frequently isolated glucose-fermenting and nonfermenting gram-negative bacilli of human origin. The E/NF kit comprises 1) BBL Crystal E/NF lids, 2) BBL Crystal bases, and 3) BBL Crystal Enteric/Stool ID inoculum fluid tubes (see Color Plate 4-5*B*). The BBL Crystal lid contains 30 dehydrated substrates on tips of plastic prongs. The BBL Crystal base has 30 reaction wells. Test inoculum is prepared with the BBL Crystal Enteric/Stool ID inoculum fluid and is used to fill all 30 wells in the BBL Crystal base. When the lid is aligned with the base and snapped in place, the test inoculum rehydrates the dried substrates and initiates test reactions. The tests used in the Crystal system include tests for fermentation, oxidation, degradation, and hydrolysis of various substrates, including chromogen-linked substrates.

Following inoculation, panels are incubated upside-down in a non-CO_2 incubator with 40% to 60% humidity for 18 to 20 hours at 35° to 37°C. After incu-

---

TABLE 4-28
CONSTRUCTION, USE, AND EVALUATION OF THE API 20E IDENTIFICATION SYSTEM

FUNCTIONAL DESIGN	OPERATING PROCEDURE	SUBSTRATES INCLUDED	EVALUATION STUDIES
The system consists of a plastic strip with 20 miniaturized cupules containing dehydrated substrates and a plastic incubation chamber with a loosely fitting lid (see Color Plate 4-5*A*). Each cupule has a small hole at the top through which the bacterial suspension can be inoculated with a pipette. Bacterial action on the substrates produces color changes that are interpreted visually.	Add 5 mL of tap water to an incubation tray to provide a humid atmosphere during incubation. Place an API 20E strip into the incubation tray. Prepare a bacterial suspension of the test organism by suspending the cells from a well-isolated colony in 5 mL of sterile 0.85% saline. The turbidity of the suspension is compared with a McFarland 0.5 standard, except for same-day identifications of the *Enterobacteriaceae* when the suspension is matched to a 1 standard. Using a Pasteur pipette, fill each cupule with the bacterial suspension through the inoculating hole. Overlay the three decarboxylase and the urease cupules with sterile mineral oil. The unit is incubated at 35°C for 5 h (same-day identification) or for 24–48 h before reading results.	ONPG Arginine dihydrolase Lysine decarboxylase Ornithine decarboxylase Citrate Hydrogen sulfide Urease Tryptophan deaminase (add 10% $FeCl_3$) Indole Voges-Proskauer (add KOH and α-naphthol) Gelatin Glucose Mannitol Inositol Sorbitol Rhamnose Sucrose Melibiose Amygdalin Arabinose	Aldridge and Hodges, International Clinical Laboratories, Nashville, TN. 90.5% of stock cultures and 96.6% of clinical isolates identified. Overall accuracy 92%. (J Clin Microbiol 13:120–125, 1981) Gooch and Hill, University of Utah, 415 cultures, same-day identification 90.2%. (J Clin Microbiol 15:885–890, 1982)

bation panels are read upside-down using the BBL Crystal light box. The wells are examined for color changes, and a 10-digit profile number is generated. The profile number and off-line test results for indole and oxidase are entered on a PC in which the BBL Crystal ID System Electronic Codebook has been installed to obtain the identification.

In an external study involving three clinical laboratories, the reproducibility of the 30 individual E/NF substrates' ranged from 96.3% to 100%. The performance of the E/NF was evaluated with both fresh clinical isolates and challenge test strains. Of 299 fresh clinical isolates tested by the laboratories' current identification methods, The BBL Crystal ID System correctly reported 96.7% including 16 instances where two or three organisms were reported and required supplemental testing to resolve. Out of 291 previously identified challenge strains confirmed by the laboratories' current identification methods, the BBL Crystal ID System correctly reported 96.9%, including eight instances where two or three organisms were reported and required supplemental testing to resolve (BBL Crystal Package Insert, May 1994). In two independent evaluations of the Crystal system with fermentative organisms largely from the family *Enterobacteriaceae*, correct identification without supplemental testing was reported to be 91.6%[268] and 92.9%[313], respectively.

RAPID ONE SYSTEM

The RapID onE system (Innovative Diagnostics Systems, Inc., Norcross GA) is a qualitative micromethod employing conventional and chromogenic substrates for the identification of medically important *Enterobacteriaceae* and other selected oxidase-negative, gram-negative bacteria isolated from human clinical specimens. The system comprises 1) RapID onE panels, and 2) RapID onE reagent. Each RapID onE panel has 18 reaction cavities molded into the periphery of a plastic disposable tray. Reaction cavities contain dehydrated reactants, and the tray allows the simultaneous inoculation of each cavity with a predetermined amount of inoculum (see Color Plate 4-5C). A suspension of the test organism in RapID inoculation Fluid-2 mL is used as the test inoculum, which rehydrates and initiates test reactions. Inoculated panels are placed into the chipboard incubation trays provided in the package and incubated at 35° to 37°C in a non-CO$_2$ incubator for 4 hours.

RapID onE panels contain 18 reaction cavities that provide 19 test scores. Tests labeled PRO, GGT, PYR (cavities 15, 16, 17) require RapID onE Reagent and are designated with a box drawn around the tests. Test 18 is bifunctional, containing two separate tests in the same cavity. This test is scored **before** the addition of reagent, providing the first test result, which is adonitol; then 2 drops of INOVA Spot Indole reagent is added to cavity 18 and the same cavity is scored again **after** the addition of reagent to provide the second test result, which is indol. The 19 test results plus oxidase are scored in the appropriate boxes of the report form and a seven-digit profile code is generated.

The organism ID is obtained by finding the profile code in the RapID onE Code Compendium.

In a study conducted at the University of Illinois Medical Center, 302 of 344 (87.8%) oxidase-negative, gram-negative bacilli tested were correctly identified to the species level, with an additional 24 (7%) organisms correctly identified to the genus or group level. Six organisms gave unacceptable or no ID, eight gave questionable IDs, and four organisms (1.1%) gave incorrect IDs.[215] Kitch and colleagues reported similar findings with an overall identification rate to species or to genus level of 95.8%, with a misidentification rate of 1.3%.[177]

ENTEROTUBE II

Of all the systems, Enterotube II (Becton Dickinson Microbiology Systems, Cockeysville MD) is the easiest to inoculate (see Color Plate 4-5D). The system takes up little space, and the risk of contamination is minimal. The color reactions are generally easy to interpret; a minor problem exists in differentiating the elevation of the wax overlay in the glucose chamber (an indicator of gas production) from artifactual shrinkage of the media during storage. A false-negative interpretation may also result if a tiny leak in the plastic allows the gas to escape as it forms. Indole and Voges-Proskauer reagents must be added with a needle and syringe through the thin plastic backing. If this is not done carefully, the added reagent can leak into other compartments, altering reactions. Thus, it is recommended that the reactions in other compartments be interpreted before adding these reagents. One additional disadvantage of the Enterotube II, compared with systems that use dry substrates, is that the incorporation of conventional agar media shortens the shelf life.

The manufacturer provides a convenient computer-coding and identification system (CCIS) that lists the possible bacterial identifications for the five-digit biotype numbers that are derived from the interpretation of color changes.

Details of the functional design, operating procedures, and substrates included are listed in Table 15-2, page 639 in the second edition of this text.

MICRO-ID

Micro-ID (Remel, Lenexa KS) is the ideal system for laboratories where identification of bacteria within 4 to 6 hours is desired. Inoculation of the system is relatively easy, and the units occupy little space during incubation or storage (see Color Plate 4-5E). Only one reagent (20% potassium hydroxide) needs to be added to one of the chambers before interpreting the results. Reactions are distinct and can be compared with a color guide. A profile register that lists the probable organism identification for the five-digit biotype numbers is supplied by the manufacturer, and computer comparisons can be made to search for the best fit. Accuracy is equal to or exceeds that of other packaged systems.

Construction details and operating procedures for this system are listed in Table 15-2, page 642, in the second edition of this text.

MINITEK

Minitek (Becton Dickinson Microbiology Systems, Cockeysville MD) can be highly recommended to microbiologists who desire freedom of choice in the selection of the characteristics for identification. The manufacturer provides approximately 40 different reagent-impregnated disks that can be selected in any combination desired by the user. This diverse choice of substrates provides the user wide flexibility in identifying groups of microorganisms other than the *Enterobacteriaceae*; considerable success has been achieved in the identification of nonfermentative bacilli, anaerobes, and medically important yeasts. Generally, the color reactions are visibly distinct, and the use of a stack of color comparator cards makes interpretation relatively easy. The manufacturer also supplies a Minicoder, a plastic grid device that permits quick classification of bacterial candidates with each biochemical profile selected.

One disadvantage of allowing complete user selectivity of identification characteristics is the difficulty in standardizing biotype numbers. Conversely, if the user selects an optimized test set, theoretically the best possible biotype number will be derived (see pages 661–667 in the second edition of this text for a review of Rypka's method for calculating separatory values). The need to purchase several pieces of equipment and supplies makes the initial investment somewhat costly. In addition, the system requires several manual manipulations in the inoculation, incubation, and interpretation steps. The need to overlay the disks and culture medium within the reaction wells with mineral oil adds an extra step to the procedure and is considered messy by many users.

Details of the functional design, operating procedures, and substrates for this system are listed in Table 15-2, page 643, in the second edition of this text.

THE REPLICATOR SYSTEM

The replicator system is another method that is used infrequently in diagnostic laboratories for identifying bacteria. This method, developed by Fuchs,[119] is easy to use, versatile, and inexpensive, thus overcoming some of the disadvantages of the packaged kits mentioned previously. The user can select any number and sequence of characteristics to be tested. Each determination costs only a few cents, in contrast with tests from commercial and conventional procedures. In addition to the *Enterobacteriaceae*, other groups of bacteria, such as the gram-positive cocci, can be studied with this technique. Quality control of this procedure is maximal because stock organisms of known reactivity can be tested along with the unknowns in each determination and not merely with only one sample selected from a batch or lot number, as occurs with other systems.

Details on the construction and operation of the replicator system are given on page 141, in the third edition of this text.

BIOLOG GN MICROPLATE

Biolog Microplate (Biolog, Inc., Hayward CA) consists of a 96-well microtiter plate that tests for the ability of a microorganism to utilize (oxidize) one or more of 95 different carbon sources in the presence of a redox indicator (tetrazolium dye). One well contains no carbon and serves as a negative control or reference well. All the necessary nutrients and biochemicals are prefilled and dried into the 96 wells of the plate. Tetrazolium violet is used to colorimetrically detect the increased respiration that occurs in a cell when it is oxidizing a carbon source (see Color Plate 4-5F). Regardless of its structure, virtually any chemical substrate that is oxidized by the cell will result in formation of NADH, leading to a flow of electrons along a pathway of electron transport. Redox dyes, such as tetrazolium, tap electrons from this flow, converting the tetrazolium to a highly colored formazan. Thus, if a cell is presented with a chemical that it can oxidize, its respiration increases and the colorless dye is irreversibly reduced to a formazan, forming a purple color. If the cell is given a chemical that it cannot oxidize, no respiratory burst occurs, and no color is formed. The test yields a pattern of purple wells that constitutes a "metabolic fingerprint" of the capacities of the inoculated organism. Bochner has published a description and overview of the system.[30] Miller and Rhoden, at the CDC, have published a preliminary evaluation on the Biolog in which they report that the system performed well with many genera, but that problems were encountered with some strains of *Klebsiella*, *Enterobacter*, and *Serratia*.[211] Holmes and colleagues studied 789 strains, including 55 gram-negative taxa encountered in the clinical laboratory. They reported significantly better results when plates were read manually, rather than when they were read by the automated reader. Plates read manually gave the following performances: oxidase-positive fermenters, five taxa, 64 strains, 92% correct, 3% not identified, and 5% incorrect; biochemically active nonfermenters, eight taxa, 122 strains, 88% correct, 6% not identified, and 6% incorrect; *Enterobacteriaceae*, 35 taxa, 511 strains, 77% correct, 8% not identified, and 15% incorrect; unreactive nonfermenters, seven taxa, 92 strains, 38% correct, 24% not identified, and 38% incorrect. These authors reported problems with identification of encapsulated strains of some *Enterobacter* and *Klebsiella* taxa, as well as the least biochemically active *Moraxella* and *Neisseria* strains.[150]

MICROSCAN SYSTEMS

The MicroScan System (Dade MicroScan Inc., West Sacramento CA) consists of plastic, standard-sized, 96-well microtiter trays in which up to 32 reagent substrates are included for the identification of the *Enterobacteriaceae* and other bacterial species (gram-positive, gram-negative, and urinary tract panels are available). Some trays, called Combo trays, also include broth microdilutions of various antibiotics in certain of the microtubes for performing susceptibility tests[83] (see Color Plate 4-5*G*). MicroScan panels are supplied either in a frozen state or contain dehydrated substrates that make shipping more convenient and allow for room temperature storage and a longer shelf life. Schieven and associates[281] found that both the frozen and dehydrated microdilution trays provided comparable organism identification and antimicrobial susceptibility results (only 1.3% and 4.2% discrepancy rates, respectively).

The microtubes are inoculated with a heavy suspension of the organism to be identified and incubated at 35°C for 15 to 18 hours. The panels can be interpreted visually, after which the biochemical results are converted into a seven- or eight-digit biotype number that can be translated into an identification with a code book supplied by the manufacturer. Alternatively, an automated tray reader can be used to detect bacterial growth or color changes by differences in light transmission. Differences in electronic pulses are automatically analyzed by a microcomputer that compares reaction patterns with an internal program to determine the likelihood of identifications. Rhoden and associates[263] found that the AutoScan-4, an automatic reader in the MicroScan system, correctly identified 95.4% of members of the *Enterobacteriaceae* (occasional false-negative readings for hydrogen sulfide and arginine dihydrolase reactions were the only problems resulting in misidentification). One disadvantage cited by the authors was that the instrument occasionally reports "very rare biotype," leaving the user unclear as to what rare biotype was indicated.

THE SCEPTOR SYSTEM

The Sceptor system (Becton Dickinson Diagnostic Instrument Systems, Towson MD) allows simultaneous hydration and inoculation of dried substrate panels in microtiter trays for identification of members of the *Enterobacteriaceae*. A broth suspension of the organism to be studied is first made (5 mL of tryptic soy broth) and then transferred to the disposable reservoir. This reservoir is placed into an automated inoculation device, and plates are simultaneously hydrated and inoculated to the substrate wells. Arginine, hydrogen sulfide, lysine, ornithine, and urease wells are overlaid with sterile mineral oil. The panels are incubated at 35°C for 18 to 24 hours. Immediately after incubation, Kovac's reagent and ferric chloride are added to the indole and tryptophan wells, respectively. Reactions are interpreted visually and entered manually into a computer module. A seven-digit biotype number and identification are provided by the computer programs. Woolfrey and associates[323] found that the Sceptor system was capable of correctly identifying 93.4% of 678 stock culture isolates to the species level.

SENSITITRE SYSTEM

The Sensititre System (AccuMed International Inc., Westlake OH) may be purchased as either a manual enteric identification system or in the form of an au-

toidentification system. The manual plate contains media for performing 23 standard biochemical tests, plus a control, which are dried in the wells of a standard-sized 96-well microtiter tray. Each tray contains four duplicate sets of biochemical wells, permitting simultaneous identification of four organisms per tray. The system contains conventional biochemical tests and is inoculated and read manually. Staneck and associates[290] reported that agreement between Sensititre and API 20E for 1415 isolates of *Enterobacteriaceae* was 94.6% at the species level.

SEMIAUTOMATED AND AUTOMATED IDENTIFICATION SYSTEMS

VITEK SYSTEM

The Vitek System (AMS) (bioMerieux Vitek Inc., Hazelwood MO) was first introduced to perform automated antimicrobial susceptibility tests, with subsequent modifications to improve accuracy.[221] In 1982, the *Enterobacteriaceae*-plus Biochemical Card (EBC+) was introduced, providing for automatic identification of the *Enterobacteriaceae* within 8 hours of incubation. Barry and Badal[21] found approximately 97% agreement of EBC+ identifications compared with those obtained by standard reference methods. These findings have been corroborated in a subsequent study by Woolfrey and associates,[322] with 95.8% agreement in identification of 364 clinical isolates. An improvement to the Gram-Negative Identification Card was made in 1996. The new version card, called the GNI+ Card has 20 additional new species added to the database and offers improved performance and increased speed of identification. Moss and coworkers reported that the GNI+ identifies glucose-fermenting organisms in 2 to 8 hours and glucose-nonfermenting organisms in 4 to 12 hours, with 40.1% of the organisms tested being identified in 3 hours.[216] The Vitek system has found wide use in clinical microbiology laboratories and has generally been accepted as a reliable approach to the rapid identification of commonly encountered gram-negative bacilli (see Color Plate 4-5*H*).[227,241,262]

The construction and operating procedures of earlier versions of the Vitek system, initially designed to perform automated antibiotic susceptibility tests, were described in some detail in the second edition of this text (Table 15-10, pages 668–670).

MICROSCAN WALKAWAY

The Walkaway (Dade MicroScan Inc., West Sacramento CA) is a fully automated instrument that incubates any combination of up to 96 conventional or Rapid MicroScan panels simultaneously, automatically adds reagents to conventional panels when required, reads and interprets panel results, and prints results, all without operator intervention. Rapid fluorescence panels in addition to the conventional MicroScan panels are available for use with the Walkaway instrument. The rapid panels use fluorescent labeled compounds and require only a 2-hour incubation for bacterial identification. Each fluorescent substrate consists of a fluorophore, either methylumbelliferone (MEU) or 7-amino-4-methyl-coumarin (AMC) attached to a phosphate, sugar, or amino acid compound. Two types of reactions occur: fluorogenic and fluorometric. In fluorogenic reactions, a specific enzyme, if present in the bacterial suspension, cleaves the fluorescent compound releasing the fluorophore, which then fluoresces. For example:

$$\underset{\text{(nonfluorescent)}}{\text{L-Alanine-AMC}} \xrightarrow[\text{Aminopeptidase}]{\text{Alanine}} \underset{\text{(fluorescent)}}{\text{Alanine}} + \underset{}{\text{AMC}}$$

Fluorometric reactions detect changes in pH such as occurs with carbohydrate fermentation. The resultant acid production causes a drop in pH and a decrease in fluorescence. In addition, eight fluorogenic rate reactions are used. These reactions measure the rate of release of the fluorophore and are used in differentiating phenotypically similar species. Results of the ID reactions are converted into 15-digit biocodes for interpretation by the computer. The Walkaway colorimetric optical system has 97 photometers illuminated by a single tungsten–halogen source through 97 optical fibers. Light from the source passes through interference filters on a color wheel and is focused on the fiberoptics, 96 of which mirror the configuration of a 96-well panel. The 97th photometer provides a baseline reading to which all photometer signals are ratioed. During each read cycle, the rotating color wheel provides readings at six different wavelengths through the visible spectrum. For biochemical reactions, the computer selects the wavelength reading that best discriminates the reaction occurring in each well. A review of the Walkaway technology has been published by Clayland and colleagues.[77] Several studies have shown that the Walkaway provides accurate identification of organisms belonging to the family *Enterobacteriaceae*.[171,224,227,241,262,326]

MicroScan's fluorogenic 2-hour Rapid Negative Identification Panel has recently been updated to significantly increase accuracy of identification and expand the number of taxa in the database. The updated panel (Rapid Gram Negative Identification Panel 3) consists of 36 newly formulated tests and a new database consisting of 138 taxa, including 19 additional new species. Achondo and associates reported that the new system has an accuracy of 98.4% (92.5% correct to species, 1.6% correct to genus, and 4.3% correct to species with additional tests) and 99.3% for clinically significant isolates (97.4% correct to species, 1.0%

correct to genus, and 0.9% correct to species with additional tests).[2]

SENSITITRE GRAM-NEGATIVE AUTOIDENTIFICATION SYSTEM

The Sensititre Gram-Negative AutoIdentification System (AccuMed International, Inc., Westlake OH) uses fluorescent technology to detect bacterial growth and enzyme activity. The system consists of 32 newly formulated biochemical tests, including selected classic biochemical media reformulated to yield a fluorescent signal, along with newly developed fluorescent tests. Each biochemical test medium along with an appropriate fluorescent indicator is dried into the individual wells of the Sensititre plate. Each plate is designed to test three separate organisms. Because these are dried plates, they may be stored at room temperature. All autoIdentification tests are read on the Sensititre AutoReader for the presence or absence of fluorescence. The results are transmitted to a computer for analysis and identification. Results may be read after 5 hours of incubation. If a satisfactory level of identification cannot be obtained at 5 hours, the plate may simply be reincubated and read after overnight incubation. Owing to the use of fluorescent technology, these plates cannot be read manually and can be read only on a correctly standardized Sensititre AutoReader. Company in-house data for 1084 isolates of *Enterobacteriaceae* show overall agreement at 5 hours to be 92.4% and at 18 hours to be 93.4% when compared with standard methods (Sensititre Technical Product Information).

In summary, commercial manufacturers continue to provide new systems and modifications of existing systems for the identification of microorganisms. To pass Food and Drug Administration standards, all of these systems must perform with an accuracy equal to or better than reference methods. Therefore, each system can be used in clinical laboratories, but the choice depends on several variables, including volume of testing, experience of the technical staff, need for definitive identifications, and cost of operation. The *Enterobacteriaceae*, as a group, are rapidly expanding and, for the most part, are biochemically very active; therefore, they are well-suited for processing by automated and semiautomated systems. Space has allowed for only a brief overview of these systems in this text. To learn more the reader is referred to the review of automated systems written by Stager and Davis.[289] The cited references may be consulted for more detailed descriptions and evaluations of performance.

R E F E R E N C E S

1. ABBOTT SL, JANDA JM: Isolation of *Yokenella regensburgei* ("*Koserella trabulsii*") from a patient with transient bacteremia and from a patient with a septic knee. J Clin Microbiol 32:2854–2855, 1994

2. ACHONDO K, BASCOMB S, BOBOLIS J, CHIPMAN A, CONNELL S, ENSCOE G, GARDNER B, MAYHEW P, NOTHAFT D, SKINNER J, STEARN L, WILLIAMS G, VOONG J, ABBOTT S, O'HARA C, SCHRECKENBERGER P: New improved Mi-

croScan Rapid Negative Identification Panel. Abstr Annu Meet Am Soc Microbiol C307, p 53, 1995

3. AEVALIOTIS A, BELLE AM, CHANIONE JP, SERRUYS E: *Kluyvera ascorbata* isolated from a baby with diarrhea. Clin Microbiol Newsl 7:51, 1985

4. AGUIRRE PM, CACHO JB, FOLGUEIRA L, LOPEZ M, GARCIA J, VELASCO AC: Rapid fluorescence method for screening *Salmonella* spp. from enteric differential agars. J Clin Microbiol 28:148–149, 1990

5. ALBALLAA SR, QADRI SMH, AL-FURAYH O, AL-QATARY K: Urinary tract infection due to *Rahnella aquatilis* in a renal transplant patient. J Clin Microbiol 30:2948–2950, 1992

6. ALBERT MJ, ALAM K, ISLAM M, MONTANARO J, RAHMAN ASMH, HAIDER K, HOSSAIN MA, KIBRIYA AKMG, TZIPORI S: *Hafnia alvei*, a probable cause of diarrhea in humans. Infect Immun 59:1507–1513, 1991

7. ALBERT MJ, FARUQUE SM, ANSARUZZAMAN M, ISLAM MM, HAIDER K, ALAM K, KABIR I, ROBINS-BROWNE R: Sharing of virulence-associated properties at the phenotypic and genetic levels between enteropathogenic *Escherichia coli* and *Hafnia alvei*. J Med Microbiol 37:310–314, 1992

8. ALEKSIC S, STEIGERWALT AG, BOCKEMUHL J ET AL: *Yersinia rohdei* sp. nov. isolated from human and dog feces and surface water. Int J Syst Bacteriol 37:327–332, 1987

9. ARCHER JR, SCHELL RF, PENNELL DR ET AL: Identification of *Yersinia* spp. with the API 20E system. J Clin Microbiol 25:2398–2399, 1987

10. ARDUINO MJ, BLAND LA, TIPPLE MA, AGUERO SM, FAVERO MS, JARVIS WR: Growth and endotoxin production of *Yersinia enterocolitica* and *Enterobacter agglomerans* in packed erythrocytes. J Clin Microbiol 27: 1483–1485, 1989

11. ARTHUR JD, PIERCE JR: *Citrobacter diversus* meningitis and brain abscess associated with *Bacteroides melaninogenicus*. Pediatr Infect Dis 3:592–593, 1984

12. ASPINALL ST, HINDLE MA, HUTCHINSON DN: Improved isolation of salmonellae from faeces using a semisolid Rappaport-Vassiliadis medium. Eur J Clin Microbiol Infect Dis 11:936–939, 1992

13. AWSARE SV, LILLO M: A case report of *Escherichia vulneris* urosepsis. Rev Infect Dis 13:1247–1248, 1991 (Letter)

14. BABU K, SONNENBERG M, KATHPALIA S, ORTEGA P, SWIATLO AL, KOCKA FE: Isolation of salmonellae from dried rattlesnake preparations. J Clin Microbiol 28: 361–362, 1990

15. BAE BHC, SUREKA SB: *Cedecea davisae* isolated from scrotal abscess. J Urol 130:148–149, 1983

16. BAE BHC, SUREKA SB, AJAMY JA: Enteric group 15 (Enterobacteriaceae) associated with pneumonia. J Clin Microbiol 14:596–597, 1981

17. BAGLEY ST, SEIDLER RJ, BRENNER DJ: *Klebsiella planticola* sp. nov.: a new species of Enterobacteriaceae found primarily in nonclinical environments. Curr Microbiol 6:105–109, 1981

18. BALE MJ, MCLAWS SM, FENN JP ET AL: Use of and cost savings with morphologic criteria and the spot indole test as a routine means of identification of *Escherichia coli*. Diagn Microbiol Infect Dis 2:187–191, 1984

19. BALE MJ, MCLAWS SM, MATSEN JM: The spot indole test for identification of swarming *Proteus*. Am J Clin Pathol 83:87–90, 1985

20. BARNES AM, QUAN TJ: Plague. In Gorbach SL, Bartlett JG, Balacklow NR (eds). Infectious Diseases, pp 1285–1291. Philadelphia, WB Saunders, 1992

21. BARRY AL, BADAL RE: Identification of Enterobacteriaceae by the AutoMicrobic system: Enterobacteriaceae biochemical cards versus Enterobacteriaceae-plus biochemical cards. J Clin Microbiol 15:575–581, 1982

22. BARRY AL, BERNSOHN KL, ADAMS AP ET AL: Improved 18-hour methyl red test. Appl Microbiol 20:866–870, 1970

23. BEAR N, KLUGMAN KP, TOBIANSKY L, KOORNHOF HJ: Wound colonization by *Ewingella americana*. J Clin Microbiol 23:650–651, 1986

24. BERCOVIER H, STEIGERWALT AG, GUIYOULE A ET AL: *Yersinia aldovae* (formerly *Yersinia enterocolitica*-like group X2): A new species of Enterobacteriaceae isolated from aquatic ecosystems. Int J Syst Bacteriol 34:166:172, 1984

25. BERCOVIER H, URSING J, BRENNER DJ, STEIGERWALT AG, FANNING GR, CARTER GP, MOLLARET HH: *Yersinia kristensenii*: a new species of Enterobacteriaceae composed of sucrose-negative strains (formerly called atypical *Yersinia enterocolitica* or *Yersinia enterocolitica*-like). Curr Microbiol 4:219–224, 1980

26. BETTELHEIM KA, EVANGELIDIS H, PEARCE JL, SOWERS E, STROCKBINE NA: Isolation of a *Citrobacter freundii* strain which carries the *Escherichia coli* 0157 antigen. J Clin Microbiol 31:760–761, 1993

27. BIERING G, KARLSSON S, CLARK NC, JONSDOTTIR KE, LUDVIGSSON P, STEINGRIMSSON O: Three cases of neonatal meningitis caused by *Enterobacter sakazakii* in powdered milk. J Clin Microbiol 27:2054–2056, 1989

28. BISSETT ML, POWERS C, ABBOTT SL, JANDA JM: Epidemiologic investigations of *Yersinia enterocolitica* and related species: sources, frequency, and serogroup distribution. J Clin Microbiol 28:910–912, 1990

29. BJUNE G, RUUD TE, ENG J: Bacterial shock due to transfusion with *Yersinia enterocolitica* infected blood. Scand J Infect Dis 16:411–412, 1984

30. BOCHNER B: "Breathprints" at the microbial level: an automated redox-based technology quickly identifies bacteria according to their metabolic capacities. ASM News 55:536–539, 1989

31. BOCHNER B: Rainbow UTI System: a rapid and simple multicolor diagnostic system for common urinary tract pathogens. Abstr Annu Meet Am Soc Microbiol C374, p 65, 1995

32. BOILEAU CR, D'HAUTEVILLE HM, SANSONETTI PJ: DNA hybridization technique to detect *Shigella* sp and enteroinvasive *Escherichia coli*. J Clin Microbiol 20:959–961, 1984

33. BOLLET C, GAINNIER M, SAINTY J-M, ORHESSER P, DE MICCO P: *Serratia fonticola* isolated from a leg abscess. J Clin Microbiol 29:834–835, 1991

34. BOTTONE EJ: Atypical *Yersinia enterocolitica*: clinical and epidemiological parameters. J Clin Microbiol 7:562–567, 1978

35. BOTTONE EJ (ED): *Yersinia enterocolitica*. Boca Raton FL, CRC Press, 1981

36. BRENNER DJ: Enterobacteriaceae. In Krieg NR, Holt JG (eds): Bergey's Manual of Systematic Bacteriology, vol 1, pp 408–420. Baltimore, Williams & Wilkins, 1984

37. BRENNER DJ, BERCOVIER H, URSING J ET AL: *Yersinia intermedia*: A new species of Enterobacteriaceae composed of rhamnose-positive, melibiose-positive, raffinose-positive strains (formerly called *Yersinia enterocolitica* or

Yersinia enterocolitica-like). Curr Microbiol 4:207:212, 1980

38. BRENNER DJ, DAVIS BR, STEIGERWALT AG ET AL: Atypical biogroups of *Escherichia coli* found in clinical specimens and description of *Escherichia hermannii* sp. nov. J Clin Microbiol 15:703–713, 1982

39. BRENNER DJ, GRIMONT PAD, STEIGERWALT AG, FANNING GR, AGERON E, RIDDLE CF: Classification of citrobacteria by DNA hybridization: designation of *Citrobacter farmeri* sp. nov., *Citrobacter youngae* sp. nov., *Citrobacter braakii* sp. nov., *Citrobacter werkmanii* sp. nov., *Citrobacter sedlakii* sp. nov., and three unnamed *Citrobacter* genomospecies. Int J Syst Bacteriol 43:645–658, 1993

40. BRENNER DJ, HICKMAN-BRENNER FW, HOLMES B, HAWKEY PM, PENNER JL, GRIMONT PAD, O'HARA CM: Replacement of NCTC 4175, the current type strain of *Proteus vulgaris*, with ATCC 29905: request for an opinion. Int J Syst Bacteriol 45:870–871, 1995

41. BRENNER DJ, McWHORTER AC, KAI A ET AL: *Enterobacter asburiae* sp. nov., a new species found in clinical specimens, and reassignment of *Erwinia dissolvens* and *Erwinia nimipressuralis* to the genus *Enterobacter* as *Enterobacter dissolvens* comb. nov. and *Enterobacter nimipressuralis* comb. nov. J Clin Microbiol 23:1114–1120, 1986

42. BRENNER DJ, McWHORTER AC, LEETE-KNUTSON JK, STEIGERWALT AG: *Escherichia vulneris*: a new species of Enterobacteriaceae associated with human wounds. J Clin Microbiol 15:1133–1140, 1982

43. BRENNER DJ, RICHARD C, STEIGERWALT AG ET AL: *Enterobacter gergoviae* sp. nov.: a new species of Enterobacteriaceae found in clinical specimens and environment. Int J Syst Bacteriol 30:1:6, 1980

44. BRENNER DJ, URSING J, BERCOVIER H ET AL: Deoxyribonucleic acid relatedness in *Yersinia enterocolitica* and *Yersinia enterocolitica*-like organisms. Curr Microbiol 4:195–200, 1980

45. BROOKER DC, LUND ME, BLAZEVIC DJ: Rapid test for lysine decarboxylase activity in Enterobacteriaceae. Appl Microbiol 26:622–623, 1973

46. CARLQUIST PR: A biochemical test for separating paracolon groups. J Bacteriol 71:339:341, 1956

47. CARPENTER CCJ: Shigellosis. In Wyngaarden JB, Smith LH (eds): Cecil Textbook of Medicine, 16th ed, pp 1517:1519. Philadelphia, WB Saunders, 1982

48. CARRERO P, GARROTE JA, PACHECO S, GARCIA AI, GIL R, CARBAJOSA SG: Report of six cases of human infection by *Serratia plymuthica*. J Clin Microbiol 33:275–276, 1995

49. CASTILLO CB, BRUCKNER DA: Comparative evaluation of the Eiken and API 20E systems and conventional methods for identification of members of the family Enterobacteriaceae. J Clin Microbiol 20:754–757, 1984

50. CENTERS FOR DISEASE CONTROL: HIP investigates *Enterobacter hormaechei* infections. CDC/NCID Focus Fol 3, No 5, 1993

51. CENTERS FOR DISEASE CONTROL: *Arizona hinshawii* septicemia associated with rattlesnake powder—California. MMWR 32:464–465, 1983

52. CENTERS FOR DISEASE CONTROL: Gastointestinal illness associated with imported Brie cheese—District of Columbia. MMWR 32:533, 1983

53. CENTERS FOR DISEASE CONTROL: Update: milkborne salmonellosis—Illinois. MMWR 34:200, 1985

54. CENTERS FOR DISEASE CONTROL: CDC Surveillance Summaries, March 1990. MMWR 39(SS-1), 1990

55. CENTERS FOR DISEASE CONTROL: Update: *Salmonella enteritidis* infections and shell eggs—United States, 1990. MMWR 39:909, 1990

56. CENTERS FOR DISEASE CONTROL: Update: *Yersinia enterocolitica* bacteremia and endotoxin shock associated with red blood cell transfusions—United States, 1991. MMWR 40:176–178, 1991

57. CENTERS FOR DISEASE CONTROL: Outbreak of *Salmonella enteritidis* infection associated with consumption of raw shell eggs, 1991. MMWR 41:369–372, 1992

58. CENTERS FOR DISEASE CONTROL: Pneumonic plague—Arizona, 1992. MMWR 41:737–739, 1992

59. CENTERS FOR DISEASE CONTROL: Outbreaks of *Salmonella enteritidis* gastroenteritis—California, 1993. MMWR 42:793–797, 1993

60. CENTERS FOR DISEASE CONTROL: Human plague—United States, 1993–1994. MMWR 43:242–246, 1994

61. CENTERS FOR DISEASE CONTROL: Update: human plague—India, 1994. MMWR 43:722–723, 1994

62. CENTERS FOR DISEASE CONTROL: Outbreak of *Salmonella enteritidis* associated wtih nationally distributed ice cream products—Minnesota, South Dakota, and Wisconsin, 1994. MMWR 43:740–741, 1994

63. CENTERS FOR DISEASE CONTROL: Summary of Notifiable Diseases, United States, 1994. MMWR Supp 43(53), 1995

64. CENTERS FOR DISEASE CONTROL: Reptile-associated salmonellosis—selected states, 1994–1995. MMWR 44:347–350, 1995

65. CENTERS FOR DISEASE CONTROL: Outbreak of acute gastoenteritis attributable to *Escherichia coli* serotype 0104:H21—Helena, Montana, 1994. MMWR 44:501–503, 1995

66. CENTERS FOR DISEASE CONTROL: Community outbreak of hemolytic uremic syndrome attributable to *Escherichia coli* 0111:NM—South Australia, 1995. MMWR 44:550–551, 557–558, 1995

67. CHAGLA HH, BOROZYK AA, ALDOM JE, ROSA SD, COLE DD: Evaluation of the L-pyrrolidonyl-α-naphthylamide hydrolysis test for the differentiation of member of the families Enterobacteriaceae and Vibrionaceae. J Clin Microbiol 31:1946–1948, 1993

68. CHAPMAN PA, SIDDONS CA, ZADIK PM, JEWES L: An improved selective medium for the isolation of *Escherichia coli* 0157. J Med Microbiol 35:107–110, 1991

69. CHAPMAN PA, WRIGHT DJ, SIDDONS CA: A comparison of immunomagnetic separation and direct culture for the isolation of verocytotoxin-producing *Escherichia coli* 0157 from bovine faeces. J Med Microbiol 40:424–427, 1994

70. CHESTER B, MOSKOWITZ LB: Rapid catalase supplemental test for identification of members of the family Enterobacteriaceae. J Clin Microbiol 25:439–441, 1987

71. CHMEL H: *Serratia odorifera* biogroup 1 causing an invasive human infection. J Clin Microbiol 26:1244–1245, 1988

72. CHRISTENSEN WB: Urea decomposition as a means of differentiating *Proteus* and paracolon cultures from each

other and from *Salmonella* and *Shigella* types. J Bacteriol 52:461–466, 1946

73. CHRISTIAENS E, HANSEN W, MOINET J: Isolament des expectorations d'un patient atteint de leucemie lymphoide chronique et de broncho-emphyseme d' une Enterobacteriaceae nouvellement decrite: *Rahnella aquatilis*. Med Maladies Infect 17:732–734, 1987

74. CLARK NC, HILL BC, O'HARA CM, STEINGRIMSSON O, COOKSEY RC: Epidemiologic typing of *Enterobacter sakazakii* in two neonatal nosocomial outbreaks. Diagn Microbiol Infect Dis 13:467–472, 1990

75. CLARK RB, JANDA JM: Isolation of *Serratia plymuthica* from a human burn site. J Clin Microbiol 21:656–657, 1985

76. CLARRIDGE JE, MUSHER DM, FAINSTEIN V ET AL: Extraintestinal human infection caused by *Edwardsiella tarda*. J Clin Microbiol 11:511–514, 1980

77. CLAYLAND BG, CLAYLAND C, TOMFOHRDE KM ET AL: Full spectrum automation for the clinical microbiology laboratory. Am Clin Lab, May 1989, pp 30–34

78. COHEN ML, POTTER M, POLLARD R, FELDMAN RA: Turtle-associated salmonellosis in the United States: effect of public health action, 1970–1976. JAMA 243:1247–1249, 1980

79. COUDRON PE, MARKOWITZ SM: *Cedecea lapagei* isolated from lung tissue. Clin Microbiol Newsl 9:171–172, 1987

80. COVER TL, ABER RC: Medical progress: *Yersinia enterocolitica*. N Engl J Med 321:16:24, 1989

81. CURLESS RG: Neonatal intracranial abscess: two cases caused by *Citrobacter* and a literature review. Ann Neurol 8:269–272, 1980

82. DARBAS H, JEAN-PIERRE H, PAILLISSON J: Case report and review of septicemia due to *Serratia ficaria*. J Clin Microbiol 32:2285–2288, 1994

83. DEGIROLAMI PC, EICHELBERGER KA, SALFITY LC ET AL: Evaluation of the AutoScan-3 devise for reading microdilution trays. J Clin Microbiol 18:1292:1295, 1983

84. DE SMEDT JM, BOLDERDIJK RF: Dynamics of *Salmonella* isolation with modified semi-solid Rappaport-Vassiliadis medium. J Food Prot 50:658–661, 1987

85. DEVENISH JA, CIEBIN BW, BRODSKY MH: Novobiocin-brilliant green–glucose agar: new medium for isolation of salmonellae. Appl Environ Microbiol 52:539–545, 1986

86. DEVREESE K, CLAEYS G, VERSCHRAEGEN G: Septicemia with *Ewingella americana*. J Clin Microbiol 30:2746–2747, 1992

87. DOMINGO D, LIMIA A, ALARCON T, SANZ JC, DEL REY MC, LOPEZ-BREA M: Nosocomial septicemia caused by *Serratia plymuthica*. J Clin Microbiol 32:575–577, 1994

88. DROW DL, MERCER L, PEACOCK JB: Splenic abscess caused by *Shigella flexneri* and *Bacteroides fragilis*. J Clin Microbiol 19:79–80, 1984

89. DUSCH H, ALTWEGG M: Comparison of Rambach agar, SM-ID medium, and Hektoen enteric agar for primary isolation of non-typhi salmonellae from stool samples. J Clin Microbiol 31:410–412, 1993

90. DUSCH H, ALTWEGG M: Evaluation of five new plating media for isolation of *Salmonella* species. J Clin Microbiol 33:802–804, 1995

91. EDBERG SC, TREPETA RW: Rapid and economical identification and antimicrobial susceptibility test methodology for urinary tract pathogens. J Clin Microbiol 18:1287–1291, 1983

92. EDERER GM, CLARK M: Motility–indole–ornithine medium. Appl Microbiol 20:849–850, 1970

93. EDWARDS PR, EWING WH: Identification of Enterobacteriaceae, 3rd ed. Minneapolis, Burgess, 1972

94. EDWARDS PR, FIFE MA: Lysine–iron agar in the detection of *Arizona* cultures. Appl Microbiol 9:478:480, 1961

95. EIDSON M, TIERNEY LA, ROOLLAG OJ ET AL: Feline plague in New Mexico: risk factors and transmission to humans. Am J Public Health 78:1333–1335, 1988

96. ELIN RJ, ROBINSON RA, LEVIN AS ET AL: Lack of clinical usefulness of the limulus test in the diagnosis of endotoxemia. N Engl J Med 293:521–524, 1975

97. ENGLER HD, TROY K, BOTTONE EJ: Bacteremia and subcutaneous abscess caused by *Proteus penneri* in a neutropenic host. J Clin Microbiol 28:1645–1646, 1990

98. EWING WH: Identification of Enterobacteriaceae, 4th ed. New York, Elsevier, 1986

99. EWING WH, MCWHORTER AC, ESCOBAR MR ET AL: *Edwardsiella*, a new genus of Enterobacteriaceae, based on a new species of *E. tarda*. Int Bull Bact Nomencl Taxon 15:33–38, 1965

100. EWING WH, ROSS AJ, BRENNER DJ, FANNING GR: *Yersinia ruckeri* sp. nov., the redmouth (RM) bacterium. Int J Syst Bacteriol 28:37–44, 1978

101. FAINSTEIN V, HOPPER RL, MILLS K, BODEY GP: Colonization by or diarrhea due to *Kluyvera* species. J Infect Dis 145:127, 1982

102. FAINSTEIN V, YANCEY R, TRIER P, BODEY GP: Overwhelming infection in a cancer patient caused by *Arizona hinshawii*: its relation to snake pill ingestion. Am J Infect Control 10:147–148, 1982

103. FALKOW S: Activity of lysine decarboxylase as an aid in the identification of *Salmonella* and *Shigella*. Am J Clin Pathol 29:598–600, 1958

104. FARMER JJ III, ASBURY MA, HICKMAN FW ET AL: *Enterobacter sakazakii*: A new species of "Enterobacteriaceae" isolated from clinical specimens. Int J Syst Bacteriol 30:569–584, 1980

105. FARMER JJ III, CARTER GP, MILLER VL, FALKOW S, WACHSMUTH IK: Pyrazinamidase, CR-MOX agar, salicin fermentation-esculin hydrolysis, and D-xylose fermentation for identifying pathogenic serotypes of *Yersinia enterocolitica*. J Clin Microbiol 30:2589–2594, 1992

106. FARMER JJ III, DAVIS BR, HICKMAN-BRENNER FW ET AL: Biochemical identification of new species and biogroups of Enterobacteriaceae isolated from clinical specimens. J Clin Microbiol 21:46:76, 1985

107. FARMER JJ III, FANNING GR, DAVIS BR, O'HARA CM, RIDDLE C, HICKMAN-BRENNER FW, ASBURY MA, LOWERY VA III, BRENNER DJ: *Escherichia fergusonii* and *Enterobacter taylorae*, two new species of Enterobacteriaceae isolated from clinical specimens. J Clin Microbiol 21:77–81, 1985

108. FARMER JJ III, FANNING GR, HUNTLEY-CARTER GP, HOLMES B, HICKMAN FW, RICHARD C, BRENNER DJ: *Kluyvera*, a new (redefined) genus in the family Enterobacteriaceae: identification of *Kluyvera ascorbata* sp. nov. and *Kluyvera cryocrescens* sp. nov. in clinical specimens. J Clin Microbiol 13:919–933, 1981

109. FARMER JJ III, MCWHORTER AC: Genus X. *Edwardsiella* Ewing and McWhorter 1965, 37[AL]. In Krieg NR, Holt JG (eds): Bergey's Manual of Systematic Bacteriology, vol 1, pp 486–491. Baltimore, Williams & Wilkins, 1984

110. FARMER JJ III, SHETH NK, HUDZINSKI JA, ROSE HD, AS-BURY MF: Bacteremia due to *Cedecea neteri* sp. nov. J Clin Microbiol 16:775–778, 1982

111. FAY GD, BARRY AL: Rapid ornithine decarboxylase test for the identification of Enterobacteriaceae. Appl Microbiol 23:710–713, 1972

112. FERRAGUT C, IZARD D, GAVINI F, KERSTERS K, DE LEY J, LECLERC H: *Klebsiella trevisanii*: a new species from water and soil. Int J Syst Bacteriol 33:133–142, 1983

113. FERRAGUT C, IZARD D, GAVINI F, LEFEBVRE B, LECLERC H: *Buttiauxella*, a new genus of the family Enterobacteriaceae. Zentralbl Bakteriol Parasitenkd Infektionskr Hyg Abt 1 Orig Reihe C 2:33–44, 1981

114. FOBERG U, FRYDEN A, KIHLSTROM E, PERSSON K, WEILAND O: *Yersinia enterocolitica* septicemia: clinical and microbiological aspects. Scand J Infect Dis 18:269–279, 1986

115. FREDERIKSEN W: Correct names of the species *Citrobacter koseri, Levinea malonatica,* and *Citrobacter diversus*: request for an opinion. Int J Syst Bacteriol 40:107–108, 1990

116. FRENEY J, FLEURETTE J, GRUER LD, DESMONCEAUX M, GAVINI F, LECLERC H: *Klebsiella trevisanii* colonization and septicaemia. Lancet 1:909, 1984

117. FRENEY J, GAVINI F, ALEXANDRE H, MADIER S, IZARD D, LECLERC H, FLEURETTE J: Nosocomial infection and colonization by *Klebsiella trevisanii*. J Clin Microbiol 23:948–950, 1986

118. FRENEY J, GAVINI F, PLOTON C, LECLERC H, FLEURETTE J: Isolation of *Escherichia fergusonii* from a patient with septicemia in France. Eur J Clin Microbiol Infect Dis 6:78, 1987 (letter)

119. FUCHS PC: The replicator method for identification and biotyping of common bacterial isolates. Lab Med 6:6–11, 1975

120. FUNKE G, HANY A, ALTWEGG M: Isolation of *Escherichia fergusonii* from four different sites in a patient with pancreatic carcinoma and cholangiosepsis. J Clin Microbiol 31:2201–2203, 1993

121. FUNKE G, ROSNER H: *Rahnella aquatilis* bacteremia in an HIV-infected intravenous drug abuser. Diag Microbiol Infect Dis 22:293–296, 1995

122. GANGAROSA EJ, MERSON MH: Epidemiological assessment of the relevance of the so-called enteropathogenic serogroups of *Escherichia coli* in diarrhea. N Engl J Med 296:1210–1213, 1977

123. GAVINI F, IZARD D, GRIMONT PAD, BEJI A, AGERON E, LECLERC H: Priority of *Klebsiella planticola* Bagley, Seidler, and Brenner 1982 over *Klebsiella trevisanii* Ferragut, Izard, Gavini, Kersters, DeLey, and Leclerc 1983. Int J Syst Bacteriol 36:486–488, 1986

124. GAVINI F, MERGAERT J, BEJI A ET AL: Transfer of *Enterobacter agglomerans* (Beijerinck 1988) Ewing and Fife 1972 to *Pantoea* gen. nov. as *Pantoea agglomerans* comb. nov. and description of *Pantoea dispersa* sp. nov. Int J Syst Bacteriol 39:337–345, 1989

124a. GIAMARELLOU H, ANTONIADOU A, KANAVOS K, PAPAIOANNOU C, KANATAKIS S, PAPADKI K: *Yersinia enterocolitica* endocarditis: case report and literature review. Eur J Clin Microbiol Infect Dis 14:126–130, 1995

125. GILL VJ, FARMER JJ III, GRIMONT PAD ET AL: *Serratia ficaria* isolated from a human clinical specimen. J Clin Microbiol 14:234–236, 1981

126. GLUSTEIN JZ, RUDENSKY B, ABRAHAMOV A: Catheter-associated sepsis caused by *Serratia odorifera* biovar 1 in an adolescent patient. Eur J Clin Microbiol Infect Dis 13:183–184, 1994

127. GOLDSTEIN EJC, LEWIS RP, MARTIN WJ ET AL: Infections caused by *Klebsiella ozaenae*: a changing disease spectrum. J Clin Microbiol 8:413–418, 1978

128. GOLDWATER PN, BETTELHEIM KA: Hemolytic uremic syndrome due to Shiga-like toxin producing *Escherichia coli* 048:H21 in South Australia. Emerg Infect Dis 1:132–133, 1995

129. GOOSSENS H, WAUTERS G, DE BOECK M, JANSSENS M, BUTZLER J-P: Semisolid selective-motility enrichment medium for isolation of salmonellae from fecal specimens. J Clin Microbiol 19:940–941, 1984

130. GORBACH SL, KEAN BH, EVANS DG ET AL: Travelers' diarrhea and toxigenic *Escherichia coli*. N Engl J Med 292:933–936, 1975

131. GOUBAU P, VAN AELST F, VERHAEGEN J, BOOGAERTS M: Septicaemia caused by *Rahnella aquatilis* in an immunocompromised patient. Eur J Clin Microbiol Infect Dis 7:697–699, 1988

132. GRAHAM DR, ANDERSON RL, ARIEL FE, EHRENKRANZ NJ, ROWE B, BOER HR, DIXON RE: Epidemic nosocomial meningitis due to *Citrobacter diversus* in neonates. J Infect Dis 144:203–209, 1981

133. GRAHAM DR, BAND JD: *Citrobacter diversus* brain abscess and meningitis in neonates. JAMA 245:1923–1925, 1981

133a. GRIFFIN PM, TAUXE RV: The epidemiology of infections caused by *Escherichia coli* 0157:H7, other enterohemorrhagic *E. coli*, and the associated hemolytic uremic syndrome. Epidemiol Rev 13:60–98, 1991

134. GRIMONT PAD, FARMER JJ III, GRIMONT F, ASBURY MA, BRENNER DJ, DEVAL C: *Ewingella americana* gen. nov. sp. nov. A new Enterobacteriaceae isolated from clinical specimens. Ann Microbiol (Paris) 134 A:39–52, 1983

135. GRIMONT PAD, GRIMONT F, FARMER JJ III, ASBURY MA: *Cedecea davisae* gen. nov., sp. nov. and *Cedecea lapagei* sp. nov., new Enterobacteriaceae from clinical specimens. Int J Syst Bacteriol 31:317–326, 1981

136. GRIMONT PAD, GRIMONT F, RICHARD C ET AL: *Edwardsiella hoshinae*, a new species of Enterobacteriaceae. Curr Microbiol 4:347–351, 1980

137. GUERRANT RL: Inflammatory enteritidis. In Mandell GL, Douglas RG Jr, Bennett JE (eds): Principles and Practice of Infectious Diseases, 2nd ed. pp 660–669. New York, John Wiley & Sons, 1985

138. HANSEN MW, GLUPCZYNSKI GY: Isolation of an unusual *Cedecea* species from a cutaneous ulcer. Eur J Clin Microbiol 3:152–153, 1984

139. HARRELL LJ, CAMERON ML, O'HARA CM: *Rahnella aquatilis*, an unusual gram-negative rod isolated from the bronchial washing of a patient with acquired immunodeficiency syndrome. J Clin Microbiol 27:1671–1672, 1989

140. HAWKE JP, McWHORTER AC, STEIGERWALT AG ET AL: *Edwardsiella ictaluri* sp. nov., the causative agent of enteric septicemia of catfish. Int J Syst Bacteriol 31:396–400, 1981

141. HEAD CB, WHITTY DA, RATNAM S: Comparative study of selective media for recovery of *Yersinia enterocolitica*. J Clin Microbiol 16:615–621, 1982

142. HEIZMANN WR, MICHEL R: *Ewingella americana* from a patient with conjunctivitis. Eur J Clin Microbiol Infect Dis 10:957–959, 1991

143. HICKMAN FW, STEIGERWALT AG, FARMER JJ III, BRENNER DJ: Identification of *Proteus penneri* sp. nov., formerly known as *Proteus vulgaris* indole negative or as *Proteus vulgaris* biogroup 1. J Clin Microbiol 15:1097–1102, 1982

144. HICKMAN-BRENNER FW, FARMER JJ III, STEIGERWALT AG ET AL: *Providencia rustigianii*: a new species in the family Enterobacteriaceae formerly known as *Providencia alcalifaciens* biogroup 3. J Clin Microbiol 17:1057–1060, 1983

145. HICKMAN-BRENNER FW, HUNTLEY-CARTER GP, FANNING GR, BRENNER DJ, FARMER JJ III: *Koserella trabulsii*, a new genus and species of Enterobacteriaceae formerly known as enteric group 45. J Clin Microbiol 21:39–42, 1985

146. HICKMAN-BRENNER FW, HUNTLEY-CARTER GP, SAITOH Y, STEIGERWALT AG, FARMER JJ III, BRENNER DJ: *Moellerella wisconsensis*, a new genus and species of Enterobacteriaceae found in human stool specimens. J Clin Microbiol 19:460–463, 1984

147. HICKMAN-BRENNER FW, VOHRA MP, HUNTLEY-CARTER GP ET AL: *Leminorella*, a new genus of Enterobacteriaceae: identification of *Leminorella grimontii* sp. nov. and *Leminorella richardii* sp. nov. found in clinical specimens. J Clin Microbiol 21:234–239, 1985

148. HODGES GR, DEGENER CE, BARNES WG: Clinical significance of *Citrobacter* isolates. Am J Clin Pathol 70:37–40, 1978

149. HOLLIS DG, HICKMAN FW, FANNING GR ET AL: *Tatumella ptyseos* gen. nov., sp. nov., a member of the family Enterobacteriaceae found in clinical specimens. J Clin Microbiol 14:79–88, 1981

150. HOLMES B, COSTAS M, GANNER M, ON SLW, STEVENS M: Evaluation of Biolog system for identification of some gram-negative bacteria of clinical importance. J Clin Microbiol 32:1970–1975, 1994

151. HOLT-HARRIS JE, TEAGUE O: A new culture medium for the isolation of *Bacillus typhosus* from stools. J Infect Dis 18:596–600, 1916

152. HOPPE JE, HERTER M, ALEKSIC S, KLINGEBIEL T, NIETHAMMER D: Catheter-related *Rahnella aquatilis* bacteremia in a pediatric bone marrow transplant recipient. J Clin Microbiol 31:1911–1912, 1993

153. HOROWITZ HW, NADELMAN RB, VAN HORN KG, WEEKES SE, GOYBURU L, WORMSER GP: *Serratia plymuthica* sepsis associated with infection of central venous catheter. J Clin Microbiol 25:1562–1563, 1987

154. HUBER TW, THOMAS JS: Detection of resistance due to inducible β-lactamase in *Enterobacter aerogenes* and *Enterobacter cloacae*. J Clin Microbiol 32:2481–2486, 1994

155. INQUE K, MIKI K, TAMURA K, SAKAZAKI R: Evaluation of L-pyrrolidonyl peptidase paper strip test for differentiation of members of the family Enterobacteriaceae, particularly *Salmonella* spp. J Clin Microbiol 34:1811–1812, 1996

156. IZARD D, FERRAGUT C, GAVINI F, KERSTERS K, DE LEY J, LECLERC H: *Klebsiella terrigena*, a new species from soil and water. Int J Syst Bacteriol 31:116–127, 1981

157. IZARD D, GAVINI F, TRINEL PA, LECLERC H: *Rahnella aquatilis*, nouveau membre de la famille des Enterobacteriaceae. Ann Microbiol 130A:163–177, 1979

158. IZARD D, GAVINI F, TRINEL, LECLERC H: Deoxyribonucleic acid relatedness between *Enterobacter cloacae* and *Enterobacter amnigenus* sp. nov. Int J Syst Bacteriol 31:35–42, 1981

159. JACOBS J, JAMAER D, VANDEVEN J, WOUTERS M, VERMYLEN C, VANDEPITTE J: *Yersinia enterocolitica* in donor blood: a case report and review. J Clin Microbiol 27:1119–1121, 1989

160. JACOBY GA, HAN P: Detection of extended-spectrum β-lactamases in clinical isolates of *Klebsiella pneumoniae* and *Escherichia coli*. J Clin Microbiol 34:908–911, 1996

161. JANDA JM, ABBOTT SL: Infections associated with the genus *Edwardsiella*: the role of *Edwardsiella tarda* in human disease. Clin Infect Dis 17:742–748, 1993

162. JANDA JM, ABBOTT SL: Expression of an iron-regulated hemolysin by *Edwardsiella tarda*. FEMS Microbial Lett 111:275–280, 1993

163. JANDA JM, ABBOTT SL, CHEUNG WKW, HANSON DF: Biochemical identification of citrobacteria in the clinical laboratory. J Clin Microbiol 32:1850–1854, 1994

164. JANDA WM, HELLERMAN DV, ZEIGER B ET AL: Isolation of *Klebsiella ozaenae* from a corneal abscess. Am J Clin Pathol 83:655–657, 1985

165. JARLIER V, NICOLAS M-H, FOURNIER G, PHILIPPON A: Extended broad-spectrum β-lactamases conferring transferable resistance to newer β-lactam agents in Enterobacteriaceae: hospital prevalence and susceptibility patterns. Rev Infect Dis 10:867–878, 1988

166. JENSEN KT, FREDERIKSEN W, HICKMAN-BRENNER FW, STEIGERWALT AG, RIDDLE CF, BRENNER DJ: Recognition of *Morganella* subspecies, with proposal of *Morganella morganii* subsp. *morganii* subsp. nov. and *Morganella morganii* subsp. *sibonii* subsp. nov. Int J Syst Bacteriol 42:613–620, 1992

167. JOKER RN, NORHOLM T, SIBONI KE: A case of neonatal meningitis caused by a yellow *Enterobacter*. Dan Med Bull 12:128–130, 1965

168. KARCH H, JANETZKI-MITTMANN C, ALEKSIC S, DATZ M: Isolation of enterohemorrhagic *Escherichia coli* 0157 strains from patients with hemolytic–uremic syndrome by using immunomagnetic separation, DNA-based methods, and direct culture. J Clin Microbiol 34: 516–519, 1996

169. KARMALI MA: Infection by verocytotoxin-producing *Escherichia coli*. Clin Microbiol Rev 2:15–38, 1989

170. KARMALI MA, STEELE BT, PETRIC M ET AL: Sporadic cases of hemolytic uremic syndrome associated with fecal cytotoxin and cytotoxin-producing *Escherichia coli*. Lancet 1:619–620, 1983

171. KELLY MT, LEICESTER C: Evaluation of the Autoscan Walkaway system for rapid identification and susceptibility testing of gram-negative bacilli. J Clin Microbiol 30:1568–1571, 1992

172. KEREN DF, RAWLINGS W, MURRAY HW, LEONARD WR: *Arizona hinshawii* osteomyelitis with antecedent enteric fever and sepsis. Am J Med 60:577–582, 1976

173. KEVILLE MW, DOERN GV: Evaluation of the DMS Rapid E system for identification of clinical isolates of the family Enterobacteriaceae. J Clin Microbiol 20:1010–1011, 1984

174. KILIAN M, BULOW P: Rapid diagnosis of Enterobacteriaceae. I. Detection of bacterial glycosidases. Acta Pathol Microbiol Scand Sect B 84:245–251, 1976

175. KING BM, ADLER DL: A previously unclassified group of Enterobacteriaceae. Am J Clin Pathol 41:230–232, 1964

176. KING S, METZGER WI: A new plating medium for the isolation of enteric pathogens: I. Hektoen enteric agar. Appl Microbiol 16:577–578, 1968

177. KITCH TT, JACOBS MR, APPELBAUM PC: Evaluation of RapID onE system for identificaiton of 379 strains in the family Enterobacteriaceae and oxidase-negative, gram-negative nonfermenters. J Clin Microbiol 32:931–934, 1994

178. KKEIMAN MB, ALLEN SD, NEAL P, REYNOLDS J: Meningoencephalitis and compartmentalization of the cerebral ventricles caused by *Enterobacter sakazakii.* J Clin Microbiol 14:352–354, 1981

179. KLINE MW: *Citrobacter* meningitis and brain abscess in infancy: epidemiology, pathogenesis, and treatment. J Pediatr 113:430–434, 1988

180. KLINE MW, MASON EO, KAPLAN SL: Characterization of *Citrobacter diversus* strains causing neonatal meningitis. J Infect Dis 157:101–105, 1988

181. KNIGHT P: Hemorrhagic *E. coli*: the danger increases. ASM News 59:247–250, 1993

182. KOSAKO Y, SAKAZAKI R: Priority of *Yokenella regensburgei* Kosako, Sakazaki, and Yoshizaki 1985 over *Koserella trabulsii* Hickman-Brenner, Huntley-Carter, Brenner, and Farmer 1985. Int J Syst Bacteriol 41:171, 1991

183. KOSARO Y, SAKAZAKI R, YOSHIZAKI E: *Yokenella regensburgei* gen. nov., sp. nov.: a new genus and species in the family Enterobacteriaceae. Jpn J Med Sci Biol 37:117–124, 1984

184. KRAJDEN S, FUKSA M, PETREA C ET AL: Expanded clinical spectrum of infections caused by *Proteus penneri.* J Clin Microbiol 25:578–579, 1987

185. LAW D: Adhesion and its role in the virulence of enteropathogenic *Escherichia coli.* Clin Microbiol Rev 7:152–173, 1994

186. LEE LA, GERBER AR, LONSWAY DR, SMITH JD, CARTER GP, PUHR ND, PARRISH CM, SIKES RK, FINTON RJ, TAUXE RV: *Yersinia enterocolitica* 0:3 infections in infants and children, associated with the household preparation of chitterlings. N Engl J Med 322:984–987, 1990

187. LEE LA, TAYLOR J, CARTER GP, QUINN B, FARMER III JJ, TAUXE RV, AND THE YERSINIA ENTEROCOLITICA COLLABORATIVE STUDY GROUP: *Yersinia enterocolitica* 0:3: an emerging cause of pediatric gastroenteritis in the United States. J Infect Dis 163:660–663, 1991

188. LEVINE MM: *Escherichia coli* that cause diarrhea: enterotoxigenic, enteropathogenic, enteroinvasive, enterohemorrhagic, and enteroadherent. J Infect Dis 155:377–389, 1987

189. LEVY RL, SAUNDERS RL: *Citrobacter* meningitis and cerebral abscess in early infancy: cure by moxalactam. Neurology 31:1575–1577, 1981

190. LIVERMORE DM: β-Lactamases in laboratory and clinical resistance. Clin Microbiol Rev 8:557–584, 1995

191. LJUNGBERG P, VALTONEN M, HARJOLA VP, KAUKORANTA-TOLVANEN SS, VAARA M: Report of four cases of *Yersinia pseudotuberculosis* septicemia and a literature review. Eur J Clin Microbiol Infect Dis 14:804–810, 1995

192. LUND ME, MATSEN JM, BLAZEVIC DJ: Biochemical and antibiotic susceptibility studies of H2S-negative *Citrobacter.* Appl Microbiol 28:22–25, 1974

193. LUTTRELL RE, RANNICK GA, SOTO-HERNANDEZ JL, VERGHESE A: *Kluyvera* species soft tissue infection: case report and review. J Clin Microbiol 26:2650–2651, 1988

194. MACCONKEY A: Lactose-fermenting bacteria in feces. J Hyg 5:333–378, 1905

195. MACFADDIN JF: Media for Isolation-Cultivation-Identification-Maintenance of Medical Bacteria, vol 1. Baltimore, Williams & Wilkins, 1985

196. MAKI DG, RHAME FS, MACKEL DC ET AL: Nationwide epidemic of septicemia caused by contaminated intravenous products: epidemiologic and clinical features. Am J Med 60:471–485, 1976

197. MANGUM ME, RADISCH D: *Cedecea* species: unusual clinical isolate. Clin Microbiol Newsl 4:117–119, 1982

198. MARAKI S, SAMONIS G, MARNELAKIS E, TSELENTIS Y: Surgical wound infection caused by *Rahnella aquatilis.* J Clin Microbiol 32:2706–2708, 1994

199. MARCH SB, RATNAM S: Sorbitol-MacConkey medium for detection of *Escherichia coli* 0157:H7 associated with hemorrhagic colitis. J Clin Microbiol 23:869–872, 1986

200. MARIANI-KURKDJIAN P, DENAMUR E, MILON A, PICARD B, CAVE H, LAMBERT-ZECHOVSKY N, LOIRAT C, GOULLET P, SANSONETTI PJ, ELION J: Identification of a clone of *Escherichia coli* 0103:H2 as a potential agent of hemolytic-uremic syndrome in France. J Clin Microbiol 31:296–301, 1993

201. MARSH PK, GORBACH SL: Invasive enterocolitis caused by *Edwardsiella tarda.* Gastroenterology 82:336–338, 1982

202. MASKELL R, PEAD L: A cluster of *Edwardsiella tarda* infection in a day-care center in Florida. J Infect Dis 162:782–783, 1990

203. MASTROIANNI A, CORONADO O, CHIODO F: *Morganella morganii* meningitis in a patient with AIDS. J Infect 29:356–357, 1994

204. MAZOYER MA, ORENGA S, DOLEANS F, FRENEY J: Evaluation of CPS ID2 medium for detection of urinary tract bacterial isolates in specimens from a rehabilitation center. J Clin Microbiol 33:1025–1027, 1995

205. MCNEIL MM, DAVIS BJ, SOLOMON SL, ANDERSON RL, SHULMAN ST, GARDNER S, KABAT K, MARTONE WJ: *Ewingella americana*: recurrent pseudobacteremia from a persistent environmental reservoir. J Clin Microbiol 25:498–500, 1987

206. MCWHORTER AC, HADDOCK RL, NOCON FA, STEIGERWALT AG, BRENNER DJ, ALEKSIC S, BOCKEMUHL J, FARMER JJ III: *Trabulsiella guamensis*, a new genus and species of the Family Enterobacteriaceae that resembles *Salmonella* subgroups 4 and 5. J Clin Microbiol 29:1480–1485, 1991.

207. MERMEL LA, SPIEGEL CA: Nosocomial sepsis due to *Serratia odorifera* biovar 1. Clin Infect Dis 14:208–210, 1992

208. METCHOCK B, LONSWAY DR, CARTER GP, LEE LA, MCGOWAN JE JR: *Yersinia enterocolitica*: a frequent seasonal stool isolate from children at an urban hospital in the southeast United States. J Clin Microbiol 29:2868–2869, 1991

209. MEYER KS, URBAN C, EAGAN JA, BERGER BJ, RAHAL JJ: Nosocomial outbreak of *Klebsiella* infection resistant to late-generation cephalosporins. Ann Intern Med 119:353–358, 1993

210. MILLER JM, ALACHI P: Evaluation of new computer-enhanced identification program for microorganisms: adaption of BioBASE for identification of members of the family Enterobacteriaceae. J Clin Microbiol 34:179–181, 1996

211. MILLER JM, RHODEN DL: Preliminary evaluation of Biolog, a carbon source utilization method for bacterial identification. J Clin Microbiol 29:1143–1147, 1991

212. MILLER RG, TATE CR, MALLINSON ET: Xylose–lysine–tergitol 4: an improved selective agar medium for the isolation of *Salmonella*. Poultry Sci 70:2429–2432, 1991 (Erratum, 71:398, 1992)

213. MOELLER V: Simplified tests for some amino acid decarboxylases and for the arginine-dihydrolase system. Acta Pathol Microbiol Immunol Scand 36:158–172, 1955

214. MONNERY I, FREYDIERE AM, BARON C, ROUSSET AM, TIGAUD S, BOUDE-CHEVALIER M, DE MONTCLOS H, GILLE Y: Evaluation of two new chromogenic media for detection of *Salmonella* in stools. Eur J Clin Microbiol Infect Dis 13:257–261, 1994

215. MONTERO M, SCHRECKENBERGER PC, HELDT N: Evaluation of the RapID onE system for identification of Enterobacteriaceae. Manuscript in preparation

216. MOSS NS, WILDER D, COMBS D, MONROE D, MAYER J, MORRIS R: Evaluation of the Vitek GNI+ Card. Abstr Annu Meet Am Soc Microbiol C389, 1996

217. MULCZYK M, SZEWCZUK A: Pyrrolidonyl peptidase in bacteria: a new colorimetric test for differentiation of Enterobacteriaceae. J Gen Microbiol 61:9–13, 1970

218. MULLER HE, BRENNER DJ, FANNING GR, GRIMONT PAD, KAMPFER P: Emended description of *Buttiauxella agrestis* with recognition of six new species of *Buttiauxella* and two new species of *Kluyvera*: *Buttiauxella ferragutiae* sp. nov., *Buttiauxella gaviniae* sp. nov., *Buttiauxella brennerae* sp. nov., *Buttiauxella izardii* sp. nov., *Buttiauxella noackiae* sp. nov., *Buttiauxella warmboldiae* sp. nov., *Kluyvera cochleae* sp. nov., and *Kluyvera georgiana* sp. nov. Int J Syst Bacteriol 46:50–63, 1996

219. MULLER HE, O'HARA CM, FANNING GR ET AL: *Providencia heimbachae*, a new species of Enterobacteriaceae isolated from animals. Int J Syst Bacteriol 36:252–256, 1986

220. MUYTJENS HL, ZANEN HC, SONDERKAMP HJ, KOLLEE LA, WACHSMUTH IK, FARMER JJ III: Analysis of eight cases of neonatal meningitis and sepsis due to *Enterobacter sakazakii*. J Clin Microbiol 18:115–120, 1983

221. NADLER HL, DOLAN C, MELE L ET AL: Accuracy and reproducibility of the AutoMicrobic system gram-negative general susceptibility-plus card for testing selected challenge organisms. J Clin Microbiol 22:355–360, 1985

222. O'BRIEN AD, HOLMES RK: Shiga and Shiga-like toxins. Microbiol Rev 51:206–220, 1987

223. OHANESSIAN JH, FOURCADE N, PRIOLET B, RICHARD C, BASHOUR G, DUGELAY M: A propos d'une infection vesiculaire par *Moellerella wisconsensis*. Med Maladies Infect 6:414–416, 1987

224. O'HARA CM, MILLER JM: Evaluation of the autoSCAN-W/A system for rapid (2-hour) identification of members of the family Enterobacteriaceae. J Clin Microbiol 30:1541–1543, 1992

225. O'HARA CM, ROMAN SB, MILLER JM: Ability of commercial identification systems to identify newly recognized species of *Citrobacter*. J Clin Microbiol 33:242–245, 1995

226. O'HARA CM, STEIGERWALT AG, HILL BC, FARMER JJ III, FANNING GR, BRENNER DJ: *Enterobacter hormaechei*, a new species of the family Enterobacteriaceae formerly known as enteric group 75. J Clin Microbiol 27:2046–2049, 1989

227. O'HARA CM, TENOVER FC, MILLER JM: Parallel comparison of accuracy of API 20E, Vitek GNI, MicroScan Walk/Away Rapid ID, and Becton Dickinson Cobas Micro ID-E/NF for identificaiton of members of the family Enterobacteriaceae and common gram-negative, non–glucose-fermenting bacilli. J Clin Microbiol 31:3165–3169, 1993

228. OKREND AJG, ROSE BE, LATTUADA CP: Use of 5-bromo-4-chloro-3-indoxyl-β-D-glucuronide in MacConkey sorbitol agar to aid in the isolation of *Escherichia coli* 0157:H7 from ground beef. J Food Prot 53:941–943, 1990

229. OLSSON M, SYK A, WOLLIN R: Identification of salmonellae with the 4-methylumbelliferyl caprilate fluorescence test. J Clin Microbiol 29:2631–2632, 1991

230. OLSVIK O, SORUM H, BIRKNESS K ET AL: Plasmid characterization of *Salmonella typhimurium* transmitted from animals to humans. J Clin Microbiol 22:336–338, 1985

231. OTANI E, BRUCKNER DA: *Leclercia adecarboxylata* isolated from a blood culture. Clin Microbiol Newsl 13:157–158, 1991

232. OVERMAN TL, PLUMLEY D, OVERMAN SB ET AL: Comparison of the API Rapid E four-hour system with the API 20E overnight system for the identification of routine clinical isolates of the family Enterobacteriaceae. J Clin Microbiol 21:542–545, 1985

233. PAI CH, SORGER S, LAFLEUR L ET AL: Efficacy of cold enrichment techniques for recovery of *Yersinia enterocolitica* from human stools. J Clin Microbiol 9:712–715, 1979

234. PARRY MF, HUTCHINSON JH, BROWN NA, WU C-H, ESTRELLER L: Gram-negative sepsis in neonates: a nursery outbreak due to hand carriage of *Citrobacter diversus*. Pediatrics 65:1105–1109, 1980

235. PATON AW, PATON JC: *Enterobacter cloacae* producing a Shiga-like toxin II-related cytotoxin associated with a case of hemolytic–uremic syndrome. J Clin Microbiol 34:463–465, 1996

236. PATON AW, RATCLIFF RM, DOYLE RM, SEYMOUR-MURRAY J, DAVOS D, LANSER JA, PATON JC: Molecular microbiological investigation of an outbreak of hemolytic–uremic syndrome caused by dry fermented sausage contaminated with Shiga-like toxin-producing *Escherichia coli*. J Clin Microbiol 34:1622–1627, 1996

237. PATTYN SR, SION JP, VERHOEVEN J: Evaluation of the LOGIC system for the rapid identification of members of the family Enterobacteriaceae in the clinical microbiology laboratory. J Clin Microbiol 28:1449–1450, 1990

238. PENNER JL: Genus XII. *Providencia* Ewing 1962, 96AL. In Krieg NR, Holt JG (eds): Bergey's Manual of Systematic Bacteriology, vol 1, pp 494–496. Baltimore, Williams & Wilkins, 1984

239. PERKINS SR, BECKETT TA, BUMP CM: *Cedecea davisae* bacteremia. J Clin Microbiol 24:675–676, 1986

240. PERRY JD, FORD M, HJERSING N, GOULD FK: Rapid conventional scheme for biochemical identification of antibiotic-resistant Enterobacteriaceae isolates from urine. J Clin Pathol 41:1010–1012, 1988

241. PFALLER MA, SAHM D, O'HARA C, CIAGLIA C, YU M, YAMANE N, SCHARNWEBER G, RHODEN D: Comparison of the

AutoSCAN-W/A rapid bacterial identification system and the Vitek AutoMicrobic System for identification of gram-negative bacilli. J Clin Microbiol 29:1422–1428, 1991

242. PFYFFER GE: *Serratia fonticola* as an infectious agent. Eur J Clin Microbiol Infect Dis 11:199–200, 1992

243. PIEN FD, BRUCE AE: *Ewingella americana*: bacteremia in an intensive care unit. Arch Intern Med 146:111–112, 1986

244. PIEN FD, FARMER JJ III, WEAVER RE: Polymicrobial bacteremia caused by *Ewingella americana* (family Enterobacteriaceae) and an unusual *Pseudomonas* species. J Clin Microbiol 18:727–729, 1983

245. PIEN FD, SHRUM S, SWENSON JM ET AL: Colonization of human wounds by *Escherichia vulneris* and *Escherichia hermannii*. J Clin Microbiol 22:283–285, 1985

246. PODSCHUN R: Isolation of *Kelbsiella terrigena* from human feces: biochemical reactions, capsule types, and antibiotic sensitivity. Zentralblat Bakteriol 275:73–78, 1991

247. PODSCHUN R, ULLMANN U: Isolation of *Klebsiella terrigena* from clinical specimens. Eur J Clin Microbiol Infect Dis 11:349–352, 1992

248. POISSON DM: Novobiocin, brilliant green, glycerol, lactose agar: a new medium for the isolation of *Salmonella* strains. Res Microbiol 143:211–216, 1992

249. POUPART MC, MOUNIER M, DENIS F, SIROT J, COUTURIER C, VILLEVAL F: A new chromogenic ready-to-use medium for *Salmonella* detection, abstr. 1254, In Abstracts of the 5th European Congress of Clinical Microbiology and Infectious Diseases, Oslo, Norway, 1991

250. PRIEST FG, SOMERVILLE HJ, COLE JA ET AL: The taxonomic position of *Obesumbacterium proteus*, a common brewery contaminant. J Gen Microbiol 75:295–307, 1973

251. QADRI SMH, ZUBAIRI S, HAWLEY HP ET AL: Simple spot test for rapid detection of urease activity. J Clin Microbiol 20:1198–1199, 1984

252. RAJ P: Pathogenesis and laboratory diagnosis of *Escherichia coli*-associated enteritis. Clin Microbiol Newsletter 15:89–93, 1993

253. RAMBACH A: New plate medium for facilitated differentiation of *Salmonella* spp. from *Proteus* spp. and other enteric bacteria. Appl Environ Microbiol 56:301–303, 1990

254. RATNAM S: Etiologic role of *Hafnia alvei* in human diarrheal illness. Infect Immun 59:4744–4745, 1991 (letter)

255. RATNAM S, BUTLER RW, MARCH S, PARSONS S, CLARKE P, BELL A, HOGAN K: *Enterobacter hafniae*-associated gastroenteritis—Newfoundland. Can Dis Weekly Rep 5:231–232, 1979

256. REED WP ET AL: Bubonic plague in the southwestern United States. Medicine 49:465–486, 1970

257. REINA J, ALOMAR P: *Enterobacter taylorae* wound infection. Clin Microbiol Newsl 11:134–135, 1989

258. REINA J, BORRELL N, LLOMPART I: Community-acquired bacteremia caused by *Serratia plymuthica*: case report and review of the literature. Diagn Microbiol Infect Dis 15:449–452, 1992

259. REINA J, HERVAS J, BORRELL N: Acute gastroenteritis caused by *Hafnia alvei* in children. Clin Infect Dis 16:443, 1993 (letter)

260. REINA J, SALVA F, GIL J, ALOMAR P: Urinary tract infection caused by *Enterobacter taylorae*. J Clin Microbiol 27:2877, 1989

261. REYNOLDS HY: Pneumonia due to *Klebsiella* (Friedlanders pneumonia). In Wyngaarden JB, Smith LH (eds): Cecil Textbook of Medicine, 16th ed, pp 1430–1432. Philadelphia, WB Saunders, 1982

262. RHOADS S, MARINELLI L, IMPERATRICE CA, NACHAMKIN I: Comparison of MicroScan WalkAway system and Vitek system for identification of gram-negative bacteria. J Clin Microbiol 33:3044–3046, 1995

263. RHODEN DL, SMITH PB, BAKER CN ET AL: AutoSCAN-4 system for identification of gram-negative bacilli. J Clin Microbiol 22:915–918, 1985

264. RICHARD C: Nouvelles Enterobacteriaceae rencontrees en bacteriologie medicale: *Moellerella wisconsensis, Koserella trabulsii, Leclercia adecarboxylata, Escherichia fergusonii, Enterobacter asburiae, Rahnella aquatilis*. Ann Biol Clin 47:231–236, 1989

265. RIDELL J, SIITONEN A, PAULIN L, LINDROOS O, KORKEALA H, ALBERT MJ: Characterization of *Hafnia alvei* by biochemical tests, random amplified polymorphic DNA PCR, and partial sequencing of 16S rRNA gene. J Clin Microbiol 33:2372–2376, 1995

266. RIDELL J, SIITONEN A, PAULIN L, MATTILA L, KORKEALA H, ALBERT MJ: *Hafnia alvei* in stool specimens from patients with diarrhea and healthy controls. J Clin Microbiol 32:2335–2337, 1994

267. RILEY LW, REMIS RS, HELGERSON SD ET AL: Hemorrhagic colitis associated with rare *Escherichia coli* serotypes. N Engl J Med 308:681–685, 1983

268. ROBINSON A, MCCARTER YS, TETREAULT J: Comparison of Crystal enteric/nonfermenter system, API 20E system, and Vitek automicrobic system for identification of gram-negative bacilli. J Clin Microbiol 33:364–370, 1995

269. RUBINSTIEN EM, KLEVJER-ANDERSON P, SMITH CA, DROUIN MT, PATTERSON JE: *Enterobacter taylorae*, a new opportunistic pathogen: report of four cases. J Clin Microbiol 31:249–254, 1993

270. RUIZ J, NUNEZ M-L, DIAZ J, LORENTE I, PEREZ J, GOMEZ J: Comparison of five plating media for isolation of *Salmonella* species from human stools. J Clin Microbiol 34:686–688, 1996

271. RUIZ J, NUNEZ M-L, SEMPERE MA, DIAZ J, GOMEZ J: Systemic infections in three infants due to a lactose-fermenting strain of *Salmonella virchow*. Eur J Clin Microbiol Infect Dis 14:454–456, 1995

272. RUIZ J, SEMPERE MA, VARELA MC, GOMEZ J: Modification of the methodology of stool culture for *Salmonella* detection. J Clin Microbiol 30:525–526, 1992

273. RUIZ J, VARELA MC, SEMPERE MA, LOPEZ ML, GOMEZ J, OLIVA J: Presumptive identification of *Salmonella enterica* using two rapid tests. Eur J Clin Microbiol Infect Dis 10:649–651, 1991

274. SACK RB: Human diarrheal disease caused by enterotoxigenic *Escherichia coli*. Annu Rev Microbiol 29:333–353, 1975

275. SAKAZAKI R, MURATA Y: The new group of Enterobacteriaceae: the Asakusa group. Jpn J Bacteriol 17:616–617, 1963

276. SANDERS CC, MOELLERING RC JR, MARTIN RR ET AL: Resistance to cefamandole: a collaborative study of emerging clinical problems. J Infect Dis 145:118–125, 1982

277. SANDERS CC, SANDERS WE JR: Emergence of resistance during drug therapy with newer beta lactam antibi-

otics: role of inducible beta lactamases and implications for the future. Rev Infect Dis 5:639–648, 1983

278. SAUTTER RL, MATTMAN LH, LEGASPI RC: *Serratia marcescens* meningitis associated with a contaminated benzalkonium chloride solution. Infect Control 5: 223–225, 1984

279. SCHAUER DB, ZABEL BA, PEDRAZA IF, O'HARA CM, STEIGERWALT AG, BRENNER DJ: Genetic and biochemical characterization of *Citrobacter rodentium* sp. nov. J Clin Microbiol 33:2064–2068, 1995

280. SCHIEVEN BC: Evaluation of Rainbow UTI system for rapid isolation and identification of urinary pathogens. Abstr Annu Meet Am Soc Microbiol C375, p. 65, 1995

281. SCHIEVEN BC, HUSSAIN Z, LANNIGAN R: Comparison of American MicroScan dry frozen microdilution trays. J Clin Microbiol 22:495–496, 1985

282. SCHONHEYDER HC, JENSEN KT, FREDERIKSEN W: Taxonomic notes: synonymy of *Enterobacter cancerogenus* (Urosevic 1966) Dickey and Zumoff 1988 and *Enterobacter taylorae* Farmer el al. 1985 and resolution of an ambiguity in the biochemical profile. Int J Syst Bacteriol 44:586–587, 1994

283. SCHRECKENBERGER PC, BLAZEVIC DJ: Rapid methods for biochemical testing of anaerobic bacteria. Appl Microbiol 28:759–762, 1974

284. SHARMA NK, DOYLE PW, GERBASI SA, JESSOP JH: Identification of *Yersinia* species by the API 20E. J Clin Microbiol 28:1443–1444, 1990

285. SIERRA-MADERO J, PRATT K, HALL GS, STEWART RW, SCERBO JJ, LONGWORTH DL: *Kluyvera* mediastinitis following open-heart surgery: a case report. J Clin Microbiol 28:2848–2849, 1990

286. SILVERBLATT FJ, WEINSTEIN R: Enterobacteriaceae. In Mandell GL, Douglas RG Jr, Bennett JE (eds): Principles and Practice of Infectious Disease, 2nd ed, pp 1226–1236. New York, John Wiley & Sons, 1985

287. SIMMONS JS: A culture medium for differentiating organisms of typhoid-colon aerogenes groups and for isolation of certain fungi. J Infect Dis 39:209–214, 1926

288. SMITH PB: Performance of Six Bacterial Identification Systems. Atlanta, Centers for Disease Control, Bacteriology Division, 1975

289. STAGER CE, DAVIS JR: Automated systems for identification of microorganisms. Clin Microbiol Rev 5:302–327, 1992

290. STANECK JL, VINCELETTE J, LAMOTHE F ET AL: Evaluation of the sensititre system for identification of Enterobacteriaceae. J Clin Microbiol 17:647–654, 1983

291. STENHOUSE MAE, MILNER LV: *Yersinia enterocolitica*: a hazard in blood transfusion. Transfusion 22:396–398, 1982

292. TAMURA K, SAKAZAKI R, KOSAKO Y, YOSHIZAKI E: *Leclercia adecarboxylata* gen. nov., comb. nov., formerly known as *Escherichia adecarboxylata*. Curr Microbiol 13:179–184, 1986

293. TARR PI: *Escherichia coli* 0157:H7: clinical, diagnostic, and epidemiological aspects of human infection. Clin Infect Dis 20:1–10, 1995

294. TAUXE RV, VANDEPITTE J, WAUTERS G, MARTIN SM, GOOSSENS V, DE MOL P, VAN NOYEN R, THIERS G: *Yersinia enterocolitica* infections and pork: the missing link. Lancet 1:1129–1132, 1987

295. TAYLOR WI: Isolation of *Shigellae*: I. Xylose lysine agars: new media for isolation of enteric pathogens. Am J Clin Pathol 44:471–475, 1965

296. TAYLOR WI, ACHANZAR D: Catalase test as an aid to the identification of Enterobacteriaceae. Appl Microbiol 24:58–61, 1972

297. THALLER R, BERLUTTI F, THALLER MC: A *Kluyvera cryocrescens* strain from a gallbladder infection. Eur J Epidemiol 4:124–126, 1988

298. THOMPSON JS, BORCZYK AA: Use of a single-tube medium, *o*-nitrophenyl-beta-D-galactopyranoside-phenylalanine-motility-sulfate, for screening of pathogenic members of the family Enterobacteriaceae. J Clin Microbiol 20:136–137, 1984

299. THOMPSON JS, HODGE DS, BORCZYK AA: Rapid biochemical test to identify verocytotoxin-positive strains of *Escherichia coli* serotype 0157. J Clin Microbiol 28:2165–2168, 1990

300. TIPPLE MA, BLAND LA, MURPHY JJ ET AL: Sepsis associated with transfusion of red cells contaminated with *Yersinia enterocolitica*. Transfusion 30:207–213, 1990

301. TREPETA RW, EDBERG SC: Methylumbelliferyl-beta-D-glucuronide-based medium for rapid isolation and identification of *Escherichia coli*. J Clin Microbiol 19: 172–174, 1984

302. TRISTRAM DA, FORBES BA: *Kluyvera*: a case report of urinary tract infection and sepsis. Pediatr Infect Dis J 7:297–298, 1988

303. TULLOCK EF JR, RYAN KJ, FORMAL SB ET AL: Invasive enteropathogenic *Escherichia coli* dysentery. Ann Intern Med 79:13–17, 1973

304. URMENYI AMC, WHITE-FRANKLIN A: Neonatal death from pigmented coliform infection. Lancet 1:313–315, 1961

305. URSING J, BRENNER DJ, BERCOVIER H ET AL: *Yersinia frederiksenii*: a new species of Enterobacteriaceae composed of rhamnose-positive strains (formerly called atypical *Yersinia enterocolitica* or *Yersinia enterocolitica*-like). Curr Microbiol 4:213–217, 1980

306. URSUA PR, UNZAGA MJ, MELERO P, ITURBURU I, EZPELETA C, CISTERNA R: *Serratia rubidaea* as an invasive pathogen. J Clin Microbiol 34:216–217, 1996

307. VANDEPITTE J, LEMMENS P, DE SWERT L: Human edwardsiellosis traced to ornamental fish. J Clin Microbiol 17:165–167, 1983

308. VERBOON-MACIOLEK M, VANDERTOP WP, PETERS ACB, ROORD JJ, GEELEN SPM: Neonatal brain abscess caused by *Morganella morganii*. Clin Infect Dis 20:471, 1995

309. VOGEL LC, FERGUSON L, GOTOFF SP: *Citrobacter* infections of the central nervous system in early infancy. J Pediatr 93:86–88, 1978

310. WAGNER SJ, FRIEDMAN LI, DODD RY: Transfusion-associated bacterial sepsis. Clin Microbiol Rev 7:290–302, 1994

311. WALLET F, FRUCHART A, BOUVET PJM, COURCOL RJ: Isolation of *Moellerella wisconsensis* from bronchial aspirate. Eur J Clin Microbiol Infect Dis 13:182–183, 1994 (letter)

312. WATERMAN SH, JUAREZ G, CARR SJ, KILMAN L: *Salmonella arizona* infections in Latinos associated with rattlesnake folk medicine. Am J Public Health 80:286–289, 1990

313. WAUTERS G, BOEL A, VOORN GP, VERHAEGEN J, MEUNIER F, JANSSENS M, VERBIST L: Evaluation of a new identifica-

tion system, Crystal enteric/non-fermenter, for gram-negative bacilli. J Clin Microbiol 33:845–849, 1995

314. WAUTERS G, JANSSENS M, STEIGERWALT AG, BRENNER DJ: *Yersinia mollaretii* sp. nov. and *Yersinia bercovieri* sp. nov., formerly called *Yersinia enterocolitica* biogroups 3A and 3B. Int J Syst Bacteriol 38:424–429, 1988

315. WEISSFELD AS, SONNENWIRTH AC: Rapid isolation of *Yersinia* spp. from feces. J Clin Microbiol 15:508–510, 1982

316. WERNER SB, WEIDMER CE, NELSON BC, ET AL.:Primary plague pneumonia contracted from a domestic cat at South Lake Tahoe, Calif. JAMA 251:929–931, 1984

317. WESTBLOM TU, COGGINS ME: Osteomyelitis caused by *Enterobacter taylorae*, formerly enteric group 19. J Clin Microbiol 25:2432–2433, 1987

318. WESTBLOM TU, MILLIGAN TW: Acute bacterial gastroenteritis caused by *Hafnia alvi*. Clin Infect Dis 14:1271–1272, 1992 (letter)

319. WILSON JP, WATERER RR, WOFFORD JD JR, CHAPMAN SW: Serious infections with *Edwardsiella tarda*, a case report and review of the literature. Arch Intern Med 149:208–210, 1989

320. WITTKE J-W, ALEKSIC S, WUTHE H-H: Isolation of *Moellerella wisconsensis* from an infected human gallbladder. Eur J Clin Microbiol 4:351–352, 1985 (letter)

321. WONG, VK: Broviac catheter infection with *Kluyvera cryocrescens*: a case report. J Clin Microbiol 25:1115–1116, 1987

322. WOOLFREY BF, LALLY RT, EDERER MN ET AL: Evaluation of the AutoMicrobic system for identification and susceptibility testing of gram-negative bacilli. J Clin Microbiol 20:1053–1059, 1984

323. WOOLFREY BF, LALLY RT, QUALL CO: Evaluation of the AutoSCAN-3 and Sceptor systems for Enterobacteriaceae identification. J Clin Microbiol 17:807–813, 1983

324. WU M-S, SHYU R-S, LAI, M-Y, HUANG G-T, CHEN D-S, WANG T-H: A predisposition toward *Edwardsiella tarda* bacteremia in individuals with preexisting liver disease. Clin Infect Dis 21:705–706, 1995

325. YONG DCT, THOMPSON JS, PRYTULA A: Rapid microbiochemical method for presumptive identification of gastroenteritis-associated members of the family Enterobacteriaceae. J Clin Microbiol 21:914–918, 1985

326. YORK MK, BROOKS GF, FISS EH: Evaluation of the autoSCAN-W/A rapid system for identification and susceptibility testing of gram-negative fermentative bacilli. J Clin Microbiol 30:2903–2910, 1992

327. ZADIK PM, CHAPMAN PA, SIDDONS CA: Use of tellurite for the selection of verocytotoxigenic *Escherichia coli* 0157. J Med Microbiol 39:155–158, 1993

328. ZBINDEN R, BLASS R: *Serratia plymuthica* osteomyelitis following a motorcycle accident. J Clin Microbiol 26:1409–1410, 1988

329. ZOBELL CE: Factors influencing the reduction of nitrates and nitrites by bacteria in semisolid media. J Bacteriol 24:273–281, 1932

The Nonfermentative Gram-Negative Bacilli

The nonfermentative gram-negative bacilli are a group of aerobic, non–spore-forming, gram-negative bacilli that either do not utilize carbohydrates as a source of energy or degrade them through metabolic pathways other than fermentation. Within this group are several genera and species of bacteria with special growth requirements that are not discussed in this chapter. The dividing line between what is a "nonfermenter" and what may otherwise be designated a "fastidious," "unusual," or "miscellaneous" non–glucose-fermenting, gram-negative bacillus (discussed in Chap. 8) is based more on convention than on well-defined genetic or phenotypic characteristics. The term **nonfermentative gram-negative bacilli** is used in this chapter to mean all aerobic gram-negative rods that show abundant growth within 24 hours on the surface of Kligler iron agar (KIA) or triple sugar iron (TSI) medium, but neither grow in nor acidify the butt of these media.

The genera of nonfermenters to be discussed in this chapter include *Achromobacter, Acidovorax, Acinetobacter, Agrobacterium, Alcaligenes, Balneatrix, Bergeyella, Bordetella, Brevundimonas, Burkholderia, Chryseobacterium, Chryseomonas, Comamonas, Empedobacter, Flavimonas, Flavobacterium, Methylobacterium, Moraxella, Ochrobactrum, Oligella, Pseudomonas, Psychrobacter, Roseomonas, Shewanella, Sphingobacterium, Stenotrophomonas, Weeksella*, and a few organisms that currently carry only Centers for Disease Control (CDC) alpha-numeric designations. Also included in this chapter are a few species of *Neisseria* that appear as gram-negative rods and must be differentiated from similarly appearing nonfermenting bacilli. The genera *Eikenella, Brucella*, and *Francisella*, although possessing the general characteristics of nonfermenters, are grouped in this text with the fastidious, gram-negative bacilli and are discussed in Chapter 8. The currently accepted organism nomenclature and a listing of previous designations are presented in Table 5-1. The synonyms for several bacterial species either previously or currently having CDC alpha-numeric designations are presented in Table 5-2.

As more information accumulates, reclassification of bacteria between genera and species and the creation of new designations must be accepted as part of scientific progress. DNA homology studies often play a larger role in the ultimate classification of bacteria than a scheme based on phenotypic characteristics alone. For example, within the genus *Pseudomonas* several biovars and pathovars are now recognized, arranged according to rRNA and DNA homologies.[230] Despite refinements, clinical microbiologists must still recognize and classify clinical laboratory isolates based on morphologic and biochemical characteristics. Microbiologists must also keep abreast of changes in bacterial nomenclature so that current names can be used in everyday practice and research data gathered from various investigations using previous designations will not be misinterpreted.

Color Plates for Chapter 5 are found between pages 80 and 81.

METABOLISM OF THE NONFERMENTERS

Bacteria that derive their energy from organic compounds are known as **chemoorganotrophs**. Most of the bacteria encountered in clinical medicine derive energy from the utilization of carbohydrates by one of several metabolic pathways. Detection and measurement of various metabolic products are necessary to identify bacterial species that may be the cause of infectious disease. Some bacteria, such as members of the genus *Moraxella*, do not metabolize carbohydrates but rather derive energy from the degradation of other organic compounds, such as amino acids, alcohols, and organic acids. Some free-living bacteria, such as the nitrogen-fixing groups or those capable of oxidizing sulfur or iron, can derive energy from simple inorganic chemicals. These so-called *chemolithotrophs* are seldom implicated as causes of disease in humans.

Space in this text permits only a brief summary of the metabolic pathways used by the nonfermenters, enough to gain a working understanding of terms such as **aerobic, anaerobic, fermentation**, and **oxidation**. These metabolic processes not only define the taxonomic niche of bacteria but also determine the tests and procedures used in the laboratory identification of microorganisms. Texts by Doelle[70] and Thimann[309] should be consulted for a more detailed discussion of bacterial metabolism and physiology, and the texts by Blazevic and Ederer[24] and MacFaddin[186] provide a review of the biochemistry of the various tests and reactions used in making identifications.

FERMENTATIVE AND OXIDATIVE METABOLISM

The bacterial degradation of carbohydrates proceeds by several metabolic pathways in which hydrogen ions (electrons) are successively transferred to compounds of higher redox potential, with the ultimate release of energy in the form of adenosine triphosphate (ATP). All six-, five-, and four-carbon carbohydrates are initially degraded to pyruvic acid, an initial intermediate. Glucose is the main carbohydrate source of carbon for bacteria, and degradation proceeds by three major pathways: the Embden–Meyerhof–Parnas, the Entner–Doudoroff, and the Warburg–Dickins (hexose monophosphate) pathways. As shown in Figure 5-1, glucose is converted to pyruvic acid in each of these three pathways by a different set of degradation steps. Bacteria use one or more of these pathways for glucose metabolism depending on their enzymatic composition and the presence or lack of oxygen.

THE EMBDEN–MEYERHOF–PARNAS PATHWAY

Because glucose is degraded without oxygen, the Embden–Meyerhof–Parnas (EMP) pathway has also been called the **glycolytic** or **anaerobic** pathway, used

(text continues on page 258)

TABLE 5-1

NOMENCLATURE FOR GRAM-NEGATIVE NONFERMENTATIVE BACILLI

CURRENT USAGE	PREVIOUS DESIGNATIONS	COMMENTS
Achromobacter groups B, E, and F	*Achromobacter xylosoxidans* *Achromobacter* sp. CDC Vd-1, Vd-2	Currently no named species in genus *Achromobacter*. Type species (*A. xylosoxidans*) moved to genus *Alcaligenes,* Vd-1 and Vd-2 moved to genus *Ochrobactrum* (synonymous with *Achromobacter* groups A, C, and D)
Acinetobacter baumannii	*Acinetobacter calcoaceticus* var. *anitratus* *Achromobacter anitratus* *Bacterium anitratum* *Herellea vaginicola* Morax-Axenfeld bacillus *Moraxella glucidolytica* var. *nonliquefaciens* *Pseudomonas calcoacetica*	Species name given to *Acinetobacter* genospecies 2. Produces acid from glucose. Can be separated from *Acinetobacter calcoaceticus* (genospecies 1) by growth at 41°C and 44°C, production of β-xylosidase, and utilization of malate (*A. baumannii* positive and *A. calcoaceticus* negative). Most *Acinetobacter* strains isolated from human clinical specimens belong to this species
Acinetobacter lwoffii	*Acinetobacter calcoaceticus* var. *lwoffi* *Achromobacter lwoffi* *Mima polymorpha* *Moraxella lwoffi*	Species name given to *Acinetobacter* genospecies 8. Non–glucose-oxidizing strain found in human clinical specimens
Agrobacterium radiobacter	CDC Vd-3 *Agrobacterium tumefaciens* *Agrobacterium biovar* 1	*Agrobacterium radiobacter* and *A. tumefaciens* are the same species; strongly urease and phenylalanine positive
Alcaligenes faecalis	CDC VI *Alcaligenes odorans*	*Alcaligenes odorans* was proposed at a later date for an organism that is a strain of the earlier named *Alcaligenes faecalis*
Alcaligenes piechaudii		New species isolated primarily from human clinical specimens, but some strains from the environment. Clinical significance is unknown. One report of otitis media caused by this organism
Alcaligenes xylosoxidans subsp. *xylosoxidans*	*Achromobacter xylosoxidans* *Alcaligenes denitrificans* subsp. *xylosoxidans* CDC IIIa and IIIb	Acidification of glucose and xylose
Alcaligenes xylosoxidans subsp. *denitrificans*	*Alcaligenes denitrificans* *Alcaligenes denitrificans* subsp. *denitrificans* CDC Vc	Rarely isolated in clinical specimens. Denitrifies nitrates.
Bergeyella zoohelcum	*Weeksella zoohelcum* CDC IIj	Rapid urea-positive. Associated with dog and cat bites
Bordetella bronchiseptica	*Alcaligenes bronchicanis* *Alcaligenes bronchiseptica* *Bordetella bronchicanis* *Brucella bronchiseptica* *Haemophilus bronchiseptica*	Rapid urea-positive
Bordetella hinzii	*Bordetella avium*–like *Alcaligenes faecalis* type II TC (turkey coryza) bacterium type II *Alcaligenes* sp. strain C_2T_2	New species isolated from respiratory tracts of chickens and turkeys. Human isolates reported from respiratory tract, ear discharge, and feces
Bordetella holmesii	CDC nonoxidizer group 2 (NO-2)	New species isolated from blood cultures. All strains produce a brown, soluble pigment on heart infusion tyrosine agar
Brevundimonas diminuta	*Pseudomonas diminuta* CDC Ia	Name derives from short wave length of flagellum

(Continued)

TABLE 5-1   *(Continued)*
NOMENCLATURE FOR GRAM-NEGATIVE NONFERMENTATIVE BACILLI

CURRENT USAGE	PREVIOUS DESIGNATIONS	COMMENTS
Brevundimonas vesicularis	*Pseudomonas vesicularis* *Corynebacterium vesiculare*	Slow growing and produces a dark yellow to orange pigment. Strong hydrolysis of esculin
Burkholderia cepacia	*Pseudomonas cepacia* *Pseudomonas multivorans* *Pseudomonas kingii* CDC EO-1	Yellow pigment; recovered from numerous water sources and wet surfaces. Respiratory pathogen in cystic fibrosis patients
Burkholderia gladioli	*Pseudomonas gladioli* *Pseudomonas marginata*	Primarily plant pathogen; has been reported from sputum of patients with cystic fibrosis
Burkholderia pickettii	*Pseudomonas pickettii* CDC Va-1, Va-2 *Pseudomonas thomasii* (Va-3)	Slow-growing, pinpoint colonies after 24 h on blood agar (BAP). Rarely associated with infection. Proposal to move species to new genus, *Ralstonia*
Burkholderia pseudomallei	*Pseudomonas pseudomallei*	Cause of melioidosis in humans
Chryseobacterium indologenes	*Flavobacterium indologenes* CDC IIb	Most frequent isolate of genus from human specimens. Dark yellow colonies
Chryseobacterium meningosepticum	*Flavobacterium meningosepticum* CDC IIa	Highly pathogenic for premature infants
Chryseomonas luteola	CDC Ve-1 *Pseudomonas luteola* *Chryseomonas polytricha*	Yellow pigmented, oxidase-negative, esculin-positive
Comamonas acidovorans	*Pseudomonas acidovorans* *Pseudomonas desmolytica* *Pseudomonas indoloxidans* *Achromobacter cystinovorum*	Orange indole reaction, owing to production of anthranilic acid from tryptone
Comamonas terrigena	Various species of *Vibrio* E. Falsen group 10 *Aquasprillum aquaticum*	Not considered a human pathogen
Comamonas testosteroni	*Pseudomonas testosteroni* *Pseudomonas desmolytica* *Pseudomonas dacunhae* *Pseudomonas cruciviae*	Uncommon isolate. Has been associated with perforated appendicitis
Empedobacter brevis	*Flavobacterium breve*	Rare human isolate of unknown significance
Flavimonas oryzihabitans	CDC Ve-2 *Pseudomonas oryzihabitans* *Pseudomonas lacunogenes*	Clinical isolates associated with septicemia and prosthetic valve endocarditis. Yellow pigment, oxidase-negative, esculin-negative
Flavobacterium odoratum	CDC M-4F	Generically misnamed
Methylobacterium mesophilicum	*Pseudomonas mesophilica* *Pseudomonas methanica* *Vibrio extorquens* *Mycoplana rubra* *Protaminobacter* sp. *Chromobacterium* sp. *Beijerinckia* sp.	Slow-growing, pink-pigmented rods; do not stain well, appear amorphous with many nonstaining vacuoles. Colonies absorb UV light
Moraxella atlantae	CDC M-3	Form spreading colonies after 48 h
Moraxella lacunata	*Moraxella liquefaciens*	Pit agar. Agent of conjunctivitis

(Continued)

TABLE 5-1 *(Continued)*
NOMENCLATURE FOR GRAM-NEGATIVE NONFERMENTATIVE BACILLI

CURRENT USAGE	PREVIOUS DESIGNATIONS	COMMENTS
Moraxella nonliquefaciens	*Bacillus duplex* nonliquefaciens	Requires serum supplement for optimum growth
Moraxella osloensis	*Mima polymorpha* var. *oxidans*	Most frequent isolate of this genus. Highly susceptible to penicillin
Moraxella phenylpyruvica	CDC M-2	Phenylalanine deaminase-positive
Neisseria weaveri	*Moraxella* sp. M-5 CDC M-5	Clinical isolates associated with dog bites
Neisseria elongata subsp. *nitroreducens*	*Moraxella* sp. M-6 CDC M-6	Catalase negative. Clinical isolates associated with endocarditis
Ochrobactrum anthropi	CDC Vd-1, Vd-2 *Achromobacter* sp. biotypes 1 and 2. *Achromobacter* groups A, C, and D	Only isolates have been from human clinical specimens. Urea and esculin positive; ONPG negative
Oligella ureolytica	CDC IV e	Rapid urea-positive and phenylalanine deaminase-positive
Oligella urethralis	CDC M-4	Clinical isolates have been from ear and urinary tract infections
Pseudomonas aeruginosa	*Pseudomonas pyocyanea* *Bacterium aeruginosa*	Belongs to fluorescent group, grows at 42°C. Most common clinical isolate
Pseudomonas fluorescens		Belongs to fluorescent group; gelatin-positive
Pseudomonas mendocina	CDC Vb-2	Rare isolate. Colonies smooth with buttery consistency
Pseudomonas putida		Belongs to fluorescent group; gelatin-negative
Pseudomonas stutzeri	CDC Vb-1	Wrinkled colonies. Ubiquitous in soil and water. Rarely associated with infection
Roseomonas spp.	CDC "pink coccoid group"	Includes three named species (*R. gilardii, R. cervicalis, R. fauriae*) and three unnamed genomospecies. Pink, often mucoid colonies that are weakly staining gram-negative, plump, coccoid rods
Shewanella putrefaciens	*Pseudomonas putrefaciens* *Alteromonas putrefaciens* *Achromobacter putrefaciens* CDC Ib-1, Ib-2	Only nonfermenter that produces H_2S in KIA and TSI media
Sphingobacterium multivorum	CDC IIk-2 *Flavobacterium multivorum*	Yellow pigment, oxidase-positive, esculin-positive, mannitol-negative, rarely associated with serious infection
Sphingobacterium spiritivorum	CDC IIk-3 *Flavobacterium spiritivorum* *Flavobacterium yabuuchiae* *Sphingobacterium versatilis*	Yellow pigment, oxidase-positive, esculin-positive, mannitol-positive. Most common sources for isolation have been blood and urine
Sphingomonas paucimobilis	*Pseudomonas paucimobilis* CDC IIk-1	Yellow pigment, oxidase-positive, esculin-positive, slow-growing. Found in a variety of clinical specimens
Stenotrophomonas maltophilia	*Xanthomonas maltophilia* *Pseudomonas maltophilia* CDC group I	Oxidase-negative, lysine- and DNAse-positive; can be recovered from almost any clinical site. May cause opportunistic infections
Weeksella virosa	CDC IIf *Flavobacterium genitale*	Mucoid and sticky; difficult to remove from agar. Clinical isolates have been associated with urinary and vaginal infections

TABLE 5-2
CDC LETTERED AND NUMBERED BACTERIAL GROUPS: SYNONYMS

CDC DESIGNATIONS	CURRENT USAGE	CDC DESIGNATIONS	CURRENT USAGE
I	*Stenotrophomonas maltophilia*	HB-1	*Eikenella corrodens*
Ia	*Brevundimonas diminuta*	HB-2	*Haemophilus aphrophilus*
Ib-1	*Shewanella putrefaciens*	HB-3,4	*Actinobacillus actinomycetemcomitans*
Ib-2	*Shewanella putrefaciens*	HB-5	*Pasteurella bettyae*
IIa	*Chryseobacterium meningosepticum*	M-1	*Kingella kingae*
IIb	*Chryseobacterium indologenes*	M-2	*Moraxella phenylpyruvica*
IIc	CDC group IIc	M-3	*Moraxella atlantae*
IId	*Cardiobacterium hominis*	M-4	*Oligella urethralis*
IIe	CDC Group IIe	M-4f	*Flavobacterium odoratum*
IIf	*Weeksella virosa*	M-5	*Neisseria weaveri*
IIg	CDC group IIg	M-6	*Neisseria elongata*
IIh	CDC group IIh		subsp. *nitroreducens*
IIi	CDC group IIi	TM-1	*Kingella denitrificans*
IIj	*Bergeyella zoohelcum*	DF	Dysgonic fermenter
IIk-1	*Sphingomonas paucimobilis*	DF-1	*Capnocytophaga ochracea*
IIk-2	*Sphingobacterium multivorum*		*Capnocytophaga gingivalis*
IIk-3	*Sphingobacterium spiritivorum*		*Capnocytophaga sputigena*
IIIa, IIIb	*Alcaligenes xylosoxidans*	DF-2	*Capnocytophaga canimorsus*
	subsp. *xylosoxidans*	DF-2-like	*Capnocytophaga cynodegmi*
IVa	*Bordetella bronchiseptica*	DF-3	Unnamed
IVb	*Bordetella parapertussis*	EO	Eugonic oxidizer
IVc	Unnamed	EO-1	*Burkholderia cepacia*
IVc-2	Unnamed	EO-2	Unnamed
IVd	Pseudomonas-like group 2	EO-3	Unnamed
IVe	*Oligella ureolytica*	EF	Eugonic fermenter
Va-1	*Burkholderia pickettii*	EF-1	*Pseudomonas*-like group 2
Va-2	*Burkholderia pickettii*	EF-3	*Vibrio vulnificus*
Va-3	*Burkholderia pickettii*	EF-4	*Pasteurella*-like
Vb-1	*Pseudomonas stutzeri*	EF-5	*Photobacterium damsela*
Vb-2	*Pseudomonas mendocina*	EF-6	*Vibrio fluvialis*
Vb-3	*Pseudomonas stutzeri*-like	EF-9	*Tatumella ptyseos*
Vc	*Alcaligenes xylosoxidans*	EF-13	*Vibrio hollisae*
	subsp. *denitrificans*	EF-19	*Comamonas terrigena*
Vd-1	*Ochrobactrum anthropi*	EF-26	*Bordetella*-like species
Vd-2	*Ochrobactrum anthropi*	NO	Nonoxidizer
Vd-3	*Agrobacterium radiobacter*	NO-1	CDC group NO-1
Ve-1	*Chryseomonas luteola*	NO-2	*Bordetella holmesii*
Ve-2	*Flavimonas oryzihabitans*	WO	Weak oxidizer
VI	*Alcaligenes faecalis*	WO-1	Unnamed

primarily by anaerobic bacteria and, to some degree, by facultatively anaerobic bacteria as well. The intermediate steps in the EMP pathway include the initial phosphorylation of glucose, conversion to fructose phosphate, and cleavage to form two molecules of glyceraldehyde phosphate, which, through a series of intermediate steps (not shown in Fig. 5-1), forms pyruvic acid. The EMP pathway is discussed more thoroughly in Chapter 4.

Historically, the EMP pathway has also been termed the **fermentative pathway**. Fermentation and anaerobic metabolism have been considered synonymous ever since Pasteur demonstrated that acids and alcohols are the major end products of carbohydrate degradation when oxygen is excluded from the system. According to a current concept, fermentative metabolism is said to exist in a glycolytic system when organic compounds serve as the final hydrogen (elec-

tron) acceptor. Thus, as shown in the EMP pathway outlined in the left column of Figure 5-1, pyruvic acid acts as an intermediate hydrogen acceptor but is then oxidized by giving up its hydrogen ions to sodium lactate to form lactic acid or to other organic salts to form one of several so-called mixed acids. These acids are the end products of glucose metabolism by the EMP pathway, accounting for the drop in pH in fermentation tests used for identifying bacteria. Bacteria that possess the appropriate enzyme systems can further degrade these mixed acids into alcohols, CO_2, or other organic compounds.

Although these biochemical principles seem somewhat removed from the daily work in the laboratory, microbiologists must have a basic understanding of bacterial metabolism when designing or interpreting test procedures that compare fermentation with oxidation. Fermentation must be determined in test systems

4

energy-yielding reactions that require molecular oxygen (or other nonorganic elements) as the terminal hydrogen (electron) acceptor.

This difference in metabolism necessitates alternative, practical approaches to the identification of oxidative and fermentative bacteria. The acids that are formed in the ED pathway (glucuronic acid and its derivatives) and those produced in the Krebs cycle (citric acid and its derivatives) are extremely weak compared with the mixed acids resulting from fermentation. Because the end product of oxidative metabolism is water, gas is not formed from carbohydrates by oxidative organisms. Therefore, test systems with more sensitive detectors of acid production must be used when studying oxidative bacteria, which are discussed in detail later in this chapter. Test systems designed to detect acid production from fermentative bacteria often cannot be applied to oxidative organisms that produce insufficient acids to convert the pH indicator.

THE WARBURG–DICKENS HEXOSE MONOPHOSPHATE PATHWAY

Facultatively anaerobic bacteria have the capacity to grow on the surface of an agar plate in the presence of oxygen or in an anaerobic environment. Just because a microorganism can grow in an aerobic environment does not necessarily mean that oxygen is metabolically used. That is, not all aerobes are oxidative. The term **aerotolerant** is more appropriate for nonoxidative bacteria that are capable of growing in the presence of oxygen but grow better in an anaerobic environment.

Many of the facultative anaerobes can use either the EMP or the ED pathway depending on the environmental conditions in which they are growing. The hexose monophosphate pathway (HMP), as shown in the right-hand column of Figure 5-1, is actually a hybrid of the EMP and ED pathways. Note that the initial steps in the degradation of glucose in the HMP pathway parallel those of the ED pathway; however, later in the HMP scheme, glyceraldehyde 3-phosphate is formed as the precursor of pyruvic acid, similar to the EMP pathway. These organisms appear fermentative in test systems, even though the EMP pathway is not strictly used.

Note in Figure 5-1 that ribulose 5-phosphate is the precursor to formation of glyceraldehyde 3-phosphate in the HMP pathway. Ribulose is a pentose and, for this reason, the HMP pathway has also been referred to as the pentose cycle. It provides the major avenue by which pentoses are metabolized by a number of bacterial species.

INITIAL CLUES THAT AN UNKNOWN ISOLATE IS A NONFERMENTER

The microbiologist may suspect that an unknown gram-negative bacillus is a member of the nonfermenter group by observing one or more of the following characteristics:

1. Lack of evidence for glucose fermentation (see Color Plate 5-1A)
2. Positive cytochrome oxidase reaction (see Color Plate 5-1B)
3. Failure to grow on MacConkey agar (see Color Plate 5-1C)

Additional characteristics used to make preliminary identification of the nonfermenters are presented in Color Plate 5-1.

LACK OF EVIDENCE FOR GLUCOSE FERMENTATION

Acids produced by nonfermenters are considerably weaker than the mixed acids derived from fermentative bacteria; thus the pH in fermentation test media, in which a nonfermenter is growing, may not drop sufficiently to convert the pH indicator. The initial clue that an unknown organism is a nonfermenter is usually the lack of acid production in either KIA or TSI media, manifest in each instance as an alkaline (red) slant and an alkaline deep (see Color Plate 5-1A). Initially, it is important that an unknown organism be classified by its mode of glucose utilization to select the correct set of biochemical characteristics to make a definitive identification. Microbiologists who use packaged commercial identification kits and bypass inoculation of the unknown organism to KIA or TSI tubes may not know whether to select a fermentative or oxidative system. Therefore, before setting up differential systems, it is recommended that the oxidative–fermentative (OF) characteristic of all unknown isolates of gram-negative bacilli be assessed by inoculating a KIA or TSI slant.

POSITIVE CYTOCHROME OXIDASE REACTION

Any colony of a gram-negative bacillus growing on blood agar or other primary isolation media that is cytochrome oxidase-positive can be suspected of belonging to the nonfermentative group (see Color Plate 5-1B). However, not all oxidase-positive, gram-negative bacilli are nonfermenters. Therefore, the mode of glucose utilization must still be measured (again demonstrating the importance of setting up a KIA or TSI tube). Cultures of oxidase-positive fermenters, such as *Pasteurella* species, *Aeromonas* species, *Plesiomonas* species, *Vibrio* species, and others, may be mistaken for nonfermenters, making identifications more difficult. The procedure for performing the cytochrome oxidase test is given in Chart 16. To test the oxidase activity of nonfermenters, the CDC recommends using a 0.5% aqueous solution of tetramethyl-*p*-phenylenediamine hydrochloride. This solution is good for 1 week if stored in a dark bottle in the refrigerator at 4° to 10°C. A few drops of reagent can be used to flood the surface of agar medium on which bacterial colonies are growing. The development of a blue color within a few seconds indicates a positive test. Negative reactions can be confirmed using the more sensitive Kovac's method, in which a loopful of organisms is mixed with a few drops of reagent on a piece of filter paper (see Color Plate 5-1*B*). The development of a dark blue color within 10 seconds indicates a positive test result.

FAILURE TO GROW ON MacCONKEY AGAR

A gram-negative bacillus that grows on blood agar but grows poorly or not at all on MacConkey agar should be suspected of belonging to the nonfermentative group. However, this guideline is far from absolute because many of the fastidious gram-negative bacilli also do not grow on MacConkey agar. The ability of bacteria to grow on MacConkey agar is determined by inspecting with reflected light the surface of plates that have been inoculated and then incubated for 24 to 48 hours. Organisms that grow well produce colonies that are 3 mm or more in diameter and easy to see. Poorly growing strains produce either widely scattered, tiny pinpoint colonies or absolutely no growth (see Color Plate 5-1*C*).

TESTS USED IN THE IDENTIFICATION OF NONFERMENTERS

UTILIZATION OF GLUCOSE

Most conventional culture media designed to detect acid production from fermentative bacteria, such as the *Enterobacteriaceae*, are not suitable for the study of nonfermentative bacilli. They do not support the growth of many strains, and the acids produced are often too weak to convert the pH indicator. Hugh and Leifson[149] were the first to design an OF medium that accommodated the metabolic properties of the nonfermentative bacilli, as outlined in Chart 58.

Note that the Hugh–Leifson OF medium contains 0.2% peptone and 1.0% carbohydrate, so that the ratio of peptone to carbohydrate is 1:5 in contrast with the 2:1 ratio found in media used for carbohydrate fermentation. The decrease in peptone minimizes the formation of oxidative products from amino acids, which tend to raise the pH of the medium and may neutralize the weak acids produced by the nonfermentative bacilli. On the other hand, the increase in carbohydrate concentration enhances acid production by the microorganism. The semisolid consistency of the agar, the use of bromthymol blue as the pH indicator, and the inclusion of a small quantity of diphosphate buffer are all designed to enhance the detection of acid.

Two tubes of each carbohydrate medium are required for the test. The medium in one tube is exposed to air; the other is overlaid with sterile mineral oil or melted paraffin (Fig. 5-2). Oxidative microorganisms produce acid only in the open tube exposed to atmospheric oxygen; fermenting organisms produce acid in both tubes; and nonsaccharolytic bacteria are inert in this medium, which remains at an alkaline pH after incubation. Color Plate 5-1*D* shows the OF reaction of an oxidative nonfermenter, with only the open tube showing the yellow color of acid production.

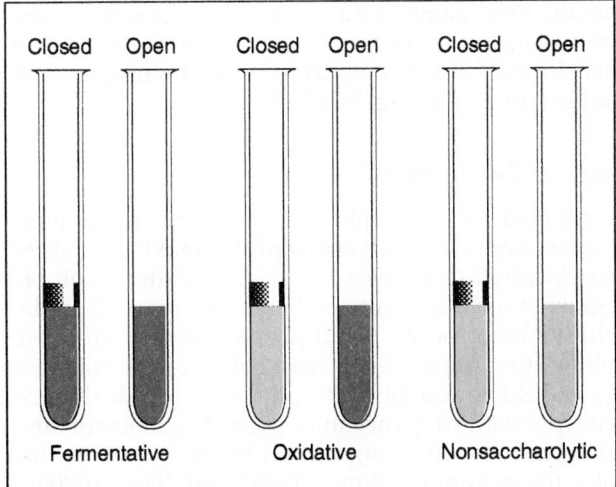

Figure 5-2.
The oxidative–fermentative (OF) test. Fermentative organisms produce acid in both the closed and open tubes (*stippled effect*); oxidative organisms provide acid only in the open tube. Asaccharolytic organisms that do not use carbohydrates produce no change in either tube.

The OF test has limitations. Slow-growing nonfermentative bacilli may not produce color changes for several days, and species that produce amides from amino acids may cause weak acid reactions to reverse with time, thereby confusing the final interpretation. It is important that the Hugh–Leifson formula be strictly followed when performing the OF test (see Chart 58).

MOTILITY

A semisolid agar medium for detecting motility of fermentative organisms may not be suitable for nonfermenting species that grow only on the surface of the agar. If a semisolid agar medium is used for nonfermentative bacilli, stab-inoculate only the upper 4 mm of the medium and make an initial reading within 4 to 6 hours. Many motile strains of nonfermentative bacilli show only an early, faint haziness near the surface of the agar, which tends to disappear with prolonged incubation. Readings should again be made at 24 and 48 hours to detect the motility of slowly growing strains. Incubation at 25°C enhances the motility of some strains. We have found that Motility B Medium with tetrazolium (available from Remel, Lenexa KS) works particularly well for demonstrating motility with the nonfermenting bacilli (see Color Plate 5-1*E*).

The hanging-drop preparation may be more accurate in detecting motility of many species of nonfermentative bacilli. In this technique, a loopful of a 6- to 24-hour, actively growing broth culture that has been incubated at 25°C is placed in the center of a No. 1 coverslip that is inverted and suspended over the concavity of a depression slide. True motility must be differentiated from brownian movement or the flow of fluid beneath the coverslip. Motile bacteria show directional movement and change in position relative to each other; when brownian movement is the cause of the motion, they maintain the same relative positions. The use of flagellar stains (see Chart 29), discussed later in this chapter, is also helpful in differentiating certain motile species (see Fig. 5-3).[52,179]

PIGMENT PRODUCTION

A number of pigments are produced by nonfermenters, some of which are helpful in making a species identification (see Color Plate 5-1F). Water-insoluble pigments include carotenoids (yellow-orange), violacein (violet or purple), and phenazines (red, maroon, yellow) that impart distinctive colors to the colonies. Water-soluble and diffusible pigments include fluorescein (pyoverdin), pyocyanin, pyorubin, melanin, and miscellaneous other pigmented byproducts that discolor the culture medium. "Tech" and "Flo" media[164] were developed to enhance formation of the water-soluble pigments pyocyanin and pyoverdin (see Color Plate 5-1G). These media have special peptones and an increased concentration of magnesium and sulfate ions to enhance pigment production. King and coworkers[164] found that the kind of peptone used in the basal medium markedly affected pigment production. Bacto peptone (Difco Laboratories, Detroit MI) proved to be superior for the production of pyocyanin but had an inhibitory effect on the elaboration of fluorescein, whereas proteose peptone 3 (Difco Laboratories) enhanced the production of fluorescein and inhibited the formation of pyocyanin. An increase in phosphate concentration causes enhanced production of fluorescein but decreases pyocyanin production. Pigment production can also be enhanced by growing organisms in gelatin-, potato-, or milk-containing media and by incubating them at 25° to 30°C. Pyoverdin may be demonstrated on Flo agar by observing fluorescence under ultraviolet light (using a Wood's lamp) or by the appearance of a yellow pigment in the media in visible light (see Color Plates 5-1G and H).

HYDROLYSIS OF UREA

Urea hydrolysis is presented in detail in Chart 72. Because many of the urea-splitting nonfermenters require enriched media for growth, Christensen's urea agar slants are used. Positive results may be achieved more rapidly by using a heavy inoculum. Bacterial species, such as *Bordetella bronchiseptica*, that avidly split urea may produce a red color change within 4 hours; weak reactors may require up to 48 hours before a positive reaction can be visualized. The appearance of a faint, delayed, pink tinge in the upper slant portion of the medium probably indicates nonspecific amino acid degradation and should be read as a negative test result (see Color Plate 5-2A).

NITRATE REDUCTION

The basic principles and procedures for performing the nitrate reduction test are presented in Chart 53. The reduction of nitrate to nitrite is only the first step in a biochemical process used by some microorganisms to re-

lease oxygen—a final hydrogen acceptor at the endpoint of oxidative metabolism. The nitrate reduction test for nonfermenters is performed similarly to that for other organisms, the endpoint being the appearance of a red color on addition of sulfanilic acid and α-naphthylamine to an overnight culture in nitrate-containing media. If a red color does not develop, either nitrate has not been reduced or reduction has proceeded beyond the nitrite stage to the formation of other compounds or to nitrogen gas (denitrification). The appearance of a red color on the addition of a small quantity of zinc dust indicates the residual presence of nitrates, denoting a negative test result; the absence of color indicates that the nitrate has been reduced to compounds other than nitrites (usually nitrogen gas), indicating that the original test was positive.

DENITRIFICATION OF NITRATES AND NITRITES

Certain nonfermenters have the capability of reducing either nitrate or nitrite (or both) to gaseous nitrogen (see Chart 30). Nitrate–nitrite broth, with an inverted Durham tube or an agar slant, may be used. Because the media contain no carbohydrates, any gas that forms is derived from the nitrate or the nitrite, indicating a positive denitrification test. The broth test is easier to interpret because the collection of gas within the inverted Durham tube is readily visualized. In agar slants, the collection of gas bubbles, usually in the depths of the butt, indicates a positive test result. Most denitrifying media contain both nitrates and nitrites. In rare instances (e.g., in the identification of *Alcaligenes faecalis* [*odorans*], which denitrifies nitrites but not nitrates), separate denitrification tests may be in order. Combination fluorescence–denitrification or fluorescence–lactose–denitrification media are available; however, the reactions may vary from those produced in the media recommended by the CDC (see Color Plate 5-2B).

INDOLE PRODUCTION

The basic principles and procedure for determination of indole production are presented in Chart 40. Minor modifications may be required when detecting indole production by certain weak-reacting nonfermenters. An enriched tryptophan-containing medium, usually heart infusion broth, may be required. Because only small quantities of indole are formed by some nonfermenters, extraction of the culture media by layering a small quantity of xylene or chloroform on the surface may be helpful. Care should be taken to add only a small quantity of extractant because even minimal dilution may lower the concentration of indole below the sensitivity of detection by either Ehrlich's or Kovac's reagent. The appearance of a fuchsia red color at the interface of the surface of the medium (or the extractant) with the reagent indicates indole formation and constitutes a positive test result. One organism, *Comamonas acidovorans*, produces a distinctive "pumpkin orange" indole reaction owing to the formation of anthranilic acid, rather than indole, from tryptophan (see Color Plate 5-2C).[191]

DECARBOXYLATION

The Moeller method for detecting decarboxylation of an amino acid (described in Chap. 4) is based on a change in pH. The development of an alkaline purple color in the test medium, following inoculation with the test organism and incubation at 35°C for 24 to 48 hours, constitutes a positive test result (see Chart 18). Many nonfermenters display only weak decarboxylase activity and may produce insufficient amines to convert the pH indicator system. This potential shortcoming in the Moeller method can be overcome by using only small quantities of substrates (1 to 2 mL) and a heavy inoculum of pregrown organisms in which a high concentration of enzymes has already accumulated. The sensitivity of detection is also increased by overlaying the culture medium with 4 mm of petrolatum. It is essential that uninoculated, amino acid–free substrate controls be used to compare the color reactions. The initial conversion of the medium to a yellow color as acids accumulate from the small amount of glucose in the medium is not seen with nonfermenters; rather, the endpoint reactions are read comparing the strong alkaline purple color reactions with the lighter blue-green hue of the controls (see Color Plate 5-2D). Tubes should be incubated at 35°C for up to 5 days before interpreting the reaction as negative. Other systems that use ninhydrin reagent as an indicator may be more sensitive in detecting decarboxylase activity because the compound reacts directly with the amines to form a purple color.

ESCULIN HYDROLYSIS

Esculin hydrolysis is used primarily as a differential characteristic to distinguish between the two *Brevundimonas* species and some of the yellow-pigmented pseudomonads. For testing of the nonfermenters an esculin medium without bile is recommended, because some nonfermenter species are inhibited by bile. Esculin agar slants are inoculated with the unknown isolate and incubated at 35°C for 24 to 48 hours. Esculin in the medium fluoresces when observed with a Wood's lamp. When esculin is hydrolyzed, the medium turns reddish black and fluorescence is lost, indicating a positive test result (see Color Plate 5-2E and Chart 26).

FLAGELLA STAINS

Although usually not required, flagellar stains are occasionally useful in identifying certain motile nonfermentative bacilli, particularly when biochemical reactions are weak or equivocal.

LEIFSON METHOD

Reliable results may be obtained using Leifson's staining technique, described in Chart 29, if the considerations described in Box 5-1 are given strict attention.[52,179]

RYU METHOD

The use of the Ryu flagella stain, which is easy to perform and gives good results, is also recom-

---

BOX 5-1. CONSIDERATIONS WHEN PREPARING A LEIFSON STAIN

1. The slides must be scrupulously clean. Slides should be soaked in acid dichromate or acid alcohol (3% concentrated hydrochloric acid in 95% ethyl alcohol) for 3 or 4 days. Final cleaning can be done immediately before use by heating the slides in the blue flame of a Bunsen burner.

2. Bacteria must be grown in a carbohydrate-free medium. A low pH may inhibit formation of flagella, and any acid formation in the medium may be detrimental. The pH of the staining solution should be maintained at 5.0 or higher.

3. Bacteria should be stained during the active log phase of growth, usually within 24 or 48 hours. Room-temperature incubation for 24 to 48 hours may be required to promote full development of flagella in some species.

4. Care should be taken not to transfer agar to the slide because it may interfere with the staining reaction. Washing the bacteria to be stained two or three times in water (lightly centrifuging between washes) before adding to the slides may help remove surface-staining inhibitors.

---

mended.[171,275] The procedure for this method is given in Chart 29.

WET-MOUNT TECHNIQUE

Heimbrook and colleagues[120] have described use of the wet-mount technique of Mayfield and Innis[195] and the stain of Ryu[275] as a rapid, simple way of staining flagella. In this approach, the test bacteria are grown on a noninhibitory medium for 16 to 24 hours. A faintly turbid suspension is made by first touching an applicator stick or wire to a colony on the plate and then touching a drop of water on a slide. A coverslip is placed over the drop, and the slide is examined for motile cells. After 5 to 10 minutes, or when about half of the cells are attached to the glass slide or coverslip, two drops of the Ryu stain (described in Chart 29) are applied to the edge of the coverslip and allowed to flow under the coverslip by capillary action. The cells are examined for the presence of flagella after 5 to 15 minutes at room temperature.

FLAGELLAR MORPHOLOGY

The number and arrangement of flagella on the bacterial cell can be an aid in identification of the species. The following types of flagellar arrangements can be observed:

Polar
    Monotrichous—single flagellum at one or both poles

Multitrichous—two or more flagella at one or both poles

Subpolar—flagella near pole with base of flagella at right angle to long axis

Lateral—flagella projecting from middle of bacterial cell

Peritrichous—flagella haphazardly arranged all around bacterial cell

Representative bacteria stained with flagellar stains are shown in Figure 5-3.

TAXONOMY, BIOCHEMICAL CHARACTERISTICS, AND CLINICAL SIGNIFICANCE OF MEDICALLY IMPORTANT GENERA OF NONFERMENTERS

In the space available here, it is possible to provide only a brief summary of the medically important nonfermenters. Several references can be consulted for an in-depth discussion of the identifying features and clinical syndromes caused by this group of organisms.[92,95,138,218,234]

Unlike the *Enterobacteriaceae* the nonfermenting gram-negative bacilli do not fit conveniently into a single family of well-characterized genera, and the correct taxonomic placement of many NFBs remains unresolved. Consequently, the study of nonfermenters is often confusing for the beginning microbiologist. The major genera of nonfermenting, gram-negative bacilli have been classified into five families (*Alcaligenaceae,*

Flavobacteriaceae, Methylococcaceae, Pseudomonadaceae, and *Rhizobiaceae*). The remaining genera of clinically important nonfermenters are as yet not assigned to a family and are grouped under the heading Organisms Whose Taxonomic Position Is Uncertain.

One approach to studying the nonfermenters is to group them on the basis of the presence or absence of motility and on the type of flagella present in strains that are motile. With this approach, the medically important nonfermenters can be grouped as in Box 5-2.

ORGANISMS THAT ARE MOTILE WITH POLAR FLAGELLA

FAMILY *PSEUDOMONADACEAE*

The genus *Pseudomonas* and some closely related genera, many of which were formerly placed in the genus *Pseudomonas*, make up what is now the *Pseudomonadaceae*.[230] Members of this family have the characteristics of being straight or slightly curved, gram-negative bacilli that are strict aerobes; most strains are motile by means of one of more polar flagella; they utilize glucose and other carbohydrates oxidatively; and are usually cytochrome oxidase-positive. The key differentiating features of the bacteria making up the *Pseudomonadaceae* are given in Table 5-3.

Two schemes for classifying organisms that belong to the family *Pseudomonadaceae* have been developed. One approach, popularized by Gilardi, is based on phenotypic characteristics and divides the pseudomonads into seven major groups: fluorescent, stutzeri,

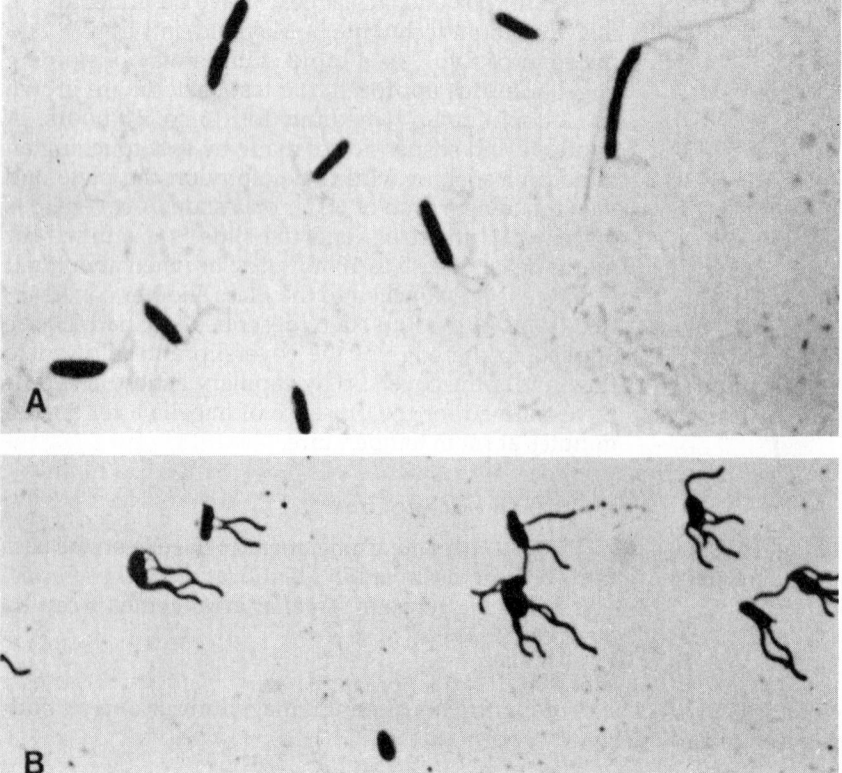

Figure 5-3. Bacteria stained with flagellar stains. (**A**) Positive flagellar stain of bacilli with polar flagella (original magnification × 900). (**B**) Positive flagellar stain of bacilli with peritrichous flagella (original magnification × 900).

Box 5-2. Medically Important Nonfermenters

Motile with Polar Flagella

Family *Pseudomonadaceae*
rRNA group I
rRNA group II
rRNA group III
rRNA group IV
rRNA group V
Unknown nucleic acid homology
Family *Methylococcaceae*
Genus *Methylobacterium*
Organisms Whose Taxonomic Position Is Uncertain
Genus *Roseomonas*
Genus *Balneatrix*

Motile with Peritrichous Flagella

Family *Alcaligenaceae*
Genus *Alcaligenes*
Genus *Bordetella*
Family *Rhizobiaceae*
Genus *Agrobacterium*
Organisms Whose Taxonomic Position Is Uncertain
Genus *Achromobacter*
Ochrobactrum anthropi
Oligella ureolytica
CDC Group IVc-2

Nonmotile, Oxidase-Positive

Family *Flavobacteriaceae*
Genus *Flavobacterium, Chryseobacterium, Empedobacter*
Genus *Weeksella, Bergeyella*
Organisms Whose Taxonomic Position Is Uncertain
Genus *Sphingobacterium*
Genus *Moraxella*
Oligella urethralis
CDC groups EO-2, EO-3, and *Psychrobacter immobilis*
Gilardi rod group 1

Nonmotile, Oxidase-Negative

Genus *Acinetobacter*
CDC group NO-1
Bordetella holmesii (CDC group NO-2)

alcaligenes, pseudomallei, acidovorans, facilis–delafieldii, and diminuta.[98] The second scheme, developed by Palleroni and others,[230] is based on rRNA–DNA homology studies and places the pseudomonads into one of five rRNA homology groups which in turn include several smaller DNA homology groups.[230] A scheme that combines the phenotypic classification of Gilardi and the genotypic classification of Palleroni is outlined in Box 5-3.

rRNA Group I. Although most members of the *Pseudomonadaceae* were originally classified in the genus *Pseudomonas*, it is now known that each of the five rRNA groups represents taxonomically distinct genetic groups, and as a result different genus names have been assigned to each of the rRNA groups. Only the members of rRNA group I will retain the genus designation of *Pseudomonas*.

FLUORESCENT GROUP. The species within this group are all characterized by the production of a water-soluble pyoverdin pigment that fluoresces white to blue-green under long-wavelength (400-nm) ultraviolet light. Production of fluorescent pigments is particularly enhanced in media with a high phosphate concentration.[164] Although all three members of this group produce pyoverdin, only one species, *P. aeruginosa*, produces the distinctive blue, water-soluble pigment pyocyanin (see Color Plate 5-1G). The key biochemical features that separate the members of the fluorescent group are given in Table 5-4.

Pseudomonas aeruginosa is the pseudomonad most frequently recovered from clinical specimens. *P. aeruginosa* infection is especially prevalent among patients with burn wounds, cystic fibrosis, acute leukemia, organ transplants, and intravenous drug addiction.[26] Infections commonly occur at any site where moisture tends to accumulate—tracheostomies, indwelling catheters, burns, the external ear ("swimmer's ear"), and weeping cutaneous wounds. The exudation of bluish pus, with a grapelike odor from the production of pyocyanin, is characteristic. *P. aeruginosa* also causes urinary tract and lower respiratory tract infections; the latter can be severe and even life-threatening in immunocompromised hosts. The organism can also cause devastating infections of the eye. Pseudomonas keratitis, infection of corneal ulcers, and endophthalmitis must be approached as a medical emergency that can be fulminant and threaten permanent loss of vision. Individual cases of endocarditis, meningitis, brain abscess, and infections of bones and joints from hematogenous spread appear with regular frequency in the literature.[26] Most cases of endocarditis require valve replacement because the infection is difficult to eradicate.[256]

P. aeruginosa produces several substances that are thought to enhance the colonization and infection of host tissue.[26] These substances together with a variety of virulence factors, including lipopolysaccharide (LPS), exotoxin A, leukocidin, extracellular slime, proteases, phospholipase, and several other enzymes (Table 5-5), make *P. aeruginosa* the most clinically significant bacteria among the NFB. An unusual mucoid morphotype of *P. aeruginosa* is frequently recovered from respiratory secretions of cystic fibrosis patients who are chronically infected with *P. aeruginosa* (see Color Plate 5-3B). The mucoid morphotype is due to the production of large amounts of a polysaccharide (called alginate) that surrounds the cell. The production of alginate is ultimately responsible for the poor prognosis and high mortality rates among patients with cystic fibrosis. Recent reviews of this subject are available.[103,194,206]

P. fluorescens and *P. putida* occur in water and soil and may exist in water sources in the hospital environ-

TABLE 5-3
KEY CHARACTERISTICS OF THE FAMILY *PSEUDOMONADACEAE*

	OXIDASE	MOTILITY	PYOVERDIN	GLUCOSE	MALTOSE	LACTOSE	MANNITOL	ARGININE	LYSINE	NO₃;NO₂	NO₃;N₂	UREA	ONPG	DNASE	ACETAMIDE	ESCULIN	POLYMYXIN
RNA Group I																	
Genus: Pseudomonas																	
Fluorescent Group																	
P. aeruginosa	+	+	+	+	V	–	V	+	–	+	V	V	–	–	+	–	S
P. fluorescens	+	+	+	+	V	–	+	+	–	V	–	V	–	–	–	–	S
P. putida	+	+	+	+	V	–	V	+	–	–	–	V	–	–	–	–	S
Stutzeri Group																	
P. stutzeri	+	+	–	+	+	–	V	–	–	+	+	V	–	–	–	–	S
P. mendocina	+	+	–	+	–	–	–	+	–	+	+	V	–	–	–	–	S
CDC group Vb-3	+	+	–	+	+	–	+	+	–	+	+	V	–	–	–	–	S
Alcaligenes Group																	
P. alcaligenes	+	+	–	–	–	–	–	–	–	V	–	V	–	–	–	NA	S
P. pseudoalcaligenes	+	+	–	–	–	–	–	V	–	+	–	–	–	–	–	–	S
Pseudomonas species group 1	+	+	–	NA	–	–	–	V	–	+	+	–	–	–	–	NA	S
RNA Group II																	
Genus: Burkholderia																	
Pseudomallei Group																	
B. pseudomallei	+	+	–	+	+	+	+	+	–	+	+	V	–	–	–	V	R
B. cepacia	w	+	–	+	+	+	+	–	+	V	–	V	V	–	V	V	R
B. gladioli	–	+	–	+	–	–	+	–	–	V	–	+	+	–	–	–	R
B. pickettii	+	+	–	+	V	V	V	–	–	V	V	+	–	–	–	–	R

RNA Group III
Genus: *Comamonas*

Acidovorans Group

RNA Group IV
Genus: *Brevundimonas*

Diminuta Group

RNA Group V
Genus: *Stenotrophomonas*

Unknown Nucleic Acid Homology
Genus: *Chryseomonas*
Genus: *Flavimonas*
Genus: *Shewanella*
Genus: *Sphingomonas*

Organism													
C. acidovorans	+	+	−	+	−	−	−	−	−	−	+	−	V
C. terrigena	+	+	−	−	−	−	−	−	−	−	−	NA	S
C. testosteroni	+	+	−	−	−	−	−	−	−	−	−	NA	S
B. diminuta	+	+	V	−	−	−	−	−	−	V	−	−	V
B. vesicularis	+	+	V	−	−	−	−	−	V	−	−	+	S
S. maltophilia	−	+	+	−	+	−	−	−	+	+	−	+	S
C. luteola	−	+	+	+	−	V	−	V	+	−	−	+	S
F. oryzihabitans	−	+	+	+	−	−	−	V	−	−	−	−	S
*S. putrefaciens**	+	+	+	−	−	−	−	−	−	+	−	−	S
S. paucimobilis	+	+	+	−	−	−	−	−	+	−	−	+	S

+, 90% or more strains positive; −, 90% or more strains negative; V, 11%–89% of strains positive; ++, strong positive reaction; NA, results not available; R, resistant; S, susceptible; shaded areas indicate key reactions.
*Other key reactions are production of hydrogen sulfide in KIA and ornithine decarboxylase.

(Data from Gilardi GI. Identification of glucose-nonfermenting gram-negative rods. New York, North General Hospital, 1990; and Gilardi GL. Pseudomonas and related genera. In: Balows A, ed. Manual of clinical microbiology, 5th ed. Washington, DC, American Society for Microbiology, 1991:429–441.)

BOX 5-3. CLASSIFICATION OF THE FAMILY *PSEUDOMONADACEAE*

rRNA Group I

Fluorescent Group
Pseudomonas aeruginosa
Pseudomonas fluorescens
Pseudomonas putida

Stutzeri Group
Pseudomonas stutzeri
Pseudomonas mendocina
CDC Group Vb-3

Alcaligenes Group
Pseudomonas alcaligenes
Pseudomonas pseudoalcaligenes
Pseudomonas species group 1

rRNA Group II

Pseudomallei Group
Burkholderia mallei
Burkholderia pseudomallei
Burkholderia cepacia
Burkholderia gladioli
Burkholderia pickettii

rRNA Group III

Acidovorans Group
Comamonas acidovorans
Comamonas terrigena
Comamonas testosteroni

Facilis-delafieldii Group
Acidovorax delafieldii
Acidovorax facilis
Acidovorax temperans

rRNA Group IV

Diminuta Group
Brevundimonas diminuta
Brevundimonas vesicularis

rRNA Group V

Stenotrophomonas maltophilia

Unknown Nucleic Acid Homology

Chryseomonas luteola
Flavimonas oryzihabitans
Sphingomonas paucimobilis
Shewanella putrefaciens
Pseudomonas-like group 2
CDC group WO-1

ment. Both may exist as normal pharyngeal flora and are rare opportunistic pathogens in humans. *P. putida* has been reported to cause catheter-related sepsis in cancer patients[3] and septic arthritis.[187,189] Both species have been associated with bacteremia from transfused blood.[159,249,282,301,307]

STUTZERI GROUP. The organisms in the stutzeri group are all soil denitrifiers and can grow anaerob-

TABLE 5-4
KEY CHARACTERISTICS OF THE FLUORESCENT GROUP

TEST	P. AERUGINOSA	P. FLUORESCENS	P. PUTIDA
Pyocyanin	+	–	–
Pyoverdin	+	+	+
NO₃ reduction	V (74)	V (19)	–
Growth at 42°C	+	–	–
Gelatin hydrolysis	V (46)	+	–
Kanamycin	R	S	S
Carbenicillin	S	R	R

+, 90% or more strains positive; –, 90% or more strains negative; V, 11–89% of strains positive; ++, strong positive reaction; numbers in parentheses are percentage of strains giving positive reaction; R, resistant; S, susceptible. Data from Ref. 97.

ically in nitrate-containing media, with production of nitrogen gas. Strains are motile by way of polar monotrichous flagella. They can grow with NH₄ as the sole source of nitrogen and acetate as the sole source of carbon for energy. Characteristics that differentiate members of the stutzeri group are given in Table 5-6.

P. stutzeri (formerly CDC group Vb-1) is ubiquitous in soil and water and has been recovered from humus, manure, straw, sewage, stagnant water, baby formula, hospital equipment, eye cosmetics, and various clinical specimens.[91,98,234] It has only rarely been associated with infections, such as otitis media,[91] conjunctivitis,[234] pneumonia,[42] septic arthritis,[188] endocarditis,[268] meningitis in an HIV-positive patient,[264] infections of synthetic vascular grafts,[88] and infections of traumatic wounds.[91,101] It is susceptible to most antibiotics. Freshly isolated colonies are adherent and have a characteristic wrinkled appearance (see Color Plate 5-3C), which may be lost after repeated laboratory subculture. *P. stutzeri* comprises a heterogeneous set of strains that include at least seven genomic groups without taxonomic status called genomovars.[273] Bennasar and associates have shown that genomovar 6 is sufficiently different from the other *P. stutzeri* strains to warrant placement in a separate species that they have named *Pseudomonas balearica*.[19] No human clinical isolates of *P. balearica* have yet been reported.

TABLE 5-5
VIRULENCE FACTORS OF *PSEUDOMONAS AERUGINOSA*

VIRULENCE FACTOR	BIOLOGIC ACTIVITY
Alginate	Capsular polysaccharide that allows infecting bacteria to adhere to lung epithelial cell surfaces and form biofilms which, in turn, protects the bacteria from antibiotics and the body's immune system
Pili	Surface appendages that allow adherence of organism to GM-1 ganglioside receptors on host epithelial cell surfaces
Neuraminidase	Removes sialic acid residues from GM-1 ganglioside receptors, facilitating binding of pili
Lipopolysaccharide	Produces endotoxin, causes sepsis syndrome: fever, shock, oliguria, leukopenia or leukocytosis, disseminated intravascular coagulation, metabolic abnormalities
Exotoxin A	Tissue destruction, inhibition of protein synthesis; interrupts cell activity and macrophage response
Enterotoxin	Interrupts normal gastrointestinal activity, leading to diarrhea
Exoenzyme S	Inhibits protein synthesis
Phospholipase C	Destroys cytoplasmic membrane; destroys pulmonary surfactant; inactivates opsonins
Elastase	Cleaves immunoglobulins and complement components, disrupts neutrophil activity
Leukocidin	Inhibits neutrophil and lymphocyte function
Pyocyanins	Suppress other bacteria and disrupt respiratory ciliary activity; cause oxidative damage to tissues, particularly oxygenated tissues such as lung

P. mendocina (formerly CDC group Vb-2) and the unnamed species CDC group Vb-3 are rarely isolated from clinical specimens. *P. mendocina* colonies are smooth and have the appearance and consistency of butter. One case of infective endocarditis has been reported in a patient following aortic valve replacement.[11] CDC group Vb-3 isolates resemble *P. stutzeri* except they are arginine positive. Potvliege and colleagues[247] have reported a case of Vb-3 septicemia in a patient with multiple myeloma.

ALCALIGENES GROUP. Organisms in the alcaligenes group are characterized by being asaccharolytic or only weakly saccharolytic in OF glucose medium. Members of this group include *P. alcaligenes*, *P. pseudoalcaligenes*, and *Pseudomonas* species CDC group 1. The latter unnamed species is similar to *P. alcaligenes*, except that *Pseudomonas* species group 1 strains reduce both nitrate and nitrite to gas.[98] Characteristics that differentiate this group from other similar alkaline pseudomonads are given in Table 5-7. Although members of this group are recovered from clinical specimens, their ability to act as human pathogens has only rarely been documented. There have been reports of *P. alcaligenes* causing eye infections, empyema, and one case of fatal endocarditis.[313]

rRNA Group II. All species in rRNA Group II have been transferred to the new genus *Burkholderia*.[104,339]

PSEUDOMALLEI GROUP. All species in this group are easily separated from other groups of pseudomonads by the property of exhibiting resistance to the polymyxin group of antibiotics (polymyxin B and colistin). The biochemical characteristics used to distinguish the members of this group are given in Table 5-8. This group comprises 13 species, including several plant-associated species (*B. andropogonis, B. caryophylli, B. cocovenenans, B. glumae, B. plantarii, B. solanacearum, B. vandii, B. vietnamiensis*)[104] that have not been associated with human disease and, therefore, are not included in Table 5-8. *B. mallei* is an obligate parasite of animals (primarily horses, mules, and donkeys) causing a respiratory tract infection known as glanders. In rare instances, it can be transmitted to humans, usually through an abrasion of the skin.[322] It is the only nonmotile species in the genus. The remaining members of this group have all been associated with human disease.

B. pseudomallei causes melioidosis, a glanders-like disease in animals and humans. This organism grows well on standard laboratory media and often produces wrinkled colonies and thus morphologically may resemble *P. stutzeri*. The organism has a specific ecologic niche, existing in soil and stagnant water in an area of latitude 20 north and south of the equator, primarily in Thailand and Vietnam. Most infections are asymptomatic and can be diagnosed only by serology. It is estimated that thousands of U.S. military personnel became infected with *B. pseudomallei* while serving in Southeast Asia in the 1960s and 1970s. Serologic surveys have revealed positive titers for this organism in 1% to 9% of U.S. soldiers returning from Vietnam.[54,167,298] Thus, with an estimated 3 million military personnel serving in Vietnam from 1965 to 1973, as many as 250,000 may have become infected with *B. pseudomallei*.[202] An important feature of this disease is its ability to produce latent infection that can reactivate

TABLE 5-6
KEY CHARACTERISTICS OF THE STUTZERI GROUP

TEST	P. STUTZERI VB-1	P. MENDOCINA VB-2	 VB-3
Oxidase	+	+	+
OF glucose	A	A	A
OF maltose	A	−	A
OF lactose	−	−	−
OF mannitol	V (70)	−	A
NO₃ reduction	+	+	+
NO₃ to gas	+	+	+
Arginine	−	+	+
Lysine	−	−	−
Starch hydrolysis	+	−	+ (75)
Polymyxin B	S	S	S
Wrinkled colonies	+	−	−

+, 90% or more strains positive; −, 90% or more strains negative; V, 11–89% of strains positive; ++, strong positive reaction; A, acid reaction; numbers in parentheses are percentage of strains giving positive reaction; S, susceptible. Data from Ref. 97.

TABLE 5-7
KEY CHARACTERISTICS OF ALKALINE PSEUDOMONADS

| | COMAMONAS | | | PSEUDOMONAS | | BREVUNDIMONAS | |
TEST	C. TERRI-GENA	C. TESTOS-TERONI	C. ACIDOVO-RANS	P. ALCALI-GENES	P. PSEUDO-ALCALIGENES	B. DIMI-NUTA	B. VESICU-LARIS
Oxidase	+	+	+	+	+	+	+
OF glucose	ALK	ALK	ALK	ALK	WK (19)	WK (29)	WK (57)
OF fructose	ALK	ALK	A	ALK	A	ALK	ALK
OF mannitol	ALK	ALK	A	ALK	ALK	ALK	ALK
NO$_3$ reduction	+	+	+	V (61)	+	−	−
NO$_3$ to gas	−	−	−	−	−	−	−
Gelatin	−	−	−	−	−	V (58)	V (38)
Esculin	−	−	−	−	−	−	+
Starch	−	−	−	V (16)	−	−	+
DNAse	−	−	−	−	−	V (12)	−
Acetamide	−	−	+	−	−	−	−
Indole	−	−	Orange*	−	−	−	−
Flagellar arrangement		Polar tuft Long wavelength (3.0 μm)		Single polar Normal wavelength (1.5 μm)		Single polar Short wavelength (0.5 μm)	

+, 90% or more strains positive; −, 90% or more strains negative; V, 11%–89% of strains positive; ++, strong positive reaction; A, acid reaction; ALK, alkaline reaction; NA, results not available; numbers in parentheses are percentage of strains giving positive reaction; R, resistant; S, susceptible; WK, weak acid.
* Pumpkin orange color develops on addition of Kovacs reagent owing to formation of anthranilic acid from tryptophan.
Data from Ref. 97.

many years after primary exposure. For this reason, melioidosis has been dubbed the "Vietnamese time bomb" because the disease may still be incubating in American veterans of the Vietnam conflict.[108,202]

Infections are acquired by contact with the organism either by inhalation of dust or direct contact through breaks in the skin. Three forms of melioidosis have been described: 1) acute disease, presenting as septicemia with metastatic lesions; 2) subacute disease, presenting as a tuberculosis-like pneumonia with cellulitis and lymphangitis; and 3) chronic disease, presenting as a localized chronic cellulitis. It is important to treat suspected cases with antibiotics before any manipulation of patients, such as draining lesions, because patients will otherwise become septic. The mortality rate is 95% in patients with acute disease who are not treated.

Definitive diagnosis of melioidosis, which has been called "the great mimicker," depends on the isolation and identification of B. pseudomallei from clinical specimens. The organism grows readily on most routine laboratory media and can be recovered from blood using standard blood culture techniques.[337] The biochemical properties useful in identifying this organism are given in Table 5-8. Laboratory workers are advised to use biologic safety hoods when working with this organism because laboratory-acquired infection with B. pseudomallei has been reported.[279] Further information on the clinical and laboratory features of melioidosis can be found in other published reviews.[62,63,178]

B. cepacia is a phytopathogen that causes onion bulb rot in plants and foot rot (jungle rot) in humans.[306] It is one of only two NFBs that are lysine decarboxylase–positive (the other being S. maltophilia). Occasionally, lysine-negative strains do occur, and these can be difficult to distinguish from B. pickettii biovar 3/thomasii. In this instance a positive result for any of the following tests—sucrose, ONPG, ornithine, esculin, or acetamide—helps identify the isolate as B. cepacia.[97] B. cepacia has been isolated from numerous water sources and wet surfaces, including detergent solutions and intravenous fluids. Disinfectants in which B. cepacia will grow include povidone-iodine, quaternary ammonium compounds, and chlorhexidine.[21,58,295] Pseudo-

TABLE 5-8

KEY CHARACTERISTICS OF THE PSEUDOMALLEI GROUP

TEST	B. PSEUDOMALLEI	B. CEPACIA	B. GLADIOLI	B. PICKETTII VA-1	VA-2	3/B. THOMASII
Oxidase	+	W+ (93)	−	+	+	+
OF glucose	A	A	A	A	A	A
OF maltose	A	A	−	A	−	A
OF lactose	A	A	−	A	−	A
OF mannitol	A	A	A	−	−	A
ONPG	−	V (79)	+	−	−	−
NO$_3$ reduction	+	V (37)	V (33)	V (87)	+	V (20)
NO$_3$ to gas	+	−	−	V (84)	+	−
Arginine	+	−	−	−	−	−
Lysine	−	+	−	−	−	−
Urea	V (43)	V (45)	+	+	+	+
Polymyxin B	R	R	R	R	R	R
Wrinkled colonies	+	−	−	−	−	−
Pigment	Cream or tan	Yellow	Green-yellow	−	−	−

+, 90% or more strains positive; −, 90% or more strains negative; V, 11%–89% of strains positive; ++, strong positive reaction; A, acid reaction; numbers in parentheses are percentage of strains giving positive reaction; R, resistant; W, weak; W+, weak positive.
Data from Refs. 97 and 98.

bacteremias (false-positive blood cultures) have been reported following the use of *B. cepacia*-contaminated disinfectant solutions.[21,58,229,233] *B. cepacia* can also grow in distilled water with a nitrogen source owing to the ability of this organism to fix CO_2 from air. Clinical infections include pneumonia and pneumonitis in patients receiving contaminated anesthetics, urinary tract infection in patients receiving contaminated irrigation fluids following catheterization or cystoscopy, septicemia following heart surgery, endocarditis caused by contaminated heart valves, conjunctivitis, and septic arthritis.[229] Peritonitis following peritoneal dialysis has been associated with povidone-iodine solution contaminated with *B. cepacia*.[233] Infections involving the central nervous system include one case of bacteremia secondary to a contaminated Holter ventriculoatrial shunt in a child with congenital hydrocephalus[15] and a case of brain abscesses secondary to chronic suppurative otitis media in an adult.[121] Since the early 1980s *B. cepacia* has emerged as a cause of opportunistic human infections, particularly in patients with chronic granulomatous disease[174,224] and cystic fibrosis.[106,109,153,291] Patients with cystic fibrosis who are colonized with *B. cepacia* have a higher mortality in the year following colonization and have a more precipitous decline in overall pulmonary function following colonization.[180] Selective media with bacteriostatic dyes, antibiotics, or low pH have been described for the selective isolation of *B. cepacia*. These include *B. cepacia* medium (PCM) containing crystal violet, polymyxin B, and ticarcillin; OFPBL medium containing polymyxin B and bacitracin; and TB-T medium containing trypan blue and tetracycline. Comparative evaluations of these media have shown that the recovery of *B. cepacia* from patients with cystic fibrosis is enhanced with their use.[23,43,103] Unlike other common pseudomonads, *B. cepacia* is resistant to aminoglycoside antibiotics but is susceptible to trimethoprim–sulfamethoxazole, which has become the drug of choice in treating *B. cepacia* infections. For further information on the biology, mechanisms of virulence, and epidemiology of *B. cepacia*, the review by Goldmann and Klinger can be consulted.[106]

B. gladioli (formerly named *P. marginata*) is primarily a plant pathogen causing "flower rot" in gladiolus and other plants. It is one of the few pseudomonads that is negative for cytochrome oxidase and produces nonfluorescent yellow colonies after 48 to 72 hours of incubation. Further differentiating characteristics are given in Table 5-8. It was reported in the sputum of 11 patients with cystic fibrosis,[50] and was a cause of pneumonia and septicemia in two patients with chronic granulomatous disease.[271]

B. pickettii is slow growing and produces only pinpoint colonies on blood agar plates after 24 hours. This species is divided into three biovariants (biovar Va-1, biovar Va-2, and biovar 3/*thomasii*) that can be differentiated on the basis of the reactions given in Table 5-8. Gillis and coworkers consider *B. pickettii* to be a genetically and phenotypically distinct species and have not included it in the emended description of the genus *Burkholderia*; therefore, the correct genetic placement of this species remains unresolved.[104] *B. pickettii* is rarely associated with human infections but has been reported to cause nosocomial infections, including bacteremia and urinary tract infections. In 1983, five infants in the special-care nursery of a hospital in Chicago became colonized with *B. pickettii* following endotracheal suctioning with saline from commercially prepared saline in 5-mL unit-dose vials. Subsequently, four additional hospitals reported respiratory colonization of infants and adults with *B. pickettii* following the use of the same brand of saline vials.[47] This outbreak demonstrates the ability of *B. pickettii* to survive and grow in commercially prepared "sterile" saline despite pertinent Food and Drug Administration (FDA) regulations and company programs for identifying such contamination. Although most reports of *B. pickettii* infection have been related to contaminated foreign bodies or contaminated supplies presumed to be sterile, one case of vertebral osteomyelitis and discitis in a patient receiving long-term hemodialysis has been reported in which an obvious contaminating source for the infection could not be found.[329]

rRNA Group III. Willems and colleagues have proposed that the organisms belonging to rRNA group III be recognized as a new bacterial family, the *Comamonadaceae*.[331]

ACIDOVORANS GROUP. This group consists of the organisms formerly named *Pseudomonas acidovorans*, *Pseudomonas testosteroni*, and *Comamonas terrigena*. In 1987, Tamaoka[305] proposed that the organisms known as *Pseudomonas acidovorans* and *P. testosteroni* be placed in the genus *Comamonas* along with the species *C. terrigena*. All are motile by way of a polar tuft of up to six flagella, with the distinctive feature of having a long wavelength (3.0 μm between the top of adjacent waves). Acid is not produced in OF glucose medium, and thus these organisms are grouped among the alkaline pseudomonads (see Table 5-7). *C. acidovorans* is the most common of this group to be isolated from clinical specimens. It can be easily distinguished by acid reactions in OF fructose and OF mannitol and is acetamide-positive. It also has the unique feature of producing an orange indole reaction, owing to the production of anthranilic acid from tryptone (see Color Plate 5-2C).[191] *C. acidovorans* has been isolated from a variety of clinical specimens and is usually considered to be nonpathogenic. There was one isolate recovered

from the blood of a patient with tuberculosis at the University of Illinois hospital. A case of *C. acidovorans* endocarditis has been described in a 42-year-old intravenous drug abuser.[145] *C. testosteroni* is an uncommon isolate in the clinical laboratory, despite its wide environmental distribution. Eighteen cases of *C. testosteroni* infections have been reviewed by Barbaro and colleagues.[12] They report that the organism was most often found in association with anatomic abnormalities of the gastrointestinal tract, with perforation of the appendix being the most common. *C. terrigena* is not considered a human pathogen, although Sonnenwirth reported the isolation of *C. terrigena* from two blood cultures of a patient with endocarditis; however, the role of the organism as a pathogen in this patient was uncertain.[296]

FACILIS–DELAFIELDII GROUP. Willems and colleagues have proposed a new genus, *Acidovorax*, which contains the following three species: *Acidovorax facilis* (formerly *Pseudomonas facilis*), *Acidovorax delafieldii* (formerly *Pseudomonas delafieldii*), and *Acidovorax temperans* (for several former *Pseudomonas* and *Alcaligenes* strains).[332] These three species form a separate group within the rRNA group III complex. Two of the species, *A. delafieldii* and *A. temperans*, have been isolated from clinical specimens; however, no information regarding the clinical significance of these organisms is available.[98,332] *Acidovorax* species are oxidase-positive, motile, and utilize carbohydrates oxidatively. For additional differentiating features, the published report by Willems and colleagues can be consulted.[332]

rRNA Group IV. All species in rRNA group IV have been transferred to the new genus *Brevundimonas* (meaning bacterium with short-wavelength flagella).[283]

DIMINUTA GROUP. This group is represented by two species, *B. diminuta* and *B. vesicularis*. They are also grouped with the alkaline pseudomonads because they are nonreactive or only weakly reactive in most carbohydrates (see Table 5-7). This group is characterized by the presence of a single, tightly coiled (wavelength of 0.6 to 1.0 μm), polar flagella. *B. vesicularis* is slow growing and usually requires 48 hours of incubation for colonies to be observed and produce a dark yellow to orange pigment. It is easily separated from all other species of alkaline pseudomonads by virtue of a strong esculin hydrolysis reaction. We have isolated *B. vesicularis* from peritoneal dialysate fluid, a renal dialysis machine, an oral abscess, and a scalp wound. Others have reported isolating this species from cervical specimens.[227] *B. diminuta* has been isolated in pure culture from the blood of three patients at the University of Illinois hospital. One patient was a diabetic, another had right middle lobe pneumonia, and a history was not obtained on the third. All isolates were nonpigmented, grew well on MacConkey agar, and were DNase positive with the UNI-N/F system (Remel, Lenexa KS). Moss and Kaltenbach have reported that glutaric acid is produced by *B. diminuta* but not by *B. vesicularis* when the organisms are grown on trypticase soy agar.[204]

rRNA GROUP V

Genus Stenotrophomonas. *Stenotrophomonas* is a new genus consisting of only one species, *S. maltophilia*, which is the current name for the organism formerly known as *Xanthomonas maltophilia* and *Pseudomonas maltophilia*.[231] It is a motile rod, possesses polar multi-trichous flagella, and can be easily distinguished from other pseudomonads by virtue of being lysine- and DNAse-positive and oxidase-negative (see Table 5-3). It vigorously attacks OF maltose but is usually negative or only weakly positive in OF glucose in 24 hours. Colonies may appear pale yellow or lavender green on blood agar medium (see Color Plate 5-3D). We have noted rare strains of *S. maltophilia* that will be slowly oxidase-positive but have all the other biochemical features characteristic of *S. maltophilia*. Students of microbiology should be aware that rare strains possessing aberrant characteristics may be recovered from clinical specimens.

S. maltophilia is ubiquitous and can be recovered from almost any clinical site. It occasionally causes opportunistic infections and is emerging as an important hospital-acquired pathogen.[160,192,208] The most common site for recovery of *S. maltophilia* is the respiratory tract, although in most patients these isolates do not appear to be clinically significant. *S. maltophilia* has been reported to cause a wide spectrum of disease, including pneumonia, bacteremia, endocarditis, cholangitis, urinary tract infection, meningitis, and serious wound infections, particularly in patients with cancer.[78,207,211,319,343] Morrison and colleagues[200] have studied the spectrum of clinical disease in patients with hospital-acquired *S. maltophilia* infections and report both an increasing rate of nosocomial isolation and a crude mortality rate of 43% in all patients from whom the organism was cultured. Risk factors associated with death for patients having an *S. maltophilia* isolate included the following: patient in intensive care unit, age older than 40 years, and a pulmonary source for the *S. maltophilia* isolate.[200] Another important feature in the rising incidence of *S. maltophilia* infections may be the unique antibiotic susceptibility profile of the organism. *S. maltophilia* is inherently resistant to most of the commonly used antipseudomonal drugs, including aminoglycosides and many β-lactam agents, including those effective against *P. aeruginosa*.[214,232,318] Thus, colonization may be favored by the use of broad-spectrum antipseudomonal therapy. Interestingly, *S. maltophilia* is inherently susceptible to trimethoprim–sulfamethoxazole, a drug that has no activity against *P. aeruginosa* nor most other *Pseudomonas* species.[49,82] In addition to the problem of inherent resistance, there is as yet no accepted standardized method for susceptibility testing of *S. maltophilia*. Some automated methods (i.e., Vitek, bioMerieux, St. Louis MO) have programmed software that will prevent the reporting of susceptibility results if the test organism is known to be *S. maltophilia*. Trailing endpoints can be observed in agar-dilution and microdilution tests, and false susceptible readings with disk diffusion assays have occurred with aminoglycosides (should be uniformly resistant) and ciprofloxacin.[123,232] Studies on the use of the E test (discussed in Chap. 15) for antimicrobial susceptibility testing of *S. maltophilia* have noted the presence of tiny microcolonies or a haze of translucent growth within the area of inhibition that if missed could lead to false susceptibility results.[232,341] To learn more, the reader is referred to the review written by Robin and Janda.[260]

OTHER PSEUDOMONADS OF UNKNOWN NUCLEIC ACID HOMOLOGY

Genus Chryseomonas. The genus *Chryseomonas* currently consists of only one species, *C. luteola*. This species has been previously known as *Chromobacterium typhiflavum*, CDC group Ve-1, *Pseudomonas luteola*, and *Pseudomonas polytricha*. The taxonomic status was resolved in 1987 with the placement of this organism into the new genus *Chryseomonas*.[143] The organism is motile by means of multitrichous polar flagella, is oxidase-negative, and grows on both MacConkey and blood agar media, producing yellow-pigmented colonies. The biochemical features that differentiate *C. luteola* from other yellow-pigmented pseudomonads are given in Table 5-9. It is a rare clinical isolate and has been recovered from a variety of clinical specimens, including wound, cervix, urine, and throat specimens.[98] Isolates recovered from clinical specimens at the University of Illinois Hospital have been from the cornea, sputum, leg, and endometrial cavity. It is often isolated with other organisms and judged not to be clinically significant. In one study, only 14 strains of *C. luteola* were found among 565 clinical isolates of nonfermenters over a 2-year period.[234] Reports of serious infections caused by *C. luteola* include bacteremia,[20,79,85,250] endocarditis,[223] osteomyelitis,[250] and peritonitis.[56,250]

Genus Flavimonas. The genus *Flavimonas* is represented by a single species, *F. oryzihabitans*. This organism has been formerly described as *Chromobacterium typhiflavum*, *Pseudomonas oryzihabitans*, and CDC group Ve-2. The taxonomic placement of this species in the new genus *Flavimonas* was made in 1987.[143] *F. oryzihabitans* has characteristics similar to *Chryseomonas luteola* in that these organisms are also motile and oxidase-negative and form yellow-pigmented colonies on blood agar medium. This organism can be differentiated from *C. luteola* by negative reactions for esculin hydrolysis and orthonitrophenyl-β-D-galactopyranoside (ONPG) and the feature of having a single polar flagellum. Additional differential characteristics are given in Table 5-9. *F. oryzihabitans* has also been recovered from a variety of clinical sites, including wounds, sputum, ear, eye, urine, peritoneal fluid, inhalation therapy equipment, and blood.[85,100,243,250] More recently, infections with this organism have been related to the presence of an intravascular catheter in immunocompromised patients.[183,266,320] At the University of Illinois Hospital, this organism has been recovered from sputum, urine, prostatic secretion, skin, and blood. *F. oryzihabitans* also appears to be an emerging pathogen in peritonitis related to continuous ambulatory peritoneal dialysis, with several cases now reported in the literature.[2,18,80] Other predisposing factors for *F. oryzi-*

TABLE 5-9
KEY CHARACTERISTICS OF YELLOW-PIGMENTED PSEUDOMONADS

TEST	SPHINGOMONAS S. PAUCIMOBILIS IIK-1	S. PARAPAUCIMOBILIS	CHRYSEOMONAS LUTEOLA VE-1	FLAVIMONAS ORYZIHABITANS VE-2	BALNEATRIX ALPICA
Oxidase	+	+	−	−	+
Growth on MacConkey	−	−	+	+	−
Motility	+	+	+	+	+
OF glucose	A	A	A	A	A
OF mannitol	−	−	A	A	A
OF rhamnose	−	A	V	V	−
NO₃ reduction	−	−	+	−	+
Indole	−	−	−	−	+
Esculin	+	+	+	−	−
ONPG	+	+	+	−	−
DNAse	+*	−	−	−	−
H₂S, lead acetate	−	+	NA	NA	−
Polymyxin	V (89)	V	S	S	S
Flagella	Single polar	Single polar	Multitrich.	Single polar	Single polar
Pigment	Deep yellow	Deep yellow	Dull yellow	Dull yellow	Yellow

+, 90% or more strains positive; −, 90% or more strains negative; V, 11%–89% of strains positive; ++, strong positive reaction; A, acid reaction; NA, results not available; numbers in parentheses are percentage of strains giving positive reaction.
* Different results reported; reaction used here is that reported by Yabuuchi et al.[340]
Data from Refs. 64, 97, and 340.

habitans infections include indwelling intravascular catheters, artificial grafts, intravenous drug abuse, severe head trauma requiring surgery, and bone marrow transplantation.[48]

Genus Sphingomonas. The new genus Sphingomonas, as originally proposed by Yabuuchi and associates in 1990, consisted of five named and two unnamed genomospecies: S. paucimobilis, S. parapaucimobilis, S. yanoikuyae, S. adhaesiva, S. capsulata, genomospecies 1, and genomospecies 2.[340] The genus description was emended in 1993 with the naming of three new species: S. macrogoltabidus, S. sanguis (formerly Sphingomonas genomospecies 1), and S. terrae (formerly Sphingomonas genomospecies 2).[302] In 1995, four new plant species were added: S. rosa (formerly Agrobacterium rhizogenes), S. pruni, S. asaccharolytica, and S. mali.[303] S. paucimobilis, formerly known as Pseudomonas paucimobilis and as CDC group IIk-1, is the most common species found in human clinical specimens. It is a gram-negative, motile rod with a polar flagellum. However, few cells are actively motile in broth culture, thus making motility a difficult characteristic to demonstrate. Motility occurs at 18° to 22°C but not at 37°C.[230] The oxidase reaction is positive, although Gilardi has reported that only 90% of the strains are oxidase-positive.[96] Colonies grown on blood agar medium are yellow pigmented; however, this species is slow growing and only small colonies may be observed after 24 hours of incubation. Growth occurs at 37°C but not at 42°C, with optimum growth occurring at 30°C.[230] Additional biochemical features are given in Table 5-9. S. paucimobilis has been isolated from a variety of clinical specimens, including blood, cerebrospinal fluid, urine, wounds, vagina, and cervix, and from the hospital environment.[135,253] Community-acquired bacteremia and peritonitis in patients receiving long-term ambulatory peritoneal dialysis have also been reported.[201] There have been a few reports of nosocomially acquired S. paucimobilis infections from contamination of hemodialysis fluids,[41] contamination during in vitro processing of bone marrow for transplantation,[177] and catheter-related sepsis.[66,276,277] There has also been a report of *S. paucimobilis* bacteremia that was accompanied by septic shock in a burn patient.[44]

Genus *Shewanella*. The newly named genus *Shewanella* is composed of three species: *S. putrefaciens* (formerly *Pseudomonas putrefaciens*), *S. hanedai*, and *S. benthica*.[185] All three are generally associated with aquatic and marine habitats; however, the type species, *S. putrefaciens*, has been recovered from human clinical specimens. Strains of *S. putrefaciens* are oxidase-positive and motile by means of polar flagella. They are easily distinguished because they are the only nonfermenters that produce hydrogen sulfide in KIA and TSI media (see Table 5-3). Colonies produce an orange-tan pigment on blood agar medium. Three biovars have been described.[98] Biovar 1 (CDC group Ib-1) is oxidative in both sucrose and maltose. Biovar 2 (CDC group Ib-2) and biovar 3 are both nonoxidative in sucrose and maltose. Biovar 2 grows in 6.5% NaCl, whereas biovars 1 and 3 do not. Biovar 1 has been recovered primarily from dairy and fish products and causes spoilage of protein foods stored at refrigerator temperatures. Biovars 2 and 3 are recovered primarily from human sources and occasionally from the environment.[98,322] Although it is an infrequent clinical isolate, *S. putrefaciens* has been associated with skin ulcers,[7,65,68] ear infections,[91,323] osteomyelitis,[246] bacteremia,[35,161,190] and peritonitis in patients undergoing continuous ambulatory peritoneal dialysis.[61] Several isolates recovered at the University of Illinois Microbiology laboratory have been from stool, sacral decubitus, ulcer of leg tissue, bile, vitreous fluid, and blood.

Unnamed Species. Some organisms possessing characteristics of the family *Pseudomonadaceae* have not been officially named. These include two organisms designated *Pseudomonas*-like group 2 and CDC group WO-1.

- *Pseudomonas-like Group 2*. This is an unclassified group of *Pseudomonas*-like organisms that had been previously included in CDC group IVd. Strains are oxidase positive and motile. Colonies on blood agar are reported to have a sticky consistency and are difficult to remove.[98] Other identifying characteristics include growth on MacConkey agar, oxidation of glucose, xylose, and mannitol, and hydrolysis of urea; and negative reactions for indole, nitrate, esculin hydrolysis, and oxidation of sucrose and maltose.[67] Human clinical isolates have been recovered from the respiratory tract, blood, spinal fluid, feces, urine, and dialysate.[98,110,162,170]
- **CDC Group WO-1**. This is the designation given to a group of weakly oxidative (WO) gram-negative rods isolated primarily from clinical specimens. They oxidize mannitol and glucose, often weakly and sometimes delayed (3 to 7 days), and reduce nitrate. Most strains are motile, with one or two polar

flagella; however, motility is usually delayed in motility medium or is detected only by wet preparation. Strains are usually oxidase- and catalase-positive. Some strains produce soluble pigment (yellow, tan, amber, olive green, or brown). Other differentiating characteristics can be found in the paper by Hollis and colleagues.[126] Isolates characterized at the CDC have been from blood (33%), CSF (10%), urine, lung, wound, and some environmental sources.[126]

FAMILY METHYLOCOCCACEAE

Genus *Methylobacterium*. *Methylobacterium* species are gram-negative, pink-pigmented bacteria that have the ability to facultatively utilize methane.[114] Nine species of *Methylobacterium* (*M. aminovorans, M. extorquens, M. fujisawaense, M. mesophilicum, M. organophilum, M. radiotolerans, M. rhodinum, M. rhodesianum,* and *M. zatmanii*) and additional unassigned biovars are recognized on the basis of carbon assimilation type, electrophoretic type, and DNA–DNA homology grouping.[114,115,312] *M. mesophilicum*, formerly classified as *Pseudomonas mesophilica* and *Vibrio extorquens*, is the species most often isolated from human clinical specimens. Isolates are reported to be oxidase-positive and motile; however, the oxidase reaction may be weak, and motility may be difficult to demonstrate. In our experience, all isolates seen have appeared nonmotile. Other key reactions include positive tests for catalase, urease, and amylase (Table 5-10). Further differentiating characteristics can be found in the paper by Urakami and colleagues.[312] Isolates are slow growing on ordinary media, with best growth occurring on Sabouraud's agar, buffered charcoal–yeast extract agar, or Middlebrook 7H11 agar.[98] Optimum growth occurs from 25° to 30°C. Colonies are dry and appear pink or coral in incandescent light (Color Plate 5-4A). Under UV light, colonies appear dark owing to absorption of UV light. Although classified as a gram-negative rod, this species often does not stain well, or it may show variable results on Gram stain. Individual cells contain large, nonstaining vacuoles that give this organism a unique microscopic appearance[294] (see Color Plate 5-4B). *M. mesophilicum* has been reported to cause chronic skin ulcers,[175] bacteremia in immunocompromised patients,[99,102,156,294] and peritonitis in a patient undergoing continuous ambulatory peritoneal dialysis.[274] Isolates have also been reported from bronchial washings[83] and from the cornea of a patient receiving corticosteroids.[76] Isolates recovered from patients at the University of Illinois Hospital have been from blood, leg tissue, and an appendectomy wound.

ORGANISMS WHOSE TAXONOMIC POSITION IS UNCERTAIN

Genus *Roseomonas*. *Roseomonas* is a newly proposed genus of pink-pigmented bacteria that phenotypically and genotypically resemble *Methylobacterium* species but are separable from the latter by their inability to oxidize methanol, to assimilate acetamide, and by lack of absorption of longwave UV light.[258] Members of the

TABLE 5-10

KEY CHARACTERISTICS OF *METHYLOBACTERIUM* AND *ROSEOMONAS* SPECIES

TEST	METHYLOBACTERIUM SP.	ROSEOMONAS SP.
Oxidase	+	+
Growth on MacConkey	–	+
Growth at 42°C	–	+
Motility	+	V
OF glucose	V	V
OF methanol	+	–
NO₃ reduction	V	V
Starch hydrolysis	+	+
Urea	+	+
Colonies appear dark when exposed to long-wave UV light	+	–
Colonial morphology	Dry, coral	Mucoid, pink
Gram stain morphology	Vacuolated rods	Coccoid rods

+, 90% or more strains positive; −, 90% or more strains negative; V, 11%–89% of strains positive; ++, strong positive reaction.
Data from Refs. 97, 258.

genus are nonfermentative, weakly staining gram-negative, plump coccoid rods, appearing in pairs or short chains, to mainly cocci with only an occasional rod (see Color Plate 5-4D). They grow on 5% sheep blood agar, chocolate agar, BCYE agar, Sabouraud's agar, and almost always (91%) on MacConkey agar. Growth occurs at 25°, 35°, and usually 42°C. Growth appears as pinpoint, pale-pink, shiny, raised, entire, and often mucoid colonies after 2 to 3 days of incubation at 35°C (Color Plate 5-4C). All strains are weakly oxidase-positive (often after 30 seconds) or oxidase-negative, catalase-positive, and urease-positive (see Table 5-10). The genus includes three named species, *R. gilardii*, *R. cervicalis*, and *R. fauriae*, and three un-named genomospecies.[258] About half of the isolates recovered have been from blood, with about 20% from wounds, exudates, and abscesses, and about 10% from genitourinary sites. One case of vertebral osteomyelitis caused by *Roseomonas* has been reported.[212] At the University of Illinois Hospital, we have recovered 21 clinical isolates of pink-pigmented bacteria, mostly from blood; 16 of these fit the description of *Roseomonas* and five have been identified as *Methylobacterium*. We have noted that the *Roseomonas* grow very well on Sabouraud's agar, producing light pink mucoid (sometimes runny) colonies. The organisms do not appear black when viewed under UV light.

Genus *Balneatrix*. *Balneatrix* is a new genus consisting of a single species, *B. alpica*.[64] This bacterium was first isolated in 1987 during an outbreak of pneumonia and meningitis among persons who attended a hot (37°C) spring spa in Southern France.[45,64,147] Thirty-five cases of pneumonia and two cases of meningitis occurred. Isolates from eight patients were recovered from blood, cerebrospinal fluid and sputum, and one from water. The bacterium is described as gram-negative, straight or curved rods, motile by a single polar flagellum, strictly aerobic, and grows at a wide range of temperatures (20° to 46°C). Colonies are 2 to 3 mm in diameter, convex, and smooth. The center of the colonies is pale yellow after 2 to 3 days and pale brown after 4 days. The organism grows on chocolate and tryptic soy agars but not on MacConkey's agar. It is oxidase-positive and nonfermentative but oxidatively utilizes glucose, mannose, fructose, maltose, sorbitol, mannitol, glycerol, and inositol. Indole is produced, and nitrate is reduced to nitrite. Gelatin is weakly hydrolyzed, and lecithinase is positive. The following substrates are not utilized: arginine, lysine, ornithine, urease, esculin, acetamide, starch, and ONPG.[45,64] *B. alpica* is reported to be susceptible to penicillin G and to all other β-lactam antibiotics and to all aminoglycosides, chloramphenicol, tetracycline, erythromycin, sulfonamides, trimethoprim, ofloxacin, and nalidixic acid. It is resistant to clindamycin and vancomycin.[45]

Organisms That Are Motile With Peritrichous Flagella

FAMILY *ALCALIGENACEAE*

This family consists of the genera *Alcaligenes* and *Bordetella*.[69] The biochemical features that differentiate the members of this family, as well as certain other nonfermenters with similar biochemical characteristics, are given in Table 5-11.

Genus *Alcaligenes*. In 1986, Kiredjian and coworkers formally proposed the new names *Alcaligenes xylosoxidans* subsp. *xylosoxidans* (formerly *Achromobacter xylosoxidans*) and *Alcaligenes xylosoxidans* subsp. *denitrificans* (formerly *Alcaligenes denitrificans*) based on rRNA homology studies.[165] They further noted that the type species of the genus, *Alcaligenes faecalis* is synonymous with "*Alcaligenes odorans*" and proposed the name for a new species, *Alcaligenes piechaudii*.[165] Members of the genus *Alcaligenes* are gram-negative rods that are oxidase-positive, grow on MacConkey agar, and are motile by means of peritrichous flagella. Additional differentiating characteristics are given in Table 5-11.

A. xylosoxidans subsp. *xylosoxidans* is easily distinguished from other *Alcaligenes* species by acidification of OF glucose and xylose (thus, the species name). It has been isolated from many types of specimens, most frequently blood, cerebrospinal fluid, bronchial washings, urine, pus, and wounds.[150,321,322] It may be an opportunistic pathogen that has been reported to cause nosocomial infections, including pneumonia, bacteremia, and meningitis, in patients with underlying disease.[199,254,297] A recent study found that *A. xylosoxidans* subsp. *xylosoxidans* colonizes the respiratory tract of intubated children and patients with cystic fibrosis and that colonization of patients with CF is associated with an exacerbation of pulmonary symptoms.[72] *A. xylosoxidans* subsp. *denitrificans* is infrequently recovered from clinical specimens; isolates have been reported from blood collection tubes, blood, ear, cerebrospinal fluid, and urine.[322]

A. faecalis is the most frequently isolated member of the *Alcaligenaceae* in the clinical laboratory. Members of this species produce strong alkaline reactions in all carbohydrate media. Most strains form characteristic colonies with a thin, spreading irregular edge (see

TABLE 5-11
Key Characteristics of *Alcaligenes*, *Bordetella*, and Related Species

TEST	ALCALIGENES A. FAECALIS (ODORANS)	A. XYLOSOXIDANS SUBSP. XYLOSOXIDANS	A. XYLOSOXIDANS SUBSP. DENITRIFICANS	A. PIECHAUDII	BORDETELLA B. HINZII	B. AVIUM	B. BRONCHI-SEPTICA	CDC GROUP IV c-2	OLIGELLA UREOLYTICA (IV e)
Oxidase	+	+	+	+	+	+	+	+	+
Growth on MacConkey	+	+	+	+	NA	+	+	+	V (79)
Motility	+	+	+	+	+	+	+	+	V (84)
OF glucose	ALK	A	ALK	ALK	ALK	ALK	ALK	ALK	ALK
OF xylose	ALK	A	ALK	ALK	ALK	ALK	ALK	ALK	ALK
NO₃ to NO₂	−	+	+	+	−	−	+	−	+
NO₃ to N₂	−	V (69)	+	−	−	−	−	−	V (58)
NO₂ to N₂	+	−	+	−	−	−	−	−	V (63)
Urea	−	−	V (31)	−	V (14)	−	+ +	+ +	+ +
PAD	−	−	−	−	NA	NA	V (25)	−	+
Acetamide	+	V (66)	V (45)	V (42)	+	+	−	−	−
6.5% NaCl	+	−	−	+	+	−	−	−	−
Malonate	+	NA	+	+	+	−	+	+	−
Flagella	Pert.	Pert.	Pert.	Pert.	Pert.	Pert.	Pert.	Pert.	P, L

+, 90% or more strains positive; −, 90% or more strains negative; V, 11%–89% of strains positive; ++, strong positive reaction; A, acid reaction; ALK, alkaline reaction; NA, results not available; numbers in parentheses are percentage of strains giving positive reaction; pert., peritrichous; P, polar; L, lateral.
Data from Refs. 97, 165, 240, 316, 330.

Color Plate 5-3A). Some strains (previously named "A. odorans") produce a characteristic fruity odor (sometimes described as the odor of green apples) and cause a greenish discoloration of blood agar medium. A key biochemical feature of this species is its ability to reduce nitrite but not nitrate. A. faecalis exists in the soil and water and has been isolated from many types of clinical specimens. Most infections are opportunistic and are acquired from moist items, such as nebulizers, respirators, and lavage fluids. Blood, sputum, and urine are common sites of recovery.

A. piechaudii was first described in 1986.[165] It can be distinguished from other species of Alcaligenes by its ability to reduce nitrate and grow in 6.5% sodium chloride (see Table 5-11). Although this species is reported to have been isolated mainly from human clinical material, there is only one report of a possible pathogenic role for this species.[235]

Genus Bordetella. The three most common human species, B. pertussis, B. parapertussis, and B. bronchiseptica, cannot be differentiated genotypically through DNA homology studies; however, phenotypically they behave quite differently. B. bronchiseptica is motile by means of peritrichous flagella and grows readily on ordinary media. B. pertussis and B. parapertussis are both nonmotile. B. pertussis requires special media for growth, whereas B. parapertussis will grow on blood and chocolate agar but not on MacConkey agar. These latter two species will not be discussed in detail here but are covered in Chapter 8 with the fastidious gram-negative rods. Colonies of B. bronchiseptica grow well on blood and MacConkey agar and in 24 hours appear as smooth translucent, colorless colonies about 1.5 mm in diameter. On Gram stain, the organisms appear small and coccobacillary. They have the distinguishing biochemical feature of rapidly converting Christensen's urea agar (see Color Plate 5-2A). Other distinguishing features are given in Table 5-11. B. bronchiseptica is found in the respiratory tract of domestic and wild mammalian animals (the name "bronchiseptica" is derived from the Greek word bronchus, meaning "trachea"). It is an infrequent isolate in the clinical laboratory, and only a few cases of human infections have been reported in the literature.[89] Pedersen and coworkers[234] reported the recovery of only 12 strains of B. bronchiseptica from a total of 565 nonfermenters, all of which were from respiratory specimens obtained from patients who were free of infections. Most symptomatic cases have been in animal caretakers who presented with mild pertussis-like symptoms. Ghosh[89] reported a case of fatal B. bronchiseptica-induced septicemia and bronchopneumonia in a malnourished alcoholic, which indicates that the organism can be virulent under the right circumstances. Woolfrey and Moody reviewed 25 cases of human B. bronchiseptica infection associated with sinusitis, tracheobronchitis, acute pneumonia, pneumonia with septicemia, septicemia, and whooping cough.[336] For the whooping cough cases, it is likely that B. bronchiseptica acted as a colonizer and not as the cause. B. bronchiseptica has been reported to cause pneumonia in patients with

AIDS,[335] and pneumonia and bacteremia following bone marrow transplantation.[16] Most strains of B. bronchiseptica are sensitive to most antibiotics, with the exception of ampicillin, cefamandole, and cefoxitin.[107]

Two new species of Bordetella have been described that may rarely infect humans. Bordetella hinzii was formerly referred to as Alcaligenes faecalis type II, or B. avium-like, and has been isolated from the respiratory tracts of chickens and turkeys in various parts of the world. Human isolates have been recovered from blood and sputum, including repeated isolations from the sputum of a patient with cystic fibrosis.[57,86a,316] B. hinzii are motile and oxidase-positive and must be distinguished from phenotypically similar organisms, as shown in Table 5-11. Bordetella holmesii is a new gram-negative species associated with septicemia.[330] This organism was formerly classified as CDC group NO-2 and is the first Bordetella species not associated with respiratory infections. They are phenotypically most similar to Acinetobacter species and CDC group NO-1. Additional morphologic and phenotypic characteristics are given under the heading "Organisms That Are Nonmotile and Oxidase-Negative."

FAMILY RHIZOBIACEAE

The only medically important member of the family Rhizobiaceae is the genus Agrobacterium. However, members of the genus Agrobacterium are phenotypically similar to saccharolytic Alcaligenes species and Ochrobactrum anthropi, from which they must be differentiated. Characteristics that are useful in separating these organisms are given in Table 5-12. CDC groups EO-2 and EO-3 are also included in Table 5-12 because they are oxidase-positive and produce acid in both OF glucose and OF xylose. However, these species are nonmotile and, therefore, are considered in more detail under the heading "Nonmotile, Oxidase-Positive Nonfermenters."

Genus Agrobacterium. The genus Agrobacterium contains several species of plant pathogens occurring worldwide in soils.[158] As a result of a large number of comparative studies, four distinct species of Agrobacterium are now recognized: A. radiobacter (formerly A. tumefaciens and CDC group Vd-3), A. rhizogenes (subsequently transferred to the genus Sphingomonas as S. rosa[303]), A. vitis,[225] and A. rubi.[278] The separation of species in the genus Agrobacterium has traditionally been based on phytopathogenic characteristics rather than on genetic criteria. In the past, two species, namely, A. tumefaciens and A. radiobacter, have been reported to be isolated from human clinical specimens. These species are indistinguishable phenotypically and were separated only on the basis of a plant tumor-inducing plasmid, which is present in A. tumefaciens and absent in A. radiobacter. Genetic studies have now shown that these two species are the same, and a proposal has been made to reject the name A. tumefaciens and to designate A. radiobacter as the type species for the genus Agrobacterium.[278] The key biochemical tests used in differentiating A. radiobacter from the closely

TABLE 5-12

CHARACTERISTICS OF *OCHROBACTRUM*, *AGROBACTERIUM*, *ACHROMOBACTER*, SACCHAROLYTIC *ALCALIGENES*, AND CDC EO GROUP

TEST	OCHROBACTRUM ANTHROPI VD-1, VD-2	AGROBACTERIUM RADIOBACTER VD-3	ALCALIGENES XYLOSOXIDANS SUBSP. XYLOSOXIDANS	ACHROMOBACTER GROUPS B	E	F	CDC GROUP EO-2	CDC GROUP EO-3
Oxidase	+	+	+	+	+	+	+	+
OF glucose	A	A	A	A	A	A	A	A
OF xylose	A	A	A	A	A	A	A	A
OF lactose	−	A	−	−	−	−	A	A
OF mannitol	V (50)	A	−	A	−	A	V (50)	WK
OF adonitol	+	+	−	−	−	A	NA	NA
OF dulcitol	+	+	−	−	−	A	NA	NA
ONPG	−	+	−	+	+		V (33)	NA
NO$_3$ to NO$_2$	+	V (84)	+	+	+	+	V (42)	−
NO$_3$ to N$_2$	+	−	V (69)	+			−	−
Urea	+	+	−	+	+	+	+ (75)	+
PAD	+	+	−	NA	NA	NA	−	NA
Esculin hydrolysis	V (40)	+	−	+	+	+	−	−
Motility	+	+	+	+	+	+	−	−
Flagella	Pert.	Pert.	Pert.	Pert.	Pert.	Pert.	−	−
Yellow pigment	−	−	−	−	−	−	−	+

+, 90% or more strains positive; −, 90% or more strains negative; V, 11%–89% of strains positive; ++, strong positive reaction; A, acid reaction; ALK, alkaline reaction; NA, results not available; WK, weak acid; Pert., peritrichous; numbers in parentheses are percentage of strains giving positive reaction.
Data from Refs. 97, 138, 205, 240.

related species *Ochrobactrum anthropi* are given in Table 5-12. Key features for this group of organisms are a rapid urease reaction and a positive test for phenylalanine deaminase. Colonies of *A. radiobacter* grow optimally at 25° to 28°C but will grow at 35°C as well. They appear circular, convex, smooth, and nonpigmented to light beige on blood agar. Colonies may appear wet looking and become extremely mucoid and pink on MacConkey with prolonged incubation (Color Plate 5-4E). *A. radiobacter* is occasionally isolated from clinical specimens but only rarely linked with human infection. In cases of reported human infection, *Agrobacterium* has been most frequently isolated from blood[25,40,73,75,77,84,117,245,248,265,333] followed by peritoneal dialysate,[119,263,265] urine,[1,265] and ascitic fluid.[251] The majority of cases have occurred in patients with transcutaneous catheters or implanted biomedical prostheses, and effective treatment often requires removal of the device.[25,73,75,77,84,117,245,248,265,333] Antimicrobial susceptibility is variable, and requires testing of individual isolates.

ORGANISMS WHOSE TAXONOMIC POSITION IS UNCERTAIN

Genus *Achromobacter*. "*Achromobacter*" is a genus without any named species and, therefore, does not have any official taxonomic status. The former type species "*Achromobacter xylosoxidans*" has been moved to the genus *Alcaligenes*.[165] The unnamed species "*Achromobacter*" Vd-1 and Vd-2 have been reassigned as *Ochrobactrum anthropi*.[139] Holmes and colleagues separated achromobacters into six groups (A–F) based on genetic patterns.[131] *Achromobacter* groups A, C, and D constitute a single species and were found to be identical to *Ochrobactrum anthropi*.[139] *Achromobacter* groups B and E constitute biotypes of a single new genus and species that has yet to be named.[129,130,134] *Achromobacter* group F is genetically distinct from groups B and E.[129,130] The biochemical tests useful for separation of *Achromobacter* groups A–F from phenotypically similar bacteria have been reported by Holmes and coworkers.[138] *Achromobacter* groups B and E can be separated from *O. anthropi* by the properties of being ONPG- and esculin-positive and failing to produce acid from adonitol and dulcitol[134] (see Table 5-12). *Achromobacter* group B has been isolated from the blood of two patients with septicemia[133] and one patient with replacement valve endocarditis.[196] Isolates of *Achromobacter* groups E and F have also been recovered from blood.[129,130]

Genus *Ochrobactrum*. *Ochrobactrum anthropi* is the name given to the urease-positive "*Achromobacter*" species formerly designated CDC group Vd-1 and Vd-2.[139] These organisms are oxidase positive, saccharolytic, and motile by means of peritrichous flagella. Key tests useful in distinguishing *O. anthropi* from related organisms include their ability to hydrolyze urea, inability to hydrolyze esculin, and a negative ONPG test. Additional biochemical tests useful in differentiating *O. anthropi* from *Agrobacterium* species and saccharolytic *Alcaligenes* species are shown in Table 5-12. Good growth is observed on routine media in 24 hours. Colonies are about 1 mm in diameter and appear circular, low convex, smooth, shining, and entire. Isolates we have observed grow readily on MacConkey agar and appear mucoid. All strains of *O. anthropi* have thus far been recovered from human clinical specimens (*anthropi* is derived from Greek and means "of a human being"). Strains have been isolated predominantly from blood, wounds, urogenital tracts or urine, respiratory tracts, ears, feces, an eye, and cerebrospinal fluid.[8,14,139,317] Of particular concern are recent reports of central venous catheter (CVC)-related sepsis caused by *O. anthropi*.[51,112,157,166] Isolation of this organism from blood should raise suspicion of CVC-related infection. *O. anthropi* are reported to be susceptible to aminoglycosides, carbenicillin, fluoroquinolones, tetracycline, and trimethoprim-sulfamethoxazole but are resistant to other antimicrobial agents.[97,157,322]

Genus *Oligella*. The genus *Oligella* consists of two species: *O. urethralis* (formerly *Moraxella urethralis* and CDC group M-4) and *O. ureolytica* (formerly CDC group IVe).[272] *O. urethralis* is similar to *Moraxella* species in that isolates are coccobacillary, oxidase-positive, nonmotile, gram-negative bacteria. Biochemical features that help differentiate *O. urethralis* from *Moraxella* species are shown in Table 5-13. As the name indicates, *O. urethralis* is most frequently recovered from urethral specimens and is considered a commensal of the genitourinary tract. There has been one report of *O. urethralis* infectious arthritis in a case clinically mimicking gonococcal arthritis.[197]

Colonies of *O. ureolytica* are first seen as slow growing on blood agar medium, producing pinpoint colonies after 24 hours but large colonies after 3 days of incubation. Colonies are white, opaque, entire, and nonhemolytic. *O. ureolytica* strains phenotypically resemble nonsaccharolytic *Alcaligenes* species, *Bordetella bronchiseptica*, and CDC group IVc-2 in that they are nonsaccharolytic, oxidase positive, and motile by means of peritrichous flagella. They differ from *Alcaligenes* species by their ability to rapidly hydrolyze urea

in Christensen's urea agar. Additional differentiating features are shown in Table 5-11. Most isolates have been obtained from human urine, often in patients with long-dwelling catheters. One case of bacteremia in a patient with obstructive uropathy has been reported.[262] One isolate was recovered from a patient at the University of Illinois hospital who presented with a facial wound with facial impetigo and cellulitis. *O. ureolytica* tends to be susceptible to most antibiotics.

CDC Group IVc-2. The unnamed species CDC group IVc-2 is an oxidase-positive, nonsaccharolytic gram-negative rod that is motile by means of peritrichous flagella. It therefore phenotypically resembles *Alcaligenes*, *Bordetella*, and *Oligella ureolytica*, from which it must be differentiated (see Table 5-11). There have been five cases of bacteremia in immunocompromised patients reportedly caused by this organism;[6,59,60,252,342] two cases of peritonitis following continuous ambulatory peritoneal dialysis, one with accompanying septicemia[342] and one with a mixed infection with IVc-2 and *Alcaligenes faecalis*;[118] and one case of tenosynovitis of the hand following a cat bite.[209] In the latter case it is not clear whether the etiology of the infectious agent was the cat bite or the tap water used to rinse the lesion.

ORGANISMS THAT ARE NONMOTILE AND OXIDASE-POSITIVE

FAMILY *FLAVOBACTERIACEAE*

Recently, Vandamme and colleagues reported that none of the established species of flavobacteria were closely related to the type species *F. aquatile*; therefore, they proposed that the generically misclassified organisms *Flavobacterium balustinum*, *F. gleum*, *F. indologenes*, *F. indoltheticum*, *F. meningosepticum*, and *F. scophthalmum* be included in a new genus, *Chryseobacterium* with *C. gleum* as the type species.[314] These same authors reported that *Flavobacterium breve* represented a distinct genetic taxon and proposed the name *Empedobacter brevis* for this species.[314] Furthermore, [*Flavobacterium*]* *odoratum* is generically misnamed and will need reclassification to a new genus.[22] French researchers working together with Vandamme's group in Belgium published an emended description of the family *Flavobacteriaceae* and an emended classification and description of the genus *Flavobacterium*.[22] The emended description of the family *Flavobacteriaceae* includes seven rRNA branches or clusters and a host of new species classifications as outlined in Box 5-4.[22]

Interestingly, none of the newly classified *Flavobacterium* species are found in human clinical specimens, and none are indole-positive—a feature that has been synonymous with the genus *Flavobacterium* in the past. The key differentiating features of the clinically significant members of the family *Flavobacteriaceae* and related bacteria are given in Tables 5-14 and 5-15. Most

---

*Brackets indicate generically misclassified bacteria.

TABLE 5-13

KEY CHARACTERISTICS OF *MORAXELLA*, *OLIGELLA URETHRALIS*, AND *MORAXELLA*-LIKE SPECIES

| | MORAXELLA | | | | | | | OLIGELLA | NEISSERIA | | GILARDI |
TEST	*LACUNATA*	*NONLIQUEFACIENS*	*CANIS*	*LINCOLNII*	*OSLOENSIS*	*PHENYLPYRUVICA* M-2	*ATLANTAE* M-3	*URETHRALIS* M-4	*WEAVERI* M-5	*ELONGATA SUBSP NITROREDUCENS** M-6	ROD GROUP 1
Oxidase	+	+	+	+	+	+	+	+	+	+	+
Catalase	+	+	+	+	+	+	+	+	+	–	+
MacConkey	–	V (17)	+	NA	V (49)	+	+	V (83)	–	V (20)	+
Motility	–	–	–	–	–	–	–	–	–	–	–
OF glucose	–	–	–	–	–	–	–	–	–	–	–
Urea	–	–	–	–	–	+	–	–	–	–	–
PAD	–	–	–	NA	–	+	–	+	w+	–	++
Gelatin hydrolysis	+	–	–	–	–	–	–	–	–	–	–
NO₃ reduced	+	+	+	–	V (26)	+	–	–	–	+	–
NO₂ reduced	–	–	V	V	–	–	V (20)	+	+	+	–
DNAse	–	–	+	–	–	–	–	–	–	–	–
Penicillin	S	S	S	S	S	S (78)	S	S	S	S	S
Cell shape	cb	cb	c	cb	cb	cb	cb	cb	r	r	r

Data obtained from references 4, 97, 113, 154, 203, 205, 240, 315.
+, 90% or more strains positive; –, 90% or more strains negative; V, 11%–89% of strains positive; ++, strong positive reaction; A, acid reaction; ALK, alkaline reaction; NA, results not available; numbers in parentheses are percent of strains giving positive reaction; R, resistant; S, susceptible; c, cocci, cb, coccobacilli, r, rods; w+, weak positive; PAD, phenylalanine deaminase
**N. elongata* subsp. *elongata* is catalase, glucose, and nitrate negative and nitrite positive. *N. elongata* subsp. *glycolytica* is catalase positive, glucose weakly positive, nitrate negative and nitrite positive. *N. elongata* subsp. *nitroreducens* is catalase negative and glucose weakly positive or negative and reduces nitrate and nitrite.[4,128]

BOX 5-4. DESCRIPTION OF THE FAMILY *FLAVOBACTERIACEAE*

Chryseobacterium–Bergeyella–Riemerella rRNA Cluster

Chryseobacterium indologenes
Chryseobacterium gleum
Chryseobacterium balustinum
Chryseobacterium indoltheticum
Chryseobacterium scophthalmum
Chryseobacterium meningosepticum
Bergeyella zoohelcum
Riemerella anatipestifer

Ornithobacterium rhinotracheale Branch

Empedobacter–Weeksella rRNA Cluster

Empedobacter brevis
Weeksella virosa

Capnocytophaga rRNA Branch

Capnocytophaga ochracea
Capnocytophaga gingivalis
Capnocytophaga sputigena

[Flavobacterium]* odoratum rRNA Branch

Flavobacterium aquatile rRNA Cluster

Flavobacterium aquatile
Flavobacterium branchiophilum
Flavobacterium columnare
Flavobacterium flevense
Flavobacterium hydatis
Flavobacterium johnsoniae
Flavobacterium pectinovorum
Flavobacterium psychrophilum
Flavobacterium saccharophilum
Flavobacterium succinicans

[Flexibacter]* maritimus rRNA Branch

* Brackets indicate generically misclassified bacteria.

species produce yellow-pigmented colonies on blood agar medium, and all are oxidase-positive. All species are nonmotile and negative for nitrate reduction, and most species fail to grow on MacConkey agar. Most species (except *Weeksella virosa*) are polymyxin-resistant, a property they share with the pseudomallei group discussed elsewhere in this chapter. Only the clinically significant members of the *Flavobacteriaceae* will be discussed further in this chapter. The taxonomic dilemma of *Flavobacterium* and *Sphingobacterium* has been reviewed in detail elsewhere.[22,288,314,338]

Chryseobacterium and Empedobacter. These former *Flavobacterium* species occur naturally in soil, water, plants, and foodstuffs. In the hospital environment they exist in water systems and wet surfaces. They are readily distinguished from other nonfermenters by their ability to produce indole in tryptophan broth (see Color Plate 5-2C). Often the indole reaction is weak and difficult to demonstrate; therefore, the more sensitive Ehrlich method (discussed earlier in this chapter) should be used. *C. indologenes* is the most frequently isolated species from human clinical specimens and is easily recognized by the production of dark yellow colonies. *C. meningosepticum*, in contrast, produces colonies with a very pale yellow pigment that may not be evident on initial examination of colonies at 24 hours. Pigment production may be augmented by incubating the culture for an additional 24 hours at room temperature. The *Chryseobacterium* species generally grow poorly, or not at all, on MacConkey agar and are

considered to be glucose oxidizers, although most strains will slowly ferment glucose after prolonged incubation. Additional characteristics separating the members of this group of organisms can be found in Table 5-14.

C. meningosepticum (formerly *Flavobacterium meningosepticum* and CDC group IIa) is the species most often associated with significant disease in humans. It is highly pathogenic for premature infants and has been associated with neonatal meningitis; it may also cause pneumonia in adults, usually in immunosuppressed patients. Although neonatal meningitis is only rarely encountered (only 100 cases were reported between 1944 and 1981),[137] it is important to diagnose the disease accurately because epidemics may occur in nurseries, and a mortality rate as high as 55% has been reported.[322] This organism was isolated from the blood of three patients at the University of Illinois Hospital during the period July 1989 to September 1990. All three were premature infants younger than 1 month old. Isolates of *C. indologenes* (formerly *F. indologenes* and CDC group IIb) recovered in the microbiology laboratory at the University of Illinois Hospital have been mostly from wounds and tracheal cultures; one isolate was recovered from the blood of a neonate delivered by cesarean section. The infant was not septic and was later discharged from the hospital. *Empedobacterium brevis* (formerly *Flavobacterium breve*) and the unnamed CDC groups IIe, IIg, IIh, and IIi are rarely recovered from clinical material, and little is known about their involvement in clinical disease. One case of meningitis

TABLE 5-14

KEY CHARACTERISTICS OF THE FAMILY *FLAVOBACTERIACEAE* AND RELATED BACTERIA THAT ARE INDOLE POSITIVE

TEST	CHRYSEOBACTERIUM MENINGOSEPTICUM IIA	INDOLOGENES IIB	CDC GROUPS IIE	IIG	IIH	III	WEEKSELLA VIROSA IIF	BERGEYELLA ZOOHELCUM IIJ	EMPEDOBACTER BREVIS
Oxidase	+	+	+	+	+	+	+	+	+
Growth on MacConkey	V (26)	−	−	+	V (11)	−	−	−	−
Motility	−	−	−	−	−	−	−	−	−
OF glucose	A*	A*	−	−	A	A	−	−	V (80)
OF mannitol	A*	−	−	−	−	−	−	−	−
Indole	+	+	+	+	+	+	+	+	+
Starch hydrolysis	−	+	+	NA	+	V (14)	−	−	V (40)
Esculin	+	+	NA	−	+	+	−	−	−
ONPG	+	V (41)	NA	NA	−	+	−	−	−
DNAse	+	−	−	−	V (78)	−	−	−	+
Urea	−	−	−	−	V (11)	−	−	++	−
Penicillin	R	R	S	NA	S (67)	S (57)	S	S	R
Polymyxin	R	R	S	S	S (22)	R	S	R	R
Pigment (yellow)	Pale	Bright	Pale	Pale	Pale	Pale	Pale	−	Pale

Data obtained from references 97, 124.
+, 90% or more strains positive; −, 90% or more strains negative; V, 11%–89% of strains positive; ++, strong positive reaction; A, acid rxn; ALK, alkaline rxn; NA, results not available; numbers in parentheses are percent of strains giving positive reaction; R, resistant; S, susceptible.
*Delayed reaction.

caused by CDC group IIe has been reported,[326] and the phenotypic characteristics of 11 clinical isolates of CDC group IIg have also been recently reported.[124]

***Weeksella* and *Bergeyella*.** The genus *Weeksella* as originally proposed contained two species, *W. virosa* (formerly CDC group IIf) and *W. zoohelcum* (formerly CDC group IIj).[141,142] Vandamme and colleagues have shown that these two species represent separate genetic taxa and thus have proposed the reclassification of one of these species, *W. zoohelcum*, as *Bergeyella zoohelcum*.[314] Both species are oxidase-positive, fail to grow on MacConkey agar, and are nonpigmented, nonsaccharolytic, and indole-positive. Both species have the unusual feature of being susceptible to penicillin, a feature that allows them to be easily differentiated from the related genera (see Table 5-14). *W. virosa* (derived from the Latin word for "slimy") forms mucoid, sticky colonies that are difficult to remove from agar. It has been recovered primarily from the urogenital tract of women, but there is as yet no evidence that it can play a pathogenic role.[141] *B. zoohelcum* is part of the normal oral and nasal

flora of dogs. It is not surprising, therefore, that the majority of human isolates have been the result of dog or cat bites.[142] A key differentiating feature of *B. zoohelcum* is the production of an intense urease reaction in Christensen's urea agar (see Table 5-14). The only evidence that it can play a pathogenic role is from a report of meningitis following multiple dog bites.[34]

[*Flavobacterium*] *odoratum*. *F. odoratum* is a generically misnamed member of the family *Flavobacteriaceae*. It is distinctive in that it typically forms effuse, spreading colonies that may be confused with the colony morphology of a *Bacillus* species. A telltale characteristic of *F. odoratum* is a characteristic fruity odor (similar to the odor of *A. faecalis*). It grows on MacConkey agar but is asaccharolytic. Additional distinguishing features are given in Table 5-15. *F. odoratum* has been reported mostly from urine, but it has also been found in wound, sputum, blood, and ear specimens.[140] Clinical infection with this organism is exceedingly rare; however, a case of rapidly progressive necrotizing fasciitis and bacteremia has been reported.[146]

KEY CHARACTERISTICS OF [FLAVOBACTERIUM] ODORATUM AND GENUS SPHINGOBACTERIUM

| TEST | [FLAVOBACTERIUM] ODORATUM M4F | SPHINGOBACTERIUM | | |
		MULTIVORUM IIK2	SPIRITIVORUM IIK3	THALPOPHILUM
Oxidase	+	+	+	+
Growth on MacConkey	V (78)	V (17)	−	V (14)
Motility	−	−	−	−
OF glucose	−	A	A	A
OF mannitol	−	−	A	−
Indole	−	−	−	−
NO₃ reduction	−	−	−	+
Gelatin hydrolysis	+	−	−	V (86)
Starch hydrolysis	−	V (79)	−	+
Esculin	−	+	+	+
ONPG	−	+	+	+
DNAse	+	−	+	+
Urea	+	+	+	+
Penicillin	S (19)	R	R	R
Polymyxin	R	R	R	R
Pigment (yellow)	Yel-Green	Pale	Pale	NA

Data obtained from reference 97.

+, 90% or more strains positive; −, 90% or more strains negative; V, 11%–89% of strains positive; ++, strong positive reaction; A, acid rxn; ALK, alkaline rxn; NA, results not available; numbers in parentheses are percent of strains giving positive reaction; R, resistant; S, susceptible.

ORGANISMS WHOSE TAXONOMIC POSITION IS UNCERTAIN

Genus *Sphingobacterium*.   The sphingobacteria are yellow-pigmented, oxidase-positive, and nonmotile. They are differentiated from Chryseobacteria and Weekesellae by their failure to produce indole from tryptophan. Eight named species and two unnamed genomospecies are currently described: *S. multivorum* (formerly *Flavobacterium multivorum*, CDC group IIk-2), *S. spiritivorum* (includes species formerly designated *Flavobacterium spiritivorum*, *F. yabuuchiae*, and CDC group IIk-3), *S. mizutae*, *S. thalpophilum*, *S. heparinum*, *S. faecium*, *S. antarcticus*, *S. piscium*, and unnamed species *Sphingobacterium* genomospecies 1 and 2.[144,289,304,338] Two species, *S. multivorum* and *S. spiritivorum*, have been most frequently recovered from human clinical specimens. They can be distinguished from the similar organism *Sphingomonas paucimobilis* (formerly IIk-1) by lack of motility and resistance to polymyxin. Additional differentiating features of these bacteria are given in Table 5-15. *S. multivorum* has been isolated from vari-

ous clinical specimens but has only rarely been associated with serious infections (peritonitis and two cases of sepsis).[86] Blood and urine have been the most common sources for the isolation of *S. spiritivorum*.[136]

Genus *Moraxella*.   The correct taxonomic placement of the genus *Moraxella* remains a controversy. It has been proposed that the genus *Branhamella* be transferred to the genus *Moraxella* in the *Neisseriaceae*, a proposal that is included in the most recent edition of *Bergey's Manual of Systematic Bacteriology*.[32] More recently, two new proposals have been made, one assigning *Moraxella* to the new family *Moraxellaceae* and another assigning *Moraxella* to the new family *Branhamaceae*. A more detailed review of the taxonomic placement of the genus *Moraxella* is given in Chapter 10 of this text.

Several key features make one suspect that an unknown nonfermenter may belong to the genus *Moraxella*. After 24 hours on blood agar, the colonies tend to be small and pinpoint (usually less than 0.5 mm in diameter), with poor or no growth on MacConkey agar. The bacterial cells appear as tiny, gram-negative diplococci or diplobacilli in gram-stained preparations. Both the cytochrome oxidase and catalase reactions are positive (the former rules out *Acinetobacter* species; the latter rules out *Kingella* species). The inability of *Moraxella* species to form acid from carbohydrates also eliminates most *Neisseria* species from consideration. However, *Moraxella catarrhalis* is also asaccharolytic and may be difficult to distinguish. Most *Moraxella* species are extremely sensitive to low concentrations of penicillin; however, β-lactamase–producing strains have been encountered.[32] Examination of gram-stained smears prepared from the outer zone of inhibition around the penicillin susceptibility disk can be used to distinguish *Neisseria* species (which retain their coccal morphology) from *Moraxella* species (which produce elongated, pleomorphic forms; see Color Plates 5-3G and H).[46] All *Moraxella* species are nonmotile.

The *Moraxella* species of medical importance are *M. lacunata*, *M. nonliquefaciens*, *M. osloensis*, *M. phenylpyruvica* (CDC group M-2), and *M. atlantae* (CDC group M-3). CDC group M-4 has been named *Oligella urethralis* and is covered elsewhere in this chapter. CDC groups M-5 and M-6 have both been placed in the genus *Neisseria*, even though their microscopic appearance is that of gram-negative rods (see Color Plates 5-4G and H). Group M-5 has been designated *Neisseria weaveri*,[128] and group M-6 has been named *Neisseria elongata* subsp. *nitroreducens*.[113] These species, along with other recently described *Moraxella* species such as *M. canis*[154] and *M. lincolnii*,[315] are difficult to distinguish from the established species of *Moraxella*. Nonhuman species include *M. bovis*, isolated from healthy cattle and other animals, including horses, and *M. caprae* isolated from healthy goats.[172] Because many strains of *Moraxella* are somewhat fastidious and biochemical reactions are often negative or equivocal, many laboratories choose to simply report members of this group as "*Moraxella* species." Table 5-13 provides some useful differential tests for those wishing to make an attempt at species identification.

Moraxella species are normal flora on mucosal surfaces and are considered to have low pathogenic potential. They occur most frequently in the respiratory tract and less commonly in the genital tract and occasionally may cause systemic infection. *M. lacunata*, which has been known since the turn of the century to cause conjunctivitis, is fastidious and requires either enriched nonpeptone media or the addition of oleic acid or rabbit serum to counteract a toxic proteolytic effect. In addition to conjunctivitis, this species has been reported to cause keratitis, chronic sinusitis, and endocarditis.[259,311] *M. nonliquefaciens* also may require serum supplements for optimal growth. It is part of the normal flora in the human upper respiratory tract and is frequently isolated from the nasal cavity. It has been isolated from the blood, eye, cerebrospinal fluid, lower respiratory tract, and other local sites[31,111,311] and has been associated with endophthalmitis[74,181] and septic arthritis.[155] *M. osloensis* and *M. phenylpyruvica* are most commonly recovered from clinical specimens and do not

require growth supplements. These species are usually not pathogenic when isolated from humans; however, isolated cases of sinusitis, conjunctivitis, bronchitis, septic arthritis, osteomyelitis, peritonitis, meningitis, endocarditis, central venous catheter infection, and septicemia have been reported.[37,81,269,300] *M. atlantae* grows slowly in culture medium, producing colonies with a tendency to form a spreading zone after 48 hours incubation.[33] There has been one report of bacteremia caused by this organism.[36] *M. canis* is a new species, the main habitat of which is the upper respiratory tracts of dogs and cats. Three human isolates have been reported: two from blood and one from a dog bite wound.[154] Isolates of *M. canis* are DNase positive and resemble *M. catarrhalis* on Gram stain; however, their colonial morphology on sheep blood agar more closely resembles that of members of the *Enterobacteriaceae* (large, smooth colonies).[154] *M. lincolnii* has been isolated mainly from the respiratory tract of humans.[315] Because all *Moraxella* species are highly sensitive to penicillin, antibiotic susceptibility testing is usually not performed on clinical isolates.

Neisseria weaveri is found as normal oral flora in dogs and is associated with human wound infections resulting from dog bites.[4,128] *N. elongata* subsp. *nitroreducens* has been reported to cause bacteremia, endocarditis, and osteomyelitis.[87,151,236,292,334] *N. elongata* subsp. *elongata* and *N. elongata* subsp. *glycolytica* are considered to be transient colonizers of the human upper respiratory tract and urogenital tract; however, *N. elongata* subsp. *elongata* has been reported to cause human endocarditis,[213] and *N. elongata* subsp. *glycolytica* has been isolated from human wounds and blood cultures.[5]

CDC Groups EO-2 and EO-3 and *Psychrobacter immobilis*. This group of eugonic oxidizers (EO) includes aerobic, gram-negative, coccoid to short, thick or slightly thick rods. All are strongly oxidase-positive, nonmotile, and indole-negative and utilize glucose, xylose, and lactose[205] (see Table 5-12). EO-2 strains have a distinctive "O"-shaped cellular morphology on Gram stain examination owing to the presence of vacuolated or peripherally stained cells (see Color Plate 5-4F).[205] This O-shaped morphology is not observed with *P. immobilis* or EO-3 strains. EO-2 strains are also reported to have an odor resembling that of a phenylethyl alcohol blood agar plate.[148] EO-3 strains are reported to have a definite yellow, nondiffusible pigment that is not observed with either *P. immobilis* or EO-2 organisms.[205] Most strains of *P. immobilis* grow lightly or not at all at 35°C and grow best at 20°C.[148] EO-2 and EO-3 have been recovered from a variety of body sites including urine, eye, blood, cerebrospinal fluid, throat, vagina, and a variety of wounds.[205] *P. immobilis* has been recovered from blood, brain tissue, urethra, poultry, wound tissue, cerebrospinal fluid, vagina, and eye.[148]

Gilardi Rod Group I. This group consists of nonfastidious, nonoxidative, gram-negative, oval to medium-length and sometimes pleomorphic rods. The cultural and biochemical characteristics of these organisms are most similar to CDC group M-5, now called *Neisseria weaveri*. All Gilardi rod group 1 strains are strongly positive in the phenylalanine deaminase reaction, producing a deep green color in the agar slant, whereas M-5 isolates, when positive, give a weak to moderate reaction. All M-5 isolates reduce 0.01% nitrite, whereas all Gilardi rod group 1 isolates are negative.[97,203] Other differentiating characteristics are given in Table 5-13. Isolates of Gilardi rod group 1 have been recovered from a variety of human sources, including leg, arm, and foot wounds; an oral lesion; urine; and blood; however, their pathogenic potential has yet to be determined.[203]

ORGANISMS THAT ARE NONMOTILE AND OXIDASE-NEGATIVE

Genus *Acinetobacter*. *Acinetobacter* species are nonmotile, oxidase-negative coccobacilli. In 1986, Bouvet and Grimont provided a new classification that distinguished 12 different groups (genomospecies) within the genus *Acinetobacter* based on DNA–DNA hybridization and nutritional characteristics.[27] In 1989, Tjernberg and Ursing[310] described three additional DNA groups coded 13 through 15; concurrently, Bouvet and Jeanjean[29] described five DNA groups of proteolytic *Acinetobacter* species that they number 13 through 17. However, two of the DNA groups described by Tjernberg and Ursing differ phenotypically from the DNA groups described by Bouvet and Jeanjean. Thus, different DNA groups have the same number, which adds to the confusion surrounding the present subdivision of the genus. Genomospecies 1 is the type species *A. calcoaceticus* and is isolated principally from soil. Genomospecies 2 is *A. baumannii* and includes those isolates previously referred to as *A. calcoaceticus* var. *anitratus*. The designation *anitratus* is considered an invalid name and should no longer be used. Genomospecies 4 is named *A. haemolyticus*; genomospecies 5 is named *A. junii*; genomospecies 7 is named *A. johnsonii*; and genomospecies 8 is named *A. lwoffii*. The remaining genomospecies are all unnamed. A scheme of phenotypic tests has been described for *Acinetobacter* genomospecies 1 through 12.[27] Because of problems in separating the saccharolytic strains belonging to DNA groups 1, 2, 3, and 13 using phenotypic tests, some laboratories have chosen to report members of this group as "*Acinetobacter calcoaceticus–A. baumannii* complex," or "saccharolytic *Acinetobacter*." Similarly, laboratories may wish to report the nonsaccharolytic members of this genus as "nonsaccharolytic *Acinetobacter*." *A. baumannii* is the most commonly found species in human clinical specimens followed by *Acinetobacter* species 3.[30] *A. johnsonii*, *A. lwoffii*, and *Acinetobacter* species 12 are nonsaccharolytic *Acinetobacter* species that occur as natural inhabitants of human skin.[30] *A. lwoffii* is the most frequently isolated of the nonsaccharolytic species.

One initial clue that a nonfermenter isolate may belong to the genus *Acinetobacter* is the gram-stained morphology: gram-negative coccobacillary cells often appear as diplococci (see Color Plate 5-3*E*). This similarity in appearance to *Neisseria gonorrhoeae* led to the archaic taxonomic genus designation "*Mima*" (to mimic). After 24 hours of growth on blood agar, the colonies are between 0.5 and 2 mm in diameter, translucent to opaque (never pigmented), convex, and entire. Most strains grow well on MacConkey agar and produce a faint pink tint (see Color Plate 5-3*F*). Presumptive identification of *Acinetobacter* species can be made on the basis of the lack of cytochrome oxidase activity, lack of motility, and resistance to penicillin.

A. baumannii is saccharolytic and acidifies most OF carbohydrates; in particular, definitive identification is made by demonstrating the rapid production of acid from lactose (1% and 10% concentrations). In contrast, *A. lwoffii* is asaccharolytic. Genomospecies 7, *A. johnsonii*, is also asaccharolytic but can be separated from all other *Acinetobacter* species by its failure to grow at 37°C. Additional differentiating features of the 12 genomospecies can be found in the paper of Bouvet and Grimont.[27]

A variety of human infections caused by *Acinetobacter* species has been reviewed by Lyons,[184] including pneumonia (most often related to endotracheal tubes or tracheostomies),[39] endocarditis, meningitis, skin and wound infections, peritonitis (in patients receiving peritoneal dialysis), and urinary tract infections. Sporadic cases of conjunctivitis, osteomyelitis, and synovitis have also been reported.[105] It is now recognized that *Acinetobacter* spp. play a significant role in the colonization and infection of hospitalized patients. They have been implicated in a variety of nosocomial infections, including bacteremia, urinary tract infection, and secondary meningitis, but their predominant role is as agents of nosocomial pneumonia, particularly ventilator-associated pneumonia in patients confined to hospital intensive care units.[20a] *A. baumannii* is the species most prevalent in clinical specimens and is the one most often responsible for hospital-acquired infections.[17,182] A biotyping system for differentiating 17 biotypes of *A. baumannii* based on utilization of six substrates has been established and may be useful for epidemiologic studies.[28] Other species, such as *A. johnsonii*, *A. lwoffii*, and genomospecies 12, seem to be natural inhabitants of the human skin and may also be commensals in the oropharynx and vagina.[30] *A. lwoffii* has been more commonly associated with meningitis than other *Acinetobacter* species.[290] *Acinetobacter* species tend to be resistant to a variety of antibiotics, although one species, *A. lwoffii*, tends to be more sensitive than the others. There is almost universal resistance to penicillin, ampicillin, and cephalothin, and most strains are resistant to chloramphenicol.[184,284] We have noticed an increased trend toward aminoglycoside resistance among the *Acinetobacter* species in recent years. Variable susceptibility to second- and third-generation cephalosporins has been found, and individual susceptibility testing must be performed to determine strain variations. Susceptibility to trimethoprim–sulfamethoxazole is also variable. Combined treatment with an aminoglycoside and ticarcillin or piperacillin is synergistic and may be effective in serious infections.

CDC Group NO-1. An unnamed species of a fastidious, nonoxidative, gram-negative rod, designated CDC group NO-1 (nonoxidizer-1), has been isolated from human wounds resulting primarily from dog or cat bites.[125] This organism is nonmotile and oxidase-negative but can be readily separated from *Acinetobacter* species by a positive nitrate reduction test.

***Bordetella holmesii* (CDC Group NO-2).** This recently named species, formerly classified as CDC group NO-2, is described as gram-negative, small coccoid and short rods, with medium-width longer rods occasionally observed. They are asaccharolytic, oxidase-negative, nonmotile, and fastidious, and they produce a brown soluble pigment.[330] The lack of oxidase activity and the production of a brown soluble pigment differentiate *B. holmesii* from *B. pertussis*, *B. bronchiseptica*, and *B. avium*; the lack of urease activity differentiates this species from *B. parapertussis*. A negative nitrate reaction differentiates it from NO-1 strains, and the production of a brown soluble pigment differentiates it from *Acinetobacter* species. *B. holmesii* has been found only in the blood of humans.[330]

APPROACH TO RECOVERY AND IDENTIFICATION OF NONFERMENTERS

LEVELS OF SERVICE IN IDENTIFICATION OF NONFERMENTERS

The level to which species identification of nonfermenters is performed depends on the size and purpose of the individual laboratory. Reference laboratories, or universities and clinics where students and residents are being trained, may be required to identify all recovered nonfermenters to the species level. Laboratories that provide services primarily for the medical community may be prepared to identify only the more frequently encountered species, sending the rare isolates to a reference laboratory. In a study of 486 strains of nonfermenters isolated in the clinical laboratories at the University of California at Los Angeles, Pickett[238] reported that a single species, namely *P. aeruginosa*, accounted for 66% of all nonfermentative bacilli isolates, followed in order by *A. baumannii* about 7%, *S. maltophilia* and *Flavobacterium* species about 4% each, and all other nonfermenter species constituted the remaining 20% in approximately equal proportions.

In the analysis of bacteriology specimens circulated by the CDC for their microbiology performance evaluation programs, Griffin and associates[116] have found that laboratories for which the volume of specimen testing is small (fewer than 80 samples per week) average about double the error rate of laboratories handling more than 1200 specimens per week. They conclude that this difference in performance is constant and that a laboratory cannot necessarily correct its performance for many of the reasons listed in Box 5-5. They recommend that laboratories limit testing to procedures that can be done well and make arrangements

BOX 5-5. FACTORS CONTRIBUTING TO THE DIFFICULTIES IN IDENTIFYING NONFERMENTERS

1. Most species are only infrequently encountered.
2. Because of this infrequency, laboratory personnel may not be familiar with many of the nonfermenters.
3. Much of the conventional culture media is not suitable for identifying nonfermenters.
4. Many species grow slowly, and biochemical reactivity is weak, requiring considerable experience to interpret equivocal reactions.
5. Quality control of culture media may be difficult, and, because of infrequent use, outdating becomes a problem.
6. Packaged commercial kit systems often have low accuracy in the identification of the more fastidious strains of nonfermenters, requiring the use of additional media.

with a reference laboratory to provide services for testing those specimens that are received infrequently. Factors that contribute to the difficulties in identifying nonfermenters are listed in Box 5-5.

Several commercial packaged systems for the identification of nonfermenters (discussed later in this chapter) are currently available;[127,169,219,222,228,261,299,327] however, because these systems depend on bacterial growth and on the formation of biochemical products in conventional media or in marginally nutritious substrates, only the more biochemically active species can be identified with an acceptable degree of accuracy. Furthermore, the biochemically active nonfermenters can be identified easily in most laboratories using a few conventional media and tests.[220]

The accuracy of performance is also improved with the use of one of several automated or semiautomated bacterial identification systems, primarily because they rely on automatic instrument readings and recording of results, eliminating the subjective bias inherent in the visual interpretation of equivocal endpoints. These instruments have the advantage of making identifications several hours faster than conventional methods. For example, Plorde and associates[244] report that the AutoMicrobic system (bioMerieux Vitek, Inc., Hazelwood MO) correctly identified, within an average time of 11 hours, 93.8% of a group of nonfermenters other than pigmented *P. aeruginosa*. These instruments, however, are costly to purchase and maintain and are designed primarily for use in laboratories with a relatively high volume of testing.

GUIDELINES FOR RECOVERY OF NONFERMENTERS

With the previous discussion in mind, each laboratory director must develop a logical approach to the identification of nonfermenters in his or her laboratory. The following guidelines are helpful in the laboratory approach to the recovery and identification of nonfermentative gram-negative bacilli:

1. Except for *P. aeruginosa* (and the rarely encountered *B. mallei* and *B. pseudomallei*), the nonfermenters have a low degree of virulence and most often cause nosocomial infections in patients who are debilitated or immunocompromised. This narrow niche of infectivity indicates that infections will be uncommon (except for the relatively high incidence of *P. aeruginosa* and *Acinetobacter baumannii*, as discussed earlier). However, because an increasingly higher proportion of hospitalized patients have serious underlying illness, nonfermenters are being recovered with increasing frequency from clinical specimens and must be considered as important agents for many infectious diseases. Specific conditions or diseases predisposing patients to infection with nonfermenters include the following:

   a. Malignancies (particularly of the reticuloendothelial system) and instrumentation and surgery—catheterizations (particularly urinary tract and indwelling intravascular), tracheostomy, lumbar puncture, dialyses, lavages, and placement of shunts and prostheses

   b. Prolonged corticosteroid, antibiotic, antimetabolic, and anticancer therapy

   c. Underlying metabolic or chronic infectious diseases (e.g., an apparent link exists between cystic fibrosis and infections caused by *B. cepacia* or mucoid *P. aeruginosa*)

   d. Burns, open wounds, and various exudative lesions

2. Most nonfermenters have their natural habitat in several environments that serve as potential reservoirs for human infections:

   a. Various water reservoirs that are prevalent in hospitals—humidifiers, mist tents and nebulizers, water baths, disinfectant and irrigation solutions, distilled water lines, hand creams, body lotions, and so on. These solutions often come in direct contact with mucous membranes and other body surfaces in the course of patient management and therapy.

   b. Implements, such as anesthetic equipment, forceps, and thermometers, that may be stored in disinfectant solutions; and mops, sponges, and towels.

   c. Moist intertriginous parts of the skin, such as the toe webs, groin, axilla, and antecubital fossa. Infections from these sources tend to be more prevalent in the summer.

   d. Various domestic animals predisposing caretakers to infection.

3. Certain nonfermenters have a propensity for causing specific infections, discussed elsewhere in this chapter. Septicemia may be found with virtually any species; pneumonitis or bronchitis, septic arthritis, urinary tract infections, postoperative and posttraumatic wound infections, and conjunctivitis may also be caused by most species of nonfermenters. Some species, particularly of *Pseudomonas*, may produce cytotoxic and lytic toxins that make some of these infections locally severe and potentially life-threatening.

4. Clinical isolates that are gram-negative bacilli on Gram stain can be suspected of being nonfermenters if they produce small colonies on blood agar, grow poorly or not at all on MacConkey agar, do not convert either the slant or the deep of KIA or TSI media, and are cytochrome oxidase-positive.

5. Many species of nonfermenters also tend to have certain patterns of multiresistance to antibiotics. These patterns are learned through experience and may provide an initial clue that one is dealing with one of the nonfermenters, or may point to a specific genus.

IDENTIFICATION OF MOST COMMON SPECIES

The identification of the three most commonly recovered clinical species, *Pseudomonas aeruginosa*, *Acinetobacter baumannii*, and *Stenotrophomonas maltophilia* is addressed first. Most strains can be identified easily on the basis of only a few observations and chemical tests. Not only does the rapid identification of these common isolates provide the physician with immediate information, but it also relieves the laboratory of performing a battery of time-consuming and expensive secondary tests.

PSEUDOMONAS AERUGINOSA

More than 95% of *P. aeruginosa* strains recovered from clinical specimens can be identified by observing the presence of the following primary characteristics:

> **Large colonies, grapelike odor**
> **Pyocyanin is produced**
> **Colonies are oxidase-positive (within 10 seconds)**

Most strains produce pyocyanin, a water-soluble green phenazine pigment that imparts a greenish color to the culture medium. In fact, it is probable that observing the presence of pyocyanin may be the only characteristic required to identify *P. aeruginosa* because no other nonfermenter synthesizes this pigment. Reyes and coworkers[255] have shown that 98% of the *P. aeruginosa* strains isolated in their laboratory produced pyocyanin on Tech agar[164] within 48 hours and suggest that the use of Tech agar is a satisfactory alternative to the use of extensive identification schemes when *P. aeruginosa* is suspected (see Color Plate 5-1G). They note that some mucoid strains of *P. aeruginosa* from patients with cystic fibrosis may not produce pigment and, therefore, may be misidentified if pigment production is the only criteria used for identification of these aberrant strains. Detecting the grapelike odor is also a helpful clue when examining the growth on agar plates. The colonies are large, may be mucoid or dry, and often spread (see Color Plate 5-3B). A few strains of *P. aeruginosa* may produce pigments with other colors—pyorubin (red), pyomelanin (brown to black), and pyoverdin (yellow).

Fluorescein pigment can be visualized by observing the growth on certain media using a long-wavelength ultraviolet light source (e.g., Wood's lamp; see Color Plate 5-1*H*). Media containing proteose peptone 3 (Difco Laboratories, Detroit MI) and cations, such as magnesium or manganese, enhance fluorescein synthesis. King's medium B, Sellers' medium, and Mueller–Hinton agar are also suitable for demonstrating fluorescence. The constricted GNF tube (Remel Laboratories, Lenexa KS) permits visual observation of the yellow pigment, and the ultraviolet light may not be needed. In our experience, combination fluorescence–lactose–denitrification (FN or FLN) media is less sensitive for ultraviolet detection of fluorescein pigment. Fluorescence may be enhanced if cultures are incubated at 20° to 30°C rather than at 35° to 37°C.[94,238] The following additional characteristics are helpful in identifying non–pigment-producing strains of *P. aeruginosa*:

Growth at 42°C
Alkalinization of acetamide
Denitrification of nitrates and nitrites
Motile with polar, monotrichous flagellum

Variants producing mucoid or dwarf colonies with atypical biochemical reactions may also be encountered, occasionally making identification difficult. Although a flagellar stain is not needed to identify most strains, assessment of flagellar morphology may be helpful in these cases.

In summary, most strains of *P. aeruginosa* can be identified easily by observing the typical large colonies, with a blue-green discoloration on primary isolation media, and further confirmed by detecting a typical grapelike odor. Demonstration of fluorescein pigment and cytochrome oxidase activity helps to confirm the final identification, and additional tests are usually not required. The typical characteristics by which *P. aeruginosa* is identified are shown in Table 5-4.

ACINETOBACTER BAUMANNII

A. baumannii is the second most frequent nonfermenter encountered in clinical laboratories but with only about one tenth the frequency of *P. aeruginosa*. The following are the characteristics by which a presumptive identification can be made:

Appear as cocci or coccobacilli on Gram stain
Grow well on MacConkey agar (colonies may have a slightly pinkish tint, a helpful characteristic when present)
Do not produce cytochrome oxidase
Exhibit rapid utilization of glucose, with production of acid
Exhibit rapid utilization of 10% lactose, with production of acid
Are nonmotile
Are penicillin resistant

The initial clue is the observation of tiny (1.0 × 0.7 μm) diplococci on Gram stains prepared directly from clinical materials. When Gram stains are prepared from agar or broth cultures, the cells may appear larger and more like coccobacilli (see Color Plate 5-3*E*). *Acinetobacter* species are not pigmented when grown on blood agar, a helpful characteristic in differentiating them from certain other nonfermenters, such as occasional oxidase-negative, nonmotile strains of *Burkholderia cepacia*. However, colonies growing on MacConkey agar may produce a faint pink tint or a deeper cornflower blue when observed on eosin methylene blue agar (see Color Plate 5-3$\overline{F}$). Resistance to penicillin helps distinguish *A. baumannii* from the highly penicillin-sensitive *Moraxella* species, which also usually appear as coccobacilli in Gram stain. Most strains of *Moraxella* species are also cytochrome oxidase-positive. *A. lwoffii* is nonsaccharolytic and can be differentiated from *A. baumannii* because it produces no acid when grown in media that contain carbohydrates.

STENOTROPHOMONAS MALTOPHILIA

S. maltophilia (formerly *Xanthomonas maltophilia*) is the third most frequently encountered nonfermenter in clinical laboratories. The following are the characteristics by which a presumptive identification can be made:

Good growth on blood and MacConkey agars
Do not produce cytochrome oxidase
Produce acid in OF maltose but may be negative in OF glucose
Lysine decarboxylase-positive
Some strains have yellow pigment

The antibiotic susceptibility pattern can also be a clue to the identification of *S. maltophilia*, which is typically resistant to most antibiotics, including the aminoglycosides, but is susceptible to trimethoprim–sulfamethoxazole.

METHODS FOR IDENTIFICATION USING CONVENTIONAL TESTS

If an unknown nonfermentative gram-negative bacillus is not *Pseudomonas aeruginosa*, *Acinetobacter baumannii*, or *Stenotrophomonas maltophilia*, additional characteristics must be determined to make a species identification. Several schemes are currently being used in clinical laboratories. In many laboratories, hybrids of the test procedures used in published schemes are used. Which approach to select is largely one of personal preference, past experience, and the local availability of the culture media required to perform the various tests, providing the criteria listed in Box 5-6 are met.

WEAVER–HOLLIS, GILARDI, AND PICKETT IDENTIFICATION SCHEMES

Except for the packaged commercial systems, the schemes designed by Pickett,[238,239–242] Gilardi,[90,92–96] and Clark, Weaver, Hollis, and associates[53,328] (based on the identification charts originally derived by Elizabeth King at the CDC)[163] have the largest databases. The authors of each of the three identification schemes (Gilardi, Pickett, and Weaver) have separately published several scores of individual identification tables, procedures, and other information relating to the nonfermenters.[95,239,328] The information has become too voluminous to include in this text, and simplification of the material is necessary to address the needs of students and new microbiologists. Therefore, the identification tables used in these schemes will not be included here; rather, only the unique approaches these researchers have devised are discussed. Interested readers are referred to the second and third editions of this text or to the references cited earlier for a complete listing of the identification tables and charts used in those systems.

THE WEAVER–HOLLIS SCHEME

In answer to the problem of how to identify nonfermenters in the clinical laboratory without doing all the tests that are done in a reference laboratory, Weaver and Hollis[328] have published a three-part guide that includes 1) an identification key for gram-negative aerobes, 2) a set of 12 identification tables, and 3) a numerical code book by which derived biotype numbers can be linked to species names. Also available from the CDC is a pamphlet, "Laboratory Methods in Special Medical Bacteriology," in which the procedures and media formulas for all of the biochemical tests cited in the Weaver–Hollis tables can be found. To correctly interpret results from a given identification table, one must use the same procedures on which the reactions are based. A full presentation of this approach and the 12 identification tables can be found in the third edition of this text.

THE GILARDI SCHEME

Gilardi's approach to the identification of nonfermentative gram-negative bacilli has evolved over the past 20 years into an extensive system that is outlined in several detailed charts and tables included in a series of publications.[90,92–96] Yet, the system is no more complex than the nonfermenters themselves, and the latest approach, directed to small and medium-sized laboratories, reflects the progressive trend toward greater simplicity and practicality.[95]

The Gilardi approach is based on two fundamental principles that have made it practical for use in clinical laboratories: 1) the media and tests are readily available in most clinical laboratories and are frequently the same as those used for the identification of other groups of bacteria, including the *Enterobacteriaceae*, and 2) identification of most clinical isolates can be made in two stages—the first, through the use of a primary battery of media and reactions that are sufficient in the majority of cases, and a secondary battery, available when the first is inadequate.[93] The reader is referred to the publications cited in the foregoing references for a full list of the differential media and scope of reactions in the primary and secondary battery of tests leading to the identification of most clinically significant nonfermenters.

THE PICKETT SCHEME

More than two decades ago, Pickett was among the first to bring some order to the identification of nonfermenters.[238,239–242] His system was designed to identify rapidly the two most frequently recovered nonfermenters: *Pseudomonas aeruginosa* and *Acinetobacter anitratus* (now called *A. baumannii*), as previously discussed. The principles listed in Box 5-8 (page 292) have also added significantly to the ease with which nonfermenters are currently approached in most clinical laboratories.

Pickett designed identification tables for several groups of nonfermenters that are similar to the Weaver–Hollis scheme. These tables were published in their entirety in the second edition of this text and are not reprinted here. Also included in the second edition are the formulas for reagents and substrates and a description of all procedures necessary to perform the differential tests required for each identification table. Because most of the substrates required to perform these tests are available in dehydrated tablet form from Key Scientific Products Co.(Round Rock, TX), the Pickett system remains a viable approach to the identification of nonfermenters, particularly in laboratories with low volume where it may be difficult to maintain differential test media within quality control standards.

In summary, the Pickett scheme for the identification of nonfermenters is viable and can be recommended. The heavy inocula and buffered single substrates are innovations that are also used in other identification systems, including the procedures for use with packaged kits discussed in the next section of this chapter. Subgrouping of the nonfermenters based on preliminary observations is also a sound exercise, both in making a presumptive identification and as a quality control check on the final answers derived from semiautomated and automated systems.

BOX 5-7. CLASSIFICATION OF CLINICALLY IMPORTANT NONFERMENTATIVE BACILLI

Oxidase-Negative, Nonmotile

Acinetobacter baumannii

Acinetobacter lwoffii

Other *Acinetobacter* species

Bordetella parapertussis

Bordetella holmesii

CDC group NO-1

Oxidase-Negative, Motile

Burkholderia cepacia (93% are weak oxidase-positive)

Burkholderia gladioli

Chryseomonas luteola

Flavimonas oryzihabitans

Sphingomonas paucimobilis (94% are oxidase-positive)

Stenotrophomonas maltophilia

Oxidase-Positive, Nonmotile

Bergeyella zoohelcum

Chryseobacterium spp.

Empedobacter brevis

Flavobacterium spp.

Moraxella spp.

Certain *Neisseria* spp.

Oligella urethralis

Sphingobacterium spp.

Weeksella virosa

Gilardi rod group 1

Oxidase-Positive, Motile

Acidovorax delafieldii

Agrobacterium radiobacter

Alcaligenes species

Balneatrix alpica

Bordetella avium

Bordetella bronchiseptica

Bordetella hinzii

Brevundimonas spp.

Burkholderia cepacia

Burkholderia pickettii

Burkholderia pseudomallei

Comamonas spp.

Methylobacterium spp.

Ochrobactrum anthropi

Oligella ureolytica

Pseudomonas aeruginosa and most other *Pseudomonas* spp.

Roseomonas spp.

Shewanella putrefaciens

Sphingomonas paucimobilis

Group IVc-2

Group Vb-3

MISCELLANEOUS SCHEMES

Two miscellaneous schemes have been published and, presumably, are being used successfully in some laboratories. Oberhofer and associates[220] have published a scheme that uses commercial media commonly available to most clinical laboratories. In this scheme, the nonfermenters are divided into two major groups, oxidative and nonoxidative. The oxidative group is further subdivided into fluorescent, nonfluorescent, peritrichous, and yellow-pigmented oxidizers. We have had no experience with this scheme; however, the approach is rational.

Romeo[267] has published dichotomous keys for the identification of nonfermenters and other miscellaneous gram-negative bacteria. Twenty-two media and tests, based primarily on formulations developed at the CDC, are used to construct 12 dichotomous keys representing various subgroups of over 100 species of bacteria. Romeo offers the keys as a means to quickly eliminate certain species from given groups and allow the rapid selection of differential tests for definitive identification of unknown isolates. Again, one can in-tuitively judge that these keys will work, provided the criteria listed in the foregoing are applied.

PRACTICAL APPROACH TO IDENTIFICATION OF NONFERMENTERS

The approach used in this text was devised by one of us (P.C. Schreckenberger)[280] and requires that the various clinically important nonfermentative bacilli be divided into four functional groups based on an immediate assessment of their motility and ability to produce cytochrome oxidase. From these two reactions, the clinically important nonfermentative bacilli can be divided into the four groups listed in Box 5-7.

Once having accomplished this subgrouping, definitive identifications can be made by referring to the identification Tables 5-16 through 5-29 and following the instructions given with the tables. The biochemical tests used in this identification guide are all conventional biochemical formulations and are available commercially from most media manufacturers. Note that in working with these tables, a given species of a nonfermenting bacillus may appear in more than one table be-

BOX 5-8. METHODS FOR IDENTIFYING NONFERMENTERS

1. The preliminary subculture of an unknown bacterial colony from primary isolation medium should be to an enriched medium on which luxuriant growth can take place. **Comment:** The contents of many differential test media are not supportive of the growth of many of the fastidious species of nonfermenters. Therefore, several days may be required for a slow-growing species to produce a detectable endpoint. By using a highly nutritious medium to propagate the bacterial colonies, considerable time can be saved by not having to wait for growth to take place in differential test substrates. Pickett prescribed the use of KIA, in which 14 mL of medium is poured into a large, 20 150-mm screw-capped tube and slanted to produce a butt of about 3 cm and a slope of 10 cm.

2. A heavy inoculum, prepared from the overnight growth of bacteria (log phase growth) on the KIA slant, should be used to perform the secondary tests necessary to determine the nutritional and biochemical characteristics. **Comment:** The heavy inoculum used in the Pickett system is an aqueous suspension of organisms having the consistency of skim milk. The inoculum is prepared by harvesting the entire lawn of growth from the surface of the KIA slant into about 3 mL of water. The rationale behind adding the heavy inoculum into the differential test substrates is to introduce a high concentration of preformed enzymes or other metabolic products that can be detected more quickly by the endpoint indicator (reactions are usually complete within 24 hours).

3. A buffered single substrate should be used for testing the acidification of carbohydrates and the alkalinization of amides and organic salts. **Comment:** The single substrates allow measurement of only one characteristic in each test without influence from other chemicals that are found in complex test media. Buffers can be selected that provide a narrow pH range to detect reactions, making certain differential test systems highly sensitive for the detection of only small quantities of products.

4. Clinically important nonfermenters should be subcategorized into several groups based on visual observations, Gram stain characteristics, and the results of rapid biochemical tests.

cause a particular organism may not be 100% positive or negative for a given characteristic; therefore, some redundancy is built into the scheme so that an unknown bacillus will be identified regardless of the test result obtained with the variable screening test. By following these tables, the microbiologist should be able to definitively identify over 95% of nonfermentative bacilli that will be recovered from clinical specimens.

COMPUTER-AIDED SCHEMES

BioBASE (BioBASE, Inc., Boston, MA) is a DOS-based computer program for computer-aided identification of microorganisms. The system enables the user to create and access hundreds of microbial databases and switch between them, depending on the primary characteristics of the microbial isolates being studied. Included with the software is the database, published by Holmes and colleagues,[138] that includes 66 taxa of nonfermenters identified using 83 phenotypic tests. Identification of bacterial isolates can be based on all or some selected tests.

COMMERCIAL KIT SYSTEMS

Packaged kit systems have been designed for, or adapted to, the identification of the nonfermentative bacilli. These kits share many of the attributes of packaged systems in general; that is, they are convenient to use, have a long shelf life, and preclude the need for fresh supplies of media and reagents. The packaged systems also provide standardized techniques that are accurate and give reproducible results equal to or better than conventional procedures, with the exceptions discussed later in this chapter.

Inherent problems in the use of many of the currently available packaged kits for identifying nonfermenters include the 1) tendency for organisms that exhibit weak or delayed biochemical activity to produce false-negative reactions, 2) less than optimal design of many systems for cultivation of certain nonfermenters, and 3) inclusion of some differential tests that may not be applicable to the identification of nonfermenters. Whereas members of the *Enterobacteriaceae* usually grow rapidly and exhibit active enzymatic activity on a variety of substrates that can readily be detected with kit systems, most nonfermenter species are slow growing and relatively inactive enzymatically. The microbiologist needs considerable experience to interpret some incomplete or weak reactions that may be encountered in the use of these systems.

It is with these perspectives in mind that the following seven kit systems are discussed. They were selected because accumulated experience has delineated their applications and limitations. These seven systems are the following:

Oxi/Ferm Tube (Becton Dickinson Microbiology Systems, Cockeysville MD)
API 20E (bioMerieux Vitek, Inc., Hazelwood MO)
API NFT (bioMerieux Vitek, Inc., Hazelwood MO)
Remel N/F System (Remel, Lenexa KS)
Crystal Enteric/Nonfermenter System (Becton Dickinson Microbiology Systems, Cockeysville MD)

(text continues on page 304)

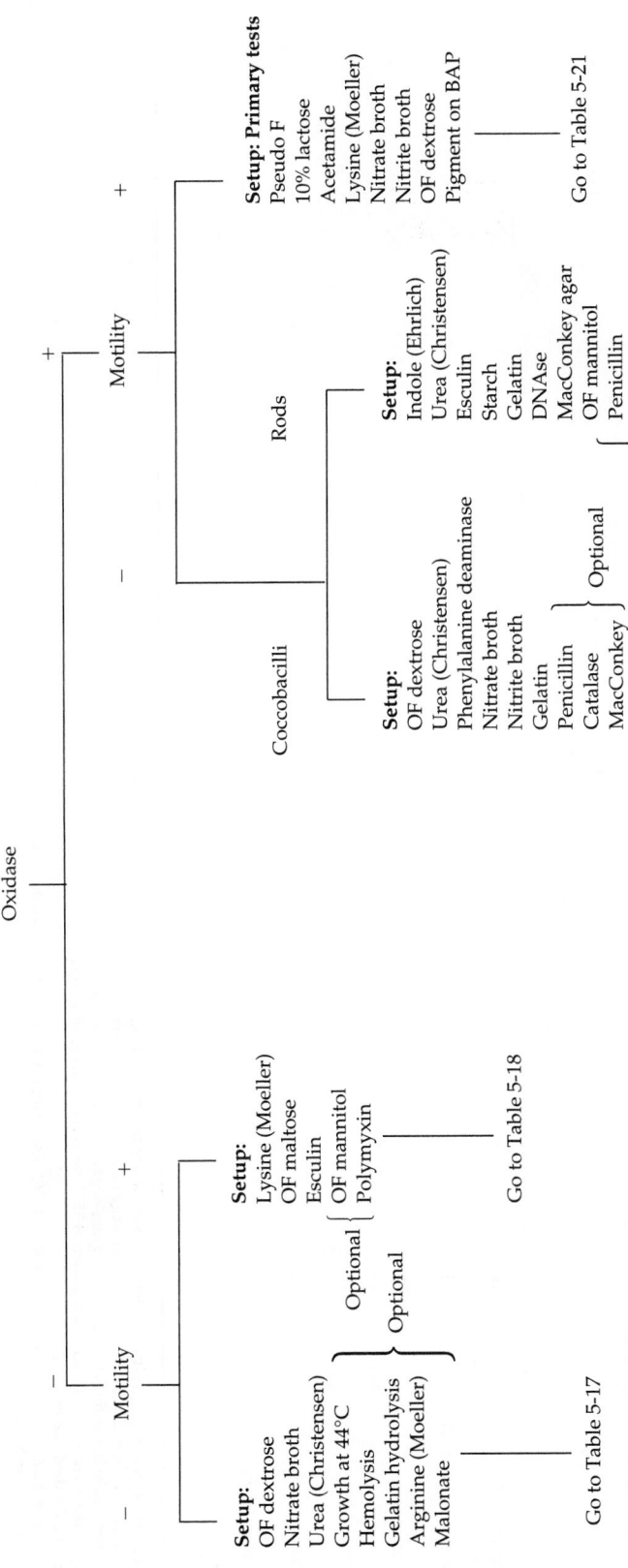

Oxidase

Motility −

Setup:
OF dextrose
Nitrate broth
Urea (Christensen)
Growth at 44°C
Hemolysis
Gelatin hydrolysis ⎫
Arginine (Moeller) ⎬ Optional
Malonate ⎭

Go to Table 5-17

Motility +

Setup:
Lysine (Moeller)
OF maltose
Esculin
OF mannitol ⎫
Polymyxin ⎬ Optional

Go to Table 5-18

Oxidase +

Motility −

Coccobacilli

Setup:
OF dextrose
Urea (Christensen)
Phenylalanine deaminase
Nitrate broth
Nitrite broth
Gelatin
Penicillin
Catalase
MacConkey ⎫ Optional

Go to Table 5-19

Rods

Setup:
Indole (Ehrlich)
Urea (Christensen)
Esculin
Starch
Gelatin
DNAse
MacConkey agar
OF mannitol ⎫
Penicillin ⎬ Optional
Polymyxin
OF dextrose ⎭

Go to Table 5-20

Motility +

Setup: Primary tests
Pseudo F
10% lactose
Acetamide
Lysine (Moeller)
Nitrate broth
Nitrite broth
OF dextrose
Pigment on BAP

Go to Table 5-21

Setup: Secondary tests
OF fructose
OF maltose
OF mannitol
OF xylose
KIA (for H₂S)
Arginine (Moeller)
ONPG
Urea (Christensen)
Phenylalanine deaminase
Esculin hydrolysis
Starch hydrolysis
Gelatin hydrolysis
6.5% NaCl
DNAse
Indole (Ehrlich)
Polymyxin
Malonate
Growth at 42°C

INSTRUCTIONS FOR USING TABLES 5-16 THRU 5-29

This approach to the identification of nonfermenters is designed to minimize the number of biochemical tests needed for identification based on a preliminary assessment of the oxidase and motility reactions of organisms to be identified. Once this information is known, a specific battery of tests is performed to complete the identification of the organism. For those organisms that are both oxidase-positive and motile, a two-step approach is used, based on the reactions obtained in a primary test battery, followed by additional supplemental tests that are specified in the designated tables. Depending on the needs and resources available, the user of this guide may wish to set up all of the tests included in the primary and secondary batteries whenever a motile, oxidase-positive nonfermenter is encountered to obtain a definitive identification in the shortest time possible. As a general rule, when working with NFBs, a heavy inoculum should be used and reactions should be held 48 h before the final reading is taken.

STEPS TO FOLLOW:

1. Determine the motility (wet mount) and oxidase reactions and follow the flow diagram in Table 5-16.
2. Set up the specified biochemical tests and go to the table indicated to complete the identification.
3. To use Tables 5-17 through 5-29, begin with the first biochemical test listed on the left-hand side of the table and locate the shaded box or boxes in the upper left-hand corner.
4. If a single box is shaded, and if the reaction given matches the reaction obtained with your specimen, you are finished. The organism identification is listed in the same row to the left of the box.
5. If multiple boxes are shaded and the reaction matches that of your specimen, use the reactions to the right of the shaded boxes to determine the correct identification.
6. If the reaction obtained with your specimen does *not* match that in the shaded box or boxes, proceed to the next column on the right and find the shaded box or boxes in this column. Repeat steps 4 and 5 until you reach a definitive identification.
7. Special consideration must be given to shaded boxes that contain a variable (V) reaction sign. In these rare cases, you must treat the variable reaction in the shaded box as both a match and a nonmatch.

TABLE 5-17
Oxidase-Negative, Nonmotile Nonfermenters

Organism*	Genomospecies	Urease	Nitrate Reduced	Brown Soluble Pigment	Growth At 37°C	Growth At 44°C	Hemolysis Sheep Blood	Gelatin Hydrolysis	OF Dextrose	Arginine	Malonate
Bordetella parapertussis		+	-	-	+	NA	+	NA	-	NA	NA
CDC NO-1		-	+	-	+	NA	-	-	-	-	NA
Bordetella holmesii (NO-2)		-	-	+†	+	-	-	-	-	-	NA
Acinetobacter johnsonii	7	-	-	-	-	-	-	-	-	V (35)	V (13)
Acinetobacter baumannii	2	-	-	-	+	+‡	-	-	+	+	+
Acinetobacter haemolyticus	4	-	-	-	+	-	+	+	V (52)	+	-
Acinetobacter spp.	6	-	-	-	+	-	+	+	V (66)	+	-
Acinetobacter spp.	10	-	-	-	+	-	-	-	+	-	-
Acinetobacter calcoaceticus	1	-	-	-	+	-	-	-	+	+	+
Acinetobacter spp.	3	-	-	-	+	-	-	-	+	+	V (87)
Acinetobacter spp.	12	-	-	-	+	-	-	-	V (33)	+	+
Acinetobacter junii	5	-	-	-	+	-	-	-	-	+	-
Acinetobacter lwoffii	8/9	-	-	-	+	-	-	-	-	-	-
Acinetobacter spp.	11	-	-	-	+	-	-	-	-	-	-

+, 90% or more of strains are positive; −, 90% or more of strains are negative; NA, results not available; V, 11%–89% strains positive; numbers in parentheses are percentage of strains giving positive reaction.
* All organisms included in this chart appear as gram-negative coccobacilli on Gram stain.
† Brown, soluble pigment produced when grown at 35°C heart infusion tyrosine agar.
‡ Must also be OF dextrose positive.

Data from Bouvet PJM et al. Int J Syst Bacteriol 36:228–240, 1986; Hollis DG et al. J Clin Microbiol 31:746–748, 1993; Weyant RS et al. J Clin Microbiol 33:1–7, 1995.

TABLE 5-18
Oxidase-Negative, Motile Nonfermenters

Organism	Lysine Decarboxylase	OF Maltose	OF Mannitol	Esculin	Polymyxin	Pigment
Stenotrophomonas maltophilia	+	+	–	+	S	Yellow-lavender
Burkholderia cepacia	+	+	+	V (67)	R	Yellow
Burkholderia gladioli	–	–	+	–	R	Yellow
Sphingomonas paucimobilis	–	+	–	+	V (89)	Deep yellow
Chryseomonas luteola	–	+	+	+	S	Dull yellow
Flavimonas oryzihabitans	–	+	+	–	S	Dull yellow

+, 90% or more strains positive; –, 90% or more strains negative; V, 11%–89% of strains positive; numbers in parentheses are percentage of strains giving positive reaction; R, resistant; S, susceptible.
Data from Gilardi GL. Identification of glucose-nonfermenting gram-negative rods, 1990.

TABLE 5-19
IDENTIFICATION OF OXIDASE-POSITIVE, NONMOTILE COCCOBACILLI

ORGANISM	CHARACTERISTIC ODOR OR APPEARANCE	OF DEXTROSE	UREASE	PHENYLALANINE DEAMINASE	NITRATE REDUCED	NITRITE REDUCED	GELATIN HYDROLYSIS	GROWTH ON MACCONKEY	CATALASE	GROWTH AT 35°C
Psychrobacter immobilis	Odor of PEA agar (roses)	+	+	+	+	NA	–	V	+	–
EO-2	O-shaped cells*	+	+	NA	V	NA	–	V	+	+
EO-3	Yellow colonies	+	+	NA	–	NA	–	V	+	+
M. phenylpyruvica (M-2)		–	+	+	V (89)	–	–	+	Weak	+
O. urethralis (M-4)	Small coccoid cells	–	–	+	–	+	–	V (83)	+	+
Neisseria weaveri (M-5)	Yellow–tan colonies	–	–	V (73)	–	V (84)	–	V (42)	+	+
Gilardi rod group 1	Light orange to salmon pink colonies	–	–	++	–	–	–	+	+	+
Neisseria elongata subsp. *nitroreducens* (M-6)		–	–	–	+	+	–	V (20)	–	+
M. lacunata		–	–	–	+	–	+	–	Weak	+
M. nonliquefaciens		–	–	–	+	–	–	V (17)	+	+
M. osloensis		–	–	–	V (26)	–	–	V (49)	Weak	+
M. atlantae (M-3)	Spreading or pitting colonies	–	–	–	–	V (20)	–	+	Weak or –	+

+, 90% or more strains positive; –, 90% or more strains negative; V, 11%–89% of strains positive; ++, strong positive reaction; NA, results not available; numbers in parentheses are percentage of strains giving positive reaction.
*Gram-stained smears show coccoid to short, thick rods that are frequently vacuolated. Cells have unstained centers, but are peripherally stained and appear as circles.

Data from Gilardi GL. Identification of glucose-nonfermenting gram-negative rods, 1990; Hudson MJ et al. J Clin Microbiol 25:1907–1910, 1987; Moss CW et al. J Clin Microbiol 31:689–691, 1993; Moss CW et al. 26:484–492, 1988.

TABLE 5-20
IDENTIFICATION OF OXIDASE-POSITIVE, NONMOTILE ROD-SHAPED BACILLI

ORGANISM	CHARACTERISTIC ODOR OR APPEARANCE	INDOLE	UREASE	ESCULIN HYDROLYSIS	GELATIN HYDROLYSIS	STARCH HYDROLYSIS	DNASE HYDROLYSIS	GROWTH ON MACCONKEY	OF MANNITOL	OF DEXTROSE	PENICILLIN	POLYMYXIN
Sphingobacterium multivorum (IIk-2)	Pale yellow	−	+	+	−	V (79)	−	V (17)	−	+	R	R
Sphingobacterium spiritivorum (IIk-3)	Pale yellow	−	+	+	−	−	+	−	+	+	R	R
Flavobacterium odoratum (M4-f)	Yellow-green Fruity odor	−	+	−	+	−	+	V (78)	−	−	S (19)	R
Bergeyella (Weeksella) zoohelcum (IIj)	No pigment	+	++	−	+	−	−	−	−	−	S	R
Weeksella virosa (IIf)	Cream colored; colonies stick to agar	+	−	−	+	−	V (13)	−	−	−	S	S
Empedobacter (Flavobacterium) brevis	Pale yellow	+	−	−	+	V (40)	+	+*	−	Delayed	R	R
CDC Group IIe	No pigment	+	−	−	−	+	−	−	−	Delayed	S	S
CDC Group IIg	No pigment	+	−	−	−	NA	−	+	−	−	NA	S
CDC Group IIh	No pigment	+	−*	+	−*	+	V (78)	−*	−	Delayed	S (67)	S (22)
CDC Group IIi	NA	+	−	+	−*	V (14)	−	−	−	Delayed	S (57)	R
Chryseobacterium (Flavobacterium) meningosepticum (IIa)	Pale yellow	+	−	+	+	−	+	V (26)	Delayed	Delayed	R	R
Chryseobacterium (Flavobacterium) indologenes (IIb)	Deep yellow	+	−	+	+	+	−	−	−	Delayed	R	R

+, 90% or more strains positive; −, 90% or more strains negative; V, 11%–89% of strains positive; ++, strong positive reaction; NA, results not available; numbers in parentheses are percentage of strains giving positive reaction; R, resistant; S, susceptible.
* Different results reported; reaction used here is that reported by CDC. Dees SB, et al. J Clin Microbiol 23:267–273, 1986.
NOTE: *Balneatrix alpica* is pale yellow and indole-positive, but is excluded from this table because it is motile (see Tables 5-26 and 5-28).
Data from Gilardi, G.L. Identification of Glucose-Nonfermenting Gram-Negative Rods, 1990; Hollis DG et al. J Clin Microbiol 33:762–764, 1995; Dees SB et al. J Clin Microbiol 23:267–273, 1986.

TABLE 5-21
Screening Tests for Species Identification of Oxidase-Positive, Motile Nonfermenters

	Fluorescence (Pseudo F agar under UV light)	10% lactose	Acetamide	Lysine (Moeller)	Pigment on blood agar	Gas from nitrate or nitrite	OF dextrose	
	+							See Table 5-22
	−	+						See Table 5-23
		−	+					See Table 5-24
			−	+				See Table 5-25
				−	+			See Table 5-26
					−	+		See Table 5-27
						−	+	See Table 5-28
							−	See Table 5-29

Directions for Table 5-21. Begin in the upper right-hand corner and proceed to the left in a step-wise fashion. When the reactions indicated match those of your unknown organism, proceed to the table indicated at the bottom of the column.

TABLE 5-22

IDENTIFICATION OF FLUORESCENT NONFERMENTERS

ORGANISM	ACETAMIDE	GROWTH 42°C	GELATIN
Pseudomonas aeruginosa	+	+	+
P. fluorescens	−	−	+
P. putida	−	−	−

+, 90% or more of strains are positive; −, 90% or more of strains are negative.

TABLE 5-23

IDENTIFICATION OF STRONGLY LACTOSE-POSITIVE NONFERMENTERS
(OXIDASE +, MOTILITY +, FLUORESCEIN −)

ORGANISM	LYSINE	OF MANNITOL	UREASE	ONPG	POLYMYXIN
Burkholderia cepacia	+	+	V (45)	V (79)	R
Burkholderia pseudomallei	−	+	V (43)	−	R
Agrobacterium radiobacter	−	+	+	+	S
Burkholderia pickettii (Va-3)	−	+	+	−	R
Burkholderia pickettii (Va-1)	−	−	+	−	R
Sphingomonas paucimobilis (IIk-1)	−	−	−	+	S (89)

+, 90% or more strains are positive; −, 90% or more of strains are negative; V, 11%–89% of strains are positive; numbers in parentheses are percentage of strains giving positive reaction; R, resistant; S, susceptible.
NOTE: *Acinetobacter baumannii* and *Sphingobacterium* species (IIk-2, IIk-3) are strongly lactose-positive, but are excluded from this table because they are nonmotile (see Tables 5-17 and 5-20)
Data from Gilardi GL. Identification of glucose-nonfermenting gram-negative rods, 1990.

TABLE 5-24
IDENTIFICATION OF ACETAMIDE-POSITIVE NONFERMENTERS
(OXIDASE +, MOTILITY +, FLUORESCEIN −, 10% LACTOSE −)

ORGANISM	ARGININE	OF DEXTROSE	OF FRUCTOSE	OF MANNITOL	NITRATE REDUCED	NITRITE TO GAS	MALONATE	NITRATE TO GAS	ORANGE INDOLE
Pseudomonas aeruginosa	+	+	V (89)	V (68)	V (74)	NA	NA	V (60)	−
Burkholderia cepacia	−	+	+	+	V (37)	NA	NA	−	−
Alcaligenes xylosoxidans subsp. *xylosoxidans*	−	+	V (9)	−	+	NA	NA	V (69)	−
Comamonas acidovorans	−	−	+	+ (92)	+	NA	NA	−	+
Alcaligenes xylosoxidans subsp. *denitrificans*	−	−	−	−	+	+	+	+	−
Alcaligenes piechaudii	−	−	−	−	+	−	+	−	−
Oligella ureolytica	−	−	−	−	+	V (63)	−	V (58)	−
Alcaligenes faecalis	−	−	−	−	−	+	+	−	−
Bordetella hinzii	−	−	−	−	−	−	+	−	−
Bordetella avium	−	−	−	−	−	−	−	−	−

+, 90% or more strains positive; −, 90% or more strains negative; V, 11%–89% of strains positive; ++, strong positive reaction; NA, results not available; numbers in parentheses are percentage of strains giving positive reaction; R, resistant; S, susceptible.
Data from Gilardi GL. Identification of glucose-nonfermenting gram-negative rods, 1990; Vandamme P, et al. Int J Syst Bacteriol 45:37–45, 1995; data for alkalinization of malonate also from Balows A et al. Manual of clinical microbiology, 5th ed, 1991.

TABLE 5-25
IDENTIFICATION OF LYSINE-POSITIVE NONFERMENTERS

ORGANISM	OF MANNITOL
Burkholderia cepacia	+
Stenotrophomonas maltophilia	−

+, 90% or more of strains are positive; −, 90% or more of strains are negative.
Note: Occasional strains of *S. maltophilia* may be oxidase-positive.

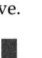

TABLE 5-26
IDENTIFICATION OF PIGMENTED NONFERMENTERS
(OXIDASE +, MOTILITY +, FLUORESCEIN −, 10% LACTOSE −, ACETAMIDE −, LYSINE −)

ORGANISM	COLOR	KIA/H₂S	OF FRUCTOSE	GAS FROM NITRATE	INDOLE	OF MANNITOL	ESCULIN HYDROLYSIS
Roseomonas spp.*	Pink	−	+	−	−	V	−
Methylobacterium spp.*	Pink	−	V (50)	−	−	−	−
Shewanella putrefaciens	Tan	+	V	−	−	−	V
Brevundimonas vesicularis	Tan/orange	−	−				+
Pseudomonas stutzeri	Yellow	−	+	+	−	V (70)	−
Balneatrix alpica	Pale yellow	−	+	−	+	+	
Burkholderia cepacia	Yellow	−	+	−	−	+	V (67)
Sphingomonas paucimobilis	Yellow	−	+	−	−	−	+

+, 90% or more strains positive; −, 90% or more strains negative; V, 11%–89% of strains positive; numbers in parentheses are percentage of strains giving positive reaction.
* *Methylobacterium* spp. appear as dark colonies under longwave UV light owing to absorption of UV light. *Roseomonas* spp. do not absorb UV light and do not appear dark.
Note: All of these pigments develop only as the culture ages. Most strains of *Flavobacterium*s spp. and *Sphingobacterium* spp. are also pigmented (yellow); however, these organisms are excluded from this table because they are nonmotile (see Table 5-20).
Data from Gilardi GL. Identification of glucose-nonfermenting gram-negative rods, 1990; Rihs JD, et al. J Clin Microbiol 31:3275-3283, 1993; Dauga C, et al. Res Microbiol 144:35-46, 1993.

TABLE 5-27
IDENTIFICATION OF DENTRIFYING NONFERMENTERS
(OXIDASE +, MOTILITY +, FLUORESCEIN −, 10% LACTOSE −, ACETAMIDE −, LYSINE −, PIGMENT −)

ORGANISM	OF DEXTROSE	POLYMYXIN	ONPG	6.5% NaCl	PHENYLALANINE DEAMINASE	ARGININE	STARCH HYDROLYSIS	OF MALTOSE	UREASE
Oligella ureolytica	−	S	−	−	+	−	−	−	++
Pseudomonas spp. CDC Group 1	−	S	−	−	−	V (50)	−	−	−
A. xylosoxidans subsp. *denitrificans*	−	S (83)	−	−	−	−	−	−	V (31)
B. pickettii (Va-1)	+	R	−	−	−	−	V (48)	+	+
B. pickettii (Va-2)	+	R	−	−	V (40)	−	V (12)	−	+
Agrobacterium radiobacter	+	S	+	−	+	−	V (16)	+	+
P. stutzeri (Vb-1)	+	S	−	+	V (55)	−	+	+	V (17)
P. mendocina (Vb-2)	+	S	−	+	V (50)	+	−	−	V (50)
CDC Vb-3	+	S	−	+	V (56)	+	V (75)	V (88)	V (31)
Ochrobactrum anthropi	+	S	−	−	+	V (36)	−	V (50)	+
P. aeruginosa	+	S	−	−	−	+	−	V (12)	V (66)
A. xylosoxidans subsp. *xylosoxidans*	+	S	−	−	−	−	−	−	−

+, 90% or more strains positive; −, 90% or more strains negative; V, 11%–89% of strains positive; numbers in parentheses are percentage of strains giving positive reaction; R, resistant; S, susceptible.
Note: *A. xylosoxidans* subsp. *denitrificans* can be separated from *Pseudomonas* spp. CDC group 1 on the basis of flagellar morphology. *Alcaligenes* has peritrichous flagella, *Pseudomonas* group 1 has a single polar flagellum.
Data from Gilardi GL. Identification of glucose-nonfermenting gram-negative rods, 1990.

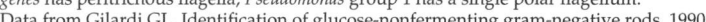

TABLE 5-28
IDENTIFICATION OF DEXTROSE-POSITIVE NONFERMENTERS
(OXIDASE +, MOTILITY +, FLUORESCEIN −, 10% LACTOSE −, ACETAMIDE −, LYSINE −, PIGMENT −, DENITRIFICATION −)

Organism	Pigment of Colonies	KIA H₂S	Indole	OF Fructose	ONPG	OF Xylose	DNase	Growth in 6.5% NaCl	Phenylalanine Deaminase	Arginine	Growth at 42°C	Gelatin Hydrolysis	Esculin Hydrolysis
Methylobacterium	Pink	−	−	V	−	V	−	−	−	−	−	−	−
Shevanella putrefaciens	−	+	−	V	−	−	+	−	−	−	V	V	−
Balneatrix alpica	Pale yellow	−	+	+	−	NA	−	−	NA	+	+	weak +	−
A. xylosoxidans subsp. xylosoxidans	−	−	−	−	−	+	−	−	−	−	V (86)	−	−
Breundimonas diminuta	−	−	−	−	−	−	V (12)	−	V (16)	−	V (19)	V (58)	+
A. radiobacter	−	−	−	+	+	+	−	−	+	−	V (13)	−	+
Pseudomonas-like Group 2	−	−	−	+	+	+	−	−	+	−	−	−	−
P. pseudoalcaligenes	−	−	−	+	−	−	−	−	V (21)	V (36)	V (75)	−	−
Acidovorax delafieldii	−	−	−	+	−	+	+	−	−	+	−	+	−
CDC Vb-3	−	−	−	+	−	+	−	+	V (56)	+	V (75)	−	V (40)
O. anthropi	−	−	−	+	−	+	−	−	+	V (36)	V (10)	−	−
B. pickettii (VA-1)	−	−	−	+	−	+	−	−	−	−	V (26)	V (77)	−
P. aeruginosa	−	−	−	+	−	V (85)	−	−	−	+	+	V (46)	−
P. fluorescens	−	−	−	+	−	+	−	−	−	+	−	+	−
P. putida	−	−	−	+	−	+	−	−	−	+	−	−	−

+, 90% or more strains positive; −, 90% or more strains negative; V, 11%–89% of strains positive; numbers in parentheses are percentage of strains giving positive reaction.
Data from Gilardi GL. Identification of glucose-nonfermenting gram-negative rods, 1990; Dauga C, et al. Res Microbiol 144:35–46, 1993.

TABLE 5-29
Identification of Dextrose-Negative Nonfermenters
(Oxidase +, Motility +, Fluorescein +, Lactose −, Acetamide −, Lysine −, Pigment −, Denitrification −, Dextrose −)

Organism	Pink-Pigmented Colonies	KIA H₂S	OF Fructose	Urease	NO₃ to NO₂	NO₂ to Gas	Starch Hydrolysis	Phenylalanine Deaminase	DNase	Arginine	Flagellar Arrangement
*Methylobacterium**	+	−	V	+	V	NA	+	−	−	−	
*Roseomonas**	+	−	+	+	−	NA	+	V (17)	−	−	
Shewanella putrefaciens	−	+	V	−	V	NA	−	−	+	−	
P. pseudoalcaligenes	−	−	+	−	+	NA	−	V (21)	−	V (36)	
O. ureolytica	−	−	−	++	+	V (63)	−	+	−	−	
B. bronchiseptica	−	−	−	++	+	−	−	V (25)	−	−	
CDC Group IVc-2	−	−	−	++	−	−	V (16)	−	−	−	
Brevundimonas diminuta	−	−	−	−	−	NA	−	V (16)	V (12)	−	Polar monotrichous
A. faecalis type II	−	−	−	−	−	−	−	V (15)	−	−	Peritrichous
P. alcaligenes	−	−	−	V (21)	V (61)	V (10)	V (16)	V (20)	−	V (7)	Polar monotrichous
C. testosteroni	−	−	−	−	+	V (11)	−	V (30)	−	−	Polar multitrichous
A. piechaudii	−	−	−	−	+	−	−	−	−	−	Peritrichous

+, 90% or more strains positive; −, 90% or more strains negative; V, 11%–89% of strains positive; ++, strong positive reaction; NA, results not available; numbers in parentheses are percentage of strains giving positive reaction.
* *Methylobacterium* spp. appear as dark colonies under longwave UV light owing to absorption of UV light.
Roseomonas spp. do not absorb UV light and do not appear dark.
Data from Gilardi GL. Identification of glucose-nonfermenting gram-negative rods, 1990.

RapID NF Plus (Innovative Diagnostic Systems, Inc., Norcross GA)
Biolog System (Biolog, Inc., Hayward CA)

THE OXI/FERM TUBE

Details of the functional design, operating procedures, and substrates included in Oxi/Ferm tube are presented in the third edition of this text.

Studies designed to evaluate the performance of the Oxi/Ferm tube in identifying clinically significant nonfermentative bacilli have shown that the more commonly encountered species—*P. aeruginosa*, *S. maltophilia*, and *Acinetobacter* species—were identified with a relatively high degree of accuracy when compared with conventional methods. The overall accuracy drops significantly, however, when all nonfermenters are considered. The overall identification accuracy of the Oxi/Ferm in these studies ranged from 50% to 95% depending on the species tested, whether readings were taken after 24 or 48 hours of incubation, and whether supplemental tests were used to obtain the correct identifications.[10,38,71,122,132,152,173,210,215,216,217,221,226,270,285] In these studies, the highest percentage of discrepancies occurred with the fastidious or rarely encountered strains and resulted most often from false-negative Oxi/Ferm reactions for citrate, hydrogen sulfide, arginine dihydrolase, nitrate reduction, OF glucose, and urease.[122,152,210,215,221] Problems in the detection of N_2 gas under the wax overlay in the denitrification chamber were also noted.[10,152,285]

The design of the Oxi/Ferm tube appears to limit its performance with slow-growing or weakly reactive organisms. The inoculating needle can hold only a relatively small amount of inoculum, and it has been demonstrated that a heavy inoculum is essential to elicit detectable biochemical products from many of the nonfermenters. Many of the nonfermenters are strict aerobes, and the environment within the confined chambers in the Oxi/Ferm tube may not support optimal growth. The test organisms are delivered into the central depths of the medium in each chamber, where they are minimally exposed to atmospheric oxygen. With surface growth lacking, it is difficult to determine if a negative reaction reflects biochemical inactivity or the inability of the organism to grow in the medium. Some of the media in the Oxi/Ferm tube are incapable of supporting the growth of the more fastidious strains of nonfermenters (e.g., citrate agar is not found in most identification systems for nonfermenters). To some extent, these shortcomings have hampered the acceptance of the Oxi/Ferm tube in many clinical laboratories.

THE API 20E SYSTEM

The API 20E system, originally designed for identification of the *Enterobacteriaceae*, has been extended to include the identification of nonfermentative bacilli as well. To maximize the use of the API 20E for nonfermenters, six additional tests are added to generate a nine-digit profile number (Table 5-30). Studies performed with nonfermenters have shown that although the API 20E system identifies *P. aeruginosa*, *S. maltophilia*, and *Acinetobacter* species with up to 99% accuracy, particularly after 48 hours of incubation, the performance with other less common nonfermenters was often less than acceptable.[10,38,71,122,198,215,216,217,226,286,325] Incorrect identifications occurred most often because of false-negative reactions for citrate, gelatin liquefaction, motility, arginine dihydrolase, ONPG, nitrate reduction, and urease tests.[10,71,122,215] In the specific study by Hofherr and associates,[122] 12.2% of 836 individual biochemical reactions differed between the API system and conventional methods (53% involved citrate utilization and gelatin liquefaction tests). In other cases, identifications were not possible because the biotype number derived from the 20E strip was not listed in the API Profile Index.[286]

As with the Oxi/Ferm tube, the API 20E strip is not designed to detect the weak metabolic activity of fastidious or weakly reactive organisms, leading to some false-negative reactions. Tests such as ONPG, citrate utilization, and arginine dihydrolase are not commonly included in conventional nonfermenter identification schemes, either because they have little discriminatory value, or because the media do not support the growth of fastidious organisms.

THE API NFT

A modification of the API 20E strip, originally developed by API System SA in France and introduced in Europe by the name API NE (nonenteric), was introduced in the United States as the DMS API NFT and is now available through bioMerieux Vitek, Inc. (Hazelwood MO) as the API NFT system. The construction of the plastic strip is the same as in the 20E system; the substrates have been changed to include eight conventional tests and 12 assimilation tests that are based on the observation of microbial growth in the presence of a single source of carbon (see Color Plate 5-2F). A description of the operating procedure and substrates included is given in Table 5-30. Positive and negative reactions are converted to a seven-digit biotype number, and organism identifications are made either from a computerized database or from a profile list provided by the manufacturer. Users of this system should note that the database is constructed on the basis of reactions obtained at an incubation temperature of 30°C (instead of the conventional 35° to 37°C). Despite the use of the word "rapid" in naming this system, it is not a rapid system in the sense that clinical microbiologists have come to use this term. In one study by Von Graevenitz and Zollinger-Iten,[324] the majority of the strains tested could not be identified until after 48 hours incubation. Most researchers recommend holding the strip 48 hours before making the final identification. Kiska et al.[168] tested 150 nonfermenters isolated from patients with cystic fibrosis and reported an overall correct identification rate of 57%, including 43% of the *B. cepacia* isolates. The overall performance of the API NFT has shown it to be one of the better-performing commercial systems for the identification of nonfermenters.[9,176,193,281,324,327]

FUNCTIONAL DESIGN	OPERATING PROCEDURE	SUBSTRATES INCLUDED	

Each system consists of a plastic strip with 20 miniaturized cupules containing dehydrated substrates and a plastic incubation chamber with a loosely fitting lid (see Color Plates 4-5A and 5-2F). Each cupule has a small hole at the top through which the bacterial suspension can be inoculated with a pipette. Bacterial action on the substrates produces turbidity or color changes that are interpreted visually.

For both systems: Add 5 mL of tap water to an incubation tray to provide a humid atmosphere during incubation. Place the strip into the incubation tray. Prepare a bacterial suspension of the test organism by suspending the cells from a well-isolated colony in 5 mL of sterile 0.85% saline. The turbidity must be equivalent to a 0.5 McFarland standard.

API 20E: With a Pasteur pipette, fill each cupule with the bacterial suspension through the inoculating hole. Overlay the three decarboxylase and the urease cupules with sterile mineral oil. The unit is incubated at 35°C for 24 or 48 h before reading results according to the following rules: after 24 h, if the glucose is positive add reagents, perform an oxidase test, and generate a 7-digit profile number to look up in the white section of the Profile Index; if glucose is negative, but three or more other reactions are positive before adding reagents, proceed as above; if glucose is negative and fewer than three other tests are positive, do not add reagents, reincubate strip for additional 24 h and inoculate OF glucose, motility medium, and MacConkey agar. After 48 h, add reagents, perform oxidase test, and generate a 9-digit profile number to look up in the blue section of the Profile Index.

Rapid NFT: With a Pasteur pipette, fill the tube portion of the first eight cupules (NO$_3$ through PNPG) with the bacterial suspension. Inoculate an ampule of AUX medium with 4 drops of the same saline suspension. Mix well. With a new sterile pipette inoculate the assimilation tests GLU through PAC (cupules with colored lines) by filling the tube and cupule until a flat liquid surface without a meniscus is obtained. Add mineral oil to the GLU, ADH, and URE cupules. Incubate strip for 24 h at 29°C–31°C. After 24 h, add nitrate reagents to NO$_3$ cupule and TRP reagent to TRP cupule. Read and record reactions. Assimilation tests are recorded as positive if there is visible growth in the cupule portion of the tube. A 7-digit profile number is generated. If a good identification is not obtained or profile number is not found in codebook, the test strip may be incubated for an additional 24 h. To do so, immediately cover the NO$_3$ and TRP cupules with mineral oil. Record the NO$_3$, TRP, and GLU test results after 24 h; do not read these tests after 48 h.

API 20E:
 ONPG
 Arginine dihydrolase
 Lysine decarboxylase
 Ornithine decarboxylase
 Citrate
 Hydrogen sulfide
 Urease
 Tryptophan deaminase (add 10% FeCl$_3$)
 Indole
 Voges-Proskauer (add KOH and α-naphthol)
 Gelatin
 Glucose
 Mannitol
 Inositol
 Sorbitol
 Rhamnose
 Sucrose
 Melibiose
 Amygdalin
 Arabinose
Supplemental Tests:
 Oxidase
 NO$_2$
 N$_2$ gas
 Motility
 MacConkey
 OF glucose-oxidative
 OF glucose-fermentative

Rapid NFT:
 Biochemical Tests:
  Nitrate reduction
  Tryptophanase
  Glucose fermentation
  Arginine dihydrolase
  Urease
  Esculin hydrolysis
  Gelatinase
  β-Galactosidase
 Assimilation Tests:
  D-Glucose
  L-Arabinose
  D-Mannose
  D-Mannitol
  N-Acetyl-D glucosamine
  Maltose
  D-Gluconate
  Caprate
  Adipate
  L-Malate
  Citrate
  Phenylacetate

The Remel N/F System

The UNI-N/F system was manufactured first by Corning, then by Flow Laboratories, and now by Remel Laboratories. The system, as described in Table 5-31 and shown in Color Plate 5-2G, includes three components:

1. A constricted gram-negative fermenter (GNF) tube that detects glucose fermentation and N_2 (below the constriction) and fluorescein production on the slant (above the constriction)
2. A nonconstricted 42P tube that is used to test for growth at 42°C and pyocyanin pigment production
3. A circular UNI-N/F Tek plate that consists of 11 independently sealed peripheral wells, containing conventional agar, with which the following characteristics can be determined: utilization of glucose, xylose, mannitol, lactose, and maltose; acetamide assimilation; hydrolysis of esculin and urea; DNase and ONPG activity. One of the peripheral wells is a carbohydrate growth control. A center well contains a medium for detecting indole and hydrogen sulfide production.

The UNI-N/F Tek plate is well constructed to test for most nonfermenters. The plate includes media that closely resembles conventional formulations and will support the growth of many of the more fastidious strains. The organism suspension is inoculated to the surface of the agar wedges, where not only are the organisms exposed to atmospheric oxygen, but the colonial growth can also be directly viewed. Thus, negative test reactions owing to no growth can be distinguished from those owing to biochemical inactivity, and the user can determine directly whether other organisms may be contaminating the inoculum.

The ability of the Remel N/F system to detect *P. aeruginosa* by the use of the supplemental constricted GNF tube and the nonconstricted 42P tube saves time. If the test organism is other than *P. aeruginosa*, 1 drop of a heavy suspension prepared from the slant of the GNF tube is delivered into each of the peripheral chambers in the UNI-N/F Tek plate, and the center well is stab-inoculated. The plate is incubated at 35°C for 24 hours, and the various reactions are interpreted visually.

About 90% of *P. aeruginosa* were identified by researchers with the two screening tubes after 24 hours incubation, increasing to approximately 98% after 48 hours incubation.[10,13,38,173,287,325] The capability to screen out *P. aeruginosa* without using a full set of biochemical tests is considered a distinct advantage by most users. Some of the problems cited with the UNI-N/F system were as follows: The screening tubes identified only about one-third of the strains of *P. fluorescens* and *P. putida*, and further testing was necessary.[10,13,38,176,287] Problems were also encountered in the interpretation of the N_2 gas reaction in the GNF tube and the indole test.[10,325] Only a low percentage of identification was possible with organisms such as *B. cepacia* and CDC group IV, and with many of the nonoxidative and nonsaccharolytic strains.[325] Supplemental tests, such as

---

TABLE 5-31
Uni N/F Tek System for Identifying Nonfermenters

Functional Design	Operating Procedure	Substrates Included

This system consists of two tubes of media poured on a slant and a wheel, including 12 peripheral and 1 central compartments containing a variety of media substrates (Color Plate 5-2G).
 	
 The two tubes are used to screen for *P. aeruginosa*. The nonconstricted tube is incubated at 42°C to observe for growth and pyocyanin pigment production; the constricted GNF tube is used to screen for fluorescence, glucose fermentation, and N_2.
 	
 The wheel is used to determine several biochemical characteristics. Each of the peripheral media compartments has a small pore through which a bacterial suspension can be inoculated. The medium in the central compartment is open to the air and is inoculated directly. A plastic lid covers the unit to prevent evaporation during incubation.
	Initially stab–inoculate the two tubes, using a straight inoculating wire that has been touched to the surface of a well-isolated colony of the test bacterium growing on an agar plate. Incubate the tubes for 18–24 h at 35°C.
	
	 If the reactions in the tubes are not consistent with *P. aeruginosa*, prepare a heavy bacterial suspension by emulsifying the entire growth from the slant of the GNF tube into 2 mL of sterile distilled water. Add 1 drop to each of the 12 peripheral wells through the inoculating pore and deeply stab-inoculate the agar medium in the center of the wheel. Replace the plastic lid on the wheel and incubate the unit at 35°C for 18–24 h. Color reactions are interpreted visually and identifications made using a logic scheme or computer program supplied by the manufacturer.
		Nonconstricted tube agar slant:
		   42°C growth and pyocyanin
		   pigment production
		 Constricted tube
		   GNF medium
		     Glucose fermentation
		     N_2
		     Fluorescence
		 Wheel
		   Peripheral compartments
		     Growth control
		     Glucose
		     Xylose
		     Mannitol
		     Lactose
		     Maltose
		     Acetamide
		     Esculin
		     Urea
		     DNAse
		     ONPG
		   Central compartment
		     Agar media:
		       Hydrogen sulfide
		       Indole

Gram stain morphology, hanging-drop motility, and flagellar stains were needed to identify these strains. The researchers, nonetheless, report that the UNI-N/F system is convenient to use, gives a high overall percentage of nonfermentative bacilli identifications in 24 hours, and performed better in identifying nonfermenters than either the Oxi/Ferm or API 20E systems.[10,13,38,173,176,287,325] Kiska and associates reported that the Uni-N/F system correctly identified 72% of the NFBs encountered in cystic fibrosis patients, including 86% of the *B. cepacia* isolates. The identification percentage for *B. cepacia* isolates was the highest among the four test kits studied.[168] We have found that the Uni-N/F system performs comparably with the Crystal Enteric/Nonfermenter and the IDS RapID NF Plus systems.[281]

THE CRYSTAL ENTERIC/NONFERMENTER SYSTEM

The Crystal Enteric/NonFermenter ID kit has been described in Chapter 4. The nonfermenter database includes 24 taxa of nonfermenters representing 10 different genera. Twenty additional taxa are included in a group called "Miscellaneous Gram-Negative Bacilli," that consists of a group of oxidase-positive species that are relatively inactive and indistinguishable from each other in the Crystal E/NF System. Included in this group are some medically relevant species of *Alcaligenes*, *Burkholderia*, *Comamonas*, *Moraxella*, *Ochrobactrum*, *Oligella*, and *Pseudomonas*. In a study by Wauters and coworkers[327] the overall correct identification of 201 nonfermenters (including 31 different species) was 75.9% with the Crystal E/NF compared with 75.3% for the API NE (same as API NFT). Of note is that only 36 of 45 *P. aeruginosa* strains were correctly identified by the Crystal E/NF compared with 41 of 45 by the API NE. The overall percentage of incorrect identifications for nonfermenters was substantially higher for the API (13.8%) than for the Crystal (6.3%). The authors noted that an advantage of Crystal over the API system is that both fermenters and nonfermenters can be tested in the same panel. In addition the API NE may require 48 hours incubation, whereas the Crystal E/NF requires only 18 hours incubation. Robinson and colleagues[261] studied 131 nonenteric bacilli on the Crystal E/NF including 11 species of nonfermenters; however, three species (*P. aeruginosa*, *A. baumannii*, *S. maltophilia*) accounted for 90% of the nonfermenters tested. The Crystal system correctly identified all of the *P. aeruginosa*, *A. baumannii*, and *S. maltophilia* species tested, but correctly identified only 8 of the 13 (61.5%) remaining nonfermenter species tested. Our own evaluation showed an overall identification rate to the species level of 62.5%.[281]

THE RapID NF PLUS SYSTEM

The RapID NF Plus System (Innovative Diagnostic Systems, Inc., Norcross GA) is a micromethod employing conventional and chromogenic substrates for the identification of medically important glucose-nonfermenting gram-negative bacteria and other selected glucose-fermenting gram-negative bacteria not belonging to the family *Enterobacteriaceae*. The tests used in the RapID NF Plus System are based on the microbial degradation of specific substrates detected by various indicator systems. The reactions employed are a combination of conventional tests and single-substrate chromogenic tests. The system is described in Table 5-32 and shown in Color Plate 5-2*H*. In the study by Kitch and colleagues,[169] 90.1 % of all strains were identified correctly to species without additional tests. Kiska and associates[168] showed that the NF Plus correctly identified 80% of the NFBs recovered from cystic fibrosis patients, including 81% of the *B. cepacia* isolates. This was the highest overall identification rate of the four commercial systems included in the study.[168] In the study by Schreckenberger and coworkers, the overall correct identification to species was 61.8%.[281] The system does not subdivide *Acinetobacter* species or *Alcaligenes xylosoxidans* into subspecies, nor does it differentiate between *P. fluorescens* and *P. putida*. The RapID NF Plus system is currently the only nonautomated 4-hour test system available for the identification of nonfermenters.

THE BIOLOG SYSTEM

The Biolog System (Biolog, Inc., Hayward CA) has been described in Chapter 4. The gram-negative database version 3.50 contains 275 species and biogroups of nonfermenting gram-negative rods. Holmes and associates[127] have evaluated the Biolog System, using 214 strains of nonfermenters representing 15 species. They report that after 4 hours of incubation, 20% of the nonfermenters were correctly identified to the species level using the automated reader; however, after 24 hours of incubation 54% and 66% of the nonfermenters were correctly identified to the species level by automated and manual reading, respectively, using version 3.01A software. The authors note that no other commercial bacterial identification system has as many taxa in a single database as that supplied by Biolog, but because there are so many, even the large number of tests available may not be adequate, in practice, for discriminating all pairs of taxa.[127]

AUTOMATED IDENTIFICATION SYSTEMS

THE VITEK SYSTEM

The Vitek System (BioMerieux Vitek, Inc., Hazelwood MO), described in Chapter 4, has also been used with success in the identification of the nonfermenters most frequently encountered in the clinical laboratory. Smith and associates[293] found an overall correlation of 89.3% correctly identified species compared with conventional methods. Plorde and coworkers[244] tested 419 NFBs including 14 genera and 35 species. Of the 356 test organisms included in the Vitek database, 86.2% were correctly identified, 10.1% were not identified,

TABLE 5-32
RAPID NF PLUS SYSTEM FOR IDENTIFYING NONFERMENTERS

FUNCTIONAL DESIGN	OPERATING PROCEDURE	SUBSTRATES INCLUDED
The system consists of 10 reaction cavities molded into the periphery of a plastic disposable tray (see Color Plate 5-2H). Reaction cavities contain dehydrated reactants, and the tray allows the simultaneous inoculation of each cavity with a predetermined amount of inoculum. When the test inoculum is added to the reaction cavity, the test substrate is rehydrated and the test reaction is initiated. After incubation for 4 h, each test cavity is examined for reactivity by noting the development of a color. In some cases, reagents must be added to the test cavities to provide a color change. The resulting pattern of positive and negative test reactions is used as the basis for identification of the test isolate by comparison of test results to reactivity of known organisms stored in a computer generated database.	**Preparation of Inocula.** Test organisms must be grown in pure culture and should be examined by Gram stain and oxidase before use in the RapID NF System. Test organisms may be removed from a variety of selective and nonselective agar growth media. Plates used for inocula preparation should preferably be 18–24 h old. Using a cotton swab or inoculating loop, remove organisms from agar plate and suspend in RapID Inoculation Fluid to achieve a visual turbidity of at least a 1 but not in excess of a 3 McFarland Turbidity Standard. Suspensions should be mixed thoroughly and used within 15 min of preparation. **Inoculation of Panels.** Peel back the panel lid over the inoculation port. With a Pasteur pipette, gently transfer the entire contents of the inoculation fluid into the upper right-hand corner of the panel. Reseal the inoculation port by pressing the peel tab back in place. After adding the test suspension, tilt the panel back away from the test cavities at approximately a 45° angle. While tilted back, gently rock the panel from side to side to evenly distribute the inoculum along the rear baffles. While maintaining a level horizontal position, slowly tilt the panel forward toward the reaction cavities until the inoculum flows along the baffles into the reaction cavities. Incubate panels at 35–37°C in a non-CO$_2$ incubator for 4 h. **Reading Panels.** Place panel on benchtop and peel back the label lid over the reaction cavities. Without the addition of any reagents, read and score cavities 1 through 10, reading from left to right and record on report form. Record color of cavity 10 (GLU) in space provided on report pad. Then add 2 drops of NF Plus Reagent to cavities 4–8, 2 drops of Innova Spot Indole Reagent to cavity 9, and 2 drops of Innova Nitrate A reagent to cavity 10. Allow 30 sec but no more than 3 min for color development. Record results in appropriate boxes on report form. Look up in Code Compendium or computer database.	Arginine dihydrolase Aliphatic thiol utilization Triglyceride hydrolysis Enzymatic hydrolysis of glycoside or phosphoester linked nitrophenyl substrates releases yellow o- or p-nitrophenol: p-Nitrophenyl-phosphoester p-Nitrophenyl-N-acetyl-β,D-glucosaminide p-Nitrophenyl-α,D-glucoside p-Nitrophenyl-β,D-glucoside o-Nitrophenyl-β,D-galactoside Urea hydrolysis Glucose utilization Enzymatic hydrolysis of substrate linked β-naphthylamide substrates releases free β-naphthylamine which is detected with the RapID NF Plus Reagent Proline β-naphthylamide Pyrrolidine β-naphthylamide γ-Glutamyl β-naphthylamide Tryptophan β-naphthylamide N-Benzyl-arginine-β-naphthylamide Tryptophan utilization with formation of indole Sodium nitrate reduction The above tests together with oxidase provide 18 test parameters

and 3.7% were misidentified. The average time to identification was 15 hours. Pfaller and coworkers[237] tested 91 NFBs, with 90.1% identified correctly. Fifteen percent were identified at 4 hours, an additional 45% were identified 5 to 8 hours, and an additional 40% were identified at 9 to 18 hours. Colonna and associates[55] tested 142 NFBs and found 79.6% agreement with the API NFT. Kiska and colleagues[168] evaluated four identification systems, including the Vitek GNI card, for

identification of NFBs from cystic fibrosis patients. A total of 150 isolates were tested including 58 B. cepacia, 30 S. maltophilia, 24 A. xylosoxidans, 14 P. aeruginosa, and 24 other NFBs. The Vitek correctly identified only 50% of the B. cepacia isolates and 60% of the isolates overall. O'Hara and coworkers[222] tested 23 nonfermenters (8 Acinetobacter, 10 P. aeruginosa, 5 S. maltophilia) and reported 100% correct identification with the Vitek GNI card and version R07.1 software.

Rhoads and associates[257] tested 80 *A. baumannii* and 39 *P. aeruginosa* and reported correct identification of 100% and 84.6%, respectively, with the Vitek GNI card and version AMS-R08.2 software. We agree with the conclusions of Smith and colleagues that the Vitek shortens the turnaround time for obtaining results, that same-day results can be issued in many instances, and work flow can be integrated to handle microorganisms belonging to many different groups, with minimal expenditure of a technologist's time, by merely using the appropriate cards. However, experience has shown that a suitable backup system must be considered for use in identifying those organisms for which the Vitek system does not provide an acceptable level of identification.

THE MICROSCAN WALKAWAY-96, WALKAWAY-40, AND AUTOSCAN-4

These three systems (manufactured by Dade Micro-Scan, West Sacramento CA), described in Chapter 4, all have an extensive database that includes many species of NFBs. Pfaller and colleagues,[237] using WalkAway-96 Rapid Gram Negative Panel, reported that 92.3% of the nonenteric bacilli were identified correctly with a likelihood of more than 85%. Tenover and colleagues[308] evaluated the Walkaway-96 (formerly called the auto-SCAN-W/A) for its ability to identify 310 well-characterized nonglucose-fermenting gram-negative bacilli. In their study, two types of identification panels were tested: the dried colorimetric Neg ID type 2 panel (DCP) and the rapid fluorometric Neg ID panel (RFP). Results with the DCP showed that 41.3% of 286 organisms were identified correctly, with a confidence of more than 85%, whereas 22.4% were misidentified with the same degree of confidence (very major errors). Fifteen percent of the organisms were reported as unidentified. Problems in identifying relatively common nonfermentative bacilli, such as *P. fluorescens*, *P. putida*, and *S. maltophilia* were reported with the DCP panel. The researchers reported better results with the RFP panels, in which 77.1% of 239 isolates were correctly identified, whereas 25% were misidentified. The researchers further noted that the results with the RFP panels were available in 2 hours; thus, if an organism cannot be identified, additional biochemical tests can be inoculated on the same day, and little time is lost in identifying the organisms. Colonna and colleagues, at UCLA, tested 142 NFBs using the 2-hour rapid Neg ID panel and reported 74.6% agreement with the API NFT.[55] O'Hara and colleagues[222] at the CDC tested 23 species of NFBs, including 8 *Acinetobacter*, 10 *P. aeruginosa*, and 5 *S. maltophilia*, and reported 100% accuracy with the Walkaway Neg combo 3 panel and version 17.02 software. Rhoads and coworkers[257] reported 97.5% and 82.1% correct identification of *A. baumannii* and *P. aeruginosa* isolates, respectively, using the Walkaway-96 system with urine combo 6 and negative combo 16 and version 20.20 software. The MicroScan rapid panels provide a 2-hour identification, thereby allowing sufficient time to set up additional supplemental testing if needed for same-day or overnight identification.

THE SENSITITRE AP80 SYSTEM

The Sensititre AP80 Identification panels (Accumed International, Inc., Westlake OH) can be inoculated and incubated off-line and then read in the Sensititre Autoreader, or can be inoculated and placed in the ARIS (Automated Reading and Incubation System) Instrument described in Chapter 4. The AP80 panel permits the identification of gram-negative bacilli in as little as 5 hours, with the option of additional overnight incubation if needed or desired. Colonna and coworkers tested 142 NFBs using the Sensititre AP80 panels and reported 71.1% agreement with the API NFT.[55] Staneck and colleagues[299] tested 144 nonenteric isolates including 135 nonfermenters representing eight species. Ninety-three percent of the isolates tested consisted of just three species (68 *P. aeruginosa*, 33 *Acinetobacter*, 25 *S. maltophilia*). Correct identification was obtained for 99.2% of these three species and for 95.1% of all nonenterics tested. The small number of nonfermenter species tested in this study makes it difficult to evaluate the performance of this system for routine clinical laboratory testing of the nonfermenters.

SELECTION OF A SYSTEM

Clinical microbiologists must evaluate parameters such as accuracy, cost effectiveness, and effects on work flow when deciding whether to use a packaged system in identifying nonfermenters. The packaged systems perform with levels of accuracy equal to or better than conventional methods in identifying *P. aeruginosa*, *Acinetobacter* species, and *S. maltophilia*; however, these metabolically active organisms can also be identified easily by using a few simple biochemical tests described earlier in this chapter. Many laboratories have adopted one of the commercial systems as a matter of convenience. However, because of the reported low sensitivity and specificity in the identification of many of the more fastidious and biochemically inactive nonfermenters, supplemental conventional differential media must still be kept on hand. Therefore, the definitive identification of most nonfermenters still requires considerable technical experience and access to a variety of fresh culture media kept under strict quality control. Because relatively few nonfermenters, particularly strains of species other than the three mentioned in the foregoing, are encountered in most medium-sized or small laboratories, the services of a reference laboratory should be seriously considered. Identifying nonfermenters is not difficult if the microbiologist is willing to devote the time and dedication necessary to achieve an acceptable level of accuracy. Packaged systems can be recommended, provided one understands their shortcomings and is willing to set up supplemental tests to identify weakly reactive or fastidious strains.

REFERENCES

1. ALOS JI, DE RAFAEL L, GONZALEZ-PALACIOS R, AGUIAR JM, ALLONA A, BAQUERO F: Urinary tract infection probably caused by *Agrobacterium radiobacter*. Eur J Clin Microbiol 4:596–597, 1985

2. AMBER IJ, REIMER LG: *Pseudomonas* sp. group Ve-2 bacterial peritonitis in a patient on continuous ambulatory peritoneal dialysis. J Clin Microbiol 25:744–745, 1987

3. ANAISSIE E, FAINSTEIN V, MILLER P, KASSAMALI H, PITLIK S, BODEY GP, ROLSTON K: *Pseudomonas putida*: newly recognized pathogen in patients with cancer. Am J Med 82:1191–1194, 1987

4. ANDERSEN BM, STEIGERWALT AG, O'CONNOR SP, HOLLIS DG, WEYANT RS, WEAVER RE, BRENNER DJ: *Neisseria weaveri* sp. nov., formerly CDC group M-5, a gram-negative bacterium associated with dog bite wounds. J Clin Microbiol 31:2456–2466, 1993

5. ANDERSEN BM, WEYANT RS, STEIGERWALT AG, MOSS CW, HOLLIS DG, WEAVER RE, ASHFORD D, BRENNER DJ: Characterization of *Neisseria elongata* subsp. *glycolytica* isolates obtained from human wound specimens and blood cultures. J Clin Microbiol 33:76–78, 1995

6. ANDERSON RR, WARNICK P, SCHRECKENBERGER PC: Recurrent CDC Group IVc-2 bacteremia in a human with acquired immune deficiency syndrome. J Clin Microbiol, submitted.

7. APPELBAUM PC, BOWEN AJ: Opportunistic infection of chronic skin ulcers with *Pseudomonas putrefaciens*. Br J Dermatol 98:229–231, 1978

8. APPELBAUM PC, CAMPBELL DB: Pancreatic abscess associated with *Achromobacter* group Vd biovar 1. J Clin Microbiol 12:282–283, 1980

9. APPELBAUM PC, LEATHERS DJ: Evaluation of the rapid NFT system for identification of gram-negative, nonfermenting rods. J Clin Microbiol 20:730–734, 1984

10. APPELBAUM PC, STAVITZ J, BENTZ MS, ET AL: Four methods for identification of gram-negative nonfermenting rods: organisms more commonly encountered in clinical specimens. J Clin Microbiol 12:271–278, 1980

11. ARAGONE MDR, MAURIZI DM, CLARA LO, ESTRADA JLN, ASCIONE A: *Pseudomonas mendocina*, an environmental bacterium isolated from a patient with human infective endocarditis. J Clin Microbiol 30:1583–1584, 1992

12. BARBARO DJ, MACKOWIAK PA, BARTH SS, ET AL: *Pseudomonas testosteroni* infections: eighteen recent cases and a review of the literature. Rev Infect Dis 9:124–129, 1987

13. BARNISHAN J, AYERS LW: Rapid identification of nonfermentative gram-negative rods by the Corning N/F system. J Clin Microbiol 9:239–243, 1979

14. BARSON WJ, CROMER BA, MARCON MJ: Puncture wound osteochondritis of the foot caused by CDC group Vd. J Clin Microbiol 25:2014–2016, 1987

15. BASSET DCJ, DICKSON JAS, HUNT GH: Infection of Holter valve by *Pseudomonas*-contaminated chlorhexidine. Lancet i:1263–1264, 1973

16. BAUWENS JE, SPACH DH, SCHACKER TW, MUSTAFA MM, BOWDEN RA: *Bordetella bronchiseptica* pneumonia and bacteremia following bone marrow transplantation. J Clin Microbiol 30:2474–2475, 1992

17. BECK-SAGUE CM, JARVIS WR, BROOK JH, CULVER DH, POTTS A, GAY E, SHOTTS BW, HILL B, ANDERSON RL, WEINSTEIN MP: Epidemic bacteremia due to *Acinetobacter baumannii* in five intensive care units. Am J Epidemiol 132:723–733, 1990

18. BENDIG JWA, MAYES PJ, EYERS DE, ET AL: *Flavimonas oryzihabitans* (*Pseudomonas oryzihabitans*; CDC Group Ve-2): An emerging pathogen in peritonitis related to continuous ambulatory peritoneal dialysis? J Clin Microbiol 27:217–218, 1989

19. BENNASAR A, ROSSELLO-MORA R, LALUCAT J, MOORE ERB: 16S rRNA gene sequence analysis relative to genomovars of *Pseudomonas stutzeri* and proposal of *Pseudomonas balearica* sp. nov. Int J Syst Bacteriol 46:200–205, 1996

20. BERGER SA, SIEGMAN–IGRA Y, STADLER J ET AL: Group VE-1 septicemia. J Clin Microbiol 17:926–927, 1983

20a. BERGOGNE-BEREZIN E, TOWNER KJ: *Acinetobacter* spp. as nosocomial pathogens: Microbiological, clinical, and epidemiological features. Clin Microbiol Rev 9:148–165, 1996

21. BERKELMAN RL, LEWIN S, ALLEN JR, ET AL: Pseudobacteremia attributed to contamination of povidone-iodine with *Pseudomonas cepacia*. Ann Intern Med 95:32–36, 1981

22. BERNARDET J-F, SEGERS P, VANCANNEYT M, BERTHE F, KERSTERS K, VANDAMME P: Cutting a Gordian knot: emended classification and description of the genus *Flavobacterium*, emended description of the family *Flavobacteriaceae*, and proposal of *Flavobacterium hydatis*, nom. nov. (basonym, *Cytophaga aquatilis* Strohl and Tait 1978). Int J Syst Bacteriol 46:128–148, 1996

23. BLACK–PAYNE C, LIERL MB, BOCCHINI JA, ET AL: Comparison of two selective media developed to isolate *Pseudomonas cepacia* from patients with cystic fibrosis. Diagn Microbiol Infect Dis 6:277–282, 1987

24. BLAZEVIC DJ, EDERER GM: Principles of Biochemical Tests in Diagnostic Microbiology. New York, John Wiley & Sons, 1975

25. BLUMBERG DA, CHERRY JD: *Agrobacterium radiobacter* and CDC group Ve-2 bacteremia. Diagn Microbiol Infect Dis 12:351–355, 1989

26. BODEY GP, BOLIVAR R, FAINSTEIN V, JADEJA L: Infections caused by *Pseudomonas aeruginosa*. Rev Infect Dis 5:279–313, 1983

27. BOUVET PJM, GRIMONT PAD: Taxonomy of the genus *Acinetobacter* with the recognition of *Acinetobacter baumannii* sp. nov., *Acinetobacter haemolyticus* sp. nov., *Acinetobacter johnsonii* sp. nov., and *Acinetobacter junii* sp. nov. and emended descriptions of *Acinetobacter calcoaceticus* and *Acinetobacter lwoffi*. Int J Syst Bacteriol 36:228–240, 1986

28. BOUVET PJM, GRIMONT PAD: Identification and biotyping of clinical isolates of *Acinetobacter*. Ann Inst Pasteur Microbiol 138:569–578, 1987

29. BOUVET PJM, JEANJEAN S: Delineation of new proteolytic genomic species of the genus *Acinetobacter*. Res Microbiol 140:291–299, 1989

30. BOUVET PJM, JEANJEAN S, VIEU J–F, ET AL: Species, biotype, and bacteriophage type determinations compared

with cell envelope protein profiles for typing *Acinetobacter* strains. J Clin Microbiol 28:170–176, 1990

31. BOVRE K: Genus II. *Moraxella* Lwoff 1939, 173 emend. Henriksen and Bovre 1968, 391AL. In Krieg NR, Holt JG (eds): Bergey's Manual of Systematic Bacteriology, vol. 1, pp 296–303. Baltimore, Williams & Wilkins, 1984

32. BOVRE K: Family VIII. *Neisseriaceae* Prevot 1933, 119AL. In Krieg NR, Holt JG (eds): Bergey's Manual of Systematic Bacteriology, vol 1, pp. 288–309. Baltimore, Williams & Wilkins, 1984

33. BOVRE K, FUGLESANG JE, HAGEN N, JANTZEN E, FROHOLM LO: *Moraxella atlantae* sp. nov. and its distinction from *Moraxella phenylpyrouvica*. Int J Syst Bacteriol 26:511–521, 1976

34. BRACIS R, SEIBERS K, JULIEN RM: Meningitis caused by Group IIj following a dog bite. West J Med 131:438–440, 1979

35. BRINK AJ, VAN STRATEN A, VAN RENSBURG AJ: *Shewanella (Pseudomonas) putrefaciens* bacteremia. Clin Infect Dis 20:1327–1332, 1995

36. BUCHMAN AL, PICKETT MJ: *Moraxella atlantae* bacteraemia in a patient with systemic lupus erythematosis. J Infect 23:197–199, 1991

37. BUCHMAN AL, PICKETT MJ, MANN L, AMENT ME: Central venous catheter infection caused by *Moraxella osloensis* in a patient receiving home parenteral nutrition. Diagn Microbiol Infect Dis 17:163–166, 1993

38. BURDASH NM, BANNISTER ER, MANOS JP, ET AL: A comparison of four commercial systems for the identification of nonfermentative gram-negative bacilli. Am J Clin Pathol 73:564–569, 1980

39. BUXTON AE, ANDERSON RL, WERDEGAR D, ET AL: Nosocomial respiratory tract infection and colonization with *Acinetobacter calcoaceticus*. Am J Med 65:507–513, 1978

40. CAIN JR: A case of septicaemia caused by *Agrobacterium radiobacter* [letter]. J Infect 16:205–206, 1988

41. CALUBIRAN OV, SCHOCH PE, CUNHA BA: *Pseudomonas paucimobilis* bacteraemia associated with haemodialysis. J Hosp Infect 15:383–388, 1990

42. CARRATALA J, SALAZAR A, MASCARO J, SANTIN M: Community-acquired pneumonia due to *Pseudomonas stutzeri* [letter]. Clin Infect Dis 14:792, 1992

43. CARSON LA, TABLAN OC, CUSICK LB, ET AL: Comparative evaluation of selective media for isolation of *Pseudomonas cepacia* from cystic fibrosis patients and environmental sources. J Clin Microbiol 26:2096–2100, 1988

44. CASADEVALL A, FREUNDLICH LF, PIROFSKI L: Septic shock caused by *Pseudomonas paucimobilis* [letter]. Clin Infect Dis 14:784, 1992

45. CASALTA JP, PELOUX Y, RAOULT D, BRUNET P, GALLAIS H: Pneumonia and meningitis caused by a new nonfermentative unknown gram-negative bacterium. J Clin Microbiol 27:1446–1448, 1989

46. CATLIN BW: Cellular elongation under the influence of antibacterial agents: way to differentiate coccobacilli from cocci. J Clin Microbiol 1:102–105, 1975

47. CENTERS FOR DISEASE CONTROL: *Pseudomonas pickettii* colonization associated with a contaminated respiratory therapy solution—Illinois. MMWR 38:495, 1983

48. CHAUDHRY HJ, SCHOCH PE, CUNHA BA: *Flavimonas oryzihabitans* (CDC Group Ve-2). Infect Control Hosp Epidemiol 13:485–488, 1992

49. CHOW AW, WONG J, BARTLETT KH: Synergistic interactions of ciprofloxacin and extended-spectrum beta-lactams or aminoglycosides against multiply drug-resistant *Pseudomonas maltophilia*. Antimicrob Agents Chemother 32:782–784, 1988

50. CHRISTENSON JC, WELCH DF, MUKWAYA G, ET AL: Recovery of *Pseudomonas gladioli* from respiratory tract specimens of patients with cystic fibrosis. J Clin Microbiol 27:270–273, 1989

51. CIESLAK TJ, ROBB ML, DRABICK CJ, FISCHER GW: Catheter-associated sepsis caused by *Ochrobactrum anthropi*: report of a case and review of related nonfermentative bacteria. Clin Infect Dis 14:902–907, 1992

52. CLARK WA: A simplified Leifson flagella stain. J Clin Microbiol 3:632–634, 1976

53. CLARK WA, HOLLIS DG, WEAVER RE, RILEY P: Identification of Unusual Pathogenic Gram-Negative Aerobic and Facultatively Anaerobic Bacteria. Atlanta, U.S. Department of Health and Human Services, Centers for Disease Control, 1984

54. CLAYTON AJ, LISELLA RS, MARTIN DG: Melioidosis: a serologic survey in military personnel. Milit Med 138:24–26, 1973

55. COLONNA P, NIKOLAI D, BRUCKNER D: Comparison of MicroScan autoSCAN-W/A, Radiometer Sensititre and Vitek systems for rapid identification of gram-negative bacilli, abstr. C-157, p. 370. Abstr 90th Annu Meet Am Soc Microbiol 1990. American Society for Microbiology, Washington DC

56. CONNOR BJ, KOPECKY RT, FRYMOYER PA, ET AL: Recurrent *Pseudomonas luteola* (CDC Group Ve-1) peritonitis in a patient undergoing continuous ambulatory peritoneal dialysis. J Clin Microbiol 25:1113–1114, 1987

57. COOKSON BT, VANDAMME P, CARLSON LC, LARSON AM, SHEFFIELD JVL, KERSTERS K, SPACH DH: Bacteremia caused by a novel *Bordetella* species, "B. hinzii." J Clin Microbiol 32:2569–2571, 1994

58. CRAVEN DE, MOODY B, CONNOLLY MG, ET AL: Pseudobacteremia caused by povidone-iodine solution contaminated with *Pseudomonas cepacia*. N Engl J Med 305:621–623, 1981

59. CROWE HM, BRECHER SM: Nosocomial septicemia with CDC group IVc-2, an unusual gram-negative bacillus. J Clin Microbiol 25:2225–2226, 1987

60. DAN M, BERGER SA, ADERKA D, LEVO Y: Septicemia caused by the gram-negative bacterium CDC IVc-2 in an immunocompromised human. J Clin Microbiol 23:803, 1986

61. DAN M, GUTMAN R, BIRO A: Peritonitis caused by *Pseudomonas putrefaciens* in patients undergoing continuous ambulatory peritoneal dialysis. Clin Infect Dis 14:359–360, 1992

62. DANCE DAB: Melioidosis. Rev Med Microbiol 1:143–150, 1990

63. DANCE DAB: Melioidosis: The tip of the iceberg. Clin Microbiol Rev 4:52–60, 1991

64. DAUGA C, GILLIS M, VANDAMME P, AGERON E, GRIMONT F, KERSTERS K, DE MAHENGE C, PELOUX Y, GRIMONT PAD: *Balneatrix alpica* gen. nov., sp. nov., a bacterium associated with pneumonia and meningitis in a spa therapy centre. Res Microbiol 144:35–46, 1993

65. DEBOIS J, DEGREEF H, VANDEPITTE J, SPAEPEN J: *Pseudomonas putrefaciens* as a cause of infection in humans. J Clin Pathol 28:993–996, 1975

66. DECKER CF, HAWKINS RE, SIMON GL: Infections with *Pseudomonas paucimobilis* [letter]. Clin Infect Dis 14:783–784, 1992

67. DEES SB, HOLLIS DG, WEAVER RE, MOSS CW: Cellular fatty acid composition of *Pseudomonas marginata* and closely associated bacteria. J Clin Microbiol 18:1073–1078, 1983

68. DEGREEF H, DEBOIS J, VANDEPITTE J: *Pseudomonas putrefaciens* as a cause of infection of venous ulcers. Dermatologica 151:296–301, 1975

69. DE LEY J, SEGERS P, KERSTERS K, ET AL: Intra- and intergeneric similarities of the *Bordetella* ribosomal ribonucleic acid cistrons: proposal for a new family, *Alcaligenaceae*. Int J Syst Bacteriol 36:405–414, 1986

70. DOELLE H: Bacterial Metabolism, 2nd ed. New York, Academic Press, 1975

71. DOWDA H: Evaluation of two rapid methods for identification of commonly encountered nonfermenting or oxidase-positive, gram-negative rods. J Clin Microbiol 6:605–609, 1977

72. DUNNE WM JR, MAISCH S: Epidemiological investigation of infections due to *Alcaligenes* species in children and patients with cystic fibrosis: use of repetitive-element-sequence polymerase chain reaction. Clin Infect Dis 20:836–841, 1995

73. DUNNE WM JR, TILLMAN J, MURRAY JC: Recovery of a strain of *Agrobacterium radiobacter* with a mucoid phenotype from an immunocompromised child with bacteremia. J Clin Microbiol 31:2541–2543, 1993

74. EBRIGH T JR, LENTINO JR, JUNI E: Endophthalmitis caused by *Moraxella nonliquefaciens*. Am J Clin Pathol 77:362–363, 1982

75. EDMOND MB, RIDDLER SA, BAXTER CM, WICKLUND BM, PASCULLE AW: *Agrobacterium radiobacter*: a recently recognized opportunistic pathogen. Clin Infect Dis 16:388–391, 1993

76. EGBERT JE, FEDER JM, RAPOZA PA, CHANDLER JW, FRANCE TD: Keratitis associated with *Pseudomonas mesophilica* in a patient taking topical corticosteroids. Am J Ophthamol 116:445–446, 1990

77. EKELUND B, JOHNSEN CR, NIELSEN PB: Septicemia with *Agrobacterium* species from a permanent vena cephalica catheter. A case report. Acta Pathol Microbiol Immunol Scand Sect B 95:323–324, 1987

78. ELTING LS, BODEY GP: Septicemia due to *Xanthomonas* species and non-*aeruginosa Pseudomonas* species: increasing incidence of catheter-related infections. Medicine 69:296–306, 1990

79. ENGEL JM, ALEXANDER FS, PACHUCKI CT: Bacteremia caused by CDC Group Ve-1 in previously healthy patient with granulomatous hepatitis. J Clin Microbiol 25:2023–2024, 1987

80. ESTEBAN J, VALERO-MORATALLA ML, ALCAZAR R, SORIANO F: Infections due to *Flavimonas oryzihabitans*: case report and literature review. Eur J Clin Microbiol Infect Dis 12:797–800, 1993

81. FEIGIN RD, SAN JOAQUIN V, MIDDELKAMP JN: Septic arthritis due to *Moraxella osloensis*. J Pediatr 75:116–117, 1969

82. FELEGIE TP, YU VL, RUMANS LW, ET AL: Susceptibility of *Pseudomonas maltophilia* to antimicrobial agents, singly and in combination. Antimicrob Agents Chemother 16:833–837, 1979

83. FLOURNOY DJ, PETRONE RL, VOTH DW: A pseudo-outbreak of *Methylobacterium mesophilica* isolated from patients undergoing bronchoscopy. Eur J Clin Microbiol Infect Dis 11:240–243, 1992

84. FRENEY J, GRUER LD, BORNSTEIN N, KIREDJIAN M, GUILVOUT I, LETOUZEY MN, COMBE C, FLEURETTE J: Septicemia caused by *Agrobacterium* sp. J Clin Microbiol 22:683–685, 1985

85. FRENEY J, HANSEN W, ETIENNE J, ET AL: Postoperative infant septicemia caused by *Pseudomonas luteola* (CDC group Ve-1) and *Pseudomonas oryzihabitans* (CDC group Ve-2). J Clin Microbiol 26:1241–1243, 1988

86. FRENEY J, HANSEN W, PLOTON C, ET AL: Septicemia caused by *Sphingobacterium multivorum*. J Clin Microbiol 25:1126–1128, 1987

86a. FUNKE G, HESS T, VON GRAEVENITZ A, VANDAMME P: Characteristics of *Bordetella hinzii* strains isolated from a cystic fibrosis patient over a 3-year period. J Clin Microbiol 34:966–969, 1996

87. GARNER J, BRIANT RH: Osteomyelitis caused by a bacterium known as M-6 [letter]. J Infect 13:298–300, 1986

88. GEORGE LJ, CUNHA BA: *Pseudomonas stutzeri* synthetic vascular graft infection. Heart Lung 19:203–205, 1990

89. GHOSH JK, TRANTER J: *Bordetella bronchiseptica* infections in man: review and case report. J Clin Pathol 32:546–548, 1979

90. GILARDI GL: Practical schema for the identification of nonfermentative gram-negative bacteria encountered in medical bacteriology. Am J Med Technol 38:65–72, 1972

91. GILARDI GL: Infrequently encountered *Pseudomonas* species causing infection in humans. Ann Intern Med 77:211–215, 1972

92. GILARDI GL (ED): Glucose Nonfermenting Gram-Negative Bacteria in Clinical Microbiology. West Palm Beach FL, CRC Press, 1978

93. GILARDI GL: Identification of *Pseudomonas* and related bacteria. In Gilardi GL (ed): Glucose Nonfermenting Gram-Negative Bacteria in Clinical Microbiology, pp 15–44. West Palm Beach FL, CRC Press, 1978

94. GILARDI GL: Identification of miscellaneous glucose nonfermenting gram-negative bacteria. In Gilardi GL (ed): Glucose Nonfermenting Gram-Negative Bacteria in Clinical Microbiology, pp 45–55. West Palm Beach FL, CRC Press, 1978

95. GILARDI GL: Nonfermentative Gram-Negative Rods: Laboratory Identification and Clinical Aspects. New York, Marcel Dekker, 1985

96. GILARDI GL: Cultural and biochemical aspects for identification of glucose-nonfermenting gram-negative rods. In Gilardi GL (ed): Nonfermentative Gram-Negative Rods: Laboratory Identification and Clinical Aspects, pp 17–84. New York, Marcel Dekker, 1985

97. GILARDI GL: Identification of Glucose-Nonfermenting Gram-Negative Rods. New York, North General Hospital, 1990

98. GILARDI GL: *Pseudomonas* and related genera. In Balows A (ed): Manual of Clinical Microbiology, 5th ed, pp 429–441. Washington DC, American Society for Microbiology, 1991

99. GILARDI GL, FAUR YC: *Pseudomonas mesophilica* and an unnamed taxon, clinical isolates of pink-pigmented oxidative bacteria. J Clin Microbiol 20:626–629, 1984

100. GILARDI GL, HIRSCHL S, MANDEL M: Characteristics of yellow-pigmented nonfermentative bacilli (groups Ve-1 and Ve-2) encountered in clinical bacteriology. J Clin Microbiol 1:384–389, 1975

101. GILARDI GL, MANKIN HJ: Infection due to *Pseudomonas stutzeri*. NY State J Med 73:2789–2791, 1973

102. GILCHRIST MJR, KRAFT JA, HAMMOND JG, ET AL: Detection of *Pseudomonas mesophilica* as a source of nosocomial infections in a bone marrow transplant unit. J Clin Microbiol 23:1052–1055, 1986

103. GILLIGAN PH: Microbiology of airway disease in patients with cystic fibrosis. Clin Microbiol Rev 4:35–51, 1991

104. GILLIS M, VAN TV, BARDIN R, GOOR M, HEBBAR P, WILLEMS A, SEGERS P, KERSTERS K, HEULIN T, FERNANDEZ MP: Polyphasic taxonomy in the genus *Burkholderia* leading to an emended description of the genus and proposition of *Burkholderia vietnamiensis* sp. nov. for N$_2$-fixing isolates from rice in Vietnam. Int J Syst Bacteriol 45:274–289, 1995

105. GLEW RH, MOELLERING RC, KUNZ LJ: Infections with *Acinetobacter calcoaceticus* (*Herellea vaginicola*): Clinical and laboratory studies. Medicine 56:79–97, 1977

106. GOLDMANN DA, KLINGER JD: *Pseudomonas cepacia*: biology, mechanisms of virulence, epidemiology. J Pediatr 108:806–812, 1986

107. GOODNOW RA: Biology of *B. bronchiseptica*. Microbiol Rev 44:722–738, 1980

108. GOSHORN RK: Recrudescent pulmonary melioidosis: a case report involving the so-called "Vietnamese time bomb." Indiana Med 80:247–249, 1987

109. GOVAN JRW, BROWN PH, MADDISON J, DOHERTY CJ, NELSON JW, DODD M, GREENING AP, WEBB AK: Evidence for transmission of *Pseudomonas cepacia* by social contact in cystic fibrosis. Lancet 342:15–19, 1993

110. GRABER CD, JERVEY LP, OSTRANDER WE, SALLEY LH, WEAVER RE: Endocarditis due to a lanthanic, unclassified gram-negative bacterium (group IVd). Am J Clin Pathol 49:220–223, 1968

111. GRAHAM DR, BAND JD, THORNSBERRY C, HOLLIS DG, WEAVER RE: Infections caused by *Moraxella*, *Moraxella urethralis*, *Moraxella*-like groups M-5 and M-6, and *Kingella kingae* in the United States, 1953–1980. Rev Infect Dis 12:423–431, 1990

112. GRANSDEN WR, EYKYN SJ: Seven cases of bacteremia due to *Ochrobactrum anthropi*. Clin Infect Dis 15:1068–1069, 1992

113. GRANT PE, BRENNER DJ, STEIGERWALT AG, HOLLIS DG, WEAVER RE: *Neisseria elongata* subsp. *nitroreducens* subsp. nov., formerly CDC group M-6, a gram-negative bacterium associated with endocarditis. J Clin Microbiol 28:2591–2596, 1990

114. GREEN PN, BOUSFIELD IJ: Emendation of *Methylobacterium* Patt, Cole, and Hanson 1976; *Methylobacterium rhodinum* (Heumann 1962) comb. nov. corrig.; *Methylobacterium radiotolerans* (Ito and Iizuka 1971) comb. nov. corrig.; and *Methylobacterium mesophilicum* (Austin and Goodfellow 1979) comb. nov. Int J Syst Bacteriol 33:875–877, 1983

115. GREEN PN, BOUSFIELD IJ, HOOD D: Three new *Methylobacterium* species: *M. rhodesianum* sp. nov., *M. zatmanii* sp. nov., and *M. fujisawaense* sp. nov. Int J Syst Bacteriol 38:124–127, 1988

116. GRIFFIN CW III, MEHAFFEY MA, COOK EC, et al: Relationship between performance in three of the Centers for Disease Control microbiology proficiency testing programs and the number of actual patient specimens tested by participating laboratories. J Clin Microbiol 23:246–250, 1986

117. HAMMERBERG O, BIALKOWSKA-HOBRZANSKA H, GOPAUL D: Isolation of *Agrobacterium radiobacter* from a central venous catheter. Eur J Clin Microbiol Infect Dis 10:450–452, 1991

118. HANSEN W, GLUPCZYNSKI Y: Group IV c-2 associated peritonitis. Clin Microbiol Newslett 7:43, 1985.

119. HARRISON GAJ, MORRIS R, HOLMES B, STEAD DG: Human infections with strains of *Agrobacterium* [letter]. J Hosp Infect 16:383–388, 1990

120. HEIMBROOK ME, WANG WLL, CAMPBELL G: Staining bacterial flagella easily. J Clin Microbiol 27:2612–2615, 1989

121. HOBSON R, GOULD I, GOVAN J: *Burkholderia (Pseudomonas) cepacia* as a cause of brain abscesses secondary to chronic suppurative otitis media. Eur J Clin Microbiol Infect Dis 14:908–911, 1995

122. HOFHERR L, VOTAVA H, BLAZEVIC DJ: Comparison of three methods for identifying nonfermenting gram-negative rods. Can J Microbiol 24:1140–1144, 1978

123. HOHL P, FREI R, AUBRY P: In vitro susceptibility of 33 clinical case isolates of *Xanthomonas maltophilia*. Inconsistent correlation of agar dilution and of disk diffusion test results. Diagn Microbiol Infect Dis 14:447–450, 1991

124. HOLLIS DG, DANESHVAR MI, MOSS CW, BAKER CN: Phenotypic characteristics, fatty acid composition, and isoprenoid quinone content of CDC group IIg bacteria. J Clin Microbiol 33:762–764, 1995

125. HOLLIS DG, MOSS CW, DANESHVAR MI, MEADOWS L, JORDAN J, BILL B: Characterization of Centers for Disease Control group NO-1, a fastidious, nonoxidative, gram-negative organism associated with dog and cat bites. J Clin Microbiol 31:746–748, 1993

126. HOLLIS DG, WEAVER RE, MOSS CW, DANESHVAR MI, WALLACE PL: Chemical and cultural characterization of CDC group WO-1, a weakly oxidative gram-negative group of organisms isolated from clinical sources. J Clin Microbiol 30:291–295, 1992

127. HOLMES B, COSTAS M, GANNER M, ON SLW, STEVENS M: Evaluation of Biolog System for identification of some gram-negative bacteria of clinical importance. J Clin Microbiol 32:1970–1975, 1994

128. HOLMES B, COSTAS M, ON SLW, VANDAMME P, FALSEN E, KERSTERS K: *Neisseria weaveri* sp. nov. (formerly CDC group M-5), from dog bite wounds of humans. Int J Syst Bacteriol 43:687–693, 1993

129. HOLMES B, COSTAS M, WOOD AC, KERSTERS K: Numerical analysis of electrophoretic protein patterns of "*Achromobacter*" group B, E and F strains from human blood. J Appl Bacteriol 68:495–504, 1990

130. HOLMES B, COSTAS M, WOOD AC, OWEN RJ, MORGAN DD: Differentiation of *Achromobacter*-like strains from human blood by DNA restriction endonuclease digest and ribosomal RNA gene probe patterns. Epidemiol Infect 105:541–551, 1990

131. HOLMES B, DAWSON CA: Numerical taxonomic studies on *Achromobacter* isolates from clinical material. In Leclerc H (ed.): Gram Negative Bacteria of Medical and Public Health Importance: Taxonomy—Identification—Applications, pp 331–341. Paris, Les Editions INSERM, 1983

132. HOLMES B, DOWLING J, LAPAGE SP: Identification of gram-negative nonfermenters and oxidase-positive fermenters by the Oxi/Ferm tube. J Clin Pathol 32:78–85, 1979

133. HOLMES B, LEWIS R, TREVETT A: Septicaemia due to *Achromobacter* group B: a report of two cases. Med Microbiol Lett 1:177–184, 1992

134. HOLMES B, MOSS CW, DANESHVAR MI: Cellular fatty acid compositions of "*Achromobacter* groups B and E." J Clin Microbiol 31:1007–1008, 1993

135. HOLMES B, OWEN RJ, EVANS A, ET AL: *Pseudomonas paucimobilis*, a new species isolated from human clinical specimens, the hospital environment, and other sources. Int J Syst Bacteriol 27:133–146, 1977

136. HOLMES B, OWEN RJ, HOLLIS DG: *Flavobacterium spiritivorum*, a new species isolated from human clinical specimens. Int J Syst Bacteriol 32:157–165, 1982

137. HOLMES B, OWEN RJ, MCMEEKIN TA: Genus *Flavobacterium*. In Krieg NR, Holt JG (eds): Bergey's Manual of Systematic Bacteriology, vol 1, pp 353–361. Baltimore, Williams & Wilkins, 1984

138. HOLMES B, PINNING CA, DAWSON CA: A probability matrix for the identification of gram-negative, aerobic, non-fermentative bacteria that grow on nutrient agar. J Gen Microbiol 132:1827–1842, 1986

139. HOLMES B, POPOFF M, KIREDJIAN M, KERSTERS K: *Ochrobactrum anthropi* gen. nov., sp. nov. from human clinical specimens and previously known as group Vd. Int J Syst Bacteriol 38:406–416, 1988

140. HOLMES B, SNELL JJS, LAPAGE SP: *Flavobacterium odoratum*: a species resistant to a wide range of antimicrobial agents. J Clin Pathol 32:73–77, 1979

141. HOLMES B, STEIGERWALT AG, WEAVER RE, BRENNER DJ: *Weeksella virosa* gen. nov., sp. nov. (formerly group IIf), found in human clinical specimens. Syst Appl Microbiol 8:185–190, 1986

142. HOLMES B, STEIGERWALT AG, WEAVER RE, BRENNER DJ: *Weeksella zoohelcum* sp. nov. (formerly group IIj), from human clinical specimens. Syst Appl Microbiol 8:191–196, 1986

143. HOLMES B, STEIGERWALT AG, WEAVER RE, BRENNER DJ: *Chryseomonas luteola* comb. nov. and *Flavimonas oryzihabitans* gen. nov., comb. nov., *Pseudomonas*-like species from human clinical specimens and formerly known, respectively, as groups Ve-1 and Ve-2. Int J Syst Bacteriol 37:245–250, 1987

144. HOLMES B, WEAVER RE, STEIGERWALT AG, BRENNER DJ: A taxonomic study of *Flavobacterium spiritivorum* and *Sphingobacterium mizutae*: proposal of *Flavobacterium yabuuchiae* sp. nov. and *Flavobacterium mizutaii* comb. nov. Int J Syst Bacteriol 38:348–353, 1988

145. HOROWITZ H, GILROY S, FEINSTEIN S, ET AL: Endocarditis associated with *Comamonas acidovorans*. J Clin Microbiol 28:143–145, 1990

146. HSUEH P-R, WU J-J, HSIUE T-R, HSIEH W-C: Bacteremic necrotizing fasciitis due to *Flavobacterium odoratum*. Clin Infect Dis 21:1337–1338, 1995

147. HUBERT B, DE MAHENGE A, GRIMONT F, RICHARD C, PELOUX Y, DE MAHENGE C, FLEURETTE J, GRIMONT PAD: An outbreak of pneumonia and meningitis caused by a previously undescribed gram-negative bacterium in a hot spring spa. Epidemiol Infect 107:373–381, 1991.

148. HUDSON MJ, HOLLIS DG, WEAVER RE, ET AL: Relationship of CDC group EO-2 and *Psychrobacter immobilis*. J Clin Microbiol 25:1907–1910, 1987

149. HUGH R, LEIFSON E: The taxonomic significance of fermentative versus oxidative metabolism of carbohydrates by various gram-negative bacteria. J Bacteriol 66:24–26, 1953

150. IGRA–SIEGMAN Y, CHMEL H, COBBS C: Clinical and laboratory characteristics of *Achromobacter xylosoxidans* infection. J Clin Microbiol 11:141–145, 1980

151. IMPERIAL HL, JOHO KL, ALCID DV: Endocarditis due to *Neisseria elongata* subspecies *nitroreducens* [letter]. Clin Infect Dis 20:1431–1432, 1995

152. ISENBERG HD, SAMPSON–SCHERER J: Clinical laboratory evaluation of a system approach to the recognition of nonfermentative or oxidase-producing gram-negative, rod-shaped bacteria. J Clin Microbiol 5:336–340, 1977

153. ISLES A, MACLUSKEY I, COREY M, GOLD R, PROBER C, FLEMING P, LEVISON H: *Pseudomonas cepacia* infection in cystic fibrosis: an emerging problem. J Pediatr 104:206–210, 1984

154. JANNES G, VANEECHOUTTE M, LANNOO M, GILLIS M, VANCANNEYT M, VANDAMME P, VERSCHRAEGEN G, HEUVERSWYN HV, ROSSAU R: Polyphasic taxonomy leading to the proposal of *Moraxella canis* sp. nov. for *Moraxella catarrhalis*-like strains. Int J Syst Bacteriol 43:438–449, 1993

155. JOHNSON DW, LUM G, NIMMO G, HAWLEY CM: *Moraxella nonliquefaciens* septic arthritis in a patient undergoing hemodialysis. Clin Infect Dis 21:1039–1040, 1995

156. KAYE KM, MACONE A, KAZANJIAN PH: Catheter infection caused by *Methylobacterium* in immunocompromised hosts: report of three cases and review of the literature. CID 14:1010–1014, 1992

157. KERN WV, OETHINGER M, KAUFHOLD A, ROZDZINSKI E, MARRE R: *Ochrobactrum anthropi* bacteremia: report of four cases and short review. Infection 21:306–310, 1993

158. KERSTERS K, DE LEY J: Genus III. *Agrobacterium* Conn 1942, 359[AL]. In Krieg NR, Holt JG (eds): Bergey's Manual of Systematic Bacteriology, vol 1, pp 244–254. Baltimore, Williams & Wilkins, 1984

159. KHABBAZ RF, ARNOW PM, HIGHSMITH AK, HERWALDT LA, CHOU T, JARVIS WR, LERCHE NW, ALLEN JR: *Pseudomonas fluorescens* bacteremia from blood transfusion. Am J Med 76:62–68, 1984

160. KHARDORI N, ELTING L, WONG E, SCHABLE B, BODEY GP: Nosocomial infections due to *Xanthomonas maltophilia* (*Pseudomonas maltophilia*) in patients with cancer. Rev Infect Dis 12:997–1003, 1990

161. KIM JH, COOPER RA, WELTY-WOLF KE, HARRELL LJ, ZWADYK P, KLOTMAN ME: *Pseudomonas putrefaciens* bacteremia. Rev Infect Dis 11:97–104, 1989

162. KING A, HOLMES B, PHILLIPS I, LAPAGE SP: A taxonomic study of clinical isolates of *Pseudomonas pickettii*,

'*P. thomasii*' and 'group IVd' bacteria. J Gen Microbiol 114:137–147, 1979

163. KING EO: The Identification of Unusual Pathogenic Gram-Negative Bacteria. Atlanta, Center for Disease Control, 1964

164. KING EO, WARD MK, RANEY DE: Two simple media for the demonstration of pyocyanin and fluorescein. J Lab Clin Med 44:301–307, 1954

165. KIREDJIAN M, HOLMES B, KERSTERS K, GUILVOUT I, DE LEY J: *Alcaligenes piechaudii*, a new species from human clinical specimens and the environment. Int J Syst Bacteriol 36:282–287, 1986

166. KISH MA, BUGGY BP, FORBES BA: Bacteremia caused by *Achromobacter* species in an immunocompromised host. J Clin Microbiol 19:947–948, 1984

167. KISHIMOTO RA, BROWN GL, BLAIR EB, ET AL: Melioidosis: serologic studies on U.S. army personnel returning from Southeast Asia. Milit Med 136:694–698, 1971

168. KISKA DL, KERR A, JONES MC, CARACCIOLO JA, ESKRIDGE B, JORDAN M, MILLER S, HUGHES D, KING N, GILLIGAN PH: Accuracy of four commercial systems for identification of *Burkholderia cepacia* and other gram-negative nonfermenting bacilli recovered from patients with cystic fibrosis. J Clin Microbiol 34:886–891, 1996

169. KITCH T, JACOBS MR, APPELBAUM PC: Evaluation of the 4-hour RapID NF Plus method for identification of 345 gram-negative non-fermentative rods. J Clin Microbiol 30:1267–1270, 1992

170. KNUTH BD, OWEN MR, LATORRACA R: Occurrence of an unclassified organism group IVd. Am J Med Technol 35:227–232, 1969

171. KODAKA H, ARMFIELD AY, LOMBARD GL, DOWELL VR: Practical procedure for demonstrating bacterial flagella. J Clin Microbiol 16:948–952, 1982

172. KODJO A, TONJUM T, RICHARD Y, BOVRE K: *Moraxella caprae* sp. nov., a new member of the classical moraxellae with very close affinity to *Moraxella bovis*. Int J Syst Bacteriol 45:467–471, 1995

173. KOESTENBLATT EK, LARONE DH, PAVLETICH KJ: Comparison of the Oxi/Ferm and N/F systems for identification of infrequently encountered nonfermentative and oxidase-positive fermentative bacilli. J Clin Microbiol 15:384–390, 1982

174. LACY DE, SPENCER DA, GOLDSTEIN A, WELLER PH, DARBYSHIRE P: Chronic granulomatous disease presenting in childhood with *Pseudomonas cepacia* septicaemia. J Infect 27:301–304, 1993

175. LAMBERT WC, PATHAN AK, IMAEDA T, ET AL: Culture of *Vibrio extorquens* from severe, chronic skin ulcers in a Puerto Rican woman. J Am Acad Dermatol 9:262–268, 1983

176. LAMPE AS, VAN DER REIJDEN TJK: Evaluation of commercial test systems for the identification of nonfermenters. Eur J Clin Microbiol 3:301–305, 1984

177. LAZARUS HM, MAGALHAES-SILVERMAN M, FOX RM, CREGER RJ, JACOBS M: Contamination during in vitro processing of bone marrow for transplantation: clinical significance. Bone Marrow Transplant 7:241–246, 1991

178. LEELARASAMEE A, BOVORNKITTI S: Melioidosis: review and update. Rev Infect Dis 11:413–425, 1989

179. LEIFSON E: Atlas of Bacterial Flagellation. New York, Academic Press, 1960

180. LEWIN LO, BYARD PJ, DAVIS PB: Effect of *Pseudomonas cepacia* colonization on survival and pulmonary function of cystic fibrosis patients. J Clin Epidemiol 43:125–131, 1990

181. LOBUE TD, DEUTSCH TA, STEIN RM: *Moraxella nonliquefaciens* endophthalmitis after trabeculectomy. Am J Ophthalmol 99:343–345, 1985

182. LORTHOLARY O, FAGON J-Y, HOI AB, SLAMA MA, PIERRE J, GIRAL P, ROSENZWEIG R, GUTMANN L, SAFAR M, ACAR J: Nosocomial acquisition of multiresistant *Acinetobacter baumannii*: risk factors and prognosis. Clin Infect Dis 20:790–796, 1995

183. LUCAS KG, KIEHN TE, SOBECK KA, ARMSTRONG D, BROWN AE: Sepsis caused by *Flavimonas oryzihabitans*. Medicine 73:209–214, 1994

184. LYONS RW: Ecology, clinical significance and antimicrobial susceptibility of *Acinetobacter* and *Moraxella*. In Gilardi GL (ed): Nonfermentative Gram-Negative Rods: Laboratory Identification and Clinical Aspects, pp 159–179. New York, Marcel Dekker, 1985

185. MACDONELL MT, COLWELL RR: Phylogeny of the *Vibrionaceae*, and recommendation for two new genera, *Listonella* and *Shewanella*. Syst Appl Microbiol 6:171–182, 1985

186. MACFADDIN JF: Biochemical Tests for Identification of Medical Bacteria, 2nd ed. Baltimore, Williams & Wilkins, 1980

187. MACFARLANE L, OPPENHEIM BA, LORRIGAN P: Septicaemia and septic arthritis due to *Pseudomonas putida* in a neutropenic patient. J Infect 23:346–347, 1991

188. MADHAVAN T: Septic arthritis with *Pseudomonas stutzeri* [letter]. Ann Intern Med 80:670–671, 1974

189. MADHAVAN T, FISHER EJ, COX F, QUINN EL: *Pseudomonas putida* and septic arthritis [letter]. Ann Intern Med 78:971–972, 1973

190. MARNE C, PALLARES R, SITGES–SERRA A: Isolation of *Pseudomonas putrefaciens* in intra-abdominal sepsis. J Clin Microbiol 17:1173–1174, 1983

191. MARRARO RV, MITCHELL JL, PAYET CR: A chromogenic characteristic of an aerobic pseudomonad species in 2% tryptone (indole) broth. J Am Med Technol 39:13–19, 1977

192. MARSHALL WF, KEATING MR, ANHALT JP, STECKELBERG JM: *Xanthomonas maltophilia*: an emerging nosocomial pathogen. Mayo Clin Proc 64:1097–1104, 1989

193. MARTIN R, SIAVOSHI F, MCDOUGAL DL: Comparison of rapid NFT system and conventional methods for identification of nonsaccharolytic gram-negative bacteria. J Clin Microbiol 24:1089–1092, 1986

194. MAY TB, SHINABARGER D, MAHARAJ R, ET AL: Alginate synthesis by *Pseudomonas aeruginosa*: a key pathogenic factor in chronic pulmonary infections of cystic fibrosis patients. Clin Microbiol Rev 4:191–206, 1991

195. MAYFIELD CI, INNIS WE: A rapid, simple method for staining bacterial flagella. Can J Microbiol 23:1311–1313, 1977

196. MCKINLEY KP, LAUNDY TJ, MASTERTON RG: *Achromobacter* group B replacement valve endocarditis. J Infect 20:262–263, 1990

197. MESNARD R, SIRE JM, DONNIO PY, RIOU JY, AVRIL JL: Septic arthritis due to *Oligella urethralis*. Eur J Clin Microbiol Infect Dis 11:195–196, 1992

198. MORRIS MJ, YOUNG VM, MOODY MR: Evaluation of a multitest system for identification of saccharolytic pseudomonads. Am J Clin Pathol 69:41–47, 1978

199. MORRISON AJ, BOYCE K: Peritonitis caused by *Alcaligenes denitrificans* subsp. *xylosoxidans*: Case report and review of the literature. J Clin Microbiol 24:879–881, 1986

200. MORRISON AJ, HOFFMANN KK, WENZEL RP: Associated mortality and clinical characteristics of nosocomial *Pseudomonas maltophilia* in a university hospital. J Clin Microbiol 24:52–55, 1986

201. MORRISON AJ, SHULMAN JA: Community-acquired bloodstream infection caused by *Pseudomonas paucimobilis*: case report and review of literature. J Clin Microbiol 24:853–855, 1986

202. MORRISON RE, LAMB AS, CRAIG DB, ET AL: Melioidosis: a reminder. Am J Med 84:965–967, 1988

203. MOSS CW, DANESHVAR MI, HOLLIS DG: Biochemical characteristics and fatty acid composition of Gilardi Rod Group 1 bacteria. J Clin Microbiol 31:689–691, 1993

204. MOSS CW, KALTENBACH CM: Production of glutaric acid: a useful criterion for differentiating *Pseudomonas diminuta* from *Pseudomonas vesiculare*. Appl Microbiol 27:437–439, 1974

205. MOSS CW, WALLACE PL, HOLLIS DG, ET AL: Cultural and chemical characterization of CDC groups EO-2, M-5, and M-6, *Moraxella (Moraxella)* species, *Oligella urethralis*, *Acinetobacter* species, and *Psychrobacter immobilis*. J Clin Microbiol 26:484–492, 1988

206. MOSS RB: Cystic fibrosis: pathogenesis, pulmonary infection, and treatment. Clin Infect Dis 21:839–851, 1995

207. MUDER RR, HARRIS AP, MULLER S, EDMOND M, CHOW JW, PAPADAKIS K, WAGENER MW, BODEY GP, STECKELBERG JM: Bacteremia due to *Stenotrophomonas (Xanthomonas) maltophilia*: a prospective, multicenter study of 91 episodes. Clin Infect Dis 22:508–512, 1996

208. MUDER RR, YU VL, DUMMER JS, VINSON C, LUMISH RM: Infections caused by *Pseudomonas maltophilia*. Arch Intern Med 147:1672–1674, 1987

209. MUSSO D, DRANCOURT M, BARDOT J, LEGRE R: Human infection due to the CDC group IVc-2 bacterium: case report and review. Clin Infect Dis 18:482–484, 1994

210. NADLER H, GEORGE H, BARR J: Accuracy and reproducibility of the Oxi-Ferm system in identifying a select group of unusual gram-negative bacilli. J Clin Microbiol 9:180–185, 1978

211. NAGAI T: Association of *Pseudomonas maltophilia* with malignant lesions. J Clin Microbiol 20:1003–1005, 1984

212. NAHASS RG, WISNESKI R, HERMAN DJ, HIRSH E, GOLDBLATT K: Vertebral osteomyelitis due to *Roseomonas* species: case report and review of the evaluation of vertebral osteomyelitis. Clin Infect Dis 21:1474–1476, 1995

213. NAWAZ T, HARDY DJ, BONNEZ W: *Neisseria elongata* subsp. *elongata*, a cause of human endocarditis complicated by pseudoaneurysm. J Clin Microbiol 34:756–758, 1996

214. NEU HC, SAHA G, CHIN N-X: Resistance of *Xanthomonas maltophilia* to antibiotics and the effect of beta-lactamase inhibitors. Diagn Microbiol Infect Dis 12:283–285, 1989

215. NORD C–E, WRETLIND B, DAHLBACK A: Evaluation of two test kits—API and Oxi/Ferm tube—for identification of oxidative–fermentative gram-negative rods. Med Microbiol Immunol 163:93–97, 1977

216. OBERHOFER TR: Comparison of the API 20E and Oxi/Ferm systems in identification of nonfermentative and oxidase-positive fermentative bacteria. J Clin Microbiol 9:220–226, 1979

217. OBERHOFER TR: Use of the API 20E, Oxi/Ferm and Minitek systems to identify nonfermentative and oxidasepositive fermentative bacteria: seven years of experience. Diagn Microbiol Infect Dis 1:241–256, 1983

218. OBERHOFER TR: Manual of Nonfermenting Gram-Negative Bacteria. New York, John Wiley & Sons, 1985

219. OBERHOFER TR: Rapid identification of glucose-nonfermenting gram-negative rods with commercial miniaturized kits. In Gilardi GL (ed): Nonfermentative Gram-Negative Rods: Laboratory Identification and Clinical Aspects, pp 85–116. New York, Marcel Dekker, 1985

220. OBERHOFER TR, ROWEN JW, CUNNINGHAM GF: Characterization and identification of gram-negative, nonfermentative bacteria. J Clin Microbiol 5:208–220, 1977

221. OBERHOFER TR, ROWEN JW, CUNNINGHAM GF, HIGBEE JW: Evaluation of the Oxi/Ferm tube system with selected gram-negative bacteria. J Clin Microbiol 6:559–566, 1977

222. O'HARA CM, TENOVER FC, MILLER JM: Parallel comparison of accuracy of API 20E, Vitek GNI, MicroScan Walk/Away Rapid ID, and Becton Dickinson Cobas Micro ID-E/NF for identification of members of the family *Enterobacteriaceae* and common gram-negative, non-glucose-fermenting bacilli. J Clin Microbiol 31:3165–3169, 1993

223. O'LEARY T, FONG IW: Prosthetic valve endocarditis caused by group Ve-1 bacteria. J Clin Microbiol 20:995, 1984

224. O'NEIL KM, HERMAN JH, MODLIN JF, MOXON ER, WINKELSTEIN JA: *Pseudomonas cepacia*: an emerging pathogen in chronic granulomatous disease. J Pediatr 108:940–942, 1986

225. OPHEL K, KERR A: *Agrobacterium vitis* sp. nov. for strains of *Agrobacterium* biovar 3 from grapevines. Int J Syst Bacteriol 40:236–241, 1990

226. OTTO LA, BLACHMAN U: Nonfermentative bacilli: evaluation of three systems for identification. J Clin Microbiol 10:147–154, 1979

227. OTTO LA, DEBOO BS, CAPERS EL, ET AL: *Pseudomonas vesicularis* from cervical specimens. J Clin Microbiol 7:341–345, 1978

228. OTTO LA, PICKETT MJ: Rapid method for identification of gram-negative, nonfermentative bacilli. J Clin Microbiol 3:566–575, 1976

229. PALLENT LJ, HUGO WB, GRANT DJW, ET AL: *Pseudomonas cepacia* as contaminant and infective agent. J Hosp Infect 4:9–13, 1983

230. PALLERONI NJ: Family I. *Pseudomonadaceae*. In Krieg NR, Holt JG (eds): Bergey's Manual of Systematic Bacteriology, vol 1, pp 141–219. Baltimore, Williams & Wilkins, 1984

231. PALLERONI NJ, BRADBURY JF: *Stenotrophomonas*, a new bacterial genus for *Xanthomonas maltophilia* (Hugh 1980) Swings et al. 1983. Int J Syst Bacteriol 43:606–609, 1993

232. PANKUCH GA, JACOBS MR, RITTENHOUSE SF, APPELBAUM PC: Susceptibilities of 123 strains of *Xanthomonas maltophilia* to eight β-lactams (including β-lactam-β-lactamase inhibitor combinations) and ciprofloxacin tested by five methods. Antimicrob Agents Chemother 38:2317–2322, 1994

233. PANLILIO AL, BECK-SAGUE M, SIEGEL JD, ANDERSON RL, YETTS SY, CLARK NC, DUER PN, THOMASSEN KA, VESS RW, HILL BC, TABLAN OC, JARVIS WR: Infections and pseudoinfections due to povidone-iodine solution contaminated with *Pseudomonas cepacia*. Clin Infect Dis 14: 1078–1083, 1992

234. PEDERSEN MM, MARSO E, PICKETT MJ: Nonfermentative bacilli associated with man: III. Pathogenicity and antibiotic susceptibility. Am J Clin Pathol 54:178–192, 1970

235. PEEL MM, HIBBERD AJ, KING BM, ET AL: *Alcaligenes piechaudii* from chronic ear discharge. J Clin Microbiol 26:1580–1581, 1988

236. PEREZ RE: Endocarditis with *Moraxella*-like M-6 after cardiac catheterization. J Clin Microbiol 24:501–502, 1986

237. PFALLER MA, SAHM D, O'HARA C, CIAGLIA C, YU M, YAMANE N, SCHARNWEBER G, RHODEN D: Comparison of the AutoSCAN-W/A rapid bacterial identification system and the Vitek AutoMicrobic system for identification of gram-negative bacilli. J Clin Microbiol 29: 1422–1428, 1991

238. PICKETT MJ: New methodology for identification of nonfermenters: rapid methods. In Gilardi GL (ed): Glucose Nonfermenting Gram-Negative Bacteria in Clinical Microbiology, pp 155–170. West Palm Beach FL, CRC Press, 1978

239. PICKETT MJ: Nonfermentative Gram-Negative Bacilli: A Syllabus for Detection and Identification. Los Angeles, Scientific Development Press, 1980

240. PICKETT MJ, HOLLIS DG, BOTTONE EJ: Miscellaneous gram-negative bacteria. In Balows A (ed): Manual of Clinical Microbiology, 5th ed, pp 410–428. Washington DC, American Society for Microbiology, 1991

241. PICKETT MJ, PEDERSEN MM: Characterization of saccharolytic nonfermentative bacteria associated with man. Can J Microbiol 16:351–362, 1970

242. PICKETT MJ, PEDERSEN MM: Nonfermentative bacilli associated with man: II. Detection and identification. Am J Clin Pathol 54:164–177, 1970

243. PIEN FD, CHUNG EYS: Group Ve infection: case report of group Ve-2 septicemia and literature review. Diagn Microbiol Infect Dis 5:177–180, 1986

244. PLORDE JJ, GATES JA, CARLSON LG, ET AL: Critical evaluation of the AutoMicrobic system gram-negative identification card for identification of glucose-nonfermenting gram-negative rods. J Clin Microbiol 23:251–257, 1986

245. PLOTKIN GR: *Agrobacterium radiobacter* prosthetic valve endocarditis. Ann Intern Med 93:839–840, 1980

246. POPE TL JR, TEAGUE WG JR, KOSSACK R, BRAY ST, FLANNERY DB: *Pseudomonas* sacroiliac osteomyelitis: diagnosis by gallium citrate Ga 67 scan. Am J Dis Child 136: 649–650, 1982

247. POTVLIEGE C, JONCKHEER J, LENCLUD C, HANSEN W: *Pseudomonas stutzeri* pneumonia and septicemia in a patient with multiple myeloma. J Clin Microbiol 25: 458–459, 1987

248. POTVLIEGE C, VANHUYNEGEM L, HANSEN W: Catheter infection caused by an unusual pathogen *Agrobacterium radiobacter*. J Clin Microbiol 27:2120–2122, 1989

249. PUCKETT A, DAVISON G, ENTWISTLE CC, BARBARA JAJ: Post-transfusion septicaemia 1980–1989: importance of donor arm cleansing. J Clin Pathol 45:155–157, 1992

250. RAHAV G, SIMHON A, MATTAN Y, MOSES AE, SACKS T: Infections with *Chryseomonas luteola* (CDC group Ve-1) and *Flavimonas oryzihabitans* (CDC group Ve-2). Medicine 74:83–88, 1995

251. RAMIREZ FC, SAEED ZA, DAROUICHE RO, SHAWAR RM, YOFFE B: *Agrobacterium tumefaciens* peritonitis mimicking tuberculosis. Clin Infect Dis 15:938–940, 1992

252. RAMOS JM, SORIANO F, BERNACER M, ESTEBAN J, ZAPARDIEL J: Infection caused by the nonfermentative gram-negative bacillus CDC group IV c-2: case report and literature review. Eur J Clin Microbiol Infect Dis 12: 456–458, 1993

253. REINA J, BASSA A, LLOMPART I, PORTELA D, BORRELL N: Infections with *Pseudomonas paucimobilis*: report of four cases and review. Rev Infect Dis 13:1072–1076, 1991

254. REVERDY ME, FRENEY J, FLEURETTE J: Nosocomial colonization and infection by *Achromobacter xylosoxidans*. J Clin Microbiol 19:140–143, 1984

255. REYES EAP, BALE MJ, CANNON WH ET AL: Identification of *Pseudomonas aeruginosa* by pyocyanin production in Tech agar. J Clin Microbiol 13:456–458, 1981

256. REYES MP, LERNER AM: Current problems in the treatment of infective endocarditis due to *Pseudomonas aeruginosa*. Rev Infect Dis 5:314, 1983

257. RHOADS S, MARINELLI L, IMPERATRICE CA, NACHAMKIN I: Comparison of MicroScan WalkAway System with Vitek System for identification of gram-negative bacteria. J Clin Microbiol 33:3044–3046, 1995

258. RIHS JD, BRENNER DJ, WEAVER RE, STEIGERWALT AG, HOLLIS DG, YU VL: *Roseomonas*, a new genus associated with bacteremia and other human infections. J Clin Microbiol 31:3275–3283, 1993

259. RINGVOLD A, VIK E, BEVANGER LS: *Moraxella lacunata* isolated from epidemic conjunctivitis among teen-aged females. Acta Ophthalmol 63:427–431, 1985

260. ROBIN T, JANDA MJ: *Pseudo-, Xantho-, Stenotrophomonas maltophilia*: an emerging pathogen in search of a genus. Clin Microbiol Nwslett 18:9–13, 1996

261. ROBINSON A, MCCARTER YS, TETREAULT J: Comparison of Crystal Enteric/Nonfermenter System, API 20E System, and Vitek Automicrobic System for identification of gram-negative bacilli. J Clin Microbiol 33:364–370, 1995

262. ROCKHILL RC, LUTWICK LI: Group IVe-like gram-negative bacillemia in a patient with obstructive uropathy. J Clin Microbiol 8:108–109, 1978

263. RODBY RA, GLICK E: *Agrobacterium radiobacter* peritonitis in two patients maintained on chronic peritoneal dialysis. Am J Kidney Dis 18:402–405, 1991

264. ROIG P, ORTI A, NAVARRO V: Meningitis due to *Pseudomonas stutzeri* in a patient infected with human immunodeficiency virus. Clin Infect Dis 22:587–588, 1996

265. ROILIDES E, MUELLER BU, LETTERIO JJ, BUTLER K, PIZZO PA: *Agrobacterium radiobacter* bacteremia in a child with human immunodeficiency virus infection. Pediatr Infect Dis J 10:337–338, 1991

266. ROMANYK J, GONZALEZ-PALACIOS R, NIETO A: A new case of bacteraemia due to *Flavimonas oryzihabitans*. J Hosp Infect 29:236–237, 1995

267. ROMEO J: A dichotomous key for the identification of miscellaneous gram-negative bacteria. Lab Med 10: 547–558, 1979

268. ROSENBERG I, LEIBOVICI L, MOR F, BLOCK C, WYSENBEEK AJ: *Pseudomonas stutzeri* causing late prosthetic valve endocarditis. J R Soc Med 80:457–459, 1987

269. ROSENTHAL SL: Clinical role of *Acinetobacter* and *Moraxella*. In Gilardi GL (ed): Glucose Nonfermenting Gram-Negative Bacteria in Clinical Microbiology, pp 105–117. West Palm Beach FL, CRC Press, 1978

270. ROSENTHAL SL, FREUDLICH LF, WASHINGTON W: Laboratory evaluation of a multitest system for identification of gram-negative organisms. Am J Clin Pathol 70:914–917, 1978

271. ROSS JP, HOLLAND SM, GILL VJ, DECARLO ES, GALLIN JI: Severe *Burkholderia (Pseudomonas) gladioli* infection in chronic granulomatous disease: report of two successfully treated cases. Clin Infect Dis 21:1291–1293, 1995

272. ROSSAU R, KERSTERS K, FALSEN E, JANTZEN E, SEGERS P, UNION A, NEHLS L, DE LEY J: *Oligella*, a new genus including *Oligella urethralis* comb. nov. (formerly *Moraxella urethralis*) and *Oligella ureolytica* sp. nov. (formerly CDC group IVe): relationship to *Taylorella equigenitalis* and related taxa. Int J Syst Bacteriol 37:198–210, 1987

273. ROSSELLO R, GARCIA-VALDES E, LALUCAT J, URSING J: Genotypic and phenotypic diversity of *Pseudomonas stutzeri*. Syst Appl Microbiol 14:150–157, 1991

274. RUTHERFORD PC, NARKOWICZ JE, WOOD CJ, ET AL: Peritonitis caused by *Pseudomonas mesophilica* in a patient undergoing continuous ambulatory peritoneal dialysis. J Clin Microbiol 26:2441–2443, 1988

275. RYU E: A simple method of staining bacterial flagella. Kitasato Arch Exp Med 14:218–219, 1937

276. SALAZAR R, MARTINO R, SUREDA A, BRUNET S, SUBIRA M, DOMINGO-ALBOS A: Catheter-related bacteremia due to *Pseudomonas paucimobilis* in neutropenic cancer patients: report of two cases [letter]. Clin Infect Dis 20:1573–1574, 1995

277. SALTISSI D, MACFARLANE DJ: Successful treatment of *Pseudomonas paucimobilis* haemodialysis catheter-related sepsis without catheter removal. Postgrad Med J 70:47–48, 1994

278. SAWADA H, IEKI J, OYAIZU H, MATSUMOTO S: Proposal for rejection of *Agrobacterium tumefaciens* and revised descriptions for the genus *Agrobacterium* and for *Agrobacterium radiobacter* and *Agrobacterium rhizogenes*. Int J Syst Bacteriol 43:694–702, 1993

279. SCHLECH WF, TURCHIK JB, WESTLAKE RE, ET AL: Laboratory-acquired infection with *Pseudomonas pseudomallei* (melioidosis). N Engl J Med 305:1133–1135, 1981

280. SCHRECKENBERGER PC: Practical Approach to the Identification of Glucose-Nonfermenting Gram-Negative Bacilli. A Guide to Identification. Denver, Colorado Association for Continuing Medical Laboratory Education, Inc., 1996

281. SCHRECKENBERGER PC, ANDERSON RR, PIERSON C, DEBUSSCHER J, BROWN W: Comparison of four commercial identificatioin systems for the identification of non-fastidious, non-fermenting, gram-negative bacilli. Manuscript in preparation

282. SCOTT J, BOULTON FE, GOVAN JRW, MILES RS, MCCLELLAND DBL, PROWSE CV: A fatal transfusion reaction associated with blood contaminated with *Pseudomonas fluorescens*. Vox Sang 54:201–204, 1988

283. SEGERS P, VANCANNEYT M, POT B, TORCK U, HOSTE B, DEWETTINCK D, FALSEN E, KERSTERS K, DE VOS P: Classification of *Pseudomonas diminuta* Leifson and Hugh 1954 and *Pseudomonas vesicularis* Busing, Doll, and Freytag 1953 in *Brevundimonas* gen. nov. as *Brevundimonas diminuta* comb. nov. and *Brevundimonas vesicularis* comb. nov., respectively. Int J Syst Bacteriol 44:499–510, 1994

284. SEIFERT H, BAGINSKI R, SCHULZE A, PULVERER G: Antimicrobial susceptibility of *Acinetobacter* species. Antimicrob Agents Chemother 37:750–753, 1993

285. SHAYEGANI M, LEE AM, MCGLYNN DM: Evaluation of the Oxi/Ferm tube system for identification of nonfermentative gram-negative bacilli. J Clin Microbiol 7:533–538, 1978

286. SHAYEGANI M, MAUPIN PS, MCGLYNN DM: Evaluation of the API 20E system for identification of nonfermentative gram-negative bacteria. J Clin Microbiol 7:539–545, 1978

287. SHAYEGANI M, MAUPIN PS, PARSONS LM, ET AL: Evaluation of the N/F system for identification of nonfermentative gram-negative bacilli using a reference laboratory population. Lab Med 12:177–182, 1981

288. SHEWAN JM: Taxonomy and ecology of *Flavobacterium* and related genera. Annu Rev Microbiol 37:233–252, 1983

289. SHIVAJI S, RAY MK, RAO NS, SAISREE L, JAGANNADHAM MV, KUMAR GS, REDDY GSN, BHARGAVA PM: *Sphingobacterium antarcticus* sp. nov., a psychrotrophic bacterium from the soils of Schirmacher Oasis, Antarctica. Int J Syst Bacteriol 42:102–106, 1992

290. SIEGMAN-IGRA Y, BAR-YOSEF S, GOREA A, AVRAM J: Nosocomial *Acinetobacter* meningitis secondary to invasive procedures: report of 25 cases and review. Clin Infect Dis 17:843–849, 1993

291. SIMMONDS EJ, CONWAY SP, GHONEIM ATM, ROSS H, LITTLEWOOD JM: *Pseudomonas cepacia*: a new pathogen in patients with cystic fibrosis referred to a large centre in the United Kingdom. Arch Dis Child 65:874–877, 1990

292. SIMOR AE, SALIT IE: Endocarditis caused by M6. J Clin Microbiol 931–933, 1983

293. SMITH SM, CUNDY KR, GILARDI GL, ET AL: Evaluation of the AutoMicrobic system for identification of glucose-nonfermenting gram-negative rods. J Clin Microbiol 15:302–307, 1982

294. SMITH SM, ENG RHK, FORRESTER C: *Pseudomonas mesophilica* infections in humans. J Clin Microbiol 21:314–317, 1985

295. SOBEL JD, HASHMAN N, REINHERZ G, ET AL: Nosocomial *Pseudomonas cepacia* infection associated with chlorhexidine contamination. Am J Med 73:183–186, 1982

296. SONNENWIRTH AC: Bacteremia with and without meningitis due to *Yersinia enterocolitica*, *Edwardsiella tarda*, *Comamonas terrigena*, and *Pseudomonas maltophilia*. Ann NY Acad Sci 174:488–502, 1970

297. SPEAR JB, FUHRER J, KIRBY BD: *Achromobacter xylosoxidans* (*Alcaligenes xylosoxidans* subsp. *xylosoxidans*) bacteremia associated with a well-water source: case report and review of the literature. J Clin Microbiol 26:598–599, 1988

298. SPOTNITZ M, RUDNITZKY J, RAMBAUD JJ: Melioidosis pneumonitis. JAMA 202:950–954, 1967

299. STANECK JL, WECKBACH LS, TILTON RC, ZABRANSKY RJ, BAYOLA-MUELLER L, O'HARA CM, MILLER JM: Collaborative evaluation of the Radiometer Sensititre AP80 for

identification of gram-negative bacilli. J Clin Microbiol 31:1179–1184, 1993

300. SUGARMAN B, CLARRIDGE J: Osteomyelitis caused by *Moraxella osloensis.* J Clin Microbiol 15:1148–1149, 1982

301. TABOR E, GERETY RJ: Five cases of pseudomonas sepsis transmitted by blood transfusions. Lancet i:1403, 1984

302. TAKEUCHI M, KAWAI F, SHIMADA Y, YOKOTA A: Taxonomic study of polyethylene glycol-utilizing bacteria: emended description of the genus *Sphingomonas* and new descriptions of *Sphingomonas macrogoltabidus* sp. nov., *Sphingomonas sanguis* sp. nov. and *Sphingomonas terrae* sp. nov. Syst Appl Microbiol 16:227–238, 1993

303. TAKEUCHI M, SAKANE T, YANAGI M, YAMASATO K, HAMANA K, YOKOTA A: Taxonomic study of bacteria isolated from plants: proposal of *Sphingomonas rosa* sp. nov., *Sphingomonas pruni* sp. nov., *Sphingomonas asaccharolytica* sp. nov., and *Sphingomonas mali* sp. nov. Int J Syst Bacteriol 45:334–341, 1995

304. TAKEUCHI M, YOKOTA A: Proposals of *Sphingobacterium faecium* sp. nov., *Sphingobacterium piscium* sp. nov., *Sphingobacterium heparinum* comb. nov., *Sphingobacterium thalpophilum* comb. nov. and two genospecies of the genus *Sphingobacterium*, and synonymy of *Flavobacterium yabuuchiae* and *Sphingobacterium spiritivorum.* J Gen Appl Microbiol 38:465–482, 1992

305. TAMAOKA J, HA D-M, KOMAGATA K: Reclassification of *Pseudomonas acidovorans* den Dooren de Jong 1926 and *Pseudomonas testosteroni* Marcus and Talalay 1956 as *Comamonas acidovorans* comb. nov. and *Comamonas testosteroni* comb. nov., with an emended description of the genus *Comamonas.* Int J Syst Bacteriol 37:52–59, 1987

306. TAPLAN D, BASSETT DCJ, MERTZ PM: Foot lesions associated with *Pseudomonas cepacia.* Lancet 2:568–571, 1971

307. TAYLOR M, KEANE CT, FALKINER FR: *Pseudomonas putida* in transfused blood. Lancet 2:107, 1984

308. TENOVER FC, MIZUKI TS, CARLSON LG: Evaluation of autoSCAN-W/A automated microbiology system for the identification of non-glucose-fermenting gram-negative bacilli. J Clin Microbiol 28:1628–1634, 1990

309. THIMANN KV: The Life of Bacteria: Their Growth, Metabolism and Relationships, 2nd ed. New York, Macmillan, 1963

310. TJERNBERG I, URSING J: Clinical strains of *Acinetobacter* classified by DNA–DNA hybridization. APMIS 97:595–605, 1989

311. TONJUM T, CAUGANT DA, BOVRE K: Differentiation of *Moraxella nonliquefaciens, M. lacunata,* and *M. bovis* by using multilocus enzyme electrophoresis and hybridization with pilin-specific DNA probes. J Clin Microbiol 30:3099–3107, 1992

312. URAKAMI T, ARAKI H, SUZUKI K-I, KOMAGATA K: Further studies of the genus *Methylobacterium* and description of *Methylobacterium aminovorans* sp. nov. Int J Syst Bacteriol 43:504–513, 1993

313. VALENSTEIN P, BARDY GH, COX CC, ZWADYK P: *Pseudomonas alcaligenes* endocarditis. Am J Clin Pathol 79:245–247, 1983

314. VANDAMME P, BERNARDET J-F, SEGERS P, KERSTERS K, HOLMES B: New perspectives in the classification of the flavobacteria: description of *Chryseobacterium* gen. nov., *Bergeyella* gen. nov., and *Empedobacter* nom. rev. Int J Syst Bacteriol 44:827–831, 1994

315. VANDAMME P, GILLIS M, VANCANNEYT M, HOSTE B, KERSTERS K, FALSEN E: *Moraxella lincolnii* sp. nov., isolated from the human respiratory tract, and reevaluation of the taxonomic position of *Moraxella osloensis.* Int J Syst Bacteriol 43:474–481, 1993

316. VANDAMME P, HOMMEZ J, VANCANNEYT M, MONSIEURS M, HOSTE B, COOKSON B, WIRSING VON KONIG CH, KERSTERS K, BLACKALL PJ: *Bordetella hinzii* sp. nov., isolated from poultry and humans. Int J Syst Bacteriol 45:37–45, 1995

317. VAN HORN KG, GEDRIS CA, AHMED T, WORMSER GP: Bacteremia and urinary tract infection associated with CDC group Vd biovar 2. J Clin Microbiol 27:201–202, 1989

318. VARTIVARIAN S, ANAISSIE E, BODEY G, SPRIGG H, ROLSTON K: A changing pattern of susceptibility of *Xanthomonas maltophilia* to antimicrobial agents: implications for therapy. Antimicrob Agents Chemother 38:624–627, 1994

319. VARTIVARIAN SE, PAPADAKIS KA, PALACIOS JA, MANNING JT, ANAISSIE EJ: Mucocutaneous and soft tissue infections caused by *Xanthomonas maltophilia.* A new spectrum. Ann Intern Med 121:969–973, 1994

320. VERHASSELT B, CLAEYS G, ELAICHOUNI A, VERSCHRAEGEN G, LAUREYS G, VANEECHOUTTE M: Case of recurrent *Flavimonas oryzihabitans* bacteremia associated with an implanted central venous catheter (Port-A-Cath): assessment of clonality by arbitrarily primed PCR. J Clin Microbiol 33:3047–3048, 1995

321. VON GRAEVENITZ A: Clinical role of infrequently encountered nonfermenters. In Gilardi GL (ed): Glucose Nonfermenting Gram-Negative Bacteria in Clinical Microbiology, pp 119–153. West Palm Beach FL, CRC Press, 1978

322. VON GRAEVENITZ A: Ecology, clinical significance, and antimicrobial susceptibility of infrequently encountered glucose-nonfermenting gram-negative rods. In Gilardi GL (ed): Nonfermentative Gram-Negative Rods: Laboratory Identification and Clinical Aspects, pp 181–232. New York, Marcel Dekker, 1985

323. VON GRAEVENITZ A, SIMON G: Potentially pathogenic, nonfermentative, H₂S-producing gram-negative rod (1b). Appl Microbiol 19:176, 1970

324. VON GRAEVENITZ A, ZOLLINGER–ITEN J: Evaluation of pertinent parameters of a new identification system for non-enteric gram-negative rods. Eur J Clin Microbiol 4:108–112, 1985

325. WARWOOD NM, BLAZEVIC DJ, HOFHERR L: Comparison of the API 20E and Corning N/F systems for identification of nonfermentative gram-negative rods. J Clin Microbiol 10:175–179, 1979

326. WATSON KC, MUSCAT I: Meningitis caused by a *Flavobacterium*-like organism (CDC IIe strain). J Infect 7:278–279, 1983

327. WAUTERS G, BOEL A, VOORN GP, VERHAEGEN J, MEUNIER F, JANSSENS M, VERBIST L: Evaluation of a new identification system, Crystal Enteric/Non-Fermenter, for gram-negative bacilli. J Clin Microbiol 33:845–849, 1995

328. WEAVER RE, HOLLIS DG: Gram-Negative Organisms: An Approach to Identification. Atlanta, U.S. Department of Health and Human Services, Centers for Disease Control, 1985

329. WERTHEIM WA, MARKOVITZ DM: Osteomyelitis and intervertebral discitis caused by *Pseudomonas pickettii.* J Clin Microbiol 30:2506–2508, 1992

330. WEYANT RS, HOLLIS DG, WEAVER RE, AMIN MFM, STEIGERWALT AG, O'CONNOR SP, WHITNEY AM, DANESHVAR MI, MOSS CW, BRENNER DJ: *Bordetella holmesii* sp. nov., a new gram-negative species associated with septicemia. J Clin Microbiol 33:1–7, 1995

331. WILLEMS A, DE LEY J, GILLIS M, KERSTERS K: *Comamonadaceae,* a new family encompassing the acidovorans rRNA complex, including *Variovorax paradoxus* gen. nov., comb. nov., for *Alcaligenes paradoxus* (Davis 1969). Int J Syst Bacteriol 41:445–450, 1991

332. WILLEMS A, FALSEN E, POT B, et al: *Acidovorax,* a new genus for *Pseudomonas facilis, Pseudomonas delafieldii,* E. Falsen (EF) Group 13, EF Group 16, and several clinical isolates, with the species *Acidovorax facilis* comb. nov., *Acidovorax delafieldii* comb. nov., and *Acidovorax temperans* sp. nov. Int J Syst Bacteriol 40:384–398, 1990

333. WILSON APR, RIDGWAY GL, RYAN KE, PATTERSON KP: Unusual pathogens in neutropenic patients. J Hosp Infect 11:398–400, 1988

334. WONG JD, JANDA JM: Association of an important *Neisseria* species, *Neisseria elongata* subsp. *nitroreducens,* with bacteremia, endocarditis, and osteomyelitis. J Clin Microbiol 30:719–720, 1992

335. WOODARD DR, CONE LA, FOSTVEDT K: *Bordetella bronchiseptica* infection in patients with AIDS. Clin Infect Dis 20:193–194, 1995

336. WOOLFREY BF, MOODY JA: Human infection associated with *Bordetella bronchiseptica.* Clin Microbiol Rev 4:243–255, 1991

337. WUTHIEKANUN V, DANCE D, CHAOWAGUL W, ET AL: Blood culture techniques for the diagnosis of melioidosis. Eur J Clin Microbiol 9:654–658, 1990

338. YABUUCHI E, KANEKO T, YANO I, ET AL: *Sphingobacterium* gen. nov., *Sphingobacterium spiritivorum* comb. nov., *Sphingobacterium multivorum* comb. nov., *Sphingobacterium mizutae* sp. nov., and *Flavobacterium indologenes* sp. nov.: glucose-nonfermenting gram-negative rods in CDC groups IIk-2 and IIb. Int J Syst Bacteriol 33:580–598, 1983

339. YABUUCHI E, KOSAKO Y, OYAIZU H, YANO I, HOTTA H, HASHIMOTO Y, EZAKI T, ARAKAWA M: Proposal of *Burkholderia* gen. nov. and transfer of seven species of the genus *Pseudomonas* homology group II to the new genus, with the type species *Burkholderia cepacia* (Palleroni and Holmes 1981) comb. nov. Microbiol Immunol 36:1251–1275, 1992

340. YABUUCHI E, YANO I, OYAIZU H, HASHIMOTO Y, EZAKI T, YAMANOTO H: Proposals of *Sphingomonas paucimobilis* gen. nov. and comb. nov., *Sphingomonas parapaucimobilis* sp. nov., *Sphingomonas yanoikuyae* sp. nov., *Sphingomonas adhaesiva* sp. nov., *Sphingomonas capsulata* comb. nov., and two genospecies of the genus *Sphingomonas.* Microbiol Immunol 34:99–119, 1990

341. YAO JDC, LOUIE M, LOUIE L, GOODFELLOW J, SIMOR AE: Comparison of E test and agar dilution for antimicrobial susceptibility testing of *Stenotrophomonas (Xanthomonas) maltophilia.* J Clin Microbiol 33:1428–1430, 1995

342. ZAPARDIEL J, BLUM G, CARAMELO C, FERNANDEZ-ROBLAS R, RODRIGUEZ-TUDELA JL, SORIANO F: Peritonitis with CDC group IV c-2 bacteria in a patient on continuous ambulatory peritoneal dialysis. Eur J Clin Microbiol Infect Dis 10:509–511, 1991

343. ZURAVLEFF JJ, YU VL: Infections caused by *Pseudomonas maltophilia* with emphasis on bacteremia: case reports and a review of the literature. Rev Infect Dis 4:1236–1246, 1982

CURVED GRAM-NEGATIVE BACILLI AND OXIDASE-POSITIVE FERMENTERS: CAMPYLOBACTERACEAE AND VIBRIONACEAE

The expanded genera of gram-negative bacilli to be discussed in this chapter are as follows:

Curved and Straight, Microaerophilic and Capnophilic Gram-Negative Bacilli
Campylobacter species
[*Bacteroides*] *ureolyticus**
Arcobacter species
Helicobacter species
Wolinella succinogenes
"*Flexispira rappini*"†
"*Gastrospirillum hominis*"
Sutterella wadsworthensis
Oxidase-Positive Fermenters
Vibrio species
Aeromonas species
Plesiomonas species
Listonella species
Shewanella species
Chromobacterium violaceum

PART I: CURVED RODS: *CAMPYLOBACTER, HELICOBACTER, WOLINELLA, ARCOBACTER* AND RELATED BACTERIA

HISTORICAL BACKGROUND

The microorganism presently classified as *Campylobacter jejuni* was discovered in 1931 by Jones and coworkers[137] as the causative agent of winter dysentery in cattle. Twenty-six years lapsed before King described a group of microaerophilic, motile curved rods isolated from the blood of children with acute dysentery, which she designated "related vibrios" because they were similar in many respects to *Vibrio fetus*.[153] King astutely mentioned that the vibrios isolated from the blood of children might be closely related to the organism described as *V. jejuni* by Jones in 1931 and that the organism might be more important as a cause of childhood diarrheal syndromes of unknown etiology than previously realized.

This was a prophetic statement; nevertheless, another 15 years passed before this association was substantiated in the laboratory. In 1972, Dekeyser and colleagues[61] isolated the "related vibrios" from the feces of patients with acute enteritis using a filtration technique that allowed the small, curved rods to pass through the membrane but retained larger fecal mi-

Color Plates for Chapter 6 are found between pages 80 and 81.
*Brackets indicate generically misnamed species.
†Organism names appearing in quotations have not been validly published and therefore do not have any official taxonomic standing.

croorganisms. Several other reports followed, linking related vibrios (*V. fetus,* subsp. *jejuni; C. jejuni*) with gastroenteritis in humans, with a distribution throughout the world.[20,21,143] This relative incidence has since been the experience in most clinical laboratories, although during the past 3 or 4 years, the rates of recovery have declined to some degree.

The history of the discovery of *Helicobacter pylori* (formerly named *Campylobacter pyloridis* and then *C. pylori*) is even more circuitous. Warren and Marshall are credited with the "discovery" of the organism in Perth, Australia, in 1982[285]; however, many previous descriptions of spiral organisms in biopsy specimens of human gastric mucosa have appeared in the literature dating back to the beginning of this century.[90,159] Only after successful cultivation of this bacterium using the unique "*Campylobacter* atmosphere" has serious attention been paid to this organism, which may be the most common cause of human gastrointestinal infection as well as the most frequent cause of gastritis.[224]

CLASSIFICATION OF *CAMPYLOBACTER* AND RELATED TAXA

Vandamme and associates,[273,276] using a variety of molecular techniques including DNA-rRNA hybridization, 16S ribosomal RNA (rRNA) sequence analysis, and immunotyping analysis, have determined that all of the named *Campylobacter* species and related taxa belong to the same phylogenetic group, which they named rRNA superfamily VI. Currently, five genera, including *Campylobacter, Arcobacter, Helicobacter, Wolinella,* and "*Flexispira*" are included in rRNA superfamily VI. Characteristics that differentiate between these related genera are listed in Table 6-1. Solnick and colleagues have also described two uncultivable human gastric spiral organisms, "*Gastrospirillum hominis*" 1 and 2, that they have identified as helicobacters by 16S rRNA analysis.[250]

Further studies have shown that bacterial species included in rRNA superfamily VI can be separated into three distinct rRNA clusters (Box 6-1).

Thompson and coworkers[269] studied the phylogenetic relationships of all species in the genera *Campylobacter* and *Wolinella* and other gram-negative bacteria by comparison of the partial 16S rRNA sequences. Their results indicated that species recognized to be in the genus *Campylobacter* made up three separate rRNA homology groups representing separate genera of organisms. They reported that only those organisms comprising rRNA group I (*C. fetus, C. coli, C. jejuni, C. lari, C. hyointestinalis, C. concisus, C. mucosalis, C. sputorum,* and *C. upsaliensis*) were the true campylobacters. Paster and Dewhirst[218] found a close relationship between *Wolinella curva, Wolinella recta, Bacteroides gracilis, Bacteroides ureolyticus* and the true campylobacters that made up the rRNA homology group I of Thompson and suggested that all members of the campylobacter cluster should be placed in the genus *Campylobacter*.

TABLE 6-1

CHARACTERISTICS FOR DIFFERENTIATING *ARCOBACTER*, *CAMPYLOBACTER*, *WOLINELLA*, *HELICOBACTER*, AND "*FLEXISPIRA*"

GENUS	NITRATE REDUCTION	GROWTH ON 0.5% GLYCINE	HYDROLYSIS OF UREA	GROWTH AT			CELL MORPHOLOGY	FLAGELLAR SHEATHS
				15°C	30°C	42°C		
Arcobacter	+	NA	V	+	+	−	Curved and spiral rods	Absent
Campylobacter	+	V	−	−	+	V	Curved and spiral rods	Absent
Wolinella	+	−	−	−	−	W	Spiral	Absent
Helicobacter	V	+	V	−	V	V	Curved and spiral rods	Present
"*Flexispira*"	−	+	+	−	−	+	Straight fusiform rods	Present
"*Gastrospirillum*"	NA	NA	NA	NA	NA	NA	Spiral	Present

+, 90% or more of strains are positive; −, 90% or more of strains are negative; V, 11%–89% of strains are positive; W, weak reaction; NA, results not available.
Modified from Vandamme P, Falsen E, Rossau R, et al: Revision of *Campylobacter*, *Helicobacter*, and *Wolinella* taxonomy: Emendation of generic descriptions and proposal of *Arcobacter* gen. nov. Int J Syst Bacteriol 41:88–103, 1991

Vandamme and colleagues[276] confirmed the findings of Thompson and coworkers[269] and Paster and Dewhirst[218] and proposed an amended description of the genus *Campylobacter* to include all organisms placed in homology group I and the transfer of *W. curva* and *W. recta* to the genus *Campylobacter* as *C. curvus* and *C. rectus*, respectively. Most recently, Vandamme and coworkers[272] proposed the reclassification of *B. gracilis* as *Campylobacter gracilis*. However, while [*B. ureolyticus*] is considered a member of the family *Campylobacteraceae*, it has not as yet been renamed and remains a species *incertae sedis* pending the isolation and characterization of additional *B. ureolyticus*-like bacteria.

The rRNA cluster II contains a homogeneous group that includes organisms for which Vandamme and associates[276] have proposed the new genus designation of *Arcobacter*. Currently included in rRNA cluster II are *Arcobacter nitrofigilis* (formerly *Campylobacter nitrogifilis*), *Arcobacter cryaerophilus* (formerly *Campylobacter cryaerophila*), *Arcobacter* (*Campylobacter*) *butzleri*, and *Arcobacter skirrowii*.[151,278]

rRNA cluster III contains members of three different genera: *Helicobacter*, *Wolinella*, "*Flexispira*," and an unnamed species, CLO-3. Vandamme and associates have emended the description of the genus *Helicobacter* and proposed the transfer of *Campylobacter cinaedi* and *C. fennelliae* to the genus *Helicobacter* as *H. cinaedi* and *H. fennelliae*, respectively.[276] *Wolinella succinogenes* remains as the only species of the genus *Wolinella*.

BOX 6-1. SUPERFAMILY VI RRNA CLUSTERS

rRNA group I—Contains the true *Campylobacter* species: *C. fetus* (type species), *C. coli*, *C. concisus*, *C. curvus*, *C. gracilis*, *C. helveticus*, *C. hyoilei*, *C. hyointestinalis*, *C. jejuni*, *C. lari*, *C. mucosalis*, *C. rectus*, *C. showae*, *C. sputorum*, *C. upsaliensis*, and the generically misnamed species [*Bacteroides ureolyticus*].

rRNA group II—Contains the *Arcobacter* species: *A. butzleri*, *A. cryaerophilus*, *A. nitrofigilis*, and *A. skirrowii*.

rRNA group III—Contains the *Helicobacter*: *H. pylori* (type species), *H. acinonyx*, *H. bilis*, *H. bizzozeronii*, *H. canis*, *H. cinaedi*, *H. felis*, *H. fennelliae*, *H. hepaticus*, *H. muridarum*, *H. mustelae*, *H. nemestrinae*, *H. pametensis*, *H. pullorum*, *Helicobacter* species strains *Mainz*; the unnamed species CLO-3; organisms previously identified as "*Flexispira rappini*," "*Gastrospirillum hominis*," and *Wolinella succinogenes*.

RRNA GROUP I (TRUE *CAMPYLOBACTER* SPECIES)

Campylobacter species are microaerophilic (require decreased O_2) and capnophilic (require increased CO_2), curved spiral bacteria, motile by means of a single unsheathed polar flagellum. These organisms are nonfermentative and nonoxidative in their metabolism, deriving energy from the use of amino acids and four- and six-carbon Krebs' cycle intermediates. These organisms used to be classified with *Vibrio* species, until DNA homology studies showed that they were unrelated to the vibrios. Even among the currently recognized *Campylobacter* species, much genotypic and phenotypic diversity exists. The organisms inhabit a wide variety of ecologic niches and environments. Most species are found in animals (cattle, swine) and cause infertility and abortion.

Before presenting the several *Campylobacter* species included in rRNA Group I, a discussion of the clinical and laboratory aspects of *C. jejuni* subsp. *jejuni*, the species most commonly recovered in clinical laboratories, is presented.

Clinical Significance. *C. jejuni* subsp. *jejuni* is the most important human pathogen among the campylobacters. It has worldwide distribution, being recovered from 4% to 35% of fecal specimens of patients with acute diarrheal disease.[22] It is also ubiquitous in domestic animals—house pets may carry the organism, and the vast majority of chickens, turkeys, and waterfowl are colonized.[102] Ingestion of raw milk,[280] partially cooked poultry,[102] or contaminated water[40] are the common sources for human infections. Enteritis with this organism is characterized by crampy abdominal pain, bloody diarrhea, chills, and fever. For most persons, the infection is self-limited and resolves in 3 to 7 days. The organism may continue to be excreted by convalescing patients for 2 weeks to 1 month. In cases of severe disease, the patient may be treated with oral erythromycin.

Although enteritis and diarrheal syndromes remain the most common manifestations of *Campylobacter* infections, other diseases have emerged during the past few years. Cases of septic arthritis, meningitis, and proctocolitis secondary to *C. jejuni* have been reported.[229] There have now been several reports that associate *C. jejuni* infection with Guillain-Barré syndrome (GBS), an acute demyelinating disease of the peripheral nerves.[160,236,251] Data from both serologic and culture studies show that between 20–40% of patients with GBS are infected with *C. jejuni* one to three weeks prior to the onset of neurological symptoms.[8] There is no relation between the severity of gastrointestinal symptoms and the likelihood of developing GBS after infection with *C. jejuni*; and in fact, even asymptomatic infections may trigger GBS.[8] In the United States and Japan, 30–80% of *C. jejuni* isolates from patients with GBS belong to Penner serotype 0:19.[8,92] A review of the epidemiology, pathogenesis, and clinical features of *C. jejuni* infection has been written by Allos and Blaser.[8]

Presumptive Identification From Stool. It may be possible to make a presumptive diagnosis of *Campylobacter* enteritis by observing characteristic gram-negative, curved, S-shaped, gull-winged, or long spiral forms in Gram-stained preparations of diarrheal stools (see Color Plate 6-1*A*). In some laboratories it is common practice to initially examine wet mounts or stained smears of all diarrheal stool specimens for polymorphonuclear leukocytes and the presence of bacterial forms suggestive of *Campylobacter* species. Stool specimens for *Campylobacter* species are not further processed in some laboratories unless polymorphonuclear leukocytes are present. The rationale for this practice is that it is unlikely that *Campylobacter* species will be recovered in clinically significant numbers in stool specimens devoid of leukocytes. The expenditure of time and use of special culture media for specimens in which there is little chance to recover significant microbes is not considered cost effective.

Methods for Laboratory Isolation. Successful isolation of *C. jejuni* from stool depends on the use of selective media (*eg.,* Campy-Thio, Campy-BAP), incubation at an elevated temperature (42°C), and the proper incubation atmosphere (5% oxygen, 10% CO_2, 85% nitrogen). A membrane filtration technique that is used with nonselective blood agar plates has been reported to be as effective as the use of antibiotic media for the isolation of *C. jejuni*.[256] This method has the advantage of allowing the isolation of antibiotic-sensitive campylobacters. For the past 2 decades, the selective culture media and special incubation conditions necessary to recover *Campylobacter* species have been used in most clinical microbiology laboratories. Indeed, in many practice settings, the rate of recovery of *Campylobacter* species exceeded the combined recovery of the time-honored enteric pathogens *Salmonella* species and *Shigella* species. For example, in a 1980 collaborative eight-hospital study in the United States, the overall isolation of *C. jejuni* from fecal specimens was greater than for *Salmonella* species and *Shigella* species combined (Table 6-2).[205]

Various procedures can be used to provide a suitable gaseous atmosphere for cultivating microaerophilic campylobacters. These include evacuation-replacement procedures, disposable gas generators, and the use of the Fortner principle. Two of these procedures, which have been used successfully by various investigators, are outlined in Table 6-3. The use of a CO^2 incubator is not recommended for cultivating campylobacters because only strains that are very aerotolerant grow in the atmosphere provided. Likewise, various investigators have emphasized that a candle extinction jar is also not recommended because the oxygen level (12% to 17%) is too high for optimal growth of campylobacters.[177,284]

Several selective media have been developed to allow for the isolation of *C. jejuni* from fecal samples. Merino and colleagues[189] evaluated the efficacy of seven selective *Campylobacter* isolation media. The names of these media, their composition, and a summary of the evaluation of each are included in Table 6-4. Butzler selective medium, Blaser medium (Campy-BAP), and Skirrow blood agar have been used in most clinical laboratories. However, Merino and colleagues[189] found that Preston *Campylobacter* blood-free medium with cefoperazone yielded the greatest number of *C. jejuni* isolations. Karmali and colleagues[144] found that a blood-free, charcoal-based selective medium (CSM), consisting of Columbia agar base, activated charcoal, hematin, sodium pyruvate, cefoperazone, vancomycin, and cycloheximide, is more selective than Skirrow's medium and has a higher isolation rate of *C. jejuni* from mixed cultures. Charcoal, hematin, ferrous sulfate, and sodium pyruvate serve as substitutes for blood in growth media for campylobacters. Casein is added to help grow certain strains of nalidixic acid-resistant thermophilic campylobacters that are environmental organisms.

Endtz and colleagues[70] compared a semisolid blood-free selective motility medium[100] with two blood-free CSM, two blood-based media (Skirrow medium and Blaser's Campy-BAP), and the membrane filter technique. They found that CSM was the

TABLE 6-2

RATE OF ISOLATION OF *CAMPYLOBACTER, SALMONELLA,* AND *SHIGELLA* FROM FECAL SPECIMENS BY HOSPITAL IN AN EIGHT-HOSPITAL STUDY CONDUCTED IN THE UNITED STATES, JANUARY–OCTOBER 1980

LOCATION OF HOSPITAL	NUMBER OF SPECIMENS EXAMINED	PERCENTAGE WITH		
		CAMPYLOBACTER	*SALMONELLA*	*SHIGELLA*
California	350	4	1.1	2.9
Colorado	351	5.7	1.4	0.9
Georgia	74	1.4	2.7	6.8
Illinois	1847	6.4	2.5	0.4
Maryland	345	2.3	9.3	1.2
Michigan	366	10.1	1.1	0.5
Oklahoma	502	1.0	2.4	2.6
Oregon	402	6.2	2.7	0.7

Data from Newell DG (ed): *Campylobacter* Epidemiology, Pathogenesis, and Biochemistry. Lancaster, MIP Press, 1982

single best medium; however, the highest isolation rates were observed when CSM was used in combination with any other media or the filter technique. Endtz and colleagues also reported that extending the incubation time from 48 to 72 hours led to an increase in the isolation rate regardless of the medium used.[70]

Rectal swabs or swab samples of the stool specimen can be inoculated directly to a small area on the surface of one of the recommended selective agar media. Formed stool specimens may also be processed by

TABLE 6-3

PROCEDURES USED BY VARIOUS INVESTIGATORS TO CREATE A MICROAEROPHILIC ENVIRONMENT SUITABLE FOR CULTIVATING *CAMPYLOBACTER* SPECIES

INVESTIGATORS	PROCEDURE
Luechtefeld et al.[177] Evacuation-replacement	Evacuated 75% of air from an anaerobic jar and refilled to atmospheric pressure with a mixture of 10% CO_2 and 90% N_2. Six plates of media were incubated in one jar.
Hebert et al.[110] Evacuation-replacement	Evacuated 75% of air from a modified pressure cooker by twice evacuating the container to −15 in. (−38 cm) Hg and refilling with a mixture of 10% CO_2 and 90% N_2 to atmospheric pressure. Plates occupied no more than one-half the volume of the container.

emulsifying a small portion (peanut sized) in phosphate-buffered saline or broth before inoculating 1 or 2 drops to the surface of the agar with a Pasteur pipette; similarly, 1 or 2 drops of liquid stool specimens can be inoculated directly.

An outline of a procedure that will allow isolation of enteric campylobacters from fecal samples is shown in Box 6-2. This technique is consistent with current information from the literature about requirements for cultivation of these bacteria and should be suitable for use in most clinical laboratories.

An alternative membrane filter technique, as described by Steele and McDermott,[256] may be used in combination with a Campy-selective medium with equivalent results (see Color Plate 6-1*B*) (Box 6-3).

Routine use of enrichment selective "Campy broth" is generally not recommended. It should be recognized, however, that Kaplan and coworkers[142] have reported that the use of Blaser Campy-Thio gave a 10% increased yield of *C. jejuni* from stool specimens. However, this increase may represent low concentrations of organisms that are of questionable clinical significance.[195] Enrichment broths may be beneficial if stool specimens are delayed in transit or left at room temperature too long. Each laboratory director must decide whether an enrichment broth will be beneficial based on local disease patterns and how well the collection and transport of quality specimens can be monitored. Since campylobacters are mcroaerophilic, they tend to grow best near the top of the tube. If a *Campylobacter* broth is used, the following procedure for subculture should be followed:

Use a Falcon brand polyethylene plastic pipette that can be inverted. Place the tip of the pipette 1 inch

TABLE 6-4
FORMULAS FOR SELECTIVE MEDIA FOR ISOLATION OF *CAMPYLOBACTER JEJUNI*

MEDIUM	BASE	ADDITIVES
Butzler's selective medium	Fluid thioglycollate medium (Difco Laboratories, Detroit MI)	Agar (3%) Sheep blood (10%) Bacitracin (25,000 IU/L) Novobiocin (5 mg/L) Colistin (10,000 IU/L) Cephalothin (15 mg/L) Actidione (50 mg/L)
Skirrow's blood agar	Blood agar base No. 2 (Oxoid)	Lysed horse blood (7%) Vancomycin (10 mg/L) Polymyxin B (2500 IU/L) Trimethoprim (5 mg/L)
Blaser's medium (Campy-BAP)	Brucella agar base (Becton Dickinson Microbiology Systems, Cockeysville MD)	Sheep blood (10%) Vancomycin (10 mg/L) Trimethoprim (5 mg/L) Polymyxin B (2500 IU/L) Cephalothin (15 mg/L) Amphotericin B (2 mg/L)
Preston *Campylobacter* selective medium	Nutrient broth No. 2 (Oxoid CM67) 1.2% New Zealand agar	5% Saponin-lysed horse blood Trimethoprim (10 µg/mL) Polymyxin B (5 IU/mL) Rifampin 10 (µg/mL) Cycloheximide (100 µg/mL)
Preston *Campylobacter* blood-free medium	Nutrient broth No. 2 (Oxoid CM67) 1.2% New Zealand agar	Bacteriologic charcoal Sodium deoxycholate Ferrous sulfate Sodium pyruvate Casein hydrolysate Cefoperazone (32 mg/L)
Butzler virion medium	Columbia agar base (Oxoid CM331)	Defibrinated sheep blood Cefoperazone (15 mg/L) Rifampin (10 mg/L) Colistin (10,000 U/L) Amphotericin B (2 mg/L)
Modified Preston medium	Nutrient broth No. 2 (Oxoid)	7% defibrinated horse blood Cefoperazone (32 mg/L) Amphotericin B (2 mg/L) Campylobacter growth supplement (Oxoid)
Charcoal-based blood-free selective medium	Columbia agar base (GIBCO)	Activated charcoal (Oxoid) Hematin (0.032 g/L) Sodium pyruvate (0.1 g/L) Vancomycin (20 mg/L) Cefoperazone (32 mg/L) Cycloheximide (100 mg/L)

Data from Karmali MA, Simer AE, Roscoe M, et al: Evaluation of a blood-free, charcoal-based, selective medium for the isolation of *Campylobacter* organisms from feces. J Clin Microbiol 23:456–459, 1986; and Merino FJ, Agulla A, Villasante PA, et al: Comparative efficacy of seven selective media for isolating *Campylobacter jejuni*. J Clin Microbiol 24:451–452, 1986

below the surface of the medium and continuously withdraw sample as you remove the pipette. Invert the pipette to facilitate mixing of the sample, place 3 drops on a Campy-BAP plate and streak for isolation. Incubate as you would a primary culture plate.

Identification From Culture. The appearance of colonies on one of the selective *Campylobacter* agars that has been incubated at 42°C in the gaseous environment described previously is already presumptive evidence that the organism is one of the thermophilic *Campy-*

BOX 6-2. PROCEDURE FOR ISOLATING *C. JEJUNI* AND OTHER ENTERIC *CAMPYLOBACTER* SPECIES FROM FECAL SPECIMENS

1. Using a fecal sample or a swab sample in Cary-Blair medium, prepare a turbid suspension of the feces in 10 mL of brain–heart infusion broth. Immediately inoculate one or two plates (two plates are preferable) of a *Campylobacter*-selective medium (best results are obtained with CSM as noted in text); streak to obtain isolated colonies; and hold in a nitrogen-holding jar (see Chapter 14) until the remaining media are inoculated.

2. Lightly centrifuge the specimen (at approximately 1000*g*) for 5 minutes.

3. Remove about 5 mL of the supernatant with a syringe and filter through a sterile 0.65-μL Millipore filter, as described by Butzler.[35] Discard the first 3 mL of fluid and use 1 or 2 drops of the remainder to inoculate two plates of chocolate agar without selective agents or a blood agar medium such as the Centers for Disease Control (CDC) anaerobe blood agar that will support the growth of *Campylobacter*. Streak for isolation.

4. Incubate one set of Campy-selective agar and chocolate agar plates at 42°C in an atmosphere of 5% O_2, 10% CO_2, and 85% N_2 and the remaining plates at 35°C to 37°C in the same gaseous atmosphere.

5. Inspect the plates after 24, 48, and 72 hours of incubation for colonies characteristic of *Campylobacter* species and identify the isolates with the techniques described in the text. Plates not showing growth after 24 or 48 hours of incubation should be returned for an additional 24 to 48 hours in the same incubator and gaseous atmospheric conditions, as described above.

BOX 6-3. STEELE AND MCDERMOTT MEMBRANE FILTER TECHNIQUE

1. Mix 1 g stool in 10 mL of sterile saline containing glass beads. Vortex for 30 seconds.

2. Place a 47-mm, 0.45 Gelman cellulose triacetate membrane filter (Gelman No. 63069) centrally onto the surface of a nonselective *Brucella* agar plate containing 5% sheep blood.

3. Place 8 to 10 drops of fecal suspension on the surface of the filter with a Pasteur pipette. Take care to ensure that the drops do not extend to the edge of the filter.

4. Remove filter and discard 30 minutes after the suspension is applied.

5. Incubate plate in Campy environment as described previously.

needed to differentiate rare nonpigmented isolates of *P. aeruginosa*.

Gram-stained preparations from colonies of *C. jejuni* after 24 to 48 hours incubation on blood agar show characteristic gram-negative, curved, "S"-shaped, gull-winged, or long spiral forms (see Color Plate 6-1*A*). Coccoid forms are more commonly seen in older cultures of *C. jejuni*, particularly after colonies have been exposed to ambient air. Since *Campylobacter* species are typically faint staining, we have adopted the practice of extending the staining time of the safranin counterstain to at least 10 minutes to allow for greater staining intensity. Also, the addition of one half gram of basic fuchsin per liter of safranin improves the intensity of the counterstain without overstaining the cellular elements.

Once isolated, both subspecies of *C. jejuni* can be easily identified since they are the only campylobacters that hydrolyze hippurate (see Color Plate 6-1*E* and Table 6-5). In addition, this species is resistant to cephalothin and susceptible to nalidixic acid (see Color Plate 6-1*F*). Hebert and associates[110] place *C. jejuni* into eight biotypes based on hippurate hydrolysis, DNA hydrolysis, and growth on charcoal-yeast extract medium. This separation may have limited clinical value in individual cases but may be important epidemiologically in tracking outbreaks.

CAMPYLOBACTER SPECIES OTHER THAN C. JEJUNI SUBSP. JEJUNI

C. coli.   *C. coli*, closely related to *C. jejuni* and also a cause of diarrhea in humans, shares several cultural characteristics with *C. jejuni*, including susceptibility to nalidixic acid and resistance to cephalothin. *C. coli* can be differentiated from *C. jejuni* by the hippurate hydrolysis test (*C. jejuni* hydrolyzes hippurate; *C. coli* does not). The report when this organism is recovered in laboratories in which the hippurate test is not performed should read, "*C. jejuni/coli*." It is estimated (*text continues on page 330*)

lobacter species (most commonly *C. jejuni*). The morphology of *Campylobacter* species on selective agar varies from flat, gray, irregular-shaped colonies that may be either dry or moist to colonies that are round and convex and glistening with entire edges (Color Plate 6-1*C,D*). There is a tendency for colonies to form confluent growth along the streak lines on the agar surface. Hemolytic reactions are not observed on blood agar. The identification can be further confirmed by performing rapid catalase and cytochrome oxidase tests (*C. jejuni*, *C. coli*, and *C. lari* are positive for both). On occasion, thermophilic bacterial species other than *Campylobacter* species, notably *Pseudomonas aeruginosa*, may break through and grow on the selective media. *P. aeruginosa* also produces cytochrome oxidase and catalase and might be confused with *Campylobacter* species; however, most strains can be differentiated by their production of pyocyanin pigment and the characteristic grape-juice odor. Examination of a wet mount of one of the suspected colonies under phase-contrast or darkfield optics may be helpful to visualize the organisms; *Campylobacter* species have a characteristic darting motility. Additional biochemical tests may be

TABLE 6-5
DIFFERENTIAL CHARACTERISTICS OF CAMPYLOBACTERS AND RELATED TAXA OF MEDICAL IMPORTANCE

ORGANISM	CATALASE	NITRATE	HYDROGEN SULFIDE TRIPLE SUGAR IRON	UREASE	INDOXYL ACETATE	HIPPURATE	GROWTH 25°C	37°C	42°C	MacCONKEY	0.1% TMAO	1.5% NaCl	1% GLYCINE	SUSCEPTIBILITY* NALIDIXIC ACID	CEPHALOTHIN
RNA Group I															
Campylobacter coli	+	+	-	-	+	-	-	+	+	+	-	-	+	S	R
C. concisus	-	+	+	-	NA	-	-	+	C	+	-	+	C	R	R
C. curvus	-	+	+	-	+	-	+	+	+	NA	NA	NA	+	C	S
C. fetus subsp. fetus	+	+	-	-	-	-	+	+	+	+	-	V	+	R	S
C. fetus subsp. venerealis	+	+	-	-	-	-	+	+	-	+	-	V	-	R	S
C. gracilis	-	+	-	-	V	-	NA	+	NA	NA	NA	NA	NA	R	S
C. helveticus	-	+	-	-	+	-	-	+	+	NA	-	NA	NA	S	S
C. hyoilei	+	+	+	-	NA	-	NA	+	+	NA	NA	NA	+	S	R
C. hyointestinalis subsp. hyointestinalis	+	+	+	-	-	-	V	+	+	+	+	-	+	R	S
C. hyointestinalis subsp. lawsonii	+	+	+	-	-	-	-	+	+	NA	NA	NA	V	R	NA
C. jejuni subsp. jejuni	+	+	-	-	+	+	-	+	+	+	-	-	+	S	R
C. jejuni subsp. doylei	V	-	-	-	+	+	-	+	W	NA	-	-	+	S	S
C. lari	+	+	-	-	-	-	C	+	+	+	+	+	C	R	R
C. mucosalis	-	+	+	-	-	-	-	+	+	+	C	C	C	C	S
C. rectus	-	+	+	-	+	-	-	+	W	NA	NA	NA	+	S	S
C. showae	+	+	+	-	+	-	-	+	+	NA	NA	NA	V	R	S

Organism													
C. sputorum biovar *bubulus*	−	+	−	−	−	−	−	C	+	+	+	R	S
C. sputorum biovar *fecalis*	+	+	−	−	−	+	+	+	+	+	+	R	S
C. sputorum biovar *sputorum*	−	+	−	−	−	+	+	+	+	C	+	V	S
C. upsaliensis	−(w)	+	−	+	−	−	+	+	−	−	C	S	S
RNA Group II													
Arcobacter butzleri	−(w)	+	−	+	+	+	−	V	+	NA	V	V	R
A. cryaerophilus	+	+	−	+	+	+	−	−	+	NA	+	V	R
A. nitrofigilis	+	+	V	−	+	−	−	−	+	NA	−	S	S
A. skirrowii	+	+	NA	−	NA	NA	NA	V	+	NA	V	S	V
RNA Group III													
Helicobacter cinaedi (CLO-1)	+	−	−	−	C	−	−	−	+	−	−	S	S
H. fennelliae (CLO-2)	+	−	−	−	−	−	−	−	+	NA	−	S	S
CLO-3	+	−	−	−	+	−	NA	+	+	NA	+	R	S
H. pullorum	+	+	−	−	−	−	NA	NA	+	NA	+	R	S
H. pylori	+	−	++	−	−	−	−	C	+	−	V	S	R
"*Flexispira rappini*"	C	−	++	−	−	NA	NA	NA	+	NA	−(w)	R	R

* Susceptibility to antibiotics determined with 30-µg disks.
+, 90% or more of strains are positive; ++, strong positive reaction; −, 90% or more of strains are negative; V, 11%–89% of strains are positive; C, contradictory reports in literature; W, weak reaction; NA, results not available; R, resistant; S, susceptible; TMAO, trimethylamine oxide. Shaded areas indicate key reactions.
Data from references 6, 11, 12, 30, 72, 78, 98, 117, 151, 213, 223, 228, 240, 253, 254, 257, 270, 273, 276, 278.

that *C. coli* accounts for 5 to 10% of cases of *Campylobacter* enteritis in humans.[198] A case of urinary tract infection caused by quinolone-resistant *C. coli* has also been reported.[217]

C. concisus.   *C. concisus* is capable of anaerobic growth and requires hydrogen or formate for growth. The organism is isolated most commonly from human gingival crevices. Lauwers and associates[167] have reported that of 153 patients from whom *Campylobacter* species were isolated, 37 had *C. concisus*. In 7 patients, the organism was found in association with an enteropathogen; however, 15 patients harbored only *C. concisus* and 11 of these had symptoms of enteritis. No clinical information was obtained on the remaining patients. All isolates were recovered only with the filter method (discussed elsewhere in this chapter). Vandamme and colleagues[274] have reported that nearly all of the *C. concisus* isolates included in their study were isolated from patients suffering from gastrointestinal disorders.

C. fetus subsp. fetus.   *C. fetus* subsp. *fetus* is primarily associated with infective abortion in cattle and sheep and is an infrequent cause of human infections. Infections usually result in systemic illness and usually affect debilitated persons with chronic hepatic, renal, or neoplastic disease, or with compromised immune function.[223] Between January 1979 and March 1981, 10 patients were reported to the San Diego Health Department with sepsis caused by *C. fetus* subsp. *fetus*.[41] All had been treated for severe underlying illness with "nutritional therapy" that had been administered in clinics in Tijuana, Mexico. The treatment consisted of a freshly prepared juice cocktail that included raw calf's liver. Physicians should be aware of the possibility of *Campylobacter* sepsis among patients who receive such nutritional therapy. *C. fetus* subsp. *fetus* has been reported to cause proctitis and proctocolitis in homosexual men[64]; premature labor and neonatal sepsis in humans[42]; septic abortion[259]; neonatal meningitis[163]; prosthetic hip joint infection[14,289]; and both native and prosthetic valve endocarditis.[76] The organism was not previously believed to cause gastroenteritis, but, because of its susceptibility to cephalothin and its failure to grow at 42°C, it may not be recovered in clinical laboratories where selective media and increased incubation temperatures are used as a screen for *C. jejuni*; therefore, its etiologic role in this infection has not been systematically assessed.[109]

C. fetus subsp. venerealis.   *C. fetus* subsp. *venerealis* comprises part of the normal genital tract flora of bulls but has not been associated with human infection.[247]

C. helveticus.   *C. helveticus* is a thermophilic catalase-negative *Campylobacter* that has been isolated from the feces of domestic cats and dogs.[253] Of note is the fact that almost half of the *Campylobacter* isolates found in cats belong to *C. helveticus*.[33] Colonies of *C. helveticus* are adherent on blood agar and can be separated from other thermophilic species (*C. jejuni*, *C. coli*, and *C. lari*)

by virtue of a negative catalase reaction. It is indoxyl acetate positive and sensitive to both nalidixic acid and cephalothin.

C. hyoilei.   *C. hyoilei* is the name for a group of similar bacteria isolated from intestinal lesions of pigs with proliferative enteritis.[6] No human isolates have been reported.

C. hyointestinalis.   *C. hyointestinalis*, closely related to *C. fetus* subsp. *fetus*, was initially found only in animals, principally as a cause of ileitis in swine,[94] but more recently has been reported from human clinical specimens. In one report, *C. hyointestinalis* was isolated from stool specimens of four persons, all of whom were experiencing non-bloody, watery diarrhea. The youngest (8 months) and the oldest (79 years) persons were female, and the other two were homosexual men.[69] A case of a 52-year-old woman with chronic myeloid leukemia and non-bloody, watery diarrhea associated with this organism has been reported from France,[192] and an isolate from the rectal culture of a homosexual man with proctitis has been reported in the United States.[77] *C. hyointestinalis* will not be recovered on many *Campylobacter* media formulations because it is susceptible to cephalosporins such as cephalothin and cefoperazone. Although it will grow at 42°C, growth is more luxuriant at 35°C.[77] The organism is also resistant to nalidixic acid, is hippurate negative, and produces hydrogen sulfide in triple sugar iron agar. The production of hydrogen sulfide in triple sugar iron agar is dependent on the test being incubated in a microaerophilic environment containing hydrogen.[94]

A group of "*C. hyointestinalis*-like" organisms obtained from porcine stomachs have recently been described. These isolates are sufficiently different from *C. hyointestinalis* to warrant creation of a separate subspecies classification, *C. hyointestinalis* subsp. *lawsonii*.[213] The creation of this new subspecies necessitates that the description of *C. hyointestinalis* be emended to *C. hyointestinalis* subsp. *hyointestinalis*. *C. hyointestinalis* subsp. *lawsonii* can be separated from subsp. *hyointestinalis* by its failure to grow in 1.5% bile. *C. hyointestinalis* subsp. *lawsonii* has been isolated from the intestines and stomachs of pigs; hamster intestines; and the feces of cattle, deer, and humans; but its pathogenicity is not known.[213]

C. jejuni subsp. doylei.   A new subspecies of *C. jejuni* has been isolated from human clinical specimens including gastric epithelium biopsies[145] and feces from children with diarrhea.[257] The pathogenicity of the organism remains unknown. *C. jejuni* subsp. *doylei* can be distinguished readily from other campylobacters because it does not reduce nitrates and hydrolyzes hippurate.[257] It is susceptible to cephalothin and therefore will not be recovered on media containing cephalosporin-type antibiotics.

C. lari.   Formerly named *C. laridis*, the organism now known as *C. lari* is thermophilic, halotolerant, and nalidixic acid resistant; otherwise, it shares several features with *C. jejuni* and *C. coli*.[246] Anaerobic growth in the presence of 0.1% trimethylamine oxide (TMAO) and failure to hydrolyze indoxyl acetate help to identify this species (reagents available from Sigma Chemical Co., St. Louis, MO). Many laboratories rely on resistance to nalidixic acid to separate *C. lari* from *C. jejuni* and *C. coli*; however, we have noted a case of *C. jejuni* infection isolated from a patient on ciprofloxacin therapy (a quinolone similar to nalidixic acid) in which resistance to nalidixic acid was developed by the *C. jejuni* isolate. *C. lari* is endemic in sea gulls but causes enteritis simulating *C. jejuni* infections in humans. The first human isolates were reported from feces of four asymptomatic persons.[16] Several cases of illness associated with *C. lari* were described by Tauxe and colleagues[266]: fecal isolation of the organism and associated enteric illness was described in five cases and terminal bacteremia in an immunocompromised host in one. Nachamkin and coworkers[200] also reported a case of terminal *C. lari* bacteremia in an immunocompromised patient. Chiu and coworkers have reported a case of chronic diarrhea and bacteremia caused by *C. lari* in a neonate.[49]

C. mucosalis.   *C. mucosalis*, formerly classified as *C. sputorum* subsp. *mucosalis*, produces a yellow pigment and is catalase negative. Phenotypically, this species is very similar to *C. sputorum* biovars *sputorum* and *bubulus* but is able to grow at 25°C. Unlike the majority of campylobacters, this species requires hydrogen and formate as an electron donor for growth, an essential requirement of *C. concisus*, *C. mucosalis*, *C. curvus*, and *C. rectus*.[273] Figura and colleagues[79] reported what was thought to be the first isolation of *C. mucosalis* from children with enteritis. However, this finding has been disputed and the isolates have been shown by molecular probe studies to be *C. concisus*.[164,166,211] These two species are difficult to separate on the basis of biochemical tests alone and it has been suggested that molecular methods must be used for the precise identification of these two species.[166] On[211] has suggested the use of several media containing various inhibitory agents for separating *C. concisus* and *C. mucosalis*. There are as yet no confirmed reports associating *C. mucosalis* with human infection.

C. showae.   *C. showae* is a recently described species isolated from human gingival crevices.[72] The organism appears as a straight rod with round ends and contains two to five unsheathed unipolar flagella—a feature that is unique among campylobacters. The organism grows in a microaerophilic atmosphere in the presence of fumarate with formate or H_2, but prefers to grow under anaerobic conditions. Because of the limited number of reliable biochemical traits which can be used to differentiate closely related *Campylobacter* species, serologic, DNA probe, or protein profile tests may be required to positively identify isolates of this species.[72] An association with human disease has not been shown.

C. sputorum.   *C. sputorum* is capable of anaerobic growth and can be recovered from the oral cavity and gingival crevices of humans. This organism is not recognized as an agent of human disease, although a few clinical isolates have been reported. Three biovars are described[235] in Box 6-4.

C. upsaliensis.   *C. upsaliensis* is catalase negative or only weakly positive and thus has been referred to as the CNW strain of *Campylobacter*. However, because weak catalase reactions may also occur for *C. jejuni* subsp. *doylei*, the CNW designation no longer holds. Except for the lack of or weak production of catalase, this organism shares several characteristics with pathogenic campylobacters. It is thermophilic (grows at 42°C) and is highly susceptible to drugs that are present in selective isolation media, making them unsuitable for the isolation of *C. upsaliensis*.[258] Goossens and coworkers[99] reported the isolation of 99 strains of *C. upsaliensis* by the filter method, with only 4 strains recovered simultaneously from selective media.

Domestic pets may serve as the reservoir of this species, which was first isolated from healthy dogs, dogs with diarrhea, and, more recently, from asymptomatic cats.[87,241] Of 12 isolates sent to the CDC, three were from stools, eight were from blood, and one was unspecified.[221] Data from some reports suggest that this organism may be an opportunistic agent of infections in children. Lastovica and associates[165] reported the recovery of *C. upsaliensis* from blood cultures of 16 patients, 10 of whom were 10 months old or younger. Walmsley and Karmali[283] reported the isolation of this organism from the stools of six children. Other reports have associated the isolation of *Campylobacter upsaliensis* from the blood of patients with serious underlying disease.[36,51,221] There has been one report of *C. upsaliensis* isolated from the blood and fetoplacental material of an 18-week pregnant woman who suffered a spontaneous abortion.[103] The patient had no underlying disease, and her only previous pregnancy was uneventful. Numerical analysis of protein profiles revealed that strains isolated from the patient and a healthy household cat were almost identical, implying that the

---

BOX 6-4. *C. SPUTORUM* BIOVARS

1. *C. sputorum* bv. *bubulus* is a commensal of cattle and has not been associated with disease in humans.

2. *C. sputorum* bv. *sputorum* is part of the normal respiratory tract flora of humans and has been isolated from stool of healthy persons. Rare cases in which this biovar is possibly clinically significant (abscess, diarrhea) have been reported.[223]

3. *C. sputorum* bv. *fecalis*, part of the normal genital flora in cattle, was formerly classified as *C. fecalis*, but has been reassigned as a biovar of *C. sputorum*. It has not been isolated from humans.

cat might have been the source of the infection.[103] The only report of *C. upsaliensis* from a site other than blood or stool was from a case of a breast abscess in which *C. upsaliensis* was recovered along with a *Peptostreptococcus* species from purulent exudate obtained through fine-needle aspiration of the infected site.[93] Sandstedt and Ursing[240] have described *C. upsaliensis*, including its phenotypic characteristics and clinical significance.

FORMER *WOLINELLA* AND *BACTEROIDES* SPECIES INCLUDED IN THE FAMILY *CAMPYLOBACTERACEAE*

Tanner and colleagues, in their studies of the taxonomy of the anaerobic, agar-pitting, gram-negative bacilli, placed the nonmotile strains into the genus *Bacteroides* and the motile strains into the group of "anaerobic vibrios" (including *Wolinella recta, W. curva,* and *Campylobacter concisus*).[264,265] The nonmotile strains are separated on the basis of urease production into *B. ureolyticus* (urease positive) and *B. gracilis* (urease negative; see Table 6-6). These species are all now included in the family *Campylobacteraceae* and are considered true campylobacters.[273,276]

C. gracilis. The name *Bacteroides gracilis* was proposed by Tanner et al.[264] for a group of agar-corroding bacteria that were originally considered to be anaerobic. In 1995, Vandamme and colleagues proposed the transfer of this organism to the genus *Campylobacter* as *C. gracilis*.[272] These bacteria are found in the gingival crevices of humans and have been isolated primarily from sites of deep tissue infection. Johnson and colleagues have reported that 83% of the specimens in which *C. gracilis* was isolated were obtained from patients with serious visceral, or head and neck infections.[135] *C. gracilis* is microaerophilic and asaccharolytic and resembles campylobacters in almost all phenotypic characteristics. Individual cells stain gram-negative and are small and unbranched, often having both tapered and rounded ends. Growth is stimulated in broth cultures by formate and fumarate. They may be differentiated from other campylobacters by the absence of flagella and the absence of oxidase activity.[264] *C. gracilis* isolates appear less susceptible to antimicrobial agents than the closely related species [*B. ureolyticus*], with only 67% of the isolates reported to be susceptible to penicillin.[135] A selective medium for isolation of *C. gracilis* has been described that contains tryptic soy agar base, formate, fumarate, nitrate, and two selective agents, nalidixic acid and teicoplanin.[171]

Bacteroides ureolyticus. Ribosomal RNA sequence analysis clearly places [*B. ureolyticus*] as a member of the family *Campylobacteraceae*, however, it is not clear whether it branches outside the *Campylobacter* cluster (and should be placed in a new genus) or inside the *Campylobacter* cluster (and should be included in the genus *Campylobacter*).[272] [*B. ureolyticus*] differs from campylobacters in its fatty acid composition, its proteolytic metabolism, and its ability to hydrolyze urea.[272] [*B. ureolyticus*] strains have been isolated from patients

with superficial ulcers, soft-tissue infections, nongonococcal nonchlamydial urethritis, and periodontal disease.[66,67,82,83] In a study by Johnson and colleagues, [*B. ureolyticus*] strains were found to be uniformly susceptible to penicillins, cephalosporins, erythromycin, clindamycin, chloramphenicol, metronidazole, and aminoglycosides.[135]

C. curvus. *C. curvus* was originally named *Wolinella curva*.[265,276] Cells stain gram negative and are short and slightly curved. Helical or straight cells may also occur. Strains exhibit rapid, darting motility and are asaccharolytic. The organism grows anaerobically and in 5% O_2 atmospheres containing H_2. No growth occurs in air enriched with 10% CO_2. All cultures require formate and fumarate for broth growth. Some strains exhibit a corroding morphology on agar media. Isolates have been recovered exclusively from human sources and include dental root canal, alveolar abscess, and blood.[265] Characteristics useful in distinguishing *C. curvus* from similar species are given in Table 6-6.

C. rectus. *C. rectus* was originally named *Wolinella recta*.[264,276] Microscopically, the cells appear small and straight with rounded ends and stain gram negative. Strains exhibit rapid, darting motility and are asaccharolytic. Growth is anaerobic; however, some strains can grow in a 5% O_2 atmosphere but not in air enriched with 10% CO_2. Growth in broth is stimulated by formate and fumarate. Nitrates and nitrites are reduced, and both oxidase and catalase are negative. Additional identifying characteristics are given in Table 6-6. *C. rectus* is found in the gingival crevices of humans.[264] Spiegel and Telford[252] reported isolating this organism along with *Actinomyces viscosus* from an actinomycotic chest wall mass. Two isolates of *C. rectus* have been recovered from patients at the University of Illinois Hospital, one from a lung nodule of a patient with an 18-year history of alcohol abuse and an 8-month history of right-sided chest pain and another from the blood culture of a patient with a lung mass.

rRNA GROUP II—THE *ARCOBACTER* GROUP

The *Arcobacter* group consists of those species referred to as the aerotolerant campylobacters because they grow in the presence of atmospheric levels of oxygen. Other characteristics useful in distinguishing aerotolerant "*Campylobacter*" species from other campylobacters include hydrolysis of indoxyl acetate; growth at 15°C, 25°C, and 36°C but not 42°C; and the inability to hydrolyze hippurate (see Table 6-5). Vandamme and colleagues have shown that the arcobacters can be separated into five major groups, which were identified by DNA-DNA hybridization data as *A. cryaerophilus* (two distinct subgroups), *A. butzleri, A. nitrofigilis,* and *A. skirrowii*.[278]

A. cryaerophilus. *A. cryaerophilus* (formerly *C. cryaerophila*)[276] grows well under aerobic conditions, although it may require microaerophilic conditions for initial isolation. Optimal growth occurs at 30°C, and the or-

TABLE 6-6

CHARACTERISTICS USEFUL FOR DIFFERENTIATING *CAMPYLOBACTER CURVUS*, *C. RECTUS*, *C. GRACILIS*, [BACTEROIDES UREOLYTICUS], AND *WOLINELLA SUCCINOGENES*

CHARACTERISTIC	C. CURVUS	C. RECTUS	C. GRACILIS	[B. UREOLYTICUS]	W. SUCCINOGENES
Source	Human clinical	Human clinical	Human clinical	Human clinical	Bovine rumen
Morphology					
Helical or curved cells dominate	+	−	−	−	+
Straight cells dominate	−	+	+	+	−
Cells with tapered ends	+	−	−	−	+
Motility	+	+	−	−	+
Urease	−	−	−	+	−
Growth in 1% glycine	+	+	NA	NA	−
Indoxyl acetate hydrolysis	+	+	V	NA	−

+, 90% or more of strains are positive; −, 90% or more of strains are negative; V, 11% to 89% of strains are positive; NA, results not available.

Modified from Tanner ACR, Listgarten MA, Ebersole JL: *Wolinella curva* sp. nov.: "*Vibrio succinogenes*" of human origin. Int J Syst Bacteriol 34:275–282, 1984.

ganism will not grow at 42°C. Biochemically, this species resembles *C. fetus* subsp. *fetus*; however, *A. cryaerophilus* is indoxyl acetate positive, whereas *C. fetus* subsp. *fetus* is not (see Table 6-5). Most strains are sensitive to nalidixic acid and resistant to cephalothin. In a report by Borczyk and colleagues[24] comparing growth of *A. cryaerophilus* on CMS, Skirrow's blood agar, and cefsulodin irgasan novobiocin (CIN) agar, it was noted that the most luxuriant growth was obtained on CIN agar incubated for 24 to 48 hours at 25°C and 36°C. Isolates resembling *A. cryaerophilus* have been recovered from humans. One case of *A. cryaerophilus* isolated from the stool of a man infected with human immunodeficiency virus (HIV) with intermittent diarrhea was reported,[268] however, this strain was subsequently found to be *A. butzleri*.[267]

A. nitrofigilis. *A. nitrofigilis* (formerly *Campylobacter nitrofigilis*)[276] is a cryophilic species that grows optimally at 25°C. It is urea positive and nonpathogenic for humans.

A. butzleri. Kiehlbauch and colleagues at the CDC[151] have reported that the strains of aerotolerant campylobacters do not make up a homogeneous group. The majority of human isolates, both from within and outside the United States, make up a distinct DNA homology group that they named *Campylobacter butzleri* (changed to *Arcobacter butzleri* following the acceptance of the new genus designation for this group of organisms)[278]. Strains of *A. butzleri* can be separated from *A. cryaerophilus* by demonstrating aerotolerance at both 30°C and 36°C (*A. cryaerophilus* is aerotolerant at 30°C but not at 36°C). In addition, *A. butzleri* grows on MacConkey agar and in glycine- and nitrate-containing media (reducing nitrate to nitrite) and in

1.5% and 3.5% NaCl. *A. cryaerophilus* gives the opposite reactions.[151] The majority of isolates from humans have been from stools of patients with diarrheal illness;[151,172,277] however, three isolates have been isolated from abdominal contents or peritoneal fluids and three isolates obtained from blood cultures.[151]

A. skirrowii. *A. skirrowii* is the newest species of *Arcobacter* to be described. Strains have been isolated mainly from the preputial fluids of bulls; other strains have been isolated from aborted fetuses and diarrheic feces from cows, pigs, and sheep. The clinical significance of this new species has not been established.[278]

rRNA GROUP III—HELICOBACTER, WOLINELLA, "FLEXISPIRA," "GASTROSPIRILLUM" AND CAMPYLOBACTER-LIKE ORGANISMS (CLOs)

(Proposed names that are not yet validated by the International Committee on Systematic Bacteriology are enclosed in quotation marks.)

This homology group currently contains four genera and one unnamed *Campylobacter*-like species. The *Helicobacter* species are strict microaerophiles with a spiral or helical morphology. Many species exhibit strong urease activity. "*Flexispira rappini*" is the name proposed for an organism that is closely related to *Helicobacter* but is straight rather than curved and fusiform shaped. The genus *Wolinella* consists of a single species, *W. succinogenes*, that is an obligate anaerobe and requires formate and fumarate for growth. Species included in the genera *Helicobacter* and "*Flexispira*" possess sheathed flagella. No other *Campylobacter* or *Wolinella* species possess sheathed flagella (see Table 6-1).

H. PYLORI

This species was initially called *Campylobacter pyloridis* and then *Campylobacter pylori*. Recent evidence suggests that this organism does not belong to the genus *Campylobacter*.[98] Features that distinguish this organism from campylobacters are its multiple sheathed flagella, its strong hydrolysis of urea, and its unique fatty acid profile (a high percentage of 14:0 acid, a low percentage of 16:0 acid, and the presence of 3-OH-18:0 acid). 16S rRNA sequencing has shown that this organism is closely related to *Wolinella succinogenes*. However, there are many differences in biochemical features and growth characteristics between *H. pylori* and *W. succinogenes* that indicate that these species should not be in the same genus. *W. succinogenes* is catalase negative, is urease negative, does not possess γ-glutamyltranspeptidase or alkaline phosphatase activity, and does not grow at 30°C or on 0.5% glycine; *H. pylori* has the opposite characteristics. For this reason Goodwin and coworkers have proposed the transfer of *C. pylori* to the new genus *Helicobacter*.[98]

H. pylori is found only on the mucus-secreting epithelial cells of the stomach. Evidence suggests that *H. pylori* is the causative agent of active chronic antral gastritis[181] and may also be a major factor in the pathogenesis of peptic ulcer disease.[224] *H. pylori* gastritis is widespread in many countries in the world and may be one of the most common chronic human infections. The case for *H. pylori* as a causative agent of duodenal ulcer remains controversial. For excellent reviews see the work of Blaser,[19] Buck,[30] Lee and Hazell,[169] and Peterson.[224]

H. pylori strains are microaerophilic (10% CO_2, 5% O_2, 85% N_2) and will also grow in air with increased (10%) CO_2 content. The optimum temperature for isolation is 35°C to 37°C, although some strains will grow at 42°C. High humidity has also been found to favor growth. Most strains take 3 to 5 days to grow, with occasional isolates requiring 7 days of incubation before growth is evident. They can be cultured on nonselective blood-containing media, producing small, translucent, gray colonies. The characteristic Gram stain (small, curved, slightly plump bacilli) and positive reactions for catalase, oxidase, and urease provide an identification.

OTHER MEDICALLY IMPORTANT HELICOBACTER SPECIES

Several species of *Helicobacter* other than *H. pylori* have been isolated from humans and are associated with human disease. These include *H. cinaedi*, *H. fennelliae*, *Helicobacter* species strain *mainz*, *H. pullorum*, "*Flexispira rappini*" (*H. rappini*), "*Gastrospirillum hominis*" (*H. heilmanni*), and the unnamed *Helicobacter* species CLO-3 (see Table 6-7).

H. cinaedi. *H. cinaedi*, originally designated as CLO-1, and formerly known as "*Campylobacter cinaedi*," has been isolated from rectal swabs taken from symptomatic as well as asymptomatic homosexual men.[78,270] This organism has also been described as a cause of bacteremia in two homosexual men with concurrent tuber-

culosis,[220] in patients with acquired immunodeficiency syndrome (AIDS),[52,60,238] and in another who was HIV seropositive but did not have AIDS.[206] Reports, however, suggest that *C. cinaedi* infections are not restricted to homosexual or bisexual men. For example, Vandamme and associates[275] have reported the isolation of *H. cinaedi* from the blood of two women without any record of sexual contact with homosexuals and from the stools of three children, two of whom were girls.

Orlicek and colleagues have reported a case of septicemia and meningitis caused by *H. cineadi* in a neonate.[214] Since *H. cinaedi* has been identified as a normal intestinal inhabitant of hamsters[95,260] and the mother of the newborn cared for pet hamsters during the first two trimesters of her pregnancy, it is likely that the hamsters served as a reservoir for the transmission of the organism to the mother and that the newborn most likely became colonized with *H. cinaedi* during the birth process.[214] Kielbauch and colleagues reported that the clinical spectrum of illness associated with *H. cinaedi* infection includes fever, bacteremia, and recurrent cellulitis, with most patients having signs of systemic infection including leukocytosis, and often thrombocytopenia.[152] These same authors report that treatment with a penicillin, tetracycline, or aminoglycoside may be more effective than treatment with cephalosporins, erythromycin or ciprofloxacin.[152] Burman and coworkers have also reported the association of skin infections and arthritis due to *H. cinaedi* bacteremia.[32] Most blood isolates are recovered in automated blood culture instruments after 5 or more days of incubation. In general, organisms are not seen on initial Gram staining of the blood culture material but can be visualized by dark-field or acridine orange staining.[152] *H. cinaedi* grows only at 37°C, shows intermediate resistance to cephalothin (30-µg disk) and reduces nitrate to nitrite. Additional genotypic and phenotypic characteristics can be found in the report by Kiehlbauch and colleagues.[150] The only known natural reservoir of *H. cinaedi* found so far is the intestinal tract of hamsters, which may serve as a reservoir of human infections.[95,260]

H. fennelliae. Originally designated CLO-2, and formerly known as "*Campylobacter fennelliae*,"[270] this organism has the distinctive odor of hypochlorite cleaning powders.[78] It is susceptible to cephalothin and does not reduce nitrates to nitrite. As with *H. cinaedi*, *H. fennelliae* has been isolated from rectal swabs taken from symptomatic and asymptomatic homosexual men.[78] There is one report of this organism being isolated from the blood of a 31-year-old bisexual man with a history of intravenous drug abuse and a positive HIV serology.[206]

CLO-3. An unnamed species originally described by Fennell and coworkers,[78] CLO-3 can be separated from the other CLOs by its ability to grow at 42°C, its resistance to cephalothin, and its inability to reduce nitrate (see Table 6-5). One isolate has been reported from a rectal swab obtained from a symptomatic homosexual man.[78]

"Flexispira rappini." *"Flexispira rappini"* is the proposed name[29] of an organism that is urease positive and possibly genomically closely related to *H. pylori*.[276] However, it is a straight organism rather than a spiral one and is fusiform with a corrugated surface owing to the presence of periplasmic fibers. It has multiple, bipolar flagella. It does not possess alkaline phosphatase or grow at 30°C but does grow at 43°C and is resistant to metronidazole (5 μg), whereas *H. pylori* has the opposite characteristics.[98] It is separated from the campylobacters by negative reactions for catalase and nitrate and an inability to grow in 1% glycine.[11] A proposal to place the organism within the genus *Helicobacter* has been made. *"F. rappini"* has been isolated from stool specimens of both humans and dogs[11,234] and from aborted ovine fetuses.[154,155] Two of the human isolates were recovered from patients with symptoms of gastroenteritis.[234]

"Gastrospirillum hominis." *Gastrospirillum hominis* is an uncultivated spiral bacterium found in human gastric mucosa that is larger and more tightly coiled than *H. pylori*. The organism is helical, 3.5–7.5 μm long and 0.9 μm in diameter with truncated ends flattened at the tips, six to eight tight spirals, and up to 12 sheathed flagella 28 nm in diameter at each pole.[185] McNulty and colleagues have proposed the name *"G. hominis."* However, Solnick and co-workers[250] have shown that *"Gastrospirillum"* is a member of the *Helicobacter* genus and have proposed the name *H. heilmannii* after Konrad Heilmann, a German histopathologist who described the first large series of patients infected with *"Gastrospirillum."*[111] Heilmann and Borchard reported the prevalence of *"Gastrospirillum"* infection in patients presenting for endoscopy to be less than 1 %.[111] *"G. hominis"* appears to be ubiquitous in domestic animals, suggesting that human infection may be acquired as a zoonosis.[65,86,112] Human infection with this bacterium may be accompanied by chronic gastritis similar to that seen with infection by *H. pylori*.[62,81,111,168,185,193]

NONHUMAN *HELICOBACTER* SPECIES

A number of *Helicobacter* species have been isolated from animals. These include *H. acinonyx*,[68] *H. bilis*,[89] *H. bizzozeronii*,[105] *H. canis*,[255] *H. felis*,[219] *H. hepaticus*,[85] *Helicobacter* species strain *Mainz*,[127] *H. muridarum*,[170] *H. mustelae*,[84,88,98] *H. nemestrinae*,[28] and *H. pullorum*.[34,254] These bacteria are generally found in the stomach or the lower gastrointestinal tract. When present in the stomach, these helicobacters are usually associated with gastritis in the host animal. Some of these strains have also been isolated from humans (see Table 6-7)

WOLINELLA SUCCINOGENES

This is the type species of the genus *Wolinella*, presently defined as being anaerobic, catalase negative, and hydrogen sulfide positive.[264] However, it has been shown that *W. succinogenes* is oxidase positive and is capable of using O_2 as a terminal electron acceptor under microaerophilic conditions (2% O_2) but not under atmospheric levels of O_2. These findings, along with additional evidence on the electron transport system, indicate that *W. succinogenes* is not an anaerobe but is an H_2-requiring microaerophile.[269] *W. succinogenes* has not been associated with human infections.

SUTTERELLA WADSWORTHENSIS

Wexler and colleagues have proposed the name *S. wadsworthensis* for a group of bacteria that were originially identified as *C. gracilis* but differed in genetic and biochemical characterisics from typical *C. gracilis* strains.[288] These organisms are gram-negative straight rods that grow in a microaerophilic atmosphere or under anaerobic conditions. They are differentiated from *C. gracilis* and *Campylobacter* species by being oxidase-, urease- and indoxyl acetate-negative, resistant to 20% bile disks and by not reducing tetrazolium tetrachloride under aerobic conditions. They have been isolated mainly from human infections of the gastrointestinal tract.[288]

DEFINITIVE IDENTIFICATION OF CAMPYLOBACTERS AND RELATED BACTERIA

The colonial morphology and Gram-stain characteristics of *C. jejuni* as described earlier also pertain to most other *Campylobacter* species. However, definitive species identification depends on the determination of the phenotypic characteristics presented in Table 6-5.

The differential susceptibility to nalidixic acid and cephalothin can be used to differentiate the more commonly encountered *Campylobacter* species according to the scheme in Box 6-5.

Luechtefeld and Wang[178] also found that resistance of *C. jejuni* to triphenyltetrazolium chloride (TTC) is helpful in distinguishing *C. fetus*. The test for hippurate hydrolysis is useful in separating *C. jejuni* from the closely related species *C. coli*. Most strains of *C. jejuni* hydrolyze hippurate to benzoic acid and glycine.[108] The rapid procedure of Hwang and Ederer for hippurate hydrolysis, described in Chapter 12, is suitable for testing clinical isolates of *Campylobacter* species. Morris and associates[194] describe a more sensitive method for detecting benzoic acid using gas liquid chromatography (GLC). This application is an extension of the procedure previously reported by Kodaka and colleagues,[158] who used hippurate formate fumarate medium to detect not only hippurate hydrolysis by GLC but the utilization of formate and fumarate as well.

Mills and Gherna[191] described the use of a rapid test for detecting hydrolysis of indoxyl acetate by *Campylobacter* species. Studies have shown that all strains of *C. jejuni*, *C. coli*, *C. curvus*, *C. helveticus*, *C. rectus*, *C. showae*, *C. upsaliensis*, *Arcobacter* butzleri, *A. cryaerophilus*, and *Helicobacter fennelliae* hydrolyze indoxyl acetate, whereas most other campylobacters are negative.[117,191,212,228] Several additional biochemical and physical characteristics may be helpful in separating the various *Campylobacter* and *Campylobacter*-like species (see Table 6-5). An extensive review of identifi-

TABLE 6-7
HELICOBACTER SPECIES AND RELATED ORGANISMS

SPECIES	HOSTS	SITE OF ISOLATION
H. acinonyx	Cheetahs	Gastric mucosa
H. bilis	Mice	Bile, liver, intestine
H. bizzozeronii	Dogs	Gastric mucosa
H. canis	Dogs, humans	Feces
H. cinaedi	Humans, hamsters	Blood, rectal swabs (humans), intestines (hamsters)
H. felis	Cats, dogs	Gastric mucosa
H. fennelliae	Humans	Blood, rectal swabs
H. hepaticus	Mice	Liver, intestine
Helicobacter species strain Mainz	Humans	Knee joint, blood
H. muridarum	Rats, mice	Intestine
H. mustelae	Ferrets	Gastric mucosa
H. nemestrinae	Pigtailed macaque monkeys	Gastric mucosa
H. pametensis	Wild birds (tern, gull), pigs	Feces
H. pullorum	Chickens, humans	Intestines, liver (chickens), feces (humans)
H. pylori	Humans, monkeys, cats	Gastric mucosa
"Flexispira rappini" ("H. rappini")	Sheep, dogs, humans	Liver (sheep), stomach (dogs), feces (humans)
"Gastrospirillum hominis" ("H. heilmannii")	Cheetahs, humans	Gastric mucosa
CLO-3	Humans	Rectal swabs

cation methods for campylobacters, helicobacters, and related organisms has been published by On.[212]

RAPID IDENTIFICATION OF CAMPYLOBACTERS FROM COLONIES AND FROM STOOL SPECIMENS

In most instances the appearance of gray, small, sometimes "spready" colonies on Campylobacter-selective agar, which exhibit characteristic "S"-shape and gull-wing morphology on Gram stain and are oxidase and catalase positive, will be sufficient to establish the diagnosis of campylobacteriosis in patients with diarrheal syndromes.

Hodge and coworkers[118] advocate the use of direct immunofluorescence techniques in the rapid screening of stool specimens from patients with an acute diarrheal syndrome. This approach has the potential for re-

moving the guesswork involved in interpreting gram-stained smears.

Because of the problems in the recovery and identification of Campylobacter species as listed previously, several more direct techniques have evolved over the past several years.

LATEX AGGLUTINATION TESTS

Latex agglutination tests are now available for the identification of Campylobacter species and related organisms. Meritec-Campy (jcl) (Meridian Diagnostics, Cincinnati, OH) is a latex agglutination assay that is used for culture isolate identification. The manufacturer claims that this test will identify C. jejuni, C. coli, and C. lari. A published study reported 100% sensitivity in detecting C. jejuni and C. coli but negative results with all six C. lari isolates tested. Two of two C.

BOX 6-5. DEFINITIVE IDENTIFICATION OF MOST COMMONLY ENCOUNTERED CAMPYLOBACTERS

	NALIDIXIC ACID	CEPHALOTHIN	TTC*	HIPPURATE HYDROLYSIS	INDOXYL ACETATE HYDROLYSIS
C. jejuni subsp. jejuni	S	R	R	+	+
C. coli	S	R	R	−	+
C. fetus subsp. fetus	R	S	S	−	−
C. lari	R	R	S	−	−

* TTC, triphenyltetrazolium chloride.

upsaliensis isolates tested also gave positive reactions. All 101 non-*Campylobacter* isolates tested gave negative reactions.[199] Campyslide (Becton Dickinson Microbiology Systems, Cockeysville, MD) is a latex agglutination assay that can be used for genus-level culture confirmation of four major *Campylobacter* pathogens, namely, *C. jejuni, C. coli, C. lari,* and *C. fetus* subsp. *fetus.* In one report by Hodinka and Gilligan,[120] a total of 50 fresh clinical isolates of *Campylobacter* species (45 *C. jejuni* and 5 *C. coli*) were examined with complete agreement between Campyslide and conventional methods. Only one of 173 non-*Campylobacter* isolates tested gave a false-positive result.

NUCLEIC ACID PROBES

Nucleic acid probes are also coming on the market for use in the identification of *Campylobacter* species. AccuProbe *Campylobacter* Culture Identification Test (Gen-Probe, Inc., San Diego, CA) is a DNA probe-based test that provides for rapid identification of *C. jejuni, C. coli,* and *C. lari* directly from bacterial colonies. The probe is non-radiometric and is labeled with a chemiluminescent acridinium ester. Reactions are read in a luminometer.

As the importance of campylobacters in patients with AIDS and other immunosuppressive conditions increases, other direct techniques using enzyme-linked immunosorbent assays[156] and DNA probes may evolve to detect specific markers for differential identifications and factors of virulence.

CULTURE AND ISOLATION OF *HELICOBACTER PYLORI*

SPECIMENS FOR RECOVERY OF *H. PYLORI*

For the diagnosis of *H. pylori*-associated gastritis, histologic staining and culturing of biopsy specimens has been considered the "gold standard."[13] Suitable specimens include gastric and duodenal biopsies. Specimens should be fresh and not delayed in transport for more than 3 hours. Specimens may be kept for up to 5 hours if stored at 4°C. Tissue should be kept moist by the addition of 2 mL or less of sterile isotonic saline.

ISOLATION PROCEDURE

Grinding of specimens in a ground-glass grinder yields heavier growth than mincing or rubbing the specimen onto an agar surface. Material should be inoculated onto a nonselective blood agar medium. At the University of Illinois Hospital Microbiology Laboratory, good growth has been obtained using Brucella, brain-heart infusion (BHI), and tryptic soy agar plates with 5% sheep or horse blood added. Poor growth is observed on commercially prepared chocolate agar plates and, therefore, this medium is not recommended. Because these bacteria are susceptible to cephalothin, *H. pylori* will not grow on Blaser's Campy-BAP or any selective medium containing cephalosporins. Many laboratories have had good results using modified Thayer-Martin agar as a selective medium for isolation of *H. pylori* in mixed cultures. Plates are incubated at 37°C in a humid, microaerophilic environment. Growth is usually observed in 3 to 5 days. Unpublished data from experiments conducted at the University of Illinois Hospital Microbiology Laboratory are shown in Table 6-8. Because of the potential hazard of using an anaerobic jar without a catalyst, we recommend the use of the Campy GasPak jar (column 2 in Table 6-8). Growth occurred in the Campy GasPak jar but not in the Poly Bag with Campy gas mixture (column 4 in Table 6-8), presumably because the water added in the former system provides the necessary humidity for growth.

IDENTIFICATION OF *H. PYLORI*

Colonies of *H. pylori* are small, gray, translucent, and weakly β-hemolytic. Gram stain reveals pale-staining, curved, gram-negative bacteria with characteristic gull-wing and "U" shapes. Presumptive identification can be made with positive reactions for oxidase and catalase and an extremely rapid (within minutes) urease reaction. Additional identifying characteristics are listed in Table 6-5.

BIOPSY UREASE TEST (CLO-TEST)

A more rapid but somewhat less sensitive and specific technique than the previously mentioned tests is the biopsy urease test (CLO-test). In this test, a medium containing urea and a pH-sensitive dye is inoculated with the mucosal biopsy specimen. If urease is present in the specimen, urea is split and ammonia causes a rise in pH and subsequent change in the color of the indicator. This test may produce false-negative results if only a small number of organisms are present or false-positive results if other urea-splitting organisms are present in the specimen.[186]

TABLE 6-8

COMPARISON OF CULTURE MEDIA AND ATMOSPHERIC CONDITIONS FOR GROWTH OF *HELICOBACTER PYLORI*

	CONDITIONS OF INCUBATION*				
AGAR MEDIA	*ANAEROBE JAR (NO CATALYST)*	*CAMPY GASPAK JAR*	*ANAEROBE JAR (CATALYST)*	*POLY BAG (CAMPY GAS MIXTURE)†*	*ATMOSPHERIC AIR WITH 5% CO₂*
Brucella with 5% sheep blood	Best growth β-hemolytic	Very good growth β-hemolytic	No growth	No growth	No growth
Tryptic soy with 5% sheep blood	Very good growth	Good growth	No growth	No growth	No growth
Brain–heart infusion with 5% horse blood	Very good growth	Good growth	No growth	No growth	No growth
Chocolate (Becton Dickinson Microbiology Systems, Cockeysville MD)	No growth	No growth	No growth	No growth	No growth
Chocolate (GIBCO)	Small colonies	Small colonies	No growth	No growth	No growth
Chocolate (freshly prepared)	Very small colonies	Very small colonies	No growth	No growth	No growth
Campy-BAP (Blaser's)	No growth	No growth	No growth	No growth	No growth

* All cultures were incubated at 37°C and read after 5 days.
† 5% O_2, 10% CO_2, 85% N_2
Data from K. Ristow, University of Illinois Hospital, Chicago IL, 1988

NONINVASIVE TESTS TO DIAGNOSE *H. PYLORI* INFECTION

H. pylori infection may be diagnosed by invasive assays that require endoscopy (culture, stain, PCR, CLO-test), or by noninvasive assays in which endoscopy is not necessary. Included in the latter category are the Urease Method and serology.

Urease Method. Two urease methods have been described. The first method, called the urea breath test, requires that the patient ingest ^{14}C-labeled urea dissolved in water, followed by collection of breath samples that are analyzed for the presence of $^{14}CO_2$ at 60 minutes. A second method utilizes radiolabelled urea containing ^{15}N.[134] After oral ingestion, radiolabelled urea is broken down into ammonia and carbon dioxide by *H. pylori* urease in the stomach. The ammonia is absorbed into the blood and excreted in the urine. The amount of [^{15}N]urea, reflecting the magnitude of *H. pylori* infection, is evaluated by measuring the abundance and excretion rate of ^{15}N in ammonia in the urine. The sensitivity of the $^{15}NH_4$ excretion test is reported to be 96% with 100% specificity when compared to patients who were *H. pylori* positive by culture and Gram stain.[134]

Serologic Methods. Serologic tests for detecting antibody to *H. pylori* have been used mainly for epidemiologic studies but can also be used to monitor the efficacy of treatment. The principle format is the ELISA test for the detection of IgG, although latex agglutination tests are available. IgA and IgM can also be detected but are less useful diagnostically. One inherent problem is attempting to establish a baseline for positivity since the prevalence of persons with elevated antibody titers is relatively high in certain populations. In an extensive study of Army recruits, Smoak et al.[249] found an overall positivity rate of 26.3%. This rate increased from 24.0% in the 17–18 age group to 43% in age group 24 to 26 years. Seropositivity for blacks was 44%, for hispanics 38%, and for whites 14%.

ACCURACY OF INVASIVE AND NONINVASIVE TESTS TO DIAGNOSE *H. PYLORI* INFECTION

Cutler and colleagues[58] evaluated the accuracy of several tests for determining *H. pylori* infection including the urea breath test (UBT), measurement of serum IgG and IgA antibody levels, and antral biopsy specimens for CLO test, histology, and Warthin-Starry stain. They found that the Warthin-Starry stain had the best sensitivity and specificity, although the CLO-test, UBT, and IgG levels were not statistically different in determining the correct diagnosis. They concluded that the noninvasive UBT and IgG serology tests are as accurate in predicting *H. pylori* status in untreated patients as the invasive tests of CLO and Warthin-Starry. The absence of chronic antral inflammation accurately excludes *H. pylori* infection.[58]

PART 2: THE FAMILIES *VIBRIONACEAE* AND "*AEROMONADACEAE*"

PHYLOGENY OF THE *VIBRIONACEAE*

The name *Vibrionaceae* was originally proposed by Veron in 1965 with the intent of grouping a number of nonenteric, fermentative, gram-negative rods that were oxidase positive and motile by means of polar flagella. This grouping was intended as a convenience for the purpose of differentiating these organisms from the *Enterobacteriaceae* and did not necessarily imply a taxonomic relationship among the included species. The *Vibrionaceae*, as presently defined in *Bergey's Manual of Systematic Bacteriology*,[15] includes the following genera: *Vibrio* (27 species), *Aeromonas* (four species), *Photobacterium* (three species), and *Plesiomonas* (one species). However, in the past decade a variety of methods for nucleic acid analysis have revolutionized microbial taxonomy and have resulted in the restructuring of this family along phylogenetic lines and the establishment of two new genera, *Listonella* and *Shewanella*, and a new family, *Aeromonadaceae*.[56,179,237] The correct phylogenic placement of the genus *Plesiomonas* remains unresolved at this time.

GENUS *VIBRIO*

Vibrio species have both historical and contemporary interest. *V. cholerae* is the etiologic agent of Asiatic cholera in humans, a potentially severe diarrheal disease that has been the scourge of humanity for centuries. The organism was first described and named by Pacini in 1854; 32 years later Koch isolated the organism, which he called "Kommabacillus" because of the characteristic curved or comma-shaped appearance of the individual bacterial cells.

Since the first pandemic in 1816 to 1817, six others have followed at about 10- to 15-year intervals through 1889; the latest occurred in 1961, involving the El Tor strain, to be discussed in a later section of this chapter. In 1989, 48,403 cases of cholera were reported to the World Health Organization from 35 countries, reflecting the widespread nature of the current pandemic.[43] In addition, a number of minor epidemics of diarrheal syndromes and extraintestinal infections caused by non-01 serogroups of *V. cholerae* and by several newly described halophilic species have been reported in the United States in several Gulf Coast states since the early 1970s.[125,141] Most infections have occurred following ingestion of contaminated and poorly cooked seafood. Wound infections have also been reported following trauma while swimming or working in infected waters or on exposure to marine animals.[125]

The point of this discussion is that clinical microbiologists cannot discount *Vibrio* species as a possible isolate from diarrheal stool specimens and must remain informed on how to recover and identify the various species. Those working in inland laboratories will have fewer potential encounters than those working in the Gulf Coast hospitals; nevertheless, with open world travel and shipping of seafoods to inland markets, everyone must remain alert.

TAXONOMY

The strains of *Vibrio cholerae* that have been recovered from classic cases of pandemic cholera agglutinate in what has been designated 01 antiserum. Strains not agglutinating in this antiserum are called either non-01 *V. cholerae* (if this species is determined biochemically) or a variety of other vibrio species names, such as *V. parahemolyticus*, *V. mimicus*, and so on. Since the non-01 species usually do not cause diarrheal syndromes as severe or potentially life threatening as 01 species, or more commonly may be associated with extraintestinal infections, early differentiation between the two groups can be of considerable clinical importance. Although 35 or more distinct *Vibrio* species have been identified, all but 11 are environmental organisms, called "marine vibrio species," and have not been associated with human infections.[132]

DESCRIPTION AND ASSOCIATED CLINICAL SYNDROMES OF *VIBRIO* SPECIES OF HUMAN IMPORTANCE

The species that are recovered from humans and potentially cause disease can be divided into two groups, namely, *Vibrio cholerae* and the non-cholera vibrios.

Vibrio cholerae. *Vibrio cholerae* is the etiologic agent of epidemic and pandemic cholera in humans. Within the species of *V. cholerae*, there is much dissimilarity among the strains in both their pathogenic and epidemic potential (Table 6-9). The strains can be divided according to differences in their cell wall composition (somatic O antigen), which forms the basis of the serotyping scheme that classifies the organisms into 139 different serogroups. All share a common flagellar (H) antigen. It was determined in the mid-1930s that all of the pandemic strains were agglutinated with a single antiserum that has been designated 01. The 01 type *V. cholerae* strains can be further separated into one of three serogroups: Inaba, Ogawa, and Hikojima. These serogroups are important for epidemiologic studies; for example, the current pandemic of cholera that began in Southeast Asia in 1961 is caused by the Ogawa serogroup. An endemic focus of cholera has been identified in the Gulf Coast region of the United States in association with a *V. cholerae* 01 Inaba serotype that is distinct from the current pandemic strain.[148] In January 1991, epidemic cholera appeared simultaneously in several coastal cites of Peru and has since been reported in Ecuador, Chile, Colombia, Brazil, and the United States. This outbreak is apparently also due to a strain other than the pandemic strain and has been identified as 01 serotype Inaba, biotype El Tor.[44]

TABLE 6-9

CHARACTERISTICS OF *VIBRIO CHOLERAE*

CLASSIFICATION METHOD	EPIDEMIC-ASSOCIATED	NOT EPIDEMIC-ASSOCIATED
Serogroups	01	Non 01 (serogroups 02-0138)*
Biotypes	Classical, El Tor	Biotypes not applicable to non-01 strains
Serotypes	Inaba, Ogawa, Hikojima	These three serotypes not applicable to non-01 strains
Toxin	Produce cholera toxin	Usually do not produce cholera toxin; sometimes produce other toxins*

* A new serogroup designated 0139 Bengal emerged in Calcutta, Bangladesh and parts of India in 1992 that produces cholera toxin in quantities similar to that produced by *V. cholerae* 01 and has spread in epidemic proportions across the Indian subcontinent.

Epidemic strains of serovar 01 may be further divided into the classic and El Tor biovars. El Tor is an actively hemolytic biotype of *V. cholerae* that was isolated at the El Tor Quarantine Station in Egypt. The El Tor strain has been found to be hardier and better capable of surviving in the environment; furthermore, chronic carriers of the El Tor strain have been reported in the literature.[146] The El Tor vibrio is now recognized as a biotype of *V. cholerae* and is responsible for most current epidemic outbreaks of classic cholera. The present pandemic of cholera that began in 1961 is caused by the El Tor biovar, as are the Gulf Coast and South American outbreaks. The classic biovar has almost disappeared except for rare isolations in India. Studies from Bangladesh indicate that the classic biotype has reemerged.[132]

CHOLERA: WORLD HISTORY. There have been seven pandemics of cholera in recorded history; the last three pandemics are known to be due to the *Vibrio cholerae* serogroup 01. The seventh pandemic of cholera, caused by the El Tor vibrio, originated in Clebes, Indonesia, in 1961 and spread worldwide over the last 35 years, reaching the South American continent in 1991. The emergence and rapid spread of cholera caused by a new serotype designated 0139 Bengal in October 1992 in nine countries (India, Bangladesh, Pakistan, Thailand, Nepal, Malaysia, Burma, Saudi Arabia, and China) suggests the possibility for the beginning of the eighth pandemic.[5a,180,261] For a synopsis of the cholera pandemics of the 19th and 20th centuries, the reader is referred to the review published by Lacey.[161]

TOXIGENIC *VIBRIO CHOLERAE* 0139 BENGAL. In October 1992, an epidemic of cholera-like illness began in Madras, India and spread to Calcutta and Bangladesh and many other places in India and in southeast Asia.[5a,196] The strain could not be identified as any of the 138 known types of *V. cholerae* and thus represents a new serogroup, 0139 (synonym Bengal to indicate its first isolation from the coastal areas of the Bay of Bengal).[5a] The strain is now associated with epidemic cholera-like illness along a 1000-mile coastline of the Bay of Bengal (from Madras, India, to Bangladesh) and appears to have largely replaced *V. cholerae* 01 strains in affected areas. The epidemic of *V. cholerae* 0139 has affected at least 11 countries in southern Asia. Specific totals for numbers of *V. cholerae* 0139 cases are unknown because affected countries do not report infections caused by 01 and 0139 separately; however, more than 100,000 cases of *V. cholerae* 0139 may have occurred. There are three important points to consider with regard to this new serotype: 1) the symptoms associated with *V. cholerae* 0139 infection suggest it is indistinguishable from cholera caused by *V. cholerae* 01 and should be treated with the same rapid fluid replacement, 2) the rapid spread of *V. cholerae* 0139 suggests that preexisting immunity to *V. cholerae* 01 offers little or no protective benefit, and travelers to affected areas should not assume that cholera vaccination is protective against the *V. cholerae* 0139 strain, and 3) laboratory identification methods for *V. cholerae* 01 depend on detection of the 01 antigen on the surface of the bacterium, and therefore do not identify this new strain.[46] The phenotypic, serologic, and toxigenic traits of *V. cholerae* 0139 Bengal have been reported by Nair and coworkers.[201]

CHOLERA: WESTERN HEMISPHERE. In January 1991, epidemic cholera, which had not been reported in South America in this century, appeared simultaneously in several coastal cities of Peru and rapidly spread throughout South and Central America.[104] Because of underreporting, the more than 1,000,000 cholera cases and 10,000 deaths (overall case-fatality rate: 0.9%) reported from Latin America through 1994 represent only a small fraction of the actual number of infections.[216] No cases of cholera have been reported from countries in the Caribbean; however, because all adjacent Latin American countries have been affected, spread to the Caribbean is likely to occur as the epidemic continues.

CHOLERA IN THE UNITED STATES. In 1973, the first case of cholera in the United States since 1911 was reported from Texas.[287] This was followed in 1978 by the report of 11 cases in Louisiana and in 1981 with two additional outbreaks in Texas involving 18 cases.[17] Crabs harvested from nearby estuaries were found to be the vehicle of infection in the Louisiana cases, while the largest of the two Texas outbreaks was traced to contamination of cooked rice following accidental rinsing with water from the environment containing the outbreak strain.[146] It is now known that 44 toxigenic *V. cholerae* 01 infections were acquired in the United States between 1973 and 1987.[132] All resulted from exposures in Louisiana and Texas near the Gulf Coast. In 1991, 26 cases of cholera were reported in the U.S.; 18 were linked to the South American outbreak.[45] In 1992,

103 cholera cases were reported in the U.S.; 75 were associated with an outbreak on board an Aerolineas Argentinas flight between Argentina and Los Angeles in February 1992. In 1993 and 1994, 22 and 47 cholera cases were reported in the U.S., respectively. Of these, 65 (94%) were associated with foreign travel. Three of these were culture-confirmed cases of *V. cholerae* 0139 in travelers to Asia.[47]

V. cholerae non-01 serotypes have been associated with isolated cases of diarrheal disease, although the majority of non-01 strains do not produce cholera toxin but appear to produce an enterotoxin different from cholera toxin. Strains have also been isolated from wounds and systemic infections. Safrin and coworkers,[239] in a review of cases of non-01 *V. cholerae* bacteremia, reported that the case-fatality rate for 13 cases in which the outcome was known was 61.5%. The majority of known cases have occurred in immunocompromised patients, particularly those with hematologic malignancy or cirrhosis. Pitrak and Gindorf[227] reported a case of bacteremic cellulitis caused by non-01 *V. cholerae* that was acquired in a freshwater inland lake in northern Illinois.

PATHOPHYSIOLOGY OF *VIBRIO CHOLERAE*-INDUCED GASTROENTERITIS. *V. cholerae* is the prototype of diarrheal syndromes in which disease is caused not by tissue invasion of microorganisms but through the production of toxins that interrupt normal intraintestinal exchanges of water and electrolytes. Toxigenic strains produce a toxin that binds to a receptor on the epithelial cell membrane and activates adenylate cyclase, causing increased levels of cyclic adenosine monophosphate (cAMP) and hypersecretion of salt and water, resulting in the characteristic "rice water" diarrhea of cholera. Box 6-6 provides a brief account of the step-by-step sequence for *V. cholerae*-induced gastroenteritis. Figure 6-1 is a schematic illustration of the mode of action of the cholera toxin. For a comprehensive review of cholera including pathogenesis and virulence factors, the reader is referred to the publication of Kaper and colleagues.[140]

TREATMENT AND PREVENTION OF *VIBRIO CHOLERAE* INFECTIONS. *V. cholerae* is rapidly killed by tetracycline; however, fluid secretion may persist for several hours after treatment from the effect of toxin already bound to the mucosal cells. Correction of fluid and electrolyte losses is essential with as much as 1 liter or more of fluid per hour required. Antibiotic therapy with trimethoprim-sulfamethoxazole or tetracycline will help shorten the duration of the diarrhea, however, strains of *V. cholerae* 0139 have been reported to be resistant to trimethoprim-sulfamethoxazole. The risk for cholera and traveler's diarrhea can be reduced by following the general rule **"boil it, cook it, peel it, or**

BOX 6-6. EVENTS LEADING TO *V. CHOLERAE*-INDUCED GASTROENTERITIS

1. Organisms ingested in contaminated water must first pass the highly acidic secretions in the stomach. An estimated 10^{10} organisms per milliliter are required to survive gastric passage in healthy persons; only about 100 organisms per milliliter are required in hypochlorhydric persons, either because of previous gastrectomy or from ingestion of antacids in treatment of gastric ulcer disease.

2. To cause disease, *V. cholerae* bacterial cells must adhere to the gastric and intestinal mucosal epithelial cells. These bacteria are motile and secrete mucin, two properties that aid in the penetration of the protective mucin layer that coats the surface of the gastroenteric mucosa. Bacterial attachment is a complex mechanism requiring the recognition by the bacterial cells of a surface marker on the epithelial cells to which they can bind.

3. *V. cholerae* produces an enterotoxin molecule composed of two subunits; an A (active) subunit and a B (binding) subunit. The A subunit is composed of two peptides: A_1 with toxin activity and A_2, which facilitates penetration of the A subunit into the cell. The B subunit binds the toxin molecule to cholera toxin specific G_{M1} ganglioside receptors on the intestinal epithelial cell membrane. There are five B subunits per toxin molecule, arranged in a ring around a central core that contains the enzyme A_1. Initial binding occurs rapidly, followed by a slow conformational change in the toxin molecule, leading to internalization of the A_1 enzyme into the host cell; thus, there is a short lag phase (15 to 60 minutes) between the time cholera-infected water is ingested and the onset of symptoms. Through a series of steps, A_1 catalyzes the ADP-ribosylation of the G_s (stimulatory) regulatory protein, locking it in the active state. The G_s protein acts to return adenylate cyclase from its inactive to active form, which in turn causes an intracellular rise in cyclic-AMP (cAMP; see Fig. 6-1).[190]

4. Cyclic AMP prevents the reabsorption of sodium ions across the brush-border membrane of the intestinal epithelial cell and the excretion of sodium bicarbonate and potassium into the bowel lumen. The intestinal chyle has high concentrations of sodium and chloride (isotonic), bicarbonate (twice that of plasma), and potassium (three to five times that of plasma). Water, therefore, is passively passed from the epithelial cells into the intestinal lumen in response to high osmotic pressure gradients, following the old adage, "where goes the sodium, there goes the water."

5. Thus, there is diffuse fluid secretion from the gut epithelial cells and the accumulation of large quantities of water in the intestinal lumen. The rate of fluid production increases between 3 and 10 hours after exposure. Fluid loss persists for up to 5 days in patients who receive no antibiotics, after which the bacterial cells are washed from the bowel by an unknown host mechanism. The result is varying degrees of dehydration and electrolyte imbalance that can lead to metabolic acidosis, hypokalemia, shock, and death in extreme cases.

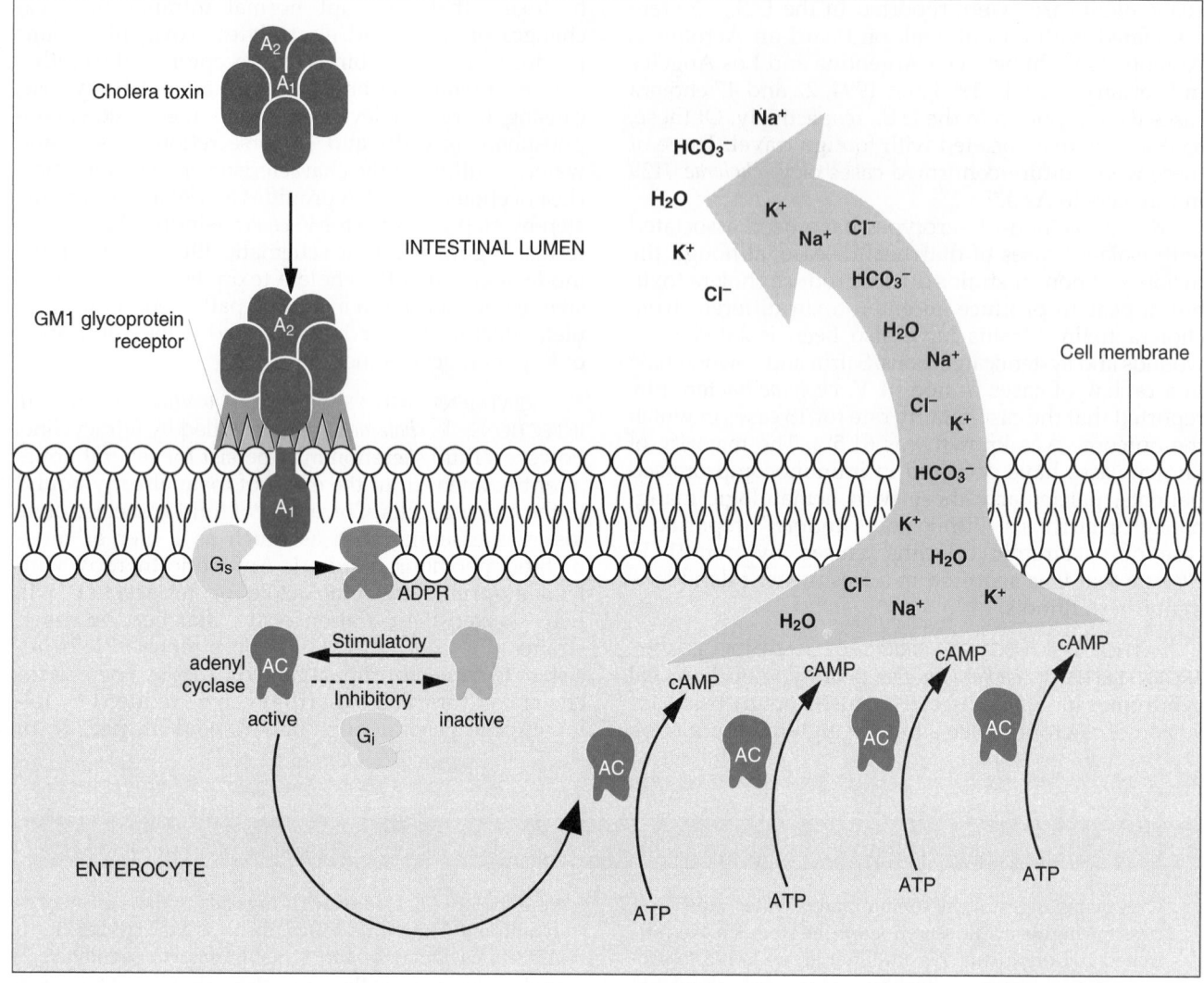

Figure 6-1
The action of cholera toxin (see Box 6-6 for details).

forget it." In particular, travelers should not consume 1) unboiled or untreated water and ice made from such water; 2) food and beverages from street vendors; 3) raw or partially cooked fish and shellfish, including ceviche; and 4) uncooked vegetables. Cold seafood salads may be particularly risky.

Non-Cholera Vibrios. Most cases of *Vibrio* infections in the United States have been caused by nonepidemic species other than *V. cholerae*. The natural habitat and geographic distribution, the culture media required for optimal recovery, the key biochemical reactions, and the clinical syndromes associated with the non-cholera species of human importance are listed in Table 6-10. The term *non-cholera* is probably a misnomer because many strains can cause severe diarrheal disease in addition to extraintestinal infections that can result in fatal septicemia. In most infections, symptoms are less severe and shorter in duration than is experienced in classic epidemic cholera.

Certain species of non-cholera vibrios can produce enterotoxins similar to those described for *V. cholerae*. In addition, some species cause invasive disease and more closely simulate *Shigella* dysentery; other species, *V. vulnificus* in particular, may invade the intestinal lymphatics and result in septicemia. Extraintestinal *Vibrio* infections are most commonly cutaneous wounds or otitis externa, where breaks in the skin have become contaminated while swimming or boating in infected marine waters or after handling contaminated raw seafood.[187,245] The following is a brief account of the microbiology and clinical syndromes associated with each of the non-cholera *Vibrio* species.

V. ALGINOLYTICUS. *V. alginolyticus* was originally classified as biotype 2 of *V. parahaemolyticus*. Most clinical isolates are recovered from superficial wounds[71,183,225,243] or the external ear.[106,132] Conjunctivitis,[174] acute gastroenteritis[231] and bacteremia[23,71,129] caused by *V. alginolyticus* have also been reported.

TABLE 6-10

CHARACTERISTICS OF CLINICALLY IMPORTANT *VIBRIO* SPECIES OTHER THAN *V. CHOLERAE*

SPECIES	NATURAL HABITAT, GEOGRAPHIC DISTRIBUTION; MODES OF HUMAN INFECTION	MEDIA FOR OPTIMAL GROWTH IN LABORATORY CULTURES	KEY BIOCHEMICAL REACTIONS		CLINICAL SYNDROMES
V. alginolyticus[132]	Habitat: Marine environment. Infection: Exposure of traumatized skin to seawater or infected animals	NaCl supplement needed for growth on nonselective media. Grows on blood agar and enteric media. Yellow colonies on thiosulfate citrate bile sucrose (TCBS) agar.	Lysine Arginine Voges-Proskauer 8%, NaCl 10% NaCl	+ − + + V	Associated with soft tissue infections; seems to also have an etiologic role in wound and ear infections.

V. damsela CDC Group EF-5 (transfer to genus *Photobacterium* proposed)[248]	Habitat: Marine environment. Infection: Exposure of broken skin or traumatic wounds to infected marine animals or contaminated seawater.	Requires 1% NaCl in nonselective culture media. Good growth on blood agar. Green colonies on TCBS agar. Optimum growth 25°C.	Arginine
			Voges-Proskauer
			Ferment:
			  Glucose
			  Mannitol
			  Galactose
			  Trehalose
				+
				+
				
				+
				−
				+
				+
					Associated with human wound infections.

V. fluvialis CDC group EF-6[263]	Habitat: Worldwide—endemic in Bangladesh. In United States—Gulf Coast, New York, and Pacific Northwest estuaries. Infection: Ingestion or contact with contaminated water.	Na⁺ supplement of culture media less critical than other halophilic *Vibrio* species. Yellow colonies on TCBS agar.	Arginine 6% NaCl Glucose (gas) Hydrolysis of esculin Aminovalerate Glutarate	+ + − − + −	Cholera-like gastroenteritis and diarrheal syndrome—watery diarrhea, vomiting, dehydration; probably enterotoxin induced.
V. furnissii[27]	Habitat: Endemic in the marine waters and estuaries in Asia. Infection: Ingestion or contact with contaminated water.	Na⁺ supplement for optimal growth in nonselective culture media. Yellow colonies on TCBS agar.	Glucose (gas) Hydrolysis of esculin Aminovalerate Glutarate	+ − − +	Isolated from patients with diarrhea and gastroenteritis, particularly tourists returning from Asia.
V. hollisae EF-13 and CDC enteric group 42[113, 230]	Habitat: Marine environment in Gulf Coast and Chesapeake Bay states. Infection: Consumption of raw seafood.	1%–2% NaCl supplement needed for growth. Poor growth on TCBS or MacConkey agars. Screen for oxidase-positive colonies on blood agar.	Indole Lysine Arginine Ornithine Motility (after 7 days) Urea	+ − − − − −	Isolated from patients with diarrhea and gastroenteritis. Invasion of bloodstream reported in persons with liver abnormalities.
V. metschnikovii CDC enteric group 16[74]	Habitat: Worldwide in fresh and brackish marine waters, rivers, sewage; also in shrimp, crabs, and lobsters. Infection: Cause of fowl cholera; exposure or ingestion of contaminated water or animals.	Grows well on most laboratory isolation media. Sodium supplement not as critical as other halophilic vibrios. Yellow colonies on TCBS agar.	Oxidase Nitrate Voges-Proskauer	− − +	Associated with rare and isolated cases of human infections: septicemia, urinary tract infections, wounds, peritonitis.

(Continued)

TABLE 6-10 *(Continued)*
CHARACTERISTICS OF CLINICALLY IMPORTANT *VIBRIO* SPECIES OTHER THAN *V. CHOLERAE*

SPECIES	NATURAL HABITAT, GEOGRAPHIC DISTRIBUTION; MODES OF HUMAN INFECTION	MEDIA FOR OPTIMAL GROWTH IN LABORATORY CULTURES	KEY BIOCHEMICAL REACTIONS		CLINICAL SYNDROMES
V. mimicus[59, 245]	Habitat: Coastal waters, and oysters and shrimp. Infection: Ingestion of undercooked seafood (particularly oysters).	Grows on enteric isolation media. Green colonies on TCBS.	Sucrose Mannitol Ornithine Lipase Voges-Proskauer Polymyxin	− + + V − S	Diarrheal syndrome related to production of heat-labile and heat-stable toxins; also swimmer's ear infections.
V. parahaemolyticus[132]	Habitat: Worldwide distribution in fresh and sea waters. Endemic in Japan. Infection: Ingestion of contaminated seafood—raw fish and shellfish.	Growth slow on nonselective media. Screen for oxidase-positive colonies on blood agar. Green colonies on TCBS agar.	Lysine Arginine Voges-Proskauer Lactose Salicin Urease Indole	+ − − − − V +	Acute gastroenteritis— nausea, vomiting, abdominal cramps, fever, chills. Positive Kanagawa test. Extraintestinal: wounds and septicemia.
V. vulnificus (Lactose-positive *Vibrio*) CDC group EF-3[73]	Habitat: Coastal water and estuaries. Infection: Ingestion of raw oysters; exposure of traumatic wounds to infected marine animals or contaminated water.	1% NaCl needed for growth. Growth good on blood agar. Green (85%) or yellow (15%) colonies on TCBS agar.	Lactose Lysine Arginine Salicin	+ + − +	Life-threatening septicemia; 50% fatality rate. High association with preexistent liver disease. Wounds are painful, with skin and muscle necrosis.

S, susceptible, 90% or greater; V, variable, 11%–89%; +, positive, 90% or greater; −, negative, 90% or greater negative

V. CARCHARIAE. *V. carchariae* is a pathogen of sharks, but has been reported in one case of human wound infection in an 11-year-old girl who was attacked by a shark while wading in knee-deep water off the South Carolina coast.[222] *V. carchariae* can be differentiated from biochemically similar species (*V. alginolyticus*, *V. parahaemolyticus*, *V. vulnificus*) by negative gelatin hydrolysis at 22°C, negative motility at 36°C, and negative ornithine decarboxylase reaction. The other species have the opposite reactions.[147]

V. CINCINNATIENSIS. The only report of human infection by this *Vibrio* species is the recovery from blood and cerebrospinal fluid of a 70-year-old patient with bacteremia and meningitis.[25] The patient was treated with ampicillin (day 1) and moxalactam for 9 days, followed by an uneventful recovery.

V. DAMSELA (PHOTOBACTERIUM DAMSELA). *V. damsela* was formerly called CDC Group EF-5. It has been reported as the cause of human wound infections, primarily after exposure to saltwater.[54,121,197] Most strains are resistant to penicillin and sensitive to gentamicin, chloramphenicol, and tetracycline. MacDonell and Colwell[179] proposed transfer of *V. damsela* to the genus *Listonella*. Subsequently, Smith and colleagues proposed that *L. damsela* should be reassigned to the genus *Photobacterium*.[248]

V. FLUVIALIS. Formerly designated as CDC Group EF-6, *V. fluvialis* has been isolated from humans with diarrhea. This species was isolated from fecal cultures of more than 500 patients with diarrhea at the Cholera Research Laboratory in Bangladesh during a 9-month period in 1976–1977.[126] In the United States, the organism has been isolated from a wound of a patient in Hawaii, from water and sediment in the New York Bay, from shellfish in Louisiana, from water and shellfish in Pacific Northwest estuaries, from an 81-year-old man from Laredo, Texas, with diarrheal illness,[263] from the stool of a 1-month old infant,[114] and from the stool of a 43-year-old man with a history of AIDS.[119]

V. FURNISSII. Formerly designated *V. fluvialis* biogroup 2, *V. furnissii* has been isolated from patients with acute gastroenteritis in at least two outbreaks of food poisoning[27] and from the stool of a 1-month old infant.[114]

V. HOLLISAE. Formerly designated CDC Group EF-13, *V. hollisae* has most commonly been isolated from stool specimens of persons with diarrhea and a history of eating raw seafood.[2,113,197] Diarrhea, abdominal pain, and leukocytosis were common symptoms. Rare cases of systemic infection caused by *V. hollisae* have been described and most often involve bacterial sepsis in persons with underlying immune deficiencies.[176,230]

Evidence suggests that *V. hollisae* may share with *V. vulnificus* a predilection for bloodstream invasion in persons with liver abnormalities.[230]

V. METSCHNIKOVII. *V. metschnikovii,* formerly CDC Enteric Group 16, is often isolated from the environment but rarely isolated from human clinical specimens. The first documented case of human infection, was from the blood of a patient with cholecystitis at Cook County Hospital in Chicago.[133] More recently, Hansen and colleagues reported two cases of *V. metschnikovii* septicemia: one fatal case involving a patient with liver cirrhosis, renal insufficiency, and diabetes; and another in an 82-year-old woman with respiratory problems and an infected leg lesion, who was treated successfully.[107] Human isolates referred to the CDC for identification include two isolates from urine and four isolates from unknown sources.[74]

V. MIMICUS. Formerly classified as sucrose-negative *V. cholerae, V. mimicus* has been isolated from shellfish and water as well as from human diarrheal stools and ear infections.[59,245]

V. PARAHAEMOLYTICUS. *V. parahaemolyticus* causes gastroenteritis in humans following ingestion of contaminated seafood, the mechanism of which has not been elucidated. Symptoms include watery and sometimes bloody diarrhea, abdominal cramps, nausea, vomiting, headache, low-grade fever, and chills. The illness is usually mild to moderate and self-limiting, with a duration of 2 to 3 days. Extraintestinal infections by *V. parahaemolyticus* have also been reported, mostly from wounds. A urea-positive biotype has appeared and has been the cause of several recent outbreaks, often associated with ingestion of contaminated raw oysters.[3,162,207,209] Janda and associates[132] reveal that 70% of the *V. parahaemolyticus* cultures submitted for identification to the Microbial Diseases Laboratory in the Berkeley, California, Department of Health Laboratory were urease positive. Similar findings have been reported in the Pacific Northwest.[149]

More than 95% of *V. parahaemolyticus* strains that have been isolated from patients with diarrhea are Kanagawa positive; that is, they hemolyze human erythrocytes on Wagatsuma agar.[139] The hemolysin is both cytotoxic and cardiotoxic. Only about 1% of strains isolated from marine environments are Kanagawa positive.[132] The implication is that Kanagawa hemolysin activity is associated with the pathogenesis of *V. parahaemolyticus* gastroenteritis. However, the association of Kanagawa hemolysin with pathogenesis has never been proven, and in fact Honda and coworkers[124] report that 11 of 12 *V. parahaemolyticus* isolates recovered from patients in a 1985 gastroenteritis outbreak in the Maldives were Kanagawa negative.

Rehydration is usually the only treatment required.

V. VULNIFICUS. Formerly CDC Group EF-3, *V. vulnificus* was first termed *lactose-positive Vibrio* by Hollis and coworkers in 1976.[121] *V. vulnificus* is a particularly virulent species associated with wound infections after exposure to contaminated sea water and primary septicemias and death following consumption of contam-

inated seafood (usually raw oysters).[48] A high fatality rate (40%–60%) is associated with septic infections.[132] The organisms reach the bloodstream by invading the intestinal mucosa. Patients with hepatic disease are particularly susceptible to septicemia.[18,73,262] One case of *V. vulnificus* infection was seen at the University of Illinois Hospital in July 1983, in a 73-year-old female with gastrointestinal bleeding. The organism was recovered from the patient's blood and pleural fluid.

Medical conditions that predispose to *V. vulnificus* bacteremia include liver dysfunction and syndromes leading to increased iron deposition: chronic cirrhosis, hepatitis, thalassemia major, hemochromatosis, and a history of heavy alcohol consumption.[132] The chief symptoms associated with sepsis are fever, chills, and vomiting, which begin about 38 hours after ingesting raw oysters. Diarrhea often is not a component of the syndrome.[132]

METHODS FOR LABORATORY ISOLATION OF *VIBRIOS*

In discussing the laboratory approach to the isolation of *Vibrio* species from clinical specimens, Farmer and colleagues[75] suggest one of the following:

1. Use normal procedures and make no specific effort to search for *Vibrio* species.
2. Use normal procedures and plating media, and look for oxidase-positive colonies.
3. Incorporate thiosulfate citrate bile sucrose (TCBS) agar as an extra plate for stool cultures and also for other likely specimens such as those from wounds, blood, eye, and ear.
4. Use other special procedures to enhance the isolation of *V. cholerae, V. parahaemolyticus,* and other *Vibrio* species.

For laboratories in the American Midwest, where positive cultures for *Vibrio* species may be few, Farmer and colleagues suggest that the first or second approaches may be most appropriate. In laboratories near oceans, particularly those located in endemic areas, the third or fourth approach is indicated. They mention several disadvantages to the routine use of TCBS agar, in addition to the increased cost for a relatively low return. Some *Vibrio* species or strains may not grow well on TCBS agar; also, Kelly did not recover any isolates of *Vibrio* species on TCBS agar during an 18-month study that did not also grow on routine media (screened for oxidase-positive colonies).[75] Our experience supports this finding—we isolated a 01 strain of *V. cholerae* from a patient just returning from a trip to India, where she had been exposed to contaminated water in an endemic area following a typhoon. No special media or enrichment broths were needed to recover good growth in this case, although the organism load was heavy. In less fulminant cases when the concentration of organisms may be low, it is helpful for laboratory personnel to be informed when clinical cases of cholera or extra-intestinal *Vibrio* infections are suspected. In these cases, the use of a selective medium or alkaline broth enrichment, to be discussed in a later section, may still be in order.

Specimen Collection, Processing, and Media Selection.
Laboratory personnel should be notified if the physician suspects a cholera syndrome or extraintestinal infections with *Vibrio* species. Specimens should be collected as early in the disease as possible. In the acute diarrheal stages of disease, specimens may be collected from the rectum with a soft rubber catheter or a rectal swab or from a small portion of the passed liquid stool. Culturing of vomitus also may be productive of organisms, particularly in the early stages of disease.

Specimens should be transported in closed containers to preserve moisture and transferred to culture media as soon as possible. *Vibrio* species are generally quite sensitive to drying, exposure to sunlight, and the development of an acid pH. They also are easily inhibited by the normal intestinal flora or contaminating organisms. If cultures cannot be set up immediately, *Vibrio* species will remain viable in Cary-Blair semisolid transport medium for an extended time. The use of buffered glycerol saline transport medium should be avoided. If a transport medium is not available, a 2 × ½-inch strip of thick blotting paper can be soaked in the fecal specimen, placed in a sealed plastic bag, and then mailed to the nearest reference laboratory.[147] Specimens suspicious for harboring *Vibrio* species should be inoculated to 5% sheep blood and MacConkey agar. Whether to also inoculate a plate of TCBS agar and/or a tube of alkaline peptone water enrichment must be determined by each laboratory supervisor depending on the prevalence of *Vibrio*-related diseases in any given locale. If TCBS agar is not used, hemolytic colonies that appear on sheep blood agar after overnight incubation should be tested for cytochrome oxidase activity. Either representative colonies can be individually touched and spot tested for the oxidase reaction using Kovac's reagent or one or two drops of Kovac's reagent can be dropped in an area on the surface of the plate where suspicious colonies are present. The rapid development of a blue color is indicative of a positive test. Oxidase-positive colonies can be transferred to TCBS agar for further species identification using biochemical and other characteristics.

Alkaline peptone water (APW) enrichment broths should be subcultured to TCBS agar for further evaluation of colonies that grow after an additional 24 to 48 hours of incubation. APW, which contains 1% peptone and 1% NaCl at pH 8.6, is a simple-to-use enrichment broth that can be recommended in situations where low concentrations of organisms in the specimen are anticipated (*eg*, in convalescent stages of disease). The high pH of the medium serves to suppress the growth of many commensal intestinal bacteria while allowing uninhibited multiplication of *V. cholerae*. Subcultures to TCBS or gelatin agar should be made within 12 to 18 hours since other organisms can begin to overgrow the broth after prolonged incubation. APW is also an excellent transport medium if specimens cannot be immediately delivered to the laboratory for processing. It is recommended that about 1 mL of liquid or 1 gram of formed stool be placed into 10 mL of APW in a screw-capped tube; alternatively, rectal swabs can be placed into a tube containing 1 to 2 ml of APW.[147]

Presumptive Identification of *Vibrio* species Based on Colonial and Microscopic Morphology. Vibrios grow readily on most isolation media; growth of all species is enhanced by adding 1% NaCl to the medium. Colonies are typically smooth, convex, creamy in consistency, and gray-white and have entire margins. Rough colonies are occasionally encountered that adhere to the agar. Certain marine vibrios are able to swarm on the surface of agar media, associated with the formation of long cells with lateral flagella. This phenomenon is not seen with most human isolates.

Microscopically, straight or curved gram-negative bacilli are observed (see Color Plate 6-2D). The curved character of the cells may be best seen in early stationary phase in broth cultures; in log phase, straight and rounded coccoid forms are intermixed. Although a presumptive diagnosis of cholera can be made by observing large numbers of curved bacilli in direct gram-stained stool specimens, recovery of the organism in culture is needed to make a definitive identification.

The differential reactions on TCBS agar are helpful in making a presumptive identification of *V. cholerae*, *V. alginolyticus*, *V. parahaemolyticus*, and *V. vulnificus*. After 18 to 24 hours of incubation on TCBS agar, *V. cholerae* grow as smooth, yellow colonies, 2 to 4 mm in diameter with an opaque center and transparent periphery (see Color Plate 6-2A). The colonies of *V. alginolyticus*, which also ferment sucrose, will also produce yellow colonies on TCBS agar; *V. parahaemolyticus* and *V. vulnificus*, which do not utilize sucrose, produce blue-green colonies (see Color Plate 6-2B). On gelatin agar, *V. cholerae* grow as transparent colonies surrounded by an opaque halo indicating liquefaction of gelatin (see Color Plate 6-2C). O'Brien and Colwell have described a modified taurocholate-tellurite gelatin agar for the differentiation of *V. cholerae* (β-galactose positive) versus *V. parahaemolyticus* (β-galactose negative) based on the hydrolysis of 4-methylumbelliferyl-β-D-galactose, in addition to determination of gelatin hydrolysis and tellurite reduction.[210]

BIOCHEMICAL CHARACTERIZATION AND LABORATORY IDENTIFICATION OF *VIBRIO* SPECIES

Members of the genus *Vibrio* are facultative anaerobes capable of both respiratory and fermentative metabolism. However, because they grow and react in carbohydrate test media designed for fermentative metabolism, they are classified with the fermenters. The natural habitat for *Vibrio* species is aquatic, in both fresh and salt water. The growth and biochemical reactivity of most species are enhanced in differential test media supplemented with 1% to 2% sodium chloride.

Most *Vibrio* species produce cytochrome oxidase, a characteristic that separates them from the Enterobacteriaceae. Therefore, *Vibrio* species are included in the group of oxidase-positive fermenters—*Aeromonas* species, *Plesiomonas* species, and *Chromobacterium* species—from which they must be differentiated (Table 6-11). Since *V. cholerae* ferments glucose, an acid-deep/alkaline-slant reaction is seen on Kligler iron agar. Since sucrose is also fermented, an acid-

TABLE 6-II

OXIDASE-POSITIVE, FERMENTATIVE, GRAM-NEGATIVE BACILLI: DIFFERENTIAL CHARACTERISTICS OF AEROMONAS HYDROPHILA, PLESIOMONAS SHIGELLOIDES, CHROMOBACTERIUM VIOLACEUM, AND VIBRIO CHOLERAE

CHARACTERISTIC	A. HYDROPHILA	P. SHIGELLOIDES	C. VIOLACEUM	V. CHOLERAE
Kligler iron agar (slant/deep/hydrogen sulfide)	K/A/−	K − A/A/−	K/A/−	K/A/−
Catalase	+	+	+	+
Esculin	+	−		
Motility	+	+	+	+
ONPG	+	+	−	+
Indole	+	+	−	+
Voges-Proskauer	(+)	−	−	(−)
Lysine decarboxylase	+	+	−	+
Ornithine decarboxylase	−	+	−	+
Carbohydrates				
Lactose	(−)	(+)	−	−
Sucrose	+	−	(−)	+
Mannitol	+	−	−	+
Inositol	−	+	−	−
Growth in peptone, 1% with				
0% NaCL	+	+	+	+
7% NaCL	−	−	−	−
11% NaCL	−	−	−	−

+, 90% or more of strains are positive; (+), 51%–89% of strains are positive; (−), 10%–50% of strains are positive; −, less than 10% of strains are positive; V, variable; K/A, alkaline/acid; K − A/A, alkaline to acid/acid; ONPG, o-nitrophenyl-β-D-galactopyranoside.

deep/acid slant reaction is seen on triple sugar iron agar. *V. cholerae* produces both lysine and ornithine decarboxylases.

Those laboratory workers who use lysine iron agar to screen stool isolates will note that *V. cholerae, A. hydrophila,* and *P. shigelloides* all produce a purple slant/purple deep reaction because of the decarboxylation of lysine. Arginine can be used to separate *V. cholerae* (negative) from both *Aeromonas* and *Plesiomonas* (positive). Most strains of *A. hydrophila* hydrolyze esculin, differentiating it from the other organisms included in Table 6-11. Differences in the utilization of lactose, sucrose, mannitol, and inositol also serve to differentiate these genera.

V. cholerae, including the El Tor biotype, can be distinguished from other *Vibrio* species by the ability to produce a positive string test (see Color Plate 6-2*E*). To perform this test, bacterial colonies are mixed with a few drops of 0.5% sodium deoxycholate on a glass slide. An inoculating loop is immersed into the mixture and pulled away from the drop. *V. cholerae* pro-

duces a long string that becomes more tenacious after 60 seconds or more (other vibrios may give an initial string reaction that diminishes or disappears 45 to 60 seconds later). A positive slide agglutination with polyvalent O antiserum is also helpful in differentiating *V. cholerae* from other closely related strains (see Color Plate 6-2*F*). The El Tor biotype can be distinguished from classic strains of *V. cholerae* by several characteristics (Table 6-12). El Tor strains are actively β-hemolytic on blood agar (see Color Plate 6-2*G*) and are capable of agglutinating chicken erythrocytes (see Color Plate 6-2*H*). The chicken erythrocytes test is performed by mixing a loopful of washed chicken erythrocytes (2.5% suspension in saline) with bacterial cells from a pure culture to be tested. Visible clumping of the erythrocytes indicates the El Tor biotype, in contrast to classic 01 strains of *V. cholerae* that do not have this property. Classic strains of *V. cholerae* are susceptible to 50 IU of polymyxin B in the disk diffusion test; El Tor strains are resistant. El Tor strains also are Voges-Proskauer positive, whereas classic strains of

TABLE 6-12
DIFFERENTIATION BETWEEN *VIBRIO CHOLERAE* BIOTYPES

TEST	CLASSIC	EL TOR
String test	+	+
β-Hemolytic on sheep blood agar	−	+
CAMP test	−	+
Voges-Proskauer test	−	+
Chicken red blood cell agglutination	−	+
Susceptibility to 50 U polymyxin B	S	R
Phage IV susceptibility	S	R

+, positive test; −, negative test; S, susceptible; R, resistant.

V. cholerae are Voges-Proskauer negative. Lesmana and coworkers recently described using a modified CAMP test to differentiate the classical biotype (CAMP negative) from the EL Tor biotype (CAMP strong positive).[173] *V. cholerae* 0139 strains also demonstrate a strong positive CAMP reaction, whereas non-01 and non-0139 isolates give a weak positive CAMP reaction. The test is performed by inoculating a beta-lysin-producing *S. aureus* strain (ATCC 25178) onto a 5% sheep blood agar plate by making a single straight line streak and then inoculating the *Vibrio* species to be tested in a line perpendicular to and a few millimeters from the *S. aureus* streak. Plates are incubated in a candle jar at 37°C for 18 to 20 hours and observed for zones of synergistic hemolysis (see Chart 7). For laboratories capable of performing phage IV susceptibility tests, El Tor strains are resistant to this phage.

As an initial first step in the identification of *Vibrio* species, Kelly and colleagues[147] have devised a dichotomous scheme for separating the *Vibrio* species into six groups based on their reactions with seven tests: requirement for 1% NaCl for growth in nutrient broth, oxidase production, reduction of nitrate to nitrite, *myo*-inositol fermentation, and production of arginine dihydrolase, lysine decarboxylase, and ornithine decarboxylase. Their scheme is reproduced in Table 6-13. Grouping the species this way will provide simple presumptive identification of most clinical isolates. Additional key reactions and clinical correlation can be obtained by consulting Table 6-10. Overman and associates[215] recommend the use of the API 20E strip for performing the biochemical tests necessary to make identifications of the more commonly encountered members of the *Vibrionaceae*.

GENERA *LISTONELLA, PHOTOBACTERIUM* AND *SHEWANELLA*

MacDonell and Colwell[179] have proposed restructuring of the *Vibrionaceae* to include the establishment of two new genera, *Listonella* and *Shewanella*, within the family. Through rather complex 5S rRNA ribonucleotide sequencing studies and cluster analysis, these authors conclude that several *Vibrio* species, notably *V. anguil-*

larum, V. pelagius, and *V. damsela* should be transferred to a proposed new genus *Listonella* as *L. anguillara, L. damsela,* and *L. pelagia.* They also conclude from these studies that *Alteromonas (Pseudomonas) putrefaciens* and *Alteromonas hanedai* should comprise the new genus *Shewanella* along with a proposed new species, *Shewanella benthica.* Subsequent to the work of MacDonnell and Colwell, Smith and colleagues proposed that *L. damsela* be reassigned to the genus *Photobacterium* as *P. damsela* based on phenotypic data.[248] Members of the genera *Listonella, Photobacterium,* and *Shewanella* are associated with marine environment and are pathogenic for fish.

Members of the genus *Shewanella* (notably *S. putrefaciens*) are straight or curved, gram-negative bacilli, motile by means of a single polar flagellum. Characteristic colonies are dome-shaped, circular, slightly viscous or mucoid, and usually red-brown or salmon-pink. They possess cytochrome oxidase activity and produce abundant hydrogen sulfide in Kligler iron agar. Nitrates are reduced to nitrites and gelatinase, ornithine decarboxylase, and DNase tests are positive. *S. putrefaciens* has been recovered from human clinical specimens and is discussed in detail in Chapter 5 of this text.

AEROMONAS AND PLESIOMONAS

In *Bergey's Manual of Systematic Bacteriology*, *Aeromonas* species are included along with *Vibrio* species and *Plesiomonas shigelloides* in the *Vibrionaceae*.[15] However, based on molecular genetic evidence, MacDonell and Colwell[56,179] have proposed the removal of *Aeromonas* species and placement in a separate family, *Aeromonadaceae*, and the removal of *Plesiomonas* to the genus *Proteus*. Phenotypic differences between *Vibrio, Aeromonas,* and *Plesiomonas* species are listed in Table 6-11.[96]

GENUS *AEROMONAS*

As the species name hydrophila ("water loving") indicates, the natural habitat of *Aeromonas* species is fresh or sea water, where they commonly cause infectious diseases in cold-blooded aquatic animals. These bacteria also reside in sink traps and drainpipes and can be recovered from tap water faucets and distilled water supplies, which are potential sources of organisms involved in nosocomial infections.

TAXONOMY

The genus *Aeromonas* consists of a large number of distinct taxa that includes at least 12 legitimate species, several other species of questionable validity,[55] and a number of unnamed hybridization groups (HG) or clusters (HG2, HG11, *Aeromonas* group 501).[1] Currently, 13 DNA hybridization groups (also called genomospecies) are recognized within the genus *Aeromonas*. However, since there is a lack of phenotypic characteristics that correlate with each specific genomospecies, some of the DNA hybridization groups

TABLE 6-13
Eight Key Differential Tests to Divide the 12 Clinically Significant *Vibrio* Species Into Six Groups

REACTIONS OF THE SPECIES IN:

	GROUP 1		GROUP 2	GROUP 3	GROUP 4	GROUP 5			GROUP 6			
Test	*V. cholerae*	*V. mimicus*	*V. metschnikovii*	*V. cincinnatiensis*	*V. hollisae*	*V. damsela*	*V. fluvialis*	*V. furnissii*	*V. alginolyticus*	*V. parahaemolyticus*	*V. vulnificus*	*V. carchariae*
Growth in nutrient broth:												
With no NaCl added	+	+	–	–	–	–	–	–	–	–	–	–
With 1% NaCl added	+	+	+	+	+	+	+	+	+	+	+	+
Oxidase	+	+	–	+	+	+	+	+	+	+	+	+
Nitrate → nitrite	+	+	–	+	+	+	+	+	+	+	+	+
myo-Inositol fermentation	–	–	V	+	–	–	–	–	–	–	–	–
Arginine dihydrolase	–	–	V	–	–	+	+	+	–	–	–	–
Lysine decarboxylase	+	+	V	V	–	V	–	–	+	+	+	+
Ornithine decarboxylase	+	+	–	–	–	–	–	–	V	+	V	–

All data are for reactions within 2 days at 35°C to 37°C: +, most strains (generally 90%–100%) are positive; –, most strains are negative (generally 0–10% positive); V, between 10%–89% are positive. Key test results are boxed.
From Kelly MT, Hickman-Brenner FW, Farmer JJ III: *Vibrio*. In Balows A (ed): Manual of Clinical Microbiology, 5th ed, pp 384–395. Washington DC, American Society for Microbiology, 1991

cannot be phenotypically separated and, therefore, some of the groups have not yet been named. The currently recognized species and the various DNA hybridization groups are summarized in Table 6-14. As it currently stands, the genus *Aeromonas* consists of ten named species, which can be grouped into two subdivisions (Box 6-7).

CLINICAL SIGNIFICANCE

A. salmonicida, the only member of the psychrophilic group, has not been recovered from humans,[281] whereas, the mesophilic group of motile species are considered to be potential human pathogens. Four categories of human infections have been described by von Graevenitz[281] (Box 6-8).

Janda and others[127a,131] have reviewed the infectious disease spectrum of *Aeromonas* species and concluded that there is strong evidence supporting *Aeromonas* species as a causative agent of diarrhea, although the data are not absolute. On one hand, they cite several reports indicating that there is little significant difference between symptomatic and asymptomatic persons who harbor *Aeromonas* species in their stools.[80,122,271] Other groups, on the other hand, cite data linking *Aeromonas* species with gastroenteritis.[31,101] Watson and associates[286] proposed that the virulence factors of *Aeromonas* species that cause intestinal infections are similar to those of other enteric pathogens, that is, adherence of bacterial cells to intestinal mucosa, toxin production and mucosal invasion. About 20% of their

patients with intestinal infections from *Aeromonas* species had symptoms of dysentery similar to those caused by *Shigella* species and by invasive strains of *Campylobacter jejuni*. Most of the invasive strains included in their study, as determined by invasiveness in cell culture, were *A. sobria*; a minority were *A. hydrophila*. The majority of *A. sobria* and *A. hydrophila* produce a cholera-like extractable toxin (Asao toxin) that causes watery diarrhea.[50,208] The previous notion

---

BOX 6-7. *AEROMONAS* SUBDIVISIONS

1. Psychrophilic group: *A. salmonicida*. The only species in this group, *A. salmonicida*, is a fish pathogen. It is nonmotile, does not grow at 37°C and, therefore, is not important in clinical microbiology.

2. Mesophilic group: *A. hydrophila* group. Members of this group grow at 37°C and are motile. This group comprises 12 DNA hybridization groups and includes several named species. It can be divided into three principal phenotypic groups (called phenons) which are equivalent to the species *A. hydrophila*, *A. caviae*, and *A. sobria*, as shown in Table 6-14.

TABLE 6-14

PHENOTYPIC GROUPING OF CURRENTLY RECOGNIZED SPECIES AND KNOWN DNA HYBRIDIZATION GROUPS IN THE GENUS *AEROMONAS*

DNA HYBRIDIZATION GROUP (GENOSPECIES)	PHENOTYPIC GROUP (PHENONS)	NAMED SPECIES
1	*A. hydrophila*	*A. hydrophila*
2		Unnamed
3		*A. salmonicida*
4	*A. caviae*	*A. caviae (A. punctata)**
5A		*A. media*
5B		*A. media*
6		*A. eucrenophila*
7	*A. sobria*	*A. sobria*
8/10†		*A. veronii* biotype *sobria*
9		*A. jandaei*
10/8†		*A. veronii* biotype *veronii*
11		*A. veronii*-like
12		*A. schubertii*
13		*Aeromonas* group 501
14		*A. trota*

* *A. punctata* has been shown to be identical to *A. caviae*.
† DNA groups 8 and 10 have been shown to be identical.
Modified from references 10 and 36a.

BOX 6-8. TYPES OF INFECTION CAUSED BY *AEROMONAS* (VON GRAEVENITZ[281])

1. *Cellulitis and wound infections:* Infections following exposure to contaminated water, soil, or food, with highest incidence in warm seasons.

2. *Acute diarrheal disease of short duration:* The diarrhea is most commonly watery in consistency with a disease syndrome that closely mimics cholera. Some strains of *A. hydrophila* and *A. sobria*, commonly biotypes that are Voges-Proskauer and lysine decarboxylase positive and arabinose negative, are enterotoxigenic and produce a hypertonic diarrhea by stimulating production of cAMP in intestinal epithelial cells (see discussion in the section on *Vibrio* species earlier in this chapter). Namdari and Bottone[203] reported on the enteropathogenic role of *A. caviae*, based on the recovery of this species as the sole organism from 14 of 17 children with watery diarrhea. Their theory was supported when in a subsequent study they demonstrated both cytotoxic activity against HEp-2 cells and enterotoxin activity through the suckling mouse assay for *A. caviae*.[204]

3. *Septicemia:* Patients with hepatobiliary disease are particularly susceptible to *A. hydrophila* septicemia in a population group that is similarly at risk to *V. vulnificus*, as discussed previously in this chapter.

4. *Miscellaneous infections:* Urinary tract, wound, hepatobiliary, meningeal, and ear infections and endocarditis and septicemia secondary to *Aeromonas hydrophila* have been reported.[281]

that *A. caviae* does not produce an enterotoxin, is not invasive, and is not considered to be a human pathogen[97] may be questioned in light of the report of Fritsche and colleagues,[91] who have found this species to be a cause of gastroenteritis. Altwegg[9] has also linked *A. caviae* with gastroenteritis in other cases. In a review of aeromonas bacteremia, Ko and Chuang reported that 68% were caused by *A. hydrophila*, 17% by *A. sobria*, and 10% by *A. caviae*.[157] Therefore, species identification within the genus *Aeromonas* may have diagnostic and prognostic value.

Other recently described *Aeromonas* species of clinical significance include *A. schubertii*[115] (formerly CDC Enteric Group 501, mannitol, sucrose and indole negative), which has been incriminated as the cause of wound infections;[39] *A. veronii*[116] (formerly CDC Enteric Group 77, ornithine decarboxylase positive), which has been reported to cause bacteremia, wound infections and diarrhea;[4,116,138] and *A. jandaei* (formerly genospecies DNA Group 9 *A. sobria*, sucrose, esculin and cellobiose negative), which has been recovered as the infectious agent in four patients.[38] *A. trota* has a unique biochemical profile, including negative reactions for esculin hydrolysis, arabinose fermentation, and the Voges-Proskauer test; positive reactions for cellobiose fermentation, lysine decarboxylation, and citrate utilization; and susceptibility to ampicillin.[37] This finding may invalidate the use of ampicillin-containing selective media (discussed in the next section) for screening stool specimens for *Aeromonas* species. *A. trota* has been isolated almost exclusively from fecal specimens. *A. allosaccharophila* is another new mesophilic *Aeromonas* species that has been isolated from diseased elvers (young eels) and from the stool of a patient with diarrhea.[182] *A. allosaccharophila* most closely resembles *A. sobria*, but may be distinguished from the latter in utilizing L-arabinose and L-histidine as sole carbon sources. In addition, this species is unique in its ability to produce acid from or utilize D-melibiose and D-raffinose, or L-rhamnose.[182] Investigators from the CDC have characterized two strains originally isolated from leg wounds that are closely related to *A. schuberti* but are indole positive and lysine decarboxylase negative. These two strains form an additional *Aeromonas* DNA hybridization group, which they call *Aeromonas* Group 501.[115]

AEROMONAS SPECIES IN MEDICINAL LEECHES

The medicinal leech *Hirudo medicinalis* has recenly enjoyed a revival as a treatment for venous congestion following microvascular or plastic surgery. Unfortunately, *Aeromonas* species are present in the leech gut, where they aid in the breakdown of ingested red blood cells. As a result, an increasing number of *Aeromonas* infections have been associated with leech application.[136] Although some of the reported patients had relatively trivial episodes of wound drainage, other patients had significant episodes of cellulitis, abscess, tissue loss, and sepsis.[5,175,188] It has been recommended that leech appplications be restricted to tissue with arterial perfusion to minimize contamination of necrotic tissue with *Aeromonas*. Furthermore, the prophylactic administration of antibiotics has been proposed when leeches are applied.[175]

LABORATORY RECOVERY OF *AEROMONAS* SPECIES FROM CLINICAL SPECIMENS

Differential or selective agars should be utilized when *Aeromonas* is suspected as the etiologic agent of gastroenteritis or when fecal specimens are submitted for workup on patients whose peak of diarrheal symptoms has subsided (Box 6-9). Most strains grow on selective enteric media as lactose fermenters and, therefore, may be overlooked as unimportant or commensal enteric organisms.

LABORATORY IDENTIFICATION OF *AEROMONAS* SPECIES

Aeromonas species are cytochrome oxidase positive and can be quickly excluded from the *Enterobacteriaceae* by performing an oxidase test. A drop or two of tetramethyl-*p*-phenylenediamine-dihydrochloride (oxidase reagent) can be placed on surface colonies and observed for the evolution of a black discoloration characteristic of the colonies of *Aeromonas* species. Mesophilic *Aeromonas* species are motile with polar rather than peritrichous flagella similar to *Pseudomonas* species; however, *Aeromonas* species can be differentiated from the latter because they utilize glucose fermentatively rather than oxidatively and most *Aeromonas* species are indole positive (*Pseudomonas* species are negative). The phenotypic characteristics of *Aeromonas* species have been reviewed by Altwegg and colleagues[10] and are summarized in Table 6-15. Janda and Duffey[131] point out that one pitfall in the identification of *Aeromonas* species is that some of the

---

BOX 6-9. SELECTIVE AGARS USED TO CULTURE *AEROMONAS*

1. Blood agar (with or without ampicillin): blood agar can be made selective by incorporation of 10 µg/mL ampicillin. Janda and associates[130] recommend the use of a selective sheep blood agar containing ampicillin (SB-A agar) to improve the recovery of *Aeromonas* species from stool specimens.

2. Alkaline peptone water (APW, pH 8.6): initially developed for isolation of *Vibrio* species, APW can be used to recover aeromonads present in low numbers (10 CFU/mL) in stools. After overnight enrichment, APW is subcultured to the agar medium of choice.

3. CIN agar: originally developed for the isolation of *Yersinia enterocolitica*, CIN agar is also suitable for recovery of *Aeromonas* from feces.

4. Enteric agars: deoxycholate, MacConkey, and xylose lysine deoxycholate gave the highest overall plating efficiencies of eight routine enteric agars tested for recovery of *Aeromonas* species from feces.[63]

TABLE 6-15

DIFFERENTIATION OF *PLESIOMONAS SHIGELLOIDES* AND CLINICALLY IMPORTANT *AEROMONAS* SPECIES

ORGANISM	β-HEMOLYSIS SHEEP BLOOD	OXIDASE	MOTILITY	DNAse	INDOLE	VOGES-PROSKAUER	DECARBOXYLASE LYSINE	DECARBOXYLASE ORNITHINE	DECARBOXYLASE ARGININE	ESCULIN	GAS FROM GLUCOSE	FERMENTATION L-ARABINOSE	FERMENTATION SUCROSE	FERMENTATION MANNITOL	FERMENTATION INOSITOL
A. hydrophila group															
A. hydrophila	+	+	+	+	+	+	+	–	+	+	+	+	+	+	–
A. caviae group															
A. caviae	–	+	+	+	+	–	–	–	+	+	–	+	+	+	–
A. media	NA	+	–	+	v	–	–	–	+	+	–	+	–	NA	NA
A. eucrenophila	NA	+	+	+	NA	–	–	–	+	+	+	v	v	+	–
A. sobria group															
A. sobria	+	+	+	+	+	+	+	–	+	–	+	v	+	+	–
A. veronii biotype sobria	+	+	+	+	+	+	+	–	+	–	v	–	+	+	–
A. veronii biotype veronii	+	+	+	+	+	+	+	+	–	+	+	+	+	+	–
A. jandaei	+	+	+	NA	+	+	+	–	+	–	+	–	–	+	–
A. schubertii	v	+	+	+	–	v	+	–	+	–	–	–	–	–	–
A. trota	+	+	+	NA	+	–	+	–	+	–	+	–	–	+	–
P. shigelloides	–	+	+	–	+	–	+	+	+	–	–	–	–	–	+

+, 90% or more of strains are positive; –, 90% or more of strains are negative; V, 11%–89% of strains are positive;
NA, results not available. Shaded areas indicate key reactions.
Data from references: 1, 7, 10, 26, 37, 115, 116, 131, 244, 281.

miniaturized, semiautomated test kit systems cannot efficiently distinguish between *Aeromonas* species and *Vibrio fluvialis*. The latter is only rarely encountered in clinical laboratories, however, and can be differentiated from *Aeromonas* species by demonstrating the ability of *V. fluvialis* to grow in 6.5% salt solutions, to produce yellow colonies on TCBS agar (sucrose positive), and to be sensitive to the vibriostatic agent 0/129.[131]

Namdari and Bottone[202] also describe the suicide phenomenon for the rapid differentiation of *Aeromonas* species. This phenomenon is expressed when unknown strains are grown in broth media containing 0.5% glucose. The supplied glucose suppresses the tricarboxylic acid cycle, resulting in accumulation of acetic acid and cell death. *A. hydrophila* is nonsuicidal, aerogenic and esculin positive; *A. sobria* is suicide variable, aerogenic and esculin negative; and *A. caviae* is suicidal, anaerogenic and esculin positive. Further studies on the biochemical characteristics and serologic properties of the genus *Aeromonas* have been published by Janda and colleagues.[128]

GENUS *PLESIOMONAS*

The term *plesiomonas* is derived from the Greek word meaning "neighbor," indicating a close association with *Aeromonas*. However, as mentioned before, *Aeromonas* species are being reclassified within their own family and *Plesiomonas* is believed to be more closely related to *Proteus* than *Aeromonas*.[179,237] For the present, *Plesiomonas* remains in the *Vibrionaceae* and *P. shigelloides* is the only species in the genus.

P. shigelloides is ubiquitous in surface waters and in soil and commonly infects various cold-blooded animals (frogs, snakes, turtles, lizards). Humans become infected primarily by ingesting contaminated or unwashed food. Although less frequently recovered from human feces than *Aeromonas* species, *Plesiomonas*-induced gastroenteritis has been reported in children[184] and in adults.[122] In the latter study, 28 of 31 patients with gastroenteritis had no other organisms to account for the acute symptoms. In Thailand a carrier rate as high as 5.5% has been reported.[226]

Plesiomonas-related gastroenteritis in humans usually manifests as a mild watery diarrhea in which the stools are free of blood and mucin. Severe colitis or a cholera-like illness may be seen in patients who are immunosuppressed or who have gastrointestinal malignancies.[233] The infection is more prevalent in the subtropical and tropical regions of the world and during the warm summer months. Pathogenicity is probably related to the production of an enteropathogenic enterotoxin; Sanyal and colleagues demonstrated that 13 clinical strains they studied produced significant fluid accumulation in the ileal loop test.[242] *P. shigelloides*-associated diarrhea has occurred in epidemics but also in isolated cases. It has been described after uncooked shellfish consumption and as a cause of travelers' diarrhea.[123] A few isolated cases of extraintestinal infections including septicemia, neonatal meningitis, cellulitis, septic arthritis, and acute cholecystitis have also

been reported.[26,53,232] There are also reports of an overwhelming postsplenectomy infection with *P. shigelloides* in a patient cured of Hodgkin's disease[57] and a *P. shigelloides*-associated persistent dysentery and pseudomembranous colitis in a 42-year-old Bangladeshi woman.[279] The clinical disease spectrum and pathogenic factors associated with *Plesiomonas* infections have been reviewed by Brenden and colleagues.[26]

LABORATORY ISOLATION AND IDENTIFICATION

P. shigelloides is a straight, rounded, short, motile gram-negative bacillus with polar, generally lophotrichous flagella (*Vibrio* species and *Aeromonas* species are monotrichous). The organism grows well on sheep blood agar and on most enteric media. Isolates are nonhemolytic on sheep blood agar and in 24 hours at 30°C to 35°C (growth is optimum at 30°C); colonies average 1.5 mm in diameter and are gray, shiny, smooth, and opaque and may be slightly raised in the center. *P. shigelloides* is readily isolated on enteric agars such as MacConkey, deoxycholate, Hektoen, and xylose lysine deoxycholate. However, ampicillin-containing selective media that are frequently used for the isolation of *Aeromonas* species are not suitable for the isolation of *P. shigelloides*.[282]

Glucose is fermented; therefore, the deep of Kligler iron agar or triple sugar iron agar tubes will appear yellow. *P. shigelloides* will appear as a non-lactose fermenter on MacConkey agar and may be confused with *Shigella* species. The cytochrome oxidase reaction is positive, and indole is produced. *P. shigelloides* decarboxylates arginine, lysine, and ornithine. It does not produce DNAse or extracellular proteases, and it ferments inositol but not mannitol. These are key characteristics by which it is separated from *Aeromonas* species. Additional key identifying characteristics are listed in Table 6-15.

P. shigelloides can be resistant to penicillin, ampicillin, carbenicillin, and other β-lactamase sensitive penicillins. Most strains are susceptible to the aminoglycosides, chloramphenicol, tetracycline, trimethoprim-sulfamethoxazole, and the quinolones, ciprofloxacin and norfloxacin.[26,232]

GENUS *CHROMOBACTERIUM*

Brief mention of the genus *Chromobacterium* is made here because some strains are oxidase-positive fermenters and can be confused with *Aeromonas* species and *Vibrio* species. *Chromobacterium violaceum* is the species most commonly encountered in clinical laboratories, although it is seldom associated with human disease. *C. violaceum* grows well on blood agar, and most strains produce abundant violet pigment that makes recognition easy. Select biochemical characteristics are shown in Table 6-11. In addition, the ability of the organism to utilize citrate, reduce nitrates, and strongly hydrolyze casein is also helpful in making a final definitive identification.

REFERENCES

1. ABBOTT SL, CHEUNG WKW, KROSKE-BYSTROM S, MALEKZADEH T, JANDA JM: Identification of *Aeromonas* strains to the genospecies level in the clinical laboratory. J Clin Microbiol 30:1262–1266, 1992

2. ABBOTT SL, JANDA JM: Severe gastroenteritis associated with *Vibrio hollisae* infection: report of two cases and review. Clin Infect Dis 18:310–312, 1994

3. ABBOTT SL, POWERS C, KAYSNER CA, TAKEDA, ISHIBASHI M, JOSEPH SW, JANDA JM: Emergence of a restricted bioserovar of *Vibrio parahaemolyticus* as the predominant cause of *Vibrio*-associated gastoenteritis on the west coast of the United States and Mexico. J. Clin Microbiol 27:2891–2893, 1989

4. ABBOTT SL, SERVE H, JANDA JM: Case of *Aeromonas veronii* (DNA Group 10) bacteremia. J Clin Microbiol 32:3091–3092, 1994

5. ABRUTYN E: Hospital-associated infection from leeches. Ann Intern Med 109:356–358, 1988

5a. ALBERT MJ: Minireview: *Vibrio cholerae* 0139 Bengal. J Clin Microbiol 32:2345–2349, 1994

6. ALDERTON MR, KOROLIK V, COLOE PJ, DEWHIRST FE, PASTER BJ: *Campylobacter hyoilei* sp. nov., associated with porcine proliferative enteritis. Int J Syst Bacteriol 45:61–66,1995

7. ALLEN DA, AUSTIN B, COLWELL RR: *Aeromonas media*, a new species isolated from river water. Int J Syst Bacteriol 33:599–604, 1983

8. ALLOS BM, BLASER MJ: *Campylobacter jejuni* and the expanding spectrum of related infections. Clin Infect Dis 20:1092–1101, 1995

9. ALTWEGG M: *Aeromonas caviae:* An enteric pathogen? Infection 13:228–230, 1985

10. ALTWEGG M, STEIGERWALT AG, ALTWEGG-BISSIG R ET AL: Biochemical identification of *Aeromonas* genospecies isolated from humans. J. Clin Microbiol 28:258–264, 1990

11. ARCHER JR, ROMERO S, RITCHIE AE ET AL: Characterization of an unclassified microaerophilic bacterium associated with gastroenteritis. J Clin Microbiol 26:101–105, 1988

12. BARRETT TJ, PATTON CM, MORRIS GK: Differentiation of *Campylobacter* species using phenotypic characterization. Lab Med 19:96–102, 1988

13. BARTHEL JS, EVERETT ED: Diagnosis of *Campylobacter pylori* infections: The "gold standard" and the alternatives. Rev Infect Dis 12:S107–S114, 1990

14. BATES CJ, CLARKE TC, SPENCER: Prosthetic hip joint infection due to *Campylobacter fetus* [letter]. J Clin Microbiol 32:2037, 1994

15. BAUMANN P, SCHUBERT RHW: Family II. *Vibrionaceae* Vernon 1965, 5245AL. In Krieg NR, Holt JG (eds): Bergey's Manual of Systematic Bacteriology, vol 1, pp 516–550. Baltimore, Williams & Wilkins, 1984

16. BENJAMIN J, LEAPER S, OWEN RJ ET AL: Description of *Campylobacter laridis*, a new species comprising the nalidixic acid resistant thermophilic *Campylobacter* (NARTC) group. Curr Microbiol 8:231–238, 1983

17. BLAKE PA, ALLEGRA DT, SYNDER JD ET AL: Cholera—a possible endemic focus in the United States. N Engl J Med 302:305–309, 1980

18. BLAKE PA, MERSON MH, WEAVER RE, HOLLIS DG, HEUBLEIN PC: Disease caused by a marine vibrio: clinical characteristics and epidemiology. N Engl J Med 300:1–4, 1979

19. BLASER MJ: *Heliobacter pylori*: its role in disease. Clin Infect Dis 15:386–393, 1992

20. BLASER MJ, BERKOWITZ ID, LAFORCE FM ET AL: *Campylobacter* enteritis: Clinical and epidemiological features. Ann Intern Med 91:179–185, 1979

21. BLASER MJ, WELLS JG, FELDMAN RA ET AL: *Campylobacter* enteritis in the United States. Ann Intern Med 98:360–365, 1983

22. BOKKENHEUSER VD, RICHARDSON NJ, BRYNER JH ET AL: Detection of enteric campylobacteriosis in children. J Clin Microbiol 9:227–232, 1979

23. BONNER JR, COKER AS, BERRYMAN CR, POLLOCK HM: Spectrum of Vibrio infections in a Gulf coast community. Ann Intern Med 99:464–469, 1983.

24. BORCZYK A, ROSA SD, LIOR H: Enhanced recognition of *Campylobacter cryaerophila* in clinical and environmental specimens. Presented before the annual meeting of the American Society for Microbiology, 1991, abstract C-267, p 386

25. BRAYTON PR, BODE RB, COLWELL RR ET AL: *Vibrio cincinnatiensis* sp. nov., a new human pathogen. J Clin Microbiol 23:104–108, 1986

26. BRENDEN RA, MILLER MA, JANDA JM: Clinical disease spectrum and pathogenic factors associated with *Plesiomonas shigelloides* infections in humans. Rev Infect Dis 10:303–316, 1988

27. BRENNER DJ, HICKMAN-BRENNER FW, LEE JV ET AL: *Vibrio furnissii* (formerly aerogenic biogroup of *Vibrio fluvialis*), a new species isolated from human feces and the environment. J Clin Microbiol 18:816–824, 1983

28. BRONSDON MA, GOODWIN CS, SLY LI ET AL: *Helicobacter nemestrinae* sp. nov., a spiral bacterium found in the stomach of a pigtailed macaque (*Macaca nemestrina*). Int J Syst Bacteriol 41:148–153, 1991

29. BRYNER JH, LITTLETON J, GATES C ET AL: Paper presented before the XIV International Congress of Microbiology, Manchester, England, 1986

30. BUCK GE: *Campylobacter pylori* and gastroduodenal disease. Clin Microbiol Rev 3:1–12, 1990

31. BURKE V, GRACEY M, ROBINSON J ET AL: The microbiology of childhood gastroenteritis: *Aeromonas* species and other infective agents. J Infect Dis 148:68–74, 1983

32. BURMAN WJ, COHN DL, REVES RR, WILSON ML: Multifocal cellulitis and monoarticular arthritis as manifestations of *Heliobacter cinaedi* bacteremia. Clin Infect Dis 20:564–570, 1995

33. BURNENS AP, ANGELOZ-WICK B, NICOLET J: Comparison of *Campylobacter* carriage rates in diarrhoeic and healthy pet animals. Zentralblatt fur Veterinarmedizin 39:175–180, 1992

34. BURNENS AP, STANLEY J, MORGENTSERN R, NICOLET J: Gastroenteritis associated with *Helicobacter pullorum* [letter]. Lancet 344:1569–1570, 1994

35. BUTZLER JP: Infections with *Campylobacter*. In Williams JD, Heremann W (eds): Modern Topics in Infectious Diseases, pp 214–239. London, Medical Books Ltd, 1978

36. CARNAHAN AM, BEADLING J, WATSKY D, FORD N: Detection of *Campylobacter upsaliensis* from a blood culture by using the BacT/Alert system. J Clin Microbiol 32:2598–2599, 1994

36a. CARNAHAN AM, BEHRAM S, JOSEPH SW: Aerokey II: a flexible key for identifying clinical *Aeromonas* species. J Clin Microbiol 29:2843–2849, 1991

37. CARNAHAN AM, CHAKRABORTY T, FANNING GR ET AL: *Aeromonas trota* sp. nov., an ampicillin-susceptible species isolated from clinical specimens. J Clin Microbiol 29:1206–1210, 1991

38. CARNAHAN AM, FANNING GR, JOSEPH SW: *Aeromonas jandaei* (formerly genospecies DNA group 9 *A. sobria*), a new sucrose-negative species isolated from clinical specimens. J Clin Microbiol 29:560–564, 1991

39. CARNAHAN AM, MARII MA, FANNING GR ET AL: Characterization of *Aeromonas shubertii* strains recently isolated from traumatic wound infections. J Clin Microbiol 27:1826–1830, 1989

40. CENTERS FOR DISEASE CONTROL: Waterborne *Campylobacter* gastroenteritis, Vermont. MMWR 27:207, 1978

41. CENTERS FOR DISEASE CONTROL: *Campylobacter* sepsis associated with "nutritional therapy"—California. MMWR 30:294–295, 1981

42. CENTERS FOR DISEASE CONTROL: Premature labor and neonatal sepsis caused by *Camplobacter fetus* subspecies *fetus*—Ontario. MMWR 33:483–489, 1984

43. CENTERS FOR DISEASE CONTROL: Cholera—Worldwide, 1989, MMWR 39:365–367, 1990

44. CENTERS FOR DISEASE CONTROL: Cholera—Peru, 1991. MMWR 40:108–110, 1991

45. CENTERS FOR DISEASE CONTROL: Cholera—New Jersey and Florida. MMWR 40:287–289, 1991

46. CENTERS FOR DISEASE CONTROL: Imported cholera associated with a newly described toxigenic *Vibrio cholera* 0139 strain—California, 1993. MMWR 42:501–503, 1993

47. CENTERS FOR DISEASE CONTROL: Update: *Vibrio cholerae* 01—western hemisphere, 1991–1994, and *V. cholerae* 0139–Asia, 1994. MMWR 44:215–219, 1995

48. CENTERS FOR DISEASE CONTROL: *Vibrio vulnificus* infections associated with eating raw oysters–Los Angeles, 1996. MMWR 45:621–624, 1996

49. CHIU C-H, KUO C-Y, OU JT: Chronic diarrhea and bacteremia caused by *Campylobacter lari* in a neonate [letter]. Clin Infect Dis 21:700–701, 1995

50. CHOPRA AK, HOUSTON CW, GENAUX CT ET AL: Evidence for production of an enterotoxin and cholera toxin cross-reactive factor by *Aeromonas hydrophila*. J Clin Microbiol 24:661–664, 1986

51. CHUSID MJ, WORTMANN DW, DUNNE WM: "*Campylobacter upsaliensis*"sepsis in a boy with acquired hypogammaglobulinemia. Diagn Microbiol Infect Dis 13:367–369, 1990

52. CIMOLAI N, GILL MJ, JONES A ET AL: "*Campylobacter cinaedi*" bacteremia: Case report and laboratory findings. J Clin Microbiol 25:942–943, 1987

53. CLAESSON BEB, HOLMLUND DEW, LINDHAGEN CA ET AL: *Plesiomonas shigelloides* in acute cholecystitis: A case report. J Clin Microbiol 20:985–987, 1984

54. CLARRIDGE JE, ZIGHELBOIM-DAUM S: Isolation and characterization of two hemolytic phenotypes of *Vibrio damsela* associated with a fatal wound infection. J Clin Microbiol 21:302–306, 1985

55. COLLINS MD, MARTINEZ-MURCIA AJ, CAI J: *Aeromonas enteropelogenes* and *Aeromonas ichthiosmia* are identical to *Aeromonas trota* and *Aeromonas veronii*, respectively, as revealed by small-subunit rRNA sequence analysis. Int J Syst Bacteriol 43:855–856, 1993

56. COLWELL RR, MacDONELL MT, DE LEY J: Proposal to recognize the family *Aeromonadaceae* fam. nov. Int J Syst Bacteriol 36:473–477, 1986

57. CURTI AJ, LIN JH, SZABO K: Overwhelming postsplenectomy infection with *Plesiomonas shigelloides* in a patient cured of Hodgkin's disease: A case report. Am J Clin Pathol 83:522–524, 1985

58. CUTLER AF, HAVSTAD S, MA CK, BLASER MJ, PEREZ-PEREZ GI, SCHUBERT TT: Accuracy of invasive and non-invasive tests to diagnose *Helicobacter pylori* infection. Gastroenterol 109:136–141, 1995

59. DAVIS BR, FANNING GR, MADDEN JM ET AL: Characterization of biochemically atypical *Vibrio cholerae* strains and designation of a new pathogenic species, *Vibrio mimicus*. J Clin Microbiol 14:631–639, 1981

60. DECKER CF, MARTIN GI, BARHAM WB, PAPARELLO SF: Bacteremia due to *Campylobacter cinaedi* in a patient infected with the human immunodeficiency virus [letter]. Clin Infect Dis 15:178–179, 1992

61. DEKEYSER P, GOSSUIN-DETRAIN M, BUTZLER JP ET AL: Acute enteritis due to related vibrio: First positive stool cultures. J Infect Dis 125:390–392, 1972

62. DENT JC, McNULTY CAM, UFF JC, WILKINSON SP, GEAR MWL: Spiral organisms in the gastric antrum. Lancet ii:96, 1987

63. DESMOND E, JANDA JM: Growth of *Aeromonas* species on enteric agars. J Clin Microbiol 23:1065–1067, 1986

64. DEVLIN HR, McINTYRE L: *Campylobacter fetus* subsp. *fetus* in homosexual males. J Clin Microbiol 18:999–1000, 1983

65. DUBOIS A, TARNAWSKI A, NEWELL DG, FIALA N, WOJCIECH D, STACHURA J, KRIVAN H, HEMAN-ACKAH LM: Gastric injury and invasion of parietal cells by spiral bacteria in rhesus monkeys. Gastroenterol 100:884–889, 1991

66. DUERDEN BI, ELEY A, GOODWIN L, MAGEE JT, HINDMARCH JM, BENNETT KW: A comparison of *Bacteroides ureolyticus* isolates from different clinical sources. J Med Microbiol 29: 63–73, 1989

67. DUERDEN BI, GOODWIN L, O'NEIL TCA: Identification of *Bacteroides* species from adult periodontal disease. J Med Microbiol 24:133–137, 1987

68. EATON KA, DEWHIRST FE, RADIN MJ, FOX JG, PASTER BJ, KRAKOWKA S, MORGAN DR: *Helicobacter acinonyx* sp. nov., isolated from cheetahs with gastritis. Int J Syst Bacteriol 43:99–106, 1993

69. EDMONDS P, PATTON CM, GRIFFIN PM ET AL: *Campylobacter hyointestinalis* associated with human gastrointestinal disease in the United States. J Clin Microbiol 25:685–691, 1987

70. ENDTZ HP, RUIJS GJHM, ZWINDERMAN AH ET AL: Comparison of six media, including a semisolid agar, for the isolation of various *Campylobacter* species from stool specimens. J Clin Microbiol 29:1007–1010, 1991

71. ENGLISH, VL, LINDBERG RB: Isolation of *Vibrio alginolyticus* from wounds and blood of a burn patient. Am J Med Technol 43:989–993, 1977

72. ETOH Y, DEWHIRST FE, PASTER BJ, YAMAMOTO A, GOTO N: *Campylobacter showae* sp. nov., isolated from the human oral cavity. Int J Syst Bacteriol 43:631–639, 1993

73. FARMER JJ III: *Vibrio* ("*Beneckea*") *vulnificus*, the bacterium associated with sepsis, septicemia and the sea. Lancet 2:903, 1979

74. FARMER JJ III, HICKMAN-BRENNER FW, FANNING GR ET AL: Characterization of *Vibrio metschnikovii* and *Vibrio gazogenes* by DNA-DNA hybridization and phenotype. J Clin Microbiol 26:1993–2000, 1988

75. FARMER JJ III, HICKMAN-BRENNER FW, KELLY MT: *Vibrio*. In Lennette EH (ed): Manual of Clinical Microbiology, 4th ed, pp 282–301. Washington, DC, American Society for Microbiology, 1985

76. FARRUGIA DC, EYKYN SJ, SMYTH EG: *Campylobacter fetus* endocarditis: two case reports and review. Clin Infect Dis 18:443–446, 1994

77. FENNELL CL, ROMPALO AM, TOTTEN PA ET AL: Isolation of "*Campylobacter hyointestinalis*" from a human. J Clin Microbiol 24:146–148, 1986

78. FENNELL CL, TOTTEN PA, QUINN TC ET AL: Characterization of *Campylobacter*-like organisms isolated from homosexual men. J Infect Dis 149:58–66, 1984

79. FIGURA N, GUGLIELMETTI P, ZANCHI A, PARTINI N, ARMELLINI D, BAYELI PF, BUGNOLI M, VERDIANI S: Two cases of *Campylobacter mucosalis* enteritis in children. J Clin Microbiol 31:727–728, 1993

80. FIGURA N, MARRI L, VERDIANI S ET AL: Prevalence, species differentiation, and toxigenicity of *Aeromonas* strains in cases of childhood gastroenteritis and in controls. J Clin Microbiol 23:595–599, 1986

81. FISHER R, SAMISCH W: "*Gastrospirillum hominis*": another four cases. Lancet i:59, 1990

82. FONTAINE EAR, BORRIELLO SP, TAYLOR-ROBINSON D, DAVIES HA: Characteristics of a gram-negative anaerobe isolated from men with nongonococcal urethritis. J Med Microbiol 17:129–140, 1984

83. FONTAINE EAR, BRYANT TN, TAYLOR-ROBINSON D, BORRIELLO SP, DAVIES HA: A numerical taxonomic study of anaerobic gram-negative bacilli classified as *Bacteroides ureolyticus* isolated from patients with nongonococcal urethritis. J Gen Microbiol 132:3137–3146, 1986

84. FOX JG, CHILVERS T, GOODWIN CS ET AL: *Campylobacter mustelae*, a new species resulting from the elevation of *Campylobacter pylori* subsp. *mustelae* to species status. Int J Syst Bacteriol 39:301–303, 1989

85. FOX JG, DEWHIRST FE, TULLY JG, PASTER BJ, YAN L, TAYLOR NS, COLLINS JR MJ, GORELICK PL, WARD JM: *Helicobacter hepaticus* sp. nov., a microaerophilic bacterium isolated from livers and intestinal mucosal scrapings from mice. J Clin Microbiol 32:1238–1245, 1994

86. FOX JG, LEE A: Gastric *Campylobacter*-like organisms: their role in gastric disease of laboratory animals. Lab Animal Sci 39:543–553, 1989

87. FOX JG, MAXWELL KO, TAYLOR NS, RUNSICK CD, EDMONDS P, BRENNER DJ: "*Campylobacter upsaliensis*" isolated from cats as identified by DNA relatedness and biochemical features. J Clin Microbiol 27:2376–2378, 1989

88. FOX JG, TAYLOR NS, EDMONDS P ET AL: *Campylobacter pylori* subsp. *mustelae* subsp. nov. isolated from the gastric mucosa of ferrets (*Mustela putorius furo*), and an emended description of *Campylobacter pylori*. Int J Syst Bacteriol 38:367–370, 1988

89. FOX JG, YAN LL, DEWHIRST FE, PASTER BJ, SHAMES B, MURPHY JC, HAYWARD A, BELCHER JC, MENDES EN: *Helicobacter bilis* sp. nov., a novel *Helicobacter* species isolated from bile, livers, and intestines of aged, inbred mice. J Clin Microbiol 33:445–454, 1995

90. FREEDBERG AS, BARRON LE: The presence of spirochetes in human gastric mucosa. Am J Dig Dis 7:443–445, 1940

91. FRITSCHE D, DAHN, R, HOFFMANN G: *Aeromonas punctata* subsp. *caviae* as the causative agent of acute gastroenteritis. Zentralbl Bakteriol Mikrobiol Hyg [A] 233: 232–235, 1975

92. FUJIMOTO S, YUKI N, ITOH T, AMAKO K: Specific serotype of *Campylobacter jejuni* associated with Guillain-Barre Syndrome [letter]. J Infect Dis 165:183, 1992

93. GAUDREAU C, LAMOTHE F: *Campylobacter upsaliensis* isolated from a breast abscess. J Clin Microbiol 30:1354–1356, 1992

94. GEBHART CJ, EDMONDS P, WARD GE ET AL: "*Campylobacter hyointestinalis*" sp. nov.: A new species of *Campylobacter* found in the intestines of pigs and other animals. J Clin Microbiol 21:715–720, 1985

95. GEBHART CJ, FENNELL CL, MURTAUGH MP, STAMM WE: *Campylobacter cinaedi* is normal intestinal flora in hamsters. J Clin Microbiol 27:1692–1694, 1989

96. GEORGE WL, JONES MJ, NAKATA MM: Phenotypic characteristics of *Aeromonas* species isolated from adult humans. J Clin Microbiol 23:1026–1029, 1986

97. GEORGE WL, NAKATA MM, THOMPSON J ET AL: *Aeromonas*-related diarrhea in adults. Arch Intern Med 145:2207–2211, 1985

98. GOODWIN CS, ARMSTRONG JA, CHILVERS T ET AL: Transfer of *Campylobacter pylori* and *Campylobacter mustelae* to *Helicobacter* gen. nov. as *Helicobacter pylori* comb. nov. and *Helicobacter mustelae* comb. nov., respectively. Int J Syst Bacteriol 39:397–405, 1989

99. GOOSSENS H, POT B, VLAES L ET AL: Characterization and description of "*Campylobacter upsaliensis*" isolated from human feces. J Clin Microbiol 28:1039–1046, 1990

100. GOOSSENS H, VLAES L, GALAND I ET AL: Semisolid blood-free selective-motility medium for the isolation of campylobacters from stool specimens. J Clin Microbiol 27:1077–1080, 1989

101. GRACEY M, BURKE V, ROBINSON J: *Aeromonas*-associated gastroenteritis. Lancet 2:1304–1306, 1982

102. GRANT IH, RICHARDSON NJ, BOKKENHEUSER VD: Broiler chickens as potential source of *Campylobacter* infections in humans. J Clin Microbiol 11:508–510, 1980

103. GURGAN R, DIKER KS: Abortion associated with *Campylobacter upsaliensis*. J Clin Microbiol 32:3093–3094, 1994

104. GUTHMANN JP: Epidemic cholera in Latin America: spread and routes of transmission. J Trop Med Hyg 98:419–427, 1995

105. HANNINEN M-L, HAPPONEN I, SAARI S, JALAVA K: Culture and characteristics of *Helicobacter bizzozeronii*, a new gastric *Helicobacter* sp. Int J Syst Bacteriol 46:160–166, 1996

106. HANSEN W, CROKAERT F, YOURASSOWSKY E: Two strains of *Vibrio* species with unusual biochemical features isolated from ear tracts. J Clin Microbiol 9:152–153, 1979

107. HANSEN W, FRENEY J, BENYAGOUB H, LETOUZEY M-N, GIGI J, WAUTERS G: Severe human infections caused by *Vibrio metschnikovii*. J Clin Microbiol 31:2529–2530, 1993

108. HARVEY SM: Hippurate hydrolysis by *Campylobacter fetus*. J Clin Microbiol 11:435–437, 1980

109. HARVEY SM, GREENWOOD JR: Probable *Campylobacter fetus* subsp. *fetus* gastroenteritis. J Clin Microbiol 18: 1278–1279, 1983

110. HEBERT GA, HOLLIS DG, WEAVER RE ET AL: 30 years of campylobacters: Biochemical characteristics and a biotyping proposal for *Campylobacter jejuni*. J Clin Microbiol 15:1065–1073, 1982

111. HEILMANN KL, BORCHARD F: Gastritis due to spiral shaped bacteria other than *Helicobacter pylori*: clinical, histological, and ultrastructural findings. Gut 32: 137–140, 1991

112. HENRY GA, LONG PH, BURNS JL, CHARBONNEAU DL: Gastric spirillosis in beagles. Am J Vet Res 48:831–836, 1987

113. HICKMAN FW, FARMER JJ III, HOLLIS DG ET AL: Identification of *Vibrio hollisae* sp. nov. from patients with diarrhea. J Clin Microbiol 15:395–401, 1982

114. HICKMAN-BRENNER FW, BRENNER DJ, STEIGERWALT AG, ET AL: *Vibrio fluvialis* and *Vibrio furnissii* isolated from a stool sample of one patient. J Clin Microbiol 20:125–127, 1984

115. HICKMAN-BRENNER FW, FANNING GR, ARDUINO MJ ET AL: *Aeromonas schubertii*, a new mannitol-negative species found in human clinical specimens. J Clin Microbiol 26:1561–1564, 1988

116. HICKMAN-BRENNER FW, MACDONALD KL, STEIGERWALT AG ET AL: *Aeromonas veronii*, a new ornithine decarboxylase-positive species that may cause diarrhea. J Clin Microbiol 25:900–906, 1987

117. HODGE DS, BORCZYK A, WAT L-L: Evaluation of the indoxyl acetate hydrolysis test for the differentiation of campylobacters. J Clin Microbiol 28:1482–1483, 1990

118. HODGE DS, PRESCOTT JF, SHEWEN PE. Direct immunofluorescence microscopy for rapid screening of *Campylobacter* enteritis. J Clin Microbiol 24:863–865, 1986

119. HODGE JR TW, LEVY CS, SMITH MA: Diarrhea associated with *Vibrio fluvialis* infection in a patient with AIDS. Clin Infect Dis 21:237–238, 1995

120. HODINKA RL, GILLIGAN PH: Evaluation of the Campyslide agglutination test for confirmatory identification of selected *Campylobacter* species. J Clin Microbiol 26: 47–49, 1988

121. HOLLIS DG, WEAVER RE, BAKER CN ET AL: Halophilic *Vibrio* species isolated from blood cultures. J Clin Microbiol 3:425–431, 1976

122. HOLMBERG SD, FARMER JJ III: *Aeromonas hydrophila* and *Plesiomonas shigelloides* as causes of intestinal infections. Rev Infect Dis 6:633–639, 1984

123. HOLMBERG SD, WACHSMUTH IK, HICKMAN-BRENNER FW ET AL: *Plesiomonas* enteric infections in the United States. Ann Intern Med 105:690–694, 1986

124. HONDA S-I, GOTO I, MINEMATSU I ET AL: Gastroenteritis due to Kanagawa-negative *Vibrio parahaemolyticus*. Lancet 1:331–332, 1987

125. HUGHES JM, HOLLIS DG, GANGAROSA EJ ET AL: Noncholera *Vibrio* infections in the United States: Clinical, epidemiological, and laboratory features. Ann Intern Med 88: 602–606, 1978

126. HUQ MI, ALAM AKMJ, BRENNER DF ET AL: Isolation of *Vibrio*-like group EF-6 from patients with diarrhea. J Clin Microbiol 11:621–624, 1980

127. HUSMANN M, GRIES C, JEHNICHEN P, WOELFEL T, GERKEN G, LUDWIG W, BHAKDI S: *Helicobacter* sp. strain *Mainz* isolated from an AIDS patient with septic arthritis: case report and nonradioactive analysis of 16S rRNA sequence. J Clin Microbiol 32: 3037–3039, 1994

127a. JANDA JM: Recent advances in the study of the taxonomy, pathogenicity and infectious syndromes associated with the genus *Aeromonas*. Clin Microbiol Rev 4: 397–410, 1991

128. JANDA JM, ABBOTT SL, KHASHE S, KELLOGG GH, SHIMADA T: Further studies on biochemical characteristics and serologic properties of the genus *Aeromonas*. J Clin Microbiol 34:1930–1933, 1996

129. JANDA JM, BRENDEN R, DEBENEDETTI JA ET AL: *Vibrio alginolyticus* bacteremia in an immunocompromised patient. Diagn Microbiol Infect Dis 5:337–340, 1986

130. JANDA JM, DIXON A, RAUCHER B ET AL: Value of blood agar for primary plating and clinical implications of simultaneous isolation of *Aeromonas hydrophila* and *Aeromonas caviae* from a patient with gastroenteritis. J Clin Microbiol 20:1221–1222, 1984

131. JANDA JM, DUFFEY PS: Mesophilic aeromonads in human disease: Current taxonomy, laboratory identification, and infectious disease spectrum. Rev Infect Dis 5:980–997, 1988

132. JANDA JM, POWERS C, BRYANT RG ET AL: Current perspectives on the epidemiology and pathogenesis of clinically significant *Vibrio* spp. Clin Microbiol Rev 1: 245–267, 1988

133. JEAN-JACQUES W, RAJASHEKARAIAH KR, FARMER JJ III ET AL: *Vibrio metschnikovii* bacteremia in a patient with cholecystitis. J Clin Microbiol 14:711–712, 1981

134. JICONG W, GUOLONG L, ZHENHUA Z, YANGLONG M, QIANG C, JINGCHUAN W, SULONG Y: $^{15}NH_4+$ excretion test: a new method for detection of *Helicobacter pylori* infection. J Clin Microbiol 30:181–184, 1992

135. JOHNSON CC, REINHARDT JF, EDELSTEIN MAC, MULLIGAN ME, GEORGE WL, FINEGOLD SM: *Bacteroides gracilis*, an important anaerobic bacterial pathogen. J Clin Microbiol 22:799–802, 1985

136. JONES BL, WILCOX MH: *Aeromonas* infections and their treatment. J Antimicrob Chemother 35:453–461, 1995

137. JONES FS, ORCUTT M, LITTLE RB: Vibrios (*Vibrio jejuni* n. sp.) associated with intestinal disorders of cows and calves. J Exp Med 53:853–864, 1931

138. JOSEPH SW, CARNAHAN AM, BRAYTON PR ET AL: *Aeromonas jandaei* and *Aeromonas veronii* dual infection of a human wound following aquatic exposure. J Clin Microbiol 29:565–569, 1991

139. JOSEPH SW, COLWELL RR, KAPER JB: *Vibrio parahaemolyticus* and related halophilic vibrios. Crit Rev Microbiol 10:77–124, 1982

140. KAPER JB, MORRIS JR JG, LEVINE MM: Cholera. Clin Microbiol Rev 8:48–86, 1995

141. KAPER JB, NATARO JP, ROBERTS NC ET AL: Molecular epidemiology of non-01 *Vibrio cholerae* and *Vibrio mimicus* in the U.S. gulf coast region. J Clin Microbiol 23: 652–654, 1986

142. KAPLAN RL, BARRETT JE, LANDAU W ET AL: The value of Campy thio in the recovery of *Campylobacter*: An analysis of three years experience. Presented before the annual meeting of the American Society for Microbiology, 1984, abstract C-77, p 249

143. KARMALI MA, FLEMING PC: *Campylobacter* enteritis. Can Med Assoc J 120:1525–1532, 1979

144. KARMALI MA, SIMOR AE, ROSCOE M ET AL: Evaluation of a blood-free, charcoal-based, selective medium for the isolation of *Campylobacter* organisms from feces. J Clin Microbiol 23:456–459, 1986

145. KASPER G, DICKGIESSER N: Isolation from gastric epithelium of *Campylobacter*-like bacteria that are distinct from "*Campylobacter pyloridis*." Lancet 1:111–112, 1985

146. KELLY MT: Cholera: A worldwide perspective. Pediatr Infect Dis 5:S101–S105, 1986

147. KELLY MT, HICKMAN-BRENNER FW, FARMER JJ III: *Vibrio.* In Balows A (ed): Manual of Clinical Microbiology, 5th ed, chap 37, pp 384–395. Washington, DC, American Society for Microbiology, 1991

148. KELLY MT, PETERSON JW, SARLES HE JR ET AL: Cholera on the Texas gulf coast. JAMA 247:1598–1599, 1982

149. KELLY MT, STROH EMD: Urease-positive, Kanagawa-negative *Vibrio parahaemolyticus* from patients and the environment in the Pacific northwest. J Clin Microbiol 27:2820–2822, 1989

150. KIEHLBAUCH JA, BRENNER DJ, CAMERON DN, STEIGERWALT AG, MAKOWSKI JM, BAKER CN, PATTON CM, WACHSMUTH IK: Genotypic and phenotypic characterization of *Helicobacter cinaedi* and *Helicobacter fennelliae* strains isolated from humans and animals. J Clin Microbiol 33: 2940–2947, 1995

151. KIEHLBAUCH JA, BRENNER DJ, NICHOLSON MA ET AL: *Campylobacter butzleri* sp. nov. isolated from humans and animals with diarrheal illness. J Clin Microbiol 29: 376–385, 1991

152. KIEHLBAUCH JA, TAUXE RV, BAKER CN, WACHSMUTH IK: *Helicobacter cinaedi*-associated bacteremia and cellultis in immunocompromised patients. Ann Inter Med 121: 90–93, 1994

153. KING EO: Human infections with *Vibrio fetus* and a closely related vibrio. J Infect Dis 101:119–128, 1957

154. KIRKBRIDE CA, GATES CE, COLLINS JE: Abortion in sheep caused by a non-classified, anaerobic, flagellated bacterium. Am J Vet Res 47:259–262, 1986

155. KIRKBRIDE CA, GATES CE, COLLINS JE ET AL: Ovine abortion associated with an anaerobic bacterium. J Am Vet Med Assoc 186:789–791, 1985

156. KLIPSTEIN FA, ENGERT RF, SHORT HB: Enzyme-linked immunosorbent assays for virulence properties of *Campylobacter jejuni* clinical isolates. J Clin Microbiol 23: 1039–1043, 1986

157. KO W-C, CHUANG Y-C: Aeromonas bacteremia: review of 59 episodes. Clin Infect Dis 20:1298–1304, 1995

158. KODAKA H, LOMBARD GL, DOWELL VR JR: Gas-liquid chromatography technique for detection of hippurate hydrolysis and conversion of fumarate to succinate by microorganisms. J Clin Microbiol 16:962–964, 1982

159. KRIENITZ W: Ueber das Auftreten von Spirochaeten verschiedener Form im Mageninhalt bei Carcinoma Ventriculi. Dtsch Med Wochenschr 22:872, 1906

160. KUROKI S, HARUTA T, YOSHIOKA M, KOBAYASHI Y, NUKINA M, NAKANISHI H: Guillain-Barre syndrome associated with *Campylobacter* infection. Pediatr Infect Dis J 10: 149–151, 1991

161. LACEY SW: Cholera: calamitous past, ominous future. Clin Infect Dis 20:1409–1419, 1995

162. LAM S, YEO M: Urease-positive *Vibrio parahaemolyticus* strain. J Clin Microbiol 12:57–59, 1980

163. LA SCOLEA LJ: *Campylobacter fetus* subsp. *fetus* meningitis in a neonate. Clin Microbiol Newsl 7:125–126, 1985

164. LASTOVICA A, LE ROUX E, WARREN R, KLUMP H: Clinical isolates of *Campylobacter mucosalis* [letter]. J Clin Microbiol 31:2835–2836, 1993

165. LASTOVICA AJ, LE ROUX E, PENNER JL: "*Campylobacter upsaliensis*" isolated from blood cultures of pediatric patients. J Clin Microbiol 27:657–659, 1989

166. LASTOVICA AJ, LE ROUX E, WARREN R, KLUMP H: Additional data on clinical isolates on *Campylobacter mucosalis* [letter]. J Clin Microbiol 32:2338–2339, 1994

167. LAUWERS S, VAN ETTERIJCK R, BREYNAERT J ET AL: Isolation of *C. upsaliensis* and *C. concisus* from human faeces. Presented before the annual meeting of the American Society for Microbiology, 1991, abstract C-266, p 386

168. LEE A: Human gastric spirilla other than *C. pylori.* In: Blaser MJ, ed. *Campylobacter pylori* in gastritis and peptic ulcer disease. New York, Igaku-Shoin Medical Publishers, pp. 225–240, 1989

169. LEE A, HAZELL SL: *Campylobacter pylori* in health and disease: An ecological perspective. Microb Ecol Health Dis 1:1–16, 1988

170. LEE A, PHILLIPS MW, O'ROURKE JL, PASTER BJ, DEWHIRST FE, FRASER GJ, FOX JG, SLY LI, ROMANIUK PJ, TRUST TJ, KOUPRACH S: *Helicobacter muridarum* sp, nov., a microareophilic helical bacterium with a novel ultrastructure isolated from the intestinal mucosa of rodents. Int J Syst Bacteriol 42:27–36, 1992

171. LEE K, BARON EJ, SUMMANEN P, FINEGOLD SM: Selective medium for isolation of *Bacteroides gracilis*. J Clin Microbiol 28:1747–1750, 1990

172. LERNER J, BRUMBERGER V, PREAC-MURSIC V: Severe diarrhea associated with *Arcobacter butzleri.* Eur J Clin Microbiol Infect Dis 13:660–662, 1994

173. LESMANA M, ALBERT MJ, SUBEKTI D, RICHIE E, TJANIADI P, WALZ SE, LEBRON CI: Simple differentiation of *Vibrio cholerae* 0139 from *V. cholerae* 01 and non-01, non-0139 by modified CAMP test. J Clin Microbiol 34:1038–1040, 1996

174. LESSNER AM, WEBB RM, RABIN B: *Vibrio alginolyticus* conjunctivitis. Arch Ophthalmol 103:229–230, 1985

175. LINEAWEAVER WC, HILL MK, BUNCKE GM, FOLLANSBEE S, BUNCKE HJ, WONG RKM, MANDERS EK, GROTTING JC, ANTHONY J, MATHES SJ: *Aeromonas hydrophila* infections following use of medical leeches in replantation and flap surgery. Ann Plast Surg 29:238–244, 1992

176. LOWRY PW, MCFARLAND LM, THREEFOOT HK: *Vibrio hollisae* septicemia after consumption of catfish [letter]. J Infect Dis 154:730–731, 1986

177. LUECHTEFELD NW, RELLER LB, BLASER MJ ET AL: Comparison of atmospheres of incubation for primary isolation of *Campylobacter fetus* subsp. *jejuni* from animal specimens: 5% oxygen versus candle jar. J Clin Microbiol 15: 53–57, 1982

178. LUECHTEFELD NW, WANG W-LL: Hippurate hydrolysis by and triphenyltetrazolium tolerance of *Campylobacter fetus.* J Clin Microbiol 15:137–140, 1982

179. MACDONELL MT, COLWELL RR: Phylogeny of the *Vibrionaceae*, and recommendation for two new genera, *Listonella* and *Shewanella.* Syst Appl Microbiol 6:171–182, 1985

180. MANDAL BK: Epedimic cholera due to a novel strain of *V. cholerae* non 01—the beginning of a new pandemic? J Infect 27:115–117, 1993

181. MARSHALL BJ: *Campylobacter pyloridis* and gastritis. J Infect Dis 153:650–657, 1986

182. MARTINEZ-MURCIA AJ, ESTEVE C, GARAY E, COLLINS MD: *Aeromonas allosaccharophila* sp. nov., a new mesophilic member of the genus *Aeromonas*. FEMS Microbiol lett 91: 199–206, 1992

183. MATSIOTA-BERNARD P, NAUCIEL C: *Vibrio alginolyticus* wound infection after exposure to sea water in an air crash. Eur J Clin Microbiol Infect Dis 12:474–475, 1993

184. MCNEELEY D, IVY P, CRAFT JC ET AL: *Plesiomonas:* Biology of the organism and diseases in children. Pediatr Infect Dis 3:176–181, 1984

185. MCNULTY CAM, DENT JC, CURRY A, UFF, JS, FORD GA, GEAR MWL, WILKINSON SP: New spiral bacterium in gastric mucosa. J Clin Pathol 42:585–591, 1989

186. MCNULTY CAM, DENT JC, UFF JS ET AL: Detection of *Campylobacter pylori* by the biopsy urease test: An assessment in 1445 patients. Gut 30:1058–1062, 1989

187. MCTIGHE AH: Pathogenic *Vibrio* species: Isolation and identification. Lab Management August 1982, pp 43–46

188. MERCER NSG, BEERE DM, BORNEMISZA AJ, THOMAS P: Medical leeches as sources of wound infection. Br Med J 294:937, 1987

189. MERINO FJ, AGULLA A, VILLASANTE PA ET AL: Comparative efficacy of seven selective media for isolating *Campylobacter jejuni*. J Clin Microbiol 24:451–452, 1986

190. MIDDLEBROOK JL, DORLAND RB: Bacterial toxins: Cellular mechanisms of action. Microbiol Rev 48:199–221, 1984

191. MILLS CK, GHERNA RL: Hydrolysis of indoxyl acetate by *Campylobacter* species. J Clin Microbiol 25:1560–1561, 1987

192. MINET J, GROSBOIS B, MEGRAUD F: *Campylobacter hyointestinalis:* An opportunistic enteropathogen? J Clin Microbiol 26:2659–2660, 1988

193. MORRIS A, ALI MR, THOMSEN L, HOLLIS B: Tightly spiral shaped bacteria in the human stomach: another cause of active chronic gastritis? Gut 31:139–143, 1990

194. MORRIS GK, EL SHERBEENY MR, PATTON CM ET AL: Comparison of four hippurate hydrolysis methods for identification of thermophilic *Campylobacter* sp. J Clin Microbiol 22:714–718, 1985

195. MORRIS GK, PATTON CM: *Campylobacter*. In Lennette EH (ed): Manual of Clinical Microbiology, 4th ed, chap 27, pp 302–308. Washington, DC, American Society for Microbiology, 1985

196. MORRIS JR JG: Vibrio cholerae 0139 Bengal: emergence of a new epidemic strain of cholera. Infect Agents Dis 4:41–46, 1995

197. MORRIS JG JR, WILSON R, HOLLIS DG ET AL: Illness caused by *Vibrio damsela* and *Vibrio hollisae*. Lancet i:1294–1296, 1982

198. NACHAMKIN I: Campylobacter infections. Current Oppinion in Infectious Diseases 6:72–76, 1993

199. NACHAMKIN I, BARBAGALLO S: Culture confirmation of *Campylobacter* spp. by latex agglutination. J Clin Microbiol 28:817–818, 1990

200. NACHAMKIN I, STOWELL C, SKALINA D ET AL: *Campylobacter laridis* causing bacteremia in an immunocompromised host. Ann Intern Med 101:55–57, 1984

201. NAIR GB, SHIMADA T, KURAZONO H ET AL: Characterization of phenotypic, serological, and toxigenic traits of *Vibrio cholerae* 0139 Bengal. J Clin Microbiol 32: 2775–2779, 1994

202. NAMDARI H, BOTTONE EJ: Suicide phenomenon in mesophilic aeromonads as a basis for species identification. J Clin Microbiol 27:788–789, 1989

203. NAMDARI H, BOTTONE EJ: Microbiological and clinical evidence supporting the role of *Aeromonas caviae* as a pediatric enteric pathogen. J Clin Microbiol 28:837–840, 1990

204. NAMDARI H, BOTTONE EJ: Cytotoxin and enterotoxin production as factors delineating enteropathogenicity of *Aeromonas caviae*. J Clin Microbiol 28:1796–1798, 1990

205. NEWELL DG (ED): *Campylobacter:* Epidemiology, pathogenesis and biochemistry. Lancaster, MIP Press, 1982

206. NG VL, HADLEY WK, FENNELL CL ET AL: Successive bacteremias with "*Campylobacter cinaedi*" and "*Campylobacter fennelliae*" in a bisexual male. J Clin Microbiol 25: 2008–2009, 1987

207. NOLAN CM, BALLARD J, KAYSNER CA ET AL: *Vibrio parahaemolyticus* gastroenteritis: An outbreak associated with raw oysters in the Pacific northwest. Diagn Microbiol Infect Dis 2:119–128, 1984

208. NOTERMANS S, HAVELAAR A, JANSEN W ET AL: Production of "Asao toxin" by *Aeromonas* strains isolated from feces and drinking water. J Clin Microbiol 23:1140–1142, 1986

209. OBERHOFER TR, PODGORE JK: Urea-hydrolyzing *Vibrio parahaemolyticus* associated with acute gastroenteritis. J Clin Microbiol 16:581–583, 1982

210. O'BRIEN M, COLWELL R: Modified taurocholate-tellurite-gelatin agar for improved differentiation of *Vibrio* species. J Clin Microbiol 22:1011–1013, 1985

211. ON SLW: Confirmation of human *Campylobacter concisus* isolates misidentified as *Campylobacter* mucosalis and suggestions for improved differentiation between the two species. J Clin Microbiol 32:2305–2306, 1994

212. ON SLW: Indentification methods for campylobacters, helicobacters, and related organisms. Clin Microbiol Rev 9: 405–422, 1996

213. ON SLW, Bloch B, Holmes B, Hoste B, Vandamme P: *Campylobacter hyointestinalis* subsp. *lawsonii* subsp. nov., isolated from the porcine stomach, and an emended description of *Campylobacter hyointestinalis*. Int J Syst Bacteriol 45:767–774, 1995

214. ORLICEK SL, WELCH DF, KUHLS T: Septicemia and meningitis caused by *Helicobacter cinaedi* in a neonate. J Clin Microbiol 31:569–571, 1993

215. OVERMAN TL, KESSLER JF, SEABOLT JP: Comparison of API 20E, API Rapid E, and API Rapid NFT for identification of members of the family *Vibrionaceae*. J Clin Microbiol 22:778–781, 1985

216. PAN-AMERICAN HEALTH ORGANIZATION. Cholera in the Americas. Epidemiol Bull 16:11–13, 1995

217. PASCUAL A, MARTINEZ-MARTINEZ L, GARCIA-GESTOSO ML, ROMERO J: Urinary tract infection caused by quinolone-resistant *Campylobacter coli*. Eur J Clin Microbiol Infect Dis 13:690–691, 1994

218. PASTER BJ, DEWHIRST FE: Phylogeny of campylobacters, wolinellas, *Bacteroides gracilis*, and *Bacteroides ureolyticus* by 16S ribosomal ribonucleic acid sequencing. Int J Syst Bacteriol 38:56–62, 1988

219. PASTER BJ, LEE A, FOX JG ET AL: Phylogeny of *Helicobacter felis* sp. nov., *Helicobacter mustelae*, and related bacteria. Int J Syst Bacteriol 41:31–38, 1991

220. PASTERNAK J, BOLIVAR R, HOPFER RL ET AL: Bacteremia caused by *Campylobacter*-like organism in two male homosexuals. Ann Intern Med 101:339–341, 1984

221. PATTON CM, SHAFFER N, EDMONDS P ET AL: Human disease associated with "*Campylobacter upsaliensis*" (catalase-negative or weakly positive *Campylobacter* species in the United States). J Clin Microbiol 27:66–73, 1989

222. PAVIA AT, BRYAN JA, MAHER KL ET AL: *Vibrio carchariae* infection after a shark bite. Ann Intern Med 111:85–86, 1989

223. PENNER JL: The genus *Campylobacter:* A decade of progress. Clin Microbiol Rev 1:157–172, 1988

224. PETERSON WL: *Helicobacter pylori* and peptic ulcer disease. N Engl J Med 324:1043–1048, 1991

225. PEZZLO M, VALTER PJ, BURNS MJ: Wound infection associated with *Vibrio alginolyticus*. Am J Clin Pathol 71:476–478, 1979

226. PITARANGSI E, ECHEVERRIA P, WHITMIRE R ET AL: Enteropathogenicity of *Aeromonas hydrophila* and *Plesiomonas shigelloides:* Prevalence among individuals with and without diarrhea in Thailand. Infect Immun 35:666–673, 1982

227. PITRAK DL, GINDORF JD: Bacteremic cellulitis caused by non-serogroup 01 *Vibrio cholerae* acquired in a freshwater inland lake. J Clin Microbiol 27:2874–2876, 1989

228. POPOVIC-UROIC T, PATTON CM, NICHOLSON MA ET AL: Evaluation of the indoxyl acetate hydrolysis test for rapid differentiation of *Campylobacter, Helicobacter,* and *Wolinella* species. J Clin Microbiol 28:2335–2339, 1990

229. QUINN TC, GOODELL SE, FENNELL C ET AL: Infections with *Campylobacter jejuni* and *Campylobacter*-like organisms in homosexual men. Ann Intern Med 101:187–192, 1984

230. RANK EL, SMITH IB, LANGER M: Bacteremia caused by *Vibrio hollisae*. J Clin Microbiol 26:375–376, 1988

231. REINA J, FERNANDEZ-BACA V, LOPEZ A: Acute gastroenteritis caused by *Vibrio alginolyticus* in an immunocompetent patient. Clin Infect Dis 21:1044–1045, 1995

232. REINHARDT JF, GEORGE WL: *Plesiomonas shigelloides*-associated diarrhea. JAMA 253:3294–3295, 1985

233. ROLSTON KVI, HOPFER RL: Diarrhea due to *Plesiomonas shigelloides* in cancer patients. J Clin Microbiol 20:597–598, 1984

234. ROMERO S, ARCHER JR, HAMACHER ME ET AL: Case report of an unclassified microaerophilic bacterium associated with gastroenteritis. J Clin Microbiol 26:142–143, 1988

235. ROOP RM II, SMIBERT RM, JOHNSON JL ET AL: DNA homology studies of the catalase-negative campylobacters and "*Campylobacter fecalis*," an emended description of *Campylobacter sputorum*, and proposal of the neotype strain of *Campylobacter sputorum*. Can J Microbiol 31:823–831, 1985

236. ROPPER AH: *Campylobacter* diarrhea and Guillain-Barre syndrome. Arch Neurol 45:655–656, 1988

237. RUIMY R, BREITTMAYER V, ELBAZE P, LAFAY B, BOUSSEMART O, GAUTHIER M, CHRISTEN R: Phylogenetic analysis and assessment of the genera *Vibrio, Photobacterium, Aeromonas,* and *Plesimonas* deduced from small-subunit rRNA sequences. J Syst Bacteriol 44:416–426, 1994

238. SACKS SL, LABRIOLA AM, GILL VJ, GORDIN FM: Use of ciprofloxacin for successful eradication of bacteremia due to *Campylobacter cinaedi* in a human immunodeficiency virus-infected person. Rev Infect Dis 13:1066–1068, 1991

239. SAFRIN S, MORRIS JG, ADAMS M ET AL: Non-01 *Vibrio cholerae* bacteremia: Case report and review. Rev Infect Dis 10:1012–1017, 1988

240. SANDSTEDT K, URSING J: Description of *Campylobacter upsaliensis* sp. nov. previously known as the CNW group. Syst Appl Microbiol 14:39–45, 1991

241. SANDSTEDT K, URSING J, WALDER M: Thermotoloerant *Campylobacter* with no or weak catalase activity isolated from dogs. Curr Microbiol 8:209–213, 1983

242. SANYAL SC, SARASWATHI B, SHARMA P: Enteropathogenicity of *Plesiomonas shigelloides*. J Med Microbiol 13:401–409, 1980

243. SCHMIDT U, CHMEL H, COBBS C: *Vibrio alginolyticus* infections in humans. J Clin Microbiol 10:666–668, 1979

244. SCHUBERT RHW, HEGAZI M: *Aeromonas eucrenophila* species nova *Aeromonas caviae*, a later and illegitimate synonym of *Aeromonas punctata*. Zentralbl Bakteriol Mikrobiol Hyg [A] 268:34–39, 1988

245. SHANDERA WX, JOHNSTON JM, DAVIS BR ET AL: Disease from infection with *Vibrio mimicus*, a newly recognized *Vibrio* species. Clinical characteristics and epidemiology. Ann Intern Med 99:169–171, 1983

246. SKIRROW MB, BENJAMIN J: "1001" Campylobacters: Cultural characteristics of intestinal campylobacters from man and animals. J Hyg (Cambridge) 85:427–442, 1980

247. SMIBERT RM: Genus *Campylobacter* Sebald and Veron 1963, 907[AL]. In Krieg NR, Holt HG (eds): Bergey's Manual of Systematic Bacteriology, vol 1, pp 111–118, Baltimore, Williams & Wilkins, 1984

248. SMITH SK, SUTTON DC, FUERST JA, REICHELT JL: Evaluation of the genus *Listonella* and reassignment of *Listonella damsela* (Love et al.) MacDonell and Colwell to the genus *Photobacterium* as *Photobacterium damsela*. Int J Syst Bacteriol 41:529–534, 1991

249. SMOAK BL, KELLEY PW, TAYLOR DN: Seroprevalence of *Helicobacter pylori* infections in a cohort of US Army recruits. Am J Epidemiol 139:513–519, 1994

250. SOLNICK JV, O'ROURKE J, LEE A, PASTER BJ, DEWHIRST FE, TOMPKINS LS: An uncultured gastric spiral organism is a newly identified *Helicobacter* in humans. J Infect Dis 168:379–385, 1993

251. SOVILLA J-Y, REGLI F, FRANCIOLI PB: Guillain-Barre syndrome following *Campylobacter jejuni* enteritis: report of three cases and review of the literature. Arch Intern Med 148: 739–741, 1988

252. SPIEGEL CA, TELFORD G: Isolation of *Wolinella recta* and *Actinomyces viscosus* from an actinomycotic chest wall mass. J Clin Microbiol 20:1187–1189, 1984

253. STANLEY J, BURNENS AP, LINTON D, ON SLW, COSTAS M, OWEN RJ: *Campylobacter helveticus* sp. nov., a new thermophilic species from domestic animals: characterization and cloning of a species-specific DNA probe. J Gen Microbiol 138:2293–2303, 1992

254. STANLEY J, LINTON D, BURNENS AP, DEWHIRST FE, ON SLW, PORTER A, OWEN RJ, COSTAS M: *Helicobacter pullorum* sp. nov.—genotype and phenotype of a new species isolated from poultry and from human patients with gastroenteritis. Microbiol 140:3441–3449, 1994

255. STANLEY J, LINTON D, BURNENS AP, DEWHIRST FE, OWEN RJ, PORTER A, ON SLW, COSTAS M: *Helicobacter canis* sp. nov., a new species from dogs: an integrated study of phenotype and genotype. J Gen Microbiol 139: 2495–2504, 1993

256. STEELE TW, MCDERMOTT SN: Technical note: The use of membrane filters applied directly to the surface of agar plates for the isolation of *Campylobacter jejuni* from feces. Pathology 16:263–265, 1984

257. STEELE TW, OWEN RJ: *Campylobacter jejuni* subsp. *doylei* subsp. nov., a subspecies of nitrate-negative campylobacters isolated from human clinical specimens. Int J Syst Bacteriol 38:316–318, 1988

258. STEELE TW, SANGSTER N, LANSER JA: DNA relatedness and biochemical features of *Campylobacter* spp. isolated in central and south Australia. J Clin Microbiol 22:71–74, 1985

259. STEINKRAUS GE, WRIGHT BD: Septic abortion with intact fetal membranes caused by *Campylobacter fetus* subsp. *fetus.* J Clin Microbiol 32:1608–1609, 1994

260. STILLS JR HF, HOOK RR, KINDEN DA: Isolation of *Campylobacter*-like organism from healthy Syrian hamsters (Mesocricetus auratus). J Clin Microbiol 27:2497–2501, 1989

261. SWERDLOW DL, RIES AA: *Vibrio cholerae* non-01—the eighth pandemic? Lancet 342:382–383, 1993

262. TACKET CO, BRENNER F, BLAKE PA: Clinical features and an epidemiological study of *Vibrio vulnificus* infections. J Infect Dis 149:558–561, 1984

263. TACKET CO, HICKMAN F, PIERCE GV ET AL: Diarrhea associated with *Vibrio fluvialis* in the United States. J. Clin Microbiol 16:991–992, 1982

264. TANNER ACR, BADGER S, LAI C-H ET AL: *Wolinella* gen. nov., *Wolinella succinogenes* (*Vibrio succinogenes* Wolin et al.) comb. nov., and description of *Bacteroides gracilis* sp. nov., *Wolinella recta* sp. nov., *Campylobacter concisus* sp. nov., and *Eikenella corrodens* from humans with periodontal disease. Int J Syst Bacteriol 31:432–445, 1981

265. TANNER ACR, LISTGARTEN MA, EBERSOLE JL: *Wolinella curva* sp. nov.: "*Vibrio succinogenes*" of human origin. Int J Syst Bacteriol 34:275–282, 1984

266. TAUXE RV, PATTON CM, EDMONDS P ET AL: Illness associated with *Campylobacter laridis,* a newly recognized *Campylobacter* species. J Clin Microbiol 21:222–225, 1985

267. TAYLOR DN, KIEHLBAUCH JA, TEE W, PITARANGSI C, ECHEVERRIA P: Isolation of group 2 aerotolerant *Campylobacter* species from Thai children with diarrhea. J Infect Dis163:1062–1067, 1991

268. TEE W, BAIRD R, DYALL-SMITH M ET AL: *Campylobacter cryaerophila* isolated from a human. J Clin Microbiol 26:2469–2473, 1988

269. THOMPSON LM III, SMIBERT RM, JOHNSON JL ET AL: Phylogenetic study of the genus *Campylobacter*. Int J Syst Bacteriol 38:190–200, 1988

270. TOTTEN PA, FENNELL CL, TENOVER FC ET AL: *Campylobacter cinaedi* (sp. nov.) and *Campylobacter fennelliae* (sp. nov): Two new *Campylobacter* species associated with enteric disease in homosexual men. J Infect Dis 151:131–139, 1985

271. TRAVIS LB, WASHINGTON JA II: The clinical significance of stool isolates of *Aeromonas.* Am J Clin Pathol 85:330–336, 1986

272. VANDAMME P, DANESHVAR MI, DEWHIRST FE, PASTER BJ, KERSTERS K, GROOSSENS H, MOSS CW: Chemotaxonomic analyses of *Bacteroides gracilis* and *Bacteroides ureolyticus* and reclassification of *B. gracilis* as *Campylobacter gracilis* comb. nov. Int J Syst Bacteriol 45:145–152, 1995

273. VANDAMME P, DE LEY J: Propsoal for a new family, *Campylobacteraceae*. Int J Syst Bacteriol 41:451–455, 1991

274. VANDAMME P, FALSEN E, POT B ET AL: Identification of EF group 22 campylobacters from gastroenteritis cases as *Campylobacter concisus.* J Clin Microbiol 27:1775–1781, 1989

275. VANDAMME P, FALSEN E, POT B ET AL: Identification of *Campylobacter cinaedi* isolated from blood and feces of children and adult females. J Clin Microbiol 28:1016–1020, 1990

276. VANDAMME P, FALSEN E, ROSSAU R ET AL: Revision of *Campylobacter, Helicobacter,* and *Wolinella* taxonomy: Emendation of generic descriptions and proposal of *Arcobacter* gen. nov. Int J Syst Bacteriol 41:88–103, 1991

277. VANDAMME P, PUGINA P, BENZI G, VAN ETTERIJCK R, VLAES L, KERSTERS K, BUTZLER J-P, LIOR H, LAUWERS S: Outbreak of recurrent abdominal cramps associated with *Arcobacter butzleri* in an Italian school. J Clin Microbiol 30:2335–2337, 1992

278. VANDAMME P, VANCANNEYT M, POT B, MELS L, BUTZLER J-P, GOOSSENS H: Polyphasic taxonomic study of the emended genus *Arcobacter* with *Arcobacter butzleri* comb. nov. and *Arcobacter skirrowii* sp. nov., an aerotolerant bacterium isolated from veterinary specimens. Int J Syst Bacteriol 42:344–356, 1992

279. VANLOON FPL, RAHIM Z, CHOWDHURY KA ET AL: Case report of *Plesiomonas shigelloides*-associated persistent dysentery and pseudomembranous colitis. J Clin Microbiol 27:1913–1915, 1989

280. VOGT RL, LITTLE AA, PATTON CM ET AL: Serotyping and serology studies of campylobacteriosis associated with consumption of raw milk. J Clin Microbiol 20:998–1000, 1984

281. VON GRAEVENITZ A, ALTWEGG A: *Aeromonas* and *Plesiomonas.* In Balows A (ed): Manual of Clinical Microbiology, 5th ed, chap 38, pp 396–401. Washington, DC, American Society for Microbiology, 1991

282. VON GRAEVENITZ A, BUCHER C: Evaluation of differential and selective media for isolation of *Aeromonas* and *Plesiomonas* spp. from human feces. J Clin Microbiol 17:16–21, 1983

283. WALMSLEY SL, KARMALI MA: Direct isolation of atypical thermophilic *Campylobacter* species from human feces on selective agar medium. J Clin Microbiol 27:668–670, 1989

284. WANG W-LL, LUECHTEFELD NW: Effect of incubation atmosphere and temperature on isolation of *Campylobacter jejuni* from human stools. Can J Microbiol 29:468–470, 1983

285. WARREN JR, MARSHALL BJ: Unidentified curved bacilli on gastric epithelium in active gastritis. Lancet 1:1273–1275, 1983

286. WATSON IM, ROBINSON JO, BURKE V ET AL: Invasiveness of *Aeromonas* spp. in relation to biotype, virulence factors, and clinical features. J Clin Microbiol 22:48–51, 1985

287. WEISSMAN JB, DEWITT WE, THOMPSON J ET AL: A case of cholera in Texas, 1973. Am J Epidemiol 100:487–498, 1974

288. WEXLER HM, REEVES D, SUMMANEN PH, MOLITORIS E, MCTEAGUE M, DUNCAN J, WILSON KH, FINEGOLD SM: *Sutterella wadsworthensis* gen. nov., sp. nov., bile-resistant microaerophilic *Campylobacter gracilis*-like clinical isolates. Int J Syst Bacteriol 46:252–258, 1996

289. YAO JDC, NG HMC, CAMPBELL I: Prosthetic hip joint infection due to *Campylobacter fetus.* J Clin Microbiol 31:3323–3324, 1993

HAEMOPHILUS

Members of the genus *Haemophilus* are small, nonmotile, gram-negative bacilli that require growth factors present in blood; the genus name is derived from the Greek words meaning "blood-loving." Some *Haemophilus* species require **X factor**, which is not a single substance but rather a group of heat-stable tetrapyrrole compounds that are provided by several iron-containing pigments (e.g., hemin, hematin). These compounds are used in the synthesis of catalases, peroxidases, and the cytochromes of the electron transport system. Most *Haemophilus* species also require **V factor**, which is nicotinamide adenine dinucleotide (NAD; coenzyme I) or nicotinamide adenine dinucleotide phosphate (NADP; coenzyme II). Both X and V factors are found within red blood cells, including the sheep erythrocytes found in blood agar formulations routinely used in clinical laboratories. Sheep blood also contains enzymes that slowly hydrolyze V factor. Consequently, V factor-dependent haemophili do not generally grow on sheep blood agar in which the erythrocytes are intact. Gentle heating during addition of

blood to the molten agar base in the preparation of chocolate agar results in lysis of erythrocytes, liberation of X and V factors, and inactivation of enzymes that hydrolyze V factor. Most laboratories rely on chocolate agar for the recovery of *Haemophilus* species from clinical specimens. *Haemophilus* species are also able to grow on blood agar containing intact 5% horse blood or rabbit blood. On these media, some *Haemophilus* species are β-hemolytic, a property that is helpful for identification.

Even though most *Haemophilus* species are unable to grow on sheep blood agar, tiny colonies of the organisms may occasionally be observed on this medium as pinpoint growth around colonies of other organisms in mixed cultures. These colonies also appear as "satellite" colonies within the hemolytic zone of a "staph streak" on sheep blood agar. The lysed erythrocytes in the agar surrounding the *Staphylococcus aureus* streak provide X factor, and the staphylococcal cells themselves secrete V factor during growth. The staph streak technique can be used to recover *Haemophilus* species from clinical specimens and is also a useful presumptive identification test (called the satellite test) for members of this genus.

Color Plates for Chapter 7 are found between pages 368 and 369.

TAXONOMY OF *HAEMOPHILUS* AND RELATED ORGANISMS

The genus *Haemophilus* is currently classified in the family *Pasteurellaceae*, which also includes members of the genera *Pasteurella* and *Actinobacillus*.[142] There are currently nine human species and five accepted or proposed animal species in the genus (Table 7-1). Although genus *Haemophilus* has traditionally been defined by the requirement of its members for X and V factors, genetic and biochemical studies have demonstrated that growth factor requirements are not exclusive features of *Haemophilus* species.[204] For example, certain V factor-dependent avian haemophili (i.e., the proposed species "*H. avium*") are genetically more closely related to the type species of the genus *Pasteurella* (*P. multocida*; see Chapter 8) than to the type species of the genus *Haemophilus* (*H. influenzae*), so these organisms have now been reclassified into three separate species in the genus *Pasteurella* as *P. avium*, *P. volantium*, and *Pasteurella* species A.[21,198] Genetic studies conducted with the animal haemophili have resulted in several taxonomic changes. "*Haemophilus pleuropneumoniae*," the cause of porcine necrotic pleuropneumonia, has been reclassified in the genus *Actinobacillus* as *A. pleuropneumoniae*.[224] "*Haemophilus equigenitalis*," the cause of contagious equine metritis, is genetically distinct from other haemophili and now belongs to the genus *Taylorella* as *T. equigenitalis*.[262] Other proposed animal haemophili, such as "*Haemophilus agni*" and "*Haemophilus somnus*" have never been validated as true *Haemophilus* species; it has been suggested that these organisms be placed in the genus *Histophilus*, along with *Histophilus ovis*, a cause of meningoencephalitis and other infections in sheep.[222,279] Currently, the animal species that are still included in the genus *Haemophilus* are *H. parasuis* (swine), *H. paragallinarum* (poultry), *H. paracuniculus* (rabbits), *H. haemoglobinophilus* (canines), and the proposed species "*H. felis*" (felines).[121,124]

The human *Haemophilus* species listed in Table 7-1 are for the most part associated with the upper respiratory tract, except for *Haemophilu ducreyi*, which is a primary pathogen of the genital tract. The remainder of this chapter will describe the infections caused by these organisms and the methods used for their isolation and identification in the clinical laboratory. The chapter concludes with a brief discussion of antimicrobial resistance trends in these microorganisms.

HAEMOPHILUS INFLUENZAE TYPE B DISEASE, IMMUNITY, AND VIRULENCE FACTORS

Infections in humans caused by *Haemophilus* species, the appropriate specimens for culture, and the clinical manifestations of these infections are summarized Table 7-2. For certain specimen types, many microbiology laboratories do not include a medium that will support the growth of *Haemophilus* species in their routine set of primary plating media. This is particularly true of respiratory tract specimens because as many as 85% of adults harbor *Haemophilus* species as a part of the normal bacterial flora of the nasopharynx and oropharynx.[187] Most of the upper respiratory tract species are nonencapsulated *H. influenzae* and *H. parainfluenzae*.[3,170] As will be described later in the chapter, these organisms may also be recovered as causes of infections under certain circumstances.

Encapsulated *H. influenzae* (capsular serotyopes a, b, c, d, e, and f) may also be found as a part of the normal upper respiratory tract flora of both children and adults. Colonization by capsular serotype b strains is found in 2% to 6% of children but may be as high as 60% among children in day care centers.[187] Therefore, recovery of *H. influenzae* from sputum specimens may reflect merely the presence of these organisms as a part of the normal nasopharyngeal flora. However, in those individuals with preexisting or chronic respiratory ailments, such as bronchitis, chronic obstructive pulmonary disease, bronchiectasis, bronchogenic carcinoma, and sinusitis, both encapsulated (typeable) and nonencapsulated (nontypeable) *H. influenzae* may cause severe respiratory tract infections.[57,65,81,148,151,189,265,272] The specific disease entities will be described later.

Most infections are caused by *H. influenzae* strains belonging to capsular serotype b. Type b is the only one of the six capsular types that contains a pentose (i.e., ribose) rather than a hexose, as the subunit carbohydrate component of the capsule, a property that may be related to virulence. The type b capsular substance is a linear polymer composed of ribose, ribitol (a 5-carbon sugar alcohol), and phosphate, or polyribosyl-ribitol-phosphate (PRP) (Figure 7-1). The reasons for the virulence of type b organisms and their ability to cause invasive and life-threatening infections remain unclear, although resistance to phagocytosis and intracellular killing by neutrophils afforded by the PRP capsule are important factors.[1] Serum anti-type b antibodies promote complement-dependent phagocytosis and killing (opsonization) of these organisms in vitro.

Although the PRP capsule is well recognized as a major virulence factor, the genetic basis of virulence in *H. influenzae* is complex and involves both capsular and noncapsular genetic determinants. The *capB* genes

---

TABLE 7-1

HUMAN AND ANIMAL SPECIES IN THE GENUS *HAEMOPHILUS*

HUMAN SPECIES	ANIMAL SPECIES
H. influenzae*	*H. parasuis* (swine)
H. parainfluenzae	*H. paragallinarum* (poultry)
H. haemolyticus	*H. paracuniculus* (rabbits)
H. parahaemolyticus	*H. haemoglobinophilus* (dogs)
H. aphrophilus	"*H. felis*" (cats)
H. paraphrophilus	
H. paraphrophaemolyticus	
H. segnis	
H. ducreyi	

*Includes the former species *H. aegyptius* as *H. influenzae* biogroup aegyptius.

TABLE 7-2

INFECTIOUS DISEASES ASSOCIATED WITH *HAEMOPHILUS* SPECIES

DISEASE	SPECIES	SPECIMENS FOR CULTURE	CLINICAL MANIFESTATIONS
Meningitis	*H. influenzae* type b (rarely other capsular types)	Cerebrospinal fluid; blood	Meningeal signs (headache, stiff neck), generally insidious onset; fever, seizures; usually seen in children 1 month to 2 years of age
Epiglottitis	*H. influenzae* type b (rarely other capsular types)	Blood; laryngeal secretions	Rapid onset and progression of sore throat; dysphagia and upper airway obstruction; red and swollen epiglottis; may require tracheostomy to establish airway
Otitis media	*H. influenzae* (usually nontypeable strains)	Swab of drainage in the ear canal; needle aspiration or myringotomy; suspected systemic disease may require collection of CSF or blood cultures	Pain and fullness in the ears; usually bilateral; bulging, opaque tympanic membranes; fever, irritability, and vomiting may be noted; concomitant systemic disease should be suspected
Acute sinusitis	*H. influenzae* (usually nontypeable strains); rarely, *H. parainfluenzae*	Sinus aspirates; surgical specimens	Frontal headaches; facial pain; swelling and redness of suborbital and periorbital tissues; sinus empyema
Acute pharyngitis or laryngeotracheobronchitis	*H. influenzae* type b	Posterior pharyngeal swab; laryngeal sections	Inflamed mucous membranes with swelling and yellow exudate; sore throat with stridor and cough; similar to croup if the laryngeal mucosa is involved
Bronchitis	*H. influenzae* (often nontypeable strains)	Sputum; transtracheal aspirates; bronchial washings	Persistent, nonproductive cough; wheezing and dyspnea; disease is usually chronic with periodic purulent exacerbations
Pneumonia	*H. influenzae* type b; nontypeable strains recovered from elderly patients	Sputum; tracheal aspirates; bronchial washings	Cough, sputum production, and pleuritic pain; distribution tends to be lobar or segmental, simulating pneumococcal pneumonia; bacteremic pneumonia caused by nontypeable strains seen in elderly patients
Endocarditis	*H. aphrophilus*; *H. paraphrophilus*; *H. parainfluenzae*; rarely, *H. influenzae*	Blood	Chills, spiking fevers, leukocytosis, and secondary complications, such as anemia, weight loss, malaise, and anorexia; mitral and aortic valves most commonly involved; high incidence of arterial embolization
Genital tract infection and postpartum bacteremia; neonatal sepsis with meningitis	*H. influenzae* (nontypeable); *H. parainfluenzae*; *H. influenzae* cryptic genospecies	Urethral and endocervical specimens; blood; fetal tissues; CSF	Urethritis characterized by thin, mucoid discharge; organisms may be recovered from cervical and blood cultures of women with postpartum fever; may also be cultured from multiple genital sites (e.g., Bartholin's glands, endometrium); placenta, amniotic fluid, and neonatal body fluids
Conjunctivitis	*H. influenzae* biogroup aegyptius	Conjunctival swab specimen	Characterized by mucopurulent conjunctival discharge; hyperemic conjunctivae, and diffusely injected sclera; spread to others by infectious secretions on towels and hands
Brazilian purpuric fever	*H. influenzae* biogroup aegyptius (BPF clone)	Blood; conjunctival swabs; skin lesions; oropharynx	Fever, abdominal pain with vomiting; petechial and hemorrhagic skin lesions; symptoms mimic meningococcal meningitis, but meningitis is not present; previous or concurrent conjuntival infection with BPF clone of *H. influenzae* biogroup aegyptius usually found
Chancroid	*H. ducreyi*	Swabs obtained from genital ulcers; aspirates from buboes; endocervical swab specimens	Sexually transmitted disease, characterized by painful, ulcerative genital lesions and enlarged, suppurative inguinal lymph nodes; may progress to abscess and fistula formation if left untreated

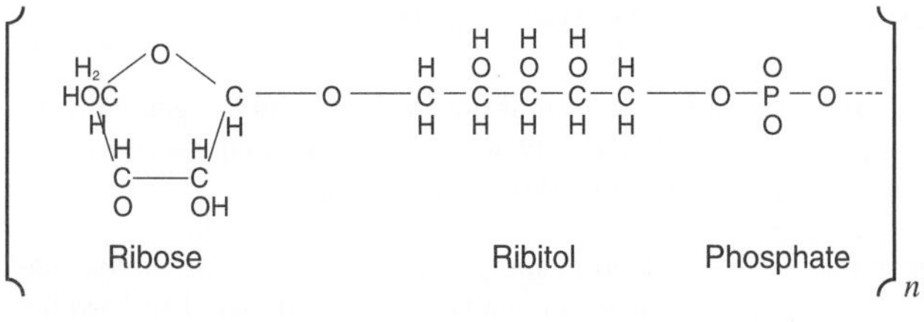

Figure 7-1.

Structure of the repeating unit of the *Haemophilus influenzae* type b capsular polysaccharide polyribose-ribitol-phosphate (PRP). This molecule consists of the five-carbon monosaccharide ribose, linked by an ester bond to ribitol, a five-carbon sugar alcohol which, in turn, is linked to a phosphate group.

that code for type b encapsulation exist in the chromosome as a duplication of two identical 17- to 18-kilobase (kb) segments that are joined by a short 1- to 1.3-kb region.[118,152] This short region contains a gene called *bexA* that codes for a protein required for export of the capsular material to the cell surface.[153] This duplicated-gene arrangement is seen in more than 98% of *H. influenzae* type b strains. In contrast, *cap* genes for types a, c, d, and f are organized as single-copy genes; capsule-deficient type b strains lack the *capB* locus duplication and possess only a single copy of this gene.[152] The theoretical evolutionary advantage imparted by the duplicated *capB* genotype is the availability of a ready template for rapid amplification of type b capsular gene sequences under environmental conditions during which it may be advantageous to produce more capsular material. An examination of 36 invasive clinical isolates of *H. influenzae* type b from Finland and 14 strains from Washington, D.C. showed that, indeed, amplification of *capB* genes occurs commonly in vivo.[117] Fifteen of the 36 Finnish strains and five of the 14 U.S. strains contained three to five copies of the *capB* gene. Strains with multiple gene copies produced more type b capsular polysaccharide; the single strain that possessed five copies made four to five times more of the type b capsular material than the wild type strain. Interestingly, encapsulation of type b organism is associated with decreased adherence to and invasion of human cells.[217,257] Type b capsule-deficient mutants resulting from loss of a copy of the duplication at the *capB* locus showed a 50-fold increase in adherence to human epithelial cells and a nearly 300-fold increase in invasive capabilities. Restoration of encapsulation by transformation resulted in a large decrease in both adherence and invasion.

Several other potential virulence factors have been identified in both typeable and nontypeable *H. influenzae* strains. Pili have been described in *H. influenzae* and have been found on both encapsulated and nontypeable strains.[95] These pili appear to mediate hemagglutination and adherence to human mucosal cells but actually inhibit mucosal cell invasion.[83] These pili are not the only cell surface structures mediating bacterial adherence to mucosal cells because nonpiliated organisms also adhere to epithelial cells and do not compete with piliated organisms for the same receptor.[160] There

is also evidence suggesting that nonpiliated cells switch to the piliated phenotype after prolonged exposure to epithelial cells.[217] Similar to many other pathogens, *H. influenzae* produces an IgA1 protease that inactivates human immunoglobulin (Ig) A1, which accounts for over 90% of the IgA present in the oropharynx.[143] More than 90% of *H. influenzae* type b strains also produce a bacteriocin called a "haemocin."[157,158] Bacteriocins are proteins that are produced by a variety of bacterial species and that are able to inhibit the growth of strains of the same or related species. Haemocin is not produced by encapsulated non-type b or nontypeable *H. influenzae* strains, although most of these organisms are susceptible to its lethal effects.[157] Haemocin production may contribute to the ability of *H. influenzae* type b strains to effectively compete with nontypeable strains in nasopharyngeal colonization.

Similar to other gram-negative bacteria, *H. influenzae* strains possess lipopolysaccharide in the cell wall outer membrane. This lipopolysaccharide consists of lipid A joined by 2-keto-3-deoxyoctulosonic acid (KDO) to a core polysaccharide polymer consisting of neutral monosaccharides, but it differs from the lipopolysaccharide of the family *Enterobacteriaceae* in that it lacks the repeating terminal side chains (the "O" or somatic antigens).[13,298] There is also evidence that two antigenically distinct types of lipid A may be found among typeable and nontypeable strains of *H. influenzae* and that these lipid A types are not found in other *Haemophilus* species.[189] For these reasons, the lipopolysaccharide of *H. influenzae* is more accurately termed a lipooligosaccharide (LOS). The neutral core LOS oligosaccharides—glucose, galactose, glucosamine, and heptose—vary in relative amounts, not only from strain to strain, but also within different generations of a given strain.[145] In vitro and in vivo studies with LOS mutants have shown that the LOS phenotype may function to modulate virulence in individual strains by genetically controlled structural modifications that essentially "switch on" or "switch off" the expression of key surface-exposed, oligosaccharide-dependent LPS epitopes.[145,146,171] The LOS of these organisms posesses all of the biological activities of endotoxin, including lymphocyte mitogenicity, lethality in the mouse model of endotoxemia, pyrogenicity in rabbits, and gelation of *Limulus* amoebocyte lysate.[87] Antibodies directed against LOS are not protective because infants with *H. influenzae* type b meningitis have antibodies to LOS at the time of infection and anti-LOS antibodies do not prevent infection on challenge in the infant rat model of meningitis.

Lastly, *H. influenzae* also possesses several outer membrane proteins, and research in this area has focused primarily on those proteins that might be useful as components of a vaccine against nontypeable *H. influenzae*, which are associated with a variety of infections in both children and adults.[13,189] Outer membrane proteins designated P2 and P6 have generated the most interest as potential vaccine antigens. P2 is the major outer membrane protein of *H. influenzae*, constituting more than 50% of the outer membrane protein content. This protein has a relative molecular weight of between 37,000 and 40,000 Da, exists in the outer membrane as a trimer, and functions as a porin protein; therefore, it is partially exposed on the surface of nontypeable strains.[188,190,192] Antibodies directed against the P2 protein are bactericidal and protective against challenge infection in the infant rat model.[188] However, considerable antigenic heterogeneity exists among P2 proteins from different strains, so analysis of P2 proteins from a variety of strains will be necessary to characterize epitopes of P2 that are highly immunogenic, yet highly conserved structurally and immunologically.[113,190] P6 is a protein that constitutes 1% to 5% of the outer membrane protein content and is present on the surface of both typeable and nontypeable strains.[203] It has a molecular weight of 16,600 Da and is actually a peptidoglycan-associated lipoprotein.[191] Antibodies directed against P6 are bactericidal and are protective against challenge in the infant rat model.[191] Amino acid sequence analysis of the P6 protein and nucleotide sequencing of the P6 gene from type b strains and nontypeable strains showed greater than 97% homology, indicating that the P6 gene is highly conserved at the genetic level.[63,203] Bactericidal antibodies directed against P6 are present in normal human serum.

HAEMOPHILUS INFLUENZAE TYPE B VACCINES

Before the introduction of effective vaccines against H. influenzae type b, this organism was associated with approximately 16,000 cases of invasive disease in children 5 years of age and younger each year.[187] Most of these infections occurred in children between the ages of 2 months and 5 years, with the majority of systemic type b infections affecting children aged 2 years and younger.[187,240] It was recognized that the presence of inadequate levels of protective, anti-PRP bactericidal antibodies at this age played a major role in the development of disease.[5] Immunity in the immediate new-

born period is probably acquired by transplacental antibodies that are lost within the first few months of life. These antibodies generally reappear later, following exposure to type b organisms or to other microbial antigens that engender cross-reactive antibodies. Most individuals who develop systemic H. influenzae type b disease have low or undetectable levels of anti-PRP capsular antibodies.

The antigenic capabilities of native, purified PRP and the protection afforded by anti-PRP antibodies were exploited in the first H. influenzae type b vaccine preparations. Purified PRP failed to elicit protective levels of antibody in infants and young children, the groups most at risk for serious illness.[28,244] Immune responses were consistently seen only in children older than 2 years of age.[223] Furthermore, the vaccine did not predictably elicit a "booster" response on subsequent antigenic challenge. Because of the poor immunogenicity of the purified capsular polysaccharide and the demonstrated lack of efficacy in children younger than 18 months of age, the H. influenzae PRP polysaccharide vaccine that was licensed in the United States in 1985 was recommended for routine use primarily in children 24 to 50 months of age. Clinical trials were subsequently undertaken with several polysaccharide–protein conjugate vaccines.[6,19,20,241,282] By using this approach, it was hoped that the immunogenicity of the PRP material would be enhanced, with the protein "carrier" acting as an adjuvant to prime the immune response. Clinical trials with the various PRP–conjugate vaccines have indeed demonstrated protective responses in progressively much younger children.[1]

As of 1994, four H. influenzae type b conjugate vaccines and one combination vaccine that combines a PRP-conjugate vaccine with diphtheria–tetanus–pertussis (DTP) have been approved by the Food and Drug Administration (Table 7-3). The four conjugate vaccines include PRP-D (ProHIBIT, Connaught Laboratories, Swiftwater PA), HbOC (HibTITER, Lederle/

TABLE 7-3
CURRENTLY AVAIABLE HAEMOPHILUS INFLUENZAE TYPE B CONJUGATE VACCINES

VACCINE	TRADE NAME	MANUFACTURER	CARBOHYDRATE	CARRIER PROTEIN
PRP-D	ProHIBIT	Connaught	Medium-sized PRP	Diphtheria toxoid
HbOC	HibTITER	Lederle/Praxis	Small-sized PRP	Nontoxic mutant diphtheria toxin (CRM$_{197}$)
PRP-OMP	PedvaxHIB	Merck, Sharpe & Dohme	Native-sized PRP	Outer membrane protein complex of Neisseria meningitidis serogroup B
PRP-T	ActHIB OmniHib	Connaught SmithKline Beecham	Native-sized PRP Native-sized PRP	Tetanus toxoid Tetanus toxoid
HbOC-DTP	Tetralmmune	Lederle-Praxis	Small-sized PRP	Nontoxic mutant diphtheria toxin (CRM$_{197}$) combined with DTP (diphtheria toxoid, tetanus toxoid, and whole-cell pertussis vaccine)

Praxis Biologicals, Rochester NY), PRP-OMP (Pedvax-HIB, Merck, Sharpe & Dohme, West Point PA), and PRP-T (ActHIB, Connaught Laboratories; OmniHib, SmithKline-Beecham Pharmaceuticals, Philadelphia PA). The single PRP–conjugate combination vaccine is HbOC-DTP (TETRAIMMUNE, Lederle-Praxis Biologicals, Rochester NY). PRP-D and HbOC vaccines consist of the *H. influenzae* type b PRP capsular polysaccharide conjugated to diphtheria toxoid (PRP-D) or to CRM_{197}, which is a "nontoxic" diphtheria toxin isolated from a mutant strain of *Corynebacterium diphtheriae* (HbOC), respectively. PRP-OMP consists of PRP linked to an outer membrane protein complex (OMP) purified from *Neisseria meningitidis*. PRP-T vaccine consists of PRP conjugated to tetanus toxoid. The licensed combination vaccine HbOC-DTP consists of HbOC combined with DTP vaccine. Unconjugated, native PRP vaccine is no longer commercially available in the United States.

As each of the conjugate vaccines have been evaluated and studied, their safety and efficacy in younger children have significantly improved. PRP-D, the first of the conjugate vaccines, was licensed in December 1987 for children at least 18 months of age. Because its immunogenicity in younger children was poor, PRP-D was not licensed for use in infants.[62,78,282] The two other subsequently licensed conjugate vaccines—HbOC and PRP-OMP—were initially recommended for use in children at least 15 months of age. Subsequently, these two vaccines were demonstrated to be efficacious in younger children, and routine use of either HbOC or PRP-OMP vaccines in infants as young as 2 months of age was recommended.[19,78,241] PRP-T was one of the first *H. influenzae* type b conjugate vaccines developed but was the last one to receive licensure in the United States. Infants given PRP-T vaccine at 2, 4, and 6 months had little or no immune response after the first vaccine dose, a moderate response following the second dose, and an anamnestic response after the third dose.[107] Furthermore, better first-dose immune responses to vaccination were observed in older children who had received DTP vaccine a few months before the PRP-T dose, suggesting that priming of the immune system with tetanus toxoid heightened the immune response on subseqent inoculation with PRP that was conjugated to tetanus toxoid.[102] This carrier–protein priming effect has been noted with all of the conjugate vaccines.[62,101,103]

In late 1993, the Committee on Infectious Diseases of the American Academy of Pediatrics and the Immunization Practices Advisory Committee of the Centers for Disease Control and Prevention (CDCP) issued recommendations for administration of *H. influenzae* type b vaccine.[39,52] General guidelines for vaccine use include the following (Box 7-1).

Although long-term experience with these vaccines in children with underlying diseases is not yet available, a few small studies suggest that they may not be as effective in such individuals. In a study of 22 premature infants of 28 weeks median gestational age, administration of PRP-OMP at 2 and 4 months of chronologic age resulted in only 27% and 55% of the infants demonstrating anti-PRP levels higher than 1 µg/mL after the first and second vaccine dose, respectively.[284] This antibody response was significantly lower than that seen in term infants. In another study of 19 human immunodeficiency (HIV-1)-infected children who were immunized with a single dose of PRP-T or HbOC at a mean age of 28 months, only 7 children had levels of anti-PRP antibodies that indicated immunity.[220] These authors postulated that the poor response to the vaccine was due to the T–cell-depleted state of the patients and the T–cell-dependent nature of the immune response to the conjugate vaccines. The antibody response to HbOC immunization in HIV-1-infected adults was previously shown to be positively correlated with the number of T-helper cells.[255]

The availability of safe and effective vaccines against *H. influenzae* type b has already dramatically altered the incidence of serious infections caused by this microorganism. From active, prospective surveillance data on the incidence of invasive *H. influenzae* disease in children living in Minnesota and Dallas County, Texas, Murphy and colleagues[194] reported that the incidence of invasive *H. influenzae* type b disease in 1991 decreased 85% in Minnesota and 92% in Dallas when compared with 1983 and 1984 baseline rates before the availability of the first native PRP polysaccharide vaccine in 1985. With use of data collected through a laboratory-based active surveillance system coordinated by the Meningitis and Special Pathogens Branch of the CDC, Adams and coworkers[1] reported a decrease in incidence of *H. influenzae* type b disease of 71% from 1985 through 1991. With data from the National Bacterial Meningitis Reporting System, these same workers also reported that the incidence of *H. influenzae* type b meningitis decreased by 82% between 1985 and 1991.[1] In a study of *H. influenzae* disease among children of U.S. Army personnel on active duty, the incidence of meningitis declined from 59 cases per 100,000 children in 1986 to 6 per 100,000 children in 1991.[27] Among children younger than than 5 years of age, the race-adjusted incidence of *H. influenzae* type b disease reported to the National Notifiable Diseases Surveillance System declined by 95% from 41 cases per 100,000 in 1987 to 2 cases per 100,000 in 1993.[40] Large ongoing vaccine studies in Los Angeles County have also reported large decreases in the incidence of disease in children younger than 60 months of age.[273,274] The incidence of *H. influenzae* type b disease in this area decreased from 43 cases per 100,000 children in 1988 to 4.4 cases per 100,000 children in 1992.

Similar decreases in the incidence of *H. influenzae* type b disease other than meningitis have also been observed. Takala and associates[267] reported that, while the number of vaccinated children in Finland steadily increased from 1987 through 1992, the number of cases of epiglottitis decreased from 50 to 60 cases seen annually in 1985 and 1986 to only 2 cases in 1992. Gorelick and Baker[99] reported that the average annual incidence of epiglottitis in Philadelphia declined from 10.9 cases per 10,000 hospital admissions before 1990 to 1.8 per 10,000 hospital admissions from 1990 through 1992,

COLOR PLATES

CHAPTERS 7–13

IDENTIFICATION OF *HAEMOPHILUS* SPECIES

A. A gram-stained slide of cerebrospinal fluid showing polymorphonuclear cells and scattered gram-negative bacilli of *Haemophilus influenzae.* These organisms characteristically appear as small, poorly staining coccobacilli on Gram stains of clinical specimens. Occasionally, longer, filamentous bacilli may be seen, as shown here.

B. Growth of moist, smooth, gray colonies of *H. influenzae* type b on chocolate agar. This medium contains hematin (X factor) and is enriched with other co-factors, such as NAD (V factor) that allow the growth of *Haemophilus* and other fastidious microorganisms.

C. Satellite growth of *Haemophilus* species around streaks of *Staphylococcus aureus* on sheep blood agar. X factor, or hemin, is provided by the lysed sheep erythrocytes surrounding the *Staphylococcus* streak, while the staphylococci themselves provide the V factor, or NAD. These factors enable the tiny, dew-drop colonies of *Haemophilus* to grow adjacent to the staphylococcus streak.

D. Growth factor test for identification of *H. influenzae.* The organism is inoculated onto a plate of trypticase–soy or brain–heart infusion agar, and disks containing X factor and V factor are placed in proximity to one another on the inoculum. After incubation in a CO_2-enriched environment, factor requirements are determined by observing organism growth relative to the two disks. In this picture, growth is observed between the X and V factor disks, indicating that the organism requires both exogenous X and exogenous V factors for growth.

E. Growth factor test for *H. parainfluenzae.* The organism is inoculated as described for plate **D**, but here, filter paper strips that are impregnated with X factor, V factor, or both X and V factors, are placed on the lawn of inoculum. After incubation, growth is observed around the V factor strip and the XV factor strip, but not around the X factor strip. This indicates that the organism requires only V factor.

F. The ALA–porphyrin agar test: This test is an alternative method for determining the X factor requirements of *Haemophilus* isolates. The agar medium contains δ-aminolevulinic acid (ALA). Organisms are inoculated onto the medium and, after overnight incubation, the growth is observed under a Wood's light (ultraviolet light). If the growth fluoresces a "brick-red" color, the organism is able to synthesize X factor (hemin) and does not require exogenous X factor. This slide shows growth of both *H. influenzae* (*left*), with its negative ALA–porphyrin test (i.e., requires exogenous hemin), and *H. parainfluenzae* (*right*), with its positive ALA–porphyrin test (i.e., synthesizes hemin from ALA).

G. Nitrate and biotyping reactions for *Haemophilus influenzae* biotype I. Both *H. influenzae* and *H. parainfluenzae* reduce nitrate to nitrite and can be grouped into distinct biotypes by their reactions in three biochemical tests—production of indole, ornithine decarboxylase, and urease. This plate shows the nitrate and biotyping reactions for *H. influenzae* biotype I. Tests shown (*left to right*) are a positive nitrate reduction test, indole production in tryptone broth following xylene extraction (positive), Moeller's decarboxylase broth base (negative), Moeller's ornithine decarboxylase broth (positive), and a urease slant (positive).

H. The MicroScan *Haemophilus–Neisseria* Identification (HNID) Panel (Dade-MicroScan, West Sacramento CA). This manual microtiter tray system identifies both *Haemophilus* and *Neisseria* species and provides biotype designations for *H. influenzae* and *H. parainfluenzae*. This slide shows a panel inoculated with *H. influenzae* biotype I (urease-positive, ornithine decarboxylase-positive, and indole-positive). (Courtesy of Dade-MicroScan.)

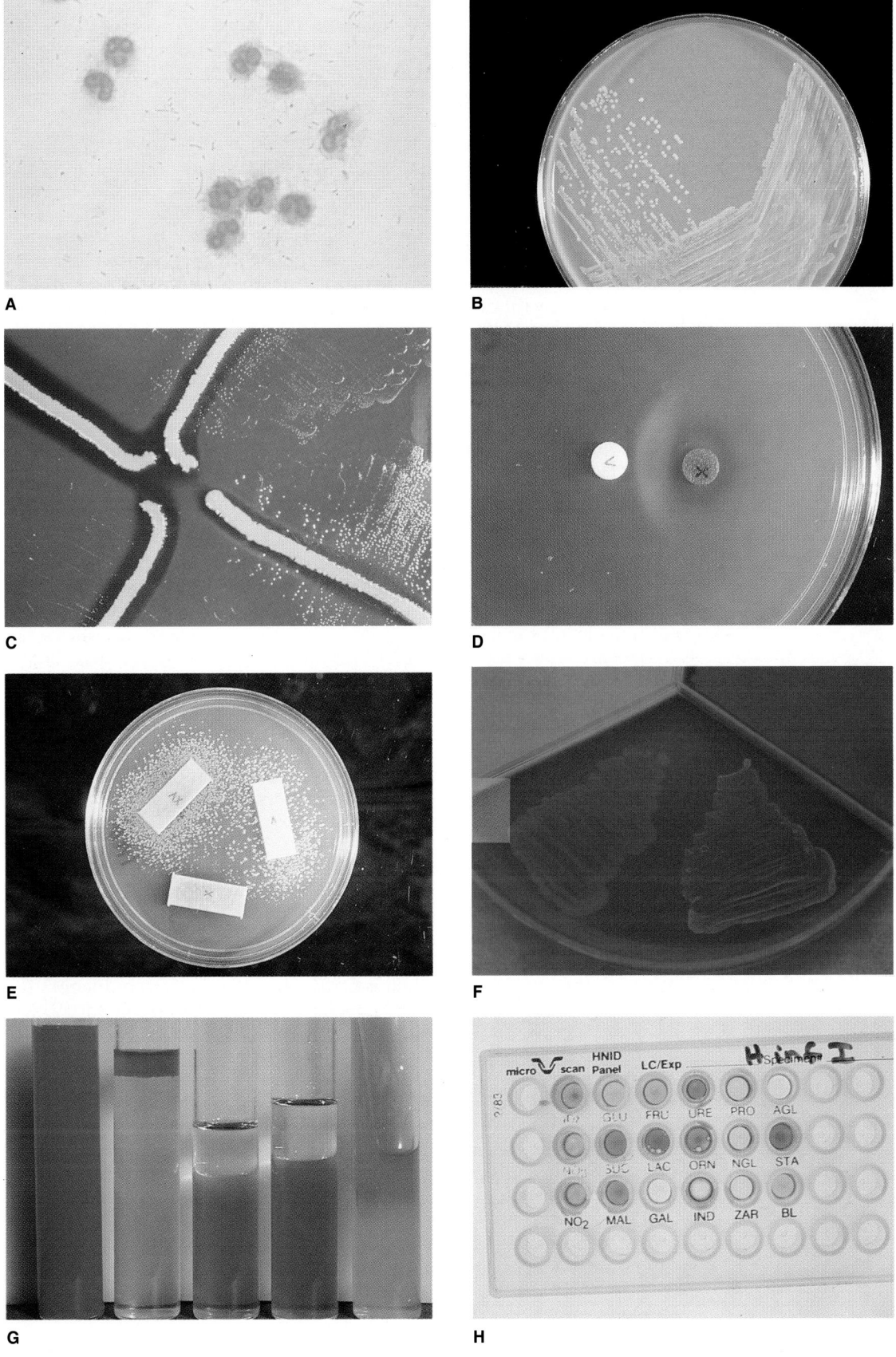

A

B

C

D

E

F

G

H

MISCELLANEOUS FASTIDIOUS GRAM-NEGATIVE BACILLI

A. Colonies of *H. aphrophilus* on chocolate agar after 48 hours growth. These colonies are characteristically small and have a slight yellow pigment. This species will also grow on sheep blood agar because X and V factors are not required for growth.

B. Gram stain of *H. aphrophilus* from culture media. This organism appears as short, pale-staining gram-negative coccobacilli, a characteristic that is shared with many of the other HACEK group bacteria.

C. Rapid carbohydrate utilization tests for *H. aphrophilus*. In this procedure, a phosphate buffered saline-phenol red solution (PBS) is dispensed in a series of tubes in 0.10 mL volumes. A single drop of a carbohydrate solution (20% w/v) is added to each tube. A heavy suspension of the organism is made in the buffer, and a single drop of the suspension is added to each of the carbohydrate-containing tubes. After incubation at 35°C for 4 hours, the reactions are read. With the production of acid, the indicator turns from red to yellow. In this frame, the tubes, from left to right, are the PBS organism suspension (no carbohydrate), PBS with glucose (G), maltose (M), sucrose (S), lactose (L), mannitol (MN), xylose (X), and mannose (MA). As can be seen in this photograph, *H. aphrophilus* produces acid from glucose, maltose, sucrose, lactose, and mannose but not from mannitol or xylose (see Table 8-1). Details of this procedure, which is also used for identifying *Neisseria* species, are given in Chart 63.

D. Other biochemical tests for identification of *H. aphrophilus*. The tubes shown in this photograph, left to right, include nitrate broth, indole-tryptone broth, Moeller's decarboxylase base, Moeller's lysine decarboxylase broth, Moeller's ornithine decarboxylase broth, and a urease agar slant. As shown here, *H. aphrophilus* is nitrate-positive but negative for indole, lysine decarboxylase, ornithine decarboxylase, and urease.

E. Colonies of *A. actinomycetemcomitans* on sheep blood agar after 72 hours growth. These colonies are small, variable in size, have irregular edges, and are usually adherent to the growth media on primary isolation. This organism, like *H. aphrophilus*, does not require X or V factors and will also grow on sheep blood agar.

F. Rapid carbohydrate utilization tests for *A. actinomycetemcomitans*. As shown here, *A. actinomycetemcomitans* produces acid from glucose (G), mannitol (MN), and mannose (MA) but not from maltose (M), sucrose (S), lactose (L), or xylose (X) (see Table 8-1). Failure to produce acid from lactose and a positive catalase test help to differentiate *A. actinomycetemcomitans* from *H. aphrophilus* (see Color Plate 8-1C above). Other biochemical reactions (i.e., nitrate reduction, decarboxylases, and urease) are the same as for *H. aphrophilus* (see Color Plate 8-1D above).

G. Gram stain of *C. hominis*. These organisms are often gram-variable but are staining uniformly gram-negative in this photomicrograph. The cells of *C. hominis* are generally longer than other HACEK bacteria and show pleomorphism (i.e., cells with pointed or swollen ends, tear drop-shaped and dumbbell-shaped cells). The characteristic palisading of the cells in "picket fence" arrangements and the clustering of cells to form compact rosettes are also evident in this picture.

H. Growth of *C. hominis* on sheep blood agar after 72 hours incubation. The colonies are small, opaque, and glistening. Some strains may also pit the agar like *E. corrodens*.

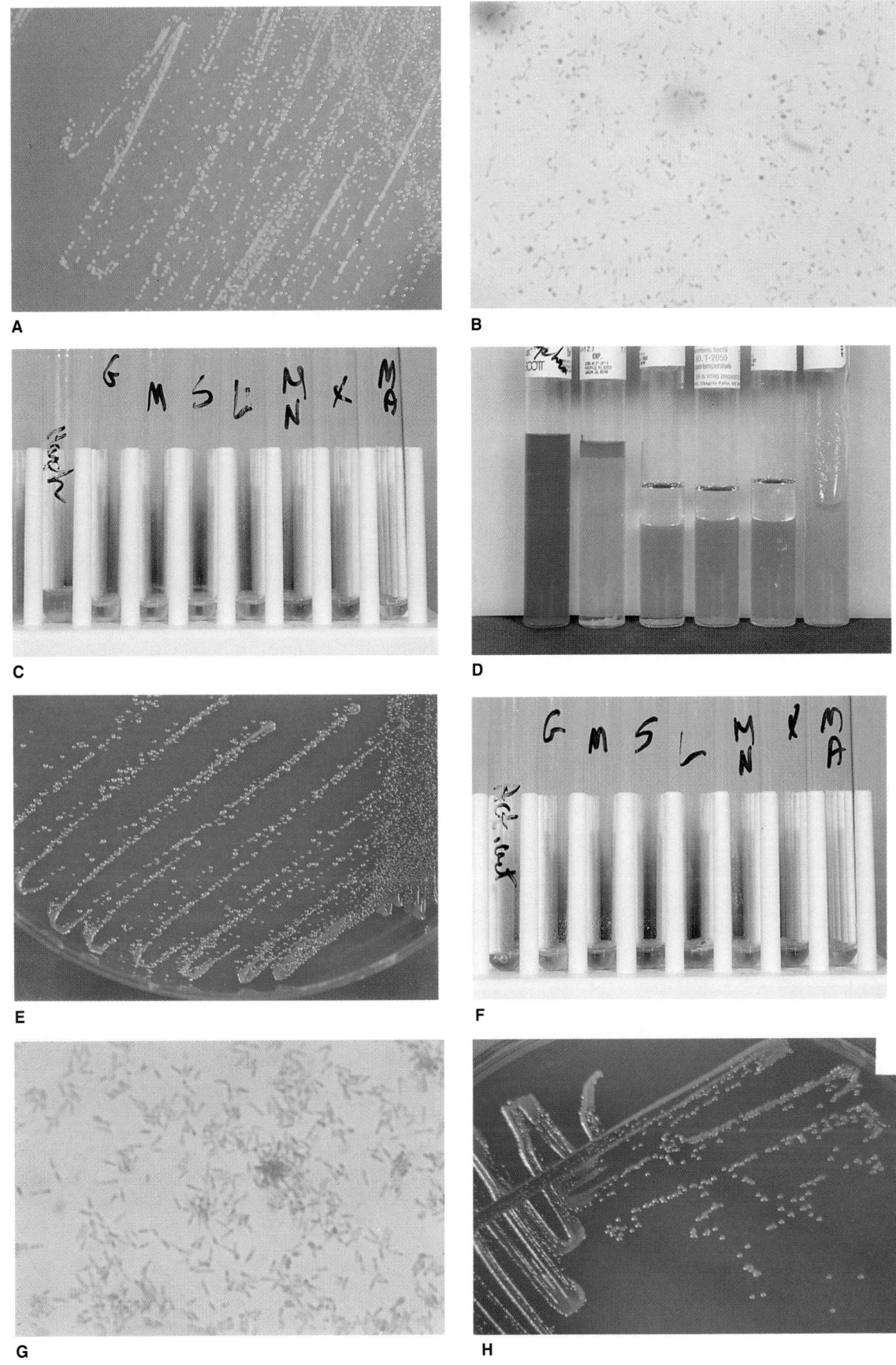

A

B

C

D

E

F

G

H

Miscellaneous Fastidious Gram-Negative Bacilli

A. Growth of *E. corrodens* on sheep blood agar. Although frequently difficult to photograph, the incident light on the plate in this photograph demonstrates the pitting of the agar surface that is characteristic of many strains of *E. corrodens*. Nonpitting strains may also be identified.

B. Biochemical reactions for *E. corrodens*. The tubes shown here are, left to right, nitrate broth; indole tryptone broth, Moeller's decarboxylase base, Moeller's lysine decarboxylase broth, Moeller's ornithine decarboxylase broth, and a urea slant. *E. corrodens* is the only member of the HACEK group that is nitrate-positive, lysine decarboxylase– and ornithine decarboxylase–positive, and urease–negative.

C. RapID NH panel inoculated with *K. denitrificans*. This commercially available identification system provides identifications of certain fastidious gram-negative organisms in 4 hours. Two identical panels are depicted in this photograph; the upper panel is before the addition of nitrate and indole reagents; the lower panel is after the addition of reagents. Positive reactions on the panel for this oxidase-positive, catalase-negative organism include prolyl aminopeptidase (PRO), glucose fermentation (GLU), and positive nitrate (NO_3) and nitrite (NO_2) reduction tests. All other tests results are negative.

D. *Capnocytophaga* species on sheep blood agar. This photograph shows the characteristic colonial morphology of these organisms, illustrating the fringe of "gliding" bacteria at the periphery of the growth. Toward the center of the areas of growth, the colonies become more mottled and rough appearing.

E. Gram stain of *Capnocytophaga* species. These organisms characteristically appear as gram-negative, slightly curved, fusiform bacteria with pointed ends. In this respect, the other species that these organisms resemble is the obligate anaerobe *Fusobacterium nucleatum*.

F. Colonies of *Capnocytophaga canimorsus* on sheep blood agar after 5 days growth. Colonies are entire, circular, convex, and shiny, as shown here.

G. Gram stain of *Capnocytophaga canimorsus*. This photograph shows the fusiform cells typical of the genus. Some of the cells in this picture are slightly curved, and this is also characteristic of the genus.

H. Colonies of CDC Group DF-3. This organism grows as pinpoint colonies after 24 hours that subsequently form larger, grey to white colonies. This photograph shows a 48-hour culture of DF-3 on sheep blood agar. Colonial growth of DF-3 has been reported to have a characteristic "sweet" odor.

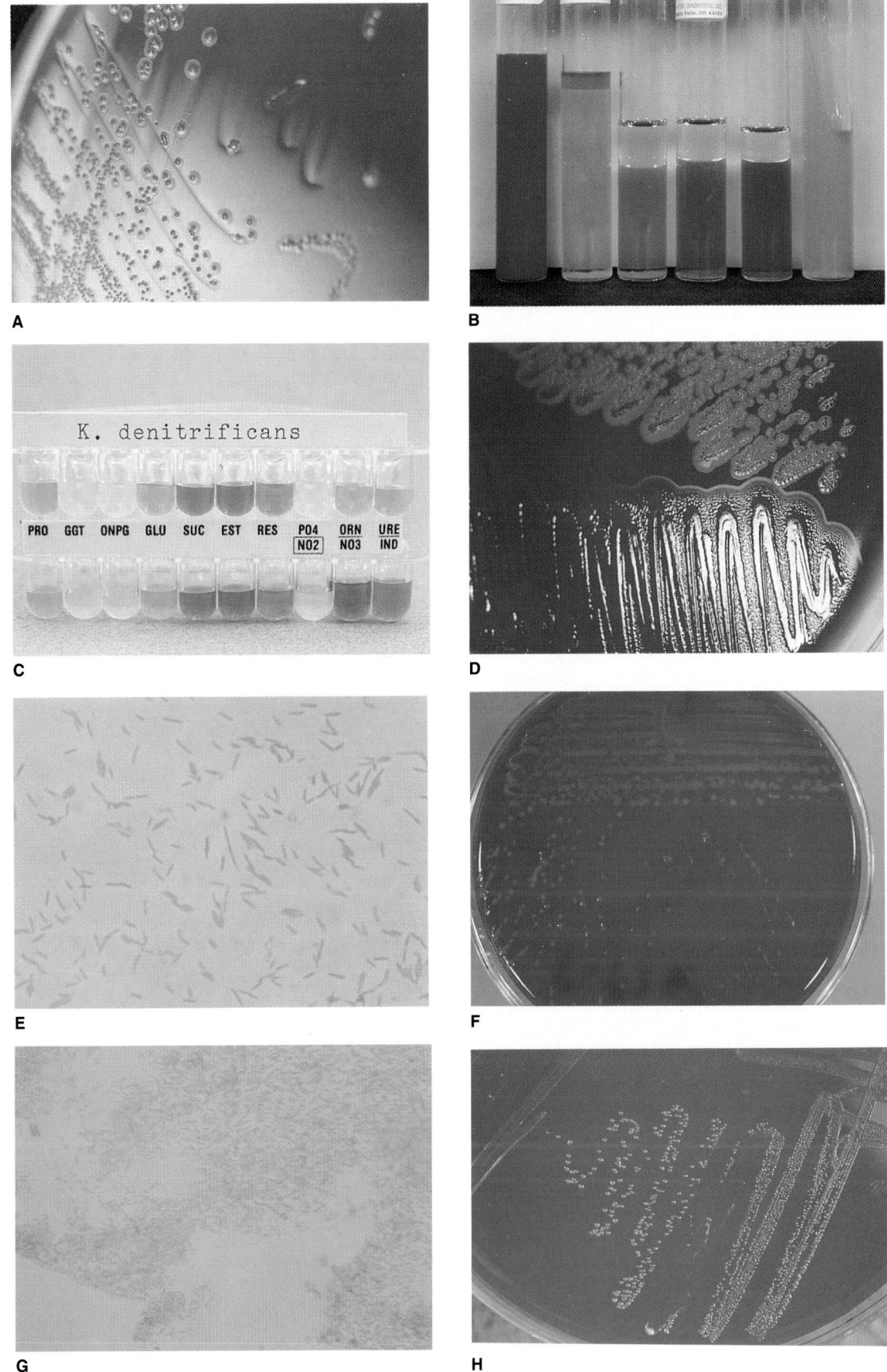

A

B

C

K. denitrificans

PRO   GGT   ONPG   GLU   SUC   EST   RES   PO4   ORN   URE
                                                NO2   NO3   IND

D

E

F

G

H

MISCELLANEOUS FASTIDIOUS GRAM-NEGATIVE BACILLI

A. Colonies of *Pasteurella multocida* growing on sheep blood agar. The isolate shown in this photograph is a mucoid *P. multocida* after 48 hours incubation. The organism is nonhemolytic and does not grow on MacConkey and other enteric media. This organism is most frequently associated with scratch and/or bite wounds from domestic animals, especially cats and dogs.

B. Spot indole test performed on filter paper using *P. multocida* as the test organism. The paper is saturated with a few drops of *p*-dimethylaminocinnamaldehyde reagent, and a few colonies of the organism are rubbed on the paper alongside a negative control organism. The appearance of a blue-green pigment at the inoculum site is a positive test, whereas the negative organism result is pale pink, as shown here.

C. Colonies of *Bordetella pertussis* growing on Bordet-Gengou agar. In this close-up photograph, the shiny "mercury droplet" morphology of the colonies is readily apparent.

D. Growth of *Bordetella pertussis* on Regan-Lowe medium. *B. pertussis* is a slow-growing, fastidious gram-negative organism that is easily inhibited by toxic materials that may be present in the agar or in the specimen itself. Regan-Lowe medium contains horse blood (10% v/v) in a charcoal agar base. The high concentration of blood and the charcoal help to neutralize the toxic materials and facilitate outgrowth of the organisms. This close-up photograph shows a pure culture of *B. pertussis* on Regan-Lowe agar after 72 hours incubation.

E. Direct fluorescent antibody (DFA) test for *B. pertussis*. The DFA test is an important adjunct to culture for the detection of *B. pertussis* in nasopharyngeal specimens. This photograph shows a positive DFA preparation, with the organisms appearing as apple-green fluorescent coccobacilli. As demonstrated here, the bacteria may appear singly or in clusters resulting from the trapping of the bacteria in mucous strands. (Photo courtesy of Marti Roe, Children's Hospital, Denver, CO).

F. *Brucella melitensis* growing on sheep blood agar. This photograph shows *B. melitensis* after 48 hours growth in CO_2 at 37°C. The colonies are slow-growing, tiny, nonpigmented, nonhemolytic, entire, convex, moist, and glistening.

G. Gram stain of *Brucella* species revealing tiny gram-negative coccobacilli. The classic description are cells that measure 0.5 to 0.7 microns by 0.6 to 1.5 microns, arranged singly, in pairs, and in small clusters.

H. Gram stain of *Francisella tularensis*. The cells of *F. tularensis* are even smaller than those of *Brucella* species, measuring 0.2 microns in width by 0.6 to 0.8 microns in length. In this photomicrograph, the cells appear as tiny, gram-negative "dots" that lie singly and in loose clusters.

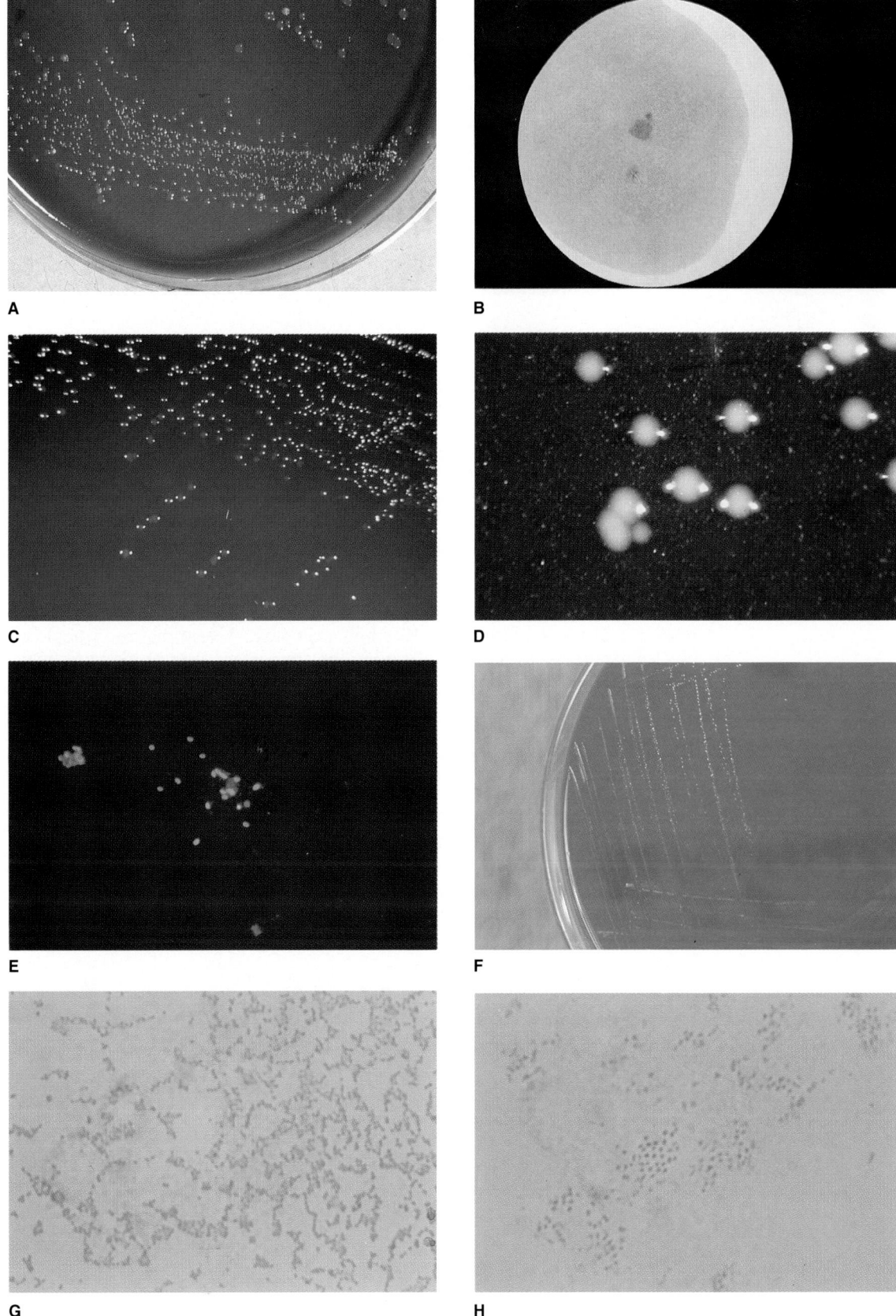

A

B

C

D

E

F

G

H

LABORATORY DIAGNOSIS OF LEGIONELLOSIS

A. Gram stain of *Legionella pneumophila* culture using basic fuchsin instead of safranin for the counterstain. The organisms are thin rods of various lengths.

B. Gram-Weigert–stained touch preparation of open-lung biopsy specimen revealing small, thin intracellular and extracellular bacilli (original magnification ×100 objective lens). Note short, blunt rods in the macrophage nearest the center of the slide. *L. pneumophila* serogroup 1 was the only organism isolated in culture; a tissue imprint of the lung was direct fluorescent antibody–positive when stained with the conjugate specific for this organism.

C. Heavy growth on buffered charcoal yeast extract agar (BCYEa) after 3 or more days of incubation and no growth on blood agar are characteristic of *Legionella* species.

D. Dissecting microscopic view of *L. pneumophila* colonies on BCYEa. Note crystalline-like internal structures within 3–5 mm colonies that have entire margins (original magnification approximately ×40).

E. Blue-white autofluorescence of *L. bozemanii* on BCYEa; photographed under long-wave ultraviolet light. Other species that autofluoresce blue-white include *L. dumoffi, L. gormanii, L. anisa, L. tucsonensis, L. cherrii, L. parisiensis,* and *L. steigerwaltii.* This characteristic is absent in *L. pneumophila, L. micdadei, L. feelei, L. longbeachae, L. oakridgensis* and in many other *Legionella* species.

F. Modified-Kinyoun acid-fast stain of *L. micdadei* grown on BCYEa. Some of the rod-shaped bacteria in the preparation are acid-fast (red), whereas some are not acid-fast (blue); thus, they are "partially acid-fast." Using the traditional Ziehl-Neelsen stain, or an auramine-rhodamine stain, they are not likely to be acid-fast (see text for details).

G. Paraffin section of lung tissue from a patient with acute Legionnaires' disease. The section shows an area of consolidation. Inflammatory exudate consisting of fibrin, many neutrophils, few macrophages, and some erythrocytes fills alveolar spaces and alveolar ducts (H&E, original magnification approx. ×200).

H. Paraffin section of lung from a different patient with a more chronic form of Legionnaires' disease. Alveoli are filled with prominent, foamy macrophages, and the interstitium is edematous. A silver impregnation stain (*e.g.*, Dieterle or Warthin-Starry [not shown]) aids in demonstrating the organisms.

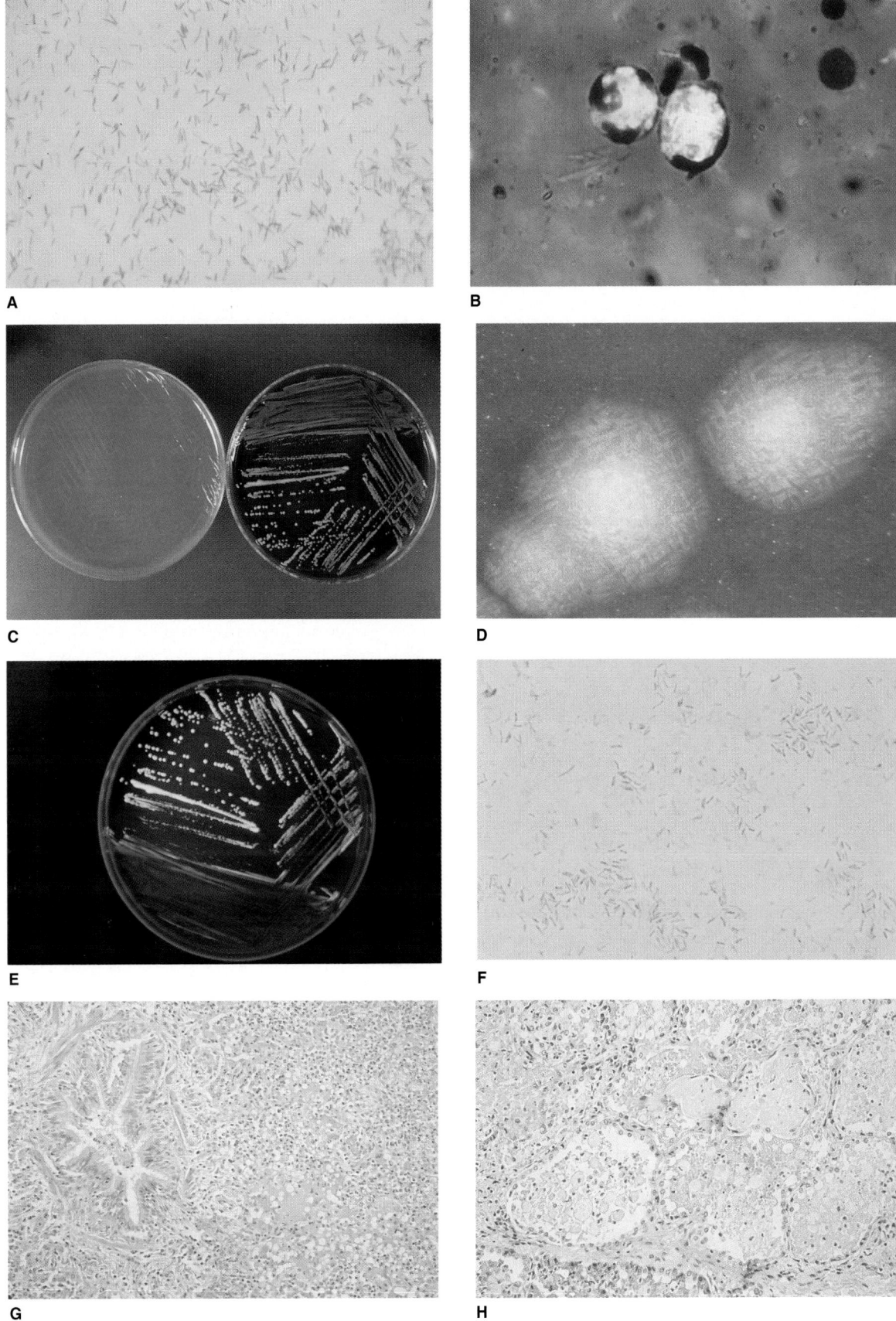

A

B

C

D

E

F

G

H

IDENTIFICATION OF *NEISSERIA* SPECIES AND *MORAXELLA CATARRHALIS*

A. Gram stain of a urethral discharge from a male with gonococcal urethritis. Note the presence of intracellular, gram-negative diplococci within pale-staining segmented neutrophils.

B. Typical colonies of *N. gonorrhoeae* on modified Thayer-Martin (MTM) medium. MTM is a chocolate agar-based formulation that contains vancomycin, colistin, and nystatin to inhibit gram-positive, gram-negative, and fungal organisms, respectively. Pathogenic *Neisseria* species, notably *N. gonorrhoeae* and *N. meningitidis*, grow well on MTM medium.

C. Conventional cystine–tryptic digest semisolid agar (CTA) for identification of *Neisseria* species. This photograph shows the typical battery of carbohydrates used for identification. The battery includes (*left* to *right*) CTA-glucose, CTA-maltose, CTA-sucrose, and CTA-lactose (the control CTA without carbohydrate is not shown). The media contain phenol-red indicator, with a color change from red to yellow indicating the production of acid. In this photograph, acid has been produced from glucose only, identifying this organism as *N. gonorrhoeae*.

D. Rapid carbohydrate utilization test for identification of *Neisseria* species (see Chart 63-1). The rapid carbohydrate utilization test is performed using a balanced salts–phenol red solution (BSS, 0.1 mL/tube), with a single drop of carbohydrate (20% aqueous solution) added for each sugar tested. A dense suspension of the organism is prepared in the BSS without carbohydrate, and a single drop of this suspension is added to each of the carbohydrate-containing tubes. The inoculated tubes are incubated at 35°C for 4 h. This photograph shows a set of sugars composed of (*left* to *right*) BSS only (for the organism suspension), BSS-glucose, BSS-maltose, BSS-sucrose, and BSS-lactose. Because acid is being produced from glucose only (color change from red to yellow), the organism is *N. gonorrhoeae*.

E. Rapid carbohydrate utilization test for identification of *N. meningitidis*. In this photograph the tubes contain (*left* to *right*) BSS with no carbohydrate, BSS-glucose (*G*), BSS-maltose (*M*), BSS-fructose (*F*), BSS-sucrose (*S*), and BSS-lactose (*L*). Acid production from glucose and maltose indicates that this organism is *N. meningitidis*.

F. Minitek *Neisseria* Test: The Minitek system uses filter paper disks that are impregnated with carbohydrates or other test reagents. After the disks are dispensed into a series of reaction wells, an organism suspension is prepared, and a small volume (0.5 mL) is added to each of the wells. Test reactions are interpreted after 4 h, although the test may be incubated overnight. The reactions shown here are (*left* to *right*), glucose (positive), maltose (positive), sucrose (negative), ONPG (positive). ONPG detects β-galactosidase, indicating that this organism is *N. lactamica*.

G. API QuadFERM+ system (bioMerieux-Vitek, Inc.) for identification of *Neisseria* species and *M. catarrhalis*. This commercial adaptation of the rapid carbohydrate utilization test includes a series of wells containing (from *left* to *right*) a carbohydrate-free control reagent (*CTRL*) and reagents for glucose (*GLU*), maltose (*MAL*), lactose (*LAC*), and sucrose (*SUC*). Wells for acidometric detection of deoxyribonuclease (DNase) for confirmation of *M. catarrhalis*, and for detection of β-lactamase (*beta-lac*) are also included on the strip. The reaction pattern shown here is characteristic of a β-lactamase-negative strain of *N. gonorrhoeae*.

H. GonoChek II tube (DuPont de Nemours, Inc.). Three chromogenic substrates are included in a single plastic tube to detect glycosidase and aminopeptidase enzymes specifically found in *N. meningitidis*, *N. lactamica*, and *N. gonorrhoeae*. The identifying patterns are blue (*upper left*)—*N. lactamica* (β-galactoside hydrolysis); yellow (*upper right*)—*N. meningitidis* (γ-glutamyl-*p*-nitroanilide hydrolysis); red (*lower left*)—*N. gonorrhoeae* (prolyl-β-naphthylamide hydrolysis). Lack of a color reaction (*lower right*) presumptively identifies the isolate as *M. catarrhalis*.

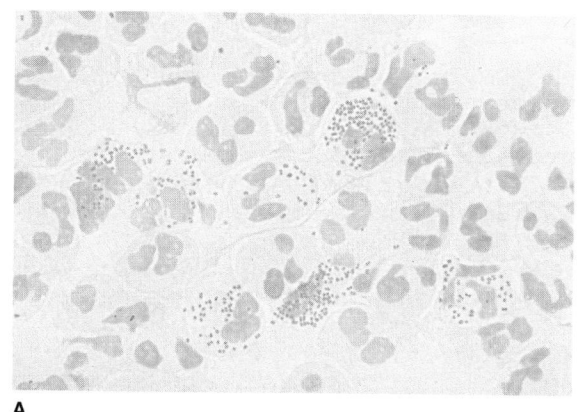

A

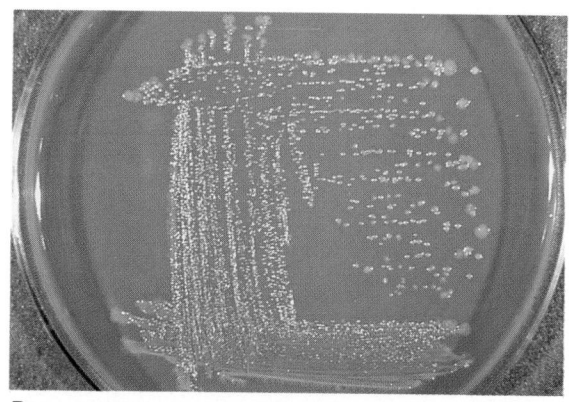

B

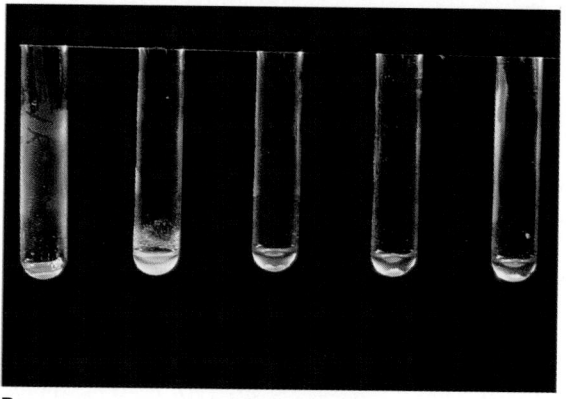

C

D

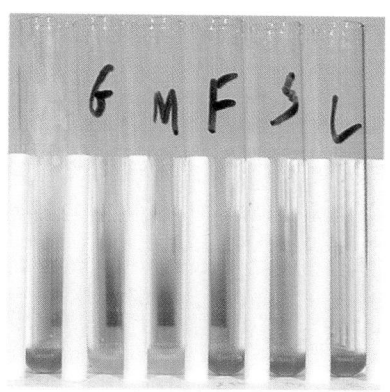

E

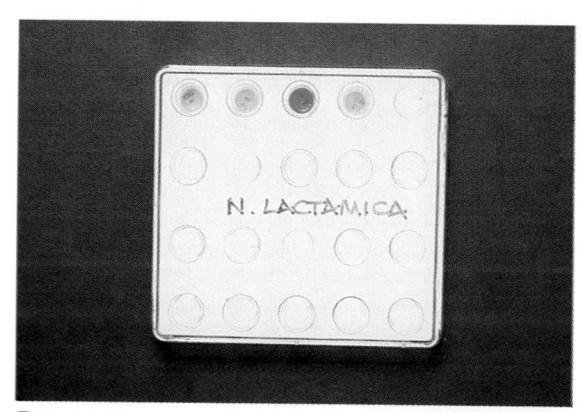

F

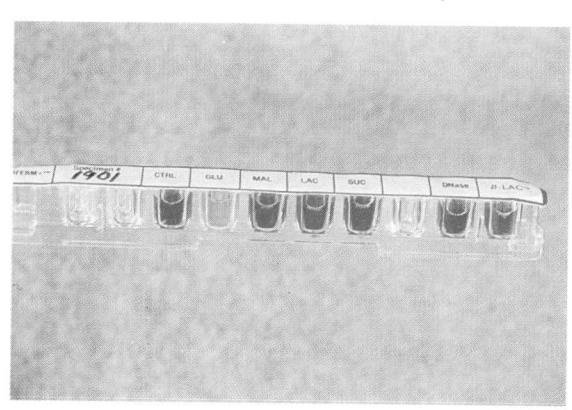

G

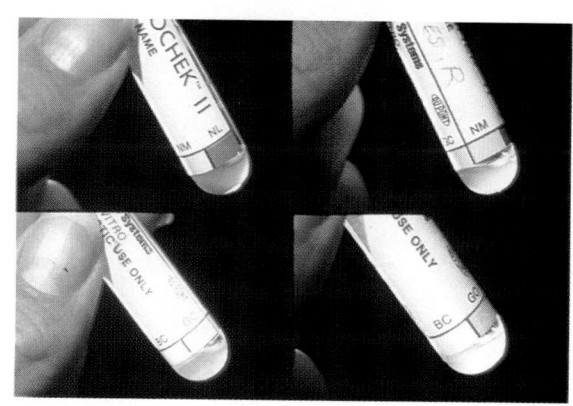

H

A. BactiCard *Neisseria* (Remel Laboratories, Lenexa KA): This identification strip contains four chromogenic enzyme substrate tests for identification of pathogenic *Neisseria* species and *M. catarrhalis*. After hydration of each of the four test circles with a drop of buffer, growth from selective media or a suitable subculture is applied onto each of the four test areas. If a blue-green color develops in the IB (butyrate esterase) test area within 2 minutes (*strip at left*), the organism is identified as *M. catarrhalis*. If no color develops in this area, the strip is incubated for an additional 13 minutes. If a blue-green color develops in the BGAL (β-galactosidase) test area (*strip at far right*) during this time, the organism is identified as *N. lactamica*. If no color develops in this area during the incubation period, a drop of a color-developing reagent is added to the PRO and GLUT test areas. Appearance of a red color in the PRO (prolyl aminopeptidase) test area identifies the isolates as *N. gonorrhoeae* (*second strip from the left*), whereas the development of a red color in the GLUT (γ-glutamyl aminopeptidase) test area identifies the isolate as *N. meningitidis* (*third strip from the left*).

B. Fluorescent antibody (FA) test for culture confirmation of *N. gonorrhoeae* (Syva Co., San Jose CA): In a positive test, apple-green fluorescent diplococci are observed, as shown in this photograph.

C. Meritec coagglutination test for identification of *N. gonorrhoeae* (Meridian Diagnostics, Cincinnati OH): This picture shows two isolates of *N. gonorrhoeae*; the first is present in circles *1* and *2*, and the second is present in circles *3* and *4*. Circles *1* and *3* contain 1 drop each of the organism suspensions and the control latex reagent, and circles *2* and *4* contain 1 drop each of the organism suspensions and the antibody-sensitized latex reagent. The expected reactions (control circles—no agglutination; test circles—positive agglutination) are demonstrated for both *N. gonorrhoeae* isolates in this photograph.

D. RapID NH system (Innovative Diagnostics Systems, Atlanta GA). The RapID NH system is a 4-hour commercial system for identification of *Neisseria* species, *Haemophilus* species, and other fastidious gram-negative bacteria. The photograph actually shows two duplicate panels inoculated with *N. meningitidis*. The top panel in the photo is the system without reagents added to the last three bi-functional test wells. The reactions that identify the isolate as *N. meningitidis* are the positive prolyl aminopeptidase (*PRO*) and γ-glutamyl aminopeptidase (*GGT*) reactions, the positive glucose (*GLU*) reaction, and the positive NO$_2$ (reduction of nitrite) test.

E. MicroScan HNID panel: The MicroScan HNID panel is a 4-hour test panel for identification of *Neisseria* and *Haemophilus* species. Positive tests on the panel shown in the photograph include positive nitrate (*NO$_3$*) and nitrite (*NO$_2$*) reduction tests, production of acid from glucose (*GLU*), sucrose (*SUC*), maltose (*MAL*), and fructose (*FRU*), and no acid from lactose (*LAC*). These characteristics identify this isolate as *N. mucosa*.

F. DNase agar with *M. catarrhalis:* Production of DNase is a confirmatory test for identifying *M. catarrhalis*. The isolate to be tested is heavily spot inoculated on an area of DNase test agar with toluidine blue O. Hydrolysis of the DNA in the medium by bacterial DNase results in a change in the color of the medium from blue to pink under and around the inoculum.

G. API QuadFERM+ inoculated with *M. catarrhalis:* The QuadFERM+ identification strip includes a DNase test along with carbohydrate utilization tests and a β-lactamase test. The photograph shows a QuadFerm+ strip inoculated with a β-lactamase-negative *M. catarrhalis* strain. The *CTRL, GLU, MAL, LAC, SUC,* and β-*lactamase* wells are negative (*red*), whereas the DNase test well is positive (*yellow*).

H. The M.Cat butyrate disk: *M. catarrhalis* strains produce a butyrate esterase enzyme that is able to hydrolyze indoxyl butyrate, which is impregnated on a filter paper disk. Inoculation of the moistened disk with growth from a colony results in hydrolysis of the compound and development of a *blue-green* color on the disk within 2 minutes. This figure shows three positive M.Cat butyrate disks.

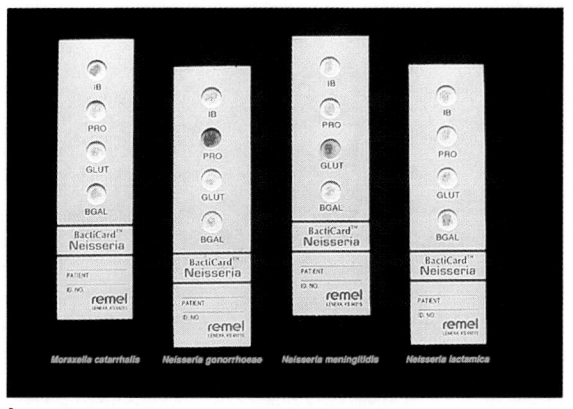

A

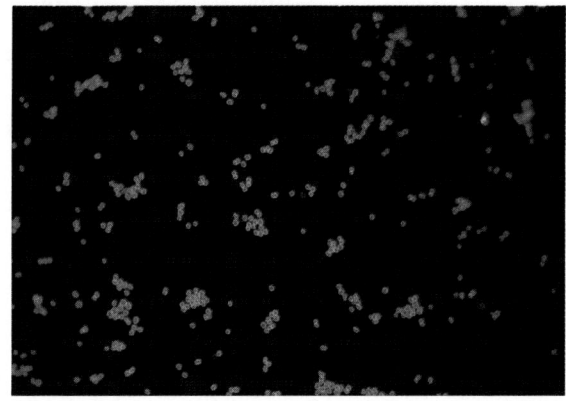

B

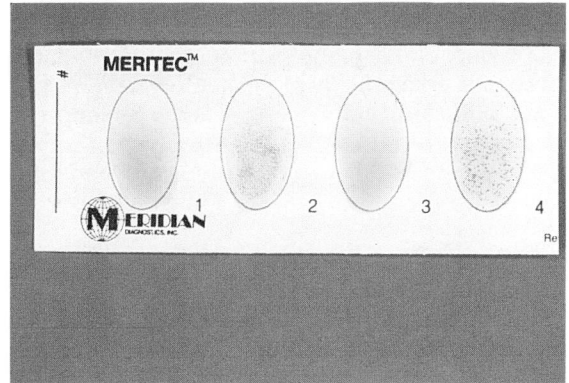

C

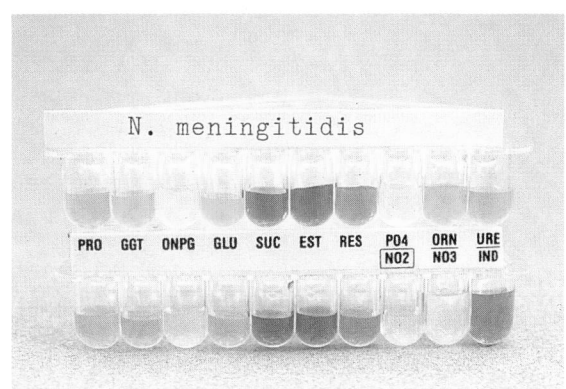

D

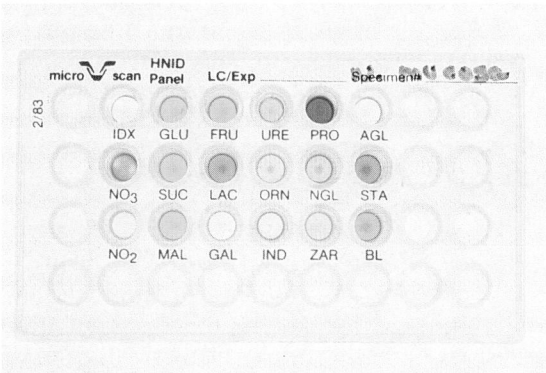

E

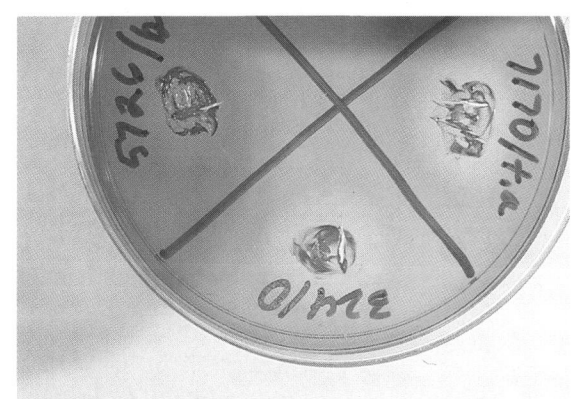

F

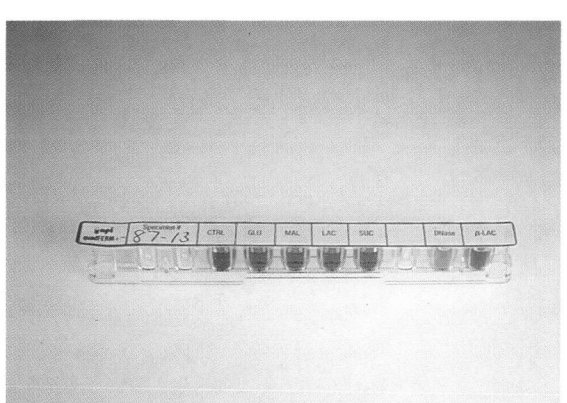

G

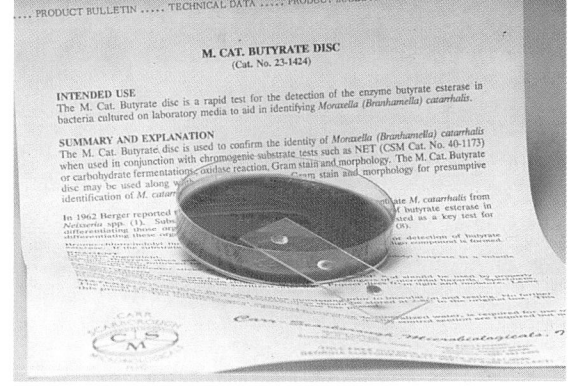

H

STAPHYLOCOCCI AND MICROCOCCI

A. Patient with a staphylococcal cellulitis of the upper lip.

B. Neonate with staphylococcal scalded skin syndrome: This syndrome is seen in newborns infected with *S. aureus* strains that produce exfoliatins (epidermolytic toxins). These toxins dissolve the mucopolysaccharide matrix of the epidermis, resulting in intraepithelial splitting of cellular linkages in the stratum granulosum. Bullous formation occurs over large areas of the body, with subsequent sloughing of the superficial skin layers, as shown here.

C. Gram stain of staphylococcal cellulitis: The organisms appear as small extracellular gram-positive cocci arranged in clusters along with the pink-staining polymorphonuclear leukocytes. (Courtesy of Schering Corp., Kenilworth NJ)

D. Colonies of *S. aureus* on sheep blood agar. This photograph shows typical colonies of *S. aureus* after a 24-hour incubation. A zone of β-hemolysis owing to the hemolytic activity of the staphylococcal α-hemolysin is seen immediately surrounding the colony. The darker red area outside of the hemolyzed area represents action of the β-hemolysin ("hot–cold" hemolysin). It is the β-hemolysin that interacts with the CAMP factor produced by group B streptococci to produce the synergistic hemolysis seen in the CAMP test for presumptive identification of group B streptococci.

E. Colonies of *Micrococcus luteus* on sheep blood agar. This species produces yellow colonies; other species may be nonpigmented or produce orange or pink-red colonies. These organisms can be differentiated from staphylococci by resistance to furazolidone, susceptibility to bacitracin, and other methods, as shown in Table 11-3.

F. Positive catalase test: The catalase test differentiates members of the *Micrococcaceae* from members of the *Streptococcaceae*. The test is performed by placing growth from a colony onto a glass slide and adding a drop of 3% hydrogen peroxide to the inoculum. Immediate and vigorous bubbling owing to the production of oxygen gas, as shown here, indicates a positive test. Micrococci and staphylococci are catalase-positive, whereas streptococci and enterococci are catalase-negative. *Stomatococcus mucilaginosus* is weakly catalase-positive or may be catalase-negative.

G. Furazolidone disk test with a *Micrococcus* species. Several tests are available for differentiating *Micrococcus* and *Staphylococcus* species. The furazolidone-susceptibility test is a reliable overnight test for making this differentiation. Micrococci are resistant to furazolidone and will usually grow right up to the edge of the furazolidone disk (*FX*, 100 μg).

H. Furazolidone disk with a *Staphylococcus* species. The growth of staphylococci is inhibited by furazolidone and will show an area of growth inhibition around the disk, as shown in this figure.

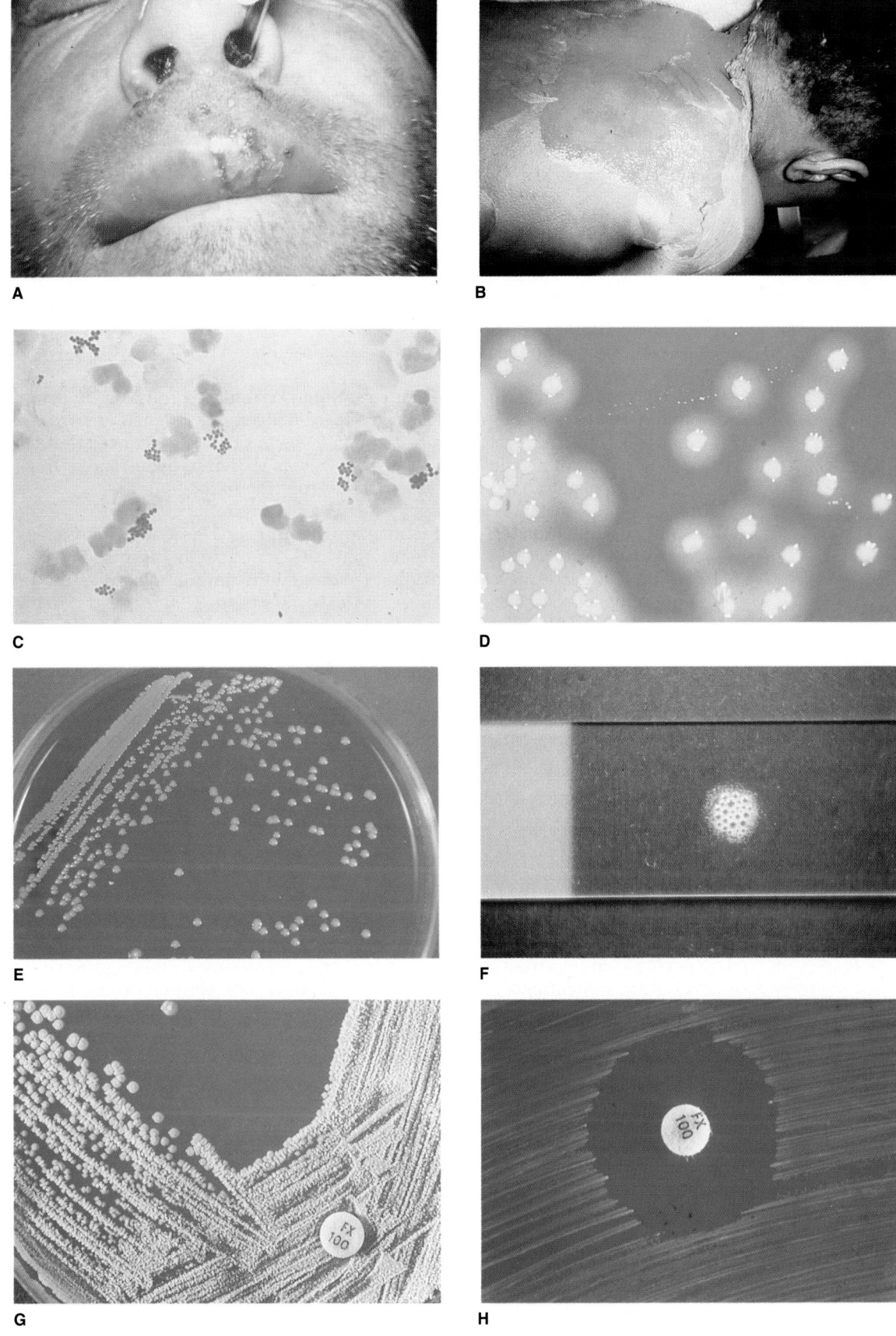

A

B

C

D

E

F

G

H

IDENTIFICATION OF STAPHYLOCOCCI

A. Modified oxidase test: This is a rapid (30-s) method for differentiating *Micrococcus* and *Staphylococcus* species. The oxidase reagent (tetramethyl-*p*-phenylenediamine dihydrochloride) is made up in dimethyl sulfoxide, which allows the reagent to penetrate the bacterial cell. The test is performed by rubbing a portion of growth onto the filter paper disk. *Micrococcus* species are modified oxidase-positive (*right*), producing a blue-purple color within 30 s, whereas *Staphylococcus* species are modified oxidase-negative (*left*), with no color development on the disk.

B. Slide coagulase test: This test is a rapid method for identifying *S. aureus*. Most strains of this species produce a cell-bound coagulase or "clumping factor" that is detected by mixing a suspension of the organism with EDTA-rabbit plasma. A saline control (*left*) must be included to assess autoagglutination. Not all *S. aureus* strains possess clumping factor, so negative slide coagulase tests must be confirmed with the tube coagulase test (see Plate 11-2**C**).

C. Tube coagulase test: In this test, extracellular coagulase produced by *S. aureus* complexes with a component in plasma, called coagulase-reacting factor. This complex, in turn, reacts with fibrinogen to form fibrin and, consequently, the development of a visible clot. A positive test is shown in the *bottom* of this figure, and a negative test is shown in the *top* portion of the figure.

D. Latex agglutination test for identification of *S. aureus:* This alternative coagulase test procedure uses latex spheres that are coated with plasma. Fibrinogen bound to the latex detects clumping factor, and the immunoglobulin, also present on the latex, detects protein A on the surface of the *S. aureus* cell. Mixing of colonial growth of *S. aureus* with the latex reagent results in rapid agglutination (*left*). A coagulase-negative staphylococcus, which produces a negative reaction, is also shown (*right*). (Courtesy of Murex Diagnostics, Norcross GA.)

E. Passive hemagglutination test for identification of *S. aureus*. This alternative coagulase test procedure uses sheep red blood cells that are coated with fibrinogen. The mixing of colonial growth of *S. aureus* with the coated red blood cells results in visible clumping of the bacteria and red blood cells, as shown in the photograph. A nonsensitized red blood cell suspension must be included as a negative control (not shown). (Courtesy of Becton-Dickinson Microbiology Systems, Cockeysville MD.)

F. Disk tests for identification of staphylococci: Although furazolidone and bacitracin disk tests are useful for differentiating micrococci from staphylococci, susceptibility to novobiocin is useful for presumptive identification of *S. saprophyticus*, an important agent of urinary tract infections. In this figure, all three tests are shown for an isolate of *S. saprophyticus*. Susceptibility to furazolidone (*FX*, 100 μg) and resistance to bacitracin (*Taxo A disk*, 0.04 U bacitracin) indicate that the organism is a *Staphylococcus*, rather than a *Micrococcus*, species. Resistance to novobiocin (*C−*, 5 μg) presumptively identifies the isolate as *S. saprophyticus*.

G. API STAPH (bioMerieux-Vitek, Inc., Hazelwood MO) for identification of staphylococci and micrococci: The strip is inoculated with an organism suspension and is incubated overnight. Interpretation of the reactions generates a biotype number that is used, along with a computer-assisted database, to identify the organism.

H. ID32 Staph (bioMerieux S.A., France) for identification of staphylococci and micrococci: This strip-format identification system, which is inoculated in a manner similar to the API STAPH (see Plate 11-2**G**) contains 26 biochemical tests to generate a biotype number that is used with a computerized database to identify the organism. As of this writing, the ID32 Staph system is not approved by the FDA for use in the United States.

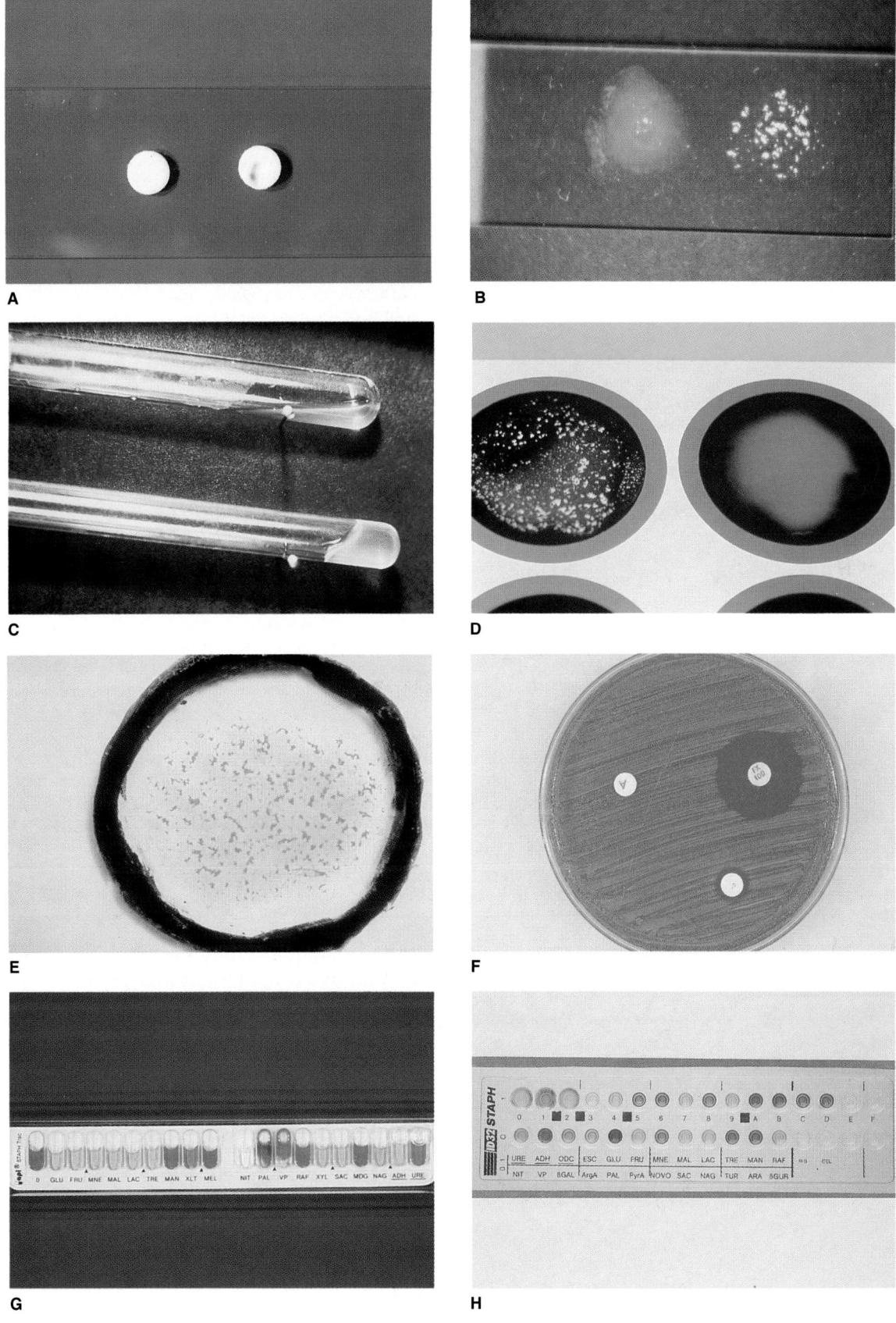

A

B

C

D

E

F

G

H

IDENTIFICATION OF STREPTOCOCCI

A. Gram stain of streptococci growing in a broth culture: As their name suggests, streptococci characteristically grow in chains. These chain forms are most frequently seen when the organisms are grown in broth. On gram-stained smears prepared from growth on agar media, the organisms usually appear in pairs or in shorter chains.

B. Gram stain of *S. pneumoniae:* This photograph shows the typical appearance of pneumococci in blood culture broth. These bacteria characteristically grow in pairs in which the cells have a slightly elongated "lanceolate" morphology. With some cells in this frame, a clear area or "halo" may be observed surrounding the organism pairs, indicating the presence of the polysaccharide capsule of *S. pneumoniae.*

C. α-Hemolytic streptococci on sheep blood agar: Streptococci initially may be classified on the basis of their hemolytic properties on sheep blood agar. Partial hemolysis of the erythrocytes results in a "greening" of the agar medium surrounding the colonies (α-hemolysis). Streptococci that are α-hemolytic include *S. pneumoniae,* the viridans group of streptococci, and most *Enterococcus* (formerly *Streptococcus*) species.

D. β-Hemolytic streptococci on sheep blood agar: β-Hemolytic streptococci produce hemolysins that lyse sheep erythrocytes, resulting in a clearing of the medium surrounding the colonies. The group A streptococcus shown here demonstrates this type of hemolysis, as do group B, C, and G streptococci. The zones of β-hemolysis surrounding colonies of group B streptococci, however, are not as large relative to the size of the colony as those seen with groups A, C, and G β-hemolytic streptococci.

E. β-Hemolytic streptococci on sheep blood agar: More intense β-hemolysis is noted in areas where the medium has been "stabbed," pushing some of the bacteria under the medium surface. The β-hemolysis in these areas is due to both streptolysin O and streptolysin S, the principal hemolysins of group A streptococci. Streptolysin O is oxygen-labile and does not show maximal activity on the surface of the agar; the surface β-hemolysis is largely due to streptolysin S, which is oxygen-stable.

F. Direct latex agglutination test for group A streptococci: Both latex agglutination and rapid enzyme immunoassays are currently available for the direct detection of group A streptococci in throat swab specimens. With the latex agglutination method shown here, the throat swab is extracted with nitrous acid. After the pH of the extract is adjusted, drops of the solution are reacted with a latex suspension coated with antigroup A antibodies, and with a control, noncoated latex suspension. Agglutination of the test (*left*), but not the control suspension (*right*), is a positive test. Although most of these tests are highly specific for the group A cell wall antigen, the sensitivities of these assays vary widely.

G. Strep A OIA (Optical Immunoassay; Biostar, Boulder CO): Strep OIA is an immunoassay for direct detection of group A streptococci in throat swab specimens. The swab is extract with acetic acid, neutralized, and then mixed with antigroup A streptococcal antibodies bound to horseradish peroxidase (HRP). A drop of this mixture is placed on the surface of an OIA slide, which is coated with antigroup A streptococcal antibodies. After a 2-minute incubation, the slide is rinsed and HRP substrate is added and allowed to react for 4 minutes. After rinsing, the test is read by examining the hue of light reflected from the reaction area on the slide. If group A streptococcal antigen is present, the slide shows a purple spot (*left*). If no antigen is present, the slide surface retains its gold color, with or without a small blue dot, as shown on here (*right*). (Courtesy of Janice Pinson, Murex Diagnostics)

H. *S. pneumoniae* colonies on sheep blood agar: Two characteristics of *S. pneumoniae* can be used for presumptive identification. At *left* is shown a typical α-hemolytic mucoid strain of *S. pneumoniae,* an appearance that is due to large amounts of capsular polysaccharide. At *right* is a close-up photograph illustrating collapse of the central portion of the colonies owing to organism autolysis, resulting in the so-called checker piece and nail head colony morphologies shown here.

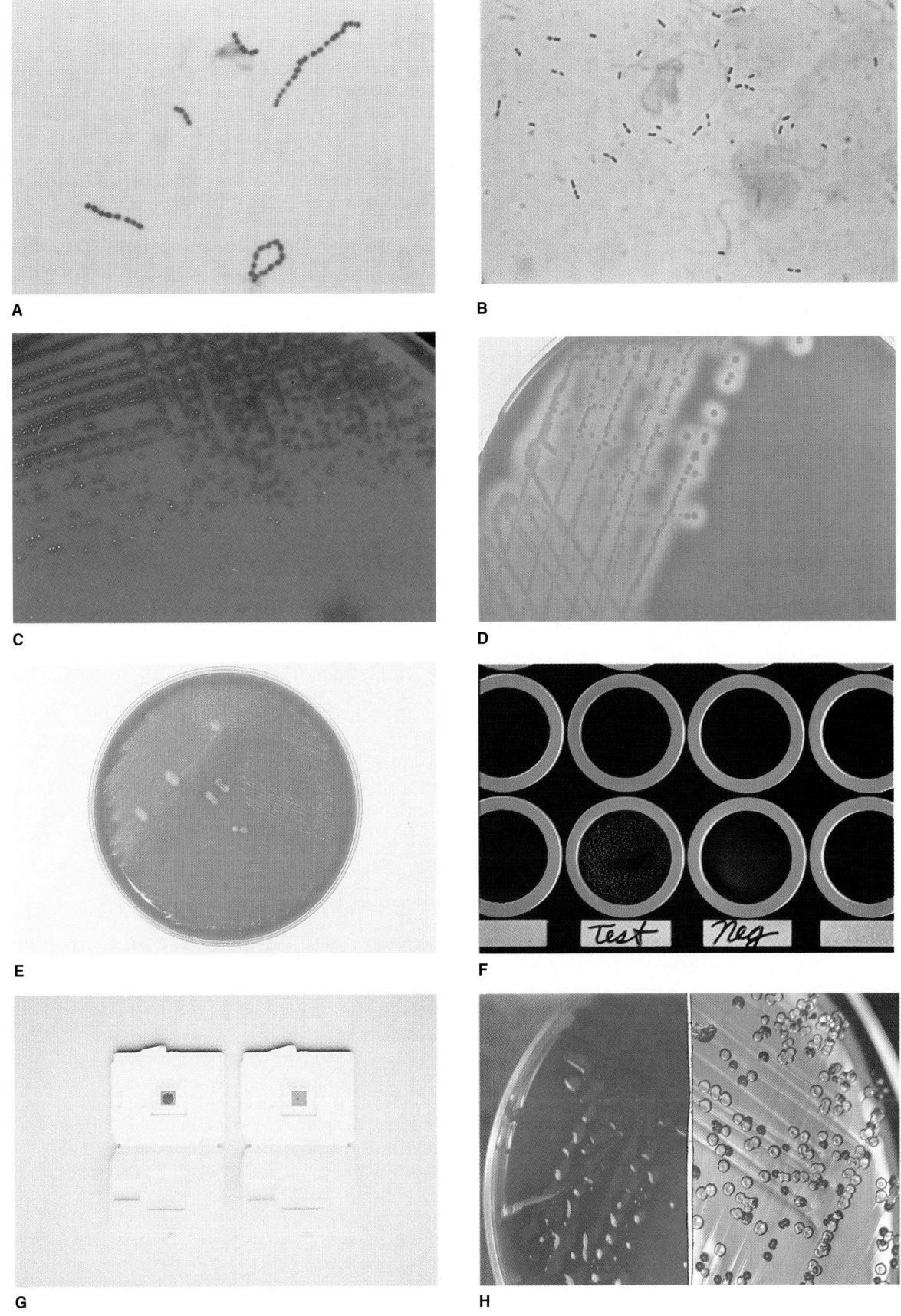

A

B

C

D

E

F

G

H

IDENTIFICATION OF STREPTOCOCCI (CONTINUED)

A. Bacitracin susceptibility test for presumptive identification of group A β-hemolytic streptococci: Group A streptococci are susceptible to low concentrations of bacitracin, and this property provides a convenient and inexpensive method for presumptively identifying these bacteria. Colonies of β-hemolytic streptococci are inoculated as a lawn onto sheep blood agar and a bacitracin differential disk (Taxo A disk, 0.04 U) is placed on the inoculum. After overnight incubation, the growth is inspected for a zone of growth inhibition around the disk. This photograph shows both a group A streptococcus (*left,* zone present) and a nongroup A streptococcus (*right,* no zone present). Some nongroup A streptococci may also be inhibited by bacitracin, so this test is frequently performed along with a sulfamethoxazole–trimethoprim susceptibility disk test (see Plate 12-2**B**).

B. Susceptibility to bacitracin and sulfamethoxazole–trimethoprim: The β-hemolytic streptococcus shown here is susceptible to bacitracin, but shows a large zone of growth inhibition around the sulfamethoxazole–trimethoprim disk (SXT). Group A streptococci are susceptible to bacitracin, but are resistant to SXT. Some nongroup A β-hemolytic streptococci (e.g., groups C, F, and G) are susceptible to bacitracin, but will be susceptible to SXT as shown here. Therefore, the performance of these two tests together increases the specificity of the presumptive identification that would be obtained by the use of the bacitracin test alone.

C. CAMP test for presumptive identification of group B streptococci: The CAMP test reaction depends on the interaction between CAMP factor, a product of the group B streptococcus, with the β-hemolysin of *S. aureus.* Possible group B streptococci are streaked at right angles to a streak of staphylococci (without the streaks touching) on a sheep blood agar plate. Following overnight incubation, an arrowhead-shaped area of synergistic hemolysis is found in the intersecting area where the CAMP factor and β-hemolysin have diffused into the medium. The photograph shows three positive CAMP reactions.

D. Bile esculin hydrolysis and salt tolerance tests: These tests are used for the presumptive identification of *Enterococcus* species and group D streptococci (*S. bovis*). The bile esculin test is performed by inoculating a slant of bile esculin medium and incubating it overnight. Enterococci and group D streptococci are able to grow in the presence of 40% bile and to hydrolyze esculin to esculetin (forming the black precipitate). The salt tolerance test is performed with a broth medium containing 6.5% NaCl. *Enterococcus* species will grow, whereas nonenterococcal group D streptococci will not grow in this medium. The photograph shows a positive reaction for both tests, identifying this organism as a group D *Enterococcus* species.

E. PYR test: Hydrolysis of L-pyrrolidonyl-α-naphthylamide (PYR) is a presumptive test for identification of group A streptococci and *Enterococcus* species that can replace the bacitracin–SXT disk tests and the salt tolerance test, respectively. In the disk test shown, colonial growth is applied to the moistened disk containing the PYR substrate. After 2 minutes, dimethylaminocinnamaldehyde reagent is applied to the disk to detect the free α-naphthylamine that is released on hydrolysis of PYR (red color). A negative PYR test is shown on the *left,* whereas a positive PYR test is shown on the *right.* (Courtesy of Janice Pinson, Murex Diagnostics)

F. BactiCard STREP (Remel Laboratories, Lenexa KA): This card-format system consists of three test circles for detection of pyrrolidonyl arylamidase (PYR), leucine aminopeptidase (LAP), and esculin hydrolysis (ESC). After rehydrating the test circles, some colonial growth is rubbed onto each of the test circles. After 10 minutes the tests are read either directly (ESC) or after addition of a developing reagent (PYR, LAP). These three tests, when used with a vancomycin susceptibility test, are helpful for the presumptive identification of streptococci, enterococci, and some of the "streptococcus-like" bacteria (i.e., aerococci, leuconostocs, pediococci, gemellae, and *Globicatella sanguis*). (Courtesy of MaryAnn Silvius, Remel Laboratories, Lenexa KA)

G. Susceptibility to optochin: Susceptibility to ethyl hydrocupreine hydrochloride (optochin) is used to differentiate *S. pneumoniae* from other viridans streptococci. α-Hemolytic colonies are subcultured to a blood agar plate and an optochin disk (*P* on the disk stands for "pneumococcus") is placed on the inoculum. The presence of a zone a of growth inhibition of 14 mm around a 6-mm disk after incubation identifies the organism as a pneumococcus. In the photograph, the mucoid organism on the *left* is optochin-susceptible (*S. pneumoniae*) and the organism on the *right* is optochin-resistant (viridans streptococcus).

H. Tri-plate for presumptive identification of streptococci: This single-plate product is designed to provide the results of several tests for the presumptive identification of streptococci and enterococci. The three sectors of the plate contain sheep blood agar, bile esculin agar, and PYR agar, respectively. Determination of hemolysis and a CAMP test are performed in the blood agar sector, and the bile esculin and PYR reactions are read from the other two sectors). The photograph shows the triplate inoculated with an *Enterococcus* species (α-hemolytic, CAMP test-negative, bile-esculin-positive, and PYR-positive).

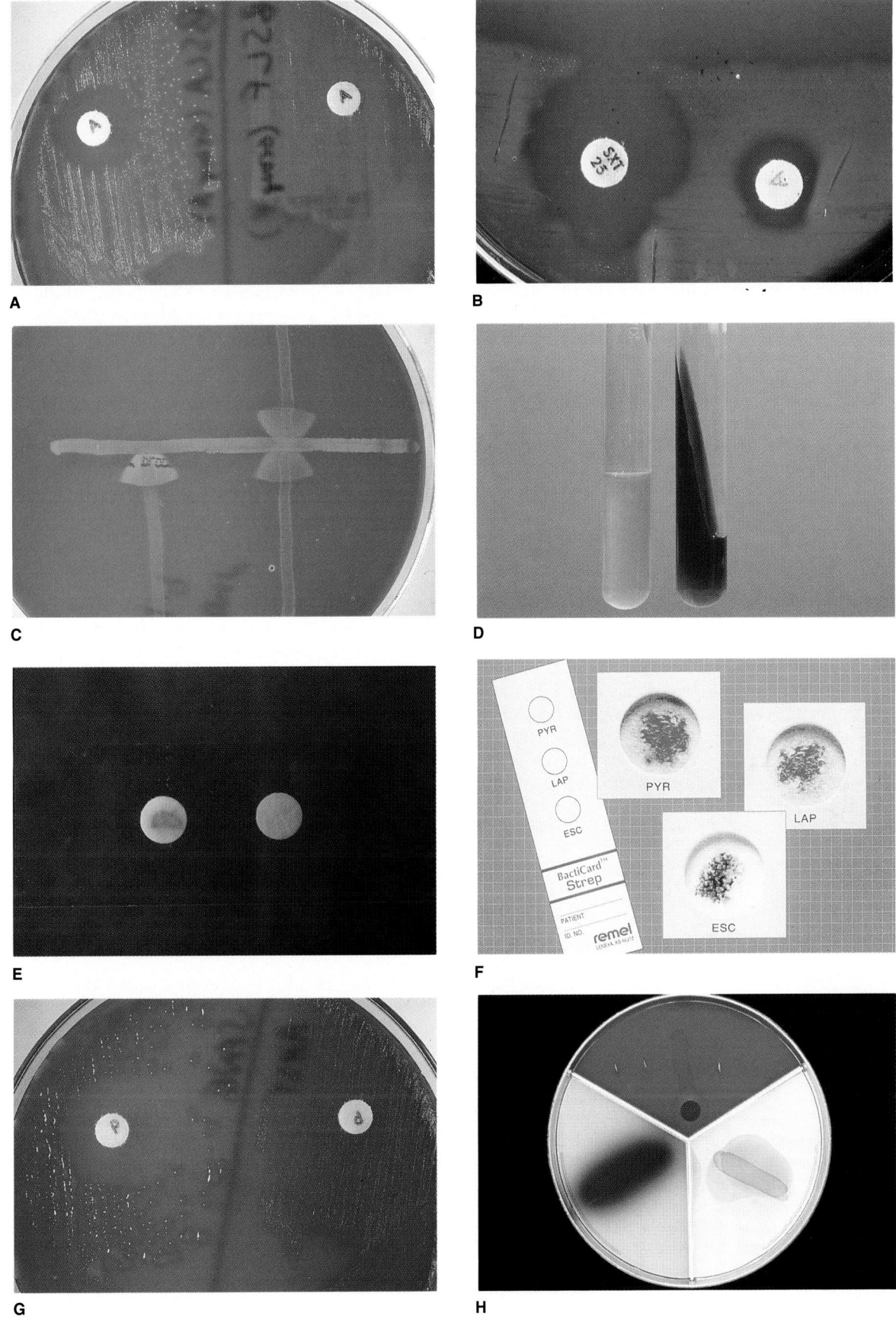

A

B

C

D

E

F

G

H

IDENTIFICATION OF STREPTOCOCCI (CONTINUED)

A. Latex agglutination for serologic grouping of streptococci: Although the Lancefield extraction method and the capillary precipitin test are the time-honored techniques for definitive identification of the groupable streptococci, other methods, such as the Streptex shown here, have been adopted in many laboratories and are considered to be standard procedures. In this test, the cell wall-grouping antigen is extracted from the bacterial cell wall enzymatically, and the extract is reacted with latex beads to which group-specific antibodies are bound. A positive test is indicated by agglutination of the latex particles in the homologous latex reagent. As shown here, agglutination has occurred with the group A reagent, but not with the group B, C, D, F, or G reagents.

B. Quellung test for identification of *S. pneumoniae:* This microscopic "precipitin test" can be used to identify or to determine capsular subtypes of pneumococci. Reaction of anticapsular antibody with the carbohydrate material of the capsule causes a microprecipitin reaction on the surface of the organism and a change in the refractive index of the capsule itself. Microscopically, the capsular appears to "swell." A small amount of methylene blue is added to the preparation to allow visualization of the cells and to provide contrast so that the subtle refractile change in the capsule can be more easily discerned.

C. Rapid STREP identification system: This kit system is one of several that is commercially available for the identification of clinically important streptococci. With this system, the chromogenic enzyme substrate tests on the first half of the strip are read 4 hours after inoculation and incubation (*top* strip); some isolates may be identified at this time. If a reliable identification is not obtained, the carbohydrate utilization tests in the second half of the strip are read after 18 to 24 hours incubation (*center* strip). Both groups of tests are then used to generate a biotype number (reaction recording sheet at *bottom*) and a computer database-assisted identification. These strips show the biochemical reactions of *S. bovis.* (Courtesy of Analytab Products, Inc., Plainview NY)

D. Nutritionally variant streptococci (NVS): NVS are streptococcal species that require thiol compounds, cysteine, or the active form of vitamin B_6 (pyridoxal or pyridoxamine) for growth on media. This requirement may be met by cross-streaking a staphylococcus across an inoculum of the probable NSV isolate, as shown in this photograph. The small streptococcal colonies are growing adjacent to the staphylococcus streak in a manner similar to that of *Haemophilus* species. The two NVS species were called *S. defectivus* and *S. adjacens,* but it has been proposed that these bacteria be transferred to the new genus *Abiotrophia* as *A. defectiva* and *A. adiacens.*

E. Gram stain of *Leuconostoc* species from a broth culture: The typical "streptococcus-like" growth of these organisms is shown.

F. Vancomycin resistance in a *Leuconostoc* species: A subculture of the organism shown in plate 12-3E was inoculated onto a sheep blood agar plate and a vancomycin disk was placed on the inoculum. After incubation, this organism grew right up to the disk, indicating resistance of this organism to vancomycin. *Leuconostoc* and *Pediococcus* are the two "streptococcus-like" bacteria that are resistant to vancomycin. Production of gas from glucose in MRS broth differentiates *Leuconostoc* species from *Pediococcus* species.

G. Rapid ID 32 Strep System (bio-Meriuex, La Balme les Grottes, France): This kit system provides 4-hour identifications of streptococci and several streptococcus-like bacteria. After inoculation and incubation, the reactions on the strip are read either manually or with an automated reader, and a computer-assisted database provides an identification. This system has the most complete database of all the systems, but is not yet available in the United States. This strip was inoculated with a strain of the viridans streptococcus *S. salivarius.* (Courtesy of bio-Meriuex-Vitek, Hazelwood MO)

H. RapID STR System (Innovative Diagnostic Systems, L.P., Norcross GA): This 15-test, cuvette-format identification system provides 4-hour identification of streptococci, enterococci, aerococci, and some species of both *Leuconostoc* and *Pediococcus.* After inoculation and incubation, the reactions for all ten tests are read directly (the *lower* cuvette). Reagents for reaction development are added to the last four wells of the cuvette, and these wells are read again to determine the four additional reactions. These 14 test results, plus the type of hemolytic reaction produced by the organism, are used to generate a biotype number for computer-assisted identification of the isolate. These cuvettes have been inoculated with an isolate of *S. mitis.* (Courtesy Jim Digh, IDS, Norcross GA)

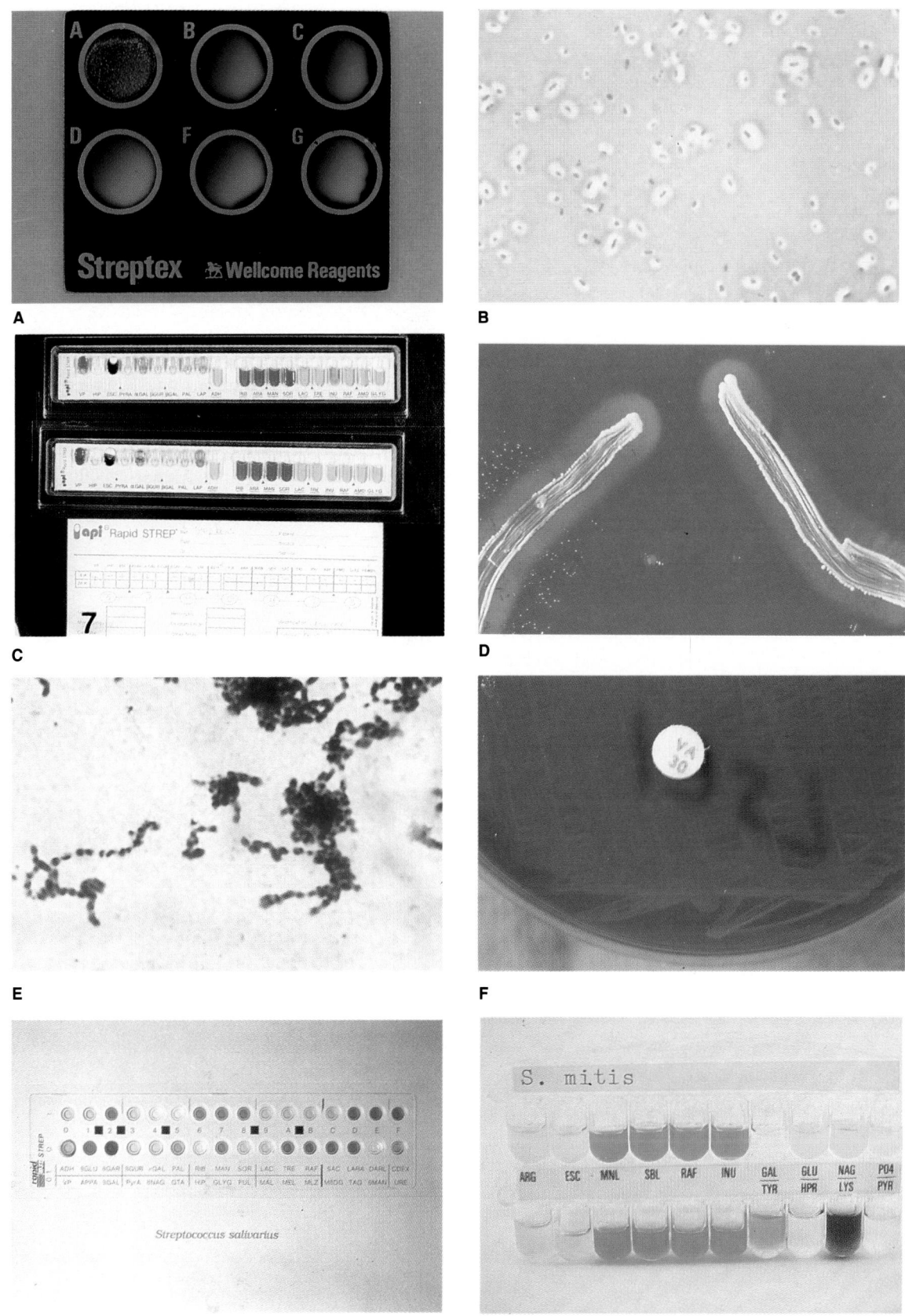

A

B

C

D

E

F

G

H

IDENTIFICATION OF AEROBIC AND FACULTATIVELY ANAEROBIC GRAM-POSITIVE
BACILLI

A. Gram stain of a broth culture of *Bacillus* species illustrating short gram-positive
bacilli containing distinct spores. This Gram stain morphology demonstrates
that not all *Bacillus* species produce the longer, characteristic "box car" cells and
that, in older cultures, the deep blue gram-positive staining of the cells may
be lost.

B. Blood agar plate on which a subculture of *Bacillus subtilis* is growing. Colonies
of *Bacillus cereus* often appear similar, and biochemical differentiation is usually
necessary. Note the dry, somewhat wrinkled nature of the colonies and the
distinct β-hemolysis. The β-hemolysis is a valuable feature in ruling out *Bacillus
anthracis*, which is not hemolytic.

C. Blood agar plate with colonies of a mucoid *Bacillus* species simulating *Pseudomonas*.
(Used previously in the Germ Ware computer program by E. Koneman; with
permission.)

D. Gram stain of *Listeria monocytogenes* grown in trypticase-soy broth at 35°C for
24 hours. The bacterial cells are short, gram-positive bacilli that may lie singly,
lie in small clusters at times with a diphtheroid arrangement, or form short
chains.

E. Sheep blood agar plate on which tiny colonies producing a "soft" β-hemolysis
are growing. This picture is consistent with one of the β-hemolytic streptococci;
however, shown here is a 48-hour growth of *Listeria monocytogenes*. Gram stains
must always be performed on any β-hemolytic, streptococcus-like colonies that
are recovered from blood cultures, cerebrospinal fluid, and genital cultures.

F. CAMP reactions of *L. monocytogenes* (the two outer vertical streaks) with *Staphylococcus aureus* (horizontal streak at top) and *Rhodococcus equi* (bottom horizontal streak). A CAMP-negative *Corynebacterium* species is streaked vertically in
the center of the plate.

G. Semisolid agar motility test medium illustrating the subsurface umbrella-like
motility pattern characteristic of *Listeria monocytogenes*. This pattern of motility
is best seen when the culture is incubated at room temperature.

H. Split frame of subcultures of *E. rhusiopathiae* on Kligler iron agar (*left*) and soft
gelatin agar (*right*). The KIA tube reveals an alk/alk reaction with production of
a small amount of hydrogen sulfide in the deep of the medium along the course
of the stab line. In soft gelatin agar, *E. rhusiopathiae* characteristically produces a
"bottle brush" extension laterally from the streak line.

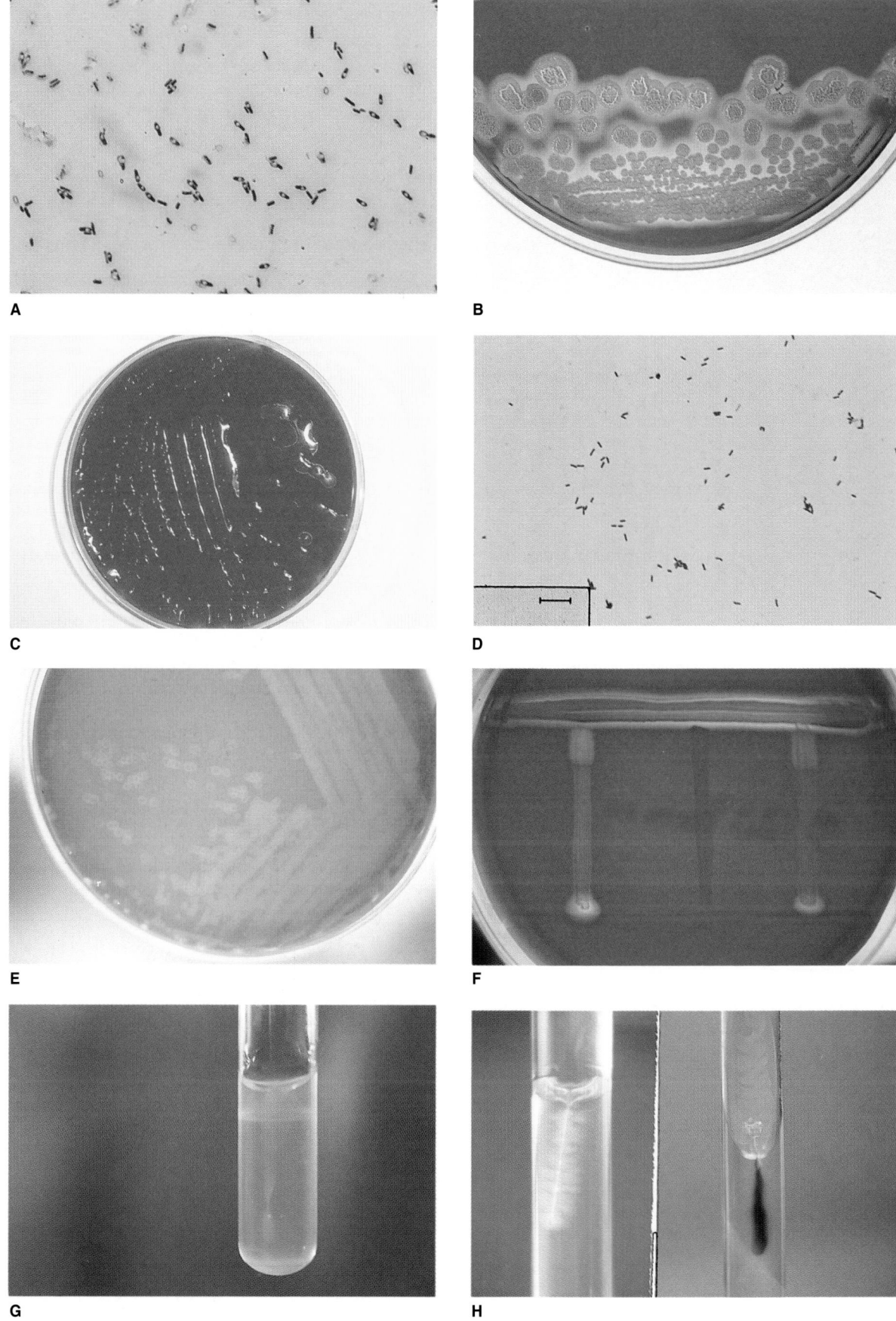

A

B

C

D

E

F

G

H

IDENTIFICATION OF AEROBIC AND FACULTATIVELY ANAEROBIC GRAM-POSITIVE
BACILLI (CONTINUED)

A. Gram stain of a smear prepared from a 24-hour broth culture of *E. rhusiopathiae* illustrating short, slender, straight, and curved gram-positive bacilli. There is a tendency for the cells to form long filaments, a feature only minimally evident in this photograph.

B. Surface of a sheep blood agar plate on which colonies of *Erysipelothrix rhusiopathiae* are growing after 24 hours of incubation at 35°C. This culture represents the smaller, convex, circular, and transparent colony type. Larger, rough colonies with a matte surface and a fimbriated edge may be formed by other strains.

C. Gram stain prepared from a smear of a 48-hour plate culture of a *Lactobacillus* species. Lactobacilli typically form long chains of rod-shaped cells.

D. Lactobacillus selective agar containing colonies of a *Lactobacillus* species. Growth on this medium of typical morphologic forms of rod-shaped bacteria in chains constitutes presumptive evidence that the isolate is a *Lactobacillus* species.

E. Gram stain preparation made from a 24-hour trypticase-soy broth culture of *Corynebacterium diphtheriae*. The cells vary from coccobacilli to short rods that may form Chinese letter or picket fence arrangements.

F. Tellurite agar illustrating several black colonies. The black colonies with sharp, discrete borders are *Staphylococcus aureus*. One large colony in the right lower corner is surrounded by a thin brown halo, consistent with the appearance of growth of *C. diphtheriae* when recovered on media containing sodium tellurite. Occasional strains of *Proteus* species can also produce colonies surrounded by a brown halo on tellurite agar; however, these can be readily distinguished from *C. diphtheriae* by the Gram stain morphology and by biochemical characteristics.

G. Colonies of *C. diphtheriae* as they appear on blood agar after 48 hours of incubation at 35°C. The isolated colonies appear white, entire, and convex; there is no β-hemolysis.

H. Gram stain of a positive blood culture from which a pure culture of *Corynebacterium jeikeium* was recovered. Note the small clusters of relatively short, gram-positive bacilli that have a distinct Chinese letter or "diphtheroidal" arrangement. *C. jeikeium* is not an uncommon isolate from blood cultures in hospitalized patients.

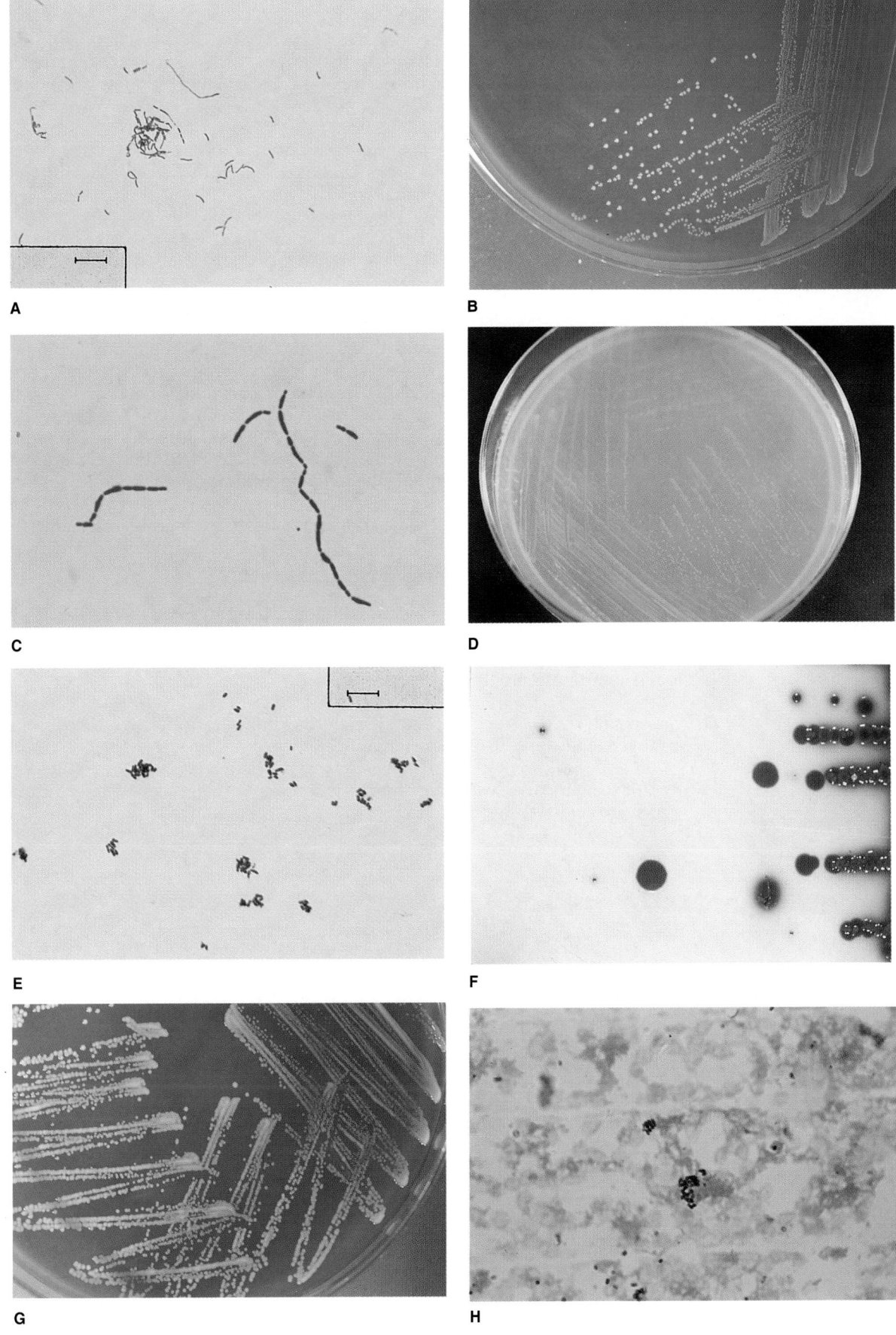

A

B

C

D

E

F

G

H

IDENTIFICATION OF AEROBIC AND FACULTATIVELY ANAEROBIC GRAM-POSITIVE
BACILLI (CONTINUED)

A. Colonies of *Corynebacterium jeikeium* as they appear on sheep blood agar after 24 hours of incubation at 35°C in 5% to 10% CO_2. Isolated colonies are white, smooth, and punctate.

B. Enhanced growth of *C. jeikeium,* one of the lipophilic species of *Corynebacterium,* on brain heart infusion (BHI) agar supplemented with Tween 80 compared with poor growth on unsupplemented BHI agar.

C. Colonies of *Actinomyces pyogenes* on sheep blood agar with striking, complete ("β") hemolysis. Colonies of *Arcanobacterium haemolyticum* also produce a similar hemolytic reaction.

D. Close-in view of *Nocardia asteroides* after 7 days of incubation at 30°C on Middlebrook 7H11 agar. Seen here is the typical orange, glabrous, wavy colonies that tend to be adherent to the agar surface. Other species produce white, dry, chalky colonies (see Color Plate 2-3J). It is noteworthy that *Nocardia* species will grow on the selective isolation media used for the recovery of *Mycobacterium* species; in fact, the laboratory diagnosis of nocardiosis is often first suspected in the mycobacteriology section of the laboratory. The detection of a distinct musty basement odor is an initial clue to the identification.

E. Partial acid-fast stain of an exudate containing acid-fast, delicate, branching filaments characteristic of *Nocardia* species. *Nocardia asteroides* was recovered from the culture obtained from this specimen.

F. Sheep blood agar plate on which a 48-hour culture of *Rhodococcus* species is growing. The colonies are relatively large, ranging from 2 to 4 mm in diameter, and are entire and smooth. Note the salmon-pink pigmentation, an initial clue to the identification of this species.

G. Gram-stain of *Rhodococcus* species illustrating short gram-positive coccobacilli arranged singly and in Chinese letter clusters.

H. Acid-fast stain of *Rhodococcus* species showing short coccobacilli, many of which are acid-fast positive.

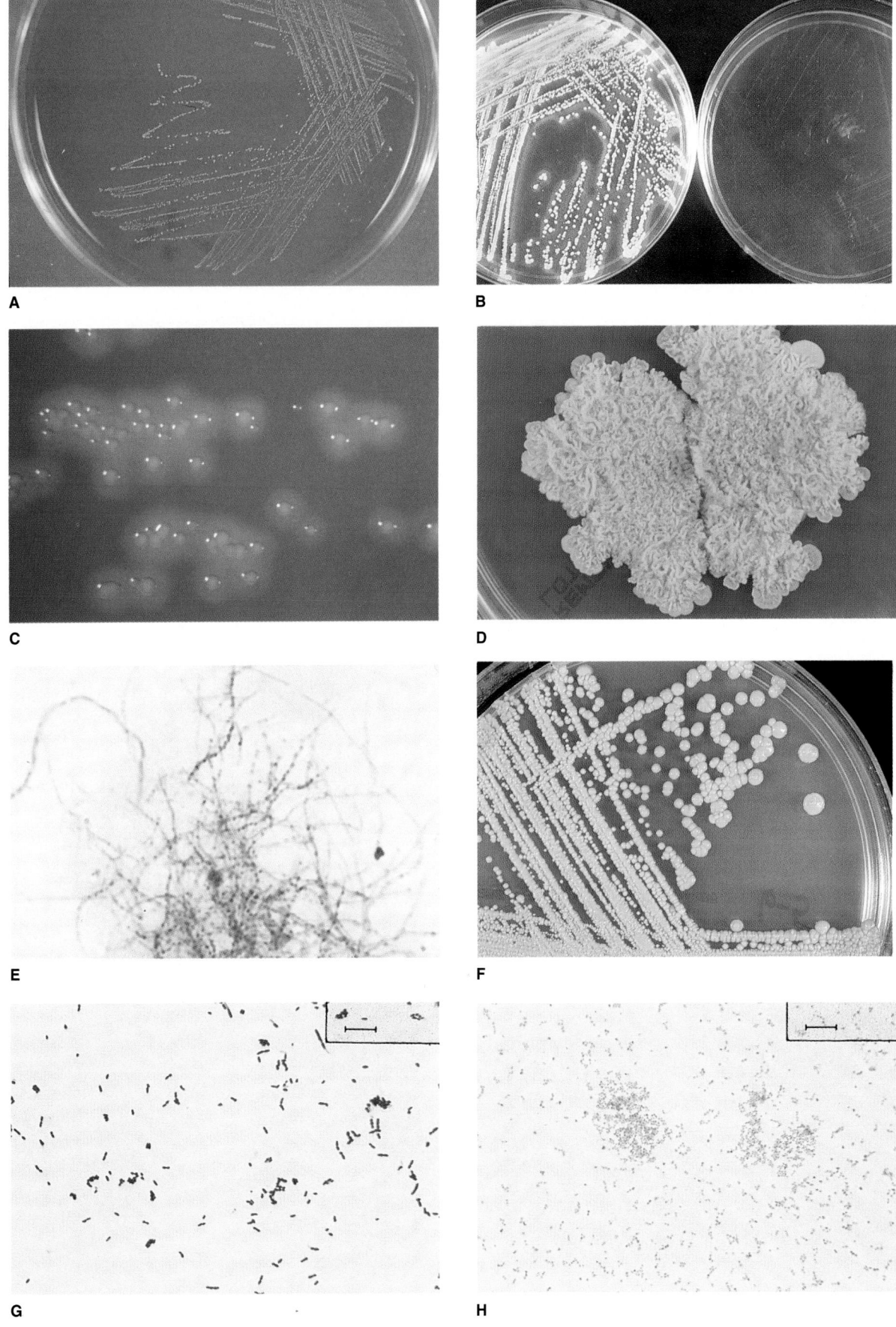

A

B

C

D

E

F

G

H

1. All children should receive one of the conjugate vaccines licensed for use in infants (HbOC, PRP-OMP, or PRP-T), beginning at 2 months of age. For the HbOC and PRP-T vaccines, three doses are given at 2-month intervals (i.e., 2, 4, and 6 months), with a fourth dose at 12 to 15 months of age. If PRP-OMP is used for the first vaccination, two doses are subsequently administered at 2-month intervals (i.e., 2 and 4 months), with a third dose at 12 to 15 months of age. For the 12- to 15-month dose, any of the conjugate vaccines may be used. These vaccines can be administered during visits when other vaccines (e.g., measles, mumps, rubella) are being given, and infants scheduled to receive both HbOC and DTP can be given the combination vaccine, HbOC-DTP. In general, conjugate vaccines should be administered in a separate syringe and at a separate site from DTP or other vaccinations.

2. For immunization of children younger than 7 months of age, either a three-dose series of HbOC or PRP-T or a two-dose series of PRP-OMP should be given at 2-month intervals using the same vaccine. A third dose of any one of the three vaccines (HbOC, PRP-T, or PRP-OMP) should be given at 12 to 15 months of age.

3. For children for whom immunization is not started until 7 to 11 months of age, HbOC, PRP-OMP, or PRP-T should be given at that time, with a second dose of the same vaccine being administered 2 months later. A third booster dose of any of the conjugate vaccines is given at 12 to 18 months of age.

4. For children in whom vaccination is started at 12 to 14 months of age, PRP-D, HbOC, PRP-OMP, or PRP-T may be given. Two doses should be administered 2 months apart.

5. For unvaccinated children age 15 months to 5 years, a single dose of any of the licensed conjugate vaccines is recommended.

6. The immunization series for premature infants is based on chronologic age and should be commenced at 2 months of age.

7. Infants who have had their primary series of immunizations for diphtheria, tetanus, and pertussis deferred to 1 year of age (e.g., children with certain neurologic disorders), PRP-OMP vaccine may present an advantage, because this vaccine is immunogenic in the absence of diphtheria or tetanus toxoids. The combination vaccine HbOC-DTP should not be used for immunization of infants in whom pertussis vaccination is contraindicated. This would include infants with a history of immediate reactions to DTP or the development of encephalopathy (alterations of consciousness, seizures) within 7 days of receipt of DTP vaccine.

8. For children 12 months to 5 years of age with underlying immunologic impairment (e.g., those with bone marrow transplants, sickle cell diseases, splenectomy, or neoplastic diseases requiring chemotherapy) who have received a primary series of injections and a booster dose at 12 months of age or older, additional doses of vaccine are not required, although some have advocated the administration of an additional dose before undergoing a cycle of chemotherapy or splenectomy. For children 12 to 59 months of age with these underlying conditions, who have not been vaccinated, two doses of any conjugate vaccine administered 2 months apart are recommended. Nonvaccinated children with sickle cell disease or asplenia who are older than 5 years of age may be given one dose of any conjugate vaccine. Two doses of any vaccine given 1 to 2 months apart are suggested for children with HIV infection, malignancies, bone marrow transplants, and IgG2 deficiency. Vaccine efficacy data on children younger than 12 months of age with immunoglobulin subclass deficiency or HIV infection is currently limited.

9. In children who have had invasive *H. influenzae* type b disease before the age of 2 years, prior immunization should be disregarded and conjugate vaccine should be readministered during convalescence, according to the age-appropriate schedules outlined in the foregoing. Children who develop *H. influenzae* disease after the age of 2 years do not require reimmunization, because infection itself induces a protective immune response in immunologically normal children of this age.

---

representing an 84% decrease in the incidence of epiglottitis caused by *H. influenzae* type b organisms.

The *H. influenzae* type b conjugate vaccines are highly efficacious and their safety has been established in several clinical trials in the U.S. and elsewhere.[58,61,62,77,97,101,137,213,219] Early surveillance data, collected during 1992, when approximately 67% of children aged 12 to 24 months had received at least one dose of conjugate vaccine, have already suggested inordinate decreases in the incidence of serious *H. influenzae* type b disease. Indeed, large decreases in incidence among children less than 18 months of age were noted long before the conjugate vaccines were in widespread use in young infants.[1,19,194] These findings suggested that the conjugate vaccines not only prevent disease by the induction of active immunity but may also decrease oropharyngeal carriage of *H. influenzae* type b. Indeed, this has been demonstrated in studies in Europe and the U.S.[183,193,264] The vaccines may provide additional protection for unvaccinated infants by reducing their risk of exposure to *H. influenzae* type b from their vaccinated older contacts. Ongoing surveillance in populations of both children and adults will be needed to see if the immunity engendered by the conjugate vaccines is long-term or whether there will be an increase in the proportion of both older children and adults who are susceptible to *H. influenzae* type b infections.

SPECIFIC *HAEMOPHILUS* INFECTIONS

MENINGITIS

Haemophilus influenzae is recovered in 45% to 48% of all cases of acute bacterial meningitis in the United States.[288] Most cases of meningitis caused by *H. influenzae* occur in infants and children younger than the age of 6 years, and this organism is the most common cause of bacterial meningitis in children between 1 month and 2 years of age, with the peak incidence between 6 and 12 months of age.[28,240] Between the ages of 2 and 6 years, *H. influenzae* and *Neisseria meningitidis* occur with equal frequency. *Hiaemophilus influenzae* meningitis is uncommon in children older than 6 years of age. More than 90% of isolates obtained from cases of meningitis belong to capsular serotype b.[28,187] Clinically, *H. influenzae* type b meningitis closely resembles meningococcal meningitis. Prior nasopharyngeal colonization in a susceptible host leads to invasion of the bloodstream and subsequent seeding of the meninges. Symptoms of an upper respiratory tract infection of viral etiology and otitis media are also common in a child with incipient meningitis.[266] Onset of meningeal signs and symptoms may be abrupt or insidious, with the latter being the most common pattern. A high index of suspicion, aggressive diagnostic approaches (i.e., lumbar puncture for collection of cerebrospinal fluid [CSF], collection of blood cultures, and early administration of appropriate antimicrobial therapy), and close communication with the laboratory are essential for proper diagnosis. Although relatively unusual, complications of *H. influenzae* type b meningitis include brain abscess, pericarditis, and abscess formation at other body sites as a result of hematogenous dissemination.[84]

Haemophilus influenzae meningitis in adults usually complicates underlying diseases or conditions, and generally results from direct extension of the organism from a contiguous focus of infection. Such conditions include CSF leakage secondary to head trauma, chronic sinusitis, and otitis media.[253] Other debilitating diseases, such as diabetes, chronic alcoholism, tracheobronchitis, pneumonia, epiglottitis, HIV infection, and other immunodeficiency states (e.g., hypogammaglobulinemia) may also predispose adults to *H. influenzae* meningitis.[57,81,82,148,265,296] In adults, approximately half of the cases of meningitis are due to nontypeable *H. influenzae* strains, whereas the other half are caused by type b and other encapsulated strains.[108,189,196,253,296]

Meningitis caused by *H. influenzae* type b is also contagious, and there is an increased risk of secondary invasive disease in household contacts 4 years of age or younger. It is recommended that families with young children who have been exposed to another family member with invasive *H. influenzae* disease receive prophylaxis with rifampin, regardless of age. Although most experts agree that prophylaxis be given when there are children in the household younger than 2 years of age, some recommend prophylaxis when there are children younger than 4 years of age in the household.[29] Rifampin is the drug of choice for prophylaxis; this drug eliminates oropharyngeal carriage of *H. influenzae* type b and, thereby, transmission of the organism by the respiratory route. Orally administered prophylactic rifampin should be given for 4 full days and should be initiated simultaneously for all household members. Household members do not require rifampin prophylaxis if all of the contacts in the household younger than 2 years of age are fully immunized.[52] All members of a household with an immunized child younger than 12 months of age (i.e., those children who have not yet received a "booster" conjugate vaccine dose) should receive rifampin. Children and staff attending day care facilities who are contacts of index cases should receive rifampin prophylaxis if the exposed children are younger than 2 years of age.[29,59] Prophylaxis should be administered regardless of the immunization status of the exposed children and should be given as soon after identification of the index case as possible.[294]

Meningitis, caused by *H. influenzae*, as a complication of CSF shunt infections has also been reported in recent years.[115,155,216,221,256,297] These infections have occurred mostly in infants and children and have involved ventriculoperitoneal, ventriculoatrial, and lumboperitoneal shunt types.[221] Unlike most of shunt infections, which are caused by *Staphylococcus epidermidis* or *S. aureus* and are attributed to intraoperative or perioperative contamination of the shunt and ventricular CSF, the pathogenesis of *H. influenzae* shunt infections apparently involves seeding of the shunt and the CSF during bacteremia. Whereas most shunt infections become clinically apparent within 2 months of placement, *H. influenzae* shunt infections have been observed to occur several months to several years after shunt placement.[221] Patients with these infections generally present with signs and symptoms of meningitis and frequently have other infections associated with childhood *H. influenzae* infections, such as otitis media. Isolates from these infections have either been capsular type b strains or have been nontypeable. Although most shunt infections caused by gram-positive bacteria require removal or replacement of the foreign body to effect cure, systemic antimicrobial therapy without shunt removal is frequently successful in eliminating *H. influenzae* type b, whereas medical therapy alone has been less successful in treatment of shunt infections caused by nontypeable strains. It has been postulated that encapsulated organisms adhere less readily to the shunt material and because of this may be more easily eradicated.[221,297]

EPIGLOTTITIS

H. influenzae type b is the most common cause of epiglottitis, a clinical entity that is the second most common manifestation of infection.[187] This infection is generally acute, with the abrupt onset of obstructive laryngeal edema. Nasotracheal intubation and vigorous administration of antimicrobial and supportive therapy may be lifesaving in cases of airway obstruction. Although posterior pharyngeal cultures may not be diagnostic because other nasopharyngeal flora may also be isolated, *H. influenzae* type b can be recovered from blood cultures in 64% to 74% of cases. Epiglottitis seldom occurs in infants, but is typically seen in children between 2 and 7 years of age. This is in contrast with other types of invasive *H. influenzae* type b infections, for which the peak incidence occurs among infants 6 months to 18 months of age. However, more recent studies suggest that this infection is occurring more often in younger children. Emmerson and colleagues[73] reported that more than 35% of children with epiglottitis were younger than 2 years of age compared with 9.6% of patients who were younger than 2 years old in previous studies. In one retrospective report, the mean age in years for 54 cases of epiglottitis that occurred from 1985 through 1990 in Philadelphia was 3.3 years.[139] The first reported case of epiglottitis was in 1936 in a 36-year-old woman with fever, dyspnea, and pharyngeal obstruction. More than 100 cases have been reported in adults, with the highest incidence occurring in men 20 to 30 years of age.[296]

OTITIS MEDIA

Streptococcus pneumoniae and *H. influenzae* are the most frequent causes of acute otitis media. This infection is seen primarily in children between 6 months and 2 years of age. More than 90% of *H. influenzae* strains recovered from middle ear aspirates of children with this infection are nontypeable, the remaining 10% being type b organisms.[278] There is some evidence that nontypeable *H. influenzae* strains may be significant causes of otitis media in adolescents and adults as well.

Patients with acute otitis media caused by *H. influenzae* generally present with ear pain with or without ear drainage. Fever and other systemic signs and symptoms may also be present, particularly in children. In fact, up to one fourth of children with otitis media caused by type b organisms have concomitant bacteremia, meningitis, or both. [187,278] Since microbiologic studies on the etiology of otitis media performed with properly collected middle ear aspirates have already delineated those organisms responsible for acute otitis media, tympanocentesis to obtain middle ear fluid for cultural diagnosis is usually not done. If drainage is present, however, it should be collected for culture. Simultaneous culture of CSF and blood may be necessary if systemic signs and symptoms are present.

SINUSITIS

Careful bacteriologic studies of patients with acute sinusitis have clearly demonstrated the role of *H. influenzae* as a principal etiologic agent in this infection, with 20% to 25% and 36% to 40% of cases of acute sinusitis being caused by *H. influenzae* in adults and children, respectively. In studies for which specimens were either obtained surgically or by needle aspiration of the maxillary sinus spaces, *H. influenzae* and *S. pneumoniae* were the organisms most frequently isolated. Evidence exists that these bacterial agents may represent secondary invaders following viral sinus infection (e.g., rhinovirus). Most isolates from patients with acute sinus infections are nonencapsulated and nontypeable.[189] Apparently, *H. influenzae* does not play an important role in the pathogenesis of chronic sinusitis; clinical features and bacteriologic studies have demonstrated that anaerobic microorganisms are primarily responsible for this clinical entity.

UPPER RESPIRATORY TRACT INFECTIONS

The role of *H. influenzae* as a cause of upper respiratory tract infections is not well established. Experimental work by Myerowitz and Michaels[199] has shed some light on the association of *H. influenzae* and acute pharyngitis. Infant rats that were first inoculated with influenza virus showed markedly increased susceptibility to mucosal colonization and invasion with *H. influenzae* when compared with an uninoculated control group. The preexisting viral infection enhanced the adherence of the bacteria to the inflamed mucosa, suppressed the animals' immune response to *H. influenzae* antigens and inhibited leukocyte functions (e.g., phagocytosis of opsonized microorganisms). Pharyngitis caused by *H. influenzae* may occur only in those patients with primary viral upper respiratory tract infections; nevertheless, these organisms may go on to cause systemic disease. Approximately two thirds of children with *H. influenzae* meningitis experience nonspecific upper respiratory symptoms or otitis media before the onset of meningeal signs and symptoms.[187,240] A crouplike syndrome may also develop in neonates and young children with *H. influenzae* pharyngitis if the larynx is involved.[254] Again, colonization by *Haemophilus* is probably superimposed on a primary viral laryngitis.

ACUTE FEBRILE TRACHEOBRONCHITIS

Chronic bronchitis is an ill-defined clinical entity characterized by a persistent, generally nonproductive cough, wheezing, and shortness of breath. Acute exacerbations of the illness result in the production of purulent sputum and may lead to a condition now called **acute febrile tracheobronchitis**.[195] The etiologic agents of this condition include *S. aureus*, group A β-hemolytic streptococci, and *H. influenzae*. Most of the isolates are nonencapsulated and serologically nontypeable.[189] Similar to epiglottitis, the onset is usually acute and includes high fever, dyspnea, and production of copious amounts of sputum. Inflammation is usually subglottic and the epiglottis shows minimal inflammation. Because *H. influenzae* colonizes the upper respiratory tract of individuals without this condition, its role in chronic bronchitis, acute suppurative exacerbations of chronic bronchitis, and even acute febrile tracheobronchitis remains unclear. Several observations and some experimental data do suggest an etiologic role for nontypeable *H. influenzae* in the pathogenesis of this condition.[189] First, these organisms are usually present in the sputum in increased numbers during acute purulent exacerbations. Second, serologic responses to cell surface antigens of nontypeable strains recovered from individual patients have been demonstrated following acute febrile exacerbations of the chronic illness. Third, antimicrobial therapy directed against these organisms has a beneficial, although transient, effect on the acute illness in many patients. Chronic bronchitis, acute exacerbations of purulent bronchitis, acute febrile tracheobronchitis, and pneumonia may represent stages in a continuum of pathologic pulmonary processes in which nontypeable *H. influenzae* strains are a primary player. There is no doubt that various host factors (e.g., immune status, other pulmonary compromises, prior or concurrent viral infections) also contribute to the pathogenesis of this ill-defined condition.

PNEUMONIA

H. influenzae pneumonia can be another manifestation of systemic *H. influenzae* infection or may develop as an extension and complication of a primary respiratory tract infection, such as chronic bronchitis or acute febrile tracheobronchitis. *H. influenzae* pneumonia in patients with systemic disease (i.e., meningitis, epiglottitis, bacteremia, otitis media) is lobar, segmental, and purulent—characteristics similar to pneumococcal pneumonia. In these patients, encapsulated type b organisms are the usual etiologic agents. Nontypeable strains of *H. influenzae* are important causes of pneumonia, with or without bacteremia, particularly in elderly patients with underlying respiratory conditions, such as chronic bronchitis, chronic obstructive pulmonary disease, and bronchiectasis, or with systemic conditions, such as immunodeficiency, diabetes, alcoholism, and neoplastic disease.[57,65,81,148,151,195,265,272] In addition, bacteremic pneumonia caused by *H. influenzae* capsular types other than type b has also been reported in patients with underlying conditions that impair local or systemic host defense mechanisms.[15,71,120,250,281] Definitive diagnosis of *H. influenzae* pneumonia is clouded by the frequent presence of the organism in the upper respiratory tract of healthy individuals. Coughed, expectorated sputum specimens may provide inadequate or misleading results; bronchial washings, bronchoscopy specimens, bronchoalveolar lavage, and transtracheal aspirates may be necessary for definitive cultural diagnosis.

BACTEREMIA

Bacteremia is a frequent and early manifestation of acute *H. influenzae* type b infection. Some children may present with primary bacteremia without meningitis, but this is considered unusual. Hematogenous spread of the microorganism, however, may result in several other clinical manifestations of infection.[187] Seeding of

the soft tissues results in cellulitis; this often appears in children as violaceous or bluish swellings on the cheeks and periorbital areas of the face. Septic arthritis and osteomyelitis may also complicate *H. influenzae* bacteremia.[276] Neonatal *H. influenzae* sepsis has also been reported, and the literature indicates that this clinical entity may be increasing.[34,90] In these cases, meningitis may or may not be present. Most of the cases of neonatal infection appear to result from maternal–fetal or maternal–perinatal transmission (discussed later). Although 90% to 95% of bacteremic *H. influenzae* infections outside of the neonatal period are due to type b organisms, only about 20% of isolates from neonatal sepsis are type b, with the majority being nontypeable.[90]

ENDOCARDITIS

Endocarditis caused by *Haemophilus* species is clinically and anatomically similar to that caused by other pyogenic bacteria. However, *H. influenzae* is an unusual agent of endocarditis.[175] *Haemophilus parainfluenzae*, *H. aphrophilus*, and *H. paraphrophilus* are the species most commonly recovered from patients with endocarditis and intravascular infections.[17,33,48,93,109,111,128,136,163,214] The incidence of this infection is highest in young to middle-aged adults and may or may not be associated with preexisting valvular disease. Although the mortality associated with properly treated *Haemophilus* endocarditis is usually about 10% to 15%, the higher rates (25% to 50%) reported in the earlier literature may have reflected difficulties in recovering these fastidious microorganisms from blood cultures, which may have resulted in inappropriate or inadequate antimicrobial therapy.

Endocarditis is the most commonly reported systemic infection associated with *H. parainfluenzae*.[93,109,128,163,177] *H. parainfluenzae* is a normal inhabitant of the nasopharynx and oropharynx, being found in 10% to 25% of cultures from normal persons. Patients with *H. parainfluenzae* endocarditis usually have a subacute presentation, with low-grade fever, malaise, chills, and respiratory tract symptoms. The organism apparently gains access into the bloodstream through the upper respiratory tract and periodontal areas, for many of the patients have had poor dentition, periodontal disease, recent dental manipulations, or oropharyngeal infections. Interestingly, preexisting or underlying valvular disease is found in only about 48% of cases, and the presence of a heart murmur may be the only suggestive finding in these patients. Peripheral stigmata of endocarditis, such as Roth's spots, Janeway lesions, and splinter hemorrhages are usually absent. Disseminated intravascular coagulation and pulmonary hemorrhage have been reported, and both hematuria and anemia may be seen with this infection.[33,163,248] *H. parainfluenzae* endocarditis is also associated with a higher incidence of vegetations on the heart valves, as detected by echocardiography, and with septic complications resulting from embolization of these vegetations to the large arteries.[214] Major arterial emboli may be seen in 30% to 85% of patients; movement of emboli to the central nervous system is the most common cause of morbidity with this infection.

H. parainfluenzae has also been implicated in cases of polymicrobial endocarditis in intravenous drug users.[232] These patients typically present with right-sided endocarditis, tricuspid valve vegetations on echocardiography, and clinical and radiographic evidence of septic pulmonary embolization. In a report by Raucher and colleagues,[232] none of ten intravenous drug users with polymicrobial endocarditis had *H. parainfluenzae* isolated from the initial blood cultures, and all patients received therapeutic agents directed against gram-positive isolates (e.g., viridans streptococci, *S. aureus*). Failure to respond to therapy prompted collection of additional blood cultures and allowed subsequent recovery of *H. parainfluenzae*. This organism has also been associated with sustained bacteremia resulting from infection of vascular implants, such as pacemaker wires.[237]

The clinical and laboratory characteristics of *H. aphrophilus* and *H. paraphrophilus* are discussed further in Chapter 8, along with the other fastidious gram-negative bacteria associated with endocarditis.

UROGENITAL, MATERNAL, AND PERINATAL INFECTIONS

Haemophilus species, particularly nontypeable *H. influenzae* and *H. parainfluenzae*, have also been recognized as probable causes of nongonococcal urethritis, obstetric and gynecologic infections (e.g., tubo-ovarian abscesses, septic abortion), female genital tract infections, postpartum bacteremia, and neonatal sepsis, with and without meningitis.[4,45,55,149,154,170,182,211,231,239,280] Sturm[260] reported that either *H. influenzae* or *H. parainfluenzae* were the only organisms (including chlamydiae and ureaplasmas) recovered from 10% of 242 episodes of nongonococcal urethritis in 234 men. These organisms were not recovered from asymptomatic men. In another study conducted in Houston between 1976 and 1981,[280] *H. influenzae* was recovered from blood cultures of 16 women with postpartum bacteremia and 36 neonates with bacteremia or meningitis. In addition, another 50 *H. influenzae* isolates, not associated with bacteremia or meningitis, were cultured from genital sites (vagina, endometrium, cervix, Bartholin's glands, fallopian tubes, male urethra, and prostatic fluid) and fetal tissues (amniotic fluid, placental tissues). Of these isolates, 94% were serologically nontypeable. In a study done in France,[231] *Haemophilus* species were recovered from genital cultures of 83 women over a 90-month period. Of these 83 women, 42 had significant genital tract infections with these bacteria, including endometritis, salpingitis, and Bartholin's gland abscesses. Genital tract infection with these organisms was linked to the presence of intrauterine devices in 62% of the patients with endometritis and in four of six patients with salpingitis, suggesting that the genital haemophili may behave as opportunistic agents in genital sites. Prenatal and perinatal acquisition of *Haemophilus* species from the maternal genital tract was also associated with prematurity, premature rupture of membranes, amnionitis, and neonatal sepsis in this and other studies.[16,55,94,154,211,280]

Results of biotyping of *H. influenzae* and *H. parainfluenzae*, a technique discussed later in this chapter, have indicated that nontypeable biotype IV *H. influenzae* and biotype I and II *H. parainfluenzae* strains are frequent inhabitants of the genital tract and may be specifically associated with localized genital tract and systemic postpartum maternal and neonatal infections.[3,170,231,280] On the other hand, another study conducted in France on the distribution of *H. influenzae* and *H. parainfluenzae* biotypes from the genital tract found that *H. parainfluenzae* biotype II was the most prevalent isolate from genital sites and that *H. influenzae* biotype IV was not a major genital tract biotype.[70]

Additional studies on serologically nontypeable *H. influenzae* strains recovered from serious urogenital, neonatal, and mother–infant infections suggest that some of these infections may be caused by a new, cryptic genospecies of *H. influenzae*.[228,230,231] This recently described genospecies types biochemically as a biotype IV strain (i.e., indole-negative, urease- and ornithine decarboxylase-positive) but is distinct by additional phenotypic and genetic criteria. These strains possess peritrichous fimbriae, have an unusual and distinctive outer membrane protein profile on polyacrylamide gel electrophoresis, express a variant P6 outer membrane protein, and display a unique enzyme pattern on multilocus enzyme electrophoresis.[230] DNA–DNA hybridization and ribosomal DNA restriction fragment length polymorphism studies indicate that isolates of this new genospecies are genetically homogeneous, suggesting a clonal derivation and, in a strict sense, share less than 70% overall genomic similarity with *H. influenzae*.[230] These same studies indicate that the new genospecies is most closely related to strains of *H. haemolyticus*. Antimicrobial susceptibility testing of these newly characterized strains indicates that, as a group, they may be more susceptible to the quinolone antibiotics (i.e., norfloxacin, enoxacin, and ciprofloxacin) than other biotype IV isolates.[229] There are as yet no readily or easily determined phenotypic characteristics that can reliably differentiate this cryptic genospecies from other *H. influenzae* biotype IV strains. This new genospecies is currently being characterized to determine those properties that may contribute to its recognized virulence in genital tract and neonatal infections.[236]

CONJUNCTIVITIS

Haemophilus species also cause a contagious, acute conjunctivitis called "pinkeye." Localized outbreaks of acute conjunctivitis occur among persons who share towels, handkerchiefs, or other objects that come in direct contact with the skin of the face or eyes. The diffuse pink color of the sclera and the presence of a serous or purulent discharge are virtually diagnostic of *Haemophilus* conjunctivitis. *Haemophilus aegyptius*, the bacterium associated with conjunctivitis, was considered to be a separate species within the genus that was phenotypically similar to *H. influenzae* biotype III. The distinctive clinical disease associated with the organism and both biochemical and serologic studies have generally been used to support the status of *H. aeygptius* as a separate species within the genus. However, genomic nucleotide studies have demonstrated more than 70% sequence homology between *H. aegyptius* and *H. influenzae*, suggesting that the two organisms are the same species. In the 1984 edition of *Bergey's Manual of Systematic Bacteriology*, *H. influenzae* and *H. aegyptius* were retained as separate species.[142] However, in the 1994 edition of *Bergey's Manual of Determinative Bacteriology*, *H. aegyptius* is considered a biovar of *H. influenzae*.[121] A unique, more highy virulent clone(s) of *H. aegyptius* called *H. influenzae* biogroup aegyptius emerged in the early 1980s as a causative agent of a newly described clinical syndrome that is now called Brazilian purpuric fever.

BRAZILIAN PURPURIC FEVER

During the last decade, a distinct subgroup of strains that are phenotypically and biochemically indistinguishable from "*H. aegyptius*" have been associated with outbreaks of a severe illness called **Brazilian purpuric fever (BPF)**.[23,24] This entity was first reported in 1984 in the rural town of Promissao in Sao Paulo State, Brazil, when 10 children (ranging in age from 3 months to 8 years) died following an acute illness that was characterized by a high fever, abdominal pain with vomiting, the development of a petechial or purpuric rash within 72 hours of the onset of fever, and eventually, vascular collapse, hypotensive shock, and death. A subsequent outbreak occurred among 10 children in the town of Serrana, also in Sao Paulo State; four of the 10 children involved in this outbreak also died. Blood cultures from these children grew "*H. aegyptius*" (nine from blood cultures and one from cerebrospinal fluid contaminated with blood).[24,114] Although the clinical syndrome resembles meningococcal bacteremia and meningitis, meningitis is not a part of the clinical presentation. During the epidemiologic investigation of the outbreaks, cases were found to have had recent or concurrent purulent conjunctivitis.[23] Since the initial South American outbreaks, sporadic cases and outbreaks have been reported in other areas of Brazil and in central and western Australia.[25,176,293] Following the initial outbreaks, surveillance mechanisms were established in BPF-endemic areas to monitor the disease and the spread of the implicated organism. Interestingly, the parts of the world where BPF has occurred lie at similar latitudes (21°S to 23°S).[293]

The "*H. aegyptius*" strains that were recovered from blood or conjunctival cultures during the initial and subsequent outbreaks of BPF have been studied extensively since their initial recognition. These BPF isolates demonstrated several characteristics that were not found in "*H. aegyptius*" strains isolated from cases of purulent conjunctivitis without BPF.[26,36,37,76,225,263,289] These characteristics included failure to react with *H. influenzae* capsular-typing sera (i.e., nontypeable), the presence of a unique 24-MDa plasmid, an unusual pattern of cell envelope proteins on polyacrylamide gel electrophoresis including the presence of a distinctive 25-kDa protein, the production of a unique secreted protein, and the ability to resist the bactericidal effects of normal human serum. These and other studies have concluded that the outbreaks of BPF in Sao Paolo were all caused by a unique clone of "*H. aegyptius*" that has been designated "*H. influenzae* biogroup aegyptius" or "BPF-associated *H. aegyptius*." However, some isolates that were recovered from subsequent outbreaks or sporadic cases of BPF in Brazil have been found to lack the 24-MDa plasmid, and strains recovered from some BPF cases in Australia also lacked some of the unusual markers that were found on *H. influenzae* biogroup aeyptius strains recovered during the initial BPF outbreaks in Brazil.

The potential virulence factors and pathogenic mechanisms of the original BPF clone and isolates recovered from the other Brazilian and Australian cases are currently under investigation. The 25-kDa protein associated with the outer membrane of the original BPF isolates has been shown to be a pilin protein.[289] This pilin protein has an amino acid composition that is unique to the BPF clone but has 71% amino acid homology with the *H. influenzae* type b pilin protein. Logically, cloning and sequencing of the pilin genes from *H. influenzae* biogroup aegyptius have demonstrated 82% sequence homology with the pilin gene of reference *H. influenzae* type b strains.[258,292] Human red blood cell agglutination and agglutination-inhibition studies have also shown that the pilin protein from *H. influenzae* biogroup aegyptius probably binds to the same red cell surface receptor as the *H. influenzae* type b pilin protein.[259] Lesse and associates[156] also found that clonal BPF strains of *H. influenzae* biogroup aegyptius possess a stable, highly conserved antigenic epitope that is expressed on the cell surface and is found on or in association with the 48-kDa P1 protein, a heat-modifiable protein that is found in the outer membrane of *H. influenzae* isolates. This epitope was not present on non–BPF-associated strains belonging to *H. influenzae* biogroup aegyptius. The relation of this unique epitope with the P1 protein and with the virulence of the BPF clone is under investigation.

Initial studies on BPF-associated isolates suggested that the organisms were encapsulated and, indeed, Carlone and coworkers[36] reported that DNA from isolates of the BPF clone hybridized to a probe for the DNA sequences involved in *H. influenzae* capsular polysaccharide synthesis (i.e., *cap* gene sequences). However, Dobson and associates[66] found that the probe used in the earlier studies contained sequences that were homologous not only with the *cap* genes of typeable *H. influenzae* strains but also contained sequences of an insertion element (IS1016) that is also present in *H. influenzae* biogroup aegyptius strains. This insertional element was found in BPF-associated *H. influenzae* biogroup aegyptius strains but not in non–BPF-associated isolates. These workers postulated that perhaps the transposition of the IS1016 gene sequences from a plasmid into the genome of the BPF clone strains may have contributed to virulence by altering the transcription and expression of gene sequences adjacent to the insertion. In vivo studies, using an infant rat model, and in vitro studies, using an immortalized human microvascular endothelial cell line, have shown that BPF-associated strains of *H. influenzae* biogroup aegyptius are more virulent and cytotoxic than non–BPF-associated strains of the same species.[238,290] Finally, multilocus enzyme electrophoresis studies have shown that *H. influenzae* biogroup aegyptius isolates form three distinct lineages within the species *H. influenzae* and that the BPF-associated isolates are not closely related genetically to non-BPF *H. influenzae* biogroup aegyptius, but do show a close genetic relation with encapsulated *H. influenzae* strains belonging to capsular serotype c.[125,197]

OTHER TYPE B, NON-TYPE B, AND NONTYPEABLE *HAEMOPHILUS INFLUENZAE* INFECTIONS

H. influenzae type b has also been reported in association with a variety of other uncommon infections; in many of the case reports, the recovery of *Haemophilus* organisms was completely unexpected. Facial and periorbital cellulitis is a frequent finding in children who have *H. influenzae* type b bacteremia, and this same syndrome has been reported in adults with bacteremia and respiratory tract infections.[69] Also, *H. influenzae* type b has been seen as a rare cause of congenital and purulent conjunctivitis and endophthalmitis.[184,218,243] It has also been associated with abdominal infections, including peritonitis, pyogenic liver abscesses, hepatobiliary tract infections, pancreatic abscess, and appendicitis.[8,35,41,207,226] In a few cases of liver abscess, the organisms were recovered from hydatid cysts.[85] In addition, *H. influenzae* has been isolated as a cause of bacteremic epididymitis and orchitis in an HIV-1-infected man.[56]

Although the overwhelming majority of systemic *Haemophilus* infections are caused by *H. influenzae* type b, other capsular serotypes and nontypeable strains have also been associated with significant disease processes.[16,30,53,64,75,98,108,120,122,159,175,277,295] These infections have included neonatal sepsis caused by capsular type c organisms; pneumonia and bacteremia in compromised adults associated with types a, d, and f; and both childhood and adult meningitis and bacteremia, by all non-type b serotypes. *H. influenzae* type f has also been reported as an unusual cause of a mycotic aneurysm in an adult and of osteomyelitis and septic arthritis in young children.[2,49,86] Nontypeable, nonencapsulated *H. influenzae* are also responsible for chronic bronchitis, febrile tracheobronchitis, pneumonia, and bacteremia, primarily in the elderly.[189,196] In several large multicenter studies, bacteremic *H. influenzae* infections were most often due to nontypeable strains.[57,65,80,81,151,272] In addition, nontypeable *H. influenzae* strains have been implicated as invasive agents in individuals with underlying disease, such as Hodgkin's disease and acute lymphocytic leukemia, and have caused systemic illness in those patients with underlying defects in immunoglobulin production.[196]

MISCELLANEOUS INFECTIONS DUE TO OTHER *HAEMOPHILUS* SPECIES

Haemophilus species other than *H. influenzae* are uncommon agents of human infections. Besides endocarditis, *H. parainfluenzae* has been associated with a variety of other types of infections, including epiglottitis, bronchitis, sinusitis, otitis media, pneumonia, empyema, peritonitis, soft-tissue cellulitis, abscesses, septic arthritis, prosthetic joint infections, genital tract infections, and rarely, meningitis and brain abscess.[9,14,44,54,89,165,167,209,283] Olk and associates[210] reported a case of *H. parainfluenzae* vertebral osteomyelitis that became clinically apparent 3 months after the patient underwent nasal septoplasty; presumably, this surgical procedure caused a bacteremia that seeded the lumbosacral vertebrae. This organism has also been isolated on rare occasions as a cause of urinary tract infection in adults[22,185] and as a cause of purulent conjunctivitis in neonates.[234] McClain and coworkers[174] reported a case of *H. parainfluenzae* purulent urethritis in a 24-year-old man that was accompanied by bacteremia with the same organism. Prostatitis caused by *H. parainfluenzae* has also been reported in a 29-year-old man with HIV-1 infection.[50] *H. parainfluenzae* was isolated as an unusual cause of peritoneal infection that was associated with the use of an intrauterine device.[92] Hepatobiliary tract infections, including liver abscess, have been reported rarely in both children and adults.[18,38,43] In these latter infections, it was postulated that *H. parainfluenzae* gained access to the hepatobiliary tree from the intestinal tract, rather than by a hematogenous route. This is supported by the lack of documented *H. parainfluenzae* bacteremia in the patients and that *H. parainfluenzae* has been recovered from the gastrointestinal tract much more frequently than other haemophili.[178]

Haemophilus aphrophilus and *H. paraphrophilus* are indigenous to the oral cavity and are seen primarily in endocarditis. Rare isolates of *H. aphrophilus* have also been recovered from brain abscesses, abdominal wounds, oral lesions, actinomycotic lesions, urinary tract infections, and human bites.[17,74,291] A case of life-threatening epiglottitis in a 6-month-old child caused by an ampicillin-resistant *H. paraphrophilus* strain has also been reported.[130] Both *H. aphrophilus* and *H. paraphrophilus* culturally resemble other fastidious gram-negative bacteria that are recovered from blood cultures, such as *Actinobacillus actinomycetemcomitans* and *Cardiobacterium hominis*. These organisms will be discussed further in Chapter 8.

Haemophilus haemolyticus, *H. parahaemolyticus*, and *H. paraphrophaemolyticus* are all members of the normal respiratory tract flora. These organisms are rarely associated with infections, although they have been recovered from cases of endocarditis, purulent oropharyngeal infections, chronic bronchitis, liver and pancreatic abscesses, cellulitis, osteitis, and empyema. *Haemophilus segnis* has been isolated from dental plaque and the upper respiratory tract. In 1981, Bullock and Devitt[31] reported on the isolation of *H. segnis* from blood and pus of a pancreatic abscess in a 29-

year-old alcoholic male. Subsequently, Welch and coworkers[287] described the isolation of *H. segnis*, in both pure and mixed cultures, from five cases of acute appendicitis. This organism was also recovered, along with anaerobic organisms, from a cutaneous umbilicus abscess of a 70-year-old woman.[46] Clearly, further investigation of these fastidious organisms is needed for a more complete appreciation of their pathogenic potential.

CHANCROID

Haemophilus ducreyi is the causative agent of chancroid, a highly contagious, sexually transmitted infection, characterized by painful genital and perianal ulcers and tender inguinal lymphadenopathy.[186] Genital lesions caused by this organism are also called "soft chancres" because, unlike the primary lesion (chancre) of syphilis, the borders of the lesion are ragged and pliable rather than sharply demarcated and indurated. In males, the lesions are generally on the penis; in females lesions may be present on the labia and within the vagina. Frequently, women with chancroid will yield positive endocervical cultures for *H. ducreyi*. The enlarged inguinal lymph nodes (buboes) may actually suppurate through the overlying skin to form draining fistulas and sinus tracts. The disease is worldwide in distribution and is endemic in South America, Africa, East and Southeast Asia, and India. Sporadic outbreaks of chancroid have been reported in the United States and Canada. Since 1981, outbreaks in the United States have occurred in California, Florida, New York, Boston, southeast Pennsylvania, and Texas.[186,242] These outbreaks have occurred almost exclusively among heterosexuals and have frequently been traced to female prostitutes, thereby accounting for the observed male/female case ratios of 3:1 to 25:1.

In undeveloped countries, infection with *H. ducreyi* is also associated with transmission of human immunodeficiency viruses (i.e., HIV-1 and HIV-2) and the acquired immunodeficiency syndrome (AIDS). Studies in Africa have provided evidence that chancroid is a risk factor for heterosexual transmission of HIV-1, the etiologic agent of AIDS.[150,249] In men, acquisition of HIV-1 was highly correlated with genital ulcers.[249] Genital ulcers caused by chancroid and other agents (e.g., syphilis) apparently render women more susceptible to infection with HIV-1 following heterosexual contact with infected men, and the presence of genital ulcers in HIV-1-infected women also increases the probability that their male sexual partners will become infected. Genital ulcers caused by chancroid and other diseases, such as lymphogranuloma venereum, apparently facilitate the passage of the virus into vaginal secretions. In Kenya, for example, it appears that perhaps one third of HIV-1 infections in prostitutes and at least half of the HIV-1 infections in their male clients are associated with concomitant infection with *H. ducreyi*.[150]

LABORATORY APPROACH TO THE DIAGNOSIS OF *HAEMOPHILUS* INFECTIONS

DIRECT EXAMINATION OF CLINICAL SPECIMENS

GRAM'S AND METHYLENE BLUE STAINS

A rapid presumptive diagnosis of *H. influenzae* infection can be made by direct examination of appropriate clinical material using the Gram's stain. If sufficient (i.e., more than 1 to 2 mL) of CSF is received, the specimen should be centrifuged to obtain a pellet of material for examination and culture. Otherwise, the uncentrifuged specimen should be examined directly. On gram-stained preparations, *Haemophilus* organisms appear as small, pale-staining, gram-negative coccobacilli (see Color Plate 7-1A). Occasionally slender filamentous cells may be observed. Because of the small size, cellular pleomorphism, and the poor staining of some strains with safranin, a simultaneously prepared smear may be stained with methylene blue to aid in the detection of these small bacterial cells. In the latter preparation, the organisms will appear as blue-black coccobacilli against a light blue-gray background. Although *H. influenzae* may be the likely pathogen on the basis of the gram-stained appearance and the patient's clinical presentation, the organisms cannot be identified from the gram-stained smear alone. Furthermore, a negative Gram's stain does not rule out the possibility of *Haemophilus* infection because very few organisms may be present in the specimen.

DETECTION OF TYPE B CAPSULAR ANTIGEN

For rapid diagnosis of *H. influenzae* type b infections, immunologic techniques are available for detection of the type b PRP capsular antigen in CSF, serum, and urine. These methods include latex particle agglutination (LA), staphylococcal protein A coagglutination (COA), and enzyme immunoassay (EIA).

The LA and COA tests for the detection of *H. influenzae* type b PRP and other bacterial capsular antigens in body fluids are now used in most clinical microbiology laboratories for bacterial antigen detection. Antibodies prepared against the *H. influenzae* PRP capsular antigen (or against capsular material of the other agents of bacterial meningitis) are bound to latex beads (LA) or to staphylococcal cells (COA) as "carriers." Mixture of the appropriate body fluid containing the antigen with the sensitized LA or COA reagent results in visible agglutination or clumping of the reagent within seconds to minutes. Commercial LA kits include the Directigen Meningitis Test (Becton-Dickinson Microbiology Systems, Cockeysville MD), the Bactigen *H. influenzae* type b (Wampole Laboratories, Cranbury NJ), and the Wellcogen Bacterial Antigen Kit (Murex Diagnostics Limited, Central Road, Temple Hill, Dartford, England). The commercial COA test is the Phadebact *H. influenzae* type b (Karo Bio AB, Huddinge, Sweden).

Several studies have compared LA and COA for their relative sensitivities and specificities in detecting

H. influenzae type b PRP antigen in various body fluids from patients with meningeal and nonmeningeal infections.[51,123,168,233,245,270,286] Most studies indicate that LA and COA are generally more sensitive and detect smaller amounts of antigen than countercurrent immunoelectrophoresis (CIE), which was the older method for detection of bacterial antigens in body fluids. In clinical studies, CIE detected antigen in 71% to 91% of CSF specimens from patients with meningitis, whereas LA and COA detected 82% to 100%. Furthermore, LA methods are apparently superior to those of CIE and COA for detection of capsular antigens in serum and urine specimens. In a study by Marcon and associates,[168] all three detection methods were performed on urine and serum specimens from 15 patients with bacteremic, nonmeningeal *H. influenzae* type b infections. Testing of these two specimen types by LA, COA, and CIE yielded collective sensitivities of 100%, 27%, and 40%, respectively. Problems with test specificity have been described with all three methods, and positive direct detection tests have been found in patients with illnesses not compatible with *H. influenzae* type b. However, LA is now probably the most sensitive, versatile, and readily accessible method for direct detection of *H. influenzae* PRP antigen in body fluids.

EIA techniques have also been applied to the direct detection of PRP antigen in body fluids. In this method, anti-PRP antibodies are bound to the plastic wells of a microtiter tray. Fluid suspected to contain PRP antigen is placed into the well, and the preparation is incubated to allow antigen–antibody complexes to form. After washing away unbound material, a specific antihuman antibody–enzyme conjugate is added to the wells. Following another incubation and wash cycle, the enzyme substrate is added, and the color developed from the action of the enzyme on the substrate is measured in a spectrophotometer. Macone and coworkers[164] compared an LA test (Bactigen) with a commercial 30-minute EIA (Seragen Diagnostics, Indianapolis IN) and found that the procedures were equally sensitive for the detection of PRP antigen in CSF, urine, and serum. The EIA test showed greater specificity than the LA test.

OTHER DIRECT DETECTION METHODS

Other methods for the direct detection of *H. influenzae* in clinical specimens have also been described. Groeneveld and associates[110] isolated, purified, and characterized a monoclonal antibody directed against P6, one of the principal outer membrane proteins of *H. influenzae*. This monoclonal antibody was conjugated to an immunoperoxidase enzyme and evaluated for its ability to detect and to identify, directly and specifically, *H. influenzae* in sputum smears. In a comparison of the direct immunoperoxidase test for *H. influenzae*, with culture, on 845 sputum specimens, the sensitivity and the specificity of the direct method were 92% and 99%, respectively. Malouin and coworkers[166] prepared and evaluated a radioactively labeled DNA probe for

direct detection of *H. influenzae* in clinical specimens. For sputum specimens, the sensitivity of the probe was directly related to the length of time that the probe was incubated with the specimen and ranged from 74% to 100% compared with culture; the specificity of the probe was high regardless of exposure time (97%). The probe also detected *H. influenzae* in a small number of positive blood and CSF specimens that were tested. Both the direct-staining procedure and the probe test detect species-specific antigen or genetic material, respectively, of *H. influenzae*, including type b strains, other capsular serotypes, and nonencapsulated, nontypeable strains. With the recognition of these non-type b organisms as important agents in infectious diseases, a species-specific, rather than a serotype-specific, direct detection method may be advantageous as these "research status" methods are adopted to routine clinical laboratory practice.

RECOVERY OF *HAEMOPHILUS* SPECIES IN CULTURE

Conventional sheep blood agar is unsuitable for recovery of *Haemophilus* species that require V factor for growth, owing to the presence of V factor-inactivating enzymes in native sheep blood.[7] Rabbit or horse blood does not contain these enzymes and an agar medium containing either of these blood products will support the growth of most *Haemophilus* species. Recent studies from Australia indicate that goat blood also is able to support the growth of both *H. influenzae* and *Streptococcus pneumoniae*, but the blood–agar mixture needs to be heated for 15 minutes at 100°C to eliminate V factor-inactivating enzyme activity.[106] Rabbit blood– or horse blood–containing media may not be available in many clinical laboratories, so other techniques or media must be used if *Haemophilus* organisms are to be isolated.

Optimal recovery of *Haemophilus* species from clinical specimens depends on proper collection and transport of such specimens, and the use of appropriate culture media and incubation environments. Because these organisms are fastidious, specimens containing them should not be exposed to drying or to extremes in temperature. Crucial specimens, such as CSF, should be hand-carried to the clinical laboratory as soon after collection as possible. Regardless of the media employed, isolation of *Haemophilus* requires incubation in a moist environment with increased CO_2 (3% to 5%). This is provided by modern CO_2 incubators or by candle extinction jars.

Primary isolation of *Haemophilus* species from clinical specimens is accomplished by using chocolate agar (see Color Plate 7-1*B*), *Haemophilus* isolation agar, or the staphylococcal streak technique (see Color Plate 7-1*C*).

CHOCOLATE AGAR

Chocolate agar is prepared by adding sheep blood to an enriched agar base medium that is at a high enough temperature (i.e., about 80°C) to lyse the red cells and to release X and V factors. Prolonged heating must be avoided to prevent inactivation of heat-labile V factor. For quality control and other technical purposes, most clinical laboratories currently purchase chocolate agar and other bacteriologic media from commercial vendors. Commercially prepared "chocolate agar" usually contains a synthetic mixture of hemin (X factor) and a "cocktail" of chemically defined growth factors added to GC (gonococcal) agar base medium. The GC agar base contains proteose peptone, cornstarch. mono- and dibasic phosphate buffers, sodium chloride, and agar. The chemically defined supplement contains NAD (V factor), vitamins (B_{12}, thiamine hydrochloride), minerals (iron, magnesium), factors that are required for or stimulate the growth of fastidious bacteria (cysteine, glutamine), and glucose. These supplements are available commercially under the trade names IsoVitalex (Becton-Dickinson Microbiology Systems) and Supplement B (Difco Laboratories, Detroit MI).

The disadvantage of using chocolate agar for primary isolation of *Haemophilus* species is that the medium does not allow the determination of hemolytic properties, which help differentiate *H. haemolyticus* and *H. parahaemolyticus* from *H. influenzae* and *H. parainfluenzae*. However, it is an excellent medium for the recovery of other fastidious organisms, such as *Neisseria meningitidis* and *N. gonorrhoeae*, from specimens that are not commonly contaminated with other organisms, such as CSF or joint fluid. Because *Haemophilus* species are common inhabitants of the upper respiratory tract (including both hemolytic and non-hemolytic species), many laboratories have adopted *Hemophilus* isolation agar for recovery of these organisms from respiratory specimens. Selective chocolate agar-based media containing various antibiotics (e.g., vancomycin, bacitracin, and clindamycin) have been described, but are not widely used.[42]

HAEMOPHILUS ISOLATION AGAR

Many commercial media companies currently market antibiotic-containing media for the selective isolation of *Haemophilus* species from respiratory tract specimens. These media contain beef heart infusion, peptones, yeast extract, and defibrinated horse blood (5%), which contains both X and V factors. In addition, bacitracin (300 µg/mL) is added to inhibit the the the other normal respiratory tract flora, including staphylococci, micrococci, neisseriae, and streptococci. Besides the selective recovery of *Haemophilus* species from heavily mixed cultures, the hemolytic properties of certain haemophili can be determined directly on primary isolation.

A selective medium for isolation and differentiation of *H. influenzae* and *H. parainfluenzae* has also been described.[268] This medium consists of hemin- and NAD-supplemented BHI agar, sucrose (10 mg/mL), phenol red indicator (100 µg/mL), and bacitracin (300 µg/mL). This medium was comparable with chocolate agar containing bacitracin for recovery of haemophili, and differentiated *H. parainfluenzae* (yellow colonies owing to acid production from sucrose) from *H. in-*

fluenzae (colorless colonies) without further testing. However, because horse blood is not present in this medium, the hemolytic reactions of haemophili cannot be ascertained.

STAPHYLOCOCCAL STREAK TECHNIQUE

Many bacteria and yeasts synthesize and secrete NAD during growth on bacteriologic media. In mixed cultures, *Haemophilus* species that require V factor may grow as pinpoint colonies around the colonies of these other microorganisms. This phenomenon is called satellitism. This property provides a technique for detecting these organisms in mixed cultures, as well as a presumptive test for genus-level identification. A colony of a possible *Haemophilus* species can be subcultured to a sheep blood agar plate and streaked as a lawn. By using an inoculating wire, a single streak of an NAD-producing organism, such as *S. aureus*, is made through the inoculum of the possible *Haemophilus* species. After overnight growth in a CO_2-enriched environment, tiny moist colonies of the haemophili may be observed within the hemolytic area adjacent to the staphylococcal growth. X factor–dependent haemophili will also grow as satellite colonies because hemin and hematin are released from the lysed red blood cells by the action of staphylococcal hemolysins (see Color Plate 7-1C). This method may be used for presumptive identification of *Haemophilus* species when species-level identification is not required or essential (e.g., upper respiratory tract specimens).

IDENTIFICATION OF HAEMOPHILUS SPECIES

IDENTIFICATION PROCEDURES

In the clinical laboratory, commonly encountered *Haemophilus* species are identified on the basis of their hemolytic reactions on horse blood agar and their growth requirements for X and V factors. The method that uses filter paper disks or strips impregnated with X factor, V factor, or both, is routinely used to determine these growth requirements. The organism to be identified is streaked as a lawn on media that is deficient in growth factors, such as trypticase-soy agar. It is important when selecting colonies from primary culture plates for this test that none of the chocolate agar or another blood-containing medium is transferred to the factor-determination plate. Suspension of the organism in factor-deficient broth before plate inoculation is one way to reduce carryover of growth factors and consequent false-positive results. The X and V factor disks or strips are placed on the agar surface about 1 to 2 cm apart. If a disk or strip containing both factors is also used, the disks may be more widely spaced on the agar surface. The plates are incubated in 3% to 5% CO_2 at 35°C for 18 to 24 hours, and the patterns of growth around the disks or strips are observed. Differentiation of *Haemophilus* species is then made on the basis of the growth patterns shown in Chart 67 and in Color Plates 7-1D and 7-1E.

Although interpretation of factor requirement tests are generally clearcut, misidentifications caused by confusing *H. influenzae* with *H. parainfluenzae* and vice versa have been reported (as high as 30%) owing to inconsistent results in X factor determinations. The following reasons were cited for these inaccuracies: 1) the presence of varying trace amounts of hemin in the basal medium used for the factor determination test; 2) the carryover of X factor in inocula taken from colonies growing on blood-containing medium; and 3) the fastidious nature of some *H. parainfluenzae* strains and the consequent difficulty in reading the factor tests for these strains. Doern and Chapin[67] evaluated the performance of trypticase-soy agar, brain-heart infusion agar, nutrient agar, and Mueller-Hinton agar in the factor disk identification of 187 *H. influenzae* isolates. They found that 95.7%, 92.5%, 56.1%, and 71.1% of isolates were correctly identified on the four media, respectively. False-positive readings of growth around V factor disks (resulting in misidentifications of *H. influenzae* as *H. parainfluenzae*) on brain-heart infusion agar, and failure of strains to grow at all on Mueller-Hinton and nutrient agars, were the principal findings of the study. Trypticase-soy agar was recommended as the medium of choice for performance of the growth factor determination procedure.

The δ-aminolevulinic acid (ALA)–porphyrin test, originally described by Kilian, bypasses many of the problems just described for the determination of X factor requirements.[140] The reaction used in this test is a direct assessment of the ability of a *Haemophilus* strain to synthesize protoporphyrin intermediates in the biosynthetic pathway to hemin from the precursor compound δ-aminolevulinic acid. Strains that require exogenous X factor for growth (i.e., *H. influenzae* and *H. haemolyticus*) are incapable of synthesizing protoporphyrins from ALA and, consequently, are negative with this test. Strains that do not require exogenous X factor for growth (i.e., *H. parainfluenzae* and *H. parahaemolyticus*) possess the enzymes that synthesize protoporphyrin compounds from the ALA substrate and, consequently, are ALA–porphyrin test-positive.

Commercially available ALA-impregnated filter paper disks (Difco Laboratories; Remel Laboratories, Lenexa KA) or growth media containing the ALA reagent (Remel Laboratories) may also be used to perform the ALA–porphyrin test.[91,161,162] With the disk method, the impregnated disk is moistened with water and inoculated with organisms from growth media. After 4 hours, the disk is observed under ultraviolet light (Wood's light). Brick-red fluorescence in the area of organism deposition indicates a positive test result; bluish fluorescence constitutes a negative test result. With the ALA agar medium, the organism is inoculated onto the medium and then is incubated overnight. The next day the growth is examined under a Wood's light for brick-red fluorescence (see Color Plate 7-1F).

Tests for hemolysis on horse blood agar and requirements for X and V factors have also been incorporated into a commercially available "quadplate" (Remel Laboratories, Lenexa KA) for *Haemophilus*

identification. In the quadplate configuration, the four areas of the sectored petri plate contain factor-supplemented Mueller-Hinton medium with horse blood, X factor-enriched medium, V factor-enriched medium, and medium containing both X and V factors, respectively. From the hemolytic reaction and the pattern of growth in the remaining quadrants, an identification of the isolate can be obtained.

SEROTYPING OF *HAEMOPHILUS INFLUENZAE*

Although most *H. influenzae* strains recovered from systemic infections belong to serotype b, the other serotypes (i.e., types a, c, d, e, and f) have also been recovered from infectious processes in both children and adults.[30,53,64,100,250,277] The easiest technique for serotyping isolates is slide agglutination.[116] A dense suspension of the organism is prepared in saline. Single drops of the suspension are placed in each of a series of circles on a glass slide, corresponding to the number of sera to be tested, plus a saline control. Type-specific antisera are added to each of the test circles, and the slide is rotated. Rapid (i.e., less than 1 minute) agglutination of organisms by a specific antiserum and the absence of agglutination in the saline control identify the isolate as a specific serotype. Polyvalent and type-specific antisera for *H. influenzae* are commercially available from Wellcome Diagnostics and Difco Laboratories.

A coagglutination culture confirmation test (Phadebact *Haemophilus* Test, Karo Bio Diagnostics AB) is also available for simultaneous identification and serotyping of *H. influenzae* type b from primary culture media. This kit contains a vial of staphylococcal cells sensitized with type b antisera (test reagent) and a second vial of staphylococci sensitized with antisera to type a, c, d, e, and f (control reagent). Colonies from the growth media are mixed with each of the two reagents on a cardboard slide. After mixing, the slide is rocked for 30 to 60 seconds. Visible agglutination of the mixture with the type b test reagent, but not the control reagent, identifies the isolate as *H. influenzae* type b. A positive reaction in the control reagent indicates that the organism belongs to capsular types a, c, d, e, or f. This test has been shown to be highly sensitive and specific for identifying type b *H. influenzae*.[104,247]

Serotyping may also be performed by incorporation of type-specific antisera in an optically clear agar medium that is supplemented with X and V factors.[12] In this format, the capsular type is detected by the formation of an antigen–antibody precipitation reaction (i.e., a "halo") surrounding the colony. This approach may be used to simultaneously serotype a large number of strains, by spot inoculating the strains on the agar surface using a Steers replicator. The antiserum agar method may also be used for detecting *H. influenzae* type b oropharyngeal carriage. When used for this purpose, bacitracin is added to inhibit other oropharyngeal organisms.[12]

Molecular methods have also been developed for capsular typing of *H. influenzae*. Falla and colleagues[79] developed a polymerase chain reaction (PCR)-based method that uses primers derived from capsule type-specific DNA sequences cloned from the capsular gene clusters (i.e., the *cap* loci) of all six *H. influenzae* serotypes. When probes and primers for the serotype-specific genes were used in conjunction with those for the capsule export gene *bexA*, capsulate, noncapsulate, and capsule-deficient type b mutants could be differentiated from one another. PCR has also been used to characterize nonencapsulated, nontypeable strains of *H. influenzae*.[131] For this, however, primers and probes were developed from randomly amplified DNA, rather than from specific genes. This technique has been applied to investigations of outbreaks of respiratory tract disease associated with nontypeable *H. influenzae* and was validated as an acceptable epidemiologic method when compared with both outer membrane protein profile and rRNA gene restriction analyses.[131]

BIOTYPING OF *HAEMOPHILUS INFLUENZAE* AND *HAEMOPHILUS PARAINFLUENZAE*

In his taxonomic study of the genus *Haemophilus*, Kilian introduced the use of biochemical tests for identifying and characterizing haemophili.[141] From the results of three tests—indole production, urease activity, and ornithine decarboxylase activity—Kilian divided *H. influenzae* strains into four **biotypes**, which were designated I through IV.[144] These biotypes were independent of the serotype of the organism; that is, organisms of different serotypes or nontypeable strains could have the same pattern of biotyping reactions. With these same tests, four additional *H. influenzae* biotypes (V, VI, VII, and VIII) have also been described.[105,205,251] Similarly, seven biotypes of *H. parainfluenzae* (designated I through IV and VI through VIII) have been delineated with the same three tests. Reactions for the identification of *Haemophilus* species, including the biotyping reactions, are shown in Table 7-4 (see Color Plate 7-1G). Biotyping may be performed with the following media:

1. *Indole test*: A heavy suspension of the organism is prepared in 0.05 M phosphate buffer (pH 8.0) containing 0.1% tryptophan. After a 4-hour incubation at 35°C, a few drops of Kovac's reagent are added, and the suspension is shaken. The appearance of red in the upper alcohol layer is a positive test result; and that of yellow is a negative test result. Heavily inoculated indole–tryptone broth, used for enterics, may also be used, with the addition of Kovac's reagent after overnight incubation.
2. *Urease test*: A balanced salts solution (0.1% KH$_2$PO$_4$, 0.1% K$_2$HPO$_4$, 0.5% NaCl, and 0.5 mL of a 2% solution of phenol red) is prepared (100 mL), adjusted to pH 7.0, and autoclaved. Filter-sterilized, aqueous urea (10 mL) is added, and the solution is dispensed onto sterile tubes in small amounts. To perform the test, a heavy suspension of the organism is prepared in the medium. The development of red in the medium after a 4-hour incubation is a positive test result. Heavily inoculated Christensen's urea agar slants may also be used for this test. Positive results are generally available after a 4-hour incubation; negative tests should be reincubated overnight.
3. *Ornithine decarboxylase test*: Standard Moeller's ornithine decarboxylase broth is used along with a tube of Moeller's decarboxylase broth base as a negative control. A heavy inoculum is used and each tube is overlayed with sterile mineral oil. Results are best read after overnight incubation, although most positive tests are apparent after 4 to 6 hours.

Biotyping of *Haemophilus* species has yielded valuable epidemiologic information, and specific biotypes have been associated with different types of infections, sources of isolation, antigenic properties, and antimicrobial resistance patterns.[100,144,173,205,281] In a survey of 130 *H. influenzae* strains from cases of meningitis, 93.1% were biotype I, and 4.6% and 2.3% were biotypes II and IV, respectively.[144] All but one strain in this series were type b. Oberhofer and Back[205] examined the biotype distribution of 464 strains of *H. influenzae* and 83 strains of *H. parainfluenzae* using a six-test battery that included the three reactions already described, hydrolysis of *o*-nitrophenyl-β-D-galactopyranoside, and acid production from sucrose and xylose. They found that *H. influenzae* biotype I was recovered principally from CSF, blood, and upper respiratory tract secretions, and that most were from infants younger than 1 year old. Biotypes II and III were most commonly recovered from conjunctival and sputum cultures and were primarily from children aged 1 to 5 years and from adults older than 20 years. Although most serotype b strains belonged to biotype I, nontypeable strains were mostly biotype II and III. Several studies have also noted the association between *H. influenzae* biotypes II and III and conjunctival infections.[3,72,205] Biotype IV *H. influenzae* strains have been documented as pathogens in obstetric, gynecologic, perinatal, and neonatal infections and have been isolated from men with nongonococcal urethritis.[45,231,260,280] A study from Canada examined the distribution of biotypes isolated simultaneously from oropharyngeal and anogenital sites in a sexually transmitted diseases clinic population.[170] *H. parainfluenzae* strains were isolated almost twice as frequently from anogenital sites as was *H. influenzae*. Among the *H. influenzae* strains, biotypes II and III were more frequent in the oropharynx, whereas biotype IV strains were more prevalent in anogenital sites. Although *H. parainfluenzae* biotypes I, II, and III were equally prevalent in the oropharynx, biotypes I and II predominated in anogenital sites.

The discovery of the new *Haemophilus*-like cryptic genospecies, associated with serious maternal and neonatal infections, that has biotyping reactions identical with *H. influenzae* biotype IV underscores the shortcomings of phenotypic methods for typing of strains. These newly described organisms can be distinguished from *H. influenzae* biotype IV strains only by molecular or genetic approaches that are not readily available in clinical microbiology laboratories. These isolates may also be less reliably identified by commercially available kit systems. Quentin and associates[227]

TABLE 7-4
CHARACTERISTICS FOR IDENTIFICATION OF HUMAN HAEMOPHILUS SPECIES

SPECIES / BIOTYPE	HEMOLYSIS	REQUIREMENT FOR: X	V	ALA TEST	INDOLE TEST	UREASE TEST	ORNITHINE DECARBOXYLASE	ACID PRODUCTION FROM: GLUCOSE	SUCROSE	LACTOSE	FRUCTOSE	RIBOSE	XYLOSE	MANNOSE
H. influenzae														
Biotype I	−	+	+	−	+	+	+	+	−	−	−	+	+	−
Biotype II	−	+	+	−	+	+	+	+	−	−	−	+	+	−
Biotype III*	−	+	+	−	−	+	−	+	−	−	−	+	+	−
Biptype IV	−	+	+	−	+	+	+	+	−	−	−	+	+	−
Biotype V	−	+	+	−	−	−	+	+	−	−	−	+	+	−
Biotype VI	−	+	+	−	+	−	+	+	−	−	−	+	+	−
Biotype VII	−	+	+	−	−	−	−	+	−	−	−	+	+	−
Biotype VIII	−	+	+	−	−	−	−	+	−	−	−	+	+	−
Biogroup aegyptius	−	+	+	−	−	+	−	+	−	−	−	+w	−	−
H. parainfluenzae†														
Biotype I	−	−	+	+	−	−	+	+	+	−	+	−	−	+
Biotype II	−	−	+	+	−	+	+	+	+	−	+	−	−	+
Biotype III	−	−	+	+	−	+	−	+	+	−	+	NA	−	+
Biotype IV	−	−	+	+	+	+	+	+	+	−	+	NA	NA	+
Biotype VI	−	−	+	+	+	−	+	+	+	−	+	NA	NA	v
Biotype VII	−	−	+	+	+	+	−	+	+	−	NA	−	−	NA
Biotype VIII	−	−	+	+	+	−	−	+	+	−	NA	−	−	NA
H. haemolyticus	+	+	+	−	v	+	−	+	−	−	+w	+	v	−
H. parahaemolyticus	+	−	+	+	−	+	v	+	+	−	+	−	−	−
H. segnis	−	−	+	+	−	−	−	+	+w	−	+w	−	−	−
H. aphrophilus	−	−	−	+	−	−	−	+	+	+	+	+	−	+
H. paraphrophilus	−	−	+	+	−	−	−	+	+	+	+	+	−	+
H. paraphrophaemolyticus	+	−	+	+	−	+	−	+	+	−	+	−	−	−
H. ducreyi	+w	+	−	−	−	−	−	−	−	−	−	−	−	−

+, positive; −, negative; +w, weak positive; v, variable; NA, not available
* Biotyping reactions are identical with those of H. influenzae biogroup aegyptius, but the biogroup aegyptius strains are xylose-negative
† Biotype V strains of H. parainfluenza are identical to H. segnis.

evaluated four commercial systems (RIM-Haemophilus 1/RIM-Haemophilus 2, API 10E, API 20E, and the HNID panel [see following section]) for their ability to identify and biotype 188 genital and neonatal isolates. Of these strains, 167 (88%) were correctly identified and biotyped, eight strains were misidentified, and 13 strains were biotyped incorrectly by at least one of the commercial systems. DNA–DNA hybridization analyses of these 21 isolates revealed that 15 of them belonged to the newly recognized cryptic genospecies of *Haemophilus.*

BIOCHEMICAL METHODS AND KIT SYSTEMS FOR *HAEMOPHILUS* IDENTIFICATION

In addition to biotyping, other biochemical methods may be used for species identification of *Haemophilus* species, and some of these biochemical properties are useful for species identification (see Table 7-4).[142] Such methods bypass some of the problems associated with determining factor requirements that were discussed earlier. As can be seen from Table 7-4, the production of acid from several carbohydrates (i.e., sucrose, fructose, ribose, xylose, and mannose) can also be used to separate *H. influenzae* from *H. parainfluenzae.* The use of a limited battery of biochemical tests, in addition to X and V factor requirements, is also essential for the identification of the infrequently encountered species, such as *H. aphrophilus, H. paraphrophilus,* and *H. segnis.* Carbohydrate utilization patterns may be determined in semisolid cysteine–tryptic digest agar containing 1% filtered, sterilized carbohydrates. These tests are heavily inoculated, and acid production is generally apparent in from 4 to 18 hours.

The RIM (Rapid Identification Method)—Haemophilus 1/RIM Haemophilus 2 system (Ortho Diagnostic Systems, Raritan NJ) is a commercially available method that uses microtubes containing buffered carbohydrates and the ALA porphyrin test to identify *Haemophilus* species. In RIM Haemophilus 1, porphyrin synthesis and utilization of dextrose, lactose, and sucrose are used for species identification, whereas the RIM Haemophilus 2 tube is used to biotype *H. influenzae* and *H. parainfluenzae* by testing for production of indole, ornithine decarboxylase, and urease. In an evaluation of this identification method,[212] 100% of 76 *H. influenzae* strains and 92% of 23 *H. parainfluenzae* strains were correctly identified. However, hemolysis on horse blood agar was required to differentiate *H. haemolyticus* from *H. influenzae* and *H. parahaemolyticus* from *H. parainfluenzae.*

Biochemical identification methods have been exploited in the development of other commercial kit systems and reagents that use modified conventional tests along with novel chromogenic enzyme substrates for both identifying and biotyping of *Haemophilus* isolates. The RapID NH panel (Innovative Diagnostics Systems, Inc., Norcross GA), the Vitek *Neisseria-Haemophilus* Identification (NHI) card (bioMerieux-Vitek, Inc., Hazelwood MO), the *Haemophilus-Neisseria* Identification (HNID) panel (Dade/MicroScan, Sacramento CA) (see Color Plate 7-1H) and the API NH strip (bioMerieux, La Balme-les Grottes, France) identify

these organisms within 4 hours of inoculation with a pure culture.[67,126,127] All of these systems will identify the species and generate a biotype based on the urease, ornithine decarboxylase, and indole tests. Several commercially available systems designed for identifying enteric bacteria (e.g., the API 20E, the Micro ID, and the Minitek System) have also been used to biotype *Haemophilus* strains.[11,72,119] Reagent-impregnated disks (Remel Laboratories) for performing urease and ornithine decarboxylase tests can also be used along with the spot indole test for rapid (1-hour) biotyping of individual isolates. In fact, the spot indole test alone can provide a presumptive identification of *H. influenzae* in respiratory tract specimens because indole-positive biotype II strains represent 40% to 70% of the *H. influenzae* strains found in these specimens.[285]

LABORATORY DIAGNOSIS OF *HAEMOPHILUS DUCREYI* INFECTION

Cotton, rayon, Dacron, or calcium alginate swabs may be used to collect specimens from chancroid ulcers. Ideally, specimens should be collected from the base and undermined margins of the ulcer. The organism is usually not recoverable from bubo pus. Transport media have not generally been evaluated for their ability to maintain clinical isolates of *H. ducreyi,* and specimens may harbor only small numbers of organisms. Therefore, media should be inoculated directly. Gram-stained smears of the suppurative exudate from the genital lesions of chancroid may be noncontributory owing to the low sensitivity (62% to 92%) and specificity (51% to 94%) of the Gram stain. When seen on the direct smears, *H. ducreyi* appears as pale staining gram-negative coccobacilli, often arranged in clustered groups ("school-of-fish") or loosely coiled, parallel chains ("railroad tracks") (Figure 7-2). They may be found inside and outside of polymorphonuclear cells. Because genital lesions and suppurative nodes or abscesses may become superinfected with other bacteria (particularly staphylococci and streptococci), diagnosis by a gram-stained smear is difficult, and culture should be attempted. Diagnosis of chancroid is frequently made on clinical and epidemiologic grounds; however, syphilis, genital herpes simplex virus infection, and lymphogranuloma venereum must be included in the differential diagnosis. A monoclonal antibody directed against *H. ducreyi* has been described and used in an indirect immunofluorescence test to detect organisms directly in smears prepared from genital ulcers.[242] DNA probes for *H. ducreyi* have also been produced and used in research settings for identification of the organism and for direct detection in specimens from experimentally infected animals.[215]

It has been historically reported that *H. ducreyi* is extremely difficult to culture and identify. However, owing to improvements in media quality, several studies have reported that isolation of the organism is relatively easy.[112,206,252,261] Aspirates from the lesion or a swab specimen from the base of a thoroughly cleansed lesion should be promptly inoculated onto growth media. Bubo aspirates will yield the organisms less often than cultures of fresh lesions. Several media have

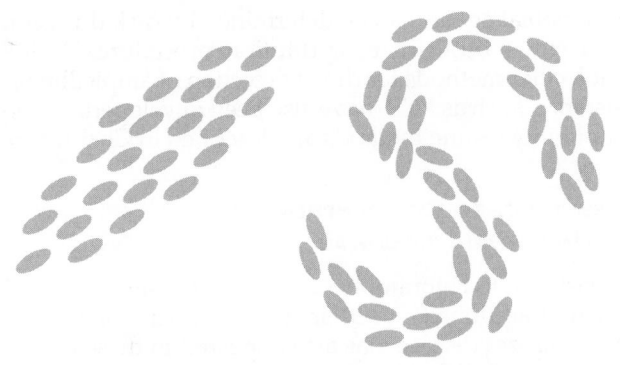

Figure 7-2.
Gram-stained morphology of *Haemophilus ducreyi*. On gram-stained smears prepared from lesions of chancroid or from colonial growth, the organisms may appear in loose clusters (i.e., "school of fish" shown *left*) or as loosely coiled clusters of gram-negative bacilli lined up in parallel (i.e., "railroad tracks," shown *right*).

been described for isolation of *H. ducreyi*. A medium containing GC agar base, 1% to 2% hemoglobin, 5% fetal calf serum, 1% IsoVitalex enrichment, and vancomycin (3 µg/mL) has been used successfully, as has Mueller-Hinton agar with 5% chocolatized horse blood, 1% IsoVitalex enrichment, and vancomycin (3 µg /mL).[186] Recently, Totten and Stamm[271] described a new clear plate and broth media for *H. ducreyi* that contains GC agar base, 1% X and V factor enrichment (PML Microbiologicals, Tualatin OR), 10% fetal bovine serum, and catalase (Sigma Chemical Co., St Louis MO). The catalase is added as a source of hemin. The broth has a similar composition, but GC broth instead of agar is used as the basal medium.

Vancomycin is added to inhibit gram-positive organisms (e.g., staphylococci and streptococci) that may be present as contaminants or superinfecting bacteria in the chancroid lesion. Commercial chocolate agar media will generally support the growth of *H. ducreyi*; vancomycin disks may be placed in various quadrants of a chocolate plate to help detect the organisms in mixed cultures. Most strains of *H. ducreyi* have vancomycin minimum inhibitory concentrations (MICs) of 32 to 128 µg/mL, but some strains have MICs as low as 4 µg/mL. Therefore, it may be advantageous to inoculate media with and without vancomycin and to collect multiple appropriate specimens. Media are incubated at 33°C to 35°C in 3% to 5% CO_2, with high humidity, and are inspected daily for 10 days. Most isolates cultured directly from clinical specimens produce visible growth in 2 to 4 days.

Colonies of *H. ducreyi* are small, nonmucoid, and gray, yellow, or tan. The colonies can characteristically be "nudged" along the agar surface with a bacteriologic loop, are difficult to pick up, and produce a nonhomogeneous, "clumpy" suspension in saline. On a Gram stain, the organisms appear as gram-negative coccobacilli, usually in close association with one another. *H. ducreyi* is catalase-negative and oxidase-positive; the oxidase reaction is usually delayed and develops only after 15 to 20 seconds with the tetramethyl-*p*-phenylenediamine dihydrochloride reagent.[186]

Because of the fastidious nature of *H. ducreyi*, growth factor requirements cannot be demonstrated with factor-impregnated disk or strip techniques. The ALA–porphyrin test is negative, indicating that exogenous hemin is required for growth. The organism is biochemically inert, except for positive nitrate reduction and alkaline phosphatase tests. Hannah and Greewood[112] tested 64 *H. ducreyi* strains with the RapID NH system; all isolates were correctly identified by this system, with the phosphatase and nitrate reduction tests being the only positive reactions for all isolates tested. In a more recent evaluation with 25 *H. ducreyi* isolates, Shawar and coworkers[246] found that all strains produced unique and consistent enzymatic reactions on the RapID ANA system (bioMerieux-Vitek, Inc.), which is a 4-hour system that is used for the identification of clinically significant anaerobic bacteria (see Chapter 14). In addition, these workers reported that *H. ducreyi* strains are also susceptible to sodium polyanetholesulfonate (SPS) as determined by a disk susceptibility method. They suggested that simple growth characteristics, SPS susceptibility, and aminopeptidase profiles obtained with the enzymatic RapID ANA system could be used for clinical laboratory identification of *H. ducreyi*. Other investigators have shown that *H. ducreyi* strains have consistant aminopeptidase profiles that may be useful for laboratory identification.[275]

Methods have also been developed for identification or direct detection of *H. ducreyi* using molecular methods. Roggen and coworkers[235] developed an EIA-based method that uses polyclonal antibodies against a 29-kDa species-specific membrane antigen and a 30- to 34-kDa immunotype-specific membrane antigen as the capture antibodies. This EIA reacted with all *H. ducreyi* isolates tested and was also able to detect the organisms directly in clinical specimens. The PCR has also been used to detect *H. ducreyi*. Chui and coworkers[47] reported on the development of a primer set and two DNA probes specific for *H. ducreyi* based on the published nucleotide sequences of the 16S rRNA of the organism. The primer set and probes were 100% sensitive in detecting 51 strains of *H. ducreyi* that were isolated on six continents over a 15-year period. The PCR-based direct detection procedure was tested on 100 clinical specimens and showed a sensitivity of 83% to 98% and a specificity of 51% to 67% depending on the number of amplification cycles.[47] Another group of investigators also developed a PCR-based assay for detection of *H. ducreyi*, but the sensitivity and specificity of the test were disappointing.[129] These workers found that failure of PCR to detect *H. ducreyi* probably resulted from nonspecific inhibition of the *Taq* DNA polymerase by material in the specimen.

ANTIMICROBIAL SUSCEPTIBILITY OF *HAEMOPHILUS* SPECIES

RESISTANCE TO AMPICILLIN IN *HAEMOPHILUS INFLUENZAE*

Until about 1973, antimicrobial susceptibility testing of *H. influenzae* was unnecessary because virtually all clinically significant isolates were susceptible to ampicillin, the drug of choice for meningitis and bacteremia caused by this organism. Ampicillin treatment failures were reported in patients with meningitis as early as 1968; these, however, were attributed to factors other than resistance of the microorganisms. By 1974, it was found that certain strains of *H. influenzae* were indeed ampicillin resistant on the basis of their ability to produce plasmid-mediated β-lactamase enzymes capable of hydrolyzing and inactivating ampicillin. The prevalence of these strains varies from one geographic area to another. A national collaborative susceptibility study found that 20% of *H. influenzae* strains obtained from medical centers throughout the country produced β-lactamase.[68] Because of this, chloramphenicol was frequently administered along with, or substituted for, ampicillin in empiric therapy of serious *H. influenzae* infections. However, strains of *H. influenzae* have been isolated that are resistant to chloramphenicol, or to both ampicillin and chloramphenicol.[10,96,138,147,208] In recent years, plasmid-mediated β-lactamase-mediated ampicillin resistance has been found in both encapsulated non-type b isolates, nontypeable *H. influenzae* strains, and *H. parainfluenzae* organisms. These organisms harbor a 3.0-MDa transposon that carries the gene for a TEM-1 type β-lactamase enzyme.[202] More recently, rare strains of *H. influenzae* that produce a second type of β-lactamase, called ROB-1, have been reported.[60] Methods for the detection of β-lactamase production are presented in Chapter 15.

In addition to β-lactamase production, some *H. influenzae* strains have been isolated that are resistant to ampicillin but do not produce β-lactamase enzymes.[169,180,208] Resistance to ampicillin in these strains is due to alterations in both the pencillin-binding proteins in the cell wall and to altered permeability of the cell membrane to the antimicrobial agents.[180] Unlike the genes coding for β-lactamase, the genes for the altered penicillin-binding proteins are located on the chromosome. Besides resistance to ampicillin, these strains also display diminished susceptibility to some cephalosporins (i.e., cefaclor, cefuroxime, aztreonam, cefixime, cefpodoxime, ceftibuten) and to β-lactam–β-lactamase inhibitor combinations (e.g., ampicillin–sulbactam, amoxicillin–clavulanate).[133,179,181] Although initial studies with these strains suggested that the disk diffusion procedure using the 10-μg ampicillin disk might not accurately detect these β-lactamase-negative, ampicillin-resistant strains, changes in the media used for the disk diffusion procedure (Haemophilus Test Medium [HTM]) and modifications of the interpretive criteria in subsequently published NCCLS interpretive standards on disk diffision and agar–broth dilution have addressed these potential problems.[134,135,181,200,201,202] Fortunately, it appears that ampicillin-resistant, β-lactamase-negative *H. influenzae* are relatively uncommon.[132] In a national collaborative study on the prevalence of antimicrobial resistance in clinical isolates of *H. influenzae*, ampicillin resistance among strains that lacked β-lactamase activity was seen in only 0.1% of 2811 clinical isolates.[68] Susceptibility of *Haemophilus* species to ampicillin and other an-

timicrobial agents can be determined by disk diffusion and either broth or agar dilution procedures.[200,201,202] Molecular methods for direct detection of ampicillin resistance, such as PCR, have also been developed.[269] Susceptibility testing methods are described in Chapter 15.

RESISTANCE TO CHLORAMPHENICOL IN *HAEMOPHILUS INFLUENZAE*

Resistance to chloramphenicol, the other antimicrobial agent traditionally used in the treatment of serious *H. influenzae* disease, has also appeared in these microorganisms.[10,32,147] Although the prevalence of these strains is not high, the microbiologist should be aware of the methods required for their detection in the clinical laboratory. Most chloramphenicol-resistant *H. influenzae* elaborate an enzyme called chloramphenicol acetyltransferase (CAT).[172] This enzyme catalyzes the transfer of two acetyl groups from acetyl coenzyme A to active sites on the chloramphenicol molecule, thereby preventing the antimicrobial from its normal function of inhibiting bacterial protein synthesis. Although CAT-producing strains of *H. influenzae* apparently produce the enzyme constitutively (i.e., under all growth conditions), CAT production by other *Haemophilus* species is inducible, requiring exposure to the drug for enzyme production.[172] The laboratory methods used for detecting CAT are described in Chapter 15.

Strains of chloramphenicol-resistant *H. influenzae* have also been found that do not produce CAT. Molecular analysis of these organisms has demonstrated a relative impermeability of the cells to chloramphenicol owing to the loss of a major outer membrane protein that serves as a porin for entrance of the drug into the bacterial cell.[32] This type of resistance also appears to be relatively uncommon. In the 1988 national collaborative study, all of the chloramphenicol-resistant (MICs ≥8 μg/mL) *H. influenzae* examined produced CAT.[68]

PATTERNS OF SUSCEPTIBILITY TO ANTIMICROBIAL AGENTS

With the large number of antimicrobial agents that have activity against both ampicillin-susceptible and ampicillin-resistant *H. influenzae*, a large armamentarium is now available to physicians for treatment of systemic infections caused by these organisms.[88] For the first- and second-generation cephalosporins, these organisms show varying degrees of susceptibility. In the 1988 collaborative study on susceptibility of *H. influenzae*, the percentage of strains susceptible to cephalothin, cephalexin, cefaclor, and cefamandole were 87.3%, 43.3%, 94.5%, and 98.7%, respectively.[68] Although erythromycin and sulfisoxazole are relatively inactive against *H. influenzae*, almost all strains remain susceptible to tetracycline, trimethoprim–sulfamethoxazole, and rifampin. New agents, such as ceftazidime, ceftizoxime, ceftriaxone, and cefuroxime not only show excellent activity against *H. influenzae*, but also are nontoxic (a major drawback of chloramphenicol) and achieve high concentrations in the CSF and blood.

REFERENCES

1. ADAMS WG, DEAVER KA, COCHI SL ET AL: Decline of childhood *Haemophilus influenzae* type b (Hib) disease in the Hib vaccine era. JAMA 269:221–226, 1993

2. ADLAKHA R, YALE SH, RATEL R ET AL: *Haemophilus influenzae* serotype f: an unusual cause of mycotic aneurysm in an adult. Mayo Clin Proc 69:467–468, 1994

3. ALBRITTON WL, BRUNTON JL, MEIER M ET AL: *Haemophilus influenzae*: comparison of respiratory tract isolates with genitourinary tract isolates. J Clin Microbiol 16:826–831, 1982

4. ALBRITTON WL, HAMMOND GW, RONALD AR: Bacteremic *Haemophilus influenzae* genitourinary tract infections in adults. Arch Intern Med 138:1819–1821, 1978

5. AMBROSINO, DM, LANDESMAN SH, GORHAM CC ET AL: Passive immunization against disease due to *Haemophilus influenzae* type b: concentrations of antibody to capsular polysaccharide in high-risk children. J Infect Dis 153:1–7, 1986

6. ANDERSON P, PICHICHERO M, INSEL R ET AL: Capsular antigens noncovalently or covalently associated with protein as vaccine to *Haemophilus influenzae* type b: comparison in two-year-old children. J Infect Dis 152:634–636, 1985

7. ARTMAN M, FRANKL G: Nicotinamide adenine dinucleotide and nicotinamide adenine dinucleotide phosphate splitting enzyme(s) of sheep and rabbit erythrocytes: their effect on the growth of *Haemophilus*. Can J Microbiol 28:696–702, 1982

8. ASTAGNEAU P, GOLDSTEIN FW, FRANCOUAL S ET AL: Appendicitis due to both *Streptococcus pneumoniae* and *Haemophilus influenzae*. Eur J Syst Bacteriol 11:559–560, 1992

9. AUTEN GM, LEVY CS, SMITH MA: *Haemophilus parainfluenzae* as a rare cause of epidural abscess: case report and review. Rev Infect Dis 13:609–612, 1993

10. AZEMUN P, STULL T, ROBERTS M: Rapid detection of chloramphenicol resistance in *Haemophilus influenzae*. Antimicrob Agents Chemother 20:168–170, 1981

11. BACK AE, OBERHOFER TR: Use of the Minitek system for biotyping *Haemophilus* species. J Clin Microbiol 7:312–313, 1978

12. BARBOUR ML, CROOK DW, MAYON-WHITE RT: An improved antiserum agar method for detecting carriage of *Haemophilus influenzae* type b. Eur J Clin Microbiol Infect Dis 12:215–217, 1993

13. BARENKAMP SJ: Outer membrane proteins and lipopolysaccharides of nontypeable *Haemophilus influenzae*. J Infect Dis 165(suppl 1):S181–S184, 1992

14. BARNSHAW JA, PHILLIPS CF: *Haemophilus parainfluenzae* meningitis in a 4 year old boy. Pediatrics 45:856–857, 1970

15. BARTLETT AV, ZUSMAN J, DAUM RS: Unusual presentations of *Haemophilus influenzae* infections in immunocompromised patients. J Pediatr 102:55–58, 1983

16. BARTON LL, DELA CRUZ R, WALENTIK C: Neonatal *Haemophilus influenzae* type c sepsis. Am J Dis Child 136:463–464, 1972

17. BIEGER RC, BREWER NS, WASHINGTON JA: *Haemophilus aphrophilus*: a microbiologic and clinical review and report of 42 cases. Medicine 57:345–355, 1978

18. BLACK CT, KUPFERSCHMID JP, WEST KW ET AL: *Haemophilus parainfluenzae* infections in children, with the report of a unique case. Rev Infect Dis 10:342–346, 1988

19. BLACK SB, SHINEFIELD HR, FIREMAN B ET AL: Efficacy in infancy of oligosaccharide conjugate *Haemophilus influenzae* type b (HbOC) vaccine in a United States population of 61,080 children. Pediatr Infect Dis J 10:97–104, 1991

20. BLACK SB, SHINEFIELD HR, KAISER-PERMANENTE PEDIATRIC VACCINE STUDY GROUP: Immunization with oligosaccharide conjugate *Haemophilus influenzae* type b (HbOC) vaccine on a large health maintenance organization population: extended follow-up and impact on *Haemophilus influenzae* disease epidemiology. Pediatr Infect Dis J 11:610–613, 1992

21. BLACKALL PJ: The avian haemophili. Rev Clin Microbiol 2:270–277, 1989

22. BLAYLOCK BL, BABER S: Urinary tract infection caused by *Haemophilus parainfluenzae*. Am J Clin Pathol 73:285–287, 1980

23. BRAZILIAN PURPURIC FEVER STUDY GROUP: Brazilian purpuric fever: epidemic purpura fulminans associated with antecedent purulent conjunctivitis. Lancet 2:757–761, 1987

24. BRAZILIAN PURPURIC FEVER STUDY GROUP: *Haemophilus aegyptius* bacteremia in Brazilian purpuric fever. Lancet 2:761–763, 1987

25. BRAZILIAN PURPURIC FEVER STUDY GROUP: Brazilian purpuric fever identified in a new region of Brazil. J Infect Dis 165(suppl 1):S16–S19, 1992

26. BRENNER DJ, MAYER LW, CARLONE GM ET AL: Biochemical, genetic, and epidemiologic characterization of *Haemophilus influenzae* biogroup *aegyptius* (*Haemophilus aegyptius*) strains associated with Brazilian purpuric fever. J Clin Microbiol 26:1524–1534, 1988

27. BROADHURST LE, ERICKSON RL, KELLEY PW: Decreases in invasive *Haemophilus influenzae* diseases in U.S. Army children, 1984–1991. JAMA 269:227–231, 1993

28. BROOME CV: Epidemiology of *Haemophilus influenzae* type b infections in the United States. Pediatr Infect Dis J 6:779–782, 1987

29. BRUNNEL PA, BASS JW, DAUM RS ET AL: Revision of recommendations for use of rifampin prophylaxis of contacts of patients with *Haemophilus influenzae* infection. Pediatrics 74:301–302, 1984

30. BUCK LL, DOUGLAS GW: Meningitis due to *Haemophilus influenzae* type e. J Clin Microbiol 4:381, 1976

31. BULLOCK DW, DEVITT PG: Pancreatic abscess and septicaemia caused by *Haemophilus segnis*. J Infect 3:82–85, 1981

32. BURNS JL, MENDELMAN PM, LEVY J ET AL: A permeability barrier as a mechanism of chloramphenicol resistance in *Haemophilus influenzae*. Antimicrob Agents Chemother 27:46–54, 1985

33. CALIO AJ, CUSUMANO S, ULLMAN RF ET AL: *Haemophilus parainfluenzae* endocarditis. Heart Lung 16:222–223, 1987

34. CAMPOGNONE P, SINGER DB: Neonatal sepsis due to nontypeable *Haemophilus influenzae*. Am J Child Dis 140:117–121, 1986

35. CANTON R, LEON A, DE LA FUENTE S ET AL: *beta*-Lactamase producing *Haemophilus influenzae* as causative agent of a liver abscess. Eur J Clin Microbiol Infect Dis 8:748–749, 1989

36. CARLONE GM, GORELKIN L, GHEESLING LL ET AL: Potential virulence-associated factors in Brazilian purpuric fever. J Clin Microbiol 27:609–614, 1989

37. CARLONE GM, SOTTNEK FO, PLIKAYTIS BD: Comparison of outer membrane protein and biochemical profiles of *Haemophilus aegyptius* and *Haemophilus influenzae* biotype III. J Clin Microbiol 22:708–713, 1985

38. CATTIER B, CAILLON J, QUENTIN R: A case of biliary tract infection caused by *Haemophilus parainfluenzae*. Eur J Clin Microbiol Infect Dis 11:197–198, 1992

39. CENTERS FOR DISEASE CONTROL AND PREVENTION: Recommendations of the Immunization Practices Advisory Committee (ACIP): Recommendations for use of *Haemophilus* b conjugate vaccines and a combined diphtheria–tetanus–pertussis and *Haemophilus* b vaccine. MMWR 42:RR-13 1993

40. CENTERS FOR DISEASE CONTROL AND PREVENTION: Progess toward elimination of *Haemophilus influenzae* type b disease among infants and children—United States, 1987–1993. MMWR 43:144–148, 1994

41. CHANG MJ, CONTRONI G: Primary peritonitis due to *Haemophilus influenzae* type b. J Clin Microbiol 18:725–726, 1983

42. CHAPIN KC, DOERN GV: Selective recovery of *Haemophilus influenzae* from specimens contaminated with upper respiratory tract flora. J Clin Microbiol 17:1163–1165, 1983

43. CHATTOPADHYAY B, SILVERSTONE PH, WINWOOD RS: Liver abscess caused by *Haemophilus parainfluenzae*. Postgrad Med J 59:788–789, 1983

44. CHOW AW, BUSHKELL LL, YOSHIKAWA TT ET AL: *Haemophilus parainfluenzae* epiglottitis with meningitis and bacteremia in an adult. Am J Med Sci 267:365–368, 1974

45. CHOWDHURY MNH, PAREK SS: Urethritis associated with *Haemophilus parainfluenzae*: a case report. Sex Transm Dis 10:45–46, 1983

46. CHRISTENSEN JJ, KIRKEGAARD E, KORNER B: *Haemophilus* isolated from unusual anatomical sites. Scand J Infect Dis 22:437–444, 1990

47. CHUI L, ALBRITTON W, PASTER B ET AL: Development of the polymerase chain reaction for diagnosis of chancroid. J Clin Microbiol 31:659–664, 1993

48. CHUNN CJ, JONES SR, MCCUTCHAN A ET AL: *Haemophilus parainfluenzae* infective endocarditis. Medicine 56:99–113, 1978

49. CHUSID MJ, SCHNEIDER JP, THOMETZ JG ET AL: Osteomyelitis and septic arthritis caused by *Haemophilus influenzae* type f in a young girl. Diagn Microbiol Infect Dis 15:157–159, 1992

50. CLAIRMONT GJ, ZON LI, GROOPMAN JE: *Haemophilus parainfluenzae* prostatitis in a homosexual man with chronic lymphadenopathy and HTLV-III infection. Am J Med 82:175–178, 1987

51. COLLINS JK, KELLY MT: Comparison of Phadebact coagglutination, Bactigen latex agglutination, and counterimmunoelectrophoresis for detection of *Haemophilus influenzae* type b antigens in spinal fluid. J Clin Microbiol 17:1005–1008, 1983

52. COMMITTEE ON INFECTIOUS DISEASES OF THE AMERICAN ACADEMY OF PEDIATRICS: *Haemophilus influenzae* type b conjugate vaccines: recommendations for immunization with recently and previously licensed vaccines. Pediatrics 92:480–488, 1993

53. CONTRONI G, RODRIGUEZ WJ, CHANG MJ: Meningitis caused by *Haemophilus influenzae* type e, biotype IV. South Med J 75:78, 1982

54. COONEY TG, HARWOOD BR, MEISNER DJ: *Haemophilus parainfluenzae* thoracic empyema. Arch Intern Med 141:940–941, 1981

55. COURTNEY SE, HALL RT: *Haemophilus influenzae* sepsis in the premature infant. Am J Dis Child 132:1039–1040, 1978

56. CROSS JT, DAVIDSON KW, BRADSHER RW JR: *Haemophilus influenzae* epididymo-orchitis and bacteremia in a man infected with the human immunodeficiency virus. Clin Infect Dis 19:768–769, 1994

57. CROWE HM, LEVITZ RE: Invasive *Haemophilus influenzae* disease in adults. Arch Intern Med 147:241–244, 1987

58. DAGAN R, BOTUJANSKY C, WATEMBERG N ET AL: Safety and immunogenicity in young infants of *Haemophilus* b–tetanus protein conjugate vaccine, mixed in the same syringe with diphtheria–tetanus–pertussis-enhanced inactivated poliovirus vaccine. Pediatr Infect Dis J 13:356–361, 1994

59. DASHEFSKY B, WALD E, LI K: Management of contacts of children in day care with invasive *Haemophilus influenzae* disease. Pediatrics 78:939–940, 1986

60. DAUM RS, MURPHEY-CORB M, SHAPIRA E ET AL: Epidemiology of ROB-1 *beta*-lactamase among ampicillin-resistant *Haemophilus influenzae* isolates in the United States. J Infect Dis 157:450–455, 1988

61. DECKER MD, EDWARDS KM, BRADLEY R ET AL: Comparative trial in infants of four conjugate *Haemophilus influenzae* type b vaccines. J Pediatr 120:184–189, 1992

62. DECKER MD, EDWARDS KM, BRADLEY R ET AL: Responses of children to booster immunization with their primary conjugate *Haemophilus influenzae* type b vaccine or with polyribosyl phosphate conjugated with diphtheria toxoid. J Pediatr 122:410–413, 1993

63. DEICH RA, METCALF BJ, FINN CW ET AL: Cloning of genes encoding a 15,000-dalton peptidoglycan-associated outer membrane lipoprotein and an antigenically related 15,000-dalton protein from *Haemophilus influenzae*. J Bacteriol 170:489–498, 1988

64. DENIS FA, CHIRON JP, CADOZ M ET AL: Meningitis caused by *Haemophilus influenzae* type c. J Pediatr 91:1064–1065, 1978

65. DEULOFEU F, NAVA JM, BELLA F ET AL: Prospective epidemiological study of invasive *Haemophilus influenzae* disease in adults. Eur J Clin Microbiol Infect Dis 13:633–638, 1994

66. DOBSON SRM, KROLL JS, MOXON ER: Insertion sequence IS11016 and absence of *Haemophilus* capsulation genes in the Brazilian purpuric fever clone of *Haemophilus influenzae* biogroup *aegyptius*. Infect Immun 60:618–622, 1992

67. DOERN GV, CHAPIN KC: Laboratory identification of *Haemophilus influenzae*: effects of basal media on the results of the satellitism test and evaluation of the RapID NH system. J Clin Microbiol 20:599–601, 1984

68. DOERN GV, JORGENSEN JH, THORNSBERRY C ET AL: National collaborative study of the prevalence of antimicrobial resistance among clinical isolates of *Haemophilus influenzae*. Antimicrob Agents Chemother 32: 180–185, 1988

69. DRAPKIN MS, WILSON ME, SHRAGER SM ET AL: Bacteremic *Haemophilus influenzae* type b cellulitis in the adult. Am J Med 63:449–452, 1977

70. DROUET EB, DENOYEL GA, BOUDE MM ET AL: Distribution of *Haemophilus influenzae* and *Haemophilus parainfluenzae* biotypes isolated from the human genitourinary tract. Eur J Clin Microbiol Infect Dis 8:951–955, 1989

71. DWORZACK DL, BLESSING LD, HODGES GR ET AL: Case report—*Haemophilus influenzae* type f pneumonia in adults. Am J Med Sci 275:87–91, 1978

72. EDBERG SE, MELTON E, SINGER JM: Rapid biochemical characterization of *Haemophilus* species by using the Micro-ID. J Clin Microbiol 11:22–26, 1980

73. EMMERSON SGP, RICHMAN B, SPAHN T: Changing patterns of epiglottitis in children. Otolaryngol Head Neck Surg 104:287–292, 1991

74. ENCK RE, BENNETT JM: Isolation of *Haemophilus aphrophilus* from an adult with acute leukemia. J Clin Microbiol 4:194–195, 1976

75. ENG RHK, CORRADO ML, CLERI D ET AL: Non-type b *Haemophilus influenzae* infections in adults with reference to biotype. J Clin Microbiol 11:669–671, 1980

76. ERWIN AL, MUNFORD RS, BRAZILIAN PURPURIC FEVER STUDY GROUP: Comparison of lipopolysaccharides from Brazilian purpuric fever isolates and conjunctivitis isolates of *Haemophilus influenzae* biogroup Aegyptius. J Clin Microbiol 27:762–767, 1989

77. ESKOLA J, KAYHTY H, TAKALA AK: A randomized, prospective field study of a conjugate vaccine in the protection of infants and young children against invasive *Haemophilus influenzae* type b disease. N Engl J Med 323:1381–1387, 1990

78. ESKOLA J, PELTOLA H, TAKALA AK ET AL: Efficacy of *Haemophilus influenzae* type b polysaccharide–diphtheria toxoid conjugate vaccine in infancy. N Engl J Med 317:717–722, 1987

79. FALLA TJ, CROOK DWM, BROPHY LN ET AL: PCR for capsular typing of *Haemophilus influenzae*. J Clin Microbiol 32:2382–2386, 1994

80. FALLA TJ, DOBSON SRM, CROOK DWM ET AL: Population-based study of non-typeable *Haemophilus influenzae* invasive disease in children and neonates. Lancet 341:851–854, 1993

81. FARLEY MM, STEPHENS DS, BRACHMAN PS ET AL: Invasive *Haemophilus influenzae* disease in adults: a prospective, population-based surveillance. Ann Intern Med 116: 806–812, 1992

82. FARLEY MM, STEPHENS DS, HARVEY RC ET AL: Incidence and clinical characteristics of invasive *Haemophilus influenzae* disease in adults. J Infect Dis 165(suppl 1): S42-S43, 1992

83. FARLEY MM, STEPHENS DS, KAPLAN SL ET AL: Pilus- and non–pilus-mediated interactions of *Haemophilus influenzae* type b with human erythrocytes and human nasopharyngeal mucosa. J Infect Dis 161:274–280, 1990

84. FELDMAN WE, SCHWARTZ J: *Haemophilus influenzae* type b brain abscess complicating meningitis: a case report. Pediatrics 72:473–475, 1983

85. FERRAN M, BUTI M, GONZALEZ A ET AL: Pyogenic liver abscess by *Haemophilus influenzae* complicating hydatid cysts. Infection 14:197, 1986

86. FISHER MC, MORTENSEN JE: Pyogenic arthritis due to *Haemophilus influenzae* type f in a child. Clin Microbiol Newslett 14:62–63, 1992

87. FLESHER AR, INSEL AR: Characterization of lipopolysaccharide of *Haemophilus influenzae*. J Infect Dis 138: 719–730, 1978

88. FOX BC, BIGGS D: Antimicrobial resistance among *Haemophilus influenzae* isolates. Clin Infect Dis 17:1978–1079, 1993

89. FRAZIER JP, ET AL: Meningitis due to *Haemophilus parainfluenzae*: report of three cases and review of the literature. Pediatr Infect Dis 1:117–119, 1981

90. FRIESEN CA, CHO CT: Characteristic features of neonatal sepsis due to *Haemophilus influenzae*. Rev Infect Dis 8:777–780, 1986

91. GADBURY JL, AMOS MA: Comparison of a new commercially prepared porphyrin test and the conventional satellite test for the identification of *Haemophilus* species that require X factor. J Clin Microbiol 23:637–639, 1986

92. GALLANT TE, MALINAK LR, GUMP DW ET AL: *Haemaophilus parainfluenzae* peritonitis associated with an intrauterine device. Am J Obstet Gyneol 129:702–703, 1977

93. GERACI JE, WILCOWSKE CJ, WILSON WR ET AL: *Haemophilus* endocarditis: report of 14 patients. Mayo Clin Proc 52:209–215, 1977

94. GIBSON M, WILLIAMS PP: *Haemophilus influenzae* amnionitis associated with prematurity and premature rupture of membranes. Obstet Gyneol 52(suppl):70s-72s, 1978

95. GILSDORF JR, CHANNG HY, MCCREA KW ET AL: Comparison of hemagglutinating pili of type b and nontypeable *Haemophilus influenzae*. J Infect Dis 165(suppl 1):S105-S106, 1992

96. GIVNER LB, ABRAMSON JS, WASILAUSKAS B: Meningitis due to *Haemophilus influenzae* type b resistant to ampicillin and chloramphenicol. Rev Infect Dis 11:329–334, 1989

97. GOLD R, SCHEIFELE D, BARRETO L ET AL: Safety and immunogenicity of *Haemophilus influenzae* vaccine (tetanus toxoid conjugate) administered concurrently or combined with diphtheria and tetanus toxoids, pertussis vaccine, and inactivated poliomyelitis vaccine to healthy infants at two, four, and six months of age. Pediatr Infect Dis J 13:348–355, 1994

98. GOMEZ-GARCES JL, AMOR E, CUBERES R ET AL: Bacteremia and biliary infection caused by *Haemophilus influenzae* type e in an adult. Eur J Clin Microbiol infect Dis 11:382–383, 1992

99. GORELICK H, BAKER MD: Epiglottitis in children, 1979–1992: effects of *Haemophilus influenzae* type b immunization. Arch Pediatr Adolesc Med 148:47–50, 1994

100. GRANATO PA, JUREK EA, WEINER LB: Biotypes of *Haemophilus influenzae*: relationship to clinical source of isolation, serotype, and antibiotic susceptibility. Am J Clin Pathol 79:73–77, 1983

101. GRANOFF DM, ANDERSON EL, OSTERHOLM MT ET AL: Differences in the immunogenicity of three *Haemophilus influenzae* type b conjugate vaccines in infants. J Pediatr 121:187–194, 1992

102. GRANOFF DM, HOLMES SJ, BELSHE RB ET AL: Effect of carrier protein priming on antibody responses to *Haemophilus influenzae* type b conjugate vaccines in infants. JAMA 272:1116–1121, 1994

103. GRANOFF DM, HOLMES SJ, OSTERHOLM MT ET AL: Induction of immunologic memory in infants primed with *Haemophilus influenzae* type b conjugate vaccines. J Infect Dis 168:663–671, 1993

104. GRASSO RJ, WEST LA, HOLBROOK NJ ET AL: Increased sensitivity of a new coagglutination test for rapid identification of *Haemophilus influenzae* type b. J Clin Microbiol 13:1122–1124, 1981

105. GRATTEN M: *Haemophilus influenzae* biotype VII. J Clin Microbiol 13:1015–1016, 1983

106. GRATTEN M, BATTISTUTTA D, TORZILLO P ET AL: Comparison of goat and horse blood as culture medium supplements for isolation and identification of *Haemophilus influenzae* and *Streptococcus pneumoniae* from upper respiratory tract secretions. J Clin Microbiol 32:2871–2872, 1994

107. GREENBERG DP, VADHEIM CM, PARTRIDGE S ET AL: Immunogenicity of *Haemophilus influenzae* type b tetanus toxoid conjugate vaccine in young infants. J Infect Dis 170:76–81, 1994

108. GREENE GR: Meningitis due to *Haemophilus influenzae* other than type b: a case report and review. Pediatrics 62:1021–1025, 1978

109. GREENE JN, SANDIN RL, VILLANUEVA L, SINNOTT JT: *Haemophilus parainfluenzae* endocarditis in a patient with mitral valve prolapse. Ann Clin Lab Sci 23:203–206, 1993

110. GROENEVELD K, VAN ALPHEN L, VAN KETEL RJ ET AL: Non-culture detection of *Haemophilus influenzae* in sputum with monoclonal antibodies specific for outer membrane lipoprotein P6. J Clin Microbiol 27:2263–2267, 1989

111. HAMED KA, DORMITZER PR, SU CK ET AL: *Haemophilus parainfluenzae* endocarditis: application of a molecular approach for identification of pathogenic bacterial species. Clin Infect Dis 19:677–683, 1994

112. HANNAH P, GREENWOOD JR: Isolation and rapid identification of *Haemophilus ducreyi*. J Clin Microbiol 7:39–43, 1982

113. HANSEN EJ, PELZEL SE, ORTH K ET AL: Structural and antigenic conservation of the P2 porin protein among strains of *Haemophilus influenzae* type b. Infect Immun 57:3270–3275, 1989

114. HARRISON LH, DESILVA GA, PITTMAN M ET AL: Epidemiology and clinical spectrum of Brazilian purpuric fever. J Clin Microbiol 27:599–604, 1989

115. HELLBUSCH LC, PENN RG: Cerebrospinal fluid shunt infections by unencapsulated *Haemophilus influenzae*. Childs Nerv Syst 5:315–317, 1989

116. HIMMELREICH CA, BARENKAMP SJ, STORCH GA: Comparison of methods for serotyping *Haemophilus influenzae*. J Clin Microbiol 21:159–160, 1986

117. HOISETH SK, CORN PG, ANDERS J: Amplification status of capsule genes in *Haemophilus influenzae* type b clinical isolates. J Infect Dis 165(suppl 1):S114, 1992

118. HOISETH SK, MOXON ER, SILVER RP: Genes involved in *Haemophilus influenzae* type b capsule expression are part of an 18-kilobase tandem duplication. Proc Natl Acad Sci USA 83:1106–1110, 1986

119. HOLMES RL, DEFRANCO LM, OTTO M: Novel method of biotyping *Haemophilus influenzae* that uses API 20E. J Clin Microbiol 15:1150–1152, 1982

120. HOLMES RL, KOZININ WP: Pneumonia and bacteremia associated with *Haemophilus influenzae* serotype d. J Clin Microbiol 18:730–732, 1983

121. HOLT JG, KRIEG NR, SNEATH PHA ET AL (EDS.): Group 5—Facultatively anaerobic gram-negative rods. In *Bergey's Manual of Determinative Bacteriology*, 9th ed. pp. 175–289. Williams & Wilkins, Baltimore, 1993

122. HUNTER JS, LEVIN RM: *Haemophilus influenzae* type f meningitis in two children. Clin Microbiol Newslett 13:6–7, 1991

123. INGRAM DL, PEARSON AW, OCCHIUTI AR: Detection of bacterial antigens in body fluids with the Wellcogen *Haemophilus influenzae* b, *Streptococcus pneumoniae*, and *Neisseria meningitidis* (ACYW135) latex agglutination tests. J Clin Microbiol 18:1119–1121, 1983

124. INZANA TJ, JOHNSON JL, SHELL L ET AL: Isolation and characterization of a newly identified *Haemophilus* species from cats: "*Haemophilus felis*." J Clin Microbiol 30:2108–2112, 1992

125. IRONO K, GRIMONT F, CASIN I: rRNA gene restriction patterns of *Haemophilus influenzae* biogroup *aegyptius* strains associated with Brazilian purpuric fever. J Clin Microbiol 26:1535–1538, 1988

126. JANDA WM, BRADNA JJ, RUTHER P: Identification of *Neisseria* spp, *Haemophilus* spp, and other fastidious gram-negative bacteria with the MicroScan *Haemophilus Neisseria* identification panel. J Clin Microbiol 27:869–873, 1989

127. JANDA WM, MALLOY PJ, SCHRECKENBERGER PC: Clinical evaluation opf the Vitek *Neisseria-Haemophilus* identification card. J Clin Microbiol 25:37–41, 1987

128. JEMSEK JG, GREENBERG SB, GENTRY LO ET AL: *Haemophilus parainfluenzae* endocarditis: two cases and a review of the literature of the past decade. Am J Med 66:51–57, 1979

129. JOHNSON SR, MARTIN DH, CAMMARATA C ET AL: Development of a polymerase chain reaction assay for detection of *Haemophilus ducreyi*. Sex Transm Dis 21:13–23, 1994

130. JONES RN, SLEPAK J, BIGELOW J: Ampicillin resistant *Haemophilus paraphrophilus* laryngo-epiglottitis. J Clin Microbiol 4:405–407, 1976

131. JORDENS JZ, LEAVES NI, ANDERSON EC ET AL: Polymerase chain reaction-based strain characterization of noncapsulate *Haemophilus influenzae*. J Clin Microbiol 31:2981–2987, 1993

132. JORGENSEN JH: Update on mechanisms and prevalence of antimicrobial resistance in *Haemophilus influenzae*. Clin Infect Dis 14:1119–1123, 1992

133. JORGENSEN JH, DOERN GV, THORNSBERRY C ET AL: Susceptibility of multiply resistant *Haemophilus influenzae* to newer antimicrobial agents. Diagn Microbiol Infect Dis 9:27–32, 1988

134. JORGENSEN JH, HOWELL AW, MAHER LA: Antimicrobial susceptibility testing of less commonly isolated

Haemophilus species using *Haemophilus* test medium. J Clin Microbiol 28:985–988, 1990

135. JORGENSEN JH, REDDING JD, MAHER LA ET AL: Improved medium for antimicrobial susceptibility testing of *Haemophilus influenzae*. J Clin Microbiol 25:2105–2113, 1987

136. JULANDER I, LINDBERG AA, SVANBOM M: *Haemophilus parainfluenzae*—an uncommon cause of septicemia and endocarditis. Scand J Infect Dis 12:85–89, 1980

137. KAPLAN SL, LAUER BA, WARD MA ET AL: Immunogenicity and safety of *Haemophilus influenzae* type b–tetanus protein conjugate vaccine alone or mixed with diphtheria–tetanus–pertussis vaccine in infants. J Pediatr 124:323–327, 1994

138. KENNY JF, ISBURG GD, MICHAELS RH: Meningitis due to *Haemophilus influenzae* type b resistant to both ampicillin and chloramphenicol. Pediatrics 66:14–16, 1980

139. KESSLER A, WETMORE RF, MARSH RR: Childhood epiglottitis in recent years. Int J Pediatr Otorhinolaryngol 25:155–162, 1993

140. KILIAN M: A rapid method for the differentiation of *Haemophilus* stains: the porphyrin test. Acta Pathol Microbiol Scand B 82:935–942, 1974

141. KILIAN M: A taxonomic study of the genus *Haemophilus* with the proposal of a new species, J Gen Microbiol 93:9–62, 1976

142. KILIAN M, BIBERSTEIN EL: Genus II. *Haemophilus*. In Krieg NR, Holt JG (eds): *Bergey's Manual of Systematic Bacteriology*, vol 1, pp 558–559. Baltimore, Williams & Wilkins, 1984

143. KILIAN M, POULSEN K: Enzymatic, serologic, and genetic polymorphism of *Haemophilus influenzae* IgA1 proteases. J Infect Dis 165(suppl 1):S192-S193, 1992

144. KILIAN M, SORENSEN I, FREDERIKSEN W: Biochemical characteristics of 130 recent clinical isolates from *Haemophilus influenzae* meningitis. J Clin Microbiol 9:409–412, 1979

145. Kimura A, Hansen EJ: Antigenic and phenotypic variations of *Haemophilus influenzae* type b lipopolysaccharides and their relationship to virulence. Infect Immun 51:69–79, 1986

146. KIMURA A, PATRICK CC, MILLER EE ET AL: *Haemophilus influenzae* type b lipopolysaccharide: stability of expression and association with virulence. Infect Immun 55:1979–1986, 1987

147. KINMOUTH AL, STORRS CN, MITCHELL RG: Meningitis due to chloramphenicol-resistant *Haemophilus influenzae* type b. Br Med J 1:694, 1978

148. KOSTMAN JR, SHERRY BL, FLIGNER CL ET AL: Invasive *Haemophilus influenzae* infections in older children and adults in Seattle. Clin Infect Dis 17:289–296, 1993

149. KRAGSBJERG P, NILSSON K, PERSSON L ET AL: Deep obstetrical and gynecologic infections caused by non-typeable *Haemophilus influenzae*. Scand J Infect Dis 25:341–346, 1993

150. KREISS JK, KOECH D, PLUMMER FA ET AL: AIDS virus infection in Nairobi prostitutes: spread of the epidemic to East Africa. N Engl J Med 314:414–418, 1986

151. KRISTENSEN K: *Haemophilus influenzae* type b infections in adults. Scand J Infect Dis 21:651–653, 1989

152. KROLL JS: The genetics of encapsulation in *Haemophilus influenzae*. J Infect Dis 165(suppl 1):S93-S96, 1992

153. KROLL JS, HOPKINS I, MOXON ER: Capsule loss in *H. influenzae* type b occurs by recombination-mediated disruption of a gene essential for polysaccharide export. Cell 53:347–356, 1988

154. LEIBERMAN JR, HAGAY ZJ, DAGAN R: Intraamniotic *Haemophilus influenzae* infection. Arch Obstet Gynecol 244:183–184, 1989

155. LERMAN SJ: *Haemophilus influenzae* infections of cerebrospinal fluid shunts. J Neurosurg 54:261–263, 1981

156. LESSE AJ, GHEESLING LL, BITTNER WE ET AL: Stable, conserved outer membrane epitope of strains of *Haemophilus influenzae* biogroup *aegyptius* associated with Brazilian purpuric fever. Infect Immun 60:1351–1357, 1992

157. LIPUMA JJ, RICHMAN H, STULL TL: Haemocin, a bacteriocin produced by *Haemophilus influenzae* type b: species distribution and role in colonization. Infect Immun 58:1600–1605, 1990

158. LIPUMA JJ, SHARETZSKY C, EDLIND TD ET AL: Haemocin production by encapsulated and nonencapsulated *Haemophilus influenzae*. J Infect Dis 165(suppl 1):S118-S119, 1992

159. LLORACH MB, FERNANDEZ DA, DAUNIS JV ET AL: *Haemophilus influenzae* septic arthritis in the adult. Clin Rheumatol 8:292–293, 1989

160. LOEB MR, CONNOR E, PENNEY D: A comparison of the adherence of fimbriated and nonfimbriated *Haemophilus influenzae* type b to human adenoids in organ culture. Infect Immun 56:484–489, 1988

161. LUND ME: Filter paper porphyrin production test for identification of *Haemophilus*. Clin Microbiol Newslett 3:27–29, 1981

162. LUND ME, BLAZEVIC D: Rapid speciation of *Haemophilus* with the porphyrin test versus the satellite test for X. J Clin Microbiol 5:142–144, 1977

163. LYNN DJ, KANE JG, PARKER RH: *Haemophilus parainfluenzae* and *influenzae* endocarditis: a review of forty cases. Medicine 56:115–128, 1977

164. MACONE AB, ARAKERE G, LETOURNEAU JM ET AL: Comparison of a new rapid enzyme-linked immunosorbent assay with latex particle agglutination for the detection of *Haemophilus influenzae* type b infections. J Clin Microbiol 21:711–714, 1985

165. MALLER R, ANSEHN S, FRYDEN A: *Haemophilus parainfluenzae* infection of the central nervous system: a report on two infants. Scand J Infect Dis 9:241–242, 1977

166. MALOUIN F, BRYAN LE, SHEWCIW P ET AL: DNA probe technology for rapid detection of *Haemophilus influenzae* in clinical specimens. J Clin Microbiol 26:2132–2138, 1988

167. MANIAN FA: Prosthetic joint infection due to *Haemophilus parainfluenzae* after dental surgery. South Med J 84:807–808, 1991

168. MARCON MJ, HAMOUDI AC, CANNON HJ: Comparative laboratory evaluation of three antigen detection methods for diagnosis of *Haemophilus influenzae* type b disease. J Clin Microbiol 19:333–337, 1984

169. MARKOWITZ SM: Isolation of an ampicillin-resistant, non-*beta*-lactamase producing strain of *Haemophilus influenzae*. Antimicrob Agents Chemother 17:80–83, 1980

170. MARTEL AY, ST-LAURENT G, DANSEREAU LA ET AL: Isolation and biochemical characterization of *Haemophilus* species isolated simultaneously from the oropharyngeal and anogenital areas. J Clin Microbiol 27:1486–1489, 1989

171. MASKELL DJ, SZABO MJ, BUTLER PD ET AL: Molecular biology of phase-variable lipopolysaccharide biosynthesis by *Haemophilus influenzae*. J Infect Dis 165(suppl 1):S90-S92, 1992

172. MATTHEWS HW, BAKER CN, THORNSBERRY C: Relationship between in vitro susceptibility test results for chloramphenicol and production of chloramphenicol acetyltransferase by *Haemophilus influenzae*, *Streptococcus pneumoniae* and *Aerococcus* species. J Clin Microbiol 26:2387–2390, 1988

173. MATTHEWS JS, REYNOLDS JA, WEESNER DE ET AL: Rapid species identification and biotyping of respiratory isolates of *Haemophilus*. J Clin Microbiol 18:472–475, 1983

174. MCCLAIN JB, ALMAZAN RD KEISER JF: *Haemophilus parainfluenzae* urethritis with accompanying bacteremia. Clin Microbiol Newslett 5:31, 1983

175. MCDONALD CL, CRAFTON EM, COVIN A ET AL: Pericarditis: a possible complication of endocarditis due to *Haemophilus influenzae*. Clin Infect Dis 18:648–649, 1994

176. MCINTYRE P, WHEATON G, ERLICH J: Brazilian purpuric fever in Central Australia. Lancet 2:112, 1987

177. MCLAREN BR, TURNER JG: *Haemophilus parainfluenzae* endocarditis. NZ Med J 106:412, 1993

178. MEGRAUD F, BEBEAR C, DABERNAT H, DELMAS C: *Haemophilus* species in the human gastrointestinal tract. Eur J Clin Microbiol Infect Dis 7:437–438, 1988

179. MENDELMAN PM: Targets of the *beta*-lactam antibiotics, penicillin binding proteins, in ampicillin-resistant, non-*beta*-lactamase-producing *Haemophilus influenzae*. J Infect Dis 165(suppl 1):S107-S109, 1992

180. MENDELMAN PM, CHAFFIN DO, CLAUSEN C ET AL: Failure to detect ampicillin-resistant, non-*beta*-lactamase-producing *Haemophilus influenzae* by standard disk susceptibility testing. Antimicrob Agents Chemother 30:274–280, 1986

181. MENDELMAN PM, CHAFFIN DO, STULL TL ET AL: Characterization of non-*beta*-lactamase-mediated ampicillin resistance in *Haemophilus influenzae*. Antimicrob Agents Chemother 26:235–244, 1984

182. MESSING M, SOTTNEK FO, BIDDLE JW ET AL: Isolation of *Haemophilus* species from the genital tract. Sex Transm Dis 10:56–61, 1983

183. MICHAELS RH, ALI O: A decline in *Haemophilus influenzae* type b meningitis. J Pediatr 122:407–409, 1994

184. MILLARD DD, YOGEV R: *Haemophilus influenzae* type b: a rare case of congenital conjunctivitis. Pediatr Infect Dis J 7:363–364, 1988

185. MORGAN MG, HAMILTON-MILLER JMT: *Haemophilus influenzae* and *Haemophilus parainfluenzae* as urinary pathogens. J Infect 20:143–145, 1990

186. MORSE SA: Chancroid and *Haemophilus ducreyi*. Clin Microbiol Rev 2:137–157, 1989

187. MOXON ER: *Haemophilus influenzae*. In Mandell GL, Bennett JE, Dolin R (eds): *Mandell, Douglas, and Bennett's Principles and Practice of Infectious Diseases*, Fourth edition, pp 2039–2045. New York, Churchill-Livingstone, 1995

188. MUNSON RS JR, SHENEP JL, BARENKAMP SJ, GRANOFF DM: Purification and comparison of outer membrane protein P2 from *Haemophilus influenzae* type b isolates. J Clin Invest 72:677–684, 1983

189. MURPHY TF, APICELLA MA: Nontypeable *Haemophilus influenzae*: a review of clinical aspects, surface antigens and human immune response to infection. Rev Infect Dis 147:838–846, 1987

190. MURPHY TF, BARTOS LC: Purification and analysis with monoclonal antibodies of P2, the major outer membrane protein of nontypeable *Haemophilus influenzae*. Infect Immun 56:1084–1089, 1988

191. MURPHY TF, BARTOS LC, RICE PA ET AL: Identificaion of a 16,600-dalton outer membrane protein on nontypeable *Haemophilus influenzae* as a target for human bactericidal antibody. J Clin Invest 78:1020–1027, 1986

192. MURPHY TF, CAMPAGNARI AA, NELSON MB, APICELLA MA: Somatic antigens of *Haemophilus influenzae* as potential vaccine components. Pediatr Infect Dis J 8:S66-S68, 1989

193. MURPHY TV, PASTOR P, MEDLEY F ET AL: Decreased *Haemophilus* colonization in children vaccinated with *Haemophilus influenzae* type b conjugate vaccine. J Pediatr 122:517–523, 1993

194. MURPHY TV, WHITE KE, PASTOR P ET AL: Declining incidence of *Haemophilus influenzae* type b disease since introduction of vaccination. JAMA 269:246–248, 1993

195. MUSHER DM, KUBITSCHEK KR, CRENNAN J ET AL: Pneumonia and acute febrile tracheobronchitis due to *Haemophilus influenzae*. Ann Intern Med 99:444–450, 1983

196. MUSHER DM, WALLACE RJ: Bacteremic infections caused by nontypeable *Haemophilus influenzae* in patients with dysgammaglobulinemia. J Clin Microbiol 17:143–145, 1983

197. MUSSER JM, SELANDER RK: Brazilian purpuric fever: evolutionary genetic relationships of the case clone of *Haemophilus influenzae* biogroup *aegyptius* to encapsulated strains of *Haemophilus influenzae*. J Infect Dis 161:130–133, 1990

198. MUTTERS P, PIECHULLA K, HINZ H-K ET AL: *Pasteurella avium* (Hinz and Kunjara 1977) comb. nov. and *Pasteurella volantium* sp. nov. Int J Syst Bacteriol 35:5–9, 1985

199. MYEROWITZ RL, MICHEALS RH: Mechanism of potentiation of experimental *Haemophilus influenzae* type b diseases in rats by influenza A virus. Lab Invest 44:434–441, 1981

200. NATIONAL COMMITTEE FOR CLINICAL LABORATORY STANDARDS: Performance Standards for Antimicrobial Disk Susceptibility Tests, 5th ed. Approved standard M2-A5. National Committee for Clinical Labvoratory Standards, Villanova PA

201. NATIONAL COMMITTEE FOR CLINICAL LABORATORY STANDARDS: Methods for Dilution Antimicrobial Susceptibility Tests for Bacteria That Gow Aerobically, 3rd ed. Approved standard M7-A3. National Committee for Clinical Laboratory Standards, Villanova PA

202. NATIONAL COMMITTEE FOR CLINICAL LABORATORY STANDARDS: Performance Standards for Antimicrobial Susceptibility Testing, 5th informational supplement. NCCLS Document M100-S5. National Committee for Clinical Laboratory Standards, Villanova, PA

203. NELSON MB, APICELLA MA, MURPHY TF ET AL: Cloning and sequencing of *Haemophilus influenzae* outer membrane protein P6. Infect Immun 56:128–134, 1988

204. NIVIN DF, O'REILLY T: Significance of V-factor dependency on the taxonomy of *Haemophilus* species and related organisms. Int J Syst Bacteriol 40:1–4, 1990

205. OBERHOFER TR, BACK AE: Biotypes of *Haemophilus influenzae* encountered in clinical laboratories. J Clin Microbiol 10:168–174, 1979

206. OBERHOFER TR, BACK AE: Isolation and cultivation of *Haemophilus ducreyi*. J Clin Microbiol 15:625–629, 1982

207. O'BRYAN TA, WHITENER CJ, KATZMAN M ET AL: Hepatobiliary infections caused by *Haemophilus* species. Clin Infect Dis 15:716–719, 1992

208. OFFIT PA, CAMPOS JM, PLOTKIN SA: Ampicillin-resistant, *beta*-lactamase–negative *Haemophilus influenzae* type b. Pediatrics 69:230–231, 1982

209. OILL PA, CHOW AW, GUZE LB: Adult bacteremic *Haemophilus parainfluenzae* infections: seven reports of cases and a review of the literature. Arch Intern Med 139:985–988, 1979

210. OLK DG, HAMILL RJ, PROCTER RA: Case report: *Haemophilus parainfluenzae* vertebral osteomyelitis. Am J Med Sci 294:114–116, 1987

211. PAAVONEN J, LEHTINEN M, TEISALA K ET AL: *Haemophilus influenzae* causes purulent salpingitis. Am J Obstet Gynecol 151:338–339, 1985

212. PALLADINO S, LEAHY BJ, NEWALL TL: Comparison of the RIM-H rapid identification kit with conventional tests for the identification of *Haemophilus* species. J Clin Microbiol 28:1862–1863, 1990

213. PARADISO PR, HOGERMAN DA, MADORE DV ET AL: Safety and immunogenicity of a combined diphtheria, tetanus, pertussis and *Haemophilus influenzae* type b vaccine in young infants. Pediatrics 92:827–832, 1993

214. PARKER SW, APICELLA MA, FULLER CM: *Haemophilus* endocarditis: two patients with complications. Arch Intern Med 143:48–51, 1983

215. PARSONS LM, SHAYEGANI M, WARING AL ET AL: DNA probes for the identification of *Haemophilus ducreyi*. J Clin Microbiol 27:1441–1445, 1989

216. PATRIARCA PA, LAUER BA: Ventriculoperitoneal shunt-associated infection due to *Haemophilus influenzae*. Pediatrics 65:1007–1009, 1980

217. PATRICK CC, PATRICK GS, KAPLAN SL ET AL: Adherence kinetics of *Haemophilus influenzae* type b to eucaryotic cells. Pediatr Res 26:500–503, 1989

218. PEAKE JE, SLAUGHTER BD: Hemorrhagic conjunctivitis and invasive *Haemophilus influenzae* type b infection. Pediatr Infect Dis J 13:230–231, 1994

219. PELTOLA H, ESKOLA J, KAYHTY H ET AL: Clinical comparison of the *Haemophilus influenzae* type b polysaccharide–diphtheria toxoid and the oligosaccharide–CRM$_{197}$ protein vaccines in infancy. Arch Pediatr Adolesc Med 148:620–625, 1994

220. PETERS VB, SOOD S: Immunity to *Haemophilus influenzae* type b polysaccharide capsule in children with human immunodeficiency virus infection immunized with a single dose of *Haemophilus* vaccine. J Pediatr 125:74–77, 1994

221. PETRAK RM, POTTAGE JC JR, HARRIS AA ET AL: *Haemophilus influenzae* meningitis in the presence of a cerebrospinal fluid shunt. Neurosurgery 18:79–81, 1986

222. PIECHULLA K, MUTTERS R, BURBACH S ET AL: Deoxyribonucleic acid relationships of "*Histophilus ovis/Haemophilus somnus*," *Haemophilus haemoglobinophilus*, and "*Actinobacillus seminis*." Int J Syst Bacteriol 36:1–7, 1986

223. PINCUS DJ, MORRISON D, ANDREWS C ET AL: Age-related response to two *Haemophilus influenzae* type b vaccines. J Pediatr 100:197–201, 1982

224. POHL S, BERTSCHINGER HU, FREDERIKSEN W ET AL: Transfer of *Haemophilus pleuropneumoniae* and the *Pasteurella haemolytica*-like organism causing porcine necrotic pleuropneumonia to the genus *Actinobacillus* (*Actinobacillus pleuropneumoniae* comb. nov.) on the basis of phenotypic and deoxyribonucleic acid relatedness. Int J Syst Bacteriol 33:510–514, 1983

225. PORTO MHO, NOEL GJ, EDELSON PJ ET AL: Resistance to serum bactericidal activity distinguishes Brazilian purpuric fever (BPF) case strains of *Haemophilus influenzae* biogroup *aegyptius* (*H. aegyptius*) from non-BPF strains. J Clin Microbiol 27:792–294, 1988

226. PURDY D, KHARDORI N, ABBAS F ET AL: Postoperative pancreatic abscess due to *Haemophilus influenzae*. Clin Infect Dis 17:49–51, 1993

227. QUENTIN R, DUBARRY I, MARTIN C ET AL: Evaluation of four commercial methods for identification and biotyping of genital and neonatal strains of *Haemophilus* species. Eur J Clin Microbiol Infect Dis 11:546–549, 1992

228. QUENTIN R, GOUDEAU A, WALLACE RJ JR ET AL: Urogenital, maternal, and neonatal isolates of *Haemophilus influenzae*: identification of unusually virulent serologically non-typeable clone families and evidence for a new *Haemophilus* species. J Gen Microbiol 136:1203–1209, 1990

229. QUENTIN R, KOUBAA N, CATTIER B ET AL: In vitro activities of five new quinolones against 88 genital and neonatal *Haemophilus* isolates. Antimicrob Agents Chemother 32:147–149, 1988

230. QUENTIN R, MARTIN C, MUSSER JM ET AL: Genetic characterization of a cryptic genospecies of *Haemophilus* causing urogenital and neonatal infections. J Clin Microbiol 31:1111–1116, 1993

231. QUENTIN R, MUSSER JM, MELLOUETT M ET AL: Typing of urogenital, maternal, and neonatal isolates of *Haemophilus influenzae* and *Haemophilus parainfluenzae* in correlation with clinical course of isolation and evidence for a genital specificity of *Haemophilus influenzae* biotype IV. J Clin Microbiol 27:2286–2294, 1989

232. RAUCHER B, DOBKIN J, MANDEL L ET AL: Occult polymicrobial endocarditis with *Haemophilus parainfluenzae* in intravenous drug abusers. Am J Med 86:169–172, 1989

233. RIERA L: Detection of *Haemophilus influenzae* type b antigenuria by Bactigen and Phadebact kits. J Clin Microbiol 21:638–640, 1985

234. ROBERTS MC, BELL TA, SANDSTROM KI AT AL: Characterization of *Haemophilus* spp isolated from infant conjunctivitis. J Med Microbiol 21:219–224, 1986

235. ROGGEN EL, PANSAERTS R, VAN DYCK E, ET AL: Antigen detection and immunological typing of *Haemophilus ducreyi* with a specific rabbit polyclonal serum. J Clin Microbiol 31:1820–1825, 1993

236. ROSENAU A, SIZARET PY, MUSSER JM ET AL: Adherence to human cells of a cryptic *Haemophilus* genospecies responsible for genital and neonatal infections. Infect Immun 61:4112–4118, 1993

237. ROSENBAUM GS, CALUBIRAN O, CUNHA BA: *Haemophilus parainfluenzae* bacteremia associated with a pacemaker wire localized by gallium scan. Heart Lung 19:271–273, 1990

238. RUBIN LG, GLOSTER ES, CARLONE GM ET AL: An infant rat model of bacteremia with Brazilian purpuric fever isolates of *Haemophilus influenzae* biogroup aegyptius. J Infect Dis 160:476–482, 1989

239. RUSIN P, ADAMS RD, PETERSEN EA ET AL: *Haemophilus influenzae*: an important cause of maternal and neonatal infections. Obstet Gynecol 77:92–96, 1991

240. SAEZ-LLORENS X, MCCRACKEN GH: Bacterial meningitis in neonates and children. In Scheld WM, Wispelwey B (eds): Infectious Diseases Clinics of North America, Volume 4, Meningitis, pp 623–644. Philadelphia, W.B. Saunders, 1990

241. SANTOSHAM M, WOLFF M, REID R ET AL: The efficacy in Navajo indians of a conjugate vaccine consisting of *Haemophilus influenzae* type b polysaccharide and *Neisseria meningitidis* outer-membrane protein complex. N Engl J Med 324:1767–1772, 1991

242. SCHALLA WO, SANDERS LL, SCHMID GP ET AL: Use of dot immunobinding and fluorescence assays to investigate clinically suspected cases of chancroid. J Infect Dis 153:879–887, 1986

243. SCHMIDT ME, SMITH MA, LEVY CS: Endophthalmitis caused by unusual gram-negative bacilli: three case reports and review. Clin Infect Dis 17:686–690, 1993

244. SHAPIRO ED, WARD H: The epidemiology and prevention of disease caused by *Haemophilus influenzae* type b. Epidemiol Rev 13:113–142, 1991

245. SHAW ED, DARKER RJ, FELDMAN WE ET AL: Clinical studies of a new latex particle agglutination test for detection of *Haemophilus influenzae* type b polyribose phosphate antigen in serum, cerebrospinal fluid and urine. J Clin Microbiol 15:1153–1156, 1982

246. SHAWAR R, SEPULVEDA J, CLARRIDGE JE: Use of the RapID-ANA system and sodium polyanetholsulfonate disk susceptibility testing in identifying *Haemophilus ducreyi*. J Clin Microbiol 28:108–111, 1990

247. SHIVELY RG, SHIGEI JT, PETERSON EM ET AL: Typing of *Haemophilus influenzae* by coagglutination and conventional slide agglutination. J Clin Microbiol 14:706–708, 1981

248. SIMON MW, MITCHELL BL, O'CONNOR WN ET AL: Glomerulonephritis, pulmonary hemorrhage, and coagulopathy associated with *Haemophilus parainfluenzae* endocarditis. Pediatr Infect Dis J 4:183–185, 1985

249. SIMONSEN JN, CAMERON DW, GAKINYA, MN ET AL: Human immunodeficiency virus infection in men with sexually transmitted diseases: experience from a center in Africa. N Engl J Med 319:274–278, 1988

250. SLATER LN, GUARNACCIA J, MAKINTUBEE S ET AL: Bacteremic disease due to *Haemophilus influenzae* capsular type f in adults: report of five cases and review. Rev Infect Dis 12:628–635, 1990

251. SOTTNEK FO, ALBRITTON WL: *Haemophilus influenzae* biotype VIII. J Clin Microbiol 20:815–816, 1984

252. SOTTNEK FO, BIDDLE JW, KRAUS SJ ET AL: Isolation and identification of *Haemophilus ducreyi* in a clinical study. J Clin Microbiol 12:170–174, 1980

253. SPAGNUOLO PJ, ELLNER JJ, LERNER PI ET AL: *Haemophilus influenzae* meningitis: the spectrum of disease in adults. Medicine 61:74–85, 1982

254. SPEER M, ROSAN RC, RUDOLPH AJ: *Haemophilus influenzae* infection in the neonate mimicking respiratory distress syndrome. J Pediatr 93:295–296, 1978

255. STEINHOFF MC, AUERBACH BS, NELSON KE ET AL: Antibody responses to *Haemophilus influenzae* type b vaccines in men with human immunodeficiency virus infection. N Engl J Med 325:1837–1842, 1991

256. STERN S, BAYSTON R, HAYWARD RJ: *Haemophilus influenzae* meningitis in the presence of cerebrospinal fluid shunts. Childs Nerv Syst 4:164–165, 1988

257. ST GEME JW III, FALKOW S: Capsule loss by *Haemophilus influenzae* type b results in enhanced adherence to and entry into human cells. J Infect Dis 165(suppl 1):S117–S118, 1992

258. ST GEME JW III, FALKOW S: Isolation, expression, and nucleotide sequence of the pilin structural gene of the Brazilian purpuric fever clone of *Haemophilus influenzae* biogroup *aegyptius*. Infect Immun 61:2233–2237, 1993

259. ST GEME JW III, GILSDORF JR, FALKOW S: Surface structures and adherence properties of diverse strains of *Haemophilus influenzae* biogroup *aegyptius*. Infect Immun 59:3366–3371, 1991

260. STURM AW: *Haemophilus influenzae* and *Haemophilus parainfluenzae* in nongonococcal urethritis. J Infect Dis 153:165–167, 1986

261. STURM AW, ZANEN HC: Characteristics of *Haemophilus ducreyi* in culture. J Clin Microbiol 19:672–674, 1984

262. SUGIMOTO C, ISAYAMA Y, SAKAZAKI R ET AL: Transfer of *Haemophilus equigenitalis* Taylor et al 1978 to the genus *Taylorella* gen. nov. as *Taylorella equigenitalis* comb. nov. Curr Microbiol 9:155–162, 1983

263. SWAMINATHAN B, MAYER LW, BIBB WF ET AL: Microbiology of Brazilian purpuric fever and diagnostic tests. J Clin Microbiol 27:605–608, 1989

264. TAKALA AK, ESKOLA J, LEINONEN M ET AL: Reduction of oropharyngeal carriage of *Haemophilus influenzae* type b (Hib) in children immunized with an Hib conjugate vaccine. J Infect Dis 164:982–986, 1991

265. TAKALA AK, ESKOLA J, VAN ALPHEN L: Spectrum of invasive *Haemophilus influenzae* type b disease in adults. Arch Intern Med 150:2573–2576, 1990

266. TAKALA AK, MEURMAN O, KLEEMOLA M ET AL: Preceding respiratory infection predisposing for primary and secondary invasive *Haemophilus influenzae* type b disease. Pediatr Infect Dis J 12:189–195, 1993

267. TAKALA AK, PELTOLA H, ESKOLA J: Disappearance of epiglottitis during large-scale vaccination with *Haemophilus influenzae* type b conjugate vaccine among children in Finland. Laryngoscope 104:731–735, 1994

268. TAYLOR DC, CRIPPS AW, CLANCY RL ET AL: Evaluation of a selective medium for the isolation and differentiation of *Haemophilus influenzae* and *Haemophilus parainfluenzae* from the respiratory tract of chronic bronchitics. Pathology 22:162–164, 1990

269. TENOVER FC, HUANG MB, RASHEED JK ET AL: Development of PCR assays to detect ampicillin resistance genes

in cerebrospinal fluid samples containing *Haemophilus influenzae*. J Clin Microbiol 32:2729–2737, 1994

270. TILTON RC, DIAS F, RYAN RW: Comparative evaluation of three commercial products and counterimmunoelectrophoresis for the detection of antigens in cerebrospinal fluid. J Clin Microbiol 20:231–234, 1984

271. TOTTEN PA, STAMM WE: Clear broth and plate media for culture of *Haemophilus ducreyi*. J Clin Microbiol 32:2019–2023, 1994

272. TROLLFORS B, CLAESSON B, LAGERGARD T ET AL: Incidence, predisposing factors, and manifestations of invasive *Haemophilus influenzae* infection in adults. Eur J Clin Microbiol 3:180–184, 1984

273. VADHEIM CM, GREENBERG DP, ERIKSEN E ET AL: Eradication of *Haemophilus influenzae* type b disease in Southern California. Arch Pediatr Adolesc Med 148:51–56, 1994

274. VADHEIM CM, GREENBERG DP, ERIKSEN E AT AL: Protection provided by *Haemophilus influenzae* type b conjugate vaccines in Los Angeles County: a case–control study. Pediatr Infect Dis J 13:274–280, 1994

275. VAN DYCK E, PIOT P: Enzyme profiles of *Haemophilus ducreyi* strains isolated on different continents. Eur J Clin Microbiol 6:40–43, 1987

276. VISSER H, MACFARLANE JD, THOMPSON J: *Haemophilus influenzae* septic arthritis in a healthy adult. Infection 21:191, 1993

277. WAGENER WC, MYEROWITZ RL, DULABON GM: Lethal meningoencephalitis and septicemia caused by *Haemophilus influenzae* type f in an adult with multiple myeloma. J Clin Microbiol 14:695–696, 1981

278. WALD ER: *Haemophilus influenzae* as a cause of acute otitis media. Pediatr Infect Dis J 8:S28-S30, 1989

279. WALKER RL, BIBERSTEIN EL, PRITCHETT RF ET AL: Deoxyribonucleic acid relatedness among *Haemophilus somnus*, *Haemophilus agni*, *Histophilus ovis*, *Actinobacillus seminis* and *Haemophilus influenzae*. Int J Syst Bacteriol 35:46–49, 1985

280. WALLACE RJ, BAKER CJ, QUINONES F ET AL: Nontypeable *Haemophilus influenzae* (biotype IV) as a neonatal, maternal, and genital pathogen. Rev Infect Dis 5:123–136, 1983

281. WALLACE RJ, MUSHER DM, SEPTIMUS EJ ET AL: *Haemophilus influenzae* infections in adults: characterization of strains by serotypes, biotypes, and *beta*-lactamase production. J Infect Dis 144:101–106, 1981

282. WARD J, BRENNEMAN G, LETSON GW ET AL: Limited efficacy of a *Haemophilus influenzae* type b conjugate vaccine in Alaska Native infants. N Engl J Med 323:1393–1401, 1990

283. WARMAN ST, REINITZ E, KLEIN RS: *Haemophilus parainfluenzae* septic arthritis in an adult. JAMA 246:868–869, 1981

284. WASHBURN LK, O'SHEA M, GILLIS DC ET AL: Response to *Haemophilus influenzae* type b conjugate vaccine in chronically ill premature infants. J Pediatr 123:791–794, 1993

285. WELCH DF, AHLIN PA, MATSEN JM: Differentiation of *Haemophilus* spp. in respiratory cultures by a spot indole test. J Clin Microbiol 15:216–219, 1982

286. WELCH DF, HENSEL D: Evaluation of Bactigen and Phadebact for detection of *Haemophilus influenzae* type b antigen in cerebrospinal fluid. J Clin Microbiol 16:905–908, 1982

287. WELCH DF, SOUTHERN PM, SCHNEIDER NR: Five cases of *Haemophilus segnis* appendicitis. J Clin Microbiol 24:851–852, 1986

288. WENGER JD, HIGHTOWER AW, FACKLAM RR ET AL: Bacterial meningitis in the United States, 1986: report of a multistate surveillance study. J Infect Dis 162:1316–1323, 1990

289. WEYANT RS, BIBB WF, STEPHENS DS ET AL: Purification and characterization of a pilin specific for Brazilian purpuric fever-associated *Haemophilus influenzae* biogroup *aegyptius* (*H. aegyptius*) strains. J Clin Microbiol 28:756–763, 1990

290. WEYANT RS, QUINN FD, UTT EA ET AL: Human microvascular endothelial cell toxicity caused by Brazilian purpuric fever-associated strains of *Haemophilus influenzae* biogroup *aegyptius*. J Infect Dis 169:430–433, 1994

291. WHITE CB, LAMPE RM, COPELAND RL ET AL: Soft tissue infection associated with *Haemophilus aphrophilus*. Pediatrics 67:434–435, 1981

292. WHITNEY AM, FARLEY MM: Cloning and sequence analysis of the structural pilin gene of Brazilian purpuric fever-associated *Haemophilus influenzae* biogroup aegyptius. Infect Immun 61:1559–1562, 1993

293. WILD BE, PEARMAN JW, CAMPBELL PB ET AL: Brazilian purpuric fever in Western Australia. Med J Aust 150:344–346, 1989

294. WILDE J, ADLER SP: Molecular epidemiology of *Haemophilus influenzae* type b: failure of rifampin prophylaxis in a day care center. Pediatr Infect Dis 5:508–505, 1986

295. WILLIAMS R, KIRKBRIDE V, CORCORAN GD: Neonatal osteomyelitis in Down's syndrome due to nonencapsulated *Haemophilus influenzae*. J Infect 29:203–205, 1994

296. WISPELWEY B, TUNKEL AR, SCHELD WM: Bacterial meningitis in adults. In Scheld WM, Wispelwey B (eds), Infectious Disease Clinics of North America, vol 4, Meningitis, pp 645–659. Philadephia, W.B. Saunders, 1990

297. WONG GWK, OPPENHEIMER SJ, VAUDRY W: CSF shunt infection by unencapsulated *Haemophilus influenzae*. Clin Infect Dis 17:519–520, 1993

298. ZAMZE SE, MOXON ER: Composition of the lipopolysaccharide from different capsular serotype strains of *Haemophilus influenzae*. J Gen Microbiol 133:1443–1451, 1987

MISCELLANEOUS FASTIDIOUS GRAM-NEGATIVE BACILLI

INTRODUCTION TO THE FASTIDIOUS GRAM-NEGATIVE BACTERIA

The fastidious gram-negative bacteria to be considered in this chapter are isolated infrequently but, nonetheless, may cause serious infections in humans. In many cases, these organisms occur in specific clinical settings, so an understanding of the disease process and the condition of the patient may help tremendously in the laboratory's efforts to recover them from clinical specimens. For example, a history of indolent, insidious symptoms with the presence of vegetations on the heart valves, as determimned by echocardiogram, is the clinical setting for endocarditis caused by the "HACEK" group of organisms. A history of recurring febrile episodes in a patient who works in the meat-packing industry may lead one to suspect *Brucella* infection. Cultures from dog bite wounds will frequently grow *Pasteurella multocida* or the fastidious organism formerly called CDC group DF-2 (*Capnocytophaga canimorsus*). Even a slight "nip" or bite from your pet gerbil may lead to serious illness with an uncommonly enountered organism called *Streptobacillus moniliformis*. Obviously, the physician caring for the patient and the microbiologist handling the specimens must be engaged in close communication for the successful diagnosis and treatment of these unusual infections.

Unlike previous chapters and the chapters to follow, in which the organisms have been fairly well characterized taxonomically, some of the bacteria that will be discussed presently are considered together on the basis of certain cultural features that delineate them from other large groups of organisms. For example, for the "HACEK" group of bacteria, their similarities include slow growth rates, requirements for a CO_2-enriched growth environment, and the clinical syndromes associated with them. *Bordetella* species are fastidious organisms that are found in humans and animals. *B. pertussis*, the species found solely in humans, causes the classic disease called "whooping cough." *Pasteurella* species, *Brucella* species, and *Francisella tularensis* are pathogens that humans acquire by contact with animals or animal products. Clearly, these organisms are diverse in their cultural characteristics, in their ecologic niches, and in the diseases that they cause.

Because of this diversity, the taxonomy, clinical significance, cultural characteristics, identification, and antimicrobial susceptibility will be discussed as each organism is presented rather than in separate sections of the text. In addition, a general laboratory approach to recovery and identification of these organisms will also be presented, including a discussion of conventional methods, modified conventional procedures, and kit systems for identifying these bacteria.

Color Plates for Chapter 8 are found between pages 368 and 369.

THE "HACEK" ORGANISMS

The organisms that compose the "HACEK" group include fastidious gram-negative bacteria that are all part of the normal human oropharyngeal or urogenital flora. Under certain circumstances they can cause serious disease. These organisms are found mainly in association with endocarditis, bacteremia, and mixed-flora wound infections. The pneumonic "HACEK" stands for *Haemophilus aphrophilus/paraphrophilus* (H), *Actinobacillus actinomycetemcomitans* (A), *Cardiobacterium hominis* (C), *Eikenella corrodens* (E), and *Kingella* species (K). All of these bacteria are slow growing, requiring 48 to 72 hours of incubation before adequate growth is apparent. When growing in blood cultures, detection of these organisms may occasionally take from a few days to 2 weeks or longer. All of them require, or are stimulated, by the presence of CO_2, necessitating incubation in a candle jar or a CO_2 incubator. Optimal growth is achieved only on enriched media, such as chocolate or blood agar, and no growth is seen on selective enteric media, such as MacConkey or EMB agar. Although not an absolute requirement, hemin in the medium generally enhances initial recovery of the organisms. Once these organisms are recovered in pure culture, identification is fairly easy if appropriate media and techniques are employed.

HAEMOPHILUS APHROPHILUS AND *HAEMOPHILUS PARAPHROPHILUS*

TAXONOMY

Haemophilus aphrophilus and *Haemophilus paraphrophilus* are members of the genus *Haemophilus* in the family *Pasteurellaceae*, which includes the three genera, *Haemophilus*, *Actinobacillus*, and *Pasteurella*. DNA–rRNA hybridization and 16S rRNA-sequencing studies have demonstrated that members of this family are most closely related to organisms in the families *Enterobacteriaceae*, *Vibrionaceae*, and *Aeromonadaceae*, with more distant relations to the families *Moraxellaceae* and *Cardiobacteriaceae* in the *gamma*-division of the *Proteobacteria*.[555,723] They were formerly designated as CDC group HB-2.[403] *H. aphrophilus* derives its name from the Greek root *aphros* or "foam"; this refers to the organism's requirement for relatively high concentrations of CO_2 ("foam-loving") for growth. This characteristic, however, does not hold true for all isolates of these organisms, particularly stock strains that have been subcultured frequently. *H. aphrophilus* is the only species in the genus that does not require either X factor or V factor for growth (see Chap. 7). Some strains may produce a weak reaction with the δ-aminolevulinic acid (ALA)–porphyrin test, indicating that some hemelike compounds are synthesized by the organism. Because it does not require X or V factors, *H. aphrophilus* will grow on sheep blood agar. *H. paraphrophilus* is biochemically similar to *H. aphrophilus* except that it requires exogenous V factor, and the ALA–porphyrin test is positive. By using multivariate analyses of lipopolysaccharide carbohydrates, fatty acids, enzymatic activities, and other chemotaxonomic data, Brondz and coworkers provided data suggesting that *H. aphrophilus* and *H. paraphrophilus* were indeed separate species that were distinct from *A. actinomycetemcomitans*.[102,103,533] Multilocus enzyme electrophoretic analysis techniques were able to differentiate *A. actinomycetemcomitans* from the other two organisms but did not demonstrate appreciable differences between *H. aphrophilus* and *H. paraphrophilus*.[121] However, data based on DNA homology, DNA–DNA hybridization, genetic transformation, and ribotyping suggest that *H. aphrophilus* and *H. paraphrophilus* may represent phenotypically different strains of the same species.[555,686,742,754]

CLINICAL SIGNIFICANCE

Both *H. aphrophilus* and *H. paraphrophilus* constitute part of the normal flora of the human upper respiratory tract. Studies using selective media have demonstrated that these bacteria are primarily found in dental plaque, particularly between the teeth and in the gingival pockets surrounding the teeth. Tempro and Slots found the organism in 36% of supragingival plaque samples and in 52% of subgingival plaque samples.[748] In neither of these samples did the numbers of organisms exceed 1% of the total bacterial count. Bacterial counts for this organism were actually found to be higher in subgingival plaque samples from healthy individuals compared with samples from adults with periodontal disease. These data suggest that *H. aphrophilus* is not a major part of the healthy periodontal flora and that the organism is not a primary periodontal pathogen.

Both *H. aphrophilus* and *H. paraphrophilus* have been implicated in a wide variety of human infectious processes.[69,249,348,364,376,459,537,557,787] Head and neck infections associated with these organisms include sinusitis, otitis media, epiglottitis, and brain abscess.[69,382] These infections probably arise from direct extension of these organisms from their normal habitat in the oral cavity.[382] However, most infections caused by *H. aphrophilus* and *H. paraphrophilus* apparently result from hematogenous dissemination and seeding of other tissues. These infections include pneumonia, empyema, septic arthritis, vertebral osteomyelitis, soft-tissue infections, endophthalmitis, meningitis, brain abscess, spinal epidural abscess, and laryngoepiglottitis.[12,57,69,124,249,376,382,459,495,537,669,677,777,799,805] *H. aphrophilus* necrotizing fasciitis, secondary to intravenous drug use, has also been documented.[168] Abdominal infections, including wound infections, hepatobiliary tract infections, abdominal abscesses, and cholecystitis, may rarely be caused by these organisms.[364,506,550] Trauma, neutropenia, malignancy, and cancer chemotherapy are apparently predisposing factors for infections with these organisms.[226]

Of the *Haemophilus* species presented in Chapter 7, *H. aphrophilus* and *H. paraphrophilus* are the most common ones recovered from patients with endocarditis. The incidence of endocarditis caused by these organisms is highest in young to middle-aged adults and may or may not be associated with preexisting valvular disease.[69,157,202,281,638,789] Arterial embolization appears to be a frequent complication; among 86 documented cases of *Haemophilus* endocarditis reviewed by Parker and asso-

ciates, 52% of the patients had major arterial emboli, which included frequent intracerebral emboli.[563] Although the mortality associated with properly treated endocarditis caused by these organisms is usually about 10% to 15%, the higher rates (25% to 50%) reported in the earlier literature may reflect difficulties in recovery of these fastidious organisms from blood cultures, with consequent inappropriate or inadequate antimicrobial therapy. Predisposing factors observed in patients with *H. aphrophilus* endocarditis included the presence of dental and oral lesions (i.e., periodontitis, dental plaque, trauma, penetrating wounds), antecedent dental manipulations or oral surgery, and diseased or damaged cardiac valves (e.g., rheumatic heart disease, congenital septal defects, or previous heart surgery).[69,281,638,789] Both native valve and prosthetic valve endocarditis caused by this bacterium have been seen in at-risk patients.[281,789] Glomerulonephritis secondary to septicemia may also occur as a complication of *H. aphrophilus* endocarditis.[787] This organism has also been reported as a cause of endocarditis in a patient receiving combination chemotherapy for acute myelocytic leukemia.[226]

CULTURAL CHARACTERISTICS AND IDENTIFICATION

These organisms grow slowly on agar medium. Colonies are small after 24 hours; 48 to 72 hours incubation is required before colony morphology can be ascertained and sufficient growth is available for preliminary identification tests. Microcolonies growing in broth tend to adhere to the sides of the tube, a characteristic these organisms share with *A. actinomycetemcomitans*. On chocolate agar colonies measure less than 0.5 to 1.0 mm after 48 hours, are convex, granular, and have a yellowish pigment (see Color Plates 8-1*A* and 8-1*B*). A distinct "grade-school paste" odor may be noted. The organisms do not grow on MacConkey agar or other selective or differential enteric media. On primary isolation, *H. aphrophilus* may require X factor (hemin); this requirement is lost after subculture. Because of the lack of factor requirements for growth, *H. aphrophilus* will grow on sheep blood agar and brain–heart infusion agar without supplementation. *H. paraphrophilus* is biochemically similar to *H. aphrophilus*, except that V factor (NAD) is required for growth (Table 8-1). Consequently, this species does not grow on sheep blood agar and will not grow on brain–heart infusion or trypticase–soy agar without NAD supplementation (e.g., a V factor disk or strip). Both *H. aphrophilus* and *H. paraphrophilus* are positive in the ALA–porphyrin test (they do not require exogenous hemin for growth), are negative for the three reactions used for biotyping of *Haemophilus* species (urease, indole, and ornithine carboxylase; see Color Plate 8-1*D*), and readily hydrolyze *o*-nitrophenyl-β-D-galactopyranoside (ONPG). Catalase is not produced, and acid is produced from both glucose and lactose (see Color Plate 8-1*C*). These characteristics differentiate *H. aphrophilus* and *H. paraphrophilus* from from *A. actinomycetemcomitans*, which is catalase-positive and does not ferment lactose. Most strains are oxidase-negative, although a delayed, weak, or equivocal oxidase reaction may be observed with some isolates. *H. para-*

TABLE 8-1

BIOCHEMICAL CHARACTERISTICS FOR IDENTIFICATION OF *HAEMOPHILUS APHROPHILUS*, *HAEMOPHILUS PARAPHROPHILUS*, *ACTINOBACILLUS ACTINOMYCETEMCOMITANS*, **AND** *ACTINOBACILLUS UREAE*

CHARACTERISTIC	H. APHROPHILUS	H. PARAPHROPHILUS	A. ACTINOMYCETEMCOMITANS	A. UREAE
Hemolysis on sheep blood	−	−	−	−
Oxidase	−*	−*	−*	+
Catalase	−	−	+	+
Reduction of NO_3 to NO_2	+	+	+	+
Requirement for X factor	−	−	−	−
Requirement for V factor	−	+	−	−
Indole	−	−	−	−
Urease	−	−	−	+
Ornithine decarboxylase	−	−	−	−
Hydrolysis of esculin	−	−	−	−
Hydrolysis of ONPG	+	+	−	−
Gas from glucose	+	+	v	−
Production of acid from				
Glucose	+	+	+	+
Maltose	+	+	+[†]	+*
Fructose	+	+	+	NA
Sucrose	+	+	−	+
Lactose	+	+	−	−
Xylose	−	−	v	−
Mannitol	−	−	v[‡]	+
Mannose	+	+	+	v
Galactose	+	−	v	−
Melibiose	−	+	−	−
Trehalose	+	+	−	−
Melezitose	−	+	NA	NA
Raffinose	+	−	−	−

+, positive reaction; −, negative reaction; v, variable reaction; NA, not available.
*Few strains may produce weak or delayed positive reactions.
†Rare strains may be maltose-negative.
‡Most strains are mannitol-positive.

phrophilus can be differentiated from *H. aphrophilus* by its requirement for V factor and by its utilization patterns for galactose, melibiose, melezitose, and raffinose. The biochemical features of *H. aphrophilus* and *H. paraphrophilus* are shown in Table 8-1 along with those of *A. actinomycetemcomitans*.

ANTIMICROBIAL SUSCEPTIBILITY

H. aphrophilus and *H. paraphrophilus* are generally susceptible to tetracycline, chloramphenicol, streptomycin, and the other aminoglycosides. Although most strains are also susceptible to penicillin and ampicillin, isolates resistant to these antimicrobials have been reported; some of these resistant isolates produced β-lac-

tamase enzymes.[382] These organisms are also susceptible to third-generation cephalosporins and quinolone antimicrobial agents. Agents such as ceftriaxone and ciprofloxacin have been curative in patients with serious central nervous system infections, brain abscess, and endocarditis.[179,669,777]

ACTINOBACILLUS ACTINOMYCETEMCOMITANS

TAXONOMY

Actinobacillus actinomycetemcomitans includes strains that were previously designated as CDC group HB-3 and HB-4.[403] This organism shares many cultural and biochemical characteristics with the haemophili. DNA hybridization, transformation studies, and immuno-diffusion methods have demonstrated that *A. actino-mycetemcomitans* is more closely related to *H. aphrophilus*, *H. paraphrophilus*, and *H. segnis* than to the other *Actinobacillus* species, which are predominantly animal rather than human isolates.[577,582,742] These animal species are also antigenically distinct from *A. actinomycetemcomitans*. In 1985, a formal proposal was made by Potts and colleagues to transfer *A. actinomycetem-comitans* to the genus *Haemophilus* as "*Haemophilus actinomycetemcomitans.*"[586] However, this proposal was subsequently rejected by the Subcommittee on *Pasteurellaceae* and Related Organisms of the International Committee on Systematic Bacteriology because *A. actinomycetemcomitans* did not show great similarity to the type species of the genus *Haemophilus* (i.e., *H. influenzae*).[365] Other workers have also argued that *A. actinomycetemcomitans* (and *H. aphrophilus*) should not be included in the genus *Haemophilus* because they do not require hemin or NAD. In the 1984 edition of *Bergey's Manual of Systematic Bacteriology*, the species is included as a member of the genus *Actinobacillus* in the family *Pasteurellaceae*.[577]

A. actinomycetemcomitans is a part of the normal flora of the oral cavity, particularly in the gingival and supragingival crevices. This species can be divided into five serotypes designated a, b, c, d, and e on the basis of reactions with type-specific monoclonal antibodies.[290,654] Studies of these serotypes with rRNA gene probes have demonstrated significant genomic heterogeneity, even among strains belonging to the same serotype.[33,654] Isolates belonging to the same serotype have been genotypically similar in the same individual, whereas isolates of the same or different serotypes are genetically nonidentical in different individuals. Patients with endocarditis caused by *A. actinomycetemcomitans* produce high titers of antibodies against the serotype-specific antigens.[578] Chemotaxonomic analysis (e.g., cellular carbohydrates, fatty acids, EDTA–lysozyme-induced lysis kinetics) also indicate that this species is fairly heterogeneous. Discrimination of different strains may also be accomplished by molecular assays such as the polymerase chain reaction (PCR).[314,589]

CLINICAL SIGNIFICANCE

A. actinomycetemcomitans is a small gram-negative coccobacillus that is associated with actinomycotic infections, endocarditis, bacteremia, wound infections, and dental infections. The organism has frequently been coisolated along with *Actinomyces* species from actinomycotic abscesses; the organism's name is derived from its "concomitant" recovery with *Actinomyces* species.[420,515,759,839] However, it has also been isolated from similar lesions in the absence of the anaerobic actinomycetes.[130,331]

The most common infection associated with *A. actinomycetemcomitans* is subacute bacterial endocarditis.[389] Several cases of endocarditis caused by this organism have been reported in the literature; most of these were in individuals with valvular damage caused by congenital heart diseases, such as congenital aortic stenosis, bicuspid aortic valve disease, ventral septal defect, atrial–ventricular septal defect, or mitral insufficiency due to rheumatic heart disease.[4,136,142,156,282,389,419,670] Prosthetic mitral valve and aortic valve endocarditis with prolonged bacteremia have also been reported in individuals with porcine valves, mechanical valve replacements, and pacemakers.[306,806,769] Localized complications of native and prosthetic valve endocarditis with this organism have included pericarditis and paravalvular abscess.[362,806] A principal predisposing factor in the development of native or prosthetic valve endocarditis with this organism is poor dentition or recent dental manipulations.[20,136,670] *A. actinomycetemcomitans* endocarditis follows a subacute indolent course. Fever, weight loss, chills, cough, and night sweats are common, and a heart murmur is usually noted. Hepatosplenomegaly and peripheral stigmata of endocarditis (conjunctival hemorrhages, splinter hemorrhages) may or may not be present. Complications of this infection include septic emboli, congestive heart failure, placement of prosthetic valves because of native valvular damage, prosthetic heart valve replacement, infectious complications of hematogenous dissemination (e.g., endophthalmitis, glomerulonephritis), and death.[282,389,437,689]

Research in the area of dental microbiology has established an important role for *A. actinomycetemcomitans* in periodontal disease. This is related to the organism's primary ecologic niche in dental plaque, periodontal pockets, and gingival sulci. The organism is specifically related to a distinct clinical entity called **localized juvenile periodontitis** (LJP).[207,464] This is a disease of older children and young adults (ages 11 to 20 years) and is characterized by rapid degeneration and destruction of the alveolar bone supporting the first permanent molars and incisors. During the development of this condition, there is minimal plaque accumulation and little or no gingival inflammation.[207] That *A. actinomycetemcomitans* may be uniquely related to the development of this condition is supported by several studies. With use of a deep gingival sampling technique and selective media, Zambon and coworkers recovered the organism from 28 of 29 patients with localized juvenile periodontitis but from only 15% of other subjects, including 28 of 134 adult patients with periodontitis, 24 of 142 patients with healthy periodontia, and five of 98 juvenile diabetics with varying degrees of clinical gingivitis.[835] Mandell and Socransky isolated *A. actinomycetemcomitans* from all of six juvenile periodontitis patients but not from any of 48 patients with either gingivitis or adult periodontitis.[464] Immunologic studies also indicate that LJP patients have elevated antibody titers against *A. actinomycetemcomitans* antigens in the saliva, crevicular fluid, and serum.[217,278] Most patients with LJP develop antibodies against a 29-kDa outer membrane protein of *A. actinomycetemcomitans* that shares considerable homology with enteric outer membrane proteins.[807,808] There is also evidence suggesting that *A. actinomycetemcomitans* may be involved in some forms of adult periodontal disease as well.[656,708]

A. actinomycetemcomitans strains recovered from these patients produce a variety of putative virulence factors in vitro. These include a potent leukotoxin, a neutrophil chemotaxis-inhibiting factor, a fibroblast-inhibiting factor, a bone–resorption-inducing toxin, collagenase, alkaline phosphatase, and a lipopolysaccharide endotoxin.[401,465,693,758,766] The leukotoxin is capable of killing neutrophils, monocytes, and T lymphocytes by inducing cell membrane damage and causing cleavage and fragmentation of chromosomal DNA, possibly by activation of endogenous nucleases.[465] Production of leukotoxin in the supragingival area may result in a localized immunosuppression, central to the development of periodontal lesions of LJP.[207] The endotoxin of *A. actinomycetemcomitans* is able to initiate bone resorption, activate complement, and induce lysosomal release from polymorphonuclear leukocytes (PMNs). Chemotaxis of PMNs is markedly reduced in LJP patients and in family members without LJP, suggesting a genetic predisposition to the development of LJP.[207] Enzymes that are able to degrade immunoglobulins G, M, and A are also produced by *A. actinomycetemcomitans*, thereby preventing opsonization by antibody.[312] *A. actinomycetemcomitans* strains also produce cell-associated and extracellular components that are able to bind the Fc region of immunoglobulin molecules.[753] The presence of these components in the gingival and crevicular fluids may cause aggregation of immunoglobulin, rendering them unavailable for opsonization of the bacteria. Finally, this organism also produces fimbriae that are thought to initiate adherence of these organisms to oropharyngeal cells.[504] The possible role of these virulence factors in clinical disease is suggested by the gradual development of serum and gingival opsonins and neutralizing antibodies directed against some of these antigenic components. The establishment of an immune response may play a role in limiting the periodontal disease process itself.[217,656] In the absence of antimicrobial therapy, failure to produce antibodies against the organism or its products may partially explain why some patients with LJP develop more severe, generalized forms of periodontal disease as adults.[807] In addition to LJP and other forms of periodontal disease, *A. actinomycetemcomitans* is also implicated in the pathogenesis of Papillon-Lefevre syndrome, which is an inherited disease characterized by hyperkeratosis of the palms and soles and extensive periodontal destruction resulting in the loss of both primary and permanent teeth.[234]

Several other types of infections caused by *A. actinomycetemcomitans* have been reported and result either from contiguous spread of the organism from its habitat in the mouth or from hematogenous spread during bacteremia. Brain abscess, cervical and submandibular lymphadenitis, soft-tissue cellulitis, tenosynovitis; subcutaneous abscess, thyroid abscess, mediastinal abscess, intra-abdominal abscess, urinary tract infections, vertebral osteomyelitis, pericarditis, and coronary arteritis associated with *A. actinomycetemcomitans* have been reported.[130,245,250,376,331,389,524,557,839] Morris and Sewell reported a case of necrotizing pneumonia caused by

A. actinomycetemcomitans and *Actinomyces israelii* in a 46-year-old man 3 months after the extraction of several teeth because of advanced periodontal disease.[515] Kuijper and colleagues reported a case of disseminated actinomycosis in which both *A. actinomycetemcomitans* and *Actinomyces meyeri* were recovered from subcutaneous skin lesions and from cerebral abscesses.[420] The patient had slowly progressive pulmonary lesions during the preceeding 6 years that were suspected, but not proved, to be the source of both organisms. Pulmonary infections with *A. actinomycetemcomitans* as the sole pathogen (i.e., in the absence of *Actinomyces* species) are rare, with only four cases reported before 1990 in the English literature. In a case reported by Yuan and coworkers, the infection involved the lung, the soft tissue of the chest wall, and the overlying ribs and sternum.[834] Septic embolization of the organism from a primary pulmonary focus may also occur.[772] Osteomyelitis and septic arthritis owing to hematogenous dissemination of this organism have also been reported.[507] The portals of entry for these various types of infections have included oral lesions, prior pulmonary infections, skin abrasions, thoracotomy sites, and urinary tract instrumentation. Endogenous endophthalmitis complicating endocarditis and bacteremia with this organism have also been reported.[437]

CULTURAL CHARACTERISTICS AND IDENTIFICATION

A. actinomycetemcomitans grows slowly on chocolate and blood agars, with visible colonies appearing after 48 to 72 hours (see Color Plate 8-1E). Growth occurs on both chocolate and blood agar media, and colonies are nonhemolytic. Colonies of *A. actinomycetemcomitans* are small, smooth, translucent, and have slightly irregular edges. Fresh clinical isolates are adherent to the agar and are difficult to emulsify. On prolonged incubation (i.e., 5 to 7 days), colonies may develop a central density that takes on the appearance of a four- or six-pointed star. On repeated subculture the surface structure of the colonies become less marked and the colonies become less adherent. As with *H. aphrophilus*, growth in broth is scant and adherent to the sides of the tube. On a Gram stain the organisms appear as pale staining, gram-negative coccobacilli. On repeated subculture longer cells may be noted on stained smears.

Characteristics for the identification of *A. actinomycetemcomitans* include lack of growth on MacConkey and other enteric agars, and positive reactions for catalase production and nitrate reduction. The organism is oxidase-negative (occasional strains may be weakly positive), urease-negative, does not produce indole, and does not require X or V factors.[707] Lysine and ornithine decarboxylase and arginine dihydrolase reactions are negative. Most strains strongly ferment glucose, fructose, and mannose (see Color Plate 8-1F). Acid production from maltose, mannitol, and xylose may vary. *A. actinomycetemcomitans* can be differentiated from *H. aphrophilus* in that the former is catalase-positive, ONPG-negative, and acid is not produced from lactose, sucrose, or trehalose (see Table 8-1).

Molecular methods for identifying *A. actinomycetemcomitans* have also been described. Genetic studies have shown that the gene for the 23S ribosomal RNA in split into two smaller forms in *A. actinomycetemcomitans*, whereas the transcript is continuous in *H. aphrophilus, H. paraphrophilus, H. segnis,* and *H. influenzae.*[590] Recognition of this atypical pattern on polyacrylamide gel electrophoresis (PAGE) of RNA can provide accurate identification and strain differentiation of *A. actinomycetemcomitans* from single colonies.[314] Amplification and probe-based detection of this rRNA-spacer region has been applied to detection of *A. actinomycetemcomitans* directly in subgingival plaque samples.[449] Amplification of the *lktA* gene, the structural gene for the *A. actinomycetemcomitans* leukotoxin, has also been used for identification and direct detection of the organism in gingival fluid samples.[251,300,755] Although typing and characterization of *A. actinomycetemcomitans* strains may be accomplished by serology, other traditional and molecular-based methods that have been used include antibiogram typing; biotyping based on fermentation of mannose, mannitol, and xylose; sodium dodecyl sulfate (SDS)–polyacrylamide gel electrophoresis of outer membrane proteins; restriction endonuclease analysis of whole chromosomal DNA, restriction fragment length polymorphisms; and ribotyping.[33,203,332,709,767] Molecular-based assays may be of particular value in differentiating atypical strains of *A. actinomycetemcomitans* (e.g., catalase-negative strains) from haemophili and for epidemiologic studies.[589]

ANTIMICROBIAL SUSCEPTIBILITY

In addition to subgingival debridement, scaling, and root planing, antimicrobial therapy directed against the bacterial agents associated with LJP appears to be essential for eradicating *A. actinomycetemcomitans* from deep periodontal pockets. In vitro studies indicate that all serotypes of *A. actinomycetemcomitans* are susceptible to tetracyline, doxycycline, cefaclor, cefuroxime, ceftriaxone, trimethoprim–sulfamethoxazole, rifampin, and ciprofloxacin.[558,560,829] Variable susceptibilities to penicillin, ampicillin, erythromycin, azithromycin, clarithromycin, and the aminoglycosides have been reported.[228,558,829] Azithromycin appears to be more active against *A. actinomycetemcomitamns* than other macrolides, including erythromycin.[558] The various *A. actinomycetemcomitans* serotypes also differ slightly in their susceptibility to antimicrobial agents.[560] In vitro studies indicate that combinations of various therapeutic agents for the treatment of *A. actinomycetemcomitans* endocarditis may be synergistic, additive, or antagonistic.[568,829] Hence, the efficacy of combination therapy cannot be predicted, and these properties must be determined for individual strains. Tetracycline and its congeners have been the drug of choice for treatment of periodontal infections with this organism; however, tetracycline resistance owing to acquisition of a plasmid-borne *tetB* determinant by *A. actinomycetemcomitans* has been reported.[633] Both agar dilution using *Haemophilus* test medium and the E test

(AB Biodisk, Solna, Sweden) have been used to determine antimicrobial susceptibilities of this fastidious pathogen.[534,559]

ACTINOBACILLUS UREAE

On the basis of genetic and phenotypic studies, it has also been proposed that several *Pasteurella* species, including *P. ureae, P. pneumotropica, P. aerogenes,* and *P. haemolytica* may actually be more closely related to the animal species of *Actinobacillus.*[7,76,197,235,531] Similarities in phenotypic traits include similar oxidase and catalase reactions, reduction of nitrate to nitrite, growth on MacConkey agar, production of urease, and fermentation of several carbohydrates. At this writing, *P. ureae* is the only species that has formally been transferred to the genus *Actinobacillus* as *Actinobacillus ureae.*[235,532]

A. ureae has been recovered only from humans. It is an uncommon commensel of the human respiratory tract and has been isolated from human infections, including bacteremia, endocarditis, meningitis, atrophic rhinitis, bronchitis, pneumonia, conjunctivitis, otitis media, and peritonitis.[68,70,85,94,313,471,546,724,826] Usually an underlying or predisposing condition is present, such as postsurgical infection, diabetes, periodontal disease, emphysema, and alcohol-associated cirrhosis of the liver. Cases of meningitis have been associated with previous skull trauma (assault, cranial surgery) and with underlying disease, including human immunodeficiency virus (HIV) infection.[68,386,826]

A. ureae is a pleomorphic gram-negative bacillus; on staining, some stains form distinct filaments. After 24 hours of growth on blood agar in a CO_2 environment, colonies are smooth, 1 mm in diameter and nonhemolytic. The organism is oxidase-positive, catalasepositive, reduces nitrate to nitrite, and does not grow on MacConkey agar. The species rapidly decomposes urea. No indole is produced, and all decarboxylase and dihydrolase reactions are negative. Acid is produced from glucose, maltose, sucrose, and mannitol; no acid is produced from lactose and xylose. The other biochemically similar *Actinobacillus* species may be differentiated from *A. ureae* by acid production from additional carbohydrates (e.g., lactose and xylose) and by the abilities of the former species to grow on MacConkey agar (see Table 8-1). The *A. ureae* strains are susceptible to most antimicrobial agents, including penicillin, ampicillin, cephalothin, cefoxitin, tetracycline, trimethoprim–sulfamethoxazole, and the aminoglycosides.

ANIMAL SPECIES IN THE GENUS ACTINOBACILLUS

In addition to *A. actinomycetemcomitans* and *A. ureae,* ten other species of *Actinobacillus* have been described. These include *A. lignieresii, A. equuli, A. suis, A. capsulatus, A. hominis, A. pleuropneumoniae, A. muris, A. rossii, A. seminis,* and the proposed species *A. delphinicola.*[53,75,261a,268,505,577,642,710,768] These species make up a part of the normal flora of certain animals and may occasionally cause disease in them. *A. lignieresii* is associated with granulomatous infections in the oral cavity ("wooden tongue" disease) and gastrointestinal tracts

TABLE 8-2

Biochemical Characteristics for Identification of *Actinobacillus* Species of Animal Origin

Species	β-Hemolysis SBA	Oxidase	Catalase	Growth on Mac	NO₃ Red	Ind	Ure	ODC	Phos
A. lignieresii	−	v⁺	v	+	+	−	+	−	+
A. equuli	−	v⁺	v	+	+	−	+	−	+
A. suis	+	v⁺	+	+	+	−	+	−	+
A. capsulatus	−	+	+	+	+	−	+	−	+
A. hominis	−	+	−	−	+	−	+	−	+
A. muris	−	+	+		+	−	+	−	−
A. pleuropneumoniae	+	v	v	−	+	−	+	−	+
A. rossiiᵃ	v	+	+	v⁺	+	−	+	−	+
A. seminis	−	v	+	−	+	−	−	v	−
A. delphinicola	−	+	−	−	+	−	−	v	+

+, >90% of strains positive
−, >90% of strains negative
v⁺, 80–89% of strains positive
v⁻, 80–90% of strains negative
vʷ, Reactions variable, but weak when positive
v, 21–79% of strains positive
+ʷ, weak-positive reaction
a, Some strains may produce gas from glucose
SBA, sheep blood agar
Mac, MacConkey agar
No₃ Red, nitrate reduction
Ind, indole production
Ure, urease production
ODC, ornithine decarboxylase
Phos, phosphatase

ONPG, o-nitrophenyl-β-D-galactopyranoside
Glu, glucose
Malt, maltose
Suc, sucrose
Lac, lactose
Xyl, xylose
Mntl, mannitol
Tre, trehalose hydrolysis
Mann, mannose
Arab, arabinose
Sorb, sorbitol
Gal, galactose
Inos, inositol
Raff, raffinose
V factor, NAD

of cattle and with pneumonic and cutaneous infections in sheep and other ungulates. *A. equuli* causes bacteremia, peritonitis, nephritis, and bone and joint infections in horses and swine.[297] It has also been isolated from systemic and localized infections in monkeys, calves, dogs, and rabbits; *A. suis* causes septicemia, pneumonia, and arthritis in in-fant and adult pigs, and can cause similar diseases in horses.[572,660] *A. capsulatus*, an encapsulated species, causes arthritis in rabbits and has been recovered from joint fluid specimens from these animals. Formerly considered to be related to the haemophili because of its V factor requirement, *A. pleuropneumoniae* is an important primary pathogen in pigs, in which it causes a highly contagious pleuropneumonia.[505] *A. muris* strains are recovered from the genital tracts of mice,[75] *A. rossii* has been recovered from the vaginas of postparturient sows and aborted piglets, and *A. seminis* causes epididymitis and sterility in sheep.[53,642,710,768] *A. delphinicola* has been isolated from sea mammals.[261a]

Human infections with animal species of *Actinobacillus* usually occur as a result of trauma associated with animals. *A. lignieresii*, *A. equuli*, and *A. suis* all have been recovered from human clinical specimens, including horse and sheep bite wounds, joint fluid, blood, and sputum.[58,199,572,577] *A. hominis* has been recovered from sputum specimens of individuals with chronic lung disease and from empyema fluid.[268] Wust and colleagues reported on two patients with hepatic failure that was due to chronic hepatitis B infection and alcoholic cirrhosis, in whom *A. hominis* septicemia occurred as the terminal event in their illness.[820] *A. rossii*, *A. seminis*, *A. capsulatus*, *A. muris*, and *A. pleuropneumoniae* have not been isolated from human clinical specimens. Characteristics for identifying *Actinobacillus* species of animal origin are presented in Table 8-2.

CARDIOBACTERIUM HOMINIS

TAXONOMY

Cardiobacterium hominis, the single species in the genus *Cardiobacterium*, was originally called CDC group IID and was christened *Cardiobacterium hominis* by Slotnick and Doughtery in 1964.[705] The latter workers demonstrated the unique biochemical features of the organism and showed that it was antigenically unrelated to a large number of other fastidious gram-negative and gram-positive bacteria. In the 1984 edi-

SPECIES	ONPG	ACID PRODUCTION FROM													REQ. FOR V FACTOR
		GLU	MALT	SUC	LAC	XYL	MNTL	TRE	MANN	ARAB	SORB	GAL	INOS	RAFF	
A. lignieresii	v	+	+	+	v	+	+	−	+	v⁻	v⁻	+	−	v	−
A. equuli	v	+	+	+	+	+	+	+	+	v⁻	v	v	−	+	−
A. suis	v⁺	+	+	+	+	+	−	+	+	v⁺	−	v⁺	−	+	−
A. capsulatus	+	+	+	+	+	+	+	+	+	−	+	+	−	+	−
A. hominis	+	+	+	+	+	+	+	+	−	−	−	+	−	+	−
A. muris	−	+	+	+	−	−	+	+	+	−	−	vʷ	vʷ	+	−
A. pleuropneumoniae	+	+	+	+	v	+	+	−	+	−	−	+ʷ	−	v	+
A. rossiᵃ	v⁺	+	v⁻	−	v	+	+	−	v	+	+	+	+	v⁻	−
A. seminis	−	+	v	−	−	−	v	−	−	v	−	v	v	−	−
A. delphinicola	−	+	−	−	−	−	−	−	+	−	−	−	−	−	−

tion of *Bergey's Manual of Systematic Bacteriology*, this organism was included with "other genera" in the section on facultatively anaerobic gram-negative bacilli.[788] In 1990, Dewhirst and coworkers examined *Cardiobacterium* strains using 16S ribosomal RNA sequence analysis and found that this organism and *Kingella indologenes* were closely related to one another and differed significantly from reference strains of other fastidious organisms.[196] They proposed a new family, the *Cardiobacteriaceae*, to include *C. hominis* and *K. indologenes*.[196] In the same publication, these authors presented genetic evidence that supported the phenotypic similarities between *C. hominis* and *K. indologenes*, and suggested that *K. indologenes* be renamed *Suttonella indologenes* and removed from the family *Neisseriaceae* into the new family *Cardiobacteriaceae*.[196]

CLINICAL SIGNIFICANCE

C. hominis has the unique characteristic of being associated almost exclusively with endocarditis.[280,380,666,817,818] It may be isolated from the human upper respiratory tract as a part of the normal flora, but, because of its slow growth rate, it is rarely noted in these specimens. The organism apparently is not found in other body sites, including the genital tract.[704] As with the other HACEK organisms, *C. hominis* enters the bloodstream and usually infects previously diseased or damaged heart valves.[143,817,818] However, *C. hominis* endocarditis has also been reported in individuals with no evidence of previous heart disease.[430,636] Prosthetic valve endocarditis associated with this organism may also occur.[592,746,817,818] The infection follows a very subacute course, with an insidious onset and vague symptoms. Consequently, the physician must have a high index of suspicion that he or she is dealing with this organism

and should inform the laboratory so that extra efforts to recover the organism may be taken. Patients frequently have a history of having had dental work performed before the the onset of symptoms of endocarditis.[591,666,818] In one case report, the patient developed prosthetic valve endocarditis following upper gastrointestinal endoscopy.[592] Complications include the development of septic emboli, mycotic aneurysms, and congestive heart failure.[430,573] *C. hominis* is rarely associated with infections other than endocarditis. In 1991, Rechtman and Nadler reported the recovery of *C. hominis* along with *Clostridium bifermentans* from an abdominal abscess and from the blood of a 65-year-old man with diabetes.[610]

CULTURAL CHARACTERISTICS AND IDENTIFICATION

Because *C. hominis* is associated with endocarditis, it will be isolated from blood cultures. The organism grows slowly and may be recovered in essentially all commercially available blood culture media. No visible change in the blood culture medium (e.g., hemolysis, pellicle formation, turbidity) will be noted, so frequent blind subculture transfer from macroscopically negative blood culture bottles to chocolate and blood agars should be performed. In our experience, the BACTEC radiometric blood culture system has been able to detect growth of the organism after 3 to 5 days. Characteristically, the growth indices on the BACTEC will increase in small increments over time when bottles become positive with this organism. Gram stains of positive blood bottles may not reveal the organism; a low-speed centrifugation to remove red blood cells and a high-speed centrifugation to pellet small numbers of organisms may aid in their visualization. On Gram staining, the organisms may appear gram-variable, with a tendency for the cells to retain the crystal violet dye at the poles. Individual cells may appear swollen at one or both ends, resulting in "tear-drop," "dumb-bell," and "lollypop-shaped" organisms. The morphology of the individual cells is dependent on the type of culture medium used. In media containing yeast extract, cells may appear as uniform, gram-negative bacilli. Frequently, the cells will assume rosette-shaped clusters or "picket fence" arrangements in their orientation with one another (see Color Plate 8-1*G*).

On blood and chocolate agars, *C. hominis* grows as very small, glistening, opaque colonies, generally after 48 to 72 hours at 35°C in 5% to 7% CO_2 (see Color Plate 8-1*H*). Some strains may also pit the agar on further incubation. No growth is observed on MacConkey agar or other enteric selective or differential agars. The organism is oxidase-positive, catalase-negative, nitrate-negative, and urease-negative. The positive oxidase

and negative nitrate reduction reactions help differentiate this organism from *H. aphrophilus* and *A. actinomycetemcomitans* but is similar to reactions seen for *Eikenella, Kingella,* and *Suttonella* (Table 8-3). The most helpful feature for identifying this organism is the production of indole. A tryptone broth should be heavily inoculated (with a swab) and incubated for 48 hours. Extraction with xylene or chloroform and use of Ehrlich's reagent rather than Kovac's reagent allows the detection of the small amounts of indole produced by this organism. The spot indole reagent (*p*-aminocinnamaldehyde) may or may not detect indole production by *C. hominis*. Hydrogen sulfide production can be detected using lead acetate strips. *C. hominis* produces acid from glucose, fructose, sucrose, mannose, and sorbitol; acid production from maltose and mannitol is variable with most strains producing positive reactions. Lactose, xylose, galactose, trehalose, and

TABLE 8-3
BIOCHEMICAL CHARACTERISTICS FOR IDENTIFICATION OF *CARDIOBACTERIUM HOMINIS, EIKENELLA CORRODENS, KINGELLA* SPECIES, AND *SUTTONELLA INDOLOGENES*

CHARACTERISTIC	C. HOMINIS	E. CORRODENS	K. KINGAE	K. DENITRIFICANS	K. ORALIS	S. INDOLOGENES
Hemolysis, sheep blood agar	−	−	+*	−	−	−
Oxidase	+	+	+	+	+	+
Catalase	−	−†	−	−	−	−
Reduction of NO_3 to NO_2	−	+	−	+	−	−
Reduction of NO_2 to gas	+	−	+	+	−	+
Indole	+	−	−	−	−	+
Urease	−	−	−	−	−	−
Ornithine decarboxylase	−	+	−	−	−	−
Hydrolysis of esculin	−	−	−	−	−	−
Hydrolysis of ONPG	−	−	−	−	−	−
Gas from glucose	−	−	−	−	−	−
Production of acid from						
Glucose	+	−	+	+	+	+
Maltose	+‡	−	+	−	−	+
Fructose	+	−	−	−	−	+
Sucrose	+	−	−	−	−	+
Lactose	−	−	−	−	−	−
Xylose	−	−	−	−	−	−
Mannitol	+‡	−	−	−	−	−
Mannose	+	−	−	−	−	+
Galactose	−	−	−	−	−	−
Trehalose	−	−	−	−	−	−
Raffinose	−	−	−	−	−	−
Sorbitol	+	−	−	−	−	−

*Most strains produce a "soft" β-hemolysis on sheep blood agar.
†Rare strains may be weakly catalase-positive.
‡Rare strains may be maltose- or mannitol-negative, or both.

raffinose are not fermented. Phenotypically, *C. hominis* is very similar to *S. indologenes* (see Table 8-3).[106]

ANTIMICROBIAL SUSCEPTIBILITY

C. hominis strains are generally susceptible to most antimicrobial agents, including penicillin, ampicillin, cephalothin, aminoglycosides, chloramphenicol, and tetracycline. Patients with *C. hominis* endocarditis are generally treated with penicillin alone or with penicillin combined with an aminoglycoside. Most patients with endocarditis caused by *C. hominis* are successfully treated with antibiotics alone, although some may require partial valve resection or valve replacement owing to hemodynamic compromise.[143,746] Penicillin-resistant strains are rare; in fact, the first report of endocarditis caused by a β-lactamase–producing strain of *C. hominis* was published in 1994.[446] This particular strain was susceptible to tetracycline, rifampin, vancomycin, and imipenem and was resistant to erythromycin, trimethoprim–sulfamethoxazole, gentamicin, amoxicillin, ticarcillin, cefotaxime, and piperacillin. Resistance to vancomycin and erythromycin is of some importance because these antimicrobial agents are occasionally used for dental prophylaxis in patients who are allergic to penicillin.[591]

EIKENELLA CORRODENS

TAXONOMY

Originally, the genus *Eikenella* defined facultative strains that were thought to be related to the anaerobic species *Bacteroides corrodens*; the obligate anaerobic species is now called *Bacteroides ureolyticus*. A key characteristic that separates these organisms from the facultative genus *Eikenella* is urease activity, with the anaerobic strains being urease-positive. *Bacteroides ureolyticus* is also susceptible to clindamycin and metronidazole (Flagyl), whereas *E. corrodens* is resistant to these agents. These faculative organisms were also termed HB-1 (*Haemophilus*-like bacteria) and are now included in the monospecific genus *Eikenella* as *Eikenella corrodens*.[91,367] On the basis of 16S ribosomal RNA sequencing and ribosomal RNA–DNA hybridization work, it was shown that *E. corrodens* is related to *Neisseria* species; currently genus *Eikenella* is a member of the newly emended family *Neisseriaceae*.[195,643]

Efforts have been made to define putative virulence factors of *E. corrodens*. In 1988, Yamazaki and his colleagues described a lectinlike protein on the surface of *E. corrodens* strains that functioned in adherence of the bacteria to human crevicular epithelial cells and interacted with a galactose-bearing receptor on the epithelial cell surface.[828] This same molecule was also able to agglutinate red blood cells. Subsequently, genes that code for two distinct hemagglutinins were cloned, characterized, and sequenced.[606] In addition, *E. corrodens* possesses pili on its surface that are also believed to function in adherence. Two of the genes that code for pilus proteins, *ecpA* and *ecpB*, are distinct from those for the hemagglutinins, and they show nucleotide sequence homology with pilin genes from *Morax-*

ella bovis.[605] Two other pilus genes, *ecpC* and *ecpD*, have been described that show considerable nucleotide sequence divergence from each other and from both *ecpA* and *ecpB*, and code for pili that demonstrate amino acid sequence homology with pili from *Neisseria gonorrhoeae* and *Pseudomonas aeruginosa*.[756] *Eikenella corrodens* also posesses a principal outer membrane protein with an apparent molecular mass of 33,000 to 42,000 Da.[462] This protein is able to trigger the release of lysosomal enzymes by macrophages and also may stimulate or depress macrophage activity in a dose-dependent manner. These bacteria also synthesize a slime layer in vivo that may function to impede phagocytosis.[593] Like other gram-negative bacteria, *E. corrodens* has an outer membrane lipopolysaccharide (LPS) that has biologic activities similar to the LPS found in enteric bacteria.[594] Similar to the outer membrane proteins, the LPS of *E. corrodens* shows considerable structural heterogeneity from strain to strain.[134] Serologically, surface antigens of *E. corrodens* show cross-reactivity with other bacterial species, including *K. kingae*, *K. denitrificans*, and *Moraxella bovis*.[134,135]

CLINICAL SIGNIFICANCE

E. corrodens is a part of the normal flora of the mouth and upper respiratory tract.[135,733] In this location the organism is associated with dental and periodontal infections (periapical abscesses, gingivitis, root canal infections), ocular infections (canaliculitis, periorbital cellulitis, corneal ulcerations, endophthalmitis, lacrimal abscesses), head and neck infections (sinusitis, brain abscesses, subdural and extradural empyema, septic cavernous sinus thrombosis, thyroid abscess, otitis media, and mastoiditis), and pleuropulmonary infections (aspiration pneumonia, mixed bacterial lung abscess, pleural fluid infection).[34,137,289,302,343,383,385,405] Pulmonary infection with *E. corrodens* is seen in the settings of immunosuppression, propensity for pulmonary aspiration, and the presence of underlying lung disease resulting in compromised local defense mechanisms.[385,732] It has also been implicated, along with obligately anaerobic species (i.e., *Actinomyces* or *Arachnia* species), in the pathogenesis of a condition called chronic diffuse sclerosing osteomyelitis, which is a mixed infection of the mandible that has distinctive radiologic and tomographic scan patterns and occurs primarily in young women.[475] By extension from periodontal, middle ear, or sinus infections, the organism may enter the central nervous system, leading to meningitis, brain or paraspinal abscesses, and subdural empyema.[100,225,289]

Bacteremia and endocarditis caused by *E. corrodens* may also occur; most of these infections have been in immunocompromised hosts, intravenous drug abusers, or individuals with previous valvular damage who had recently had extensive dental work.[289,554,714] Prosthetic valve endocarditis and infections of indwelling vascular prostheses associated with *E. corrodens* have also been reported.[181] *E. corrodens* bacteremia, with or without endocarditis, may also occur in individuals with underlying disease (e.g., rheumatoid arthritis, hematologic malignancies).[239] In recent years, *E. corro-*

dens has been isolated from cutaneous and subcutaneous abscesses and from cellulitis associated with the injection of drugs ("skin popping"), when needles are lubricated with saliva before introduction of the needle into the skin, or when saliva is used to dissolve the drug before injection, or to cleanse the skin following injection.[19,301,554,714] This organism may also be isolated from infections of the hand following "clenched fist injuries" resulting from fist fights.[295,381] Traumatic implantation of the organism into the subcutaneous tissue by this or other mechanisms (e.g., puncture wounds, human bite wounds, chronic paronychia related to nail biting) may result in extension of the organism into the bone, resulting in osteomyelitis and septic arthritis.[381,655,695] In these settings the organism is often recovered in mixed culture with other facultative organisms (α- and β-hemolytic streptococci, *Staphylococcus aureus*, coagulase-negative staphylococci, enteric gram-negative bacilli, and obligate anaerobes [*Peptostreptococcus* species, oral *Bacteroides*, *Prevotella*, and *Porphyromonas* species]). Cases of bacteremic *E. corrodens* infection resulting in cellulitis, septic arthritis, vertebral osteomyelitis, intervertebral diskitis, paraspinal abscess, and sacroiliitis have also been reported.[215,252,547,596] *E. corrodens* has also been isolated from a patient with Brodie's abscess, which is a chronic localized bone abscess found on the distal tibia and usually caused by *S. aureus*.[426] *E. corrodens* may also be recovered from the gastrointestinal tract and in this milieu may be present in mixed culture with facultative and anaerobic gut flora in the settings of abdominal abscesses and peritonitis.[728] The organism has also been isolated in pure culture from splenic and pancreatic abscesses.[415,575,603,728] It has also been isolated from gynecologic infections, mostly in cases of endometritis and cervicitis, resulting from colonization of intrauterine devices,[378,733] and from an amniocentesis specimen of a 25-year-old woman with premature labor and chorioamnionitis.[378]

CULTURAL CHARACTERISTICS AND IDENTIFICATION

E. corrodens can be recovered on blood and chocolate agar and does not grow on MacConkey agar. Colonies are small (0.5 to 1.0 mm) after 48 hours. About 50% of isolates may "pit" the agar as they grow, and both pitting and nonpitting variants may be observed in the same culture (see Color Plate 8-2A). A pale yellow pigment (observed best on a white swab swept through growth on a chocolate agar plate) is usually produced, and most strains have an odor suggestive of sodium hypochlorite (i.e., Clorox bleach) when grown on commercial chocolate and blood agars. On a gram-stained slide the organisms appear as regular, slender gram-negative bacilli or coccobacilli with rounded ends.

Biochemical characteristics of both pitting and nonpitting *E. corrodens* strains are uniform. The organisms are oxidase-positive and catalase-negative, although rare strains may be weakly catalase-positive. The organism reduces nitrate to nitrite and does not require X or V factors, although hemin is necessary for aerobic growth.[367] Nonpitting isolates may be mistaken for

Haemophilus species and, when tested with X and V factor disks, display growth around the X, but not around the V, disk. Indole and urease are not produced, but most strains are lysine decarboxylase- and ornithine decarboxylase-positive (see Color Plate 8-2B). Unlike the other organisms in the HACEK group, *E. corrodens* does not produce acid from carbohydrates. Consequently, in some texts the organism is grouped with the nonfermentative bacteria, although its cultural characteristics correspond more to those of the fastidious gram-negative bacteria. The phenotypic characteristics of *E. corrodens* are presented in Table 8-3, along with the other oxidase-positive, catalase-negative fastidious HACEK bacteria.

As with many of the organisms involved in periodontal infection, molecular approaches for detection, identification, and typing of *E. corrodens* have also been explored. *E. corrodens*–specific DNA probes, as well as probes for other periodontal pathogens, have been designed by analysis of 16S rRNA, identification of unique nucleotide sequences, and chemical synthesis of probe molecules that are complementary to these species-specific sequences.[204] These probes have been used for direct detection of the organism in subgingival plaque samples of patients with gingivitis, periodontitis, and HIV-associated periodontal disease.[452,528] Epidemiologic methods, including SDS-PAGE, pulsed-field gel electrophoresis, and restriction endonuclease analysis, have also been applied to *E. corrodens* to determine relatedness to other bacteria and strain differences among different *E. corrodens* isolates.[132,133,727]

ANTIMICROBIAL SUSCEPTIBILITY

Most *E. corrodens* strains are susceptible to ampicillin, ticarcillin, carbenicillin, tetracycline, and chloramphenicol and are resistant to the penicillinase-resistant penicillins (e.g., methicillin, dicloxacillin, nafcillin, and oxacillin), clindamycin, lincomycin, vancomycin, erythromycin, metronidazole, and the aminoglycosides. Penicillin susceptibility may vary from strain to strain. Most isolates are variably susceptible to the first-generation cephalosporins. Goldstein and coworkers found that cefazolin was the most active of these agents, whereas cephalothin showed moderate activity.[296] The second-generation cephalosporin cefamandole showed poor activity against *E. corrodens*. This organism is also susceptible to cefoxitin, cefuroxime, cetriaxone, ciprofloxacin, and the carbopenems (imipenem and meropenem).[147] Although they are rare, β-lactamase-positive strains of *E. corrodens* have been reported.[296,429] The β-lactamase enzyme in *E. corrodens* is highly cell-associated, shows little activity against cephalosporins, and is strongly inhibited by clavulanate and sulbactam.[429]

KINGELLA SPECIES AND *SUTTONELLA INDOLOGENES*

TAXONOMY

The type species of the genus *Kingella*, *K. kingae*, was originally described in the 1960s by Elizabeth King and at that time was called CDC group M-1.

Early descriptions of several strains suggested that this organism was related to the moraxellae, except that they were catalase-negative.[711] The organism was renamed *Moraxella kingii* and, subsequently, this name was taxonomically amended to *Moraxella kingae*.[92] In 1976, Henriksen and Bovre recommended that *M. kingae* be removed from the genus *Moraxella* and renamed as the new genus and species *Kingella kingae* in the family *Neisseriaceae*.[344] This was done because of substantial genetic unrelatedness to the moraxellae, differences in fatty acid content, and differences in a variety of phenotypic characteristics, including catalase activity, saccharolytic capabilities, and hemolytic reactions. Also in 1976, Snell and LaPage proposed the transfer of two other moraxella-like, oxidase-positive, catalase-negative, saccharolytic species to the genus *Kingella*.[712] These new species included the organism previously identified as the "TM-1" group, described by Hollis and colleagues (*Kingella denitrificans*), and indole-positive strains that had originally been isolated from cases of conjunctivitis (*Kingella indologenes*).[352,712] Other oxidase-positive, catalase-negative organisms that must be differentiated from the *Kingella* species include *C. hominis* and *E. corrodens* (see Table 8-3).

Nucleic acid relatedness studies have now determined that *K. indologenes* is more closely related to *C. hominis* than to the other two *Kingella* species or to the other members of the family *Neisseriaceae*.[196] However, although *C. hominis* and *K. indologenes* are very similar phenotypically, the G–C content of their DNA differs enough to warrant separate species status. On the basis of these data, it was proposed that *K. indologenes* be removed from the family *Neisseriaceae*, renamed *Suttonella indologenes* (after the Australian microbiologist R. G. A. Sutton) and placed with *C. hominis* in the family *Cardiobacteriaceae*.[196] The other two *Kingella* species remain in the newly emended family *Neisseriaceae*.[195,643] In 1993, Dewhirst and colleagues described a new species of *Kingella* that was recovered from human dental plaque of a patient with adult periodontitis.[194] This new species was named *Kingella orale*; this name subsequently was emended as *Kingella oralis*.

CLINICAL SIGNIFICANCE

Although they are part of the normal upper respiratory and genitourinary tract flora of humans, *Kingella* species, and *K. kingae* in particular, may occasionally be isolated from significant infections. *K. kingae* appears to have a specific tissue tropism for cardiac, valvular, joint space, and skeletal tissue; therefore, it has been associated primarily with bacteremia, endocarditis, and bone and joint infections.[146,260,518,552,773,822] The portal of entry for the organism into the bloodstream is probably by a breach in the oropharyngeal mucosa.[260] Many patients are noted to have poor oral hygiene, pharyngitis, or mucosal ulcerations resulting from treatment for other conditions (e.g., radiation therapy).[773,824] In one reported case, the patient experienced acute gastroenteritis before the onset of systemic symptoms, raising the question of possible foodborne transmission.[260] *K. kingae* endocarditis, as with the

other fastidious bacteria discussed thus far, occurs primarily in those persons with underlying heart disease (congenital malformation, rheumatic heart disease, mitral valve prolapse) or cardiac prostheses, although cases in persons with no previous heart disease have been reported.[552,773] Cardiac complications, including pericarditis, pericardial abscess, embolic phenomena, mycotic aneurysm, cerebral infarction, and congestive heart failure, may also occur in the clinical course of *K. kingae* disease.[773] Bacteremia caused by *K. kingae* has also been reported as the immediate cause of death in a patient with acquired immunodeficiency syndrome (AIDS) from India.[761]

Among bone and joint infections, septic arthritis with osteomyelitis is the most common clinical presentation.[185,271,428,518,564,609,773,776,824] These localized infections result from hematogenous spread of the organism. The joints most frequently involved in arthritis are the knees and hip. Usually, *K. kingae* osteomyelitis affects the femur, other long bones, and the vertebrae, leading to spondylitis and intervertebral diskitis; however, osteomyelitis of the small bones of the heel has also been reported.[825] Interestingly, *K. kingae* intervertebral diskitis and osteomyelitis are most often seen in infants and young children, usually 5 years of age and younger.[128,305,428,824] Some of these children may also have significant underlying conditions, such as acute lymphocytic leukemia or congenital heart disease. Although rare, bone and joint infections caused by *K. kingae*, including intervertebral diskitis, have also been diagnosed in adults.[493]

Septicemia with *K. kingae* may also mimic systemic neisserial infections (i.e., meningococcemia or disseminated gonococcal infection) in its clinical presentation. Redfield and coworkers[611] reported a case of *K. kingae* bacteremia in a 4-year-old boy with acute lymphocytic leukemia who presented with skin lesions and joint involvement suggestive of disseminated gonococcal infection (see Chapter 10). Acute *K. kingae* meningitis in a female patient with sickle cell anemia, *K. kingae* bacteremia presenting as meningococcemia in a male patient with alcoholic liver disease, and a "DGI-like" arthritis–dermatitis syndrome caused by *K. kingae* septicemia in a previously healthy 21-year-old woman have been reported.[690,757] Additional complications of *K. kingae* bacteremia and bone infections include meningitis, paraspinal abscess, hematogenous endophthalmitis, and corneal abscess.[117,509,785,812]

Kingella denitrificans and *S. indologenes* have rarely been isolated from clinically significant infections: *K. denitrificans* has been cultured from the upper respiratory and genitourinary tracts, where it constitutes a part of the normal flora. A small number of publications document *K. denitificans* as a cause of septicemia and endocarditis.[104,293,336,396,738] In these reports, patients ranged from 22 to 66 years of age, and all but one had either preexisting valvular disease or had prosthetic valves in place. Many of the patients had undergone dental procedures without prophylaxis or had concomitant respiratory tract infections. This organism has also been recovered from empyema fluid of a patient with bronchogenic carcinoma and from the bone marrow of an AIDS patient.[501,508] It was also isolated along with group B streptococci from the amniotic fluid of a 23-year-old woman with chorioamnionitis.[457] *S. indologenes* has been isolated from human eye infections and was first reported in association with a case of prosthetic valve endocarditis in 1987.[375,711,737,763] *K. oralis* has not been associated with any infectious process.

CULTURAL CHARACTERISTICS AND IDENTIFICATION

Kingella species are plump gram-negative bacilli or coccobacilli that sometimes occur in pairs or short chains. They are oxidase-positive and, unlike *Neisseria* and *Moraxella* species, catalase-negative. All species grow on chocolate and blood agars and do not grow on MacConkey agar or other enteric media. Multiple colony types may be produced in a single culture. *K. kingae* is β-hemolytic on sheep blood agar; the hemolytic reaction is "soft," resembling group B streptococci and may be noted only in areas of confluent growth or after the removal of the colony from the agar surface. Both *K. kingae* and *K. denitrificans* may pit or corrode the agar surface, particularly on primary isolation. The ability to pit the agar is related to the presence of pili on these two organisms; non-pitting colonial variant lack surface pili.[791] *S. indologenes* is distinguished by its ability to produce indole. Similar to *C. hominis*, this characteristic should be determined in tryptone broth, with xylene extraction and addition of Ehrlich's indole reagent. *K. denitrificans* was originally called TM-1 and was first recognized by its ability to grow on Thayer-Martin medium.[352] It will also produce acid from glucose in supplemented media, rapid carbohydrate degradation tests, and various kit systems; it is also prolyl-aminopeptidase-positive (see Color Plate 8-2C). Because of these characteristics, *K. denitrificans* may be misidentified as *N. gonorrhoeae*, particularly in specimens from the genitourinary tract.[350,371,372] This organism, unlike the other species in the genus, reduces nitrate to nitrite, and most strains will also reduce nitrite to nitrogen gas on prolonged incubation. *K. oralis* produces acid from glucose only, but may be differentiated from *K. denitrificans* by its failure to reduce nitrate and nitrite and the absence of prolylaminopeptidase activity.[194] *S. indologenes* may be differentiated from *C. hominis*, which it closely resembles, by appearance on Gram stain, positive alkaline phosphatase activity, and failure to produce acid from mannitol and sorbitol.[106,196] *E. corrodens* may be differentiated from both *C. hominis* and *Kingella* species by its Gram stain morphology, failure to ferment carbohydrates, and its positive ornithine and lysine decarboxylase reactions. Biochemical reactions for identification of *Kingella* species and *S. indologenes* are presented in Table 8-3.

Although identification of these organisms is straightforward once they are isolated, some workers have reported difficulty in the recovery of *K. kingae* from clinical specimens, particularly joint fluid specimens, from patients with arthritis and osteomyelitis. Yagupsky and coworkers found that direct plating of aspirates was much less sensitive for recovering *K. kingae* than inoculation of BACTEC blood culture media.[823] Among 100 specimens cultured by both methods, 34 grew significant organisms; 10 of the 11 *K. kingae* isolates that were obtained grew only in the BACTEC medium and were not recovered on direct plating. The discrepancy in the isolation rate of *K. kingae* was not observed for other organisms causing bone and joint infections.

ANTIMICROBIAL SUSCEPTIBILITY

K. kingae strains are usually susceptible to penicillin, ampicillin, oxacillin, cephalosporins of all generations, chloramphenicol, the aminoglycosides, trimethoprim–sulfamethoxazole, and ciprofloxacin. Some strains may be relatively resistant to erythromycin, and most strains are resistant to clindamycin, lincomycin, and vancomycin.[377] Isolates of *K. denitrificans* have antimicrobial susceptibilities similar to *K. kingae*; growth of *K. denitrificans* on Thayer-Martin agar indicates that they are resistant to vancomycin and colistin.[352] The *K. indologenes* endocarditis isolate reported by Jenny and coworkers was susceptible to ampicillin, cefazolin, and tobramycin.[375] In 1993, Sordillo and colleagues recovered a *K. kingae* strain from the blood of a 29-year-old AIDS patient that produced β-lactamase and was highly resistant to ampicillin, cefazolin, and ticarcillin but was susceptible to β-lactamase resistant agents and combination drugs containing β-lactamase inhibitors (clavulanate and sulbactam).[717]

OTHER MISCELLANEOUS FASTIDIOUS GRAM-NEGATIVE BACTERIA

HUMAN CAPNOCYTOPHAGA SPECIES

TAXONOMY

Capnocytophaga species have a long and interesting history. Strains belonging to this genus were originally described by Prevot in 1956 at the Pasteur Institute. At that time they were thought to be indole-negative, fermentative variants of the anaerobic gram-negative fusiform organism *Fusobacterium nucleatum*, and they were named "*F. nucleatus* var. *ochraceus*." In 1962 Seball, also of the Pasteur Institute, analyzed the guanosine plus cytosine content of these same strains and concluded that these organisms were more closely related to a group of bacteria called the *Ristella* species than to the fusobacteria, and proposed that *F. nucleatus* var. *ochraceus* strains be reclassified as *Ristella ochracea*. At the same time in the United States, Loesche was examining several isolates of "*Bacteroides oralis*" from the human oral cavity and found that some of these strains had "fusiform" morphologies suggestive of fusobacteria. He suggested the epithet "*Bacteroides oralis* var. *elongatus*" for these organisms. Although the original strains studied by Prevot have been lost, further examination of the *Ristella ochracea* strains of Seball and the *Bacteroides oralis* var. *elongatus* strains of Loesche demonstrated that these were the same organism.

Holdeman and Moore suggested they be renamed "*Bacteroides ochraceus.*"

Also, during the early 1960s, Elizabeth O. King at the CDC was investigating a group of thin, fusiform gram-negative bacilli that had been recovered from human clinical specimens. These strains were designated CDC group DF-1, the "DF" meaning "dysgonic fermenter," referring to the poor fermentative capabilities of these organisms in medium not supplemented with serum. These strains were not anaerobic in their metabolism, but showed a distinct requirement for CO_2 for growth on agar media.

During the late 1970s workers at the University of Massachusetts and at the Forsyth Dental Center in Boston published a series of articles on a group of fusiform, gram-negative bacilli that required CO_2 for both aerobic and anaerobic growth and that demonstrated gliding motility.[357,439,715,802] These organisms appeared to have a role in the pathogenesis of human periodontal diseases and were named *Capnocytophaga* species, reflecting the organism's "consumption" or requirement for CO_2 for growth. Laboratory groups working simultaneously at UCLA and the Wadsworth VA Hospital compared strains of all these species and concluded that the *Capnocytophaga* species of the Boston investigators, Dr. King's CDC group DF-1, and Holdeman and Moore's *Bacteroides ochraceus* (Seball's *Ristella ochracea* and Loesche's *Bacteroides oralis* var. *elongatus*) were different names for the same group of organisms and that the type species name be *Capnocytophaga ochracea.*[542,803] Related isolates studied at the same time were named *Capnocytophaga sputigena* and *Capnocytophaga gingivalis.* Subsequent research studies using other methods (e.g., gas–liquid chromatography of cellular fatty acids and chromogenic enzyme substrate determinations of aminopeptidase profiles) supported the species status of *Capnocytophaga*, the synonomy of the various "species" described by United States and European scientists, and the inclusion of three separate species within the genus.[184] In *Bergey's Manual of Systematic Bacteriology*, *Capnocytophaga* species are included in Class *Flexibacteriae*, Order *Cytophagales*, Family *Cytophagaceae* along with several genera of nonphotosynthetic, nonfruiting, gliding bacteria.[356] Five human species are now included in the genus *Capnocytphaga*: *C. ochracea, C. sputigena, C. gingivalis, C. haemolytica*, and *C. granulosa.*[356,827] The latter two species were described and named in 1994 and represent previously unclassified strains recovered from human dental plaque.[827]

CLINICAL SIGNIFICANCE

Capnocytophaga species are gliding, gram-negative bacteria that are a part of the normal oropharyngeal flora. They are implicated as playing a role (along with *A. actinomycetemcomitans*) in the pathogenesis of localized juvenile periodontitis, a particularly aggressive disease that leads to alveolar bone destruction, and in other forms of periodontal disease. In recent years, *Capnoctyophaga* species have also been reported as a cause of sepsis in patients with malignancy, granulo-cytopenia, and other severe underlying illnesses (e.g., myeloblastic leukemia, acute lymphocytic leukemia, adenocarcinoma, multiple myeloma, Hodgkin's disease, endometrial carcinoma).[23,71,257,273,286,299] In virtually all cases, bacteremic episodes with this organism coincided with periods of profound granulocytopenia caused by the underlying disease (particularly hematologic malignancies) or by the administration of cytotoxic chemotherapeutic agents. Oral ulcerations and bleeding gums have been characteristically found in these patients, thus establishing the route of entry for the organism into the bloodstream.[46,273] The organism is most frequently isolated from respiratory sources (gingival crevices, the oropharynx, periodontal pockets, saliva) and is occasionally isolated from blood and cerebrospinal fluid. Rarely, the organism may be recovered from the lower respiratory tract, lung abscesses, wound infections, pleural or peritoneal fluids, joint fluid, osteomyelitis, and endophthalmitis.[224,519,562,647,810] Occasionally *Capnocytophaga* species may be isolated from infections of the female genital tract, where they may cause serious intrauterine or perinatal infections (e.g., endometritis, amnionitis, chorioamnionitis) and neonatal sepsis.[233,244,366,482,488,494] Cases of *Capnocytophaga* endocarditis, cervical lymphadenitis, empyema, lung abscess, sinusitis, conjunctivitis, subphrenic abscess, osteomyelitis, and clenched-fist injuries have also been reported in both immunocompromised and nonimmunocompromised hosts.[112,478,562,687] In 1995, the first case of *Capnocytophaga* species (*C. sputigena*) as a cause of continuous ambulatory peritoneal dialysis–related peritonitis was documented in a 73-year-old man with end-stage renal disease.[236]

Because of the recognized role of human *Capnocytophaga* species in periodontal disease, these organisms have been extensively examined to identify factors related to virulence. Studies on isolates recovered from oral lesions have shown that *Capnocytophaga* species produce large amounts of various aminopeptidases.[438,538,706] These enzymes may act as virulence factors for the organism directly by causing degradation of subgingival and periodontal tissue, and indirectly by the action of these enzymes on proteins in dental plaque that result in small molecules having known inflammatory potential in periodontal disease (e.g., bradykinin). Such small molecules may then cause increases in vascular permeability, polymorphonuclear cell accumulation, and pain. Both *C. ochracea* and *C. sputigena* produce neuraminidase, an enzyme produced by many other microorganisms and considered to contribute to virulence.[511] In both periodontal disease and septicemia, *Capnocytophaga* species also produce a dialyzable substance that has a direct toxic effect on neutrophils.[694] This substance alters the microscopic appearance of these cells and markedly inhibits neutrophil chemotaxis in vitro.[766] In vivo, this inhibitory substance may act locally in periodontal disease to abrogate polymorphonuclear cell function in those patients who are already immunocompromised. The organisms also produce proteolytic enzymes that hydrolyze IgA1 and IgG, thereby disabling the immune response on mucosal surfaces.[265,312,402] Extracellu-

TABLE 8-4

BIOCHEMICAL CHARACTERISTICS OF *Capnocytophaga ochracea*, *C. gingivalis*, *C. sputigena*, *C. haemolytica*, AND *C. granulosa*

CHARACTERISTIC	C. OCHRACEA	C. GINGIVALIS	C. SPUTIGENA	C. HAEMOLYTICA	C. GRANULOSA
Hemolysis on sheep blood agar	−	−	−	β (lost on subculture)	−
Oxidase	−	−	−	−	−
Catalase	−	−	−	−	−
Gliding motility	+	+	+	+	+
Growth on MacConkey agar	−	−	−	−	−
Reduction of NO_3 to NO_2	−	v	−	+	−
Reduction of NO_2 to gas	−	−	−	−	−
Indole	−	−	−	−	−
Urease	−	−	−	−	−
Arginine dihydrolase	−	−	−	−	−
Lysine decarboxylase	−	−	−	−	−
Ornithine decarboxylase	−	−	−	−	−
Hydrolysis of esculin	v	−	−	+	−
Hydrolysis of glycogen	v	−	−	+	−
Hydrolysis of starch	+	−	−	+	+
Hydrolysis of dextran	+	v	−	v	−
Gas from glucose	−	−	−	−	−
Production of acid from					
Glucose	+	+	+	+	+
Maltose	+	+	+	+	+
Fructose	v*	v	v†	NA	NA
Sucrose	+	+	+	+	+
Lactose	+	v	−	+	+
Xylose	−	−	−	−	−
Mannitol	−	−	−	−	−
Trehalose	−	−	−	NA	NA
Mannose	+	+	+	+	+
Raffinose	v	v	v	NA	NA
Galactose	v*	−	−	NA	NA
Ribose	−	−	−	−	−
Arabinose	−	−	−	NA	NA
Salicin	−	−	−	NA	NA
Sorbitol	−	−	−	−	−
L-Alanyl-aminopeptidase	2+	2+	3+	−	1+
L-Arginine-aminopeptidase	2+	2+	3+	−	2+
L-γ-glutamylaminopeptidase	1+	1+	1+	−	1+
L-Leucyl-aminopeptidase	2+	2+	3+	−	2+
L-Lysyl-aminopeptidase	2+	2+	3+	−	2+
N-α-benzoyl-DL-arginylaminopeptidase	−	1+	−	−	−

+, positive reaction; −, negative reaction; v, variable reaction; NA, not available; 1+–4+, intensity of aminopeptidase reactions.
*, most strains positive.
†, most strains negative.

lar polysaccharides produced by these organisms may also contribute to virulence by inhibiting the response of T lymphocytes to mitogens and antigens.[89] Finally, the LPS of *Capnocytophaga* species may render some strains resistant to the bactericidal effects of normal human serum.[809]

CULTURAL CHARACTERISTICS AND IDENTIFICATION

The organisms are slow-growing, with colonies becoming visible generally after 48 hours of incubation and developing a characteristic morphology after this time. All species require a CO_2-enriched environment for growth; this may be provided in a CO_2 incubator or a candle jar. The colonies of the organism are yellow, tan, or slightly pinkish and have marginal fingerlike projections (gliding motility) that appear as a film surrounding the central area of the colony (see Color Plate 8-2D). The central part of the colonies also have a moist, mottled or "sweaty" appearance. The organism grows on blood and chocolate agar but not on MacConkey agar. Good growth may also be observed on modified Thayer-Martin agar because of its resistance to vancomycin, colistin, and trimethoprim. The organisms are gram-negative, fusiform, and may appear straight or slightly curved (see Color Plate 8-2E). Pleomorphism and variations in the size of the cells is characteristic, with swollen or large coccal cells being seen in older cultures. All species are catalase-negative, oxidase-negative, and produce acid from glucose, maltose, sucrose and mannose, but not from ribose, xylose, mannitol, or sorbitol.[418,715] Indole and urease are not produced and all decarboxylase reactions are negative. Species identification is achieved by an expanded battery of fermentation tests and by physiologic properties (e.g., nitrate and nitrite reduction, starch and dextran hydrolysis, and so forth). The newly described species *C. haemolytica* is β-hemolytic on sheep blood and is the only human hemolytic species.[827] *C. granulosa* strains form intracellular granular inclusions that stain with carbolfuchsin when the organisms are grown in peptone–yeast glucose broth under anaerobic conditions.[827] These two newly described species can also be differentiated from the three previously described human *Capnocytophaga* species by determination of various aminopeptidase activities.[827] Biochemical characteristics of the five species of *Capnocytophaga* are shown in Table 8-4.

ANTIMICROBIAL SUSCEPTIBILITY

Most strains are susceptible to penicillin, ampicillin, cefaclor, clindamycin, chloramphenicol, carbenicillin, cefaperazone, and tetracycline.[256,736] Many strains also demonstrate susceptibility to metronidazole, erythromycin, and cefamandole. Variable susceptibility may be seen for the various types of first-generation cephalosporins (cephalothin, cefazolin, cephalexin, and cephradine). Most isolates are also susceptible to cefotaxime, ceftazidime, cefuroxime, ceftizoxime, ceftriaxone, the ureidopenicillins, and the quinolones.[28,337,639,640,651] Good antimicrobial activity is also seen with clindamycin and imipenem, whereas some strains may be resistant to aztreonam. *Capnocytophaga* species are generally resistant to aminoglycosides (kanamycin, gentamicin, tobramycin, amikacin, netilmicin, and neomycin), trimethoprim, colistin, and vancomycin, although some strains may be susceptible.[337,639,640,651] In recent years, *Capnocytophaga* strains have been isolated that are able to produce β-lactamase enzymes.[262,639,640] These β-lactamase–producing strains are highly resistant to penicillin and amoxicillin; addition of clavulanate results in a 64-fold decrease in the amoxicillin MIC for over 90% of the β-lactamase–producing strains.[640] These strains are highly resistant to cefazolin and are more resistant to cefuroxime, cefotaxime, and ceftazidime than β-lactamase–negative strains.[639,640] The β-lactamase–producing strains, similar to the nonproducing strains, remain susceptible to clindamycin, imipenem, and ciprofloxacin; resistant to aminoglycosides, and are variably susceptible to vancomycin and metronidazole.[640] However, Gomez-Garces and associates reported a case of fatal bacteremia caused by a ciprofloxacin-resistant β-lactamase–producing strain of *C. sputigena* that was resistant to all β-lactams (except cefoxitin) and aminoglycosides but was susceptible to tetracycline, erythromycin, clindamycin, aztreonam, and imipenem.[299] Generally, immunocompromised and granulocytopenic patients are empirically treated with a combination of a β-lactam antibiotic and an aminoglycoside, and they usually require cidal levels of antimicrobials for an optimal therapeutic response. Therefore, rapid recognition of the salient features of this organism by the microbiologist is important. The intrinsic resistance of *Capnocytophaga* species to aminoglycosides and the production of β-lactamase enzymes by some clinical isolates (detected by the nitrocefin test) should be reported to the physician as soon as possible.

CANINE *CAPNOCYTOPHAGA* SPECIES: *CAPNOCYTOPHAGA CANIMORSUS* (CDC GROUP DF-2) AND *CAPNOCYTOPHAGA CYNODEGMI* (CDC GROUP DF-2–LIKE)

TAXONOMY

The CDC group DF-2 was originally isolated in 1976 from blood and spinal fluid cultures of a patient who had become symptomatic after suffering a dog bite.[84] Subsequently, several case reports describing similar organisms were published and, through 1987, over 150 isolates of the organism, designated DF-2 (for dysgonic fermenter) were sent to the Special Bacteriology Branch of the CDC.[96,111,177,247,346,473] On the basis of genetic relatedness and phenotypic characteristics, DF-2 and a group of "DF-2–like" organisms have been recently classified as *Capnocytophaga* species.[96] The CDC group DF-2 is now called *Capnocytophaga canimorsus* (Latin for "dog bite") and the "DF-2–like" strains are now called *Capnocytophaga cynodegmi* (Greek for "dog bite").[96] Although these organisms are genotypically and phenotypically different from the previously described *Capnocytophaga* species, they are similar to them in gram-staining morphology, cellular fatty acids, gliding-type motility, and cultural conditions for growth.

CLINICAL SIGNIFICANCE

The DF-2 infections are generally associated with dog bites or close contact with dogs.[80,148,177,247,334,346,632] Susceptible hosts generally have underlying diseases or conditions that predispose them to severe infection with the organism. These conditions include hepatic disease secondary to alcoholism, previous splenectomy related to other medical circumstances, Hodgkin's disease, hairy cell leukemia, pulmonary fibrosis, malabsorption syndrome, renal disease, chronic obstructive pulmonary disease, peptic ulcer disease, Waldenstrom's macroglobulinemia, and the use of systemic or topical corticosteroids.[125,131,335,346,387,473,540,632] The frequently noted association of systemic DF-2 infection with asplenia strongly suggests that the reticuloendothelial system plays an important role in containing the infection.[131,247,335,387] Major clinical features of these infections have included wound infection with cellulitis, meningitis, fulminant bacteremia with septic shock, renal failure, hemorrhagic skin lesions reminiscent of meningococcal disease, pneumonia with empyema, and bacterial endocarditis.[15,80,125,177,182,247,334,346,632] Disseminated intravascular coagulation, purpura fulminans, and symmetrical peripheral gangrene, similar to that seen in meningococcal disease, have also been associated with fulminant C. canimorsus sepsis.[148,363,421] Unusual presentations of C. canimorsus sepsis have included precipitous hypotension complicated by adult respiratory distress syndrome, unrelenting secretory diarrhea, musculocutaneous mononeuropathy, and thrombotic thrombocytopenic purpura without disseminated intravascular coagulation.[45,148,363,387,570,668] C. canimorsus has been isolated from the oropharynx and saliva of dogs, and in at least one case of sepsis the strain recovered from the patient's blood was also recovered from gingival swab specimens from the patient's dog.[473] Eye infections, including angular blepharitis, chronic corneal ulcers, and corneal ulcer with perforation caused by C. canimorsus have also been reported.[192,288,400] In one case, the patient had sustained a scratch on the cornea, from his dog, which was treated with, among other things, topical prednisone. C. canimorsus infections have also been reported occasionally in immunocompetent hosts and in individuals with no known contact with dogs or other animals.[148,334] Interestingly, a few cases of C. canimorsus infection, including keratitis and systemic infection, have occurred in individuals who sustained bites or scratches from

TABLE 8-5

BIOCHEMICAL CHARACTERISTICS OF *CAPNOCYTOPHAGA CANIMORSUS* (DF-2), *C. CYNODEGMI* (DF-2–LIKE), AND OTHER *CAPNOCYTOPHAGA* SPECIES

CHARACTERISTIC	C. CANIMORSUS	C. CYNODEGMI	CAPNOCYTOPHAGA SPP*
Hemolysis on sheep blood agar	−	−	−
Oxidase	+	+	−
Catalase	+	+	−
Gliding motility	+	+	+
Growth on MacConkey agar	−	−	−
Reduction of NO$_3$ to NO$_2$	−	v	v
Reduction of NO$_2$ to gas	v	v	−
Indole	−	−	−
Urease	−	−	−
Arginine dihydrolase	+	+	−
Lysine decarboxylase	−	−	−
Ornithine decarboxylase	−	−	−
Hydrolysis of esculin	v	+	v
Hydrolysis of ONPG	+	+	v
Production of acid from			
Glucose	+	+	+
Maltose	+	+	+
Fructose	v	+	v
Sucrose	−	+	+
Lactose	+	+	v
Xylose	−	−	−
Mannitol	−	−	−
Mannose	v	+	+
Raffinose	−	+	v
Inulin	−	+	NA
Galactose	+	v	v
Melibiose	−	+	−
Hydrolysis of glycogen	+	v	v
Hydrolysis of starch	+	+	v

C. ochracea, C. gingivalis, and *C. sputigena.*
+, positive reaction; −, negative reaction; v, variable reaction; NA, not available.

domestic cats.[119,460,566] Cases have also been reported in persons working with tigers, bears, and coyotes.

CULTURAL CHARACTERISTICS AND IDENTIFICATION

C. canimorsus is usually recovered from blood cultures, although other specimens (wound cultures, aspirates from cellulitis) may also be submitted. In cases of high-grade bacteremia, organisms may actually be observed on smears of perpheral blood.[569] The organism has been recovered in several types of blood culture media, and growth is generally slow. The lysis–centrifugation method (Isolator) has also been used successfully for isolation.[752] In most reports cultures become positive 3 to 7 days after collection. The organism grows on both blood and chocolate agar that is incubated at 35°C and in a CO_2 incubator or a candle jar with increased humidity.[342] Poor growth on routine sheep blood agar has been attributed to the use of a trypicase–soy base; better growth is seen when a heart infusion base is employed. Heltberg and coworkers found that media supplemented with cysteine supported the best growth.[342] Commercial supplemented chocolate agars containing IsoVitalex (which contains cysteine) or other similar enrichments are satisfactory. Pinpoint colonies appear after 3 or 4 days of incubation. After a few more days the colonies appear circular, smooth, and convex (see Color Plate 8-2F). On a gram-stained slide the bacteria appear as thin, fusiform bacilli that are 2 to 4 μm in length (see Color Plate 8-2G). Some cells may appear slightly curved. Similar to the other fastidious bacteria discussed thus far, no growth is observed on MacConkey agar. Both *C. canimorsus* and *C. cynodegmi* are catalase- and oxidase-positive. These two reactions differentiate them from the other *Capnocytophaga* species, which are both oxidase- and catalase-negative. Both species are also arginine dihydrolase-positive and ONPG-positive. Lysine and ornithine decarboxylase tests are negative. The two organisms are differentiated by carbohydrate utilization tests, with the latter organism producing acid from a wider variety of sugars. Table 8-5 lists the biochemical reactions of *C. canimorsus* and *C. cynodegmi* along with the general biochemical characteristics of the other *Capnocytophaga* species discussed previously. The term *dysgonic* means that biochemical test media for identification, including the basal medium for carbohydrate fermentation, should be supplemented with serum (3 to 5 drops/5 mL broth) to obtain reliable and consistent reactions.

ANTIMICROBIAL SUSCEPTIBILITY

Slow growth of *C. canimorsus* on agar medium and failure of some strains to grow in certain types of broth media have generally precluded adequate studies of the antimicrobial susceptibility of this organism. Nonstandardized studies with disk diffusion procedures designed for more rapidly growing bacteria had previously reported that *C. canimorsus* strains were susceptible to most antimicrobials, but were resistant to aminoglycosides.[646] In 1988, Verghese and associates reported results of a broth dilution technique that used Schaedler broth as the growth medium.[775] All eight *C. canimorsus* strains tested were susceptible to all antibiotics except aztreonam. These antimicrobial agents included penicillin, erythromycin, ticarcillin, piperacillin, cefazolin, cefaperazone, cefotaxime, ceftazidime, gentamicin, amikacin, chloramphenicol, trimethoprim–sulfamethoxazole, and ciprofloxacin. Antibiotics that are generally more active against gram-positive organisms, such as vancomycin, clindamycin, erythromycin, and rifampin, were also active against *C. canimorsus*. These data support the clinical efficacy observed with penicillin (mean penicillin MIC = 0.04 μg/mL ± 0.01 μg/mL for all strains tested).

CDC GROUP DF-3

The CDC group DF-3 is an extremely rare isolate. In fact, the first reports of this organism in association with human disease were published in 1988. This case involved multiple isolations of the organism in pure culture from the stool of an elderly woman with common variable hypogammaglobulinemia of long standing.[781] The second case, also reported in 1988, occurred in a 24-year-old male patient with a relapse of acute lymphocytic leukemia.[31] During intensive chemotherapy and irradiation, the patient became profoundly granulocytopenic, and during this period multiple blood cultures were drawn to determine the etiology of low-grade fevers. The organism was isolated from blood cultures collected during this time. In 1991, Gill and coworkers at the National Cancer Institute screened 690 stool specimens submitted for culture and found 11 specimens with moderate to heavy growth of DF-3.[284] Of these 11 patients, four had a history of prolonged diarrhea and were treated; diarrhea had been documented in the other seven patients, but the infections (and the organisms) were cleared without treatment.[284] Blum and colleagues recovered DF-3 from the stool of eight patients during a year-long period.[83] All patients were immunocompromised or had severe underlying disease, including three patients with HIV infection and two with inflammatory bowel disease. In this report, it was noted that the clinical spectrum of DF-3 ranged from a chronic diarrhea with a clinical response to anti-DF-3 therapy to an asymptomatic carrier state.[83] Other investigators have also noted the association of enteric DF-3 infection with both HIV coinfection and common variable hypogammaglobulinemia.[340] DF-3 has also been isolated from a soft-tissue abscess in a diabetic patient and was coisolated with *Escherichia coli* from a postoperative urinary tract infection in an 81-year-old woman.[44,679]

DF-3 is most easily recovered from stool specimens using cefoperazone-vancomycin-amphotericin blood agar incubated at 35°C in 5% to 7% CO_2. The organism grows relatively slowly, with pinpoint colonies being visible after a 24-hour incubation. After 48 to 72 hours the colonies are gray-white, smooth, and nonhemolytic (see Color Plate 8-2H). On Gram stain, the organisms appear as gram-negative coccobacilli. Several reports also mention that a sweet odor is produced by the organism on agar media.[31,64,83,284,781] Both oxidase and catalase reactions are negative and nitrate is not reduced.

The organism produces acid fermentatively from glucose, xylose, and maltose; most strains also produce acid from sucrose and lactose, do not produce acid from mannitol, and hydrolyze esculin (Table 8-6). Gas–liquid chromatography has also been helpful in indentifying clinical isolates. All DF-3 strains consistently demonstrate the presence of 12- and 13-methyltetradecanoate, with minor amounts of tetradecanoate and hexadecanoate, in their cell wall.[64,83,175]

Antimicrobial susceptibility of these DF-3 isolates was determined by disk diffusion and broth dilution methods.[31,83,284,340,781] DF-3 strains are resistant to several agents, including penicillin, ampicillin, ampicillin–sulbactam, aztreonam, aminoglycosides, cephalosporins (including cephalothin, cefoxitin, ceftriaxone, cefoperazone, and ceftazidime), erythromycin, ciprofloxacin, and vancomycin. Most isolates are susceptible to trimethoprim–sulfamethoxazole and chloramphenicol, and variably susceptible to piperacillin, clindamycin, tetracycline, and imipenem.

CDC GROUP EF-4A AND EF-4B

Formerly a group of uncertain taxonomic affiliation, these bacteria have recently been classified as unnamed members of the family *Neisseriaceae*.[643] CDC group EF-4 (eugonic fermenter 4) is part of the normal oral flora of cats and dogs, and it may also cause purulent cutaneous and pulmonary infections in these animals.[166] EF-4 has been isolated from human wounds resulting from scratches and bites from cats and dogs.[39] This organism has also been isolated from the blood of a 65-year-old woman with metastatic small-cell carcinoid of the liver. Although she owned and lived with a dog, she did not have a history of a dog bite.[214] EF-4 was also coisolated along with *Pasteurella multocida* from an eye laceration and vitreous fluid of an 8-year-old girl shortly after being scratched on the face by her pet cat.[770]

CDC group EF-4 is a gram-negative coccobacillus that grows on both blood and chocolate agars; some strains may also grow on MacConkey agar. After a 24-hour incubation, the colonies are about 1 mm in diameter, opaque, smooth, have an entire edge, and are nonhemolytic or weakly α-hemolytic. Some strains have a distinct popcorn-like odor and may display a yellow pigment. In the single bacteremic case reported, the organism was detected radiometrically on the BACTEC system after 2 days of incubation. The organism is nonmotile, oxidase-positive, catalase-positive, and reduces nitrate to nitrite. Some strains may also reduce nitrite to nitrogen gas. The organism does not produce urease or indole. The EF-4 strains are further divided into groups EF-4a and EF-4b on the basis of carbohydrate utilization. The EF-4a strains ferment glucose, do not produce acids from other carbohydrates, and are arginine dihydrolase-positive[333]; EF-4b strains similarly produce acid only from glucose, but this acid is produced oxidatively, rather than fermentatively. EF-4b strains also do not reduce nitrate all the way to gas and are arginine dihydrolase-negative.[333] Biochemical characteristics for identification of group EF-4 strains are shown in Table 8-6.

Most EF-4 isolates are susceptible to penicillin, ampicillin, cefazolin, chloramphenicol, tetracycline, erythromycin, clarithromycin, trimethoprim–sulfamethoxazole, the quinolones, and the aminoglycosides.[294]

TABLE 8-6

BIOCHEMICAL CHARACTERISTICS FOR IDENTIFICATION OF CDC GROUPS DF-3, EF-4A, AND EF-4B

CHARACTERISTIC	DF-3	EF-4A	EF-4B
Hemolysis, sheep blood agar	−	−*	−*
Oxidase	−	+	+
Catalase	−	+	+
Growth on MacConkey agar	−	v	v
Reduction of NO$_3$ to NO$_2$	−	+	+
Reduction of NO$_2$ to gas	NA	v	−
Indole	v†	−	−
Urease	−	−	−
Arginine dihydrolase	NA	+	−
Lysine decarboxylase	−	−	−
Ornithine decarboxylase	−	−	−
Esculin hydrolysis	+	−	−
Gas from glucose	−	−	−
Production of acid from			
Glucose	+	+‡	+§
Maltose	+	−	−
Fructose	NA	−	−
Sucrose	+	−	−
Lactose	+	−	−
Xylose	−	−	−
Mannitol	−	−	−
Mannose	−	−	−

+, positive reaction; −, negative reaction; v, variable reaction; NA, not available.
*Some strains may show weak α-hemolysis on sheep blood agar.
†In one report the organism was indole-positive; in the second report the organism was indole-negative.
‡Acid produced from glucose by fermentation.
§Acid produced from glucose by oxidation.

STREPTOBACILLUS MONILIFORMIS

CLINICAL SIGNIFICANCE

Streptobacillus moniliformis is a fastidious gram-negative bacillus that is normally found in the oropharynx of rodents and can be transmitted to man by bites from these animals. Rats are the natural reservoir of *S. moniliformis* and play a key role in organism transmission. The organism is found in the upper respiratory tracts of wild rats, laboratory rats and mice, and domesticated rodents (e.g., guinea pigs and gerbils) and may cause disease in these animals.[404,413,801] The organism may also be carried by animals that catch or feed on rodents, such as dogs or cats. *S. moniliformis* is a fastidious, pleomorphic, gram-negative bacillus that tends to form long, thin, filamentous single cells.[667] These thin (about 1 μm), filamentous cells may be over 100 μm in length and may fold into loops and coils. On prolonged incubation, bulbous or sausage-shaped swelling may appear along the filament, causing the organism to resemble a string of beads. On enriched, serum-containing media, the organisms appear as regular, thin, fusiform bacteria, with rounded or pointed ends. The organism may also lose its cell wall and exist as an "L-form." In fact, there is genetic, phenotypic, serologic, and structural evidence suggesting that this organism is taxonomically related to the mycoplasmas and ureaplasmas, which also lack a typical bacterial cell wall.[819] *S. moniliformis* is microaerophilic and growth in liquid medium usually requires supplementation with serum (10% to 20%), blood, or ascites fluid.

In humans, the organism causes a disease called "rat-bite fever" or Haverhill fever when it is acquired by ingestion of the organism. The latter name comes from Haverhill, Massachusetts, where this organism was recovered from blood cultures of several patients during a local outbreak of the disease.[431,579] After an incubation period of 7 to 10 days following the bite of a rat or the ingestion of food or water contaminated with rat excrement, there is an abrupt onset of high fever, chills, headache, muscle aches, vomiting, and other constitutional symptoms. A few days after disease onset, a rash appears on the extremities (including the palms and soles), and some patients may develop severe joint pain or frank arthritis.[412,463,653] Typically the rash is pink-red and maculopapular, although it may also be pustular, petechial, or purpuric.[588] The disease may resolve spontaneously with no residual symptoms, or may develop into a chronic, periodically febrile condition. Several complications (e.g., endocarditis, pericarditis, pneumonia, pleural effusion, septicemia, brain abscess, amnionitis, prostatitis, pancreatitis, and cutaneous abscess) may also occur in the course of the disease, and arthritic symptoms may persist for years after resolution or treatment of the infection.[116,200,243,463,652,653,771] Without a clue to the origin of infection, rat-bite fever or Haverhill fever may resemble viral infection, syphilis, leptospirosis, disseminated gonococcal infection, meningococcemia, typhoid, or Rocky Mountain spotted fever.[584,819] Diagnosis may also be problematic because cases have been reported in patients with no history of rodent bites or direct exposure to rodents.[254] Because of the fastidious nature of the organism and the difficulties involved with culture, retrospective diagnoses of *S. moniliformis* infection have been made on occasion by serologic techniques, including detection of serum agglutinins and complement-fixing antibodies against the bacillary form of the organism.[601] However, serologic tests for this infection are not readily available, and most serologic approaches have been used to assess the presence of the organism in laboratory rodent colonies.[90]

CULTURAL CHARACTERISTICS AND IDENTIFICATION

Diagnosis of rat-bite or Haverhill fever is made by recovery of the organism from blood cultures.[220,691,692] Because the organism is inhibited by the anticoagulant sodium polyanethol sulfonate (SPS), blood (10 mL) must be anticoagulated with citrate (10 mL sodium citrate, 2.5%) before processing.[431,692] The citrated blood cells are sedimented by centrifugation and the packed cells are inoculated onto agar medium (heart infusion agar) containing 10% to 20% sterile decomplemented horse serum and 0.5% yeast extract. The inoculum is gently spread over the agar surface. A broth medium of similar ingredients (heart infusion broth with 10% to 20% serum and yeast extract) is also inoculated with the packed cells. Isolation of *S. moniliformis* has also been accomplished using a biphasic medium of trypticase–soy broth containing a trypticase–soy agar slant. Media is incubated at 35°C in a candle jar or a CO_2 incubator. Other specimens (citrated joint fluid, aspirates, abscess material, or other) may be cultured in the same manner. In broth medium the organism grows as small "puff balls" near the bottom of the tube or bottle and overlying the red cells and stroma. On serum-enriched agar medium, growth may appear within 2 to 3 days, or may require a week or more. Colonies are small, white, smooth, and buttery in consistency. The L-phase variants form spontaneously under or around the existing colonies and have the typical "fried egg" morphology that is seen with *Mycoplasma* species (see Chap. 16).

Identification of *S. moniliformis* is accomplished by observing the typical gram-negative, filamentous morphology on gram-staining and by performing biochemical identification tests in serum-supplemented medium.[220,667] Carbohydrate utilization tests may be performed in nutrient broth containing 1% filter-sterilized carbohydrates and 0.5% sterile horse serum. These tests should be incubated for 3 weeks before reading, although reliable and reproducible results have been obtained when cultures were incubated for only 1 week before test interpretation. Rapid identification of the organism may also be accomplished by fatty acid profile analyses using gas–liquid chromatography and by detection of enzymatic activities for various aminopeptidases and glycosidases using the API-ZYM strip.[220,644] The reactions of *S. moniliformis* in various biochemical identification tests are shown in Table 8-7.

TABLE 8-7

BIOCHEMICAL CHARACTERISTICS FOR IDENTIFICATION OF *STREPTOBACILLUS MONILIFORMIS*

CHARACTERISTIC	REACTION
Oxidase	−
Catalase	−
Nitrate reduction	−
Indole	−
Urease	−
Esculin hydrolysis	+
Production of H_2S (lead acetate)	+
Alkaline phosphatase	+
Gas production from glucose	−
Acid production from	
Glucose	+
Maltose	+
Fructose	+
Sucrose	v
Lactose	v
Xylose	−
Mannitol	−
Mannose	+

+, positive; −, negative; v, variable reaction.

ANTIMICROBIAL SUSCEPTIBILITY

In vitro antimicrobial susceptibility data indicate that *S. moniliformis* is susceptible to penicillin, ampicillin, extended-spectrum and penicillinase-resistant penicillins (azlocillin, mezlocillin, piperacillin, oxacillin), cephalosporins (cefazolin, cefixime, cefotaxime, cefoxitin, cefpirome, ceftazidime), erythromycin, clindamycin, tetracyline, rifampin, imipenem, and vancomycin.[220,819] The organisn is intermediate in susceptibility to the aminoglycosides, chloramphenicol, and ciprofloxacin, and is generally resistant to nalidixate, norfloxacin, colistin, and trimethoprim–sulfamethoxazole.[220,819] The drug of choice for treatment is penicillin, although cephalothin and tetracycline have also shown clinical efficacy.

PASTEURELLA SPECIES

TAXONOMY AND CHARACTERISTICS OF THE GENUS

Pasteurella species, along with *Haemophilus* species and *Actinobacillus* species, are members of the family *Pasteurellaceae*.[7,120,197,466,582] In recent years, these genera have been under intense investigation by taxonomists to determine the relations among the three genera and the proper generic assignment of various species.[145,187,197] Examination of 16S rRNA sequences and DNA–DNA hybridization studies have shown that some existing species of *Pasteurella*—namely, *P. pneumotropica*, *P. aerogenes*, and *P. haemolytica*—are not very closely related to the type species of *Pasteurella*, or to each other, and probably belong in the genus *Actinobacillus*.[529,710] One former *Pasteurella* species, *P. ureae*, has already been formally reassigned to the genus *Actinobacillus* as *A. ureae*.[532] These genetic studies also resulted in the transfer of *Haemophilus pleuropneumoniae* to the genus *Actinobacillus* and the transfer of "*Haemophilus avium*" and other unclassified V factor-dependent isolates to the genus *Pasteurella* (i.e., *P. avium*, *P. volantium*, and *Pasteurella* species A and B).[530,583] In addition, several new species of *Pasteurella*, most of which are found in animals, have been described.[77,529,623,675,710] Table 8-8 lists the *Pasteurella* species that are currently recognized. Fortunately, human clinical isolates represent only a few of the bewildering number of species now included in the genus.[657]

All members of the genus *Pasteurella* have certain phenotypic characteristics in common.[120,529,657] They are all nonmotile, gram-negative, facultatively anaerobic coccobacilli or rods. Most species are oxidase-positive, catalase-positive, and alkaline phosphatase-positive, and reduce nitrate to nitrite. Most species produce acid from glucose, fructose, mannose, and sucrose, and none of them hydrolyze starch or salicin. They are all generally susceptible to penicillins, cephalosporins, and tetracyclines. Members of the genus *Pasteurella* and the nonhuman species of *Actinobacillus* (i.e., *A. lignieresii*, *A. equuli*, *A. suis*, *A. capsulatus*, *A. muris*, *A. pleuropneumoniae*, *A. rossii*, and *A. seminis*) are often difficult to distinguish from one another on the basis of phenotypic characteristics (see Table 8-2).[657] Similar to the pasteurellae, these *Actinobacillus* species are characteristically oxidase- and catalase-positive, gram-negative coccobacilli that reduce nitrate to nitrite. Several members of both genera also produce urease.

The habitats and clinical significance of *Pasteurella* species are described in Table 8-8, and the biochemical characteristics that are useful for their identification are presented in Tables 8-9 and 8-10. The characteristics of the related nonhuman *Actinobacillus* species are shown in Table 8-2. The present discussion will be restricted to those organisms in the genus *Pasteurella* and the *Pasteurella* (*Actinobacillus*) group that have been associated with human disease. The biochemical characteristics of the animal pasteurellae are included for completeness and as a basis for comparison with species already recognized in human clinical microbiology.[529,623,675,710,713] It is probably only a matter of time before some of the unusual animal species are isolated from human disease.

PASTEURELLA MULTOCIDA

Clinical Significance. *P. multocida* is the species that is most frequently recovered from human specimens and is also recovered from a wide variety of animals. The organism can commonly be cultured from the oral cavities of healthy domesticated cats (50% to 70%) and dogs (40% to 66%), but it is also found in a wide variety of other animals, including cattle, horses, swine, sheep, fowl, rodents, rabbits, monkeys, lions, panthers, lynx, birds, reindeer, buffalo, and Tasmanian devils.[39,279] In some animals, this organism causes serious infections. Among cattle, *P. multocida* causes "shipping fever" and hemorrhagic septicemia, resulting from secondary infection of animals that are already compromised by respiratory myxovirus infection. It also causes a cholera-like disease in fowl; atrophic rhinitis in swine; and pleuritis, pneumonia, abscess formation, chronic rhinitis, otitis media, and septicemia in laboratory rabbits. Serious infections (i.e., bacteremia, meningitis, purulent arthritis) have been seen in patients who have been bitten by lions and tigers.[109]

In humans, *P. multocida* causes several types of infections; most of these follow some sort of contact with domesticated animals. Local wound infections in humans are associated with cat bites, cat scratches or dog bites.[2,30] Local wound infections are characterized by rapid development of pain, erythema, swelling, cellulitis with or without abscess formation, and purulent or serosanguinous drainage at the site of the wound.[105,790] Systemic signs of infection may or may not be present.[790] Occasionally, this organism may be found in wounds that are not associated with animal bites or obvious animal exposure. Serious localized complications most frequently follow cat bites, in which the wound may be deep, forceful, and traumatic to underlying tissues. Because the wound is generally on the hand, bone and joint complications are usually seen at this site. Traumatic implantation or extension of the cellulitis from the bite wound site may lead to local osteomyelitis, tenosynovitis, and septic arthritis.[30,790] Bone and joint infections may also result from hematogenous seeding of the joint spaces; in fact, *P. multo-*

TABLE 8-8
CURRENT *PASTEURELLA* SPECIES AND *PASTEURELLA* (*ACTINOBACILLUS*) SPECIES

SPECIES/SUBSPECIES	HABITAT AND CLINICAL SIGNIFICANCE IN HUMANS (IF ANY)
P. multocida subsp. *multocida*	Respiratory tract of nonhuman mammals, birds; clinical isolate from infections in humans
P. multocida subsp. *septica*	Same as above
P. multocida subsp. *gallicida*	Same as above; also associated with fowl cholera
P. pneumotropica (*A. pneumotropica*)	Respiratory tract of guinea pigs, rats, hamsters, cats, and dogs; rarely isolated from humans
P. haemolytica (*A. haemolytica*)	Pneumonic infections in cattle; mastitis in ewes; septicemia in goats and sheep; rare human isolates reported
P. aerogenes	Normal flora in intestinal tract of swine; human infection following a swine bite
Pasteurella sp. new species 1 (called *Pasturella* "gas")	Upper respiratory tract flora of dogs and cats; associated with dog- and cat-bite wounds; human endocarditis also reported
P. dagmatis	Respiratory tract of dogs and cats; animal bite wounds and systemic infections in humans
P. gallinarum	Respiratory tracts of chickens and hens
P. canis	Respiratory tract of dogs; dog-bite wound in humans; respiratory tract of calves
P. stomatis	Respiratory tracts of dogs and cats
P. anatis	Intestinal tract flora of ducks
P. langaa	Respiratory tract flora of chickens and other fowl
P. avium	Respiratory tract flora of healthy fowl
P. volantium	Respiratory tract flora of healthy fowl
P. bettyae	Human Bartholin's gland and human finger abscesses (formerly CDC group HB-5)
P. lymphangitidis	Bovine lymphangitis
P. mairi	Abortion in sows and sepsis in piglets
P. testudinis	Parasitic in certain species of desert tortoises
P. trehalosii	Septicemia in adolescent lambs
P. caballi	Equine isolate causing pneumonia, wound infection; single human case reported
P. granulomatis	Progressive granulomatis disease of cattle

cida arthritis is often associated with preexisting joint diseases, rheumatoid arthritis, and the use of corticosteroids.[42,423,790] Hematogenous spread of *P. multocida* may also result in infected joint prostheses, including knee and total hip arthroplasties.[93,269,318] The bacterium has been isolated from decubitus ulcers and from postsurgical abdominal and orthopedic wound infections. Ocular infections with *P. multocida* usually occur following corneal lacerations from a cat scratch.[347]

P. multocida may also be isolated from the respiratory tract, where it may exist as a commensal agent, or as a cause of pneumonia, empyema, lung abscess, bronchitis, sinusitis, tonsillitis, and otitis media.[87,88,210,414,731,790]

The organism may be found in respiratory tract secretions from individuals with no respiratory tract disease or symptoms; frequently, such individuals have a history of occupational or recreational exposure to animals. Most patients usually have some preexisting compromise of the lungs or upper airways (e.g., chronic obstructive pulmonary disease, chronic bronchitis or sinusitis, bronchiectasis, lung carcinoma, or AIDS).[210,724,731] Symptoms of *P. multocida* pneumonia include an insidious or abrupt onset with fever, malaise, shortness of breath, and pleuritic chest pain. On a chest radiograph, lobar consolidation, with mostly lower lobe involvement, is the most common presentation.[414]

TABLE 8-9
BIOCHEMICAL CHARACTERISTICS OF *PASTEURELLA MULTOCIDA* AND THE *PASTEURELLA* (*ACTINOBACILUS*) GROUP

SPECIES/SUBSPECIES	HEMOLYSIS	OXIDASE	CATALASE	GROWTH ON MACCONKEY AGAR	INDOLE	UREASE	ODC	ACID PRODUCTION FROM									
								GLU	MALT	LAC	XYL	MNTL	TREH	ARAB	SORB	DULC	GAL
P. multocida																	
subsp. *multocida*	−	+	+	−	+	−	+	+	−	−*	v	+	v	−	+	−	+
subsp. *septica*	−	+	+	−	+	−	+	+	−	−*	+	+	+	−	−	−	+
subsp. *gallicida*	−	+	+	−	+	−	+	+	−	−*	+	+	−	v	+	+	+
P. (A.) pneumotropica	−	+	+	v	+	+	+	+	+	v†	+‡	−	+	−	−	−	+
P. (A.) haemolytica	v§	+	+	v	−	−	v	+	+	v†	v†	+	+	−	+	v	+
P. aerogenes	−	+	+	+	−	+	v	+//	+	v†	v#	−	−	−	−	−	NA
Pasteurella new sp. 1	−	+	+	−	+	v	−	+**	+	−	−	−	NA	NA	NA	NA	NA

*Rare strains may be lactose positive
†Most reactions are negative for the indicated organism
‡Rare strains may be negative
§72% of strains are *beta*-hemolytic; property may be lost on subculture
//Gas produced from glucose by most strains
#Most strains are positive
**Some strains produce small amounts of gas from carbohydrate
ODC, ornithine decarboxylase; Glu, glucose; Malt, maltose; Lac, lactose; Xyl, xylose; Mntl, mannitol; Treh, trehalose; Arab, arabinose; Sorb, sorbitol; Dulc, dulcitol; Gal, galactose.

Complications include the development of pleural effusion and empyema.[87,88,414,731] An unusual case of *P. multocida* tonsillitis was reported following accidental ingestion of a culture that was being used to induce pneumonia in piglets.[838] Another case of severe, recurrent *P. multocida* tonsillitis was also reported in a woman whose cat had the cute habit of biting her toothpaste tubes and licking her toothbrush.[602]

Bacteremia caused by *P. multocida* may occur by spread of the organism from a localized bite wound, or it may originate from an infected site elsewhere. Occasionally, the initial wound may be so innocuous (e.g., a minor scratch from a dog's paw) that it is ignored until signs and symptoms of sepsis supervene.[232] Bacteremia with this organism occurs predominantly in the settings of preexisting liver disease (e.g., cirrhosis) or other underlying conditions, such as solid neoplasms, hematologic malignancies, systemic lupus erythematosus, and HIV infection.[41,101,114,246,283,370,516,599,729] However, profound sepsis caused by *P. multocida* has been seen following animal bites in individuals with no underlying disease.[649] In patients with bacteremia, hematogenous dissemination resulting in other infected sites occurs in over 75% of patients, and results in intra-abdominal infections, meningitis, pneumonia, septic arthritis and bursitis, and vertebral osteomyelitis.[422,423,447,516,599] Endocarditis, purulent pericarditis, mycotic aneurysms, and prosthetic valve infections resulting from bacteremia have been reported but are quite rare.[358,444,696] Central nervous system infections caused by *P. multocida* have included meningitis, subdural empyema, and brain abscess.[216,422,447,499,750] It is an infrequent cause of intra-abdominal infections, including postsurgical wound infections, spontaneous bacterial peritonitis, appendicitis, and intra-abdominal and hepatic abscesses.[167,283,359,370,600,762] Continuous ambulatory peritoneal dialysis–associated peritonitis caused by *P. multocida* is quite rare but has been reported.[223,567] *P. multocida* may also be a cause of pelvic infections in women. These infections are usually hematogenous in origin and include diffuse female genital tract infection, tuboovarian abscess, Bartholin's gland abscess, intrauterine infection followed by septic abortion, chorionitis, chorioamnionitis with neonatal sepsis and meningitis, and upper and lower urinary tract infections.[108,750,782,790] Again, most patients from which this organism has been isolated have had some sort of underlying disease or immune compromise, including previous cranial trauma, neurosurgery, hepatic cirrhosis, postoperative wound infection, cervical carcinoma, and congenital genitourinary tract malformations. Most reports have also documented that these patients had past or current exposure to animals, usually, cats or dogs.

Cultural Characteristics and Identification. *P. multocida* is generally not difficult to isolate and identify, although knowledge of the specimen type and a history of exposure to animals (e.g., "cat-bite wound" on the requisition) increases the index of suspicion that this organism may be present. The organism grows well on chocolate and sheep blood agar on which it forms smooth, gray colonies that are 0.5 to 2.0 mm after 24 hours of incubation in CO_2 (see Color Plate 8-3A). The organism is nonhemolytic and does not grow on MacConkey agar, EMB agar, or other types of selective or differential enteric media. Isolates from respiratory tract specimens may be mucoid. A characteristic odor (similar to an *E. coli*, but more pungent) is frequently noted, perhaps owing to the formation of large amounts of indole by the organism. It is oxidase-positive, catalase-positive, ornithine decarboxylase-positive, indole-positive, and urease-negative. The spot indole test using the *p*-aminocinnamaldehyde reagent is generally strongly positive (see Color Plate 8-3B). *P. multocida* produces acid but no gas from glucose, sucrose, and mannitol but not from maltose or lactose. For typical isolates recovered from likely sources, such as a cat bite or scratch, the recovery of oxidase-positive, gram-negative bacilli that are strongly spot indole-positive and fail to grow on MacConkey agar is usually sufficient to make an identification of the organism as *P. multocida*. *P. multocida* strains may be further broken down into three subspecies (*P. multocida*, *P. septica*, and *P. gallicida*) based on acid production from sorbitol and dulcitol (see Table 8-9). Identification to subspecies is of interest in the study of veterinary isolates but is not particularly relevant or important for human clinical isolates. Human isolates have also been broken down into biotypes on the basis of differential fermentation reactions for xylose, sorbitol, and trehalose.[549] Research-based assays have also been developed to assay toxicity of different *P. multocida* strains.[253,536]

Antimicrobial Susceptibility. Antimicrobial susceptibility testing and clinical response of infected patients indicate that *P. multocida* isolates are generally susceptible to a wide variety of antimicrobial agents.[294,730] The organism is susceptible to penicillin, ampicillin, broad-spectrum penicillins (e.g., carbenicillin, ticarcillin, piperacillin, mezlocillin), second-generation cephalosporins (cefotaxime, cefoperazone), third-generation cephalosporins (cefuroxime, ceftazidime, ceftizoxime), tetracycline, and chloramphenicol. Less activity has been noted for the first-generation cephalosporins, such as cephalothin and cefazolin, and the semisynthetic penicillins, such as methicillin and oxacillin.[294]

P. multocida strains may be moderately resistant to erythromycin and the aminoglycosides and are resistant to vancomycin and clindamycin.[294,730] Clarithromycin has greater activity against *P. multocida* than erythromycin.[294] For most antimicrobial agents, the (MIC) and the minimum bactericidal concentration (MBC) are the same. Although disk diffusion susceptibility test results generally correlate with those obtained by agar and broth dilution techniques, discrepancies have been noted primarily with aminoglycosides and erythromycin. The disk diffusion results generally indicate a greater degree of resistance to these drugs than the more quantitative procedures. Because of this, penicillins and the newer cephalosporins tend to be the mainstay for treatment of infections caused by *P. multocida*.

TABLE 8-10

BIOCHEMICAL CHARACTERISTICS FOR IDENTIFICATION OF OTHER *PASTEURELLA* SPECIES

SPECIES	β-HEMOLYSIS	OXIDASE	CATALASE	GROWTH ON MAC	NO₃ RED	IND	URE	ODC	PHOS
P. dagmatis*	−	+	+	−	+	+	+	−	+
P. gallinarum	−	+	+	−	+	−	−	−	+
P. canis	−	+	+	−	+	v	−	+	+
P. stomatis	−	+	+	−	+	+ʷ	−	−	+
P. anatis	−	+ʷ	+	+ʷ	+	−	−	−	+
P. langaa	−	+ʷ	−	−	+	−	−	−	+
P. avium	−	+	+ʷ	−	+	−	−	−	+
P. bettyae*	−	v	v	v	+	+	−	−	+
P. lymphagitidis	−	−	+	v	−	−	+	−	+
P. mairi	v	+	v⁺	v	+	−	+	v⁺	+
P. testudinis	+	+	+	v	−	+	−	−	−
P. trehalosi	v⁺	+	−	+	+	−	−	−	+
P. caballi	−	+	−	−	+	−	−	v	+
P. granulomatis	+	+	+ʷ	+	+	−	−	−	+
Pasteurella									
Species A	−	+	+	−	NA	−	−	−	NA
Species B	−	+	+	−	NA	+	−	+	NA

+, >90% of strains positive
−, >90% of strains negative
+ʷ, Weak positive reaction
v⁺, 80–89% of strains positive
v⁻, 80–89% of strains negative
v, 21–79% of strains positive
vʷ⁺, variable, but positive reactions weak.
NA, Not available
*These species may produce small amounts of gas from pyranoside hydrolysis of glucose.
SBA, sheep blood agar
Mac, MacConkey agar
No₃ Red, nitrate reduction
Ind, indole production
Ure, urease production
ODC, ornithine decarboxylase

Phos, phosphatase
ONPG, o-nitrophenyl-β-D-galactopyranoside
Glu, glucose
Malt, maltose
Suc, sucrose
Lac, lactose
Xyl, xylose
Mntl, mannitol
Tre, trehalose
Mann, mannose
Arab, arabinose
Sorb, sorbitol
Gal, galactose
Inos, inositol
Raff, raffinose
V factor, NAD

PASTEURELLA PNEUMOTROPICA
(ACTINOBACILLUS PNEUMOTROPICA)

Pasteurella pneumotropica is part of the respiratory tract flora of dogs, cats, rats, and mice. In laboratory rodents, the organism causes lower respiratory tract infections. Humans acquire the organism by traumatic exposure to animals, such as dog and cat bites. Human infections attributed to *P. pneumotropica* include meningitis, bacteremia with shock, bone and joint infections, wound infection and cellulitis, and upper respiratory tract infection.[32,164,270,492,503,634] Bilateral interstitial pneumonia caused by *P. pneumotropica* has also

been documented in a 27-year-old patient with AIDS who lived at home with several dogs.[172] Specimens yielding positive cultures have included wound drainage, bone fragments, joint fluid, throat swabs, urine, pleural fluid, and blood.

After 24 hours of incubation on blood agar, colonies of *P. pneumotropica* are variable in size (0.5 to 1 mm in diameter), smooth, convex, and nonhemolytic. They are urease-positive, indole-positive and ornithine decarboxylase-positive (see Table 8-9). The latter two identification tests help to differentiate *P. pneumotropica* from *A. ureae*, which is negative for the two reac-

SPECIES	ONPG	ACID PRODUCTION FROM													V FACTOR REQUIREMENT
		GLU	MALT	SUC	LAC	XYL	MNTL	TRE	MANN	ARAB	SORB	GAL	INOS	RAFF	
P. dagmatis*	–	+	+	+	–	–	–	+	+	–	–	+	–	+^{w}	–
P. gallinarum	–	+	+	+	–	v	–	+	+	–	–	+	–	v$^+$	–
P. canis	–	+	–	+	–	v$^-$	–	v	+	–	–	+	–	–	–
P. stomatis	–	+	–	+	–	–	–	+	+	–	–	+	–	–	–
P. anatis	+	+	–	+	+	+	+	+	+	–	–	+	–	+^{w}	–
P. langaa	+	+	–	+	+	–	+	+	+	–	–	+	–	–	–
P. avium	–	+	–	–	v	v	–	–	+	–	–	+	–	–	v
P. bettyae*	–	+	v	–	–	–	–	–	v	–	–	–	–	–	–
P. lymphagitidis	–	+	v	v	–	–	+	+	+	+	v	+	–	–	–
P. mairi	v	+	v	+	v$^-$	+	v$^+$	v$^-$	+	+	v$^+$	+	v	–	–
P. testudinis	v$^+$	+	v$^+$	+	v$^-$	+	v	v	–	v	v	v$^+$	+	v	–
P. trehalosi	–	+	+	+	–	–	+	+	+	–	+	–	v	–	–
P. caballi	+	+	+	+	+	+	+	–	+	–	–	+	–	+	–
P. granulomatis	+	+	+^{w}	+	+^{w}	–	+^{w}	–	–	–	+	+	–	NA	–
Pasteurella Species A	NA	+	v	NA	v^{w+}	v	v	+	NA	+	–	NA	NA	–	+
Species B	NA	+	+	NA	–	+	–	+	NA	–	–	NA	NA	–	–

tions. Some strains of *P. pneumotropica* will grow on MacConkey agar. The positive urease test and differential reactions for maltose and mannitol help differentiate this organism from *P. multocida*.

Another species that is closely related to *P. pneumotropica* has the provisional name *Pasteurella* sp. new species 1 or *Pasteurella* "gas."[120] It has also been isolated from animal bites, miscellaneous specimens from humans, and oropharyngeal specimens from dogs and cats. This organism resembles *P. pneumotropica* in cultural characteristics and biochemical reactions. Colonies tend to be slightly larger than those of *P. pneumotropica* after 24 hours of incubation. Similar to *P. pneumotropica*, it is indole-, urease-, and maltose-positive, but it can be differentiated by lack of ornithine decarboxylase activity and failure to produce acid from xylose. Urease, ornithine decarboxylase and acid production from maltose are helpful for differentiating this species from *P. multocida*. Urease-negative "*P. pneumotropica*–like" isolates have also been referred to as *Pasteurella* species taxon 16.[78] Some strains of *Pasteurella* "gas" produce small amounts of gas from glucose and other carbohydrates. Some strains of this species, plus some other *P. pneumotropica*-like organ-

isms have been reclassified as *P. dagmatis* (see Tables 8-8 and 8-10).

P. pneumotropica isolates are generally susceptible to penicillin, ampicillin, first-, second-, and third-generation cephalosporins (cefotaxime, cefuroxime), piperacillin, tetracycline, erythromycin, chloramphenicol, and ciprofloxacin. Most strains are susceptible to the aminoglycosides and trimethoprim–sulfamethoxazole.[172]

PASTEURELLA HAEMOLYTICA (ACTINOBACILLUS HAEMOLYTICUS)

Pasteurella haemolytica, along with *P. multocida*, are prominent pathogens in domesticated animals, causing severe diseases and major economic losses in the cattle, sheep, swine, and poultry industries. Strains of *P. haemolytica* can be divided into two biotypes, designated biotype A (cattle-associated) and biotype T (sheep-associated).[120] Biotype A strains produce acid from arabinose and xylose but no acid from trehalose and salicin. Biotype B strains produce acid from trehalose and salicin, but not from arabinose and xylose. These biotypes are each further divided into serotypes.

Biotype A strains cause bovine pneumonic pasteurellosis, a severe fibronecrotic pneumonia of cattle.[800] Rare human infections have been reported, and these have usually resulted from occupational or recreational exposure to animals. Rivera and colleagues reported a case of aortic graft infection that was due to both *P. haemolytica* biotype A and group C β-hemolytic streptococci in a 50-year-old man.[628] This patient had no contact with cattle or other farm animals. Biotype T strains cause septicemia in lambs and have not been isolated from human infections.

Although the name suggests the hemolytic character of the organism, this feature is generally observed only with fresh isolates. The species does not produce either indole or urease, and most strains grow on MacConkey agar. Acid is usually produced from glucose, maltose, and sucrose, whereas other fermentation results vary from strain to strain (see Table 8-9).

Given the limited number of isolates tested, *P. haemolytica* is susceptible to penicillin, ampicillin, erythromycin, chloramphenicol, and the aminoglycosides.

PASTEURELLA AEROGENES

Pasteurella aerogenes is a part of the oropharyngeal and intestinal flora of swine. Rare human infections have reportedly followed bites or other occupational exposure to these animals.[49,483] This organism is also associated with abortion and stillbirth in animals, including pigs, dogs, and rabbits.[483,749] Also, *P. aerogenes* has been recovered from the ears and throat of a stillborn child delivered by a women in the 31st week of pregnancy.[751] The same organism was isolated from vaginal cultures following the delivery. On investigation, the authors learned that the woman worked as an assistant on a pig farm in Denmark. It was not known whether the organism infected the fetus hematogenously or by ascending genital tract infection.

This species produces smooth, convex, circular, nonhemolytic colonies on blood agar and also grows on MacConkey agar. It is indole-negative and urease-positive; most isolates also produce ornithine decarboxylase (see Table 8-9). As the name implies, this species is "aerogenic," meaning that gas is produced from glucose during fermentation. Susceptibility information on this species is not available.

OTHER *PASTEURELLA* SPECIES ISOLATED FROM HUMAN INFECTIONS

Pasteurella dagmatis. *P. dagmatis* is a part of the oral flora of dogs and cats and is associated with bites and scratches from these animals.[604] In a series of 32 bacterial isolates from dog-bite wounds submitted to an Australian reference laboratory, three were identified as *P. dagmatis*.[571] Of 159 *Pasteurella* strains submitted to a veterinary laboratory in Denmark, five isolates were identified as *P. dagmatis*. These strains were isolated from a case of cellulitis (1), a groin abscess (1), a throat abscess (1), and dog-bite wounds (2).[355] This organism has also been isolated from cat-bite wounds.[837] It is a rare cause of endocarditis, with two cases reported in

the literature.[320,716] In one of these reports, endocarditis was complicated by vertebral osteomyelitis.[716] This patient was a 55-year-old female who worked in an animal welfare agency and had sustained multiple cat bites and scratches from strays. *P. dagmatis* pneumonia was also documented in a 54-year-old female patient with squamous cell carcinoma of the pharynx, from whom the organism was isolated in pure culture from a sputum specimen.[604] This patient also kept close company with a dog as a part of the support system offered by her social worker. Bacteremia caused by *P. dagmatis* was documented in a 50-year-old male with a long-standing history of diabetes. This patient had developed *P. multocida* cellulitis of the toe and bacteremia 1 year earlier. At that time, his infection was traced to his dachshund, which had licked an open blister on the patient's foot. On his second hospital admission, *P. dagmatis* was recovered from blood cultures; again the infection was likely due to loving licks from his Yorkshire terrier.[240] The *P. dagmatis* isolates from these human infections have been susceptible to penicillin, ampicillin, ticarcillin, cephalosporins and cephamycins, aminoglycosides, tetracycline, ciprofloxacin, and trimethoprim–sulfamethoxazole.[240,604,716]

Pasteurella canis and Pasteurella stomatis. Both *P. stomatis* and *P. canis* have also been isolated from wound infections resulting from dog bites.[355,587] *P. canis* strains are divided into two biotypes; biotype 1 is found in the oral cavity of dogs, whereas biotype 2 has been recovered from calves.[529] In the study conducted by Holst and colleagues, 28 of 159 strains examined were identified as *P. canis*; all of these were from dog-bite wounds and belonged to biotype 1.[355] Of the 159 strains, 10 were identified as *P. stomatis*; eight were from dog-bite wounds, and two were from abscesses. In the 8 *P. stomatis* wound infections, *P. multocida* or *P. canis* were coisolated along with *P. stomatis*. Both *P. canis* and *P. stomatis* are susceptible to ampicillin, cephalothin, the aminoglycosides, tetracycline, cefotaxime, the quinolones, and piperacillin.[355,587]

Pasteurella caballi. *P. caballi* is an inhabitant of the upper respiratory tract of horses. It has also been isolated in pure or mixed culture from equine infections, including pneumonia, peritonitis, wounds, abscesses, and genital tract infections.[675] The only documented case of human *P. caballi* infection was an inflammatory, boil-like fluctuant finger lesion that occurred, without any previous traumatic injury, in a 28-year-old veterinarian who worked with horses and ponies.[77] Culture of pus from the wound following incision and drainage grew a pure culture of *P. caballi*. *P. caballi* stains are broadly susceptible to antimicrobial agents; some strains, however, are resistant to lincomycin, streptomycin, and sulfonamides and are intermediate in susceptibility to penicillin G.[675] The isolate obtained from the veterinarian was susceptible to all antimicrobials tested except penicillin and the sulfonamides.[77]

Pasteurella bettyae. *P. bettyae* was formerly known as CDC group HB-5. The name of the organism was changed to *P. bettii* and then modified to *P. bettyae* in keeping with the rules of binomial nomenclature. This organism has been isolated primarily from the genitourinary tract and related specimens (i.e., vagina, cervix, urethra, Bartholin's glands, and amniotic fluid).[38,659] In 1989, a cluster of five patients with urethritis, pelvic inflammatory disease, or Bartholin's gland abscesses was identified in Tennessee, from whom *P. bettyae* was isolated as the etiologic agent. This outbreak suggested that the organism may be a sexually transmitted pathogen.[38] Also, it may be associated with genital ulcer disease. In a study performed in Rwanda, the organism was isolated from 25 (3.6%) of 675 patients (204 women and 471 men) with genital ulcer disease but from only one of 983 patients without genital ulcer disease.[86] Of 145 men with a urethal discharge but without genital ulcers, *P. bettyae* was isolated from only one patient. Occasionally, *P. bettyae* has also been isolated from blood, wounds, perianal lesions and abscesses.[38]

P. bettyae is a gram-negative coccobacillus that grows on both blood agar and chocolate agar; its ability to grow on MacConkey agar is variable. After 24 hours of incubation in a CO_2 environment, colonies are pinpoint, nonhemolytic, smooth, and white. The organism is oxidase-variable, weak, or delayed, although positive results are usually obtained with the tetramethylphenylene diamine reagent. The catalase reaction is often negative. Nitrate is reduced to nitrite, but not to gas, and urease is not produced. Acid is formed from glucose (along with gas), fructose, and mannose, but not from maltose, sucrose, lactose, mannitol, or xylose. The organism produces indole after overnight incubation in tryptone broth. As with *C. hominis* the amount of indole formed may be small, so xylene extraction of the broth and use of Ehrlich's indole reagent are often required for its detection.

Isolates of *P. bettyae* are usually suscepible to the cephalosporins, aztreonam, imipenem, fluoroquinolones, aminoglycosides, trimethoprim, and trimethoprim–sulfamethoxazole but are resistant to erythromycin, clindamycin, vancomycin, and tetracycline. All five isolates recovered in the Tennessee cluster were susceptible to ampicillin, whereas seven of the 24 isolates tested from the Rwanda study were ampicillin-resistant and produced a β-lactamase.[38,86]

The biochemical characteristics of *P. dagmatis, P. canis, P. stomatis, P. bettyae,* and *P. caballi* are presented in Table 8-10 along with those of other animal pasteurellae.

BORDETELLA SPECIES

BACKGROUND AND TAXONOMY OF *BORDETELLA* SPECIES

The genus *Bordetella* contains six species: *B. pertussis, B. parapertussis, B. bronchiseptica, B. avium,* and two recently described species, *B. hinzii* and *B. holmesii* (former CDC group NO-2).[395,580,764,798] Genetic studies have shown that these organisms are quite closely related to each other. In fact, DNA hybridization techniques indicate that the species may not be different enough to justify the assignment of individual species, although definite genetic, phenotypic, and immunologic differences exist among them.[397,398,406] In the past, various members of the genus have been classified with other bacterial species, including *Haemophilus, Brucella,* and *Alcaligenes.* In the 1984 edition of *Bergey's Manual of Determinative Bacteriology,* both *Bordetella* and *Brucella* species are listed as genera of uncertain affiliation. In 1986, De Ley and coworkers proposed a new family, called *Alcaligenaceae* to include *Alcaligenes* and *Bordetella* species.[189,394] The genetic relatedness of *Bordetella* species to the genus *Alcaligenes* is further supported by the finding that *B. pertussis* and *B. bronchiseptica* both produce a siderophore called alcaligin that is identical with that produced by *Alcaligenes denitrificans.*[513] Humans are the only host of *B. pertussis* and *B. parapertussis. B. bronchiseptica* is found in a wide variety of animals (e.g., rabbits, nonhuman primates, dogs, cats, swine, foxes, and opossums) and is occasionally found in humans.[221] As the name suggests, *B. avium* is found in birds, particularly turkeys, in which it causes rhinotracheitis.[395] The newly named species *B. hinzii* was formerly referred to as *B. avium*–like bacterium, turkey coryza bacterium type II, *Alcaligenes faecalis* type II, and *Alcaligenes* species strain C_2T_2, and was formally assigned to the genus *Bordetella* in 1995.[63,79,625] *B. holmesii* was formerly called CDC nonoxidizer group 2 (NO-2). This organism has been recovered primarily from blood cultures of young adults. Characterization of these isolates by DNA–DNA hybridization, 16S rRNA sequencing, and cellular fatty acid–ubiquinone analysis established that group NO-2 strains are most closely related to organisms in the genus *Bordetella.*[798]

Members of the genus *Bordetella* are small, gram-negative coccobacilli on primary isolation. On subculture, they tend to become more pleomorphic. They are obligately aerobic, grow optimally at 35° to 37°C, do not utilize carbohydrates, and are inactive in most biochemical tests. They are nonmotile except for *B. bronchiseptica, B. avium,* and *B. hinzii,* which possess peritrichous flagella. These organisms do not require hemin or NAD. However, primary isolation of *B. pertussis,* in particular, requires the addition of charcoal, ion-exchange resins, or 15% to 20% blood to neutralize the growth-inhibiting effects of such substances as unsaturated fatty acids, sulfides, peroxides, and heavy metals.[361] *B. parapertussis* is somewhat less exacting in its growth requirements, but isolation still requires the use of the specialized media used for pertussis. The remaining species are less fastidious and will grow on routinely used agar media, including blood, chocolate, and MacConkey agars.

CLINICAL SIGNIFICANCE AND VIRULENCE FACTORS OF *BORDETELLA PERTUSSIS*

B. pertussis causes the syndrome called pertussis or "whooping cough."[266] The organism is acquired by droplet infection and is highly contagious, with an attack rate higher than 90% in nonimmunized individuals. Currently, about half of the reported cases of pertussis occur in unvaccinated or incompletely vaccinated infants, and studies have demonstrated that adults with symptomatic but unrecognized pertussis are frequently the source of the organism for these pediatric cases.[183,242] The atypical or mild pertussis that is seen in adults, particularly in the United States, is attributed to the fact that most adults were immunized as children and that waning immunologic recall results in a modified, less severe illness.[631] Studies of pertussis infection in adults have used serologic methods to demonstrate significant titer increases against unique antigens of *B. pertussis*. In a study of 130 university students with a cough of 6 days duration or longer reporting to the student health service, 26% had serologic evidence of recent *B. pertussis* infection.[502] In another study, 51 health care workers were annually evaluated over a 5-year period (1984 to 1989) for rises in antibody titers to four pertussis-specific antigens (PT, FHA, pertactin, and fimbriae). Of these individuals, 90% had a significant increase in antibody titer to one or more of the antigens between 2 consecutive years during the 5-year period of the study.[193] In a study performed with 246 German adults with a coughing illness of longer than 14 days, evidence of *B. pertussis* infection was found in 64 (26%); five had positive nasopharyngeal cultures, and 59 were diagnosed on the basis of serology or PCR.[678] Although pertussis in adults is usually either asymptomatic or atypical in its presentation, full-blown pertussis, with coughing paroxysms, vomiting, and encephalopathy has also been documented.[330]

B. pertussis has also been isolated in recent years from adults with underlying disease such as HIV infection. Ng and coworkers isolated *B. pertussis* from bronchoalveolar lavage and transbronchial biopsy specimens of three patients with AIDS.[545] These organisms were recovered on media for isolation of *Legionella*. Doebbeling and associates reported the isolation of *B. pertussis* from the upper respiratory tract of a 25-year-old HIV-positive patient with a 4-month history of paroxysmal cough; a similar case was also reported in a 60-year-old patient with AIDS in Belgium.[155,205] Despite these case reports, pertussis is believed to be relatively rare in HIV-infected individuals, with an estimated prevalence of nasopharyngeal carriage of less than 6.5 cases per 10,000 patients.[153] In a very unusual case, *B. pertussis* was isolated from a blood culture of a 31-year-old man with Wegener's granulomatosis, a condition associated with chronic pneumonia and the development of pulmonary nodules and cavitary lung lesions.[373] Pertussis has also been recovered from the respiratory tracts of infants with other underlying problems, such as necrotizing enterocolitis, chronic lung disease, and adenoviral pneumonia.[309,688]

Clinical pertussis in unvaccinated children can be divided into three stages. The **prodromal** or **catarrhal stage** begins 5 to 10 days after acquistion of the organism and is characterized by nonspecific "cold" or "flu" symptoms. The disease is highly communicable at this stage because large numbers of organisms are present in the upper respiratory tract. Cultures collected at this time have the greatest likelihood of being positive. A cough appears late in this stage and increases in persistence, severity, and frequency. This evolves into the **paroxysmal stage** after 7 to 14 days. This stage is characterized by the "staccato cough" with the prolonged inspiratory "whoop" heard at the end of the coughing spell. Inspiratory efforts are futile during the coughing paroxysm, and the whoop is caused by the inspiration of air through the swollen and narrowed glottis. The coughing spell is frequently accompanied by cyanosis and vomiting. This stage may be so severe that patients sometimes require intermittent ventilatory assistance. Complications that may occur during the course of the disease include secondary bacterial infections and otitis media; central nervous system symptoms, such as convulsions and high fever, particularly with the presence of intervening secondary infections; encephalopathy; and inguinal hernia and rectal prolapse associated with the severe coughing.[272] The cause of encephalopathy associated with complicated pertussis is unknown, owing to the unavailability of a suitable animal model, but suggested mechanisms include anoxia secondary to the coughing paroxysms, hypoglycemia secondary to the toxic effects of PT, and intracerebral hemorrhage. The **convalescent stage** generally begins within 4 weeks of onset and, during this time, there is a decrease in the frequency and severity of the coughing spells.

B. pertussis produces an array of virulence factors that may play a role in the pathogenesis of pertussis. Regulation of these various factors at the genetic level represents one of the better-studied systems in molecular biology.[54,608] **Pertussis toxin** (PT; also called lymphocytosis-promoting factor, pertussigen, islet-activating factor, and histamine-sensitizing factor) is a major virulence factor of *B. pertussis*.[510] This toxin is a single 105- to 117-kDa protein that has a wide spectrum of biologic activity and is produced only by *B. pertussis*. It is a hexamer, consisting of an enzymatic, toxic moiety (A protomer) and a nontoxic moiety (B oligomer). The B oligomer is responsible for binding of the toxin to susceptible cells and transporting the A protomer across the eucaryotic cell membrane. The A subunit contains a single polypeptide, designated S1, that has ADP-ribosyltransferase activity.[390] This enzyme transfers ADP-ribose groups from NAD to the G_i (inhibitory) regulatory proteins that normally function in cell signal transduction. The B subunit is composed of two dimers—polypeptides S2 and S4 and polypeptides S3 and S4—joined by another polypeptide called S5. The biologic effects of PT include the sensitization of mice to histamine, the production of lymphocytosis, activation of pancreatic islet cells, and stimulation of immune responses.[629] Antibody directed against PT is protective for mice when challenged by either intracerebral or respiratory tract inoculation. The genes for the PT peptides are arranged as an operon; this operon is present in *B. pertussis*, *B. parapertussis*, and *B. bronchiseptica*, but the genes are neither transcribed nor translated in the latter two species.[26,469] The activity of PT is believed to be responsible for many of the clinical signs and symptoms of pertussis, although this has not been unequivocally demonstrated.[267,811] Antibody directed against PT is also protective in animal models of pertussis.

Filamentous hemagglutinin (FHA) is a cell surface adhesin of 220 kDa that has hemagglutinating activity and mediates adhesion of *B. pertussis* to eucaryotic cells in vitro and to the ciliated cells of the upper respiratory tract.[619] Antibody against FHA provides some immunity against respiratory, but not intracerebral, challenge, presumably by inhibiting attachment of the organisms. **Pertactin** is an outer membrane protein of *B. pertussis* that may function along with FHA to mediate attachment of the bacterium by helping the FHA molecule achieve a conformation that maximizes bacterium-cell binding.[25] This protein was originally called P69 or 69K protein; the true molecular weight has been determined to be about 60.5 kDa after it was found that pertactin was derived from posttranslational processing of a 93-kDa precursor.[608] *B. pertussis* also produces an **adenylate cyclase hemolysin** (AC-H), a bifunctional protein that is secreted into the medium and possesses both adenylate cyclase and hemolytic activities.[399] The protein is able to bind to susceptible cells and is translocated into the cell intact. Inside the target cell, the molecule is proteolytically cleaved. Activation of the adenylate cyclase activity by the eucaryotic protein calmodulin results in intracellular accumulation of cyclic-AMP. This accumulation may suppress expression of the local immune response by inhibiting neutrophil chemotaxis and phagocytosis.[608] **Tracheal cytotoxin** (TCT) is a molecule of about 921 Da that is composed of fragments of the cell wall peptidoglycan.[162] This molecule has been fully characterized and shown to consist of a disaccharide tetrapeptide containing glucosamine, muramic acid, alanine, glutamic acid, and diaminopimelic acid in a 1:1:2:1:1 ratio.[161] This toxin specifically damages the ciliated epithelial cells, which line the airways where the organism attaches, and may be responsible for the characteristic cough of clinical pertussis. It also adversely affects polymorphonuclear cell function at low concentrations, and is toxic to these cells at higher concentrations.[173] In addition, there is also in vitro evidence that *B. pertussis* produces a **heat-labile toxin** (HLT; or dermonecrotic toxin) that is a single polypeptide of about 140 kDa. This protein induces contraction of blood vessels and hemorrhagic necrosis in mice and guinea pigs, but its role in pathogenesis, if any, is unknown.[608] Finally, similar to other gram-negative bacteria, *B. pertussis* possesses **lipopolysaccharide** (LPS; or endotoxin) in its cell wall outer membrane. Again, the role of LPS in the pathogenesis of pertussis is unknown.

Bordetella species also possess heat-stable somatic antigens, termed "O" agglutinogens, that are common to all species. In addition, 14 heat-labile capsular agglutinogens, called factors, have been described for *Bordetella* species. These agglutinogens are associated with **fimbriae** and apparently are also involved in the mediation of attachment to target cells. Factors 1 through 6 are specific for *B. pertussis*, factor 7 is common to all members of the genus, factor 14 is specific for *B. parapertussis*, and factor 12 is specific for *B. bronchiseptica*.

PERTUSSIS VACCINES

Despite the availability of an effective vaccine, pertussis continues to be a problem of worldwide importance. Before the introduction of the whole-cell vaccine, 100,000 to 280,000 cases and 5,000 to 10,000 deaths were attributable to pertussis each year.[139] At this time, the disease was primarily seen in children 1 to 5 years of age; younger infants were spared owing to the presence of transplacental antibody from previous exposure or disease in the adult. With the introduction of the whole-cell killed vaccine into routine childhood immunization schedules in the 1950s, the yearly incidence of disease dwindled. However, because most adults do not receive booster vaccinations, many children are now born without passively transferred antibody. In the period from 1982 to 1985, more than half of the reported cases of pertussis occurred in children younger than 1 year old.[242] Added to this are the large number of susceptible adults whose vaccine-induced immunity has waned.

The pertussis vaccine itself has been an area of controversy in the medical arena for several years. The current vaccine is a killed, whole-cell vaccine that is administered along with diphtheria and tetanus toxoids (the DPT or "three-in-one" vaccine). This vaccine is administered in three intramuscular doses at 2-month intervals beginning at age 6 to 8 weeks, with booster doses given at 6 to 12 months and 4 to 6 years of age. The vaccine is 80% to 100% efficacious, and widespread use has been associated with the decline in numbers of reported cases in countries employing mandatory immunization. Additional evidence of efficacy has, unfortunately, accrued as a result of diminished immunization programs in some countries. In Denmark, an upswing in the number of cases occurred a few years after alterations were made in the vaccine preparation, with the use of smaller amounts of antigen. Diminished public acceptance of immunization in Great Britain since the mid-1970s resulted in pertussis reaching epidemic proportions among children younger than 5 years of age in the late 1970s.

Publicity surrounding cases of severe encephalopathy and permanent neurologic sequelae that were temporally related to receipt of DPT vaccine has accelerated efforts to develop acellular or "subunit" vaccines. The isolation and characterization of the subcellular components and virulence factors of *B. pertussis* have enabled the manufacture of several acellular vaccines consisting of one or more antigens.[218] Since 1981, six different subunit pertussis vaccines, administered as "DPT" inoculations (diphtheria toxoid–tetanus toxoid–pertussis subunits), have been licensed for immunization of children in Japan.[520] The vaccines in use in Japan vary in their composition, but all contain PT and FHA. In the United States, the safety and efficacy of at least 13 different acellular subunits vaccines are under evaluation.[218] These putative vaccines have included two monocomponent formulations containing PT; four two-component formulations containing PT and FHA antigens; five three-component vaccines containing PT, FHA, and pertactin or fimbriae; and two four-component vaccines containing PT, FHA, pertactin, and fimbrial antigens (Table 8-11). A vaccine trial conducted in Sweden with nearly 400 children used two component vaccines—PT only and PT-FHA—and compared the efficacy with placebo inoculation (the whole-cell vaccine was not included because of concerns about adverse reactions).[734] The efficacies of the PT and PT-FHA vaccines in this study were 65% and 77%, respectively; these data were disappointing and did not lead to licensure of either of these vaccines in Sweden. Several of these vaccines are undergoing further evaluation in other efficacy trials.[218]

Separate issues that are related to the efficacy of these subunit vaccines in children are those of adult pertussis and pertussis in young infants. Although *B. pertussis* is not a significant cause of respiratory illness in most adults, epidemiologic studies have repeatedly implicated infected adults as the source and transmitter of the organism to the child.[55,169,541] In addition, outbreaks of pertussis have occurred among adult caregivers exposed to children with pertussis in day care situations. Because whole-vaccine reactogenicity may be more severe in adults than in children, subcellular component vaccines must also be investigated for their immunogenicity in previously vaccinated or unvaccinated adults. A study of an acellular pertussis vaccine, combined with diphtheria and tetanus toxoid, in

adults found minimal adverse effects; brisk antibody responses to PT, FHA, pertactin, and fimbrial antigens present in the vaccine; and no interference of the pertussis components with the immune responses to either tetanus or diphtheria toxoids.[219] Pertussis may also be seen in young infants because of suboptimal levels of transplacental antibodies from pertussis-susceptible mothers. A study of an acellular pertussis vaccine in young infants showed that the vaccine did not prevent infection in these children but did substantially ameliorate the development of severe symptoms.[21]

Before moving on to a discussion of isolation techniques for *B. pertussis* and other *Bordetella* species, it is necessary to address briefly the pathogenetic capabilities of *B. parapertussis*, *B. bronchiseptica*, and the newly described species *B. hinzii* and *B. holmesii*.

CLINICAL SIGNIFICANCE OF OTHER *BORDETELLA* SPECIES

B. parapertussis is also associated with a pertussis-like illness in humans, but it is generally less severe in clinical presentation.[341] However, outbreaks of *B. parapertussis* have been reported in which the illness has been quite severe and resulted in death, particularly in very young children.[451] Wirsing von Konig and Finger

		SUBCELLULAR COMPONENT			
MANUFACTURER	NUMBER OF VACCINES	PERTUSSIS TOXIN	FILAMENTOUS HEMAGGLUTININ	PERTACTIN	FIMBRIAE
Massachusetts Department of Public Health (Boston MA)	1	X			
Michigan Department of Public Health (Lansing MI)	2	X	X		
Sclavo (Siena, Italy)	3	X			
	4	X	X	X	
Smith-Kline Biologics (Rixensart, Belgium)	5	X	X		
	6	X	X	X	
Connaught/Biken (Swiftwater PA)	7	X	X		
Connaught Canada (Willowdale)	8	X	X		X
	9	X	X	X	X
Pasteur Merieux (Lyon, France)	10	X	X		
Lederle/Takeda (Pearl River, NY)	11	X	X	X	
	12	X	X	X	X
Center for Applied Microbiologic Research (Porton Down, UK)	13	X	X		X

compared the severity of disease in 33 children with *P. parapertusis* infection with 331 patients with *B. pertussis* infection and found that the frequency of paroxysmal coughing, whooping, and vomiting were almost identical in both groups.[811] Heininger and colleagues also compared *B. pertussis* infection in 76 patients with *B. parapertussis* infection in 38 patients matched by age and sex.[341] They also found that the illness caused by *B. parapertussis* was typical of pertussis but was much less severe and, that unlike pertussis, lymphocytosis was not a characteristic of the infection, presumably owing to the absence of the lymphocytosis-promoting activity of PT. Decreased pathogenicity in *B. parapertussis* may indeed be due to lack of expression of PT and other virulence factors. Interestingly, when genes coding for certain pertussis virulence factors (e.g., PT and FHA) are transferred into *B. parapertussis* by genetic techniques, the organism becomes capable of producing pertussis-like characteristics in vitro (e.g., anaphylaxis, histamine sensitivity, and leukocytosis), suggesting that the presence of virulence genes and their regulation may be the primary difference between these genetically "identical" species.

B. bronchiseptica causes respiratory tract infections in various animal species (e.g., tracheobronchitis or "kennel cough" in dogs, atrophic rhinitis in pigs, pneumonia and otitis media in rabbits and guinea pigs) and may be isolated as a commensal from the human upper respiratory tract.[221] It may also cause infections primarily in immunocompromised hosts.[816] Cases of sepsis, meningitis following head trauma, peritonitis, and especially pneumonia caused by *B. bronchiseptica* have been reported in patients with underlying liver disease, alcoholism, asplenia, Hodgkin's disease, hematologic malignancy, chronic renal failure, chronic asthma, systemic lupus erythematosus, or severe hypertension.[113,129,391,561,735,816] Reina and colleagues reported a case of pneumonia caused by *B. bronchiseptica* in a 37-year-old patient who had sustained serious chest injury in an automobile accident and required intubation.[617] The patient developed infiltrates (as seen on chest radiographs) within 72 hours, and culture of the endotracheal aspirate grew the organism in pure culture. More recent case reports further document the opportunistic nature of this organism. Bauwens and associates described a case of bacteremia and pneumonia in 20-year-old woman following bone marrow transplantation for acute myelogenous leukemia.[51] Since 1991, several cases of *B. bronchiseptica* pneumonia have also been reported in patients with AIDS.[13,180,186,497,543,815] Rare reports of endocarditis caused by *B. bronchiseptica* have also appeared in the literature. In one such case, the patient presented with fever and a dermatitis around a recent surgical incision. It turned out that the patient's dog frequently nipped and licked the area of dermatitis surrounding the incision, suggesting a canine origin for the organism.[697] In fact, this organism was formerly called *B. bronchicanis* because of its residence in the upper respiratory tract of dogs.

Both *B. hinzii* and *B. holmesii* have been recovered from human clinical specimens. *B. hinzii* has been isolated from sputum and from four of four blood cultures collected from a 42-year-old patient with AIDS who did not have any respiratory tract symptoms.[163,764] *B. holmesii* has been isolated from blood cultures of patients with acute febrile illnesses, endocarditis, sickle cell anemia complicated by arthritis, diabetes, prior splenectomies, Hodgkin's disease, and respiratory insufficiency.[798] The strains described in the initial report of Weyant and coworkers had been isolated in Switzerland, Saudi Arabia, and the United States. *B. avium* has not been isolated from human specimens or infections.

CULTURE AND ISOLATION OF *BORDETELLA PERTUSSIS*

Since *B. pertussis* preferentially attaches to the ciliated epithelium in the upper respiratory tract, the specimen of choice is a nasopharyngeal swab or a nasopharyngeal aspirate.[266,470] For collection of nasopharngeal swabs, two specimens are usually collected by passing a small-tipped, nasopharyngeal swab posteriorly through each nostril until the tip reaches the posterior nasopharynx. The swabs are left in place for 30 seconds to 1 minute to allow organisms to adsorb onto the swab. Fine-tipped, calcium alginate (Ultrafine Calgiswab, Inolex Corp.) or Dacron swabs (Spectrum Laboratories, Inc., Los Angeles CA) on the end of a fine, flexible aluminum wire are the optimal specimen collection devices.[266,641,832] Cotton-tipped swabs should not be used because cotton material is actually inhibitory to the organism. In addition, PCR-based assays for direct detection of *B. pertussis* may be inhibited by calcium alginate fibers and aluminum; specimens processed for detection of *B. pertussis* by PCR should be collected with Dacron swabs with plastic shafts.[780] Nasopharngeal aspirates are collected by passing an infant-sized feeding tube attached to a mucus trap into the posterior pharynx along the floor of the nasopharynx and applying gentle suction once the tube is in place.[326] Nasopharyngeal swabs collected along with an aspirate may provide the highest yield of positive cultures, and regular throat cultures for isolation of *B. pertussis* are not appropriate.[56] Special media is required for the isolation of *B. pertussis*. The classic medium used for this organism is Bordet-Gengou (BG) agar. This medium is prepared from pototoes to impart a high starch content to it. The starch neutralizes toxic materials that may be present in the agar or in the specimen itself. Peptones are ommitted from the medium, because these proteins are also inhibitory. The BG agar also contains glycerol as a stabilizing agent. Although "home made" BG agar base is superior, dehydrated basal medium is commercially available (Difco Bordet-Gengou Agar Base, 0048, Difco Laboratories, Detroit MI). The base is prepared ahead and stored under refrigeration. If a patient is suspected of having pertussis, the laboratory must be notified in advance of receiving the specimen, because the final medium must be freshly made. To prepare the medium for use, the potato–glycerol agar base is melted, and 30 mL of defibrinated sheep blood per 100 mL of agar base medium (approx. 23% blood: w/v) is added. Methicillin (final concentration of 2.5 µg/mL) or cephalexin (final concentration of 40 μg/mL) should be added to some of the medium to inhibit contaminant gram-positive organisms that may be present in the specimen. Both nonselective and selective medium should be inoculated, because some *B. pertussis* strains may be slightly inhibited by methicillin or cephalexin.

In 1977, Regan and Lowe described a medium containing charcoal and horse blood that has demonstrated superiority to BG agar in several studies.[266,613] Although originally described as a transport–enrichment medium, Regan-Lowe agar formulations are available both as a semisolid transport–enrichment medium and as a solid medium for organism isolation. The formula for Regan-Lowe (RL) medium (per liter distilled water) is shown in Box 8-1.

The semisolid transport/enrichment medium is identical in formula to the isolation medium shown in Box 8-1, except that the charcoal agar is present in half-strength (i.e., 25.5 g/L), and is dispensed into sterile screw-capped tubes rather than into 100-mm petri dishes. It is also recommended that some of the medium be prepared without cephalexin so that both selective and nonselective medium is available for recovery of the organisms.

Optimally, media should be directly inoculated at the time of specimen collection onto both selective (methicillin- or cephalexin-containing) and nonselective media. If a transport system is used, the Regan-Lowe (RL) semisolid medium is optimal, because Stuart and Amies transport medium formulations are not suitable for maintaining the viability of *B. pertussis*. Specimens transported in semisolid RL medium can be subcultured on receipt to RL isolation medium or BG medium with and without cephalexin (or methicillin). The transport medium is then incubated along with the primary plate and subcultured to RL agar after 48 hours enrichment, at 35°C in 5% to 7% CO_2. All plates should be held for at least 7 days.

Various other media formulations for isolating *B. pertussis* have been reported in the literature.[22,360,361,425,514] Many of these have been modifications of the Regan-Lowe formula; that is, a charcoal agar base supplemented with defibrinated blood plus antibiotics, such as lincomycin. Hoppe and Schlagenhauf found that horse blood encouraged abundant, more rapid growth of *B. pertussis* than sheep blood, and that both were clearly superior to human blood.[360] The organism will also grow on buffered charcoal yeast extract (BCYE) agar, the medium used for the isolation of *Legionella* species. Ng and colleagues unexpectedly isolated *B.*

pertussis from bronchoalveolar lavage and transbronchial biopsy specimens of three AIDS patients on BCYE agar in their search for *Legionella* organisms in these patients.[545] A blood-free medium called cyclodextrin solid medium (CSM) has also been described.[22] This medium contains a compound called heptakis (2,6-*O*-dimethyl)-β-cyclodextrin in a synthetic broth base containing glutamate, proline, balanced salts, TRIS buffer, casamino acids, and L-cysteine. Heptakis cyclodextrin stimulates the growth of *B. pertussis* and suppresses the growth of the normal oropharyngeal flora. This medium can also be made selective by the inclusion of cephalexin (5 μg/mL final concentration). In a study of 40 specimens from 29 patients with clinical pertussis, *B. pertussis* was recovered from 100% of the specimens cultured on selective CSM medium, but from only 65% of the specimens cultured on selective BG agar. The CSM medium was also demonstrated to have a longer refrigerated shelf life than BG agar.

DIRECT FLUORESCENT ANTIBODY TEST

In addition to culture, direct fluorescent antibody (DFA) tests are used to detect *B. pertussis* directly on smears prepared from nasopharyngeal specimens. Although DFA tests do provide rapid results, it is well accepted that culture on appropriate media is more sensitive than DFA.[285,329,832] Depending on when in the clinical course the specimens are collected, the DFA test may not detect small numbers of organisms that will be picked up on culture. Some workers have found the DFA test to be unacceptably insensitive and nonspecific. Halperin and associates found that only six of 20 cases positive by culture were DFA-positive, and that only four of the 12 DFA-positive, culture-negative cases were confirmed by serologic testing of acute and convalescent serum specimens.[329] Added to this are the inherent difficulties with interpretation and subjectivity of fluorescence techniques. Furthermore, the polyclonal *Legionella* antisera for direct fluorescent antibody detection of these organisms will also react with some *B. pertussis* and *B. bronchiseptica* strains, resulting in false-positive immunofluorescence results for *Legionella* species.[61,379,544] The DFA test for detection of *B. pertussis* should be used in conjunction with culture, not in place of it.

Nasopharyngeal swab specimens collected at the same time as culture specimens are placed in a sterile tube containing a small amount (0.5 mL) of casamino acids. After vigourous mixing, four to eight smears are prepared. Layering of drops of the material, allowing drying between drops, should yield a smear that has a visible film of material on it. After drying and heat fixing, the slides may be stained. Properly titered *B. pertussis* and *B. parapertussis* conjugates should be used; because of the high specificity of the conjugates, one can be used as the nonspecific negative-staining control for the other in the staining procedure. Both conjugates are available only from Difco Laboratories. Positive and negative control smears are prepared from stock cultures of the organisms grown on antibiotic-free BG or RL medium. On DFA, the organisms appear as small coccobacilli with bright, apple-green periph-

---

BOX 8-1. FORMULA FOR RL MEDIUM (PER 1L DISTILLED WATER)

Charcoal agar (Oxoid Cm 119)	51 g
Horse blood, defibrinated	100 mL
Cephalexin	0.04 g
Amphotericin B (optional)	0.05 g
Final pH 7.4	

eral fluorescence (see Color Plate 8-3E). They may appear singly, in pairs, or in clusters. In smears prepared from highly tenacious specimens, the organisms may appear adherent to the mucous strands. Gram stains of simultaneously prepared smears help confirm the coccobacillary morphology of organisms observed to fluoresce with the reagent. Gram-stained or DFA-stained organisms taken from antibiotic-containing medium may appear more elongated and filamentous owing to antibiotic effects on the organism.

CULTURAL CHARACTERISTICS AND IDENTIFICATION OF BORDETELLA SPECIES

On culture, colonies of B. pertussis may be observed after 2 to 4 days. Growth is usually apparent sooner on antibiotic-free medium, but this is not always true. Plates should be examined under a dissecting microscope (10×) with oblique incident light to determine colony characteristics. Fresh clinical isolates of B. pertussis on BG agar appear as smooth, shiny colonies with a high, domed profile. Classically, they are described as resembling small droplets of mercury (see Color Plate 8-3C). Colonies on BG may be slightly β-hemolytic, particularly in the more confluent areas of growth or after prolonged incubation. On RL agar medium, colonies are small, domed, and shiny, with a white mother-of-pearl opalescence (see Color Plate 8-3D). B. parapertussis colonies grow more rapidly, are more β-hemolytic, and are gray or slightly brown. B. bronchiseptica colonies are apparent within 24 hours, are large and more flat, and have a dull, rather than a shiny, appearance. The latter species resembles a nonfermentative gram-negative rod (such as an Alcaligenes species) in the appearance of its colonies and the production of a distinct "nonfermenter" odor. The gram-stained morphology of these organisms also differ. B. pertussis appears as small, pale-staining, coccobacilli, whereas B. parapertussis and B. bronchiseptica are more definitely rod-shaped. Because of the pale staining of the organisms, the safranin counterstain should be left on the slide for at least 2 minutes.

Once isolated, B. pertussis is generally identified by the fluorescent antibody test because the organism is so inert in biochemical identification tests (Table 8-12). Serologic methods may be used to identify B. parapertussis as well, but biochemical methods may provide a presumptive identification. B. pertussis, B. bronchiseptica, and B. hinzii are oxidase-positive, whereas B. parapertussis and B. holmesii are oxidase-negative; B. parapertussis, B. bronchiseptica, B. hinzii, and B. holmesii are catalase-positive, whereas B. pertussis is variable for catalase production. Both B. parapertussis and B. bronchiseptica are urease-positive, with the latter species producing a positive test in less than 4 hours. B. hinzii is variable for urease production, whereas both B. avium and B. holmesii are urease-negative. Both B. parapertussis and B. holmesii produce a soluble brown pigment on certain agar media, whereas B. pertussis, B. bronchiseptica, and B. avium do not. Other characteristics for the identification of Bordetella species are shown in Table 8-12.

NEW TECHNOLOGIES FOR DETECTION AND IDENTIFICATION OF BORDETELLA PERTUSSIS

New technologies are also being applied to the identification and the direct detection of B. pertussis in clinical specimens.[267,321,322,323] Monoclonal antibodies developed against B. pertussis LPS and FHA have been used in dot-blot and enzyme-linked immunosorbent assay (ELISA) formats for identification of B. pertussis from isolated colonies.[321,322,661] Various rapid methods for direct detection of B. pertussis antigens and virulence factors in nasopharyngeal specimens have also been described. Monoclonal antibodies prepared against B. pertussis PT and FHA proteins and against B. pertussis LPS have been developed and tested in enzyme-immunoassay formats as "antigen-capture" tests for direct detection of these pertussis-specific virulence factors in clinical specimens.[267,321,323] In vitro tissue culture assays, such as the Chinese hamster ovary cell cytotoxicity test, performed directly on upper respiratory tract specimens, have also been described as rapid, sensitive, and specific assays for diagnosis of pertussis.[328] Purified PT and FHA proteins are also being exploited, not only as candidates for acellular pertussis vaccines, but also as antigens for use in antibody detection assays as diagnostic tools and for immune status surveys.[310]

With the genetic characterization of B. pertussis and its virulence factors (e.g., PT and FHA) and the cloning of the genes for these proteins, genus- or species-specific probes have been created and used for direct detection of organisms in nasopharyngeal specimens or for culture confirmation.[618] Assays using probes following PCR amplification techniques have, generally, been highly sensitive and specific.[287] Primers and probes have been developed for detection of unique repeated gene elements, B. pertussis–specific insertion sequences, the pertussis toxin gene promoter region, the adenylate cyclase gene, and the structural genes for unique B. pertussis porin proteins.[37,72,208,238,287,315,339,450,491,673,674,765] Molecular techniques, such as pulsed-field gel electrophoresis, have also been used to characterize and compare B. pertussis strains recovered in outbreaks of pertussis.[191]

SEROLOGIC TESTS FOR DIAGNOSIS OF PERTUSSIS

Serologic tests for pertussis have attracted a great deal of scientific interest in recent years owing to the development and testing of acellular pertussis vaccines. Until quite recently, serologic tests for pertussis were performed with inactivated whole cells or with crude acellular extracts of B. pertussis as antigens; interpretation of serologic tests using these antigens was often difficult. With the development of techniques for isolation and purification of discrete pertussis antigens, such as PT and FHA, serologic methods to determine the immune responses to these specific antigens following clinical infection or immunization have been developed.[496,698] Tests for antibodies to specific B. pertussis antigens are currently used to evaluate the ability of subunit components of the organism to elicit an antibody response in experimental animals and in vac-

TABLE 8-12
Biochemical Characteristics for Identification of *Bordetella* Species

Characteristic	B. pertussis	B. parapertussis	B. bronchiseptica	B. avium	B. hinzii	B. holmesii
Catalase	v	+	+	+	+	+
Oxidase	+	–	+	+	+	–
Motility	–	–	+	+*	+	–
Nitrate reduction	–	–	+	–†	–	–
Urease		+ (24 h)	+ (4 h)	–	v	–
Growth on citrate	–	+	+	+	+	NA
Brown pigment in heart infusion agar with L-tyrosine (1 g/L)	–	+	–	–	–	+
Growth on						
BG agar	3–6 d	1–3 d	1–2 d	2 d	2 d	2 d
Chocolate agar	–	1–3 d	1–2 d	2 d	2 d	2 d
MacConkey agar	–	–	+	+	NA	3–7 d
Salmonella-Shigella agar	–	–	+	+	NA	NA
Regan-Lowe agar	3–6 d	2–3 d	1–2 d	1–2 d	2 d	2 d

*Motility more pronounced at 25°C.
†In serum-supplemented media, nitrate is reduced.
d, days

cine efficacy trials.[138,327] Serology has also been used to diagnose recently acquired pertussis owing to the difficulties in isolating the organism and the frequent presentation of the patient at a time in the course of the disease during which organisms may no longer be present in the nasopharynx.

Several components of *B. pertussis* are immunogenic and engender brisk antibody responses. Guiso and colleagues used Western blot analysis to examine the host reponse to several *B. pertussis* antigens, including PT, FHA, H-AC, and pertactin, in 27 children with suspected pertussis.[319] Of these children, 19 were diagnosed as having pertussis by serology, and 10 of these 19 children were culture-positive. Convalescent sera from all 19 patients were positive for anti-PT, anti-FHA, and antiH-AC antibodies by Western immunoblot, whereas only one convalescent serum specimen demonstrated anti-pertactin antibodies. He and his coworkers examined pooled and purified antigens of *B. pertussis* in an enzyme-linked immunoassay (EIA) format to determine the antigen or antigens that would provide the most sensitive test having a specificity of at least 99%.[338] They found that the sensitivities of the EIA using PT alone, FHA alone, or pertactin alone were 92%, 85%, and 62%, respectively; the sensitivity of the EIA with a pool of these antigens was 85%. The adenylate cyclase of *B. pertussis* has also been purified and used as the antigen in a EIA-based serologic test, which showed that high titers of anti-AC antibodies are produced after infection and after immunization with whole-cell vaccines.[241] Functional assays for antibody-mediated inhibition of biologic effects of these toxins have also been developed. For example, Kaslow and coworkers described direct and indirect methods for measuring the inhibition of PT-mediated ADP-ribosyltransferase activity following both immunization and infection with *B. pertussis*.[390]

ANTIMICROBIAL SUSCEPTIBILITY AND TREATMENT OF PERTUSSIS

Pertussis is generally treated with erythromycin for a period of at least 2 weeks to prevent relapse. Administration of this antibiotic, even during the paroxysmal stage, shortens the severity and the duration of illness. In 1995, however, the first case of pertussis caused by an erythromycin-resistant *B. pertussis* strain was reported in a 2-month-old child in Yuma, Arizona.[448] After the child failed to improve clinically on a 12-day course of erythromycin, disk testing of the isolate showed no zones of inhibition around the erythromycin, clarithromycin, and clindamycin disks. Agar dilution testing revealed an erythromycin MIC of higher than 64 μg/mL. In vitro, *B. pertussis* is susceptible to a wide variety of antimicrobial agents, including ampicillin–amoxicillin, trimethoprim–sulfamethoxazole, rifampin, ciprofloxacin, ofloxacin, and temafloxacin.[424,739] These other drugs have been used and will eliminate the organism from the respiratory tract, but clinical experience indicates that erythromycin is superior. In addition, most strains are resistant to tetracycline.

The other *Bordetella* species are more resistant to antimicrobial agents than *B. pertussis*. As a part of the

Multicenter Pertussis Surveillance Project, agar dilution antimicrobial susceptibility data were collected on 46 *B. parapertussis* and 11 *B. bronchiseptica* isolates.[424] Although the *B. parapertussis* strains were susceptible to erythromycin, trimethoprim–sulfamethoxazole, and ciprofloxacin, most were resistant to amoxicillin, and all were resistant to rifampin and tetracycline. Among the *B. bronchiseptica* isolates, 82% were susceptible to trimethoprim–sulfamethoxazole, and 27% were susceptible to ciprofloxacin. All strains were resistant to amoxicillin, erythromycin, rifampin, and tetracycline.

BRUCELLA SPECIES

EPIDEMIOLOGY OF BRUCELLOSIS

Brucellosis (infection with *Brucella* species) is worldwide in distribution and has been known historically as undulant fever, Bang's disease, Gibralter fever, Mediterranean fever, and Malta fever. The organism was first isolated in 1887 by Sir David Bruce, who recovered a suspect organism from the spleens of British soldiers dying of Malta fever. It was later found that goat's milk and products produced from it (e.g., goat cheese) were the source of the infection in these soldiers. Subsequently, several other similar organisms were recovered from cattle and sows and from humans exposed to these animals and their products. The disease, therefore, is a zoonosis and is of great economic importance to the livestock industry in certain parts of the world. In developed countries, some human infections are associated with meatpacking and dairy-related occupations.[831] In the United States, most of the reported cases have come from California, Iowa, Virginia, and Texas, reflecting the animal husbandry, cattle, and dairy industries central to the economy of those states.

The incidence of human brucellosis in the United States has declined steadily as a result of control measures implemented in the livestock industry. These measures include vaccination of young animals and slaughter of older animals with serologic evidence of infection.[831] When the Federal–State Cooperative Brucellosis Eradication Program and routine dairy pasteurization began in 1945, over 5000 human cases were reported to the CDC annually. In 1981, the reported domestic incidence of human brucellosis had dropped to 185 cases, and since that time fewer than 200 cases per year have been reported. However, human brucellosis is underdiagnosed and underreported, with estimates that at least 25 cases go unrecognized for every case that is diagnosed.[598] With the increasing popularity of international travel, cases of brucellosis are being seen in the United States that are imported from areas of the world where the disease is still endemic.[598] *Brucella melitensis*, the organism most commonly implicated, is found in the Mediterranean, the Arabian Gulf, the Indian subcontinent, Latin America, Asia, and parts of Mexico. *Brucella abortus* is found worldwide, and *B. suis* is endemic in the southern United States, Southeast Asia, and Latin America; *B. canis* infections are seen in Latin America, Central Europe, and Japan.

Over the last 5 to 10 years, increasing numbers of brucellosis cases have been diagnosed in Texas and California among individuals who have ingested Mexican cheese prepared from unpasteurized goat's milk.[747] Similar cases are being seen among travelers to Italy, France, Greece, Spain, and Mexico after their return to this country.[29] Here, *B. melitensis* infection, particularly, is primarily food-borne and is associated with consumption of unpasteurized dairy products (milk, cheese, yogurt). Brucellosis may pose an occupational hazard to laboratory workers handling cultures of the organism, as a result of laboratory accidents, such as spills or aerosolization.[6,317,472,512,553,725] Occasionally, this infection is diagnosed in unusual settings or circumstances. For example, Grave and Sturm reported on an outbreak of *B. melitensis* infections associated with the use of a cosmetic facial "beauty" treatment consisting of bovine fetal and placental cells.[311]

Brucella infection is a zoonosis; that is, a disease that humans acquire from animals or from animal products. A wide variety of animals may be infected with brucellae, including goats, sheep, cattle, swine, dogs, buffalo, caribou, and reindeer. The organisms are transmitted among the animals through the gastrointestinal tract, skin, and mucous membranes. Organisms reach the lymph nodes and bacteremia occurs. In some animals (e.g., *B. abortus* infection in cattle), the organisms proliferate in the uterus and in the mammary glands. Growth of the organism in the chorionic membranes of the pregnant animal leads to abortion.[118] Many animals recover from the infection spontaneously but continue to shed the bacteria for varying times in urine, vaginal secretions, and milk. The six recognized species in the genus are named for the animals that they primarily infect: *B. abortus* (cattle), *B. melitensis* (sheep, goats), *B. suis* (swine), *B. canis* (dogs, especially beagles), *B. ovis* (rams), and *B. neotomae* (wood rats). The first four species are associated with human disease. *B. melitensis* is considered the most virulent species, followed by *B. suis* and *B. abortus*. The protean complications associated with these species (e.g., meningitis, endocarditis, hepatic and splenic abscesses, osteomyelitis, arthritis) are not generally seen in human *B. canis* infections.[81]

TAXONOMY

The taxonomy of *Brucella* species, like that of *Bordetella*, is still unclear and unresolved. In the 1957 edition of *Bergey's Manual*, *Brucella* species were listed in the family *Brucellaceae*. However, in the subsequent two editions of the same manual (1974 and 1984), the family *Brucellaceae* was not recognized, and *Brucella* (like *Bordetella*) was listed as a genus of uncertain affiliation. De Ley and coworkers examined *Brucella* species when they proposed the family *Alcaligenaceae* for the bordetellae and found that *Brucella* species were significantly different genetically and should not be included in the family *Alcaligenaceae*.[189] Subsequent ribosomal ribonucleic acid:DNA hybridization studies by the same group indicated that *Brucella* species are related to CDC Group Vd (*Ochrobactrum anthropi*) and *Phyllobac-*

terium species, which are chemoautotrophic pathogens of tropical plants.[188,354] With use of the same technology, *Brucella* species were shown to be genetically distinct from, and unrelated to, *Haemophilus*, *Bordetella*, *Alcaligenes*, *Francisella*, and *Moraxella* species, and to the *Enterobacteriaceae*. In fact, Verger and colleagues used DNA–DNA hybridization studies to investigate 51 *Brucella* strains of all species and found them to be identical.[774] Given these data, this group proposed that all species be considered biovars of *Brucella melitensis* (i.e., *B. melitensis* biovars *abortus*, *suis*, and *canis*). However, because of the differences in the animal reservoirs and in the severity of clinical disease associated with the different species, this proposal has not been widely accepted.

VIRULENCE OF *BRUCELLA* SPECIES

Brucella species are one of the organisms that undergo antigenic variation or "dissociation" on subculture. Morphologically, the colonies switch from a "smooth" to a "rough" morphology that results in a loss of virulence and diminished reactivity with *Brucella*-specific antibodies. On the molecular level, antigenic variation is the result of decreased expression of genes encoding the additional glycosylation of the polysaccharide moieties of the cell wall lipopolysaccharide (LPS).[417] The LPS of *B. melitensis*, *B. abortus*, and *B. suis* contains two major antigenic determinants called A (for "abortus") and M (for "melitensis").[107] The A and M antigenic determinants are not found in *B. canis*. These determinants are not species-restricted, and both may be expressed to varying degrees on the same cell. As a result, a great deal of serologic cross-reactivity may be seen among these three species. Organisms that are in the smooth phase are resistant to intracellular killing by polymorphonuclear cells (PMNs), presumably by inhibiting lysosomal degranulation and the respiratory burst associated with activation of PMNs.[624] Other than the antigenic variation of LPS and its relation to virulence, *Brucella* species do not produce exotoxins, and very little else is known about additional virulence mechanisms in *Brucella* species.

Brucella species are facultative intracellular organisms, and the disease spectrum is partially explained by the ability of the organism to evade host defense mechanisms by virtue of its intracellular existence. Brucellae are transmitted to humans by three principal routes: direct contact with infected animal tissues, ingestion of contaminated meats or dairy products, and inhalation of aerosolized organisms.[598,831] Once in the host, the organisms are phagocytosed but are able to survive within these cells, presumably by inactivating the intracellular myeloperoxidase–peroxide defense mechanisms. The organisms are carried into the lymph nodes and the bloodstream and become sequestered in various parts of the reticuloendothelial system, such as liver sinusoids, spleen, and bone marrow. In these sites, the PMNs eventually degenerate and release the intracellular organisms. The bacteria, in turn, are endocytosed by macrophages and monocytes; the bacteria continue to multiply within these cells and, eventually, the cells are killed, thus releasing the organisms. It is thought that the "undulant" fever pattern seen in brucellosis corresponds with the periodic release of bacteria and bacterial components, such as LPS, from phagocytic cells. Release of bacteria into the peripheral circulation results in hematogenous seeding of other organs and tissues, thereby leading to the protean clinical manifestations of human brucellosis. Relapses and recurrences of brucellosis are kept in check, to some degree, by a balance between the virulence of the organism and the presence of an intact, functional cellular immune response. As with other intracellular pathogens, humoral antibodies are produced, but cellular immune defense mechanisms are required to contain the intracellular bacteria. The spectrum of disease depends on many factors, including the immune status of the host, the presence of other underlying diseases or conditions, and the species of infecting organisms. The greater virulence of *B. melitensis* and *B. suis* has been supported by in vivo studies with experimentally infected animals and by in vitro work examining phagocytosis, intracellular survival, and lymphocyte responses to the different species. Diseases caused by *B. abortus* and *B. canis* are insidious in their onset but tend to cause milder constitutional symptoms and less severe complications.

CLINICAL SPECTRUM OF *BRUCELLA* INFECTIONS

Brucella infections may be difficult to diagnose because of the wide spectrum of clinical manifestations associated with them.[598,831] Following an incubation period of about 2 to 3 weeks (with a range of from 1 week to 2 or 3 months), the onset of symptoms may be abrupt or may develop over a period of several days to more than a week. Fever, night sweats, chills, and malaise, often accompanied by severe headache, myalgias, and arthralgias are the nonspecific symptoms seen in most cases of brucellosis. Lymphadenopathy, splenomegaly, and hepatomegaly may also be present; cutaneous manifestations (including erythema nodosum-like lesions and maculopapular or papulonodular rashes) may also be noted in some patients. The name "undulant fever" is synonymous with brucellosis (especially that caused by *B. melitensis*) because of the periodic fevers that may occur over weeks, months, or even years.[831] Fevers tend to occur in the evening and night, with normal temperatures maintained during the day, over a period of 2 to 3 weeks. After this, several days may ensue when the patient is afebrile and feels relatively well, only to experience another cycle of waxing and waning fevers. These symptoms may come and go over prolonged periods owing to the containment of the organisms in granulomas in tissue and the subsequent release of these organisms (or organism components, such as LPS) back into the circulation. Therefore, the disease presents nonspecifically and assumes the characteristics of a debilitating, chronic illness. These patients are frequently pancultured to determine an etiology for a "fever of unknown origin."[521]

In some patients, acute and chronic brucellosis may lead to complications that affect several organ systems. These complications include invasion of the skeletal system, the central nervous system, the respiratory tract, the gastrointestinal tract, the cardiovascular system (native or prosthetic valve endocarditis with septic emboli), and the skin.[9,144,198,308,368,517,522,535,598,831] Bone and joint involvement, including peripheral joint arthritis, bursitis, sacroiliitis, spondylitis, and osteomyelitis, is the most commonly described complication of brucellosis and is seen most often with *B. melitensis* infection.[10,59,158,487] Arthritis and sacroiliitis are associated with acute disease and in pediatric patients, whereas spondylitis, vertebral osteomyelitis, and paravertebral abscess are seen more frequently in chronic infections and in older persons.[9,159,841] Neurobrucellosis presents initially as encephalitis or meningitis, and patients will have CSF pleocytosis, elevated protein, and low glucose levels in the CSF. Patients with acute meningitis usually present with headache, vomiting, fever, and nuchal rigidity, and some patients may develop papilledema, visual symptoms, and cranial nerve palsy. Thrombosis of blood vessels may lead to cerebral infarction and hemorrhage, encephalitis, myelitis, and peripheral neuropathy.[490] Epidural spinal abscesses, paraspinal abscesses, and brain abscesses are rare, but do occur occasionally.[35,388,574,664] Brucella infection of the central nervous system with colonization of a ventriculoperitoneal shunt has also been documented as the source of the organism in a patient who developed *B. melitensis* peritonitis.[14] Pulmonary infections with *Brucella* may result from hematogenous dissemination and seeding of the lungs, or from direct inhalation of the organisms in aerosols. Clinical manifestations of pulmonary brucellosis may include hilar lymphadenopathy, interstitial pneumonitis, empyema, and pleural effusion.[393] Gastrointestinal and hepatobiliary symptoms occur as a manifestation of acute systemic infections, so patients may experience nausea, weight loss, and vomiting. Long-standing infections may result in more extensive gastrointestinal disease, including colitis, enterocolitis, or spontaneous peritonitis.[190,384,427,585] Liver involvement may be reflected only by elevations in liver enzymes but is usually more extensive, particularly in *B. melitensis* and *B. suis* infections. Infections with these two species are associated with the formation of caseating hepatic granulomas and microabscesses, whereas *B. abortus* tends to produce noncaseating granulomas in the liver. Brucellae may also infect the genitourinary tract, usually as a consequence of systemic infection, where thay may cause epididymitis, orchitis, and renal granulomas. Although these organisms cause abortion in infected animals by localization in the chorioamniotic membranes of the placenta, there is little evidence supporting a role for them in spontaneous abortion in humans.[556] However, the organisms may rarely be isolated from amniotic fluid and placental tissues of women with brucellosis.[831] Cardiovascular brucellosis is a rare complication, occurring in less than 2% of infected patients, and includes native and prosthetic-valve endocarditis, mycocarditis, pericarditis, septic embolization, and

aortic aneuryms.[127] Interestingly, brucellar endocarditis is the main cause of death related to this disease.[368] Ulcerative mucocutaneous skin lesions and subcutaneous abscesses are rarely manifestations of brucellosis.[585] Unusual complications of brucella infection include thyroiditis, arthroplasty-associated infections, optic neuritis, endogenous endophthalmitis, uveitis, and focal suppurative soft-tissue abscesses.[1,3,11,154,277,598,779]

Various types of hematologic dyscrasias may be present owing to the residency of the organism in the reticuloendothelial system, including the lymph nodes, the bone marrow, and the spleen. These may include granuloma and abscess formation directly in these tissues or peripheral hematologic manifestations.[36] Small, poorly defined noncaseating granulomas may be found in the bone marrow in about 70% of patients, along with nonspecifically reactive histiocytes.[8] Leukopenia, pancytopenia, microangiopathic hemolytic anemia, and severe thrombocytopenia, all have been observed in patients with brucellosis.[8,170,201] On occasion, hematologic abnormalities may predominate in early infection, thereby masking the infectious etiology of the disease and mimicking primary hematologic diseases.[170,201] These hematologic abnormalities are transient and normalize following successful antimicrobial therapy for the bacterial infection.

SEROLOGIC DIAGNOSIS OF *BRUCELLA* INFECTIONS

Serology is also helpful for diagnosis of brucellosis, with the standard tube agglutination test (STA) being the most widely used. This test can detect both immunoglobulin M (IgM) and IgG and, consequently, can be helpful in diagnosing acute infection, relapsing infection, and chronic disease.[830] The STA uses a standardized commercial *B. abortus* antigen (Difco), is performed as a tube dilution test, and detects agglutinogens of the IgG and IgM classes. Incorporation of dithiothreitol or 2-mercaptoethanol into the tube test inactivates IgM, thereby providing an IgG-specific agglutinin titer. Most patients with active brucellosis will have STA titers of 160 or higher; these titers subsequently fall with adequate therapy. Many of the serologic assays currently in use were developed to monitor brucellae activity in animal herds.[82]

As with many other serologic tests, other less labor-intensive and less subjective methods such as EIA have been exploited for serologic diagnosis of *Brucella* infections. Enzyme immunoassays for detecting IgM, IgG, and IgA antibodies against *Brucella* have been described that use whole *B. abortus* cells, *B. abortus* smooth LPS, *B. abortus* protein extracts, and smooth LPS from *B. melitensis* as the solid-phase antigen.[27,523,830] Ariza and coworkers compared the standard tube agglutination tests with EIA methods for detection of *Brucella*-specific IgG, IgM, and IgA in 761 sera obtained from 75 patients with brucellosis. The EIA methods in this study used *B. abortus* LPS (smooth antigen) as the antigen. These workers found that the EIA methods were just as sensitive and more specific than standard serologic tests for brucellosis. Initial IgM titers were higher in patients who presented to their physician earlier in the clinical course, whereas patients who had been ill for some time before seeking medical attention tended to have high IgG titers and lower IgM titers. With receipt of adequate antimicrobial therapy, the serum IgG titers decreased four- to eightfold over the subsequent 3 to 6 months. Subsequent increases in EIA IgG and IgA were seen in patients with relapsing disease. Persistence of high levels of IgG or a slower decrease in titers following treatment in patients without relapse was associated with the presence of focal infection.[27] Serologic methods for *Brucella* diagnosis in animals have also been described.[82]

Goldbaum and coworkers in Argentina recently characterized an 18-kDa cytoplasmic protein from *Brucella* species that was present in all smooth and rough *Brucella* species examined.[291] Sera from patients who had active infections with *Brucella* reacted with this antigen in an EIA-based assay, whereas results from patients who did not have brucellosis or who had inactive disease were negative in this antibody test. This test could also differentiate healthy vaccinated cattle from vaccinated cattle who had been infected with a wild-type, disease-producing strain. Other serologic tests for diagnosis of brucellosis include the complement fixation test, precipitin tests, and indirect fluorescent antibody techniques.[830]

ISOLATION AND CULTURAL CHARACTERISTICS

Because *Brucella* species infect the reticuloendothelial system, the specimens of choice in suspected cases of brucellosis primarily include blood and bone marrow specimens. In one study of 50 patients who were eventually diagnosed with brucellosis, cultures of blood and bone marrow were positive in 70% and 92% of the patients, respectively.[304] The high rate of positive bone marrow cultures is consistent with the sequestration of these bacteria in the reticuloendothelial system. Other specimens (e.g., tissue, biopsies, CSF, or other) may occasionally be submitted for culture from those patients suspected of having complicated disease.

Because of the documented risk of laboratory-acquired infections caused by *Brucella* species, all work with specimens suspected of harboring *Brucella* and all manipulations of *Brucella* cultures should be performed in a biologic safety cabinet, with recommended precautions for Biosafety Level 3 organisms (e.g., mycobacteria, *Francisella tularensis*).[122] Procedures that are known to generate aerosols (aspiration of liquid with syringes, mixing on a "vortex" mixer, vigorous bulb pipetting, and such) should be kept to a minimum. Obviously, to comply with these guidelines, close communication among the laboratory director, the technologists, and the physicians caring for patients with "possible" brucellosis is necessary. The clinician should alert the clinical laboratory personnel when a diagnosis of brucellosis is being considered so that the laboratory staff can take the necessary safety precautions.[317]

For the isolation of *Brucella* species from blood and bone marrow specimen cultures, it was originally recommended that blood be inoculated in Castenada bottles. These are bottles in which a slant of enriched agar medium is partially submerged in a broth medium into which the blood is inoculated (i.e., the medium is "biphasic"). Subculture of such bottles is performed by washing the blood–broth mixture over the slant. Because of the slow growth of the organism, blood cultures and supplemental broth cultures should be incubated at 35°C for 4 to 6 weeks, with frequent blind subcultures to chocolate and blood agar (see Color Plates 8-3F and 8-3G).[840] Radiometric detection by the BACTEC system may or may not detect the organism and, if so, it may require at least a 10-day incubation before a positive growth index value is obtained. In our laboratory, we have recovered *Brucella* species from BACTEC blood cultures after 5 to 7 days of incubation. Yagupsky evaluated the ability of the nonradiometric BACTEC 9240 instrument to detect growth of *Brucella* species and found that 21 (78.8%) of 27 positive cultures were detected by the 9240 instrument within 7 days; the remainder were detected by blind subculture after 2 to 3 weeks of incubation.[821] The organism has also been successfully recovered after a 12-day incubation using the Septi-Chek system, for which the aerobic blood culture bottle is fitted with a "paddle" containing chocolate and blood agar media and "subcultures" are performed by inverting the bottle so the medium washes over the agar paddle.[308] Faster recovery of *Brucella* species from blood cultures has also been accomplished with the isolator lysis–centrifugation method.[539]

IDENTIFICATION OF *BRUCELLA* SPECIES

Brucella species are identified on the basis of carbon dioxide requirements for growth, biochemical tests (H_2S and urease production), growth in the presence of thionin and basic fuchsin dyes, and agglutination in antisera (Table 8-13). A presumptive identification of a "possible *Brucella* species" can be made when a slow-growing, faintly staining, minute coccobacillus is recovered from blood or bone marrow cultures of a "compatible" patient; that is, one with a history of possible occupational exposure, "exotic" travel, or ingestion of uncooked meats or unpasteurized dairy products. *Brucella* species grow slowly on blood and chocolate agars, but not on MacConkey, EMB, or other "enteric" media. Good growth will also be obtained on buffered charcoal–yeast extract agar used for isolation of *Legionella* species.[597] Both the oxidase and catalase tests are positive for all *Brucella* species.

Conventional identification methods for *Brucella* species include the requirement of CO_2 for growth, production of urease and H_2S (using lead acetate strips), and sensitivity to the dyes basic fuchsin, thionin, and thionin blue (see Table 8-13). Dye sensitivity is used not only to aid in identifying the species, but, with *B. abortus* and *B. suis*, it is also used in determining the biovar of the organism. *B. abortus* and *B. suis* are subdivided into biovars on the basis of biochemical and serologic differences, whereas the biovars (actually serovars) of *B. melitensis* are defined solely on the basis of serologic differences because they

TABLE 8-13
BIOCHEMICAL CHARACTERISTICS FOR THE IDENTIFICATION OF *BRUCELLA* SPECIES

					GROWTH IN THE PRESENCE OF DYES				SEROLOGIC AGGLUTINATION*			
					BASIC FUCHSIN	THIONIN		THIONIN BLUE				
SPECIES	BIOTYPE	CO$_2$ REQUIREMENT	H$_2$S	UREASE	20 µg	20 µg	40 µg	2 µg/mL	A	M	R	COMMON HOST
B. melitensis	1	–	–	Variable	+	+	+	+	–	+	–	Sheep
	2	–	–	Variable	+	+	+	+	+	–	–	Sheep
	3	–	–	Variable	+	+	+	+	+	+	–	Sheep
B. abortus	1	+/v	+	1–2 h	+	–	–	+	+	–	–	Cattle
	2	+/v	+	1–2 h	–	–	–	–	+	–	–	Cattle
	3	+/v	+	1–2 h	+	+	+	+	+	–	–	Cattle
	4	+/v	+	1–2 h	+/v	–	–	+	–	+	–	Cattle
	5	–	–	1–2 h	+	–	+	+	–	+	–	Cattle
	6	–	+/v	1–2 h	+	–	+	+	+	–	–	Cattle
	7	–	+	1–2 h	+	–	+	+	–	+	–	Cattle
B. suis	1	–	+	0–30 min	–/v	+	+	–/v	+	–	–	Pigs
	2	–	–	0–30 min	–	–	+	–	+	–	–	Pigs, horses
	3	–	–	0–30 min	+	+	+	+	+	–	–	Pigs
	4	–	–	0–30 min	–/v	+	+	–	+	+	–	Reindeer
	5	–	–	0–30 min	–	+	+	NA	–	+	–	Rodents
B. canis		–	–	0–30 min	–	+	+	–/v	–	–	+	Dogs
B. ovis		+	–	–	–/v	+	+	–	–	–	+	Sheep
B. neotomae		–	+	0–30 min	–	–	–	+	+	–	–	Wood rat

+, positive; –, negative; +/v, variable, but most strains positive; –/v, variable, but most strains negative; NA, not available.
*A, monospecific *B. abortus* antiserum; M, monospecific *B. melitensis* antiserum; R, Anti-rough *Brucella* serum.

are classically resistant to basic fuchsin, thionin, and thionin blue. The recognition of serologically confirmed strains of *B. melitensis* that are thionin-sensitive suggests that the conventional identification scheme needs to be modified and that new, less cumbersome identification methods are needed.[165] *B. melitensis*, *B. suis*, and *B. abortus* all produce urease; with a heavy inoculum, *B. suis* strains usually will be urease-positive on Christensen's urea medium within 5 minutes. Identification of *Brucella* species has also been accomplished by coagglutination and colony dot-blot using a genus-specific monoclonal antibody that detects the A or M antigens of *B. melitensis*, *B. abortus*, and *B. suis*.[637,778] Molecular methods with PCR have also been devised for identifying these organisms. Herman and DeRidder described a dot-blot hybridization test for identification of *Brucella* species using synthetic primers and probes for a conserved, genus-specific DNA sequence.[345] In 1994, Bricker and Halling at the U.S. Department of Agriculture developed a PCR test that was able to identify and differentiate several *Brucella* species and biovars, including *B. abortus* biovars 1, 2, and 4, all three biovars of *B. melitensis*, *B. suis* biovar 1, and all *B. ovis* biovars.[99] These species and biovars constitute most of the species and biovars seen in the United States, both in animals and in human infections.

Brucella species are not yet included in the databases of any of the commercially available kit systems for identifying gram-negative organisms, and the inadvertent use of these kits may delay diagnosis and treatment. *Brucella* organisms have been misidentified as *Moraxella phenylpyruvica* by the API 20NE nonenteric identification system, as *Moraxella* species by the MicroScan Negative COMBO type 5 system (Dade-MicroScan, West Sacramento CA), and as *Haemophilus influenzae* biotype IV by the *Haemophilus–Neisseria* identification (HNID) panel (Dade-MicroScan).[47,50] In one case, the technologist who inoculated an API 20NE strip with a *B. melitensis* isolate subsequently developed brucellosis.[50] Preliminary studies on the identification of *Brucella* species with the Biolog carbon substrate utilization identification system indicated that all *Brucella* species oxidized three of the 95 substrates on the panel, and that *B. melitensis*, *B. abortus*, and *B. suis* could be differentiated from one another by differential oxidation of seven additional substrates.[813]

TREATMENT OF BRUCELLOSIS

The treatment of human brucellosis is a controversial area because of the spectrum of disease, the possibility of chronic infection, and the development of complications.[598] Despite in vitro susceptibility to a wide variety of antimicrobial agents, these results do not directly translate into good clinical efficacies and outcomes in the patient. Successful treatment requires prolonged chemotherapy, usually with a combination of agents. With some regimens, this may lead to problems with patient compliance. Because brucellae are facultative intracellular pathogens, at least one of the antimicrobial agents should have good intracellular penetration. Traditionally, oral tetracycline for 6 weeks,

combined with intramuscular streptomycin daily for 2 to 3 weeks was the recommended therapy for brucellosis.[831] Gentamicin has been given in place of streptomycin, but both drugs require daily intramuscular administration. The use of doxycycline (a tetracycline derivative having greater solubility in lipids and a longer serum half-life) and rifampin administered orally for at least 6 weeks is a currently recommended treatment regimen.[432] Treatment of brucellosis with newer cephalosporin monotherapy, such as ceftriaxone, has resulted in failures and cannot be recommended.[433] The quinolone antibiotics show good activity against *Brucella* species in vitro, with ofloxacin being the most active.[52] A randomized, prospective study evaluated the efficacy of ciprofloxacin versus rifampin plus doxycycline in the treatment of acute brucellosis. After treatment for 45 days, five of the six patients treated with ciprofloxacin relapsed, despite in vitro susceptibility and low MICs of the *B. melitensis* isolates.[434] In a Turkish study, the clinical efficacy of a combination of ofloxacin and rifampin for 6 weeks was comparable with that achieved with the doxycycline–rifampin combination.[5] Quinolone agents and the newer cephalosporins may show better clinical efficacy when incorporated in combination therapy with other agents.

Treatment of neurobrucellosis and endocarditis also requires combination therapy. In neurobrucellosis, streptomycin regimens are contraindicated because this drug does not reach therapeutic levels in the central nervous system. For this infection, combination therapy with two or three drugs—that is, doxycycline, rifampin, and trimethoprim–sulfamethoxazole—that penetrate the CNS and are active against the infecting isolate is recommended.[490] Adequate therapy of brucellar endocarditis, similar to that caused by other bacterial agents, requires that bactericidal levels of antimicrobial agents be administered. The combination of doxycycline with rifampin and trimethoprim–sulfamethoxazole has been used successfully in the treatment of brucellar endocarditis.[490] Although cases of endocarditis caused by brucellae have been cured with antimicrobial chemotherapy alone, it is generally believed that surgical intervention (i.e., valve replacement) combined with antibiotic therapy is the best approach.[831]

FRANCISELLA TULARENSIS

EPIDEMIOLOGY OF TULAREMIA

Tularemia, the disease caused by the fastidious, gram-negative coccobacillus *Francisella tularensis*, is also a disease of animals that humans acquire by contact with them.[110,237,248] Reservoirs of the bacterium in nature include rabbits, rodents, squirrels, muskrats, beavers, voles, deer, and raccoons; domestic animals, such as cattle, sheep, swine, horses, and even cats and dogs, may also become infected.[43,489] Certain animals, such as dogs, swine, horses and cattle are fairly resistant to infection, whereas sheep and cats are relatively susceptible.[110] The organism is transmitted among animals by ticks and biting flys, such as deerflys. Transovarial transmission of *F. tularensis* occurs in the tick, thereby providing a constant source of the organism in the environment. Infections in humans are most commonly acquired by bites from infected ticks or deerflys or by direct contact with blood or internal organs of infected animals (e.g., as would occur when skinning game). Unusual sources of infection have included bites from squirrels and spiders.[458,645] Eating contaminated animal meat, ingestion of contaminated water, or inhalation of the organism in aerosols may also lead to infection. There are also several reports of human infections acquired from exposure to, or bites from, domestic cats.[43] The organism is highly contagious—as few as 10 organisms administered subcutaneously or 25 organisms given by the aerosol route are enough to cause infection, and the bacterium can easily penetrate minute breaks in the skin.[237,248] Cases of tularemia have resulted from laboratory accidents that have occurred during processing of infected specimens, isolation of the organism, or working with large numbers of the organisms in research. Although the disease has been reported throughout the United States, most cases now occur in the southern and south-central states, including Missouri, Kansas, Arkansas, Oklahoma, and Texas. Over the last 25 years, the only cases reported from Canada have occurred in Quebec.[255]

TAXONOMY

Tularemia was first described in 1911 by McCoy as a cause of a plaguelike disease in rodents during his investigations of possible bubonic plague in the rodent population of San Francisco following the devastating earthquake of 1906.[484] McCoy and Chapin subsequently isolated the causative agent and named it *Bacterium tularense* after Tulare County, California, the site of their laboratory.[485] From 1912 through 1925, Edward Francis was studying the human disease called "deer fly fever" and made the connection between this illness and the "plaguelike disease" described by McCoy in rodents. He investigated the modes of transmission, studied the causative agent, and coined the name "tularemia."[264] For his pioneering work on this disease, he received the 1959 Nobel Prize in science, and the name of the organism was changed from *Bacterium tularense* to *Francisella tularensis* in his honor.

Similar to several other organisms described in this chapter, the taxonomic position of *Francisella* is uncertain. Currently, it has no familial classification.[222] Over the years, it has been provisionally classified as genus "*Bacterium*" and included with the brucellae and pasteurellae. However, genetic, phenotypic, and cell wall analyses have demonstrated no relation to *Brucella* or *Pasteurella* species, or to the tick-borne members of the genus *Yersinia* (i.e., *Y. pestis*). *Francisella* was accepted as a new genus in the mid-1960s. The *F. tularensis* strains can be further subdivided into *F. tularensis* biovar *tularensis* (or Jellison type A) and *F. tularensis* biovar *palaearctica* (or Jellison type B). The biovar *F. tularensis tularensis* predominates in North America and is not found in Europe, is associated with

ticks and rabbits, is quite virulent in both rabbits and humans, and is recognized by acid production from glycerol and posession of citrulline ureidase.[468,662] Biovar *F. tularensis palaearctica* has been isolated in Europe, Asia, Japan, and North America, is associated with waterborne infection of rodents, tick, and mosquito vectors, and is less pathogenic in humans.[369] Disease caused by this biovar may be more common in the United States than previously thought.[760] Both biovars have been isolated from diseased cats.[43] In addition to the two well-recognized biovars just described, additional biovars have also been proposed. *F. tularensis* biovar *mediaasiatica* was suggested for strains isolated in the central Asian focus of the Soviet Union, and *F. tularensis* biovar *palaearctica japonica* was the name given for isolates from Japan.[662] Initially, all four of the biovars were proposed as different subspecies by Soviet scientists, but this has not been generally accepted. Differentiation of these biovars from each other will be described later.

A second *Francisella* species, isolated from water in Utah in 1951 and also previously classified as a *Pasteurella* species, was renamed as *Francisella novicida* in 1959.[222,436] Genetic studies now indicate that *F. novicida* is probably identical with *F. tularensis* and, instead of being a separate species, probably consitutes a third biovar of *F. tularensis* (biovar *novicida*).[351] A "third" (but actually second) *Francisella* species, *F. philomiragia* includes bacterial strains formerly called "philomiragia bacteria" that were mistakenly included with the yersiniae as "*Y. philomiragia*."[351] These organisms show genetic and antigenic relatedness to *F. tularensis* biogroups and have similar cell wall fatty acid and ubiquinone constituents. Analysis of the 16S rRNA of these organisms has corroborated the present differentiation of the genus into two species—*F. tularensis* and *F. philomiragia*.[259] Furthermore, these studies have demonstrated that *F. novicida* is more properly consider another biovar of *F. tularensis*, rather than a separate species, because the degree of 16S rRNA similarity is 99.6%.[259] An interesting thing about *F. philomiragia* is that it is a rare cause of disease in two specific groups: individuals with chronic granulomatous disease and near-drowning victims.

CLINICAL SPECTRUM OF TULAREMIA

The factors that are responsible for the virulence of *F. tularensis* are unknown. The organism produces no identifiable exotoxins but apparently posesses a capsule containing carbohydrate, protein, and lipid. The LPS of the organism has a unique structure, induces less cellular toxicity, and is less active in the the *Limulus* amoebocyte lysate assay for endotoxin than other gram-negative bacteria.[663] In experimental infections established in mice, the organisms can be recovered only from tissue of the reticuloendothelial system and from the cellular components of the peripheral blood.[261] This may explain the infrequent recovery of this organism from blood cultures collected by venipuncture. Natural infection or immunization with *F. tularensis* LVS (live vaccine strain) engenders long-lasting cell-mediated and humoral resistance to reinfection, with the cell-mediated immune response being the most important protective mechanism.[745] Persistence of cell-mediated, protective immunity, with a concomitant decline in humoral immunity, has been demonstrated in individuals who were naturally infected 25 years earlier.[231] Studies performed with mutants of the LVS strain suggest that the principal virulence factor of *F. tularensis* is the ability to invade and multiply within macrophages and other cells of the reticuloendothelial system.[67]

Clinical tularemia can be divided into six major syndromes that are delineated by the mode of organism acquisition.[110,237,248,635] **Ulceroglandular tularemia** is the most common form (70% to 85% of cases). The patient presents with an ulcerated skin lesion, usually at the site of a tick bite, along with painful regional lymphadenopathy. Other symptoms (e.g., headache, fever, chills, sweating, coughing) also are present. **Glandular tularemia** (2% to 12% of cases) is characterized by lymphadenopathy and fever, but no skin lesion may be readily apparent. **Typhoidal tularemia** (7% to 14% of cases) presents with an abrupt onset of fever, chills, headache, vomiting, and diarrhea, with no initial skin lesion or lymphadenopathy. Typhoidal tularemia is the only form in which diarrhea is usually seen.[110,248] In this form, blood and sputum cultures may be positive, and the mortality rate is usually high. **Oculoglandular tularemia** (1% to 2% of cases) results from inoculation of the organism into the conjunctivae, with severe conjunctivitis and regional lympadenopathy. **Oropharyngeal tularemia** (2% to 4% of cases) describes those patients in whom the primary lesion is in the oropharynx, and the patient presents with severe headache and bilateral tonsillitis, or an exudative pharyngitis suggestive of severe streptococcal pharyngitis, diphtheria, or Vincent's disease. Deep cervical lymphadenitis, usually in the form of an isolated, persistent swollen lymph node, appears after 1 or 2 weeks.[349,548] **Pneumonic tularemia** (8% to 13% of cases) may occur as a complication of all of the other forms, owing to seeding of the pulmonary tract during bacteremia, or as a clinical entity resulting from inhalation of the organisms in an aerosol. Radiographic examinations may show involvement of one or more lobes, with pleural effusions, pneumonic infiltrates, abscess formation, and hilar lymphadenopathy. The disease tends to be more severe in patients with other underlying conditions, such as malnourishment, alcoholism, and renal disease, and complications such as hepatosplenomegaly, renal failure, and rhabdomyolysis occur more frequently in these individuals. Pneumonic tularemia is usually seen in adults and is associated with farming activities, such as handling hay or threshing.[740] This association is likely due to the presence of rodent feces or remains in hay.[349] Suppuration of enlarged lymph nodes may be a late complication in up to 50% of patients with lymphadenopathy.[369]

Although the clinical forms of tularemia have been well described, cases have been reported in which manifestations of several clinical types appear in the same individual. Plourde and coworkers reported a case of glandular tularemia, with some features of typhoidal disease, in a child who had sustained an insect bite on the left shoulder blade.[581] Inguinal lymphadenopathy rather than lymphadenopathy near the site of the insect bite was found, and the patient developed abdominal distention and severe, watery diarrhea, both of which are features of typhoidal disease. Meningitis is a rare complication of *F. tularensis* infection, with only seven documented cases reported in the literature between 1931 and 1986.[178,455] These patients usually had significant nonmeningeal disease (glandular or typhoidal tularemia), CSF findings that were consistent with a bacterial meningitis (i.e., low glucose with high protein levels), and showed mononuclear cells as the predominent cell type on Gram stain of the CSF.

ISOLATION AND CULTURAL CHARACTERISTICS

Because this organism can penetrate through small breaks in the skin, it is considered potentially dangerous to handle specimens or cultures of the organism. As with brucellar infections, the disease may not be suspected, and considerable time may be spent handling specimens and cultures before this diagnosis is entertained. If the clinical history suggests the possibility of tularemia, all specimens and cultures should be processed in a biologic saftey cabinet, gloves should be worn during all procedures, and any procedures that may generate aerosols should be avoided.[122]

Because tularemia may not be suggested until late in the clinical course and because culture for the organism is not always successful, serology is sometimes used in establishing a diagnosis. The conventional serologic test is the tube agglutination (TA) test. This procedure has been adapted to a microagglutination (MA) procedure using safranin-stained, formalinized *F. tularensis* organisms as the antigen. Sato and coworkers demonstrated that the MA test was more sensitive than the standard TA test, detecting anti-*F. tularensis* antibodies of the IgM class, 9 days earlier than the TA test.[665] Enzyme-linked immunosorbent assays for detection of tularemia-specific antibodies are also being developed, using purified outer membrane protein antigens of the organism that seem to evoke strong immune responses regardless of clinical presentation.[66]

F. tularensis may be isolated from primary ulcers, lymph node aspirates and biopsies, sputum, bone marrow, and tissue biopsies (liver, spleen). The organisms have also been isolated from the peripheral blood; this is uncommon and usually occurs in the setting of preexisting underlying disease and in patients with the typhoidal form, although the organism has been recovered from peripheral blood in patients with other clinical forms.[349,581,595,650,760,784] In case reports describing *F. tularensis* bacteremia, growth of the organism was found after 3 to 7 days of incubation using the BACTEC radiometric system. In one case report, the organism was not recovered from BACTEC blood cultures, but was isolated on chocolate agar from the blood after 5 days using the DuPont Isolator (lysis–centrifugation technique).[650]

F. tularensis is a small, pale-staining, gram-negative coccobacillus (see Color Plate 8-3*H*). Classically, the organism has a growth requirement for the amino acids cysteine and cystine, and the preferred medium for isolation was called blood–cysteine agar. However, *F. tularensis* will grow on commercially available chocolate agar and Thayer-Martin agar because these hemin-containing media are supplemented with a growth enrichment (e.g., IsoVitelex, BD Microbiology Systems) that contains cysteine and other nutrients required by fastidious bacteria.[784] Similar to the brucellae, this organism is also able to grow on buffered charcoal–yeast extract agar, the medium used for isolation of *Legionella* species.[597,797] In 1994, Bernard and coworkers at the National Laboratory for Bacteriology in Ontario, Canada reported on seven isolates, submitted to the Canadian reference laboratory as *Haemophilus* species or as unidentified fastidious gram-negative bacteria, that were identified as *F. tularensis*.[65] These strains lacked the cysteine requirement of the classic *F. tularensis* strains. These atypical isolates were oxidase- and catalase-negative, agglutinated strongly in *Francisella* agglutinating serum (Difco Laboratories) and were unreactive in all other phenotypic tests, including those used for biovar determinations. Cellular fatty acid analysis of these strains revealed the presence of a large amount of 3-hydroxyoctadecanoate (3OH-18:O), a fatty acid that is unique to *F. tularensis* and is not found in other bacteria.[222,374] Consequently, these organisms may be identified readily by cellular fatty acid analysis using the Microbial Identification (MIDI) System and Library Generation System (LGS) software (MIDI, Newark NJ).

F. tularensis is obligately aerobic; growth is stimulated by increased CO_2 and may require 2 to 5 days before colonies are visible on agar medium. Colonies on chocolate agar are about 2 mm in diameter after a 3-day incubation in a CO_2 atmosphere and have a greenish appearance. Characteristics for presumptive identification of *Francisella* species are shown in Table 8-14. The *F. tularensis* biovars are oxidase-negative, weakly catalase-positive, grow poorly (if at all) on MacConkey agar, and are fairly inert biochemically. Species identification is usually confirmed by agglutination tests using specific antisera. Studies using spiked blood cultures and experimentally infected mice have confirmed the usefulness of a PCR-based assay for detection and identification of *F. tularensis*.[453] This assay was able to detect both biovars of *F. tularensis* at sensitivities equal to 1 colony-forming unit (CFU)/mL of blood.

Because strains belonging to the different *F. tularensis* biovars (bv.) are antigenically homogenous, the different biovars are differentiated from one another on the basis of phenotypic criteria or biovar-specific probes for 16S rRNA.[258] Strains of *F. tularensis* bv. *tularensis* produce acid in media containing either glucose or glycerol as a carbon source, and hybridize with an oligonucleotide probe for *F. tularensis* bv. *tularensis*-specific 16S rRNA sequences. The *F. tularensis* bv. *palaearctica* strains produce acid from glucose, but not from glycerol and hybridize with a probe that is specific for the *F. tularensis* bv. *palaearctica* (Jellison group

B) 16S rRNA sequences. Both *F. tularensis* bv. *mediaasiatica* and *F. tularensis* bv. *palaearctica japonica* strains hybridize with the *F. tularensis* bv. *tularensis*-specific probe; however, the *F. tularensis* bv. *mediaasiatica* strains produce acid from glycerol only, whereas *F. tularensis* bv. *palaearctica japonica* strains acidify media containing either glucose or glycerol (see Table 8-14). Citrulline ureidase, an enzyme that correlates with virulence of *F. tularensis*, is found in virulent strains of *F. tularensis* bv. *tularensis*, some *F. tularensis* bv. *palaearctica* strains, and *F. tularensis* bv. *mediaasiatica* strains.[468,662] The enzyme is not found in attenuated *F. tularensis* bv. *tularensis* strains and in most *F. tularensis* bv. *palaearctica* strains with low virulence.

TREATMENT OF TULAREMIA

The drug of choice for treatment of tularemia is the aminoglycoside streptomycin; gentamicin is an acceptable alternative.[227,237,369,476] However, clinical relapse after treatment with gentamicin has been reported.[227,626] Other regimens, such as tetracyline and chloramphenicol, have been used but are associated with a higher rate of relapse, especially if these drugs are administered early in the clinical course.[237] The initial clinical response to treatment with tetracycline is dramatic (i.e., patients defervesce rapidly), but relapse rates after therapy with this drug are over 12%, twice as much as the relapse rate seen with gentamicin therapy.[227] Intravenous therapy with erythromycin has also been used successfully.[797]

Many of the newer agents, including other aminoglycosides and some of the third-generation cephalosporins (ceftriaxone, cefotaxime) are active against *F. tularensis* in vitro.[40,671] On the other hand, a recent report on the in vitro susceptibility of Scandinavian isolates of *F. tularensis* found that all 22 strains tested were resistant not only to penicillin and cephalothin, but also to cefuroxime, ceftazidime, aztreonam, imipenem, and meropenem, with MICs of higher than 32 µg/mL for all drugs.[671] Clinical experience with the use of some third-generation cephalosporins for tularemia indicates that they are not effective. Cross and Jacobs reported on eight cases of documented failure of outpatient use of ceftriaxone in the treatment of tularemia.[171] Even though MICs of ceftazidime are lower for *F. tularensis* than those of ceftriaxone, there is currently no evidence to suggest that this drug would be useful either.[227] There is little experience reported with the use of other drugs, such as the fluoroquinolones, imipenem, or even amikacin, for the treatment of tularemia. A single case report has documented successful treatment of pneumonic tularemia with a 14-day course of imipenem–cilastatin.[443] In vitro and clinical outcome data also suggest that the fluoroquinolones ciproprfloxacin and norfloxacin may be useful for treatment of tularemia.[227,672,741] Syrjala and colleagues reported on three patients with pneumonic tularemia and one with ulceroglandular tularemia who were successfully treated with ciprofloxacin; one other patient with ulceroglandular tularemia responded to norfloxacin therapy.[741]

TABLE 8-14
BIOCHEMICAL CHARACTERISTICS FOR IDENTIFICATION OF *FRANCISELLA TULARENSIS* BIOGROUPS AND *F. PHILOMIRAGIA*

CHARACTERISTICS	F. TULARENSIS BIOGROUP TULARENSIS	F. TULARENSIS BIOGROUP PALAEARCTICA	F. TULARENSIS BIOGROUP NOVICIDA	F. TULARENSIS BIOGROUP MEDIAASIATICA	F. TULARENSIS BIOGROUP PALEARCTICA-JAPONICA	F. PHILOMIRAGIA
Oxidase	−	−	−	−	−	$-/+^w$
Motility	−	−	−	−	$-/+^w$	−
Growth on MacConkey agar	v	−	v	NA	NA	v
H$_2$S in TSI agar	−	−	−	−	−	$+^w$
Growth in nutrient broth w/6.5% NaCl	−	−	v	NA	NA	v
Urease	−	−	−	−	−	−
Nitrate reduction	−	−	−	−	−	−
Acid production from						
Glucose	+	+	$+^w$	−	+	$+^w$
Sucrose	−	−	$+^w$	NA	NA	$+^w$
Glycerol	+	−	+	+	+	NA
Maltose	+	+	−	NA	NA	$+^w$
Citrulline ureidase	$+^-$	$-^+$	+	+	−	NA

+, positive; −, negative; $+^-$, most strains positive, with rare strains negative; $-^+$, most strains negative, rare strains positive; v, variable; NA, not available; $+^w$, weakly positive; $-/+^w$, negative or weakly positive,

BARTONELLA (*ROCHALIMAEA*) SPECIES

TAXONOMY

In the 1984 edition of *Bergey's Manual of Systematic Bacteriology*, the order *Rickettsiales* included three families: *Rickettsiaceae*, *Bartonellaceae*, and *Anaplasmataceae*.[627,794] The family *Rickettsiaceae* included three genera: the genus *Rickettsia*, the genus *Coxiella*, and the genus *Rochalimaea*. Although the rickettsias and coxiellas could not be cultivated outside of specific host cells, members of the genus *Rochalimaea* were rod-shaped organisms that could be cultivated in host cell-free media. The family *Bartonellaceae* included two genera—the genus *Bartonella* and the genus *Grahamella*.[627] Members of the genus *Bartonella* were capable of infecting humans and characteristically grew in close association with the surfaces of vertebrate erythrocytes, including those of humans, whereas members of the genus *Grahamella* preferentially grew within the erythocytes of vertebrates, but did not infect humans. Only a single species of *Bartonella* (*B. bacilliformis*) two species of *Grahamella* (*G. talpae* and *G. peromysci*), and two species of *Rochalimaea* (*R. quintana* and *R. vinsonii*) were described in the 1984 edition of *Bergey's Manual of Systematic Bacteriology*.[627] *R. quintana* is the cause of trench fever in humans; *R. vinsonii* has been isolated only from voles that live on Grosse Isle, Quebec, Canada.[792,793] All of these organisms are members of the α-2 subgroup of the class *Proteobacteria*, which includes the rickettsiae, erlichiae, and *Afipia* species.[621,723]

In the early 1990s, several new clinical entities in compromised hosts, particularly patients with HIV infection, were described in association with organisms that could be seen on stained sections of biopsy material, but that were extremely fastidious and difficult to grow.[680] Isolation and characterization of these novel bacteria by molecular and genetic techniques prompted a reexamination of taxonomic considerations when it was found that these organisms were closely related to members of the genus *Rochalimaea*, specifically *R. quintana*.[174,702,796] These new organisms were given the names *Rochalimaea henselae* and *Rochalimaea elizabethae*. Subsequently in 1993, elegant taxonomic studies by Brenner and colleagues confirmed that species in the genus *Rochalimaea* were more closely related to *Bartonella bacilliformis*, the type species of the genus, and that the genus *Rochalimaea* be formally unified with the genus *Bartonella*.[98] Consequently, all of the members of the genus *Rochalimaea* have been transferred to the genus *Bartonella* as *Bartonella quintana* comb. nov., *Bartonella vinsonii* comb. nov., *Bartonella henselae* comb. nov., and *Bartonella elizabethae* comb. nov. (Table 8-15).[98]

In 1995, three new proposed *Grahamella* species were described, along with 16S rRNA analyses and comparisons with the two extant *Grahamella* species and *Bartonella* species.[74] On the basis of genetic and phenotypic criteria, Birtles and his colleagues at the Central Public Health Laboratory in London proposed that the genus *Grahamella* be unified with the genus

TABLE 8-15
TABLE 8-15
CHANGES AND PROPOSED CHANGES IN THE CLASSIFICATION OF *ROCHALIMAEA* AND *BARTONELLA* SPECIES

BERGEY'S MANUAL, 1984	BRENNER ET AL, 1993*; BIRTLES ET AL, 1995†; BREITSCHWERDT ET AL, 1995‡
Family *Rickettsiaceae*	Family *Rickettsiaceae*
Genus *Rickettsia*	Genus *Rickettsia*
Genus *Rochalimaea*	
R. quintana	
R. vinsonii	
Genus *Coxiella*	Genus *Coxiella*
Family *Bartonellaceae*	Family *Bartonellaceae*
Genus *Bartonella*	Genus *Bartonella*
B. bacilliformis	B. bacilliformis
	B. quintana
	B. vinsonii
	B. vinsonii subspecies berkoffii
	B. henselae
	B. elizabethae
Genus *Grahamella*	
G. talpae	B. talpae
G. peromysci	B. peromysci
	B. grahamii
	B. taylorii
	B. dochiae

*Brenner et al[98] proposed that the genus *Rochalimaea* and the family *Bartonellacaeae* be removed from the order *Rickettsiales,* thereby emending the order *Rickettsiales* to exclude motile organisms and organisms that are able to grow on bacteriologic media. Brenner et al also proposed that members of the genus *Rochalimaea* be removed from the family *Rickettsiaceae* and added to the family *Bartonellaceae* as emended members of the genus *Bartonella.* They also proposed that the names of the new *Rochalimaea* species, *R. henselae* and *R. elizabethae* be emended to *Bartonella henselae* and *Bartonella elizabethae,* respectively.
†Birtles et al[74] proposed that extant *Grahamella* species, *G. talpae* and *G. peromysci,* be transferred to the genus *Bartonella* as *B. talpae* and *B. peromysci,* respectively. Birtles et al also described three new *Bartonella* species from small mammals (i.e., *B. grahamii, B. taylorii,* and *B. doshiae*).
‡Breitschwerdt et al[95] described a novel *Bartonella* isolate from a dog with endocarditis and proposed the name *Bartonella vinsonii* subspecies *berkoffii* for this isolate.

Bartonella, with the latter name taking precedence, according to rules of nomenclature.[74] Therefore, the genus *Bartonella* now contains the four species listed in the foregoing, the two original former *Grahamella* species (*B. talpae* comb. nov., *B. peromysci* comb. nov.), and three newly described species, *B. grahamii* sp. nov., *B. taylorii* sp. nov., and *B. doshiae* sp. nov.[74] The following discussion will concern those *Bartonella* species that have been associated with human infections: *B. bacilliformis, B. quintana, B. henselae,* and *B. elizabethae* (see Table 8-15). The other newly described species are found in small mammals.[74]

CLINICAL SIGNIFICANCE

Bartonella species are associated primarily with infections in the compromised host, particularly those patients with HIV-1 infection. Infections with these organisms now encompass several conditions, including cat-scratch disease, bacillary angiomatosis with cuta-

neous or systemic involvement, peliosis hepatis, relapsing fever with bacteremia, and endocarditis. The type species of the genus *Bartonella, B. bacilliformis* causes Oroya fever, a geographically restricted febrile illness. *B. quintana* is the classic agent of trench fever, a louse-borne, debilitating febrile illness that is rarely seen today, despite the fact that it affected a great many military personnel during World War I.

Oroya Fever and Verruga Peruana. These two clinical entities are both manifestations of infection with *B. bacilliformis.*[551] These infections are geographically restricted because of the limited habitats of the sandfly vectors belonging to the genus *Phlebotomus.* Infections are seen in river valleys of the Andes mountains at altitudes between approximately 610 and 2438 m (2000 and 8000 ft) in Peru, Ecuador, and Columbia.[630] This infection is also known as Carrion's disease after Daniel Carrion, a Peruvian medical student who developed the disease after inoculating himself with material from an infectious lesion.

Following the bite of an infected vector, symptoms of Oroya fever develop in from 3 weeks to 3 months. Onset may be abrupt or insidious. The patient may have anorexia, headache, malaise, and a slight fever lasting 2 to 7 days or more. When the onset is abrupt, the patient may present with fever, severe headache, chills, and mental status changes. Severe anemia ensues owing to destruction of red cells by the organisms. As the disease progresses, muscle and joint pain may become severe; dypsnea and angina may develop, as well as delirium and coma. During this phase, the organisms may be isolated from the blood.[630] Following this "critical" stage, the organisms disappear from the circulation, the fever normalizes, and the anemia corrects itself.[630]

After resolution of the Oroya fever, pain in the bones, joints, and muscles may persist to the stage of veruga development. This stage is characterized by the appearance of nodular lesions on exposed parts of the body, on mucous membranes, or in internal organs.[24] These nodules develop over a period of 1 to 2 months and may persist for months to years. The lesions are red to purple in color, are nontender if not secondarily infected, and may appear in crops. The "verrugas" may be sessile, miliary, nodular, pedunculated, or confluent.[24] Joint pain and fever usually subside after appearance of the skin lesions. Anemia is usually not present during this stage of the disease. *B. bacilliformis* can be cultured from the cutaneous lesions and occasionally from the blood and bone marrow during the verruga stage.

Treatment of *B. bacilliformis* infections with chloramphenicol, penicillin, tetracycline, or streptomycin produces a clinical response within 24 hours, although organisms may persist for longer in the blood.

Bacillary Angiomatosis. Bacillary angiomatosis (BA) is a bacterial infection that results in widespread unusual vascular proliferation and is seen most commonly in patients with HIV disease, although cases have been reported in transplant patients and in individuals receiving cancer chemotherapy.[149,411,440,527] Rare cases of BA have been diagnosed in immunocompetent persons.[150,744] The disease is distinct from Kaposi's sarcoma (KS) and other vascular neoplasms in that, clinically, lesions begin as small papules that gradually enlarge to form rounded red to violaceous purple nodules.[151] Individual lesions may ulcerate and crust over. On some body surfaces, the lesions may develop as flat, hyperpigmented, indurated plaques. Some lesions are located more deeply in the subcutaneous tissues (e.g., liver, or spleen) and the bone.[726] Visceral involvement may occur as disseminated vascular lesions or as bacillary peliosis hepatis when the liver is involved. Lesions of extracutaneous BA have been documented in mucosal surfaces of the upper and lower respiratory tract, the heart, the diaphragm, the biliary tract, liver and spleen, lymph nodes, bone marrow, and the central nervous system.[126,152,160,416,445,700,722,726]

Histologically, the BA lesions are composed of large, cuboidal, endothelial cells lining blood vessels. These cells extend into the vascular lumen and are associated with aggregates of purplish granular material representing clusters of bacteria.[442] Often there is also a dense inflammatory infiltrate of neutrophils. The BA lesions can be histologically differentiated from KS lesions in that there are no bizarre jagged blood vessels, as seen in KS, and the inflammatory cell infiltrate in the lesions consists of lymphocytes, histiocytes, and neutrophils as opposed to plasma cells.[152,718] When tissue sections from lesion biopsies are stained with the Warthin-Starry silver stain, numerous clumps of interstitial bacteria are seen. B. henselae and, in some cases, B. quintana have been isolated from the blood, skin lesions, bone, visceral organs, and brain of patients with BA.[410,620,622,703,722,796] At one time, BA was thought to be caused by Afipia felis, the organism initially associated with cat-scratch disease (CSD; discussed later); however, this has been shown not to be true. As with CSD, a strong epidemiologic association has been documented between BA and bites or scratches from domestic cats.[743] Because B. henselae is the likely cause of CSD, some clinicians believe that BA may be another manifestation of CSD in the compromised host.[409] In addition, BA lesions histologically and clinically resemble the lesions of late-stage verruga peruana, which is caused by B. bacilliformis.[275] In vitro examination of these Bartonella organisms has established that they are able to stimulate angiogenesis, the physiologic process that results in the formation of new blood vessels, and to affect the migration and proliferation of endothelial cells.[274,275,407]

All patients with recognized BA should be treated. Erythromycin is the drug of choice in the treatment of cutaneous BA, using a dose of 500 mg four times a day for at least 6 weeks.[648] If the BA lesions are confined to the skin, they may be excised surgically. Longer courses of antimicrobial therapy may be necessary if recurrence occurs after cessation of therapy. Parenteral therapy may be required to treat relapses of cutaneous and disseminated infections. Other antibiotics (e.g., rifampin, doxycycline, minocycline, tetracycline, azithromycin, chloramphenicol, trimethoprimsulfamethoxazole, vancomycin, norfloxacin,

ciprofloxacin with gentamicin) have been anecdotally reported as effective therapy.[525] Drugs that inhibit cell wall biosynthesis (e.g., penicillins and cephalosporins) usually fail to cure BA.

Peliosis. Before the AIDS epidemic, the condition known as peliosis of the internal visceral organs was rare. Peliosis is characterized by the presence of cystic, blood-filled lesions that are scattered throughout the parenchyma of the involved organ.[680] Before the epidemic of HIV infection, this rare condition was usually seen in patients with other chronic debilitating conditions, such as malignancies or tuberculosis. Increasing numbers of cases of peliosis, most commonly involving the liver (peliosis hepatis) and spleen, have been reported in association with HIV infection.[411,576,685] Most patients with hepatic or splenic peliosis also have BA, and bacteria similar to those seen on Warthin-Starry-stained biopsies of BA are also seen within the blood-filled cysts that are present in the internal organs, particularly in the liver and spleen. Most patients with bacillary peliosis hepatis present with weight loss, abdominal pain, intractable nausea, anemia, diarrhea, fever, hepatosplenomegaly, lymphadenopathy, and elevated alkaline phosphatase levels. Parenchymal bacillary peliosis of other internal organs (heart, larynx, lungs, adrenals, cervix, ovaries, pineal gland, and choroid plexus) have been reported. Again, the agents associated with this syndrome include B. henselae and B. quintana.[410,703] Peliosis of the internal organs is believed by some to be another manifestation of BA. The association of BA and peliosis with CSD has been demonstrated by case–control studies on the epidemiology of BA and peliosis, in which traumatic contact (i.e., bites and scratches) with cats was highly associated with the development of disease.[743]

Fever and Bacteremia. B. henselae bacteremia has been described in HIV-infected patients, patients with AIDS, recipients of allogeneic transplants, and immunocompetent hosts with no known risk factors for immunosuppressive diseases.[614,702] HIV-infected patients generally present with fever, weight loss, malaise, and fatigue; relapse following therapy often occurs in immunocompromised individuals. In HIV-infected patients, B. henselae may also cause a generalized inflammatory disease of the reticuloendothelial system.[701] These organisms may be detected histopathologically or by molecular techniques in necrotic, inflammatory lesions in the spleen, liver, heart, bone marrow, and lymph nodes.[701] Immunocompetent, HIV-negative individuals have an abrupt onset of a febrile illness, with accompanying joint and muscle pain; some patients may manifest signs and symptoms of central nervous system involvement (i.e., headache, photophobia, and meningismus). Fever and bacteremia caused by B. quintana have been documented in 10 homeless, inner-city patients who were HIV antibody–negative but had chronic alcoholism as an underlying disease.[721] All of these men presented with fever; two had splenomegaly; and three had reported a recent cat scratch. Immunocompetent patients usually have a rapid response to a short (10 days or less) course of therapy and generally do not relapse. However, Lucey and colleagues reported on two immunocompetent patients who had relapsing illness with positive blood cultures for *B. henselae*.[456] Interestingly, both of these patients had experienced tick bites before becoming ill. Although insect vectors are known to be involved in the transmision of both *B. quintana* (lice) and *B. bacilliformis* (sandflys), these two cases were the first in which transmission of *B. henselae* by insects was epidemiologically suggested. These workers also found that faster recovery of the organism was obtained using the lysis–centrifugation procedure than with broth or biphasic blood culture media.[456]

Endocarditis. *Bartonella* species have been isolated as causes of "culture-negative" endocarditis.[720] Endocarditis caused by *B. quintana* was first reported in 1993 in a 50-year-old, HIV-1–infected homosexual man.[719] Subsequently, *B. quintana* was documented as a cause of bacteremia in 10 febrile patients in Seattle; two of these patients developed endocarditis.[721] All of these patients were HIV-negative and had chronic alcoholism as their underlying disease; most were homeless and lived on the street. *B. quintana* was also documented as a cause of endocarditis in three homeless, alcoholic men in France.[212] In the Seattle cases, one patient required replacement of the aortic valve. Even

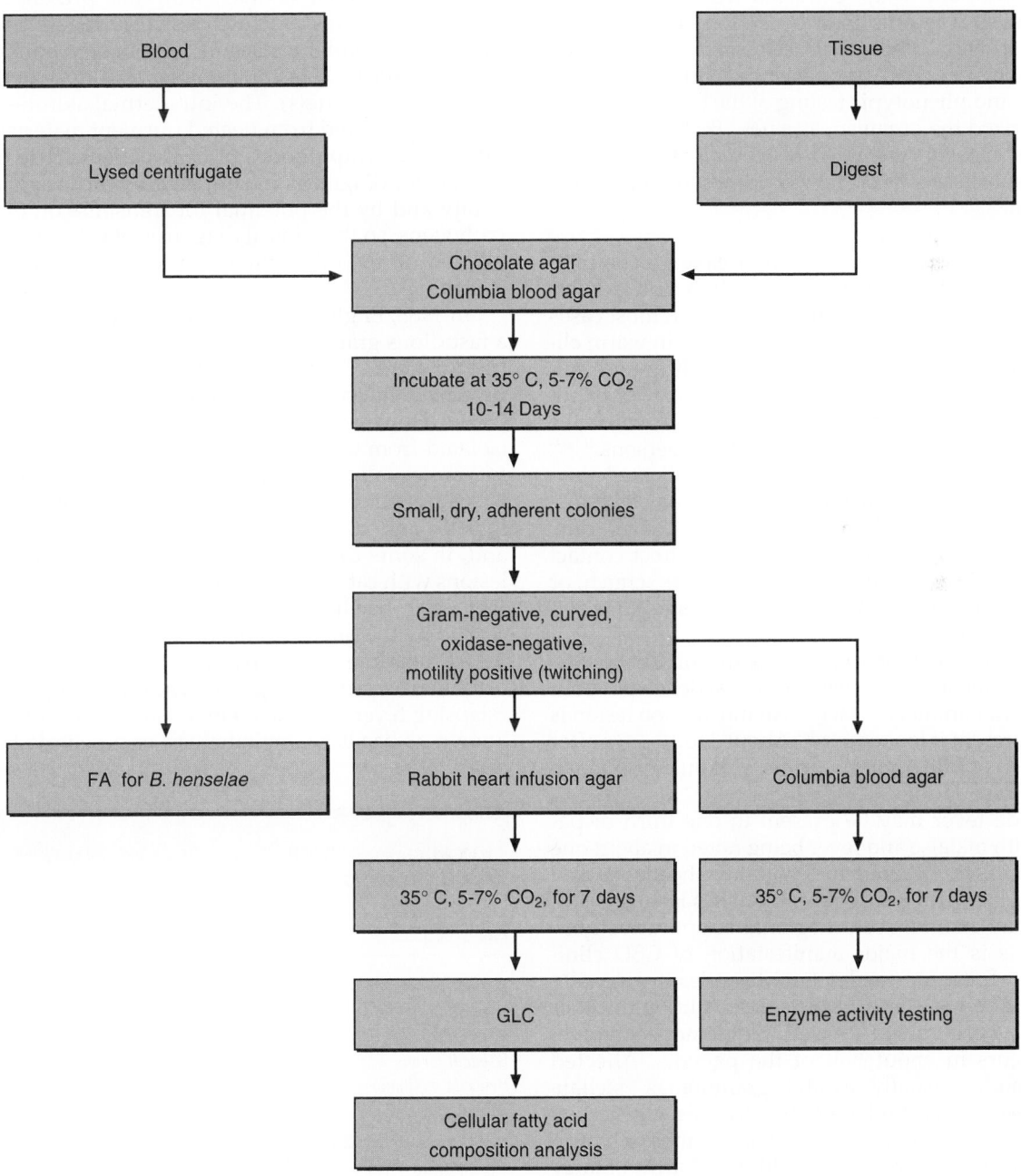

Figure 8-1.
Laboratory diagnosis of *Bartonella* infections. (After Welch et al, J Clin Microbiol 31:2381–2386, 1993)

after 21 days of therapy, *B. quintana* was detected in the tissues by PCR.[721] Also in 1993, Hadfield and coworkers described the first case of endocarditis caused by *B. henselae* in a 59-year-old HIV-negative man with a history of alcohol abuse.[324] A subsequent case of *B. henselae* endocarditis was reported in 1995 in a previously healthy 41-year-old man.[353] Both of these patients required valve replacement surgery. The first and only report of *B. elizabethae* was as a cause of endocarditis in an immunocompetent 31-year-old man.[174] Lastly, Breitschwerdt and colleagues, in North Carolina, described a case of endocarditis involving the aortic and mitral valves in a 3-year-old spayed Labrador retriever.[95] A fastidious gram-negative bacillus was isolated from the dog's blood using the lysis–centrifugation method, and DNA extracted from the involved heart valves was amplified by PCR technology and compared with other *Bartonella* species. DNA hybridization, 16S rRNA sequencing, cellular fatty acid analysis, and phenotypic testing of the bacterial isolate characterized the organism as a new *Bartonella* species that most closely resembled *B. vinsonii*. The name *B. vinsonii* subspecies *berkhoffii* was proposed for this new organism.[95]

Cat-Scratch Disease. Cat-scratch disease is a common cause of lymphadenopathy in children and adolescents. It occurs throughout the world, with most cases occurring between September and March; in warm climates, peak occurrences may occur in July and August.[680] About 90% of patients have a history of exposure to cats, and a cat scratch or a cat bite will have occurred in about 75% to 80% of these persons.[461,836] Kittens seem to be more frequently implicated than adult cats, suggesting that the CSD agent may be transmissible from cat to human for only a limited time period. Transmission appears to be by direct contact because the disease generally follows a bite, scratch, or lick from a young cat. Cats themselves show no evidence of illness.

The most common clinical feature of CSD is the chronic, regional lymphadenopathy that develops about 2 weeks after animal contact.[680] An inoculation lesion is usually present if looked for.[461] About 3 to 10 days after the scratch or bite occurs, a primary papule or pustule forms. These lesions persist for about 2 to 3 weeks. Low-grade fever may be present in one third of patients, with malaise and fever being noted in about one fourth of cases.[176] About 10% will have headache and muscle aches with a sore throat. Rashes lasting 1 to 2 weeks may also be seen. Regional suppurative lymphadenitis is the major manifestation of CSD clinically.[206,303] Enlarged tender lymph nodes are usually found in the head and neck regions, although other sites may be involved as well. Single-node involvement occurs in about half of the patients. Affected lymph nodes usually exhibit granulomas, stellate microabscesses, and follicular hyperplasia. Clusters of bacillary organisms are often seen in sections of lymph node biopsies that are stained with the Warthin-Starry silver impregnation stain. The enlarged lymph nodes eventually regress after 2 to 4 months. Atypical manifestations of CSD include the oculoglandular syndrome of Parinaud, which presents as an ocular granuloma or conjunctivitis with preauricular lymphadenopathy, osteomyelitis, epitrochlear mass mimicking rhabdomyosarcoma, and hepatic and splenic granulomas.[263,292] CSD encephalopathy is a rare complication, characterized by convulsions, combative behavior, and coma.[123,325]

Since CSD was first described, the putative agent of this disease has been sought. With the observation of bacillary organisms on silver stains of affected tissues, a bacterial etiology was strongly suspected. Because of the apparent inability to cultivate this agent, the diagnosis of CSD was largely clinical. Diagnosis of CSD was made if the patient presented with lymphadenitis and fulfilled three of four diagnostic criteria: that is, a history of animal contact with the presence of a scratch, a positive cat-scratch skin test, negative results for other potential causes of lymphadenopathy, and characteristic CSD histopathology on biopsy of the affected lymph node(s). The intradermal skin test antigen was prepared from heated purulent material aspirated from lymph nodes of CSD patients. Use of this antigen for diagnosis is hampered by the lack of availability and by the potential for transmission of other pathogens, so the clinical diagnosis of CSD largely depended on the other clinical criteria described in the foregoing.

In 1988, English and Wear reported the isolation of a fastidious gram-negative bacillus from the tissues of CSD patients.[230] Brenner and colleagues at the CDC proposed the name *Afipia felis* for this putative agent of CSD.[97] However, this organism has only rarely been isolated from CSD patients, and antibodies against *A. felis* are usually absent in CSD patients. The finding of Warthin-Starry-positive bacillary organisms in these hepatic and disseminated angiomatous skin lesions and, in some cases, the temporal association of these lesions with cat bites or scratches led some to speculate that CSD, bacillary angiomatosis, and peliosis were caused by the same organism.[149,307,392,441,467,498,500,681]

At the same time as research on the putative agent of CSD was progressing, the syndromes of persistent, relapsing fever and bacteremia and the clinical entities known as bacillary angiomatosis and peliosis hepatis

TABLE 8-16

Key Microscan Rapid Anaerobe Panel Reactions for Identifying *Bartonella* Species*

Organism	BPO₄	LYA	PRO	URE
B. henselae	+	+	+	−
B. quintana	v†	−	+	−
B. vinsonii	+	−	−	−
B. bacilliformis	+	+	−	−
Brucella melitensis	−	−	+	+
Afipia spp.	NA	NA	NA	+

*As per reference 795.
†67% of strains are negative.
BPO₄, bis-*p*-nitrophenyl phosphate; LYA, L-lysine-β-naphthylamide (acid); PRO, L-proline-β-naphthylamide; URE, urease.

were being described in patients with HIV infection.[411] *Rochalimaea* species, subsequently emended to the *Bartonella* species, were demonstrated to be the primary etiologic agents of BA and peliosis by culture studies, molecular techniques (e.g., PCR), and serologic studies.[474,622] By using highly conserved oligonucleotide primers from the bacterial 16S rRNA genes, Relman and colleagues were able to demonstrate and amplify bacterial DNA sequences in BA tissues from AIDS patients and showed that these sequences were genotypically related to *Bartonella* species, specifically *B. quintana*.[622] Slater and his colleagues recovered a *Bartonella*-like organism from blood cultures of febrile immunocompromised adults that had 16S rRNA gene sequences that were identical with those described by Relman's group.[702] In 1992, Regnery and coworkers isolated and characterized this new "*Rochalimaea*" species, *R. henselae*.[614] By IFA techniques, Regnery and colleagues also demonstrated that patients with BA and CSD had high antibody titers to *B. henselae*.[616] This organism was also isolated from the lymph nodes of two patients with CSD.[206] Culture for *B. henselae* has also been successful in other patients with disseminated CSD.[676] Goral and others have used PCR to demonstrate the presence of *B. henselae* DNA and the absence

of *B. quintana* and *A. felis* DNA in purulent material from the supperative lymph nodes of patients with CSD.[62,303,783] With use of PCR amplification of 16S rRNA and subsequent sequence analysis of the amplified material, Anderson and coworkers were actually able to demonstrate nucleotide sequences of *B. henselae* in lots of CSD skin test antigen from two different sources, and in clinical specimens from patients with clinical CSD.[16,18] A 17-kDa protein has been isolated, by recombinant DNA technology, from *B. henselae* that is specifically reactive with sera from patients with CSD and may have value as a diagnostic serologic reagent.[17] EIA-based serologic assays for detection of IgG, IgM, and IgA antibodies against *B. henselae* have also been developed.[48] With the difficulties involved in culture of the organism, serology for *B. henselae* may be extremely helpful in making diagnostic and therapeutic decisions.[209,229,292,303,325,607,616] Some serologic tests may also be able to distinguish antibodies directed against different *Bartonella* species (i.e., *B. henselae* and *B. quintana*).[699]

The role of *B. henselae* in CSD has been further strengthened by epidemiologic studies on *B. henselae* infection in domestic cats.[316] In a study conducted in San Francisco on the prevalence of infection in cats, Koehler and coworkers reported that 41% of blood specimens from 61 impounded or pet cats were culture-positive for *B. henselae*.[408] These workers found that kittens were more likely to be bacteremic with the organism than older cats, and that these asymptomatic animals remained bacteremic for several months. A seroprevalence study conducted on banked serum from 592 cats in the Baltimore area yielded a prevalence of *B. henselae* antibodies of 14.7%.[140] Chomel and colleagues studied 205 cats living in Northern California and found that 39.5% of them had sustained *B. henselae* bacteremia; 52% of these bacteremic cats had more than 1000 CFU of bacteria per milliliter of blood cultured.[141] Among these 205 animals, 81% tested positive for antibodies against *B. henselae*, and bacteremic cats tended to have higher antibody titers than nonbacteremic cats. These workers and others have made the suggestion that *B. henselae*–seronegative cats may be more appropriate pets for immunocompromised individuals because of the risks of transmission and the severity of disease in compromised patients.[141,615]

Miscellaneous Infections. Since the discovery of the association of *Bartonella* species with CSD, BA, and peliosis hepatis, several other manifestations of *B. henselae* infection have been reported in both immunocompromised and immunocompetent hosts.[814] In the vast majority of these infections, an association with cats, usually those younger than 1 year old, has been documented, lending further credence to the possibility that clinical manifestations of *B. henselae* infection represent a continuum in the presentation of CSD. These clinical manifestations have include neuroretinitis, with and without the oculoglandular syndrome of Parinaud, a chronic fatigue–like syndrome, aseptic meningitis or encephalitis, isolated unilateral and diffuse lymphadenitis, and neurologic disease associated with rapidly progressive dementia.[486,684,814] The associa-

TABLE 8-17
BIOCHEMICAL TESTS FOR IDENTIFICATION OF BARTONELLA SPECIES*

TEST	B. HENSELAE	B. QUINTANA	B. VINSONII
Growth, MacConkey agar	–	–	–
Hemin dependence	+	+	+
Oxidase	–	–	–
Catalase	–	–	–
Nitrate reduction	–	–	–
Indole production	–	–	–
Arginine dihydrolase	–	–	–
Acetoin (VP)	–	+	–
Gelatin hydrolysis	–	–	–
Esculin hydrolysis	+	+	–
Hippurate hydrolysis	+	–	+
Acid from			
Glucose	–	–	–
Maltose	–	+	–
Sucrose	–	+	–
Lactose	+	–	–
Susceptibility to			
Vancomycin	+	+	+
Colistin	–	–	–
Urease	–	–	–
Pyrazinamidase	–	+	+
PYR			–
Alkaline phosphatase	–	–	+
β-Glucuronidase	–	–	–
α-Galactosidase	–	–	–
β-Galactosidase	–	–	–
α-Glucosidase	–	–	–
Leucine arylamidase	+	+	–

*As per reference 213.

tion of *Bartonella* with AIDS-related dementia has been further elucidated by a serologic study conducted in Los Angeles, by Schwartzman and colleagues, in which both cat ownership and neuropsychologic decline and dementia were associated significantly with the presence of IgM antibodies to *B. henselae*.[683] Caniza and coworkers described a case of opportunistic pulmonary infection caused by *B. henselae* in a 19-year-old female kidney transplant recipient.[115] Tissue from pulmonary nodules of this patient were negative on culture but contained 16S rRNA specific for *B. henselae* by PCR. All eight of the domestic cats that lived with the patient had positive blood cultures for *B. henselae*; PCR analysis of these isolates established that the feline isolates were identical with that found in the lung tissue of the patient.[115] Lastly, Golnick and coworkers reported four patients who presented with substantial loss in visual acuity resulting from intraocular and retinal inflammation and optic nerve swelling; although no organisms were isolated, all four patients had elevated titers against *B. henselae* or *B. quinatana* and all responded to treatment with ciprofloxacin or doxycycline.[298] All four patients had contact with cats and kittens, although none reported bites or scratches. Although both organisms have been investigated as possible etiologic agents, neither *B. henselae* nor *A. felis* are associated with "chronic fatigue syndrome."[60]

DETECTION, ISOLATION, AND IDENTIFICATION

Slater and his colleagues were the first to successfully cultivate *B. henselae* in the laboratory.[702] The organism grows best on chocolate agar and Columbia agar with 5% sheep or rabbit blood. Blood-supplemented BHI and tryptic-soy agars also support growth. Heme appears to be an essential nutrient for these organisms. Characteristically, *B. henselae* colonies are white, dry, adherent, "cauliflower-like," embedded in the agar, and morphologically heterogeneous. With multiple passages, the colonies become less dry, less adherent, larger, and tend to grow faster. During primary isolation, visible colonies usually appear in 5 to 15 days after incubation at 35° to 37°C in 5% CO_2. Plates should be held for a minimum of 2 to 3 weeks. Isolates do not grow anaerobically or at temperatures of 25°C or 42°C. Isolates appear to require hemin and 5% to 7% CO_2. On Gram stain, the organisms appear as small, slightly curved bacilli measuring about 2 to 2.5 μm in length by 0.5 to 0.6 μm, and display "twitching" motility when mounted in saline. Isolates of *B. henselae* are nonreactive in many of the routine biochemical identification tests, including oxidase, catalase, indole, urease, decarboxylase, and nitrate reduction tests.

In their report on the isolation of *R. henselae* from a child with bacteremia, Welch and colleagues at the University of Oklahoma Health Sciences Center presented a scheme for the microbiologic diagnosis of *Bartonella* infections.[795] (Fig. 8-1). Isolator blood cultures or tissue homogenates are plated onto fresh chocolate and Columbia blood agars and incubated at 35°C in CO_2 for a minimum of 14 days. Isolates may also be recovered in the BACTEC high-volume aerobic resin PLUS 26 bottle, although the organism may not register a growth index threshold for positivity. The acridine orange stain is preferred for detection of the organisms in broth media blood cultures.[435] Dry, adherent colonies that are detected after approximately 10 days of incubation and are oxidase-, catalase-, and urease-negative may be *B. henselae*. Confirmatory identification is possible by cellular fatty acid analysis, by *B. henselae* fluorescent antibody, or by use of enzymatic substrates in commercial identification kits (see later discussion).[795] In addition to culture and isolation, *B. henselae* may also be detected in tissues by immunocytochemical methods.[612] The other recently described *Bartonella* species, *B. elizabethae*, phenotypically resembles *B. henselae*, except that it causes weak or partial hemolysis when plated on heart infusion agar with 5% rabbit blood.[174] *B. henselae* has also been cultivated on a red blood cell–free, defined medium containing brucella agar or broth, 6% to 5% Fildes enrichment, and hemin (250 μg/mL).[682]

In addition to detection, molecular and immunologic methods have also been used to characterize and subtype isolates of *Bartonella* species. These methods have included immunofluorescence, SDS–PAGE, Western blot, restriction fragment length polymorphism, 16S rRNA sequencing, and pulsed-field gel electrophoresis.[477,481] Several of these methods were able to differentiate *Bartonella* species from one another, but species identification was most easily obtained by immunofluorescence with species-specific murine antisera.[481]

Bartonella species may be identified by gas–liquid chromatographic analysis of cellular fatty acids.[796] All *Bartonella* species contain greater than 50% $C_{18:1}$, 16–25% $C_{18:0}$, and 16–22% $C_{16:0}$, with minor amounts of $C_{13:1}$ and $C_{17:0}$ fatty acids. The *B. henselae* isolates lack cellular fatty acids $C_{15:0}$ and $C_{12:0}$, which are present in isolates of *B. vinsonii* and *B. bacilliformis*, respectively. *B. quintana* could be differentiated from most *B. henselae* isolates by the presence of less than 20% $C_{18:0}$ in *B. quintana* and higher than 20% $C_{18:0}$ in *B. henselae*. The cellular fatty acid composition of *B. elizabethae* is most similar to that of *B. vinsonii* and includes $C_{15:0}$ (not found in *B. henselae* or *B. quintana*) and larger amounts (21%) of $C_{17:0}$ than *B. henselae* (3%), *B. quintana* (1%), and *B. visonii* (9%). *B. elizabethae* also contained smaller amounts of cellular fatty acid $C_{16:0}$ (13%) than the other species, which contain from 17% to 20% $C_{16:0}$ cellular fatty acids.[174]

Welch and colleagues also examined the reactivities of *B. henselae*, along with *B. quintana* and *B. vinsonii*, on several identification panels that use chromogenic enzymatic substrates (Microscan Rapid Anaerobe panel, Vitek *Neisseria–Haemophilus* Identification card, IDS RapID ANA II panel, API AnIDENT panel, Microscan HNID Panel, and the API Rapid STREP).[795] All of these systems (except the Rapid STREP) gave reactions that were unique within their own databases, but only the Microscan Rapid Anaerobe Panel was able to separate *B. henselae* and *B. quintana* at the species level. This panel distinguished all species tested, generating unique biotyping codes for each species. The reactivity of *Bartonella* species with key tests on this panel are shown in Table 8-16. In a similar type of study, Drancourt and Raoult examined strains of *B. henselae*, *B. quintana*, and *B. vinsonii* for other phenotypic tests that may be used for identifying these organisms.[213] These workers used hemin-supplemented tryptic soy broth to inoculate the API Rapid STREP and the Rapid CORYNE strips and performed a variety of spot and susceptibility tests (Table 8-17). All three species were oxidase- and catalase-negative and were capnophilic and microaerophilic. *B. henselae* strains exhibited leucyl arylamidase (LAP) activity, hydrolyzed esculin and hippurate, and produced acid from lactose; *B. quintana* exhibited positive VP, LAP, and pyrazinamidase activity, were esculin hydrolysis-positive, and produced acid from maltose and sucrose. *B. vinsonii* demonstrated alkaline phosphatase and pyrazinamidase activity, and hippurate hydrolysis. Curiously, all three species were found to be susceptible to vancomycin and resistant to colistin.

ANTIMICROBIAL SUSCEPTIBILITY

By using an agar dilution method, Maurin and Raoult tested the in vitro susceptibility of *B. henselae*, *B. quinatana*, and *B. vinsonii* to a variety of antimicrobial agents.[480] These organisms were susceptible to ampicillin, third-generation cephalosporins (cefotaxime, ceftriaxone), tetracyclines (doxycycline, minocycline), macrolides, rifampin, trimethoprim–sulfamethoxazole, and aminoglycosides (gentamicin, amikacin). The MICs for oxacillin, cephalothin, clindamycin, chloramphenicol, and the fluoroquinolones (ciprofloxacin, perfloxacin, ofloxacin) were near the maximum concentrations of drug available in the serum.

AFIPIA SPECIES

TAXONOMY AND CLINICAL SIGNIFICANCE

Organisms subsequently assigned to the new genus *Afipia* were first isolated from lymph node aspirates of patients with cat-scratch disease (CSD) by using a cell culture method.[73] Brenner and associates proposed that these organisms were the causative agent of CSD and named the type strain *Afipia felis* (after the *Armed Forces Institute of Pathology*, where the organism was originally isolated).[97] A second, similar organism was recovered from a tibial biopsy of a 69-year-old man at the Cleveland Clinic. A third biochemically and genetically similar organism was subsequently recovered from sputum, bone marrow, and a wrist abscess. These three species have been assigned to the genus *Afipia*, as *A. felis*, *A. clevelandensis*, and *A. broomeae*, respectively.[97] In addition, three unnamed *Afipia* genospecies have also been described. These three genospecies, termed *Afipia* genospecies 1, 2, and 3, have been isolated from a human pleural fluid specimen, a human bronchial wash specimen, and water, respectively. These organisms, similar to *Bartonella*, belong in the α-2 subgroup of the class *Proteobacteria*.[723] With the isolation of *B. henselae* and the evidence indicating that most, if not all, cases of CSD are due to this bacterium, the role of *A. felis* in CSD is now uncertain.[211] Monoclonal antibodies and serologic tests for *Afipia* species have also been developed, but with the evidence that has accumulated for *B. henselae* as the cause of CSD, it is felt that the performance of routine

A. felis serology does not improve the sensitivity and specificity of the laboratory diagnosis of CSD.[526,565,833]

ISOLATION AND IDENTIFICATION

Afipia species are gram-negative, oxidase-positive, bacilli that are motile owing to possession of a single polar, subpolar, or lateral flagellum. At present, three species (*A. felis*, *A. clevelandensis*, *A. broomeae*) and three unamed genospecies (*Afipia* genospecies 1, 2, and 3, respectively) have been described. *A. felis* is the most fastidious of the species identified to date. The organisms grow on buffered charcoal–yeast extract agar, on blood agar, and in nutrient broth but do not grow in the presence of 6.5% NaCl in broth and rarely grow on MacConkey agar. Good growth is obtained after incubation at 25°C and 30°C for 3 to 4 days. Scant growth is obtained after incubation at 35°C, and no growth is observed at 42°C. All described species and unnamed genospecies are urease-positive.

After 72 hours growth on blood agar, colonies of *Afipia* species are gray-white, glistening, convex and opaque with an entire edge. All species and genospecies are oxidase- and urease-positive and are negative in reactions for hemolysis, gas production from nitrate, indole production, H_2S production (TSI method), gelatin hydrolysis, esculin hydrolysis, and are nonfermentative. Acid is not produced oxidatively from glucose, lactose, sucrose, or maltose. *A. felis* is catalase-, citrate-, and D-mannitol-negative, reduces nitrate, and produces acid oxidatively from D-xylose in a delayed, weak reaction (Table 8-18). *A. clevelandensis* exhibits all genus characteristics except that delayed, scant growth may occur on MacConkey agar. The species is catalase-negative, and negative in tests for nitrate reduction, growth on citrate, and acid production from mannitol and xylose. *A. broomeae* exhibits all of the genus characteristics, is weakly catalase-positive, and shows delayed, weak acid production from xylose. The organism is negative in tests for nitrate reduction, utilization of citrate, and acid production from mannitol (see Table 8-18).

Organisms belonging to *Afipia* genospecies 1 are weakly catalase-positive, citrate-positive, weakly positive for acid production from xylose and mannitol, and negative for nitrate reduction. *Afipia* genospecies 2 is also weakly catalase-positive, and weakly xylose-positive. It does not reduce nitrate, grow on citrate, or produce acid from mannitol. *Afipia* genospecies 3 exhibits the characteristics of the genus, is weakly catalase-positive, and produces a delayed, weakly positive reaction with xylose. It is also nitrate reduction-, citrate-, and mannitol-negative. Genospecies 3 is H_2S positive by the lead acetate method only (see Table 8-18).

ANTIMICROBIAL SUSCEPTIBILITY

A. felis is resistant to ampicillin, cefamandole, cefazolin, cefoperazone, cephalothin, clindamycin, erythromycin, penicillin, tetracycline, and ciprofloxacin.[97,479] Intermediate susceptibility to piperacillin, sulfamethoxazole–trimethoprim, ticarcillin, and vancomycin has been reported.[97,479] It is susceptible to the aminoglycosides (gentamicin, netilmicin, and tobromycin), imipenem, and rifampin.

TABLE 8-18
Biochemical Tests for Identification of *Afipia* Species and Genospecies

Test	A. FELIS	A. CLEVELANDENSIS	A. BROOMEAE	AFIPIA GENOSP. 1	AFIPIA GENOSP. 2	AFIPIA GENOSP. 3
Hemolysis	−	−	−	−	−	−
Oxidase	+	+	+	+	+	+
Catalase	−	−	+ʷ	+ʷ	+ʷ	+ʷ
Growth at 25°C	+	+	+	+	+	+
Growth at 30°C	+	+	+	+	+	+
Growth at 35°C	+ʷ	+ʷ	+ʷ	+	+	+ʷ
Growth at 42°C	−	−	−	−	−	−
Motility	+	+	+	+	+	+
Nitrate reduction	+	−	−	−	−	−
Gas from nitrate	−	−	−	−	−	−
Growth, nutrient broth	+	+ˢˡ	+	+	+	+
Growth, 6.5% NaCl	−	−	−	−	−	−
Growth, MacConkey agar	−	+ˢˡ	−	−	−	−
Urease	+	+	+	+	+	+
H₂S, lead acetate	−	−	−	−	−	+ʷ
H₂S, TSI agar	−	−	−	−	−	−
Gelatin hydrolysis	−	−	−	−	−	−
Indole production	−	−	−	−	−	−
Esculin hydrolysis	−	−	−	−	−	−
Simmon's citrate	−	−	−	+	−	−
Gas, D-glucose	−	−	−	−	−	−
Acid production from						
Glucose	−	−	−	−	−	−
Maltose	−	−	−	−	−	−
Sucrose	−	−	−	−	−	−
Lactose	−	−	−	−	−	−
D-Mannitol	−	−	−	+ʷ	−	−
D-Xylose	+ʷ	−	+ʷ	+ʷ	+ʷ	+ʷ

+, positive; −, negative; +ʷ, weak positive; +ˢˡ, positive but delayed.

GENERAL APPROACH TO THE ISOLATION AND IDENTIFICATION OF THE FASTIDIOUS GRAM-NEGATIVE BACTERIA

The hallmark of many of these fastidious bacteria is their slow rate of growth and, hence, their recovery from clinical specimens that routinely have shorter turnaround times. Isolates from blood cultures may re-quire several days or, occasionally, weeks to grow. Therefore, communication with the physician concerning the patient and the tentative diagnosis is essential. Just knowing the patient may have a clinical diagnosis of endocarditis or suspected endocarditis may serve as a signal to hold the blood cultures for longer than 7 to 10 days (rule-of-thumb is 4 weeks). A history of travel or ingestion of unpasteurized milk is a good "flag" for incubating blood cultures for several weeks and performing blind subcultures (in a biologic safety cabinet) to look for brucellae.

Radiometric methods have worked surprisingly well for detecting these organisms in blood cultures. Fastidious bacteria (especially the HACEK organisms and brucellae) should be suspected when the growth index on the BACTEC radiometric or spectrophotometric instrument rises slowly, rather than abruptly, with sequential readings on the instrument. Gram stain of the blood culture broth directly may not allow visualization of the organisms. Aspiration of a sample from the bottle, low-speed centrifugation to remove red cells, and a high-speed centrifugation of the broth to produce a concentrated bacterial pellet allows easier visualization of the organisms and their Gram stain morphology and characteristics. Care should be taken during the performance of such manipulations to prevent aerosols and splashes. Alternatively, other methods to enhance detection and visualization of the organisms, such as the acridine orange stain, should be employed.

Other than *Capnocytophaga* species, with its characteristic, large "spready" colony, the fastidious gram-negative bacilli are usually initially recognized by their slow growth and tiny colonies. At this point the Gram stain will confirm the bacterial morphology and staining characteristics. Once the colonies are large enough to work with, oxidase and catalase tests may be performed. The organism should also be subcultured to MacConkey agar and incubated for 48 hours. This reaction is scored as "growth" or "no growth."

For the **oxidase test**, tetramethyl-*p*-phenylenediamine dihydrochloride reagent should be used. Fresh reagent should be dropped on a piece of filter paper, and some of the organisms, picked up with a white cotton swab, should be rubbed on the moist reagent. The test reaction should be read on the swab. The swab test may frequently be observed to be positive, whereas the inoculum placed on the paper may appear negative. Rapid oxidase reactions will develop within 10 to 15 seconds; delayed or weak oxidase reactions develop over 30 seconds to 1 minute.

The **catalase test** is performed by placing some of the growth from a chocolate plate onto a glass slide and placing a drop of 3% hydrogen peroxide on the organisms. This should be observed closely for the formation of bubbles. Catalase tests performed from blood agar may be difficult to interpret owing to the endogenous catalase activity present in sheep red blood cells.

We have found that subculture of the organisms to a few chocolate agar plates and incubation for 24 to 48 hours provides enough inoculum for a variety of test procedures. For **nitrate reduction** and **indole production**, nitrate broth and tryptone broth, respectively, should be inoculated with a sterile swab to achieve a turbidity equivalent to a number 1 or 2 McFarland standard and incubated for 48 hours before the addition of reagents. The nitrate reagents A and B are added as for enterics, with crystalline zinc being added to confirm negative reactions or the conversion of nitrite to gas. Alternatively, a Durham tube may be used.

The tryptone broth is extracted with xylene and the reaction is developed with Ehrlich's reagent instead of Kovac's reagent. For weakly indole-positive organisms such as *C. hominis* and *S. indologenes*, the spot indole reagent may not be sensitive enough. For the **urease test**, the surface of a Christensen's urea agar slant is inoculated heavily with the organism in a small area and incubated for 48 hours in CO_2. **X and V factor requirements** are determined as for *Haemophilus* species, using factor-impregnated strips or disks on brain–heart infusion or tryptic–soy agar. This plate should also be incubated in a CO_2 incubator or in a candle jar.

Acid production from carbohydrates may be determined using conventional or modified rapid methods. Purple broth base or cystine–tryptic digest semi-solid agar containing 1% carbohydrates may be used. Incubation must be continued for 5 to 7 days before reactions are called negative. Prolonged incubation may be circumvented by using a heavy inoculum prepared in a carbohydrate-free broth for each carbohydrate tube. A modification of the **rapid fermentation test procedure**, originally described for identifying *Neisseria* species, may also be used.[350] This method provides carbohydrate utilization reactions after 4 hours and is extremely useful and economical. At the University of Illinois, we have used this procedure to determine acid production from glucose, maltose, sucrose, lactose, xylose, mannitol, and mannose by fastidious bacteria. Additional carbohydrates can be added as required. As with the *Neisseria* procedure, it is recommended that carbohydrates be reagent-grade quality (e.g., Sigma Biochemical, Fisher, or Mallinkrodt).

Commercial kit systems are also available for assistance in identifying many of the fastidious gram-negative species. The **RapID NH system** (Innovative Diagnostics, Atlanta GA) includes *H. aphrophilus* and *H. paraphrophilus*, *A. actinomycetemcomitans*, *C. hominis*, *E. corrodens*, *Kingella* species, and *P. multocida* in its database. However, the newly reformatted panel has not been extensively evaluated. The **Vitek *Neisseria–Haemophilus* Identification (NHI) Card** (Vitek Systems, Hazelwood MO) includes all the HACEK group organisms in its database. In the single published evaluation, the NHI card provided definitive identifications for these organisms or indicated the correct identification among a choice of two or three possible identifications.[372] The performance of selected modified conventional tests is suggested by the database of the computer-assisted identification system. The **MicroScan *Haemophilus–Neisseria* Identification (HNID) panel** (American MicroScan, Sacramento CA) currently lists only *H. aphrophilus* and *H. paraphrophilus* in its database. However, Janda and coworkers tested several strains of fastidious gram-negative species (including *A. actinomycetemcomitans*, *C. hominis*, *E. corrodens*, and *Kingella* species) and found that unique biochemical profiles were produced.[371] Agreement was noted between the modified conventional tests on the panel (e.g., carbohydrate fermentations, indole, urease, ornithine decarboxylase) and conventional identification procedures. Unfortunately, these kit systems do not perform well with isolates normally found in

animals other than humans, with the exception of
P. multocida.[658,786] Additional work needs to be done to
expand the databases of these systems as more of these
species are recovered from human clinical specimens.

REFERENCES

1. ABD-ELRAZEK M: *Brucella* optic neuritis. Arch Intern Med 151:776–778, 1991
2. ACAY MC, ORAL ET, YENIGUM M ET AL: *Pasteurella multocida* ulceration on the penis. Int J Dermatol 32:519–520, 1993
3. AGARWAL S, KADHI SKM, ROONEY RJ: Brucellosis complicating bilateral total knee arthroplasty. Clin Orthop 267:179–181, 1991
4. AH FAT LNC, PATEL BR, PICKENS S: *Actinobacillus actinomycetemcomitans* endocarditis in hypertrophic obstructive cardiomyopathy. J Infect 6:81–84, 1983
5. AKOVA M, UZUN O, AKALIN HE ET AL: Quinolones in treatment of human brucellosis: comparative trial of ofloxacin-rifampin versus doxycycline-rifampin. Antimicrob Agents Chemother 37:1831–1834, 1993
6. AL-ASKA AK, CHAGLA AH: Laboratory-acquired brucellosis. J Hosp Infect 14:69–71, 1989
7. ALBRITTON WL, SETLOW JK, THOMAS ML ET AL: Relatedness within the family *Pasteurellaceae* as determined by genetic transformation. Int J Syst Bacteriol 36:103–106, 1986
8. AL-EISSA YA, ASSUHAIMI SA, AL-FAWAZ IM ET AL: Pancytopenia in children with brucellosis: clinical manifestations and bone marrow findings. Acta Haematol 89:132–136, 1993
9. AL-EISSA YA, KAMBAL AM, AL-NASSER MN ET AL: Childhood brucellosis: a study of 102 cases. Pediatr Infect Dis J 9:74–79, 1990
10. AL-EISSA YA, KAMBAL AM, ALRABEEAH AA ET AL: Osteoarticular brucellosis in children. Ann Rheum Dis 49:896–900, 1990
11. AL-FARAN MF: *Brucella melitensis* endogenous endophthalmitis. Ophthalmologica 201:19–22, 1990
12. ALVAREZ O, MORALES J, MCCARTNEY DL ET AL: *Haemophilus aphrophilus* endophthalmitis associated with a filtering bleb. Arch Ophthalmol 109:618–620, 1991
13. AMADOR C, CHINER E, CALPE JL ET AL: Pneumonia due to *Bordetella bronchiseptica* in a patient with AIDS. Rev Infect Dis 13:771–772, 1991
14. ANDERSEN HK, MORTENSEN A: Unrecognized neurobrucellosis giving rise to *Brucella melitensis* peritonitis via a ventriculoperitoneal shunt. Eur J Clin Microbiol Infect Dis 11:953–954, 1992
15. ANDERSEN JK, PEDERSEN M: Infective endocarditis with involvement of the tricuspid valve due to *Capnocytophaga canimorsus*. Eur J Clin Microbiol Infect Dis 11:831–832, 1992
16. ANDERSON B, KELLY C, THRELKEL R ET AL: Detection of *Rochalimaea henselae* in cat-scratch disease skin test antigens. J Infect Dis 168:1034–1036, 1993
17. ANDERSON B, LU E, JONES D ET AL: Characterization of a 17-kilodalton antigen of *Bartonella henselae* reactive with sera from patients with cat scratch disease. J Clin Microbiol 33:2358–2365, 1995
18. ANDERSON B, SIMS K, REGNERY R ET AL: Detection of *Rochalimaea henselae* DNA in specimens from cat scratch disease patients by PCR. J Clin Microbiol 32:942–948, 1994
19. ANGUS BJ, GREEN ST, MCKINLEY JJ ET AL: *Eikenella corrodens* septicaemia among drug injectors: a possible association with "licking wounds." J Infect 28:102–103, 1994
20. ANOLIK R, BERKOWITZ RJ, CAMPOS JM ET AL: *Actinobacillus* endocarditis associated with periodontal disease. Clin Pediatr 20:653–655, 1981
21. AOYAMA T, IWATA T, IWAI Y ET AL: Efficacy of acellular pertussis vaccine in young infants. J Infect Dis 167:483–386, 1993
22. AOYAMA T, MURASE Y, IWATA T ET AL: Comparison of blood-free (cyclodextrin solid medium) with Bordet-Gengou medium for clinical isolation of *Bordetella pertussis*. J Clin Microbiol 23:1046–1048, 1986
23. APPELBAUM PC, BALLARD JO, EYSTER ME: Septicemia due to *Capnocytophaga* (*Bacteroides ochraceus*) in Hodgkin's disease. Ann Intern Med 90:716–717, 1979
24. ARIAS-STELLA J, LIEBERMAN PH, ERLANDSON RA ET AL: Histology, immunochemicstry, and ultrastructure of the verruga in Carrion's disease. Am J Surg Pathol 10:595–610, 1986
25. ARICO B, NUTI S, SCARLATO V ET AL: Adhesion of *Bordetella pertussis* to eucaryotic cells requires a time-dependent export and maturation of filamentous hemagglutinin. Proc Natl Acad Sci USA 90:9204–9208, 1993
26. ARICO B, RAPPUOLI R: *Bordetella parapertussis* and *Bordetella bronchiseptica* contain transcriptionally silent pertussis toxin genes. J Bacteriol 169:2847–2853, 1987
27. ARIZA J, PELLICER T, PALLARES R ET AL: Specific antibody profile in human brucellosis. Clin Infect Dis 14:131–140, 1992
28. ARLET G, SANSON-LE PORS M-J, CASIN IM ET AL: In vitro susceptibility of 96 *Capnocytophaga* strains, including a *beta*-lactamase producer, to new *beta*-lactam antibiotics and six quinolones. Antimicrob Agents Chemother 31:1283–1284, 1987
29. ARNOW PM, SMARON M, ORMISTE V: Brucellosis in a group of travelers to Spain. JAMA 251:505–507, 1984
30. ARONS MS, FERNANDO L, POLAYES IM: *Pasteurella multocida*—the major cause of hand infections following domestic animal bites. J Hand Surg 7:47–52, 1982
31. ARONSON NE, ZBICK CJ: Dysgonic fermenter 3 bacteremia in a neutropenic patient with acute lymphocytic leukemia. J Clin Microbiol 26:2213–2215, 1988
32. ASHDOWN LR. MOTTARELLY IW: Acute painful cellulitis caused by a *Pasteurella pneumotropica*-like bacterium in Northern Queensland. Med J Aust 152:333–334, 1990
33. ASIKAINEN S, CHEN C, SLOTS J: *Actinobacillus actinomycetemcomitans* genotypes in relation to serotypes and periodontal status. Oral Microbiol Immunol 10:65–68, 1995
34. ASSEFA D, DALITZ E, HANDRICK W ET AL: Septic cavernous sinus thrombosis following infection of ethmoidal and maxillary sinuses: a case report. Int J Pediatr Otorhinolaryngol 29:249–255, 1994

35. AYALA-GAYTAN JJ, ORTEGON-BAQUEIRO H, DE LA MAZA M: *Brucella melitensis* cerebellar abscess. J Infect Dis 160: 730–732, 1989

36. AYSHA MH, SHAYIB MA: Pancytopenia and other haematological findings in brucellosis. Scand J Haematol 36: 335–338, 1986

37. BACKMAN A, JOHANSSON B, OLCEN P: Nested PCR optimized for detection of *Bordetella pertussis* in clinical nasopharyngeal samples. J Clin Microbiol 32:2544–2548, 1994

38. BADDOUR LM, GELFAND MS, WEAVER RE ET AL: CDC group HB-5 as a cause of genitourinary tract infection in adults. J Clin Microbiol 27:801–805, 1989

39. BAILIE WE, STOWE EC, SCHMITT AM: Aerobic flora of oral and nasal fluids of canines with reference to bacteria associated with bites. J Clin Microbiol 7:223–231, 1978

40. BAKER CN, HOLLIS DG, THORNSBERRY C: Antimicrobial susceptibility testing of *Francisella tularensis* using a modified Mueller-Hinton broth. J Clin Microbiol 22: 212–215, 1985

41. BAKER D, STAHLMAN GC: *Pasteurella multocida* infection in a patient with AIDS. J Tenn Med Assoc 84:325–326, 1991

42. BAKER JL, ODDIS CV, MEDSGER TA: *Pasteurella multocida* polyarticular septic arthritis. J Rheumatol 14:355–357, 1987

43. BALDWIN CJ, PANCIERA RJ, MORTON RJ ET AL: Acute tularemia in three domestic cats. J Am Vet Med Assoc 11:1602–1605, 1991

44. BANGSBORG JM, FREDERIKSEN W, BRUUN B: Dysgonic fermenter 3-associated abscess in a diabetic patient. J Infect 20:237–240, 1990

45. BANNERJEE TK, GRUBB W, OTERO C ET AL: Musculocutaneous mononeuropathy complicating *Capnocytophaga canimorsus* infection. Neurology 43:2411–2412, 1993

46. BAQUERO F, FERNANDEZ J, DRONDA F ET AL: Capnophilic and anaerobic bacteremia in neutropenic patients: an oral source. Rev Infect Dis 12(suppl 2):S157–S160, 1990

47. BARHAM WB, CHURCH P, BROWN JE ET AL: Misidentification of *Brucella* species with use of rapid bacterial identification systems. Clin Infect Dis 17:1068–1069, 1993

48. BARKA NE, HADFIELD T, PATNAIK M ET AL: EIA for detection of *Rochalimaea henselae*-reactive IgG, IgM, and IgA antibodies in patients with suspected cat scratch disease. J Infect Dis 167:1503–1504, 1993

49. BARNHAM M: Pig bite injuries and infection: report of seven human cases. Epidemiol Infect 101:641–645, 1988

50. BATCHELOR BI, BRINDLE RJ, GILKS GF ET AL: Biochemical misidentification of *Brucella melitensis* and subsequent laboratory-acquired infections. J Hosp Infect 22:159–162, 1992

51. BAUWENS JE, SPACH DH, SCHACKER TW ET AL: *Bordetella bronchiseptica* pneumonia and bacteremia following bone marrow transplantation. J Clin Microbiol 30: 2474–2475, 1992

52. BAYKAL M, AKALIN HE, FIRAT M ET AL: In vitro activity and clinical efficacy of ofloxacin in infections due to *Brucella melitensis*. Rev Infect Dis 11(suppl 3):S993–S994, 1989

53. BAYNES ID, SIMMONS GC: Ovine epididymitis caused by *Actinobacillus seminis* n. sp. Aust Vet J 36:454–459, 1960

54. BEIER D, SCHWARZ B, FUCHS TM ET AL: *In vivo* characterization of the unorthodox BvgS two-component sensor protein of *Bordetella pertussis*. J Mol Biol 248:596–610, 1995

55. BEITER A, LEWIS K, PINEDA E ET AL: Unrecognized maternal peripartum pertussis with subsequent fatal neonatal pertussis. Obstet Gynecol 82:691–693, 1989

56. BEJUK D, BEGOVAC J, BACE A ET AL: Culture of *Bordetella pertussis* from three upper respiratory tract specimens. Pediatr Infect Dis J 14:64–65, 1995

57. BEJUK D, KUZMAN I, SOLDO I ET AL: Vertebral osteomyelitis caused by *Haemophilus aphrophilus*. Eur J Clin Microbiol Infect Dis 12:643–644, 1993

58. BENAOUDIA F, ESCANDE F, SIMONET M: Infection due to *Actinobacillus lignieresii* after a horse bite. Eur J Clin Microbiol Infect Dis 13:439–440, 1994

59. BENJAMIN B, KHAN MRH: Hip involvement in childhood brucellosis. J Bone Joint Surg Br 76B:544–547, 1994

60. BENNETT AL, FAGLIOLI L, KOMAROFF AL ET AL: Persistent infection with *Bartonella* (*Rochalimaea*) *henselae* or *Afipia felis* is unlikely to be a cause of chronic fatigue syndrome. Clin Infect Dis 19:804–805, 1994

61. BENSON RF, LANIER-THACKER W, PLIKAYTIS BB ET AL: Cross-reactions in *Legionella* antisera with *Bordetella pertussis* strains. J Clin Microbiol 25:594–596, 1987

62. BERGMANS AMC, GROOTHEDDE J-W, SCHELLEKENS JFP ET AL: Etiology of cat scratch disease: comparison of polymerase chain reaction detection of *Bartonella* (formerly *Rochalimaea*) and *Afipia felis* DNA with serology and skin tests. J Infect Dis 171:916–923, 1995

63. BERKHOFF HA, RIDDLE GD: Differentiation of *Alcaligenes*-like bacteria of avian origin and comparison with *Alcaligenes* spp. reference strains. J Clin Microbiol 19: 477–481, 1984

64. BERNARD K, COOPER C, TESSIER S ET AL: Use of chemotaxonomy as an aid to differentiate among *Capnocytophaga* species, CDC group DF-3, and aerotolerant strains of *Leptotrichia buccalis*. J Clin Microbiol 29:2263–2265, 1991

65. BERNARD K, TESSIER S, WINSTANLEY J ET AL: Early recognition of atypical *Francisella tularensis* strains lacking a cysteine requirement. J Clin Microbiol 32:551–553, 1994

66. BEVANGER L, MAELAND JA, NAESS AI: Competitive enzyme immunoassay for antibodies to a 43,000-molecular-weight *Francisella tularensis* outer membrane protein for the diagnosis of tularemia. J Clin Microbiol 27: 922–926, 1989

67. BHATNAGAR N, GETACHEW E, STRALEY S ET AL: Reduced virulence of rifampicin-resistant mutants of *Francisella tularensis*. J Infect Dis 170:841–847, 1994

68. BIA F, MARIER R, COLLINS WF ET AL: Meningitis and bacteremia caused by *Pasteurella ureae*: report of a case following intracranial surgery. Scand J Infect Dis 10: 251–253, 1978

69. BIEGER RC, BREWER NS, WASHINGTON JA: *Haemophilus aphrophilus*: a microbiologic and clinical review and report of 42 cases. Medicine 57:345–355, 1978

70. BIGEL ML, BERARDI-GRASSIAS LD, FURIOLL J: Isolation of *Actinobacillus ureae* (*Pasteurella ureae*) from a patient with otitis media. Eur J Clin Microbiol Infect Dis 7: 206–207, 1988

71. BILGRAMI S, BERGSTROM SK, PETERSON DE ET AL: Capnocytophaga bacteremia in a patient with Hodgkin's dis-

ease following bone marrow transplantation: case report and review. Clin Infect Dis 14:1045–1049, 1992

72. BIRKEBAEK NH, HERON I, SKJODT K: *Bordetella pertussis* diagnosed by polymerase chain reaction. APMIS 102: 291–294, 1994

73. BIRKNESS KA, GEORGE VG, WHITE EH ET AL: Intracellular growth of *Afipia felis*, a putative etiologic agent of cat scratch disease. Infect Immun 60:2281–2287, 1992

74. BIRTLES RJ, HARRISON TG, SAUNDERS NA ET AL: Proposals to unify the genera *Grahamella* and *Bartonella*, with descriptions of *Bartonella talpae* comb. nov., *Bartonella peromysci* comb. nov., and three new species, *Bartonella grahamii* sp. nov., *Bartonella taylori* sp. nov., and *Bartonella doshiae* sp. nov. Int J Syst Bacteriol 45:1–8, 1995

75. BISGAARD M: *Actinobacillus muris* sp. nov. isolated from mice. APMIS Sect B 94:1–8, 1986

76. BISGAARD M, FALSEN E: Reinvestigation and reclassification of a collection of 56 human isolates of *Pasteurellaceae*. APMIS Sect B 94:215–222, 1986

77. BISGAARD M, HELTBERG O, FREDERIKSEN W: Isolation of *Pasteurella caballi* from an infected wound on a veterinary surgeon. APMIS 99:291–294, 1991

78. BISGAARD M, MUTTERS R: Characterization of some previously unclassified "*Pasteurella*" spp. obtained from the oral cavity of dogs and cats and description of a new species tentatively classified with the family *Pasteurellaceae* Pohl 1981 and provisionally called taxon 16. APMIS Sect B 94:177–184, 1986

79. BLACKALL PJ, DOHENY CM: Isolation and characterisation of *Bordetella avium* and related species and an evaluation of their role in respiratory diseases in poultry. Aust Vet J 64:235–239, 1987

80. BLANCHE P, SICARD D, MEYNIARD O ET AL: *Capnocytophaga canimorsus* lymphocytic meningitis in an immunocompetent man who was bitten by a dog. Clin Infect Dis 18:654–655, 1994

81. BLANKENSHIP RM, SANFORD JP: *Brucella canis*: a cause of undulant fever. Am J Med 59:424–426, 1975

82. BLASCO JM, MARIN C, DE BAGUES MJ ET AL: Evaluation of allergic and serological tests for diagnosing *Brucella melitensis* infection in sheep. J Clin Microbiol 32: 1835–1840, 1994

83. BLUM RN, BERRY CD, PHILLIPS MG ET AL: Clinical illnesses associated with isolation of dysgonic fermenter 3 from stool samples. J Clin Microbiol 30:396–400, 1992

84. BOBO RA, NEWTON EJ: A previously undescribed gram-negative bacillus causing septicemia and meningitis. Am J Clin Pathol 65:564–569, 1976

85. BOGAERTS J, LEPAGE P, KESTELYN P ET AL: Neonatal conjunctivitis caused by *Pasteurella ureae*. Eur J Clin Microbiol 4:427–428, 1985

86. BOGAERTS J, VERHAEGEN J, TELLO WM ET AL: Characterization, in vitro susceptibility, and clinical significance of CDC group HB-5 from Rwanda. J Clin Microbiol 28: 2196–2199, 1990

87. BOHNER BJ, EMORY WB, BLALOCK JB: *Pasteurella multocida* empyema: successful treatment with open thoracostomy. J La State Med Soc 142:27–29, 1990

88. BOLDT J, GRAHAM B, RATNER H: *Pasteurella multocida* empyema. Clin Microbiol Newslett 6:67–68, 1984

89. BOLTON RW, KLUEVER EA, DYER JK: In vitro immunosuppression mediated by an extracellular polysaccharide from *Capnocytophaga ochracea*: influence of macrophages. J Periodontal Res 20:251–259, 1985

90. BOOT R, BAKKER RHG, THUIS H ET AL: An enzyme-linked immunosorbent assay (ELISA) for monitoring rodent colonies for *Streptobacillus moniliformis* antibodies. Lab Anim 27:350–357, 1993

91. BOTTONE EJ, KITTICK J, SCHNEIERSON SS: Isolation of bacillus HB-1 from human clinical sources. Am J Clin Pathol 59:560–566, 1973

92. BOVRE K, HENRIKSEN SD, JONSSON V: Correction of the specific epithet *kingii* in the combinations *Moraxella kingii* Henriksen and Bovre 1968 and *Pseudomonas kingii* Jonsson 1970 to *kingae*. Int J Syst Bacteriol 24:307, 1974

93. BRAITHWAITE BD, GIDDINS G: *Pasteurella multocida* infection of a total hip arthroplasty: a case report. J Arthroplasty 7:309–310, 1992

94. BRASS EP, WRAY LM, MCDUFF T: *Pasteurella ureae* meningitis associated with endocarditis. Eur Neurol 22: 138–141, 1983

95. BREITSCHWERDT EB, KORDICK DL, MALARKEY DE ET AL: Endocarditis in a dog due to infection with a novel *Bartonella* subspecies. J Clin Microbiol 33:154–160, 1995

96. BRENNER DJ, HOLLIS DG, FANNING R ET AL: *Capnocytophaga canimorsus* sp. nov. (formerly CDC group DF-2), a cause of septicemia following dog bite, and *C. cynodegmi* sp. nov., a cause of localized wound infection following dog bite. J Clin Microbiol 27:231–235, 1989

97. BRENNER DJ, HOLLIS DG, MOSS CW ET AL: Proposal of *Afipia* gen. nov., with *Afipia felis* sp. nov., (formerly the cat-scratch disease bacillus), *Afipia clevelandensis* sp. nov. (formerly the Cleveland Clinic Foundation strain), *Afipia broomeae* sp. nov., and three unnamed genospecies. J Clin Microbiol 29:2450–2460, 1991

98. BRENNER DJ, O'CONNOR SP, WINKLER HH ET AL: Proposals to unify the genera *Bartonella* and *Rochalimaea*, with descriptions of *Bartonella quintana* comb. nov., *Bartonella vinsonii* comb. nov., *Bartonella henselae* comb. nov., and *Bartonella elizabethae* comb. nov., and to remove the Family *Bartonellaceae* from the Order *Rickettsiales*. Int J Syst Bacteriol 43:777–786, 1993

99. BRICKER BJ, HALLING SM: Differentiation of *Brucella abortus* bv. 1, 2, and 4, *Brucella melitensis*, *Brucella ovis*, and *Brucella suis* bv. 1 by PCR. J Clin Microbiol. 32: 2660–2666, 1994

100. BRILL CB, PEARLSTEIN LS, KAPLAN JM ET AL: CNS infection caused by *Eikenella corrodens*. Arch Neurol 39: 431–432, 1982

101. BRIVET F, GUIBERT M, BARTHELEMY P ET AL: *Pasteurella multocida* sepsis after hemorrhagic shock in a cirrhotic patient: possible role of endoscopic procedures and gastrointestinal translocation. Clin Infect Dis 18:842–843, 1994

102. BRONDZ I, OLSEN I: Multivariate analyses of carbohydrate data from lipopolysaccharides of *Actinobacillus* (*Haemophilus*) *actinomycetemcomitans*, *Haemophilus aphrophilus*, and *Haemophilus paraphrophilus*. Int J Syst Bacteriol 40:405–408, 1990

103. BRONDZ I, OLSEN I, SJOSTROM M: Multivariate analysis of quantitative chemical and enzymic characterization data in classification of *Actinobacillus*, *Haemophilus*, and *Pasteurella* spp. J Gen Microbiol 136:507–513, 1990

104. BROWN AM, ROTHBURN MM, ROBERTS C ET AL: Septicaemia and probable endocarditis caused by *Kingella denitrificans*. J Infect 15:225–228, 1987

105. BRUE C, CHOSIDOW O: *Pasteurella multocida* wound infection and cellulitis. Int J Dermatol 33:471–473, 1994

106. BRUUN B, YING Y, KIRKEGAARD E ET AL: Phenotypic differentiation of *Cardiobacterium hominis*, *Kingella indologenes*, and CDC group EF-4: Eur J Clin Microbiol 3:230–235, 1984

107. BUNDLE DR, CHERWONOGRODZKY JW, GIDNEY JW ET AL: Definition of *Brucella* A and M epitopes by monoclonal typing reagents and synthetic oligosaccharides. Infect Immun 57:2829–2836, 1992

108. BURDASH N, BLOCK BA, BECHER P: *Pasteurella multocida* from a tubo-ovarian abscess. Clin Microbiol Newslett 11:95–96, 1989

109. BURDGE DR, SCHEIFELE D, SPEERT DP: Serious *Pasteurella multocida* infections from lion and tiger bites. JAMA 253:3296–3297, 1985

110. BURNETT JW: Tularemia. Cutis 54:77–78, 1994

111. BUTLER T, WEAVER RE, RAMANI V ET AL: Unidentified gram-negative rod infection: a new disease of man. Ann Intern Med 86:1–5, 1977

112. BUU-HOI AY, JOUNDY S, ACAR JF: Endocarditis caused by *Capnocytophaga ochracea*. J Clin Microbiol 26:1061–1062, 1988

113. BYRD LH, ANAMA L, GUTKIN M ET AL: *Bordetella bronchiseptica* peritonitis associated with continuous ambulatory peritoneal dialysis. J Clin Microbiol 14:232–233, 1981

114. CALDEIRA L, DUTSCHMANN L, CARMO G ET AL: Fatal *Pasteurella multocida* infection in a systemic lupus erythematosus patient. Infection 21:254–255, 1993

115. CANIZA MA, GRANGER DL, WILSON KH ET AL: *Bartonella henselae*: etiology of pulmonary nodules in a patient with depressed cell-mediated immunity. Clin Infect Dis 20:1505–1511, 1995

116. CARBECK RB, MURPHY JF, BRITT EM: Streptobacillary rat-bite fever with massive pericardial effusion. JAMA 201:133–134, 1967

117. CARDEN SM, COLVILLE DJ, GONIS G ET AL: *Kingella kingae* endophthalmitis in an infant. Aust NZ J Ophthalmol 19:217–220, 1991

118. CARMICHAEL LE, KENNY RM: Canine abortion caused by brucellosis. J Am Vet Med Assoc 152:605–616, 1968

119. CARPENTER PD, HEPPNER BT, GNANN JW: DF-2 bacteremia following cat bites: report of two cases. Am J Med 82:621–623, 1987

120. CARTER GR: Genus I. *Pasteurella* Trevisan 1887. 94^AL. Nom. cons. Opin. 13, Jud. Comm. 1954, 153. In Krieg NR, Holt JG (eds), *Bergey's Manual of Systematic Bacteriology*, Vol 1, pp 552–557. Baltimore, Williams & Wilkins, 1984

121. CAUGANT DA, SELANDER RK, OLSEN I: Differentiation between *Actinobacillus* (*Haemophilus*) *actinomycetemcomitans*, *Haemophilus aphrophilus*, and *Haemophilus paraphrophilus* by multilocus enzyme electrophoresis. J Gen Microbiol 136:2135–2141, 1990

122. CENTERS FOR DISEASE CONTROL: Biosafety in microbiological and biomedical laboratories, 2nd ed. Atlanta GA, Centers for Disease Control, 1988

123. CENTERS FOR DISEASE CONTROL AND PREVENTION: Encephalitis associated with cat scratch disease—Broward and Palm Beach Counties, Florida, 1994. MMWR 43:909–916, 1994

124. CHADWICK PR, MALNICK H, EBIZIE AO: *Haemophilus paraphrophilus* infection: a pitfall in laboratory diagnosis. J Infect 30:67–69, 1995

125. CHAMBERS GW, WESTBLOM TU: Pleural infection caused by *Capnocytophaga canimorsus*, formerly CDC group DF-2. Clin Infect Dis 15:325–326, 1992

126. CHAN JKC, LEWIN KJ, TEITELBAUM S ET AL: Histopathology of bacillary angiomatosis of lymph node. Am J Surg Pathol 15:430–437, 1991

127. CHAN R, HARDIMAN RP: Endocarditis caused by *Brucella melitensis*. Med J Aust 158:631–632, 1993

128. CHANAL C, TIGET F, CHAPIUS P ET AL: Spondylitis and osteomyelitis caused by *Kingella kingae* in children. J Clin Microbiol 25:2407–2409, 1987

129. CHANG KC, ZAKHEIM RM, CHO CT ET AL: Post-traumatic purulent meningitis due to *Bordetella bronchiseptica*. J Pediatr 86:639–640, 1975

130. CHAO C-L, CHANG S-C, SHEU J-C ET AL: Transdiaphragmatic *Actinobacillus actinomycetemcomitans* infection: case report. Clin Infect Dis 19:958–960, 1994

131. CHAUDHURI AK, HARTLEY RB, MADDOCKS AC: Waterhouse-Friderichsen syndrome caused by a DF-2 bacterium in a splenectomized patient. J Clin Pathol 34:172–173, 1981

132. CHEN C-KC, POTTS TV, WILSON ME: DNA homologies shared among *E. corrodens* isolates and other corroding bacilli from the oral cavity. J Periodont Res 25:106–112, 1990

133. CHEN C-CK, SUNDAY GJ, ZAMBON JJ ET AL: Restriction endonuclease analysis of *Eikenella corrodens*. J Clin Microbiol 28:1265–1270, 1990

134. CHEN C-KC, WILSON ME: Outer membrane protein and lipopolysaccharide heterogeneity among *Eikenella corrodens* isolates. J Infect Dis 162:664–671, 1990

135. CHEN C-KC, WILSON ME: *Eikenella corrodens* in human oral and non-oral infections. J Periodont Res 63:941–953, 1992

136. CHEN Y-C, CHANG S-C, LUH K-T ET AL: *Actinobacillus actinomycetemcomitans* endocarditis: a report of four cases and review of the literature. Q J Med 81:871–878, 1991

137. CHENG AF, MAN DWK, FRENCH GL: Thyroid abscess caused by *Eikenella corrodens*. J Infect 16:181–185, 1988

138. CHERRY JD, BEER T, CHARTRAND SA ET AL: Comparison of values of antibody to *Bordetella pertussis* antigens in young German and American men. Clin Infect Dis 20:1271–1274, 1995

139. CHERRY JD, BRUNELL PA, GOLDEN GS ET AL: Report of the Task Forse on Pertussis and Pertussis Immunization—1988. Pediatrics 81(suppl):933–984, 1988

140. CHILDS JE, ROONEY JA, COOPER JL ET AL: Epidemiologic observations on infection with *Rochalimaea* species among cats living in Baltimore, Md. J Am Vet Med Assoc 204:1775–1778, 1994

141. CHOMEL BB, ABBOTT RC, KASTEN RW ET AL: *Bartonella henselae* in domestic cats in California: risk factors and association between bacteremia and antibody titers. J Clin Microbiol 33:2445–2450, 1995

142. CHOWDHURY MNH, AL-NOZHA M, HUSIAN IS ET AL: Endocarditis due to *Actinobacillus actinomycetemcomitans*. J Infect 10:158–162, 1985

143. CHRISTEN RD: *Cardiobacterium hominis* endocarditis in a patient with a hypersensitivity reaction to penicillin. Successful treatment with partial resection of the posterior mitral valve leaflet and antibiotic therapy with cefazolin. Infection 18:291–293, 1990

144. CHRISTIANSON HB, PANKEY GA, APPLEWHITE ML: Ulcers of skin due to *Brucella suis*. Report of a case. Arch Dermatol 98:175–176, 1968

145. CHUBA PJ, BOCK R, GRAF G ET AL: Comparison of 16S RNA sequences from the Family *Pasteurellaceae*: phylogenetic relatedness by cluster analysis. J Gen Microbiol 134:1923–1930, 1988

146. CLAESSON B, FALSEN E, KJELLMAN B: *Kingella kingae* infections: a review and a presentation of data from 10 Swedish cases. Scand J Infect Dis 17:233–243, 1985

147. CLARK RB, JOYCE SE: Activity of meropenem and other antimicrobial agents against uncommon gram-negative organisms. J Antimicrob Chemother 32:233–237, 1993

148. CLARKE K, DEVONSHIRE D, VEITCH A ET AL: Dog-bite induced *Capnocytophaga canimorsus* septicaemia. Aust NZ J Med 22:86–87, 1992

149. COCKERELL CJ: Bacillary angiomatosis and related diseases caused by *Rochalimaea*. J Am Acad Dermatol 32:783–790, 1995

150. COCKERELL CJ, BERGSTRESSER PR, MYRIE-WILLIAMS C ET AL: Bacillary epithelioid angiomatosis occurring in an immunocompetent individual. Arch Dermatol 126:787–790, 1990

151. COCKERELL CJ, LEBOIT PE: Bacillary angiomatosis: a newly characterized, pseudoneoplastic, infectious, cutaneous vascular disorder. J Am Acad Dermatol 22:501–512, 1990

152. COCKERELL CJ, TIERNO PM, FRIEDMAN-KIEN AE: Clinical, histologic, microbiologic, abd biochemical characterization of the causative agent of bacillary (epithelioid) angiomatosis, a rickettsial illness with features of bartonellosis. J Invest Dermatol 97:812–817, 1991

153. COHN SE, KNORR KL, GILLIGAN PH ET AL: Pertussis is rare in human immunodeficiency virus disease. Am Rev Respir Dis 147:411–413, 1993

154. COKCA F, MECO O, ARASIL E ET AL: An intramedullary dermoid cyst abscess due to *Brucella abortus* biotype 3 at T11-L2 spinal levels. Infection 22:359–360, 1994

155. COLEBUNDERS R, VAEL C, BLOT K ET AL: *Bordetella pertussis* as a cause of chronic respiratory infection in an AIDS patient. Eur J Clin Microbiol Infect Dis 13:313–315, 1994

156. COLLAZOS J, DIAZ F, AYARZA R ET AL: *Actinobacillus actinomycetemcomitans*: a cause of pulmonary-valve endocarditis of 18 month's duration with unusual manifestations. Clin Infect Dis 18:115–116, 1994

157. COLL-VINENT B, SURIS X, LOPEZ-SOTO A ET AL: *Haemophilus aphrophilus* endocarditis: case report and review. Clin Infect Dis 20:1381–1383, 1995

158. COLMENERO JD, CISNEROS JM, ORJUELA DL ET AL: Clinical course and prognosis of brucella spondylitis. Infection 20:38–42, 1992

159. COLMENERO JD, REGUERA JM, CABRERA FP ET AL: Serology, clinical manifestations and treatment of brucellosis in different age groups. Infection 18:152–156, 1990

160. CONRAD SE, JACOBS D, GEE J ET AL: Pseudoneoplastic infection of bone in acquired immunodeficiency syndrome. J Bone Joint Surg (Am) 73:774–777, 1991

161. COOKSON BT, CHO HL, HERWALDT LA ET AL: Biological activities and chemical composition of purified tracheal cytotoxin of *Bordetella pertussis*. Infect Immun 57:2223–2229, 1989

162. COOKSON BT, GOLDMAN WE: Tracheal cytotoxin: a conserved virulence determinant of all *Bordetella* species. J Cell Biochem 11(suppl B):124, 1987

163. COOKSON BT, VANDAMME P, CARLSON C ET AL: Bacteremia caused by a novel *Bordetella* species, "*B. hinzii*." J Clin Microbiol 32:2569–2571, 1994

164. COOPER A, MARTIN R, TIBBLES JAR: *Pasteurella* meningitis. Neurology 23:1097–1100, 1973

165. CORBEL MJ: Identification of dye-sensitive strains of *Brucella melitensis*. J Clin Microbiol 29:1066–1068, 1991

166. CORBOZ L, OSSENT P, GRUBER H: Isolation and characterization of group EF-4 bacteria from various lesions in cat, dog, and badger. Int J Med Microbiol Virol Parasitol Infect Dis 279:140–145, 1993

167. CORREIA J, CONN H: Spontaneous bacterial peritonitis in cirrhosis; endemic or epidemic. Med Clin North Am 59:964–974, 1975

168. CRAWFORD SA, EVANS JA, CRAWFORD GE: Necrotizing fasciitis associated with *Haemophilus aphrophilus*. Arch Intern Med 138:1714–1715, 1978

169. CROMER BA, GOYDOS J, HACKELL J ET AL: Unrecognized pertussis infection in adolescents. Am J Dis Child 147:575–577, 1993

170. CROSBY E, LLOSA L, QUESADA MM ET AL: Hematologic changes in brucellosis. J Infect Dis 150:419–424, 1984

171. CROSS JT, JACOBS RF: Tularemia treatment failures with outpatient use of ceftriaxone. Clin infect Dis 17:976–980, 1993

172. CUADATO-GOMEZ LM, ARRANZ-CASO JA, CUADROS-GONZALEZ J: *Pasteurella pneumotropica* pneumonia in a patient with AIDS. Clin Infect Dis 21:445–446, 1995

173. CUNDELL DR, KANTHAKUMAR K, TAYLOR GW ET AL: Effect of tracheal cytotoxin from *Bordetella pertussis* on human neutrophil function in vitro. Infect Immun 62:639–643, 1994

174. DALY JS, WORTHINGTON MG, BRENNER DJ ET AL: *Rochalimaea elizabethae* sp. nov., isolated from a patient with endocarditis. J Clin Microbiol 31:872–881, 1993

175. DANESHVAR MI, HOLLIS DG, MOSS CW: Chemical characterization of clinical isolates which are similar to CDC group DF-3 bacteria. J Clin Microbiol 29:2351–2353, 1991

176. DANGMAN BC, ALBANESE BA, KACICA MA ET AL: Cat scratch disease in two children presenting with fever of unknown origin: imaging features and association with a new causative agent, *Rochalimaea henselae*. Pediatrics 95:767–770, 1995

177. DANKNER WM, DAVIS CE, THOMPSON MA: DF-2 bacteremia following a dog bite in a 4-month-old child. Pediatr Infect Dis 6:695–696, 1987

178. DAVID JK JR, OWENS JN JR: Tularemic meningitis: report of a case and summary of previously reported cases. Am J Dis Child 67:44–51, 1944

179. DAWSON SJ, WHITE LA: Treatment of *Haemophilus aphrophilus* endocarditis with ciprofloxacin. J Infect 24:317–320, 1992

180. DECKER GR, LAVELLE JP, KUMAR PN ET AL: Pneumonia due to *Bordetella bronchiseptica* in a patient with AIDS. Rev Infect Dis 13:1250–1251, 1991

181. DECKER MD, GRAHAM BS, HUNTER EB ET AL: Endocarditis and infections of intravascular devices due to *Eikenella corrodens*. Am J Med Sci 292:209–212, 1986

182. DECOSTER H, SNOECK J, PATTYN S: *Capnocytophaga canimorsus* endocarditis. Eur Heart J 13:140–142, 1992

183. DEEN JL, MINK CM, CHERRY JD ET AL: Household contact study of *Bordetella pertussis* infections. Clin Infect Dis 21:1211–1219, 1995

184. DEES SB, KARR DE, HOLLIS D: Cellular fatty acids of *Capnocytophaga* species. J Clin Microbiol 16:779–783, 1982

185. DE GROOT R, GLOVER D, CLAUSEN C ET AL: Bone and joint infections caused by *Kingella kingae*: six cases and review of the literature. Rev Infect Dis 10:998–1004, 1988

186. DE LA FUENTE J, ALBO C, RODRIGUEZ A ET AL: *Bordetella bronchiseptica* pneumonia in a patient with AIDS. Thorax 49:719–720, 1994

187. DE LEY J, MANNHEIM W, MUTTERS R ET AL: Inter- and intrafamilial similarities of rRNA cistrons of the *Pasteurellaceae*. Int J Syst Bacteriol 40:126–137, 1990

188. DE LEY J, MANNHEIM W, SEGERS P ET AL: Ribosomal ribonucleic acid cistron similarities and taxonomic neighborhood of *Brucella* and CDC group Vd. Int J Syst Bacteriol 37:35–42, 1987

189. DE LEY J, SEGERS P, KERSTERS K ET AL: Intra- and intergeneric similarities of the *Bordetella* ribosomal ribonucleic acid cistrons: proposal for a new family, *Alcaligenaceae*. Int J Syst Bacteriol 26:405–414, 1986

190. DEMIRKAN F, AKALIN HE, SIMSEK H ET AL: Spontaneous peritonitis due to *Brucella melitensis* in a patient with cirrhosis. Eur J Clin Microbiol Infect Dis 12:66–67, 1993

191. DE MOISSAC YR, RONALD SL, PEPPLER MS: Use of pulsed field gel electrophoresis for epidemiological study of *Bordetella pertussis* in a whooping cough outbreak. J Clin Microbiol 32:398–402, 1994

192. DE SMET MD, CHAN CC, NUSSENBLATT RB ET AL: *Capnocytophaga canimorsus* as the cause of a chronic corneal infection. Am J Ophthalmol 109:240–242, 1990

193. DEVILLE JG, CHERRY JD, CHRISTENSON PD ET AL: Frequency of unrecognized *Bordetella pertussis* infections in adults. Clin Infect Dis 21:639–642, 1995

194. DEWHIRST FE, CHEN C-K, PASTER BJ ET AL: Phylogeny of species in the Family *Neisseriaceae* isolated from human dental plaque and description of *Kingella orale* sp. nov. Int J Syst Bacteriol 43:490–499, 1993

195. DEWHIRST FE, PASTER BJ, BRIGHT PL: *Chromobacterium, Eikenella, Kingella, Neisseria, Simonsiella,* and *Vitreoscilla* species comprise a major branch of the *beta* group *Proteobacteria* by 16S ribosomal ribonucleic acid sequence comparison: transfer of *Eikenella* and *Simonsiella* to the family *Neisseriaceae* (emend.). Int J Syst Bacteriol 39:258–266, 1990.

196. DEWHIRST FE, PASTER BJ, LA FONTAINE S ET AL: Transfer of *Kingella indologenes* (Snell and Lapage 1976) to the genus *Suttonella* gen. nov. as *Suttonella indologenes* comb. nov.; transfer of *Bacteroides nodosus* (Beveridge 1941) to the genus *Dichelobacter* gen. nov. as *Dichelobacter nodosus* comb. nov.; and assignment of the genera *Cardiobacterium, Dichelobacter,* and *Suttonella* to *Cardiobacteriaceae* fam. nov. in the *gamma* division of *Proteobacteria* on the basis of 16S rRNA sequence comparisons. Int J Syst Bacteriol 40:426–433, 1990

197. DEWHIRST FE, PASTER BJ, OLSEN I ET AL: Phylogeny of 54 representative strains of species in the Family *Pasteurellaceae* as determined by comparison of 16S rRNA sequences. J Bacteriol 174:2002–2013, 1992

198. DHAR R, DHAR PM, GAFOOR M: Recurrent epidermal cyst infection caused by *Brucella melitensis* in a diabetic patient. J Clin Microbiol 26:1040–1041, 1988

199. DIBB WL, DIGRANES A, TONJUM S: *Actinobacillus lignieresii* infection after a horse bite. Br Med J 283:583–584, 1981

200. DIJKMANS BAC, THOMEER RTWN, VIELVOYE GJ ET AL: Brain abscess due to *Streptobacillus moniliformis* and *Actinobacterium meyeri*. Infection 12:262–264, 1984

201. DI MARIO A, SICA S, ZINI G ET AL: Microangiopathic hemolytic anemia and severe thrombocytopenia in *Brucella* infection. Ann Hematol 70:59–60, 1995

202. DIMMITT SB, CHRISTIANSEN K, NEWMAN M: *Haemophilus paraphrophilus*—an unusual cause of endocarditis. Aust NZ J Med 24:581, 1994

203. DIRIENZO JM, MCKAY TL: Identification and characterization of genetic cluster groups of *Actinobacillus actinomycetemcomitans* isolated from the human oral cavity. J Clin Microbiol 32:75–81, 1994

204. DIX K, WATANABE SM, MCARDLE S ET AL: Species-specific oligodeoxynucleotide probes for the identification of periodontal bacteria. J Clin Microbiol 28:319–323, 1990

205. DOEBBELING BN, FEILMEIER ML, HERWALDT LA: Pertussis in an adult man infected with the human immunodeficiency virus. J Infect Dis 161:1296–1298, 1990

206. DOLAN MJ, WONG MT, REGNERY RL ET AL: Syndrome of *Rochalimaea henselae* adenitis suggesting cat scratch disease. Ann Intern Med 118:331–336, 1993

207. DONLY KJ, ASHKENAZI M: Juvenile periodontitis: a review of pathogenesis, diagnosis, and treatment. J Clin Pediatr Dent 16:73–78, 1992

208. DOUGLAS E, COOTE JG, PARTON R ET AL: Identification of *Bordetella pertussis* in nasopharyngeal swabs by PCR amplification of a region of the adenylate cyclase gene. J Mol Microbiol 38:140–144, 1993

209. DOYLE D, EPPES SC, KLEIN JD: Atypical cat-scratch disease: diagnosis by a serologic test for *Rochalimaea* species. South Med J 87:485–487, 1994

210. DRABICK JJ, GASSER RA, SAUNDERS NB ET AL: *Pasteurella multocida* pneumonia in a man with AIDS and nontraumatic feline exposure. Chest 10:37–11, 1993

211. DRANCOURT M, DONNET A, PELLETIER J ET AL: Acute meningoencephalitis associated with seroconversion to "*Afipia felis.*" Lancet 340:558, 1992

212. DRANCOURT M, MAINARDI JL, BROUQUI P ET AL: *Bartonella (Rochalimaea) henselae* endocarditis in three homeless men. N Engl J Med 332:419–423, 1995

213. DRANCOURT M, RAOULT D: Proposed tests for the routine identification of *Rochalimaea* species. Eur J Clin Microbiol Infect Dis 12:710–713, 1993

214. DUL MJ, SHLAES DM, LERNER PI: EF-4 bacteremia in a patient with hepatic carcinoid. J Clin Microbiol 18:1260–1261, 1983

215. DUPON M, D'IVERNOIS C, MALOU M ET AL: Sacro-iliac joint infection caused by *Eikenella corrodens*. Eur J Clin Microbiol Infect Dis 10:529–530, 1991

216. EASTON J, LISTER J, PAKASH C: Meningitis due to *Pasteurella multocida*. Br Med J 1:366–374, 1970

217. EBERSOLE JL, CAPPELLI D: Gingival crevicular fluid antibody to *Actinobacillus actinomycetemcomitans* in periodontal disease. Oral Microbiol Immunol 9:335–344, 1994

218. EDWARDS KM: Acellular pertussis vaccines—a solution to the pertussis problem? J Infect Dis 168:15–20, 1993

219. EDWARDS KM, DECKER MD, GRAHAM BS ET AL: Immunization of adults with acellular pertussis vaccine. JAMA 269:53–56, 1993

220. EDWARDS R, FINCH RG: Characterization and antibiotic susceptibilities of *Streptobacillus moniliformis*. J Med Microbiol 21:39–42, 1986

221. EHRHARDT M, LYNCH KM, TYSON GM ET AL: *Bordetella bronchiseptica*: pathogen vs. commensal. Clin Microbiol Newslett 8:26–27, 1986

222. EIGELSBACH HT, MCGANN VG: Genus *Francisella* Dorofe'ev 1947m, 176^AL. In Krieg NR, Holt JG (eds), *Bergey's Manual of Systematic Bacteriology*, Vol 1, pp 394–399. Baltimore, Williams & Wilkins, 1984

223. ELSEY RM, CARSON RW, DuBOSE TD: *Pasteurella multocida* peritonitis in an HIV-positive patient on continuous cycling peritoneal dialysis. Am J Nephrol 11:61–63, 1991

224. ELSTER AD, MACONE AB, KASSER JR: Osteomyelitis caused by *Capnocytophaga ochracea*. J Pediatr Orthop 3:613–615, 1983

225. EMMERSON AM, MILLS F: Recurrent meningitis and brain abscess caused by *Eikenella corrodens*. Postgrad Med J 54:343–348, 1976

226. ENCK RE, BENNETT JM: Isolation of *Haemophilus aphrophilus* from an adult with acute leukemia. J Clin Microbiol 4:194–195, 1976

227. ENDERLIN G, MORALES L, JACOBS RF ET AL: Streptomycin and alternative agents for the treatment of tularemia: review of the literature. Clin Infect Dis 19:42–47, 1994

228. ENG RK, SMITH SM, GOLDSTEIN EJC ET AL: Failure of vancomycin prophylaxis and treatment for *Actinobacillus actinomycetemcomitans* endocarditis. Antimicrob Agents Chemother 29:699–700, 1986

229. ENGBAEK K, KOCH C: Antibody response in rabbits infected with *Rochalimaea henselae, Rochalimaea quintana,* and *Afipia felis*. APMIS 102:943–949, 1994

230. ENGLISH CK, WEAR DJ, MARGILETH AM ET AL: Cat scratch disease. Isolation and culture of the bacterial agent. JAMA 259:1347–1352, 1988

231. ERICSSON M, SANDSTROM G, SJOSTEDT A ET AL: Persistence of cell-mediated immunity and decline of humoral immunity to the intracellular bacterium *Francisella tularensis* 25 years after natural infection. J Infect Dis 170:110–114, 1994

232. ERNST AA, SANDERS WM: A case of unexpected *Pasteurella multocida* bacteremia. J Emerg Med 8:437–440, 1990

233. ERNST JM. WAUSILAUSKAS B: *Capnocytophaga* in the amniotic fluid of a woman in preterm labor with intact membranes. Am J Obstet Gynecol 153:648–649, 1985

234. ERONAT N, UCAR F, KILINC G: Papillon Lefevre syndrome: treatment of two cases with a clinical microbiological and histopathological investigation. J Clin Pediatr Dent 17:99–104, 1993

235. ESCANDE F, GRIMONT F, GRIMONT PAD ET AL: Deoxyribonucleic acid relatedness among strains of *Actinobacillus* spp. and *Pasteurella ureae*. Int J Syst Bacteriol 34:309–315, 1984

236. ESTEBAN J, ALBALATE M, CARAMELO C ET AL: Peritonitis involving a *Capnocytophaga* species in a patient undergoing continuous ambulatory peritoneal dialysis. J Clin Microbiol 33:2471–2472, 1995

237. EVANS ME, GREGORY DW, SCHAFFNER W ET AL: Tularemia: a 30-year experience with 88 cases. Medicine 64:251–269, 1985

238. EWANOWICH CA, CHUI LW-L, PARANCHYCH MG ET AL: Major outbreak of pertussis in Northern Alberta, Canada: analysis of discrepant direct fluorescent-antibody and culture results by using polymerase chain reaction methodology. J Clin Microbiol 31:1715–1725, 1993

239. FAINSTEIN V, LUNA MA, BODEY GP: Endocarditis due to *Eikenella corrodens* in a patient with acute lymphocytic leukemia. Cancer 48:40–42, 1981

240. FAJFAR-WHETSTONE CJT, COLEMAN L, BIGGS DR ET AL: *Pasteurella multocida* septicemia and subsequent *Pasteurella dagmatis* septicemia in a diabetic patient. J Clin Microbiol 33:202–204, 1995

241. FARFEL Z, KONEN S, WIERTZ E ET AL: Antibodies to *Bordetella pertussis* adenylate cyclase are produced in man during pertussis infection and after vaccination. J Med Microbiol 32:173–177, 1990

242. FARIZO KM, COCHI SL, ZELL ER ET AL: Epidemiological features of pertussis in the United States, 1980–1989. Clin Infect Dis 14:708–719, 1992

243. FARO S, WALKER C, PIERSON RL: Amnionitis with intact amniotic membranes involving *Streptobacillus moniliformis*. Obstet Gynecol 55(suppl):9S–11S, 1980

244. FELDMAN JD, KONTAXIS EN, SHERMAN MP: Congenital bacteremia due to *Capnocytophaga*. Pediatr Infect Dis 4:415–416, 1985

245. FENICHEL S, BODINO C, KOCKA F: Isolation of *Actinobacillus actinomycetemcomitans* from a skin lesion. Eur J Clin Microbiol 4:428–429, 1985

246. FERNANDEZ-ESPARRACH G, MASCARO J, ROTA R ET AL: Septicemia, peritonitis, and empyema due to *Pasteurella multocida* in a cirrhotic patient. Clin Infect Dis 18:486, 1994

247. FINDLING JW, POHLMANN GP, ROSE HD: Fulminant gram-negative bacillemia (DF-2) following a dog bite in an asplenic woman. Am J Med 68:154–156, 1980

248. FINLEY CR, HAMILTON BW, HAMILTON TR: Tularemia: a review. Missouri Med 83:741–743, 1986

249. FISCHBEIN CA, BECKETT KM, ROSENTHAL A: *Haemophilus aphrophilus* brain abscess associated with congenital heart disease. J Pediatr 83:631–633, 1973

250. FISCHER P, DRAPKIN MS, HAROLD G: *Actinobacillus actinomycetemcomitans* infection. Rev Infect Dis 11:1032, 1989

251. FLEMMIG TF, RUDIGER S, HOFMAN U ET AL: Identification of *Actinobacillus actinomycetemcomitans* in subgingival plaque by PCR. J Clin Microbiol 33:3102–3105, 1995

252. FLESHER SA, BOTTONE EJ: *Eikenella corrodens* cellulitis and arthritis of the knee. J Clin Microbiol 27:2606–2608, 1989

253. FOGED NT, NIELSEN JP, PEDERSEN KB: Differentiation of toxigenic from non-toxigenic isolates of *Pasteurella multocida* by enzyme-linked immunosorbent assay. J Clin Microbiol 26:1419–1420, 1988

254. FORDHAM JN, MCKAY-FERGUSON E, DAVIES A ET AL: Rat bite fever without the bite. Ann Rheum Dis 51:411–412, 1992

255. FORD-JONES L, DELAGE G, POWELL KR ET AL: "Muskrat fever": two outbreaks of tularemia near Montreal. Can Med Assoc J 127:298–299, 1982

256. FORLENZA SW, NEWMAN MG, HORIKOSHI AL ET AL: Antimicrobial susceptibility of *Capnocytophaga*. Antimicrob Agents Chemother 19:144–146, 1981

257. FORLENZA SW, NEWMAN NG, LIPSEY AI ET AL: *Capnocytophaga* sepsis: a newly recognized entity in granulocytopenic patients. Lancet i:567–568, 1980

258. FORSMAN M, SANDSTROM G, JAURIN B: Identification of *Francisella* species and discrimination of type A and type B strains of *F. tularensis* by 16S rRNA analysis. Appl Environ Microbiol 56:949–955, 1990

259. FORSMAN M, SANDSTROM G, SJOSTEDT A: Analysis of 16S DNA sequence of *Francisella* stains and utilization for determination of the phylogeny of the genus and for identification of strains by PCR. Int J Syst Bacteriol 44:38–46, 1994

260. FORSTL H, RUCKDESCHEL G, LANG M ET AL: Septicemia caused by *Kingella kingae*. Eur J Clin Microbiol 3:267–269, 1984

261. FORTIER AH, SLAYTER MV, ZIEMBA R ET AL: Live vaccine strain of *Francisella tularensis*: infection and immunity in mice. Infect Immun 59:2922–2928, 1991

261a. FOSTER G, ROSS HM, MALNICK H ET AL: *Actinobacillus delphinicola* sp. nov., a new member of the Family *Pasteurellaceae* Pohl (1979) 1981 isolated from sea mammals. Int J Syst Bacteriol 46:648–652, 1996.

262. FOWERAKER JE, HAWKEY PM, HERITAGE J ET AL: Novel *beta*-lactamase from *Capnocytophaga* sp. Antimicrob Agents Chemother 34:1501–1504, 1990

263. FOX BC, GURTLER RA: Cat-scratch disease mimicking rhabdomyosarcoma. Orthop Rev 22:1148–1149, 1993

264. FRANCIS E: Tularemia. JAMA 84:1243–1250, 1925

265. FRANDSEN EVG, REINHOLDT J, KJELDSEN M ET AL: In vivo cleavage of immunoglobulin A1 by immunoglobulin A1 proteases from *Prevotella* and *Capnocytophaga* species. Oral Microbiol Immunol 10:291–296, 1995

266. FRIEDMAN RL: Pertussis: the disease and new diagnostic methods. Clin Microbiol Rev 1:365–376, 1988

267. FRIEDMAN RL, PAULAITIS S, MCMILLAN JW: Development of a rapid diagnostic test for pertussis: direct detection of pertussis toxin in respiratory secretions. J Clin Microbiol 27:2466–2470, 1989

268. FRIIS-MOLLER A: A new *Actinobacillus* species from the human respiratory tract: *Actinobacillus hominis* nov. sp. In Kilian M, Frederiksen W, Biberstein EL (eds), *Haemophilus, Pasteurella, and Actinobacillus*, pp 151–160. London, Academic Press, 1981

269. GABUZDA GM, BARNETT PR: *Pasteurella* infection in a total knee arthroplasty. Orthop Rev 21:601–605, 1992

270. GADBERRY JL, ZIPPER R, TAYLOR JA ET AL: *Pasteurella pneumotropica* isolated from bone and joint infections. J Clin Microbiol 19:926–927, 1984

271. GAMBLE JG, RINSKY LA: *Kingella kingae* infections in healthy children. J Pediatr Orthop 8:445–449, 1988

272. GAN VN, MURPHY TV: Pertussis in hospitalized children. Am J Dis Child 144:1130–1134, 1990

273. GANDOLA C, BUTLER T, BADGER S ET AL: Septicemia caused by *Capnocytophaga* in a granulocytopenic patient with glossitis. Arch Intern Med 140:851–852, 1980

274. GARCIA FU, WOJTA J, BROADLEY KN ET AL: *Bartonella bacilliformis* stimulate endothelial cells in vitro and is angiogenic in vitro. Am J Pathol 136:1125–1135, 1990

275. GARCIA FU, WOJTA J, HOOVER RL: Interactions between live *Bartonella bacilliformis* and endothelial cells. J Infect Dis 165:1138–1141, 1992

276. GARLAND RM, PRITCHARD MG: *Actinobacillus actinomycetemcomitans* causing a mediastinal abscess. Thorax 38:472–473, 1983

277. GASSER I, ALMIRANTE B, FERNENDEZ-PEREZ F ET AL: Bilateral mammary abscess and uveitis caused by *Brucella melitensis*—report of a case. Infection 19:44–45, 1991

278. GENCO RJ, ZAMBON JJ, MURRAY PA: Serum and gingival fluid antibodies as adjuncts in the diagnosis of *A. actinomycetemcomitans*-associated periodontal disease. J Periodontol 56:41–50, 1985

279. GEORGHIOU PR, MOLLEE TF, TILSE MH: *Pasteurella multocida* infection after a Tasmanian devil bite. Clin Infect Dis 14:1266–1267, 1992

280. GERACI JE, GREIPP PR, WILKOWSKE CJ ET AL: *Cardiobacterium hominis* endocarditis: four cases with clinical and laboratory observations. Mayo Clin Proc 53:49–53, 1978

281. GERACI JE, WILCOWSKE CJ, WILSON WR ET AL: *Haemophilus* endocarditis: report of 14 patients. Mayo Clin Proc 52:209–215, 1977

282. GERACI JE, WILSON WR, WASHINGTON JA: Infective endocarditis caused by *Actinobacillus actinomycetemcomitans*: report of four cases. Mayo Clin Proc 55:415–419, 1980

283. GERDING DN, KHAN MY, EWING JW ET AL: *Pasteurella multocida* peritonitis in hepatic cirrhosis with ascites. Gastroenterology 70:413–415, 1977

284. GILL VJ, TRAVIS LB, WILLIAMS DY: Clinical and microbiological observations on CDC group DF-3, a gram-negative coccobacillus. J Clin Microbiol 29:1589–1592, 1991

285. GILLIGAN PH, FISHER MC: Importance of culture in laboratory diagnosis of *Bordetella pertussis* infections. J Clin Microbiol 20:891–893, 1984

286. GILLIGAN PH, MCCARTHY LR, BISSETT BK: *Capnocytophaga ochracea* septicemia. J Clin Microbiol 13:643–645, 1981

287. GLARE EM, PATON JC, PREMIER RR ET AL: Analysis of a repetitive DNA sequence from *Bordetella pertussis* and its application to the diagnosis of pertussis using the polymerase chain reaction. J Clin Microbiol 28:1982–1987, 1990

288. GLASSER DB: Angular blepharitis caused by gram-negative bacillus DF-2. Am J Ophthalmol 102:119–120, 1986

289. GLASSMAN AB, SIMPSON JS: *Eikenella corrodens*: a clinical problem. J Am Dent Assoc 91:1237–1241, 1975

290. GMUR R, MCNABB H, VAN STEENBERGEN TJM ET AL: Seroclassification of hitherto nontypeable *Actinobacillus actinomycetemcomitans* strains: evidence for a new serotype e. Oral Microbiol Immunol 8:116–120, 1993

291. GOLDBAUM FA, LEONI J, WALLACH JC ET AL: Characterization of an 18-kilodalton *Brucella* cytoplasmic protein which appears to be a serological marker of active infection in both human and bovine brucellosis. J Clin Microbiol 31:2141–2145, 1993

292. GOLDEN SE: Hepatosplenic cat-scratch disease associated with elevated anti-*Rochalimaea* antibody titers. Pediatr Infect Dis J 12:868–871, 1993

293. GOLDMAN IS, ELLNER PD, FRANCKE EL ET AL: Infective endocarditis due to *Kingella denitrificans*. Ann Intern Med 93:152–153, 1980

294. GOLDSTEIN EJC, CITRON DM: Comparative susceptibilities of 173 aerobic and anaerobic bite wound isolates to sparfloxacin, temafloxacin, clarithromycin, and older agents. Antimicrob Agents Chemother 37:1150–1153, 1993

295. GOLDSTEIN EJC, MILLER TA, CITRON DM ET AL: Infections following clenched fist injury: a new perspective. J Hand Surg 3:455–457, 1978

296. GOLDSTEIN EJC, SUTTER VL, FINEGOLD SM: Susceptibility of *Eikenella corrodens* to ten cephalosporins. Antimicrob Agents Chemother 14:639–641, 1978

297. GOLLAND LC, HODGSON DR, HODGSON JL ET AL: Peritonitis associated with *Actinobacillus equuli* in horses: 15 cases (1982–1992). J Am Vet Med Assoc 205:340–343, 1994

298. GOLNIK KC, MAROTTO ME, FANOUS MM ET AL: Ophthalmic manifestations of *Rochalimaea* species. Am J Ophthalmol 118:145–151, 1994

299. GOMEZ-GARCES J-L, ALOS J-I, SANCHEZ J ET AL: Bacteremia by multidrug-resistant *Capnocytophaga sputigena*. J Clin Microbiol 32:1067–1069, 1994

300. GONCHAROFF P, FIGURSKI DH, STEVENS RH ET AL: Identification of *Actinobacillus actinomycetemcomitans*: polymerase chain reaction amplification of *lktA*-specific sequences. Oral Microbiol Immunol 8:105–110, 1993

301. GONZALEZ MH, GARST J, NOURBASH P ET AL: Abscesses of the upper extremity from drug abuse by injection. J Hand Surg Am 18:868–870, 1993

302. GOODMAN AD: *Eikenella corrodens* isolated in oral infections of dental origin. Oral Surg 44:128–134, 1977

303. GORAL S, ANDERSON B, HAGER C ET AL: Detection of *Rochalimaea henselae* DNA by polymerase chain reaction from supperative nodes of children with cat-scratch disease. Pediatr Infect Dis J 13:994–997, 1994

304. GOTUZZO E, CARRILLO C, GUERRA J ET AL: An evaluation of diagnostic methods for brucellosis: the value of bone marrow culture. J Infect Dis 153:122–125, 1986

305. GOUTZMANIS JJ, GONIS G, GILBERT GL: *Kingella kingae* infection in children: ten cases and a review of the literature. Pediatr Infect Dis J 10:677–683, 1991

306. GRACE CJ, LEVITZ H, KATZ-POLLAK H ET AL: *Actinobacillus actinomycetemcomitans* prosthetic valve endocarditis. Rev Infect Dis 10:922–929, 1988

307. GRADON JD, STEIN DS: Association between *Rochalimaea* infection and cat-scratch disease. Clin Infect Dis 17:287–288, 1993

308. GRADUS MS, NG C, PRIES R ET AL: An unsuspected case of brucellosis mimicking appendicitis in a child. Clin Microbiol Newslett 10:188–190, 1988

309. GRAHNQUIST L, ERIKSSON M: Pertussis and necrotizing enterocolitis in a previously healthy neonate. Pediatr Infect Dis J 12:698–699, 1993

310. GRANSTROM G, WRETLIND B, SALENSTEDT C-R ET AL: Evaluation of serologic assays for diagnosis of whooping cough. J Clin Microbiol 26:1818–1823, 1988

311. GRAVE W, STURM AW: Brucellosis associated with a beauty parlour. Lancet 1:1326–1327, 1983

312. GREGORY RL, KIM DE, KINDLE JC ET AL: Immunoglobulin-degrading enzymes in localized juvenile periodontitis. J Periodontal Res 27:176–183, 1992

313. GREWAL P, FONSECA K, ANDREWS HJ: *Pasteurella ureae* meningitis and septicemia. J Infect 7:74–76, 1983

314. GRIFFEN AL, LEYS EJ, FUERST PA: Strain identification of *Actinobacillus actinomycetemcomitans* using the polymerase chain reaction. Oral Microbiol Immunol 7:240–243, 1992

315. GRIMPREL E, BEGUE P, ANJAK I ET AL: Comparison of polymerase chain reaction, culture, and Western immunoblot serology for diagnosis of *Bordetella pertussis* infection. J Clin Microbiol 31:2745–2750, 1993

316. GROVES MG, HARRINGTON KS: *Rochalimaea henselae* infections: newly recognized zoonoses transmitted by domestic cats. J Am Vet Med Assoc 204:267–271, 1994

317. GRUNER E, BERNASCONI E, GALEAZZI L ET AL: Brucellosis: an occupational hazard for medical laboratory personnel. Report of five cases. Infection 22:33–36, 1994

318. GUION TL, SCULCO TP: *Pasteurella multocida* infection in total knee arthroplasty. J Arthroplasty 7:157–160, 1992

319. GUISO N, GRIMPREL E, ANJAK I ET AL: Western blot analysis of antibody responses of young infants to pertussis infection. Eur J Clin Microbiol Infect Dis 12:506–600, 1993

320. GUMP DW, HOLDEN RA: Endocarditis caused by a new species of *Pasteurella*. Ann Intern Med 76:275–278, 1972

321. GUSTAFSSON B, ASKELOF P: Monoclonal antibody-based sandwich enzyme-linked immunosorbent assay for detection of *Bordetella pertussis* filamentous hemagglutinin. J Clin Microbiol 26:2077–2082, 1988

322. GUSTAFSSON B, ASKELOF P: Rapid detection of *Bordetella pertussis* by a monoclonal antibody-based colony blot assay. J Clin Microbiol 27:628–631, 1989

323. GUSTAFSSON B, LINDQUIST U, ANDERSSON M: Production and characterization of monoclonal antibodies directed against *Bordetella pertussis* lipopolysaccharide. J Clin Microbiol 26:188–193, 1988

324. HADFIELD TL, WARREN R, KASS M ET AL: Endocarditis caused by *Rochalimaea henselae*. Hum Pathol 24:1140–1141, 1993

325. HADLEY S, ALBRECHT MA, TARSY D: Cat-scratch encephalopathy: a cause of status epilepticus and coma in a healthy young adult. Neurology 45:196, 1995

326. HALLANDER HO, REIZENSTEIN E, RENEMAR B ET AL: Comparison of nasopharyngeal aspirates with swabs for culture of *Bordetella pertussis*. J Clin Microbiol 31:50–52, 1993

327. HALLANDER HO, STORSAETER J, MOLLBY R: Evaluation of serology and nasopharyngeal cultures for diagnosis of pertussis in a vaccine efficacy trial. J Infect Dis 163:1046–1054, 1991

328. HALPERIN SA, BORTOLUSSI R, KASINA A ET AL: Use of a Chinese hamster ovary cell cytotoxicity assay for the rapid diagnosis of pertussis. J Clin Microbiol 28:32–38, 1990

329. HALPERIN SA, BORTOLUSSI R, WORT J: Evaluation of culture, immunofluorescence, and serology for the diagnosis of pertussis. J Clin Microbiol 27:752–757, 1989

330. HALPERIN SA, MARRIE TJ: Pertussis encephalopathy in an adult: case report and review. Rev Infect Dis 13:1043–1047, 1991

331. HAMMERBERG O, GREGSON DB, GOPAUL D ET AL: Recurrent cervical and submandibular lymphadenitis due to *Actinobacillus actinomycetemcomitans*. Clin Infect Dis 17:1077–1078, 1993

332. HAN N, HOOVER CI, WINKLER JR ET AL: Identification of genomic clonal types of *Actinobacillus actinomycetemcomitans* by restriction endonuclease analysis. J Clin Microbiol 29:1574–1578, 1991

333. HANNER TL, ALLEN JW, ROBERTSON-BYERS A ET AL: Characterization of eugonic fermenter group EF-4 by polyacrylamide gel electrophoresis and protein immunoblot analysis. Am J Vet Res 52:1065–1068, 1991

334. HANTSON P, GAUTIER P, VEKEMANS MC ET AL: Fatal *Capnocytophaga canimorsus* septicemia in a previously healthy woman. Ann Emerg Med 20:93–94, 1991

335. HARTLEY JW, MARTIN ED, GOTHARD WP ET AL: Fulminant *Capnocytophaga canimorsus* (DF-2) septicaemia and diffuse intravascular coagulation in hairy cell leukemia with splenectomy. J Infect 29:229–230, 1994

336. HASSAN IJ, HAYEK L: Endocarditis caused by *Kingella denitrificans*. J Infect 27:291–295, 1993

337. HAWKEY PM, SMITH SD, HAYNES J ET AL: In vitro susceptibility of *Capnocytophaga* species to antimicrobial agents. Antimicrob Agents Chemother 31:331–332, 1987

338. HE Q, MERTSOLA J, HIMANEN JP ET AL: Evaluation of pooled and individual components of *Bordetella pertussis* as antigens in an enzyme immunoassay for diagnosis of pertussis. Eur J Clin Microbiol Infect Dis 12:690–695, 1993

339. HE Q, MERTSOLA J, SOINI H ET AL: Comparison of polymerase chain reaction with culture and enzyme immunoassay for diagnosis of pertussis. J Clin Microbiol 31:642–645, 1993

340. HEINER AM, DISARIO JA, CARROLL K ET AL: Dysgonic fermenter-3: a bacterium associated with diarrhea in immunocompromised hosts. Am J Gastroenterol 87:1629–1630, 1992

341. HEININGER U, STEHR K, SCHMITT-GROHE S ET AL: Clinical characteristics of illness caused by *Bordetella parapertussis* compared with illness caused by *Bordetella pertussis*. Pediatr Infect Dis J 13:306–309, 1994

342. HELTBERG O, BUSK HE, BREMMELGAARD A ET AL: The cultivation and rapid enzyme identification of DF-2. Eur J Clin Microbiol 3:241–243, 1984

343. HEMADY R, ZIMMERMAN A, KATZEN BW ET AL: Orbital cellulitis caused by *Eikenella corrodens*. Am J Ophthalmol 114:584–588, 1992

344. HENRIKSEN SD, BOVRE K: Transfer of *Moraxella kingae* Henriksen and Bovre to the genus *Kingella* gen. nov. in the family *Neisseriaceae*. Int J Syst Bacteriol 26:447–450, 1976

345. HERMAN L, DE RIDDER H: Identification of *Brucella* spp. by using the polymerase chain reaction. Appl Env Microbiol 58:2099–2101, 1992

346. HICKLIN H, VERGHESE A, ALVAREZ S: Dysgonic fermenter 2 septicemia. Rev Infect Dis 9:884–890, 1987

347. HO AC, RAPUANO CJ: *Pasteurella multocida* keratitis and corneal laceration from a cat scratch. Ophthalmic Surg 24:346–348, 1993

348. HO JL, SOUKIASIAN S, HO WH: *Haemophilus aphrophilus* osteomyelitis spread from endogenous flora. Am J Med 76:159–161, 1984

349. HOEL T, SCHEEL O, NORDAHL SHG ET AL: Water- and airborne *Francisella tularensis* biovar *palaearctica* isolated from human blood. Infection 19:348–350, 1991

350. HOLLIS DG, SOTTNEK FO, BROWN WJ ET AL: Use of the rapid carbohydrate fermentation test in determining carbohydrate reactions of fastidious bacteria in clinical laboratories. J Clin Microbiol 12:520–623, 1980

351. HOLLIS DG, WEAVER RE, STEIGERWALT AG ET AL: *Francisella philomiragia* comb. nov. (formerly *Yersinia philomiragia*) and *Francisella tularensis* biogroup *novicida* (formerly *Francisella novicida*) associated with human disease. J Clin Microbiol 27:1601–1608, 1989

352. HOLLIS DG, WIGGINS GL, WEAVER RE: An unclassified gram-negative rod isolated from the pharynx on Thayer-Martin medium (selective agar). Appl Microbiol 24:772–777, 1972

353. HOLMES AH, GREENOUGH TC, BALADY GJ ET AL: *Bartonella henselae* endocarditis in an immunocompetent adult. Clin Infect Dis 21:1004–1007, 1995

354. HOLMES B, POPOFF M, KIREDJIAN M ET AL: *Ochrobactrum anthropi* gen. nov., sp. nov. from human clinical specimens and previously known as group Vd. Int J Syst Bacteriol 38:406–416, 1988

355. HOLST E, ROLLOF J, LARSSON L ET AL: Characterization and distribution of *Pasteurella* species recovered from infected humans. J Clin Microbiol 30:2984–2987, 1992

356. HOLT SC, KINDER SA: Genus II. *Capnocytophaga* Leadbetter, Holt and Socransky 1982, 266^VP Effective publication: Leadbetter, Holt and Socransky, (1979,13). In Staley JT, Bryant MP, Pfennig N (eds), *Bergey's Manual of Systematic Bacteriology*, Vol 3, pp 2050–2058. Baltimore, Williams & Wilkins, 1989

357. HOLT SC, LEADBETTER ER, SOCRANSKY SS: *Capnocytophaga*: a new genus of gram-negative gliding bacteria. II. Morphology and ultrastructure. Arch Microbiol 122:17–27, 1979

358. HOMBAL SM, DINCSOY HP: *Pasteurella multocida* endocarditis. Am J Clin Pathol 98:565–568, 1992

359. HONBERG PZ, FREDRICKSEN W: Isolation of *Pasteurella multocida* in a patient with spontaneous peritonitis and liver cirrhosis. Eur J Clin Microbiol 5:340–342, 1986

360. HOPPE JE, SCHLAGENHAUF M: Comparison of three kinds of blood and two incubation atmospheres for cultivation of *Bordetella pertussis* on charcoal agar. J Clin Microbiol 27:2115–2117, 1989

361. HOPPE JE, SCHWADERER J: Comparison of four charcoal media for the isolation of *Bordetella pertussis*. J Clin Microbiol 27:1097–1098, 1989

362. HOROWITZ EA, PUGSLEY MP, TURBES PG ET AL: Pericarditis caused by *Actinobacillus actinomycetemcomitans*. J Infect Dis 155:152–153, 1987

363. HOWELL JM, WOODWARD GR: Precipitous hypotension in the emergency department caused by *Capnocytophaga canimorsus* sp. nov. sepsis. Am J Emerg Med 8:312–314, 1990

364. HUCK W, BRITT MR: *Haemophilus aphrophilus* cholecystitis. Am J Clin Pathol 69:361–363, 1978

365. INTERNATIONAL COMMITTEE ON SYSTEMATIC BACTERIOLOGY SUBCOMMITTEE ON *PASTEURELLACEAE* AND RELATED ORGANISMS: Minutes of the meeting, September 6 and 10, 1986. Int J Syst Bacteriol 37:474, 1986

366. IRALU JV, ROBERTS D, KAZANJIAN PH: Chorioamnionitis caused by *Capnocytophaga*: case report and review. Clin Infect Dis 17:457–461, 1993

367. JACKSON FL, GOODMAN Y: Genus *Eikenella* Jackson and Goodman 1972, 74[AL]. In Krieg NR, Holt JG, *Bergey's Manual of Systematic Bacteriology*, Vol 1, pp 591–597. Baltimore, Williams & Wilkins, 1984

368. JACOBS F, ABRAMOWICZ D, VEREERSTRAETEN P ET AL: Brucella endocarditis: the role of combined medical and surgical treatment. Rev Infect Dis 12:740–744, 1990

369. JACOBS RF, CONDREY YM, YAMAUCHI T: Tularemia in adults and children: a changing presentation. Pediatrics 76:818–822, 1985

370. JACOBSON JA, MINER P, DUFFY O: *Pasteurella multocida* bacteremia associated with peritonitis and cirrhosis. Am J Gastroenterol 68:489–491, 1977

371. JANDA WM, BRADNA JJ, RUTHER P: Identification of *Neisseria* spp., *Haemophilus* spp., and other fastidious gram-negative bacteria with the MicroScan *Haemophilus–Neisseria* identification panel. J Clin Microbiol 27:869–873, 1989

372. JANDA WM, MALLOY PJ, SCHRECKENBERGER PC: Clinical evaluation of the Vitek *Neisseria–Haemophilus* identification card. J Clin Microbiol 25:37–41, 1987

373. JANDA WM, SANTOS E, STEVENS J ET AL: Unexpected isolation of *Bordetella pertussis* from a blood culture. J Clin Microbiol 32:2851–2853, 1994

374. JANTZEN E, BERDAL BP, OMLAND T: Cellular fatty acid composition of *Francisella tularensis*. J Clin Microbiol 10:928–930, 1979

375. JENNY DB, LETENDRE PW, IVERSON G: Endocarditis caused by *Kingella indologenes*. Rev Infect Dis 9:787–788, 1987

376. JENSEN KT, HOJBJERG T: Meningitis and brain abscess due to *Haemophilus paraphrophilus*. Eur J Clin Microbiol 4:419–421, 1985

377. JENSEN KT, SCHONHEYDER H, THOMSEN VF: In vitro activity of beta-lactam and other antimicrobial agents against *Kingella kingae*. J Antimicrob Chemother 33:635–640, 1994

378. JEPPSON KG, REIMER LG: *Eikenella corrodens* chorioamnionitis. Obstet Gynecol 78:503–505, 1991

379. JIMENEZ-LUCHO V, SHULMAN M, JOHNSON J: *Bordetella bronchiseptica* in an AIDS patient cross-reacts with *Legionella* antisera. J Clin Microbiol 32:3095–3096, 1994

380. JOBANPUTRA PS, MOYSEY J: Endocarditis due to *Cardiobacterium hominis*. J Clin Pathol 30:1033–1036, 1977

381. JOHNSON SM, PANKEY GA: *Eikenella corrodens* osteomyelitis, arthritis, and cellulitis of the hand. South Med J 69:535–539, 1976

382. JONES RN, SLEPACK J, BIGELOW J: Ampicillin-resistant *Haemophilus paraphrophilus* laryngo-epiglottitis. J Clin Microbiol 4:405–407, 1976

383. JORDAN DR, AGAPITOS PJ, MCCUNN PD: *Eikenella corrodens* canaliculitis. Am J Ophthalmol 115:823–824, 1993

384. JORENS PG, MICHIELSEN PP, VAN DEN ENDEN EJ ET AL: A rare cause of colitis—*Brucella melitensis*. Dis Colon Rectum 34:194–196, 1991

385. JOSHI N, O'BRYAN T, APPELBAUM PC: Pleuropulmonary infections caused by *Eikenella corrodens*. Rev Infect Dis 13:207–212, 1991

386. KAKA S, LUNZ R, KLUGMAN KP: *Actinobacillus* (*Pasteurella*) *ureae* meningitis in a HIV-positive patient. Diagn Microbiol Infect Dis 20:105–107, 1994

387. KALB R, KAPLAN MH, TENENBAUM MJ ET AL: Cutaneous infection of dog bite wounds associated with fulminant DF-2 septicemia. Am J Med 78:687–690, 1985

388. KALELIOGLU M, CEYLAN S, KOKSAL I ET AL: Brain abscess caused by *Brucella abortus* and *Staphylococcus aureus* in a child. Infection 18:386–387, 1990

389. KAPLAN AH, WEBER DJ, ODDONE EZ ET AL: Infection due to *Actinobacillus actinomycetemcomitans*: 15 cases and review. Rev Infect Dis 11:46–63, 1989

390. KASLOW HR, PLATLER BW, BLUMBERG DA ET AL: Detection of antibodies inhibiting the ADP-ribosyltransferase activity of pertussis toxin in human serum. J Clin Microbiol 30:1380–1387, 1992

391. KATZENSTEIN DA, CIOFALO L, JORDAN MC: *Bordetella bronchiseptica* bacteremia. West Med J 140:96–98, 1984

392. KEMPER CA, LOMBARD CM, DERESINSKI SC ET AL: Visceral bacillary epithelioid angiomatosis: possible manifestations of disseminated cat scratch disease in the immunocompromised host: a report of two cases. Am J Med 89:216–222, 1990

393. KEREM E, DIAV O, NAVON P ET AL: Pleural fluid characteristics in pulmonary brucellosis. Thorax 49:89–90, 1994

394. KERSTERS K, DE LEY J: Genus *Alcaligenes* Castellani and Chalmers 1919, 936[AL]. In Krieg NR, Holt JG (eds), *Bergey's Manual of Systematic Bacteriology*, Vol 1, pp 361–373. Baltimore, Williams & Wilkins, 1984

395. KERSTERS K, HINZ K-H, HERTLE A ET AL: *Bordetella avium* sp. nov., isolated from the respiratory tracts of turkeys and other birds. Int J Syst Bacteriol 34:56–70, 1984

396. KHAN JA, SHARP S, MANN KB ET AL: Case report: *Kingella denitrificans* prosthetic endocarditis. Am J Med Sci 291:187–189, 1993

397. KHATTAK MN, MATTHEWS RC: Genetic relatedness of *Bordetella* species as determined by macrorestriction digests resolved by pulsed-field gel electrophoresis. Int J Syst Bacteriol 43:695–664, 1993

398. KHELEF N, DANVE B, QUENTIN-MILLET MJ ET AL: *Bordetella pertussis* and *Bordetella parapertussis*: two immunologically distinct species. Infect Immun 61:486–490, 1993

399. KHELEF N, SAKAMOTO H, GUISO N: Both adenylate cyclase and hemolytic activities are required by *Bordetella pertussis* to initiate infection. Microb Pathog 12:227–235, 1992

400. KIEL RJ, CRANE LR, AGUILAR WA ET AL: Corneal perforation caused by dysgonic fermenter-2. JAMA 23:3269–3270, 1987

401. KILEY P, HOLT SC: Characterization of the lipopolysaccharide from *Actinobacillus actinomycetemcomitans* Y4 and N27. Infect Immun 30:862–873, 1980

402. KILIAN M: Degradation of immunoglobulins A1, A2, and G by suspected principal periodontal pathogens. Infect Immun 34:757–765, 1981

403. KING EO, TATUM HW: *Actnobacillus actinomycetemcomitans* and *Haemophilus aphrophilus*. J Infect Dis 111:85–94, 1962

404. KIRCHNER BK, LAKE SG, WIGHTMAN SR: Isolation of *Streptobacillus moniliformis* from a guinea pig with granulomatous pneumonia. Lab Anim Sci 42:519–521, 1992

405. KLEIN B, COUCH J, THOMPSON J: Ocular infections associated with *Eikenella corrodens*. Am J Ophthalmol 109:127–131, 1990

406. KLOOS WE, MOHAPATRA N, DOBROGOSZ WJ ET AL: Deoxyribonucleotide sequence relationships among *Bordetella* species. Int J Syst Bacteriol 31:173–176, 1981

407. KOEHLER JE: Bacillary angiomatosis: investigation of the unusual interactions between *Rochalimaea* bacilli and endothelial cells. J Lab Clin Med 124:475–477, 1994

408. KOEHLER JE, GLASER CA, TAPPERO JW: *Rochalimaea henselae* infection: a new zoonosis with the domestic cat as reservoir. JAMA 271:531–535, 1994

409. KOEHLER JE, LEBOIT PE, EGBERT BM ET AL: Cutaneous vascular lesions and disseminated cat scratch disease in patients with the acquired immunodeficiency syndrome (AIDS) and AIDS-related complex. Ann Intern Med 109:449–455, 1988

410. KOEHLER JE, QUINN FD, BERGER TG ET AL: Isolation of *Rochalimaea* species from cutaneous and osseus lesions of bacillary angiomatosis. N Engl J Med 325:1625–1631, 1992

411. KOEHLER JE, TAPPERO JW: Bacillary angiomatosis and bacillary peliosis in patients infected with human immunodeficiency virus. Clin Infect Dis 17:612–624, 1993

412. KONSTANTOPOULOS K, SKARPAS P, HITJAZIS F ET AL: Rat bite fever in a Greek child. Scand J Infect Dis 24:531–533, 1992

413. KOOPMAN JP, VAN DEN BRINK, VENNIX PPCA: Isolation of *Streptobacillus moniliformis* from the middle ear of rats. Lab Anim 25:35–39, 1991

414. KOPITA JM, HANDSHOE D, KUSSIN PS ET AL: Cat germs! Pleuropulmonary pasteurella infection in an old man. NC Med J 54:308–311, 1993

415. KRALOVIC SM, HUTCHINS MG, SMULIAN AG: Pancreatic abscess due to *Eikenella corrodens* in association with severe ethanolism. Clin Infect Dis 20:198–199, 1995

416. KREKORIAN TD, RADNER AB, ALCORN JM ET AL: Biliary obstruction caused by epithelioid angiomatosis in a patient with AIDS. Am J Med 89:820–822, 1990

417. KREUTZER DL, ROBERTSON DC: Surface macromolecules and virulence in intracellular parasitism: comparison of the cell envelope components of smooth and rough strains of *Brucella abortus*. Infect Immun 23:819–828, 1979

418. KRISTIANSEN JE, BRENNELGAARD A, BUSK HE ET AL: Rapid identification of *Capnocytophaga* isolated from septicemic patients. Eur J Clin Microbiol 3:236–240, 1984

419. KRISTINSSON KG, THORGEIRSSON G, HOLBROOK WP: *Actinobacillus actinomycetemcomitans* and endocarditis. J Infect Dis 157:599, 1988

420. KUIJPER EJ, WIGGERTS HO, JONKER GJ ET AL: Disseminated actinomycosis due to *Actinomyces meyeri* and *Actinobacillus actinomycetemcomitans*. Scand J Infect Dis 24:667–672, 1992

421. KULLBERG B-J, WASTENDORP RGJ, VAN'T WOUT JW ET AL: Purpura fulminans and symmetrical peripheral gangrene caused by *Capnocytophaga canimorsus* (formerly DF-2) septicemia—a complication of dogbite. Medicine 70:287–292, 1991

422. KUMAR A, DEVLIN AR, VELLAND H: *Pasteurella multocida* meningitis in an adult: case report and review. Rev Infect Dis 12:440–448, 1990

423. KUMAR A, KANNAMPUZHA P: Septic arthritis due to *Pasteurella multocida*. South Med J 85:329–330, 1992

424. KURZYNSKI TA, BOEHM DM, ROTT-PETRI JA ET AL: Antimicrobial susceptibilities of *Bordetella* species isolated in a multicenter pertussis surveillance project. Antimicrob Agents Chemother 32:137–140, 1988

425. KURZYNSKI TA, BOEHM DM, ROTT-PETRI JA ET AL: Comparison of modified Bordet-Gengou and modified Regan-Lowe media for the isolation of *Bordetella pertussis* and *Bordetella parapertussis*. J Clin Microbiol 26:2661–2663, 1988

426. KYI MS, AL WALI W, GILLESPIE SH ET AL: Brodie's abscess caused by *Eikenella corrodens*. J Infect 23:213–214, 1991

427. LABRUNE P, JABIR B, MAGNY JF ET AL: Recurrent enterocolitis-like symptoms as the possible presenting manifestations of neonatal *Brucella melitensis* infection. Acta Paediatr Scand 79:707–709, 1990

428. LACOUR M, DUARTE M, BEUTLER A ET AL: Osteoarticular infections due to *Kingella kingae* in children. Eur J Pediatr 150:612–618, 1991

429. LACROIX J-M, WALKER C: Characterization of a *beta*-lactamase found in *Eikenella corrodens*. Antimicrob Agents Chemother 35:886–891, 1991

430. LAGUNA J, DERBY BM, CHASE R: *Cardiobacterium hominis* endocarditis with cerebral mycotic aneurysm. Arch Neurol 32:638–639, 1975

431. LAMBE DW: *Streptobacillus moniliformis* isolated from a case of Haverhill fever: biochemical characterization and inhibitory effect of sodium polyanethol sulfonate. Am J Clin Pathol 60:854–860, 1973

432. LANDINEZ R, LINARES J, LOZA E ET AL: In vitro activity of azithromycin and tetracycline against 358 clinical isolates of *Brucella melitensis*. Eur J Clin Microbiol Infect Dis 11:265–167, 1992

433. LANG R, DAGAN R, POTASMAN I ET AL: Failure of ceftriaxone in the treatment of acute brucellosis. Clin Infect Dis 14:506–509, 1992

434. LANG R, RAZ R, SACKS T ET AL: Failure of prolonged treatment with ciprofloxacin in acute infections due to *Brucella melitensis*. J Antimicrob Chemother 26:841–846, 1990

435. LARSON AM, DOUGHERTY MJ, NOWOWIFISKI DJ ET AL: Detection of *Bartonella (Rochalimaea) quintana* by routine acridine orange staining of broth blood cultures. J Clin Microbiol 32:1492–1496, 1994

436. LARSON CL, WICHT W, JELLISON WL: An organism resembling *P. tularensis* from water. Public Health Rep 70:2530258, 1955

437. LASS JH, VARLEY MP, FRANK KE ET AL: *Actinobacillus actinomycetemcomitans* endophthalmitis with subacute endocarditis. Ann Ophthalmol 16:54–61, 1984

438. LAUGHON BE, SYED SA, LOESCHE WJ: API ZYM system for identification of *Bacteroides* spp., *Capnocytophaga* spp., and spirochetes of oral origin. J Clin Microbiol 15:97–102, 1982

439. LEADBETTER ER, HOLT SC, SOCRANSKY SS: *Capnocytophaga*: a new genus of gram-negative gliding bacteria. I. General characteristics, taxonomic considerations, and significance. Arch Microbiol 122:9–16, 1979

440. LEBOIT PE: The expanding clinical spectrum of a new disease: bacillary angiomatosis. Arch Dermatol 126:808–811, 1990

441. LEBOIT PE, BERGER TG, EGBERT EM ET AL: Epithelioid haemangioma-like vascular proliferation in AIDS: man-

ifestation of cat scratch disease bacillus infection? Lancet 1:960–963, 1988

442. LeBoit PE, Berger TG, Egbert EM et al: Bacillary angiomatosis: the histopathology and differential diagnosis of a pseudoneoplastic infection in patients with human immunodeficiency virus disease. Am J Surg Pathol 13:909–920, 1989

443. Lee H-C, Horowitz E, Linder W: Treatment of tularemia with imipenem/cilastatin sodium. South Med J 84:1277–1278, 1991

444. Lehmann V, Knotsen SB, Ragnhildstveit F et al: Endocarditis caused by *Pasteurella multocida*. Scand J Infect Dis 9:247–248, 1977

445. Leong SS, Cazen RA, Yu GSM et al: Abdominal visceral poliosis associated with bacillary angiomatosis. Arch Pathol Lab Med 116:866–871, 1992

446. Le Quellec A, Bessis D, Perez C et al: Endocarditis due to a *beta*-lactamase-producing *Cardiobacterium hominis*. Clin Infect Dis 19:994–995, 1994

447. Levin JM, Talan DA: Erythromycin failure with subsequent *Pasteurella multocida* meningitis and septic arthritis in a cat-bite victim. Ann Emerg Med 19:1458–1461, 1990

448. Lewis K, Saubolle MA, Tenover FC et al: Pertussis caused by an erythromycin-resistant strain of *Bordetella pertussis*. Pediatr Infect Dis J 14:388–391, 1995

449. Leys EJ, Griffen AL, Strong SJ et al: Detection and strain identification of *Actinobacillus actinomycetemcomitans* by nested PCR. J Clin Microbiol 32:1288–1294, 1994

450. Li Z, Jansen DL, Finn TM et al: Identification of *Bordetella pertussis* infection by shared-primer PCR. J Clin Microbiol 32:783–789, 1994

451. Linnemann CC, Perry EB: *Bordetella parapertussis*: recent experience and a review of the literature. Am J Dis Child 131:560–563, 1977

452. Lippke JA, Peros WJ, Keville MW et al: DNA probe detection of *Eikenella corrodens*, *Wolinella recta*, and *Fusobacterium nucleatum* in subgingival plaque. Oral Microbiol Immunol 6:81–87, 1991

453. Long GWE, Oprandy JJ, Narayanan RB et al: Detection of *Francisella tularensis* in blood by polymerase chain reaction. J Clin Microbiol 31:152–154, 1993

454. Long SS, Welkon CJ, Clark JL: Widespread silent transmission of pertussis in families: antibody correlates of infection and symptomatology. J Infect Dis 161:480–486, 1990

455. Lovell VM, Cho CT, Lindsey NJ et al: *Francisella tularensis* meningitis: a rare clinical entity. J Infect Dis 154:916–917, 1986

456. Lucey D, Dolan MJ, Moss CW et al: Relapsing illness due to *Rochalimaea henselae* in immunocompetent hosts; implications for therapy and new epidemiological associations. Clin Infect Dis 14:683–688, 1992

457. Maccato M, McLean W, Riddle G et al: Isolation of *Kingella denitrificans* from amniotic fluid in a woman with chorioamnionitis: a case report. J Reprod Med 36:685–687, 1991

458. Magee JS, Steele RW, Kelly NR et al: Tularemia transmitted by a squirrel bite. Pediatr Infect Dis J 8:123–125, 1989

459. Maggiore G, Scotta MS, deGiacomo C et al: Bacteremia and meningitis associated with *Haemophilus aphrophilus* infection in a previously healthy child. Infection 10:375, 1982

460. Mahrer S, Raik E: *Capnocytophaga canimorsus* septicemia associated with cat scratch. Pathology 24:194–196, 1992

461. Malatack JJ, Jaffe R: Granulomatous hepatitis in three children due to cat-scratch disease without peripheral adenopathy. Am J Dis Child 147:949–953, 1993

462. Maliszewski CR, Shuster CW, Badger SJ: A type-specific antigen of *Eikenella corrodens* is the major outer membrane protein. Infect Immun 42:208–213, 1983

463. Mandel DR: Streptobacillary fever, an unusual cause of infectious arthritis. Cleve Clin Proc 51:203–205, 1985

464. Mandell RL, Socransky SS: A selective medium for *Actinobacillus actinomycetemcomitans* and the incidence of the organism in juvenile periodontitis. J Periodontol 52:593–598, 1981

465. Mangan DF, Taichman NS, Lally ET et al: Lethal effects of *Actinobacillus actinomycetemcomitans* leukotoxin on human T lymphocytes. Infect Immun 59:3267–3272, 1991

466. Mannheim W: Family III. *Pasteurellaceae* Pohl 1981a, 382 VP. In Krieg NR, Holt JG (eds), *Bergey's Manual of Systematic Bacteriology*, Vol 1, pp 557–558. Baltimore, Williams & Wilkins, 1984

467. Marasco WA, Lester S, Parsonnet P: Unusual presentation of cat-scratch disease in a patient positive for antibody to the human immunodeficiency virus. Rev Infect Dis 11:793–803, 1989

468. Marchette NJ, Nicholes PS: Virulence and citrulline ureidase activity of *Pasteurella tularensis*. J Bacteriol 82:26–32, 1961

469. Marchitto KS, Smith SG, Locht C et al: Nucleotide sequence homology to pertussis toxin gene in *Bordetella bronchiseptica* and *Bordetella parapertussis*. Infect Immun 55:497–501, 1987

470. Marcon MJ, Hamoudi AC, Cannon HJ et al: Comparison of throat and nasopharyngeal swab specimens for culture diagnosis of *Bordetella pertussis* infection. J Clin Microbiol 25:1109–1110, 1987

471. Marriott DJ, Brady LM: *Pasteurella ureae* meningitis. Med J Aust 2:455–456, 1983

472. Martin-Mazuelos E, Nogales MC, Florez C et al: Outbreak of *Brucella melitensis* among microbiology laboratory workers. J Clin Microbiol 32:2035–2036, 1994

473. Martone WJ, Zuehl RW, Minson GE et al: Postsplenectomy sepsis with DF-2: report of a case with isolation of the organism from the patient's dog. Ann Intern Med 93:457–458, 1980

474. Marullo S, Jaccard A, Roulot D et al: Identification of the *Rochalimaea henselae* 16S rRNA sequence in the liver of a French patient with bacillary peliosis hepatis. J Infect Dis 166:1462–1464, 1992

475. Marx RE, Carlson ER, Smith BR et al: Isolation of *Actinomyces* species and *Eikenella corrodens* from patients with chronic diffuse sclerosing osteomyelitis. J Oral Maxillofac Surg 52:26–33, 1994

476. Mason WL, Eigelsbach HT, Little SF et al: Treatment of tularemia, including pulmonary tularemia, with gentamicin. Am Rev Respir Dis 12:39–45, 1980

477. Matar GM, Swaminathan B, Hunter SB et al: Polymerase chain reaction-based restriction fragment length

polymorphism analysis of a fragment of the ribosomal operon from *Rochalimaea* species for subtyping. J Clin Microbiol 31:1730–1734, 1993

478. MATLOW A, VELLAND H: *Capnocytophaga*: a pathogen in immunocompetent hosts. J Infect Dis 152:233–234, 1985

479. MAURIN M, LEPOCHER H, MALLET D ET AL: Antibiotic susceptibilities of *Afipia felis* in axenic medium and in cells. Antimicrob Agents Chemother 37:1410–1413, 1993

480. MAURIN M, RAOULT D: Antimicrobial susceptibility of *Rochalimaea quintana, Rochalimaea vinsonii,* and the newly recognized *Rochalimaea henselae.* J Antimicrob Chemother 32:587–594, 1993

481. MAURIN M, ROUX V, STEIN A ET AL: Isolation and characterization by immunofluorescence, sodium dodecyl sulfate–polyacrylamide gel electrophoresis, Western blot, restriction fragment length polymorphism-PCR, 16S rRNA gene sequencing, and pulsed-field gel electrophoresis of *Rochalimaea quintana* from a patient with bacillary angiomatosis. J Clin Microbiol 32:1166–1171, 1994

482. MAYATEPEK E, ZILOW E, POHL S: Severe intrauterine infection due to *Capnocytophaga ochracea.* Biol Neonate 60: 184–186, 1991

483. MCALLISTER HA, CARTER GR: An aerogenic *Pasteurella*-like organism recovered from swine. Am J Vet Res 35: 917–922, 1974

484. MCCOY GW: A plague-like disease of rodents. Public Health Bull 43:53–71, 1911

485. MCCOY GW, CHAPIN CW: Further observations on a plague-like disease of rodents with a preliminary note on the causative agent, *Bacterium tularense.* J Infect Dis 10:61–72, 1912

486. MCCRARY B, COCKERHAM W, PIERCE P: Neuroretinitis in cat-scratch disease associated with the macular star. Pediatr Infect Dis J 13:838–839, 1994

487. MCDERMOTT M, O'CONNELL B, MULVIHILL TE ET AL: Chronic *Brucella* infection of the supra-patellar bursa with sinus formation. J Clin Pathol 47:764–766, 1994

488. MCDONALD H, GORDON DL: *Capnocytophaga* species: a cause of amniotic fluid infection and preterm labour. Pathology 20:74–76, 1988

489. MCKEEVER S, SCHUBERT JH, MOODY MD ET AL: Natural occurrence of tularemia in marsupials, carnivores, lagomorphs, and large rodents in southwestern Georgia and northwestern Florida. J Infect Dis 103:120–126, 1958

490. MCLEAN DR, RUSSELL N, KHAN MY: Neurobrucellosis: clinical and therapeutic features. Clin Infect Dis 15: 582–590, 1992

491. MEADE BD, BOLLEN A: Recommendations for use of the polymerase chain reaction in the diagnosis of *Bordetella pertussis* infections. J Med Microbiol 41:51–55, 1994

492. MEDLEY SA: A dog bite wound infected with *Pasteurella pneumotropica.* Med J Aust 2:224–225, 1977

493. MEIS JF, SAUERWEIN RW, GYSSENS IC ET AL: *Kingella kingae* intervertebral diskitis in an adult. Clin Infect Dis 15:530–532, 1992

494. MERCER LJ: *Capnocytophaga* isolated from the endometrium as a cause of neonatal sepsis. J Reprod Med 30:67–68, 1985

495. MERINO D, SAAVEDRA J, PUJOL E ET AL: *Haemophilus aphrophilus* as a rare cause of arthritis. Clin Infect Dis 19:320–322, 1994

496. MERTSOLA J, RUUSKANEN O, KURONEN T ET AL: Serologic diagnosis of pertussis: evaluation of pertussis toxin and other antigens in enzyme-linked immunosorbent assay. J Infect Dis 161:966–971, 1990

497. MESNARD R, GUISO N, MICHELET C ET AL: Isolation of *Bordetella bronchiseptica* from a patient with AIDS. Eur J Clin Microbiol Infect Dis 12:304–306, 1993

498. MILAM MW, BALERDI MJ, TONEY JF ET AL: Epithelioid angiomatosis secondary to disseminated cat-scratch disease involving the bone marrow and skin of a patient with acquired immunodeficiency syndrome. Am J Med 88:180–183, 1989

499. MILLER JJ, GRAY BM: *Pasteurella multocida* meningitis presenting as a fever withhout a source in a young infant. Pediatr Infect Dis J 14:331–332, 1995

500. MIN K-W, REED JA, WELCH DF ET AL: Morphologically variable bacilli of cat scratch disease are identified by immunocytochemical labeling with antibodies to *Rochalimaea henselae.* Am J Clin Pathol 101:607–610, 1994

501. MINAMOTO GY, SORDILLO EM: *Kingella denitrificans* as a cause of granulomatous disease in a patient with AIDS. Clin Infect Dis 15:1052–1053, 1992

502. MINK CM, CHERRY JD, CHRISTENSON P ET AL: A search for *Bordetella pertussis* infection in university students. Clin Infect Dis 14:464–471, 1992

503. MINTON EJ: *Pasteurella pneumotropica*: meningitis following a dog bite. Postgrad Med J 66:125–126, 1990

504. MINTZ KP, FIVES-TAYLOR PM: Adhesion of *Actinobacillus actinomycetemcomitans* to a human oral cell line. Infect Immun 62:3672–3678, 1994

505. MITTAL KR, BOURDON S, BERROUARD M: Evaluation of counterimmunoelectrophoresis for serotyping *Actinobacillus pleuropneumoniae* isolates and detection of type-specific antigens in lungs of infected pigs. J Clin Microbiol 31:2339–2342, 1993

506. MOLINA F, DURAN MT, MIGUEZ E ET AL: Isolation of *Haemophilus paraphrophilus* from an abdominal abscess. Eur J Clin Microbiol Infect Dis 12:722–723, 1993

507. MOLINA F, ECHANIZ A, DURAN MT ET AL: Infectious arthritis of the knee due to *Actinobacillus actinomycetemcomitans.* Eur J Clin Microbiol Infect Dis 13:687–689, 1994

508. MOLINA R, BARO T, TORNE J ET AL: Empyema caused by *Kingella denitrificans* and *Peptostreptococcus* spp. in a patient with bronchogenic carcinoma. Eur Respir J 1: 870–871, 1988

509. MOLLEE T, KELLY P, TILEE M: Isolation of *Kingella kingae* from a corneal ulcer. J Clin Microbiol 30:2516–2517, 1992

510. MONACK D, MUNOZ JJ, PEACOCK MG ET AL: Expression of pertussis toxin correlates with pathogenesis in *Bordetella* species, J Infect Dis 159:205–210, 1989

511. MONCLA BJ, BRAHAM P, HILLIER SL: Sialidase (neuraminidase) activity among gram-negative anaerobic and capnophilic bacteria. J Clin Microbiol 28:422–425, 1990

512. MONTES J, RODRIGUEZ A, MARTIN T ET AL: Laboratory-acquired meningitis caused by *Brucella abortus* strain 19. J Infect Dis 154:915–916, 1986

513. MOORE CH, FOSTER L-A, GERBIG DG ET AL: Identification of alcaligin as the siderophore produced by *Bordetella pertussis* and *B. bronchiseptica.* J Bacteriol 177:1116–1118, 1995

514. MORRILL WE, BARBAREE JM, FIELDS BS, ET AL: Effects of temperature and medium on recovery of *Bordetella pertussis* from nasopharyngeal swabs. J Clin Microbiol 26:1814–1817, 1988

515. MORRIS JF, SEWELL DL: Necrotizing pneumonia caused by mixed infection with *Actinobacillus actinomycetemcomitans* and *Actinomyces israelii*: case report and review. Clin Infect Dis 18:450–452, 1994

516. MORRIS JT, MCALLISTER CK: Bacteremia due to *Pasteurella multocida*. South Med J 85:442–443, 1992

517. MORRIS SJ, GREENWALD RA, TURNER RL ET AL: Brucella-induced cholecystitis. Am J Gastroenterol 71:481–484, 1979

518. MORRISON VA, WAGNER KF: Clinical manifestations of *Kingella kingae* infections: case report and review. Rev Infect Dis 11:776–782, 1989

519. MORTENSON JE, LeMAISTRE A, MORRE DG ET AL: Peritonitis involving *Capnocytophaga ochracea*. Diagn Microbiol Infect Dis 3:359–362, 1985

520. MORTIMER EA JR, KIMURA M, CHERRY JD ET AL: Protective efficacy of the Takeda acellular pertussis vaccine combined with diphtheria and tetanus toxoids following household exposure of Japanese children. Am J Dis Child 144:899–904, 1990

521. MOUAKET AE, EL-GHANIM MM, ABD-EL-AL YK ET AL: Prolonged unexplained pyrexia: a review of 221 paediatric cases from Kuwait. Infection 18:226–229, 1990

522. MOUSA ARM, MUHTASAB SA, ALMUDALLAL DS ET AL: Osteoarticular complications of brucellosis: a study of 169 cases. Rev Infect Dis 9:531–543, 1987

523. MOYER NP, EVINS GM, PIGOTT NE ET AL: Comparison of serologic screening tests for brucellosis. J Clin Microbiol 25:1969–1972, 1987

524. MUHLE I, RAU J, RUSKIN J: Vertebral osteomyelitis due to *Actinobacillus actinomycetemcomitans*. JAMA 241:1824–1825, 1979

525. MUI BSK, MULLIGAN ME, GEORGE WL: Response of HIV-associated disseminated cat-scratch disease to treatment with doxycycline. Am J Med 89:229–231, 1990

526. MULLER HE: Detection of antibodies to *Afipia* species by the microagglutination test. Eur J Clin Microbiol Infect Dis 12:951–954, 1993

527. MULVANY NJ, BILLSON VR: Bacillary angiomatosis of the spleen. Pathology 25:398–401, 1993

528. MURRAY PA, WINKLER JR, PEROS WJ ET AL: DNA probe detection of periodontal pathogens in HIV-associated periodontal lesions. Oral Microbiol Immunol 6:34–40, 1991

529. MUTTERS R, IHM P, POHL S ET AL: Reclassification of the genus *Pasteurella trevisan* 1887 on the basis of deoxyribonucleic acid homology, with proposals for the new species *Pasteurella dagmatis*, *Pasteurella canis*, *Pasteurella stomatis*, *Pasteurella anatis*, and *Pasteurella langaa*. Int J Syst Bacteriol 35:309–322, 1985

530. MUTTERS R, PEICHULLA K, HINZ K-H ET AL: *Pasteurella avium* (Hinz and Kunjara) comb. nov. and *Pasteurella volantium* sp. nov. Int J Syst Bacteriol 35:509, 1985

531. MUTTERS R, PEICHULLA K, MANNHEIM W: Phenotypic differentiation of *Pasteurella sensu stricto* and *Actinobacillus* group. Eur J Clin Microbiol 3:225–229, 1984

532. MUTTERS R, POHL S, MANNHEIM W: Transfer of *Pasteurella ureae* Jones 1962 to the genus *Actinobacillus* Brumpt 1910: *Actinobacillus ureae* comb. nov. Int J Syst Bacteriol 36:343–344, 1986

533. MYHRVOLD CV, BRONDZ I, OLSEN I: Application of multivariate analyses of enzymic data to classification of members of the *Actinobacillus–Haemophilus–Pasteurella* group. Int J Syst Bacteriol 42:12–18, 1992

534. NACHNANI S, SCUTERI A, NEWMAN MG ET AL: E-test: a new technique for antimicrobial susceptibility testing for periodontal microorganisms. J Periodontol 63:576–583, 1992

535. NADLER H, DOLAN C, FORGACS P ET AL: *Brucella suis*: an unusual cause of supperative lymphadenitis in an outpatient. J Clin Microbiol 16:575–576, 1982

536. NAGAI S, SOMENO S, YAGIHASHI T: Differentiation of toxigenic from nontoxigenic isolates of *Pasteurella multocida* by PCR. J Clin Microbiol 32:1004–1010, 1994

537. NAHASS RG, COOK S, WEINSTEIN MP: Vertebral osteomyelitis due to *Haemophilus aphrophilus*: treatment with ceftriaxone. J Infect Dis 159:811–812, 1989

538. NAKAMURA M, SLOTS J: Aminopeptidase activity of *Capnocytophaga*. J Periodontal Res 17:597–603, 1982

539. NAVAS E, GUERRERO A, COBO J ET AL: Faster isolation of *Brucella* spp. from blood by Isolator compared with BACTEC NR. Diagn Microbiol Infect Dis 16:79–81, 1993

540. NDON JA: *Capnocytophaga canimorsus* septicemia caused by a dog bite in a hairy cell leukemia patient. J Clin Microbiol 30:211–213, 1992

541. NELSON JD: The changing epidemiology of pertussis in young infants: the role of adults as reservoirs of infection. Am J Dis Child 132:371–373, 1978

542. NEWMAN MG, SUTTER VL, PICKETT MJ ET AL: Detection, identification, and comparison of *Capnocytophaga*, *Bacteroides ochraceus*, and DF-1. J Clin Microbiol 10:557–562, 1979

543. NG VL, BOGGS JM, YORK MK ET AL: Recovery of *Bordetella bronchiseptica* from patients with AIDS. Clin Infect Dis 15:376–377, 1992

544. NG VL, WEIR L. YORK MK ET AL: *Bordetella pertussis* versus Non-L. *pneumophila Legionella* spp.: a continuing diagnostic challenge. J Clin Microbiol 30:3300–3301, 1992

545. NG VL, YORK M, HADLEY WK: Unexpected isolation of *Bordetella pertussis* from patients with acquired immunodeficiency syndrome. J Clin Microbiol 27:337–338, 1989

546. NOBLE RC, MAREK BJ, OVERMAN SB: Spontaneous bacterial peritonitis caused by *Pasteurella ureae*. J Clin Microbiol 25:442–444, 1987

547. NOORDEEN MHH, GODFREY LW: Case report of an unusual cause of low back pain: intervertebral diskitis caused by *Eikenella corrodens*. Clin Orthop 280:175–178, 1992

548. NORDAHL SHG, HOEL T, SCHEEL O ET AL: Tularemia: a differential diagnosis in oto-rhino-laryngology. J Laryngol Otol 107:127–129, 1993

549. OBERHOFER TR: Characteristics and biotypes of *Pasteurella multocida* isolated from humans. J Clin Microbiol 13:566–571, 1981

550. O'BRYAN TA, WHITENER CJ, KATZMAN M ET AL: Hepatobiliary infections caused by *Haemophilus* species. Clin Infect Dis 15:716–719, 1992

551. O'CONNOR SP, DORSCH M, STEIGERWALT AG ET AL: 16S rRNA sequences of *Bartonella bacilliformis* and cat-

scratch disease bacillus reveal phylogenetic relationships with the *alpha*-2 subgroup of the class *Proteobacteria*. J Clin Microbiol 29:2144–2150, 1991

552. ODUM L, JENSEN KT, SLOTSBJERG TD: Endocarditis due to *Kingella kingae*. Eur J Clin Microbiol 3:263–266, 1984

553. OLLE'-GOIG JE, CANELA-SOLER J: An outbreak of *Brucella melitensis* infection by airborne transmission among laboratory workers. Am J Public Health 77:335–338, 1987

554. OLOPOENIA LA, MODY V, REYNOLDS M: *Eikenella corrodens* endocarditis in an intravenous drug user: case report and literature review. J Natl Med Assoc 86: 313–315, 1994

555. OLSEN I: Recent approaches to the chemotaxonomy of the *Actinobacillus–Haemophilus–Pasteurella* group (family *Pasteurellaceae*). Oral Microbiol Immunol 8:327–336, 1993

556. OSCHERWITZ SL: Brucellar bacteremia in pregnancy. Clin Infect Dis 21:714–715, 1995

557. PAGE MI, KING EO: Infection due to *Actinobacillus actinomycetemcomitans* and *Haemophilus aphrophilus*. N Engl J Med 275:181–188, 1966

558. PAJUKANTA R, ASIKAINEN S, SAARELA M ET AL: In vitro activity of azithromycin compared with that of erythromycin against *Actinobacillus actinomycetemcomitans*. Antimicrob Agents Chemother 36:1241–1243, 1992

559. PAJUKANTA R, ASIKAINEN S, SAARELA M ET AL: Evaluation of the E test for antimicrobial susceptibility testing of *Actinobacillus actinomycetemcomitans*. Oral Microbiol Immunol 7:376–377, 1992

560. PAJUKANTA R, ASIKAINEN S, SAARELA M ET AL: In vitro antimicrobial susceptibility of different serotypes of *Actinobacillus actinomycetemcomitans*. Scand J Dent Res 101: 299–303, 1993

561. PAPASIAN CJ, DOWNS NJ, TALLEY RL ET AL: *Bordetella bronchiseptica* bronchitis. J Clin Microbiol 25:575–577, 1987

562. PARENTI DM, SNYDMAN DR: *Capnocytophaga* species: infections in nonimmunocompromised and immunocompromised hosts. J Infect Dis 151:140–147, 1985

563. PARKER SW, APICELLA, MA, FULLER CM: *Haemophilus* endocarditis: two patients with complications. Arch Intern Med 143:48–51, 1983

564. PATEL NJ, MOORE TL, WEISS TD ET AL: *Kingella kingae* infectious arthritis: case report and review of literature of *Kingella* and *Moraxella* infections. Arthritis Rheum 26: 557–559, 1983

565. PATNAIK M, PETER JB: Cat-scratch disease, *Bartonella henselae*, and the usefulness of routine serological testing for *Afipia felis*. Clin Infect Dis 21:1064, 1995

566. PATON BG, ORMEROD LD, PEPPE J ET AL: Evidence for a feline reservoir for dysgonic fermenter 2 keratitis. J Clin Microbiol 26:2439–2440, 1988

567. PAUL RV, ROSTAND SG: Cat bite peritonitis: *Pasteurella multocida* peritonitis following feline contamination of peritoneal dialysis tubing. Am J Kidney Dis 10:318–319, 1987

568. PAVICIC MJAMP, VAN WINKELHOFF AJ, DEGRAFF J: In vitro susceptibilities of *Actinobacillus actinomycetemcomitans* to a number of antimicrobial combinations. Antimicrob Agents Chemother 36:2634–2638, 1992

569. PEDERSEN G, SCHONHEYDER HC, NIELSEN LF: *Capnocytophaga canimorsus* bacteraemia demonstrated by a positive peripheral blood smear. APMIS 101:572–574, 1993

570. PEEK RM, TRUSS C: Secretory diarrhea following a dog bite. Dig Dis Sci 36:1151–1153, 1991

571. PEEL MM: Dog-associated bacterial infections in humans: isolates submitted to an Australian reference laboratory, 1981–1992. Pathology 25:379–384, 1993

572. PEEL MM, HORNIDGE KA, LUPPINO M ET AL: *Actinobacillus* spp. and related bacteria in infected wounds of humans bitten by horses and sheep. J Clin Microbiol 29: 2535–2538, 1991

573. PERDUE GD, GORNEY ER, FERRIER F: Embolomycotic aneurysm associated with bacterial endocarditis due to *Cardiobacterium hominis*. Am Surg 34:901–904, 1968

574. PEREZ-CALVO J, MATAMALA C, SANJOAQUIN I ET AL: Epidural abscess due to acute *Brucella melitensis* infection. Arch Intern Med 154:1410–1411, 1994

575. PEREZ-POMATA MT, DOMINGUEZ J, HORCAJO P ET AL: Spleen abscess caused by *Eikenella corrodens*. Eur J Clin Microbiol Infect Dis 11:162–163, 1992

576. PERKOCHA LA, GEAGHAN SM, BENEDICT YES TS ET AL: Clinical and pathological features of bacillary peliosis hepatis in association with human immunodeficiency virus infection. N Engl J Med 323:1581–1586, 1990

577. PHILLIPS JE: Genus III. *Actinobacillus* Brumpt 1910, 849[AL]. In Krieg NR, Holt JG (eds), *Bergey's Manual of Systematic Bacteriology*, Vol 1, pp 570–575. Baltimore, Williams & Wilkins, 1984

578. PIERCE CS, BARTHOLOMEW WR, AMSTERDAM DD ET AL: Endocarditis due to *Actinobacillus actinomycetemcomitans* serotype c and patient immune response. J Infect Dis 149, 479, 1984

579. PILSWORTH R: Haverhill fever. Lancet 2:236–237, 1983

580. PITTMAN M: Genus *Bordetella* Moreno-Lopez 1952, 178[AL]. In Krieg NR, Holt JG (eds), *Bergey's Manual of Determinative Bacteriology*, Vol 1, pp 388–393. Baltimore, Williams & Wilkins, 1984

581. PLOURDE PJ, EMBREE J, FRIESEN F ET AL: Glandular tularemia with typhoidal features in a Manitoba child. Can Med Assoc J 146:1953–1955, 1992

582. POHL S: DNA relatedness among members of *Haemophilus*, *Pasteurella*, and *Actinobacillus*. In Kilian M, Frederiksen W, Biberstein EL (eds), *Haemophilus, Pasteurella, and Actinobacillus*, pp 245–253. London, Academic Press, 1981

583. POHL S, BERTSCHINGER U, FREDERIKSEN W ET AL: Transfer of *Haemophilus pleuropneumoniae* and the *Pasteurella haemolytica*-like organism causing porcine necrotic pleuropneumonia in the genus *Actinobacillus* (*Actinobacillus pleuropneumoniae* comb. nov.) on the basis of phenotypic and deoxyribonucleic acid relatedness. Int J Syst Bacteriol 33:510–514, 1983

584. PORTNOY BL, SATTERWHITE TK, DYCKMAN JK: Rat bite fever misdiagnosed as Rocky Mountain spotted fever. South Med J 72:607–609, 1979

585. POTASMAN I, EVEN L, BANAI M ET AL: Brucellosis: an unusual diagnosis for a seronegative patient with abscesses, osteomyelitis, and ulcerative colitis. Rev Infect Dis 13:1039–1042, 1991

586. POTTS TV, ZAMBON JJ, GENCO RJ: Reassignment of *Actinobacillus actinomycetemcomitans* to the genus *Haemophilus* as *Haemophilus actinomycetemcomitans* comb. nov. Int J Syst Bacteriol 35:337–341, 1985

587. POUEDRAS P, DONNIO PY, LE TULZO Y ET AL: *Pasteurella stomatis* infection following a dog bite. Eur J Clin Microbiol Infect Dis 12:65, 1993

588. PRAGER L, FRENCK RW: *Streptobacillus moniliformis* infection in a child with chickenpox. Pediatr Infect Dis J 13:417–418, 1994

589. PREUS HR, HARASZTHY VI, ZAMBON JJ ET AL: Differentiation of strains of *Actinobacillus actinomycetemcomitans* by arbitrarily primed polymerase chain reaction. J Clin Microbiol 31:2773–2776, 1993

590. PREUS HR, SUNDAY GJ, HARASZTHY VI ET AL: Rapid identification of *Actinobacillus actinomycetemcomitans* based on analysis of 23S ribosomal RNA. Oral Microbiol Immunol 7:372–375, 1992

591. PRIOR RB, SPAGNA VA, PERKINS RL: Endocarditis due to a strain of *Cardiobacterium hominis* resistant to erythromycin and vancomycin. Chest 75:85–86, 1979

592. PRITCHARD TM, FOUST RT, CANTEY JR ET AL: Prosthetic valve endocarditis due to *Cardiobacterium hominis* occurring after upper gastrointestinal endoscopy. Am J Med 90:516–518, 1991

593. PROGULSKE A, HOLT SC: Transmission-scanning electron microscopic observations of selected *Eikenella corrodens* strains. J Bacteriol 143:1003–1018, 1980

594. PROGULSKE A, MISHELL R, TRUMMEL C ET AL: Biological activities of *Eikenella corrodens* outer membrane and lipopolysaccharide. Infect Immun 43:178–182, 1984

595. PROVENZA JM, KLOTZ SA, PENN RL: Isolation of *Francisella tularensis* from blood. J Clin Microbiol 24:453–455, 1986

596. RAAB MG, LUTZ RA, STAUFFER ES: *Eikenella corrodens* vertebral osteomyelitis: a case report and literature review. Clin Orthop 293:144–147, 1993

597. RAAD I, RAND K, GASKINS D: Buffered charcoal-yeast extract medium for the isolation of brucellae. J Clin Microbiol 28:1671–1672, 1990

598. RADOLF JD: Brucellosis: don't let it get your goat. Am J Med Sci 307:64–75, 1994

599. RAFFI F, BARNER J, BARON D ET AL: *Pasteurella multocida* bacteremia: report of 13 cases over 12 years and review of the literature. Scand J Infect Dis 19:385–393, 1987

600. RAFFI F, DAVID A, MOUZARD A ET AL: *Pasteurella multocida* appendiceal peritonitis: report of three cases and review of the literature. Pediatr Infect Dis J 5:695–698, 1986

601. RAFFIN BJ, FREEMARK M: Streptobacillary rat-bite fever: a pediatric problem. Pediatrics 64:214–217, 1979

602. RAMDEEN GD, SMITH RJ, SMITH EA ET AL: *Pasteurella multocida* tonsillitis: case report and review. Clin Infect Dis 20:1055–1057, 1995

603. RAMOS JM, PACHO E, GARCIA-VALLE B ET AL: Splenic abscess due to *Eikenella corrodens*. Postgrad Med J 70: 848–849, 1994

604. RANK EL, MANDOUR M, ZIMMERMAN SE: Problems with species identification of *Pasteurella* sp., new species 1: two case reports. Clin Microbiol Newslett 6:166–167, 1984

605. RAO VK, PROGULSKE-FOX A: Cloning and sequencing of two type 4 (*N*-methylphenylalanine) pilin genes from *Eikenella corrodens*. J Gen Microbiol 139:651–660, 1993

606. RAO VK, WHITLOCK JA, PROGULSKE-FOX A: Cloning, characterization, and sequencing of two haemagglu-tinin genes from *Eikenella corrodens*. J Gen Microbiol 139: 639–650, 1993

607. RAOULT D, DUPONT HT, ENEA-MUTILLOD M: Positive predictive value of *Rochalimaea henselae* antibodies in the diagnosis of cat-scratch disease. Clin Infect Dis 19:355, 1994

608. RAPPUOLI R: Pathogenicity mechanisms of *Bordetella*. Curr Top Microbiol Immunol 192:319–336, 1994

609. RAYMOND J, BERGEREYT M, BARGY F ET AL: Isolation of two strains of *Kingella kingae* associated with septic arthritis. J Clin Microbiol 24:1100–1101, 1986

610. RECHTMAN DJ, NADLER JP: Abdominal abscess due to *Cardiobacterium hominis* and *Clostridium bifermentans*. Rev Infect Dis 13:418–419, 1991

611. REDFIELD DC, OVERTURF GD, EWING ND ET AL: Bacteremia, arthritis, and skin lesions due to *Kingella kingae*. Arch Dis Child 55:411–414, 1980

612. REED JA, BRIGATI DJ, FLYNN SD ET AL: Immunocytochemical identification of *Rochalimaea henselae* in bacillary (epithelioid) angiomatosis, parenchymal bacillary peliosis, and persistent fever with bacteremia. Am J Surg Pathol 16:650–657, 1992

613. REGAN J, LOWE F: Enrichment medium for the isolation of *Bordetella pertussis*. J Clin Microbiol 6:303–309, 1977

614. REGNERY RL, ANDERSON BE, CLARRIDGE JE ET AL: Characterization of a novel *Rochalimaea* species, *R. henselae* sp. nov., isolated from blood of a febrile, human immunodeficiency virus-positive patient. J Clin Microbiol 30: 265–274, 1992

615. REGNERY RL, MARTIN M, OLSON JG: Naturally occurring *"Rochalimaea henselae"* infection in domestic cats. Lancet 340:557–558, 1992

616. REGNERY RL, OLSON JG, PERKINS BA ET AL: Serological response to *"Rochalimaea henselae"* antigen in suspected cat-scratch disease. Lancet 339:1443–1445, 1992

617. REINA J, BASSA A, LLOMPART I ET AL: Pneumonia caused by *Bordetella bronchiseptica* in a patient with a thoracic trauma. Infection 19:46–48, 1991

618. REIZENSTEIN E, LOFDAHL S, GRANSTROM M ET AL: Evaluation of an improved DNA probe for diagnosis of pertussis. Diagn Microbiol Infect Dis 15:569–673, 1992

619. RELMAN DA, DOMENIGHINI M, TUOMANEN E ET AL: Filamentous hemagglutinin of *Bordetella pertussis*: nucleotide sequence and crucial role in adherence. Proc Natl Acad Sci USA 86:2637–2641, 1989

620. RELMAN DA, FALKOW S, LEBOIT PE ET AL: The organism causing bacillary angiomatosis, peliosis hepatis, and fever and bacteremia in immunocompromised patients. N Engl J Med 324:1514, 1991

621. RELMAN DA, LEPP PW, SADLER N ET AL: Phylogenetic relationships among the agent of bacillary angiomatosis, *Bartonella bacilliformis*, and other *alpha*-proteobacteria. Mol Microbiol 6:1801–1807, 1990

622. RELMAN DA, LOUTIT JS, SCHMIDT TM ET AL: The agent of bacillary angiomatosis: an approach to the identification of uncultured pathogens. N Engl J Med 323:1573–1580, 1990

623. RIBEIRO GA, CARTER GR, FREDERIKSEN W ET AL: *Pasteurella haemolytica*-like bacterium from a progressive granuloma of cattle in Brazil. J Clin Microbiol 27:1401–1402, 1989

624. RILEY LK, ROBERTSON DR: Ingestion and survival of *Brucella abortus* in human and bovine polymorphonuclear leukocytes. Infect Immun 46:224–230, 1984

625. RIMLER RB, SIMMONS DG: Differentiation among bacteria isolated from turkeys with coryza (rhinotracheitis). Avian Dis 27:491–500, 1983

626. RISI GF, PLOMBO DJ: Relapse of tularemia after aminoglycoside therapy: case report and discussion of therapeutic options. Clin Infect Dis 20:174–175, 1995

627. RISTIC M, KREIER JP: Family II. *Bartonellaceae* Gieszczykiewicz 1939, 25^AL. In Krieg NR, Holt JG (eds.), *Bergey's Manual of Systematic Bacteriology*, Vol 1, pp 717–719. Baltimore, Williams & Wilkins, 1984

628. RIVERA M, HUNTER GC, BROOKER J ET AL: Aortic graft infection due to *Pasteurella haemolytica* and group C beta-hemolytic streptococcus. Clin Infect Dis 19:941–943, 1994

629. ROBBINS JB, PITTMAN M, TROLLFORS B ET AL: *Primum non nocere*: a pharmacologically inert pertussis toxoid alone should be the next pertussis vaccine. Pediatr Infect Dis J 12:795–807, 1993

630. ROBERTS NJ JR: *Bartonella bacilliformis* (Bartonellosis). In Mandell GL, Bennett JE, Dolin R (eds.), *Mandell, Douglas, and Bennett's Principles and Practice of Infectious Diseases*, 4th ed, pp 2209–2210. New York, Churchill-Livingstone, 1995

631. ROBERTSON PW, GOLDBERG H, JARVIE BH ET AL: *Bordetella pertussis* infection: a cause of persistent cough in adults. Med J Aust 147:522–525, 1987

632. ROBLOT P, BAZILLOU M, GROLIER G ET AL: Septicemia due to *Capnocytophaga canimorsus* after a dog bite in a cirrhotic patient. Eur J Clin Microbiol Infect Dis 12:302–303, 1993

633. ROE DE, BRAHAM PH, WEINBERG A ET AL: Characterization of tetracycline resistance in *Actinobacillus actinomycetemcomitans*. Oral Microbiol Immunol 10:227–232, 1995

634. ROGERS BT, ANDERSON JC, PALMER CA ET AL: Septicaemia due to *Pasteurella pneumotropica*. J Clin Pathol 26:396–398, 1973

635. ROHRBACH BW, WESTERMAN E, ISTRE GR: Epidemiology and clinical characteristics of tularemia in Oklahoma, 1979–1985. South Med J 84:1091–1096, 1991

636. RONNEVIK PK, NEESS HC: Septicemia caused by *Cardiobacterium hominis*: a case report. Acta Pathol Microbiol Scand Sect B 89:243–244, 1981

637. ROOP RM, PRESTON-MOORE D, BAGCHI T ET AL: Rapid identification of smooth *Brucella* species with a monoclonal antibody. J Clin Microbiol 25:2090–2093, 1987

638. ROOT TE, SILVA EA, EDWARDS LD ET AL: *Haemophilus aphrophilus* endocarditis with a probable primary dental focus of infection. Chest 80:109–110, 1981

639. ROSCOE D, CLARKE A: Resistance of *Capnocytophaga* species to *beta*-lactam antibiotics. Clin Infect Dis 17:284–285, 1993

640. ROSCOE DL, ZEMCOV SJV, THORNBER D ET AL: Antimicrobial susceptibilities and *beta*-lactamase characterization of *Capnocytophaga* species. Antimicrob Agents Chemother 36:2197–2200, 1992

641. ROSS PW, CUMMING CG: Isolation of *Bordetella pertussis* from swabs. Br Med J 282:23–26, 1981

642. ROSS RF, HALL JE, ORNING AP ET AL: Characterization of an *Actinobacillus* isolated from the sow vagina. Int J Syst Bacteriol 22:39–46, 1972

643. ROSSAU R, VANDENBUSSCHE G, THIELEMANS S ET AL: Ribosomal ribonucleic acid cistron similarities and deoxyribonucleic acid homologies of *Neisseria, Kingella, Eikenella, Simonsiella, Alysiella*, and Centers for Disease Control Groups EF-4 and M-5 in the emended family *Neisseriaceae*. Int J Syst Bacteriol 39:185–198, 1989.

644. ROWBOTHAM TJ: Rapid identification of *Streptobacillus moniliformis*. Lancet 2:567, 1983

645. ROWLAND MD, GRIFFITHS DW: The spider as a possible source of tularemia. JAMA 260:33, 1988

646. RUBIN SJ: DF-2, a fastidious fermentative, gram-negative rod. Eur J Clin Microbiol 3:253–257, 1984

647. RUBSAMEN PE, MCLEISH WM, PFLUGFELDER S ET AL: *Capnocytophaga* endophthalmitis. Ophthalmology 100:456–459, 1993

648. RUDIKOFF D, PHELP RG, GORDON RE ET AL: Acquired immunodeficiency syndrome-related bacillary vascular proliferation (epithelioid angiomatosis): rapid response to erythromycin therapy. Arch Dermatol 125:706–707, 1989

649. RUIZ-IRASTORZA G, GAREA C, ALONSO JJ ET AL: Septic shock due to *Pasteurella multocida* subspecies in a previously healthy woman. Clin Infect Dis 21:232–234, 1995

650. RULE D, MILLER-CATCHPOLE R, WEDELL HG ET AL: Tularemia: a present-day problem. Clin Microbiol Newslett 12:141–143, 1990

651. RUMMENS J-L, GORDTS B, VAN LANDUYT HW: In vitro susceptibility of *Capnocytophaga* species to 29 antimicrobial agents. Antimicrob Agents Chemother 30:739–742, 1986

652. RUPP ME: *Streptobacillus moniliformis* endocarditis: case report and review. Clin Infect Dis 14:769–772, 1992

653. RYGG M, BRUUN CF: Rat bite fever (*Streptobacillus moniliformis*) with septicemia in a child. Scand J Infect Dis 24:535–540, 1992

654. SAARELA M, ASIKAINEN S, JOUSIMIES-SOMER H ET AL: Hybridization patterns of *Actinobacillus actinomycetemcomitans* serotypes a–e detected with an rRNA gene probe. Oral Microbiol Immunol 8:111–115, 1993

655. SAGERMAN SD, LOURIE GM: *Eikenella* osteomyelitis in a chronic nail biter: a case report. J Hand Surg Am 20:71–72, 1995

656. SAITO A, HOSAKA Y, NAKAGAWA T ET AL: Significance of serum antibody against surface antigens of *Actinobacillus actinomycetemcomitans* in patients with adult periodontitis. Oral Microbiol Immunol 8:146–153, 1993

657. SAKAZAKII R, YOSHIZAKI E, TAMURA K ET AL: Increased frequency of isolation of *Pasteurella* and *Actinobacillus* species and related organisms. Eur J Clin Microbiol 3:244–248, 1984

658. SALMON SA, WATTS JL, YANCEY JR RJ: Evaluation of the RapID NH system for identification of *Haemophiluis somnus, Pasteurella multocida, Pasteurella haemolytica*, and *Actinobacillus pleuropneumoniae* isolated from cattle and pigs with respiratory disease. J Clin Microbiol 31:1362–1363, 1993

659. SALOPATEK A: Infected Bartholin abscess caused by HB-5. Can J Med Technol 37:86–87, 1975

660. SAMITZ EM, BIBERSTEIN EL: *Actinobacillus suis*-like organisms and evidence of hemolytic strains of *Actinobacillus lignieresii* in horses. Am J Vet Res 52:1245–1251, 1991

661. SANDEN GN, CASSIDAY PK, BARBAREE JM: Rapid immunoblot technique for identifying *Bordetella pertussis*. J Clin Microbiol 31:170–172, 1993

662. SANDSTROM, SJOSTEDT A, FORSMAN M ET AL: Characterization and classification of strains of *Francisella tularensis* isolated in the central Asian focus of the Soviet Union and Japan. J Clin Microbiol 30:172–175, 1992

663. SANDSTROM G, SJOSTEDT A, JOHANSSON T ET AL: Immunogenicity and toxicity of lipopolysaccharide from *Francisella tularensis* LVS. FEMS Microbiol Immunol 5: 201–210, 1993

664. SANTINI C, BAIOCCHI P, BERARDELLI A ET AL: A case of brain abscess due to *Brucella melitensis*. Clin Infect Dis 19:977–978, 1994

665. SATO T, FUJITA H, OHARA Y ET AL: Microagglutination test for early and specific serodiagnosis of tularemia. J Clin Microbiol 28:2372–2374, 1990

666. SAVAGE DD, KAGAN RL, YOUNG NA ET AL: *Cardiobacterium hominis* endocarditis: description of two patients and characterization of the organism. J Clin Microbiol 5:75–80, 1977

667. SAVAGE N: Genus *Streptobacillus* Levaditi, Nicolau, and Poincloux 1925, 1188^AL. In Krieg NR, Holt JG (eds), *Bergey's Manual of Systematic Bacteriology*, Vol 1, pp 598–600. Baltimore, Williams & Wilkins, 1984

668. SCARLETT JD, WILLIAMSON HG, DADSON PJ ET AL: A syndrome resembling thrombotic purpura associated with *Capnocytophaga canimorsus* septicemia. Am J Med 90: 127–128, 1991

669. SCERPELLA EG, WU S, OEFINGER PE: Case report of spinal epidural abscess caused by *Haemophilus paraphrophilus*. J Clin Microbiol 32:563–564, 1994

670. SCHACK SH, SMITH RW, PENN RG ET AL: Endocarditis caused by *Actinobacillus actinomycetemcomitans*. J Clin Microbiol 20:579–581, 1984

671. SCHEEL O, HOEL T, SANDVIK T ET AL: Susceptibility pattern of Scandinavian *Francisella tularensis* isolated with regard to oral and parenteral antimicrobial agents. APMIS 101:33–36, 1993

672. SCHEEL O, REIERSON R, HOEL T: Treatment of tularemia with ciprofloxacin. Eur J Clin Microbiol Infect Dis 11: 447–448, 1992

673. SCHLAPFER G, CHERRY JD, HEININGER U ET AL: Polymerase chain reaction identification of *Bordetella pertussis* infections in vaccinees and family members in a pertussis vaccine efficacy trial in Germany. Pediatr Infect Dis J 14:209–214, 1995

674. SCHLAPFER G, SENN HP, BERGER R ET AL: Use of the polymerase chain reaction to detect *Bordetella pertussis* in patients with mild or atypical symptoms of infection. Eur J Clin Microbiol Infect Dis 12:459–463, 1993

675. SCHLATER LK, BRENNER DJ, STEIGERWALT AG ET AL: *Pasteurella caballi*, a new species from equine clinical specimens. J Clin Microbiol 27:2169–2174, 1989

676. SCHLOSSBERG D, MORAD Y, KROUSE TB ET AL: Culture proven disseminated cat-scratch disease in acquired immunodeficiency syndrome. Arch Intern Med 149:1437–1439, 1989

677. SCHMIDT ME, SMITH MA, LEVY CS: Endophthalmitis caused by unusual gram-negative bacilli: three case reports and review. Clin Infect Dis 17:686–690, 1993

678. SCHMITT-GROHE S, CHERRY JD, HEININGER U ET AL: Pertussis in German adults. Clin Infect Dis 21:860–866, 1995

679. SCHONHEYDER H, EJLERTSON T, FREDERIKSEN W: Isolation of a dysgonic fermenter (DF-3) from urine of a patient. Eur J Clin Microbiol Infect Dis 10:530–531, 1991

680. SCHWARTZMAN WA: Infections due to *Rochalimaea*: the expanding clinical spectrum. Clin Infect Dis 15:893–902, 1992

681. SCHWARTZMAN WA, MARCHEVSKY A, MEYER RD: Epithelioid angiomatosis or cat-scratch disease with splenic and hepatic abnormalities in AIDS; case report and review of the literature. Scand J Infect Dis 22:121–133, 1990

682. SCHWARTZMAN WA, NESBIT CA, BARON EJ: Development and evaluation of a blood-free medium for determining growth curves and optimizing growth of *Rochalimaea henselae*. J Clin Microbiol 31:1882–1885, 1993

683. SCHWARTZMAN WA, PATNAIK M, ANGULO FJ ET AL: *Bartonella (Rochalimaea)* antibodies, dementia, and cat ownership among men infected with human immunodeficiency virus. Clin Infect Dis 21:954–959, 1995

684. SCHWARTZMAN WA, PATNAIK M, BARKA NE ET AL: *Rochalimaea* antibodies in HIV-associated neurologic disease. Neurology 44:1312–1316, 1994

685. SCOAZEC J, MARCHE C, GIRARD P ET AL: Peliosis hepatis and sinusoidal dilitation during infection by the human immunodeficiency virus (HIV). Am J Pathol 131:38–47, 1988

686. SEDLACEK I, GERNER-SMIDT P, SCHMIDT J ET AL: Genetic relationship of *Haemophilus aphrophilus, H. paraphrophilus*, and *Actinobacillus actinomycetemcomitans* studies by ribotyping. Int J Med Microbiol Virol Parasitol Infect Dis 279:51–59, 1993

687. SEGER R, KLOETI J, VON GRAVENITZ A ET AL: Cervical abscess due to *Capnocytophaga ochracea*. Pediatr Infect Dis 1:170–172, 1982

688. SEVERIEN C, TEIG N, RIEDAL F ET AL: Severe pneumonia and chronic lung disease in a young child with adenovirus and *Bordetella pertussis* infection. Pediatr Infect Dis J 14:400–401, 1995

689. SHAH GM, WINER RL: Glomerulonephritis associated with endocarditis caused by *Actinobacillus actinomycetemcomitans*. Am J Kidney Dis 1:113–115, 1981

690. SHANSON DC, GAZZARD BG: *Kingella kingae* septicaemia with a clinical presentation resembling disseminated gonococcal infection. Br Med J 289:730–731, 1984

691. SHANSON DC, GAZZARD BG, MIDGLEY J ET AL: *Streptobacillus moniliformis* isolated from blood in four cases of Haverhill fever. First outbreak in Britain. Lancet 2:92–94, 1983

692. SHANSON DC, PRATT J, GREENE P: Comparison of media with and without "Panemede" for the isolation of *Streptobacillus moniliformis* from blood cultures and observations on the inhibitory effect of sodium polyanethol sulfonate. J Med Microbiol 19:181–186, 1985

693. SHENECKER BJ, KUSHNER ME, TSAI C-C: Inhibition of fibroblast proliferation by *Actinobacillus actinomycetemcomitans*. Infect Immun 38:986–992, 1982

694. SHURIN SB, SOCRANSKY SS, SWEENEY E ET AL: A neutrophil disorder induced by *Capnocytophaga*, a dental microorganism. N Engl J Med 301:849–854, 1979

695. SIEGEL IM: Identification of non-metallic foreign bodies in soft tissue: *Eikenella corrodens* metatarsal osteomyelitis due to a retained toothpick. J Bone Joint Surg 74A:1408–1410, 1992

696. SINGH CP, SPURREL JRR: *Pasteurella multocida* endocarditis. Br Med J 286:1862–1863, 1983

697. Sinnott JT, Blazejowski C, Bazzini MD: *Bordetella bronchiseptica* endocarditis: a tale of a boy and his dog. Clin Microbiol Newslett 11:111–112, 1989

698. Skelton SK, Wong KH: Simple, efficient purification of filamentous hemagglutinin and pertussis toxin from *Bordetella pertussis* by hydrophobic and affinity interaction. J Clin Microbiol 28:1062–1065, 1990

699. Slater LN, Coody DW, Woolridge LK et al: Murine antibody responses distinguish *Rochalimaea henselae* from *Rochalimaea quintana*. J Clin Microbiol 30:1722–1727, 1992

700. Slater LN, Min KW: Polypoid endobronchial lesions: a manifestation of bacillary angiomatosis. Chest 102:972–974, 1992

701. Slater LN, Pitha JV, Herrera L et al: *Rochalimaea henselae* infection in acquired immunodeficiency syndrome causing inflammatory disease without angiomatosis or peliosis. Arch Pathol Lab Med 118:33–38, 1994

702. Slater LN, Welch DF, Hensel D et al: A newly recognized fastidious gram-negative pathogen as a cause of fever and bacteremia. N Engl J Med 323:1587–1593, 1990

703. Slater LN, Welch DF, Min K-W: *Rochalimaea henselae* causes bacillary angiomatosis and peliosis hepatis. Arch Intern Med 152:602–606, 1992

704. Slotnick IJ: *Cardiobacterim hominis* in genitourinary specimens. J Bacteriol 95:1175, 1986

705. Slotnick IJ, Dougherty M: Further characterization of an unclassified group of bacteria causing endocarditis in man: *Cardiobacterium hominis* gen. et sp. nov. Antonie Leeuwenhoek J Microbiol Serol 30:261–272, 1964

706. Slots J: Enzymatic characteristics of some oral and nonoral gram-negative bacteria with the API-ZYM system. J Clin Microbiol 14:288–294, 1981

707. Slots J: Salient biochemical characteristics of *Actinobacillus actinomycetemcomitans*. Arch Microbiol 131:60–67, 1982

708. Slots J: Bacterial specificity in adult periodontitis—a summary of recent work. J Clin Periodontol 13:912–917, 1986

709. Slots J, Liu YB, DiRienzo JM et al: Evaluating two methods for fingerprinting genomes of *Actinobacillus actinomycetemcomitans*. Oral Microbiol Immunol 8:337–343, 1993

710. Sneath PHA, Stevens M: *Actinobacillus rossii* sp. nov., *Actinobacillus seminis* sp. nov. nom. rev., *Pasteurella bettii* sp. nov., *Pasteurella lympangitidis* sp nov., *Pasteurella mairi* sp. nov., and *Pasteurella trehalosi* sp. nov. Int J Syst Bacteriol 40:148–153, 1990

711. Snell JJS: Genus IV. *Kingella* Henriksen and Bovre 1976, 449[AL]. In Krieg NR, Holt JG (eds), *Bergey's Manual of Systematic Bacteriology*, Vol 1, pp 307–309. Baltimore, Williams & Wilkins, 1984

712. Snell JJS, LaPage SP: Transfer of some saccharolytic *Moraxella* species to *Kingella* Henriksen and Bovre 1976, with descriptions of *Kingella indologenes* sp. nov. and *Kingella denitrificans* sp. nov. Int J Syst Bacteriol 26:451–458, 1976

713. Snipes KP, Biberstein EL: *Pasteurella testudinis* sp. nov.: a parasite of desert tortoises (*Gopherus agassizi*). Int J Syst Bacteriol 32:201–210, 1982

714. Sobel JD, Carrizosa J, Ziobrowski TF et al: Polymicrobial endocarditis involving *Eikenella corrodens*. Am J Med Sci 282:41–44, 1981

715. Socransky SS, Holt SC, Leadbetter EP et al: *Capnocytophaga*: a new genus of gram-negative gliding bacteria. III. Physiological characterization. Arch Microbiol 122:29–33, 1979

716. Sorbello AF, O'Donnell J, Kaiser-Smith J et al: Infective endocarditis due to *Pasteurella dagmatis*: case report and review. Clin Infect Dis 18:226–228, 1994

717. Sordillo EM, Rendel M, Sood R et al: Septicemia due to *beta*-lactamase-positive *Kingella kingae*. Clin Infect Dis 17:818–819, 1993

718. Spach DH: Bacillary angiomatosis. Int J Dermatol 31:19–24, 1992

719. Spach DH, Callis KP, Paauw DS et al: Endocarditis caused by *Rochalimaea quintana* in a patient infected with human immunodeficiency virus. J Clin Microbiol 31:692–694, 1993

720. Spach DH, Kanter AS, Daniels NA et al: *Bartonella* (*Rochalimaea*) species as a cause of apparent "culture-negative" endocarditis. Clin Infect Dis 20:1044–1047, 1995

721. Spach DH, Kanter AS, Doughertry MJ et al: *Bartonella* (*Rochalimaea*) *quintana* bacteremia in inner-city patients with chronic alcoholism. N Engl J Med 332:424–428, 1995

722. Spach DH, Panther LA, Thorning DR et al: Intracerebral bacillary angiomatosis in a patient infected with human immunodeficiency virus. Ann Intern Med 116:740–742, 1992

723. Stackbrandt E, Murray RGE, Truper HG: *Proteobacteria* classis nov., a name for the phylogenetic taxon that includes the "purple bacteria and their relatives." Int J Syst Bacteriol 38:321–325, 1988

724. Starkebaum GA, Plorde JJ: Pasteurella pneumonia: report of a case and review of the literature. J Clin Microbiol 5:332–335, 1977

725. Staszkiewicz J, Lewis CM, Colville J et al: Outbreak of *Brucella melitensis* among microbiology laboratory workers in a community hospital. J Clin Microbiol 29:287–290, 1991

726. Steeper TA, Rosenstein H, Weiser J et al: Bacillary angiomatosis involving the liver, spleen, and skin in an AIDS patient with concurrent Kaposi's sarcoma. Am J Clin Pathol 97:713–718, 1992

727. Steffens L, Franke S, Nickel S et al: DNA fingerprinting of *Eikenella corrodens* by pulsed-field gel electrophoresis. Oral Microbiol Immunol 9:95–08, 1994

728. Stein A, Teysseire N, Capobianco C et al: *Eikenella corrodens*, a rare cause of pancreatic abscess: two case reports and review. Clin Infect Dis 17:273–275, 1993

729. Stein AA, Fialk MA, Blevins A et al: *Pasteurella multocida* septicemia. Experience at a cancer hospital. JAMA 249:508–509, 1983

730. Stevens DL, Higbee JW, Oberhofer TR et al: Antibiotic susceptibilities of human isolates of *Pasteurella multocida*. Antimicrob Agents Chemother 16:322–324, 1979

731. Steyer BJ, Sobonya RE: *Pasteurella multocida* lung abscess: a case report and review of the literature. Arch Intern Med 144:1081–1082, 1984

732. St John MA, Belda AA, Matlow A et al: *Eikenella corrodens* empyema in children. Am J Dis Child 135:415–417, 1981

733. STOLOFF AL, GILLIES ML: Infections with *Eikenella corrodens* in a general hospital: a report of 33 cases. Rev Infect Dis 8:50–53, 1986

734. STORSAETER J, HALLANDER H, FARRINGTON CP ET AL: Secondary analyses of the efficacy of two acellular pertussis vaccines evaluated in a Swedish phase III trial. Vaccine 8:457–461, 1990

735. STROLL DB, MURPHEY SA, BALLAS SK: *Bordetella bronchiseptica* infection in stage IV Hodgkin's disease. Postgrad Med J 57:723–724, 1981

736. SUTTER VL, PYEATT D, KWOK YY: In vitro susceptibility of *Capnocytophaga* strains to 18 antimicrobial agents. Antimicrob Agents Chemother 20:270–271, 1981

737. SUTTON RGA, O'KEEFFE MF, BUNDOCK MA ET AL: Isolation of a new *Moraxella* from a corneal abscess. J Med Microbiol 5:148–150, 1972

738. SWANN RA, HOLMES B: Infective endocarditis caused by *Kingella denitrificans*. J Clin Pathol 37:1384–1387, 1984

739. SWANSON RN, HARDY DJ, CHU DTW ET AL: Activity of temafloxacin against respiratory pathogens. Antimicrob Agents Chemother 35:423–429, 1991

740. SYRJALA H, KUJALA P, MYLLYLA V ET AL: Airborne transmission of tularemia in farmers. Scand J Infect Dis 17: 371–375, 1985

741. SYRJALA H, SCHILDT R, RAISAINEN S: In vitro susceptibility susceptibility of *Francisella tularensis* to fluoroquinolones and treatment of tularemia with norfloxacin and ciprofloxacin. Eur J Clin Microbiol Infect Dis 10: 68–70, 1991

742. TANNER ACR, VISCONTI RA, SOCRANSKY SS ET AL: Classification and identification of *Actinobacillus actinomycetemcomitans* and *Haemophilus aphrophilus* by cluster analysis and deoxyribonucleic acid hybridizations. J Periodontal Res 17:585–596, 1982

743. TAPPERO JW, MOHLE-BOETANI J, KOEHLER JE ET AL: The epidemiology of bacillary angiomatosis and bacillary peliosis. JAMA 269:770–775, 1993

744. TAPPERO JW, KOEHLER JE, BERGER TG ET AL: Bacillary angiomatosis and bacillary splenitis in immunocompetent adults. Ann Intern Med 118:363–365, 1993

745. TARNVIK A: Nature of protective immunity to *Francisella tularensis*. Rev Infect Dis 11:440–451, 1989

746. TAVERAS JM, CAMPO R, SEGAL N ET AL: Apparent culture-negative endocarditis of the prosthetic valve caused by *Cardiobacterium hominis*. South Med J 86:1439–1440, 1993

747. TAYLOR JP, PURDUE JN: The changing epidemiology of human brucellosis in Texas, 1976–1986. Am J Epidemiol 130:160–165, 1989

748. TEMPRO PJ, SLOTS J: Selective medium for the isolation of *Haemophilus aphrophilus* from the human periodontium and other oral sites and the low proportion of the organism in the oral flora. J Clin Microbiol 23:777–782, 1986

749. THIGPEN JE, CLEMENTS ME, GUPTA BN: Isolation of *Pasteurella aerogenes* from the uterus of a rabbit following abortion. Lab Anim Sci 28:444–447, 1978

750. THOMPSON CM, PAPPU L, LEVKOFF AH ET AL: Neonatal septicemia and meningitis due to *Pasteurella multocida*. Pediatr Infect Dis 3:559–561, 1984

751. THORSEN P, MOLLER BR, ARPI M ET AL: *Pasteurella aerogenes* isolated from stillbirth and mother. Lancet 343: 485–486, 1994

752. TISON DL, LATIMER JM: Lysis centrifugation-direct plating technique for isolation of group DF-2 from the blood of a dog bite victim. J Infect Dis 153:1001–1002, 1986

753. TOLLO K, HELGELAND K: Fc-binding components: a virulence factor in *Actinobacillus actinomycetemcomitans*? Oral Microbiol Immunol 6:373–377, 1991

754. TONJUM T, BUKHOLM G, BOVRE K: Identification of *Haemophilus aphrophilus* and *Actinobacillus actinomycetemcomitans* by DNA–DNA hybridization and genetic transformation. J Clin Microbiol 28:1994–1998, 1990

755. TONJUM T, HAAS R: Identification of *Actinobacillus actinomycetemcomitans* by leukotoxin gene-specific hybridization and polymerase chain reaction assays. J Clin Microbiol 31:1856–1859, 1993

756. TONJUM T, WEIR S, BOVRE K ET AL: Sequence divergence in two tandemly located pilin genes of *Eikenella corrodens*. Infect Immun 61:1909–1916, 1993

757. TOSHNIWAL R, DRAGHI TC, KOCKA FE ET AL: Manifestations of *Kingella kingae* infections in adults: resemblance to neisserial infections. Diagn Microbiol Infect Dis 5: 81–85, 1986

758. TSAI C-C, SHENEKER BJ, DIRIENZO JM ET AL: Extraction and isolation of a leukotoxin from *Actinobacillus actinomycetemcomitans* with polymyxin B. Infect Immun 43: 700–705, 1984

759. TYRRELL J, NOONE P, PRICHARD JS: Thoracic actinomycosis complicated by *Actinobacillus actinomycetemcomitans*: case report and review of literature. Respir Med 86: 341–343, 1992

760. UHARI M, SYRJALA H, SALMINEN A: Tularemia in children caused by *Francisella tularensis* biovar *palaearctica*. Pediatr Infect Dis J 9:80–83, 1990

761. URS S, D'SILVA BSV, JEENA CP ET AL: *Kingella kingae* septicaemia in association with HIV disease. Trop Doct 24: 127, 1994

762. VAKIL N, ADIYODY J, TRESER G ET AL: *Pasteurella multocida* septicemia and peritonitis in a patients with cirrhosis: case report and review of the literature. Am J Gastroenterol 80:565–568, 1985

763. VAN BIJSTERVELD OP: New *Moraxella* strain isolates from angular conjunctivitis. Appl Microbiol 20:405–408, 1970

764. VANDAMME P, HOMMEZ J, VANCANNEYT M ET AL: *Bordetella hinzii* sp. nov., isolated from poultry and humans. Int J Syst Bacteriol 45:37–45, 1995

765. VAN DER ZEE A, AGTERBERG C, PEETERS M ET AL: Polymerase chain reaction assay for pertussis: simultaneous detection and discrimination of *Bordetella pertussis* and *Bordetella parapertussis*. J Clin Microbiol 31:2134–2140, 1993

766. VAN DYKE TE, BARTHOLOMEW E, GENCO RJ ET AL: Inhibition of neutrophil chemotaxis by soluble bacterial products. J Periodontol 53:502–508, 1982

767. VAN STEENBERGAN TJM, BOSCH-TIJHOF CJ, VAN WINKELHOFF AJ ET AL: Comparison of six typing methods for *Actinobacillus actinomycetemcomitans*. J Clin Microbiol 32:2769–2774, 1994

768. VAN TONDER EM: Infection of rams with *Actinobacillus seminis*. J S Afr Vet Assoc 44:235–240, 1973

769. VAN WINKELHOFF AJ, OVERBEEK BP, PAVICIC MJAMP ET AL: Long-standing bacteremia caused by oral *Actinobacillus actinomycetemcomitans* in a patient with a pacemaker. Clin Infect Dis 16:216–218, 1993

770. VARTIAN CV, SEPTIMUS EJ: Endophthalmitis due to *Pasteurella multocida* and CDC EF-4. J Infect Dis 160:733, 1989

771. VASSEUR E, JOLY P, NOUVELLON M ET AL: Cutaneous abscess: a rare complication of *Streptobacillus moniliformis* infection. Br J Dermatol 129:95–96, 1993

772. VENKATARAMANI A, SANTO-DOMINGO NE, MAIN DM: *Actinobacillus actinomycetemcomitans* pneumonia with possible septic embolization. Chest 105:645–646, 1994

773. VERBRUGGEN A-M, HAUGLUSTAINE D, SCHILDERMANS F ET AL: Infections caused by *Kingella kingae*: reports of four cases and review. J Infect 133–142, 1986

774. VERGER J-M, GRIMONT F, GRIMONT PAD ET AL: *Brucella*, a monospecific genus as shown by deoxyribonucleic acid hybridization. Int J Syst Bacteriol 35:292–295, 1985

775. VERGHESE A, HAMATI F, BERK S ET AL: Susceptibility of dysgonic fermenter 2 to antimicrobial agents in vitro. Antimicrob Agents Chemother 32:78–80, 1988

776. VINCENT J, PODEWELL C, FRANKLIN GW ET AL: Septic arthritis due to *Kingella* (*Moraxella*) *kingae*: case report and review of the literature. J Rheumatol 8:501–503, 1981

777. VISVANATHAN K, JONES PD: Ciprofloxacin treatment of *Haemophilus paraphrophilus* brain abscess. J Infect 22: 306–307, 1991

778. VIZCAINO N, FERNANDEZ-LAGO L: A rapid and sensitive method for the identification of *Brucella* species with a monoclonal antibody. Res Microbiol 143:513–518, 1992

779. VON GRAEVENITZ A, COLLA F: Thyroiditis due to *Brucella melitensis*—report of two cases. Infection 18:179–180, 1990

780. WADOWSKY RM, LAUS S, LIBERT T ET AL: Inhibition of PCR-based assay for *Bordetella pertussis* by using calcium alginate fiber and aluminum shaft components of a nasopharyngeal swab. J Clin Microbiol 32:1054–1057, 1994

781. WAGNER DK, WRIGHT JJ, ANSHER AF ET AL: Dysgonic fermenter 3-associated gastrointestinal disease in a patient with common variable hypogammaglobulinemia. Am J Med 84:315–318, 1988

782. WALDOR M, ROBERTS D, KAZANJIAN P: In utero infection due to *Pasteurella multocida* in the first trimester of pregnancy: case report and review. Clin Infect Dis 14:497–500, 1992

783. WALDVOGEL K, REGNERY RL, ANDERSON BE ET AL: Disseminated cat-scratch disease: detection of *Rochalimaea henselae* in affected tissue. Eur J Pediatr 153:23–27, 1994

784. WANAGER RA: Primary pneumonic tularemia with positive blood cultures. Clin Microbiol Newslett 6:120–122, 1984

785. WATERSPIEL JN: *Kingella kingae* meningitis with bilateral infarcts of the basal ganglia. Infection 11:307–308, 1983

786. WATTS JL, YANCEY RJ: Identification of veterinary pathogens by use of commercial identification systems and new trends in antimicrobial susceptibility testing of veterinary pathogens. Clin Microbiol Rev 7:346–356, 1994

787. WAUTERS JP, FERGUSON RK, MICHAUD PA ET AL: Glomerulonephritis associated with *Haemophilus aphrophilus* endocarditis. Clin Nephrol 9:73–76, 1978

788. WEAVER RE: Genus *Cardiobacterium* Slotnick and Dougherty 1964, 271[AL]. In Krieg NR, Holt JG (eds),

Bergey's Manual of Systematic Bacteriology, Vol 1, pp 583–585. Baltimore, Williams & Wilkins, 1984

789. WEBB CH, HOGG GM: *Haemophilus aphrophilus* endocarditis. Br J Clin Prac 44:329–331, 1990

790. WEBER DJ, WOLFSON JS, SWARTZ MN ET AL: *Pasteurella multocida* infections: report of 34 cases and review of the literature. Medicine 63:133–154, 1984

791. WEIR S, MARRS CF: Identification of type 4 pili in *Kingella denitrificans*. Infect Immun 60:3437–3441, 1992

792. WEISS E, DASCH GA: Differential characteristics of strains of *Rochalimaea*: *Rochalimaea vinsonii* sp nov., the Canadian vole agent. Int J Syst Bacteriol 32:305–314, 1982

793. WEISS E, DASCH GA, WOODMAN DR ET AL: Vole agent identified as a strain of the trench fever rickettsia, *Rochalimaea quintana*. Infect Immun 19:1013–1020, 1978

794. WEISS E, MOULDER JW: Genus II. *Rochalimaea* (Macchiavello 1947) Krieg 1961. 162[AL]. In Krieg NR, Holt JG (eds.), *Bergeys's Manual of Systematic Bacteriology*, Vol 1, pp 698–701. Baltimore, Williams & Wilkins, 1984

795. WELCH DF, HENSEL DM, PICKETT DA ET AL: Bacteremia due to *Rochalimaea henselae* in a child: practical identification of isolates in the clinical laboratory. J Clin Microbiol 31:2381–2386, 1993

796. WELCH DF, PICKETT DA, SLATER LN ET AL: *Rochalimaea henselae* sp. nov., a cause of septicemia, bacillary angiomatosis, and parenchymal bacillary peliosis. J Clin Microbiol 30:275–280, 1992

797. WESTERMAN EL, MCDONALD J: Tularemia pneumonia mimicking legionnaires' disease: isolation of organism on CYE agar and successful treatment with erythromycin. South Med J 76:1169–1170, 1983

798. WEYANT RS, HOLLIS DG, WEAVER RE ET AL: *Bordetella holmesii* sp. nov., a new gram-negative species associated with septicemia. J Clin Microbiol 33:1–7, 1995

799. WHITE CB, LAMPE RM, COPELAND RL ET AL: Soft tissue infection with *Haemophilus aphrophilus*. Pediatrics 67: 434–435, 1981

800. WHITELEY LO, MAHESWAREN SK, WEISS DJ ET AL: *Pasteurella haemolytica* A1 and bovine respiratory disease: pathogenesis. J Vet Intern Med 6:11–22, 1992

801. WILKINS EGL, MILLAR JGB, COCKCROFT PM ET AL: Ratbite fever in a gerbil breeder. J Infect. 16:177–180, 1988

802. WILLIAMS BL, HAMMOND BF: *Capnocytophaga*: new genus of gram-negative gliding bacteria. IV. DNA base composition and sequence homology. Arch Microbiol 122: 35–39, 1979

803. WILLIAMS BL, HOLLIS D, HOLDEMANN LV: Synonymy of strains of Centers for Disease Control group DF-1 with species of *Capnocytophaga*. J Clin Microbiol 10:550–556, 1979

804. WILLIAMS JD, MASKELL JP, SHAIN H ET AL: Comparative in-vitro activity of azithromycin, macrolides (erythromycin, clarithromycin and spiramycin) and streptogramin RP 59500 against oral organisms. J Antimicrob Chemother 30:27–37, 1992

805. WILSON CM, REISS-LEVY EA, STURGESS AD ET AL: *Haemophilus paraphrophilus* vertebral osteomyelitis. Med J Aust 160:512–514, 1994

806. WILSON ME: Prosthetic valve endocarditis and paravalvular abscess caused by *Actinobacillus actinomycetemcomitans*. Rev Infect Dis 11:665–667, 1989

807. WILSON ME: IgG antibody response of localized juvenile periodontitis patients to the 29 kilodalton outer membrane protein of *Actinobacillus actinomycetemcomitans*. J Periodontol 62:211–218, 1991

808. WILSON ME: The heat-modifiable outer membrane protein of *Actinobacillus actinomycetemcomitans*: relationship to OmpA proteins. Infect Immun 59:2505–2507, 1991

809. WILSON ME, JONAK-URBANCZYK JT, BRONSON PM ET AL: *Capnocytophaga* species: increased resistance of clinical isolates to serum bactericidal action. J Infect Dis 156:99–106, 1987

810. WINN RE, CHASE WF, LAUDERDALE PW ET AL: Septic arthritis involving *Capnocytophaga ochracea*. J Clin Microbiol 19:538–540, 1983

811. WIRSING VON KONIG CH, FINGER H: Role of pertussis toxin in causing symptoms of *Bordetella parapertussis* infection. Eur J Clin Microbiol Infect Dis 13:455–458, 1994

812. WONG AS, DYKE J, PERRY D ET AL: Paraspinal mass associated with intervertebral disk infection secondary to *Moraxella kingii*. J Pediatr 86–88, 1978

813. WONG JD, JANDA JM, DUFFEY PS: Preliminary studies on the use of carbon substrate utilization patterns for identification of *Brucella* species. Diagn Microbiol Infect Dis 15:109–113, 1992

814. WONG MT, DOLAN MJ, LATTUADA CP JR ET AL: Neuroretinitis, aseptic meningitis, and lymphadenitis associated with *Bartonella* (*Rochalimaea*) *henselae* infection in immunocompetent patients and patients infected with human immunodeficiency virus type 1. Clin Infect Dis 21:352–360, 1995

815. WOODARD DR, CONE LA, FOSTVEDT K: *Bordetella bronchiseptica* infection in patients with AIDS. Clin Infect Dis 20:193–194, 1995

816. WOOLFREY RR, MOODY JA: Human infections associated with *Bordetella bronchiseptica*. Clin Microbiol Rev 4:243–255, 1991

817. WORMSER GP, BOTTONE EJ, TUDY J ET AL: *Cardiobacterium hominis*: review of prior infections and report of endocarditis on a fascia lata prosthetic heart valve. Am J Med Sci 276:117–126, 1978

818. WORMSER GP, BOTTONE EJ: *Cardiobacterium hominis*: review of microbiologic and clinical features. Rev Infect Dis 5:680–691, 1983

819. WULLENWEBER M: *Streptobacillus moniliformis*—a zoonotic pathogen. Taxonomic considerations, host species, diagnosis, therapy, geographical distribution. Lab Anim 29:1–15, 1995

820. WUST J, GUBLER J, MANNHEIM W ET AL: *Actinobacillus hominis* as a causative agent of septicemia in hepatic failure. Eur J Clin Microbiol Infect Dis 10:693–694, 1991

821. YAGUPSKY P: Detection of *Brucella melitensis* by BACTEC NR660 blood culture system. J Clin Microbiol 32:1899–1901, 1994

822. YAGUPSKY P, DAGAN R: *Kingella kingae* bacteremia in children. Pediatr Infect Dis J 12:1148–1149, 1994

823. YAGUPSKY P, DAGAN R, HOWARD CW ET AL: High prevalence of *Kingella kingae* in joint fluid from children with septic arthritis revealed by the BACTEC blood culture system. J Clin Microbiol 30:1278–1281, 1992

824. YAGUPSKY P, DAGAN R, HOWARD CB ET AL: Clinical features and epidemiology of invasive *Kingella kingae* infections in southern Israel. Pediatrics 92:800–804, 1993

825. YAGUPSKY P, HOWARD CB, EINHORN M ET AL: *Kingella kingae* osteomyelitis of the calcaneus in young children. Pediatr Infect Dis J 12:540–541, 1993

826. YAGUPSKY P, SIMO A: *Pasteurella ureae* meningitis as complication of skull fractures. Eur J Clin Microbiol 4:589–590, 1985

827. YAMAMOTO T, KAJIURA S, HIRAI Y ET AL: *Capnocytophaga haemolytica* sp. nov. and *Capnocytophaga granulosa* sp. nov., from human dental plaque. Int J Syst Bacteriol 44:324–329, 1994

828. YAMAZAKI Y, EBISU S, OKADA H: Partial purification of a bacterial lectin-like substance from *Eikenella corrodens*. Infect Immun 56:191–196, 1988

829. YOGEV R, SHULMAN D, SHULMAN ST ET AL: In vitro activity of antibiotics alone and in combination against *Actinobacillus actinomycetemcomitans*. Antimicrob Agents Chemother 29:179–181, 1986

830. YOUNG EJ: Serologic diagnosis of human brucellosis: analysis of 214 cases by agglutination tests and review of the literature. Rev Infect Dis 13:359–372, 1991

831. YOUNG EJ: An overview of human brucellosis. Clin Infect Dis 21:283–290, 1995

832. YOUNG SA, ANDERSON GL, MITCHELL PD: Laboratory observations during an outbreak of pertussis. Clin Microbiol Newslett 9:176–179, 1987

833. YU X, RAOULT D: Monoclonal antibodies to *Afipia felis*—a putative agent of cat scratch disease. Am J Clin Pathol 101:603–606, 1994

834. YUAN A, YANG PCH, LEE LN ET AL: *Actinobacillus actinomycetemcomitans* pneumonia with chest wall involvement and rib destruction. Chest 101:1450–1451, 1992

835. ZAMBON JJ, CHRISTERSSON LA, SLOTS J: *Actinobacillus actinomycetemcomitans* in human periodontal disease: prevalence in patient groups and distribution of biotypes and serotypes within families. J Periodontal 54:707–711, 1983

836. ZANGWILL KM, HAMILTON DH, PERKINS BA ET AL: Cat scratch disease in Connecticut: epidemiology, risk factors, and evaluation of a new diagnostic test. N Engl J Med 329:8–13, 1993

837. ZBINDEN R, SOMMERHALDER P, VON WARTBURG U: Co-isolation of *Pasteurella dagmatis* and *Pasteurella multocida* from cat-bite wounds. Eur J Clin Microbiol Infect Dis 7:203–204, 1988

838. ZHAO G, GALINA L, HANYANUN W ET AL: Human tonsillitis associated with porcine *Pasteurella multocida* ingestion. Lancet 342:491, 1993

839. ZIJLSTRA EE, SWART GR, GODFROY FJM ET AL: Pericarditis, pneumonia, and brain abscess due to a combined *Actinomyces-Actinobacillus actinomycetemcomitans* infection. J Infect 25:83–87, 1992

840. ZIMMERMAN SJ, GILLIKIN S, SOFAT N ET AL: Case report and seeded blood culture study of *Brucella* bacteremia. J Clin Microbiol 28:2139–2141, 1990

841. ZWASS A, FELDMAN F: Case report 875: Multifocal osteomyelitis—a manifestation of chronic brucellosis. Skeletal Radiol 23:660–663, 1994

LEGIONELLA

During the summer of 1976, an explosive outbreak of pneumonia of unknown etiology occurred among persons who attended an American Legion convention in Philadelphia.[53] Individuals who developed the multisystem illness that included pneumonia were said to have *legionnaires' disease.*[20] A total of 182 cases was documented; 29 of these patients died. By early January 1977, the etiologic agent had been isolated by Dr. Joseph McDade of the Centers for Disease Control (CDC).[84] Thus, a major medical mystery was solved and a new family of bacteria, the *Legionellaceae,* was discovered. For those interested in more details, the history of legionnaires' disease has been reviewed by Winn.[131]

TAXONOMY AND CHARACTERISTICS OF THE GENUS *LEGIONELLA*

In 1979, Brenner, Steigerwalt, and McDade classified the bacterium that caused the Philadelphia outbreak of legionnaires' disease as *Legionella pneumophila,* in the family *Legionellaceae.*[18] At present, there are 41 validly published species of *Legionella* that have been isolated from either human clinical materials, environmental sources, or both (Table 9-1).[60,62] At this writing, one of the species most recently described is *L. lytica* (for-

merly called *Sarcobium lyticum*); this is an obligate intracellular parasite of certain strains of Acanthamoebae and other free-living amoebae.[29,62]

Legionella species are non–spore-forming, narrow, gram-negative rods, 0.3 to 0.9 μm in width that vary from short forms 1.5 to 2 μm in length to longer filamentous forms.[17,18] They are usually short and thin or coccobacillary when seen in direct smears of clinical specimens but more variable in length following growth in culture media, with forms greater than 20 μm long not unusual. Legionellae stain much more readily with the Diff-Quik, Giemsa, or Gram-Weigert stains than they do with Gram stain in touch preparations of fresh tissue imprints, smears of bronchial alveolar lavage fluid, or sputum. Except for three species that are nonmotile, *L. oakridgensis, L. nautarum,* and *L. londinensis,* the remainder of *Legionella* species are motile by means of one or more polar or subpolar flagella.[62,102] The *Legionellaceae* are aerobic and nutritionally fastidious. They require L-cysteine and iron salts for growth, which are provided in buffered charcoal yeast extract agar (BCYEa), but do not grow on the usual blood agar and differential agar media commonly used for respiratory specimens in clinical microbiology laboratories. Although R. E. Weaver first cultivated *L. pneumophila* on Mueller-Hinton agar supplemented with 1% IsoVitalex and 1% hemoglobin and isolates may grow very slowly on the chocolate agar used for gonococcus isolation as well, growth is much better and more rapid on BCYEa.[46,68]

Color Plates for Chapter 9 are found between pages 368 and 369.

TABLE 9-1
Species of the Genus Legionella

Isolated From Humans	Not Isolated From Humans
L. pneumophila	L. adelaidensis
subsp. pneumophila	L. brunensis
subsp. fraseri	L. cherrii
subsp. pascullei	L. erythra
L. anisa	L. fairfieldensis
L. birminghamensis	L. geestiana
L. bozemanii	L. gratiana
L. cincinnatiensis	L. israelensis
L. dumoffii	L. jamestowniensis
L. feeleii	L. londiniensis
L. gormanii	L. lytica
L. hackeliae	L. moravica
L. jordanis	L. nautarum
L. lansingensis	L. oakridgensis
L. longbeachae	L. parisiensis
L. maceachernii	L. quarterirensis
L. micdadei	L. quinlivanii
L. sainthelensi	L. rubrilucens
L. tucsonensis	L. santicrucis
L. wadsworthii	L. shakespearei
	L. spiritensis
	L. steigerwaltii
	L. waltersii
	L. worsleiensis

Based on references 60, 62, and 133.

Growth on BCYEa with no growth on blood agar is one of the most useful **presumptive clues** that an isolate could be a species of Legionella. Another gram-negative organism that also grows on BCYE but not on ordinary blood agar is Francisella tularensis.[17] In contrast to Francisella species, which produce acid from carbohydrates, Legionella species neither ferment nor oxidize carbohydrates. Similarly, certain thermophilic spore-forming bacilli and Bordetella pertussis are other bacteria capable of growing on BCYEa; differences in morphology, serologic features, and cellular fatty acids aid in differentiating them.[133] Legionella species produce characteristic branched-chain fatty acids in their cell walls.[76,87,88] Most species are weakly catalase and peroxidase positive.[17] With the exceptions of L. micdadei, L. feelei, L. maceachernii, L. fairfieldensis, and L. lansingensis, gelatin is liquefied. The sodium hippurate hydrolysis test, which is positive for L. pneumophila and negative for the majority of Legionella species isolated from clinical materials, provides a useful presumptive procedure for differentiation between L. pneumophila and the other Legionella species. Phenotypic characterization of Legionella isolates using biochemical tests is of only limited value for presumptive identification of isolates to the species level. Serotyping of isolates using immunofluorescent antibody testing, however, is a practical way to differentiate isolates presumptively as species of Legionella. Definitive identification of Legionella species requires nucleic acid studies and other chemotaxonomic reference procedures (see Chap. 1).[17,32,34,98]

CLINICAL AND PATHOLOGIC SPECTRUM OF LEGIONELLOSIS

Legionnaires' disease occurs both sporadically in the form of community-acquired pneumonia[20,42,43,131] and in epidemics.[12] In addition to legionnaires' disease, a mild form of illness called Pontiac fever occurs. Illness may also involve anatomic regions of the body outside the chest cavity. Thus, the term **legionellosis,** including legionnaires' disease, Pontiac fever, and extrapulmonary involvement with Legionella species, is used in this chapter to refer to any infection caused by bacteria of the family Legionellaceae. Approximately 85% of the documented cases of legionellosis have been caused by L. pneumophila. Serogroups 1 and 6 of L. pneumophila have, by themselves, accounted for up to 75% of the legionellae reported to cause human illness.[100] In addition to L. pneumophila, many other species have been isolated from clinical specimens collected from humans (see Table 9-1). Of these other species, L. micdadei has been the species most commonly implicated in pneumonia, followed less often in isolated cases by L. bozemanii. Implicated even less frequently have been L. dumoffii, L. longbeachae, L. jordanis, L. gormanii, L. feeleii, L. hackeliae, L. maceachernii, L. wadsworthii, L. birminghamensis, L. cincinnatiensis, L. oakridgensis, L. anisa, and L. tucsonensis.[11,100,118,119]

Legionellosis has most commonly been recognized as a form of pneumonia.[135] The earliest symptoms typically include a rundown feeling, muscle aches, and a slight headache. During the first day, patients commonly experience a rapid onset of dry cough and elevated temperature (e.g., 102°F to 104°F or higher is not uncommon) with chills. Abdominal pain and gastrointestinal symptoms (e.g., nausea, vomiting, and diarrhea) occur in many patients. A summary of clinical manifestations is given in Table 9-2. Chest roentgenograms typically show patchy infiltrates at the onset that may progress to five-lobe consolidation.[52,53,131,135] Infiltrates are bilateral in two thirds of patients, and abscess cavities may be present, particularly in immunocompromised patients. Laboratory findings commonly include, in varying combinations, a moderate leukocytosis with a left shift, proteinuria, hyponatremia, azotemia, elevated serum glutamic oxaloacetic transaminase (also called aspartate aminotransferase, or AST), and a high erythrocyte sedimentation rate. As mentioned previously, legionellosis may also take the form of a mild, self-limited illness of short duration, known as Pontiac fever, with elevated temperature, myalgia, malaise, and headache, but with few or no respiratory findings and no pneumonia.[52,55,135] Table 9-2 provides a comparison of the clinical aspects of legionnaires' disease and Pontiac fever.

In recent years, the clinical spectrum of legionellosis has expanded. The illness may involve essentially any organ system of the body, with or without pneumonia. Examples of selected manifestations of extrapulmonary involvement follow. Bacteremia has been reported, but data on its frequency are lacking.[32,101] Nearly half the patients with legionnaires' disease show central nervous system manifestations such as headache, lethargy, confusion, stupor, and other less

TABLE 9-2

CLINICAL MANIFESTATIONS IN TWO KINDS OF LEGIONELLOSIS

	LEGIONNAIRES' DISEASE	PONTIAC FEVER
Mortality	15%–30%	0%
Incubation period	2–10 days	1–2 days
Symptoms	Fever, chills, cough, myalgia, headache, chest pain, sputum, and diarrhea (and confusion or other mental states in some)	Similar to influenza: fever, chills, and myalgia (and cough, chest pain, and confusion in some)
Lung	Pneumonia and pleural effusion (lung abscess in some)	Pleuritic pain; no pneumonia, no lung abscess
Kidney	Renal failure (proteinuria, azotemia, and hematuria in some)	No renal manifestations
Liver	Modest liver function abnormalities	No liver function abnormalities
Gastrointestinal tract	Watery diarrhea, abdominal pain, and nausea and vomiting	No abnormalities
Central nervous system	Somnolence, delirium, disorientation, confusion, and obtundation (seizure rarely documented)	No central nervous system manifestations

Modified from Refs. 52, 131, 134, and 135.

frequent manifestations, including ataxia, coma, and seizures.[65] Other patients have had focal signs and symptoms suggesting brain abscess or encephalitis mimicking herpes encephalitis.[6,99] *Legionella* species have been detected by the direct fluorescent antibody test in cerebrospinal fluid of one patient and in brain tissue of another who died of legionellosis.[15] A painful, nonpruritic, macular rash, limited to the pretibial surfaces of the legs, has been reported; however, dermal manifestations are uncommon.[61] *L. pneumophila* serogroup 1 has been demonstrated in lymph nodes, spleen, kidney, and bone marrow and has been documented in acute myocarditis,[126,132] prosthetic valve endocarditis,[83] pericarditis,[82] and hemodialysis fistula infections.[131] Arnow and associates[7] reported on the isolation of *L. pneumophila* serogroup 3, mixed with multiple species of anaerobic bacteria, from a perirectal abscess. *L. pneumophila* serogroup 4 was shown by direct immunofluorescence in lesions of acute pyelonephritis in a patient who had both pneumonia and pyelonephritis associated with this organism.[28] *Legionella micdadei* was the only organism isolated from a cutaneous leg abscess of a 62-year-old woman who had been receiving prednisone and cyclophosphamide for rapidly progressive glomerulonephritis.[5] However, in general, reports of extrapulmonary manifestations have been more commonly associated with *L. pneumophila* than with other species. For a review of the manifestations of illness produced by *Legionella* species other than *L. pneumophila*, the report by Fang and colleagues[43] and Chapter by Muder and Yu[89] are recommended.

PREDISPOSING FACTORS

Persons who have legionnaires' disease are usually middle-aged or older (mean age about 55 years); however, the disease can occur in persons of any age, including children.

Legionellosis must be included in the differential diagnosis of immunosuppressed patients who develop fever and pulmonary infiltrates,[59,106] or in patients who develop pneumonia not responsive to penicillins, cephalosporins, or aminoglycosides, or in any patient with severe pneumonia, especially when there is no other readily apparent alternative diagnosis. In hemodialysis, renal transplant and cardiac transplant patients and other surgical patients, for example, legionnaires' disease has been a major cause of morbidity and mortality.[75,135]

Other potential predisposing conditions include diabetes mellitis, ethanolism, chronic obstructive pulmonary disease, and cardiovascular disease. Cigarette smoking was suggested as a predisposing factor in the Philadelphia outbreak and in some subsequent outbreaks. Another predisposing factor is exposure to concentrated virulent *Legionella* organisms in the environment. Thus, legionellosis has occurred with higher frequencies among travelers to an epidemic site such as a hotel or hospital with an ongoing hyperendemic problem or in a highly endemic area and in hospitalized patients who have developed pneumonia during hospitalization.[20,39,131,135]

PATHOLOGY AND PATHOGENETIC CONSIDERATIONS

Pathologic features of human infection with several of the species of *Legionella* other than *L. pneumophila* are similar to those found in *L. pneumophila* infections. At autopsy, varying patterns and degrees of consolidation are found. Most species produce a severe confluent lobar pneumonia, with or without abscesses (see Color Plate 9-1G and H).[12,132]

Histologically, pulmonary infiltrates containing neutrophils, macrophages, large amounts of fibrin in alveolar spaces, and septic vasculitis of small blood vessels have been observed. The histopathology is that of bacterial pneumonia and differs from pneumonia caused by *Chlamydia, Mycoplasma,* or viruses.[23,132] In addition to findings of focal bronchopneumonia or lobar patterns of pneumonia, some patients show necrotizing pneumonitis with microabscesses or abscesses of larger size (*i.e.,* ≥1 cm). Pulmonary fibrosis may occur as a long-term sequela with persistence of scar tissue in the lungs, and this contributes to persistent chronic problems with pulmonary function in some patients who survive acute legionnaires' disease.[24,132] Legionellae do not stain with hematoxylin and eosin in formalin-fixed paraffin sections but can be demonstrated easily with Dieterle or Warthin-Starry silver impregnation procedures. Silver impregnation techniques are nonspecific and stain virtually all microorganisms present in addition to *Legionella.*

As mentioned previously, *Legionella* can usually be demonstrated in fresh imprints of lung biopsy material stained with Giemsa's or Gram-Weigert stain (see Color Plate 9-1*B*) and can sometimes be seen in fresh imprints using routine Gram stain procedures with basic fuchsin used as a counterstain (see Color Plate 9-1*A*) (SD Allen, unpublished observations). The finding of weakly acid-fast bacilli using a modified Kinyoun stain may be a clue to the presence of *L. micdadei.*[132] The electron micrographic appearance of *L. pneumophila* has been published.[23] The organisms are facultative intracellular pathogens and may be found within macrophages and neutrophils. *Legionella* may be seen in phagocytic vacuoles or free within the cytoplasm of phagocytic cells. Extracellular bacteria may also be present. Because the ultrastructural features of *Legionella* species are not unique, electron microscopic features do not differentiate *Legionella* species from other small gram-negative bacteria.

Considerable progress has been made toward an understanding of the pathogenesis of legionellosis.[64] The organisms are facultative intracellular pathogens and reside within cells of the monocyte-macrophage system (*e.g.,* mainly monocytes and alveolar macrophages) and neutrophils, or extracellularly. Within macrophages, Legionellae inhibit phagolysosomal fusion and acidification of the phagosome; they continue multiplying until the host cell ruptures, thus releasing the organisms which can infect other phagocytic cells.[63,64] The organisms do not multiply in neutrophils. As reviewed by Horwitz, the specific virulence factors involved are not clearly defined, and cell-mediated immunity (not humoral immunity) plays a key role in the host's defense against the Legionellae.[64]

EPIDEMIOLOGIC AND ECOLOGIC ASPECTS OF LEGIONELLOSIS

Legionella species are ubiquitous in both natural and man-made environments. Legionnaires' disease and Pontiac fever may be contracted by exposure to a wide variety of environmental sources, but there is no convincing evidence of person-to-person transmission. Thus, there is no evidence that patients who have legionnaires' disease are "contagious." Furthermore, cultures of *Legionella* species have not proven to be of

any more hazard to laboratory personnel than those bacteria routinely isolated in the clinical microbiology laboratory. Inhalation of aerosolized organisms from environmental sources or possibly the aspiration of organisms present in water or in oropharyngeal contents are the most likely routes of spread.[75,134]

INCIDENCE

Legionellosis has been documented in countries around the world, but the morbidity and mortality associated with both the epidemics and sporadic cases of legionellosis are underreported in public health statistics. Not only do most countries lack a disease-oriented surveillance system for tracking the disease, but clinicians and microbiology laboratories may overlook and not diagnose the disease (*e.g.,* because of lack of awareness, because the clinical manifestations are similar to those seen in other bacterial pneumonias, or because of failure to use proper laboratory diagnostic methods). Better surveillance programs are needed to determine accurately the incidence of legionnaires' disease and Pontiac fever.

In general, it has been estimated that less than 1% to 5% of cases of pneumonia are caused by *Legionella* species, but this is probably an oversimplification.[33] In outbreaks of legionnaires' disease, attack rates for the exposed high-risk population have been as high as 30%.[134] *Legionella* species (6.7% of etiologic agents) ranked as the third most common etiologic agents (following *Streptococcus pneumoniae,* 15.3%, and *Haemophilus influenzae,* 10.9%) for community-acquired pneumonia among 359 patients admitted to university, community, and Veterans Administration hospitals examined in a recent U.S. multicenter study.[42] In other countries, the frequency of sporadic cases of community-acquired pneumonias caused by *Legionella* species varied from 2% in the United Kingdom to 5% in Germany and 10% in France.[104,134] The incidence of Pontiac fever in the general population is not known. Outside an outbreak setting, sporadic cases of Pontiac fever are probably almost always unrecognized.

NOSOCOMIAL OUTBREAKS OF LEGIONELLOSIS

Within hospitalized populations are patients who may be compromised and are very susceptible to infections in general. These patients are at risk of acquiring legionellosis should there be concentrated exposure to the organisms.

The usual source of *Legionella* in hospitalized patients is water (mainly the hot water system), especially from the showers or baths,[40] and from cooling towers that are part of the buildings' air-conditioning systems.[1,54] Other documented sources have included nasogastric tubes (with microaspiration of *Legionellae* in contaminated water), humidifiers, respiratory therapy equipment (*e.g.,* masks and hand-held nebulizers washed with contaminated tap water), whirlpools, and other less common sources.[33,41] Early diagnosis of legionellosis and epidemiologic surveillance of cases within the hospital are needed not only for prompt and effective therapy but to aid in instituting control measures to prevent subsequent cases. With the high mortality of nosocomial legionnaires' disease (range, 30%–50%) it would seem prudent that efforts be taken to prevent the spread of *Legionella* species from the hospital environment to patients who are likely to be most susceptible to infection (see the last section of this chapter).

LEGIONELLOSIS IN TRAVELERS

Since the 1976 outbreak of legionnaires' disease, which occurred among travelers to Philadelphia, travel-associated epidemics and sporadic cases of legionnaires' disease have been recognized in many countries in all continents.[134] The true incidence of travel-associated cases is not clear. Cases are likely to be underreported due not only to underdiagnosis and lack of awareness of the epidemiologic significance but also conceivably related to concerns about adverse publicity to tourism.[134] Nonetheless, clusters and sporadic cases occur each year, associated especially with hotels and with hotel water systems contaminated with legionellae.[1] Clusters of cases have also been observed among travelers who have been on board cruise ships.

Cases and clusters of travel-associated *Legionella* infection should be reported to state and federal public health agencies and should lead to investigations of the source and magnitude of the outbreak to prevent further spread among the traveling public.

LEGIONELLACEAE IN THE ENVIRONMENT

As mentioned earlier, species of the genus *Legionella* are present in diverse natural and man-made habitats. Numerous studies have been focused on the ecology of *Legionella* species in man-made habitats such as water cooling towers and potable (*e.g.* drinking) water systems within buildings. Man-made habitats probably serve as "amplifiers" or disseminators of legionellae and these habitats play a major role in the epidemiology and control of legionellosis.

NATURAL HABITATS

Legionella pneumophila was first isolated from the natural environment by George K. Morris and his colleagues at the CDC.[86] As part of an investigation of a large outbreak of legionnaires' disease associated with travelers who visited the Memorial Union Building on the Indiana University Campus at Bloomington, Indiana, *L. pneumophila* was isolated from water of a small creek (called the "Jordan River") and soil from the banks of the Jordan. Subsequently in 1979, Carl B. Fliermans, W.B. Cherry, and others were the first to isolate *L. pneumophila* from non–epidemic-associated aquatic natural habitats.[51] Since that time, *Legionella* species have been found in natural waters from around the world and are known to be widespread in lakes, ponds, and streams. They have been isolated from aquatic habitats with temperatures ranging from 5.7°C to 63°C[50] and in hot spring water used for hy-

drotherapy.[14] There appear to be higher concentrations of *Legionella* species in warmer waters (*e.g.*, 30°C to 45°C) than in water at cooler temperatures.[124] In Puerto Rico, legionellae were recovered from marine waters and from epiphytes in trees.[94]

Although soil (*i.e.*, wind-blown dust from an excavation site) was implicated epidemiologically (but not studied microbiologically) for *Legionella* in one of the earlier outbreaks of legionnaires' disease,[20,52] there have been few reports of attempts to isolate *Legionella* species from soil. *Legionella* species including *L. pneumophila* and *L. bozemanii* have been isolated from samples of wet soil.[86] More recently, Steele and colleagues isolated *L. pneumophila, L. longbeachae* serogroup 1, and *L. micadadei* from potting soils in Australia.[113] *L. longbeachae* serogroup 1 was also isolated from natural soil and from pine sawdust. Epidemiologic and microbiologic studies from South Australia in association with an outbreak of legionellosis due to *L. longbeachae* serogroup 1 suggested that soil, and not water, could be the natural habitat of *L. longbeachae* serogroup 1 and that soil could be the source of this organism in human disease. In this study, gardening in soil, rather than exposure to water contaminated with *L. longbeachae*, appeared to be the major environmental risk factor associated with legionellosis.[112,113] Much more work on the ecology of *Legionella* in natural aquatic and terrestrial habitats is needed.

MAN-MADE (ARTIFICIAL) AQUATIC HABITATS

It has become clear that legionellae are ubiquitous in man-made water systems, both in the absence as well as in the presence of clinically demonstrated legionellosis. *Legionella* species are frequently present in water cooling towers and have been found in tap water, shower water, hot water tanks, the insides of shower heads, rubber gaskets, and metal surfaces within plumbing systems used for domestic potable water supplies. Potable water has been implicated as the most likely source of the organism in many epidemics and sporadic cases of legionellosis that were not epidemiologically associated with cooling towers or faulty air conditioning/heat exchange systems.[8,27,48,52,90,109,112]

Whirlpool spas have also been implicated in cases of legionellosis.[41,56] When whirlpools are inadequately chlorinated, conditions may favor the growth of legionellae and organisms may be aerosolized into the atmosphere and inhaled.

In 1990, the CDC reported an outbreak of community-acquired legionnaires' disease involving 33 persons that was associated with a grocery store mist machine. The mist machine continuously generated a tap water aerosol (probably containing *L. pneumophila*) in respirable (<5 µm) droplets over the produce display. The system used ultrasonic transducers located in the humidifier's tap water reservoir to create the mist. The Food and Drug Administration (FDA) has issued guidelines for the weekly disassembly, cleaning, and washing (using a hypochlorite solution) of such devices, but more studies are needed to determine the microbiology of such humidifiers and the factors that lead to contamination and colonization of these machines by *Legionella* species.[22]

Although legionellae have been isolated from shower heads and shower water on repeated occasions, the epidemiologic evidence that bathing or showering in such water leads to legionellosis has been rather weak.[52,90] Supportive evidence reported by Breiman and associates from an outbreak investigation of nosocomial legionnaires' disease at a hospital in South Dakota strengthened the hypothesis that aerosolized shower water can serve as the vehicle for spread of *Legionella pneumophila* to patients.[16]

Nosocomial legionnaires' disease has also been specifically linked to the use of tap water to clean medication nebulizers and other respiratory therapy equipment. In a report by Mastro and colleagues, the use of tap water contaminated with *L. pneumophila* to wash medication nebulizers was a major factor that led to an outbreak of nosocomial legionnaires' disease in patients with chronic obstructive pulmonary disease.[80]

Of recent concern, some cases of nosocomial legionnaires' disease have been linked to microaspiration of water contaminated with *Legionella* species in patients with nasogastric tubes.[13,33,78,79] Therefore, if the organism is present within hospital water, it would seem prudent to irrigate NG tubes with sterile water.[33]

Thus, there have been numerous reports that associated the presence of *L. pneumophila* in institutional potable hot water with the occurrence of legionellosis. Legionellae appear to survive the usual chlorination procedures of municipal water treatment facilities and thus, not unexpectedly, may be present in potable water supplied to homes, apartment buildings, hotels, hospitals, and other buildings.[3,77,115,116] Potable hot water, especially if it does not exceed 55°C, has contained heavy concentrations of *Legionella* in some instances. In addition to water temperature, the construction of the plumbing system also seems to play an important role; for example, the presence of certain kinds of resins in gaskets, the presence of dead ends or cul-de-sacs, where there is stasis, obstruction, or stagnation in water flow, and the presence of biofilms or slime layers on the surface of pipes containing other commensal bacteria, protozoa, and algae may favor the presence of legionellae.[77,111,117,134,135]

Factors that promote the growth of legionellae in plumbing systems are poorly known in spite of a large accumulation of literature. Legionellae are fastidious organisms that require enriched media for growth in the laboratory, and it is unlikely that drinking water supplies all their nutritional requirements for growth and energy. Rowbotham was the first to report that *Legionella* species multiply in close association with free-living aquatic and soil amebae of the genera *Acanthamoeba* and *Naegleria*.[103] Others have confirmed and extended these observations, not only with *Acanthamoeba* and *Naegleria*, but also with other amebae such as *Hartmanella* and the ciliate *Tetrahymena*.[47,48,92,123] Thus, amebae or ciliates phagocytize legionellae, as they do other bacteria in nature, and the legionellae then survive and multiply within nutritionally deficient habitats by living parasitically within the protozoan. In ad-

dition, it has been suggested that the amoebae, which form cysts, might offer further protection to legionellae within the cysts against the effects of chlorine.[70,111]

LABORATORY DIAGNOSIS

Major steps in the laboratory diagnosis or confirmation of legionellosis include the following:

Selection, collection, and transport of specimens
Direct examination of clinical specimens
    Gross examination
    Microscopic examination (including the direct fluorescent antibody [DFA] test)
    Nucleic acid probes
    Immunoassays for direct detection of *Legionella* antigen in urine and other body fluids
Isolation of *Legionella* from clinical specimens using nonselective and selective media
Identification of *Legionella* species
Antimicrobial susceptibility and treatment
Positive indirect fluorescent antibody (IFA) test (demonstration of a fourfold or greater rise in serum antibody titer)
Reporting of results

SELECTION, COLLECTION, AND TRANSPORT OF CLINICAL SPECIMENS

The broad clinical spectrum and severe morbidity and mortality of legionnaires' disease emphasize the need for rapid and accurate laboratory diagnosis. When legionellosis is suspected clinically, lower respiratory tract specimens should be collected for both culture and direct fluorescent antibody (DFA) testing. Appropriate specimens include expectorated sputum, materials collected using bronchoscopy (*e.g.*, bronchial brush, biopsy, lavage, or washings), transtracheal aspirates, closed- and open-lung biopsy material, fine needle aspirates of lung, and pleural fluid. In the microbiology laboratory at Indiana University Hospital, for example, *Legionella* culture and DFA are not done routinely on expectorated sputum samples but only on specimens accompanied by a special request for a *Legionella* examination.

Primary isolation of *Legionella* species on solid media has been successful from closed- and open-lung biopsy material, pleural fluid, and transtracheal aspirates, bronchial alveolar lavage samples, and sputum. A reasonably semi-effective selective medium is available for the primary isolation of *L. pneumophila* from sputum and contaminated bronchial materials.[30,31,45,127]

Specimens should be carefully collected to avoid aerosolization and transported to the laboratory at ambient temperature in sterile leakproof containers, preferably within 2 hours after collection. Specimens to be sent to a reference laboratory should be refrigerated or packed on wet ice if a delay of less than 2 days is anticipated. Specimens that are to be stored for days or weeks should be maintained at −70°C or colder. These may be shipped on dry ice. Specimens that must be shipped to a reference laboratory should be packaged and mailed in accordance with federal regulations (see Chap. 2). If specimens are being submitted only for pathologic study and DFA examination, and are to be fixed in buffered neutral formalin prior to shipment, they *should not be* refrigerated or frozen during transport.

L. pneumophila has been isolated from blood cultures on a few occasions using conventional media supplemented with L-cysteine and ferric pyrophosphate, or using BACTEC (Becton Dickinson Instrument Systems, Sparks, MD) radiometric aerobic and anaerobic media without any special supplements.[36,101] Blind subculture of the Bactec aerobic and anaerobic bottles onto BCYEa appears to be necessary for isolation of Legionellae.[101] As mentioned previously, Legionellae may also be encountered (rarely) in extrapulmonary sites. However, the practical value (or the clinical relevance) of seeking *Legionella* in blood cultures or extrapulmonary sites has not been established. In addition to the above, urine (preferably an early morning sample) should be collected if a radioimmunoassay, enzyme-linked immunosorbent assay, or latex agglutination test for *Legionella* antigen is available.

In addition, it is recommended that an acute-phase serum sample be collected early because other tests that may enable a more rapid diagnosis lack sensitivity.[31,37] A follow-up serum specimen should be collected within 2 to 6 weeks after collection of the acute phase specimen, so that a fourfold rise in antibody titer against *Legionella* can be demonstrated, which aids in establishing a retrospective diagnosis.[127] Unfortunately, the development of a diagnostic fourfold rise in antibody titer can be slow and may occur in no more than 75% to 80% of patients who ultimately are shown to have legionnaires' disease.[31,127] In addition, some persons have seroconverted but remained asymptomatic (probably related to subclinical infection).

DIRECT EXAMINATION OF CLINICAL SPECIMENS

GROSS EXAMINATION AND MICROSCOPIC EXAMINATION OF STAINED MATERIALS

Gross examination of samples of lung may aid the pathologist in selecting the best areas for culture or DFA staining. Direct smears of exudates or touch preparations (dab smears) of fresh lung biopsy material should be prepared. Frozen sections of lung samples are also useful in diagnosis. Shortly after sections are cut, they should be placed in 10% neutral buffered formalin if *Legionella* DFA stains are desired. Frozen sections and touch preparations should be placed in methanol for fixation if Gram stain, hematoxylin and eosin, Giemsa's, "Diff-Quik," or modified-Kinyoun acid-fast stains are desired. The Giemsa stain is preferred over the other non-DFA stains for demonstrating legionellae and other bacteria in fresh touch preparations of lung or bronchoscopic materials.

MICROSCOPIC EXAMINATION OF STAINED MATERIALS

Various specimens (*e.g.*, transtracheal aspirates, pleural fluids, aspirates from thoracic empyema, fine-needle aspirates of lung, and touch preparations of lungs) can be stained with Gram stain. Methanol fixation is better than heat fixation, and the intensity of staining can be improved by increasing the time of safranin staining to 10 minutes or longer. Alternatively, 0.05% carbolfuchsin has been added to the safranin by some workers to improve the intensity of staining with the counterstain.[130] The Gram-Weigert, "Diff-Quik," or Giemsa stain may reveal more organisms than can be seen with routine Gram staining. In formalin-fixed, paraffin-embedded histologic sections, *Legionella* organisms cannot be readily seen in the hematoxylin and eosin (H&E), Gram, Brown–Brenn, Brown–Hopp, or MacCallum–Goodpasture stained preparations. Likewise, we have been unable to demonstrate the organism in permanent sections with an overnight Giemsa stain, Gomori methenamine silver (GMS) stain, periodic acid-Schiff stain, or other stains routinely used in histology. In the modified Dieterle silver impregnation stain the organisms stain black to dark brown.[12,132] The morphology of *L. pneumophila* is shown in Color Plates 9-1 *A, B,* and *F.*

At the Indiana University Medical Center, *Legionella* testing (*i.e.*, DFA and culture) is performed on samples collected using bronchoscopy (*e.g.*, bronchoalveolar lavage and/or a bronchial biopsy), or by a surgical procedure (*e.g.*, open lung biopsy, needle biopsy of the lung, etc.) as part of an **"immunosuppressed protocol"** (ISP).[4] Clinicians may request an ISP as part of a clinical microbiologic consultation for immunosuppressed patients who have pulmonary infiltrates of possible infectious etiology. The ISP includes frozen sections stained by H&E, Giemsa, GMS, and a modified Kinyoun acid-fast stain, touch preparations ("dab smears") of tissue, and/or smears from liquid specimens. Following methanol fixation, touch preparations are stained using "Diff-Quick," Giemsa, GMS, the Legionella DFA, a modified-Kinyoun acid-fast stain, and, if warranted, a Gram stain. In addition, an auramine-rhodamine acid-fast stain is done (see Chap. 17). Cultures done on such specimens, using all necessary special media and processing, are for aerobic and anaerobic bacteria, *Legionella*, fungi, *Mycobacterium*, viruses, *Mycoplasma* and *Chlamydia* if warranted clinically. *Legionella* is not uncommon in these patients, who may have either a community-acquired illness, or possibly, a nosocomial infection.

DIRECT EXAMINATION USING A DIRECT FLUORESCENT ANTIBODY (DFA) PROCEDURE

Direct immunofluorescence assays, originally developed by Cherry and colleagues at the CDC,[25,26] have been used successfully for rapid detection of *Legionella* species in clinical specimens from the respiratory tract. Compared with cultures using currently available media and processing methods, the DFA has a low sensitivity (25%–70%).[32,133] However, provided the DFA is done carefully and meticulously by an experienced microbiologist who uses a good fluorescence microscope, the specificity of the DFA test has been high (>95%).[32,133] The DFA test requires close attention to detail and precautions to ensure that all steps are performed properly. Although immunologic cross-reactions have been documented with some bacteria, it has been our experience that most cross-reactions result from 1) processing a positive control slide in the same container as that prepared from a patient's specimen (in the Indiana University Hospital microbiology laboratories, each positive control slide, as well as each patient slide is processed in a separate clean, disposable cup); 2) the microscopist's acceptance of fluorescing morphologic forms such as cocci or debris that are not typical of Legionella species; and 3) the contamination of rinse water, reagents, or slides by environmental Legionella species.[130] Various reagents used in the DFA test may have to be filter-sterilized, and the microscope slides may have to be specially cleaned to avoid false-positive staining with environmental contaminants.

Some strains of staphylococci (due to staphylococcal protein A), pneumococci, and streptococci may fluoresce because of natural antibodies in the conjugate or because of nonspecific reaction of IgG with bacterial cell wall components of these organisms. Some species of *Pseudomonas*, including *P. fluorescens*, and *P. aeruginosa*, *Stenotrophomonas maltophilia*, *Bordetella pertussis*, plus a few stains of *Bacteroides fragilis*, and *Francisella tularensis*[26,31,35,133] have been shown to fluoresce with the Legionella conjugates. It is, therefore, necessary to be familiar with the morphologic and staining characteristics of Legionella to recognize the staining of cross-reacting organisms. Any morphologically atypical organisms should not be called Legionella species. Smears containing atypical fluorescing organisms should be shown to the supervisor or director of the laboratory when the technologist has questions regarding interpretation.

Commercial suppliers of fluorescein isothiocyanate (FITC)-conjugated polyvalent antisera, as well as control sera and other reagents for Legionella DFA testing include SciMedx (Denville, NJ), Genetic Systems (Seattle, WA), and others. Genetic Systems markets a monoclonal antibody conjugate that has the advantage of decreasing the number of false-positive reactions while retaining the ability to react with most serotypes of *L. pneumophila*.[31] As a note of caution, the Genetic Systems monoclonal DFA conjugate failed to detect *L. pneumophila* in hot and cold storage tank water and in swab samples from showers and a water tap[122]; thus, it cannot be recommended for DFA studies of potable water or other samples from man-made water systems and its performance in natural habitat water studies is uncertain.

In performing the DFA test, specific antibody in the form of FITC-labeled polyvalent antiserum (conjugate) directed against the antigen(s) to be detected is usually purchased commercially. The directions of the manufacturer of the kit should be followed exactly. Antigen (present on or in Legionella organisms) is fixed on a slide, and then overlain with FITC-labeled antibody. The antigen binds the globulin in the FITC-labeled antibody, forming an antigen-antibody complex (not washed away when gently rinsed with buffer) that is visible by the excitation of the FITC with ultraviolet light. When the antigen(s) of a Legionella species has reacted with FITC-conjugated antibody, exposure to ultraviolet light causes the FITC to emit longer wavelengths of light in the yellow-green region of the color spectrum, and the bacteria can be seen (using a fluorescence microscope) as brilliantly fluorescing yellow-green rods.

NUCLEIC ACID PROBE FOR LEGIONELLA SPECIES

A DNA probe test kit for detection of Legionella is now commercially available from Gen-Probe, Inc. (San Diego, CA). The kit, which contains a genus-specific [125]-I labeled cDNA probe, was developed for in-solution hybridization of Legionella RNA in clinical specimens. The sensitivity of the DNA probe test is similar to that of the DFA procedure, and the specificity slightly better (*i.e.*, 99%–100%).[34,98]

The sensitivity and specificity of the probe appear comparable to that of the DFA test; therefore, some laboratories may wish to substitute the probe test kit for the DFA test. The probe was found to identify all Legionella species correctly to the genus level when colonies were taken from plate cultures, and it did not cross-react with any bacteria other than legionellae in culture.[31,34] However, the probe test is not sufficiently sensitive to replace culture for Legionella species. A drawback of the probe test is the cost (*i.e.*, the use of a radioactive probe with a short half-life and the need for a gamma counter).

The application of the polymerase chain reaction (PCR) to detect DNA of Legionella species is a subject of considerable research interest. Experimentaly, PCR procedures have been applied to detect Legionella species in human pulmonary materials (*e.g.*, bronchoalveolar lavage fluid); the results have generally been promising, but more data are needed before these methods can be recommended for use in the clinical laboratory.[69,74,81] In addition, PCR methods are now being used to detect Legionella species in environmental water samples during epidemiologic investigations or as part of other environmental studies.[9,85,95–97]

ANTIGEN DETECTION IN URINE AND BODY FLUIDS

It has been known for many years that some patients with pneumonia caused by *Streptococcus pneumoniae* excrete a polysaccharide substance in their urine that can be detected with immunologic procedures.[73] Procedures for detecting Legionella antigens in urine, developed by Kohler and associates of the Indiana University Medical Center, include radioimmunoassay, enzyme-linked immunosorbent assay, and latex agglutination.[73] A commercially available RIA kit for detection of Legionella antigenuria shows good promise as a rapid aid to diagnosis.[2] Although its sensitivity is about 80% and specificity very high, limiting factors include its ability to detect antigenuria produced only by *L. pneumophila* serogroup 1, cross-reactions with a number of other serogroups, the use of radiolabeled reagents having a short half-life, and urinary excretion of the antigen for months to nearly a year.[71,72,133] Thus, patients who do not necessarily have acute legionnaires' disease can have a positive test result for *Legionella* urinary antigen. At present, EIAs and latex agglutination assays for *Legionella* antigenuria are either not available commercially, or their performance has not been adequate for use in the laboratory.[133]

ISOLATION OF *LEGIONELLA* SPECIES FROM CLINICAL SPECIMENS

Bacteriologic culture of *Legionella* is the preferred (so-called "gold standard") way to diagnose legionellosis.[33,133] According to Edelstein, culture is one and one-half to three times more sensitive than the DFA test.[31] *Legionella* species are not routinely isolated from the upper respiratory tract normal flora, although the DFA test for *L. pneumophila* was positive in a few healthy individuals.[19]

The recommended nonselective solid medium for isolation of legionellae is buffered charcoal yeast extract agar (BCYEa), which contains L-cysteine, ferric pyrophosphate, ACES (N-[2-acetamido]-2-aminoethanesulfonic acid) buffer, α-ketoglutaric acid, and activated charcoal (BCYEa).[30,45] The medium is available commercially from several manufacturers. In addition to BCYEa, it is recommended that one or more selective media be used to avoid overgrowth by normal flora and the possibility that other organisms may inhibit the growth of *Legionella*. Antibiotics have been added to the BCYEa base, resulting in reasonably effective selective media. One useful selective medium contains BCYEa base supplemented with cefamandole, polymyxin B, and anisomycin (BMPAa); a second contains glycine, vancomycin, polymyxin B, and anisomycin (referred to as "modified Wadowsky-Yee" or MWY medium). The cefamandole in BMPAa may inhibit *Legionella* species that do not produce β-lactamase, whereas the MWY medium is not as selective as BMPAa.[31] BCYEa-based selective media are widely available commercially. Because the selective media may inhibit some legionellae, such media should be used in conjunction with nonselective BCYEa.

BIOPSY, SURGICAL REMOVAL, AND AUTOPSY TISSUE

To inoculate BCYEa or BMPAa media, the fresh-cut surface of lung should be gently dabbed in the first quadrant and a sterile inoculating loop used to transfer this inoculum to the other quadrants for primary isolation. A sterile tissue grinder can be used to homogenize 1- to 2-mm pieces of minced tissue in 0.5 to 1 mL of a sterile broth (such as trypticase soy broth or enriched thioglycolate medium). After homogenization, the plating medium is inoculated with approximately 0.1 mL of the homogenate and streaked for isolation. In addition, six slides for DFA testing should be prepared from the same specimen (as described previously).

PLEURAL FLUID AND TRANSTRACHEAL ASPIRATES

Pleural fluid and transtracheal aspirates are inoculated directly onto the selective and nonselective media as for tissue homogenates. The BCYEa and BMPAa plates are sealed in CO_2-permeable plastic bags (two plates per bag) and incubated in a 5% to 10% CO_2 incubator at 35°C and examined every 2 to 3 days for up to 2 weeks. The reasons for the CO_2-permeable bags are to prevent contamination of plates, which is more likely to occur during long-term incubation than in short-term incubation, and to protect laboratory personnel from exposure to potentially dangerous organisms other than *Legionella* (*e.g.*, *Francisella tularensis*), which may also grow well on BCYEa. The other media for lower respiratory tract specimens are inoculated and incubated in the usual way (see Chap. 2). The same specimen used for culture is further processed by making six smears, on separate slides, for DFA staining.

ACID-WASH DECONTAMINATION PROCEDURE FOR SPUTUM AND OTHER CONTAMINATED SPECIMENS

The selective media currently available for primary isolation of Legionellae are not especially selective, thus permitting breakthrough growth of certain unwanted organisms (*e.g.*, *Bacillus* species, *Pseudomonas*). In addition, as mentioned previously, growth of Legionellae on BCYEa (even with media containing antibiotics) may be inhibited by other bacteria in clinical specimens. Treatment of contaminated respiratory specimens such as sputum, bronchial wash, bronchial lavage, and tracheal aspirates with an acid-wash solution prior to inoculation of BCYEa and BMPAa plates aids in the inhibition of normal flora, thus improving conditions for *Legionella* to grow.[21] The protocol outlined in Box 9-1 is recommended for processing specimens that contain normal flora (for the DFA test and culture; both tests can be done on the same specimen).

BLOOD CULTURES

Collection of blood for *Legionella* culture may occasionally be useful in certain clinical settings.[31,36,101] The method used at Indiana University is to collect 8 to 10 mL of blood (per venipuncture) in a 10-mL lysis centrifuge tube (Wampole Laboratories, Cranbury, NJ) (see Chap. 3). The isolator tube is then centrifuged and processed according to the manufacturer's directions for routine blood cultures, except that the sample is inoculated onto BCYEa and is streaked for isolation. The plate is placed in a plastic bag and incubated in 5% to 10% CO_2 at 35°C for 2 weeks and examined every 2 to 3 days for growth. Alternatively, biphasic blood culture bottles have been used successfully by others, as have BACTEC aerobic and anaerobic broth media.[36,101] In the latter case, BACTEC bottles may or may not show a positive growth index. There is a good chance that growth will not be detected except by blind subculture to BCYEa. The BCYEa is incubated as previously described. (Prolonged incubation of the Bactec broth cultures [*e.g.*, up to 2 weeks] will probably be required in some instances.)

1. Before performing the acid treatment of the specimen, prepare six smears for DFA testing.

2. Inoculate one BCYEa and one BMPAa plate with 3 to 5 drops of untreated respiratory specimen and streak for isolation.

3. Add 0.5 mL of respiratory specimen to 4.5 mL of acid solution (0.2M KCl-HCl) in a screw-cap tube.
   a. Tightly seal the tube and thoroughly mix by vortexing under a safety hood.
   b. Allow the suspension to stand at room temperature for 5 minutes.

4. Inoculate a second set of BCYEa and BMPAa plates with 3 to 5 drops of the acid-specimen mixture prepared in step 3 and streak for isolation. Mark plates with an "A" to identify plates inoculated after acid treatment.

5. Place the four inoculated plates in CO_2-permeable plastic bags (two per bag) and incubate in CO_2 at 35°C for 2 weeks. Examine every 2 to 3 days for growth.

IDENTIFICATION OF LEGIONELLA SPECIES

Colonies of *Legionella* typically appear on BCYEa after 2 to 3 days of incubation in areas that have been heavily inoculated. However, if only a few organisms are present, and if the plates have been lightly inoculated, isolated colonies may take several more days to develop. The colonies are variable in size (punctate or up to 3 to 4 mm). They are glistening, convex, circular, and slightly irregular and have an entire margin (see Color Plate 9-1C). When examined through a dissecting microscope (7X to 15X), *Legionella* colonies appear to have crystalline internal structures within the colonies or a speckled, opalescent appearance similar to that of *Fusobacterium nucleatum* (see Chap. 14, Color Plates 9-1, C and D). *L. bozemanii, L. dumoffii,* and *L. gormanii* show a blue-white fluorescence under long-wave (366 nm) ultraviolet light (see Color Plate 9-1E).[68] Additional, more recently named, species with a blue-white fluorescence are *L. anisa, L. tusconensis, L. cherrii, L. parisiensis,* and *L. steigerwaltii.*[133] Colonies suspected of being *Legionella* should be subcultured onto an ordinary unsupplemented 5% sheep blood agar plate or L-cysteine–deficient BCYEa and onto the supplemented BCYEa medium. Organisms that grow on 5% sheep blood, L-cysteine–deficient BCYEa, or other routine media (such as MacConkey agar) are probably not *Legionella*. Pure culture isolates of gram-negative bacilli with typical colony characteristics of *Legionella* that grow on BCYEa or BMPAa medium after 48 hours or longer of incubation, but do not grow on L-cysteine–deficient BCYEa or routine laboratory media, should be further characterized. Most such isolates belong to *L. pneumophila* serogroup 1. The most convenient laboratory test for confirming a suspected *Legionella* isolate is the DFA test, or alternatively, a DNA probe. Colonies can be tested with the fluorescent-antibody conjugates mentioned previously to serogroup the isolate.

However, it is quite likely that organisms will be found that resemble *Legionella* but do not react with the serologic reagents used in the DFA test. These may be further characterized using the tests listed in Tables 9-3 and 9-4. An isolate with physical and biochemical properties similar to those of *Legionella* that does not react with the serologic reagents supplied with the DFA kit could represent a new species or serogroup and should be sent to a reference laboratory for definitive characterization and confirmation. However, there are non-*Legionella* species that require L-cysteine and fail to grow on blood agar and may resemble *Legionella* on BCYEa.[133] Tests used in definitive characterization of *Legionella* species in some reference or research laboratories include serologic tests, gas-liquid chromatography of cellular fatty acids, and nucleic acid genetic studies. As mentioned earlier, the commercially developed ^{125}I-labeled cDNA probe, designed to detect rRNA from legionellae, was shown to differentiate between the genus *Legionella* and non-*Legionella* organisms grown in culture.[31,34] Selected characteristics for laboratory recognition of *Legionella* species are shown in Color Plate 9-1.

ANTIMICROBIAL SUSCEPTIBILITY AND TREATMENT

The mortality rate among patients with legionellosis caused by *L. pneumophila* has varied from 0% to 30%, depending on the clinical setting and patient population. Erythromycin has been effective in reducing the case-mortality rate and historically has been the drug of choice for legionellosis.[52,131,135] Because *Legionella* species are facultative intracellular pathogens, which replicate inside monocytes and macrophages, antimicrobial agents that are concentrated within *Legionella*-infected cells are most likely to be successful in treatment. The newer macrolide antimicrobial agents (*e.g.,* azithromycin and clarithromycin), and the fluoroquinolones (*e.g.,* ciprofloxacin and pefloxacin) are more active in vitro and in experimental models than erythromycin, although clinical experience with these agents is still limited.[33,135] Rifampin is known to be very active *in vitro*[121] and could be given in addition to erythromycin to some patients who are seriously ill or fail to respond to erythromycin alone, but rifampin should not be given alone. Alternatively, doxycycline in combination with rifampin has been recommended for moderately or severely ill patients. Trimethoprim-sulfamethoxazole with or without rifampin is another potential option. The penicillins (*e.g.,* penicillin, carbenicillin, oxacillin), first- (*e.g.,* cephalothin, cefazolin), second- (*e.g.,* cefamandole, cefoxitin), and presumably the third-generation cephalosporins, aminoglycosides (*e.g.,* gentamicin, tobramycin, amikacin), and vancomycin are not effective in treatment. *In vitro* antimicrobial susceptibility testing of *Legionella* isolates has

TABLE 9-3
Selected Characteristics of *Legionella* Species Implicated in Human Illnesses*

Species	No. of Serogroups	Browning of YE With Tyrosine‡	Gelatin Liquefaction	Hippurate Hydrolysis	Motility	Oxidase	Beta-Lactamase	Autofluorescence Long-Wave Length (366 mm) UV Light
L. pneumophila†	14	+	+	+	+	+/−	+	−
L. micdadei	1	−	−	−	+	+	−	+BW
L. bozemanii	2	+‡	+	−	+	+/−	+/−	+BW
L. dumoffii	1	+	+	−	+	−	+/−	−
L. longbeachae	2	+	+	−	+	+	+	+BW
L. gormanii	1	+	+	−	+	−	+	−
L. jordanis	1	+	+	−	+	+	+	−
L. feeleii	2	+(w)	−	+/−	+	−	−	+BW
L. anisa	1	+	+	−	+	+	+	−
L. oakridgensis	1	ND	+	−	−	−	+(w)	−
L. cincinnatiensis	1	−	+	−	+	+	−	−
L. wadsworthii	1	−	+	−	+	−	+	−
L. hackeliae	2	+	+	−	+	+	+	+BW
L. tucsonensis	1	ND	+	−	+	−	+	−
L. maceachernii	1	+	+	−	+	+/−	−	−
L. birminghamensis	1	ND	+	−	+	+	+	+YG
L. sainthelensi	1	+	+	−	+	+	+	−
L. lansingensis	1	−	−	−	+	+	−	−

* All species are gram-negative, show no growth on unsupplemented blood agar, and require l-cysteine (present in BCYEa agar—see text) for primary isolation (except for laboratory adapted strains of *L. oakridgensis*, which lose the requirement for l-cysteine), and are catalase or peroxidase positive. None reduce nitrate to nitrite, produce acid from D-glucose, or produce urease. Adapted from references 17, 60, 62, and 133.

† There are now three subspecies of *L. pneumophila*—*L. pneumophila* subsp. *pneumophila*, subsp. *pascullei* and subsp. *fraseri*.

‡ YE, charcoal-treated yeast extract agar.

+, positive; −, negative; +(w), weak reaction; +/−, variable; ND, no data; BW, bluish-white autofluorescence; R, reddish autofluorescence; YG, yellow-green autofluorescence.

TABLE 9-4
MAJOR CELLULAR FATTY ACIDS OF LEGIONELLA SPECIES ISOLATED FROM HUMANS*

SPECIES	CELLULAR FATTY ACIDS†
L. pneumophila	i-$C_{16:0}$
L. micdadei	a-$C_{15:0}$
L. bozemanii	a-$C_{15:0}$
L. dumoffii	a-$C_{15:0}$
L. longbeachae	i-$C_{16:0}$
L. gormanii	a-$C_{15:0}$
L. jordanis	a-$C_{15:0}$
L. feeleii	a-$C_{15:0}$, n-$C_{16:1}$
L. anisa	a-$C_{15:0}$
L. oakridgensis	i-$C_{16:0}$
L. cincinnatiensis	i-$C_{16:0}$, i-C_{16h}
L. wadsworthii	a-$C_{15:0}$
L. hackeliae	a-$C_{15:0}$
L. tucsonensis	a-$C_{15:0}$, n-C_{14h}
L. maceachernii	a-$C_{15:0}$
L. birminghamensis	a-$C_{15:0}$, i-C_{14h}
L. sainthelensi	i-$C_{16:0}$
L. lansingensis	a-$C_{17:0}$, a-C_{15h}

* The major cellular fatty acids (determined by gas-liquid chromatography) of the *Legionella* species isolated from humans are listed. These bacteria are unusual compared with the other gram-negative bacteria because of their relatively large amounts of cellular branched-chain acids. The most abundant acid of *L. pneumophila* and some strains of *L. longbeachae* is i-16:0. However, strains of *L. longbeachae* may have either i-16:0 or 16:1 as the major acid, or the two acids may be present in roughly equal amounts as the two most abundant acids. On the other hand, the major fatty acid of *L. bozemanii*, *L. micdadei*, *L. dumoffii*, *L. gormanii*, *L. jordanis*, and certain others is a saturated, branched-chain, 15-carbon acid (a-15:0).
† Numbers to the left of the colon represent the number of carbon atoms contained in each of the different fatty acids; numbers to the right of the colon are the number of double bonds; *i* indicates a methyl (-CH₃) branch at the iso (next to last) carbon atom; *a* indicates a methyl branch at the anteiso (second from last) carbon atom.
Based on references 25, 76, 87, and 88.

not been standardized and does not correlate with the clinical response to antibiotic therapy in patients.[131] Therefore, performance of *in vitro* antimicrobial susceptibility testing on *Legionella* isolates in the hospital diagnostic laboratory is not recommended because the results are not readily interpretable by either the microbiologist or the clinician.

SERUM INDIRECT IMMUNOFLUORESCENT ANTIBODY TEST

The serum indirect immunofluorescent antibody (IFA) test is highly recommended as an aid for diagnosis of legionellosis, particularly for patients who do not or cannot provide adequate respiratory specimens (such as sputum) for culture and the DFA test. The sensitivity of the IFA test is 75% to 80%, and the specificity is 96%.[31,37,120,128,129] However, clinicians must wait 2 to 6 weeks for patients to develop a fourfold rise in antibody titer. Reagents for *Legionella* serodiagnostic tests should be capable of detecting antibodies of IgG, IgM, and IgA classes. In some patients, a rise in IgM titer may occur without a detectable rise in IgG or IgA titers or may occur earlier in the course of illness than a rise in IgG titer.[136]

As documented by Wilkinson and colleagues, the serum IFA test using *Legionella* antigens has the potential for cross-reacting with serum of patients who have certain other kinds of infections.[128,129] Sera of patients who had outbreak-associated *Mycoplasma pneumoniae* infections cross-reacted with *L. longbeachae* serogroup 2 and *L. jordanis*. Sera of patients with Q fever cross-reacted with antigens of *L. longbeachae* serogroup 2 and *L. jordanis*. Also, cross-reactions were noted between sera of patients who had outbreak-associated tularemia (*Francisella tularensis*) and *L. jordanis* antigen. In addition, false-positive cross-reactions have been observed in patients with *Bacteroides fragilis*, *Proteus vulgaris*, *Rickettsia* species, and *Citrobacter* species.[31,58]

Seroconversions (fourfold increase in antibody titer) to reciprocal titers of 1:128 or greater are required for serodiagnosis of recent infection with *Legionella*.[128] Single elevated reciprocal IFA titers of 256 or greater may be suggestive of *Legionella* infection during an outbreak. However, in sporadic cases of pneumonia, a 1:256 or higher titer does not necessarily indicate recent infection because titers of 1:256 and higher can persist in healthy persons with no current clinical evidence of legionellosis.

ENVIRONMENTAL MICROBIOLOGY STUDIES

ISOLATION OF LEGIONELLA FROM ENVIRONMENTAL SAMPLES

The ubiquitous presence of *Legionella* species in both natural and man-made environmental waters, in the absence of patients with clinical illness, has been observed repeatedly and argues against routine microbiologic culture of environmental water. On the other hand, considerable evidence has accumulated that links potable water as the source of the organism in many patients who have had infection with *L. pneumophila*. Institutional hot water has been implicated frequently in legionellosis[125]; however, more studies are needed on the magnitude of *Legionella* contamination in home potable water and hot water systems, and the frequency of association with legionellosis.[33] Given the high probability that large numbers of healthy persons are frequently exposed to these organisms in nature, in homes, in the workplace, and in private and public buildings of all sorts, it appears that many legionellae in natural and municipal waters are either not highly virulent, that exposure to the organism is minimal in extent, or that most persons are not susceptible hosts; or perhaps all are true.[52] Thus, microbiologic enumeration of *Legionella* species in potable or other waters (such as cooling towers) has no clinical or epidemiologic relevance to disease in humans unless cases are documented clinically.[131] Unfortunately, there are not sufficiently adequate markers of virulence that will distinguish between environmental isolates that are "pathogenic" from those that are unlikely to be pathogens, nor are there appropriate tests that predict which human hosts will develop legionellosis versus who will be resistant when exposed to *Legionella* in the environment. Furthermore, the degree and extent of exposure to the organism cannot be measured accurately.[52] Therefore, microbiologic surveillance of environmental waters is especially difficult to interpret in absence of cases of the disease (and even in the presence of documented cases as well). On the other hand, the clinical and epidemiologic surveillance of patients (*e.g.*, by hospital infection control nurses) is recommended as part of a program to prevent nosocomial legionellosis.[131]

In outbreaks of nosocomial legionellosis, hyperchlorination of the hospital water to a level between 2 and 6 mg/liter of free residual chlorine and raising the temperature of the hot water to more than 70°C or a combination of hyperchlorination and heat flushing are methods that have proven effective for suppressing the growth of *Legionella*.[91,110,111] To accomplish heat flushing or thermal eradication, the hot water is circulated throughout the building water system at a temperature of 70°C to 75°C. All shower heads and faucets are flushed with hot water with the objective to kill the *Legionella* in these sites. Protocols for hyperchlorination and thermal eradication have been published elsewhere.[91,110,111] Unfortunately, there is a risk of scalding from the hot water and precautions should be taken to minimize this possibility (*e.g.*, warning signs, heating the water for relatively short periods of time when most patients are asleep). (Regulations in some states require that the water temperature in hospitals be less than 120°F [48.9°C] to prevent scalding of patients.) Continuous chlorination (*i.e.*, to achieve 1.5 part per million free residual chlorine levels) may be unduly corrosive and destructive for some plumbing systems and equipment; there is also a potential risk of toxic exposure to trihalomethane.[52] If the heat and/or chlorination treatments are not done continuously, treatment should be recurrent because recolonization of the water is highly predictable and tends to recur following cessation of either heat shock or chlorination.[110] Other methods including ultraviolet light sterilization, ozonation, addition of amebicidal agents, and addition of trace metal ions (*e.g.*, silver, copper) are being investigated as alternative water system treatments.[16,134]

If nosocomial cases of infection with *Legionella* are documented, a highly focused microbiologic investigation of environmental samples may be undertaken to aid in determining the most likely source of the *Legionella*. Control measures such as heat and/or chlorination may be designed in an effort to eliminate or suppress the organism, and follow-up environmental cultures may help determine the effectiveness of these measures.[131] For hospitals with an outbreak or a hyperendemic *Legionella* problem, periodic microbiologic surveillance of the environment, combined with ongoing or repetitive control measures, should be considered unless it can be shown that no new cases of legionellosis have occurred.

The methods outlined in the protocol of Barbaree and co-workers,[10] in the CDC procedure manual of Gorman and co-workers,[57] and by Feeley[44] are recommended for persons who wish to isolate and identify *Legionella* species from environmental water. In this protocol, water samples (1 to 2 liters) are collected and concentrated using 0.2-μm (pore size) polycarbonate filters. Viable counts are performed with and without prior acid treatment on BCYEa and medium that contains BCYEa base supplemented with glycine polymyxin B, vancomycin, and anisomycin.

TYPING OF *LEGIONELLA* ISOLATES

Because of the extreme ubiquity of *L. pneumophila* serogroup 1 in the environment, serogrouping with the DFA reagents described previously has had only limited epidemiologic usefulness in investigating the source of different strains. Therefore, a number of investigators have developed methods to type or subgroup within different strains of *L. pneumophila* serogroup 1. Analyses of subtypes within *L. pneumophila* serogroup 1 using panels of monoclonal antibodies,[66,67] genetic structural analysis of *L. pneumophila* using a multilocus enzyme electrophoresis technique,[38,108] and determination of plasmid contents[93] of different isolates from different sources have all been investigated. More recently developed techniques have included electrophoresis of *L. pneumophila* outer membrane proteins[114] and a typing method based on the use of cloned biotinylated DNA probes for analysis of restriction fragment length polymorphisms (RFLPs).[107] One of the more promising typing methods is random amplified polymorphic DNA (RAPD) profiling of *Legionella pneumophila* by PCR; this method appears to be faster and costs less than RFLP typing. RAPD profiling has been reported to be more discriminatory than RFLP typing of some *Legionella* isolates, and is capable of detecting differences among isolates with identical RFLP types.[105] The usefulness of these procedures for epidemiologic investigations remains to be determined.

REFERENCES

1. ADDISS DG, DAVIS JP, LAVENTURE M ET AL: Community-acquired legionnaires' disease associated with a cooling tower: Evidence for longer-distance transport of *Legionella pneumophila*. Am J Epidemiol 130:557–568, 1989

2. AGUERO–ROSENFELD M, EDELSTEIN PH: Retrospective evaluation of the DuPont radioimmunoassay kit for detection of *Legionella pneumophila* serogroup 1 antigenuria in humans. J Clin Microbiol 26:1775–1778, 1988

3. ALARY M, JOLY JR: Risk factors for contamination of domestic hot water systems by legionellae. Appl Environ Microbiol 57:2360–2367, 1991

4. ALLEN SD, WILSON ER: *Legionella* Testing Procedures. Indiana University Hospital Clinical Laboratory Procedure Manual. Indianapolis, Indiana University School of Medicine, 1986

5. AMPEL NM, RUBEN FL, NORDEN CW: Cutaneous abscess caused by *Legionella micdadei* in an immunosuppressed patient. Ann Intern Med 102:630–632, 1985

6. ANDERSON BB, SOGAARD I: Legionnaire's disease and brain abscess. Neurology 37:333–334, 1987

7. ARNOW PM, BOYKO EF, FRIEDMAN EL: Perirectal abscess caused by *Legionella pneumophila* and mixed anaerobic bacteria. Ann Intern Med 98:184–185, 1983

8. ARNOW PM, CHOU T, WEIL D, ET AL: Nosocomial legionnaires' disease caused by aerosolized tap water from respiratory devices. J Infect Dis 146: 460–467, 1982.

9. ATLAS RM, WILLIAMS JF, HUNTINGTON MK: *Legionella* contamination of dental-unit waters. Appl Environ Microbiol 61:1208–1213, 1995

10. BARBAREE JM, GORMAN GW, MARTIN WT ET AL: Protocol for sampling environmental sites for *Legionella*. Appl Environ Microbiol 53:1454–1458, 1987

11. BENSON RF, THACKER WL, FANG FC, KANTER B, ET AL: *Legionella sainthelensi* serogroup 2 isolated from patients with pneumonia. Res Microbiol 141:453–463, 1990

12. BLACKMON JA, CHANDLER FW, CHERRY WB, ENGLAND AC III ET AL: Legionellosis. Am J Pathol 103:429–465, 1981

13. BLATT SP, PARKINSON MD, PACE E, HOFFMAN P ET AL: Nosocomial Legionnaires' disease: aspiration as a primary mode of disease acquisition [see comments]. Am J Med 95:16–22, 1993

14. BORNSTEIN N, MARMET D, SURGOT M, NOWICKI M ET AL: Exposure to *Legionellaceae* at a hot spring spa: A prospective clinical and serological study. Epidemiol Infect 102:31–36, 1989

15. BOUZA E, RODRIGUEZ–CREIXEMS M: Legionnaires' disease in Spain. In Thornsberry C, Balows A, Feeley JC, Jakubowski W (eds): *Legionella*: Proceedings of the 2nd International Symposium, pp 15–17. Washington, DC, American Society for Microbiology, 1984

16. BREIMAN RF, FIELDS BS, SANDEN GN ET AL: Association of shower use with legionnaires' disease: Possible role of amoebae. JAMA 263:2924–2926, 1990

17. BRENNER DJ, FEELEY JC, WEAVER RE: Family VII. *Legionellaceae* Brenner, Steigerwalt and McDade 1979. 658. In Kreig NR, Holt JG (eds): Bergey's Manual of Systematic Bacteriology, vol 1. Baltimore, Williams & Wilkins, 1984

18. BRENNER DJ, STEIGERWALT AG, MCDADE JE: Classification of the legionnaires' bacterium: *Legionella pneumophila*, genus novum, species nova, of the family *Legionellaceae*, familia nova. Ann Intern Med 90:656–658, 1979

19. BRIDGE JA, EDELSTEIN PH: Oropharyngeal colonization with *Legionella pneumophila*. J Clin Microbiol 18: 1108–1112, 1983

20. BROOME CV, FRASER DW: Epidemiologic aspects of legionellosis. Epidemiol Rev 1:1–16, 1979

21. BUESHING WJ, BRUST RA, AYERS LW: Enhanced primary isolation of *Legionella pneumophila* from clinical specimens by low *p*H treatment. J Clin Microbiol 17: 1153–1155, 1983

22. CENTERS FOR DISEASE CONTROL: Legionnaires' disease outbreak associated with a grocery store mist machine—Louisiana, 1989. MMWR 39:108–110, 1990

23. CHANDLER FW, BLACKMON JHA, HICKLIN MD ET AL: Electron microscopy of the legionnaires' disease bacterium. In Jones GL, Herbert GA (eds): "Legionnaires' ": The Disease, the Bacterium, and Methodology, pp 42–46. US Department of Health, Education and Welfare publication No. (CDC) 79-8375. Atlanta, Centers for Disease Control, 1979

24. CHASTRE J, RAGHU G, SOLER P ET AL: Pulmonary fibrosis following pneumonia due to acute legionnaires' disease: Clinical, ultrastructural and immunofluorescent study. Chest 91:57–62, 1987

25. CHERRY WB, MCKINNEY RM: Detection of legionnaires' disease bacteria in clinical specimens. In Jones GL, Herbert GA (eds): "Legionnaires' ": The Disease, the Bacterium and Methodology, pp 91–103. US Department of Health, Education and Welfare publication No. (CDC) 79-8375. Atlanta, Centers for Disease Control, 1979

26. CHERRY WB, PITTMAN B, HARRIS PP, HEBERT GA ET AL: Detection of legionnaires' disease bacteria by direct immunofluorescent staining. J Clin Microbiol 8:329–338, 1978

27. CORDES LG, WIESENTHAL AM, GORMAN GW, PHAIR JP ET AL: Isolation of *Legionella pneumophila* from hospital shower heads. Ann Intern Med 94:195–197, 1981

28. DORMAN SA, HARDIN NJ, WINN WC JR: Pyelonephritis associated with *Legionella pneumophila*, serogroup 4. Ann Intern Med 93:835–837, 1980

29. DROZANSKI W: *Sacrobium lyticum* gen. nov., sp. nov., an obligate intra-cellular bacterial parasite of small free-living amoebae. Int J Syst Bacteriol 41:82–87, 1991

30. EDELSTEIN PH: Improved semi-selective medium for isolation of *L. pneumophila* from clinical and environmental specimens. J Clin Microbiol 14:298–303, 1981

31. EDELSTEIN PH: Laboratory diagnosis of infections caused by Legionellae. Eur J Clin Microbiol 6:4–10, 1987

32. EDELSTEIN PH: Laboratory diagnosis of Legionnaires' disease: an update from 1984. In Babaree J, Breiman RF, Dufour AP (eds): *Legionella*: current status and emerging perspectives, pp 7–11. Washington, DC, American Society for Microbiology, 1993

33. EDELSTEIN PH: Legionnaires' disease. Clin Infect Dis 16:741–747, 1993

34. EDELSTEIN PH, BRYAN RN, ENNS RK, KOHNE DE ET AL: Retrospective study of Gen-Probe Rapid Diagnostic System for detection of legionellae in frozen clinical respiratory tract samples. J Clin Microbiol 25:1022–1026, 1987

35. EDELSTEIN PH, MCKINNEY RM, MEYER RD ET AL: Immunologic diagnosis of legionnaires' disease: Cross-reactions with anaerobes and microaerophilic organisms and infections caused by them. J Infect Dis 141:652–655, 1980

36. EDELSTEIN PH, MEYER RD, FINEGOLD SM: Isolation of *Legionella pneumophila* from blood. Lancet 1:750–751, 1979

37. EDELSTEIN PH, MEYER RD, FINEGOLD SM: Laboratory diagnosis of legionnaires' disease. Am Rev Respir Dis 121:317–327, 1980

38. EDELSTEIN PH, NAKAHAMA C, TOBIN JO ET AL: Paleoepidemiologic investigation of legionnaires' disease at Wadsworth Veterans Administration Hospital by using three typing methods for comparison of legionellae from clinical and environmental sources. J Clin Microbiol 23:1121–1126, 1986

39. ENGLAND AC III, FRASER DW, PLIKAYTIS DB ET AL: Sporadic legionellosis in the United States: The first thousand cases. Ann Intern Med 94:64–170, 1981

40. EZZEDDINE H, VANOSSEL C, DELMEE M, WAUTERS G ET AL: *Legionella* spp. in a hospital hot water system: Effect of control measures. J Hosp Infect 13:121–131, 1989

41. FALLON RJ, ROWBOTHAM TJ: Microbiological investigations into an outbreak of Pontiac fever due to *Legionella micdadei* associated with use of a whirlpool. J Clin Pathol 43:479–483, 1990

42. FANG GD, FINE M, ORLOFF J, ARISUMI D ET AL: New and emerging etiologies for community-acquired pneumonia with implications for therapy: A prospective multicenter study of 359 cases. Medicine 69:307–316, 1990

43. FANG GD, YU VL, VICKERS BS: Disease due to the Legionellaceae (other than *Legionella pneumophila*): Historical, microbiological, clinical and epidemiological review. Medicine 68:116–132, 1989

44. FEELEY JC: State of the art lecture. Current microbiological methods used in analysis of environmental specimens for *Legionella* spp. In: Proceeding of the Second International Symposium on *Legionella*, pp 283–284. Washington, DC, American Society for Microbiology, 1984

45. FEELEY JC, GIBSON RJ, GORMAN GW ET AL: Charcoal yeast extract agar: Primary isolation media for *L. pneumophila*. J Clin Microbiol 10:437–441, 1979

46. FEELEY JC, GORMAN GW, WEAVER RE ET AL: Primary isolation media for legionnaires' disease. J Clin Microbiol 8:320–325, 1978

47. FIELDS BS, FIELDS SR, LOY JN, WHITE EH ET AL: Attachment and entry of *Legionella pneumophila* in *Hartmannella vermiformis*. J Infect Dis 167:1146–1150, 1993

48. FIELDS BS, SANDEN GN, BARBAREE JM ET AL: Intracellular multiplication of *Legionella pneumophila* in amoebae isolated from hospital hot water tanks. Curr Microbiol 18:131–137, 1989

49. FINKELSTEIN R, PALUTKE WA, WENTWORTH BB, GEIGER JG ET AL: Colonization of the respiratory tract with *Legionella* species. Isr J Med Sci 29:277–279, 1993

50. FLIERMANS CB, CHERRY WB, ORRISON LH ET AL: Ecological distribution of *Legionella pneumophila*. Appl Environ Microbiol 41:9–16, 1981

51. FLIERMANS CB, CHERRY WB, ORRISON LH ET AL: Isolation of *Legionella pneumophila* from non-epidemic-related habitats. Appl Environ Microbiol 37:1239–1242, 1979

52. FRASER DW, MCDADE JE: Legionellosis. Sci Am 241:82–99, 1979

53. FRAZIER DW, TSAI T, ORENSTEIN W ET AL: Legionnaires' disease I: Description of an epidemic of pneumonia. N Engl J Med 297:1189–1197, 1977

54. GARBE PL, DAVIS BJ, WEISFELD JS ET AL: Nosocomial legionnaires' disease: Epidemiologic demonstration of cooling towers as a source. JAMA 254:521–524, 1985

55. GLICK TH, GREGG MB, BERMAN B ET AL: Pontiac fever: An epidemic of unknown etiology in a health department: I. Clinical and epidemiologic aspects. Am J Epidemiol 107:149–160, 1978

56. GOLDBERG DJ, WRENCH JG, COLLIER PW, FALLON RF ET AL: Lochgoilhead fever: Outbreak of nonpneumonic legionellosis due to *Legionella micdadei*. Lancet 1: 316–318, 1989

57. GORMAN GW, BARBAREE JM, FEELEY JC: Procedures for Recovery of *Legionella* From Water. CDC Manual. Atlanta, Centers for Disease Control, 1983

58. GRAY JJ, WARD KN, WARREN RE, FARRINGTON M: Serological cross-reaction between *Legionella pneumophila* and *Citrobacter freundii* in indirect immunofluorescence and rapid microagglutination tests. J Clin Microbiol 29:200–201, 1991

59. GUMP DW, FRANK RO, WINN WC JR ET AL: Legionnaires' disease in patients with associated serious disease. Ann Intern Med 90:638–542, 1979

60. HARRISON TG, SAUNDERS NA: Taxonomy and typing of legionellae. Rev Med Microbiol 5:19–90, 1994

61. HELMS CM, JOHNSON W, DONALDSON MF ET AL: Pretibial rash in *Legionella pneumophila* pneumonia. JAMA 245:1758–1759, 1981

62. HOOKEY JV, SAUNDERS NA, FRY NK, BIRTLES RJ ET AL: Phylogeny of *Legionellaceae* based on small-subunit ribosomal DNA sequences and proposal of *Legionella lytica* comb. nov. for *Legionella*-like amoebal pathogens. Int J Syst Bacteriol 46:526–531, 1996

63. HORWITZ MA: Interactions between macrophages and *Legionella pneumophia*. Curr Top Microbiol Immunol 181:265–282, 1992

64. HORWITZ MA: Toward an understanding of host and bacterial molecules mediating *Legionella pneumophila* pathogenesis. In Barbaree JM, Breiman RF, Dufour AP (eds): *Legionella*: current Status and emerging perspectives, pp 55–62. Washington, DC, American Society for Microbiology, 1993

65. JOHNSON JD, RAFF MY, VAN ARSDALL JA: Neurologic manifestations of legionnaires' disease. Medicine 63: 303–310, 1984

66. JOLY JR, MCKINNEY RM, TOBIN JO ET AL: Development of a standardized subgrouping scheme for *Legionella pneumophila* serogroup 1 using monoclonal antibodies. J Clin Microbiol 23:768–771, 1986

67. JOLY JR, WINN WC: Correlation of subtypes of *Legionella pneumophila* defined by monoclonal antibodies with epidemiological classification of cases and environmental sources. J Infect Dis 150:667–671, 1984

68. JONES GT, HEBERT GA (EDS): "Legionnaires": The Disease, the Bacterium and Methodology. US Department of Health, Education and Welfare publication No. (CDC) 79-8375. Atlanta, Centers for Disease Control, 1979

69. KESSLER HH, REINTHALER FF, PSCHAID A, PIERER K ET AL: Rapid detection of *Legionella* species in bronchoalveolar lavage fluids with the EnviroAmp Legionella PCR amplification and detection kit. J Clin Microbiol 31: 3325–3328, 1993

70. KING CH, SHOTTS EB, WOOLEY RE, PORTER KG ET AL: Survival of coliforms and bacterial pathogens within protozoa during chlorination. Appl Environ Microbiol 54:3023–3033, 1988

71. KOHLER RB, WHEAT LJ, FRENCH ML, MEENHORST PL ET AL: Cross-reactive urinary antigens among patients infected with *Legionella pneumophila* serogroups 1 and 4 and the Leiden 1 strain. J Infect Dis 152:1007–1012, 1985

72. KOHLER RB, WINN WC JR, WHEAT LJ: Onset and duration of urinary antigen excretion in Legionnaires' disease. J Clin Microbiol 20:605–607, 1984

73. KOHLER RB, ZIMMERMAN SE, WILSON EW ET AL: Rapid radioimmunoassay diagnosis of legionnaires' disease: Detection and partial characterization of urinary antigen. Ann Intern Med 94:601–605, 1981

74. KOIDE M, SAITO A: Diagnosis of *Legionella pneumophila* infection by polymerase chain reaction. Clin Infect Dis 21:199–201, 1995

75. KORVICK JA, YU VL: Legionnaires' disease: An emerging surgical problem. Ann Thorac Surg 43:341–347, 1987

76. LAMBERT MA, MOSS CW: Cellular fatty acid composition and isoprenoid quinone contents of 23 *Legionella* species. J Clin Microbiol 27:465–473, 1989

77. LEE TC, STOUT JE, YU VL: Factors predisposing to *Legionella pneumophila* colonization in residential water systems. Arch Environ Health 43:59–62, 1988

78. MARRIE TJ, BEZANSON G, HALDANE DJ, BURBRIDGE S: Colonization of the respiratory tract with *Legionella pneumophila* for 63 days before the onset of pneumonia. J Infect 24:81–86, 1992

79. MARRIE TJ, HALDANE, MACDONALD S, CLARKE K ET AL: Control of endemic nosocomial legionnaires' disease by using sterile potable water for high risk patients. Epidemiol Infect 107:591–605, 1991

80. MASTRO TD, FIELDS BS, BREIMAN RF ET AL: Nosocomial legionnaires' disease and use of medication nebulizers. J Infect Dis 163:667–670, 1991

81. MATSIOTA-BERNARD P, PITSOUNI E, LEGAKIS N, NAUCIEL C: Evaluation of commercial amplification kit for detection of *Legionella pneumophila* in clinical specimens. J Clin Microbiol 32:1503–1505, 1994

82. MAYOCK R, SKALE B, KOHLER RB: *Legionella pneumophila* pericarditis proved by culture of pericardial fluid. Am J Med 75:534–536, 1983

83. MCCABE RE, BALDWIN JC, MCGREGOR CA ET AL: Prosthetic valve endocarditis caused by *Legionella pneumophila*. Ann Intern Med 100:525–527, 1984

84. MCDADE JE, SHEPARD CC, FRASER DW ET AL: Legionnaires' disease: Isolation of a bacterium and demonstration of its role in other respiratory disease. N Engl J Med 297:1197–1203, 1977

85. MILLER LA, BEEBE JL, BUTLER JC, MARTIN W ET AL: Use of polymerase chain reaction in an epidemiological investigation of Pontiac fever. J Infect Dis 168:769–772,1993

86. MORRIS GK, PATTON CM, FEELEY JC, JOHNSON SE ET AL: Isolation of the legionnaires' disease bacterium from environmental samples. Ann Intern Med 90:664–666, 1979

87. MOSS CW: Gas-liquid chromatography as an analytical tool in microbiology. J Chromatogr 203:337–346, 1981

88. MOSS CW, KARR DE, DEES SB: Cellular fatty acid composition of *Legionella longbeachae* sp nov. J Clin Microbiol 14:692–694, 1981

89. MUDER RR, YU VL: Other *Legionella* species. In Mandell GL, Bennett JE, Dolin R (eds): Mandell, Douglas and Bennett's principle and practice of infectious diseases, vol 2, pp 2097–2103. New York, Churchill Livingstone, 1995

90. MUDER RR, YU VL, WOO AH: Mode of transmission of *Legionella pneumophila*: A critical review. Arch Intern Med 146:1607–1612, 1986

91. MURACA MS, YU VL, GOETZ A: Disinfection of water distribution systems for *Legionella*: A review of application procedures and methodologies. Infect Control Hosp Epidemiol 11:79–88, 1990

92. NEWSOME AL, BAKER RL, MILLER RD, ARNOLD RR: Interactions between *Naegleria fowleri* and *Legionella pneumophila*. Infect Immun 50:449–452, 1985

93. NOLTE FS, CONLIN CA, ROISIN AJ ET AL: Plasmids as epidemiological markers in nosocomial legionnaires' disease. J Infect Dis 149:251–256, 1984

94. ORTIZ–ROGUE CM, HAZEN TC: Abundance and distribution of Legionellaceae in Puerto Rican waters. Appl Environ Microbiol 53:2231–2236, 1987

95. OSHIRO KK, PICONE T, OLSON BH: Modification of reagents in the EnviroAmp kit to increase recovery of *Legionella* organisms in water. Can J Microbiol 40: 495–499, 1994

96. PALMER CJ, BONILLA GF, ROLL B, PASZKO-KOLVA C ET AL: Detection of *Legionella* species in reclaimed water and air with the EnviroAmp Legionella PCR kit and direct fluorescent antibody staining. Appl Environ Microbiol 61:407–412, 1995

97. PALMER CJ, TSAI YL, PASZKO-KOLVA C, MAYER C ET AL: Detection of *Legionella* species in sewage and ocean water by polymerase chain reaction, direct fluorescent-antibody, and plate culture methods. Appl Environ Microbiol 59:3618–3624, 1993

98. PASCULLE AW, VETO GE, KRYSTOFIAK S ET AL: Laboratory and clinical evaluation of a commercial DNA probe for the detection of *Legionella* spp. J Clin Microbiol 27: 2350–2358, 1989

99. POTASMAN S, LIBERSON A, KRIMERMAN S: *Legionella* infection mimicking herpes encephalitis. Crit Care Med 18: 453–454, 1990

100. REINGOLD AL, THOMASON BM, BRAKE FB ET AL: *Legionella pneumophila* in the United States: The distribution of serogroups and species causing human illness. J Infect Dis 149:819, 1984

101. RIHS JD, YU BL, ZURAVLEFF JJ ET AL: Isolation of *Legionella pneumophila* from blood with the BACTEC system: A prospective study yielding positive results. J Clin Microbiol 22:422–424, 1985

102. RODGERS FG, PASCULLE AW: *Legionella*. In Balows A, Hausler WJ Jr, Herrmann KL et al (eds): Manual of Clinical Microbiology, pp 442–453. Washington, DC, American Society for Microbiology, 1991

103. ROWBOTHAM TJ: Preliminary report on the pathogenicity of *Legionella pneumophila* for freshwater and soil amoebae. J Clin Pathol 33:1179–1183, 1980

104. RUF B, SCHURMAN D, HORBACH I, FEHRENBACH FJ ET AL: The incidence of *Legionella* pneumonia: A 1-year prospective study in a large community hospital. Lung 167:11–22, 1989

105. SANDERY M, COBLE J, MCKERSIE-DONNOLLEY S: Random amplified DNA (RAPD) profiling of *Legionella pneumophila*. Lett Appl Microbiol 19:184–187, 1994

106. SARAVOLATZ LD, BURCH KH, FISHER E ET AL: The compromised host and legionnaires' disease. Ann Intern Med 90:533–537, 1979

107. SAUNDERS NA, HARRISON TG, HATHTHOTUWA A ET AL: A method for typing strains of *Legionella pneumophila* serogroup 1 by analysis of restriction fragment length polymorphisms. J Med Microbiol 31:45–55, 1990

108. SELANDER RK, MCKINNEY RM, WHITTAM TS ET AL: Genetic structure of populations of *Legionella pneumophila*. J Bacteriol 163:1021–1037, 1985

109. SHANDS KN, HO JL, MEYER RD ET AL: Potable water as a source of legionnaires' disease. JAMA 253:1412–1416, 1985

110. SNYDER MB, SIWICKI M, ET AL: Reduction in *Legionella pneumophila* through heat flushing followed by continous supplemental chlorination of hospital hot water. J Infect Dis 162:127–132, 1990

111. STATES SJ, CONLEY LF, KUTCHA JM, WOLFORD RS: Chlorine, *pH*, and control of *Legionella* in hospital plumbing systems. JAMA 261:1882–1883, 1989

112. STEELE TW, LANSER J, SANGSTER N: Isolation of *Legionella longbeachae* serogroup 1 from potting mixes. Appl Environ Microbiol 56:49–53, 1990

113. STEELE TW, MOORE CV, SANGSTER N: Distribution of *Legionella longbeachae* serogroup 1 and other Legionellae in potting soils in Australia. Appl Environ Microbiol 56:2984–2988, 1990

114. STOUT JE, JOLY J, PARA M ET AL: Comparison of molecular methods for subtyping patients and epidemiologically linked environmental isolates of *Legionella pneumophila*. J Infect Dis 157:486–495, 1988

115. STOUT JE, YU VL, MURACA P, JOLY J ET AL: Potable water as a cause of sporadic cases of community-acquired legionnaires' disease. N Engl J Med 326:151–155, 1992

116. STOUT JE, YU VL, YEE YC, VACCARELLO S ET AL: *Legionella pneumophila* in residential water supplies: environmental surveillance with clinical assessment for Legionnaires' disease. Ann Occupational Hyg 32:63–67, 1988

117. SYKES JM, BRAZIER AM: Assessment and control of risks from legionnaires' disease. Ann Occup Hyg 32:63–67, 1988

118. THACKER WL, BENSON RF, SCHIFMAN RB, PUGH E ET AL: *Legionella tucsonensis* sp. nov. isolated from a renal transplant recipient. J. Clin Microbiol 27:1831–1834, 1989

119. THACKER WL, DYKE JW, BENSON RF, HAVLICHEK DH JR, ET AL: *Legionella lansingensis* sp. nov. isolated from a patient with pneumonia and underlying chronic lymphocytic leukemia. J Clin Microbiol 30:2398–2401, 1992

120. THACKER WL, WILKINSON HW, BENSON RF: Comparison of slide agglutination test and direct immunofluorescence assay for identification of *Legionella* isolates. J Clin Microbiol 18:1113–1118, 1983

121. THORNSBERRY C, BAKER CM, KIRVIN LA: *In vitro* activity of antimicrobial agents of legionnaires' disease bacterium. Antimicrob Agents Chemother 13:78–80, 1978

122. VICKERS RM, STOUT JE, YU VL: Failure of a diagnostic monoclonal immunofluorescent reagent to detect *Legionella pneumophila* in environmental samples. Appl Environ Microbiol 56:2912–2914, 1990

123. WADOWSKY RM, BUTLER LJ, COOK MK ET AL: Growth-supporting activity for *Legionella pneumophila* in tap water cultures and implication of hartmannellid amoebae as growth factors. Appl Environ Microbiol 54:2677–2682, 1988

124. WADOWSKY RM, WOLFORS R, MCNAMARA AM ET AL: Effect of temperature, *pH*, and oxygen level on the multiplication of naturally occurring *Legionella pneumophila* in potable water. Appl Environ Microbiol 49:1197–1205, 1985

125. WADOWSKY RM, YEE RB, MEZMAR L ET AL: Hot water systems as sources of *Legionella pneumophila* in hospital and nonhospital plumbing fixtures. Appl Environ Microbiol 43:1104–1110, 1982

126. WHITE HJ, FELTON WW, SUN CN: Extrapulmonary histopathologic manifestations of legionnaires' disease: Evidence for myocarditis and bacteremia. Arch Pathol Lab Med 104:287–289, 1980

127. WILKINSON HW: Hospital-Laboratory Diagnosis of *Legionella* Infections, rev. ed. Atlanta, Centers for Disease Control, January 1988

128. WILKINSON HW, CRUCE DD, BROOME CV: Validation of *Legionella pneumophila* indirect immunofluorescence assay with epidemic sera. J Clin Microbiol 13:139–146, 1981

129. WILKINSON HW, REINGOLD AL, BRAKE BJ ET AL: Reactivity of serum from patients with suspected legionellosis against 29 antigens of Legionellaceae and *Legionella*-like organism by indirect immunofluorescence assay. J Infect Dis 147:23–31, 1983

130. WINN WC JR: Legionellosis. In Wentworth BB (ed): Diagnostic Procedures for Bacterial Infections, pp 318–334. Washington, DC, American Public Health Association, 1987

131. WINN WC JR: Legionnaires' disease: Historical perspective. Clin Microbiol Rev 1:60–81, 1988

132. WINN WC JR, MYEROWITZ RL: The pathology of the *Legionella* pneumonias: A review of 74 cases and the literature. Hum Pathol 12:401–422, 1981

133. WINN WC JR: *Legionella*. In Murray PR, Baron EJ, Pfaller MA et al (eds): Manual of Clinical Microbiology (6 ed), pp 533–544. Washington, DC, ASM Press, 1995

134. WORLD HEALTH ORGANIZATION: Epidemiology, prevention and control of legionellosis: Memorandum from a WHO meeting. Bull WHO 68:155–164, 1990

135. YU VL: *Legionella pneumophila* (legionnaires' disease). In Principles and Practice of Infectious Diseases, 3rd ed, pp 1764–1774. New York, John Wiley & Sons, 1990

136. ZIMMERMAN SE, FRENCH ML, ALLEN SD ET AL: Immunoglobulin M antibody titers in the diagnosis of legionnaires' disease. J Clin Microbiol 16:1007–1011, 1982

NEISSERIA SPECIES AND MORAXELLA CATARRHALIS

Gonorrhea was recognized at least as early as the time of Galen (second century A.D.), who named the disease after the Greek words *gonor* ("seed") and *rhoia* ("flow"), suggesting that the disease was related to the flow of semen. Gonorrhea was recognized as a sexually transmitted infection by the 13th century but was not distinguished from syphilis until the mid-19th century. *Neisseria gonorrhoeae*, the etiologic agent of gonorrhea, was first observed in 1879 by Neisser in purulent urethral and conjunctival exudates. Subsequent isolation of the organism, inoculation into human volunteers, and reisolation of the organism by

Color Plates for Chapter 10 are found between pages 368 and 369.

Bumm in 1885 proved the causal relationship between the organism and the disease.

Epidemic cerebrospinal meningitis was known early in the 19th century, but the etiologic agent was not described until 1884, when Marchiofava and Celli observed the organism in meningeal exudates. In 1887, Weichselbaum isolated the organism, now called *Neisseria meningitidis*, in pure culture and first described its characteristics and etiologic role in six patients with acute cerebrospinal meningitis. Additional work by Kiefer in 1896 and Albrecht in 1901 established the existence of the meningococcal carrier state in healthy individuals.[51] Over the period from 1928 through 1930 and in 1941, outbreaks of meningococcal disease in Chile and U.S. cities (Detroit and Milwaukee) focused scientific attention on this organism. With subsequent outbreaks among military recruits in the United States and abroad, a greater understanding of the epidemiology, pathogenesis, chemoprophylaxis, and prospects for vaccine development emerged.[141,396] These issues are still the focus of meningococcal research today.

Although the procedures for the isolation of *Neisseria* species from clinical specimens have not changed over the last several years, new methods for rapid identification and direct detection have modified the laboratory approach to these fastidious microorganisms and the infections they cause. The gonococcus, in particular, has been an especially successful and resourceful human pathogen. This bacterium is capable of causing localized urogenital, rectal, oropharyngeal, and systemic disease.[410,411] Similarly, the meningococcus is no longer restricted to the oropharynx as its reservoir in human populations; this organism has been recovered from genital and rectal sites as well.[215] In addition, the "nonpathogenic" or "saprophytic" *Neisseria* species that constitute a part of the normal oropharyngeal flora may, on occasion, cause life-threatening illness, such as endocarditis and bacteremia.[192,468] Therefore, the identity of *Neisseria* species can no longer be presumed on the basis of the site of isolation. For these reasons, definitive biochemical or serologic identification of isolates is now required in most clinical microbiology laboratories.

Changing patterns of antibiotic resistance in *N. gonorrhoeae* have been observed in recent years.[201] In 1976, penicillinase-producing strains of *N. gonorrhoeae* were first imported into the United States, and now these organisms are endemic in this country. The subsequent appearance of chromosomally mediated penicillin resistance and plasmid-mediated high-level tetracyline resistance in gonococci has significantly altered the therapeutic and public health approaches to treatment of gonococcal disease. Isolation of penicillinase-producing meningococci and the recovery of "nonpathogenic" and newly recognized *Neisseria* species from immunocompromised patients must also be considered by the microbiologist in formulating an approach to the detection and identification of *Neisseria* species and "neisseria-like" bacteria in clinical specimens.[47,107,134,192]

INTRODUCTION TO THE FAMILY *NEISSERIACEAE*

TAXONOMY OF THE FAMILY *NEISSERIACEAE*

In the 1984 edition of *Bergey's Manual of Systematic Bacteriology*, the family *Neisseriaceae* included four genera: *Neisseria, Moraxella, Kingella,* and *Acinetobacter*.[41] In this volume, the genus *Neisseria* consisted of 11 species that are considered as "true neisseriae" and three animal species, collectively called the "false neisseriae" (*N. caviae, N. ovis,* and *N. cuniculi*) that were considered to be *species incertae sedis*.[442,446] The genus *Moraxella* was subdivided into two subgenera: the subgenus *Moraxella* and the subgenus *Branhamella*.[40] Six species—M. (M.) *lacunata*, M. (M.) *bovis*, M. (M.) *nonliquefaciens*, M. (M.)

atlantae, M. (M.) *phenylpyruvica,* and M. (M.) *osloensis*—were placed into the genus *Moraxella* subgenus *Moraxella,* and four species—M. (B.) *catarrhalis,* M. (B.) *caviae,* M. (B.) *ovis,* and M. (B.) *cuniculi*—were placed in the subgenus *Branhamella*.[40,42] "*Moraxella urethralis*" was considered an organism of uncertain affiliation. The family also included three *Kingella* species (*K. kingae, K. denitrificans,* and *K. indologenes*) and *Acinetobacter* phenotypic groups.[41] *Psychrobacter immobilis* was added to the family *Neisseriaceae* in 1986.[231]

In 1988, using several molecular genetic techniques new to bacterial taxonomy, Stackebrandt and associates described the class *Proteobacteria* and its phylogenetic RNA subclasses (α, β, τ, and δ).[415] The application of such techniques, including DNA–ribosomal (rRNA) hybridization studies, DNA–DNA hybridization studies, and 16S rRNA sequence analysis, has resulted in substantial changes in the taxonomy of the family *Neisseriaceae*.[103,374] These techniques have demonstrated that the true neisseriae, *Kingella kingae, Kingella denitrificans,* and "*Moraxella urethralis*" belong to the β-subclass of the class *Proteobacteria*.[374] The latter species has been shown to be unrelated to the true moraxellae and is now called *Oligella urethralis,* the type strain of the new genus *Oligella*.[371,374] *Acinetobacter, Moraxella,* the false neisseriae, and *Branhamella catarrhalis* belong to the τ-subclass of the class *Proteobacteria*. Furthermore, these same techniques have revealed that the genera *Eikenella; Simonsiella; Alysiella;* and CDC groups EF-4A, EF-4B, M-5, and M-6 also belong to the emended family *Neisseriaceae*.[372,374] The CDC groups M-5 and M-6, formerly considered as "moraxella-like" species, have now been reclassified as *N. weaveri* and as a subspecies of *N. elongata* (*N. elongata* subsp. *nitroreducens*), respectively.[7,162,200] Although the genus *Kingella* is retained in the new scheme, one species, *K. indologenes,* has been transferred to a new family (the *Cardiobacteriaceae*) as the new species *Suttonella indologenes*.[104] The nonneisserial species in the family *Neisseriaceae* were described in the chapter on fastidious gram-negative bacilli (see Chap. 8) and will not be discussed further here. *Psychrobacter immobilis* was also excluded from the family *Neisseriaceae* by the work of Rossau and colleagues.[372]

The taxonomic status of M. (B.) *catarrhalis,* the other *Moraxella* species, and the false neisseriae are still subjects of debate and disagreement. Rossau and colleagues[373] recognized a large group within the τ-subclass of the *Proteobacteria* that was called the "*Moraxellaceae* rRNA cluster." This cluster contained the genus *Acinetobacter* and the *Moraxella–Psychrobacter* group. The latter group was divided into the *Moraxella lacunata* subgroup (containing the classic moraxellae—M. *lacunata* subsp. *lacunata,* M. *lacunata* subsp. *liquefaciens,* M. *bovis,* M. *liquefaciens*—the false neisseriae, and M. *catarrhalis*), the *Moraxella osloensis* subgroup, the *Moraxella atlantae* subgroup, and the *Psychrobacter–Moraxella phenylpyruvica* subgroup. These investigators have proposed a new family, the family *Moraxellaceae,* for this rRNA cluster.[373] A second proposal, based on the work of Catlin, created a new family called the family *Branhamaceae*.[68,72] This family would include the genus *Branhamella* (not recognized in the family

Moraxellaceae of Rossau and associates) and the genus *Moraxella*. Genus *Branhamella* would include *B. catarrhalis*, and the false neisseriae (*B. ovis, B. cuniculi,* and *B. caviae*), whereas the genus *Moraxella* would include all *Moraxella* species (*M. bovis, M. lacunata, N. nonliquefaciens*) and the moraxella-like species (*M. osloensis, M. phenylpyruvica,* and *M. atlantae*). The genus *Acinetobacter* is not accommodated in Catlin's proposal.

Despite its cultural and phenotypic similarities to the saprophytic *Neisseria* species and the familiarity of the name "*Branhamella catarrhalis*" to most practicing clinical microbiologists, the name of this organism will likely be accepted as *Moraxella catarrhalis*. Although many texts still classify them with the moraxellae, the false neisseriae are now generally considered to be *Neisseria* species of animal origin, along with *N. weaveri, N. canis, N. denitrificans, N. macacae,* and the newly described species *Neisseria iguanae*.[446] A new canine species called *Moraxella canis* has been described that is genotypically distinct from the true moraxellae and is closely related to *M. catarrhalis* and to the false neisseriae.[225] In addition, the confusion that still surrounds the taxonomic positions of extant and newly described *Moraxella* species has not been resolved.[225] *M. catarrhalis* and the false neisseriae will be discussed in detail in this chapter along with the *Neisseria* species. The other *Moraxella* species are considered with the nonfermentative gram-negative bacilli in Chapter 5. Table 10-1 summarizes the old classification and the newly emended classification system for the family *Neisseriaceae*.[128,372,374]

GENERAL CHARACTERISTICS OF THE GENUS *NEISSERIA* AND *MORAXELLA CATARRHALIS*

Members of the genus *Neisseria* are coccal or rod-shaped gram-negative organisms that frequently occur in pairs or short chains. The coccal organisms have adjacent sides that are flattened, giving them a coffee bean shape. All species in the genus *Neisseria* inhabit mucous membrane surfaces of warm-blooded hosts. These organisms are nonmotile, do not form spores, and most grow optimally at 35°C to 37°C. The organisms are capnophilic and grow best in a moist environment. *Neisseria* spp. produce acid from carbohydrates oxidatively; acid production from various carbohydrates constitutes part of the reference identification of these species. Currently, *Neisseria* species (except for the three *N. elongata* subspecies and *N. weaveri*) are the only true coccal members of the family *Neisseriaceae*. The *N. elongata* subspecies and *N. weaveri* are medium to large, plump rods that sometimes occur in pairs or short chains.[7,43,200] All species in the genus are oxidase-positive and (except for *N. elongata* subspecies *elongata* and *N. elongata* subspecies *nitroreducens*) are catalase-positive.[43,162] Members of the genus that are found in humans include *N. gonorrhoeae, N. meningitidis, N. lactamica, N. sicca, N. subflava* (including biovars *subflava, flava,* and *perflava*) *N. mucosa, N. flavescens, N. cinerea, N. polysaccharea,* and *N. elongata* subspecies.[249] *Neisseria kochii*, a rarely isolated organism that is considered a subspecies of *N. gonorrhoeae*, is both phenotypically and genetically related to *N. gonorrhoeae*.[296] Among the animal species, *N. canis* and *N. weaveri* are found as part of the normal respiratory tract flora of dogs; *N. denitrificans, N. animalis,* and *N. caviae* are found in the upper respiratory tract of guinea pigs; *N. ovis* is part of the oral flora of sheep and goats; and *N. cuniculi* is found in the upper respiratory tracts of rabbits.[7,40,42,200,442,446] The clinical significance, cultural characteristics, and procedures for differentiating these organisms will be discussed later in this chapter.

VIRULENCE FACTORS OF THE PATHOGENIC *NEISSERIA* AND *MORAXELLA CATARRHALIS*

As in the other gram-negative bacteria, *Neisseria* species possess an inner cytoplasmic membrane, a thin peptidoglycan layer, and an outer membrane containing lipooligosaccharide (LOS), proteins, and phospholipid (Fig. 10–1). Unlike several other gram-negative bacteria (e.g., the *Enterobacteriaceae*), gonococcal and meningococcal lipooligosaccharides lack the repeating "O" somatic antigen side chains external to the core polysaccharide.[167] The gonococcal LOS core polysaccharide undergoes antigenic variation in molecular structure at a fairly high frequency, resulting in the exposure of different core LOS epitopes at the cell surface.[12,390] Structural variation of LOS may influence bacterial adherence and attachment and may affect killing of the cells by normal human serum.[389] The LOS of *N. meningitidis* also shows structural and antigenic diversity, and at least 12 LOS serotypes have been described.[287] Components of the gonococcal peptidoglycan may also function as virulence factors in that these components are cytotoxic in explanted Fallopian tube cultures and may also contribute to gonococcal pathology by activating the complement cascade.[139]

Surface structures of the pathogenic *Neisseria* have been the subjects of intense microbiologic investigations for some time in an attempt to identify immunogenic structures that might be exploited in the development of vaccines. Both *N. gonorrhoeae* and *N. meningitidis* possess pili, which are hairlike protein polymers that project from the surface of the bacterial cell and partially mediate attachment of the organisms to mucosal surfaces.[186] Piliated gonococci adhere to susceptible cells and can initiate infection; antibodies directed against gonococcal pili can inhibit adherence.[447] It is also thought that pili may function to overcome electrostatic repulsion between the negatively charged mucosal surface and the similarly charged bacterial cells.[186] Gonococcal pili may also deter ingestion and destruction of gonococci by neutrophils, and they may be involved in the exchange of genetic material. Gonococcal pili are composed of pilin protein subunits that have an apparent molecular weight of 16.5 to 21.5 kDa.[394] Although less readily demonstrable, freshly isolated meningococci are also piliated, and the pili mediate attachment of the organisms to the mucosal cells of the nasopharynx.[339] Organisms found in the cerebrospinal fluid are piliated in vivo, but it is not known whether meningococcal pili play any role in the

CLASSIFICATION OF ORGANISMS WITHIN THE FAMILY *NEISSERIACEAE*

GENUS AND SPECIES IN *BERGEY'S MANUAL* 1984[41]	GENUS AND SPECIES IN PROPOSED SCHEME 1989[372]	COMMENTS
Neisseria spp.	*Neisseria* spp.	
N. gonorrhoeae	N. gonorrhoeae	
	"N. kochii"	Not included in 1989 scheme,[372] but accepted in other reports[243,296]
N. meningitidis	N. meningitidis	
N. lactamica	N. lactamica	
N. sicca	N. sicca	
N. subflava	N. subflava	Biovars N. flava, N. subflava, and N. perflava recognized in 1989 scheme
N. mucosa	N. mucosa	
N. flavescens	N. flavescens	
N. cinerea	N. cinerea	
	N. polysaccharea	Species described by Riou[360]
	N. macacae	Species found in monkeys
N. elongata subsp. elongata	N. elongata subsp. elongata	
N. elongata subsp. glycolytica	N. elongata subsp. glycolytica	
	N. elongata subsp. nitroreducens	Formerly CDC group M-6[162]
	N. weaveri	Former CDC group M-5[7, 200]
N. canis	N. canis	Respiratory flora, cats
N. denitrificans	N. denitrificans	Respiratory flora, guinea pigs
	N. iguanae	Respiratory flora, iguanas
Kingella spp.	*Kingella* spp.	
K. kingae	K. kingae	
K. denitrificans	K. denitrificans	
K. indologenes	Not included	Now classified as *Suttonella indologenes* in the Family *Cardiobacteriaceae* (see Chap. 8)[104]
Acinetobacter spp.	Not included	Family affiliation uncertain
Moraxella spp.	Not included	Family affiliation uncertain Family *Moraxellaceae*[373] and Family *Branhamaceae*[72] proposed
"*Psychrobacter immobilis*"	Not included	Added to the family *Neisseriaceae* by Bovre in 1986, excluded by Rossau et al,[372] and placed in family *Moraxellaceae*[373]
	Eikenella spp.	Not formerly included in a designated family (see Chap. 8)
	Simonsiella spp. *Alysiella* spp.	*Simonsiella* spp. and *Alysiella* spp. are aerobic, gram-negative gliding bacteria that are normally found in the oral cavities of humans and animals; nonpathogenic
	CDC Group EF-4a and CDC Group EF-4b	These organisms are found as normal flora in the oral cavities of dogs and cats and may be isolated from infected dog- and cat-bite or scratch wounds (see Chap. 8).

ability of the organism to transgress the blood–brain barrier or to interact with meningeal tissues.[186]

Gonococcal pili undergo both phase variation and antigenic variation. In vitro, **phase variation** between the piliated (P+ and P++) and nonpiliated (P−) state occurs at a high frequency; in this situation the *pil* genes (the structural genes for pilus proteins) may be nonexpressed (i.e., pilus proteins are not produced), or the pilus proteins that are synthesized by the organism cannot be assembled into functional pili. Pili also may undergo **antigenic variation**, in which the *pil* genes, of which there are at least 20 copies per cell, undergo re-

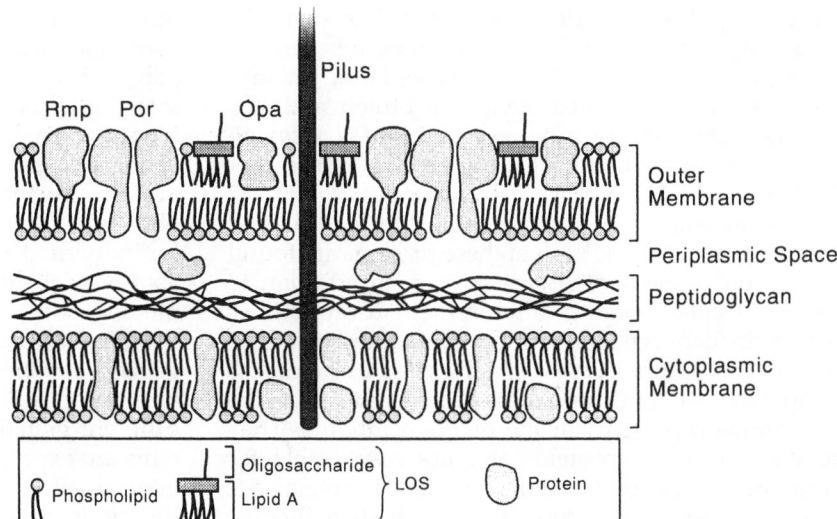

Figure 10-1.
Schematic representation of the surface structure of *N. gonorrhoeae*, showing the major components that contribute to pathogenicity and antimicrobial resistance. Opa, Por, and Rmp are the designations of the major outer membrane proteins (see text); LOS denotes lipooligosaccharide.

combinational events with each other to produce new antigenic types of pili. In a given strain at any given time, only a single pilus gene is functional, so only one pilus type is expressed. The total number of pilus types that may result from recombinational events among the 20 or so *pil* genes suggests that the array of different antigenic pilus types theoretically may be quite large. Additional studies also suggest that quantitative *pil* gene expression in *N. gonorrhoeae* may respond to positive and negative transcriptional regulation by signal-transducing proteins that are formed in response to various environmental stimuli, such as pH, osmolarity, and temperature. Pili, along with gonococcal outer membrane proteins, continue to be investigated as candidate antigens for development of gonococcal vaccines.[431]

N. gonorrhoeae bacterial cells also contain various proteins that are present on the surface of the outer membrane or that span the entire outer membrane (see Fig. 10–1). Gonococcal outer membrane proteins demonstrate or impart many biologic activities, including the elicitation of antibody formation and cell-mediated immune responses, decreased leukocyte association, and conference of resistance to the bactericidal effects of normal human serum.[410] In the cells of *N. gonorrhoeae*, some of these proteins are species-, strain-, and type-specific and have been exploited as possible antigens for the development of antigonococcal vaccines.[431] Porin protein, termed **Por** or **protein I**, is a heat-stable, LOS-associated protein of 32 to 36 kDa. This protein spans the width of the outer membrane and functions in the entrance and exit of small molecules to and from the periplasmic space.[410] Monoclonal antibodies directed against epitopes of Por are currently the basis for various serologic-typing schemes for gonococci.[251,385] These antibodies are also used in commercially available kits for identification of *N. gonorrhoeae* by staphylococcal coagglutination (discussed later).[6,223]

N. gonorrhoeae express outer membrane **opacity (Opa) proteins** (formerly called protein II) that also

function along with pili in mucosal adherence. Opa proteins have apparent molecular weights of 20 to 28 kDa.[425] The organisms possess 10 to 12 complete *Opa* genes in the chromosome, more than one of which may be expressed simultaneously. Regulation of *Opa* gene expression depends on the presence of a five-nucleotide sequence (CTCTT) occuring in triplicate (or a multiple of three times) at the 3′ end of the structural gene.[419] Generation of variability in the number of copies of the five-nucleotide sequence occurs during the process of DNA replication; subsequent transcription and translation of the genetic information results in a translational frame shift that results in the expression of up to three different Opa types.[91,92] A third type of gonococcal protein, called **protein III** or **Rmp** (reduction modifiable protein) has an apparent molecular weight of 30 to 31 kDa, is closely associated with LOS and Por, shows little inter- and intrastrain variation, and shares considerable antigenic identity with an *Escherichia coli* outer membrane protein called OmpA (outer membrane protein A).[156,350] Antibodies directed against OmpA bind to Rmp on the gonococcal cell surface and block binding of anti-LOS and anti-Por antibodies. The binding of these antibodies greatly diminishes the bactericidal effects of normal human serum on gonococci.[350] In addition to Por, Opa, and Rmp proteins, several other outer membrane proteins have been described in *N. gonorrhoeae*. Some of these proteins function as receptors for human transferrin and lactoferrin and probably act in acquiring the necessary iron for bacterial metabolism.[458]

Virulent *N. meningitidis* organisms possess polysaccharide capsules external to the outer membrane on the surface of the bacterial cells; 13 different capsular **serogroups** have been described (see later discussion). The capsules render the organisms resistant to phagocytosis, particularly in the absence of opsonizing antibodies.[11] Several protein antigens are also associated with the outer membrane of *N. meningitidis* strains. Certain of these proteins, along with the LOS serotypes (mentioned earlier), impart type-specific antigenicity along with the group-specific antigenicity associated with the polysaccharide capsule.[142,143] For example, serogroup B and C meningococci can each be further differentiated into 15 distinct serotypes based on antigenically distinctive outer membrane protein and LOS antigens. The outer membrane proteins of *N. meningitidis* can be divided into five classes based on their molecular weights: class 1 (44 to 47 kDa), class 2 (40 to 42 kDa), class 3 (37 to 39 kDa), class 4 (33 to 34 kDa), and class 5 (26 to 30 kDa).[143] All of these proteins are found on the outer membrane surface and, in addition to their molecular weights, differ in their susceptibilities to trypsin, deoxycholate, and heat denaturation. All *N. meningitidis* strains possess either a class 2 or a class 3 Omp, but never both, and these proteins constitute the predominant proteins in the outer membrane. They function as porin proteins and are responsible for serotype specificity. Class 1 and class 5 proteins are found in most meningococci, although both qualitative and quantitative differences in their expression have been noted. The typing system that is used for epidemiologic studies of meningococci is based on the polysaccharide grouping antigen along with antigenic differences between the class 2 or class 3 proteins and the LOS determinants present.[11,143,390] Antigenic determinants found on proteins 1 and 5, if present, are used to designate subserotypes. For example, a meningococcus of serotype C:2b:P1.3;P5.2;L3,7 is a group C meningococcus expressing a serotype "b" class 2 protein, a serotype 3 class 1 protein, a serotype 2 class 5 protein, and LOS types 3 and 7.[143]

Pathogenic *Neisseria* spp. also produce other factors that are believed to contribute to virulence. Both gonococci and meningococci produce an immunoglobulin A (IgA) protease capable of splitting humoral and secretory IgA1 into Fab and Fc fragments, potentially neutralizing the effects of secretory IgA and abrogating mucosal resistance to infection.[315] The meningococcal IgA protease is immunogenic, and antibodies to this enzyme appear during both infection and asymptomatic nasopharyngeal carriage.[52] The capsular material of *N. meningitidis* serogroup B strains is immunochemically indistinguishable from the neuraminic acid found in the human central nervous system; consequently, this organism's capsule is not recognized as foreign by the human immune system and is completely nonimmunogenic.[138]

The fastidious nature of *N. gonorrhoeae* and *N. meningitidis* is reflected in their nutritional requirements for growth and the methods these organisms use to obtain required nutrients. For example, *N. gonorrhoeae* strains will not grow in vitro unless the amino acid cysteine is present.[410] In fact, *N. gonorrhoeae*'s requirements for discrete amino acids, vitamins, purines, and pyrimidines have been employed as a method for typing gonococcal isolates, called **auxotyping** (discussed later in this chapter).[70,245,309,385] Nutritional and atmospheric conditions also contribute to the virulence of both gonococci and meningococci. Colonization and subsequent infection of mucosal surfaces by these organisms require iron, and both of these organisms have genetically regulated enzymatic methods for re-

leasing iron from transferrin and lactoferrin, thereby making the free iron available for bacterial metabolism.[81] Gonococcal mutants lacking these enzymatic capabilities are avirulent in animal models of gonococcal infection. A hemoglobin-binding protein has also been identified on the surface of *N. meningitidis* strains, indicating that hemin may also attach to, and be transported directly into, the bacterial cytoplasm, thereby obtaining the iron needed for growth.[269] Requirements for individual amino acids or other trace nutrients may also restrict the abilities of different gonococcal and meningococcal strains to cause certain clinical syndromes. *N. gonorrhoeae* strains also have the ability to grow anaerobically in the presence of nitrite as an electron acceptor.[242,244] Under these conditions, new and different genetically regulated outer membrane proteins are expressed.[86] This property may contribute to gonococcal virulence by allowing the organism to proliferate in anaerobic milieus, such as the endocervix, the rectum, the genital tract, and the pharynx, and would also explain the pivotal role of this organism in pelvic inflammatory disease, in which the organism may be recovered in culture along with obligately anaerobic bacteria.[81]

The virulence factors of *M. catarrhalis* are also under investigation because of the demonstrated pathogenicity of this species.[71] Most clinically significant isolates produce β-lactamase enzymes, which render these organisms resistant to ampicillin and amoxicillin. The elaboration of these enzymes contributes to the organism's virulence because isolates recovered from clinical disease produce more of these enzymes and have higher minimal inhibitory concentration values for ampicillin than commensal strains.[450] In vitro studies indicate that the *M. catarrhalis* β-lactamases may indirectly function in virulence by inactivating penicillin or ampicillin given for other respiratory tract infections, such as pneumococcal pneumonia.[197] *M. catarrhalis* strains are piliated, and the gene coding for the pili is related to the pilin gene of *M. bovis*, again reinforcing the close genetic (and, therefore, taxonomic) relation of *M. catarrhalis* to the other moraxellae.[289] Some workers have found that these pili mediate adherence to pharyngeal epithelial cells, whereas others have not been able to demonstrate differences in adherence among piliated and nonpiliated strains.[1,357]

In efforts to identify potential antigens for use in vaccine development, some surface-associated, highly conserved, outer membrane protein antigens have been identified.[317] Helminen and colleagues[189] identified a protein, designated UspA, that was present on every isolate of *M. catarrhalis* examined. The UspA protein has an apparent molecular weight of 300 to 400 kDa and may be closely associated with the outer membrane LOS. Passive immunization of mice with a monoclonal antibody reactive with UspA and subsequent endobronchial bacterial challenge resulted in enhanced pulmonary clearance of the challenge strain in an animal model.[286] In addition, convalescent sera from patients with culture-confirmed *M. catarrhalis* pneumonia contained antibodies directed against UspA on Western blot analysis. Another surface-expressed protein, designated CopB, has an apparent molecular weight of about 81 kDa and is found on about 70% of strains.[188] Antibody to this antigen also enhances pulmonary clearance of challenge *M. catarrhalis* organisms in the mouse model. Mutants that lack this protein fail to survive and do not initiate respiratory tract infections in mice, suggesting a role for the CopB protein in the establishment of a pulmonary focus of infection.[190] This same protein may also render some strains of the organism resistant to the bactericidal effects of normal human serum.[190] As with the pathogenic *Neisseria*, *M. catarrhalis* also posesses membrane-associated proteins that are able to bind lactoferrin and transferrin, thereby providing a means for the organism to acquire iron for growth.[317] Strains that are able to bind complement to the cell surface have also been described. More studies need to be done to elucidate the mechanisms whereby *M. catarrhalis* is able to cause serious human infections.

Most species in the genus *Neisseria* are a part of the commensal flora of the human upper respiratory tract. However, these organisms are being reported more and more frequently as etiologic agents of significant infectious processes. With the demonstrated ability of genetic exchange by conjugation and transformation among both the pathogenic and saprophytic *Neisseria*, the acquisition of plasmid-mediated virulence factors, such as antimicrobial resistance, is a likely eventuality.[108] The clinical significance of the various species of *Neisseria* will now be considered in further detail.

CLINICAL SIGNIFICANCE OF *NEISSERIA* SPECIES

NEISSERIA GONORRHOEAE

N. gonorrhoeae is the causative agent of gonorrhea, a bacterial infection of tremendous public health significance. In the United States, the incidence of gonorrhea steadily increased during the 1960s and early 1970s, with the highest incidence—over 460 cases per 100,000 population—occurring in 1975.[179] The "gonorrhea epidemic" that occurred during this time was attributable to several factors, including an increasing at-risk population of young adults, importation of less susceptible gonococcal strains along with the return of servicemen from the Vietnam conflict, increasing use of nonbarrier contraceptive methods (i.e., the birth control pill and intrauterine devices), and improved screening and outreach and contact tracing.[230] Since the early 1980s and into the 1990s, the incidence of gonorrhea has steadily declined. This trend was largely due to changes in sexual behaviors, particularly among gay and bisexual men, in response to the epidemic of human immunodeficiency virus (HIV) infection and to more effective case-finding among women. However, the incidence of gonorrhea is still high among sexually active teenagers and young adults, as a group, and this incidence has actually increased slightly over the last several years.[179] Risk factors for gonorrhea that have been recognized over years of study include low socioeconomic status, residence in urban areas, and past histories of gonorrhea and other sexually transmitted diseases. Gonococcal infection has increasingly be-

come a disease of the poor and disenfranchised and, as with HIV infection, epidemiologic associations have been noted between gonorrhea, the use of crack cocaine and intravenous drugs, and the exchange of sex for money and drugs.[230]

In males, *N. gonorrhoeae* causes an acute urethritis with dysuria and urethral discharge (Fig. 10–2).[179,230] The incubation period between acquisition of the organism and the onset of symptoms ranges from 1 to 10 days, with the average being about 3 to 5 days. Most men with gonorrhea have acute symptoms, but asymptomatic infections in men have been reported.[95] Infections in men are all asymptomatic during the prodromal stages of infection, and conversely, 95% to 99% of men with urethral gonococcal infection will experience a discharge at some time. The discharge is purulent in 75% of cases, cloudy in 20%, and mucoid in about 5%; the consistency of the discharge at presentation is affected by the length of time that the infection has been incubating and whether the patient has recently urinated.[230] About 4% of men presenting to sexually transmitted disease clinics with urethral gonorrhea are truly asymptomatic and have no signs or symptoms.[95,179] If left untreated, ascending infection in men may result in gonococcal epididymitis, epididymo-orchitis, prostatitis, periurethral abscess, and urethral stricture, although these complications are rarely seen in current practice. Homosexual and bisexual men may also acquire oropharyngeal and rectal gonococcal infections by engaging in unprotected oral or anal intercourse with an infected partner. Oropharyngeal gonococcal infection is usually asymptomatic. Rectal gonococcal infections are usually asymptomatic, but some individuals may experience acute proctitis with a mucopurulent discharge, bleeding, and tenesmus.[179]

In females, the primary infection is present in the endocervix, with concomitant urethral infection occur-

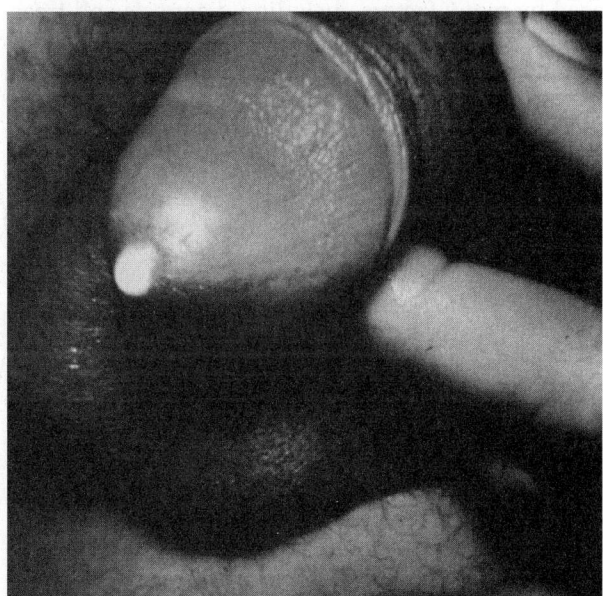

Figure 10-2.
Male with purulent urethral discharge characteristic of *Neisseria gonorrhoeae* infection.

ring in 70% to 90%. Patients may present with cervico-vaginal discharge, dysuria, abnormal or intermen-strual bleeding, and abdominal or pelvic pain; the latter may indicate the presence of upper genital tract disease. Most women who become symptomatic do so within 8 to 10 days after organism acquisition. Although it has often been stated that most women with genital gonococcal infection are asymptomatic, this is probably not true. This assertion was based on the detection of infected women during widespread screening, and it did not account for those women who presented to physicians or emergency rooms with a spectrum of symptoms referable to the genital tract (e.g., vaginal discharge, dyspareunia, menorrhagia) or the lower abdomen.[179,230,281] In women, symptoms of uncomplicated endocervical infection often resemble those of other conditions, such as cystitis or vaginal infections. Only 10% to 20% of infected women, however, will present with an obvious mucopurulent endocervical discharge. Infection of the Bartholin's glands and the periurethral glands of the external female genitalia may be seen in about one third of women with genital tract infection. Women may also acquire pharyngeal or rectal gonococcal infections by engaging in oro- and anogenital sexual practices; in some cases the anal canal may become secondarily infected by cervical secretions owing to the proximity of the rectum to the vagina.

Ascending gonococcal infection may occur in 10% to 20% of infected women and results in acute salpingitis, which can lead to scarring of the fallopian tubes, ectopic pregnancies, and sterility.[179,230] Symptoms of gonococcal salpingitis include lower abdominal pain, abnormal cervical discharge and bleeding, pain on motion, fever, and peripheral leukocytosis. Salpingitis caused by *N. gonorrhoeae* generally occurs early, rather than late, in infection and either during or shortly after menstruation. The development of salpingitis is influenced by many factors, including diagnosis and treatment for other genital tract infections, the use of oral contraceptives, characteristics of infecting strains, and the immune competence of the host. Obstruction of the fallopian tubes, leading to infertility, occurs in 10% to 20% of women following acute gonococcal salpingitis.

In a small percentage (approximately 0.5% to 3%) of infected individuals, gonococci may invade the bloodstream, resulting in disseminated gonococcal infection (DGI).[179,238] This infection is characterized by fever, hemorrhagic skin lesions (usually located on the hands or feet), tenosynovitis, polyarthralgias, and frank arthritis. The skin lesions are generally painful and appear as a necrotic pustule on an erythematous base (Fig. 10–3). On rare occasions, cutaneous involvement may be extensive. Mastrolonardo and associates[294] reported a case of DGI in a 24-year-old woman who presented with extensive vesicobullous, hemorrhagic, and necrotic lesions on the buttocks and lower limbs. In 30% to 40% of cases, organisms from the bloodstream may localize in one or more joints to cause a purulent and destructive gonococcal arthritis, commonly involving the knee, elbow, wrist, fingers, or ankle joints.[466] Occasionally, other joints may be in-

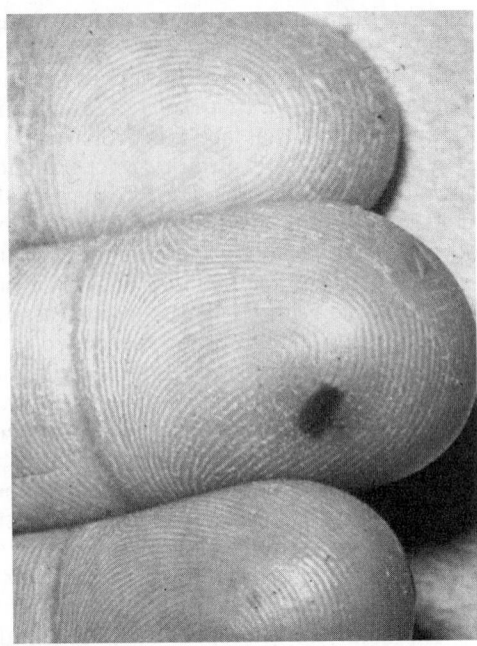

Figure 10-3.
Characteristic skin lesion of disseminated gonococcal infection on finger. Skin lesions are usually located on the extremities.

volved.[49,268] Complications of DGI include permanent joint damage, perihepatitis, endocarditis, and rarely, meningitis.[238,354,455] Perihepatitis, also called the Fitz-Hugh-Curtis syndrome, occurs when gonococci hematogenously seed the peritoneum, resulting in the formation of adhesions between the peritoneal mucosa and the surface of the liver. Gonococcal endocarditis occurs in about 1% to 2% of patients with disseminated infection and is characterized by a rapid and destructive course.[455] Pericarditis and pericardial effusions are also rare complications of DGI,[88,464] and adult respiratory distress syndrome has been reported in association with gonococcal bacteremia.[23] Gonococcal meningitis is a rare complication of disseminated infection.[354] Clinical entities that must be differentiated from DGI include Reiter's syndrome, pyogenic and crystal-induced arthritis, syphylitic and tuberculous arthritis, rheumatoid arthritis, Lyme disease, and rheumatic fever.[238] DGI occurs more frequently in females than males and is often temporally related to menstruation. Repeated bouts of DGI have also been observed in individuals with certain complement deficiencies.[369] Orogenital and anogenital sexual contacts may also result in oropharyngeal and anorectal gonococcal infections, respectively,[215] and systemic dissemination from localized infections at these sites may occur. Studies of isolates recovered from cases of DGI have shown that these particular strains have unusual characteristics, including unique nutritional requirements, resistance to the bactericidal action of normal human serum, and exquisite susceptibility to penicillin.[122,245,309,393]

In recent years, reports of unusual gonococcal infections have increasingly appeared in the literature. Ocular gonococcal infections, once seen primarily among neonates who acquired the organism during passage through an infected birth canal ("ophthalmia neonatorum"), are now being reported more frequently among adults who become inoculated with infected genital secretions.[453] Laboratory personnel who work with cultures of the organism may also become accidently infected if care is not taken to protect the eyes.[55] Infection of the eye results in periorbital cellulitis, a profuse purulent discharge, conjunctival injection, eyelid edema and erythema, and epithelial and stromal keratitis. Inadequate treatment of eye infections can lead to ulcerative keratitis, corneal perforation, and blindness.[433,453] Rare reports of primary cutaneous gonococcal infection, resulting from inoculation of a preexisting injury or lesion, have also appeared in the literature, including a case of gonococcal mastitis in a male.[32,397] Gonococcal scalp abscesses have been reported in neonates as a complication of intrauterine fetal monitoring.[16,340] Atypical presentations and clinical courses may be seen in patients with underlying diseases, including HIV infection.[314] Risher and McFadden reported a case of *N. gonorrhoeae* mycotic aneurysm of the ascending aorta in a 38-year-old woman with systemic lupus erythematosus that required prolonged antimicrobial therapy and surgical resection.[362] Strongin and coworkers[422] reported on a 27-year-old HIV-positive homosexual man who presented with gonococcal arthritis of the hip and a single sternoclavicular joint. In 1994, Bodsworth and associates reported the first case of gonococcal infection of the "neovagina" of a male-to-female transexual.[31] Lastly, Burnett and colleagues[57] reported a very unusual case of gonococcal ventriculoperitoneal shunt infection in a 17-year-old female. The authors postulated that the peritoneal end of the shunt, which yielded the heaviest growth of the organism, may have become contaminated with gonococci during menstruation, when menstrual blood may reflux through the fallopian tubes and enter the peritoneal cavity.

Gonococcal infections are not always symptomatic, and a reservoir of infected, asymptomatic individuals maintains this organism in the general population.[95,230] It is essential, therefore, that individuals at high risk for acquiring gonorrhea (and other sexually transmitted diseases) be screened periodically for gonorrhea and other infections. The appearance of AIDS and the recognition of HIV as a sexually transmitted agent has significantly decreased the incidence and prevalence of all sexually transmitted diseases among gay men, the group most at risk for all sexually transmitted diseases just over a decade ago.

Historically, gonococcal infections in children included only ophthalmia neonatorum, which is ocular gonorrhea transmitted to the infant during passage through the infected cervix.[275] Transmission of gonorrhea from adults to children by fomites (e.g., shared towels, and such) was proposed as a mode of transmission in older children. However, studies have concluded that children acquire gonococcal infection by sexual contact with an infected individual.[208] In 1983, the Committee on Early Childhood, Adoption, and Dependent Care of the American Academy of Pediatrics stated that, in children with documented gonococcal

infection, it should be assumed that sexual contact was the mode of acquisition and that such infections indicate sexual abuse.[90] With a careful, multidisciplinary approach, histories of sexual contacts could usually be obtained from abused children.[208] When a child with gonorrhea is identified, investigation of both adult caretakers and older siblings frequently reveals infected adults and other infected children.[3]

Gonococcal infections in children resemble those in adults, with some notable differences. *N. gonorrhoeae* causes a vaginitis, rather than a cervicitis, in prepubertal girls. The epithelium of the prepubertal vagina is composed of columnar epithelial cells, which are the cell types that *N. gonorrhoeae* preferentially infects. With the onset of puberty, these columnar epithelial cells are replaced by a thick, stratified squamous epithelium that is not susceptible to gonococcal infection.[179] Female children with genital gonococcal infection generally present with a vaginal discharge. Urethral infection in male children, if present, resembles gonococcal urethritis in adults. Pharyngeal and rectal gonococcal infections, as in adults, are usually asymptomatic in children.[3,208]

NEISSERIA MENINGITIDIS

N. meningitidis is a primary pathogen that causes a spectrum of infectious processes, ranging from occult sepsis with rapid recovery, to fulminant overwhelming disease resulting in death.[11] Individual patients may manifest only limited aspects of the clinical spectrum; others may progress across this spectrum, sometimes with alarming rapidity. The most serious clinical manifestation of meningococcal disease is meningitis; in fact, *N. meningitidis* is the second leading cause of community-acquired meningitis in the United States.[118,165] The classic signs of meningitis, such as confusion, headache, fever, and nuchal rigidity, may be seen only in about half of the patients.[11] Vomiting may also be a part of the clinical presentation, particularly in children. Meningitis may occur with or without meningococcemia. Meningococcemia and widespread dissemination of the organism are heralded by the rapid development of small hemorrhagic skin lesions called **petechiae**. Initially, these petechiae appear on the mucous membranes (e.g., the conjunctivae), the trunk, and the lower extremities. These lesions are indicators of bleeding complications and coagulopathies that are caused by the organism. Fulminant, rapidly progressive disease may result in coalescence of petechial lesions to form areas of cutaneous hemorrhagic necrosis. A nonpruritic, rubellalike rash has also been reported to occur in some cases of meningococcal disease.[467] About 10% of patients with meningococcemia develop **purpura fulminans**, resulting in extensive areas of tissue destruction secondary to coagulopathy; aggressive monitoring of coagulation parameters and replacement of coagulation factors may benefit some of these patients.[346] Diffuse neurologic involvement, rather than focal signs and symptoms, and myocardial involvement are seen more frequently with meningococcal meningitis than with other types of bacterial meningitis. Cardiac abnormalities, including purulent pericarditis with tamponade, are also a frequent complication during convalescence from meningococcal disease. The presence of shock, a low white blood cell count, a rash, and altered mental status on presentation are associated with a poor clinical outcome in these patients.[426] Death may supervene as a result of disseminated intravascular coagulation (DIC). In these fatal cases, autopsies often reveal terminal myocarditis or the lesions of DIC, with microthrombi and thromboses observed in many organs. The classic finding of acute hemorrhage into the adrenal glands represents the anatomic hallmark of the Waterhouse-Friderichsen syndrome. Despite the availability of excellent therapeutic agents, meningitis and sepsis caused by *N. meningitidis* still may have a mortality rate of up to 30%. Among survivors of infection, about 10% will have sensorineural deafness.[172,295]

N. meningitidis may also cause acute and chronic bloodstream infection (meningococcemia) without meningitis.[11] In the acute form, the patient usually presents with a slight fever and symptoms of a respiratory tract infection. Meningococci are recovered from blood cultures, but the patient is usually clinically well by this time, and no therapy or a short course of therapy is administered. With chronic meningococcemia, the patient is generally symptomatic, with fever, rash, and occasionally arthritis. This form of meningococcal disease, with or without recurrent meningitis, has been noted to recur in some patients, and such individuals frequently have underlying deficiencies in certain complement components (a picture similar to that seen with the gonococcus), particularly the terminal components of the cascade.[80,126,137,270,328,369] Meningococcemia has also been reported as a complication of upper gastrointestinal endoscopy; in this case, the organism was probably introduced from the upper respiratory tract into the bloodstream by mucosal damage that occurred during passage of the endoscope through the mouth and down into the intestine.[4] *N. meningitidis* sepsis has also documented as a complication of preterm labor in a 19-year-old woman, although complement studies were not performed.[322]

In recent years, primary meningococcal conjunctivitis has been recognized as a distinct clinical entity.[9] Conjunctival infection secondary to meningococcal meningitis has been recognized for a long time as a complication of systemic disease. Primary conjunctivitis caused by *N. meningitidis* has been reported in neonates, older children, and adults.[20] In two thirds of cases, the infection is limited to only one eye. In a review of 84 cases of primary meningococcal conjunctivitis, systemic meningococcal disease (i.e., meningitis or meningococcemia) developed in 17.8%; among these patients, the mortality was 13.3%.[20] Systemic infection occurred more frequently among those patients who received topical, rather than systemic, antimicrobial therapy; in fact, the risk of developing systemic disease was almost 20-fold greater for patients receiving topical therapy versus systemic therapy. Complications of the infection that were limited to the eye included corneal ulcers, keratitis, subconjunctival

hemorrhage, and iritis. In a report of three cases of primary meningococcal conjunctivitis in the United Kingdom, a younger sibling of the index case developed meningococcal meningitis, prompting the authors of this report to suggest that prophylaxis for close contacts of cases of primary meningococcal conjunctivitis is warranted.[416] In addition to infection of the eye, either primarily or secondarily, the development of transient cataracts in conjunction with the onset of rash and fever has been reported in association with meningococcal disease.[181]

N. meningitidis may also cause other infections, some of which result from hematogenous dissemination. Blood-borne spread of the organism may seed other internal organs, leading to complications such as osteomyelitis, arthritis, pericarditis, endophthalmitis, and peritonitis.[11,48,204,271,292] Meningococcal pneumonia apparently may occur by the hematogenous route or by aspiration and direct invasion of the lung parenchyma. Meningococcal pneumonia may occur in previously healthy young adults with no underlying diseases and in older persons with preexisting pulmonary compromise, such as systemic lupus erythematosus and AIDS.[48,193,211] Diagnosis of meningococcal pneumonia is complicated by the presence of the organism in the oro- and nasopharynx. In a study of 68 military recruits with meningococcal pneumonia proved by culture of transtracheal aspirates, fever, rales, and lobar infiltrates were common. The patients were moderately ill, and there were no fatalities.[257] *N. meningitidis* may occasionally be isolated from the male urethra, the female genital tract, and the anal canal. In these sites, it may cause infections that are clinically indistinguishable from gonococcal infections, such as acute purulent urethritis, cervicitis, salpingitis, and proctitis.[66,82,151,174,184,215,234,240,402,461] It is believed that orogenital, anogenital, and oroanal sexual practices may be responsible for the presence of meningococci in these anogenital sites.[185,215,462] Lastly, *N. meningitidis* is one of a long list of organisms that have been recovered from patients with peritonitis and bacteremia complicating continuous ambulatory peritoneal dialysis.[36]

The epidemiology of serious meningococcal disease is an area of considerable interest, and many unanswered questions surround this organism and the types of diseases it causes. Endemic meningococcal disease occurs at rates of 1 to 3 cases per 100,000 persons in the United States, and in 10 to 25 cases per 100,000 persons in developing countries.[396] Periodically, *N. meningitidis* infections will occur in epidemic forms, with attack rates higher than 500:100,000. Although there are currently 13 meningococcal capsular polysaccharide serogroups (A, B, C, D, H, I, K, L, X, Y, Z, W135, and 29E) recognized, most serious infections are caused by organisms belonging to serogroups A, B, C, Y, and W135.[48,130,144,396] Attack rates are highest among children aged 3 months to 1 year and among young adults, although occasional infections may be seen in the elderly. Group A and group C meningococci are frequently the cause of major epidemic disease, particularly in undeveloped countries and among the poorer segments of society, perhaps reflecting certain risk factors associated with transmission, such as crowding and poor sanitation.[166,427] Recent epidemics caused by serogroup A strains have occurred in Nairobi, Kenya, Nepal, Saudi Arabia, Chad, and Ethiopia.[169,338] Group B meningococci are a major cause of endemic, sporadic disease in developed countries. During the last three decades, strains of this serogroup have caused sporadic outbreaks in the Netherlands, Denmark, Norway, Great Britain, Canada, Iceland, Cuba, and Brazil.[14,73,255,384,391,392] In recent years, clusters of infections caused by serogroup C *N. meningitidis* have emerged in Iowa City, Iowa; Urbana-Champaign, Illinois; Los Angeles, California; Ontario, Quebec, and Saskatchewan, Canada; Italy, Denmark, and Brazil.[15,30,120,213,293,359,367,376,421,427,471] Groups B, C, Y, and W135 are the predominant serogroups now associated with clinical disease in the United States; group B and group C strains account for about 50% and 20% of sporadic disease, respectively.[396]

The pathogenesis of meningococcal disease is poorly understood and, although much has been reported on the descriptive epidemiology of the organism and the diseases it causes, very little is known about the dynamics of disease production. Humans are the only natural host for *N. meningitidis*, and the organism is spread by respiratory droplets. The organism may be asymptomatically carried in the oropharynx and nasopharynx of a variable percentage of individuals, and the rate of carriage is related to several factors, such as age, socioeconomic class, and the presence of actual disease in a community.[51] Carriage of meningococci in the nasopharynx may be transient, intermittent, or chronic. In general, carriage rates tend to be about 8% to 20%, with older children and young adults having higher carriage rates (20% to 40%) than young children.[74,326] The duration of carriage may also vary with the individual and the serogroup of the colonizing strain. During periods when disease is present in a community, the carriage rates may not be very different from observed rates when no clinical disease is being reported, but the proportion of individuals carrying the more virulent strain has been noted to increase.[11,396] Contrary to what has been promulgated for years, the rate of meningococcal carriage does not appear to be seasonal, although most meningococcal disease in developed countries tends to occur during late winter and early spring. Crowded living conditions facilitate respiratory spread of meningococci, and this crowding affects both the transmission of the organism and the occurrence of overt disease. This has been amply demonstrated by the large outbreaks that have occurred on military bases over the years, where large numbers of young, susceptible adults live together in close quarters for prolonged periods. Among such closed populations, carriage rates may approach 100%. Carriage strains may be encapsulated (groupable) or nonencapsulated (nongroupable) and result in the formation of serogroup-specific antibodies and broadly cross-reactive antibodies against several other outer membrane antigens. Even individuals who are colonized with nonserogroupable strains develop high titers of antibodies against groupable strains, probably owing to the presence of shared antigenic determinants. In one study of 38 individuals who carried nongroupable strains in the nasopharynx, 2% to 52% of the men developed group-specific antibodies, depending on the serogroup examined.[349] In most hosts, infection of the upper respiratory tract results in the formation of serogroup-specific serum bactericidal antibodies within 7 to 10 days.[11] This response does not eliminate the carriage state, but it may protect the host from overt disease.

In some individuals, the meningococcal strain that becomes established in the upper respiratory tract goes on to enter the bloodstream and initiate systemic disease. It appears that invasive *N. meningitidis* disease occurs in those persons who are newly infected with a strain against which the individual lacks bactericidal meningococcal serogroup-specific antibodies. In a study among military personnel, Edwards and coworkers[121] found that 86% of 31 patients had negative nasopharyngeal cultures during the 2 weeks before becoming ill, and that four patients were culture-negative the day before disease onset. Concurrent viral or mycoplasmal infection of the upper respiratory tract may also facilitate systemic invasion by the organism because both sporadic and epidemic outbreaks of meningococcal disease have also been associated with concurrent outbreaks of respiratory viral and mycoplasmal infections.[307,478] The risk of meningococcal disease is also higher among those individuals with deficiencies in the terminal complement components (e.g., C5, C6, C7, C8, and C) or the properdin system.[270,369,408] Other underlying conditions, such as hepatic failure, systemic lupus erythematosus, multiple myeloma, and asplenia may also predispose to serious meningococcal disease.[11]

Because the virulence of *N. meningitidis* is closely associated with the group-specific capsular polysaccharides of the organism, it has been possible to develop vaccines to protect against meningococcal disease.[141] Univalent group A and group C polysaccharide vaccines have been developed, as has a quadrivalent vaccine incorporating group A, C, Y, and W135 capsular material.[141] These vaccines are able to elicit an immune response in both children and adults. However, the vaccines are generally poorly immunogenic in children younger than 2 years of age.[27,235,272,333,334] It has also been noted that, particularly in young children, the elicited antibody titer falls fairly rapidly over time.[235] Currently, the quadrivalent vaccine is recommended only for individuals at high risk (e.g., those with complement deficiencies, travelers to areas that are highly endemic for meningococcal disease, military recruits, and those individuals living in an outbreak situation). Because of the overall low risk for infection in the United States and the failure to provide lasting immunity, the vaccine is not recommended for use in children.

Coupled with the poor immunogenicity of the purified meningococcal polysaccharide vaccines is the lack of immunogenicity of *N. meningitidis* serogroup B antigens. This serogroup is the one most commonly seen in the United States, but vaccines prepared from group B strains are poorly immunogenic even in adults. This is believed to result from the close resemblance of the group B capsular material to antigens found in human brain tissue; the capsule is recognized as "self" by the immune system, so there is no immune response to the group B organism's capsular material.[138] Current efforts to develop group B vaccines have centered around the organism's outer membrane protein (OMP) antigens. The OMPs of group B meningococci are immunogenic in both children and adults, but this immunity was demonstrated to be suboptimal in a double-blind placebo-controlled study.[142] To complicate matters, immunity to group B OMPs is type- rather than group-specific, so any potential vaccine would have to include the OMPs of several group B serotypes involved in disease production. Ways to increase the immunogenicity of both the type B capsular antigens and OMPs and the native capsular polysaccharides of the other meningococcal serogroups are under investigation. These efforts involve conjugating the polysaccharide material to protein carriers to provide an "adjuvant" for enhancement of the native antigenicity of the molecules.[27,141,142] Another approach to vaccine development involves the use of other antigens that are not considered a part of the meningococcal outer membrane complex. For example, the transferrin-binding proteins TBP-1 and TBP-2, which are expressed by meningococci during growth in vivo, have been demonstrated to be immunogenic in mice, and sera from eight patients convalescing from meningococcal disease caused by group A, B, and C N. meningitidis reacted immunologically with the TBP-2 protein purified from both the the homologous strain and representative heterologous strains.[2]

A few serogroup B meningococcal vaccines have been developed and field tested in parts of the world with high rates of both epidemic and endemic disease.[29,303,308] In an attempt to control an epidemic of group B disease in greater Sao Paolo State, Brazil, a Cuban-produced vaccine was given to over 2 million children aged 3 months to 6 years during 1989 and 1990. This vaccine, called the Cuban BC vaccine, consisted of purified, LOS-depleted, serogroup B outer membrane proteins of molecular weight 65 to 95 kDa. Purified group C polysaccharide was also included to provide protection against group C meningococci and to help solubilize the group B proteins. As reported with earlier group B vaccines, efficacy varied by age of the vaccinees. Among children 48 months and older, 74% had a protective immune response, whereas only 37% of children younger than 24 months of age had an effective immune response to the vaccine. In Norway, a group B vaccine efficacy trial was conducted using a vaccine containing group B polysaccharide, type (class 3) and subtype (class 1) protein antigens, and LOS immunotype antigens.[29] Vaccine recipients were 171,800 persons 13 to 21 years of age. The vaccine demonstrated only 57.2% efficacy in preventing meningococcal disease. Clearly, additional studies need to be done in formulating an effective vaccine against group B strains of N. meningitidis.

The risk of secondary meningococcal disease in close contacts of a primary case of meningitis or meningococcemia is 500- to 800-fold greater than that of the general population.[67,302] Therefore, it has become common medical practice to provide prophylactic antimicrobial therapy to these contacts. During the 1940s and 1950s, sulfonamides were found efficacious in eradicating the meningococcal carrier state and in preventing disease. However, during the 1960s resistance to the sulfonamides developed in N. meningitidis strains. High doses of penicillin transiently eliminate meningococci from the nasopharynx, but the organisms rapidly reestablish themselves after treatment is discontinued. Currently, oral rifampin is administered to eradicate carriage, although this drug does fail to eradicate the organisms in 10% to 20% of carriers.[51,94,396] Rapid emergence of rifampin resistance among meningococci has also been noted, even during the time of drug administration. In fact, a case of meningococcal meningitis caused by a rifampin-resistant strain was reported in a child who was receiving prophylactic rifampin at the time of disease onset.[94] Both ciprofloxacin and ofloxacin are also effective in eradicating the carrier state for prolonged periods, even after a single oral dose.[146,149,347]

OTHER NEISSERIA SPECIES

Neisseria lactamica is an organism that is of special concern because it is able to grow on selective media for gonococci and meningococci and must be differentiated from these organisms. It is found more frequently in the oropharnyges of children than in adults. In a study of 2969 infants and children, Gold and associates[153] found that the the carriage rates of N. lactamica increased from 3.8% at 3 months of age to a peak rate of 21% at 18 months of age, followed by a decrease to 1.8% by ages 14 to 17 years. These same workers also demonstrated that carriage of N. lactamica may stimulate the production of bactericidal antibodies against N. meningitidis groups A, B, and C because of antigenic cross-reactivity between the two organisms.[153] N. lactamica has been isolated as a rare cause of meningitis in both adults and children; the adult case was associated with a fracture of the cribiform plate.[101,164,182,264,463] It has also been associated with recurrent otitis media and with septicemia in a 7-year-old child during immunosuppressive therapy for acute lymphocytic leukemia.[327,388] This organism has been recovered from the endocervix.[226] In addition, N. lactamica strains that are resistant to penicillin have been isolated in recent years. These strains have an altered penicillin-binding protein (PBP 2) that is similar to the PBP 2 found in relatively penicllin-resistant strains of N. meningitidis, suggesting that commensal species, such as N. lactamica, could be the source of genetic resistance determinants currently being found in meningococci.[283,381]

Neisseria subflava (biovars *flava*, *subflava*, and *perflava*), N. mucosa, N. sicca, and N. flavescens have been most frequently reported in association with native and prosthetic valve endocarditis.[10,18,50,85,96,99,105,116,147,183,187,191,209,280,343,398,403,406,428,435,444] In cases of native-valve endocarditis, prior cardiac structural abnormalities caused by other underlying diseases (e.g., rheumatic fever) were frequently present. In many of the case reports, the use of intravenous drugs was a significant risk factor for these infections, in that oral secretions may be used as a solvent or to clean or lubricate the needle before injection.[18,96,403,428,435] Myocardial abscess formation has been documented as a complication of *N. mucosa* endocarditis.[136]

In addition to endocarditis, these normally saprophytic organisms have been isolated as causes of other significant infections. *N. subflava* has been isolated from joint fluid of a child with septic arthritis, from abscesses of the Bartholin's glands, as a cause of septicemia in a 63-year-old man with multiple myeloma, and as a cause of bacteremia and meningitis in a child.[100,325,348,472] At the University of Illinois, a *N. subflava* bv. *perflava* strain was also repeatedly recovered from urine cultures of a 10-year-old boy with congenital structural abnormalities of the urinary bladder.[220] *N. mucosa* strains have been isolated as unusual causes of meningitis, ocular infections, crepitant cellulitis, and bacteremia associated with dialysis in a 33-year-old man with end-stage renal disease.[152,278,404,420] *N. sicca* has been isolated as a rare cause of pneumonia and bronchiectasis, osteomyelitis, septic bursitis, Bartholin's gland abscess, and peritonitis in patients maintained on long-term peritoneal dialysis.[24,110,168,176,203,285,321,404] *N. subflava* bv. *perflava* and *N. sicca* have also been isolated from blood cultures of patients with end-stage HIV disease.[311] Rare strains of these organisms may present therapeutic dilemmas because some may be penicillin-resistant owing to elaboration of β-lactamase enzymes. In these cases, the isolates must be identified to species, and susceptibility tests should be performed.

Neisseria cinerea is a saprophytic species of the upper respiratory tract that is of particular interest because of its cultural resemblance to *N. gonorrhoeae*, its occasional recovery from genital sites, and its association with syndromes similar to those caused by gonococci, such as ophthalmia neonatorum and proctitis.[17,39,45,115,246,252] This organism has also been recovered as the cause of nosocomial pneumonia in a patient with AIDS and as an agent causing lymphadenitis.[47,87] In 1995, *N. cinerea* was isolated from blood and CSF cultures from a 17-year-old male following a fist fight in which he suffered significant facial trauma.[240a] The "species" *N. gonorrhoeae* subspecies *kochii* (or "*N. kochii*") has been isolated from patients with conjunctivitis in rural Egypt; no isolates have been described from the United States.[296] *Neisseria polysaccharea* is another respiratory tract commensal species. The carriage rate of this organism is about 0.5%, and it has not yet been described as part of a pathologic process.[38,61,360] *Neisseria canis* and *N. denitrificans* are animal strains isolated from the upper respiratory tracts of cats and guinea pigs, respectively. *Neisseria denitrificans* has not been associated with human disease, but *N. canis* has been recovered from human wounds resulting from cat bites.[171,196]

The rod-shaped members of the genus *Neisseria* include the three subspecies of *N. elongata* (subsp. *elon-gata*, subsp. *glycolytica*, and subsp. *nitroreducens*) and *N. weaveri*.[7,8,43,162,200] Up until 1990, *N. elongata* included only two subspecies, *N. elongata* subsp. *elongata* and *N. elongata* subsp. *glycolytica*. These organisms are normally found in the human upper respiratory tract. Neither of these subspecies had been implicated in human infections until 1995, when *N. elongata* subsp. *glycolytica* was isolated from wound specimens of three patients and from blood cultures of a 57-year-old man with subacute bacterial endocarditis and aortic insufficiency.[8] *N. elongata* subsp. *nitroreducens* was formerly called CDC group M-6.[162] This "moraxella-like" bacterium was shown to be related to the *Neisseria* species, in general, and to *N. elongata* subspecies isolates, in particular, on the basis of genetic studies, cellular fatty acid composition, and phenotypic properties. *N. elongata* subsp. *nitroreducens* is also found normally in the oropharynx of humans and has been reported as an opportunistic agent of bacteremia and endocarditis and as a cause of osteomyelitis following oral surgery.[145,158,162,256,336,405,423,469] It has also been isolated from urine and appendiceal tissue.[162] *Neisseria weaveri*, the rod-shaped organism that was formerly called CDC group M-5, is part of the upper respiratory tract flora of dogs and may be isolated from human wounds resulting from dog bites.[7,200]

CLINICAL SIGNIFICANCE OF *MORAXELLA CATARRHALIS*

During the last 10 years, the organism formerly called "*Neisseria catarrhalis*," "*Branhamella catarrhalis*," "*Branhamella (Moraxella) catarrhalis*," and now *M. catarrhalis* has received a great deal of attention as an emerging human pathogen.[25,71] Before 1990, it was believed that *M. catarrhalis* was a part of the normal human upper respiratory tract flora; over the years this assertion was made in many textbooks and case reports without any supporting evidence. Studies by Vaneechouette and colleagues[440] and Knapp and Hook[246] have now shown that the organism is found in the upper respiratory tracts of only about 1.5% to 5.4% of healthy adults and actually is more common in the respiratory tracts of healthy children (50.8%) and elderly adults (26.5%). A recent study from Denmark also reported that *M. catarrhalis* was not a significant member of the nasopharyngeal flora of adults and was rarely present in children younger than 1 month of age.[124] However, 36% of children aged 1 to 48 months had *M. catarrhalis* as a part of their respiratory tract flora. In this same age group, the prevalence of *M. catarrhalis* in children presenting with respiratory tract infections was 68%. A study of nasopharyngeal colonization with *M. catarrhalis* during the first 2 years of life showed that 66% of 120 serially cultured children become colonized during the first year and that 77.5% were colonized by the end of the second year.[131] Higher colonization rates have also been seen in preschool children with asthma (70%) than in healthy children (33%).[400] When isolated from adults with respiratory tract disease, the organism is more frequently found in specimens judged to represent lower respiratory tract secretions than in those specimens determined to have large amounts of oropharyngeal contamination. The organism is not, therefore, a significant part of the normal upper respiratory tract flora and may be involved in respiratory tract infections more frequently than previously thought.[440] The more frequent recovery of this organism from the respiratory tracts of children and the elderly supports its role in certain childhood infections (otitis media, acute sinusitis) and in lower respiratory tract infections (bronchitis, pneumonia) in older individuals.[131,440]

Infections of the respiratory tract and adjacent anatomic areas account for the majority of clinical conditions involving *M. catarrhalis* as an etiologic agent. These infections include otitis media, sinusitis, bronchitis, and pneumonia.[89,173,259,288,441] Although otitis media caused by this organism may occur in any age group, most studies have centered on this organism's role in pediatric infection. In a study by Van Hare and coworkers,[441] *M. catarrhalis* was the only bacterial pathogen isolated from middle ear fluid of 40 (11%) of 355 children with acute otitis media and was coisolated with either *Haemophilus influenzae* or *Streptococcus pneumoniae* in 21 (6%) of the patients. In vitro studies have shown that *M. catarrhalis* strains demonstrate increased adherence to nasopharyngeal epithelial cells of otitis-prone children than to cells from non–otitis-prone children.[418] Serial culture studies of otitis-prone children over the first 2 years of life have also shown that these children have consistently higher rates of colonization with *M. catarrhalis* than other children.[131] The bacteriologic findings with acute otitis media are mirrored in studies of acute sinusitis in the same age groups. In carefully collected maxillary sinus aspirates from children with acute sinusitis, *M. catarrhalis* may be isolated in either pure or mixed cultures from 2% to 16% of patients.[288] Acute sinus infections in adults have also been associated with this organism but with less frequency than in children.

Lower respiratory tract infections caused by *M. catarrhalis* occur predominantly in immunocompromised hosts, particularly those individuals with chronic obstructive pulmonary disease.[89,173,299,387,473] Immunologic abnormalities because of underlying diseases, such as diabetes or alcoholism, are also important contributory factors. *M. catarrhalis* is most frequently associated with clinical findings of acute bronchitis, with pneumonia being seen less often.[228] Patients with bronchitis caused by this organism usually present with increasing production of purulent sputum and mild respiratory distress without fever. Pneumonic involvement is heralded by the appearance of low-grade fever, dyspnea, and production of increasing amounts of purulent sputum.[387] Progression to respiratory failure has been observed in some patients. Radiologically, the disease usually appears as patchly infiltrates in both lungs, although lobar involvement with and without subpleural abscess formation has also been documented.[123,173] *M. catarrhalis* bacteremia and empyema secondary to pneumonia are uncommon. Epiglottitis caused by *M. catarrhalis* has also been reported as a complication of acute myeloid leukemia in a 65-year-old diabetic man.[445]

Despite its frequent involvement in otitis media and sinusitis in children, *M. catarrhalis* is an infrequent cause of community-acquired lower respiratory tract infection in this group.[84,258] In children with pneumonia, *M. catarrhalis* may behave as a primary pathogen or as a secondary pathogen superimposed on an antecedent viral infection (e.g., respiratory syncytial virus).[135] On rare occasions, *M. catarrhalis* may cause fulminant tracheitis and lower respiratory tract disease in apparently healthy children.[407] Fulminant pneumonia caused by *M. catarrhalis* has also been reported in preterm infants requiring ventilatory assistance.[119]

M. catarrhalis also has been isolated from patients with bacteremia, endocarditis, meningitis, conjunctivitis, eye infections, urogenital tract infections, wound infections, septic arthritis, nosocomial respiratory tract infections, and continous ambulatory peritoneal dialysis–associated peritonitis.[59,71,89,111,163,210,284,300,355,449] Bacteremia and endocarditis have usually occurred in individuals who were immunosuppressed by underlying diseases (leukemia, lymphomas, immunoglobulin deficiency states, AIDS), treatment for other conditions, or various types of invasive procedures (e.g., balloon angioplasty).[71,383,386,470] Predisposing conditions for *M. catarrhalis* bacteremia in infants include underlying disease (e.g., leukemia), neutropenia, respiratory insufficiency, prematurity or very young age, and congenital neurologic abnormalities.[34] Rare cases of meningeal infections with *M. catarrhalis* usually occurred after surgical procedures of the head and neck or involved infected ventriculoperitoneal shunts.[93,318] Conjunctival infections caused by *M. catarrhalis* have been documented in both the neonatal period and later in childhood. A scleral buckle infection and *M. catarrhalis* endophthalmitis secondary to glaucoma filtering surgery have also been documented.[59,279] "Ophthalmia neonatorum" caused by this organism is believed to result either from acquisition of the organism at birth from the mother's colonized genital tract or from respiratory tract secretions of the child's caretakers.[71] Recovery of this organism from the genital tract of either men or women is rare, but *M. catarrhalis* has been reported as a cause of a gonorrhea-like urethritis in a few cases.[111] It is an extremely rare cause of urinary tract infections.[125] Because of its close resemblance to *Neisseria* species and the frequency of isolation of this organism in the clinical laboratory, methods for identifying *M. catarrhalis* will be discussed following those used for the *Neisseria* species.

ISOLATION OF THE PATHOGENIC *NEISSERIA* SPECIES

ISOLATION OF *NEISSERIA GONORRHOEAE*

SPECIMEN COLLECTION

As with other pathogenic microorganisms, successful isolation depends on the collection of proper specimens, and this is particularly important for the recovery of *N. gonorrhoeae*. Because this organism can cause infection at a variety of body sites, collection of appropriate specimens for culture and diagnosis is dependent on the sex and sexual practices of the patient and on the clinical presentation. In all cases, specimens from genital sites (male urethra, female endocervix) should be collected. If the patient has a history of orogenital or anogenital sexual contacts, collection of oropharyngeal or anal canal specimens is also appropriate. In suspected cases of disseminated gonococcal infection, blood cultures and specimens from genital and extragenital sites should be obtained. Appropriate sites for culture are summarized in Table 10-2.

Specimens should be collected with Dacron or rayon swabs. Some lots of calcium alginate may be toxic to certain gonococcal strains.[265] Cotton swabs may also be used; however, some brands of cotton contain fatty acids that may be inhibitory for gonococci. Therefore, calcium alginate and cotton swabs should be used only if the specimen is inoculated directly onto growth media or is transported in nonnutritive media containing charcoal to absorb or neutralize inhibitory materials. Instruments used to aid in the proper collection of specimens (e.g., vaginal speculums) should be lubricated only with warm water or saline because various water- and oil-based lubricants may also be inhibitory. Direct smears for Gram stain should be prepared from urethral and endocervical sites and should be collected with a separate swab. For smear preparation, the swab should be rolled gently over the surface of a glass slide in one direction only. This technique will minimize distortion and breakage of polymorphonuclear leukocytes and will preserve the characteristic appearance of the microorganisms (Color Plate 10-1A). Smears from normally sterile or minimally contaminated sites (e.g., joint fluid, skin lesions) should also be prepared. Table 10-3 describes collection procedures for the recovery of *N. gonorrhoeae* from different anatomic sites.

The role of the clinical microbiology laboratory in diagnosing gonococcal infection in a child is crucial and involves the proper handling of appropriately collected specimens and the accurate identification of isolated organisms. Specimens should be obtained from the vagina or urethra, the oropharynx, and the rectum and inoculated onto media as described in the following.

SPECIMEN TRANSPORT

Although maximal recovery of gonococci is obtained when specimens are plated directly onto growth medium after collection, this technique might not always be possible or practical, particularly in busy clinics or hospital emergency rooms. For these situations, various types of transport systems are available:

Nonnutritive Swab Transport Systems. Stuart's or Amie's buffered semisolid transport medium can be used for the transport of swab specimens for *N. gonorrhoeae*. These systems are easy to use, are readily available in most clinic and hospital situations, and require no special equipment or storage conditions. Specimens sent to the laboratory in swab transport systems must be processed within 6 hours of collection, however, because there is a decrease in the numbers of viable organisms after this time. With these systems, long delays in transport and exposure to extremes in temperature (e.g., refrigeration) may compromise successful recovery of the organism. Transport medium containing activated charcoal is preferable if cotton swabs are used for the collection of the specimen. Some of the newer semisolid transport formulations (e.g., APO-Swab, Apotex, Inc., Windsor, Ontario) are also satisfactory for maintaining viability of *N. gonorrhoeae* for short periods.

Culture Media Transport Systems. Transport of specimens on culture media presents certain advantages and several systems for this purpose are commercially available. These include JEMBEC (James E. Martin *b*iological *e*nvironmental *c*hamber) plates containing various formulations of selective media and the Gono-Pak (Becton Dickinson [BD] Microbiology Systems, Cockeysville MD).[102,290] With these systems, media are inoculated with the specimen and placed in an imperme-

TABLE 10-2		
BODY SITES TO CULTURE FOR *NEISSERIA GONORRHOEAE*		
PATIENT	**PRIMARY SITE(S)**	**SECONDARY SITE**
Female	Endocervix	Rectum, urethra, pharynx
Male, heterosexual	Urethra	Pharynx
Male, homosexual/bisexual	Urethra, rectum, pharynx	
Female, disseminated infection	Blood, endocervix, rectum	Pharynx, skin lesions,* joint fluid[†]
Male, disseminated infection	Blood, urethra	Pharynx, rectum, skin lesions,* joint fluid[†]

*If present.
[†]Culture if arthritis present.

TABLE 10-3

S<small>PECIMEN</small> C<small>OLLECTION</small> P<small>ROCEDURES FOR</small> D<small>IAGNOSIS OF</small> G<small>ONOCOCCAL</small> I<small>NFECTIONS</small>

B<small>ODY</small> S<small>ITE</small>	C<small>OLLECTION</small> P<small>ROCEDURE</small>
Male urethra	Purulent discharge may be expressed by stripping the penis anteriorly and collecting the material on a swab. Specimens from asymptomatic males are obtained by inserting a calcium alginate nasopharyngeal swab 2–3 cm into the urethra. The swab is gently rotated as it is withdrawn.
Endocervix	After the speculum is in place, remove any cervical mucus with cotton or gauze. Insert the swab and collect the specimen with a gentle side-to-side motion. Allow time for the organisms to absorb onto the swab surface. Sample any purulent cervical discharge that may be present.
Rectum	Insert the swab 4–5 cm into the anal canal and gently move it from side to side to sample the anal crypts. Allow a few seconds for the organisms to adsorb onto the swab, and gently rotate the swab during withdrawal. If heavy fecal contamination is observed on the swab, collect another specimen with a fresh swab.
Oropharynx	With the aid of a tongue depressor, firmly swab the tonsillar areas and the posterior pharynx.
Blood	After venipuncture, inoculate suitable blood culture media (tryptic soy broth, Columbia broth) containing sodium polyanethol sulfonate (SPS). If SPS Vacutainer tubes are used for blood collection, transfer the blood specimen from the tube into culture media as soon as possible, because exposure to high concentrations of SPS may be inhibitory to gonococci.
Joint fluid	Material should be aspirated with a needle and syringe and hand-carried to the laboratory.
Skin lesions	Punch biopsy specimens are collected and placed in a sterile container with a small amount of broth or sterile saline and hand-carried to the laboratory.
Conjunctivae	Collect conjunctival discharge from the inner aspect of the lower eyelid with a small nasopharyngeal swab. Prepare smears for Gram stain as described above.

able plastic bag with a bicarbonate–citric acid pellet. Contact of the pellet with moisture (by evaporation of water from the medium during incubation [JEMBEC] or by crushing an ampoule of water adjacent to the pellet [Gono-Pak]) generates a CO_2-enriched environment within the bag. Incubation for at least 18 to 24 hours at 35°C before transport to a reference laboratory allows outgrowth of the organisms and minimizes the loss of viability that may be encountered with swab transport systems.

SELECTIVE CULTURE MEDIA

A variety of enriched selective media for culture of *N. gonorrhoeae* are available and include modified Thayer-Martin (MTM) medium, Martin-Lewis (ML) medium, New York City (NYC) medium, and GC-Lect medium (BD Microbiology Systems). All of these formulations contain antimicrobial agents that inhibit other microorganisms and allow the selective recovery of both *N. gonorrhoeae* and *N. meningitidis*. Table 10-4 shows the concentrations of antimicrobial agents present in MTM, ML, NYC, and GC-Lect agar media. Vancomycin and colistin, antimicrobials present in all four formulations, inhibit gram-positive and gram-negative bacteria (including saprophytic *Neisseria* species), respectively. Trimethoprim is added to inhibit the swarming of *Proteus* species present in rectal and, occasionally, in cervicovaginal specimens.[401] Nystatin, amphotericin B, or anisomycin is added to inhibit yeasts and molds.[291] MTM and ML are chocolate agar-

based media that are supplemented with growth factors for fastidious microorganisms, whereas NYC medium is a clear peptone–corn starch agar-based medium containing yeast dialysate, citrated horse plasma, and lysed horse erythrocytes.[133,291] All of these media allow selective recovery of *N. gonorrhoeae* from body sites harboring a large endogenous bacterial flora. The NYC medium will also support the growth of genital mycoplasmas and ureaplasmas. All of these media are commercially available in either petri dishes or JEMBEC plates. Their formulas are available in general media references. Various modifications of selective

TABLE 10-4

A<small>NTIMICROBIAL</small> A<small>GENTS IN</small> S<small>ELECTIVE</small> N<small>EISSERIA</small> M<small>EDIA</small>

A<small>NTIMICROBIAL</small> A<small>GENT</small> (μ/mL)	M<small>EDIA</small>			
	MTM	*ML*	*NYC*	*GC-LECT*
Vancomycin	3	4	2	2
Lincomycin	—	—	—	1
Colistin	7.5	7.5	5.5	7.5
Nystatin	12.5	—	—	—
Anisomycin	—	20	—	—
Amphotericin B	—	—	1.2	1.5
Trimethoprim	5	5	5	5

MTM, Modified Thayer-Martin medium; ML, Martin-Lewis medium; NYC, New York City medium.

media have also been described, such as a hemoglobin-free formulation of NYC agar.[160]

GC-Lect agar (BD Microbiology Systems) is another more recently developed, agar-based formulation for isolation of pathogenic *Neisseria*.[129] In addition to vancomycin, colistin, amphotericin B, and trimethoprim, lincomycin is also present (see Table 10-4). Evaluations indicate that GC-Lect medium may be superior to MTM in recovery of *N. gonorrhoeae* from clinical specimens, and that breakthrough growth of other organisms (particularly yeasts and gram-positive cocci) may occur less frequently. In addition, *Capnocytophaga* species, an organism normally present in the oropharynx, is also greatly inhibited on GC-Lect medium (see Chap. 8). Because of its "spready" growth patterns, recovery of gonococci from throat cultures may be compromised in the presence of *Capnocytophaga* organisms (see later discussion).

Strains of *N. gonorrhoeae* with increased susceptibility to vancomycin have also been reported.[305,465] These strains may account for a variable percentage of isolates depending on the geographic area. The appearance of these strains has prompted studies on the efficacy of media with and without vancomycin for the recovery of gonococci. In a study conducted in Seattle by Bonin and coworkers,[35] 92% of cervical gonococcal infections were detected with chocolate agar compared with 98% on MTM. Comparing MTM with a vancomycin-free selective medium (VFSM; MTM without vancomycin), 96% of 306 endocervical infections were detected with VFSM, whereas 98% were detected with MTM. The diagnostic yield was increased by 1.5% and 2.4% for 206 male urethral and 83 endocervical infections, respectively, when two sequential specimens were obtained from the patient and inoculated onto a biplate containing MTM in both halves. Therefore, MTM appears to be superior to either chocolate agar or VFSM for diagnosis of male urethral and endocervical gonococcal infections. Because the prevalence of vancomycin-susceptible gonococci varies from place to place, it is probably prudent to inoculate male and female genital specimens onto both selective (e.g., MTM) and nonselective (chocolate agar) media. Inoculation of a selective media only will also not allow recovery of other possible genital tract pathogens, such as *Haemophilus* species (see Chap. 7) or *Pasteurella bettyae* (the former CDC group HB-5) (see Chap. 8).

INOCULATION AND INCUBATION OF CULTURE MEDIA

Media for isolation of *Neisseria* should be at room temperature before inoculation and should not be excessively dry or moist. If excessive moisture is present on the lid of the plates, place them upside-down and slightly ajar in an air incubator at 35°C for 20 to 30 minutes. The "stacker plates" (BD Microbiology Systems) tend to seal up if excessive moisture is present, and growth of the organisms is retarded. Specimens collected on swabs are firmly rolled in a "Z" pattern on selective media and cross-streaked with a bacteriologic loop. If nonselective media are also inoculated, these plates should be streaked for isolation. The plates are incubated in a CO_2 incubator or a candle extinction jar at 35° to 37°C. The CO_2 level of the incubator should be 3% to 7% and should not exceed this, for some organisms will actually be inhibited at higher CO_2 concentrations. The CO_2 level in a candle extinction jar is about 3%. The atmosphere should be moist and, with candle jars, the moisture evaporating from the medium is usually sufficient for organisms' growth. The CO_2 incubators not equipped with humidifiers may be kept moist by placing a pan of water on the lower shelf. If candle jars are used, candles should be made of white wax or bees' wax; scented or colored candles release volatile products during burning and extinction that may inhibit the growth of the organisms.

ISOLATION OF *NEISSERIA MENINGITIDIS*

SPECIMEN COLLECTION AND TRANSPORT

Specimens helpful in the diagnosis of meningococcal disease include cerebrospinal fluid, blood, aspirates and biopsy specimens, and nasopharyngeal and oropharyngeal swabs. Occasionally, meningococci may be sought in sputum and transtracheal aspirates. Genital isolates of *N. meningitidis* may be recovered using the collection and inoculation procedures described for *N. gonorrhoeae*. Specimen collection and processing procedures are summarized in Table 10-5. Incubation conditions for the isolation of *N. meningitidis* are the same as those described for *N. gonorrhoeae*. Meningococci grow well on all selective media for the pathogenic neisseriae and vancomycin-susceptible strains have not been described. Contrary to widely held beliefs, most strains of *N. gonorrhoeae* will grow on commercially available sheep blood agar, albeit not as well as on chocolate agar. Recovery of both gonococci and meningococci from blood cultures may be adversely affected by the anticoagulant sodium polyanethol sulfonate (SPS) that is present in blood culture media. This effect may be neutralized by addition of sterile gelatin (1% final concentration) to the media or by processing the blood specimen by lysis–centrifugation (i.e., Isolator).[127,329,399]

IDENTIFICATION OF PATHOGENIC *NEISSERIA* SPECIES

PRESUMPTIVE IDENTIFICATION OF *NEISSERIA GONORRHOEAE*

COLONY MORPHOLOGY

Gonococci produce several colony types in culture. In Kellogg's scheme, these types are termed T1 through T5 and are described in terms of colony size and other colonial characteristics (coloration, topography of the colonies, reflection of light, and so forth).[237] On the individual cellular level, organisms comprising colony types P+ and P++ (formerly T1 and T2, respectively) possess pili on the cell surface, whereas cells in colony type P− (T3, T4, and T5) lack pili.[410] An-

TABLE 10-5

SPECIMEN COLLECTION PROCEDURES FOR ISOLATION OF NEISSERIA MENINGITIDIS

SPECIMEN	COLLECTION PROCEDURE
Cerebrospinal fluid	In cases of suspected meningococcal meningitis, as much spinal fluid as possible (at least 1 mL) should be sent for culture, because small numbers of organisms may be present. The CSF specimens should be hand-carried to the laboratory after collection and must not be refrigerated. The CSF should be centrifuged, and the supernatant saved for use in antigen detection procedures. Part of the pellet should be used to prepare a smear for Gram stain, and the rest should be inoculated onto chocolate and blood agar. A supplemented back-up broth (e.g., brain–heart infusion broth with 1% IsoVitalex) should also be inoculated with some of the pellet.
Blood	Blood should be cultured as described for gonococci. Direct inoculation of blood culture bottles is preferred over SPS Vacutainer tubes owing to the recognized inhibitory effects of SPS on meningococci. This inhibition may be overcome by the addition of 1% (final volume) sterile gelatin to the blood culture medium. It has also been demonstrated that lysed blood can neutralize the inhibitory and cidal effects of SPS on meningococci, and that the lysis of cells in the Wampole Isolator system overcomes the SPS effects on these organisms.
Petechiae	Specimens from petechial skin lesions may be collected by injection and aspiration of a small amount of sterile saline at the edge of the lesion, using a tuberculin syringe. Aspirates are cultured directly on chocolate and blood agars. Because some of the lesions are a result of immunologic phenomena, culture of skin lesions may be noncontributory for diagnosis.
Nasopharyngeal swabs	Nasopharyngeal swabs are particularly important for detecting colonization of individuals who are close contacts to cases of meningococcal disease and for carrier surveys. For these specimens, a fine swab on a flexible metal wire (e.g., a calcium alginate nasopharyngal swab) is passed through the oropharynx and behind the uvula, where the nasopharynx is sampled. Usually, carefully collected throat swabs will provide the same information. These specimens are inoculated onto a selective medium such as MTM agar.
Biopsies	Biopsy specimens should be hand-carried to the laboratory in sterile containers. Specimens should be moistened with sterile saline or broth and should not be refrigerated. In the laboratory, tissue specimens should be aseptically teased apart and cultured on chocolate and blood agar. A portion of the specimen should also be placed in a suitably supplemented backup broth medium.
Aspirates	Aspirates from closed spaces are collected with a needle and syringe and are inoculated onto chocolate and blood agars and into a suitable backup broth.

other descriptive system also addresses colony opacity characteristics determined by examination of growth on a transparent medium using magnification and substage illumination. Opaque colonies, regardless of size, are termed O+ and O++, whereas transparent colonies are termed O−. The colonial T types described by Kellogg and coworkers[237] can be recognized on routine MTM or chocolate agar cultures because appropriate transparent medium for determining the opacity characteristics of the colonies is not routinely available.

Isolates obtained on primary cultures are predominantly of the P+ and P++ colony types. These colonies tend to be small, glistening, and raised (Color Plate 10-1B). With subculture of individual piliated colonies the culture can be maintained in this colonial type. Organism suspensions prepared from 18- to 24-hour cultures containing primarily P+ and P++ colony types tend to be smooth and homogeneous. With nonselective subculture (i.e., a "sweep" of growth), the other colony types will become more evident, with all colonies eventually becoming the nonpiliated varieties. These types are larger, flatter, and do not have the characteristic glistening highlights of the piliated colony types. Cultures containing predominantly the

large colony types frequently do not form smooth suspensions, as the colonies become gummy and rubbery owing to autolysis and release of cellular DNA. The presence of all of these colony types on a subculture from a primary plate may frequently give the appearance of a mixed culture. Careful scrutiny and subculture with the use of a dissecting microscope (10×) enables one to become familiar with these colony types. Variation in colony type is invariably seen with fresh isolates of N. gonorrhoeae and occasional isolates of N. meningitidis. Atypical gonococci (i.e., those with multiple nutritional requirements such as the arginine–hypoxanthine–uracil [AHU]-requiring strains) also produce various colony types, but these develop more slowly and require the use of a dissecting microscope for detection and colony type characterization.[309]

GRAM STAIN AND OXIDASE TEST

Primary plates for isolation of N. gonorrhoeae should be examined after 24, 48, and 72 hours incubation using a hand lens or, preferably, a dissecting microscope. Smears prepared from suspicious colonies should be examined with the Gram stain, and an oxidase test should be performed. The Gram stain of the colony should show uniform, characteristic gram-negative diplococci. Some of the organisms may appear as tetrads, particularly on smears prepared from young colonies. Organisms on smears prepared from older cultures may appear swollen and display a wide variation in counterstaining intensity. Smears prepared from partially autolyzed colonies may be uninterpretable. Examination by Gram stain is essential for presumptive identification because other organisms may occasionally grow on selective media, particularly from oropharyngeal specimens (discussed later).

The best oxidase test results are obtained with the tetramethyl derivative of the oxidase reagent (N',N',N',N'-tetramethyl-*p*-phenylenediamine dihydrochloride, 1% aqueous solution). This solution is placed on a piece of filter paper and a portion of the colonial growth is rubbed onto the reagent with a platinum loop, a cotton swab, or a wooden applicator stick. With fresh cultures a dark purple color will appear within 10 seconds. Excellent results are obtained with the oxidase reagents that are packaged in crushable glass ampoules (e.g., Difco Oxidase Reagent, Difco Laboratories, Detroit MI).

SUPEROXOL TEST

Superoxol is another helpful test for the rapid presumptive identification of *N. gonorrhoeae*.[335,382] Superoxol is 30% hydrogen peroxide (not the 3% solution routinely used for the catalase test). *N. gonorrhoeae* strains produce immediate, brisk bubbling when some of the colony material is emulsified with the reagent on a glass slide. Both *N. meningitidis* and *N. lactamica*, the other species that grow on selective media, produce weak, delayed bubbling. In a study using this test on organisms recovered on selective media, all 201 gonococci tested produced immediate, vigorous bubbling in superoxol, whereas 241 of 242 meningococci and one of two *N. lactamica* strains produced negative or delayed, weak positive reactions.[382]

DIFFERENTIATION OF OTHER ORGANISMS ON SELECTIVE MEDIA

Both the presumptive and confirmatory identification of *Neisseria* species is dependent on the ability to differentiate these organisms from others that may also grow on selective media. These organisms include *Kingella denitrificans*, *Moraxella* species (other than *M. catarrhalis*), *Acinetobacter* species, and *Capnocytophaga* species. *K. denitrificans* grows well on MTM medium and produces colony types that resemble those of *N. gonorrhoeae*.[199] A rapid test that is useful in presumptively identifying gonococci and differentiating them from *K. denitrificans* is the **catalase test.** Gonococci will produce vigorous bubbling when growth from the plate is immersed in 3% hydrogen peroxide (H_2O_2): *K. denitrificans* produces a negative catalase reaction. *Moraxella* species, similar to gonococci, are oxidase-positive and catalase-positive. These organisms can be differentiated from *Neisseria* by the **penicillin disk test.**[69] The organism is subcultured to a trypticase–soy blood agar plate and streaked as a lawn to obtain confluent growth. A penicillin susceptibility disk (10 units) is then placed on the inoculum. After overnight incubation in CO_2, a Gram stain is prepared from growth at the edge of the zone of inhibition. *Neisseria* species and *M. catarrhalis* will retain their diplococcal morphology, although the cells may appear swollen. Coccobacillary *Moraxella* species will form long filaments or spindle-shaped cells under the influence of subinhibitory concentrations of penicillin. *Acinetobacter* species can be differentiated by their negative oxidase reaction. *Capnocytophaga* species appear as pale-staining, gram-negative, slightly curved, fusiform bacteria and are both oxidase-negative and catalase-negative. On prolonged incubation (i.e., longer than 48 hours) these organisms tend to spread owing to their gliding motility and may impede recovery of gonococci from oropharyngeal specimens (see earlier discussion of GC-Lect agar).

PRESUMPTIVE CRITERIA FOR IDENTIFICATION OF *NEISSERIA GONORRHOEAE*

All isolates of oxidase-positive, gram-negative diplococci that are recovered from urogenital sites and that grow on selective media may be **presumptively** identified as *N. gonorrhoeae*. The superoxol test described in the foregoing provides an additional presumptive test for identifying these isolates. However, confirmatory identification tests are recommended for all isolates and are required for identification of isolates from extragenital sites (i.e., throat, rectum, blood, joint fluid, cerebrospinal fluid). Furthermore, suspect gonococci isolated from children should also be confirmed by at least two different methods that involve different principles.[249,460] These may include carbohydrate utilization tests, immunologic methods (e.g., monoclonal antibody fluorescence tests; coagglutination tests), enzymatic procedures (e.g., chromogenic detection of specific enzyme activities) or the DNA probe culture confirmation test. This is extremely important because certain social and medical–legal issues are raised following release of the results.[460]

In sexually transmitted disease clinics the diagnosis of gonococcal urethritis in adult males is frequently made by the observation of gram-negative intracellular diplococci on a smear preprepared from the urethral discharge (see Color Plate 10-1*A*). When properly performed, the Gram stain is highly sensitive and specific for diagnosis of genital gonorrhea in men.[230,241] In females, Gram stain of a carefully collected endocervical specimen may also be very helpful in diagnosis (see section on specimen collection). Gram-stained smears of such specimens have a sensitivity of 50% to 70%, depending on the adequacy of the specimen and the patient population. An endocervical smear showing gram-negative intracellular diplococci, particularly from a woman with other signs and symptoms of gonococcal infection, is highly predictive.[281] In asymptomatic women, however, the predictive value of the Gram stain is much lower. At any rate, the Gram stain should not be relied on for diagnosis of endocervical or extragenital infections, and culture is necessary for making a diagnosis of gonococcal infection at these sites.

IDENTIFICATION TESTS FOR *NEISSERIA* SPECIES

Confirmatory tests for gonococci, meningococci, and other *Neisseria* species include carbohydrate utilization tests, chromogenic enzyme substrate tests, immunologic tests employing fluorescent antibody or staphylococcal coagglutination, and a DNA probe test for culture confirmation of *N. gonorrhoeae*.

CARBOHYDRATE UTILIZATION TESTS

Conventional CTA Carbohydrates. The conventional technique for the identification of *Neisseria* species employs cystine–tryptic digest semisolid agar-base (CTA) medium containing 1% carbohydrate and a phenol red pH indicator (Color Plate 10-1C). The usual test battery includes CTA-glucose, -maltose, -sucrose, and -lactose, plus a carbohydrate-free CTA control. The lactose structural analogue, o-nitrophenyl-β-D-galactopyranoside (ONPG), may be substituted for the lactose tube, and the addition of fructose to the test battery is helpful for identifying the various *N. subflava* biovars.[243] Some commercial CTA formulations may be supplemented with ascitic fluid to support the growth of more fastidious organisms. The CTA media are inoculated with a dense suspension of the organism to be identified from a pure 18- to 24-hour culture on chocolate agar. The inoculum is either prepared in 0.5 mL of saline and divided among the tubes, or each tube is individually inoculated with a loopful of the organism. The inoculum is restricted to the top ½ inch of the agar-deep tubes. The tubes are incubated in a non-CO_2 incubator at 35°C with the caps tightened firmly. With a heavy inoculum, most isolates produce a detectable change in the color of the phenol red indicator within 24 hours. If the inoculum is heavy enough, many strains will change the indicator within 4 hours. However, some fastidious gonococcal strains may require 24 to 72 hours to produce sufficient acid to change the indicator. Because CTA media containing 1% carbohydrate is used primarily for detection of acid by fermentative organisms, the small amounts of acid produced oxidatively by some strains of *Neisseria* species may not be detected.

Rapid Carbohydrate Utilization Test. This test is a non–growth-dependent method for the detection of acid production from carbohydrates. In this method, small volumes of a balanced salts solution (BSS; pH 7.0) with phenol red indicator are dispensed in nonsterile tubes to which single drops of 20% filter-sterilized carbohydrates are added (Color Plates 10-1D and 10-1E). A dense suspension of the organism is prepared in the BSS with a bacteriologic loop; this suspension may be mixed on a Vortex mixer to disperse clumps. One drop of this suspension is added to each of the carbohydrate-containing tubes. The tubes are incubated for 4 hours at 35°C in a non-CO_2 incubator or a water bath. This method is very economical, the reagents are easy to prepare and inoculate, and the results are clearcut. Details for this method are presented in Chart 63. The key to this technique is the use of "reagent grade" carbohydrates. Maltose obtained from some bacteriologic

media companies may produce positive or equivocal results for *N. gonorrhoeae* in the rapid carbohydrate degradation test, presumably owing to the presence of contaminant glucose. Inocula for this procedure may be obtained from the primary culture if sufficient colonies are present and if the growth is less than 24 hours old. Because bacterial growth does not occur in the test medium, small numbers of contaminants that may be present do not interfere with results. However, incubation cannot be continued overnight.

Commercial Carbohydrate Utilization Tests. Several commercial vendors currently market kits that use rapid fermentation test methods.

MINITEK *NEISSERIA* TEST. In the Minitek system (BD Microbiology Systems), paper disks impregnated with the appropriate carbohydrates are dispensed into individual wells of a plastic tray (Color Plate 10-1F). A small volume (0.05 mL) of a heavy suspension of the organism prepared in broth is pipetted into each disk-containing well. Plates are incubated without CO_2 and observed hourly. Most positive reactions occur within 4 hours; the remainder are read after overnight incubation.[312] Use of this system requires Minitek equipment (plates, pipet gun and tips, humidor, and disk dispenser) and is most convenient for those laboratories that use the Minitek system for the identification of other microorganisms. This system has been available for a long time and has generally produced carbohydrate utilization test results for *Neisseria* species that are equivalent to reference methods.[106] However, weak-positive glucose reactions have been noted with the Minitek system for some strains of *N. cinerea* and may result in their misidentification as *N. gonorrhoeae*.[45,115]

RIM–*NEISSERIA* TEST (RAPID IDENTIFICATION METHOD–*NEISSERIA*). In this kit system (Austin Biological Laboratories, Austin TX), small quantities (2 to 3 drops) of buffered, 2% carbohydrate–phenol red solutions (glucose, maltose, sucrose, lactose) and a buffer control lacking carbohydrate are added to five nonsterile, specially buffered microtubes included in the kit. Inocula from a pure 18- to 24-hour culture of oxidase-positive, gram-negative diplococci, growing on selective media or a chocolate agar subculture, are delivered into each of the tubes with small disposable plastic loops. After inoculation the tubes are agitated on a Vortex mixer for 10 seconds and incubated in air at 35°C for 1 hour. Acid production is indicated by a change in the phenol red indicator from red-pink to yellow or yellow-orange. Negative carbohydrate reactions remain red-pink or turn slightly pink-orange. In an evaluation of this system done at the University of Illinois, the RIM–*Neisseria* system identified 98% of 176 *N. gonorrhoeae*, 99% of 173 *N. meningitidis*, 94% of 48 *N. lactamica*, and 100% of 12 *M. catarrhalis* within 60 minutes.[222] Of those organisms correctly identified by the kit after 1 hour, 94% of the gonococci, 99% of the meningococci, and 84% of the *N. lactamica* strains were correctly identified after only 30 minutes. Other workers have also reported good agreement of the RIM–*Neisseria* test with conventional methods.[114,148,263,365] A similarly inoculated DNase test is also available separately for confirmation of *M. catarrhalis*.

API QUAD-FERM+. This product (bioMerieux-Vitek, Inc., Hazelwood MO) consists of a plastic strip with seven microcupules containing dehydrated buffers with a phenol red indicator (Color Plates 10-1G and 10-2G). The microcupules contain glucose, maltose, sucrose, and lactose, with a fifth control cupule lacking carbohydrate. The sixth cupule contains penicillin and phenol red for the acidometric determination of β-lactamase production by *N. gonorrhoeae* and *M. catarrhalis*, and the seventh cupule contains an acidometric test for detection of DNase production by *M. catarrhalis*. Following inoculation with a dense (MacFarland no. 3) organism suspension prepared in saline and incubation for 2 hours at 35°C, reactions are read and interpreted. The API QuadFERM+ provides reliable results compared with conventional systems, and the addition of the DNase test allows rapid identification of *M. catarrhalis* strains. The API Quad-FERM+ has shown excellent agreement with reference methods for identifying both *Neisseria* species and *M. catarrhalis*.[114,157,224]

OTHER CARBOHYDRATE UTILIZATION METHODS. The *Neisseria*-Kwik test kit (Micro-Biologics, St. Cloud MN), and the Gonobio Test (I.A.F. Production, Inc., Laval, Quebec, Canada) are also commercial modifications of the rapid carbohydrate test procedure. The *Neisseria*-Kwik uses a tray containing dehydrated carbohydrates in separate wells. Each well is inoculated with a heavy suspension of the organism prepared in buffer, and results are read after 3 to 4 hours by noting changes in the colors of indicators. The Gonobio Test is a 2-hour method that requires heavy inoculation of microtubes containing carbohydrate substrates. Both of these systems have been evaluated and compare well with conventional methods.[106]

CHROMOGENIC ENZYME SUBSTRATE TESTS

The enzymatic identification systems use specific biochemical substrates that, after hydrolysis by bacterial enzymes, yield a colored end product that is detected directly (e.g., a yellow nitrophenol or nitroaniline product) or after the addition of a diazo dye-coupling reagent (i.e., cinnamaldehyde reagent for detection of free β-naphthylamide). The use of these systems is restricted to those species that are able to grow on selective media (MTM, ML, NYC, or GC-Lect media; i.e., *N. gonorrhoeae*, *N. meningitidis*, and *N. lactamica*). Because some strains of *M. catarrhalis* grow on selective media, these systems will also provide a presumptive identification of this organism. The enzymatic activities that are detected in these systems include β-galactosidase, τ-glutamylaminopeptidase, and prolyl–hydroxyprolyl aminopeptidase (Table 10-6). β-galactosidase and τ-glutamylaminopeptidase are specific for *N. lactamica* and *N. meningitidis*, respectively. Absence of these activities and presence of prolyl–hydroxyprolyl aminopeptidase identifies an organism as *N. gonorrhoeae*. *M. catarrhalis* lacks all three of these activities. The commercial systems that use this approach are the Gonochek II, BactiCard Neisseria, and the Neisstrip.

Gonochek II. The Gonochek II (DuPont deNemours Co., Wilmington DE) is a single tube that contains the three dehydrated chromogenic substrates (Color Plate 10-1H). After rehydration with 4 drops of phosphate-buffered saline (pH 7.4), five to ten colonies of oxidase-positive, gram-negative diplococci from a pure culture growing on selective medium, or a suitable subculture, are emulsified in the tube with a wooden applicator stick. The tube is capped with the stopper and incubated at 35°C for 30 minutes. Specific color reactions in the bacterial suspension confirm the isolate as *N. meningitidis* (hydrolysis of τ-glutamyl-*p*-nitroanilide; yellow) or *N. lactamica* (hydrolysis of 5-bromo-4-chloro-3-indoyl-β-D-galactopyranoside; blue). If the suspension is colorless at the end of the incubation period, the stopper is split apart and the top part of the stopper is inserted into the tube. The tube is then inverted so that the bacterial suspension comes in contact with the diazo dye-coupler (*o*-aminoazotoluene diazonium salt [Fast Garnet]) present on the stopper. The detection of β-naphthylamine released by bacterial hydroxyprolyl aminopeptidase activity (red) identifies the isolate as *N. gonorrhoeae*. The absence of a colored product at the

---

TABLE 10-6
ENZYME ACTIVITIES USED FOR IDENTIFICATION OF THE PATHOGENIC *NEISSERIA* SPECIES

SPECIES	β-GALACTOSIDASE	γ-GLUTAMYL-AMINOPEPTIDASE	HYDROXYPROLYL-AMINOPEPTIDASE	BUTYRATE-ESTERASE
N. lactmica	+	−	+	−
N. meningitidis	−	+	v	−
N. gonorrhoeae	−	−	+	−
M. catarrhalis	−	−	−	+

+, positive reaction; −, negative reaction; v, variable reaction.

completion of the testing and reading steps provides a presumptive identification of *M. catarrhalis*. In our evaluation,[222] the Gonochek II identified 99% of 176 gonococci, 97% of 173 meningococci, and 100% of 48 *N. lactamica* and 10 *M. catarrhalis*, respectively. Several other investigators have also evaluated Gonochek II and have found it reliable for identifying these organisms.[54,106,456]

BactiCard Neisseria. The BactiCard Neisseria (Remel Laboratories, Lenexa KA) uses four chromogenic substrates that are impregnated on four individual test circles within a cardboard holder (Color Plate 10-2*A*). After moistening each of the four circles with a single drop of rehydrating fluid, several colonies of the organism taken from selective media (or from a subculture from selective media) are rubbed onto each of the four test areas. After incubation on the bench top for 2 minutes, the indoxyl butyrate esterase substrate circle (IB; 5-bromo-4-chloro-3-indolyl butyrate) is inspected for the appearance of a blue to blue-green color. If this test is positive, the organism can be identified as *M. catarrhalis*, and no further testing is necessary. If the IB test is negative, the card is incubated on the bench for an additional 13 minutes (total test time: 15 minutes). After this time, the β-galactosidase substrate circle (BGAL; 5-bromo-4-chloro-3-indolyl-β-D-galactopyranoside) is inspected for the presence of a blue-green color. If this test is positive, the organism can be identified as *N. lactamica*, and no further testing is necessary. If the BGAL test is negative, a single drop of color developer reagent is placed on the prolyl aminopeptidase (PRO; L-proline-β-naphthylamide) and the τ-glutamylaminopeptidase (GLUT; τ-glutamyl-β-naphthylamide) test circles. These two tests are read as positive if a definite pink or red develops within 30 seconds of reagent addition. A positive PRO reaction identifies the isolate as *N. gonorrhoeae*, whereas a positive GLUT reaction identifies the organism as *N. meningitidis*. The PRO reaction may also be positive for some *N. meningitidis* strains. At the University of Illinois, the BactiCard Neisseria test was compared with conventional identification procedures for 558 isolates. The BactiCard Neisseria identified 100% of 254 *N. gonorrhoeae*, 100% of 125 *N. meningitidis*, 98.2% of 54 *N. lactamica*, and 98.4% of 125 *M. catarrhalis* strains.[218] A third product, called Neisstrip (Lab M Ltd., Bury, United Kingdom) is very similar to the BactiCard, but does not have the indoxyl butyrate reagent for identifying *M. catarrhalis*. Dealler and colleagues reported that the Neisstrip identified 93 of 95 gonococcal strains; 2 of 400 nongonococcal strains were misidentified with the strip.[98]

IMMUNOLOGIC METHODS FOR CULTURE CONFIRMATION OF *NEISSERIA GONORRHOEAE*

Fluorescent Monoclonal Antibody Test. Identification of *N. gonorrhoeae* by fluorescent antibody (FA) techniques is fast and can identify both living and nonviable organisms. Older FA methods employed fluorescein-conjugated polyclonal antigonococcal anti-

bodies that were raised in rabbits. Nongonococcal isolates cross-reacted with this reagent and some gonococcal strains reacted weakly or not at all. The current FA procedure uses monoclonal antibodies that recognize epitopes on the Por outer membrane protein (the old protein I), the principal outer membrane protein of *N. gonorrhoeae*.[33,223,266,457] The commercial monoclonal FA test (*Neisseria gonorrhoeae* Culture Confirmation Test; Syva Co., San Jose CA) is performed by preparing a light suspension of the organism in 5 μL of water on an FA slide, allowing the suspension to dry, heat fixing the specimen, overlaying the smear with the FA reagent, and incubating the smear for 15 minutes. The smear is rinsed, air-dried, mounted with a cover slip, and examined with a fluorescence microscope. Gonococci appear as apple-green fluorescent diplococci (Color Plate 10-2*B*).

When the Syva reagent was initially introduced in 1986 to 1987, sensitivities and specificities of 100% were reported.[114,266,457] In 1989, Walton[452] reported the isolation of two FA-negative, β-lactamase-positive *N. gonorrhoeae* strains from two sexual partners. Boehm and associates[33] reported 100% sensitivity and specificity for the test but mentioned that an FA-negative, β-lactamase-positive strain was isolated subsequent to the completion of their study. In 1993, Janda and colleagues[223] found that the FA test correctly identified 95.4% of 151 β-lactamase negative strains but only 74.4% of 43 β-lactamase positive strains. In another 1993 study, Beebe and coworkers[22] found that 18 (4.6%) of 395 gonococcal strains isolated during 1991 and 1992 were FA-negative; six of the 18 strains were β-lactamase-positive. Serotyping data indicate that β-lactamase–producing and non-β-lactamase–producing strains that are negative with the Syva FA reagent belong to a variety of serovars and serotypes.[22,223] The current anti-Por monoclonal antibody mixture used in the Syva FA test needs to be augmented with additional antibodies that recognize epitopes on the *N. gonorrhoeae* strains not identified by the present reagent.

The advantages of the Syva FA test include its rapidity, the ability to test colonies directly from primary cultures, and the small amount of growth required for test performance. The Syva FA test is not intended for direct detection and identification of organisms on smears from patient specimens.

Coagglutination Tests. The coagglutination tests make use of the ability of protein A on *Staphylococcus aureus* cells to bind IgG molecules by their Fc region. Binding of antigonococcal antibody to killed *S. aureus* cells, and subsequent mixture with a suspension of gonococci causes visible agglutination of the suspension. Three coagglutination tests for the identification of *N. gonorrhoeae* are currently available:

PHADEBACT GC OMNI TEST. The Phadebact coagglutination test (GC OMNI test; Karo-Bio, Huddinge, Sweden) employs monoclonal antibodies to gonococcal Por (protein I), rather than polyclonal antibodies that were used in the older, original version of this test.[222] A suspension (0.5 McFarland standard) is prepared in buffered saline (pH 7.2 to 7.4) and is boiled for 5 minutes. After cooling, the suspension is mixed with test and control reagents on a cardboard slide. Agglutination of the suspension with the test, but not with the control reagent, within 1 minute is a positive test. A blue dye is incorporated in the reagents to help visualize agglutination against the white background of the card.

In general, this monoclonal antibody-based test is much improved over the former polyclonal antibody-based product.[33,65,106,223] Several favorable evaluations have been published, with reported sensitivities of 98% to 100% and specificities of 99% to 100%.[6,65,106,114,223] Organism suspensions heavier than the specified McFarland density, however, may yield false-positive results. In addition, the use of saline with a pH less than or greater than 7.4 has also been reported to produce false-positive results with some strains of *N. lactamica*, *N. cinerea*, and *M. catarrhalis*.[65,106,223,243]

GONOGEN I TEST. The GonoGen I (New Horizons Diagnostics, Columbia MD) coagglutination test also uses staphylococcal cells coated with monoclonal antibodies directed against the outer membrane protein I of several gonococcal serovars.[304] The test is performed, as described for the Phadebact system, using a boiled organism suspension (McFarland no. 3). Results are usually clearcut and appear within 15 to 30 seconds of mixing the test reagent and suspension. The kit contains test and control coagglutination reagents, as well as both positive and negative gonococcal test control suspensions. Evaluations of this test have reported sensitivities of 86% to 100% and specificities of 99% to 100%.[6,223,236,267,304]

MERITEC GC TEST. This coagglutination test (Meridian Diagnostics, Cincinnati OH) is very similar to the GonoGen I in test specifications and procedure. These reagents contain a red dye to enhance detection and interpretation of test results. Janda and associates[223] reported a sensitivity of 92.3% and a specificity of 99% for the Meritec GC test (Color Plate 10-2C).

Other Immunologic Tests. Another immunologic test system for identification of *N. gonorrhoeae* is the GonoGen II (New Horizons Diagnostics, Columbia MD). The GonoGen II uses protein I monoclonal antibodies that are conjugated to colloidal gold as the detection reagent. A suspension (McFarland no. 1) is prepared in 0.5 mL of an organism lysing solution, and 1 drop of the antibody reagent is added. After 5 minutes, 2 drops of the suspension are passed through a membrane filter that retains antigen–antibody complexes. Retention and concentration of the complex on the filter turns the filter red, identifying the organism as *N. gonorrhoeae*. Nongonococcal isolates result in the filter remaining white or pale pink. Janda and associates[223] found that the GonoGen II identified 91.8% of 194 *N. gonorrhoeae* strains; five strains were negative and 11 strains produced equivocal color reactions on the membrane. In addition, a meningococcal strain and two *N. lactamica* isolates repeatedly produced false-positive test results. Kellogg and Orwig[236] found that the GonoGen II iden-

tified 99.6% of 248 gonococcal strains, but seven of 22 *N. menignitidis* strains produced false-positive test results, leading these investigators to suggest that positive GonoGen II test results need to be confirmed by another method.

Carballo and colleagues also described a culture confirmation enzyme immunoassay for *N. gonorrhoeae*.[64] The test is performed in microtiter wells coated with monoclonal antibodies against commonly shared epitopes of the Por proteins (protein I). A well is inoculated with a suspension of the organism to be identified, and following incubation and washing, an anti-Por protein monoclonal antibody conjugated to the enzyme urease is added. After another incubation and wash step, urease substrate solution is added, resulting in a color reaction if the organism is *N. gonorrhoeae*. When this test was compared with conventional procedures with 276 gonococci and 85 nongonococcal isolates, the sensitivity and specificity of the urease-based test were 97.5% and 100%, respectively.[64] This test is not commercially available.

MULTITEST IDENTIFICATION SYSTEMS

Four kit systems are available that can be used not only for identifying *Neisseria* species but also for identifying other fastidious gram-negative organisms. These systems are the RapID NH (*Neisseria–Haemophilus*) system (Innovative Diagnostic Systems, Atlanta GA: Color Plate 10-2D) the Vitek NHI (*Neisseria–Haemophilus* Identification) card (bio-Merieux-Vitek, Inc., Hazelwood MO), the *Haemophilus–Neisseria* identification (HNID) panel (Dade/American Microscan, Sacramento CA: Color plate 10-2E), and the API NH system (bioMerieux, La Balme-les-Grottes, France).[19,114,216,217] All of these systems use modified conventional tests (e.g., acid production from carbohydrates, urease, indole, ornithine decarboxylase) and the chromogenic substrates described in the foregoing to provide either 2-hour or 4-hour identifications of *Neisseria*, *Haemophilus*, and other fastidious gram-negative bacteria encountered in clinical specimens. The Vitek NHI card generally provides excellent results for the pathogenic *Neisseria* species, and is also able to identify *N. cinerea*.[217] However, *M. catarrhalis* strains cannot be differentiated from other *Moraxella* species with the tests currently present on the card. The MicroScan HNID panel does not include *N. cinerea* in its database, and these organisms are misidentified as either *N. gonorrhoeae* or as *M. catarrhalis* when tested on this system.[216] In addition, some *N. meningitidis* strains do not produce clearcut reactions with key identification tests on the panel (i.e., acid production from maltose or from τ-glutamylaminopeptidase activity), resulting in misidentifications. The reformatted IDS RapID NH contains tests (e.g., nitrite reduction and an esterase substrate) that will presumably allow reliable identification of both *N. cinerea* and *M. catarrhalis*. A single evaluation of this system indicated that the RapID NH was reliable for identifying *Neisseria* species, but that some reactions were difficult to interpret.[114] In the study by Barbe and coworkers,[19] the API NH system was able to identify gonococci, meningococci, *N. lactamica*, and *M. catarrhalis* within 2 hours, whereas other *Neisseria* species required additional tests for correct species identification.

PROBE TECHNOLOGY FOR CULTURE CONFIRMATION AND DIRECT DETECTION OF *N. GONORRHOEAE*

Nucleic acid probes for culture confirmation were originally developed in research settings. In 1983, Totten and associates[430] developed a radiolabeled probe directed against the 2.6 MDa cryptic plasmid of *N. gonorrhoeae* and found the test to be highly sensitive. However, gonococcal strains that did not harbor this cryptic plasmid failed to react with the plasmid-directed probe. Subsequently, probes that hybridize specifically with rRNA of *N. gonorrhoeae* have shown much greater sensitvity.[375] In 1990, Rossau and coworkers[370] described a radiolabeled rRNA oligonucleotide probe and compared it with a similarly labeled cryptic plasmid probe. Although the rRNA probe was 100% sensitive and specific, the cryptic plasmid probe was equally specific, but less sensitive. However, the use of radiolabeled reagents and their entailed autoradiographic detection methods precludes the adaptability of these tests to routine clinical laboratory use. The development of colorimetric, fluorescent, and chemiluminescent hybridization detection methods have greatly facilitated the introduction of probe technology into diagnostic laboratories.[62]

Commercial probes for culture confirmation of *N. gonorrhoeae* initially included the OrthoProbe (Ortho Diagnostics, Raritan NJ) and the Gen-Probe AccuProbe (Gen-Probe, Inc., San Diego CA). Although some investigators reported reliable results with the OrthoProbe test, others found that the test was neither sensitive nor specific enough.[261,356] Ridderhof and colleagues[356] found that, although 127 of 134 *N. gonorrhoeae* were correctly identified, 12 of 34 nongonococcal *Neisseria* species, 1 *M. catarrhalis* isolate, and 1 *Moraxella urethralis* isolate were also positive with the OrthoProbe. The OrthoProbe test was subsequently removed from the market.

The Accuprobe *Neisseria gonorrhoeae* Culture Confirmation Test identifies the organism by the detection of specific rRNA sequences that are unique to *N. gonorrhoeae*. In the test, the organism is lysed and mixed with a chemiluminescent-labeled single-stranded DNA probe that is specifically complementary to gonococcal rRNA. After the hybridization occurs, the DNA probe–rRNA double-stranded complex is selected by a chemical process, and the presence of the probe in the double-stranded material is detected by addition of detection reagents that hydrolyze the chemiluminescent tag on the probe, thereby releasing light energy. This energy is detected in a chemiluminometer instrument, and the result is reported as positive or negative. In an evaluation conducted at the University of Illinois examining monoclonal antibody coagglutination procedures, the fluorescent antibody test, and the AccuProbe for *N. gonorrhoeae* identification, the latter test was the only procedure that was 100% accurate in

identifying *N. gonorrhoeae*.[223] Similar results for the AccuProbe test have been reported by others.[274,477] This test may be particularly useful for confirming those isolates that may not be easily identified by other confirmatory test procedures.

Probe technology is also used in the only currently available test for the direct detection of gonococci in urogenital specimens. The PACE (probe assay—chemiluminescence enhanced) 2NG system is a nonisotopic chemiluminescent DNA probe that hybridizes specifically with gonococcal rRNA. Specimens are collected as for culture and are placed in a transport–lysing solution. A sample of the specimen is mixed with the acridinium ester-linked probe. Following incubation, hybridized nucleic acid is separated from nonhybridized material. The acridinium ester-labeled probe–rRNA complex is assayed in a semiautomated chemiluminometer by the addition of an alkaline hydrogen peroxide solution. This hydrolyzes the ester linkage of the probe label, causing a release of light, which is detected in a chemiluminometer instrument. The amount of light released is directly proportional to the amount of gonococcal rRNA present in the specimen. The assay requires about 2 hours to perform.

Published evaluations of the PACE 2NG system suggest that the probe system may actually be more sensitive than culture, owing to the fastidious nature of the organisms.[79,175,277,448] This problem is more acute for laboratories that receive cultures of gonococci from remote sites, such as municipal sexually transmitted disease clinics. In all of the studies, probe competition assays were used to confirm whether culture-negative–probe-positive specimens were due to false-negative cultures or to false-positive probe results. Chapin-Robinson and coworkers[79] compared the PACE 2 with culture on 795 endocervical specimens and found that the resolved sensitivity and specificity of the assay were 100% and 99.5%, respectively. A similar study was conducted by Hale and associates[175] in three public health laboratories on 271 endocervial and 165 male urethral specimens. Twenty of 27 probe-positive–culture-negative specimens were resolved as false-negative cultures by probe competition; the resolved sensitivity and specificity of the PACE 2NG were 99.4% and 99.6%, respectively. Finally, a large study of the PACE 2 direct detection system, conducted in the Netherlands on 1750 specimens, reported a sensitivity of 97.1% and a specificity of 99.1%.[448] Hanks and coworkers[180] evaluated the PACE 2NG system as a test-of-cure and found that it was reliable for this application as soon as 6 days after treatment. The PACE 2NG system has also been evaluated for the detection of *N. gonorrhoeae* in pharyngeal and rectal specimens. The overall accuracy of the PACE 2 system for evaluating these specimens was 99.4%, with a sensitivity of 87.5% and a specificity of 99.7%.[273]

In addition to the PACE 2NG and the PACE 2CT (for direct detection of *Chlamydia trachomatis*), Gen-Probe, Inc. has also marketed the PACE 2C. The PACE 2C is a combination probe assay for simultaneous detection of *N. gonorrhoeae* and *C. trachomatis* in a single patient specimen. Specimens that are reactive in the

PACE 2C assay are further tested with the PACE 2NG and PACE 2CT assays to determine which (or both) of the pathogens is present. This combination assay has demonstrated accuracy similar to the stand-alone PACE 2 assays.[212]

The polymerase chain reaction (PCR) and other molecular techniques have also been applied to the direct detection of *N. gonorrhoeae* in clinical specimens. Ho and coworkers[194] designed a PCR assay for *N. gonorrhoeae* using primers that flanked the *cppB* gene, a nucleotide sequence of an integrated cryptic plasmid. This PCR test detected gonococci in 100% of 34 culture-positive urethral specimens. Birkenmeyer and Armstrong[28] evaluated an amplification technique called the ligase chain reaction (LCR) that uses two probes for detection of multicopy *Opa* genes and one probe for the detecton of multicopy *pil* genes of *N. gonorrhoeae*. Evaluation of 100 urogenital specimens and comparison with culture showed the LCR test to be 100% sensitive and 97.8% specific for the direct detection of *N. gonorrhoeae*.[28] The LCR assay has also been applied to the detection of *N. gonorrhoeae* in urine specimens from females. Examination of 283 urine specimens from a Birmingham, Alabama STD clinic resulted in a test sensitivity of 94.6% and a specificity of 100% in comparison with culture.[409] PCR has also been applied to the detection of gonococci in synovial fluid.[276,316]

CULTURAL CHARACTERISTICS OF *NEISSERIA* SPECIES AND *MORAXELLA CATARRHALIS*

The following sections present helpful features for the laboratory identification and characterization of the gram-negative cocci. Suggestions for the performance of differential and confirmatory tests described in detail in the previous section plus additional test procedures are also outlined. All of the characteristics for identification of *Neisseria* species and *M. catarrhalis* are shown in Table 10-7.

NEISSERIA GONORRHOEAE

Although the identification systems discussed in the previous section of this chapter and the biochemical characteristics in Table 10-7 are reliable for the routine identification of *N. gonorrhoeae* in the clinical laboratory, other techniques have contributed greatly to our understanding of the biology and epidemiology of the gonococcus. Techniques such as **auxotyping** and **serotyping** have been helpful in assessing the potential virulence, invasiveness, antimicrobial susceptibility, and genetic constitution of various strains of gonococci. Strains of gonococci that have specific requirements for certain nutritional growth factors are known as auxotypes.[70,250] Although as many as 15 different growth factors (such as requirements for valine, leucine, lysine, arginine, proline, hypoxanthine, citrulline, or others) may be assessed in auxotyping studies, strains requiring the triad of arginine, hypoxanthine, and uracil (AHU strains) have been the most closely studied. These strains are of particular interest because they are commonly recovered from patients with disseminated gonococcal infection (DGI) and are highly susceptible to penicillin.[245,309] The AHU strains and auxotypes that have been recovered from systemic infections are frequently resistant to the normal bactericidal action of human serum, which may partially explain their ability to enter the bloodstream.[393] AHU strains are also associated with asymptomatic urethral infections in men; in one study, 96% of asymptomatic men were infected with this auxotype.[95] The AHU strains grow as atypical colonies on agar media; some may require 72 hours or more of incubation before visible growth is observed.[309]

Studies on the immunologic characteristics of the gonococcus have included the characterization of the organism's outer membrane proteins and the development of monoclonal antibodies against epitopes of Por protein (protein I), the principal outer membrane protein of *N. gonorrhoeae*.[150,251] These antibodies can be adsorbed onto staphylococcal cells for use as coagglutination reagents. Several gonococcal-typing schemes have been developed using these techniques. For example, the typing scheme developed by Knapp and coworkers and currently used by the CDC consists of 12 coagglutination reagents. From the coagglutination pattern of a given isolate with these 12 reagents, 46 distinct patterns or **serovars** have been described.[250] These typing reagents have also been adapted to an enzyme immunoassay in which the endpoints were less subjective and more reproducible.[63] Applications of these typing schemes have included 1) the study of regional differences and temporal changes in gonococci nationwide and within communities, 2) the examination of serovar–auxotype relations, 3) the study of gonococcal serovars as indicators or predictors of virulence, 4) the use of serovar determinations to assess relapse versus reinfection in individual patients, and 5) the use of serovar determinations as a tool in forensic pathology relating to sexual assault and abuse.[150,243,250] A six-reagent kit for gonococcal typing (Gonotype; New Horizons Diagnostics) is also commercially available.[223] In addition to auxotyping and serotyping, other techniques for epidemiologic differentiation of gonococcal strains include antibiogram characteristics, plasmid analysis, riboprobing, isoenzyme analysis, and restriction endonuclease analysis with pulsed-field gel electrophoresis.[323,324,342]

Because of the medical–legal issues that are raised after isolating *N. gonorrhoeae* from a child, and the frequent recovery of gonococci from both genital and nongenital body sites, proper identification of isolates is imperative. Whittington and associates[460] reported on 40 bacterial isolates from children younger than 15 years of age that had been identified as *N. gonorrhoeae* and that were referred to the CDC for confirmation. Fourteen (35%) of these strains had been misidentified by the originating laboratory, including 4 *N. cinerea*, 3 *N. lactamica*, 2 *N. meningitidis*, 3 *M. catarrhalis*, 1 *K. denitrificans*, and an unidentified nongonococcal *Neisseria* species. In 10 of the 14 cases, the organisms were isolated from children for whom there was no supporting evidence of sexual abuse.

TABLE 10-7

CHARACTERISTICS FOR IDENTIFICATION OF *NEISSERIA* SPECIES, *MORAXELLA CATARRHALIS*, AND THE "FALSE *NEISSERIA*"

SPECIES	OXIDASE	CATALASE	GROWTH			ACID PRODUCTION FROM		
			SELECTIVE MEDIA, 35°C	CHOCOLATE AGAR, 22°C	NUTRIENT AGAR, 35°C	GLUCOSE	MALTOSE	FRUCTOSE
N. gonorrhoeae	+	+	+	−	−	+	−	−
N. meningitidis	+	+	+	−	−	+	+	−
N. lactamica	+	+	+	−	−	+	+	−
N. cinerea	+	+	−†	−	−	−	−	−
N. polysaccharea	+	+	v	−	+	+	+	−
N. sicca	+	+	−	+	+	+	+	+
N. subflava								
bv. *subflava*	+	+	−	+	+	+	+	−
bv. *flava*	+	+	−	+	+	+	+	+
bv. *perflava*	+	+	−‡	+	+	+	+	+
N. mucosa	+	+	−	+	+	+	+	+
N. flavescens	+	+	−	−	+	−	−	−
"*N. kochii*"	+	+	+	−	−	+	−	−
N. elongata								
ssp. *elongata*	+	−	−	+	+	−	−	−
ssp. *glycolytica*	+	+	−	+	+	+ʷ	−	−
ssp. *nitroreducens*	+	−	−	+	+	−/+ʷ	−	−
N. weaveri	+	+	−	+	+	−	−	−
N. canis	+	+	NA	NA	NA	−	−	−
N. denitrificans	+	+	−	NA	NA	+	−	+
N. macacae	+	+	−	NA	NA	+	+	+
N. caviae	+	+	NA	NA	NA	−	−	−
N. ovis	+	+	NA	NA	NA	−	−	−
N. cuniculi	+	+	NA	NA	NA	−	−	−
N. iguanae	+	+	NA	NA	NA	v	−	NA
Moraxella catarrhalis	+	+	v	+	+	−	−	−

+, positive reaction; −, negative reaction; v, variable reaction; +ʷ, weak positive reaction; −/+ʷ, negative to weakly positive reaction; NA, data not available.
*Reactions shown are for media with 0.1% nitrite, *N. gonorrhoeae* will reduce 0.01% nitrite.
†Some strains recovered on selective media.
‡Some strains grow on selective media.

In many instances, the laboratories reporting these isolates were using the commercial kits described earlier for identification of *N. gonorrhoeae*. As mentioned, some commercial carbohydrate utilization test systems may produce false-positive glucose reactions for *N. cinerea*, which could lead to the misidentification of this species as *N. gonorrhoeae*.[45,46] Coagglutination tests, although generally quite reliable, may produce false-negative results with some gonococcal strains and may also show false-positive results with some isolates of other *Neisseria* or related species, including *N. lactamica*, *N. cinerea*, and *M. catarrhalis*. Procedural details for

SPECIES	SUCROSE	LACTOSE	POLYSACCHARIDE FROM SUCROSE	REDUCTION OF NO₃	NO₂*	DNASE	TRIBUTYRIN HYDROLYSIS	HABITAT
N. gonorrhoeae	−	−	−	−	−	−	−	Humans
N. meningitidis	−	−	−	−	v	−	−	Humans
N. lactamica	−	+	−	−	v	−	−	Humans
N. cinerea	−	−	−	−	v	−	−	Humans
N. polysaccharea	−	−	+	−	v	−	−	Humans
N. sicca	+	−	+	−	+	−	−	Humans
N. subflava								
bv. *subflava*	−	−	−	−	+	−	−	Humans
bv. *flava*	−	−	−	−	+	−	−	Humans
bv. *perflava*	+	−	+	−	+	−	−	Humans
N. mucosa	+	−	+	+	+	−	−	Humans
N. flavescens	−	−	+	−	+	−	−	Humans
"*N. kochii*"	−	−	−	−	−	−	−	Humans (rare)
N. elongata								
ssp. *elongata*	−	−	−	−	+	−	−	Humans
ssp. *glycolytica*	−	−	−	−	+	−	−	Humans
ssp. *nitroreducens*	−	−	−	+	+	−	−	Humans
N. weaveri	−	−	−	−	+	−	−	Dogs
N. canis	−	−	−	+	−	NA	−	Dogs
N. denitrificans	+	−	+	−	+	NA	−	Guinea pigs
N. macacae	+	NA	+	−	+	NA	NA	Nonhuman primates
N. caviae	−	−	−	+	+	NA	+	Guinea pigs
N. ovis	−	−	−	+	−	NA	+	Sheep/cattle
N. cuniculi	−	−	−	−	−	NA	+	Rabbits
N. iguanae	v	NA	+	+	v	NA	NA	Iguanas
Moraxella catarrhalis	−	−	−	+	+	+	+	Humans

these tests (e.g., densitiy of the test suspension, type and pH of the suspending fluid) differ among manufacturers, and package insert instructions must be followed closely. Enzymatic tests for detection of gonococcal prolyl aminopeptidase must be used only for those neisserial isolates that are able to grow well on selective media. Some *N. cinerea* strains and occasional isolates of *N. subflava* bv. *perflava* may be recovered on selective media and may also be positive for prolyl aminopeptidase in commercial systems.[221] Isolates recovered from oropharyngeal sites may be particularly troublesome. *N. lactamica*, a species that grows well on selective media and that may be misidentified as *N. gonorrhoeae*, colonizes the oropharynges of almost 60% of children between the ages of 1 and 4 years.[153] If a laboratory is unable to establish a definitive identification, the isolate should be sent to a reference laboratory for further testing. If possible, the isolate should also be saved. This can be accomplished by removing the growth from a few chocolate agar plates, suspending the growth in 1 mL of decomplemented horse serum: brain–heart infusion broth (1:1), and storing at −70°C.

N<small>EISSERIA MENINGITIDIS</small>

On gram-stained smears prepared from clinical specimens, particularly CSF, meningococci appear as gram-negative diplococci both inside and outside of polymorphonuclear cells (PMNs). Organisms may display considerable size variation and tend to resist decolorization. Heavily encapsulated strains may have a distinct pink halo around the cells. Because the presence of inflammatory cells has prognostic value (e.g., with fulminant, rapidly fatal disease, many organisms and few inflammatory cells are present), the Gram stain report to the physician should include quantitation of both organisms and PMNs. In addition to Gram stain and culture of the CSF, the laboratory may also perform direct antigen detection tests for meningococcal capsular polysaccharides.[262] The direct antigen tests currently available will detect capsular antigens of groups A, B, C, Y, and W135. These reagents are available from several vendors (latex tests: Hynson, Westcott, and Dunning, Baltimore MD; Burroughs-Wellcome Corp., Research Triangle Park NC; Coagglutination tests: Pharmacia Diagnostics). Even though positive test results with these reagents are helpful for early diagnosis, a negative test does not rule out meningitis caused by any of the organisms that commonly occur. These tests should always be performed in conjunction with a Gram stain and culture on both enriched solid media and in a suitable enriched broth (e.g., brain–heart infusion broth with IsoVitalex).

Meningococci grow well on both blood and chocolate agars, as well as on the selective media for the pathogenic *Neisseria*. The CSF specimens should be cultured on nonselective media (as described in Table 10-5), whereas specimens that may harbor other organisms (e.g., oropharyngeal and nasopharyngeal swab specimens) should be inoculated onto both selective and nonselective media. Plates are incubated in 5% to 7% CO_2 at 35°C and inspected after 24, 48, and 72 hours. For CSF specimens on which no growth is evident on the primary plates, the enriched backup broth should be subcultured to a solid medium before a final report is issued.

Identification procedures for meningococci (and gonococci as well) produce the best results when inoculated from fresh 18- to 24-hour subcultures on chocolate or blood agar. In carbohydrate utilization confirmatory tests, the reaction in the maltose tube will frequently be much more intense than that in the glucose tube because maltose is degraded by the organism to two glucose molecules, which are then metabolized. Glucose-negative, maltose-negative, and asaccharolytic *N. meningitidis* strains have been isolated.[159,337,378,454] If such a biochemically aberrant strain is recovered, a chromogenic substrate confirmatory test or serogrouping of the isolate by the slide-agglutination technique should be performed.

Slide agglutination is the most commonly used technique for serogrouping meningococci. A dense suspension of the organism is prepared in 0.5 to 1.0 mL of phosphate-buffered saline (PBS), pH 7.2, from a 12- to 18-hour subculture on trypticase–soy blood agar. One drop of this suspension is mixed with 1 drop of meningococcal antisera on a sectored slide, and the slide is rotated for 2 to 4 minutes. Groupable strains will generally agglutinate strongly within this time. Although isolates from systemic infections will usually agglutinate rapidly, those from carriers may fail to agglutinate (nongroupable strains) or may autoagglutinate in the PBS. Use of younger cultures from blood agar (6 to 8 hours) or use of a serum-enriched media, such as trypticase–soy agar containing 10% decomplemented horse serum, may resolve these problems. Antisera for the major meningococcal serogroups is available from Burroughs-Wellcome Corp. and from Difco Laboratories. Some of these nongroupable strains may actually be *N. polysaccharea*; testing for production of polysaccharide from sucrose will help identify this species (see later discussion).[38] In addition to slide agglutination, serogrouping of meningococci may also been done by a whole-cell, indirect enzyme immunoassay and by a dot-blotting assay using monoclonal antibodies against serogroups A, B, C, Y, and W135. Rosenqvist and associates[368] found that the latter two techniques were more sensitive, more specific, and easier to interpret than slide-agglutination tests, but their applicability was limited by the availability of monoclonal, serogroup-specific reagents.

In addition to serogroup determinations, *N. meningitidis* isolates may also be serotyped and subserotyped on the basis of their outer membrane protein and LOS antigens (described earlier in this chapter). These techniques are used mainly for investigations of epidemics and sporadic outbreaks of endemic disease and are not amenable to routine clinical microbiology laboratories. In addition to these serologic techniques, several molecular techniques have been applied to investigations of meningococcal disease and to the epidemiology of *N. meningitidis* strains. These techniques include multilocus enzyme electrophoresis, restriction enzyme fragment length polymorphism analysis, rRNA probe technology (ribotyping), PCR amplicon restriction endonuclease analysis of the chromosomal *dhps* (dihydropteroatesynthase) and *porA* genes of *N. meningitidis*, and pulsed field gel electrophoresis.[58,170,239,260,332,421,429,474]

O<small>THER</small> N<small>EISSERIA</small> S<small>PECIES</small>

N<small>EISSERIA LACTAMICA</small>

N. lactamica resembles *N. meningitidis* in colony morphology and was initially thought to be a lactose-positive variant of *N. meningitidis*.[198] This species is resident in the throat and is found more frequently in children than in adults.[153] It grows on selective media and produces acid from glucose, maltose, and lactose. ONPG is also hydrolyzed and can be used as a substitute for lactose in the test battery. Some strains of this organism have been reported to cause false-positive reactions with some commercial coagglutination tests (e.g., the Phadebact GC OMNI test).[222]

NEISSERIA CINEREA

N. cinerea, a recently described species, has generated considerable interest because it produces colonies that resemble the large-colony types of *N. gonorrhoeae* and, with certain identification systems, may yield results consistent with *N. gonorrhoeae*.[45,46] Although this organism is part of the commensal flora of the upper respiratory tract, it has been isolated from other sites as well. In fact, the initial publication on this organism by Knapp and coworkers[252] described strains that had been isolated from cervical cultures on Martin-Lewis medium. Dossett and associates[115] also reported on the isolation of this organism from a rectal culture from an 8-year-old child with proctitis. The organism was misidentified as *N. gonorrhoeae* by the API NeiDENT and the BACTEC *Neisseria* differentiation kit (the latter two identification systems are no longer available).

N. cinerea grows on both blood and chocolate agar. On chocolate agar, after 24 hours incubation, colonies are about 1 mm in diameter and are smooth with entire edges. The organism does not produce acid from carbohydrates in either CTA-base media or the rapid carbohydrate degradation test. Weak positive reactions with glucose after overnight incubation have been reported with the Minitek system,[45] and its positive hydroxyprolyl aminopeptidase reaction may also produce misidentifications of *N. cinerea* as *N. gonorrhoeae*.[216,218,221] Most *N. cinerea* isolates, however, do not grow well on selective media; this characteristic precludes the testing of this organism on chromogenic substrate tests such as the Gonochek II and the BactiCard-Neisseria. *Neisseria cinerea* can be differentiated from the asaccharolytic species *N. flavescens* by its inability to produce polysaccharide from sucrose (see later discussion) and the lack of a discernable yellow pigment. This species can also be separated from *M. catarrhalis*, another asaccharolytic species, by its negative nitrate reduction, DNase, and tributyrin hydrolysis reactions (see Table 10-7).

A helpful test for differentiating *N. cinerea* from *N. gonorrhoeae* is the **colistin susceptibility test**. A suspension of the organism is prepared in broth (corresponding to a 0.5 MacFarland turbidity standard), and is swabbed on a chocolate or blood agar plate as for a Bauer-Kirby disk diffusion susceptibility test. A 10-μg colistin disk is placed, and the plate is incubated in CO_2 for 18 to 24 hours. *N. cinerea* is colistin-susceptible and will have a zone that is larger than or equal to 10 mm around the disk. Generally, *N. gonorrhoeae* will grow up to the edge of the disk.

NEISSERIA FLAVESCENS

N. flavescens is found in the respiratory tract and is rarely associated with infectious processes. This organism grows as smooth, yellowish colonies on both blood and chocolate agar. In addition to growth on nutrient agar at 35°C, most strains will also grow at room tem-

perature on chocolate or blood agar. This organism is able to synthesize iodine-positive polysaccharides from sucrose (see later discussion) and can be differentiated from *M. catarrhalis* by its inability to reduce nitrate and its negative DNase and tributyrin hydrolysis reactions.

NEISSERIA SUBFLAVA BIOVARS, NEISSERIA SICCA, AND NEISSERIA MUCOSA

Identification of the "nonpathogenic" *Neisseria* species is not generally necessary unless the organism is determined to be clinically significant, or if the organism is isolated from a systemic site (e.g., blood, CSF) or in pure culture. Identification is based on colony morphology, growth on simple nutrient medium, inability to grow on selective media, acid production from carbohydrates, reduction of nitrate and nitrite, and synthesis of a starchlike polysaccharide from sucrose. **Nitrate reduction** and **nitrite reduction** are determined in medium (tryptic–soy or heart infusion broth) containing 0.1% (w/v) KNO_3 and 0.01% (w/v) KNO_2, respectively.[242,243] **Polysaccharide synthesis** is determined by inoculating the organism onto brain–heart infusion agar containing 5% sucrose. Medium lacking sucrose is inoculated as a negative control. After incubation at 35°C for 48 hours, the plates are flooded with Gram's or Lugol's iodine (1:4 dilution). A positive test is indicated by the development of a deep blue color in and around the colonies synthesizing polysaccharide. We have also obtained excellent results by adding regular Gram's iodine (1 to 2 drops) to the sucrose-containing tube in the rapid carbohydrate degradation technique after 4 hours incubation. If positive, a deep blue color appears in the tube. This is compared with the tan color seen in the other carbohydrate tubes (e.g., the maltose tube) after addition of Gram's iodine.

N. subflava can be subdivided into three biovars (biovars *subflava*, *flava*, and *perflava*) on the basis of acid production from fructose and sucrose and synthesis of iodine-positive polysaccharide from sucrose (see Table 10-7). All three biovars reduce nitrite, but not nitrate. *N. mucosa* has a carbohydrate utilization pattern similar to *N. subflava* bv. *perflava* and also produces the iodine-positive polysaccharide, but reduces both nitrate and nitrite. All of these organisms also display varying degrees of yellow pigmentation. The *N. sicca* strains are biochemically identical with *N. subflava* bv. *perflava*, but they characteristically form dry, adherent, leathery colonies on agar media that cannot be emulsified readily.

NEISSERIA POLYSACCHAREA

N. polysaccharea is a newly described species that is found in the human oropharynx. It is an oxidase-positive, catalase-positive, gram-negative diplococcus that forms smooth yellow colonies.[360] In the orginal description of this organism, the ability to grow on selective media (e.g., MTM agar) was a key characteristic.[360] Subsequent studies indicate, however, that growth on selective media for the pathogenic *Neisseria* is a variable characteristic of *N. polysaccharea* because of the colistin susceptibility of some strains.[5] Strains that are able to grow on selective media have colistin MICs of 64 μg/mL or higher, whereas strains that are inhibited have colistin MICs of 1 μg/mL or less. The organisms are resistant to vancomycin. At 24 hours the organism forms colonies of about 2 mm in diameter on chocolate or blood agars. Acid is produced from glucose and maltose but not from fructose or lactose. Acid production from sucrose is variable and appears to depend on the types of media used to determine this characteristic. The extracellular polysaccharide that is produced by *N. polysaccharea* from sucrose is a D-glucan that is acidic, and production of various amounts of the material by different strains may explain the variable nature of the sucrose reaction.[361] Nitrate is not reduced, whereas nitrite frequently is reduced. Strains of this organism can be differentiated from *N. meningitidis* by the polysaccharide synthesis test and by τ-glutamyl-aminopeptidase. *N. polysaccharea* produces iodine-positive polysaccharide from sucrose and is τ-glutamyl-aminopeptidase-negative, whereas *N. meningitidis* does not produce iodine-positive polysaccharide from sucrose and is τ-glutamylaminopeptidase-positive.[5,38] Similar to *N. gonorrhoeae*, *N. lactamica*, and some *N. meningitidis* strains, *N. polysaccharea* is L-hydroxyprolyl-aminopeptidase-positive.[5,61] It requires cysteine for growth and does not grow on nutrient agar or on chocolate agar at 22°C. Although this organism's cultural characteristics resemble *N. meningitidis*, its outer membrane protein profiles resemble *N. lactamica* more than the pathogenic species.[61]

NEISSERIA ELONGATA SUBSPECIES

N. elongata subspecies *elongata*, *glycolytica*, and *nitroreducens* are rod-shaped members of the genus *Neisseria*. The first two subspecies were recognized in the last edition of *Bergey's Manual of Systematic Bacteriology* as *Neisseria* species, whereas the last subspecies, formerly known as CDC group M-6, was recently reclassified in the genus.[43,162,442,469] All subspecies are members of the human upper respiratory tract flora and all have been isolated from infectious processes.[145,336,405,469] These subspecies can be differentiated on the basis of catalase reactivity, acid production from glucose, and reduction of nitrate (see Table 10-7).

NEISSERIA GONORRHOEAE SUBSPECIES KOCHII ("NEISSERIA KOCHII")

In 1986, seven isolates of an unusual *Neisseria* were recovered from conjunctival cultures of children in two rural villages in Egypt.[296] These isolates grew on chocolate and modified Thayer-Martin medium and produced large, smooth colonies resembling meningococci. Similar to gonococci, these organisms required the amino acid cysteine for growth. The isolates were oxidase-positive, produced acid from glucose only, and were τ-glutamylaminopeptidase-negative. They did not react with fluorescent gonococcal monoclonal antibody reagents and failed to react with monoclonal coagglutination reagents used for serovar determina-

tions for *N. gonorrhoeae*. On further analysis, these strains had different surface proteins than the gonococcal strains to which they were compared. However, plasmid analysis showed significant homology with the plasmids commonly found in gonococcal strains. The DNA homology experiments showed sufficient similarity to both *N. gonorrhoeae* and *N. meningitidis*; on this basis, the workers felt that these isolates did not represent a new species but rather a subspecies of *N. gonorrhoeae*. Because these isolates would probably be identified as *N. gonorrhoeae* in a clinical laboratory and because their site of isolation and carbohydrate utilization pattern were similar to those associated with gonococci, these isolates have been named *N. gonorrhoeae* subsp. *kochii* or "*N. kochii*."[296] This species has not yet been formally adopted.

ATYPICAL AND NONHUMAN NEISSERIA SPECIES

Neisseria species with atypical or unusual biochemical or serologic profiles are being increasingly recognized. Hodge and coworkers[195] isolated an organism that was a meningococcus biochemically, yet reacted with monoclonal antibody immunofluorescence and coagglutination reagents for *N. gonorrhoeae*. Janda and colleagues isolated *N. subflava* bv. *perflava* strains from oropharyngeal cultures of homosexual men that grew luxuriantly on selective media (modified Thayer-Martin agar).[221,222] In chromogenic enzyme substrate tests, these organisms were identified as *N. gonorrhoeae* based on positive hydroxyprolylaminopeptidase reactions and negative β-galactosidase and τ-glutamylaminopeptidase reactions. More complete characterization of neisserial isolates, particularly from immunocompromised patients, may uncover other aberrant and unusual isolates in the future.

On occasion, the clinical microbiology laboratory may recover *Neisseria* species of animal origin from human infections, such as bite wounds from animals. Isolates may include *N. weaveri*, *N. canis*, *N. denitrificans*, and members of the "false neisseriae." All of these organisms exhibit typical gram-negative diplococcal morphology except for *N. weaveri*, which is a gram-negative rod. The biochemical reactions for these organisms are also presented in Table 10-7.

CULTURAL CHARACTERISTICS AND IDENTIFICATION OF MORAXELLA CATARRHALIS

M. catarrhalis grows well on both blood and chocolate agars, and some strains will also grow well on MTM and other selective media. Colonies are generally gray-to-white, opaque, and smooth. A selective medium incorporating acetazolamide as an inhibitor of other respiratory tract flora has also been described.[439] The organism is asaccharolytic in carbohydrate degradation tests and may actually turn peptone-based identification media alkaline. Most strains reduce nitrate and nitrite and produce DNase.[109] The DNase activity is detected by heavily spot-inoculating a plate of DNase test medium containing toluidine blue 0 on an area the size of a dime (Color Plate 10-2*F*). After overnight incubation, hydrolysis of the DNA is detected by a change in the color of the media around and under the inoculum from blue to pink. *S. aureus* and *S. epidermidis* strains are also inoculated onto the plate as positive and negative test controls, respectively. A 2-hour acidometric DNase test is included on the API QuadFERM+ strip (Color Plate 2-10*G*). In our evaluation of this system, all *M. catarrhalis* strains tested were DNase-positive after 2 hours incubation.[224]

M. catarrhalis may also be distinguished from *Neisseria* species by its ability to hydrolyze ester-linked butyrate groups (butyrate esterase).[412] This enzyme activity is detected with a substrate called tributyrin. A rapid fluorescent tributyrin hydrolysis test that uses 4-methylumbelliferyl butyrate as a substrate was reported by Vaneechoutte and coworkers.[438] In this study, all 62 *M. catarrhalis* strains were positive with this test within 5 minutes, whereas all other *Neisseria* species tested were negative. Janda and Ruther[219] evaluated a rapid tributyrin hydrolysis test called BCAT CONFIRM (Scott Laboratories). This test uses a microcupule containing a disk impregnated with tributyrin. Eight drops of a balanced salts–phenol red solution are added to the cupule, and several colonies of the isolate are then emulsified in the cupule. A change in the color of the indicator from red to yellow indicates hydrolysis of tributyrin and a positive test. In this study, all 68 *M. catarrhalis* strains were positive on the BCAT CONFIRM within 30 minutes, whereas all *Neisseria* species were negative. A very rapid (2.5 minute) and reliable indoxyl-butyrate hydrolysis spot test has also been described and is commercially available (Remel Laboratories; Carr-Scarbourough, Stone Mountain GA: Color Plate 10-2*H*).[97,282] This same test is also included on the BactiCard-Neisseria along with the three other chromogenic substrates for *Neisseria* identification (see Color Plate 10-2*A*).[218] The RapID NH system also contains a fatty acid ester hydrolysis test to assist in the identification of *M. catarrhalis*. Indoxyl acetate, which is used for the identification of *Campylobacter* species, can also be used as a substrate for the esterase enzyme of *M. catarrhalis*.[412]

Most clinically significant *M. catarrhalis* strains also produce an inducible, cell-associated β-lactamase.[113] Because of its inducible nature, rapid acidometric β-lactamase tests (i.e., those that rely on conversion of hydrolysis of penicillin to penicilloic acid) may yield false-negative results. Best results are obtained with the iodometric method or with the chromogenic cephalosporin test.[306]

With the recognition of *M. catarrhalis* as a primary pathogen in certain clinical settings and the suspicion that nosocomial infections with this organism may indeed occur, methods for strain typing have been investigated.[207,310] These methods include enzymatic biotyping, polyacrylamide gel electrophoresis of whole-cell proteins, immunoblotting, and restriction endonuclease analysis.[298,310,331] These methods have been applied to investigations of outbreaks of respiratory tract disease in critical care units in the United States and abroad.[330,355]

ANTIMICROBIAL SUSCEPTIBILITY OF *NEISSERIA* SPECIES AND *MORAXELLA CATARRHALIS*

NEISSERIA GONORRHOEAE

Before 1976, antimicrobial susceptibility testing of *N. gonorrhoeae* was not generally performed. At that time, however, strains of penicillinase-producing *N. gonorrhoeae* (PPNG) imported from Asia, Africa, and the Philippines were reported in the United States. These isolates contain a plasmid (extrachromosomal DNA) that carries the genes for a β-lactamase enzyme.[108,201] Between 1976 and 1979, PPNG were associated with sporadic outbreaks in the United States. Between 1979 and 1982, however, the number of cases of gonorrhea caused by PPNG strains increased 15-fold, with large outbreaks occurring in New York City, Los Angeles, and Miami. The PPNG strains have now become endemic in several metropolitan areas of the United States.[459]

With the appearance of disease caused by PPNG strains, spectinomycin became the drug of choice for the treatment of these infections. By 1981, however, four spectinomycin-resistant *N. gonorrhoeae* isolates had been reported, and subsequently, spectinomycin-resistant PPNG isolates also appeared.[13,344,479] Resistance to spectinomycin is due to a single-step ribosomal mutation that results in high-level resistance (i.e., MICs of 256 µg/mL or higher).

In 1983, a localized outbreak caused by penicillin-resistant, β-lactamase-negative gonococci was reported from North Carolina.[75] These strains lacked the β-lactamase plasmid and were negative with tests for β-lactamase detection. The plasmid composition of these strains was not appreciably different from other penicillin-susceptible gonococci. The high-level resistance in these organisms is due to a combination of chromosomal mutations at several genetic loci known to contribute to antibiotic resistance; these strains were designated chromosomally mediated-resistant *N. gonorrhoeae* (CMRNG).[132] Initial CMRNG isolates were detected by disk diffusion testing and subsequent agar dilution susceptibility testing of organisms recovered from patients who were not cured after treatment with penicillin or ampicillin. By October 1984, 446 cases of CMRNG infection had been reported to the CDC from 23 states that had been screening for this type of resistance.[351] The CMRNG strains generally have MICs for penicillin higher than 1.0 µg/mL, with 75% of these having MICs higher than 2.0 µg/mL. Most strains also show moderate resistance to tetracycline (MICs at least 2.0 µg/mL) and decreased susceptibility to erythromycin, cefoxitin, and trimethoprim–sulfamethoxazole. The CMRNG isolates are usually susceptible to both spectinomycin and ceftriaxone. They will generally grow on media containing 1.0 µg/mL penicillin and will show zones smaller than 25 mm around a 10-U penicillin disk.[351]

In 1985, the CDC reported the isolation of 12 *N. gonorrhoeae* strains from Georgia, Pennsylvania, and New Hampshire that were penicillin-susceptible but showed high-level tetracycline resistance (tetracycline-resistant *N. gonorrhoeae* [TRNG]).[76] Again, these isolates were recovered after treatment failures with oral tetracyclines. Agar dilution susceptibility testing showed high-level resistance to tetracycline (MICs of 16 to 32 µg/mL) and doxycycline (MICs = 8 to 24 µg/mL), but susceptibility to penicillin (MICs = 0.008 to 0.25 µg/mL), spectinomycin, and cefotaxime. These strains were also moderately resistant to cefoxitin. Studies have now determined that tetracycline-resistant *N. gonorrhoeae* harbor a 25.2 MDa plasmid resulting from the insertion of a tetracycline-resistance determinant (*tetM*) into the 24.5 MDa conjugative plasmid found in some gonococcal strains.[254,313] This gene is located on a transposon and has also been found in streptococci, *Mycoplasma hominis*, *Ureaplasma urealyticum*, *Gardnerella vaginalis*, *Kingella denitrificans*, *Eikenella corrodens*, and *N. meningitidis*.[247,364,432] The conjugative plasmid carrying the *tetM* determinant can be transferred to suitable recipient strains of *N. gonorrhoeae* by both genetic transformation and conjugation.[108] The *tetM* determinant is believed to code for a protein or proteins that interact with the gonococcal ribosome to prevent inhibition of protein synthesis by tetracycline.

With the recognition and characterization of PPNG, CMRNG, and TRNG strains, workers at the CDC have delineated five resistance phenotypes in *N. gonorrhoeae* strains.[352] These include 1) penicillin-susceptible strains (MICs lower than 2.0 µg/mL), 2) penicillinase-producing *N. gonorrhoeae* strains (PPNG, β-lactamase positive), 3) high-level, plasmid-mediated tetracycline resistant strains (TRNG, MICs of 2.0 µg/mL or higher) possessing the *tetM* determinant, 4) strains with chromosomally mediated resistance to penicillin (CMRNG, MICs of 2.0 µg/mL or higher), and 5) strains with high-level, plasmid-mediated resistance to both penicillin and tetracycline (PPNG, β-lactamase positive and having the *tetM* determinant). The appearance and spread of other resistance determinants among these five resistance phenotypes forms the basis of ongoing gonococcal surveillance conducted throughout the United States by the CDC.[155,395]

Because of increasing resistance of *N. gonorrhoeae* to previously recommended antimicrobial agents and based on several controlled clinical efficacy trials, the U.S. Public Health Service has recommended that all patients with uncomplicated gonococcal infection receive one of four single-dose treatment regimens.[77,117,154,177,178,202,297,341,345,366,417,443] These include ceftriaxone (125 mg IM), cefixime (400 mg orally), ciprofloxacin (500 mg orally), or ofloxacin (400 mg orally). Each of these four therapies also includes doxycycline (100 mg orally, twice a day for 7 days) for treatment of coinfecting *Chlamydia trachomatis*. Although not included in the formal treatment guidelines, azithromycin (1.0 g given orally, single dose) is also active against both *N. gonorrhoeae* and *C. trachomatis*.[177,417] Pregnant women should be treated with ceftriaxone (250 mg IM) followed by 7 to 10 days of erythromycin,

because the oral cephalosporins have not been studied in this population, and the quinolones and tetracyclines are contraindicated in pregnant women. Additional regimens for inpatient and outpatient treatment of salpingitis and disseminated gonococcal infections are also included in the PHS Treatment Guidelines.[77]

Subsequent to the publication of the 1993 PHS Treatment Guidelines and the recommendation of the fluoroquinolones as acceptable therapy for uncomplicated gonorrhea, gonococcal isolates with decreased susceptibility to ciprofloxacin and ofloxacin have been isolated. From January 1992 through June 1993, 22 isolates of *N. gonorrhoeae* that had ciprofloxacin MICs of 0.125 µg/mL or higher were isolated (suseptible strains have MICs of 0.06 µg/mL or less) from men with uncomplicated gonorrhea in Cleveland, Ohio.[78,253] These strains displayed intermediate susceptibility or resistance to penicillin, but were β-lactamase-negative; all strains were susceptible to ceftriaxone and cefixime. From January 1992 through January 1994, PPNG strains were isolated in Hawaii that also displayed decreased susceptibility to the fluoroquinolones. Some of these strains had ciprofloxacin MICs as high as 2.0 µg/mL.[78,248] These strains were recovered from patients who has traveled to or were sexual contacts of individuals who had recently traveled to Southeast Asia. These strains were resistant to penicillin and many were also resistant to tetracycline; all strains were susceptible to ceftriaxone and cefixime. Quinolone-resistant gonococcal isolates have also been reported in the United Kingdom.[161] The rapid emergence of resistance to the fluoroquinolones in *N. gonorrhoeae* suggests that the usefulness of these agents for treatment of gonorrhea will need to be reassessed in the not too distant future. Additional surveillance of gonococcal antimicrobial susceptibility in selected patient groups (e.g., women with pelvic inflammatory disease or other complications) who may receive other antimicrobial agents (e.g., cefoxitin, clindamycin, metronidazole, and gentamicin) is also necessary to prevent the emergence of clinically relevant resistance.[353]

The CDC has also made recommendations on the indications and methods for antimicrobial susceptibility testing of *N. gonorrhoeae*. These recommendations relate more to ongoing surveillance of gonococcal resistance patterns rather than to individual patient management. A multicenter study has been published in which disk diffusion and agar dilution interpretive criteria for these drugs were determined, and the guidelines for testing and interpretation have been published by the National Committee on Clinical Laboratory Standards (NCCLS).[227,319,320] In addition to disk diffusion and agar dilution, the E test has also been used to determine antimicrobial susceptibilities of *N. gonorrhoeae*.[437,476] The E test strips consist of a plastic carrier strip with a predefined continuous antibiotic gradient immobilized on one side. Procedural details and interpretive criteria for the performance of susceptibility tests on *N. gonorrhoeae* isolates are presented in Chapter 15.

NEISSERIA MENINGITIDIS

Routine susceptibility testing of meningococci is generally not performed because most strains remain susceptible to penicillin. However, the patterns of antimicrobial susceptibility of this organism also appear to be changing. In 1983, Dillon and associates[107] isolated a β-lactamase–producing meningococcal strain that harbored the same β-lactamase plasmid as many PPNG strains. This organism was coisolated with a PPNG from a urogenital specimen. In 1988, β-lactamase–producing meningococci were also reported in two patients with meningitis in South Africa, and other isolates have been recovered from patients in Spain.[37,140] In addition, *N. meningitidis* strains that are not β-lactamase-positive, but have diminished susceptibility to penicillin (i.e., penicillin MICs of 0.10 to 1.0 μg/mL) have also been reported in Spain and the United Kingdom.[60,358,377,379,414,424] This diminished susceptibility appears to be due to decreased binding of penicillin by a specific meningococcal cell wall penicillin-binding protein (PBP 2).[301] The alteration in the affinity of PBP 2 for penicillin results from an altered nucleotide sequence of the PBP 2 gene, *penA*.[480] Operationally, penicillin-susceptible *N. meningitidis* strains have penicillin MICs of 0.05 μg/mL or lower, whereas relatively resistant strains have penicillin MICs that range from 0.10 μg/mL to 1.0 μg/mL.[380] Similar low-affinity forms of PBP 2 are also seen in penicillin-resistant strains of other *Neisseria* species, including *N. lactamica*, *N. flavescens*, *N. polysaccharea*, and *N. gonorrhoeae*. The altered, low-affinity forms of PBP 2 in these *N. meningitidis* strains apparently arose from recombinational events that resulted in the replacement of parts of the native meningococcal *penA* gene with corresponding genetic material from the commensal *Neisseria* species.[44,380,381,413] Since the initial reports from Spain in 1985, relatively penicillin-resistant *N. meningitidis* strains have been reported in the United States, England, Sweden, and Canada.[30,56,214,358,424,434] Most of the relatively resistant meningococci that have been reported in the literature have belonged to either serogroup B or C.[26,30] The acquisition of the *tetM* tetracycline resistance determinant by *N. meningitidis* has already been mentioned.[432]

Meningococcal isolates from patients who are not responding well to antimicrobial therapy warrant a β-lactamase test and a disk diffusion test performed as described for *N. gonorrhoeae* (see Chapter 15). Since most clinical microbiology laboratories are not equipped to perform agar dilution tests, any presumptively penicillin-resistant meningococci should be sent to a reference laboratory for an agar dilution susceptibility test. Alternatively, the E test may also prove valuable in determining the antimicrobial susceptibility of individual meningococcal isolates.[205]

OTHER NEISSERIA SPECIES

Because zone size criteria for other *Neisseria* species have not been established, the method of choice for determining susceptibility to antimicrobial agents is the agar dilution method. There are anecdotal reports that the disk diffusion procedure, agar dilution procedure, and interpretive criteria published by NCCLS for gonococci also may be used for other *Neisseria* species.[319,320] Although these organisms will generally grow well on Mueller-Hinton agar, some strains may require medium supplementation provided by additives such as IsoVitalex.

MORAXELLA CATARRHALIS

The appearance and spread of resistance to antimicrobial agents among the pathogenic *Neisseria* are also reflected in the antimicrobial susceptibility of *M. catarrhalis* isolates. Before the mid-1970s, this organism was broadly susceptible to antimicrobial agents. β-lactamase-positive *M. catarrhalis* were first isolated in 1976; by the end of the 1970s, about 75% of strains produced β-lactamase enzymes. Jorgensen and coworkers studied 378 *M. catarrhalis* isolates that were collected during 1987 and 1988 and found that 84% of them produced β-lactamase.[229]

All *M. catarrhalis* strains should be tested for β-lactamase production. A study by Doern and Tubert[113] demonstrated that the chromogenic cephalosporin (nitrocefin) disk and tube tests had superior sensitivity for detection of β-lactamase when compared with tests using pyridinium-2-azo-*p*-dimethylaniline cephalosporin (PADAC), tube and disk acidometric and iodometric procedures.[113]

Broth dilution ampicillin susceptibility tests on *M. catarrhalis* isolates may produce confusing results. Some β-lactamase–producing strains will have high ampicillin MICs (12.5 to 25.0 μg/mL), whereas others will have low ampicillin MICs (0.10 to 0.40 μg/mL). Ampicillin broth dilution tests for the latter strains are inoculum dependent.[112,450,475] With smaller inocula (10^4 CFU/mL), these strains appear susceptible to ampicillin and other β-lactam antibiotics. With higher inocula (10^7 CFU/mL), these strains have higher MICs and are resistant. This inoculum effect was observed for ampicillin, penicillin G, cephalothin, cefamandole, cefuroxime, and cefaclor.

Studies of *M. catarrhalis* β-lactamase enzymes by purification and isoelectric focusing procedures have shown that three types of enzymes are found in strains of this organism.[450] Two of these enzymes—called BRO-1 (or Ravisio-type) and BRO-2 (or 1908-type enzymes)—seem to be the most common, and a third, called BRO-3, has recently been described.[83,206,451] Strains that produce BRO-1 enzymes account for about 90% of the β-lactamase–producing *M. catarrhalis* isolated from clinical specimens, and BRO-2–producing strains account for the remaining 10%.[450] Strains that produce the BRO-1-type enzyme possess significantly greater enzymatic activity than do strains that produce the BRO-2-type enzyme. It is likely that β-lactamase–producing *M. catarrhalis* strains for which ampicillin MICs are low produce the BRO-2-type enzyme. Patients who have been infected with β-lactamase–producing *M. catarrhalis* strains have also responded clinically to ampicillin and penicillin; it is possible that these infections were caused by BRO-2 enzyme-producing strains. The genes for β-lactamase production appear to be located on the chromosome or on a transposon that can be transferred by a conjugative mechanism.[232,233,451] Isolates of *M. catarrhalis* are generally susceptible to second- and third-generation cephalosporins (including several oral agents, such as cefixime and cefaclor), azithromycim, clarithromycin, erythromycin, trimethoprim–sulfamethoxazole, and β-lactam drug–β-lactamase inhibitor combinations.[21,229] Rare tetracycline- or erythromycin-resistant isolates of *M. catarrhalis* have been reported.[53,363]

More detailed information on antimicrobial susceptibility testing of these organisms is presented in Chapter 15.

REFERENCES

1. AHMED K: Fimbriae of *Branhamella catarrhalis* as possible mediators of adherence to pharyngeal epithelial cells. APMIS 100:1066–1072, 1992

2. ALA'ALDEEN DAA, STEVENSON P, GRIFFITHS E ET AL: Immune responses in humans and animals to meningococcal transferrin-binding proteins: implications for vaccine design. Infect Immun 62:2984–2990, 1994

3. ALEXANDER WJ, GRIFFITH H, HOUSCH JG ET AL: Infections in sexual contacts and associates of children with gonorrhea. Sex Transm Dis 11:156–158, 1984

4. AL-ZAMIL F, AL-BALLAA S, NAZER H ET AL: Meningococcaemia: a life-threatening complication of upper gastrointestinal endoscopy. J Infect 28:73–75, 1994

5. ANAND CM, ASHTON F, SHAW H ET AL: Variability in growth of *Neisseria polysaccharea* on colistin-containing selective media for *Neisseria* spp. J Clin Microbiol 29:2434–2437, 1991

6. ANAND CM, GUBASH SM, SHAW H: Serologic confirmation of *Neisseria gonorrhoeae* by monoclonal antibody-based coagglutination reagents. J Clin Microbiol 26:2283–2286, 1988

7. ANDERSEN BM, STEIGERWALT AG, O'CONNOR SP ET AL: *Neisseria weaveri* sp. nov., formerly CDC group M-5, a gram-negative bacterium associated with dog bite wounds. J Clin Microbiol 31:2456–2466, 1993

8. ANDERSEN BM, WEYANT RS, STEIGERWALT AG ET AL: Characterization of *Neisseria elongata* subsp. *glycolytica* isolates obtained from human wound specimens and blood cultures. J Clin Microbiol 33:76–78, 1995

9. ANDERSEN J, LIND I: Characterization of *Neisseria meningitidis* isolates and clinical features of meningococcal conjunctivitis in ten patients. Eur J Clin Microbiol Infect Dis 13:388–393, 1994

10. ANDERSON MD, MILLER LK: Endocarditis due to *Neisseria mucosa*. Clin Infect Dis 16:184, 1993

11. APICELLA MA: *Neisseria meningitidis*. In Mandell GL, Bennett JE, Dolin R (eds.), *Mandell, Douglas, and Bennett's Principles and Practice of Infectious Diseases*, 4th ed, pp 1896–1909. New York, Churchill Livingstone, 1990

12. APICELLA MA, SHERO M, JARVIS GA ET AL: Phenotypic variation in epitope expression of *Neisseria gonorrhoeae* lipooligosaccharide. Infect Immun 55:1755–1751, 1987

13. ASHFORD WA, POTTS DW, ADAMS HJU ET AL: Spectinomycin-resistant penicillinase-producing *Neisseria gonorrhoeae*. Lancet 2:1035–1037, 1981

14. ASHTON FE, MANCINO L, RYAN AJ ET AL: Serotypes and subtypes of *Neisseria meningitidis* serogroup B strains associated with meningococcal disease in Canada, 1977–1989. Can J Microbiol 37:613–617, 1991

15. ASHTON FE, RYAN JA, BORCZYK A ET AL: Emergence of a virulent clone of *Neisseria meningitidis* serotype 2a that is associated with meningococcal group C disease in Canada. J Clin Microbiol 29:2489–2493, 1991

16. ASNIS DS, BRENNESSEL DJ: Gonococcal scalp abscess: a risk of intrauterine monitoring. Clin Pediatr (Phila) 31:316–317, 1992

17. AU Y-K, REYNOLDS MD, RAMBIN ED ET AL: *Neisseria cinerea* purulent conjunctivitis. Am J Ophthalmol 109:96–97, 1990

18. BACON AE, PAI PG, SCHABERG DR: *Neisseria mucosa* endocarditis. J Infect Dis 162:1199–1201, 1990

19. BARBE G, BABOLAT M, BOEUFGRAS JM ET AL: Evaluation of API NH, a new 2-hour system for identification of *Neisseria* and *Haemophilus* species and *Moraxella catarrhalis* in a routine clinical laboratory. J Clin Microbiol 32:187–189, 1994

20. BARQUET N, GASSER I, DOMINGO P ET AL: Primary meningococcal conjunctivitis: report of 21 patients and review. Rev Infect Dis 12:838–847, 1990

21. BARRY AL, PFALLER MA, FUCHS PC ET AL: In vitro activities of 12 orally administered antimicrobial agents against four species of bacterial respiratory pathogens from U.S. medical centers in 1992 and 1993. Antimicrob Agents Chemother 38:2419–2425, 1994

22. BEEBE JL, RAU MP, FLAGEOLLE S ET AL: Incidence of *Neisseria gonorrhoeae* isolates negative by Syva direct fluorescent-antibody test but positive by Gen-Probe Accuprobe test in a sexually transmitted disease clinic population. J Clin Microbiol 31:2535–2537, 1993

23. BELDING ME, CARBONE J: Gonococcemia associated with adult respiratory distress syndrome. Rev Infect Dis 13:1105–1107, 1991

24. BERGER SA, GOREA A, PEYSSER MR ET AL: Bartholin's gland abscess caused by *Neisseria sicca*. J Clin Microbiol 26:1589, 1988

25. BERK SL: From *Micrococcus* to *Moraxella*: the reemergence of *Branhamella catarrhalis*. Arch Intern Med 150:2254–2257, 1990

26. BERRON S, VAZQUEZ JA: Increase in moderate penicillin resistance and serogroup C in meningococcal strains isolated in Spain. Is there any relationship? Clin Infect Dis 18:161–165, 1994

27. BEUVERY EC, MIEDEMA F, VAN DELFT R ET AL: Preparation and immunochemical characterization of meningococcal group C polysaccharide–tetanus toxoid conjugates as a new generation of vaccines. Infect Immun 40:39–45, 1983

28. BIRKENMEYER L, ARMSTRONG AS: Preliminary evaluation of the ligase chain reaction for specific detection of *Neisseria gonorrhoeae*. J Clin Microbiol 30:3089–3094, 1992

29. BJUNE G, HOIBY EA, GRONNESBY JK ET AL: Effect of outer membrane vesicle vaccine against group B meningococcal disease in Norway. Lancet 338:1093–1096, 1991

30. BLONDEAU JM, ASHTON FE, ISACCSON M ET AL: *Neisseria meningitidis* with decreased susceptibility to penicillin in Saskatchewan, Canada. J Clin Microbiol 33:1784–1786, 1995

31. BODSWORTH NJ, PRICE R, DAVIES SC: Gonococcal infection of the neovagina in a male-to-female transsexual. Sex Transm Dis 21:211–212, 1994

32. BODSWORTH NJ, PRICE R, NELSON MJ: A case of gonococcal mastitis in a male. Genitourin Med 69:222–223, 1993

33. BOEHM DM, BERNHARDT M, KURZYNSKI TA ET AL: Evaluation of two commercial procedures for rapid identification of *Neisseria gonorrhoeae* using a reference panel of antigenically diverse gonococci. J Clin Microbiol 28:2099–2100, 1990

34. BONADIO WA: *Branhamella catarrhalis* bacteremia in children. Pediatr Infect Dis J 7:738–739, 1988

35. BONIN P, TANINO TT, HANDSFIELD HH: Isolation of *Neisseria gonorrhoeae* on selective and non-selective media in a sexually-transmitted diseases clinic. J Clin Microbiol 19:218–220, 1984

36. BOSCH MA, BORDES A, LAFARGA B ET AL: *Neisseria meningitidis* serogroup B in a continuous ambulatory peritoneal dialysis patient. Clin Microbiol Newslett 14:188–189, 1992

37. BOTHA P: Penicillin-resistant *Neisseria meningitidis* in southern Africa. Lancet 1:54, 1988

38. BOUQUETE MT, MARCOS C, SAEZ-NIETO JA: Characterization of *Neisseria polysacchareae* sp. nov. (Riou, 1983) in previously identified noncapsulated strains of *Neisseria meningitidis*. J Clin Microbiol 23:973–975, 1986

39. BOURBEAU P, HOLLA V, PEIMONTESE S: Ophthalmia neonatorum caused by *Neisseria cinerea*. J Clin Microbiol 28:1640–1641, 1990

40. BOVRE K: Proposal to divide the genus *Moraxella* Lwoff 1939 emend. Henriksen and Bovre 1968 into two subgenera, subgenus *Moraxella* (Lwoff 1939) Bovre 1979 and subgenus *Branhamella* (Catlin 1970) Bovre 1979. Int J Syst Bacteriol 29:403–406, 1979

41. BOVRE K: Family VIII. *Neisseriaceae* Prevot 1933, 119AL. In Krieg NR, Holt JG (eds), *Bergey's Manual of Systematic Bacteriology*, Vol 1, pp 288–290. Baltimore, Williams & Wilkins, 1984

42. BOVRE K: Genus II. *Moraxella* Lwoff 1939, 173 emend. Henriksen and Bovre 1968, 391. In Krieg NR, Holt JG (eds), *Bergey's Manual of Systematic Bacteriology*, Vol 1, pp 296–303. Baltimore, Williams & Wilkins, 1984

43. BOVRE K, HOLTEN E: *Neisseria elongata* sp. nov., a rod-shaped member of the genus *Neisseria*. Re-evaluation of cell shape as a criterion for classification. J Gen Microbiol 60:67–75, 1970

44. BOWLER LD, ZHANG Q-Y, RIOU J-Y ET AL: Interspecies recombination between the *penA* genes of *Neisseria meningitidis* and commensal *Neisseria* species during the emergence of penicillin resistance in *N. meningitidis*: natural events and laboratory simulation. J Bacteriol 176:333–337, 1994

45. BOYCE JM, MITCHELL EB: Difficulties in differentiating *Neisseria cinerea* from *Neisseria gonorrhoeae* in rapid systems used for identifying pathogenic *Neisseria* species. J Clin Microbiol 22:731–734, 1985

46. BOYCE JM, MITCHELL EB, KNAPP JS ET AL: Production of 14C-labeled gas in BACTEC *Neisseria* differentiation kits by *Neisseria cinerea*. J Clin Microbiol 22:416–418, 1985

47. BOYCE JM, TAYLOR MR, MITCHELL EB ET AL: Nosocomial pneumonia caused by a glucose-metabolizing strain of *Neisseria cinerea*. J Clin Microbiol 21:1–3, 1985

48. BRANDSTETTER RD, BLAIKR RJ, ROBERTS RB: *Neisseria meningitidis* serogroup W-135 disease in adults. JAMA 246:2060–2061, 1981

49. BRIGHTON RW, WILDING K: Delayed diagnosis of gonococcal arthritis of the foot caused by *beta*-lactamase-producing *Neisseria gonorrhoeae*. Med J Aust 156:368, 1992

50. BRODIE E, ADLER JL, DALY AK: Bacterial endocarditis due to an unusual species of encapsulated *Neisseria*: *Neisseria mucosa* endocarditis. Am J Dis Child 122:433–437, 1971

51. BROOME CV: The carrier state: *Neisseria meningitidis*. J Antimicrob Chemother 18(suppl A):25–34, 1986

52. BROOKS GF, LAMMEL CJ, BLAKE MS ET AL: Antibodies against IgA1 protease are stimulated both by clinical disease and asymptomatic carriage of serogroup A *Neisseria meningitidis*. J Infect Dis 166:1316–1321, 1992

53. BROWN BA, WALLACE RJ JR, FLANAGAN CW ET AL: Tetracycline and erythromycin resistance among clinical isolates of *Moraxella catarrhalis*. Antimicrob Agents Chemother 33:1631–1633, 1989

54. BROWN JD, THOMAS KR: Rapid enzyme system for the identification of *Neisseria* spp. J Clin Microbiol 21:857–858, 1985

55. BRUINS SC, TIGHT RR: Laboratory-acquired gonococcal comjunctivitis. JAMA 241:274, 1979

56. BRUNEN A, PEETERMANS W, VERHAGEN J ET AL: Meningitis due to *Neisseria meningitidis* with intermediate susceptibility to penicillin. Eur J Clin Microbiol Infect Dis 12:969–970, 1993

57. BURNETT IA, DENTON K, SUTCLIFFE J: Cerebrospinal fluid shunt infection: an unusual case. J Infect 22:205–206, 1990

58. BYGRAVES JA, MAIDEN MCJ: Analysis of the clonal relationships between strains of *Neisseria meningitidis* by pulsed field gel electrophoresis. J Gen Microbiol 138:523–531, 1992

59. CALANAN D, RUBSAMEN PE: *Moraxella* infection of a scleral buckle. Am J Ophthalmol 114:637–638, 1992

60. CAMPOS J, MENDELMAN PM, SAKU MU ET AL: Detection of relatively penicillin G-resistant *Neisseria meningitidis* by disk susceptibility testing. Antimicrob Agents Chemother 31:1478, 1987.

61. CANN KJ, ROGERS TR: The phenotypic relationship of *Neisseria polysacharea* to commensal and pathogenic *Neisseria* ssp. J Mol Microbiol 39:351–354, 1989

62. CANO RJ, PALOMARES JC, TORRES MJ ET AL: Evaluation of a fluorescent DNA hybridization assay for the detection of *Neisseria gonorrhoeae*. Eur J Clin Microbiol Infect Dis 11:602–609, 1992

63. CARBALLO M, DILLON JR: Evaluation of an enzyme immunoassay and a modified coagglutination assay for

typing gonococcal isolates with monoclonal antibodies. Sex Transm Dis 19:219–224, 1992

64. CARBALLO M, DILLON JR, LUSSIER M ET AL: Evaluation of a urease-based confirmatory enzyme-linked immunosorbenty assay for diagnosis of *Neisseria gonorrhoeae*. J Clin Microbiol 30:2181–2183, 1992

65. CARLSON BL, CALNAN MB, GOODMAN RE ET AL: Phadebact monoclonal GC OMNI test for confirmation of *Neisseria gonorrhoeae*. J Clin Microbiol 25:1982–1984, 1987

66. CARLSON BL, FUIMARA NJ, KELLY R ET AL: Isolation of *Neisseria meningitidis* from anogenital specimens from homosexual men. Sex Transm Dis 7:70–73, 1980

67. CARTWRIGHT KAV, STUART JM, ROBINSON PM: Meningococcal carriage in close contacts of cases. Epidemiol Infect 106:133–141, 1991

68. CATLIN BW: Transfer of the organism named *Neisseria catarrhalis* to *Branhamella* gen. nov. Int J Syst Bacteriol 20:155–159, 1970

69. CATLIN BW: Cellular elongation under the influence of antibacterial agents: way to differentiate coccobacilli from cocci. J Clin Microbiol 1:102–105, 1975

70. CATLIN BW: Nutritional profiles of *Neisseria gonorrhoeae*, *Neisseria meningitidis*, and *Neisseria lactamica* in chemically defined media and the use of growth requirements for gonococcal typing. J Infect Dis 128:178–194, 1975

71. CATLIN BW: *Branhamella catarrhalis*: an organism gaining respect as a pathogen. Clin Microbiol Rev 3:293–330, 1990

72. CATLIN BW: *Branhamaceae* fam. nov., a proposed family to accommodate the genera *Branhamella* and *Moraxella*. Int J Syst Bacteriol 41:320–323, 1991

73. CAUGANT DA, BOL P, HOIBY EA ET AL: Clones of serogroup B *Neisseria meningitidis* causing systemic disease in the Netherlands, 1958–1986. J Infect Dis 162: 867–874, 1990

74. CAUGANT DA, HOIBY EA, MAGNUS P ET AL: Asymptomatic carriage of *Neisseria meningitidis* in a randomly sampled population. J Clin Microbiol 32:323–330, 1994

75. CENTERS FOR DISEASE CONTROL: Chromosomally-mediated resistant *Neisseria gonorrhoeae*—United States. MMWR 33:408–410, 1984

76. CENTERS FOR DISEASE CONTROL: Tetracycline-resistant *Neisseria gonorrhoeae*—Georgia, Pennsylvania, New Hampshire. MMWR 34:563–570, 1985

77. CENTERS FOR DISEASE CONTROL AND PREVENTION: 1993 sexually transmitted diseases treatment guidelines. MMWR 42(suppl RR-14):47–83, 1993

78. CENTERS FOR DISEASE CONTROL AND PREVENTION: Decreased susceptibility of *Neisseria gonorrhoeae* to fluoroquinolones—Ohio and Hawaii, 1992–1994. MMWR 43:325–327, 1994

79. CHAPIN-ROBERSTON K, REECE EA, EDBERG SC: Evaluation of the Gen-Probe PACE II assay for the direct detection of *Neisseria gonorrhoeae* in endocervical specimens. Diagn Microbiol Infect Dis 15:645–649, 1992

80. CHAUDHURI AKR, BANATVALA, CAUGANT DA ET AL: Phenotypically similar clones of serogroup B *Neisseria meningitidis* causing recurrent meningitis in a patient with total C5 deficiency. J Infect 26:236–238, 1994

81. CHEN C-Y, GENCO CA, ROCK JP ET AL: Physiology and metabolism of *Neisseria gonorrhoeae* and *Neisseria menin-

gitidis: implications for pathogenesis. Clin Microbiol Rev 2(suppl):S35–S40, 1989

82. CHER DJ, MAXWELL WJ, FRUSZTAJER N ET AL: A case of pelvic inflammatory disease associated with *Neisseria meningitidis* bacteremia. Clin Infect Dis 17:134–135, 1993

83. CHRISTENSEN JJ, KEIDING J, SCHUMACHER H ET AL: Recognition of a new *Branhamella catarrhalis* beta-lactamase—BRO 3. J Antimicrob Chemother 28:774–775, 1991

84. CLAESSON BA, LEINONEN M: *Moraxella catarrhalis*—an uncommon cause of community-acquired pneumonia in Swedish children. Scand J Infect Dis 26:399–402, 1994

85. CLARK H, PATTON RD: Post-cardiotomy endocarditis due to *Neisseria perflava* on a prosthetic aortic valve. Ann Intern Med 68:386, 1968

86. CLARK VL, CAMPBELL LA, PALERMO DA ET AL: Induction and repression of outer membrane proteins by anaerobic growth of *Neisseria gonorrhoeae*. Infect Immun 55: 1359–1364, 1987

87. CLAUSEN CR, KNAPP JS, TOTTEN PA: Lymphadenitis due to *Neisseria cinerea*. Lancet 1:908, 1984

88. COE MD, HAMER DH, LEVY CS ET AL: Gonococcal pericarditis with tamponade in a patient with systemic lupus erythematosus. Arthritis Rheum 33:1438–1441, 1990

89. COLLAZOS J, DE MIGUEL J, AYARZA R: *Moraxella catarrhalis* bacteremic pneumonia in adults: two cases and review of the literature. Eur J Clin Microbiol Infect Dis 11: 237–240, 1992

90. COMMITTEE ON EARLY CHILDHOOD, ADOPTION, AND DEPENDENT CARE: Gonorrhea in prepubertal children. Pediatrics 71:553, 1983

91. CONNELL TD, BLACK WJ, KAWULA TH ET AL: Recombination among protein II genes of *Neisseria gonorrhoeae* generates new coding sequences and increases structural variability in the protein II family. Mol Microbiol 2: 227–236, 1988

92. CONNELL TD, SHAFFER D, CANNON JG: Characterization of the repertoire of hypervariable regions in the protein II (*Opa*) gene family of *Neisseria gonorrhoeae*. Mol Microbiol 4:439–449, 1990

93. COOKE RP, WILLIAMS R, BANNISTER CM: Shunt-associated ventriculitis caused by *Branhamella catarrhalis*. J Hosp Infect 15:197–198, 1990

94. COOPER ER, ELLISON RT, SMITH GS ET AL: Rifampin-resistant meningococcal disease in a contact patient given prophylactic rifampin. J Pediatr 107:93, 1985

95. CRAWFORD G, KNAPP JS, HALE J: Asymptomatic gonorrhea in men: caused by gonococci with unique nutritional requirements. Science 196:1352–1353, 1977

96. DAVIS CL, TOWNS M, HENRICH WL ET AL: *Neisseria mucosa* endocarditis following drug abuse. Case report and review of the literature. Arch Intern Med 143:583–385, 1983

97. DEALLER SF, ABBOTT M, CROUGHAN MJ ET AL: Identification of *Branhamella catarrhalis* in 2.5 min with an indoxyl butyrate strip test. J Clin Microbiol 27:1390–1391, 1989

98. DEALLER SF, GOUGH KR, CAMPBELL L ET AL: Identification of *Neisseria gonorrhoeae* using the Neisstrip rapid enzyme detection test. J Clin Pathol 44:376–379, 1991

99. DEGER R, LUDMIR J: *Neisseria sicca* endocarditis complicating pregnancy—a case report. J Reprod Med 37:473–475, 1992

100. DEMMLER GJ, COUCH RS, TABER LH: *Neisseria subflava* bacteremia and meningitis in a child: report of a case and review of the literature. Pediatr Infect Dis 4:286, 1985

101. DENNING DW, GILL SS: *Neisseria lactamica* meningitis following skull trauma. Rev Infect Dis 13:216–218, 1991

102. DeVAUX DL, EVANS GL, ARNDT CW ET AL: Comparison of the Gono-Pak system with the candle extinction jar for recovery of *Neisseria gonorrhoeae*. J Clin Microbiol 25:571–572, 1987

103. DEWHIRST FE, PASTER BJ, BRIGHT PL: *Chromobacterium*, *Eikenella*, *Kingella*, *Neisseria*, *Simonsiella*, and *Vitreoscilla* species comprise a major branch of the *beta* group *Protobacteria* by 16S ribosomal nucleic acid sequence comparison: transfer of *Eikenella* and *Simonsiella* to the Family *Neisseriaceae* (emend.). Int J Syst Bacteriol 39:258–266, 1989

104. DEWHIRST FE, PASTER BJ, LA FONTAINE S ET AL: Transfer of *Kingella indologenes* (Snell and LaPage 1976) to the genus *Suttonella* gen. nov. as *Suttonella indologenes* comb. nov.; transfer of *Bacteroides nodosus* (Beveridge 1941) to the genus *Dichelobacter* gen. nov. as *Dichelobacter nodosus* comb. nov.; and assignment of the genera *Cardiobacterium*, *Dichelobacter*, and *Suttonella* to *Cardiobacteriaceae* fam. nov. in the *gamma* division of *Proteobacteria* on the basis of 16S rRNA sequence comparisons. Int J Syst Bacteriol 40:426–433, 1990

105. DIAZ FJ, FERNANDEZ-GUERRERO ML: Endocarditis due to *Neisseria mucosa* complicated by myocardial abscess. J Infect 18:294–295, 1989

106. DILLON JR, CARBALLO M, PAUZE M: Evaluation of eight methods for identification of pathogenic *Neisseria* species: Neisseria-Kwik, RIM-N, Gonobio Test, Minitek, Gonochek II, GonoGen, Phadebact Monoclonal GC OMNI test, and Syva MicroTrak test. J Clin Microbiol 26:493–497, 1988

107. DILLON JR, PAUZE M, YEUNG K-H: Spread of penicillinase-producing and transfer plasmids from the gonococcus to *Neisseria meningitidis*. Lancet 1:779–781, 1983

108. DILLON JR, YEUNG K-H: *beta*-Lactamase plasmids and chromosomally mediated antibiotic resistance in pathogenic *Neisseria* species. Clin Microbiol Rev 2(suppl): S125–S133, 1989

109. DOERN GV: *Branhamella catarrhalis*: phenotypic characteristics. Am J Med 88(suppl 5A):33S–35S, 1990

110. DOERN GV, BLACKLOW NR, GANTZ NM ET AL: *Neisseria sicca* osteomyelitis. J Clin Microbiol 16:595–597, 1982

111. DOERN GV, GANTZ NM: Isolation of *Branhamella* (*Neisseria*) *catarrhalis* from men with urethritis. Sex Transm Dis 9:202–204, 1982

112. DOERN GV, TUBERT TA: Effect of inoculum size on results of macrotube broth dilution susceptibility tests with *Branhamella catarrhalis*. J Clin Microbiol 25:1576–1578, 1987

113. DOERN GV, TUBERT TA: Detection of *beta*-lactamase activity among clinical isolates of *Branhamella catarrhalis* with six different *beta*-lactamase assays. J Clin Microbiol 25:1380–1383, 1987

114. DOLTER J, BRYANT L, JANDA JM: Evaluation of five rapid systems for the identification of *Neisseria gonorrhoeae*. Diagn Microbiol Infect Dis 13:265–267, 1990

115. DOSSETT JH, APPLEBAUM PC, KNAPP JS ET AL: Proctitis associated with *Neisseria cinerea* misidentified as *Neisseria gonorrhoeae* in a child. J Clin Microbiol 21:575–577, 1985

116. DOWLING JN, LEE W, SACCO RJ ET AL.: Endocarditis caused by *Neisseria mucosa* in Marfan's syndrome. Ann Intern Med 81:641–643, 1974

117. DUNNETT DM, MOYER MA: Cefixime in the treatment of uncomplicated gonorrhea. Sex Transm Dis 19:92–93, 1992

118. DURAND ML, CALDERWOOD SB, WEBER DJ ET AL: Acute bacterial meningitis in adults. N Engl J Med 328: 21–28, 1993

119. DYSON C, POONYTH HD, WATKINSON M ET AL: Life-threatening *Branhamella catarrhalis* pneumonia in young infants. J Infect 21:305–307, 1990

120. EDMOND MB, HOLLIS RJ, HOUSTON AK ET AL: Molecular epidemiology of an outbreak of meningococcal disease in a university community. J Clin Microbiol 33:2209–2211, 1995

121. EDWARDS EA, DEVINE LF, SENGBUSCH CH ET AL: Immunological investigations of meningococcal disease. III. Brevity of group C acquisition prior to disease occurrence. Scand J Infect Dis 9:105–110, 1987

122. EISENSTEIN BI, LEE TJ, SPARLING PF: Penicillin sensitivity and serum resistance are independent attributes of strains of *Neisseria gonorrhoeae* causing disseminated gonococcal infections. Infect Immun 15:834–841, 1977

123. EJLERTSEN T, SCHONHEUDER HC: *Branhamella catarrhalis* as a cause of multiple subpleural abscess. Scand J Infect Dis 23:117–118, 1991

124. EJLERTSEN T, THISTED E, EDDESON F ET AL: *Branhamella catarrhalis* in children and adults. A study of prevalence, time of colonisation, and association with upper and lower respiratory tract infection. J Infect 29:23–31, 1994

125. ELBASHIER AM, DESHPANDE H: Recurrent urinary tract infection with hematuria caused by *Moraxella* (*Branhamella*) *catarrhalis*. J Infect 22: 1993

126. ELLISON RT, KOHLER PF, CURD JG ET AL: Prevalence of congenital or acquired complement deficiency in patients with sporadic meningococcal disease. N Engl J Med 308:913–916, 1983

127. ENG J, HOLTEN E: Gelatin neutralization of the inhibitory effect of sodium polyanethol sulfonate on *Neisseria meningitidis* in blood culture media. J Clin Microbiol 6:1–3, 1977

128. ENRIGHT MC, CARTER PE, MacLEAN IA ET AL: Phylogenetic relationship between some members of the genera *Neisseria*, *Acinetobacter*, *Moraxella*, and *Kingella* based on partial 16S ribosomal DNA sequence analysis. Int J Syst Bacteriol 44:387–391, 1994

129. EVANS GL, KOPYTA DL, CROUSE K: New selective medium for the isolation of *Neisseria gonorrhoeae*. J Clin Microbiol 27:2471–2474, 1989

130. EVANS JR, ARTENSTEIN MS, HUNTER DH: Prevalence of meningococcal serogroups and description of three new groups. Am J Epidemiol 87:643–646, 1968

131. FADEN H, HARABUCHI Y, HONG JJ ET AL: Epidemiology of *Moraxella catarrhalis* in children during the first two years of life: relationship to otitis media. J Infect Dis 169:1312–1317, 1994

132. FARUKI H, KOHMESCHER RN, McKINNEY WP ET AL: A community-based outbreak of infection with penicillin-

resistant *Neisseria gonorrhoeae* not producing *beta*-lactamase (chromosomally mediated resistance). N Engl J Med 313:607–611, 1985

133. FAUR YC, WEISBURD MH, WILSON ME ET AL: A new medium for the isolation of pathogenic *Neisseria* (NYC medium). Health Lab Sci 10:44–54, 1973

134. FEDER HM, GARIBALDI RA: The significance of nongonococcal, nonmeningococcal *Neisseria* isolates from blood cultures. Rev Infect Dis 6:181–188, 1984

135. FENTON AC, FOWERAKER JE, PEARSON GA ET AL: Bronchopulmonary infection with *Moraxella catarrhalis* in infants requiring extracorporeal membrane oxygenation. Pediatr Pulmonol 17:393–395, 1994

136. FERNANDEZ-GUERRERO ML, BARROS C, RODRIGUEZ TEDULA JL: Endocarditis due to *Neisseria mucosa* complicated by myocardial abscess. J Infect 18:294–295, 1989

137. FIJEN CAP, KUIJPER EJ, TJIA HG ET AL: Complement deficiency predisposes for meningitis due to nongroupable meningococci and *Neisseria*-related bacteria. Clin Infect Dis 18:780–784, 1994

138. FINNE J, LEINONEN M, MAKELA PH: Antigenic similarities between brain components and bacteria causing meningitis. Lancet 2:355, 1983

139. FLEMING TJ, WALLSMITH DE, ROSENTHAL RS: Arthropathic properties of gonococcal peptidoglycan fragments: implications for the pathogenesis of disseminated gonococcal disease. Infect Immun 52:600–608, 1986

140. FONTANALS D, PINEDA V, PONS I ET AL: Penicillin-resistant *beta*-lactamase-producing *Neisseria meningitidis* in Spain. Eur J Clin Microbiol Infect Dis 8:90–91, 1989

141. FRASCH CE: Vaccines for prevention of meningococcal disease. Clin Microbiol Rev 2(suppl):S134–S138, 1989

142. FRASCH CE, ZAHRADNIK JM, WANG LY ET AL: Antibody response in adults to an aluminum hydroxide adsorbed *Neisseria meningitidis* serotype 2b protein group B–polysaccharide vaccine. J Infect Dis 158:710–718, 1988

143. FRASCH CE, ZOLLINGER WD, POOLMAN JT: Proposed scheme for identification of serotypes of *Neisseria meningitidis*. In Schoolnik GK (ed.), *The Pathogenic Neisseriae*, pp. 519–524. American Society for Microbiology, Washington DC, 1985

144. GALAID EI, CHERUBIN CE, MARR JS: Meningococcal disease in New York City, 1973–1978. Recognition of groups Y and W135 as frequent pathogens. JAMA 224:2167–2171, 1980

145. GARNER J, BRIANT RH: Osteomyelitis caused by a bacterium known as M-6. J Infect 13:298–300, 1986

146. GAUNT PN, LAMBERT PE: Single-dose ciprofloxacin for the eradication of pharyngeal carriage of *Neisseria meningitidis*. J Antimicrob Chemother 21:489–496, 1988

147. GAY RM, SEVIER RE: *Neisseria sicca* endocarditis: report of a case and review of the literature. J Clin Microbiol 8:729–732, 1978

148. GERMER JJ, WASHINGTON JA: Evaluation of a rapid identification method for *Neisseria* spp. J Clin Microbiol 21:987–988, 1985

149. GILJA OH, HALSTENSEN A, DIGRANES A ET AL: Use of single-dose ofloxacin to eradicate tonsillopharyngeal carriage of *Neisseria meningitidis*. Antimicrob Agents Chemother 37:2024–2026, 1993

150. GILL MJ: Serotyping *Neisseria gonorrhoeae*: a report of the fourth international workshop. Genitourin Med 67:53–57, 1991

151. GILLES RG, MONIF MD: Recovery of *Neisseria meningitidis* from the cul-de-sac of a woman with endometritis–salpingitis–peritonitis. Am J Obstet Gynecol 139:108–109, 1981

152. GINI GA: Ocular infection in a newborn caused by *Neisseria mucosa*. J Clin Microbiol 25:1574–1575, 1987

153. GOLD R, GOLDSCHNEIDER I, LEPOW ML ET AL: Carriage of *Neisseria meningitidis* and *Neisseria lactamica* in infants and children. J Infect Dis 137:112–121, 1978

154. GOLDSTEIN AMB, CLARK JH, WICKLER MA: Comparison of single-dose ceftizoxime or ceftriaxone in the treatment of uncomplicated urethral gonorrhea. Sex Transm Dis 18:180–182, 1991

155. GORWITZ RJ, NAKASHIMA AK, MORAN JS ET AL: Sentinel surveillance for antimicrobial resistance in *Neisseria gonorrhoeae*—United States, 1988–1991. MMWR 42(suppl):29–39, 1993

156. GOTSCHLICH EC, SEIFF M, BLAKE MS: The DNA sequence of the structural gene of gonococcal protein III. and the flanking region containing a repetitive sequence: homology of protein III with enterobacterial *ompA* proteins. J Exp Med 165:471–481, 1987

157. GRADUS MS, NG CM, SILVER KJ: Comparison of the QuadFERM+ 2-hr identification system with conventional carbohydrate degradation tests for confirmatory identification of *Neisseria gonorrhoeae*. Sex Transm Dis 16:57–59, 1989

158. GRAHAM DR, BAND JD, THORNSBERRY C ET AL: Infections caused by *Moraxella*, *Moraxella urethralis*, *Moraxella*-like groups M-5 and M-6, and *Kingella kingae* in the United States, 1953–1980. Rev Infect Dis 12:423–431, 1990

159. GRANATO PA, HOWARD R, WILKINSON B ET AL: Meningitis caused by maltose-negative variant of *Neisseria meningitidis*. J Clin Microbiol 11:270–273, 1980

160. GRANATO PA, SCHNEIBLE-SMITH C, WEINER LB: Primary isolation of *Neisseria gonorrhoeae* on hemoglobin-free New York City medium. J Clin Microbiol 14:206–209, 1981

161. GRANSDEN WR, WARREN C, PHILLIPS I: 4-Quinolone-resistant *Neisseria gonorrhoeae* in the United Kingdom. J Med Microbiol 34:23–27, 1991

162. GRANT PE, BRENNER DJ, STEIGERWALT AG ET AL: *Neisseria elongata* subsp. *nitroreducens* subsp. nov., formerly CDC group M-6, a gram-negative bacterium associated with endocarditis. J Clin Microbiol 28:2591–2596, 1990

163. GRAY LD, VAN SCOY RE, ANHALT JP ET AL: Wound infection caused by *Branhamella catarrhalis*. J Clin Microbiol 27:818–820, 1989

164. GREENBERG LW, KLEINERMAN E: *Neisseria lactamica* meningitis. J Pediatr 93:1061–1062, 1978

165. GREENLEE JE: Approaches to diagnosis of meningitis: cerebrospinal fluid evaluation. In Scheld WM, Wispelwey B (eds), *Infectious Disease Clinics of North America*, Vol 4, Meningitis, pp 583–598. Philadelphia, W.B. Saunders, 1990

166. GREENWOOD BM, GREENWOOD AM, BRADLEY AK ET AL: Factors influencing the susceptibility to meningococcal disease during an epidemic in the Gambia. West Afr J Infect 14:167–184, 1987

167. GRIFFISS JM, SCHNEIDER H, MANDRELL RE ET AL: Lipooligosaccharides: the principal glycolipids of the neisserial outer membrane. Rev Infect Dis 10:S87–S95, 1988

168. GRIS P, VINCKE G, DELMEZ JP ET AL: *Neisseria sicca* pneumonia and bronchiectasis. Eur Respir J 2:685–687, 1989

169. GUIBOURDENCHE M, CAUGANT DA, HERVE V ET AL: Characteristics of serogroup A *Neisseria meningitidis* strains isolated in the Central African Republic in February. Eur J Clin Microbiol Infect Dis 13:174–177, 1994.

170. GUIBOURDENCHE M, DARCHIS J-P, BOISIVON A ET AL: Enzyme electrophoresis, sero- and subtyping, and outer membrane protein characterization of two *Neisseria meningitidis* strains involved in laboratory acquired infections. J Clin Microbiol 32:701–704, 1994

171. GUIBOURDENCHE M, LAMBERT T, RIOU JY: Isolation of *Neisseria canis* in mixed culture from a patient after a cat bite. J Clin Microbiol 27:1673–1674, 1989

172. HABIB RG, GIRGIS NI, YASSIN MW ET AL: Hearing impairment in meningococcal meningitis. Scand J Infect Dis 11:121–123, 1979

173. HAGER H, VERGHESE A, ALVAREZ S ET AL: *Branhamella catarrhalis* respiratory infections. Rev Infect Dis 9:1140–1149, 1987

174. HAGMAN M, FORSLIN L, MOI H ET AL: *Neisseria meningitidis* in specimens from urogenital sites: is increased awareness necessary. Sex Transm Dis 18:228–231, 1991

175. HALE YM, MELTON ME, LEWIS JS ET AL: Evaluation of the PACE 2 *Neisseria gonorrhoeae* assay by three public health laboratories. J Clin Microbiol 31:451–453, 1993

176. HALLA JT: Septic olecranon bursitis caused by *Neisseria sicca*. J Rheumatol 17:1240–1241, 1990

177. HANDSFIELD HH, DALU ZA, MARTIN DH ET AL: Multicenter trial of single-dose azithromycin vs. ceftriaxone in the treatment of uncomplicated gonorrhea. Sex Transm Dis 21:107–111, 1994

178. HANDSFIELD HH, MCCORMACK WM, HOOK EW ET AL: A comparison of single-dose cefixime with ceftriaxone as treatment for uncomplicated gonorrhea. N Engl J Med 325:1337–1341, 1991

179. HANDSFIELD HH, SPARLING PF: *Neisseria gonorrhoeae*. In Mandell GL, Bennett JE, Dolin R (eds), *Mandell, Douglas, and Bennett's Principles and Practice of Infectious Diseases*, pp 1909–1926. New York, Churchill-Livingstone, 1995

180. HANKS JW, SCOTT CT, BUTLER CE ET AL: Evaluation of a DNA probe assay (Gen-Probe PACE 2) as the test of cure for *Neisseria gonorrhoeae* genital infections. J Pediatr 125:161–162, 1994

181. HANNA LS, GIRGIS NI, FARID Z ET AL: Transient cataracts in a young child with meningococcal meningitis. Pediatr Infect Dis J 8:802–803, 1989

182. HANSMAN D: Meningitis caused by *Neisseria lactamica*. N Engl J Med 299:491, 1978

183. HARRIS LF: *Neisseria subflava* endocarditis. Arch Intern Med 141:545–546, 1981

184. HARTMANN AA, ELSNER P: Urethritis caused by *Neisseria meningitidis* group B: a case report. Sex Transm Dis 15:150–151, 1988

185. HAY PE, MURPHY SM, CHINN RJS: Acute urethritis due to *Neisseria meningitidis* group A acquired by oro-genital contact: case report. Genitourin Med 65:285–286, 1989

186. HECKELS JE: Structure and function of pili of pathogenic *Neisseria* species. Clin Microbiol Rev 2(suppl):S66–S73, 1989

187. HEIDDAL S, SVERRISSON JT, YNGVASON FE ET AL: Native valve endocarditis due to *Neisseria sicca*: case report and review. Clin Infect Dis 16:667–670, 1993

188. HELMINEN ME, MACIVER I, LATIMER JL ET AL: A major outer membrane protein of *Moraxella catarrhalis* is a target for antibodies that enhance pulmonary clearance of the pathogen in an animal model. Infect Immun 61:2003–2010, 1993

189. HELMINEN ME, MACIVER I, LATIMER JL ET AL: A large, antigenically conserved protein on the surface of *Moraxella catarrhalis* is a target for protective antibodies. J Infect Dis 170:867–872, 1994

190. HELMINEN ME, MACIVER I, PARIS M ET AL: A mutation affecting expression of a major outer membrane protein of *Moraxella catarrhalis* alters serum resistance and survival in vivo. J Infect Dis 168:194–201, 1993

191. HENNESSEY R, REINHART JH, MCGUCKIN MB: Endocarditis caused by *Neisseria mucosa* in a patient with a prosthetic heart valve. Am J Med Technol 47:909–911, 1981

192. HERBERT DA, RUSKIN J: Are the "non-pathogenic" neisseriae pathogenic? Am J Clin Pathol 75:739–741, 1981

193. HERRUZ PG, ASPA FJ, MARTINEZ R ET AL: *Neisseria meningitidis* pneumonia in a patient with AIDS. Clin Microbiol Newslett 12:188–189, 1990

194. HO BSW, FENG WG, WONG BKC ET AL: Polymerase chain reaction for the detection of *Neisseria gonorrhoeae* in clinical samples. J Clin Pathol 45:439–442, 1992

195. HODGE DS, ASHTON FE, TERRO R ET AL: Organism resembling *Neisseria gonorrhoeae* and *Neisseria meningitidis*. J Clin Microbiol 25:1546–1547, 1987

196. HOKE C, VEDROS NA: Characterization of atypical aerobic gram-negative cocci isolated from humans. J Clin Microbiol 15:906–914, 1982

197. HOL C, VAN DIJKE EEM, VERDUIN CM ET AL: Experimental evidence for *Moraxella*-induced penicillin neutralization in pneumococcal pneumonia. J Infect Dis 170:1613–1616, 1994

198. HOLLIS DG, WIGGINS GL, WEAVER RE: *Neisseria lactamica* sp. nov., a lactose-fermenting species resembling *Neisseria meningitidis*. Appl Microbiol 17:71–77, 1969

199. HOLLIS DG, WIGGINS WL, WEAVER RE: An unclassified gram-negative rod isolated from the pharynx on Thayer-Martin medium (selective agar). Appl Microbiol 24:772–777, 1972

200. HOLMES B, COSTAS M, ON SLW ET AL: *Neisseria weaveri* sp. nov. (formerly CDC group M-5), from dog bite wounds of humans. Int J Syst Bacteriol 43:687–693, 1993

201. HOOK EW, BRADY WE, REICHART CA ET AL: Determinants of emergence of antibiotic-resistant *Neisseria gonorrhoeae*. J Infect Dis 159:900–907, 1989

202. HOOK EW, JONES RB, MARTIN DH ET AL: Comparison of ciprofloxacin and ceftriaxone as single-dose therapy for uncomplicated gonorrhea in women. Antimicrob Agents Chemother 37:1670–1673, 1993

203. HORNYIK G, PIATT JH JR: Cerebrospinal fluid shunt infection by *Neisseria sicca*. Pediatr Neurosurg 21:189–191, 1994

204. HUGHES J, GOLDSMITH C, SHIELDS MD ET AL: Primary meningococcal pericarditis with tamponade in an infant. J Infect 29:339–341, 1994

205. HUGHES JH, BIEDENBACH DJ, ERWIN ME ET AL: E test as susceptibility test and epidemiologic tool for evaluation of Neisseria meningitidis isolates. J Clin Microbiol 31:3255–3259, 1993

206. IKEDA F, YOKOTA Y, MINE Y ET AL: Characterization of BRO enzymes and beta-lactamase transfer of Moraxella (Branhamella) catarrhalis isolated in Japan. Chemotherapy 39:88–95, 1993

207. IKRAM RB, NIXON M, AITKEN J ET AL: A prospective study of isolation of Moraxella catarrhalis in a hospital during the winter months. J Hosp Infect 25:7–14, 1993

208. INGRAM DL, WHITE ST, DURFEE MF ET AL: Sexual contact in children with gonorrhea. Am J Dis Child 136:994–996, 1982

209. INGRAM RJH, CORNERE B, ELLIS-PEGLER RB: Endocarditis due to Neisseria mucosa: two case reports and review. Clin Infect Dis 15:312–324, 1992

210. IOANNIDIS JPA, WORTHINGTON M, GRIFFITHS JK ET AL: Spectrum and significance of bacteremia due to Moraxella catarrhalis. Clin Infect Dis 21:390–397, 1995

211. IRWIN RS, WOELK WK, COUDON III WL: Primary meningococcal pneumonia. Ann Intern Med 82:493–498, 1975

212. IWEN PC, WALKER RA, WARREN KL ET AL: Evaluation of nucleic acid-based test (PACE 2C) for simultaneous detection of Chlamydia trachomatis and Neisseria gonorrhoeae in endocervical specimens. J Clin Microbiol 33:2587–2591, 1995

213. JACKSON LA, SCHUCHAT A, REEVES MW ET AL: Serogroup C meningococcal outbreaks in the United States: an emerging threat. JAMA 273:383–389, 1995

214. JACKSON LA, TENOVER FC, BAKER C ET AL: Prevalence of Neisseria meningitidis relatively resistant to penicillin in the United States, 1991. J Infect Dis 169:438–441, 1994

215. JANDA WM, BOHNHOFF M, MORELLO JA ET AL: Prevalence and site-pathogen studies of Neisseria meningitidis and N. gonorrhoeae in homosexual men. JAMA 244:2060–2064, 1980

216. JANDA WM, BRADNA JJ, RUTHER P: Identification of Neisseria spp., Haemophilus spp., and other fastidious gram-negative bacteria with the MicroScan Haemophilus–Neisseria identification panel. J Clin Microbiol 27:869–873, 1989

217. JANDA WM, MALLOY PJ, SCHRECKENBERGER PC: Clinical evaluation of the Vitek Neisseria–Haemophilus identification card. J Clin Microbiol 25:37–41, 1987

218. JANDA WM, MONTERO M: Premarket evaluation of the BactiCard Neisseria. Abstracts of the 95th General Meeting of the American Society for Microbiology. Abstract C-303, p 53, 1995

219. JANDA WM, RUTHER P: B.CAT CONFIRM: a rapid test for confirmation of Branhamella catarrhalis. J Clin Microbiol 27:1130–1131, 1989

220. JANDA WM, SENSUNG C, TODD KM ET AL: Asymptomatic Neisseria subflava biovar. perflava bacteriuria in a child with obstructive uropathy. Eur J Clin Microbiol Infect Dis 12:540–542, 1993

221. JANDA WM, SOBIESKI V: Evaluation of a ten-minute chromogenic substrate test for identification of pathogenic Neisseria species and Branhamella catarrhalis. Eur J Clin Microbiol Infect Dis 7:25–29, 1987

222. JANDA WM, ULANDAY MG, BOHNHOFF M ET AL: Evaluation of the RIM-N, Gonochek II, and Phadebact systems for the identification of pathogenic Neisseria spp. and Branhamella catarrhalis. J Clin Microbiol 21:734–737, 1985

223. JANDA WM, WILCOSKI LM, MANDEL KL ET AL: Comparison of monoclonal antibody-based methods and a ribosomal ribonucleic acid probe test for Neisserai gonorrhoeae culture confirmation. Eur J Clin Microbiol Infect Dis 12:177–184, 1993

224. JANDA WM, ZIGLER KL, BRADNA JJ: API QuadFERM+ with rapid DNase for identification of Neisseria spp. and Branhamella catarrhalis. J Clin Microbiol 25:203–206, 1987

225. JANNES G, VANEECHOUTTE M, LANNOO M ET AL: Polyphasic taxonomy leading to the proposal of Moraxella canis sp. nov. for Moraxella catarrhalis-like strains. Int J Syst Bacteriol 43:438–449, 1993

226. JEPHCOTT AE, MORTON RS: Isolation of Neisseria lactamica from a genital site. Lancet 2:739–740, 1972

227. JONES RN, GAVAN TL, THORNSBERRY C ET AL: Standardization of disk diffusion and agar dilution susceptibility tests for Neisseria gonorrhoeae: interpretive criteria and quality control guidelines for ceftriaxone, penicillin, spectinomycin, and tetracycline. J Clin Microbiol 27:2758–2766, 1989

228. JONSSON I, HOLME T, KROOK A: Significance of isolation of Moraxella catarrhalis in routine cultures from the respiratory tract in adults: antibody response studied in a whole cell EIA. Scand J Infect Dis 26:553–558, 1994

229. JORGENSEN JH, DOERN GV, MAHAR LA ET AL: Antimicrobial resistance among respiratory isolates of Haemophilus influenzae, Moraxella catarrhalis, and Streptococcus pneumoniae in the United States. Antimicrob Agents Chemother 34:2075–2080, 1990

230. JUDSON FN: Gonorrhea. Med Clin North Am 74:1353–1366, 1990

231. JUNI E, HEYM GA: Psychrobacter immobilis gen. nov., sp. nov.: genospecies composed of gram-negative, aerobic, oxidase-positive coccobacilli. Int J Syst Bacteriol 36:366–391, 1986

232. KAMME C, VANG M, STAHL S: Transfer of beta-lactamase production in Branhamella catarrhalis. Scand J Infect Dis 15:225–226, 1983

233. KAMME C, VANG M, STAHL M: Intrageneric and intergeneric transfer of Branhamella catarrhalis beta-lactamase production. Scand J Infect Dis 16:153–155, 1984

234. KAROLUS JJ, GANDELMAN AL, NOLAN BA: Urethritis caused by Neisseria meningitidis. J Clin Microbiol 12:284–285, 1980

235. KAYHTY H, KARENKO V, PELTOLA H ET AL: Serum antibodies to capsular polysaccharide vaccine of group A Neisseria meningitidis followed for three years in infants and children. J Infect Dis 142:861–868, 1980

236. KELLOGG JA, ORWIG LK: Comparison of GonoGen, GonoGen II, and MicroTrak direct fluorescent antibody test with carbohydrate fermentation for confirmation of culture isolates of Neisseria gonorrhoeae. J Clin Microbiol 33:474–476, 1995

237. KELLOGG DS, PEACOCK WL, DEACON WE ET AL: Neisseria gonorrhoeae I. Virulence genetically linked to clonal variation. J Bacteriol 94:1274–1279, 1963

238. Kerle KK, Mascola JR, Miller TA: Disseminated gonococcal infection. Am Fam Physician 45:209–214, 1992

239. Kertesz DA., Byrne SK, Chow AW: Characterization of *Neisseria meningitidis* by polymerase chain reaction and restriction endonuclease digestion of the *porA* gene. J Clin Microbiol 31:2594–2598, 1993

240. Keys TF, Hecht RH, Chow AW: Endocervical *Neisseria meningitidis* with meningococcemia. N Engl J Med 285:505–506, 1971

240a. Kirchgesner V, Plesiat P, DuPont MJ et al: Meningitis and septicemia due to *Neisseria cinerea*. Clin Infect Dis 21:1351, 1995

241. Kleris GS, Arnold AJ: Differential diagnosis of urethritis: predictive value and therapeutic implications of the urethral smear. Sex Transm Dis 8:810–816, 1981

242. Knapp JS: Reduction of nitrite by *Neisseria gonorrhoeae*. Int J Syst Bacteriol 34:376–377, 1984

243. Knapp JS: Historical perspectives and identification of *Neisseria* and related species. Clin Microbiol Rev 1:415–431, 1988

244. Knapp JS, Clark VL: Anaerobic growth of *Neisseria gonorrhoeae* coupled to nitrite reduction. Infect Immun 46:176–181, 1984

245. Knapp JS, Holmes KK: Disseminated gonococcal infections caused by *Neisseria gonorrhoeae* strains with unique nutritional requirements. J Infect Dis 132:204–208, 1975

246. Knapp JS, Hook EW: Prevalence and persistence of *Neisseria cinerea* and other *Neisseria* spp. in adults. J Clin Microbiol 26:896–900, 1988

247. Knapp JS, Johnson SR, Zenilman JM et al: High-level tetracycline resistance resulting from *TetM* in strains of *Neisseria* spp., *Kingella denitrificans*, and *Eikenella corrodens*. Antimicrob Agents Chemother 32:765–767, 1988

248. Knapp JS, Ohye R, Neal SW et al: Emerging in vitro resistance to quinolones in penicillinase-producing *Neisseria gonorrhoeae* strains in Hawaii. Antimicrob Agents Chemother 38:2200–2203, 1994

249. Knapp JS, Rice RJ: *Neisseria* and *Branhamella*, In Murray PR, Baron EJ, Pfaller MA et al (eds), *Manual of Clinical Microbiology*, 6th ed, pp 324–340. Washington DC, ASM Press, 1995

250. Knapp JS, Sandstrom EG, Holmes KK: Overview of epidemiologic and clinical applications of auxotype/serovar classification of *Neisseria gonorrhoeae*. In Schoolnik GK (ed), *The Pathogenic Neisseriae*, pp 6–12. Washington DC, American Society for Microbiology, 1985.

251. Knapp JS, Tam MR, Nowinski RC et al: Serological classification of *Neisseria gonorrhoeae* with use of monoclonal antibodies to gonococcal outer membrane protein I. J Infect Dis 150:44–48, 1984

252. Knapp JS, Totten PA, Mulks MH et al: Characterization of *Neisseria cinerea*, a non-pathogenic species isolated on Martin-Lewis medium selective for pathogenic *Neisseria* spp. J Clin Microbiol 19:63–67, 1984

253. Knapp JS, Washington JA, Doyle LJ et al: Persistence of *Neisseria gonorrhoeae* strains with decreased susceptibilities to ciprofloxacin and ofloxacin in Cleveland, Ohio, from 1992 through 1993. Antimicrob Agents Chemother 38:2194–2196, 1994

254. Knapp JS, Zenilman JM, Biddle JW et al: Frequency and distribution in the United States of strains of *Neisseria gonorrhoeae* with plasmid-mediated, high-level resistance to tetracycline. J Infect Dis 155:819–822, 1987

255. Knight AI, Cartwright KAV, McFadden J: Identification of a UK outbreak strain of *Neisseria meningitidis* with a DNA probe. Lancet 335:1182–1184, 1990

256. Kociuba K, Munro R, Daley D: M-6 endocarditis: report of an Australian case. Pathology 25:310–312, 1993

257. Koppes GM, Ellenbogen C, Gebhart RJ: Group Y meningococcal disease in United States Air Force recruits. Am J Med 62:661–666, 1977

258. Korppi M, Katila ML, Jaaskelainen J et al: Role of *Moraxella* (*Branhamella*) *catarrhalis* as a respiratory pathogen in children. Acta Paediatr 81:993–996, 1992

259. Kovatch AL, Wald ER, Michaels RH: *beta*-Lactamase-producing *Branhamella catarrhalis* causing otitis media in children. J Pediatr 102:261–264, 1983

260. Kristiansen B-E, Fermer C, Jenkins A et al: PCR amplicon restriction endonuclease analysis of the chromosomal *dhps* gene of *Neisseria meningitidis*: a method for studying spread of the disease-causing strain in contacts of patients with meningococcal disease. J Clin Microbiol 33:1174–1179, 1995

261. Kuritza AP, Edberg SC, Chapis C et al: Identification of *Neisseria gonorrhoeae* with the ORTHOProbe DNA test. Diagn Microbiol Infect Dis 12:129–132, 1989

262. Kurzynski TA, Kimball JL, Polyak MB: Evaluation of the Phadebact and Bactigen reagents for detection of *Neisseria meningitidis* in cerebrospinal fluid. J Clin Microbiol 21:989–990, 1985

263. Lairscey RC, Kelly MT: Evaluation of a one-hour test for identification of *Neisseria* species. J Clin Microbiol 22:238–240, 1985

264. Lauer BA, Fisher E: *Neisseria lactamica* meningitis. Am J Dis Child 130:198–199, 1976

265. Lauer BA, Masters HB: Toxic effect of calcium alginate swabs on *Neisseria gonorrhoeae*. J Clin Microbiol 26:54–56, 1988

266. Laughon BE, Ehret JM, Tanino TT et al: Fluorescent monoclonal antibody for confirmation of *Neisseria gonorrhoeae* cultures. J Clin Microbiol 25:2388–2390, 1987

267. Lawton WD, Battaglioli GJ: GonoGen coagglutination test for *Neisseria gonorrhoeae*. J Clin Microbiol 18:1264–1265, 1983

268. Lee AH, Chin AE, Ramanujam T et al: Gonococcal septic arthritis of the hip. J Rheumatol 18:1932–1933, 1991

269. Lee BC, Hill P: Identification of an outer-membrane haemoglobin binding protein in *Neisseria meningitidis*. J Gen Microbiol 138:2647–2656, 1992

270. Lee TJ, Snyderman R, Patterson J: *Neisseria meningitidis* bacteremia in association with deficiency of the sixth component of complement. Infect Immun 24:656–658, 1979

271. Leggiadro RJ, Lazar LF: Spontaneous bacterial peritonitis due to *Neisseria meningitidis* serogroup Z in an infant with liver failure. Clin Pediatr 30:350–352, 1991

272. Lepow ML, Beeler J, Randolph M et al: Reactogenicity and immunogenicity of a quadrivalent combined meningococcal polysaccharide vaccine in children. J Infect Dis 154:1033–1036, 1986

273. Lewis JS, Fakile O, Foss E et al: Direct DNA probe assay for *Neisseria gonorrhoeae* in pharyngeal and rectal specimens. J Clin Microbiol 31:2783–2785, 1993

274. LEWIS JS, KRANIG-BROWN D, TRAINOR DA: DNA probe confirmatory test for *Neisseria gonorrhoeae*. J Clin Microbiol 28:2349–2350, 1990

275. LEWIS LS, GLAUSER TA, JOFFE MD: Gonococcal conjunctivitis in prepubertal children. Am J Dis Child 144:546–548, 1990

276. LIEBLING MR, ARKFELD DG, MICHELINI GA ET AL: Identification of *Neisseria gonorrhoeae* in synovial fluid using the polymerase chain reaction. Arth Rheum 37:702–709, 1994

277. LIMBERGER RJ, BIEGA R, EVANCOE A ET AL: Evaluation of culture and the Gen-Probe PACE 2 assay for detection of *Neisseria gonorrhoeae* and *Chlamydia trachomatis* in endocervical specimens transported to a state health laboratory. J Clin Microbiol 30:1162–1166, 1992

278. LINQUIST PR, LINQUIST JA: *Neisseria mucosa* bursitis: a rare case of gas in soft tissue. Clin Orthop 231:222–224, 1988

279. LIPMAN RM, DEUTSCH TA: Late-onset *Moraxella catarrhalis* endophthalmitis after filtering surgery. Can J Ophthalmol 27:249–250, 1992

280. LOPEZ-VELEZ R, FORTUN J, DE PABLO C ET AL: Native valve endocarditis due to *Neisseria sicca*. Clin Infect Dis 18:660–661, 1994

281. LOSSICK JG, SMELTZER MP, CURRAN JW: The value of the cervical Gram stain in the diagnosis of gonorrhea in women in a sexually transmitted diseases clinic. Sex Transm Dis 9:124–127, 1982

282. LOUIE M, ONGSANSOY EG, FORWARD KR: Rapid identification of *Branhamella catarrhalis*: a comparison of five rapid methods. Diagn Microbiol Infect Dis 13:205–208, 1990

283. LUJAN R, ZHANG Q-Y, SAEZ-NIETO JA ET AL: Penicillin-resistant isolates of *Neisseria lactamica* produce altered forms of penicillin-binding protein 2 that arose by interspecies horizontal gene transfer. Antimicrob Agents Chemother 35:300–304, 1991

284. MACARTHUR RD: *Branhamella catarrhalis* peritonitis in two continuous ambulatory peritoneal dialysis patients. Perit Dial Int 11:185, 1990

285. MACIA M, VEGA N, ELCUAZ R ET AL: *Neisseria mucosa* peritonitis in CAPD: another case of "non-pathogenic" neisseriae infection. Perit Dial Int 13:72–73, 1993

286. MACIVER I, UNHANAND M, MCCRACKEN JR GH ET AL: Effect of immunization on pulmonary clearance of *Moraxella catarrhalis* in an animal model. J Infect Dis 168:469–472, 1993

287. MANDRELL RE, ZOLLINGER WD: Lipopolysaccharide serotyping of *Neisseria meningitidis* by hemagglutination inhibition. Infect Immun 16:471–475, 1977

288. MARCHANT CD: Spectrum of disease due to *Branhamella catarrhalis* in children with particular reference to acute otitis media. Am J Med 88(suppl 5A):15S–19S, 1990

289. MARRS CF: Pili (fimbriae) of *Branhamella* species. Am J Med 88(suppl 5A):36S–40S, 1990

290. MARTIN JE, JACKSON RL: A biological environmental chamber for the culture of *Neisseria gonorrhoeae*. J Am Vener Dis Assoc 2:28–30, 1975

291. MARTIN JE, LEWIS JS: Anisomycin: improved antimycotic activity in modified Thayer-Martin medium. Public Health Lab 35:62–63, 1977

292. MASON W, IGDALOF S, FRIEDMAN R ET AL: Meningococcal sepsis with endophthalmitis. Am J Dis Child 133:1151–1152, 1979

293. MASTRANTONIO P, CONGIU ME, SELANDER RK ET AL: Genetic relationships among strains of *Neisseria meningitidis* causing disease in Italy, 1984–1987. Epidemiol Infect 106:143–150, 1991

294. MASTROLONARDO M, LOCONSOLE F, CONTE A ET AL: Cutaneous vasculitis as the sole manifestation of disseminated gonococcal infection: case report. Genitourin Med 70:130–131, 1994

295. MAYATEPEK E, GRAUER M, HANSCH GM ET AL: Deafness, complement deficiencies and immunoglobulin status in patients with meningococcal disease due to uncommon serogroups. Pediatr Infect Dis J 12:808–811, 1993

296. MAZLOUM H, TOTTEN PA, BROOKS GF ET AL: An unusual *Neisseria* isolated from conjunctival cultures in rural Egypt. J Infect Dis 154:212–224, 1986

297. MCCORMACK WM, MOGABGAB WJ, JONES RB ET AL: Multicenter comparative study of cefotaxime and ceftriaxone for treatment of uncomplicated gonorrhea. Sex Transm Dis 20:269–273, 1993

298. MCKENZIE H, MORGAN MG, JORDENS JZ ET AL: Characterization of hospital isolates of *Moraxella (Branhamella) catarrhalis* by SDS–PAGE of whole cell proteins, immunoblotting and restriction endonuclease analysis. J Med Microbiol 37:70–76, 1992

299. MCNEELY DJ, KITCHENS CS, KLUGE RM: Fatal *Neisseria (Branhamella) catarrhalis* pneumonia in an immunodeficient host. Am Rev Respir Dis 114:399–406, 1976

300. MELENDEZ PR, JOHNSON RH: Bacteremia and septic arthritis caused by *Moraxella catarrhalis*. Rev Infect Dis 13:428–429, 1991

301. MENDELMAN PM, CAMPOS J, CHAFFIN DO ET AL: Relative penicillin G resistance in *Neisseria meningitidis* and reduced afinity of penicillin-binding protein 2. Antimicrob Agents Chemother 32:706–709, 1988

302. MENINGOCOCCAL DISEASE SURVEILLANCE GROUP: Analysis of endemic meningococcal disease by serogroup and evaluation of chemoprophylaxis. J Infect Dis 134:201–204, 1976

303. MILAGRES LG, RAMOS SR, SACCHI CT ET AL: Immune response of Brazilian children to a *Neisseria meningitidis* serogroup b outer membrane protein vaccine: comparison with efficacy. Infect Immun 62:4419–4424, 1994

304. MINSHEW BH, BEARDSLEY JL, KNAPP JS: Evaluation of GonoGen coagglutination test for serodiagnosis of *Neisseria gonorrhoeae*: identification of problem isolates by auxotyping, serotyping, and with a fluorescent antibody reagent. Diagn Microbiol Infect Dis 3:41–46, 1985

305. MIRRETT S, RELLER LB, KNAPP JS: *Neisseria gonorrhoeae* strains inhibited by vancomycin in selective media and correlation with auxotype. J Clin Microbiol 14:94–99, 1981

306. MONTGOMERY K, RAYMUNDO L, DREW WL: Chromogenic cephalosporin spot test to detect *beta*-lactamase in clinically significant bacteria. J Clin Microbiol 9:205–207, 1979

307. MOORE PS, HIERHOLZER J, DEWITT W ET AL: Respiratory viruses and mycoplasma as cofactors for epidemic group A meningococcal meningitis. JAMA 264:1271–1275, 1990

308. MORAES JC, PERKINS BA, CAMARGO MCC ET AL: Protective efficacy of a serogroup B meningococcal vaccine in Sao Paulo, Brazil. Lancet 340:1074–1078, 1992

309. MORELLO JA, LERNER SA, BOHNHOFF M: Characteristics of atypical *Neisseria gonorrhoeae* from disseminated and localized infections. Infect Immun 13:1510–1516, 1976

310. MORGAN MG, MCKENZIE H, ENRIGHT MC ET AL: Use of molecular methods to characterize *Moraxella catarrhalis* strains in a suspected outbreak of nosocomial infection. Eur J Clin Microbiol Infect Dis 11:305–312, 1992

311. MORLA N, GUIBOURDENCHE M, RIOU J-Y: *Neisseria* spp. and AIDS. J Clin Microbiol 30:2290–2294, 1992

312. MORSE SA, BARTENSTEIN L: Adaptation of the Minitek system for the rapid identification of *Neisseria gonorrhoeae*. J Clin Microbiol 3:8–13, 1976

313. MORSE SA, JOHNSON SR, BIDDLE JW ET AL: High-level tetracycline resistance in *Neisseria gonorrhoeae* is a result of acquisition of streptococcal *tetM* determinant. Antimicrob Agents Chemother 30:664–670, 1986

314. MOYLE G, BARTON SE, MIDGLEY J ET AL: Gonococcal arthritis caused by auxotype P in a man with HIV infection. Genitourin Med 66:91–92, 1990

315. MULKS MH, PLAUT AG: IgA protease production as a characteristic distinguishing pathogenic from harmless *Neisseriaceae*. N Engl J Med 299:973–976, 1978

316. MURALIDHAR B, RUMORE PM, STEINMAN CR: Use of the polymerase chain reaction to study arthritis due to *Neisseria gonorrhoeae*. Arthritis Rheum 37:710–717, 1994

317. MURPHY TF: Studies on the outer membrane proteins of *Branhamella catarrhalis*. Am J Med 88(suppl 5A):41S–45S, 1990

318. NAQVI SH, KILPATRICK B, BOUHASIN J: *Branhamella catarrhalis* meningitis following otolaryngologic surgery. APMIS Suppl 3:74–75, 1988

319. NATIONAL COMMITTEE FOR CLINICAL LABORATORY STANDARDS: Performance standards for antimicrobial disk susceptibility tests. Approved Standard M2-A5, 5th ed. Villanova PA, 1993

320. NATIONAL COMMITTEE FOR CLINICAL LABORATORY STANDARDS: Methods for dilution antimicrobial susceptibility tests for bacteria that grow aerobically. Approved Standard M7-A3, 3rd ed. Villanova PA, 1993

321. NEU AM, CASE B, LEDERMAN HM ET AL: *Neisseria sicca* peritonitis in a patient maintained on chronic peritoneal dialysis. Pediatr Nephrol 8:601–602, 1994

322. NEUBERT AG, SCHWARTZ PA: *Neisseria meningitidis* sepsis as a complication of labor. J Reprod Med 39:749–751, 1994

323. NG, L-K, CARBALLO M, DILLON JR: Differentiation of *Neisseria gonorrhoeae* isolates requiring proline, citrulline, and uracil by plasmid content, serotyping, and pulsed-field gel electrophoresis. J Clin Microbiol 33:1039–1041, 1995

324. NG L-K, DILLON JR: Typing by serovar, antibiogram, plasmid content, ribotyping, and isoenzyme typing to determine whether *Neisseria gonorrhoeae* isolates requiring proline, citrulline, and uracil for growth are clonal. J Clin Microbiol 31:1555–1561, 1993

325. OBEID EMH: *Neisseria subflava* causing septic arthritis of the ankle of a child. J Infect 27:100–101, 1993

326. OLSEN SF, DJURHUUS B, RASMUSSEN K ET AL: Pharyngeal carriage of *Neisseria meningitidis* and *Neisseria lactamica* in households with infants within areas with high and low incidences of meningococcal disease. Epidemiol Infect 106:445–457, 1991

327. ORDEN B, AMERIGO MA: Acute otitis media caused by *Neisseria lactamica*. Eur J Clin Microbiol Infect Dis 10:986–987, 1991

328. ORREN A, CAUGANT DA, FIJEN CAP ET AL: Characterization of strains of *Neisseria meningitidis* recovered from complement-sufficient and complement-deficient patients in the Western Cape Province, South Africa. J Clin Microbiol 32:2185–2191, 1994

329. PAI CH, SORGER S: Enhancement of recovery of *Neisseria meningitidis* by gelatin in blood culture media. J Clin Microbiol 14:20–23, 1981

330. PATTERSON TF, PATTERSON EJ, MASECAR BL ET AL: A nosocomial outbreak of *Branhamella catarrhalis* confirmed by restriction endonuclease analysis. J Infect Dis 157:996–1001, 1988

331. PEIRIS V, HEALD J: Rapid method for differentiating strains of *Branhamella catarrhalis*. J Clin Pathol 45:532–534, 1992

332. PEIXUAN Z, XUJING H, LI X: Typing *Neisseria meningitidis* by analysis of restriction fragment length polymorphisms in the gene encoding the class 1 outer membrane protein: application to assessment of epidemics through the last four decades in China. J Clin Microbiol 33:458–462, 1995

333. PELTOLA H, MAKELA PH. KAYHTY H ET AL: Clinical efficacy of meningococcus group A capsular polysaccharide vaccine in children three months to five years of age. N Engl J Med 297:686–691, 1977

334. PELTOLA H, SAFARY A, KAYHTY H ET AL: Evaluation of 2 tetravalent (ACYW135) meningococcal vaccines in infants and small children—a clinical study comparing immunogenicity of O-acetyl-negative and O-acetyl-positive group C polysaccharides. Pediatrics 76:91–96, 1985

335. PEREZ JL, PULIDO A, GOMEZ E ET AL: Superoxol and aminopeptidase tests for identification of pathogenic *Neisseria* species and *Moraxella (Branhamella) catarrhalis*. Eur J Clin Microbiol Infect Dis 9:421–424, 1990

336. PEREZ RE: Endocarditis with *Moraxella*-like M-6 after cardiac catheterization. J Clin Microbiol 24:501–502, 1986

337. PHILLIPS EA, SCHULTZ TR, TAPSALL JW ET AL: Maltose-negative *Neisseria meningitidis* isolated from a case of male urethritis. J Clin Microbiol 27:2851–2852, 1989

338. PINNER R, ONYANGO F, PERKINS BA ET AL: Epidemic meningococcal disease in Nairobi, Kenya, 1989. J Infect Dis 166:359–364, 1992

339. PINNER R, SPELLMAN P, STEPHENS DS: Evidence for functionally distinct pili expressed by *Neisseria meningitidis*. Infect Immun 59:3169–3175, 1991

340. PLAVIDAL FJ, WERCH A: Gonococcal fetal scalp abscess: a case report. Am J Obstet Gynecol 127:437–438, 1977

341. PLOURDE PJ, TYNDALL M, AGOKI E ET AL: Single-dose cefixime versus single-dose ceftriaxone in the treatment of antimicrobial-resistant *Neisseria gonorrhoeae* infection. J Infect Dis 166:919–922, 1992

342. POH CL, LAU QC: Subtyping of *Neisseria gonorrhoeae* auxotype–serovar groups by pulsed-field gel electrophoresis. J Med Microbiol 38:366–370, 1993

343. POLLACK S, MOGTADER A, LANGE M: *Neisseria subflava* endocarditis: case report and review of the literature. Am J Med 76:752–758, 1984

344. PON E, BATCHELOR RA, HOWELL HB ET AL: An unusual case of penicillinase-producing *Neisseria gonorrhoeae* resistant to spectinomycin in California. Sex Transm Dis 13:47–49, 1986

345. PORTILLO I, LUTZ B, MONTALVO M ET AL: Oral cefixime versus intramuscular ceftriaxone in patients with uncomplicated gonococcal infections. Sex Transm Dis 19: 94–98, 1992

346. POWARS D, LARSEN R, JOHNSON J ET AL: Epidemic meningococcemia and purpura fulminans with induced protein C deficiency. Clin Infect Dis 17:254–261, 1993

347. PUGSLEY PM, DWORZACK DL, HOROWITZ EA ET AL: Efficacy of ciprofloxacin in the treatment of nasopharyngeal carriers of *Neisseria meningitidis*. J Infect Dis 156: 211–213, 1987

348. QUENTIN R, PIERRE F, DUBOIS M ET AL: Frequent isolation of capnophilic bacteria in aspirate from Bartholin's gland abscesses and cysts. Eur J Clin Microbiol Infect Dis 9:138–141, 1990

349. RELLER BL, MACGREGOR RR, BEATY HN: Bactericidal antibody after colonization with *Neisseria meningitidis*. J Infect Dis 127:56–62, 1973

350. RICE PA, VAYO HE, TAM MR ET AL: Immunoglobulin G antibodies directed against protein III block killing of serum-resistant *Neisseria gonorrhoeae* by immune serum. J Exp Med 164:1735–1748, 1986

351. RICE RJ, BIDDLE JW, JEAN-LOUIS YA ET AL: Chromosomally-mediated resistance in *Neisseria gonorrhoeae* in the United States: results of surveillance and reporting, 1983–1984. J Infect Dis 153:340–345, 1986

352. RICE RJ, KNAPP JS: Antimicrobial susceptibilities of *Neisseria gonorrhoeae* strains representing five distinct resistance phenotypes. Antimicrob Agents Chemother 38: 155–158, 1994

353. RICE RJ, KNAPP JS: Susceptibility of *Neisseria gonorrhoeae* associated with pelvic inflammatory disease to cefoxitin, ceftriaxone, clindamycin, gentamicin, doxycycline, azithromycin, and other antimicrobial agents. Antimicrob Agents Chemother 38:1688–1691, 1994

354. RICE RJ, SCHALLA WO, WHITTINGTON WL ET AL: Phenotypic characterstics of *Neisseria gonorrhoeae* isolated from three cases of meningitis. J Infect Dis 153:362–365, 1986

355. RICHARDS SJ, GREENING AP, ENRIGHT MC ET AL: Outbreak of *Moraxella catarrhalis* in a respiratory unit. Thorax 48:91–92, 1993

356. RIDDERHOF JC, VAUGHAN M, TINNEY A ET AL: Two confirmatory tests for identification of *Neisseria gonorrhoeae* from primary culture. J Clin Microbiol 28:619–620, 1990

357. RIKITOMI N, ANDERSSON B, MATSUMOTO K ET AL: Mechanism of adherence of *Moraxella (Branhamella) catarrhalis*. Scand J Infect Dis 23:559–567, 1991

358. RILEY G, BROWN S, KRISHNAN C: Penicillin resistance in *Neisseria meningitidis*. Lancet 324:997, 1990

359. RINGUETTE L, LORANGE M, RYAN A ET AL: Meningococcal infections in the province of Quebec, Canada, during the period 1991 to 1992. J Clin Microbiol 33:53–57, 1995

360. RIOU JY, GUIBOURDENCHE M: *Neisseria polysaccharea* sp. nov. Int J Syst Bacteriol 37:163–165, 1987

361. RIOU JY, GUIBOURDENCHE M, PERRY MB ET AL: Structure of the extracellular D-glucan produced by *Neisseria polysaccharea*. Can J Microbiol 32:909–911, 1986

362. RISHER WH, MCFADDEN PM: *Neisseria gonorrhoeae* mycotic ascending aortic aneurysm. Ann Thorac Surg 57: 748–750, 1994

363. ROBERTS MC, BROWN BA, STEINGRUBE VA ET AL: Genetic basis of tetracycline resistance in *Moraxella (Branhamella) catarrhalis*. Antimicrob Agents Chemother 34: 1816–1818, 1990

364. ROBERTS MC, KNAPP JS: Host range of the conjugative 25.2 megadalton tetracycline resistance plasmid from *Neisseria gonorrhoeae* and related species. Antimicrob Agents Chemother 32:488–491, 1988

365. ROBINSON A, GRIFFITH SB, MOORE DG ET AL: Evaluation of the RIM system and Gonogen test for identification of *Neisseria gonorrhoeae* from clinical specimens. Diagn Microbiol Infect Dis 3:125–130, 1985

366. ROMPALO AM, COLLETTA L, CAINE VA ET AL: Efficacy of 250 mg trospectomycin sulfate IM vs. 250 mg ceftriaxone IM for treatment of uncomplicated gonorrhea. Sex Transm Dis 21:213–216, 1994

367. RONNE T, BERTHELSEN L, BUHL L ET AL: Comparative studies on pharyngeal carriage of *Neisseria meningitidis* during a localized outbreak of serogroup C meningococcal disease. Scand J Infect Dis 25:331–339, 1993

368. ROSENQVIST E, WEDEGE E, HOIBY EA ET AL: Serogroup determination of *Neisseria meningitidis* by whole-cell ELISA, dot-blotting, and agglutination. APMIS 98: 501–506, 1990

369. ROSS SC, DENSEN P: Complement deficiency states and infection: epidemiology, pathogenesis and consequences of neisserial and other infections in an immune deficiency. Medicine 63:243–273, 1984

370. ROSSAU R, DUHAMEL M, VAN DYCK E ET AL: Evaluation of an rRNA-derived oligonucleotide probe for culture confirmation of *Neisseria gonorrhoeae*. J Clin Microbiol 28:944–948, 1990

371. ROSSAU R, KERSTERS K, FALSEN E ET AL: *Oligella*, a new genus including *Oligella urethralis* comb. nov. (formerly *Moraxella urethralis*) and *Oligella ureolytica* sp. nov. (formerly CDC group IVe): relationship to *Taylorella equigenitalis* and related taxa. Int J Syst Bacteriol 37: 198–210, 1987

372. ROSSAU R, VANDENBUSSCHE G, THIELEMANS S ET AL: Ribosomal ribonucleic acid cistron similarities and deoxyribonucleic acid homologies of *Neisseria*, *Kingella*, *Eikenella*, *Simonsiella*, *Alysiella*, and Centers for Disease Control groups EF-4 and M-5 in the emended Family *Neisseriaceae*. Int J Syst Bacteriol 39:185–198, 1989

373. ROSSAU R, VAN LANDSCHOOT A, GILLIS M ET AL: Taxonomy of *Moraxellaceae* fam. nov., a new bacterial family to accommodate the genera *Moraxella*, *Acinetobacter*, *Psychrobacter* and related organisms. Int J Syst Bacteriol 41:310–319, 1991

374. ROSSAU R, VAN LANDSCHOOT A, MANNHEIM W ET AL: Inter- and intrageneric similarities of ribosomal nucleic acid cistrons of the *Neisseriaceae*. Int J Syst Bacteriol 26:323–332, 1986

375. ROSSAU R, VANMECHELEN E, DELEY J ET AL: Specific *Neisseria gonorrhoeae* DNA probes derived from ribosomal RNA. J Gen Microbiol 135:1735–1745, 1989

376. SACCHI CT, TONDELLA MLC, DE LEMOS APS ET AL: Characterization of epidemic *Neisseria meningitidis* serogroup C strains in several Brazilian states. J Clin Microbiol 32:1783–1787, 1994

377. SAEZ-NIETO JA, CAMPOS J: Penicillin-resistant strains of *Neisseria meningitidis* in Spain. Lancet 1:1452–1453, 1988

378. SAEZ-NIETO JA, FENOLL A, VASQUEZ J ET AL: Prevalence of maltose-negative *Neisseria meningitidis* variants during an epidemic period in Spain. J Clin Microbiol 15:78–81, 1982

379. SAEZ-NIETO JA, FONTANALS D, DE JALON JG ET AL: Isolation of *Neisseria meningitidis* strains with increase of penicillin minimal inhibitory concentrations. Epidemiol Infect 99:463–469, 1987

380. SAEZ-NIETO JA, LUJAN R, BERRON S ET AL: Epidemiology and molecular basis of penicillin-resistant *Neisseria meningitidis* in Spain: a 5-year history (1985–1989). Clin Infect Dis 14:394–402, 1992

381. SAEZ NIETO JA, LUJAN R, MARTINEZ-SUAREZ JV ET AL: *Neisseria lactamica* and *Neisseria polysacchorea* as possible sources of meningococcal *beta*-lactam resistance by genetic transformation. Antimicrob Agents Chemother 34:2269–2272, 1990

382. SAGINUR R, CLECNER B, PORTNOY J ET AL: Superoxol (catalase) test for identification of *Neisseria gonorrhoeae*. J Clin Microbiol 15:475–477, 1982

383. SAITO H, ANNAISSIE EJ, KHARDORI N ET AL: *Branhamella catarrhalis* septicemia in patients with leukemia. Cancer 61:3215–3217, 1988

384. SAMUELSSON S, GUSTAVSEN S, RONNE T: Epidemiology of meningococcal disease in Denmark, 1980–1988. Scand J Infect Dis 23:723–730, 1991

385. SANDSTROM EG, RUDEN A-K: Markers of *Neisseria gonorrhoeae* for epidemiological studies. Scand J Infect Dis Suppl 69:149–156, 1990

386. SANYAL SK, WILSON N, TWUM-DANSO K ET AL: *Moraxella* endocarditis following balloon angioplasty of aortic coarctation. Am Heart J 119:1421–1423, 1991

387. SARUBBI FA, MYERS JW, WILLIAMS JJ ET AL: Respiratory infections caused by *Branhamella catarrhalis*. Am J Med 88(suppl 5A):9S–14S, 1990

388. SCHIFMAN RB, RYAN KJ: *Neisseria lactamica* septicemia in an immunocompromised patient. J Clin Microbiol 17:935–937, 1983

389. SCHNEIDER H, GRIFFISS JM, MANDRELL RE ET AL: Elaboration of a 3.6-kilodalton lipooligosaccharide, antibody against which is absent from human sera, is associated with serum resistance of *Neisseria gonorrhoeae*. Infect Immun 50:672–677, 1985

390. SCHNEIDER H, HAMMACK CA, APICELLA MA ET AL: Instability of expression of lipooligosaccharides and their epitopes in *Neisseria gonorrhoeae*. Infect Immun 56:942–946, 1988

391. SCHOLTEN RJPM, BIJLMER HA, POOLMAN JT ET AL: Meningococcal disease in the Netherlands, 1958–1990: a steady increase in the incidence since 1982 partially caused by new serotypes and subtypes of *Neisseria meningitidis*. Clin Infect Dis 16:237–246, 1993

392. SCHOLTEN RJPM, POOLMAN JT, VALKENBURG HA ET AL: Phenotypic and genotypic changes in a new clone complex of *Neisseria meningitidis* causing disease in the Netherlands, 1958–1990. J Infect Dis 169:673–676, 1994

393. SCHOOLNIK GK, BUCHANEN TM, HOLMES KK: Gonococci causing disseminated gonococcal infections are resistant to the bactericidal action of normal human serum. J Clin Invest 58:1163–1173, 1976

394. SCHOOLNIK GK, FERNANDEZ R, TAI J-Y: Gonococcal pili: primary structure and receptor binding domain. J Exp Med 159:1351–1370, 1984

395. SCHWARCZ SK, ZENILMAN JM, SCHNELL D ET AL: National surveillance of antimicrobial resistance in *Neisseria gonorrhoeae*. JAMA 264:1413–1417, 1990

396. SCHWARTZ B, MOORE PS, BROOME CV: Global epidemiology of meningococcal disease. Clin Microbiol Rev 2 (suppl):S118–S124, 1989

397. SCOTT MJ, SCOTT MJ: Primary cutaneous *Neisseria gonorrhoeae* infection. Arch Dermatol 118:351–352, 1982

398. SCOTT RM: Bacterial endocarditis due to *Neisseria flava*. J Pediatr 78:673–675, 1971

399. SCRIBNER RK: Neutralization of the inhibitory effect of sodium polyanethol sulfonate on *Neisseria meningitidis* in blood cultures processed with the DuPont Isolator system. J Clin Microbiol 20:40–42, 1984

400. SEDDON PC, SUNDERLAND D, O'HALLORAN SM ET AL: *Branhamella catarrhalis* colonization in pre-school asthmatics. Pediatr Pulmonol 13:133–135, 1992

401. SETH A: Use of trimethoprim to prevent overgrowth by *Proteus* in the cultivation of *Neisseria gonorrhoeae*. Br J Vener Dis 46:201–202, 1970

402. SHANMUGARATNAM K, PATTMAN RS: Acute urethritis due to *Neisseria meningitidis*. Genitourin Med 65:401–403, 1989

403. SHAWAR RM, LAROCCO MT, REVES RR: *Neisseria sicca* and *Streptococcus sanguis* I endocarditis in an intravenous drug user. Clin Microbiol Newslett 13:142–144, 1991

404. SHOOTER JR, HOWLES MJ, BASELSKI VS: Neisserial infections in dialysis patients. Clin Microbiol Newslett 12:15–16, 1990

405. SIMOR AE, SALIT IE: Endocarditis caused by M-6. J Clin Microbiol 17:931–933, 1983

406. SINAVE CP, RATZAN KR: Infective endocarditis caused by *Neisseria flavescens*. Am J Med 82:163–164, 1987

407. SINGH RP, MARWAHA RK: Fulminant *Branhamella catarrhalis* tracheitis. Ann Trop Paediatr 10:221–222, 1990

408. SJOHOLM AG, KUIJPER EJ, TIJSSEN CC ET AL: Dysfunctional properdin in a Dutch family with meningococcal disease. N Engl J Med 319:33–37, 1988

409. SMITH KR, CHING S, LEE H ET AL: Evaluation of ligase chain reaction for use with urine for identification of *Neisseria gonorrhoeae* in females attending a sexually transmitted disease clinic. J Clin Microbiol 33:455–457, 1995

410. SPARLING PF: Biology of *Neisseria gonorrhoeae*. In Holmes KK, Mardh P-A, Sparling PF, Weisner PJ (eds), *Sexually Transmitted Diseases*, 2nd ed, pp 131–147. New York, McGraw-Hill, 1990

411. SPARLING PF, TSAI J, CORNELISSEN CN: Gonococci are survivors. Scand J Infect Dis Suppl 69:125–136, 1990

412. SPEELEVELD E, FOSSEPRE J-M, GORDTS B ET AL: Comparison of three rapid methods, trybutyrine, 4-methylumbelliferyl butyrate, and indoxyl acetate, for rapid identification of *Moraxella catarrhalis*. J Clin Microbiol 32:1362–1363, 1994

413. SPRATT BG, ZHANG Q-Y, JONES DM ET AL: Recruitment of a penicillin-binding protein gene from *Neisseria flavescens* during the emergence of penicillin resistance in *Neisseria meningitidis*. Proc Natl Acad Sci USA 86: 8988–8992, 1989

414. SPROTT MS, KERANS AM, FIELD JM: Penicillin insensitive *Neisseria meningitidis*. Lancet 1:1167, 1988

415. STACKEBRANDT E, MURRAY RGE, TRUPER HG: *Proteobacteria* classis nov. a name for the phylogenetic taxon that includes the "purple bacteria and their relatives." Int J Syst Bacteriol 38:321–325, 1988

416. STANSFIELD RE, MASTERSON RG, DALE BAS ET AL: Primary meningococcal conjunctivitis and the need for prophylaxis in close contacts. J Infect 29:211–214, 1994

417. STEINGRIMSSON O, OLAFSSON JH, THORARINSSON H ET AL: Single dose azithromycin treatment of gonorrhea and infections caused by *C. trachomatis* and *U. urealyticum* in men. Sex Transm Dis 21:43–46, 1994

418. STENFORS L-E, RAISANEN S: Abundant attachment of bacteria to nasopharyngeal epithelium in otitis-prone children. J Infect Dis 165:1148–1150, 1992

419. STERN A, BROWN M, NICKEL P ET AL: Opacity genes in *Neisseria gonorrhoeae*: control of phase and antigenic variation. Cell 47:61–71, 1986

420. STOTKA JL, RUPP ME, MEIER FA ET AL: Meningitis due to *Neisseria mucosa*: case report and review. Rev Infect Dis 13:837–841, 1991

421. STRATHDEE CA, TYLER SD, RYAN JA ET AL: Genomic fingerprinting of *Neisseria meningitidis* associated with group C meningococcal disease in Canada. J Clin Microbiol 31:2506–2508, 1993

422. STRONGIN IS, KALE SA, RAYMOND MK ET AL: An unusual presentation of gonococcal arthritis in an HIV positive patient. Ann Rheum Dis 50:572–573, 1991

423. STRUILLOU L, RAFFI F, BARRIER JH: Endocarditis caused by *Neisseria elongata* subspecies *nitroreducens*: case report and literature review. Eur J Clin Microbiol Infect Dis 12:625–627, 1993

424. SUTCLIFFE EM, JONES DM, EL-SHEIKH S ET AL: Penicillin-insensitive meningococci in the U.K. Lancet 1:657–658, 1988

425. SWANSON J: Colony opacity and protein II compositions of gonococci. Infect Immun 37:359–368, 1982

426. TESORO LJ, SELBST SM: Factors affecting outcome in meningococcal infections. Am J Dis Child 145:218–220, 1991

427. THOMAS JC, BENDANA NS, WATERMAN SH ET AL: Risk factors for carriage of meningococcus in the Los Angeles County men's jail system. Am J Epidemiol 133:286–295, 1991

428. THORNHILL-JONES M, LI MW, CANAWATI HN ET AL: *Neisseria sicca* endocarditis in intravenous drug abusers. West J Med 142:255–256, 1985

429. TONDELLA MLC, SACCHI CT, NEVES BC: Ribotyping as an additional molecular marker for studying *Neisseria meningitidis* serogroup B epidemic strains. J Clin Microbiol 32:2745–2748, 1994

430. TOTTEN PA, HOLMES KK, HANDSFIELD HH ET AL: DNA hybridization technique for the detection of *Neisseria gonorrhoeae* in men with urethritis. J Infect Dis 148: 462–471, 1983

431. TRAMONT EC: Gonococcal vaccines. Clin Microbiol Rev 2(suppl):S74–S77, 1989

432. TURNER A, JEPHCOTT AE, GOUGH KR: Tetracycline-resistant meningococci. Lancet 1:1454, 1988

433. ULLMAN S, ROUSSEL TJ, FORSTER RK: Gonococcal kerato-conjunctivitis. Surv Ophthalmol 32:199–208, 1987

434. URIZ S, PINEDA V, GRAU M ET AL: *Neisseria meningitidis* with reduced sensitivity to penicillin: observation in 10 children. Scand J Infect Dis 23:171–174, 1991

435. VALENZUELA GA, DAVIS TD, PIZZANI E ET AL: Infective endocarditis due to *Neisseria sicca* and associated with intravenous drug abuse. South Med J 85:929, 1992

436. VANDAMME P, GILLIS M, VANCANNEYT M ET AL: *Moraxella lincolnii* sp. nov., isolated from the human respiratory tract, and reevaluation of the taxonomic position of *Moraxella osloensis*. Int J Syst Bacteriol 43:474–481, 1993

437. VAN DYCK E, SMET H, PIOT P: Comparison of E test with agar dilution for antimicrobial susceptibility testing of *Neisseria gonorrhoeae*. J Clin Microbiol 32:1586–1588, 1994

438. VANEECHOUTTE M, VERSCHRAEGEN G, CLAEYS G ET AL: Rapid identification of *Branhamella catarrhalis* with 4-methylumbelliferyl butyrate. J Clin Microbiol 26: 1227–1228, 1988

439. VANEECHOUTTE M, VERSCHRAEGEN G, CLAEYS G ET AL: Selective medium for *Branhamella catarrhalis* with acetazolamide as a specific inhibitor of *Neisseria* species. J Clin Microbiol 26:2544–2548, 1988

440. VANEECHOUTTE M, VERSCHRAEGEN G, CLAEYS G ET AL: Respiratory tract carrier rates of *Moraxella* (*Branhamella*) *catarrhalis* in adults and children and interpretation of the isolation of *M. catarrhalis* from sputum. J Clin Microbiol 28:2674–2680, 1990

441. VAN HARE GF, SHURIN PA, MARCHANT CD ET AL: Acute otitis media caused by *Branhamella catarrhalis*: biology and therapy. Rev Infect Dis 9:16–27, 1987

442. VEDROS NA: Genus I. *Neisseria* Trevisan 1885, 105AL. In Krieg NR, Holt JG (eds), *Bergey's Manual of Systematic Bacteriology*, vol 1, pp 190–196. Baltimore, Williams & Wilkins, 1984

443. VERDON MS, DOUGLAS JR JM, WIGGINS SD ET AL: Treatment of uncomplicated gonorrhea with single doses of 200 mg cefixime. Sex Transm Dis 20:290–293, 1993

444. VERNALEO JR, MATHEW A, CLERI DJ ET AL: *Neisseria sicca* endocarditis with embolic phenomena. Diagn Microbiol Infect Dis 15:165–167, 1992

445. VERNHAM GA, CROWTHER JA: Acute myeloid leukaemia presenting with acute *Branhamella catarrhalis* epiglottitis. J Infect 26:93–95, 1993

446. VERON M, LENVOISE-FURET A, COUSTERE C ET AL: Relatedness of three species of "false neisseriae," *Neisseria caviae*, *Neisseria cuniculi*, and *Neisseria ovis*, by DNA–DNA hybridizations and fatty acid analysis. Int J Syst Bacteriol 43:210–220, 1993

447. VIRJI M, HECKELS JE: The role of common and type-specific pilus antigenic domains in adhesion and virulence of gonococci for human epithelial cells. J Gen Microbiol 130:1089–1095, 1984

448. VLASPOLDER F, MUTSAERS JAEM, BLOG F ET AL: Value of a DNA probe assay (Gen-Probe) compared with that of culture for diagnosis of gonococcal infection. J Clin Microbiol 31:107–110, 1993

449. WALLACE MR, OLDFIELD EC: *Moraxella (Branhamella) catarrhalis* bacteremia: a case report and literature review. Arch Intern Med 150:1332–1334, 1990

450. WALLACE RJ JR, NASH DR, STEINGRUBE VA: Antibiotic susceptibilities and drug resistance in *Moraxella (Branhamella) catarrhalis*. Am J Med 88(suppl 5A):46S–50S, 1990

451. WALLACE RJ JR, STEINGRUBE VA, NASH DR ET AL: BRO *beta*-lactamases of of *Branhamella catarrhalis* and *Moraxella* subgenus *moraxella*, including evidence for chromosomal *beta*-lactamase transfer by conjugation in *B. catarrhalis*, *M. nonliquefaciens*, and *M. lacunata*. Antimicrob Agents Chemother 33:1845–1854, 1989

452. WALTON DT: Fluorescent antibody-negative penicillinase-producing *Neisseria gonorrhoeae*. J Clin Microbiol 27:1885–1886, 1989

453. WAN WL, FARKAS GC, MAY WN ET AL: The clinical characteristics and course of adult gonococcal conjunctivitis. Am J Ophthalmol 102:575–583, 1986

454. WATANAKUNAKORN C, THOMSON RB: Septicemia due to a maltose-positive, glucose-negative strain of group C *Neisseria meningitidis*. J Clin Microbiol 18:436–437, 1983

455. WEISS PJ, KENNEDY CA, MCCANN DF ET AL: Fulminant endocarditis due to infection with penicillinase-producing *Neisseria gonorrhoeae*. Sex Transm Dis 19:288–290, 1992

456. WELBORN PP, UYEDA CT, ELLISON-BIRANG N: Evaluation of Gonochek II as a rapid identification system for pathogenic *Neisseria* species. J Clin Microbiol 20:680–683, 1984

457. WELCH WD, CARTWRIGHT G: Fluorescent monoclonal antibody compared with carbohydrate utilization for rapid identification of *Neisseria gonorrhoeae*. J Clin Microbiol 26:293–296, 1988

458. WEST SE, SPARLING PF: Response of *Neisseria gonorrhoeae* to iron limitation: alterations in expression of membrane proteins without apparent siderophore production. Infect Immun 14:388–394, 1985

459. WHITTINGTON WL, KNAPP JS: Trends in resistance of *Neisseria gonorrhoeae* to antimicrobial agents in the United States. Sex Transm Dis 15:202–210, 1988

460. WHITTINGTON WL, RICE RJ, BIDDLE JW ET AL: Incorrect identification of *Neisseria gonorrhoeae* from infants and children. Pediatr Infect Dis J 7:3–10, 1988

461. WILLIAM DC, FELMAN YM, CORSARO MC: *Neisseria meningitidis* probable pathogen in two related cases of urethritis, epididymitis, and acute pelvic inflammatory disease. JAMA 242:1653–1654, 1979

462. WILSON APR, WOLFF J, ATIA W: Acute urethritis due to *Neisseria meningitidis* group A acquired by orogenital contact: a case report. Genitourin Med 65:122–123, 1989

463. WILSON HD, OVERMAN TL: Septicemia due to *Neisseria lactamica*. J Clin Microbiol 4:214–215, 1976

464. WILSON J, ZAMAN AG, SIMMONS AV: Gonococcal arthritis complicated by acute pericarditis and pericardial effusion. Br Heart J 63:134–135, 1990

465. WINDALL JJ, HALL MM, WASHINGTON JA ET AL: Inhibitory effects of vancomycin on *Neisseria gonorrhoeae* in Thayer-Martin medium. J Infect Dis 142:775, 1980

466. WISE CM, MORRIS CR, WAUSILAUSKAS BL ET AL: Gonococcal arthritis in an era of increasing penicillin resistance: presentations and outcomes in 41 recent cases (1985–1991). Arch Intern Med 154:2690–2695, 1994

467. WOLFE RE, BIRBARA CA: Meningococcal infections at an Army training center. Am J Med 44:243–255, 1968

468. WONG JD: Pathogenic "non-pathogenic" *Neisseria* spp. Clin Microbiol Newslett 16:41–44, 1994

469. WONG JD, JANDA JM: Association of an important *Neisseria* species, *Neisseria elongata* subsp. *nitroreducens*, with bacteremia, endocarditis, and osteomyelitis. J Clin Microbiol 30:719–720, 1992

470. WONG VK, ROSS LA: *Branhamella catarrhalis* septicemia in an infant with AIDS. Scand J Infect Dis 20:559–560, 1988

471. WOODS JP, KERSULYTE D, TOLAN RW ET AL: Use of arbitrarily primed polymerase chain reaction analysis to type disease and carrier strains of *Neisseria meningitidis* during a university outbreak. J Infect Dis 169:1384–1389, 1994

472. WRIGHT DN, LIU F: *Neisseria subflava* as a cause of bacteremia. Clin Microbiol Newslett 6:58–59, 1984

473. WRIGHT PW, WALLACE RJ, SHEPHERD JR: A descriptive study of 42 cases of *Branhamella catarrhalis* pneumonia. Am J Med 88(suppl 5A):2S–8S, 1990

474. YAKUBU DE, ABADI FJR, PENNINGTON TH: Molecular epidemiology of recent United Kingdon isolates of *Neisseria meningitidis* serogroup C. Epidemiol Infect 113:53–65, 1994

475. YEO SF, LIVERMORE DM: Effect of inoculum size on the in-vitro susceptibility to *beta*-lactam antibiotics of *Moraxella catarrhalis* isolates of different *beta*-lactamase types. J Med Microbiol 40:252–255, 1994

476. YEUNG K-H, NG L-K, DILLON JR: 1993. Evaluation of E test for testing antimicrobial susceptibilities of *Neisseria gonorrhoeae* isolates with different growth media. J Clin Microbiol 31:3053–3055, 1993

477. YOUNG LS, MOYES A: Comparative evaluation of AccuProbe culture identification test for *Neisseria gonorrhoeae* and other rapid methods. J Clin Microbiol 31:1996–1999, 1993

478. YOUNG LS, LAFORCE FM, HEAD JJ ET AL: A simultaneous outbreak of meningococcal and influenza infections. N Engl J Med 287:5–9, 1972

479. ZENILMAN JM, NIMS LJ, MENEGUS MA ET AL: Spectinomycin-resistant gonococcal infections in the United States. J Infect Dis 156:1002–1004, 1987

480. ZHANG QY, JONES DM, SAEZ-NIETO JA ET AL: Genetic diversity of penicillin-binding protein 2 genes of penicillin-resistant strains of *Neisseria meningitidis* revealed by fingerprinting of amplified DNA. Antimicrob Agents Chemother 34:1523–1528, 1990

THE GRAM-POSITIVE COCCI:
PART I: STAPHYLOCOCCI AND RELATED ORGANISMS

With the exception of the *Enterobacteriaceae*, gram-positive bacteria, particularly the cocci, are the microorganisms most frequently isolated from clinical specimens in the microbiology laboratory. These bacteria are widespread in nature and can be recovered from the environment or as commensel inhabitants of the skin, mucous membranes, and other body sites in humans and animals. The ubiquitous distribution of several gram-positive bacteria in nature makes the interpretation of their recovery from patient specimens somewhat difficult, unless there are classic clinical manifestations of an infectious disease process. The gram-positive cocci cause a variety of diseases, including folliculitis, furuncles, carbuncles, abscesses (staphylococci); pharyngitis, endocarditis, erysipelas and cellulitis (streptococci); and pneumonia and bacteremia (pneumococci). Therefore, their recovery from specimens should always be correlated with the clinical condition of the patient before their role in the etiology of an infectious process can be established.

Although gram-positive bacteria may cause infection by multiplication both locally and systemically, some organisms may multiply at a localized site and exert their pathogenic effects by producing exotoxins or enzymes that act at distant sites. Staphylococcal toxins are responsible for food poisoning, scalded skin syndrome, and toxic shock syndrome. The newly described streptococcal toxic shock syndrome (see Chap. 12) is another example of a disease in which the signs and symptoms of infection and the pathologic features of disease are largely due to the effects of exotoxins. Gram-negative bacteria, on the other hand, possess endotoxin, which is the lipid portion of the outer membrane lipopolysaccharide (LPS). Systemic infections with gram-negative bacteria may lead to endotoxic shock, which is characterized by hypotension, vascular collapse, and sometimes death. This occurs most frequently when gram-negative organisms gain entrance to the bloodstream.

With the increasing numbers of staphylococcal species being recognized in human infections and the finding of resistance to multiple antimicrobial agents in both the common and the uncommon isolates, it is imperative that the clinical microbiologist be familiar with current methods for characterizing these organisms. Several of the newly described animal staphylococcal species may also be important in veterinary practice, and this is reflected in the growing veterinary literature on the subject. Among the streptococci, changes in the spectrum of disease and increasing antimicrobial resistance among these bacteria necessitate a broad knowledge of this group of organisms. In addition, the isolation of other gram-positive, "streptococcus-like" bacteria from serious infections over the last few years requires that these organisms be recognized and identified as well. In this chapter, the clinical significance and laboratory procedures for isolation

Color Plates for Chapter 11 are found between pages 368 and 369.

and identification of the staphylococci and related organisms will be presented. In Chapter 12, the streptococci and streptococcus-like bacteria will be discussed. Antimicrobial susceptibility testing of these bacterial groups will be addressed in Chapter 15.

THE FAMILY *MICROCOCCACEAE*: TAXONOMY AND CLINICAL SIGNIFICANCE

According to the 1986 edition of *Bergey's Manual of Systematic Bacteriology*, the family *Micrococcaceae* includes four genera: *Planococcus*, *Micrococcus*, *Stomatococcus*, and *Staphylococcus*.[27,28,171,178,179] Nucleic acid homology studies and analysis of other properties (e.g., cell wall composition, cellular fatty acids) have demonstrated that these organisms are not as closely related as once thought. Micrococci are related genetically to the arthrobacters and the actinomycetes, whereas the staphylococci show genetic relatedness to the streptococci, enterococci, lactobacilli, and the genus *Bacillus*. The members of this family can be differentiated from members of the family *Streptococcaceae* by the catalase test (see later discussion). Members of the family *Micrococcaceae* are catalase-positive, whereas members of the family *Streptococcaceae* are catalase-negative.

Planococcus species are asaccharolytic, motile, gram-positive cocci that live in marine environments.[179] They have been isolated from seawater, estuaries, brine tanks, ocean fauna and flora, and frozen seafood. Cells of planococci are arranged in pairs or tetrads, with each cell possessing one to three flagella. Most strains also produce a yellow-orange pigment on nutrient agar. Planococci are asaccharolytic and halotolerant, being able to grow in media containing from less than 1% to more than 15% NaCl. There are currently two species in the genus: *P. citreus* and *P. kocuri*. *Planococcus halophilus*, a former member of the genus, has been transferred to the new genus *Marinococcus*, which are halophilic organisms that require at least 7.5% NaCl for growth. *P. citreus* may be differentiated from *P. kocuri* by the ability of the former species to grow on nutrient agar containing 12% NaCl.[130] They have not been implicated in human infections.

Members of the genus *Micrococcus* are found in the environment and as transient flora on the skin of humans and several other mammals. Some species produce carotenoid pigments, and colonies of these species appear bright yellow or pink on agar media. Certain micrococcal species have been used in industry as bioassay organisms for the detection of antimicrobial agents in animal feeds, cosmetics, and body fluids. They are occasionally isolated from human clinical specimens, in which they usually represent contaminants from the skin or mucous membrane surfaces or from the environment, although they may cause opportunistic infections in appropriate hosts.[82,281,289,334] Recently, Magee and coworkers[201] reported two cases of Hickman catheter-related sepsis, three cases of continuous ambulatory peritoneal dialysis (CAPD)-related peritonitis, and a case of ventriculoperitoneal shunt-associated meningitis that were caused by *Micrococccus* species. There are nine species in the genus *Micrococcus*: *M. luteus, M. lylae, M. varians, M. roseus, M. agilis, M. kristinae, M. nishinomiyaensis, M. sedentarius,* and *M. halobius*.[173,178]

In late 1995, Stackebrandt and associates performed 16S ribosomal DNA sequence analysis on the nine recognized *Micrococcus* species and proposed several changes in the taxonomy of these organisms.[177,291] According to these workers, *Micrococcus luteus* and *Micrococcus lylae* are the only species retained in the genus *Micrococcus*; *M. roseus, M. varians,* and *M. kristinae* now belong to the genus *Kocuria* as *K. roseus, K. varians,* and *K. kristinae,* respectively. *M. halobius, M. nishinomiyaensis,* and *M. sedentarius* are now placed in three separate genera as *Nesterenkonia halobia, Kytococcus nishinomiyaensis,* and *Dermacoccus sedentarius,* respectively. *Micrococcus agilis* has been reclassified in the genus *Arthrobacter* as *A. agilis*.[177] In the rest of this chapter, these organisms will be referred to as micrococci and related species.

Stomatococcus mucilaginosus (formerly *Micrococcus mucilaginosus*), the single member of the genus *Stomatococcus,* is an encapsulated gram-positive coccus that is a part of the normal human respiratory tract flora.[27,28] The first human infection with this organism was reported in 1978 in a patient who developed endocarditis following cardiac catheterization.[261] Since then, several case reports of both native valve and prosthetic valve endocarditis caused by *S. mucilaginosus* have appeared in the literature; in many of these cases, infection was associated with the use of intravenous drugs.[56,131,241,248,252] *S. mucilaginosus* sepsis has been reported in association with head and neck trauma, central and peripheral access devices, cancer chemotherapy, cardiac catheterization following myocardial infarction, and continuous ambulatory peritoneal dialysis.[220,243] *S. mucilaginosus* also has emerged as a significant pathogen in both adults and children with underlying malignancies (including leukemia, lymphoma, breast cancer, Hodgkin's disease, squamous cell carcinoma, osteosarcoma, and rhabdomyosarcoma), and in recipients of bone marrow transplants.[11,12,23,122,160,185,193,217,227,290,331] Infections in these patients have included transient and sustained bacteremias, peripheral and central line-associated sepsis, and meningitis. Recovery of *S. mucilaginosus* from these patients was associated with severe neutropenia as a result of underlying disease, immunosuppression, or cytotoxic chemotherapy. Colonized indwelling access devices (e.g, intravenous or intra-arterial lines, Brouviac and Hickman catheters) were the source of the organism in some patients, whereas mucosal or esophageal ulcerations secondary to cytotoxic chemotherapy, periodontal disease, or dental infections or procedures were believed to be possible sources in others. Other case reports also suggest an expanding disease spectrum for this organism. A case of severe *S. mucilaginosus* endophthalmitis following intraocular lens implantation and requiring evisceration of the eye has also been reported.[303] *S. mucilaginosus* has also been isolated from the bile of a 64-year-old man with cholangitis.[115]

S. mucilaginosus is nonmotile and, unlike other members of the Family *Micrococcaceae,* is only weakly catalase-positive and may be catalase-negative. Lack of growth on nutrient agar containing 5% NaCl helps to differentiate *S. mucilaginosus* from *Micrococcus* and *Staphylococcus* species.[27,28] Additional characteristics of *S. mucilaginosus* will be discussed later in this chapter.

The genus *Staphylococcus* is currently composed of 33 species, 17 of which may be encountered in human clinical specimens (Table 11-1).[49,69,70,87,111,112,113,142,155,162,168,170,171,172,175,235,266,267,268,270,304,319,330,342] Staphylococci are generally found on the skin and mucous membranes of humans and other animals. In some instances, this association is amazingly specific. For example, *S. capitis* is found primarily as a part of the human normal flora of the skin and sebaceous glands of the scalp, forehead, and neck, whereas *S. auricularis* is found primarily in the external auditory canal.[168,170] Many species are found only in certain animals; some of them are recognized veterinary pathogens. *Staphylococcus hyicus* causes an infectious dermatitis in swine, and *S. intermedius* has been isolated from several types of infections in dogs, including skin infections, mastitis, wounds, and reproductive tract infections.[69,111,112] The latter species has also been isolated from dog-bite wounds in humans.[301,302] *Staphylococcus delphini* and *S. felis* cause infectious processes in dolphins and domesticated cats, respectively.[142,319] Humans may become colonized or infected with these organisms by frequent or close contact with animals (e.g., veterinarians, zoo workers, farmers). Some of the pathogenic staphylococci in both humans and animals produce an enzyme called **coagulase,** and detection of this enzyme is used in the laboratory to identify these organisms.[111,319] Among the staphylococci, the coagulase-positive species *S. aureus* and two coagulase-negative species, *S. epidermidis* and *S. saprophyticus,* are seen frequently in human infections.

STAPHYLOCOCCUS AUREUS SUBSP. AUREUS

Staphylococcus aureus subsp. *aureus* (herein called *S. aureus*) is by far the most important human pathogen among the staphylococci. It is found in the external environment and in the anterior nares of 20% to 40% of adults. Other sites of colonization include intertriginous skin folds, the perineum, the axillae, and the vagina. Although this organism is frequently a part of the normal human microflora, it can cause significant opportunistic infections under the appropriate conditions.[324] Factors that may predispose an individual to serious *S. aureus* infections include the following:

- Defects in leukocyte chemotaxis, either congenital (e.g., Wiskott-Aldrich syndrome, Down syndrome, Job's syndrome) or acquired (e.g., diabetes mellitus, rheumatoid arthritis)
- Defects in opsonization by antibodies (e.g., hypogammaglobulinemia)
- Defects in intracellular killing of bacteria following phagocytosis (e.g., chronic granulomatous disease)
- Skin injuries (e.g., burns, surgical incisions, eczema)
- Presence of foreign bodies (e.g., sutures, intravenous lines, prosthetic devices)

TABLE 11-1
HUMAN, ANIMAL, AND ENVIRONMENTAL *STAPHYLOCOCCUS* SPECIES

SPECIES	COMMENTS
Staphylocci Found in Man and Nonhuman Primates	
S. aureus	See text
S. epidermidis	See text
S. saprophyticus	See text
S. haemolyticus[269]	A part of the human normal skin flora, *S. haemolyticus* is also found in nonhuman primates. It has been recovered from human clinical specimens. Strains of *S. haemolyticus* that are resistant to vancomycin (MICs of $\geq$ 8 μg/mL) have been reported recently in the clinical setting of prolonged vancomycin administration, suggesting selection of resistant clones of previously susceptible organisms.[125,318]
S. warneri[168]	This species represents about 1% of the staphylococci normally found on human skin. It is now a well-recognized cause of catheter-related bacteremia, native valve endocarditis, hematogenous veretebral osteomyelitis, and ventriculoperitoneal shunt-associated meningitis.[42,60,154,158,258,309,337] Isolates recovered from humans are now called *S. warneri* subsp. 1, whereas isolates from nonhuman primates are called *S. warneri* subsp. 2.
S. hominis[168]	This species is found on human skin, and it has been isolated as a cause of bacteremia in cancer patients.[38]
S. simulans[168]	Found on skin and in the urethras of healthy women, *S. simulans* has been isolated as a cause of septicemia, osteomyelitis, and septic arthritis following open reduction of a fractured fibula;[204] as a cause of native valve endocarditis;[148, 213] and as a cause of osteomyelitis of the pubic bone in a 77-year-old woman.[297] *S. simulans* possesses a capsule that inhibits phagocytosis in vitro and contributes to virulence in vivo.[226]
S. lugdunensis[87]	First described in 1988, has rapidly established itself as a significant human pathogen. It has been associated mainly with native and prosthetic valve endocarditis, skin and soft-tissue cellulitis, peritonitis, infected hip prostheses, osteomyelitis, vascular line infections, and breast abscesses.[21,55,77,87,123,195,201,284,317,323] A case of *S. lugdunensis* arthritis of the knee as a complication of arthroscopy has also been reported.[229]
S. capitis[168]	As part of the normal human flora, *S. capitis* is found surrounding the sebaceous glands on the scalp and forehead. Since 1992, this species has been reported as a cause of native valve endocarditis in five patients.[18,189,194,203] Recently, the species has been divided into two subspecies, *S. capitis* subsp. *capitis* and *S. capitis* subsp. *ureolyticus*.[20] The latter subspecies is urease-positive.
S. schleiferi[87]	First described in 1988, *S. schleiferi* has been isolated from several human infections, including brain empyema, wound infections, bacteremia complicating vertebral osteitis, infection of a hip prosthesis, and indwelling catheter infection.[87,150,190] The species has recently been divided into two subspecies; human isolates have been designated *S. schleiferi* subsp. *schleiferi* and canine isolates have been designated *S. schleiferi* subsp. *coagulans*. The canine isolates are associated with external otitis in dogs.[143]
S. pasteuri[49]	As a newly described species that is found in human and animal clinical specimens and in food, it has not yet been associated with infectious processes and is phenotypically similar to *S. warneri*.[49]
S. auricularis[170]	This species is found in the human external auditory canal, is rarely implicated in infections.
S. cohnii[270]	This species has been divided into two subspecies, designated *S. cohnii* subsp. *cohnii* and *S. cohnii* subsp. *urealyticum*.[175] The former subspecies has been isolated only from humans, whereas the latter urease-positive subspecies has been isolated from both human and nonhuman primates. Both of these organisms are normal skin flora.
S. xylosus[270]	This organsim is found in both human and nonhuman primates, it has been reported as a cause of human lower and upper urinary tract infections and endocarditis associated with intravenous drug use.[57,312] This organism was also isolated from the blood and bile of an 11-year-old cardiac and hepatic transplant patient.[210]
S. saccharolyticus[162]	An anaerobic species, previously called *Peptococcus saccharolyticus*, was transferred to the genus *Staphylococcus* based on oligonucleotide analysis of 16S ribosomal RNA. It is found on human mucous membranes. The single case of endocarditis caused by this organism was reported in 1990.[333]
S. caprae[70]	Originally isolated from goats, it has recently been found on human skin and in human clinical specimens.[155]
S. pulvereri[342]	A proposed species first described in 1995 as a new coagulase-negative, novobiocin-resistant species, is found in humans and chickens. One of the original five isolates described was recovered from a human hip infection.[342]

(Continued)

TABLE 11-1 *(Continued)*
HUMAN, ANIMAL, AND ENVIRONMENTAL *STAPHYLOCOCCUS* SPECIES

SPECIES	COMMENTS
Staphylocci Found in Other Animals	
S. intermedius[111]	Found as a part of the flora of dogs, minks, horses, and cats, it may cause cutaneous, urinary tract, bone, and central nervous system infections in several animal species. *S. intermedius* is the predominant coagulase-positive staphylococcus recovered from normal and infected canine skin. This organism has been isolated from humans with infected dog bite wounds.[24,300,301,302]
S. hyicus[69]	Found in pigs, cattle, and cows' milk, it is associated with exudative epidermitis, an acute disease of suckling and weaned pigs.
S. chromogenes[69, 112]	Formerly a subspecies of *S. hyicus*, it causes cutaneous infections in cattle.
S. sciuri[172]	Normally found in rodents and other small mammals, particularly squirrels.
S. gallinarum[70]	This species is found in poultry and is nonpathogenic.
S. lentus[267]	Part of the normal skin flora of sheep and goats.
S. equorum[268]	A rare equine species of undetermined pathogenic significance.
S. delphini[319]	A coagulase-positive species, it causes purulent skin lesions in dolphins.
S. felis[142]	It causes otitis, cystitis, abscesses, wounds, and other cutaneous infections in cats.
S. muscae[113]	A newly described species found as a transient part of the body surface flora of flies that inhabit cow barns, but it is not found on flies inhabiting human dwellings.
S. piscifermentans[304]	Found in fish, fermented fish products, and soy mash.
S. vitulus[330]	First described in 1994, is found as a part of the flora of horses, voles, and pilot whales. It has also been isolated from meat products, including lamb, chicken, ground beef, and veal.
Other Staphylococcal Species (mostly environmental)	
S. carnosus[266]	Used as a starter culture in the processing of meats, such as salami and sausage.
S. caseolyticus[269]	A saprophytic species found in milk and other dairy products and as a part of the flora of cattle and whales.
S. kloosii[268]	Found in mammals, it is of uncertain clinical significance and taxonomic status.
S. arlettae[268]	Found on mammals and birds, it is of undetermined clinical significance and taxonomic status.

- Infection with other agents, particularly viruses (e.g., influenza)
- Chronic underlying diseases, such as malignancy, alcoholism, and heart disease
- Therapeutic or prophylactic antimicrobial administration

Under these circumstances, *S. aureus* may cause a variety of infectious processes, ranging from relatively benign skin infections to life-threatening systemic illnesses.[324] Skin infections include simple folliculitis (superficial infection surrounding the hair follicles: Color Plate 11-1*A*) and impetigo (a superficial skin infection frequently seen in children), as well as furuncles and carbuncles involving subcutaneous tissues and causing systemic symptoms, such as fever. *S. aureus* is frequently isolated from postsurgical wound infections, which may serve as a nidus for the development of systemic infections.[7] Community-acquired staphylococcal bronchopneumonia is usually seen in elderly individuals and is associated with viral pneumonia as a predisposing factor. Nosocomial pneumonia caused by *S. aureus* occurs in the clinical settings of obstructive pulmonary disease, intubation, and aspiration. Underlying malignant diseases are recognized as important risk factors for the development of *S. aureus* bacteremia.[46,116] Bacteremia may also "seed" distant sites throughout the body, leading to endocarditis, osteomyelitis, pyoarthritis, and metastatic abscess formation, particularly in the skin, the subcutaneous tissues, lungs, liver, kidneys, and brain. Staphylococcal meningitis occurs in patients with central nervous system abnormalities related to trauma, surgery, malignancy, and hydrocephalus, and this organism is the second most common cause of ventriculoperitoneal shunt--

associated meningitis.[163] It is also one of many microorganisms associated with peritonitis in patients receiving CAPD.[240] Staphylococcal toxins are also responsible for toxic epidermal necrolysis (staphylococcal scalded skin syndrome) and toxic shock syndrome.[30,238,255,273,280] S. aureus strains may also cause food poisoning owing to their elaboration of exotoxins during growth in contaminated foods.

S. aureus possesses several properties that are believed to contribute to its ability to cause disease. These virulence factors are not found in all strains of S. aureus, however, and this organism continues to be a constant source of surprise as new and different pathogenic properties are discovered. These properties include the following.

CAPSULE FORMATION

Some strains of S. aureus produce an exopolysaccharide that may prevent ingestion of the organism by polymorphonuclear cells (Fig. 11-1). These exopolysaccharides have been observed by electron microscopic examination of S. aureus–infected pacemaker leads, peritoneal catheters, and intravenous lines and have been demonstrated immunologically in vitro.[129,151] This material may promote the adherence of the organisms to host cells and to prosthetic devices. Clinical isolates of S. aureus have been classified into eight types based on capsular polysaccharide immunotyping, and 70% to 80% of significant clinical isolates belong to capsular serotypes 5 or 8.[8,37,156] These two capsular types, particularly type 8, are also associated with other S. aureus virulence factors, such as the production of toxic shock syndrome toxin.[191] In addition, a predominant number of S. aureus strains that are resistant to oxacillin, the most widely used antistaphylococcal penicillin, express the serotype 5 capsular polysaccharide.[40,84] Capsular types 5 and 8 have also been found among animal isolates of S. aureus.[246,247]

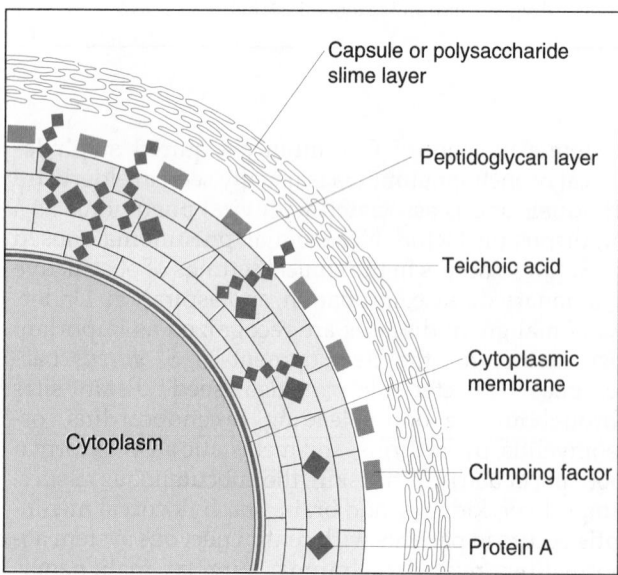

Figure 11-1.
Staphylococcal cell wall structure.

Capsule or polysaccharide slime layer

Peptidoglycan layer

Teichoic acid

Cytoplasmic membrane

Clumping factor

Protein A

Cytoplasm

PROTEIN A

S. aureus cell walls contain this unique protein that has the ability to bind the Fc region of immunoglobulin G (IgG) molecules. Protein A is bound to the cell wall peptidoglycan and is also shed into the medium during growth (see Fig. 11-1). Protein A functions as a virulence factor by interfering with opsonization and ingestion of the organisms by polymorphonuclear cells, activating complement, and eliciting immediate and delayed type hypersensitivity reactions.[324] Protein A is immunogenic, and antibodies against it are found in individuals with serious S. aureus infections. The presence of protein A on S. aureus provides the basis for coagglutination test procedures that are used in many clinical laboratories for organism identification (e.g., gonococci, streptococcal grouping) and for detection of bacterial antigens in body fluids.

CELL WALL CONSTITUENTS

S. aureus cell walls contain peptidoglycans (crosslinked polymers of N-acetylglucosamine and N-acetylmuramic acid; see Chap. 1), which are similar to those found in other gram-positive bacteria, and teichoic acids, which are unique ribitol (five-carbon monosaccharides)–phosphate polymers. Teichoic acids function in the specific adherence of gram-positive bacteria to mucosal surfaces. In addition to their role in providing rigidity and resilience to the staphylococcal cell wall, peptidoglycans and teichoic acids also have several biologic activities that are thought to contribute to virulence.[324] These properties include the ability to activate complement, to inhibit chemotaxis of inflammatory cells, and to stimulate antibody production. Serologic tests for the detection of antibodies to these molecules have been investigated for their possible diagnostic or prognostic value; results have been disappointing because of considerable overlap of antibody titers among infected and noninfected individuals, the wide spectrum of infection and disease caused by S. aureus, and the host-dependent variability of the immune response because of age, other infections, and general immunocompetence.[47,332]

ENZYMES

S. aureus produces several enzymes that may contribute to its virulence. **Catalase** production by these organisms may function to inactivate toxic hydrogen peroxide and free radicals formed by the myeloperoxidase system within phagocytic cells after ingestion of the microorganisms. Both **free** and **bound coagulase** (also called **clumping factor**) may act to coat the bacterial cells with fibrin, rendering them resistant to opsonization and phagocytosis. **Fibrinolysins** may break down fibrin clots and allow spread of infection to contiguous tissues. Similarly, **hyaluronidase** hydrolyzes the intercellular matrix of mucopolysaccharides in tissue and, thus, may act to spread the organisms to adjacent areas. Strains of S. aureus causing chronic furunculosis are producers of potent **lipases** that may help to spread the organisms in cutaneous and subcutaneous tissues. A **phosphatidylinositol-specific phospholipase C** has been described that is associated with strains recovered from patients with adult respiratory distress syndrome and disseminated intravascular coagulation.[206] Tissues affected by this enzyme become more susceptible to damage and destruction by bioactive complement components and products during complement activation. Immunologic and substrate-specificity studies indicate that at least three different types of β-lactamase enzymes are produced by *S. aureus*. Production of these enzymes may be inducible (i.e., they are produced only in the presence of β-lactam antimicrobial agents) or constitutive (i.e., they are produced continually) and render these organisms resistant to penicillin and ampicillin. Genes coding for these enzymes usually reside on plasmids (extrachromosomal DNA) that also carry genes for resistance to several antibiotics, such as erythromycin and tetracycline.[324] These resistance genes may be transferred to other bacteria by transformation and transduction.

HEMOLYSINS

S. aureus hemolysins have several biologic activities. **α-Hemolysin** has lethal effects on a wide variety of cell types, including human polymorphonuclear cells, and will lyse erythrocytes from several animal species. The toxin is dermonecrotic on subcutaneous injection and is lethal for animals when administered intravenously. It is also a potent neurotoxin. This toxin is responsible for the zone of hemolyzed red blood cells observed around colonies of some *S. aureus* strains growing on sheep blood agar. **β-hemolysin** is a sphingomyelinase (acts on the complex lipocarbohydrate sphingomyelin) that is active on a variety of cells. It is a "hot–cold" hemolysin (i.e., its hemolytic properties are enhanced by subsequent exposure of the red blood cells to cold temperatures). The β-hemolysin, along with the CAMP factor produced by group B streptococci, is responsible for the synergistic hemolysis observed in a positive CAMP test for presumptive identification of group B streptococci (see Chap. 12). **τ-hemolysin** and **δ-hemolysin** are found in some *S. aureus* strains and also cause lysis of a variety of cell types. The δ-hemolysin acts primarily as a surfactant and also is able to activate adenylate cyclase, resulting in cyclic-AMP production (a mode of action similar to cholera toxin; see Chap. 6). This enzymatic activity may play a role in the diarrhea seen with certain staphylococcal diseases such as toxic shock syndrome and staphylococcal food poisoning.

TOXINS

Leucocidin is an exotoxin that exerts a direct toxic effect on human polymorphonuclear cell membranes, causing degranulation of the cytoplasm, cell swelling, and lysis. The toxin has two components that interact synergistically with each other to produce a profound though reversible granulocytopenia in rabbits. The mode of action of this toxin involves the formation of pores that alter cellular permeability to potassium and other cations. **Exfoliatins** or **epidermolytic toxins** are produced by some staphylococcal strains and consist of two proteins, designated **ET-A** and **ET-B**, each of 24,000 Da relative molecular weight.[324] The two molecules are biochemically and immunologically distinct but have similar biologic activities. ET-A is a thermostable protein for which the structural gene is chromosomal, although ET-B is heat-labile and of plasmid origin. These proteins have proteolytic activity and dissolve the mucopolysaccharide matrix of the epidermis, resulting in intraepithelial splitting of cellular linkages in the stratum granulosum.[61,299] Strains producing either one or both of these toxins are responsible for the **"staphylococcal scalded skin syndrome."** In this condition, bullous formation occurs over large areas of the body, with subsequent sloughing of the superficial skin layers (Color Plate 11-1*B*). This results in the exposure of large areas of denuded and raw skin. The disease is usually seen in neonates and infants. Both toxins are antigenic, and antibodies against them are protective. **Enterotoxins A through E** are heat-stable molecules that are responsible for the clinical features of staphylococcal food poisoning. The exact mode of action of these enterotoxins is unknown, but they increase intestinal peristalsis. Ingestion of preformed enterotoxins in food supporting staphylococcal growth (e.g., bakery goods, custards, potato salad, processed meats, ice cream) results in vomiting and diarrhea within 2 to 8 hours. These toxic conditions are self-limited and require only supportive therapy. Immunologic detection methods and nucleic acid probes have been developed for the exfoliatins and the enterotoxins.[74,132,225,238,255,339] Immunologic methods detect the toxins directly, whereas the probes detect the structural genes within the bacterial cell that code for the toxins themselves.

Toxic shock syndrome (TSS) was first described by Todd and associates in 1978.[308] It is a multisystem illness characterized by a clinical syndrome that includes fever, hypotension, orthostatic dizziness, erythroderma (blanching rash), and varying degrees of vomiting, diarrhea, renal failure, headache, chills, sore throat, and conjunctivitis.[324] Initially, the disease was noted most frequently in women, with onset mainly occurring during menstruation. Investigations of the initial cases noted an association between the onset of disease and the use of hyperabsorbable tampons. Subsequently, TSS has been reported in both males and females as a complication of staphylococcal abscesses, osteomyelitis, postsurgical wound infections, and postinfluenza pneumonia.[30] The case definition for TSS is presented in Table 11-2.

Soon after the illness was described, it was postulated that TSS was caused by a toxin. In 1981, two groups reported the isolation and characterization of unique toxins produced by *S. aureus* isolates from TSS patients.[29,30,273] These two proteins were designated **pyrogenic exotoxin type C** and **staphylococcal enterotoxin F**. Further studies indicated that these two were identical, and the toxin is now designated **toxic shock syndrome toxin 1 (TSST-1)**. Although this toxin has a broad range of biologic activity, its role in the pathogenesis of TSS is unclear. A most provocative feature

TABLE 11-2
TOXIC SHOCK SYNDROME CASE DEFINITION

Fever	Temperature 38.9°C or higher
Rash	Diffuse macular erythroderma
Desquamation	1–2 weeks (usually 10–14 days) after onset of illness; particularly of palms, soles, fingers, and toes
Hypotension	Systolic blood pressure 90 mm Hg or higher for adults For children, higher than 5th percentile by age for those younger than 16 years Orthostatic syncope or orthostatic dizziness

Involvement of three or more of the following organ systems

Gastrointestinal	Vomiting or diarrhea at onset of illness
Muscular	Severe myalgia or creatinine phosphokinase higher than twice the upper limit of normal
Mucous membranes	Vaginal, oropharyngeal, or conjunctival hyperemia
Renal	BUN or serum creatinine higher than twice the upper limit of normal *or* more than five white blood cells per high-power field in the urine in the absence of a urinary tract infection.
Hepatic	Total bilirubin, SGOT, or SGPT higher than twice the upper limit of normal.
Hematologic	Platelets 100,000 μL, or fewer
CNS	Disorientation or alterations in consciousness without focal neurologic signs when fever and hypotension are absent.

Negative results on the following tests

Blood, throat, and spinal fluid cultures; but blood cultures may be positive for *S. aureus.*
Serologic tests for Rocky Mountain spotted fever, leptospirosis, and measles.

MMWR 29:441–445, 1980; MMWR 31:201–204, 1982.

of its activity is its ability to potentiate the lethal response to minute amounts of gram-negative endotoxin in animal models. TSST-1 and the staphylococcal enterotoxins and exfoliatins are also "superantigens," which means that they are able to bypass the usual mononuclear cell antigen-processing steps and bind directly to monocytes and lymphocytes, resulting in the release of lymphokines and monokines. The systemic release of these cytokines may explain the rapid appearance of multisystem involvement seen with TSS.

The role of TSST-1 in the disease is also supported by the acute onset of symptoms, with vascular congestion developing over a 1- to 2-day period. With the increase in capillary leakage and the system-wide decrease in vascular resistance, there is loss of intravascular fluids into the interstitial spaces. Fluid loss is also exacerbated by the presence of diarrhea in some patients. Loss of intravascular volume leads to hypotension and tissue hypoxia. TSST-1 also appears to have some direct toxic effects on the myocardium, skeletal muscle, liver, and kidney tissue.[324] Other conditions that may be included in the differential diagnosis of TSS include other toxin-mediated infections, (e.g., scalded skin syndrome, gastroenteritis, scarlet fever), local infections with shock or acute abdominal pain (e.g., infectious gastroenteritis, salpingitis, septic abortion, acute urinary tract infections), and multisystem illnesses of infectious (e.g., septic shock associated with pneumococci, meningococci, or *Haemophilis influenzae* type b; rubeola, Rocky Mountain spotted fever, tick-borne typhus, leptospirosis, *Legionella* infection;

toxoplasmosis; and adenoviral or enteroviral syndromes) and noninfectious (Kawasaki's disease, systemic lupus erythematosus, acute rheumatic fever, rheumatoid arthritis, drug reactions) etiologies. Additional studies also suggested that some coagulase-negative staphylococci may also produce TSST-1, and cases of TSS caused by these organisms have been reported.[58,153] A toxin similar to TSST-1 has also been identified in *S. aureus* strains isolated from sheep, goats, and cows.[128,161]

Diagnosis of TSS is generally based on the clinical signs and symptoms according to the case definition. A reverse passive latex agglutination test using latex beads sensitized with anti-TSST-1 antibodies has been described for detection of toxin production in vitro.[141] This test is performed on serial dilutions of culture filtrates from staphylococcal isolates. Miwa and associates[221] developed an enzyme immunoassay for detection of TSST-1 in serum from patients with proved or suspected TSS. Although the mean concentration of TSST-1 serum from healthy indviduals was less than 30 pg/mL, the mean and maximum quantities detected in TSS patients were 440 pg/mL and 5450 pg/mL, respectively. Neill and coworkers[225] described the synthesis and application of a radioactive oligonucleotide TSST-1 probe. This probe hybridized with the bacterial structural genes that coded for TSST-1. Whereas methods for toxin detection (e.g., latex agglutination, colony immunoblot techniques, enzyme immunoassays) are dependent on the presence of TSST-1 at or above the level of detection for the assay and on the proper bacterial growth conditions for toxin production, the probe was able to detect the genetic capability of individual strains to produce TSST-1, regardless of the ability of the individual strains to produce toxin in vitro.[141,225,280]

S. aureus subsp. *anaerobius* causes abscess formation in sheep, but has not been isolated from human infections or clinical specimens.[67]

COAGULASE-NEGATIVE STAPHYLOCOCCI

In the past, coagulase-negative staphylococci were generally considered to be contaminants having little clinical significance. Over the last two decades, however, these organisms have become recognized as important agents of human disease.[14,33,75,76,208,244,337] Although several different species of coagulase-negative staphylococci have been described (see Table 11-1), relatively few of them cause infections in humans. However, as more laboratories have attempted to identify the coagulase-negative staphylococci, infections caused by other species are being recognized more frequently.[87,117,150,301,333] The types of infections associated with coagulase-negative staphylococci include the following:

- Nosocomial and community-acquired urinary tract infections[133]
- Infections of indwelling devices (e.g., prosthetic heart valves, intravenous catheters, joint prostheses, intrathecal pump implants, hemodialysis and cerebrospinal shunts, pacemakers, peritoneal dialysis catheters)[26,81]
- Bacteremia in compromised hosts (premature infants, patients with cardiovascular or neoplastic diseases, patients with hematologic malignancies, burn patients, trauma patients, transplant recipients, patients with congenital defects)[6,25,38,52,81,209,337]
- Native and prosthetic valve endocarditis[44]
- Osteomyelitis (postsurgical wound infections, protheses-associated infections, trauma-associated infections)
- Postsurgical endophthalmitis

STAPHYLOCOCCUS EPIDERMIDIS

When clinical findings are correlated with the isolation of coagulase-negative staphylococci, *S. epidermidis* is by far the most frequently recovered organism, accounting for 50% to over 80% of isolates.[9] Infections caused by *S. epidermidis* include endocarditis of native and prosthetic valves, intravenous catheter infections, CSF shunt infections, peritoneal dialysis catheter—associated peritonitis, bacteremia, osteomyelitis, wound infections, vascular graft infections, prosthetic joint infections, mediastinitis, and urinary tract infections.[9,10,15,114,140,157,159,200,244,322] Scanning and transmission electron microscopic studies and immunologic examination of *S. epidermidis* strains from infections of indwelling medical devices have shown that these bacteria produce cell surface and extracellular macromolecules that initiate and, subsequently, enhance bacterial adhesion to the plastic surfaces of foreign bodies. Initial, specific adherence of some *S. epidermidis* strains

appears to be mediated by a capsular polysaccharide–adhesin called **PS/A**. PS/A is a high molecular weight (greater than 500,000 Da) galactose–arabinose (1:1) polymer.[222,309] Purified PS/A can block adherence of PS/A-producing *S. epidermidis* to plastic catheters in vitro, and antibodies directed against PS/A also appear to block adherence to biomaterials. There is some evidence suggesting that a protein-containing polymer with a molecular weight of 220 kDa may also function to promote adherence to plastic in some *S. epidermidis* strains.[307]

Following initial adhesion to biomaterials, the pathogenesis of *S. epidermidis* infection apparently involves specific interaction with various serum and tissue components of the host. In fact, interactions with host connective tissue proteins, such as collagen and laminen, and serum-derived proteins, such as fibronectin and vitronectin, are probably among the initial steps in tissue colonization and establishment of postsurgical wound infection in the absence of foreign bodies, such as catheters or shunts.[124,230] After the initiation of adherence, it appears that the next step in colonization of surfaces by *S. epidermidis* involves the production of a **glycocalyx**, which is also called **extracellular slime substance (ESS)**.[335] ESS forms a biofilm on plastic surfaces that contains several layers of bacteria. Its matrix may serve to protect the organisms from antimicrobial agents administered to treat these infections, hence the necessity for removal of the foreign body to effect cure. ESS also has significant biologic activities, including inhibition of human peripheral T-lymphocyte or monocyte proliferation by induction of prostaglandin E_2 production and interference with B-cell blastogenesis, immunoglobulin production, and coagulation[43,106,295] ESS also appears to adversely affect opsonization and phagocytosis by inhibiting polymorphonuclear cell (PMNs) chemotaxis, inducing PMN degranulation, inhibiting oxygen-dependent metabolic activities of PMNs that normally occur during phagocytosis and subsequent intracellular killing, and interfering with bacterial cell surface–opsonin (i.e., immunoglobulin G or complement) interactions that are prerequisites for processing by phagocytic cells.[80,147] Production of ESS by *S. epidermidis* in vitro is partially dependent on cultural conditions, such as pH, CO_2 tension, the presence of calcium, magnesium, and phosphate, the protein composition of the growth medium, and the presence of agar in the medium.[22,50,51,68,73] Growth of ESS-producing *S. epidermidis* strains in a chemically defined medium indicates that ESS is composed of glycerol phosphate, D-alanine, *N*-acetylglucosamine, and glucose and may be a modified or specialized glycerol teichoic acid.[136,137,138] It appears that similar ESS-like substances may be produced by other coagulase-negative staphylococci, including *S. saprophyticus*, *S. simulans*, and *S. lugdunensis*.[127,226,295]

In an effort to investigate slime production by *S. epidermidis* as a virulence marker, several workers have described in vitro techniques for determining slime production and bacterial adherence as a model for prostheses-associated infections.[53,54,62,65,69,71,144,234,262,341] In a study using an in vitro technique to assay the ability of *S. epidermidis* strains to adhere to plastic, isolates from an outbreak of intravenous-related sepsis and CSF shunt infections were more adherent than those isolated from blood cultures, CSF contaminants, or those isolated from patients with bacterial endocarditis.[54] A simple broth tube test for slime production by *S. epidermidis* has been described by Ishak and associates[144] for routine use in the clinical microbiology laboratory. The test organism is incubated in a tube of tryptic soy broth overnight at 35°C in ambient air. After an 18- to 24-hour incubation, the broth is gently poured off, and the tube is examined for a thin film of slime on its inner wall. The absence of a film or the mere presence of a ring at the liquid–air interface is interpreted as negative. The addition of several drops of safranin or toluidine blue O to the culture medium shortly before decanting imparts a more contrasting appearance to the slime. This test was performed on 27 blood culture isolates of *S. epidermidis*. Fourteen of these were considered significant on clinical grounds, but 13 were judged to be contaminants. The slime production tube test was positive for 13 of the 14 clinically significant strains, whereas only three of the 13 contaminant organisms were slime-positive.[144] On the other hand, other investigators have not been able to demonstrate an association between ESS-positive, adherent strains and adverse clinical outcome in patients with *S. epidermidis* bacteremia.[14,180] Consequently, the role of *S. epidermidis* ESS as a marker of virulence has been questioned and the validity of in vitro techniques for determining slime production and adherence have been criticized.[4,73,180,336]

ESS may function in allowing the adherent organisms to persist on foreign bodies and to evade host defenses involved in bacterial clearance and killing.[251] Other possible virulence factors (e.g., hemolysins, lipases, and proteases) of *S. epidermidis* may also play an as yet undetermined role in the pathogenesis of serious infections. *S. epidermidis* strains may also undergo phenotypic variation, as evidenced by the generation of different and distinctive colonial morphotypes that are stable on subculture.[14,66] The contribution of phenotypic variation to pathogenicity and the underlying genetic mechanisms that are responsible for these phenomena are not known.

STAPHYLOCOCCUS SAPROPHYTICUS

The coagulase-negative species *S. saprophyticus* deserves special mention because this species is a well-documented pathogen causing primarily acute urinary tract infections in young healthy, sexually active women.[107,120,133,207,326] In this population, *S. saprophyticus* is the second most common cause of cystitis after *Escherichia coli*.[216] In urine specimens from these patients, the organism is frequently present in quantities of fewer than 100,000 CFU/mL but will be detected in sequential specimens from infected patients. Patients with this infection usually present with dysuria, pyuria, and hematuria. Upper urinary tract infections (e.g., pyelonephritis) may be seen in 41% to 86% of patients, and occasionally *S. saprophyticus* bacteremia

may be seen as a complication of upper urinary tract infection.[99,102,192,263] This organism has also been implicated as a cause of urethritis in men and women (i.e., the acute urethral syndrome), catheter-associated urinary tract infections, prostatitis in elderly men, and, rarely, bacteremia, sepsis, and endocarditis.[31,99,102,134,236,263,286] *S. saprophyticus* has been demonstrated as a cause of acute, symptomatic urinary tract infections in both male and female children and teenagers in the absence of urinary tract structural abnormalities.[1,310] Although unrelated to urinary tract infection, an outbreak of *S. saprophyticus* bacteremia and sepsis related to contamination of total parenteral nutrition supplements has also been reported.[198]

The source of *S. saprophyticus* in the pathogenesis of urinary tract infections has also been investigated. Rupp and coworkers[264] studied the prevalence of urogenital colonization in 276 women and found that the rectum was the most frequent site of colonization by *S. saprophyticus* (40%), followed by the urethra (30%), the urine (20%), and the cervix (10%). In this study, follow-up of the colonized women for almost 7 months did not reveal any women progressing on to symptomatic urinary tract infection with *S. saprophyticus*. In another study of 14 women with *S. saprophyticus* urinary tract infection, the same isolate was found in the stool of six women, suggesting that the rectal canal may be a principal reservoir for this organism.[121]

Several potential virulence factors of *S. saprophyticus* have been delineated in recent years. In vitro studies on the adherence of this species to various cell types have shown that *S. saprophyticus* adheres to uroepithelial, urethral, and periurethral cells in greater numbers than other staphylococci and does not adhere to other cell types, including skin and buccal mucosal cells.[205,216] This uroepithelial tissue tropism may partially explain the high frequency of urinary tract infections caused by this organism. Urease, a recognized virulence factor for other urogenital pathogens (e.g., *Proteus* spp., *Corynebacterium ureolyticum*), is also produced by *S. saprophyticus* and contributes to bladder tissue invasion in animal models of urinary tract infection.[89,91] Slime production has not been a consistent attribute of *S. saprophyticus* strains.[256] Heljm and Lundell-Etherden[127] found that, whereas only nine of 30 *S. saprophyticus* strains produced slime in trypticase–soy broth, all 30 strains produced slime in urine. These workers proposed that both the presence of urine and urease production were essential for slime production by this organism. A 95-kDa fibriller protein associated with the surface of *S. saprophyticus* strains has also been identified as a putative virulence factor.[90] This protein, designated **Ssp** (for *S. saprophyticus* surface-associated protein), may be involved in initial interactions with and adherence to uroepithelial cells. A 160-kDa **hemagglutinin** has also been demonstrated on the surface of *S. saprophyticus* cells; its role in organism virulence is as yet unclear.[88] Lastly, Schneider and Riley[274] reported that 79% of 100 urinary isolates of *S. saprophyticus* displayed strong cell surface hydrophobicity in a two-phase aqueous–hydrocarbon partition assay. Because cell surface hydrophobic interactions between bacteria and mammalian cells promote adherence, hydrophobic surface structures of *S. saprophyticus* may function in the initial interaction of these organisms with uroepithelial cells.

OTHER COAGULASE-NEGATIVE STAPHYLOCOCCI

Other staphylococcal species are found in both humans and animals as part of the normal flora and as causes of several types of infections. Some species are found in the environment and are used in various industries, including food processing. Although coagulase-negative species other than *S. epidermidis* and *S. saprophyticus* are frequently found as contaminants in clinical specimens, medical progress has created an important role for many of the other coagulase-negative staphylococci in human infections and disease. Several other species have now been reported as causes of human infections, principally in wounds, urinary tract infections, bacteremia, osteomyelitis, catheter-related sepsis, and both native valve and prosthetic valve endocarditis.[6,9,10,15,38,44,64,324] These agents are being recognized increasingly as important opportunistic pathogens in immunocompromised patients, including premature neonates, neutropenic cancer patients, elderly persons with serious underlying diseases, and hospitalized patients following invasive procedures and with indwelling plastic devices. Infections with many of these other species are acquired in the hospital setting. Implicated species include *S. haemolyticus, S. hominis, S. warneri, S. simulans, S. lugdunensis, S. schleiferi,* and *S. saccharolyticus.*[38,75,76,77,87,98,148,165,182,201,208,263,298,301,333] Some of these agents, such as *S. schleiferi* and *S. warneri*, produce a variety of extracellular products (i.e., glycocalyx, DNase, lipase, esterase, protease, and α- and β-hemolysins) that contribute to virulence. *S. haemolyticus* has demanded increased interest recently because of the emergence of vancomycin resistance in this species.[199,275,276,277,320] The ecologic niches and clinical significance of staphylococci other than *S. aureus, S. epidermidis,* and *S. saprophyticus* are summarized in Table 11-1.

DIFFERENTIATION OF THE MEMBERS OF THE FAMILY *MICROCOCCACEAE*

DIRECT GRAM-STAINED SMEARS

On direct Gram-stained smears from clinical specimens, staphylococci appear as gram-positive or gram-variable cocci ranging in size from 0.5 µm to larger than 1.0 µm in diameter. The organisms may appear singly, in pairs, in short chains, or in clusters, both within and outside of polymorphonuclear cells (Color Plate 11-1C). Variations in cell size and Gram reaction are probably due to the action of the inflammatory cells and their hydrolytic enzymes on the bacterial cells. On direct smears, pairs and short chains of organisms cannot be differentiated from streptococci, micrococci, or peptostreptococci, although streptococci frequently appear as chains of diplococci, rather than as chains of discreet, individual cells. Reports of direct

smears should include quantitation of cell types and microorganisms (e.g., "many PMNs, moderate gram-positive cocci"). If the Gram stain appearance is more typical, a report of "gram-positive cocci resembling staphylococci" can be issued, with culture confirmation to follow.

COLONY MORPHOLOGY

Micrococcus and *Staphylococcus* species form distinctive colonies on sheep blood agar. Micrococci generally grow more slowly, often requiring 48 hours of incubation before typical colony morphology can be discerned. After this time, micrococcal colonies are 1 to 2 mm in diameter, are dull in appearance, and have a high convex profile with entire edges. Some strains produce pigments and will appear yellow, pink, orange, or tan, whereas others will be off-white or bone white. Colonies of most staphylococcal species grow more rapidly and are 1 to 2 mm in diameter after a 24-hour incubation, although some (e.g., *S. warneri, S. simulans*) may form smaller colonies during this time. Colonies are usually smooth, butyrous, and have a low convex profile with an entire edge. Colonies of some *S. aureus* strains may be pigmented yellow or yellow-orange, whereas other strains may produce off-white or gray colonies. The latter strains may resemble group D streptococci and enterococci (catalase-negative). Pigment production in both *S. aureus* and among the coagulase-negative staphylococci may become apparent or more pronounced after incubation at room temperature. Often, strains of some staphylococcal species will show considerable variation in the size of colonies on the same culture plate, giving the appearance of a mixed culture. Some *S. aureus* and some coagulase-negative species may have a distinct or hazy zone of β-hemolysis around the colonies; this hemolytic property may become apparent only after prolonged incubation (Color Plate 11-1D).

Colonies of *S. mucilaginosus* are gray to white and may be mucoid in appearance. They tend to adhere to the agar and, when removed from the media, are difficult to emulsify. Colonies of *Micrococcus, Nesterenkonia, Dermacoccus,* and *Kocuria* species and *A. agilis* may be smooth or matte in appearance. Some species are nonpigmented (*M. lylae, N. halobia*), or may produce yellow (*M. luteus, K. sedentarius, K. varians*), orange (*D. nishinomiyaensis, K. kristinae*), or pink to red (*K. rosea, A. agilis*) colonies on agar media (Color Plate 11-1E). Pigmentation usually becomes more obvious or intense if plates are incubated at room temperature for several days.

THE CATALASE TEST

The *Micrococcaceae* are differentiated from the *Streptococcaceae* by the **catalase test**. This test detects the presence of cytochrome oxidase enzymes in the *Micrococcaceae* (Chart 10). The test is performed with 3% hydrogen peroxide (H_2O_2) on a glass slide. Immediate and vigorous bubbling indicates conversion of the H_2O_2 to water and oxygen gas (Color Plate 11-1F). Ideally, the catalase test should be performed from a medium that does not contain blood because red blood cells themselves may produce a weakly positive catalase reaction. However, because most clinical laboratories recover staphylococci on either nonselective or selective blood-containing media (e.g., sheep blood agar and CNA agar, respectively), care should be taken to sample only the tops of colonies for the catalase test to avoid carryover of blood and possible false-positive reactions. This can be done most expeditiously with a wooden applicator stick. Rare strains of staphylococci may be catalase-negative,[313] and some enterococci (i.e., fecal streptococci; see Chap. 12), produce a "pseudocatalase" and are weakly reactive with H_2O_2. S. mucilaginosus is usually catalase-negative or weakly positive.[27,28]

METHODS FOR DIFFERENTIATING MICROCOCCI AND STAPHYLOCOCCI

Several methods are available for differentiating *Micrococcus* and *Staphylococcus* species, the two catalase-positive genera most frequently seen in the clinical laboratory. Some require special media and prolonged incubation, whereas others are commercially available and provide results within 18 to 24 hours or less. Table 11-3 lists the test methods and results for *Micrococcus* and *Staphylococcus* species. These procedures include the following.

FERMENTATION OF GLUCOSE

The glucose fermentation test[171] is performed in a manner similar to the oxidation–fermentation (OF) tests for nonfermentative gram-negative bacilli (see Chap. 5). The OF medium for staphylococci contains additional nutrients, such as yeast extract, to fulfill the more exacting growth requirements of staphylococci. This method, which is considered the reference procedure for differentiation of the *Micrococcaceae*,[171] requires prolonged incubation and is not readily adaptable or amenable to routine laboratory use.

SUSCEPTIBILITY TO LYSOSTAPHIN

Lysostaphin is an endopeptidase that cleaves the glycine-rich pentapeptide cross-bridges in the staphylococcal cell wall peptidoglycan. This activity renders the cells susceptible to osmotic lysis.[92,135,282] Certain staphylococcal species (i.e., S. aureus, S. simulans, S. cohnii, and S. xylosus) are more susceptible to lysostaphin than others (e.g., S. hominis, S. saprophyticus, and S. haemolyticus); hence, standardization and interpretation of this test are sometimes difficult.[282] A tube test for lysostaphin susceptibility is commercially available from Remel (Remel Laboratories, Lenexa KA). A heavy suspension of the organism is prepared in 0.2 mL of sterile saline, after which 0.2 mL of the Remel lysostaphin solution is added. The suspension is incubated at 35°C for 2 hours. The clearing of the suspension indicates susceptibility to lysostaphin. Lysostaphin susceptibility can also be determined using a filter paper–disk diffusion method.[245] A plate of Mueller-Hinton agar is inoculated with the organism to be tested (0.5 McFarland turbidity standard) and a disk impregnated with 10 µg of lysostaphin filter-sterilized solution, 287 U/mL) is placed on the plate. The plate is incubated for 24 hours at 35°C. *Staphylococcus* species will generally show zones of inhibition of 10 to 16 mm in diameter. *Micrococcus* and related species will show no zones.

To obtain optimal results with the lysostaphin susceptibility test, the organism should be grown on a beef peptone-based medium, rather than on one that is casein peptone-based. The crucial factor is the glycine content of the medium because glycine is an important part of the staphylococcal cell wall and is essential for the action of lysostaphin.

TABLE 11-3

METHODS FOR THE DIFFERENTIATION OF *MICROCOCCUS* AND *STAPHYLOCOCCUS* SPECIES

	REACTION FOR	
METHOD	*MICROCOCCUS*	*STAPHYLOCOCCUS*
Acid production from glucose under anaerobic conditions	−	+
Lysostaphin	R	S
Production of acid from glucose aerobically in the presence of 0.4 µg/mL erythromycin	−	+
Furazolidone (100 µg furazolidone disk)	R	S
Modified oxidase test	+	−
Bacitracin (0.04 U Taxo A disk)	S	R

+, positive; −, negative; S, susceptible; R, resistant

PRODUCTION OF ACID FROM GLYCEROL IN THE PRESENCE OF ERYTHROMYCIN

In this test,[271] medium containing glycerol (1%) and erythromycin (0.4 μg/mL) is prepared with an enriched agar base containing bromcresol purple indicator and poured into petri plates. Several colonies of the isolate are streaked as a single line on the medium, and the plate is incubated for up to 3 days at 35°C. Staphylococci will produce acid on this medium, but micrococci will not.[271]

SUSCEPTIBILITY TO FURAZOLIDONE

The furazolidone test[16,321] is performed as a disk susceptibility procedure using commercially available disks (FX disk, 100 μg, Becton-Dickinson Microbiology Systems [BDMS], Cockeysville MD). The procedure for this test is described in detail in Chart 33 and in Color Plates 11-1G and 11-1H. Staphylococci are inhibited by furazolidone and show zones of 15 mm or more, whereas micrococci and related species are resistant and show zones of 6 mm (no zone) to 9 mm.[16] However, coagulase-negative staphylococci that are resistant to furazolidone may be seen occasionally.

MODIFIED OXIDASE TEST

This test[16,79] is also commercially available from Remel (Microdase Test Disks). Filter paper disks impregnated with tetramethyl-*p*-phenylenediamine dihydrochloride (oxidase reagent) in dimethyl sulfoxide (DMSO) are used. The DMSO renders the cells permeable to the reagent. A colony from the growth medium is removed with an applicator stick and rubbed onto the disk. The development of a blue-purple color within 30 seconds is a positive test (Color Plate 11-2A). No color development within this time is a negative test. *Micrococcus* species, *N. halobia*, *D. nishinomiyaensis*, and *A. agilis* are modified oxidase-positive, but some strains of *K. sedentarius*, *K. rosea*, and *K. varians* are modified oxidase-negative.[177,291] All *Staphylococcus* species are modified oxidase-negative except for strains of *S. caseolyticus*, *S. sciuri*, *S. lentus*, and *S. vitulus* (Tables 11-4 and 11-5).

SUSCEPTIBILITY TO BACITRACIN

The bacitracin susceptibility procedure[16,78] employs the same bacitracin disk used for the presumptive identification of group A β-hemolytic streptococci. A lawn of growth is prepared on a Mueller-Hinton agar or a blood agar plate as described in the foregoing for the FX disk test, and a bacitracin differential disk (Taxo A, 0.04 U of bacitracin, BDMS) is placed on the inoculum. After overnight incubation, zone sizes are measured. Staphylococci are resistant and grow to the edge of the disk, whereas micrococci and related species are susceptible, producing zones of 10 mm or larger.[16]

The choice of the method used in a given laboratory depends on the type of work performed (e.g., reference laboratory, environmental microbiology, clinical laboratory). In most clinical microbiology laboratories, the modified oxidase test, the furazolidone disk test, and the Taxo A bacitracin disk test are probably the most logical choices because they are rapid, reliable, inexpensive, and commercially available.

IDENTIFICATION OF *STAPHYLOCOCCUS AUREUS*

The single most reliable characteristic for identifying *S. aureus* is the coagulase test. The conventional coagulase test may be performed by the following slide or tube procedures.

SLIDE COAGULASE TEST

Most strains of *S. aureus* have a **bound coagulase** or **"clumping factor"** on the surface of the cell wall. This factor reacts directly with fibrinogen in plasma, causing rapid cell agglutination (Color Plate 11-2B). Performance of this test is described in detail in Chart 13. The test can be performed with growth from blood agar, CNA agar, or other nonselective nutrient media but should not be performed from media having a high salt content (e.g., mannitol salts agar) because the high salt content causes some strains to autoagglutinate. Any strain that is negative with the slide coagulase test must be confirmed with a tube coagulase test because strains deficient in clumping factor will usually produce free coagulase. Some strains of the hu-man coagulase-negative species *S. lugdunensis* and *S. schleiferi* subsp. *schleiferi* also produce clumping factor and may be positive with the slide test.[87,117,318]

TUBE COAGULASE TEST

The coagulase detected by this method is secreted extracellularly and reacts with a substance in the plasma called **"coagulase-reacting factor (CRF)"** to form a complex which, in turn, reacts with fibrinogen to form fibrin (clot formation; see Chart 13 and Color Plate 11-2C). Tests that are negative after a 4-hour incubation at 35°C should be held at room temperature and read again after 18 to 24 hours because some strains will produce fibrinolysin on prolonged incubation at 35°C, causing dissolution of the clot during the incubation period.[184] Rare *S. aureus* strains may be coagulase-negative, and some animal isolates (*S. intermedius*, *S. hyicus*, *S. delphini*, and *S. schleiferi* subsp. *coagulans*) may be tube coagulase-positive.[69,111,112,318,319]

Recently, *S. schleiferi* subsp. *schleiferi* strains that were both clumping factor–negative and tube coagulase–positive have been recovered from human infections.[318] These isolates also produced a heat-stable DNase (see later discussion) and, therefore, could be misidentified as *S. aureus*. These strains can be differentiated from *S. aureus* by failure to produce acid from maltose, lactose, mannitol, sucrose, and turanose. In addition, *S. schleiferi* subsp. *coagulans*, an organism that causes canine external otitis, has been found in human infections and may also be misidentified as clumping factor–negative strains of *S. aureus*. This subspecies can be differentiated from *S. aureus* by carbohydrate utilization tests (see Table 11-4).[318]

The recommended medium for both the slide and the tube coagulase procedures is rabbit plasma with EDTA. Citrated plasma should not be used because organisms that are able to metabolize citrate (e.g., *Enterococcus* species) will yield positive results if they are inadvertently mistaken for staphylococci. This error can be avoided by always performing a catalase test first. Human plasma (e.g., outdated material from blood banks) contains variable amounts of CRF and antistaphylococcal antibodies and should not be used.

The tube coagulase test is still the reference procedure for identification of *S. aureus*. Although it is generally performed with isolates taken from agar media, it may also be inoculated with positive blood culture broths or pelleted organisms centrifuged from these culture broths. McDonald and Chapin[214] recently reevaluated a 2-hour tube coagulase procedure for identification of *S. aureus* in positive blood cultures. Inoculation of the coagulase test directly with a positive culture medium was compared with an inoculum obtained by centrifugation and resuspension of the organisms from the blood culture medium. In addition, both the culture broth and the bacterial pellet were also tested with two commercial latex agglutination tests (see later discussion). For 180 clinical and seeded blood cultures, the 2-hour tube coagulase test showed sensitivities of 86.4% and 84.4%, with 100% specificity, when inoculated directly with positive blood culture broth and with a bacterial pellet, respectively. The latex agglutination tests were 6.8% to 8.6% sensitive and only 95.9% specific when inoculated with positive blood culture broth or bacterial pellets, respectively.[214]

ALTERNATIVE COAGULASE TEST PROCEDURES

LATEX AGGLUTINATION

These procedures use latex beads coated with plasma. Fibrinogen bound to the latex detects clumping factor. In addition, immunoglobulin molecules also present on the beads detect protein A, the staphylococcal cell wall protein that is able to bind IgG molecules by the Fc region. Mixing of the test reagent with colonial material from an agar plate results in rapid clumping of the latex–organism suspension (Color Plate 11-2D). Several products that use this approach are commercially available and include StaphAurex (Murex, Norcross GA), Slidex Staph (bioMerieux-Vitek, Hazelwood MO), Staphylatex (Dade/MicroScan, West Sacramento CA), Accu-Staph (Carr-Scarborough, Stone Mountain GA), Staph Rapid (Roche, Nutley NJ), and Veri-Staph (Zeus Technologies, Raritan NJ) In addition, some strains of *S. lugdunensis* and *S. schleiferi* subsp. *schleiferi* produce clumping factor and may be positive with these rapid procedures.[87]

PASSIVE HEMAGGLUTINATION

The passive hemagglutination test procedures use sheep red blood cells that are sensitized with fibrinogen to detect clumping factor on the surface of *S. aureus* cells (Color Plate 11-2E). Three commercial kits—Staphyloslide (BDMS), Hemastaph (Remel) and Staphyslide (bioMerieux SA, France)—are available. Some workers prefer these tests to the latex agglutination tests because a nonsensitized red blood cell suspension is included as a negative control for each test.

Several evaluations comparing latex and passive hemagglutination kits with the 4-hour and 24-hour tube coagulase tests have been published. These kits have sensitivities and specificities of 94% to 100% and 93% to 100%, respectively.[2,3,17,32,152,211,224,231,250,259] Sensitivities ranging from as low as 6% to 62% have been observed when these tests have been used directly on blood cultures showing gram-positive cocci in clusters on gram-stained smear.[214,287] Some investigators have reported that false-negative latex agglutination and passive hemagglutination results may be encountered when methicillin- or oxacillin-resistant *S. aureus* are tested.[2,242,250,260,327] For example, Piper and coworker[242] found that only 82% to 86% of these strains were identified when tested with three of the latex agglutination and one of the hemagglutination procedures. In another study comparing reactivity with the rapid coagulase tests, capsular serotypes, and oxacillin-susceptibility, all isolates that were negative with the agglutination tests were capsular serotype 5, and all of these, except one strain, were oxacillin-resistant.[83] Therefore, failure of *S. aureus* strains to react with the rapid coagulase procedures may likely be due to the presence of the serotype 5 capsule on the cell surface, rather than to methicillin resistance. Interestingly, capsular serotype 5 strains also appear to be the predominant serotype among methicillin-resistant isolates.[84] The presence of this capsule may interfere with accessibility of the test reagents to the clumping factor and protein A present on the bacterial cell wall.

Kuusela and colleagues[183] examined 79 strains of methicillin-resistant *S. aureus*; 14 of these strains failed to agglutinate (i.e., "aggl−") with two latex tests and one hemagglutination test. The other 65 strains were "aggl+". Sodium dodecyl sulfate–polyacrylamide gel electrophoresis (SDS–PAGE) examination of lysostaphin digests of these strains revealed a 230-kDa protein that was present on all aggl− strains, but was absent in all aggl+ strains. Antibodies directed against the purified 230-kDa protein agglutinated all aggl− strains, indicating the surface location of this protein. In aggl− strains, this protein may interfere with detection of cell-associated clumping factor and protein A. Finally, some *S. saprophyticus* strains may also produce false-positive results with rapid latex or hemmagglutination coagulase tests.[107] This can be explained by the presence of a hemagglutinin that is found on the surface of *S. saprophyticus* strains.[88]

Fournier and coworkers[85] recently reported on a new latex agglutination test called "Pastorex Staph-Plus" (Sanofi-Diagnostics Pasteur, France). This reagent consists of a 2:1 mixture of latex beads coated with fibrinogen and IgG for the detection of clumping factor and protein A, respectively, plus latex beads coated with monoclonal antibodies directed against serotype 5 and serotype 8 capsular polysaccharides. The latter components of this reagent would presumably identify those strains not reliably identified by the regular latex agglutination reagents. In the study by Fournier and associates,[85] this new reagent was compared with Staphyslide (a French hemagglutination reagent), StaphAurex (Murex), and Pastorex-Staph (a French equivalent of the StaphAurex). Of 220 *S. aureus* strains (61 of which were oxacillin-resistant) and 128 coagulase-negative staphylococci tested, the Pastorex Staph-Plus identified 98.6% of the *S. aureus* strains compared with 91.8%, 91.4%, and 84.5% for the Pastorex-Staph, the Staphyslide, and the StaphAurex tests, respectively. None of the coagulase-negative staphylococci reacted with the new reagents. When the 61 oxacillin-resistant strains were examined separately, the Pastorex Staph-Plus identified 95.1%, compared with 73.8%, 72.1%, and 49.2% obtained with the Pastorex Staph, the Staphyslide, and the StaphAurex tests, respectively. Because capsular types 5 and 8 predominate among clinical isolates, that capsular type 5 strains predominate among oxacillin-resistant strains, and that these latter strains may not be reliably identified by existing latex or passive hemagglutination tests, the incorporation of monoclonal antibodies against these capsular types in a latex preparation offers a theoretical and a real advantage in identifying *S. aureus*.

Other studies have suggested that *S. aureus* strains that do not agglutinate with the latex reagents are genetically deficient for both clumping factor and protein A. Schwarzkopf and colleagues[279] examined 50 oxacillin-resistant, clumping factor- and protein A-negative strains in Germany and found that all had similar antibiograms, were nontypeable with an international set of bacteriophages, and possessed a 30-kilobase plasmid that was similar for all strains on restriction enzyme analysis. These data suggested that these deficient *S. aureus* strains belonged to a single clone. Amplification and restriction enzyme analysis of the coagulase genes of these strains revealed a single 650-base–pair product in the deficient strains, whereas similar analysis of coagulase-positive, oxacillin-resistant strains showed different restriction patterns, indicating substantial differences in coagulase gene loci.[278] Polymerase chain reaction (PCR) amplification of the protein A genes indicated that the protein A-negative strains possessed genes that coded for four IgG-binding domains, whereas wild-type strains possessed genes coding for five binding domains, suggesting that the missing protein A gene sequence is required for latex agglutination reactivity.[278]

OTHER COAGULASE TEST PROCEDURES

Another alternative to the traditional coagulase test is the StaphASE test (bioMerieux-Vitek, Inc.). This modified slide/tube coagulase test is performed in a microcupule similar to that used for other API kit systems (e.g., the API 20E, see Chap. 4). Dehydrated rabbit plasma in the cupule is rehydrated with sterile water, and several colonies are emulsified in the

medium. Clumping of the suspension within 1 minute is a positive test, whereas a milky, smooth suspension is negative. The negative test cupule is then incubated for 5 hours at 35°C and read for clot formation at that time.

A fluorogenic coagulase test is included as a test for *S. aureus* in the RapiDEC Staph (bioMerieux-Vitek, Inc) identification system (see later discussion). This test, which is performed by inoculating a small cupule containing the substrate, detects what the manufacturer calls "aurease" (coagulase). Aurease is a proteolytic enzyme of coagulation that reacts with prothrombin to form a complex called staphylothrombin. Staphylothrombin then enzymatically cleaves a fluorogenic peptide present in the test cupule, thereby releasing a peptide and a radical that fluoresces under ultraviolet light. Greater fluorescence in the test cupule relative to a control cupule lacking the substrate provides an identification of *S. aureus*. The aurease test on the RapiDEC Staph has been demonstrated to be a highly sensitive and specific test.[94,146,211,219] Mitchell and coworkers[219] evaluated the RapIDEC aurease test for identifying *S. aureus* directly in blood cultures; 27 of 28 *S. aureus* were correctly identified within 2 hours using this test; none of the coagulase-negative staphylococci produced false-positive results when the aurease test was inoculated with bacterial suspensions from positive blood cultures.

ADDITIONAL CONFIRMATORY TESTS

DEOXYRIBONUCLEASE TEST

Some *S. aureus* strains may produce weak or equivocal tube coagulase reactions, and rare isolates may indeed be coagulase-negative. In these circumstances, it may be helpful to perform other tests that correlate highly with coagulase production. *S. aureus* produces both DNase and a thermostable endonuclease.[109,187] Both of these enzymes hydrolyze nucleic acid (i.e., DNA). The DNase can be detected by heavily spot-inoculating several colonies of the organism on DNase test medium containing the metachromatic dye toluidine blue O (commercially available from several vendors). After a 24-hour incubation at 35°C, the medium under and around the inoculum turns from azure blue to pink, indicating hydrolysis of the DNA. The content of toluidine blue O in the medium should not exceed 0.005% because the blue color imparted to the agar by higher concentrations may mask detection of DNase activity.[325] Spot inoculation is necessary because some *S. aureus* strains do not grow well on the media, and growth is not required for detection of DNase activity.

THERMOSTABLE ENDONUCLEASE TEST

For this test, the same DNase test medium is used, only 3-mm holes are cut into the agar with a sterile cork borer and the wells are filled with a 24-hour broth culture of the test organism that has been boiled in a water bath for 15 minutes. The plate is incubated overnight at 35°C. *S. aureus* strains will show a pink zone surrounding the well containing the boiled suspension.

MANNITOL FERMENTATION

In addition to the forgoing tests, *S. aureus*, unlike *S. epidermidis* and several other coagulase-negative species, is able to ferment mannitol. This property is exploited in epidemiologic studies to detect *S. aureus* in soil, feces, and in screening nasal carriers of *S. aureus*. The medium used is **mannitol salt agar**. This medium contains mannitol (1%), 7.5% NaCl, phenol red, and peptones. The high salt concentration discourages the growth of other organisms (except enterococci) and selectively recovers staphylococci. *S. aureus* can be detected by the presence of a yellow zone around isolated colonies, indicating acid production from mannitol. However, other infrequently isolated staphylococcal species may also produce acid from mannitol; consequently, mannitol-positive organisms recovered on this medium should be checked for coagulase production as well.

OTHER METHODS FOR IDENTIFICATION
OF *STAPHYLOCOCCUS AUREUS*

A different approach to identification of *S. aureus* that also uses a latex agglutination procedure was reported by Larsson and Sjoquist.[188] This method used latex beads coated with chicken antiprotein A antibodies. Because protein A is present on the surface of *S. aureus* cells and is also secreted into the growth media, this test could presumably be used for detecting protein A in liquid specimens, such as blood culture broths, as well as for identifying isolates growing on solid media.

Ayres and Duda[13] recently reported that alphazurine A, a bluish-green anionic triphenylmethane dye, was able to specifically inhibit growth of *S. aureus*. With a disk diffusion procedure, all of 126 strains of *S. aureus* tested showed a zone of inhibition around disks that were soaked in a solution of alphazurine A dye (Aldrich Chemical Co., Milwaukee WI). None of 38 *S. epidermidis* strains and 28 *S. saprophyticus* strains were inhibited by the dye. Unfortunately, other species of coagulase-negative staphylococci were not tested for susceptibility to this dye; hence, further studies are needed to determine the sensitivity and specificity of this test for identifying *S. aureus*.

Detection of the presence of enzymes unique to *S. aureus* has also been exploited as a way to identify *S. aureus*. Guzman and coworkers[110] developed an enzyme immunoassay for identifying *S. aureus* that uses simultaneous detection of protein A and *S. aureus* endo-β-*N*-acetylglucosaminidase (SaG), an enzyme produced by all isolates of this species. By using a monoclonal capture antibody directed against SaG, this enzyme immunoassay could identify *S. aureus* strains by simultaneous detection of SaG (by binding of the bacterial enzyme to the Fab sites of the antibody) and protein A (by binding to the Fc region). This assay performed better than either latex agglutination or passive hemagglutination when compared with these commerically available products.[108] The test showed 100%

sensitivity and specificity and was particularly helpful for identifying those strains that lacked detectable clumping factor, protein A, or both.

Molecular biology techniques, such as DNA probe methods and PCR, have also been used for identification of *S. aureus*. Davis and Fuller[63] found that the AccuProbe for *S. aureus* culture confirmation (GenProbe, San Diego CA) performed well for the direct identification of *S. aureus* in blood cultures that showed gram-positive cocci in clusters on Gram stain. In a similar study, Skulnick[287] reported a sensitivity of 95% and a specificity of 98.5% when the *S. aureus* AccuProbe test was performed directly on blood culture broths. Primers and probes for amplification and detection of the *nuc* gene of *S. aureus* have also been synthesized and examined for their usefulness in culture confirmation and direct detection.[39] The *nuc* gene codes for the thermostable endonuclease of *S. aureus*. For identification, the lower limit of sensitivity of the PCR assay was 5 to 20 CFU of the organism. Using staphylococcus-free clinical specimens that were seeded with serial dilutions of *S. aureus*, the lower limit for direct detection of *S. aureus* by the PCR assay ranged from 10 to 20 CFU up to 1000 CFU, depending on the type of clinical specimen. The PCR-based assay was 100% specific for *S. aureus*.[39] PCR methods have also been developed for detectionof the *mecA* gene. The *mecA* gene is the structural gene for a low-affinity penicillin-binding protein (PBP 2' or PBP 2a) that is found in oxacillin-resistant *S. aureus* strains.[95,284,314] However, the presence of *mecA* genes is not specific for *S. aureus*, for these studies also demonstrated that *mecA* was found not only in oxacillin-resistant *S. aureus*, but also in oxacillin-resistant strains of several coagulase-negative species.[223]

DIFFERENTIATION OF COAGULASE-POSITIVE
STAPHYLOCOCCI OF VETERINARY ORIGIN

In veterinary medicine, three coagulase-positive cocci—*S. aureus* (both subspecies *aureus* and *anaerobius*), some *S. hyicus* strains, and *S. intermedius*—have been implicated as causes of bovine mastitis. These organisms all produce free coagulase, as indicated by positive tube tests after 4 to 24 hours of incubation. Roberson and associates[257] examined 80 strains of each of these species to investigate simple tests that could differentiate them. *S. aureus* strains grew on P agar and on P agar with acriflavin (7 µg/mL), were VP-positive, and produced acid from mannitol under anaerobic conditions. *S. hyicus* and *S. intermedius* failed to grow on P agar or on P agar with acriflavin and did not produce acetoin or ferment mannitol; *S. intermedius* strains were β-galactosidase–positive, whereas *S. hyicus* strains were β-galactosidase–negative.

S. schleiferi subsp. *coagulans* causes infections in both dogs and humans; these strains are clumping factor-negative and tube coagulase-positive (the opposite reactions for these two tests are seen in strains of

S. schleiferi subsp. *schleiferi*). Both *S. schleiferi* subsp. *schleiferi* and subsp. *coagulans* can be differentiated from *S. aureus* by the lack of acid production from maltose and trehalose (see Table 11-4). *S. delphini* is also coagulase-positive, but this species is associated only with marine environments and cutaneous infections in dolphins.[319] Other species that are recovered from animals are coagulase-negative.

IDENTIFICATION OF COAGULASE-NEGATIVE STAPHYLOCOCCI

As described earlier, *S. epidermidis* and *S. saprophyticus* are the most frequently isolated and clinically significant coagulase-negative staphylococci in clinical laboratories working with specimens of human origin. Because of the recognized clinical significance of *S. saprophyticus* in urinary tract infections and the importance of *S. epidermidis* as an agent causing serious infections, it is advantageous for laboratories to employ methods for confirmatory identification of these two species. In addition, kit systems are available that enable the laboratory to identify not only *S. epidermidis* and *S. saprophyticus* but also several of the other human, animal, and environmental staphylococci. Although several coagulase-negative staphylococcal species have been described and many of them have been recovered from human clinical specimens, relatively few species are seen with any regularity in actual practice. Kleeman and associates[164] recently published the results of species identification on 500 coagulase-negative isolates recovered from specimens submitted to the microbiology laboratory of Rex Hospital, a 400-bed community hospital in Raleigh, North Carolina. *S. epidermidis* accounted for 64.5% of the isolates, followed in decreasing frequency by *S. haemolyticus* (13.4%), *S. hominis* (7.4%), *S. warneri* (4.0%), *S. lugdunensis* (2.8%), *S. simulans* (2.4%), *S. capitis* subsp *capitis* (2.0%), and *S. capitis* subsp. *ureolyticus* (1.6%). *Staphylococcus saprophyticus*, *S. cohnii* subsp. *urealyticum*, *S. cohnii* subsp. *cohnii*, and *S. auricularis* each accounted for less than 1% of significant isolates recovered in the laboratory. This species distribution reflects the literature that has accumulated on the clinical significance of the individual species.

PRODUCTION OF PHOSPHATASE FOR IDENTIFICATION OF STAPHYLOCOCCUS EPIDERMIDIS

In traditional schemes for identifying coagulase-negative staphylococci, phosphatase activity was reported to be positive for *S. epidermidis* and *S. xylosus* strains and negative for other coagulase-negative staphylococci.[187,288] Subsequent studies have shown, however, that other staphylococcal species may also produce phosphatase enzymes. By using four different methods, Langlois and coworkers[187] found phosphatase activity in all *S. aureus*, coagulase-positive *S. hyicus* and *S. intermedius* strains, and in most

strains of *S. epidermidis*, *S. chromogenes*, coagulase-negative *S. hyicus*, *S. sciuri*, *S. simulans*, *S. xylosus*, and *S. warneri/hominis* after 24 and 48 hours of incubation. Production of phosphatase activity was affected by pH and by the presence of inorganic phosphate (P_i) in the growth medium. Soro and associates[288] found that all strains of various staphylococcal species were phosphatase-positive when testing was done at pH 8.0 and when the organisms were grown in the absence of P_i. When grown on media supplemented with 0.3% P_i, only *S. aureus*, *S. epidermidis*, and *S. xylosus* strains were phosphatase-positive. These workers concluded that phosphatase activity was a more common property among human staphylococcal isolates than was previously thought and that this activity may be constitutive in some species and repressed by phosphates in others.[288]

There are now no commercially available standalone tests for detection of phosphatase activity in staphylococci, although several commercial kit systems (e.g., API Staph-IDENT, API STAPH, ID32 Staph, and RapiDEC Staph) include a phosphatase test in the biochemical test battery. Geary and Stevens[93] reported a simple agar method (PNP agar) that used Mueller-Hinton agar buffered at ph 5.6–5.8 and containing *p*-nitrophenyl phosphate (0.495 mg/mL). The medium is spot-inoculated and is read after 18 to 24 hours of incubation. The presence of a bright yellow color under and around the inoculum is a positive test. Geary and Stevens identified 305 coagulase-negative isolates to species and tested them with PNP agar.[93] They found that 83% of 170 *S. epidermidis*, 17% of seven *S. cohnii*, and 75% of four *S. xylosus* strains were PNP positive, whereas 124 isolates representing six other species (including 38 *S. saprophyticus* strains) were PNP-negative.

SUSCEPTIBILITY TO DESFERRIOXAMINE FOR IDENTIFICATION OF STAPHYLOCOCCUS EPIDERMIDIS AND STAPHYLOCOCCUS HOMINIS

In 1991 and 1993, Lindsay and coworkers[196,197] reported a new test for specific identification of *S. epidermidis* and *S. hominis*. The test determines susceptibility to desferrioxamine, which is a siderophore that is produced by *Streptomyces pilosus* and is used clinically to treat acute and chronic iron overload. The test is performed as a disk diffusion test similar to the furazolidone and bacitracin susceptibility tests. After preparing a suspension of the organism corresponding to a 0.5 McFarland turbidity standard, a plate of BHI agar is inoculated with the suspension, and a 1-mg desferrioxamine disk (Desferal, Ciba-Geigy, Switzerland) is placed on the inoculum. After overnight incubation at 35°C, the plate is inspected for a zone of growth inhibition around the disk. In their original study, Lindsay and Riley[197] found that, among 95 coagulase-negative staphylococci, all 57 *S. epidermidis* and four *S. hominis* isolates were susceptible to desferrioxamine, whereas all 34 other isolates were resistant. In a subsequent study of 161 coagulase-negative staphylococci, all *S. epidermidis* and *S. hominis* strains were susceptible to desferrioxamine, but all of the remaining staphylococci were resistant.[196] Although desferrioxamine is commercially available, standardized susceptibility test disks must as yet be prepared in-house.

SUSCEPTIBILITY TO NOVOBIOCIN FOR IDENTIFICATION
OF *STAPHYLOCOCCUS SAPROPHYTICUS*

Four human staphylococcal species (*S. saprophyticus, S. cohnii* subspecies, *S. xylosus*, and *S. pulvereri*) and seven animal species (*S. sciuri, S. lentus, S. gallinarum, S. kloosii, S. equorum, S. arlettae*, and *S. vitulus*) are resistant to novobiocin, with MICs of 1.6 µg/mL or higher.[169,172,267,268,270,342] Because novobiocin-resistant species other than *S. saprophyticus* are infrequently encountered in human clinical specimens, the novobiocin susceptibility test provides a useful method for *S. saprophyticus* identification. The novobiocin test is performed as a disk susceptibility test using a novobiocin disk (5 µg) and is described in detail in Chart 55 (Color Plate 11-2*F*). Strains resistant to novobiocin will show zones measuring 6 mm (no zone) to 12 mm; susceptible strains will have zones of 16 mm to 27 mm. This test was originally described using a medium called P agar, which is not available commercially. However, studies with the routine media mentioned in the foregoing have shown that comparable results are obtained.[101]

In an effort to assess the reliability and accuracy of the novobiocin susceptibility test, McTaggart and Elliott[215] examined 36 presumptive *S. saprophyticus* strains (i.e., novobiocin-resistant organisms from urine specimens of patients with urinary tract infections) with a commercial identification system (API Staph-IDENT, see later discussion) and with expanded batteries of additional substrates, including carbohydrate utilization tests, 7-amino-4-methylumbelliferone derivatives of inorganic and organic esters and glycosides, and 7-amino-4-methylcoumarin derivatives of amino acids. Of the 36 strains, 21 (58%) were identified as *S. saprophyticus*, three strains could not be identified, nine strains had characteristics that were attributable to more than one novobiocin-resistant species, and three strains were identified as *S. epidermidis, S. hominis*, and *S. simulans*, respectively. Even strains that were identified as *S. saprophyticus* by the Staph-IDENT produced a spectrum of reactivities with the other chromogenic substrates, illustrating the heterogeneity of organisms called "*S. saprophyticus*" and suggesting that organisms called *S. saprophyticus* may actually represent a heterogeneous group of novobiocin-resistant, genotypically and phenotypically related strains. These workers concluded that additional tests are needed for reliable presumptive identification of *S. saprophyticus* other than, or in addition to, the novobiocin susceptibility test. Occasional human isolates that are not *S. saprophyticus, S. cohnii* subspecies, or *S. xylosus* may also

be resistant to novobiocin. In an evaluation of the RapiDEC-Staph, Janda and associates[146] found that, although all *S. saprophyticus* isolates were resistant to novobiocin, five (7%) of 74 *S. epidermidis* strains were also novobiocin-resistant.

TREHALOSE–MANNITOL–PHOSPHATASE AGAR
FOR IDENTIFICATION OF *STAPHYLOCOCCUS EPIDERMIDIS*
AND *STAPHYLOCOCCUS SAPROPHYTICUS*

Trehalose–mannitol–phosphatase agar (TMPA) was formulated to assist in the detection and differentiation of *S. epidermidis* and *S. saprophyticus*.[292] *S. epidermidis* does not produce acid from either trehalose or mannitol, and most strains (90%–96%) are phosphatase-positive. *S. saprophyticus* strains are variable for acid production from both trehalose and mannitol and are phosphatase-negative. Other human species of coagulase-negative staphylococci produce variable trehalose, mannitol, and phosphatase reactions. Acid production on TMPA is indicated by a color change in the medium from purple to yellow, and alkaline phosphatase activity is detected by spotting colonies from the medium (which contains phenolphthalein diphosphate) onto a piece of filter paper moistened with 1 N ammonium hydroxide. Phosphatase-positive colonies produce a pink color on the filter paper. With this medium, in conjunction with a novobiocin disk susceptibility test, *S. epidermidis* and *S. saprophyticus* can be reliably differentiated and identified. TMPA contains (final concentrations) 1% filter-sterilized trehalose, 1% filter-sterilized mannitol, and 0.01% filter-sterilized phenolphthalein diphosphate in autoclaved and cooled purple agar base medium. A trehalose–mannitol broth has also been described by Knapp and Washington.[176] This broth, which comprises 2% mannitol and 2% trehalose in 0.2 mL of purple broth base, was able to differentiate *S. epidermidis* from other coagulase-negative staphylococci within 2 hours.

FLUOROGENIC/CHROMOGENIC METHOD
FOR IDENTIFICATION OF *STAPHYLOCOCCUS AUREUS*,
STAPHYLOCOCCUS EPIDERMIDIS, AND *STAPHYLOCOCCUS*
SAPROPHYTICUS

RAPIDEC STAPH

RapiDEC Staph (bioMerieux-Vitek, Hazelwood MO) is a kit system that identifies *S. aureus, S. epidermidis*, and *S. saprophyticus* within 2 hours. The isolate to be identified is emulsified in water, and the suspension is dispensed into four cupules. The first cupule is a control, and the others contain a fluorescent coagulase substrate (see previous "aurease" test description), an alkaline phosphatase substrate (PAL), and a β-galactosidase substrate (BGAL), respectively. After a 2-hour incubation, the cupules are observed under an ultraviolet light (wavelength = 365 nm). If greater fluorescence is observed in the second cupule relative to the first control cupule, the isolate is identified as *S. aureus*. If this test is negative, the other two cupules are read either directly (cupule 3) or after the addition of a detection reagent (cupule 4). A positive reaction in cupule 3 or cupule 4 identifies the isolate as *S. epidermidis* (alkaline phosphatase–positive) or *S. saprophyticus* (β-galactosidase–positive), respectively. Positive results in both the PAL and BGAL tests provide a presumptive identification of *S. xylosus/S. intermedius*. In a recently published evaluation, RapiDEC Staph correctly identified 100% of 130 *S. aureus* strains, whereas only 70% of 74 *S. epidermidis* strains and 81% of 32 *S. saprophyticus* strains were correctly identified.[146] Among 62 other coagulase-negative isolates tested, four *S. sciuri* strains were misidentified as *S. epidermidis*, and eight isolates (one *S. hominis*, three *S. cohnii* subsp. *urealyticum*, three *S. simulans*, and one *S. kloosii*) were misidentified as *S. saprophyticus*. Even though the PAL test on the RapiDEC Staph appears to be relatively specific for detection of the phosphatase of *S. epidermidis*, strains of this species that are phosphatase-negative or that produce low levels of the enzyme will not be identified as *S. epidermidis* by RapiDEC Staph. Consequently, the sensitivity and performance of RapiDEC Staph for identifying *S. epidermidis* depends on the relative prevalence of PAL-positive and PAL-negative strains in a population.[146]

CONVENTIONAL IDENTIFICATION PROCEDURES

In 1975, Kloos and Schleifer published a scheme for the biochemical identification of coagulase-negative staphylococci.[169] This scheme uses the coagulase test for identifying *S. aureus* and employs a large battery of physiologic and biochemical tests for differentiating the coagulase-negative species. The scheme was updated and expanded by Kloos and Lambe in 1991,[167] but several new species have been described since then and are not currently included. The conventional method is time-consuming, labor intensive, and not amenable to implementation as a routine procedure in a clinical laboratory. Reference laboratories wishing to use this procedure should consult several of the references at the end of the chapter for media formulations and inoculation procedures. Figure 11-2 shows a dichotomous key that will enable identification of a majority of clinical isolates by the conventional method, although additional tests may be necessary on occasion. Biochemical reactions for identification of staphylococci are presented in Table 11-4 (novobiocin-susceptible staphylococci) and Table 11-5 (novobiocin-resistant staphylococci). Briefly, biochemical tests are performed using enteric media, such as nitrate broth, urease slants, and arginine dihydrolase media. Carbohydrate utilization tests are performed in purple broth agar containing 1% sterile carbohydrates. Supplementation with yeast extract (1% to 2%) may be necessary to encourage growth of more fastidious strains. In addition to biochemical tests and acid production from carbohydrates, Hebert and associates have shown that susceptibility to certain antimicrobial agents, such as polymyxin B (300-U disk) and bacitracin (10-U disk),

and the pyrrolidonyl arylamidase (PYR) test (also used for identification of enterococci; see Chap. 12), are also helpful for identifying coagulase-negative staphylococci.[117,118,119] These reactions are incorporated into Tables 11-4 and 11-5 as well.

Recently, Rhoden and associates[253] at the CDC formulated a modified conventional approach to identification of the *Micrococcaceae* using conventional carbohydrate utilization and biochemical tests along with selected chromogenic enzyme substrate tests from the API Staph-IDENT system (see later discussion). This approach differs from previous reference identification methods in that a numeric coding system was designed for the conventional test batteries to generate a database similar to those for commercial systems rather than using a "best fit" analysis based on reactions included in identification tables. Screening tests were used to identify morphology (Gram stain), family designation (catalase test), genus grouping (glucose fermentation), and presence of bound and free coagulase (slide and tube coagulase, StaphAurex latex agglutination test). A battery of 18 conventional primary tests were then inoculated for identification. A confirmatory battery of 11 additional tests was used to resolve the identity of problem isolates and rare or unusual biotypes that were generated from the primary test battery. By using 147 reference strains, 388 well-characterized control strains, and 289 clinical isolates, this method identified more than 95% of the *Staphylococcus*, *Micrococcus*, and *Stomatococcus* species tested.[253]

COMMERCIAL IDENTIFICATION SYSTEMS

Currently, several commercial kits are available for the identification of coagulase-negative staphylococci. All of these kits use modified carbohydrate fermentation tests, adaptations of standard bacteriologic identification tests (e.g., nitrate reduction, urease, Voges-Proskauer), and chromogenic enzyme substrate tests for organism identification. These systems are adapted to the particular format used by the manufacturer (e.g., strip with small cupules, microtiter trays, plastic cards, and so on).

API STAPH-IDENT

The API Staph-IDENT (BioMerieux-Vitek, Inc) product uses a battery of 10 miniaturized biochemical tests that are inoculated with a heavy suspension of the organism to be identified. Species identification is determined by the generation of a four-digit octal code derived from the positive tests on the strip and the database. Additional tests (e.g., acid from xylose, novobiocin susceptibility) may be required for identifying some strains. Currently, the database of the system includes 17 species or subspecies of staphylococci, micrococci, and *Stomatococcus mucilaginosus*. Organisms that are called *S. mucilaginosus* on Staph-IDENT require confirmation; recommendations include lysostaphin susceptibility to separate the organism from

(text continues on page 562)

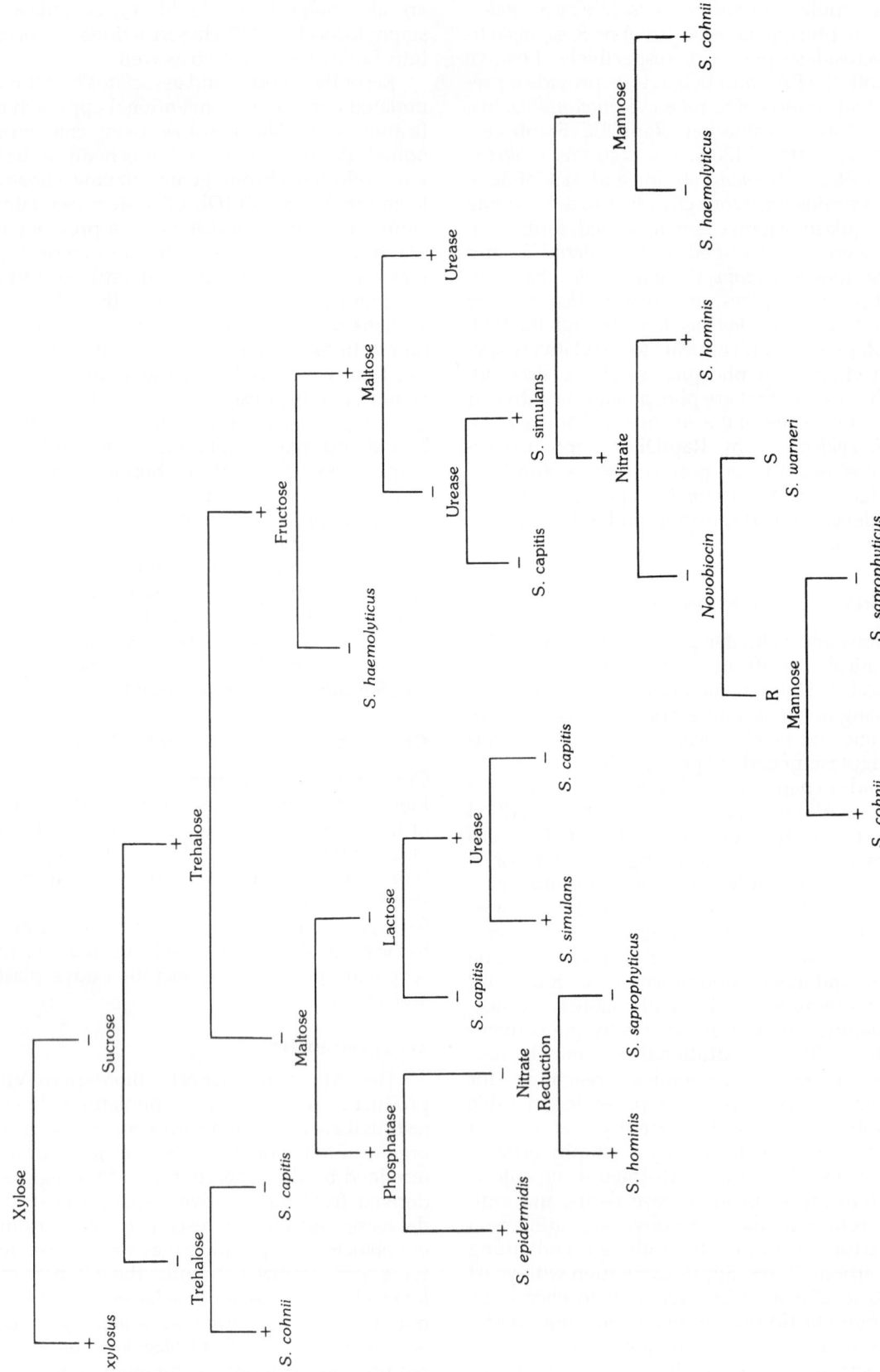

Figure 11-2.
Dichotomous key for identification of the more common human coagulase-negative staphylococci.

TABLE 11-4
CHARACTERISTICS FOR IDENTIFICATION OF NOVOBIOCIN-SUSCEPTIBLE STAPHYLOCOCCI

SPECIES	COAGULASE	CLUMPING FACTOR	ANAEROBIC GROWTH IN THIOGLYCOLLATE	HEAT-STABLE ENDONUCLEASE	ALKALINE PHOSPHATASE	ARGININE DIHYDROLASE	ORNITHINE DECARBOXYLASE	PYRROLIDONYL ARYLAMIDASE	ACETOIN PRODUCTION	NITRATE REDUCTION	UREASE	β-GLUCOSIDASE	β-GLUCURONIDASE	β-GALACTOSIDASE	POLYMYXIN B	BACITRACIN	MODIFIED OXIDASE	MALTOSE	FRUCTOSE	SUCROSE	LACTOSE	D-MANNITOL	D-MANNOSE	RAFFINOSE	D-TREHELOSE	D-CELLOBIOSE	D-XYLOSE	XYLITOL	RIBOSE	D-TURANOSE	L-ARABINOSE
S. aureus subsp. *aureus*	+	+	+	+	+	+	–	–	+	+	v	+	–	–	R	S	–	+	+	+	+	+	+	–	+	–	–	–	+	+	–
S. aureus subsp. *anaerobius*	+	–	+sl	+	+	NA	NA	NA	–	–	NA	–	–	–	NA	NA	–	+	+	+	–	NA	–	–	–	–	–	–	+	+	–
S. epidermidis	–	–	+	–	+	v	vsl	–	+	+	+	v	–	–	R	S	–	+	+	+	v	–	+sl	–	–	–	–	–	v	vsl	–
S. haemolyticus	–	–	+sl	–	–	+	–	+	+	+	–	v	v	–	S	R	–	+	v	+	v	v	–	–	+	–	–	–	v	vsl	–
S. hominis	–	–	–	–	–	v	–	–	v	v	+	–	–	–	S	S	–	+	+	+sl	v	–	–	–	v	–	–	–	–	+	–
S. capitis ssp. *capitis*	–	–	+sl	–	–	v	–	–	v	v	+	–	–	–	S	S	–	–	+	+sl	–	+	+	–	–	–	–	–	–	–	–
S. capitis ssp. *ureolyticus*	–	–	+sl	–	–	+	–	v	v	+	+	–	–	–	NA	NA	–	+	+	+	vsl	+	+	–	–	–	–	–	–	–	–
S. warneri	–	–	+	–	–	v	–	–	+	v	+	+	v	–	S	S	–	+sl	+	+	v	v	–	–	+	–	–	–	v	vsl	–
S. auricularis	–	–	+sl	–	–	v	–	v	–	vsl	–	–	–	v	S	S/R	–	+sl	+	v	–	–	–	–	+sl	–	–	–	–	vsl	–
S. simulans	–	–	+	–	v	+	–	+	v	+	+	–	v	+	S	S	–	+sl	+	+	+	+	v	–	v	–	–	–	v	–	–

(Continued)

TABLE 11-4 (Continued)
CHARACTERISTICS FOR IDENTIFICATION OF NOVOBIOCIN-SUSCEPTIBLE STAPHYLOCOCCI

SPECIES	COAGULASE	CLUMPING FACTOR	ANAEROBIC GROWTH IN THIOGLYCOLLATE	HEAT-STABLE ENDONUCLEASE	ALKALINE PHOSPHATASE	ARGININE DIHYDROLASE	ORNITHINE DECARBOXYLASE	PYRROLIDONYL ARYLAMIDASE	ACETOIN PRODUCTION	NITRATE REDUCTION	UREASE	β-GLUCOSIDASE	β-GLUCURONIDASE	β-GALACTOSIDASE	POLYMYXIN B	BACITRACIN	MODIFIED OXIDASE	MALTOSE	FRUCTOSE	SUCROSE	LACTOSE	D-MANNITOL	D-MANNOSE	RAFFINOSE	D-TREHELOSE	D-CELLOBIOSE	D-XYLOSE	XYLITOL	RIBOSE	D-TURANOSE	L-ARABINOSE
S. lugdunensis	−	+	+	−	−	−	+	+	+	+	v	+	−	−	S/R	S/R	−	+	+	+	+	−	−	−	+	−	−	−	−	v^sl	−
S. schleiferi spp. schleiferi	−	+	+	+	+	+	−	+	+	+	−	−	−	+	S	S	−	−	+^sl	−	−	−	+	−	v	−	−	NA	−	−	−
spp. coagulans	+	−	+	+	+	+	−	NA	+	+	NA	NA	NA	NA	NA	NA	−	−	NA	v	v	v	+	−	−	−	−	NA	NA	−	−
S. saccharolyticus	−	−	+	−	v	+	NA	NA	NA	+	NA	−	−	−	NA	NA	−	−	NA	+	−	−	+^sl	−	−	−	−	NA	NA	NA	−
S. hyicus	v	−	+	+	+	+	−	−	−	+	v	v	+	−	R	S	−	v^wt	+	+	+	−	+	−	+	−	−	−	+	−	−
S. chromogenes	−	−	+	−	+	+	−	v	−	+	+	v	−	−	R	S	−	v	+	+	+	v	+	−	+	−	−	−	+	v	−
S. intermedius	+	v	+^sl	+	+	v	−	v	−	+	+	v	−	+	S	S	−	v^wt	+	+	v	v^sl	+	−	+	−	−	−	+	v	−
S. caprae	−	−	+^sl	−	+^sl	+	−	v	+	+	+	−	−	−	S	S	−	v^sl	−	−	+	v	+	−	+^sl	−	−	−	−	−	−
S. delphini	+	−	+^sl	−	+	+	NA	NA	−	+	+	NA	NA	NA	NA	NA	−	+	+	+	+	+^sl	+	NA	−	NA	−	−	NA	NA	−
S. felis	−	−	+	−	+	+	NA	NA	−	+	+	−	−	+	NA	NA	−	−	NA	v	+	+	+	−	+	−	−	−	v	NA	−
S. carnosus	−	−	+	−	+	+	−	+	+	+	−	−	−	+	S	S	+	−	+	−	v	+	+	−	v	−	−	−	NA	−	−
S. caseolyticus	−	−	+^sl	NA	−	v	−	+	−	+	−	−	−	−	S	S	−	+	+	v	+	−	−	NA	v	−	−	−	+	−	−
S. muscae	−	−	+	−	+	−	−	NA	−	+	+	NA	−	−	NA	NA	−	−	NA	+	+	−	−	−	+	−	+	+	NA	+	−
S. piscifermentans	−	−	+	−	+	+	NA	NA	−	+	+	+	−	v^w+	NA	NA	−	v	NA	v	v	v	−	−	+	−	−	NA	NA	−	−
S. pasteuri	−	−	+	−	−	v	−	−	v	v	+	+	+	−	NA	NA	−	v^sl	NA	+	v	v	−	−	+	−	−	NA	NA	v^sl	−

+, ≥90% of strains positive; −, ≥90% of strains negative; +^sl, ≥90% of strains positive, reaction slow; v, 11–89% of strains positive; v^sl, 11–89% of strains positive, reaction slow; NA, data not available.

Polymixin (300 unit disk): S, ≥ 10 mm; R, < 10 mm.

Bacitracin (10 unit disk): S, ≥ 11 mm; R, < 11 mm.

v^w+, variable but weak reaction when positive.

TABLE 11-5
CHARACTERISTICS FOR IDENTIFICATION OF NOVOBIOCIN-RESISTANT STAPHYLOCOCCI

SPECIES	Coagulase	Clumping Factor	Anaerobic Growth in Thioglycolate	Heat-stable Endonuclease	Alkaline Phosphatase	Arginine Dihydrolase	Ornithine Decarboxylase	Pyrrolidonyl Arylamidase	Acetoin Production	Nitrate Reduction	Urease	β-Glucosidase	β-Glucuronidase	β-Galactosidase	Polymyxin B	Bacitracin	Modified Oxidase	Maltose	Fructose	Sucrose	Lactose	D-Mannitol	D-Mannose	Raffinose	D-Trehelose	D-Cellobiose	D-Xylose	Xylitol	Ribose	D-Turanose	L-Arabinose
																		Acid Production From												
S. saprophyticus	−	−	+sl	−	−	−	−	−	+	−	+	v	−	+	S	S/R	−	+	+	+	v	v	−	−	+	−	−	v	−	+	−
S. cohnii																															
spp. cohnii	−	−	v	−	−	−	−	v	v	−	−	−	−	−	S	S/R	−	v^{sl}	+	−	−	v	v^{sl}	−	+	−	−	v^{sl}	−	−	−
spp. urealyticum	−	−	+sl	−	+	−	−	v	v	−	+	−	+	+	NA	NA	−	+^{sl}	+	−	+	+	+	−	+	−	−	v^{sl}	−	−	−
S. xylosus	−	−	+	−	v	−	−	v	v	v	+	+	+	+	S	S/R	−	+	+	+	v	+	+	−	+	−	+	v^{sl}	+	v	v
S. sciuri	−	−	+sl	−	+	−	−	−	−	+	+	+	−	−	S	R	+	v^{sl}	+	+	v^{sl}	+	v^{sl}	−	+	+	v^{sl}	−	+	+^{sl}	v
S. gallinarum	−	−	+sl	−	+^{sl}	−	−	−	−	+	+	+	v	v	S	S	−	+	+	+	v	+	+	−	+	+	+	v	+	+	+
S. lentus	−	−	+sl	−	+^{sl}	−	−	−	−	+	−	+	−	−	S	S	+	v	+^{sl}	+	v	+	+^{sl}	+	+	+	+^{sl}	−	+	+^{sl}	v^{sl}
S. arlettae	−	−	−	−	+^{sl}	−	−	−	−	−	−	NA	+	−	NA	NA	−	+	+	+	+	+	+	+	+	−	+	−	+	+	+
S. kloosii	−	−	−	−	v	−	−	v	v	−	v	v	v	v	S	S	−	v	+	+	v^{sl}	+	−	−	+	−	v^{sl}	v	+	+	v
S. equorum	−	−	−	−	+^{sl}	−	−	−	−	+	+	NA	+	−	NA	NA	−	v	+	+	v	+	+	−	+	v^{sl}	+	−	+	v	+
S. vitulus	−	−	−	−	−	−	−	−	−	+	−	v	−	−	NA	NA	+	−	+	+	−	v	v	−	v^{sl}	v	v	−	NA	−	−
S. pulvereri	−	−	−	NA	v	v	−	v	v	+⁻	v	NA	v	v	NA	NA	NA	+	+	+	v	v	v	−	v	−	NA	NA	−	−	−

See legend Table 11–4 for explanation of symbols.

staphylococci, and catalase and growth in salt broth to separate the organism from *M. kristinae.* Staph-IDENT has been extensively evaluated and agreement with conventional procedures has ranged from 43% to 95% depending on the species tested.[5,59,72,96,97,104,126,139,149,174,228,328] Rhoden and Miller[254] at the CDC recently published a 4-year prospective study comparing the API Staph-IDENT with reference methods on 1106 isolates and found an overall agreement of 81.1%. The percentage agreements for the five most common isolates were 97.1% for *S. epidermidis,* 82.5% for *S. hominis,* 77.2% for *S. aureus,* 75.8% for *S. haemolyticus,* and 64.1% for *S. warneri.* These workers concluded that the Staph-IDENT system is inadequate for identifying both the commonly encountered and uncommon species in the family *Micrococcaceae.*

API STAPH

API STAPH (formerly API Staph-Trac, bio-Merieux-Vitek, Inc.) is an 18- to 24-hour identification system for both micrococci and staphylococci. This system contains 19 tests arranged in a strip format and is inoculated with a suspension of the organism prepared in a peptone–yeast extract broth medium provided with the kit. After reading the biochemical reactions, a seven-digit octal code is generated and identification of the organism is obtained with the computer-assisted database (Color Plate 11-2*G*). The database consists of 25 taxa and includes staphylococci of human and veterinary origin, *Micrococcus* species, and *Stomatococcus mucilaginosus.* Although the database of this system is large, it has not been extensively evaluated.[97,186,212] A recent study by Perl and colleagues[233] found that the API STAPH system correctly identified 73% of 277 coagulase-negative staphylococci. Although 94% of 94 *S. epidermidis* isolates were correctly identified, the system performed poorly with less common isolates such as *S. haemolyticus* (85% correct), *S. hominis* (75% correct), *S. simulans* (67% correct), and *S. warneri* (22% correct).

ID32 STAPH

ID32 Staph (bioMerieux S.A., France) is a 24-hour strip system for identifying the *Micrococcaceae.* It contains 32 cupules and currently has 26 biochemical tests, allowing room for expansion of the test battery. The system may be read manually to generate a profile number that is interpreted by a computer-assisted database (Color Plate 11-2*H*). Alternatively, the strip can be used with the automated bioMerieux ATB system, which includes a densitometer, an inoculator, a reader, a microcomputer, and a printer. The ID32 Staph has the most extensive database of all the systems, with all human staphylococcal species (except *S. saccharolyticus*) and several animal and environmental species being included. The system also identifies six *Micrococcus* species and *S. mucilaginosus.* An international collaborative evaluation with 792 strains conducted in eight laboratories found that the ID32 Staph correctly identified 95.5% of the isolates

tested; 83.5% were identified without further testing, and, for an additional 12% of strains, the correct identification was among the proposed choices.[41] Only 1.2% of isolates were misidentified, and 3.3% were not identified by the ID32 Staph. Other European investigators challenged the system with a collection of 42 isolates that could not be classified by other available phenotypic procedures and found that only 22 (52%) could be identified by the ID32 Staph.[48] This system has not yet been FDA approved and, therefore, is not available for use in clinical laboratories in the United States.

VITEK GRAM-POSITIVE IDENTIFICATION (GPI) CARD

The Vitek GPI card (bioMeriuex-Vitek, Inc.) is a gram-positive organism identification card designed for use with the automated Vitek bacterial identification–susceptibility testing system. The card contains 30 microwells (28 test wells and 2 control wells) containing substrates for the identification of *Staphylococcus* species (11 human and 4 veterinary species), *Streptococcus* species, and several gram-positive bacillary species (e.g., *Corynebacterium* species, *Erysipelothrix rhusiopathiae,* and *Listeria monocytogenes*). A suspension of the organism is prepared in saline, and the card is attached to the bacterial suspension by a transfer tube and placed in the filling module of the instrument. The card is inoculated by a vacuum-release method. The card is then placed in the reader–incubator module of the Vitek instrument, where it is optically scanned and read periodically. Identification of coagulase-negative staphylococci generally requires 10 to 13 hours. Bannerman and coworkers[19] recently evaluated the updated GPI database with 500 clinical isolates. The overall agreement between the GPI card and conventional methods was 89%. The card identified 92% of *S. epidermidis,* 95% of *S. haemolyticus,* 88% of *S. capitis* subsp. *capitis,* and 100% of *S. saprophyticus* strains tested. Organisms that are not currently in the database, such as *S. lugdunensis,* were either misidentified or unidentified by the GPI card. In the 1994 evaluation by Perl and associates,[233] the GPI card correctly identified only 67% of 185 isolates. These workers pointed out that the poorer performance of the GPI card in their study may have been due to the preponderance of "non-*S. epidermidis*" staphylococci among the 277 isolates tested.

MICROSCAN RAPID POS COMBO PANEL

The new MicroScan Rapid Pos Combo Panel (Dade/MicroScan, West Sacramento CA) is a microtiter-plate format system that uses fluorogenic substrates and a fluorescent pH indicator to detect various bacterial enzymatic activities.[166] The panel contains 34 substrate wells, 22 of which contain metabolites that are conjugated to fluorophores. Twelve of the 22 wells contain 4-methylumbelliferyl-conjugated substrates, and 10 contain 7-amido-4-methylcoumarin-conjugated substrates. The remaining 12 wells contain various carbohydrates and urea along with a fluorescent pH indicator. The system is inoculated with a suspension of the organism and is incubated and read in the autoSCAN Walk/Away instument. Identifications are available 2 hours after panel inoculation. In a Canadian evaluation of this system, the MicroScan Rapid Pos Combo panel correctly identified 91.6% of 239 staphylococcal isolates.[294] For an additional 3.8% of the isolates, the correct identification was listed among the species choices provided by the database. Another evaluation from Portland, Oregon found that the Rapid Pos panel identified only 50.5% of 233 isolates, with an additional 24.9% having the correct identification among the possibilities generated by the database.[103]

MICROSCAN POS ID PANEL

The MicroScan Pos ID Panel (Dade/MicroScan, West Sacramento CA) system offers combination identification and susceptibility testing capabilities for gram-positive organisms, including micrococci, staphylococci, streptococci, enterococci, and listeriae. The panel contains 27 miniaturized conventional biochemical identification tests, 18 of which are used for the *Micrococcaceae*. The lyophilized panels are thawed, inoculated, incubated for 24 to 48 hours, and read manually or with the autoSCAN Walk/Away automated system. The test results compute into a six-digit code, and the database of the MicroScan system provides an identification. In one evaluation, the panel provided accurate identification of *S. epidermidis* and *S. saprophyticus* but only after a 48-hour incubation.[139] Other *Staphylococcus* species were identified less reliably within the same time period. A more recent MicroScan Pos ID panel evaluation reported that the system identified only 53.6% of 233 staphylococcal isolates, with an additional 24.9% of isolates having the correct identification listed among possible choices by the computer-assisted database.[103]

MINITEK GRAM-POSITIVE PANEL

The Minitek system (BD Microbiology Systems) uses filter paper disks that are impregnated with various test substrates and carbohydrates.[59] This system is designed for identification of micrococci, staphylococci, and streptococci. Disks are dispensed into the wells of a plastic tray, and each well is inoculated with 0.05 mL of a broth suspension of the organism, and the tray is incubated in a humidor for 18 to 24 hours. Interpretation of color reactions after the addition of reagents to some of the tests results in the generation of a seven-digit code. A code book is consulted for the identification. A comparative evaluation of this system against both the Staph-IDENT and conventional methods found that Minitek correctly identified 86% of 78 clinically significant coagulase-negative isolates from children with cancer.[59] Although Minitek identified 96% of

54 *S. epidermidis* isolates, the small number of other species tested in the study (23 isolates representing 6 other species) did not permit an assessment of the system's accuracy. Because the Minitek Gram-Positive Panel also addresses the identification of streptococci and micrococci, test selection for the variety of staphylococcal species is not optimal.

SCEPTOR GRAM-POSITIVE MIC/ID PANEL

The Sceptor Panel (BD Microbiology Systems) is a combination identification–antimicrobial susceptibility system in which the antimicrobial agents and the biochemical test media are dried in the wells of a microtiter plate. The panel is inoculated with an organism suspension by the Sceptor automatic inoculator, and they are read manually after incubation. Test results are entered into the system's computer for the identification. The Sceptor test battery is essentially the same as that of the Minitek Gram-Positive kit. The performance of this system for identifying staphylococci has not been evaluated.

STAF-SISTEM 18-R

The Staf-Sistem 18-R (Liofilchem s.r.l. Roseto degli Abruzzi, Teramo, Italy) consists of a plastic tray containing 18 modified conventional substrates. The wells are inoculated with an organism suspension using a multichannel pipette, and the panel is incubated and read after 18 to 24 hours. Piccolomini and colleagues[237] evaluated this system with 523 strains belonging to 16 human *Staphylococcus* species and found that 491 strains (93.9%) were correctly identified, with another 28 strains (5.4%) requiring additional supplemental tests for complete identification. As with many of these kit systems, the authors point out the need for database adjustment and more discriminating test selection to correctly identify important isolates such as *S. lugdunensis* and *S. schleiferi*.

STAPH-ZYM

The Staph-Zym (ROSCO, Taastrup, Denmark) is a new Scandinavian identification system that is composed of a plastic strip of 10 minitubes that contain dehydrated chromogenic and modified conventional substrates. The individual microtubes are inoculated with an aliquot of a bacterial suspension prepared in saline, and the results are read after overnight incubation. This system has been evaluated for its ability to identify isolates from bovine intramammary infections but has not been investigated for identifying human staphylococcal isolates.[329]

MICROBIAL IDENTIFICATION SYSTEM

The Microbial Identification System (MIS or MIDI, Microbial ID Inc., Newark DE) uses high-resolution

CHARACTERISTICS FOR IDENTIFICATION OF FORMER *MICROCOCCUS* SPECIES

| SPECIES | CELL ARRANGEMENT | | | | CATALASE | PIGMENTATION | OXIDASE | MOTILITY | ARGININE DIHYDROLASE |
	PAIRS	TETRADS	CUBES	CLUSTERS					
Kytococcus sedentarius	−	+	+	−	+	Creamy white/ yellow	−+	−	+
Nesterenkonia halobia	+	+	−	+	+	Non-pigmented	+	−	−
Dermacoccus nishinomiyaensis	+	+	−	+	+	Orange	+	−	−
Kocuria rosea	+	+	−	+	+	Pink-to-red	+w+	−	−
Kocuria varians	−	+	−	+	+	Yellow	−	−	−
Kocuria kristinae	−	+	−	+	+	Pale creme to orange	+	−	−
Micrococcus luteus	+	+	+	+	+	Yellow	+	−	−
Micrococcus lylae	+	+	+	+	+	White	+	−	−
Arthrobacter agilis	+	+	−	+	+	Rose-red	+	+	−

+, positive reaction; −, negative reaction; v, variable reaction; −w+, most strains negative, few strains weakly positive; −+, most strains negative, rare strains positive; +−, most strains positive, rare strains negative.

gas-liquid chromatography (GLC) of cellular fatty acid derivatives for the identification of bacteria.[34] The database of the system is composed of libraries containing the analyses of cellular fatty acid profiles of various bacteria and compares the composition of individual isolates with those in the database using covariance matrix–pattern recognition software. A similarity index is used to express the relatedness of a profile of an unknown organism to representative profiles of known organisms. In a comparative evaluation of the MIS with conventional procedures for identifying staphylococci, the MIS system showed complete agreement with conventional methods for 87.8% of 470 isolates tested.[293] The system identified all strains of *S. epidermidis*, *S. intermedius*, *S. cohnii*, *S. lugdunensis*, *S. schleiferi*, *S. simulans*, *S. sciuri*, and *S. xylosus*. *S. hominis* and *S. saprophyticus* strains accounted for over half of the misidentifications obtained with the system. The GLC approach used in the MIS shows promise as an alternative method for species identification of the staphylococci.

BIOLOG MICROPLATE IDENTIFICATION SYSTEM

The Biolog Microplate Identification System (Biolog, Inc., Hayward CA) identifies microorganisms on the basis of oxidation of a variety of substrates. The system uses a 96-well microtiter tray with 95 substrates plus a control well lacking substrate. The plate is inoculated with a suspension of the organism and is incubated for 4 or 24 hours. If the organism oxidizes a substrate in an individual well, the respiration of the organism during oxidative substrate assimila-

tion causes the reduction of a tetrazolium indicator dye, turning the well from colorless to purple. Currently, the Biolog MicroPlate System includes the GN MicroPlate for identifying 569 gram-negative species and the GP Biolog MicroPlate, which includes 225 gram-positive organisms in its database. Miller and Biddle at the CDC and Quenzer and McLaughlin at the University of New Mexico performed a joint evaluation of the GP Biolog MicroPlate for identification of 113 isolates belonging to the family *Micrococcaceae*, including 33 type strains of staphylococci, 5 strains of *Micrococcus* species, and 1 strain of *S. mucilaginosus*.[218] These workers found the overall accuracy of the system to be 69% and 73% at the CDC and the New Mexico laboratories, respectively. These results indicate that the Biolog system is not yet accurate enough to be used as a routine method for identifying the coagulase-negative staphylococci and related organisms.

MOLECULAR TYPING AXND IDENTIFICATION METHODS FOR STAPHYLOCOCCI

Several approaches using both traditional and newly developed molecular methods have also been used to identify staphylococci and to characterize strains in epidemiologic studies and in outbreaks of unusual or multiresistant strains. Until recently, epidemiologic studies were based on phenotypic markers, such as unusual carbohydrate utilization or biochemical reaction patterns, antimicrobial susceptibility, serotyping, biotyping, or susceptibility to certain types of bacte-

SPECIES	NITRATE REDUCT.	UREASE	HYDROLYSIS OF			ACID AEROBICALLY FROM:				
			ESCULIN	STARCH	GELATIN	GLUCOSE	GLYCEROL	LACTOSE	MANNOSE	XYLOSE
Kytococcus sedentarius	v	−	−	−	+	−	−	−	−	−
Nesterenkonia halobia	−	−	−	+	−	+	+	+	−	+
Dermacoccus nishinomiyaensis	v	+⁻	−	v	+	v	−	−	−	−
Kocuria rosea	+	−	−	v	−	v	−	−	−	+
Kocuria varians	+	+	−	v	v	+	−	−	−	+
Kocuria kristinae	−	v	+	−	−	+	+	−⁺	+	−
Micrococcus luteus	−	−	−	−	+	−	−	−	−	−
Micrococcus lylae	−	−	−	−	+	−	−	−	−	−
Arthrobacter agilis	−	−	+	+	+	−	−	−	−	−

riophages.[165] Other approaches, such as whole-cell protein analysis using SDS–PAGE, gas-liquid chromatography, high-presssure liquid chromatography, and mass spectrometry, are more discriminating for recognizing similarities and differences among strains but are expensive and time-consuming to perform.[34,239,306] SDS-PAGE of total cell protein and penicillin-binding proteins and gas-liquid chromatography of cellular fatty acids have shown 92% to more than 95% agreement with phenotypic reference procedures.[181,239]

Newer molecular and genetic techniques have gained widespread popularity as highly discriminatory and relatively inexpensive methods for epidemiologic typing and characterization of strains. These methods include restriction enzyme fragment length polymorphism analysis of plasmid, ribosomal, and chromosomal nucleic acids; pulsed-field gel electrophoresis of total DNA; ribotyping; and polymerase chain reaction–nucleic acid probe hybridization procedures.[32,35,36,45,64,86,100,105,145,181,232,249,265,272,296,305,315,316,340] These procedures have been used to investigate outbreaks of oxacillin-resistant *S. aureus* in neonatal intensive care units, the spread of vancomycin-resistant *S. haemolyticus* in patients and caregivers, and phenotypic variation of coagulase-negative staphylococci recovered from serious infections.[64,66,105,139,340] Such techniques have also been useful in studies designed to identify colonized individuals and to trace the sources of organisms responsible for infections, such as the relation between carriage of a particular *S. aureus* strain in the nares of patients and caregivers and

the subsequent development of CAPD-related peritonitis.[240] These methods are also being applied to taxonomic analysis of microorganisms and, in this regard, have already revolutionized our concepts of organism relatedness, classification, and identification.[145,232]

IDENTIFICATION OF *MICROCOCCUS* AND RELATED SPECIES

Micrococci and the former micrococcal species are not generally identified to species level in clinical laboratories because they are rarely clinically significant. By using the tests described in the foregoing and in Table 11-3, laboratories may issue reports of "*Micrococcus* species" without further testing. However, with the recognition of these agents as opportunistic pathogens, it may on occasion be necessary to identify these organisms to species.[82,202,281,289,334] Identification criteria for the newly reclassified members of the former genus *Micrococcus* are presented in Table 11-6. These organisms are also included in the databases of some of the commercial kit systems used in laboratories.

IDENTIFICATION OF *STOMATOCOCCUS MUCILAGINOSUS*

Stomatococcus mucilaginosus is a resident of the human upper respiratory tract and has been isolated from blood cultures of patients with endocarditis sec-

TABLE 11-7
BIOCHEMICAL CHARACTERISTICS OF
STOMATOCOCCUS MUCILAGINOSUS

CHARACTERISTIC	REACTION
Acetoin production (VP test)	+
Hydrolysis of gelatin	+
Growth under anaerobic conditions	+
Catalase	v
Growth on nutrient agar with 5% NaCl	−
Coagulase	−
Alkaline phosphatase	−
Acid production from	
Glucose	+
Sucrose	+
Fructose	+
Salicin	+
Mannose	v
Trehalose	v
Mannitol	−
Sorbitol	−

+, positive; −, negative; v, variable.

ondary to cardiac catheterization and intravenous drug use.[23,56,241,243,250,252,261] *S. mucilaginosus* colonies are generally mucoid, clear to white, and adherent to the agar surface. They appear on gram-stained smears as large gram-positive cocci arranged in pairs or clusters. They are weakly catalase-positive, although some strains are catalase-negative. *S. mucilaginosus* can be differentiated from *Micrococcus* and *Staphylococcus* species by their failure to grow on nutrient agar medium containing 5% NaCl and by the presence of a capsule.[27,28] These organisms are also included in the databases of the API Staph-IDENT, the API STAPH, and ID32 STAPH systems. Other biochemical characteristics are shown in Table 11-7.

Medium used for enteric identification can be inoculated to determine biochemical reactions for this organism, and carbohydrate utilization tests may be performed with purple broth-based or cystine tryptic digest agar-based media containing 1% filter sterilized carbohydrates.

LABORATORY APPROACH TO THE IDENTIFICATION OF STAPHYLOCOCCI

Because staphylococci are among the most frequently isolated organisms in the clinical laboratory, decisions must be made on "how far to go" in identifying them. This is especially true for the coagulase-negative organisms. Many laboratories have adopted rapid coagulase procedures (i.e., latex or hemagglutination tests), so these tests may quickly be performed on colonies that "look like" staphylococci and are catalase-positive. If the colonies are coagulase-positive, the organism is identified as *S. aureus*. For isolates that are coagulase-negative, a furazolidone or bacitracin disk test or the modified oxidase test may be performed to differentiate coagulase-negative staphylococci from *Micrococcus* species. Significant staphylococcal isolates from urine cultures should also be tested for susceptibility to novobiocin to identify *S. saprophyticus*. Complete species identification using a kit method or the reference procedure should be reserved for clinically significant isolates. These may include isolates that have been recovered from multiple sets of blood cultures, from infected intraveous catheters (where the patient may have the same isolate in multiple blood cultures), or from other normally sterile sites where what appears to be the same coagulase-negative staphylococcus has been repeatedly isolated. Decisions involving further identification of these organisms should be made on a case-by-case basis with input from both the laboratory and the physicians caring for the patient.

REFERENCES

1. ABRAHAMSSON K, HANSSON S, JODAL U, LINCOLN K: *Staphylococcus saprophyticus* urinary tract infections in children. Eur J Pediatr 152:69–71, 1993

2. ADAMS J, VAN ENK R: Use of commercial particle agglutination systems for the rapid identification of methicillin-susceptible and methicillin-resistant *Staphylococcus aureus*. Eur J Clin Microbiol Infect Dis 13:86–89, 1994

3. ALDRIDGE KE, KOGOS C, SANDERS CV ET AL: Comparison of rapid identification assays for *Staphylococcus aureus*. J Clin Microbiol 19:703–704, 1984

4. ALEXANDER W, RIMLAND D: Lack of correlation of slime production wih pathogenicity in continuous ambulatory peritoneal dialysis peritonitis caused by coagulase-negative staphylococci. Diagn Microbiol Infect Dis 8:215–220, 1987

5. ALMEIDA RJ, JORGENSEN, JH: Identification of coagulase-negative staphylococci with the API Staph-IDENT system. J Clin Microbiol 18:254–257, 1983

6. ANDAY E, TALBOT G: Coagulase-negative staphylococcal bacteremia—a rising threat in the newborn infant. Ann Clin Lab Sci 13:246–251, 1985

7. ANIA BJ: *Staphylococcus aureus* meningitis after short-term epidural analgesia. Clin Infect Dis 18:844–845, 1994

8. ARBEIT RD, KARAKAWA WW, VANN WF ET AL: Predominance of two newly described capsular polysaccharide types among clinical isolates of *Staphylococcus aureus*. Diagn Microbiol Infect Dis 85–91, 1984

9. ARCHER GL: *Staphylococcus epidermidis* and other coagulase-negative staphylococci. In Mandell GL, Bennett JE, Dolin R (eds), *Mandell, Douglas, and Bennett's Principles and Practice of Infectious Diseases*, 4th ed, pp. 1777–1784. New York, Churchill-Livingstone, 1995

10. ARCHER GL, TENENBAUM MJ: Antibiotic-resistant *Staphylococcus epidermidis* in patients undergoing cardiac surgery. Antimicrob Agents Chemother 17:269–272, 1980

11. ASCHER DP, BASH MC, ZBICK C ET AL: *Stomatococcus mucilaginosus* catheter-related infection in an adolescent with osteosarcoma. South Med J 84:409–410, 1991

12. ASCHER DP, ZBICK C, WHITE C ET AL: Infections due to *Stomatococcus mucilaginosus*: 10 cases and review. Rev Infect Dis 13:1048–1052, 1991

13. AYRES WW, DUDA J: Differential diagnosis of *Staphylococcus aureus* from *Staphylococcus epidermidis* and *Staphylococcus saprophyticus* by alphazurine A dye. Milit Med 158:571–572, 1993

14. BADDOUR LM, BARKER LP, CHRISTENSEN GD ET AL: Phenotypic variation of *Staphylococcus epidermidis* in infection of transvenous endocardial pacemaker electrodes. J Clin Microbiol 28:676–679, 1990

15. BADDOUR L, PHILLIPS T, BISNO A: Coagulase-negative staphylococcal endocarditis. Arch Intern Med 46:118–121, 1986

16. BAKER JS: Comparison of various methods for differentiation of staphylococci and micrococci. J Clin Microbiol 19:875–879, 1984

17. BAKER JS, BORMAN MA, BOUDREAU DH: Evaluation of various rapid agglutination methods for the identification of *Staphylococcus aureus*. J Clin Microbiol 21:726–729, 1985

18. BANDRES JC, DAROUICHE RO: *Staphylococcus capitis* endocarditis: a new cause of an old disease. Clin Infect Dis 14:366–367, 1992

19. BANNERMAN TL, KLEEMAN KT, KLOOS WE: Evaluation of the Vitek Systems gram-positive identification card for species identification of coagulase-negative staphylococci. J Clin Microbiol 31:1322–1325, 1993

20. BANNERMAN TL, KLOOS WE: *Staphylococcus capitis* subsp. *ureolyticus* subsp. nov. from human skin. Int J Syst Bacteriol 41:144–147, 1991

21. BARKER KF, O'DRISCOLL JC, BHARGAVA A: *Staphylococcus lugdunensis*. J Clin Pathol 44:873–874, 1991

22. BARKER LP, SIMPSON WA, CHRISTENSEN GD: Differential production of slime under aerobic and anaerobic conditions. J Clin Microbiol 28:2578–2579, 1990

23. BARLOW JF, VOGELE KA, DZINTARS PF: Septicemia with *Stomatococcus mucilaginosus*. Clin Microbiol Newslett 8:22, 1986

24. BARNHAM M, HOLMES B: Isolation of CDC group M-5 and *Staphylococcus intermedius* from infected dog bites. J Infect 25:332–334, 1992

25. BAUMGART S, HALL SE, CAMPOS JM ET AL: Sepsis with coagulase-negative cocci in critically ill newborns. Am J Dis Child 137:461–463, 1983

26. BENNETT MI, TAI YMA, SYMONDS JM: Staphylococcal meningitis following Synchromed intrathecal pump implant: a case report. Pain 56:243–244, 1994

27. BERGAN T, KOCUR M: *Stomatococcus mucilaginosus* gen. nov., sp. nov., emend. rev., a member of the family *Micrococcaceae*. Int J Syst Bacteriol 32:374–377, 1982

28. BERGAN T, KOCUR M: Genus II. *Stomatococcus*. In Sneath PHA, Nair NS, Holt JG (eds), *Bergey's Manual of Systematic Bacteriology*, vol 2, pp 1008–1010. Baltimore, Williams & Wilkins, 1986

29. BERGDOLL MS, REISER RF, CRASS BA ET AL: A new staphylococcal enterotoxin, enterotoxin F, associated with toxic shock syndrome *Staphylococcus aureus* isolates. Lancet 1:1017–1021, 1981

30. BERGDOLL MS, SCHLIEVERT PM: Toxic shock syndrome toxin. Lancet 2:691, 1984.

31. BERGMAN B, WEDREN H, HOLM SE: *Staphylococcus saprophyticus* in males with symptoms of chronic prostatitis. Urology 34:241–245, 1989

32. BERKE A, TILTON RC: Evaluation of rapid coagulase methods for the identification of *Staphylococcus aureus*. J Clin Microbiol 23:916–919, 1986

33. BIALKOWSKA-HOBRZANSKA H, JASKOT D, HAMMERBERG O: Evaluation of restriction endonuclease fingerprinting of chromosomal DNA and plasmid profile analysis for characterization of multiresistant coagulase-negative staphylococci in bacteremic neonates. J Clin Microbiol 28:269–275, 1990

34. BIRNBAUM D, HERWALDT L, LOW DE ET AL: Efficacy of Microbial Identification System for epidemiologic typing of coagulase-negative staphylococci. J Clin Microbiol 32:2113–2119, 1994

35. BLANC DS, LUGEON C, WENGER A ET AL: Quantatitive antibiogram typing using inhibition zone diameters compared with ribotyping for epidemiological typing of methicillin-resistant *Staphylococcus aureus*. J Clin Microbiol 32:2505–2509, 1994

36. BLUMBERG HM, RIMLAND D, KIEHLBAUCH JA ET AL: Epidemiological typing of *Staphylococcus aureus* by DNA restriction fragment length polymorphisms of rRNA genes: elucidation of the clonal nature of a group of bacteriophage-nontypeable, ciprofloxacin-resistant, methicillin-susceptible *S. aureus* isolates. J Clin Microbiol 30:362–369, 1992

37. BOUTONNIER A, NATO F, BOUVET A ET AL: Direct testing of blood cultures for detection of the serotype 5 and 8 capsular polysaccharides of *Staphylococcus aureus*. J Clin Microbiol 27:989–993, 1989

38. BOWMAN RA, BUCK M: *Staphylococcus hominis* septicaemia in patients with cancer. Med J Aust 140:26–27, 1984

39. BRAKSTAD OG, AASBAKK K, MAELAND JA: Detection of *Staphylococcus aureus* by polymerase chain reaction amplification of the *nuc* gene. J Clin Microbiol 30:1654–1660, 1992

40. BRANGER C, GOULLET P, BOUTONNIER A ET AL: Correlation between esterase electrophoretic types and capsular polysaccharide types 5 and 8 among methicillin-susceptible and methicillin-resistant strains of *Staphylococcus aureus*. J Clin Microbiol 28:150–151, 1990

41. BRUN Y, BES M, BOEUFGRAS JM ET AL: International collaborative evaluation of the ATB 32 Staph gallery for identification of the *Staphylococcus* species. Zentrabl Bakteriol 273:319–326, 1990

42. BRYAN CS, PARISI JT, STRIKE DG: Vertebral osteomyelitis due to *Staphylococcus warneri* attributed to a Hickman catheter. Diagn Microbiol Infect Dis 8:57–59, 1987

43. BYKOWSKA K, LUDWICKA A, WEGRZYNOWICZ Z ET AL: Anticoagulant properties of extracellular slime substance produced by *Staphylococcus epidermidis*. Thromb Hemost 54:853–856, 1985

44. CAPUTO G, ARCHER G, CALDERWOOD S ET AL: Native valve endocarditis due to coagulase-negative staphylococci: clinical and microbiologic features. Am J Med 83:619–625, 1987

45. CARLES-NURIT MJ, CHRISTOPHLE B, BROCHE S ET AL: DNA polymorphisms in methicillin-susceptible and

methicillin-resistant strains of *Staphylococcus aureus.* J Clin Microbiol 30:2092–2096, 1992

46. CARNEY DN, FOSSIECK BE, PARKER RH ET AL: Bacteremia due to *Staphylococcus aureus* in patients with cancer: report on 45 cases and a review of the literature. Rev Infect Dis 4:1–12, 1982

47. CARRUTHERS MM, JENKINS KE, KABAT WJ ET AL: Detection of antibody to staphylococcal lipoteichoic acid with a micro-enzyme linked immunosorbent assay. J Clin Microbiol 19:552–554, 1984

48. CHESNEAU O, AUBERT S, MORVAN A ET AL: Usefulness of the ID32 Staph System and a method based on rRNA gene restriction site polymorphism analysis for species and subspecies identification of staphylococcal clinical isolates. J Clin Microbiol 30:2346–2352, 1992

49. CHESNEAU O, MORVAN A, GRIMONT F ET AL: *Staphylococcus pasteuri* sp. nov. isolated from human, animal, and food specimens. Int J Syst Bacteriol 43:237–244, 1993

50. CHRISTENSEN GD, BADDOUR LM, SIMPSON WA: Phenotypic variation of *Staphylococcus epidermidis* slime production in vitro and in vivo. Infect Immun 55:2870–2877, 1987

51. CHRISTENSEN GD, BARKER LP, MAWHINNEY TP ET AL: Identification of an antigenic marker of slime production for *Staphylococcus epidermidis.* Infect Immun 58:2906–2911, 1990

52. CHRISTENSEN GD, BISNO A, PARISI J ET AL: Nosocomial septicemia due to multiply antibiotic resistant *Staphylococcus epidermidis.* Ann Intern Med 96:1–10, 1992

53. CHRISTENSEN GD, SIMPSON WA, BISNO AL ET AL: Adherence of slime-producing strains of *Staphylococcus epidermidis* to smooth surfaces. Infect Immun 37:318–326. 1982

54. CHRISTENSEN GD, SIMPSON WA, YOUNGER JJ ET AL: Adherence of coagulase-negative staphylococci to plastic tissue culture plates: a quantitative model for adherence of staphylococci to medical devices. J Clin Microbiol 22:996–1006, 1985

55. CORMICAN MG, EL BOURI K, CORBETT-FEENEY G ET AL: *Staphylococcus lugdunensis* endocarditis. J Infect 24:335–336, 1992

56. COUDRON PE, MARKOWITZ SM, MOHANTY LB ET AL: Isolation of *Stomatococcus mucilaginosus* from drug user with endocarditis. J Clin Microbiol 25:1359–1363, 1987

57. COURAL SA, WEST BC: Endocarditis caused by *Staphylococcus xylosus* associated with intravenous drug abuse. J Infect Dis 149:826–827, 1984

58. CRASS BA, BERGDOLL MS: Involvement of coagulase-negative staphylococci in toxic shock syndrome. J Clin Microbiol 23:43–45, 1986

59. CROUCH SF, PEARSON TA, PARHAM DM: Comparison of modified Minitek system with Staph-IDENT system for species identification of coagulase-negative staphylococci. J Clin Microbiol 25:1626–1628, 1987

60. DAN M, MARIEN G, GOLDSAND G: Endocarditis caused by *Staphylococcus warneri* on a normal aortic heart valve following vasectomy. Can Med Assoc J 131:211–213, 1984

61. DANCER SJ, GARRATT R, SALDANHA J ET AL: The epidermolytic toxins are serine proteases. FEBS Lett 268:129–131, 1990

62. DAVENPORT DS, MASSANARI RM, PFALLER MA ET AL: Usefulness of a test for slime production as a marker for clinically significant infections with coagulase negative staphylococci. J Infect Dis 153:332–339, 1986

63. DAVIS TE, FULLER DD: Direct identification of bacterial isolates in blood cultures by using a DNA probe. J Clin Microbiol 29:2193–2196, 1991

64. DEGENER JE, HECK MEO, VAN LEEUWEN WJ ET AL: Nosocomial infection by *Staphylococcus haemolyticus* and typing methods for epidemiological study. J Clin Microbiol 32:2260–2265, 1994

65. DEIGHTON MA, BALKAU B: Adherence measured by microtiter assay as a virulence marker for *Staphylococcus epidermidis* infections. J Clin Microbiol 28:2442–2447, 1990

66. DEIGHTON M, PEARSON S, CAPSTICK J ET AL: Phenotypic variation of *Staphylococcus epidermidis* isolated from a patient with native valve endocarditis. J Clin Microbiol 30:2385–2390, 1992

67. DE LA FUENTE R, SUAREZ G, SCHLEIFER JH: *Staphylococcus aureus* subsp. *anaerobius* subsp. nov., the causal agent of abscess disease of sheep. Int J Syst Bacteriol 35:99–102, 1985

68. DENYER SP, DAVIES MC, EVANS JA ET AL: Influence of carbon dioxide on the surface characteristics and adherence potential of coagulase-negative staphylococci. J Clin Microbiol 28:1813–1817, 1990

69. DEVRIESE LA, HAJEK V, OEDING P ET AL: *Staphylococcus hyicus* (Sompolinsky 1953) comb. nov. and *Staphylococcus hyicus* subsp. *chromogenes* subsp. nov. Int J Syst Bacteriol 28:482–490, 1978

70. DEVRIESE LA, POUTREL B, KILPPER-BALZ R ET AL: *Staphylococcus gallinarum* and *Staphylococcus caprae*, two new species from animals. Int J Syst Bacteriol. 33:480–486, 1983

71. DIAZ-MITOMA F, HARDING GKM, HOBAN DJ ET AL: Clinical significance of a test for slime production in ventriculoperitoneal shunt infections caused by coagulase-negative staphylococci. J Infect Dis 156:555–560, 1987

72. DOERN LK, EARLS JE, JEZNACH PA ET AL: Species identification and biotyping of staphylococci by the API Staph-IDENT system. J Clin Microbiol 17:260–263, 1983

73. DREWRY DT, GALBRAITH L, WILKINSON BJ ET AL: Staphylococcal slime: a cautionary tale. J Clin Microbiol 28:1292–1296, 1990

74. EDWIN C: Quantitative determination of staphylococcal enterotoxin A by an enzyme-linked immunosorbent assay using a combination of polyclonal and monoclonal antibodies and biotin–streptavidin interaction. J Clin Microbiol 27:1496–1501, 1989

75. EISENBERG ES, AMBALU M, SZYLAGI G ET AL: Colonization of the skin and development of peritonitis due to coagulase-negative staphylococci in patients undergoing peritoneal dialysis. J Infect Dis 156:478–482, 1987

76. ENG RHK, WANG C, PERSON A ET AL: Species identification of coagulase-negative staphylococcal isolates from blood cultures. J Clin Microbiol 15:439–442, 1982

77. ETIENNE J, PANGON B, LEPORT C ET AL: *Staphylococcus lugdunensis* endocarditis. Lancet 1:390, 1989

78. FALK D, GUERING SJ: Differentiation of *Staphylococcus* and *Micrococcus* spp. with the Taxo A bacitracin disk. J Clin Microbiol 18:719–720, 1983

79. FALLER A, SCHLEIFER KH: Modified oxidase and benzidine tests for separation of staphylococci and micrococci. J Clin Microbiol 13:1031–1035, 1981

80. FERGUSON DA JR, VERINGA EM, MAYBERRY WR ET AL: *Bacteroides* and *Staphylococcus* glycocalyx: chemical analysis and the effects on chemiluminescence and chemotaxis of human polymorphonuclear leucocytes. Microbios 69:53–65, 1992

81. FIDALGO S, VASQUEZ F, MENDOZA M ET AL: Bacteremia due to *Staphylococcus epidermidis*: microbiologic, epidemiologic, clinical, and prognostic features. Rev Infect Dis 12:520–528, 1990

82. FOSSE T, PELOUX Y, GRANTHIL B ET AL: Meningitis due to *Micrococcus luteus*. Infection 13:280–281, 1985

83. FOURNIER JM, BOUTONNIER A, BOUVET A: *Staphylococcus aureus* strains which are not identified by rapid agglutination procedures are of capsular serotype 5. J Clin Microbiol 27:1372–1374, 1989

84. FOURNIER JM, BOUVET A, BOUTONNIER A ET AL: Predominance of capsular type 5 among oxacillin-resistant *Staphylococcus aureus*. J Clin Microbiol 25:1932–1933, 1987

85. FOURNIER JM, BOUVET A, MATHIEU D ET AL: New latex reagent using monoclonal antibodies to capsular polysaccharide for reliable identification of both oxacillin-susceptible and oxacillin-resistant *Staphylococcus aureus*. J Clin Microbiol 31:1342–1344, 1993

86. FRENAY HME, THEELEN JPG, SCHOULS M ET AL: Discrimination of epidemic and nonepidemic methicillin-resistant *Staphylococcus aureus* strains on the basis of protein A gene polymorphism. J Clin Microbiol 32:846–847, 1994

87. FRENEY J, BRUN Y, BES M ET AL: *Staphylococcus lugdunensis* sp. nov. and *Staphylococcus schleiferi* sp. nov., two species from human clinical specimens. Int J Syst Bacteriol 38:168–172, 1988

88. GATERMANN S, HEINZ-GEORG WM, WANNER G: *Staphylococcus saprophyticus* hemagglutinin is a 160-kilodalton surface polypeptide. Infect Immun 60:4127–4132, 1992

89. GATERMANN S, JOHN J, MARRE R: *Staphylococcus saprophyticus* urease: characterization and contribution to uropathogenicity in unobstructed urinary tract infection of rats. Infect Immun 57:110–116, 1989

90. GATERMANN S, KREFT B, MARRE R ET AL: Identification and characterization of a surface-associated protein (Ssp) of *Staphylococcus saprophyticus*. Infect Immun 60: 1055–1060, 1992

91. GATERMANN S, MARRE R: Cloning and expression of *Staphylococcus saprophyticus* urease gene sequences in *Staphylococcus carnosus* and contribution of the enzyme to virulence. Infect Immun 57:2998–3002, 1989

92. GEARY C, STEVENS M: Rapid lysostaphin test to differentiate *Staphylococcus* and *Micrococcus* species. J Clin Microbiol 23:1044–1045, 1986

93. GEARY C, STEVENS M: Detection of phosphatase production by *Staphylococcus* species: a new method. Med Lab Sci 46:291–294, 1989

94. GEARY C, STEVENS M: A rapid test to detect the most clinically significant *Staphylococcus* species. Med Lab Sci 48: 99–105, 1991

95. GEHA DJ, UHL JR, GUSTAFERRO A ET AL: Multiplex PCR for identification of methicillin-resistant staphylococci in the clinical laboratory. J Clin Microbiol 32:1768–1772, 1994

96. GEMMELL CG, DAWSON JE: Identification of coagulase-negative staphylococci with the API Staph-IDENT system. J Clin Microbiol 16:874–877, 1982

97. GIGER P, CHARILAOU CC, CUNDY KR: Comparison of the API Staph-IDENT and the DMS Staph-TRAC systems with conventional methods used for identification of coagulase-negative staphylococci. J Clin Microbiol 19: 68–72, 1984

98. GILL VJ, SELEPAK AT, WILLIAMS EC: Species identification and antibiotic susceptibilities of coagulase-negative staphylococci isolated from clinical specimens. J Clin Microbiol 18:1314–1319, 1983

99. GLIMAKER M, GRANERT C, KROOK A: Septicemia caused by *Staphylococcus saprophyticus*. Scand J Infect Dis 20: 347–348, 1988

100. GOH SH, BRYNE SK, ZHANG JL ET AL: Molecular typing of *Staphylococcus aureus* on the basis of coagulase gene polymorphisms. J Clin Microbiol 30:1642–1645, 1992

101. GOLDSTEIN J, SCHULMAN R, KELLEY E ET AL: Effect of different media on determination of novobiocin resistance for differentiation of coagulase-negative staphylococci. J Clin Microbiol 18:592–595, 1983

102. GOLLEDGE CL: *Staphylococcus saprophyticus* bacteremia. J Infect Dis 157:215, 1988

103. GRANT CE, SEWELL DL, PFALLER M ET AL: Evaluation of two commercial systems for identification of coagulase-negative staphylococci to species level. Diagn Microbiol Infect Dis 18-1-5, 1994

104. GRASMICK AE, NAITO N, BRUCKNER DA: Clinical comparison of the AutoMicrobic system gram-positive identification card, API Staph-IDENT, and conventional methods in the identification of coagulase-negative *Staphylococcus* spp. J Clin Microbiol 18:1323–1328, 1983

105. GRATTARD F, ETIENNE J, POZZETTO B ET AL: Characterization of unrelated strains of *Staphylococcus schleiferi* by using ribosomal DNA fingerprinting, DNA restriction patterns, and plasmid profiles. J Clin Microbiol 31: 812–818, 1993

106. GRAY ED, PETERS G, VERSTEGEN M, REGELMANN WE: Effects of extracellular slime from *Staphylococcus epidermidis* on the cellular immune response. Lancet 1:365–367, 1984

107. GREGSON DB, LOW DE, SKULNICK M ET AL: Problems with rapid agglutination of *Staphylococcus aureus* when *Staphylococcus saprophyticus* is being tested. J Clin Microbiol 26:1398–1399, 1988

108. GUARDATI MC, GUZMAN CA, PIATTI G ET AL: Rapid methods for identification of *Staphylococcus aureus* when both human and animal staphylococci are tested: comparison with a new immunoenzymatic assay. J Clin Microbiol 31:1606–1608, 1993

109. GUDDING R: Differentiation of staphylococci on the basis of nuclease properties. J Clin Microbiol 18:1098–1101, 1983

110. GUZMAN CA, GUARDATI MC, FENOGLIO D ET AL: Novel immunoenzymatic assay for identification of coagulase- and protein A-negative *Staphylococcus aureus* strains. J Clin Microbiol 30:1194–1197, 1992

111. HAJEK V: *Staphylococcus intermedius*, a new species isolated from animals. Int J Syst Bacteriol 26:401–408, 1976

112. HAJEK V, DEVREISE LA, MORDARSKI M ET AL: Elevation of *Staphylococcus hyicus* subsp. *chromogenes* (Devreise et al, 1978) to species status: *Staphylococcus chromogenes* (Devreise et al, 1978) comb. nov. Syst Appl Microbiol 8:169–173, 1986

113. HAJEK V, LUDWIG W, SCHLEIFER KH ET AL: *Staphylococcus muscae*, a new species isolated from flies. Int J Syst Bacteriol 42:97–101, 1992

114. HAMORY BH, PARISI JT: *Staphylococcus epidermidis*: a significant nosocomial pathogen. Am J Infect Control 15:59–74, 1987

115. HARJOLA VP, VALTONEN M, SIVONEN A: Association of *Stomatococcus mucilaginosus* with cholangitis. Eur J Clin Microbiol Infect Dis 13:606–608, 1994

116. HARTSTEIN AI, MULLIGAN ME, MORTHLAND VH ET AL: Recurrent *Staphylococcus aureus* bacteremia. J Clin Microbiol 30:670–674, 1992

117. HEBERT GA: Hemolysins and other characteristics that help differentiate and biotype *Staphylococcus lugdunensis* and *Staphylococcus schleiferi*. J Clin Microbiol 28:2425–2431, 1990

118. HEBERT GA, COOKSEY RC, CLARK NC ET AL: Biotyping coagulase-negative staphylococci. J Clin Microbiol 26:1950–1956, 1988

119. HEBERT GA, CROWDER CG, HANCOCK GA ET AL: Characteristics of coagulase-negative staphylococci that help differentiate these species from other members of the Family *Micrococcaceae*. J Clin Microbiol 26:1939–1946, 1988

120. HEDMAN P, RINGERTZ O: Urinary tract infections caused by *Staphylococcus saprophyticus*. A matched case-control study. J Infect 23:145–153, 1991

121. HEDMAN P, RINGERTZ O, OLSSON K, WOLLIN R: Plasmid-identified *Staphylococcus saprophyticus* isolated from the rectum of patients with urinary tract infections. Scand J Infect Dis 23:569–572, 1991

122. HENWICK S, KOEHLER M, PATRICK CC: Complications of bacteremia due to *Stomatococcus mucilaginosus* in neutropenic children. Clin Infect Dis 17:667–671, 1993

123. HERCHLINE TE, AYERS LW: Occurrence of *Staphylococcus lugdunensis* in consecutive clinical cultures and relationship of isolation to infection. J Clin Microbiol 29:419–421, 1991

124. HERRMANN M, VAUDEAUX PE, PITTET D ET AL: Fibronectin, fibrinogen, and laminin act as mediators for adherence of clinical staphylococcal isolates to foreign materials. J Infect Dis 158:693–701, 1988

125. HERWALDT L, BOYKEN L, PFALLER M: In vitro selection of resistance to vancomycin in bloodstream isolates of *Staphylococcus haemolyticus* and *Staphylococcus epidermidis*. Eur J Clin Microbiol Infect Dis 10:1007–1012, 1991

126. HILL RB, SANDBERG G, GUNN BA ET AL: Reproducibility of three identification systems for biotyping of coagulase-negative staphylococci. Am J Clin Pathol 101:443–445, 1994

127. HJELM E, LUNDELL-ETHERDEN I: Slime production by *Staphylococcus saprophyticus*. Infect Immun 59:445–448, 1991

128. HO G, CAMPBELL WH, BERGDOLL MS ET AL: Production of a toxic shock syndrome toxin variant by *Staphylococcus aureus* strains associated with sheep, goats, and cows. J Clin Microbiol 27:1946–1948, 1989

129. HOCHKEPPEL HK, BRAUN DG, VISCHER W ET AL: Serotyping and electron microscopy studies of *Staphylococcus aureus* clinical isolates with monoclonal antibodies to capsular serotypes 5 and 8. J Clin Microbiol 25:526–530, 1987

130. HOLT JG, KRIEG NR, SNEATH PHA ET AL (EDS): Group 17. Gram-positive cocci, pp. 527–558. In *Bergey's Manual of Determinative Bacteriology*, 9th ed. Baltimore, Williams & Wilkins, 1994

131. HOPKINS RJ, SCHWALBE RS, DONNENBERGE M: Infections due to *Stomatococcus mucilaginosus*: report of two new cases and review. Clin Infect Dis 14:1264, 1992

132. HOSOTSUBO K, HOSOTSUBO H, NISHIJIMA MK ET AL: Rapid screening for *Staphylococcus aureus* infection by measuring enterotoxin B. J Clin Microbiol 27:2794–2798, 1989

133. HOVELIUS B, MARDH PA: *Staphylococcus saprophyticus* as a common cause of urinary tract infections. Rev Infect Dis 6:328–337, 1984

134. HOVELIUS B, THELIN I, MARDH PA: *Staphylococcus saprophyticus* in the aetiology of nongonococcal urethritis. Br J Vener Dis 55:369–374, 1979

135. HUBER MM, HUBER TW: Susceptibility of methicillin-resistant *Staphylococcus aureus* to lysostaphin. J Clin Microbiol 27:1122–1124, 1989

136. HUSSAIN M, HASTINGS JGM, WHITE PJ: A chemically defined medium for slime production by coagulase-negative staphylococci. J Med Microbiol 34:143–147, 1991

137. HUSSAIN M, HASTINGS JGM, WHITE PJ: Isolation and composition of the extracellular slime made by coagulase-negative staphylococci in a chemically defined medium. J Infect Dis 163:534–541, 1991

138. HUSSAIN M, HASTINGS JGM, WHITE PJ: Comparison of cell-wall teichoic acid with high-molecular-weight extracellular slime material from *Staphylococcus epidermidis*. J Med Microbiol 37:368–375, 1991

139. HUSSAIN Z, STOAKES L, STEVENS DL ET AL: Comparison of the MicroScan system with the API Staph-IDENT system for species identification of coagulase-negative staphylococci. J Clin Microbiol 23:126–128, 1986

140. HUTTON JP, HAMORY BH, PARISI JT ET AL: *Staphylococcus epidermidis* arthritis following catheter-induced bacteremia in a neutropenic patient. Diagn Microbiol Infect Dis 3:119–124, 1985

141. IGARASHI MA, FUJIKAWA H, SHIGAKI M ET AL: Latex agglutination test for staphylococcal toxic shock syndrome toxin. J Clin Microbiol 23:509–512, 1986

142. IGIMI S, KAWAMURA S, TAKAHASHI E ET AL: *Staphylococcus felis*, a new species from clinical specimens from cats. Int J Syst Bacteriol 39:373–377, 1989

143. IGIMI S, TAKAHASHI E, MITSUOKA T: *Staphylococcus schleiferi* subsp. *coagulans* subsp. nov., isolated from the external auditory meatus of dogs with external ear otitis. Int J Syst Bacteriol 40:409–411, 1990

144. ISHAK MA, GROSCHEL DHM, MANDELL GL ET AL: Association of slime with the pathogenicity of coagulase-negative staphylococci causing nosocomial septicemia. J Clin Microbiol 22:1025–1029, 1985

145. IZARD NC, HACHLER H, GREHN M, KAYSER FH: Ribotyping of coagulase-negative staphylococci with special emphasis on intraspecific typing of *Staphylococcus epidermidis*. J Clin Microbiol 30:817–823, 1992

146. JANDA WM, RISTOW K, NOVAK D: Evaluation of Rapi-DEC Staph for identification of *Staphylococcus aureus*, *Staphylococcus epidermidis*, and *Staphylococcus saprophyticus*. J Clin Microbiol 32:2056–2059, 1994

147. JANSEN B, SCHUMACHER-PERDREAU F, PETERS G ET AL: New aspects in the pathogenesis and prevention of polymer-associated, foreign-body infections caused by coagulase-negative staphylococci. J Invest Surg 2:361–380, 1989

148. JANSEN B, SCHUMACHER-PERDREAU F, PETERS G ET AL: Native valve endocarditis caused by *Staphylococcus simulans*. Eur J Clin Microbiol Infect Dis 11:268–269, 1992

149. JASPER E, INFANTE F, DELLINGER JD: Accuracy of the API Staph-Ident system for identification of *Staphylococcus* species from milk. Am J Vet Res 46:1263–1267, 1985

150. JEAN-PIERRE H, DARBAS H, JEAN-ROUSSENQ ET AL: Pathogenicity in two cases of *Staphylococcus schleiferi*, a recently described species. J Clin Microbiol 27:2110–2111, 1989

151. JOHNE B, JARP J, HAAHEIM LR: *Staphylococcus aureus* exopolysaccharide in vivo demonstrated by immunomagnetic separation and electron microscopy. J Clin Microbiol 27:1631–1635, 1989

152. JUNGKIND DJ, TORHAN NJ, KORMAN KE ET AL: Comparison of two commercially available test methods with conventional coagulase tests for identification of *Staphylococcus aureus*. J Clin Microbiol 19:191–193, 1984

153. KAHLER RC, BOYCE JM, BERGDOLL MS ET AL: Case report: toxic shock syndrome associated with TSST-1-producing coagulase-negative staphylococci. Am J Med Sci 292:310–312, 1986

154. KAMATH U, SINGER C, ISENBERG HD: Clinical significance of *Staphylococcus warneri* bacteremia. J Clin Microbiol 30:261–264, 1992

155. KANDA K, SUZUKI E, HIRAMATSU K ET AL: Identification of a methicillin-resistant strain of *Staphylococcus caprae* from a human clinical specimen. Antimicrob Agents Chemother 35:174–176, 1991

156. KARAKAWA WW, FOURNIER JM, VANN WF ET AL: Methods for serological typing of the capsular polysaccharides of *Staphylococcus aureus*. J Clin Microbiol 22:445–447, 1985

157. KARCHMER AW, ARCHER GL, DISMUKES WE: *Staphylococcus epidermidis* causing prosthetic valve endocarditis: microbiologic and clinical observations as guides to therapy. Ann Intern Med 98:447–455, 1983

158. KARTHIGASU KT, BOWMAN RA, GRAVE DI: Vertebral osteomyelitis caused by *Staphylococcus warneri*. Ann Rheum Dis 45:1029–1030, 1986

159. KAUFFMAN CA, SHEAGREN JN, QUIE PG: *Staphylococcus epidermidis* mediastinitis and disseminated intravascular coagulation. Ann Intern Med 100:60–61, 1984

160. KAUFHOLD A, REINERT RR, KERN W: Bacteremia caused by *Stomatococcus mucilaginosus*: report of seven cases and review of the literature. Infection 20:213–220, 1992

161. KENNY K, REISER RF, BASTIDA-CORCUERA FD ET AL: Production of enterotoxins and toxic shock syndrome toxin by bovine mammary isolates of *Staphylococcus aureus*. J Clin Microbiol 31:706–707, 1993

162. KILPPER-BALZ R, SCHLEIFER KH: Transfer of *Peptococcus saccharolyticus* (Foubert and Douglas) to the genus *Staphylococcus*: *Staphylococcus saccharolyticus* (Foubert and Douglas) comb. nov. Zentralbl Bakteriol Parasitenkd Infektionskr Hyg Abt 1 Orig 2:324–331, 1981

163. KIM JH, VAN DER HORST C, MULROW CD ET AL: *Staphylococcus aureus* meningitis: review of 28 cases. Rev Infect Dis 11:698–706, 1989

164. KLEEMAN KT, BANNERMAN TL, KLOOS WE: Species distribution of coagulase-negative staphylococcal isolates at a community hospital and implications for selection of staphylococcal identification procedures. J Clin Microbiol 31:1318–1321, 1993

165. KLOOS WE, BANNERMAN TL: Update on clinical significance of coagulase-negative staphylococci. Clin Microbiol Rev 7:117–140, 1994

166. KLOOS WE, GEORGE CG: Identification of *Staphylococcus* species and subspecies with the MicroScan Pos ID and Rapid Pos ID panel systems. J Clin Microbiol 29:738–744, 1991

167. KLOOS WE, LAMBE DW JR: *Staphylococcus*. In Balows A, Hausler WJ Jr, Herrman KL, et al (eds.), *Manual of Clinical Microbiology*, 5th ed, pp 222–237. Washington DC, American Society for Microbiology, 1991

168. KLOOS WE, SCHLEIFER KH: Isolation and characterization of staphylococci from human skin II. Description of four new species: *Staphylococcus warneri*, *Staphylococcus capitis*, *Staphylococcus hominis*, and *Staphylococcus simulans*. Int J Syst Bacteriol 25:62–79, 1975

169. KLOOS WE, SCHLEIFER KH: Simplified scheme for routine identification of human *Staphylococcus* species. J Clin Micobiol 1:82–87, 1975

170. KLOOS WE, SCHLEIFER KH: *Staphylococcus auricularis* sp. nov.: an inhabitant of the human external ear. Int J Syst Bacteriol 33:9–14, 1983

171. KLOOS WE, SCHLEIFER KH:. Genus IV. *Staphylococcus* Rosenbach 1984, 19AL (Nom. Cons. Opin. 17 Jud. Comm. 1958, 163). In Sneath PHA, Mair NS, Sharpe ME, Holt JG (eds), *Bergey's Manual of Systematic Bacteriology*, vol 2, pp 1013–1035. Baltimore, Williams & Wilkins, 1986

172. KLOOS WE, SCHLEIFER KH, SMITH RF: Characterization of *Staphylococcus sciuri* sp. nov. and its subspecies. Int J Syst Bacteriol 26:22–37, 1976

173. KLOOS WE, TORNABENE TG, SCHLEIFER KH: Isolation and characterization of micrococci from human skin, including two new species: *Micrococcus lylae* and *Micrococcus kristinae*. Int J Syst Bacteriol 24:79–101, 1974

174. KLOOS WE, WOLFSHOHL JF: Identification of *Staphylococcus* species with the API Staph-IDENT system. J Clin Microbiol 16:509–516, 1982

175. KLOOS WE, WOLFSOHL JF: *Staphylococcus cohnii* subspecies: *Staphylococcus cohnii* subsp. *cohnii* subsp. nov. and *Staphylococcus cohnii* subsp. *urealyticum* subsp. nov. Int J Syst Bacteriol 41:284–289, 1991

176. KNAPP CC, WASHINGTON JA: Evaluation of trehalose–mannitol broth for differentiation of *Staphylococcus epidermidis* from other coagulase-negative staphylococcal species. J Clin Microbiol 27:2624–2625, 1989

177. KOCH C, SCHUMANN P, STACKEBRANDT E: Reclassification of *Micrococcis agilis* (Ali-Cohen 1889) to the genus *Arthrobacter* as *Arthrobacter agilis* comb. nov. and emendation of the genus *Arthrobacter*. Int J Syst Bacteriol 45:837–839, 1995

178. KOCUR M: Genus I. *Micrococcus*. In Sneath PHA, Nair NS, Holt JG (eds), *Bergey's Manual of Systematic Bacteriology*, vol 2, pp 1004–1008. Baltimore, Williams & Wilkins, 1986

179. KOCUR M: Genus III. *Planococcus*. In Sneath PHA, Nair NS, Holt JG (eds), *Bergey's Manuals of Systematic Bacteriology*, vol 2, pp 1011–1013. Baltimore, Williams & Wilkins, 1986

180. KOTILAINEN P: Association of coagulase-negative staphylococcal slime production and adherence with the development and outcome of adult septicemias. J Clin Microbiol 28:2779–2785, 1990

181. KOTILAINEN P, HUOVINEN P, EEROLA E: Application of gas–liquid chromatographic analysis of cellular fatty acids for species identification and typing of coagulase-negative staphylococci. J Clin Microbiol 29:315–322, 1991

182. KRALOVIC SM, MELIN-ALDANA H, SMITH KK, LINNEMANN CC JR: *Staphylococcus lugdunensis* endocarditis after tooth extraction. Clin Infect Dis 20:715–716, 1995

183. KUUSELA P, HILDEN P, SAVOLAINEN K ET AL: Rapid detection of methicillin-resistant *Staphylococcus aureus* strains not identified by slide agglutination tests. J Clin Microbiol 32:143–147, 1994

184. LANDAU W, KAPLAN RL: Room temperature coagulase production by *Staphylococcus aureus* strains. Clin Microbiol Newslett 2:10, 1980

185. LANGBAUM M, EYAL FG: *Stomatococcus mucilaginosus* septicemia and meningitis in a premature infant. Pediatr Infect Dis J 11:334–335, 1992

186. LANGLOIS BE, HARMON RJ, AKERS K: Identification of *Staphylococcus* species of bovine origin with the DMS Staph-TRAC system. J Clin Microbiol 20:277–230, 1984

187. LANGLOIS BE, HARMON RJ, AKERS K ET AL: Comparison of methods for determining DNase and phosphatase activities by staphylococci. J Clin Microbiol 27:1127–1129, 1989

188. LARSSON A, SJOQUIST J: Novel latex agglutination method with anti-protein A for detection of *Staphylococcus aureus* infections. J Clin Microbiol 27:2856–2857, 1989

189. LATORRE M, ROJO PM, FRANCO R, CISTERNA R: Endocarditis due to *Staphylococcus capitis* subspecies *ureolyticus*. Clin Infect Dis 16:343–344, 1993

190. LATORRE M, ROJO PM, UNZAGA MJ, CISTERNA R: *Staphylococcus schleiferi*: a new opportunistic pathogen. Clin Infect Dis 16:589–590, 1993

191. LEE JC, LIU M-J, PARSONNET J ET AL: Expression of type 8 capsular polysaccharide and production of toxic shock syndrome toxin 1 are associated among vaginal isolates of *Staphylococcus aureus*. J Clin Microbiol 28:2612–2615, 1990

192. LEE W, CARPENTER RJ, PHILLIPS LE, FARO S: Pyelonephritis and sepsis due to *Staphylococcus saprophyticus*. J Infect Dis 155:1079–1080, 1987

193. LEMOZY J, HUGUET F, CHOMARAT M ET AL: Source of infection in *Stomatococcus mucilaginosus* septicaemia. Lancet 1:416, 1990

194. LINA B, CELARD M, VANDENESCH F ET AL: Infective endocarditis due to *Staphylococcus capitis*. Clin Infect Dis 15:173–174, 1992

195. LINA B, VANDENESCH F, REVERDY ME ET AL: Non-puerperal breast infection due to *Staphylococcus lugdunensis*. Eur J Clin Microbiol Infect Dis 13:686–687, 1994

196. LINDSAY JA, ARAVENA-ROMAN MA, RILEY TV: Identification of *Staphylococcus epidermidis* and *Staphylococcus hominis* from blood cultures by testing susceptibility to desferrioxamine. Eur J Clin Microbiol Infect Dis 12:127–131, 1993

197. LINDSAY JA, RILEY TV: Susceptibility to desferrioxamine: a new test for the identification of *Staphylococcus epidermidis*. J Med Microbiol 35:45–48, 1991

198. LLOP JM, MANGUES I, PEREZ JL ET AL: *Staphylococcus saprophyticus* sepsis related to total parenteral nutrition admixtures contamination. J Parent Ent Nutr 17:575–577, 1993

199. LOW DE, SCHMIDT BK, KIRPALANI HM ET AL: An endemic strain of *Staphylococcus haemolyticus* colonizing and causing bacteremia in neonatal intensive care unit patients. Pediatrics 89:696–700, 1992

200. LOWY F, HAMMER S: *Staphylococcus epidermidis* infections. Ann Intern Med 99:834–839, 1983

201. LUDLUM H, PHILLIPS I: *Staphylococcus lugdunensis* peritonitis. Lancet 1:1394, 1989

202. MAGEE JT, BURNETT IA, HINDMARCH JM, SPENCER RC: *Micrococcus* and *Stomatococcus* spp. from human infections. J Hosp Infect 16:67–73, 1990

203. MAINARDI JL, LORTHOLARY O, BUU-HOI A ET AL: Native valve endocarditis caused by *Staphylococcus capitis*. Eur J Clin Microbiol Infect Dis 12:789–791, 1993

204. MALES BM, BARTHOLOMEW WR, AMSTERDAM D: *Staphylococcus simulans* septicemia in a patient with chronic osteomyelitis and pyoarthritis. J Clin Microbiol 21:255–257, 1985

205. MARDH P-A, COLLEN S, HOVELIUS B: Attachment of bacteria to exfoliated cells from the urinary tract. Invest Urol 16:322–325, 1979

206. MARQUES MB, WELLER PF, PARSONNET J ET AL: Phosphatidylinositol-specific phospholipase C, a possible virulence factor of *Staphylococcus aureus*. J Clin Microbiol 27:2451–2454, 1989

207. MARRIE TJ, KWAN C, NOBLE MA ET AL.: *Staphylococcus saprophyticus* as a cause of urinary tract infections. J Clin Microbiol 16:427–431, 1982

208. MARSIK FJ, BRAKE S: Species identification and susceptibility to 17 antibiotics of coagulase-negative staphylococci isolated from clinical specimens. J Clin Microbiol 15:640–645, 1982

209. MARTIN MA, PFALLER MA, WENZEL RP: Coagulase-negative staphylococcal bacteremia. Ann Intern Med 110:9–16, 1989

210. MARTINEZ-MARTINEZ L, CUERVEZ-MONS V, ALONSO-PULPON L ET AL: *Staphylococcus xylosus* from a patient with cardiac and hepatic transplants. Clin Microbiol Newslett 10:47–48, 1988

211. MATHIEU D, PICARD V: Comparative evaluation of five agglutination techniques and a new miniaturized system for rapid identification of methicillin-resistant strains of *Staphylococcus aureus*. Zentralbl Bakteriol 276:46–53, 1991

212. MATTHEWS KR, OLIVER P, KING SH: Comparison of Vitek gram-positive identification system with the API Staph-TRAC system for species identification of staphylococci of bovine origin. J Clin Microbiol 28:1649–1651, 1990

213. MCCARTHY JS, STANLEY PA, MAYALL B: A case of *Staphylococcus simulans* endocarditis affecting a native heart valve. J Infect 22:211–212, 1991

214. MCDONALD CL, CHAPIN K: Rapid identification of *Staphylococcus aureus* from blood culture bottles by a classic two-hour tube coagulase test. J Clin Microbiol 33:50–52, 1995

215. MCTAGGART LA, ELLIOTT TSJ: Is resistance to novobiocin a reliable test for confirmation of the identification of *Staphylococcus saprophyticus*? J Med Microbiol 30:253–266, 1989

216. McTaggart LA, Rigby RC, Elliott TSJ: The pathogenesis of urinary tract infections associated with *Escherichia coli*, *Staphylococcus saprophyticus*, and *S. epidermidis*. J Med Microbiol 32:135–141, 1990

217. McWhinney PHM, Kibbler CC, Gillespie SH: *Stomatococcus mucilaginosus*: an emerging pathogen in neutropenic patients. Clin Infect Dis 14:641–646, 1992

218. Miller JM, Biddle JW, Quenzer VK et al: Evaluation of the biology for identification of members of the Family *Micrococcaceae*. J Clin Microbiol 31:3170–3173, 1993

219. Mitchell CJ, Geary C, Stevens M: Detection of *Staphylococcus aureus* in blood cultures: evaluation of a two-hour method. Med Lab Sci 48:106–109, 1991

220. Mitchell PS, Huston BJ, Jones RN et al: *Stomatococcus mucilaginosus* bacteremias—typical case presentations, simplified diagnostic criteria, and a literature review. Diagn Microbiol Infect Dis 13:521–525, 1990

221. Miwa K, Fukuyama M, Kunitomo T et al: Rapid assay for detection of toxic shock syndrome toxin 1 from human sera. J Clin Microbiol 32:539–542, 1994

222. Muller E, Hubner J, Gutierrez N et al: Isolation and characterization of transposon mutants of *Staphylococcus epidermidis* deficient in capsular polysaccharide/adhesin and slime. Infect Immun 61:551–558, 1993

223. Murakami K, Minamide W, Wada K et al: Identification of methicillin-resistant strains of staphylococci by polymerase chain reaction. J Clin Microbiol 29:2240–2244, 1991

224. Myrick BA, Ellner PD: Evaluation of the latex slide agglutination test for identification of *Staphylococcus aureus*. J Clin Microbiol 15:275–277, 1982

225. Neill RJ, Fanning GR, Delahoz F et al: Oligonucleotide probes for detection and differentiation of *Staphylococcus aureus* strains containing genes for enterotoxins A, B, and C and toxic shock syndrome toxin 1. J Clin Microbiol 28:1514–1518, 1990

226. Ohshima Y, Schumacher-Perdreau F, Peters G et al: Antiphagocytic effect of the capsule of *Staphylococcus simulans*. Infect Immun 58:1350–1354, 1990

227. Oppenheim BA, Weightman NC, Prendeville J: Fatal *Stomatococcus mucilaginosus* septicaemia in a neutropenic host. Eur J Clin Microbiol Infect Dis 8:1004–1005, 1989

228. Overman TL, Overley JK: Reproducibility of API Staph-IDENT system identifications of coagulase-negative staphylococci isolated from blood cultures. J Clin Microbiol 28:2585–2586, 1990

229. Palazzo E, Pierre J, Besbes N: *Staphylococcus lugdunensis* arthritis: a complication of arthroscopy. J Rheumatol 19:327–328, 1992

230. Paulsson M, Ljungh A, Wadstrom T: Rapid identification of fibronectin, vitronectin, laminin, and collagen cell surface binding proteins on coagulase-negative staphylococci by particle agglutination assays. J Clin Microbiol 30:2006–2012, 1992

231. Pennell DR, Rott-Petri JA, Kurzynski TA: Evaluation of three commercial agglutination tests for the identification of *Staphylococcus aureus*. J Clin Microbiol 20:614–617, 1984

232. Pennington TH, Harker C, Thomson-Carter F: Identification of coagulase-negative staphylococci by using sodium dodecyl sulfate–polyacrylamide gel electrophoresis and rRNA restriction patterns. J Clin Microbiol 29:390–392, 1991

233. Perl TM, Rhomberg PR, Bale MJ et al: Comparison of identification systems for *Staphylococcus epidermidis* and other coagulase-negative *Staphylococcus* species. Diagn Microbiol Infect Dis 18:151–155, 1994

234. Pfaller M, Davenport D, Bale M et al: Development of the quantitative microtest for slime production by coagulase-negative staphylococci. Eur J Clin Microbiol Infect Dis 7:30–33, 1988

235. Pfaller MA, Herwaldt LA: Laboratory, clinical, and epidemiological aspects of coagulase-negative staphylococci. Clin Microbiol Rev 1:281–299, 1988

236. Pfau A: Bacterial prostatitis caused by *Staphylococcus saprophyticus*. Urology 21:102–103, 1983

237. Piccolomini R, Catamo G, Picciani C et al: Evaluation of Staf-Sistem 18-R for identification of staphylococcal clinical isolates to the species level. J Clin Microbiol 32:649–653, 1994

238. Piemont Y, Haubensack M, Monteil H: Enzyme-linked immunosorbent assays for *Staphylococcus aureus* exfoliative toxins A and B and some applications. J Clin Microbiol 20:1114–1121, 1984

239. Pierre J, Gutmann L, Bornet M et al: Identification of coagulase-negative staphylococci by electrophoretic profile of total proteins and analysis of penicillin-binding proteins. J Clin Microbiol 28:443–446, 1990

240. Pignatari A, Pfaller M, Hollis R et al: *Staphylococcus aureus* colonization and infection in patients on continuous ambulatory peritoneal dialysis. J Clin Microbiol 28:1898–1902, 1990

241. Pinsky RL, Piscitelli V, Patterson JE: Endocarditis caused by relatively penicillin-resistant *Stomatococcus mucilaginosus*. J Clin Microbiol 27:215–216, 1989

242. Piper J, Hadfield T, McClesky F et al: Efficacies of rapid agglutination tests for identification of methicillin-resistant strains of *Staphylococcus aureus*. J Clin Microbiol 26:1907–1909, 1988

243. Poirier LP, Gaudreau CL: *Stomatococcus mucilaginosus* catheter-associated infection with septicemia. J Clin Microbiol 27:1125–1126, 1989

244. Ponce de Leon S, Wenzel RP: Hospital-acquired bloodstream infections with *Staphylococcus epidermidis*: review of 100 cases. Am J Med 77:639–644, 1984

245. Poutrel B, Caffin JP: Lystostaphin disk test for routine presumptive identification of staphylococci. J Clin Microbiol 13:1023–1025, 1981

246. Poutrel B, Mendolia C, Sutra L et al: Reactivity of coagulase-negative staphylococci isolated from cow and goat milk with monoclonal antibodies to *Staphylococcus aureus* capsular polysaccharide types 5 and 8. J Clin Microbiol 28:358–360, 1990

247. Poutrel B, Sutra L: Type 5 and 8 capsular polysaccharides are expressed by *Staphylococcus aureus* isolates from rabbits, poultry, pigs, and horses. J Clin Microbiol 31:467–469, 1993

248. Praz J, Kjoller E, Espersen F: *Stomatococcus mucilaginosus* endocarditis. Eur J Clin Microbiol 4:422–424, 1985

249. Prevost G, Jaulhac B, Piemont Y: DNA fingerprinting by pulsed field electrophoresis is more effective than ribotyping in distinguishing among methicillin-resistant *Staphylococcus aureus* isolates. J Clin Microbiol 30:967–973, 1992

250. QADRI SMH, AKHTER J, QADRI SGM: Latex agglutination and hemagglutination tests for the rapid identification of methicillin sensitive and methicillin resistant *Staphylococcus aureus*. J Hyg Epidemiol Microbiol Immunol 35:65–71, 1991

251. QUIE PG, BELANI KK: Coagulase-negative staphylococcal adherence and persistence. J Infect Dis 156:543–547, 1987

252. RELMAN DA, RUOFF K, FARRARO MJ: *Stomatococcus mucilaginosus* endocarditis in an intravenous drug abuser. J Infect Dis 5:1080–1082, 1987

253. RHODEN DL, HANCOCK GA, MILLER JM: Numerical approach to reference identification of *Staphylococcus, Stomatococcus,* and *Micrococcus.* J Clin Microbiol 31:490–493, 1993

254. RHODEN DL, MILLER JM: Four-year prospective study of Staph-IDENT system and conventional method for reference identification of *Staphylococcus, Stomatococcus,* and *Micrococcus* spp. J Clin Microbiol 33:96–98, 1995

255. RIFAI S, BARBANCON V, PREVOST G ET AL: Synthetic exfoliative toxin A and B DNA probes for detection of toxigenic *Staphylococcus aureus* strains. J Clin Microbiol 27:504–506, 1989

256. RILEY TV, SCHNEIDER PF: Infrequency of slime production by urinary isolates of *Staphylococcus saprophyticus.* J Infect 24:63–66, 1992

257. ROBERSON JR, FOX LK, HANCOCCK DD ET AL: Evaluation of methods for differentiation of coagulase-positive staphylococci. J Clin Microbiol 30:3217–3219, 1992

258. ROSCOE D, FORBES J, STEINBOK P, ANDERSON JD: Infection due to *Staphylococcus warneri.* Clin Infect Dis 15:1053, 1992

259. ROSSNEY AS, ENGLISH LF, KEANE CT: Coagulase testing compared with commercial kits for routinely identifying *Staphylococcus aureus.* J Clin Pathol 43:246–252, 1990

260. RUANE RJ, MORGAN MM, CITRON DM ET AL: Failure of rapid agglutination methods to detect oxacillin-resistant *Staphylococcus aureus.* J Clin Microbiol 24:490–491, 1986

261. RUBIN SJ, LYONS RW, MURCIA AJ: Endocarditis associated with cardiac catheterization due to gram-positive coccus designated *Micrococcus mucilaginosus incertae sedis.* J Clin Microbiol 7:546–549, 1978

262. RUPP ME, ARCHER GL: Hemagglutination and adherence to plastic by *Staphylococcus epidermidis.* Infect Immun 60:4322–4327, 1992

263. RUPP ME, ARCHER GL: Coagulase-negative staphylococci: pathogens associated with medical progress. Clin Infect Dis 19:231–245, 1994

264. RUPP ME, SOPER DE, ARCHER GL: Colonization of the female genital tract with *Staphylococcus saprophyticus.* J Clin Microbiol 30:2975–2979, 1992

265. SAULNIER P, BOURNEIX C, PREVOST G ET AL: Random amplified polymorphic DNA assay is less discriminant than pulsed field gel electrophoresis for typing strains of methicillin-resistant *Staphylococcus aureus.* J Clin Microbiol 31:982–985, 1993

266. SCHLEIFER KH, FISCHER U: Desription of a new species in the genus *Staphylococcus: Staphylococcus carnosus.* Int J Syst Bacteriol 32:153–156, 1982

267. SCHLEIFER KH, GEYER U, KILPPER-BALZ R ET AL: Elevation of *Staphylococcus sciuri* subsp. *lentus* (Kloos et al.) to species status: *Staphylococcus lentus* (Kloos et al.) comb. nov. Syst Appl Microbiol 4:382–387, 1983

268. SCHLEIFER KH, KILPPER-BALZ R, DEVRIESE LA: *Staphylococcus arlettae* sp. nov., *S. equorum* sp. nov., and *S. kloosii* sp. nov.: three new coagulase-negative, novobiocin-resistant species from animals. Syst Appl Microbiol 5:501–509, 1984

269. SCHLEIFER KH, KILPPER-BALZ R, FISCHER U ET AL: Identification of "*Micrococcus candidus*" ATCC 14852 as a strain of *Staphylococcus epidermidis* and of "*Micrococcus caseolyticus*" ATCC 13548 and *Micrococcus varians* ATCC 29750 as members of a new species, *Staphylococcus caseolyticus.* Int J Syst Bacteriol 32:15–20, 1982

270. SCHLEIFER KH, KLOOS WE: 1975. Isolation and characterization of staphylococci from human skin I. Amended descriptions of *Staphylococcus epidermidis* and *Staphylococcus saprophyticus* and descriptions of three new species: *Staphylococcus cohnii, Staphylococcus haemolyticus,* and *Staphylococcus xylosus.* Int J Syst Bacteriol 25:50–61, 1975

271. SCHLEIFER KH, KLOOS WE: A simple test system for the separation of staphylococci and micrococci. J Clin Microbiol 1:337–338, 1975

272. SCHLICHTING C, BRANGER C, FOURNIER JM ET AL: Typing of *Staphylococcus aureus* by pulsed field gel electrophoresis, zymotyping, capsular typing, and phage typing: resolution of clonal relationships. J Clin Microbiol 31:227–232, 1993

273. SCHLIEVERT PM, SHANDS KN, DAN BB ET AL: Identification and characterization of an exotoxin from *Staphylococcus aureus* associated with toxic shock syndrome. J Infect Dis 143:509–516, 1981

274. SCHNEIDER PF, RILEY TV: Cell-surface hydrophobicity of *Staphylococcus saprophyticus.* Epidemiol Infect 106:71–75, 1991

275. SCHWALBE RS, RITZ WJ, VERMA PR ET AL: Selection for vancomycin resistance in clinical isolates of *Staphylococcus haemolyticus.* J Infect Dis 161:45–51, 1990

276. SCHWALBE RS, STAPLETON JT, GILLIGAN PH: Emergence of vancomycin resistance in coagulase-negative staphylococci. N Engl J Med 316:927–931, 1987

277. SCHWALBE RS, RITZ WJ, VERMA PR ET AL: Selection for vancomycin resistance in clinical isolates of *Staphylococcus haemolyticus.* J Infect Dis 161:45–51, 1990

278. SCHWARZKOPF A, KARCH H: Genetic variation in *Staphylococcus aureus* coagulase genes: potential and limits for use as epidemiological marker. J Clin Microbiol 32:2407–2412, 1994

279. SCHWARZKOPF A, KARCH H, SCHMIDT H ET AL: Phenotypical and genotypical characterization of epidemic clumping factor-negative, oxacillin-resistant *Staphylococcus aureus.* J Clin Microbiol 31:2281–2285, 1993

280. SEE RH, ADILMAN S, BARTLETT KH ET AL: Colony immunoblot assay for the detection of staphylococcal toxic shock syndrome toxin (TSST-1) with anti-TSST-1 F(ab')₂ fragments. J Clin Microbiol 27:2050–2053, 1989

281. SELLADURAI BM, SIVAKUMARAN MS, SUBRAMANIAN A ET AL: Intracranial supperation caused by *Micrococcus luteus.* Br J Neurosurg 7:205–208, 1993

282. SEVERANCE PJ, KAUFMAN CA, SHEAGREN JH: Rapid identification of *Staphylococcus aureus* by using lysostaphin sensitivity. J Clin Microbiol 11:724–727, 1980

283. SHEPPARD M, JANKOWSKI S: *Staphylococcus lugdunensis* endocarditis. J Infect 25:116–117, 1992

284. SHIMAOKA M, YOH M, SEGAWA A ET AL: Development of enzyme-labeled oligonucleotide probe for detection of *mecA* gene in methicillin-resistant *Staphylococcus aureus*. J Clin Microbiol 32:1866–1869, 1994

285. SHUTTLEWORTH R, COLBY WD: *Staphylococcus lugdunensis* endocarditis. J Clin Microbiol 30:1948–1952, 1992

286. SINGH VR, RAAD I: Fatal *Staphylococcus saprophyticus* native valve endocarditis in an intravenous drug addict. J Infect Dis 162:784–785, 1990

287. SKULNICK M, SIMOR AE, PATEL MP ET AL: Evaluation of three methods for the rapid identification of *Staphylococcus aureus* in blood cultures. Diagn Microbiol Infect Dis 19:5–8, 1994

288. SORO O, GRAZI G, VARALDO PE ET AL: Phosphatase activity of staphylococci is constitutive in some species and repressed by phosphates in others. J Clin Microbiol 28:2707–2710, 1990

289. SOUHAMI L, FELD R, TUFFNELL PG ET AL: *Micrococcus luteus* pneumonia: a case report and review of the literature. Med Pediatr Oncol 7:309–314, 1979

290. SOUILLET G, CHOMARAT M, BARBE G ET AL: *Stomatococcus mucilaginosus* meningitis in a child with leukemia. Clin Infect Dis 15:1045, 1992

291. STACKBRANDT E, KOCH C, GVOZDIAK O ET AL: Taxonomic dissection of the genus *Micrococcus: Kocuria* gen. nov., *Nesterenkonia* gen. nov., *Kytococcus* gen. nov., *Dermacoccus* gen. nov., and *Micrococcus* Cohn 1872 gen. amend. Int J Syst Bacteriol 45:682–692, 1995

292. STEVENS DL, JONES C: Use of trehalose–mannitol–phosphatase agar to differentiate *Staphylococcus aureus* and *Staphylococcus saprophyticus*. J Clin Microbiol 20:977–980, 1984

293. STOAKES L, JOHN MA, LANNIGAN R ET AL: Gas–liquid chromatography of cellular fatty acids for identification of staphylococci. J Clin Microbiol 32:1908–1910, 1994

294. STOAKES L, SCHIEVEN BC, OFORI E ET AL: Evaluation of the MicroScan Rapid Pos Combo panels for identification of staphylococci. J Clin Microbiol 30:93–95, 1992

295. STOUT RD, FERGUSON KP, LI Y, LAMBE DW JR: Staphylococcal exopolysaccharides inhibit lymphocyte proliferative responses by activation of monocyte prostaglandin production. Infect Immun 60:922–927, 1992

296. STRUELENS MJ, BAX R, DEPLANO A ET AL: Corcordant clonal delineation of methicillin-resistant *Staphylococcus aureus* by macrorestriction analysis and polymerase chain reaction genomic fingerprinting. J Clin Microbiol 31:1964–1970, 1993

297. STURGESS I, MARTIN FC, EYKYN S: Pubic osteomyelitis caused by *Staphylococcus simulans*. Postgrad Med J 69: 927–929, 1993

298. SURANI S, CHANDNA H, WEINSTEIN RA: Breast abscess: coagulase-negative staphylococci as a sole pathogen. Clin Infect Dis 17:701–704, 1993

299. TAKAGI Y, FUTAMURA S, ASADA Y: Action site of exfoliative toxin on keratinocytes. J Invest Dermatol 94:52–56, 1990

300. TALEN DA, GOLDSTEIN EJC, STAATZ D ET AL: *Staphylococcus intermedius*: clinical presentation of a new human dog bite pathogen. Ann Emerg Med 18:410–413, 1989

301. TALEN DA, STAATZ, D, STAATZ A ET AL: *Staphylococcus intermedius* in canine gingiva and canine-inflicted wound infections: a newly recognized zoonotic pathogen. J Clin Microbiol 27:78–81, 1989

302. TALEN DA, STAATZ D, STAATZ A ET AL: Frequency of *Staphylococcus intermedius* as human nasopharyngeal flora. J Clin Microbiol 27:2393, 1989

303. TAN R, WHITE V, SERVAIS G ET AL: Postoperative endophthalmitis caused by *Stomatococcus mucilaginosus*. Clin Infect Dis 18:492–493, 1994

304. TANASUPAWAT S, HASHIMOTO Y, EZAKI T ET AL: *Staphylococcus piscifermentans* sp. nov. from fermented fish in Thailand. Int J Syst Bacteriol 42:577–581, 1992

305. TENOVER FC, ARBEIT R, ARCHER G ET AL: Comparison of traditional and molecular methods of typing isolates of *Staphylococcus aureus*. J Clin Microbiol 32:407–415, 1994

306. THOMSON-CARTER FM, PENNINGTON TH: Characterization of coagulase-negative staphylococci by sodium dodecyl sulfate–polyacrylamide gel electrophoresis and immunoblot analysis. J Clin Microbiol 27:2199–2203, 1989

307. TIMMERMAN CP, FLEER A, BESNIER JM ET AL: Characterization of a proteinaceous adhesin of *Staphylococcus epidermidis* which mediates attachment to polystyrene. Infect Immun 59:4187–4192, 1991

308. TODD J, FISHAUT M: Toxic shock syndrome associated with phage-group-1 staphylococci. Lancet 2:1116–1118, 1978

309. TOJO M, YAMASHITA N, GOLDMANN DA ET AL: Isolation and characterization of a capsular polysaccharide adhesin from *Staphylococcus epidermidis*. J Infect Dis 157: 713–722, 1988

310. TOLAYMAT A, AL-JAYOUSI Z: *Staphylococcus saprophyticus* urinary tract infection in male children. Child Nephrol Urol 11:100–102, 1991

311. TORRE D, FERRARO G, FIORI GP ET AL: Ventriculoatrial shunt infection caused by *Staphylococcus warneri*: case report and review. Clin Infect Dis 14:49–52, 1992

312. TSELENIS-KOTSOWILIS AD, KOLIOMICHALIS MP, PAPAVASILOV TT: Acute pyelonephritis caused by *Staphylococcus xylosus*. J Clin Microbiol 16:593–594, 1982

313. TU KK, PALUTKE WA: Isolation and characterization of a catalase-negative strain of *Staphylococcus aureus*. J Clin Microbiol 3:77–78, 1976

314. UBUKATA K, NAKAGAMI S, NITTA A ET AL: Rapid detection of the *mecA* gene in methicillin-resistant staphylococci by enzymatic detection of polymerase chain reaction products. J Clin Microbiol 30:1728–1733, 1992

315. UNAL S, HOSKINS J, FLOKOWITSCH JE ET AL: Detection of methicillin-resistant staphylococci by using the polymerase chain reaction. J Clin Microbiol 30:1685–1691, 1992

316. VAN BELKUM A, BAX R, PEERBOOMS P ET AL: Comparison of phage typing and DNA fingerprinting by polymerase chain reaction for discrimination of methicillin-resistant *Staphylococcus aureus* strains. J Clin Microbiol 31:798–803, 1993

317. VANDENESCH F, ETIENNE J, REVERDY ME ET AL: Endocarditis due to *Staphylcococcus lugdunensis*: report of 11 cases and review. Clin Infect Dis 17:871–876, 1993

318. VANDENESCH F, LeBEAU C, BES M ET AL: Clotting activity in *Staphylococcus schleiferi* subspecies from human patients. J Clin Microbiol 32:388–392, 1994

319. VARALDO PE, KILPPER-BALZ R, BIAVASCO F ET AL: *Staphylococcus delphini* sp. nov., a coagulase-positive species isolated from dolphins. Int J Syst Bacteriol 38:436–439, 1988

320. VEACH LA, PFALLER MA, BENNETT M ET AL: Vancomycin resistance in *Staphylococcus haemolyticus* causing colonization and bloodstream infection. J Clin Microbiol 28:2064–2068, 1990

321. VON RHEINBABEN KE, HADLOCK RM: Rapid distinction between micrococci and staphylococci with furazolidone agar. Antonie Leeuvenhoek J Microbiol Serol 47: 41–51, 1981

322. WADE JC, SCHIMPF SC, NEWMAN KA: *Staphylococcus epidermidis*: an increasing cause of infection in patients with granulocytopenia. Ann Intern Med 96:1–10, 1982

323. WAGHORN DJ: *Staphylococcus lugdunensis* as a cause of breast abscess. Clin Infect Dis 19:814–815, 1994

324. WALDVOGEL FA: Chapter 173. *Staphylococcus aureus* (including toxic shock syndrome). In Mandell GL, Bennett JE, Dolin R (eds), *Mandell, Douglas, and Bennett's Principles and Practice of Infectious Diseases*, 4th ed, pp 1754–1777. New York, Churchill-Livingstone, 1995

325. WALLER JR, HODEL SL, NUTI RN: Improvement of two toluidine blue O-mediated techniques for DNase detection. J Clin Microbiol 21:195–199, 1985

326. WALLMARK GI, ANEMARK I, TELANDER B: *Staphylococcus saprophyticus*: a frequent cause of urinary tract infections among female outpatients. J Infect Dis 138:791–797, 1978

327. WANGER AR, MORRIS SL, ERICSSON C ET AL: Latex agglutination-negative methicillin-resistant *Staphylococcus aureus* recovered from neonates: epidemiologic features and comparison of typing methods. J Clin Microbiol 30:2583–2588, 1992

328. WATTS JL, PANKEY W, NICKERSON SC: Evaluation of the Staph-Ident and STAPH-ase systems for identification of staphylococci from bovine intramammary infections. J Clin Microbiol 20:448–452, 1984

329. WATTS JL, WASHBURN PJ: Evaluation of the Staph-Zym system with staphylococci isolated from bovine intramammary infections. J Clin Microbiol 29:59–61, 1991

330. WEBSTER JA, BANNERMAN TL, HUBNER RJ ET AL: Identification of the *Staphylococcus sciuri* species group with *Eco*R1 fragments containing rRNA sequences and description of *Staphylococcus vitulus* sp. nov. Int J Syst Bacteriol 44:454–460, 1994

331. WEINBLATT ME, SAHDEV I, BERMAN M: *Stomatococcus mucilaginosus* infections in children with leukemia. Pediatr Infect Dis J 9:678–679, 1990

332. WERGELAND HI, HAAHEIM LR, NATAS OB ET AL: Antibodies to staphylococcal peptidoglycan and its peptide epitopes, teichoic acid, and lipoteichoic acid in sera from blood donors and patients with staphylococcal infections. J Clin Microbiol 27:1286–1291, 1989

333. WESTBLOM TU, GORSE GJ, MILLIGAN TW ET AL: Anaerobic endocarditis caused by *Staphylococcus saccharolyticus*. J Clin Microbiol 28:2818–2819, 1990

334. WHARTON M, RICE JR, McCALLUM R ET AL: Septic arthritis due to *Micrococcus luteus*. J Rheumatol 13:659–660, 1986

335. WILLCOX MH, HUSSAIN M, FAULKNER MK ET AL: Slime production and adherence by coagulase-negative staphylococci. J Hosp Infect 18:327–331, 1991

336. WILCOX MH, SMITH DGE, EVANS JA ET AL: Influence of carbon dioxide on growth and antibiotic susceptibility of coagulase-negative staphylococci cultured in human peritoneal dialysate. J Clin Microbiol 28:2183–2186, 1990

337. WINSTON DJ, DUDNICK DV, CHAPIN M ET AL: Coagulase-negative staphylococcal bacteremia in patients receiving immunosuppressive therapy. Arch Intern Med 143: 32–36, 1983

338. WOOD CA, SEWELL DL, STRAUSBAUGH LJ: Vertebral osteomyelitis and native valve endocarditis caused by *Staphylococcus warneri*. Diagn Microbiol Infect Dis 12: 261–263, 1989

339. WUEPPER KD, HASS BAKER D, DIMOND RL: Measurement of the staphylococcal epidermolytic toxin: a comparison of bioassay, radial immunodiffusion, and radioimmunoassay. J Invest Dermatol 67:526–531, 1976

340. YOUMANS GR, DAVIS TE, FULLER DD: Use of chemiluminescent DNA probes in the rapid detection of oxacillin resistance in clinically isolated strains of *Staphylococcus aureus*. Diagn Microbiol Infect Dis 16:99–104, 1993

341. YOUNGER JJ, CHRISTENSEN GD, BARTLEY DL ET AL: Coagulase-negative staphylococci isolated from cerebrospinal fluid shunts: importance of slime production, species identification, and shunt removal to clinical outcome. J Infect Dis 156:548–554, 1987

342. ZAKRZEWSKA-CZERWINSKA J, GASZEWSKA-MASTALARZ A, LIS B ET AL: *Staphylococcus pulvereri* sp. nov., isolated from human and animal specimens. Int J Syst Bacteriol 45:169–172, 1995

THE GRAM-POSITIVE COCCI
PART II: STREPTOCOCCI, ENTEROCOCCI, AND THE "STREPTOCOCCUS-LIKE" BACTERIA

THE "FAMILY *STREPTOCOCCACEAE*": TAXONOMY AND CLINICAL SIGNIFICANCE

In traditional taxonomic schemes, the streptococci belong to the family *Streptococcaceae*. These organisms are gram-positive, catalase-negative bacteria that tend to grow in pairs and chains. The detection of cytochrome enzymes with the catalase test distinguishes members of the family *Micrococcaceae* (catalase-positive) from the members of the family *Streptoccaceae* (catalase-negative). In recent years, the taxonomy of the streptococci and streptococcus-like bacteria has undergone extensive revision and expansion. The taxonomic status of the "family *Streptococcaceae*" has been questioned, and the number of different streptococcal and streptococcus-like species has grown. Several changes have also occurred in the taxonomy of the enterococcal group D streptococci, with the creation of the new genus *Enterococcus* and the description of several new human and animal species that are genetically and phenotypically related to the enterococci. The recognition of "minute colony streptococci," their role in disease, and the relation of these organisms to the "large colony," groupable β-hemolytic streptococci has also muddied the waters of the "comfortable" streptococcal classifications that we have grown used to over the years. Added to this are several new species belonging to previously described genera, plus the discovery of several new streptococcus-like genera such as *Leuconostoc*, *Pediococcus*, *Alloiococcus*, *Vagococcus*, *Globicatella*, *Tetragenococcus*, and *Helcococcus*. These changes have more than academic significance for clinical microbiologists as we move into the 21st century because previously uncommon organisms belonging to the streptococci and the streptococcus-like bacteria are being recovered from human infections with increasing regularity.

In the 1984 edition of *Bergey's Manual of Systematic Bacteriology*, the family *Streptococcaceae* was divided into 10 genera, including *Streptococcus* (Table 12-1).[576] Since the publication of *Bergey's Manual*, several modifications concerning the taxonomy of the streptococci and streptococcus-like bacteria have been proposed and adopted (Box 12-1).

The genera listed in Table 12-1 and described in points 1 through 4 in Box 12-1 can also be placed into a useful taxonomic framework for the clinical laboratory on the basis of their growth requirements relative to atmospheric oxygen. This chapter will deal with those organisms listed as facultative anaerobes. The organisms listed in group 2 are obligate anaerobes, and only those species belonging to the genus *Peptostreptococcus* and the genus *Peptococcus* are found in humans. The other genera in group 2 include species that are normal gastrointestinal tract flora in animals. These are listed in Box 12-2.

As mentioned previously and as will be noted in the subsequent discussions of these various species, the taxonomy and nomenclature of these and other

Color Plates for Chapter 12 are found between pages 368 and 369.

TABLE 12-1

STREPTOCOCCAL NOMENCLATURE IN *BERGEY'S MANUAL OF SYSTEMATIC BACTERIOLOGY, 1984*

Family *Deinococcaceae*
  Genus *Deinococcus*

Other Genera (*Streptococcaceae*)
  Genus *Streptococcus*
  Genus *Leuconostoc*
  Genus *Aerococcus*
  Genus *Pediococcus*
  Genus *Peptococcus*
  Genus *Peptostreptococcus*
  Genus *Gemella*
  Genus *Ruminococcus*
  Genus *Coprococcus*
  Genus *Sarcina*

microorganisms have been profoundly affected by the application of genetic techniques. These include DNA–DNA hybridization, DNA–ribosomal RNA (rRNA) hybridization, and small subunit (16S) rRNA sequencing. Small subunit (16S) rRNA sequencing has become the most powerful approach for delineating the phylogenetic interrelations of microorganisms. This method was initially used to validate the division of the *Streptococcaceae* into the *Streptococcus*, *Enterococcus*, and *Lactococcus* genera and is now being applied to individual species to determine related groups of organisms within the three genera.[599,600] In 1991, Bentley and coworkers[53] applied partial 16S rRNA sequencing to the major streptococcal species to determine inter- and intrageneric relations among them. With use of the same methodologies, Kawamura and associates[387] extended these studies to some of the newly described viridans streptococci. Given their work, the genus *Streptococcus* can be operationally divided into seven groups, as shown in Table 12-2. Whereas the "pyogenic cocci" (i.e., groups A, B, and C streptococci) tended to cluster together phylogenetically, the viridans streptococci, found in the upper respiratory tract, fell into several different phylogenetic groups. It is interesting to note that *S. pneumoniae*, a classically pyogenic pathogen, is genetically more closely related to the viridans streptococcal species *S. mitis*, *S. gordonii*, *S. oralis*, *S. sanguis*, *S. parasanguis* than to the other "classic" pyogenic cocci in group I (see Table 12-2).

GENERAL CHARACTERISTICS OF STREPTOCOCCI

Streptococci are facultative anaerobes; in fact, some strains will grow better under anaerobic conditions. Many isolates are also stimulated by increased CO_2. Medically important streptococci, enterococci, and aerococci are **homofermentative**, meaning that the sole product of glucose fermentation is lactic acid. Streptococci are also oxidase-negative, a property that, together with the Gram stain, differentiates streptococci

BOX 12-1. MODIFICATIONS TO *BERGEY'S MANUAL TAXONOMY*

1. All species formerly classified in the genus *Peptococcus* have been incorporated into the genus *Peptostreptococcus*, with the exception of one species, *Peptococcus niger*.[443] On the basis of DNA homology studies, DNA base composition, and whole-cell fatty acid profiles, *Peptococcus* species (*P. asaccharolyticus, P. prevotii, P. magnus, P. indolicus*) were more closely related to *Peptostreptococcus anaerobius,* the type species of the genus *Peptostreptococcus,* than to *P. niger,* the type species of the genus *Peptococcus*.[215] In addition, four new *Peptostreptococcus* species (*P. hydrogenalis, P. lacrimalis, P. lactolyticus,* and *P. vaginalis*) have been described.[214, 436] The anaerobic cocci will be discussed further in Chapter 14.

2. On the basis of DNA–ribosomal RNA (rRNA) hybridization studies and rRNA sequence analysis, organisms formerly included in the genus *Streptococcus* have been subdivided into three genera: *Streptococcus, Enterococcus,* and *Lactococcus*.[599, 600] The genus *Streptococcus sensu stricto* (i.e., in the strictest sense), comprises the majority of the various species, including the pyogenic streptococci, the nonenterococcal group D streptococci, the viridans streptococci, and the pneumococci. The genus *Enterococcus* includes the former group D enterococci, and the genus *Lactococcus* (lactic acid streptococci) includes the streptococci that carry the Lancefield group N antigen. In *Bergey's Manual,* the latter organisms are listed as "lactic acid streptococci."[576] The three genera can be differentiated by growth at various temperatures. *Enterococcus* species grow at both 10°C and 45°C, whereas the streptococci grow over a narrower temperature range (about 25° to 37°C) and usually do not grow at either of the extreme temperatures. *Lactococcus* species show optimal growth at 30°C and are able to grow at 10°C; only about 50% of strains will show good growth at 45°C.[221] *Enterococcus* spp. and *Lactococcus* spp. can also be differentiated from one another by demonstrating the group D antigen in the former and the group N antigen in the latter. However, only about 80% of the members of the genus *Enterococcus* and about 60% of the members of the genus *Lactococcus* possess demonstrable (or extractable) grouping antigens. Definitive separation of the *Lactococcus* and *Enterococcus* genera can also be accomplished by the Gen-Probe AccuProbe *Enterococcus* culture confirmation test (Gen-Probe, San Diego CA). There are currently seven recognized *Lactococcus* species and subspecies. Methods for their identification are included in Table 12-22.

3. The number of species assigned to the genus *Enterococcus* has been greatly expanded. Application of genetic techniques has demonstrated that several of the new *Enterococcus* species do not conform to the old definition of the "enterococcal group D streptococci" (i.e., possession of the group D antigen, growth on bile-esculin agar, growth in 6.5% NaCl, hydrolysis of PYR, etc.). These will be discussed in detail later.

4. Several new streptococcus-like organisms that are found in human clinical specimens have been described. In addition to *Aerococcus* species, *Leuconostoc* species, *Pediococcus* species, and *Gemella* species, newly described genera that are genetically related and phenotypically similar to the streptococci include *Alloiococcus* species, *Vagococcus* species, *Tetragenococcus* species, *Globicatella* species, and *Helcococcus* species.

from *Neisseria* species. Table 12-3 compares certain basic characteristics of the streptococci and other gram-positive cocci and bacilli.

Members of the genus *Streptococcus* characteristically grow in chains (or chains of diplococci) when grown in broth media. This characteristic is shared with the enterococci, the lactococci, and some of the newly recognized or proposed genera (i.e., *Leuconostoc* species, *Vagococcus* species, and *Globicatella* species). Other streptococcus-like bacteria (i.e., aerococci, *Alloiococcus* species, *Gemella* species, *Pediococcus* species, *Tetragenococcus* species, and *Helcococcus* species) grow as pairs or tetrads in broth. Assessment of the cellular arrangement is best made by performing a Gram stain from a culture of the organism growing in thioglycolate broth. When this broth is used, the smear preparation must be fixed in methanol after air-drying, rather than heat-fixed, to prevent the bacteria from "washing off" the slide during the staining process.

The cell wall composition of the streptococci is similar to that of other gram-positive bacteria, being composed primarily of peptidoglycan, in which are embedded a variety of carbohydrates, teichoic acids, lipoproteins, and surface protein antigens (see Chap. 1). Some streptococcal species may be serologically classified on the basis of cell surface carbohydrate antigens. The pioneering work of Rebecca Lancefield established the **Lancefield grouping system** for the β-hemolytic streptococci.[419] The antigens detected in the Lancefield grouping system are either cell wall polysaccharides (as in the human group A, B, C, F, and G streptococci) or are cell wall lipoteichoic acids (group D streptococci and *Enterococcus* species). Originally, these cell wall–grouping antigens were extracted with dilute hydrochloric or nitrous acid, formamide, or autoclaving, and groups were determined by capillary precipitin reactions. Commercially available streptococcal-grouping kits use enzymatic extraction techniques and either coagglutination or latex particle agglutination for antigen detection. Other streptococci, particularly members of the viridans group, do not possess any of the recognized Lancefield cell wall–

grouping antigens, although some strains may possess similar antigens that will cross-react with β-hemolytic streptococcal group-specific antisera. Well-studied viridans streptococci, such as the cariogenic organism *S. mutans*, have been divided into serotypes based on their own cell wall carbohydrate antigens. The various serotypes of *S. mutans* have subsequently been elevated to species status and now comprise the so-called *S. mutans* group of oral streptococci (see later discussion).

VIRULENCE FACTORS OF STREPTOCOCCI

Pathogenic streptococci have several characteristics that contribute to their virulence. The virulence mechanisms of the group A, β-hemolytic streptococci (*S. pyogenes*) have been studied most extensively. The major group A **cell wall antigen** is a complex polysaccharide consisting of L-rhamnose and *N*-acetyl-D-glucosamine in a 2:1 ratio.[63] The antigen is covalently attached to the peptidoglycan. The role of the cell wall–grouping antigen as a virulence factor is not known, although the peptidoglycan material itself has biologic activity, including the induction of fever, dermal and cardiac necrosis in animals, lysis of erythrocytes and platelets, and enhancement of nonspecific resistance. Some group A strains possess a capsule composed of **hyaluronic acid**. Chemically, this capsular material is indistinguishable from the ground substance of connective tissue, which may explain the lack of immunogenicity of this substance in the infected host. In vitro, the capsule is generally lost as the organism enters the stationary phase of growth; this loss is probably due to the elaboration of **hyaluronidase** during the latter stages of the logarithmic growth phase. The hyaluronic acid capsule functions to prevent opsonization of the organism and, in this way, functions as a virulence determinant.

The major virulence factor of the group A streptococcus is a cell surface antigen designated **M protein**.[63]

M proteins are acid- and heat-stable, trypsin-labile, fibrillar proteins associated with the outer surface of the cell wall. The M protein is anchored in the cell membrane, extends through the peptidoglycan layer, and projects from the surface of the bacterial cell (Fig. 12-1). Strains that are rich in M protein are resistant to phagocytosis and intracellular killing by polymorphonuclear cells; cells lacking demonstrable M protein are readily phagocytosed and killed.[420] There are currently more than 80 recognized M serotypes, and immunity to group A streptococcal infection is M–type-specific.[379] M typing is generally performed on hot acid extracts (Lancefield extracts) of group A streptococci using capillary precipitin or agarose gel immunodiffusion techniques. Unfortunately, many strains are nontypeable; either appropriate M antiserum is not available, or the M protein of a given strain may not be optimally expressed under the conditions of cultivation.[560] Nucleic acid probe techniques have been used to identify M protein–specific DNA sequences in serologically M-nontypeable strains. These M protein–specific DNA sequences apparently represent distinct M types for which antisera either are not available or are not produced under the cultural condition employed.[560] M protein genes have also been identified using oligonucleotide probes corresponding to the NH_2-terminal sequences of specific M types. Probes that were able to hybridize to dot-blotted genomic DNA from group A streptococcal strains were able to identify a variety of M types and were equally sensitive and more specific than conventional serologic M-typing procedures.[385]

Because protective antibody against group A streptococcal infection is M–type-specific, M protein has been a focus of vaccine research for many years. M antigens exist in the cell wall as α-helical-coiled dimers with a highly variable NH_2-terminal portion and a more conserved COOH-terminal portion.[537] The immunodominant epitopes responsible for M-type variability and, hence, type-specific immunity, reside in the NH_2-terminal portion of the molecule. Amino acid sequence analysis of M proteins of many types has identified a portion of the M protein molecule that is common among several M protein types; that is, this sequence of amino acids is highly conserved.[547] Sera from individuals living in different geographic areas with high rates of streptococcal infection reacted with this conserved M peptide in an enzyme-linked immunosorbent assay (ELISA). Furthermore, antibodies directed against this peptide were able to opsonize streptococci belonging to a variety of M types. This highly conserved part of the M protein molecule is being investigated further as a possible candidate vaccine against group A streptococcal infection and rheumatic fever.

Opacity factor (OF) describes another M protein–associated cell surface antigen of group A streptococci that is a putative virulence factor.[558] OF is an α-lipoproteinase that is able to opacify (render opaque) media containing horse serum.[379] This factor is produced by 29 of the 80 or so different M types and can be detected in those M types even if M–type-specific reactivity is lost or undetectable (i.e., the presence of OF is associated

TABLE 12-2
STREPTOCOCCAL SPECIES GROUPS BASED ON SMALL-SUBUNIT rRNA SEQUENCE ANALYSIS

GROUP	GROUP DESIGNATION	MEMBERS
I	Pyogenic group	*S. pyogenes*—group A streptococci *S. agalactiae*—group B streptococci *S. equi, S. dysgalactiae*—group C streptococci Group G streptococci *S. uberis*—nongroupable; swine *S. parauberis*—nongroupable; swine *S. iniae*—nongroupable; freshwater dolphins *S. canis*—Lancefield groups L and M; canines *S. porcinus*—Lancefield groups E, P, U, and V; swine, humans *S. intestinalis*—nongroupable or cross-react with group G antisera *S. phocae*—nongroupable; harbor seals
II	"*S. bovis*" group	*S. bovis*—group D streptococci; humans, animals *S. equinus*—group D streptococci; horses, occasionally humans *S. alactolyticus*—proposed name for *S. bovis*-like isolates from pigs and chickens
III	"*S. mitis*" group	*S. mitis* *S. gordonii* *S. pneumoniae* *S. oralis* *S. sanguis* *S. parasanguis*
IV	"*S. mutans*" group	*S. mutans*—principal species in human dental plaque and caries; formerly *S. mutans* serotypes e and c *S. sobrinus*—oral flora in some humans; role in dental caries likely; formerly *S. mutans* serotypes d and g *S. cricetus*—oral flora and dental plaque of hamsters; rarely found in humans; formerly *S. mutans* serotype a *S. macacae*—oral flora and dental plaque of monkeys; reacts with serotype c antisera *S. rattus*—oral flora and dental plaque of rats; rare in humans; formerly *S. mutans* serotype b *S. downeii*—oral flora and dental plaque of monkeys; reacts with *S. mutans* serotype c antisera *S. ferus*—oral flora and dental plaque of wild rats; reacts with *S. mutans* serotype c antisera
V	"*S. salivarius*" group	*S. salivarius* *S. thermophilus* *S. vestibularis*
VI	"*S. milleri*" group	*S. anginosus* *S. constellatus* *S. intermedius*
VII	Unaffiliated species group	*S. acidominimus*—included with the viridans streptococci *S. suis* (α-hemolytic; Lancefield groups R, S, RS, and T) *S. pleomorphus*—obligately anaerobic streptococcus

Data from Refs. 53 and 387.

only with specific M types). Therefore, OF-positive and OF-negative reactions are consistently associated with specific M types. Group A streptococci also may possess **T** and **R antigens**. T antigens are acid- and heat-stable antigens that may be restricted to a single M type or that may be shared by several different M types.[63] Neither the T nor R antigen is associated with virulence, and these antigens are now rarely used in current typing systems, since the description of OF typing. In addition to these serologic typing methods, group A streptococci may also be typed by phenotypic biotyping with commercial identification systems, multilocus

enzyme electrophoresis, DNA restriction enzyme fragment length polymorphisms, rRNA gene restriction fragment length polymorphisms (ribotyping), and random amplified polymorphic DNA analysis.[77,88,317,497,611]

Group A streptococci produce two hemolysins: streptolysin O and streptolysin S. **Streptolysin O** is oxygen-labile, antigenic, inhibited by cholesterol, and toxic to a variety of cell types, including leukocytes, monocytes, and cultured cells. Because of its oxygen lability, streptolysin O is primarily responsible for the β-hemolysis seen around subsurface colonies of group A streptococci in pour plates or in the stabbed regions

TABLE 12-3

COMPARISON OF STREPTOCOCCI AND OTHER MAJOR GRAM-POSITIVE BACTERIAL GROUPS

ORGANISM	GRAM STAIN	ATMOSPHERE	CATALASE	MOTILITY	SPORES	VANCOMYCIN
Streptococci	GPC	Facultative	−	−	−	S
Enterococci	GPC	Facultative	−	−/+	−	S/R
Staphylococci	GPC	Facultative	+	−	−	S
Peptococci/peptostreptococci	GPC	Anaerobic	−	−	−	S
Corynebacterium spp.	GPR	Facultative	+	v	−	S
Listeria spp.	GPR	Facultative	+	+	−	S
Erysipelothrix spp.	GPR	Aerobic	−	−	−	R
Arcanobacterium spp.	GPR	Facultative	−	−	−	S
Bacillus spp.	GPR	Aerobic	+	+	+	S
Lactobacillus spp.	GPR	Facultative	−	−	−	R/S
Leuconostoc spp.	GPC	Facultative	−	−	−	R
Pediococcus spp.	GPC	Facultative	−	−	−	R

GPC, gram-positive cocci; GPR, gram-positive rod; +, positive reaction or characteristic; −, negative reaction or characteristic; S, susceptible; R, resistant.

of inoculated sheep blood agar plates. Streptolysin O is also produced by some group C and group G streptococci.[280] Measurement of antibodies against streptolysin O (antistreptolysin O [ASO] titers) in serum is useful for retrospective diagnosis of recent pharyngeal streptococcal infections. The ASO response following skin infections is poor, presumably because of inactivation of the antigen by cholesterol present in skin. In such cases, anti-DNaseB titers are more reliable (see later discussion). **Streptolysin S** (SLS) is oxygen-stable, nonantigenic, and also toxic to a variety of cell types. SLS is largely bound to the cell and may cause the leukotoxic action of group A streptococci, as evidenced by the killing of a certain proportion of the leukocytes that phagocytose the streptococci. SLS is active in both surface and subsurface hemolysis when the organisms are grown on sheep blood agar. Both SLO and SLS can induce injury to nonerythrocytic cell types, causing the formation of slits and pores in the cell membrane and subsequent leakage of cellular contents.

Group A streptococci also produce several extracellular products; many of these play a real or theoretical role in the virulence of the organism. **Streptococcal pyrogenic exotoxins (SPEs)** are responsible for the rash of scarlet fever and are also believed to be principal virulence determinants in the pathogenesis of the streptococcal toxic shock-like syndrome.[601] Three immunologically distinct SPEs, designated SPE types A, B, and C, have been well described, and the genes that encode them have been identified and character-

ized.[298,299,338,509,694] A fourth SPE, designated type D, has been reported but has not yet been completely characterized.[471] The genes for streptococcal pyrogenic exotoxins A and C (*speA* and *speC*) are encoded on a streptococcal lysogenic bacteriophage, whereas the gene for the type B exotoxin (*speB*) is chromosomal. It appears that the *speB* gene is found in all group A streptococci, whereas the other two genes may or may not be present. These organisms also produce four immunologically and electrophoretically distinct **deoxyribonucleases**, designated DNase A, B, C, and D. Antibodies against DNase B (anti-DNase B) are helpful, along with ASO titers, for serologic documentation of prior group A streptococcal pharyngeal or skin infections. **Hyaluronidase** produced by group A streptococci depolymerizes the ground substance of connective tissue, resulting in contiguous spread of the organism. **Streptokinases** produced by group A streptococci hydrolyze fibrin clots and may function in virulence by preventing the formation of fibrin barriers at the periphery of spreading streptococcal lesions. The contribution of these enzymes and toxins to infection is uncertain. Many of these factors are produced by other β-hemolytic streptococci as well.

The group B streptococcus (*S. agalactiae*) contains a Lancefield-grouping antigen, a type-specific cell-surface polysaccharide and protein antigens. The group antigen of these organisms is composed of a rhamnose–glucosamine polymer attached to the peptidoglycan layer. Type specificity is provided by both

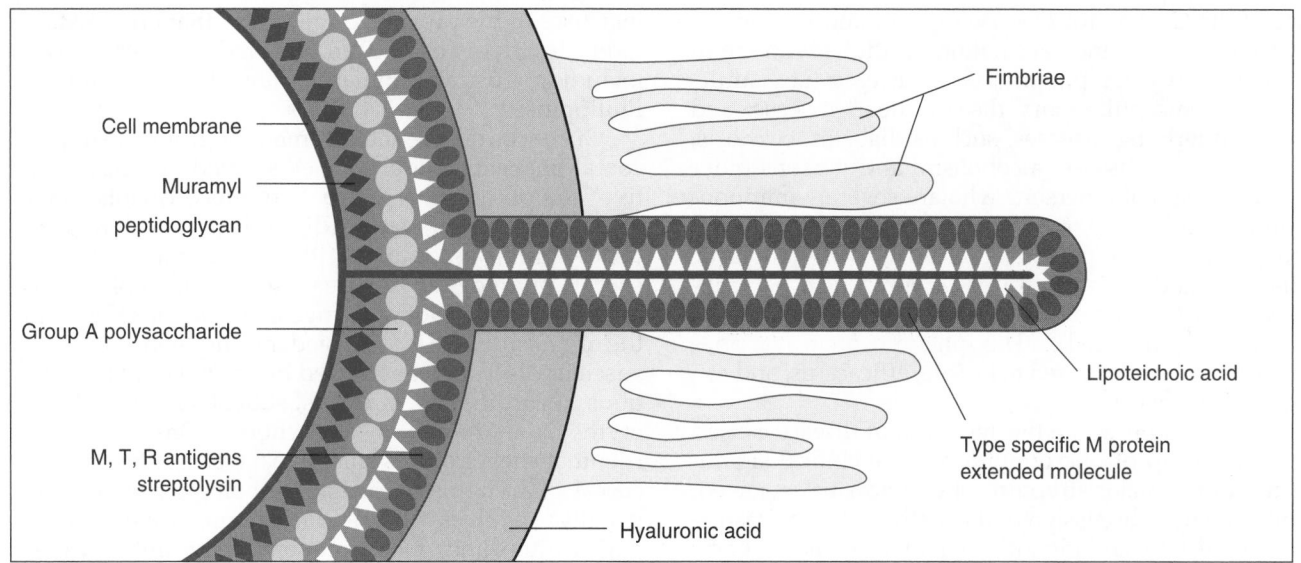

Figure 12-1
The major known antigenic determinants on the surface of virulent, encapsulated group A streptococci.

capsular polysaccharide and protein antigens. The polysaccharide capsular antigens are designated Ia, Ib, II, III, IV, V, and VI, and the protein antigen is designated by the single letter *c*.[314,347,374,682] This c antigen is found in all Ia and Ib strains, in 60% of type II strains, and is rarely found in type III strains (not enough serotype IV, V, or VI strains have been examined for the presence of the c antigen). Therefore, serotype designations for c–antigen-containing strains are expressed as Ia/c, Ib/c, and II/c. Lack of antibodies to these type-specific antigens is a crucial factor in the risk of development of group B streptococcal disease. Type III strains of group B streptococci account for 60% of isolates from cases of neonatal sepsis and over 80% of isolates from infants with meningitis, suggesting that this group B streptococcal serotype posesses enhanced virulence.[181] The structural component of the type III capsule that appears to be associated with augmented virulence is the presence of *N*-acetylneuraminic acid (sialic acid). The presence of this molecule on the surface of the organism inhibits activation of the alternative complement cascade and prevents phagocytosis; removal of sialic acid with neuraminidase leads to complement activation, phagocytosis, and intracellular killing of the organisms.[198,200,701]

The virulence of *S. pneumoniae* is primarily related to its ability to resist ingestion and killing by phagocytic cells, although other virulence factors have been described.[495] This resistance is related to primarily the **polysaccharide capsule** of the organism. Inhibition of capsule production by genetic techniques renders these organisms avirulent in animal models.[691] There are over 84 capsular types of *S. pneumoniae*; 23 of these types account for over 88% of pneumococcal bacteremia and meningitis.[495] Initial adherence of pneumococci apparently is not mediated by capsular material but is related to a bacterial **adhesin** that interacts

with disaccharide receptors on pharyngeal epithelial cell surfaces.[15] Other cellular products of *S. pneumoniae*, such as the α-hemolysin, autolysin, and cell surface molecules, may also play a role in pneumococcal virulence. Mutants that are defective in the production of these various components have diminished virulence in animal models, and immunization with purified products results in the production of specific antibodies that confer partial resistance to challenge infection.[75] **Pneumolysin**, a thiol-activated protein produced by *S. pneumoniae*, interacts with the cell membrane of a variety of host cells, inhibits the bactericidal activity of phagocytic cells, and arrests ciliary motility, thereby compromising bacterial clearance. This toxin is also able to activate an acute inflammatory response by the activation of the classic complement pathway. Mutants that lack the ability to produce pneumolysin have diminished virulence in animal models, and immunization with purified pneumolysin provides partial protection on challenge with virulent, pneumolysin-producing strains.[60,524] **Autolysin**, a cell wall enzyme responsible for pneumococcal lysis during the stationary growth phase, may function in pathogenesis by causing lytic dispersal of both pneumolysin and α-hemolysin.[59] A **pneumococcal surface protein (PspA)** that functions in virulence has also been described.[466] Antibodies directed against PspA from a given pneumococcal strain protect experimental animals against challenge with both the homologous strain and heterologous strains, and mutants that are defective in PspA production are avirulent.

The currently available pneumococcal vaccines—Pneumovax (Merck, Sharpe, and Dohme) and Pnu-Imune (Lederle)—are composed of a mixture of 23 pneumococcal capsular polysaccharides; antibodies directed against these polysaccharides are protective.[496] The Immunization Practices Advisory Committee of the Centers for Disease Control and Prevention (CDC) recommends vaccination of adults who are at increased risk for pneumococcal disease (i.e., adults with chronic pulmonary disease, heart disease, and with underlying diseases, such as diabetes, cirrhosis, chronic renal disease, alcoholism; and persons older than 65 years old, persons who are severely immunocompromised [e.g., transplant patients, HIV-infected patients, asplenic persons, and those with neoplastic disease], and societal groups recognized to be at increased risk for pneumococcal disease [e.g., American Indian populations]).[2] The pneumococcal vaccines have been demonstrated to be safe, efficacious, and relatively inexpensive.

To fully appreciate the spectrum of disease caused by this group of microorganisms, the clinical significance of the major streptococci will now be reviewed, followed by a discussion of the methods for their isolation, detection, and identification in the clinical laboratory.

GROUP A β-HEMOLYTIC STREPTOCOCCI (*STREPTOCOCCUS PYOGENES*)

Humans are the natural reservoir for group A, β-hemolytic streptococci, and the organism is transmitted from person to person by the respiratory route. The most common infection caused by group A streptococci is streptococcal pharyngitis. Most cases of pharyngitis are seen in school-aged children (5 to 15 years old) during the winter or spring. Following an initial incubation period of 2 to 4 days, onset is generally abrupt, with fever, sore throat, headache, malaise, and abdominal pain. The posterior pharynx is usually inflamed and swollen, and a grayish-white exudate may be present on the tonsils. The anterior cervical lymph nodes are usually tender and swollen. The presence of rhinorrhea, hoarseness, cough, or diarrhea speaks against group A streptococcal infection, instead suggesting a viral or mycoplasmal etiology.[618] Infection with strains that elaborate pyrogenic exotoxins A, B, or C may also cause a scarlatiniform rash (i.e., classic scarlet fever). Complications of group A streptococcal pharyngitis may be suppurative (peritonsillar abscess, retropharyngeal abscess, suppurative cervical adenitis, otitis media, sinusitis, mastoiditis, bacteremia), nonsuppurative (acute and chronic rheumatic fever, glomerulonephritis), or toxin-mediated (streptococcal toxic shock–like syndrome).[617] In the absence of complications, streptococcal pharyngitis is self-limited in nature. However, treatment (ideally, culture followed by antimicrobial therapy) is usually sought. About 15% of individuals with streptococcal pharyngitis may become asymptomatic carriers of the organisms following treatment.[63] Currently, recommendations for treatment of streptococcal pharyngitis include oral penicillin V for 10 days, intramuscular benzathine penicillin G (600,000 to 1.2 million units), oral erythromycin estolate for 10 days, oral azithromycin (for those older than 15 years old) for 4 days, or oral cefadroxil for 10 days.[401] Group A β-hemolytic streptococci remain quite susceptible to penicillin G, although

increases in the prevalence of strains that are resistant to erythromycin have been reported in several areas, including Australia, Finland, Hawaii, Japan, and the Philippines.[145,612]

Of concern in the management of group A streptococcal pharyngitis are the well-studied "nonsuppurative" complications of group A streptococcal infections, **acute rheumatic fever** (ARF) and **glomerulonephritis**.[62,64] ARF is associated with prior group A streptococcal pharyngitis, whereas glomerulonephritis is associated with prior pharyngeal or skin infection with the organism. ARF is a delayed, multisystem collagen–vascular disease characterized by the major manifestations of carditis, polyarthritis, subcutaneous nodules, erythema marginatum, and chorea. Onset of acute rheumatic fever occurs from 2 to 5 weeks after streptococcal pharyngitis.[64] Cardiac pathologic presentation usually involves the endocardium, myocardium, pericardium and, most frequently, the mitral valve; clinically this pathologic manifestation appears as characteristic heart murmurs, cardiac enlargement, congestive heart failure, or, rarely, intractable cardiac arrest and death. The arthritis is usually migratory, involves multiple joints (especially the knees, elbows, ankles, and wrists), and resolves spontaneously. Subcutaneous, firm, painless nodules appear at the same time as carditis and are usually found on the extremities near the bony areas of the feet and hands. Erythema marginatum lesions are erythematous eruptions with red, raised, serpiginous borders and central areas of clearing that usually appear on the trunk, arms, and legs. Chorea is a neurologic manifestation that is characterized by muscular spasms, incoordination, and muscle weakness that develop during ARF or after several months. Attacks of ARF generally last 3 to 6 months. The differential diagnosis of this illness is broad owing to the protean manifestations of the syndrome and includes rheumatoid arthritis, systemic lupus erythematosus, sickle cell disease, rubella, septic arthritis, disseminated gonococcal infection, Lyme disease, bacterial endocarditis, and myocarditis. Laboratory findings associated with ARF include elevated sedimentation rate, elevated C-reactive protein, and the occurrence of an antecedent streptococcal infection, as evidenced by a positive throat culture or positive direct antigen test for group A streptococci, or by elevated or rising streptococcal antibody titers (e.g., ASO, anti-DNaseB, antihyaluronidase).[158] Therapy for ARF includes analgesics, salicylates, and corticosteroids for treatment of fever and inflammation, plus supportive therapy to prevent cardiac failure.[64]

Acute glomerulonephritis is an inflammatory disease of the renal glomerulus that is associated with diffuse glomerular lesions, hypertension, hematuria, and proteinuria.[64] Glomerular lesions can be demonstrated to contain depositions of complement components (especially C3), properdin, and immunoglobulin by immunofluorescence techniques.[477] Rheumatic fever may appear 1 to 5 weeks following streptococcal pharyngitis, whereas glomerulonephritis may occur as soon as 10 days following pharyngitis or longer than 3 weeks following skin infections.[19] Clinically, the disease is characterized by malaise, weakness, anorexia, headache, edema, and circulatory congestion, as evidenced by hypertension and encephalopathy. Laboratory findings include anemia, an elevated sedimentation rate, decreased C3 and total complement, hematuria, and proteinuria. Urinalysis reveals red blood cells, leukocytes, and casts. Antecedent group A streptococcal infection is usually demonstrable by recovery of organisms from the throat or from skin lesions or by elevation of antistreptococcal antibodies. ASO responses following streptococcal skin infections are not reliably elevated, and titers for anti-DNaseB or anti-hyaluronidase should be performed.[65]

Several theories have been advanced concerning the mechanism by which group A streptococci induce ARF and glomerulonephritis. The most tenable theory is that the streptococci induce the formation of antistreptococcal antibodies against capsular (hyaluronic acid), cell wall (antigroup-carbohydrate, anti-M, and other associated proteins), and cell membrane antigens that cross-react with various antigenic moieties in myocardial, endocardial, and valvular heart tissue, the myocardial sarcolemma, skeletal muscle, and the joints. Indeed, certain group A streptococcal M types—M1, M3, M5, M16, and M18—have been shown to be "rheumatogenic."[639] These strains are usually OF-negative and have a mucoid colonial morphology on primary isolation. Antigenic epitopes of some of these M types have been demonstrated to share determinants with human cardiac muscle, sarcolemma membrane proteins, and synovial membranes.[33,159,160] Other workers have shown similar immunologic cross-reactions between the polysaccharide antigen of group A streptococci and certain heart valve glycoproteins, between streptococcal hyaluronic acid (i.e., the capsular material) and human hyaluronic acid, and between streptococcal cell membranes and the caudate and subthalamic neuronal nuclei in the human central nervous system.[247,289,357,607] The latter may explain the role of antecedent streptococcal infection in the neurologic components of ARF. "Nephritogenic" group A streptococcal M types have also been identified: types M-2, M-49, M-55, M-57, M59, M-60, and M-61 have been associated with glomerulonephritis following skin infections, whereas types M-1, M-4, M-12, and M-25 are most frequently implicated following pharyngeal infections. Although cross-reactions between nephritogenic streptococcal strains and renal tissues have been demonstrated,[66,297] the pathologic abnormalities of nephritis may actually be due to the deposition of preformed immune complexes containing streptococcal antigens and host antibodies in the glomerular tissues.[662,669]

Since the end of World War II, the incidence of streptococcal pharyngitis in North America and Western Europe has remained fairly stable, whereas the incidence of poststreptococcal sequelae has decreased dramatically.[452,550,673] Beginning in 1985, however, "outbreaks" of rheumatic fever have been reported in the Salt Lake City area, Colorado, North Carolina, Pittsburgh, Tennessee, Missouri, West Virginia, Texas, Ohio, and New York.[96,112,113,114,115,286,316,319,431,458,684,703,704] In these outbreaks, some individuals did not recall having had a streptococcal infection. In such cases, and in the diagnosis of the nonsuppurative sequelae, serologic studies (serum antibodies to streptolysin O, serum antibodies to anti-DNase B) are helpful for retrospective documentation of previous group A streptococcal infection. Among the patients who did have positive pharyngeal cultures for group A streptococci, it was noted that many were mucoid strains belonging to M types 1, 3, 6, and 18; these strains had not been recovered with any great frequency before 1985.[63]

Shortly after the reports of resurgent rheumatic fever caused by these recognized rheumatogenic M serotypes appeared in the literature, severe invasive group A streptococcal infections associated with a **toxic shock–like syndrome (TSLS)** started to be reported from European and American medical centers.[43,90,118,144,253,319,452,633,638] In one of the initial publications, Stevens and coworkers reported on 20 patients from the Rocky Mountain region of the United States who presented with various types of group A streptococcal soft-tissue infections (pharyngitis, cellulitis, suppurative thrombophlebitis, peritonitis, necrotizing fasciitis, postpartum myometritis, localized wound infection) and went on to develop additional symptoms that were similar to those found in patients with classic staphylococcal toxic shock syndrome.[633,634] These clinical characteristics included hypotension, renal dysfunction, hypoalbuminuria, thromocytopenia, hypocalcemia, and respiratory failure. All of the patients had positive cultures for group A streptococci, including 12 patients with positive blood cultures. Of the 20 patients, 19 went into shock, and six died as a result of their infections. Interestingly, eight of the 10 group A streptococcal strains that were available for subsequent study produced streptococcal pyrogenic exotoxin A (SPE A), the toxin associated with scarlet fever. This was of particular interest because strains that produce this toxin have been infrequently isolated in the United States since 1976. Most of the strains associated with these severe infections have been type M-1, but several other M types (i.e., M-2, M-3, M-5, M-12, M-18, M-28) have also been implicated.

Many of the authors of these reports suggested that the streptococcal pyrogenic exotoxins may play an important role in the pathogenesis of TSLS.[338] Hauser and colleagues[339] examined 34 TSLS group A streptococcal isolates and found that 74% were either type M1 or M3. Although 53% produced SPE A, 85% contained the *speA* gene that codes for SPE A. All strains contained the gene coding for SPE B (*speB*), and 21% contained the gene coding for SPE C (*speC*). These workers concluded that SPE A was strongly associated with group A streptococci that are capable of causing TSLS, although they postulated that other factors may also be involved because not all strains recovered from patients with TSLS contained the *speA* gene. Recently, Musser and coworkers[498] examined the M types and the presence of genes coding for SPE A (*speA* genotype) and SPE C (*speC* genotype) in a collection of group A streptococcal isolates from cases of pharyngitis occurring in nine different states. More than 50% of these isolates that expressed the M1 or M3 serotype hybridized specifically with a probe for *speA*, indicating that strains with the potential for causing severe streptococcal disease were well represented among those causing community-acquired pharyngitis. Others have now shown that SPE A, similar to the staphylococcal enterotoxins and the staphylococcal toxic shock syndrome toxin 1 (TSST-1), is a "superantigen" that is capable of inducing the release of various cytokines and lymphokines.[236,321,601] These molecules, in turn, mediate the profound systemic effects that promote rapid systemic invasion by the organisms and precipitate the multiorgan system involvement that characterizes the syndrome.

At the same time that TSLS was being recognized, increases in the incidence of other serious group A streptococcal infections, especially bacteremias and serious soft-tissue infections, were being observed in both adult and pediatric populations in the United States and abroad.[90,118,243,634] This increase in severe infections has been reported among intravenous drug users in Philadelphia, adults in the Denver and Los Angeles areas, and among children in Winston-Salem, North Carolina and Denver, Colorado.[115,286,434,651,704] Familial clusters and outbreaks centered in hospitals and nursing homes have also been reported.[609] Although bacteremia and sepsis have been the most common presentations, other severe infections have included cellulitis, necrotizing fasciitis, myositis, osteomyelitis, pharyngitis, pneumonia, empyema, retroperitoneal abscess, peritonitis, and meningitis.[116,376,440,500,635,725] Intrapartum transmission of group A streptococci, leading to severe and often fatal group A streptococcal disease in the neonate has also been observed.[518] Some of these infections have occurred in association with the presence of catheters and other indwelling medical devices.[455] Group A streptococci have also joined the growing list of other microorganisms implicated in continuous ambulatory peritoneal dialysis–associated peritonitis.[111] Because of the severity of these infections and the high mortality associated with them, aggressive medical and surgical interventions have been necessary and lifesaving in many patients.[725] With the recognition of these severe streptococcal infections and the emergence of TSLS, the group A streptococcus has reestablished itself as an organism to be reckoned with in the 21st century.

GROUP B β-HEMOLYTIC STREPTOCOCCI (*STREPTOCOCCUS AGALACTIAE*)

Group B β-hemolytic streptococci are a major cause of disease in the neonatal and perinatal periods. Women become colonized with the organism in the vagina and the rectum, and asymptomatic vaginal colonization is found in 5% to 35% of pregnant women; up to 60% of the colonized women will carry the organism intermittently.[18,81] Indeed, colonization of the vagina may actually reflect contamination from the rectum, with the gastrointestinal tract being the principal reservoir of the organisms.[180] The newborn becomes colonized by vertical transmission from the colonized mother, either in utero or during delivery. In addition, the neonate may become colonized by nosocomial exposure to the organism after birth. Among colonized infants, disease may occur in one to four infants per 1000 live births.[198] Neonatal disease with group B streptococci follows two patterns, termed early-onset disease and late-onset disease.

Early-onset disease occurs with an incidence of 0.7:1000 to 3.7:1000 live births and is associated with in utero or perinatal organism acquisition.[198,695] The organism is acquired either by ascending infection in utero before delivery, through ruptured fetal membranes, or during passage through a birth canal that is colonized with group B streptococci. Although a substantial proportion of these infants (approximately 50%) will be colonized with group B streptococci, only 1% to 2% of them become infected.[198,242] Onset of disease occurs during the first 5 days of life; in more than half the cases, infants become ill within the first 12 to 20 hours after birth.[256] The disease spectrum includes bacteremia, pneumonia, meningitis, septic shock, and neutropenia. Although more than 50% of cases occur in term infants, a higher attack rate and greater morbidity are associated with preterm infants.[241] Mortality owing to early-onset disease in term infants ranges from 2% to 8%; higher mortality rates are seen in premature infants and are inversely proportional to the birth weight of the neonate.[605,729] Maternal factors that increase the risk for early-onset infection of the neonate include premature labor, prolonged rupture of the fetal membranes, postpartum bacteremia, maternal amnionitis, heavy vaginal colonization with group B streptococci, and group B streptococcal bacteriuria.[14,181,211,256]

Late-onset disease occurs with an incidence of 0.5:1000 to 1.8:1000 live births.[198] Disease becomes clinically evident 7 days to 3 months (average 3 to 4 weeks) after birth. Whereas about half of the late-onset infections are acquired from the birth canal of colonized mothers, the remaining cases result from postnatal organism acquisition from the mother or other caregivers or nosocomially.[520] Bacteremia with accompanying meningitis is the predominant clinical presentation.[198] Mortality associated with late-onset disease is about 10% to 15%. Up to 50% of children with late-onset meningitis will have permanent neurologic complications and sequelae.[683] The distribution of group B streptococcal serotypes also varies with early- versus late-onset disease.[34] Among neonates with early-onset disease without meningitis, the serotype distribution is equally divided among types I, II, and III. Among similarly infected neonates with meningitis, serotype III strains predominate. In late-onset disease, in which meningitis is the common clinical presentation, serotype III strains account for over 90% of the isolates. On the other hand, group B streptococcal meningitis in adults is primarily associated with serotype II organisms. Methods for subtyping strains associated with outbreaks have also been described.[293]

Diagnosis of systemic group B streptococcal disease is accomplished by culture of the organisms from appropriately collected specimens or by detection of group B streptococcal capsular antigen in cerebrospinal fluid, serum, and urine. Since 1979, latex agglutination tests or rapid enzyme immunoassay methods have been used in many laboratories for rapid diagnosis of systemic group B streptococcal infections. Currently available latex agglutination tests include the Wellcogen Strep B (Murex Diagnostics, Research Triangle Park NC), Bactigen Group B Streptococcus (Wampole Laboratories, Cranbury NJ) and the Directigen Group B Strep test kit (Becton-Dickinson Microbiology Systems, Cockeysville MD). The enzyme immunoassay kit is the ICON Strep B assay (Hybritech Inc., San Diego CA). Sensitivities of the latex agglutination products range from the mid-80% to 100%, although some studies have reported sensitivities as low as 27% to 54%.[35,45,264,320,325,360] Corresponding specificities of the latex agglutination tests range from 80% to 100%.[35,264,325,360] The sensitivity and specificity of these assays depend on several factors, including the type of specimen tested, whether the specimens are concentrated before testing, and the times during the clinical course that the specimens being tested are collected from the patient. In a recent evaluation of the three latex tests and the ICON immunoassay for detection of group B streptococcal antigen in urine, the sensitivities of the Directigen, Bactigen, Wellcogen, and ICON assays were 84%, 76%, 43%, and 59%, respectively, when unconcentrated urine specimens were tested.[315] Retesting of the urine specimens after they had been concentrated 25-fold resulted in sensitivities of 98%, 92%, 68%, 89% for the four assays, respectively. Specificities of all of the assays exceeded 99.5% for both concentrated and unconcentrated specimens. Because of the high cost of these assays and the relatively low yield of positive results, many laboratories are reconsidering the continued use of these assays as a way to cut costs.

A central focus of pediatric research is the prevention of group B streptococcal disease in the newborn infant.[510] Because infants born to heavily colonized mothers are more likely to develop early-onset disease and because infants who acquire a large bacterial inoculum during birth have significantly increased likelihoods of developing both early- and late-onset disease, the identification of colonized mothers has become a central focus for chemoprophylactic prevention strategies. Antepartum administration of antimicrobial therapy fails to eradicate group B streptococcal colonization at delivery in almost 70% of women.[268] However, organism transmission, neonatal early-onset infection, and postpartum maternal complications can be largely prevented by intrapartum administration of intravenous ampicillin during labor.[82] Even this chemoprophylactic approach prevents only about 70% to 75% of early-onset disease and has no apparent effect on the development of late-onset disese.[82] Intrapartum antimicrobial therapy for high-risk pregnancies with heavy group B streptococcal colonization has reduced vertical transmission to the newborn infant.[382]

In general, conventional antenatal vaginal cultures collected during pregnancy have been effective in predicting vaginal colonization at term. About 60% to 70% of women with positive vaginal cultures for group B streptococci in the second trimester will be colonized at term, but up to 30% of women with negative cultures during the second trimester will be culture-positive for group B streptococci at delivery. The validity of the premise that the risk of neonatal group B streptococcal infection is greater for infants born to women with heavy vaginal colonization has also been confounded by a few clinical reports. In an evaluation of a rapid enzyme immunoassay (EIA) kit for direct detection of group B streptococci in vaginal specimens, Towers and coworkers reported that two of nine infants born to mothers with light colonization (and negative rapid EIA results) developed fatal early-onset disease.[655] In a study of another method for rapid detection of group B streptococcal colonization, Morales and Lim reported that, among 37 women with light colonization and negative rapid screening tests, six delivered babies with early-onset sepsis.[486] Therefore, the development of accurate methods for rapid, sensitive, and specific detection of group B streptococcal colonization in women at or near the time of delivery has become a central focus of clinical microbiologic research.

Methods for detection of vaginal colonization with group B streptococci include culture amplification, latex agglutination, and enzyme immunoassay techniques. In the culture amplification technique, vaginal swabs are placed in a selective broth medium that is incubated overnight and then either subcultured to agar media or tested directly by latex–coagglutination methods. Such techniques are very sensitive in that both heavy and light colonization are detected, but rapid results are not available. However, this method can be modified to identify heavily colonized women. In two studies, Lim and coworkers demonstrated that women who were heavily colonized could be identified by group B streptococcal coagglutination testing after vaginal swabs were incubated for 5 hours in a selective broth medium.[437,438] The commercially available tests for detection of group B streptococci directly in vaginal swab specimens vary significantly in sensitivity (11% to 88%) when compared with overnight broth techniques and, in general, will identify only those women who are heavily colonized with group B streptococci.[13,311,322,410,444,549,685,728,730,731] The direct tests for group B streptococci include latex particle agglutination tests, EIAs, or DNA probe tests performed on nitrous acid or enzyme extracts of vaginal swabs.

Group B streptococci also cause significant infections in postpartum women. These organisms are associated with about 20% of postpartum endometritis, 25% of bacteremias following cesarean section, and about 25% to 30% of cases of asymptomatic bacteriuria during and after pregnancy. Bacteriuria with group B streptococci alone has been associated with adverse pregnancy outcome and increased rates of premature labor and premature rupture of fetal membranes.[484,723] Complications of bacteremia in these patients include meningitis, endocarditis, cellulitis, fasciitis, and intra-abdominal abscess.[9,198,254,640] In older children and nonpregnant adults, group B streptococci cause a variety of other clinical manifestations.[435] Group B streptococcal pneumonia occurs in debilitated hosts with underlying diseases, such as diabetes, and may be complicated by the development of empyema and pleural effusions.[277,676] Skin and soft-tissue infections are also found in compromised hosts and range in severity from cellulitis and abscesses to pyomyositis and necrotizing fasciitis.[465,566] Group B streptococcal endocarditis occurs in both men and women and may be either acute or subacute in presentation. Preexisting cardiac abnormalities are usually present before disease onset and, once established, large vegetations usually develop, with the mitral valve being the most commonly affected. Complications caused by embolic phenomena or rapid destruction of valvular tissue may necessitate valve replacement.[266,610] Endocarditis in neonates and infants occurs rarely but resembles adult cases with extensive valvular destruction and the occurrence of embolic phenomena.[3,42,624] Group B streptococcal arthritis usually presents as fever and joint pain following or concomitant with bacteremia. Antimicrobial therapy with aspiration or open drainage of infected joints and removal of prosthetic devices, if present, are necessary to effect cure. Group B streptococci are also the major cause of osteomyelitis in infants; hematogenous seeding of bone is the likely source of the organism in infants.[199,641] In adults, osteomyelitis may occur in areas of adjacent arthritis or infected decubital ulcers or as a result of hematogenous seeding from another site of infection.[295,468] Vertebral osteomyelitis caused by group B streptococci is rare, usually results from hematogenous seeding from another focus of infection or from the gastrointestinal tract, and is seen in debilitated patients with underlying diseases, such as diabetes, chronic renal failure, malignancy, or immunosuppression.[203,235] Vertebral osteomyelitis has also been reported as a rare complication of bacteremia in the postpartum period.[57,439] Group B streptococcal meningitis is rare and occurs in individuals with chronic underlying diseases, such as diabetes, alcoholic liver disease, neurologic impairment, malignancy, renal failure, and cardiovascular or pulmonary disease.[193,229] Group B streptococcal meningitis following severe head trauma or associated with cerebrospinal rhinorrhea has also been reported.[672] Group B streptococcal bacteremia, endocarditis, and meningitis in patients with gastrointestinal, colonic, and pancreatic malignancies have suggested an association similar to that of *S. bovis* and colonic pathology and malignancy.[275,722] Group B streptococcal conjunctivitis, keratitis, and hematogenous endophthalmitis are rare, but severe infections that usually occur in previously damaged eyes and result in significant abnormalities that may lead to decreased visual acuity or blindness have been reported.[228,514]

Besides being a well-recognized cause of urinary tract infection in pregnant women, this organism is also a cause of cystitis and pyelonephritis in men, nonpregnant women, and children. In these groups, the risk factors for urinary tract infection caused by group B streptococci include underlying disease (especially diabetes) and structural abnormalities of the urinary tract.[87,229,490] Pyelonephritis and renal abscess are potential complications of both ascending infection and hematogenous dissemination of group B streptococci.[727]

Lastly, group B streptococci may also be capable of causing the toxic shock–like syndrome (TSLS) associated with group A streptococci. Schlievert and colleagues[602] reported a case of a 27-year-old woman who presented with a toxic shock–like illness consisting of fever, hypotension, an erythematous rash, desquamation, and multiorgan system involvement. Although her blood cultures were negative, group B β-hemolytic streptococci were isolated from urine and vaginal cultures. Further study of these isolates demonstrated that they produced a toxic substance that had the properties associated with pyrogenic exotoxins; the substance caused fever, enhanced susceptibility to endotoxin in experimental animals, and acted as a potent lymphocyte mitogen.

GROUP C β-HEMOLYTIC STREPTOCOCCI

The group C β-hemolytic streptococci currently include three species: *S. equisimilis*, *S. zooepidemicus*, and *S. equi*. All of these organisms carry the Lancefield group C carbohydrate antigen in their cell wall and produce hemolysins that are similar to those of group A streptococci.[280] A fourth species designated *S. dysgalactiae* carries the group C antigen, but it is α- or nonhemolytic.[272] Genetic studies have demonstrated extensive similarities between *S. equi* and *S. zooepidemicus*, but the organisms differ in a few phenotypic characteristics and in the presence of certain enzymatic activities. On the basis of genetic relatedness studies, Farrow and Collins[231] have recommended that *S. zooepidemicus* be reclassified as a subspecies of *S. equi* (i.e., *S. equi* subsp. *zooepidemicus*). Similar studies have shown considerable similarities between *S. equisimilis* and *S. dysgalactiae*, with the only consistent phenotypic difference being the β-hemolytic character of the former species.[231,397] Adding to this taxonomic confusion are the "minute" or "small-colony" β-hemolytic, α-hemolytic, or nonhemolytic streptococci of the *S. milleri* group that may carry the group C polysaccharide antigen (see later discussion).[667] These organisms differ from the "large-colony" group C organisms genetically and phenotypically.[213,425] Case-control studies indicate that large-colony group C organisms may cause pharyngitis, whereas the *S. milleri* group organisms carrying the group C (or the group G) antigen do not.[129]

S. equisimilis, the most common human isolate, has been recovered from the pharynges of carriers and from those with exudative pharyngitis and tonsillitis.[148,255,341,474,663,664] It also causes several other human infections, including sepsis in neutropenic hosts, puerperal sepsis, cellulitis, necrotizing fasciitis, pneumonia, epiglottitis, empyema, bacteremia, meningitis, brain abscess, osteomyelitis, septic arthritis, endocarditis, endophthalmitis, and even the streptococcal TSLS.[24,28,41,55,107,296,389,417,504,516,554,592,626,629] The organism has also been recovered from intra-abdominal abscesses in cases of cholecystitis and appendicitis. Many of the patients with these infections have underlying diseases, including chronic cardiopulmonary disease, diabetes, immunosuppression, dermatologic conditions, neoplasms, and alcoholism.[85,619] This species also causes a severe infection in piglets. *S. zooepidemicus* causes various types of diseases in animals, including bovine mastitis, respiratory infections in horses, and genital tract infections in poultry. This species has also been implicated in human infections, including pneumonia, bacteremia, endocarditis, meningitis, septic arthritis, abdominal aortic aneurysm, deep vein thrombosis, nephritis, and cervical lymphadenitis.[36,37,133,422,734] Outbreaks of human pharyngitis caused by *S. zooepidemicus* have also been reported. These outbreaks have been traced to unpasteurized cows' milk and homemade cheese that contained the organism.[37,257,579] In some of the affected individuals, poststreptococcal glomerulonephritis was also observed.[257] *S. equi* is the cause of a respiratory tract infection in horses called "strangles." Strangles is characterized by a high fever, a mucopurulent nasal discharge, and abscesses in the submandibular and retropharyngeal lymph nodes that eventually rupture and drain into the respiratory tract of the infected animal.[653] This organism is extremely rare in humans.[55] *S. dysgalactiae* causes bovine mastitis and purulent arthritis in lambs and goats. Case reports of meningitis in a premature infant and in a 73-year-old man with alcoholic liver disease caused by *S. dysgalactiae* have been published.[417,485]

GROUP D STREPTOCOCCI (*STREPTOCOCCUS BOVIS* AND *STREPTOCOCCUS EQUINUS*)

These streptococci possess the group D lipoteichoic acid antigen in their cell walls. Although these organisms are β-hemolytic on rabbit blood agar, they are usually α- or nonhemolytic on the sheep blood agar used routinely in clinical laboratories. Some former group D species are predominant normal inhabitants of the human gastrointestinal tract and were termed "enterococci," whereas other species that possess the group D antigen and compose only a small part of the normal enteric flora were termed "nonenterococci." The practical consideration behind the division of these organisms into two groups was that the enterococci are generally more resistant to penicillin, cephalosporins, and the aminoglycosides than the nonenterococcal group D streptococci.[204,251] During the mid- and late 1980s, the taxonomy of the group D streptococci changed dramatically. The application of molecular genetic techniques led to the division of the group D streptococci into two separate genera. Enterococcal species are now placed in the separate genus *Enterococcus*, whereas the group D streptococci now includes only two species, *Streptococcus bovis* and *Streptococcus equinus*. *S. bovis* is associated with humans and human infections, whereas *S. equinus* is the predominant streptococcal species found in the alimentary tract of horses. *S. equinus* is a rare cause of bacteremia and endocarditis in humans.[207,284]

Although not routinely performed, certain physiologic characteristics allow the differentiation of *S. bovis* strains into two biotypes, termed *S. bovis* or *S. bovis* I and *S. bovis* variant or *S. bovis* II. *S. bovis* II strains have also been separated into two subbiotypes called *S. bovis* II/1 and *S. bovis* II/2. It has also been proposed that the three *S. bovis* biotypes may actually represent two species: *S. bovis* (comprised of biotype II/1 strains) and *S. inulinaceus* (comprised of biotype I and II/2 strains). This proposal, however, has not been generally accepted.

S. bovis bacteremia and both native and prosthetic valve endocarditis have been associated with carcinoma of the colon in humans, and the organism may be recovered from both feces and blood in patients with this malignancy.[192,265,334,353,402,470,493,505,562,687] *S. bovis* is found significantly more often in the stool of patients with colorectal malignancies than in that of healthy controls or those with benign intestinal polyps.[403,735] A bacteriologic survey of patients with colon cancer and other bowel diseases showed that 56% of patients with colon cancer had *S. bovis* in their feces compared with 10% of control patients with no bowel disorders.[403] Zarkin and coworkers found that *S. bovis* bacteremia was also associated with hepatic disease and dysfunction.[735] Fifty-eight percent of patients with *S. bovis* endocarditis and 46% of those with bacteremia had colonic disease. Liver disease was found in 52% of the patients with endocarditis and 57% of those with bacteremia. Both colon and liver disease were found in 27% of the patients who developed endocarditis. Wilson and others have also reported an association between *S. bovis* endocarditis and diseases of the colon other than carcinoma.[334,336,721] Among 21 patients with *S. bovis* endocarditis, 62% had colonic disease that was not restricted to carcinoma; 24% had inflammatory bowel disease, 14% had diverticulitis, 10% had colonic polyps, 10% had colonic villous adenomas, and 5% had colonic carcinoma.[721] An association between disseminated *S. bovis* infections and both idiopathic ulcerative colitis and chronic radiation enterocolitis has also been found.[370,489] It has been postulated that either the underlying colonic disease or changes in hepatic secretion of bile or immunoglobulins into the intestinal lumen may promote the overgrowth of *S. bovis* and the movement of the organisms from the intestine into the portal venous circulation. Failure of the compromised reticuloendothelial system of the liver to contain the organisms results in bacteremia and endocarditis. Patients with *S. bovis* bacteremia, endocarditis, or meningitis should have a complete colonoscopy to detect occult gastrointestinal lesions.[451]

Bacteremia and hematogenous dissemination of *S. bovis* may result in a variety of other clinical presentations. *S. bovis* meningitis and brain abscess have been diagnosed in patients who subsequently were found to have occult villous adenomas and carcinomas of the colon.[190,209,368,696] *S. bovis* meningitis has also been reported in patients with no underlying malignancies.[239,246,273,404,548] Jain and associates reported an unusual case of *S. bovis* meningitis in an HIV-infected patient, who also had severe colitis and gastrointestinal bleeding secondary to *Strongyloides stercoralis* infection.[371] Presumably, the mucosal ulcerations created by strongyloides allowed the *S. bovis* organisms access to the blood stream. Other infections asssociated with

S. bovis have included acute spondylodiskitis, osteomyelitis, and brain abscess.[433,454,536]

S. bovis is also found in several animal species, in which it is generally considered to be a harmless inhabitant of the gastrointestinal tract. In fact, the type strain of *S. bovis* was originally recovered from cow dung and differs from human clinical isolates in several physiologic tests.[406] Some strains appear to be important causes of septicemia in pigeons.[167] *S. bovis*-like strains have also been isolated from the gastrointestinal tracts of pigs and chickens and have been provisionally named *S. alactolyticus*.[234]

Although most strains of *S. bovis* are susceptible to penicillin, strains that are relatively resistant to penicillin have also been reported.

GROUP F β-HEMOLYTIC STREPTOCOCCI

Organisms of this group have been called "*S. milleri*" in the British taxonomic scheme and *S. anginosus*, *S. constellatus*, and *S. intermedius* in American taxonomic schemes (see later discussion of the *Streptococcus milleri* group). These organisms may be α-, β-, or non-hemolytic. These streptococci characteristically grow as minute colonies on agar media. The colonies are pinpoints after 24 hours and, if β-hemolytic, have a large zone of hemolysis that extends well beyond the margin of the colony. Group F β-hemolytic streptococci are recognized causes of severe suppurative infections, including cellulitis, deep tissue abscesses, bacteremia, osteomyelitis, and endocarditis.[300] Many patients infected with these organisms have significant underlying disease. Other minute-colony β-hemolytic streptococci may carry the group A, C, or G antigen or may be nongroupable.

GROUP G β-HEMOLYTIC STREPTOCOCCI

Group G streptococci constitute a part of the normal human gastrointestinal, vaginal, oropharyngeal, and skin flora. Infections caused by these organisms include pharyngitis, otitis media, pleuropulmonary infection, cellulitis, septic arthritis, osteomyelitis, septic thrombophlebitis, bacteremia, endocarditis, and meningitis.[31,94,364,671,690,732] Severe infections of bone and joint prostheses caused by these organisms have also been reported.[94] Group G streptococcal cellulitis at sites of parenteral injection and bacteremia with subsequent hematogenous complications have been reported frequently in intravenous drug users.[156,288,426] Bacteremia with this organism is also seen in the clinical settings of underlying malignancies, puerperal sepsis, septic abortion, chronic pulmonary disease, and congestive heart failure. Group G streptococcal meningitis and sepsis has also been reported in a patient with AIDS.[555]

OTHER β-HEMOLYTIC STREPTOCOCCI
AND *SPECIES INCERTAE SEDIS*

Other pyogenic β-hemolytic streptococci have been described that carry other Lancefield cell wall antigens and that cause infections in animals other than humans.[332] These include *S. canis*, *S. porcinus*, *S. iniae*, *S. intestinalis*, and *S. phocae*. *S. canis* is found primarily in canines and carries Lancefield group L or M antigens. *S. porcinus* strains belong to Lancefield groups E, P, U, or V and cause infections in swine. In 1995, Facklam and colleagues[222] reported on 13 isolates of *S. porcinus* that had been recovered from humans and forwarded to the CDC over the previous 10 years. Of these 13 isolates, five were from the female genital tract (vagina, cervix), three were from placental tissues, two were recovered from blood, and one isolate each was recovered from skin, urine, and an infected wound. Nine of these 13 isolates reacted with the new provisional group antigen C1, three reacted with Lancefield group P antiserum, and one isolate was nongroupable. *S. iniae* is a β-hemolytic streptococcus that causes abscesses in freshwater dolphins.[332] This species does not react with any Lancefield antisera. *S. shiloi*, a β-hemolytic streptococcal species that causes meningoencephalitis in trout, is identical biochemically and genetically to *S. iniae*.[202] The β-hemolytic species *S. intestinalis* is a predominant member of the colonic flora of pigs and is one of the only urease-positive streptococcal species that has been described.[571] In the original description of this organism, 29 of 130 strains examined reacted with Lancefield group G antisera. *S. phocae* is a newly described species of β-hemolytic streptococcus that causes pleuropulmonary infections in harbor seals and gray seals. In the original description of this species, 22 strains were characterized.[623] Five of the 22 strains reacted with Lancefield group C antisera, but the remaining 17 were nongroupable. The same five strains reacted with the Streptex group C latex reagent, 13 strains reacted with the Streptex group F latex reagent, and four failed to react with any Streptex reagent.

Several other "species" of streptococci have been described in the human medical and veterinary literature. The taxonomic status of many of these species is as yet uncertain. In *Bergey's Manual of Systematic Bacteriology*, *S. bovis*, *S. equinus*, and *S. acidominimus* are listed in a section titled "Other Streptococci." These organisms are now considered along with the viridans streptococci, particularly because the group D enterococci were split off into their own genus. Another species, *S. thermophilus*, shares characteristics with *S. bovis*, group B streptococci, *S. equisimilis*, and *S. acidominimus*. More recent DNA hybridization studies indicate a close genetic relation between *S. thermophilus* and *S. salivarius*; this organism may be incorporated as a subspecies of *S. salivarius* or may be a species distinct from *S. salivarius*.[230,597]

Several "species" are listed in *Bergey's Manual* as *species incertae sedis* (species of uncertain affiliation). These include "*S. alactolyticus*," "*S. cecorum*," "*S. garviae*," and "*S. plantarum*." With genetic analysis, several of these organisms have now been placed in groups with genetically related streptococci (see earlier discussion on 16S rRNA sequencing of streptococci) or have been placed as new species in the genus *Enterococcus*. *S. alactolyticus* describes strains from pigs and chickens that genotypically and phenotypically resemble *S. bovis* and *S. equinus*. *S. cecorum* is now included with the enterococci as *Enterococcus cecorum*, a species that is found in the intestines of pigeons.[174,176] *S. garviae* and *S. plantarum* have now been assigned to the genus *Lactobacillus*.

This section of the manual also lists a genus called "*Melissococcus*," containing a single species, "*M. pluton*." This organism causes a disease of bees called "European foulbrood." In 1994, using 16S rRNA sequence data, Cai and Collins[100] demonstrated that *M. pluton* was most closely related to the genus *Enterococcus*. Since the naming of this organism in the genus *Melissococcus* predated the description of the genus *Enterococcus*, incorporation of *M. pluton* among the enterococci would, according to the rules of nomenclature, necessitate that all of the enterococcal species be transferred to the genus *Melissococcus*. Because of the familiarity of the enterococci to both clinicians and microbiologists, Cai and Collins recommended that *M. pluton* remain as the only species in the genus *Melissococcus*.[100]

STREPTOCOCCUS PNEUMONIAE

S. pneumoniae is the major cause of community-acquired bacterial pneumonia. The organism may be harbored in the upper respiratory tract of 5% to 10% of adults, although carriage rates higher than 60% have been reported in closed populations.[494,495] Infants usually become colonized at about 3 to 4 months of age and remain colonized for about 4 months with a given serotype; in adults, colonization and carriage persist from 1 month up to 12 to 18 months.[309] Serious infections with *S. pneumoniae* usually occur in infants younger than 2 years of age and in late middle-aged and elderly adults.[494] Colonization of infants with pneumococci is related to the absence of specific anticapsular antibody and the poorly immunogenic serotypes that are common in this age group.[189,308] The susceptibility of elderly persons to pneumococcal disease reflects aging of the immune system and consequent diminished production of antibodies, along with general changes in levels of activity, compromised mucociliary clearance mechanisms, malnutrition, or debilitation owing to other underlying chronic diseases such as diabetes and alcoholism.[95]

The principal virulence factor in *S. pneumoniae* is the polysaccharide capsule, and anticapsular antibodies are effective in providing protection against pneumococcal infections.[494] The capsule material allows the pneumococcus to escape ingestion and killing by host phagocytic cells. More than 80 antigenically distinct capsular types are recognized, with certain types being more virulent than others.[346] Bacteremic infections are associated predominantly with capsular types 3, 4, 14, and 19. Other serotypes associated with severe pulmonary disease with or without bacteremia include serotypes 1, 2, 5, and 8. Humans develop anticapsular antibodies during acute infections, carriage, or following immunization with pneumococcal vaccine.[496] The currently available pneumococcal vaccine contains capsular polysaccharide from each of the 23 serotypes most frequently associated with disease. The vaccine

provides a substantial degree of protection in most subjects, although responses to the polysaccharide antigens are reduced in those persons with underlying diseases or conditions (e.g., lymphoma, HIV infection, renal transplantation, splenectomy). In the appropriate host, *S. pneumoniae* may gain access to the alveolar spaces by aspiration or inhalation and eventually may cause a lobar pneumonia, with consolidation and bacteremia. Conditions that are recognized to predispose adults to pneumococcal disease include underlying bronchopulmonary disease or conditions that compromise humoral immunity.[95] Therefore, the incidence and severity of pneumococcal disease are increased among those persons with defects in upper respiratory tract clearance mechanisms (smokers, those with asthma, chronic bronchitis, chronic obstructive pulmonary disease, or with bronchogenic or squamous cell carcinoma of the lung). Viral respiratory tract infections also predispose to pneumococcal infection of the respiratory tract because these agents also damage the bronchial clearance mechanisms. Conditions that abrogate the humoral immune response (e.g., myeloma, lymphoma, chronic lymphocytic leukemia, hepatic cirrhosis, HIV infection, complement component deficiencies) probably have the greatest influence on individual susceptibility to pneumococcal infection. The onset of pneumococcal disease is generally abrupt, even in patients in whom a prior respiratory viral infection, with its attendant symptoms of nonproductive cough and low-grade fever, is the principal predisposing factor. Symptomatology of acute pneumococcal pneumonia includes cough and copious sputum production, which reflects the intense alveolar inflammatory response to the rapidly dividing pneumococci. In elderly patients, this presentation may be altered; in these patients, the presentation may vary from a minimal cough, with an actual decrease in temperature, to a fulminant presentation, leading rapidly to shock and death. Blood cultures are positive in 20% to 30% of patients with pneumococcal pneumonia. Complications of pneumococcal pneumonia include lung abscess, pericardial infections, empyema, pleural effusions, and endocarditis.[494] The case fatality rate for pneumococcal pneumonia is about 5% but may approach 20% to 30% when accompanied by bacteremia. Pneumococcal bacteremia without pulmonary involvement is an entity that occurs in immunologically compromised hosts. Underlying diseases or conditions that predispose patients to pneumococcal bacteremia include splenectomy, acute myelogenous leukemia, bone marrow transplantation, sickle cell disease, HIV infection, and short bowel syndrome.[281,287,415,511,556,559]

S. pneumoniae is also the most common cause of bacterial meningitis in adults; with the increasing use of the conjugate vaccines for *Haemophilus influenzae* type b, the pneumococcus is also the most common agent in infants and toddlers.[495] In adults, the pneumococcus accounts for about 15% of cases of meningitis in the United States and has an associated mortality of 20% to 25%.[596,699] *S. pneumoniae* meningitis usually occurs as a result of seeding of the meninges during bacteremia. *S. pneumoniae* is also the leading cause of meningitis following skull fractures. Head trauma resulting in basilar skull fracture with leakage of cerebrospinal fluid interrupts the integrity of the dura mater and may allow direct entry of organisms into the central nervous system from an adjacent site of infection (e.g., sinusitis, mastoiditis, otitis media).[495] *S. pneumoniae* accounts for 20% to 50% of cases of acute otitis media and has also been associated with sinusitis and mastoiditis.[69]

This organism is an infrequent cause of endocarditis, peritonitis, septic arthritis, and pelvic infections in women. Pneumococci account for less than 3% of cases of bacterial endocarditis. Most patients have underlying disease, such as diabetes and alcoholism, and other foci of pneumococcal illness such as meningitis or pneumonia.[545] Pneumococcal endocarditis follows an acute course, is associated with the formation of aortic perivalvular abscesses, and has a mortality rate in excess of 50%.[276] Primary peritonitis caused by the pneumococci was once a frequently seen clinical entity in children but is now seen primarily in adults with cirrhosis along with enteric gram-negative bacilli. Septic arthritis caused by *S. pneumoniae* is seen mostly in children with sickle cell disease.[643] In some women, *S. pneumoniae* may be a transient part of the vaginal flora and pelvic, obstetric, and gynecologic infections can occur, particularly with predisposing conditions, such as the presence of an intrauterine device or recent gynecologic surgery.[191,702]

S. pneumoniae has also been recognized as a significant cause of soft-tissue infections, such as facial and periorbital cellulitis, fasciitis, rhabdomyolysis, and abscesses. Most of these have occurred in hosts with underlying conditions, such as systemic lupus erythematosus, end-stage renal disease, rheumatoid arthritis, or HIV infection, and an association with connective tissue disorders has been noted by several investigators.[182,283,306,424,522,527,573,627,631] *S. pneumoniae* is also an important pathogen in patients with HIV infections. Infections tend to occur early in the course of HIV infection (often before a diagnosis of such infection has even been considered), are unusually severe, and often have unusual clinical presentations along with bacteremia.[532] Rodriguez-Barradas reported five cases of severe pneumococcal infections in HIV-infected patients; presentations included pneumonia with recurrent pleural effusions, pyopneumothorax complicated by a bronchopleural fistula, purpura fulminans with peripheral gangrene of the extremities, pneumococcal mediastinitis with adjacent chest wall soft-tissue infection, and pneumococcal brain abscess.[573]

Currently, the major concern surrounding *S. pneumoniae* is the emergence of resistance to antimicrobial agents, especially penicillin.[102,405] Pneumococci with decreased resistance to penicillin were first reported in 1967 and, since then, isolates with high-level resistance to penicillin and other agents have been reported from several areas throughout the world.[20,606] Penicillin resistance in *S. pneumoniae* is associated with altered penicillin-binding proteins (PBPs) that have a decreased affinity for binding penicillin to the bacterial cell wall.[369,736] Strains with penicillin minimal inhibitory concentrations (MICs) of 0.06 µg/mL or less are considered susceptible, those with MICs of 0.1 to 1 µg/mL are considered intermediately resistant, and those with MICs higher than 1 µg/mL are considered resistant.[367,405] During the period 1987 and 1988, rates of pneumococcal resistance to penicillin in the United States were between 4% and 5%; in 1990 to 1991, more than 15% of strains had penicillin MICs of 0.12 to 1 µg/mL and 2.6% had MICs higher than 1 µg/mL.[380,652] Strains that are resistant to penicillin G are also more resistant to other penicillins and cephalosporins of all generations, and treatment failures for serious pneumococcal infections have been reported with previously useful agents such as cefotaxime, cefuroxime, and ceftriaxone.[102,110,367,377,553] Besides the penicillins and cephalosporins, pneumococcal resistance to several other antimicrobial agents, including chloramphenicol, macrolides, quinolones, sulfonamides, and tetracylines, has been reported.[369]

Additional information on *S. pneumoniae* and methods for antimicrobial susceptibility testing are found in Chapter 15.

VIRIDANS STREPTOCOCCI

The viridans group of organisms includes several species of α- and nonhemolytic streptococci, most of which constitute part of the normal upper respiratory tract and urogenital tract flora.[258,331] These streptococci are seen in 30% to 40% of cases of subacute bacterial endocarditis, and in this setting cause a sustained bacteremia, leading to their recovery from multiple sets of blood cultures.[567,688] Viridans streptococcal endocarditis occurs most frequently in individuals with preexisting native valvular disease; they may also be associated with infection of prosthetic valves. Viridans streptococcal endocarditis presents insidiously, with fever, fatigue, and weight loss being the most common findings. Heart murmurs, peripheral stigmata of endocarditis (e.g., splinter and conjunctival hemorrhages, petechiae), and vegetations on echocardiogram are also frequently present. Complications of viridans streptococcal endocarditis include paravalvular abscesses and glomerulonephritis associated with circulating immune complexes.[513] Reference identifications of viridans streptococcal species that are associated with subacute bacterial endocarditis indicate that *S. sanguis*, *S. oralis*, *S. gordonii*, *S. mitis*, *S. mutans*, and *S. salivarius* have been significant causes of this infection.[187,366,688] The oropharynx is the probable source of bacteria in most of these infections; poor oral hygiene and periodontal disease are often noted in these patients. Other procedures, such as fiberoptic sigmoidoscopy, may also cause a transient bacteremia that may infect previously damaged heart valves.[507] The presence of an infected atrial myxoma has also been described as the cause of sustained bacteremia with viridans streptococci.[649]

Although transient bacteremias with these organisms are generally cleared in the normal host without any adverse sequelae, prolonged bacteremia with viridans streptococci, particularly in neutropenic patients undergoing cancer chemotherapy, has become recognized as a distinct clinical entity.[32,70,71,688] Bacteremia in these patients is associated with aggressive cytotoxic chemotherapy administered for the treatment of leukemias or solid tumors (e.g., small cell carcinoma of the bronchus, breast cancer, stomach cancer) and for bone marrow transplantation.[32,46,93,130,632] Risk factors for the development of viridans streptococcal bacteremia in these immunocompromised patients include the administration of high doses of cytotoxic agents (e.g., cytosine arabinoside), the presence of oral mucosal ulcerations secondary to cytotoxic chemotherapy or radiation, the absence of previous antimicrobial therapy, and severe neutropenia.[71] The oral mucosal lesions probably serve as the portal of entry for these organisms into the blood stream. Viridans streptococcal bacteremia in these patients may be complicated by the development of adult respiratory distress syndrome (ARDS), hypotension, shock, and bacterial endocarditis.[70,71,391,472] Viridans streptococcal species that have been associated with bacteremia primarily include *S. mitis, S. oralis, S. salivarius,* and *S. sanguis*.[46,70,71,93,130,632] Bacteremic infections with viridans streptococci have also been reported in low-birth-weight term and preterm neonates.[1] The mothers of these neonates frequently have several risk factors that adversely affect pregnancy outcome, including chorioamnionitis, premature rupture of fetal membranes, premature onset of labor, and urinary tract infection at the time of delivery.

Viridans streptococci may also be isolated on rare occasions from other serious infections, such as meningitis and pneumonia, particularly in compromised hosts. Meningitis caused by viridans streptococci may occur in both adults and children, and the clinical presentation differs little from that of the other pyogenic meningitides (i.e., nuchal rigidity, seizures, meningeal inflammation, and altered mental status).[61,157] The source of the organism in most cases is endogenous; congenital structural abnormalities of the head and neck, head and neck infections, endocarditis, extracranial infections, and previous head trauma or neurosurgical procedures have been associated with the development of meningitis, but definite sources of infection may not be pinpointed in up to a third of cases.[411] Recurrent viridans streptococcal meningitis has been documented in children with structural abnormalities of the inner ear and mastoid sinuses.[478] Meningitis and bacteremia caused by *S. mitis* and *S. salivarius* have been reported following lumbar puncture, upper gastrointestinal endoscopy, and cauterization for a gastric bleed.[68,106,501,654] Similarly, a case of recurrent *S. sanguis* meningitis was reported in a 15-year-old boy with a ventriculoperitoneal shunt.[12] Colville and associates[143] reported the first case of meningitis caused by *S. oralis* in a healthy 12-year-old girl following extraction of a deciduous canine tooth as part of her orthodontic treatments. *S. salivarius* was isolated as a cause of meningitis in a previously healthy 73-year-old woman who was subsequently found to have an asymptomatic colonic adenocarcinoma, suggesting an association of this "*S. bovis*-like" species with occult neoplastic dis-

ease.[432] The rare isolate *S. acidominimus* has also been reported as a cause of meningitis, pericarditis, and pneumonia in a previously healthy 41-year-old man.[11]

Bacteremic viridans streptococcal pneumonia has also been reported but is rare. Marrie reported on seven patients with community-acquired viridans streptococcal pneumonia.[453] All seven patients were older (49 to 80 years old), had several predisposing conditions (including alcoholism, resected carcinoma of the lung, hypothyroidism, diabetes mellitus), and were bacteremic. Viridans streptococcal isolates from these patients included *S. mitis, S. sanguis, S. intermedius,* and *S. uberis.* Sarker and colleagues[593] reported three cases of community-acquired viridans streptococcal pneumonia with concomitant positive blood cultures in previously healthy adults. Empyema and lung abscesses associated with viridans streptococcal pneumonia are also relatively rare clinical entities.[108,546] Miscellaneous infections caused by various species of viridans streptococci have included epiglottitis, septic arthritis, and vertebral osteomyelitis secondary to bacteremia, pericarditis, and infectious crystalline keratitis.[11,72,91,108,361,467,525,578,660]

Many species of viridans streptococci inhabiting the oral cavity have emerged as significant pathogens associated predominantly with the initiation and pathogenesis of dental caries. *S. mutans, S. sobrinus,* and other members of the "*S. mutans* group" of oral streptococci are able to produce enzymes called **glucosyltransferases**, which hydrolyze dietary sucrose (a disaccharide of glucose and fructose) and connect the glucose moieties together in α-1,6 and α-1,4 glycosidic linkages to form insoluble glucans.[416] These glucans enable these organisms to adhere to the smooth surfaces of the teeth and form the matrix of dental plaque. Specific and nonspecific attachment of *S. mutans* and other organisms to the insoluble, adherent glucans and subsequent formation of acid leads to demineralization of the tooth enamel and the initiation of carious lesions. Other oral streptococci, including *S. sanguis, S. salivarius,* and possibly *S. gordonii,* are also able to synthesize these polysaccharides, but only the "mutans strep" display sucrose-induced enhancement of oral colonization.[441,666,677] In addition, the mutans streptococci also appear to produce a greater amount of acid from carbohydrates than other oral bacteria because they are able to ferment a wide variety of sugars, and they are more acid-tolerant than other oral streptococci.[335,441] These organisms also synthesize intracellular polysaccharides that can be metabolized to acid in the absence of exogenous fermentable carbohydrates, enabling these organisms to produce significant amounts of acid even "between meals."[441] Other oral streptococci, including *S. vestibularis,* are not able to initiate dental caries in animal models.[716] The mutans streptococci originally described a single species—*S. mutans*—that was divided into eight serotypes designated *a* through *h* based on the serological specificity of cell wall carbohydrate antigens.[323] Subsequently, these various serotypes were assigned separate species status.[150,151] *S. mutans* (which include serogroups c, e, and f) and *S. sobrinus* (serogroups d and g) are those members of the mutans group that predominate in humans, with the other species being found in various animals (see Table 12-2).[48,150,151,711] Monclonal antibodies against *S. mutans* that are used along with colony immunoblot techniques have been developed by workers in dental microbiology for identification and enumeration of these organisms in saliva and dental plaque specimens.[173]

Before the 1980s, the various species of viridans streptococci were described entirely in terms of their phenotypic characteristics. Analysis of the viridans streptococci by molecular and genetic techniques and with expanded batteries of phenotypic tests has considerably altered the taxonomy of these organisms. Major changes that have occurred as a result of these analyses include emended descriptions of well-recognized species such as *S. mitis* and *S. sanguis*, the discovery and description of several new species of oral viridans streptococci (e.g., *S. vestibularis*, *S. gordonii*, *S. parasanguis*, *S. oralis*, and *S. crista*), the division of the various serotypes of the *S. mutans* group into distinct species, and the taxonomic reassignment of the viridans "streptococcus" *S. morbillorum* as a second species in the genus *Gemella*.[48,150–153,327,381,395,400,707,709,711]

Some of the new viridans *Streptococcus* species have particularly interesting aspects to their ecology that, at present, only suggest their putative roles in the initiation of pathology. A particularly interesting new viridans streptococcus that has been described is *S. crista*.[327] This species resembles the "old" *S. sanguis* I, except that the organisms have tufts of short fibrils located in a lateral position on the cell surface rather then having sparse, peritrichously arranged fibrils. These organisms appear to specifically coaggregate with *Corynebacterium matruchotii* (the old *Bacterionema matruchotii*) both in vitro and in vivo within dental plaque. On electron microscopy, this specific interaction appears as a "corn-on-the-cob" arrangement, with the straight *C. matruchotii* bacilli being the cob, and the adherent streptococci being the kernels of corn. These strains were previously called "*S. sanguis* I with tufts of fibrils," the "CR-group," and the "tufted fibril group."[327] This species is the only one that demonstrates the coaggregation just described, and the organism is phenotypically distinguishable from other viridans streptococci. The role of the specific interaction between *S. crista* and *C. matruchotii* in the pathogenesis of plaque formation is unknown.

Not all of the viridans streptococci are found in human infections. *S. mitis*, *S. sanguis*, *S. salivarius*, *S. bovis*, and the organisms composing the *S. milleri* group are the most frequent isolates from human infections such as endocarditis. Although reported from human specimens, *S. uberis* and *S. parauberis* are primarily animal isolates and cause bovine mastitis.[54,350,373,718] The frequency of some of the newly described species (e.g., *S. oralis*, *S. gordonii*, *S. vestibularis*, *S. crista*, *S. parasanguis*) in clinical specimens is not known and awaits further investigations as methods for their reliable identification become more readily available to clinical microbiology laboratories.[400,707,709]

In years past, the viridans streptococci were generally susceptible to penicillin, ampicillin, and most other antimicrobial agents. However, in recent years, susceptibility surveys of viridans streptococci have clearly shown that resistance to penicillins, cephalosporins, aminoglycosides, and other classes of antimicrobial agents has increased. Potgeiter and colleagues reported the antimicrobial susceptibilities of 211 viridans streptococci recovered from blood cultures.[544] Although all isolates were susceptible to cefotaxime, ceftriaxone, imipenem, and vancomycin, 38% were resistant to penicillin (MICs 0.25 µg/mL or higher), 41% were resistant to erythromycin, and 7% were resistant to both erythromycin and tetracycline. Five *S. mitis* strains were resistant to penicillin (MICs of 16 to 32 µg/mL) and also showed increased resistance (MICs of 64 to 128 µg/mL) or high-level resistance (MICs 500 µg/mL or higher) to gentamicin and tobramycin. Kaufhold and Potgeiter reported on four blood culture isolates of *S. mitis* that were resistant to penicillin (MICs 16 to 32 µg/mL); two of these were resistant to gentamicin (MIC 128 µg/mL), and two demonstrated high-level gentamicin resistance (MIC higher than 1000 µg/mL).[386] Polymerase chain reaction (PCR) and probe analysis of these strains showed that the *S. mitis* strains contained the same structural gene that codes for gentamicin resistance in strains of *E. faecalis* and *E. faecium* and that this genetic determinant was integrated into the chromosome and was not borne on a plasmid. Wilcox and coworkers[715] examined 44 isolates of viridans streptococci recovered from cases of endocarditis and found that 20% of them were resistant to penicillin. These resistant strains were also more resistant to the cephalosporins.

THE "STREPTOCOCCUS MILLERI" GROUP (STREPTOCOCCUS ANGINOSUS, STREPTOCOCCUS CONSTELLATUS, AND STREPTOCOCCUS INTERMEDIUS)

Among the viridans streptococci, a group of organisms that has gone through repeated taxonomic revisions is the *S. milleri* group, so named in the British taxonomic literature. In the CDC scheme for identification of viridans streptococci, *S. milleri* strains corresponded to two α-hemolytic or nonhemolytic minute-colony species (*S. intermedius* and *S. constellatus*) and to minute-colony β-hemolytic streptococci (*S. anginosus*) that may or may not carry Lancefield group antigens (group A, C, F, or G). In 1987, Coykendall and coworkers proposed that all members of the *S. milleri* group (the three CDC species) were actually only a single species based on DNA hybridization studies.[155] All of these organisms would, therefore, be called *S. anginosus*, which was the original name proposed for these bacteria. Then, in 1990 and 1991, Whiley and Beighton presented additional genetic and phenotypic data supporting the distinct nature of these organisms and proposed that *S. anginosus*, *S. intermedius*, and *S. constellatus* be reinstated as separate species.[705] These workers and others have also documented that *S. intermedius* is associated more frequently with liver and brain abscesses than the other two species, and that *S. anginosus* is seen in infections having either gastrointestinal or genitourinary sources.[292,706] The shifting sand of bacterial nomenclature illustrated by these organisms again represents the expansion of genetic methods into bacterial taxonomy.

The three species composing the *Streptococcus milleri* group—*S. intermedius*, *S. constellatus*, and *S. anginosus*—are recognized for their propensity to cause purulent, deep tissue abscesses, bacteremia, endocarditis, intra-abdominal infections, pulmonary infections, central nervous system infections, and oral infections.[249,300,365,483,539,587,620,628] These organisms are part of the normal oropharyngeal flora and may be cultivated from the throat, the nasopharynx, and the gingival crevices. They may also be found normally in the gastrointestinal tract and in the vagina. The recognized virulence of this group may be related to the presence of a capsule on some strains, production of an immunosuppressive protein, and the production of a variety of hydrolytic and glycosoaminoglycan-degrading enzymes (e.g., neuraminidase, DNase, chondroitin sulfate depolymerase, and hyaluronidase).[23,50,355,585] Bacteremia with members of this group is attributable to a focus of infection elsewhere, with the gastrointestinal and the upper respiratory tracts being the likely sources. These organisms, similar to some of the other viridans streptococcal species discussed in the foregoing, are associated with bacteremia in patients with underlying neoplastic disease who are being treated with cytotoxic regimens, although fulminant bacteremia in previously healthy individuals may also occur.[149,249,365] *S. milleri* group organisms account for about 8% of cases of endocarditis caused by viridans streptococci. However, unlike endocarditis caused by other viridans streptococcal species, normal and previously damaged heart valves appear to be equally susceptible to infection by these more virulent streptococci.

Pleuropulmonary infections and head and neck infections caused by *S. milleri* usually occur in the form of mixed-flora abscesses, and these abscesses serve as a focus for bacteremia. Pleuropulmonary infection usually results from aspiration, leading to pneumonia that is often complicated by empyema and the formation of lung abscesses.[577] These organisms are also associated with dental and periapical abscesses and other suppurative infections in the mouth. Fisher and Russell isolated milleri group streptococci from 37% of 45 patients with dentoalveolar periapical abscesses; all but one of these isolates was *S. anginosus*.[248] Spread of the organism from infected sites in the oropharynx may occur by direct extension to involve the soft tissues of the head and neck and the central nervous system. Consequently, *S. milleri* organisms may be recovered in pure or mixed culture from cases of chronic sinusitis, brain abscesses, submandibular abscesses, middle and inner ear fluid, cervical abscesses, epidural abscesses, and subdural empyema fluid.

Up to 40% of infections associated with the *S. milleri* group are intra-abdominal infections that occur following surgery, appendectomy, or as a result of colonic perforation caused by trauma or other gastrointestinal lesions (e.g., colonic carcinoma).[539] Intra-abdominal infection may result in abscesses that yield mixed aerobes and anaerobes on culture. In fact, evidence from animal models suggests that the pathogenic potential of these streptococci is enhanced by synergistic growth with anaerobic bacteria.[615] Intra-abdominal infections are associated with peritonitis and the formation of appendicular, hepatic, subphrenic, and pancreatic abscesses.[128,274] Mucosal bowel trauma and disease apparently facilitate the invasion of the blood stream by the organisms. Tresadern and associates reported on *S. milleri* infections in 23 general surgery patients, many of whom had undergone colorectal procedures, and concluded that the use of preoperative antibiotics, such as gentamicin and metronidazole, may actually promote the emergence of these organisms as pathogens in this anatomic sight.[656] *S. milleri* group organisms are occasionally recovered from gynecologic, obstetric, urogenital, and neonatal infections, including pelvic abscesses, colorectal carcinoma, tuboovarian abscesses, and lesions of the external genitalia.[564] Suppurative metastatic abscesses are a relatively frequent complication of *S. milleri* bacteremia. Abscesses may arise in the liver, joint spaces, spleen, bone, and myocardium. In addition, these bacteria are the causative agents in from 8% to over 30% of all skin and subcutaneous infections. Stocker and coworkers reported on two intravenous drug users with bacteremia and antecubital abscesses caused by *S. milleri* at the sites of drug injection.[637]

S. intermedius, *S. anginosus*, and *S. constellatus* are generally susceptible to penicillin, ampicillin, cefotaxime, vancomycin, trimethoprim, and ciprofloxacin.[292] Some strains may be resistant to erythromycin and clindamycin.

THE NUTRITIONALLY VARIANT STREPTOCOCCI (*ABIOTROPHIA* SPECIES)

Nutritionally variant streptococci are viridans streptococci that require thiol compounds, cysteine, or the active form of vitamin B_6—pyridoxal or pyridoxamine—for growth in media.[104,105] These isolates have variously been called nutritionally variant, nutritionally deficient, thiol-requiring, pyridoxal-requiring, and "satelliting" streptococci.[595] From use of media supplemented with pyridoxal, a taxonomic relation was suggested to exist between nutritionally variant streptococci, *S. mitis*, and *S. sanguis* II.[105] DNA relatedness studies comparing nutritionally variant streptococci with other species of viridans streptococci, however, have shown that two DNA hybridization groups, representing two different species, comprise the members of the nutritionally variant streptococci. These two groups fit the genus description of *Streptococcus* but are unrelated to other viridans streptococci. In 1989, the two nutritonally variant streptococcal species were given the names *Streptococcus defectivus* and *Streptococcus adjacens*.[78] Further analysis of the rRNA gene restriction patterns of these organisms by the same group of researchers confirmed that they indeed represented two distinct species and that the rRNA intraspecies variation seen with *S. defectivus* suggests that there may be two subspecies of *S. defectivus*. In 1995, Kawamura and associates in Japan performed

16S rRNA sequence analysis of these two species and found that they were not related to any species belonging to the genus *Streptococcus*. These workers proposed the new genus *Abiotrophia* to accommodate the former nutritionally variant streptococci, with the new species names being *Abiotrophia adiacens* and *Abiotrophia defectiva*.[388]

Abiotrophia species are a part of the normal flora of the upper respiratory, urogenital, and gastrointestinal tracts and may also be found in disease processes. They have been recovered primarily from patients with endocarditis, although isolates from other sites (e.g., respiratory tract, vaginal discharge, conjunctivae, cutaneous wounds, pleural fluid, middle ear aspirates, brain abscess, pancreatic abscess) have also been reported.[39,76,78,105,464,515] They have been associated with intestinal and postpartum sepsis, osteomyelitis, pneumonia, and neoplastic diseases. These organisms produce a variety of extracellular factors in vitro, including neuraminidase and several aminopeptidases, that may contribute to their virulence.[49] Because of their clinical significance and their exacting cultural requirements, it is essential that the clinical microbiologist be familiar with the clinical settings in which they occur and the laboratory methods that are necessary for their isolation from patient specimens.

STREPTOCOCCUS SUIS

Streptococcus suis deserves special mention because of its economic importance and its recognition as an important zoonotic pathogen.[570] This organism was originally recognized as a cause of meningitis, sepsis, and purulent arthritis in young pigs.[349] These animals become colonized in the tonsils and nasal passages between 5 and 10 weeks of age; carriage rates among healthy animals may be as high as 80%.[26] A study recently performed in Australia showed that over 70% of pigs slaughtered for human consumption in that country were carriers of *S. suis*.[569,570] In sick animals, the organism initially causes anorexia and fever; meningeal involvement is manifested by the onset of seizures, paralysis, and death.

The first human cases of *S. suis* infection were reported in 1968 from Denmark; by 1989, 108 human cases of *S. suis* infection had been reported in the literature. Most cases have occurred in Hong Kong, the Netherlands, Denmark, Great Britain, France, Canada, Belgium, Germany, and Sweden. Although most of these cases involved individuals who had occupational exposure to pigs, those cases reported from Hong Kong have been attributed to the heavy consumption of pork in that country.[117] In fact, *S. suis* is now the most common cause of meningitis in Hong Kong. The organism has also been isolated from swine herds in the United States (e.g., Minnesota and Nebraska).[210] In 1991, Trottier and colleagues in Quebec reported the first case of human endocarditis caused by *S. suis* in North America.[658]

S. suis disease occurs mainly in individuals who are exposed to or work with swine and includes abattoir and slaughterhouse workers, pig farmers, meat inspectors, veterinarians, and others in the food-processing industry who work with pork preparations.[92,185,568] The organism is believed to enter the host percutaneously through cuts, scratches, or abrasions in the skin. Entry of the organisms through the nasopharynx and the gastrointestinal tract has also been proposed.[27] After organism acquisition, the onset of disease is heralded by an "influenza-like" prodrome, with the rapid development of bacteremia and meningitis.[27,329,340,446,448] Overwhelming bacteremia without the development of meningitis may also occur.[92,340] The most common sequela of meningeal infection is cochlear–vestibular involvement resulting in ataxia and dizziness.[195] Involvement of the eighth cranial nerve is also commonly seen and results in unilateral or bilateral hearing loss.[604] Complications result from seeding of distant sites during bacteremia and may include arthritis, spondylodiscitis, endophthalmitis, pneumonia, and gastroenteritis.[25,185,448,469] Several cases of *S. suis* endocarditis have also been reported.[185,352,528,658] The organism is susceptible to penicillin, which is the drug of choice for treating systemic *S. suis* infection.

S. suis was officially recognized as an extant *Streptococcus* species in 1987.[398] Strains are groupable by Lancefield antisera into groups R, S, RS, and T or are ungroupable.[172,409,529,530] The organism also possesses the group D lipoteichoic antigen; consequently, it was thought to be a group D streptococcus or an *Enterococcus* species. This, however, has not been substantiated by genetic techniques. Reactivity with group D antisera is believed to be due to a spurious cross-reaction and is not helpful in identifying the organism. *S. suis* also possesses a capsule, and to date 34 different capsular serotypes, designated serotypes 1 through 34, have been described.[302,303,348,531] *S. suis* serotype 1 causes meningitis in piglets younger than 6 weeks of age. This serotype includes those strains belonging to Lancefield group S. The *S. suis* capsular serotype 2 is also associated with systemic disease in pigs 3 to 20 weeks of age, and it is the only serotype that has been reported to cause systemic disease in humans. This serotype encompasses the Lancefield group R streptococci. Other serotypes having Lancefield groups RS (reacts with both R and S antisera) and T reactivity may be found in both asymptomatic and diseased pigs. In the series of human cases reported in 1988 by Arends and Zanen from The Netherlands, 28 of 30 strains recovered from human infections were capsular serotype 2, one was serotype 4, and one was nontypable.[27] Serotypes can be determined by slide agglutination, immunodiffusion, or coagglutination.[301] Various methods for genomic fingerprinting have demonstrated considerable heterogeneity among strains having the same capsular serotype.[326,481,482] Virulent *S. suis* type 2 strains produce a hemagglutinin, a thiol activated streptolysin O-like hemolysin (suilysin), a cell wall–associated 136-kDa protein, and a 110-kDa extracellular protein that are not found in other serotypes and are believed to function as virulence factors.[237,304,363,674]

THE "STREPTOCOCCUS-LIKE" BACTERIA

ENTEROCOCCUS SPECIES

The genus *Enterococcus* includes the enterococcal members previously classified with the group D streptococci.[598] These organisms are normal residents of the gastrointestinal and biliary tracts and, in lower numbers, of the vagina and male urethra. They are becoming increasingly important agents of human disease, largely because of their resistance to antimicrobial agents to which other streptococci are generally susceptible.[492] Tests of enterococci in vitro have demonstrated that these organisms have penicillin MICs that are 10- to 100-fold higher than other streptococci. Enterococci are important causes of both community-acquired and nosocomial infections; in fact, within the last 6 years enterococci have become the second most common cause of nosocomial infections in the United States and the third most common cause of nosocomial bacteremia.[480,594] Because of their resistance to penicillins and cephalosporins of several generations, the acquisition of high-level resistance to aminoglycosides, and now the recent emergence of vancomycin resistance, these bacteria are often involved in serious superinfections among patients receiving these antimicrobial agents (see later discussion).

The taxonomy of *Enterococcus* species has undergone considerable change since the mid-1980s. Before the advent and widespread use of genetic techniques for taxonomic analysis, enterococci were distinguished from streptococci and related taxa by their ability to grow at 10°C and 45°C, growth in the presence of 6.5% NaCl, growth at pH 9.6, ability to hydrolyze esculin in the presence of 40% bile, and production of pyrrolidonyl arylamidase (PYR). More than 90% of strains also contained the Lancefield group D lipoteichoic antigen in their cell wall. Current taxonomic studies have subsequently revealed several species that are members of the genus *Enterococcus* by genetic criteria, but that lack many of the phenotypic characteristics typical of the genus.[720] Fortunately, most of these species are not commonly found in human clinical specimens. *E. faecalis* is the most common isolate, being associated with 80% to 90% of human enterococcal infections. *E. faecium* ranks second and is isolated from 10% to 15% of infections. Other enterococcal species, including *E. avium*, *E. casseliflavus*, *E. durans*, *E. gallinarum*, *E. raffinosus*, *E. hirae*, *E. malodoratus*, and *E. mundtii*, are infrequently isolated from human infections.[120,136,138,139,165,219,313,383,475,523,542,584,670] The other species are rarely encountered in human clinical specimens or are primarily found in the gastrointestinal tracts of various animals.[86,140,174,175,177,232,418,456,541,572,719] However, reports of other *Enterococcus* species from human infections will be seen from time to time in the literature. In the era of the compromised host, the clinical microbiologist should be aware of these other species and the methods for their identification. Members of the genus *Enterococcus* are described in Table 12-4.

Unlike several of the streptococcal species discussed thus far, the factors that determine the pathogenicity of the enterococci are not well understood.[375] Some strains of *E. faecalis* and *E. faecium* produce a **cytolysin** that acts as a hemolysin against human, rabbit, equine, and bovine erythrocytes (but not sheep erythrocytes) and is toxic for certain eukaryotic cell types.[122,358] **Aggregation substance** is a surface-bound, plasmid-encoded protein that promotes clumping of the organisms to facilitate the exchange of plasmids.[122,194] This substance is also believed to function in enterococcal adherence to intestinal and renal epithelial cells and to cardiac vegetations in an experimental endocarditis model.[122,267,412] *E. faecalis* strains also produce **pheromones**, which are small peptides that are secreted by the organism and that promote the conjugative transfer of plasmid DNA between strains.[131,132] It also appears that these same molecules may act as chemoattractants for neutrophils, thereby helping to augment the inflammatory response to infection.[208] **Lipoteichoic acids** constitute the group D antigen of enterococci and may also function in virulence by inducing the production of tumor necrosis factor (TNF) and interferon, leading to modulation of the immune response.[661,714] Some *E. faecalis* strains apparently also produce a plasmid-encoded, 7.4-kDa **bacteriocin**, called AS-48, that has lytic activity for a wide spectrum of gram-positive and gram-negative bacteria.[375] Lastly, some *E. faecalis* strains produce various extracellular enzymes, such as **gelatinase** and **hyaluronidase**.[449,575]

Enterococcus species cause complicated urinary tract infections, bacteremia, endocarditis, intra-abdominal and pelvic infections, wound and soft-tissue infections, neonatal sepsis, and, rarely, meningitis. Enterococci have been associated with cystitis, pyelonephritis, prostatitis, and perinephric abscesses; most of these are nosocomial in origin, or are associated with structural abnormalities or instrumentation of the urinary tract.[413,488] Risk factors for the development of bacteremia include immunosuppression or debilitation because of prematurity, diabetes, malignancy, and deep-seated infections (e.g., secondarily infected decubitus ulcers), prior gastrointestinal, genitourinary, or respiratory tract instrumentation, long-term hospitalization, and the use of broad-spectrum antibiotics having little or no antienterococcal activity (e.g., cephalosporins).[305,318,689] The organisms generally gain entry into the bloodstream through the urinary tract, intra-abdominal or pelvic sepsis, wounds, decubitus ulcers, or intravenous access devices. Enterococci also cause 5% to 20% of all cases of endocarditis, and they are the fifth most common cause of prosthetic valve endocarditis.[473,492] Endocarditis usually occurs in older patients with underlying valvular disease or with prosthetic valves and is generally subacute in clinical presentation.[473,563,675] In intra-abdominal and pelvic infections, enterococci usually are found admixed with other indigenous aerobic and anaerobic organisms; pure spontaneous enterococcal peritonitis and enterococcal peritonitis associated with continuous ambulatory peritoneal dialysis have also been reported.[186,492,503]

TABLE 12-4
MEMBERS OF THE GENUS *ENTEROCOCCUS*

SPECIES	COMMENTS
E. faecalis	Most frequent isolate from human clinical specimens and from the human gastrointestinal tract; also found in the intestinal tracts of poultry, cattle, pigs, dogs, horses, sheep, and goats.
E. faecium	Also found in human clinical specimens; generally more resistant to antimicrobial agents than *E. faecalis*; also found in the gastrointestinal tracts of various species of animals.
E. avium	Isolated from avian, canine, and human gastrointestinal tracts; strains may carry both Lancefield group D and group Q carbohydrate antigens; this species (and *E. malodoratus*) are the two enterococcal species that produce H_2S.
E. durans	Rare clinical isolate; found mainly in milk and other dairy products.
E. casseliflavus	Recovered from plants, soil, and rarely, from the feces of chickens; originally classified as a subspecies of *E. faecium*; produces a yellow pigment and is also motile; opportunistic agent in human infections.
E. gallinarum	Isolated from chicken feces; originally classified as *Streptococcus gallinarum* "chicken group D"; one of the two motile *Enterococcus* species; has also been isolated from an infection in a hemodialysis patient.
E. malodoratus	Isolated from Gouda cheese and unpasteurized milk products; name means "ill smelling"; also produces H_2S.
E. mundtii	Yellow-pigmented, nonmotile organisms; isolated from plants, soil, and the gastrointestinal tracts of cattle, pigs, and horses; named after J. O. Mundt, an American microbiologist.
E. hirae	Causes growth depression in chickens; isolated from chicken crops and feces, and the gastrointestinal tracts of cattle, pigs, dogs, horses, sheep, goats, and rabbits; type strain (*E. hirae* ATCC 8043) has complex nutritional requirements and is used in the food industry as a bioassay organism for amino acids and vitamins.
E. raffinosus	Originally considered to be related to *E. avium* (along with *E. solitarius* and *E. pseudoavium*); named for its ability to produce acid from raffinose; recovered from human infections, including blood cultures, urine, and abscesses.
E. pseudoavium	Genetic relatedness studies and certain phenotypic characteristics differentiate this species from *E. avium*; type strain isolated from a case of bovine mastitis
E. dispar	Species originally thought to be a biochemical variant of *E. hirae*, but analysis of 16S rRNA indicated that this organism is indeed a previously undescribed species; recovered from human specimens, including stool and synovial fluid.
E. sulfureus	Newly described, yellow-pigmented species; recovered from plants; has not been isolated from humans (yet).
E. flavescens	Newly described, yellow-pigmented, motile species; has been isolated from several specimens of human origin, including blood, abscess material, and bone (osteomyelitis); closely related to other yellow-pigmented enterococcal species (i.e., *E. casseliflavus*, *E. mundtii*, and *E. sulfureus*).
E. cecorum	Newly reclassified former streptococcal species found in intestines of chickens; lacks the group D antigen, is PYR-negative, and is unable to grow in salt broth; similar to *E. columbae*, it may be confused with *E. avium* and with *S. bovis*.
E. columbae	New reclassified streptococcal species isolated from the intestinal tract of pigeons; closely related to *E. cecorum* and *E. avium*; characterized by being unable to grow in 6.5% NaCl and being PYR-negative.
E. saccharolyticus	Originally called *S. saccharolyticus*; described a group of *S. bovis*-like strains recovered from cows; genetic analysis has shown that it is more closely related to the enterococci than the streptococci; has certain phenotypic characteristics that are similar to *Enterococcus* species (e.g., growth at 10°C and 45°C, growth in 6.5% NaCl), but does not react with group D antisera; proposed that this species be moved from the viridans streptococcus group to the genus *Enterococcus* as *E. saccharolyticus*.
"*E. solitarius*"	Delineated as an *Enterococcus* species by DNA homology studies; only a single isolate (the type strain 885/78) has been described; this strain was recovered from an "ear exudate" (the species of the organism to which the "ear" was attached was not specified in the report); does not react with the genus-specific rRNA probe (AccuProbe *Enterococcus*, Gen Probe, San Diego CA); 16S rRNA sequence studies indicate that this species is most closely related to the newly described species *Tetragenococcus halophilus*.
"*E. seriolicida*"	Causes "streptococcicosis" in yellow-tail fish; has not been isolated from humans or human clinical specimens; 16S rRNA sequencing suggests that this species is identical with that of *Lactococcus garvieae* and, therefore, is not a member of the genus *Enterococcus*.

Enterococcal bacteremia or intra-abdominal abscesses containing enterococci may also develop as a complication of cesarian section, endometritis, or acute pelvic inflammatory disease.[428] Enterococci are rarely isolated from postoperative wound infections after penetrating abdominal trauma if no gastrointestinal perforation has occurred.[503] Enterococci are usually found in wound and soft-tissue infections with other facultative and anaerobic bacteria, and complications associated with such infections (e.g., enterococcal osteomyelitis) are rarely due to enterococci unless they are present as superinfecting agents.[492] Neonatal enterococcal sepsis has an acute, early-onset presentation, characterized by fever and respiratory distress accompanied by bacteremia and meningitis.[44] Premature neonates are at greater risk of developing serious nosocomial enterococcal infections, particularly if peripheral access devices or feeding tubes are in place.[445] Enterococcal meningitis is a rare manifestation of enterococcal infection. Adults with enterococcal meningitis have serious underlying disease, such as malignancy, diabetes, or renal failure, or are receiving treatment with immunosuppressive agents. About one third of patients with enterococcal meningitis have an antecedent history of trauma to the central nervous system (e.g., accidents, surgery, shunt placement), and about one third have enterococcal infection at another site.[442,636] Respiratory tract infection caused by enterococci are rare and only seen in severely debilitated patients.[56]

The resistance of enterococci to a variety of antimicrobial agents does indeed contribute to their pathogenicity. These organisms display intrinsic low-level resistance to the aminoglycosides and lincosamides, have relatively high MICs for penicillins and cephalosporins, and are resistant to the action of sulfonamide agents in vivo.[492] The higher MICs for the β-lactam agents are due to diminished affinity of cell wall penicillin-binding proteins for these agents, whereas low-level aminoglycoside resistance is due to decreased penetrability of the enterococcal cell wall.[204] Although enterococci appear susceptible to sulfonamides in vitro, they are able to circumvent the block in folate synthesis in vivo.

Serious infections associated with enterococci are usually treated with a combination of penicillin or ampicillin with an aminoglycoside. The emergence of high-level resistance to aminoglycosides (i.e., streptomycin MICs higher than 2000 μg/mL; gentamicin MICs higher than 500 μg/mL) in enterococci, particularly E. faecalis and E. faecium, seriously affected the therapeutic approach to and clinical response of patients with bacteremia, endocarditis, and other serious infections.[17,97] High-level aminoglycoside resistance has disseminated among several enterococcal species and has been documented in strains of E. avium, E. casseliflavus, E. gallinarum, E. raffinosus, and E. mundtii.[591] Strains displaying high-level resistance to aminoglycosides are not killed by the synergistic activity of the β-lactam agent along with an aminoglycoside. This high-level resistance is transposon-mediated and can be transferred to other organisms.[204] Bactericidal synergism between penicillin and aminoglycosides requires

that the organism not only have MICs for aminoglycosides lower than the values cited in the foregoing but that the serum concentration of penicillin be near or exceed the MIC; increasing β-lactam resistance among enterococci along with high aminoglycoside MICs further abrogate synergism. High-level resistance to both streptomycin and gentamicin effectively excludes synergistic killing by penicillin–aminoglycoside combination therapy. Because of the lack of reliable penicillin–aminoglycoside synergistic activity among high-level aminoglycoside-resistant enterococci and the emergence of methicillin-resistant S. aureus, vancomycin became a first-line drug effective against both staphylococci and enterococci.

Until the early 1980s, the susceptibility of enterococci to ampicillin and vancomycin remained fairly predictable. Since that time, Enterococcus species resistant to ampicillin or vancomycin have been reported with increasing frequency. Resistance to ampicillin in some E. faecalis strains was demonstrated to be due to production of β-lactamase enzymes.[526] Subsequently, ampicillin resistance in strains of E. faecium, E. gallinarum, and E. raffinosus was reported; with these organisms, resistance was due to decreased penicillin-binding affinity of the cell wall penicillin-binding proteins.[120,204,463] The appearance of vancomycin-resistant strains of E. faecalis and E. faecium heralded a major change in the enterococci. Vancomycin-resistant enterococci, or VRE, have been characterized as having Van A, Van B or Van C phenotypes. E. faecalis and E. faecium isolates that have the vanA genotype characteristically display inducible, transposon-mediated, high-level resistance to both vancomycin (MIC higher than 64 μg/mL) and teicoplanin (MIC of 16 μg/mL or higher), both of which are glycopeptide-class antimicrobial agents.[427,502,590] The vanA gene cluster encodes a D-alanine-D-alanine ligase that synthesizes peptidoglycan precursors with reduced affinities for both vancomycin and teicoplanin.[551] Strains with the vanB genotype have acquired inducible resistance to various concentrations of vancomycin (MICs 8 to 64 μg/mL) but remain susceptible to teicoplanin (MIC 1 μg/mL or lower), although rare vanB strains may also be resistant to the latter antibiotic.[342] Isolates expressing the vanB genotype also include E. faecalis and E. faecium strains. Isolates that have the vanC genotype display intrinsic, constitutive, low-level resistance to vancomycin (MIC ≥ 8, and ≤ 32) and are susceptible to teicoplamin (MIC ≤ 1 μg/mL); this genotype is intrinsic in strains of E. casseliflavus and E. gallinarum, is not transferred by conjugation to other organisms, and is chromosomal in origin.[551,678] Enterococci with the VanA phenotype are most worrisome because these strains are able to transfer vanA resistance markers by a conjugation mechanism to other enterococci and other gram-positive organisms, including Staphylococcus aureus.[80,83,121,506] However, in 1993 and 1994, strains with the vanB class genotype were shown to be able to transfer their vancomycin resistance genes as well.[80,551] Epidemiologic investigations of nosocomial outbreaks caused by VRE have been aided by the development of DNA probes for direct detection of resistance loci.[726]

Identification of *Enterococcus* species is discussed later in this chapter, and methods for susceptibility testing are discussed in detail in Chapter 15.

AEROCOCCUS AND HELCOCOCCUS SPECIES

Aerococci are streptococcus-like organisms that are found in the environment, usually in association with water, and they may be recovered from air, dust, soil, vegetation, meat products, and the hospital environment.[212,390,521] They are known to cause a fatal disease in lobsters, but in humans they are primarily opportunists. Aerococci have been isolated from patients with a number of clinical conditions, including endocarditis, bacteremia, meningitis, septic arthritis, osteomyelitis, and wound infections.[372,392,499,521,538,647,665] Aerococci are included occasionally in proficiency surveys and can easily be confused with the viridans streptococci and enterococci. Aerococci have a characteristic tendency to form tetrads when grown in broth media. The organisms tend to be microaerophilic, and sparse or no growth is observed under anaerobic conditions. Until recently, all aerococci were considered to belong to one species called *Aerococcus viridans*.[212] Isolates that were previously assigned to the genus *Pediococcus* as *P. urinae-equi* have been shown to be closely related phylogenetically to *A. viridans*.[142]

In 1989, Christensen and colleagues in Copenhagen reported on a group of 29 patients with suspected urinary tract infections from whom "*Aerococcus*-like organisms" (ALOs) were recovered from urine specimens.[125,126] In 11 of these patients, this organism was isolated in pure culture (more than 10^6 CFU/mL). The patients (20 women and 9 men) ranged in age from 49 to 88 years old, and half of them had either local or systemic conditions (e.g., diabetes, urinary tract and nonurinary tract malignancies, urolithiasis) that may have predisposed them to infection with opportunistic organisms. Patients with septicemia and endocarditis caused by ALOs are usually elderly, have some type of underlying disease (e.g., myocardial infarction, prostate cancer, diabetes), and have ALOs recovered from both the blood and the urine.[123,124] Phenotypic characterization of these ALO strains demonstrated that they indeed differed from *A. viridans* strains in several respects.[6,126] On the basis of differing phenotypic criteria and phylogenetic analysis of 16S rRNA sequence data from reference strains of *A. viridans*, Aguirre and Collins proposed that ALOs be classified as the new species *Aerococcus urinae*.[6] Strains examined at the CDC have shown less than 10% relatedness between the ALOs and *A. viridans*, suggesting that these organisms may not belong to the genus *Aerococcus*.[221] Since the naming of this new species, additional cases of septicemia and endocarditis caused by *A. urinae* have appeared.[343,414] Strains of *A. viridans* are usually susceptible to penicillin, macrolides, sulfonamides, and trimethoprim. Isolates of *A. urinae* are usually susceptible to penicillin and erythromycin and resistant to the aminoglycosides and sulfonamides.[125,414]

During an examination of several isolates from human clinical sources, Collins and coworkers[137] encountered nine strains of facultative, gram-positive, catalase-negative cocci that resembled aerococci but produced variable growth in 6.5% NaCl broth.[137] Seven of the nine strains were recovered from wounds on the feet or legs, and two isolates were from cultures of breast masses. The other unusual feature of these organisms was that they were lipophilic; growth on agar media and in broth was enhanced by the presence of serum or Tween 80. These organisms were shown to be a new genus and species of gram-positive cocci, both by genetic analysis and by phenotypic criteria. They have been assigned to the new genus *Helcococcus* and have been given the species name *H. kunzii*. Additional studies on the ecology of this new organism suggest an association with the bacterial flora of the lower extremities and a propensity to be isolated from wound infections and cellulitis along with more virulent organisms, such as *S. aureus*.[101]

LEUCONOSTOC SPECIES

Leuconostoc species are gram-positive, nonmotile, non–spore-forming, heterofermentative, facultative cocci that are found in the environment (i.e., on plants, soil, and such).[270] These organisms have economic importance because of their use in the dairy and pickling industries and in wine making. In recent years, these organisms have been isolated from human infections, most of them occurring in immunocompromised hosts.[58,282,285,290,310,312,362] They have been isolated from blood cultures of patients with underlying malignancies and indwelling intravenous catheters and have also been isolated from hepatic and intra-abdominal abscesses, gastrostomy and tracheostomy sites, odontogenic abscesses, breast abscesses, and draining fistulas.[40,58,290,328,333,700] *Leuconostoc* species have been recovered as opportunistic agents causing bacteremia and pulmonary infections in bone marrow recipients and AIDS patients.[240,282,285,534] A *Leuconostoc* species was also isolated from the cerebrospinal fluid of a previously healthy 16-year-old girl, in whom the organism caused a purulent meningeal infection.[146] Friedland and colleagues[263] also reported a case of purulent meningitis due to *L. mesenteroides* in a 1-month-old female infant. Carapetis and coworkers[103] described two cases of bacteremia caused by *Leuconostoc* species (specifically, *L. lactis* and *L. pseudomesenteroides*) in children with necrotizing enterocolitis who were receiving long-term parenteral nutrition. In one of these cases, the same *L. lactis* strain was recovered from the patient's gastrostomy tube site. Finally, bacteremia caused by *L. mesenteroides* and *Enterobacter sakazakii* was reported in association with contaminated infant formula.[508]

The genus *Leuconostoc* consists of the type species *L. mesenteroides* and eight other species including *L. pseudomesenteroides*, *L. lactis*, *L. citreum*, *L. gelidum*, *L. carnosum*, *L. fallax*, *L. argentinum*, and *L. oenos*.[179,233,269,270,457,613] The organisms formerly designated *L. cremoris* and *L. dextranicum* are now included as subspecies of *L. mesenteroides*. Organisms belonging to the former species *L. paramesenteroides* probably will be reclassified in the new genus *Weisella* as *Weisella paramesenteroides*.[141] Similarly, genetic sequencing and hybridization studies and electrophoretic analysis of enzyme activities of *L. oenos* strains has revealed that these organisms form a distinct branch away from the other *Leuconostoc* species. Therefore, it has been proposed that these organisms be transferred to the new genus *Oenococcus* as *Oenococcus oeni*.[178] *L. mesenteroides* subspecies and *L. lactis* are found primarily in milk and milk products, whereas *L. (O.) oenos* is isolated only from wine and related habitats.[269,270] *L. pseudomesenteroides* and *L. citreum* are found on plants, vegetables, and in dairy products. *L. gelidum* and *L. carnosum* are found in meats (beef, pork, bacon, ham). *L. fallax* is found in pickled cabbage (sauerkraut), and *L. argentinum* has been isolated from raw milk (from Argentina, of course).[179] *Leuconostoc* species that have been isolated from human clinical material to date include *L. mesenteroides*, *L. (Weissela) paramesenteroides*, *L. pseudomesenteroides*, *L. citreum*, and *L. lactis*.

These organisms may be misidentified as pneumococci, species of viridans streptococci (especially *S. sanguis* II), or lactobacilli.[98] Similar to lactobacilli and pediococci, but unlike most other gram-positive bacteria, *Leuconostoc* species are intrinsically resistant to vancomycin. In some case reports, patients were being treated with vancomycin when infections with these organisms became clinically apparent. The characteristics of *Leuconostoc* species that help to differentiate them from the other streptococcus-like bacteria are their resistance to vancomycin and the formation of gas from glucose during growth in MRS broth (discussed later). Therapy for serious *Leuconostoc* infections includes penicillin and aminoglycosides; most isolates are susceptible to tetracyclines, imipenem, clindamycin, and gentamicin.

PEDIOCOCCUS AND TETRAGENOCOCCUS SPECIES

Pediococcus species are gram-positive cocci that, similar to the streptococci, produce lactic acid as the sole product of glucose fermentation. These organisms are found naturally on plants and are important in the brewing and food industries.[271] Pediococci may be found in beers and ales and are also used in food, such as sausage and cheese, for processing and preservation. They are included as flavor enhancers in processed vegetables and soy products. As are the micrococci and *E. hirae*, pediococci are also employed in biotechnology as indicator strains for vitamin bioassays. In *Bergey's Manual of Systematic Bacteriology*, eight species are listed as belonging to the genus: *P. acidilactici*, *P. damnosus*, *P. dextrinicus*, *P. inopinatus*, *P. parvulus*, *P. pentosaceus*, *P. urinae-equi*, and *P. halophilus*. Isolates of *P. urinae-equi* phenotypically resemble *A. viridans* and a DNA probe specific for *A. viridans* also reacts with *P. urinae-equi*, indicating that these two organisms are the same.[142,307] Genetic studies using 16S rRNA and DNA–DNA hybridization indicate that *P. halophilus* represents a line of descent that is separate from both pediococci and aerococci and that is more closely related to the enterococci. Because of these genetic data, isolates that were previously called

P. halophilus have been placed in the new genus *Tetragenococcus*, with the type species being *Tetragenococcus halophilus*.[142] Interestingly, *T. halophilus* is susceptible to vancomycin, whereas the other pediococci are vancomycin-resistant.

The Bacterial Reference Laboratory of the Respiratory Diseases Branch at the CDC has received isolates of pediococci from a variety of human clinical specimens, including saliva, stool, urine, wounds, abscesses, and blood.[459] These bacteria have usually been isolated from patients with various underlying conditions, including hematologic malignancies, cardiovascular disease, chronic lung disease, gastroschisis, pancreatitis, and diabetes.[30,147,459,565,621] Several patients also had previous abdominal surgery or had nasogastric tubes or central venous catheters for total perenteral nutrition in place for prolonged periods. Pediococci recovered from blood cultures were usually single, positive cultures among several cultures positive with other organisms. In a study of 26 patients who were undergoing total bowel decontamination with gentamicin–vancomycin–colimycin preparatory to remission induction therapy or bone marrow transplantation, Maugein and colleagues found *Pedicoccus* species in 89% of the stool specimens collected from these patients.[461] Similar to *Leuconostoc* species, these organisms are resistant to vancomycin; many patients first manifest symptoms of infection while being treated with this antimicrobial agent.[459,642] In one report, *P. acidilactici* was identified in multiple blood cultures from a 53-year-old man with acute myeloblastic leukemia.[291] At the time of the first positive blood culture, this patient had been receiving vancomycin for 14 days along with ceftazidime, metronidazole, and cancer chemotherapy. Isolates of pediococci from clinical specimens have been identified as either *P. acidilactici* or *P. pentosaceus*.[147,291,312,459] Pediococci are generally susceptible to penicillin G, erythromycin, clindamycin, gentamicin, and imipenem.[644]

GEMELLA SPECIES

The genus *Gemella* includes two species, *G. haemolysans* and *G. morbillorum*.[583] Although *G. haemolysans* has been recognized for some time, *G. morbillorum* is a recent addition to the genus.[399] *G. haemolysans* is an easily decolorized gram-positive coccus that characteristically appears as diplococci with adjacent sides flattened. Because of these properties, it was previously included with the gram-negative cocci in the genus *Neisseria*. Cell wall analysis demonstrated that the organism did have a gram-positive type cell wall, although it is much thinner than that of other gram-positive organisms. Nucleic acid hybridization studies showed no relatedness to members of the family *Neisseriaceae*. These data, along with the negative catalase reaction, relegated this species to the family *Streptococcaceae*. Unlike the streptococci, however, growth is poor under anaerobic conditions. *G. morbillorum* was previously classified with the streptococci as *Streptococcus morbillorum* and was included among the viridans streptococci in the Facklam scheme.[216] Genetic analysis of *S. morbillorum* strains indicated that the organism was more closely related to *G. haemolysans* than to the streptococci and peptostreptococci.[399,443,713] Gas–liquid chromatography studies showed that, in addition to lactic acid, some strains also form acetic acid, formic acid, succinic acid, pyruvate, and ethanol in small amounts. These additional properties also serve to differentiate this species from the homofermentative streptococci. Consequently, *S. morbillorum* has been reclassified into the genus *Gemella* as *G. morbillorum*.[399]

Members of the genus *Gemella* are infrequently isolated from clinical specimens. However, their similarity to the viridans streptococci has probably resulted in their being underrecognized and misidentified. *G. haemolysans* is part of the upper respiratory tract flora, whereas *G. morbillorum* can be found in the human respiratory and gastrointestinal tracts. Both species have been implicated as occasional causes of human infections, particularly bacteremia and endocarditis.[51,84,262,384,460,487] Cases of meningitis, septic arthritis, and an infected knee arthroplasty associated with *Gemella* species have also been reported.[29,166,201,462,479,512,680] *Gemella* species are usually susceptible to a wide variety of antimicrobial agents, including penicillin, ampicillin, rifampin, and vancomycin, but low-level resistance to aminoglycosides and trimethoprim may be observed in some isolates.[99] However, a strain of *G. haemolysans* that was recovered from a blood culture was found to have decreased susceptibility to penicillin and was frankly resistant to vancomycin, teicoplanin, erythromycin, and tetracycline.[557]

ALLOIOCOCCUS, VAGOCOCCUS, AND GLOBICATELLA SPECIES

In 1989, Faden and Dryja[227] reported on the recovery of a slow-growing, large, gram-positive coccus from 10 children with chronic otitis media with effusion. The children ranged in age from 10 months to almost 3 years, and each of them had two to five previous episodes of otitis media. Middle ear aspirates from these children consisted of serous, mucoid, or frankly purulent fluid; inflammatory cells were observed in all specimens. Large, gram-positive, coccal organisms could also be seen on gram-stained smears in most cases. The organism was recovered in pure culture from 11 ear aspirates and in mixed culture with nontypable *Haemophilus influenzae*, diphtheroids, micrococci, or coagulase-negative staphylococci in five specimens. One of the children examined in the study had this organism isolated from three separate middle ear specimens collected over an 8-month period. On culture, these organisms grew extremely slowly, leading the authors to suggest that perhaps they had been missed in the past because culture plates had not been incubated long enough. Because of the association of this slow-growing gram-positive coccus with chronic otitis media, Faden and Dryja[227] recommended that middle ear aspirates submitted for culture should be incubated for at least 5 days to facilitate detection of these bacteria. In addition to isolates from middle ear fluids, the CDC has received strains of *A. otitidis* that

were recovered from blood cultures and from sputum.[221] Aguirre and Collins[4] subsequently characterized this unusual coccus and named it *Alloiococcus otitis*. A revision of the name of this organism from *A. otitis* to *A. otitidis* was subsequently suggested and approved in keeping with the rules of binomial nomenclature.[681] No information is available on the antimicrobial susceptibility of *A. otitidis*.

During a taxonomic investigation of the "group N lactic streptococci," or lactococci, several motile cocci that also carried the Lancefield group N antigen were found among the strains being examined. These motile organisms had been recovered from chicken feces and river water. With 16S rRNA sequence analysis, it was shown that the lactococci were clearly separate from the streptococci and enterococci and that the motile "lactococcus-like" strains were phylogenetically unrelated to *Lactococcus* species *sensu stricto*. Furthermore, these strains were also found to be phenotypically distinct. Collins and associates[135] have placed these organisms into the new genus *Vagococcus* ("wandering coccus"). The motile group N lactococcus-like isolates in the genus *Vagococcus* are now named *Vagococcus fluvialis* ("belonging to a river"). Strains of *V. fluvialis* have also been recovered from cutaneous lesions and tonsils of pigs, cattle, horses, and domestic cats.[543] The CDC has reported receipt of two *V. fluvialis*, one from a blood culture and the other from peritoneal fluid of a renal dialysis patient.[221]

Subsequently, during a genetic study of atypical lactobacilli isolated from poultry meat (members of the new genus *Carnobacterium*), two isolates from adult rainbow trout were described that were distinct from the poultry isolates.[686] These two strains showed the highest degree of 16S rRNA sequence homology with strains of *V. fluvialis*, forming a genetic cluster that was phylogenetically close to, but distinct from, the carnobacteria, the streptococci, the lactococci, and the enterococci. These two salmonid isolates have been assigned to the genus *Vagococcus* as *Vagococcus salmoninarum*. Subsequently, this organism was shown to cause peritoneal infections in salmon and brown trout.[603] *V. fluvialis* is a very rare human clinical isolate; *V. salmoninarum* has not as yet been isolated from human clinical specimens.

In 1992, Collins and associates[134] described nine unique human clinical isolates (five from blood cultures, three from urine cultures, and one from CSF). Phenotypic traits indicated that these strains were not members of the *Streptococcus*, *Lactococcus*, *Enterococcus*, or *Aerococcus* groups. Furthermore, genetic investigations clearly showed a distinct line of descent for these isolates within the "lactic acid group" of bacteria. These strains have been assigned to the new genus *Globicatella* (meaning a short chain composed of spherical cells). All of these strains were phenotypically similar and have been given the species name *Globicatella sanguis*. Isolates of *G. sanguis* that have been submitted to the CDC have been from blood cultures, urine cultures, a wound culture, and a CSF specimen obtained during an autopsy.[221]

THE GENUS *LACTOCOCCUS*

The genus *Lactococcus* consists of the "lactic acid streptococci" or "milk streptococci." Historically, these organisms carry the Lancefield group N antigen, although only about 80% of lactococcal isolates will carry extractable antigen in their cell wall. Lactococci are rare clinical isolates that have been recovered from blood, urine, and wound specimens.[447,450,724] Lactococci should be considered as opportunistic pathogens of low virulence.[8] Members of the genus *Lactococcus* include *L. lactis* subsp. *lactis*, *L. lactis* susp. *cremoris*, *L. lactis* subsp. *hordniae*, *L. garviae*, *L. plantarum*, *L. raffinolactis*, and *L. xyloses*.

IDENTIFICATION OF STREPTOCOCCI AND THE "STREPTOCOCCUS-LIKE" BACTERIA

DIRECT GRAM-STAINED SMEARS

Gram-stained smears of clinical specimens that yield streptococci on culture will generally show gram-positive or gram-variable cocci arranged in pairs and chains (see Color Plate 12-1*A*). Chains of cells in both specimens and broth cultures tend to appear as chains of pairs of cells rather than as chains of individual cells. Individual cell shapes range from those that resemble diplococci to those that appear coccobacillary or coryneform. This morphology is often observed on smears from broth cultures and from solid media as well. Viridans streptococci, in particular, tend to have cells that appear more elongated. *S. pneumoniae* will most often appear as pairs of lanceolate-shaped cells (see Color Plate 12-1*B*). On smears of specimens yielding mucoid, heavily encapsulated strains, the capsule may appear as a pink halo or as a nonstaining area surrounding the cells in relief against a pink background surrounding the organism.

CULTURE MEDIA

Specimens that may be expected to yield streptococci on culture should be plated onto a suitable blood-containing medium that has a peptone base rich enough to support these fastidious organisms. The agar base medium should be a peptone infusion medium (e.g., tryptic–soy, proteose peptone, Todd-Hewitt) without added carbohydrates. Although the colonies will generally be larger on glucose-containing media (e.g., Columbia base medium) after 24 hours, acid produced from glucose utilization inactivates the streptolysin S of group A streptococci and may interfere with the interpretation of the hemolytic qualities of the organism. Sheep blood is added to the basal medium at a 5% concentration as the indicator cells for hemolysis. Lower concentrations of blood in the media make the hemolytic reaction difficult to discern, whereas higher concentrations may obscure hemolysis entirely. On sheep blood agar, streptococci belonging to groups A, B, C, F and G are β-hemolytic (to be described in the

following), whereas the majority of *Enterococcus* species and group D streptococci are α- or non-hemolytic. Except for group D and occasional group B strains, nonhemolytic groupable streptococci are rare. Sheep blood agar does not support the growth of *Haemophilus haemolyticus* or *Haemophilus parahaemolyticus*; hence small, β-hemolytic colonies recovered from specimens on sheep blood agar are usually streptococci. The growing literature on *Arcanobacterium haemolyticum* as a cause of pharyngitis may require changes in the laboratory approach to throat cultures, for this organism is β-hemolytic and catalase-negative but is a gram-positive rod.

Selective agar may also enhance the recovery of group A streptococci from throat cultures. The formulations that are most often used and that are commercially available employ a tryptic–soy agar base containing 5% sheep blood and sulfamethoxazole (23.75 μg/mL)–trimethoprim (1.25 μg/mL).[197,697] Much of the normal flora of the oropharynx (e.g., viridans streptococci, micrococci, staphylococci, and neisseriae) will be inhibited on this medium. Use of this selective medium enhances recovery of group A and B streptococci and allows visualization of β-hemolysis without the "background" of other organism growth. Commercially available selective media include Streptococcus Selective Agar (ssA; BD Microbiology Systems, Cockeysville MD) and Strep A Isolation Agar (Remel Laboratories, Lenexa KS). In a side-by-side evaluation, Pacifico and coworkers[517] compared the recovery of group A streptococci on selective streptococcal media (ssA) and regular sheep blood agar incubated under different incubation conditions (in air, in CO_2, and in anaerobic atmosphere). The highest yield of positive cultures in this study was obtained using selective medium incubated under anaerobic conditions for 48 hours. Most laboratories incubate media for isolation of group A streptococci for 48 hours in a CO_2-enriched environment, assuming that only cultures from patients with small numbers of organisms or from those who are group A streptococcal carriers will grow under anaerobic conditions.[16] However, even patients with small numbers of organisms may have an immune response, suggesting that they are infected and not just carrying the organism.[517] Small numbers of organisms on a culture plate in a patient with clinical streptococcal pharyngitis may also reflect inadequate specimen collection.

Streptococci recovered from human clinical specimens are identified on the basis of their hemolytic qualities, serologic tests for the detection of cell wall or capsular antigens, and physiologic and biochemical tests. Some of the tests performed in the laboratory for identification of these organisms provide **presumptive** results, whereas others provide **definitive** results. Before proceeding with identification tests, however, one must be sure that the gram-positive cocci under consideration are catalase-negative, placing them in the *Streptococcus* and streptococcal-like bacterial groups. The catalase test is discussed in detail in Chapter 11.

HEMOLYSIS ON BLOOD AGAR

Four types of hemolysis may be produced by streptococci on sheep blood agar (Box 12-3). Observation and correct interpretation of the hemolytic properties of streptococci is very important because the performance of subsequent tests is predicated on this initial evaluation.

Hemolysis is best observed by examining colonies grown under anaerobic conditions or by inspecting subsurface colonies in pour plates or streak-stab plates because, for group A streptococci, maximal activity of both the oxygen-labile (SLO) and oxygen-stable (SLS) hemolysins is observed only under anaerobic conditions. Oxygen-labile hemolysins are also produced by group C and some group G strains, so detection of hemolysis by these organisms is also enhanced by anaerobic incubation. Although routine anaerobic incubation of specimens expected to yield streptococci is not recommended, steps can be taken to maximize detection of hemolysis under aerobic or capnophilic incubation. This is the point of the "streak-and-stab" technique that is used for inoculating throat swab specimens on blood agar for diagnosis of streptococcal pharyngitis (Fig. 12-2; and see Color Plate 12-1E). This technique forces some of the inoculum under the agar, thereby creating a relatively anaerobic environment. Areas of the plate not inoculated with specimen should also be stabbed. Plates should be incubated at 35°C in air or in 5% to 7% CO_2. Although some laboratorians advocate one incubation environment over the other for throat cultures, the recovery of β-hemolytic

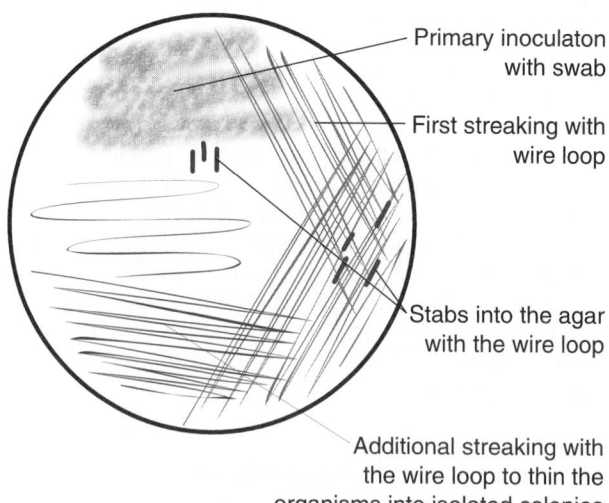

Figure 12-2
Streak–stab technique for isolation of β-hemolytic streptococci.

streptococci from patients with streptococcal pharyngitis will not generally be compromised under either environmental condition.[697]

NONCULTURE, DIRECT DETECTION TECHNIQUES FOR GROUP A STREPTOCOCCI

Nonculture techniques for direct detection of group A streptococci on throat swab specimens are in wide use in both clinical laboratories and physicians' offices. The streptococcal-grouping antigen is extracted from the throat swab using either nitrous acid or enzymatic treatment, followed by a procedure to detect the extracted antigen. Most kits use latex agglutination or enzyme immunoassay (EIA) methods for antigen detection (see Color Plate 12-1F). Tests that are based on enzyme immunoassay techniques offer the advantage of having more sharply defined endpoints.[183,608] Commercial enzyme immunoassay tests include the TestPack Strep A-Plus (Abbott Laboratories, North Chicago IL) and the CARDS O.S. (Pacific Biotech, Inc., San Diego CA). Although the specificity of both latex agglutination and EIA kits is quite high (usually more than 98%), the sensitivities of the various kits for group A streptococcal detection vary widely (between 68% and 95%).[16,163,217,278,345,354,423,552,574,650]

Another technique used for direct detection of group A streptococcal antigen relies on a solid-phase liposome immunoassay. This technique is used in the Q Test Strep kit (Becton-Dickinson and Co., Franklin Lakes NJ). Instead of using a conjugate composed of anti-group–A streptococcal antibodies conjugated to an enzyme, this test uses anti-group–A streptococcal antibodies conjugated to a liposome (an artificial phospholipid sphere) containing the dye rhodamine sulfate. The endpoint signal in this system is generated by the release of the rhodamine sulfate dye on reaction of the antistreptococcal antibodies with the antigen extract from the swab. The liposome method has been

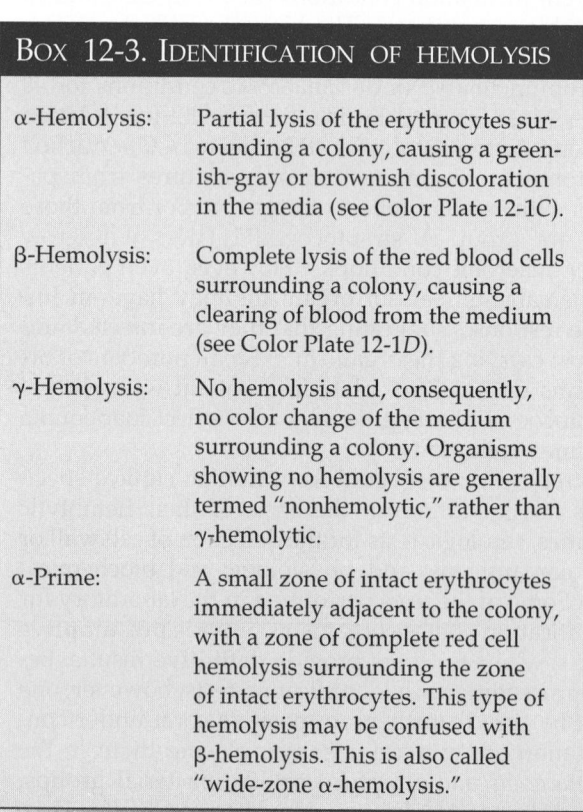

BOX 12-3. IDENTIFICATION OF HEMOLYSIS	
α-Hemolysis:	Partial lysis of the erythrocytes surrounding a colony, causing a greenish-gray or brownish discoloration in the media (see Color Plate 12-1C).
β-Hemolysis:	Complete lysis of the red blood cells surrounding a colony, causing a clearing of blood from the medium (see Color Plate 12-1D).
γ-Hemolysis:	No hemolysis and, consequently, no color change of the medium surrounding a colony. Organisms showing no hemolysis are generally termed "nonhemolytic," rather than γ-hemolytic.
α-Prime:	A small zone of intact erythrocytes immediately adjacent to the colony, with a zone of complete red cell hemolysis surrounding the zone of intact erythrocytes. This type of hemolysis may be confused with β-hemolysis. This is also called "wide-zone α-hemolysis."

evaluated; the sensitivity and specificity were 91% and 83%, respectively.[279,356]

A newly developed test for direct detection of group A streptococci uses an optical immunoassay rather than latex agglutination or membrane filter techniques. This test, called the "Strep A OIA" (for optical immunoassay; Biostar, Inc., Boulder CO), is performed on a slide that allows the direct visualization of a physical change in the thickness of thin films resulting from the binding reactions between antigens and antibodies (see Color Plate 12-1G). After collection of a throat swab specimen, the group A streptococcal antigen is extracted with acetic acid (0.3 M). The extract is neutralized, and then a horseradish peroxidase-labeled rabbit anti-group–A streptococcal antibody is added to the extract. The mixture is than deposited on the surface of the OIA slide; a 2-minute incubation allows the immune complex to bind to the anti-group–A streptococcal antibodies fixed on the slide surface. Unbound material is then washed off the slide. An enzyme substrate (tetramethyl benzidine containing hydrogen peroxide) is then dropped on the slide and allowed to react for 4 minutes. After another washing step, the reaction is read by examining the hue of light reflected from the reaction spot on the slide. If group A streptococcal antigen is present in the original swab specimen, the reaction area on the slide appears as a purple spot. If antigen is not present, the slide surface retains its golden color. In various studies on the Strep A OIA, the sensitivity and specificity of this test have ranged from 81.0% to 98.9% and 95.0% to 98.6%, respectively.[161,162,170,330,345]

DNA probe technology has also been used for direct detection of group A streptococci in throat swab specimens. The Group A Streptococcus Direct Test (Gen-Probe, San Diego CA) is a nonisotopic method that uses a DNA probe to detect the complementary rRNA sequences of group A streptococci directly in an extract from a throat swab. This test has been evaluated by several groups, and sensitvities and specificities of 85.7% to 93.5% and 98.0% to 99.7% have been reported, respectively.[344,540,630]

Although all of these tests are highly specific, it is generally felt that the variable sensitivity is a cause for concern. Regardless of the test kits' assay method or the manufacturers' claims for a given test kit or technique, it is recommended that two throat swabs be collected. Culture should be performed with the second swab on those specimens yielding negative rapid detection results with the first swab.

COLONY MORPHOLOGY AND CATALASE TESTING

After 18 to 24 hour's incubation on blood agar, group A streptococcal colonies are about 0.5 mm in diameter, translucent or transparent, and have a smooth or matte surface. The zone of β-hemolysis is usually 2 to 4 times the diameter of the colony. The colonies are domed and have an entire edge. Groups C and G also have a similar appearance, although colonies of some group G strains may have a golden cast on close inspection and the hemolytic zones are usually very large. Group B streptococci form larger colonies on agar medium,

the margin of hemolysis around the colony is comparatively smaller for group B streptococci than for the other β-hemolytic streptococci, and the hemolysis is generally "softer" and less obvious. A significant proportion of group B streptococci (up to 11%) may be nonhemolytic. Group D streptococcal colonies tend to be larger than those of group A, being 0.5 to 1.0 mm after overnight incubation. Group D isolates are α- or nonhemolytic on sheep blood agar. The colonies are usually gray, smooth, and have an entire edge. Group F streptococci form very small, pinpoint colonies with a large zone of β-hemolysis. These extremely small colonies are called "minute colonies"; they are also very characteristic of the S. milleri group organisms. Minute β-hemolytic colonies are generally pinpoint after 24 hours' incubation, yet will have a rather large, florid zone of β-hemolysis. The S. milleri group organisms growing on solid media also have a distinct sweet, caramel ("butterscotch") or honeysuckle odor owing to the production of diacetyl.[119] This characteristic can be noted with α-hemolytic, β-hemolytic, and nonhemolytic members of this group.

S. pneumoniae displays a spectrum of colony types, the appearance of which depends on the degree of encapsulation. These colonies are generally surrounded by a large zone of intense green α-hemolysis. Colonies of heavily encapsulated strains may be several millimeters in diameter, are very mucoid, appear gray, and may resemble drops of oil on the agar surface. Colonies of the less heavily encapsulated strains are smaller (see Color Plate 12-1H). On prolonged incubation, the central portion of the colony may collapse, giving the characteristic "checker piece" appearance. Some colonies may collapse altogether, giving the appearance of a flat nail-head on the surface of the agar.

Other species of viridans streptococci form colonies of various sizes and textures. Some may be smooth and have an entire edge, whereas others may appear rough, with the formation of a scalloped edge on prolonged incubation. Colonies of Aerococcus, Pediococcus, Gemella, Leuconostoc, Tetragenococcus, Vagococcus, Globicatella, Helcococcus, and the facultative Lactobacillus species strongly resemble viridans streptococci or group D streptococci in their appearance, and they are either α-hemolytic or nonhemolytic.

Members of the streptococci and streptococcus-like bacterial groups are catalase-negative, except for Alloiococcus otitidis. This organism is streptococcus-like in its colony morphology but is catalase-positive. Some enterococcal strains (particularly E. faecalis strains) produce a "pseudocatalase" that is responsible for the weak-positive catalase reaction that is seen with some strains, particularly on primary isolation. The strength of this reaction may diminish after a few serial subcultures.

RECOGNITION AND PRELIMINARY CHARACTERIZATION OF STREPTOCOCCI AND THE STREPTOCOCCUS-LIKE BACTERIA

The determination of hemolysis and the performance of a catalase test used to be the only tests that were required to preliminarily characterize streptococci. However, with the recognition of several groups of streptococcus-like bacteria in human infections, it is also necessary to perform additional tests, particularly for those isolates recovered from sterile body fluids. Some of these organisms are intrinsically resistant to vancomycin and related cyclic glycopeptide antibiotics (e.g., ristocetin, aracidin, and teicoplanin).[378] The apparent increase in the recognition and isolation of these organisms may be partly related to the emergence of methicillin-resistant *S. aureus* and the consequent use of vancomycin as a first-line antibiotic, particularly in severely debilitated hosts. These and other "look-alike" organisms may be preliminarily differentiated from *Streptococcus* and *Enterococcus* species and from one another with the tests shown in Table 12-5.

On sheep blood agar, these organisms resemble viridans streptococci or enterococci; all of them are α-hemolytic or nonhemolytic. Characteristic streptococcal Gram stain morphology (i.e., chains of cocci) in thioglycolate broth is seen with the streptococci, enterococci, lactococci, *Leuconostoc* species, *Vagococcus* species, and *Globicatella* species, whereas gram-positive cocci arranged predominantly in pairs or tetrads are more characteristic of the aerococci, *Alloiococcus* species, *Gemella* species, *Pediococcus* species, *Tetragenococcus* species, and *Helcococcus* species. Facultative lactobacilli will generally show the typical rod-shaped morphology, whereas other species will appear coccal.

On media containing blood, some isolates may produce a weak catalase reaction with 3% H_2O_2; therefore, strains showing this reaction should be subcultured onto blood-free medium and retested for catalase activity. It is noteworthy that the only species among the streptococcus-like bacteria that is truly catalase-positive is *Alloiococcus otitidis*.

Viridans or nonhemolytic streptococci from sterile body fluids should be screened for susceptibility to vancomycin using the regular 30-μg disk on a sheep blood agar plate incubated at 35°C for 18 to 24 hours. Occasional isolates may require prolonged incubation (i.e., up to 72 hours) for test interpretation. Organisms that are resistant to vancomycin generally have MICs higher than 250 μg/mL and will grow right up to the edge of the disk. The presence of any zone around the disk indicates susceptibility to vancomycin.

Production of **gas from glucose**, a helpful test for differentiation of *Leuconostoc* species from the other organisms, is best determined in *Lactobacillus* Mann, Rogosa, and Sharpe (MRS) broth (Difco Laboratories, Detroit MI) overlayed with petrolatum.[171] The formation of bubbles under the petrolatum seal indicates gas production and the heterofermentative nature of their metabolism. The MRS broth is incubated for up to 7 days. Other tests that are helpful for preliminary characterization of the streptococcus-like organisms include **pyrrolidonyl arylamidase (PYR), leucine aminopepti-**

TABLE 12-5
Characteristics for Preliminary Characterization of Streptococci and Streptococcus-Like Bacteria

Genus	Vancomycin	Catalase	Gas from Glucose	LAP	PYR	Esculin Hydrolysis	Growth 6.5% NaCl	Arginine Dihydrolase	Growth at 10°C	45°C
Streptococcus	S	−	−	+	−	v	v	v	−	−+
Enterococcus	S	−	−	+	+	+	+	v	+	+
Lactococcus	S	−	−	+	+	+−	v	−	+	−
Aerococcus	S	−	−	v	v	−	+	−	v	−
Leuconostoc	R	−	+	−	−	v	v	+	+	v
Pediococcus	R	−	−	+	−	+−	v	v	−	v
Gemella	S	−	−	v	v	−	−	−	−	−
Alloiococcus	S	+	−	+	+	−	+	−	−	−
Vagococcus	S	−	−	+	+−	+	+−	v	+	−
Tetragenacoccus	S	−	−	+	−	NA	NA	NA	−	−
Globicatella	S	−	−	−	+	+	+	−	−	−
Helcococcus	S	−	−	−	+	+	v	−	NA	NA

+, positive reaction; −, negative reaction; +−, most strains positive; −+, most strains negative; v, variable reaction; NA, data not available.

dase (LAP), and **salt tolerance** tests. The latter test is performed in heart infusion broth containing 6.5% NaCl and is incubated up to 14 days before being called negative. The presence of growth is the endpoint, as in the salt tolerance test for identification of enterococci. The PYR and LAP tests are available as rapid disk tests from several manufacturers (e.g., Remel, Carr-Scarborough) and are also on some of the kit systems (e.g., API Rapid STREP). The BactiCard Streptococcus test (Remel Laboratories) includes PYR, LAP, and an esculin hydrolysis test. This card, when used with vancomycin susceptibility results, can provide preliminary characterization of *Enterococcus, Lactococcus, Aerococcus, Gemella, Leuconostoc, Pediococcus,* and *Globicatella* species.

Occasionally, more uncommon tests may be helpful to augment traditional tests or to confirm identifications obtained with kit systems. For the **growth temperature tests**, a water bath set at 45°C and a 10°C refrigerator are recommended. Growth, if any, is observed after 24 to 48 hours of incubation. **Motility** is determined in regular semisolid motility agar medium, with or without the addition of tetrazolium. This test should be incubated for up to 48 hours at room temperature. The **VP test for acetylmethyl carbinol** that is used for streptococci is performed in heavily inoculated VP broth incubated overnight. After addition of α-naphthol and sodium hydroxide reagents, the tube is shaken or vortexed and incubated at room temperature for 30 minutes. Red, pink, and colorless reactions at this time correspond to positive, weakly positive, and negative reactions, respectively.

PRESUMPTIVE IDENTIFICATION OF STREPTOCOCCI

β-Hemolytic streptococci, pneumococci, group D streptococci, and enterococci are definitively identified using serologic procedures (discussed later) that detect either the Lancefield group antigens (groups A, B, C, D, F, and G) or the capsular polysaccharide antigens (*S. pneumoniae*) of the organisms. Species identification of group D streptococci, *Enterococcus* species, and the viridans streptococci is accomplished primarily by biochemical, physiologic, and enzymatic tests. Many laboratories, however, use a handful of **presumptive** tests that correlate highly with the serologic methods, yet are less expensive to perform. Results of presumptive tests for the major streptococcal groups are summarized in Table 12-6. Detailed procedures for performance and interpretation of the more commonly used presumptive tests are described in Charts 3, 4, 5, 7, 56, 61 and 65.

SUSCEPTIBILITY TO BACITRACIN

The bacitracin susceptibility test is used for the presumptive identification of group A β-hemolytic streptococci. The test is performed on a blood agar medium with a bacitracin differential disk (e.g., TAXO A Bacitracin Disk, 0.04 unit, BD Microbiology Systems, Cockeysville MD). The procedure is described in detail in Chart 3. Any zone of inhibition around the disk is considered a positive test (see Color Plate 12-2*A*). Although this test is simple, inexpensive, and fairly accurate for presumptive identification of group A streptococci, it is not highly specific. Over 10% of group C and G streptococcal strains are also susceptible to bacitracin, as are about 5% of group B strains. Consequently, this test is often performed along with the sulfamethoxazole–trimethoprim (SXT) susceptibility test because groups C and G streptococci are usually susceptible to SXT, whereas groups A and B streptococci are resistant. Some workers have advocated the use of bacitracin disks directly on primary, nonselective blood agar for rapid detection and identification of group A streptococci in throat cultures. However, this

---

TABLE 12-6
PRESUMPTIVE IDENTIFICATION OF CLINICALLY SIGNIFICANT STREPTOCOCCI

ORGANISM	HEMOLYSIS	BACITRACIN	SXT	CAMP TEST	HYDROLYSIS OF HIPPURATE	PYR	BILE ESCULIN	GROWTH IN 6.5% NACL	OPTOCHIN	BILE SOLUBILITY
Group A	β	S	R	–	–	+	–	–	R	–
Group B	β, none	R	R	+	+	–	–	v	R	–
Groups C, F, G	β	v	S	–	–	–	–	–	R	–
Group D										
Enterococci	α, β, none	R	R	–	v	+	+	+	R	–
Nonenterococci	α, none	R	S	–	–	–	+	–	R	–
Viridans streptococci	α, none	v	S	–	v	–	v	–	R	–
Pneumococcus	α	v	S	–	–	–	–	–	S	+

+, positive reaction; –, negative reaction; v, variable reaction; S, susceptible; R, resistant.

method will identify only 50% to 60% of isolates. Placement of bacitracin disks on primary plates containing selective media is considerably more sensitive. The laboratory report should reflect the use of a presumptive method; "β-hemolytic streptococci, presumptively group A by bacitracin" or "β-hemolytic streptococci, presumptively not group A by bacitracin."

SUSCEPTIBILITY TO SULFAMETHOXAZOLE–TRIMETHOPRIM

The SXT test distinguishes groups A and B streptococci from other β-hemolytic streptococci. When used in conjunction with the bacitracin test, the SXT susceptibility test helps screen out those non-A, non-B streptococci that may be susceptible to bacitracin because both group A and B strains are SXT-resistant, whereas groups C, F, and G are SXT-susceptible (see Color Plate 12-2B). The test is performed the same as the bacitracin test, except that a commercial disk containing 1.25 μg trimethoprim and 23.75 μg of sulfamethoxazole is used. Any zone of inhibition indicates susceptibility to SXT (see Chart 3).

CAMP TEST AND PIGMENT PRODUCTION

The CAMP test (named for Christie, Atkins, and Munch-Petersen) is used to presumptively identify group B streptococci (see Chart 7) and is performed using a β-hemolysin-producing strain of *S. aureus* (ATCC #25923).[127] Group B streptococci secrete a protein called "CAMP factor" that interacts with the β-hemolysin produced and secreted by *S. aureus* to cause enhanced or synergistic hemolysis. This appears as an arrowhead-shaped area of increased hemolysis in the area where the two streaks of growth are closest (see Color Plate 12-2C).[164] This test is highly sensitive, and even nonhemolytic group B strains will be CAMP-positive. A small percentage of group A streptococci will also be CAMP-positive, as will some *Listeria monocytogenes* strains. This test is frequently used in conjunction with the bacitracin and SXT tests on the same blood agar plate to presumptively identify these organisms. A summary of the interpretations of these three tests is shown in Table 12-7. Reports should state "presumptive β-hemolytic group B streptococci by CAMP test."

The CAMP test is still widely used for presumptive identification of group B streptococci, but other physiologic characteristics of the organism have been exploited as possible identification methods.[648] Group B streptococci produce a red-orange carotenoid pigment in certain types of culture media. This property has been exploited for presumptive identification of group B streptococci, and several workers have published media formulations for this purpose.[169,476,645] Recently, de la Rosa and his colleagues in Spain reported on a medium called NGM (new Granada medium).[168] This medium contains proteose peptone, soluble starch, glucose, pyruvate, and agar as the basal medium, with sodium methotrexate as a pigment enhancer and col-

istin as a selective agent. When female genital tract specimens were plated on NGM and incubated anaerobically, 95% of the group B streptococci were detected by the growth of red-orange colonies after 18 hours' incubation. Dispensing the NGM in agar deep tubes detected 98% of the group B streptococci within 12 hours. Pigmentation was less obvious or intense when plates were incubated aerobically, but this difference was not noted with tubed NGM. This test, however, is not yet commercially available.

HYDROLYSIS OF SODIUM HIPPURATE

Group B streptococci are also able to hydrolyze hippurate to its components, glycine and benzoic acid. To perform the test, broth containing sodium hippurate is inoculated with the organism and incubated overnight at 35°C. The cells are centrifuged and the supernatant is removed. Ferric chloride reagent (0.2 mL; $FeCl_3 \cdot 6H_2O$, 12 g, in 100 mL 2% aqueous HCl) is then added to the supernatant (0.8 mL), with the formation of a heavy precipitate. If the precipitate remains after 10 minutes, benzoic acid is present and the test is positive for hippurate hydrolysis. Alternatively, ninhydrin reagent may be added to the supernatant to detect free glycine.[359] In this method, the formation of a deep blue color is positive. Hippurate-positive, β-hemolytic streptococci are reported as "presumptive group B streptococci by hippurate hydrolysis."

BILE-ESCULIN TEST

This test is used for the presumptive identification of *Enterococcus* species and group D streptococci (*S. bovis* and *S. equinus*). It is generally performed on an agar slant or in a plate (Chart 4). Organisms that are bile-esculin–positive are able to grow in the presence of 40% bile and to hydrolyze esculin. Most *Enterococcus* species and group D streptococci will blacken bile-esculin medium within 24 hours (see Color Plate 12-2D); rare strains may require a 48-hour incubation before hydrolysis is apparent. Care should be taken to use bile-esculin agar formulations that contain the requisite 40% bile; some manufacturers' products contain less bile than this amount, resulting in misidentification of some viridans streptococci as group D streptococci or enterococci.

TABLE 12-7
INTERPRETATION OF BACITRACIN, SXT, AND CAMP TEST RESULTS

ORGANISM	BACITRACIN	SXT	CAMP TEST
Presumptive group A	S	R	Negative
Presumptive group B	R	R	Positive
Non-group A or B	R	S	Negative
Non-group A or B	S	S	Negative

S, susceptible; R, resistant.

SALT TOLERANCE TEST

The salt tolerance test (6.5% NaCl broth) separates *Enterococcus* species from the group D nonenterococcal streptococci *S. bovis* and *S. equinus* (see Chart 65). The organism to be identified is inoculated into an infusion-based agar or broth containing 6.5% NaCl. After overnight incubation, the medium is observed for the presence of growth, indicating tolerance to 6.5% salt. *Enterococcus* species will be salt-tolerant (see Color Plate 12-2D); *S. bovis* will not grow.

PYRROLIDONYL ARYLAMIDASE TEST

The PYR hydrolysis test (Chart 61) is a presumptive test for both group A and group D enterococcal streptococci.[226] It replaces the bacitracin test and the salt tolerance test for group A streptococci and *Enterococcus* species, respectively. The enzyme that is detected is called pyrrolidonyl arylamidase. Broth containing PYR (L-pyrrolidonyl-β-naphthylamide) is inoculated with the organism and incubated at 35°C for 4 hours. During this time PYR is hydrolyzed. Free β-naphthylamide is then detected by addition of the diazo dye coupler, *N,N*-dimethylaminocinnamaldehyde. A red color develops if PYR has been hydrolyzed (see Color Plate 12-2E). This test is highly sensitive and specific for group A streptococci and most *Enterococcus* species. Several adaptations of the PYR hydrolysis test are commercially available and provide rapid results (15 minutes or less). Other organisms (e.g., most lactococci, *A. viridans*, *G. hemolysans*, the nutritionally variant streptococci, and some staphylococci) are also PYR-positive.

LEUCINE AMINOPEPTIDASE TEST

Production of leucine aminopeptidase (LAP), along with PYR, is helpful for identifying streptococci, enterococci, and some of the streptococcus-like organisms. This test is available as a disk spot test (Remel Laboratories; Carr-Scarborough Microbiologicals, Decatur, GA), as a part of a three-test presumptive identification system (Remel Bacti-Card Strep; see Color Plate 12-2F) or on 4-hour or overnight panels for streptococcal identification (the API Rapid STREP).[224] Disks are moistened and heavily inoculated with colonial material from an agar plate (this may require that plates of very slow-growing isolates be incubated 2 to 3 days before sufficient inoculum is available for testing). After 10 minutes, a drop of the detection reagent is added to the disk. Development of a red color on the disk after 3 minutes indicates a positive LAP reaction; a yellow color is a negative test; and a pink color is coded as a weakly positive test. The LAP test is positive for all streptococci and enterococci, the latter also being PYR-positive.

SUSCEPTIBILITY TO OPTOCHIN

Susceptibility to optochin (ethyl hydrocupreine hydrochloride) is used to differentiate *S. pneumoniae* from the other viridans streptococci (see Chart 56). As with the bacitracin and SXT tests, the optochin susceptibility test is performed on blood agar media. Unlike the former two tests, however, zones of inhibition must be measured before interpretation. A zone of 14 mm or wider around the 6-mm disk indicates susceptibility to optochin and identifies the organism as a pneumococcus (see Color Plate 12-2G). If the zone is smaller than 14 mm, an alternative identification test (e.g., serology or bile solubility) should be performed because some nonpneumococcal viridans streptococci and aerococci may show small zones of inhibition. Viridans streptococci and group D enterococci are generally optochin-resistant. Optochin-resistant *S. pneumoniae* isolates have been reported but are rarely encountered.[238,491] In addition to this rapid phenotypic method, several molecular methods have been developed for direct detection, identification, and characterization of *S. pneumoniae*.[337,430,582,679] Most of these are PCR-based techniques.

BILE SOLUBILITY TEST

The bile solubility test is another test for identification of *S. pneumoniae*. The test can be performed on a broth or saline suspension of the organism or directly on a plate. Both procedures are described in Chart 5. Deoxycholate, the "bile" reagent used in these procedures, activates the autolytic enzymes of the organism.

COMMERCIAL PRESUMPTIVE TESTS

Commercially produced triplates are available for the presumptive identification of β-hemolytic streptococcal groups A and B, the group D streptococci, and *Enterococcus* species. The Strep-ID Tri-Plate (Remel, Lenexa KA) contains three compartments: a sheep blood agar quadrant for assessment of hemolysis and performance of the CAMP and SXT tests, a bile esculin agar quadrant, and a PYR medium quadrant. After inoculation and overnight incubation, the tests are interpreted as shown in Table 12-8 and in Color Plate 12-2H.

SEROLOGIC IDENTIFICATION OF β-HEMOLYTIC STREPTOCOCCI

The pioneering work of Rebecca Lancefield set the stage for the serologic classification of human streptococci. This classification is based on the detection of the group-specific carbohydrate antigen from the cell wall of the organism.[419] Groupable streptococci that cause disease in humans belong to Lancefield groups A, B, C, D, F, and G. Only β-hemolytic streptococci and the α- or nonhemolytic group D organisms can be classified with this scheme. To detect the cell wall antigens of these organisms, the antigen must first be extracted from the cell wall and solubilized. This may be accomplished by acid extraction (e.g., nitrous acid), autoclave extraction (Rantz-Randall method), or by enzymatic extraction. Once extracted, the antigen may be detected by a variety of methods.

CAPILLARY PRECIPITIN TEST

In this method used by Lancefield, the extracted antigen is layered over group-specific antisera in a capillary tube.[419] The formation of a precipitin reaction at

TABLE 12-8
INTERPRETATION OF REACTIONS IN THE STREP-ID QUAD-PLATE

ORGANISM	HEMOLYSIS	CAMP TEST	SXT	PYR TEST	GROWTH ON BE AGAR
Presumptive group A	β	−	R	+	−
Presumptive group B	β, none	+	R	−	−
Non-groups A or B	β	−	S	−	−
Enterococcus species	α, β, none	−	R/S	+	+
Group D streptococci	α, none	−	R/S	−	+
Viridans streptococci	α, none	−	R/S	−	−ʷ⁺

+, positive reaction; −, negative reaction; S, susceptible; R, resistant; −ʷ⁺, occasional weak positive reaction seen with some isolates; R/S, resistant or susceptible.

the extract–antiserum interface provides the group designation of the organism.

COAGGLUTINATION

In this technique, the antigen extract is reacted with *S. aureus* cells sensitized with group-specific antisera.[324] Visible agglutination of the staphylococcal cells coated with a specific antiserum provides the group designation of the organism. Commercial coagglutination test kits are available (Phadebact Streptococcus, Karo Bio Diagnostics AB, Huddinge, Sweden; Meritec Strep, Meridian Diagnostics, Cincinniati OH).

LATEX AGGLUTINATION

The latex agglutination tests employ polystyrene latex beads as the carriers for the group-specific antisera that are reacted with the organism extract.[67,163,220] Commercial kits for this method are widely used as well (Streptex, Murex, Norcross GA; Patho-Dₓ Strep Grouping Kit, Diagnostic Products Corporation, Los Angeles CA; Slidex Strep, bioMerieux-Vitek, Inc., Hazelwood MO). The Streptex procedure has essentially replaced the Lancefield extraction–capillary precipitin technique as the reference method for serogrouping of β-hemolytic streptococci (see Color Plate 12-3A). The proper assessment of hemolysis is essential for test reliability, and cross-reactions with other organisms have been reported. For example, Lee and Wetherall demonstrated that some *S. pneumoniae* strains may-cross react with the group C streptococcal latex reagent.[429] This error may occur when organisms are tested directly from blood culture bottles without first determining the hemolytic character of the isolate. Some of the commercial reagents may also have difficulty detecting the group D antigen in *Enterococcus* species. Truant and Satishchandran examined eight strains of vancomycin-resistant enterococci with the Streptex and PathoDₓ reagents and found that the antigen was detected in all eight isolates with the PathoDₓ group D reagent, whereas none were positive with the Streptex procedure.[659] Testing of over 200 isolates of vancomycin-susceptible enterococci in the same laboratory showed no difference in the sensitivity of the two serologic tests.

SEROLOGIC TESTS FOR IDENTIFICATION OF *STREPTOCOCCUS PNEUMONIAE*

Definitive identification of *S. pneumoniae* involves the serologic detection of pneumococcal capsular polysaccharides using specific antisera. This is complicated because there are more than 83 different capsular serotypes. Omniserum, a Scandinavian product, is capable of detecting all pneumococcal serotypes. Such antiserum pools have been used to develop commercial coagglutination (Phadebact Pneumococcus, Karo Bio) and latex agglutination tests (Pneumoslide, BD Microbiology Systems) for rapid serologic identification of *S. pneumoniae*.[625,698] Specific identification and assignment to an individual capsular serotype is accomplished with the **Quellung test**.

The Quellung test may employ a serum pool, as well as type-specific antisera. A light suspension of the organism is prepared in saline, and a loopful of this suspension is mixed with a loopful of antiserum and a loopful of methylene blue on a glass slide. A glass cover slip is applied, and the slide is incubated at room temperature for 10 minutes. The slide is examined under the high dry objective and under oil immersion, with decreased light. Owing to a microprecipitin reaction occurring on the surface of the organism, the refractive index of the capsule changes and takes on a "swollen," more visible appearance as a halo around the blue-stained bacterial cells (see Color Plate 12-3B). Microscopic organism agglutination may also be observed, particularly with heavily encapsulated strains. Quellung results must be compared microscopically with a similar preparation made with saline instead of antisera.

BIOCHEMICAL CHARACTERISTICS FOR IDENTIFICATION OF GROUPABLE STREPTOCOCCI

The groupable streptococci can be identified to species on the basis of physiologic characteristics. Several of these reactions are used in the various kit systems for identifying the β-hemolytic streptococci. Although most clinical laboratories dealing with specimens from humans use serologic methods for identification of these organisms, workers in veterinary microbiology may find these tests helpful because Lancefield antisera for groups other than A, B, C, F, and G are not readily available. Phenotypic characteristics for the identification of groupable streptococci are presented in Table 12-9.

IDENTIFICATION OF THE VIRIDANS STREPTOCOCCI

The viridans streptococci other than *S. pneumoniae* encompass several species of α-hemolytic and non-hemolytic organisms (see Table 12-2). Unlike the human β-hemolytic streptococci, these organisms, with the exception of most *S. bovis* biotypes and *S. equinus*, lack specific Lancefield serologic group antigens, although some may carry antigens that cross-react with these antisera. Unlike the pneumococci, they are optochin-resistant and bile-insoluble. Under certain circumstances, such as in cases of endocarditis, it may be clinically helpful to identify these organisms. Individuals with preexisting valvular damage may have recurrent episodes of endocarditis or experience relapse following inadequate treatment. A knowledge of the identity and the antimicrobial susceptibility of these isolates may help sort out problems such as treatment failures, reinfections, and antimicrobial tolerance.

The conventional method that has been used in the United States for identifying the viridans streptococci was described by Dr. Facklam at the CDC in 1977.[216] This method involved the performance of a battery of physiologic and carbohydrate fermentation tests. The application of nucleic acid hybridization techniques and the use of novel chromogenic enzyme substrates for the detection of enzymatic activities in these bacteria have significantly altered viridans streptococcal taxonomy.[153,259,393,394] Usually, the databases for kit systems that are available for streptococcal identification do not yet reflect the taxonomic changes that have been accepted. In addition, most of the systems have not yet incorporated the newly accepted or proposed species (i.e., *S. vestibularis, S. gordonii, S. crista, S. sobrinus,* or *S. parasanguis*) or the emended descriptions of existing species (i.e., *S. sanguis, S. mitis,* and *S. oralis*) in their databases. It is noteworthy that one of the systems, the API Rapid STREP (see Color Plate 12-3C), is being used in the current taxonomic literature to assist in the delineation of phenotypic characteristics of new, proposed species and emended descriptions of older species.[259]

Some new phenotypic characteristics that are not amenable to incorporation into kit systems have been described by workers in oral microbiology. Some species of viridans streptococci may be discriminated by their ability to bind salivary amylase. This test is performed by suspending and incubating the organisms in clarified saliva. After incubation, the organisms are removed by centrifugation, and the supernatant is assayed for amylase activity. Decreased or absent amylase activity in the supernatant relative to a control that

---

TABLE 12-9
BIOCHEMICAL CHARACTERISTICS OF THE β-HEMOLYTIC GROUPABLE STREPTOCOCCI

CHARACTERISTIC	S. PYOGENES	S. AGALACTIAE	S. EQUI	S. DYSGALACTIAE	STREPTOCOCCUS GROUP G	S. INIAE	S. PORCINUS	S. PHOCAE
Hemolysis	β	β	β	α, γ	β	β	β	β
Hydrolysis of								
Arginine	+	+	+	+	+	NA	+	−
Esculin	v	−	v	−	−	+	+	−
Hippurate	−	+	−	−	v	−	−	−
PYR	+	−	−	−	−	−	−	−
Production of								
Acetoin (VP)	−	+	−	−	−	NA	+	−
Alkaline phosphatase	+	+	+	+	+	NA	+	+
α-Galactosidase	−	v	−	−	−	−	−	−
β-Glucuronidase	v	v	+	+	+	NA	+	
Acid Produced from								
Inulin	−	−	−	−	−	−	−	−
Lactose	+	v	−	+	+	+	v	−
Mannitol	−	−	−	−	−	+	+	−
Raffinose	−	−	−	−	−	−	−	−
Ribose	−	+	−	+	+	+	+	+
Salicin	+	v	+	v	NA	+	+	−
Sorbitol	−	−	−	v	−	−	+	−
Trehalose	+	+	−	+	+	+	+	−
Lancefield group	A	B	C	C	G	None	E, P, U, V	−/F/C
Bacitracin (0.04 U disk)	S	S/R	R	R	R	R	R	R

+, positive reaction; −, negative reaction; v, variable reaction; NA, data not available; S, susceptible; R, resistant;
S/R, both sensitive and resistant strains noted.

lacks organisms indicates that the organisms bound the enzyme and is a positive test, whereas no change in the amount of amylase relative to a control without organisms is a negative test. Douglas and colleagues at the Department of Oral Pathology at the University of Sheffield (England) found that strains of *S. mitis* and *S. crista* were able to bind salivary amylase, whereas strains of *S. sanguis* and *S. oralis* did not.[188] Kilian and Hyvad[396] extended these studies and found that 86% of 22 *S. gordonii* strains, 52% of 23 *S. mitis* strains, 33% of 10 *S. salivarius* strains, and 17% of 24 *S. anginosus* strains were able to bind salivary amylase. Strains of *S. mutans*, *S. vestibularis*, *S. oralis*, and *S. sanguis* were negative in this test.

For convenience, the viridans streptococci can be placed in groups in a manner similar to the three species that compose the *S. milleri* group, and certain common biochemical features can be used to identify these groups. The viridans streptococci can be divided into the "*S. mutans*" group (the human isolates *S. mutans* and *S. sobrinus* plus the other animal species), the "*S. salivarius*" group (*S. salivarius* and *S. vestibularis*), the "*S. mitis*" group (*S. mitis* and *S. oralis*), and the "*S. sanguis*" group (*S. sanguis*, *S. gordonii*, *S. parasanguis*, and *S. crista*). These groups can be delineated by the production of acetoin (VP test), hydrolysis of esculin, production of arginine dihydrolase and urease, and acid production from mannitol and sorbitol (Table 12-10).

Because of the association with colonic carcinoma, identification of the "nonenterococcal" group D streptococcus *S. bovis* is particularly important. As do most of the *Enterococcus* species, *S. bovis* strains possess the group D antigen, hydrolyze esculin in the presence of 40% bile, grow at 45°C but do not grow in 6.5% NaCl broth, do not possess PYR, and do not grow at 10°C. Most isolates of *S. bovis* I and *S. bovis* II/1 ferment mannitol, lactose, raffinose, salicin, melibiose, trehalose, and inulin. Arabinose and sorbitol are not fermented. In the Rapid STREP system, *S. bovis* I and II/2 strains acidify amygdalin and glycogen. *S. bovis* variant (*S. bovis* biotype II/1) strains usually do not ferment mannitol, but do acidify starch (amygdalin). These organisms may be confused with *S. salivarius* strains, which they resemble in several physiologic and biochemical characteristics.[588] Characteristics that are helpful for identifying *S. bovis* and *S. bovis* variant and for differentiating these organisms from the biochemically similar *S. salivarius* are shown in Table 12-11.[154] Some strains of *S. salivarius* also produce urease, which is helpful in differentiating this organism from *S. bovis*.[622] Starch hydrolysis can be detected with Mueller-Hinton agar plates that are streaked with the organism and incubated for 48 hours. The plates are then flooded with Gram's iodine. Colorless areas under and surrounding organism growth indicate hydrolysis of starch, whereas the maintenance of the blue or purple color

TABLE 12-10

DIFFERENTIATION OF VIRIDANS STREPTOCOCCAL GROUPS

VIRIDANS GROUP	ARGININE HYDROLYSIS	ESCULIN HYDROLYSIS	VP REACTION	ACID FROM MANNITOL	ACID FROM SORBITOL	UREASE PRODUCTION	GROUP MEMBERS	COMMENTS
"*S. mutans*" group	−	+	+	+	+	−	*S. mutans* *S. sobrinus* *S. cricetus* *S. rattus*	*S. rattus* is rare in human clinical specimens and is arginine hydrolysis-positive
"*S. sanguis*" group	+	+	−	−	−	−	*S. sanguis* *S. parasanguis* *S. gordonii* *S. crista*	Strains of *S. crista* are esculin-negative and may also be arginine-negative
"*S. mitis*" group	−	−	−	−	−	−	*S. mitis* *S. oralis*	
"*S. salivarius*" group	−	+	+	−	−	v	*S. salivarius* *S. vestibularis*	Strains of *S. vestibularis* may be VP-negative

+, positive reaction; −, negative reaction; v, variable reaction.

TABLE 12-11

CHARACTERISTICS FOR IDENTIFICATION OF
STREPTOCOCCUS BOVIS, *STREPTOCOCCUS BOVIS* VARIANT AND
DIFFERENTIATION OF THESE SPECIES FROM *STREPTOCOCCUS SALIVARIUS*

CHARACTERISTIC	S. BOVIS	S. BOVIS VARIANT	S. SALIVARIUS
Hemolysis	γ, α	α, γ	α
Growth, BE agar	+	+	−⁺
Esculin hydrolysis	+	+	+
Growth, 6.5% NaCl	−	−	−
PYR	−	−	−
Group D antigen	+	+	−
Acetoin (VP)	+	+	+
Arginine dihydrolase	−	−	−
Starch hydrolysis	+	−	−
Urease	−	−	+
Acid produced from			
Mannitol	+	−	−
Lactose	+	+	+
Raffinose	+	+	+⁻
Inulin	+⁻	−	+

+, positive; −, negative; +⁻, most strains positive; −⁺, most strains negative.

around the colonies indicates no hydrolysis of starch. Alternatively, starch plates (various manufacturers) can be used. The Rapid STREP identification system splits *S. bovis* strains into *S. bovis* I, *S. bovis* II/1, and *S. bovis* II/2. On the strip, *S. bovis* I strains are mannitol-positive and amygdalin-positive. *S. bovis* II/1 and *S. bovis* II/2 are mannitol-negative, with II/1 strains being amygdalin-positive and II/2 strains being amygdalin-negative.

Panosian and Edberg[519] reported a rapid (30-minute) test procedure that used PYR hydrolysis along with two enzyme substrates—*p*-nitrophenyl-α-D-galactopyranoside (PGAL) and 4-methylumbelliferyl-β-D-glucoside (MGLU) in the presence of 2.5% sodium deoxycholate—for identifying *S. bovis*. *S. bovis* strains were both PGAL- and MGLU-positive and were PYR-negative. Enterococci were either PGAL- and MGLU-positive or just MGLU-positive, but all were PYR-positive. Other viridans streptococci, including strains of *S. pneumoniae*, produced negative reactions for all three substrates.

A DNA probe for identifying *S. bovis* has also been developed by cloning the *S. bovis* amylase gene.[712] This probe was able to specifically hybridize with DNA from human clinical isolates of *S. bovis* and from isolates recovered from the bovine rumen and from cow feces. Interestingly, this probe also hybridized with DNA from three strains of *S. salivarius*.

In 1991, Beighton and coworkers in the Department of Oral Microbiology at London Hospital Medical College published a scheme for the identification of all the currently recognized members of the viridans streptococci.[47] This scheme uses conventional 24-hour carbohydrate fermentation tests plus a battery of 4-methy-

lumbelliferyl-linked substrates for the rapid (3-hour) determination of glycosidic enzymes. Table 12-12 is an amalgamation of several identification schemes for the viridans streptococci.[47,216,244,259,707,709] The dichotomous key in Figure 12-3 incorporates the "grouping" tests from Table 12-10 and additional tests from Table 12-12 for identifying the "typical" individual species within a group. Until commercial vendors update the databases of individual commercial systems to include the newer species and phenotypic tests, microbiologists will have to use a "best fit" approach to species-level identification of the viridans streptococci. Nonphenotypic methods for characterizing these organisms, such as pyrrolysis–gas chromatograhy and Fourier-transform infrared spectroscopy, have also shown promise as adjunct methods for identification.[260,668] In addition to phenotypic identification methods, molecular methods, such as rRNA sequence analysis (ribotyping), restriction fragment length polymorphisms, and PCR- and nucleic acid probe–based methods, have also been developed for identifying this group of microorganisms.[52,54,245,580,581,589]

IDENTIFICATION OF THE *STREPTOCOCCUS MILLERI* GROUP

The three species that compose the *S. milleri* group of streptococci—*S. anginosus*, *S. constellatus*, and *S. intermedius*— produce small pinpoint colonies on blood agar and may be α-, β-, or nonhemolytic. For β-hemolytic strains, the size of the hemolytic zone is several times the diameter of the colony. An initial clue that an isolate may be a member of this group is the presence of a sweet odor that has been described as "caramel, butterscotch, or honeysuckle." This is due to the production of the metabolite diacetyl.[119] Isolates may carry group A, C, F, or G antigens or may be nongroupable.[616] The individual species may be differentiated by the biochemical and enzymatic tests shown in Table 12-13.[407,705,708,710] Many of the tests shown in Table 12-13 are found in the commercially available kit systems. The Rapid STREP and the RapID STR kits will identify these organisms, with the suggestion that β-hemolytic strains be serogrouped.

The *S. milleri* group organisms may also be identified by a dedicated commercially available system called the Fluo-Card Milleri (Key Scientific, Round Rock, TX).[250] This test consists of a small filter paper strip with three reagent-impregnated circles containing 4-methylumbelliferyl-β-D-fucoside, 4-methylumbelliferyl-β-D-glucoside, and 4-methylumbelliferyl-α-D-glucoside for detection of β-D-fucosidase, β-glucosidase, and α-glucosidase, respectively. The test circles are moistened with water, and several colonies of the isolate are rubbed on each of the test circles. After a 15-minute incubation at 35°C, the circles are inspected for fluorescence under a Wood's lamp (long wave UV light). Fluorescence observed in the first test circle only, the second test circle only, or the third test circle only provides an identification of *S. intermedius* (β-D-fucosidase-positive), *S. anginosus* (β-glucosidase-positive), or *S. constellatus* (α-glucosidase positive), respectively. In an evaluation of this system

TABLE 12-12

CHARACTERISTICS FOR IDENTIFICATION OF THE VIRIDANS STREPTOCOCCI

	HEMOLYSIS, SBA	ESCULIN HYDROLYSIS	ARGININE DIHYDROLASE	HIPPURATE HYDROLYSIS	STARCH HYDROLYSIS	UREASE	ACETOIN (VP)	GROWTH, 6.5% NaCl	PYR	AMYGDALIN	ARBUTIN	CELLOBIOSE	INULIN	LACTOSE	MANNITOL	MELEZITOSE	MELIBIOSE
										ACID PRODUCED FROM:							
S sanguis bio. 1	α	+	+	−	V	−	−	−	−	−	+	+	+⁻	+	−	−	+
S. sanguis bio. 2	α	+	+	−	V	−	−	−	−	+	+	+	+⁻	+	−	−	V
S. sanguis bio. 3	α	−⁺	+	−	V	−	−	−	−	−	V	−⁺	+⁻	+	−	−	−
S. parasanguis	α	−⁺	+	−	+	−	−	−	−	−⁺	V	V	−	+	−	−	+⁻
S. mitis	α	−	−	−	+⁻	−	−	−	−	−	V	V	+⁻	−	−	−	+
S. oralis	α	−⁺	−	−	+	−	−	−	−	−⁺	−⁺	−⁺	−	+	−	−	V
S gordonii	α	+	+	−	+⁻	−	−	−	−	+	+	+	+	+	−	−	−⁺
S. crista	α	−	+⁻	−	NA	−	−	−	−	+	NA	−	+⁻	−	−	−	−
S. vestibularis	α	+⁻	−	−	+⁻	+	+	−	−	V	+⁻	V	−	+⁻	−	−	−
S. salivarius	γ	+	−	−	+	V	V	−	−	−⁺	+	+	+⁻	+⁻	−	−	−⁺
S. mutans	α, γ	+⁻	−	−	+	−	+	−	−	+⁻	+	+	+	+	+	−	+⁻
S. sobrinus	α, γ	−	−	−	NA	−	NA	−	−	−	−	NA	+⁻	+⁻	+ˢˡ	−	−
*S. uberis/parauberis**	α, γ	+	+	V	−	−	+	−	+	+	+	+	V	+	+	−	−
S. acidominimus	α	−	−⁺	+	−	−	−	−	−⁺	−	NA	NA	−	+ˢˡ	V	NA	NA

* *S. uberis* and *S. parauberis* cannot be differentiated by physiologic tests.
+, positive; −, negative; +⁻, most strains positive, some negative; −⁺, most strains negative, some positive; NA, data not available; +ˢˡ, positive reaction, but slow or delayed; V, variable.

performed by Flynn and Ruoff, the Fluo-Card Milleri identified 88% of 17 *S. intermedius* strains, 98% of 50 *S. anginosus* strains, and 97% of 31 *S. constellatus* strains.[250]

ISOLATION AND IDENTIFICATION OF THE NUTRITIONALLY VARIANT STREPTOCOCCI ("*ABIOTROPHIA* SPECIES")

These organisms should be suspected when direct Gram stains of specimens or of positive blood cultures show streptococcal organisms that fail to grow on sub-sequent culture or subculture. Commercial blood culture medium does contain pyridoxal and will support the growth of these organisms. Subculture onto blood agar and the placement of a staphylococcal streak as is done in the satellite test for *Haemophilus* spp. will ensure growth of the nutritionally variant streptococci adjacent to the staph streak (see Color Plate 12-3*D*). Alternatively, disks impregnated with pyridoxal may also be placed on the subculture plate, with subsequent growth of the organisms appearing as satellite colonies surrounding the disk.

	N-ACETYLGLUCOSAMINE	RAFFINOSE	SALICIN	SORBITOL	STARCH	SUCROSE	TREHALOSE	α-GLUCOSIDASE	β-GLUCOSIDASE	α-GALACTOSIDASE	β-GALACTOSIDASE	α-L-FUCOSIDASE	β-D-FUCOSIDASE	α-ARABINOSIDASE	β-N-ACETYLGLUCOSAMINIDASE	β-N-ACETYLGALACTOSAMINIDASE	SIALIDASE	β-GLUCURONIDASE	ALKALINE PHOSPHATASE
S sanguis bio. 1	+	+	+	V	−	+	+	−	$-^+$	V	−	−	—	—	—	—	—	—	—
S. sanguis bio. 2	+	+	+	$+^-$	−	+	+	−	+	+	$-^+$	−	+	−	$-^+$	−	−	−	—
S. sanguis bio. 3	+	−	+	−	−	+	+	−	V	−	+	−	$+^-$	−	+	—	—	—	—
S. parasanguis	+	$+^-$	+	$-^+$	−	+	V	+	$-^+$	+	+	$-^+$	$-^+$	$-^+$	+	+	−	−	$+^-$
S. mitis	+	+	$-^+$	$-^+$	−	+	$-^+$	+	−	$+^-$	V	−	−	−	−	−	$-^+$	−	V
S. oralis	+	V	−	−	−	$+^-$	$-^+$	+	−	$-^+$	V	−	−	−	+	+	+	−	+
S gordonii	+	$-^+$	+	−	−	+	+	$-^+$	+	$-^+$	V	+	−	−	+	$+^-$	−	−	+
S. crista	+	−	NA	−	−	NA	+	−	−	−	$-^+$	+	−	−	+	+	−	−	−
S. vestibularis	$+^-$	−	+	−	−	+	−	V	−	−	+	−	−	+	−	−	−	−	NA
S. salivarius	$-^+$	$-^+$	+	−	−	+	$-^+$	V	V	$-^+$	$+^-$	−	$+^-$	+	−	−	−	−	+
S. mutans	+	+	+	+	−	+	+	+	+	$+^-$	V	−	−	−	−	−	−	−	−
S. sobrinus	−	$-^+$	NA	$-^+$	−	+	+	+	−	−	NA	−	−	−	−	−	−	−	NA
*S. uberis/parauberis**	+	V	+	+	−	+	+	V	NA	NA	NA	NA	NA	NA	NA	NA	NA	−	+
S. acidominimus	NA	−	NA	−	NA	NA	$+^{sl}$	NA	NA	−	$-^+$	NA	NA	NA	NA	NA	NA	$+^-$	+

The nutritionally variant streptococci have been genetically characterized and given the species names *A. defectiva* and *A. adiacens*.[388] If grown on pyridoxal-supplemented (10 mg pyridoxal hydrochloride per liter) or cysteine-supplemented (100 mg L-cysteine per liter) media, these organisms can be identified with the biochemical tests shown in Table 12-14.[78,79] Again, many of these tests are found on the commercial kit systems (e.g., the Rapid STREP). Similar to the other streptococci, these two species are LAP-positive, but a key test in differentiating these organisms from

other viridans streptococci is the PYR test (pyrrolidonyl-arylamidase); the nutritionally variant streptococcal species are PYR-positive, whereas viridans streptococci other than *Enterococcus* species are PYR-negative. Similar to other streptococci, they are homofermentative, with lactic acid as the sole end-product of glucose fermentation. They are also optochin-resistant and vancomycin-susceptible. It should also be kept in mind that occasional isolates of other viridans streptococci (e.g., *S. mitis*) may also display nutritional variance.[614]

IDENTIFICATION OF VIRIDANS STREPTOCOCCI

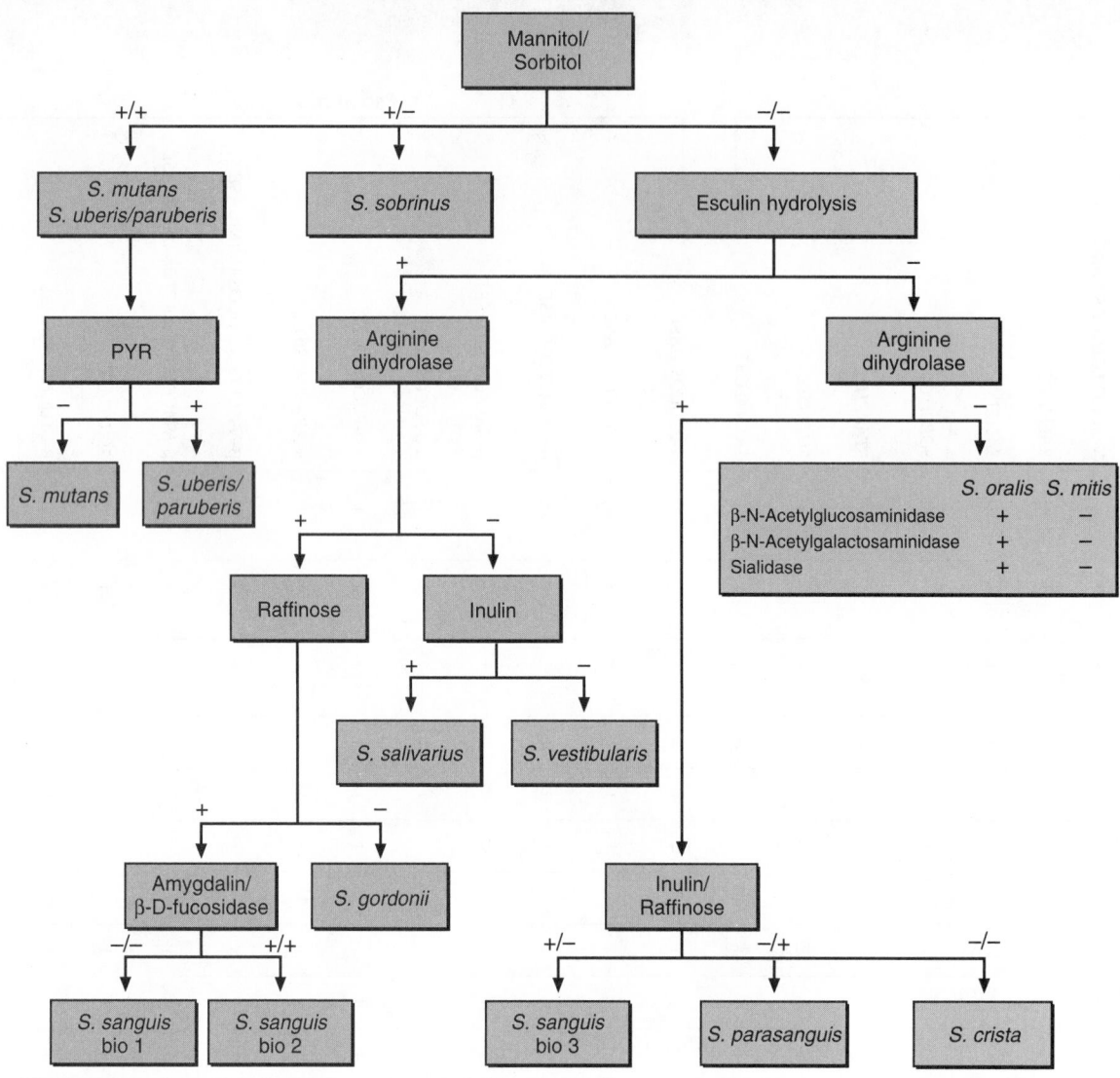

Figure 12-3
Flowchart for identification of viridans streptococci.

IDENTIFICATION OF *STREPTOCOCCUS SUIS*

S. suis should be suspected in those patients with systemic signs of sepsis and meningitis who have had contact with pigs or porcine products. The organism is a typical-looking, catalase-negative, nonmotile, gram-positive coccus that occurs singly, in pairs, or in short chains. It is α-hemolytic on sheep blood agar (β-hemolytic on horse blood agar), resistant to optochin, and does not grow in 6.5% NaCl broth. Some strains will grow in the presence of 40% bile, and all strains are able to hydrolyze esculin. Additional characteristics that are helpful for identification of *S. suis* are presented in Table 12-15.[646] This important animal pathogen is included in the database of the Rapid STREP system (see later discussion).

IDENTIFICATION OF *ENTEROCOCCUS* SPECIES

Identification of *Enterococcus* species is accomplished by biochemical and physiologic tests. Only about 80% of *Enterococcus* species react with antiserum against Lancefield group D by capillary precipitin or latex agglutination. However, most *Enterococcus* species hydrolyze esculin in the presence of bile, grow in broth containing 6.5% NaCl, and are PYR-positive. Although *E. faecalis* and *E. faecium* constitute those species that are most commonly recovered from clinical specimens, the incidence of the other species and their roles in specific disease processes are unknown. Facklam and Collins[219] have proposed a stepwise method for identifying *Enterococcus* species. Isolates that fit the criteria listed in the foregoing are inoculated into several test

TABLE 12-13

CHARACTERISTICS FOR IDENTIFICATION OF *S. ANGINOSUS*, *S. INTERMEDIUS*, AND *S. CONSTELLATUS*

CHARACTERISTIC	S. ANGINOSUS	S. INTERMEDIUS	S. CONSTELLATUS
Lancefield group	None, F >A >G > C	None (rare)	None, F > A > C
Hemolysis	α, γ	γ, α	β, α, γ
Catalase	−	−	−
Growth enhanced by CO_2	+	+	+
Arginine dihydrolase	+	+	+
Esculin hydrolysis	+	+	+
Acetoin (VP)	+	+	+
Hippurate hydrolysis	−	−	−
Urease	−	−	−
Leucine arylamidase (LAP)	+	+	+
Pyrrolidonyl arylamidase (PYR)	−	−	−
Alkaline phosphatase	+	+	+
Acid production from			
Amygdalin	+	+⁻	v
Arabinose	−	−	−
Cellobiose	+	+⁻	−⁺
Glucose	+	+	+
Glycerol	−	−	−
Inulin	−	−	−
Lactose	+⁻	+	v
Mannitol	−⁺	−	−
Melibiose	−⁺	−⁺	−⁺
Raffinose	−⁺	−	−
Salicin	+⁻	+⁻	+⁻
Sorbitol	−	−	−
Trehalose	+⁻	+	+⁻
Production of:			
α-Glucosidase	−⁺	+	+⁻
β-Glucosidase	+	v	−
α-Galactosidase	−⁺	−	−
β-Galactosidase	−	+	−⁺
β-D-Fucosidase	−	+	−
β-Glucuronidase	−	−	−
β-*N*-Acetylglucosaminidase	−	+	−
β-*N*-Acetylgalactosaminidase	−	+	−
Sialidase	−	+	−
Hyaluronidase	−⁺	+	+
H_2O_2 production	−⁺	−	−

+, positive; −, negative; v, variable; +⁻, most strains positive; −⁺, most strains negative.

media and are divided into three groups based on those reactions. Individual species within each group are further differentiated into separate species on the basis of additional tests or characteristics. More recently, Knudtson and Hartman[408] at Iowa State University examined 59 strains of 13 *Enterococcus* species with conventional methods and two kit systems (including the API Rapid Strep system and the MicroScan Pos ID panel). These workers found several discrepancies between published reactions for individual tests, reactions in their own conventional tests, and individual test results obtained with the two kit systems. By using combinations of various conventional and kit-based tests, these workers also published multiphasic dichotomous keys for identifying these organisms. A flowchart for identifying the clinically significant *Enterococcus* species is presented in Figure 12-4.[219,408]

For identification of enterococci by conventional procedures, carbohydrate fermentation tests and pyruvate utilization are determined in heart infusion broth base media containing bromcresol purple and 1% filter-sterilized carbohydrates or 1% pyruvate. Deamination of arginine is determined using Moeller's decarboxylase broth, and motility is determined in semisolid motility medium. Detection of the yellow pigment produced by *E. casseliflavus*, *E. gallinarum*, and *E. mundtii* is acheived by sweeping up some of the growth on a white Dacron swab and observing the colonial material on the swab for a yellow or yellow-orange color. Cartwright and coworkers found that the

TABLE 12-14
CHARACTERISTICS FOR IDENTIFICATION OF "ABIOTROPHIA DEFECTIVA" AND "ABIOTROPHIA ADIACENS"

CHARACTERISTIC	A. DEFECTIVA	A. ADIACENS
PYR test	+	+
Leucine aminopeptidase	+	+
Alkaline phosphatase	−	−
α-Galactosidase	+	−
β-Galactosidase	+	−
β-Glucuronidase	−	v
β-Glucosidase	−	v
Hippurate hydrolysis	−	−
Arginine dihydrolase	−	−
Acid production from:		
Trehalose	+	−
Inulin	−	v
Lactose	v	−
Raffinose	v	−
Starch	−	v

+, positive; −, negative; v, variable.

TABLE 12-15
CHARACTERISTICS FOR IDENTIFICATION OF STREPTOCOCCUS SUIS

CHARACTERISTIC	REACTION
Hemolysis on sheep blood agar	α
Esculin hydrolysis	+
Growth, 6.5% NaCl	−
Growth, 10°C	−
Growth, 45°C	−
Growth in 40% bile	v
Group D antigen	+
Leucine arylamidase	+
Arginine dihydrolase	+
Starch hydrolysis	+
Glycogen hydrolysis	+
Hippurate hydrolysis	−
Acetoin production	−
Alkaline phosphatase	−
α-Galactosidase	+
β-Galactosidase	v
β-Glucuronidase	+
Acid produced from	
Arabinose	−
Glucose	+
Glycerol	−
Inulin	+
Lactose	+
Maltose	+
Mannitol	−
Melezitose	−
Melibiose	v
Raffinose	v
Ribose	−
Salicin	+
Sorbitol	−
Sucrose	+

+, positive; −, negative; v, variable.

use of both motility and pigment detection tests together with a commercial test system greatly improved the reliability and accuracy of enterococcal identification in the clinical laboratory.[109]

Identification of enterococci to species level may be helpful and sometimes crucial for proper patient management and for epidemiologic purposes. It is recognized that *E. faecium* isolates tend to be even more resistant to penicillin and ampicillin than *E. faecalis* isolates, and vancomycin-resistance is seen most often in *E. faecium*. Ford and colleagues described a medium called cephalexin–aztreonam–arabinose agar that could be used in epidemiologic studies to detect the presence of *E. faecium* in stools of hospitalized patients who are at risk for serious enterococcal infections.[252] This medium contained arabinose (10 g/L), aztreonam (75 mg/L), cephalexin (50 mg/L), and phenol-red indicator (2%) in a Columbia agar base (40 g/L). *E. faecium* grew on this media as white colonies with yellow haloes, indicating acid production from arabinose, while *E. faecalis* grew as clear colonies with no haloes, indicating lack of arabinose utilization. Several other media fomulations have also been devised for direct detection of VRE in stool specimens of at-risk patients.[421]

Many laboratories rely on kit systems for identifying enterococci. Most of the kit systems described later in the chapter also perform very well for identifying the more common species. Table 12-16 is a compendium of the biochemical characteristics of all accepted or proposed *Enterococcus* species described in the American and European literature. Genetic and molecular methods for identification of *Enterococcus* species and for genotypic characterization of phenotypically derived antimicrobial susceptibilities have also been developed and include DNA hybridization

methods, contour-clamped homogeneous electric field electrophoresis, ribotyping, pulsed-field gel electrophoresis, and PCR.[184,196,294]

IDENTIFICATION OF AEROCOCCUS AND HELCOCOCCUS SPECIES

Aerococci closely resemble the viridans streptococci or enterococci. They are usually α-hemolytic. Currently, there are two species in the genus *Aerococcus*: *A. viridans* and *A. urinae*. Strains of *A. viridans* characteristically appear as tetrads on gram-stained smears, whereas *A. urinae* isolates occur mostly in clusters. On agar media, strains of *A. viridans* form large colonies that resemble those of enterococci. Both of these species will grow in 6.5% NaCl. Some strains of *A. viridans* are bile–esculin-positive, whereas *A. urinae* strains are negative. Isolates of *A. viridans* are PYR-positive and LAP-negative, but *A. urinae* strains are PYR-negative and LAP-posi-

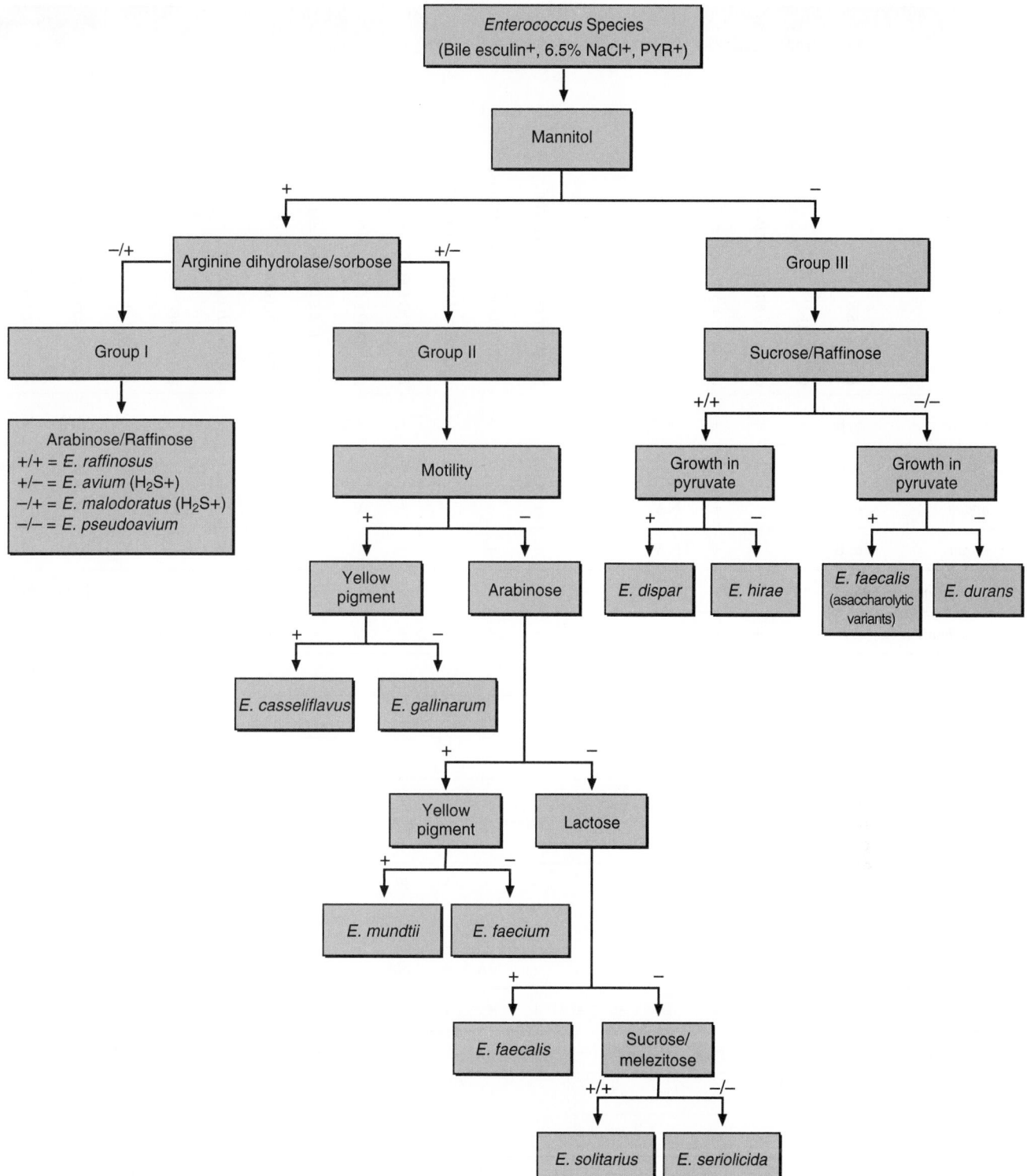

Figure 12-4
Flowchart for biochemical identification of *Enterococcus* species (after reference 219).

tive. Other tests that differentiate *A. viridans* and *A. urinae* include production of β-galactosidase and β-glucuronidase, hydrolysis of hippurate, and acid production from maltose, lactose, trehalose, and sorbitol (Table 12-17). PCR- and DNA probe-based

assays have been developed for identification of both *A. viridans* and *A. urinae*.[7,73,307]

Another aerococcus-like species that has recently been described is *Helcococcus kunzii*. Unlike most aerococci, this species produces variable growth in 6.5%

TABLE 12-16
Characteristics for Identification of *Enterococcus* Species

	HEMOLYSIS ON SBA	GROUP D ANTIGEN	GROWTH, BILE ESCULIN AGAR	GROWTH, 6.5% NaCl BROTH	GROWTH AT 10°C	GROWTH AT 45°C	MOTILITY	PIGMENT ON SBA (YELLOW)	PYRROLIDONYLARYLAMIDASE (PYR)	LEUCINE AMINOPEPTIDASE (LAP)	ESCULIN HYDROLYSIS	HIPPURATE HYDROLYSIS	ARGININE DIHYDROLASE	α-GALACTOSIDASE	β-GALACTOSIDASE	β-GLUCURONIDASE	H₂S PRODUCTION	ACETOIN PRODUCTION (VP)	ALKALINE PHOSPHATASE
E. faecalis	γ, β	+⁻	+	+	+	+	−⁺	−	+	+	+⁻	+⁻	+	−	−	−	−	NA	NA
E. faecium	γ, α	+⁻	+	+	+	+	−⁺	−	+	+	+⁻	−⁺	+	−	+	−	−	NA	NA
E. avium	α, γ	+⁻	+	+	NA	+	−	−	+	+	+	V	−	−	−⁺	−	+	V	NA
E. durans	α, β	+⁻	+	+	NA	+	−	−	+	+	+	V	+	−	V	−	−	NA	NA
E. gallinarum	α, β	+	+	+	+	+	+	−	+	+	+	+⁻	+	+	+	V	−	NA	NA
E. malodoratus	γ	+	+	+	NA	−⁺	−	−	+	+	+	V	−	+	+	NA	+	−	NA
E. casseliflavus	α	+	+	+	NA	+	+	+	+	+	+	−	+⁻	+	+	−	−	+	NA
E. mundtii	γ	+⁻	+	+	+	+	−	+	+	+	+	−	+	+⁻	+	−	NA	+	−
E. hirae	γ	+⁻	+	+	+	+	−	−	+	+	+	−⁺	+	NA	+	−	NA	NA	−
E. raffinosus	α, γ	+⁻	+	+	+ʷ	+	−	−	+	+	+	−⁺	−	−	−	−	NA	+	−
E. pseudoavium	α	−	+	−	+	+	−	−	+	+	+	+⁻	−	−	+	−	NA	+	−
E. solitarius	α	+	+	+	+	+	−	−	+	+	+	+	+	+	−	−	NA	V	−
E. dispar	α, γ	NA	+	+	+	−	−	−	+	+	+	V	+	+	+	−	NA	NA	−
E. seriolicida	α	−	NA	+	NA	+	−	−	NA	+	NA	−	+	NA	NA	NA	−	+	+
E. sulfureus	α	−	+	+	+	−	−	+	+	+	+	−	−	+	+	−	NA	NA	−
E. flavescens	γ	+	NA	NA	−⁺	+⁻	+	+	+	+	+	−	+	+	+	−	NA	+	−
E. columbae	α, γ	−	+	−	NA	NA	−	−	+	+	−	−	+	V	−	NA	+	+
E. cecorum	α	−	NA	−⁺	−	+	−	−	+	+	+	−	−	−⁺	−⁺	+	NA	+	+
E. saccharolyticus	α	−	NA	+ʷ	+	+	−	−	+	+	+	−	−	+	+	−	NA	−	−

+, positive; −, negative; +⁻, most strains positive, some negative; −⁺, most strains negative, some positive;
V, variable; +ʷ, positive, but weak or delayed; NA, data not available.

NaCl, and growth is stimulated by serum or Tween 80. On the API Rapid Strep system, *H. kunzii* produces a profile that corresponds to a "doubtful" identification of *A. viridans* (profile 4100413). Isolates of *H. kunzii* are nonhemolytic and do not grow at either 10°C or 45°C. The organism is PYR-positive, LAP-negative, produces acid from glucose, maltose, lactose, and trehalose, and does not produce β-galactosidase or β-glucuronidase. All of these organisms are vancomycin-susceptible. Characteristics for identifying *A. viridans*, *A. urinae*, and *H. kunzii* are shown in Table 12-17.

	ADONITOL	AMIDON	AMYGDALIN	L-ARABINOSE	GLUCOSE	GLYCEROL	GLYCOGEN	INOSITOL	INULIN	MANNITOL	MELIBIOSE	MELEZITOSE	LACTOSE	RAFFINOSE	RIBOSE	SORBITOL	SORBOSE	SUCROSE	D-TAGATOSE	TREHALOSE	D-XYLOSE	XYLITOL
												ACID PRODUCTION FROM:										
E. faecalis	−	−⁺	+	−	+	+⁻	−	−	−	+	−	+⁻	+	−	+	+⁻	−	+⁻	+	+	−	−
E. faecium	−	−	+	+	+	V	−	−	−	+⁻	+⁻	−	+	−	+	−	−	V	−⁺	+	−⁺	−
E. avium	+	−	NA	+	+	V	−	NA	−	+	V	+⁻	NA	−	+	+⁻	−	+⁻	+	+	−	+
E. durans	−	−	NA	−	+	−	−	NA	−	−⁺	V	−	NA	−	+	−	−	−	−⁺	+⁻	−	−
E. gallinarum	−	+⁻	+	+	+	+⁻	−⁺	−⁺	V	+	+	−⁺	+	+	+	−	−	+	+⁻	+	+	−
E. malodoratus	+	−	NA	−	+	V	−	NA	−	+	+	−	NA	+	NA	+	+	+	+	+	V	+
E. casseliflavus	−	+ʷ	NA	+	+	V	−	NA	+⁻	+	+	−	NA	+⁻	+	−	−	+	−⁺	+	+	−
E. mundtii	−	−⁺	+	+	+	V	−	−	−⁺	+	+	−	+	+⁻	+	+⁻	−	+	−	+	+	−
E. hirae	−	NA	+	−	+	−⁺	−	−	−	−	+⁻	V	+	V	+	−	−	+	−⁺	−⁺	−	−
E. raffinosus	NA	V	NA	+	+	+	−	NA	−	+	+	+	+	+	+	+	+	+	NA	+	NA	NA
E. pseudoavium	NA	−	NA	−	+	−	−	NA	−	+	−	−	+	−	+	+	+	−	NA	+	NA	NA
E. solitarius	−	−	+	−	+	+	−	−	−	+	−⁺	+	−	NA	−	+	−	+	+	+	−	−
E. dispar	NA	−	NA	−	+	+	−	NA	−	−	+	NA	+	+	+	−	−	+	NA	+	NA	NA
E. seriolicida	−	NA	NA	NA	+	−	−	−	NA	+	−	−	−	−	NA	+	NA	−	NA	+	−	NA
E. sulfureus	−	NA	+	−	+	−	−	−	−	+	+	+	+	+	+	NA	+	−	+	−	−	−
E. flavescens	−	−	+	+	+	−	−	+	+	NA	−	+	+	−	−	−	−	+	−	+	+	−
E. columbae	−	+	V	+	+	−	−	−	+	+	+	V	V	+	+	+	−	+	V	+	+	V
E. cecorum	−	NA	+	−	+	−	V	−	+	−	+	+	+	+	+	−	−	+	−⁺	+	−	−
E. saccharolyticus	−	+	+	−	+	−	−	+	+	+	+	+	+	+	+	+	+	−⁺	+	−	+	−

IDENTIFICATION OF *LEUCONOSTOC*, *PEDIOCOCCUS*, AND *TETRAGENOCOCCUS* SPECIES

Leuconostoc species are gram-positive, catalase-negative, lactic acid-producing cocci that are resistant to vancomycin and produce CO_2 gas from glucose.[223]

These bacteria may be differentiated from the gas-producing lactobacilli by careful scrutiny of gram-stained smears made from thioglycolate broth (see Color Plates 12-3E and 12-3F). *Leuconostoc* species do not grow at 45°C and are arginine dihydrolase-negative, PYR-negative, and LAP-negative. Production of gas

TABLE 12-17

CHARACTERISTICS FOR IDENTIFICATION OF *AEROCOCCUS VIRIDANS*, *AEROCOCCUS URINAE*, AND *HELCOCOCCUS KUNZII*

CHARACTERISTIC	A. VIRIDANS	A. URINAE	H. KUNZII
Gram stain	Pairs, tetrads	Pairs, tetrads	Pairs, short chains, clusters
Relation to oxygen	Microaerophilic	Microaerophilic	Facultative
Hemolysis	α	α	Nonhemolytic
Catalase	−	−	−
Growth, BE agar	−[a]	−	−
Growth, 6.5% NaCl	+	+	v
PYR	+	−	+
LAP	−	+	+
Growth at 10°C	+	−	−
Growth at 45°C	−	−	−
Esculin hydrolysis	−	−	+
Arginine dihydrolase	−	−	−
Hippurate hydrolysis	−	v	−
β-Galactosidase	+	−	−
β-Glucuronidase	−	+	−
Acid production from			
Glucose	+	+	+
Maltose	+	−	+
Lactose	+	−	+
Trehalose	+	−	+
Sorbitol	−	+	−
Acetoin (VP)	−	−	−
Nitrate reduction	−	−	−
Motility	−	−	−
Growth stimulated by serum or Tween 80	−	−	+

+, positive; −, negative; v, variable; NA, data not available; [a]Rare bile-esculin-positive strains have been reported.

from glucose is best determined in *Lactobacillus* MRS (Mann-Rogosa-Sharpe) broth (Difco Laboratories, Detroit MI) overlayed with sterile petrolatum. The formation of bubbles under the petrolatum seal indicates gas production and confirms their heterofermentative metabolism. The eight *Leuconostoc* species are further identified by a battery of biochemical tests (Table 12-18).[38,270] *Leuconostoc* species have also been identified by sodium dodecyl sulfate–polyacryamide gel electrophoresis (SDS–PAGE) analysis of soluble whole-cell proteins.[205,206]

Pediococcus species are also intrinsically vancomycin-resistant gram-positive cocci. However, they are generally homofermentative, similar to the streptococci and, unlike *Leuconostoc* species, they do not produce gas from glucose in MRS broth.[223] The organisms appear as gram-positive cocci in pairs, clusters, and tetrads, and they are catalase-negative. Growth occurs over a temperature range of 25°C to 50°C. On plates, they resemble viridans streptococci in their colony morphology. They may be confused with group D streptococci or enterococci because they are bile–esculin-positive, they possess the Lancefield group D antigen, and some strains grow in the presence of 6.5% NaCl. Pediococci are PYR-negative and LAP-positive.

The species that have been recovered from human infections include *P. acidilactici* and *P. pentosaceus*. These organisms may be difficult to differentiate from one another, with maltose fermentation—positive for *P. pentosaceus* and negative for *P. acidilactici*—being the most reliable test for separation of the two. Tankovic and associates noted, however, that the two species could be separated by susceptibility to novobiocin.[644] All 25 *P. acidilactici* strains were susceptible to novobiocin (5-μg disk zone diameters of 16 mm or larger), whereas all nine *P. pentosaceus* strains were resistant to novobiocin (zone diameters 10 mm or smaller).[644] Both of these species are susceptible to β-lactams, clindamycin, rifampin, erythromycin, gentamicin, and imipenem and are resistant to vancomycin, teicoplanin, and the fluoroquinolones.[644]

In *Bergey's Manual*, eight species of *Pediococcus* are described; *P. acidilactici*, *P. pentosaceus*, *P. dextrinicus*, *P. damnosus*, *P. parvulus*, *P. inopinatus*, *P. halophilus*, and *P. urinae-equi*. *P. urinae-equi* has been shown to be identical with *A. viridans*.[307] *P. halophilus* appears to be quite different from both the pediococci and the aerococci and is phylogenetically closer to the enterococci. Because of this, it has been proposed that *P. halophilus* be reclassified into the new genus *Tetragenococcus* as *T.*

TABLE 12-18

Characteristics for Identification of Leuconostoc Species

Characteristic	L. MESENTEROIDES ss. MESENTEROIDES	L. MESENTEROIDES ss. DEXTRANICUM	L. MESENTEROIDES ss. CREMORIS	L. (W.) PARAMESENTEROIDES	L. PSEUDOMESENTEROIDES	L. CITREUM	L. LACTIS	L. OENOS (O. OENOS)	L. GELIDUM	L. CARNOSUM	L. FALLAX	L. ARGENTINUM
Hemolysis, SBA	−	−	−	−	−	−	−	−	−	−	−	−
Lemon-yellow pigment	NA	NA	$-^{+}$	−	$-^{+}$	+	−	−	−	−	−	−
Growth, 10°C	$+^{-}$	+	NA	NA	+	+	NA	$+^{-}$	+	+	+	+
Growth, 37°C	+	NA	−	$+^{-}$	+	$+^{-}$	+	$+^{-}$	$-^{+}$	$-^{+}$	+	+
Growth, 45°C	−	−	NA	NA	−	−	$-^{+}$	NA	−	−	−	−
Esculin hydrolysis	$+^{-}$	$+^{-}$	−	$+^{-}$	+	+	−	+	+	$-^{+}$	NA	−
Dextran from sucrose	+	+	−	−	NA	NA	−	−	V	+	NA	−
Acid produced from												
Amygdalin	V	V	−	−	$-^{+}$	$+^{-}$	−	NA	+	−	−	−
L-Arabinose	$+^{-}$	−	−	+	$+^{-}$	+	$-^{+}$	V	+	+	−	V
Arbutin	V	−	−	−	$-^{+}$	+	−	NA	+	V	−	−
Cellobiose	$+^{-}$	V	−	V	$+^{-}$	+	−	V	+	+	+	V
Fructose	+	+	V	+	+	+	+	+	+	+	+	$+^{-}$
Galactose	$+^{-}$	V	$+^{-}$	+	+	$-^{+}$	+	V	NA	NA	NA	V
β-Gentobiose	V	NA	−	$-^{+}$	V	+	−	NA	NA	NA	NA	−
Gluconate	V	NA	−	+	V	+	+	NA	−	+	+	+
Glucose	+	+	+	+	+	+	+	+	+	+	+	+
Lactose	V	+	V	−	V	+	+	+	−	−	−	+
Maltose	+	+	$-^{+}$	+	+	+	+	+	+	V	+	V
Mannitol	$+^{sl}$	V	−	$+^{sl}$	$-^{+}$	V	−	V	V	−	$+^{sl}$	+
Mannose	+	V	V	+	+	+	+	V	+	V	+	+
Melibiose	+	V	$-^{+}$	+	$+^{-}$	−	+	−	+	V	−	$+^{-}$
Raffinose	$+^{-}$	+	$-^{+}$	+	$+^{-}$	−	$+^{-}$	−	+	−	−	−
Ribose	$+^{-}$	NA	−	$-^{+}$	+	+	$-^{+}$	NA	V	V	+	+
Salicin	+	V	−	+	V	+	−	+	+	V	−	−
Starch	−	−	−	−	$+^{sl}$	+	−	NA	NA	NA	NA	−
Sucrose	+	+	−	+	$+^{-}$	+	+	−	+	+	+	+
Trehalose	+	+	V	+	+	+	V	+	NA	+	$+^{sl}$	V
Turanose	$+^{-}$	NA	V	+	$+^{-}$	+	−	NA	NA	NA	+	V
Xylose	+	V	$-^{+}$	+	+	$-^{+}$	−	V	−	−	−	V
Habitat	Dairy products, vegetation	Dairy products	Dairy products	Dairy products	Plants, vegetation, dairy products	Plants	Dairy products	Wine	Meat and meat products	Meat and meat products	Pickled cabbage (sauerkraut)	Argentinean raw milk

+, positive; −, negative; $+^{sl}$, positive reaction but slow or delayed; NA, data not available; V, variable; NTD, not to date; $-^{+}$, most strains negative, some positive; $+^{-}$, most strains positive, some negative.

halophilus. From data given in the original description of this species, *T. halophilus* characteristically grow as pairs or tetrads (hence, the name) and, occasionally, as clusters, do not grow at 10°C or at 45°C, are nonmotile, grow in 6.5% NaCl (actually will grow in up to 10% NaCl), grow on BE agar, and are arginine dihydrolase-negative. Most strains produce acid from arabinose, glucose, glycerol, maltose, ribose, sucrose, and trehalose, and do not produce acid from lactose, mannose, mannitol, and sorbitol. Unlike the other pediococci, *T. halophilus* is susceptible to vancomycin. Additional characteristics for identifying *T. halophilus* and the remaining six species of pediococci are shown in Table 12-19.

IDENTIFICATION OF GEMELLA SPECIES

There are two species in the genus *Gemella*: *G. hemolysans* and *G. morbillorum*. *G. morbillorum* was formerly called *Streptococcus morbillorum* and was classified with the viridans streptococci. *Gemella* species are α- or nonhemolytic on sheep blood agar and resemble colonies of viridans streptococci. *G. hemolysans* differs from *G. morbillorum* in basic growth characteristics: the former species grows better under aerobic conditions, whereas the latter species grows better under anaerobic conditions. Both species are stimulated by incubation in a CO_2-enriched environment. Because of their thin cell walls, these bacteria easily decolorize on gram-staining and may appear as gram-negative cocci in pairs, tetrads, clusters, and short chains.[561] The individual cells in these arrangements may show considerable variations in size. Both species, similar to streptococci, produce lactic acid as the major end product of glucose fermentation. Biochemically, these organisms resemble one another closely, but they can be differentiated from one another by nitrite reduction, with *G. hemolysans* being nitrite reduction-positive and *G. morbillorum* being nitrite reduction-negative(Table 12-20). Growth is enhanced by the presence of fermentable carbohydrates and by the addition of Tween 80 to the growth media. Because of limited numbers of clinical isolates, the performance of kit systems for identifying these bacteria cannot be assessed critically, although they are included in the databases of the Vitek GPI card, the RapID STR, and the API Rapid Strep system.

IDENTIFICATION OF ALLOIOCOCCUS, VAGOCOCCUS, AND GLOBICATELLA SPECIES

A. otitidis has been isolated from tympanocentesis specimens obtained from the middle ear of children with chronic otitis media, from blood cultures, and from sputum.[4,74,221,227] The organism grows slowly, with visible colonies apparent only after 2 to 3 days. Gram-stained smears from broth or agar media show cocci arranged in pairs, tetrads, and sometimes clusters. Optimal growth occurs at 35° to 37°C, and no growth occurs at either 10° or 45°C. Colonies appear off-white, pinpoint, and nonhemolytic, although α-hemolysis and slightly yellow pigmentation may be observed after several days' incubation.[74] Fresh clinical isolates of *A. otitidis* will grow on blood agar but may not grow on chocolate agar. Luxuriant growth in broth containing 0.5% Tween or 0.07% lecithin suggests that the organism may require lipid for optimal growth.[74] Unlike the other organisms considered in this chapter, *A. otitidis* is catalase-positive; this reaction may be quite weak or delayed. Acid is not produced from any carbohydrates, and the organism is aerobic rather than facultative in its metabolism. *A. otitidis* grows on bile–esculin agar but does not hydrolyze esculin and also grows sparsely and slowly in 6.5% NaCl broth. PYR, LAP, and β-galactosidase are produced, and hippurate is hydrolyzed by some isolates. Aguirre and Collins have described a PCR-probe test for specific identification of *A. otitidis*.[5] Bosley and colleagues[74] performed antimicrobial susceptibility studies on 19 *A. otitidis* strains and found that all 19 strains were resistant to trimethoprim–sulfamethoxazole, and 18 of 19 were resistant to erythromycin. The MICs for penicillin

TABLE 12-19
CHARACTERISTICS FOR IDENTIFICATION OF *PEDIOCOCCUS* SPP. AND *TETRAGENOCOCCUS HALOPHILUS*

SPECIES	GROWTH AT 45°C	ACID PRODUCTION FROM							
		GLUCOSE	GLYCEROL	STARCH	MALTOSE	ARABINOSE	DEXTRIN	XYLOSE	MELEZITOSE
*P. acidilactici**	+	+	−	−	−	v	−	+	−
*P. pentosaceus**	v	+	−	−	+	+	−	v	−
P. dextrinicus	−	+	−	+	+	−	+	−	−
P. damnosus	−	+	−	−	v	−	−	−	v
P. parvulus	−	+	−	−	+	−	−	−	−
P. inopinatus	−	+	−	−	+	−	v	−	−
T. halophilus	−	+	+	−	+	+	−	−	+

+, positive; −, negative; v, variable.
* These two species have been recovered from human clinical specimens. *P. acidilactici* is susceptible to novobiocin (5 µg disk, zones ≥ 16 mm), whereas *P. pentosaceus* is resistant to novobiocin (zone ≤ 10 mm).

TABLE 12-20
CHARACTERISTICS FOR IDENTIFICATION OF GEMELLA HEMOLYSANS AND GEMELLA MORBILLORUM

CHARACTERISTIC	G. HEMOLYSANS	G. MORBILLORUM
Esculin hydrolysis	−	−
Arginine dihydrolase	−	−
Leucine aminopeptidase	v	+
PYR test	v	−
Reduction of nitrate	−	−
Reduction of nitrite	+	−
Acid production from		
Glucose	+	+
Maltose	+^{w}	+^{w}
Mannitol	v	+^{w}

+, positive; −, negative; v, variable; +^{w}, positive, but reaction delayed or weak.

and ampicillin ranged from susceptible to intermediately resistant (MIC range for penicillin, 0.06 to 0.12 µg/mL; ampicillin MIC range, 0.12 to 0.5 µg/mL), with the same degree of relative resistance being seen for ceftriaxone and cefixime. None of the strains they examined produced β-lactamases.[74]

The genus *Vagococcus* was initially described as motile, group N lactococci, with the type strain being *V. fluvialis*. *V. fluvialis* is streptococcus-like in its colony morphology and is α- or nonhemolytic, facultative and homofermentative in its metabolism, and is catalase-negative. On Gram stain, the organisms appear as spherical to ovoid cells, arranged in pairs or chains. According to the original description by Collins and coauthors, *V. fluvialis* are motile cocci that produce peritrichous flagella. Motility can be demonstrated with motility medium incubated at room temperature. The organism grows at 10° and 40°C but does not grow at 45°C. In the original description of *V. fluvialis* by Collins and colleagues, this organism was reported to be LAP-negative, PYR-variable, and negative for growth in 6.5% NaCl broth, but strains submitted to the CDC have been both PYR- and LAP-positive and have demonstrated growth in 6.5% NaCl broth medium.[221] Strains of *V. fluvialis* have been recovered from pigs, cats, and horses; these strains were VP-, alkaline phosphatase- and LAP-positive, and some of the strains were nonmotile.[543] The organism is VP, hippurate, and gelatin hydrolysis negative.

V. salmoninarum isolates have been recovered only from diseased rainbow trout, Atlantic salmon, and brown trout with peritonitis, so, at least for the time being, its appearance in human clinical specimens is unlikely.[603,686] *V. salmoninarum* is not motile (even though the name "vagococcus" means "wandering berry"). Besides motility, the two *Vagococcus* species can also be differentiated by acid production from glycerol, mannitol, and sorbitol, inability of *V. salmoninarum* to grow at 40°C, and the production of H_2S by *V. salmoninarum* but not by *V. fluvialis*.[686]

G. sanguis strains, on the other hand, have been recovered from human specimens and may represent those occasional isolates for which the biochemical characteristics do not seem to "fit." The organisms appear as gram-positive cocci in pairs and short chains. Colonies on sheep blood agar are streptococcus-like and are α-hemolytic. They differ from the enterococci and the lactococci in that they do not grow at 10°C or at 45°C. Similar to the enterococci, *G. sanguis* is able to grow in 6.5% NaCl and produces pyrrolidonyl arylamidase; unlike both the enterococci and the streptococci, leucine aminopeptidase is not produced.[134] These reactions also differentiate *G. sanguis* from other viridans streptococci in that the latter species are PYR-negative, LAP-positive, and do not grow in 6.5% NaCl broth. Esculin is hydrolyzed, and some strains may grow on bile–esculin agar. The BactiCard STREP (Remel Laboratories), which includes rapid PYR, LAP, and esculin hydrolysis tests in a card format, can be used for this purpose. Unlike the aerococci, *G. sanguis* produces distinct chains in broth media instead of tetrads. This growth characteristic must be determined to differentiate this organism from *A. viridans*, which it phenotypically resembles.

A summary of the biochemical characteristics for identifying *A. otitis*, *V. fluvialis*, *V. salmoninarum*, and *G. sanguis* is presented in Table 12-21.

IDENTIFICATION OF *LACTOCOCCUS* SPECIES

Because of the superficial resemblance to enterococci or the viridans streptococci, these organisms were (and are) probably misidentified as atypical streptococci or enterococci in the clinical laboratory. Lactococci, unlike enterococci, should not grow at 45°C. The lactococci show many of the characteristics of both streptococci and enterococci; many strains are PYR-, LAP-, BE-, and 6.5% NaCl-positive, and are able to grow at 10°C. A "tip off" to the possibility that one is dealing with a possible *Lactococcus* species is the generation of a list of characteristics that do not fit either streptococci or enterococci.[221] Most clinical isolates of lactococci submitted to the CDC have been either *L. lactis* subsp. *lactis* or *L. garviae*.[221] These two species can be differentiated from common *Enterococcus* species in that both species produce acid from mannitol but do not produce acid from raffinose, sorbitol, or arabinose. *Lactococcus* species and "*Streptococcus lactis–S. cremoris*" are included in the databases of the ID 32 Strep and the API Rapid STREP kits, respectively (see the following section). Biochemical characteristics for identifying *Lactococcus* species are presented in Table 12-22.

KIT SYSTEMS FOR IDENTIFYING STREPTOCOCCI, ENTEROCOCCI, AND SELECTED STREPTOCOCCUS-LIKE BACTERIA

Fortunately, the development of kit systems that incorporate similar types of physiologic and enzymatic tests

TABLE 12-21

CHARACTERISTICS FOR IDENTIFICATION OF *ALLOIOCOCCUS OTITIS*, *VAGOCOCCUS* SPP., AND *GLOBICATELLA SANGUIS*

CHARACTERISTIC	A. OTITIS	V. FLUVIALIS	V. SALMONINARUM	G. SANGUIS
Cell arrangement	Pairs, tetrads	Singles, pairs, short chains	Singles, pairs	Pairs, short chains
Hemolysis	α	α, nonhemolytic	α, nonhemolytic	α
Catalase	+	−	−	−
Relation to oxygen	Aerobic	Facult.	Facult.	Facult.
Growth at 10°C	−	+	+	−
Growth at 45°C	−	−	−	−
Growth, BE agar	+	NA	NA	v
Growth, 6.5% NaCl	+	+*	NA	+
PYR	+	+*	NA	+
Leucine aminopeptidase	+	+*	NA	−
Arginine dihydrolase	−	v	−	−
Esculin hydrolysis	−	+	+	+
Hippurate hydrolysis	v	−	NA	+
H₂S production	NA	−	+	−
Motility	−	+	−	−
α-Galactosidase	NA	−	NA	NA
β-Galactosidase	+	v	NA	NA
β-Glucuronidase	NA	−	NA	NA
Acid production from				
Arabinose	−	−	−	−
Fructose	−	+	+	NA
Galactose	−	−	−	NA
Glucose/gas	−/−	+/−	+/−	+/−
Glycerol	−	+	−	−
Inulin	−	−	−	NA
Lactose	−	−	−	+
Maltose	−	+	+	+
Mannitol	−	+	−	+
Mannose	−	+	+	NA
Ribose	−	+	+	+
Raffinose	−	−	−	+
Sorbitol	−	+	−	+
Sucrose	−	v	+	+
Trehalose	−	+	+	+
Isolated from	Middle ear	River water, human specimens	Salmonid fish	Human specimens

+, positive; −, negative; v, variable; NA, data not available.
* In the original description of *V. fluvialis,* these three tests were negative, but strains submitted to the CDC have been LAP-, PYR-, and 6.5% NaCl-positive.

for streptococcal identification have been of great help in species identification of the viridans streptococci, *Enterococcus* species, and the group D streptococci. The biochemical reactions included in the kit systems are used to generate an organism biotype number that corresponds to the organism's identity. Although these systems include the β-hemolytic streptococci in their databases, these organisms are best handled using other methods, such as the presumptive tests described earlier or the rapid streptococcal-grouping kits that are available. However, caution should also be exercised with the commercial identification kits. For example, the Rapid STREP strip will misidentify *Leuconostoc* organisms as species of viridans streptococci, so vancomycin-resistance and other preliminary test

results must be considered along with the biochemical reactions that are observed on the strip. Commercial systems for the identification of streptococci include the following.

API RAPID STREP

This strip format system (bioMerieux-Vitek, Hazelwood MO) includes 20 tests, including physiologic tests, chromogenic enzyme substrate tests, and carbohydrate utilization tests. The unique thing about this system is that the strip can be read twice. If an identification is not obtained after 4 hours' incubation using the physiologic and chromogenic substrates, the strip is reincubated and read after overnight incuba-

TABLE 12-22
CHARACTERISTICS FOR IDENTIFICATION OF LACTOCOCCUS SPECIES

SPECIES SUBSPECIES	ARGININE HYDROLYSIS	HIPPURATE HYDROLYSIS	HYDROLYSIS OF PYR	VP REACTION	Acid from								
					GLUCOSE	LACTOSE	MALTOSE	SUCROSE	MANNITOL	SORBITOL	RAFFINOSE	TREHALOSE
L. lactis												
subsp. *lactis*	+	−	v	+⁻	+	+	+	+⁻	+	−	−	+
subsp. *cremoris*	−	+	−	+	+	+	−	−	−	−	−	−
subsp. *hordniae*	+	−	−	+	+	−	−	+	−	−	−	+
L. garveiae	+	−	+	+	+	v	+	v	+	−	−	+
L. plantarum	−	−	−	+	+	−	+	+	+	+	−	+
L. raffinolactis	−	−	−	+	+	+	+	−	v	−	+	−
L. xyloses	+	−	−	+	+	−	+	+	+	−	−	+

+, positive reaction; −, negative reaction; +⁻, most strains positive, rare negative reactions; −⁺, most strains negative, rare positive reactions; v, variable reactions.

627

tion to include acid production from 10 carbohydrates (see Color Plate 12-3C). Evaluations have shown that this system provides excellent identifications for the group D streptococci and will identify 74% to 92% of the viridans streptococci and *S. milleri* group organisms.[10,21,351,586] The Rapid Strep system also has been evaluated for identifying some veterinary pathogens, specifically the agents of bovine mastitis (group B streptococci, *S. dysgalactiae*, *S. uberis*, *S. equi*, and *S. equinus*) and is also a reliable system for species identification of these organisms.[693] The database of the system is fairly extensive and includes groupable β-hemolytic streptococci, *Enterococcus* species (*E. faecalis*, *E. faecium*, *E. gallinarum*, *E. avium*, and *E. durans*), viridans streptococci, lactococci, aerococci, *Gemella* species, *S. bovis* strains, and *Listeria monocytogenes*. The Rapid STREP system is now the most widely available commercial system for identifying the streptococci and streptococcus-like bacteria. Identification of strains that have been completely characterized by conventional biochemical tests and genetic analysis (e.g., DNA relatedness, 16S rRNA sequencing) indicate that the Rapid STREP system is reproducible and complements existing genetic studies. In some cases, tests on the strip actually revealed phenotypic differences not seen with conventional methods. In other instances, the presence of phenotypic differences between strains on the Rapid STREP system could be demonstrated to be genotypically distinct when nucleic acid studies were performed. The biochemical reactions for many organisms shown in the tables of this chapter reflect the recent studies during which genetic analysis and the description of new species were performed along with the Rapid STREP characterization. The biggest problem with the Rapid STREP is that the database has not been updated or expanded to include several of the newer species (e.g., *S. vestibularis*, *S. gordonii*, *S. crista*).

RAPID ID 32 STREP SYSTEM

This system (bioMerieux, La Balme les Grottes, France) is a 32-test strip format identification system for the streptococci and streptococcus-like bacteria. The database of this system is very extensive and includes the groupable streptococci, several *Enterococcus* species, and the viridans streptococci (including newly described species such as the "mutans group" oral streptococci, *S. oralis*, *S. gordonii*, and *S. vestibularis*). A suspension of the bacterium to be identified is prepared in sterile water to a turbidity equivalent to a McFarland 4 standard and 55 μL of the suspension is placed into each of the 32 cupules. The strip is then incubated at 35° to 37°C for 4 hours and either read manually using a code book or with the automated reader (ATB 1520 Reader linked with an ATB 1545 computer, bioMerieux; see Color Plate 12-3G). In a recent evaluation of the Rapid ID 32 Strep system with 433 strains belonging to the genera *Streptococcus*, *Enterococcus*, *Lactococcus*, *Aerococcus*, *Gemella*, *Leuconostoc*, *Erysipelothrix*, *Gardnerella*, and *Listeria*, 95.3% of strains were correctly identified.[261] Additional tests were required for identification of 25.1% of the strains. Only

16 isolates (3.7%) were not identified, and only four isolates (1.0%) were misidentified. Another evaluation by Kikuchi and coworkers reported that the ID 32 Strep system identified 87% of 156 viridans streptococcal strains and that most misidentification involved strains of *S. oralis*, *S. mitis*, and *S. gordonii*.[393] The Rapid ID 32 Strep system is not yet available in the United States.

RAPID STR

This system (Innovative Diagnostic Systems, Norcross GA) employs a small cuvette containing 10 wells, four of which are bifunctional, resulting in a total of 14 biochemical tests (used in conjunction with the hemolytic reaction of the isolate). Tests include physiologic determinations (arginine dihydrolase, esculin hydrolysis), carbohydrate utilization tests, and chromogenic enzyme substrate hydrolysis (see Color Plate 12-3H). The system is inoculated with a suspension of the organism (McFarland 1 turbidity standard) prepared in a fluid purchased along with the kit, and the tests are read after 4-hour incubation at 35°C in a non-CO_2 incubator. In a large evaluation of over 200 viridans streptococcal isolates, the RapID STR identified 100% of the group D organisms and 85% of the viridans streptococci.[225] The RapID STR performed less well in another study at UCLA, where only 50% of 203 viridans streptococci were correctly identified.[351] The database of this system was recently updated and now includes the β-hemolytic streptococci group A, B, and C/G, group D streptococci (*S. bovis*, *S. bovis* variant, *S. equinus*), the *S. milleri* group (*S. anginosus*, *S. constellatus*, *S. intermedius*), *Enterococcus* species (*E. faecalis*, *E. faecium*, *E. avium*, *E. cassiliflavus/mundtii*, *E. durans/ hirae*, *E. gallinarum*, and *E. malodoratus*), viridans streptococcal species (*S. acidominimus*, *S. mitis*, *S. mutans*, *S. salivarius/vestibularis*, *S. sanguis/gordonii*), *S. pneumoniae*, the aerococci, and *Gemella morbillorum*.[22,733] The updated database now also includes *Leuconostoc* species (*L. citreum*, *L. lactis*, *L. mesenteroides* group) and *Pediococcus* species (*P. acidilactici*, *P. pentosaceus*).

VITEK GRAM-POSITIVE IDENTIFICATION (GPI) CARD

This card (Vitek Systems, Inc.) is the same one used for identifying the coagulase-negative staphylococci and certain non–sporeforming facultative gram-positive bacilli. The card contains 27 tests and two controls and provides automated identifications in from 4 to 13 hours. In the initial evaluations, the GPI card provided excellent results for the group D organisms but performed less well for identifying the viridans streptococci.[218] In an evaluation by Peterson and colleagues, performed at the University of California at Irvine, the GPI card correctly identified 72% of 109 clinical viridans streptococcal isolates.[534] This card has been modified slightly since its initial release and the database has been updated. The modified card with the expanded database has not been evaluated. The data-base for streptococcal identification includes the β-hemolytic streptococci, group D streptococci, *Enterococcus* species (*E. faecalis*, *E. faecium*, *E. avium*, *E. du-*

rans), some species of viridans streptococci, *S. anginosus*, and *Aerococcus* species. Less frequently isolated, but clinically important *Enterococcus* species, such as *E. casseliflavus*, are not included in the GPI database and may be misidentified as *E. faecium*.[89] As with the other systems, the more recently described species of viridans streptoccci are not yet included in the database.

MICROSCAN GRAM-POSITIVE BREAKPOINT COMBO PANEL

This 18-hour system provides simultaneous identification and antimicrobial susceptibility results in a microtiter format. Tritz and colleagues evaluated this system for its ability to identify enterococci and found that both *E. faecalis* and *E. faecium* were reliably identified, but less common enterococcal species were misidentified.[657]

MINITEK GRAM-POSITIVE KIT

This system (from BBL) employs filter paper disks that are impregnated with various substrates. The disks are dispensed into wells in a plastic tray, and the wells are inoculated with a suspension of the organism prepared in a broth provided with the kit. Watts evaluated this system for identifying streptococcal strains recovered from bovine mastitis and found that only 34.6% of 127 isolates were correctly identified, with more than 95% of *S. uberis* strains being misidentified as enterococci.[692] This system has not been evaluated extensively with human isolates. A semiautomated version of this system (BBL Sceptor) is also available, but its performance has not been examined.

Other microtiter format systems for streptococcal identification are available from American MicroScan (Sacramento CA) and from MicroMedia (San Jose CA), but these have not been evaluated.

REFERENCES

1. ADAMS JT, FAIX RG: *Streptococcus mitis* infection in newborns. J Perinatol 14:473–478, 1994
2. ADVISORY COMMITTEE ON IMMUNIZATION PRACTICES OF THE CENTERS FOR DISEASE CONTROL AND PREVENTION: Pneumococcal polysaccharide vaccine. MMWR 38:64–74, 1989
3. AGARWALA BN: Group B streptococcal endocarditis in a neonate. Pediatr Cardiol 9:51–53, 1988
4. AGUIRRE M, COLLINS MD: Phylogenetic analysis of *Alloiococcus otitis* gen. nov. sp. nov., an organism from human middle ear fluid. Int J Syst Bacteriol 42:79–83, 1992
5. AGUIRRE M, COLLINS MD: Development of a polymerase chain reaction-probe test for identification of *Alloiococcus otitis*. J Clin Microbiol 30:2177–2180, 1992
6. AGUIRRE M, COLLINS MD: Phylogenetic analysis of some *Aerococcus*-like organisms from urinary tract infections: description of *Aerococcus urinae* sp. nov. J Gen Microbiol 138:401–405, 1992
7. AGUIRRE M, COLLINS MD: Development of polymerase chain reaction test for specific identification of the urinary tract pathogen *Aerococcus urinae*. J Clin Microbiol 31:1350–1353, 1993
8. AGUIRRE M, COLLINS MD: Lactic acid bacteria and human clinical infection. J Appl Microbiol 75:95–107, 1993
9. AHARONI A, POTASMAN I, LEVITAN Z ET AL: Postpartum maternal group B streptococcal meningitis. Rev Infect Dis 12:273–276, 1990
10. AHMET Z, WARREN M, HOUANG ET: Species identification of members of the *Streptococcus milleri* group isolated from the vagina by ID32 Strep system and differential phenotypic characteristics. J Clin Microbiol 33:1592–1595, 1995
11. AKAIKE T, SUGA M, ANDO M ET AL: *Streptococcus acidominimus* infections in a human. Jpn J Med 27:317–320, 1988
12. ALBA D, ZAPATER P, TORRES E: Recurrent *Streptococcus sanguis* meningitis in a patient with a ventriculoperitoneal shunt. Clin Infect Dis 19:808, 1994
13. ALTAIE SS, DRYJA D: Detection of group B *Streptococcus*: comparison of solid and liquid culture media with and without selective antibiotics. Diagn Microbiol Infect Dis 18:141–144, 1994
14. ANCONA RJ, FERRIERI P, WILLIAMS PP: Maternal factors that enhance the acquisition of group B streptococci by newborn infants. J Med Microbiol 13:273–280, 1980
15. ANDERSSON B, DAHMEN J, FREJD T ET AL: Identification of an active disaccharide unit of a glycoconjugate receptor for pneumococci attaching to human pharyngeal epithelial cells. J Exp Med 158:559–569, 1983
16. ANHALT JP, HEITER BJ, NAUMOVITZ DW ET AL: Comparison of three methods for detection of group A streptococci in throat swabs. J Clin Microbiol 30:2135–2138, 1992
17. ANTALEK MD, MYLOTTE JM, LESSE AJ ET AL: Clinical and molecular epidemiology of *Enterococcus faecalis* bacteremia, with special reference to strains with high-level resistance to gentamicin. Clin Infect Dis 20:103–109, 1995
18. ANTHONY BF, EISENSTADT R, CARTER J ET AL: Genital and intestinal carriage of group B streptococci during pregnancy. J Infect Dis 143:761–766, 1977
19. ANTHONY BF, KAPLAN EL, WANNAMAKER LW ET AL: Attack rates of acute nephritis after type 49 streptococcal infection of the skin and the respiratory tract. J Clin Invest 48:1697–1704, 1969
20. APPELBAUM PC: Antimicrobial resistance in *Streptococcus pneumoniae*: an overview. Clin Infect Dis 15:77–83, 1992
21. APPELBAUM PC, CHARUSHIYA PD, JACOBS MR ET AL: Evaluation of the Rapid Strep system for species identification of streptococci. J Clin Microbiol 19:588–591, 1984
22. APPLEBAUM PC, JACOBS MR, PALKO WM ET AL: Accuracy and reproducibility of the IDS RapID STR system for species identification of streptococci. J Clin Microbiol 23:843–846, 1986
23. ARALA-CHAVES MP, RIBEIRO AS, SANTAREM MMG ET AL: Strong mitogenic effect for murine B lymphocytes of an immunosuppressor substance released by *Streptococcus intermedius*. Infect Immun 54:543–548, 1986

24. ARDITI M, SHULMAN ST, DAVIS AT ET AL: Group C *beta*-hemolytic streptococcal infections in children: nine pediatric cases and review. Rev Infect Dis 11:34–45, 1989

25. AREND SM, VAN BUCHEM MA, VAN OGTROP ML ET AL: Septicaemia, meningitis, and spondylodiscitis caused by *Streptococcus suis* type 2. Infection 23:128, 1995

26. ARENDS JP, HARTWIG N, RUDOLPHY M ET AL: Carrier rate of *Streptococcus suis* capsular type 2 in palatine tonsils of slaughtered pigs. J Clin Microbiol 20:945–947, 1984

27. ARENDS JP, ZANEN HC: Meningitis caused by *Streptococcus suis* in humans. Rev Infect Dis 10:131–137, 1988

28. ASCIUTTO R, DRENNAN J, FITZGERALD V ET AL: Group C streptococcal arthritis and osteomyelitis in an adolescent with a hereditary sensory neuropathy. Pediatr Infect Dis J 4:553–554, 1985

29. ASPEVALL O, HILLEBRANT E, LINDEROTH B ET AL: Meningitis due to *Gemella haemolysans* after neurosurgical treatment of trigeminal neuralgia. Scand J Infect Dis 23:503–505, 1991

30. ATKINS JT, TILLMAN J, TAN TQ ET AL: *Pediococcus pentosaceus* catheter-associated infection in an infant with gastroschisis. Pediatr Infect Dis J 13:75–76, 1994

31. AUCKENTHALER R, HERMANS PE, WASHINGTON JA: Group G streptococcal bacteremia: clinical study and review of the literature. Rev Infect Dis 33:196–204, 1983

32. AWADA A, VAN DER AUWERA P, MEUNIER F ET AL: Streptococcal and enterococcal bacteremia in patients with cancer. Clin Infect Dis 15:33–48, 1992

33. BAIRD RW, BRONZE MS, KRAUS W ET AL: Epitopes of group A streptococcal M proteins shared with antigens of articular cartilage and synovium. J Immunol 146:3132–3137, 1991

34. BAKER CJ, BARRETT FF: Group B streptococcal infection in infants: the importance of the various serotypes. JAMA 230:1158–1160, 1974

35. BAKER CJ, RENCH MA: Commercial latex agglutination for detection of group B streptococcal antigen in body fluids. J Pediatr 102:393–395, 1983

36. BARNHAM M, LJUNGGREN A, MCINTYRE M: Human infection with *Streptococcus zooepidemicus* (Lancefield group C): three case reports. Epidemiol Infect 98:183–190, 1987

37. BARNHAM M, THORNTON TJ, LANGE K: Nephritis caused by *Streptococcus zooepidemicus* (Lancefield group C). Lancet 1:45–946, 1983

38. BARREAU C, WAGENER G: Characterization of *Leuconostoc lactis* strains from human sources. J Clin Microbiol 28:1728–1733, 1990

39. BARRIOS H, BUMP CM: Conjunctivitis caused by a nutritionally variant *Streptococcus*. J Clin Microbiol 23:379–380, 1986

40. BARRY H, CLANCY MT, BRADY A ET AL: Isolation of a *Leuconostoc* species from a retroareolar breast abscess. J Infect 27:208–210, 1993

41. BARSON W: Group C streptococcal osteomyelitis. J Pediatr Orthop 6:346–348, 1986

42. BARTON CW, CROWLEY DC, UZARK K ET AL: A neonatal survivor of group B *beta*-hemolytic streptococcal endocarditis. Am J Perinatol 1:214–215, 1984

43. BARTTER T, DASCAL A, CARROLL K ET AL: "Toxic strep syndrome": manifestation of group A streptococcal infection. Arch Intern Med 148:1421–1424, 1988

44. BAVIKATTE K, SCHREINER RL, LEMONS JA ET AL: Group D streptococcal septicemia in the neonate. Am J Dis Child 133:493–496, 1979

45. BECKER JA, ASCHER DP, MENDIOLA J ET AL: False-negative urine latex particle agglutination testing in neonates with group B streptococcal bacteremia. Clin Pediatr 32:467–471, 1993

46. BEIGHTON D, CARR AD, OPPENHEIM BA: Identification of viridans streptococci associated with bacteremia in neutropenic cancer patients. J Med Microbiol 40:202–204, 1994

47. BEIGHTON D, HARDIE JM, WHILEY RA: A scheme for the identification of viridans streptococci. J Med Microbiol 35:367–372, 1991

48. BEIGHTON D, HAYDAY H, RUSSELL RRB ET AL: *Streptococcus macacae* sp. nov. from dental plaque of monkeys (*Macaca fasicularis*). Int J Syst Bacteriol 34:332–335, 1984

49. BEIGHTON D, HOMER KA, BOUVET A ET AL: Analysis of enzymatic activities for differentiation of two species of nutritionally variant streptococci, *Streptococcus defectivus* and *Streptococcus adjacens*. J Clin Microbiol 33:1584–1587, 1995

50. BEIGHTON D, WHILEY RA: Sialidase activity of the "*Streptococcus milleri* group" and other viridans group streptococci. J Clin Microbiol 28:1431–1433, 1990

51. BELL E, MCCARTNEY AC: *Gemella morbillorum* endocarditis in an intravenous drug abuser. J Infect 25:110–112, 1992

52. BENTLEY RW, LEIGH JA: Development of PCR-based hybridization protocol for identification of streptococcal species. J Clin Microbiol 33:1296–1301, 1995

53. BENTLEY RW, LEIGH JA, COLLINS MD: Intrageneric structure of *Streptococcus* based on comparative analysis of small-subunit rRNA sequences. Int J Syst Bacteriol 41:487–494, 1991

54. BENTLEY RW, LEIGH JA, COLLINS MD: Development and use of species-specific oligonucleotide probes for differentiation of *Streptococcus uberis* and *Streptococcus parauberis*. J Clin Microbiol 31:57–60, 1993

55. BERENGUER J, SAMPEDRO I, CERCENADO E ET AL: Group C *beta*-hemolytic streptococcus bacteremia. Diagn Microbiol Infect Dis 15:151–155, 1992

56. BERK SL, VERGHESE A, HOLTZCLAW SA ET AL: Enterococcal pneumonia. Occurrence in patients receiving broad-spectrum antibiotic regimens and enteral feeding. Am J Med 74:153–154, 1983

57. BERKOWITZ K, MCCAFFREY R: Postpartum osteomyelitis caused by group B streptococcus. Am J Obstet Gynecol 163:1200–1201, 1990

58. BERNALDO DE QUIROS JCL, MUNOZ P, CERCENADO E ET AL: *Leuconostoc* species as a cause of bacteremia: two case reports and a literature review. Eur J Clin Microbiol Infect Dis 10:505–509, 1991

59. BERRY AM, LOCK RA, HANSMAN D ET AL: Contribution of autolysin to virulence of *Streptococcus pneumoniae*. Infect Immun 57:2324–2330, 1989

60. BERRY AM, YOTHER J, BRILES DE ET AL: Reduced virulence of a defined pneumolysin-negative mutant of *Streptococcus pneumoniae*. Infect Immun 57:2037–2042, 1989

61. BIGNARDI GE, ISSACS D: Neonatal meningitis due to *Streptococcus mitis*. Rev Infect Dis 11:86–88, 1989

62. BISNO AL: Group A streptococcal infections and acute rheumatic fever. N Engl J Med 325:783–793, 1991

63. BISNO AL: *Streptococcus pyogenes*. In Mandell GL, Bennett JE, Dolin R (eds): *Mandell, Douglas, and Bennett's Principles and Practice of Infectious Diseases*, 4th ed, pp 1786–1799. New York, Churchill Liningstone, 1995

64. BISNO AL: Nonsuppurative poststreptococcal sequelae: rheumatic fever and glomerulonephritis. In Mandell GL, Bennett JE, Dolin R (eds), *Mandell, Douglas, and Bennett's Principles and Practice of Infectious Diseases*, 4th ed, pp 1799–1810. New York, Churchill-Livingstone, 1995

65. BISNO AL, OFEK I: Serologic diagnosis of streptococcus infection. Comparison of a rapid hemagglutination technique with conventional antibody tests. Am J Dis Child 127:676–681, 1974

66. BISNO AL, WOOD JW, LAWSON J ET AL: Antigens in urine of patients with glomerulonephritis and in normal human serum which cross-react with group A streptococci: identification and partial characterization. J Lab Clin Med 91:500–513, 1978

67. BIXLER-FORELL E, MARTIN WJ, MOODY MAX D: Clinical evaluation of the improved Streptex method for grouping streptococci. Diagn Microbiol Infect Dis 2:113–118, 1984

68. BLACKMORE TK, MORLEY HR, GORDON DL: *Streptococcus mitis*-induced bacteremia and meningitis after spinal anesthesia. Anesthesiology 78:592–594, 1993

69. BLUESTONE CD, STEPHENSON JS, MARTIN LM: Ten-year review of otitis media pathogens. Pediatr Infect Dis J 11:S7–S11, 1992

70. BOCHUD P-Y, CALANDRA T, FRANCIOLI P: Bacteremia due to viridans streptococci in neutropenic patients: a review. Am J Med 97:256–264, 1994

71. BOCHUD P-Y, EGGIMAN P, CALANDRA T ET AL: Bacteremia due to viridans streptococcus in neutropenic patients with cancer: clinical spectrum and risk factors. Clin Infect Dis 18:25–31, 1994

72. BOS AP, FETTER WPF, BAERTS W ET AL: Streptococcal pharyngitis and epiglottitis in a newborn infant. Eur J Pediatr 151:874–875, 1992

73. BOSLEY GS, WALLACE PL, MOSS CW ET AL: Phenotypic characterization, cellular fatty acid composition, and DNA relatedness of aerococci and comparison to related genera. J Clin Microbiol 28:416–422, 1990

74. BOSLEY GS, WHITNEY AM, PRUCKLER JM ET AL: Characterization of ear fluid isolates of *Alloiococcus otitidis* from patients with recurrent otitis media. J Clin Microbiol 33:2876–2880, 1995

75. BOULNOIS GJ: Pneumococcal proteins and the pathogenesis of disease caused by *Streptococcus pneumoniae*. J Gen Microbiol 138:249–259, 1992

76. BOUVET A: Human endocarditis due to nutritionally variant streptococci: *Streptococcus adjacens* and *Streptococcus defectivus*. Eur Heart J 16(suppl B):24–27, 1995

77. BOUVET A, GESLIN P, KRIZ-KUZEMENSKA P ET AL: Restricted association between biotypes and serotypes with group A streptococci. J Clin Microbiol 32:1312–1317, 1994

78. BOUVET A, GRIMONT F, GRIMONT PAD: *Streptococcus defectivus* sp. nov. and *Streptococcus adjacens* sp. nov., nutritionally variant streptococci from human clinical specimens. Int J Syst Bacteriol 39:290–294, 1989

79. BOUVET A, GRIMONT F, GRIMONT PAD: Intraspecies variations in nutritionally variant streptococci: rRNA gene restriction patterns of *Streptococcus defectivus* and *Streptococcus adjacens*. Int J Syst Bacteriol 41:483–486, 1991

80. BOYCE JM, OPAL DSM, CHOW JW ET AL: Outbreak of multidrug-resistant *Enterococcus faecium* with transferable *vanB* class vancomycin resistance. J Clin Microbiol 32:1148–1153, 1994

81. BOYER KM, GADZELLA CA, BURD LI ET AL: Selective intrapartum chemoprophylaxis of neonatal group B streptococcal early-onset disease. I. Epidemiologic rationale. J Infect Dis 148:795–801, 1983

82. BOYER KM, GOTOFF SP: Prevention of early-onset neonatal group B streptococcal disease with selective intrapartum chemoprophylaxis. N Engl J Med 314:1665–1669, 1986

83. BOYLE JF, SOUMAKIS SA, RENDO A ET AL: Epidemiologic analysis and genotypic characterization of a nosocomial outbreak of vancomycin-resistant enterococci. J Clin Microbiol 31:1280–1285, 1993

84. BRACK MJ, AVERY PG, HUBNER PJB ET AL: *Gemella haemolysans*: a rare and unusual cause of infective endocarditis. Postgrad Med J 67:210, 1991

85. BRADLEY S, GORDON J, BAUMGARTNER D ET AL: Group C streptococcal bacteremia: analysis of 88 cases. Rev Infect Dis 13:270–280, 1991

86. BRIDGE PD, SNEATH PHA: *Streptococcus gallinarum* sp. nov. and *Streptococcus oralis* sp. nov. Int J Syst Bacteriol 32:410–415, 1982

87. BROOK I: Urinary tract infection caused by group B streptococcus in infancy and childhood. Urology 17:428–430, 1981

88. BRUNEAU S, DE MONTCLOS H, DROUET E ET AL: rRNA gene restriction patterns of *Streptococcus pyogenes*: epidemiological applications and relation to serotypes. J Clin Microbiol 32:2953–2958, 1994

89. BRYCE EA, ZEMCOV SJV, CLARKE AM: Species identification and antibiotic resistance patterns of the enterococci. Eur J Clin Microbiol Infect Dis 10:745–747, 1991

90. BUCHER A, MARTIN PR, HOIBY EA ET AL: Spectrum of disease in bacteremic patients during a *Streptococcus pyogenes* serotype M-1 epidemic in Norway in 1988. Eur J Clin Microbiol Infect Dis 11:416–426, 1992

91. BUCHMAN AL: Streptococcus viridans osteomyelitis with endocarditis presenting as acute onset lower back pain. J Emerg Med 8:291–295, 1990

92. BUNGENER W, BIALEK R: Fatal *Streptococcus suis* septicemia in an abattoir worker. Eur J Clin Microbiol Infect Dis 8:306–308, 1989

93. BURDEN AD, OPPENHEIM BA, CROWTHER D ET AL: Viridans streptococcal bacteraemia in patients with haematological and solid malignancies. Eur J Cancer 27:409–411, 1991

94. BURKERT T, WATANAKUNAKORN C: Group G streptococcus septic arthritis and osteomyelitis: report and literature review. J Rheumatol 18:904–907, 1991

95. BURMAN LA, NORRBY R, TROLLFORS B: Invasive pneumococcal infections: incidence, predisposing factors, and prognosis. Rev Infect Dis 7:133–142, 1985

96. BURNS DL, GINSBURG CM: Recrudescence of acute rheumatic fever in Dallas, Texas. Pediatr Res 21(suppl):256A, 1987

97. BUSCHELMAN BJ, BALE MJ, JONES RN: Species identification and determination of high-level aminoglycoside resistance among enterococci: comparison study of sterile body fluid isolates, 1985–1991. Diagn Microbiol Infect Dis 16:119–122, 1993

98. BUU-HOI A, BRANGER C, ACAR JF: Vancomycin-resistant streptococci or *Leuconostoc* sp. Antimicrob Agents Chemother 28:458–460, 1985

99. BUU-HOI A, SAPOETRA A, BRANGER C ET AL: Antimicrobial susceptibility of *Gemella hemolysans* isolated from patients with subacute endocarditis. Eur J Clin Microbiol 1:102–106, 1982

100. CAI J, COLLINS MD: Evidence for a close phylogenetic relationship between *Melissococcus pluton*, the causative agent of European foulbrood disease, and the genus *Enterococcus*. Int J Syst Bacteriol 44:365–367, 1994

101. CALIENDO AM, JORDAN CD, RUOFF KL: *Helcococcus*: a new genus of catalase-negative, gram-positive cocci isolated from clinical specimens. J Clin Microbiol 33:1638–1639, 1995

102. CAPUTO GM, APPELBAUM PC, LIU HH: Infections due to penicillin-resistant pneumococci: clinical, epidemiologic, and microbiologic features. Arch Intern Med 153:1301–1310, 1993

103. CARAPETIS J, BISHOP S, DAVIS J ET AL: *Leuconostoc* sepsis in association with continuous enteral feeding: two case reports and a review. Pediatr Infect Dis J 13:816–823, 1994

104. CAREY RB: Vitamin B$_6$-dependent *Streptococcus mitior* (*mitis*). J Infect Dis 131:722–726, 1975

105. CAREY RB, GROSS KC, ROBERTS RB: Vitamin B$_6$ dependent *Streptococcus mitior* (*mitis*) isolated from patients with systemic infections. J Infect Dis 131:722–726, 1975

106. CARLEY NH: *Streptococcus salivarius* bacteremia and meningitis following upper gastrointestinal endoscopy and cauterization for gastric bleeding. Clin Infect Dis 14:947–948, 1992

107. CARMELI Y, RUOFF KL: Report of cases of and taxonomic considerations for large-colony-forming Lancefield group C streptococcal bacteremia. J Clin Microbiol 33:2114–2117, 1995

108. CARRASCOSA M, PEREZ-CASTRILLON JL, SAMPEDRO I ET AL: Lung abscess due to *Streptococcus mitis*: case report and review. Clin Infect Dis 19:781–783, 1994

109. CARTWRIGHT CP, STOCK F, FAHLE GA ET AL: Comparison of pigment production and motility tests with PCR for reliable identification of intrinsically vancomycin-resistant enterococci. J Clin Microbiol 33:1931–1933, 1995

110. CATALAN MJ, FERNANDEZ JM, VAZQUEZ A ET AL: Failure of cefotaxime in the treatment of meningitis due to relatively resistant *Streptococcus pneumoniae*. Clin Infect Dis 18:766–769, 1994

111. CAVALIERI SJ, ALLAIS JM, SCHLIEVERT PM ET AL: Group A streptococcal peritonitis in a patient undergoing continuous ambulatory peritoneal dialysis. Am J Med 86:249–250, 1989

112. CENTERS FOR DISEASE CONTROL AND PREVENTION: Acute rheumatic fever—Utah. MMWR 35:105–118, 1987

113. CENTERS FOR DISEASE CONTROL AND PREVENTION: Acute rheumatic fever at a Navy training center—San Diego. MMWR 37:101–104, 1988

114. CENTERS FOR DISEASE CONTROL AND PREVENTION: Acute rheumatic fever among Army trainees—Fort Leonard Wood, Missouri, 1987–1988. MMWR 37:519–522, 1988

115. CENTERS FOR DISEASE CONTROL AND PREVENTION: Group A *beta*-hemolytic streptococcal bacteremia—Colorado, 1989. MMWR 39:3–11, 1990

116. CHAPNICK EK, GRADON JD, LUTWICK LI ET AL: Streptococcal toxic shock syndrome due to noninvasive pharyngitis. Clin Infect Dis 14:1074–1077, 1992

117. CHAU PY, HUANG CY, KAY R: *Streptococcus suis* meningitis: an important underdiagnosed disease in Hong Kong. Med J Aust 1:414–417, 1983

118. CHERCHI GB, KAPLAN EL, SCHLIEVERT PM ET AL: First reported case of *Streptococcus pyogenes* infection with toxic shock-like syndrome in Italy. Eur J Clin Microbiol Infect Dis 11:836–838, 1992

119. CHEW TA, SMITH JMB: Detection of diacetyl (caramel odor) in presumptive identification of the "*Streptococcus milleri*" group. J Clin Microbiol 30:3028–3029, 1992

120. CHIRURGI VA, OSTER SE, GOLDBERG AA ET AL: Ampicillin-resistant *Enterococcus raffinosus* in an acute-care hospital: case–control study and antimicrobial susceptibilities. J Clin Microbiol 29:2663–2665, 1991

121. CHOW JW, KURITZA A, SHLAES DM ET AL: Clonal spread of vancomycin-resistant *Enterococcus faecium* between patients in three hospitals in two states. J Clin Microbiol 31:1609–1611, 1993

122. CHOW JW, THAL LA, PERRI MB ET AL: Plasmid-associated hemolysin and aggregation substance production contributes to virulence in experimental enterococcal endocarditis. Antimicrob Agents Chemother 37:2472–2477, 1993

123. CHRISTENSEN JJ, GUTSCHIK E, FRISS-MOLLER A ET AL: Urosepticemia and fatal endocarditis caused by *Aerococcus*-like organisms. Scand J Infect Dis 23:717–721, 1991

124. CHRISTENSEN JJ, JENSEN IP, FAERK J ET AL: Bacteremia/septicemia due to *Aerococcus*-like organisms: report of seventeen cases. Clin Infect Dis 21: 943–947, 1995

125. CHRISTENSEN JJ, KORNER B, KJAERGAARD H: *Aerococcus*-like organism—an unnoticed urinary tract pathogen. APMIS 97:539–546, 1989

126. CHRISTENSEN JJ, VIBITS H, URSING J ET AL: *Aerococcus*-like organism, a newly recognized urinary tract pathogen. J Clin Microbiol 29:1049–1053, 1991

127. CHRISTIE R, ATKINS NE, MUNCH-PETERSEN E: A note on a lytic phenomenon shown by group B streptococci. Aust J Exp Biol Med Sci 22:197–200, 1944

128. CHUA D, REINHART HH, SOBEL JD: Liver abscess caused by *Streptococcus milleri*. Rev Infect Dis 11:197–202, 1989

129. CIMOLAI N, MORRISON BJ, MACCULLOCH L ET AL: *beta*-Haemolytic non-group A streptococci and pharyngitis: a case-control study. Eur J Pediatr 150:776–779, 1991

130. CLASSEN DC, BURKE JP, FORD CD ET AL: *Streptococcus mitis* sepsis in bone marrow transplant patients receiving oral antimicrobial prophylaxis. Am J Med 89:441–446, 1990

131. CLEWELL DB: Movable genetic elements and antibiotic resistance in enterococci. Eur J Clin Microbiol Infect Dis 9:90–102, 1990

132. CLEWELL DB: Bacterial sex pheromone-induced plasmid transfer. Cell 73:9–12, 1993

133. COLLAZOS J, ECHEVARRIA MJ, AYARZA R ET AL: *Streptococcus zooepidemicus* septic arthritis: case report and review of group C streptococcal arthritis. Clin Infect Dis 15:744–746, 1992

134. COLLINS MD, AGUIRRE M, FACKLAM RR ET AL: *Globicatella sanguis* gen. nov., sp. nov., a new gram-positive, catalase-negative bacterium from human sources. J Appl Microbiol 73:433–437, 1992

135. COLLINS MD, ASH C, FARROW JAE ET AL: 16S ribosomal ribonucleic acid sequence analysis of lactococci and related taxa: description of *Vagococcus fluvialis* gen. nov. sp. nov. J Appl Microbiol 67:453–460, 1989

136. COLLINS MD, FACKLAM RR, FARROW JAE ET AL: *Enterococcus raffinosus* sp. nov., *Enterococcus solitarius* sp. nov., and *Enterococcus pseudoavium* sp. nov. FEMS Microbiol Lett 57:283–288, 1989

137. COLLINS MD, FACKLAM RR, RODRIGUES UM ET AL: Phylogenetic analysis of some *Aerococcus*-like organisms from clinical sources: description of *Helcococcus kunzii* gen. nov. sp. nov. Int J Syst Bacteriol 43:425–429, 1993

138. COLLINS MD, FARROW JAE, JONES D: *Enterococcus mundtii* sp. nov. Int J Syst Bacteriol 36:8–12, 1986

139. COLLINS MD, JONES D, FARROW JAE ET AL: *Enterococcus avium* nom. rev., comb. nov.; *E. casseliflavus* nom. rev., comb. nov.; *E. durans* nom. rev., comb. nov.; *E. gallinarum* nom. rev., comb. nov., and *E. malodoratus* sp. nov. Int J Syst Bacteriol 34:220–223, 1984

140. COLLINS MD, RODRIGUES UM, PIGGOTT NE ET AL: *Enterococcus dispar* sp. nov., a new *Enterococcus* species from human sources. Lett Appl Microbiol 12:95–98, 1991

141. COLLINS MD, SAMELIS J, METAZOPOULOS J ET AL: Taxonomic studies of some *Leuconostoc*-like organisms from fermented sausages—description of a new genus *Weissella* for the *Leuconostoc paramesenteroides* group of species. J Appl Microbiol 75:595–603, 1993

142. COLLINS MD, WILLIAMS AM, WALLBANKS S: The phylogeny of *Aerococcus* and *Pediococcus* as determined by 16S rRNA sequence analysis: description of *Tetragenococcus* gen. nov. FEMS Microbiol Lett 70:255–262, 1990

143. COLVILLE A, DAVIES W, HENEGHAN M ET AL: A rare complication of dental treatment: *Streptococcus oralis* meningitis. Br Dent J 175:133–134, 1993

144. CONE LA, WOODARD DR, SCHLIEVERT PM ET AL: Clinical and bacteriologic observations of a toxic shock-like syndrome due to *Streptococcus pyogenes*. N Engl J Med 317:146–149, 1987

145. COONAN KM, KAPLAN EL: In vitro susceptibility of recent North American group A streptococcal isolates to eleven oral antibiotics. Pediatr Infect Dis J 13:630–635, 1994

146. COOVADIA YM, SOLWA Z, VAN DEN ENDE J: Meningitis caused by vancomycin-resistant *Leuconostoc* sp. J Clin Microbiol 25:1784–1785, 1987

147. CORCORAN GD, GIBBONS N, MULVIHILL TE: Septicaemia caused by *Pediococcus pentosaceus*: a new opportunistic pathogen. J Infect 23:179–182, 1991

148. CORSON AP, GARIGUSA VF, CHRETIEN JH: Group C beta-hemolytic streptococci causing pharyngitis and scarlet fever. South Med J 82:1119–1121, 1989

149. COX RA, CHEN K, COYKENDALL AL ET AL: Fatal infection in neonates of 26 weeks gestation due to *Streptococcus milleri*: report of two cases. J Clin Pathol 40:190–193, 1987

150. COYKENDALL AL: Proposal to elevate the subspecies of *Streptococcus mutans* to species status based on their molecular composition. Int J Syst Bacteriol 27:26–30, 1977

151. COYKENDALL AL: *Streptococcus sobrinus* nom. rev. and *Streptococcus ferus* nom. rev.: habitat of these and other mutans streptococci. Int J Syst Bacteriol 33:883–885, 1983

152. COYKENDALL AL: Rejection of the type strain of *Streptococcus mitis* (Andrews and Horder 1906): request for an opinion. Int J Syst Bacteriol 39:207–209, 1989

153. COYKENDALL AL: Classification and identification of the viridans streptococci. Clin Microbiol Rev 2:315–328, 1989

154. COYKENDALL AL, GUSTAFSON KB: Deoxyribonucleic acid hybridizations among strains of *Streptococcus salivarius* and *Streptococcus bovis*. Int J Syst Bacteriol 35:274–280, 1985

155. COYKENDALL AL, WESBECHER PM, GUSTAFSON KB: "*Streptococcus milleri*," *Streptococcus constellatus*, and *Streptococcus intermedius* are later synonyms of *Streptococcus anginosus*. Int J Syst Bacteriol 37:222–228, 1987

156. CRAVEN DE, RIXINGER AI, BISNO AL ET AL: Bacteremia caused by group G streptococci in parenteral drug abusers: epidemiological and clinical aspects. J Infect Dis 153:988–992, 1986

157. CUNNEY RJ, FENTON S, FIELDING JF ET AL: *Streptococcus mitis* meningitis in an adult. J Infect 27:96–97, 1993

158. DAJANI AS, AYOUB E, BIERMAN FZ ET AL: Guidelines for the diagnosis of rheumatic fever: Jones criteria, updated 1992. Circulation 87:302–307, 1993

159. DALE JB, BEACHEY EH: Protective antigenic determinant of streptococcal M protein shared with sarcolemmal membrane protein of human heart. J Exp Med 156:1165–1176, 1982

160. DALE JB, BEACHEY EH: Epitopes of streptococcal M proteins shared with cardiac myosin. J Exp Med 162:583–591, 1985

161. DALE JC, VETTER EA, CONTEZAC JM ET AL: Evaluation of two rapid antigen assays, BioStar Strep A OIA and Pacific Biotech CARD O.S. and culture for detection of group A streptococci in throat swabs. J Clin Microbiol 32:2698–2701, 1994

162. DALY JA, KORGENSKI EK, MUNSON AC ET AL: Optical immunoassay for streptococcal pharyngitis: evaluation of accuracy with routine and mucoid strains associated with acute rheumatic fever outbreak in the intermountain area of the United States. J Clin Microbiol 32:531–532, 1994

163. DALY JA, SESKIN KC: Evaluation of rapid, commercial latex techniques for serogrouping beta-hemolytic streptococci. J Clin Microbiol 26:2429–2431, 1988

164. DARLING CL: Standardization and evaluation of the CAMP reaction for the prompt, presumptive identification of *Streptococcus agalactiae* (Lancefield group B) in clinical material. J Clin Microbiol 1:171–174, 1975

165. DEALLER SF, GRACE RJ, NORFOLK DR: *Enterococcus avium* septicemia in an immunocompromised patient. Eur J Clin Microbiol Infect Dis 9:367–368, 1990

166. DEBAST SB, KOOT R, MEIS JFGM: Infections caused by *Gemella morbillorum*. Lancet 342:560, 1993

167. DEHERDT P, HAESEBROUCK F, DEVRIESE LA ET AL: Biochemical and antigenic properties of *Streptococcus bovis* isolated from pigeons. J Clin Microbiol 30:2432–2434, 1992

168. DE LA ROSA M, PEREZ M, CARAZO C ET AL: New Granada medium for detection and identification of group B streptococci. J Clin Microbiol 30:1019–1021, 1992

169. DE LA ROSA M, VILLARREAL R, VEGA D ET AL: Granada medium for detection and identification of group B streptococci. J Clin Microbiol 18:779–785, 1983

170. DELLA-LATTA P, WHITTIER S, HOSMER M ET AL: Rapid detection of group A streptococcal pharyngitis in a pediatric population with optical immunoassay. Pediatr Infect Dis J 13:742–743, 1994

171. DEMAN JC, ROGOSA M, SHARPE ME: A medium for the cultivation of lactobacilli. J Appl Microbiol 23:130–135, 1960

172. DE MOOR CE: Septicaemic infections in pigs caused by haemolytic streptococci of new Lancefield groups designated R, S, and T. Antonie Leeuwenhoek J Microbiol Serol 29:272–280, 1963

173. DE SOET JJ, DE GRAF J: Monoclonal antibodies for enumeration and identification of mutans streptococci in epidemiological studies. Arch Oral Biol 35:165S–168S, 1990

174. DEVRIESE LA, CEYSSENS K, HAESEBROUCK F: Characteristics of *Enterococcus cecorum* strains from the intestines of different animal species. Lett Appl Microbiol 12:137–139, 1991

175. DEVRIESE LA, CEYSSENS K, RODRIGUES UM ET AL: *Enterococcus columbae*, a species from pigeon intestines. FEMS Microbiol Lett 71:247–252, 1990

176. DEVRIESE LA, DUTTA GN, FARROW JAE ET AL: *Streptococcus cecorum*, a new species isolated from chickens. Int J Syst Bacteriol 33:772–776, 1983

177. DEVRIESE LA, VAN DE KERCKHOVE A, KILPPER-BALZ R ET AL: Characterization and identification of *Enterococcus* species isolated from the intestines of animals. Int J Syst Bacteriol 37:257–259, 1987

178. DICKS LMT, DELLAGLIO F, COLLINS MD: Proposal to reclassify *Leuconostoc oenos* as *Oenococcus oeni* [corrig.] gen. nov. comb. nov. Int J Syst Bacteriol 45:395–397, 1995

179. DICKS LMT, FANTUZZI L, GONZALES FC ET AL: *Leuconostoc argentinum* sp. nov., isolated from Argentine raw milk. Int J Syst Bacteriol 43:347–351, 1993

180. DILLON HC JR, GRAY E, PASS MA ET AL: Anorectal and vaginal carriage of group B streptococci during pregnancy. J Infect Dis 145:794–799, 1982

181. DILLON HC JR, KHARE S, GRAY BM: Group B streptococcal carriage and disease: a 6–year prospective study. J Pediatr 110:31–36, 1987

182. DINUBILE MJ, ALBORNOZ MA, STUMACHER RJ ET AL: Pneumococcal soft-tissue infections: possible association with connective tissue diseases. J Infect Dis 163:897–900, 1991

183. DOBKIN D, SCHULMAN ST: Evaluation of an ELISA for group A streptococcal antigen for diagnosis of pharyngitis. J Pediatr 110:566–569, 1987

184. DONABEDIAN S, CHOW JW, SHLAES DM ET AL: DNA hybridization and contour-clamped homogeneous electric field electrophoresis for identification of enterococci to the species level. J Clin Microbiol 33:141–145, 1995

185. DOUBE A, CALIN A: Bacterial endocarditis presenting as acute monoarthritis. Ann Rheum Dis 47:598–599, 1988

186. DOUGHERTY SH: Role of enterococcus in intraabdominal sepsis. Am J Surg 148:308–312, 1984

187. DOUGLAS CWI, HEATH J, HAMPTON KK ET AL: Identity of viridans streptococci isolated from cases of infective endocarditis. J Med Microbiol 39:179–182, 1993

188. DOUGLAS CWI, PEASE AA, WHILEY RA: Amylase-binding as a discriminator among oral streptococci. FEMS Microbiol Lett 66:193–198, 1990

189. DOUGLAS RM, PATON JC, DUNCAN SJ ET AL: Antibody response to pneumococcal vaccination in children younger than five years of age. J Infect Dis 148:131–137, 1983

190. DUBROW R, EDBERG S, WIKFORS E ET AL: Fecal carriage of *Streptococcus bovis* and colorectal adenomas. Gastroenterology 101:721–725, 1991

191. DUFF P, GIBBS RS: Acute intraamniotic infection due to *Streptococcus pneumoniae*. Obstet Gynecol 61(suppl):25S–27S, 1983

192. DUNHAM WR, SIMPSON JH, FEEST TG ET AL: *Streptococcus bovis* endocarditis and colorectal disease. Lancet 2:421–422, 1980

193. DUNNE DW, QUAGLIARELLO V: Group B streptococcal meningitis in adults. Medicine 72:1–10, 1993

194. DUNNY GM: Genetic functions and cell–cell interactions in the pheromone-inducible plasmid transfer system of *Enterococcus faecalis*. Plasmid 4:689–696, 1990

195. DUPAS D, VIGNON M, GERAUT C: *Streptococcus suis* meningitis: a severe, noncompensated occupational disease. J Occup Med 34:1102–1105, 1992

196. DUTKA-MALEN S, EVERS S, COURVALIN P: Detection of glycopeptide resistance genotypes and identification to the species level of clinically relevant enterococci by PCR. J Clin Microbiol 33:24–27, 1995

197. DYKSTRA MA, MCLAUGHLIN JC, BARTLETT RC: Comparison of media and techniques for detection of group A streptococci in throat swab specimens. J Clin Microbiol 9:236–238, 1979

198. EDWARDS MS, BAKER CJ: *Streptococcus agalactiae* (group B streptococcus). In Mandell GL, Bennett JE, Dolin R (eds), *Mandell, Douglas, and Bennett's Principles and Practice of Infectious Diseases*, 4th ed, pp 1835–1845. New York, Churchill Livingstone, 1995

199. EDWARDS MS, BAKER CJ, WAGNER ML ET AL: An etiologic shift in infantile osteomyelitis: the emergence of the group B streptococcus. J Pediatr 93:578–583, 1978

200. EDWARDS MS, KASPER DL, JENNINGS HJ ET AL: Capsular sialic acid prevents activation of the alternative complement pathway by type III, group B streptococci. J Immunol 128:1278–1283, 1982

201. EGGELMEIJER F, PETIT P, DIJKMANS BA: Total knee arthroplasty infection due to *Gemella haemolysans*. Br J Rheumatol 31:67–69, 1992

202. ELDAR A, FRELIER PF, ASSENTA L ET AL: *Streptococcus shiloi*, the name for an agent causing septicemic infection in fish, is a junior synonym of *Streptococcus iniae*. Int J Syst Bacteriol 45:840–842, 1995

203. ELHANEN G, RAZ R: Group B streptococcal vertebral osteomyelitis in an adult. Infection 21:397–399, 1993

204. ELIOPOULOS GM: Increasing problems in the therapy of enterococcal infections. Eur J Clin Microbiol Infect Dis 12:409–412, 1993

205. ELLIOTT JA, COLLINS MD, PIGOTT NE ET AL: Differentiation of *Lactococcus lactis* and *Lactococcus garvieae* from humans by comparison of whole-cell protein patterns. J Clin Microbiol 29:2731–2734, 1991

206. ELLIOTT JA, FACKLAM RR: Identification of *Leuconostoc* spp. by analysis of soluble whole cell protein patterns. J Clin Microbiol 31:1030–1033, 1993

207. ELLIOTT PM, WILLIAMS H, BROOKSBY IAB: A case of infective endocarditis in a farmer caused by *Streptococcus equinus*. Eur Heart J 14:1291–1293, 1993

208. EMBER JA, HUGLI TE: Characterization of the human neutrophil response to sex pheromones from *Streptococcus faecalis*. Am J Pathol 134:797–805, 1989

209. EMILIANI VJ, CHODOS JE, COMER GM ET AL: *Streptococcus bovis* brain abscess associated with an occult colonic villous adenoma. Am J Gastroenterol 85:78–80, 1990

210. ERICKSON D, DOSTER AR, POKORNY TS: Isolation of *Streptococcus suis* from swine in Nebraska. J Am Vet Assoc 185:666–668, 1984

211. EVALDSON GR, MALMBORG A-S, NORD CE: Premature rupture of the membranes and ascending infection. Br J Obstet Gynaecol 89:793–801, 1982

212. EVANS JB: Genus *Aerococcus*. In Sneath PHA, Mair NS, Sharpe ME, Holt JG (eds), *Bergey's Manual of Systematic Bacteriology*, vol 2, p. 1080. Baltimore, Williams & Wilkins, 1986

213. EZAKI T, FACKLAM RR, TAKEUCHI N ET AL: Genetic relatedness between the type strain of *Streptococcus anginosus* and minute-colony-forming *beta*-hemolytic streptococci carrying different Lancefield grouping antigens. Int J Syst Bacteriol 36:345–347, 1986

214. EZAKI T, LIU SL, HASHIMOTO Y ET AL: *Peptostreptococcus hydrogenalis* sp. nov. from human fecal and vaginal flora. Int J Syst Bacteriol 40:305–306, 1990

215. EZAKI T, YAMAMOTO N, NINOMIYA K ET AL: Transfer of *Peptococcus indolicus, Peptococcus asaccharolyticus, Peptococcus prevotii,* and *Peptococcus magnus* to the genus *Peptostreptococcus* and proprosal of *Peptostreptococcus tetradius* sp. nov. Int J Syst Bacteriol 33:683–698, 1983

216. FACKLAM RR: Physiological differentiation of viridans streptococci. J Clin Microbiol 5:184–201, 1977

217. FACKLAM RR: Specificity study of kits for detection of group A streptococci directly from throat swabs. J Clin Microbiol 25:504–508, 1987

218. FACKLAM RR, BOSLEY GS, RHODEN D ET AL: Comparative evaluation of the API 20S and AutoMicrobic gram positive identification systems for non-*beta*-hemolytic streptococci and aerococci. J Clin Microbiol 21:535–541, 1985

219. FACKLAM RR, COLLINS MD: Identification of *Enterococcus* species isolated from human infections by a conventional test scheme. J Clin Microbiol 27:731–734, 1989

220. FACKLAM RR, COOKSEY RC, WORTHAM EC: Evaluation of commercial latex agglutination reagents for grouping streptococci. J Clin Microbiol 10:641–646, 1979

221. FACKLAM R, ELLIOTT JA: Identification, classification, and clinical relevance of catalase-negative, gram-positive cocci, excluding streptococci and enterococci. Clin Microbiol Rev 8:479–495, 1995

222. FACKLAM R, ELLIOTT J, PIGOTT N ET AL: Identification of *Streptococcus porcinus* from human sources. J Clin Microbiol 33:385–388, 1995

223. FACKLAM R, HOLLIS D, COLLINS MD: Identification of gram-positive coccal and coccobacillary vancomycin-resistant bacteria. J Clin Microbiol 27:724–730, 1989

224. FACKLAM R, PIGOTT N, FRANKLIN R ET AL: Evaluation of three disk tests for identification of enterococci, leuconostocs, and pediococci. J Clin Microbiol 33:885–887, 1995

225. FACKLAM RR, RHODEN DL, SMITH PB: Evaluation of the RapID STR system for identification of clinical isolates of *Streptococcus* species. J Clin Microbiol 20:894–898, 1984

226. FACKLAM RR, THACKER LG, FOX B ET AL: Presumptive identification of streptococci with a new test system. J Clin Microbiol 15:987–990, 1982

227. FADEN H, DRYJA D: Recovery of a unique bacterial organism in human middle ear fluid and its possible role in chronic otitis media. J Clin Microbiol 27:2488–2491, 1989

228. FARBER BP, WEINBAUM DL, DUMMER JS: Metastatic bacterial endophthalmitis. Arch Intern Med 145:62–64, 1985

229. FARLEY MM, HARVEY C, STULL T ET AL: A population-based assessment of invasive disease due to group B streptococcus in non-pregnant adults. N Engl J Med 328:1807–1811, 1993

230. FARROW JAE, COLLINS MD: DNA base composition, DNA-DNA homology, and long-chain fatty acid studies on *Streptococcus thermophilus* and *Streptococcus salivarius*. J Gen Microbiol 130:357–362, 1984

231. FARROW JAE, COLLINS MD: Taxonomic studies on streptococci of serological groups C, G, and L and possibly related taxa. Syst Appl Microbiol 5:483–493, 1984

232. FARROW JAE, COLLINS MD: *Enterococcus hirae*, a new species that includes amino acid assay strain NCDO 1258 and strains causing growth depression in young chickens. Int J Syst Bacteriol 35:73–75, 1985

233. FARROW JAE, FACKLAM RR, COLLINS MD: Nucleic acid homologies of some vancomycin-resistant leuconostocs and description of *Leuconostoc citreum* sp. nov. and *Leuconostoc pseudomesenteroides* sp. nov. Int J Syst Bacteriol 39:279–283, 1989

234. FARROW JAE, KRUZE J, PHILLIPS BA ET AL: Taxonomic studies on *Streptococcus bovis* and *Streptococcus equinus*: description of *Streptococcus alactolyticus* sp. nov. and *Streptococcus saccharolyticus* sp. nov. Syst Appl Microbiol 5:467–483, 1982

235. FASANO FJ, GRAHAM DR, STAUFFER ES: Vertebral osteomyelitis secondary to *Streptococcus agalactiae*. Clin Orthop 256:101–104, 1990

236. FAST DJ, SCHLIEVERT PM, NELSON RD: Toxic shock syndrome-associated staphylococcal and streptococcal pyrogenic toxins are potent inducers of tumor necrosis factor production. Infect Immun 57:291–294, 1989

237. FEDER I, CHENGAPPA MM, FENWICK B ET AL: Partial characterization of *Streptococcus suis* type 2 hemolysin. J Clin Microbiol 32:1256–1260, 1994

238. FENOLL A, MARTINEZ-SUAREZ JV, MUNOZ R ET AL: Identification of atypical strains of *Streptococcus pneumoniae* by a specific DNA probe. Eur J Clin Microbiol Infect Dis 9:396–401, 1990

239. FERRER JC, PADILLA JJV, IGUAL RI ET AL: *Streptococcus bovis* meningitis: no association with colonic malignancy. Clin Infect Dis 17:527–528, 1993

240. FERRER S, DEMIGUEL G, DOMINGO P ET AL: Pulmonary infection due to *Leuconostoc* species in a patient with AIDS. Clin Infect Dis 21:225–226, 1995

241. FERRIERI P: Neonatal susceptibility and immunity to major bacterial pathogens. Rev Infect Dis 12(suppl 4): S394–S400, 1990

242. FERRIERI P, CLEARY PP, SEEDS SE: Epidemiology of group B streptococcal carriage in pregnant women and newborn infants. J Med Microbiol 13:273–280, 1976

243. FERRIERI P, KAPLAN EL: Invasive group A streptococcal infections. Infect Dis Clin North Am 6:149–161, 1992

244. FERTALLY SS, FACKLAM R: Comparison of physiologic tests used to identify non–*beta*-hemolytic aerococci, enterococci, and streptococci. J Clin Microbiol 25: 1845–1850, 1987

245. FIEHN N-E, GUTSCHIK E, LARSEN T ET AL: Identity of streptococcal blood isolates and oral isolates from two patients with infective endocarditis. J Clin Microbiol 33:1399–1401, 1995

246. FIKAR C, LEY J: *Streptococcus bovis* meningitis in a neonate. Am J Dis Child 113:1149–1150, 1979

247. FILLIT HM, MCCARTY M, BLAKE M: Induction of antibodies to hyaluronic acid by immunization of rabbits with encapsulated streptococci. J Exp Med 164:762–776, 1986

248. FISHER LE, RUSSELL RRB: The isolation and characterization of milleri group streptococci from dental periapical abscesses. J Dent Res 72:1191–1193, 1993

249. FLANAGAN PG, MILLS RG: Fulminant septicaemia due to *Streptococcus milleri* infection in a previously healthy adult. Eur J Clin Microbiol Infect Dis 13:247–248, 1994

250. FLYNN CE, RUOFF KL: Identification of "*Streptococcus milleri*" group isolates to the species level with a commercially available rapid test system. J Clin Microbiol 33:2704–2706, 1995

251. FONTANA R, AMALFITANO G, ROSSI L ET AL: Mechanism of resistance to growth inhibition and killing by *beta*-lactam antibiotics in enterococci. Clin Infect Dis 15:486–489, 1992

252. FORD M, PERRY JD, GOULD FK: Use of cephalexin–aztreonam–arabinose agar for selective isolation of *Enterococcus faecium*. J Clin Microbiol 32:2999–3001, 1994

253. FORNI AL, KAPLAN EL, SCHLIEVERT PM ET AL: Clinical and microbiological characteristics of severe group A streptococcus infections and streptococcal toxic shock syndrome. Clin Infect Dis 21:333–340, 1995

254. FOX BC: Delayed-onset postpartum meningitis due to group B streptococcus. Clin Infect Dis 19:350–351, 1994

255. FOX K, TURNER J, FOX A: Role of *beta*-hemolytic group C streptococci in pharyngitis: incidence and biochemical characteristics of *Streptococcus equisimilis* and *Streptococcus anginosus* in patients and healthy controls. J Clin Microbiol 31:804–807, 1993

256. FRANCIOSI RA, KNOSTMAN JD, ZIMMERMAN RA: Group B streptococcal neonatal and infant infections. J Pediatr 82:707–718, 1973

257. FRANCIS AJ, NIMMO GR, EFSTRATIOU A ET AL: Investigation of milk-borne *Streptococcus zooepidemicus* infection associated with glomerulonephritis in Australia. J Infect 27:317–323, 1993

258. FRANDSEN EVG, PEDRAZZOL V, KILIAN M: Ecology of viridans streptococci in the oral cavity and pharynx. Oral Microbiol Immunol 6:129–133, 1991

259. FRENCH GL, TALSANIA H, CHARLTON JRH ET AL: A physiological classification of the viridans streptococci by use of the API-20 STREP system. J Med Microbiol 28:275–286, 1989

260. FRENCH GL, TALSANIA H, PHILLIPS I: Identification of viridans streptococci by pyrrolysis-gas chromatography. J Med Microbiol 29:19–27, 1989

261. FRENEY J, BLAND S, ETIENNE J ET AL: Description and evaluation of the semi-automated 4-hour rapid ID 32 Strep method for identification of streptococci and members of related genera. J Clin Microbiol 30:2657–2661, 1992

262. FRESARD S, MICHEL VP, RUEDA X ET AL: *Gemella hemolysans* endocarditis. Clin Infect Dis 16:586–587, 1993

263. FRIEDLAND IR, SNIPELISKY M, KHOOSAL M: Meningitis in a neonate caused by *Leuconostoc* sp. J Clin Microbiol 28:2125–2126, 1990

264. FRIEDMAN CA, WENDER DF, RAWSON JE: Rapid diagnosis of group B streptococcal infection utilizing a commercially available latex agglutination assay. Pediatrics 73:27–30, 1984

265. FRIEDRICH IA, WORMSER GP, GOTTFIED EB: The association of remote *Streptococcus bovis* bacteremia with colonic neoplasia. Am J Gastroenterol 77:82–84, 1982

266. GALLAGHER PG, WATANAKUNAKORN C: Group B streptococcal endocarditis: report of seven cases and review of the literature, 1962–1985. Rev Infect Dis 8:175–188, 1986

267. GALLI D, WIRTH R: Comparative analysis of *Enterococcus faecalis* sex pheromone plasmids identifies a single homologous DNA region which codes for aggregation substance. J Bacteriol 173:3029–3033, 1991

268. GARDNER SE, YOW MD, LEEDS LJ ET AL: Failure of penicillin to eradicate group B streptococcal colonization in the pregnant woman. Am J Obstet Gynecol 135: 1062–1065, 1979

269. GARVIE EI: *Leuconostoc oenos* sp. nov. J Gen Microbiol 48:431–438, 1967

270. GARVIE EI: Genus *Leuconostoc* van Teighem 1878, 198 emend. mut. charc. Hucker and Pederson 1930, 66[AL]. In Sneath PHA, Mair NS, Sharpe ME (eds), *Bergey's Manual of Systematic Bacteriology*, vol 2, pp 1071–1075. Baltimore, Williams & Wilkins, 1986

271. GARVIE EI: Genus *Pediococcus* Claussen 1903, 86[AL]. In Sneath PHA, Mair NS, Sharpe ME (eds), *Bergey's Manual of Systematic Bacteriology*, vol 2, pp 1075–1079. Baltimore, Williams & Wilkins, 1986

272. GARVIE EI, FARROW JAE, BRAMLEY AJ: *Streptococcus dysgalactiae* (Diernhofer) nom. rev. Int J Syst Bacteriol 33:404–405, 1983

273. GAVRYCK WA, SATTLER FR: Meningitis caused by *Streptococcus bovis*. Arch Neurol 39:307–308, 1982

274. GELFAND MS, HODGKISS T, SIMMONS BR: Multiple hepatic abscesses caused by *Streptococcus milleri* in association with an intrauterine device. Rev Infect Dis 11:983–987, 1989

275. GELFAND MS, HUGHEY JR, SLOAS DD: Group B streptococcal bacteremia associated with adenocarcinoma of the stomach. Clin Infect Dis 19:364, 1994

276. GELFAND MS, THRELKELD MG: Subacute bacterial endocarditis secondary to *Streptococcus pneumoniae*. Am J Med 93:91, 1992

277. GEORGE AL JR, SAVAGE AM: Fatal group B streptococcal empyema in an adult. South Med J 80:1436–1438, 1987

278. GERBER MA: Comparison of throat cultures and rapid strep tests for diagnosis of streptococcal pharyngitis. Pediatr Infect Dis 8:820–824, 1989

279. GERBER MA, RANDOLPH MF, DEMEO KK: Liposome immunoassay for rapid identification of group A streptococci directly from throat swabs. J Clin Microbiol 28:1463–1464, 1990

280. GERLACH D, KOHLER W, GUNTHER E ET AL: Purification and characteristics of streptolysin O secreted by *Streptococcus equisimilis* (group C). Infect Immun 61:2727–2731, 1993

281. GESNER M, DESIDERIO D, KIM M ET AL: *Streptococcus pneumoniae* in human immunodeficiency virus type 1-infected children. Pediatr Infect Dis J 13:697–703, 1994

282. GIACOMETTI A, RANALDI R, SIQUINI FM ET AL: *Leuconostoc citreum* isolated from lung in an AIDS patient. Lancet 342:622, 1993

283. GILLESPIE SH, ELLMAN C, SMITH MD ET AL: Detection of *Streptococcus pneumoniae* in sputum samples by PCR. J Clin Microbiol 32:1308–1311, 1994

284. GILON D, MOSES A: Carcinoma of the colon presenting as *Streptococcus equinus* bacteremia. Am J Med 86:135–136, 1989

285. GIRAUD P, ATTAL M, LEMOUZY J ET AL: *Leuconostoc*: a potential pathogen in bone marrow transplantation. Lancet 341:1481–1482, 1993

286. GIVNER LB, ABRAMSON JS, WASILAUSKAS B: Apparent increase in the incidence of invasive group A streptococcal disease in children. J Pediatr 118:341–346, 1991

287. GODEAU B, BACHIR D, SCHAEFFER A ET AL: Severe pneumococcal sepsis and meningitis in human immunodeficiency virus-infected adults with sickle cell disease. Clin Infect Dis 15:327–329, 1992

288. GOLDSHLACK P, BLACKBURN G: Lancefield group G streptococcus septic arthritis in a heroin user: report of a case. J Am Osteopath Assoc 84:60–61, 1984

289. GOLDSTEIN I, REBEYROTTE P, PARLEBAS J ET AL: Isolation from heart valves of glycopeptides which share immunological properties with *Streptococcus haemolyticus* group A polysaccharides. Nature 219:866–868, 1968

290. GOLLEDGE CL: Infection due to *Leuconostoc* species. Rev Infect Dis 13:184–185, 1991

291. GOLLEDGE CL, STRINGEMORE N, ARAVENA M ET AL: Septicemia caused by vancomycin-resistant *Pediococcus acidilactici*. J Clin Microbiol 28:1678–1679, 1990

292. GOMEZ-GARCES J-L, ALOS J-I, COGOLLOS R: Bacteriological characteristics and antimicrobial susceptibility of 70 clinically significant isolates of the *Streptococcus milleri* group. Diagn Microbiol Infect Dis 19:69–73, 1994

293. GORDILLO ME, SINGH KV, BAKER CJ ET AL: Typing of group B streptococci: comparison of pulsed-field gel electrophoresis and conventional electrophoresis. J Clin Microbiol 31:1430–1434, 1993

294. GORDILLO ME, SINGH KV, MURRAY BE: Comparison of ribotyping and pulsed-field gel electrophoresis for subspecies differentiation of strains of *Enterococcus faecalis*. J Clin Microbiol 31:1570–1574, 1993

295. GORDON DM, OSTER CN: Hematogenous group B streptococcal osteomyelitis in an adult. South Med J 77:643–645, 1984

296. GORMAN PW, COLLINS DN: Group C streptococcal arthritis: a case report of equine transmission. Orthopedics 10:615–616, 1987

297. GORONCY-BERMES P, DALE JB, BEACHEY EH ET AL: Monoclonal antibody to human renal glomeruli cross-reacts with streptococcal M-protein. Infect Immun 55:2416–2419, 1987

298. GOSHORN SC, BOHACH GA, SCHLIEVERT PM: Cloning and characterization of the gene, *speC*, for pyrogenic exotoxin type C from *Streptococcus pyogenes*. Mol Gen Genet 212:66–70, 1988

299. GOSHORN SC, SCHLIEVERT PM: Nucleotide sequence of streptococcal pyrogenic exotoxin type C. Infect Immun 56:2518, 1988

300. GOSSLING J: Occurrence and pathogenicity of the *Streptococcus milleri* group. Rev Infect Dis 10:257–275, 1988

301. GOTTSCHALK M, HIGGINS R, BOUDREAU M: Use of polyvalent coagglutination reagents for serotyping of *Streptococcus suis*. J Clin Microbiol 31:2192–2194, 1993

302. GOTTSCHALK M, HIGGINS R, JACQUES M ET AL: Description of 14 new capsular types of *Streptococcus suis*. J Clin Microbiol 27:2633–2636, 1989

303. GOTTSCHALK M, HIGGINS R, JACQUES M ET AL: Characterization of six new capsular types (23 through 28) of *Streptococcus suis*. J Clin Microbiol 29:2590–2594, 1991

304. GOTTSCHALK M, LEBRUN A, JACQUES M ET AL: Hemagglutination properties of *Streptococcus suis*. J Clin Microbiol 28:2156–2158, 1990

305. GRANINGER W, RAGETTE R: Nosocomial bacteremia due to *Enterococcus faecalis* without endocarditis. Clin Infect Dis 15:49–57, 1992

306. GRANOWITZ EV, DONALDSON WR, SKOLNICK PR: Gas-forming soft tissue abscess caused by *Streptococcus pneumoniae*. Am J Med 93:105–107, 1992

307. GRANT KA, DICKINSON JH, COLLINS MD ET AL: Rapid identification of *Aerococcus viridans* using the polymerase chain reaction and an oligonucleotide probe. FEMS Microbiol Lett 95:63–68, 1992

308. GRAY BM, CONVERSE GM III, DILLON HC JR: Epidemiologic studies of *Streptococcus pneumoniae* in infants: acquisition, carriage, and infection during the first 24 months of life. J Infect Dis 142:923–933, 1980

309. GRAY BM, DILLON HC JR: Epidemiological studies of *Streptococcus pneumoniae* in infants: antibody to types 3, 6, 14, and 23 in the first two years of life. J Infect Dis 158:948–955, 1988

310. GREEN M, BARBADORA K, MICHAELS M: Recovery of vancomycin-resistant gram-positive cocci from pediatric liver transplant recipients. J Clin Microbiol 29:2503–2506, 1991

311. GREEN M, DASHEFSKY B, WALD ER ET AL: Comparison of two antigen assays for rapid detection of group B streptococcal colonization. J Clin Microbiol 31:78–82, 1993

312. GREEN M, WADOWSKY RW, BARBADORA K: Recovery of vancomycin-resistant gram-positive cocci from children. J Clin Microbiol 28:484–488, 1990

313. GREEN PA, CAMPBELL JR: Transient, asymptomatic bacteremia due to *Enterococcus avium* in a 33-month-old child. Clin Infect Dis 19:561, 1994

314. GREENBERG DN, ASCHER DP, YODER BA ET AL: Group B streptococcus serotype V. J Pediatr 123:494–495, 1993

315. GREENBERG DN, ASCHER DP, YODER BA ET AL: Sensitivity and specificity of rapid diagnostic tests for detection of group B streptococcal antigen in bacteremic neonates. J Clin Microbiol 33:193–198, 1995

316. GRIFFITH SP, GERSONY WM: Acute rheumatic fever in New York City (1969–1988): a comparative study of two decades. J Pediatr 116:882–887, 1990

317. GRUTEKE P, VAN BELKUM A, SCHOULS LM ET AL: Outbreak of group A streptococci in a burn center: use of pheno- and genotypic procedures for strain tracking. J Clin Microbiol 34:114–118, 1996

318. GULLBERG RM, HOMANN SR, PHAIR JP: Enterococcal bacteremia: analysis of 75 episodes. Rev Infect Dis 11: 74–85, 1989

319. GUNZENHAUSER JD, LONGFIELD JN, BRUNDAGE JF ET AL: Epidemic streptococcal disease among army trainees, July 1989 through June 1991. J Infect Dis 172:124–131, 1995

320. HACHEY WE, WISWELL TE: Limitations in the usefulness of urine latex particle agglutination and hematologic measurements in diagnosing neonatal sepsis during the first week of life. J Perinatol 12:240–245, 1992

321. HACKETT SP, STEVENS DL: Superantigens associated with staphylococcal and streptococcal toxic shock syndrome are potent inducers of tumor necrosis factor-*beta* synthesis. J Infect Dis 168:232–235, 1993

322. HAGAY ZJ, MISKIN A, GOLDCHMIT R ET AL: Evaluation of two rapid tests for detection of maternal endocervical group B streptococcus: enzyme-linked immunosorbent assay and Gram stain. Obstet Gynecol 82:84–87, 1993

323. HAMADA S, SLADE HD: Biology, immunology, and cariogenicity of *Streptococcus mutans*. Microbiol Rev 44: 331–384, 1980

324. HAMILTON JR: Comparison of Meritec-Strep with Streptex for direct colony grouping of *beta*-hemolytic streptococci from primary isolation and subculture plates. J Clin Microbiol 26:692–695, 1988

325. HAMOUDI AC, MARCON MJ, CANNON HJ ET AL: Comparison of three major antigen detection methods for the diagnosis of group B streptococcal sepsis in neonates. Pediatr Infect Dis 2:432–435, 1983

326. HAMPSON DJ, TROTT DJ, CLARKE IL ET AL: Population structure of Australian isolates of *Streptococcus suis*. J Clin Microbiol 31:2895–2900, 1993

327. HANDLEY PS, COYKENDALL A, BEIGHTON D ET AL: *Streptococcus crista* sp. nov., a viridans streptococcus with tufted fibrils, isolated from the human oral cavity and throat. Int J Syst Bacteriol 41:543–547, 1991

328. HANDWERGER S, HOROWITZ H, COBURN K ET AL: Infection due to *Leuconostoc* species: six cases and review. Rev Infect Dis 12:602–610, 1990

329. HANTSON P, VEKEMANS MC, GAUTHER P ET AL: Fatal *Streptococcus suis* meningitis in man. Acta Neurol Belg 91:165–168, 1991

330. HARBECK RJ, TEAGUE J, CROSSEN GR ET AL: Novel, rapid optical immunoassay technique for detection of group A streptococci from pharyngeal specimens: comparison with standard culture methods. J Clin Microbiol 31: 839–844, 1993

331. HARDIE JM: Oral streptococci. In Sneath PHA, Mair NS, Sharpe ME (eds), *Bergey's Manual of Systematic Bacteriology*, vol 2, pp 1054–1063. Baltimore, Williams & Wilkins, 1986

332. HARDIE JM: Other streptococci. In Sneath PHA, Mair NS, Sharpe ME (eds), *Bergey's Manual of Systematic Bacteriology*, vol 2, pp 1054–1063. Baltimore, Williams & Wilkins, 1986

333. HARDY S, RUOFF KL, CATLIN EA ET AL: Catheter-associated infection with a vancomycin-resistant gram-positive coccus of the *Leuconostoc* sp. Pediatr Infect Dis J 7:519–520, 1988

334. HARLEY WB, GIBBS C, HORTON JM: *Streptococcus bovis* meningitis associated with a colonic villous adenoma. Clin Infect Dis 14:979–980, 1992

335. HARPER DS, LOESCHE WJ: Growth and acid tolerance of human dental plaque bacteria. Arch Oral Biol 29: 843–848, 1984

336. HARRINGTON P, FINKELMAN D, BALART L, ET AL: *Streptococcus bovis* septicemia and pancreatic adenocarcinoma. Ann Intern Med 92:441–442, 1980

337. HASSAN-KING M, BALDEH I, SECKA O ET AL: Detection of *Streptococcus pneumoniae* DNA in blood cultures by PCR. J Clin Microbiol 32:1721–1724, 1994

338. HAUSER AR, SCHLIEVERT PM: Nucleotide sequence of the streptococcal pyrogenic exotoxin type B gene and relationship between toxin and the streptococcal proteinase precursor. J Bacteriol 172:4536–4542, 1990

339. HAUSER AR, STEVENS DL, KAPLAN EL ET AL: Molecular analysis of pyrogenic exotoxins from *Streptococcus pyogenes* isolates associated with toxic shock-like syndrome. J Clin Microbiol 29:1562–1567, 1991

340. HAY PE, CUNNIFE JG, KRAMER G ET AL: Two cases of *Streptococcus suis* meningitis. Br J Ind Med 46:352–353, 1989

341. HAYDEN GF, TURNER JC, KISELICA D ET AL: Latex agglutination testing directly from throat swabs for rapid detection of *beta*-hemolytic streptococci from Lancefield serogroup C. J Clin Microbiol 30:716–718, 1992

342. HAYDEN MK, TRENHOLME GM, SCHULTZ JE ET AL: In vivo development of teicoplanin resistance in a VanB *Enterococcus faecium* isolate. J Infect Dis 167:1224–1227, 1993

343. HEILESEN AM: Septicaemia due to *Aerococcus urinae*. Scand J Infect Dis 26:759–760, 1994

344. HEITER BJ, BOURBEAU PP: Comparison of the Gen-Probe group A streptococcus direct test with culture and a rapid streptococcal antigen assay for diagnosis of streptococcal pharyngitis. J Clin Microbiol 31:2070–2073, 1993

345. HEITER BJ, BOURBEAU PP: Comparison of two rapid streptococcal antigen detection assays with culture for diagnosis of streptococcal pharyngitis. J Clin Microbiol 33:1408–1410, 1995

346. HENRICHSEN J: Six newly recognized types of *Streptococcus pneumoniae*. J Clin Microbiol 33:2759–2760, 1995

347. HENRICHSEN J, FERRIERI P, JELINKOVA J ET AL: Nomenclature of antigens of group B streptococci. Int J Syst Bacteriol 34:500, 1984

348. HIGGINS R, GOTTSCHALK M, BOUDREAU M ET AL: Description of six new capsular types (29–34) of *Streptococcus suis*. J Vet Diagn Invest 7:405–406, 1995

349. HIGGINS R, GOTTSCHALK M, MITTAL MK ET AL: *Streptococcus suis* infections in swine: a 16-month study. Can J Vet Res 54:170–173, 1990

350. HILL AW, LEIGH JA: DNA fingerprinting of *Streptococcus uberis*: a useful tool for epidemiology of bovine mastitis. Epidemiol Infect 103:165–271, 1989

351. HINNEBUSCH CJ, NIKOLAI DM, BRUCKNER DA: Comparison of API Rapid STREP, Baxter-MicroScan Rapid Pos ID panel, BBL Minitek Differential Identification sys-

tem, IDS RapID STR system, and Vitek GPI to conventional biochemical tests for identification of viridans streptococci. Am J Clin Pathol 96:459–463, 1991

352. HO AKC, WOO KS, TSE KK ET AL: Infective endocarditis caused by *Streptococcus suis* serotype 2. J Infect 21: 209–211, 1990

353. HOEN B, BRIANCON S, DELAHAYE F ET AL: Tumors of the colon increase the risk of developing *Streptococcus bovis* endocarditis: case–control study. Clin Infect Dis 19:361–362, 1994

354. HOFFMANN S: Detection of group A streptococcal antigen from throat swabs with five diagnostic kits in general practice. Diagn Microbiol Infect Dis 13:209–215, 1990

355. HOMER KA, DENBOW L, WHILEY RA ET AL: Chondroitin sulfate depolymerase and hyaluronidase activities of viridans streptococci determined by a sensitive spectrophotometric assay. J Clin Microbiol 31:1648–1651, 1993

356. HUCK W, REED BD, FRENCH T ET AL: Comparison of the Directigen 1-2-3 Group A Strep Test with culture for detection of group A *beta*-hemolytic streptococci. J Clin Microbiol 27:1715–1718, 1989

357. HUSBY G, VAN DE RIJN I, ZABRISKIE JB ET AL: Antibodies reacting with cytoplasm of subthalamic and caudate nuclei neurons in chorea and rheumatic fever. J Exp Med 144:1094–1100, 1976

358. HUYCKE MM, JOYCE WA, GILMORE MS: *Enterococcus faecalis* cytolysin without effect on the intestinal growth of susceptible enterococci in mice. J Infect Dis 172:273–276, 1995

359. HWANG M, EDERER GM: Rapid hippurate hydrolysis method for presumptive identification of group B streptococci. J Clin Microbiol 1:114–115, 1975

360. INGRAM DL, SUGGS DM, PEARSON AW: Detection of group B streptococcal antigen in early-onset and late-onset group B streptococcal disease with the Wellcogen Strep B latex agglutination test. J Clin Microbiol 16: 656–658, 1982

361. IRVINE MCG, SOLOMONS NB: Atypical supraglottitis caused by *Streptococcus sanguis*. J Laryngol Otol 104: 430–431, 1990

362. ISENBERG HD, VELLOZI EM, SHAPIRO J ET AL: Clinical laboratory challenges in the recognition of *Leuconostoc* spp. J Clin Microbiol 26:479–484, 1988

363. JACOBS AAC, LOEFFEN PLW, VAN DEN BERG AJG ET AL: Identification, purification, and characterization of a thiol-activated hemolysin (suilysin) of *Streptococcus suis*. Infect Immun 62:1742–1748, 1994

364. JACOBS JA, DE KROM MCT, KELLENS JTC ET AL: Meningitis and sepsis due to group G streptococcus. Eur J Clin Microbiol Infect Dis 12:224–225, 1993

365. JACOBS JA, PIETERSEN HG, STOBBERINGH EE ET AL: Bacteremia involving the "*Streptococcus milleri*" group: analysis of 19 cases. Clin Infect Dis 19:704–713, 1994

366. JACOBS JA, STAPPERS JLN, SELS JP: Endocarditis due to *Streptococcus oralis* in a patient with a colon tumour. Eur J Clin Microbiol Infect Dis 14:557–558, 1995

367. JACOBS MR: Treatment and diagnosis of infections caused by drug-resistant *Streptococcus pneumoniae*. Clin Infect Dis 15:119–127, 1992

368. JACOBSON MA, ANDERSON ET: *Streptococcus bovis* meningitis. J Neurol Neurosurg Psychiatry 50:940–941, 1987

369. JACOBY GA: Prevalence and resistance mechanisms of common bacterial respiratory pathogens. Clin Infect Dis 18:951–957, 1994

370. JADEJA L, KANTARJIAN H, BOLIVAR R: *Streptococcus bovis* bacteremia and meningitis associated with chronic radiation entercolitis. South Med J 76:1588–1589, 1983

371. JAIN AK, AGARWAL SK, EL-SADR W: *Streptococcus bovis* bacteremia and meningitis associated with *Strongyloides stercoralis* colitis in a patient infected with human immunodeficiency virus. Clin Infect Dis 18:253–254, 1994

372. JANOSEK J, ECKERT J, HUDAC A: *Aerococcus viridans* as a causative agent of infectious endocarditis. J Hyg Epidemiol Microbiol Immunol 24:92–96, 1980

373. JAYARAO BM, DORE JJ, JR, BAUMBACH GA ET AL: Differentiation of *Streptococcus uberis* from *Streptococcus paruberis* by polymerase chain reaction and restriction fragment length polymorphism analysis of 16S ribosomal DNA. J Clin Microbiol 29:2774–2778, 1991

374. JELINKOVA J, MOTLOVA J: Worldwide distribution of two new serotypes of group B streptococci: type IV and provisional type V. J Clin Microbiol 21:361–362, 1985

375. JETT BD, HUYCKE MM, GILMORE MS: Virulence of enterococci. Clin Microbiol Rev 7:462–478, 1994

376. JEVON GP, DUNNE WM, JR, HAWKINS HK ET AL: Fatal group A streptococcal meningitis and toxic shock-like syndrome: case report. Clin Infect Dis 18:91–93, 1994

377. JOHN CC: Treatment failure with use of third-generation cephalosporin for penicillin-resistant pneumococcal meningitis: case report and review. Clin Infect Dis 18:188–193, 1994

378. JOHNSON AP, UTTLEY AHC, WOODFORD N ET AL: Resistance to vancomycin and teicoplanin: an emerging clinical problem. Clin Microbiol Rev 3:280–291, 1990

379. JOHNSON DR, KAPLAN EL: A review of the correlation of T-agglutination patterns and M-protein typing and opacity factor production in the identification of group A streptococci. J Med Microbiol 38:311–315, 1993

380. JORGENSEN JH, DOERN GV, MAHER LA ET AL: Antimicrobial resistance among respiratory isolates of *Haemophilus influenzae*, *Moraxella catarrhalis*, and *Streptococcus pneumoniae* in the United States. Antimicrob Agents Chemother 34:2075–2080, 1990

381. JUDICIAL COMMISSION OF THE INTERNATIONAL COMMITTEE ON SYSTEMATIC BACTERIOLOGY: Opinion 66: Designation of strains NS 51 (NCTC 12261) in place of strain NCTC 3165 as the type strain of *Streptococcus mitis* Andrews and Horder 1906. Int J Syst Bacteriol 43:391, 1993

382. KATZ VL, MOOS M-K, CEFALO RC ET AL: Group B streptococci: results of a protocol of antepartum screening and intrapartum treatment. Am J Obstet Gynecol 170:521–526, 1994

383. KAUFHOLD A, FERRIERI P: Isolation of *Enterococcus mundtii* from normally sterile body sites in two patients. J Clin Microbiol 29:1075–1077, 1991

384. KAUFHOLD A, FRANZEN D, LUTTICKEN R: Endocarditis caused by *Gemella haemolysans*. Infection 17:385–387, 1989

385. KAUFHOLD A, PODBIELSKI A, JOHNSON DR ET AL: M protein gene typing of *Streptococcus pyogenes* by nonradioactively labeled oligonucleotide probes. J Clin Microbiol 30:2391–2394, 1992

386. KAUFHOLD A, POTGIETER E: Chromosomally mediated high-level gentamicin-resistance in *Streptococcus mitis.* Antimicrob Agents Chemother 37:2740–2742, 1993

387. KAWAMURA Y, HOU X-C, SULTANA F ET AL: Determination of 16S rRNA sequences of *Streptococcus mitis* and *Streptococcus gordonii* and phylogenetic relationships among members of the genus *Streptococcus.* Int J Syst Bacteriol 45:406–408, 1995

388. KAWAMURA Y, HOU X-G, SULTANA F ET AL: Transfer of *Streptococcus adjacens* and *Streptococcus defectivus* to *Abiotrophia* gen. nov. and *Abiotrophia adiacens* comb. nov. and *Abiotrophia defectiva* comb. nov. Int J Syst Bacteriol 45:798–803, 1995

389. KEISER P, CAMPBELL W: "Toxic strep syndrome" associated with group C streptococcus. Arch Intern Med 152:882–884, 1992

390. KERBAUGH MA, EVANS JB: *Aerococcus viridans* in the hospital environment. Appl Microbiol 16:519–523, 1968

391. KERN W, KURRLE E, SCHMEISER T: Streptococcal bacteraemia in adult patients with leukaemia undergoing aggressive chemotherapy: a review of 55 cases. Infection 18:138–145, 1990

392. KERN W, VANEK E: *Aerococcus* bacteremia associated with granulocytopenia. Eur J Clin Microbiol 6:670–673, 1987

393. KIKUCHI K, ENARI T, TOTSUKA K-I ET AL: Comparison of phenotypic characteristics, DNA–DNA hybridization results, and results with a commercial rapid biochemical and enzymatic reaction system for identification of viridans group streptococci. J Clin Microbiol 33:1215–1222, 1995

394. KILIAN M, MIKKELSON L, HENRICHSEN J: Taxonomic study of viridans streptococci: description of *Streptococcus gordonii* sp. nov. and amended descriptions of *Streptococcus sanguis* (White and Niven 1946), *Streptococcus oralis* (Bridge and Sneath 1982), and *Streptococcus mitis* (Andrews and Horder 1906). Int J Syst Bacteriol 39:471–484, 1989

395. KILIAN M, MIKKELSON L, HENRICHSEN J: Replacement of the type strain of *Streptococcus mitis.* Int J Syst Bacteriol 39:498–499, 1989

396. KILIAN M, NYVAD B: Ability to bind salivary *alpha*-amylase discriminates certain viridans group streptococcal species. J Clin Microbiol 28:2567–2577, 1990

397. KILPPER-BALZ R, SCHLEIFER KH: Nucleic acid hybridization and cell wall composition studies of pyogenic streptococci. FEMS Microbiol Lett 24:355–364, 1984

398. KILPPER-BALZ R, SCHLEIFER KH: *Streptococcus suis* sp. nov. nom. rev. Int J Syst Bacteriol 37:160–162, 1987

399. KILPPER-BALZ R, SCHLEIFER KH: Transfer of *Streptococcus morbillorum* to the genus *Gemella* as *Gemella morbillorum* comb. nov. Int J Syst Bacteriol 38:442–443, 1988

400. KILPPER-BALZ R, WENZIG P, SCHLEIFER KH: Molecular relationships and classification of some viridans streptococci as *Streptococcus oralis* and emended description of *Streptococcus oralis* (Bridge and Sneath 1982). Int J Syst Bacteriol 35:482–488, 1985

401. KLEIN JO: Management of streptococcal pharyngitis. Pediatr Infect Dis J 13:572–575, 1994

402. KLEIN RS, CATALANO MT, EDBERG SC ET AL: *Streptococcus bovis* septicemia and carcinoma of the colon. Ann Intern Med 91:560–562, 1979

403. KLEIN RS, RECCA RA, CATALANO MT ET AL: Association of *Streptococcus bovis* with carcinoma of the colon. N Engl J Med 296:800–802, 1977

404. KLEIN RS, WARMAN SW, KNACKMUHS GG ET AL: Lack of association of *Streptococcus bovis* with noncolonic gastrointestinal carcinoma. Am J Gastroenterol 82:540–543, 1987

405. KLUGMAN KP: Pneumococcal resistance to antibiotics. Clin Microbiol Rev 3:171–196, 1990

406. KNIGHT RG, SHLAES DM: Physiological characteristics and deoxyribonucleic acid relatedness of *Streptococcus bovis* and *Streptococcus bovis* (var.). Int J Syst Bacteriol 35:357–361, 1985

407. KNIGHT RG, SHLAES DM: Physiological characteristics and deoxyribonucleic acid relatedness of *Streptococcus intermedius* strains. Int J Syst Bacteriol 38:19–24, 1988

408. KNUDTSON LM, HARTMAN PA: Routine procedures for isolation and identification of enterococci and fecal streptococci. Appl Env Microbiol 58:3027–3031, 1992

409. KOEHNE G, MADDUX RL, CORNELL WD: Lancefield group R streptococci associated with pneumonia in swine. J Vet Res 40:1640–1641, 1979

410. KONTNICK CM, EDBERG SC: Direct detection of group B streptococci from vaginal specimens compared with quantitative culture. J Clin Microbiol 28:336–339, 1990

411. KOOREVAAR CT, SCHERPENZEEL PGN, NEIJENS HJ ET AL: Childhood meningitis caused by enterococci and viridans streptococci. Infection 20:118–121, 1992

412. KREFT B, MARRE R, SCHRAMM U ET AL: Aggregation substance of *Enterococcus faecalis* mediates adhesion to cultured renal tubular cells. Infect Immun 60:25–30, 1992

413. KRIEGER JN, KAISER DL, WENZEL RP: Urinary tract etiology of bloodstream infections in hospitalized patients. J Infect Dis 148:57–62, 1983

414. KRISTENSEN B, NIELSEN G: Endocarditis caused by *Aerococcus urinae*, a newly recognized pathogen. Eur J Clin Microbiol Infect Dis 14:49–51, 1995

415. KUHLS TL, VIERING TP, LEACH CT ET AL: Relapsing pneumococcal bacteremia in immunocompromised patients. Clin Infect Dis 14:1050–1054, 1992

416. KURAMITSU HK: Virulence factors of mutans streptococci: role of molecular genetics. Crit Rev Oral Biol Med 4:159–176, 1993

417. KUSKIE MR: Group C streptococcal infections. Pediatr Infect Dis J 6:856–859, 1987

418. KUSUDA R, KAWAI K, SALATI F ET AL: *Enterococcus seriolicida* sp. nov., a fish pathogen. Int J Syst Bacteriol 41:406–409, 1991

419. LANCEFIELD RC: A serological differentiation of human and other groups of *beta*-hemolytic streptococci. J Exp Med 57:571–595, 1933

420. LANCEFIELD RC: Current knowledge of type-specific M antigens of group A streptococci. J Immunol 89:307–313, 1962

421. LANDMAN D, QUALE JM, ODYNA E ET AL: Comparison of five selective media for identifying fecal carriage of vancomycin-resistant enterococci. J Clin Microbiol 34:751–752, 1996

422. LATTORE M, ALVAREZ M, FERNANDEZ JM ET AL: A case of meningitis due to "*Streptococcus zooepidemicus.*" Clin Infect Dis 17:932–933, 1993

423. LAUBSCHER B, VAN MELLE G, DREYFUSS N ET AL: Evaluation of a new immunologic test kit for rapid detection of group A streptococci, the Abbott Testpack Strep A Plus. J Clin Microbiol 33:260–261, 1995

424. LAWLOR MT, CROWE HM, QUINTILIANI R: Cellulitis due to *Streptococcus pneumoniae*: case report and review. Clin Infect Dis 14:247–250, 1992

425. LAWRENCE J, YAJKO DM, HADLEY WK: Incidence and characterization of *beta*-hemolytic *Streptococcus milleri* and differentiation from *S. pyogenes* (group A), *S. equisimilis* (group C), and large colony group G streptococci. J Clin Microbiol 22:772–777, 1985

426. LEBAR WD, BARNOSKY AR: Group G streptococcal septic arthritis and bacteremia in a parenteral drug abuser. Clin Microbiol Newslett 10:135, 1988

427. LECLERQ R, DUTKA-MALEN S, BRISSON-NOEL A ET AL: Resistance of enterococci to aminoglycosides and glycopeptides. Clin Infect Dis 15:495–501, 1992

428. LEDGER WJ, NORMAN M, GEE C ET AL: Bacteremia on an obstetric–gynecologic service. Am J Obstet Gynecol 121:205–212, 1975

429. LEE P-C, WETHERALL BL: Cross-reaction between *Streptococcus pneumoniae* and group C streptococcal latex reagent. J Clin Microbiol 25:152–153, 1987

430. LEFEVRE JC, FAUCON G, SICARD AM ET AL: DNA fingerprinting of *Streptococcus pneumoniae* strains by pulsed-field gel electrophoresis. J Clin Microbiol 31:2724–2728, 1993

431. LEGGIADRO RJ, BIRNBAUM SE, CHASE NA ET AL: A resurgence of acute rheumatic fever in a mid-South children's hospital. South Med J 83:1418–1420, 1990

432. LEGIER JF: *Streptococcus salivarius* meningitis and colonic carcinoma. South Med J 84:1058–1059, 1991

433. LEIBOVITCH G, MAARAVI Y, SHALEV O: Multiple brain abscesses caused by *Streptococcus bovis*. J Infect 23:195–196, 1991

434. LENTNEK AL, GIGER O, O'ROURKE E: Group A *beta*-hemolytic streptococcal bacteremia and intravenous drug abuse: a growing clinical problem? Arch Intern Med 150:89–93, 1990

435. LERNER PI, GOPALAKRISHNA KV, WOLINSKY E ET AL: Group B streptococcus (*S. agalactiae*) bacteremia in adults: analysis of 32 cases and review of the literature. Medicine 56:457–473, 1977

436. LI N, HASHIMOTO Y, ADNAN S ET AL: Three new species of the genus *Peptostreptococcus* isolated from humans: *Peptostreptococcus vaginalis* sp. nov., *Peptostreptococcus lacrimalis* sp. nov., and *Peptostreptococcus lactolyticus* sp. nov. Int J Syst Bacteriol 42:602–605, 1992

437. LIM DV, MORALES WJ, WALSH AF: Reduction of morbidity and mortality rates for neonatal group B streptococcal disease through early diagnosis and chemoprophylaxis. J Clin Microbiol 23:489–492, 1986

438. LIM DV, MORALES WJ, WALSH AF: Lim group B strep broth and coagglutination for rapid identification of group B streptococci in preterm pregnant women. J Clin Microbiol 25:452–453, 1987

439. LISCHKE JH, MCCREIGHT PHB: Maternal group B streptococcal vertebral osteomyelitis: an unusual complication of vaginal delivery. Obstet Gynecol 76:489–491, 1990

440. LLIBRE JM, PUIG P, ALOY A ET AL: Silent spontaneous retroperitoneal abscess caused by M-type 18 *Streptococcus pyogenes*. Eur J Clin Microbiol Infect Dis 11:205–206, 1992

441. LOESCHE WJ: Role of *Streptococcus mutans* in human dental decay. Microbiol Rev 50:353–380, 1986

442. LOSONSKY GA, WOLF A, SCHWALBE RS ET AL: Successful treatment of meningitis due to multiply resistant *Enterococcus faecium* with a combination of intrathecal teicoplanin and intravenous antimicrobial agents. Clin Infect Dis 19:163–165, 1994

443. LUDWIG W, WEIZENEGGER M, KILPPER-BALZ R ET AL: Phylogenetic relationships of anaerobic streptococci. Int J Syst Bacteriol 38:15–18, 1988

444. LUGENBILL C, CLARK RB, FAGNANT RJ ET AL: Comparison of the cervicovaginal Gram stain and rapid latex agglutination slide test for identification of group B streptococci. J Perinatol 10:403–405, 1993

445. LUGINBUHL LM, ROTBART HA, FACKLAM RR ET AL: Neonatal enterococcal sepsis: case–control study and description of an outbreak. Pediatr Infect Dis 6: 1022–1030, 1987

446. LUTTICKEN R, TEMME N, HAHN G ET AL: Meningitis caused by *Streptococcus suis*: case report and review of the literature. Infection 14:181–185, 1986

447. MACKEY T, LEJEUNE V, JANSSENS M ET AL: Identification of vancomycin-resistant lactic acid bacteria isolated from humans. J Clin Microbiol 31:2499–2501, 1993

448. MAHER D: *Streptococcus suis* septicaemia presenting as severe, acute gastro-enteritis. J Infect 21:303–304, 1990

449. MAKINEN P, CLEWELL DB, AN F ET AL: Purification and substrate specificity of a strongly hydrophobic extracellular metalloendopeptidase ("gelatinase") from *Streptococcus faecalis* (strain OG1-10). J Biol Chem 264: 3325–3334, 1989

450. MANNION PT, ROTHBURN MM: Diagnosis of bacterial endocarditis caused by *Streptococcus lactis* assisted by immunoblotting of serum antibodies. J Infect 21:317–326, 1990

451. MANZELLA JP: *Streptococcus bovis* bacteremia: diagnosis of neoplasms by colonoscopy. South Med J 74:999–1000, 1981

452. MARKOWITZ M: Changing epidemiology of group A streptococcal infections. Pediatr Infect Dis J 13:557–560, 1994

453. MARRIE TJ: Bacteremic community-acquired pneumonia due to viridans group streptococci. Clin Invest Med 16:38–44, 1993

454. MARSAL S, CASTRO-GUARDIOLA A, CLEMENTE C ET AL: *Streptococcus bovis* endocarditis presenting as acute spondylodiscitis. Br J Rheumatol 33:403–404, 1994

455. MARTIN MA, HEBDEN JN, BUSTAMANTE CI ET AL: Group A streptococcal bacteremias associated with intravenous catheters. Infect Control Hosp Epidemiol 11:542–544, 1990

456. MARTINEZ-MURCIA AJ, COLLINS MD: *Enterococcus sulfureus*, a new yellow-pigmented *Enterococcus* species. FEMS Microbiol Lett 80:69–74, 1991

457. MARTINEZ-MURCIA AJ, COLLINS MD: A phylogenetic analysis of an atypical leuconostoc: description of *Leuconostoc fallax* sp. nov. FEMS Microbiol Lett 82:55–60, 1991

458. MASON T, FISHER M, KUJALA G: Acute rheumatic fever in West Virginia: not just a disease of children. Arch Intern Med 151:133–136, 1991

459. MASTRO TD, SPIKA JS, LOZANO P ET AL: Vancomycin-resistant *Pediococcus acidilactici*: nine cases of bacteremia. J Infect Dis 161:956–960, 1990

460. MATSIS PP, EASTHOPE RN: *Gemella haemolysans* endocarditis. Aust NZ J Med 24:417–418, 1994

461. MAUGEIN J, CROUZIT P, CONY MAKHOUL P ET AL: Characterization and antibiotic susceptibility of *Pediococcus acidilactici* strains isolated from neutropenic patients. Eur J Clin Microbiol Infect Dis 11:383–385, 1992

462. MAY T, AMIEL C, LION C ET AL: Meningitis due to *Gemella haemolysans*. Eur J Clin Microbiol Infect Dis 12:644–645, 1993

463. MCCARTHY AE, VICTOR G, RAMOTAR K ET AL: Risk factors for acquiring ampicillin-resistant enterococci and clinical outcomes at a Canadian tertiary-care hospital. J Clin Microbiol 32:2671–2676, 1994

464. MCCARTHY L, BOTTONE EJ: Bacteremia and endocarditis caused by satelliting streptococci. Am J Clin Pathol 61:585–591, 1974

465. MCCARTY JM, HABER J: Group B streptococcal soft tissue infections beyond the neonatal period. West Med J 147:558–560, 1987

466. MCDANIEL LS, SHEFFIELD JS, DELUCCHI P ET AL: PspA, a surface protein of *Streptococcus pneumoniae*, is capable of eliciting protection against pneumococci of more than one serotype. Infect Immun 59:222–228, 1991

467. MCDONNELL PJ, KWITKO S, MCDONNELL JM ET AL: Characterization of infectious crystalline keratitis caused by a human isolate of *Streptococcus mitis*. Arch Ophthalmol 109:1147–1151, 1991

468. MCGUIRE T, GERJARUSAK P, HINTHORN P ET AL: Osteomyelitis caused by *beta*-hemolytic streptococcus group B. JAMA 238:2054–2055, 1977

469. MCLENDON BF, BRON AJ, MITCHELL CJ: *Streptococcus suis* type II (group R) as a cause of endophthalmitis. Br J Ophthalmol 62:729–731, 1978

470. MCMAHON AJM, AULD CD, DALE BAS ET AL: *Streptococcus bovis* septicaemia associated with uncomplicated colonic carcinoma. Br J Surg 78:883–885, 1991

471. MCMILLAN RA, BLOOMSTER TA, SAEED AM ET AL: Characterization of a fourth streptococcal pyrogenic exotoxin (SPE D). FEMS Microbiol Lett 44:317–320, 1987

472. MCWHINNEY PHM, GILLESPIE SH, KIBBLER CC ET AL: *Streptococcus mitis* and ARDS in neutropenic patients. Lancet 337:429, 1991

473. MEGRAN DW: Enterococcal endocarditis. Clin Infect Dis 15:63–71, 1992

474. MEIER FA, CENTOR RM, GRAHAM L ET AL: Clinical and microbiologic evidence for endemic pharyngitis among adults due to group C streptococci. Arch Intern Med 150:825–829, 1990

475. MELLMAN RL, SPISAK GM, BURAKOFF R: *Enterococcus avium* bacteremia in association with ulcerative colitis. Am J Gastroenterol 87:375–378, 1992

476. MERRIT K, JACOBS NJ: Improved medium for detecting pigment production by group B streptococci. J Clin Microbiol 4:379–380, 1976

477. MICHAEL AF, DRUMMOND KN, GOOD RA ET AL: Acute poststreptococcal glomerulonephritis: immune deposit disease. J Clin Invest 45:237–248, 1966

478. MICHEL RS, DEFLORA E, JEFFERIES J ET AL: Recurrent meningitis in a child with inner ear dysplasia. Pediatr Infect Dis J 11:336–338, 1992

479. MITCHELL RG, TEDDY PJ: Meningitis due to *Gemella haemolysans* after radiofrequency trigeminal rhizotomy. J Clin Pathol 38:558–560, 1985

480. MOELLERING RC JR: Emergence of *Enterococcus* as a significant pathogen. Clin Infect Dis 14:1173–1178, 1992

481. MOGOLLON JD, PIJOAN C, MURTAUGH MP ET AL: Characterization of prototype and clinically defined strains of *Streptococcus suis* by genomic fingerprinting. J Clin Microbiol 28:2462–2466, 1990

482. MOGOLLON JD, PIJOAN C, MURTAUGH MP ET AL: Identification of epidemic strains of *Streptococcus suis* by genomic fingerprinting. J Clin Microbiol 29:782–787, 1991

483. MOLINA JM, LEPORT C, BURE A ET AL: Clinical and bacterial features of infections caused by *Streptococcus milleri*. Scand J Infect Dis 23:659–666, 1991

484. MOLLER M, THOMSEN AC, BORCH K ET AL: Rupture of fetal membranes and premature delivery associated with group B streptococci in urine of pregnant women. Lancet 2:69–70, 1984

485. MOLLISON LC, DONALDSON E: Group C streptococcal meningitis. Med J Aust 152:319–320, 1990

486. MORALES WJ, LIM DV: Reduction in group B streptococcal maternal and neonatal infections in preterm pregnancies with premature rupture of membranes through a rapid identification test. Am J Obstet Gynecol 157:13–16, 1987

487. MOREA P, TONI M, BRESSAN M ET AL: Prosthetic valve endocarditis caused by *Gemella haemolysans*. Infection 19:446, 1991

488. MORRISON AJ JR, WENZEL RP: Nosocomial urinary tract infections due to enterococcus; ten years' experience at a university hospital. Arch Intern Med 146:1549–1551, 1986

489. MOSHKOWITZ M, ARBER N, WAJSMAN R ET AL: *Streptococcus bovis* endocarditis as a presenting manifestation of idiopathic ulcerative colitis. Postgrad Med J 68:930–931, 1992

490. MUNOZ P, COQUE T, CREIXEMS MR ET AL: Group B *Streptococcus*: a cause of urinary tract infection in nonpregnant adults. Clin Infect Dis 14:492–496, 1992

491. MUNOZ R, FENOLL A, VICIOSO D ET AL: Optochin-resistant variants of *Streptococcus pneumoniae*. Diagn Microbiol Infect Dis 13:63–66, 1989

492. MURRAY BE: The life and times of the enterococcus. Clin Microbiol Rev 3:46–65, 1990

493. MURRAY HW, ROBERTS RB: *Streptococcus bovis* bacteremia and underlying gastrointestinal diseases. Arch Intern Med 138:1097–1099, 1978

494. MUSHER DM: Infections caused by *Streptococcus pneumoniae*: clinical spectrum, pathogenesis, immunity, and treatment. Clin Infect Dis 14:801–809, 1992

495. MUSHER DM: *Streptococcus pneumoniae*. In Mandell GL, Bennett JE, Dolin R (eds): *Mandell, Douglas, and Bennett's Principles and Practice of Infectious Diseases*, 4th ed, pp 1811–1826. New York, Churchill Livingstone, 1995

496. MUSHER DM, GROOVER JE, ROWLAND JM ET AL: Antibody to capsular polysaccharides of *Streptococcus pneumoniae*: prevalence, persistence, and response to revaccination. Clin Infect Dis 17:66–73, 1993

497. MUSSER JM, GRAY BM, SCHLIEVERT M, ET AL: *Streptococcus pyogenes* pharyngitis: characterization of strains by multilocus enzyme genotype, M and T protein serotype,

and pyrogenic exotoxin gene probing. J Clin Microbiol 30:600–603, 1992

498. MUSSER JM, HAUSER AR, KIM MH ET AL: *Streptococcus pyogenes* causing toxic shock-like syndrome and other invasive diseases: clonal diversity and pyrogenic exotoxin expression. Proc Natl Acad Sci USA 88:2668–2672, 1991

499. NATHAVITHARANA KA, ARSECULERATNE SN, APONSO HA ET AL: Acute meningitis in early childhood caused by *Aerococcus viridans.* Br Med J 286:1248, 1983

500. NATHAVITHARANA KA, WATKINSON M: Neonatal pleural empyema caused by group A streptococcus. Pediatr Infect Dis J 13:671–672, 1994

501. NEWTON JA, JR, LESNIK IK, KENNEDY CA: *Streptococcus salivarius* meningitis following spinal anesthesia. Clin Infect Dis 18:840–841, 1994

502. NICAS TI, WY CYE, HOBBS JN JR, ET AL: Characterization of vancomycin resistance in *Enterococcus faecium* and *Enterococcus faecalis.* Antimicrob Agents Chemother 33: 1121–1124, 1989

503. NICHOLS RL, MUZIK AC: Enterococcal infections in surgical patients: the mystery continues. Clin Infect Dis 15:72–76, 1992

504. NIELSEN SV, KOLMOS HJ: Bacteremia due to different groups of *beta*-hemolytic streptococci: a two-year survey and presentation of a case of recurring infection due to *Streptococcus "equisimilis."* Infection 21:358–361, 1993

505. NOBLE CJ, UTTLEY AHC, FALK RH ET AL: *Streptococcus bovis* endocarditis and colonic cancer. Lancet 1:766, 1978

506. NOBLE WC, VIRANI Z, CREE RGA: Co-transfer of vancomycin and other resistance genes from *Enterococcus faecalis* NCTC 12201 to *Staphylococcus aureus.* FEMS Microbiol Lett 93:195–198, 1992

507. NORFLEET RG: Infectious endocarditis after fiberoptic sigmoidoscopy. J Clin Gastroenterol 13:448–451, 1991

508. NORIEGA FR, KOTLOFF KL, MARTIN MA ET AL: Nosocomial bacteremia caused by *Enterobacter sakazakii* and *Leuconostoc mesenteroides* resulting from extrinsic contamination of infant formula. Pediatr Infect Dis J 9: 447–449, 1990

509. NORRBY-TEGLUND A, HOLM SE, NORGREN M: Detection and nucleotide sequence analysis of the *speC* gene in Swedish clinical group A streptococcal isolates. J Clin Microbiol 32:705–709, 1994

510. NOYA FJD, BAKER CJ: Prevention of group B streptococcal infection. Infect Dis Clin North Am 6:41–55, 1992

511. OLOPOENIA L, FREDERICK W, GREAVES W ET AL: Pneumococcal sepsis and meningitis in adults with sickle cell disease. South Med J 83:1002–1004, 1990

512. OMRAN Y, WOOD CA: Endovascular infection and septic arthritis caused by *Gemella morbillorum.* Diagn Microbiol Infect Dis 16:131–134, 1993

513. ORFILA C, LEPERT J-C, MODESTO A ET AL: Rapidly progressive glomerulonephritis associated with bacterial endocarditis: efficacy of antibiotic therapy alone. Am J Nephrol 13:218–222, 1993

514. ORMEROD LD, PATON BG: Severe group B streptococcal eye infections in adults. J Infect 18:29–34, 1989

515. ORMEROD LD, RUOFF KL, MEISLER DM ET AL: Infectious crystalline keratopathy: role of nutritionally variant streptococci and other bacterial factors. Ophthalmology 98:159–169, 1991

516. ORTEL TL, KALLIANOS J, GALLIS HA: Group C streptococcal arthritis: case report and review. Rev Infect Dis 12:829–837, 1990

517. PACIFICO L, RANUCCI A, RAVAGNAN G ET AL: Relative value of selective group A streptococcal agar incubated under different atmospheres. J Clin Microbiol 33: 2480–2482, 1995

518. PANARO NR, LUTWICK LI, CHAPNICK EK: Intrapartum transmission of group A *Streptococcus.* Clin Infect Dis 17:79–81, 1993

519. PANOSIAN KJ, EDBERG SC: Rapid identification of *Streptococcus bovis* by using combination constitutive enzyme substrate hydrolyses. J Clin Microbiol 27:1719–1722, 1989

520. PAREDES A, WONG P, MASON EO JR ET AL: Nosocomial transmission of group B streptococci in a newborn nursery. Pediatrics 59:679–682, 1976

521. PARK JW, GROSSMAN O: *Aerococcus viridans* infection. Case report and review. Clin Pediatr 29:525–526, 1990

522. PATEL M, AHRENS JC, MOYER DV ET AL: Pneumococcal soft-tissue infections: a problem deserving more recognition. Clin Infect Dis 19:149–151, 1994

523. PATEL R, KEATING MR, COCKERILL FR III ET AL: Bacteremia due to *Enterococcus avium.* Clin Infect Dis 17: 1006–1011, 1993

524. PATON JC, LOCK RA, LEE C-J ET AL: Purificiation and immunogenicity of genetically toxoided derivatives of pneumolysin and their conjugation to *Streptococcus pneumoniae* type 19F polysaccharide. Infect Immun 59: 2297–2304, 1991

525. PATRICK MR, LEWIS D: Short of a length: *Streptococcus sanguis* knee infection from dental source. Br J Rheumatol 31:569, 1992

526. PATTERSON JE, MASECAR BL, ZERVOS MJ: Characterization and comparison of two penicillinase-producing strains of *Streptococcus (Enterococcus) faecalis.* Antimicrob Agents Chemother 32:122–124, 1988

527. PEETERMANS WE, BUYSE B, VANHOOF J: Pyogenic abscess of the gluteal muscle due to *Streptococcus pneumoniae.* Clin Infect Dis 17:939, 1993

528. PEETERMANS WEC, MOFFIE BG, THOMPSON J: Bacterial endocarditis caused by *Streptococcus suis* type 2. J Infect Dis 159:595–596, 1989

529. PERCH B, KJEMS E: Group R streptococci in man: group R streptococci as etiologic agent in a case of purulent meningitis. APMS B 79:549–550, 1971

530. PERCH B, KRISTJANSEN P, SKADHAUGE K: Group R streptococci pathogenic for man: two cases of meningitis and one fatal case of sepsis. APMIS 74:69–76, 1968

531. PERCH B, PEDERSEN KB, HENRICHSEN J: Serology of encapsulated streptococci pathogenic for pigs: six new serotypes of *Streptococcus suis.* J Clin Microbiol 17: 993–996, 1983

532. PESANTI EL, LYONS RW, VERILLI M ET AL: Infection with the human immunodeficiency virus (HIV) as a risk factor for bacteremic illness due to *Streptococcus pneumoniae.* Conn Med 52:703–704, 1988

533. PETERS NS, EYKYN SJ, RUDD SG: Pneumococcal cellulitis: a rare manifestation of pneumococcaemia in adults. J Infect 19:57–59, 1989

534. PETERS VB, BOTTONE EJ, BARZILAI A ET AL: *Leuconostoc* species bacteremia in a child with acquired immunodeficiency syndrome. Clin Pediatr (Phila) 31:699–701, 1992

535. PETERSON EM, SHIGEI JT, WOOLARD A ET AL: Identification of viridans streptococci by three commercial systems. Am J Clin Pathol 90:87–91, 1988

536. PEYSER A, LIEBERGALL M, BAR-ON E ET AL: *Streptococcus bovis* osteomyelitis of the ileum. Clin Infect Dis 19:205–206, 1994

537. PHILLIPS GN JR, FLICKER PF, COHEN C ET AL: Streptococcal M protein: *alpha*-helical coiled-coil structure and arrangement on the cell surface. Proc Natl Acad Sci USA 78:4689–4693, 1981

538. PIEN FD, WILSON WR, KUNZ K ET AL: *Aerococcus viridans* endocarditis. Mayo Clin Proc 59:47–48, 1984

539. PISCITELLI SC, SCHWED J, SCHRECKENBERGER P ET AL: *Streptococcus milleri* group: renewed interest in an elusive pathogen. Eur J Clin Microbiol Infect Dis 11:491–498, 1992

540. POKORSKI SJ, VETTER EA, WOLLAN PC ET AL: Comparison of Gen-Probe group A streptococcus direct test with culture for diagnosing streptococcal pharyngitis. J Clin Microbiol 32:1440–1443, 1994

541. POMPEI R, BERLUTTI F, THALLER MC ET AL: *Enterococcus flavescens* sp. nov., a new species of enterococci of clinical origin. Int J Syst Bacteriol 42:365–369, 1992

542. POMPEI R, LAMPIS G, BERLUTTI F ET AL: Characterization of yellow-pigmented enterococci from severe human infections. J Clin Microbiol 29:2884–2886, 1991

543. POT B, DEVRIESE LA, HOMMEZ J ET AL: Characterization and identification of *Vagococcus fluvialis* strains isolated from domestic animals. J Appl Bacteriol 77:362–369, 1994

544. POTGIETER E, CARMICHAEL M, KOORNHOF HJ AT AL: In vitro antimicrobial susceptibility of viridans streptococci isolated from blood cultures. Eur J Clin Microbiol Infect Dis 11:543–546, 1992

545. POWDERLY WG, STANLEY SL JR, MEDOFF G: Pneumococcal endocarditis: report of a series and review of the literature. Rev Infect Dis 8:786–791, 1986

546. PRATTER MR, IRWIN RS: Viridans streptococcal pulmonary parenchymal infections. JAMA 243:2515–2517, 1980

547. PRUKSAKORN S, CURRIE B, BRANDT E ET AL: Towards a vaccine for rheumatic fever: identification of a conserved target epitope on M protein of group A streptococci. Lancet 344:639–642, 1994

548. PURDY RA, CASSIDY B, MARRIE TJ: *Streptococcus bovis* meningitis: report of two cases. Neurology 40:1782–1784, 1990

549. QUENTIN R, DUBARRY I, GIGNIER C ET AL: Evaluation of a rapid latex test for direct detection of *Streptococcus agalactiae* in various obstetrical and gynaecological disorders. Eur J Clin Microbiol Infect Dis 12:51–54, 1993

550. QUINN RW: Comprehensive review of morbidity and mortality trends for rheumatic fever, streptococcal disease, and scarlet fever: the decline of rheumatic fever. Rev Infect Dis 11:928–953, 1989

551. QUINTILIANI R JR, EVERS S, COURVALIN P: The *vanB* gene confers various levels of self-transferable resistance to vancomycin in enterococci. J Infect Dis 167:1220–1223, 1993

552. RADETSKY M, WHEELER RC, ROE MH ET AL: Comparative evaluation of kits for rapid diagnosis of group A streptococcal disease. Pediatr Infect Dis 4:274–281, 1985

553. RAHMANN S, SMITH MA, ALPERSTEIN P ET AL: A case of bacteremia due to resistant *Streptococcus pneumoniae*. Clin Infect Dis 14:1140–1141, 1992

554. RAMASWAMY G, NG A, QUINLAN L ET AL: *Streptococcus equisimilis* (group C) as a cause of ophthalmic infection. Am J Clin Pathol 79:385–387, 1983

555. RAVIGLIONE MC, TIERNO PM, OTTUSO P ET AL: Group G streptococcal meningitis and sepsis in a patient with AIDS. Diagn Microbiol Infect Dis 13:261–264, 1990

556. REDD SC, RUTHERFORD GW III, SANDE MA ET AL: The role of human immunodeficiency virus infection in pneumococcal bacteremia in San Francisco residents. J Infect Dis 162:1012–1017, 1990

557. REED C, EFSTRATIOU A, MORRISON D ET AL: Glycopeptide-resistant *Gemella haemolysans* from blood. Lancet 342:927–928, 1993

558. REHDER CD, JOHNSON DR, KAPLAN EL: Comparison of methods for obtaining serum opacity factor from group A streptococci. J Clin Microbiol 33:2963–2967, 1995

559. REINERT RR, BUSSING A, KIERDORF H ET AL: Recurrent systemic pneumococcal infection in an immunocompromised patient. Eur J Clin Microbiol Infect Dis 13:304–307, 1994

560. RELF WA, MARTIN DR, SRIPRAKASH KS: Identification of sequence types among the M-nontypeable group A streptococci. J Clin Microbiol 30:3190–3194, 1992

561. REYN A: Genus *Gemella* Berger 1960, 253[AL]. In Sneath PHA, Mair NS, Sharpe ME (eds), *Bergey's Manual of Systematic Bacteriology*, vol 2, pp 1081–1082. Baltimore, Williams & Wilkins, 1986

562. REYNOLDS JG, SILVA E, McCORMACK WM: Association of *Streptococcus bovis* bacteremia with bowel disease. J Clin Microbiol 17:696–697, 1983

563. RICE LB, CALDERWOOD SB, ELIOPOULOS GM ET AL: Enterococcal endocarditis: a comparison of prosthetic and native valve disease. Rev Infect Dis 13:1–7, 1991

564. RICH MW, RADWANY SM: "*Streptococcus milleri*" septicemia in a patient with colorectal carcinoma. Eur J Clin Microbiol Infect Dis 12:225, 1993

565. RIEBEL WJ, WASHINGTON JA: Clinical and microbiologic characteristics of pediococci. J Clin Microbiol 28:1348–1355, 1990

566. RIEFLER J, MOLAVI A, SCHWARTZ D ET AL: Necrotizing fasciitis in adults due to group B *Streptococcus*. Arch Intern Med 148:727–729, 1988

567. ROBERTS RB, KREIGER AG, SCHILLER NI ET AL: Viridans streptococcal endocarditis: the role of various species, including pyridoxal-dependent streptococci. Rev Infect Dis 1:955–965, 1979

568. ROBERTSON ID, BLACKMORE DK: Occupational exposure to *Streptococcus suis* type 2. Epidemiol Infect 103:157–164, 1989

569. ROBERTSON ID, BLACKMORE DK: Prevalence of *Streptococcus suis* types 1 and 2 in domestic pigs in Australia and New Zealand. Vet Rec 124:391–394, 1989

570. ROBERTSON ID, DAVIES PR: *Streptococcus suis* type 2—an underdiagnosed zoonotic agent? Med J Aust 151:238, 1989

571. ROBINSON IM, STROMLEY JM, VAREL VH ET AL: *Streptococcus intestinalis*, a new species from the colons and feces of pigs. Int J Syst Bacteriol 38:245–248, 1988

572. RODRIGUES U, COLLINS MD: Phylogenetic analysis of *Streptococcus saccharolyticus* based on 16S rRNA sequencing. FEMS Microbiol Lett 71:231–234, 1990

573. RODRIGUEZ-BARRADAS MC, MUSHER DM, HAMILL RJ ET AL: Unusual manifestations of pneumococcal infection in human immunodeficiency virus-infected individuals: the past revisited. Clin Infect Dis 14:192–199, 1992

574. ROE M, KISHIYAMA C, DAVIDSON K ET AL: Comparison of BioStar Strep A OIA optical immune assay, Abbott Test-Pack Plus Strep A, and culture with selective media for diagnosis of group A streptococcal pharyngitis. J Clin Microbiol 33:1551–1553, 1995

575. ROSAN B, WILLIAMS NB: Hyaluronidase production by oral enterococci. Arch Oral Biol 9:291–298, 1964

576. ROTTA J: Pyogenic hemolytic streptococci. In Sneath PHA, Mair NS, Sharpe ME (eds), *Bergey's Manual of Systematic Bacteriology*, vol 2, pp 1047–1064. Baltimore, Williams & Wilkins, 1986

577. ROY WJ, ROY TM, DAVIS GJ: Thoracic empyema due to *Streptococcus intermedius*. KMA Journal 89:558–562, 1991

578. RUBIN MM, SANFILIPPO RJ, SADOFF RS: Vertebral osteomyelitis secondary to an oral infection. J Oral Maxillofac Surg 49:897–900, 1991

579. RUDENSKY B, ISACSOHN M: *beta*-Hemolytic group C streptococci and pharyngitis. Rev Infect Dis 11:668, 1989

580. RUDNEY JD, LARSON CJ: Species identification of oral viridans streptococci by restriction fragment polymorphism analysis of rRNA genes. J Clin Microbiol 31:2467–2473, 1993

581. RUDNEY JD, LARSON CJ: Use of restriction fragment polymorphism analysis of rRNA genes to assign species to unknown clinical isolates of oral viridans streptococci. J Clin Microbiol 32:437–443, 1994

582. RUDOLPH KM, PARKINSON AJ, BLACK CM ET AL: Evaluation of polymerase chain reaction for diagnosis of pneumococcal pneumonia. J Clin Microbiol 31:2661–2666, 1993

583. RUOFF KL: *Gemella*: a tale of two species (and five genera). Clin Microbiol Newsl 12:1–4, 1990

584. RUOFF KL, DE LA MAZA L, MURTAUGH MJ ET AL: Species identities of enterococci from clinical specimens. J Clin Microbiol 28:435–437, 1990

585. RUOFF KL, FERRARO MJ: Hydrolytic enzymes of "*Streptococcus milleri*." J Clin Microbiol 25:1645–1647, 1987

586. RUOFF KL, KUNZ LJ: Use of the Rapid STREP system for identification of viridans streptococcal species. J Clin Microbiol 18:1138–1140, 1983

587. RUOFF KL, KUNZ LJ, FERRARO MJ: Occurrence of *Streptococcus milleri* among *beta*-hemolytic streptococci isolated from clinical specimens. J Clin Microbiol 22:149–151, 1985

588. RUOFF KL, MILLER SI, GARNER CV ET AL: Bacteremia with *Streptococcus bovis* and *Streptococcus salivarius*: clinical correlates of more accurate identification of isolates. J Clin Microbiol 27:305–308, 1989

589. SAARELA M, ALALUUSUA S, TAKEI T ET AL: Genetic diversity within isolates of the mutans streptococci recognized by an rRNA gene probe. J Clin Microbiol 31:584–587, 1993

590. SADER HS, PFALLER MA, TENOVER FC ET AL: Evaluation and characterization of multiresistant *Enterococcus faecium* from 12 U.S. medical centers. J Clin Microbiol 32:2840–2842, 1994

591. SAHM DF, BOONLAYANGOOR S, SCHULZ JE: Detection of high-level aminoglycoside resistance in enterococci other than *Enterococcus faecalis*. J Clin Microbiol 29:2595–2598, 1991

592. SALATA RA, LERNER PI, SHLAES DM ET AL: Infections due to Lancefield group C streptococci. Medicine 68:225–239, 1989

593. SARKER TK, MURARKA RS, GILARDI GL: Primary *Streptococcus viridans* pneumonia. Chest 96:831–834, 1989

594. SCHABERG DR, CULVER DH, GAYNES RP: Major trends in the microbial etiology of nosocomial infections. Am J Med 91(suppl 3B):72S-75S, 1991

595. SCHILLER NL, ROBERTS RB: Vitamin B_6 requirements of nutritionally variant *Streptococcus mitior*. J Clin Microbiol 15:740–743, 1982

596. SCHLECH WF III, WARD JI, BAND JD ET AL: Bacterial meningitis in the United States, 1978–1981. The national bacterial meningitis surveillance study. JAMA 253:1749–1754, 1985

597. SCHLEIFER KH, EHRMANN M, KRUSCH U ET AL: Revival of the species *Streptococcus thermophilus* (ex. Orla-Jensen, 1919) nom. rev. Syst Appl Microbiol 14:386–388, 1991

598. SCHLEIFER KH, KILPPER-BALZ R: Transfer of *Streptococcus faecalis* and *Streptococcus faecium* to the genus *Enterococcus* nom. rev. as *Enterococcus faecalis* comb. nov. and *Enterococcus faecium* comb. nov. Int J Syst Bacteriol 34:31–34, 1984

599. SCHLEIFER KH, KILPPER-BALZ R: Molecular and chemotaxonomic approaches to the classification of streptococci, enterococci, and lactococci: a review. Syst Appl Microbiol 10:1–9, 1987

600. SCHLEIFER KH, KRAUS J, DVORAK C ET AL: Transfer of *Streptococcus lactis* and related streptococci to the genus *Lactococcus* gen nov. Syst Appl Microbiol 6:183–195, 1985

601. SCHLIEVERT PM: Role of superantigens in human disease. J Infect Dis 167:997–1002, 1993

602. SCHLIEVERT PM, GOCKE JA, DERINGER JR: Group B streptococcal toxic shock-like syndrome: report of a case and purification of an associated pyrogenic toxin. Clin Infect Dis 17:26–31, 1993

603. SCHMIDTKE LM, CARSON J: Characteristics of *Vagococcus salmoninarum* isolated from diseased salmonid fish. J Appl Bacteriol 77:229–236, 1994

604. SCHNEERSON JM, CHATTOPADHYAY B, MURPHY MFG ET AL: Permanent perceptive deafness due to *Streptococcus suis* type II infection. J Laryngol Otol 94:425–427, 1980

605. SCHUCHAT A, OXTOBY M, COCHI S ET AL: Population-based risk factors for neonatal group B streptococcal disease: results of a cohort study in metropolitan Atlanta. J Infect Dis 162:672–677, 1990

606. SCHUTZE GE, KAPLAN SL, JACOB RF: Resistant pneumococcus: a worldwide problem. Infection 22:233–237, 1994

607. SCHWAB JH, CROMARTIE WJ: Immunological studies on a C polysaccharide complex of group A streptococci having a direct toxic effect on connective tissue. J Exp Med 111:295–307, 1960

608. SCHWABE LD, SMALL MT, RANDALL SL: Comparison of TestPack Strep A test kit with culture technique for detection of group A streptococci. J Clin Microbiol 25:309–311, 1987

609. SCHWARTZ B, ELLIOTT JA, BUTLER JC ET AL: Clusters of invasive group A streptococcal infections in family, hospital, and nursing home settings. Clin Infect Dis 15:277–284, 1992

610. SCULLY BE, SPRIGGS D, NEU HC: *Streptococcus agalactiae* (group B) endocarditis—a description of twelve cases and review of the literature. Infection 15:169–176, 1987

611. SEPPALA H, HE Q, OSTERBLAD M ET AL: Typing of group A streptococci by random amplified polymorphic DNA analysis. J Clin Microbiol 32:1945–1948, 1994

612. SEPPALA H, NISSINEN A, JARVINEN H ET AL: Resistance to erythromycin in group A streptococci. N Engl J Med 326:292–297, 1992

613. SHAW BG, HARDING CD: *Leuconostoc gelidum* sp nov. and *Leuconostoc carnosum* sp. nov. from chill-stored meats. Int J Syst Bacteriol 39:217–223, 1989

614. SHEA KW, SCHOCH PE, KLEIN NC ET AL: Liver abscess due to pyridoxal-dependent *Streptococcus mitis*. Clin Infect Dis 21:238–289, 1995

615. SHINZATO T, SAITO A: A mechanism of pathogenicity of "*Streptococcus milleri* group" in pulmonary infection: synergy with an anaerobe. J Med Microbiol 40:118–123, 1994

616. SHLAES DM, LERNER PI, WOLINSKY E ET AL: Infections due to Lancefield group F and related streptococci (*S. milleri*, *S. anginosus*). Medicine 60:197–207, 1981

617. SHULMAN ST: Complications of streptococcal pharyngitis. Pediatr Infect Dis J 13:S70–S74, 1994

618. SHULMAN ST: Streptococcal pharyngitis: diagnostic considerations. Pediatr Infect Dis J 13:567–571, 1994

619. SIEFKIN AD, PETERSON DL, HANSEN B: *Streptococcus equisimilis* pneumonia in a compromised host. J Clin Microbiol 17:306–308, 1983

620. SINGH KP, MORRIS A, LANG SDR ET AL: Clinically significant *Streptococcus anginosus* (*Streptococcus milleri*) infections: a review of 186 cases. NZ Med J 101:813–816, 1988

621. SIRE JM, DONNIO PY, MESNARD R ET AL: Septicemia and hepatic abscess caused by *Pediococcus acidilactici*. Eur J Clin Microbiol Infect Dis 11:623–625, 1992

622. SISSONS CH, HANCOCK EM: Urease activity in *Streptococcus salivarius* at low pH. Arch Oral Biol 38:507–516, 1993

623. SKAAR I, GAUSTAD P, TONJUM T ET AL: *Streptococcus phocae* sp. nov., a new species isolated from clinical specimens from seals. Int J Syst Bacteriol 44:646–650, 1994

624. SLEDGE D, AUSTIN E, SOBCZYK W ET AL: Group B streptococcal endocarditis involving the tricuspid valve in a 7–month-old infant. Clin Infect Dis 19:166–168, 1994

625. SMITH SK, WASHINGTON JA II: Evaluation of the Pneumoslide latex agglutination kit test for identification of *Streptococcus pneumoniae*. J Clin Microbiol 20:592–593, 1984

626. SOBRINO J, BOSCH X, WENNBERG P ET AL: Septic arthritis secondary to group C streptococcus typed as *Streptococcus equisimilis*. J Rheumatol 18:485–486, 1991

627. SPATARO V, MARONE C: Rhabdomyolysis associated with bacteremia due to *Streptococcus pneumoniae*: case report and review. Clin Infect Dis 17:1063–1064, 1993

628. SPENCER RC, NANAYAKARRA CS, COUP AJ: Fulminant neonatal sepsis due to *Streptococcus milleri*. J Infect 11:88–89, 1982

629. STAMM AM, COBBS CG: Group C streptococcal pneumonia: report of a fatal case and review of the literature. Rev Infect Dis 2:889–898, 1980

630. STEED LL, KORGENSKI EK, DALY JA: Rapid detection of *Streptococcus pyogenes* in pediatric patient specimens by DNA probe. J Clin Microbiol 31:2996–3000, 1993

631. STEINER JL, SEPTIMUS EJ, VARTIAN CV: Infection of the psoas muscle secondary to *Streptococcus pneumoniae* infection. Clin Infect Dis 15:1047–1048, 1992

632. STEINER M, VILLABLANCA J, KERSEY J ET AL: Viridans streptococcal shock in bone marrow transplantation patients. Am J Hematol 42:354–358, 1993

633. STEVENS DL: Invasive group A streptococcus infections. Clin Infect Dis 14:2–13, 1992

634. STEVENS DL: Invasive group A streptococcal infections: the past, present, and future. Pediatr Infect Dis J 13:561–566, 1994

635. STEVENS DL, TANNER MH, WINSHIP J ET AL: Severe group A streptococcal infections associated with a toxic shock-like syndrome and scarlet fever toxin A. N Engl J Med 321:1–7, 1989

636. STEVENSON KB, MURRAY EW, SARUBBI FA: Enterococcal meningitis: report of four cases and review. Clin Infect Dis 18:233–239, 1994

637. STOCKER E, CORTES E, PEMA K ET AL: *Streptococcus milleri* as a cause of antecubital abscess and bacteremia in intravenous drug abusers. South Med J 87:95–96, 1994

638. STOLLERMAN GH: Changing group A streptococci: the reappearance of streptococcal "toxic shock." Arch Intern Med 148:1268–1270, 1988

639. STOLLERMAN GH: Rheumatogenic streptococci and autoimmunity. Clin Immunol Immunopathol 61:131–142, 1991

640. SUTTON GP, SMIRZ LR, CLARK DH ET AL: Group B streptococcal necrotizing fasciitis arising from an episiotomy. Obstet Gynecol 66:733–736, 1985

641. SWARZTRAUBER K, COHEN I: Nonhemolytic group B streptococcal osteomyelitis: identification and treatment in a five-week-old infant.

642. SWENSON JM, FACKLAM RR, THORNSBERRY C: Antimicrobial susceptibility of vancomycin-resistant *Leuconostoc*, *Pediococcus*, and *Lactobacillus* species. Antimicrob Agents Chemother 34:543–549, 1990

643. SYROGIANNOPOULOS GA, McCRAKEN GH JR, NELSON JD: Osteoarticular infections in children with sickle cell disease. Pediatrics 78:1090–1096, 1986

644. TANKOVIC J, LECLERCQ R, DUVAL J: Antimicrobial susceptibility of *Pediococcus* spp. and genetic basis of macrolide resistance in *Pediococcus acidilactici* HM3020. Antimicrob Agents Chemother 37:789–792, 1993

645. TAPSALL JW: Pigment production by Lancefield-group-B streptococci (*Streptococcus agalactiae*). J Med Microbiol 21:75–81, 1986

646. TARRADAS C, ARENAS A, MALDONADO A ET AL: Identification of *Streptococcus suis* isolated from swine: proposal for biochemical parameters. J Clin Microbiol 32:578–580, 1994

647. TAYLOR PW, TRUEBLOOD MC: Septic arthritis due to *Aerococcus viridans*. J Rheumatol 12:1004–1005, 1985

648. TEIXEIRA LA, FIGUEIREDO AMS, BENCHETRIT LC: Liquid medium for rapid presumptive identification of group B streptococci. J Clin Microbiol 30:506–508, 1992

649. TEN BERG JM, ELBERS HRJ, DEFAUW JJAM ET AL: Endocarditis on a left atrial myxoma. Eur Heart J 13:1592–1593, 1992

650. TENJARLA G, JUMAR A, DYKE JW: TestPack Strep A kit for the rapid detection of group A streptococci on 11,088 throat swabs in a clinical pathology laboratory. Am J Clin Pathol 96:759–761, 1991

651. THOMAS JC, CARR SJ, FUJIOKA K ET AL: Community-acquired group A streptococcal deaths in Los Angeles County. J Infect Dis 160:1086–1087, 1989

652. THORNSBERRY C, MARLER JK, RICH TJ: Increased penicillin resistance in recent U.S. isolates of Streptococcus pneumoniae. In Abstracts of the 92nd General Meeting of the American Society for Microbiology, C-268, p 465. Washington DC, American Society for Microbiology, 1995

653. TIMONEY JF: Strangles. Vet Clin North Am Equine Pract 9:365–374, 1993

654. TORRES E, ALBA D, FRANK A ET AL: Iatrogenic meningitis due to Streptococcus salivarius following a spinal tap. Clin Infect Dis 17:525–526, 1993

655. TOWERS CV, GARITE TJ, FRIEDMAN WW ET AL: Comparison of a rapid enzyme-linked immunosorbent assay test and the Gram stain for detection of group B Streptococcus in high-risk antepartum patients. Am J Obstet Gynecol 163:965–967, 1990

656. TRESADERN JC, FARRAND RJ, IRVING MH: Streptococcus milleri and surgical sepsis. Annu Rev Coll Surg (Engl) 65:78–79, 1983

657. TRITZ DM, IWEN PC, WOODS GL: Evaluation of MicroScan for identification of Enterococcus species. J Clin Microbiol 28:1477–1478, 1990

658. TROTTIER S, HIGGINS R, BROCHU G ET AL: A case of human endocarditis due to Streptococcus suis in North America. Rev Infect Dis 13:1251–1252, 1991

659. TRUANT AL, SATISHCHANDRAN V: Comparison of Streptex versus PathoDx for group D typing of vancomycin-resistant Enterococcus. Diagn Microbiol Infect Dis 16:89–91, 1993

660. TSAI C-Y, WU T-H, YANG C-C ET AL: Streptococcus sanguis osteomyelitis of the L2,3 lumbar vertebrae in seronegative rheumatoid arthritis. Clin Exp Rheumatol 12:93–94, 1994

661. TSUTSUI O, KOKEGUCHI S, MATSUMURA T ET AL: Relationship of the chemical structure and immunobiological activities of lipoteichoic acid from Streptococcus faecalis (Enterococcus hirae) ATCC 9790. FEMS Microbiol Immunol 3:211–218, 1991

662. TUNG KSK, WOODROFFE AJ, AHLIN TD ET AL: Application of the solid phase C1q and Raji cell radioimmune assays for the detection of circulating immune complexes in glomerulonephritis. J Clin Invest 62:61–72, 1978

663. TURNER JC, FOX A, FOX K ET AL: Role of group C beta-hemolytic streptococci in pharyngitis: epidemiologic study of clinical features associated with isolation of group C streptococci. J Clin Microbiol 31:808–811, 1993

664. TURNER JC, HAYDEN GF, KISELICA D ET AL: Association of group C beta-hemolytic streptococci with endemic pharyngitis among college students. JAMA 264:2644–2647, 1990

665. UNTEREKER WJ, HANNA BA: Endocarditis and osteomyelitis caused by Aerococcus viridans. Mt Sinai J Med 43:248–252, 1976

666. VACCA-SMITH AM, JONES CA, LEVINE MJ ET AL: Glucosyltransferase mediates adhesion of Streptococcus gordonii to human epithelial cells in vitro. Infect Immun 62:2187–2194, 1994

667. VANCE DW JR: Group C streptococci: "Streptococcus equisimilis" or Streptococcus anginosus. Clin Infect Dis 14:616, 1992

668. VAN DER MEI, NAUMANN D, BUSSCHER HJ: Grouping of oral streptococcal species using Fourier-transform infrared spectroscopy in comparison with classical microbiological identification. Arch Oral Biol 38:1013–1019, 1993

669. VAN DE TIJN I, FILLIT H, BRANDEIS WE ET AL: Serial studies on circulating immune complexes in post-streptococcal sequelae. Clin Exp Immunol 34:318–325, 1978

670. VAN GOETHEM GF, LOUWAGIE BM, SIMOENS MJ ET AL: Enterococcus casseliflavus septicaemia in a patient with acute myeloid leukemia. Eur J Clin Microbiol Infect Dis 13:519–520, 1994

671. VARTIAN C, LERNER PI, SHLAES DM ET AL: Infections due to Lancefield group G streptococci. Medicine 64:75–88, 1985

672. VARTIAN CV, SEPTIMUS EJ: Meningitis caused by group B Streptococcus in association with cerebrospinal rhinorrhea. Clin Infect Dis 14:1261–1262, 1992

673. VEASY LG, WIEDMEIER SE, ORSMOND GS: Resurgence of acute rheumatic fever in the intermountain area of the United States. N Engl J Med 316:421–427, 1987

674. VECHT U, WISSELINK HJ, JELLEMA ML ET AL: Identification of two proteins associated with virulence of Streptococcus suis type 2. Infect Immun 59:3156–3162, 1991

675. VENDITTI M, BIAVASCO F, VARALDO PE ET AL: Catheter-related endocarditis due to glycopeptide-resistant Enterococcus faecalis in a transplanted heart. Clin Infect Dis 17:524–525, 1993

676. VERGHESE A, BERK SL, BOELEN LJ ET AL: Group B streptococcal pneumonia in the elderly. Arch Intern Med 142:1642–1645, 1982

677. VICKERMAN MM, CLEWELL DB, JONES GW: Sucrose-promoted accumulation of growing glucosyltransferase variants of Streptococcus gordonii on hydroxyapatite surfaces. Infect Immun 59:3523–3530, 1991

678. VINCENT S, KNIGHT RG, GREEN M ET AL: Vancomycin susceptibility and identification of motile enterococci. J Clin Microbiol 29:2335–2337, 1991

679. VIROLAINEN A, SALO P, JERO J ET AL: Comparison of PCR assay with bacterial culture for detecting Streptococcus pneumoniae in middle ear fluid of children with acute otitis media. J Clin Microbiol 32:2667–2670, 1994

680. VON ESSEN R, IKAVALKO M, FORSBLOM B: Isolation of Gemella morbillorum from joint fluid. Lancet 342:177–178, 1993

681. VON GRAEVENITZ A: Revised nomenclature of Alloiococcus otitis. J Clin Microbiol 31:472, 1993

682. VON HUNOLSTEIN C, D'ASCENZI S, WAGNER B ET AL: Immunochemistry of capsular type polysaccharide and virulence properties of type VI Streptococcus agalactiae (group B streptococci). Infect Immun 61:1272–1280, 1993

683. WALD ER, BERGMAN I, TAYLOR HG ET AL: Long-term outcome of group B streptococcal meningitis. Pediatrics 77:217–221, 1986

684. WALD ER, DASHEFSKY B, FEIDT C ET AL: Acute rheumatic fever in western Pennsylvania and the tri-state area. Pediatrics 80:371–374, 1987

685. WALD ER, DASHEFSKY B, GREEN M ET AL: Rapid detection of group B streptococci directly from vaginal swabs. J Clin Microbiol 8:410–412, 1987

686. WALLBANKS S, MARTINEZ-MURCIA AJ, FRYER JL ET AL: 16S rRNA sequence determination for members of the genus *Carnobacterium* and related lactic acid bacteria and description of *Vagococcus salmoninarum*. Int J Syst Bacteriol 40:224–230, 1990

687. WARREN J, LOUIE KG, GREENSPAHN BR ET AL: *Streptococcus bovis* endocarditis on a prosthetic heart valve with a colonic neoplasm. N Engl J Med 304:1239–1240, 1981

688. WATANAKUNIKORN C, PANTELAKIS J: *alpha*-Hemolytic streptococcal bacteremia: a review of 203 episodes during 1980–1991. Scand J Infect Dis 25:403–408, 1993

689. WATANAKUNIKORN C, PATEL R: Comparison of patients with enterococcal bacteremia due to strains with and without high-level resistance to gentamicin. Clin Infect Dis 17:74–78, 1993

690. WATSKY KL, KOLLISCH N, DENSEN P: Group G streptococcal bacteremia: the clinical experience at Boston University Medical Center and a critical review of the literature. Arch Intern Med 145:58–61, 1985

691. WATSON DA, MUSHER DM: Interruption of capsule production in *Streptococcus pneumoniae* serotype 3 by insertion of transposon *Tn916*. Infect Immun 58:3135–3138, 1990

692. WATTS JL: Evaluation of the Minitek Gram-Positive set for identification of streptococci isolated from bovine mammary glands. J Clin Microbiol 27:1008–1010, 1989

693. WATTS JL: Evaluation of the Rapid STREP system for identification of gram-positive, catalase-negative cocci isolated from bovine intramammary infections. J Dairy Sci 72:2728–2732, 1989

694. WEEKS CR, FERRETTI JJ: Nucleotide sequence of the type A streptococcal exotoxin (erythrogenic toxin) gene from *Streptococcus pyogenes* bacteriophage T12. Infect Immun 52:144, 1986

695. WEISMAN LE, STOLL BJ, CRUESS DF ET AL: Early-onset group B streptococcal sepsis: a current assessment. J Pediatr 121:428–433, 1992

696. WEITBERG AB, ANNESE C, GINSBERG MB: *Streptococcus bovis* meningitis and carcinoma of the colon. Johns Hopkins Med J 148:260–261, 1981

697. WELCH DF, HENSEL D, PICKETT D ET AL: Comparative evaluation of selective and nonselective culture techniques for isolation of group A *beta*-hemolytic streptococci. Am J Clin Pathol 95:587–590, 1991

698. WELLSTOOD S: Evaluation of a latex test for rapid detection of pneumococcal antigens in sputum. Eur J Clin Microbiol Infect Dis 11:448–451, 1992

699. WENGER JD, HIGHTOWER AW, FACKLAM RR ET AL: Bacterial meningitis in the United States, 1986: report of a multistate surveillance study. J Infect Dis 162:1316–1323, 1990

700. WENOCUR HS, SMITH MA, VELLOZI EM ET AL: Odontogenic infection secondary to *Leuconostoc* species. J Clin Microbiol 26:1893–1894, 1988

701. WESSELS MR, HAFT R, HEGGEN LM ET AL: Identification of a genetic locus essential for capsule sialylation in type III group B streptococci. Infect Immun 60:392–400, 1992

702. WESTH H, SKIBSTED L, KORNER B: *Streptococcus pneumoniae* infections of the female genital tract and the newborn child. Rev Infect Dis 12:416–422, 1990

703. WESTLAKE RM, GRAHAM TP, EDWARDS KM: An outbreak of acute rheumatic fever in Tennessee. Pediatr Infect Dis J 9:97–100, 1990

704. WHEELER MC, ROE MH, KAPLAN EL ET AL: Outbreak of group A streptococcal septicemia in children: clinical, epidemiologic, and microbiological correlates. JAMA 266:533–537, 1991

705. WHILEY RA, BEIGHTON D: Emended descriptions and recognition of *Streptococcus constellatus*, *Streptococcus intermedius*, and *Streptococcus anginosus* as distinct species. Int J Syst Bacteriol 41:1–5, 1991

706. WHILEY RA, BEIGHTON D, WINSTANLEY TG, ET AL: *Streptococcus intermedius*, *Streptococcus constellatus*, and *Streptococcus anginosus* (the *Streptococcus milleri* group): association with different body sites and clinical infections. J Clin Microbiol 30:243–244, 1992

707. WHILEY RA, FRASER HY, DOUGLAS CWI ET AL: *Streptococcus parasanguis* sp. nov., an atypical viridans streptococcus from human clinical specimens. FEMS Microbiol Lett 68:115–122, 1990

708. WHILEY RA, FRASER H, HARDIE JM ET AL: Phenotypic differentiation of *Streptococcus intermedius*, *Streptococcus constellatus*, and *Streptococcus anginosus* strains within the "*Streptococcus milleri*" group. J Clin Microbiol 28:1497–1501, 1990

709. WHILEY RA, HARDIE JM: *Streptococcus vestibularis* sp. nov. from the human oral cavity. Int J Syst Bacteriol 38:335–339, 1988

710. WHILEY RA, HARDIE JM: DNA–DNA hybridization studies and phenotypic characteristics of strains within the "*Streptococcus milleri* group." J Gen Microbiol 135:2623–2633, 1989

711. WHILEY RA, RUSSELL RRB, HARDIE JM ET AL: *Streptococcus downeii* sp. nov. for strains previously described as *Streptococcus mutans* serotype h. Int J Syst Bacteriol 38:25–29, 1988

712. WHITEHEAD TR, COTTA MA: Development of a DNA probe for *Streptococcus bovis* by using a cloned amylase gene. J Clin Microbiol 31:2387–2391, 1993

713. WHITNEY AM, O'CONNOR SP: Phylogenetic relationship of *Gemella morbillorum* to *Gemella haemolysans*. Int J Syst Bacteriol 43:832–838, 1993

714. WICKEN AJ, ELLIOTT SD, BADDILEY J: The identity of streptococcal group D antigen with teichoic acid. J Gen Microbiol 31:231–239, 1963

715. WILCOX MH, WINSTANLEY TG, DOUGLAS CWI ET AL: Susceptibility of *alpha*-hemolytic streptococci causing endocarditis to benzylpenicillin and ten cephalosporins. J Antimicrob Chemother 32:63–69, 1993

716. WILLCOX MDP, KNOX KW, GREEN RM ET AL: An examination of strains of the bacterium *Streptococcus vestibularis* for relative cariogenicity in gnotobiotic rats and adhesion *in vitro*. Arch Oral Biol 36:327–333, 1991

717. WILLEY BM, KREISWIRTH BN, SIMOR AE ET AL: Identification and characterization of multiple species of vancomycin-resistant enterococci, including an evaluation of Vitek software version 7.1. J Clin Microbiol 31:2777–2779, 1993

718. WILLIAMS AM, COLLINS MD: Molecular taxonomic studies on *Streptococcus uberis* types I and II. Description of *Streptococcus parauberis* sp. nov. J Appl Bacteriol 68: 485–490, 1990

719. WILLIAMS AM, FARROW JAE, COLLINS MD: Reverse transcriptase sequencing of 16S ribosomal RNA from *Streptococcus cecorum*. Lett Appl Microbiol 8:185–189, 1989

720. WILLIAMS AM, RODRIGUES UM, COLLINS MD: Intrageneric relationships of enterococci as determined by reverse transcriptase sequencing of small subunit rRNA. Res Microbiol 142:67–74, 1990

721. WILSON WR, THOMPSON RL, WILKOWSKE CJ ET AL: Short-term therapy for streptococcal infective endocardtiis. JAMA 245:360–363, 1981

722. WISEMAN A, RENE P, CRELINSTEN GL: *Streptococcus agalactiae* endocarditis: an association with villous adenomas of the large intestine. Ann Intern Med 103: 893–894, 1985

723. WOOD EG, DILLON HC: A prospective study of group B streptococcal bacteriuria in pregnancy. Am J Obstet Gynecol 140:515

724. WOOD HF, JACOBS K, MCCARTY M: *Streptococcus lactis* isolated from a patient with subacute bacterial endocarditis. Am J Med 18:345–347, 1985

725. WOOD TF, POTTER MA, JONASSON O: Streptococcal toxic shock-like syndrome: the importance of surgical intervention. Ann Surg 217:109–114, 1993

726. WOODFORD N, MORRISON D, JOHNSON AP ET AL: Application of DNA probes for rRNA and *vanA* genes to investigation of a nosocomial cluster of vancomycin-resistant enterococci. J Clin Microbiol 31:653–658, 1993

727. WOODS CR, EDWARDS MS: Renal abscess caused by group B *Streptococcus*. Clin Infect Dis 18:662–663, 1994

728. WUST J, HEBISCH G, PETERS K: Evaluation of two enzyme immunoassays for rapid detection of group B streptococci in pregnant women. Eur J Clin Microbiol Infect Dis 12:124–127, 1993

729. YAGUPSKY P, MENEGUS MA, POWELL KR: The changing spectrum of group B streptococcal disease in infants: an eleven-year experience in a tertiary care hospital. Pediatr Infect Dis J 10:801–808, 1991

730. YANCEY MK, ARMER T, CLARK P ET AL: Assessment of rapid identification tests for genital carriage of group B streptococci. Obstet Gynecol 80:1038–1047, 1992

731. YANCEY MK, CLARK P, ARMER T ET AL: Use of a DNA probe for the rapid detection of group B streptococci in obstetric patients. Obstet Gynecol 81:635–640, 1993

732. YANELLI B, GUREVICH I, SCHOCH PE ET AL: Group G streptococcal bacteremia. Clin Microbiol Newslett 9:86–87, 1987

733. YOU MS, FACKLAM RR: New test system for identification of *Aerococcus*, *Enterococcus*, and *Streptococcus*. J Clin Microbiol 24:607–611, 1986

734. YUEN KY, SETO WH, CHOI CH ET AL: *Streptococcus zooepidemicus* (Lancefield group C) septicaemia in Hong Kong. J Infect 21:241–250, 1990

735. ZARKIN BA, LILLEMOE KD, CAMERON JL ET AL: The triad of *Streptococcus bovis* bacteremia, colonic pathology, and liver disease. Ann Surg 211:786–791, 1990

736. ZIGHELBOIM S, TOMASZ A: Penicillin-binding proteins of multiply-antibiotic resistant South African strains of *Streptococcus pneumoniae*. Antimicrob Agents Chemother 17:434–442, 1980

THE AEROBIC GRAM-POSITIVE BACILLI

The gram-positive bacteria covered in this chapter are divided into the following four groups:

- Spore-forming, aerobic or facultatively anaerobic bacilli
- Morphologically, regular, non–spore-forming bacilli

- Irregular or coryneform, non–spore-forming bacilli
- Nocardioforms and aerobic actinomycetes

There is some overlap between the genera of gram-positive rods covered herein and those included in Chapter 14 on the anaerobic bacteria. This is unavoidable because some aerotolerant anaerobes and facultatively anaerobic bacteria that grow in the presence of air have been classified within genera traditionally

Color Plates for Chapter 13 are found between pages 368 and 369.

reserved for anaerobes. For example, those formerly referred to as CDC coryneform groups 1 and 2, have now been reclassified as *Actinomyces bernardiae* and *A. neuii* subsp. *neuii* and *A. neuii* subsp. *anitratus*, respectively.[123] *Corynebacterium pyogenes* is now called *A. pyogenes*.[67] Aerotolerant species of the genus *Clostridium* (i.e., *C. tertium*, *C. histolyticum*, and *C. carnis*), discussed in Chapter 14, pose a similar problem and might be confused with species of *Bacillus*. Even though the spore-forming bacilli that grow aerobically are classified in the genus *Bacillus*, some *Bacillus* species may grow best under anaerobic conditions, or at least on initial isolation. Some species of the genus *Lactobacillus* grow as obligate anaerobes, yet many others grow well aerobically. In spite of overlap within the two chapters, we have elected to discuss the following genera in Chapter 14: *Actinomyces*, *Bifidobacterium*, *Clostridium*, *Eubacterium*, and *Propionibacterium*. The genus *Lactobacillus* is described in this chapter, although just as strong a rationale might be offered for its placement in Chapter 14. The genus *Mycobacterium* (see Chap. 17) contains strongly acid-fast rods that are closely related to the genera *Corynebacterium*, *Rhodococcus*, and *Norcardia*. *Mycobacterium* species may or may not stain with Gram stain, but taxonomically are considered to be gram-positive and, on occasion, might be confused with the corynebacteria or nocardioforms unless appropriate differential tests are done. Aerobic and facultatively anaerobic rods are commonly isolated in the clinical microbiology laboratory. They are ubiquitous, inhabiting terrestrial and aquatic habitats, and many are part of the normal skin and mucous membrane flora of humans and various animals.

The virulence of the gram-positive bacilli is highly variable. For example, *Bacillus anthracis* is one of the most highly pathogenic microorganisms known to mankind (Table 13-1). Almost all gram-positive rods isolated in hospital laboratories are of the genera *Bacillus*, *Corynebacterium*, and *Lactobacillus*. Many of these isolates (e.g., *Bacillus cereus*, other *Bacillus* species, and various *Corynebacterium* species other than *C. diphtheriae*) are common laboratory contaminants. On the other hand, many of them have the potential to be opportunistic pathogens, capable of producing disease only in persons with compromised host resistance related to underlying disorders. Thus, in the setting of an immunocompromised patient who has clinical signs of sepsis, the finding of a nonanthrax *Bacillus* species, or one of the *Corynebacterium* species other than *C. diphtheriae* in two or more sets of positive blood cultures may be highly clinically important, rather than representative of contamination.

TABLE 13-1

PRESENT AND FORMER NAMES OR COMMENTS ON THE AEROBIC GRAM-POSITIVE BACILLI

PRESENT NAME	FORMER NAME/COMMENT	PRESENT NAME	FORMER NAME/COMMENT
Genus *Actinomyces*		Genus *Brevibacterium*	CDC coryneform groups B-1 and
A. *bernardiae*	CDC coryneform group 2	B. *casei*	B-3
A. *neuii* subsp. *neuii*	CDC coryneform group 1	B. *epidermidis*	
A. *neuii* subsp. *anitratus*	CC coryneform-like group 1	B. *mcbrellneri*	
A. *pyogenes*	*Corynebacterium pyogenes*		
		Genus *Corynebacterium*	
Genus *Arcanobacterium*		C. *afermentans*-like	CDC coryneform group ANF-1-like
A. *haemolyticum*	*Corynebacterium haemolyticum*	bacteria	
		C. *afermentans* subsp.	CDC coryneform group ANF-1 in
Genus *Aureobacterium*	Includes some taxa previously	*afermentans*	part
	classified as *Arthrobacter*, *Curto-*	C. *afermentans* subsp.	CDC coryneform group ANF-1 in
	bacterium and *Microbacterium* and	*lipophilum*	part
	some "*Corynebacterium aquaticum*"	C. *amycolatum*	C. *xerosis*, C. *minutissimum*, C.
			striatum and CDC coryneform
Genus *Bacillus*			Group I_2 and Group F_2
B. *alvei*		"C. *aquaticum*"	Not a valid species
B. *anthracis*	Causative agent of anthrax	C. *argentoratense*	New species
B. *brevis*		C. *auris*	CDC coryneform group ANF-1-like
B. *cereus*	Can cause food poisoning		in part
B. *circulans*		C. *bovis*	Cow flora
B. *coagulans*		C. *cystitidis*	
B. *licheniformis*		C. *diphtheriae*	Causative agent of diphtheria
B. *macerans*		C. *glutamicum*	*Brevibacterium divaricatum*,
B. *megaterium*			"B. *flavum*," "B. *lactofermentum*"
B. *pumilus*			and *Corynebacterium lilum*
B. *sphaericus*		C. *jeikeium*	CDC coryneform group JK
B. *subtilis*		C. *kutscheri*	Rodent flora
B. *thuringiensis*		C. *macginleyi*	CDC coryneform group G-1 in part

(Continued)

TABLE 13-1 *(Continued)*
PRESENT AND FORMER NAMES OR COMMENTS ON THE AEROBIC GRAM-POSITIVE BACILLI

PRESENT NAME	FORMER NAME/COMMENT	PRESENT NAME	FORMER NAME/COMMENT
Genus *Corynebacterium* (cont'd)		L. innocua	Nonpathogen
C. matruchotii	*Bacterionema matruchotii*	L. ivanovii	*L. monocytogenes* serovar 5, *L. bulgaria*
C. mycetoides		L. monocytogenes	Causative agent of listeriosis
C. pilosum		L. seeligeri	Nonpathogen
C. pseudodiphtheriticum	*C. hofmanii*	L. welshimeri	Nonpathogen
C. propinquum	CDC coryneform group ANF-3		
C. pseudotuberculosis	Associated with infection in livestock	Genus *Microbacterium*	CDC coryneform group A-4, A-5 in part
C. renale	Cattle flora	M. arborescens	CDC coryneform group A-4 in part
C. seminale	New species	M. imperiale	CDC coryneform group A-4 in part
C. ulcerans	Can cause diphtheria-like illness	M. abscessus	*Mycobacterium chelonae* subsp. *abscessus*
C. urealyticum	*Corynebacterium* group D2, CDC coryneform group D2		
		Genus *Nocardia*	
Genus *Dermabacter*		N. asteroides	
D. hominis	CDC fermentative coryneform groups 3 and 5	N. brasiliensis	
		N. carnea	
		N. farcinica	
Genus *Dermatophilus*		N. nova	
D. congolensis		N. otitidiscaviarum	*N. caviae*
		N. pseudobrasiliensis	New species
Genus *Erysipelothrix*		N. transvalensis	
E. rhusiopathiae	Causative agent of erysipeloid; *E. insidiosa*	Genus *Norcardiopsis*	New genus—*Actinomadura* in part
		N. dassonvillei	
Genus *Gardnerella*			
G. vaginalis	*Haemophilus vaginalis, Corynebacterium vaginalis*	Genus *Oerskovia*	
		O. turbata	CDC coryneform groups A-3 and A-4
Genus *Gordona*	New genus	O. xanthineolyticum	CDC coryneform groups A-1 and A-2
G. aichiensis	*Rhodococcus aichiensis, Tsukamura aichiessii*		
G. bronchialis	*R. bronchialis*	Genus *Rhodococcus*	
G. rubropertincta	*R. rubropertinatus*	R. equi	*Corynebacterium equi*
G. spuita	*R. chubuensis*		
G. terrae	*R. terrae*	Genus *Rothia*	
		R. dentocariosa	*Nocardia dentocariosus*
Genus *Kurthia*			
K. bessonii		Genus *Streptomyces*	
K. gibsonii		S. anulatus	*Streptomyces griseus*
K. sibirca		S. paraguayensis	Soil and decaying vegetation
K. zopfii		S. albus	
		S. coelicolor	
Genus *Lactobacillus*		S. lavendulae	
L. acidophilus		S. rimosus	
L. amylovorus	L. acidophilus group A3	S. somaliensis	
L. casei		S. violaceoruber	
L. crispatus			
L. gasseri		Genus *Tsukamurella*	
L. johnsonii		T. inchonesis	New species
L. oris		T. pulmonis	New species
L. reuteri		T. paurometabola	*Gordona aurantiaca*
L. vaginalis			
		Genus *Turicella*	
Genus *Listeria*		T. otitidis	*Corynebacterium* group ANF-1-like in part, *Rhodococcus aurantiazus*
L. dentrificans	Uncertain taxonomic affiliation		
L. grayi	*L. murrayi*		

This was not intended to be an all inclusive list. Several species of no or doubtful relevance to the clinical laboratory have not been included.
Based on information compiled for taxa published in (a) the International Journal of Systematic Bacteriology, Volumes 30–46: 1980–1996 and (b) Chapters 27, 28, 29 and 30 of the ASM Manual of Clinical Microbiology (60), the list compiled by Bruckner and Colonna (34a), and the report by Funke et al (117).

It is essential for the clinical microbiologist to be able to isolate and learn to recognize the various commonly encountered aerobic and facultatively anaerobic gram-positive bacilli. The microbiologist must also become familiar with the key differential characteristics that differentiate between the species that are of classic medical importance (Table 13-2) from those that are rarely, if ever, pathogenic for humans. Gram-positive rods should be identified to the species level when their presence in clinical specimens carries potential clinical significance. Thus, isolates from body fluids other than urine (e.g., blood, cere-

TABLE 13-2

SOME DISEASES OF HUMANS CAUSED BY, OR ASSOCIATED WITH, AEROBIC AND FACULTATIVELY ANAEROBIC GRAM-POSITIVE RODS

DISEASE	SPECIES OR GROUP OF ORGANISMS	MAJOR BODY SITES INVOLVED AND ASSOCIATED DISORDERS
Anthrax	*Bacillus anthracis*	Skin, rarely lungs, more rarely intestinal tract
Actinomycosis	*Actinomyces israelii* and *A. naeslundii* are the most common species. (They include obligate anaerobes and facultative anaerobes and are covered in Chapter 14.)	Cervicofacial, thoracic, intra-abdominal, and intrauterine
Actinomycetoma	*Actinomadura madurae, A. pelletierii, Nocardia asteroides, N. brasiliensis, Nocardiopsis dassonvillei, Streptomyces somaliensis,* others	Body surfaces, especially feet, legs, and upper extremities
Diphtheria	*Corynebacterium diphtheriae*	Infections localized to throat, occasionally nose, and rarely wounds. Local production of toxin causes systemic disease.
Endocarditis	*Corynebacterium jeikeium* and other "non-diphtheria" *Corynebacterium* species, *Listeria monocytogenes,* "Nonanthrax" *Bacillus* species, *Lactobacillus* species, *Erysipelothrix rhusiopathiae, Kurthia bessonii, Oerskovia turbata*	Infection of the heart valves by gram-positive rods is rare and usually occurs on prosthetic valves or scarred (fibrotic) valves
Erysipeloid	*Erysipelothrix rhusiopathiae*	Usually skin (especially fingers or hand), but patient may also have septicemia, arthritis, or endocarditis
Food-borne gastroenteritis	*Bacillus cereus*	Gastrointestinal tract
Hypersensitivity pneumonitis	*Thermoactinomyces vulgaris, Micropolyspora faeni, Saccharomonospora viridis*	Lung
Listeriosis	*Listeria monocytogenes*	Food-borne gastroenteritis Asymptomatic carriers (intestinal) Septicemia (pregnant, neonate, and immunosuppressed patients) Granulomatosis infantiseptica (transplacental infection and abortion?) Meningitis (cerebritis, meningoencephalitis) Focal lesions (skin lesions, conjunctivitis, lymphadenitis, endocarditis, peritonitis, osteomyelitis, pneumonitis, brain abscess)
Leprosy	*Mycobacterium leprae*	Skin
Mycobacterioses (and tuberculosis)	Various species of *Mycobacterium,* including *M. tuberculosis, M. avium* complex, and others	Lungs, lymph nodes, skin, gastrointestinal tract
Nocardiosis	*Nocardia asteroides;* rarely *N. brasiliensis, N. caviae, N. farcinica*	Lungs most common; also, disseminated form may involve lung, central nervous system, kidney, and other sites. Superficial form involves skin, especially of extremities.

(Continued)

TABLE 13-2 *(Continued)*

SOME DISEASES OF HUMANS CAUSED BY, OR ASSOCIATED WITH, AEROBIC AND FACULTATIVELY ANAEROBIC GRAM-POSITIVE RODS

DISEASE	SPECIES OR GROUP OF ORGANISMS	MAJOR BODY SITES INVOLVED AND ASSOCIATED DISORDERS
Miscellaneous infections	*Corynebacterium jeikeium*	Septicemia caused by multiply antibiotic-resistant organisms in immunocompromised patients, endocarditis, pneumonia, wound infections
	Corynebacterium *urealyticum*	Alkaline-encrusted cystitis, urinary tract infections with multiple antibiotic-resistant bacteria
	"*Corynebacterium ulcerans*"	Sore throat following consumption of raw milk; diphtheria-like disease
	Corynebacterium pseudodiphtheriticum	Endocarditis (prosthetic valve), pneumonia, lung abscess, lymphadenopathy, urinary tract infections
	"*Corynebacerium aquaticum*"	Rare cases of meningitis, urinary tract infection, peritonitis, bacteremia
	"*Corynebacterium minutissimum*"	Rare cases of erythrasma (a superficial skin infection) and septicemia
	Arcanobacterium hemolyticum	Pharyngitis sometimes with diphtheria-like pseudomembranes, wound infections, septicemia
	Actinomyces pyogenes	Skin infections, septicemia, endocarditis, pneumonia
	Rhodococcus equi	Bronchopneumonia in horses; most infections in humans follow exposure to livestock; isolates commonly from patients with acquired immunodeficiency syndrome, pneumonia, bacteremia; osteomyelitis; wounds

brospinal fluid, pleural fluid, and such) should be identified. Except in special circumstances, aerobic gram-positive rods do not require identification to the species level when isolated from specimens contaminated with normal flora, but do require identification to species when isolated from properly selected specimens collected from infected sites of immunocompromised patients. These specimens, not infrequently, will contain *Corynebacterium jeikeium* or other *Corynebacterium* species that may be resistant to multiple antibiotics. These organisms and many other opportunistic species discussed in this chapter can cause life-threatening infections that may be difficult to treat and manage clinically.

SPORE-FORMING, AEROBIC, OR FACULTATIVELY ANAEROBIC BACILLI

BACILLUS SPECIES

The genus *Bacillus*, the type genus of the family *Bacillaceae*, currently comprises more than 60 species of aerobic or facultatively anaerobic gram-positive bacilli that produce endospores (see Color Plate 13-1*A*).[300] The bacterial cells range from 0.5×1.2 to 2.5×10 μm in diameter. These organisms usually grow well on blood agar, producing large, spreading, gray-white colonies, with irregular margins. Many clinical isolates are β-hemolytic, a helpful characteristic in differentiating various *Bacillus* species from *B. anthracis*, which is not hemolytic (see Color Plate 13-1*B*). Catalase is produced by most species, and sporulation is not inhibited by aerobic incubation, positive characteristics that aid in

distinguishing *Bacillus* from the genus *Clostridium* (see Chap. 14).

Most *Bacillus* species encountered in the clinical laboratory are saprophytic contaminants or members of the normal flora. They fall into three broad groups, depending on the morphology of the spore and sporangium, as originally proposed in 1952 by Smith and colleagues,[299] further refined by Gordon and associates in 1973,[145] and summarized by Turnbull and Kramer in 1991.[336] These groupings are listed in Box 13-1.

Most *Bacillus* species encountered in the clinical laboratory are in group 1. An approach to their identification is discussed below and is summarized in the algorithms presented in Figure 13-1 and Table 13-3.

Although rarely encountered in the United States, *B. anthracis* has historically been the most important member of this genus, causing anthrax in animals, and rarely, in humans. From 1974 to 1980, only 13 cases of anthrax were reported by the Centers for Disease Control and Prevention (CDC) in the United States; this trend continued during 1981 through 1989, when only 4 cases were reported.[46,49] *B. cereus*, another species of importance to humans, has been associated with outbreaks of human food poisoning.[327] In addition, *B. cereus* and several other species have been reported to cause a variety of invasive infections in immunocompromised individuals. These infections caused by *B. cereus* and other species are much more common than anthrax.[336]

HABITAT

Bacillus species are ubiquitous, inhabiting soil, water, and airborne dust. Thermophilic and psy-

BOX 13-1. *BACILLUS* SPECIES ENCOUNTERED IN THE CLINICAL LAB

Group 1

Subgroup (large cell):

    Bacillus cereus

    Bacillus cereus var *mycoides*

    Bacillus megaterium

    Bacillus anthracis

    Bacillus thuringiensis

Large cell subgroup (cell width >1 μm) that produce central or terminal ellipsoid or cylindrical spores that do not distend the sporangium

Subgroup (small cell):

    Bacillus subtilis

    Bacillus pumilus

    Bacillus licheniformis

Cell width <1 μm, protoplasmic poly-β-hydroxy-butyrate not found Gram-variable, and swollen sporangia, with central or terminal ellipsoid spores

Group 2

    Bacillus circulans

    Bacillus macerans

    Bacillus polymyxa

    Bacillus popillae

    Bacillus larvae

    Bacillus lentimorbus

    Bacillus alvei

    Bacillus stearothermophilus

    Bacillus brevis

Group 3

    Bacillus sphaericus

Heterogeneous gram-variable, sporangia swollen with terminal or subterminal spores

chrophilic members of the genus can grow at temperatures as high as 75°C or as low as 58°C and can flourish at extremes of acidity and alkalinity, ranging from pH 2 to 10. *Bacillus* species, therefore, can be recovered from a wide variety of ecologic niches. Some species may be part of the normal intestinal microbiota of humans and other animals.

DISEASES CAUSED BY *BACILLUS* SPECIES

Anthrax. Although anthrax is rare in the United States, principally because the disease has been controlled in animals, it remains enzootic in certain foreign countries (e.g., Turkey, Iran, Pakistan, and Sudan).[188] The organism has three well-defined cycles: 1) multiplication of spores in the soil; 2) animal infection; and 3) infection in humans.[187] The propensity for *B. anthracis* spores to undergo periodic bursts of local multiplication in the soil, under favorable environmental conditions, increases the chance of infection in grazing animals. A soil pH higher than 6.0, soils rich in organic matter, and changes in the soil microenvironment after periods of rainfall and drought are thought to favor multiplication of spores. Anthrax spores can remain infectious for decades, an important factor to consider in the epidemiology and control of this disease. This property was demonstrated by the well-known biologic warfare experiments conducted on the island of Gruinard, off the western coast of Scotland.[209] An estimated 4×10^{14} spores were exploded over the island; annual tests for more than 20 years demonstrated persistence of fully virulent spores. The infective spores were eliminated in 1987 following disinfection of the area with a mixture of formaldehyde and seawater.

Anthrax is primarily a disease of herbivorous animals and can be transmitted to humans by direct contact with certain animal products, principally wool and hair. Anthrax still poses a threat to the world because of its occurrence in areas where poor health practices remain and the potential of importing materials contaminated with spores from these countries. For example, bones, hides, and other materials from dying animals (infected with anthrax spores) have been ground into fertilizer or used to supplement animal feeds. Thus, spore contamination in these materi-

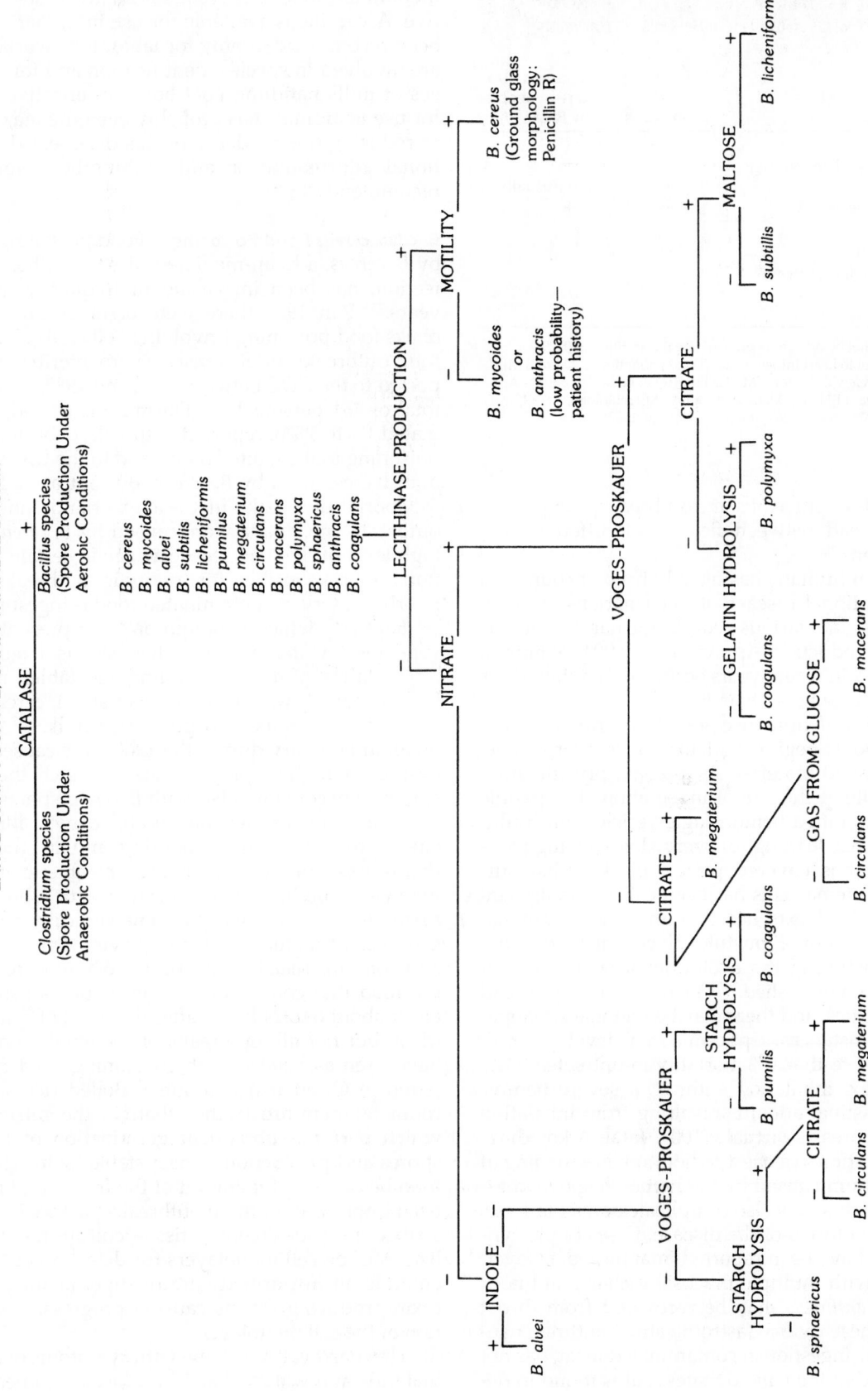

Figure 13-1
Flow chart for identification of *Bacillus* spp.

657

TABLE 13-3
SOME KEY CHARACTERISTICS FOR DISTINGUISHING BETWEEN
BACILLUS ANTHRACIS **AND OTHER SPECIES OF** *BACILLUS*

CHARACTERISTIC	B. ANTHRACIS	B. CEREUS AND OTHER SPECIES OF BACILLUS
Hemolysis (sheep blood agar)	−	+
Motility	−	+ (usually)
Gelatin hydrolysis (7 days)	−	+
Salicin fermentation	−	+
Growth on phenylethyl alcohol blood agar*	−	+

* Phenylethyl alcohol blood agar is prepared by the addition of 0.3% phenylethyl alcohol to heart infusion agar (Difco Laboratories, Detroit, MI). (Modified from Feeley JC, Patton CM: Bacillus. In Lennette EH, Balows A, Hausler WJ Jr, Truant JP [eds]: Manual of Clinical Microbiology, chap 13. Washington DC, American Society for Microbiology, 1980)

als has been the source of some outbreaks, and poses a threat of spread between fields and different geographic regions.[188]

Anthrax in humans has usually been encountered as an occupational disease of veterinarians, agricultural workers, and various people who handle animals and animal products.[336] Approximately 90% of human cases reported in recent years occurred in millworkers handling imported goat hair.[103,336]

About 95% of human cases of anthrax are cutaneous infections, beginning 1 to 5 days after contact with the infected materials as a small, pruritic, nonpainful papule at the site of inoculation. The papule then develops into a hemorrhagic vesicle, which ultimately ruptures, leading to a very slow-healing painless ulcer that is covered with a black eschar surrounded by edema. This has been called a malignant pustule in various texts; however, the lesion is not malignant and is not a pustule. Excellent color photographs illustrating the evolution of cutaneous anthrax have been published.[187] The infection may spread to the lymphatics, and there may be regional adenopathy. In some instances, septicemia may develop.

In contrast to the 20% mortality in untreated cutaneous anthrax, inhalation anthrax, a severe hemorrhagic mediastinal adenitis resulting from inhalation of anthrax spores, is virtually 100% fatal. A key diagnostic observation in a chest radiograph is widening of the mediastinum caused by the hemorrhagic mediastinitis. Meningitis may also complicate both cutaneous and inhalation forms of the disease. Cases of pharyngeal anthrax have been reported, manifested as fever, pharyngitis with multiple mucosal eschars, and neck swelling. *B. anthracis* may be recovered from throat cultures in these cases. Gastrointestinal anthrax, usually caused by ingestion of contaminated meat, has not been reported in the United States, but is found in developing nations. Rapid onset of abdominal pain and hemorrhagic ascites are common manifestations. Gram-positive bacilli may be seen in gram-stained preparations of paracentesis fluid.

Penicillin is usually the drug of choice in the treatment of anthrax; tetracycline is an acceptable alternative. A vaccine is available for use in humans but has been recommended only for laboratory workers who are involved in species identification and for employees of mills handling goat hair. An effective vaccine for use in animals has probably been the major factor in reducing the incidence of this disease.[103] For additional information on anthrax, another reference is recommended.[188]

***Bacillus cereus* Food Poisoning.** Food poisoning caused by *B. cereus*, a toxin-mediated disease, rather than infection, has been increasing in frequency in recent years.[25,327] In 1982 there were eight outbreaks of *B. cereus* food poisoning (involving 200 cases).[47] Twenty-four outbreaks of *B. cereus* gastroenteritis were reported to the CDC between 1982 and 1987, involving a total of 461 persons.[47,48,50] During this period, an estimated 1% to 3% of reported outbreaks of bacterial food poisoning in the United States and in the United Kingdom were caused by *B. cereus*. By contrast, 22% of all foodborne outbreaks in the Netherlands and 7% of outbreaks in Canada were caused by *B. cereus*.[94,184] A high level of *B. cereus* fecal carriage in certain populations is responsible for periodic outbreaks when poorly preserved contaminated food is ingested.

B. cereus, which is ubiquitous and present in soil, vegetation, water, and dust, has been isolated from a large variety of foods, including vegetables, meats (a large outbreak was traced to beef stew), cereals, pasteurized fresh milk, and powdered milk.[25,47] An outbreak in Hungary during the 1960s was caused by ingestion of highly spiced meats in which the added spices were contaminated with *B. cereus* spores.[184]

Two toxins are responsible for clinical illness: an emetic toxin that causes vomiting, and an enterotoxin that is associated with diarrhea. The emetic or vomiting syndrome has been associated with a heat-stable toxin of *B. cereus*. This syndrome clinically resembles staphylococcal food poisoning; symptoms of nausea and vomiting usually develop 1 to 6 hours after ingesting food that contains the toxin. Patients usually recover about 6 to 24 hours after the onset of symptoms. Most, but not all, outbreaks of the emetic syndrome have been associated with consuming fried rice prepared in Oriental restaurants.[47] Boiled rice stored at room temperature (rather than in the refrigerator), which permits subsequent germination of *B. cereus* spores and production of heat-stable toxin within the food before the preparation of the fried rice, has often been implicated in these outbreaks. Jackson[163] has described a rapid-screening tissue culture test that utilizes McCoy cell monolayers for detection of *B. cereus* enterotoxin in purified culture supernatants. Enterotoxin-producing strains cause a progressive destruction of the cell monolayer.

The diarrheal syndrome with symptoms of abdominal pain and watery diarrhea, caused by a heat-labile toxin, clinically resembles *Clostridium perfringens* food poisoning and has an average incubation time of 10 to 12 hours. The flagellar (H) serotypes most commonly involved in the diarrheal syndrome are 1, 2, 6, 8, 10, 12, and 19.[132] Recovery is usually within 12 hours after onset. Implicated foods associated with the diarrheal syndrome have included poultry, cooked meats, mashed potatoes, various soups, and desserts. Because it is nearly impossible to eliminate *B. cereus* spores from foods, the best practice to prevent this type of food poisoning is to properly refrigerate foods to minimize the possibility of toxin production during storage. Because *B. cereus* is part of the normal fecal flora, the isolation of *B. cereus* from a patient's feces is not clinically relevant, and does not implicate *B. cereus* as a cause of gastrointestinal or invasive illness. The diagnosis of *B. cereus* food poisoning can be confirmed by demonstrating 10^5 or more organisms per gram of food that has been implicated epidemiologically. Negative culture results do not necessarily rule out *B. cereus* in fried rice associated with the emetic form of illness, because the quick-heating of the fried rice may have eliminated the organism but not the heat-stable toxin.[47,93] Serotyping of *B. cereus* isolates from food samples, which can be performed in some reference or research laboratories, is beyond the resources of most clinical laboratories, but is required for further confirmation of *B. cereus* in a foodborne outbreak.

Opportunistic Infections Caused by Other *Bacillus* species. Through the years, it has been the practice of many clinical laboratories to simply discard isolates of *Bacillus* species, other than *B. anthracis*, as contaminants (i.e., from skin or air). However, not all isolates are contaminants or harmless saprophytes. Serious opportunistic infections, associated with significant morbidity and mortality, have been caused by a variety of *Bacillus* species. The most frequently encountered species that causes opportunistic *Bacillus* infections is *B. cereus*. The invasive disease is not related to the food-poisoning syndromes described previously. In addition to *B. cereus*, *Bacillus* species, which may be clinically significant occasionally and viewed as potential opportunistic pathogens, include *B. subtilis*, *B. sphaericus*, *B. megaterium*, *B. pumilus*, *B. circulans*, *B. licheniformis*, *B. mycoides*, *B. macerans*, *B. coagulans*, and *B. thuringiensis*.[21,102,250,297,317,333,336]

Drobniewski has defined six broad groups into which clinical infections caused by *B. cereus* fall:[94] 1) local infections, particularly of burns, traumatic or postsurgical wounds, and the eye; 2) bacteremia and septicemia; 3) central nervous system, including meningitis, brain abscesses, and shunt-associated infections; 4) respiratory infections; 5) endocarditis and pericarditis; and 6) food poisoning, including emetic and diarrheal syndromes.

Local infections most commonly complicate postsurgical or traumatic wounds, burns, and the eye. Pathogenicity should be considered when large numbers of gram-positive bacilli are seen microscopically, particularly when present in surgical biopsy specimens. Khavari and coworkers[179] found the periodic acid–Schiff stain particularly useful in the detection of *B. cereus* cells in cutaneous biopsy specimens. Cutaneous infections have also been reported, from orthopedic departments, caused by the application of plaster of Paris casts or gauze rolls that were contaminated

with *B. cereus* spores.[278] Skin abrasions caused by road contact related to motor vehicle accidents, particularly involving motorcycles, commonly lead to infections with various *Bacillus* species.[362] Keratitis, endophthalmitis, and panophthalmitis are the eye infections most commonly associated with *B. cereus*, the incidence of which has increased in recent years, particularly among immunocompromised patients and intravenous drug abusers.[87,94]

Most *B. cereus* septicemias and bacteremias have occurred in intravenous drug users and in patients receiving hemodialysis or continuous intravenous infusions.[258,354] The majority of bacteremias are transient and clinically insignificant. Cases of *B. cereus* endocarditis are rare and are usually associated with intravenous drug use or with an underlying valvular disease.[114,313] Antimicrobial therapy is usually effective, although in some instances valve replacement may be necessary. Central nervous system infections most commonly occur in association with conditions that reduce immunity or that provide direct access (shunts, spinal anesthesia), particularly in neonates and pediatric patients.[353] Brain abscesses have been reported, but are rare.[164] Most cases have occurred secondary to infections elsewhere. Bert and associates[28] report a recent case of brain abscess caused by *B. macerans* following penetration of the periorbital tissue with a wooden stick that became lodged as a foreign body in the underlying brain. Pulmonary infections also are rare, but can be severe and potentially life-threatening. Pneumonia, lung abscess, and pleuritis have most commonly been reported.[21] In a recent review article, Drobniewski[94] has tabulated, referenced, and given clinical details of over 30 case reports of systemic *B. cereus* infections.

The types of infections involving other *Bacillus* species have included septicemia, endocarditis, osteomyelitis, myonecrosis simulating clostridial gas gangrene (involving *B. cereus*), necrotizing fasciitis, bronchopneumonia, necrotizing pneumonia, empyema, meningitis, peritonitis, and endophthalmitis. These life-threatening infections have been associated with parenteral drug abuse, various operative procedures, hemodialysis, traumatic wounds, burns, immunosuppression, and other predisposing factors. Granulocytopenic bone marrow transplant and other organ transplant recipients, patients receiving corticosteroids, and patients being treated with various antineoplastic chemotherapeutic agents are examples of patients who appear to have the highest risk.

In practice, decisions concerning the clinical significance of bacillus isolates are often difficult to make, in part because of the wide distribution of bacillus spores in the environment. These spores may survive treatment with common disinfectants, and the spores of many species are resistant to boiling (100°C). Thus, there is the potential for culture results to suggest infection or pseudoinfection because of the survival of spores in ethanol, isopropyl alcohol, or hexachlorophene used to decontaminate skin or other surfaces, and at least one false outbreak, related to pseudoinfection with *Bacillus* species, was traced to spore contamination of fiberoptic bronchoscopy equipment.[134]

In the latter example, it was observed that *Bacillus* species were isolated with higher frequency from bronchial washings (through a bronchoscope) than in the past. However, there was no clinical evidence of infection in the patients, either before or after the procedure. In this instance, the presence of *Bacillus* species had no clinical importance. The spores had remained in the bronchoscopy equipment after routine cleaning. It is not uncommon to find low numbers of *Bacillus* species remaining in respiratory therapy equipment after the equipment has been disassembled and washed with soap and hot water (at pasteurization temperature; 75°C for 10 min). In the cleaning of fiberoptic bronchoscopes and ancillary equipment following use (in a patient), all parts of the instrument should be disassembled completely before being cleaned. The disassembled equipment should be thoroughly cleaned and rinsed with tap water, then soaked in 2% glutaraldehyde (Cidex), followed again by a tap water rinse.[134] It has been reported that thorough soaking of all bacteria-contaminated surfaces for 10 hours is required to achieve sterilization. Glutaraldehyde kills not only vegetative bacterial cells, but is also sporicidal, if there is sufficient contact time. Following this treatment, the equipment should be stored under dry conditions.

Assessing the potential clinical significance of isolates of *Bacillus* species, or of other organisms that may either be contaminants or opportunistic pathogens (including coagulase-negative staphylococci, *Corynebacterium* species, and *Propionibacterium* species), underscores the need for close communication between the microbiologist and the clinician who is taking care of the patient. Some clinical and laboratory clues that may aid in making these determinations include the following: 1) presence of *Bacillus* colonies (of the species that has questionable significance) on the streak lines of agar plate cultures (and not outside the streaks); 2) isolation of the same species from two or more blood culture specimens (collected from different venipuncture sites); 3) repeated isolation of the identical species from other normally sterile sites; 4) presence of morphologic forms, suggestive of the organism that was isolated, along with acute inflammatory cells, in a direct smear of the specimen that was culture positive; and 5) clinical evidence of infection in a compromised patient, such as a parenteral drug-abuser or an immunosuppressed individual, that is not explained by infection with another etiologic agent.[93]

Bacillus species are commonly isolated in mixed culture from superficial skin lesions, wounds, drainage sites, and specimens that may have come in contact with skin and mucous membrane flora. In most instances such as these, it is reasonable for the microbiologist to rule out *B. anthracis* (e.g., presence of β-hemolysis would be inconsistent with *B. anthracis*) and simply identify the isolate to the genus (but not species) level. The significance of *Bacillus* species in mixed cultures is often very difficult to determine. As Doyle and coauthors[93] pointed out, most such isolates probably are contaminants, or are representative of superficial contamination, unless there is evidence to the contrary. The direct gram-stained smear (as indicated in the foregoing item 4 may aid in these kinds of interpretations. Further identification to the species level

when there is evidence of contamination is costly and not usually relevant clinically.

SPECIMEN COLLECTION AND PROCESSING FOR CULTURE

Anthrax. If anthrax is suspected, the state public health laboratory and the Centers for Disease Control and Prevention (CDC; Atlanta GA; telephone 404 639-3311) should be notified immediately. Specimens that may be collected include material from cutaneous lesions and blood, or any other material that may be infected. Laboratory safety is of utmost importance when working with any material thought to contain *B. anthracis*.[93] All specimens and cultures should be processed and examined with great care in a biologic safety cabinet.[93] Every precaution should be taken to avoid the production of aerosols of the infected material. Laboratory personnel should wear protective coats or gowns, masks, and surgical gloves when processing the samples. This safety apparel should be autoclaved before it is reused, or it should be discarded. When the work is finished, all surfaces in the biologic safety cabinet and laboratory workbenches must be decontaminated with 5% hypochlorite or 5% phenol, and all instruments used for processing the specimen must be autoclaved. Persons who work directly with spore suspensions, contaminated animal tissues, or contaminated hair must be properly immunized.[103]

In cutaneous anthrax infections, specimens to collect include swab samples of the serous fluid of vesicles or of material beneath the edge of the black eschar, plus three sets of blood cultures (before administration of antimicrobial agents). With inhalation anthrax, a sputum sample and blood cultures (also three sets) should be obtained. If gastrointestinal anthrax is suspected, gastric aspirates, feces, or food may be cultured, along with blood cultures.

***Bacillus cereus* Food Poisoning.** Epidemiologically implicated food should be collected when *B. cereus* food poisoning is suspected. Because *B. cereus* may be present in stools of healthy individuals, and because a serotyping or other typing system is not readily available to clinical laboratories, the simple isolation and identification of *B. cereus* from stools of ill patients provides insufficient evidence to implicate *B. cereus* in persons suspected of having food poisoning. On the other hand, it may be worthwhile to isolate the organism from feces of ill persons (involved in an outbreak) when the stools of appropriate matched controls (in an epidemiologic investigation) can be shown not to contain the organism. A sufficiently large specimen sample (e.g., 25 to 50 g) to perform all the laboratory studies required should be collected. Refrigeration in a clean, sealed, leak-proof container should be done if storage is required. Shipment to the state health department laboratory or to the CDC (as per their instructions) should be undertaken only after prior notification and discussion of the outbreak situation with authorities at these agencies.

Other *Bacillus* species Infections. No special collection and handling procedures, beyond those recommended in Chapter 2, are required.

ISOLATION AND IDENTIFICATION OF *BACILLUS* SPECIES

Bacillus anthracis. *B. anthracis* cells are large, gram-positive bacilli, measuring 1 to 1.3 µm by 3 to 10 µm, and the individual cells have square or concave ends. Ovoid, subterminal endospores that do not cause any significant swelling of the cells may be observed. The spores appear as unstained areas within the bacterial cells in gram-stained preparations. Free spores with no visible sporangium may also be found. Endospores may be observed in direct smears prepared from animal or human tissue; however, they are best demonstrated after the organisms have grown in artificial media. Capsules, however, do not form in artificial culture media, but are found only in smears prepared from infected tissues.[93]

B. anthracis grows well on ordinary blood agar within 18 to 24 hours at 35°C. Typically the colonies are flat and irregular, 4 to 5 mm in diameter, and have a slightly undulate margin when grown on heart infusion blood agar. The organism is not hemolytic on sheep blood agar, a helpful feature in differentiating *B. anthracis* from α- or β-hemolytic isolates of other *Bacillus* species (see Color Plate 13-1*B*). Under the dissecting microscope, numerous undulated outgrowths consisting of long filamentous chains of bacilli may be seen (so-called Medusa-head appearance). Although characteristic for *B. anthracis*, Medusa-head colonies are not unique to this species, can be found in certain other *Bacillus* species, and are also characteristic of colonies of *Clostridium sporogenes* (see Chap. 14).

The biochemical characteristics that aid in differentiating *B. anthracis* from other species of *Bacillus* are shown in Tables 13-3 and 13-4. In addition, *B. anthracis* can be separated from *B. cereus*, *B. mycoides*, and *B. thuringiensis*, using the API-20E and API-50CH systems plus morphologic appearance and a few additional characteristics.[203] Any *Bacillus* isolate that is not hemolytic on blood agar, that has the morphologic features suggestive of *B. anthracis* in a gram-stained preparation, and has the presumptive identification characteristics in Table 13-3 should be submitted immediately to the state public health laboratory or the CDC for final confirmation.

***Bacillus cereus* and Other *Bacillus* species.** The heat-shock and the ethanol spore selection procedures described for *Clostridium* species (see Chap. 14) provide excellent methods for quantitative recovery of *Bacillus* species from feces and other specimens (including foods) containing mixed populations of microorganisms. Also, spore selection techniques aid in the demonstration of endospore production in culture.[183] Following heat treatment (e.g., 70°C for 10 min) or alcohol treatment (one part sample mixed with one part absolute ethanol for 1 hour at room temperature) of a homogenized clinical specimen,* or food collected in the outbreak of food-

borne illness, plate out 0.1-mL samples of a series of dilutions (e.g., 10^{-1}, 10^{-2}, 10^{-3}, 10^{-4}, and 10^{-5} dilutions in buffered gelatin diluent) onto sheep blood agar (SAP) plates. Also, a series of dilutions of sample that have not been pretreated with heat or ethanol should be plated onto phenylethyl alcohol (PEA) blood agar. Incubate the plates aerobically at 35°C for 18 to 24 hours and count the colonies of suspected *Bacillus* species per gram dry weight of sample. *Bacillus* spore counts higher than $10^5/g$ of feces or of epidemiologically implicated food (compared with lower counts in control samples) would be of potential significance.

Colonies of *B. cereus*, after overnight growth on SAP or PEA plates, are frequently (not always) surrounded by a large zone of β-hemolysis. *B. cereus* colonies are variable in size, depending on growth conditions, but are often about 3 to 8 mm in diameter, raised, irregular, with a grayish to greenish frosted-glass appearance, and undulate margins. The key biochemical characteristics by which *B. cerus* can be suspected are listed in Box 13-2.

Colonies that are larger and have hairy, rhizoid, rootlike outgrowths from the colony margin that spread over the surface of the agar, should suggest *B. mycoides* (formerly *B. cereus* var. *mycoides*), which is a nonmotile species. The colonies of many other *Bacillus* species encountered clinically are also very commonly β-hemolytic, tend to be large with a frosted-glass appearance initially, but may become opaque, and their colors vary.[145,300] Many species have round or irregular, raised, flat colonies with entire to undulate or rhizoid edges. Colonies of *B. licheniformis* are often dry, spreading, and have a lichenlike appearance. Other colonies may be mucoid, resembling *Pseudomonas* species (see Color Plate 13-1*C*); others form smooth colonies that resemble colonies of *Enterobacteriaceae* on blood agar.

Although *B. cereus* does not grow on MacConkey agar, occasional strains of some *Bacillus* species will grow poorly on MacConkey; hence, they may be mistaken for a gram-negative bacillus. Gram stains can aid in differentiation, especially if done after a short incubation period; unfortunately, some *Bacillus* species are gram-variable and thus, may stain gram-negative. A KOH string test (see Chap. 4) may be of further aid in distinguishing isolates of an uncertain Gram reaction. More detailed descriptions of the colonies and growth characteristics of various *Bacillus* species are given elsewhere.[145,300]

Further characteristics for differentiation of *Bacillus* species are given in Tables 13-3 and 13-4. Figure 13-1 is an algorithm that can facilitate the identification of the various *Bacillus* species, using several biochemical characteristics that have been selected from published identification charts. The tests included in the algorithm were selected on the basis of the highest separatory values determined by the number of times each test can distinguish between all possible pair comparisons. Lecithinase activity is the only test included in the algorithm with a low separatory value; however, it is placed at the top because it is *(text continues on page 664)*

---

* For example, to homogenize for the *spore selection procedure*, mince the sample into several 1-mm pieces using sterile scissors, then grind in a mortar and pestle or a Ten-Broeck grinder in an equal volume of buffered gelatin diluent (see Chap. 14), vortex within a biologic safety cabinet, aerobically at 35°C, for 18 to 24 hours, and count the colonies of suspected *Bacillus* species per gram dry weight of sample.

TABLE 13-4
DIFFERENTIAL CHARACTERISTICS OF SELECTED *BACILLUS* SPECIES ENCOUNTERED IN CLINICAL LABORATORIES

Species	Spores* Morphology	Spores* Location	Motility	Rods ≥ 1 μM in Width	Action on Blood Agar	Lecithinase‡‡	Gas From Glucose	Carbohydrate Base Used§	Acid From Glucose	Xylose	Mannitol	Lactose	Sucrose	Maltose	Salicin	Starch Hydrolysis	Growth in Nutrient Broth With 6% NaCl	Urea Agar Christensen	Nitrate Reduction	Indole	TSI Slant/Butt	TSI H₂S-Butt¶	TSI H₂S-Paper	VP†	Gelatin Hydrolysis	Esculin Hydrolysis	Growth at 42°C
*B. anthracis***	O	C, PC	−	+	− or LG	+	−	F	+	−	−	−	+	+	−		−	−	+	−	V/A	−	V	V	+[7]	V	+
B. cereus†† and *B. mycoides*‡‡	O, N	C, PC	+	+	V	+	−	F	+	−	−	−	V	+	+	V	V	V	V	−	V/A	−	V	V	+	V	V
B. megaterium	O, N	C, PC	V	+	V	−	−	F	+	−	+	V	+	V	V	+	V	V	−	−	V/V	−	+	V	+	V	V
B. licheniformis	O, N	C, PC	V	−	B	+	−	F	+	+	+	−	+	+		+	+	V	+	−	V/A	−	V	−	+	+	+
B. subtilis	O, N	C, PC	V	−	V	−	−	F	+	+	+	−	+	V	−	V	+	V	V	−	V/A	−	V	V	V	+	+
B. firmus	O, N	C, ST	+	−	V		−	F	+	−	+	V	+	+	+	V	V	−	V	−	V/V	−	V	V	+	V	+
B. pumilus	O, N	C, PC	+	−	V	−	−	F	+	V	+	−	+	−		−	+	−	−	−	V/V	−	V	−	V	+	+
B. (possible) *macerans*	O, S	ST, T	V	−	−		+	F	+	V	+	+	+	+	+	+	−	V	+	−	A/A	−	V	−		+	V
B. polymyxa	O, S	C, ST, T	+	−	V	−	+	F	+	V	V	+	+	+	+	+	V		+	−	A/A	−	V	+		+	+
B. circulans§§	O, S	ST, T	+	−	V	−	−	F	+	+	+	+	+	+	+	+	V	−	V	−	A/A	−	V	−	−	+	V
B. stearothermophilus	O, S	ST, T	+	V	V	−	−	F	+	+	−	V	+	+		+	−	V	+	−	A/A	−	+	−		+	+
B. laterosporus	O, S¶¶	C, PC	+	−	V	−	−	F	+	−	+	−	−	+			−	−	+	V	Alk/A	−	V	−	+	+	+

662

Species	Spores*	Sporangium			Action on blood agar†													TSI		VP¶		
B. alvei	O,S***	C,ST,T	+	V	−	F	+	+	−	−	+	+	V	+	+	V	+	A/V	V/+	V	+	+
B. (possible) brevis	O,S	C,ST,T	+	−	−	OF	V	−	−	+	−	V	V	−	V	V	−	Alk/Alk	−/V	V	V	+
B. (possible) sphaericus	R,S	ST, T	+	V	V	OF	−	V	V	V	−	−	V	−	V	V	−	Alk/Alk	−/V	−	−	V
B. coagulans	O,N	ST, T	+	−	−	F	+	−	−	−	−	−	+	−	−	+	−	A/A	−/+	+	−	+
B. thuringiensis†††	O,N	C,PC	+	+	B	F	+	(+W)	+	−	+	+	+	−	+	+	−	A/A	−/+	−	−	+
B. lentus	O,N	C,PC	+	+	−	F W	W	+	−	−	W	W	W	W	−	+	−	A/A	−/+	−	+	−

+, 90% or more positive in 1 or 2 days; −, no reaction (90% or more); V, 11%–89% positive; (+), some reactions delayed; W, weak; A, acid reaction in triple sugar iron (TSI) agar; Alk, alkaline reaction in TSI; 7, delayed 3–7 days. Blank spaces indicate that no data are available.

* Spores: O, oval or cylindrical; R, round; S, spores swell cells; N, spores do not appreciably swell cells; C, central; PC, paracentral; T, terminal; ST, subterminal.

† Action on blood agar: −, no beta hemolysis; LG, lavender color beneath area of heavy growth; B, β-hemolysis; V, variable.

‡ Lecithinase reaction determined using egg yolk agar (see Chapter 14).

§ Carbohydrate base used: see details for F, fermentation base media, *and* OF media in Chapter 4 (as described for gram-negative bacilli by R. Weaver, D. Hollis, and colleagues of the CDC Special Bacteriology Laboratory).

¶ VP, Voges-Proskauer medium: see Chapter 3 for details.

** *B. anthracis* key characteristics include no β-hemolysis on sheep blood agar (SAP) susceptible to 10 units penicillin (PCN disk test), lecithinase −, or (occas. +, usually narrow zone). Also, *B. anthracis* can be differentiated from *B. cereus* using the API system. Data from Logan NA, Carman JA, Melling H, Berkeley RCW: Identification of *Bacillus anthracis* by API tests. J Med Microbiol 20:75–78, 1985.

†† *B. cereus* strains often, but not always, are β-hemolytic on SAP and there is often lavender-green coloration under areas of heavy growth; *B. cereus* is resistant to 10 units PCN and produces a wide zone of lecithinase in egg yolk agar.

‡‡ *B. mycoides* differs from *B. cereus* by production of spreading rhizoid colonies by *B. mycoides*. Also, *B. mycoides* is nonmotile.

§§ *B. circulans* colonies may circulate (when viewed through dissecting microscope, one may see active circular movement within the colony).

‖ *B. stearothermophilus* grows at 65°C. For descriptions of additional thermophilic species that grow at 65°C, see 1986 edition of *Bergey's Manual of Systematic Bacteriology*, vol 2.

¶¶ *B. laterosporus* forms an oval spore with a C-shaped or canoe-shaped body attached to the edge of the spore.

*** *B. alvei* forms free spores parallel in rows.

††† *B. thuringiensis* is an insect pathogen; it produces parasporal crystals that are not produced by the other species it resembles, namely *B. cereus*, *B. mycoides*, and *B. anthracis*.

(Data from Hollis DG, Weaver RE: Gram Positive Organisms: A Guide to Identification. Atlanta, Centers for Disease Control, 1981; Gordon RE, Haynes WC, Pang CH-N: The Genus *Bacillus*, U.S. Department of Agriculture Handbook No. 427. Washington DC, U.S. Government Printing Office, 1973; and Sneath PA, Mair NS, Sharpe ME, Holt JG: Bergey's Manual of Systematic Bacteriology, vol 2. Baltimore, Williams & Wilkins, 1986)

a key reaction in the separation of *B. cereus* (positive) from most other *Bacillus* species (negative). Thus, if an unknown isolate has lecithinase activity, *B. cereus* can be presumptively identified, with the observation of colony morphology, hemolytic activity, and motility as confirmatory tests.

Various molecular techniques are also being used in research laboratories for the identification and strain analysis of *Bacillus* species. Recently published examples of these new approaches include the characterization of different strains of *B. thuringiensis* by rRNA gene restriction fragment length polymorphisms,[251] the in situ hybridization of 16S rRNA segments for differentiating various strains of *B. polymyxa* and *B. macerans*,[172] and the use of a specific DNA probe for the identification of *B. licheniformis*.[30] DNA hybridization studies have also been used to characterize several new *Bacillus* species, the clinical significance of which is yet to be determined. Included are *B. brevis*, *B. migulanus*, *B. choshinensis*, *B. parabrevis*, and *B. galactophilus*.[322] Further discussion of the applications of these molecular techniques in the identification of new and old *Bacillus* species is beyond the scope of this text.

SUSCEPTIBILITY OF *BACILLUS* SPECIES TO ANTIMICROBIAL AGENTS

Although there is variation among different species, *Bacillus* species, with the exception of *B. anthracis*, are generally considered resistant to the older penicillins and cephalosporins including the third-generation cephalosporins. β-Lactamase production has been documented in some species, particularly *B. cereus*. Most strains are susceptible to the aminoglycosides, clindamycin, vancomycin, chloramphenicol, and erythromycin.[94] Some authors[21] consider vancomycin to be the drug of choice for serious *Bacillus* infections.

REGULAR, NON–SPORE-FORMING RODS

The major primary headings of this chapter provide a practical guide for separating gram-positive organisms based on similarities of microscopic characteristics. Thus, the cells of organisms discussed under this heading—the genera *Listeria*, *Erysipelothrix*, *Lactobacillus*, and *Kurthia*—tend to be more regular in shape than the cells of bacteria discussed under the following primary heading: Irregular or Coryneform, Non–spore-forming

Rods. Because of overlap and variability in the morphologic characteristics of organisms discussed under each of these primary headings, readers who wish to identify gram-positive rods should be familiar with the differential characteristics of organisms grouped under the primary heading: Nocardioforms and Aerobic Actinomycetes, as well as those covered under the other primary headings.

Three additional genera, *Brochothrix*, *Caryophanon*, and *Renibacterium*, are included with the "Regular, Non-sporing Gram-Positive Rods" in Section 14 of *Bergey's Manual*.[174] These are mentioned briefly because clinical microbiologists who are involved in environmental work (*e.g.*, as part of an epidemiologic investigation) should be aware that these organisms may be encountered in certain environmental specimens. Thus, they might have to be differentiated from *Listeria* or another potential human pathogen in environmental samples. *Brochothrix*, which has been isolated from meat products (similar to *Listeria* and *Kurthia*), is nonpathogenic for humans and not likely to be isolated from clinical specimens. However, in an epidemiologic study of meat products, *Brochothrix*, *Listeria*, and *Kurthia* would likely have to be differentiated from one another. *Brochothrix*, similarly to *Listeria*, is a catalase-positive, facultative anaerobe; however, it is nonmotile at 22°C and is unable to grow at 37°C. *Kurthia* is a strict aerobe, and does not ferment carbohydrates, two features that distinguish it from *Brochothrix* and *Listeria*. *Caryophanon*, which is unique in that it is a multicellular (trichromes produced), gram-positive, peritrichously flagellated, strictly aerobic, catalase-positive rod that is found in cattle feces, has not been reported from clinical specimens of humans. *Renibacterium*, a catalase-positive, strictly aerobic rod, with a temperature optimum for growth of 15° to 18°C (no growth at 37°C), is a pathogen in salmonid fish (*e.g.*, various species of salmon and trout). *Bergey's Manual* is a recommended reference for those who would like to know more about these interesting genera, which contain bacteria that have not been associated with disease in humans.[174]

LISTERIA

The genus *Listeria* contains the following species: *L. monocytogenes*, *L. ivanovii*, *L. seeligeri*, *L. welshimeri*, *L. innocua*, *L. grayi*, and *L. denitrificans*.[289] Only *L. monocytogenes* and *L. ivanovii* (formerly called *L. bulgarica* and *L. monocytogenes* serovar 4) are associated with disease in humans. *L. monocytogenes* is the clinically important species most commonly encountered in clinical laboratories, and its pathogenicity for humans is well established. The isolation of *L. ivanovii* from blood cultures and other clinical materials from humans has been documented rarely, but the clinical significance of *L. ivanovii* remains uncertain.[195] Although *Listeria* species other than *L. monocytogenes* are frequently present in various foods, food plants, decaying vegetation, soil, water, and sewage, their pathogenic potential for humans is far less than that of *L. monocytogenes*; therefore, these other species will not be discussed further.

HABITAT

L. monocytogenes has been isolated from a wide variety of sources, including freshwater, saltwater, sewage, soil, dust, silage, fertilizers, and decaying vegetation; animal feeds, raw foods of animal origin, including fresh and frozen poultry, red meat, and meat products; fish; raw dairy products, including milk, cheese, and ice cream; raw fruits and vegetables; and from feces of both healthy and symptomatic humans as well as other animals. *Listeria* is difficult to isolate from stools; thus, reports that only 1% to 5% of the U.S. population carry the organism in their feces[2] may underestimate its presence within the gastrointestinal flora.[357] The organism has been demonstrated in more than 40 different species of mammals (including cattle and sheep) and 17 species of birds (including both wild and domestic fowl), and has been recovered from flies, ticks, and crustaceans.[129] Soil and decaying vegetable matter, in which it can grow saprophytically, are considered to be the primary habitats of *L. monocytogenes*.[320] Probably because the organism is so ubiquitous, it frequently contaminates foods during production or processing.[249,320,359]

EPIDEMIOLOGIC AND CLINICAL ASPECTS

In spite of its widespread presence in the environment and in many foods, most people are at low risk for developing infections with *L. monocytogenes*. The organism is rarely isolated from clinical specimens in hospital diagnostic microbiology laboratories. Nonetheless, these infections may be severe. Listeriosis occurs both in epidemics of foodborne illness and as sporadic cases.[286-288] The annual incidence of listeriosis in Europe has ranged from 0.1 to 11.3 cases per million population.[239] In the United States, the incidence reported in 1992 was 7.4 cases per million population.[287] This rate translates to an estimated 1850 cases of listeriosis per year.

Approximately one-fourth (23%) to nearly three-fourths (70%) of infections with *L. monocytogenes* result in death.[2,200,287] Significantly, the case–fatality rate of listeriosis is higher than that of other foodborne illnesses.[287] However, the mortality varies considerably with the different clinical syndromes. For example, healthy, pregnant women may have a mild, self-limited, "flulike" illness, or they may have sepsis with more severe manifestations. The highest mortality is generally seen in granulomatosis infantisepticum, and in immunosuppressed patients who have meningitis.

The incubation period of listeriosis averages about 3 to 4 weeks, with a range of 3 to 90 days.[2] Foods implicated as sources of *L. monocytogenes* in infected patients have included coleslaw or cabbage, pasteurized milk, and soft cheeses (including Mexican-style feta cheeses), undercooked chicken, turkey hot dogs, fish and shellfish, mushrooms, sliced meats and block cheeses packaged at store delicatessan counters, and vegetables.[192]

Persons with increased risk for listeriosis include pregnant women and their conceptus, the elderly, and individuals who have immunosuppressive conditions. In one study, about one-third of the patients with listeriosis were pregnant, whereas nearly all of the remaining individuals had at least one underlying medical condition that increased their risk for acquiring listeriosis.[287] Thus, malignancy, receipt of corticosteroids, and HIV infection or AIDS were the most common underlying immunosuppressive conditions associated with listeriosis in nonpregnant patients. Other reports have also documented that the prevalence of listeriosis is higher in persons infected with HIV or with AIDS than in the general population.[101] In patients with listeriosis who have underlying malignancy, various forms of hematologic malignancy (e.g., leukemia, lymphoma, and multiple myeloma) appear more common than solid tumors.[295] Additional underlying conditions or factors predisposing to listeriosis have included heart disease, diabetes mellitus, renal disease, liver disease, continuous dialysis, and organ transplantation (renal or bone marrow). Interestingly, 15% of the patients with listerosis, reviewed by Skogberg, were not pregnant, and had been previously healthy with no documented underlying illness.[295]

Although foodborne transmission of *L. monocytogenes* accounts for most cases of epidemic and sporadic listeriosis, other routes of spread have played a role in some settings. Thus, there have been a few, non–food-associated nosocomial outbreaks of listeriosis, mostly in newborn nurseries.[129,130,320] In most cases of early-onset neonatal listeriosis, the infant is infected in utero, presumably by transplacental infection from the mother who is bacteremic, and likely acquired the infection through a foodborne mode of transmission. On the other hand, ascending infection, presumably involving *Listeria* acquired from the vagina, has been described in neonates with early-onset illness.[129] Late-onset neonatal listeriosis, which involves full-term infants who are born healthy from healthy mothers, presumably is transmitted to the infant from a contaminated birth canal.[129] There have been outbreaks of nosocomial, late-onset listeriosis, associated with delivery room contamination and transmission.[129] One nosocomial outbreak in a nursery was caused by bathing neonates with mineral oil.[288]

L. monocytogenes causes meningoencephalitis in cattle and sheep, and causes stillbirths in a variety of animals. Primary cutaneous listeriosis has been documented among veterinarians who acquired the organism from contact with infected animals.[320] Laboratory workers could acquire listeriosis as a result of direct inoculation. In addition to skin-associated infections, ocular infectons acquired by direct contact have been documented.[10]

Epidemiologic Typing and Subtyping of *L. monocytogenes*. As reviewed elsewhere, various typing methods have been studied for typing and subtyping *L. monocytogenes* for potential use in epidemiologic investigations.[130,320] Based on somatic (O) and flagellar (H) antigens, there are 11 serotypes of *L. monocytogenes*. However, three of them (1/2a, 1/2b, and 4b) cause most of the infections; thus, serotyping is of limited value. Phage typing and multilocus enzyme electrophoresis have been used successfully in several epidemiologic studies. Other promising methods for typing or subtyping strains of *L. monocytogenes* include the characterization of chromosomal DNA by restriction endonuclease analysis or by ribosomal DNA gene restriction patterns (ribotyping), random amplified polymorphic DNA (RAPD) typing, and pulsed-field gel electrophoresis (PFGE). Ribotyping may not have adequate discriminating ability for some strains, and PFGE is not suitable for routine typing applications. RAPD typing appears to be one of the more promising new methods for subtyping *L. monocytogenes*.

Clinical and Pathologic Aspects of Listeriosis. *Bacterium monocytogenes* was first described by Murray and associates[231] in the setting of infections of laboratory rabbits. The organism was associated with peripheral blood monocytes. *L. monocytogenes* is now known to be one of the classic facultative intracellular pathogens, along with species of *Mycobacterium*, *Brucella*, *Legionella*, *Salmonella*, and others, thus having the ability to persist in cells of the monocyte–macrophage system. This same organism, now called *L. monocytogenes*, was later found to cause meningoencephalitis in sheep and cattle (called circling disease in sheep).[133] It has also been recognized as a cause of abortions in ruminants, as well as humans, as a result of infection within the placenta.[9]

During pregnancy, infections have occurred more often in the third trimester. The pregnant patient usually has a transient illness with nonspecific, mild to moderate symptoms, including fever, headache, vomiting (and possibly other gastrointestinal complaints), and may mention that she has back pain. The symptoms and signs are often self-limiting, and the patient may not request treatment. The only diagnostic test is usually a positive blood culture. In other cases, the infection is more severe, with clinical signs of sepsis and meningitis. In some women, the infection may precipitate labor, resulting in a dead fetus or a premature infected fetus (e.g., in granulomatosis infantiseptica).[9,329]

Prenatal listeriosis, or granulomatosis infantiseptica, is a distinctive form of illness in the newborn period. The infection almost always involves the placenta and fetal membranes, which should be examined by the pathologist and cultured for *Listeria*. Samples from the reproductive tract of the mother should also be cultured by the clinician. Examination of the placenta usually reveals multiple, well-demarcated, acute abscesses, or so-called macroabscesses (approximately 0.5 to 3 cm in diameter), composed of aggregates of necrotic villi, with neutrophilic exudate within and outside of villi (acute villitis).[329] Grossly, the abscesses are most frequently confused with ischemic infarcts, but microscopic examination reveals that the neutrophilic infiltration is more prominent than that found in infarcts. In chronic lesions, there may be areas of granulation tissue and mononuclear infiltrates, but true epithelioid granulomas are not found.[360]

Most infected infants are severely ill, although some may just appear weak and develop respiratory distress or circulatory insufficiency.[10] Infected infants develop widespread abscesses in many organs, including brain, lungs, liver, spleen, kidneys, bones, skin, and soft tissues.[10] In addition to the placenta, appropriate specimens to be selected for culture may include amniotic fluid, meconium, blood of the infant and the mother, cerebrospinal fluid (CSF) of the infant, the mother's vagina and lochia, the infant's throat and skin lesions, and if conjunctivitis is suspected, exudate from the conjunctival sac.

In older children and adults, septicemia and meningitis are the most common clinical manifestations of listeriosis. However, some patients may have asymptomatic bacteremia. Cerebrospinal fluid findings in *Listeria* meningitis are quite variable.[238,311] In addition to meningitis (or meningoencephalitis) and bloodstream infections, *L. monocytogenes* causes several kinds of focal infections (see Table 13-1).[11,238,294] These include skin infections, endophthalmitis, endocarditis, lymphadenitis, arthritis, osteomyelitis, brain abscess, peritonitis, and cholecystitis. Listerial pneumonitis has been reported, mostly in immunosuppressed patients, but it is not common.[92]

Strains of *L. monocytogenes* vary in their in vitro susceptibility to various antimicrobial agents.[52] Currently, antimicrobial agents recommended for treatment of listeriosis are ampicillin or penicillin G, often in combination with an aminoglycoside (e.g., gentamicin).[10] Patients with listeriosis usually should be treated for at least 3 weeks (with ampicillin plus an aminoglycoside); shorter treatment may result in relapse.[311] For patients who are hypersensitive to penicillin or ampicillin, sulfamethoxazole in combination with trimethoprim is an alternative. Thus, Winslow and Steele successfully treated a 76-year-old man who had peritonitis with sulfamethoxazole–trimethoprim.[361] It appears that cephalosporins, and perhaps chloramphenicol, are ineffective in the treatment of immunosuppressed patients who have listeriosis, despite in vitro susceptibility test results that may suggest that an isolate is susceptible.[54] At present, *L. monocytogenes* can no longer be assumed to be susceptible to tetracycline, minocycline, or trimethoprim.[52] The emergence of strains resistant to trimethoprim raises concerns about the use of sulfamethoxazole–trimethoprim, because this combination may not be synergistic against these organisms. Vancomycin is an alternative for treatment of patients with septicemia[8] or endocarditis.[168] Because vancomycin does not cross the blood–brain barrier, it would not be effective for patients with meningitis if administered intravenously. Based on the results of in vitro susceptibility testing, imipenem is another potential alternative for treating patients who have sepsis.[8]

COLLECTION, TRANSPORT, AND PROCESSING OF SPECIMENS FOR CULTURE

Blood, CSF, amniotic fluid, placenta, genital tract specimens, stool specimens (which are preferred rather than rectal swabs), or other materials for culture are collected, transported, and processed as outlined in Chapter 3. Because *L. monocytogenes* may be difficult to isolate from certain clinical specimens, particularly from tissues removed at surgery or at autopsy, a cold enrichment technique has long been recommended.[148]

This involves mixing contaminated materials with trypticase–soy broth (alternatively, tryptose broth; e.g., at a ratio of one part specimen with nine parts broth) and then the specimen–broth combination is held at a low temperature (4°C) for several days to 2 months and is subcultured onto solid media at frequent intervals until recovery has been accomplished. Sheep blood (trypticase–soy) agar and Columbia base colistin–nalidixic acid agar (CNA) have been used for the solid media in the clinical microbiology laboratory at the Indiana University Medical Center for these subcultures. Other selective enrichment procedures are currently used at the CDC for the isolation of *L. monocytogenes* from foods or from clinical specimens collected from nonsterile sites during outbreak investigations.[320] These include the U.S. Department of Agriculture method and the Netherlands Government Food Inspection Service method.

MICROSCOPIC EXAMINATION OF SMEAR PREPARATIONS

L. monocytogenes is a non–spore-forming, short, gram-positive bacillus with cells varying from 0.4 to 0.5 µm by 1.0 to 2.0 µm. It is somewhat smaller than other species of aerobic gram-positive bacilli. The cells are coccobacillary; on occasion, diplobacilli occurring in short chains may be observed (see Color Plate 13-1D). When examining smears of CSF, it is important for microbiologists to be aware that *L. monocytogenes*, an important cause of bacterial meningitis, although it is a less common cause than *Neisseria meningitidis*, *Streptococcus pneumoniae*, group B streptococcus, and *Haemophilus influenzae*. In gram-stained smears of CSF sediments, the organism may occur intracellularly or extracellularly, at times occurring in pairs, in which event, the organisms can be mistaken for pneumococci. If the gram-stained preparation is overdecolorized, the bacterial cells of *L. monocytogenes* may appear gram-negative and can be confused with *Haemophilus*. In other smear preparations, the organisms may assume the pleomorphic, palisade forms of diphtheroids.

PRIMARY ISOLATION AND CULTURAL CHARACTERISTICS

On sheep blood agar (or CNA plates), incubated at 35°C for 24 hours in ambient air, the growth is generally light. Growth may also be obtained on sheep blood agar plates incubated in 5% to 10% CO_2 or anaerobically. The colonies are small, translucent, and gray, and most strains produce a narrow zone of β-hemolysis that usually does not extend much beyond the margins of the colonies (see Color Plate 13-1E). The hemolysin is the major virulence factor of of *L. monocytogenes*.[320] Two other species of *Listeria*, namely *L. seeligeri* and *L. ivanovii*, are β-hemolytic, and it is important to be able to differentiate them from *L. monocytogenes* (Table 13-5).

L. seeligeri, which is nonpathogenic, produces a narrow zone of hemolysis similar to that of *L. monocytogenes*. *L. ivanovii* produces a much wider zone of hemolysis. On occasion this β-hemolysis may be confused

with that produced by β-hemolytic streptococci (particularly group B streptococci; see Table 13-5), and a Gram stain should always be performed when this type of colony is recovered in cultures of spinal fluid, blood, or vaginal secretions. *L. monocytogenes* is never α-hemolytic and does not form white colonies, characteristics helpful in differentiating it from other species of gram-positive bacilli. Additional characteristics by which *L. monocytogenes* may be identified are listed in Box 13-3.

The results of these reactions are compared with those of other gram-positive bacilli in Table 13-5.

The catalase test is performed by adding 3% H_2O_2 to growth on brain–heart infusion agar. *L. monocytogenes* is catalase-positive, whereas streptococci and lactobacilli are not.

Motility can be determined either in a wet mount or in semisolid motility medium. When examined in wet-mount preparations, the bacterial cells of *L. monocytogenes*, that have been grown in a 6-hour broth culture at 20°C, exhibit a tumbling or head-over-heels motility. The use of a phase-contrast microscope aids in the microscopic examination of these preparations. The motility of *L. monocytogenes* in semisolid agar should be determined at room temperature. An umbrellalike zone of growth 2 to 5 mm below the surface of the medium is characteristic (see Color Plate 13-1G). Motility at 35°C incubation is either absent or extremely sluggish.

It is important to distinguish between *L. monocytogenes* and *Streptococcus agalactiae*, both of which are β-hemolytic, CAMP test–positive, and hydrolyze sodium hippurate. In the CAMP test (done with *Staphylococcus aureus*, as described in Chap. 12), a rectangular, rather than an arrowhead-shaped, zone of accentuated hemolysis is more commonly seen with *L. monocytogenes* (see Color Plate 13-1F). Although the CAMP test can be used to enhance or verify the hemolytic activity of *L. monocytogenes*, the test is most useful in the differentiation between *L. monocytogenes* and the other species of *Listeria*, and is ordinarily not required to differentiate *L. monocytogenes* from *S. agalactiae* (see Chap. 12) or from the other genera discussed in this chapter. *S. agalactiae* is nonmotile, forms cocci in chains, is catalase-negative, and does not hy-

---

BOX 13-3. IDENTIFICATION OF *L. MONOCYTOGENES*

Positive reaction for catalase in almost all strains

Optimal motility at 25°C

Growth at 4°C

Narrow zone of β-hemolysis on blood agar

Fermentation of glucose, trehalose, and salicin

Hydrolysis of esculin

Negative reaction for H_2S

TABLE 13-5
DIFFERENTIATION OF *LISTERIA* AND *ERYSIPELOTHRIX* FROM CERTAIN OTHER ORGANISMS THAT MAY BE SIMILAR MORPHOLOGICALLY

ORGANISM	CELLULAR MORPHOLOGY	STRICT AEROBE	β-HEMOLYSIS	CATALASE	MOTILITY	H₂S/TSI	ESCULIN	FERMENTATION OF			OTHER CHARACTERISTICS
								GLUCOSE	MANNITOL	SALICIN	
Listeria monocytogenes	Short, thin, coccobacillary to diphtheroidal	−	+	+	+ (25°C)	−	+	+	−	+	"Umbrella" growth in stab culture; translucent colonies
Erysipelothrix rhusiopathiae	Same as above, but may form long filaments	−	−	−	−	+	−	+	−	−	"Bottle brush" growth in stab culture
Lactobacillus species	Long, slender to short coccobacilli; chain formation common	−	−	−	−	−	+	+	+ or −	+ or −	"Good growth" on tomato juice agar
Kurthia species	Long, parallel chains of rods (0.8 to 1.2 mm wide × 2 to 4 mm long); old cultures contain coccoid cells formed by fragmentation of rods	+	−	+	+	− (or V)	−	−	−	−	"Bird-feather" growth in stab culture; rhizoid colonies
Corynebacterium species	Medium size, diphtheroidal	V	V	+	−	−	−	+	+	−	Opaque colonies
C. jeikeium (Group JK)	Pleomorphic, short coccobacilli and long bacillary forms	−	−	+	−	−	−	+	−	−	Opaque colonies
Enterococcus species	Long to short chains of cocci; produce rodlike cells under some conditions	−	V	−	−	−	+				Both *L. monocytogenes* and *Enterococcus* species grow in 6.5% NaCl
Group B *Streptococcus*	Long to short chains of cocci; produce rodlike cells under some conditions	−	+	−	−	−	−				Both *L. monocytogenes* and group B streptococci may be CAMP + organisms that may be similar morphologically

+, 90% or more strains positive; V, 11%–89% strains positive; −, 1%–10% strains positive.
Other bacteria that can be confused with those included in this table are *Propionibacterium* and *Actinomyces* species, because some of these organisms grow in 5% to 10% CO₂ or in air. Their identification is discussed in Chapter 13. The identification of obligate aerobes that produce long, branching filaments, such as *Nocardia*, *Streptomyces*, and *Actinomadura* species, is discussed in the last section of this chapter.
(Data from Hollis DG, Weaver RE: Gram-Positive Organisms: A Guide to Identification. Atlanta, Centers for Disease Control, 1981; Keddie RM, Shaw S: *Kurthia*: Genus *Kurthia* Trevisan 1885, 92[AL] Nom. cons. Opin. 13 Jud. Comm. 1954, 152. In Sneath PHA, Mair NS, Sharpe ME, Holt JG [eds]: Bergey's Manual of Systematic Bacteriology, Vol 2, pp 1255–1258. Baltimore, Williams & Wilkins, 1986)

drolyze esculin; thus *S. agalactiae* differs from *L. mono-cytogenes* in each of these characteristics.

ERYSIPELOTHRIX

E. rhusiopathiae is a short, slim, gram-positive rod of major economic importance, principally because it causes septicemia and arthritis in swine, calves, lambs, turkeys, ducks, and other farm animals.[55] Classified with the "Regular, Nonsporing Rods" in the 1986 edition of *Bergey's Manual*,[166] *E. rhusiopathiae* is the only species of this genus that infects humans. *E. tonsillarum*, isolated from the tonsils of swine, other animal sources, and water, is the only other species of the genus.[55] *E. tonsillarum* is distinguished from *E. rhusiopathiae* by fermentation of saccharose, by lack of DNA–DNA homology, by a lack of pathogenicity for either pigs or humans, and by serologic differences,[323] and will not be discussed further. Similar to anthax and listeriosis, infection of humans with *E. rhusiopathiae* is rarely documented and has traditionally been categorized as one of the zoonoses.

HABITAT

E. rhusiopathiae is widely distributed in nature and has been isolated from soil, food, and water, presumably contaminated by infected animals. Various animal hosts have been found for this organism, including cattle, horses, dogs, rodents, poultry, other birds, several species of fish, and shellfish. It has been isolated from the gastrointestinal tracts of healthy swine; domestic pigs are believed to be the major reservoir.[254]

DISEASES

As reviewed by Reboli and Farrar, Loeffler established *E. rhusiopathiae* as the cause of "swine erysipelas" in 1886.[254] It was not known to be pathogenic for humans until in 1909, when Rosenbach reported that *E. rhusiopathiae* had been isolated from skin lesions of a patient. Rosenbach created the term "erysipeloid" to avoid confusion with "human erysipelas," a skin infection caused by *Streptococcus pyogenes*.[255]

Erysipeloid, a form of cellulitis, usually involves the skin of the hands and fingers. It is largely an occupational disease of persons who handle meat, poultry, fish, or crustaceans. *E. rhusiopathiae* is thought to enter the skin through minor abrasions, scratches, or punctures, leading to raised, erythematous areas of inflammation of the hands and fingers. The lesions are painful and tend to spread peripherally while the central areas fade. The organism is able to survive for long periods outside the animal body in the soil and is not killed by salting, smoking, or pickling procedures used for the preservation of meats. In rare instances, severe systemic infection of humans occur with manifestations of septicemia and endocarditis. As reviewed by Reboli and Farrar,[254] there are reports of at least 50 cases of systemic infection involving *E. rhusiopathiae*; 90% of these had endocarditis as a major manifestation. Over one-third of the patients had a history of a skin lesion or a concomitant skin lesion characteristic of erysipeloid, and nearly two-thirds of the patients

had previously normal heart valves before developing *E. rhusiopathiae* endocarditis.[254] Most of the patients who had endocarditis were not known to be immunocompromised; however, approximately one-third had a history of alcohol abuse. Although *E. rhusiopathiae* produces neuraminidase and hyaluronidase, the clinical significance of these enzymes is unclear and not much is known about the pathogenesis of *E. rhusiopathiae* disease.

COLLECTION AND PROCESSING OF CLINICAL SPECIMENS FOR CULTURE

In patients with clinical erysipeloid, it is best to obtain a biopsy through the full thickness of the infected skin at the advancing margin of the lesion. The skin surface should be first cleansed and disinfected with alcohol and povidone–iodine before the biopsy procedure. Blood specimens should be obtained in suspected cases of endocarditis or septicemia.

Selective media are not required for the isolation of the organism from skin or tissue aspirates, provided that the skin surface is properly decontaminated during collection. The organism grows well on routinely used blood agar media. Cutaneous biopsy specimens should be placed in an infusion broth containing 1% glucose and incubated aerobically under 5% to 10% CO_2 at 35°C. The broth is then subcultured to a routine blood agar plate at 24-hour intervals.

IDENTIFICATION OF E. RHUSIOPATHIAE

Both smooth and rough colonies develop on blood agar. The smooth colonies are smaller, measuring 0.5 to 1 mm in diameter, and are convex, circular, and transparent. The larger rough colonies show a matte surface, with a fimbriated edge. Greenish discoloration of the blood medium adjacent to the colonies may be seen after prolonged incubation.

Cells from smooth colonies typically appear as short, slender, straight, or slightly curved gram-positive rods, measuring 0.2 to 0.4 μm by 1.0 to 2.5 μm. There is also a tendency for the cells to form long filaments (4 to 15 μm in length).

E. rhusiopathiae is nonmotile, does not produce catalase, and produces either α-hemolysis or no hemolysis on blood agar, which helps to distinguish it from *Listeria* species. The important biochemical characteristics for the identification of *E. rhusiopathiae* are listed in Table 13-5.

The ability of this organism to produce H_2S in Kligler iron agar (KIA) or triple sugar iron (TSI) agar is a helpful feature for differentiating it from the other gram-positive bacilli (see Color Plate 13-1*H*). The fermentation reactions for *E. rhusiopathiae* should be determined in a fermentation-based medium. In addition, another helpful characteristic in the identification of this organism is the test tube brush pattern of growth exhibited in gelatin stab cultures (see Color Plate 13-1*H*).[351]

The treatment and antimicrobial susceptibility of *E. rhusiopthiae* infection has been reviewed in more detail elsewhere.[143,254,255] Most isolates are highly susceptible to penicillin G (the drug of choice), ampicillin, methicillin or nafcillin, and cephalothin. In a study of ten isolates (nine from swine; one from a human) from Italy, penicillin and imipenem were the most active agents. Other antimicrobial agents with good activity were piperacillin, cefotaxime, ciprofloxacin, pefloxacin, and clindamycin.[143,254,255,340] Most isolates are resistant to vancomycin, teicoplanin, trimethoprim–sulfamethoxazole, and various aminoglycosides; they show variable susceptibility to erythromycin, chloramphenicol, and tetracycline. The resistance to vancomycin and aminoglycosides is of clinical interest and importance because the empirical treatment of systemic infections (e.g., endocarditis and septicemia) involving other gram-positive bacteria frequently involves vancomycin with or without an aminoglycoside. Thus, *E. rhusiopthiae* is an exception to the observation that most species of clinically encountered gram-positive bacteria are susceptible to vancomycin (as discussed in the next section, *Lactobacillus* may also be resistant to vancomycin). This fact underscores the need for prompt identification and susceptibility testing of gram-positive bacteria in the diagnostic laboratory, especially in patients with systemic infections.

LACTOBACILLUS

The genus *Lactobacillus* consists of non–spore-forming, gram-positive bacilli that are classified in the family *Lactobacillaceae*. The genus is defined in part by the metabolic products produced, and most species are homofermentative; that is, they form lactic acid from glucose as the major fermentation product. Heterofermentative species may be encountered that produce about 50% lactic acid and varying amounts of CO_2, acetic acid, and ethanol from glucose.

HABITAT

Lactobacilli are widely distributed in nature and are ubiquitous in humans. They inhabit the mouth, gastrointestinal tract, vagina, and other sites. Several older textbooks have used the term "Doderlein's bacillus" for a variety of human vaginal strains of *Lactobacillus*. Sonnenwirth, as cited in previous editions of this text, pointed out that the Doderlein's bacilli include *L. acidophilus*, *L. casei*, *L. fermenti*, *L. cellobiosus*, and *Leuconostoc mesenteroides*.[182] In most instances, identification of these organisms to the species level is unnecessary because they usually have little clinical significance. However, it is important to differentiate lactobacilli from streptococci, which can show rod-shaped forms on solid media.

DISEASES

Lactobcilli are commonly encountered in the clinical laboratory as an important component of the human indigenous flora, as commensals, or as isolates of little or doubtful significance. They have rarely been implicated in clinically significant bacteremia, pneumonia, endocarditis, meningitis, or in focal or localized infections.[151,253,291,318]

Although vancomycin has been commonly thought of as a drug of choice for treating infections involving gram-positive bacteria, *Lactobacillus* species have shown a high level of resistance to this compound.[135,321] The treatment of choice is currently a penicillin combined with an aminoglycoside (e.g., gentamicin).[151,318] Other antimicrobial agents with good activity against vancomysin-resistant *Lactobacillus* species include imipenem, chloramphenicol, minocycline, and gentamicin.[321]

LABORATORY IDENTIFICATION OF LACTOBACILLI

The lactobacilli are non–spore-forming, rod-shaped bacteria, varying from long and slender forms to short coccobacilli, often producing chains (see Color Plate 13-2C). Pleomorphic forms are at times encountered, with some tendency to form palisades. Most species are nonmotile.

The lactobacilli are generally grown on blood agar and chocolate agar media. Good growth is also obtained on Rogosa's selective tomato juice agar medium (LBS medium, Becton Dickinson Microbiology Systems),[19] which has an acid pH. Additional characteristics for differentiating the lactobacilli from other species of gram-positive bacilli are shown in Table 13-5 and in Chapter 14. The negative catalase reaction, the production of major quantities of lactic acid (as determined by gas–liquid chromatography), and the lack of lateral outgrowth from the stab line in a gelatin tube are among the most helpful differentiating features. The use of enriched thioglycolate broth is helpful to allow differentiation of lactobacilli from streptococci; the latter form chains of cocci.

KURTHIA

K. bessonii has been recovered from blood cultures and excised aortic valve tissue of a patient with endocarditis. As referred to by Pancoast and coworkers, isolates of this species in the past have been from feces, a pilonidal cyst, sputum, and an eye.[242] The pathogenic potential of *K. bessonii* had not been previously recognized. The genus *Kurthia* contains regular, unbranched, relatively large, rod-shaped bacteria with rounded ends, occurring in chains. Older cultures (3 to 7 days) contain coccoid cells formed by fragmentation of the rods. They are motile by peritrichous flagella, non–spore-forming, gram-positive, non–acid-fast, obligately aerobic, catalase-positive, and oxidase-negative, and neither reduce nitrate nor produce acid from carbohydrates (see Table 13-5). Further characteristics are given elsewhere.[176]

IRREGULAR OR CORYNEFORM, NON–SPORE-FORMING BACILLI

In the ninth edition of *Bergey's Manual of Determinative Bacteriology*,[158] a large and diverse collection of genera is discussed under the title "Irregular, Nonsporing Gram-Positive Rods." Included are irregular-shaped or pleomorphic, non–spore-forming, gram-positive rods, most of which are nonmotile. Examples of "aerobes" listed in this group include the following (habitats and pathogenicity indicated in parentheses): *Arthrobacter* (soil); *Aureobacterium* (dairy, sewage, soil, insect sources); *Brevibacterium* (cheese, skin); *Caseobacter* (isolated from cheese); *Clavibacter* (plants, plant pathogens); *Curtobacterium* (plants, soil, oil brine; one species is a plant pathogen); and *Microbacterium* (dairy, sausage, insects). Except for *Brevibacterium*, which may be isolated in the clinical laboratory from the skin as a member of the skin flora and from other body sites,[116] none of the other genera are pathogenic for humans; therefore, they will not be discussed further. Section 20 of *Bergey's Manual*[158] includes the following genera as "... facultatively anaerobic, irregular, nonsporing gram-positive rods":

Actinomyces (oral and other cavities of human and animals; human and animal pathogens)

Agromyces (soil)

Arachnia (transferred to *Propionibacterium*; oral cavity; human pathogen)

Arcanobacterium (humans and animals; human and animal pathogens)

Cellulomonas (soil and rotting vegetation)

Corynebacterium (humans and animals; human and animal pathogens)

Dermabacter (human skin)

Exiguobacterium (potato-processing effluent)

Gardnerella (urogenital tract of humans; nonspecific bacterial vaginosis)

Jonesia (unknown)

Propionibacterium (dairy products, human skin; some species are human pathogens)

Rarobacter (alcoholic beverage factories)

Turicella (human middle ear fluid; otitis media in humans[121])

Rothia (oral cavity; opportunistic pathogen infrequently isolated from human materials)

Of these genera, the genera *Agromyces*, *Cellulomonas*, *Exiguobacterium*, *Jonesia*, and *Rarobacter* will not be discussed further, because they are not pathogenic for humans. *Actinomyces*, *Propionibacterium*, and *Arachnia* (*Arachnia propionica* was moved to the genus *Propionibacterium*) have traditionally been classified with the anerobes; therefore, we have included them in Chapter 14, along with *Bifidobacterium*, *Clostridium*, *Eubacterium*, *Lachnospira*, the obligately anaerobic species of the genus *Lactobacillus*, and *Mobiluncus*.

OBSERVATION OF "CORYNEFORM" OR DIPHTHEROID GRAM-POSITIVE BACILLI IN SMEARS OF CLINICAL SPECIMENS OR IN PRIMARY ISOLATION MEDIA

The diphtheroid bacterial cells are of varying shapes and sizes, ranging from coccoid to definite rod forms. They often stain unevenly with the Gram stain procedure. Chinese figures or picket-fence arrangements of these cells, presumably owing to "snapping" after the cells divide, are frequently observed in smears (see

Color Plate 13-2*E* and *H*). Members of the genera *Bacillus*, *Clostridium*, *Lactobacillus*, and *Mycobacterium* rarely exhibit diphtheroidal morphology.

Some members of the genus *Streptococcus*, not a bacillus, may appear elongated and pleomorphic in some smears, but usually do not form the characteristic picket-fence arrangements of the cells. The following aerobic or facultatively anaerobic organisms may demonstrate the diphtheroid appearance in Gram stains: *Corynebacterium*, *Arcanobacterium* (formerly *Corynebacterium*), *Brevibacterium*, *Rothia*, *Listeria*, *Erysipelothrix*, *Dermabacter*, *Turicella*, *Nocardia*, and the other aerobic actinomycetes. The anaerobes discussed in Chapter 14 that can show this appearance include *Actinomyces*, *Bifidobacterium*, *Eubacterium*, and *Propionibacterium*. Bifid or branching forms may also be seen with some species. Tables 13-6 to 13-7 can aid in differentiating the clinically enountered gram-positive bacilli that have a diphtheroid appearance.

FURTHER DIFFERENTIATION OF NON–SPORE-FORMING GRAM-POSITIVE BACILLI TO THE GENUS LEVEL IN THE CLINICAL LABORATORY

Microbiologists should be aware that *Mycobacterium* species sometimes stain gram-positive in direct smears. The mycobacteria are acid-fast when examined in smears stained with auramine-O, auramine–rhodamine, Ziehl–Neelsen, or modified Kinyoun acid-fast stains (see Chap. 17). Only the non–endospore-forming, facultatively anaerobic, microaerophilic, and aerobic bacteria are discussed in the remainder of this chapter. Those formerly called *Corynebacterium pyogenes* (now *Actinomyces pyogenes*) and *C. haemolyticum* (now called *Arcanobacterim haemolyticum*) are addressed herein.

Differentiating this group of facultatively anaerobic organisms to the genus level can be accomplished by observing several morphologic and biochemical characteristics, which are outlined in Tables 13-5 through 13-7. Also, the determination of metabolic products by gas–liquid chromatography (GLC), quite useful in the identification and classification of the anaerobic bacteria (see Chap. 14), aids in the differentiation of these facultatively anaerobic, gram-positive bacilli. For example, the genera *Lactobacillus*, *Listeria*, and *Rothia* produce large quantities of lactic acid; whereas *Corynebacterium* species are metabolically heterogeneous with respect to various short-chain fatty acids they produce.[256,324] Fortunately, for laboratories that lack the equipment, GLC is not required for differentiation of some of the more common aerobic and facultativeley anaerobic gram-positive rods. However, GLC analysis of cellular fatty acids and high-pressure liquid chromatography (HPLC) analyses for mycolic acids and menaquinones aid reference, referral, and research laboratories in definitive identification of the gram-positive bacilli. The following references are recommended for those who are interested in 1) GLC analysis of cellular fatty acids,[26,27,38,122,171,342] and 2) HPLC analysis of mycolic acids[35,36,88,98,343] and 3) menaquinones.[18,23,66,72,365]

SPECIES	LIPOPHILIC	NITRATE REDUCTION	UREASE	PYRAZINAMIDASE	ALK. PHOS.	ACID FROM GLUCOSE	MALTOSE	SUCROSE
C. accolens	+	+	−	V	−	+	−	−
C. afermentans subsp. afermentans	−	−	−	+	+	−	−	−
C. afermentans subsp. lipophilum	+	−	−	+	+	−	−	−
C. amycolatum†	−	V	V	+	+	+	V	V
C. argentoratense	−	−	−	+	V	+	−	−
C. auris	−	−	−	+	+	−	−	−
C. bovis	+	−	−	V	+	+	−	−
C. cystitidis	−	−	+	+	−	+	−	−
C. diphtheriae	−	V	−	−	−	+	+	−
C. flavescens	−	−	−	−	−	+	−	−
C. glucuronolyticum†	−	V	V	+	V	+	V	+
C. jeikeium	+	−	−	+	+	+	V	−
C. kutscheri	−	+	+	+	−	+	+	+
C. macginleyi	+	+	+	+	+	+	−	+
C. minutissimum†	−	−	−	+	+	+	V	−
C. matruchotii	ND	+	−	+	ND	V	V	V
C. pilosum	+	+	+	+	−	+	−	−
C. propinquum	−	+	−	V	V	−	−	−
C. pseudodiphtheriticum	−	+	+	+	V	−	−	−
C. pseudotuberculosis	−	V	+	−	V	+	+	V
C. renale	−	−	+	+	−	+	V	−
C. seminale†	−	V	V	+	−	+	V	+
C. striatum†	−	+	−	+	+	+	−	+
C. urealyticum	+	−	+	+	V	−	−	−
C. xerosis†	−	+	−	+	+	+	+	+

* Data were compiled from the following references: 60, 117, 118, 260, 261, 263, 264, 290, and 350.
Abbreviations are as follows: +, positive reaction; −, negative reaction; V, variable; and ND, no data. Carbohydrate fermentation tests performed in peptone-meat extract broth fermentation base.
All isolates are catalase positive, nonmotile, and negative for esculin hydrolysis (except *C. kutscheri*, which is esculin positive), negative for xylose (except for *C. cystitidis*, which is xylose positive), and negative for mannitol and lactose.
† *C. amycolatum* produces propionic acid and the majority of strains lack α-glucosidase activity; it thus differs from *C. xerosis*, which is negative for propionate and is positive for α-glucosidase. In addition, *C. minutissimum* and *C. striatum*, which do not produce propionic acid, both decompose tyrosine, whereas *C. amycolatum* is tyrosine negative. *C. amycolatum* can be differentiated from *C. glucuronolyticum* and *C. seminale* by its absence of β-glucuronidase activity (ref #350).

CORYNEBACTERIUM

CLASSIFICATION

In the 1986 edition of *Bergey's Manual of Systematic Bacteriology*, it was noted that the genus *Corynebacterium* included a heterogeneous group of bacteria, and that it was in marked need of revision.[64,158,167] Subsequently, there have been many improvements in the taxonomy, and several of the species have been placed in other genera. For example, the aerobic plant pathogens containing 2,4-diaminobutyric acid in their cell walls were moved to the new genus *Clavibacter*.[158] Through the years, a chemotaxonomic approach provided the basis for a more narrow definition of the genus.[64-67,70-72,158]

The genus *Corynebacterium* now contains gram-positive, straight or slightly curved, thin rods that are tapered or sometimes have club-shaped ends. Endospores are not formed. One species, *C. matruchotii*, forms "whip-handle" shapes of cells. Snapping division results in "V," or "birds in flight" formations, palisades of parallel cells, or "Chinese letter" arrangements of cells. They do not branch, are not acid-fast, and with the exception of *C. aquaticum*, are nonmotile. Metachromatic granules within the cells are common. The genus includes both aerobic and facultatively anaerobic species; most ferment glucose and other carbohydrates, and most are catalase-positive.[64,158]

During the last decade, taxonomists have been redefining the genus *Corynebacterium* to restrict it to contain species that have 1) chemotype IV cell walls that contain *meso*-diaminopimelic acid (*meso*-DAP), arabinose, and galactose; 2) mycolic acids of approximately 22 to 36 carbon atoms in length ("corynomycolic acids"); 3) straight-chain saturated and monounsaturated cellular fatty acids; 4) dihydrogenated menaquinones (i.e., forms of vitamin K found in bacteria) with eight or nine isoprene units; and 5) have a G + C content of approximately 51 to 68 mol%. However, the genus still contains some species that do not meet this definition, and they will proabably be reclassified relatively soon. Results of two recent phylogenetic studies, based on analysis of small-subunit ribosomal DNA sequences in one laboratory,[277] and on 16S rRNA gene sequence analyses in another laboratory,[244] indicate that the genus *Corynebacterium* is closely related to the following medically important genera: *Mycobacterium*, *Nocardia*, and *Rhodococcus*, and a few others of doubtful or no medical relevance. Pascual suggested that if this association of genera were at the rank of a family, it could be designated the family *Mycobacteriaceae*.[244]

The coryneform bacteria include several species that have been reclassified into genera other than *Corynebacterium*. The organism formerly called *C. haemolyticum* is now *Arcanobacterium haemolyticum*.[71] *C. pyogenes* is now *Actinomyces pyogenes*.[67] Organisms formerly classified as *C. equi* are currently in the genus *Rhodococcus* as *R. equi*.[139] The CDC group E coryneform bacilli are considered to be aerotolerant *Bifidobacterium adolescentis*.[154] The former *Bacterionema matruchotii* is now *Corynebacterium matruchotii*.[64] The name "*Corynebacterium minutissimum*," a skin pathogen that causes erythrasma in humans, was revived for this organism.[162] The organisms formerly referred to as CDC group JK are now *Corynbacterium jeikeium*. Since the 4th edition of this book was published there have been several additional nomenclature changes in the coryneform, nonsporing bacilli (see Table 13-1).

HABITAT

The corynebacteria are widely distributed in nature and are commonly found in the soil and water, and reside on the skin and mucous membranes of humans and other animals. Except for *C. diphtheriae*, *Corynebacterium* species are usually considered to be contaminants when recovered in the clinical laboratory. On the other hand, the repeated isolation of *Corynebacterium* species from blood, CSF, and other body fluids that are normally sterile suggests that the organism may be the cause of an infectious process. *C. diphtheriae* infection usually involves the upper respiratory tract, but this species has also been recovered from wounds, the skin of infected persons, and the oropharynx of healthy carriers. This species is not found in animals.

DISEASES

Diphtheria. Diphtheria is an acute, contagious, febrile illness caused by *C. diphtheriae*.[15,207] The disease is characterized by a combination of local inflammation with pseudomembrane formation of the oropharynx and damage to the heart and peripheral nerves caused by the action of a potent exotoxin. In this country, the disease occurs primarily in the south and in the Pacific Northwest, although sporadic cases can occur anywhere in the United States. An association between full immunization of the population and a decrease in the incidence of diphtheria has been noted. The annual incidence of the disease in the United States declined from 200 cases per 100,000 population in 1920 to about 0.001 cases per 100,000 population in 1980 (only 2 cases were reported in the United States in 1994).[51] Recently, there has been an ongoing epidemic of diphtheria in 14 of the 15 countries of the former Soviet Union.[7,51,90] Two cases involved U.S. citizens residing in the former Soviet Union. In 1994, there was no report of importation of diphtheria into the United States related to these outbreaks.[51]

C. diphtheriae is spread primarily by convalescent and healthy carriers by the respiratory route. During infection, *C. diphtheriae* grows in the nasopharynx, or elsewhere in the upper respiratory tract, and elaborates an exotoxin that causes necrosis and superficial inflammation of the mucosa. A grayish pseudomembrane is formed, which is an exudate composed of neutrophils, necrotic epthelial cells, erythrocytes, and numerous bacteria embedded in a meshwork of fibrin. The organisms do not invade the submucosal tissue. The exotoxin produced locally in the throat is absorbed through the mucosa, and is carried in the circulation to distant organs. The major sites of action of the toxin are the heart and peripheral nervous system, although other organs and tissues also may be affected.

(text continues on page 676)

TABLE 13-7
SOME DIFFERENTIAL CHARACTERISTICS OF OTHER CORYNEFORM BACTERIA*

Organism	β-Hemolysis on sheep blood	Catalase	Motility	Nitrate reduction	Urease	Esculin hydrolysis	Glucose	Xylose	Mannitol	Lactose	Sucrose	Maltose	Other Characteristics
Actinomyces bernardiae	−	−	−	−	−	−	+	−	−	−	−	+	
A. naeslundii	−	−	−	V	+	+	+	V	V	+	+	+	CAMP−
A. neuii subsp. neuii	−	+	−	+	−	−	+	+	+	+	+	+	CAMP+
A. neuii subsp. anitratus	−	+	−	−	−	−	+	+	+	+	+	+	CAMP+
A. odontolyticus	−	−	−	+	+	V	+	V	−	V	+	V	Red after 1 wk at 30°C on blood agar; CAMP−
A. pyogenes	+	−	−	−	−	−	+	+	V	+	V	V	CAMP−; gelatin+
A. viscosus	−	+	−	+	V	V	+	V	−	+	+	+	CAMP−
Arcanobacterium haemolyticum	+	−	−	−	−	−	+	−	−	+	V	+	Gelatin−
Aurebacterium liquefaciens	−	+	V	−	−	+	+	−	−	+	+	+	Strong lemon yellow; gelatin+; (oxidative metabolism)
Brevibacterium casei	−	+	−	−	−	−	−	−	−	−	−	−	Tan colonies
B. epidermidis	−	+	−	+	−	−	−	−	−	−	−	−	Brown colonies
B. linens	−	+	−	+	−	−	−	−	−	−	−	−	Yellow or brown
Exiguobacterium aurantiacum (Brevibacterium acetylicum)	V	+	+	+	−	+	+	−	+	−	+	+	Dirty yellow/brown colonies
Dermabacter hominis	−	+	−	−	−	+	+	+	−	+	+	+	Yellow colonies
Mycobacterium fortuitum	−	+	−	V	V	V	+	−	V	−	−	−	Acid-fast

Organism											Comments
Oerskovia turbata	−	+	+	V	+	+	+	+	+	+	Yellow colonies; xanthine hydrolysis−
O. xanthineolytica	−	+	+	+	V	+	+	+	+	+	Yellow colonies; xanthine+
Rhodococcus equi	−	−	V	V	V	+	V	−	+	V	Pink colonies; CAMP+; partially acid fast (mod. Kinyoun stain)
Rothia dentocariosa	−	+	+	+	−	+	−	+	−	+	Normal inhabitant of human oral cavity; acetate and lactate are its major short-chain fatty acids
Turicella otitidis	−	−	−	−	−	−	−	−	−	−	CAMP+
CDC coryneform Group E	−	−	+	−	−	+	V	−	+	+	
(aerotolerant *Bifidobacterium adolescentis?*)	−	−	+	−	−	−	−	−	+		
CDC coryneform Group G-2	−	−	+	−	−	+	−	+	−	V	
"*Corynebacterium aquaticum*"	−	+	+	−	+	+	V	V	+	−	Yellow colonies; gelatin− (oxidizer)
Cellulomonas spp.	V	+	+	+	+	+	−	V	+	+	Yellow pigmented; includes some clinical strains of CDC coryneform groups A-3 (mannitol−) and A-4 (mannitol+)
Microbacterium spp.	−	−	V	+	+	+	+	V	+	+	Yellow or orange colonies; strains able to ferment all 5 carbohydrates resemble CDC coryneform group A-4; those unable to ferment xylose resemble CDC coryndrom group A-5; not cellulolytic

* Data were compiled from the following references: 60, 117, 199a, 120, 123, 124, 156a, 157 and 182.
Abbreviations are as follows: +, positive reaction; −, negative reaction; V, variable; and ND, no data. Carbohydrate fermentation tests performed in peptone-meat extract broth fermentation base.

Diphtheria carries a 10% to 30% mortality rate, and death results most commonly secondary to congestive heart failure (CHF) and cardiac arrhythmias caused by toxic myocarditis. Obstruction of the airway is a severe complication, especially when the pseudomembrane involves the larynx or trachea.

Diphtheria toxin is produced only by strains of *C. diphtheriae* that have been infected by a specific bacteriophage called β-phage. Nontoxigenic strains of *C. diphtheriae* are commonly isolated from carriers, particularly during a diphtheria outbreak. Such strains may cause pharyngitis, but do not produce the systemic manifestations of diphtheria. Therefore, the laboratory confirmation of diphtheria includes not only recovery of the organism in culture, but animal testing for toxigenic effects. The biochemical criteria for identification of *C. diphtheriae* and other corynebacteria are listed in Table 13-6.

Other conditions that must be differentiated from diphtheria include streptococcal pharyngitis, adenovirus infection, infectious mononucleosis, and Vincent's disease. The physician usually must make a presumptive diagnosis of diphtheria from clinical criteria, and immediately initiate therapy without waiting for laboratory confirmation.

Some strains of *C. ulcerans*, recovered on occasion from the throat of persons with a diphtheria-like disease, can also elaborate diphtheria toxin. Some strains of *C. ulcerans* elaborate a second toxic substance that is not an exotoxin.

SELECTION, COLLECTION, AND TRANSPORT OF CLINICAL SPECIMENS FOR CULTURE

The selection, collection, transport, and processing of specimens for corynebacteria and related bacteria other than *C. diphtheriae* require no unique or special considerations over and above the general approach and procedures given in Chapter 3. When diphtheria is suspected clinically, the swab should be rubbed vigorously over any inflammatory lesion to obtain suitable material for laboratory examination. Nasopharyngeal specimens, not material from the anterior nares, should be submitted for culture in addition to the throat swab. If the swab cannot be transported immediately to the laboratory, the specimen should be inoculated directly on the Loeffler's serum medium or tellurite medium, as described in the following section. If the personnel working in a given laboratory are not experienced in the recovery and identification of *C. diphtheriae*, the specimens should be sent to a reference laboratory, such as a state health department laboratory. Such specimens should be shipped dry in packets or tubes containing a desiccant, such as silica gel.[60,78]

PROCESSING OF THROAT AND NASOPHARYNGEAL SPECIMENS WHEN DIPHTHERIA IS SUSPECTED

Figure 13-2 is an overview of one approach that can be used in the processing of clinical specimens in which the presence of *C. diphtheriae* is suspected. The laboratory may be asked to process specimens for *C. diphtheriae* from acutely ill patients, from patients who are recovering from diphtheria, from healthy carriers, or rarely, from patients with suspected skin or wound diphtheria.

Smears should be prepared from the clinical specimen, one stained by the Gram method and the other with Loeffler's methylene blue stain (Albert's stain). Loeffler's methylene blue stain is described in Chart 43. Direct examination of smears is valuable because early presumptive information may aid the clinician long before organisms have grown in culture.

The direct Gram stain of a smear prepared from a throat swab in a suspected case of diphtheria is valuable in differentiating Vincent's disease (acute necrotizing ulcerative gingivostomatitis), a condition that may clinically resemble diphtheria, from true diphtheria.[105] The presence of large numbers of fusiform gram-negative bacteria and spirochetes and the absence of diphtheroidal gram-positive bacilli suggest Vincent's disease. However, it may be difficult to see these faint-staining anaerobic bacteria with the usual Gram procedure; an acridine orange, Giemsa stain, or a darkfield examination (performed on a wet mount) may aid in interpretation of the direct microscopic examination.

Traditionally, the bacterial cells of the corynebacteria can best be visualized in the direct smear stained with Loeffler methylene blue. The characteristic V, L, and Y arrangements of the cells may be seen, but most importantly, one should search for the typical deep-blue-staining metachromatic granules of corynebacteria. Unfortunately, the morphologic characteristics of *C. diphtheriae* in the methylene blue smear preparation are not distinctive from other corynebacteria that constitute the commensal flora of the throat and nasopharynx. Therefore, the results of direct microscopic examination can be reported only as "gram-positive pleomorphic bacilli present, morphologically resembling *C. diphtheriae*," and the physician must determine whether this finding is clinically relevant. In most instances, additional cultural, biochemical, and toxigenicity studies must be performed before a definitive diagnosis can be made.

SELECTION AND USE OF PRIMARY ISOLATION MEDIA: CULTURAL CHARACTERISTICS OF *C. DIPHTHERIAE*

Primary recovery of *C. diphtheriae* from clinical specimens requires the use of selective and nonselective culture media. As illustrated in Figure 13-2, the recommended media include a blood agar plate (the medium employed for the routine cultivation of β-hemolytic streptococci is adequate.); a slant of Loeffler serum medium; medium containing potassium tellurite (Tinsdale agar or cystine–tellurite blood agar).

Blood Agar Plate. All throat and nasopharyngeal specimens should be inoculated to blood agar when diphtheria is clinically suspected. It is important that these specimens be examined for the presence of group A β-hemolytic streptococci because the patient may have streptococcal pharyngitis or a mixed strepto-

Swab Specimen (Throat or Nasopharynx)

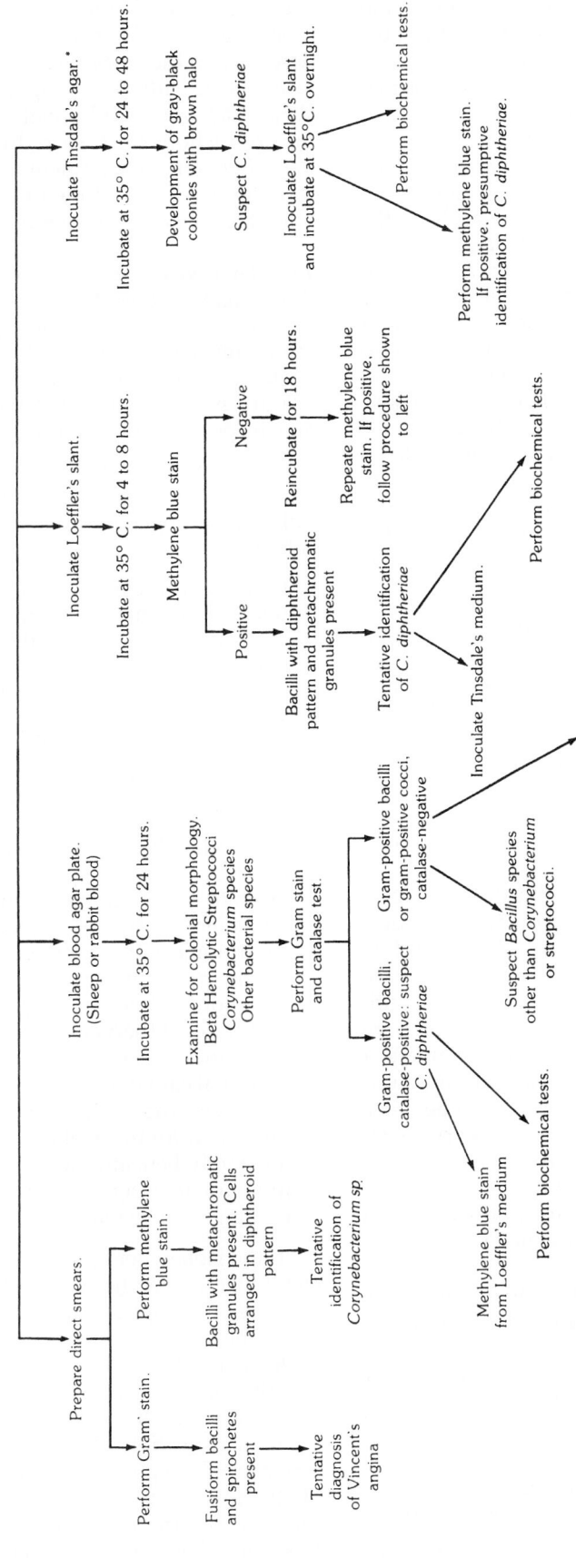

*Use within 3 days of preparation.

Figure 13-2
Schema for specimen processing in the laboratory diagnosis of diphtheria.

coccal–diphtherial infection. Some strains of *C. diphtheriae* are hemolytic; however, differences in Gram stain morphology readily distinguish these species from the hemolytic streptococci. Blood agar also serves as a valuable backup to recover strains of *C. diphtheriae* that do not grow on tellurite-containing media.

Loeffler Serum Medium. Loeffler serum medium may be used both for the direct recovery of species of *Corynebacterium* from clinical specimens and for the subculture of colonies suggestive of *C. diphtheriae* to tellurite media. Growth on Loeffler medium is used to enhance the granule formation as seen in methylene blue stains to demonstrate the characteristic cellular morphology of *C. diphtheriae*. However, in contrast to the Tinsdale medium, the colonies on Loeffler medium show no characteristic differential features to distinguish the corynebacteria from other aerobic gram-positive bacilli. Consequently, primary colonies isolated on Loeffler medium are usually transferred to tellurite medium or subjected to other biochemical tests or toxigenicity studies for definitive identification of the organism. The preparation and use of Loeffler medium is reviewed in Chart 44.[19]

Potassium Tellurite Medium. A medium containing potassium tellurite should be used for the primary recovery of *C. diphtheriae* from clinical materials in cases in whom the diagnosis of diphtheria is clinically suspected. Potassium tellurite inhibits the growth of most of the normal flora of the upper respiratory tract, allowing *C. diphtheriae* and other saprophytic corynebacteria to grow. All corynebacteria produce grayish-black colonies on tellurite medium after 24 to 48 hours of incubation at 35°C.

Tinsdale medium and cystine–tellurite (CT) blood agar are the two tellurite-containing media most commonly used in clinical laboratories.[115,126] If possible, both should be used. CT medium is simple to prepare and has a long shelf life (1 month), in contrast with Tinsdale medium, which is more difficult to prepare and must be used within 2 or 3 days. If it is impractical to use both media, the modified Tinsdale medium should be selected because *C. diphtheriae* can be more readily differentiated from the saprophytic corynebacteria on the basis of a brown halo around the black *C. diphtheriae* colonies (see Color Plates 13-2*F*). The preparation and use of Tinsdale medium is presented in Chart 69, and the preparation and use of CT blood agar is presented in Chart 15.

If an organism is suspected of being *C. diphtheriae* or *C. ulcerans*, based on characteristic colony morphology on tellurite medium, or the cellular morphology observed in methylene blue-stained smears, a series of biochemical tests must be performed to confirm the tentative identification.

BIOCHEMICAL CHARACTERISTICS OF THE *CORYNEBACTERIUM* SPECIES AND RELATED BACTERIA

The media and methods recommended for the biochemical characterization of the clinically important species of *Corynebacterium* and related bacteria have been described by others (see Table 13-6). The colonial morphology of *C. diphtheriae* on Tinsdale medium, as described in the foregoing, is the most important characteristic in differentiating it from other species of *Corynebacterium*. Additional characteristics, including the production of urease, reduction of nitrate, liquefaction of gelatin, and fermentation reactions for various carbohydrates, as outlined in Table 13-6, aid in identifying the species of the genus *Corynebacterium*.

Tests for Toxigenicity. Nontoxigenic strains of *C. diphtheriae* may be carried in a person's throat or nasopharynx; therefore, for epidemiologic and clinical reasons, the definitive laboratory identification of pathogenic strains must include tests for toxigenicity. In vivo and in vitro methods are available, and one or the other may be performed as follows:

IN VIVO TOXIGENICITY TEST FOR *C. DIPHTHERIAE* (FRASER AND WELD).[110] The in vivo toxin test for identification of pathogenic strains of *C. diphtheriae* is outlined below.

1. From a pure culture of an isolate grown on Loeffler's serum medium, inoculate a 10-mL tube of brain–heart infusion broth (pH 7.8 to 8.0), and incubate at 35°C for 48 hours.
2. Clip the hair close from the back and sides of a white rabbit or light-skinned guinea pig. After the hair is removed, mark the skin off into 2-cm^2 areas with a marking pencil.
3. A syringe graduated to 0.1 mL and fitted with an 0.5-in., 24-gauge needle is filled with 1 to 2 mL of the broth culture to be tested.
4. Inject the rabbit or guinea pig with 0.2 mL of each broth to be tested intracutaneously. The square immediately below each injection site will be used for control injections. Refrigerate the syringes containing the remaining portions of broth suspensions
5. Five hours after the test injections, administer 500 units of diphtheria antitoxin, intraperitoneally, into the guinea pig, if a guinea pig was used, or into the marginal ear vein, if a rabbit was used. Wait 30 minutes. With the refrigerated syringe, inject 0.2 mL of broth culture intracutaneously into the square immediately beneath the corresponding test site. Preliminary readings can be made in 24 hours; final readings can be made at 48 hours.

If the isolate being tested is a toxigenic strain of *C. diphtheriae*, a necrotic area, usually about 5 to 10 mm in diameter, will appear at the site of the first injection, while the corresponding control site will show only a pinkish nodule without evidence of necrosis. Any culture that does not elicit the response does not contain a toxigenic strain of *C. diphtheriae*.

A modification of the in vivo test has been described.[356] Two guinea pigs are used for this test. One of the animals is injected intraperitoneally with 250 units of diphtheria antitoxin. After waiting 2 hours, this animal is injected subcutaneously or intraperitoneally with 4 mL of the broth culture containing the test organism. The second guinea pig is injected directly with 4 mL of the broth culture without prior administration of the diphtheria antitoxin.

If the isolate is a toxigenic strain of *C. diphtheriae*, the unprotected guinea pig will die within 24 to 96 hours, whereas the animal that has received the antitoxin will remain healthy. If both animals die, the organism is probably not *C. diphtheriae*. If neither animal dies, the organism is most likely a nontoxigenic strain of *C. diphtheriae* or one of the nonpathogenic (or strictly opportunistic) species of *Corynebacterium*.

MODIFIED ELEK IN VITRO TOXIGENICITY TEST FOR *C. DIPHTHERIAE*. Add 2 mL of sterile rabbit serum and 1 mL of 0.03% potassium tellurite to 10 mL of KL virulence agar (Difco) that has been warmed to 55°C in a water bath. Pipette 10 mL of medium into a petri dish and rotate 20 times to mix. Before the medium solidifies, place a 1- by 8-cm filter paper strip that has been saturated with diphtheria antitoxin (diluted to contain 100 units/mL of antitoxin) across the center diameter of the plate. This strip should sink through the medium and rest on the bottom of the plate. Sterile forceps can be used to submerge the strip. Allow the medium to solidify and then place the plate in the incubator with the lid ajar to allow the surface moisture to evaporate. Inoculate the plate within 2 hours after drying by streaking a 24-hour culture of a known toxin-producing strain of *C. diphtheriae* at right angles to the antitoxin strip. Similarly streak a negative control strain. Streak the unknown cultures to be tested parallel to the streaks of the control cultures. Incubate the plate for 24 to 48 hours at 35°C. Examine for white lines of precipitation that extend out from the line of bacterial growth, forming an angle of about 45°. These white precipitin lines form where the toxin from pathogenic strains of *C. diphtheriae* combines with the antitoxin from the paper strip, thereby identifying the strains of *C. diphtheriae* that produce the toxin.

OTHER *CORYNEBACTERIUM* SPECIES AND RELATED BACTERIA

Coryneform bacteria, other than *C. diphtheriae*, are frequently isolated from a variety of clinical specimens. They should be identified (see Tables 13-5 to 13-7) to the genus level and, if clinically relevant, to the species level when isolated in pure culture; when isolated from blood, CSF, and other usually sterile body fluids; when isolated repeatedly from specimens; when isolated in high number (e.g., more than 10^4 colony forming units [CFU]/mL of urine with no more than one other organism present); or when isolated as the predominant organism from a mixed infection.[60,78] In addition, yellow (possible *Oerskovia* spp.) or salmon-pink (possible *Rhodococcus* spp.) colonies and colonies with hemolysis (possible *Arcanobacterium haemolyticum*, *Actinomyces pyogenes*, or *Listeria monocytogenes*) should be picked for identification. If Tables 13-6 and 13-7 are used, biochemical tests should be performed using enteric fermentation base containing Andrade or brom-

cresol purple indicator.[185] The addition of 1 to 2 drops of sterile rabbit serum to the biochemical test media is necessary for several species (e.g., *C. jeikeium*, "*C. bovis*," "*C. pseudogenitalium*," *C. genitalium*, *C. matruchotii*, CDC groups E, F, G, and 2 [*Actinomyces bernardiae*], and *Actinomyces pyogenes*).[185]

Commercial packaged kit systems have been described for characterization of some of the medically important *Corynebacterium* species. These include the Rapid Identification Method (RIM; Austin Biological Laboratories, Inc., Austin TX), the Minitek System (Becton Dickinson Microbiology Systems, Cockeysville MD),[147,177,296] and the API Rapid Coryne Strip (bioMerieux-Vitek, Inc., Hazelwood MO).

In recent evaluations of the Rapid Coryne, the system was simple to use and showed promise, although only 65.8% of the strains tested by Freney and coworkers were identified;[113] thus, additional supplemental tests were required for identification of approximately 32% of the isolates. In contrast, Gavin and colleagues[128] found that all but 4% of the isolates they tested could be identified with the Rapid Coryne strips without supplemental testing. As these authors pointed out, differences in the protocols used in the two laboratories provide possible explanations for these differences in results. These authors emphasize that in their evaluation, the manufacturer's directions in the package insert were closely followed related to not incubating the strips for more than 24 hours, wheras Freney and coworkers reincubated the Rapid Coryne strips for an additional 24 hours when growth on the check plates was insufficient.[113] Another point that may be significant is that Gavin's group used Columbia agar medium to prepare the inoculum, again as recommended by the manufacturer, wheras Freney's used trypticase–soy agar supplemented with horse blood. It is possible that the strains selected for testing in the two laboratories may also have influenced the different outcomes. This commercial kit is not necessarily more rapid than the conventional approach because a 24- to 48-hour incubation period is required, but it could provide a practical alternative to the traditional biochemical methods now used in large tubes. In our collaborative study at the Denver Veterans Administration Hospital (DVAH) and at Indiana University Medical Center (IUMC), the Rapid Coryne strip identified 86% to 87% of the isolates correctly using inocula prepared from Columbia agar.[31] Significantly, more than 90% of the strains of *C. diphtheriae*, *C. jeikeium*, *C. minutissimum*, and *C. pseudodiphtheriticum*, were identified correctly. In our study, species less likely to be identified correctly included *C. xerosis*, *C. striatum*, *C. aquaticum*, and several of the CDC coryneform group organisms, including those designated CDC group ANF, B, D2, and G1. As recommended in the package insert, Columbia agar was better (87% correct identifications) than trypticase–soy agar (82% correct identifications) for preparation of the inoculum.[31] Thus, if the Rapid Coryne is to be used, results are more likely to be correct if the manufacturer's directions are followed exactly.

CORYNEBACTERIUM JEIKEIUM (FORMERLY CDC GROUP JK)

Other than *C. diphtheriae*, the most clinically important species of *Corynebacterium* to isolate and identify in the clinical laboratory, and also the most commonly encountered species isolated from blood and other normally sterile body fluids (other than urine), is *C. jeikeium*.[358] In 1976, Hande and colleagues reported four cases of life-threatening septicemia in immunocompromised patients caused by a coryneform bacterium that was highly resistant to multiple antibiotics.[155] Subsequently, similar organisms were isolated from blood of oncology patients; caused bacteremia in 32 of 284 marrow transplant patients;[312] were seen in an outbreak setting;[252] and caused septicemia in even an immunocompetent patient.[85] In 1979, Riley and colleagues of the CDC characterized and identified 95 diphtheroid bacteria that had been isolated from a variety of clinical specimens, most of which were from blood, genitourinary specimens, CSF specimens, miscellaneous wounds, and a variety of other sources.[268] They considered these organisms to be unique and designated them group JK. They stated in this report that organisms isolated repeatedly from four cases of diphtheroid bacterial endocarditis, in 1964 by Davis and colleagues, were members of this group.[268] Other reports have since documented that group JK organisms can cause infections in a wide variety of locations including bacterial endocarditis (most commonly involving a prosthetic valve), cavitating or noncavitating pneumonia, CSF shunt infections, osteomyelitis, liver abscesses, peritonitis, skin infections, and surgical wound infections.[29,78,214,215,223,335,338,349,355]

Although it is still rare, there are increasing numbers of reports indicating that corynebacterial species are important causes of life-threatening endocarditis. In a recent review of the literature, Petit and colleagues reported that there have been 126 cases of corynebacterial endocarditis, 53 of which were in patients who had prosthetic valves, and 73 of which were in patients with native valves. The most common *Corynebacterium* species that causes prosthetic valve endocarditis is *C. jeikeium*, followed by *C. pseudodiphtheriticum*, nontoxigenic strains of *Corynebacterium diphtheriae*, *C. xerosis*, and rare case reports involving other coryneform bacteria, including *Arcanobacterium hemolyticum* and *Actinomyces pyogenes*.[247] In native valve corynebacterial endocarditis, *C. diphtheriae* is more common than *C. jeikeium* and *C. pseudodiphtheriticum*.[247] Most of these species are members of the skin or nasopharyngeal flora, and colonization of these sites with the organism before developing the infection probably plays a role in many instances.

Factors that predispose patients to infections with *C. jeikeium* include prolonged hospitalization, prolonged neutropenia, the receipt of multiple antibiotics, and disruption of the skin (e.g., by an indwelling catheter or surgically).[32] Although *C. jeikeium* is not usually found in the skin flora of healthy, nonhospitalized patients, it is commonly encountered in the cutaneous microbiota of those who are hospitalized,[307] particularly those treated with antibiotics.[32] Most patients

with *C. jeikeium* are probably colonized before becoming infected.[32] These bacteria have emerged as a potential cause of serious nosocomial infections in immunocompromised hosts (e.g., patients with hematologic or oncologic disorders who are receiving chemotherapy; bone marrow transplant recipients who have indwelling central venous catheters; and patients with AIDS)[32,78,252,325]; although not all patients are immunocompromised.

Appoximately a fourth of the patients with *C. jeikeium* infections have skin manifestations.[86,170] These are of two types: 1) focal lesions in areas of skin disruption, and less common 2) secondary papular eruptions (skin rashes) scattered over the trunk, extremities, or face in patients who have *C. jeikeium* septicemia. Skin biopsies of the second category of lesions reveal grains of bacteria within the dermis composed of rod-shaped bacteria in an eosinophilic matrix, surrounded by an inflammatory cell infiltrate. These lesions are similar in histologic appearance to those of human botryomycosis (usually caused by *Staphylococcus aureus* and *Pseudomonas aeruginosa*).[170]

In gram-stained smears, *C. jeikeium* isolates are pleomorphic, nonsporulative, gram-positive rods that vary from short coccobacilli to long bacillary forms. They are nonmotile. Colonies are punctate, smooth, and whitish on sheep blood agar after 18 to 24 hours of incubation in a 5% to 10% CO_2 incubator at 30°C. *C. jeikeium* is one of the lipid-requiring species of *Corynebacterium*;[265] it produces turbid growth in brain–heart infusion broth supplemented with 1% Tween 80, in contrast to an absence of visible growth in the unsupplemented medium. A negative test for nitrate reduction, a negative urease test, and acid production from glucose, plus resistance to many antibiotics, are additional key characteristics of this species. Further characteristics are given in Tables 13-5 and 13-6.

A key reason why *C. jeikeium* is so important clinically is its resistance to multiple antibiotics. In most studies, the majority of *C. jeikeium* isolates were reported to be susceptible to vancomycin, but resistant to most antibiotics that are commonly used to treat infections involving gram-positive bacteria.[32] Thus, the results of antibiotic susceptibility testing of a pleomorphic coryneform rod that is susceptible only to vancomycin may be the best clue to its identity.

CORYNEBACTERIUM UREALYTICUM (CDC GROUP D2)

C. urealyticum, formerly CDC group D-2, is also a lipid-requiring, multiantibiotic-resistant microorganism, with a coryneform or diphtheroid morphology. *C. urealyticum* differs from *C. jeikeium* in that *C. urealyticum* is urease-positive and is a well-documented cause of alkaline-encrusted cystitis and other urinary tract infections that are difficult to treat, and have been hospital-acquired in some instances.[1,89,227,241,279,302–304,306,315,344] Similar to *C. jeikeium*, isolates of *C. urealyticum* may be susceptible only to vancomycin or possibly to one of the quinolones. Alkaline-encrusted cystitis is a chronic inflammatory condition in which ammonium magnesium phosphate (AMP) is deposited in a previously damaged bladder wall, resulting in ulceration. The condition is caused by organisms that split urea to form ammonia, which leads to alkalinization of the urine, resulting in the deposition of AMP crystalline crusts in the bladder wall. Factors associated with these infections include concurrent illness (e.g., immunosuppression), urologic procedures, bladder lesions, previous urinary tract infection, previous antibiotic treatment, and older than 65 years of age.[315] In addition, it has also been suggested that the organism may be of etiologic significance in struvite renal stone formation.[273] Although *C. urealyticum* isolates have been most frequently associated with urinary tract infections, other clinical settings have included patients with bacteremia, endocarditis, pneumonia, peritonitis, and osteomyelitis.[78]

Urinary tract infections caused by *Corynebacterium* species are not commonly documented,[201] and could be easily overlooked. Thus, microbiologists should be aware that *C. urealyticum* grows slowly, requiring 48 to 72 hours for colonies to form on agar plates, and thus would be missed if the culture plates are examined after overnight incubation and discarded as negative before a full 48- to 72-hour incubation. A second problem is the coryneform or diphtheroid morphology, which could be interpreted falsely as representing contamination from skin or mucous membrane flora.[273]

C. urealyticum is strongly urease-positive and does not ferment carbohydrates, key characteristics that separate it from *C. jeikeium*. As for *C. jeikeium*, the resistance of these organisms to multiple antimicrobial agents is noteworthy. *C. urealyticum* strains are resistant to most β-lactams, clindamycin, erythromycin, azithromycin, a number of quinolones, gentamicin, and other antimicrobial agents.[125,248,308] As with infections involving *C. jeikeium*, vancomycin is considered the drug of choice for treating infections involving *C. urealyticum*.

CORYNEBACTERIUM XEROSIS–C. STRIATUM GROUP

C. xerosis and *C. striatum* are discussed under the same heading because of taxonomic ambiguity. Organisms now classified as *C. xerosis* and as *C. striatum* are genetically heterogeneous.[76,77] There were six different DNA homology groups among ten strains purchased from the ATCC and the NCTC;[76,77] three strains of *C. xerosis* were indistinguishable from *C. striatum* by cellular fatty acid analyses and DNA hybridization.

C. xerosis (most strains are probably *C. amycolatum*; see footnote to Table 13-6) is a common commensal that colonizes the normal human skin, nasopharynx, and conjunctival sac. It can serve as food for *Acanthamoeba* species (see Chap. 20), and there is a hypothesis that it could play a role in contact lens-associated *Acanthamoeba* keratitis.[14] This organism is a rare cause of human infections that include clinically significant bacteremia,[230] endocarditis,[97] sternal wound infections,[180] mediastinitis,[204] pneumonia,[348] and vertebral osteomyelitis.[186] Most infections are in immunocompromised patients. According to Wallet et al.,[348] *C. xerosis* is usually susceptable to penicillin, cephalosporins, and

vancomycin, but resistance to multiple antibiotics has been reported.[348]

C. striatum was originally isolated from the human nasopharynx, and also from the milk of cows with mastitis;[64] it has been described as a normal inhabitant of the skin and the anterior nares.[78] Organisms called *C. striatum* have been isolated from blood cultured from a patient with AIDS, and another neutropenic patient who was septic.[84,334] In 1994, the first known case of endocarditis attributed to this organism was reported.[275] Other sources of isolates identified as *C. striatum* have included samples from patients with pneumonia,[210] sputum from a patient with chronic obstructive pulmonary disease,[75] a central venous catheter tip, peritoneal fluid, an excised granuloma from a finger, conjunctiva, the uterus, placenta, and urine from a 31-year-old woman with premature rupture of amniotic membranes,[350] and wound exudates, bronchial aspirates, endotracheal tubes, urine samples, and other materials.[211] These organisms have been reported to be susceptible to imipenem, vancomycin, ampicillin, and certain cephalosporins, but resistant to clindamycin, erythromycin, tetracycline, and fosfomycin.[211] In contrast, Martinez-Martinez and associates report that *C. xerosis* is commonly resistant to ampicillin and cephalothin.[211]

In gram-stained smears, both *C. xerosis* and *C. striatum* are pleomorphic, irregular, may produce club forms, and barred rods. On trypticase–soy blood agar, *C. xerosis* may produce yellowish-tan, slightly dry colonies (0.2 to 1 mm in diameter), creamy gray-white colonies (2 mm in diameter), or punctate, translucent gray colonies, and does not produce a halo on Tinsdale agar. Colonies of *C. striatum*, which are similar, differ from those of *C. xerosis* (nonhemolytic); thus, colonies of *C. striatum* may be "slightly hemolytic."[64] *C. xerosis* resembles *C. striatum* biochemically in that all strains of both species produce catalase and ferment glucose and sucrose. Although the CDC scheme for differentiation of coryneform bacilli of Hollis and Weaver[157] indicates *C. xerosis* ferments maltose, whereas *C. striatum* does not, the reactions given in *Bergey's Manual* are in disagreement.[64,77] Our tables in this text are based on the CDC tables and the report of Coyle and associates,[77] not on *Bergey's Manual*.

CORYNEBACTERIUM MINUTISSIMUM

C. minutissimum is thought to be the causative agent of erythrasma, a superficial skin infection characterized by small, brown-red macular areas between the toes, between the fingers, and in the axillae.[32,78] As reviewed elsewhere, there have been a few anecdotal case reports of infections other than erythrasma in humans, including a 42-year-old woman with severe breast abscesses, a case of peritonitis in a patient undergoing peritoneal dialysis, a case of fatal septicemia in an elderly man with myeloid leukemia, three other cases of bacteremia, and a case of endocarditis involving a patient with mitral valve prolapse.[78] Although *C. minutissimum* and *C. xerosis* are similar biochemically, the former does not reduce nitrate; *C. xerosis* does.

CORYNEBACTERIUM ULCERANS

In 1995, as proposed by Riegel and coworkers,[266] the name C. ulcerans was validated when it appeared in List No. 54 of the *International Journal of Systematic Bacteriology*.[202] C. ulcerans is closely related genetically to C. diphtheriae and C. pseudotuberculosis.[244] Before 1995, C. ulcerans was not considered a valid species.[60] C. ulcerans produces mastitis in cattle, and it has been isolated from a few human cases following consumption of raw milk.[245] Human isolates of C. ulcerans have most frequently been from the respiratory tract, especially the throat, and human infections have tended to occur in persons exposed to cattle. C. ulcerans infections have presented as a pharyngitis or as a diphtheria-like illness, including pseudomembrane formation, with toxic involvement of the central nervous system or heart similar to diphtheria.[245] C. ulcerans, which differs from C. diphtheriae by a negative test for nitrate reduction and production of urease activity, is otherwise similar to C. diphtheriae. On Tinsdale agar, C. ulcerans produces brown-black colonies, with halos indistinguishable from those of C. diphtheriae. Some strains have produced diphtheria toxin, presumably because they carried the "β" or a related phage.[245]

CORYNEBACTERIUM PSEUDOTUBERCULOSIS

This microorganism is associated with infections in livestock, including suppurative lymphadenitis, abscesses, and pneumonia.[201] C. pseudotuberculosis is extremely rare in humans; most infections have occurred in individuals who developed a suppurative granulomatous lymphadenitis following contact with animals, their hides, or other products, or after drinking raw milk.[32,159,259] Strains of C. pseudotuberculosis, similar to C. ulcerans, can be lysogenized with bacteriophage and produce diphtheria toxin. However, there are no reports of diphtheria caused by C. pseudotuberculosis. C. pseudotuberculosis and C. ulcerans produce phospholipase D, which can be detected by inhibition of the CAMP phenomenon or with the reverse CAMP test.[17,18]

CORYNEBACTERIUM PSEUDODIPHTHERITICUM

This organism, which does very little in biochemical tests, is best known as a cause of endocarditis, and is commonly encountered in the normal flora of the human nasopharynx. Although corynebacterial endocarditis is rare, C. pseudodiphtheriticum is second only to C. jeikeium as a cause of corynebacterial endocarditis.[37,199,228] It has also been reported to be an uncommon cause of respiratory infections. Recently, the clinical and microbiologic features of several patients with lower respiratory tract infections (including necrotizing tracheitis, tracheobronchitis or bronchitis, or pneumonia) involving C. pseudodiphtheriticum were reported.[4,32,78] Preexisting chronic pulmonary disease, congestive heart failure, diabetes mellitus, or malignancy were the most common underlying conditions associated with these infections. In addition to bronchitis and pneumonia, a case of lung abscess in a patient with AIDS-related complex, a case involving a urinary tract infection in a patient with a transplanted kidney, suppurative lymphadenopathy, septic arthritis, and vertebral osteomyelitis have involved C. pseudodiphtheriticum. This species does not produce acid from carbohydrates; it reduces nitrate and hydrolyzes urea. Strain variation in susceptibility to antimicrobial agents is sufficiently high that antimicrobial susceptibility testing of isolates is recommended to guide the clinician in selection of antibiotics for treatment of individual patients.[32]

CORYNEBACTERIUM AQUATICUM

C. aquaticum was first isolated from distilled water by Liefson in 1962, and presumably can be found in freshwater.[201] There are a few reports of this organism as a cause of human disease. These include a case of meningitis in a neonate, a urinary tract infection in another neonate, two cases of peritonitis in patients receiving continuous ambulatory peritoneal dialysis, and bacteremia in two patients.[20,106,175,225,326] C. aquaticum is the only species of Corynebacterium that is motile. It is esculin-positive, but nonhemolytic and should be differentiated from Listeria monocytogenes, which is also esculin-positive, but is hemolytic. C. aquaticum is a strict aerobe and produces acid from mannitol; L. monocytogenes is microaerophilic and does not produce acid from mannitol.

MISCELLANEOUS CORYNEBACTERIUM SPECIES AND CDC CORYNEBACTERIUM GROUP ORGANISMS

For many years, Hollis and Weaver, of the Special Bacteriology Section, Centers for Disease Control, received, characterized, and painstakingly catalogued the phenotypic characteristics of gram-positive, coryneform or "Corynebacterium"-like rods in several groups of related strains.[157,185] Accordingly, these include organisms designated as "CDC group A-3, A-4, A-5, ANF-1, ANF-3, B-1, B-3, D-2, E, F-1, F-2, G-1, G-2, I-1, I-2, J-K, and group 1 and group 2." In recent years, the data they so painstakingly collected and compiled,[157,185] and the reference strains in their collection, have been providing a valuable foundation for major improvements in the classification of the irregular coryneform nonsporulative rods. Thus, these microbiologists, who are now retired, deserve much credit for their many outstanding contributions to this current exploding field of taxonomic change.

C. afermentans subsp. afermentans and C. afermentans subsp. lipophilum (CDC Corynebacterium Group ANF-1) is a new species with two subspecies that was proposed based on rRNA gene restriction patterns and DNA–DNA relatedness studies of strains that previously were in the CDC Coryneform Group ANF-1.[261] Although the type strains of both subspecies were isolated from human blood cultures, their clinical significance is unknown. Subsequently, C. afermentans subsp. lipophilum ("fat loving") was implicated in a human case of prosthetic valve endocarditis.[290] These organisms are catalase-positive, urease-negative, do not reduce nitrate, and do not ferment carbohydrates. Enhanced growth on 1% Tween 80-supplemented sheep blood agar compared with poor or no growth on un-supplemented blood agar was reported to be characteristic of the lipophilic subspecies, whereas the other subspecies grow well on both media.[261]

C. auris is another newly named species that was also derived from CDC *Corynebacterium* ANF-1 like organisms.[118] *C. auris* was proposed on the basis of 16S rRNA gene sequence analysis and on phenotypic characteristics. Although the organisms have been isolated only from children with ear infections, their clinical significance remains unknown. This species resembles *C. afermentans*, but the colonies of *C. auris* differ by being dry, becoming slightly yellowish with time, and having weak adherence to agar. Thus, *C. auris* differs from *C. afermentans* and *Turicella otitidis* colonies, which are creamy and do not adhere to agar.[118]

C. propinquum, formerly called *Corynebacterium* group ANF-3 by Hollis and Weaver of the CDC, has been isolated infrequently from human sources, including sputum, throat, nasopharynx, nose, blood, and miscellaneous other sites.[157,262] Petit and coworkers recently reported a case of native aortic valve endocarditis caused by this organism in a 52-year-old man, along with an in-depth review of corynebacterial endocarditis. *C. propinquum*, which is catalase-positive, nitrate-positive, urease-negative, and does not ferment carbohydrates, is probably most easily confused with *C. pseudodiphtheriticum* that gives similar reactions, except the latter is urease-positive.[247]

C. macginleyi, formerly called CDC *Corynebacterium* group G-1, is a lipophilic species that has been isolated most frequently from human eyes. It has also been isolated from a few blood cultures, a surgically removed heart valve from one patient with bacterial endocarditis, a patient receiving hemodialysis, and miscellaneous other sites.[157] *C. macginleyi* is a nonmotile, pleomorphic, coryneform, non–acid-fast rod that requires lipid for growth (i.e., as can be demonstrated by enhanced growth on trypticase–soy sheep blood agar or brain–heart infusion broth supplemented with 1% Tween 80).[265] In addition, the organism is catalase-positive, nitrate-positive, urea-negative, pyrazinamidase-positive, alkaline phosphatase-positive, and ferments glucose and sucrose but not maltose.

An additional lipophilic group of catalase-positive, urea-negative, fermentative coryneform bacilli, originally characterized by D. G. Hollis, R. E. Weaver, and others of the Special Pathogens Section of the CDC is *Corynebacterium* group G-2.[12,78,358] From 1982 through 1991 at the Clinical Pathology Department microbiology laboratory of the National Institutes of Health, CDC *Corynebacterium* group G-2 was the second most common species identified (after *C. jeikeium*).[358] Most of these isolates were from intravenous catheter sites and blood. An additional isolate has been reported from a patient with prosthetic valve endocarditis.[12] At the CDC, other sources of isolates have included eyes, cerebrospinal fluid, throat, urethra, and miscellaneous other sites.[157] Previously, Hollis and Weaver used nitrate reduction to differentiate between groups G-1 (nitrate-positive) and G-2 (nitrate-negative). However, Riegel and associates reported that both nitrate-positive and nitrate-negative strains are included in G-2, and recommended that they be grouped together simply as "CDC coryneform group G."[265] Thus, according to Reigel and coworkers,[265] group G organisms are pyrazinamidase-positive and maltose-variable, whereas *C. macginleyi* is pyrazinamidase-negative and maltose-negative.

C. argentoratense, isolated exclusively from the human throat, is a new species that was proposed based on analyses of cell wall amino acid and sugar content, mycolic acids, cellular fatty acids, the mole percentage of guanine + cytosine, DNA–DNA hybridization, and on small-subunit rDNA gene sequencing.[263] Although it has been isolated from the throats of patients with tonsillitis, the clinical significance of this new species is unknown. This species is catalase-positive, urease-negative, nitrate-negative, and can be differentiated from other *Corynebacterium* species by its mycolic acid pattern, its fermentation of glucose but not sucrose or maltose, and enzyme reactions obtained with the API-Coryne system.[263]

C. seminale is a new species isolated from genital tract infections of adult male patients.[264] Isolated from semen specimens from infertile men who had been diagnosed as having prostatitis, their clinical significance remains unestablished. Characteristics that aid in differentiating *C. seminale* from other corynebacteria include the following: 1) poor growth on sheep blood agar supplemented with 1% Tween 80, but good growth on sheep blood agar; 2) a positive CAMP (done with *Staphylococcus aureus*), fermentation of glucose and sucrose, and β-glucuronidase activity as determined using Rosco tablets (Rosco: Eurobio, Les Ullis, France).[264]

C. matruchotii, once called *Bacterionema matruchotii*, has been isolated from the human oral cavity,[62] and from human eye infections.[357] The cells are in the form of bacilli and nonseptate and septate filaments that may show rudimentary branching. Interestingly, a filament will be attached to a bacillus; thus, they have a "whip and handle" arrangement.

C. kutscheri is known primarily as a pathogen for mice and rats, but has been isolated from two humans with illness believed to be related to the organism. One was a case of chorioamnionitis and funisitis; the other was a case of infectious arthritis in a 68-year-old woman with polymyalgia rheumatica.[107,157,185,220]

Lipid-Requiring or Lipophilic Corynebacteria.   Aerobic diphtheroids (or irregular coryneform nonsporulative rods) are major components of the human microflora in certain skin sites.[196,213] The growth of some of these bacteria is stimulated markedly when lipid (e.g., Tween 80) is added to culture media, thus giving rise to two groups of diphtheroids: the "lipophilic" group and the "nonlipophilic" group.[213] McGinley and colleagues demonstrated that these so-called lipophilic diphtheroids actually required lipid for growth. Thus, Riegel and coworkers refer to the corynebacteria that exhibit a lipid requirement for optimal growth as "lipid requiring," rather than "lipophilic."[260,261,265]

The method, as described by Riegel and coauthors,[263] to assess the lipid requirement of corynebacteria was to compare the growth of the organism in brain–heart infusion (BHI) broth supplemented with

1% (v/v) Tween 80, compared with growth in BHI without the Tween 80. Incubation was for 72 hours at 37°C (aerobic). The lipid-requiring bacteria exhibited good growth in BHI supplemented with the Tween 80, in contrast with the unsupplemented BHI that remained visibly clear (no visible evidence of growth). In addition, lipid-requiring corynebacteria grown aerobically at 37°C on trypticase–soy agar supplemented with 5% (v/v) sheep blood and 1% (v/v) Tween 80, formed large (2- to 4-mm) colonies at 48-hours incubation. In contrast, colonies on the same medium without the Tween 80 were much smaller. Tween 80 (polyoxyethylene sorbitan monooleate) is a detergent that contains a number of different 14- to 18-carbon fatty acids.[78] From the method of Riegel and coworkers,[265] the lipid-requiring *Corynebacterium* species are summarized in Box 13-4.

The taxonomic status of "*C. genitalium*" and "*C. pseudogenitalium*," which have no current standing in nomenclature, requires clarification. Some strains of *C. genitalium* are synonyms of *C. jeikeium*, and some strains of *C. pseudogenitalium* apparently are related to CDC group F-1.[260,265] In addition, the *C. diphtheriae* var. *intermedius* requires lipid for growth.[185]

At the CDC, lipid stimulation of growth is determined in enteric fermentation base medium that has been supplemented by adding 2 drops of rabbit serum to 3 mL of medium.[185] Data are lacking relative to the correlation of results between the CDC method and the Tween 80 method used by Riegel and coworkers (as described in the foregoing).

BOX 13-4. LIPID-REQUIRING CORYNEBACTERIA—POTENTIALLY PATHOGENIC FOR HUMANS

Corynebacterium jeikeium (antibiotic-resistant; the most common species, especially in bacteremia, endocarditis)

Corynebacterium urealyticum (alkaline-encrusted cystitis and other urinary tract infections of humans)

Corynebacterium macginleyi (CDC group G-1; eye infections, blood, miscellaneous human sources)

Corynebacterium afermentans subsp. *lipophilum* (CDC group ANF-1; ear, blood, miscellaneous human sources)

CDC *Corynebacterium* group G (blood, eyes, miscellaneous sources)

CDC *Corynebacterium* group F-1 (urogenital, urine, miscellaneous sources)[305]

Corynebacterium accolens (CDC group 6; eye, blood, other human clinical materials; significance not known; satellite growth near colonies of *Staphylococcus aureus*)[236]

Corynebacterium bovis (cattle; no convincing case of human infection since 1970s)[78, 201]

BOX 13-5. NON–LIPID-REQUIRING CORYNEBACTERIA— PATHOGENIC SIGNIFICANCE FOR HUMANS UNLIKELY

Corynebacterium renale (cattle and goats)[63, 64]

Corynebacterium cystitidis (cows)[64]

Corynebacterium pilosum (cattle)[64]

Corynebacterium mycetoides (1942 report of tropical ulcers in humans, but not documented since that time)[64]

Corynebacterium flavescens (cheese)[64]

Corynebacterium vitarumen (rumen of a cow)[64]

Corynebacterium glutamicum (sewage)[64]

Corynebacterium callunae (isolated from heather)[64]

Corynebacterium amycolatum (1988 description of "new mycolic acid-less" species from human skin; no evidence of involvement in an infected site)[63]

Other *Corynebacterium* species that do not require lipid for growth are unlikely to be encountered as human pathogens. Although at this writing, the following are valid species of *Corynebacterium* with standing in nomenclature, and most are listed in the 9th edition of *Bergey's Manual*,[158] there is no evidence that they are encountered as pathogens in humans (Box 13-5).

MEDICALLY IMPORTANT CORYNEBACTERIA TRANSFERRED TO OTHER GENERA

ARCANOBACTERIUM HAEMOLYTICUM

A. haemolyticum (formerly *C. haemolyticum*),[71] has been isolated mostly from young adults (15 to 25 years old) with symptomatic pharyngitis, fever, occasionally accompanied by a cutaneous rash, sometimes with pseudomembranes on the pharynx and tonsils, and submandibular lymphadenopathy.[41,208] In addition, *A. haemolyticum* has also been isolated from various wound sites, including cutaneous ulcers and cellulitis, patients with septicemia, endocarditis, brain abscesses and abscesses in other sites, and vertebral osteomyelitis.[22,59,91,100,104,109,146,201,208,271,363] It has been difficult to establish the significance of *A. haemolyticum* as a cause of acute pharyngitis because β-hemolytic streptococci have also been found at the same time from many patients,[41] and viruses, which were not sought in some studies, could not be ruled out as causes of the sore throats.[208] The organism produces at least one toxin, a phospholipase D that is similar to that of *C. pseudotuberculosis*, and this could potentially play a role in pathogenesis of infections.[81] *A. haemolyticum* has a pleomorphic coryneform morphology, and at times may be granular or beaded, resembling small streptococci. It is nonmotile and is not acid-fast. The microscopic features are distinctive. Gram-stained smears prepared from colonies after overnight incubation reveal thin, irregular, club-shaped, curved rods with "V" formations, and there may be rudimentary branching.[59] As they age (24 to 48 hours of incubation), the cells no longer appear club-shaped, become granular or beaded, stain unevenly, and resemble short chains of small cocci.[60,64] When grown in some broth media, they are more likely to form regular or elongated rods, and they may have pointed ends. It is important to be aware that *A. haemolyticum*, like the genus *Streptococcus*, is catalase-negative, and the colonies of *A. haemolyticum* might be confused with colonies of β-hemolytic streptococci on blood agar. *A. haemolyticum* grows more slowly and produces less distinctive hemolysis than β-hemolytic streptococci. After 18 to 24 hours of incubation on trypticase–soy agar with sheep blood, colonies are approximately 0.1 to 0.4 mm in diameters, with a narrow zone of hemolysis, which may be difficult to see.[59,185] Cummings and associates found that a minimum of 48 hours of incubation was needed to be able to see β-hemolysis and pitting;[82] thus, colonies are about 0.5 mm in diameter at 48 hours with small zones of β-hemolysis (about 0.8 mm).[82] It is said that dark pits can be seen in the agar after colonies are scraped away.[82] *A. haemolyticum* differs from most other coryneform bacteria by being both catalase-negative and hemolytic, characteristics it shares with *Actinomyces pyogenes*. Differentiation between *A. haemolyticum* and *Actinomyces pyogenes* can be accomplished using the Rapid Coryne system,[128] or using a 4-hour α-mannosidase test (Rosco Diagnostica, Taastrup, Denmark).[39] *A. haemolyticum* and *Listeria monocytogenes* are α-mannosidase-positive, whereas *A. pyogenes*, *Corynebacterium* species, *Rhodococcus equi*, and *Erysipelothrix rhusiopathiae* are negative. For further details on differentiation, see Table 13-7 and additional references.[59,60,82,157,185] The antimicrobial susceptibility of *A. haemolyticum* appears to be highly predictable; in one study, all strains tested were susceptible to phenoxymethylpenicillin, cephalexin, cefuroxime, cefotaxime, erythromycin, azithromycin, clindamycin, vancomycin, and ciprofloxacin, but they all were resistant to trimethoprim–sulfamethoxazole.[40]

ACTINOMYCES PYOGENES

A. pyogenes (formerly *C. pyogenes*), similar to *Arcanobacterium hemolyticum*, is a rare cause of infection in humans. Although the cellular morphology of *A. pyogenes* is similar to that of *A. haemolyticum*, and both are β-hemolytic on sheep blood agar, the colonies of *A. pyogenes* are whitish and larger than those of *A. haemolyticum*, with wider areas of hemolysis around the colonies. According to Krech and Hollis, older (3 to 7 days) colonies of *A. pyogenes* may become "brick red."[185] Both species are catalase-negative and similar biochemically. Gelatin hydrolysis and xylose (*A. pyogenes* is gelatin-positive and xylose-negative; *A. haemolyticum* is gelatin-negative and produces acid from xylose) are the key conventional biochemical tests that aid in differentiating them. The Rapid Coryne system provides a simple and reliable alternative to conventional biochemical

testing for identification of *A. pyogenes*,[113,128,197,309] as does the α-mannosidase test[39] mentioned earlier. *A. pyogenes* is a common pathogen in veterinary medicine (causes infections in pigs, cattle, sheep, goats, and other domestic animals). Infection of humans involving *A. pyogenes* is rare and is thought to represent a zoonosis when it occurs.[32] Human infections with *A. pyogenes* have included an annual outbreak of leg ulcers in children in Thailand; skin infections complicated by septicemia, endocarditis, otitis media, mastoiditis, peritonitis, and intra-abdominal abscesses; osteomyelitis, septic arthritis, pneumonia, empyema, cystitis, and ulcerative vulvovaginitis.[32]

Actinomyces neuii subsp. *neuii* and *A. neuii* subsp. *anitratus* (CDC Coryneform Group 1 and 1-like organisms), a recently named species and subspecies, has been isolated from a variety of human clinical materials, including abscesses, a patient with fatal septicemia, eyes, and miscellaneous other sources, but no cases typical of actinomycosis have been described.[234] The cells tend to be diphtheroidal, may be arranged in "V" and "Y" shapes and in clusters, or in the form of coccobacilli, and they are nonmotile and not acid-fast. The cellular fatty acids, cell wall composition, and membrane characteristics of *A. neuii* differ from those of *Corynebacterium* species in that *A. neuii* lacks *meso*-diaminopimelic acid and mycolic acids. Both subspecies of *A. neuii* are catalase-positive (similar to *Actinomyces viscosus*), nonhemolytic on sheep blood agar, urease-negative, esculin hydrolysis-negative, and ferment glucose, maltose, sucrose, mannitol, and xylose. Both, similar to *Arcanobacterium haemolyticum*, give a positive reverse CAMP reaction.[119] According to Funke and associates,[123] *A. neuii* subsp. *neuii* is nitrate-positive, whereas *A. neuii* subsp. *anitratus* is nitrate-negative.

Actinomyces bernardiae (CDC Coryneform Group 2), a newly named species for bacteria previously belonging to CDC group 2, forms irregular, nonmotile, coryneform rods with a predominance of coccobacilli, sometimes in clusters, and without branching.[120] It can be differentiated from other species based on fermentation of only glucose and maltose, and negative reactions for the following: catalase, β-hemolysis, nitrate reduction, urease, hydrolysis of gelatin and esculin, sucrose, maltose, and xylose.[120,185,234] Although its clinical significance is unknown, *A. bernardiae* has been isolated from a variety of human sources including blood, wounds, abscesses, bone, urine, and bladder.[234]

Dermabacter hominis (CDC Coryneform Groups 3 and 5), another new genus composed of irregular, coryneform rods, has been isolated from human skin, blood cultures, wounds, an abscess of the mandible, and other sites.[122] The clinical significance of this species has not been established. It has been suggested that human skin and mucous membranes serve as a reservoir. For further information, other references are recommended.[60,122]

***Aureobacterium* species Versus "*Corynebacterium aquaticum*"; Yellow-Pigmented, Catalase-Positive Coryneform Rods That May Be Motile.** As reviewed recently by Funke and colleagues,[124] the genus *Aureobacterium*, which contains irregular short, thin rods that form bright yellow colonies, was established by Collins and associates in 1983[69] to accomodate some species that had previously been classified in the genera *Arthrobacter*, *Curtobacterium*, and *Microbacterium*. Similar to "*C. aquaticm*," *Aureobacterium* species are catalase-positive, form yellow colonies and may be motile. Seven isolates from human clinical materials (e.g., blood cultures, maxillary sinus, CSF, wounds, and an epidural abscess), that had been tentatively identified as "*C. aquaticum*," were reidentified as *Aureobacterium* species. "*C. aquaticum*," which is listed in the CDC tables of Hollis and Weaver,[157] is not currently considered a valid species of the genus *Corynebacterium* because it has 2,4-diaminobutyric acid within the cell wall (rather than *meso*-diaminopimelic acid); yet it has not been renamed. The reactions in the CDC charts do not differentiate between *C. aquaticum* and *Aureobacterium* species. Therefore, when gram-positive rods with yellow-pigmented colonies are isolated from clinical materials, positive reactions for gelatin and casein hydrolysis would be consistent with a species of *Aureobacterium*. In contrast, *C. aquaticum* should give negative reactions.[124]

Turicella otitidis is a recently named species that accomodates certain gram-positive, coryneform rods that have been isolated from middle-ear fluids from patients with otitis media.[121] The cells are nonmotile diphtheroids that may occur singly, in V-shaped arrangements or in palisades. On sheep blood agar incubated aerobically at 37°C for 48 hours, colonies are nonhemolytic, circular and convex, creamy, and 1 to 2 mm in diameter. They are catalase-positive and produce negative reactions in all the following: urease, nitrate reduction, indole production, and esculin hydrolysis. They do not produce acid from glucose or other carbohydrate test media. Similar to the genera *Corynebacterium* and *Nocardia*, their cell wall contains *meso*-diaminopimelic acid, and they also produce tuberculostearic acid. *Turicella* does not produce mycolic acids, and produces MK-(10) and MK-(11) as the major menaquinones; it thus differs from *Corynebacterium* and *Nocardia* species, which produce mycolic acids and different menaquinones.[121]

BREVIBACTERIUM SPECIES

The genus *Brevibacterium* has recently begun to appear more relevant to clinical microbiologists as a result of studies indicating that *Brevibacterium* species are probably involved in infections in humans.[117,152,153,198,237] Through the years, the CDC Special Bacteriology Reference Laboratory received isolates of nonfermentative coryneform bacteria, which they identified as CDC groups B-1 and B-2, from a wide variety of sources.[157] In 1994, Gruner and coworkers reported that both groups contained strains belonging to *B. casei*, a species not previously reported from human clinical specimens. Most strains of *B. casei* were isolated from blood, cerebrospinal fluid, or other normally sterile body sites.[153] In addition, Funke and Carlotti reported[116,117] that *Brevibacterium* species had been isolated from many blood

cultures and normally sterile body fluids. Other isolates were from human skin, infected toe webs (tinea pedis), a corneal ulcer, and a variety of additional sites. Currently, the genus *Brevibacterium* contains five species (*B. casei*, *B. epidermidis*, *B. linens*, *B. iodinum*, and *B. mcbrellneri*); of these, *B. casei* was by far the most common species identified in the two laboratories.[153] The major habitat of *Brevibacterium* species is milk and other dairy products, and some species contribute to both the aroma and color of cheeses (e.g., *B. linens*, which forms orange colonies). In addition, it is possible that *B. casei*, *B. epidermidis*, and possibly others reside on or in the human skin as members of the normal flora. The cells of *Brevibacterium* species are characterized by a marked rod–coccus cycle in which, short, thin, irregular, nonmotile rods predominate in young, fresh culture, and coccoid forms predominate in older culture. After 2 to 3 days of incubation, the colonies reach about 2 mm in diameter, are grayish-white, and produce a striking "Limburger cheese-like" odor, or an odor that some say is akin to "body odor."[153] Other colony pigments (e.g., yellowish or orange-red) and odors may be observed. Rapid Coryne tests for nitrate reduction, pyrazinamidase, mannose, ribose, and xanthine utilization may aid in differentiation between species.[212] If available, cellular fatty acid analysis can aide in identification of *Brevibacterium* species.[74,117,153]

ROTHIA DENTOCARIOSA

Another of the lesser-known gram-positive bacilli that has been recently reported to cause septicemia, infective endocarditis, or pneumonia in immunocompromised patients is *R. dentocariosa*.[5,161,246,274,283,316,352] This organism, along with *C. matruchotii*, was previously considered to be an aerobic actinomycete. These organisms occur as normal flora in the human oropharynx. *Rothia* species and *C. matruchotii* have been associated with dental caries and periodontal disease, but their role in these conditions remains speculative. *R. dentocariosa* is an aerobic or facultatively anaerobic, non–spore-forming, nonmotile, pleomorphic, gram-positive, coccoid- to rod-shaped bacterium that also forms branched filaments. It produces catalase on media lacking hemin. This aids in differentiating *R. dentocariosa* from *Lactobacillus* and *Bifidobacterium* species (see Chap. 14), which are catalase-negative. *Actinomyces viscosus* and *A. neuii* are the only catalase-positive species of the genus *Actinomyces* that are encountered clinically (see Table 13-7). Most strains of *A. viscosus* ferment lactose and none ferment mannitol, whereas *Rothia* species ferment neither. *Propionibacterium propionicum* (*Arachnia propionicum*; see Chap. 14) is morphologically similar, but is catalase-negative and ferments both lactose and mannitol. *R. dentocariosa* should be differentiated from *C. matruchotii*, which is also catalase-positive and does not ferment lactose or mannitol. *C. matruchotii* forms whip-handle cells and produces metachromatic granules, whereas *Rothia* does not. *R. dentocariosa*, curiously, produces rodlike forms on agar and spheroidal forms in broth, whereas *C. matruchotii* does not.[16]

GARDNERELLA VAGINALIS

The Gram stain reaction of *Gardnerella* is gram-negative to weakly gram-positive. Because of the variable Gram reactions, this organism currently designated *G. vaginalis* was previously included in the genera *Corynebacterium* and *Haemophilus*. In the 1986 edition of *Bergey's Manual*, Pickett and Greenwood[150] make the concluding remark, "because of the unusual cell wall of *Gardnerella* and the apparent lack of a genetic relationship to other genera with comparable mol% G + C values, the genus is not presently assignable to any existing family." Although in many clinical laboratories the workup of *G. vaginalis* is more closely linked with the fastidious gram-negative bacilli and appears in many identification charts and in the databases of commercial systems designed for the identification of these fastidious organisms, a brief description of this organism will be presented here.

Culture of *G. vaginalis* is best accomplished using semiselective media, most commonly either human blood bilayer–Tween (HBT) agar or V agar. Both are commercially available. HBT agar is Columbia CNA agar base containing human blood poured as a layer over agar containing Tween 80. V agar contains Columbia CNA base including proteose peptone 3 and human blood. Both media are commercially available, but are expensive to purchase. Media containing human blood is used because *G. vaginalis* is β-hemolytic on this medium, but not on media containing other animal sources of blood. The organism grows best at 35°C in a 5% to 7% CO_2 atmosphere. Cultures usually take longer than 24 hours to grow, with tiny, β-hemolytic colonies appearing on one of the human blood-containing selective media after 48 to 72 hours of incubation.

Presumptive identification of an unknown isolate may be sufficient in most clinical settings and can be made based on the typical cellular morphology described earlier, by finding small gram-variable coccobacilli in Gram stains, and by demonstrating the lack of oxidase and catalase reactivity. For isolates from certain body sites, including from blood cultures, more definitive identification may be required. In addition to the negative oxidase and catalase reactions, most strains hydrolyze sodium hippurate and produce acid from glucose, maltose, sucrose, and starch, but not from mannitol. Carbohydrate tests should not be performed using large inocula from cultures no older than 24 hours. *G. vaginalis* is susceptible to sodium polyanetholsulfonate (SPS), and an SPS disk susceptibility test may be useful in helping to make a definitive species identification. *G. vaginalis* is also susceptible to metronidazole (50-g disk), trimethoprim (5 g), and to sulfonamide (1 mg), in contrast to the lactobacilli and other unclassified catalase-negative coryneforms, which may be recovered from vaginal secretions and which are generally resistant to these antibiotics. The biochemical characteristics of *G. vaginalis* are shown in Table 13-8.

G. vaginalis is associated with bacterial vaginosis, but can also be isolated from women without any signs

TABLE 13-8
BIOCHEMICAL CHARACTERISTICS OF *GARDNERELLA VAGINALIS*

BIOCHEMICAL TEST	REACTION
β-Hemolysis on human blood bilayer-Tween (HBT) agar	+
Oxidase	−
Catalase	−
Hippurate hydrolysis	+
Acid production from:	
Glucose	+
Maltose	+
Sucrose	+
Mannitol	−
Starch	+
Zone of inhibition with:	
Metronidazole (50 μg disk)	+
Trimethoprim	+
Sulfonamide	+

or symptoms of infection. Because of this, routine culture of vaginal specimens for *G. vaginalis* should be discouraged. The vaginal infections are limited to the production of a discharge with an offensive odor, presumably resulting from the breakdown of proteinaceous products of parasitized degenerating squamous epithelial cells that are sloughed into the vaginal secretions. Segmented neutrophils are not a prominent component of the vaginal secretion, suggesting that organisms do not invade the subepithelial tissue. For this reason, the condition is called "vaginosis," rather than "vaginitis." The observation in stained smears of vaginal secretions of large numbers of squamous epithelial cells heavily colonized with surface pleomorphic bacilli is one accepted method for making a presumptive diagnosis.

Another nonculture method for making a presumptive diagnosis is based on the liberation of a fishlike odor when a drop of 10% KOH is added to the vaginal fluid from patients with *G. vaginalis* infections (the so-called whiff test). This reaction reflects high concentrations of amines found in the vaginal secretions of symptomatic women, but not in those of normal women. The production of the amines at a more basic pH also explains why women with *G. vaginalis* vaginosis particularly complain of foul-smelling vaginal discharge following intercourse, because the seminal ejaculate is alkaline. In fact, *G. vaginalis* vaginosis is considered a sexually transmitted disease because the organism can be recovered in high concentrations from male sexual partners of females who incur reinfection after successful treatment of previous infections.

G. vaginalis has been recovered from various extragenital sites, such as blood, urine, the male urethra, perinephric abscess, pharynx, and intra-abdominal fluid.[149] Josephson and Thomason have cited several reported cases in the literature on the role of *G. vaginalis* as a cause of urinary tract infection.[169] They recovered *G. vaginalis* from 2.3% of 14,178 urine specimens submitted from patients at the University of Wisconsin (Milwaukee) Medical Center. When *G. vaginalis* was recovered in pure culture in concentrations of organisms higher than 10^4/mL, 60% of the patients they studied were asymptomatic. Approximately 95% of their patients were women in whom urethritis is more likely to occur because of the close proximity of the urethra to the colonized vaginal mucosa. Pregnancy and a history of urinary tract disease or recent diagnostic procedures involving instrumentation were predisposing factors. At the Denver Veterans Affairs Hospital, which serves largely a male population, *G. vaginalis* is not an infrequent isolate from urine specimens, often reflecting cases of acute and chronic prostatitis.

SUSCEPTIBILITY OF IRREGULAR AND CORYNEFORM BACILLI TO ANTIMICROBIAL AGENTS

The most important agent used to treat patients who have diphtheria is diphtheria antitoxin. In addition, penicillin or erythromycin may be used to eliminate *C. diphtheriae* from the upper respiratory tract, or to eliminate the carrier state.[207]

Erythromycin, or alternatively penicillin, a first-generation cephalosporin, or vancomycin is usually the drug of choice for treatment of disease caused by most species of nondiphtheria corynebacteria and their allies (e.g., *Rhodococcus equi* and *Arcanobacterium haemolyticum*), with the exception of *C. jeikeium*, *C. urealyticum*, and other organisms that may be resistant to these antimicrobial agents. The drug of choice for serious infections caused by *C. jeikeium* and *C. urealyticum* is vancomycin.[32]

NOCARDIOFORMS AND AEROBIC ACTINOMYCETES

Included in this section are clinically encountered aerobic gram-positive bacteria that are usually more filamentous and branched than the bacteria discussed previously, commonly producing a funguslike mycelium that fragments or breaks up into rod-shaped and short coccoid forms. These organisms, when isolated in many clinical laboratories, are referred to the "mycology section" or the "mycobacteriology section," rather than in the routine bacteriology laboratory for identification. This often occurs because most species grow more slowly than other aerobic and facultatively anaerobic bacteria, and they can be isolated on commonly used fungus media (e.g., Sabouraud dextrose agar) or mycobacteriology recovery media (e.g., Middlebrook synthetic agars and Lowenstein-Jensen medium). However, these aerobic, branching, filamentous gram-positive rods are bacteria, not fungi. True fungi have a eucaryotic cellular organization. In contrast with the fungi, the procaryotic nocardioforms and aerobic actinomycetes do not have a membrane-enclosed nucleus; they lack intracellular organelles that eucaryotic organism have (e.g., no mitochondria); their cell walls contain muramic acid, diaminopimelic acid, or lysine (which fungi lack); they are inhibited by antibacterial antibiotics, and not by antifungal agents; and they differ in other fundamental characteristics. Also, in contrast with the cell diameter of filamentous

fungi, the branching hyphae of *Nocardia* (for example) are more narrow: 0.5 to 1.2 μm in diameter.

The aerobic actinomycetes are commonly termed "nocardioform," a term that is used simply for convenience and is as imprecise a term as "coryneform" or "diphtheroid. *Nocardia* species serve as the point of reference for this group, which includes organisms belonging to several closely related genera including *Streptomyces*, *Nocardiopsis*, *Actinomadura*, *Rhodococcus*, *Oerskovia*, and *Dermatophilus*. *Streptomyces* and *Actinomadura* species resemble *Nocardia* species in many cultural characteristics; however, differ in that they form a specialized aerial mycelium that produces spores, often in chains, rather than a substrate mycelium that undergoes fragmentation. Organisms in the genus *Nocardiopsis* produce a substrate mycelium that fragments on aging into bacillary and coccoid elements, in addition to an aerial mycelium that produces long chains of coccoid spores. *Dermatophilus* species produces a rudimentary substrate mycelium that eventually becomes both longitudinally and transversely septate, ultimately fragmenting into motile "spores." There is also a certain overlap morphologically and phylogenetically with the coryneform bacteria and the anaerobic actinomycetes (e.g., *Actinomyces*, *Arachnia*, and *Bifidobacterium*; see Chap. 14). The salient characteristics of these organisms are summarized in Table 13-9.

The terms defined in Box 13-6 are used in differentiating these bacteria.

THE AEROBIC ACTINOMYCETES: *NOCARDIA*, *STREPTOMYCES*, *NOCARDIOPSIS*, *ACTINOMADURA*

These nocardioform bacteria include organisms that are recognized human pathogens, as well as several species that are primarily found in the environment. The nocardioforms and aerobic actinomycetes are widely distributed in terrestrial and aquatic ecosystems throughout the world.[142] *Nocardia asteroides* is found normally in soil, compost, and other forms of decaying vegetation. *N. brasiliensis*, which also has a worldwide distribution in soil, is present in many areas of North and South America (including the United States), but is highly endemic in parts of Brazil, Central America, and Mexico.[298] Because foods may be contaminated with *Nocardia* species, gastric cultures are not clinically relevant specimens to attempt to isolate the organism from patients. In addition, *N. asteroides* has been isolated from various diseased animals, including cattle and fish, and as referred to by Rippon, has been isolated from normal human skin.[269]

These organisms can be recognized in the laboratory because they form glabrous, tough, adherent, waxy, or dry chalky colonies that grow after 3 days to 2 weeks of incubation. Tan, pink, orange, or gray pigments may be observed. The odor of a musty basement or freshly turned soil is an important clue by which they can be recognized. The optimum temperature for growth is 30°C to 36°C, both in the CO_2 incubator (as for the culture of mycobacteria) or in ambient air (as in the incubator used for fungal cultures). As will be discussed later, they grow well on culture media such as Lowenstein-Jensen and Middlebrook synthetic agars and on most fungal recovery media that is free of cycloheximide.

TABLE 13-9
TAXONOMIC GROUPING OF CLINICALLY SIGNIFICANT AEROBIC ACTINOMYCETES

GROUP AND GENERA	CHARACTERISTICS
Nocardioform group *Nocardia* species	Substrate mycelium that fragments into bacillary and coccoid elements; limited aerial mycelium may occur with some strains; cell wall contains *meso*-diaminopimelic acid (DAP), arabinose, galactose, and nocardiomycolic acid.
Rhodococcus species	Produce a substrate mycelium that undergoes rapid fragmentation into bacillary and coccoid elements; smooth surface colonies consist of coccoid elements almost exclusively; *meso*-DAP, arabinose, galactose, and nocardiomycolic acid are present in cell wall.
Oerskovia species	Only substrate mycelium present that fragments into motile elements; no *meso*-DAP present.
Streptomycete group *Streptomyces* species	Aerial mycelium with long chains of spores formed; *levo*-DAP is present in cell wall.
Maduromycete group *Actinomadura* species	Aerial mycelium produces short chains of spores; *levo*-DAP and the unique carbohydrate madurose are present in the cell wall.
Thermomonospora group *Nocardiopsis* species	Aerial hyphae produces long chains of spores; *meso*-DAP is present, but no other diagnostic or characteristic cell wall carbohydrates are present.
Loculated sporangia group (convenience designation only) *Dermatophilus* species	Rudimentary substrate mycelium fragments longitudinally and transversely to form motile spores; *meso*-DAP is present in cell wall.

All species are gram-positive, although *Nocardia* species, in particular, tend to stain with a beaded, gram-variable pattern. Thus, the finding of gram-positive or gram-variable, beaded, delicate (1 μm in diameter), branching organisms should alert one to the

BOX 13-6. TERMS USED TO DIFFERENTIATE AEROBIC ACTINOMYCETES

Substrate mycelium: This refers to the cells that grow on and then into the surface of the medium. These organisms characteristically form branching cells ("hyphae") that grow together to form tough, leathery colonies. This growth may also be called the vegetative mycelium.

Fragmentation: The substrate mycelium of these organisms are generally composed of chains of long bacilli that, on growth and aging, start to "break up" into individual bacilli-shaped (bacillary) and coccus-shaped (coccoid) cells.

Aerial hyphae: Some species actually produce cells that grow upright and away from the agar surface. More mature aerial hyphae will be found in the center of the colony, with more rudimentary aerial hyphae being found on the periphery of the colony. On aging, the aerial hyphae fragment into coccoid "spores," giving older colonies a velvety or powdery appearance. For one species (*Dermatophiulus congoliensis*), the spores that are produced on the aerial mycelium are motile.

presence of one of these nocardioform organisms, and isolation plates should be held and reincubated for several days to ensure recovery. The branching of the bacterial cells, their "partial" acid-fastness (acid-fast reaction only when a low concentration, inorganic acid instead of acid alcohol is used as the decolorizer), and the detection of a musty odor produced by the mature colonies, are the practical characteristics by which *Nocardia* species are most commonly separated from *Mycobacterium* species in clinical laboratories. These properties are variable, and not always reliable. Future applications of molecular techniques promise to make this differentiation simpler and more accurate. Recently published applications include 16S rRNA gene amplification and sequencing,[56] polymerase chain reaction (PCR), restriction fragment-length polymorphism (RFLP),[205] and DNA amplification and restriction endonuclease analysis, particularly observing for the absence of a recognition site for the endonuclease *Bst*EII in *Nocardia* species (present in mycobacteria),[314] have provided rapid and sensitive methods for differentiating *Nocardia* species from rapidly growing *Mycobacterium* species.

Because the application of these techniques remain largely in research laboratories, the identification in most clinical laboratories of the aerobic actinomycetes and their differentiation from other closely related organisms is still based on the observation of physiologic characteristics. An overview of the more commonly used physiologic and biochemical characteristics are found in Table 13-10. The specific characteristics will be presented in more detail under the discussions of

TABLE 13-10
BIOCHEMICAL AND PHYSIOLOGIC TESTS FOR THE IDENTIFICATION OF MEDICALLY IMPORTANT AEROBIC ACTINOMYCETES

ORGANISM	MODIFIED ACID FAST	LYSOZYME	DECOMPOSITION OF CASEIN	TYROSINE	XANTHINE	HYPOXANTHINE	UREASE	GELATIN HYDROLYSIS	ACID PRODUCED FROM LACTOSE	XYLOSE	ARABINOSE	NITRATE REDUCTION
Nocardia asteroides	+	R	–	–	–	–	+	–	–	–	–	+
Nocardia brasiliensis	+	R	+	+	–	+	+	+	–	–	–	+
Nocardia otitidiscaviarum (N. caviae)	+	R	–	–	+	+	+	–	–	–	–	+
Nocardia transvaliensis	+	R	–	+	–	+	+	–	–	–	–	+
Nocardia coeliaca	+	S	–	V	+	+	+	NA	+	+	+	–
Actinomadura madurae	–	S	+	+	–	+	–	+	+	+	+	+
Actinomadura pelletieri	–	S	+	+	–	+	–	+	–	–	–	+
Streptomyces somaliensis	–	S	+	+	–	–	–	+	–	–	–	–
Streptomyces griseus	–	S	+	+	+	+	V	+	–	–	–	–
Streptomyces albus	–	S	+	+	+	+	+	+	–	–	–	–
Nocardiopsis dassonvillei	–	S	+	+	+	+	+	+	–	+	+	+
Streptomyces species	–	S	+	+	+	+	V	+	V	V	V	V

+, positive; –, negative; V, variable; R, resistant; S, susceptible; NA, not available.

each organism group, and can be found in the references cited.[140–142,156,189,269]

NOCARDIA

Nocardiosis is an infectious disease most commonly caused by *N. asteroides* (over 90% of cases), less commonly by *N. brasiliensis* and *N. otitidiscaviarum* (formerly *N. caviae*),[83,111,194,270,298] and even less frequently by *N. farcinica*. The incidence of nocardiosis in the United States has been estimated to be close to 1000 new cases per year; it is likely that more occur, but are not recognized.[83] Humans become infected by inhaling contaminated airborne dust particles or by traumatic implantation of the bacterium into the subcutaneous tissues (actinomycotic mycetomas).

EPIDEMIOLOGIC, CLINICAL, AND PATHOLOGIC ASPECTS

Nocardia asteroides. Given numerous taxonomic methods, including DNA homology and immunology studies, *N. asteroides* is markedly heterogeneous and encompasses a complex of organisms.[141] Most recently, Steingrube and associates,[314] using DNA amplification and restriction fragment length polymorphism (RFLP) analysis of endonuclease (*Msp*I and *Bsa*HI) products derived from an amplified 439-bp segment of the 65-kDa heat-shock protein gene of several strains of bacterial isolates from the *N. asteroides* complex, have defined four separate unnamed groups, currently designated Type I, Type II, Type IV, and Type VI. The clinical significance of these separate groups remains to be determined; however, they do show differences in antimicrobial susceptibility profiles against amikacin, cefamandole, and the aminoglycosides gentamicin, kanamycin, and tobramycin. Specifically, the Type IV and *N. transvalensis* isolates studied were amikacin-resistant and also resistant to gentamicin, kanamycin, and tobramycin. These isolates utilized citrate and assimilated galactose and trehalose, additional clues to their identification.

N. farcinica and *N. nova* also belong to the *N. asteroides* complex. The ability to grow at 45°C and resistance to erythromycin, cefotaxime, and tobramycin serve to distinguish *N. farcinica* (antibiotic-resistant) from *N. asteroides*.[43] Observation of the development of a milky white opacity around colonies growing on Middlebrook agar also serves to separate *N. farcinica* (opacification) from other members of the *N. asteroides* complex and from other *Nocardia* species, all of which are negative.[43,108] *N. nova* can be identified in the laboratory by observing its unique susceptibility to ampicillin and erythromycin, the demonstration of α- and β-esterase activity, and the turning of arylsulfatase media in 2 weeks.[346]

In a series of 200 cases of *Nocardia* species infections presented by Wallace and coauthors,[346] the isolates that they designated *N. farcinica* were from patients with severe illness, 56% of whom had disseminated infections. Most of these patients had underlying disease or were immunosuppressed. Since their introduction of *N. farcinica* as a new species, several additional case reports have appeared in the literature. Miralles described a case of disseminated disease in a patient with AIDS,[221] with the diagnosis being made by a renal biopsy. The strain isolated was initially identified as *N. asteroides*; however, the correct identification was made after the strain was found to be resistant to gentamicin, tobramycin, and cephalosporins. Miralles, therefore, recommends that third-generation cephalosporins should not be used empirically in the treatment of *Nocardia* infections until susceptibility tests have been performed.[221] Schiff and coworkers report a case of a deep abscess of the face with underlying osteomyelitis in a nonimmunocompromised patient who had incurred a facial laceration.[285] The infection resolved following intramuscular treatment with amikacin.

N. nova has a clinical disease spectrum similar to that of *N. asteroides*, with which it is closely aligned. Pneumonia, cutaneous infections, and brain abscesses have been caused by *N. nova*, particularly following trauma, use of cortisteroids, and following organ transplants. Wallace and associates, from their own experience, estimate that up to 20% of clinical isolates identified as *N. asteroides* in many laboratories may in fact be *N. nova* if differential tests are performed.[346] *N. nova* has recently been implicated along with *Aspergillus fumigatus* in a patient with pneumonia following cardiac transplantation.[224] Oral therapy with clarithromycin was successful in this case.

N. asteroides is an opportunistic pathogen in individuals whose host defenses are compromised (e.g., by leukemias, malignant lymphomas, solid tumors, asthma, bronchiectasis, tuberculosis, chronic obstructive pulmonary disease, hemochromatosis, ulcerative colitis, alcoholism, cirrhosis, and corticosteroid treatment; renal and cardiac transplant recipients seem to be particularly at risk).[53,83,269] The organism is capable of living inside macrophages by inhibiting phagosome–lysosome fusion and by their ability to produce catalase and superoxide dismutase, which inactivate the myeloperoxidase system of these phagocytic cells. T-cell–mediated immunity plays a key role in defense against these organisms.[194]

Many individuals with nocardiosis have no known underlying impairment in their host defenses.[83,194] Nocardiosis is an acute, subacute, or chronic disease, which usually begins in the respiratory tract. It is acquired by inhalation of airborne conidia from the soil or other environmental sources, which results in a primary pneumonitis. Manifestations include fever, a cough productive of mucopurulent sputum, and nonresolving infiltrates of varying appearance on chest radiographs. There may be progressive bronchopneumonia, localized or diffuse infiltrates, extensive consolidation, single or multiple abscesses, pleural effusions, empyema, and sinus tracts with involvement of the chest wall. Granuloma formation and presence of giant cells has been described with *Nocardia* species, but in our experience granulomas are not typical of pulmonary involvement with these species.

From the lungs, hematogenous (bloodstream) dissemination of the organisms occurs in about 50% of patients, and disseminated infection can involve virtually any organ.[83,194] A case of blood-borne, disseminated nocardiosis in a patient with AIDS has been recently reported by Vanderstigel.[339] Metastatic brain abscesses develop in about a third of patients, resulting in headaches, changing mental status, seizures, focal neurologic deficits, or other neurologic abnormalities. Interestingly, blood cultures (in spite of hematogenous spread of the organism) and CSF cultures almost invariably fail to demonstrate the organism. Histopathologic findings include acute granulocytic inflammation, with abscess formation and necrosis.

The bacterial cells of *Nocardia* species are not usually seen in hematoxylin and eosin-stained sections, and may not be seen in periodic acid–Schiff stains. They are quite readily seen in Gomori methenamine-silver, Gram-Weigert, Giemsa, tissue Gram stains, Brown and Brenn, or Brown-Hopps Gram stains. In a tissue Gram stain, the organisms are usually observed as thin, beaded, branched filamentous rods. The modified Kinyoun acid-fast stain (in which destaining is done with 1% aqueous H_2SO_4, instead of the usual acid alcohol that is used in the Ziehl–Neelsen method) is useful for direct smears and frozen sections, whereas the Fite-Ferraco acid-fast stain is recommended for paraffin sections.[99] With these stains, *Nocardia* species are acid-fast (or "partially acid-fast"), *Mycobacterium* spp. are strongly acid-fast, whereas *Actinomyces israelii* and the other anaerobic actinomycetes are not acid-fast (see Table 13-10).

Evidence has been mounting that *N. asteroides* is sometimes (how often is not certain) a saprophytic member of the respiratory tract flora (at least transiently);[194,270] some patients may have sputum cultures positive for *Nocardia* who have no clinical evidence of nocardiosis.[111] The respiratory tracts of some individuals who have cavitary tuberculosis, malignancy, cystic fibrosis, asthma, or other underlying diseases, may simply be colonized with *Nocardia* species. Even the recovery of *Nocardia* species from blood cultures may not be significant. Of nine cases of *Nocardia* bacteremia reported by Esteban and associates,[100] *N. asteroides* was thought to be clinically relevant in only two of four cases; the remaining isolates were considered insignificant or undetermined. All patients were cured. These authors conclude that *Nocardia* species may be a contaminant and the significance of any given isolate remains a matter of clinical judgement.

Nocardia brasiliensis. *N. brasiliensis* is a common cause of subcutaneous infections and mycetoma in South America, much of Latin America, and Mexico. In the 1960s, 85% to 95% of reported mycetomas in Mexico were caused by *N. brasiliensis.*[137] More currently, Castro and associates also report that *N. brasiliensis* was by far the most common actinomycete isolated from 41 cases seen in Sao Paulo, Brazil between 1978 and 1989.[44] The feet and the legs were the most common sites of involvement. Most patients were from rural areas in the northeast regions of the country, and the majority were field laborers. Significant infections of skin and soft tissues with *N. brasiliensis* was also found in 35 patients included in a study of nocardiosis in Queensland, Australia.[131] A case of disseminated disease in a patient living in the United States has been reported.[181] The patient had been treated for several years with dexamethasone. Pneumonia and septic arthritis were the primary sources of infection. Interesting cases of sporotrichoid lymphocutaneous infections with *N. brasiliensis* have been reported, one following a cat scratch[280] (perhaps establishing cats as another mode for transmission of this organism); an-

other presenting as multiple subcutaneous nodules and abscesses on the extensor aspect of the forearm in a patient with systemic lupus erythematosus,[366] and a third affecting the face and arm following skin abrasions that had occurred 2 weeks previously.[235] Rippon had previously drawn attention to the lymphocutaneous syndrome that simulates sporotrichosis.[269]

N. brasiliensis is also taxonomically heterogeneous. *N. pseudobrasiliensis* is the current proposed designation[276] for an unnamed taxon of *N. brasiliensis* previously described by Wallace and coworkers,[345] representing strains that were frequently involved in extracutaneous and disseminated disease. *N. pseudobrasiliensis* differs from *N. brasiliensis* sensu stricto by being capable of hydrolyzing adenine, and having different β-lactamase patterns on isoelectric focusing and restriction patterns of a 439-bp fragment of the 65-kDa heat-shock protein gene. Most of the strains of the unnamed taxon (*N. pseudobrasiliensis*) studied by Wallace and associates[345] were susceptible to ciprofloxacin and clarithromycin, and resistant to minocycline, a profile opposite that of the *N. brasiliensis* sensu stricto strains. Therefore, when an organism suggestive of *N. brasiliensis* is recovered from extracutaneous sources, a specific identification of *N. pseudobrasiliensis* may be in order.

Nocardia otitidiscaviarum (caviae). Several cases of cutaneous and soft-tissue infections with *N. otitidiscaviarum* have also been reported.[33,45,58,319] From the older literature, Brown and coauthors[33] and Causey[45] independently have reported cases caused by what was then called *N. caviae* (currently, *N. otitidiscaviarum*). Two recent cases reported from France by Freland and associates[112] were found in patients recently immigrating from Vietnam and Zimbabwe, respectively, indicating the wide distribution of this organism. These infections commonly occur following trauma, most often in persons who are immunocompetent, and may mimic other cutaneous infections, thereby delaying the diagnosis and treatment.[58] Suzuki and coworkers report[319] the first case of lymphocutaneous nocardiosis from Japan, involving a 78-year-old woman who had received long-term prednisone therapy for bronchial asthma. A case of disseminated disease in a heart transplant patient beginning as a deep thigh abscess ("Madura thigh") has also been reported,[293] indicating the spectrum of disease that may be caused by this species.

Miscellaneous *Nocardia* species. Several other *Nocardia* species are listed in the 1986 edition of *Bergey's Manual*;[140] however, these are generally considered soil and water contaminants, and they have not been associated with diseases in humans. One exception are recent reports of human infections caused by *N. transvalensis.*[284] *N. transvalensis* is similar to *N. asteroides* type IV, being amikacin resistant, which is unusual for *Nocardia* species. McNeil and coauthors[217] reviewed 16 cases, the isolates from whom had been referred to the CDC for study. Infections were definitely established in 10 of these patients, 75% of whom were immunosuppressed or receiving immunosuppressive drugs. Most isolates were from sputum specimens; 3 patients with disseminated disease died. The increasing resistance of *N. transvalensis* to amikacin was cited as an emerging problem. The patient reported by Schiff and coworkers[284] was the first case of lymphocutaneous infection, in whom a cure was effected by administration of amikacin and cefotaxime.

Mycetoma.   Traumatic implantation of the organism into the deep subcutaneous tissue may result in an indolent condition called actinomycotic mycetoma, a term that distinguishes this condition from the eumycotic ("true") mycetomas caused by certain species of fungi. The species most commonly involved include *Actinomadura madurae, A. pelletieri, Streptomyces somaliensis, N. brasiliensis, N. caviae, N. asteroides,* and less commonly, species of *Nocardiopsis, Dermatophilus,* and other genera.[99,269] The lesions caused by these organisms may become extensive, consisting of suppurating abscesses, granulomas, and the formation of sinus tracts. Grains and granules, usually measuring less than 1 mm in diameter, may often be observed within the purulent material. They are usually white or yellow, varying in color, depending on the age of the lesion and the species involved. Fibrosis is usually seen in chronic cases, but not nearly to the extent that is typical of actinomycosis (caused by *Actinomyces israelii*).

PRIMARY ISOLATION OF *NOCARDIA* SPECIES AND OTHER AEROBIC ACTINOMYCETES

N. asteroides and other *Nocardia* species are aerobic organisms that grow on a variety of ordinary media including blood agar, brain–heart infusion agar and on Sabouraud dextrose agar without antibiotics (e.g., they are inhibited by chloramphenicol, penicillin, and streptomycin). *N. asteroides* grows well at 25°C, 35°to 37°C, and at 42° to 45°C. Incubation at 42° to 45°C permits growth of *N. asteroides* whereas many other bacteria will be inhibited. Growth on ordinary laboratory media may take from 4 days to 6 weeks of incubation. Growth is enhanced by incubation in 10% CO_2.

Murray and coworkers[233] have also demonstrated that *Nocardia* species can be recovered from contaminated specimens using modified Thayer-Martin (MTM) medium; Shawar and associates[292] have demonstrated the more rapid recovery of larger colonies from contaminated specimens using a chemically defined medium containing paraffin (paraffin-baiting technique). By this technique, a paraffin-coated glass rod is inserted into a carbon-free broth mixed with the sputum specimen. In positive cultures growth appears on the rod just above the surface of the broth. Ayyar and associates[13] found that paraffin agar serves as an inexpensive selective medium for isolation of *Nocardia* species, being superior to either MTM or the paraffin bait technique. This improved recovery reflects that *Nocardia* species can use paraffin as the sole source of carbon.

Selective buffered charcoal–yeast extract medium (BCYE, commonly used for the recovery of *Legionella* species from respirator specimens) also facilitates the recovery of *Nocardia* species from sputum and other specimens that may be contaminated with mixed bacteria.[127,178,341] The use of selective BCYE agar, to which polymyxin B, anisomycin, and vancomycin have been added, and pretreatment of the specimen by an acid wash improved recovery of *Nocardia*

species from 8% to 33% for the former and to 67% for the latter.[178]

N. asteroides can survive the usual *N*-acetylcysteine digestion procedure (without NaOH) that is used for sputum or bronchial washings.[232] It is recommended that cultures of sputum and bronchial washings for isolation of *Nocardia* (when nocardiosis is suspected) be done both before and after the digestion procedure). Some strains grow well on the media that are used for primary isolation of mycobacteria (e.g., 7H1O or Lowenstein-Jensen [LJ] media). Colonies on LJ media often develop within 1 to 2 weeks. They may be similar in appearance to atypical mycobacteria (see Chap. 17). However, *Mycobacterium* species do not produce aerial hyphae, are strongly acid-fast using a Ziehl–Neelsen or auramine–rhodamine stain, and many are arylsulfatase-positive, whereas *Nocardia* species are not acid-fast with these procedures, but are partially acid-fast using the modified Kinyoun stain, and they are negative in the arylsulfatase test. In addition, another difference is that the branched hyphae of *Nocardia* that may not always be seen in smears prepared from growth on solid media can sometimes be demonstrated from growth in broth cultures, whereas mycobacteria do not usually branch (even though the rods may be elongated). One noteworthy exception is one of the rapidly growing species of *Mycobacterium, M. fortuitum,* which has been observed to produce branching filaments in smears of pus, or may produce filamentous colonial forms. *M. fortuitum* differs from *Nocardia* species according to the characteristics described in the foregoing.

DIFFERENTIATION OF *NOCARDIA* FROM ADDITIONAL GENERA OF AEROBIC ACTINOMYCETES

Infections of humans with the genera *Streptomyces, Nocardiopsis, Rhodococcus, Actinomadura, Orskovia,* and *Dermatophilus* appear to be rare in the United States, although good incidence data are lacking.[99,139,269,298,337] Some differential characteristics that may aid in differentiating *Nocardia* from these aerobic actinomycetes and other related bacteria are given in Tables 13-10 and 13-13.[141]

The laboratory identification of *Nocardia* and *Streptomyces* species can be made using the following criteria: The typical colonies of *Nocardia* and *Streptomyces* species are dry to chalky in consistency, usually heaped or folded, and range in color from yellow to gray-white (see Color Plate 13-3D). *Nocardia* species are more commonly some shade of yellow, whereas *Streptomyces* species are most frequently gray-white. Both groups produce colonies with a pungent musty-basement odor.

A Gram stain of a portion of a suspected colony shows delicate, branching filaments no more than 1 μm in diameter (see Color Plate 13-3E). *Nocardia* species are partially acid-fast (i.e., they do not decolorize when treated with 1% H_2SO_4 or 3% HCl instead of the more active acid-alcohol decolorizer used in the Ziehl–Neelsen or Kinyoun stains), whereas *Streptomyces* species are not partially acid-fast. Acid-fastness may be enhanced by growing the organism on certain media, such as Middlebrook 7H11 agar (Box 13-7). If the unknown organism is not acid-fast, a report of "nonacid-fast aerobic actinomycete" can be made.

Growth in the presence of lysozyme is useful in identifying *Nocardia* species (see Table 13-10), particularly those strains that are acid-fast–negative. All *Nocardia* species are resistant to lysozyme and will grow in its presence in 5 to 20 days. A control tube of glycerol broth without lysozyme and both positive and negative controls should be performed with each test. The test is performed as outlined in Box 13-8.

HYDROLYSIS OF CASEIN, TYROSINE, XANTHINE, AND HYPOXANTHINE

The differential ability of the various *Nocardia* species, and related aerobic actinomyces, to hydrolyze casein, tyrosine, xanthine, and hypoxanthine is one of the mainstays of making identifications in most clinical laboratories. The procedure is described in Chart 38, and the patterns of reaction are shown in Table 13-10. The differential plates are inoculated with the unknown organism for up to 2 weeks at 30°C and observed for hydrolysis (clearing of the medium around the colonies). An example of hydrolysis by a colony of *Streptomyces* species is shown in Fig. 13-3.

Nocardia and *Streptomyces* species can be differentiated by inoculating plates of casein, tyrosine, xanthine, and hypoxanthine agars, incubating them for up to 2 weeks at 30°C, and observing for hydrolysis (clearing of the medium around the colonies; see Fig. 13-3). The reactions of several species of *Nocardia* and *Streptomyces* on these media are listed in Table 13-10. An example of casein hydrolysis by a colony of *Streptomyces* is shown in Figure 13-3.

If the results of these tests are equivocal, thin-layer chromatography may be helpful. Differences in the cell wall composition are used in some research laboratories or reference laboratories for taxonomic purposes.[141,272,279] Most of the nocardioform organisms, including *Nocardia* and *Rhodococcus*, have a type IV cell wall composition (the significant constituents are *meso*-

diaminopimelic acid [DAP], arabinose, and galactose). *Streptomyces* species have type I cell walls. *Oerskovia* species have type VI (with *levo*-DAP and no diagnostic carbohydrates). Other chemotaxonomic tests, in addition to determining cell wall type, include analyses of menaquinones, long-chain fatty acids, phospholipids, and mycolic acids.[36,335] These studies are not practical, nor are they necessary for differentiation of *Nocardia* in the clinical microbiology laboratory. If definitive iden-

BOX 13-8. LYSOZYME TEST FOR THE IDENTIFICATION OF *NOCARDIA* SPECIES

1. Prepare glycerol broth by adding 5 g peptone and 70 mL of glycerol to 1000 mL of distilled water (reduce amounts proportionally if smaller quantities are desired). Sterilize by autoclaving at 15 psi for 15 minutes.
2. Prepare lysozyme solution by dissolving 100 mg lysozyme powder in 100 mL 0.01 N HCl.
3. Combine 95 mL of glycerol broth with 5 mL of lysozyme solution and dispense in 5-mL aliquots into screw-capped tubes. Use 5-mL aliquots of glycerol broth without lysozyme for the growth control.
4. Prepare a light suspension of the unknown organism in sterile saline. Using a Pasteur pipette, inoculate 1 or 2 drops into the lysozyme and control tube (keep the inoculum light).
5. Incubate at 25°C. Examine each tube for growth in 7 to 14 days. Growth will appear as a pellicle on the surface, as a sediment, or as both. The tubes can be gently shaken to observe bread crumb-like particles in the tubes showing positive growth.
6. An organism resistant to lysozyme will grow in both the lysozyme tube and the control; an organism that is susceptible will grow only in the control tube.

BOX 13-7. MODIFIED ACID-FAST STAIN FOR *NOCARDIA* SPECIES

1. Make a smear of the organism from growth media and heat fix.
2. Flood the slide with Kinyoun carbolfuchsin for 5 minutes.
3. Pour off the excess stain.
4. Decolorize with a 1% aqueous solution of sulfuric acid.
5. Wash with tap water.
6. Counterstain with methylene blue for 1 minute.
7. Rinse with water and dry. Examine under oil immersion optics.

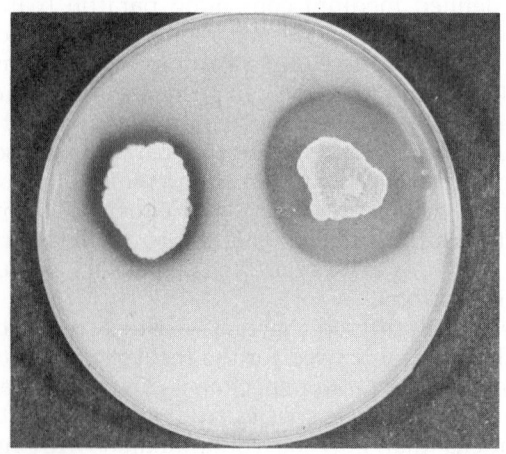

Figure 13-3
Casein agar plate illustrating the hydrolytic action of two species of *Streptomyces*.

tification is necessary, laboratories may wish to send isolates to a reference laboratory.

Mishra and colleagues[222] have devised a key for more detailed differentiation of the nocardiae and the streptomycetes than is presented in Table 13-10. Their differential table is particularly useful in that it lists percentages of strains positive for a large battery of biochemical tests, morphologic features, and various physiologic characteristics. Emerging technologies for the direct detection of *Nocardia* species in clinical specimens include enzyme immunoassay (EIA) techniques,[6] the use of monoclonal antibodies using cell extracts of *N. asteroides* and *N. brasiliensis*,[165] recombinant DNA probes,[34] and various molecular techniques, including gene sequencing[56] and polymerase chain reaction and restriction fragment-length polymorphism (PCR-RFLP) analyses.[205] These techniques are currently being used primarily in research or large reference laboratories; microbiologists must remain alert to the future availability of commercial products.

The Genus *Streptomyces*. *Streptomyces* species are environmental organisms of the soil that have significant importance in the industrial and pharmaceutical fields. A few species cause human infections and have been isolated from sputum, other respiratory specimens, superficial wounds, skin, and other specimens. In a study of 366 aerobic actinomyces isolates from clinical mycetomas submitted for study at the CDC in the late 1980s, only *N. asteroides* and *A. madurae* were recovered more frequently than *Streptomyces* species.[218] *S. somaliensis* causes actinomycotic mycetoma, and has virtually a worldwide distribution, having been recovered from cases of mycetoma in Saudi Arabia, Nigeria, Niger, Sudan, Somolia, South Africa, Venezuela, India, and Mexico.[216] A high proportion of these cases involved the head and neck, producing what is known as "Madura skull." Several cases have also been diagnosed in the United States.[328] Grains from mycetoma lesions are large (2 to 4 mm) and yellow-brown. *S. griseus*, an organism causing subcutaneous mycetomas in felines and dolphin, also has been recovered from human mycetomas.

Streptomyces species typically form dry, chalky gray-white colonies that emit a pungent musty-basement odor. Beaded, branching, gram-positive filaments are observed microscopically; however, the partial acid-fast stain is negative. *Streptomyces* species are sensitive to lysozyme and will not grow in lysozyme broth. They typically rapidly hydrolyze casein (see Fig. 13-3 and Table 13-10) and more slowly hydrolyze xanthine and tyrosine. In contrast to *Nocardia* species, *Streptomyces* species do not reduce nitrate to nitrite.

The Genus *Nocardiopsis*. *N. dassonvillei*, which forms zigzag chains of spores within a sheathlike structure, has a type IIIC cell wall in which *meso*-DAP and galactose are major constituents. The genus *Nocardiopsis* was split off from the genus *Actinomadura* to accommodate related organisms that lack the unique cell wall carbohydrate madurose. Seven species have been assigned to the genus; however, only *N. dassonvillei* (with its two

subspecies, *dassonvillei* and *prasina*), ordinarily a soil saprophyte, has been recovered from animals and from cases of human actinomycotic mycetoma.[270] This species hydrolyses casein, tyrosine, and xanthine (just the opposite of *N. asteroides*).

The Genus *Rhodococcus*. *R. equi* was previously known as *Corynebacterium equi*. It has also been called "*Mycobacterium rhodochrous*" and has been referred to as the "rhodochrous" complex.[139] The organism does not form aerial hyphae, but forms smooth, glistening, salmon-pink to red-orange colonies, and forms diphtheroid rods with traces of branching in early stages of growth. Similar to other *Rhodococcus* and *Nocardia* species, the rod-shaped cells fragment into coccoid cells.[138,139] As are the *Nocardia* species, *Rhodococcus* species may be partially acid-fast using the modified Kinyoun stain. Further characteristics of *R. equi* are given in Table 13-11.

R. equi is the cause of pulmonary disease in foals and other domestic animals. Between 1967 and the early 1980s, only a handful of human infections were reported. Human infections are believed to result from contact with animal carriers (e.g., cattle, pig, horses, or cattle manure), presumably by a respiratory route.[337] The rhodococci are widely distributed in soil and may account for the source of infection in persons who do not recall animal contacts. Human infections most commonly occur in the immunocompromised, primarily those with defects in cell-mediated immunity, and in patients with lymphoma, Hodgkin's disease, leukemia, AIDS, and following transplantation.[24,206,240,281,337] In fact, McNeil and Brown cite over 100 cases of *R. equi* infections in patients with AIDS.[216]

Pulmonary infections may mimic tuberculosis, become slowly progressive, and cavitate.[32,42,126,136,206,337] Invasive pneumonia with cavity formation is particularly noted in patients with AIDS, with a high propensity for the infection to disseminate to the brain, liver, spleen, and other organs.[216] Other *R. equi* infection sites recently reported include a case of endoph-

TABLE 13-11

DIFFERENTIAL CHARACTERISTICS OF *R. EQUI* AND *R. AURANTIACUS*

CHARACTERISTIC	*R. EQUI*	*R. AURANTIACUS*
Weak or partial acid fast	–	+
Rough colonies	–	+
Salmon-pink/coral colonies	+	–
Orange or brown colonies	–	+
Catalase	+	+
Motility	–	–
Urease	V	+
Nitrate reduction	V	–
Orthonitrophenyl-β-D-galactopyranoside	–	+
Acid produced from glucose	–	+

+, positive; –, negative; V, variable

thalmitis,[95] osteomyelitis,[240] pleura with effusion,[190] and a wound in a nonimmunocompromised patient.[229]

Isolates are frequently resistant to penicillins and cephalosporins; however, most strains are susceptible to erythromycin, chloramphenicol, vancomycin, and the aminoglycosides.

Other *Rhodococcus* species may be agents of opportunistic infections in humans. *R. aurantiacus* has been isolated from the sputum of patients with chronic pulmonary disease,[331] from the CSF of a patient with hairy cell leukemia, and from a severe gangrenous tenosynovitis lesion with multiple subcutaneous abscesses in a woman with de Quervain disease.[330] This species is also resistant to multiple antibacterial and antimycobacterial antibiotics. *R. sputi*, a cause of mesenteric lymphadenitis in swine,[332] has been isolated from the sputum of humans, but has not been associated with disease.

The Genus *Actinomadura*. *Actinomadura* species contain *meso*-DAP in their cell walls (cell wall type IIIB; madurose is a major carbohydrate component). They form variously pigmented, (whitish to yellowish, pink to reddish), waxy, cerebriform, somewhat tough, membranous colonies, with a branched, aerial mycelium (bearing short chains of conidia).[99,270,301] *Actinomadurae* are not acid-fast. *A. madurae* and *A. pelletieri* are the only two species of clinical importance. Both species are sensitive to lysozyme and hydrolyze casein, tyrosine, and hypoxanthine (see Table 13-10). They both also hydrolyze esculin, a characteristic helpful in separating them from other aerobic actinomycetes, which do not possess this property. Most strains of *A. pellitieri* are asaccharolytic, assimilating only glucose and trehalose; *A. madurae* strains are saccharolytic and utilize most carboydrates commonly tested in clinical laboratories.[216]

Most human infections are caused by *A. madurae* and *A. pelletieri*, characterized by granulocytic infiltrates within craterlike openings in skin and subcutaneous tissue, most commonly of the lower legs. In a study of 366 isolates of aerobic actinomycetes from mycetomas submitted to the CDC in the late 1980s, *A. madurae* was second (11.5%) in incidence only to *Nocardia asteroides* (26%).[218] Formation of sinus tracts is characteristic, and bone involvement is common.[99,270] Grains, consisting of masses of branching filaments, are formed within the involved tissue, surrounded by purulent exudate. The grains of *A. madurae* are large (1 to 5 mm) and yellowish; those of *A. pelletieri* are small (300 to 500 μm) and garnet red in ("red grain mycetoma"). Most infections occur in tropical countries, particularly in India and Tunisia (*A. madurae*) and in Senegal, Chad, and Somalia (*A. pelletieri*). Recent case studies of *A. madurae* infections include a case of *A. madurae* peritonitis in a patient undergoing continuous peritoneal dialysis;[364] and a case of disseminated *A. madurae* infection in a patient with AIDS,[219] who was also a habitual heroin user.

The Genus *Oerskovia*. Sottnek and coauthors[310] reported on the characteristics of 57 clinical isolates, belonging to the genus *Oerskovia*, referred to the CDC

from hospital and public health laboratories throughout the country. Five of these cases were from heart valves or cardiac isolates, nine were blood isolates, one was from the cerebrospinal fluid and the remainder from sites such as urine, traumatic and surgical wounds, eye drainage, pleural fluids, pilonidal cysts and infant formula. Rihs and coworkers[267] recently reported a case of *O. xanthineolytica* peritonitis in a patient receiving peritoneal dialysis, and reviewed several other cases in the literature. Included in their review were two cases caused by *O. turbata*, one case of endocarditis reported in 1975[257] in a 68-year-old homograph cardiac valve recipient, and a case of bacteremia in a 3-year-old child associated with a Broviac catheter.[193] A second case of *O. turbata* endocarditis was also reported.[243] Rihs and coauthors[267] cited two other cases in which *O. xanthineolytica* was recovered from clinical specimens, one from the vitreous humor in a case of traumatic endophthalmitis in a 47-year-old man[160] and the other from the cerebrospinal fluid of a 38-year-old woman with meningitis resulting from an infected ventriculoperitoneal shunt.[173] The species was not indicated in a urine isolate from a 47-year-old woman with pyelonephrosis nor from a blood isolate from a 40-year-old woman with Crohn's disease and bacteremia associated with a Hickman catheter.[80]

The genus includes two species, *O. turbata* and *O. xanthineolytica*, formerly classified as CDC Coryneform Groups A-3 and A-4 and A-1 and A-2, respectively.[310] *Oerskovia* species are aerobic, gram-positive, nocardia-like bacteria that are found in the soil. They form yellow-pigmented colonies on heart infusion agar or other media.[191] Branched hyphae are produced that break up into motile rods which are non–acid-fast. Additional characteristics are given in Tables 13-12 and 13-13.

TABLE 13-12
CHARACTERISTICS OF *OERSKOVIA* SPECIES

CHARACTERISTIC	O. TURBATA	O. XANTHINEOLYTICA
Vegetative hyphae	+	+
Motility	+	+
OF glucose	F	F[a]
Nitrate reduction	V	+
Acid produced from:		
Maltose	+	+
Sucrose	+	+
Lactose	+	+
Mannitol	–	–
Xylose	+	+
Hydrolysis of:		
Casein	+	+
Xanthine	–	+
Tyrosine	–	–
Hypoxanthine	–	+
Cell wall containing:		
meso-diaminopimelic		
acid (DAP)	–	–
Galactose	+	+

+, positive; –, negative; V, variable; F, fermentative

TABLE 13-13

ADDITIONAL DIFFERENTIAL CHARACTERISTICS: NOCARDIA, OTHER ACTINOMYCETES, AND RELATED GENERA THAT MAY BE ENCOUNTERED IN THE CLINICAL LABORATORY

GENUS	RELATION TO OXYGEN*	AERIAL MYCELIUM†	CONIDIA	BRANCHING FILAMENTS (MICROSCOPIC)	FRAGMENTATION OF MYCELIA IN OLDER CULTURES§	CATALASE	STRONGLY ACID-FAST**	BOTH PARTIALLY ACID-FAST†† AND ARYLSULFATASE−‡ ARYLSULFATASE+	MOTILITY
Actinomadura	A	+	+	+	−	+	−	−	−
Actinomyces	OA, F, M	−	−	+	−	D¶	−	−	−
Arcanobacterium	A, F	−	−	−	−	−	−	−	−
Bacterionema	A, F	−	−	+	−	+	−	−	−
Bifidobacterium	OA	−	−	−‡	−	−	−	−	−
Corynebacterium	A, F	−	−	−	−	+	−	−	−
Dermatophilus	A, M	−	−	+	−‖	+	−	−	+
Mycobacterium	A	−	−	+‡	−	+	+	+	−
Nocardia	A	+	+	+	+	+	−	−	−
Nocardiopsis	A	+	+	+	D	+	−	−	−
Oerskovia	A, F	−	−	+	+	D	−	−	+
Propionibacterium	OA, F, M	−	−	+‡	−	D	−	−	−
Rhodococcus	A	−	−	+	+	+	−	+	−
Rothia	A, M	−	−	+	+	+	−	−	−
Streptomyces	A	+	+	+	−	+	−	−	−

−, 90% or more of strains negative; +, 90% or more of strains are positive; D, 11%–89% of strains are positive
* Relation to oxygen: A, aerobic; F, facultative anaerobe; M, microaerophilic; OA, obligate anaerobe
† Aerial mycelium: +, produced either persistently or transiently; −, not produced.
‡ Branching filaments (microscopic): The bifurcated cells ordinarily produced by *Bifidobacterium* are not considered to be true branches. Most strains of *Propionibacterium* isolated clinically do not branch; the occasional strains that branch might be confused with *Actinomyces* or *Arachnia*. Most clinically encountered *Mycobacterium* do not branch. However, *M. fortuitum*, a rapid grower, may form branching hyphae and resemble *Nocardia*.
§ Fragmentation of mycelium in older cultures; the filaments tend to break up into short rod or coccoid elements.
¶ *Dermatophilus congloensis*, a skin parasite and agent of exudative dermatitis in animals (rarely in humans), forms mycelial filaments that divide both transversely and longitudinally to form packets of up to eight motile coccoid cells.
‖ D, *Actinomyces viscosus* and two species of nonmedical importance, *A. howelii* and *A. hordeovulneris*, are the only species of *Actinomyces* that are catalase positive.
** *Mycobacterium* species are strongly acid fast when stained with Ziehl-Neelsen, auramine-rhodamine, or modified Kinyoun stains. In contrast, *Nocardia* species and *Rhodococcus* species are only weakly or partially acid fast and stain only with a modified acid-fast stain (see text).
‡ Arylsulfatase test (3 day). See Chapter 17 on the mycobacteria.
(Data from Sneath PHA, Mair NS, Sharpe ME, Holt G: Bergey's Manual of Systematic Bacteriology, vol. 2. Baltimore, Williams & Wilkins, 1986; Buchanan RE, Gibbons NE: Bergey's Manual of Determinative Bacteriology, 8th ed. Baltimore, Williams & Wilkins, 1974; and Rippon JW: Medical Mycology, 2nd ed. Philadelphia, WB Saunders, 1982)

697

The Genus *Dermatophilus*. *D. congloensis* is an interesting actinomycete that causes a pustular, exudative dermatitis known as dermatophiliases (or foot rot; or pitted keratolysis; or streptotrichosis) in many species of animals (including cattle, sheep, horses, goats, deer, swine, squirrels, and domestic cats), and infrequently in humans. The exact mode of transmission is unknown, although most infections occur following direct contact with infected materials, and possibly from the bites of ectoparasites and flying insects. Pathologists may encounter these organisms within hair follicles or keratin layers of the soles of the feet in the forms of masses of non–acid-fast, branching, septate filaments. The branching filaments, which are 0.5 to 1.5 μm in diameter, divide both longitudinally and transversely, forming packets of eight coccoid- or cuboidal-shaped cells (or spores) which become motile.[144,189,270] Cell walls are type III. The organisms are aerobic and grow optimally at 37°C. They form rough, β-hemolytic colonies on horse blood agar, but fail to grow on Sabouraud dextrose agar. Colonies on heart infusion agar are often whitish-gray after 18 to 24 hours of incubation, later becoming orange to yellow with prolonged incubation.[189] The organism ferments glucose, but not xylose, mannitol, lactose, sucrose, or maltose (using CDC fermentation carbohydrate base medium), and are catalase- and urease-positive, but nitrate-negative.[157]

SUSCEPTIBILITY OF *NOCARDIA* AND RELATED BACTERIA TO ANTIMICROBIAL AGENTS

The drugs of choice for treatment of nocardiosis, even in immunosuppressed patients, are still the sulfonamides (e.g., sulfadiazine, sulfisoxazole, and triple-sulfonamide combinations). Despite considerable initial enthusiasm about treatment with the trimethoprim–sulfamethoxazole (TMP–SMX) combination, there have been reports of treatment failure and relapses, and TMP–SMX may not be as effective as a single sulfonamide used alone.[194,270] In vitro studies may be needed to aid in the selection of antimicrobial agents for patients who are hypersensitive to sulfonamides. Minocycline and amikacin look promising in in vitro studies and in limited clinical trials as alternative drugs. Wallace and coworkers found five antibiotic resistance patterns for 95% of 200 *N. asteroides* strains studied.[347] Nineteen percent were of resistance type 5; that is, resistant to cefotaxime and cefamandole (also tobramycin), a drug resistance pattern that is identical for *N. farcinica*. This species often is associated with serious human infections; therefore, a *Nocardia* isolate showing this type 5 drug resistance pattern should be further biochemically characterized.

Pencillin G, the drug of choice for treating actinomycosis (see Chap. 14), is not effective in the treatment of nocardiosis. For treatment of actinomycetoma, either trimethoprim–sulfamethoxazole, or dapsone in combination with streptomycin sulfate has been recommended.[194,270] *Rhodococcus equi* appears to be susceptible to vancomycin, erythromycin, aminoglycosides, and chloramphenicol.[32] However, experience with treatment is very limited. Optimal treatment for dermatophiliases in humans does not appear well established; however, the organism appears susceptible (in vitro) to sulfonamides and other antimicrobial agents.[270]

REFERENCES

1. AGUADO JM, PONTE C, SORIANO F: Bacteriuria with a multiply resistant species of *Corynebacterium* (*Corynebacterium* group D2): An unnoticed cause of urinary tract infection. J Infect Dis 156:144–150, 1987

2. ALTEKRUSE S, HYMAN F, KLONTZ K, ET AL: Foodborne bacterial infections in individuals with the human immunodeficiency virus. South Med J 87:169–173, 1994

3. ALTMAIER KR, SHERMAN DM, SCHELLING SH, ET AL: Osteomyelitis and disseminated infection caused *by Corynebacterium renale* in a goat. J Am Vet Med Assoc 204:934–937, 1994

4. ANDAVOLU RH, JAGADHA V, LUE Y, MCLEAN T: Lung abscess involving *Corynebacterium pseudodiphtheriticum* in a patient with AIDS-related complex. NY State J Med 86:594–596, 1986

5. ANDERSON MD, KENNEDY CA, WALSH TP, BOWLER WA: Prosthetic valve endocarditis due to *Rothia dentocariosa* [letter]. Clin Infect Dis 17:945–946, 1993

6. ANGELES AM, SUGAR AM: Rapid diagnosis of nocardiosis with an enzyme immunoassay. J Infect Dis 155:292–296, 1987

7. ANTOS H, MOLLISON LC, RICHARDS MJ, ET AL: Diphtheria: Another risk of travel. J Infect 25:307–310, 1992

8. APPLEMAN MD, CHERUBIN CE, HESELTINE PN, STRATTON CW: Susceptibility testing of *Listeria monocytogenes*. A reassessment of bactericidal activity as a predictor for clinical outcome. Diagn Microbiol Infect Dis 14:311–317, 1991

9. ARMSTRONG D: *Listeria monocytogenes*. In Mandell GL, Douglas RG Jr, Bennett JE (eds): Principles and Practice of Infectious Diseases (2nd ed.), pp 1177–1182. New York, John Wiley & Sons, 1985

10. ARMSTRONG D: *Listeria monocytogenes*. In Mandell GL, Bennett JE, Dolin R (eds): Principles and Practice of Infectious Diseases, vol 2 (4th ed.), pp 1880–1885. New York, Churchill Livingstone, 1995

11. ARMSTRONG RW, FUNG PC: Brainstem encephalitis (rhombencephalitis) due to *Listeria monocytogenes*: Case report and review. Clin Infect Dis 16:689–702, 1993

12. AUSTIN GE, HILL EO: Endocarditis due to *Corynebacterium* CDC group G2. J Infect Dis 147:1106, 1983

13. AYYAR S, TENDOLKAR U, DEODHAR L: A comparison of three media for isolation of *Nocardia* species from clinical specimens. J Postgrad Med 38:70–72, 1992

14. BADENOCH PR, ADAMS M, COSTER DJ: Corneal virulence, cytopathic effect on human keratocytes and genetic characterization of *Acanthamoeba*. Int J Parasitol 25:229–239, 1995

15. BARKSDALE L: *Corynebacterium diphtheriae* and its relatives. Bacteriol Rev 4:378–422, 1970

16. BARKSDALE L: Identifying *Rothia dentocariosa*. Ann Intern Med 91:786–788, 1979

17. BARKSDALE L, LINDER R, SULEA IT, POLLICE M: Phospholipase D activity of *Corynebacterium pseudotuberculosis* (*Corynebacterium ovis*) and *Corynebacterium ulcerans*, a distinctive marker within the genus *Corynebacterium*. J Clin Microbiol 13:335–343, 1981

18. BARTON MD, GOODFELLOW M, MINNIKIN DE: Lipid composition in the classification of *Rhodococcus equi*. Int J Med Microbiol 272:154–170, 1989

19. BBL: BBL Manual of Products and Laboratory Procedures (5th ed.). Cockeysville MD, Becton Dickinson Microbiology Systems, 1973

20. BECKWITH DG, JAHRE JA, HAGGERTY S: Isolation of *Corynebacterium aquaticum* from spinal fluid of an infant with meningitis. J Clin Microbiol 23:375–376, 1986

21. BEKEMEYER WB, ZIMMERMAN GA: Life-threatening complications associated with *Bacillus cereus* pneumonia. Am Rev Respir Dis 131:466–469, 1985

22. BEN-YAACOB D, WARON M, BOLDUR I, ET AL: Septicemia due to *Corynebacterium haemolyticum*. Isr J Med Sci 20:431–433, 1984

23. BENDINGER B, KROPPENSTEDT RM, KLATTE S, ALTENDORF K: Chemotaxonomic differentiation of coryneform bacteria isolated from biofilters. Int J Syst Bacteriol 42:474–486, 1992

24. BERG R, CHMEL H, MAYO J, ARMSTRONG D: *Corynebacterium equi* infection complicating neoplastic disease. Am J Clin Pathol 68:73–77, 1977

25. BERGDOLL MS: *Bacillus cereus* foodborne disease. Clin Microbiol Newslett 3:85–87, 1981

26. BERNARD K, BELLEFEUILLE M, HOLLIS DG, ET AL: Cellular fatty acid composition and phenotypic and cultural characterization of CDC fermentative coryneform groups 3 and 5. J Clin Microbiol 32:1217–1222, 1994

27. BERNARD KA, BELLEFEUILLE M, EWAN EP: Cellular fatty acid composition as an adjunct to the identification of asporogenous, aerobic gram-positive rods. J Clin Microbiol 29:83–89, 1991

28. BERT F, OUAHES O, LAMBERT-ZECHOVSKY N: Brain abscess due to *Bacillus macerans* following a penetrating periorbital injury. J Clin Microbiol 33:1950–1953, 1995

29. BOC SF, MARTONE JD: Osteomyelitis caused by *Corynebacterium jeikeium* [letter]. J Am Podiatr Med Assoc 85:338–339, 1995

30. BOLLET C, VIGNOLI C, DE MICCO P: Molecular cloning of a specific DNA probe for the identification of *Bacillus licheniformis*. Microbiologica 15:291–295, 1992

31. BORLING SL, KONEMAN EW, HARRIS EE, ALLEN SD: Identification of *Corynebacterium* species with the Rapid Coryne system. Abstr Am Soc Microbiol Gen Meet 93: Abstr C-330, 1993

32. BROWN AE: Other corynebacteria and *Rhodococcus*. In Mandell GL, Bennett JE, Dolin R (eds): Principles and Practice of Infectious Diseases, vol 2 (4th ed.), pp 1872–1880. New York, Churchill Livingstone, 1995

33. BROWN RA, JAND WM, HELLERMEN DV: Pulmonary *Nocardia caviae* infection. Clin Microbiol Newslett 4:65–66, 1982

34. BROWNELL GH, BELCHER KE: DNA probes for the identification of *Nocardia asteroides*. J Clin Microbiol 28:2082–2086, 1990

34a. Bruckner DA, Colonna P: Nomenclature for aerobic and facultative bacteria. Clin Infect Dis 21:263–272, 1995

35. BUTLER WR, AHEARN DG, KILBURN JO: High-performance liquid chromatography of mycolic acids as a tool in the identification of *Corynebacterium*, *Nocardia*, *Rhodococcus*, and *Mycobacterium* species. J Clin Microbiol 23:182–185, 1986

36. BUTLER WR, KILBURN JO, KUBICA GP: High-performance liquid chromatography analysis of mycolic acids as an aid in laboratory identification of *Rhodococcus* and *Nocardia* species. J Clin Microbiol 25:2126–2131, 1987

37. CABANA EM, KELLY WR, DANIEL RC, O'BOYLE D: A case of bovine valvular endocarditis caused by *Corynebacterium pseudodiphtheriticum*. Vet Rec 126:41–42, 1990

38. CARLSON P, EEROLA E, KONTIAINEN S: Additional tests to differentiate *Arcanobacterium haemolyticum* and *Actinomyces pyogenes*. Int J Med Microbiol Virol Parasitol Infect Dis 282:232–236, 1995

39. CARLSON P, KONTIAINEN S: alpha-Mannosidase: A rapid test for identification of *Arcanobacterium haemolyticum* [see comments]. J Clin Microbiol 32:854–855, 1994

40. CARLSON P, KONTIAINEN S, RENKONEN OV: Antimicrobial susceptibility of *Arcanobacterium haemolyticum*. Antimicrob Agents Chemother 38:142–143, 1994

41. CARLSON P, RENKONEN OV, KONTIAINEN S: *Arcanobacterium haemolyticum* and streptococcal pharyngitis. Scand J Infect Dis 26:283–287, 1994

42. CARPENTER JL, BLOM J: *Corynebacterium equi* pneumonia in a patient with Hodgkin's disease. Am Rev Respir Dis 114:235–239, 1976

43. CARSON M, HELLYAR A: Opacification of Middlebrook agar as an aid in distinguishing *Nocardia farcinica* within the *Nocardia asteroides* complex. J Clin Microbiol 32:2270–2271, 1994

44. CASTRO LG, BELDA JUNIOR W, SALEBIAN A, CUCE LC: Mycetoma: A retrospective study of 41 cases seen in Sao Paulo, Brazil, from 1978 to 1989. Mycoses 36:89–95, 1993

45. CAUSEY WA: *Nocardia caviae*: A report of 13 new isolations with clinical correlation. Appl Microbiol 28:193–198, 1974

46. CENTERS FOR DISEASE CONTROL: Reported morbidity and mortality in the United States, 1983: Annual summary. MMWR 32, 1984

47. CENTERS FOR DISEASE CONTROL: *Bacillus cereus*—Maine. MMWR 35:408–410, 1986

48. CENTERS FOR DISEASE CONTROL: CDC Surveillance Summaries. CDC Surveillance Summaries 35, 1986

49. CENTERS FOR DISEASE CONTROL: Summary of notifiable diseases, United States, 1989. MMWR 38:1–59, 1989

50. CENTERS FOR DISEASE CONTROL: CDC Surveillance Summaries, March 1990. MMWR 39(SS-1), 1990

51. CENTERS FOR DISEASE CONTROL: Summary of notifiable diseases, United States, 1994. MMWR 43:1–80, 1994

52. CHARPENTIER E, GERBAUD G, JACQUET C, ET AL: Incidence of antibiotic resistance in *Listeria* species. J Infect Dis 172:277–281, 1995

53. CHAZEN G: *Nocardia*. Infect Control 8:260–263, 1987

54. CHERUBIN CE, APPLEMAN MD, HESELTINE PNR, ET AL: Epidemiological spectrum and current treatment of listeriosis. Rev Infect Dis 13:1108–1114, 1991

55. CHOOROMONEY KN, HAMPSON DJ, EAMENS GJ, TURNER MJ: Analysis of *Erysipelothrix rhusiopathiae* and *Erysipelothrix tonsillarum* by multilocus enzyme electrophoresis. J Clin Microbiol 32:371–376, 1994

56. CHUN J, GOODFELLOW M: A phylogenetic analysis of the genus *Nocardia* with 16S rRNA gene sequences. Int J Syst Bacteriol 45:240–245, 1995

57. CIMOLAI N, ROGERS P, SEEAR M: *Corynebacterium pseudo-diphtheriticum* pneumonitis in a leukaemic child. Thorax 47:838–839, 1992

58. CLARK NM, BRAUN DK, PASTERNAK A, CHENOWETH CE: Primary cutaneous *Nocardia otitidiscaviarum* infection: Case report and review. Clin Infect Dis 20:1266–1270, 1995

59. CLARRIDGE JE: The recognition and significance of *Arcanobacterium haemolyticum*. Clin Microbiol Newslett 11:41–45, 1989

60. CLARRIDGE JE, SPIEGEL CA: *Corynebacterium* and miscellaneous irregular gram-positive rods, *Erysipelothrix*, and *Gardnerella*. In Murray PR, Baron EJ, Pfaller MA, et al (eds): Manual of Clinical Microbiology (6th ed.), pp 357–378. Washington DC, ASM Press, 1995

61. COHEN Y, FORCE G, GROS I, ET AL: *Corynebacterium pseudodiphtheriticum* pulmonary infection in AIDS patients [letter]. Lancet 340:114–115, 1992

62. COLLINS MD: Reclassification of *Bacterionema matruchotii* (Mendel) in the genus *Corynebacterium*, as *Corynebacterium matruchotii* comb. nov. Zentralbl Bakteriol Parasitenkd Infectionskr Hyg Abt 1 Orig C3:364–367, 1982

63. COLLINS MD, BURTON RA, JONES D: *Corynebacterium amycolatum* sp. nov. a new mycolic acid-less *Corynebacterium* species from human skin. FEMS Microbiol Lett 49:349–352, 1988

64. COLLINS MD, CUMMINS CS: Genus *Corynebacterium* Lehmann and Neumann 1896, 350^{AL}. In Sneath PHA, Mair NS, Sharpe ME, et al (eds): Bergey's Manual of Systematic Bacteriology, vol 2, pp 1266–1283. Baltimore, Williams & Wilkins, 1986

65. COLLINS MD, GOODFELLOW M, MINNIKIN DE: Isoprenoid quinones in the classification of coryneform and related bacteria. J Gen Microbiol 110:127–136, 1979

66. COLLINS MD, GOODFELLOW M, MINNIKIN DE, ALDERSON G: Menaquinone composition of mycolic acid-containing actinomycetes and some sporoactinomycetes. J Appl Bacteriol 58:77–86, 1985

67. COLLINS MD, JONES D: Reclassification of *Corynebacterium pyogenes* (Glage) in the genus *Actinomyces*, as *Actinomyces pyogenes* comb.nov. J Gen Microbiol 128:901–903, 1982

68. COLLINS MD, JONES D: *Corynebacterium minutissimum* sp. nov., mon. rev. Int J Syst Bacteriol 33:870–871, 1983

69. COLLINS MD, JONES D, KEDDIE RM, ET AL: Classification of some coryneform bacteria in a new genus *Aureobacterium*. Syst Appl Microbiol 4:236–252, 1983

70. COLLINS MD, JONES D, KROPPENSTEDT RM, SCHLEIFER KH: Chemical studies as a guide to the classification of *Corynebacterium pyogenes* and "*Corynebacterium haemolyticum*." J Gen Microbiol 128:335–341, 1982

71. COLLINS MD, JONES D, SCHOFIELD GM: Reclassification of "*Corynebacterium haemolyticum*" (MacLean, Liebow & Rosenberg) in the genus *Arcanobacterium* gen.nov. as *Arcanobacterium haemolyticum* nom.rev., comb.nov. J Gen Microbiol 128:1279–1281, 1982

72. COLLINS MD, PIROUZ T, GOODFELLOW M, MINNIKIN DE: Distribution of menaquinones in actinomycetes and corynebacteria. J Gen Microbiol 100:221–230, 1977

73. COLT HG, MORRIS JF, MARSTON BJ, SEWELL DL: Necrotizing tracheitis caused by *Corynebacterium pseudodiphtheriticum*: Unique case and review. Rev Infect Dis 13:73–76, 1991

74. CONLY J, STEIN K: Reduction of vitamin K_2 concentrations in human liver associated with the use of broad spectrum antimicrobials. Clin Invest Med 17:531–539, 1994

75. COWLING P, HALL L: *Corynebacterium striatum*: A clinically significant isolate from sputum in chronic obstructive airways disease [letter]. J Infect 26:335–336, 1993

76. COYLE MB, LEONARD RB, NOWOWIEJSKI DJ: Pursuit of the *Corynebacterium striatum* type strain. Int J Syst Bacteriol 43:848–851, 1993

77. COYLE MB, LEONARD RB, NOWOWIEJSKI DJ, ET AL: Evidence of multiple taxa within commercially available reference strains of *Corynebacterium xerosis*. J Clin Microbiol 31:1788–1793, 1993

78. COYLE MB, LIPSKY BA: Coryneform bacteria in infectious diseases: Clinical and laboratory aspects. Clin Microbiol Rev 3:227–246, 1990

79. CRAIG TJ, MAGUIRE FE, WALLACE MR: Tracheobronchitis due to *Corynebacterium pseudodiphtheriticum*. South Med J 84:504–506, 1991

80. CRUICKSHANK JG, GAWLER AH, SHALDON C: *Oerskovia* species: Rare opportunistic pathogens. J Med Microbiol 12:513–515, 1979

81. CUEVAS WA, SONGER JG: *Arcanobacterium haemolyticum* phospholipase D is genetically and functionally similar to *Corynebacterium pseudotuberculosis* phospholipase D. Infect Immun 61:4310–4316, 1993

82. CUMMINGS LA, WU WK, LARSON AM, ET AL: Effects of media, atmosphere, and incubation time on colonial morphology of *Arcanobacterium haemolyticum*. J Clin Microbiol 31:3223–3226, 1993

83. CURRY WA: Human nocardiosis. A clinical review with selected case reports. Arch Intern Med 140:818–826, 1980

84. DALL L, BARNES WG, HURFORD D: Septicaemia in a granulocytopenic patient caused by *Corynebacterium striatum*. Postgrad Med J 65:247–248, 1989

85. DAN M, BERGER SA, LEVO Y, CAMPUS A: *Corynebacterium group* JK septicemia: Community-acquired infection in an apparently immunocompetent patient. Isr J Med Sci 20:1107–1108, 1984

86. DAN M, SOMER I, KNOBEL B, GUTMAN R: Cutaneous manifestations of infection with *Corynebacterium group* JK. Rev Infect Dis 10:1204–1207, 1988

87. DAVEY RT, TAUBER WB: Posttraumatic endophalmitis: The emerging role of *Bacillus cereus* infections. Rev Infect Dis 9:110–123, 1993

88. DE BRIEL D, COUDERC F, RIEGEL P, ET AL: High-performance liquid chromatography of corynomycolic acids as a tool in identification of *Corynebacterium* species and related organisms. J Clin Microbiol 30:1407–1417, 1992

89. DE BRIEL D, LANGS JC, ROUGERON G, ET AL: Multiresistant corynebacteria in bacteriuria: A comparative study of the role of *Corynebacterium* group D2 and *Corynebacterium jeikeium*. J Hosp Infect 17:35–43, 1991

90. DE ZOYSA A, EFSTRATIOU A, GEORGE RC, ET AL: Molecular epidemiology of *Corynebacterium diphtheriae* from northwestern Russia and surrounding countries studied by using ribotyping and pulsed-field gel electrophoresis. J Clin Microbiol 33:1080–1083, 1995

91. DETHY M, HANTSON P, VAN BOSTERHAUT B, ET AL: [Septicemia caused by *Arcanobacterium haemolyticum*

(*Corynebacterium haemolyticum*) and *Streptococcus milleri*]. Acta Clin Belg 41:115–118, 1986

92. DOMINGO P, SERRA J, SAMBEAT MA, AUSINA V: Pneumonia due to *Listeria monocytogenes* [letter; comment]. Clin Infect Dis 14:787–789, 1992

93. DOYLE RJ, KELLER KF, EZZEL JW: *Bacillus*. In Lennette EH, Balows AW, Hausler WJ Jr, et al (eds): Manual of Clinical Microbiolgoy (4th ed.), pp 211–215. Washington DC, American Society for Microbiology, 1985

94. DROBNIEWSKI FA: *Bacillus cereus* and related species. Clin Microbiol Rev 6:324–338, 1993

95. EBERSOLE LL, PATURZO JL: Endophthalmitis caused by *Rhodococcus equi* Prescott serotype 4. J Clin Microbiol 26:1221–1222, 1988

96. ELEK SD: The plate virulence test for diphtheria. J Clin Pathol 2:250–258, 1949

97. ELIAKIM R, SILKOFF P, LUGASSY G, MICHEL J: *Corynebacterium xerosis* endocarditis. Arch Intern Med 143:1995, 1983

98. EMBLEY TM, STACKEBRANDT E: The molecular phylogeny and systematics of the actinomycetes. Annu Rev Microbiol 48:257–289, 1994

99. EMMONS CW, ET AL: Medical Mycology (3rd ed.). Philadelphia, Lea & Febiger, 1977

100. ESTEBAN J, ZAPARDIEL J, SORIANO F: Two cases of soft-tissue infection caused by *Arcanobacterium haemolyticum* [letter]. Clin Infect Dis 18:835–836, 1994

101. EWERT DP, LIEB L, HAYES PS, ET AL: *Listeria monocytogenes* infection and serotype distribution among HIV-infected persons in Los Angeles County, 1985–1992. J Acquir Immune Defic Syndr Hum Retrovirol 8:461–465, 1995

102. FARRAR WE: Serious infections due to "non-pathogenic" organisms of the genus *Bacillus*: Review of their status as pathogens. Am J Med 34:134–141, 1963

103. FEELEY JC, PATTON CM: *Bacillus*. In Lennette EH, Balows A, Hausler WJ Jr, et al (eds): Manual of Clinical Microbiology (3rd ed.), pp 145–149. Washington DC, American Society for Microbiolgoy, 1980

104. FELL HW, NAGINGTON J, NAYLOR GR, OLDS RJ: *Corynebacterium haemolyticum* infections in Cambridgeshire. J Hyg (Lond) 79:269–274, 1977

105. FINEGOLD SM: Anaerobic Bacteria in Human Diseases. New York, Academic Press, 1977

106. FISCHER RA, PETERS G, GEHRMANN J, JURGENS H: *Corynebacterium aquaticum* septicemia with acute lymphoblastic leukemia [letter]. Pediatr Infect Dis J 13:836–837, 1994

107. FITTER WF, DE SA DJ, RICHARDSON H: Chorioamnionitis and funisitis due to *Corynebacterium kutscheri*. Arch Dis Child 54:710–712, 1979

108. FLORES M, DESMOND E: Opacification of Middlebrook agar as an aid in identification of *Nocardia farcinica*. J Clin Microbiol 31:3040–3041, 1993

109. FORD JG, YEATTS RP, GIVNER LB: Orbital cellulitis, subperiosteal abscess, sinusitis, and septicemia caused by *Arcanobacterium haemolyticum*. Am J Ophthalmol 120:261–262, 1995

110. FRASER DT, WELD CB: The intracutaneous "virulence test" for *Corynebacterium diphtheriae*. Trans R Soc Can Sect V 10:343–345, 1926

111. FRAZIER AR, ROSENOW ECD, ROBERTS GD: Nocardiosis. A review of 25 cases occurring during 24 months. Mayo Clin Proc 50:657–663, 1975

112. FRELAND C, FUR JL, NEMIROVSKY-TREBUCQ B, ET AL: Primary cutaneous nocardiosis caused by *Nocardia otitidiscaviarum*: Two cases and a review of the literature. J Trop Med Hyg 98:395–403, 1995

113. FRENEY J, DUPERRON MT, COURTIER C, ET AL: Evaluation of API Coryne in comparison with conventional methods for identifying coryneform bacteria. J Clin Microbiol 29:38–41, 1991

114. FRICCHIONE LF, SEPKOWITZ DV, GRADON JD, BERKOWITZ LB: Pericarditis due to *Bacillus cereus* in an intravenous drug user [letter]. Rev Infect Dis 13:774, 1991

115. FROBISHER M: Cystine-tellurite agar for *C. diphtheriae*. J Infect Dis 60:99–105, 1937

116. FUNKE G, CARLOTTI A: Differentiation of *Brevibacterium* spp. encountered in clinical specimens. J Clin Microbiol 32:1729–1732, 1994

117. FUNKE G, LAWSON PA, BERNARD KA, ET AL: Most *Corynebacterium xerosis* strains identified in the routine clinical laboratory correspond to *Corynebacterium amycolatum*. J Clin Microbiol 34:1124–1128, 1996

118. FUNKE G, LAWSON PA, COLLINS MD: Heterogeneity within human-derived Centers for Disease Control and Prevention (CDC) coryneform group ANF-1-like bacteria and description of *Corynebacterium auris* sp. nov. Int J Syst Bacteriol 45:735–739, 1995

119. FUNKE G, LUCCHINI GM, PFYFFER GE, ET AL: Characteristics of CDC group 1 and group 1-like coryneform bacteria isolated from clinical specimens. J Clin Microbiol 31:2907–2912, 1993

120. FUNKE G, RAMOS CP, FERNANDEZ-GARAYZABAL JF, ET AL: Description of human-derived Centers for Disease Control coryneform group 2 bacteria as *Actinomyces bernardiae* sp. nov. Int J Syst Bacteriol 45:57–60, 1995

121. FUNKE G, STUBBS S, ALTWEGG M, ET AL: *Turicella otitidis* gen. nov., sp. nov., a coryneform bacterium isolated from patients with otitis media. Int J Syst Bacteriol 44:270–273, 1994

122. FUNKE G, STUBBS S, PFYFFER GE, ET AL: Characteristics of CDC group 3 and group 5 coryneform bacteria isolated from clinical specimens and assignment to the genus *Dermabacter*. J Clin Microbiol 32:1223–1228, 1994

123. FUNKE G, STUBBS S, VON GRAEVENITZ A, COLLINS MD: Assignment of human-derived CDC group 1 coryneform bacteria and CDC group 1-like coryneform bacteria to the genus *Actinomyces* as *Actinomyces neuii* subsp. neuii sp. nov., subsp. nov., and *Actinomyces neuii* subsp. anitratus subsp. nov. Int J Syst Bacteriol 44:167–171, 1994

124. FUNKE G, VON GRAEVENITZ A, WEISS N: Primary identification of *Aureobacterium* spp. isolated from clinical specimens as "*Corynebacterium aquaticum*." J Clin Microbiol 32:2686–2691, 1994

125. GARCIA-RODRIGUEZ JA, GARCIA SANCHEZ JE, MUNOZ BELLIDO JL, ET AL: In vitro activity of 79 antimicrobial agents against *Corynebacterium* group D2. Antimicrob Agents Chemother 35:2140–2143, 1991

126. GARDNER SE, PEARSON T, HUGHES WT: Pneumonitis due to *Corynebacterium equi*. Chest 70:92–94, 1976

127. GARRETT MA, HOLMES HT, NOLTE FS: Selective buffered charcoal–yeast extract medium for isolation of nocardiae from mixed cultures. J Clin Microbiol 30:1891–1892, 1992

128. GAVIN SE, LEONARD RB, BRISELDEN AM, COYLE MB: Evaluation of the Rapid CORYNE identification system for *Corynebacterium* species and other coryneforms. J Clin Microbiol 30:1692–1695, 1992

129. GELLIN BG, BROOME CV: Listeriosis [see comments]. JAMA 261:1313–1320, 1989

130. GELLIN BG, BROOME CV, BIBB WF, ET AL: The epidemiology of listeriosis in the United States—1986. Listeriosis Study Group. Am J Epidemiol 133:392–401, 1991

131. GEORGHIOU PR, BLACKLOCK ZM: Infection with *Nocardia* species in Queensland. A review of 102 clinical isolates. Med J Aust 156:692–697, 1992

132. GILBERT RJ, PARRY JM: Serotypes of *Bacillus cereus* from outbreaks of food poisoning and from routine foods. J Hyg 78:69–74, 1977

133. GILL DA: Circling disease: A new meningoencephalitis of sheep in New Zealand, with notes on a new species of pathogenic organism. Vet J 89:258–270, 1933

134. GOLDSTEIN B, ABRUTYN E: Pseudo-outbreak of *Bacillus* species: Related to fibreoptic bronchoscopy. J Hosp Infect 6:194–200, 1985

135. GOLLEDGE C: Vancomycin resistant lactobacilli. J Hosp Infect 11:292–295, 1988

136. GOLUB B, FALK G, SPINK WW: Lung abscess due to *Corynebacterium equi*. Report of first human infection. Ann Intern Med 66:1174–1177, 1967

137. GONZALEZ-OCHOA A: Mycetoma caused by *Nocardia brasiliensis* with a note on the isolation of the causative organism from soil. Lab Invest 11:1118–1123, 1962

138. GOODFELLOW M: Genus *Rhodococcus* Zopf 1891, 28[AL]. In Sneath PHA, Mair NS, Sharpe ME, et al (eds): Bergey's Manual of Systematic Bacteriology, vol 2, pp 1472–1481. Baltimore, Williams & Wilkins, 1986

139. GOODFELLOW M, ALDERSON G: The actinomycete-genus *Rhodococcus*: A home for the "rhodochrous" complex. J Gen Microbiol 100:99–122, 1977

140. GOODFELLOW M, LECHAVALIER MD: Genus *Nocardia* Trevisan 1889 9[AL]. In Sneath PHA, Mair NS, Sharpe E, et al (eds): Bergey's Manual of Systematic Bacteriology, vol 2, pp 1459–1465. Baltimore, Willians & Wilkins, 1986

141. GOODFELLOW M, LECHEVALIER MP: Genus *Nocardia* Trevisan 1889, 9[AL]. In Williams ST, Sharpe ME, Holt JG (eds): Bergey's Manual of Systematic Bacteriology, vol 4, pp 2350–2361. Baltimore, Williams & Wilkins, 1989

142. GOODFELLOW M, WILLIAMS ST: Ecology of actinomycetes. Annu Rev Microbiol 37:189–216, 1983

143. GORBY GL, PEACOCK JE JR: *Erysipelothrix rhusiopathiae* endocarditis: Microbiologic, epidemiologic, and clinical features of an occupational disease. Rev Infect Dis 10:317–325, 1988

144. GORDON MA: Aerobic pathogenic *Actinomycetaceae*. In Lennette EH, Balows A, Hausler B, et al (eds): Manual of Clinical Microbiology (4th ed.), pp 249–262. Washington DC, American Society for Microbiology, 1985

145. GORDON RE, HAYNES WC, PANG CNN: The genus *Bacillus*. US Department of Agriculture, Agriculture Handbook No. 427, 1973

146. GOUDSWAARD J, VAN DE MERWE DW, VAN DER SLUYS P, DOORN H: *Corynebacterium haemolyticum* septicemia in a girl with mononucleosis infectiosa. Scand J Infect Dis 20:339–340, 1988

147. GRASMICK AE, BRUCKNER DA: Comparison of rapid identification method and conventional substrates for identification of *Corynebacterium* group JK isolates. J Clin Microbiol 25:1111–1112, 1987

148. GRAY ML, KILLINGER AH: *Listeria monocytogenes* and listeric infections. Bacteriol Rev 30:309–382, 1966

149. GREENWOOD JR: *Gardnerella vaginalis* infections. In Bottone EJ (ed): Unusual Microorganisms: Gram-Negative Fastidiious Species, pp 87–102. New York, Marcel Decker, 1983

150. GREENWOOD JR, PICKETT MJ: Genus *Gardnerella* Greenwood and Pickett 1980, 170[VP]. In Sneath PHA, Mair NS, Sharpe ME, et al (eds): Bergey's Manual of Systematic Bacteriology, vol 2, pp 1283–1286. Baltimore, Williams & Wilkins, 1986

151. GRIFFITHS JK, DALY JS, DODGE RA: Two cases of endocarditis due to *Lactobacillus* species: Antimicrobial susceptibility, review, and discussion of therapy. Clin Infect Dis 15:250–255, 1992

152. GRUNER E, PFYFFER GE, VON GRAEVENITZ A: Characterization of *Brevibacterium* spp. from clinical specimens. J Clin Microbiol 31:1408–1412, 1993

153. GRUNER E, STEIGERWALT AG, HOLLIS DG, ET AL: Human infections caused by *Brevibacterium casei*, formerly CDC groups B-1 and B-3. J Clin Microbiol 32:1511–1518, 1994

154. GUILLARD F, APPELBAUM PC, SPARROW FB: Pyelonephritis and septicemia due to gram-positive rods similar to *Corynebacterium* group E (aerotolerant *Bifidobacterium adolescentis*). Ann Intern Med 92:635–636, 1980

155. HANDE KR, WITEBSKY FG, BROWN MS, ET AL: Sepsis with a new species of *Corynebacterium*. Ann Intern Med 85:423–426, 1976

156. HOLLICK GE: Isolation and identification of thermophilic actinomycetes associated with hypersensitivity pneumonitis. Clin Microbiol Newslett 8:29–32, 1986

157. HOLLIS DG, WEAVER RE: Gram-positive organisms: A guide to identification. Special Bacteriology Laboratory, pp 1–10. Atlanta, Centers for Disease Control, 1981 (reprinted 1986)

158. HOLT JG, KRIEG NR, SNEATH PHA, ET AL: Bergey's Manual of Determinative Bacteriology (9th ed). Philadelphia, Williams & Wilkins, 1994

159. HOUSE RW, SCHOUSBOE M, ALLEN JP, GRANT CC: *Corynebacterium ovis* (*pseudo-tuberculosis*) lymphadenitis in a sheep farmer: A new occupational disease in New Zealand. NZ Med J 99:659–662, 1986

160. HUSSAIN Z, GONDER JR, LANNIGAN R, STOAKES L: Endophthalmitis due to *Oerskovia xanthineolytica*. Can J Ophthalmol 22:234–236, 1987

161. ISAACSON JH, GRENKO RT: *Rothia dentocariosa* endocarditis complicated by brain abscess. Am J Med 84:352–354, 1988

162. JACKMAN PJH, PITCHER DG, PELCZYNSKA S, BORMAN P: Classification of corynebacteria associated with endocarditis (group JK) as *Corynebacterium jeikeium* sp. nov. Syst Appl Microbiol 9:83–90, 1987

163. JACKSON SG: Rapid screening test for enterotoxin-producing *Bacillus cereus*. J Clin Microbiol 31:972–974, 1993

164. JENSON HB, LEVY SR, DUNCAN C, MCINTOSH S: Treatment of multiple brain abscesses caused by *Bacillus cereus*. Pediatr Infect Dis J 8:795–798, 1989

165. JIMENEZ T, DIAZ AM, ZLOTNIK H: Monoclonal antibodies to *Nocardia asteroides* and *Nocardia brasiliensis* antigens. J Clin Microbiol 28:87–91, 1990

166. JONES D: Genus *Erysipelothrix* Rosenboch 1909. In Sneath PHA, Mair NS, Sharpe ME, et al (eds): Bergey's Manual of Systematic Bacteriology, vol 2, pp 1245–1249. Baltimore, Williams & Wilkins, 1986

167. JONES D, COLLINS MD: Section 15: Irregular, nonsporing gram-positive rods. In Sneath PHA, Mair NS, Sharpe ME, et al (eds): Bergey's Manual of Systematic Bacteriology, vol 2, pp 1261–1434. Baltimore, Williams & Wilkins, 1986

168. JONES EM, MACGOWAN AP: Antimicrobial chemotherapy of human infection due to *Listeria monocytogenes*. Eur J Clin Microbiol Infect Dis 14:165–175, 1995

169. JOSEPHSON SL, THOMASON JL: The role of *Gardnerella vaginalis* in urinary tract infections. Clin Microbiol Newslett 8:42–43, 1986

170. JUCGLA A, SAIS G, CARRATALA J, ET AL: A papular eruption secondary to infection with *Corynebacterium jeikeium*, with histopathological features mimicking botryomycosis. Br J Dermatol 133:801–804, 1995

171. JULAK J, RYSKA M, KORUNA I, MENCIKOVA E: Cellular fatty acids and fatty aldehydes of *Listeria* and *Erysipelothrix*. Int J Med Microbiol 272:171–180, 1989

172. JURTSHUK RJ, BLICK M, BRESSER J, ET AL: Rapid in situ hybridization technique using 16S rRNA segments for detecting and differentiating the closely related gram-positive organisms *Bacillus polymyxa* and *Bacillus macerans*. Appl Environ Microbiol 58:2571–2578, 1992

173. KAILITH EJ, GOLDSTEIN E, WAGNER FH: Case report: Meningitis caused by *Oerskovia xanthineolytica*. Am J Med Sci 295:216–217, 1988

174. KANDLER O, WEISS N: Section 14: Regular, nonsporing gram-positive rods. In Sneath PHA, Mair NS, Sharpe ME, et al (eds): Bergey's Manual of Systematic Bacteriology, vol 2, pp 1208–1260. Baltimore, Williams & Wilkins, 1986

175. KAPLAN A, ISRAEL F: *Corynebacterium aquaticum* infection in a patient with chronic granulomatous disease. Am J Med Sci 296:57–58, 1988

176. KEDDIE RM, SHAW SL: Genus *Kurthia* Trevisan 1885, 92[AL] Nom. cons. Opin. 12 Jed. Comm. 1954, 152. In Sneath PHA, Mair NS, Sharpe ME, et al (eds): Bergey's Manual of Systematic Bacteriology, vol 2, pp 1255. Baltimore, Williams & Wilkins, 1986

177. KELLY MC, SMITH ID, ANSTEY RJ, ET AL: Rapid identification of antibiotic-resistant corynebacteria with the API 20S system. J Clin Microbiol 19:245–247, 1984

178. KERR E, SNELL H, BLACK BL, ET AL: Isolation of *Nocardia asteroides* from respiratory specimens by using selective buffered charcoal–yeast extract agar. J Clin Microbiol 30:1320–1322, 1992

179. KHAVARI PA, BOLOGNIA JL, EISEN R, ET AL: Periodic acid–Schiff-positive organisms in primary cutaneous *Bacillus cereus* infection. Case report and an investigation of the periodic acid–Schiff staining properties of bacteria. Arch Dermatol 127:543–546, 1991

180. KING CT: Sternal wound infection due to *Corynebacterium xerosis* [letter; comment]. Clin Infect Dis 19:1171–1172, 1994

181. KOLL BS, BROWN AE, KIEHN TE, ARMSTRONG D: Disseminated *Nocardia brasiliensis* infection with septic arthritis [see comments]. Clin Infect Dis 15:469–472, 1992

182. KONEMAN EW, ALLEN SD, JANDA WM, ET AL: Color Atlas and Textbook of Diagnostic Microbiology (4th ed.). Philadelphia, JB Lippincott, 1992

183. KORANSKY JR, ALLEN SD, DOWELL VR JR: Use of ethanol for selective isolation of sporeforming microorganisms. Appl Environ Microbiol 35:762–765, 1978

184. KRAMER JM, TURNBULL PCB, MUNSHI G, GILBERT RJ: *Bacillus cereus* and other *Bacillus* species. In Doyle MP (ed): Foodborne Bacterial Pathogens, pp 21–70. New York, Marcel Dekker, 1989

185. KRECH T, HOLLIS DG: *Corynebacterium* and related organisms. In Balows A, Hausler WJ Jr, Herrmann KL, et al (eds): Manual of Clinical Microbiology (5th ed.), pp 277–286. Washington DC, American Society for Microbiology, 1991

186. KRISH G, BEAVER W, SARUBBI F, VERGHESE A: *Corynebacterium xerosis* as a cause of vertebral osteomyelitis. J Clin Microbiol 27:2869–2870, 1989

187. LAFORCE FM: Anthrax. Clin Infect Dis 19:1009–1013; quiz 1014, 1994

188. LAFORCE MF: *Bacillus anthracis* (anthrax). In Mandell GL, Douglas RG, Bennett JE (eds): Principles and Practice of Infectious Diseases (3rd ed.), pp 1593–1595. New York, Churchill Livingstone, 1990

189. LAND G, MCGINNIS MR, STANECK J, GATSON A: Aerobic pathogenic *Actinomycetales*. In Balows A, Hausler WJ Jr, Herrmann KL, et al (eds): Manual of Clinical Microbiology (5th ed.), pp 340–359. Washington DC, American Society for Microbiology, 1991

190. LEBAR WD, PENSLER MI: Pleural effusion due to *Rhodococcus equi* [letter]. J Infect Dis 154:919–920, 1986

191. LECHEVALIER HA, LECHEVALIER MP: Genus *Oerskovia* Prauser, Lechevalier and Lechevalier 1970, 534; emended Lechevalier 1972, 263[AL]. In Sneath PHA, Mair NS, Sharpe ME, et al (eds): Bergey's Manual of Systematic Bacteriology, vol 2, pp 1489–1491. Baltimore, Williams & Wilkins, 1986

192. LENNON D, LEWIS B, MANTELL C, ET AL: Epidemic perinatal listeriosis. Pediatr Infect Dis 3:30–34, 1984

193. LEPROWSE CR, MCNEIL MM, MCCARTY JM: Catheter-related bacteremia caused by *Oerskovia turbata*. J Clin Microbiol 27:571–572, 1989

194. LERNER PI: *Nocardia* species. In Mandell GL, Bennett JE, Dolin R (eds): Principles and Practice of Infectious Diseases, vol 2 (4th ed.), pp 2273–2280. New York, John Wiley & Sons, 1995

195. LESSING MP, CURTIS GD, BOWLER IC: *Listeria ivanovii* infection [letter]. J Infect 29:230–231, 1994

196. LEYDEN JJ, MCGINLEY KJ, HOLZLE E, ET AL: The microbiology of the human axilla and its relationship to axillary odor. J Invest Dermatol 77:413–416, 1981

197. LEYDEN JJ, MCGINLEY KJ, KLIGMAN AM: Tetracycline and minocycline treatment. Arch Dermatol 118:19–22, 1982

198. LINA B, CARLOTTI A, LESAINT V, ET AL: Persistent bacteremia due to *Brevibacterium* species in an immunocompromised patient [letter]. Clin Infect Dis 18:487–488, 1994

199. LINDNER PS, HARDY DJ, MURPHY TF: Endocarditis due to *Corynebacterium pseudodiphtheriticum*. NY State J Med 86:102–104, 1986

200. LINNAN MJ, MASCOLA L, LOU XD, ET AL: Epidemic listeriosis associated with Mexican-style cheese. N Engl J Med 319:823–828, 1988

201. LIPSKY BA, GOLDBERGER AC, TOMPKINS LS, PLORDE JJ: Infections caused by nondiphtheria corynebacteria. Rev Infect Dis 4:1220–1235, 1982

202. LIST N: Validation of the publication of new names and new combinations previously effectively published outside the IJSB. Int J Syst Bacteriol 45:619–620, 1995

203. LOGAN NA, CARMAN JA, MELLING J, BERKELEY RC: Identification of *Bacillus anthracis* by API tests. J Med Microbiol 20:75–85, 1985

204. LORTHOLARY O, BUU-HOI A, FAGON JY, ET AL: Mediastinitis due to multiple resistant *Corynebacterium xerosis* [letter; see comments]. Clin Infect Dis 16:172, 1993

205. LUNGU O, DELLA LATTA P, WEITZMAN I, SILVERSTEIN S: Differentiation of *Nocardia* from rapidly growing *Mycobacterium* species by PCR-RFLP analysis. Diagn Microbiol Infect Dis 18:13–18, 1994

206. MACGREGOR JH, SAMUELSON WM, SANE DC, GODWIN JD: Opportunistic lung infection caused by *Rhodococcus (Corynebacterium) equi*. Radiology 160:83–84, 1986

207. MACGREGOR RR: *Corynebacterium diphtheriae*. In Mandell GL, Bennett JE, Dolin R (eds): Principles and Practice of Infectious Diseases, vol 2 (4th ed.), pp 1865–1872. New York, Churchill Livingstone, 1995

208. MACKENZIE A, FUITE LA, CHAN FT, ET AL: Incidence and pathogenicity of *Arcanobacterium haemolyticum* during a 2-year study in Ottawa. Clin Infect Dis 21:177–181, 1995

209. MANCHEE RJ, BROSTER MG, STAGG AJ, ET AL: Out of Gruinard Island. In Turnbull PCB (ed): Proceedings of the International Workshop on Anthrax, pp 1–105, Salisbury Medical Bulletin, 1990

210. MARTINEZ-MARTINEZ L, SUAREZ AI, ORTEGA MC, RODRIGUEZ-JIMENEZ R: Fatal pulmonary infection caused by *Corynebacterium striatum* [letter]. Clin Infect Dis 19:806–807, 1994

211. MARTINEZ-MARTINEZ L, SUAREZ AI, WINSTANLEY J, ET AL: Phenotypic characteristics of 31 strains of *Corynebacterium striatum* isolated from clinical samples. J Clin Microbiol 33:2458–2461, 1995

212. MCBRIDE ME, ELLNER KM, BLACK HS, ET AL: A new *Brevibacterium* sp. isolated from infected genital hair of patients with white piedra. J Med Microbiol 39:255–261, 1993

213. MCGINLEY KJ, LABOWS JN, ZECHMAN JM, ET AL: Analysis of cellular components, biochemical reactions, and habitat of human cutaneous lipophilic diphtheroids. J Invest Dermatol 85:374–377, 1985

214. MCGOWAN JE JR: JK coryneforms: A continuing problem for hospital infection control. J Hosp Infect 11:358–366, 1988

215. MCNAUGHTON RD, VILLANUEVA RR, DONNELLY R, ET AL: Cavitating pneumonia caused by *Corynebacterium* group JK. J Clin Microbiol 26:2216–2217, 1988

216. MCNEIL MM, BROWN JM: The medically important aerobic actinomycetes: Epidemiology and microbiology. Clin Microbiol Rev 7:357–417, 1994

217. MCNEIL MM, BROWN JM, GEORGHIOU PR, ET AL: Infections due to *Nocardia transvalensis*: Clinical spectrum and antimicrobial therapy. Clin Infect Dis 15:453–463, 1992

218. MCNEIL MM, BROWN JM, JARVIS WR, AJELLO L: Comparison of species distribution and antimicrobial susceptibility of aerobic actinomycetes from clinical specimens. Rev Infect Dis 12:778–783, 1990

219. MCNEIL MM, BROWN JM, SCALISE G, PIERSIMONI C: Nonmycetomic *Actinomadura madurae* infection in a patient with AIDS. J Clin Microbiol 30:1008–1010, 1992

220. MESSINA OD, MALDONADO-COCCO JA, PESCIO A, ET AL: *Corynebacterium kutscheri* septic arthritis [letter]. Arthritis Rheum 32:1053, 1989

221. MIRALLES GD: Disseminated *Nocardia farcinica* infection in an AIDS patient. Eur J Clin Microbiol Infect Dis 13:497–500, 1994

222. MISHRA SK, GORDON RE, BARNETT DA: Identification of nocardiae and streptomycetes of medical importance. J Clin Microbiol 11:728–736, 1980

223. MOFFIE BG, VEENENDAAL RA, THOMPSON J: Native valve endocarditis due to *Corynebacterium* group JK. Neth J Med 37:236–238, 1990

224. MONTEFORTE JS, WOOD CA: Pneumonia caused by *Nocardia nova* and *Aspergillus fumigatus* after cardiac transplantation. Eur J Clin Microbiol Infect Dis 12:112–114, 1993

225. MOORE C, NORTON R: *Corynebacterium aquaticum* septicaemia in a neutropenic patient. J Clin Pathol 48:971–972, 1995

226. MOORE M, PARSONS EI: A study of modified Tinsdale's medium for one primary isolation of *Corynebacterium diphtheriae*. J Infect Dis 102:88–93, 1958

227. MORALES JM, AGUADO JM, DIAZ-GONZALEZ R, ET AL: Alkaline-encrusted pyelitis/cystitis and urinary tract infection due to *Corynebacterium urealyticum*: A new severe complication after renal transplantation. Transplant Proc 24:81–82, 1992

228. MORRIS A, GUILD I: Endocarditis due to *Corynebacterium pseudodiphtheriticum*: Five case reports, review, and antibiotic susceptibilities of nine strains [see comments]. Rev Infect Dis 13:887–892, 1991

229. MULLER F, SCHAAL KP, VON GRAEVENITZ A, ET AL: Characterization of *Rhodococcus equi*-like bacterium isolated from a wound infection in a noncompromised host. J Clin Microbiol 26:618–620, 1988

230. MUNNELLY P, O'BRIEN AA, MOORE DP, ET AL: *Corynebacterium xerosis* septicaemia in a haemodialysis patient. Nephrol Dial Transplant 3:87–88, 1988

231. MURRAY EGD, WEBB RA, SWANN MBR: A disease of rabbits characterized by a large nomonuclear leucocytosis, caused by a hitherto undescribed bacillus, *Bacterium monocytogenes* (n. sp.). J Pathol Bacteriol 29:407–439, 1926

232. MURRAY PR, HEEREN RL, NILES AC: Effect of decontamination procedures on recovery of *Nocardia* spp. J Clin Microbiol 25:2010–2011, 1987

233. MURRAY PR, NILES AC, HEEREN RL: Modified Thayer-Martin medium for recovery of *Nocardia* species from contaminated specimens. J Clin Microbiol 26:1219–1220, 1988

234. NA'WAS TE, HOLLIS DG, MOSS CW, WEAVER RE: Comparison of biochemical, morphologic, and chemical characteristics of Centers for Disease Control fermentative coryneform groups 1, 2, and A-4. J Clin Microbiol 25:1354–1358, 1987

235. NAKA W, MIYAKAWA S, NIIZEKI H, FUKUDA T ET AL: Unusually located lymphocutaneous nocardiosis caused by *Nocardia brasiliensis*. Br J Dermatol 132:609–613, 1995

236. NEUBAUER M, SOUREK J, RYE M, ET AL: *Corynebacterium accolens* sp. nov., a gram-positive rod exhibiting satellitism, from clinical material. Syst Appl Microbiol 14:46–51, 1991

237. NEUMEISTER B, MANDEL T, GRUNER E, PFYFFER GE: *Brevibacterium* species as a cause of osteomyelitis in a neonate. Infection 21:177–178, 1993

238. NIEMAN RE, LORBER B: Listeriosis in adults: A changing pattern. Report of eight cases and review of the literature, 1968–1978. Rev Infect Dis 2:207–227, 1980

239. NOLLA-SALAS J, ANTO JM, ALMELA M, ET AL: Incidence of listeriosis in Barcelona, Spain, in 1990. The Collaborative Study Group of Listeriosis of Barcelona. Eur J Clin Microbiol Infect Dis 12:157–161, 1993

240. NOVAK RM, POLISKY EL, JANDA WM, LIBERTIN CR: Osteomyelitis caused by *Rhodococcus equi* in a renal transplant recipient. Infection 16:186–188, 1988

241. OHL CA, TRIBBLE DR: *Corynebacterium* group D2 infection of a complex renal cyst in a debilitated patient [letter]. Clin Infect Dis 14:1160–1161, 1992

242. PANCOAST SJ, ELLNER PD, JAHRE JA, NEU HC: Endocarditis due to *Kurthia bessonii*. Ann Intern Med 90:936–937, 1979

243. PAPE J, SINGER C, KIEHN TE, ET AL: Infective endocarditis caused by *Rothia dentocariosa*. Ann Intern Med 91:746–747, 1979

244. PASCUAL C, LAWSON PA, FARROW JA, ET AL: Phylogenetic analysis of the genus *Corynebacterium* based on 16S rRNA gene sequences. Int J Syst Bacteriol 45:724–728, 1995

245. PERS C: Infection due to "*Corynebacterium ulcerans,*" producing diphtheria toxin—a case report from Denmark. Acta Pathol Microbiol Immunol Scand [B] 95:361–362, 1987

246. PERS C, KRISTIANSEN JE, JONSSON V, HANSEN NE: *Rothia dentocariosa* septicaemia in a patient with chronic lymphocytic leukaemia and toxic granulocytopenia. Dan Med Bull 34:322–323, 1987

247. PETIT PL, BOK JW, THOMPSON J, ET AL: Native-valve endocarditis due to CDC coryneform group ANF-3: Report of a case and review of corynebacterial endocarditis. Clin Infect Dis 19:897–901, 1994

248. PHILIPPON A, BIMET F: In vitro susceptibility of *Corynebacterium* group D2 and *Corynebacterium jeikeium* to twelve antibiotics. Eur J Clin Microbiol Infect Dis 9:892–895, 1990

249. PINNER RW, SCHUCHAT A, SWAMINATHAN B, ET AL: Role of foods in sporadic listeriosis. II. Microbiologic and epidemiologic investigation. The Listeria Study Group [see comments]. JAMA 267:2046–2050, 1992

250. PORETZ DM: Other *Bacillus* species. In Mandell GL, Douglas RJ Jr, Bennett JE (eds): Principles and Practice of Infectious Diseases (2nd ed.), pp 1184. New York, John Wiley & Sons, 1985

251. PRIEST FG, KAJI DA, ROSATO YB, CANHOS VP: Characterization of *Bacillus thuringiensis* and related bacteria by ribosomal RNA gene restriction fragment length polymorphisms. Microbiology 140:1015–1022, 1994

252. QUINN JP, ARNOW PM, WEIL D, ROSENBLUTH J: Outbreak of JK diphtheroid infections associated with environmental contamination. J Clin Microbiol 19:668–671, 1984

253. RAHMAN M: Chest infection caused by *Lactobacillus casei* ss *rhamnosus*. Br Med J Clin Res Ed 284:471–472, 1982

254. REBOLI AC, FARRAR WE: *Erysipelothrix rhusiopathiae*: An occupational pathogen. Clin Microbiol Rev 2:354–359, 1989

255. REBOLI AC, FARRAR WE: *Erysipelothrix rhusiopathiae*. In Mandell GL, Bennett JE, Dolin R (eds): Principles and Practice of Infectious Diseases, vol 2 (4th ed.), pp 1894–1896. New York, Churchill Livingstone, 1995

256. REDDY CA, KAO M: Value of acid metabolic products in identification of certain corynebacteria. J Clin Microbiol 7:428–433, 1978

257. RELLER LB, MADDOUX GL, ECKMAN MR, PAPPAS G: Bacterial endocarditis caused by *Oerskovia turbata*. Ann Intern Med 83:664–666, 1975

258. RICHARD V, VAN DER AUWERA P, SNOECK R, ET AL: Nosocomial bacteremia caused by *Bacillus* species. Eur J Clin Microbiol Infect Dis 7:783–785, 1988

259. RICHARDS M, HURSE A: *Corynebacterium pseudotuberculosis* abscesses in a young butcher [letter]. Aust NZ J Med 15:85–86, 1985

260. RIEGEL P, DE BRIEL D, PREVOST G, ET AL: Genomic diversity among *Corynebacterium jeikeium* strains and comparison with biochemical characteristics and antimicrobial susceptibilities. J Clin Microbiol 32:1860–1865, 1994

261. RIEGEL P, DE BRIEL D, PREVOST G, ET AL: Taxonomic study of *Corynebacterium* group ANF-1 strains: Proposal of *Corynebacterium afermentans* sp. nov. containing the subspecies *C. afermentans* subsp. *afermentans* subsp. nov. and *C. afermentans* subsp. *lipophilum* subsp. nov. Int J Syst Bacteriol 43:287–292, 1993

262. RIEGEL P, DEBRIEL D, PREVOST G, ET AL: Proposal of *Corynebacterium propinquum* sp. nov. for *Corynebacterium* group ANF-3 strains. FEMS Microbiol Lett 113:229–234, 1993

263. RIEGEL P, RUIMY R, DE BRIEL D, ET AL: *Corynebacterium argentoratense* sp. nov., from the human throat. Int J Syst Bacteriol 45:533–537, 1995

264. RIEGEL P, RUIMY R, DE BRIEL D, ET AL: *Corynebacterium seminale* sp. nov., a new species associated with genital infections in male patients. J Clin Microbiol 33:2244–2249, 1995

265. RIEGEL P, RUIMY R, DE BRIEL D, ET AL: Genomic diversity and phylogenetic relationships among lipid-requiring diphtheroids from humans and characterization of *Corynebacterium macginleyi* sp. nov. Int J Syst Bacteriol 45:128–133, 1995

266. RIEGEL P, RUIMY R, DE BRIEL D, ET AL: Taxonomy of *Corynebacterium diphtheriae* and related taxa, with recognition of *Corynebacterium ulcerans* sp. nov. nom. rev. FEMS Microbiol Lett 126:271–276, 1995

267. RIHS JD, MCNEIL MM, BROWN JM, YU VL: *Oerskovia xanthineolytica* implicated in peritonitis associated with peritoneal dialysis: Case report and review of *Oerskovia* infections in humans. J Clin Microbiol 28:1934–1937, 1990

268. RILEY PS, HOLLIS DG, UTTER GB, ET AL: Characterization and identification of 95 diphtheroid (group JK) cultures isolated from clinical specimens. J Clin Microbiol 9: 418–424, 1979

269. RIPPON JSW: Nocardiosis. In Medical Mycology: The Pathogenic Fungi and the Pathogenic Actinomycetes (3rd ed.), pp 53–68. Philadelphia, WB Saunders, 1988

270. RIPPON JW: Medical Mycology: The Pathogenic Fungi and the Pathogenic Actinomycetes (3rd ed.). Philadelphia, WB Saunders, 1988

271. RITTER E, KASCHNER A, BECKER C, ET AL: Isolation of *Arcanobacterium haemolyticum* from an infected foot wound [letter]. Eur J Clin Microbiol Infect Dis 12: 473–474, 1993

272. ROBERTS GD: Mycobacteria and *Nocardia*. In Washington JA II (ed): Laboratory Procedures in Clinical Microbiology (2nd ed.). New York, Springer-Verlag, 1985

273. ROBINSON RG, DICKIE AS, ROSE TF, STAPLETON AMF: Struvite renal calculi caused by *Corynebacterium* group D2. Aust NZ J Surg 65:294–295, 1995

274. RUBEN SJ: *Rothia dentocariosa* endocarditis. West J Med 159:690–691, 1993

275. RUFAEL DW, COHN SE: Native valve endocarditis due to *Corynebacterium striatum*: Case report and review [see comments]. Clin Infect Dis 19:1054–1061, 1994

276. RUIMY R, BOIRON P, BOIVIN V, CHRISTEN R: A phylogeny of the genus *Nocardia* deduced from the analysis of small-subunit ribosomal DNA sequences, including transfer of *Nocardia amarae* to the genus *Gordona* as *Gordona amarae* comb. nov. FEMS Microbiol Lett 123: 261–267, 1994

277. RUIMY R, RIEGEL P, BOIRON P, ET AL: Phylogeny of the genus *Corynebacterium* deduced from analyses of small-subunit ribosomal DNA sequences. Int J Syst Bacteriol 45:740–746, 1995

278. RUTALA WA, SAVITEER SM, THOMANN CA, WILSON MB: Plaster-associated *Bacillus cereus* wound infection. A case report. Orthopedics 9:575–577, 1986

279. RYAN M, MURRAY PR: Prevalence of *Corynebacterium urealyticum* in urine specimens collected at a university-affiliated medical center. J Clin Microbiol 32:1395–1396, 1994

280. SACHS MK: Lymphocutaneous *Nocardia brasiliensis* infection acquired from a cat scratch: Case report and review. Clin Infect Dis 15:710–711, 1992

281. SANE DC, DURACK DT: Infection with *Rhodococcus equi* in AIDS [letter]. N Engl J Med 314:56–57, 1986

282. SAVDIE E, PIGOTT P, JENNIS F: Lung abscess due to *Corynebacterium equi* in a renal transplant recipient. Med J Aust 1:817–819, 1977

283. SCHIFF MJ, KAPLAN MH: *Rothia dentocariosa* pneumonia in an immunocompromised patient. Lung 165:279–282, 1987

284. SCHIFF TA, GOLDMAN R, SANCHEZ M, ET AL: Primary lymphocutaneous nocardiosis caused by an unusual species of *Nocardia*: *Nocardia transvalensis*. J Am Acad Dermatol 28:336–340, 1993

285. SCHIFF TA, MCNEIL MM, BROWN JM: Cutaneous *Nocardia farcinica* infection in a nonimmunocompromised patient: Case report and review. Clin Infect Dis 16:756–760, 1993

286. SCHLECH WFD, LAVIGNE PM, BORTOLUSSI RA, ET AL: Epidemic listeriosis—evidence for transmission by food. N Engl J Med 308:203–206, 1983

287. SCHUCHAT A, DEAVER KA, WENGER JD, ET AL: Role of foods in sporadic listeriosis. I. Case–control study of dietary risk factors. The Listeria Study Group [see comments]. JAMA 267:2041–2045, 1992

288. SCHUCHAT A, SWAMINATHAN B, BROOME CV: Epidemiology of human listeriosis [published erratum appears in Clin Microbiol Rev 1991 Jul;4(3):396]. Clin Microbiol Rev 4:169–183, 1991

289. SEELIGER HPR, JONES D: Genus *Listeria* Pirie 1940, 383[AL]. In Sneath Ph, Mair NS, Sharpe ME, et al (eds): Bergey's Manual of Systemic Bacteriology, vol 2 (8th ed.), pp 1235–1245. Baltimore, Williams & Wilkins, 1986

290. SEWELL DL, COYLE MB, FUNKE G: Prosthetic valve endocarditis caused by *Corynebacterium afermentans* subsp. *lipophilum* (CDC coryneform group ANF-1). J Clin Microbiol 33:759–761, 1995

291. SHARPE ME, HILL LR, LAPAGE SP: Pathogenic lactobacilli. J Med Microbiol 6:281–286, 1973

292. SHAWAR RM, MOORE DG, LAROCCO MT: Cultivation of *Nocardia* spp. on chemically defined media for selective recovery of isolates from clinical specimens. J Clin Microbiol 28:508–512, 1990

293. SIMMONS BP, GELFAND MS, ROBERTS GD: *Nocardia otitidiscaviarum* (*caviae*) infection in a heart transplant patient presented as having a thigh abscess (Madura thigh). J Heart Lung Transplant 11:824–826, 1992

294. SIVALINGAM JJ, MARTIN P, FRAIMOW HS, ET AL: *Listeria monocytogenes* peritonitis: Case report and literature review. Am J Gastroenterol 87:1839–1845, 1992

295. SKOGBERG K, SYRJANEN J, JAHKOLA M, ET AL: Clinical presentation and outcome of listeriosis in patients with and without immunosuppressive therapy [see comments]. Clin Infect Dis 14:815–821, 1992

296. SLIFKIN M, GIL GM, ENGWALL C: Rapid identification of group JK and other corynebacteria with the Minitek system. J Clin Microbiol 24:177–180, 1986

297. SLIMAN R, REHM S, SHLAES DM: Serious infections caused by *Bacillus* species. Medicine 66:218–223, 1987

298. SMEGO RA JR, GALLIS HA: The clinical spectrum of *Nocardia brasiliensis* infection in the United States. Rev Infect Dis 6:164–180, 1984

299. SMITH NR, GORDON RE, CLARK FE: Aerobic spore forming bacteria. US Department of Agriculture Monograph 16. Washington DC, Government Printing Office, 1952

300. SNEATH PHA: Endospore forming gram positive rods and cocci. In Sneath PHA, Mair NS, Sharpe ME (eds): Bergey's Manual of Systematic Bacteriology, vol 2, pp 1104–1105. Baltimore, Williams & Wilkins, 1986

301. SNEATH PHA, MAIR NS, SHARPE ME, HOLTE JG: Bergey's Manual of Systematic Bacteriology, vol 2. Baltimore, Williams & Wilkins, 1986

302. SOFRAS F, YIANNOPOULOU K, KOSTAKOPOULOS A, DIMOPOULOS C: *Corynebacterium*-induced cystitis with mucosal incrustations. J Urol 139:810, 1988

303. SORIANO F, AGUADO JM, PONTE C, ET AL: Urinary tract infection caused by *Corynebacterium* group D2: Report of 82 cases and review. Rev Infect Dis 12:1019–1034, 1990

304. SORIANO F, FERNANDEZ-ROBLAS R, ZAPARDIEL J, ET AL: Increasing incidence of *Corynebacterium* group D2 strains resistant to norfloxacin and ciprofloxacin [letter]. Eur J Clin Microbiol Infect Dis 8:1117–1118, 1989

305. SORIANO F, PONTE C: A case of urinary tract infection caused by *Corynebacterium urealyticum* and coryneform group F1. Eur J Clin Microbiol Infect Dis 11:626–628, 1992

306. SORIANO F, PONTE C, SANTAMARIA M, ET AL: *Corynebacterium* group D2 as a cause of alkaline-encrusted cystitis: Report of four cases and characterization of the organisms. J Clin Microbiol 21:788–792, 1985

307. SORIANO F, RODRIGUEZ-TUDELA JL, FERNANDEZ-ROBLAS R, ET AL: Skin colonization by *Corynebacterium* groups D2 and JK in hospitalized patients. J Clin Microbiol 26:1878–1880, 1988

308. SORIANO F, ZAPARDIEL J, NIETO E: Antimicrobial susceptibilities of *Corynebacterium* species and other non–spore-forming gram-positive bacilli to 18 antimicrobial agents. Antimicrob Agents Chemother 39:208–214, 1995

309. SOTO A, ZAPARDIEL J, SORIANO F: Evaluation of API Coryne system for identifying coryneform bacteria. J Clin Pathol 47:756–759, 1994

310. SOTTNEK FO, BORWN JM, WEAVER RE, ET AL: Recognition of *Oerskovia* species in the clinical laboratory: Characterization of 35 isolates. Int J Syst Bacteriol 27:263–270, 1977

311. STAMM AM, DISMUKES WE, SIMMONS BP, ET AL: Listeriosis in renal transplant recipients: Report of an outbreak and review of 102 cases. Rev Infect Dis 4:665–682, 1982

312. STAMM WE: Other corynebacteria. In Mandell GL, Douglas RF, Jr, Bennet JE (eds): Principles and Practice of Infectious Diseases (2nd ed.), pp 1174–1177. New York, John Wiley & sons, 1985

313. STEEN MK, BRUNO-MURTHA LA, CHAUX G, ET AL: *Bacillus cereus* endocarditis: Report of a case and review. Clin Infect Dis 14:945–946, 1992

314. STEINGRUBE VA, BROWN BA, GIBSON JL, ET AL: DNA amplification and restriction endonuclease analysis for differentiation of 12 species and taxa of *Nocardia*, including recognition of four new taxa within the *Nocardia asteroides* complex. J Clin Microbiol 33:3096–3101, 1995

315. STEWART RG, NOWBATH V, CARMICHAEL M, KLUGMAN KP: *Corynebacterium* group D2 urinary tract infection. S Afr Med J 83:95–96, 1993

316. SUDDUTH EJ, ROZICH JD, FARRAR WE: *Rothia dentocariosa* endocarditis complicated by perivalvular abscess. Clin Infect Dis 17:772–775, 1993

317. SUGAR AM, MCCLOSKEY RV: *Bacillus licheniformis* sepsis. JAMA 238:1180–1181, 1977

318. SUSSMAN JI, BARON EJ, GOLDBERG SM, ET AL: Clinical manifestations and therapy of *Lactobacillus* endocarditis: Report of a case and review of the literature. Rev Infect Dis 8:771–776, 1986

319. SUZUKI Y, TOYAMA K, UTSUGI K, ET AL: Primary lymphocutaneous nocardiosis due to *Nocardia otitidiscaviarum*: The first case report from Japan. J Dermatol 22:344–347, 1995

320. SWAMINATHAN B, ROCOURT J, BILLE J: *Listeria*. In Murray PR, Baron EJ, Pfaller MA, et al (eds): Manual of Clinical Microbiology (6th ed.), pp 341–348. Washington DC, ASM Press, 1995

321. SWENSON MM, FACKLAM RR, THORNSBERRY C: Antimicrobial susceptibility of vancomycin-resistant *Leuconostoc*, *Pediococcus* and *Lactobacillus* species. Antimicrob Agents Chemother 34:543–549, 1990

322. TAKAGI H, SHIDA O, KADOWAKI K, ET AL: Characterization of *Bacillus brevis* with descriptions of *Bacillus migulanus* sp. nov., *Bacillus choshinensis* sp. nov., *Bacillus parabrevis* sp. nov., and *Bacillus galactophilus* sp. nov. Int J Syst Bacteriol 43:221–231, 1993

323. TAKAHASHI T, FUJISAWA T, TAMURA Y, ET AL: DNA relatedness among *Erysipelothrix rhusiopathiae* strains representing all twenty-three serovars and *Erysipelothrix tonsillarum*. Int J Syst Bacteriol 42:469–473, 1992

324. TASMAN A, BRANWYK AC: Experiments on metabolism with diphtheria bacillus. J Infect Dis 63:10–20, 1938

325. TELANDER B, LERNER R, PALMBLAD J, RINGERTZ O: *Corynebacterium* group JK in a hematological ward: Infections, colonization and environmental contamination. Scand J Infect Dis 20:55–61, 1988

326. TENDLER C, BOTTONE EJ: *Corynebacterium aquaticum* urinary tract infection in a neonate, and concepts regarding the role of the organism as a neonatal pathogen. J Clin Microbiol 27:343–345, 1989

327. TERRANOVA W, BLAKE PA: *Bacillus cereus* food poisoning. N Engl J Med 298:143–144, 1978

328. TIGHT RR, BARTLETT MS: Actinomycetoma in the United States. Rev Infect Dis 3:1139–1150, 1981

329. TOPALOVSKI M, YANG SS, BOONPASAT Y: Listeriosis of the placenta: Clinicopathologic study of seven cases. Am J Obstet Gynecol 169:616–620, 1993

330. TSUKAMURA M, HIKOSAKA K, NISHIMURA K, HARA S: Severe progressive subcutaneous abscesses and necrotizing tenosynovitis caused by *Rhodococcus aurantiacus*. J Clin Microbiol 26:201–205, 1988

331. TSUKAMURA M, KAWAKAMI K: Lung infection caused by *Gordona aurantiaca* (*Rhodococcus aurantiacus*). J Clin Microbiol 16:604–607, 1982

332. TSUKAMURA M, KOMATSUZAKI C, SAKAI R, ET AL: Mesenteric lymphadenitis of swine caused by *Rhodococcus sputi*. J Clin Microbiol 26:155–157, 1988

333. TUAZON CU, MURRAY HW, LEVY C, ET AL: Serious infections from *Bacillus* sp. JAMA 241:1137–1140, 1979

334. TUMBARELLO M, TACCONELLI E, DEL FORNO A, ET AL: *Corynebacterium striatum* bacteremia in a patient with AIDS [letter]. Clin Infect Dis 18:1007–1008, 1994

335. TURETT GS, FAZAL BA, JOHNSTON BE, TELZAK EE: Liver abscess due to *Corynebacterium jeikeium* in a patient with AIDS [letter]. Clin Infect Dis 17:514–515, 1993

336. TURNBULL PCB, KRAMER JM: *Bacillus*. In Balows A, Hausler WJ Jr, Herrmann KL, et al (eds): Manual of Clinical Microbiology (5th ed.), pp 296–303. Washington DC, American Society for Microbiology, 1991

337. VAN ETTA LL, FILICE GA, FERGUSON RM, GERDING DN: *Corynebacterium equi*: A review of 12 cases of human infection. Rev Infect Dis 5:1012–1018, 1983

338. VANBOSTERHAUT B, SURMONT I, VANDEVEN J, ET AL: *Corynebacterium jeikeium* (group JK diphtheroids) endocarditis. A report of five cases. Diag Microbiol Infect Dis 12:265–268, 1989

339. VANDERSTIGEL M, LECLERCQ R, BRUN-BUISSON C, ET AL: Blood-borne pulmonary infection with *Nocardia asteroides* in a heroin addict. J Clin Microbiol 23:175–176, 1986

340. VENDITTI M, GELFUSA V, TARASI A, ET AL: Antimicrobial susceptibilities of *Erysipelothrix rhusiopathiae*. Antimicrob Agents Chemother 34:2038–2040, 1990

341. VICKERS RM, RIHS JD, YU VL: Clinical demonstration of isolation of *Nocardia asteroides* on buffered charcoal–yeast extract media [published erratum appears in J Clin Microbiol 1992 Jul;30(7):1905]. J Clin Microbiol 30:227–228, 1992

342. VON GRAEVENITZ A, OSTERHOUT G, DICK J: Grouping of some clinically relevant gram-positive rods by automated fatty acid analysis: Diagnostic implications. APMIS 99:147–154, 1991

343. VON GRAEVENITZ A, PUNTER V, GRUNER E, ET AL: Identification of coryneform and other gram-positive rods with several methods. APMIS 102:381–389, 1994

344. WALKDEN D, KLUGMAN KP, VALLY S, NAIDOO P: Urinary tract infection with *Corynebacterium urealyticum* in South Africa. Eur J Clin Microbiol Infect Dis 12:18–24, 1993

345. WALLACE RJ JR, BROWN BA, BLACKLOCK Z, ET AL: New *Nocardia* taxon among isolates of *Nocardia brasiliensis* associated with invasive disease. J Clin Microbiol 33:1528–1533, 1995

346. WALLACE RJ JR, BROWN BA, TSUKAMURA M, ET AL: Clinical and laboratory features of *Nocardia nova*. J Clin Microbiol 29:2407–2411, 1991

347. WALLACE RJ JR, TSUKAMURA M, BROWN BA, ET AL: Cefotaxime-resistant *Nocardia asteroides* strains are isolates of the controversial species *Nocardia farcinica*. J Clin Microbiol 28:2726–2732, 1990

348. WALLET F, MARQUETTE CH, COURCOL RJ: Multiresistant *Corynebacterium xerosis* as a cause of pneumonia in a patient with acute leukemia [letter; see comments]. Clin Infect Dis 18:845–846, 1994

349. WATERS BL: Pathology of culture-proven JK *Corynebacterium pneumonia*. An autopsy case report. Am J Clin Pathol 91:616–619, 1989

350. WATKINS DA, CHAHINE A, CREGER RJ, ET AL: *Corynebacterium striatum*: A diphtheroid with pathogenic potential. Clin Infect Dis 17:21–25, 1993

351. WEAVER RE: *Erysipelothrix*. In Lennette EH, Balows A, Hausler WJ Jr, et al (eds): Manual for Clinical Microbiology (4th ed.). Washington DC, American Society for Microbiology, 1985

352. WEERSINK AJ, ROZENBERG-ARSKA M, WESTERHOF PW, VERHOEF J: *Rothia dentocariosa* endocarditis complicated by an abdominal aneurysm [letter]. Clin Infect Dis 18:489–490, 1994

353. WEISSE ME, BASS JW, JARRETT RV, VINCENT JM: Nonanthrax *Bacillus* infections of the central nervous system. Pediatr Infect Dis J 10:243–246, 1991

354. WELLER PF, NICHOLSON A, BRASLOW N: The spectrum of *Bacillus* bacteremias in heroin addicts. Arch Intern Med 139:293–294, 1979

355. WELLER TM, SMITH PM, CROOK DW: *Corynebacterium jeikeium* osteomyelitis following total hip joint replacement [letter]. J Infect 29:113–114, 1994

356. WIGGINS GL, SOTTNEK FO, HERMANN G: Diptheria and other corynebacterial infections. In Balows A, Hausler WJ Jr (eds): Diagnostic Procedures for Bacterial, Mycotic and Parasitic Infections (6th ed.). Washington DC, American Public Health Association, 1981

357. WILHELMUS KR, ROBINSON NM, JONES DB: *Bacterionema matruchotii* ocular infections. Am J Ophthalmol 87:143–147, 1979

358. WILLIAMS DY, SELEPAK ST, GILL VJ: Identification of clinical isolates of nondiphtherial *Corynebacterium* species and their antibiotic susceptibility patterns. Diagn Microbiol Infect Dis 17:23–28, 1993

359. WILSON IG: Occurrence of *Listeria* species in ready to eat foods. Epidemiol Infect 115:519–526, 1995

360. WINN WC JR, KISSANE JM: Bacterial diseases. In Damjanov I, Linder J (eds): Anderson's Pathology, vol 1 (10th ed.), pp 747–842. St. Louis, Mosby, 1996

361. WINSLOW DL, STEELE ML: *Listeria* bacteremia and peritonitis associated with a peritoneovenous shunt: Successful treatment with sulfamethoxazole and trimethoprim. J Infect Dis 149:820, 1984

362. WONG MT, DOLAN MJ: Significant infections due to *Bacillus* species following abrasions associated with motor vehicle-related trauma. Clin Infect Dis 15:855–857, 1992

363. WORTHINGTON MG, DALY BD, SMITH FE: *Corynebacterium hemolyticum* endocarditis on a native valve. South Med J 78:1261–1262, 1985

364. WUST J, LANZENDORFER H, VON GRAEVENITZ A, ET AL: Peritonitis caused by *Actinomadura madurae* in a patient on CAPD [letter]. Eur J Clin Microbiol Infect Dis 9:700–701, 1990

365. YASSIN AF, BRZEZINKA H, SCHAAL KP, HG ET AL: Menaquinone composition in the classification and identification of aerobic actinomycetes. Zentralbl Bakteriol Mikrobiol Hyg [A] 267:339–356, 1988

366. YOSHIDA M, SUGIYAMA Y, HARADA M, ET AL: Lymphocutaneous nocardiosis with multiple subcutaneous nodules distributed over the extensor aspect of the forearm. Report of a case. Acta Derm Venereol 74:447–448, 1994

THE ANAEROBIC BACTERIA

RELATION OF BACTERIA TO OXYGEN

Although defined in various ways by different authors, a practical working definition is that the **obligately anaerobic bacteria** are those bacteria that grow in the absence of free oxygen but fail to multiply in the presence of oxygen on the surface of nutritionally adequate solid media incubated in room air or in a CO_2 incubator (containing 5% to 10% CO_2 in air). The amount of O_2 in a CO_2 incubator, or in a candle extinction jar, is considerable (about 18% to 19%). In practice, anaerobic bacteria are most often recognized in the clinical laboratory following aerotolerance tests of colonies that grew on primary isolation plates incubated anaerobically (see later discussion). Thus, most anaerobes iden-

Color Plates for Chapter 14 are found between pages 784 and 785.

tified in the clinical laboratory grow initially on anaerobe blood agar, on one of the selective anaerobic media, or in an enrichment broth incubated anaerobically but not on blood agar or chocolate agar plates incubated aerobically or in a CO_2 incubator.

It is an oversimplification to discuss the anaerobes as if they uniformly fit into one large group, just as it is an oversimplification (and incorrect) to refer to all bacteria that grow in room air as aerobes. Thus, several terms, including *obligate aerobe, facultative anaerobe, microaerophile, aerotolerant anaerobe,* and *obligate anaerobe* (strict and moderate), have been used to subdivide bacteria based on their relation to oxygen. These terms reflect a continuous spectrum of bacteria, from those that cannot tolerate oxygen to those that require it for growth.

Obligate aerobes, including species of *Micrococcus* and *Pseudomonas,* require molecular oxygen as a terminal electron acceptor, resulting in the formation of water and do not obtain energy by fermentative pathways. However, it is not uncommon to find *P. aeruginosa* growing scantily on anaerobically incubated media in the clinical laboratory because these bacteria can use nitrate in the medium as a terminal electron acceptor (through anaerobic respiration) in place of O_2. In contrast, molecular oxygen varies in its toxicity for different species of anaerobic bacteria, and it is not a terminal electron acceptor for these bacteria. In general, the clinically important anaerobes obtain their energy through fermentative pathways in which organic compounds, such as organic acids, alcohols, and other products, serve as final electron acceptors.

Anaerobes, on the other hand, are divided into two major groups: the obligate anaerobes (defined previously) and the aerotolerant anaerobes. The obligate anaerobes have been further subdivided into two groups based on their ability to grow in the presence of or to tolerate oxygen. Strict obligate anaerobes are not capable of growth on agar surfaces exposed to O_2 levels higher than 0.5%. Atmospheric oxygen is highly toxic for these organisms for reasons that are not entirely known. Examples of these bacteria include *Clostridium haemolyticum, C. novyi* type B, *Selenomonas ruminatium,* and *Treponema denticola.* The second group of obligate anaerobes, the moderate obligate anaerobes, are bacteria that can grow when exposed to oxygen levels ranging from about 2% to 8% (average 3%). Examples of these bacteria include members of the *Bacteroides fragilis* and the pigmented *Prevotella–Porphyromonas* groups (formerly called the pigmented *Bacteroides* group), *Fusobacterium nucleatum,* and *C. perfringens.*[116]

The term *aerotolerant anaerobe* is used by some microbiologists to describe anaerobic bacteria that will show limited or scant growth on agar in room air or in a 5% to 10% CO_2 incubator but show good growth under anaerobic conditions. Examples of these bacteria include *Clostridium carnis, C. histolyticum,* and *C. tertium.* Most of the anaerobes isolated from properly selected and collected specimens in the clinical laboratory fit into the moderate obligate anaerobe category. These organisms are more tolerant to the toxic effects of oxygen than the strict obligate anaerobes but are still killed by oxygen, unless anaerobic conditions are maintained properly during specimen collection and transport to the laboratory and during the steps required for processing of specimens and isolation and identification, as discussed in later sections of the chapter. Strict obligate anaerobes are rare in infections of humans, but both the moderate and the strict obligate anaerobes are found in a variety of nonpathogenic habitats (e.g., feces and the oropharynx) as part of the normal flora.

The facultative anaerobes (e.g., *Escherichia coli* and *Staphylococcus aureus*) grow under either aerobic or anaerobic conditions. They use oxygen as a terminal electron acceptor or, less efficiently, can obtain their energy through fermentation reactions under anaerobic conditions. Grown aerobically, facultative anaerobes obtain much more energy (38 ATP) when they completely catabolize a molecule of glucose to CO_2 and H_2O, than when grown anaerobically. Under anaerobic conditions, fermentative metabolism of the glucose molecule yields only two to three ATP.[34]

The microaerophiles require oxygen as a terminal electron acceptor, yet these bacteria do not grow on the surface of solid media in an aerobic incubator (21% O_2) and grow minimally if at all under anaerobic conditions. An example of a microaerophile is *Campylobacter jejuni,* which grows optimally in 5% O_2 (the gas mixture of the incubation environment commonly used for recovering this organism in clinical laboratories is 5% O_2, 10% CO_2, and 85% N_2).

Through the years, bacteriologists working on the development of improved media and systems for cultivation of anaerobes have focused on two fundamental limiting factors that may affect the growth of anaerobes. The first and most important of these is the inhibitory effects of atmospheric oxygen and its toxic derivatives. The second limiting factor of concern is the oxidation–reduction potential (E_h) of the culture medium.

OXYGEN TOLERANCE

Some of the strictest obligate anaerobes (e.g., *Clostridium haemolyticum* and *C. novyi* type B) are killed when exposed to atmospheric oxygen on the open laboratory bench for 10 minutes or longer. On the other hand, most of the moderate obligate anaerobes encountered in human infections tolerate exposure to oxygen for longer times. The reasons anaerobes vary in their tolerance to oxygen are probably multiple, but one idea is that the oxygen tolerance of many moderate obligate anaerobes depends on their production of superoxide dismutase, catalases, and possibly peroxidase enzymes that are protective against toxic oxygen reduction products.[28,34,76,84,136,166,197]

A popular notion is that exposure to atmospheric O_2 results in a series of reactions within the bacterial cells, possibly reactions mediated by flavoproteins, which result in production of the negatively charged superoxide radical (O_2^-), hydrogen peroxide (H_2O_2), and other toxic oxygen reduction products.[28,136] The superoxide anion and H_2O_2 may react together to produce free hydroxyl radicals (OH·), the most powerful biologic oxidants known, and there may also be the production of toxic singlet oxygen ($^1O_2$) through the reaction of superoxide anions with free hydroxyl radicals. Superoxide dismutase catalyzes the conversion of superoxide radicals to less toxic hydrogen peroxide and molecular oxygen. Catalase catalyzes the conversion of hydrogen peroxide to form water and oxygen. Several species of oxygen-tolerant, moderate obligate anaerobes produce superoxide dismutase (SOD), and the level of SOD produced correlates with the level of oxygen tolerance and virulence of the organism.[197] In another study, several strains of the genus *Bacteroides*, several anaerobic cocci, anaerobic non–spore-forming gram-positive rods, and clostridia produced SOD, but no correlation was found between the source of the organism, the presumed level of pathogenicity, and the SOD level produced.[76] Several species of anaerobes produce catalase (e.g., members of the *Bacteroides fragilis* group, *Propionibacterium acnes*, and others), as well as SOD, but some anaerobes that are relatively oxygen tolerant or aerotolerant (e.g., *Clostridium tertium*) produce neither SOD nor catalase. Rolfe and coworkers observed that the degree of oxygen tolerance of anaerobic bacteria is related to the proportion of the bacterial cells in the population that survive following exposure to oxygen.[167] In practice, it is often essential to use large inocula when inoculating or subculturing anaerobic culture media, which probably serves to minimize the harmful effects of multiple toxic oxygen growth-limiting factors. Clearly, much more work is needed on the mechanisms of oxygen tolerance and intolerance of anaerobic bacteria.

OXIDATION–REDUCTION POTENTIAL

The oxidation–reduction potential (abbreviated "redox" potential or E_h) of a culture medium, expressed in volts or millivolts, can be measured by using a platinum wire electrode along with a standard reference electrode connected to a pH meter. The E_h is affected by pH (or the hydrogen ion concentration); thus, redox potential is commonly expressed at neutral pH (pH 7) as E_h. Reducing agents, such as thioglycolate and L-cysteine, may be added to anaerobic transport media and to certain culture media to help maintain reduced conditions (or a low E_h) in the medium. A positive oxidation–reduction potential (e.g., as indicated by pink color of resazurin indicator in certain media, or a blue color of methylene blue indicator in other media) means that the medium is oxidized. In nature, the upper limit of E_h is +820 mV, which might be found in some environments that have considerable oxygenation. Oxidizing conditions prevail in healthy human tissue that is well-oxygenated and has an intact blood supply (e.g., the E_h is about +150 mV). In contrast, the lower limit of E_h in nature is about −420 mV. An anaerobic environment (e.g., an abscess or necrotic tissue) or a culture medium rich in hydrogen might have such a low E_h. The large bowel of humans, which contains enormous numbers of strict obligate anaerobes,

has an E_h of about −250 mV.[34] What is the relative significance of the oxidation–reduction potential versus atmospheric oxygen in relation to survival and growth of anaerobic bacteria? As reviewed several years ago by Hentges and Maier,[84] there are older reports indicating that certain anaerobes would not grow above a certain low E_h level and that some obligate anaerobes would grow in room air if the E_h of the medium was kept sufficiently low. In an excellent study reported by Walden and Hentges in 1975, some of the myths about the effects of E_h on anaerobic bacteria were dispelled.[209] These workers studied the differential effects of O_2 and redox potential on the growth of *C. perfringens*, *B. fragilis*, and *P. magnus*. Oxygen inhibited multiplication of these three anaerobes whether the medium was at a negative redox potential (E_h = −50 mV), poised by the addition of dithiothreitol ([DTT] a reducing agent), or at a positive redox potential (E_h near +500 mV) in aerated medium without DTT. In the absence of O_2, these organisms were able to multiply, even when the E_h was maintained at +325 mV, by the addition of potassium ferricyanide (an oxidizing agent). From their work, a practical conclusion was drawn that the purging of oxygen from the cultural environment, to avoid oxygen toxicity, is probably more important than the establishment of a low E_h.[209] Thus, the rapid achievement and maintenance of a low oxygen tension, or the absence of oxygen, is an essential requirement for the successful cultivation of anaerobes in modern anaerobic systems (e.g., anaerobic jars and glove boxes used for incubation of anaerobes in the clinical laboratory).

HABITATS

Anaerobic bacteria are widespread in soil, marshes, lake and river sediments, the oceans, sewage, foods, and animals. In humans, anaerobic bacteria normally are prevalent in the oral cavity around the teeth, in the gastrointestinal tract, especially in the colon, where they outnumber coliforms by at least 1000:1, in the orifices of the genitourinary tract, and on the skin.[61,69,186,209] Most of these anaerobic habitats have both a low oxygen tension and reduced oxidation–reduction potential (E_h) resulting from the metabolic activity of microorganisms that consume oxygen through respiration.[34] If the oxygen is not replaced, anaerobic conditions are maintained in the environment.

A brief summary of commonly encountered anerobes in the normal flora of the human body is given in Box 14-1.

CLASSIFICATION AND NOMENCLATURE

The anaerobes include essentially all morphologic forms of bacteria. Based on their ability to form spores and on the morphologic characteristics observed in gram-stained preparations, the anaerobic bacteria are broadly classified as shown in Table 14-1. Several of the genera in this list are found only in nonpathogenic habitats and have not been shown to occur in diseases

BOX 14-1. ANAEROBES FOUND IN NORMAL HUMAN FLORA

Oral Cavity and Upper Respiratory Passages

Pigmented *Prevotella* species; *Porphyromonas* spp.

Nonpigmented *Prevotella* spp. (especially *P. oralis*)

Bacteroides spp. (e.g., *B. ureolyticus*)

Fusobacterium spp. (especially *F. nucleatum*)

Peptostreptococcus spp. (anaerobic streptococci)

Veillonella spp.

Actinomyces and *Propionibacterium* spp.

Stomach (During Fasting)

Lactobacilli

Small Intestine (Proximal Portion)

Streptococci

Lactobacilli

Large Bowel (and Terminal Ileum)

Bacteroides fragilis group

Porphyromonas spp.

Fusobacterium spp.

Anaerobic cocci—many species

Clostridium spp.

Eubacterium spp.

Bifidobacterium spp.

Propionibacterium spp.

Genitourinary Tract, Vagina, and Cervix

Pigmented *Prevotella* spp.; *Porphyromonas* spp.

Nonpigmented *Prevotella*

Bacteroides spp.

Peptostreptococcus spp.

Clostridium spp.

Veillonella spp.

Lactobacillus spp.

Eubacterium spp.

Propionibacterium spp.

Urethra (Male and Female)

Propionibacterium spp.

Peptostreptococcus spp.

Bacteroides (*Prevotella*) spp.

Fusobacterium spp.

Skin

Propionibacterium spp.

Peptostreptococcus spp.

of humans. Most of these genera will not be discussed further. Additional information on the classification and nomenclature of anaerobes commonly involved in human illnesses is given in Table 14-3 and Table 14-12 and in the identification section of this chapter.

HUMAN INFECTIONS

Anaerobic infections in humans and various animals can involve virtually any organ when conditions are suitable. Some of the more commonly involved sites are shown in Figure 14-1. On the basis of other reports in the literature, the relative incidence of anaerobes in infections is listed in Table 14-2.[23,61,67,69]

Most deep-seated abscesses and necrotizing lesions involving anaerobes are polymicrobial and may include obligate aerobes, facultative anaerobes, or microaerophiles as concomitant microorganisms.[67,69] These microorganisms, acting in concert with trauma, vascular stasis, or tissue necrosis, lower the oxygen tension and the oxidation–reduction potential in tissues, and provide favorable conditions for obligate anaerobes to multiply. Historically, infections and diseases involving anaerobes from exogenous sources are the ones that have been best known (Box 14-2).

Within the past few decades, however, endogenous anaerobic infections have become far more common. There are two probable explanations. One is that laboratory recovery of anaerobic bacteria has improved, so that endogenous infections are no longer misdiagnosed or overlooked as they were in the past. The other is that a larger proportion of the patient population is receiving immunosuppressive drugs for malignancy and other disorders, resulting in compromised host resistance.[61,67,69] Primary anaerobic infections easily become established in areas of tissue damage, and bacteremia, metastatic spread of bacteria with formation of distant abscesses, and a progressive chain of events, sometimes resulting in a fatal outcome, may occur. The more common endogenous anaerobic infections are listed in Box 14-3.

It is essential to isolate and identify anaerobic bacteria because 1) these infections are associated with high morbidity and mortality and 2) the treatment of the infection varies with the bacterial species involved. Antibiotic therapy for certain anaerobic infections is different from that used for many infections caused by aerobic or facultatively anaerobic bacteria.[63,67] Prompt surgical intervention, including debridement of necrotic tissue or amputation of a limb, may be of extreme importance, particularly in cases of clostridial gas gan-

TABLE 14-1

CLASSIFICATION OF THE GENERA OF ANAEROBIC BACTERIA

Spores Formed

Gram-positive bacilli
  Clostridium*†
  Desulfotomaculum
  Caloramator†
  Filifactor†
  Moorella†
  Oxobacter†
  Oxalophagus†

Spores not Formed

Gram-positive bacilli
  Acetobacterium
  Actinomyces*
  Arcanobacterium*
  Atopobium*
  Bifidobacterium*
  Eubacterium*
  Lachnospira
  Lactobacillus*
  Methanobacterium
  Propionibacterium*

Gram-positive cocci
  Coprococcus
  Gemmiger
  Peptococcus
  Peptostreptococcus*
  Ruminococcus
  Sarcina
  Staphylococcus*
  Streptococcus*
  Gemella*

Gram-negative bacilli (curved, spiral and spirochete forms are included)
  Acetivibrio
  Anaerovibrio
  Anaerorhabdus
  Anaerobiospirillum
  Anaerobacter
  Bacteroides*
  Bilophila*
  Borrelia
  Butyrivibrio‡
  Capnocytophaga

Capsularis
Campylobacter*
Catonella*
Centipeda
Cristispira
Desulfobacter
Desulfobulbus
Desulfococcus
Desulfosarcina
Desulfomonas
Desulfuromonas
Desulfovibrio
Dialister*
Dichelobacter
Fibrobacter
Fusobacterium*
Hallella*
Helicobacter
Johnsonella*
Ilyobacter
Leptotrichia
Megamonas
Mitsuokella
Mobiluncus*

Oribaculum*
Pectinatus
Porphyromonas*
Prevotella*
Propionigenium
Propionispira
Rikenella
Roseburia
Ruminobacter
Sebaldella
Selenomonas
Serpula
Spirochaeta
Succinimonas
Succinivibrio
Sutterella*
Tissierella
Treponema
Wolinella

Gram-negative cocci
  Acidaminococcus
  Megasphaera
  Veillonella*

* In the majority of properly collected clinical specimens, only the genera indicated with a * will need to be considered by the clinical microbiologist. However, on rare occasions, serious illness may involve *Anaerobiospirillum, Succinivibrio, Wolinella,* or one of the other genera above that is not listed in Table 14-3.

† The genus *Clostridium* is now under major taxonomic revision. Thus, in 1994, five new genera of spore-forming anaerobes were proposed by Collins et al.[40] None of these is known to be pathogenic for humans.

‡ *Butyrivibrio* is discussed with the gram-negative bacilli in Vol. 1 and with the irregular non–spore-forming gram-positive anaerobic rods in Vol. 2 of Bergey's Manual [Sneath, 1986[161]; Krieg, 1984[109]]. Although they are gram-negative with the Gram stain, some strains have atypical gram-positive cell wall features by electron microscopy. Adapted and modified from Bergey's Manual of Systematic Bacteriology [Krieg, 1984[109]; Sneath, 1986[161]] and from very recent volumes (Volumes 34–46) of the International Journal of Systematic Bacteriology that contain numerous publications related to recent changes in anaerobe taxonomy.

grene or in loculated abscesses where antibiotics may be ineffective until the exudate is drained.

Before the mid-1960s, clostridial infections predominated; at present, 85% of anaerobes isolated from properly selected clinical specimens are accounted for by *Bacteroides, Prevotella, Porphyromonas, Fusobacterium, Peptostreptococcus* species, and the gram-positive, non–spore-forming bacilli (Table 14-3).

The most common disease-producing, gram-negative, non–spore-forming bacilli in humans are the *Bacteroides fragilis* and pigmented *Prevotella–Porphyromonas* (formerly the pigmented *Bacteroides*) groups and *Fusobacterium nucleatum*. The percentage distribution of 5398 isolates of anaerobic bacteria recovered from materials submitted to the laboratory at the Indiana University Medical Center (IUMC) during 1988 through 1990 is given in Table 14-3. *B. fragilis, B. thetaiotaomicron,* and other species of the *B. fragilis* group are particularly important because they may be isolated from a variety of life-threatening infections and because of their resistance to the action of penicillin and its analogues; their increasing resistance to many cephalosporins, including the third-generation cephalosporins; the tetracyclines; the aminoglycosides; and several of the newer quinolones.[1,12,65,68,215]

Penicillin G was historically the antibiotic of choice for clinical infections caused by most anaerobic bacteria. Currently, in addition to the *B. fragilis* group, *Fusobacterium mortiferum, F. varium,* members of the pigmented *Prevotella–Porphyromonas* group, *Prevotella bivia, P. disiens,* and some *Clostridium* species are now resistant to penicillin G, some of its analogues, and many of the cephalosporins. Although the clostridia are recovered from anaerobic infections less frequently than *Bacteroides* species, *Fusobacterium* species, and the anaerobic cocci, they can be responsible for life-threatening illness.

The more common species of *Clostridium* isolated from clinical sources include *C. perfringens, C. ramosum, C. difficile, C. clostridioforme, C. innocuum, C. septicum, C. sordellii, C. cadaveris, C. paraputrificum, C. sporogenes, C. tertium, C. bifermentans, C. butyricum,* and *C. subterminale* (see Table 14-3). Many of these species are of unknown clinical importance; their significance usually varies with the clinical setting.

Isolation of a *Clostridium* species from a wound, blood culture, or other body fluid does not necessarily have clinical significance. *C. perfringens,* the most frequently isolated *Clostridium* species, is a common inhabitant of the large bowel; it and other clostridia tran-

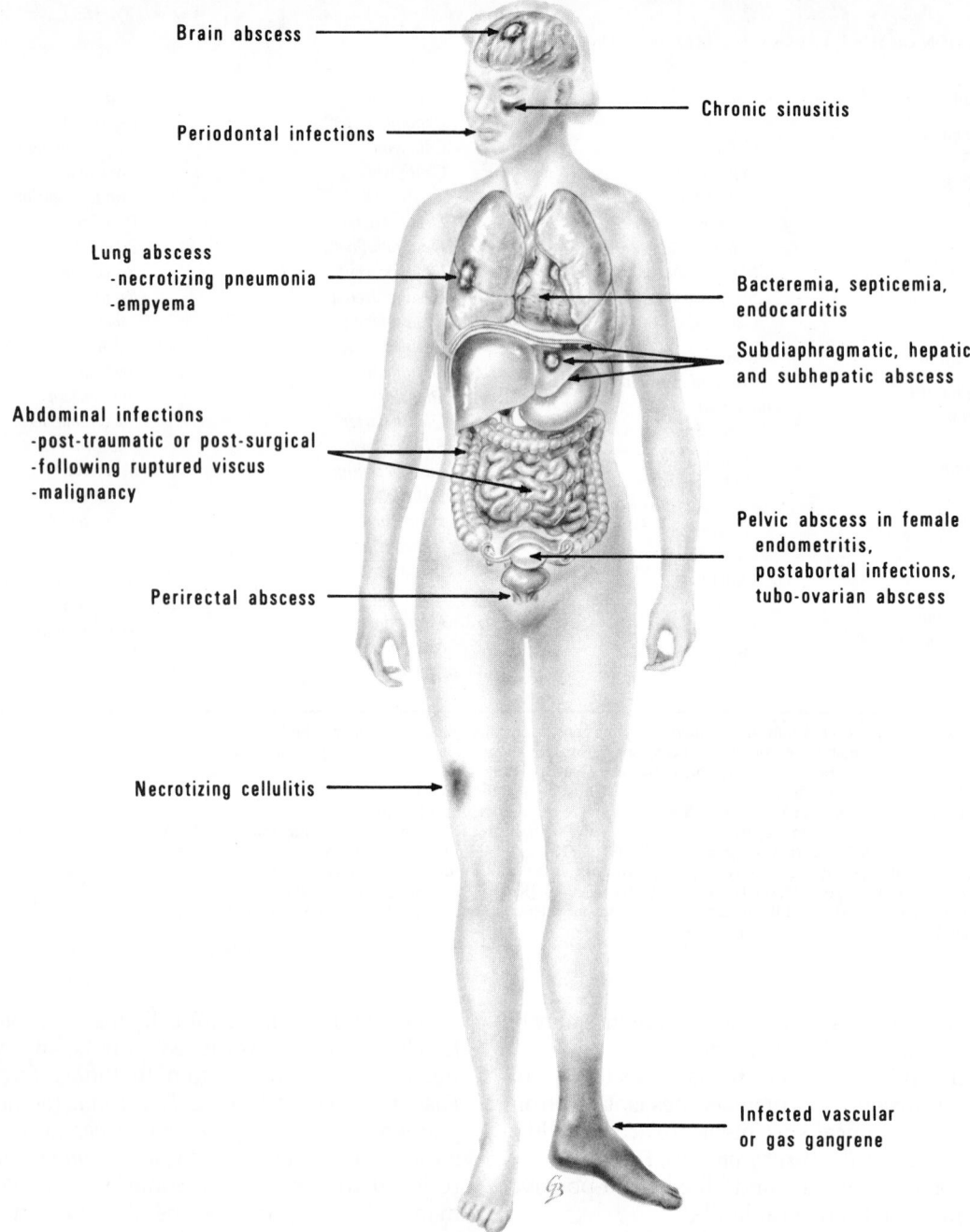

Brain abscess

Periodontal infections

Chronic sinusitis

Lung abscess
  -necrotizing pneumonia
  -empyema

Bacteremia, septicemia,
endocarditis

Subdiaphragmatic, hepatic
and subhepatic abscess

Abdominal infections
  -post-traumatic or post-surgical
  -following ruptured viscus
  -malignancy

Pelvic abscess in female
  endometritis,
  postabortal infections,
  tubo-ovarian abscess

Perirectal abscess

Necrotizing cellulitis

Infected vascular
or gas gangrene

Figure 14-1
Common locations of infections involving anaerobic bacteria.

siently contaminate the skin of the perianal area and other skin surfaces. *C. perfringens* is not always pathogenic. However, it, along with *C. botulinum, C. difficile, C. septicum*, and a few other clostridia are associated with major diseases and are discussed later in this chapter.

At least six species of the gram-positive, non–spore-forming bacilli can cause actinomycosis in humans: *Actinomyces israelii, A. naeslundii, A. viscosus, A. odontolyticus, A. meyeri*, and *Propionibacterium propionicum* (formerly *Arachnia propionica*).[4,183] Although encoun-

tered in relatively low frequency in routine specimens, these species are well-documented pathogens. Actinomycosis is a chronic granulomatous disease characterized by suppurative lesions, abscesses, and draining sinus tracts.[183] The disease most often presents as cervicofacial, thoracic, abdominal, or pelvic actinomycosis but can occur in other regions of the body.[4,69,183]

Bifidobacterium eriksonii (now recognized taxonomically as *Bifidobacterium dentium*), a potential cause of pulmonary anaerobic infections, is the only documented pathogenic species of this genus.[4,61] *Propioni-*

TABLE 14-2
INCIDENCE OF ANAEROBES IN INFECTIONS

TYPE OF INFECTION	INCIDENCE (%)
Aspiration pneumonia, lung abscess, necrotizing pneumonia	62–93
Bacteremia	9–10
Brain abscess	60–89
Dental infection, chronic sinusitis	52–100
Thoracic empyema	76
Intra-abdominal/pelvic sepsis	60–100
Osteomyelitis	40
Miscellaneous soft-tissue infections:	
Breast abscess	53–83
Postappendectomy and elective colon surgery wounds	79–95
Perirectal abscess	77
Soft-tissue and cutaneous abscesses	60–62
Nonclostridial crepitant celluitis	75
Gas gangrene (clostridial myonecrosis)	100
Pilonidal sinus	88
Diabetic foot ulcers, infected diabetic gangrene	85–95
Urinary tract infection	≤1

After Finegold SM, George WL (eds): Anaerobic Infections in Humans. San Diego CA, Academic Press, 1989; Bartlett JG: Anaerobic bacteria: general concepts. In Mandell GL, Douglas RG, Bennett JE (eds): Principles and Practices of Infectious Diseases, 3rd ed, pp 1828–1842. New York, Churchill-Livingstone, 1990; and Finegold SM: Anaerobic bacteria: general concepts. In Mandell GL, Bennett JE, Dolin R (eds): Principles and Practice of Infectious Diseases, 4th ed, pp 2156–2208. New York, Churchill-Livingstone, 1995.

bacterium acnes, usually a contaminant in clinical specimens, has been recovered from cases of endocarditis and other diseases, frequently those associated with implanted prosthetic devices.

The anaerobic cocci most commonly encountered in clinical specimens include *Peptostreptococcus magnus*, *P. asaccharolyticus, P. prevotii, P. anaerobius*, and *Streptococcus intermedius*. There is little doubt that some of the anaerobic cocci are pathogenic for humans in certain clinical settings. At the Mayo Clinic, *P. magnus* was recovered from 10% of anaerobic cultures collected from patients with suspected infections and was the most frequently isolated anaerobic gram-positive coccus.[32] It was usually involved in bone and joint, soft tissue, foot ulcer, and abdominal infections.

Anaerobic and microaerophilic cocci are also important in brain abscess, chronic maxillary sinusitis, and anaerobic pleuropulmonary and pelvic infections. To underscore their clinical importance, increasing numbers of *P. magnus, P. asaccharolyticus, P. prevotii*, and other species have been showing resistance to penicillin G, clindamycin, and metronidazole (Table 14-4).

ISOLATION OF ANAEROBIC BACTERIA

The steps involved in the laboratory diagnosis of anaerobic bacterial infections are similar to those described in Chapters 2 and 3. It is particularly important that attention be paid to the proper selection, collec-

BOX 14-2. ANAEROBIC INFECTIONS OF EXOGENOUS ORIGIN

Clostridium difficile hospital-acquired (nosocomial) diarrhea
Food-borne botulism
Infant botulism
Wound botulism
C. perfringens gastroenteritis
Myonecrosis (gas gangrene)
Tetanus
Crepitant cellulitis
Benign superficial infections
Infections following animal or human bites
Septic abortion

tion, and transport of clinical specimens for recovering anaerobic bacteria. The processing of specimens, selection of media, inoculation and incubation methods, and inspection of positive cultures are laboratory procedures that must be carefully quality controlled. Failure to perform any one step correctly may lead to erroneous results, thus creating the potential to supply misinformation to the physician.

BOX 14-3. ANAEROBIC INFECTIONS OF ENDOGENOUS ORIGIN

Abscess of any organ
Actinomycosis
Antibiotic-associated diarrhea and colitis
Aspiration pneumonia
Complications of appendicitis or cholecystitis
Crepitant and noncrepitant cellulitis
Clostridial myonecrosis
Dental and periodontal infections
Endocarditis
Meningitis, usually following brain abscess
Necrotizing pneumonia
Osteomyelitis
Otitis media
Peritonitis
Septic arthritis
Sinusitis
Subdural empyema
Tetanus
Thoracic empyema

TABLE 14-3

CLINICAL ISOLATES OF ANAEROBIC BACTERIA IDENTIFIED BY THE INDIANA UNIVERSITY MEDICAL CENTER ANAEROBE LABORATORY, 1988–1990*

ORGANISMS OR GROUP	NUMBER	PERCENTAGE	ORGANISMS OR GROUP	NUMBER	PERCENTAGE
Bacteroides	1348	25	*P. prevotii*	210	4
B. fragilis "group" total	1068	20	*P. productus*	3	<1
B. caccae	6	<1	*P. tetradius*	7	<1
B. distasonis	62	1	Peptostreptococcus spp.	124	2
B. fragilis	545	10			
B. fragilis "other"	22	<1	*Streptococcus*	119	2
B. ovatus	151	3	S. constellatus	3	<1
B. stercoris	3	<1	S. intermedius	75	1
B. thetaiotaomicron	108	2	Streptococcus spp.	23	<1
B. uniformis	50	1			
B. vulgatus	121	2	*Gemella morbillorum*	18	<1
B. eggerthii	1	<1			
B. gracilis	8	<1	*Staphylococcus saccharolyticus*	20	<1
B. splanchnicus	12	<1			
B. ureolyticus	63	1	*Veillonella* spp.	157	3
Bacteroides spp.	196	4			
Porphyromonas asaccharolytica	40	1	*Actinomyces*	40	1
			A. israelii	3	<1
Prevotella	399	7	A. meyeri	1	<1
P. bivia	76	1	A. naeslundii	3	<1
P. disiens	9	<1	A. odontolyticus	7	<1
P. intermedia	12	<1	Actinomyces spp.	26	<1
P. loescheii	2	<1			
P. melaninogenica	64	1	*Eubacterium*	272	5
P. melaninogenica "group"	94	2	E. aerofaciens	1	<1
P. oralis	7	<1	E. brachy	4	<1
P. oralis "group"	109	2	E. contortum	6	<1
P. oris	1	<1	E. lentum	84	2
P. oris/buccae	20	<1	E. limosum	14	<1
P. veroralis	1	<1	E. nitritogenes	1	<1
P. zoogleoformans	3	<1	E. saburreum	2	<1
			Eubacterium spp.	160	3
Fusobacterium	262	4			
F. gonidiaformans	1	<1	*Propionibacterium*	681	13
F. mortiferum	9	<1	P. acnes	599	11
F. naviforme	15	<1	P. propionicum	1	<1
F. necrophorum	17	<1	P. avidium	1	<1
F. necrogenes	3	<1	P. granulosum	6	<1
F. nucleatum	167	3	P. lymphophilum	2	<1
F. periodonticum	1	<1	Propionibacterium spp.	32	1
F. russii	10	<1			
F. varium	10	<1	*Bifidobacterium*	48	1
Fusobacterium spp.	29	1	B. adolescentis	2	<1
			B. bifidum	3	<1
Miscellaneous Organisms	20	,1	B. breve	5	<1
Campylobacter spp.	1	<1	B. catenulatum	1	<1
Capnocytophaga spp.	10	<1	B. dentium	1	<1
Curved gram-negative rod	2	<1	B. infantis	1	<1
Mitsuokella multiacidus	1	<1	B. longum/magnum	3	<1
Leptotrichia buccalis	3	<1	Bifidobacterium spp.	32	1
Selenomonas spp.	1	<1			
Mobiluncus spp.	2	<1	*Lactobacillus*	150	3
			L. acidophilus	3	<1
Peptococcus niger	4	<1	L. casei	3	<1
			L. catenaformis	1	<1
Peptostreptococcus	1171	22	L. fermentum	1	<1
P. anaerobius	146	3	L. minutus	1	<1
P. asaccharolyticus	247	5	L. plantarum	3	<1
P. indolicus	2	<1	L. rhamnosus	2	<1
P. magnus	304	6	Lactobacillus spp.	137	3
P. micros	128	2			

(Continued)

TABLE 14-3 *(Continued)*
CLINICAL ISOLATES OF ANAEROBIC BACTERIA IDENTIFIED BY THE INDIANA UNIVERSITY
MEDICAL CENTER ANAEROBE LABORATORY, 1988–1990*

ORGANISMS OR GROUP	NUMBER	PERCENTAGE	ORGANISMS OR GROUP	NUMBER	PERCENTAGE
Clostridium	706	13	C. malenominatum	4	<1
C. barati	1	<1	C. paraputrificum	11	<1
C. bifermentans	21	<1	C. perfringens	118	2
C. botulinum type A	1	<1	C. ramosum	92	2
C. butyricum	33	1	C. septicum	12	<1
C. cadaveris	22	<1	C. sordellii	3	<1
C. carnis	1	<1	C. sphenoides	1	<1
C. clostridioforme	96	2	C. sporogenes	10	<1
C. coccoides	1	<1	C. sporogenes/botulinum	1	<1
C. cocleatum	2	<1	C. subterminale	6	<1
C. difficile†	59	1	C. symbiosum	1	<1
C. ghonii	1	<1	C. tertium	11	<1
C. glycolicum	10	<1	C. tetani	2	<1
C. indolis	2	<1	*Clostridium* spp.	80	1
C. innocuum	103	2	**Grand Total**	5398	
C. limosum	1	<1			

* Allen SD and Siders JA, Unpublished data; organisms isolated from properly collected specimens.
† The *C. difficile* isolates listed in the table were from blood, body fluids other than urine, abscesses, or other, and
not from stool specimens.

Because Chapters 2 and 3 cover each of these steps in detail, with the exception of anaerobic blood cultures, only a few comments pertaining specifically to the anaerobic bacteria are included here.

SELECTION OF SPECIMENS FOR CULTURE

With few exceptions, all materials collected from sites not harboring an indigenous flora, such as body fluids other than urine, exudates from deep abscesses, transtracheal aspirates or direct lung aspirates, and tissue biopsies, should be cultured for anaerobic bacteria.[11] However, because anaerobes normally inhabit the skin and mucous membranes as part of the normal indigenous flora, the specimens listed in Table 14-5 are virtually always unacceptable for anaerobic culture because the results cannot be interpreted.

COLLECTION AND TRANSPORT OF SPECIMENS

When collecting specimens from mucous membranes or the skin, stringent precautions must be taken to decontaminate the surface properly. A surgical soap scrub, followed by application of 70% ethyl or isopropyl alcohol and tincture of iodine, and then removal of the iodine with alcohol, is recommended. However, some patients are allergic to tincture of iodine.

Alternatively, an alcohol scrub followed by 10% povidone-iodine (Betadine) is also satisfactory, provided that the Betadine is allowed to remain on the skin for at least 2 minutes before the specimen is collected.

A needle and syringe should be used whenever possible for collecting specimens for anaerobic culture. Collection of swab specimens should be discouraged because they dry out and also because they expose anaerobes, if present, to ambient oxygen. Once the specimens are collected, particular precautions should be taken to protect them from oxygen exposure and to deliver them to the laboratory promptly.

ANAEROBIC BLOOD CULTURE (SUMMARY OF GUIDELINES FOR TRADITIONAL BROTH AND INSTRUMENTED SYSTEMS)

Blood culture techniques should permit optimal recovery of obligate anaerobes as well as aerobes and facultative anaerobes. For many years, anaerobes were encountered in about 9% to 20% of all positive blood culture sets at a number of medical centers. Recently, however, the percentage of gram-positive cocci (e.g., staphylococci, enterococci, streptococci) and *Enterobacteriaceae* has increased at the Indiana University Medical Center (IUMC), probably as a result of shifting antimicrobial treatments and greater proportions of tertiary care, immunocompromised patients. Thus, the incidence of anaerobic bacteremia has decreased at several medical centers including IUMC.[12,13,43,45,111,119,150,152,169,182] Interestingly, a relative increase in numbers of patients with bacteremia involving species of the *Bacteroides fragilis* group that were less common during the 1970s and 1980s, and are now more resistant to antibiotics, has been documented recently at IUMC. In addition, increased numbers of *Fusobacterium mortiferum*, *Clostridium* species, *Leptotrichia buccalis*, *Lactobacillus* species, and *Actinomyces* species are now being encountered, reflecting the emergence of anaerobes now resistant to several widely used antimicrobial agents.[13] It is likely these changes in resistance patterns will lead to re-

(text continues on page 720)

TABLE 14-4
PERCENTAGES OF ANAEROBES SUSCEPTIBLE TO CONCENTRATIONS OF ANTIMICROBIAL AGENTS AT MINIMAL INHIBITORY CONCENTRATION BREAKPOINTS INDICATING SUSCEPTIBILITY*

BACTERIA (NO. STRAINS TESTED)	AMPICILLIN/ SULBACTAM 16/8**	CEFOPERAZONE 32**	CEFOTAXIME 32**	CEFOTETAN 32**	CEFOXITIN 32**	CEFTRIAXONE 32**
Bacteroides fragilis (277)	97	22	61	83	91	42
Bacteroides ovatus (86)	100	47	58	23	80	14
Bacteroides thetaiotaomicron (79)	99	23	42	33	86	5
Bacteroides vulgatus (75)	96	42	52	69	90	4
Bacteroides distasonis (21)	86	52	43	10	81	24
Bacteroides uniformis (24)	100	71	58	58	88	46
Prevotella melaninogenica "group" (17)	94	94	94	94	100	88
Prevotella bivia/disiens (18)	100	94	100	100	100	94
Prevotella oralis "group" (23)	100	96	93	100	100	93
Fusobacterium necrophorum (10)	100	100	100	100	100	100
Fusobacterium nucleatum (29)	97	100	100	100	100	100
Fusobacterium varium (6)	100	100	100	100	100	100
Actinomyces (8)	100	88	88	88	88	100
Eubacterium lentum (19)	100	37	47	58	89	47
Eubacterium (26)	100	96	96	85	92	96
Propionibacterium acnes (161)	100	100	100	100	100	100
Lactobacillus (70)	100	83	80	10	21	36
Clostridium perfringens (57)	100	100	100	98	100	100
Clostridium ramosum (44)	100	100	98	91	96	98
Clostridium difficile (37)	100	86	51	100	29	89
Clostridium septicum (4)	100	100	100	100	100	100
Clostridium butyricum (5)	100	100	100	100	100	100
Clostridium clostridioforme (33)	100	85	70	97	100	91
Clostridium innocuum (50)	100	100	100	8	32	100
Peptostreptococcus anaerobius (31)	100	68	94	68	97	90
Peptostreptococcus asaccharolyticus (56)	100	100	100	100	100	100
Peptostreptococcus magnus (91)	100	99	99	100	99	99
Peptostreptococcus micros (40)	100	98	98	98	98	98
Peptostreptococcus prevotii (43)	100	93	95	100	100	98
Streptococcus intermedius (13)	100	100	100	100	100	100
Veillonella (82)	99	89	99	99	99	99

Data given is from the Indiana University Medical Center Anaerobe Lab, November 1995 thru May 1996.
* Breakpoints listed are based on the NCCLS document; based on microbroth dilution methods given in NCCLS. Methods for antimicrobial susceptibility testing of anaerobic bacteria—3rd ed. Approved Standard. NCCLS Document M11-A3, Villanova, PA, vol. 13, No. 26, December 1993. NCCLS. Performance standards for antimicrobial susceptibility testing; fifth informational supplement. NCCLS document M100-S5. Villanova, PA, vol. 14, No. 16, December 1994.
** The numbers appearing beneath each antimicrobial agent is in µg/ml.
(The data in the table represent percents of strains of each species inhibited at susceptible and intermediate end points. Maximum doses of antimicrobial agents are generally recommended for treatment of anaerobic infections in order to achieve the best possible antimicrobial levels in abscesses, necrotic or poorly perfused tissues.)

Chloram-phenicol 16**	Clindamycin 4**	Imipenem 8**	Metro-nidazole 16**	Penicillin G 8**	Piperacillin 64**	Piperacillin/ Tazobactam 64/4**	Ticarcillin/ Clavulanate 64/2**	Amoxicillin/ Clavulanal 8/4**
100	87	99	100	7	77	99	98	97
100	72	100	100	4	73	100	100	97
100	63	100	100	4	73	100	99	97
100	69	100	100	20	52	100	100	98
100	81	100	100	19	38	96	76	93
100	71	100	100	4	71	100	100	100
100	100	100	94	82	100	100	94	82
100	100	100	100	61	94	100	94	92
100	86	100	100	75	93	100	100	100
100	100	100	100	100	100	100	100	100
100	100	100	100	93	93	100	100	94
100	84	100	100	100	100	100	100	100
100	75	100	25	88	88	88	88	100
100	100	100	95	100	89	100	100	100
100	92	100	85	96	96	100	92	94
100	98	100	13	100	100	100	100	100
90	94	99	4	97	100	100	90	100
100	91	100	100	100	100	100	100	100
100	91	100	100	97	100	100	100	100
100	84	100	100	100	100	100	100	100
100	100	100	100	100	100	100	100	100
100	80	100	100	100	100	100	100	100
100	100	100	100	85	100	100	94	100
100	92	100	100	100	100	100	100	100
100	100	100	97	78	94	100	74	92
100	98	100	100	98	100	100	100	96
100	89	100	90	98	99	99	99	98
100	98	100	98	98	98	100	100	100
100	98	100	98	93	95	100	100	100
100	100	100	38	100	100	100	100	100
99	96	98	98	89	95	95	96	95

TABLE 14-5

SPECIMENS THAT SHOULD NOT BE CULTURED
FOR ANAEROBIC BACTERIA

Throat or nasopharyngeal swabs
Gingival swabs
Sputum or bronchoscopic specimens
Gastric contents, small-bowel contents, feces, rectal swabs,
    colocutaneous fistulae, colostomy stomata*
Surfaces of decubitus ulcers, swab samples of encrusted walls of
    abscesses, mucosal linings, and eschars
Material adjacent to skin or mucous membranes other than the
    above that have not been properly decontaminated
Voided urine
Vaginal or cervical swabs

---

* When indicated clinically, specimens from these sources may be used for
the diagnosis of botulism and for intestinal disease caused by *Clostridium
difficile* and *C. perfringens*.

---

newed interest in the laboratory diagnosis of anaerobic bacteremia.

Similar to the collection of the other specimens, the skin over the venipuncture site should first be prepared using alcohol and povidone-iodine. Contamination with skin flora (e.g., especially *Propionibacterium acnes* and coagulase-negative staphylococci) should be in less than 3% of all blood specimens cultured; also, blood for culture should not be drawn through indwelling venous or arterial catheter lines unless it can not be obtained by venipuncture.[164] The blood specimen volume recommended from adult patients is 15 to 30 mL per venipuncture if a traditional broth system is used. If the BACTEC (Becton Dickinson Microbiology Systems, Sparks MD) system is used, 15 mL of blood from a single venipuncture can be divided equally into three bottles; or a 20-mL blood sample can be divided into four bottles (5 mL/bottle). One to two of these bottles would be for anaerobic culture—the remainder for aerobic incubation. Alternatively, 8 to 10 mL of blood can be inoculated into each Bactec Plus (26 aerobic or 27 anaerobic) bottle. For neonates and older children, smaller volumes must be collected (e.g., less than 0.5 mL for an infant; 2 to 5 mL for an older child). Collection of more than two to three blood specimens per 24-hour period to diagnose a suspected episode of bacteremia is not required and is not recommended.[164]

Several traditional broth media formulations, available in unvented bottles under vacuum with CO_2, appear to be satisfactory for isolation of anaerobes (e.g., Difco broth, Becton Dickinson enriched thioglycolate medium 0135C formulation, trypticase–soy broth, supplemented peptone broth, brain–heart infusion broth, *Brucella* broth, Columbia broth, and others).[164,211,212] These media are usually dispensed in volumes of about 40 to 100 mL per bottle. The BACTEC media recommended for anaerobes include the following: 1) radiometric systems (e.g., BACTEC 460) 7D anaerobic or 17D anaerobic resin broth; 2) nonradiometric systems (e.g., BACTEC NR 660; BACTEC NR 720; BACTEC NR 860) NR 7A anaerobic broth, NR 17A anaerobic resin

broth or BACTEC Plus 27 (formerly "NR27," or "high volume") broth with resin. Except for the BACTEC Plus 26/27 bottles which hold 25 mL, and the "Peds Plus" bottle which holds 20 mL (for use with children), the other BACTEC bottles hold 30 mL of culture medium per bottle. (Another source of radiometric media that can be used with the Bactec 460 instrument is Baxter-Microscan, but published evaluations of these media are lacking.) For traditional blood culture media, the recommended blood to broth volume ratio is 1:5 to 1:10.[164] However, the volume of media was decreased from 30 mL in the traditional BACTEC bottles to 25 mL in the BACTEC Plus 26/27 bottles to accommodate a higher blood volume. Thus, the inoculation of 10 mL into a BACTEC Plus bottle creates a dilution factor of only 1:3.5; the resins in the Bactec Plus media offset the problem of residual antimicrobial activity that might be present in patients' blood.[108]

Although the addition of sodium polyanethol sulfonate (SPS) to blood culture media enhances the recovery of most bacteria, including anaerobes, it may be inhibitory to some bacteria, such as the pathogenic *Neisseria* species. *Peptostreptococcus anaerobius* is the only anaerobe known to be inhibited by SPS in blood culture media. *P. anaerobius* is so uncommon in blood cultures that special attempts to isolate it using special supplemented media (e.g., by adding 1.2% gelatin to overcome the SPS effect) are not very cost-effective.

The atmospheres of incubation for broth blood cultures should include at least one anaerobic bottle incubated unvented, and at least one aerobic bottle should be transiently vented per blood culture set (if a traditional broth system is used). The BACTEC broth culture systems have special aerobic and anaerobic atmospheres. Both aerobic and anaerobic bottles should be shaken during incubation and should be incubated at 35°C for 5 to 7 days. Non-BACTEC traditional broth bottles should be inspected visually for growth (e.g., for turbidity, gas production, hemolysis, colonies in the sediment, and so forth) twice daily during the first 72 hours; once daily thereafter. The BACTEC NR media should be inspected twice daily during the first 48 hours; then once daily. Gram stains and blind subcultures of non-BACTEC traditional media should be performed aerobically during the first 6 to 12 hours of incubation regardless of whether macroscopic evidence of growth is seen.[29,164] The relatively low yield of blind anaerobic subcultures, reported by Murray and Sondag[151] and Paisley and coauthors,[159] argued against the need for this procedure on macroscopically negative blood cultures. However, data obtained using traditional broth media at Indiana University Hospital[8] indicated that about 30% of anaerobes were detected during the first 18 hours of incubation that would not have been observed by macroscopic inspection (using blind subculture of supplemented and prereduced brain–heart infusion medium); also, at least 5% of significant isolates would have been missed without blind subculture. The director of the microbiology laboratory must decide whether blind anaerobic subcultures should be done in a given hospital laboratory and must make the decision whether the cost of blind anaerobic subculture takes precedence over the perceived relevance to patient care. Negative cultures should be held for 5 to 7 days before they are reported as negative.

Blind subcultures are not required for the aerobic or anaerobic bottles in the BACTEC, BacT/Alert, or ESP instrumented systems. When either the aerobic or anaerobic bottles show macroscapic evidence of growth, they should be subcultured onto chocolate agar (incubated in a 5% to 10% CO_2–air incubator) and anaerobe blood agar (incubated anaerobically). Also, the use of selective plating media for anaerobic subculture (such as phenylethyl alcohol anaerobe blood agar or kanamycin–vancomycin blood agar), in addition to nonselective anaerobe blood agar, is recommended to aid in recovery of anaerobes in the setting of polymicrobial bacteremia. Anaerobes are isolated on occasion from the aerobic bottles (as well as from anaerobic bottles). Failure to perform anaerobic subcultures of macroscopically positive aerobic bottles is an *unacceptable* practice. In recovering anaerobic bacteria, the lysis–centrifugation (ISOLATOR; Wampole) system[212] and the Septichek (Roche) blood culture system[221] (discussed in Chaps. 2 and 3), thus far, have performed only suboptimally compared with the traditional and Bactec broth systems for anaerobic blood culture. It is recommended that laboratories using either of these systems also use a traditional or an instrumented broth culture system (in addition) for anaerobic blood cultures.[83,102,214]

Additional instrumented blood culture systems include the BACTEC 9240, the BacT/Alert (Organon Teknica), the ESP (Difco), and the BioArgos (Sanofi Diagnostics Pasteur, Marnes-la-Coquette, France). Although the BACTEC 9240, the BacT/Alert, and the ESP appear to perform in a manner comparably with the BACTEC NR 660 in terms of overall yield and time to recovery, data on the performance of these systems for the recovery of anaerobes per se are lacking.[149,157,169,212,222].

DIRECT EXAMINATION OF CLINICAL MATERIALS

Gross examination of specimens is particularly valuable in bringing to light the possible presence of anaerobes. A foul odor, purulent appearance of fluid specimens, and the presence of necrotic tissue and gas or sulfur granules are all valuable clues.

The importance of microscopic examination of clinical specimens has been emphasized by several authors, and the information derived may give immediate presumptive evidence that anaerobes are present.[48,91,195] In preparing slides for a Gram stain, methanol fixation is much better than traditional heat fixation. The background and cellular characteristics of the smear should be observed; and the Gram reaction; the size, shape, and arrangement of bacteria; and the relative number of organisms present should be recorded. The presence of spores, their shape and position in the bacterial cell, and other distinctive morphologic features, such as branching, filaments with spherical bodies, pointed ends, and granular forms, should be noted. Although the Gram stain is ordinarily satisfactory for determining cellular characteristics, the

Giemsa and Wright's stains may occasionally reveal valuable additional information. Acridine orange stains are most worthwhile for detecting bacteria in blood cultures, cerebrospinal fluid (CSF), pleural fluid, joint fluid, and exudates.[112] The morphology of several anaerobes in stained preparations examined microscopically is illustrated in the photomicrographs included in Color Plates 14-1, 14-2, 14-3, and 14-4 and in the Color Plates of Chapter 2.

The presence of numerous squamous epithelial cells without inflammatory cells in specimens from skin wounds or from the respiratory or urogenital tracts usually indicates poor quality, superficially collected material that probably will yield mixtures of insignificant organisms from the normal flora or contaminants. At IUMC, the extent of identification is limited when a direct microscopic examination reveals samples of poor quality. The clinicians should be notified of the direct examination results and the problem of specimen quality discussed in a timely fashion before discarding the primary culture plates. Microbiologists should work closely with clinicians in an effort to enhance the quality and the clinical relevance of the specimens processed and the results reported.

Immunologic tests for the direct detection of anaerobe antigens have had only limited successful applications. Fluorescent antibodies in kits developed commercially for *Bacteroides* species several years ago were hampered in general by nonspecificity and cross-reactions, with insufficient sensitivity to aid in direct identification of organisms in fresh specimens. A *Clostridium difficile* cytotoxin neutralization assay, based on the use of specific antisera coupled with clinical findings, is considered to be the gold standard test procedure against which other *C. difficile* diagnostic tests should be compared. Alternative immunologic procedures for the direct detection of *C. difficile* antigen or toxin in fecal samples include the CDT latex agglutination test (Becton Dickinson), and various enzyme immunoassay (EIA) systems, now marketed by several companies. The rapid CDT latex agglutination test, which reacts with a glutamate dehydrogenase of *C. difficile*,[128] has been a highly useful test for *Clostridium difficile*-associated disease (CDAD), despite concerns about its lack of specificity.[127,140] Although the test reacts with nontoxigenic *C. difficile*, and cross-reacts with *Peptostreptococcus anaerobius*, certain clostridia, and other anaerobes, this has not created a major problem in clinical practice.

Another rapid immunologic procedure that detects the glutamate dehydrogenase of *C. difficile* in feces, the Immunocard (Meridian Diagnostics), is available in an EIA format. Preliminary data based on a multicenter trial conducted at three medical centers revealed that the Immunocard was much more sensitive than the CDT latex agglutination test, $p<0.05$, probably because of the inherent technical differences between an enzyme immunoassay and a latex agglutination procedure.[9]

Theoretically, both the sensitivity and specificity of direct *C. difficile* toxin testing in feces should be greatly improved using an EIA to detect the enterotoxin (toxin A) or the cytotoxin (toxin B), or both, produced by the organism in feces. As discussed in a later section of this chapter, both toxins are believed to be involved in the pathogenesis of CDAD. At this writing, the six commercially available EIA products for the detection of toxins A or B, or both, are as follows:the TechLab Tox-A Test, the Meridian Laboratories Premier Toxin A Test, the bioMerieux VIDAS *C. difficile* Toxin A test, the Cambridge Cytoclone A+B EIA, the Bartels Prima Toxin A EIA, and the Becton Dickinson Toxin CD EIA. Of these, only the Cytoclone A+B EIA detects both toxins A and B of *C. difficile.* Each of the other five systems detects toxin A, but not toxin B. All of these EIA procedures for detecting *C. difficile* toxin(s) in feces are rapid (e.g., 1- to 3-hour turnaround time), easy to use, and offer promising alternatives to the traditional cytotoxin neutralization assays. More detailed information about the performance of these commercial systems, and other information on methods for diagnosing *C. difficile* disease have been reviewed elsewhere.[12,126,158]

Use of gas–liquid chromatography (GLC) to detect anaerobes in exudates and body fluids has been advocated by some, but has not had wide popularity.[75] The value of this procedure is increased by careful direct microscopic examination of material from the same specimens. A major amount of butyric acid in a specimen that contains only thin, pointed, gram-negative rods would suggest *Fusobacterium* species. A major peak of succinate and the presence of only gram-negative rods would suggest *Bacteroides, Prevotella,* or *Porphyromonas* species. A major propionate peak in a positive blood culture containing pleomorphic, non–spore-forming gram-positive rods (so-called diphtheroids) would be most consistent with *Propionibacterium* species. However, direct GLC provides only presumptive clues; and should be interpreted cautiously in polymicrobial infections.

SELECTION AND USE OF MEDIA

The media used for recovering anaerobes from specimens should include nonselective, selective, and enrichment types, as illustrated in Table 14-6. Other media may also be included or substituted for those listed in Table 14-6. For example, chopped meat glucose medium is commonly used instead of enriched thioglycolate medium; colistin–nalidixic acid (CNA) agar may be used instead of phenylethyl alcohol (PEA) agar. Either paromomycin–vancomycin blood agar or kanamycin–vancomycin blood agar can be used for the selective isolation of the gram-negative non–spore-forming anaerobes. Bacteroides bile esculin agar is recommended in the *Wadsworth Anaerobic Bacteriology Manual* for the selection and presumptive identification of the *Bacteroides fragilis* group[195] and has also been found useful as a selective medium for *Bilophila wadsworthia.*[20] Results obtained with plating media formulations such as Schaedler, Columbia, Brucella, or others may not be entirely comparable with the morphology and growth characteristics of anaerobes seen on the Centers for Disease Control (CDC) anaerobe blood agar-based media formulations (see Color Plates 14-1 through 14-4).

The anaerobe blood agar used at the CDC and at Indiana University is recommended as a nonselective medium. It contains 5% defibrinated rabbit or sheep blood added to trypticase–soy agar (Becton Dickinson Microbiology Systems; BDMS, Cockeysville MD), with L-cystine, yeast extract (Difco, Detroit MI), vitamin K_1, and hemin added.[52] The formula is found in Box 14-4.

Plates of this medium are commercially available from Carr-Scarborough Microbiologicals (Stone Mountain GA); Becton Dickinson Microbiology Systems (Cockeysville MD); and Remel (Lenexa KA). Provided they do not dry out, commercially prepared anaerobe blood agar plates can be stored in the refrigerator within cellophane bags for at least 6 weeks.[117]

Before use, the plates are held for 4 to 16 hours in an anaerobic jar or an anaerobic glove box in an atmosphere of 85% N_2, 10% H_2, and 5% CO_2. An added benefit of the CDC anaerobe blood agar described earlier is that the added L-cystine in the medium permits growth of certain thiol-dependent or sulfur-containing amino acid-requiring bacteria, such as *Fusobacterium necrophorum,* and fastidious, thiol-dependent streptococci that have been isolated from patients with endocarditis.[6] This medium also supports excellent growth of the strict anaerobes *Clostridium novyi* type B and *C. haemolyticum.*

The phenylethyl alcohol blood agar is prepared by supplementing the anaerobe blood agar, described previously, with 0.25% phenylethyl alcohol. Similarly, the kanamycin–vancomycin or the paromomycin–vancomycin blood agar is prepared by adding 100 µg of kanamycin or paromomycin and 7.5 µg of vancomycin per milliliter of the blood agar medium.

The enriched thioglycolate medium (BBL-135C with hemin and vitamin K_1 supplement) is primarily recommended as a back-up to the plating media.[52] This medium is particularly helpful for cultivating slow-growing species of *Actinomyces.* Chopped meat glucose broth, a good alternative to enriched thioglycolate medium, is useful for isolation of *Clostridium* species by the spore selection technique and as a holding medium for anaerobic cultures in general. Prereduced anaerobically sterilized (PRAS) media in roll tubes are recommended in the Virginia Polytechnic Institute (VPI) anaerobe laboratory manual for isolating anaerobes.[91] These media are available from

---

BOX 14-4. CDC ANAEROBE BLOOD AGAR

INGREDIENT	AMOUNT
Trypticase soy agar (BDMS)	15 g
Phytone (BDMS)	5 g
Sodium chloride	5 g
Agar	20 g
Yeast extract (Difco)	5 g
Hemin	5 mg
Vitamin K_1 (3-phytylmenadione)	10 mg
L-Cystine	400 mg
Demineralized water	1 L
Blood (sheep or rabbit), defibrinated	50 mL

MEDIUM	MAJOR INGREDIENTS AND COMMENTS	PURPOSE
CDC Anaerobe Blood Agar (AnBAP)	Trypticase soy agar base with 5% sheep blood; supplemented with yeast extract, hemin, vitamin K_1 and L-cystine for anaerobes requiring additional growth factors (e.g., *Prevotella melaninogenica, Fusobacterium necrophorum,* and others). Additional media bases, including Brucella, brain–heart infusion, Schaedler, and Columbia blood agar support excellent growth of many anaerobes, but morphology and other characteristics tend to differ on these media.	Nonselective blood agar-plating medium for primary isolation of essentially all types of anaerobes found in clinical materials (see text and Color Plates 14-1 through 14-4).
Anaerobe Phenylethyl Alcohol Blood Agar (PEA)	In addition to containing the same ingredients as the CDC Anaerobe Blood Agar formulation above, the medium has phenylethyl alcohol (2.5 g/L). PEA inhibits the swarming of *Proteus* spp. and inhibits the growth of many other gram-negative facultatively anaerobic bacteria, including most *Enterobacteriaceae.* PEA is volatile. Plates should be tightly sealed in cellophane or plastic bags and stored at 4°C. A batch of plates that no longer inhibits the swarming of *Proteus* should be discarded, regardless of the expiration date.	PEA medium aids in selective isolation of anaerobes from infected materials containing a mixture of bacteria. It should support good growth of most gram-positive and gram-negative obligately anaerobic bacteria. Facultatively anaerobic gram-positive bacteria such as staphylococci, streptococci, *Bacillus* spp., and coryneform bacteria also grow well on it.
Anaerobe Kanamycin–Vancomycin Blood Agar (KV)	Contains the same CDC Anaerobe Blood Agar formulation as AnBAP above, but in addition, contains 100 mg/L of kanamycin and 7.5 mg/L of vancomycin. The kanamycin inhibits many (but not all) facultatively anaerobic gram-negative rods and the vancomycin inhibits gram-positive bacteria in general (including most gram-positive anaerobes and nonanaerobes). Vancomycin in this concentration can also inhibit the *Porphyromonas* spp.	KV medium is useful for selective isolation of most *Bacteroides* spp., *Prevotella* spp., *Fusobacterium* spp., and *Veillonella* spp. from clinical specimens containing mixed aerobic and anaerobic bacteria.
Anaerobe Paromomycin–Vancomycin Laked Blood Agar (PV)	Laked PV medium is similar to the formulation above, except KV that 100 mg/L of paromomycin is substituted for the kanamycin. Also in PV, the blood is laked before it is added (by freezing and thawing the blood). Performance is similar to KV, except that the paromomycin may inhibit some additional facultative anaerobes that are resistant to kanamycin such as some strains of *Klebsiella* spp. Similar to KV agar, laked PV should inhibit growth of gram-positive organisms in general. The laked blood may aid in early recognition of pigmented *Prevotella.*	Laked PV is an excellent medium for selective primary isolation of organisms in the *Bacteroides fragilis* group, the pigmented and nonpigmented *Prevotella* spp., *Fusobacterium nucleatum, F. necrophorum, F. mortiferum, Veillonella,* and other obligately anaerobic gram-negative non–spore-forming anaerobes. It is not necessary to use both KV and PV; rather, it is reasonable to select one or the other of these media, based on preferences of the microbiologist.
Cycloserine–Cefoxitin Fructose Agar (CCFA)	Trypticase–soy or proteose peptone base containing fructose and neutral red indicator. In addition, cycloserine (500 mg/L) and cefoxitin (16 mg/L) are added to inhibit intestinal flora. *C. difficile,* at 48 h of incubation, forms 4 mm or larger yellowish rhizoid colonies that have birefringent crystalline internal structures ("speckled opalescence"). *C. difficile* colonies show yellow-green fluorescence under long-wave UV light (their odor is reminiscent of horse manure). *C. difficile* is negative for both lipase and lecithinase activity.	CCFA is for selective isolation of *C. difficile* from stool specimens or other intestinal materials. However, growth on CCFA is not specific for only *C. difficile;* therefore, identification of pure culture isolates is still required. (It is common to find breakthrough growth on the medium of unwanted *Enterobacteriaceae, Bacillus* spp., staphylococci and other clostridia).
Enriched Thioglycollate Medium (THIO)	THIO is an enriched liquid medium prepared by supplementing the BBL-0135C Formula Thioglycollate Medium (without indicator) with hemin and vitamin K_1.	This is a noninhibitory broth that is especially useful for primary isolation of actinomycetes. THIO is also an excellent supplement or backup to solid plating media for isolation of slow-growing or fastidious organisms. It should support good growth of essentially all anaerobes commonly found in clinical materials.

* All the media in this table are available in prepared form from several manufacturers (see text). All but CCFA are described in detail by Dowell, Lombard, and colleagues in an excellent CDC manual (1977). The publication by George, et al. (J Clin Microbiol 9:214–219) is recommended for those who desire more information on CCFA. Also, publications by Bartley and Dowell, Lab Med Vol. 22, No. 5 and Marler et al. (J Clin Microbiol 30:514–516, 1992) are recommended.

おはか을 stop

Carr-Scarborough Microbiologicals (Stone Mountain GA).

Other special-purpose selective media for primary isolation of anaerobes in normal flora studies have been described in detail by Summanen and colleagues in the *Wadsworth Manual*.[195] In addition, Smith and Moore described new selective media and a cold enrichment technique to aid in isolation of *Mobiluncus* species from vaginal specimens.[184] Eley and coworkers reported on a selective and differential medium for isolation of *Bacteroides ureolyticus*.[55] Lee and coworkers developed a new selective medium for *Bacteroides gracilis*.[115] Malnick and associates formulated a new selective medium for isolating *Anaerobiospirillum* spp. from feces.[130] Additional special-purpose selective media and isolation procedures have been developed for the isolation and enumeration of *Clostridium difficile*, *C. perfringens*, and *C. botulinum* from feces (or food samples).[5,27,195]

In a previous study, Siders and associates (unpublished data) examined the performance of CDC-anaerobe blood agar that had been prepared by three commercial manufacturers (i.e., Carr-Scarborough Microbiologicals, Stone Mountain GA; BDMS, Cockeysville MD; and Gibco, Columbus IN). The Carr-Scarborough medium showed better quantitative and qualitative performance for the recovery of several gram-negative and gram-positive anaerobes, but the media from all three manufacturers were satisfactory.

ANAEROBIC SYSTEMS FOR CULTIVATION OF ANAEROBIC BACTERIA

Comparative studies have shown that the following systems are satisfactory for the cultivation of anaerobic bacteria commonly associated with human disease if used properly:[103,168] Evacuation-replacement; GasPak (Becton Dickinson Microbiology Systems) or Oxoid (Oxoid USA, Inc., Columbia MD); disposable gas generator method; anaerobic glove box techniques; roll tube and roll–streak tube with PRAS media.

To ensure optimal results, the general principles listed in Box 14-5 must be followed.

ANAEROBIC JAR TECHNIQUES

Some of the different jars used for cultivating anaerobic bacteria have included the Brewer, Baird-Tatlock, GasPak, McIntosh-Fildes, Oxoid, and Torbal jars. The GasPak jar, illustrated in Figure 14-2, is the system most commonly used in clinical laboratories in the United States.

The Oxoid jar (Fig. 14-3) has a metal lid, Schrader valves and a pressure gauge. Otherwise, it is used similarly to the other jars.

The basic principle of these jars is the same; namely, removal of oxygen from the chamber by reaction with hydrogen added to the system in the presence of the catalyst. Oxygen is reduced to water as follows:

$$\text{Catalyst}$$
$$2H_2 + O_2 \longleftrightarrow 2H_2O$$

The use of an active catalyst in each system is important. The older Brewer jar technique used a palladium catalyst in the lid of the jar (a modified McIntosh-Fildes jar), which had to be heated with an electric current to be fully active. The GasPak jar uses a "cold" catalyst, composed of palladium-coated alumina pellets, which does not require heating. The cold catalyst is more convenient to use and has no explosion hazard. The cold palladium catalyst can be inactivated in the jar by the production of hydrogen sulfide or other volatile metabolic products of the bacteria. It is recommended that the catalyst pellets be replaced with new or rejuvenated pellets each time the jar is used.[11,48] The pellets can be rejuvenated or restored to full activity by heating them in a dry-heat oven at 160° to 170°C for 2 hours. After heating, the pellets are stored at room temperature in a clean, dry container or in a dessicator until the time of use.

Anaerobic conditions can be produced in jar systems with either the disposable hydrogen–carbon dioxide generator (GasPak, Oxoid) or by the evacuation–replacement procedure. The evacuation–replacement procedure, in which the air in the jar is removed and replaced with a mixture of 85% N_2, 10% H_2, and 5% CO_2 is more economical than gas generators and allows anaerobic conditions to be established more rapidly. Any airtight container can be used, including a GasPak jar with a vented lid, a Brewer jar, Oxoid jar, or even a modified pressure cooker.

Whaley and Gorman described an inexpensive device for evacuating and gasing jars or other systems.[217] This device can be used with an in-house vacuum, thereby eliminating the need for a vacuum pump when the evacuation–replacement procedure is used. Air is evacuated from the jar by drawing a vacuum of 20 to 24 in. Hg (51 to 61 cm Hg). This procedure is repeated three times. The jar is then filled with N_2 after the first two evacuations and the final replacement is made with the 85% N_2, 10% H_2 and 5% CO_2 gas mixture.

The disposable H_2 and CO_2 generators are used by opening the generator envelope and placing it into the jar to be used. Approximately 10 mL of water is added

> **BOX 14-5. PRINCIPLES FOR OPTIMUM RECOVERY OF ANAEROBES**
>
> 1. Proper collection and transport of the clinical specimens
> 2. Processing of specimens with minimal exposure to atmospheric oxygen
> 3. Use of fresh or prereduced media
> 4. Proper use of an anaerobic system with inclusion of an active catalyst to allow removal of oxygen (from jar or glove box system)

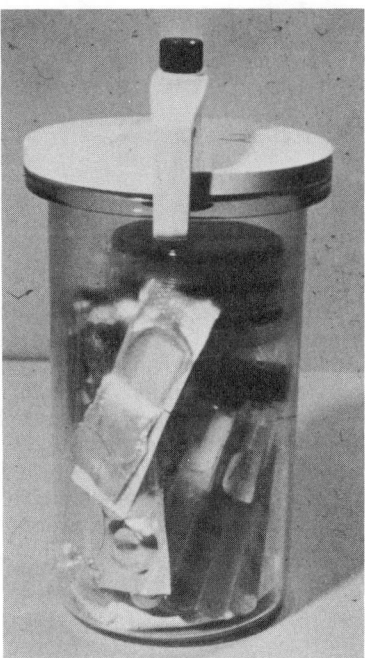

Figure 14-2
The GasPak (Becton Dickinson Microbiology Systems, Cockeysville, MD) anaerobic system: The jar contains inoculated plates, broth tubes, a GasPak hydrogen and carbon dioxide generator envelope, a disposable methylene blue indicator strip, and a catalyst basket in the lid.

to allow the generation of hydrogen and carbon dioxide, and the lid is tightly sealed. If the lid is not warm to the touch within 40 minutes after it is sealed, or if condensation does not appear on the inner surface of the glass within 25 minutes, the jar should be opened and the generator envelope discarded and replaced with a new generator. A defective gasket in the lid that allows escape of gas or inactivated catalyst pellets are the two most common causes of failure of this system.

Anaerobic conditions should always be monitored when using either of the two jar techniques by including an oxidation–reduction indicator. Methylene blue strips are available commercially for this purpose (BBL Microbiology Systems, Cockeysville MD). Alternatively, a 13- by 100-mm test tube containing a few milliliters of methylene blue–$NaHCO_3$–glucose mixture can be placed in the jar.[48] Methylene blue is blue when oxidized, clear when reduced. The color changes at about +11.0 mV. Thus, if anaerobic conditions are achieved, the methylene blue indicator solution will gradually turn colorless and will remain that way if there are no leaks that allow additional oxygen to enter the system. If the solution turns blue after being colorless, this indicates that anaerobic conditions were not maintained and the culture results may not be valid.

The GasPak 100 Anaerobic system has been analyzed relative to O_2 and CO_2 concentrations, time of appearance of water condensate, catalyst temperature, and E_h of commercially prepared plated media at various time intervals at 20° to 25°C.[171] The O_2 concentration was 0.2% to 0.6% within 60 minutes after activat-

ing the generator and less than 0.2% at 100 minutes. The CO_2 concentration was 4.6% to 6.2% at 60 minutes after activation. The E_h of the three different media tested varied from +60 mV (Columbia agar with 5% sheep blood) to +500 mV (Schaedler agar with 5% sheep blood) at zero time. The E_h ranged from −30 mV to −229 mV after 60 minutes and ranged from −115 mV to −300 mV after 100 minutes. This indicates rapid reduction of the media, even though the methylene blue indicator did not become decolorized in less than 6 hours at 25°C. At 35°C, the methylene blue usually becomes reduced in about 5 hours, and it is likely that the media is reduced more rapidly at 35°C than at 25°C. However, if ambient air enters the system, the methylene blue indicator changes to blue within minutes.

USE OF THE ANAEROBIC GLOVE BOX

An anaerobic glove box is a self-contained anaerobic system that allows the microbiologist to process specimens and perform most bacteriologic techniques for

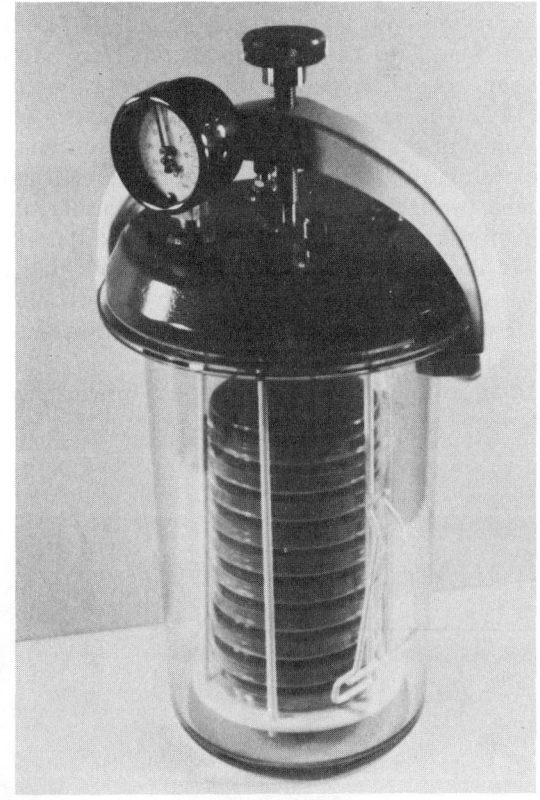

Figure 14-3
The Oxoid Anaerobic Jar (Oxoid USA, Columbia, MD) contains a 3.5-L polycarbonate jar closed by a heavy-duty metal lid and metal clamp. The lid center has two Schrader valves and a plus or minus pressure gauge, with two valves to facilitate the evacuation–replacement (E/R) technique. There is also a safety valve in the lid to prevent extra gas pressure caused by incorrect use of the E/R technique. A sachet containing a low-temperature catalyst is clipped to the undersurface of the lid. In lieu of using the E/R technique, the jar can be used with the Oxoid Generating Kit available from the manufacturer.

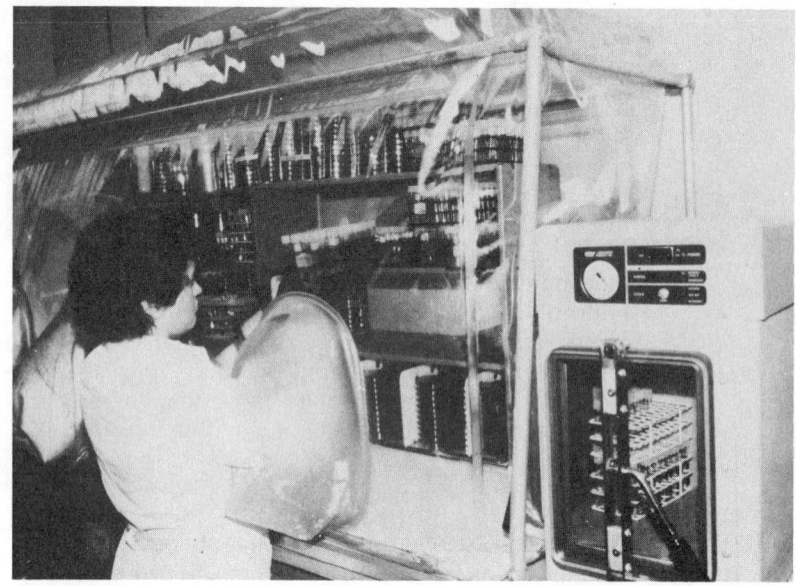

Figure 14-4
The anaerobic glove box (Coy Laboratory Products, Inc., Ann Arbor, MI): Materials are passed in and out of the large, flexible plastic chamber through an automatic entry lock. Anaerobic conditions are maintained by constant recirculation of the atmosphere within the plastic chamber (85% N_2, 10% H_2, 5% CO_2) through a palladium catalyst. Cultures are incubated either within a separate incubator inside the glove box, or by maintaining the entire chamber at 35°C through use of heated catalyst boxes.

isolation and identification of anaerobic bacteria without exposure to air. Glove boxes suitable for cultivation of anaerobes can be constructed from various materials, including steel, acrylic plastic, or fiberglass (Fig. 14-4). The flexible vinyl plastic anaerobic chamber developed at the University of Michigan has enjoyed wide popularity,[15] and a modification of this design is available in varying sizes from the Coy Manufacturing Co., Ann Arbor, Michigan. A glove box of different design is shown in Figure 14-5. In addition, a rigid, "gloveless," glove box is marketed by Anaerobe Systems (San Jose, CA) and Toucan Technologies (Cincinnati, OH).

An anaerobic glove box, if properly constructed, is economical to operate because it permits the use of conventional-plating media and the cost of gases for operation of the system is minimal. Once set up, the major expense is for the 85% N_2, 10% H_2, 5% CO_2 gas mixture used to replace the air in the entry lock when materials are passed into the glove box chamber.

THE ROLL–STREAK SYSTEM

The roll–streak system, developed by Moore and associates of the VPI Anaerobe Laboratory,[91] is a modification of the roll-tube technique developed by Hungate and associates for culturing anaerobic bacteria from the rumen of cows and other herbivorous animals. Equipment for the VPI anaerobic culture system is available commercially from Bellco Glass Corp. (Vineland NJ).

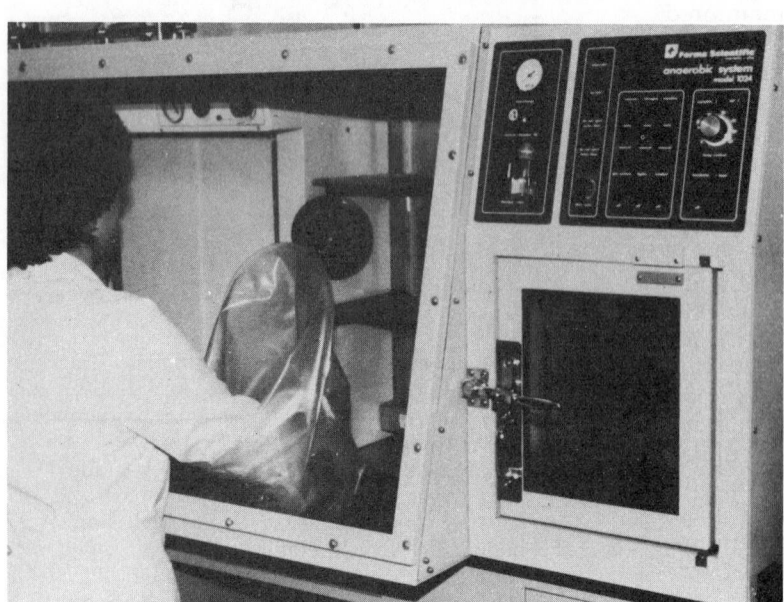

Figure 14-5
The Forma Model 1024 anaerobic glove box (Forma Scientific, Marietta, OH): This system has an automatic entry lock. During routine daily operation, atmospheric air is bubbled through a methylene blue–glucose–HEPES buffer solution, which aids in monitoring O_2 leaks, or determining if the catalyst is not working properly.

The roll–streak system uses PRAS media prepared in tubes with rubber stoppers. After autoclaving, the tubes of agar media are cooled in a rolling machine, which results in a thin coating of the inner surfaces of the tubes with solidified medium. Both the roll–streak tubes and the PRAS liquid media require the addition of a reducing agent, such as L-cysteine hydrochloride, which is added just before autoclaving to help maintain a low oxidation–reduction potential within the system. All inoculating and subculturing of the PRAS solid and liquid media are performed under a stream of oxygen-free CO_2, which minimizes exposure to air and helps maintain a reduced oxidation–reduction potential in the media before and after growth of the obligate anaerobes. The Hungate technique requires less equipment than the roll–streak technique for inoculating liquid media. A needle and syringe are used to inoculate PRAS media in Hungate tubes through a rubber stopper–screw-cap closure assembly. PRAS media in Hungate tubes are available from Carr-Scarborough Microbiologicals, Inc. (Stone Mountain GA).

ANAEROBIC DISPOSABLE PLASTIC BAGS

The Bio-Bag system, originally developed by Marion Scientific (Kansas City MO) is now available form Becton Dickinson Microbiology Systems (Sparks MD). A second system, called the "Anaerobic Pouch System Catalyst-Free," is marketed by Difco Laboratories (Detroit MI). A third anaerobic disposable bag system, called the Anaerocult A, is manufactured in Germany (Merck, Darmstadt, FRG).

The anaerobic Bio-Bag consists of a clear, plastic bag (sold in varying sizes capable of holding one to three, 100-mm–diameter petri dishes), an H_2–CO_2 gas generator that generates an atmosphere when water is added to it (analogous to the generator used in a Gas-Pak jar), cold palladium catalyst pellets, and a resazurin indicator. The bag is heat-sealed following activation of the generator to permit maintenance of anaerobic conditions, according to the same principle described for the GasPak jar system.

On the other hand, the Difco Anaerobic Pouch and the Anaerocult both achieve anaerobic conditions differently, without catalyst, to remove oxygen from the atmosphere. In these disposable systems, water is added to sodium carbonate, resulting in production of CO_2 and H_2. Oxygen is removed from within the sealed plastic pouch by combining with iron powder to produce iron oxides. In one study, the Bio-Bag was reported to be less effective than the Difco Anaerobic Pouch for recovery of anaerobes from clinical specimens, whereas the latter system was comparable with the anaerobic chamber methods that were used.[53] In another study, no apparent differences were seen between the performance of the Anaerocult A and the GasPak Plus jar system during a quantitative in vitro culture comparison.[82] Thus, the Anaerobic Pouch and Anae-

rocult systems may be practical alternatives to glove box or anaerobic jar systems for the incubation of anaerobes when only one or two plates are to be incubated.

USE OF THE ANAEROBIC HOLDING JAR

A modification of the Martin holding jar procedure is a convenient and inexpensive adjunct to the jar and glove box anaerobic systems that allows primary plating, inspection of cultures, and subculture of colonies at the bench, with only minimal exposure of anaerobic bacteria to atmospheric oxygen.[6,134] The holding jar assembly is illustrated in Figure 14-6, and its use is briefly described in Box 14-6.

Inexpensive, commercial-grade N_2 can be used in the holding jar system. Open the small needle valve on the gas manifold (see Fig. 14-6) and set the gas tank regulator to 4 psi for 20 to 30 seconds to rapidly purge the jar of air. Then turn the regulator pressure down to about 0.5 to 1 psi and regulate the flow to each jar at 50 to 100 mL/min, using the small needle valve on the manifold. This is equivalent to a flow rate of one to two bubbles per second when the rubber tubing in the jar is placed just beneath the surface of water in a beaker. Alternatively, CO_2 passed through a tube of heated copper catalyst (Sargent furnace) can be used in the holding jars instead of N_2.[6,134]

BOX 14-6. ANAEROBIC HOLDING JAR PROCEDURE

1. Three holding jars are used, the first to hold uninoculated media, the second for plates on which are growing colonies to be subcultured, and the third to receive freshly inoculated plates of media.

2. Commercially prepared agar plates or agar media freshly prepared in the laboratory can be used. These may be held in a refrigerator for up to 6 weeks if bagged in cellophane.

3. The plates to be used on any given day should first be placed in an anaerobic glove box or an anaerobic jar for 4 to 15 hours before use to reduce the media.

4. As needed, the reduced media are placed in the first holding jar and continuously flushed with a gentle stream of N_2.

5. The plates of reduced media are surface inoculated, one at a time, in ambient air and immediately placed in the third holding jar, which is also flushed with N_2. The second holding jar is used to hold any plates removed from the GasPak jar that require subculture.

6. After the jar containing the newly inoculated plates is filled, the plates can be transferred to a conventional anaerobic system, such as a GasPak jar, or into an anaerobic glove box for incubation at 35°C.

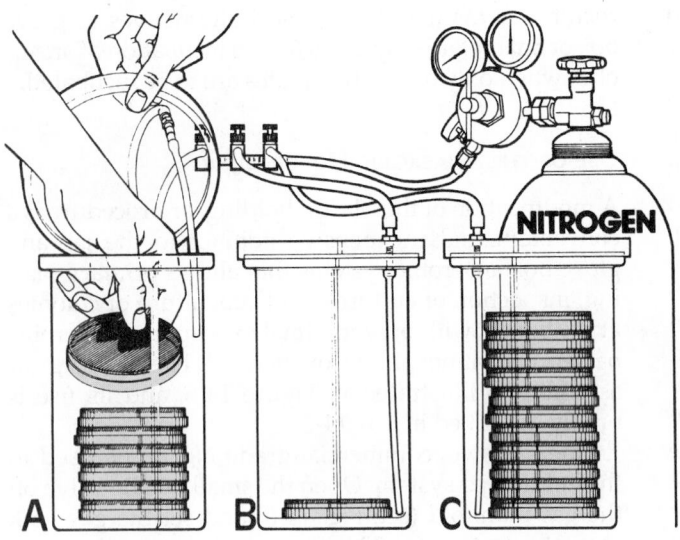

Figure 14-6
Schematic of the anaerobic-holding jar system: The flow rate of nitrogen to each jar is regulated by the needle valves on the manifold (three-gang valve, available where aquarium supplies are sold). Jars *A, B,* and *C* contain uninoculated plates, plates with colonies to be subcultured, and freshly inoculated plates, respectively.

INCUBATION OF CULTURES

In most instances, 35°to 37°C is the temperature most satisfactory for primary isolation of anaerobic bacteria from clinical specimens. Plates inoculated at the bench and placed in anaerobic jars should be incubated for at least 48 hours, and reincubated for another 2 to 4 days to allow slow-growing organisms to form colonies; some anaerobes, such as certain species of *Actinomyces* and *Eubacterium,* grow rather slowly, and colonies may not be detected if jars are opened sooner. Also, if the jar is opened too soon, some of the slow-growing organisms may be killed by oxygen exposure. In emergency situations, duplicate sets of plating media can be incubated in two different jars, one set incubated for 18 to 24 hours and the other for 3 to 5 days. This procedure allows rapid isolation of fast-growing anaerobes in the 18- to 24-hour jar and the later recovery of slow growers in the jars left for delayed incubation. If clostridial myonecrosis is suspected clinically, plates can be inspected as early as 6 to 12 hours after inoculation.

Prolonged exposure of freshly inoculated plates to ambient air must be avoided. Certain anaerobes commonly encountered in clinical specimens, such as *Peptostreptococcus anaerobius,* may either fail to grow or may exhibit a prolonged lag in growth when freshly inoculated plates are held in ambient air for as short a time as 2 hours. Thus, if a holding jar procedure is not used, inoculated plates must be immediately placed in an anaerobic system (anaerobic jar or anaerobic glove box) to allow effective cultivation of these anaerobes.

Enriched thioglycolate and chopped meat glucose media should also be inoculated with clinical materials incubated in an anaerobic system to allow maximum recovery of anaerobes. PRAS media in rubber-stoppered tubes can also be used. It is not necessary to boil the tubes of enriched thioglycolate or chopped meat glucose broth if they are prepared in tight-fitting screw-cap tubes and gased in a glove box after autoclaving. Unless growth is apparent visually, broth cultures should be held a minimum of 5 to 7 days before discarding them as negative.

INSPECTION AND SUBCULTURE OF COLONIES

After incubation, plates removed from 5% to 10% CO_2 atmospheres should be examined with a hand lens or preferably a dissecting microscope. If anaerobic jars are used, a holding jar system should be employed at the time of colony examination and subculture, to minimize exposure of oxygen-sensitive isolates to air. The anaerobic glove box and the anaerobic disposable bag systems (Fig. 14-7), allow inspection of colonies in the absence of air.

Use of the stereoscopic dissecting microscope during examination of colonies is extremely helpful because several anaerobes have distinctive colonial features.[48] The dissecting microscope is also a valuable aid during the subculture of colonies to obtain pure culture isolates.

During the inspection of colonies, any action on the medium, such as hemolysis of blood agar or clearing of egg yolk agar, as well as the size and distinctive features of the colonies should be recorded. A number of characteristic colonies of anaerobes are illustrated in Color Plates 14-1, 14-2, 14-3, and 14-4. When recording colony characteristics, the following should be noted: the age of the culture and the name of the medium; the diameter in millimeters of each colony, in addition to its color, surface features (glistening, dull), density (opaque, translucent), consistency (butyrous, viscid, membranous, brittle), and other descriptive features (see Fig. 2-17).

Gram-stained smears of colonies from the anaerobic and CO_2-incubated plates should also be examined. Do not assume on the basis of colony and microscopic features only that colonies on plates that have been in-

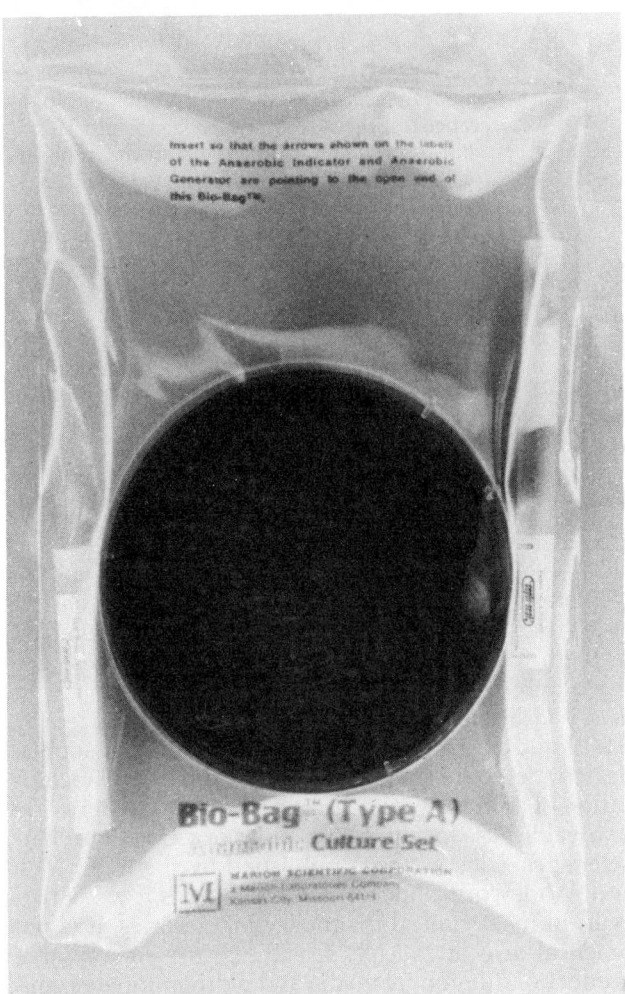

Figure 14-7
The Bio-Bag Anaerobic Culture Set (Becton Dickinson Microbiology Systems, Cockeysville, MD): This culture set includes a plate of CDC–anaerobic blood agar contained within an oxygen-impermeable bag. The system contains its own gas-generating kit and cold catalyst.

After incubation, Gram stain the enriched thioglycolate and chopped meat glucose subcultures. If the organisms appear to be in pure culture, they can be used to inoculate appropriate differential media for identification of isolates.

Examine enriched thioglycolate and chopped meat glucose cultures that were inoculated with the original specimen, along with all primary isolation plates. If no growth is evident on the primary anaerobic plates, or if the colonies isolated fail to account for all the morphologic types found in the direct gram-stained smear of the specimen, each broth medium should be subcultured to two anaerobe blood agar plates, one for anaerobic incubation and the other incubated in a 5% to 10% CO_2 air incubator. Alternatively, a chocolate agar plate can be used for the subculture plate to be incubated in the 5% to 10% CO_2–air incubator. These subculture plates should then be examined as described previously.

AEROTOLERANCE TESTS

Each colony type from the anaerobic isolation plate is subcultured to an aerobic (5% to 10% CO_2, or candle jar) and anaerobic blood agar plate for overnight incubation.

Haemophilus influenzae, which grows on anaerobe blood agar anaerobically, but not on ordinary blood agar aerobically, can be mistaken for an anaerobe. This can be avoided by inoculating a chocolate agar plate (in place of the aerobic blood agar plate) for incubation in a 5% to 10% CO_2–air incubator. It may be expedient to inoculate quadrants or sixths of the chocolate agar plate for testing the aerotolerance of four to six colonies from a primary isolation plate (Fig. 14-8). However, this should be done only if colonies are well separated or were picked from a purity plate. Otherwise, single plates should be streaked with each isolate to transfer a pure culture and avoid contamination.

PRELIMINARY REPORTING OF RESULTS

Organisms that are shown to be obligate anaerobes should be reported to the clinician immediately, together with the results from observing a gram-stained preparation and characteristics of colonies. However, it is not justified to report the presence of an obligate anaerobe until aerotolerance studies have been completed.

Unfortunately, 3 days or longer are often required for these studies to be completed. Clinicians should be made aware that this lengthy time cannot be avoided with some slow-growing anaerobes (e.g., some species of *Actinomyces* and *Propionibacterium*). Fortunately, the colonial and microscopic morphology of certain anaerobic bacteria is often so distinctive that *preliminary* or *presumptive* reports of these isolates can be made before aerotolerance studies. Examples include *Clostridium perfringens*, members of the *Bacteroides fragilis* group, the pigmenting *Prevotella* and *Porphyromonas* group, and others.

cubated in an anaerobic system are obligate anaerobes. Although the morphology and colony characteristics of certain anaerobes are distinctive, it is often impossible to distinguish some facultative anaerobes from obligate anaerobes without aerotolerance tests, even when the CO_2-incubated plates show no growth.

The number of different colony types on the anaerobe plates should be determined, and a semiquantitative estimate of the number of each type should be recorded (light, moderate, or heavy growth). With a needle or a sterile Pasteur capillary pipette, transfer each different colony to another anaerobe blood agar plate to obtain a pure culture and an aerobic blood agar plate for aerotolerance testing (described later). If colonies are well separated on the primary isolation plate, a tube of enrichment broth, such as enriched thioglycolate or chopped meat glucose medium, should be inoculated to provide a source of inoculum for differential tests.

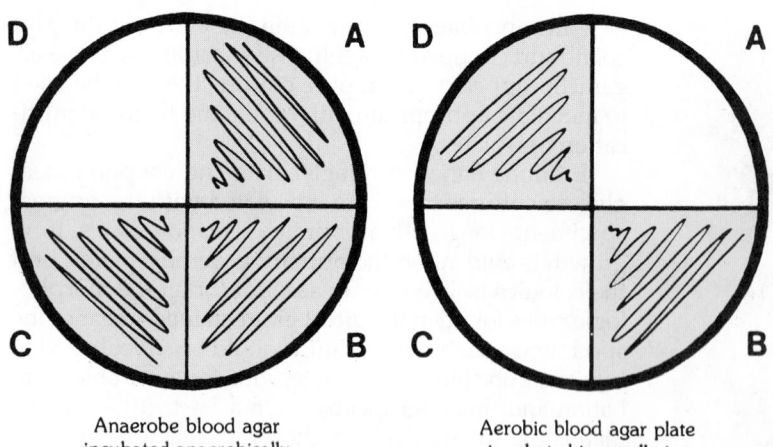

Anaerobe blood agar
incubated anaerobically

Aerobic blood agar plate
incubated in candle jar

Figure 14-8
Quadrant plating technique used for aerotolerance testing of four anaerobe isolates: The *left plate* has been incubated in an anaerobe jar for 18 to 24 hours, whereas the plate on the *right* was incubated in a candle jar. Isolates *A* and *C* are obligate anaerobes. Isolate *B* is facultatively anaerobic. Isolate *D* is either a microaerophile or an obligate anaerobe and should be further tested for its ability to grow in ambient air, compared with the environment containing increased CO_2. A candle jar is not adequate for testing *Campylobacter jejuni*; this species grows optimally in 5% to 10% CO_2, 10% CO_2, and 85% N_2.

DETERMINATION OF CULTURAL AND BIOCHEMICAL CHARACTERISTICS FOR DIFFERENTIATION OF ANAEROBE ISOLATES

Once the presence of anaerobes has been confirmed by aerotolerance tests and a description of morphologic features has been reported, the next priority is to identify the pure-culture isolates as rapidly and as accurately as possible and to report the results to the clinician within a relevant time. Although probably more than 500 species of anaerobes are currently recognized by taxonomists, the task of identifying anaerobes for the clinical microbiologist is not nearly as formidable as it might seem because only a relatively few are involved in anaerobic infections with any frequency (see Table 14-3).

PRESUMPTIVE IDENTIFICATION

Nearly all clinically significant isolates are moderate obligate or aerotolerant anaerobes and, with practice, are not particularly difficult to isolate and identify. In addition to organisms of the *Bacteroides fragilis* group, the pigmented *Prevotella–Porphyromonas* group, *F. nucleatum*, and the anaerobic cocci that are quite frequently isolated, certain other, less common anaerobes nonetheless have major pathogenic potential. Consequently, it is important to be familiar with and be able to recognize *Actinomyces israelii, A. naeslundii, A. meyeri, Propionibacterium propionicum*, and *Bifidobacterium dentium* (formerly *B. eriksonii*), all of which may cause serious acute suppurative and chronic inflammatory disease; *Prevotella bivia* and *Prevotella disiens*, which are commonly resistant to various penicillins and cephalosporins; *Fusobacterium necrophorum*, which may be highly virulent; *F. mortiferum* and *F. varium*, which vary in susceptibility to certain penicillins, cephalosporins, and clindamycin; *C. septicum*, an organism frequently associated with carcinoma of the colon or hematopoietic malignancy when isolated from patients' blood; the "histotoxic" clostridia in addition to *C. perfringens*, which can cause gas gangrene and various wound infections; *C. difficile*, a major cause of antibiotic-associ-

ated diarrhea and colitis; and *C. tetani* and *C. botulinum*, because of the diseases they cause.[5,23,64,67]

Reference laboratories commonly use large batteries of tests in characterizing anaerobe isolates referred to them for identification or confirmation. These are listed in Box 14-7.

In addition, new species are being recognized by use of nucleic acid homology studies and other sophisticated methods. The data derived from the characterization of cultures with a large number of tests provide a valuable base for compiling tables of differential characteristics, such as those published by the CDC, VPI, and Wadsworth Anaerobe Laboratories.[48,91,195] However, in most clinical diagnostic laboratories, it is not practical or economically feasible to use such a large number of differential media and biochemical determinations to identify isolates from clinical specimens.

Fortunately, certain characteristics (Box 14-8) are especially useful in the identification of anaerobes. These characteristics form the basis of a practical ap-

---

BOX 14-7. CHARACTERIZATION OF ANAEROBIC BACTERIA

Relation to O_2
Colony morphology
Gram stain reaction
Microscopic features
Motility
Growth in liquid media
Biochemical tests
Metabolic products (GLC)
Antibiotic susceptibility
Serologic tests
Toxicity, toxin neutralization, pathogenicity in animals
Polyacrylamide gel electrophoresis of soluble proteins
Cell wall long-chain fatty acids; menaquinones

BOX 14-8. SOME CARDINAL IDENTIFYING CHARACTERISTICS OF ANAEROBES

Relation to O_2

Colonial characteristics

Pigment

Hemolysis

Pitting of medium

Gram stain reaction

Morphology

Spores

Motility

Flagella

Miscellaneous

Growth in thioglycolate broth, catalase, lecithinase, lipase; reactions on milk medium; production of indole; hydrolysis of starch, esculin, and gelatin; reduction of nitrate; fermentation of key carbohydrates (e.g., glucose, mannitol, lactose, rhamnose); growth in presence of bile, penicillin, rifampin, and kanamycin; inhibition by sodium polyanetholsulfonate; production of toxins; metabolic products

---

proach for identifying anaerobe isolates that are commonly encountered in the clinical laboratory and additional species that either are less common or are potential major pathogens, even if they are rare.

USE OF DIFFERENTIAL AGAR MEDIA

Several important characteristics for identifying anaerobic bacteria can be obtained with pure cultures on CDC anaerobe blood agar and in enriched thioglycolate medium. These characteristics, outlined in Table 14-7, provide important clues for differentiating anaerobes in general. Additional characteristics are determined by use of differential disks, which are added to freshly inoculated anaerobe blood agar plates. A 2-U penicillin disk, 1000-g kanamycin disk, and 15-g rifampin disk (available from Becton Dickinson Microbiology Systems) aid in the differentiation of anaerobic, non–spore-forming, gram-negative bacilli. Colistin and vancomycin disks may also be extremely useful, as described elsewhere.[195] A sodium polyanetholsulfonate disk test is a practical way to separate *Peptostreptococcus anaerobius* from other anaerobic cocci. A nitrate disk test is a convenient method to demonstrate nitrate reduction during the workup of anaerobic bacteria (in general).

PRESUMPTO PLATES

Three types of quadrant plates (Presumpto 1, 2, and 3) containing 12 differential agar media have been developed by Dowell and associates into a system that al-

lows determination of 20 different characteristics (see Table 14-7) of anaerobe isolates at a minimal cost.[50] The information derived from using the three-quadrant plates, along with the other characteristics obtained from anaerobe blood agar and enriched thioglycolate medium plus metabolic product analysis using GLC, permits definitive identification of many clinically significant anaerobic bacteria that are encountered in the laboratory. In addition, the quadrant plates, especially the Presumpto 1 and 2 plates, can be used to supplement several of the commercial-packaged kit systems, as well as traditional broth identification systems, with important tests or characteristics these nonagar systems lack.

The basal medium in the Presumpto quadrant plate system is Lombard-Dowell (LD) medium. LD agar is a specially designed medium that supports growth of a wide variety of anaerobes, including fastidious ones. It is noteworthy that LD broth (the same medium without agar or with only a small amount) is the inoculum broth for both the Minitek (Becton Dickinson Microbiology Systems, Sparks MD) and API systems (Analytab Products, Inc., Plainview NY).

The Presumpto 1 plate is a four-quadrant petri dish containing the following media: LD agar, LD esculin agar, LD egg yolk agar, and LD bile agar. Details on the use of the Presumpto 1 plate were first published by Dowell and Lombard of the CDC.[49] It was first used for presumptive identification of *Bacteroides* and *Fusobacterium* (without Presumpto plates 2 and 3), but has since been useful for identifying other anaerobic bacteria.

The Presumpto 2 plate contains LD glucose agar, LD DNA agar, LD milk agar, and LD starch agar.[193] It is useful for characterization of clostridia; the anaerobic, non–spore-forming, gram-negative and gram-positive bacilli; and the anaerobic cocci. Similar to the Presumpto 1 plate, it can be used along with packaged micromethod kits that lack the tests it contains, or along with conventional tube tests.

The Presumpto 3 plate contains LD gelatin agar, LD mannitol agar, LD lactose agar, and LD rhamnose agar. Use of LD gelatin agar and the use of the carbohydrates in this quadrant plate has been described.[50]

Characteristics that can be determined with each of the three quadrant plates are shown in Table 14-7. Formulations and preparation of the media and reagents used in the quadrant plate system are given in detail elsewhere.[50–52,107]

Inoculation and Reading of Presumpto Plates. The procedures for inoculation of the media in the Presumpto quadrant plates, the method of incubation, and the use of differential inhibitory and antibiotic disk tests are outlined in Box 14-9.

Observation and Interpretation of Results. After incubation, examine the quadrant plates, the anaerobe blood agar plates containing the antibiotic disks, and the SPS and nitrate differentiation disks.

TABLE 14-7

Media and Characteristics of Cultures That Can Be Determined Using the Differential Agar Media System for Identifying Anaerobes

MEDIA	CHARACTERISTICS
Blood agar	Relation to O_2^*, colonial characteristics, hemolysis, pigment, fluorescence with UV light (Wood's lamp), pitting of agar, cellular morphology, Gram stain reaction, spores, motility (wet mount); inhibition by penicillin, rifampin, and kanamycin
Enriched thioglycolate medium	Appearance of growth, rapidity of growth, gas production, odor, cellular morphology
Presumpto 1 plate	
LD agar	Indole, growth on LD medium, catalase[†]
LD esculin agar	Esculin hydrolysis, H_2S, catalase
LD egg yolk agar	Lipase, lecithinase, proteolysis
LD bile agar	Growth in presence of 20% bile (2% oxgall), insoluble precipitate under and immediately surrounding growth
Presumpto 2 plate	
LD glucose agar	Glucose fermentation; stimulation of growth by fermentable carbohydrate
LD starch agar	Starch hydrolysis
LD milk agar	Casein hydrolysis
LD DNA agar	Deoxyribonuclease activity
Presumpto 3 plate	
LD mannitol agar	Mannitol fermentation
LD lactose agar	Lactose fermentation
LD rhamnose agar	Rhamnose fermentation
LD gelatin	Gelatin hydrolysis

* By comparing growth on anaerobe plate with blood agar (or chocolate agar) incubated in 5% to 10% CO_2 incubator (or candle jar) or in room air.
† The catalase test can be performed by adding 3% hydrogen peroxide to the growth on LD agar, but the reactions of catalase-positive cultures are more vigorous on LD esculin agar.

Presumpto Quadrant Plate 1 (see Color Plate 14-5)

LD AGAR. Note and record the degree of growth on LD agar (light, moderate, heavy). Test for indole by adding 2 drops of *p*-dimethyl-aminocinnamaldehyde reagent to the paper disk on the medium. Observe for the development of a blue or bluish-green color in the disk within 30 seconds, which is a positive reaction for indole. Development of another color (pink, red, violet) or no color is negative for indole. A lavender to violet color is a positive reaction for indole derivative(s).

LD EGG YOLK AGAR. Formation of a zone of insoluble precipitate in the medium surrounding the bacterial colonies is a positive reaction for lecithinase production. This is best seen with transmitted light.

The presence of an iridescent sheen (a pearly layer on the surface of colonies and on the medium immediately surrounding the bacterial growth, best demonstrated with reflected light) indicates lipase production. If the reaction is questionable, add a few drops of water and look for a film that floats on top of water.

Clearing of the medium in the vicinity of the bacterial growth indicates proteolysis, as exhibited by certain proteolytic clostridia.

LD ESCULIN AGAR. A positive test for esculin hydrolysis is indicated by the development of a reddish brown to dark brown color in the esculin agar surrounding the bacterial growth after exposure of the quadrant plate cultures to air for at least 15 minutes. Further evidence for esculin hydrolysis can be obtained by examining the esculin agar quadrant under a Wood's lamp. Esculin agar exhibits a bright blue fluorescence under the ultraviolet light that is not present after the esculin is hydrolyzed.

Blackening of the bacterial colonies on the esculin agar indicates H_2S production. The blackening dissipates very rapidly after exposure to air. Therefore, the bacterial growth should be observed for blackening under anaerobic conditions (anaerobic glove box) or immediately after opening anaerobic jars to air. To test for hydrogen peroxide degradation as an indication of catalase, expose the plates to air for at least 30 minutes and then flood the esculin agar quadrant with a few drops of fresh 3% H_2O_2. Sustained bubbling after addition of the H_2O_2 is a positive reaction for catalase. In some cases, rapid bubbling may not be evident until after 30 seconds to 1 minute.

LD BILE AGAR. Compare the degree of bacterial growth on the LD bile agar with that on the plain LD agar and record as I (growth less than on the LD agar control) or E (growth equal to or greater than on the LD agar control). Using transmitted light, look for the

BOX 14-9. USE OF PRESUMPTO QUADRANT PLATES

1. Prepare the inoculum from fresh growth of a pure culture of the anaerobe isolate. Use either a turbid cell suspension (McFarland 3) in LD broth prepared from isolated colonies, or a 24- to 48-hour enriched thioglycolate medium subculture from an isolated colony (alternatively, a 24- to 48-hour chopped meat glucose broth subculture can be used).
2. Inoculate the quadrant plates as follows:
    a. Saturate one sterile swab (for each quadrant plate to be inoculated) in either the cell suspension or broth culture.
    b. Streak the middle portion of each quadrant with the swab containing bacteria.
3. Place a sterile, blank, ½-in. diameter paper disk on the LD agar near the outer periphery of the quadrant. This disk is used in the test for indole after incubation of the plates.

In addition to setting up the Presumpto plates, also:

1. Inoculate the surface of an anaerobe blood agar plate evenly with a sterile swab that has been dipped in the cell suspension or broth culture.
2. Place the antibiotic disks (penicillin, 2-U; rifampin, 15-µg; kanamycin, 1000-µg) on the blood agar with sterile forceps. Space the disks evenly such that overlapping zones of inhibition will not be a problem.
3. Place the sodium polyanetholsulfonate (SPS) and nitrate disks on a second anaerobe blood agar plate, if they are used in addition to the antibiotic disks. To prepare the SPS disk, pipette 20 µL of 5% SPS (available in 10-mL vials of 5% SPS solution known as GROBAX; Roche Diagnostics, Nutley NJ) onto ¼-in. (0.635-cm) sterile blank disks (Difco Laboratories, Detroit MI) and dry. SPS disks are stable at room temperature for 6 months. To prepare the nitrate disk, dissolve 30 g KNO_3 and 0.1 g sodium molybdate ($Na_2MoO_4 \cdot 2H_2O$) in 100 mL distilled water and filter-sterilize the solution using a 0.45-µm membrane filter. Then add 20 µL of this reagent to ¼-in. (0.635-cm) sterile blank disks and dry at room temperature for at least 72 hours.

presence or lack of an insoluble white precipitate underneath or immediately surrounding the bacterial growth. If in doubt, inspect under a stereomicroscope using transmitted light.

Presumpto Quadrant Plate 2 (see Color Plate 14-5)

LD GLUCOSE AGAR. Fermentation of glucose is indicated by acid production or a yellow color in and around the growth in the medium. A blue color around the growth is a negative reaction. Some bacteria reduce the indicator; therefore, it is sometimes necessary to flood the quadrant with dilute bromthymol blue reagent to see whether acid has been produced.

Glucose stimulation can be observed by comparing the amount of bacterial growth on LD glucose agar with that on plain LD agar.

LD STARCH AGAR. To detect hydrolysis of starch, flood the quadrant with Gram's iodine solution; clearing around the growth indicates a positive reaction. A brownish color indicates unhydrolyzed starch and is a negative reaction.

LD MILK AGAR. A clear zone around the growth in the quadrant indicates hydrolysis of casein (i.e., digestion of milk proteins) and a positive reaction. If casein is unhydrolyzed, the medium remains cloudy (a negative reaction).

LD DNA AGAR. A pink to reddish zone around the growth on the quadrant indicates a positive reaction for the degradation of DNA (i.e., deoxyribonuclease activity). If the medium remains blue around the growth, DNA was not degraded and the reaction is negative.

Presumpto Quadrant Plate 3

LD GELATIN AGAR. To detect the hydrolysis of gelatin, flood the quadrant with acidified mercuric chloride reagent. This reagent binds to unhydrolyzed gelatin. A zone of complete clearing around the growth on the quadrant indicates gelatin has been hydrolyzed and is recorded as a positive test.

LD MANNITOL AGAR, LD LACTOSE AGAR, AND LD RHAMNOSE AGAR. Examine and interpret these quadrants as described for LD glucose agar.

ANTIMICROBIAL SUSCEPTIBILITY PLATES

GROWTH INHIBITION ON ANAEROBE BLOOD AGAR USING ANTIBIOTIC DISK TEST

Zones of inhibition around the antibiotic disks are observed and recorded as follows:

Penicillin, 2-U disk: sensitive (S) if zone of growth inhibition is 12 mm or wider in diameter; and resistant (R) if the zone is less than 12 mm.
Rifampin, 15-µg disk: sensitive (S) if zone of growth inhibition is 15 mm or larger; and resistant (R) if zone is less than 12 mm.
Kanamycin, 1000-µg disk: sensitive (S) if zone of growth inhibition is 12 mm or wider; and resistant (R) if zone is less than 12 mm.

USE OF SPS AND NITRATE DISK TESTS

SPS Disk Test. Measure the zone of inhibition around the ¼-in. disk. A 12-mm or larger zone of inhibition is recorded as sensitive (S).

Nitrate Disk Test. Test for nitrate reduction by adding 1 drop of nitrate A reagent (sulfanilic acid) and 1 drop of nitrate B reagent (1,6 Cleave's acid) to the disk.[195] A pink or red color indicates that nitrate has been reduced to nitrite. If the disk was colorless after addition of reagents A and B, sprinkle zinc dust on the disk to confirm a negative reaction. The development of a red color after zinc dust is added confirms that nitrate is still present in the disk (a negative reaction).

For summaries of characteristics for the identification of various species of anaerobes using differential tests in or on agar media see Tables 14-14 to 14-16 and 14-18 to 14-25.

The anaerobe blood agar, Presumpto quadrant plates, and other media described in this section are available commercially (Carr-Scarborough Microbiologicals, Inc., Stone Mountain GA) or can be prepared in the laboratory. Details for preparation of the media and reagents may be found elsewhere.[49–52,107] If prepared in one's own laboratory, there is the option of putting a single differential medium in a plate and not using quadrant petri dishes. This approach increases the flexibility of the system for microbiologists who would prefer to use other combinations of tests.

CHARACTERIZATION OF ANAEROBES USING CONVENTIONAL BIOCHEMICAL TESTS IN LARGE TUBES

It is not possible in this text to discuss all the procedures that are available for biochemical characterization of anaerobes. Conventional tube culture procedures are covered briefly in the following. For further details, refer to the laboratory manuals on anaerobic bacteriology.[48,52,91,146,196]

Instead of the differential tests in agar media described, one may use PRAS media in large test tubes for determining biochemical characteristics. These are inoculated either through a rubber diaphragm in Hungate tubes or with a special gasing device according to procedures of the VPI manual.[91] PRAS media can be prepared in the laboratory or can be obtained from commercial sources (Carr-Scarborough Microbiologicals, Inc., Stone Mountain GA). If PRAS media are used for characterization of isolates, the identification tables of Holdeman and associates[91] and Moore and colleagues should also be used.[91,93,146]

The pH of PRAS PY-based carbohydrate fermentation tests is determined directly by using a pH meter; a long, thin, combination electrode is inserted into each culture tube. According to the VPI manual, a pH of 5.5 to 6.0 is recorded as weak acid, whereas a pH lower than 5.5 is strong acid. Note that the pH of PY carbohydrate cultures should be compared with that of plain PY cultures (without carbohydrate). The pH of PY broth ranges between 6.2 and 6.4 when inoculated under CO_2. Also, some organisms apparently may produce acid from peptones in plain PY medium.[91] Furthermore, the pH of uninoculated PRAS PY-arabinose, PY-ribose, or PY-xylose may be as low as 5.9 after the medium has been held 1 to 2 days under a CO_2 atmosphere; thus, the pH of cultures in these media is not interpreted as acid unless it is lower than 5.7.[91,182a]

The conventional media of Dowell and associates are commercially available in 15- × 90-mm screw-cap

tubes (Carr-Scarborough Microbiologicals, Inc., Stone Mountain GA). Details on preparation and use of these media are published elsewhere.[48,52] If these differential media are used, one should refer to the identification tables of Dowell and Hawkins.[48] With either the VPI or CDC conventional system, biochemicals can be read after overnight incubation of certain rapid-growing cultures of anaerobes (e.g., some *B. fragilis* and clostridia), or after good growth is seen (usually 48 hours, but longer for slow-growing species). The fermentation tests are read by using bromthymol blue (yellow at pH 6.0) or can be read using a pH meter (a pH less than 6.0 is considered acid). In our experience some of the so-called rapid micromethod systems are not really more rapid.

ALTERNATIVE PROCEDURES

Use of conventional media in Hungate or other large tubes is relatively time-consuming, and the media are costly to prepare or purchase. Therefore, various investigators have described alternative procedures for characterizing isolates and identification schemas based on smaller volumes of media in containers that can be manipulated with reasonable speed at the bench.[3,7,14,46,143,191] In addition, descriptions of several rapid tests for preliminary grouping of isolates are given in the *Wadsworth Anaerobic Bacteriology Manual* and elsewhere.[3,7,14,46,143,191,195] These include the use of bacteroides bile esculin agar for selective isolation as well as presumptive identification of *B. fragilis* group organisms, the use of a battery of antibiotic disk tests somewhat different than those listed in Table 14-7, an indole spot test (the procedure differs from that used with the Presumpto 1 plate), a rapid gelatin hydrolysis test using unexposed Pan X film in a turbid broth suspension, rapid urease test, the Nagler reaction, and others.

THE NAGLER TEST AND THE CAMP TEST FOR *C. PERFRINGENS*

Historically, the Nagler test has been used for the presumptive identification of *C. perfringens*. Although most of the clostridia isolated in the clinical laboratory that give a positive reaction are *C. perfringens*, the antitoxin used in the test is nonspecific. *C. bifermentans*, *C. sordellii*, and *C. barati* (formerly *C. paraperfringens*) are also Nagler-positive, and additional tests are still necessary to separate them. During the past few years, popularity of the Nagler test has waned because the antitoxin has not been widely available. Additional details describing the Nagler test are given in previous editions of this text.

An alternative to the Nagler test, used in some laboratories, is the so-called reverse CAMP test.[35,79] To perform the test, inoculate an anaerobe blood agar plate with a single streak of an unknown organism that is possibly a *C. perfringens* isolate. Next, make a single streak at a 90° angle to within 1 to 2 mm of the first streak, using an inoculum of a group B β-hemolytic *Streptococcus*. An arrowhead of synergistic hemolysis, with the tip of the arrow pointing from the *Streptococcus* toward the *C. perfringens*, is a positive test. Both false-positive and false-negative results may occur. Additional data on the specificity of this test for clinical isolates of *C. perfringens* are needed. In our view, most laboratories experienced in anaerobic bacteriology and the additional morphologic and cultural characteristics of *C. perfringens* may find the Nagler test and the reverse CAMP test, while perhaps novel, to be unnecessary.

GLUTAMIC ACID DECARBOXYLASE MICROTUBE TEST

A rapid glutamic acid decarboxylase (GDC) microtube test (Carr-Scarborough Microbiologicals, Inc., Stone Mountain GA) was investigated in detail by Banks and associate,[18] who established a database for use in presumptive identification of clinically encountered anaerobic bacteria. The GDC test was positive for only a relatively few anaerobes. Species of bile-stimulated *Bacteroides*, including the *B. fragilis* group, were likely to be positive, whereas *Prevotella* spp., *Porphyromonas* spp. and *Fusobacterium nucleatum* showed negative results. Variable reactions were seen with *F. varium* and *F. necrophorum*, whereas *F. mortiferum* was usually, but not always, negative. Of several species of *Peptostreptococcus* tested, the only one with a positive reaction was *P. micros*. Nearly 100% of *C. perfringens*, *C. barati*, and *C. sordellii* were GDC positive, whereas only 25% of *C. difficile* strains were positive; otherwise, a wide variety of other *Clostridium* species gave negative reactions. All strains of *Eubacterium limosum* and about half of the *Propionibacterium acnes* strains tested gave positive reactions; however, the database for non–spore-forming gram-positive bacilli is not yet very large.

The commercially available GDC test product consists of a small microdilution tube (6 by 50 mm) containing the substrate within a semisolid medium. The microdilution tube containing the substrate is packaged within a second, larger screw-cap carrier tube (13 by 82 mm) that maintains sterility (during shipment and storage), prevents drying of the substrate, and provides support for the microdilution tube. The tubes are stored in the dark at 2° to 4°C and have a 3-month expiration date. To perform the test, a heavy inoculum is prepared from a fresh, pure culture of an anaerobe isolate. By using a small inoculating loop the inoculum is stabbed into and mixed within the upper one-fourth of the GDC substrate semisolid medium. Following inoculation, the screw-cap is replaced loosely on the outer carrier tube containing the microdilution substrate tube and incubation is carried out aerobically at 35°C for up to 4 hours. A color change in the microdilution tube from green to deep blue indicates a positive test. No change from green or a light blue indicates a negative reaction.

PACKAGED MICROSYSTEMS

Since the early 1970s, two commercial-packaged micromethod kits have been widely used in clincal laboratories for identification of anaerobes, namely the API-20A (bioMerieux Vitek, Hazelwood MO) and the Minitek (Becton Dickinson Microbiology Systems, Cockeysville MD).

The construction and use of these systems have been reviewed by Stargel and coworkers.[191] Although these kits can be inoculated rapidly and the reactions read quickly, they are not necessarily more rapid than the conventional tests described previously. Also, they are convenient, but many essential characteristics for identifying anaerobes can not be determined with the kits per se. The lack of sufficient tests in these kits prompted Dowell and colleagues develop the Presumpto system described previously.

COMMERCIAL PACKAGED KITS FOR IDENTIFICATION OF ANAEROBES AFTER 4 HOURS OF AEROBIC INCUBATION

Several manufacturers have marketed packaged kits that test for preformed enzymes. Most of these systems use a battery of chromogenic substrates to rapidly test for various amino peptidases and glycosidases. Each system requires the preparation of a heavy cell suspension from the surface of a purity plate culture. These packaged kits enable the microbiologist to determine multiple enzymatic characteristics of a pure culture isolate after 4 hours or less of aerobic incubation. Except for the API-ZYM kit,[131] all of these packaged systems provide numeric codes, computed databases and identification tables to aid in identification once an isolate has been characterized using the system. In addition to the API-ZYM (bioMérieux-Vitek), the list of products includes the following: API An-Ident (bio-Mérieux-Vitek, Hazelwood MO); IDS RapID-ANA II (Innovative Diagnostic Systems, Inc., Atlanta GA); Vitek Anaerobe Identification (ANI) Card (bio-Mérieux-Vitek, Hazelwood MO); MicroScan Rapid Anaerobe Identification System (Baxter Microscan, Sacramento CA); ATB 32A Anaerobes ID (bioMérieux-Vitek, Hazelwood MO); or the Rapid ID 32A (bio-Mérieux, Marcy l'Etoile, France).

These kits are popular with microbiologists and are being used widely in diagnostic microbiology laboratories. In general, they are simple to use and less time-consuming than conventional methods. Several of the systems have been evaluated in many different laboratories. As has been recently reviewed elsewhere, the identification accuracies of these systems have generally been disappointing (range of about 60% to 70%).[12] However, manufacturers continue to update and improve their products, and it is hoped that identification accuracies will be improved in the future.

On the other hand, many of the commonly encountered species of the *B. fragilis* group are identified accurately with almost all of the systems. The IDS-RapID ANA and the ATB 32A Anaerobes ID systems have even been highly successful for identification of certain difficult to identify species within the pigmented *Prevotella–Porphyromonas* group.[44,162,204,206]

The API AN-Ident is one of the earlier 4-hour systems developed with a database for identification of anaerobes; a brief description follows: The An-Ident has a 20-microcupule panel of dehydrated substrates to perform a combination of 21 miniaturized conventional and chromogenic tests. The substrates in the panel are reconstituted by adding a turbid suspension (24- to 48-hour culture) from a nonselective medium (such as anaerobe blood agar). The final turbidity of the inoculum suspension should be equivalent to a McFarland 5 (Ba_2SO_4) turbidity standard. To achieve the suspension, fresh colonies of a pure culture on CDC-anaerobe blood agar, brucella blood agar, or Columbia blood agar are transferred with a sterile cotton swab to a tube of sterile water (which can be vortexed as necessary to achieve a homogeneous suspension). The An-Ident is incubated aerobically for 4 hours at 35° to 37°C in a non-CO_2 incubator. After incubation, microcupules marked "ADG, ARB, BDG, FUC, PHS, GAL, NPG, INA, and ARG" are read without adding any reagent. Then Kovacs' reagent is added to the "IND" well to test for indole production; 3% H_2O_2 is added to the "ADG" well to test for catalase; and "cinnamaldehyde" reagent is added to the LEU, PRO, PYR, TYR, ARL, ALA, HIS, PHA, and GLY microcupules; color reactions are interpreted according to a "Reaction Guide" color chart provided by the manufacturer. The manufacturer provides differential tables and a computer-based code book for identification.

The ability to differentiate some of the more commonly encountered anaerobes after 4 hours of aerobic incubation, compared with the 24 to 48 hours required for the API-20A and Minitek Anaerobe II is an attractive advantage of the AnIdent and the newer rapid systems. However, the requirement to harvest sufficient numbers of colonies in pure culture to produce inocula equivalent to a McFarland 5 turbidity standard tends to negate the advantage of the rapid incubation time for slow-growing and fastidious strains. Although this 4-hour system showed higher overall accuracy of identification than the API-20A and Minitek, it must be supplemented with additional tests for accurate and definitive identification of selected groups of anaerobes (e.g., use of egg yolk agar and GLC for clostridia other than *C. perfringens*; the use of rapidity of growth and growth appearance in liquid as well as solid media, several additional supplemental tests, plus GLC for the anaerobic gram-positive non–spore-forming rods; the use of 20% bile, esculin, selected conventional carbohydrate tests for *Bacteroides* spp., the use of GLC and egg yolk reactions for differentiation of *Fusobacterium* spp., or other tests). It is still necessary to observe and interpret correctly Gram reactions, microscopic and colonial morphology, the results of aerotolerance tests, and to always use pure cultures when attempting to differentiate anaerobes with the commercial 4-hour packaged systems.

The IDS RapID ANA II, an upgraded and improved version of the IDS RapID ANA (described in the third edition of this book), was given a revised test selection to address new taxa and previous problem areas. The RapID ANA II tests for 18 preformed enzymes in ten wells, eight of which are bifunctional. As with other rapid systems, there are chromogenic substrates to test for certain glycosidases and aminopeptidases. In addition, the system includes tests for urease activity, the formation of indole from tryptophane, and the hydrolysis of a phosphate ester. The inoculum, prepared from a pure culture suspension of a fresh isolate, should be equivalent to a McFarland 3 (Ba_2SO_4) turbidity standard.

The manufacturer's literature permits the preparation of inocula from pure cultures grown on CDC-anaerobe blood agar, brucella blood agar, Columbia blood agar, trypticase–soy blood agar, phenylethyl alcohol blood agar, laked blood kanamycin–vancomycin blood agar, and bacteroides bile esculin blood agar but not Schaedler blood agar or cycloserine–cefoxitin–fructose agar. One problem with the long list of media that can be used to prepare culture inocula is that trypticase–soy blood agar (TSA), by itself, is not enriched with vitamin K, L-cystine, or yeast extract (all found in CDC-anaerobe blood agar); thus, TSA may not be adequately enriched to meet the nutritional requirements of the pigmented *Prevotella–Porphyromonas* groups (some of which require both hemin and vitamin K for growth), or of certain other anaerobe species. Likewise, growth of anaerobes on selective media such as bacteroides bile esculin (BBE) agar may be different (physiologically) than that on nonselective agar. Also, viable colonies will not always be transferable from BBE to another medium. Unfortunately, there is little published information on the effect of growth medium used for inoculum preparation on the enzymatic test results obtained with this and other commercially packaged rapid test kits. It would seem better to prepare the inoculum from the same nonselective medium base used by the manufacturer in creating the manufacturer's identification database.[12,132]

The inoculated IDS RapID II panels are incubated aerobically for 4 hours in the absence of CO_2 in a 35°C incubator, and the reactions should be interpreted according to the manufacturer's directions. With this system, the formation of indole from tryptophan is determined by using *p*-dimethylamino-cinnamaldehyde (DMAC) reagent. In the API An-Ident, in contrast, either Kovac's reagent or DMAC is used to detect indole formation. In the Microscan 4-hour system, Ehrlich's reagent is used. Only the reagents recommended by each manufacturer should be used with each kit; otherwise, results may not be correct.

In general, the Vitek Anaerobe Identification (ANI) System, the Microscan system, and the ATB 32A Anaerobes ID system, similar to the An-Ident and IDS RapID-ANA II, have been the subjects of many evaluations; with widely differing results.[12] These systems were comparable with the API AN-Ident and RapID-ANA II and performed best with *B. fragilis*, certain other species of the *B. fragilis* group, and with *C. perfringens*. Most of the packaged systems have shown difficulty in identifying the less commonly encountered anaerobic gram-negative bacilli, other *Clostridium* species, the anaerobic non–spore-forming gram-positive bacilli,[142] and the anaerobic cocci.[12] When a kit produces an identification of a rare species, one should not accept this identification without repeat testing with alternative procedures, or perhaps confirmation from a reference laboratory when relevant clinically.

In the design of commercial kits, manufacturers have attempted to create one card or kit that could identify a wide variety of species from many different genera of anaerobes, rather than to use the approach taken with aerobic bacteria in which differently designed kits were developed primarily for the facultatively anaerobic gram-negative rods, other kits were developed for the staphylococci, and different kits were developed for other groups of facultatively anaerobic bacteria. Therefore, the anaerobe kits require the use of additional supplemental tests (such as those described in the Presumpto system) to identify the less common species with accuracy. Thus, it can not be overemphasized that the determination of colonial characteristics and microscopic features of isolates, catalase, lipase, and lecithinase on egg yolk agar, growth in the presence of bile, the reduction of nitrate, inhibition by sodium polyanetholsulfonate, inhibition by certain antibiotics (e.g., vancomycin, kanamycin, and others), and metabolic products (as determined using gas–liquid chromatography) are required to improve the identification accuracies of the kits. Additional information on the performance of the "4-hour" kits has been recently published elsewhere.[12,142]

CHARACTERIZATION OF ANAEROBES USING DIFFERENTIAL TESTS IN MICROTITER TRAYS

The use of a multipoint inoculating device to inoculate multiple wells of microtiter trays with a single inoculum suspension of an anaerobe isolate was described by Allen and colleagues.[10] This approach permits simultaneous small-well biochemical characterization using miniaturized conventional tests and broth microdilution antimicrobial susceptibility testing of an anaerobe isolate in 96-well microtiter trays. Additional trays can be added to expand the system as needed to accomodate new drugs for susceptibility testing. This system is useful both for research and clinical laboratory applications, has a low materials cost, and provides advantages in time savings because of the automation used to manufacture the trays, and the computed rapid data-processing capability.

A microtiter system of a different design is available from Baxter Microscan (Sacramento CA). A limited evaluation on 237 strains showed identification accuracy results comparable with those obtained with several other rapid 4-hour systems.[192]

DETERMINATION OF METABOLIC PRODUCTS BY GAS–LIQUID CHROMATOGRAPHY

Analysis of metabolic products by gas–liquid chromatography (GLC) is a practical, inexpensive procedure that is easily performed by personnel in the clinical laboratory.[182b] Metabolic products, released into a broth culture medium during anaerobic growth, are key characteristics of anaerobic bacteria and many facultatively anaerobic bacteria. Together with determin-

ing the relation to oxygen, most anaerobic bacteria can be identified to the genus level based on presence or lack of spores, Gram reaction, cellular morphology, and results of GLC analysis. This technique improves the speed and accuracy of identification; cost actually decreases because of the time saved.[148]

Facultative anaerobes use aerobic respiration in their production of energy from glucose, but in addition, they are capable of obtaining energy by fermentation reactions. Obligate anaerobes are similar to facultative anaerobes in terms of the pathways used for fermentation reactions. Similar to the obligate aerobes and facultative anaerobes, some obligate anaerobes also use anaerobic respiration as a means of obtaining energy, but the obligate anaerobes do not use aerobic respiration, and oxygen is not a terminal electron acceptor for them. When grown in a liquid medium containing glucose, many of the obligate anaerobes isolated in the clinical laboratory produce pyruvate from glucose by way of the Embden–Meyerhoff and other pathways. However, many anaerobic bacteria obtain energy in media that are deficient in glucose or other carbohydrates by fermenting one or more amino acids. For example, *C. sporogenes* ferments alanine and glycine (the Strickland reaction) to produce acetate, CO_2, and NH_3.[34] There is a direct relation between the amounts of peptone and glucose in a medium and the production of branched, short-chain, fatty acids (e.g., isobutyrate, isovalerate, isocaproate) by certain anaerobes.[118] Fermentation products produced by bacteria from organic compounds, such as pyruvic acid, vary among different genera and species of obligate anaerobes and among facultatively anaerobic microorganisms.

The fermentation patterns of microorganisms have long been used for taxonomic groupings.[34] Certain yeasts such as *Saccharomyces* carry out an alcoholic fermentation in which the metabolic products consist mainly of ethanol and CO_2. The lactic acid bacteria, which include the genera *Lactobacillus* and *Streptococcus*, are well known for their characteristic pattern of fermentation in which lactic acid accumulates as the major product. *Escherichia coli* and certain other *Enterobacteriaceae* are metabolically characterized by their mixed-acid fermentation in which acetate, lactate, and succinate are formed in significant amounts, along with ethanol, CO_2, and H_2. Other members of the *Enterobacteriaceae*, for example, *Enterobacter aerogenes*, produce a butanediol type of fermentation; major products include 2,3-butanediol, ethanol, CO_2, and H_2, and smaller amounts of acetate, lactate, and succinate are formed. The presence of this type of fermentation is ordinarily determined in the clinical laboratory by the Voges-Proskauer test (see Chart 75). The butyric acid fermentation, in which butyric acid, limited amounts of acetic acid, CO_2, and H_2 are produced, is carried out by certain species of *Clostridium* (e.g., *C. butyricum*). The butyric acid fermentation pattern is one of about 14 groupings or subdivisions that can be made of this genus, based on metabolic product analysis alone. On the other hand, many of the other genera of anaerobes are readily defined based on a single major metabolic pattern (e.g., propionic acid for the genus *Propionibacterium*).

Definitions of genera based on metabolic pathways has held up scientifically because metabolic pathways represent genetically stable or conserved traits of bacteria.[148] The schemas in Tables 14-8 and 14-9 illustrate the value of metabolic product analysis for differentiating genera of anaerobic bacteria.

Although GLC analysis is not mandatory for presumptive identification of the *B. fragilis* group, the pigmenting anaerobic gram-negative bacilli, *F. nucleatum*, *C. perfringens*, *P. anaerobius*, and a few other anaerobes commonly recovered from clinical specimens, it is necessary for definitive identification of many species of *Bacteroides* and *Fusobacterium*, for most *Actinomyces*,

Bifidobacterium, Clostridium, Eubacterium, Lactobacillus, Propionibacterium, and for nearly all of the anaerobic cocci.[182b]

Gas chromatographs are now relatively inexpensive, safe, simple to operate, and reliable, and are commercially available from various scientific instrument manufacturing companies. Two gas chromatographs and their specifications are listed in Table 14-10. In general, thermal conductivity detectors are more commonly used; however, hydrogen flame ionization detectors can also be used effectively.[182b] Recorders should have a full 1-mV response within 1 second. The most commonly used carrier gas is helium.

TABLE 14-8

DIFFERENTIATION OF ANAEROBIC, GRAM-NEGATIVE, NONSPOREFORMING RODS TO THE GENUS LEVEL

I. Nonmotile or motile with peritrichous flagella; straight or coccobacillary rods
  A. Proposal by Shah and Collins[174] to include only the highly fermentative and bile-resistant species resembling *B. fragilis* (i.e., *B. distasonis, B. caccae, B. ovatus, B. thetaiotaomicron, B. merdae, B. vulgatus, B. uniformis, B. eggerthii,* and *B. stercoris*). Several other species remain in this genus and are awaiting further studies to determine their correct place (e.g., *B. capillosus, B. coagulans, B. cellulosolvens, B. pectinophilus, B. tectum, B. ureolyticus,* and others). Until the latter group is moved this genus remains heterogenous. .... *Bacteroides**
  B. Most often black-pigmented colonies; produces acetic, butyric, and succinic acids, with minor amounts of propionic, isobutyric, and isovaleric acids. All are asaccharolytic and indole positive. .... *Porphyromonas*†
  C. Nonpigmented to pigmented colonies; bile-inhibited and saccharolytic; usually oral flora .... *Prevotella**
  D. Bile-resistant, catalase-positive, nitrate-reduced, and urease-positive .... *Bilophila*†
  E. Found as a part of the human normal flora, but rarely encountered in properly selected clinical specimen .... *Anaerorhabdus*‡
       Fibrobacter‡
       Megamonas‡
       Mitsuokella‡
       Tissierella‡
       Pectinatus‡
       Rikenella‡
       Roseburia‡
       Ruminobacter‡
       Sebaldella‡
  F. Found in animals and nature.
  G. Produces major amounts of butyric acid (but little or no isoacids) as the major metabolic product; succinic acid is not produced; all species are nonmotile .... *Fusobacterium**
  H. Lactic acid is the only major product; *L. buccalis,* the only species, is nonmotile. .... *Leptotrichia*†
  I. Acetic acid is the major acid metabolic product; produces hydrogen sulfide; reduces sulfate; *D. pigra,* the only species, is nonmotile. .... *Desulfomonas*‡
II. Motile, peritrichous flagella not produced
  A. Curved rods with monotrichous or lophotrichous polar flagella or subpolar flagella; butyric acid is major product of fermentation. .... *Butyrivibrio*†
  B. Succinic and acetic acids are major products of fermentation.
    1. Short, straight rods to coccobacilli; a single polar flagellum; found only in bovine rumen. .... *Succinimonas*‡
    2. Curved, helically twisted rods with pointed ends; vibrating-type motility by a single polar flagellum .... *Succinivibrio*†
    3. Helical, curved rods; bipolar tufts of flagella .... *Anaerobiospirillum*†
  C. Microaerophilic; oxidase-positive; curved and spiral rods; single polar flagellum, with absence of a flagellar sheath; carbohydrates not fermented; produce succinic acid from fumaric acid .... *Campylobacter*§
       Wollinella#
  D. Curved rods, with multiple subterminal flagella; fermentative in peptone yeast glycogen broth, supplemented with rabbit serum; succinic and acetic acids as major fermentation products, with or without lactic acid; oxidase-negative. .... *Mobiluncus*†
  E. Propionic and acetic acids as major fermentation products
    1. Tufts of flagella on concave side of crescent-shaped cells .... *Selenomonas*†
    2. Single polar flagellum; lipolytic; curved rods .... *Anaerovibrio*†
    3. Flagella are inserted in a spiral along the cell .... *Centipeda*‡

* Commonly found in clinical specimens.
† Rarely found in clinical specimens.
‡ Normal flora of only humans or other animals only
§ *Campylobacter gracilis* is oxidase-negative and lacks flagella, but has "twitching motility"; it differs from other *Campylobacter* species in these two respects.
# *Wolinella succinogenes,* isolated from the bovine rumen and now the only species remaining in *Wolinella,* is difficult to differentiate from species of the genus *Campylobacter.*
Based on references 56, 92, 93, 107, 145, 147, 174, 190, 198, 207, 209.

TABLE 14-9

TABLE 14-9
DIFFERENTIATION OF ANAEROBIC, GRAM-POSITIVE RODS ENCOUNTERED IN HUMAN SPECIMENS TO THE GENUS LEVEL

I. Bacterial endospores produced   *Clostridium*
II. Endospores not produced
    A. Produce major amounts of propionic and acetic acids; catalase usually produced; irregular- or regular-shaped
        rods, coccoid cells; occasional branching   *Propionibacterium*
    B. Produce acetic and lactic acids (>1:1 ratio); very irregular rods with bifid forms and branching.   *Bifidobacterium*
    C. Produce lactic acid as sole major product
        1. Short to long and slender rods; chain formation common; irregular rods uncommon; usually grow on
            tomato juice agar at pH ≤4.5 (see Chap. 13).   *Lactobacillus*
        2. Irregular rods predominant; filamentous forms with some branching.   *Actinomyces*
    D. Produce 1) moderate acetic and major succinic, 2) major lactic and major succinic, or 3) a major amount of lactic
        acids (see II.C.2 above). Irregular rods; filaments with branching.   *Actinomyces*
    E. Produce mixture of acid metabolic products, including butyric acid and others, acetic and formic acids, or no
        major acids; obligate anaerobes; pleomorphic diphtheroid cells common, or uniform.   *Eubacterium*

Adapted from Allen SD: Gram-positive, nonsporeforming anaerobic bacilli. In Lennette EH, Balows A, Hausler WJ Jr, Shadomy EJ (eds): Manual of Clinical Microbiology, 4th ed, pp 461–472. Washington DC, American Society for Microbiology, 1985; Jones D, Collins MD: Irregular, nonsporing gram-positive rods. In Sneath PHA, Mair NS, Sharpe MG, Holt JG (eds): Bergey's Manual of Systematic Bacteriology, pp 1261–1434. Baltimore, Williams & Wilkins, 1986.

Column packing materials that are satisfactory for determining metabolic products include 15% Sp-1220:1% H_3PO_4 on 100/120 Chromasorb W; AW (Supelco Inc., Bellefonte PA); 10% SP-1000:1% H_3PO_4 on 100/120 Chromasorb W; AW (Supelco Inc., Bellefonte PA).

Equipment and procedures for determining metabolic products by GLC are described in more detail elsewhere.[91,118,195]

IDENTIFICATION OF VOLATILE FATTY ACIDS

The procedure is used for identifying short-chain, volatile fatty acids that are soluble in ether. The acids detected with this procedure include acetic, propionic, isobutyric, butyric, isovaleric, valeric, isocaproic, and caproic.[182b] The procedure is explained in Box 14-10.

Volatile fatty acids can be identified by comparing elution times of products in extracts with those of a

TABLE 14-10
SPECIFICATIONS FOR TWO COMMERCIAL GAS–LIQUID CHROMATOGRAPHS

CHROMATOGRAPH	TYPE OF DETECTOR	TYPE OF COLUMN	COLUMN MATERIAL	COLUMN TEMPERATURE	INJECTION PORT TEMPERATURE	CARRIER GAS	FLOW RATE	ATTENUATION
Fisher Series 2400*	Thermal conductivity	6-ft × ¼-in. stainless steel	Volatile acids: 15% SP 1220/1% H_3PO_4 on 100/120 Chromasorb WAW, Supelco Inc., Bellefonte Pa. Nonvolatile acids: 10% SP 1000/1% H_3PO_4 on 100/120 Chromasorb WAW, Supelco, Inc., Bellefonte Pa.	145°C	210°C	Helium	100 mL/min	×2
Gow-Mac Model Series 550†	Thermal conductivity	6-ft × ¼-in. stainless steel	Same as above	135°C–140°C	200°C	Helium	120 mL/min	×2

* Fisher Scientific Co., Pittsburgh PA 15219
† Gow-Mac Co., Boundbrook NJ 08805

BOX 14-10. IDENTIFYING VOLATILE FATTY ACIDS

1. Inoculate tubes containing 7- to 8-mL of prereduced peptone–yeast extract–glucose (PYG) broth with a few drops (0.05 to 0.1 mL) of an actively growing culture.

2. Incubate under anaerobic conditions for 48 hours, or until adequate growth is obtained.

3. Transfer 2 mL of the culture to a clean, 13- by 100-mm screw-cap tube.

4. Acidify the culture to pH 2.0 or lower by adding 0.2 mL of 50% (v/v) aqueous H_2SO_4.

5. Add 1 mL of ethyl ether, tighten the cap, and mix by gently inverting the tube about 20 times.

6. Centrifuge briefly in a clinical centrifuge (1500 to 2000 rpm) to break the ether–culture emulsion.

7. Place the ether–culture mixture in a freezer at −20°C or lower or in an alcohol–dry ice bath until the aqueous portion (bottom) is frozen.

8. Rapidly pour off the ether layer into a clean screw-cap tube. If desired, add one or two anhydrous $CaCl_2$ pellets to the ether extract to allow removal of residual water.

9. Inject 14 µL of the extract into the column of a gas chromatograph packed with Sp-1220.

propionic, isobutyric, butyric, isovaleric, valeric, isocaproic, and caproic acids. The nonvolatile acid standard should contain at least pyruvic, lactic, fumaric, succinic, hydrocinnamic, and phenylacetic acids. A tube of uninoculated medium should be examined in the same manner, because various lots of PYG broth may contain significant quantities of these acids.

Lombard and associates have found that several other liquid media as well as PYG broth can be used for analysis of acidic metabolic products.[118] These media include enriched thioglycolate broth, chopped meat glucose, Lombard–Dowell glucose broth, and modified Schaedler broth (BBL). When grown in these other broth media, however, results for a given organism may differ from those attained in PYG. Thus, caution should be exercised in interpreting products from different media when the identification tables have been prepared from a PYG database. A further note of caution is warranted: the amount of acetic, lactic, and other acids present in certain liquid media, such as chopped meat glucose broth, may make it difficult or, at times, impossible to determine if the acetic or lactic acid peak was produced by the unknown isolate or simply by the uninoculated medium.[118]

Chromatographic tracings of a volatile acid standard; PYG broth cultures of *Fusobacterium mortiferum*, *Clostridium difficile*, and *Peptostreptococcus anaerobius*; and a nonvolatile acid standard are shown in Figures 14-9 through 14-13. The metabolic products of common species of anaerobic gram-negative rods are listed in Table 14-11.

known acid mixture (volatile fatty acid standard) chromatographed under the same conditions on the same day. A representative standard tracing is shown in Fig. 14-9, and examples of the GLC results for three anaerobe isolates are shown in Figures 14-10 through 14-12.

ANALYSIS OF NONVOLATILE ACIDS

Pyruvic, lactic, fumaric, succinic, hydrocinnamic, and phenylacetic acids are not detected with the ether extraction procedure for volatile fatty acids (see preceding section).[182b] These nonvolatile acids are identified after preparation of methylated derivatives. The procedure is outlined in Box 14-11.

Analysis of chloroform extracts is performed using the same chromatographic conditions as those for the volatile acids. Identify nonvolatile or methylated acids by comparing elution times of products in extracts with those of known acids chromatographed on the same day. After testing approximately 20 methylated samples, recondition the packing material by injecting 14 µL of methanol into the gas chromatograph.

GAS–LIQUID CHROMATOGRAPHY CONTROLS

Standard solutions containing 1 mEq/100 mL of each volatile acid or nonvolatile acid should be examined each time unknowns are tested. The volatile acid standard should contain at least the following acids: acetic,

IDENTIFICATION OF ANAEROBIC BACTERIA

The species of anaerobic bacteria most frequently isolated from properly selected and collected clinical specimens at a large university medical center are listed in Table 14-3. Table 14-12 lists changes in the nomenclature of anaerobic bacteria that have occurred during the

BOX 14-11. IDENTIFYING NONVOLATILE FATTY ACIDS

1. Transfer 1 mL of the original PYG culture to a clean 13- by 100-mm screw-cap tube.

2. Add 0.4 mL of H_2SO_4 (v/v) and 2 mL of methanol.

3. Place the tube in a 55°C water bath for 1 hour or overnight.

4. Add 1 mL of distilled water and 0.5 mL of chloroform, and centrifuge briefly to break any emulsion in the chloroform layer (chloroform will be in the bottom of the tube).

5. Fill a syringe with the chloroform extract after placing the tip of the needle beneath the aqueous layer.

6. Wipe off the outside of the needle with a clean tissue and inject 14 µL into a GLC column packed with SP-1000.

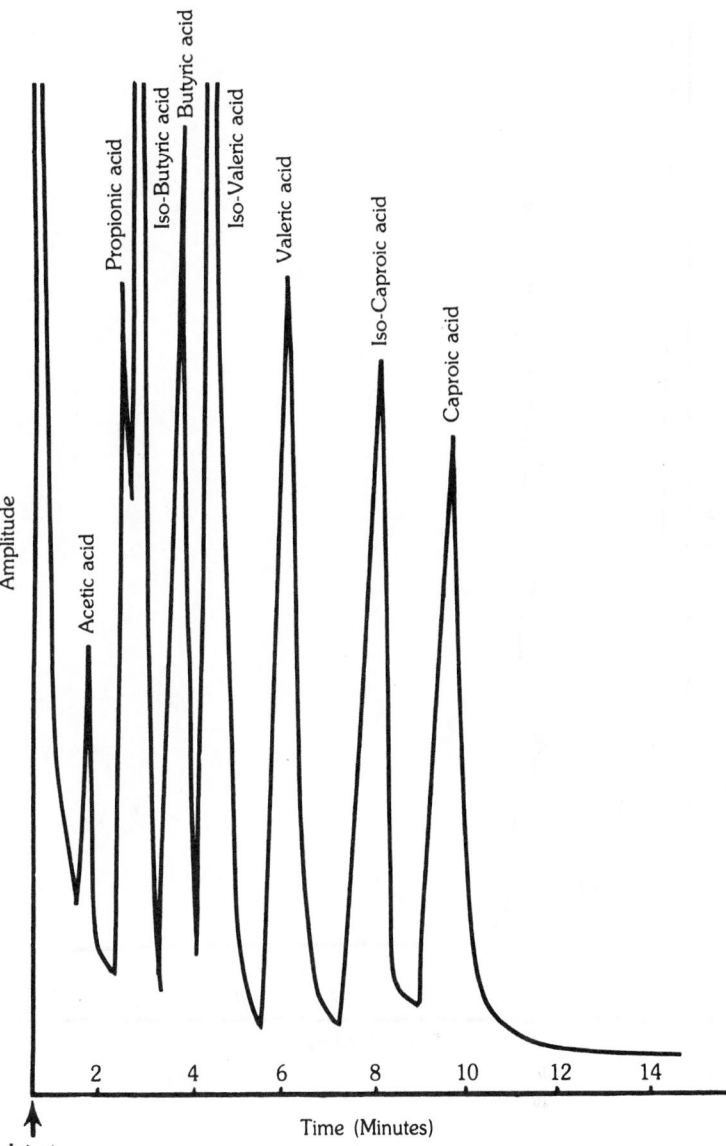

Figure 14-9
A typical volatile acid standard chromatogram:
The time elapsed between the injection of an
ether extract of the standard solution and the
peak for each acid (retention time) is used to
identify the acids. Note, for example, that the
retention time for acetic acid is 1.8 minutes and
for valeric acid is 6 minutes (instrument used:
Dohrmann Anabac, Clinical Analysis Products
Co., Sunnyvale CA; Detector: thermal conductivity; column packing: 15%, SP-1220/1% H_3PO_4 on
100/120 Chromasorb W/AW from Supelco Inc.,
Bellefonte PA)

past decade. Even though there have been numerous
changes in the taxonomic classification of anaerobes,
and numerous species are described in the current literature, only a limited number of species are encountered
with any frequency. Only about 12 to 15 groups or
species account for about 75% or more of the isolates
from properly collected species. These include the *Bacteroides fragilis* group, the pigmented *Prevotella–Porphyromonas* group, *Fusobacterium nucleatum, Peptostreptococcus magnus, P. anaerobius, P. asaccharolyticus, P.
prevotii, Propionibacterium acnes, Eubacterium lentum,
Clostridium perfringens, C. ramosum,* and *Veillonella* spp.
Laboratory personnel should be familiar with these
species, because they are so common and often clinically significant. It is also especially important that clinical microbiologists know about and be able to recognized *Fusobacterium necrophorum, Actinomyces israelii,
Propionibacterium propionicum, C. septicum, C. difficile, C.
botulinum, C. tetani,* and a few other species (discussed
later in the text) because these organisms may be highly

pathogenic for patients (even though they are not so
common).

Beyond considerations of the need to be familiar
with the common and medically significant anaerobes, it has been proposed that microbiologists in
clinical laboratories may wish to limit the extent of
anaerobe identification, based on levels of capability.[2,12] As proposed previously, laboratories with limited capability (level 1 or extent 1) should be able to
isolate anaerobes in pure culture and to evaluate
microscopic and colonial morphology. Together with
results of aerotolerance testing, this information
would then be reported to the clinician (as a preliminary report). If clinically relevant, based on 1) the clinical situation as viewed by the clinician; 2) a direct
gram-stained smear of a wound or abscess, peritoneal fluid, or other, showing evidence of acute inflammation (such as numerous polymorphonuclear
leukocytes, but a lack of squamous epithelial cells) or
necrosis; 3) microscopic evidence of clostridial my-

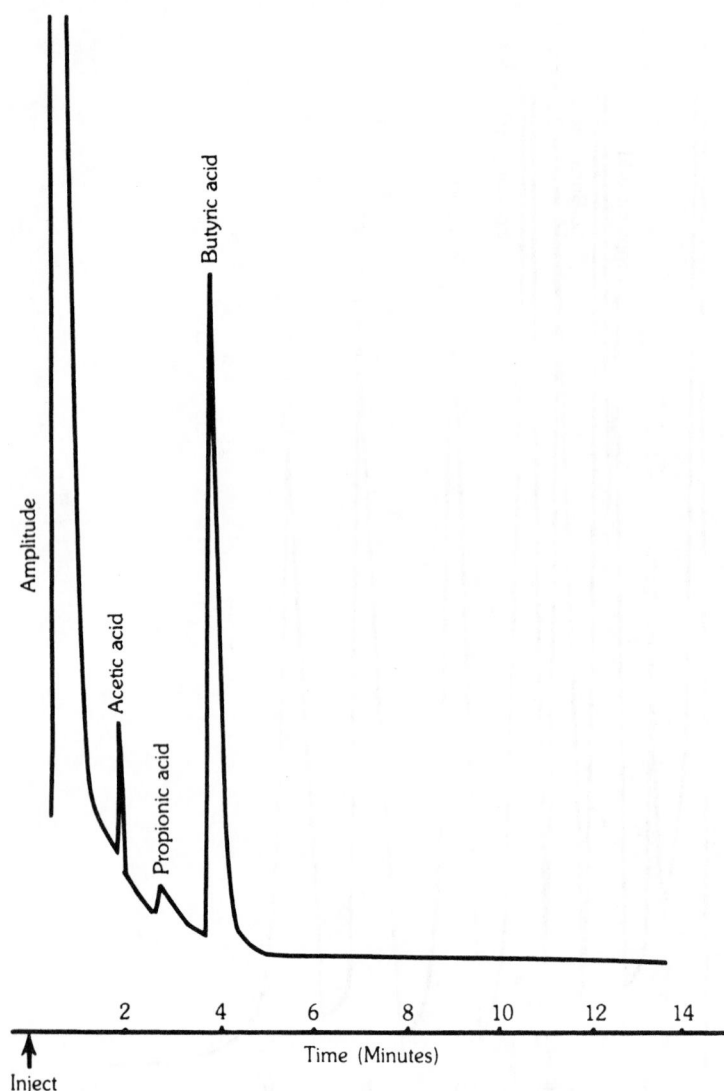

Figure 14-10
Volatile acid chromatogram of a 48-hour peptone–yeast extract–glucose broth culture of *Fusobacterium mortiferum:* The retention times of the products in the broth culture are compared with those of the standard tracing (see Fig. 14-9) to identify the unknown acids. The peaks indicate major amounts of butyric and acetic acids, but only a minor amount of propionate for this culture. The same instrument and operating conditions were used for the tracing in Fig. 14-9.

onecrosis (see Color Plate 14-3D); 4) sulfur granules suggestive of actinomycetes (see Color Plate 14-2C and D); 5) positive blood cultures or other positive body fluid cultures (e.g., pleural fluid, spinal fluid, joint fluid), the isolates, together with direct smears, should be transported to a reference laboratory and processed further. Alternatively, laboratories with even the capability of definitive identification (level 4) of anaerobe isolates may wish to limit the extent of processing to level 1 when there is no clinical relevance to take the identification further. One example would be of a peritoneal swab sample obtained at operation from a patient within hours of a penetrating knife or gunshot wound to the abdomen. Predictably, perforation of the large bowel or distal small intestine results in fecal spillage into the abdomen. Samples obtained at this time will probably show many mixed bacterial morphologic forms and few polymorphonuclear leukocytes in gram-stained smears and will grow a mixture of normal bowel flora. Identification of these organisms would have no clinical usefulness and would be inordinately expensive.

The second level of capability that was proposed would require, in addition to level 1, some identification capability.[2,12] Specifically, the differentiation of the *B. fragilis* group from the other gram-negative anaerobes and identification of *C. perfringens* would be performed. Similar to the first level of identification, isolates and direct smears from clinically relevant cases would be transported to a reference laboratory for further identification of isolates.

The third level of capability that was proposed would require the presumptive identification of most of the 12 or so common anaerobe groups and species mentioned previously. This third category or extent of identification can be accomplished without the use of gas chromatography. As mentioned in the discussion of GLC procedures, the common and clinically important anaerobes that can be presumptively identified, using a few simple rapid tests, include the *B. fragilis* group, the pigmented *Prevotella–Porphyromonas* groups (when pigment is formed), *F. nucleatum, P. anaerobius, P. asaccharolyticus, P. acnes, C. perfringens, C. ramosum, A. israelii,* and several not so

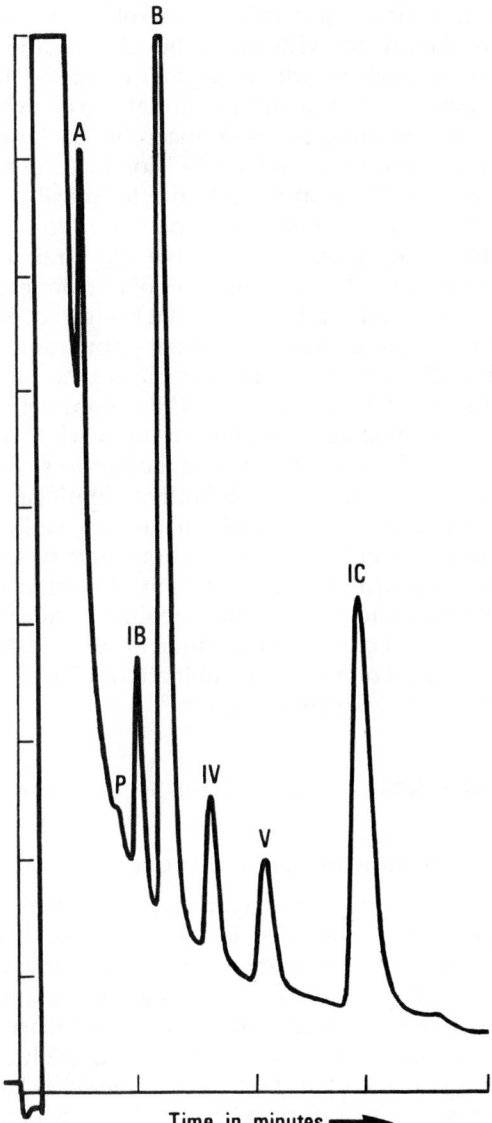

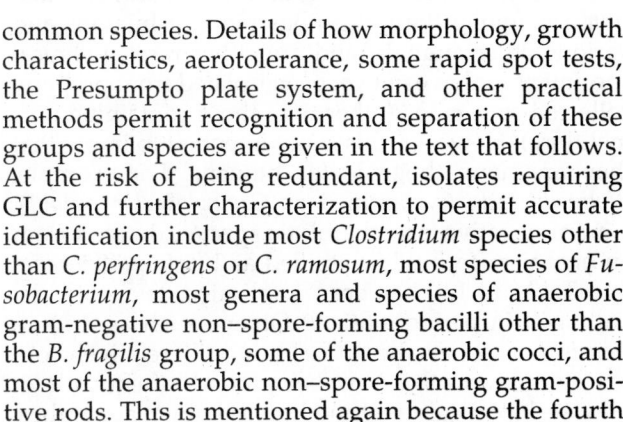

Figure 14-11
Example of a volatile acid chromatograph of a 48-hour peptone–yeast extract–glucose broth culture of *Clostridium difficile: A,* acetic acid; *P,* propionic acid; *IB,* isobutyric acid; *B,* butyric acid; *IV,* isovaleric acid; *V,* valeric acid; *IC,* isocaproic acid.

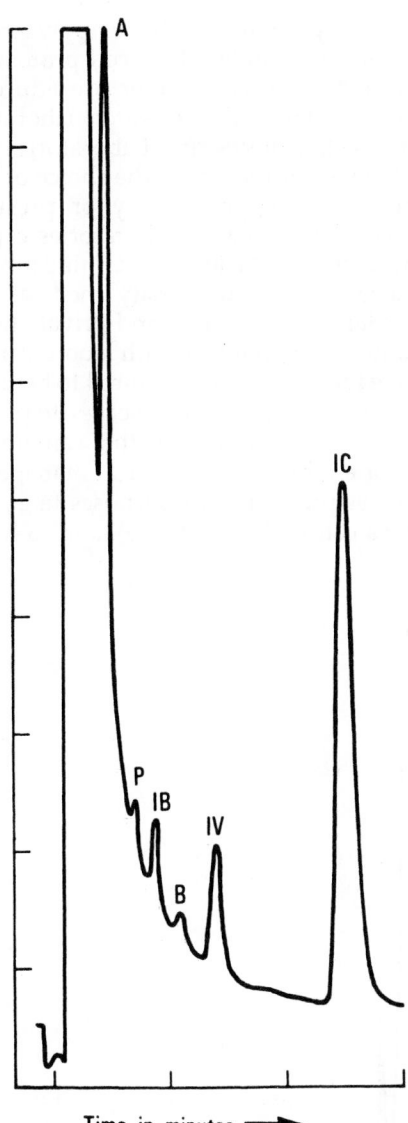

Figure 14-12
Example of a volatile acid chromatograph tracing of a 48-hr peptone–yeast extract–glucose broth culture of *Peptostreptococcus anaerobius: A,* acetic acid; *P,* propionic acid; *IB,* isobutyric acid; *B,* butyric acid; *IV,* isovaleric acid; *IC,* isocaproic acid.

common species. Details of how morphology, growth characteristics, aerotolerance, some rapid spot tests, the Presumpto plate system, and other practical methods permit recognition and separation of these groups and species are given in the text that follows. At the risk of being redundant, isolates requiring GLC and further characterization to permit accurate identification include most *Clostridium* species other than *C. perfringens* or *C. ramosum*, most species of *Fusobacterium*, most genera and species of anaerobic gram-negative non–spore-forming bacilli other than the *B. fragilis* group, some of the anaerobic cocci, and most of the anaerobic non–spore-forming gram-positive rods. This is mentioned again because the fourth

level of identification (or definitive identification), including the tests done in the previous levels, also includes GLC for organisms that require it. In addition to determining morphology, growth characteristics, relation to oxygen, preliminary spot tests, use of the Presumpto system, and GLC, definitive identification (level 4) includes determining whatever additional characteristics are needed (within reason) to arrive at an accurate identification to species (including those species that are not frequently isolated). Thus, additional characteristics might be obtained by traditional broth biochemical tests, the use of certain rapid enzyme tests (e.g., available in the API-ZYM, RapID-ANA II, Vitek ANI, or one of the other API rapid systems), toxicity testing, slab gel polyacrylamide electrophoresis of soluble whole-cell proteins, long-chain fatty acid analysis, or other procedures (such as referral of isolates to a research laboratory for genetic analysis), as necessary. Laboratories capable of definitive identification have the choice of limiting identifications to the preliminary or presumptive levels described previously. Laboratories capable of performing definitive or level 4 identification might include those at large university medical centers, many of the larger community and private hospitals, and state and federal public health laboratories.

Definitive identification is required to better define the role of anaerobic bacteria in diseases, to provide an accurate microbiologic diagnosis that can aid in optimal choice of antibiotics and clinical management of the patient, for public health purposes (e.g., nosocomial diarrhea caused by *C. difficile*), and to help edu-

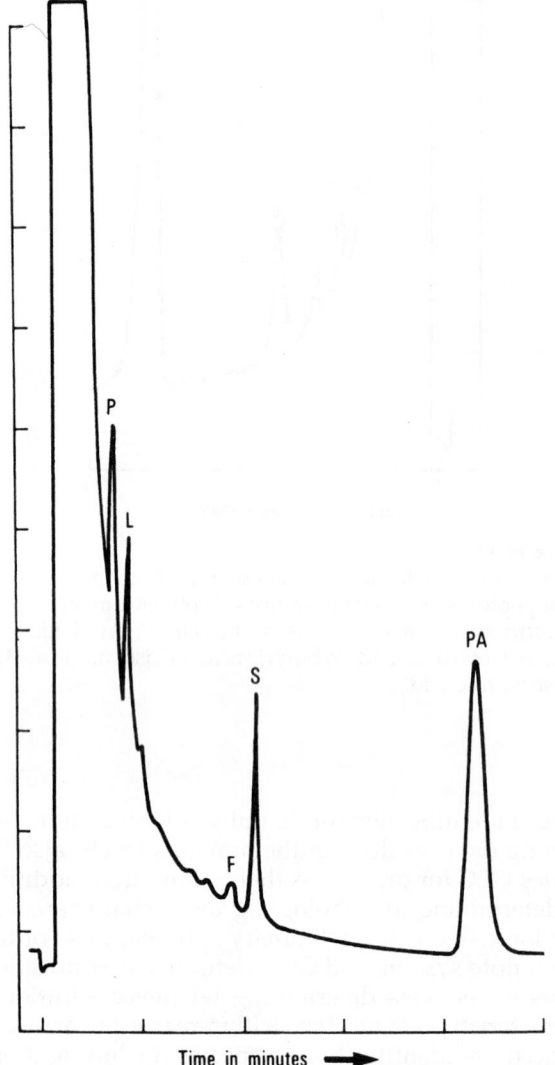

Figure 14-13
A typical nonvolatile acid standard chromatogram: The column was packed with 10% SP. 1000/1% H₃PO₄ on 100/120 chromasorb W/AW (Supelco Inc., Bellefonte PA). *P*, pyruvic acid; *L*, lactic acid; *F*, fumaric acid; *S*, succinic acid; *PA*, phenylacetic acid.

cate both clinicians and clinical microbiologists. How far one should go with anaerobe identification depends on several considerations that will differ in different laboratories. Not all laboratories can be expected to perform the same levels of anaerobic bacteriologic studies. Factors that influence decision making for the extent of identification include the technical competence and experience of the people who work in the laboratory, the resources available (e.g., reimbursement of the laboratory, the number of personnel available, supplies and capital equipment budgeted, as well as other considerations), the patient population being served, and the needs of the clinicians who have responsibility for their patients.[2,12] Clinical microbiology laboratories must be competent in the work that they do and should not hesitate to use the services of reference laboratories for aid in definitive identification or for reference confirmation of isolates, as well as antimicrobial susceptibility testing, toxigenicity testing, or other procedures when relevant clinically, if the referring laboratory lacks this capability. Additional approaches and current information on anaerobe identification, based on various combinations of tests at different levels, is given elsewhere.[56,195]

ANAEROBIC GRAM-NEGATIVE NON–SPORE-FORMING BACILLI

CLASSIFICATION AND NOMENCLATURE

The anaerobic, gram-negative, non–spore-forming bacteria are now classified in the genera as listed in Table 14-1. Key characteristics for differentiation of these are given in Table 14-8. The anaerobic gram-negative bacilli are among the normal flora of the oropharynx, lower digestive tract, vagina, cervix, urethra, and external genitalia. Only *Bacteroides, Prevotella, Porphyromonas,* and *Fusobacterium* among these genera are commonly isolated from properly selected and collected specimens (i.e., those specimens without contamination with normal flora) from humans with significant infections. Thus, the gram-negative organisms *Leptotrichia buccalis, Desulfomonas pigra, Butyrivibrio fibrisolvens, Succinovibrio dextrinosolvens, Anaerovibrio lipolytica, Anaerobiospirillum succiniciproducens, Selenomonas sputigena, Succinimonas amylolytica, Treponema denticola, Mobiluncus mulieris,* and *Campylobacter sputorum* are among the indigenous biota of humans and various other animals, and are either rare in clinical specimens, or have not yet been isolated from properly collected specimens (other than those containing normal flora). However, this is not intended to imply that they are nonpathogenic for humans. For example, *Wolinella recta* (reclassified as *Campylobacter recta*[208]), a gram-negative, asaccharolytic species, derived from an organism formerly classified as *Vibrio succinogenes* (see Table 14-12), has been implicated as a potential pathogen in periodontitis.[198] Others, such as *Anaerobiospirillum succiniciproducens,* are still relatively obscure organisms that have been found infrequently in positive blood cultures, and little is known about their role in health and disease.[139,160]

TABLE 14-11
METABOLIC PRODUCTS OF *BACTEROIDES*, *PORPHYROMONAS*, *PREVOTELLA*, AND *FUSOBACTERIUM* SPECIES IN PEPTONE–YEAST EXTRACT–GLUCOSE BROTH CULTURES AFTER 48 HOURS AT 35°C*

SPECIES OR GROUP	A	P	IB	B	IV	V	IC	C	L	S	PA[s]	PROPIONATE FROM THREONINE
Bacteroides												
Bacteroides group												
CDC F₂	+	–	–	–	–	–	–	–	–	V		
B. capillosus	+	V	–	–	–	–	–	–	–	+		
B. distasonis	+	+/–	–	–	V	–	–	–	+/–	+	+	
B. fragilis	+	+/–	V	–	V	–	–	–	+	+	+	
B. ovatus	+	+	V	–	V	–	–	–	V	+	+	
B. splanchnicus	+	+	+	+	V	–	–	–	V	S		
B. thetaiotaomicron	+	+/–	V	–	V	–	–	–	V	+	+	
B. uniformis	+	+/–	V	–	V	–	–	–	+	+		
B. ureolyticus	+	–	–	–	–	–	–	–	–	+		
B. vulgatus	+	+	V	–	–	V	–	–	+	+	–	
Porphyromonas												
asaccharolytica†	+	+	+	+	+	–	–	–	–	+	–	
P. gingivalis	+	+	+	+	+	–	–	–	–	+	+	
Prevotella bivia	+	–	V	–	+/–	–	–	–	–	+		
P. disiens	+	V	V	–	V	–	–	–	–	+		
P. intermedia	+	V	V	–	+	–	–	–	–	+	–	
Fusobacterium												
F. gonidiaformans	+	+	–	+	–	–	–	–	–	–		+
F. mortiferum	+	+/–	–	+	–	–	–/+	–	–	–		+
F. naviforme	+	V	–	+	–	–	–	–	–	–		–
F. necrophorum	+	+	–	+	–	–	–	–	–	–		+
F. nucleatum	+	+	–	+	–	–	–	–	–	–/+		+
F. varium	+	+	–	+	–	–	–	–	+	–/+		+

* The species listed in this table are those that can be differentiated using the differential agar media system (see Tables 14–4 and 14–12). The asaccharolytic, black-pigmented *Poryphyromonas*, *P. asaccharolyticus* and *P. gingivalis*, can be presumptively differentiated by presence or lack of phenylacetic (PA) acid and additional tests described in the text.
† Data on differentiation of certain *Bacteroides fragilis* group organisms and black pigmented species using phenylacetic (PA) acid is from Mayrand[134a] and Shah and Collins.[173]
A, acetic; P, propionic; IB, isobutyric; B, butyric; IV, isovaleric; IC, isocaproic; C, caproic; L, lactic; PA, phenylacetic acid; S, succinic acid; +, major peak; –, no major peak; +/–, usually a major peak, but may be negative; –/+, usually negative, but may be present; V, variable.
After Dowell VR, Lombard GL: Presumptive Identification of Anerobic Nonsporeforming Gram-negative Bacilli. DHEW Publication, p. 13, Atlanta, Centers for Disease Control, 1977.

PRESUMPTIVE OR PRELIMINARY GROUP IDENTIFICATION OF *BACTEROIDES*, *PREVOTELLA*, *PORPHYROMONAS*, AND *FUSOBACTERIUM*

The first major goal of identification should be to determine whether anaerobic bacteria are present and to isolate them in pure culture.[2] The presence of anaerobic gram-negative rods suggestive of *Bacteroides*, *Prevotella*, *Porphyromonas*, or *Fusobacterium* spp. (based on determining their relation to oxygen), together with the Gram stain results and colony observations, should be promptly reported to the clinician. Presumptive or preliminary identification of the *B. fragilis* group, and the *Prevotella–Porphyromonas* group, along with other obligately anaerobic, gram-negative rods, can easily be done using differential characteristics obtained with the Presumpto 1 quadrant plate and anaerobe blood agar (Tables 14-14 and 14-15). Additional characteris-

tics are provided in Tables 14-11, 14-13, 14-16, and 14-17. Further clues for group differentiation of various species based on key characteristics are provided in Table 14-18. Note that the common anaerobic gram-negative, non–spore-forming bacilli encountered clinically (see Tables 14-15 and 14-16) are all nonmotile. In practice, it is neither practical nor necessary to determine motility and perform flagella stains to differentiate the other genera of anaerobic gram-negative bacilli (see Table 14-8), unless the differential characteristics of an isolate (in pure culture) do not clearly fit those of species listed in Tables 14-11 and 14-13 through 14-18.

Identification of *Bacteroides*: The *Bacteroides fragilis* Group. Organisms of the *B. fragilis* group are the anaerobic bacteria most often isolated from infections

(text continues on page 749)

TABLE 14-12

PRESENT AND FORMER NAMES OF ANAEROBIC BACTERIA

PRESENT NAME	FORMER NAME/COMMENT	PRESENT NAME	FORMER NAME/COMMENT
Anaerobic Gram-Negative Rods		P. oulora	Bacteroides oulorum
		P. ruminicola	Bacteroides ruminicola
Genus Bacteroides—Bacteroides fragilis Group		P. tannerae	New species—humans; ~40% of strains pigmented
Bacteroides caccae	"3452A"—human fecal flora	P. veroralis	Bacteroides veroralis
B. distasonis	Occasional isolates in human infections	P. zoogleoformis	Bacteroides zoogleoformis
B. eggerthii	Fecal flora—not common in infections	**Genus Porphyromonas**	
B. fragilis	The most common anaerobe in human infections	Porphyromonas asaccharolytica	Bacteroides asaccharolyticus—various clinical infections of humans; pigmented
B. merdae	"T4-1"—human fecal flora	P. cangingivalis	New species—dogs
B. ovatus	Human fecal flora—occasionally infections	P. canoris	New species—dogs
		P. cansulci	New species—dogs
B. stercoris	"Subsp. A"—human fecal flora	P. catoniae	Oribaculum catoniae—human oral cavity; not pigmented
B. thetaiotaomicron	The second most common Bacteroides in human infections	P. circumdentaria	New species—cats
		P. crevioricanis	New species—dogs
B. uniformis	Occasional isolates in human infections	P. endodontalis	Bacteroides endodontalis—humans; pigmented
B. vulgatus	Common in human fecal flora—occasional isolates in infections	P. gingivalis	Bacteroides gingivalis—human root canal and other dental/oral infections; pigmented
Other species remaining in the genus Bacteroides, but not of the Bacteroides fragilis Group		P. gingivicanis	New species—dogs
B. capillosus	Uncommon in wounds	P. levii	Bacteroides levii—cattle
B. coagulans	Rare in clinical specimens	P. macacae	Bacteroides macacae—monkeys Porphyromonas salivosa—cats Bacteroides salivosus—cats
B. cellulosolvens	New species—sewage sludge		
B. pectinophilus	New species—human fecal flora		
B. forsythus	New species—human oral cavity	**Genus Fusobacterium**	
B. galacturonicus	New species—human fecal flora	F. alocis	New species—human gingival sulci
B. heparinolyticus	New species—human and animal oral flora	F. gonidiaformans	Human infections
		F. mortiferum	Human infections
B. putredinis	Rare—human intra-abdominal infections	F. naviforme	Human infections
		F. necrogenes	Human feces—animals
B. splanchnicus	Resembles B. fragilis group	F. necrophorum ss. funduliforme	New subsp.—necrotic lesions
B. tectum	New species—dogs and cats		
B. ureolyticus	Bacteroides corrodens—related to genus Campylobacter	F. necrophorum ss. necrophorum	F. necrophorum—various necrotizing lesions
B. xylanolyticus	New species—cattle manure	F. nucleatum ss. animalis	New subsp.
Genus Prevotella		F. nucleatum ss. fusiforme	New subsp.—CNS, head and neck, respiratory infections
P. bivia	Bacteroides bivius—GU tract infections	F. nucleatum ss. nucleatum	New subsp.—CNS, head and neck, respiratory infections
P. buccae	Bacteroides buccae—head and neck, chest infections	F. nucleatum ss. polymorphorum	F. nucleatum—as above
P. buccalis	Bacteroides buccalis		
P. corporis	Bacteroides corporis—humans; pigmented	F. nucleatum ss. vincentii	F. nucleatum—as above
P. dentalis	Mistuokella dentalis and Hallela seregens	F. perfoetans	Pig feces
P. denticola	Bacteroides denticola—humans; pigmented	F. periodonticum	New species
		F. prausnitzii	Human fecal flora—more closely related to some Eubacterium spp. than to Fusobacterium
P. disiens	Bacteroides disiens—GU tract infections		
P. enoeca	New species—human oral cavity; not pigmented	F. pseudonecrophorum	F. necrophorum biovar C—not pathogenic for mice
P. heparinolytica	Bacteroides heparinolyticus	F. russii	Human feces
P. intermedia	Bacteroides intermedius—common in humans; head and neck, abdominal, pelvic sites; pigmented	F. simiae	Mouth of stump-tailed macaque
		F. sulci	New species—gingival sulci
		F. ulcerans	New species—cutaneous ulcers
P. loescheii	Bacteroides loescheii—humans; pigmented	F. varium	Various human infections
P. melaninogenica	Bacteroides melaninogenicus—various human infection sites; pigmented		
P. nigrescens	Formerly genotype II of P. intermedia—humans; pigmented		
P. oralis	Bacteroides oralis		
P. oris	Bacteroides oris		

(Continued)

TABLE 14-12 *(Continued)*
PRESENT AND FORMER NAMES OF ANAEROBIC BACTERIA

PRESENT NAME	FORMER NAME/COMMENT
Other genera of anaerobic gram-negative rods	
Anaerobiospirillum succiniciproducens	
Anaerorhabdus furcosus	*Bacteroides furcosus*
Bilophilia wadsworthia	New species—human appendix
Genus *Campylobacter*	
C. concisus	
C. curvus	*Wolinella curva*
C. gracilis	*Bacteroides gracilis*
C. mucosalis	
C. rectus	*Wolinella recta*
C. showae	
C. sputorum	
Genus *Capnocytophaga*	
C. canimorsus	CDC group DF-2
C. cynodegmi	New species
C. gingivalis	New species
C. granulosa	New species—dental plaque
C. haemolytica	New species—dental plaque
C. ochracea	*Bacteroides ocharaceus*
C. sputigena	New species
Others	
Catonella morbi	New species
Centipeda periodontii	New species
Desulfomonas pigra	
Desulfovibrio desulfuricans	
Dialister pneumosintes	*Bacteroides pneumosintes*
Dichelobacter nodosus	*Bacteroides nodosus*—foot rot in sheep and cattle
Falcivibrio grandis	"*Vibrio mulieris*"
F. vaginalis	"*Vibrio mulieris*"
Fibrobacter intestinalis	New species
F. succinogenes	*Bacteroides succinogenes*
Johnsonella ignava	New species
Leptotrichia buccalis	
Megamonas hypermegas	*Bacteroides hypermegas*
M. mutiacidus	*B. multiacidus*
Oxalobacter formigenes	New species—human colon
Pectinatus cerevisiiphilus	New species—brewery
P. frisingensis	New species—brewery
Propionigenium modestum	New species—anaerobic fresh water and marine muds; human saliva
Rikenella microfusus	*B. microfusus*
Ruminobacter amylophilus	*B. amylophilus*
Sebaldella termitidis	*B. termitidis*
Genus *Selenomonas*	
S. artemidis	New species—human gingival crevice
S. dianae	New species—human oral flora
S. flueggei	New species—human gingival crevice
S. infelix	New species—human gingival crevice
S. lacticifex	New species—brewery
S. noxia	New species—human gingival crevice
Serpula hyodysenteria	*Treponema hyodysenteria*—swine intestine
S. innocens	*T. innocess*—swine intestine
Sutterella wadsworthensis	New species
Tissierella praecuta	*Bacteroides praecutus*
Treponoma pectinovorum	New species
T. saccharophilum	New species—bovine rumen

PRESENT NAME	FORMER NAME/COMMENT
T. socranskii ss. *buccale*	New species—human oral flora
T. socranskii ss. *paredis*	New species—human oral flora
T. socranskii ss. *socranskii*	New species—human oral flora
Zymophilus paucivorans	New species—brewery
Z. raffinosivorans	New species—brewery
Anaerobic Cocci	
Gram-positive cocci	
Genus *Peptostreptococcus*	
P. anaerobius	
P. asaccharolyticus	*Peptococcus asaccharolyticus*
P. barnesae	New species—chicken feces
P. heliotrinreducens	New species—sheep rumen
P. hydrogenalis	New species—human vaginal and fecal flora
P. indolicus	*P. indolicus*
P. lacrimalis	
P. lactolyticus	
P. magnus	*P. magnus* *P. variabilis*
P. micros	
P. prevotii	*P. prevotii*
P. tetradius	*Gaffkya anaerobia*
P. vaginalis	
Peptococcus niger	
Gemella morbillorum	*Streptococcus morbillorum*
Genus *Streptococcus*	
S. anginosus	"*S. milleri*" group
S. constellatus	"*S. milleri*" group
S. intermedius	"*S. MG-intermedius*," "*S. MG*"
S. intestinalis	New species—pig feces
Genus *Staphylococcus*	
Staphylococcus aureus ss. *anaerobius*	New species—sheep abscess
S. saccharolyticus	*Peptococcus saccharolyticus*
Genus *Ruminococcus*	
R. hansenii	*Streptococcus hansenii*
R. productus	*Peptostreptococcus productus*
Sarcina ventriculi	Diseased stomach—colon
Gram-negative cocci	
Acidaminococcus fermentans	
Megasphaera elsdenii	
Megasphaera cerevisiae	New species—spoiled beer
Veillonella parvula	
Anaerobic Gram-Positive, Non–Spore-Forming Rods	
Genus *Actinomyces*	
A. bernardiae	New species—CDC coryneform group 2
A. bovis	Actinomycosis in cattle—not in humans
A. denticolens	New species—cow dental plaque
A. georgiae	New species—human gingival crevices
A. gerencseriae	New species—human periodontal flora
A. hordeovulneris	New species—canine infections
A. howellii	New species—cow dental plaque
A. hyovaginalis	New species— pig vagina
A. israelii	Major cause of human actinomycosis

(Continued)

TABLE 14-12 *(Continued)*
PRESENT AND FORMER NAMES OF ANAEROBIC BACTERIA

PRESENT NAME	FORMER NAME/COMMENT
A. meyeri	Human periodontal sulcus—abscesses of brain; head and neck infections
A. naeslundii	A cause of human actinomycosis
A. neuii ss. *neuii*	New species—CDC coryneform group 1; from human sources
A. neuii ss. *anitratus*	New subsp.—CDC coryneform group 1-"like", from human sources
A. odontolyticus	Human oral cavity—rare cause of actinomycosis
A. pyogenes	*Corynebacterium pyogenes*—human sources
A. slackii	New species—cow dental plaque
A. suis	*Eubacterium suis*—pig
A. viscosus	Human oral cavity and cervicovaginal sources; actinomycosis occasionally
Genus *Atopobium*	
A. minutum	*Lactobacillus minutus*
A. parvulum	*Streptococcus parvulus* / *Peptostreptococcus parvulus*
A. rimae	*Lactobacillus rimae*
Genus *Bifidobacterium*	
B. breve	
B. denticolens	New species—dental caries
B. dentium	*Bifidobacterium ericksonii*
B. gallicum	New species—human feces
B. inopinatum	New species—dental caries
B. longum	
B. merycicum	New species—rumen of cattle
B. ruminatum	New species—rumen of cattle
Genus *Eubacterium*	
E. acidaminophilum	New species—anaerobic mud
E. aerofaciens	
E. alactolyticum	
E. angustum	New species—sewage sludge
E. brachy	
E. combesii	
E. callanderi	New species—anaerobic wood digestor
E. contortum	
E. desmolens	New species—cat feces
E. fossor	New species—horse oral flora
E. oxidoreducans	New species—rumen of cow
E. lentum	
E. limosum	
E. moniliforme	
E. nodatum	
E. nitrogenes	
E. uniforme	New species—rumen of sheep
E. saburreum	
E. saphenum	
E. tenue	
E. timidum	
E. xylanophilum	New species—rumen of sheep
E. yurii ss. *margaretiae*	New species—human dental plaque
E. yurii ss. *schtitka*	New species—human dental plaque
E. yurii ss. *yurii*	New species—human dental plaque
Genus *Lactobacillus*	
L. acidophilus	
L. brevis	
L. catenaforme	

PRESENT NAME	FORMER NAME/COMMENT
L. jensenii	
L. oris	New species—human saliva
L. rimae	New species—human gingival crevices
L. uli	New species—human gingival crevices
Genus *Mobiluncus*	
M. curtisii ss. *curtisii*	
M. curtisii ss. *homesii*	
M. mulieris	
Genus *Propionibacterium*	
P. acnes	
P. avidum	
P. granulosum	
P. lymphophilum	
P. propionicum	*Arachnia propionica* / *Actinomyces propionicus*—rare cause of human actinomycosis
Gram-Positive Spore-Forming Rods	
***Clostridium*: Human**	
C. argentinense	*C. botulinum* type G and some nontoxigenic *C. hastiforme* and *C. subterminale*
C. baratii	*C. barati* / *C. paraperfringens* / *C. perenne*
C. bifermentans	
C. botulinum	
C. butyricum	*C. pseudotetanicum*
C. cadaveris	
C. carnis	
C. clostridioforme	*C. clostridiiforme*
C. cochlearium	
C. difficile	
C. fallax	
C. ghoni	
C. glycolicum	
C. haemolyticum	
C. hastiforme	
C. histolyticum	
C. indolis	
C. innocuum	
C. irregulare	
C. limosum	
C. malenominatum	
C. methylpentosum	New species—human fecal flora
C. novyi	
C. orbiscindens	New species—human fecal flora
C. oroticum	
C. paraputrificum	
C. perfringens	*C. welchii*
C. putrificum	
C. ramosum	*Eubacterium filamentosum* / *Ramibacterium ramosum* / *Actinomyces ramosus* / *Eubacterium ramosus*
C. scindens	New species—human fecal flora
C. septicum	
C. sordellii	
C. sphenoides	

TABLE 14-12 *(Continued)*
PRESENT AND FORMER NAMES OF ANAEROBIC BACTERIA

PRESENT NAME	FORMER NAME/COMMENT
C. sporogenes	
C. symbiosum	*Fusobacterium symbiosum*
C. tertium	
C. tetani	
C. tetanomorphorum	Revived name—human infections
Clostridium: **Animal and Other Sources**	
C. aerotolerans	New species—soil
C. aldrichii	New species—wood-fermenting digestion
C. celerecrescens	New species—cow manure
C. cellulofermentans	New species—sewage sludge digestion
C. colinum	New species—foul intestine
C. cylindrosporum	Revived name—soil and chicken intestines
C. disporicum	New species—rat cecal contents
C. fervidus	New species—geothermal spring
C. homopropionicum	New species—digestion sludge
C. intestinalis	New species—feces of cattle and pigs
C. josui	New species—compost heap
C. lentocellum	New species—mud bank
C. litorale	New species—marine sediment
C. magnum	New species—digestion sludge and anaerobic freshwater sediments

PRESENT NAME	FORMER NAME/COMMENT
C. oxalicum	New species—anaerobic freshwater sediments
C. pfennigii	New species—cattle rumen
C. populeti	New species—popular wood fermentation
C. proteolyticum	New species—chicken manure digestion
C. roseum	New species—soil
C. thermobutyricum	New species—horse manure compost
C. thermocopriae	New species—camel feces and soil compost
C. thermopalmarium	New species—palm wine
C. thermopapyrolyticum	New species—riverside mud
C. xylanolyticum	New species—decayed wood chips
Other genera of spore-forming rods	
Desulfotomaculum species	Ubiquitous in environment
Caloramator fervidus	*Clostridium fervidus*—hot spring
Filifactor villosus	*C. villosum*—cats
Moorella thermoacetica	*C. thermoacetica*
Oxobacter pfennigii	*C. pfennigii*—rumen fluid
Oxalophagus oxalicus	*C. oxalicum*—sediment

This was not intended to be an all-inclusive list. A number of species of no or doubtful clinical relevance have not been included, especially in the genera *Bacteroides, Lactobacillus,* and *Clostridium.*
Based on information compiled from 1) the following references: [56, 111a, 186a, 194, and 195] and from 2) taxa published in the International Journal of Systematic Bacteriology, Volumes 30–46; 1980–1996.

of humans, and these bacteria are particularly important clinically (see Tables 14-3 and 14-4). They are a part of the indigenous microbiota of the intestinal tract of most persons, but are seldom found in the mouth. Through the years, numerous species names have been used for this group (e.g., *B. convexus, B. convexa, B. pseudoinsolita, B. inequalis, B. incommunis, B. uncata*), and likewise, several genus names, but now the group includes only those listed in Table 14-12.

The previously unnamed DNA homology group VPI "3452A," which closely resembles *B. distasonis* phenotypically, was given the name *B. caccae* by Johnson and colleagues.[99] Most strains of *B. caccae* have been isolated from feces; only a few have been found in human clinical specimens. Two other DNA homology groups, VPI "T4-1" and "B5-21," were named *B. merdae* and *B. stercoris*, respectively. These species also bear a close phenotypic similarity to *B. fragilis* and all the other species of the *B. fragilis* group. *B. merdae* and *B. stercoris* have both been isolated from fecal samples and have been isolated rarely from clinical samples contaminated with feces or intestinal contents (Siders JA, personal communication).

B. fragilis is the most common species of the group found in clinical specimens, but it is not often isolated from feces during studies of the intestinal flora. On the other hand, *B. ovatus* is not as frequently isolated from

properly collected specimens, but is common in fecal materials. However, compromised patients with polymicrobial bacteremia secondary to massive trauma or necrosis of the bowel are occasionally seen from whom *B. ovatus* is isolated from the blood. The chances of isolating *B. ovatus, B. caccae, B. merdae,* or *B. stercoris* from properly collected, nonintestinal specimens are so low that isolates believed to show the differential characteristics of these species should be brought to the attention of the laboratory supervisor or director. *B. thetaiotaomicron* is the second most common species of this group in clinical infections (Table 14-3). For information on pathogenic properties and infections caused by the *B. fragilis* group, the reader is referred to Finegold and George[69] and Smith and Williams.[186]

Organisms of the *B. fragilis* group are nonmotile, gram-negative rods with rounded ends, and are 0.5 to 0.8 μm in diameter by 1.5 to 9 μm long.[186] Cells from broth culture tend to be pleomorphic, often with vacuoles. Many strains are encapsulated; the pathogenic significance of their capsules is unclear. Colonies of *B. fragilis* on CDC-anaerobe blood agar are 1 to 4 mm in diameter, nonhemolytic, gray, entire, and semiopaque, with concentric whorls or ringlike structures inside the colonies (see Color Plate 14-1). Colonies of other species of the group are similar in size and shape, but
(text continues on page 756)

TABLE 14-13

CHARACTERISTICS HELPFUL IN DIFFERENTIATION OF BACTEROIDES FRAGILIS GROUP AND CLOSELY RELATED SPECIES THAT GROW WELL IN 20% BILE

SPECIES	PRODUCTION OF		FERMENTATION OF									
	INDOLE	CATALASE	ARABINOSE	CELLOBIOSE	GLUCOSE	MELEZITOSE	RHAMNOSE	RIBOSE	SALICIN	SUCROSE	TREHALOSE	XYLAN
B. fragilis group												
A. Indole-negative subgroup												
B. caccae	−	−	+	+	+	+	+/−	+	+	+	+	−
B. distasonis	−	+	−	+	+	+	+/−	+/−	+	+	+	−
B. fragilis	−	+	−	−/w	+	−	−	−	−	+	−	−
B. merdae	−	−	−/+	−	+	+	−/+	−	w	+	+	−
B. vulgatus	−	V	+	−	+	−	+	−/+	−	+	−	−/+
B. Indole-positive subgroup												
B. ovatus	+	+	+	+	+	+/−	+	+	+	+	+	+
B. stercoris	+	−	−/+	−	+	−	+	−/w	−	+	−	−
B. thetaiotaomicron	+	+	+	+	+	V	+	+	−/+	+	+	−
B. uniformis	+	−	+	+	+	−	−/+	−/+	+/−	+	−	ND
B. eggerthii	+	V	+	−/w	+	−	w/−	−	−	−	−	+
Other Related Bacteroides spp.												
B. splanchnicus	+	−	+	−	+	−	−	−	−	−	−	ND

+, Positive reaction for 90% or more of strains (includes weak and strong reactions); +/−, 51%–89% strains positive; −/+, 10–50% strains positive; −, less than 10% strains positive; V, variable reactions; w, weak reactions; ND, data not available. After Holdeman et al[93], Johnson et al[99], and Allen and Siders, unpublished data.

TABLE 14-14

Presumptive or Preliminary Identification of Obligately Anaerobic Gram-Negative Bacilli

Groups or Species	Anaerobe Blood Agar							Presumpto 1 Quadrant Plate				Catalase (LD Esculin Agar)	Growth on Bile Agar
	Red Fluorescence (UV Light)	Brown-Black Colonies	Colonies <1 mm in Diameter	Agar Pitted	Penicillin (2-U Disk)	Rifampin (15 UG Disk)	Kanamycin 1-µG Disk	Indole	Lipase	Esculin	H₂S		
B. fragilis group	-	-	-	-	R	S	R	V	-	+/-	-	V	E
Pigmenting Porphyromonas–Prevotella	+	+	-	-	S or R	S	R	+	-/+	-	-	-	I or E
B. ureolyticus	-	-	+	+	S	S	S	-	-	-	-	-	I
Bacteroides CDC group F₂	-	-	+	-	S	S	S	-	-	-	-	-	I
Fusobacterium mortiferum	-	-	-	-	R or S	R	S	-	-	+	+	-	E
F. necrophorum	-	-	-	-	S	S	S	+	+	-	+	-	I
F. nucleatum	-	-	-	-	S	S	S	+	-	-	-	-	I
F. varium	-	-	-	-	R or S	R	S	+	-	-	+	-	E

R, growth not inhibited; S, growth inhibited; LD, Lombard-Dowell; V, variable reaction; +, positive reaction of 90%–100% of strains tested; –, negative reaction of 90%–100% of strains tested; +/– or –/+, reaction of 11%–25% of strains tested; E, growth ≥ growth on LD agar; I, growth inhibited (compared with LD agar).

TABLE 14-15
SOME KEY DIFFERENTIAL CHARACTERISTICS OF COMMONLY ISOLATED BACTEROIDES AND FUSOBACTERIUM SPECIES AVAILABLE ON CDC ANAEROBE BLOOD AGAR

SPECIES	RELATION TO O_2	COLONY CHARACTERISTICS	HEMOLYSIS SHEEP BLOOD	BRICK-RED FLUORESCENCE	BLACK PIGMENT	PITTING OF AGAR	CELLULAR MORPHOLOGY	GRAM-NEGATIVE, SPORES MOTILITY	PENICILLIN (2-U DISK)	RIFAMPIN (15-μg DISK)	KANAMYCIN 1-μg DISK	NITRATE REDUCTION
B. distasonis	OA	Small to medium, convex, semiopaque, entire edge	–	–	–	–	Small rods, variable length	–	R	S	R	–
B. fragilis	OA	Small to medium, convex, mottled surface, concentric rings, entire edge	–	–	–	–	Small rods, variable length	–	R	S	R	–
B. ovatus	OA	Small to medium, convex, opaque, entire edge	–	–	–	–	Small rods, variable length	–	R	S	R	–
B. thetaiotaomicron	OA	Small to medium, convex, opaque, entire edge	–	–	–	–	Small rods, variable length	–	R	S	R	–
B. uniformis	OA	Small to medium, convex, opaque, entire edge	–	–	–	–	Small rods, variable length	–	R	S	R	–
B. ureolyticus	OA	Pinpoint, convex, irregular edge	–	–	–	+	Small, slim rods, variable length	–	S	S	S	+
B. vulgatus	OA	Small to medium, convex, semiopaque, entire edge	–	–	–	–	Small rods, variable length	–	R	S	R	–
Porphyromonas asaccharolytica– P. gingivalis group	OA	Small to medium, convex, entire edge	+	+	+	–	Tiny coccoid rods	–	S	S	R	–
Prevotella bivia	OA	Small to medium, convex, entire edge	–	–	–	–	Tiny coccoid rods, vary in length	–	R	S	R	–

Organism		Colony morphology				Cell morphology					
P. disiens	OA	Small to medium, convex, entire edge	–	–	–	Tiny coccoid rods, vary in length	–	R	S	R	–
P. intermedia	OA	Small to medium, convex, edge	+	+	+	Tiny coccoid rods	–	S or R	S	R	–
Fusobacterium											
F. mortiferum	OA	Small to medium, fried egg†	–	–	–	Highly pleomorphic rods, filaments, large round bodies	–	R or S	R	S	–
F. naviforme	OA	Small, low-convex mottled, entire	–	–	–	Pleomorphic slim rods, some with pointed ends	–	S	S	S	–
F. necrophorum	OA	Small to medium, raised with opaque centers	–*	–	–	Highly variable in length and width	–	S	S	S	–
F. nucleatum	OA	Small to medium, speckled opalescence.‡ Occasionally colonies will resemble bread crumbs (rough colony form)	Green	–	–	Slim filamentous rods, even diameter, usually with pointed ends	–	S	S	S	–
F. varium	OA	Small to medium, fried egg†	–	–	–	Small rods, variable length, rounded ends	–	R or S	R	S	–

OA, obligate anaerobe; +, positive reaction in 90% of strains tested; –, negative reactions in 90% of strains tested; R, resistant; S, sensitive.

* *F. necrophorum* hemolyzes rabbit, but not sheep, red blood cells.
† Fried egg; raised opaque center with translucent, entire edge.
‡ Speckled opalescence: colonies of *F. nucleatum* show flecking (in the colonies) when viewed through the dissecting microscope with reflected light; they usually are not hemolytic, but may cause greenish discoloration of the blood agar on exposure to oxygen.

After Dowell VR, Allen SD: Anaerobic bacterial infections. In Balows A, Hausler WJ Jr (eds): Diagnostic Procedures for Bacterial, Mycotic, and Parasitic Infections, 6th ed, pp. 174–219. Washington, DC.

TABLE 14-16

SOME KEY CHARACTERISTICS OF COMMONLY ISOLATED ANAEROBIC, GRAM-NEGATIVE RODS ON CDC DIFFERENTIAL AGAR MEDIA

SPECIES	NO. OF STRAINS EXAMINED	INDOLE	INDOLE DERIVATIVE	ESCULIN HYDROLYSIS	H₂S	CATALASE	LECITHINASE	LIPASE	GROWTH ON BILE AGAR	GLUCOSE FERMENTATION	STARCH HYDROLYSIS	MILK PROTEOLYSIS	DNASE	GELATIN HYDROLYSIS	MANNITOL FERMENTATION	LACTOSE FERMENTATION	RHAMNOSE FERMENTATION
		Presumpto 1 Plate								_Presumpto 2 Plate_					_Presumpto 3 Plate_		
B. distasonis	21	-	-	+	-	+/-	-	-	E	+	-	-/+	-	-	-	+	+
B. fragilis	135	-	-	+	-	+	-	-	E-ppt	+	-/+	-/+	-	-	-	+	+
B. ovatus	5	+/-	-	+	-	V	-	-	E-ppt	+	V	V	V	-	+/-	+	-
B. thetaiotaomicron	71	+	-	+	-	+	-	-	E	+	-/+	-/+	+/-	-	-	+	+
B. uniformis	5	+	-	+/-	-	-	-	-	E	+	-	V	V	-	-	+	-/+
B. vulgatus	23	-	-	-/+	-	-	-	-	E	+	-	-	-	-	-	+	+
B. splanchnicus	2	+	-	+	V	-	-	-	E	+	-	-	-	V	-	+	-
B. ureolyticus	1	-	-	-	-	-	-	-	V	-	-	-/+	-	-/+	-	-	-
Campylobacter gracilis	10	-	-	V	-	-	-	-	V	-	-	-	-/+	-	-	-	-
Porphyromonas asaccharolytica	6	+/-	-	-	-	-	-	-/+	NG	-	-	+/-	-/+	V	-	-	-
P. gingivalis	13	+	-	-	V	-	-	-	NG	-	-/+	+	-	+	-	-	-
Prevotella bivia	14	-	-	-	-	-	-	-	NG	+	-/+	+/-	+/-	V	-/+	+	-/+
P. disiens	3	-	-	-	-	-	-	-	V	+/-	+	+	V	+	-	-	-
P. denticola	5	-	-	-/+	-	-	-	-	NG	+	+	+	+/-	-/+	-	+	-
P. intermedia/nigrescens	16	+	-	-	-	-	-	+	NG	+/-	+/-	+	+	+	-	+	-
P. melaninogenica	10	-	-	+	-	-	-	-	NG	+	+	-	+/-	V	-	+	-
P. oralis	2	-	-	+	-	-	-	-	NG	V	V	-	V	-	-	V	V
P. oris/buccae	9	-	-	+	-	-	-	-	NG	+	+	+/-	+	-	-	+	-/+
P. veroralis	2	-	V	+	-	-	-	-	NG	+	+	-	V	-	-	+	V
Fusobacterium gonidiaformans	6	+/-	-	-	-/+	-	-	-	NG	-/+	-	-	-	-	-	-	-
F. mortiferum	5	-/+	-	+	-	-	-	-	E	+	-	-	-	-	-	V	-
F. naviforme	6	+	-	-	-	-	-	-	NG	-/+	-	-	-	-	-	-	-
F. necrophorum	18	+	-	-	V	-	-	+	NG	V	-	+	-/+	-/+	-	+	-/+
F. nucleatum	31	+	-	-	V	-	-	-	NG	V	-	-	-	-	-	+	-
F. varium	6	V	-	-	V	-	-	-	E	+	-	-	-	-	-	-	-

+, positive reaction in >90% strains; -, negative reaction in >90% strains; +/-, most strains positive, occasional strain negative; -/+, most strains negative, occasional strain positive; V, variable; I, growth inhibited; E, growth equal to control without bile; E', equal growth with an occasional strain inhibited; E-ppt, equal growth with a precipitate adjacent to or under growth; NG, no growth.
Adapted from Whaley DN, Wiggs LS, Miller PH, Srivastava PU, Miller JM: Use of Presumpto plates to identify anaerobic bacteria. J Clin Microbiol 33:1196–1202, 1995 and previous editions of this book.

TABLE 14-17

Characteristics of Glucose-Fermenting, Bile-Sensitive, Pigmented and Nonpigmented *Prevotella* spp. Isolated From Clinical Specimens*

	FERMENTATION OF									ESCULIN HYDROLYSIS	INDOLE
	AMYGDALIN	ARABINOSE	CELLOBIOSE	LACTOSE	MELIBIOSE	RAFFINOSE	SALICIN	SUCROSE	XYLOSE		
May be pigmented											
P. corporis	-**	-	-	-	-	-	-	-	-	-	-
P. denticola	-	-	V	+	-	+	V	+	-	+	-
P. intermedia	-	-	-	-	-	V	-	+	-	-	+
P. loescheii	-	-	+	+	V	+	V	+	-	+	-/+
P. melaninogenica	-	-	V	+	-/+	+	-	+	-	V	-
P. nigrescens	-	-	-	-	-	NT	-	+	-	-	+
P. tannerae	-	-	-	V	-	V	-	V	-	V	-
Not pigmented											
P. bivia	-	-	-	+	-	-	-	-	-	-	-
P. buccae	+/-	+	+	+	+	+	+	+	+	+	-
P. buccalis	NT	-	+	+	+	+	+	+	-	+	-
P. dentalis	NT	+	+	+	w	+	-	w	-	-	-
P. disiens	-	-	-	-	-	-	-	-	-	-	-
P. enoeca	-	-	-	+	-	-	-	-	V	V	-
*P. heparinolytica****	NT	+	+	+	NT	-	+	+	+	+	+
P. oralis	+	-	+	+	+	+	+	+	+	+	-
P. oris	+/-	+	+	+	V	+	+	+	+	+	-
P. oulora	NT	-	-	+	w/+	+	-	+	-	+	-
P. veroralis	-	-	V	+	w	+	V	+	V	V	-
*P. zoogleoformans****	-/w	V	V	V	V	V	V	+	V	V	+/-

* Biochemical features modified from Holdeman, Kelly and Moore (1984, Bergey's Manual of Systematic Bacteriology), Shah and Collins (1990, Int J System Bacteriol 40:205–208), Shah and Ghorbia (1992, Int J System Bacteriol 42:542–546), Moore and Moore (1994, Int J System Bacteriol 44:599–602), and Williams and Collins (1995, Int J System Bacteriol 45:832–836).

**-, negative reaction; +, positive reaction; V, variable; +/-, most strains positive; -/+, most strains negative; NT, not tested; +/w, most strains positive, some weakly positive; w/+, most weakly positive; w, weak reaction.

***Broth cultures have a glutinous or sticky sediment.

TABLE 14-18
CHARACTERISTICS THAT ARE ESPECIALLY USEFUL FOR IDENTIFYING COMMONLY ENCOUNTERED
BACTEROIDES, PORPHYROMONAS, PREVOTELLA, AND *FUSOBACTERIUM* SPECIES

CHARACTERISTIC	SPECIES
Brick-red fluorescence (with long-wave UV light) or brown-black pigment	*Prevotella melaninogenica* group,* *Porphyromonas* spp.
Good growth on 20% bile; resistant to penicillin (2-U disk), kanamycin (1-mg disk); and inhibited by rifampin (15-µg disk)	*Bacteroides fragilis* group*
Catalase produced on LD esculin agar	*B. fragilis, B. thetaiotaomicron, B. distasonis, B. ovatus*
Lipase produced on LD egg yolk agar	*Prevotella intermedia, F. necrophorum*
Asaccharolytic (glucose or other carbohydrates not fermented)	*Bacteroides* CDC group F_2, *Porphyromonas asaccharolytica, P. gingivalis, B. capillosis* (this species is rare), *B. ureolyticus, F. gonidiaformans* (rare), *F. naviforme, F. nucleatum*
Agar pitted; urease-positive	*B. ureolyticus*
Gelatin hydrolyzed; milk digested	*Prevotella bivia, P. disiens, P. intermedia*
DNase-positive; enhanced growth on 20% bile	*B. thetaiotaomicron, B. uniformis, B. ovatus*
Resistant to rifampin; esculin hydrolyzed	*F. mortiferum*
Resistant to rifampin; esculin not hydrolyzed	*F. varium*
Long, thin, filamentous rods; internal speckling of colonies; propionate produced from threonine	*F. nucleatum*

* See text for listing of species included.

differ in their internal structures. A key characteristic of species of the *B. fragilis* group is that growth is enhanced by bile (see Tables 14-12 and 14-13). They are all resistant to penicillin and kanamycin, but sensitive to rifampin by the disk technique (see Table 14-14). All are saccharolytic, and their carbohydrate fermentation patterns (along with indole) help differentiate between the species (see Table 14-13). Detailed characteristics of the species are given in Tables 14-11, 14-13, 14-15, and 14-16. There are two species of *Bacteroides* in Table 14-13 that do not ferment sucrose, *B. eggerthii* and *B. splanchnicus,* and these share several phenotypic characteristics. In their proposal to restrict the genus *Bacteroides* to *B. fragilis* and closely related species, Shah and Collins included *B. eggerthii,* but not *B. splanchnicus,* in the *B. fragilis* group.[174] For practical purposes, both species are rare in properly selected and collected clinical materials. Thus, the differentiation between *B. eggerthii* and *B. splanchnicus* is seldom an issue in the clinical laboratory. For additional detailed characteristics of *B. splanchnicus* see Tables 14-13 and 14-16. For a further description of *B. splanchnicus* and *B. eggerthii,* the chapter in *Bergey's Manual* by Holdeman and colleagues is recommended.[93]

Pigmenting Anaerobic Gram-Negative Bacilli. Shah and Collins proposed that the genus *Bacteroides* be restricted

to the *B. fragilis* group and related species, which actively ferment glucose (pH less than 5.4; highly saccharolytic), grow in the presence of 20% bile, and hydrolyze esculin.[174] Their major acid metabolic products from glucose are acetic and succinic acids, and smaller amounts of other short-chain fatty acids may be produced.[174] Thus, the pigmenting anaerobic gram-negative bacilli are no longer classified in the genus *Bacteroides.* The moderately saccharolytic, pigmenting species were placed in the genus *Prevotella.* In 1988, the asaccharolytic, pigmented *Bacteroides,* all isolated from humans, were reclassified in the genus *Porphyromonas* as *P. asaccharolytica, P. gingivalis,* and *P. endodontalis.*[173] The following pigmenting species are encountered in clinical specimens from humans: *Prevotella melaninogenica, P. corporis, P. denticola, P. intermedia, P. nigrescens, P. loescheii, P. tannerae, Porphyromonas asaccharolytica, P. gingivalis,* and *P. endodontalis.*[144,173,175,177,178,218] Many species of *Prevotella* are commonly isolated from the oral cavity, from infections involving the head and neck and lower respiratory tract, and from the urogenital tract. Most *Porphyromonas* strains isolated from the oral cavity probably are *P. gingivalis;*[206] most of the nonoral clinical isolates of *Porphyromonas* isolated from other anatomic regions of humans are probably *P. asaccharolytica,* whereas *P. endodontalis* strains have been isolated from infected root canals.[173]

Since 1992, the genus *Porphyromonas* has changed markedly, with the addition of 9 additional species, for a grand total now of 12 species (see Tables 14-12 and 14-17). Five of the new species were isolated from oral cavities of dogs only (*P. canoris, P. cangingivalis, P. cansulci, P. gingivicanis,* and *P. crevioricanis*),[41,89,124] one has been isolated from the oral cavities of cats only (*P. circumdentaria*),[122] another has been isolated from both monkeys and cats (*P. macacae,* which includes those previously called *P. salivosa*),[120,122,123] another is from cattle (*P. levii*),[176] and one of the nine new species was isolated from the human oral cavity (*P. catoniae,* previously called *Oribaculum catoniae* by Moore and Moore).[145,219] Presently, although their clinical importance in humans is unknown, the species isolated from the mouths of dogs, cats, and monkeys might be encountered in bite wound infections.

In 1975, not only did Willems and Collins reclassify *Oribaculum catoniae* (Moore and Moore 1994) as *Porphyromonas catoniae,* but they emended the genus *Porphyromonas* as well. In accordance with their emended description, some species are now included that are saccharolytic (*P. levii, P. macacae,* and *P. catoniae*), and *P. catoniae* does not form pigment.[219]

Presumptive clues for the recognition of anaerobic gram-negative bacilli that belong to the genus *Porphyromonas* include the formation of tan to buff colonies that fluoresce brick-red under long-wave ultraviolet light or brown-black colonies (most species); inhibition of growth in the presence of vancomycin (i.e., failure to grow on kanamycin–vancomycin blood agar); inhibition by bile; inhibition by penicillin and rifampin, but resistant to kanamycin; formation of indole; and failure of most species to ferment glucose or other carbohydrates. Definitive identification of *Porphyromonas* to the species level is difficult. Some key differential characteristics of the three asaccharolytic, pigmented, and catalase-negative species encountered in human illnesses are listed in Box 14-12.

Thus, the determination of enzyme activities through the use of a rapid, 4-hour test system (i.e., the ATB 32A Anaerobes ID or RapID ANA II) is a practical aid to identify *Porphyromonas* species encountered in

humans.[44,204–206] Additional characteristics of *Porphyromonas* species are given in Table 14-17.

In contrast with *Porphyromonas,* all of the pigmented species of *Prevotella* ferment glucose and other carbohydrates (see Tables 14-16 and 14-17). It is emphasized that the "pigmenting" *Prevotella* group described in Table 14-17 may take from 2 days to 3 weeks to form pigment on CDC-anaerobe blood agar, or may even fail to produce pigmented colonies. *P. intermedia* is distinctive in that it forms black colonies, produces indole, is lipase positive on egg yolk agar, and ferments sucrose. *P. nigrescens* is a new species derived from a genetically distinct group of strains formerly included in *P. intermedia.*[177] Some of these strains were from patients with periodontitis; others were from healthy individuals. Whereas both *P. nigrescens* and *P. intermedia* form brown to black colonies on blood agar, produce indole, and ferment sucrose, only *P. intermedia* produces lipase. *P. corporis,* formerly classified as *Bacteroides melaninogenicus* subsp. *intermedius,* differs from *P. intermedia* in that *P. corporis* does not produce indole, is lipase negative, and does not ferment sucrose (see Table 14-17). *P. bivia* and *P. disiens* are very similar phenotypically to *P. intermidia* and *P. corporis. P. bivia* is found in the urogenital tract and mouth, and *P. disiens* is commonly isolated from the urogenital tract. They are saccharolytic, and can easily be confused when *P. intermedia* and *P. corporis* fail to produce pigment. In addition, it has been reported by Ueno that *P. bivia* may produce pigment under certain conditions (personal communication, September 1990). Four other species of saccharolytic, pigmenting *Prevotella* species may be isolated from humans—*P. melaninogenica, P. loescheii, P. denticola,* and *P. tannerae.* Each usually ferments lactose, in contrast with *P. intermedia, P. nigrescens,* and *P. corporis,* which are lactose-negative. *P. denticola* is slow to produce pigment; some strains may not produce pigment even after 3 weeks of incubation. *P. denticola* ferments esculin (acid produced) and ribose, characteristics that help separate it from *P. melaninogenica* (which is negative for these characteristics).[93] *P. loescheii* also does not ferment esculin; in contrast with both *P. denticola* and *P. melaninogenica,* and is cellobiose-positive. Most strains of *P. tannerae* do not hydrolyze esculin (86% of strains negative for esculin), and most (69%) do not ferment sucrose. Another pigmented organism, *Porphyromonas levii,* previously called *B. melaninogenicus* subsp. *levii* and later *Bacteroides levii,* to our knowledge, has been isolated only from ruminants and will not be further discussed.[176] A major problem in identifying the pigmented group to species is that they are often fastidious, slow growing, and may require anywhere from 2 days to a full 3 weeks to form pigment (on laked rabbit blood or on sheep blood agar). The pigmented *Prevotella–Porphyromonas* group are part of the normal flora of the oropharynx, nose, and gastrointestinal and genitourinary tracts. They are the second most common group of anaerobic bacteria encountered in human infections (Table 14-3). In some clinical situa-

BOX 14-12. CHARACTERISTICS FOR IDENTIFICATION OF *PORPHYROMONAS* SPP.

1. *P. gingivalis:* Produces phenylacetic acid (see Table 14-11) and agglutinates sheep red blood cells;[173] produces β-galactose-6-phosphatase, and N-acetyl-β-glucosaminidase, but not α-fucosidase; can be tested in the ATB 32A Anaerobes ID System (API-bioMérieux, Inc., La Balme les Grottes, France).[204, 206]

2. *P. asaccharolytica:* not as the foregoing species; produces α-flucosidase; can be tested in the ATB 32A Anaerobes ID System.[204, 206]

3. *P. endodontalis:* not as either of the foregoing species.

tions—for example, orofacial lesions and anaerobic pleuropulmonary infections—they are more common than the *B. fragilis* group. Certain species, in particular *Prevotella intermedia* (and possibly *P. nigrescens*), are of special clinical interest because they commonly produce β-lactamase and may be resistant in vitro to penicillin G and other antibiotics (see Table 14-4). Before pigmentation, young colonies often exhibit a brick-red fluorescence when examined under long-wave (365 nm) ultraviolet light. In gram-stained preparations, the cells are short, coccoid, gram-negative rods, usually 0.3 to 0.4 μm in diameter by 0.6 to 1 μm long (see Color Plate 14-1). In the Presumpto plate system, these species are inhibited by bile, usually (but not always) sensitive by the 2-U penicillin disk test, sensitive to rifampin, and resistant to kanamycin. Further characteristics for differentiation include those given in Table 14-17, or may be determined using tests for enzymatic activities.[44,144,178,204-206]

Other species of Prevotella.   *P. bivia* and *P. disiens* are species that phenotypically resemble *P. intermedia*, *P. nigrescins*, and *P. corporis*. They are inhibited by bile, usually resistant to penicillin, susceptible to rifampin, and resistant to kanamycin. Acetate and succinate are major metabolic products. Besides their usual lack of pigment on CDC-anaerobe blood agar held 5 to 7 days, *P. bivia* and *P. disiens* differ from *P. intermedia–nigrescens* in being indole negative and lipase negative. In addition, *P. bivia* ferments lactose, whereas neither *P. disiens* nor *P. intermedia–nigrescens* ferments lactose.[92] A nonpigmented *P. corporis* would appear virtually identical to *P. disiens* (see Table 14-17). Similar to the *B. fragilis* and pigmented *Prevotella–Porphyromonas* groups, *P. bivia* and *P. disiens* are resistant to several antibiotics (see Table 14-4). They have been isolated from blood, head and neck infections, genitourinary tract infections in both males and females, and other infection sites. Characteristics useful for separating *P. bivia* and *P. disiens* from phenotypically similar *P. oralis* and related species are given in Table 14-17. In addition to *Prevotella tannerae*, Moore and associates recently described another new species that inhabits the human gingival crevice, *P. enoeca*, and emended the description of *P. zoogleoformans*.[144] Both species have been isolated from patients with periodontitis, neither forms pigment on blood agar, and both ferment a variety of carbohydrates. Key features that aid in distinguishing *P. enoeca* from other species of *Prevotella* are its inability to digest gelatin, its failure to ferment sucrose, and its cellular fatty acid profile. Fermentation of cellobiose and lactose, lack of pigment, and its cellular fatty acid profile, are key characteristics that aid in differentiating *P. zoogleoformans* from other indole-positive *Prevotella* species, especially *P. intermedia* and *P. nigrescens*, with which it shares phenotypic characteristics.[144] An additional taxonomic change made in 1995 was the reclassification of *Hallella seregens* and *Mitsuokella dentalis* as *Prevotella dentalis*.[218] Isolated from dental root canals, the colonies of *P. dentalis* are not pigmented; they differ from those of other *Prevotella* species by having a "characteristic water drop appearance."[218]

Prevotella oralis and Related species.   Major changes in the taxonomic classification of organisms previously called *B. oralis* and *B. ruminicola* (human strains) have been made on the basis of DNA homology studies.[90] In addition, some of the isolates identified as "*B. oralis*" in the past undoubtedly were members of the *B. melaninogenicus* group that had not formed pigment, especially *Prevotella denticola* (discussed previously). *P. buccalis, P. veroralis,* and *P. oralis* were all previously called *B. oralis.* They are all inhibited in 20% bile medium, indole-negative, positive for esculin hydrolysis, and ferment several carbohydrates.[93] Differential tests that aid in separating these species include fermentation of salicin, amygdalin, and xylan, and hydrolysis of starch (see Table 14-17). If they fail to produce pigment, *P. denticola* and *P. melaninogenica* can be easily confused with *P. buccalis, P. veroralis,* and *P. oralis.* However, the latter three species ferment cellobiose; *P. denticola* and *P. melaninogenica* are cellobiose-negative. *P. oris* and *P. buccae* are two species that have been isolated from periodontal infections and various other infection sites in humans.[95] Many strains of these species were previously called *B. ruminicola* (human strains). In 1994, Avgustin and associates proposed that *P. (Bacteroides) ruminicola* strains isolated from the rumen, should be redefined more narrowly, based on genotypic characteristics. It is not clear whether nonrumen isolates phenotypically similar to *P. ruminicola* (e.g., from pig guts or human feces) will correspond genetically to *P. ruminicola*, or perhaps will represent new species.[17,175] Similar to *P. buccalis, P. veroralis,* and *P. oralis, P. oris* and *P. buccae* are inhibited by bile, are indole-negative, are positive for esculin hydrolysis, and ferment glucose plus additional carbohydrates. The production of acid from either arabinose or xylose separates *P. oris* and *P. buccae* from *P. oralis.*[95] The fermentation of salicin helps to separate *P. buccae* and *P. oris* from *P. buccalis* and *P. veroralis*, which are salicin-negative. A positive test for β-glucosidase activity by *P. buccae*, but negative for *P. oris*, aids in separating these species.[93] Reactions obtained using the RapID-ANA II system may also be useful as a supplement to the tests in Table 14-17, to help differentiate these species.[44,218]

Bacteroides ureolyticus and Other Asaccharolytic Nitrate-Positive species.   *B. ureolyticus* (formerly *B. corrodens*), is a microaerophilic (but previously thought to be anaerobic), fastidious, relatively small gram-negative rod (about 0.5 μm in diameter by 1.5 to 2 μm in length) that produces pitting of anaerobe blood agar. This species is likely to be reclassified relatively soon. The cells do not produce flagella and are nonmotile. Characteristically, the colonies may be of two types: 1) 0.5 to 1 mm in diameter after 2 or more days incubation, circular, convex, and translucent, with entire or erose margins; or 2) thin, flat, spreading, irregular translucent colonies that extend out from a slightly raised central area. These latter colony types produce depressions or "pits" within the surface of agar, perhaps resembling the "corrosion" of pitted sheet metal. *B. ureolyticus* is inhibited by penicillin (2-U disk), rifampin (15-μg disk), and kanamycin (1000-μg disk), and does not grow in the presence of 20% bile, nor does it ferment any carbohydrates (i.e., it is asaccharolytic). *Campylobacter gracilis*, formerly called *Bacteroides gracilis*,[207] is also microaerophilic, has growth characteristics similar to those of *B. ureolyticus*. A positive test for urease activity separates *B. ureolyticus* from *C. gracilis* and phenotypically similar species of *Campylobacter* and *Wollinella succinogenes* (the only remaining species after *W. curva* and *W. rectus* were reclassified as *Campylobacter curvus* and *C. rectus*), which are all urease negative. *B. gracilis* does not form flagella and is nonmotile, in contradistinction to both *Campylobacter* spp. and *W. succinogenes*. *C. recta*, for example, is actively motile (by means of a single polar flagellum).[195] According to a report by Johnson and colleagues,[97] *B. ureolyticus* was most frequently isolated from superficial soft-tissue or bone infections that tended to be mild. *C. gracilis* (*B. gracilis*), in contrast, was commonly isolated from "serious" deep-seated infections, including head and neck infections, pleuropulmonary infections, and infected sites within the abdomen and pelvis. *B. ureolyticus* was uniformly susceptible to the various penicillins, cephalosporins, and other antimicrobial agents tested (included clindamycin, chloramphenicol, metronidazole, and even aminoglycosides), whereas the *C. gracilis* isolates were commonly resistant to the penicillins, cephalosporins, and clindamycin.[97] Thus, these authors demonstrated evidence that *C. gracilis* may be a more virulent organism for humans than *B. ureolyticus*, and that its frequent resistance to antimicrobial agents may contribute to its clinical importance. The clinical importance of *C. concisus* and *C. recta*, which share some features with *B. ureolyticus* and *C. gracilis*, has not been established.

Examples of other *Bacteroides* spp. or former *Bacteroides* species for which the clinical significance is not well known or established include *B. amylophilus*, *B. coagulans*, *B. eggerthii*, *B. hypermegas* (now called *Megamonas hypermegas*), *B. multiacidus* (now called *Mitsuokella multiacidus*), *B. nodosus*, *B. pneumosintes*, *B. praeacutus* (now called *Tissierella praeacuta*), *B. putredinis*, *B. splanchnicus*, and others.[56,106,195] Most of these species are encountered only on rare occasions in human clinical specimens. Detailed characteristics of these and other little-known species of *Bacteroides* are given in the *VPI Manual*[91] and in *Bergey's Manual*.[93] For an excellent review of their role in infections and their susceptibility to antimicrobial agents, see Kirby and coauthors.[106]

Bilophila species. During a study of bacteria isolated from appendicitis specimens and human feces, a unique new anaerobic gram-negative bacillus was isolated on bacteroides bile esculin agar by Baron and associates of the VA Wadsworth Medical Center in Los Angeles.[21] This new species was reported to show the characteristics listed in Box 14-13.

BOX 14-13. CHARACTERISTICS OF *BILOPHILA* SPP.

Gram-negative, non–spore-forming, nonmotile, pleomorphic rods; 0.7 to 1.1 μm in width by 1 to 10 μm in length

Growth enhanced by 20% bile and by 1% pyruvate; grow slowly on bacteroides bile esculin (BBE); colonies on BBE after 4 days of incubation were described as 1- to 2-mm (diameter), either as circular, erose, umbonate, and translucent with dark black centers, or as irregular, low convex, opaque black colonies

Colonies on brucella agar formed slowly (4 to 7 days), were punctate, less than 1-mm–diameter, circular, erose, translucent, and gray

Strongly catalase-positive (using 15% H_2O_2)

Asaccharolytic

Urease-positive

H_2S-positive, desulfoviridin-positive

Nitrate-positive

Negative for the hydrolysis of esculin or starch

Indole-negative; gelatin not liquefied; no reactions produced in milk or on egg-yolk agar; oxidase-negative

β-lactamase-negative (nitrocefin test), but nonetheless, resistant to β-lactam antibiotics

Acetate is the major metabolic product; lactate not detected; minor or trace amounts of succinate produced in peptone–yeast glucose (supplemented by pyruvate)

Although *B. wadsworthia* is similar to the *Bacteroides fragilis* group and to certain *Fusobacterium* species that grow in the presence of 20% bile, several of the phenotypic properties of *B. wadsworthia* are different from those of the *Bacteroides fragilis* group and *Fusobacterium* spp. *Bilophila wadsworthia* differs from the *B. fragilis* group by its failure to ferment carbohydrates, its production of urease and its failure to produce a major amount of succinic acid. The production of strong catalase activity and its lack of butyric acid production are key characteristics that separate *B. wadsworthia* from *Fusobacterium* species.

Fusobacterium. The genus *Fusobacterium* includes several species that were formerly classified in *Sphaerophorus* and *Fusiformis* by Prevot.[186] Production of butyric acid as the major metabolic product (see Fig. 14-10), without much isobutyric or isovaleric acid, separates *Fusobacterium* from *Bacteroides*, *Prevotella*, *Porphyromonas*, and *Leptotrichia*. *Fusobacterium* species are normally found in the gastrointestinal, genitourinary, and upper respiratory tracts. Fusobacteria are commonly involved in serious infections in various body sites. They were described in 54 cases of bacteremia by Felner and Dowell.[60]

F. nucleatum and members of the *Prevotella–Porphyromonas* group are the organisms most frequently involved in anaerobic pleuropulmonary infections (e.g., aspiration pneumonia, lung abscess, necrotizing pneumonia, thoracic empyema). Fusobacteria are also fairly common pathogens in brain abscess, chronic sinusitis, metastatic osteomyelitis, septic arthritis, liver abscess, and other intra-abdominal infections.[61]

F. nucleatum is the most common species found in clincal materials. Recent attention has been called to severe systemic infections with a high mortality caused by *F. nucleatum* in hematologic patients with neutropenia and mucositis following chemotherapy.[113] Thus, early recognition of *F. nucleatum* in clinical materials, particularly during direct microscopic examination of freshly collected exudates or body fluids, can be important. The spindle-shaped cells are long, slender filaments, with tapered ends (see Color Plate 14-1). Sometimes there are spherical swellings. Cells are usually 5 to 10 μm long, but shorter forms are often seen. Colonies on anaerobe blood agar are 1 to 2 mm in diameter, slightly convex with slightly irregular margins, and have a characteristic internal flecking that was aptly called speckled opalescence by the late G. L. Lombard (see Color Plate 14-1). Biochemically, *F. nucleatum* is relatively inactive (see Table 14-16). Based on electrophoretic patterns of whole-cell proteins and DNA homology studies, it was proposed in 1990 that *F. nucleatum* be subdivided into three subspecies: *F. nucleatum* subsp. *nucleatum*, *F. nucleatum* subsp. *polymorphum*, and *F. nucleatum* subsp. *vincentii*.[54] In 1992, Gharbia and Shah proposed that two additional subspecies should be recognized, *F. nucleatum* subsp. *fusiforme* and *F. nucleatum* subsp. *animalis*.[74] Traditional phenotypic methods do not yet differentiate between these subspecies.

F. necrophorum has the ability to cause serious infections (e.g., liver abscess), and it is not unusual to isolate it alone (in pure culture) from soft-tissue lesions.[186] The cells measure about 0.6 by 5 μm and are pleomorphic, often with curved forms and spherical areas within cells (see Color Plate 14-1). They also produce free coccoid bodies. Most strains produce lipase on LD egg yolk agar. *F. necrophorum* has been divided into three varieties (or biovars: A, B, and C). A new species, *Fusobacterium pseudonecrophorum* was proposed for *F. necrophorum* biovar C.[181] *F. necrophorum* is pathogenic, producing liver abscesses in mice and is susceptible to penicillin (500 U/mL), whereas the new species does not produce abscesses in mice and is highly resistant to penicillin (500 U/mL).[181]

F. mortiferum and *F. varium* isolates are often resistant to clindamycin (see Table 14-4), and they may produce β-lactamase.[63] The cells are 0.5 to 2 μm wide by 2 to 10 μm long, highly pleomorphic, coccoid to filamentous, with spherical swellings near the center or one end of unevenly stained rods. Colonies on blood agar are 1 to 2 mm in diameter and have a distinctive fried-egg appearance, with raised, opaque centers and a flat, translucent margin. *F. mortiferum* and *F. varium* are resistant to rifampin (15-μg disk), which helps separate them from other *Fusobacterium*, *Bacteroides*, *Porphyromonas*, and *Prevotella* species. The two *Fusobacterium* species can be differentiated with tests for esculin hydrolysis and lactose fermentation (see Table 14-16).

Other *Fusobacterium* species may be encountered rarely in infections. The characteristics of *F. gonidiaformans* and *F. naviforme* obtained using the Presumpto plate system are shown in Table 14-16. For additional characteristics of these and other species, the following references are recommended:[66,91,93,195]

***Mobiluncus* and Bacterial Vaginosis.** *Mobiluncus* has been of interest because it has been isolated from vaginal samples of women with nonspecific vaginitis (or bacterial vaginosis).[86,88,188,190] In 1984, Spiegel and Roberts proposed the name *Mobiluncus* for a new genus of gram-variable or gram-negative, motile, curved, nonsporing anaerobic rods, which occur singly or in pairs, and with a "gull wing" appearance.[190] Electron micrographs revealed multilayered cell walls lacking an outer membrane that were probably more typical of gram-positive cell walls than gram-negative; nonetheless, the organisms tend to stain gram-variable in young culture and gram-negative in older culture. The name *Mobiluncus* was derived from the words *mobilis* (meaning capable of movement) and *uncus* (which means hook).[190] The organisms are motile by means of multiple subpolar flagella. *Mobiluncus* has been found in urogenital tract specimens of women who had nonspecific bacterial vaginosis, as well as urogenital tract specimens of asymptomatic women without vaginosis and in urogenital secretions of asymptomatic heterosexual males.[88] Although the role of *Mobiluncus* spp. in nonspecific bacterial vaginosis remains controversial, the organism is one of many genera of anaerobes that colonizes the vagina in both health and disease.[190] Bacterial vaginosis involves an overgrowth of multiple bacteria, including *Gardnerella vaginalis* (discussed in Chap. 13), *Mycoplasma hominis*, *Mobiluncus* spp., *Prevotella bivia*, *P. disiens*, other *Prevotella* spp., *Peptostreptococcus anaerobius*, *P. asaccharolyticus*, *P. magnus*, and other anaerobic cocci, plus anaerobic gram-positive rods including *Propionibacterium* spp.[188,200] Therefore, vaginosis is probably a synergistic infection in which many organisms play a role. As reviewed elsewhere,[86,88,188] the diagnosis of bacterial vaginosis is still based on demonstrating three of the following four criteria, originally described by Gardner and Dukes: 1) a "thin" (but profuse) vaginal discharge, 2) a pH higher than 4.5, 3) an odor usually described as "fishy" (especially with the addition of 10% potassium hydroxide), and 4) the demonstration of "clue cells" by microscopic examination. Clue cells are squamous epithelial cells of the vagina with myriads of small rods adherent to their surfaces. Clue cells may be observed in wet-mounts or in gram-stained smears (or in Papanicalaou-stained preparations). *Gardnerella vaginalis* can be isolated from vaginal discharges of women who have bacterial vaginosis, as well as from asymptomatic women without the condition. Data are not so clear-cut as to whether *Mobiluncus* spp. are part of the "normal" vaginal flora in absence of bacterial vaginosis. They are not always isolated from patients with vaginosis, so culture of these organisms has not replaced the original Gardner and Dukes criteria (as outlined previously) for diagnosis. In addition, direct gas–liquid chromatography (GLC) of vaginal fluid samples has been used in studies of vaginosis. Direct GLC is more time-consuming and expensive, but has not been more accurate or as sensitive as the Gardner and Dukes clinical criteria for establishing a diagnosis. The idea behind the use of GLC is to demonstrate a major amount of succinate in vaginal fluid of vaginosis patients (related to an overgrowth of *Bacteroides* spp. and other anaerobes). In contrast, *Lactobacillus* spp., which can grow and predominate in the normal vagina at pH less than 4.5, produce lactate as a major product.

The rate of isolating *Mobiluncus* from vaginal specimens that are wet-mount or gram-stain positive for curved rods has often been low (e.g., about 10% to 30% of patients).[188,189,200] Culture of *Mobiluncus* is time-consuming, costly, difficult to accomplish (for technical reasons), and in one study, required on the average, 1 month for primary isolation, plus an additional week for identification of the isolates.[165] *Mobiluncus* spp. grow on several kinds of nonselective plating media, including anaerobe blood agar (e.g., brain–heart infusion, brucella and CDC-anaerobe blood agar-based media) and chocolate agar. Colonies, after 3 to 5 days of incubation, are 2 to 4 mm in diameter, colorless, translucent, smooth and flat, sometimes with a spreading appearance. The cells are less than 0.5 µm in width by about 1.5 to 3 µm in length. Succinate and acetate are major products (with or without minor amounts of lactate) after growth in peptone–yeast extract broth supplemented with glycogen and 2% rabbit serum (see Table 14-8). Differentiation between the three subspecies originally described by Spiegel and Roberts (*M. curtisii* subsp. *curtisii*, *M. curtisii* subsp. *holmesii*, and *M. mulieris*), based on differences in morphology, growth in presence of arginine, hippurate hydrolysis, nitrate reduction, and other characteristics[190] is difficult. From results of partial 16S rRNA gene sequences and the results of Southern blot analyses, Tiveljung and associates "confirmed" the division of the genus *Mobiluncus* into the species *M. curtisii* and *M. mulieris*.[201] However, the division of *M. curtisii* into *M. curtisii* subsp. *curtisii* and *M. curtisii* subsp. *holmesii* was not supported by their genetic data.

IDENTIFICATION OF THE ANAEROBIC COCCI

The anaerobic cocci, compared with the anaerobic gram-negative bacilli, are the second most common group of anaerobes encountered in human infections (see Table 14-3). Similar to the anaerobic gram-negative rods, they are frequently encountered in the clinical laboratory in blood cultures, other body fluids, and in a wide variety of wound and abscess specimens. In the eighth edition of *Bergey's Manual of Determinative Bacteriology*, anaerobic gram-positive cocci were classified in the family *Peptococcaceae* in the following genera: *Peptococcus*, *Peptostreptococcus*, *Ruminococcus*, and *Sarcina*.[107] The gram-negative anaerobic cocci were listed in three genera in the family *Veillonellaceae* as follows: *Veillonella*, *Acidaminococcus*, and *Megasphaera*. Later, in 1974, Holdeman and Moore proposed that a

new genus, *Coprococcus*, be added to the family *Peptococcaceae*.[94] They also proposed two new *Ruminococcus* species and a new *Streptococcus* species. They recommended the transfer of *Peptostreptococcus intermedius*, *Peptostreptococcus morbillorum*, and *Peptococcus constellatus* to the genus *Streptococcus*, because these species produce lactic acid as the only major metabolic product. In 1981, *Peptococcus saccharolyticus* was transferred to the genus *Staphylococcus*.[105] Thus, *S. saccharolyticus* is considered to be an anaerobic species of the genus *Staphylococcus*. In 1983, major changes in the taxonomic classification of the anaerobic cocci were made, based on the percentage G+C data and DNA homology studies of Ezaki and colleagues.[58] Except for *P. niger*, all former species of the genus *Peptococcus* were transferred to the genus *Peptostreptococcus*. Currently, the gram-positive cocci that belong to the genus *Peptostreptococcus* include *P. anaerobius*, *P. asaccharolyticus*, *P. indolicus*, *P. magnus*, *P. micros*, *P. prevotii*, *P. productus*, *P. tetradius*, *P. hydrogenalis*, and others listed in Table 14-12.[57,58,146,147] Another species, *P. heliotrinreducens* has been isolated from the rumen of sheep and *P. barnesae* has been isolated from chicken feces; neither has been reported from human clinical materials, and they will not be discussed further. *P. tetradius* probably includes organisms formerly referred to as *Gaffkya anaerobia*.[91] In addition, the former *Peptostreptococcus parvulus* is now *Streptococcus parvulus*.[36] Other anaerobic streptococci are *S. hansenii*, *S. intermedius*, and *S. pleomorphus*. Those formerly called *Streptococcus morbillorum* are now *Gemella morbillorum*.[104]

Until recently, *Veillonella parvula* was the only species of *Veillonella* recognized. In 1982, however, six additional species, *V. dispar*, *V. atypica*, *V. rodentium*, *V. ratti*, *V. criceti*, and *V. caviae*, were proposed.[135] Of these, *V. parvula* still appears to be the most common in specimens from humans.

Although representatives of the previoulsy mentioned genera of anaerobic cocci may be part of the normal microbiota of various sites in humans and other animals, only the *Peptostreptococcus* species listed in Table 14-3, *Streptococcus intermedius*, *Staphylococcus saccharolyticus*, and *Veillonella parvula* are encountered with any significant frequency from properly collected and processed clinical specimens. Identifying characteristics of 14 of the most commonly encountered species are given in Tables 14-19 and 14-20. For additional information, the chapter by Moore and colleagues in *Bergey's Manual of Systematic Bacteriology* is recommended.[147] A typical volatile acid chromatogram tracing of *Peptostreptococus anaerobius* is shown in Figure 14-12. The susceptibility of anaerobic cocci (isolated at the Indiana University Medical Center) to antimicrobial agents is given in Table 14-4.

IDENTIFICATION OF THE ANAEROBIC NON–SPORE-FORMING GRAM-POSITIVE BACILLI

Included in this group of anaerobes are members of the genera *Actinomyces*, *Bifidobacterium*, *Eubacterium*, *Lactobacillus*, and *Propionibacterium*. Numerous changes
(text continues on page 764)

TABLE 14-19
Some Key Characteristics of Anaerobic Cocci Commonly Isolated from Clinical Specimens

SPECIES	GRAM REACTION	BLACK PIGMENT	INDOLE	NITRATE	COAGULASE	UREASE	INHIBITED BY SPS*	ALK. PHOS.	FERMENTATION OF GLUCOSE	LACTOSE	MALTOSE	ACID METABOLIC PRODUCTS IN PYG, 48 H, 35°C
Peptococcus niger	+**	+	–	–	–	–	–	NT	–	–	–	A, (P), IB, B, IV, (V), C
Peptostreptococcus												
P. asaccharolyticus	+	–	+	–	–	–	–	–	–	–	–	A, (P), B
P. hydrogenalis	+	–	+	–	–	–	–	+	+	NT	–	A, B
P. indolicus	+	–	+	+	+	–	–	+	–	–	–	A, (P), B
P. anaerobius	+	–	–	–	–	–	+	–	w/–	–	w/–	A, (IB), (B), (IV), IC
P. prevotii	+	–	–	–/+	–	–/+	–	+	–	–	–	A, (P), B
P. tetradius	+	–	–	–	–	+	–	–	+***	–	+	A, B
P. magnus	+	–	–	–	–	–	–	–	–	–	–	A
P. micros†	+	–	–	–	–	–	–	+	–	–	–	A
P. productus	+	–	–	–	–	–	–	NT	+	+	+	A
Staphylococcus saccharolyticus	+	–	–	+	–	–	–	NT	+	–	–	A
Streptococcus intermedius	+	–	–	–	–	–	–	NT	+	+	+	A, L
Gemella morbillorum	+	–	–	–	–	–	–	NT	+	–	w	A, L
Veillonella spp.	–	–	–	+	–	–	–	NT	–	–	–	A, P

* SPS, Sodium polyanethol sulfonate.
** +, positive reaction; –, negative reaction; w, weakly fermentative; –/+, occasional strains positive; w/–, most strains weakly fermentative, but occasional strains negative; A, acetic acid; P, propionic acid; IB, isobutyric acid; B, butyric acid; IV, isovaleric acid; V, valeric acid; IC, isocaproic acid; C, caproic acid; L, lactic acid; ( ), variable acid; NT, not tested.
*** *P. tetradius* strains lose their ability to ferment sugars rapidly after subculturing so it is not uncommon for these reactions to be negative.
† Most strains of *P. micros* will produce a very slight β-hemolysis on CDC Anaerobe Blood Agar (Carr-Scarborough) which helps distinguish it from *P. magnus* (Allen and Siders, unpublished data).

TABLE 14-20
REACTIONS OF ANAEROBIC COCCI ON CDC DIFFERENTIAL AGAR MEDIA

SPECIES	NO. OF STRAINS EXAMINED	PRESUMPTO 1 PLATE							PRESUMPTO 2 PLATE				PRESUMPTO 3 PLATE			
		INDOLE	ESCULIN HYDROLYSIS	H₂S	CATALASE	LECITHINASE	LIPASE	GROWTH ON BILE AGAR	GLUCOSE FERMENTATION	STARCH HYDROLYSIS	MILK PROTEOLYSIS	DNASE	GELATIN HYDROLYSIS	MANNITOL FERMENTATION	LACTOSE FERMENTATION	RHAMNOSE FERMENTATION
Peptostreptococcus																
P. anaerobius	21	–	–	V	–	–	–	V	V	–	–	–	–	–	–	–
P. asaccharolyticus	22	+	–	–	–	–	–	V	–	–	–	–	–	–	–	–
P. magnus	21	–	–	–	–/+	–	–	I	–	–	–	–	–	–	–	–
P. micros	1	–	–	–	–	–	–	NG	–	–	–	–	–	–	–	–
P. prevotii	15	–	–	–	–	–	–	V	–	–	–	–	–	–	–	–
Streptococcus																
S. intermedius	9	–	+	–	–	–	–	I	+	–	–	–	–	–	+	–
Staphylococcus																
S. saccharolyticus	2	–	–	–	+	–	–	V	+	–	–	–	–	–	–	–
Veillonella spp.	6	–	–	–	–/+	–	–	I	–	–	–	–	–	–	–	–

+, positive reaction in >90% of strains; –, negative reaction in >90% of strains; –/+, most strains negative, occasional strain positive; I, growth inhibited; V, variable; NG, no growth.
Adapted from Whaley DN, Wiggs LS, Miller PH, Srivastava PU, Miller JM: Use of Presumpto plates to identify anaerobic bacteria. J Clin Microbiol 33:1196–1202, 1995, and previous editions of this book.

763

have been made in the taxonomy of these bacteria through the years (see Table 14-12).[4,42,56,70,71,125,194,195] Important characteristics of species of non–spore-forming, gram-positive bacilli are given in Tables 14-21 and 14-22. The microscopic morphology and colonial characteristics of *Actinomyces israelii* and a *Eubacterium* species are shown in Color Plate 14-2.

Identification of the anaerobic, gram-positive, non–spore-forming bacilli requires the use of GLC for metabolic product analysis. Cellular morphology of many of these organisms tends to vary with the type of culture medium and growth conditions. On morphologic grounds alone, they can sometimes be confused with several other genera, including *Clostridium*, *Corynebacterium*, *Lactobacillus*, *Leptotrichia*, *Listeria*, *Nocardia*, *Peptostreptococcus*, and *Streptococcus*. Thus, GLC results and morphologic characteristics, considered together, aid in practical differentiation (see Tables 14-9 and 14-21).

At times some strains of anaerobic bacilli resemble cocci, particularly in gram-stained preparations of young colonies on blood agar. In addition, some streptococci, such as *S. mutans*, *S. intermedius*, *S. constellatus*, and *Gemella morbillorum* and certain peptostreptococci, may appear rod-shaped when cells from colonies on blood agar are examined microscopically. On the other hand, these bacteria usually form long chains of cells in enriched thioglycolate broth and other liquid media. It should be remembered that many gram-positive bacteria tend to become gram-negative as they age. Also, some clostridia (e.g., *C. perfringens*, *C. ramosum*, and *C. clostridioforme*) fail to produce spores in media routinely used in the clinical laboratory, whereas other clostridia do so as they age. Thus, gram-stained preparations of very young cultures may aid in demonstration of gram-variability, and observation of smears from older cultures may aid in demonstrating spores of clostridia.

PROPIONIBACTERIUM SPECIES

P. acnes is by far the most common gram-positive, non–spore-forming anaerobic rod encountered in clinical specimens. It is part of the normal flora of the skin, nasopharynx, oral cavity, and gastrointestinal and genitourinary tracts. It is frequently a contaminant of blood cultures. However, it occasionally causes endocarditis, central nervous system shunt infections, and other infections. *P. avidum* and *P. granulosum* are seldom encountered in the clinical laboratory, and are usually not clinically significant. The cells of *P. acnes* usually measure 0.3 to 1.3 µm in diameter by 1 to 10 µm in length.[186] Their morphology has often been described as diphtheroid in appearance. The cells are markedly pleomorphic and occur in varying shapes and sizes, ranging from coccoid to definite rods. Cells are often unevenly stained by Gram's procedure. Similar to the corynebacteria, the cells reveal Chinese letters, birds-in-flight, and picket fence arrangements, presumably because of "snapping" after they divide. *P. acnes* typically grows as an obligate anaerobe; however, some strains show good growth in a candle jar

(but better growth anaerobically), and have been described as aerotolerant or microaerophilic. Colonies of *P. acnes* on anaerobe blood agar are 1 to 2 mm in diameter, circular, entire, convex, glistening, and opaque. Some strains produce a narrow zone of hemolysis. *P. acnes* can be recognized without the use of GLC when it produces both indole and catalase. However, not all strains produce indole; nor do all strains produce catalase. In addition, *Actinomyces viscosus*, which has a similar morphology on some media, produces catalase.

Propionibacterium propionicum. In 1988, *Arachnia propionica* was reclassified as *P. propionicum*.[39] Previously, *Arachnia propionica* had been created to accomodate the bacteria once called *Actinomyces propionicus*. This species, although its pathogenicity and morphologic characteristics resemble those of certain species of *Actinomyces*, differs from *Actinomyces* spp. by producing propionic acid as a major metabolic product and by its cell wall murein content and menaquinone composition that resemble those of *Propionibacterium* spp. *P. propionicum* should still be considered as a potential etiologic agent of human actinomycosis. The organisms have been incriminated in cases involving cervicofacial "actinomycosis," pulmonary abscess formation with or without thoracic empyema, a neck abscess, a finger wound infection following a human bite, a renal abscess, and a few cases of lacrimal canalicultis.[33] *P. propionicum* is morphologically indistinguishable, in tissue and in culture, from *Actinomyces israelii*. Both *P. propionicum* and *A. israelii* form pleomorphic "diptheroidal" rods and long, branched, filaments (described in more detail in the section on *Actinomyces* spp.). Both species are microaerophilic to anaerobic and grow optimally under anaerobic conditions.

EUBACTERIUM SPECIES

Eubacterium species are not nearly as common as *P. acnes*. When isolated from wounds and abscesses, they are often mixed with other bacteria. Their pathogenic significance in clinical specimens is often uncertain; however, similar to *P. acnes*, they may cause endocarditis and other infections. *E. lentum* is the species isolated most often. It shows very little biochemical activity.

A report by Hill and colleagues[87] focused attention on one of the more recently described species, *E. nodatum*, which shares morphologic similarity with *Actinomyces* species. This species has been isolated from a wide variety of clinical sources that are similar to the specimen sites that are expected to contain species of *Actinomyces*. In contrast with *A. israelii* and other actinomycetes, described in the following section, which ferment carbohydrates and produce acetic, lactic, and succinic acids as major metabolic products, *E. nodatum* does not ferment carbohydrates and produces only acetic and butyric acids.

ACTINOMYCES SPECIES

The bacteria that can cause actinomycosis in humans include *A. israelii*, *A. naeslundii*, *A. odontolyticus*, *A. viscosus*, *A. meyeri*, *A. pyogenes* (formerly *Cornyebac-*

TABLE 14-21
Some Key Differential Characteristics of Anaerobic, Gram-Positive Non–Spore-Forming Bacilli

Species	Relation to Oxygen	Rapidity of Growth	Colonies on Blood Agar	Red Pigment on Blood Agar	Appearance in Enriched Thioglycolate Broth	Cellular Morphology in Enriched Thioglycolate Broth	Nitrate Reduction	Metabolic Products in PYG Broth, 48 H, 35°C
A. israelii	M or OA	Slow	Rough	−	Granular or diffuse	Branching filaments or diphtheroidal	V	A, L, S
A. naeslundii	F	Moderate	Smooth	−	Diffuse	Diphtheroidal, branching	+ −	A, L, S
A. odontolyticus	M or OA	Moderate	Smooth	+	Diffuse	Diphtheroidal, branching	+	A, L, S
A. viscosus	F	Rapid	Smooth	−	Diffuse	Diphtheroidal, branching	+	A, L, S
A. meyeri	OA, F		Smooth	−	Diffuse	Diphtheroidal, branching	−	A, L, S
A. pyogenes	F		Smooth	−	Diffuse	Diphtheroidal, coccoidal	−	A, L, S
Bifidobacterium dentium	OA	Rapid	Smooth	−	Diffuse	Thin rods, bifid ends, bulbous ends	−	A, L
Eubacterium alactolyticum	OA	Slow	Smooth	−	Diffuse	Thin rods, V-forms, cross-stick arrangements	−	A, B, C
E. lentum	OA	Moderate	Smooth	−	Diffuse	Short coccoidal rods, diphtheroidal	V	A
E. limosum	OA	Rapid	Smooth	−	Diffuse	Plump rods, bulbous and bifid forms	V	A, B (acid products from a non-glucose-containing broth are A, IB, B, IV)
Lactobacillus catenaforme	OA	Rapid	Smooth	−	Diffuse (granular)	Short rods in chains or singly	−	A, L
Propionibacterium avidum	F	Rapid	Smooth	−	Diffuse	Diphtheroidal	V	A, P
P. acnes	OA^F	Moderate	Smooth	−	Diffuse (granular)	Diphtheroidal	+	A, P
P. granulosum	F	Rapid	Smooth	−	Diffuse	Diphtheroidal	−	A, P
P. propionicum	M or OA	Slow	Rough	−	Granular or diffuse	Branching filaments or diphtheroidal	+	A, P

+, positive reaction for 90%–100% of strains tested; −, negative reaction for 90%–100% of strains tested; superscript, reaction shown with 11%–25% of strains tested; V, variable reaction; parentheses, variable; F, facultatively anaerobic; M, microaerophilic; OA, obligately anaerobic; A, acetic acid, B, butyric acid; C, caproic acid; L, lactic acid; P, propionic acid; S, succinic acid; IB, isobutyric acid; IC, isocaproic acid.
Modified from Dowell VR: Clinical Veterinary Anaerobic Bacteriology. DHEW Publication, pp. 1–25. Atlanta, Center for Disease Control, 1977, and adapted from the following references: Allen SD, Gram-positive, nonspore-forming anaerobic bacilli. In Lennette EH, Balows A, Hausler WJ Jr, Shadomy EJ (eds): Manual of Clinical Microbiology, 4th ed, pp 461–472. Washington DC, American Society for Microbiology, 1985; Jones D, Collins MD: Irregular, nonsporing gram-positive rods. In Sneath PHA, Mair NS, Sharpe MG, Holt JG (eds): Bergey's Manual of Systematic Bacteriology, pp 1261–1434. Baltimore, Williams & Wilkins, 1986.

TABLE 14-22
REACTIONS OF GRAM-POSITIVE, NON–SPORE-FORMING BACILLI ON CDC DIFFERENTIAL AGAR MEDIA

SPECIES	No. of Strains Examined	Indole	Indole Derivative	Esculin Hydrolysis	H_2S	Catalase	Lecithinase	Lipase	Growth on Bile Agar	Glucose Fermentation	Starch Hydrolysis	Milk Proteolysis	DNase	Gelatin Hydrolysis	Mannitol Fermentation	Lactose Fermentation	Rhamnose Fermentation
						Presumpto 1 Plate				Presumpto 2 Plate				Presumpto 3 Plate			
Actinomyces																	
A. israelii	12	+/–	–	+	–	–	–	–	V	+	–	–/+	–/+	–	V	–/+	–/+
A. meyeri	39	–	–	–	–	–	–	–	I^{NG}	+/–	–	–	–/+	–	–	V	–
A. naeslundii	31	–	–	+/–	–	–	–	–	V	+	–	–	–	–	–/+	+/–	–
A. odontolyticus	56	–	–	V	–	–	–	–	V	+	–	–	–	–	–	V	–/+
A. pyogenes	12	–	–	–	–	–	–	–	I^{NG}	+	–	+	–/+	+/–	–	–/+	–/+
A. viscosus	25	–	–	V	–	+/–	–	–	NG^{I}	+	–	–	–	–	–	V	–
Bifidobacterium																	
B. adolescentis	8	–	–	V	–	–	–	–	E	+	–/+	–	–	–	–/+	+	–
B. bifidum	4	–	–	–	–	–	–	–	E	+	–	–	–	–	–	+	–
B. breve	4	–	–	+/–	–	–	–	–	E	+	–/+	–	–	–	V	+	–
*B. dentium**	3	–	–	–	–/+	–	–	–	E	+	V	–	–	–	+	+/–	–
B. infantis/longum	3	–	–	–	–	–	–	–	E	+	V	–	–	–	–	+	–
Eubacterium																	
E. aerofaciens	3	–	–	–/+	–	–	–	–	E	+	–	+/–	–	–	–	+	–
E. alactolyticum	4	–	–	–	–	–	–	–	I	V	–	–	–	–	–	–	–
E. brachy	2	–	–	–	–	–	–	–	NG	–	–	–	–	–	–	–	–
E. lentum	33	–	–	–	–/+	V	–	–	E^{I}	–	–	–	–	–	–	–	–
E. limosum	8	–	–	–	+	–	–	–	E	+	V	–	–	–	+	–	–
E. nodatum	3	–	–	–	–	–	–	–	NG	–	–	–	–	–	–	–	–
E. saburreum	2	V	–	V	–	–	–	–	NG	–	–	–	–	–	–	–	–
E. timidum	3	–	–	–	–	–	–	–	NG	–	–	–	–	–	–	+	–
Propionibacterium																	
P. acnes	144	+/–	–	–	–	+	–	–/+	V	+	–	+/–	–	V	–	+	–
P. avidum	5	–	–	+/–	–	+	–	+/–	E	+	–	V	–	+/–	–	V	–
P. granulosum	7	–	–	–	–	+	–	–/+	V	+	–	V	–/+	–/+	–/+	–/+	–
P. propionicum	10	–	–	–	–	–	–	–	I	V	–	–	–	–	V	V	–

+, positive reaction in >90% of strains; –, negative reaction in >90% of strains; +/–, most strains positive, occasional strain negative; –/+, most strains negative with an occasional strain positive; V, variable; E, growth equal to control without bile; E^{I}, equal growth with an occasional strain inhibited; I, growth inhibited; I^{NG}, inhibited growth with occasional strains not growing.
* Formerly called *B. eriksonii*.
Adapted from Whaley DN, Wiggs LS, Miller PH, Srivastava PU, Miller JM: Use of Presumpto plates to identify anaerobic bacteria. J Clin Microbiol 33:1196–1202, 1995, and previous editions of this book.

terium pyogenes), *Propionibacterium propionicum*, and *Bifidobacterium dentium* (includes those formerly called *B. eriksonii*—in part).[4,183] These bacteria are part of the normal flora of the mouth, and many of them can be found in the genitourinary tract. *A. israelii* is the most common species in clinical infections. However, actinomycosis (with lesions in tissue) is currently rare. In gram-stained smears prepared from lesions, one may observe characteristic sulfur granules, which are granular microcolonies of the organism surrounded by purulent exudate. The cells of *A. israelii* are gram-positive rods, usually 1 μm in diameter, but they are extremely variable in length. The cells may be short diphtheroid rods, club-shaped, branched, or unbranched filaments (see Color Plate 14-2). Rough colonies composed of branched rods or filaments usually develop slowly on blood agar. Young colonies (2 to 3 days old), when viewed with the dissecting microscope, appear as thin, radiating filaments, known as spider colonies. When the colonies are about 7 to 14 days old, they are often raised, heaped-up, white, opaque, and glistening; have irregular or lobate margins; and are called molar tooth colonies (see Color Plate 14-2). However, smooth strains (about one-third of *A. israelii*) produce colonies more rapidly than rough strains. Smooth strains may produce 1- to 2-mm, circular, slightly raised white, opaque, smooth, glistening colonies after only 2 to 3 days of incubation. *A. naeslundii* may also produce smooth or rough colonies. Colonies of *A. viscosus* are most often 0.5 to 2 mm in diameter, entire, convex, grayish, and translucent. *A. odontolyticus* colonies may develop a red color on blood agar after 7 to 14 days of anaerobic incubation, or after the plates have been left out in room air at ambient temperature for several days. The cellular and colony characteristics of *P. propionicum* are similar to those of the other actinomyces.[4,183]

Besides morphology, colony characteristics, and metabolic products, characteristics useful for identification of the actinomycetes include their relation to oxygen, appearance, and rapidity of growth in enriched thioglycolate medium; indole production, esculin and gelatin hydrolysis, and fermentation of certain carbohydrates.

In addition, fluorescent antibody procedures have been used for many years by reference laboratories of the CDC, by some state health department laboratories, and by others for serologic identification and typing of *Actinomyces*, *Bifidobacterium*, and *Propionibacterium*. Although additional species of *Actinomyces* and other genera of anaerobic gram-positive rods have been described since the fourth edition of this book was published, the clincial significance of most of these remains unclear (see Table 14-12). For further detailed descriptions of these gram-positive anaerobic bacteria, the reader is urged to see additional references.[42,70,71,77,85,98,125,170,183,187,223,224]

Bifidobacterium dentium now includes those formerly called *A. eriksonii* and later *B. eriksonii*. It is part of the normal microflora of the mouth and gastrointestinal tract, and has been found in polymicrobial infections of the lower respiratory tract. The morphology of *B. dentium* is somewhat similar to that of *Actino-* *myces*, but it differs in not producing branched filaments in thioglycolate medium. Gram-stained smears prepared from solid media or broth cultures show gram-positive diphtheroidal forms that are much more variable in size and shape than *P. acnes*. Cells vary from coccoid forms to long, often curved forms, with characteristic swollen ends, or bifid forms that are regularly produced by *B. dentium*. None of the other *Bifidobacterium* spp. are known to be pathogenic for humans.[4]

The genus *Lactobacillus* is described elsewhere (see Chap. 13).

IDENTIFICATION OF *CLOSTRIDIUM* SPECIES

The anaerobic gram-positive, spore-forming bacilli encountered in human clinical materials are members of the genus *Clostridium*. In 1994, Collins and associates,[40] on the basis of 16S rRNA gene sequences determined by PCR direct sequencing, found that the genus *Clostridium* is extremely heterogeneous. Thus, they named five new genera of spore-forming rods.[40] Included were the following: *Caloramator*, *Filifactor*, *Moorella*, *Oxobacter*, and *Oxalophagus* species (see Table 14-12). In addition, 11 new species combinations were proposed. Fortunately, none of these new generic and species designations appear to be relevant to infectious diseases of humans. Nonetheless, clinical microbiologists should be aware that changes in the taxonomic classification and nomenclature of the genus *Clostridium* could occur in the future.

Currently, species of *Clostridium* encountered clinically vary in their relations to oxygen and in their anabolic and catabolic physiologic activities. Certain clostridia, for example *C. haemolyticum* and *C. novyi* type B, are among the strictest of obligate anaerobes. At the other end of the spectrum, *C. histolyticum*, *C. tertium*, and *C. carnis* are aerotolerant, and form colonies on anaerobe blood agar plates incubated in a candle jar or in a 5% to 10% CO_2 incubator. In the clinical laboratory the problem sometimes arises of determining whether an isolate is an aerotolerant *Clostridium* or a facultatively anaerobic *Bacillus*. Aerotolerant clostridia rarely form spores when grown aerobically and are catalase-negative, whereas species of the genus *Bacillus* rarely form spores when grown under anaerobic conditions, and they produce catalase.[186]

Although the clostridia are considered gram-positive, many are gram-negative by the time smears of growing cultures are prepared. For example, *C. ramosum* and *C. clostridioforme* are usually gram-negative.

The demonstration of spores is frequently difficult with some species: for example, *C. perfringens*, *C. ramosum*, and *C. clostridioforme*. Demonstration of spore production is not necessary for identifying these three species. They have several other distinctive properties. To demonstrate spores, gram-stained preparations are usually sufficient; special spore stains generally offer no particular advantage. However, examination of wet-mounts with a phase contrast microscope is useful when spores are mature and refractile. In our experience, the best way to demonstrate production of spores is to inoculate a cooked-meat agar slant and incubate anaerobically for 5 to 7 days at 30°C. The cells from the growth on the slant are then observed in a gram-stained preparation or in a wet mount by phase contrast microscopy. In addition, a heat-shock or alcohol spore selection technique may be used.[109] Identifying characteristics for most of the clostridia encountered in human infections are given in Tables 14-23 through 14-25.

Some of the key reactions for identifying *C. perfringens* are illustrated in Color Plate 14-3. The double zone of hemolysis on blood agar, production of lecithinase on egg-yolk agar, and stormy fermentation of litmus milk (or proteolysis of milk agar) are characteristic of this species. The cells of *C. perfringens* are usually 0.8 to 1.5 μm in diameter by 2 to 4 μm long and have blunt ends. They are often described as boxcar-shaped. However, cells examined during early growth in broth culture tend to be short and coccoid, whereas older cultures contain longer cells that may be almost filamentous. After overnight incubation on blood agar, colonies are usually 1 to 3 mm in diameter, but may reach a diameter of 4 to 15 mm after prolonged incubation. Colonies are usually flat, somewhat rhizoid, and raised centrally. Some colonies tend to spread, but they do not swarm. *C. perfringens* is nonmotile.

C. perfringens is by far the most commonly isolated species of *Clostridium* from human sources. However, clostridia account for only about 10% to 12% of the anaerobic bacteria isolated from properly selected and collected clinical specimens. *C. perfringens* and other clostridia are commonly found among the normal flora of the gastrointestinal tract. They also transiently inhabit the skin. Many clostridia isolated from clinical specimens, even blood cultures, are accidental contaminants and may have no clinical significance. In other circumstances, the presence of certain clostridia in a lesion can have dire consequences to the host. Thus, the pathogenic properties of clostridia may be manifested only in special circumstances, and communication between the microbiologist and the attending physician is usually necessary to assess the significance of a given isolate. *C. perfringens* is also encountered in myonecrosis (gas gangrene), gangrenous cholecystitis, septicemia, and intravascular hemolysis following abortion and anaerobic pleuropulmonary infections; it is a major cause of food poisoning in the United States, and is also one cause of antibiotic-associated diarrhea, and a major worldwide cause of necrotizing enterocolitis, involving children and adults.[5,30,72,141,153,161,186,213]

HISTOTOXIC CLOSTRIDIA INVOLVED IN CLOSTRIDIAL MYONECROSIS OR GAS GANGRENE

The clostridia most often involved in gas gangrene are *C. perfringens* (80%), *C. novyi* (40%), and *C. septicum* (20%), followed occasionally by *C. histolyticum* and *C. sordellii*.[186] Clostridial myonecrosis (gas gangrene) is a clinical entity that involves rapid invasion and liquefactive necrosis of muscle, with gas formation and clinical signs of toxicity. Nonetheless, close liaison between the microbiology laboratory and clinical staff is often an urgent necessity for confirmation of the clinical diagnosis. Gram-stained smears of aspirated mate-

rial from myonecrosis reveal a necrotic background with a lack of inflammatory cells and presence of morphologic forms resembling *C. perfringens* or other clostridia. In other conditions, such as simple wound infection or anaerobic cellulitis (in which there may also be gas in tissue), muscle cell outlines or presence of granulocytes and mixed morphologic forms of bacteria in gram-stained smears of lesions would be evidence against clostridial myonecrosis. For further details on the histotoxic clostridia, several references are available.[5,25,61,186,220]

Intestinal Diseases Involving *C. perfringens*. *C. perfringens*, ranking behind *Salmonella* spp. and *Staphylococcus aureus*, has been the third most common etiologic agent of foodborne disease in the United States for many years.[38] Most of the *C. perfringens* foodborne outbreaks in the United States have involved strains of toxin type A.[5,38] *C. perfringens* food poisoning results from eating contaminated beef, turkey, chicken, pork, gravy, and other foods containing large numbers of the organism. Patients develop crampy abdominal pain, usually within 7 to 15 hours after eating the suspected food. In most cases, there is diarrhea, with foamy, "foul-smelling" stools, but there is little vomiting or fever. Illness occurs after about 10^8 viable vegetative *C. perfringens* cells reach the small intestine and undergo sporulation. A potent enterotoxin (a protein of about 34,000 Da), produced in the gut while the spores are being formed, causes the diarrhea. The illness tends to be mild and self-limited, and patients usually recover in 2 to 3 days from the onset. Quantitative anaerobic cultures on selective plating media, demonstrating at least 10^5 *C. perfringens* organisms in the epidemiologically implicated food, and spore counts showing 10^6 or more *C. perfringens* spores per gram of feces collected within 24 hours of onset of symptoms, are done to confirm the diagnosis in an outbreak investigation. In addition, serotyping of the isolates is performed to demonstrate that the same serotype of *C. perfringens* is present in epidemiologically implicated food and in the feces of ill persons, but not in controls. Serologic typing must be performed in established laboratories that are satisfactorily equipped to perform this service (such as at the CDC).[5,48,179]

A kit for the detection of *C. perfringens* enterotoxin has been marketed by Oxoid (Oxoid Limited, Wade Road, Basingstoke, Hampshire, RG240PN, England). The supernatant of a saline homogenate of feces is tested for enterotoxin using a reversed passive latex agglutination procedure, according to directions provided by the manufacturer. Data are lacking on the sensitivity, specificity, and accuracy of the test.

Necrotizing bowel disease (NBD), caused by *C. perfringens*, is much more serious than the foodborne illness just described. NBD is characterized by the sudden onset of abdominal cramps and abdominal distention, vomiting, bloody diarrhea, and shock that is related to fluid and electrolyte problems, and acute inflammation and focal or widespread necrosis of the intestinal mucosa. The disease, recognized in postwar Germany, called *Darmbrand* (meaning "fire bowels")

TABLE 14-23

SOME KEY CHARACTERISTICS OF *CLOSTRIDIUM* SPECIES ASSOCIATED WITH DISEASE IN HUMANS

SPECIES*	AEROTOLERANT	DOUBLE ZONE HEMOLYSIS	TERMINAL SPORES	MOTILITY	VOLATILE METABOLIC PRODUCTS (GLC) IN PYG, 48 H, 35°C	OTHER
C. bifermentans	–	–	–	+	A, IC, (P), (IB), (B), (IV)	Urease-negative; indole-positive
C. botulinum[†]	–	–	–	+	A, (P), (IB), B, IV, (V), (IC)	Lipase-positive
C. butyricum	–	–	–	+	A, B	Very saccharolytic
C. difficile	–	–	–	+	A, IB, B, IV, IC	
C. innocuum	–	–	+	–	A, B	Lactose- and maltose-negative
C. limosum	–	–	–	+	A	Asaccharolytic; gelatin-positive
C. novyi type A	–	–	–	+	A, P, B	Rarely encountered in clinical species
C. perfringens	–	+	–	–	A, B, (P)	Spores seldom observed
C. ramosum	–	–	+	–	A	Spores seldom observed; frequently gram-negative
C. septicum	–	–	–	+	A, B	Saccharolytic, but sucrose-negative
C. sordellii	–	–	–	+	A, IC, (P), (IB), (IV)	Urease-positive; indole-positive
C. sporogenes[†]	–	–	–	+	A, P, IB, B, IB, V, IC	Lipase-positive
C. subterminale	–	–	–	+	A, IB, B, IV, (P)	Asaccharolytic; gelatin-positive
C. tetani	–	–	+	+	A, (P), B	May appear gram-negative
C. tertium	+	–	+	+	A, B	No spores under aerobic conditions

+, positive reaction for 90%–100% of strains tested; –, negative reaction for 90%–100% of strains tested; V, variable reaction; parentheses, variable; A, acetic acid; P, propionic acid; IB, isobutyric acid; IV, isovaleric acid; V, valeric acid; IC, isocaproic acid.

* For additional information on definitive identification of these species and other clostridia that may be encountered in clinical specimens, see Allen SD, Baron EJ. *Clostridium.* In Balows A, Hausler WJ Jr, Herrmann K Jr, et al. (eds): Manual of Clinical Microbiology, 5th ed, p. 505. Washington DC, American Society for Microbiology, 1991; Onderdonk AB, Allen SD. *Clostridium.* In Murray PR, Baron EJ, Pfaller MA, Tenover FC, Yolken RH (eds): Manual of Clinical Microbiology, 6th ed, pp. 574–586. Washington DC, ASM Press, 1995; Dowell VR Jr, Lombard GL. Laboratory Methods in Anaerobic Bacteriology, DHEW Publication No. (CDC) 78-8772. Atlanta, Centers for Disease Control, 1977; Holdeman LV, Cato EP, Moore WEC. Anaerobe Laboratory Manual. Blacksburg, Virginia, Polytechnic Institute and State University, 1977; Cato EP, George WL, Finegold SM. Genus *Clostridium* Prazmowski 1880, 23[AL]. In Sneath PHA, Mair NS, Sharpe ME, Holt GH (eds): Bergey's Manual of Systematic Bacteriology, vol. 2, pp. 1141–1200. Baltimore, Williams & Wilkins, 1986. Summanen P, Baron EJ, Citron DM, et al: Wadsworth Anaerobic Bacteriology Manual, 5th ed. Belmont, Star Publishing, 1993.

[†] Toxin neutralization tests required for definitive identification.

TABLE 14-24 REACTIONS OF *CLOSTRIDIUM* SPECIES ON CDC DIFFERENTIAL AGAR MEDIA

SPECIES	NO. OF STRAINS EXAMINED	PRESUMPTO 1 PLATE								PRESUMPTO 2 PLATE				PRESUMPTO 3 PLATE			
		INDOLE	INDOLE DERIVATIVE	ESCULIN HYDROLYSIS	H₂S	CATALASE	LECITHINASE	LIPASE	GROWTH ON BILE AGAR	GLUCOSE FERMENTATION	STARCH HYDROLYSIS	MILK PROTEOLYSIS	DNASE	GELATIN HYDROLYSIS	MANNITOL FERMENTATION	LACTOSE FERMENTATION	RHAMNOSE FERMENTATION
C. baratii	8	−	−	+	−	−	+	−	E	+	V	V	−	−	−	+/−	−
C. bifermentans	16	+	−	+	−	−	+	−	E	+	−	+/−	+	+	−	−	−
C. butyricum	31	−	−	+	−	−	−	−	I	+	+/−	−	−	−	−	+	−
C. cadaveris	6	+/−	−/+	−	V	−	−	−	E^NG	+	+/−	+/−	+	−/+	−	−	V
C. clostridioforme	18	−/+	−	V	−	−	−	−	V	+/−	−	−	−/+	−	−	+/−	−
C. difficile	490	−	−	+	−	−	−	−	E	+	−	−	−	−	+	−	−
C. histolyticum	5	−	−	−	−	−	−	−	V	−	−	+	+	+/−	−	−	−
C. innocuum	18	−	−	+	−	−	−	−	E	+	−	−	−	−	+/−	−	−
C. limosum	2	−	−	−	−	−	−	−	NG	V	V	V	V	−	−	−	−
C. malenominatum	7	+	−	−	V	−	−	−	I^E	−	−	−	−/+	−	−	−	−
C. paraputrificum	13	−	−	+	−	−	−	−	E	+	−/+	−	−	+	−	+	−
C. perfringens	79	−	−	V	−/+	−	+	−	E	+	+/−	V	+	+	−	+	−
C. ramosum	16	−	−	+	−	−	−	−	E	+	−	−	−	−	V	+	V
C. septicum	56	−	−	+/−	−	−	−	−	E	+	−	−	+	+/−	−	+/−	−
C. sordellii	32	+	−	−	V	−	+/−	−	E	+	−	+	−	+	−	−	−
C. sphenoides	8	+/−	−	V	−	−	−	−	V	+	−	−	V	−	V	V	V
C. sporogenes	52	−	+	+	−	−	−/+	+	E	+	−	+	−/+	+	−	−	−
C. subterminale	7	−	−	−	V	−	−	−	V	−	−/+	V	−/+	+/−	−	−	−
C. symbosium	2	−	−	−	−	−	−	−	V	V	−	−	−	−	V	+	−
C. tertium	44	−	−	+	−	−	−	−	E	+	V	−	+/−	−	+	+	−
C. tetani	27	+/−	−	−	V	−	−	−/+	E^I	−	−	V	V	+	−	−	−

+, positive reaction in >90% of strains; −, negative reaction in >90% of strains; +/−, most strains positive, occasional strain negative; −/+, most strains negative, occasional strain positive; V, variable; E, growth equal to control without bile; E^I, equal growth with occasional strain inhibited; E^NG, equal growth with occasional strains not growing; NG, no growth; I^E, most strains inhibited with equal growth for occasional strains.

Adapted from Whaley DN, Wiggs LS, Miller PH, Srivastava PU, Miller JM: Use of Presumpto plates to identify anaerobic bacteria. J Clin Microbiol 33:1196–1202, 1995, and previous editions of this book.

TABLE 14-25
CHARACTERISTICS THAT ARE ESPECIALLY USEFUL FOR IDENTIFYING SOME *CLOSTRIDIUM* SPECIES

CHARACTERISTIC	SPECIES
Aerotolerant	*C. histolyticum, C. tertium, C. carnis*
Nonmotile	*C. innocuum, C. perfringens, C. ramosum*
Terminal spores	*C. baratii, C. cadaveris, C. innocuum, C. ramosum, C. tertium, C. tetani*
Lecithinase produced on egg-yolk agar	*C. bifermentans, C. limosum, C. novyi, C. perfringens, C. sordellii, C. subterminale, C. barati, C. haemolyticum*
Lipase produced on egg-yolk agar	*C. botulinum, C. novyi* type A, *C. sporogenes*
Asaccharolytic and proteolytic (i.e., gelatin-positive)	*C. histolyticum, C. limosum, C. subterminale, C. tetani, C. malenominatum* (weak to negative gelatin)
Urease-positive	*C. sordellii* (*C. bifermentans*, which it resembles, is urease-negative)
Do not hydrolyze gelatin	*C. butyricum, C. clostridioforme, C. malenominatum, C. paraputrificum, C. baratii, C. ramosum*
Mannitol fermented	*C. difficile, C. innocuum, C. ramosum, C. sphenoides, C. symbiosum, C. tertium*
Rhamnose fermented	*C. clostridioforme, C. ramosum, C. sporogenes*
Saccharolytic and proteolytic	*C. bifermentans, C. botulinum, C. cadaveri, C. difficile, C. haemolyticum, C. novyi, C. perfringens, C. putrificum, C. septicum, C. sordellii, C. sporogenes*
Saccharolytic and nonproteolytic	*C. baratii, C. beiierinckii, C. butyricum, C. clostridioforme, C. glycolicum, C. innocuum, C. paraputrificum, C. ramosum, C. tertium*

was a severe form of necrotizing enterocolitis with an associated mortality of approximately 40%. "Pig bel," a form of necrotizing enteritis seen mainly in children in the highlands of Papua New Guinea, has been associated with mortality of about 30% to 60%.[141,180,210] Sporadic cases of *C. perfringens* NBD have been reported from many countries around the world, including Europe and the United States.[96] Factors believed to be important predisposing conditions to NBD include the consumption of excessive amounts of rich food or foods containing trypsin inhibitors (e.g., sweet potatoes and peanuts) by malnourished individuals. *C. perfringens* type C has been implicated in both Darmbrand and the pig bel syndrome and in NBD in Western countries during recent times.[172] It has been suggested that *C. perfringens* type A also plays a role in some cases of NBD, particularly in Western countries.[203] In Papua New Guinea, the native highlanders typically develop the disease after consuming large amounts of poorly cooked pork at a pig feast. A heavy inoculum of *C. perfringens* type C is ingested with the meal, the organism proliferates in the small intestine, where it produces β-toxin. Low levels of pancreatic proteolytic enzymes, associated with the usual low protein diet of the highlanders, but a diet rich in sweet potatoes, may permit the β-toxin of *C. perfringens* to act on the small intestine without the β-toxin being destroyed by pancreatic trypsin or other proteases. There is both a clinical and

pathologic spectrum in terms of the severity of NBD. Some patients may survive with supportive care and decompression of the bowel; others may require resection of the involved intestinal segment; still others are inoperable and die with extensive gangrenous necrosis of the small and large bowel. The differential diagnosis includes pseudomembranous colitis (whether or not associated with *C. difficile*), acute shigellosis, foodborne illness caused by various etiologic agents (including *Escherichia coli, Campylobacter jejuni*, and others), acute ulcerative colitis, and obstruction of the bowel (by adhesions, volvulus, or other). In suspected cases, efforts to culture *C. perfringens* type A and C (e.g., blood cultures, peritoneal cultures if there is peritonitis, and intestinal contents of surgical removal or necropsy specimens) should be made. A reference laboratory (such as the CDC), where typing of isolates can be accomplished, should be consulted. Paired sera should be obtained for serologic studies (e.g., to attempt to show a rise in serum antibody titer to β-toxin). A rise in antibody titer would be consistent with either type B or type C *C. perfringens* disease.[210]

MISCELLANEOUS CLOSTRIDIA IN OTHER CLINICAL SETTINGS

Clostridium ramosum. *C. ramosum* has in the past been called *Eubacterium filamentosum, Catenabacterium filamentosum, Actinomyces ramosus, Fusiformis ramosus,*

Ramibacterium ramosus, and other names.[186] In 1971, it was found to produce terminal spores and was placed in the genus *Clostridium*.[37] It is a prominent member of the large-bowel flora, and is the second most common *Clostridium* isolated from properly collected clinical specimens. It is particularly common in intra-abdominal infections following trauma. *C. ramosum* is especially important clinically because of its resistance to penicillin G, clindamycin, and other antibiotics (see Table 14-4). Although it has been found in severe infections from virtually all body sites, *C. ramosum* can easily be misidentified or overlooked, because it usually stains as a gram-negative rod, and its terminal spores are frequently hard to demonstrate.

Cells of *C. ramosum* are usually less than 0.6 μm in diameter by 2 to 5 μm long but are extremely pleomorphic, sometimes producing short chains or long filaments. On blood agar, colonies are often 1 to 2 mm in diameter, usually nonhemolytic, slightly irregular or circular, entire, low convex, and translucent. Isolates of *C. ramosum* are characteristically resistant to rifampin by the 15-μg disk method discussed earlier, but are inhibited by the 2-U penicillin disk and the 1-mg kanamycin disk (similar to *F. mortiferum* and *F. varium*). *C. ramosum* is indole-negative (*F. mortiferum* and *F. varium* are indole-positive); shows enhanced growth on bile agar; hydrolyzes esculin; and is negative for catalase, lipase, and lecithinase. It is among the few clostridia that ferment mannitol (see Table 14-25). Acetic, lactic, and succinic acids are the major metabolic products.

Although *C. septicum* is not nearly as common as *C. perfringens* and *C. ramosum*, it is especially important to recognize in the clinical laboratory. *C. septicum* is usually isolated from serious, often fatal infections. *C. septicum* bacteremia, for unknown reasons, is often associated with underlying malignancy, particularly carcinoma of the colon or cecum, carcinoma of the breast, and hematologic malignancies (e.g., leukemia–lymphoma).[110] The cells are usually about 0.6 μm wide, and 3 to 6 μm long. It tends to be pleomorphic, sometimes producing long, thin filaments. Chain formation is common, as are intensely staining citron (lemon-shaped) forms. Spores are oval and subterminal, and distend the organism. After 48 hours of incubation on blood agar, colonies are 2 to 5 mm in diameter, surrounded by a 1- to 4-mm zone of complete hemolysis; they are flat, slightly raised, gray, glistening, and semitranslucent, and have markedly irregular to rhizoid margins, often surrounded by a zone of swarming. Extremely motile strains may swarm across a wide area of the plate. Stiff blood agar, which contains 4% to 6% instead of the usual 1.5% agar, is sometimes used in plating media to minimize swarming. Some key characteristics of *C. septicum* are that it hydrolyzes gelatin; does not produce indole, lipase, or lecithinase; and ferments lactose, but not mannitol, rhamnose, or sucrose. Acetic and butyric acids are the major metabolic products.

CLOSTRIDIUM DIFFICILE–ASSOCIATED INTESTINAL DISEASE

C. difficile, first isolated in 1935,[78] was believed to be nonpathogenic for humans until the late 1970s, when it was implicated as a causative agent in antibiotic-associated diarrhea (AAD) and pseudomembranous colitis (PMC).[22,24,26,59] Benign, self-limited diarrhea frequently develops in hospitalized patients who are being treated with antibiotics. The mild diarrhea often subsides following discontinuation of the antibiotic, and the cause of the diarrhea is not determined. In other patients, the intestinal symptoms may be more severe, and the diarrhea may persist. These patients may have antibiotic-associated colitis (AAC) or life-threatening PMC.[22,137] *C. difficile* probably causes most cases of PMC.[121,138] However, as reviewed by Fekety, PMC is infrequently caused by *Staphylococcus aureus* or by *C. perfringens*.[59] Also, as reviewed elsewhere, Borriello and associates have seen an association between enterotoxigenic *C. perfringens* and antibiotic-associated diarrhea in the United Kingdom.[30,31] In addition to PMC, *C. difficile* has been estimated to cause some "60% to 75% of antibiotic-associated cases of colitis, and 11% to 33% of cases of AAD."[138] Whether *C. perfringens* causes AAD in the United States with any frequency has not been established. The severity of illness as well as pathologic findings are highly variable, depending on whether the patient has PMC, AAC, AAD without anatomic evidence of colitis, or is simply colonized with *C. difficile* (or is an asymptomatic carrier). The pathologic findings in PMC and AAC have been adequately reviewed elsewhere.[163]

Factors that may be involved in *C. difficile*–associated disease include 1) toxin A (also termed D-1),[19] first described by Taylor and colleagues,[199] which is an enterotoxin capable of producing fluid accumulation in rabbit ligated ileal loop assays; 2) toxin B (also called D-2),[19] which is a potent cytotoxin capable of producing cytopathogenic effects in several tissue culture cell lines; and 3) a "motility-altering factor," which stimulates smooth-muscle contractions of intestine and is distinct from toxins A and B.[19,101,114,199] Toxin A is also cytotoxic in certain cell lines, but is not as cytotoxic as toxin B in the cell lines used for over a decade for toxin B testing.[126,129] Several reviews of *C. difficile* and its toxins are recommended.[24,26,72,81,126]

C. difficile is ubiquitous in nature and has been isolated from soil, water, intestinal contents of various animals, the vagina and urethra of humans, and feces of many healthy infants, but from the stools of only about 3% of healthy adult volunteers. However, the organism is more prevalent in the feces of some hospitalized adults who do not have diarrhea or colitis. It has been found in the feces of about 13% to 30% of hospitalized adults, who were colonized, but had no evidence of disease caused by *C. difficile* or of antecedent antibiotic treatment. However, *C. difficile* is also frequently implicated as the causative agent of hospital-acquired diarrhea and colitis.[73,137,202] Although *C. difficile* is commonly found in the feces of many healthy infants, some infants with severe and protracted diarrhea, associated with antecedent antibiotic therapy, have had pseudomembranous colitis and at the same time, *C. difficile* cytotoxin present in their feces without any other putative etiologic agent. These patients have often responded clinically to oral vancomycin treatment (Schaeffer J, personal communication, 1986).

Antimicrobial agents implicated in *C. difficile*-associated gastrointestinal illness have included numerous aminoglycosides, penicillins, cephalosporins, second- and third-generation β-lactam compounds, clindamycin, erythromycin, lincomycin, metronidazole, rifampin, trimethoprim–sulfamethoxazole, and amphotericin B.[24,72,202]

In addition, *C. difficile* has been involved in the following clinical settings without an association with antimicrobial therapy: 1) pseudomembranous colitis; 2) diarrhea associated with methotrexate treatment and other anticancer chemotherapeutic agents; 3) relapses of nonspecific inflammatory bowel disease (e.g., Crohn's disease or ulcerative colitis); 4) obstruction or strangulation of the bowel; and 5) in a few cases of sudden infant death syndrome.[16] However, the role of *C. difficile* in these conditions, if any, has not been clarified. For more information on the clinical findings and clinical diagnosis of AAD, AAC, and PMC, the reader is referred to other sources.[24,59,72,138]

Collection and Transport of Specimens Containing *C. difficile*.

Ordinarily, passed liquid or semisolid, unformed fecal specimens (about 5 to 50 g or 5 to 50 mL, if liquid) are the preferred specimens for laboratory diagnosis. Swab specimens, because of the small volume obtained, are inadequate. Formed stool specimens are inappropriate unless an epidemiologic study of stool carriage is being conducted. Other suitable specimens include biopsy material or lumen contents obtained by colonoscopy and involved bowel (surgical removal; autopsy). However, lumen contents or biopsy material from colonoscopic procedures may excessively dilute the sample, or the quantity obtained by biopsy may be insufficient for the laboratory work required. Leakproof plastic containers should be used for transport of specimens. If specimens are to be processed by the laboratory on the same day as collected, transportation at room temperature will suffice. If a specimen arrives late in the day and cannot be processed until the following day, it can be held in the refrigerator without demonstrable loss of cytotoxic activity. Optimally, specimens should not remain at room temperature longer than 2 hours before either being processed or refrigerated. However, for shipment of specimens to a reference laboratory for a toxin assay, we recommend they be shipped on dry ice. On the other hand, an anaerobic transport container (transported at 25°C) should be used for specimens to be processed for isolation and identification of *C. difficile*. Specimens to be processed for the *C. difficile* latex agglutination test (Culturette Brand CDT *C. difficile* test; Becton Dickinson Microbiology Systems, Sparks MD) should not be frozen, because the antigen detected is unstable on freezing.

Laboratory Diagnosis of *C. difficile*.

As discussed in the direct examination section of this chapter, diagnostic testing in cases of suspected *C. difficile*–associated disease can be accomplished in the laboratory by either demonstrating the cytotoxin, isolation and identification of toxin-producing *C. difficile* from stool specimens, by performing a latex agglutination test or an EIA for the glutamate dehydrogenase of *C. difficile*, by an EIA test for the enterotoxin or cytotoxin produced by the organism in feces, or by a combination of methods. A brief description of a practical procedure for detection of the cytotoxin of *C. difficile* is outlined in Box 14-14.

C. difficile can be isolated by the use of a spore selection technique (i.e., heat shock or alcohol spore selection procedures) and by use of selective plating media, such as phenylethyl alcohol (PEA) blood agar (Carr-Scarborough Microbiologicals, Stone Mountain GA), or cycloserine–cefoxitin, egg yolk, fructose agar (CCFA) plus nonselective CDC-anaerobe blood agar.[5,109,133] Detailed descriptions of the alcohol and heat treatment spore selection procedures are given elsewhere.[5,109,158] If either of these procedures is used, the alcohol or heat-treated sample is inoculated onto CDC-anaerobe blood agar (AnBAP) (or on egg yolk agar) after the treatment. Following 48 hours of incubation anaerobically, colonies of *C. difficile* on AnBAP are nonhemolytic,

---

BOX 14-14. ASSAY FOR TOXIN IN FECES BY TISSUE CULTURE CYTOTOXICITY PROCEDURE[1]

1. Centrifuge liquid stool or extract of formed stool (2000 *g* for 20 minutes or 10,000 *g* for 10 minutes).

2. Filter through 0.45-μm membrane filter.

3. Add 0.1 mL of cell-free supernatant plus 0.1 mL buffered gelatin diluent (pH 7.0 to 7.2) or PBS to a tissue culture tube. Commercially available human diploid lung fibroblasts (WI-38 cells) are convenient to use.

4. Observe the tissue culture cells for cytotoxicity at 4, 24, and 48 hours (most are positive at 24 hours).

5. For the antitoxin neutralization test, add 0.1 mL of *C. difficile* antitoxin (TechLab, Blacksburg VA) to 0.1 mL cell-free supernatant and carry out steps 1 and 4. Rounding of WI-38 cells (so-called actinomorphic change) or other cytopathic effects should not be seen if toxin that is present in the stool is neutralized.

6. The toxin titer is determined using serial twofold or tenfold dilutions of the filtered fecal sample in buffered gelatin diluent (pH 7.0 to 7.2) or PBS. Correlation between the toxin titers and severity of illness is very crude.

---

[1] Commercial kits for performing *C. difficile* cytotoxin neutralization assays are available from at least two manufacturers (Bartels Diagnostics; Bio-Whittaker/Wampole). The kits can be purchased complete with human foreskin fibroblasts in microbroth dilution trays, and they provide the necessary antitoxin and other reagents to accomplish the cytotoxin neutralization assay.

about 2 to 4 mm in diameter, grayish-translucent, slightly raised, flat, and spreading, with rhizoid margins. As seen through a dissecting microscope, the colonies show an iridescent, "speckled–opalescent" appearance. *C. difficile* is negative for lipase and lecithinase on egg yolk agar.

In addition to the spore selection procedure, a plate of PEA medium and a CCFA plate should be inoculated with untreated stool (or stool suspension prepared in buffered gelatin diluent). After 48 hours of incubation, colonies of *C. difficile* on PEA medium will be virtually identical with those on AnBAP (described earlier). The appearance of *C. difficile* colonies on CCFA medium is described in Table 14-6. Recently, Marler and colleagues found major differences in the performance of CCFA medium that had been prepared by three different manufacturers.[133] The CCFA prepared by Carr-Scarborough Microbiologicals, (Stone Mountain GA) was quite satisfactory and can be recommended. In addition, there was no significant difference between the alcohol spore selection procedure and CCFA prepared by Carr-Scarborough in terms of recovery of *C. difficile* from fresh fecal specimens.[133] Bartley and Dowell evaluated additional selective media formulations for the primary isolation of *C. difficile*.[27]

Identification of *C. difficile* is described in several manuals.[5,22,48,158,161,195] In addition to the colony characteristics already described, there is a distinctive odor. The gram-positive to gram-variable rods have subterminal spores and, in early broth culture, are motile. Metabolic product analysis reveals acetic, propionic, isobutyric, butyric, isovaleric, valeric, and isocaproic acids (see Table 14-23). Esculin and gelatin are hydrolyzed. Indole, nitrate, and urease are negative. Most strains ferment glucose, mannitol, and mannose. Salicin and xylose are variable (see Tables 14-24 and 14-25).

BOTULISM

Botulism is a life-threatening neuroparalytic disease caused by antigenically distinct, heat-labile, protein toxins of *C. botulinum*.[47,80,185] Although seven toxin types (A, B, C, D, E, F, and G) are produced by different strains of *C. botulinum*, most cases of botulism in humans are caused by types A, B, E, and F. Of these, type F is the least common. Types C and D are associated with botulism in birds and mammals, but not humans. Type C can be subdivided into two types, C1 and C2.[80] Although type G organisms, now called *C. argentinense*, as referred to by Hatheway,[81] have been isolated from autopsy samples of a few individuals who died suddenly, it is not clear whether type G organisms cause botulism in humans. Regardless of which antigenic type (A, B, D, or E), botulinal toxin acts primarily by binding to synaptic vesicles of cholinergic nerves, thereby preventing the release of acetylcholine at the peripheral nerve endings (including neuromuscular junctions), and patients develop acute, flaccid, descending paralysis.[47] The paralysis begins with bilateral impairment of cranial nerves, resulting in paralysis of muscles of the face (including eyelids), head, and throat. The paralysis then descends symmetrically to involve the muscles of the thorax, diaphragm, and extremities. Patients may die of respiratory paralysis unless they have proper respiratory intensive care, including mechanical ventilation; death may also result from secondary pneumonia (caused by nonbotulinal organisms).[5,47,61,185]

Four different categories of botulism are recognized by the CDC. The first of these is the classic foodborne botulism, typically seen in adults, resulting from the ingestion of preformed toxin in contaminated food. The second category, wound botulism, is the rarest form; it results from production of botulinal toxin in vivo after *C. botulinum* has multiplied in an infected wound. The third category, infant botulism, is the most common; it results from in vivo multiplication of *C. botulinum* with production of the neurotoxin within the infant gut. The fourth category, "classification undetermined," is for cases of botulism in individuals who are older than 12 months in whom no food or wound source of *C. botulinum* can be implicated.[47] Home-processed foods, rather than commercially processed foods, have been involved in most of the outbreaks of foodborne botulism. The foods most often implicated have been vegetables (e.g., home-canned tomatoes, tomato juice, green beans, greens, peppers, corn, beets, spinach), fish (e.g., home-processed tuna fish, smoked salmon, fish eggs, commercially processed tuna, smoked whitefish, and others), fruits (home-canned apple butter, blackberries, and such), and miscellaneous foods (e.g., beef stew, chili, spaghetti sauce, luncheon meats, and so on).

Infant botulism was recognized as a distinct clinical entity in 1976.[16] From 1976 to 1988, 760 cases were diagnosed.[107] Infant botulism has been reported from many different states, with the greatest number of cases in California.[80] Most cases reported west of the Mississippi River have been type A; the majority of those east of it have been type B. Affected infants have ranged from 6 days to 11.7 months in age, and both sexes have been affected equally.[80] Almost all racial and ethnic groups have been affected. The infants ingest spores, but not preformed toxin (preformed toxin is ingested in foodborne botulism), from soil, household dust, honey, or another source. Within the gut, *C. botulinum* multiplies and elaborates toxin. Clinical features include constipation (usually the first sign), listlessness, difficulty in sucking and swallowing, an altered cry, hypotonia, and muscle weakness. Eventually the baby appears "floppy," loses head control, and may develop ptosis, ophthalmoplegia, flaccid facial expression, dysphagia, and other neurologic signs. Respiratory arrest or respiratory insufficiency necessitating respiratory therapy occur. A small number of infants with laboratory-confirmed infant botulism have died. Infant botulism has accounted for about 4% of cases of sudden infant death syndrome.[16]

The diagnosis of classic foodborne botulism is confirmed in reference laboratories, such as the CDC, by demonstrating botulinal toxin in serum, feces, gastric contents, or vomitus. Also, the organism may be isolated from the patient's feces.[47] The detection of botulinal toxin in epidemiologically implicated food, with or without isolating the organism, is useful for ascertaining what food was involved in the outbreak. About 15 to 20 mL of serum and 25 to 50 g of feces should be collected for shipment to the appropriate reference laboratory (as directed by the appropriate state or federal public health official who is capable of providing epidemiologic and laboratory aid in the investigation). In suspected wound botulism, serum, exudate, or swab samples from the wound should be collected, along with tissue (e.g., at autopsy), and feces should also be collected.

When infant botulism is suspected, serum (2 to 3 mL) and as much stool as possible (ideally, 25 to 50 g) should be collected in a leak-proof plastic container, and refrigerated or placed on ice for shipment. However, many, if not most, of these infants are constipated early in the illness, and stool may not be available. Therefore, the clinician must decide whether the risk of obtaining an anorectal swab specimen is clinically warranted for the laboratory to isolate *C. botulinum* from this source.

Some, but not all, state health department laboratories provide diagnostic services for botulism. With prior approval of the CDC, telephone (409)639-3753, and the local state health department laboratory, specimens may be submitted to the CDC for laboratory diagnosis. Confirmation of the clinical diagnosis of botulism requires demonstration of botulinal toxin (mouse neutralization test) in serum or feces, or of *C. botulinum* in feces.[5,47,80] Isolation and identification of the organism is by conventional cultural biochemical procedures and the toxin neutralization test. Toxin has only rarely been detected in serum of an affected infant. It is recommended that culture and toxin testing for *C. botulinum* be done only by properly equipped reference laboratories for this specialized testing. For further details, the interested reader is referred to the publications by Allen and Baron, Dowell, or Hathaway.[5,47,80]

TETANUS

Tetanus is an infectious disease, caused by *C. tetani*, that largely involves unimmunized persons in the United States—mostly of the rural South.[5] It is a dramatic illness characterized by spastic contractions of voluntary muscles and hyperreflexia, caused by a protoplasmic, heat-labile protein toxin (tetanospasmin) elaborated by *C. tetani*.[5,47,61] Tetanus shares some similarity to diphtheria, in that the infection (and the organism) remains localized (usually a minor penetrating wound), and the toxin is absorbed, producing major systemic effects. The spores of *C. tetani*, similar to those of *C. botulinum*, are widely distributed in the soil, as well as in aquatic environments. Tetanus usually results from spore contamination of puncture wounds, lacerations, or even crush injuries.[5,47,61] Fecal contamination of the umbilical cord has been the source of *C. tetani* in some cases of neonatal tetanus. Following a localized penetrating injury, there may be a deep-seated mixed infection involving anaerobes plus nonanaerobes in devitalized tissue, resulting in a low oxygen tension and low oxidation–reduction potential, thus providing favorable conditions for *C. tetani* spores to germinate and for the vegetative cells to multiply and release the tetanospasmin upon autolysis of the bacterial cells.[47] Tetanospasmin attaches to peripheral motor nerve endings, and it travels along nerves to the central nervous system (CNS). The toxin binds to gangliosides in the CNS, and blocks inhibitory impulses to the motor neurons. Patients have prolonged muscle spasms of both flexor and extensor muscles. Tetanospasmin attaches to binding sites at myoneural junctions, thus inhibiting the release of acetylcholine. This is like the attachment of botulinal toxin to myoneural junctions, except that the binding sites for tetanospasmin and for botulinal toxin are different.[47] As indicated previously, patients with tetanus have spastic muscle contractions, difficulty opening the jaw (called lockjaw, "trismus"), a characteristic smile called "risus sardonicus," and contractions of back muscles, resulting in backward arching. Patients are extremely irritable, and develop tetanic seizures (brought about by violent, painful muscle contractions following some minor stimulus, such as a noise). Diagnosis of tetanus is based largely on the clinical findings, not on laboratory studies. The antecedent wound is often minor or trivial. Direct gram-stained smears and anaerobic cultures of the wound site are often negative, failing to reveal the organism. *C. tetani* forms round, terminal spores, produces spreading or swarming growth on anaerobe blood agar, produces major amounts of acetate and butyrate, with only a minor amount of propionate, is lipase- and lecithinase-negative on egg yolk agar, and is asaccharolytic. For more information on *C. tetani*, the books by Finegold and George[69] and Smith and Williams,[186] and the review articles by Dowell[47] and Hatheway[81] are recommended.

ANTIMICROBIAL SUSCEPTIBILITY TESTING OF ANAEROBIC BACTERIA

Successful management of diseases involving anaerobic bacteria requires selection of and treatment with appropriate antimicrobial agents, often in conjunction with removal of bacteria by drainage of abscesses, elimination of foreign bodies, by debridement of necrotic tissue, and other surgical measures. It was once believed that most anaerobes had predictable antimicrobial susceptibility patterns and that accurate identification of isolates was all that was necessary for one to predict the susceptibility of individual isolates to various antibiotics. This is an oversimplification. Although some antimicrobial agents are active against almost all anaerobic bacteria (including ampicillin–sulbactam, chloramphenicol, imipenem, and ticarcillin–clavulanate), several other antimicrobial agents that might be selected for use in treatment are not nearly as predictable in their activities against selected genera and species of anaerobes. For example, the penicillins and ureidopenicillins, the second- and third-generation cephalosporins, and clindamycin may or may *not* be active against certain commonly encountered species of anaerobic gram-negative bacilli and clostridia.[215,216]

Nonetheless, it is usually necessary for the attending physician to start antimicrobial therapy empirically, before results of identification and susceptibility testing are available. Therefore, tabulated susceptibility and treatment results reported in the literature or in the local hospital, and clinical experience of the physician may, of necessity, be the basis for the initial choice of antibiotics. However, there is enough variability in the susceptibility patterns of clinically significant anaerobes that in vitro susceptibility testing of individual isolates is indicated at times to aid clinicians with the management of serious infections and those that require prolonged therapy, such as brain abscess, endocarditis, lung abscess, infections involving joints, infections involving prosthetic devices, vascular grafts, recurrent or refractory bacteremia, osteomyelitis, or when patients fail to respond to empirical therapy.[62,64,155]

Another indication for testing is the setting in which there has not been a clear-cut clinical precedent on which to base treatment decisions. In addition, clinical microbiologists experienced with anaerobe work are encouraged to investigate the activities of newly marketed or investigational antimicrobial agents on anaerobes isolated in their hospital laboratory. Also, there is a need to monitor susceptibility patterns of anaerobes at the local community and hospital levels and in multiple medical centers around the United States and in various countries around the world.[62,64,155,215,216]

Organisms to be considered for antimicrobial susceptibility testing, because of their virulence, or because they are commonly resistant to certain antimicrobial agents include species of the *Bacteroides fragilis* group, species of the pigmented *Prevotella–Porphyromonas* group, *Campylobacter* (*Bacteroides*) *gracilis*, the *Prevotella oralis* group, *Fusobacterium mortiferum*, *F. varium* and *F. necrophorum*, *Clostridium perfringens*, *C. ramosum*, *C. clostridioforme*, and nonintestinal isolates (e.g., from blood cultures) of *C. difficile*.

As illustrated in Table 14-4 in the data from a single, large midwestern medical center, there have been some striking changes in anaerobe susceptibility patterns since the last edition of this book was published.[107] At the breakpoints indicated in Table 14-4, many of the *B. fragilis* group isolates are no longer susceptible to third- generation cephalosporins (e.g., cefoperazone, cefotaxime, ceftriaxone) and penicillins, including piperacillin. Interestingly, we now find striking differences in the activities of the two second-generation cephalosporins tested against the *B. fragilis* group, with cefoxitin now more active than cefotetan. During 1988 through 1990, the activities of these compounds against species of the *B. fragilis* group were similar. Of the β-lactam–β-lactamase inhibitor combinations tested, piperacillin–tazobactam is the most active against anaerobes in general, possibly because it is not on the hospital formulary at IUMC. Other combinations, including ampicillin–sulbactam, ticarcillin–clavulanate, and amoxicillin–clavulanate, appear somewhat less active than was true during the survey performed in 1988 through 1990. We now have a few strains of the *B. fragilis* group that are resistant to imipenem. Although clindamycin was active against

86% of *B. fragilis* strains at the breakpoint tested, it was no longer active against most strains of *B. thetaiotaomicron* or *B. distasonis*.[107] In addition, we are witnessing a trend toward increased resistance to the β-lactam compounds and clindamycin among other anaerobes, including species of *Prevotella*, *Lactobacillus*, *Clostridium*, and the anaerobic cocci.

SUSCEPTIBILITY OF ANAEROBES TO VARIOUS ANTIMICROBIAL AGENTS

Table 14-4 summarizes current antimicrobial susceptibility data on anaerobes isolated from properly selected clinical specimens at IUMC. The data were obtained on fresh clinical isolates using a microdilution method with Wilkins-Chalgren broth, according to a previously described procedure,[14,100,107] which is performed according to the recommendations of the NCCLS for testing anaerobic bacteria.[155] These percentage data were tabulated to conform to the current NCCLS guidelines for minimal inhibitory concentration (MIC) breakpoints indicating susceptibility.[156]

METHODS FOR ANTIMICROBIAL SUSCEPTIBILITY TESTING OF ANAEROBES

The agar dilution and broth dilution methods for antimicrobial susceptibility testing discussed in Chapter 15 also apply in principle to the anaerobes. However, the broth disk elution and disk agar diffusion techniques should not be used for anaerobe testing, despite their convenience. Most anaerobes other than some *B. fragilis* group and *Clostridium* spp. grow too slowly for the disk diffusion procedure to work; the Bauer-Kirby interpretive charts were not designed for anaerobes, and interpretive charts based on standardized media and methods for disk-diffusion testing of anaerobes are lacking; also, there has been poor correlation between zone size measurements and the results from MIC dilution tests.

NCCLS AGAR DILUTION METHOD

In 1972, a collaborative group formed as a subcommittee of the National Committee for Clinical Laboratory Standards (NCCLS) began developing a standardized method for the antimicrobial susceptibility testing of anaerobes. In 1976, their preliminary studies were presented (as referred to previously).[107] The procedure they developed ultimately became the NCCLS reference agar dilution procedure for anaerobe susceptibility testing. It need not necessarily be used in clinical laboratories. It serves as the reference standard for evaluating the accuracy and precision of other methods that may be used. In 1990, the NCCLS subcommittee approved their recommended methods for antimicrobial susceptibility testing of anaerobes.[154] The methods include the reference agar dilution procedure, the Wadsworth agar dilution procedure, a limited agar dilution procedure, a broth microdilution procedure, and a broth dilution procedure. The more recently approved NCCLS document provides detailed descriptions of each recommended method, describes MIC breakpoints indicating susceptibility, designates control strains (*B. thetaiotaomicron* ATCC 29741, *C. perfringens* ATCC 13124, and *E. lentum* ATCC 43055), and provides acceptable ranges of MICs for control strains for the reference agar dilution method.[155]

In the NCCLS agar dilution method, desired concentrations of antimicrobics are mixed with molten Wilkins-Chalgren agar and poured into petri plates. Each plate contains one concentration of one antimicrobic. Up to 36 different bacteria can be tested on each plate by spot inoculation with a Steers replicator (or similar device). After a 48-hour incubation in an anaerobic glove box or GasPak jar (Becton Dickinson Microbiology Systems, Cockeysville MD), the MIC of each drug that inhibits growth is determined. Unfortunately, it is not always necessary or practical to test numerous organisms simultaneously in a clinical laboratory, and this approach becomes less cost-effective if only a few isolates are to be tested. Also, it is extremely difficult to test swarming clostridia with this system. The recommendations in the current NCCLS document should be followed by those wishing to use the agar dilution method.

MICROTUBE BROTH DILUTION METHOD

In the microtube dilution (MD) procedure, MICs of different antimicrobials for anaerobic bacteria are determined in microtiter trays.[14,100,155] Broth media that have been found to be satisfactory as the basal medium include brain–heart infusion broth, modified Schaedler broth, and Wilkins-Chalgren (WC) agar in which the agar has been omitted (Anaerobe Broth, MIC, Difco Laboratories, Detroit MI). All three media have performed successfully in studies in which they were used in the MD procedure and in comparison with the NCCLS reference agar dilution procedure. At IUMC

the Difco Anaerobe Broth is used. In our procedure, the commercially available medium is purchased in dehydrated form and then prepared as the basal medium broth. Broths (as prepared) containing different concentrations of antimicrobials are dispensed in 0.1-mL volumes into 96-well plastic microdilution trays by use of a semiautomated dispensing instrument (Sandy Springs Dispenser, Bellco Glass Co., Vineland NJ).

A commonly used range of antimicrobial concentrations is as follows: 0.5, 1, 2, 4, 8, 16, 32, and 64 µg/mL (eight dilutions), but this must be modified for certain drugs (e.g., ticarcillin and piperacillin, in which 128 µg/mL and 256 µg/mL are also used). Microtiter plates are sealed in plastic bags (to prevent dehydration) and frozen (−70°C) until used. Plates are thawed in room air, then inoculated with a 1:100 dilution of a turbid, actively growing (overnight) Schaedler broth culture, using a disposable plastic replicator (Dynatech Laboratories, Inc., Alexandria VA). After a 48-hour incubation anaerobically, the MIC for each drug is read (using a Dynatech view-box) as the lowest concentration of antimicrobic that completely prevented growth (clear well).[155]

The MD procedure is less cumbersome than macro broth tube dilution procedures. MD systems are commercially available from a few companies (MicroMedia Systems, Potomac MD; American Microscan, Sacramento CA), but can easily be prepared in-house. If plates are frozen at −70°C, they have a long shelf life without detectable deterioration of antimicrobics (about 4 to 6 months). The MD system has an advantage for smaller laboratories over agar dilution replica-plating procedures in that one organism is inoculated per plate, and the MD system has a relatively low cost. For a description and further details describing this and other recommended procedures, the interested reader is referred to the current NCCLS document.[155]

REFERENCES

1. ALDRIDGE KE, GELFAND M, RELLER LB, ET AL: A five-year multicenter study of the susceptibility of the *Bacteroides fragilis* group isolates to cephalosporins, cephamins, penicillins, clindamycin, and metronidazole in the United States. Diagn Microbiol Infect Dis 18:235–241, 1994

2. ALLEN SD: Identification of anaerobic bacteria: how far to go. Clin Microbiol Newslett 1:3–5, 1979

3. ALLEN SD: Systems for rapid identification of anaerobic bacteria. In Tilton RC (ed): Rapid Methods and Automation in Microbiology, pp 214–217. Washington DC, American Society for Microbiology, 1982

4. ALLEN SD: Gram-positive, nonsporeforming anaerobic bacilli. In Lennette EH, Balows A, Hausler WJ Jr, et al (eds): Manual of Clinical Microbiology, 4th ed, pp 461–472. Washington DC, American Society for Microbiology, 1985

5. ALLEN SD, BARON EJ: *Clostridium*. In Balows A, Hausler WJ Jr, Herrmann K Jr, et al (eds): Manual of Clincal Microbiology, 5th ed, pp 505. Washington DC, American Society for Microbiology, 1991

6. ALLEN SD, LOMBARD GL, ARMFIELD AY, ET AL: Development and evaluation of an improved anaerobic holding jar procedure, Abstr Ann Meet Am Soc Microbiol, Abstr C142, 1977

7. ALLEN SD, SIDERS J, MARLER L, O'BRYAN N: Rapid identification of anaerobes. In Sanna A, Morace G (eds): New Horizons in Microbiology, pp 233–240. New York, Elsevier Science Publishers, 1984

8. ALLEN SD, SIDERS JA: Unpublished data, 1991

9. ALLEN SD, SIDERS JA, GRANT Y, ET AL : Multicenter evaluation of the Meridian Immunocard for detection of *Clostridium difficile* in feces. Abstr Ann Meet Am Soc Microbiol, Abstr C144, 1993

10. ALLEN SD, SIDERS JA, JOHNSON KS, GERLACH EH: Simultaneous biochemical characterization and antimicrobial susceptibility testing of anaerobic bacteria in microdilution trays. In Tilton RC (ed): Rapid Methods and Automation in Microbiology, pp 266–270. Washington DC, American Society for Microbiology, 1982

11. ALLEN SD, SIDERS JA, MARLER LM: Isolation and examination of anaerobic bacteria. In Lennette EH, Balows A, Hausler WJ Jr, et al (eds): Manual of Clinical Microbiology, 4th ed, pp 413–443. Washington DC, American Society for Clinical Microbiology, 1985

12. ALLEN SD, SIDERS JA, MARLER LM: Current issues and problems in dealing with anaerobes in the clinical laboratory. Clin Lab Med 15:333–364, 1995

13. ALLEN SD, SIDERS JA, MCCRACKEN RA, FILL JA: Anaerobic bacteremia: a 24 year survey revealing new trends in species isolated in the '90's. Paper presented at the Anaerobe Society of the Americas Congress on Anaerobic Bacteria and Anaerobic Infections, Chicago IL, 1996

14. ALLEN SD, SIDERS JA, O'BRYAN N, ET AL: Microtube plate procedure for biochemical characterization and antimicrobial susceptibility testing of anaerobic bacteria. In Borriello SP, Hardie JM (eds): Recent Advances in Anaerobic Bacteriology, pp 294–296. Boston, Martinus Nihjoff Publishers, 1987

15. ARANKI A, SYED SA, KENNEY EB, FRETER R: Isolation of anaerobic bacteria from human gingiva and mouse cecum by means of a simplified glove box procedure. Appl Microbiol 17:568–576, 1969

16. ARNON SS: Infant botulism. In Finegold SM, George WL (eds): Anaerobic Infections in Humans, pp 601–609. New York, Academic Press, 1989

17. AVGUSTIN G, WRIGHT F, FLINT HJ: Genetic diversity and phylogenetic relationships among strains of *Prevotella* (*Bacteroides*) *ruminicola* from the rumen. Int J Syst Bacteriol 44:246–255, 1994

18. BANKS ER, ALLEN SD, SIDERS JA, ET AL: Characterization of anaerobic bacteria by using a commercially available rapid tube test for glutamic acid decarboxylase. J Clin Microbiol 27:361–363, 1989

19. BANNO Y, KOBAYASHI T, KONO H, WATANABE K, ET AL: Biochemical characterization and biologic actions of two toxins (D-1 and D-2) from *Clostridium difficile*. Rev Infect Dis 6:S11–20, 1984

20. BARON EJ, CURREN M, HENDERSON G, ET AL: *Bilophila wadsworthia* isolates from clinical specimens. J Clin Microbiol 30:1882–1884, 1992

21. BARON EJ, SUMMANEN P, DOWNES J, ET AL: *Bilophila wadsworthia*, gen. nov. and sp. nov., a unique gram-negative anaerobic rod recovered from appendicitis specimens and human faeces. J Gen Microbiol 135:3405–3411, 1989

22. BARTLETT JG: Antibiotic-associated colitis. Disease-A-Month 30:1–54, 1984

23. BARTLETT JG: Anaerobic bacteria: general concepts. In Mandell GL, Douglas RG Jr, Bennett JE (eds): Principles and Practices of Infectious Diseases, 3rd ed, pp 1828–1842. New York, Churchill Livingstone, 1990

24. BARTLETT JG: *Clostridium difficile*: clinical considerations. Rev Infect Dis 12:S243–251, 1990

25. BARTLETT JG: Gas gangrene (other *Clostridium*-associated diseases). In Mandell GL, Douglas RG Jr, Bennett

JE (eds): Principles and Practice of Infectious Diseases, 3rd ed, pp 1850–1860. New York, Churchill Livingstone, 1990

26. BARTLETT JG: *Clostridium difficile*: history of its role as an enteric pathogen and the current state of knowledge about the organism. Clin Infect Dis 18:S265–272, 1994

27. BARTLEY SL, DOWELL VR JR: Comparison of media for the isolation of *Clostridium difficile* from fecal specimens. Lab Med 22:335–338, 1991

28. BEAMAN L, BEAMAN BL: The role of oxygen and its derivatives in microbial pathogenesis and host defense. Annu Rev Microbiol 38:27–48, 1984

29. BLAZEVIC DJ, MCCARTHY LR, MORELLO JA: Editorial: Minimum guidelines for blood cultures. Clin Microbiol Newslett 4:85–86, 1982

30. BORRIELLO SP: Clostridial disease of the gut [review]. Clin Infect Dis 209(Suppl 2):S242–250, 1995

31. BORRIELLO SP, BARCLAY FE, WELCH AR, ET AL: Epidemiology of diarrhoea caused by enterotoxigenic *Clostridium perfringens*. J Med Microbiol 20:363–372, 1985

32. BOURGAULT AM, ROSENBLATT JE, FITZGERALD RH: *Peptococcus magnus*: a significant human pathogen. Ann Intern Med 93:244–248, 1980

33. BROCK DW, GEORG LK, BROWN JM, HICKLIN MD: Actinomycosis caused by *Arachnia propionica*: report of 11 cases. Am J Clin Pathol 59:66–77, 1973

34. BROCK TD, MADIGAN MT, MARTINKO JM, PARKER J: Biology of Microorganisms, 7th ed. Englewood Cliffs NJ, Prentice Hall, 1994

35. BUCHANAN AG: Clinical laboratory evaluation of a reverse CAMP test for presumptive identification of *Clostridium perfringens*. J Clin Microbiol 16:761–762, 1982

36. CATO EP: Transfer of *Peptostreptococcus parvulus* (Weinberg, Nativelle, and Prevot 1937) Smith 1957 to the genus *Streptococcus*: *Streptococcus parvulus* (Weinberg, nativelle and prevot 1937) comb. nov., nom. rev., emend. Int J Syst Bacteriol 33:82–84, 1983

37. CATO EP, GEORGE WL, FINEGOLD SM: Genus *Clostridium*, Prazmowski 1880, 23AL. In Sneath PHA, Mair NS, Sharpe ME, et al (eds): Bergey's Manual of Systematic Bacteriology, vol 2, pp 1141–1200. Baltimore, Williams & Wilkins, 1986

38. CENTERS FOR DISEASE CONTROL: Foodborne disease outbreaks, annual summary, 1982. CDC Surveillance Summaries 35:7SS–16SS, 1986

39. CHARFREITAG O, COLLINS MD, STACKEBRANDT E: Reclassification of *Arachnia propionica* as *Propionibacterium propionicus* comb. nov. Int J Syst Bacteriol 38:354–357, 1988

40. COLLINS MD, LAWSON PA, WILLEMS A, ET AL: The phylogeny of the genus *Clostridium*: proposal of five new genera and eleven new species combinations. Int J Syst Bacteriol 44:812–826, 1994

41. COLLINS MD, LOVE DN, KARJALAINEN J, ET AL: Phylogenetic analysis of members of the genus *Porphyromonas* and description of *Porphyromonas cangingivalis* sp. nov. and *Porphyromonas cansulci* sp. nov. Int J Syst Bacteriol 44:674–679, 1994

42. COLLINS MD, STUBBS S, HOMMEZ J, DEVRIESE LA: Molecular taxonomic studies of *Actinomyces*-like bacteria isolated from purulent lesions in pigs and description of *Actinomyces hyovaginalis* sp. nov. Int J Syst Bacteriol 43:471–473, 1993

43. CREGAN P, FISS EH, SULLIVAN A, ET AL: Comparison of two BACTEC anaerobic culture media for recovery of anaerobic bacteria. Diagn Microbiol Infect Dis 17: 239–242, 1993

44. DELLINGER CA, MOORE LV: Use of the RapID-ANA System to screen for enzyme activities that differ among species of bile-inhibited *Bacteroides*. J Clin Microbiol 23:289–293, 1986

45. DORSHER CW, ROSENBLATT JE, WILSON WR, ILSTRUP DM: Anaerobic bacteremia: decreasing rate over a 15-year period (see comments). Rev Infect Dis 13:633–636, 1991

46. DOWELL VR JR: Clinical veterinary anaerobic bacteriology. DHEW, Atlanta, Centers for Disease Control, 1977

47. DOWELL VR JR: Botulism and tetanus: selected epidemiologic and microbiologic aspects. Rev Infect Dis 6: S202–207, 1984

48. DOWELL VR JR, LOMBARD GL: Laboratory methods in anaerobic bacteriology, DHEW Publication 78-8772. Atlanta, Centers for Disease Control, 1977

49. DOWELL VR JR, LOMBARD GL: Presumptive identification of anaerobic non-spore-forming gram-negative bacilli. Atlanta, Centers for Disease Control, 1977

50. DOWELL VR JR, LOMBARD GL: Differential agar media for identification of anaerobic bacteria. In Tilton RC (ed): Rapid Methods and Automation in Microbiology, pp 258–262. Washington DC, American Society for Microbiology, 1982

51. DOWELL VR JR, LOMBARD GL: Procedures for preliminary identification of bacteria. DHEW, Atlanta, Centers for Disease Control, 1984

52. DOWELL VR JR, LOMBARD GL, THOMPSON FS, ARMFIELD AY: Media for isolation, characterization, and identification of obligately anaerobic bacteria. Atlanta, Centers for Disease Control, 1977

53. DOWNES J, MANGELS JI, HOLDEN J, ET AL: Evaluation of two single-plate incubation systems and the anaerobic chamber for the cultivation of anaerobic bacteria. J Clin Microbiol 28:246–248, 1990

54. DZINK JL, SHEENAN MT, SOCRANSKY SS: Proposal of three subspecies of *Fusobacterium nucleatum* Knorr 1922: *Fusobacterium nucleatum* subsp. *nucleatum* subsp. nov., comb. nov.; *Fusobacterium nucleatum* subsp. *polymorphum* subsp. nov., nom. rev., comb. nov.; and *Fusobacterium nucleatum* subsp. *vincentii* subsp. nov., nom. rev., comb. nov. Int J Syst Bacteriol 40:74–78, 1990

55. ELEY A, CLARRY T, BENNETT KW: Selective and differential medium for isolation of *Bacteroides ureolyticus* from clinical specimens. Eur J Clin Microbiol Infect Dis 8:83–85, 1989

56. ENGELKIRK PG, DUBEN-ENGELKIRK J, DOWELL VR JR: Principles and Practice of Clinical Anaerobic Bacteriology. Belmont, Star Publishing, 1992

57. EZAKI T, LIU SL, HASHIMOTO Y, YABUUCHI E: *Peptostreptococcus hydrogenalis* sp. nov. from human fecal and vaginal flora. Int J Syst Bacteriol 40:305–306, 1990

58. EZAKI T, YAMAMOTO N, NINOMIYA K, ET AL: Transfer of *Peptococcus indolicus*, *Peptococcus asaccharolyticus*, *Peptococcus prevotii* and *Peptococcus magnus* to the genus *Peptostreptococcus* and proposal of *Peptostreptococcus tetradius* sp. nov. Int J Syst Bacteriol 33:683–698, 1983

59. FEKETY R: Recent advances in management of bacterial diarrhea. Rev Infect Dis 5:246–257, 1983

60. FELNER JM, DOWELL VR JR: "*Bacteroides*" bacteremia. Am J Med 50:787–796, 1971

61. FINEGOLD SM: Anaerobic Bacteria in Human Disease. New York, Academic Press, 1977

62. FINEGOLD SM: The National Committee for Clinical Laboratory Standards Working Group on Anaerobic Susceptibility Testing: susceptibility testing of anaerobic bacteria. J Clin Microbiol 26:1253–1256, 1988

63. FINEGOLD SM: Therapy of anaerobic infections. In Finegold SM, George WL (eds): Anaerobic Infections in Humans, pp 793–818. New York, Academic Press, 1989

64. FINEGOLD SM: Anaerobes: problems and controversies in bacteriology, infections, and susceptibility testing. Rev Infect Dis 12:S223–230, 1990

65. FINEGOLD SM: Clinical relevance of antimicrobial susceptibility testing. Eur J Clin Microbiol Infect Dis 11: 1021–1024, 1992

66. FINEGOLD SM: Host factors predisposing to anaerobic infections. FEMS Immunol Med Microbiol 6:159–163, 1993

67. FINEGOLD SM: Anaerobic bacteria: general concepts. In Mandell GL, Bennett JE, Dolin R (eds): Mandell, Douglas and Bennett's Principles and Practice of Infectious Diseases, vol 2, 4th ed, pp 2156. New York, Churchill Livingstone, 1995

68. FINEGOLD SM: Overview of clinically important anaerobes. Clin Infect Dis 20:205–207, 1995

69. FINEGOLD SM, GEORGE WL: Anaerobic Infections in Humans. San Diego, Academic Press, 1989

70. FUNKE G, RAMOS CP, FERNANDEZ-GARAYZABAL JF, ET AL: Description of human-derived Centers for Disease Control coryneform group 2 bacteria as *Actinomyces bernardiae* sp. nov. Int J Syst Bacteriol 45:57–60, 1995

71. FUNKE G, STUBBS S, VON GRAEVENITZ A, COLLINS MD: Assignment of human-derived CDC group 1 coryneform bacteria and CDC group 1-like coryneform bacteria to the genus *Actinomyces* as *Actinomyces neuii* subsp. *neuii* sp. nov., subsp. nov., and *Actinomyces neuii* subsp. *anitratus* subsp. nov. Int J Syst Bacteriol 44:167–171, 1994

72. GERDING DN, JOHNSON S, PETERSON LR, ET AL: *Clostridium difficile*-associated diarrhea and colitis. Infect Control Hosp Epidemiol 16:459–477, 1995

73. GERDING DN, OLSON MM, PETERSON LR, ET AL: *Clostridium difficile*-associated diarrhea and colitis in adults. A prospective case-controlled epidemiologic study. Arch Intern Med 146:95–100, 1986

74. GHARBIA SE, SHAH HN: *Fusobacterium nucleatum* subsp. *fusiforme* subsp. nov. and *Fusobacterium nucleatum* subsp. *animalis* subsp. nov. as additional subspecies within *Fusobacterium nucleatum*. Int J Syst Bacteriol 42:296–298, 1992

75. GORBACH SL, MAYHEW JW, BARTLETT JG, ET AL: Rapid diagnosis of anaerobic infections by direct gas–liquid chromatography of clinical speciments. J Clin Invest 57:478–484, 1976

76. GREGORY EM, MOORE WEC, HOLDEMAN LV: Super-oxide dismutase in anaerobes: survey. Appl Environ Microbiol 35:988–991, 1978

77. GUERIN-FAUBLEE V, FLANDROIS JP, BROYE E, ET AL: *Actinomyces pyogenes*: susceptibility of 103 clinical animal isolates to 22 antimicrobial agents. Vet Res 24:251–259, 1993

78. HALL IC, O'TOOLE E: Intestinal flora in new-born infants: with a description of a new pathogenic anaerobe, *Bacillus difficilis*. Am J Dis Child :390–402, 1935

79. HANSEN MV, ELLIOTT LP: New presumptive identification test for *Clostridium perfringens*: reverse CAMP test. J Clin Microbiol 12:617–619, 1980

80. HATHEWAY CL: Botulism. In Balows A, Hausler WJ Jr, Ohashi M, et al (eds): Laboratory Diagnosis of Infectious Diseases: Principles and Practice, vol 1, pp 111–133. New York, Springer, 1988

81. HATHEWAY CL: Toxigenic clostridia. Clin Microbiol Rev 3:66–98, 1990

82. HEIZMANN WR, WERNER H: GasPak versus Anaerocult A: two carbon dioxide/hydrogen systems for cultivation of anaerobes. Zentralbl Bakteriol Hyg A 270: 511–516, 1989

83. HENRY NK, MCLIMANS CA, WRIGHT AJ, ET AL: Microbiological and clinical evaluation of the isolator lysis–centrifugation blood culture tube. J Clin Microbiol 17:864–869, 1983

84. HENTGES DJ, MAIER BR: Theoretical basis for anaerobic methodology. Am J Clin Nutr 25:1299–1305, 1972

85. HILL GB: *Eubacterium nodatum* mimics *Actinomyces* in intrauterine device-associated infections and other settings within the female genital tract. Obstet Gynecol 79:534–538, 1992

86. HILL GB: The microbiology of bacterial vaginosis. Am J Obstet Gynecol 169:450–454, 1993

87. HILL GB, AYERS OM, KOHAN AP: Characteristics and sites of infection of *Eubacterium nodatum, Eubacterium timidum, Eubacterium brachy*, and other asaccharolytic eubacteria. J Clin Microbiol 25:1540–1545, 1987

88. HILLER SL, ESCHENBACH DA: Bacterial vaginosis: role of *Mobiluncus* species. Infect Dis Newslett 5:65–68, 1984

89. HIRASAWA M, TAKADA K: *Porphyromonas gingivicanis* sp. nov. and *Porphyromonas crevioricanis* sp. nov., isolated from beagles. Int J Syst Bacteriol 44:637–640, 1994

90. HOLDEMAN LV, CATO EP, MOORE WE: Taxonomy of anaerobes: present state of the art. Rev Infect Dis 6: S3–10, 1984

91. HOLDEMAN LV, CATO EP, MOORE WEC: Anaerobe Laboratory Manual. Blacksburg, Virginia Polytechnic Institute and State University, 1977

92. HOLDEMAN LV, JOHNSON JL: *Bacteroides disiens* sp. nov. and *Bacteroides bivius* sp. nov. from human clinical infections. Int J Syst Bacteriol 27:337–345, 1977

93. HOLDEMAN LV, KELLEY RW, MOORE WEC: Anaerobic gram-negative straight, curved, and helical rods. Family 1. Bacteroidaceae Pribram 1933, 10AL. In Krieg NR, Holt JG (eds): Bergey's Manual of Systemic Bacteriology, pp 602–662. Baltimore, Williams & Wilkins, 1984

94. HOLDEMAN LV, MOORE WE: New genus *Coprococcus*: twelve new species and emended descriptions of four previously described species of bacteria from human species. Int J Syst Bacteriol 24:260–277, 1974

95. HOLDEMAN LV, MOORE WEC, CHURN PJ, JOHNSON JL: *Bacteroides oris* and *Bacteroides buccae*: new species from human periodontitis and other human infections. Int J Syst Bacteriol 32:125–131, 1982

96. JARKOWSKI TL, WOLF PL: Unusual gas bacillus infections including necrotic enteritis. JAMA 181:845–850, 1962

97. JOHNSON CC, REINHARDT JF, EDELSTEIN MA, ET AL: *Bacteroides gracilis*, an important anaerobic bacterial pathogen. J Clin Microbiol 22:799–802, 1985

98. JOHNSON JL, MOORE LV, KANEKO B, MOORE WE: *Actinomyces georgiae* sp. nov., *Actinomyces gerencseriae* sp. nov., designation of two genospecies of *Actinomyces naeslundii*, and inclusion of *A. naeslundii* serotypes II and III and *Actinomyces viscosus* serotype II in *A. naeslundii* genospecies 2. Int J Syst Bacteriol 40:273–286, 1990

99. JOHNSON JL, MOORE WEC, MOORE LVH: *Bacteroides caccae* sp. nov., *Bacteroides merdae* sp. nov., and *Bacteroides stercoris* sp. nov. isolated from human feces. Int J Syst Bacteriol 36:499–501, 1986

100. JONES RN, FUCHS PC, THORNSEBERRY C, RHODES N: Antimicrobial susceptibility tests for anaerobic bacteria: comparison of Wilkins-Chalgren agar reference method and micro-dilution method and determination of stability of antimicrobics frozen in broth. Curr Microbiol 1:81–83, 1978

101. JUSTUS PG, MARTIN JL, GOLDBERG DA, ET AL: Myoelectric effects of *Clostridium difficile*: motility-altering factors distinct from its cytotoxin and enterotoxin in rabbits. Gastroenterology 83:836–843, 1982

102. KELLY MT, FOJTASEK MF, ABBOTT TM, ET AL: Clinical evaluation of a lysis–centrifugation technique for the detection of septicemia. JAMA 250:2185–2188, 1983

103. KILLGORE GE, STARR SE, DEL BENE VE, ET AL: Comparison of three anaerobic systems for the isolation of anaerobic bacteria from clinical specimens. Am J Clin Pathol 59:552–559, 1973

104. KILPER-BALZ R, WNEZIG P, SCHLEIFER KH: Molecular relationship and classification of some viridans streptococci as *Streptococcus oralis* and emended description of *Streptococcus oralis* (Bridge and Sneath, 1982). Int J Syst Bacteriol 35:482–488, 1984

105. KILPPER-BALZ R, SCHLEIFER KH: Transfer *Peptococcus saccharolyticus* Foubert and Douglas to the genus *Staphylococcus: Staphylococcus saccharolyticus* (Foubert and Douglas) comb. nov. Zentralbl Baketeriol Parasitenkd Infektionskr Hyg 2:324–331, 1981

106. KIRBY BD, GEORGE WL, SUTTER VL, ET AL: Gram-negative anaerobic bacilli: their role in infection and patterns of susceptibility to antimicrobial agents. I. Little-known *Bacteroides* species. Rev Infect Dis 2:914–951, 1980

107. KONEMAN EW, ALLEN SD, JANDA WM, ET AL: Color Atlas and Textbook of Diagnostic Microbiology, 4th ed. Philadelphia, JB Lippincott, 1992

108. KOONTZ FP, FLINT KK, REYNOLDS JK, ALLEN SD: Multicenter comparison of the high volume (10 mL) NR BACTEC PLUS system and the standard (5 mL) NR BACTEC system. Diag Microbiol Infect Dis 14:111–118, 1991

109. KORANSKY JR, ALLEN SD, DOWELL VR JR: Use of ethanol for selective isolation of sporeforming microorganisms. Appl Environ Microbiol 35:762–765, 1978

110. KORANSKY JR, STARGEL MD, DOWELL VR JR: *Clostridium septicum* bacteremia. Its clinical significance. Am J Med 66:63–66, 1979

111. KORNOWSKI R, SCHWARTZ D, AVERBUCH M, ET AL: Anaerobic bacteremia: a retrospective four-year analysis in general medicine and cancer patients. Infection 21: 241–244, 1993

111a. KRIEG NR, HOLD JG: Bergey's Manual of Systematic Baceriology, vol 1. Baltimore: Williams & Wilkins, 1984

112. KRONVALL G, MYHRE E: Differential staining of bacteria in clinical specimens using acridine orange buffered at low pH. Acta Pathol Microbiol Scand B Microbiol 85:249–254, 1977

113. LANDSAAT PM, VAN DER LELIE H, BONGAERTS G, KUIJPER EJ: *Fusobacterium nucleatum*, a new invasive pathogen in neutropenic patients? Scand J Infect Dis 27:83–84, 1995

114. LAUGHON BE, VISCIDI RP, GDOVIN SL, ET AL: Enzyme immunoassays for detection of *Clostridium difficile* toxins A and B in fecal specimens. J Infect Dis 149:781–788, 1984

115. LEE K, BARON EJ, SUMMANEN P, FINEGOLD SM: Selective medium for isolation of *Bacteroides gracilis*. J Clin Microbiol 28:1747–1750, 1990

116. LOESCHE WJ: Oxygen sensitivity of various anaerobic bacteria. Appl Microbiol 18:723–727, 1969

117. LOMBARD GL, ARMFIELD AY, STARGEL MD, FOX JB: The effect of storage of blood agar medium on the growth of certain obligate anaerobes. Abstr Annu Meet Am Soc Microbiol, Abstr C95, 1976

118. LOMBARD GL, DOWELL VR JR: Gas Liquid Chromatography: Analysis of Acid Products of Bacteria. Atlanta, Centers for Disease Control, 1982

119. LOMBARDI DP, ENGLEBERG NC: Anaerobic bacteremia: incidence, patient characteristics, and clinical significance. Am J Med 92:53–60, 1992

120. LOVE DN: *Porphyromonas macacae* comb. nov., a consequence of *Bacteroides macacae* being a senior synonym of *Porphyromonas salivosa*. Int J Syst Bacteriol 45:90–92, 1995

121. LOVE DN, BAILEY GD: Chromosomal DNA probes for the identification of *Bacteroides tectum* and *Bacteroides fragilis* from the oral cavity of cats. Vet Microbiol 34:89–95, 1993

122. LOVE DN, BAILEY GD, COLLINGS S, BRISCOE DA: Description of *Porphyromonas circumdentaria* sp. nov. and reassignment of *Bacteroides salivosus* (Love, Johnson, Jones, and Calverley 1987) as *Porphyromonas* (Shah and Collins 1988) *salivosa* comb. nov [published errata appear in Int J Syst Bacteriol 1992;42(4):660 and 1993;43(3):630]. Int J Syst Bacteriol 42:434–438, 1992

123. LOVE DN, JOHNSON JL, JONES RF, CALVERLEY A: *Bacteroides salivosus* sp. nov., an asaccharolytic, black-pigmented species from cats. Int J Syst Bacteriol 37:307–309, 1987

124. LOVE DN, KARJALAINEN J, KANERVO A, ET AL: *Porphyromonas canoris* sp. nov., an asaccharolytic, black-pigmented species from the gingival sulcus of dogs. Int J Syst Bacteriol 44:204–208, 1994

125. LUDWIG W, KIRCHHOF G, WEIZENEGGER M, WEISS N: Phylogenetic evidence for the transfer of *Eubacterium suis* to the genus *Actinomyces* as *Actinomyces suis* comb. nov. Int J Syst Bacteriol 42:161–165, 1992

126. LYERLY DM: *Clostridium difficile* testing. Clin Microbiol Newslett 17:17, 1995

127. LYERLY DM, BALL DW, TOTH J, WILKINS TD: Characterization of cross-reactive proteins detected by Culturette Brand Rapid Latex Test for *Clostridium difficile*. J Clin Microbiol 26:397–400, 1988

128. LYERLY DM, BARROSO LA, WILKINS TD: Identification of the latex test-reactive protein of *Clostridium difficile* as glutamate dehydrogenase. J Clin Microbiol 29:2639–2642, 1991

129. LYERLY DM, KRIVAN HC, WILKINS TD: *Clostridium difficile*: its disease and toxins. Clin Microbiol Rev 1:1–18, 1988

130. MALNICK H, WILLIAMS K, PHIL-EBOSIE J, LEVY AS: Description of a medium for isolating *Anaerobiospirillum* spp., a possible cause of zoonotic disease, from diarrheal feces and blood of humans and use of the medium in a survey of human, canine, and feline feces. J Clin Microbiol 28:1380–1384, 1990

131. MARLER L, ALLEN S, SIDERS J: Rapid enzymatic characterization of clinically encountered anaerobic bacteria with the API ZYM system. Eur J Clin Microbiol 3:294–300, 1984

132. MARLER LM, SIDERS JA, WOLTERS LC, ET AL: Evaluation of the new RapID-ANA II system for the identification of clinical anaerobic isolates. J Clin Microbiol 29:874–878, 1991

133. MARLER LM, SIDERS JA, WOLTERS LC, ET AL: Comparison of five cultural procedures for isolation of *Clostridium difficile* from stools. J Clin Microbiol 30:514–516, 1992

134. MARTIN WJ: Practical method for isolation of anaerobic bacteria in the clinical laboratory. Appl Microbiol 22, 1971

134a. MAYRAND D: Identification of clinical isolates of selected species of *Bacteroides*: production of phenylacetic acid. Can J. Microbiol 25:927–928, 1979.

135. MAYS TD, HOLDEMAN LV, MOORE WEC, ET AL: Taxonomy of the genus *Veillonella* Prevot. Int J Syst Bacteriol 32:28–36, 1982

136. MCCORD JM, KEELE BBJ, FRIDOVICH: An enzyme-based theory of obligate anaerobiosis: the physiologic function of superoxide dismutase. Proc Natl Acad Sci USA 68:1024–1027, 1971

137. MCFARLAND LV, MULLIGAN ME, KWOK RY, STAMM WE: Nosocomial acquisition of *Clostridium difficile* infection. N Engl J Med 320:204–210, 1989

138. MCFARLAND LV, STAMM WE: Review of *Clostridium difficile*-associated diseases. Am J Infect Control 14:99–109, 1986

139. MCNEIL MM, MARTONE WJ, DOWELL VR JR: Bacteremia with *Anaerobiospirillum succiniciproducens*. Rev Infect Dis 9:737–742, 1987

140. MILES BL, SIDERS JA, ALLEN SD: Evaluation of a commercial latex test for *Clostridium difficile* for reactivity with *C. difficile* and cross-reactions with other bacteria. J Clin Microbiol 26:2452–2455, 1988

141. MILLAR JS: Enteritis necroticans: a review. Trop Gastroenterol 10:3–8, 1989

142. MILLER PH, WIGGS LS, MILLER JM: Evaluation of API An-IDENT and RapID ANA II systems for identification of *Actinomyces* species from clinical specimens. J Clin Microbiol 33:329–330, 1995

143. MILLS CK, GRIMES BY, GHERNA RL: Three rapid methods compared with a conventional method for detection of urease production in anaerobic bacteria. J Clin Microbiol 25:2209–2210, 1987

144. MOORE LV, JOHNSON JL, MOORE WE: Descriptions of *Prevotella tannerae* sp. nov. and *Prevotella enoeca* sp. nov.

from the human gingival crevice and emendation of the description of *Prevotella zoogleoformans*. Int J Syst Bacteriol 44:599–602, 1994

145. MOORE LV, MOORE WE: *Oribaculum catoniae* gen. nov., sp. nov.; *Catonella morbi* gen. nov., sp. nov.; *Hallella seregens* gen. nov., sp. nov.; *Johnsonella ignava* gen. nov., sp. nov.; and *Dialister pneumosintes* gen. nov., comb. nov., nom. rev., Anaerobic gram-negative bacilli from the human gingival crevice. Int J Syst Bacteriol 44:187–192, 1994

146. MOORE LVH, CATO EP, MOORE WEC: Anaerobe Laboratory Manual Update: Supplements to the VPI Anaerobe Laboratory Manual, 4th ed. Blacksburg, Virginia Polytechnic Institute and State University, 1987

147. MOORE LVH, JOHNSON JL, MOORE WEC: Genus *Peptostreptococcus* Kluyver and van Niel 1936, 401AL. In Sneath PHA, Mair NS, Sharpe ME, et al (eds): Bergey's Manual of Systematic Bacteriology, vol 2, pp 1083–1092. Baltimore, Williams & Wilkins, 1986

148. MOORE WEC: Chromatography for the clincial laboratory: all you wanted to know (and possibly more). API Species 4:21–28, 1980

149. MORELLO JA, LEITCH C, NITZ S, ET AL: Detection of bacteremia by Difco ESP blood culture system. J Clin Microbiol 32:811–818, 1994

150. MORRIS AJ, WILSON ML, MIRRETT S, RELLER LB: Rationale for selective use of anaerobic blood cultures. J Clin Microbiol 31:2110–2113, 1993

151. MURRAY PR, SONDAG JE: Evaluation of routine subcultures of macroscopically negative blood cultures for detection of anaerobes. J Clin Microbiol 8:427–430, 1978

152. MURRAY PR, TRAYNOR P, HOPSON D: Critical assessment of blood culture techniques: analysis of recovery of obligate and facultative anaerobes, strict aerobic bacteria, and fungi in aerobic and anaerobic blood culture bottles. J Clin Microbiol 30:1462–1468, 1992

153. MURRELL TG, WALKER PD: The pigbel story of Papua New Guinea. Trans R Soc Trop Med Hyg 85:119–122, 1991

154. NCCLS: Methods for antimicrobial susceptibility testing of anaerobic bacteria. Approved standard, NCCLS publication M11-A2. Villanova PA, National Committee for Clincal Laboratory Standards, 1990

155. NCCLS: Methods for antimicrobial susceptibility testing of anaerobic bacteria. Approved standard., vol 13 no. 26, 3rd ed. Villanova PA, National Committee for Clinical Laboratory Standards, 1993

156. NCCLS: Performance standards for antimicrobial susceptibility testing; fifth informational supplement. NCCLS Document M100-S3, vol 14 no. 16. Villanova PA, National Committee for Clinical Laboratory Standards, 1994

157. NOLTE FS, WILLIAMS JM, JERRIS RC, ET AL: Multicenter clinical evaluation of a continuous monitoring blood culture system using fluorescent-sensor technology (BACTEC 9240). J Clin Microbiol 31:552–557, 1993

158. ONDERDONK AB, ALLEN SD: *Clostridium*. In Murray PR, Baron EJ, Pfaller MA, et al (eds): Manual of Clinical Microbiology, 6th ed, pp 574–586. Washington DC, ASM Press, 1995

159. PAISLEY JW, ROSENBLATT JE, HALL M, WASHINGTON JAD: Evaluation of a routine anaerobic subculture of blood cultures for detection of anaerobic bacteremia. J Clin Microbiol 8:764–766, 1978

160. PARK CH, HIXON DL, ENDLICH JF, ET AL: *Anaerobiospirillum succiniciproducens*. Two case reports. Am J Clin Pathol 85:73–76, 1986

161. PETERSON LR, KELLY PJ: The role of the clinical microbiology laboratory in the management of *Clostridium difficile*-associated diarrhea. Infect Dis Clin North Am 7:277–293, 1993

162. PHILLIPS I: New methods for identification of obligate anaerobes. Rev Infect Dis 12:S127–132, 1990

163. PRICE AB: Histopathology of clostridial gut diseases in man. In Borriello SP (ed): Clostridia in Gastrointestinal Disease, pp 177–193. Boca Raton FL, CRC Press, 1985

164. RELLER LB, MURRAY PR, MACLOWRY JD: Cumitech IA, Blood Cultures II. Washington DC, American Society for Microbiology, 1982

165. ROBERTS MC, HILLIER SL, SCHOENKNECHT FD, HOLMES KK: Comparison of Gram stain, DNA probe, and culture for the identification of species of *Mobiluncus* in female genital specimens. J Infect Dis 152:74–77, 1985

166. ROLFE RD, HENTGES DJ, BARRETT JT, CAMPBELL BJ: Oxygen tolerance of human intestinal anaerobes. Am J Clin Nutr 30:1762–1769, 1977

167. ROLFE RD, HENTGES DJ, CAMPBELL BJ, BARRETT JT: Factors related to the oxygen tolerance of anaerobic bacteria. Appl Environ Microbiol 36:303–313, 1978

168. ROSENBLATT JE, FALLON A, FINEGOLD SM: Comparison of methods for isolation of anaerobic bacteria from clinical specimens. Appl Microbiol 25:77–85, 1973

169. RYAN MR, MURRAY PR: Laboratory detection of anaerobic bacteremia. Clin Lab Med 14:107–117, 1994

170. SCHAAL KP, LEE HJ: Actinomycete infections in humans—a review. Gene 115:201–211, 1992

171. SEIP WF, EVANS GL: Atmospheric analysis and redox potentials of culture media in the GasPak System. J Clin Microbiol 11:226–233, 1980

172. SEVERIN WP, DE LA FUENTE AA, STRINGER MF: *Clostridium perfringens* type C causing necrotising enteritis. J Clin Pathol 37:942–944, 1984

173. SHAH HN, COLLINS DM: Proposal for re-classification of *Bacteroides asaccharolyticus*, *Bacteroides gingivalis*, and *Bacteroides endodontalis* in a new genus, *Porphyromonas*. Int J Syst Bacteriol 38:128–131, 1988

174. SHAH HN, COLLINS DM: Proposal to restrict the genus *Bacteroides* (Castellani and Chalmers) to *Bacteroides fragilis* and closely related species. Int J Syst Bacteriol 39: 85–87, 1989

175. SHAH HN, COLLINS DM: *Prevotella*, a new genus to include *Bacteroides melaninogenicus* and related species formerly classified in the genus *Bacteroides*. Int J Syst Bacteriol 40:205–208, 1990

176. SHAH HN, COLLINS MD, OLSEN I, PASTER BJ ET AL: Reclassification of *Bacteroides levii* (Holdeman, Cato, and Moore) in the genus *Porphyromonas*, as *Porphyromonas levii* comb. nov. Int J Syst Bacteriol 45:586–588, 1995

177. SHAH HN, GHARBIA SE: Biochemical and chemical studies on strains designated *Prevotella intermedia* and proposal of a new pigmented species, *Prevotella nigrescens* sp. nov. Int J Syst Bacteriol 42:542–546, 1992

178. SHAH HN, GHARBIA SE: Proposal of a new species *Prevotella nigrescens* sp. nov. among strains previously

classified as *Prevotella intermedia*. FEMS Immunol Med Microbiol 6:97, 1993

179. SHANDERA WX, TACKET CO, BLAKE PA: Food poisoning due to *Clostridium perfringens* in the United States. J Infect Dis 147:167–170, 1983

180. SHEPHERD A: Clinical features and operative treatment of pigbel—enteritis necroticans. Papua New Guinea Med J 22:18–23, 1979

181. SHINJO T, HIRAIWA K, MIYAZATO S: Recognition of biovar C of *Fusobacterium necrophorum* (Flugge) Moore and Holdeman as *Fusobacterium pseudonecrophorum* sp. nov., nom. rev. (ex Prevot 1940). Int J Syst Bacteriol 40:71–73, 1990

182. SIBONI A, GRAVERSEN K, OLSEN H: Significant decrease of gram-negative anaerobic bacteremia in a major hospital from 1967–73 to 1981–89: an effect of the introduction of metronidazole? Scand J Infect Dis 25:347–351, 1993

182a. SIDERS JA: Prereduced anaerobically sterilized biochemicals. In Isenberg HD (ed): Clinical Microbiology Handbook. Washington, DC: American Society for Microbiology, 2.6.1–2.6.10, 1992

182b. SIDERS JA: Gas-liquid chromatography. In Isenberg HD (ed): Clinical Microbiology Procedures Handbook. Washington, DC: American Society for Microbiology, 2.7.1–2.7.6, 1992

183. SLACK JM, GENERCSER MA: *Actinomyces*, Filamentous Bacteria Biology and Pathogenicity. Minneapolis, Burgess Publishing, 1975

184. SMITH HJ, MOORE HB: Isolation of *Mobiluncus* species from clinical specimens by using cold enrichment and selective media. J Clin Microbiol 26:1134–1137, 1988

185. SMITH LDS: Botulism: The Organism, Its Toxins, the Disease. Springfield, Charles C Thomas, 1977

186. SMITH LDS, WILLIAMS BL: The Pathogenic Anaerobic Bacteria, 3rd ed. Springfield, Charles C Thomas, 1984

186a. SNEATH PHA, MAIR NS, SHARPE ME, HOLT JG: Bergey's Manual of Systematic Bacteriology, vol 2. Baltimore: Williams & Wilkins, 1986

187. SOTO A, ZAPARDIEL J, SORIANO F: Evaluation of API Coryne system for identifying coryneform bacteria. J Clin Pathol 47:756–759, 1994

188. SPIEGEL CA: Bacterial vaginosis. Clin Microbiol Rev 4:485–502, 1991

189. SPIEGEL CA, ESCHENBACH DA, AMSEL R, HOLMES KK: Curved anaerobic bacteria in bacterial (nonspecific) vaginosis and their response to antimicrobial therapy. J Infect Dis 148:817–822, 1983

190. SPIEGEL CA, ROBERTS M: *Mobiluncus* gen. nov., *Mobiluncus cutisii* subsp. *curtisii* sp. nov., and *Mobiluncus mulieris* sp. nov., curved rods from the human vagina. Int J Syst Bacteriol 34:177–184, 1984

191. STARGEL MD, LOMBARD GL, DOWELL VR JR: Alternative procedures for identification of anaerobic bacteria. Am J Med Technol 44:709–722, 1978

192. STOAKES L, KELLY T, MANARIN K, ET AL: Accuracy and reproducibility of the MicroScan rapid anaerobe identification system with an automated reader. J Clin Microbiol 28:1135–1138, 1990

193. STORY S, DOWELL VR JR: Development of a Presumpto plate for identification of clostridia. Abstr Ann Meet Am Soc Microbiol, Abstr C24, 1978

194. SUMMANEN P: Recent taxonomic changes for anaerobic gram-positive and selected gram-negative organisms. Clin Infect Dis 16:S168–174, 1993

195. SUMMANEN P, BARON EJ, CITRON DM, ET AL: Wadsworth Anaerobic Bacteriology Manual, 5th ed. Belmont, Star Publishing, 1993

196. SUTTER VL, CITRON DM, EDELSTEIN MAC, FINEGOLD SM: Wadsworth Anaerobic Bacteriology Manual, 4th ed. Belmont, Star Publishing, 1985

197. TALLY FP, GOLDIN BR, JACOBUS NV, GORBACH SL: Superoxide dismutase in anaerobic bacteria of clinical significance. Infect Immun 16:20–25, 1977

198. TANNER ACR, BADGER S, LAI CH, ET AL: *Wolinella* gen. nov. *Wolinella succinogenes* (*Vibrio succinogenes* Wolin et al.) comb. nov., and description of *Bacteriodes gracilis* sp. nov. *Wolinella recta* sp. nov., *Campylobacter concious* sp. nov., and *Eikenella corrodens* from humans with periodontal diseases. Int J Syst Bacteriol 31:432–445, 1981

199. TAYLOR NS, THORNE GM, BARTLETT JG: Comparison of two toxins produced by *Clostridium difficile*. Infect Immun 34:1036–1043, 1981

200. THOMASON JL, SCHRECKENBERGER PC, SPELLACY WN, ET AL: Clinical and microbiological characterization of patients with nonspecific vaginosis associated with motile, curved anaerobic rods. J Infect Dis 149:801–809, 1984

201. TIVELJUNG A, FORSUM U, MONSTEIN HJ: Classification of the genus *Mobiluncus* based on comparative partial 16S rRNA gene analysis. Int J Syst Bacteriol 46:332–336, 1996

202. TRNKA YM, LAMONT JT: *Clostridium difficile* colitis. Adv Intern Med 29:85–107, 1984

203. VAN KESSEL LJ, VERBRUGH HA, STRINGER MF, HOEKSTRA JB: Necrotizing enteritis associated with toxigenic type A *Clostridium perfringens* [letter]. J Infect Dis 151:974–975, 1985

204. VAN WINKELHOFF AJ, CLEMENT M, DE GRAAFF J: Rapid characterization of oral and nonoral pigmented *Bacteroides* species with the ATB Anaerobes ID system. J Clin Microbiol 26:1063–1065, 1988

205. VAN WINKELHOFF AJ, VAN STEENBERGEN TJ, KIPPUW N, DE GRAAFF J: Further characterization of *Bacteroides endodontalis*, an asaccharolytic black-pigmented *Bacteroides* species from the oral cavity. J Clin Microbiol 22:75–79, 1985

206. VAN WINKELHOFF AJ, VAN STEENBERGEN TJ, KIPPUW N, DE GRAAFF J: Enzymatic characterization of oral and nonoral black-pigmented *Bacteroides* species. Antonie Van Leeuwenhoek 52:163–171, 1986

207. VANDAMME P, DANESHVAR MI, DEWHIRST FE, ET AL: Chemotaxonomic analyses of *Bacteroides gracilis* and *Bacteroides ureolyticus* and reclassification of *B. gracilis* as *Campylobacter gracilis* comb. nov. Int J Syst Bacteriol 45:145–152, 1995

208. VANDAMME P, FALSEN E, ROSSAU R, ET AL: Revision of *Campylobacter*, *Helicobacter*, and *Wolinella* taxonomy: emendation of generic descriptions and proposal of *Arcobacter* gen. nov. Int J Syst Bacteriol 41:88–103, 1991

209. WALDEN WC, HENTGES DJ: Differential effects of oxygen and oxidation–reduction potential on the multiplication of three species of anaerobic intestinal bacteria. Appl Microbiol 30:781–785, 1975

210. WALKER PD: Pig-Bel. In Borriello SP (ed): Clostridia in Gastrointestinal Disease, pp 94–115. Boca Raton FL, CRC Press, 1985

211. WASHINGTON J II: Anaerobic blood cultures. In Lennette EH, Spaulding EH, Truant JP (eds): Manual of Clinical Microbiology, 2nd ed, pp 402–404. Washington DC, American Society for Microbiology, 1974

212. WASHINGTON JA: Evolving concepts on the laboratory diagnosis of septicemia. Infect Dis Clin Pract 2:65, 1993

213. WATSON DA, ANDREW JH, BANTING S, ET AL: Pig-bel but no pig: enteritis necroticans acquired in Australia. Med J Aust 155:47–50, 1991

214. WEINSTEIN MP, RELLER LB, MIRRETT S, ET AL: Controlled evaluation of trypticase soy broth in agar slide and conventional blood culture systems. J Clin Microbiol 21: 626–629, 1985

215. WEXLER HM: Susceptibility testing of anaerobic bacteria: myth, magic, or method? Clin Microbiol Rev 4: 470–484, 1991

216. WEXLER HM: Susceptibility testing of anaerobic bacteria—the state of the art. Clin Infect Dis 16:S328–333, 1993

217. WHALEY DN, GORMAN GW: An inexpensive device for evacuating and gassing anaerobic systems with in-house vacuum. J Clin Microbiol 5:668–669, 1977

218. WILLEMS A, COLLINS MD: 16S rRNA gene similarities indicate that *Hallella seregens* (Moore and Moore) and *Mitsuokella dentalis* (Haapsalo et al.) are genealogically highly related and are members of the genus *Prevotella*: emended description of the genus *Prevotella* (Shah and Collins) and description of *Prevotella dentalis* comb. nov. Int J Syst Bacteriol 45:832–836, 1995

219. WILLEMS A, COLLINS MD: Reclassification of *Oribaculum catoniae* (Moore and Moore 1994) as *Porphyromonas catoniae* comb. nov. and emendation of the genus *Porphyromonas*. Int J Syst Bacteriol 45:578–581, 1995

220. WILLIS AT: Clostridia of Wound Infections. London, Butterworths, 1969

221. WILSON ML, HARRELL LJ, MIRRETT S, ET AL: Controlled evaluation of BACTEC PLUS 27 and Roche Septi-Chek anaerobic blood culture bottles. J Clin Microbiol 30:63–66, 1992

222. WILSON ML, WEINSTEIN MP, REIMER LG, ET AL: Controlled comparison of the BacT/Alert and BACTEC 660/730 nonradiometric blood culture systems. J Clin Microbiol 30:323–329, 1992

223. WUST J, STUBBS S, WEISS N, ET AL: Assignment of *Actinomyces pyogenes*-like (CDC coryneform group E) bacteria to the genus *Actinomyces* as *Actinomyces radingae* sp. nov. and *Actinomyces turicensis* sp. nov. Lett Appl Microbiol 20:76–81, 1995

224. YEUNG MK: Complete nucleotide sequence of the *Actinomyces viscosus* T14V sialidase gene: presence of a conserved repeating sequence among strains of *Actinomyces* spp. Infect Immun 61:109–116, 1993

COLOR PLATES

CHAPTERS 14–21

IDENTIFICATION OF ANAEROBIC BACTERIA: GRAM-NEGATIVE BACILLI

A. *Bacteroides fragilis.* Gram stain of cells in 48-hour thioglycollate broth culture.

B. *B. fragilis.* Colonies on anaerobe blood agar after 48 hours of incubation at 35°C.

C. *Prevotella melaninogenica.* Gram stains of cells from a 48-hour colony on blood agar.

D. *P. melaninogenica.* Black colonies on blood agar after 5 days of incubation at 35°C.

E. *Fusobacterium nucleatum.* Gram stain of cells from a 48-hour colony on anaerobe blood agar. Note long, gram-negative bacilli with pointed ends.

F. *F. nucleatum.* Characteristic colonies on anaerobe blood agar after 48 hours of incubation at 35°C, illustrating the opalescent effect.

G. *F. necrophorum.* Gram stain of cells from a 48-hour colony on anaerobe blood agar. Note pleomorphism.

H. *F. necrophorum.* Colonies on anaerobe blood agar after 48 hours of incubation at 35°C.

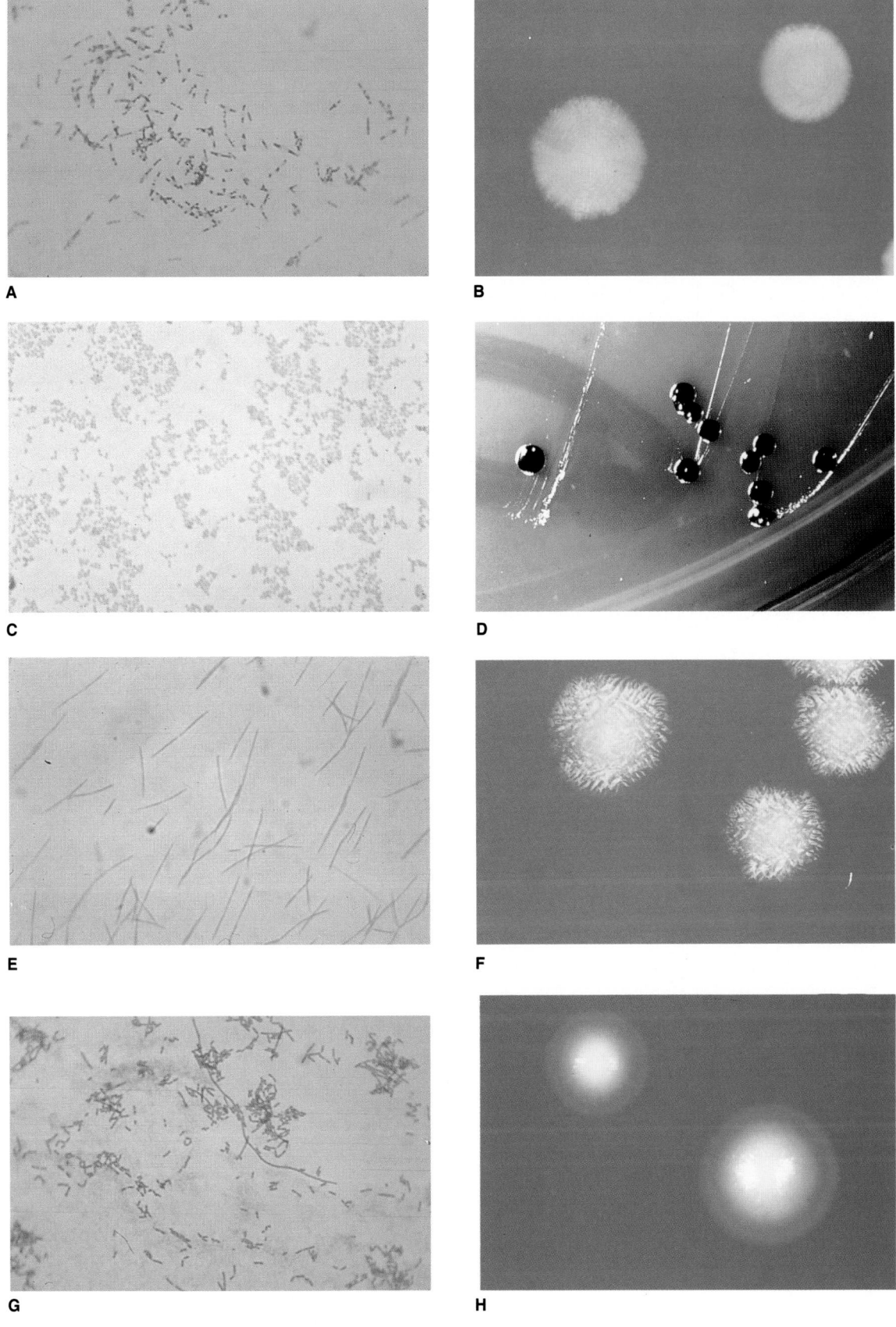

A

B

C

D

E

F

G

H

IDENTIFICATION OF ANAEROBIC BACTERIA: GRAM-POSITIVE, NONSPORING
ORGANISMS

A. Gram-stained direct smear of a purulent exudate showing degenerated neutrophils and a mixture of gram-negative rods of different sizes. The smallest
coccobacilli suggest one of the pigmented *Prevotella-Porphyromonas* species; the
larger, pleomorphic rods suggest a member of the *Bacteroides fragilis* group.

B. Gram-stained direct smear of a purulent exudate from an intra-abdominal abscess showing segmented neutrophils, gram-positive cocci in pairs and short
chains, and tiny gram-negative rods. Anaerobic infections usually contain a
mixed bacterial flora.

C. Dissecting microscope view of actinomycotic "sulfur granules" (×10). (Exudate
from an abdominal wound infection was photographed within a Petri dish.)

D. Appearance of a gram-stained smear from the same specimen as in **C**, showing
"sulfur granule" with thin, branching filaments of an *Actinomyces* species
(×800).

E. *Actinomyces israelii.* Gram-stained preparation of growth from a colony on
blood agar. Note branching of cells.

F. *A. israelii.* Characteristic "molar tooth" colonies produced on brain-heart infusion agar after 7 days of anaerobic incubation at 35°C.

G. *Eubacterium alactolyticum.* Gram stain of cells from growth in enriched thioglycollate broth after 48 hours of incubation at 35°C.

H. *E. alactolyticum.* Forty-eight-hour colonies on anaerobic blood agar.

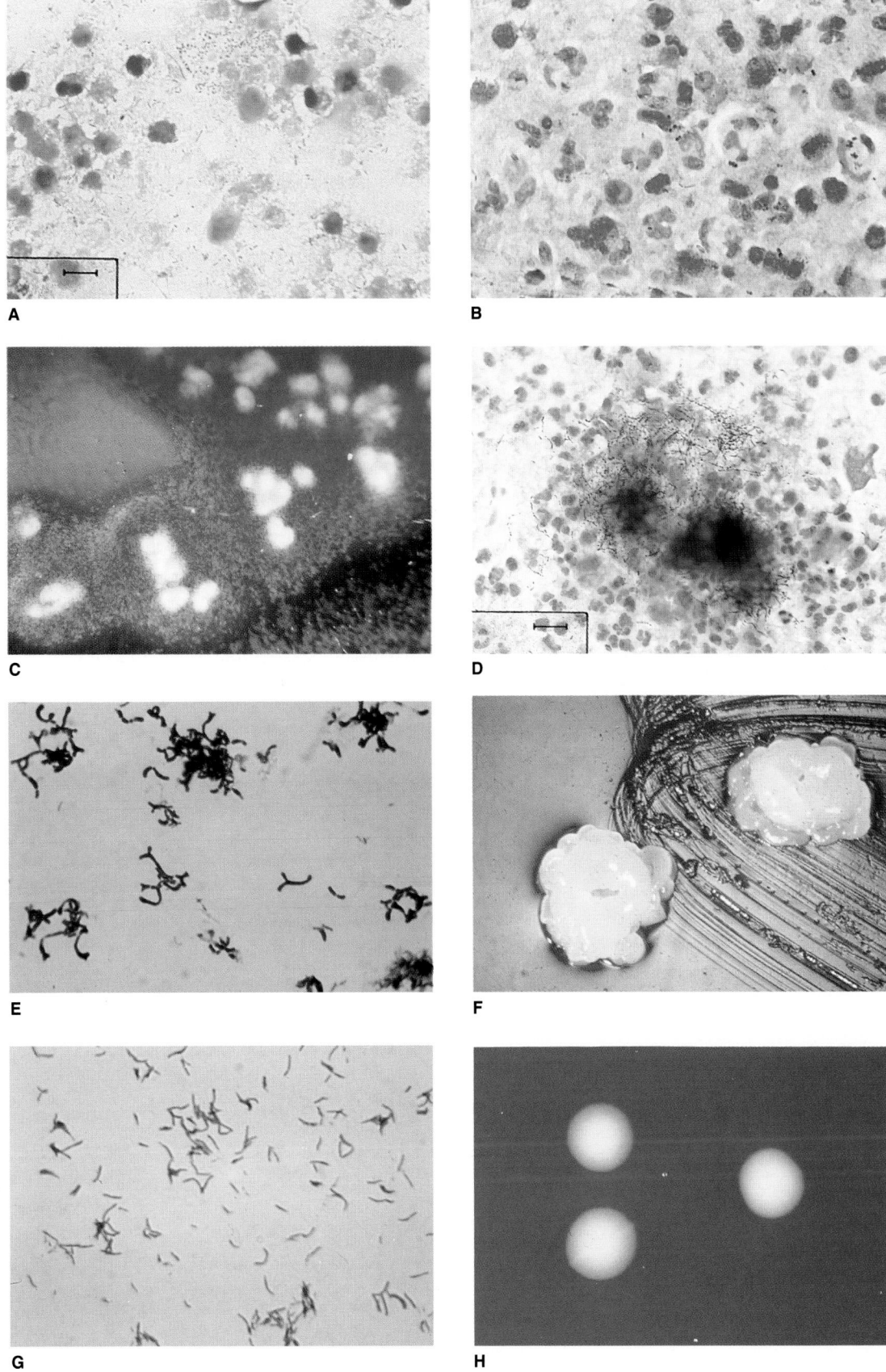

A

B

C

D

E

F

G

H

IDENTIFICATION OF ANAEROBIC BACTERIA: CLOSTRIDIA

A. *Clostridium perfringens.* Gram stain of cells from a 24-hour colony on blood agar. Note lack of spores and of some cells that tend to stain red (gram-negative).

B. *C. perfringens.* Gram stain of cells from a 24-hour thioglycollate broth culture. Note lack of spores and presence of a few filamentous forms.

C. Typical appearance of *C. perfringens* on blood agar after a 24-hour incubation at 35°C. Note the double zone of hemolysis. The inner zone of complete hemolysis is due to theta-toxin and the outer zone of incomplete hemolysis to alpha-toxin (lecithinase activity).

D. *C. perfringens.* Direct Gram stain of a muscle tissue aspirate from a patient with gas gangrene myonecrosis. There is a necrotic background, without intact inflammatory cells or muscle cells, and relatively large "box car"-shaped gram-positive rods and a gram-negative rod that is either a gram-variable *C. perfringens* cell or another organism.

E. Colonies of *C. perfringens* on modified McClung egg yolk agar. The precipitate surrounding the colonies indicates lecithinase activity of alpha-toxin produced by the organism.

F. Lipase production on egg yolk agar. A few clostridia, such as *C. botulinum, C. sporogenes,* and *C. novyi* type A, exhibit lipase activity on egg yolk agar, as shown here. Note the iridescent pearly layer on the surface of the colonies extending onto the surface of the medium immediately surrounding them.

G. *C. septicum.* Rough, irregular, flat, rhizoid, spreading colony on a 48-hour anaerobe blood agar plate.

H. Direct gram-stained smear of a positive blood culture that contained *C. septicum.* Numerous ovoid or citron-shaped, subterminal spores are present.

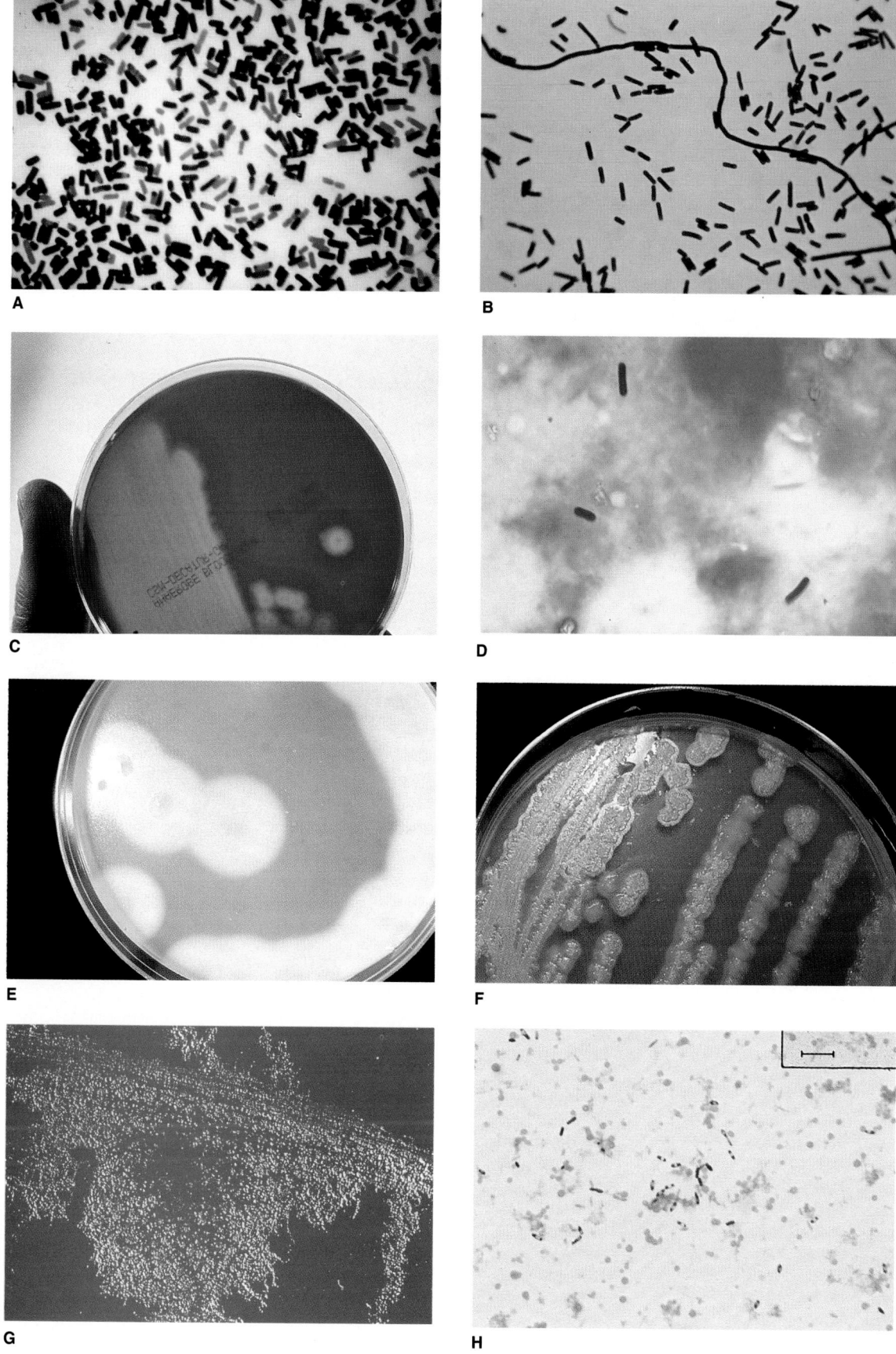

A

B

C

D

E

F

G

H

IDENTIFICATION OF ANAEROBIC BACTERIA: CLOSTRIDIA (CONTINUED)

A. Colonies of *C. tetani* on stiff blood agar (4% agar), which is used to inhibit the swarming of the microorganism so that it can be isolated from other bacteria present in mixed cultures.

B. *C. tetani*. Gram stain of cells from a chopped meat glucose broth culture. Some of the cells have round, terminal spores, which are characteristic of *C. tetani*.

C. *C. sporogenes*. "Medusa-head" colonies on 48-hour anaerobe blood agar.

D. *C. ramosum*. Gram stain from a thioglycollate broth culture after 48 hours of incubation.

E. *C. difficile* on anaerobe blood agar after 48 hours of incubation (original magnification ×2.8).

F. *C. difficile* on cycloserine-cefoxitin fructose agar after 48 hours of incubation.

G. *C. sordellii* on anaerobe blood agar following prolonged anaerobic incubation. Colony is 5 × 10 mm.

H. *C. sordellii*. Gram stain from 2-day-old blood agar plate reveals clumps of free spores and bacteria distended with ovoid subterminal spores.

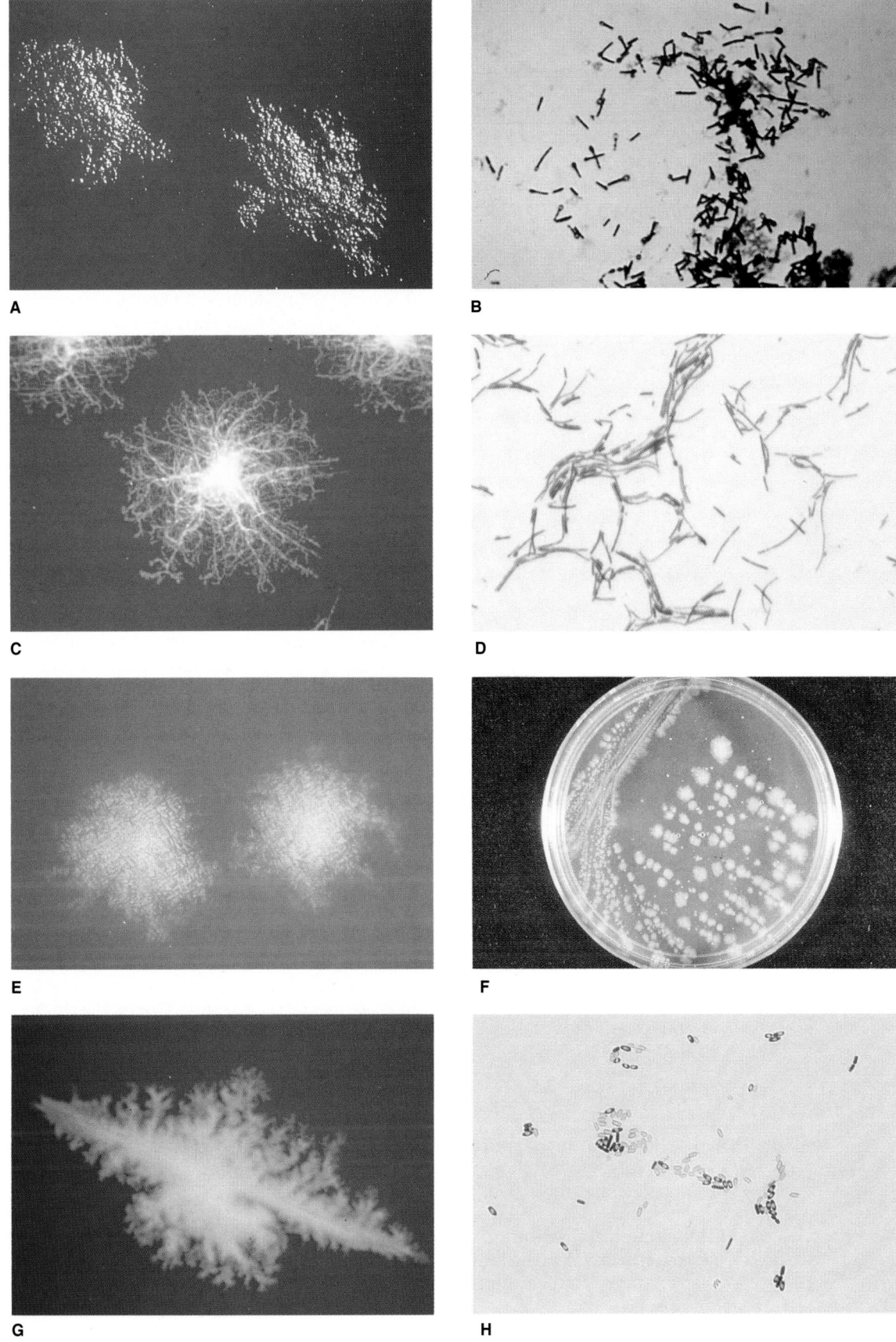

A

B

C

D

E

F

G

H

IDENTIFICATION OF ANAEROBIC BACTERIA: USE OF PRESUMPTO QUADRANT PLATES
AND DISKS ON ANAEROBE BLOOD AGAR

A. Overview appearance of three quadrant plates (described in detail in the text).

B. A Presumpto 1 quadrant plate and a plate of CDC anaerobe blood agar. After inoculation with an active broth culture or cell suspension of the isolate to be identified, antibiotic disks (penicillin, 2 units; rifampin, 15 g; kanamycin, 1000 g) are placed on the blood agar medium, and a blank filter-paper disk is placed on the LD agar portion of the quadrant plate for use in detection of indole production. The Presumpto 1 plate contains the following media: LD agar, LD esculin agar, LD egg yolk agar, and LD bile agar.

C. Growth of *Bacteroides fragilis* on Presumpto 1 plate after 48 hours of incubation at 35°C. On the first quadrant (*top, far right*), LD agar shows moderate growth. Indole production can be detected by adding a drop of paradimethylaminocinnamaldehyde to the paper disk (see **F**). The LD esculin agar to the left of the LD agar is diffusely dark because of the hydrolysis of the esculin.* The LD egg yolk agar underneath the esculin agar shows good growth but no lecithinase, lipase, or proteolytic activity. There is abundant growth in the LD bile agar (*bottom, far right*), and a characteristic precipitate was produced in the medium by this strain.

D. Antibiotic disk tests. A zone of growth inhibition is seen around the 15-g rifampin disk, but no growth inhibition is seen around the 2-unit penicillin disk or the 1000-g kanamycin disk. This pattern is characteristic of the *B. fragilis* group.

E. Reactions of *B. thetaiotamicron* on the Presumpto 1 quadrant plate. The first quadrant (*top, far right*) shows a weak, positive indole reaction, as indicated by the pale blue color of the disk on LD agar after addition of paradimethylaminocinnamaldehyde reagent. Black (amber) appearance of esculin agar (*left of first quadrant*) indicates esculin hydrolysis. There is adequate growth but no lecithinase, lipase, or proteolysis on LD egg yolk agar (*bottom, far left*). There is good growth on LD bile agar but no precipitate as exhibited by *B. fragilis* (*bottom, far right*).

F. Reactions of *Fusobacterium necrophorum* on the Presumpto 1 quadrant plate after 48 hours of incubation at 35°C. The first quadrant (*bottom, far right*) shows strong indole reaction as evidenced by the dark blue color of the paper disk on LD agar after the addition of paradimethylaminocinnamaldehyde reagent. Growth is inhibited on LD bile agar (*top, right*). Although not visible in this photograph because of the lighting arrangement, there is good growth in LD egg yolk agar (*top, far left*) and characteristic lipase activity as evidenced by an iridescent sheen—a pearly layer—on the surface of the colonies and in the medium immediately surrounding the bacterial growth. This is best demonstrated with reflected light. On LD esculin agar (*bottom, left*), the *F. necrophorum* shows good growth and hydrogen sulfide production, as evidenced by the black appearance of the colonies, but no darkening of the medium to suggest esculin hydrolysis.

G. Presumpto 2 quadrant plate (uninoculated). The plate contains the following quadrants: LD starch agar, LD glucose agar, LD-DNA agar, and LD milk agar (*clockwise, starting at 12 o'clock with LD starch agar*).

H. Presumpto 2 quadrant plate following inoculation, incubation, and addition of reagents. Note positive reactions for hydrolysis, deoxyribonuclease activity, and glucose fermentation.

In these photographs, the LD esculin agar appears black on hydrolysis of esculin owing to the black background. In transmitted light, the agar appears deep amber when esculin is hydrolyzed.

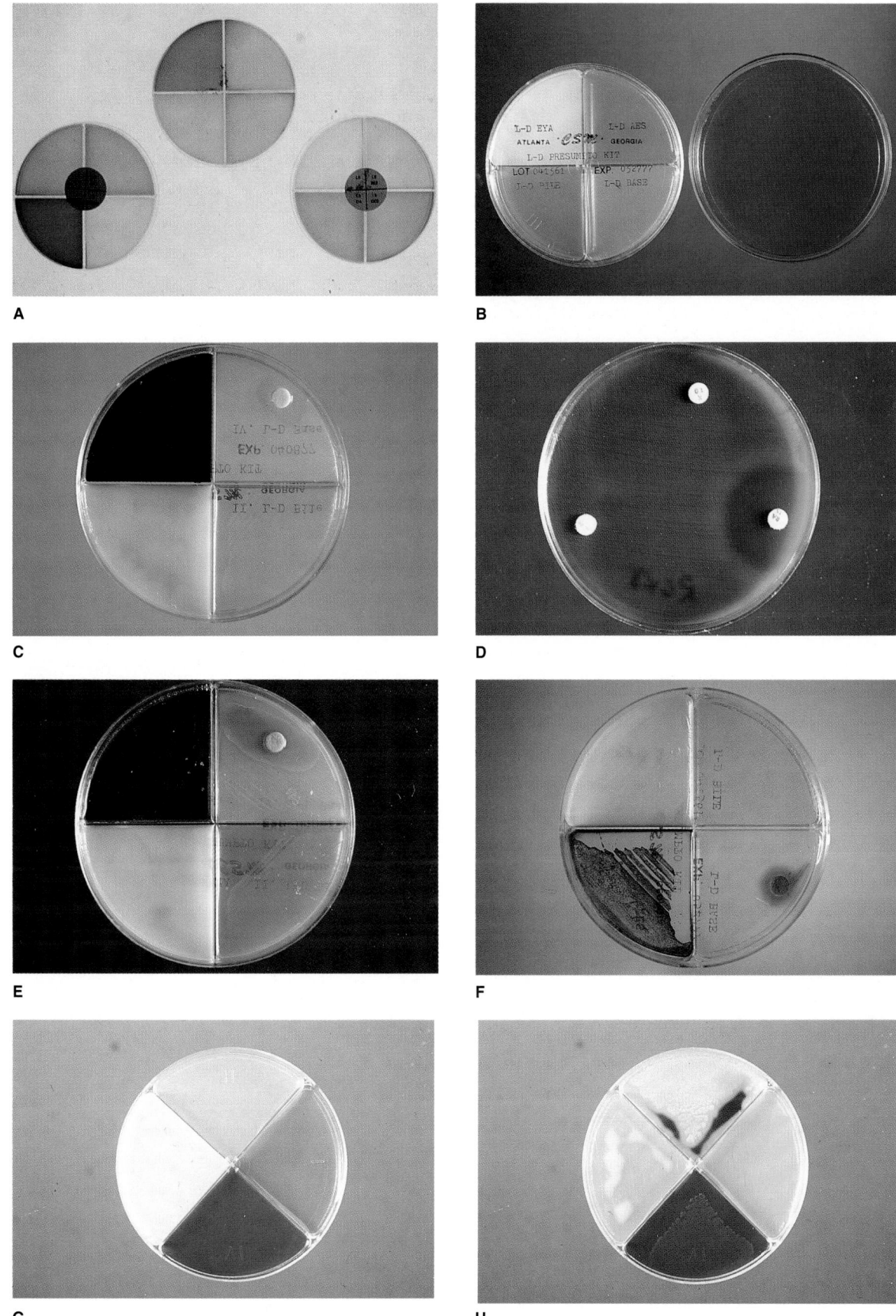

A

B

C

D

E

F

G

H

HUMAN MYCOPLASMAS

A. Colony of *M. pneumoniae* on mycoplasma agar. This picture shows a single colony to which guinea pig red blood cells have become adsorbed. *M. pneumoniae* is the only species that demonstrates this hemadsorbing property. (Photo courtesy of Health and Education Resources, Inc., Bethesda, MD)

B. Colonies of *M. hominis* and *U. urealyticum* growing on Shepard's A7B differential agar. *M. hominis* colonies have the typical "fried egg" morphology; the blue color is due to the Diene's stain. *U. urealyticum* colonies are smaller, more dense, and have a brownish coloration because of urease activity, which results in precipitation of manganese oxide in the colony. (Photo courtesy of Health and Education Resources, Inc., Bethesda, MD)

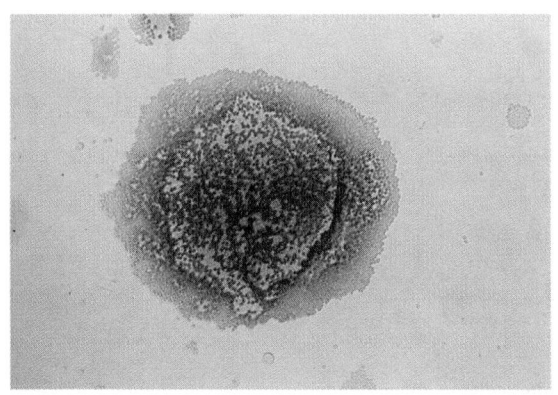 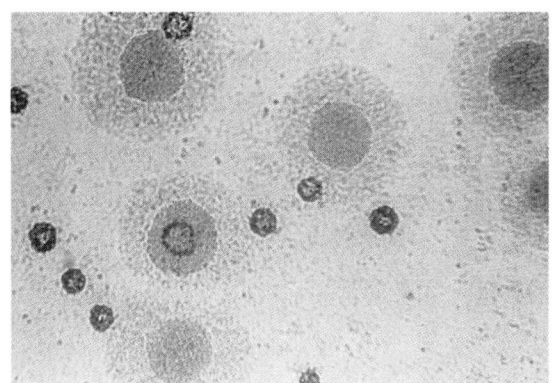

A   B

THE LABORATORY IDENTIFICATION OF *MYCOBACTERIUM TUBERCULOSIS*

A. Photomicrograph of a smear prepared from a colony similar to that illustrated in Color Panel **C**, stained with auramine–rhodamine. Note the bright yellow fluorescence of the very short, slightly curved bacilli. Although the cellular morphology is suggestive of *M. tuberculosis*, examination under higher-power optics and culture confirmation must be made before a definitive species identification can be made.

B. Photomicrograph of a Kinyoun acid-fast stain of a smear prepared from material obtained from a necrotic tuberculoma of the lung. Note the relatively short, thin, beaded, slightly curved, red-staining acid-fast bacilli. Although species identifications cannot be made from acid-fast smears alone, the appearance here is highly consistent with *M. tuberculosis*.

C. A microcolony growing on the surface of Middlebrook 7H10 agar, observed microscopically under low-power optics. Note that the bacterial cells are arranged in an undulating, serpiginous pattern. This indicates the production of cording factor, as illustrated in the acid-fast stain shown in Color Plate 17-1I.

D. A niacin accumulation test: The tubes contain a filter paper strip impregnated with cyanogen bromide. The fluid in the tube on the *right* had been extracted from the surface of Lowenstein-Jensen culture medium after colonial growth of an unknown *Mycobacterium* species, compared with a negative water control on the left. The development of a yellow color on the strip and in the underlying fluid indicates the presence of niacin. *M. tuberculosis* has the unique property of accumulating niacin when colonies are grown on Lowenstein-Jensen medium, a property shared by the less commonly encountered *M. simiae* and occasional strains of *M. marinum*.

E. Tubes illustrating the nitrate reduction test: The tube on the *right* had been inoculated with an unknown *Mycobacterium* species compared with an uninoculated control on the *left*. The development of a red color after addition of sulfonamide and α-naphthylethylenediamine reagents indicates the presence of nitrites and a positive test. *M. tuberculosis* is an active nitrate reducer.

F. A quadrant plate containing Middlebrook 7H10 agar in which thiophene-2-carboxylic acid hydrazide (T_2H) had been incorporated. The three quadrants in which growth is observed are different strains of *M. tuberculosis* (resistant to T_2H); the quadrant without growth was inoculated with a strain of *M. bovis*. The ability to grow or not grow on medium containing T_2H is helpful in separating *M. tuberculosis* from *M. bovis*, respectively.

G. A flask of Lowenstein-Jensen medium on which are growing colonies of *M. tuberculosis* after a 22-day incubation at 35°C in a 10% CO_2 incubator. The colonies seen here are distinctly rough in consistency; however, they have more of a yellow pigmentation than the buff-colored colonies usually observed.

H. Colonies of a subculture of *M. tuberculosis* growing on Middlebrook 7H10 agar after a 25-day incubation at 35°C in 10% CO_2 incubator. The colonies have a rough, buff appearance, characteristic for the species.

I. Photomicrograph of a Kinyoun acid-fast stain prepared from the broth of a BACTEC 12A blood culture vial after a 10-day incubation at 35°C. Numerous acid-fast bacilli are seen, arranged in parallel sheaths. When the aggregation of bacterial cells, as illustrated here, is observed in smears prepared from a broth preparation, one can make a presumptive identification of *M. tuberculosis*, because the phenomenon is due to the production of cording factor, thought to be a virulence factor.

J. Photomicrograph of a Gram stain prepared from a smear of pleural fluid from a case of empyema in a patient with AIDS. Note the relatively long, slender, delicately beaded, poorly staining bacilli. Because of their thick waxy outer coating, the bacterial cells of mycobacteria do not stain well with gentian violet, the primary stain used in the Gram stain. Note the distinct halo around the bacilli, a clue that the organism is encapsulated and suggestive of a *Mycobacterium* species. *M. tuberculosis* grew out in culture in this case.

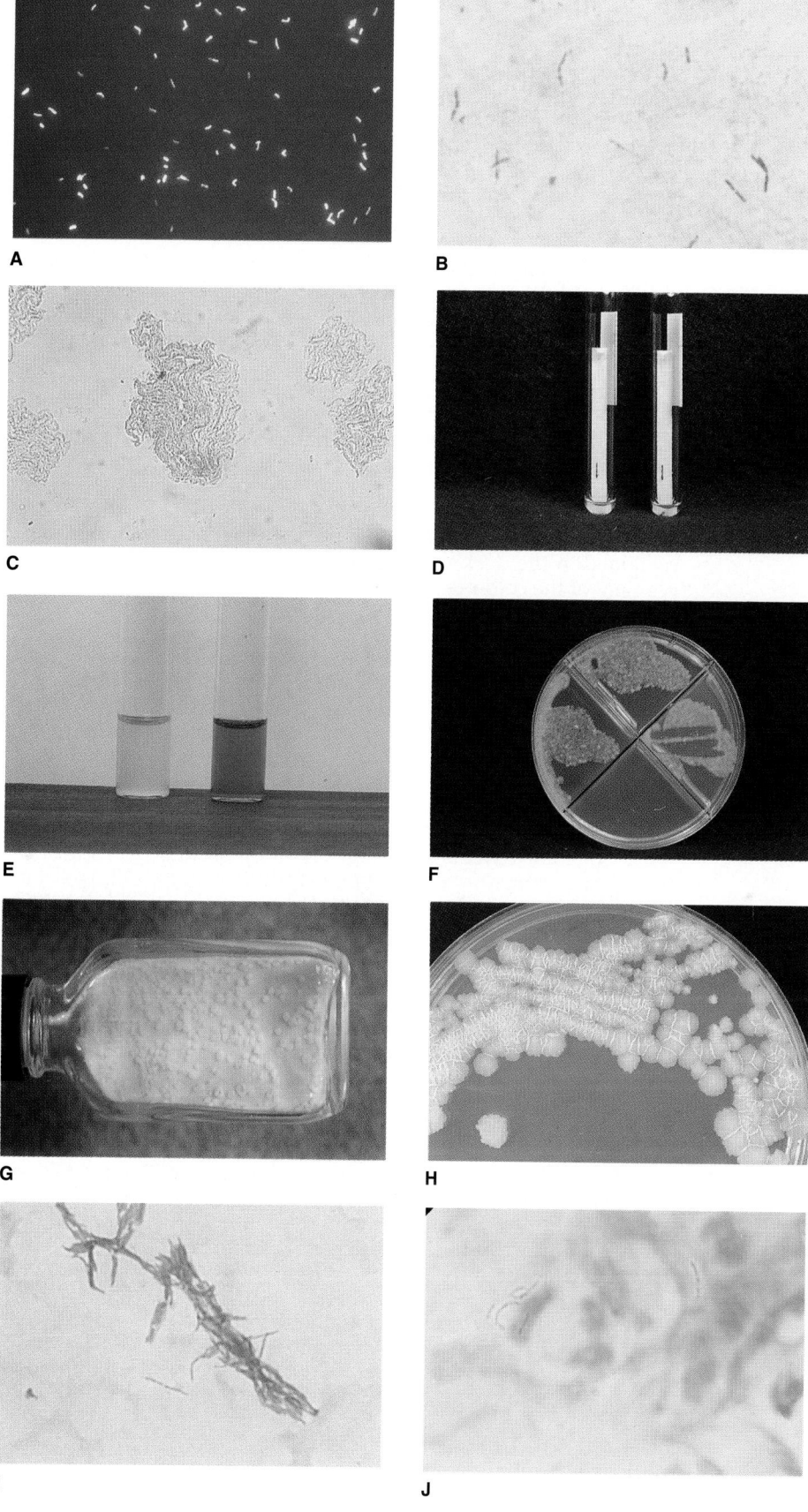

A

B

C

D

E

F

G

H

I

J

LABORATORY IDENTIFICATION OF *MYCOBACTERIUM* SPECIES OTHER THAN
M. TUBERCULOSIS

A. Photomicrograph of microcolonies of *M. avium* growing on Middlebrook 7H10 agar after a 6-day incubation at 35°C in 10% CO_2: The flat, thin, translucent microcolonies, with a central darker umbonate elevation, suggestive of a fried egg, are characteristic of the smooth strains of *M. avium* commonly recovered from AIDS patients. The observation of this type of microcolony may be helpful in directing one to perform an *M. avium–intracellulare* nucleic acid probe in the rapid culture confirmation of an unknown isolate.

B. Close-in photomicrograph of a single microcolony of *M. avium–intracellulare,* again illustrating the thin, translucent colony described in Color Plate 17-2**A**: The rhizoid-like peripheral extensions, as illustrated here, are often seen and provide an added clue to the presumptive identification of *M. avium–intracellulare* complex organisms.

C. Two Middlebrook 7H10 agar plates, each inoculated with the same subculture of *M. kansasii:* The plate on the *left* was exposed to light; the one on the *right* remained in the dark until just before the photograph was taken. The yellow pigment of the colonies in the light-exposed plate is characteristic of a photochromogen.

D. Two Middlebrook 7H10 agar plates each inoculated with the same subculture of *M. scrofulaceum:* The plate on the *left* was exposed to light; the one on the *right* remained in the dark until just before the photograph was taken. The yellow pigment of the colonies in both the light-exposed and non–light-exposed plates is characteristic of a scotochromogen.

E. A Middlebrook 7H10 agar plate previously inoculated with a strain of *M. gordonae: M. gordonae* is a scotochromogen and characteristically produces a deep yellow pigment, as illustrated here.

F. Several tubes containing varying concentrations of buffered sodium nitrate inoculated with various strains of *Mycobacterium* species to illustrate 1+ (*second tube from left*) through 4+ (*right-hand tube*) reactions: Red color develops after the addition of sulfanilamide and N-naphthylethylenediamine reagents, the intensity of color reflecting the concentration of nitrites produced. The quantitative nitrate reduction test may be helpful in differentiating strains of *M. tuberculosis* (4+ positive) from *M. bovis* (1+ positive) and *M. kansasii* (4+) positive from other photochromogens (negative to 1+ positive).

G. Two tubes containing Tween-80 reagent: The *left* tube had been inoculated with a negative control strain, the tube on the *right* with a subculture of *M. kansasii.* The development of a red color (*right tube*) after incubation for 3 to 10 days is a positive test, indicating the ability of the test strain to hydrolyze Tween 80. The color change from yellow to red in this assay is not due to a shift in pH, rather it results from a change in optical density as oleic acid and polyolxyethylated sorbitol are produced as breakdown products of Tween hydrolysis.

H. Two tubes of Lowenstein-Jensen deeps previously inoculated with a catalase-negative control (*left tube*) and a subculture of *M. kansasii* (*right tube*): Note the tall area of bubble formation in the right tube after addition of hydrogen peroxide to the surface of the agar, exceeding 45 mm, indicative of a positive test and strong catalase activity.

I. A positive catalase test: Immediately before the photograph was taken, a few drops of hydrogen peroxide were placed on isolated colonies of the photochromogenic colonies of *M. kansasii.* The evolution of rapid bubbles, as illustrated here, indicates a positive test indicating active catalase activity.

J. Two tubes of Dubos broth base, the *right* containing tripotassium phenolphthalein disulfate reagent (arylsulfatase reagent) compared with a negative control tube on the *left* devoid of reagent: Both tubes had been previously inoculated with a subculture of a strain of *M. fortuitum.* The development of a pink color after addition of sodium carbonate reagent in the *left* tube indicates a positive test and arylsulfatase activity of the test strain.

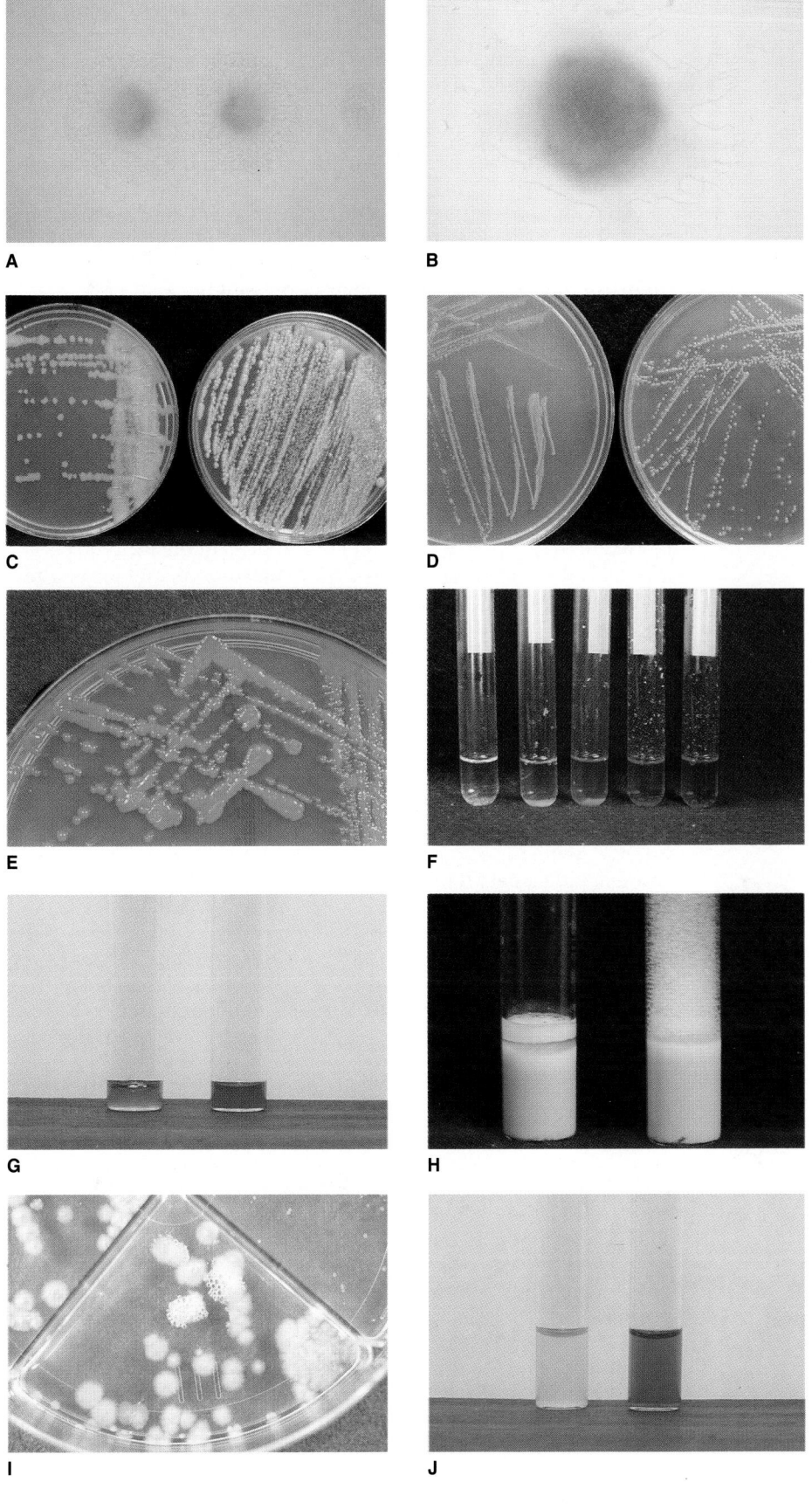

A

B

C

D

E

F

G

H

I

J

K. Two tubes of urea broth previously inoculated with a negative control (*left tube*) and a subculture of *M. gordonae* (*right*): Mycobacterial strains having urease activity will turn the broth a pink within several hours (strong positive) to a few days, owing to the release of ammonia and alkalinization of the medium. Assessment of urease activity may be helpful in separating *M. gordonae* (strong positive) from other scotochromogens, and *M. fortuitum–chelonae* complex from other rapid growers.

L. Two tubes of Dubos broth base, the *left* containing pyrazinamide and the *right* tube a negative control devoid of reagent: Both tubes had previously been inoculated with a subculture of a strain of *M. avium*. The development of a pink-red band at the reagent layer toward the surface of the agar in the *left* tube, after addition of ferrous ammonium sulfate reagent, indicates a positive test and the ability of this strain to deaminate pyrazinamide.

M. Photomicrograph of an acid-fast smear prepared from a subculture of *M. kansasii*: The bacterial cells of *M. kansasii* are described as rectangular, straight, and banded, which is reasonably represented here. Because of variation between strains and between other species, a presumptive identification of *Mycobacterium* species based on acid-fast stain morphology is risky at best.

N. A Middlebrook 7H10 agar plate previously inoculated with a subculture of a classic strain of *M. avium*: The classic strains of *M. avium* were originally included in the group III nonphotochromogens in the Runyon classification. Note that the colonies here are relatively small, smooth, and gray-white, without evidence of pigmentation.

O. A Middlebrook 7H10 agar plate previously inoculated with a strain of *M. avium–intracellulare* (MAI) complex recovered from a patient with AIDS. Many of the MAI strains recovered from patients with AIDS have this distinct yellow pigmentation. The peculiar doughnut-shaped colonies have been produced by most of the strains recovered at the Denver Veterans Hospital during the early 1990s, but is probably not a distinctive characteristic for all strains.

P. Low-power photomicrograph of a liver biopsy from a patient with AIDS also infected with *M. avium–intracellulare*: Note the tight intracellular clusters of short, acid-fast bacilli in the central part of the photograph.

Q. A Middlebrook 7H10 agar plate inoculated 3 days before with a strain of *M. fortuitum* and incubated at 35°C in 10% CO_2: The colonies average 1 to 2 mm in diameter, are entire, smooth, moist, and devoid of pigmentation. The *M. fortuitum–chelonae* complex of organisms were originally assigned to Runyoun group IV, the rapid growers.

R. A modified MacConkey agar plate (devoid of crystal violet) on which are growing colonies taken from a subculture of *M. fortuitum*: Strains belonging to the *M. fortuitum–chelonae* have the unique ability to grow on modified MacConkey agar. The colonies average 2 mm in diameter, are entire, moist, and have a slight pink-yellow tinge, pigment derived from the agar.

S. A 5% sheep blood agar plate with a 48-hour growth of *M. fortuitum*: Strains belonging to the *M. fortuitum–chelonae* complex will grow on routine 5% sheep blood agar within 48 to 72 hours and may cause confusion with other gram-positive bacillary organisms if a partial acid-fast stain is not performed.

T. Photomicrograph of a Gram stain of a smear prepared from an isolated colony illustrated in Color Plate 17-2**H**: The bacterial cells appear as short, slender almost filamentous, faintly staining gram-positive coccobacilli. Microscopists must be alerted to this microscopic picture and not make a presumptive misidentification of an *Actinomyces* species or atypical corynebacterium. A partial acid-fast stain of a second smear will be helpful in making the correct identification.

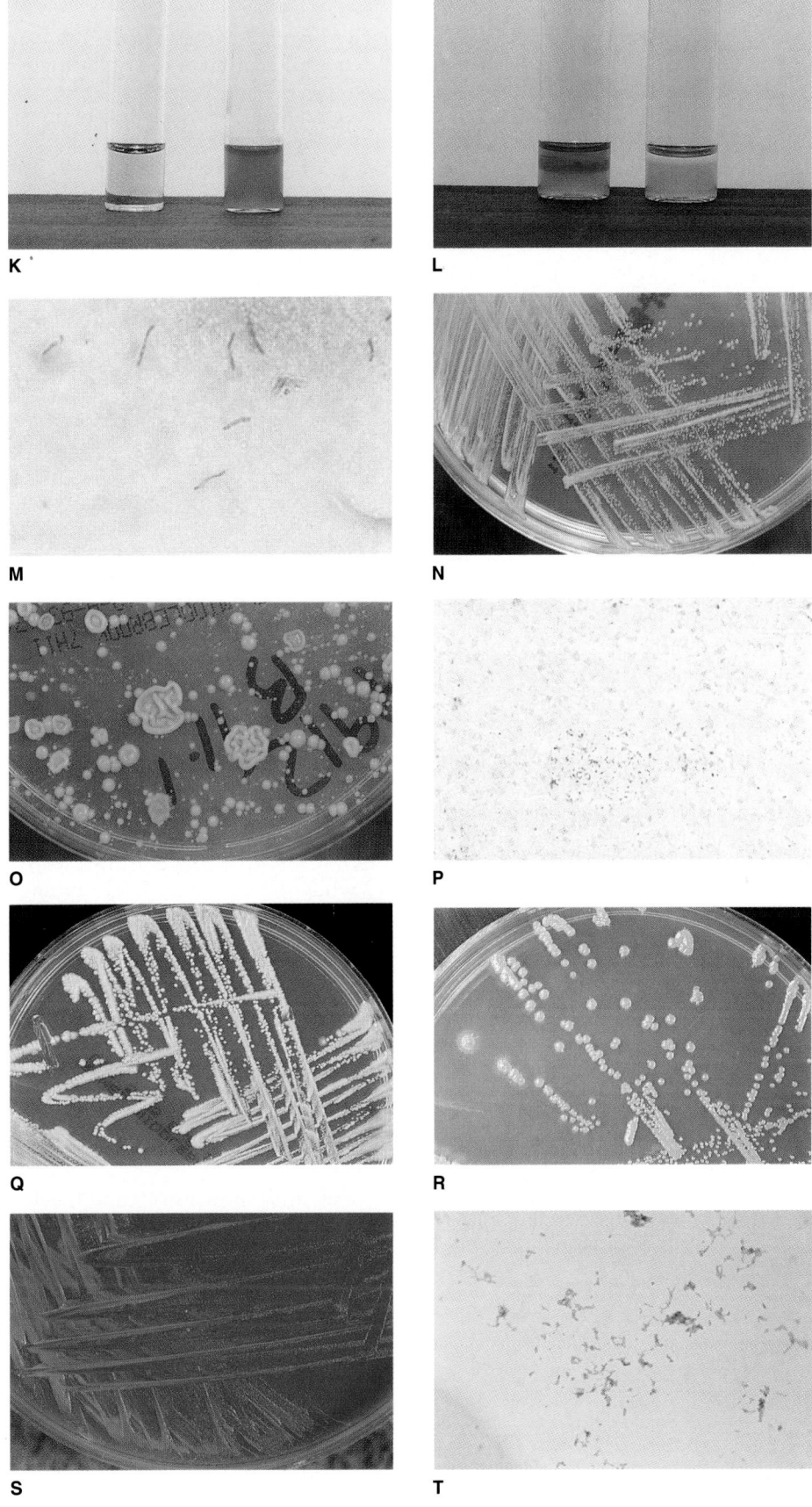

K

L

M

N

O

P

Q

R

S

T

CLINICAL MANIFESTATIONS OF SELECT MYCOBACTERIAL DISEASES

A. Photograph of an X-ray of the chest from a patient with pulmonary tuberculosis. Note the extensive area of dense infiltration of the right upper lobe.

B. A solitary nodular lesion with well-defined margins is seen in the upper segment of the *left lower* lung field. A coin lesion of pulmonary coccidioidomycosis must be included in the differential diagnosis of such a lesion. This turned out to be a tuberculoma.

C. A resected lobe of lung illustrating centrally a well-circumscribed, 2.5-cm–diameter, white, firm-appearing nodule. This histologically was a tuberculoma, similar to what may have been removed from the patient whose chest radiograph is shown in Frame **B**.

D. Photomicrograph of a hematoxylin and eosin-stained section taken through a tuberculoma illustrating varying degrees of background fibrosis and a cellular infiltration composed of lymphocytes and macrophages, many of the latter forming characteristic Langhans giant cells.

E. The base of the brain in a patient dying with tuberculous meningitis: The pia arachnoid covering the base of the brain, particularly in the area of the optic chiasm, appears cloudy, as a manifestation of the chronic inflammatory reaction.

F. A case of cutaneous tuberculosis of the fifth digit: The lesion shown here appears active and inflammatory. In fact, a radiograph revealed bone and joint involvement of the middle and distal phalanx. Lesions of the fingers similar to that shown here were, at one time, common among individuals who milked cows.

G. This posterior neck demonstrates an enlarged, postauricular lymph node with healed draining sinuses along the route of the lymphatic drainage: This is a classic picture of "scrofula" or tuberculous lymphadenitis, typically caused by *M. scrofulaceum* and other mycobacteria other than *M. tuberculosis*. The route of infection is oral, and commonly occurs in two age groups during periods of teething—young children 3 to 7 when secondary teeth are coming in and in the late teens when molars are being cut.

H. The anterior portion of the neck illustrating multiple healed sinus tracts in a case of chronic tuberculous lymphadenitis. Again, the route of infection is oral, with drainage of infecting mycobacteria along the lymphatic channels.

I. Low-power photomicrograph of a section of small bowel stained with a carbol-fuchsin-based acid-fast stain: The pink mottling seen in the submucosa is dense aggregates of acid-fast bacilli from a case of intestinal tuberculosis caused by *M. avium–intracellulare* in a patient with AIDS.

J. High-power photomicrograph of an area shown in Frame **I**, better illustrating the dense intracellular aggregates of acid-fast bacilli. This histopathologic picture is similar to the "lepra cells" seen in patients with Hanson's disease (leprosy).

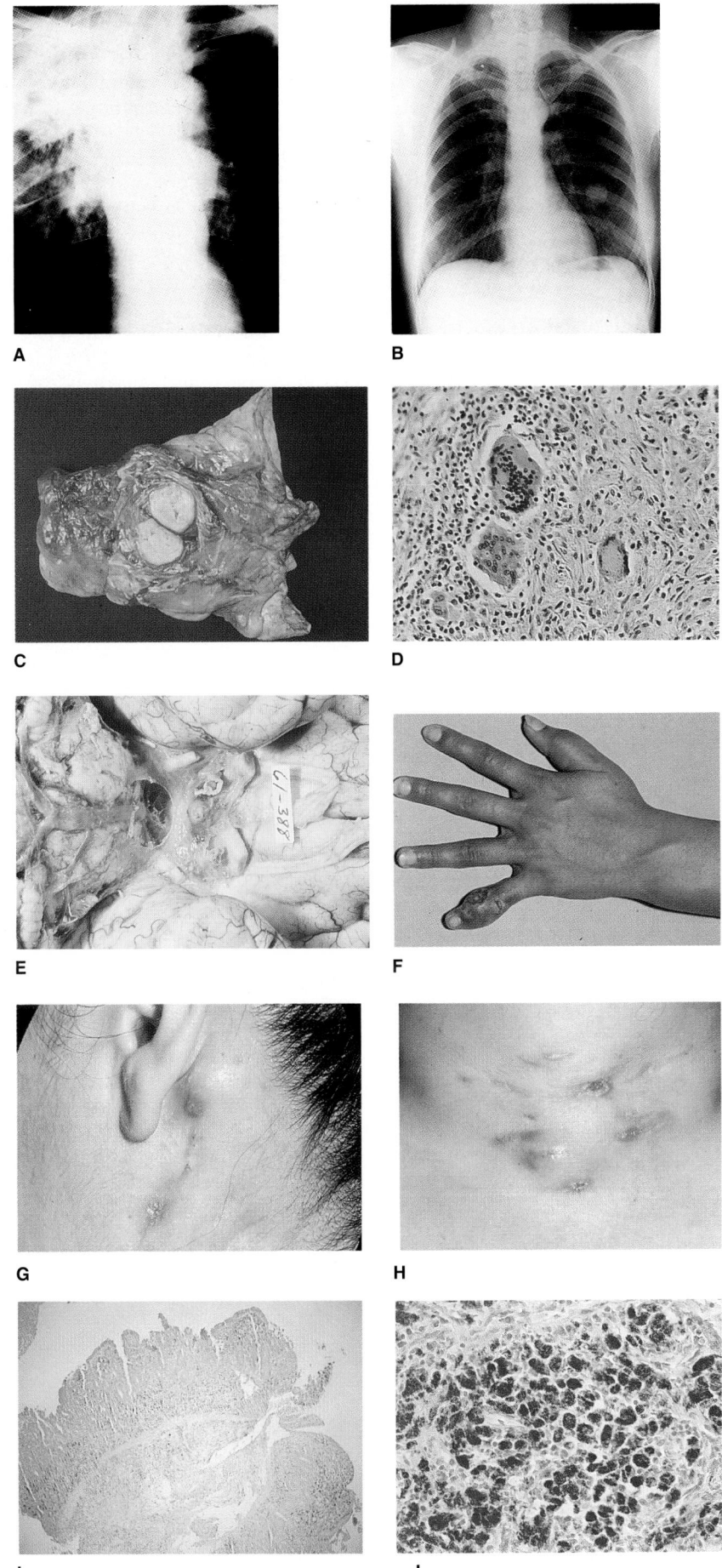

LABORATORY DIAGNOSIS OF SPIROCHETAL DISEASES

A. *Treponema pallidum:* This photomicrograph shows a Warthin-Starry stain of a histologic section of placenta from a case of congenital syphilis. The tight spiral coils of the spirochete are clearly evident (original magnification ×1000).

B. *Treponema pallidum:* This control for the FTA-ABS test demonstrates 4+ staining of the spirochetes. The helical shape is evident, and the tightly coiled spirals can be visualized in some of the bacterial cells. This photomicrograph is an indirect immunofluorescence preparation of *T. pallidum* using fluorescein-conjugated antihuman globulin (original magnification ×600). (Courtesy of Burton Wilcke, PhD and Mary Celotti, Vermont Department of Public Health)

C. Wright-stained peripheral blood smear from a case of *Borrelia* infection: The loose coils of the *Borrelia* organisms are evident, but the thin structure is easy to overlook. These spirochetes may be detected when examining smears for malaria or for cellular morphology, even if the physician does not suspect the diagnosis (original magnification ×1000). (Courtesy of Thomas Fritsche, MD, PhD)

D. An acridine orange stain of peripheral blood demonstrates *Borrelia* spp. dramatically. If the diagnosis is suspected, this technique, which may be more sensitive than Giemsa or Wright's stains, may be employed (original magnification ×1000). (Courtesy of Brian Lauer, MD)

E. *Ixodes scapularis* (*dammini*) tick: This adult female hard-bodied tick contains a dorsal shield and a clearly visible capitulum. *I. scapularis* is the most common vector of Lyme disease in the eastern United States. When the spirochete is transmitted by the larval and nymphal stages, the patient is less likely to recognize the event than when the adult is the vector. (Courtesy of Paul Duray, MD)

F. *Borrelia burgdorferi* in a culture pellet stained with a monoclonal antibody to OspA protein conjugated to streptavidin–alkaline phosphatase. The typical polymorphism of *B. burgdorferi* is demonstrated. (Courtesy of Paul Duray, MD)

G. A histologic section of dog kidney stained with a silver impregnation stain (Warthin-Starry) demonstrates several renal tubules in longitudinal orientation. Even at low power, the masses of *Leptospira* organisms are evident as blackening of the surface of the tubular epithelium. It is clear that this privileged site, where the leptospires are protected from host defenses, can serve as a productive source for spread of infection as the leptospira-contaminated urine is passed onto the ground (original magnification ×1000). (Courtesy of David Miller, DVM, MS)

H. Tubes of polysorbate 80–bovine albumin (PSO-BA) semisolid medium: An uninoculated tube is shown on the *left*. The tube on the *right* was inoculated with *Leptospira interrogans*. The subsurface growth in semisolid culture media is typical of leptospires, such as *L. interrogans* sv. *pomona*. Growth appears as a gray-white horizontal band about 1 cm below the medium surface after incubation for 2 to 6 weeks at room temperature. The band grows denser with continued incubation, but may be very scant with fastidious isolates, such as with *L. interrogans* sv. *hardjo.* (Courtesy of David Miller, DVM, MS)

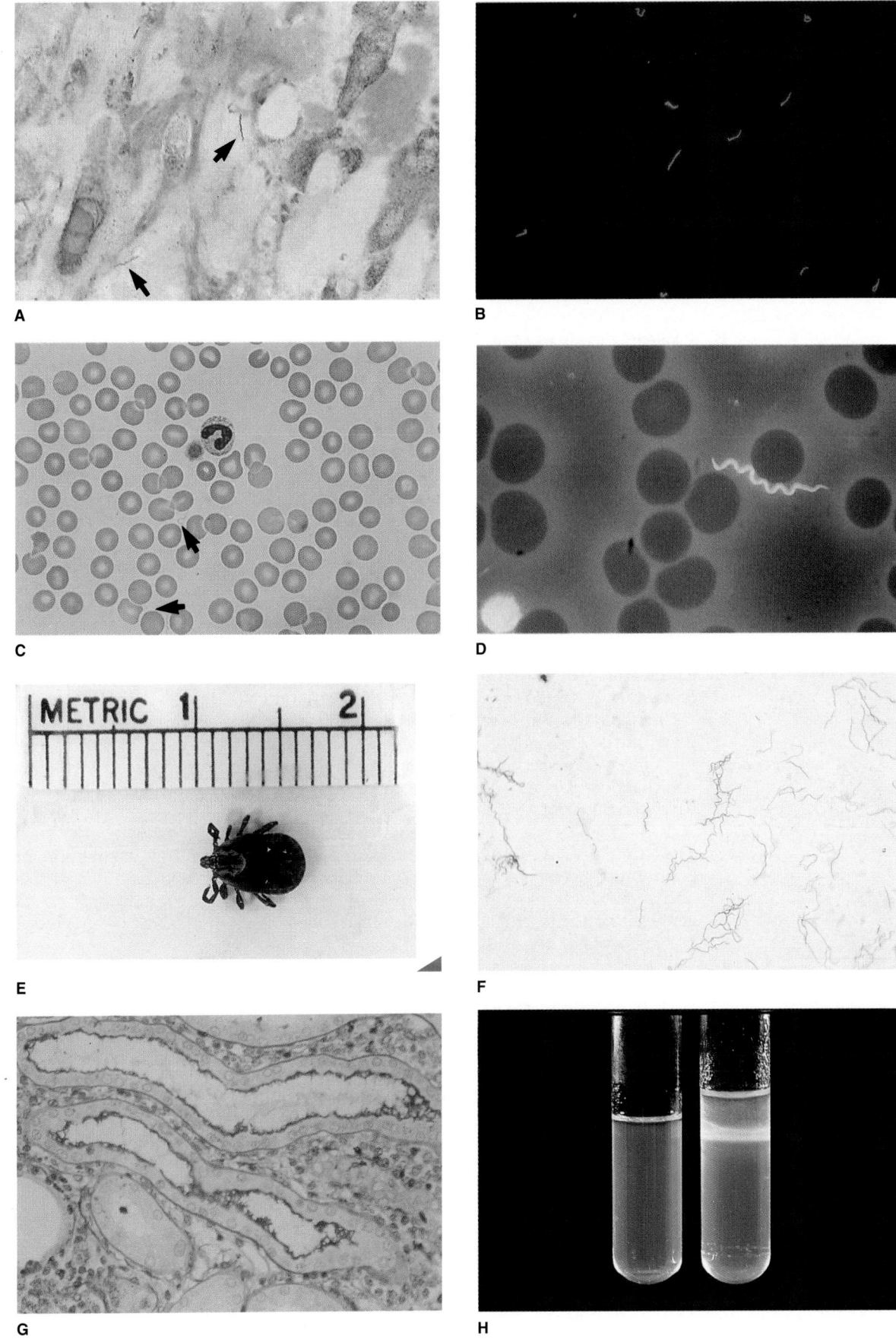

A

B

C

D

E

F

G

H

COLONY MORPHOLOGY OF *ZYGOMYCETES* SPECIES AND SELECT *ASPERGILLUS* SPECIES

Members of the *Zygomycetes* and certain *Aspergillus* species are commonly encountered in clinical laboratories as agents of opportunistic infections. These fungi grow rapidly in culture, particularly the *Zygomycetes* species, which can fill a culture plate within 48 hours. Of the aspergilli, *A. fumigatus*, *A. flavus*, *A. niger*, and *A. terreus* are most commonly recovered from specimens obtained from patients with aspergillosis. Other species, when recovered, are usually not identified to the species level. *A. nidulans* and *A. glaucus* are two uncommonly encountered species that often produce cleistothecia, the telomorphic form that contain ascospores.

A. A Sabouraud's dextrose agar plate inoculated with a *Zygomyces* species: Notice that the entire plate is filled with a wooly, gray-white surface mycelium.

B. Close in view of a colony of a *Zygomyces* species after 96 hours of incubation: As a *Zygomyces* species colony matures, it takes on a gray-brown color, often with black, pepperlike stipples, indicating the production sporangia.

C. The surface of a colony of *Aspergillus fumigatus* after a 5-day incubation on Sabouraud's dextrose agar: Mature colonies of *A. fumigatus* are generally powdery or granular, and have some shade of green from the production of pigmented conidia. The growing margin often appears as a white apron, as illustrated here.

D. The surface of a colony of *Aspergillus flavus* growing on Sabouraud's dextrose agar: The texture of mature colonies is usually granular from the production of conidia; and, as the species name suggests, some shade of yellow pigmentation is characteristic.

E. The surface of a colony of *Aspergillus niger* after a 4-day incubation on Sabouraud's dextrose agar: The deep brown to black, densely stippled surface is characteristic. The black surface pigmentation of *A. niger* can be distinguished from one of the dematiaceous fungi by observing the reverse side. The reverse of *A. niger* is a light gray or buff color as the pigmentation is caused by surface conidia; the reverse of dematiaceous fungi is jet black, as the vegetative hyphae carry the pigment.

F. The surface of a colony of *Aspergillus terreus* after a 6-day incubation on Sabouraud's dextrose agar: *A. terreus* characteristically has a granular surface and some shade of yellow or brown pigmentation. Rugae radiating from the center are often seen, and the concentric zones of light and dark pigmentation as seen here are not unusual.

G. The surface of an albino strain of *Aspergillus nidulans*: Although most strains have some light pigmentation, albino strains of most *Aspergillus* species may occasionally be encountered and must be kept in the differential identification. The granular surface, with radiating rugae, is also common.

H. The surface of a colony of *Aspergillus glaucus:* The green and yellow variegated appearance seen here is not specific, because other *Aspergillus* species may have a similar appearance. Microscopic examination is necessary to make a species identification.

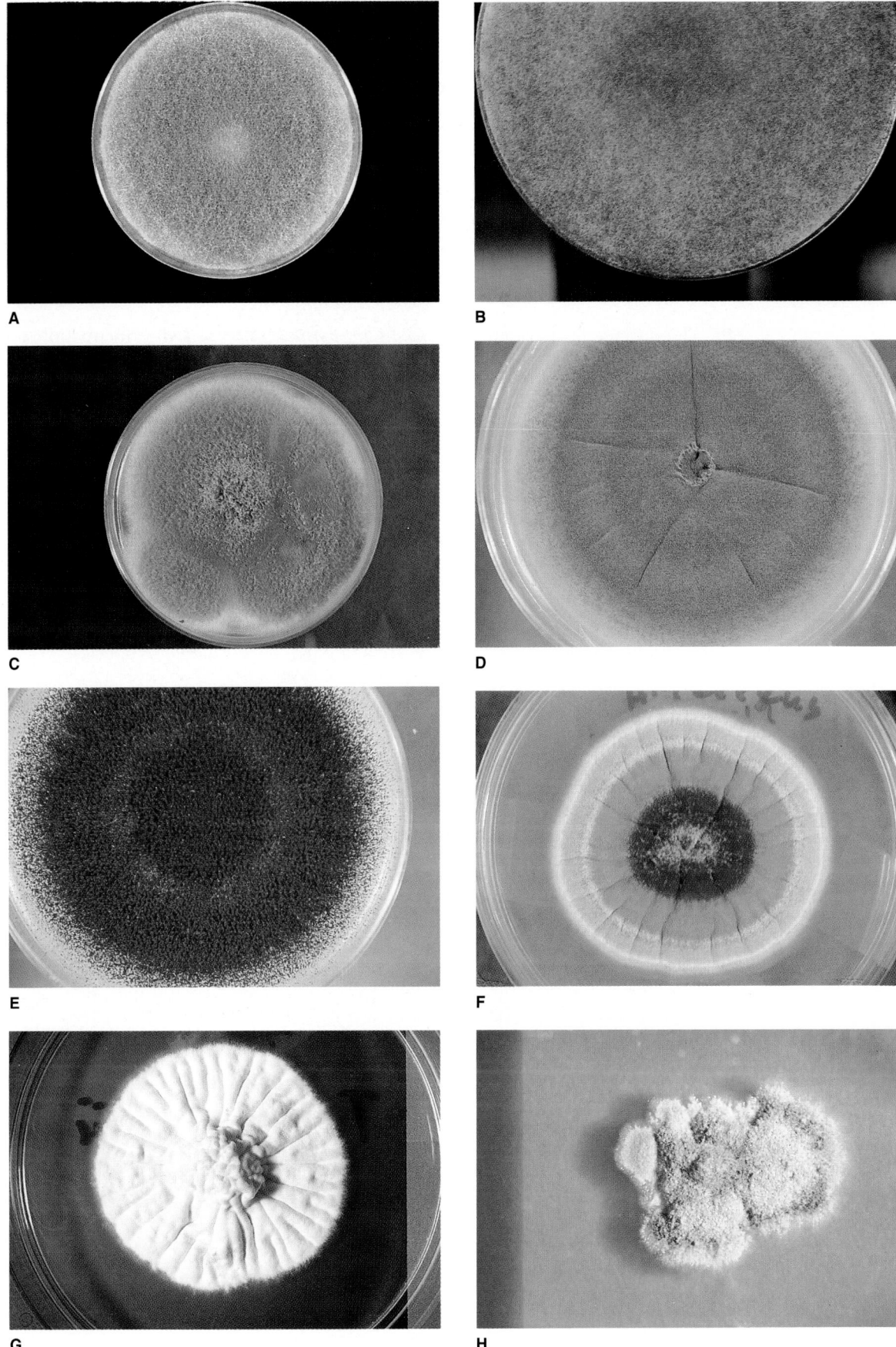

A

B

C

D

E

F

G

H

COLONY MORPHOLOGY OF COMMONLY ENCOUNTERED HYALINE MOLDS

The colonies of the hyaline fungi have a varied appearance. Most display light pastel or deeper pigmentation, with combinations of green, yellow, orange, and brown hues commonly observed. The texture of the colonies may be smooth (glabrous), granular, cottony, or wooly, depending on their maturity and degree of sporulation. Microscopic studies must be performed to confirm the genus and species identification.

A. The surface of a colony of *Penicillium* species after a 5-day incubation on Sabouraud's dextrose agar, illustrating the distinctive green color, granular surface, radial rugae and white apron at the periphery. Although most strains of *Penicillium* species display some shade of green, yellow variants are sometimes seen.

B. The surface of a colony of *Penicillium marneffei* after a 4-day incubation on Sabouraud's dextrose agar, illustrating the distinctive red pigmentation of a portion of the colony: Note that the pigment has leached out into the agar, which has a light wine red coloration. The surface tends to be granular to fluffy depending on the degree of sporulation; note the distinct white apron at the margin of peripheral new growth.

C. The surface of a colony of *Paecilomyces* species: The colonies of *Paecilomyces* species are usually granular and often have a yellow-brown pigmentation, as illustrated here. Other strains, however, may have a light pastel green, green-yellow, or bluish appearance.

D. The surface of a colony of *Scopulariopsis* species after 5 days of growth on Sabouraud's dextrose agar: The yellow pigmentation, granular texture, and radiating rugae, as illustrated here, are hallmarks of *Scopulariopsis* species.

E. The surface of a colony of *Acremonium* species after 5 days of incubation on Sabouraud's dextrose agar: The colonies of *Acremonium* species usually have a smooth, almost yeast-like appearance, as illustrated here, owing to the extremely delicate nature of the hyphae and fruiting bodies. Light pastel yellow, light green, and peach-red hues may be observed.

F. The surface of a typical colony of *Fusarium* species after 6 days of growth on Sabouraud's dextrose agar: *Fusarium* species can be suspected when a rapidly growing, granular or fluffy colony, with a distinct rose-red, lavender, or purple pigmentation is observed.

G. The surface of a typical fluffy, "house mouse gray" colony of *Scedosporium apiosperum* (anamorphic form of *Pseudallescheria boydii*) after 5 days of incubation on Sabouraud's dextrose agar: A rapidly growing colony with the mouse gray appearance, as illustrated here, always suggests *Scedosporium* species. The unique pigmentation is caused by darkly pigmented conidia.

H. A colony of *Gliocladium* species after 5 days of growth on Sabouraud's dextrose agar: The green pigment, extension of the colony from border to border without a well defined growing margin and granular texture (so-called green lawn) is unique for *Gliocladium* and *Trichoderma* species. The latter more frequently may show a yellow, rather than a green, pigmentation.

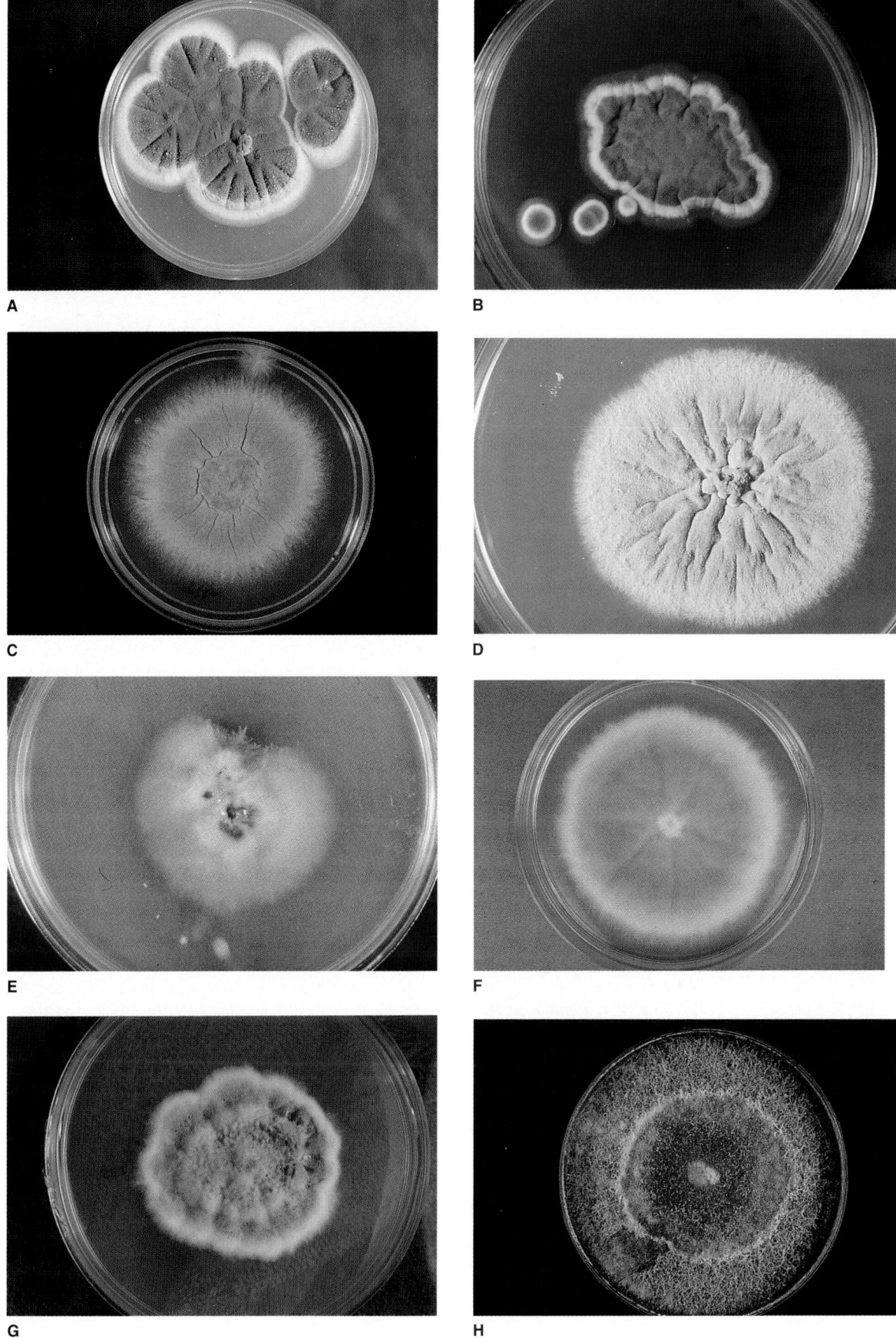

A

B

C

D

E

F

G

H

COLONY MORPHOLOGY OF COMMONLY ENCOUNTERED DEMATIACEOUS MOLDS

The dematiaceous (dark) molds are characterized by the growth of deep green, brown, or black colonies, with black pigmentation on the reverse surface. Most environmental species grow rapidly, producing mature colonies within 5 days. Slower-growing species, at times requiring 2 weeks or more before mature colonies are observed, are often recovered from clinical specimens taken from patients with mycetomas or chromomycosis. Photographs of representative colonies of select dematiaceous molds growing on Sabouraud's dextrose agar are illustrated here.

A. Fluffy, gray-black surface of a colony of *Alternaria* species after 6 days growth: The appearance shown here is not distinctive for *Alternaria* species, but may also be observed with other species of environmental dematiaceous molds.

B. Reverse surface of a dematiaceous mold illustrating the dark appearance caused by the dark brown pigmentation of the vegetative hyphae.

C. Surface view of a subculture of *Ulocladium* species, illustrating a wooly, dark brown to black pigmentation: Although frequently seen with certain strains of dematiaceous fungi, the light and darker concentric rings observed here are not distinctive for any given species.

D. Surface view of a colony of *Phialophora verrucosum* after 14 days incubation: This particular strain has a dark gray-black hue, with a hairlike texture. Microscopic study is necessary, because other slow-growing species may produce similar-appearing colonies.

E. Surface view of a colony of *Fonsecaea pedrosoi* after 16 days incubation: The colony is quite small, typical for the species, and the typical dark brown-black pigmentation is evident. This strain has a flatter, almost suedelike consistency.

F. Surface view of a colony of a more rapidly growing (5 days), environmental strain of *Cladosporium* species illustrating a dark green, suedelike surface interrupted by irregular rugae: Environmental strains of *Cladosporium* species may appear dark green, as shown here, or may be gray, gray-brown, or brown-black, simulating other dematiaceous fungi.

G. Surface view of another variant of an environmental *Cladosporium* species showing a dark gray, leatherlike consistency: Colony texture among the dematiaceous molds range from wooly, to downy or hairlike, to suedelike, to leathery.

H. Appearance of the flat, smooth, yeastlike surface of *Aureobasidium pullulans* after 6 days incubation. *Aureobasidium* spp. should be first on the list when a "black yeast," similar to that illustrated here, is observed; however, certain strains of *Exophiala wernickii* (so-called *Phaeoannelomyces* synanamorphs) must also be considered, which will develop a low, hairlike mycelium with true hyphae after several additional days of incubation.

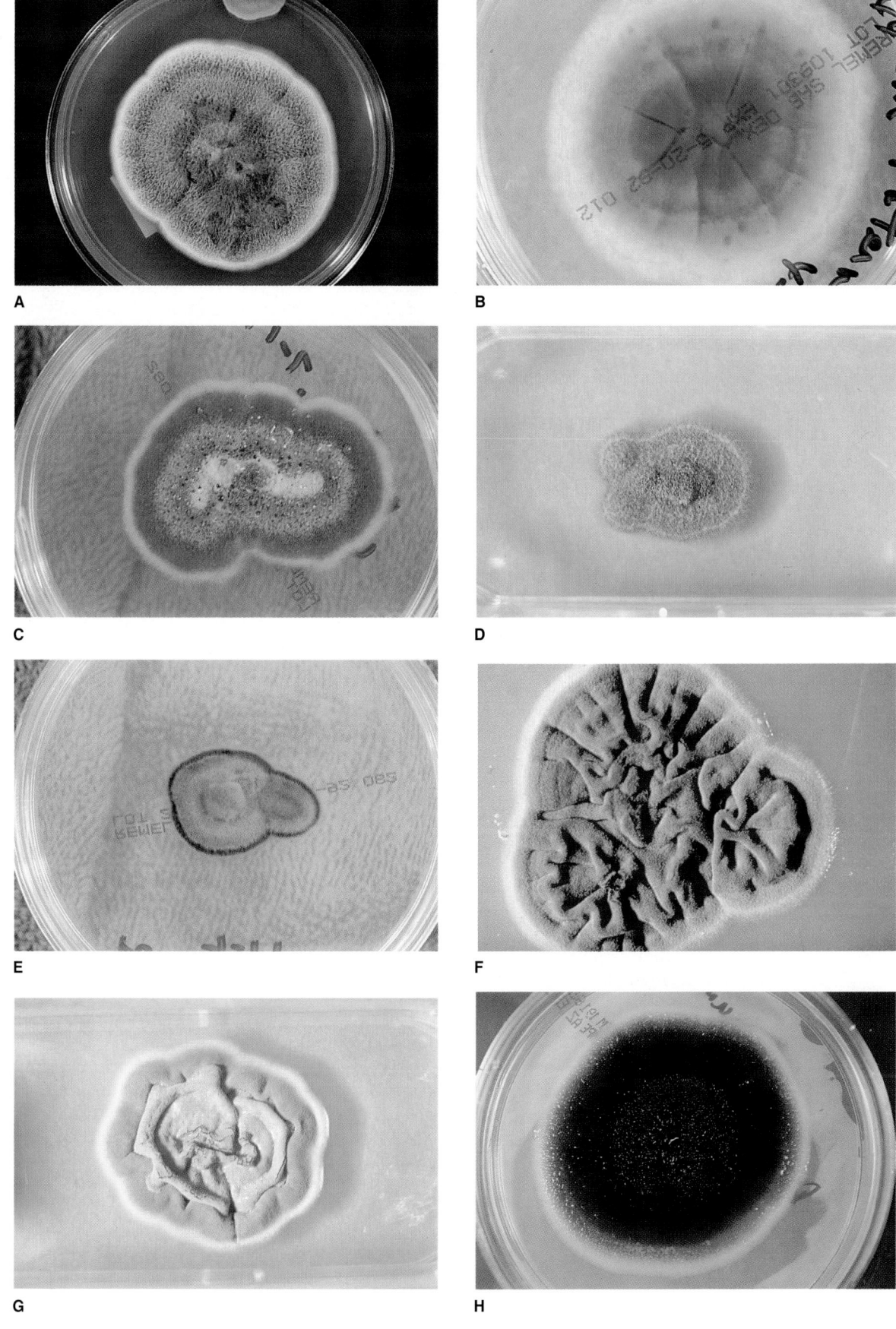

A

B

C

D

E

F

G

H

COLONY MORPHOLOGY OF DERMATOPHYTES

The colonies representative of the dermatophytic molds on artificial culture media are not distinctive. There is sufficient strain variation and differences in appearance of the same strain, depending on the type of culture medium used and the environmental conditions during incubation, that colonial morphology is not a reliable criterion for making presumptive identifications. Microscopic studies are almost always necessary to derive a definitive identification. Illustrated here are photographs of the colonies of select dermatophytes growing on Sabouraud's dextrose agar at 30°C, chosen to show certain characteristics that may offer clues to making a presumptive identification.

A. Colony of *Microsporum canis* after 5 days incubation: The colonies tend to be fluffy or, at times, granular if conidiation is heavy. The lemon-yellow apron seen here, with pigment also extending to the reverse surface, is one clue suggesting *M. canis*.

B. Surface of a powdery, off-yellow colony of *Microsporum gypseum* after 6 days incubation: *M. gypseum* tends to sporulate heavily; therefore, it is more prone to produce granular colonies than *M. canis*.

C. Surface of a smooth, white variant of *Trichophyton mentagrophytes* with no evidence of background pigmentation of the agar: The colony illustrated here is not distinctive, and microscopic study is required to make an identification.

D. Surface of a fluffy variant of *Trichophyton mentagrophytes* demonstrating a reddish pigmentation of the background agar: Wine-red pigmentation is one feature that suggests *T. rubrum*; however, certain strains of *T. mentagrophytes* may also produce reddish pigment when growing on Sabouraud's dextrose agar. Pigmentation, however, is never as intense as with *T. rubrum* when colonies are grown on cornmeal or potato dextrose agar.

E. Reverse of a colony of *Trichophyton rubrum* growing on potato dextrose agar. The deep wine-red pigmentation is characteristic of the species, and is particularly intense when the colony is grown on potato dextrose or cornmeal agar.

F. Comparative growth of *T. mentagrophytes* (*bottom*) and *T. rubrum* (*top*) on cornmeal agar, illustrating the distinct difference in pigmentation between the two species.

G. Surface of a small colony of *Trichophyton tonsurans* after 14 days incubation: *T. tonsurans* grows slower on Sabouraud's dextrose agar. Most strains produce some shade of yellow-brown pigment. The surface tends to be granular, and radial rugae are frequently seen. Except for the slower growth, the colonies of *T. tonsurans* appear similar to *Scopulariopsis* species and *Aspergillus terreus*.

H. Surface of *Epidermophyton floccosum* after 6 days incubation: This colony appears more fluffy than granular and has an off-yellow pigmentation. Classic colonies of *E. floccosum* are described as khaki green. The colony texture tends to be more fluffy than granular, as microconidia are not produced by this genus.

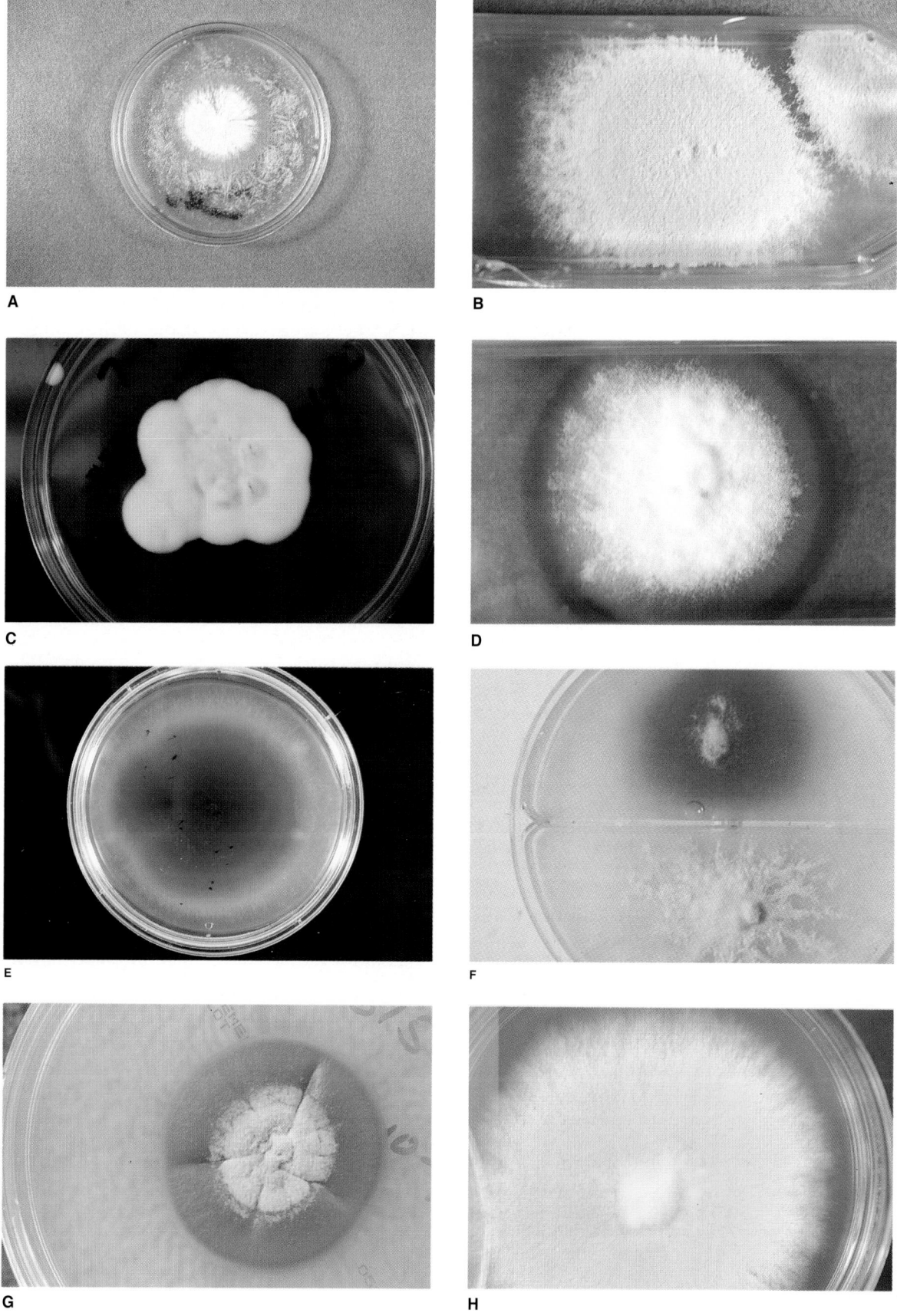

COLONY MORPHOLOGY OF DIMORPHIC FUNGI

The dimorphic fungi, so called because they grow in a mold form at 25° to 30°C (room temperature) and a yeast form at 37°C, are pathogenic in humans and are the agents of the deep-seated mycoses. Although the definitive species identification depends on microscopic study, confirmation that a given species belongs to the dimorphic group depends on demonstrating both the mold and yeast forms in laboratory isolates. The mold form may be converted to the yeast form by incubating subcultures on enriched media at 37°C and observing microscopically for the appearance of yeast forms typical of the species. With the advent of exoantigen extraction techniques and nucleic acid probe assays, conversion tests are performed only infrequently in most clinical laboratories.

A. Surface colony of a dimorphic mold illustrating both the yeast form (*centrally*) and the mold form (*peripherally*): This colony was incubated for 14 days at 30°C. When this mixture of yeast and mold texture is observed, one of the dimorphic fungi can be suspected, particularly if the colony is relatively slow growing and the mold appears more hairlike or cobweb in consistency.

B. Colonies of *Blastomyces dermatitidis* growing on 5% sheep blood agar after 5 days incubation: Note the cobweb appearance of these colonies, one clue that the isolate may be a dimorphic fungus and alerting one to take special precautions when preparing subcultures or microscopic mounts to avoid a laboratory-acquired infection.

C. Appearance of colonies of *Blastomyces dermatitidis* incubated at 37°C, during a mold-to-yeast conversion: There is an intermediate form of the colonies between mold and yeast, known as the "prickly stage." Note the rather coarse spicules formed by these white colonies.

D. Colonies of *Histoplasma capsulatum* on brain-heart infusion agar after 25 days incubation at 30°C. The colonies appear white and cobweb in consistency. These colonies are nondescript, and microscopic examination is nessary to make an identification.

E. Surface of a 5% sheep blood agar plate incubated at 37°C on which are growing small, yellowish yeast colonies of *Histoplasma capsulatum* after successful conversion from the mold form: The yeast forms are similar to other true yeasts, except that growth is very slow and the colonies remain quite small.

F. Surface of colonies of *Coccidioides immitis* growing on 5% sheep blood agar after 7 days incubation: The colonies are gray-white and have a delicate hairlike texture. Colonies of *C. immitis* growing on blood agar often show a red discoloration from leaching of hemoglobin from the culture medium (not shown in this illustration).

G. Surface of a smooth, gray-brown yeast colony of *Sporothrix schenckii*: Because of the extremely delicate sporulation of *S. schenckii*, colonies often appear more yeastlike than moldlike, even when incubated at 25° to 30°C. After prolonged incubation, colonies of *S. schenckii* tend to darken considerably, becoming almost jet black with some strains (see Plate 19-5H).

H. Tubes of brain–heart infusion agar, one containing cycloheximide, on which are growing the yeast (*top*) and mold (*bottom*) forms of *S. schenckii*. Because of the delicate nature of the hyphae and fruiting structures, the mold colony appears quite yeastlike. The colonies tend to darken with maturity, becoming distinctly black in some cases, as illustrated here.

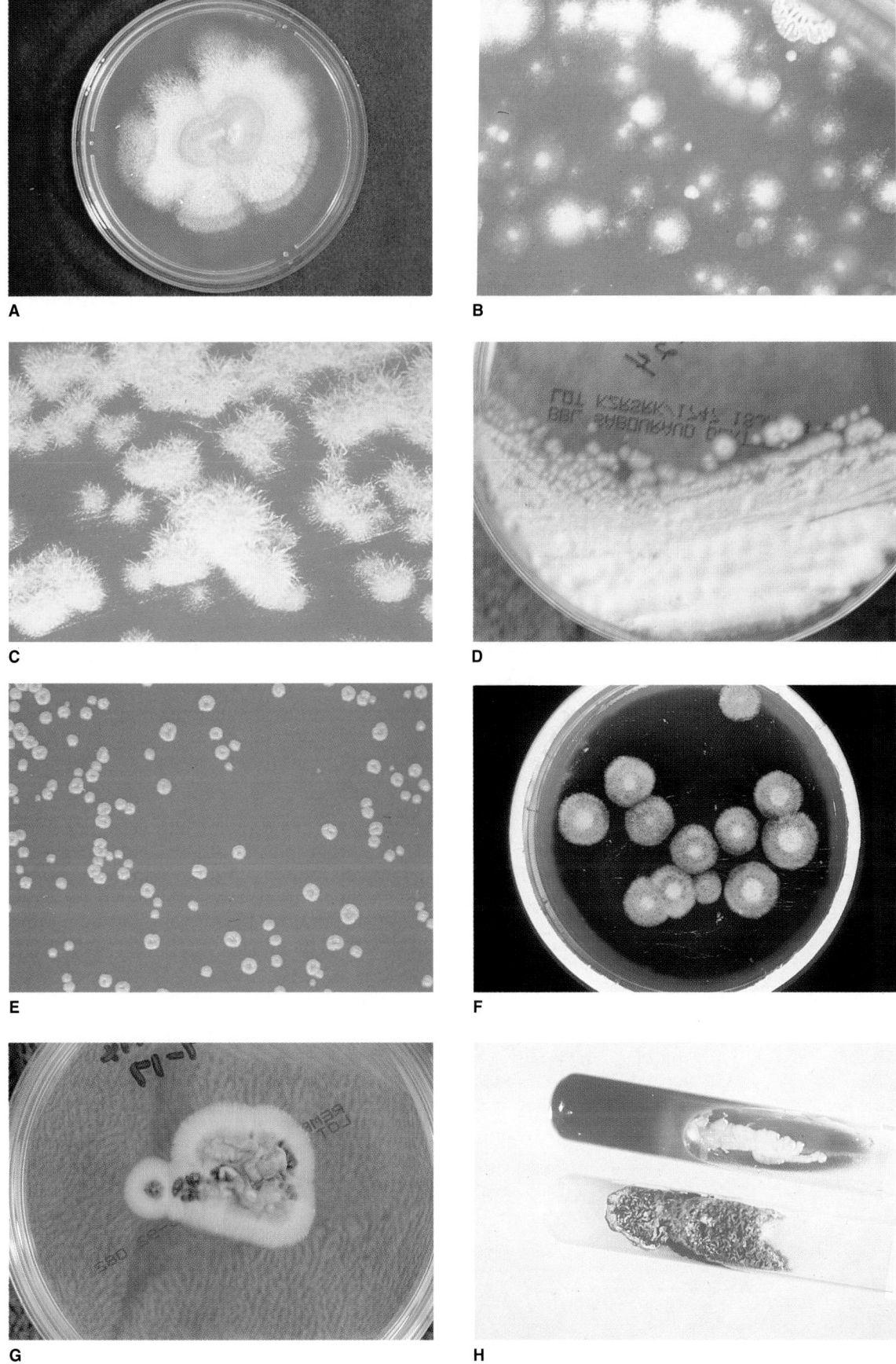

A

B

C

D

E

F

G

H

Morphology of Commonly Recovered Yeasts

The laboratory identification of medically important yeasts involves visual assessment of colonial characteristics and the interpretation of results of carbohydrate fermentation and assimilation tests.

A. Surface of a smooth, off-white yeast colony obtained from a subculture of *Candida albicans* after 3 days incubation: The colony shown here is not distinctive for *C. albicans*, but may be seen with other *Candida* species and yeasts of other species. Further studies are required when a yeastlike colony, as illustrated here, is recovered in the microbiology laboratory.

B. Surface of 5% sheep blood agar plate on which are growing white colonies of a yeast. The footlike extensions from the margins of the colonies are typically produced by *C. albicans*.

C. Colonies of *Cryptococcus neoformans* on Sabouraud's dextrose agar after 4 days incubation: The distinct mucoid consistency of the colonies is indicative of a capsule-forming yeast, suggesting *Cryptococcus* species. Further tests are required to identify *C. neoformans*.

D. Colonies of *Cryptococcus neoformans* growing on niger seed (birdseed) agar: The maroon-red pigmentation of the colonies when growing on this medium is characteristic of *C. neoformans*, distinguishing this species from other *Cryptococcus* species that are incapable of producing darkly pigmented colonies.

E. Colonies of *Torulopsis (Candida) glabrata* growing on Sabouraud's dextrose agar after 3 days incubation at 30°C: *T. glabrata* is suggested when small, more translucent yeast colonies are observed, although further studies are necessary to confirm the identification.

F. Colonies of *Rhodotorula* species illustrating the distinctive orange-red pigmentation characteristic of this genus: Some strains of *Cryptococcus* species may also produce a reddish pigmentation; therefore, additional studies may be necessary to confirm a definitive identification.

G. Surface of a blood agar plate on which are growing the yeastlike colonies of *Malassezia furfur* only in the area where virgin olive oil had been spread: *M. furfur* is a lipophilic yeast commonly found on human skin. A medium rich in oil (such as spreading virgin olive oil on the surface, as shown here) is necessary for the recovery of this yeast. Laboratory personnel must be notified if cases of tinea versicolor are suspected so that an oil overly preparation can be made.

H. Photomicrograph of an acid-fast–stained smear prepared from an isolated colony of *Saccharomyces cerevisiae* growing on the surface of ascospore agar: The spherical, red-staining (acid-fast) bodies seen here are ascospores. *Hansenula anomala* also produces acid-fast–staining ascospores when grown on ascospore agar; however, they are cap-shaped, rather than spherical, in outline.

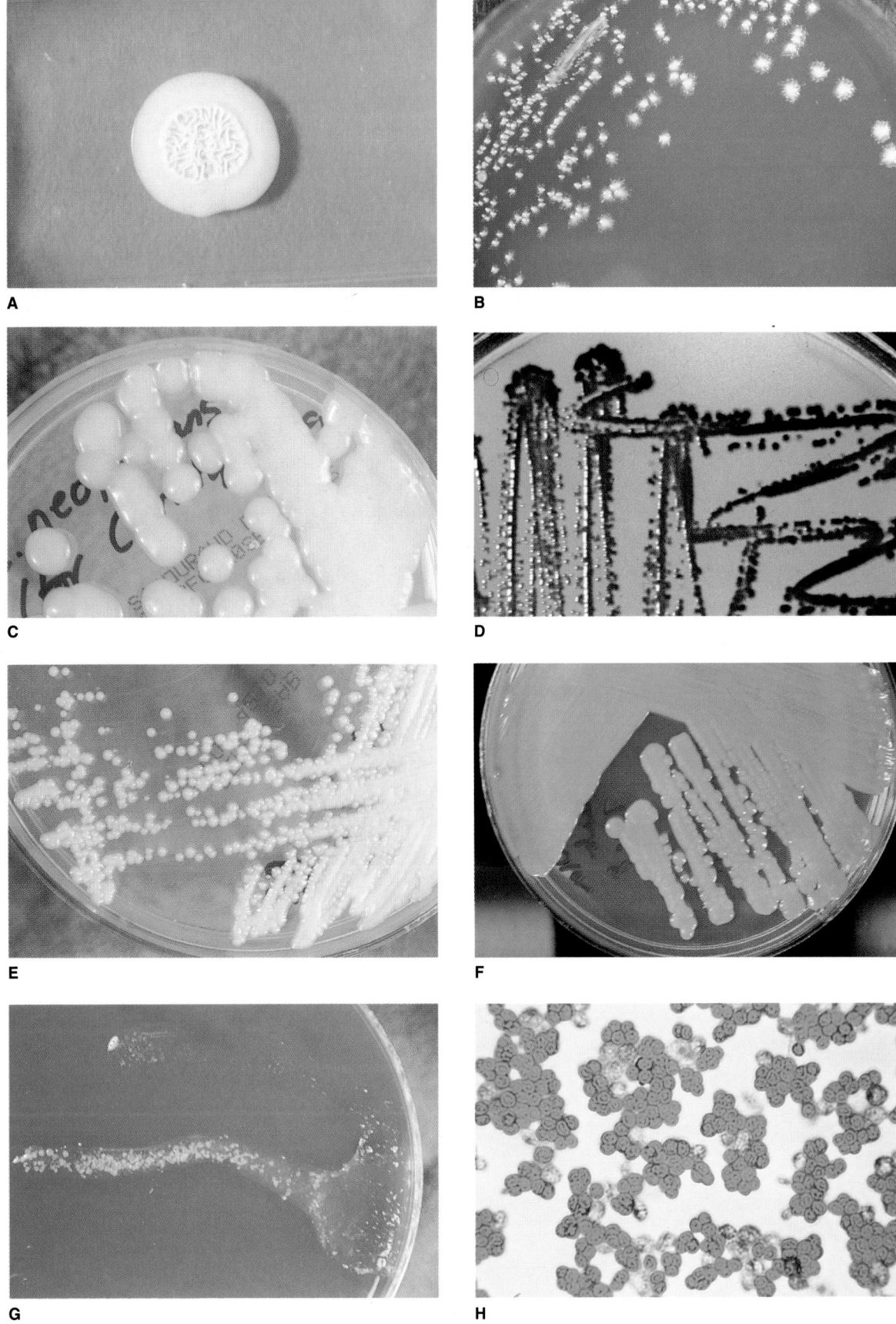

A

B

C

D

E

F

G

H

LABORATORY IDENTIFICATION OF INTESTINAL AMOEBA

A. Photomicrograph of a fecal smear stained with iron hematoxylin illustrating a single trophozoite of *Entamoeba histolytica* with a spherical nucleus containing a tiny, compact, centrally placed karyosome, and even, beadlike distribution of chromatin along the nuclear membrane (the entamoeba-type nucleus). The extension of a single pseudopod reflects purposeful, directional motility (×1000).

B. Close-in view of a trichrome-stained fecal smear illustrating a trophozoite of *E. histolytica*. Note the single nucleus with a centrally placed karyosome and even distribution of chromatin around the nuclear membrane. The cytoplasm has a homogeneous, "clean" appearance (×1000).

C. Photomicrograph of a trichrome-stained smear of fecal material including a single cyst of *Iodamoeba butschlii*. Note the nucleus with a large karyosome surrounded by an empty space, with no visible nuclear membrane (so-called ball-in-socket nucleus). Note the large vacuole in the cytoplasm, another feature aiding in the identification of *I. butschlii* (×400).

D. Split-frame photomicrograph comparing a cyst of *I. butschlii* (D1) with a uninucleate precyst of *E. histolytica* (D2). Note that each cyst contains a cytoplasmic vacuole; however, the two forms can be distinguished by the ball-in-socket type nucleus for the *I. butschlii* cyst, compared with the entamoeba-type nucleus with delicate distribution of chromatin around the nuclear membranes of the *E. histolytica* cyst.

E. Photomicrograph of an iron–hematoxylin-stained fecal smear illustrating a single trophozoite of *E. coli*. Note the large karyosome, the uneven distribution of chromatin along the nuclear membrane and the coarse, "junky" cytoplasm containing undigested debris and several irregular-sized vacuoles. The trophozoites of *E. coli* also tend to be larger than those of *E. histolytica,* ranging on the average from 14 to 25 μm in diameter.

F. Photomicrograph of a fecal smear stained with iron hematoxylin illustrating a cyst of *E. histolytica* containing two distinct, rod-shaped, dark staining, intracytoplasmic chromatoidal bars. The chromatoidal bars of *E. histolytica* cysts are typically rod-shaped and have smooth, rounded ends, in contrast with the splintered ends characteristic of *Entamoeba coli*. Note three indistinct entamoeba-like nuclei in the background (×400).

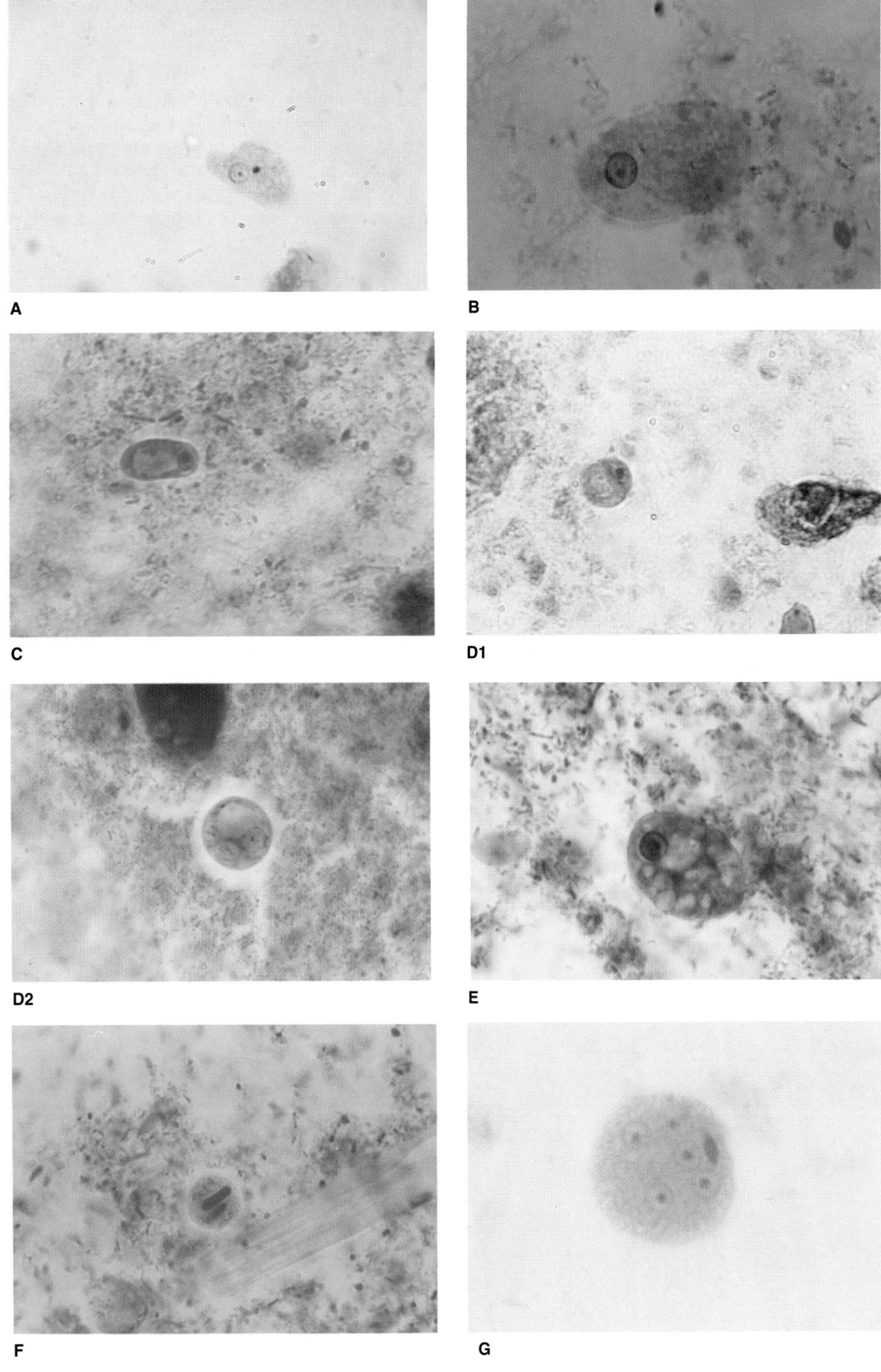

A

B

C

D1

D2

E

F

G

G. Photomicrograph of a trichrome-stained smear illustrating a single cyst of *Entamoeba coli*. Note the five distinct nuclei (any number exceeding four rules out *E. histolytica*), the karyosomes of which are large, although the chromatin is delicate and evenly distributed. Note also the single chromatoidal bar with pointed, rather than rounded, ends.

H. Split photomicrograph of trichrome-stained smears illustrating a trophozoite (*left* frame) and cyst (*right* frame) of *Endolimax nana*. The trophozoite possesses a single nucleus with a large karyosome, indistinct nuclear membrane (ball-in-socket) and a few small food vacuoles in the cytoplasm. The cyst has four nuclei, each with a prominent central karyosome, appearing as "owl eyes." Both the trophozoites and cysts of *E. nana* are very small, ranging from 5 to 8 μm in diameter.

I. Photomicrograph of a hematoxylin and eosin-stained section of colon mucosa, taken from a case of active intestinal amebiasis, demonstrating many infiltrating *E. histolytica* trophozoites. The trophozoites seen here are the light-staining, irregular-shaped spherical bodies, some of which show distinct entamoeba-type nuclei (×400).

J. Split photomicrograph of trichrome-stained smears illustrating two variants of *Blastocystis hominis*. The cyst-like forms of *B. hominis* are described as having a central body or vacuole and nuclear chromatin irregularly placed between the central body and the nuclear membrane, as illustrated in these split frames.

K. Photomicrograph of an iodine wet mount preparation illustrating a cyst of *E. histolytica*. The cyst is distinctly spherical, contains three distinct nuclei and a fourth that is more obscure, each showing beaded peripheral chromatin (×1000).

L. Photomicrograph of a direct iodine mount of fecal material illustrating a single cyst of *Entamoeba coli*. Five nuclei are distinctly visible; any number of nuclei exceeding five rules out *E. histolytica*. The individual nuclei, however, show tiny central karyosomes and a relatively even distribution of chromatin along the nuclear membrane, secondary features more consistent with *E. histolytica*.

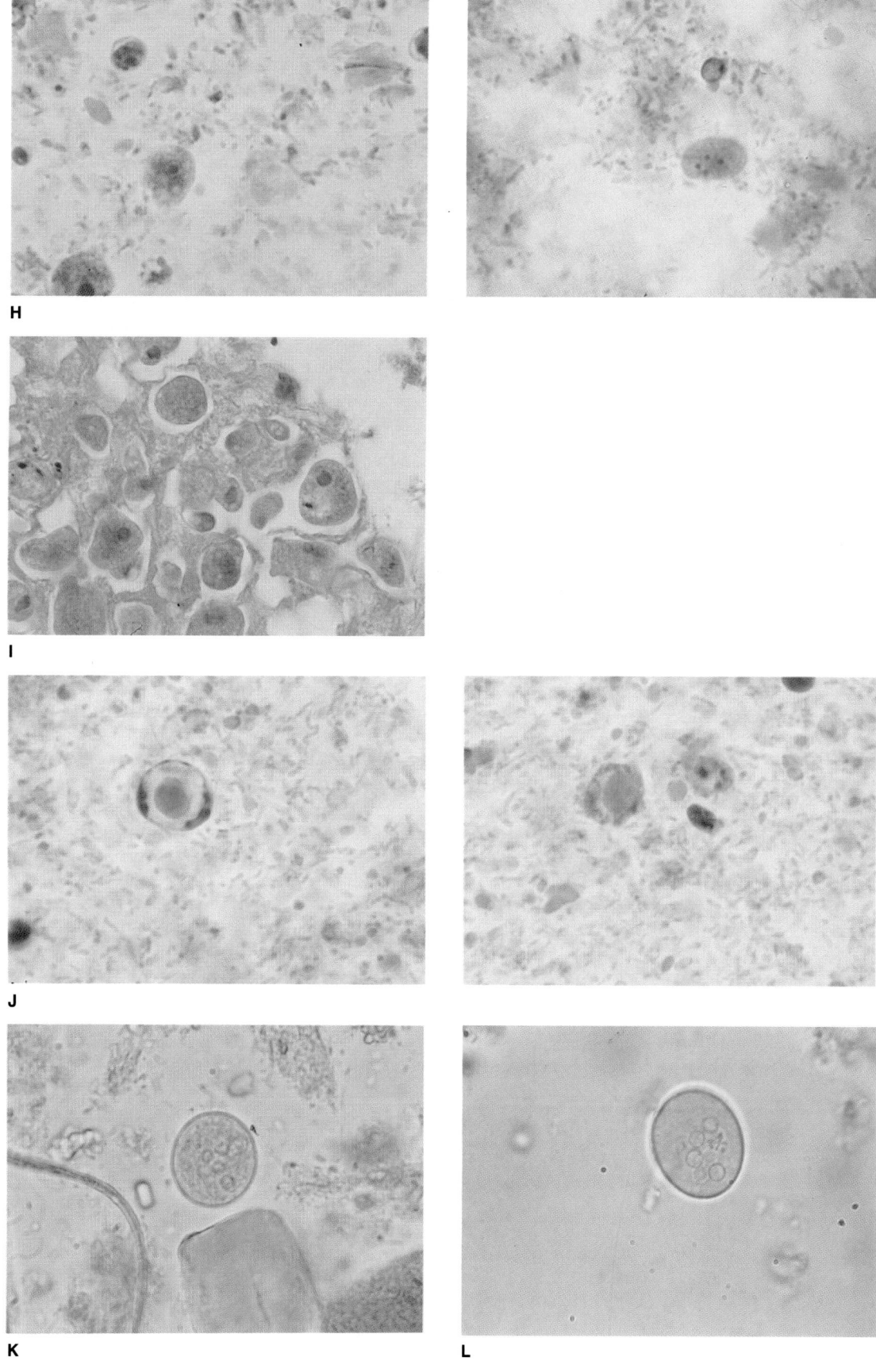

H

I

J

K

L

Laboratory Identification of Intestinal Protozoa Other Than Amoeba

A. Photomicrograph of an H&E-stained section of small bowel mucosa showing histologically normal appearing superficial columnar epithelial cells. A typical trophozoite of *Giardia lamblia* is observed hovering over the brush border of the epithelial cells. *G. lamblia* trophozoites are known to attach to the intestinal epithelial cells; however, the exact mechanism by which they cause diarrhea and malabsorption is not known.

B. Photomicrograph of a trichrome-stained smear of intestinal debris illustrating a *G. lamblia* trophozoite recognized by its distinctly oval to elliptical shape, the two nuclei, with prominent central karyosomes, lying anteriorly on either side of the rodlike axostyle, which runs the length of the organism, and the eosinophilic-staining parabasal body (the "mustache") lying posteriorly on the axostyle. These features provide the so-called monkey face appearance. *G. lamblia* trophozoites have six flagella, two each at anterior, posterior, and caudal positions, only three of which are visible in this photomicrograph.

C. Trichrome-stained smear of intestinal debris including two *G. lamblia* cysts. The cysts are oval, range from 9 to 12 µm in diameter and typically include double the number of organelles seen in the trophozoite. Each cyst has four nuclei, only two or three of which are usually seen in a single plane of focus, two axostyles, multiple parabasal bodies, and a smooth cyst wall.

D. Photomicrograph of two trophozoites of *Chilomastix mesnili,* one seen on end, the other from a lateral view. The trophozoite is typically pear-shaped and can be readily identified by observing the extreme anterior placement of a single nucleus, the posterior protrusion of the axostyle, and a spiral groove, which is difficult to observe in most preparations. A tuft of three anterior flagella, adjacent to the nucleus, is an additional identifying feature that is not commonly seen in most microscopic mounts.

E. Photomicrograph of a cyst of *C. mesnili.* A single nucleus, with central karyosome and a distinct cytostome, appearing as a well-outlined clear area in the cyst shown here, are easily observed. The outline of the cytostome, described as appearing as a shepherd's crook, is seen in this photomicrograph. Cysts typically are lemon-shaped, have a smooth cell wall, range from 6 to 10 µm in diameter and, in addition to the cytostome, often have an anterior knob that is helpful in making an identification.

F. Photomicrograph of a *Trichomonas hominis* trophozoite illustrating its typical tear-drop shape and single nucleus placed anteriorly, but not against the cell wall, as seen with *Chilomastix mesnili* (see Plate 20-2**D** for comparison). The longitudinally running axostyle is visible in this photomicrograph, as is a single posterior flagellum. *T. hominis* typically has three to five anterior and one posterior flagella and an undulating membrane that runs along the full length of the body, a structure that is seen only in preparations made from cultures.

G. Photomicrograph of a trophozoite of *Dientamoeba fragilis,* demonstrating the two distinctive nuclei, each with a large karyosome and indistinct nuclear membranes. The cytoplasm of this trophozoite is finely granular and shows early evidence of disintegration, as reflected by the species name.

H. Photomicrograph of a direct saline mount including a trophozoite of *Balantidium coli.* The trophozoites typically range from 40 to 70 µm wide by 50 to 100 µm long, are oval in outline, and have a smooth cell wall that is covered with short cilia over the entire circumference. The cilia and an indistinct macronucleus are seen in this photomicrograph; the cytostome is not visible here.

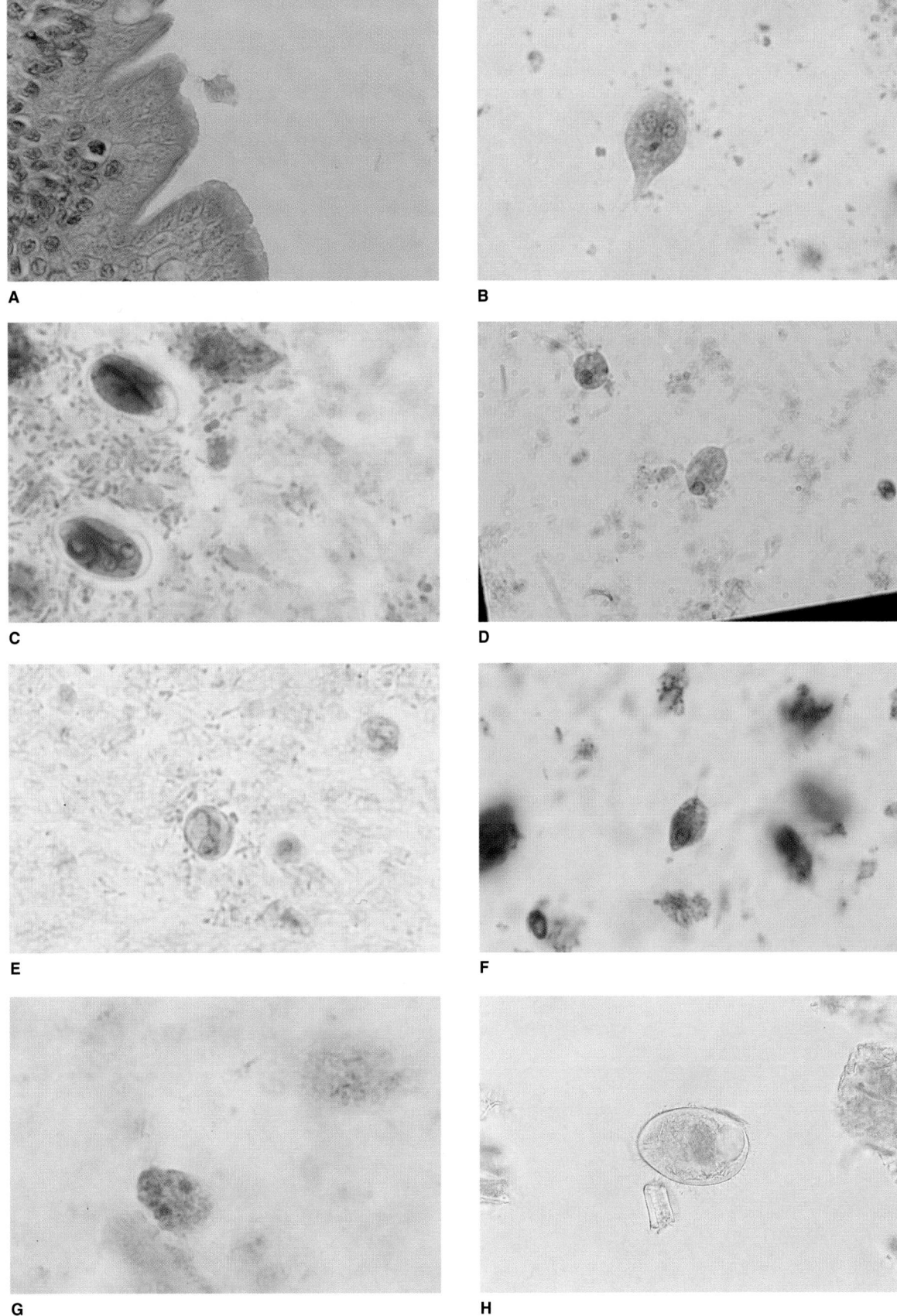

A

B

C

D

E

F

G

H

I. Photomicrograph of an H&E-stained intestinal biopsy illustrating many trophozoites of *B. coli.* Note the distinct macronuclei which, along with the large size, are helpful features in making an identification.

J. Split-frame photomicrograph of an H&E-stained small-bowel biopsy (*left* frame) revealing numerous oocysts of *Cryptosporidium parvum*, appearing as tiny spherical excrescences along the brush borders of the columnar epithelial cells. A presumptive diagnosis of cryptosporidiosis can be made by intestinal biopsy, as seen here; however, it is more commonly made by observing the acid-fast–staining oocysts in fecal smears, shown in the *right* frame. The two spherical, red-staining, acid-fast oocysts measure 5 μm in diameter and appear somewhat mottled, without an internal structure when stained with carbolfuchsin stain.

K. Photomicrograph of fecal material including a single spherical, acid-fast oocyst of cyclospora species. These oocysts average 8 to 10 μm, about twice the size of the oocysts of *Cryptosporidium parvum*, and have ill-defined internal structures that take on a dark, filamentous stain.

L. Photomicrograph of a smear stained by the modified Weber trichrome technique showing numerous 1- to 2-μm, light pink-staining spores of *Enterocytozoon* species, one of the microsporidia that commonly is detected in the gastrointestinal tract and other organs in patients with AIDS. The spores often have a central, transverse, deeper pink-staining bar, a helpful identifying feature when examining specimens with light microscopy.

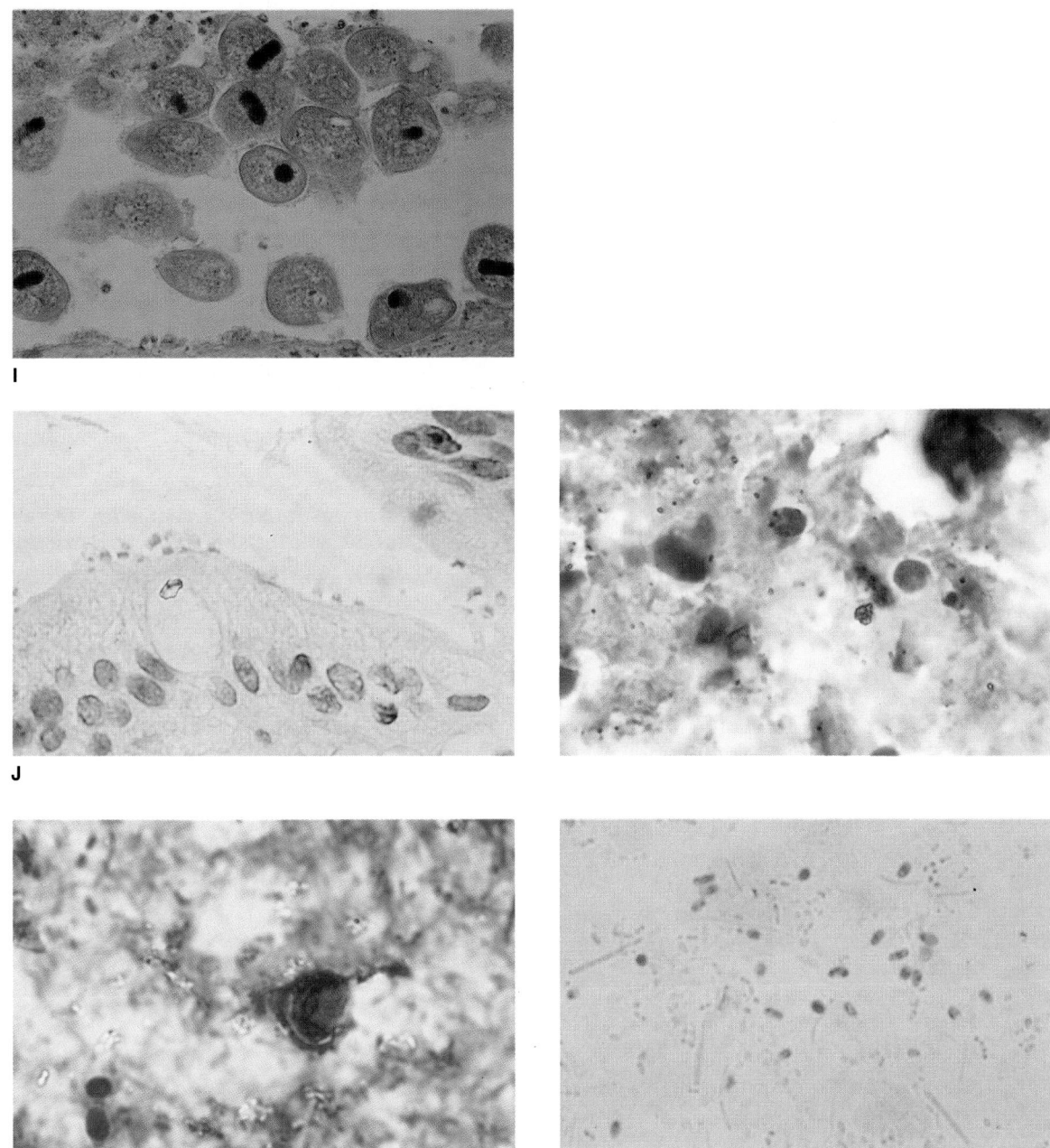

I

J

K

L

LABORATORY IDENTIFICATION OF INTESTINAL NEMATODES

A. Photograph of a stool specimen inhabited by several adult *Ascaris lumbricoides* worms. Adult males are generally shorter than females, averaging 20 to 25 cm in length, as opposed to 25 to 30 cm. The males also have a curved tail. The light pink, smooth, unsegmented cuticle is a helpful feature in distinguishing ascarids from common earthworms, which on occasion may find their way into sewage systems.

B. Fertilized, bile-stained, yellow-brown, slightly ovoid *A. lumbricoides* egg, demonstrating the characteristic thick shell, covered by an undulating albuminous coat and internal cleavage in an early stage of development. Fertilized *A. lumbricoides* eggs average 60 by 45 μm in diameter.

C. Split photograph illustrating a spherical *A. lumbricoides* egg (*left*), with a relatively smooth outer shell externally and a well-developed larva internally. The larva is in the process of hatching in the *right* frame, breaking through the nonoperculated thick-walled shell.

D. An adult *Trichuris trichiura* adult worm demonstrating the characteristic long, attenuated whiplike anterior segment and the shorter, thicker more handlelike posterior portion. These worms are relatively small, measuring 35 to 45 mm in length.

E. Typical bile-stained, yellow-brown *T. trichiura* egg demonstrating the characteristic barrel-shape and polar hyaline "plugs."

F. Photograph of the anterior end of an *Enterobius vermicularis* adult worm, demonstrating the characteristic transparent wings (alae) on either side of the mouth parts.

G. Photomicrograph of a transparency tape preparation demonstrating numerous ovoid, asymmetric eggs flattened on one side, with doubly refractile, smooth shells and a well-developed larva within some. Transparency tape mounts obtained by pressing the sticky side to the perianal skin is a common method for confirming a diagnosis of pinworm infection.

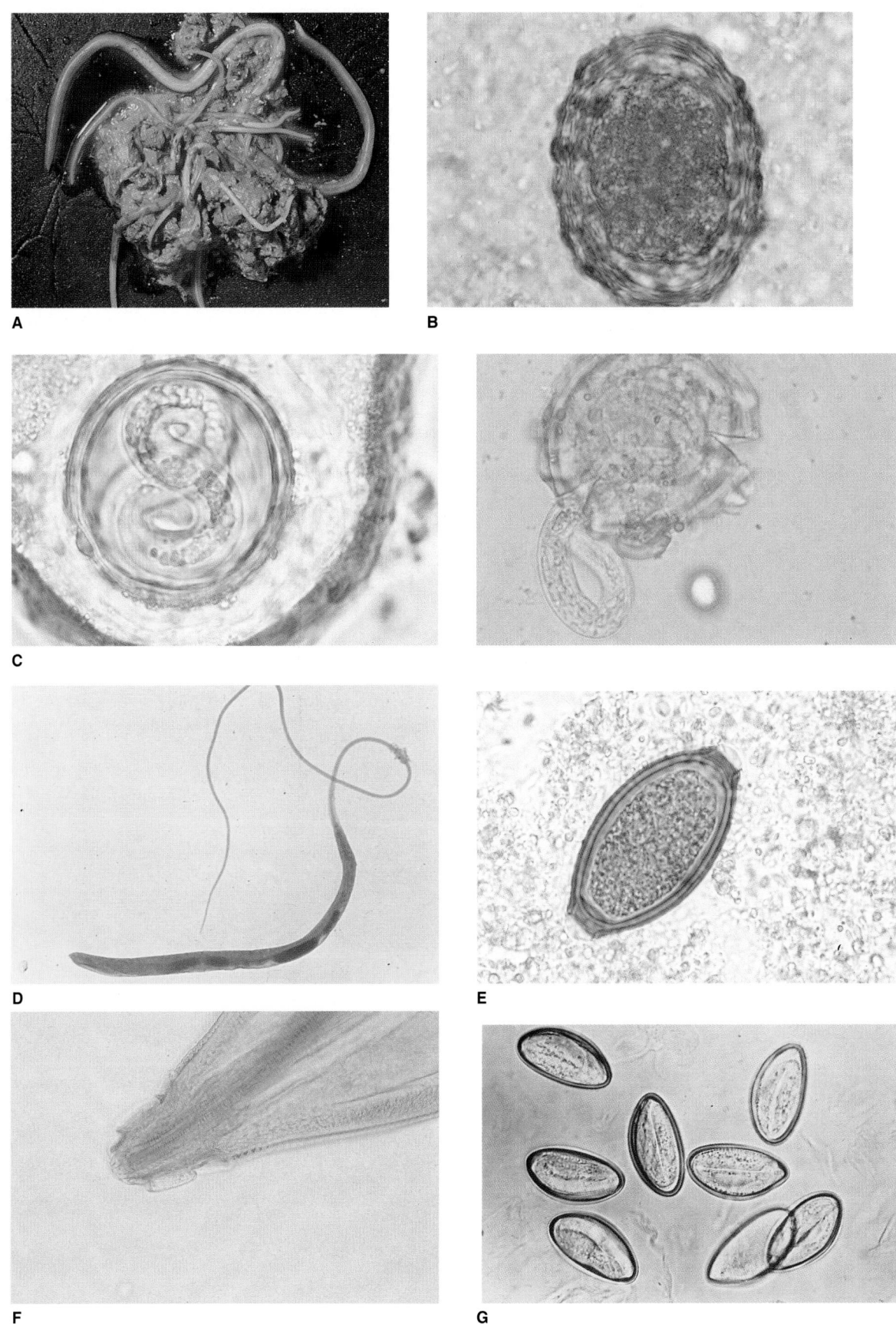

A

B

C

D

E

F

G

H. Photomicrograph of an H&E-stained section of appendix inhabited by an adult *E. vermicularis* worm cut in cross section. The identification of *E. vermicularis* is made in tissue sections by observing the lateral spikes on opposite sides of the worm.

I. Photomicrograph of a direct iodine mount of fecal material, including a typical oval-shaped, thin, smooth-shelled hookworm egg, with the characteristic internal cleavage pulling away from the inner shell producing an empty space. Although these ova cannot be morphologically distinguished from those of *Strongyloides stercoralis*, the latter virtually always hatch by the time they are passed, and eggs of the latter are almost never seen. Hookworm eggs range from 40 to 60 μm in greatest dimensions.

J. Split-frame photomicrographs of the mouth part of an *Ancylostoma duodenale* adult worm demonstrating the characteristic two pairs of chitinous teeth (*left*) and the cutting plates of *Necator americanus* (*right*). These mouth parts are well suited for the deep attachment to the intestinal mucosa and the fracture of capillaries to milk blood from the circulation.

K. Split-frame photomicrograph illustrating the short buccal cavity of a *S. stercoralis* rhabditiform larva (*left*) with the long buccal cavity of a hookworm rhabditiform larva (*right*). Although the differentiation is usually easy to make morphologically, the exercise rarely is necessary when examining stool specimens, as hookworm ova rarely hatch within the intestine.

L. Photomicrograph of an H&E-stained section of small intestine in which can be seen burrowing into the lamina propria several round, smooth *S. stercoralis* filariform larvae in a case of self-infection strongyloidiasis. In patients with strongyloides who develop a compromised immune system, the cycle from oviposition, to rhabditiform larva, to filariform larva may be sufficiently short that self-infection may occur within the intestine before stools are produced.

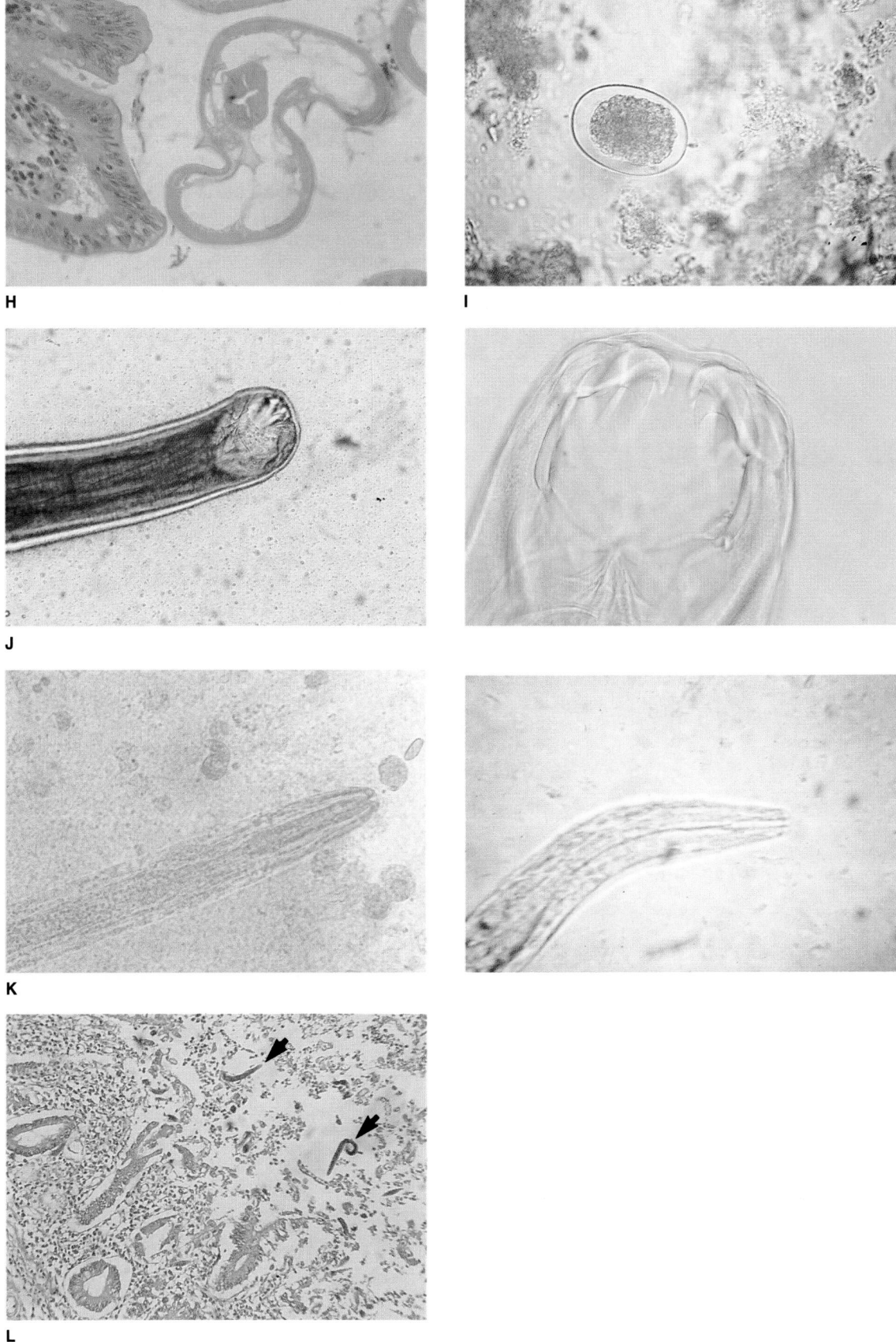

H

I

J

K

L

LABORATORY IDENTIFICATION OF INTESTINAL CESTODES

A. An adult *Taenia saginata* tapeworm illustrating the small scolex and several foot-long strobila containing a long chain of proglottids.

B. The scolex of a *T. solium* tapeworm demonstrating the four suckers characteristic of the genus and the protruding, armed rostellum with circular rows of hooklets characteristic of the species.

C. A *T. solium* proglottid that had been injected with India ink through the genital pore to outline the branching uterine segments: The proglottids of *T. solium* typically have fewer than 13 lateral uterine segments, in contrast with *T. saginata*, which has numerous segments, often approaching 20 or more.

D. Photomicrograph of *Taenia* species eggs demonstrating the spherical shape and thick, smooth shell, with radial striations: When mature, the eggs contain a hexacanth embryo with six hooklets, not seen in the immature eggs shown here.

E. Split-frame photographs of a piece of measly pork (*left* frame) including several small cystic spaces inhabited by a cysticercus larva (bladder worm) demonstrated in the photomicrograph in the *right* frame: Cysticerci form in various tissues in humans, particularly in the central nervous system, following ingestion of *T. solium* eggs.

F. Photomicrograph of a brain biopsy in a human case of cysticercosis demonstrating the cystic, fluid-filled space (bladder) occupied by a *T. solium* cysticercus worm cut in cross section: Observe the inner membrane produced by the cysticercus, as opposed to the thicker reactive, inflammatory capsule produced by the host.

G. Photomicrograph of a *Diphyllobothrium latum* egg demonstrating the thin, smooth shell nicked in two places near the narrower end at the site of an operculum: The operculum is flat, an important differential feature from the similar-appearing, but shouldered, operculated egg of *Paragonimus westermani*. The cleavage extends to the inner shell, without leaving an empty space. These eggs average 60 to 75 µm long by 40 to 50 µm wide.

H. A *Diphyllobothrium latum* proglottid, wider than broad (latum) and enclosing a nondescript coiled uterus appearing as a compact rosette.

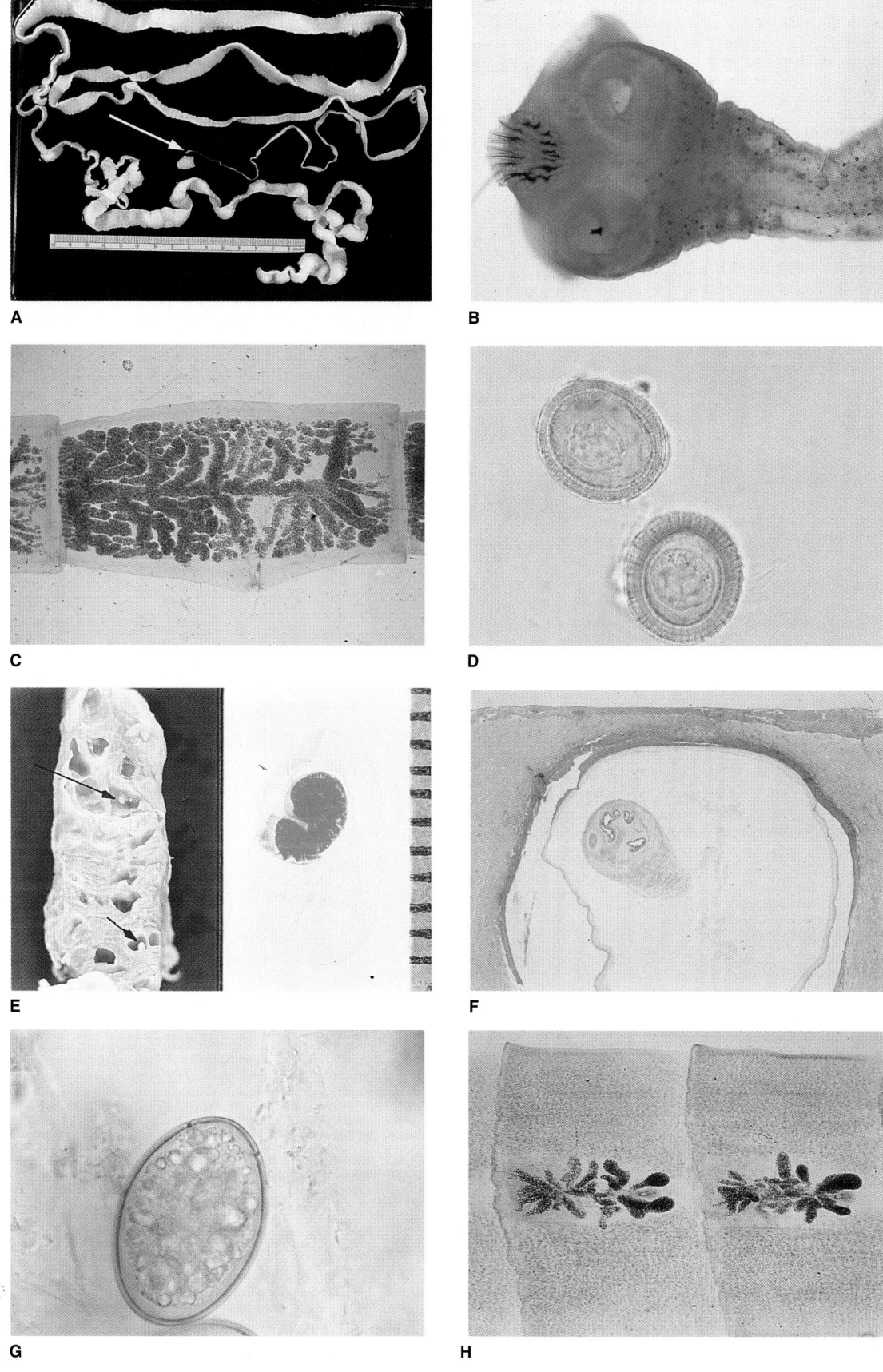

A

B

C

D

E

F

G

H

I. The spatula-shaped scolex of *D. latum* demonstrating the central, longitudinal groove (bothrium) flanked by elevated folds on either side.

J. Split-frame photographs of *Hymenolepis nana*, illustrating an adult worm (*left* frame) with a scolex possessing a protruding, armed rostellum. An *H. nana* egg is shown in the *right* frame, demonstrating the characteristic smooth, outer thickened shell and an inner membrane enclosing an onchosphere (hooklets are faintly visible). Note the polar filaments extending from the inner membrane into the clear space.

K. A *Dipylidium caninum* proglottid, demonstrating a genital pore on either side (thus the genus name): The proglottid is longer than wide. Proglottids of other tapeworms characteristically possess only one lateral genital pore, which alternates from one side to the other from one segment to the next. Thus, the double genital pore per proglottid is a unique feature.

L. Photomicrograph of an egg packet of *D. caninum* demonstrating an aggregate of spherical eggs held in a matrix: These eggs are immature as internal hooklets are not observed, which develop as the eggs mature.

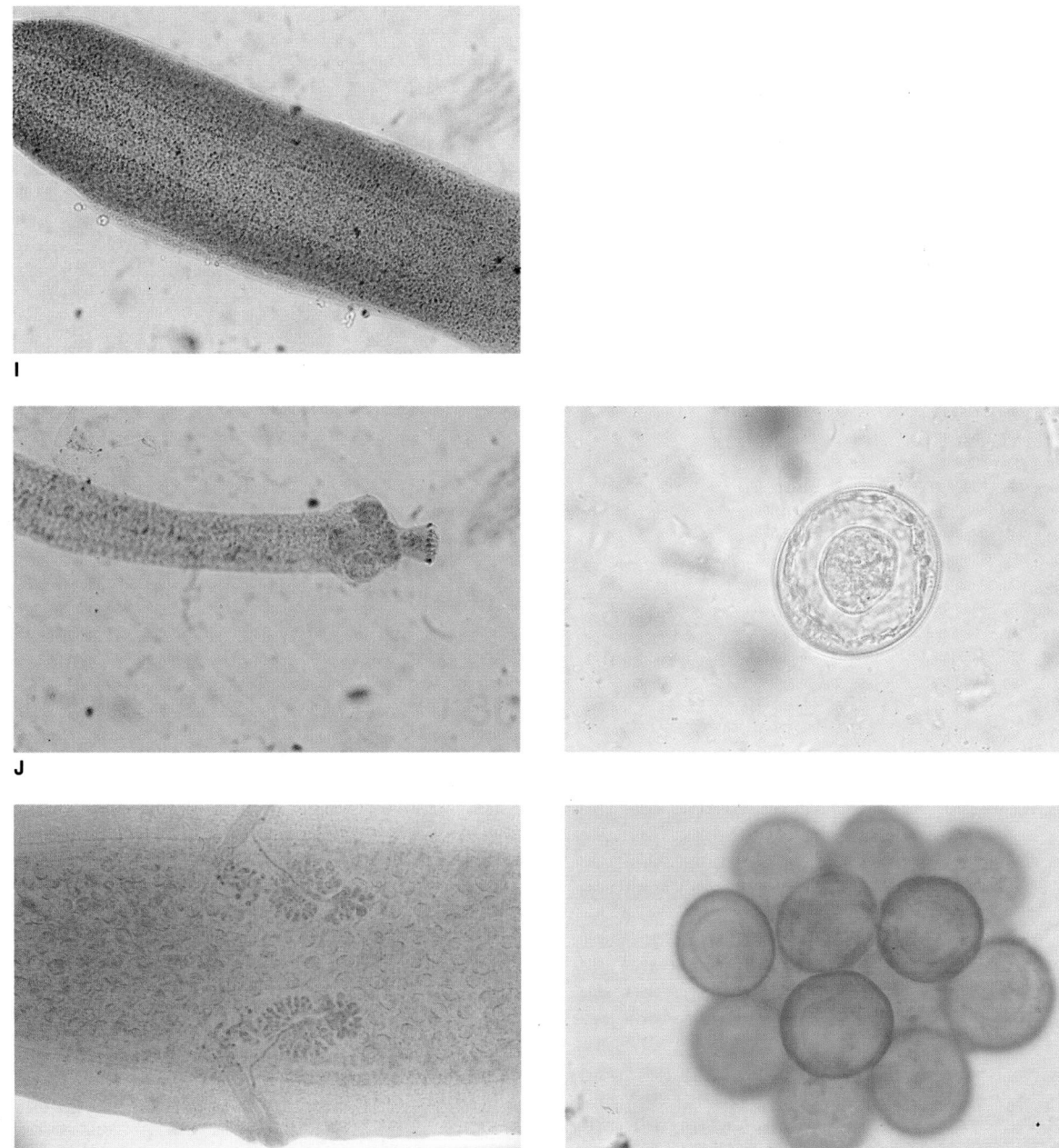

I

J

K

L

LABORATORY IDENTIFICATION OF TREMATODES

A. Photomicrograph of freely swimming, forked tail cercariae of *Schistosoma* species, with their ability to directly penetrate skin on contact, which serve as the infective form for humans.

B. Adult flukes of *Schistosoma* species demonstrating a lighter-staining male with a longitudinal gynecophoric canal within which the copulating female, darker staining and detached in this picture, resides during copulation. Adult males average 20 to 30 mm in length; females 7 to 14 mm. These flukes are threadlike allowing them to occupy the lumens of venules without causing blockage of the blood flow.

C. Photomicrograph of an egg of *S. mansoni*, with its characteristic smooth, thin wall and prominent lateral spine: These eggs are relatively very large, ranging from about 115 to 180 μm long by 45 to 70 μm wide.

D. Photomicrograph of an egg of *S. haematobium*, demonstrating a thin, smooth shell and the characteristic delicate terminal spine: These eggs are relatively large, ranging from 110 to 170 μm long and 40 to 70 μm wide.

E. Photomicrograph of an egg of *S. japonicum*, which is spherical to slightly oval in outline, has a smooth, relatively thick shell, and cleavage that extends to the inner shell. A small lateral knob may be seen in some eggs (not shown in this illustration).

F. An adult fluke of *Fasciola hepatica:* These flukes are hermaphroditic and possess both female and male reproductive organs. The anterior portion of *F. hepatica* projects into a cone-shaped nose, just posterior to which is the anterior sucker. Immediately posterior to the sucker, and darkly staining in this photograph, is the branching convoluted uterus. Immediately posterior to the uterus is the ventral sucker. The bulk of the posterior portion of the fluke includes the branching testes, appearing as a pink-staining meshwork in this photograph. These flukes measure about 3 by 1 cm (the size of a glass slide).

G. An adult fluke of *Fasciolopsis buski*, which is also hermaphroditic and has structures similar to those described for *F. hepatica* (see Plate 20-5F), except that the cephalic end is rounded and does not have the conical protrusion. These flukes range from about 2 to 7.5 cm long by 0.8 to 2 cm wide.

H. Photomicrograph of an egg of *F. hepatica* (appearing identical with those of *Fasciolopsis buski*), demonstrating a thin, smooth wall and an internal cleavage that extends to the inner shell membrane: Notice the nick in either side of the shell toward the narrower end of the egg, representing the operculum, a lidlike structure that opens at the time the larva hatches. These eggs are large, averaging about 150 by 80 μm.

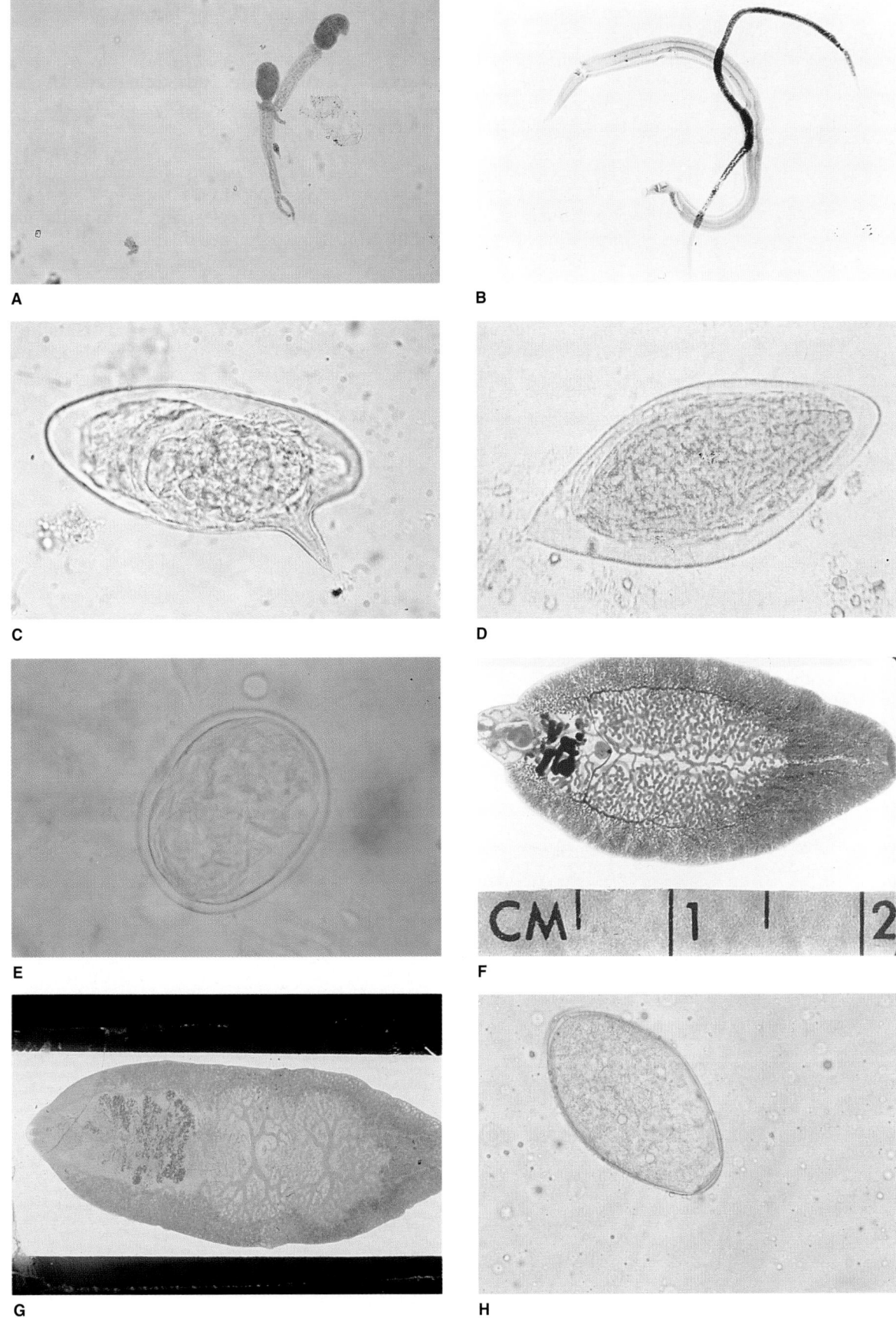

A

B

C

D

E

F

CM | 1 | 2

G

H

I. An adult fluke of *Clonorchis sinensis* demonstrating the long, bottle-shaped cephalic end with a prominent terminal sucker, dark brown-staining uterus anterior, and the extensively branched, lighter pink-staining testes posteriorly.

J. Photomicrograph of an H&E-stained section of a dilated bile duct in which reside three *C. sinensis* adult flukes cut in cross section. Although a mild chronic inflammatory infiltrate is noted in the surrounding submucosa, extensive fibrosis and lumen occlusion is not evident here.

K. Split photomicrograph of fertilized eggs of *C. sinensis*, illustrating a thin, smooth wall, with a prominent, shouldered operculum at one end. Note the small knob at the posterior end of the egg in the *right* frame, an additional feature helpful in making an identification. These eggs are relatively small, ranging from 25 to 35 µm long by 14 to 17 µm wide.

L. Photomicrograph of an egg of *Paragonimus westermani*. The shell is smooth, relatively thin, and interrupted at one end by a prominent, shouldered operculum. These eggs are relatively large, ranging from 65 to 120 µm long by 40 to 70 µm wide. They are essentially the same size as and have a similar appearance to the eggs of *Diphyllobothrium latum*, and differ only in the lateral extension, or shoulder, of the operculum.

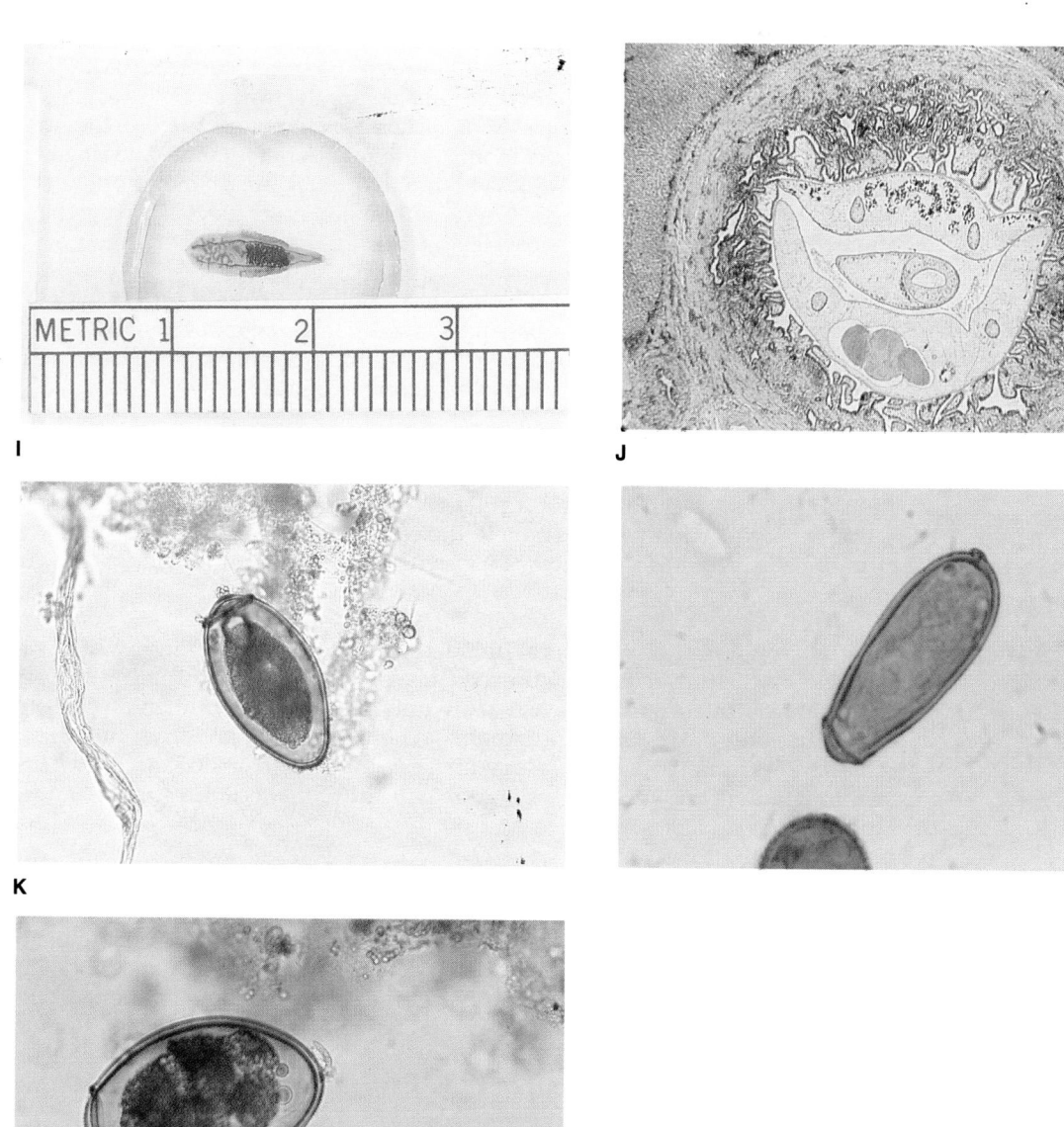

I

J

K

L

LABORATORY IDENTIFICATION OF BLOOD PARASITES

A. Photomicrographs of a peripheral blood smear illustrating erythrocytes invaded by small ring forms of *Plasmodium falciparum*, often attached to the inner surface of the red cell membrane in an "applique" arrangement. The rings are quite small, typically measuring less than one-quarter the diameter of the erythrocyte, and the infection here is heavy, with many erythrocytes involved and often with two or more rings in each cell.

B. Photomicrograph of a peripheral blood smear obtained from a patient with falciparum malaria, illustrating a banana-shaped gametocyte (*lower field*), a form that is diagnostic of *P. falciparum* when seen in the peripheral blood. A small ring form is seen within the erythrocyte at the top margin.

C. Photomicrograph of a peripheral blood smear, including one enlarged, pale erythrocyte inhabited by a ring form (trophozoite) of *P. vivax*. Note the distinct stippling of the erythrocyte cytoplasm, and granules that are known as Schüffner's dots which, in addition to the enlargement and pale appearance of the red cells, provide the features necessary for the identification of *P. vivax* infection.

D. Photomicrograph of a peripheral blood smear demonstrating in the center of the field a schizont of *P. vivax*. In the process of maturation, the trophozoite breaks into numerous fragments, known as merozoites, to form a schizont. Schizonts with more than 13 segments, as shown here, are characteristic of *P. vivax* infection. Note that the erythrocyte is enlarged, pale, and a few tiny Schüffner's dots are noted in the cytoplasm, additional criteria supporting the identification of *P. vivax*.

E. Photomicrograph of a peripheral blood smear illustrating in the center of the field a gametocyte of *P. vivax*. Any parasitic form that occupies more than one-half the diameter of the erythrocyte and has a single nucleus is a gametocyte. Male and female gametocytes are the sexual forms in the life cycle which, when taken up by the mosquito during a blood meal, mate and form the infective sporozoites. In this photograph, notice that the infected erythrocyte is enlarged and pale, and also contains finely granular, brown-staining malarial pigment, additional features helpful in making the diagnosis of vivax malarial infection.

F. Split-frame photomicrograph of a peripheral blood smear illustrating in the *left* frame an erythrocyte infected with a developing trophozoite of *P. malariae*. Notice that the infected erythrocyte is not enlarged and retains a coloration similar to the surrounding red cells. The cytoplasm of the trophozoites of *P. malariae* is condensed, and typically takes on a band form that extends from one side of the cell to the other. In the *right* frame is a schizont that has fewer than 13 segments, another helpful feature in the identification of *P. malariae* infection.

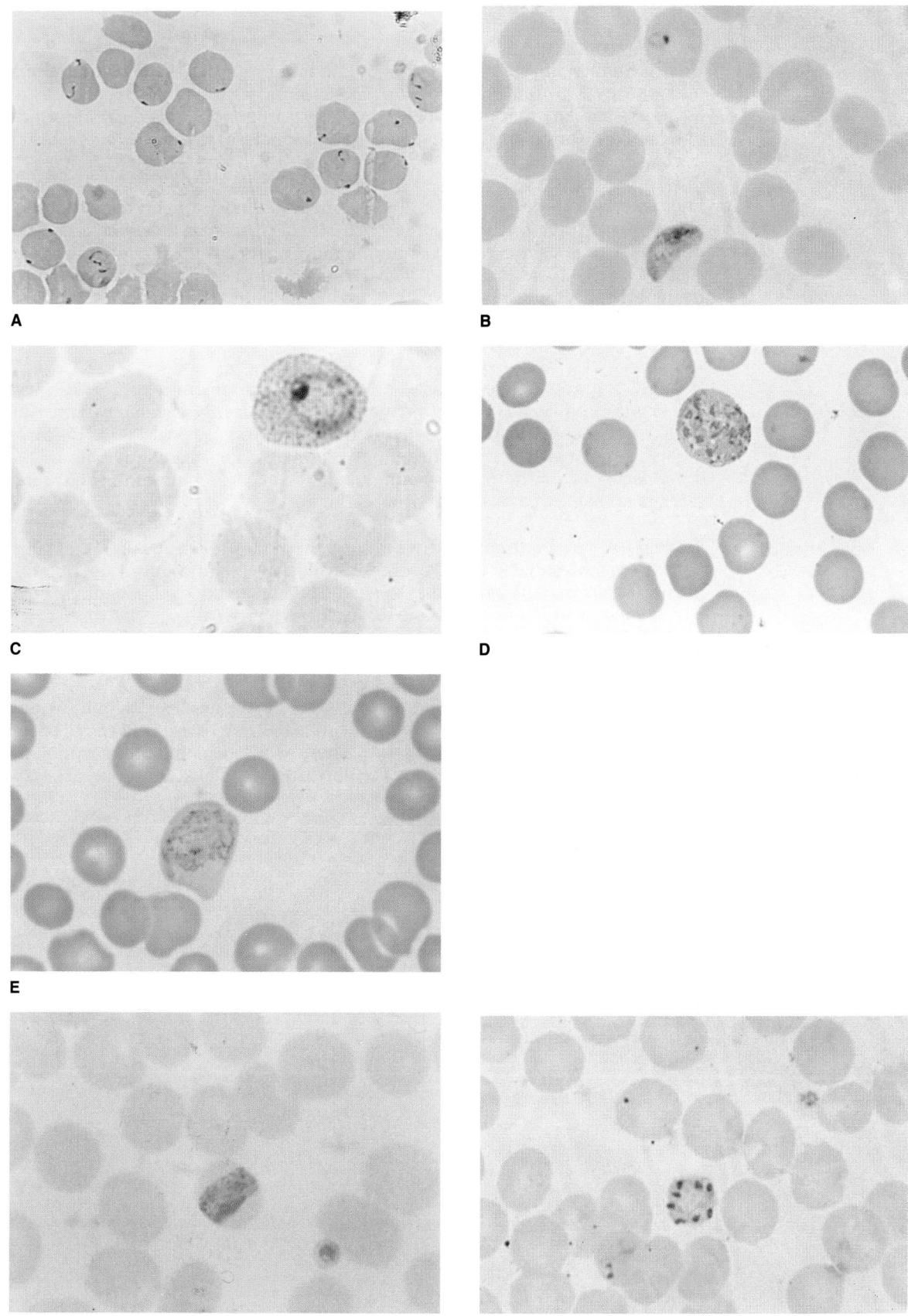

A

B

C

D

E

F

G. Photograph of the lower legs of a patient infected with *L. tropica*. The ulcerating cutaneous lesions represent the results of the granulomatous inflammation caused by the infecting organisms.

H. Giemsa-stained impression smear showing background macrophages and numerous tiny 2–3 μm amastigotes of *Leishmania* species. These tiny parasitic forms are similar in appearance to the yeast forms of *Histoplasma capsulatum* but can be distinguished by the rod-shaped kinetoplast lying adjacent to the nucleus.

I. Photomicrograph of a peripheral blood smear demonstrating a heavy infiltration of extracellular trypanosomes from a case of African trypanosomiasis. Each individual organism is long, slender, spindle-shaped, and ranges from 15 to 30 μm long by 1.5 to 4 μm wide. The darker-staining dotlike structure seen posteriorly is the kinetoplast from which a single flagellum originates. The flagellum extends along the length of an undulating membrane and extends for some distance anterior to the organism.

J. Photomicrograph of a peripheral blood smear demonstrating "C"-form trypanosomes from a case of South American trypanosomiasis (Chagas' disease). Each trypanosome has a deeper-staining, dotlike structure posteriorly, the kinetoplast, from which a single flagellum originates. The flagellum follows the outer border of an undulating membrane that runs the length of the body, and extends for some distance from the anterior end.

K. Photograph of a triatomid (reduviid) bug, the vector for transmission of Chagas' disease. Metacyclic trypanosomes develop in the hind gut of the bug following ingestion of trypanosomes when the bug bit an infected patient. The trypanosomes reenter the subcutaneous tissue when fecal material discharged from the bug is scratched into the wound at the bite site in a second unsuspecting host.

L. Photomicrograph of an H&E-stained section of heart muscle, with one swollen fiber seen from *top* to *bottom center* that is inhabited by dense collections of the amastogotic forms of *Trypanosoma cruzi*. These forms are similar in morphology to the amastigotes of *Leishmania* species illustrated in plates 20-6**G** and 6**H**. Cardiac involvement in patients with Chagas' disease commonly results in heart failure and death.

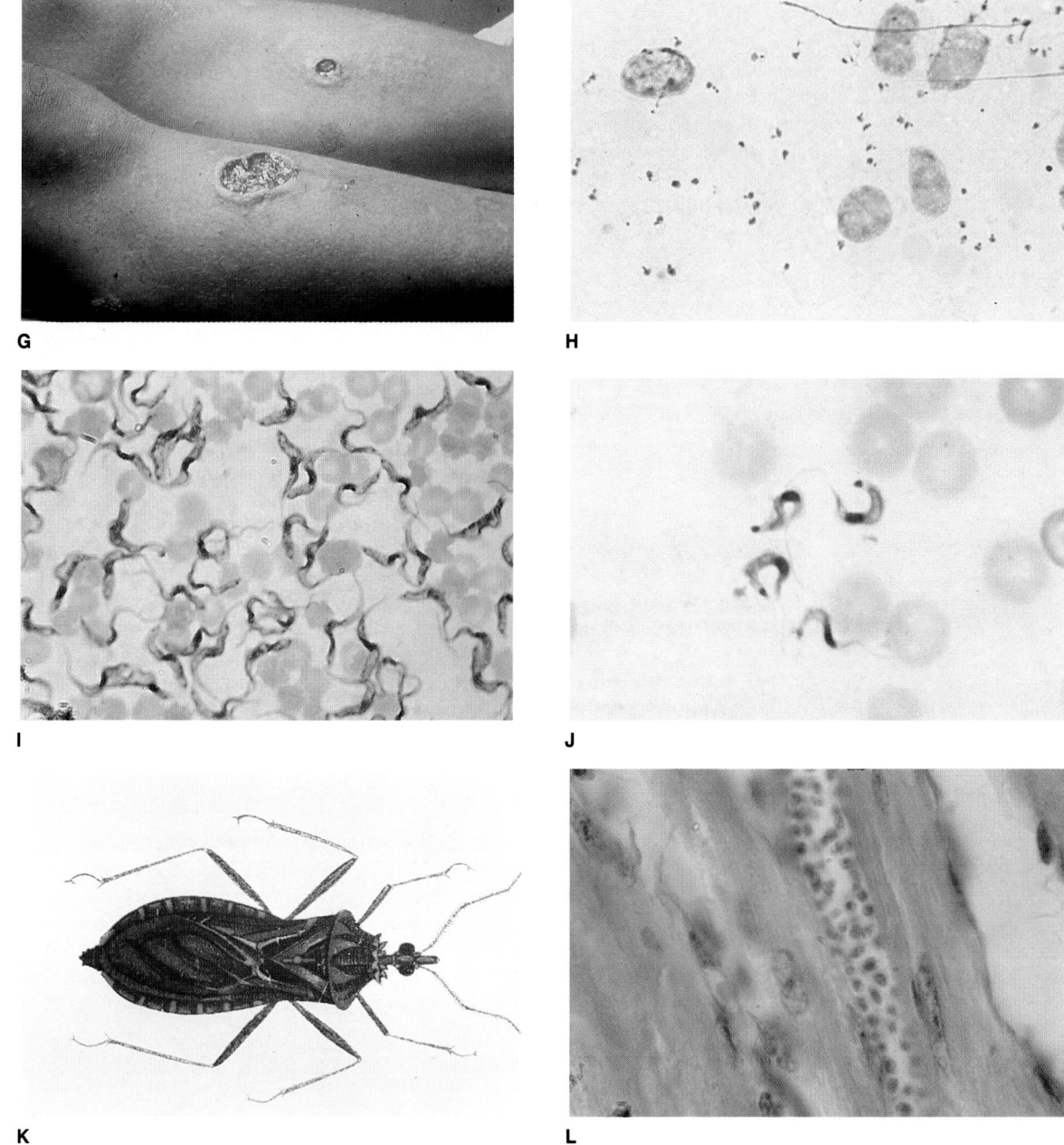

G

H

I

J

K

L

LABORATORY IDENTIFICATION OF TISSUE PARASITES

A. Photomicrograph of a peripheral blood smear demonstrating a sheathed micro-filaria. Microfilariae are extracellular parasites that measure about 245 to 295 μm in length and between 7 and 10 μm wide. They are released into the circulation from gravid female worms that reside within lymphatic channels in infected parts of the body. The microfilaria of species pathogenic for humans have a sheath, as well illustrated in this photograph. As the column of nuclei seen in the parasite illustrated in this photograph does not appear to extend to the tip of the tail, the most likely species is *Wuchereria bancrofti*.

B. Photomicrograph of a peripheral blood smear illustrating the tail section of a microfilaria and the nuclear arrangement in the tail portion of a microfilaria. Notice the two detached nuclei extending into the tail section, a feature characteristic of *Brugia malayi*.

C. Photomicrograph of a peripheral blood smear demonstrating a microfilaria of *Loa loa*, with the column of nuclei characteristically extending to the tip of the tail section.

D. Photomicrograph of an H&E-stained section of a subcutaneous nodule including in cross section the body of a female filarial worm, *Onchocerca volvulus*. Within the cavity of this organism are numerous microfilariae, which ultimately are released into the surrounding tissue. The microfilariae of *O. volvulus* do not circulate in the peripheral blood.

E. Photograph of a dog heart heavily infested with the adult worms of *Dirofilaria immitis*. Canines serve as the definitive host for this tissue nematode. In humans, who may serve as inadvertent accidental hosts, the larval forms never reach the heart, being stopped in the lungs where they produce a granulomatous inflammatory reaction.

F. Photomicrograph of a Giemsa-stained impression smear demonstrating numerous blue-staining tachyzoites of *Toxoplasma gondii*. Each tachyzoite measures about 3 by 6 μm, is pyriform or bow-shaped, has a nucleus and various internal organelles, including mitochondria, endoplasmic reticulum, and a Golgi apparatus, as seen in electron micrographic prints. The tachyzoites are the infective form of the parasite and can transmigrate the placenta of pregnant women, leading to congenital infections in unborn fetuses.

G. Photomicrograph of an H&E-stained section of a brain biopsy from a patient with cerebral toxoplasmosis. Demonstrated in this photograph are three cysts, ranging between 10 and 20 μm in diameter, within which are packed a myriad of tiny blue-staining tachyzoites. While in the cyst form the disease is arrested; however, with loss of immunity, the cyst wall breaks down, releasing the tachyzoites, leading to progressive reinfection.

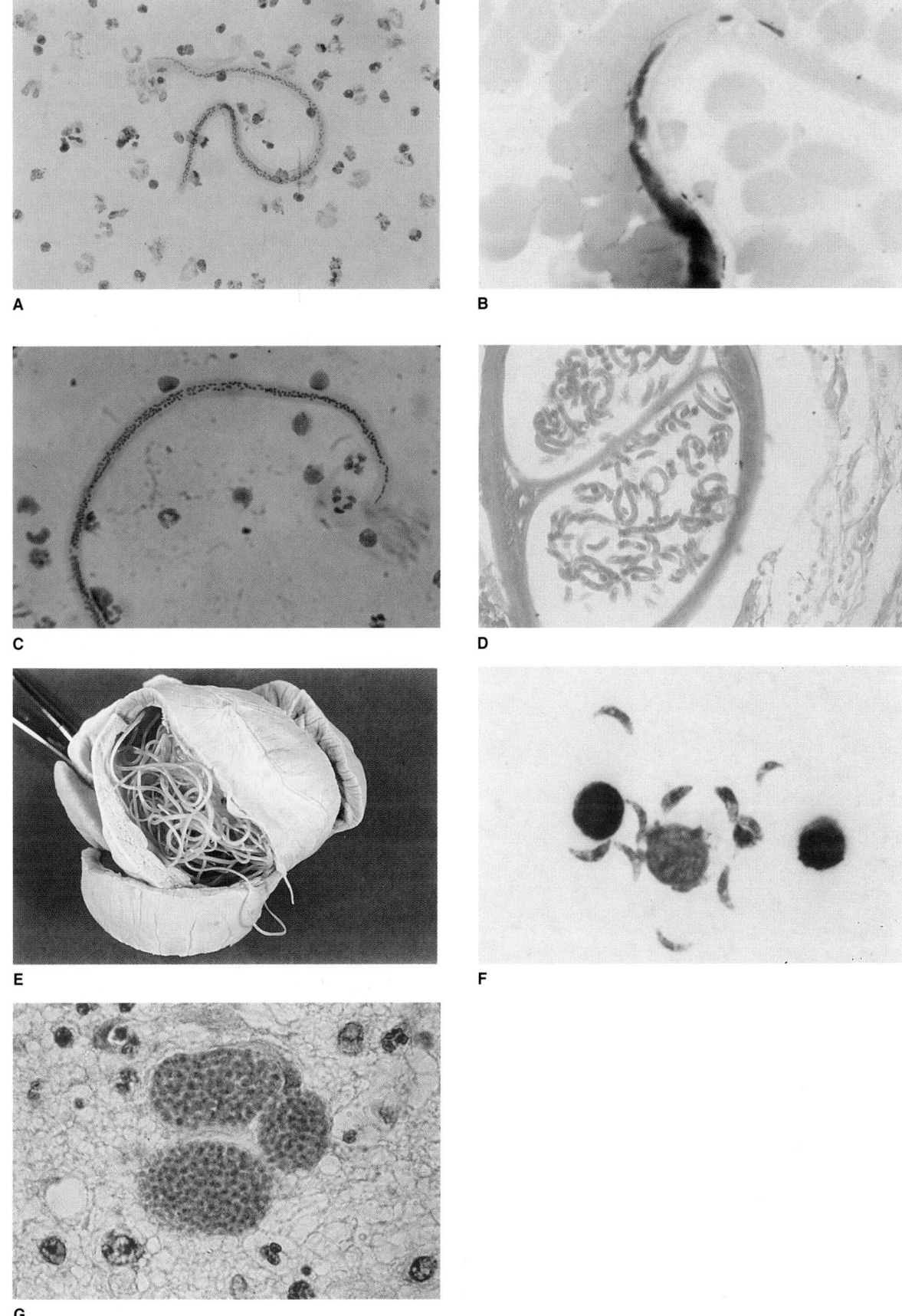

A

B

C

D

E

F

G

H. Split-frame photomicrograph of a methenamine silver-stained smear (*left*) prepared from material obtained from a bronchoalveolar lavage specimen. Seen are numerous gray-black spherical organisms of *Pneumocystis carinii*. The silver stain highlights the cyst cell wall and does not stain the intracellular organisms. However, thickened areas of the cell wall may appear as a dark dot in the center of the cell as seen in this photograph, or as opposing parentheses. In the *right* frame is a photomicrograph of a rapid trichrome (Diff-Quick) stain of material obtained from bronchoalveolar lavage fluid from a patient with *P. carinii* pulmonary infection. Although this stain is rapid, locating and identifying the organisms requires some experience. The cell walls do not stain; rather, the tiny intracellular trophozoites become visible. The pneumocysts are located within aggregates of degenerate material, as shown in this photograph. Note the clear spherical areas within which are aggregates of up to eight tiny bodies, representing the trophozoites.

I. Photomicrograph of pressed muscle tissue from a patient with trichinosis. The preparation is stained with safranin and shows several characteristic spiral-shaped larvae, each enclosed within an ill-defined cystic space.

J. Split-frame photomicrograph of an H&E-stained section of brain (*left*) illustrating a hydatid cyst from a patient with echinococcosis. The cyst wall has a thin membrane derived from the parasite and a thicker reactive fibrous capsule produced by the host. The inner parasite membrane is a germinal membrane from which daughter embryos, each with an inverted scolex, develop. Three of these are shown in this photograph, each having an inverted scolex, two of which also have brown-staining hooklets. In the *right* frame is illustrated a single protoscolex ("hydatid sand") of *Echinococcus granulosis*. Note the inverted rostellum and the prominent row of hooklets, representing the anlage of the armed rostellum of the adult worm.

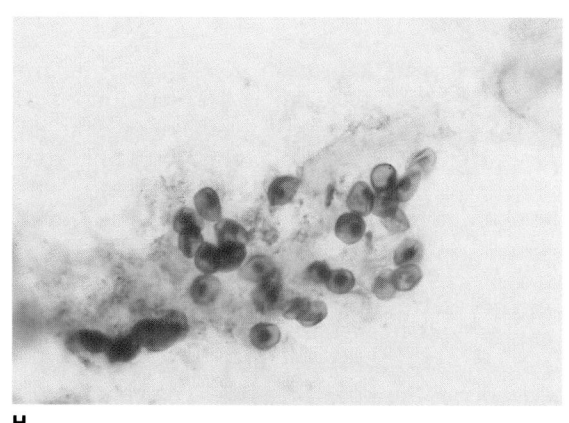

H

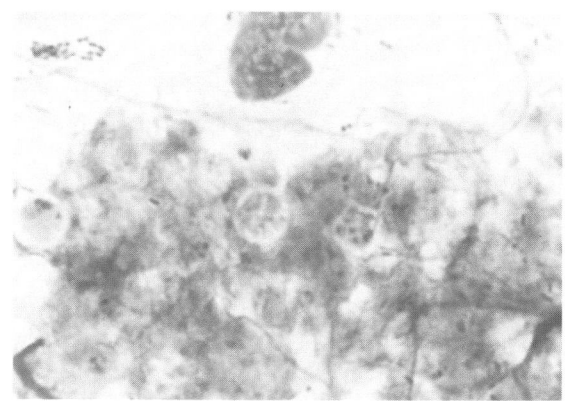

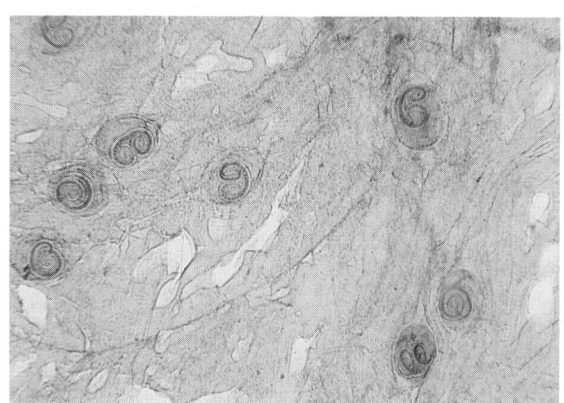

I

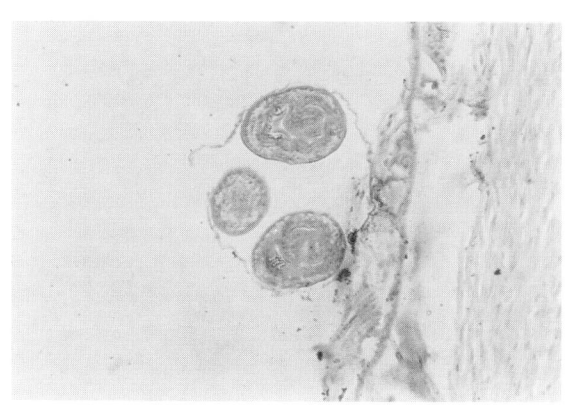

J

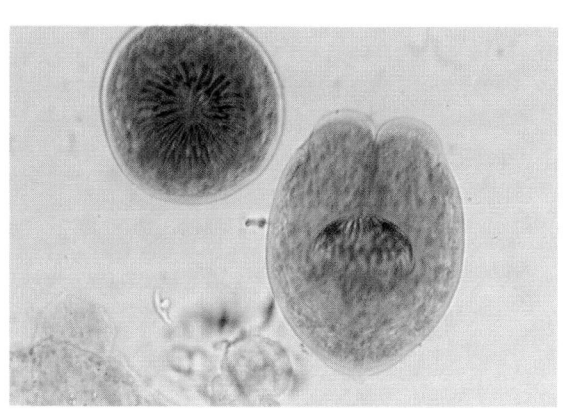

LABORATORY IDENTIFICATION OF SELECTED ECTOPARASITES

A. Dorsal view of *Ixodes* spp. The mouth parts of hard ticks are clearly visible from above, and the characteristic shieldlike scutum is evident. The scutum of *Ixodes* spp. does not have prominent or colorful markings. The size of an immature and a mature tick is illustrated by a dime. (Courtesy of Gerald Mandell, MD)

B. Ventral view of *Ixodes* spp. The characteristic semicircular groove around the anus is evident.

C. Dorsal view of *Dermacentor* spp. These hard ticks have prominent markings on the scutum. The mouthparts are clearly visible from above.

D. Dorsal view of *Amblyomma americanum*, the Lone Star tick. The characteristic white marking ("lone star") is evident, and the mouth parts are clearly visible. (Courtesy of David Spach, MD, and New England Journal of Medicine.[35] Used with permission)

E. Dorsal view of *Ornithodorus* spp. This soft tick lacks a scutum, and the mouthparts are not visible from above.

F. *Sarcoptes scabei* in its burrow. The mite has deposited eggs in its new-found home, adding to the discomfort of its victim.

G. *Dermatobia hominis:* The human bot fly has been extracted from a pustular lesion. The flask shape, tapered neck, and encircling spines of the larva are evident. The neck was damaged at the time of surgical extraction.

H. Ventral view of *Cimex* spp., the bedbug. The orange-brown color and characteristic shape provide identifying features.

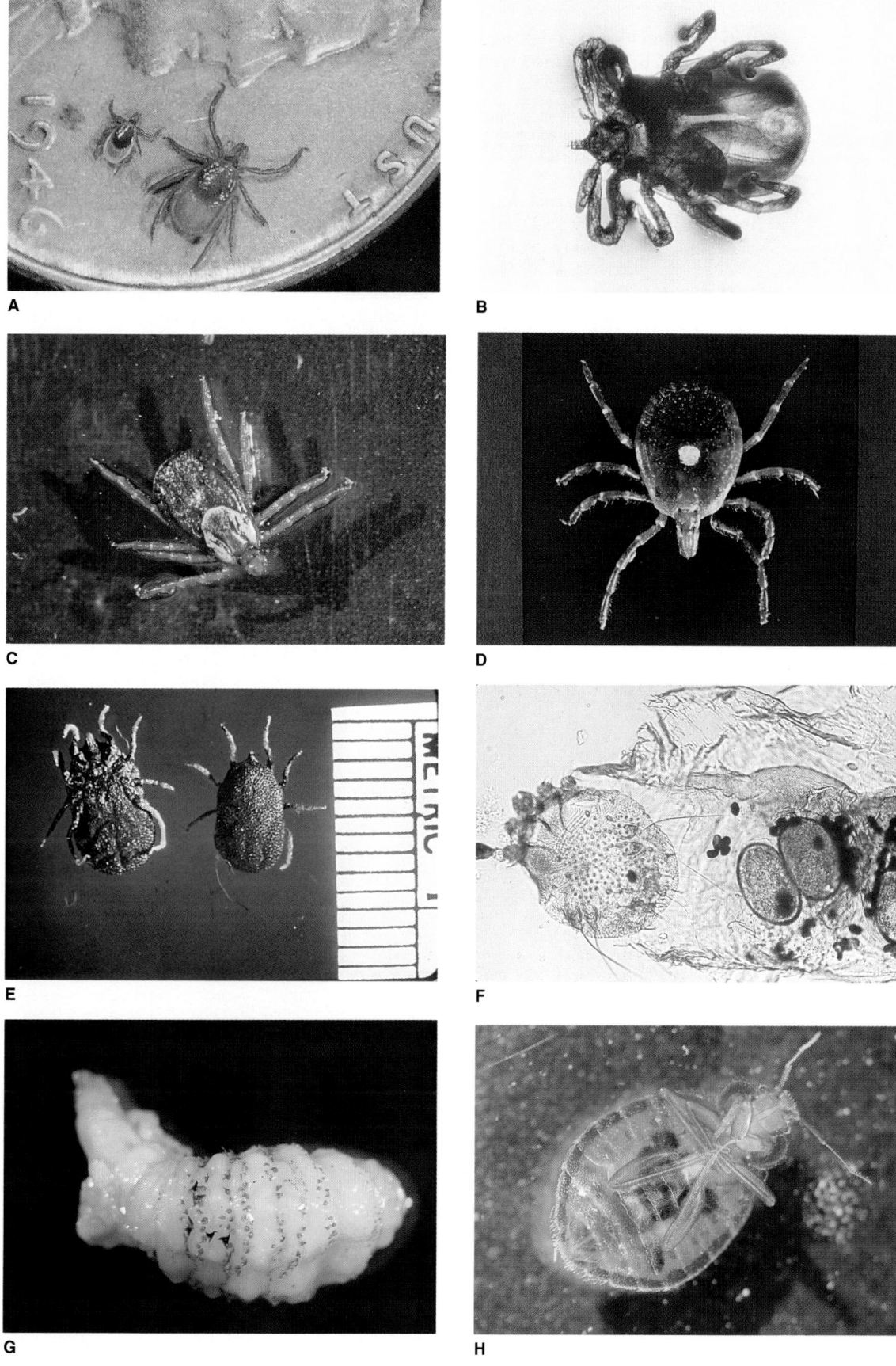

A

B

C

D

E

F

G

H

LABORATORY IDENTIFICATION OF SELECTED ECTOPARASITES (CONTINUED)

A. Dorsal view of *Triatoma* spp., a reduviid or kissing bug: The elongated body and long, thin head are characteristic. A pair of wings is evident.

B. *Tunga penetrans*, the jigger flea: Most fleas bite their host quickly and depart for completion of their life cycle, but the jigger flea remains embedded in the skin, where its eggs develop.

C. Female *Ctenocephalides* spp., the dog or cat flea: The long, muscular legs hang from the body and make the flea a prodigious jumper. The "hunched" appearance of the body is evident.

D. Female *Pediculosus humanus*, the human body louse: The long slender body supports three pairs of legs, each of which has clawlike hooks at the terminus.

E. Nit of a head louse: The egg is firmly attached to a hair shaft.

F. Female *Phthirus pubis*, the crab louse: The squat body and awesome pincers on three pairs of legs make the derivation of the popular name clear. The louse hangs onto a hair shaft, which also supports a nit.

G. *Loxosceles reclusa*, the brown recluse spider. The brown color and characteristic head marking distinguish this venomous spider. (Courtesy of Robert Suter, PhD)

H. Black widow spider: The deep black color and characteristic red, hourglass-shaped marking on the ventral side are clearly visible. (Courtesy of Robert Suter, PhD)

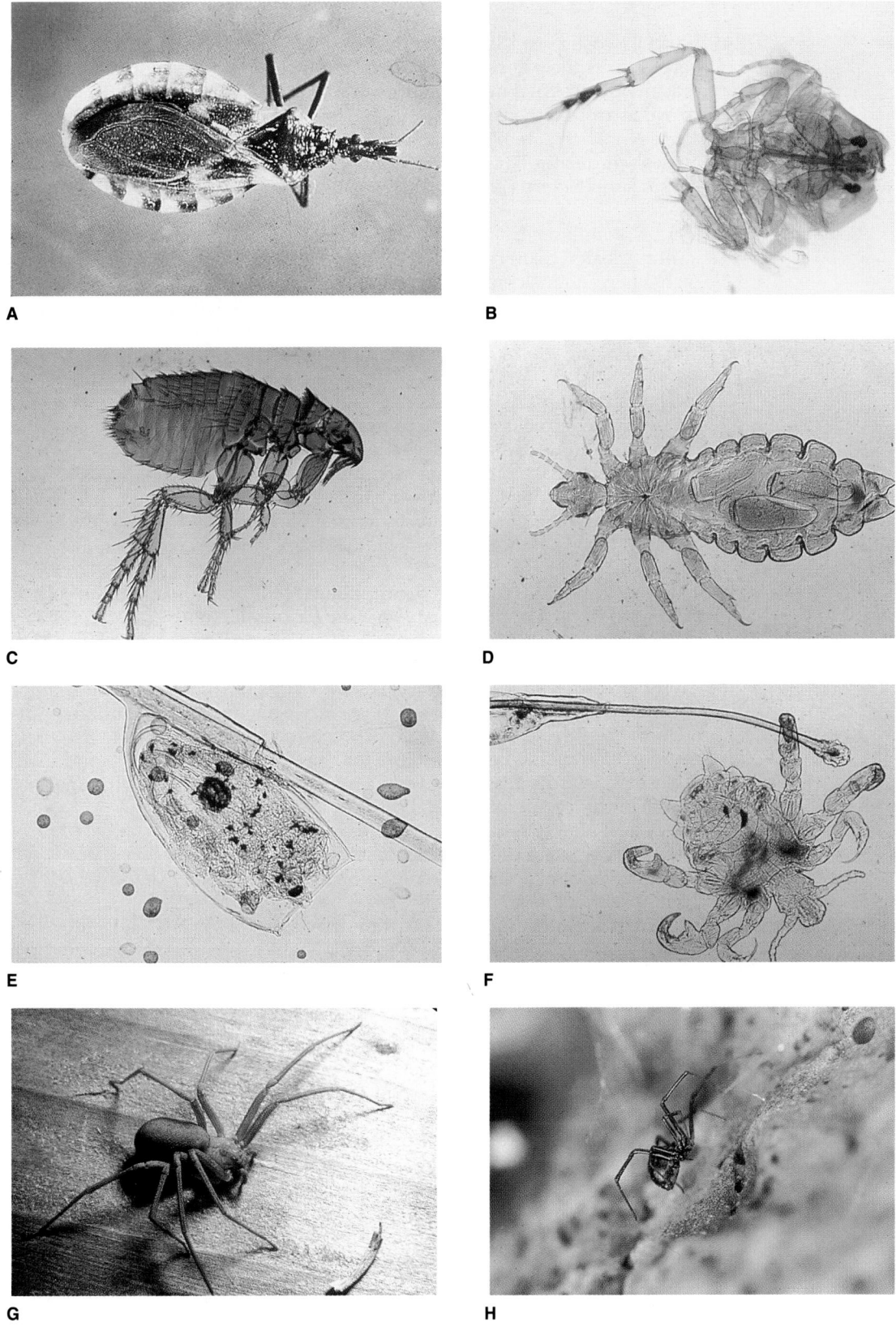

A

B

C

D

E

F

G

H

VIRAL INCLUSION

A. Varicella-zoster virus hepatitis. The nuclei of several hepatocytes contain typical herpes virus inclusions. The mass of the inclusion is eosinophilic and colored red, and the residual nuclear chromatin, which is basophilic and colored blue, is crowded around the rim of the nuclear membrane. The inclusion stands out because of an artifactual clear halo between the inclusion and the peripheralized nuclear chromatin. This artifact is caused by formalin fixation. The inclusions of herpes simplex virus and varicella-zoster virus cannot be distinguished. (H&E)

B. Herpes simplex cervicitis. The Papanicolaou stain demonstrates numerous multinucleated giant cells in a cervical scraping. The nuclei are molded against each other, and inclusions are present. The inclusions appear homogeneous and nuclear chromatin is peripheralized to the rim of the nuclear membrane. The cytologic preparation was fixed promptly in ethanol, and the formalin halo artifact is not present. A mature squamous epithelial cell stains pink.

C. Herpes simplex vesicular lesion—Tsanck test. These cells were scraped from the base of a herpetic vesicle. The multinucleated cell is characteristic of herpes infection, but one cannot differentiate the effects of herpes simplex virus from those of varicella-zoster virus. The multiple nuclei are molded and homogeneous, but inclusions are difficult to see in air-dried smears that have been stained with a Giemsa or similar stain. The direct scrapings can also be stained by the Papanicolaou method or with hematoxylin and eosin.

D. Cytomegalovirus sialadenitis. The epithelial cells of a salivary gland contain the inclusions of cytomegalovirus. The large basophilic (blue or purple) inclusions fill much of the nucleus. In some cells there are artifactual clear halos between the inclusion and the nuclear membrane that are produced by formalin fixation. Granular cytoplasmic inclusions are also visible in some cells. The architecture of the salivary gland is distorted by an intense lymphocytic infiltrate. Enlargement of the infected cells and nuclei inspired the name of the virus. Salivary gland virus was the original name for the virus, and salivary gland inclusion disease was the original name for the infection, because of the prominence of infection of this organ in neonatal disease. (H&E)

E. Adenovirus pneumonia. In this case of adenovirus infection there is a large amount of proteinaceous exudate (which is eosinophilic) in the air spaces, but there are few inflammatory cells. The nuclei of the infected respiratory epithelial cells are completely replaced by viral deoxyribonucleic acid, which produces a dense basophilic inclusion. Early inclusions may resemble those of herpes simplex virus. The mature inclusions, as seen here, fill the nucleus and obliterate the outline of the nuclear membrane. They are referred to as *smudge cells*. (H&E)

F. Measles virus pneumonia. Several large multinucleated giant cells are in the airways of this patient with measles pneumonia. The multiple nuclei contain eosinophilic nuclear inclusions that resemble those of herpes simplex virus. The nuclear chromatin is pushed to the rim of the nuclear membrane, but the formalin clear halo artifact is not present in this section. In addition, in this case there are also eosinophilic cytoplasmic inclusions, some of which are coalescent and/or surrounded by a clear space. (H&E)

G. Respiratory syncytial virus infection. Monolayer of HEp-2 cells infected with respiratory syncytial virus. Two large syncytial giant cells have formed in the monolayer. There are no inclusions in the nuclei of the cells, but several brightly eosinophilic intracytoplasmic inclusions can be seen. (H&E)

H. Rabies encephalitis. Two neurons each have an eosinophilic intracytoplasmic inclusion, which is known as a *Negri body*. Some vacuoles are evident in the inclusion. The irregular appearance comes from an admixture of normal cytoplasmic structures with masses of viral ribonucleic acid (H&E). (Courtesy of Daniel Perl, MD).

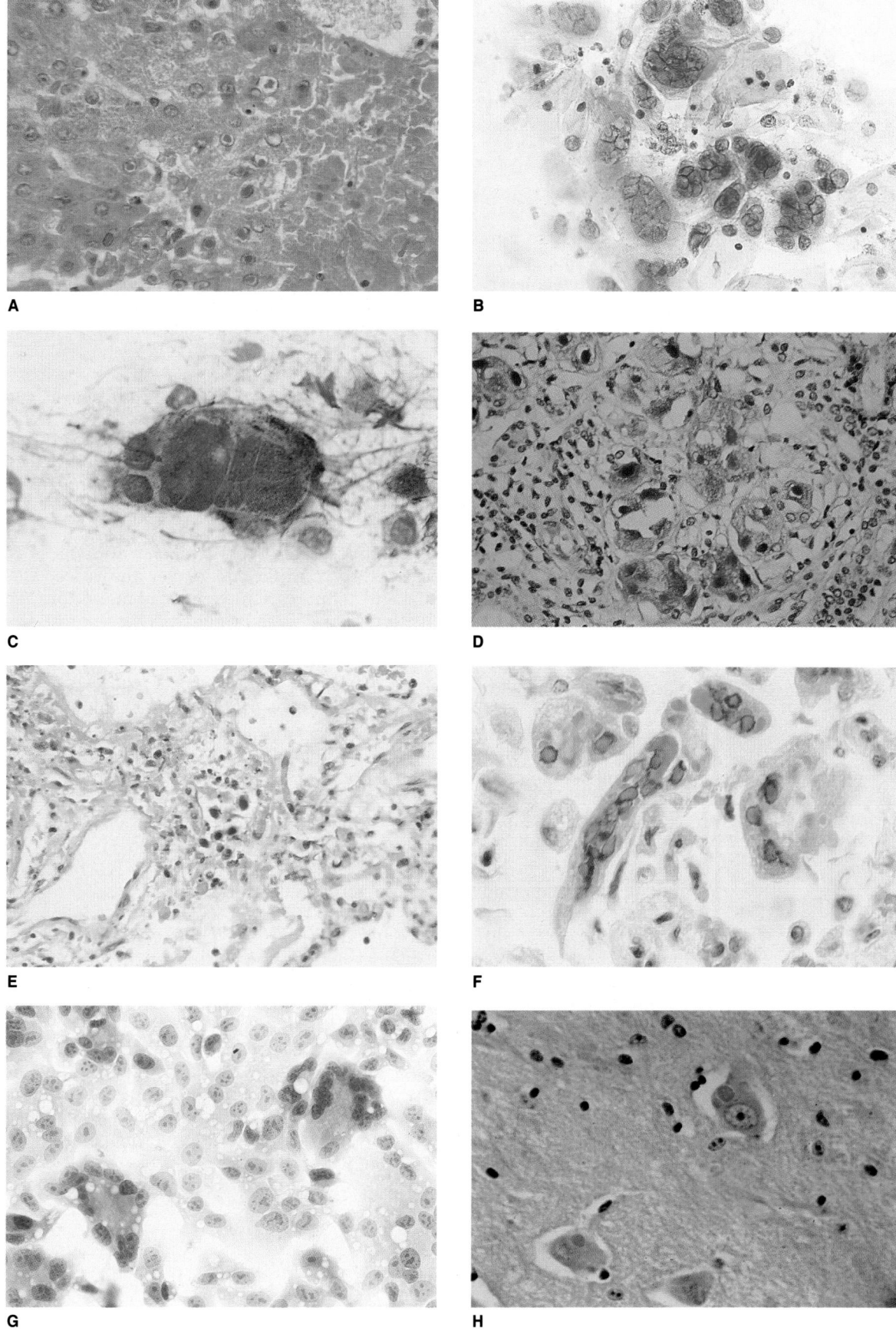

A

B

C

D

E

F

G

H

DIAGNOSIS OF INFECTIONS CAUSED BY VIRUSES, *CHLAMYDIA*, AND *EHRLICHIA*

A. *Chlamydia trachomatis* inclusion conjunctivitis. An epithelial cell that contains a chlamydial inclusion body is depicted. The cell has degenerated, leaving only the nucleus and the large inclusion. The large inclusion is molded around or capped over the underlying nucleus. Smear stained by the Giemsa method. (Photograph reproduced with permission of Julius Schachter and Publishing Sciences Group, Inc.)

B. *C. trachomatis* cervicitis. Innumerable elementary bodies are present in this very heavy infection. The Evans blue counterstain causes the cells to fluoresce red, and the inclusions appear yellow in the photomicrograph. In areas with less background material or without a counterstain the fluoresceinated antibody causes the elementary bodies to fluoresce apple green. A very heavily infected cell is present in the center of the photograph. Such cases are little challenge, but detecting positive specimens in which only a few elementary bodies are present is considerably more difficult.

C. McCoy cell monolayer infected with *C. trachomatis*. The specimen was centrifuged onto this monolayer of cycloheximide-treated McCoy cells, which were incubated for 48 hours. The cells have been stained with a fluorescein-conjugated monoclonal antibody to a major outer membrane protein (MOMP) of *C. trachomatis*. Multiple intracytoplasmic inclusions, which correspond to the inclusion demonstrated in **A** above, stain bright green.

D. HEp-2 cells infected with herpes simplex virus, type 1. When cytopathic effect became evident, the cells were scraped from the monolayer and placed on a slide. The cells have been stained with a fluorescein-conjugated monoclonal antibody to herpes simplex virus, type 1. There is bright, specific fluorescence, which is both nuclear and cytoplasmic.

E. Nasal aspirate infected with respiratory syncytial virus. Two cells in the smear show bright green cytoplasmic fluorescence. In addition to diffuse fluorescence, the discrete, punctate fluorescence represents viral inclusions, which are characteristic of this virus and help to confirm the specificity of the fluorescence. (FITC-conjugated monoclonal antibody to respiratory syncytial virus)

F. Cytomegalovirus-infected human diploid fibroblasts in a shell vial. The elongated fibroblast cells are colored by the counterstain. The infected cells are distinguished by the bright green fluorescence of the oval nuclei. (FITC-conjugated antibody to cytomegalovirus early-intermediate antigen)

G. Human monocytic ehrlichiosis caused by *Ehrlichia chaffeensis*. A circulating mononuclear cell contains a distinct cytoplasmic inclusion (morula) that is made up of individual bacterial cells. Inclusions are rarely seen in cases of monocytic ehrlichiosis (Wright stain. Slide contributed by J. Stephen Dumler, M.D.).

H. Human granulocytic ehrlichiosis caused by an unnamed *Ehrlichia* sp. A distinct bluish inclusion is present in the cytoplasm of a circulating neutrophil. The frequency with which inclusions are found in human granulocytic ehrlichiosis is unclear. (Wright stain. Slide contributed by J. Stephen Dumler, M.D.).

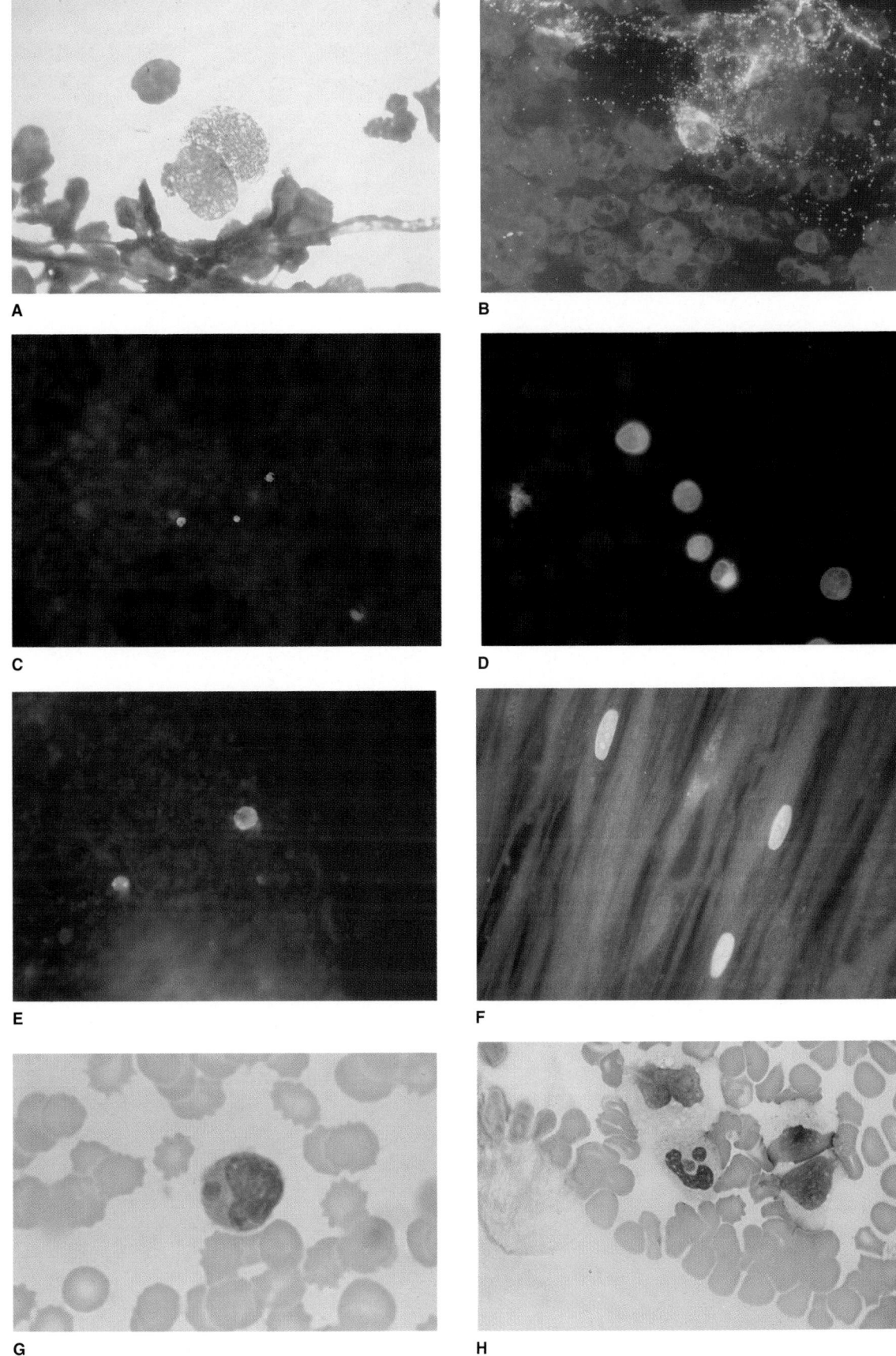

A

B

C

D

E

F

G

H

ANTIMICROBIAL SUSCEPTIBILITY TESTING

The primary role of clinical microbiology laboratory personnel is to provide information with which physicians can diagnose and treat infectious diseases. If a communicable disease is present, the identification of a specific pathogen is of utmost importance to a hospital epidemiologist or public health care worker. Identification of a microbe that has been recovered from a clinical specimen often benefits the patient by definitively identifying a puzzling disease and assisting in the provisional selection of chemotherapy. However, the two most important pieces of information for a clinician are 1) whether an infectious agent is present and 2) which antimicrobial agent should provide adequate therapy.

These priorities were derived from one of the great medical advances of this century—the discovery of penicillin.[70] In 1928, Alexander Fleming observed that a contaminant mold was growing in a culture dish that had been carelessly left open to the air. In addition, staphylococcal colonies growing adjacent to the mold were undergoing lysis (Fig. 15-1). Fleming correctly concluded that the mold, later identified as a strain of *Penicillium notatum,* was producing a diffusible bacteriolytic substance capable of killing staphylococci. Fleming's unknown antibiotic, which was later named penicillin, heralded the advent of the modern antibiotic era. The practical application of Fleming's discovery did not begin until 1939, when Florey and Chain developed a practical technique by which the antimicrobial extract of *Penicillium* could be obtained in sufficient purity and quantity for use in humans.

The need for antimicrobial susceptibility testing became evident soon after antibiotics became commercially available. Before World War II, penicillin production was limited and extremely expensive. During World War II, additional antibiotics were discovered and patterns of susceptibility against various organisms were established. Through his long-time interest in soil microbes Waksman discovered streptomycin in 1943, and Dubos discovered gramicidin and tyrocidin soon thereafter. Duggar's research resulted in the discovery of chlortetracycline (aureomycin) by Lederle Laboratories (Pearl River, NY) in 1944. Although these new antibiotics were truly "wonder drugs" at the time of their introduction, it was not long before resistant bacterial strains emerged. Susceptibility testing became a practical necessity.

Initial optimism that antibiotics would put an end to bacterial infection has given way to reluctant acceptance that chemotherapeutic resources must be managed wisely to control disease.[185] A few bacteria, such as *Streptococcus pyogenes* (group A β-hemolytic streptococci), have maintained their predictable susceptibility to penicillin. This persistent susceptibility is, unfortunately, the exception rather than the rule. Bacteria have been so inventive that strains have been isolated that require the presence of a therapeutic antibiotic for growth![75] The ingenuity of the chemists in the pharma-

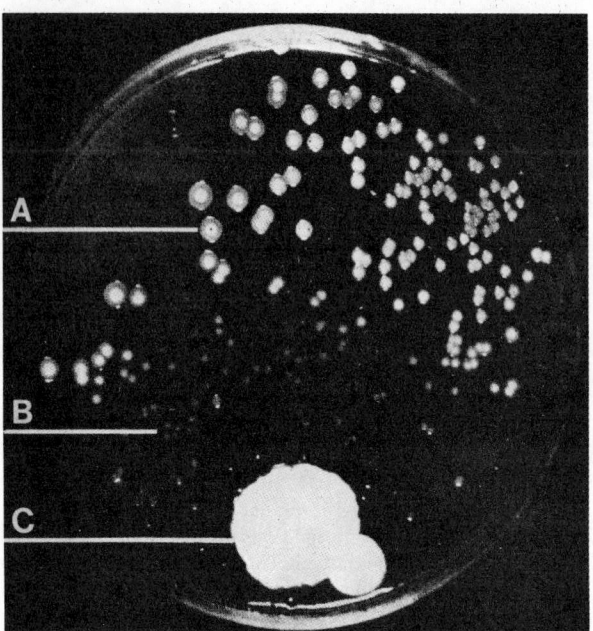

Figure 15-1
Reproduced photograph of Fleming's discovery of the antibiotic action of *Penicillium*. Colonies of *Staphylococcus* are seen growing at *A*; a contaminating colony of *Penicillium* is growing at *C*. The *Staphylococcus* colonies around the fungus colony in area *B* are poorly developed and are undergoing lysis secondary to an antibiotic substance produced by the mold. This unknown substance was later called penicillin.

ceutical industry has also been great and is reflected in the large number of antibiotics available to physicians (Table 15-1).

BACTERIAL RESISTANCE TO ANTIMICROBIAL AGENTS

The mechanisms of bacterial resistance are complex, varied, and not completely understood. Interested readers should consult Lorian's *Antibiotics in Clinical Medicine*[152] or an excellent discussion in Mandell's *Principles and Practice of Infectious Diseases.*[165] A comprehensive review is provided by Jacoby and Archer,[116] who have tabulated the major resistance mechanisms of the most important human pathogens. The tools of molecular biology have added greatly to our understanding of resistance mechanisms. For the clinical microbiologist the result can sometimes be intimidating and unfriendly terminology and extremely complex ideas. It is worth taking the time to understand at least the basics, however, both because of the beauty of the biologic systems and also because of the increased sophistication with which day-to-day clinical decisions can be made.

TABLE 15-1
CLASSIFICATION OF ANTIBIOTICS

CLASS	GROUP	EXAMPLES
β-Lactams	Natural penicillins	Penicillin G, penicillin V
	Penicillinase-resistant penicillins (PRP)	Nafcillin, methicillin
	PRP: isoxazolyl penicillins	Oxacillin, cloxacillin, dicloxacillin
	Amino penicillins	Ampicillin, amoxicillin
	Carboxy penicillins	Carbenicillin, ticarcillin
	Ureidopenicillins	Piperacillin, azlocillin, mezlocillin
	First-generation cephalosporins	Cephalothin, cefazolin, cephradine, cephapirin
	Second-generation cephalosporins	Cefamandole, cefuroxime, cefonicid, cefaclor
	Cephamycins	Cefoxitin, cefotetan, cefmetazole
	Third-generation cephalosporins	Ceftriaxone, cefotaxime, ceftizoxime, cefoperazone, cefpirome, cefpiramide
	Monobactams	Aztreonam
	Carbapenems	Imipenem, meropenem
	β-Lactamase inhibitors	Clavulanate, sulbactam, tazobactam
Aminoglycosides		Streptomycin, gentamicin, tobramycin, netilmicin, kanamycin, amikacin
Macrolides		Erythromycin, clarithromycin, azithromycin
Lincosamides		Lincomycin, clindamycin
Glycopeptides		Vancomycin, teicoplanin
Quinolones		Norfloxacin, ciprofloxacin, ofloxacin

MECHANISTIC VARIABLES

To understand the mechanisms of bacterial resistance it is necessary to understand bacterial physiology, the pharmacology of antimicrobial drugs, and the molecular biology of infectious agents. Some of the important variables needed to understand resistance mechanisms are listed in Table 15-2.

The genes for the resistance mechanism may be located either on the chromosome or on an extrachromosomal element called a plasmid. Plasmids are circularized pieces of DNA that act independently of the chromosome. The practical significance of the difference is that the chromosomal DNA is relatively stable whereas the plasmid DNA is easily mobilized from one strain to another, one species to another, or even one genus to another. In addition, the linking of resistance genes for multiple antibiotics on a plasmid allows the bulk transfer of resistance that characterizes many newly resistant organisms.[226]

The most common mechanism by which resistance genes are transferred is conjugation. An additional genetic transfer factor is necessary before a plasmid that carries a resistance gene can move from one organism to another. The most recently delineated transfer mechanism is the transposon (transposable genetic element).[239] Transposons can carry portions of plasmids. More importantly, they can also carry a piece of the chromosome from one bacterium to another by conjugal transfer (conjugative transposon or "jumping gene"). Transfer of antibiotic resistance across a major barrier between gram-positive and gram-negative bacteria has been documented.[39]

A resistance mechanism may be expressed continuously whether an inciting challenge is present or not. This state is referred to as constitutive expression. In contrast, some genes must be "induced" to produce their product by exposure to the challenge substance. Staphylococcal β-lactamase (penicillinase) is an exam-

TABLE 15-2
VARIABLES IN THE EXPRESSION AND TRANSFER OF BACTERIAL RESISTANCE

CHARACTERISTIC	VARIABLE	COMMENTS
Location	Chromosomal	Genetic stability; expression often constitutive
	Extrachromosomal	Plasmids easily mobilized for transfer from bacterial cell to cell
	Transposon	Can move genetic material between chromosome and plasmid or between bacterial cells
Transfer	Conjugation	Either plasmids (R-factor) or transposons
	Transduction	Transfer by bacteriophage
	Transformation	Direct transfer of DNA between compatible species
Expression	Constitutive	Produced with or without exposure to stimulus
	Inducible	Produced only after exposure to stimulus
	Constitutive–inducible	Produced at low level without stimulus; production greatly increased after stimulation

ple of an inducible enzyme. It is present on a plasmid and is not produced unless the bacteria are exposed to a β-lactam antibiotic, such as penicillin, after which production of the enzyme is turned on. Many β-lactamases of gram-negative bacteria are present on the chromosome and are produced constitutively, but may be induced to produce greater levels of enzyme.

Some enzymes are secreted actively into the extracellular environment, where they can exert their antibacterial action. The β-lactamases of staphyloccci are secreted. In contrast, most of the enzymes of gram-negative bacteria are cell bound so that they exert their effects only if the antibiotic enters the bacterial cell wall.

Finally, some resistance mechanisms are expressed homogeneously, while others are expressed heterogeneously. Homogeneous or uniform expression of a factor facilitates detection of the factor in the laboratory. If only a small fraction of the bacteria expresses the resistance mechanism (heterogeneous expression or heteroresistance), sampling error may compromise detection of the resistance in the laboratory.

MECHANISMS OF RESISTANCE

The mechanisms by which resistance is expressed in bacteria are summarized in Table 15-3 and Figure 15-2. Transport of antibiotics to their site of action will be considered first, because it is important for all compounds and all bacteria. Other mechanisms of resistance will be considered separately for antibiotics that are active against cell walls (the β-lactam antibiotics, the single most important group of antimicrobial agents, and the glycopeptides) and for antimicrobial agents that work by other mechanisms. It should be emphasized at the outset that virtually any resistance mechanism may be found in most bacteria and that multiple mechanisms are often found in a single or-

ganism (Table 15-4). It is impossible to overestimate the importance of multiple, often complementary mechanisms of resistance in bacterial species. When a pharmaceutical representative boasts that the antibiotic from his company should be used because of its effectiveness against prevalent resistant strains, be assured that it will only be a matter of time before the bacteria develop resistance to this product also.

TRANSPORT OF ANTIMICROBIAL AGENTS ACROSS THE CELL WALL AND CELL MEMBRANES

Accumulation of antibiotics at their site of action in the bacterial cell is the sum of transport into the cell, inactivation during the transport process, and clearance of antibiotic from the cell. The process of forward movement across the membrane(s) will be considered first. To understand transport of molecules to the active site it is necessary to consider the structural differences between gram-positive and gram-negative bacteria. Bacteria are prokaryotic organisms, and both gram-positive and gram-negative species contain a mixture of nucleic acids, ribosomes, and other cellular machinery in their cytoplasm (Fig. 15-3). Gram-positive bacteria have a single cell membrane with a generous external layer of peptidoglycan (Fig. 15-3A and Fig. 15-4). For β-lactam and glycopeptide antibiotics, which probably do not have to traverse the plasma membrane to exert their antimicrobial activity, transport across membranes of gram-positive bacteria is not an issue at all.

Gram-negative bacteria possess an inner plasma membrane and an outer cell membrane, between which is an attenuated peptidoglycan layer (Fig. 15-3B and Fig. 15-5). Permeability of membranes to antibiotics and transport of the molecules across the barriers are most important for gram-negative bacteria, which

TABLE 15-3
MECHANISMS OF BACTERIAL RESISTANCE TO ANTIMICROBIAL AGENTS

MECHANISM	ANTIBIOTIC GROUP	EXAMPLES
Enzymatic inactivation	β-Lactams	β-Lactamases: penicillinases; cephalosporinases; carbapemenases
	Aminoglycosides	Aminoglycoside-modifying enzymes of gram-negative and gram-positive bacteria
Altered receptors	β-Lactams	Altered penicillin-binding proteins of gram-negative and gram-positive bacteria
	Ribosomal alterations	Tetracyclines, erythromycin, aminoglycosides
	DNA gyrase alterations	Quinolones
	Altered bacterial enzymes	Sulfamethoxazole, trimethoprim
Altered antibiotic transport	Alterations in outer membrane proteins (porins)	Gram-negative bacteria; decreased influx
	Reduced proton motive force	Aminoglycosides and gram-negative bacteria; decreased influx
	Active transport from bacterial cell	Tetracyclines; erythromycin; active efflux

have two membrane hurdles for antimicrobial agents that have targets inside the cell.

The outer cell membrane, which is a crucial barrier for all antimicrobial agents, will be considered first. Several excellent reviews of the subject have been published.[148,190,192] The simplest method for entry of drugs into the cell is direct diffusion across the lipid membrane, but even very hydrophobic substances do not cross the lipid bilayer efficiently. The reason for this block to diffusion is in part the asymmetric, polarized nature of the bacterial outer cell membrane, which has lipopolysaccharide with lipid A and an attached oligosaccharide on the outer aspect of the membrane only.

Porin Proteins and Diffusion Through the Outer Membrane.   For many antibiotics, including the β-lactam group, the primary means of transport across the outer membrane of enteric bacteria are a remarkable group of membrane proteins, called porins (Fig. 15-5).[191,192,297] Two major porin proteins have been identified in *E. coli*, the most extensively studied species: a large porin channel designated Omp F (outer membrane protein F) and a small channel porin named Omp C.[297] A third channel called PhoE is produced in mutants that lack both Omp F and Omp C, but this channel does not appear to be important for antibiotic movement.[191] Factors such as the charge on the molecule and the hydrophobicity of the compound play an important role (Fig. 15-6). Negatively charged molecules move more slowly across the membrane than do more positively charged molecules or zwitterions (compounds with balanced positive and negative charges). Presumably the negative charges cause the antibiotic to "hang up" as it crosses the negatively charged porin channel. The

exclusion of hydrophobic compounds from the aqueous environment of the porin may explain the lack of efficacy of the hydrophobic compound methicillin against gram-negative bacteria. Likewise, β-lactam antibiotics with large bulky side chains, such as mezlocillin, piperacillin, and cefoperazone, also cross the membrane poorly. The "best performer" among the β-lactam antibiotics is imipenem, which is a zwitterionic, hydrophilic compound with a very compact structure.[297] It has been proposed that the explanation for susceptibility of *Enterobacter cloacae* to imipenem in the presence of resistance to third-generation cephalosporins is the greater accessibility of imipenem to targets, mediated by rapid transit probably through several porin channels.[206]

The influence of porins on susceptibility is well illustrated by an interesting case reported by Medeiros and colleagues (Fig. 15-7).[170] These researchers isolated a strain of *Salmonella typhimurium* that contained two porin proteins, OmpF and OmpC (isolate 1). A variant strain isolated from the same patient produced only the OmpF protein (isolate 2). Both strains produced a similar β-lactamase. In low osmolality media, strain 1 produced proteins F and C whereas strain 2 produced only protein F, the large channel porin. Under conditions of high osmolality, such as might occur in the patient's tissues, synthesis of the OmpF protein was repressed in both strains. On closure of the OmpF porin, expression of OmpC continued in strain 1 while in strain 2 there were no remaining transport channels (porins), so transport of the antibiotic across the membrane ceased and bacterial resistance resulted.

The porin proteins of other enteric gram-negative bacteria appear to behave in a similar fashion to those

A
Enzymatic Cleavage

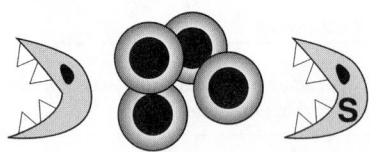

Examples: Beta lactamase
        Aminoglycoside Modifying Enzymes

B
Altered Receptors (Binding Proteins)

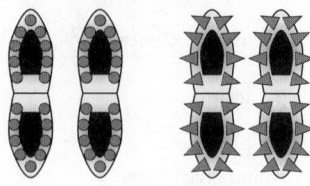

Examples: Pneumococcal Resistance to PCN
        Staphylococcal Resistance to Methicillin

C
Altered Permeability

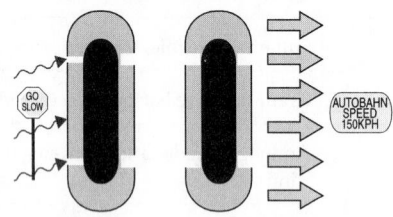

Examples: Pseudomonas and Aminoglycosides (Influx)
        Tetracycline and Multible Antibiotics (Efflux)

D
Bypass of Inhibitions

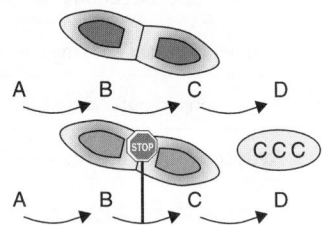

Example: Enterococci and Bactrim (Auxotroph)

Figure 15-2
The four most important classes of antimicrobial resistance to antibiotics are illustrated. (**A**) Enzymatic inactivation of antimicrobial agents is represented by the voracious sharks of β-lactamase (*S*) released from staphylococcal cells. Other classes of antibiotics are degraded by other enzymes, such as the aminoglycoside-modifying enzymes or chloramphenicol acetyltransferase. (**B**) The second most important mechanism is the change in receptors for antibiotic attachment to critical structures, here represented by alteration of normal binding proteins (*circles*) on the cell membranes of gram-positive bacteria to binding proteins with reduced affinity for antibiotics (*triangles*). Changes in the affinity of receptors for other antibiotics, such as DNA gyrase and quinolones or ribosomes and aminoglycosides, are also important. (**C**) A third class of mechanism is represented by the effect of membrane permeability on resistance to several classes of antibiotics in gram-negative bacteria. The gram-negative bacillus on the *left* restricts entry of antibiotics by changes in transport proteins, such as porins. The bacillus on the *right* is pumping antibiotics out of the cell so fast that they cannot accumulate in the cytoplasm. (**D**) Lastly, bypass of a metabolic block imposed by antimicrobial agents is illustrated by trimethoprim–sulfamethoxasole and enterococci. The metabolic block produced by the antibiotics between steps *B* and *C* is obviated when the bacteria obtain preformed compound *C in vivo*.

of *E. coli*. The porins of *Pseudomonas aeruginosa*, however, do not behave in the same way.[151] The only antibiotic for which resistance in *P. aeruginosa* by means of altered membrane transport is clearly explained is imipenem. In some situations this antibiotic gains entry, not through the main porin protein, but through a specific transport protein, designated D2.[217] It appears, however, that the presence of a chromosomal Class C β-lactamase is necessary for resistance in addition to the altered porin protein.[149]

Antibiotics other than β-lactam compounds may also depend on porin channels for access to the cell. Resistance to chloramphenicol, which is usually caused by enzymatic degradation, may also be mediated by altered porin proteins in enteric bacteria[270] and *Haemophilus influenzae*.[27] Similarly, resistance to aminoglycosides may be mediated by alterations in porin

proteins, although the primary mechanism for resistance is enzymatic degredation.[89] Resistance to quinolones, which is principally mediated by changes in the structure of the target enzyme, may also be caused by alterations in membrane proteins.[232]

Specific transport proteins have evolved in bacteria for transport of large molecules, such as vitamins, across the cell membrane. If antimicrobial agents could be devised that availed themselves of this ready-made superhighway into the bacterial cell, they would have a major competitive advantage. Unfortunately it has been difficult to develop such compounds that are also clinically useful.

For some bacteria that must gain entrance to the bacterial cytoplasm a second barrier may exist at the inner plasma membrane. Crossing the second membrane is accomplished by a process that requires expenditure of

TABLE 15-4
MECHANISMS OF ANTIMICROBIAL RESISTANCE IN CLINICALLY IMPORTANT BACTERIA

BACTERIAL TYPE	ANTIBIOTIC GROUP	COMMON MECHANISM(S)	OTHER MECHANISM(S)
Staphylococcus spp.	Penicillins	β-Lactamase (penicillinase)	Altered penicillin-binding proteins
	Penicillinase-resistant penicillins	Altered penicillin-binding proteins	Borderline: Altered penicillin-binding proteins; modification of normal proteins; methicillinase; hyperproduction of β-lactamase
	Quinolones	Active efflux; altered DNA gyrase	Poor transport across membrane
	Erythromycin	Altered ribosomal targets	Active efflux of antibiotic
Streptococcus pneumoniae	β-Lactams	Altered penicillin-binding proteins	
	Erythromycin	Altered ribosomal targets	
Enterococcus spp.	β-Lactams	Low-affinity penicillin-binding proteins	β-Lactamase
	Aminoglycosides	Low-level: Poor transport across membrane High-level: Aminoglycoside-modifying enzymes	Altered ribosomal binding sites
	Glycopeptides	Altered binding proteins	
Haemophilus influenzae	Penicillins	β-Lactamase (penicillinase)	Altered penicillin-binding proteins
	Chloramphenicol	Chloramphenicol acetyltransferase	Altered membrane transport
Neisseria gonorrhoeae	Penicillins	β-Lactamase (penicillinase)	Altered penicillin-binding protein
Neisseria meningitidis	Penicillins		β-Lactamase (penicillinase); altered penicillin-binding proteins
Enterobacteriaceae	β-Lactams	Poor diffusion or altered porins; β-lactamases	Altered penicillin-binding proteins; low proton motive force; extended-spectrum β-lactamases
	Aminoglycosides	Poor diffusion or altered porins; aminoglycoside-modifying enzymes	
	Quinolones	Altered DNA gyrase	Altered transport through outer membrane
	Tetracyclines	Active efflux	
	Trimethoprim–Sulfamethoxazole	Altered enzyme targets	
Pseudomonads	β-Lactams	Poor diffusion or altered porins; β-lactamases	Altered penicillin-binding proteins; low proton motive force; extended-spectrum β-lactamases
	Aminoglycosides	Poor diffusion or altered porins; aminoglycoside-modifying enzymes	
	Quinolones	Altered DNA gyrase	Altered transport through outer membrane

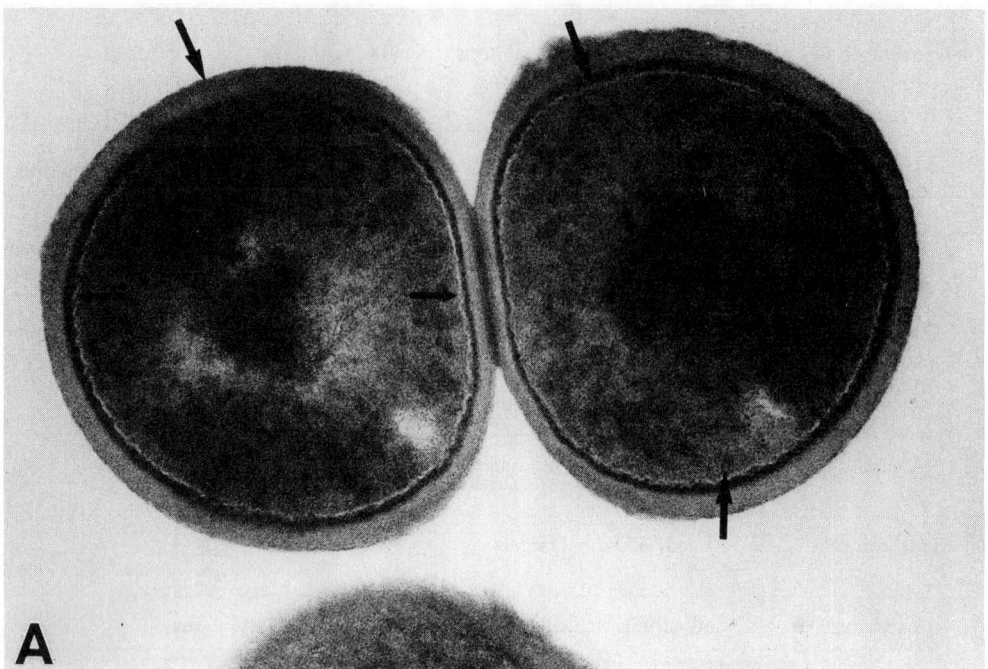

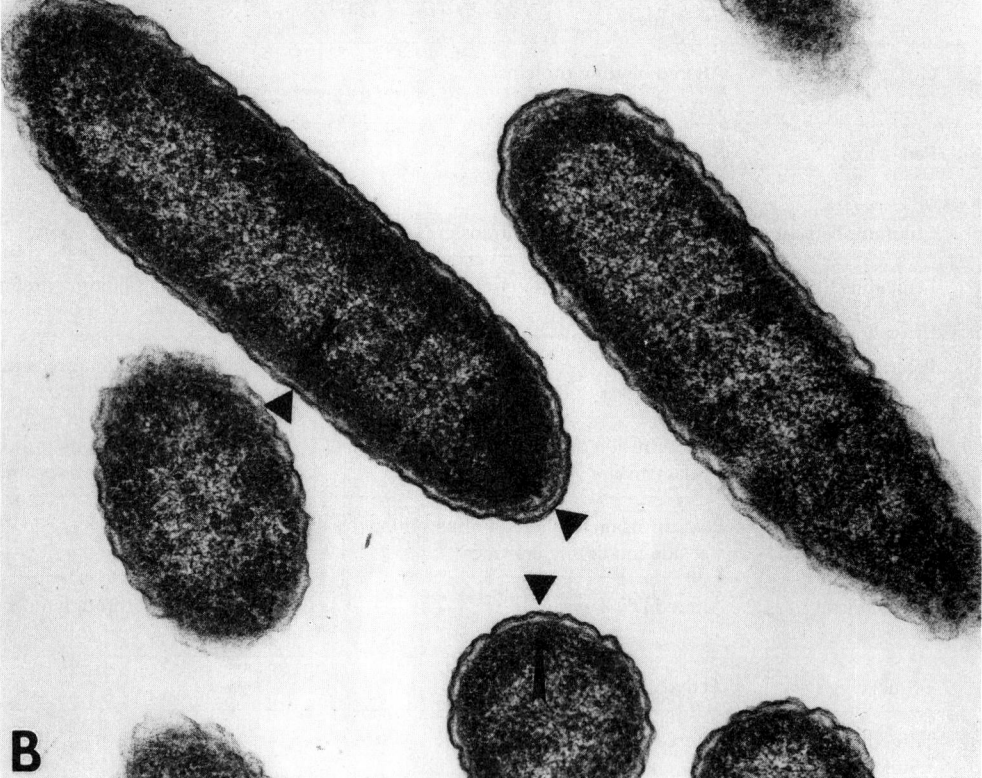

Figure 15-3
Ultrastructure of bacteria. (**A**) *Staphylococcus aureus.* Two gram-positive cocci are in the final stages of division. The bacterial cell membrane (*arrows*) is surrounded by a thick peptidoglycan layer that is freely accessible to antibiotics. ×30,000 (**B**) *Pseudomonas aeruginosa.* These gram-negative bacilli have an internal cytoplasmic membrane (*arrows*) and an outer cell membrane (*arrowheads*). Between these two membranes lies the periplasmic space that contains the peptidoglycan. β-Lactam antibiotics must cross the cell membrane before they reach the peptidoglycan. ×35,000

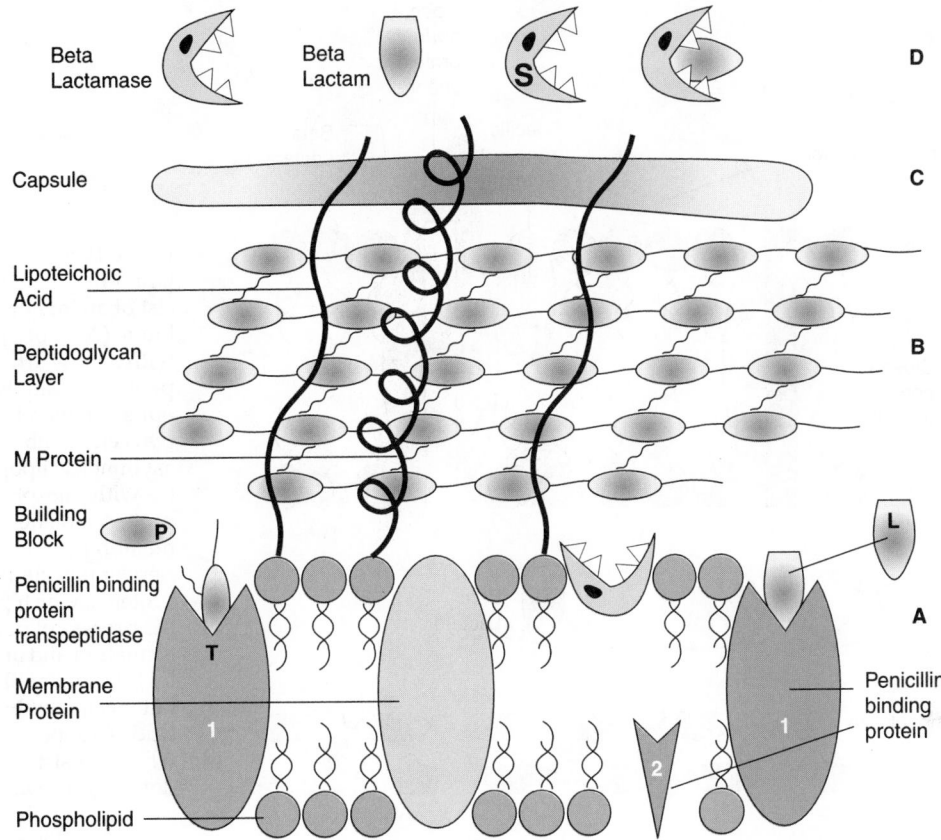

Figure 15-4

The cell wall of gram-positive bacteria consists, from inside out, of (**A**) a lipoprotein cell membrane, (**B**) a peptidoglycan cell wall, (**C**) a polysaccharide capsule (in some strains of some species, such as *Streptococcus pneumoniae*), and (**D**) the extracellular environment. The cell membrane *A* contains phospholipid, membrane proteins (including M protein in *Streptococcus pyogenes*), lipoteichoic acid in staphylococci, and a variety of penicillin-binding proteins, including β-lactamase, illustrated by the pac-men with shark's teeth (*S*). In gram-positive bacteria the β-lactamases are secreted into the extracellular environment (*D*), where they can inactivate β-lactam antibiotics. The peptidoglycan building blocks (*P*) in the cell wall (*B*) are integrated into the peptidoglycan by penicillin-binding transpeptidase in the membrane (*A*). β-Lactam antibiotics (*L*) also interact with these proteins in the membrane (*A*) and interfere with the process.

energy and a minimal negative charge in the cytoplasm, the proton motive force, in order to "pull" aminoglycoside antibiotics into the cytoplasm. This transport mechanism has been demonstrated in both gram-positive[159] and gram-negative bacteria.[26] Mutant *Enterobacteriaceae* have been described that are resistant to antibiotics in vitro because of deficiencies in this transport mechanism, but their clinical significance is unclear.[227] These variants appear as small colonies on agar media, but they may revert to normal colonial morphology.

Active Transport of Antibiotics Out of the Bacterial Cell. For some bacteria an important mechanism of resistance is active removal of antibiotics from the bacterial cell, so that the intracellular concentrations of antibiotics never reach a sufficiently high level to exert effective antimicrobial activity. This energy-dependent efflux mechanism is a prime defense for bacteria against tetracyclines[167] and macrolides,[88] two groups of antibiotics that interfere with protein synthesis at the ribo-

somal level. Similarly, removal of the antibiotic is a resistance mechanism of staphylococci against the quinolones, which interfere with DNA gyrase.[186] The transporter may effectively remove multiple types of antibiotic, as in the case of an outer membrane protein (OprK) that is involved in secretion of siderophores in *Pseudomonas aeruginosa*.[215] Mutant strains that overproduced the protein demonstrated resistance to multiple antibiotics, including ciprofloxacin, nalidixic acid, tetracycline, and chloramphenicol. Strains that had lost the ability to produce the transporter protein showed enhanced susceptibility to the antibiotics.

ANTIBIOTICS THAT INTERFERE WITH FORMATION OF BACTERIAL CELL WALLS: THE β-LACTAM AND GLYCOPEPTIDE ANTIBIOTICS

The Superfamily of Penicillin-Recognizing Enzymes and Antibiotics Active at Cell Membranes. Before trying to understand individual mechanisms of resistance it is

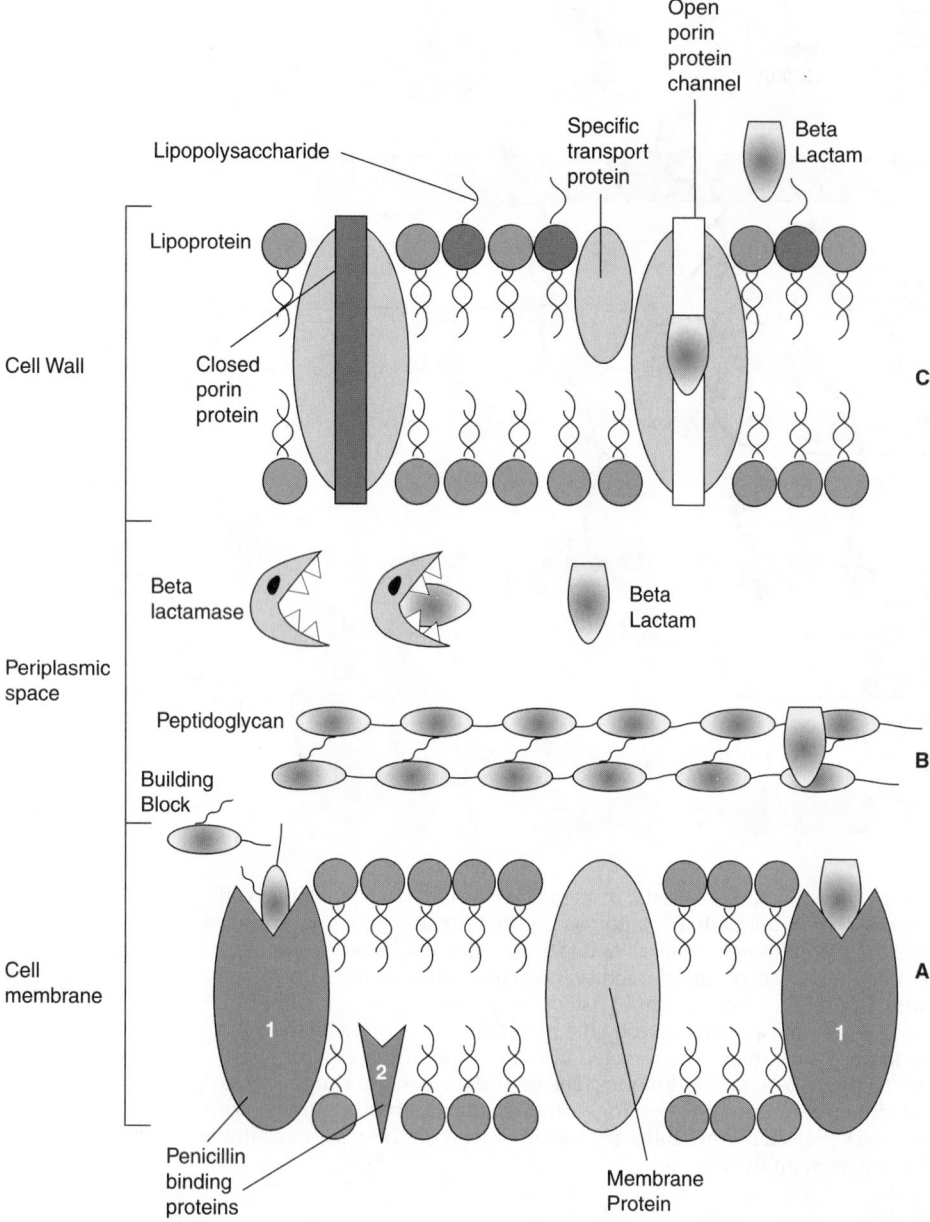

Figure 15-5
Gram-negative bacteria consist of an inner plasma membrane (**A**), a periplasmic space with a loose arrangement of peptidoglycan (**B**), and an outer cell membrane (**C**). The two cell membranes consist of asymmetric lipoprotein bilayers with phospholipids and protein moieties. The plasma membrane (*A*) contains a variety of penicillin-binding proteins, which participate in the process of peptidoglycan formation and are inhibited by β-lactam antibiotics. The outer cell membrane (*C*) includes lipopolysaccharide, which consists of lipid A (endotoxin), a covalently bound core, and a polysaccharide chain that determines the O somatic antigen used in many serologic typing schemes. The outer membrane also includes important transport proteins, including specific transporters and the important porin proteins of several sizes and types. β-Lactamase in gram-negative bacteria is limited to the periplasmic space, where it can inactivate antibiotics as they pass through; the β-lactamase is not secreted into the external environment.

important to consider the evolving concept of a superfamily of penicillin-recognizing enzymes and their relationship to the structure of bacterial cells. These interactions are integral to understanding the most important group of antimicrobial agents, the β-lactam family of antibiotics. As often happens in biology the complexity of the processes and interactions become more evident as we learn more about them. What appears at first glance to be an isolated process may eventually be seen as part of a much larger and more complex biologic system, much as a single dot in a Seurat painting can be appreciated as part of a beautiful work of art when one backs away and looks at the whole canvas.

THE PENICILLIN AND VANCOMYCIN-BINDING PROTEINS. Peptidoglycan, which provides rigidity and functional stability to the bacterial cell, consists of

strands of alternating amino sugars, *N*-acetylglucosamine and *N*-acetylmuramic acid, cross-linked by peptides. As discussed earlier, the peptidoglycan layer of gram-positive bacteria is a thick layer external to the single cell membrane (Fig. 15-3*A* and Fig. 15-4), whereas the peptidoglycan layer of gram-negative bacteria, which is attenuated, is located between the plasma membrane and the outer cell membrane (Fig. 15-3*B* and Fig. 15-5). The biosynthesis of peptidoglycan consists of many steps that begin in the cytoplasm and end outside the cell membrane. The final stage in the process is the transpeptidation of the developing peptidoglycan molecule, in which a terminal glycine residue on a pentaglycine side chain is linked to d-alanine on an adjacent strand, releasing a second d-alanine molecule in the process. A glycosylase and carboxylase also appear to be involved in the process, but their roles are less clear.[156] The transpeptidase, which is

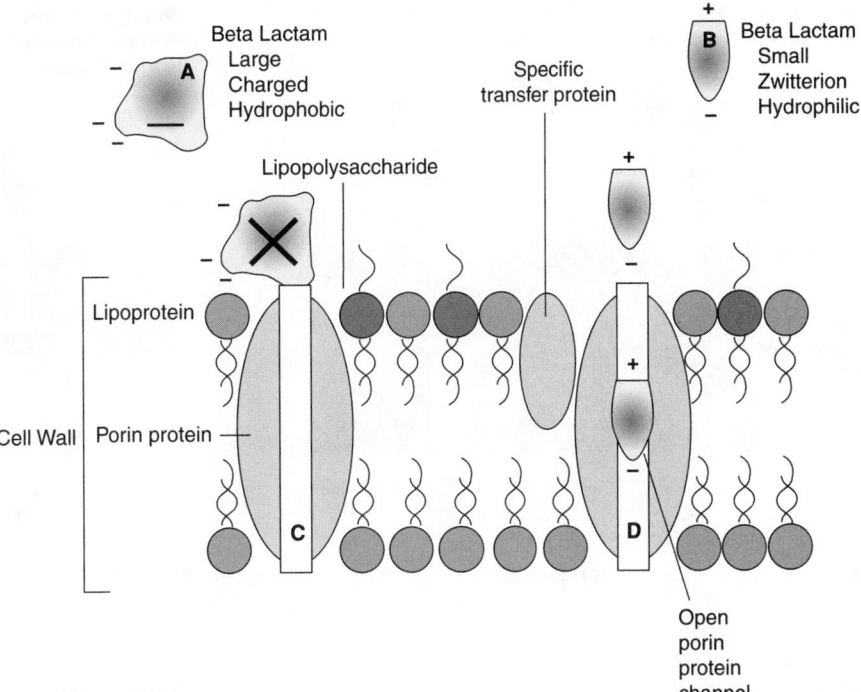

Figure 15-6
Factors influencing movement of antibiotics through the porin proteins of gram-negative bacteria: The outer cell membrane (see layer *C* of Fig. 15-5) is depicted. Two antibiotics with different characteristics are depicted. Antibiotic *A*, which is large, hydrophobic, and has multiple negative charges, is excluded by the porin channel (*C*). Antibiotic (*B*), which is compact, has balanced charges (zwitterionic) and is hydrophilic, moves through porin channel *D* without any difficulty.

bound to the cell membrane, is one of a family of enzymes known as penicillin-binding proteins, which in turn are part of the superfamily of penicillin-recognizing enzymes.[169] In addition to the transpeptidases, other penicillin-binding proteins participate in the formation of the bacterial cell wall. These binding proteins are attached to the cell membrane in gram-positive bacteria and to the inner plasma membrane in gram-negative species. The distinct function of different penicillin-binding proteins has been illustrated dramatically in *Escherichia coli*, where interference with different proteins produces different morphologic effects as the synthesis of cell walls is impaired (Fig. 15-8).[245] In bacillary organisms different binding proteins appear to function in the formation of cross-walls at cell division (protein 2 in *E. coli*) and in elongation of the cells after division (protein 3 in *E. coli*).[245] Penicillin-binding proteins are numbered according to their molecular weight, protein 1 having the highest molecular weight. The numbering system is specific for each species, so that penicillin-binding protein 1 in *Escherichia coli* is not the same as protein 1 in *Klebsiella pneumoniae* or *Streptococcus pneumoniae*. The high molecular weight compounds function as the transpeptidases that are essential for formation of peptidoglycan.[77,246] The low molecular weight compounds appear to function as d-alanine carboxypeptidases, and their biologic significance is unclear.

β-lactam antibiotics exert their effects by interfering with the formation of peptidoglycan, a mechanism that is shared with the glycopeptide agents, such as vancomycin.[268,282] Many years ago it was recognized that a structural similarity between the penicillin molecule and the d-alanine–d-alanine terminus of the peptidoglycan chain was integral to the antibacterial action of the compound.[266] Kelly and colleagues have elucidated the three-dimensional structure of the transpeptidase penicillin-binding protein and observed directly its interaction with penicillins and cephalosporins, definitively establishing the identity of the penicillin-binding site and the transpeptidase enzyme.[131] In essence penicillin fools the penicillin-binding protein into thinking it is the next building block to be added to the peptidoglycan chain. Once inserted, the penicillin molecule abrogates further elongation of the peptidoglycan. Various members of the large β-lactam group of antibiotics have differing affinities for individual penicillin-binding proteins. The efficacy of compounds against bacteria is, in part, determined by the degree to which they are bound. Aztreonam, which is a β-lactam antibiotic, does not interact with the binding proteins of gram-positive bacteria and is the only ineffective member of the group against these organisms. Bactericidal activity may require the interaction of a β-lactam antibiotic with more than one penicillin-binding protein.[92] Satta and colleagues demonstrated that resistance to *E. coli* increased as more critical binding proteins were saturated. Saturation of nonessential binding proteins had no effect on antimicrobial susceptibility.[234] The action of autolytic enzymes may also be important for the bactericidal activity of β-lactam antibiotics.[72]

The other major class of antibiotics that actively interferes with the synthesis of bacterial cell walls is the glycopeptide group, represented by vancomycin and teicoplanin. In contrast to β-lactam antibiotics, which block the activity of the cell membrane-bound peptidases, the glycopeptides bind noncovalently to the d-alanyl-d-alanyl terminus of a pentapeptide peptidoglycan precursor.[181] The antibiotic has structural and

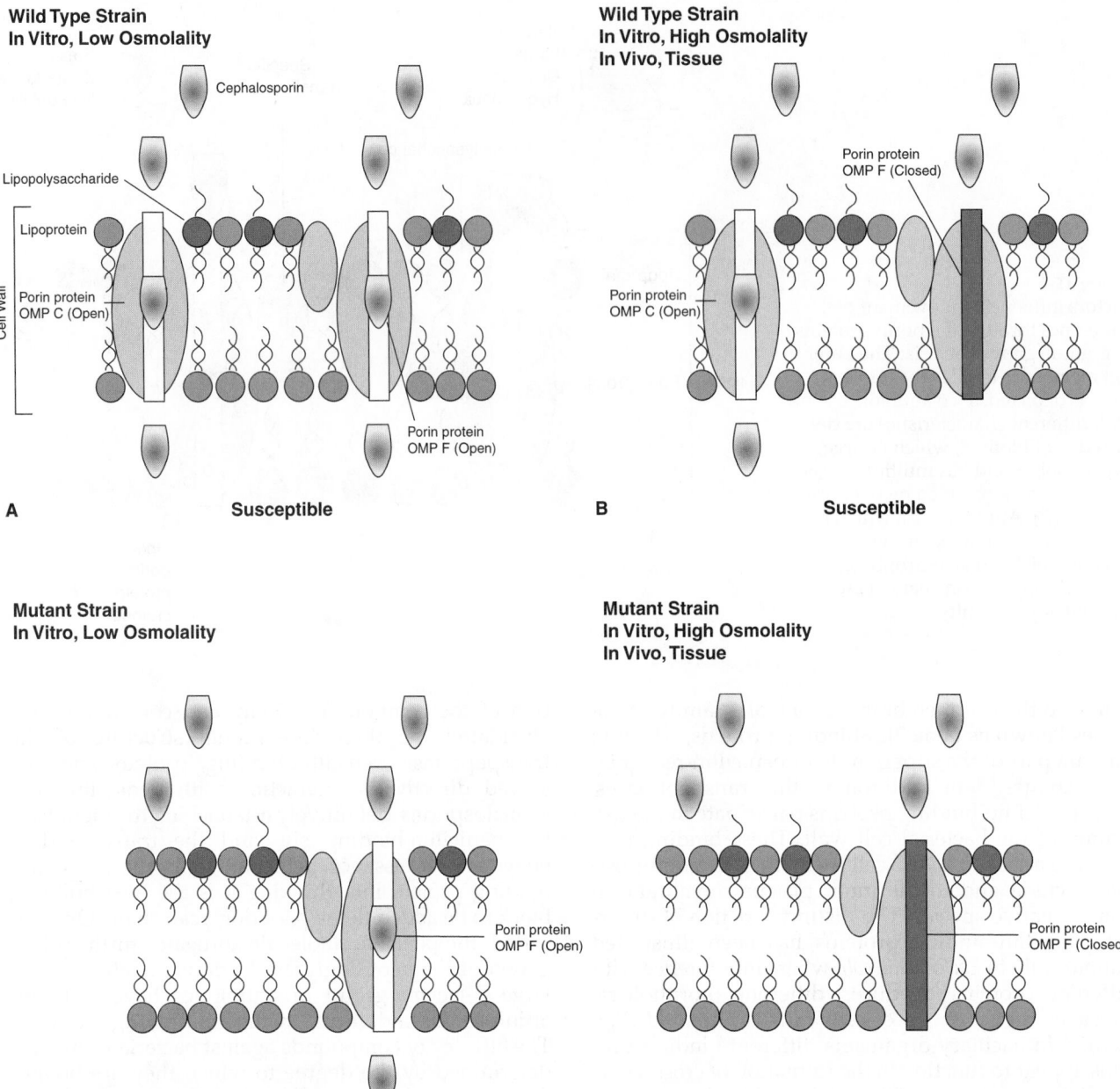

Figure 15-7

The critical importance of porin proteins in antimicrobial resistance as illustrated by a mutant strain of *Salmonella typhimurium*:[170] The outer cell membrane is illustrated for four combinations of bacterium and environment. In panel **A** the wild-type strain grown in low-osmolality medium in the laboratory has two porin channels: a small channel porin (OmpC) and a large-channel porin (OmpF). The cephalosporin has free access to its binding sites on the inner plasma membrane (not shown) and the strain is susceptible. In panel **B** the wild-type strain has been grown in high-osmolality media in the laboratory, mimicking the conditions in vivo. The large-channel porin (*OmpF*) has closed down, but the small-channel porin is still available for the cephalosporin, and the strain remains susceptible. In panel **C** a mutant strain has lost its small-channel porin (*OmpC*), but it still has the *OmpF* porin when grown in low-osmolality media in the laboratory. The cephalosporin can transverse the membrane through *OmpF* and the mutant strain is susceptible in vitro. Panel **D** demonstrates the mutant strain in high-osmolality media or in vivo. The *OmpF* protein shuts down, as it did in the wild-type strain under similar conditions, but there is now no *OmpC* porin available for the antibiotic. With no means for entering the cell the cephalosporin is ineffective and the mutant strain is now resistant.

Figure 15-8

Effects of three penicillin-binding proteins on the structure of *Escherichia coli*: The inner plasma membrane of *E. coli* (corresponding to layer *A* in Figure 15-5) is depicted. Three different penicillin-binding proteins are numbered *1* through *3*, in order of decreasing molecular weight. A variant of protein *1* is also present. β-Lactam antibiotics that interact with protein *1* cause the bacillus to lyse rapidly. Interaction with protein *2* causes formation of coccal cells (*C*), which eventually progress to lysis. Antibiotics that interact with protein *3* do not cause lysis, but cause a defect in information of crosswalls so that the bacterial cells elongate and assume bizarre shapes (*E*). Penicillin-binding proteins 4 through 6 (*not shown*) are not essential and do not produce obvious changes when antibiotics interact with them.[245]

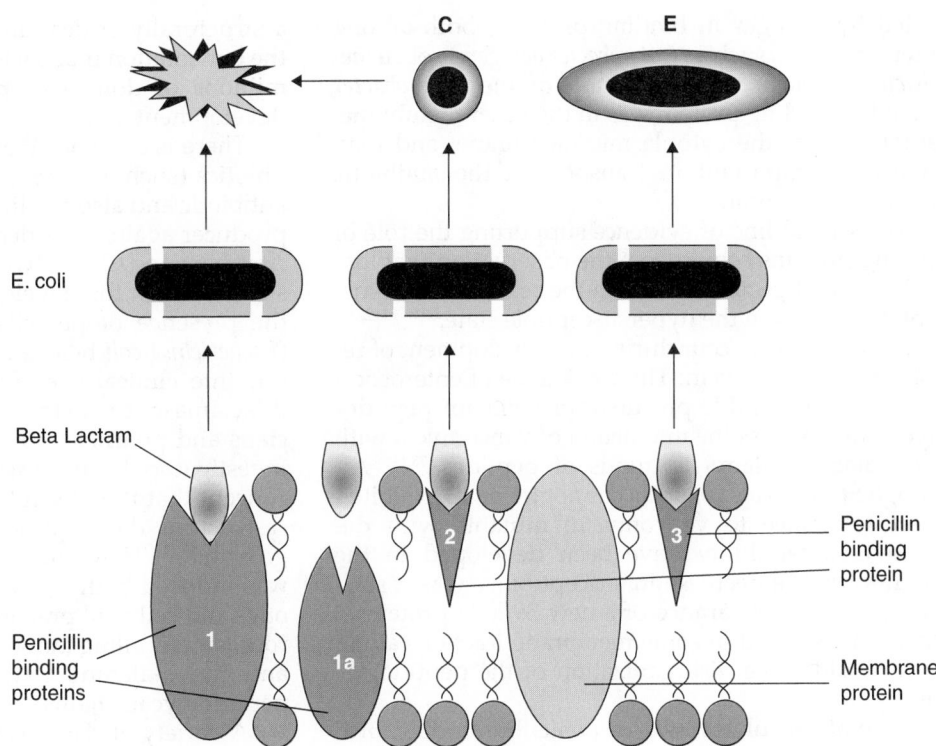

functional similarities to a d-alanyl-d-alanyl peptidase that participates in the elongation of the peptidoglycan chain.[138] Binding of the antibiotic to the precursor protein may block access of the crucial building block to the peptidase by steric interference.

MODIFICATION OF TARGET ENZYMES: BINDING PROTEINS AND ANTIBIOTIC RESISTANCE. An important mechanism for resistance of bacteria to β-lactam antibiotics is an alteration of penicillin-binding proteins so that the antibiotic no longer has access to the enlarging peptidoglycan chain. Altered proteins are indicated by addition of a suffix, which may either be a letter or a prime (') designation, to the numbering scheme. For instance, the mechanism for high-level resistance of *Staphylococcus aureus* to penicillinase-resistant penicillins is the production of a variant of penicillin-binding protein 2 (PBP 2) to a variant that is designated PBP 2a. Alternatively, there may be a loss of the binding proteins that have the highest affinity for the antibiotic.

The evidence supporting the role of altered binding proteins comes from two sources. First, the presence of the altered proteins is associated with the appearance of resistance. Exposure of staphylococci to methicillin induced an alteration of penicillin-binding protein 2 (PBP 2) to a variant (PBP 2a).[100,273] Variants that lost resistance did not contain the variant binding protein.[100,273] Similarly, isolates of *Streptococcus pneumoniae* that were resistant to penicillin exhibited decreased affinity of penicillin for whole bacterial cells, membrane preparations, and two major penicillin-binding proteins.[95] Similar results have been reported for viridans streptococci in South Africa.[65] Conversely, the transition

from resistance to hypersusceptibility was associated with the loss of a low-affinity binding protein. The resulting binding protein of high affinity was then associated with susceptibility to the bound antibiotic.

The alterations in binding proteins may be a one-step process, controlled by a single gene, such as the MecA gene that codes for variant PBP 2a in *Staphylococcus aureus*.[273] In the case of *Streptococcus pneumoniae*, however, alterations of multiple binding proteins result in a multi-step process of increasing resistance.[115]

Alterations in binding proteins are more important for resistance of gram-positive bacteria to β-lactam antibiotics than for enteric gram-negative bacteria and *Pseudomonas* spp. Changes in binding proteins do have major effects on some gram-negative bacteria and some β-lactam antibiotics, however. The mechanism by which *Haemophilus influenzae* and *Neisseria gonorrhoeae* that do not produce β-lactamase are resistant to β-lactam antibiotics is the alteration of binding proteins.[54,199] Even *N. meningitidis*, which for so many years remained uniformly susceptible to penicillin, has developed altered binding proteins that have produced resistance to penicillin.[301] The clinical importance of these binding proteins is well illustrated by a patient in whom nontypable *H. influenzae* produced meningitis. The patient was treated unsuccessfully with cefuroxime. The isolate did not produce β-lactamase and did not contain permeability barriers but did contain proteins that bound cefuroxime poorly.[171] Even among the *Enterobacteriaceae* changes in binding proteins may be important. Changes in PBP 3 of *Escherichia coli* were associated with resistance to cephalexin and some other cephalosporin antibiotics.[104] Similarly, resistance to imipenem may be mediated by changes in binding proteins, both among enteric bacteria, such as *Enterobacter aerogenes*, or *Acinetobacter baumanii*.[36,85] In the case of the *Enterobacter* strain the binding protein was in the outer membrane, rather than at the cytoplasmic membrane, and may have been important in transport of the antibiotic across the membrane.

The second line of evidence supporting the role of binding proteins comes from the observation that loss of the variant protein results in the restoration of susceptibility or even the hypersusceptible state.[65,73,100,273]

Similar events occur during the development of resistance to vancomycin. The vanA gene of enterococci encodes depsipeptide precursor proteins for peptidoglycan that bypass the interaction of vancomycin with the D-alanyl-D-alanyl terminus of peptides.[138,144] Although *Staphylococcus aureus* has not (to date) exhibited overt resistance to vancomycin, mutants with decreased susceptibility have been developed in the laboratory. The decrease in susceptibility was associated with the appearance of a new 39 kDa protein in the cytoplasm and in some membrane fractions along with considerable disorganization of the peptidoglycan layer.[42]

Several useful reviews of penicillin-binding proteins as resistance mechanisms are available.[155,244]

ANTIBIOTIC-MODIFYING ENZYMES: THE β-LACTAMASES. Another major group of penicillin-recognizing proteins is the class of enzymes known as β-lactamases. It is now clear that the β-lactamases and the penicillin-binding proteins have a common, although distant evolutionary origin.[246] Both classes of compound must interact with β-lactam antibiotics in order to perform their function. Similar amino acid sequences have been demonstrated in penicillin-binding proteins of high and low molecular weight and certain types of β-lactamase. In addition, similarities in conformation and three dimensional structure have been documented. Interestingly, some penicillin-binding proteins can function as a β-lactamase, albeit not as efficiently or with as great clinical importance as "professional" β-lactamases.[169,189] Furthermore, the mechanism of action of both β-lactamases and the transpeptidase penicillin-binding protein is cleavage of an amide bond by an acyl-enzyme mechanism.[19]

β-lactamases are a family of enzymes, which range in importance from the almost exclusive mechanism of staphylococcal resistance to penicillin at one extreme to clinically insignificant constituents of the cell wall in some enteric bacteria. Any β-lactam antibiotic or group of antibiotics may be inactivated by these enzymes. The number of different enzymes now exceeds 170 and the growth spurt shows no signs of slowing down.[169] Just as the specificity of penicillin-binding proteins for β-lactam antibiotics is a factor in determination of the susceptibility of the bacterium to the antibiotic, so the specificity of the β-lactamase for a β-lactam antibiotic is an important determinant in the efficiency with which the enzyme hydrolyzes the antibiotic. A point mutation in one or more amino acids can change the specificity of the molecule if it occurs in a structurally critical area of the enzyme,[21,29] causing the lamentation that bacteria can with one stroke undo millions of dollars of pharmaceutical research and development.

There is evidence that the microbial sources of antibiotics (such as *Streptomyces* spp.) produce both the antibiotic and also modifying enzymes that protect the producer against self-destruction. It is interesting that Abraham and Chain, two of the scientists who were instrumental in the development of penicillin, reported the presence of penicillinase in a strain of *Bacillus (Escherichia) coli* before the introduction of the antibiotic into clinical use.[1] Clearly nature did not invent β-lactamases solely to bedevil infectious disease physicians and pharmaceutical companies. Two groups of investigators have presented evidence to support the concept that the physiologic role of β-lactamases is to restructure the peptidoglycan during bacterial cell growth.[19,271] They found that synthesis of β-lactamase was induced both by the presence of β-lactam antibiotics and cell wall precursors in the extracellular environment, recalling the structural similarity of penicillin and the d-alanine-d-alanine dipeptide terminus of peptidoglycan chains.

A variety of classification schemes has been developed, leading to some confusion in nomenclature. A useful early classification scheme was provided by Richmond and Sykes,[224] but the number and variety of enzymes have proliferated beyond the boundaries of the scheme. A more modern scheme based on molecular structure (Table 15-5) proposed by Ambler[3] includes of necessity only those enzymes that have been characterized. The most important group is Class A which are serine proteases that have either preference for penicillins or broad-spectrum activity. They are found either on chromosomes or on plasmids and, therefore, easily transferable from one bacterium to another. They may be produced constitutively or may require induction. In this group are the staphylococcal enzymes and many of the most important β-lactamases of gram-negative bacteria. Class C enzymes are primarily cephalosporinases, either constitutive or inducible, that are found on the chromosomes of gram-negative bacteria. Class B enzymes (metalloenzymes) and Class D enzymes (oxacillinases) are less important clinically. Recently a new classification of β-lactamases, the Bush-Jacoby-Medeiros scheme has been developed to integrate functional and molecular characteristics (Table 15-6).[29]

Some β-lactamases, such as those produced by *Staphylococcus aureus*, have been stable over several decades. These enzymes have a rather narrow spectrum of activity aimed at penicillin molecules. The broader spectrum, plasmid-mediated β-lactamases of gram-negative bacteria, such as TEM-1 and SHV-1, were also stable for many years. Beginning in the early 1980s, however, a series of enzymatic variants appeared that had a broadened spectrum of activity against many of the newly developed β-lactam antibiotics. These extended-spectrum β-lactamases were first found in Europe, most commonly in isolates of *Klebsiella* spp., less commonly in *Escherichia coli*.[212] The num-

TABLE 15-5
CLASSIFICATION OF β-LACTAMASES

CLASS	EXAMPLES	LOCATION	BACTERIA
Gram-Positive β-Lactamases			
Staphylococcal	Serologic types	Plasmids	*Staphylococcus aureus; S. epidermidis*
Enterococcal	A–D	Plasmid	*Enterococcus faecalis*
Streptococcal		Plasmid	*Streptococcus uberis*
Gram-Negative β-Lactamases			
Class A	TEM-1 and 2	Plasmid; broad-spectrum	*Enterobacteriaceae* *Neisseria gonorrhoeae* *Haemophilus influenzae* *Vibrio cholerae*
	SHV-1	Plasmid; broad-spectrum	*Enterobacteriaceae;* also found on chromosomes of *Klebsiella pneumoniae*
	OXA-1	Plasmid; oxacil-linase	*Escherichia coli*
	PSE-1	Plasmid; carbenicil-linase in *Pseudomonas* spp.	*Enterobacteriaceae;* most common type in *P. aeruginosa*
	BRO-1	Plasmid; carbenicillinase	*Branhamella; Moraxella*
Class B		Cephalosporinase	*Bacillus cereus*
Class C	Broad-spectrum	Chromosome	*Klebsiella pneumoniae; Proteus vulgaris; K. oxytoca; K. aerogenes* K-1
	Cephalosporinase	Chromosome	*Escherichia coli, Bacteroides fragilis*
	Inducible	Chromosome	*Enterobacter aerogenes, E. cloacae, Providencia rettgeri, Pseudomonas aeruginosa, Serratia marcescens, Acinetobacter baumanii*
	Carbapenemase (Imipenem)	Chromosome	*Xanthomonas maltophilia, Bacteroides fragilis, Serratia marcescens, Enterobacter cloacae*
Class D	Oxacillinases	—	—

Adapted from references 29, 168, 169.

ber of enzymes continues to increase.[117] The new enzymes and their precursors, such as TEM-1 and SHV-1, are located on plasmids, but may have been derived originally from a chromosomal enzyme. Many of the new β-lactamases differ from each other only in a single amino acid substitution, but the changes have profound implications for clinical management of infectious diseases.[37,169] The characteristics of the extended-spectrum enzymes are summarized in Table 15-7.

β-LACTAMASE INHIBITORS. The final piece in the penicillin-recognizing protein puzzle is the introduction of β-lactamase inhibitors.[28,150] These compounds resemble β-lactam antibiotics sufficiently well that they can bind to the β-lactamase, either reversibly or irreversibly, protecting the antibiotic from destruction. When they are most effective, they serve as suicide bombers, sopping up all available enzyme.[150] It should not be surprising that these compounds, which must mimic β-lactams in order to function, also have limited antibacterial activity in their own right. In fact, aztreonam, which was developed as a β-lactam antibiotic was later discovered to have additional activity as an inhibitor of β-lactamase.[28] The three inhibitors of β-lactamase activity that have found a place in clinical medicine are clavulanic acid, sulbactam, and tazobactam. All three inhibitors are effective against staphylococcal penicillinase and have variable effectiveness against the chromosomal enzymes of gram-negative bacteria. Clavulanate and tazobactam are superior to sulbactam in activity against plasmid-mediated β-lactamases of gram-negative organisms, including the extended-spectrum β-lactamases.[204] There is no significant difference between clavulanate and tazobactam, although the spectrum of their activity is different. Some extended spectrum enzymes are resistant to the activity of all three compounds.

TABLE 15-6

THE BUSH-JACOBY-MEDEIROS FUNCTIONAL CLASSIFICATION SCHEME FOR β-LACTAMASES

GROUP	ENZYME TYPE	INHIBITION BY CLAVULANATE	MOLECULAR CLASS	NUMBER OF ENZYMES	EXAMPLES
1	Cephalosporinase	No	C	53	*Enterobacter cloacae* P99, MIR-1
2a	Penicillinase	Yes	A	20	*Staphylococcus aureus, Streptomyces albus*
2b	Broad-spectrum	Yes	A	16	TEM-1, SHV-1
2be	Extended-spectrum	Yes	A	38	TEM-3, SHV-2, *Klebsiella oxytoca* K-1
2br	Inhibitor-resistant	Diminished	A	9	TEM-30, TRC-1
2c	Carbenicillinase	Yes	A	15	PSE-1, CARB-3, BRO-1
2d	Cloxacillinase	Yes	D or A	18	OXA-1, PSE-2, *Streptomyces cacaoi*
2e	Cephalosporinase	Yes	A	19	*Proteus vulgaris, Bacteroides fragilis* CepA
2f	Carbapenemase	Yes	A	3	*Enterobacter cloacae* IMI-1, NMC-A
3	Metalloenzyme	No	B	15	*Stenotrophomonas (Xanthomonas) maltophilia* L1
4	Penicillinase	No		7	*Burkholderia (Pseudomonas) cepacia*

Adapted from References 29, 168, and 169.

β-LACTAMASES AND ANTIMICROBIAL RESISTANCE. β-lactamases of gram-positive bacteria, represented predominantly by the staphylococci, are for the most part inducible Class A enzymes that are formed at the cell membrane, but are also secreted extracellularly (Fig. 15-4). The practical implications of these characteristics are twofold. First, the bacteria must be exposed to the β-lactam antibiotic before the enzyme is produced in large quantities. In the laboratory it is possible to kill the bacteria with large quantities of antibiotic before enzymatic induction occurs, producing a false impression of susceptibility. Theoretically, small numbers of staphylococci might also be killed in vivo before induction of β-lactamase, but this eventuality has not been documented. Second, the extracellular production of β-lactamase could protect co-infecting bacteria that do not produce the enzyme. It has been hypothesized that relapses of streptococcal pharyngitis after treatment with penicillin might be caused by this mechanism,[25] but other investigators have not been able to document a relationship between the presence of bacteria that produce β-lactamase and the outcome of treatment.[256]

The β-lactamases of gram-negative bacteria are more complicated. Most enteric bacteria contain constitutive chromosomal enzymes that are produced at a low level and vary with the species. Induction of these Class C chromosomal enzymes, primarily cephalosporinases, to higher levels increases the level of resistance and expands the effective coverage of the enzymes to enzymes that are resistant to the action of β-lactams, such as the third-generation cephalosporins and the cephapenems.[264] The appearance of inducible Class A β-lactamases that function as penicillinases and/or cephalosporinases broadened the arsenal of bacterial weapons.[169] The location of enzymes such as TEM-1 and SHV-1 on plasmids facilitated the spread of the enzymes among diverse species. Several developments have further increased the capability of bacteria to inactivate new antibiotics, such as the third-generation (β-lactamase-resistant) cephalosporins and carbapenems. First, overproduction of inducible chromosomal or plasmid enzymes may inactivate antibiotics such as imipenem or third-generation cephalosporins that were resistant to degradation by normal quantities of enzyme.[103,209] Second, the ex-

TABLE 15-7

CHARACTERISTICS OF THE MOST COMMON PLASMID-MEDIATED EXTENDED-SPECTRUM β-LACTAMASES

Class A cephalosporinases carried on plasmids
Klebsiella spp. most common, followed by *Escherichia coli*
Described first in Germany and France
All enzymes active against cephalothin
Imipenem and cefoxitin not hydrolyzed
Comparative activity against cefotaxime and ceftazidime varies with enzyme
Some enzymes active against aztreonam
Resistance may not be detected by standard susceptibility tests
Demonstration of inhibition of activity by β-lactamase inhibitors

tended-spectrum β-lactamases inactivate many of the third-generation cephalosporins, although the carbapenems are relatively resistant to these versatile enzymes.[169] Finally, gram-negative bacteria have been sufficiently resourceful to produce β-lactamases that specifically inactivate antibiotics, such as imipenem, that are resistant to the activity of most other enzymes.[194,281] In fact, the bacteria have been able to craft enzymes that are active against virtually any antibiotic that the chemists have been able to produce!

Several factors determine the effectiveness of combinations of inhibitors, antibiotics, enzymes and specific bacterial strains. These factors include the extent to which the antibiotics or inhibitors induce β-lactamase activity, the amount of enzyme produced, and the effectiveness of the inhibitor against the specific type of β-lactamase produced.[28,150] Antibiotics that are efficient inducers of β-lactamases often sew the seeds of destruction not only of themselves, but of their friends and relatives.[233] Among the extended-spectrum β-lactamases some are blocked by various inhibitors, while others are unaffected by their presence.[20,169,281]

ANTIBIOTICS THAT DO NOT EXERT THEIR EFFECT ON CELL WALLS

Production of Modifying Enzymes.   Modifying enzymes are also important for some antibiotics that exert their effects within the cytoplasm of the bacterial cells. The primary mechanism for resistance to aminoglycosides is modifying enzymes. There are three general types of processes: 1) phosphorylation, 2) acetylation, and 3) adenylation. All aminoglycoside antibiotics are at risk to inactivation by one of these enzymes.[164,213] Although all three types of enzymes are found in all types of bacteria, the enzymes of gram-positive and gram-negative organisms are different. The enzymes in gram-negative bacteria that inactivate streptomycin and kanamycin have become so widely distributed that these antibiotics have fallen out of common clinical use. Amikacin is least vulnerable to these inactivating enzymes but may be rendered ineffective by other mechanisms, particularly in *Pseudomonas aeruginosa*. Aminoglycoside resistance has developed in epidemic proportions at hospitals around the world.[164]

Erythromycin and chloramphenicol may also be inactivated enzymatically. In the case of chloramphenicol, the acetyltransferase enzyme is responsible for most clinical resistance.[81] A minor mechanism for resistance to tetracyclines is enzymatic inactivation.[257]

Alteration of Targets.   Changes in affinity of ribosomal targets for enzymes are important for resistance to some antimicrobial agents, particularly tetracycline, erythromycin, quinolones, aminoglycosides, trimethoprim, and sulfamethoxazole. Although the primary resistance mechanism for tetracyclines is the efflux mechanism as discussed earlier, protection of ribosomes by a soluble protein has also been described as an important secondary mechanism.[257] Alterations in the ribosomal site of action of macrolides and lincosamides, such as erythromycin and clindamycin, are

important mechanisms for resistance to this group of antibiotics.[142,287] Mutation in the DNA gyrase target of quinolone antibiotics is the most important mechanism for resistance to this important new group of antibiotics in both gram-positive and gram-negative bacteria,[247,291] although resistance may also be mediated by barriers in diffusion through the cell wall. Aminoglycoside resistance may be mediated by alterations in ribosomal targets as well as by enzymatic inactivation. When this mechanism is operative, there may actually be an accumulation of (ineffective) antibiotic within the bacterial cell.[2] A major mechanism for resistance to both sulfamethoxazole and trimethoprim is alteration of the sequential target enzymes in the biochemical pathway for formation of nucleic acids, dihydropteroate synthetase for sulfonamides and dihydrofolate reductase for trimethoprim.[112]

Bypass of Resistance Mechanisms.   Auxotrophic mutants that require thymine for growth may be able to circumvent the activity of trimethoprim and sulfamethoxazole in vitro by utilizing available substrates and alternative pathways.[205] The most clinically important example of a bypass mechanism is the ability of naturally occurring strains of *Enterococcus* sp. to utilize compounds such as folinic acid for growth in vivo in the presence of trimethoprim-sulfamethoxazole.[91,300] Strains may appear susceptible in vitro, although they do not respond to chemotherapy in vivo. The in vitro result can be converted from susceptible to resistant by addition of folinic acid to the testing medium. Enterococci should not, therefore, be tested against trimethoprim-sulfamethoxazole.

INTERACTIONS AMONG RESISTANCE MECHANISMS

Many bacteria have developed multiple resistance mechanisms and they are often complementary. The best example of synergistic defenses is the combination of barriers to diffusion of β-lactam antibiotics through the outer cell membrane of gram-negative bacteria and production of β-lactamases in the confined space of the peptidoglycan layer between the two membranes (Fig. 15-5). As a result the effectiveness with which the enzymes can degrade the antibiotic is considerably enhanced. A military analogy can be used to illustrate the utility of the bacterial strategy. Gram-positive bacteria that allow relatively free access to the inner cell membrane, but can secrete enzyme into the extracellular environment (Fig. 15-4) are analogous to defenders that have heavy-duty long-range artillery, but face an opposing army arrayed on an open plain. In contrast, gram-negative bacteria have only single-shot rifles, but they have positioned their sharpshooters to pick off the enemy soldiers as they march single-file through the mountain pass of the porin channels and peptidoglycan layer. The effect of the combined strategy is well-illustrated by *Serratia marcescens*, which is usually susceptible to third-generation cephalosporins and carbapenems.[103] An isolate that produced large amounts of a chromosomal β-lactamase possessed low-level resistance to these antibiotics. When barriers to passage of antibiotic through the outer membrane were added to the β-lactamase, however, the isolate became highly resistant to the antibiotics.

The complementation phenomenon can also be illustrated by looking at inoculum effects in the interaction between various gram-negative bacteria and β-lactam antibiotics (Fig. 15-9). A β-lactamase producing strain of *Haemophilus influenzae*, which has minimal

barriers to transport of ampicillin across the membrane, is effectively killed if the ratio of bacteria to antibiotic molecules is small. If the ratio is increased, however, antibiotic molecules are not able to reach all the bacteria, so that some organisms escape damage and are able to multiply. This phenomenon is known as an inoculum effect, which has potential important implications for testing in the laboratory. In contrast,

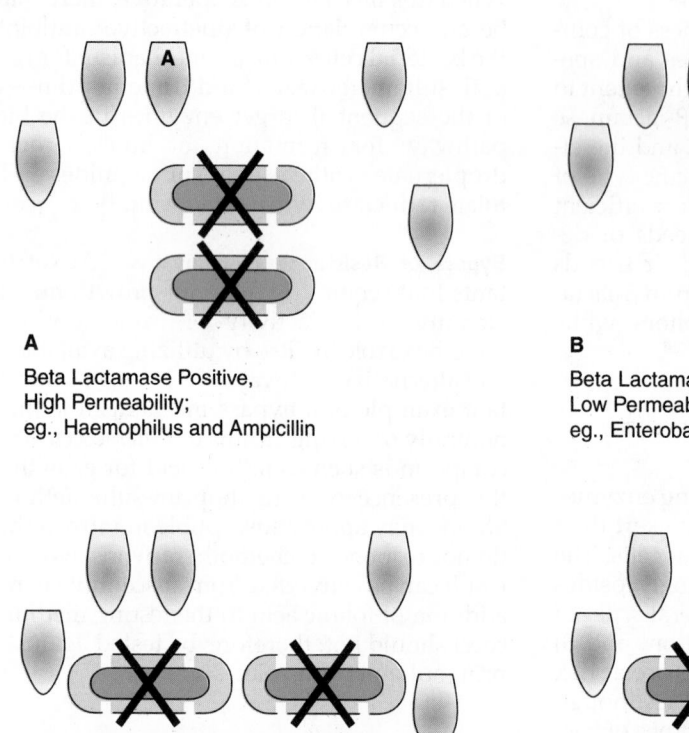

A

Beta Lactamase Positive,
High Permeability;
eg., Haemophilus and Ampicillin

B

Beta Lactamase Positive,
Low Permeability;
eg., Enterobacter and Ampicillin

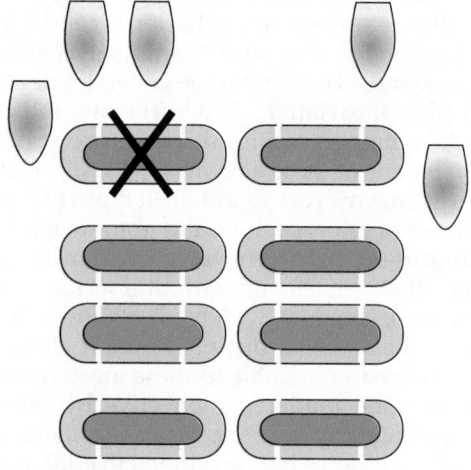

C

Beta Lactamase Positive,
High Permeability;
Inoculum Effect

D

Beta Lactamase Positive,
Low Permeability;
No Inoculum Effect

Figure 15-9
Complementary activity of β-lactamase and barriers to diffusion through outer membranes, as illustrated by inoculum effects in gram-negative bacteria: In panel **A** a β-lactamase-producing strain of *Haemophilus influenzae* allows free diffusion of ampicillin (*A*) across the cell wall. Despite the presence of the enzyme the antibiotic is able to kill a small number of bacteria (*X*). In panel **C**, however, the presence of a large number of bacteria overcomes the effect of the antibiotic; a portion of the bacterial population escapes injury and is able to replicate. In contrast, panels **B** and **D** illustrate a strain of *Enterobacter cloacae*, which also produces β-lactamase, but additionally restricts entry of the antibiotic to its site of action on the inner plasma membrane. As a result a portion of the bacterial population is able to escape antibiotic killing and replicate, whether the inoculum is large or small. There is an inoculum effect with *H. influenzae* and ampicillin, but not with *Enterobacter* and ampicillin. The importance of combining two resistance mechanisms—production of inactivating enzymes and restriction of antibiotic transport across the outer cell membrane—is critical for the dichotomous result. Other causes of inoculum effects are discussed in the text.

enteric bacteria that have significant barriers to passage of the antibiotic across the membrane are resistant to bactericidal activity even when few bacteria are present. There is no inoculum effect.

On the other side scientists have used their knowledge of the mechanisms of action of antibiotics to construct synergistic combinations that can defeat bacterial resistance mechanisms. The combination of sulfamethoxazole and trimethoprim is a good example of the efficacy of employing two drugs that act at different points in an important bacterial biochemical pathway. Similarly, combination of β-lactam antibiotics and inhibitors of β-lactamase has obvious logic as a therapeutic strategy. Finally, the combination of aminoglycoside and β-lactam antibiotics for serious enterococcal infection, which was used initially empirically,[111] has a rational basis once one understands the mechanisms of action of antibiotics and bacterial resistance (Fig. 15-10). Enterococci are intrinsically resistant to aminoglycoside antibiotics, which do not cross the bacterial cell wall efficiently. The addition of β-lactam antibiotics, however, sufficiently disorganizes the cell wall peptidoglycan that the aminoglycosides can penetrate into the cytoplasm and gain access to their ribosomal targets. The enterococci have, in turn, responded by developing several mechanisms for resistance to the synergistic combination: binding protein alterations and β-lactamase for the penicillins and high-level resistance to the aminoglycosides by enzymatic degradation or ribosomal alterations, as discussed on page 837.

LABORATORY GUIDANCE OF ANTIMICROBIAL THERAPY

A chemotherapeutic drug is a chemical compound that is used in the treatment of a disease. The compound may come from natural sources or may have been synthesized by a chemist in the laboratory. The disease may be of any type, including infectious and neoplastic processes. An antibiotic is an antimicrobial agent that is derived from a microorganism; an antimicrobial agent is a drug that acts primarily against infectious organisms.

Microbiologists can be of great assistance to clinicians. They can evaluate the *in vitro* interactions between an isolated microbe and antimicrobial agents that would be appropriate for treatment of an infection *in vivo*. Their work in the laboratory can provide data to help the clinician decide whether the selected doses of an antibiotic are adequate.

In this chapter, the evaluation of antimicrobial agents that are active against aerobic and facultatively anaerobic bacteria is discussed. Testing of anaerobic bacteria, mycobacteria, and fungi is discussed in Chapters 14, 17, and 19, respectively.

Antimicrobial test procedures are summarized in Table 15-8, which includes a brief description of each test and a list of specimens that the laboratory must have in hand. The tests may be divided conveniently into two groups: (1) tests that *predict* the effectiveness of therapy and (2) tests that *monitor* the effectiveness of therapy.

Several types of antimicrobial susceptibility (or sensitivity) tests have been devised. The two reference tests are the macroscopic broth dilution and agar dilution procedures. Both are designed to quantitate the lowest concentration of an antibiotic that inhibits visible *in vitro* growth of the microbe—the minimum inhibitory concentration (MIC). The test used most frequently to guide antibiotic therapy is the disk diffusion procedure (Bauer-Kirby test), in which clinical interpretations are derived from correlations with the reference test. In recent years, an increasing number of laboratories have routinely used a miniaturized broth test (microdilution broth test) or an automated commercial system. The broth microdilution test has become so prevalent and so well studied that it has become the reference standard for many investigators.

The remaining antibiotic test procedures will be discussed more briefly for several reasons. With the exception of monitoring serum aminoglycoside levels, there are few well-documented clinical indications for these tests, and their use is limited to large referral medical centers. The test procedures are listed in Box 15-1.

The most useful means for assessing the adequacy of antimicrobial therapy in many infections are the clinical response of the patient to treatment and, if needed, the demonstration by repeated culture that the infecting organism either has been eliminated (bacterial cure) or persists (bacterial failure). Unfortunately, a bacterial cure does not always ensure a successful clinical outcome.

It is important to emphasize that antibiotic susceptibility tests are intended to be a guide for the clinician, not a guarantee that an antimicrobial agent will be effective in therapy. A goal of microbiologists has been, and should continue to be, the provision of standardized *in vitro* tests that can be reproduced from day to day and from laboratory to laboratory. Without reproducibility there is no scientific basis for therapy. However, in striving for standardization it is possible that the variability of each infection and each patient is not addressed. The factors that determine the outcome of an infectious process are complex and, in many instances, are incompletely addressed by *in vitro* tests.[279] The examples that follow may clarify the elusiveness of an absolute correlation between laboratory interactions and clinical outcome.

pH: Microbial susceptibility tests are standardized at physiologic *p*H (7.2 to 7.4), yet unphysiologic levels of *p*H often develop at the sites of purulent infections (such as bacterial meningitis[250] or abscesses[102]). Some antibiotics, such as the penicillins and cephalosporins, function well at a wide range of *p*H. Tetracyclines function better in more acidic environments and might actually perform better in an acidic inflammatory exudate than in laboratory culture media. In contrast, aminoglycosides and macrolides, such as erythromycin, are less effective in acidic environments than at neutral *p*H. Although high

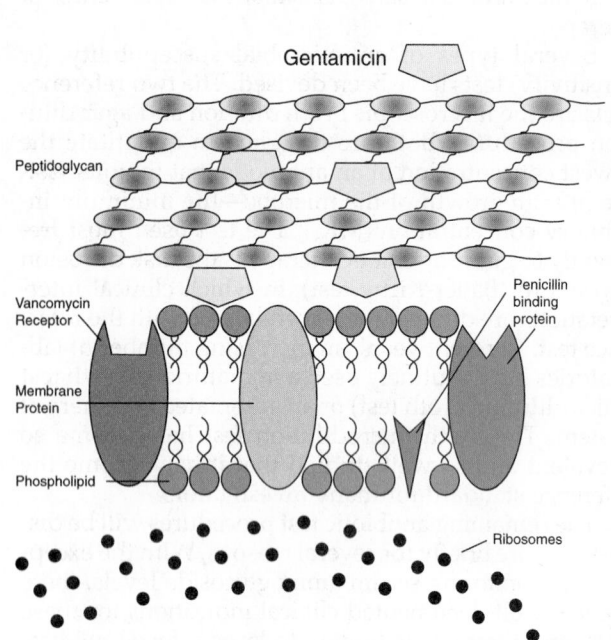

A   **Intrinsic Low Level Aminoglycoside Resistance**

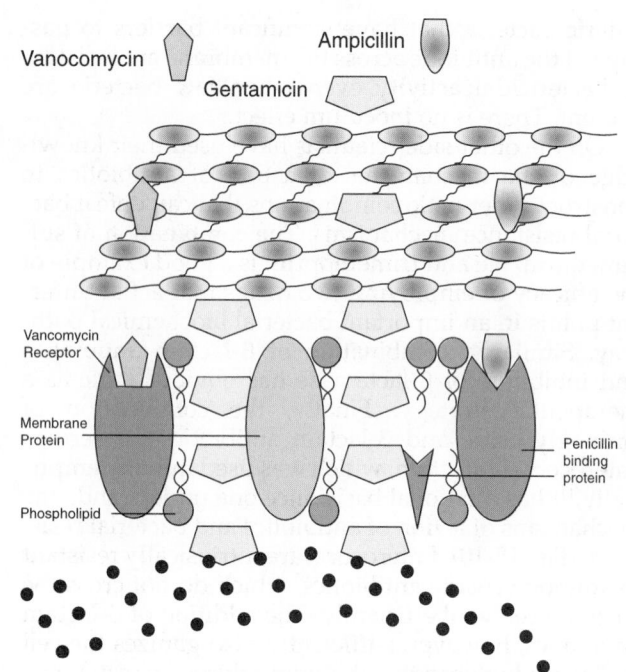

B   **Beta Lactam-Aminoglycoside Synergy**

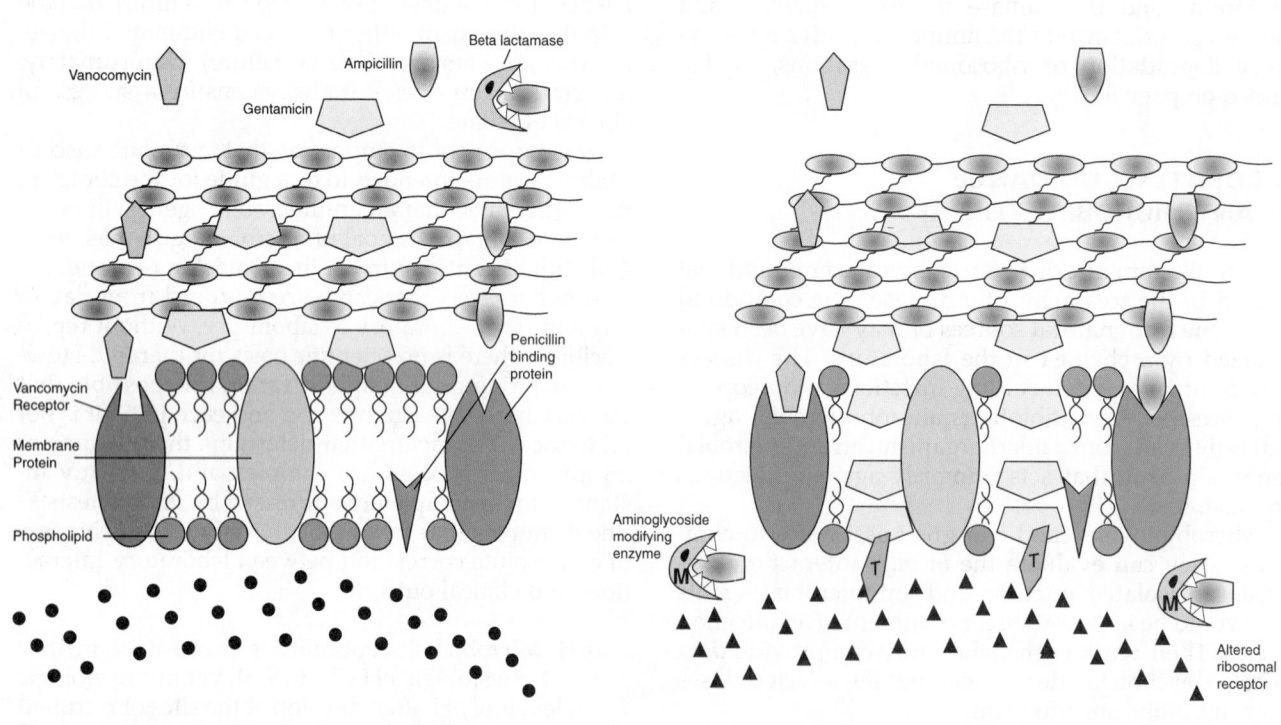

C   **Penicillin and Vancomycin Resistance**

D   **High Level Aminoglycoside Resistance**

TABLE 15-8
GUIDANCE OF ANTIMICROBIAL THERAPY

PROCEDURE	DEFINITION	SPECIMENS	INDICATIONS
Minimum inhibitory concentration (MIC, broth or agar)	Lowest concentration of antibiotic that inhibits visible growth	Microbial isolate	Antimicrobial susceptibility of isolates if etiologic role established and susceptibility is not predictable
Disk diffusion	Diameter of inhibition of growth around paper disk impregnated with antibiotic	Microbial isolate	Simplified method to approximate MIC with interpretative correlates
Minimum bactericidal concentration	Lowest concentration of antibiotic that kills 99.9% of the inoculum	Microbial isolate	Streptococcal endocarditis; potentially for osteomyelitis; potentially tolerant isolates if unresponsive to therapy
Antimicrobial levels	Concentration (μg/mL) of antibiotic in serum	Peak serum Trough serum	Unpredictability of peak levels or potential for toxicity
Serum bactericidal titers	Dilution of serum that kills 99.9% of the inoculum	Peak serum Trough serum Microbial isolate	Bacterial endocarditis; osteomyelitis; gram-negative sepsis in immunosuppressed patients
Synergy tests	Synergistic activity of multiple antibiotics	Microbial isolate	Research procedure for development of therapeutic regimens; rarely, confirmation of synergy against individual isolates

concentrations of aminoglycosides may be achieved in the urinary tract, the drugs will not function optimally if the pH of the urine is low.

Cations: With certain combinations of bacterium and antibiotic, most notably *Pseudomonas aeruginosa* and aminoglycosides, the concentration of divalent cations, particularly calcium (Ca^{2+}) and magnesium (Mg^{2+}), has a dramatic effect on the apparent *in vitro* susceptibility. A result that ranges from susceptible to resistant can be achieved by varying the cation concentration,[220]

because of changes in transport of the antibiotic across the cell membrane. Agar and broth media vary greatly in the concentration of divalent cations. By convention, testing is done under physiologic conditions.

Inoculum: For some combinations of bacterium and antibiotic, the inoculum is of great importance in determining the *in vitro* susceptibility.[64] Enzymatic inactivation of β-lactam antibiotics, such as the penicillins and cephalosporins, is an important mechanism of bacterial resistance.

◀ **Figure 15-10**
The microbial response of enterococci to the synergistic activity of aminoglycoside and β-lactam antibiotics: In each panel the single-cell membrane and surrounding peptidoglycan cell wall (compare Figure 15-4) of an enterococcus surrounds a cytoplasm that contains ribosomes. Panel **A** demonstrates the intrinsic resistance of enterococci to gentamicin, which does not cross the cell membrane efficiently and thus never reaches its target, the bacterial ribosome. In panel **B** a β-lactam antibiotic has disorganized the cell membrane, "poking holes" in the membrane so that the aminoglycoside can pour through to reach its ribosomal target. The combination of β-lactam and aminoglycoside, neither of which is fully effective alone, produces a synergistic antimicrobial action. In panel **C**, however, the resilient enterococcus has produced β-lactamase, negating the effect of the β-lactam antibiotic and reproducing the situation found in panel *A*. Once again the aminoglycoside is unable to reach the ribosomal target. Panel **D** demonstrates another microbial strategy. In this case the β-lactam is still effective and the aminoglycoside is able to reach its ribosomal target. Altered ribosomes, however, block the antibacterial activity of the aminoglycoside (*T*) once it reaches the target. Synergistic activity is no longer present. Alteratively, aminoglycoside-modifying enzymes (*M*) inactivate the antibiotic before it reaches the ribosome. Synergistic activity is again lost, because the bacteria have acquired high-level resistance to the aminoglycoside. Obviously, the bacterial resistance mechanisms depicted in panels *C* and *D* could both be operative in the same strain, producing a double whammy.

BOX 15-1. MISCELLANEOUS ANTIBIOTIC TEST PROCEDURES

1. Determination of bactericidal activity as well as inhibitory activity of antibiotics against bacterial isolates
2. Measurement of antibacterial activity of drugs in combination, also known as synergy testing
3. Quantitation of antibiotic levels in body fluids, especially serum
4. Determination of serum bactericidal activity, sometimes referred to as the Schlichter test

---

These enzymes are always expressed in some bacteria but must be induced by the presence of the antibiotic in other bacteria. If small numbers of *Staphylococcus aureus*, which contains an inducible β-lactamase, are incubated *in vitro* with penicillin, the bacteria may be killed before the enzyme can be produced in effective quantities. In contrast, large numbers of bacteria in an active, clinical infection may survive to produce the inactivating enzyme and destroy the antibiotic. In this case, a false impression of bacterial susceptibility and false sense of security might be produced by the laboratory test.

When staphylococci and β-lactamase-resistant penicillins, such as methicillin, interact, only a small fraction of bacteria express resistance (heteroresistance). Therefore, if the inoculum is small, the resistant bacterial cells may not be included. The number of bacteria in infected patients varies greatly, so that the standardized inocula used in the laboratory represent a reasonable compromise rather than a reproduction of *in vivo* conditions.

Finally, the interaction between β-lactamases and the membranes of gram-negative bacteria may result in inoculum effects, as illustrated in Figure 15-9.

Clinical pharmacology: The penetration of antibiotics into sites of infection is another important variable that cannot be addressed *in vitro*. High concentrations of antimicrobial agents may be achieved in sites where they are excreted from the body, usually the urine or the bile. In contrast, low concentrations relative to serum may be found in tissues, such as prostatic fluid, bone, or cerebrospinal fluid. The ineffectiveness of many antibiotics, such as the aminoglycosides, in the treatment of *Legionella* infections, despite their excellent activity *in vitro*, is probably caused by the poor penetration of the antibiotics into macrophages where the bacteria are growing.[174]

Some interactions favor resolution of infection, even if the antimicrobial therapy is suboptimal. The inflammatory and immune defenses of the patient are essential to a successful clinical outcome. It is clear that low concentrations of antibiotics, below the concentration necessary to kill the bacterium, may enhance the ability of phagocytic cells to ingest and kill an infecting microorganism.[108]

Many infections, particularly those caused by obligately anaerobic bacteria, are synergistic; that is, the bacteria depend on each other for survival. Such an infection may be cured by drugs that are ineffective against some of the infecting bacteria if the essential participants are eliminated.[225] Considering all the factors that influence the outcome of an infection, it is imperative that the laboratory provide physicians with the "track record" of the antibiotic to guide them in the selection of appropriate antibiotic therapy. Well-designed clinical studies have demonstrated a correlation of outcome with the appropriateness of therapy.[284] Physicians must, therefore, correlate the results of antibiotic susceptibility tests and clinical experience when selecting therapeutic regimens for patients with similar infections.

TESTS FOR DETERMINING INHIBITORY ACTIVITY OF ANTIBIOTICS

INDICATIONS

Tests of inhibitory activity of antibiotics are designed for bacteria that grow well after overnight incubation in air and have unpredictable susceptibilities. Fastidious bacteria, which grow more slowly or require nutritional or atmospheric supplements, should be tested with a dilution test only if careful use of control bacterial strains demonstrates the absence of inhibitory effects on the interactions. The disk diffusion test may be modified for such organisms if the procedure has been validated by comparison to reference tests and to clinical experience.[187]

Microbiologists should resist pressure from clinicians to extend the procedures beyond their established limits. Many mistakes were made by participants in the proficiency testing surveys of the College of American Pathologists in the determination of the susceptibility of *Listeria monocytogenes* to penicillin and ampicillin because the published guidelines were not designed for this bacterium.[120] Further studies made it possible to establish valid guidelines for *Listeria* species, and results of the surveys have improved.

The list of bacteria that have consistently predictable susceptibilities is, unfortunately, becoming shorter. The prevalence of β-lactamase-producing strains of *Haemophilus influenzae* and *Neisseria gonorrhoeae* is sufficiently high that susceptibility to penicillin analogues can no longer be assumed.[50] Pneumococci that are relatively resistant to penicillin (MIC = 0.12 μg/ml to 1.0 μg/ml) or have high-level resistance (MIC > 1.0 μg/ml) are increasingly common in the United States, and pneumococcal strains isolated from serious infections should be tested for resistance.[113] Almost alone *Streptococcus pyogenes* remains susceptible to penicillin.

Only isolates producing an infection should be tested. Bacteria recovered from a normally sterile body fluid are usually pathogenic. If the potentially pathogenic bacterium is isolated from a site that contains colonizing flora, such as the upper respiratory tract or the skin, the culture should be scrutinized more closely before a susceptibility test is performed, particularly if multiple species of organisms are present. Examination of a Gram-stained smear may document the inclusion of squamous epithelial cells, which suggests contamination by colonized secretions, or the absence of segmented neutrophils, which indicates the lack of an inflammatory response. In situations in which the microbiologist cannot determine the suitability of a susceptibility test, consultation with the clinician is appropriate.

CHOICE OF TEST

In most situations either a disk diffusion or a microdilution broth test is adequate to guide clinical therapy. Advantages of dilution tests are that they provide more quantitative information and may be applied to a wider range of isolates than the diffusion test. However, there is definite potential for misinterpretation of a quantitative result if physicians do not understand how to use the information and the laboratory fails to provide sufficient guidance in interpretation. The disk diffusion test has a long and successful track record. The choice of which method to use will depend on local needs and resources. For evaluation of susceptibility tests most investigators use the following convention:

- very major error—characterization of a resistant isolate as susceptible
- major error—characterization of a susceptible isolate as resistant
- minor error—characterization of a susceptible or resistant isolate as intermediate, or characterization of an intermediate isolate as susceptible or resistant.

SELECTION OF ANTIMICROBIAL AGENTS

The final selection of antibiotics for the hospital formulary should be decided in consultation with members of the medical staff. Lists of antimicrobial agents that have been suggested by the National Committee for Clinical Laboratory Standards (NCCLS) is detailed in Tables 15-9 and 15-10.* Note that many antibiotics are

---

* Permission to use portions of M100-S6 (Performance Standards for Antimicrobial Susceptibility Testing: Sixth Informational Supplement) has been granted by the NCCLS. M110-S6 updates M2-A5 (Performance Standards for Antimicrobial Susceptibility Tests—Fifth Edition; Approved Standard) and M7-A3 (Methods for Dilution Antimicrobial Susceptibility Tests for Bacteria that Grow Aerobically—Third Edition; Approved Standard). The interpretive data are valid only if the methodology in M2-A5 and M7-A3 is followed. NCCLS frequently updates the M2 and M7 tables through new edition of the standards and supplements. Users should refer to the most recent editions. The current standards may be obtained from NCCLS, 940 West Valley Road, Suite 1400, Wayne, PA 19087, US).

grouped by class because the spectrum of activity is similar. The recent recommendations of the NCCLS address selective testing and selective reporting, recognizing that the issues are complex and vary from institution to institution. Washington has provided a guide to the antimicrobial groupings (Table 15-11).[280] It is not necessary to test each antibiotic in the list. Patterns of antibiotic usage and bacterial resistance in each community should be known and considered when selecting antibiotics for testing. Distinctions may be made between antibiotics that are tested routinely and those for which results are reported routinely to physicians.

STANDARDIZATION

The major improvement in laboratory guidance of susceptibility testing over the past several decades has come from the development of standardized procedures that have been widely adopted. It is extremely important to adhere to the recommended protocols if reproducible results are to be achieved. The NCCLS publishes standards for these and other tests on a continuing basis. (Copies of the *Performance Standards for Antimicrobial Disk Susceptibility Tests*[182] and the *Methods for Dilution Antimicrobial Susceptibility Tests for Bacteria that Grow Aerobically*[183] may be obtained on request by writing the NCCLS at 940 West Valley Road, Suite 1400, Wayne, PA 19087-1898). It is important that revised procedures and current recommendations be promptly promulgated in all clinical laboratories. An institutional membership in the NCCLS ensures the timely receipt of all new and revised recommendations. Washington has summarized the resources and processes of this national consensus organization that affect clinical microbiologists.[280]

The following are some of the important facets of susceptibility testing that have been standardized.

GROWTH MEDIUM

Mueller-Hinton broth and agar have been selected for testing aerobic and facultatively anaerobic bacterial isolates. These formulations most closely approximate the criteria for a reproducible medium. They contain dehydrated beef infusion, acid digest of casein, and cornstarch. Most pathogens grow satisfactorily, and the media have minimal inhibitory effect on sulfonamides, trimethoprim, and tetracycline.[11] Large quantities of thymidine are present in some lots of media. Some organisms can use the thymidine to bypass the mechanism of action of trimethoprim and grow, even though they are innately resistant to the antibiotic. Enterococci are particularly affected; isolated colonies may appear within the established zone of inhibition around disks that contain trimethoprim.

It is obvious from examining the formula that even Mueller-Hinton medium is not chemically defined.[141] Agar is a natural compound that is prepared from red seaweed. Variation occurs in the composition of agar

(Text continues on page 811)

TABLE 15-9
SUGGESTED GROUPINGS OF US FDA-APPROVED ANTIMICROBIAL AGENTS THAT SHOULD BE CONSIDERED FOR ROUTINE TESTING AND REPORTING ON NONFASTIDIOUS ORGANISMS BY CLINICAL MICROBIOLOGY LABORATORIES

ENTEROBACTERIACEAE[a]	PSEUDOMONAS AERUGINOSA AND OTHER NON-ENTEROBACTERIACEAE[g]	STAPHYLOCOCCUS SPP.	ENTEROCOCCUS SPP.[k]
Group A Primary Test and Report Ampicillin[a,b]	Mezlocillin or ticarcillin Piperacillin	Penicillin[j]	Penicillin[j] or ampicillin
Cefazolin[b,c] Cephalothin[b,c]	Gentamicin	Oxacillin[j] or methicillin[j]	
Gentamicin[b]	Ceftazidime		
Group B[n] Primary Report Selectively Mezlocillin or piperacillin Ticarcillin	Ticarcillin/clavulanic acid[h]	Vancomycin	Vancomycin[m]
Amoxicillin/clavulanic acid or ampicillin/sulbactam **Piperacillin/tazobactam** Ticarcillin/clavulanic acid	Cefoperazone Aztreonam	Clindamycin[f]	
Cefmetazole Cefoperazone[a] Cefotetan Cefoxitin	Imipenem	Azithromycin[f] or clarithromycin[f] or erythromycin[f]	
	Amikacin		
Cefamandole or cefonicid or cefuroxime	Tobramycin	Trimethoprim/ sulfamethoxazole	
Cefotaxime[a,d] or ceftizoxime[a] or ceftriaxone[a,d]	Ciprofloxacin		
Imipenem	Trimethoprim/ sulfamethoxazole[h]		
Amikacin			
Ciprofloxacin[a,b]			
Trimethoprim/sulfamethoxazole[a, b]			
Group C[o] Supplemental Report Selectively Ceftazidime Aztreonam	Cefotaxime or ceftriaxone	Gentamicin	Gentamicin (high-level resistance screen only)
(Both are helpful indicators of extended-spectrum β-lactamases.)[e]	Netilmicin		Streptomycin (high-level resistance screen only)
Kanamycin	Chloramphenicol[f,h]		
Netilmicin		Ciprofloxacin or ofloxacin	
Tobramycin		Chloramphenicol[f]	
Tetracycline[b]		Rifampin	
Chloramphenicol[a,f]		Tetracycline[i]	

(Continued)

TABLE 15-9 *(Continued)*

SUGGESTED GROUPINGS OF US FDA-APPROVED ANTIMICROBIAL AGENTS THAT SHOULD BE CONSIDERED FOR ROUTINE TESTING AND REPORTING ON NONFASTIDIOUS ORGANISMS BY CLINICAL MICROBIOLOGY LABORATORIES

ENTEROBACTERIACEAE[a]	PSEUDOMONAS AERUGINOSA AND OTHER NON-ENTEROBACTERIACEAE[g]	STAPHYLOCOCCUS SPP.	ENTEROCOCCUS SPP.[k]
Group D Supplemental For Urine Only Carbenicillin	Carbenicillin	Lomefloxacin or norfloxacin	Ciprofloxacin Norfloxacin
Cinoxacin Lomefloxacin or norfloxacin[a] or ofloxacin	Ceftizoxime	Nitrofurantoin	Nitrofurantoin
	Tetracycline[h,i]		
Loracarbef	Lomefloxacin or norfloxacin or ofloxacin	Sulfisoxazole	Tetracycline
Nitrofurantoin			
Sulfisoxazole	Sulfisoxazole	Trimethoprim	
Trimethoprim			

NOTE 1: Selection of the most appropriate antimicrobial agents to test and to report is a decision best made by each clinical laboratory in consultation with infectious disease practitioners, the pharmacy, and the pharmacy and infection control committees of the medical staff. The lists for each organism group comprise agents of proven efficacy that show acceptable *in vitro* test performance. Considerations in the assignment of agents to Groups A, B, C, and D include clinical efficacy, prevalence of resistance, minimizing emergence of resistance, cost, and current consensus recommendations for first-choice and alternative drugs, in addition to the specific comments in footnotes "m"and "n." Tests of selected agents may be useful for infection control purposes.

NOTE 2: The boxes in the table designate clusters of comparable agents that need not be duplicated in testing because interpretive results are usually similar and clinical efficacy comparable. In addition, an "or" designates a related group of agents that has an almost identical spectrum of activity and interpretive results, and for which cross-resistance and susceptibility are nearly complete. Therefore, usually only one of the agents within each selection box (cluster or related group) need be selected for testing. Agents reported must be tested, unless reporting based on testing another agent provides a more accurate result (e.g., susceptibility of staphylococci to cefazolin or cephalothin based on oxacillin testing), and they usually should match those included in the hospital formulary; or else the report should include footnotes indicating the agents that usually have comparable interpretive results. Last, unexpected results should be considered for reporting (e.g., resistance of Enterobacteriaceae to third-generation cephalosporins or imipenem).

NOTE 3: Information in boldface type is considered tentative for 1 year.

[a] For isolates of *Salmonella* and *Shigella* spp., only ampicillin, a quinolone, and trimethoprim/sulfamethoxazole should be tested and reported routinely. In addition, chloramphenicol and a third-generation cephalosporin should be tested and reported for extra-intestinal isolates of *Salmonella* spp.

[b] May also be appropriate for inclusion in a panel for testing of urinary tract isolates along with the agents in Group D.

[c] **Cephalothin can be used to represent cephalothin, cephapirin, cephradine, cephalexin, cefaclor, and cefadroxil. Cefazolin, cefuroxime, cefpodoxime, cefprozil, and lorcarbef (urinary isolates only) may be tested individually because they may be active when cephalothin is not.**

[d] Should be reported on isolates from cerebrospinal fluids (CSF) along with agents in Group A.

[e] Strains of *Klebsiella* spp. and *Escherichia coli* may be clinically resistant to cephalosporin and aztreonam therapy by virtue of extended-spectrum β-lactamase production, despite apparent *in vitro* susceptibility to some of these agents. Some of these strains may be recognized by intermediate or resistant results to ceftazidime or aztreonam (or to cefotaxime, **cefpodoxime**, ceftriaxone, **or** ceftizoxime) and often are resistant to other agents, such as aminoglycosides and trimethoprim/sulfamethoxazole. The identification and susceptibility of such strains should be verified by retesting or submission to a reference laboratory. Until more data are available, laboratories may choose to report such strains as resistant to all cephalosporins and aztreonam.

[f] Not routinely tested against organisms isolated from the urinary tract.

[g] Non-*Enterobacteriaceae* includes *Acinetobacter* spp., **Stenotrophomonas** maltophilia, and *Pseudomonas* spp.

[h] May be indicated for primary testing of some *Pseudomonas* spp. other than *P. aeruginosa*, *S. maltophilia* (moxalactam may also be tested), and *Acinetobacter* spp. (ampicillin/sulbactam may be tested for *Acinetobacter* spp. resistant to other agents).

[i] Doxycycline or minocycline may be tested in place of, or in addition to, tetracycline for some isolates of *Staphylococcus aureus* and nonfermentative, gram-negative bacilli (e.g., *Acinetobacter* spp.) but should not be used to predict tetracycline susceptibility.

[j] Penicillin-susceptible staphylococci are also susceptible to other penicillins, cephems, and carbapenems approved for use by the FDA for staphylococcal infections. Penicillin-resistant, oxacillin-susceptible strains are resistant to β-lactamase-labile penicillins but susceptible to other β-lactamase-stable penicillins, β-lactamase inhibitor combinations, relevant cephems, and carbapenems. Oxacillin-resistant staphylococci are resistant to all currently available β-lactam antibiotics. Thus, susceptibility or resistance to a wide array of β-lactam antibiotics may be deduced from testing only penicillin and oxacillin. Routine testing of other penicillins, β-lactamase inhibitor combinations, cephems, and carbapenems is not needed.

[k] Antimicrobial agents not listed in this column, such as the cephalosporins, aminoglycosides, clindamycin, and trimethoprim/sulfamethoxazole, should not be tested and/or reported against enterococci because the reporting of these results can be dangerously misleading (except for screening for high-level aminoglycoside resistance).

[l] Penicillin susceptibility may be used to predict the susceptibility to ampicillin, amoxicillin, acylampicillins, ampicillin/sulbactam, amoxicillin/clavulanic acid, piperacillin, and piperacillin/tazobactam for non-β-lactamase-producing enterococci. However, combination therapy of penicillin or ampicillin, plus an aminoglycoside, is usually indicated for serious enterococcal infections, such as endocarditis. For blood and CSF isolates, a β-lactamase test is also recommended.

[m] Combination therapy with vancomycin plus an aminoglycoside is usually indicated for serious enterococcal infections, such as endocarditis.

[n] Group B represents agents that may warrant primary testing but which should be reported only selectively, such as when the organism is resistant to agents of the same family in Group A. Other indications for reporting the result might include selected specimen sources (e.g., **selected** third-generation cephalosporins for isolates of enteric bacteria from CSF or trimethoprim/sulfamethoxazole for urinary tract isolates), stated allergy or intolerance or failure to respond to an agent in Group A, polymicrobial infections, infections involving multiple sites with different microorganisms, or reports to infection control for epidemiologic aid.

[o] Group C represents alternative or supplemental antimicrobial agents that may require testing in those institutions harboring endemic or epidemic strains resistant to one or more of the primary drugs (especially in the same family, e.g., β-lactams or aminoglycosides), or for treatment of unusual organisms (e.g., chloramphenicol for some *Pseudomonas* spp.), or reporting to infection control as an epidemiologic aid.

NCCLS Vol. 15, No. 14, 1995.

TABLE 15-10
SUGGESTED GROUPINGS OF US FDA-APPROVED ANTIMICROBIAL AGENTS THAT SHOULD
BE CONSIDERED FOR ROUTINE TESTING AND REPORTING ON FASTIDIOUS ORGANISMS
BY CLINICAL MICROBIOLOGY LABORATORIES

HAEMOPHILUS SPP.[a,b]	NEISSERIA GONORRHOEAE[d]	STREPTOCOCCUS PNEUMONIAE	STREPTOCOCCUS SPP. OTHER THAN S. PNEUMONIAE
Group A Primary Test and Report Ampicillin[a,c]		Penicillin[e]	Penicillin[h] or ampicillin[h]
		Erythromycin[f,g]	
Trimethoprim/ sulfamethoxazole		Trimethoprim/ sulfamethoxazole[f]	Erythromycin[g,i]
Group B[j] Primary Report Selectively Amoxicillin/ clavulanic acid[b] or ampicillin/sulbactam		Cefotaxime or ceftriaxone	Vancomycin
Azithromycin[b] or clarithromycin[b]			
Cefaclor[b] or cefprozil[b] or loracarbef[b] Cefixime[b] or cefpodoxime[b]		Vancomycin	
Cefuroxime			
Cefotaxime[a] or ceftazidime[a] or ceftizoxime[a] or ceftriaxone[a]		Tetracycline[f]	Chloramphenicol[i]
Chloramphenicol[a]		Chloramphenicol	Clindamycin[i]
Tetracycline[b]			
Group C[k] Supplemental Report Selectively Cefonicid	Penicillin	Ofloxacin[f]	Cefotaxime or ceftriaxone
Imipenem	Cefixime or cefotaxime or cefpodoxime or ceftizoxime or ceftriaxone	**Amoxicillin[f] or amoxicillin/clavulanic acid[f]**	Azithromycin[g,i] Clarithromycin[g,i]
Aztreonam	Cefmetazole Cefotetan Cefoxitin Cefuroxime	**Cefuroxime** **Imipenem**	
Ciprofloxacin or lomefloxacin[b] or ofloxacin	Spectinomycin		Ofloxacin
	Tetracycline		
Rifampin	Ciprofloxacin or ofloxacin		

among manufacturers and even among lots produced by a single company, depending on the source of the seaweed. Attempts to minimize the variation among lots of Mueller-Hinton agar continue. A reference standard for manufacturers may provide greater reproducibility.[214] A specially formulated medium for testing of *Haemophilus influenzae* has been developed and recommended by the NCCLS for routine use.[126] This *Haemophilus* test medium can also be used for *Haemophilus* spp, as described later.[124]

pH

The pH of the medium should be between 7.2 and 7.4 at room temperature. The pH of broth media may be tested directly with a pH electrode, and agar media may be tested by macerating enough agar so that the tip of the electrode can be submerged, by allowing a portion of agar to solidify around the electrode, or by using a properly calibrated surface electrode.

SERUM

Antibiotics differ greatly in the degree to which they bind to proteins. In the bloodstream, free antibiotic is in equilibrium with serum protein-bound antibiotic. Free and protein-bound antibiotic can be measured, but it is not clear which is the more useful result. In the laboratory, different values can be obtained for highly protein-bound antibiotics if serum is added to the medium. The NCCLS method does not include added serum because of the difficulty in standardization of the product and uncertainty about how to interpret the results. Perl and colleagues studied the effect of serum on 11 broad-spectrum antibiotics used to treat nosocomial gram-negative bacillary infections.[208] The results were identical with 9 of the 11 antibiotics. Only in the case of ceftriaxone (>95% protein bound) and cefoperazone (90% protein bound) were there substantial differences when serum was incorporated into the reference procedure.

CATION CONCENTRATION

As previously discussed, the concentration of the divalent cations Ca^{2+} and Mg^{2+} affects the susceptibility results when certain combinations of bacterial species and antibiotic are tested.[220] Barry has postulated that the mechanism by which cation concentration affects the activity of *Pseudomonas aeruginosa*, for example, involves the permeability of the bacterial cell wall.[11] The lipopolysaccharides in the cell wall of *P. aeruginosa* are cross-linked with divalent cations, providing stability. When the organisms are grown in

◄ NOTE 1: Selection of the most appropriate antimicrobial agents to test and to report is a decision best made by each clinical laboratory in consultation with the infectious disease practitioners, the pharmacy, and the pharmacy and infection control committees of the medical staff. The lists for each organism group comprise agents of proven efficacy that show acceptable *in vitro* test performance. Considerations in the assignment of agents to Groups A, B, C, and D include clinical efficacy, prevalence of resistance, minimizing emergence of resistance, cost, and current consensus recommendations for first-choice and alternative drugs, in addition to the specific comments in footnotes "j" and "k." Tests on selected agents may be useful for infection control purposes.

NOTE 2: The boxes in the table designate clusters of comparable agents that need not be duplicated in testing because interpretive results are usually similar and clinical efficacy comparable. In addition, an "or" designates a related group of agents that has an almost identical spectrum of activity and interpretive results, and for which cross-resistance and susceptibility are nearly complete. Therefore, usually only one of the agents within each selection box (cluster or related group) need be selected for testing. Agents reported must be tested, unless reporting based on testing another agent provides a more accurate result, and they usually should match those included in the hospital formulary; or else the report should include footnotes indicating the agents that usually show comparable interpretive results. Last, unexpected results should be considered for reporting.

NOTE 3: Information in boldface type is considered tentative for 1 year.

a Only results of testing with ampicillin, one of the third-generation cephalosporins, and chloramphenicol should be reported routinely with all blood and cerebrospinal fluid isolates of *Haemophilus influenzae* recovered from patients with life-threatening infections (e.g., meningitis, bacteremia, epiglottitis, and facial cellulitis).

b The results of tests with agents that are administered by the oral route only should be reported only with isolates of *Haemophilus* spp. from localized, non-life-threatening infections (e.g., uncomplicated cases of otitis media and sinusitis, and selected bronchopulmonary infections).

c The results of ampicillin susceptibility tests should be used to predict the activity of amoxicillin. The majority of isolates of *H. influenzae* that are resistant to ampicillin and amoxicillin produce a TEM-type β-lactamase. In most cases, a direct β-lactamase test can provide a rapid means of detecting ampicillin and amoxicillin resistance.

d A β-lactamase test will detect one form of penicillin resistance in *N. gonorrhoeae* and also may be used to provide epidemiologic information. Strains with chromosomally mediated resistance can be detected only by additional susceptibility testing, such as the disk diffusion method or the agar dilution MIC method.

e **If the penicillin result is intermediate or resistant, cefotaxime or ceftriaxone MICs should also be reported.**

f Only results of testing with penicillin, cefotaxime, ceftriaxone, chloramphenicol, and vancomycin should be reported routinely with blood and CSF isolates of *S. pneumoniae* recovered from patients with life-threatening infections (e.g., meningitis, bacteremia).

g Susceptibility and resistance to azithromycin and clarithromycin can be predicted by testing erythromycin.

h Penicillin or ampicillin intermediate isolates may require combined therapy with an aminoglycoside for bactericidal action.

i Not routinely tested against organisms isolated from the urinary tract.

j Group B represents agents that may warrant primary testing but which should be reported only selectively, such as when the organism is resistant to agents of the same class in Group A. Other indications for reporting the result might include selected specimen sources (e.g., third-generation cephalosporin for isolates of *H. influenzae* from CSF), stated allergy or intolerance or failure to respond to an agent in Group A, polymicrobial infections, infections involving multiple sites with different microorganisms, or reports to infection control for epidemiologic aid.

k Group C represents alternative or supplemental antimicrobial agents that may require testing in those institutions harboring endemic or epidemic strains resistant to one or more of the primary drugs (especially in the same class, e.g., β-lactams), or for treatment of unusual organisms, or reporting to infection control as an epidemiologic aid.

NCCLS Vol. 15, No. 14, 1995.

TABLE 15-11
GROUPING OF RECOMMENDED ANTIBIOTICS FOR TESTING AND REPORTING

GROUP	CATEGORY	TYPE OF ANTIMICROBIAL AGENT
A	Primary test and report	Include in routine panel and report routinely
B	Primary test; report selectively	Second-line or backup antibiotics for group A, because of greater expense or toxicity, appropriateness for a specific site, or clinical failure with a group A antibiotic. Results may be needed but on a selective basis.
C	Supplemental testing; selective reporting	Testing in institutions with specific bacterial resistance problems, or in patients who are allergic to other antibiotics, or in unusual infections
D	Supplemental	Testing of lower urinary tract infections only

Adapted from reference 280.

media deficient in cations, cell-wall permeability to the aminoglycoside antibiotics and other compounds is increased. The organisms, therefore, are more sensitive to the action of the aminoglycosides, producing falsely low MIC results or large inhibitory zone sizes. Mueller-Hinton broth has very low concentrations of divalent cations and should be supplemented to physiologic concentrations (20 to 35 µg/liter Mg^{2+} and 50 to 100 µg/liter Ca^{2+}). Some batches of Mueller-Hinton agar may actually have an abnormally high concentration of these cations, so that small inhibitory zones are produced when *P. aeruginosa* is tested against aminoglycosides. Such lots, which can be identified by testing with reference strains of known reactivity, should be discarded.

Detection of resistance of certain strains of staphylococci to semisynthetic penicillins is improved by including 2% NaCl in the broth media or 4% NaCl in the agar media.[38,265] The recommended concentration of NaCl for agar media has recently been revised to 2%.[8]

ATMOSPHERE

Agar or broth is incubated in an ambient air incubator. A CO_2 incubator should not be used for routine tests. The carbonic acid formed on the surface of the agar or in the broth can cause a decrease in pH, which can affect the antibacterial activity of certain antibiotics, as previously discussed. In laboratories with a small workload and where only a CO_2 incubator is available, it is acceptable to place the susceptibility plates or tubes in a sealed jar to prevent access of the CO_2 from the incubator.

TEMPERATURE

Plates and tubes should be incubated routinely at 35°C. At higher temperatures, the detection of oxacillin-resistant staphylococci is compromised. If oxacillin resistance is suspected and not manifested at 35°C, the plates or tubes may be incubated at 30°C.

INOCULUM

The inoculum is usually prepared from a broth culture that has been incubated for 4 to 6 hours, when growth is considered to be in the logarithmic phase. Several similar-appearing colonies should be sampled to minimize variation in the bacterial population. The density of the suspension is adjusted to approximately 10^8 colony-forming units (CFU) per milliliter by comparing its turbidity to a McFarland 0.5 $BaSO_4$ standard. The standard is prepared by adding 0.5 ml of 0.048 M $BaCl_2$ (1.175% w/v $BaCl_2 \cdot H_2O$) to 99.5 ml of 0.36 N H_2SO_4. Aliquots of 4 to 6 ml of the barium sulfate turbidity standard are distributed to screw-capped tubes of the same size, sealed tightly, and stored in the dark at room temperature. Nephelometers may be used to determine turbidity. Commonly, the degree of cloudiness in the broth is compared with the standard, visualizing the two against a white background on which black lines have been drawn. Further adjustments to the inoculum depend on the type of test employed. Alternatively, commercially available devices for preparing a standardized inoculum have worked well.[12]

If time does not permit incubation for 4 to 6 hours, young colonies may be removed from the surface of an agar plate that has been incubated overnight and diluted to the proper density. This method is recommended when staphylococci are tested for resistance to methicillin and when testing isolates of *Streptococcus pneumoniae* and *Haemophilus influenzae*.

It is useful to document the number of organisms in the inoculum periodically by inoculating serial dilutions of the suspension onto agar plates.

ANTIBIOTICS

Reference antibiotic powders for use in dilution tests should be obtained from the manufacturer or from the U.S. Pharmacopeia in Rockville, Maryland. These reference powders are documented with an assay of antimicrobial activity. For example, the label may indicate that the powder contains 1075 µg of active chemical in each 1000 µg of powder. The amount of powder weighed must be adjusted for the activity of each lot. Vials should not be obtained from the hospital pharmacy because they may contain fillers and are not assayed for biologic activity. The antibiotics should be stored in a desiccator as indicated for each agent. Many antibiotics, especially those of the β-lactam class, are more stable at temperatures below −20°C. Suspensions of antibiotic should be stored at −20°C or less, preferably at −70°C; they should not be refrozen after dispensing. Imipenem, which is particularly affected by freezing and thawing,[290] should be reconstituted each time a batch of plates or tubes is prepared. A frost-free freezer should not be used because repeated cycles of freezing and thawing occur.

Antimicrobial-impregnated disks should be stored at −20°C or lower in an anhydrous condition. Under guidelines established by the U.S. Food and Drug Administration, manufacturers of antibiotic disks must carefully control the concentration of antibiotics in the disks to within 60% to 120% of the stated content; the actual variation is usually considerably less. A small working supply may be maintained at refrigerator temperatures in a desiccator. Disks should always be allowed to warm to room temperature before opening the desiccator, so that condensation of moisture from the air does not partially rehydrate the disks. Spurious resistance of *Staphylcoccus aureus* to oxacillin has resulted from use of a defective lot of disks.[23]

QUALITY CONTROL

Rigorous quality control is important for antimicrobial susceptibility testing because of the large numbers of variables that may affect the results. Some of the physical and chemical characteristics of the media, such as pH and depth of agar, may be monitored, but the final control is provided by a series of reference bacterial strains, including *Escherichia coli* (ATCC #25922), *Pseudomonas aeruginosa* (ATCC #27853), *Staphylococcus aureus* (ATCC #29213 for dilution tests; ATCC #25923 for disk tests), *Streptococcus faecalis* (ATCC #29212) for dilution tests, *Haemophilus influenzae* (ATCC 49247 and ATCC 49766) for tests performed on *Haemophilus* Test Medium, and *Neisseria gonorrhoeae* (ATCC 49226) for which expected results have been established. A strain of *Enterococcus faecalis* (ATCC 29212 or ATCC 33186) may be used to test Mueller-Hinton agar or broth for the appropriateness of thymidine and thymine levels. These reference strains are available from the American Type Culture Collection in Washington, DC, or from various commercial sources. The ideal control strains have susceptibility end points in the mid range of antimicrobial concentrations tested and have minimal tendencies to change susceptibility patterns over time.

These reference strains must be stored in a condition that minimizes the possibility of mutation. They may be stored frozen (below −20°C or preferably below −60°C) after suspension in a stabilizer, such as defibrinated whole blood, 50% fetal calf serum in bacteriologic broth, or 10% glycerol in broth. Alternatively, the strains may be lyophilized. For short-term storage, the bacteria may be grown on soybean-casein digest agar and stored at 2°C to 8°C. Fresh slants should be prepared every 2 weeks, and a new stock culture should be obtained when aberrant results are noted. A fresh subculture should be prepared each day that the control strain is used.

INTERPRETATION OF RESULTS

A clinician who receives the results of a dilution susceptibility test knows the concentrations of a group of drugs that inhibited growth of the pathogen under carefully defined conditions in the laboratory. To make a rational selection of the most appropriate antibiotic for a patient, the physician needs at least three other pieces of information: 1) the pharmacokinetics of the antimicrobial agent, including the peak level that can be expected at the site of infection and the rapidity with which that level will decrease, that is, the half-life (Table 15-12); 2) how the isolated bacterium compares to other isolates of the same species; and 3) any available clinical data on the *in vivo* response of similar isolates in similar situations.

Without complete knowledge of these factors, it is easy to misinterpret the raw data. For instance, a β-lactam antibiotic such as ampicillin, with an MIC of 2 μg/ml for an isolate of *E. coli,* might be considered less effective than an aminoglycoside antibiotic, such as gentamicin, with an MIC of 0.5 μg/ml. In fact, the achievable levels of drug in serum are far greater for ampicillin than for gentamicin and the risk of toxicity is much lower in the absence of a history of allergic reactions to the drug. The appropriate choice of therapy would, therefore, be ampicillin, and not the antibiotic with the "lowest MIC."

The laboratory must assist the clinician in making a rational selection of therapy by providing suggested interpretations of the quantitative results. The recommendations address the expected response in serum and in body fluids or tissues where concentrations similar to serum accumulate. The physician must remember that higher levels of certain drugs accumulate in certain sites, such as urine or bile; an organism that is classified as "resistant" by the criteria for serum may well be treatable if it is in the lower urinary tract. For example, an isolate of *E. coli* with an MIC of 32 μg/ml for ampicillin would be considered resistant in serum where relatively low concentrations of drug are present. In contrast, concentrations of ampicillin in the hundreds of micrograms per milliliter would be expected in the urine; one would expect to use ampicillin successfully for an infection of the lower urinary tract, even though the isolate is intrinsically rather resistant. Assuming that ampicillin is the least costly and least toxic antibiotic available, the clinician must decide whether the patient has an infection that involves the parenchyma of the kidney (pyelonephritis), in which case ampicillin would be inappropriate, or whether the infection is in the urinary bladder, in which case ampicillin may well be effective even against this resistant organism. Obviously, the severity of the infection and the potential damage to the patient if a miscalculation is made also impact on the decision.

Similarly, an isolate of *E. coli* with an MIC of 8 μg/ml to cefazolin would be considered susceptible in serum or most tissues. Cefazolin penetrates through the meninges very poorly, however, and this antibiotic should not be used to treat a patient with meningitis, no matter what the MIC. In fact, if the isolate comes from the cerebrospinal fluid, the laboratory should not even report results with this antibiotic.

Computer-generated interpretations of individual test results, including construction of a "therapeutic ratio" (MIC value:peak serum level), have been suggested.[289] To be valid, such interpretative programs must take other operative factors, including clinical experience, into account.

Three categories of antibiotic susceptibility are recognized by the NCCLS for dilution tests (Table 15-13). *(Text continues on page 816)*

TABLE 15-12

ACHIEVABLE ANTIBIOTIC LEVELS IN SERUM

ANTIBIOTIC	DOSE AND ROUTE OF ADMINISTRATION (SINGLE = S OR MULTIPLE = M DOSES)	SERUM CONCENTRATION MEAN (RANGE) (μg/mL)	SERUM HALF-LIFE (h)
Ampicillin	500 mg PO (M)	2.9 (0.03–10.0)	1.1
	2000 mg IV (M)	59 (10–164)	1.1
Amikacin	7.5 mg/kg IV (S)	31.2 ± 2.3	2.0
Carbenicillin	5000 mg IV (S)	187 (155–218)	1.5
Cefaclor	1000 mg PO (S)	21 (7–34)	0.7
Cefazolin	1000 mg IV (S)	76.3 (49–138)	1.8
Cefotaxime	1000 mg IV (M)	19.4 (8.6–48.2)	1.2
Cefoxitin	2000 mg IV (M)	86 (20–160)	0.8
Cephalexin	1000 mg PO (S)	10.6 (9–11)	0.8
Ceftazidime	2000 mg IV (S)	125 ± 20 S.D.	1.9
Ceftizoxime	1000 mg IV (S)	24.1 + 4.4 S.D.	1.0
Cephalothin	1000 mg IV (S)	12.7 (4–46)	0.5
Chloramphenicol	500 mg IV (S)	1.4 (1.25–5)	2.5
Clindamycin	300 mg PO (M)	2.1	2.0
	600 mg IV (S)	11.3 (6–19)	2.0
Doxcycline	100 mg PO (M)	3.5 (1.2–6.0)	20
Erythromycin stearate	500 mg PO (M)	2.2 (0.3–5.0)	1.5
Gentamicin	80 mg IM (M)	6.3 (3–12)	2.0
Imipenem–cilastatin	500 mg IV	40	1.0
Methicillin	2000 mg IV (M)	23.3 (13.2–>50)	0.5
Nafcillin	62–140 mg/kg/day IV (M)	37 (5.8–92)	1.0
Piperacillin	2000 mg IV (M)	85.2 (54–108)	1.1
Tobramycin	1.7 mg/kg IV (M)	8.0 (5.6–12.0)	2.0
Tetracycline	500 mg PO (M)	3.7 (2.1–4.6)	10
Ticarcillin	5000 mg IV (S)	186 (118–242)	1.2
Trimethoprim	160 mg PO (M)	3.1 ± 0.8	8–10
	5 mg/kg IV (S)	3.7 (3.0–4.1)	8–10
Vancomycin	500 mg IV (S)	7.5 (5.2–10.0)	6.0

Note the large variations in achievable levels even within these single studies. Variability is even greater among different studies, reflecting differences in doses and time and methods of measurements and whether single or multiple doses had been given. The estimations provided in this and similar tables should not be used, therefore, as a simple means of determining the susceptibility category of individual bacterial isolates; other factors that affect antimicrobial susceptibility must be considered.

Gerding DN, Peterson LR, Hughes CE, et al: Extravascular antimicrobial distribution in man. In: Lorian V (ed): Antibiotics in Laboratory Medicine, 2nd ed, pp 938–994. Baltimore, Williams & Wilkins, 1986.

TABLE 15-13

Minimum Inhibitory Concentration (MIC) Interpretive Standards (µg/mL) for Organisms Other Than *Haemophilus* spp., *Neisseria gonorrhoeae*, and Streptococci

Antimicrobial Agent	Susceptible[o]	Intermediate[p]	Resistant
β-Lactam Penicillins			
Ampicillin[a]			
when testing Enterobacteriaceae	≤8	16	≥32
when testing staphylococci[b,c] and *Moraxella catarrhalis*[d]	≤0.25	—	≥0.5
when testing *Listeria monocytogenes*	≤2	—	≥4
when testing enterococci[e]	≤8	—	≥16
Azilocillin when testing *Pseudomonas aeruginosa*[f]	≤64	—	≥128
Carbenicillin			
when testing *P. aeruginosa*	≤128	256	≥512
when testing other gram-negative organisms	≤16	32	≥64
Methicillin			
when testing staphylococci[g,h]	≤8	—	≥16
Mezlocillin			
when testing *P. aeruginosa*[f]	≤4	—	≥128
when testing other gram-negative organisms	≤16	32–64	≥128
Nafcillin			
when testing staphylococci[g,h]	≤2	—	≥4
Oxacillin			
when testing staphylococci[g,h]	≤2	—	≥4
Penicillin			
when testing staphylococci[b,c] and *M. catarrhalis*[d]	≤0.12	—	≥0.25
when testing *L. monocytogenes*	≤2	—	≥4
when testing enterococci[e]	≤8	—	≥16
Others			
Chloramphenicol	≤8	16	≥32
Clindamycin	≤0.5	1–2	≥4
Nitrofurantoin[j]	≤32	64	≥128
Rifampin	≤1	2	≥4
Sulfonamides[j,m]	≤256	—	≥512
Trimethoprim[j]	≤8	—	≥16
Trimethoprim/sulfamethoxazole[n]	≤2/38	—	≥4/76

NOTE: Information in boldface type is considered tentative for 1 year.
[a] Class representative for ampicillin, amoxicillin, bacampicillin, cyclacillin, and hetacillin.
[b] Resistant strains of *Staphylococcus aureus* produce β-lactamase and the testing of penicillin instead of ampicillin is preferred. Penicillin should be used to test the susceptibility of all staphylococci to all penicillinase-sensitive penicillins, such as ampicillin, amoxicillin, azlocillin, bacampicillin, hetacillin, carbenicillin, mezlocillin, piperacillin, and ticarcillin. Results may also be applied to phenoxymethyl penicillin or phenethicillin. Only one category of susceptibility is appropriate for penicillinase-negative staphylococci. A penicillin MIC of ≤0.03 µg/mL usually implies lack of β-lactamase production and MICs of ≥0.25 µg/mL should be considered resistant; staphylococci with MICs between these values may or may not produce the enzyme. Laboratories should perform an induced β-lactamase test on strains with these MICs.

Susceptible implies that the organism should respond to usual doses of the antimicrobial agent administered by an appropriate route, including orally. *Intermediate* implies that the isolate may be inhibited by concentrations of drug that are achieved when the maximum parenteral doses are given; the antibiotic may be selected, but consideration should be given to other choices that may provide more optimal therapy. *Resistant* indicates that the bacterium is not inhibited by achievable concentrations of drug and, therefore, the drug should not be selected for therapy, except in certain body fluids where high concentrations of the antibiotic may accumulate. The number of "major and very major errors" —those that transpose susceptible and resistant— should be kept to the absolute minimum.

If the laboratory performs a disk diffusion test, the standardized method and interpretations suggested by the NCCLS should be reported (Table 15-14). Occasionally, a physician may derive useful information from the closeness of the actual zone size to the MIC breakpoints, but this information is rarely reported.

A laboratory that performs dilution susceptibility tests may report the interpretative correlate alone, that is, susceptible, intermediate, or resistant, or may report the MIC value along with the interpretative correlate. Increasingly, many institutions have chosen to report only the interpretation, although they actually determine an MIC, because of the potential for misinterpretation of the numerical value by clinicians. The MIC values are reserved for knowledgeable users, such as infectious disease physicians. If the MIC is included in the report, the physicians must be educated as to its purpose. A convenient mechanism is to publish the data on achievable antibiotic levels and the relation of MIC to interpretative correlate in a form that is easily accessible to physicians.

SELECTION OF ANTIBIOTICS TO BE REPORTED

Only antibiotics appropriate for the infection should be included in a report. Drugs that are active only in the urinary tract should not be reported if the isolate comes from another site. Antibiotics that do not penetrate into a site, such as cefazolin or cephalothin in the meninges, should not be reported for organisms isolated from that site. Use of chloramphenicol for urinary tract infections is inappropriate because it is not excreted in the urine; its use should not be encouraged by including the susceptibility results in a laboratory report. There are unfortunately very few of these absolute prohibitions. Most of the decisions should be made in consultation with members of the medical staff and pharmacy. All accredited hospitals have pharmacy and therapeutics committees (or the equivalent) that provide a useful forum for coordinated effort. Several reasonable strategies, depending on local policy, needs, and resources, are listed in Box 15-2 (page 818).

MACRODILUTION BROTH SUSCEPTIBILITY TEST

The macrodilution broth susceptibility test was among the first to be developed and still serves as a reference method. Serial dilutions of antimicrobial agent are made in broth or in agar, after which a standardized bacterial suspension is added. Figure 15-11 shows 10 test tubes that contain cation supplemented Mueller-Hinton broth. Quantities of antibiotic are serially diluted from 100 µg/ml to 0.4 µg/ml. Tube number 10 is free of antibiotic and serves as a growth control. Each of the 10 tubes is inoculated with a calibrated suspension of the microorganism to be tested and incubated at 35°C for 18 hours. At the end of the incubation period, the tubes are visually examined for turbidity. Note in Figure 15-11 that the five tubes to the left are clear; the five to the right appear cloudy. Cloudiness indicates that bacterial growth has not been inhibited by the concentration of antibiotic contained in the medium.

Figure 15-12 (page 819) illustrates that the breakpoint of growth inhibition in Figure 15-11 is between tubes 5 and 6, or between 6.25 µg/ml and 3.12 µg/ml of antibiotic. This breakpoint represents the MIC, defined as the lowest concentration of antibiotic in micrograms per milliliter that prevents the *in vitro* growth of bacteria. Thus, in the example shown in Figures 15-11 and 15-12, the MIC lies somewhere between 6.25 µg/ml and 3.12 µg/ml. However, by convention, the MIC is interpreted as the concentration of the antibiotic, contained in the first tube in the series, that inhibits visible growth. Therefore, in this example, the MIC is 6.25 µg/ml.

The adaptation of this test to small volumes for routine testing is described in a later section.

AGAR DILUTION SUSCEPTIBILITY TEST

The agar dilution procedure, which is the second reference method, has been successfully adapted for routine use in large laboratories by testing only selected concentrations of antibiotic. A standardized suspension of bacteria is inoculated onto a series of agar plates, each containing a different concentration of antibiotic, encompassing the therapeutic range of the drug. For example, if the therapeutic range for a given antibiotic is 2 to 12 µg/ml, a series of agar plates containing 1, 4, 8, 16, and 32 µg/ml of antibiotic might be used to determine the susceptibility of the organism being tested. If the organism grows on the first three plates but not in the plate containing 16 µg/ml of antibiotic, an MIC value of 16 µg/ml can be established, similar to the interpretation of the end point in the broth dilution technique.

Agar dilution plates ready for interpretation are shown in Figure 15-13 (page 819). Note that those microorganisms that are sensitive to the concentration of antibiotic contained in any given agar plate do not produce a circle of growth at the inoculum site, whereas those that are resistant appear as circular colonies. The agar plates are marked with a grid so that each microorganism can be identified by a number and the results entered on the worksheet.

To facilitate testing of a large volume of cultures, an instrument known as the Steers replicator is used (Fig. 15-14, page 820). The main feature of the instrument is a spring-loaded head that is fitted with 32 to 36 flat-surfaced inoculating pins, each about 3 mm in

TABLE 15-14
ZONE DIAMETER INTERPRETIVE STANDARDS AND EQUIVALENT MINIMUM INHIBITORY CONCENTRATION (MIC) BREAKPOINTS FOR ORGANISMS OTHER THAN *HAEMOPHILUS* SPP., *NEISSERIA GONORRHOEAE*, AND STREPTOCOCCI

ANTIMICROBIAL AGENT	DISK CONTENT	ZONE DIAMETER, NEAREST WHOLE mm			EQUIVALENT MIC BREAKPOINTS[t] (µg/mL)	
		RESISTANT	INTERMEDIATE[q]	SUSCEPTIBLE[s]	RESISTANT	SUSCEPTIBLE
β-Lactam Penicillins						
Ampicillin[a]						
when testing gram-negative enteric organisms	10 µg	≤13	14–6	≥17	≥32	≤8
when testing staphylococci[b,c]	10 µg	≤28	—	≥29	β-Lactamase[b]	≤0.25
when testing enterococci[d]	10 µg	≤16	—	≥17[d]	≥16	—
when testing *L. monocytogenes*	10 µg	≤19	—	≥20	≥4	≤2
Azilocillin when testing *Pseudomonas aeruginosa*[e]	75 µg	≤17	—	≥18	≥128	≤64
Carbenicillin[b]						
when testing *P. aeruginosa*	100 µg	≤13	14–16	≥17	≥512	≤128
when testing other gram-negative organisms	100 µg	≤19	20–22	≥23	≥64	≤16
Methicillin when testing staphylococci[f, g]	5 µg	≤9	0–13	≥14	≥16	≤8
Mezlocillin[b]						
when testing *P. aeruginosa*[e]	75 µg	≤15	—	≥16	≥128	≤64
when testing other gram-negative organisms	75 µg	≤17	18–20	≥21	≥128	≤16
Nafcillin when testing staphylococci[f, g]	1 µg	≤10	11–12	≥13	—	≤1
Oxacillin when testing staphylococci[f, g]	1 µg	≤10	11–12	≥13	≥4	≤2
Penicillin						
when testing staphylococci[b,c]	10 units	≤28	—	≥29	β-Lactamase[b]	≤0.1
when testing enterococci[d]	10 units	≤14	—	≥15[d]	≥16	—
when testing *L. monocytogenes*	10 units	≤19	—	≥20	≥4	≤2
Others						
Chloramphenicol	30 µg	≤12	13–17	≥18	≥32	≤8
Clindamycin	2 µg	≤14	15–20	≥21	≥4	≤0.5
Nitrofurantoin[k]	300 µg	≤14	15–16	≥17	≥128	≤32
Rifampin	5 µg	≤16	17–19	≥20	≥4	≤1
Sulfonamides[k,p]	250 or 300 µg	≤12	13–16	≥17	≥350	≤100
Trimethoprim[k,p]	5 µg	≤10	11–15	≥16	≥16	≤4
Trimethoprim/ sulfamethoxazole[p]	1.25/23.75 µg	≤10	11–15	≥16	≥8/152	≤2/38

NOTE: Information in boldface type is considered tentative for 1 year.

[a] Class disk for ampicillin, amoxicillin, bacampicillin, cyclacillin, and hetacillin.

[b] Resistant strains of *Staphylococcus aureus* produce β-lactamase and the testing of the 10-unit penicillin disk is preferred. Penicillin should be used to test the susceptibility of all penicillinase-sensitive penicillins, such as ampicillin, amoxicillin, azlocillin, bacampicillin, hetacillin, carbenicillin, mezlocillin, piperacillin, and ticarcillin. Results may also be applied to phenoxymethyl penicillin or phenethicillin.

[c] Staphylococci exhibiting resistance to methicillin, oxacillin, or nafcillin should be reported as also resistant to other penicillins, cephalosporins, carbacephems, carbapenems, and β-lactamase inhibitor combinations despite apparent *in vitro* susceptibility of some strains to the latter agents. This is because infections with methicillin-resistant staphylococci have not responded favorably to therapy with β-lactam antibiotics.

diameter. The head is attached to a piston and spring-loaded cylinder mechanism by which it can be moved up and down in a vertical plane. The counterpart is an aluminum seed plate containing 32 to 36 wells. These wells are tooled in such a manner that when the seed plate is properly aligned within the guide at the base of the replicator, each of the inoculating pins on the movable head fits exactly into the wells. Each well in the seed plate provides a receptacle into which different bacterial suspensions can be placed.

The agar dilution susceptibility plate is inoculated by placing the seed tray with its multiple suspensions directly under the inoculating head. The head is lowered so that the pins extend fully into each of the wells, thus sampling approximately 0.003 ml of each bacterial suspension on the surface of each inoculating pin. Next, the head is raised and an agar plate is moved into position under the prongs, which in turn are lowered so that the flat surface of each inoculating pin just touches the agar surface. The head is again raised, and the seed plate is moved back into position for inoculation of the next agar plate. The procedure is repeated for all of the antibiotic plates to be tested. After all the plates have been inoculated, they are incubated at 35°C for 18 hours.

DISK DIFFUSION SUSCEPTIBILITY TEST

Figure 15-15 illustrates the basic principle of the disk diffusion method of antimicrobial susceptibility testing.[11] As soon as the antibiotic-impregnated disk comes in contact with the moist agar surface, water is absorbed into the filter paper and the antibiotic diffuses into the surrounding medium. The rate of extraction of the antibiotic out of the disk is greater than its outward diffusion into the medium, so that the concentration immediately adjacent to the disk may exceed that in the disk itself. As the distance from the

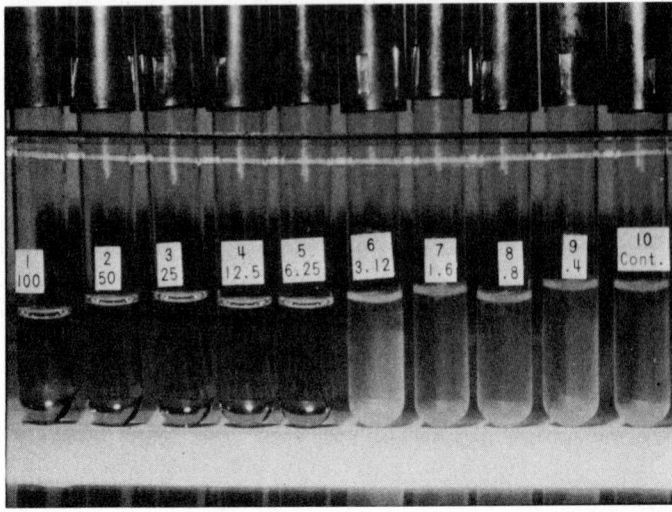

Figure 15-11
Illustration of broth dilution antibiotic susceptibility test in which the antibiotic to be tested is serially diluted in a range between 100 µg/mL and 0.4 µg/mL. Tube number *10* serves as a positive control.

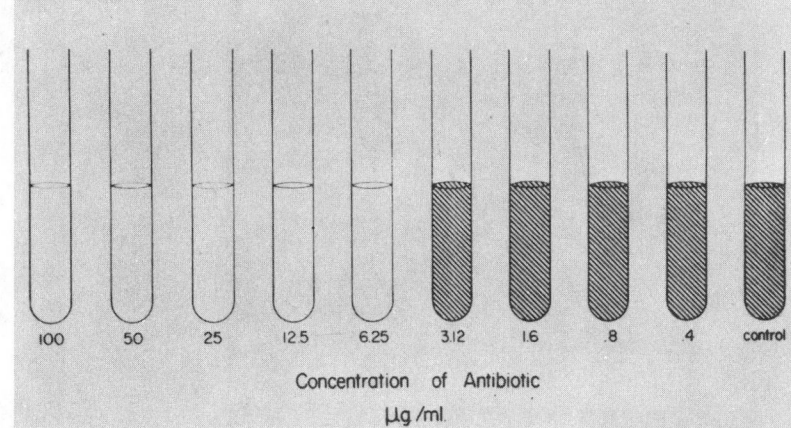

Figure 15-12
Line drawing of the broth dilution susceptibility test shown in Figure 15-11: The minimum inhibitory concentration for the test illustrated here is 6.25 μg/mL.

disk increases, however, there is a logarithmic reduction in the antibiotic concentration. If the plate has
been previously inoculated with a bacterial suspension, simultaneous growth of bacteria occurs on the
surface of the agar. When a critical cell mass of bacteria
is reached, the inhibitory activity of the antibiotic is
overcome and bacterial growth occurs. The time (critical time) required to reach the critical cell mass (4 to 10
hours for commonly tested bacteria) is characteristic of
each species but is influenced by the composition of
the medium and temperature of incubation. The lateral
extent of antimicrobial diffusion before the critical time
is reached will be affected by the depth of the agar because diffusion occurs in three dimensions. The points
at which the critical cell mass is reached appear as a
sharply marginated circle of bacterial growth, with the
middle of the disk forming the center of the circle if the
test has been performed properly (Fig. 15-16, page
820). The concentration of diffused antibiotic at this interface of growing and inhibited bacteria is known as
the critical concentration and approximates the MIC
obtained in dilution tests. Although direct calculation
of the inhibitory concentration is not done in practice,
the MIC can actually be calculated with reasonable accuracy if the characteristics of antimicrobial diffusion
and bacterial growth are known.[11]

EARLY DEVELOPMENTS

With the advent of several new antibiotics during
the 1940s, tube dilution methods were no longer practical for the large volume of work required. In 1943,
Foster and Woodruff placed a paper strip that had
been impregnated with antibiotics on the surface of an
agar plate that had been inoculated previously.[74] Multiple antibiotics could be tested simply by this method.

The so-called zone versus no zone method was
used initially for interpretation of results. The development of an inhibitory zone of any size around a single
disk was considered evidence that the organism was
susceptible to the antibiotic. Resistant bacteria were
classified as such if they grew right up to the margin of
the disk.

Initially it was believed that zone sizes around
disks impregnated with various antibiotics could be
correlated with the relative susceptibility of the organism to those antibiotics; that is, the larger the zone, the
more effective the antibiotic should be therapeutically.
As more was learned of the mechanisms by which diffusion occurred and inhibitory zones were formed, it
became apparent that factors influencing the diffusion
rate *in vitro* did not necessarily correlate with antimicrobial activity *in vivo*.

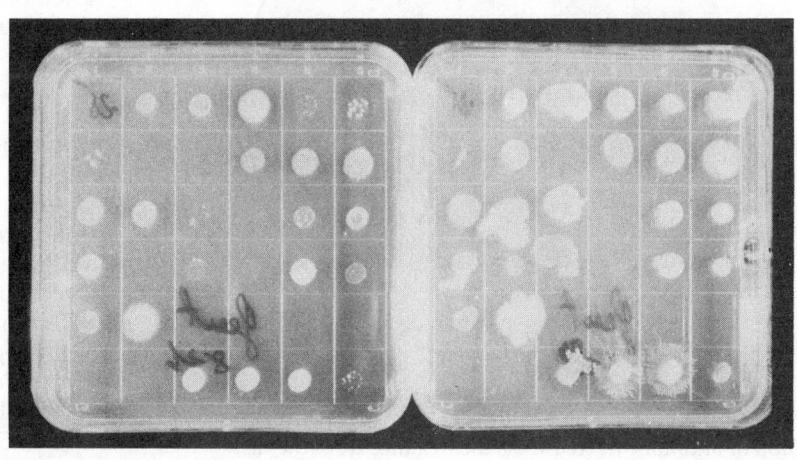

Figure 15-13
Agar dilution antimicrobial susceptibility
plates that have been inoculated with several
species of bacteria from a Steers replicator:
Sensitive organisms are inhibited by the concentration of antibiotic contained in the
plate, and no growth is evident at the points
of inoculation; resistant organisms appear as
distinct colonies of bacterial growth.

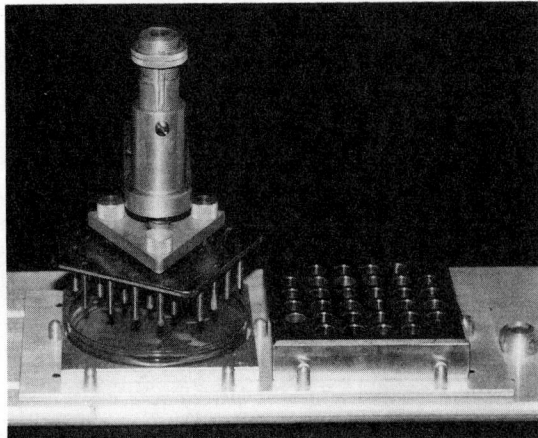

Figure 15-14
Steers replicator: The inoculating head and prongs are fixed. A sliding tray alternately positions a template containing the inoculum and an agar plate under the head. The parts can be disassembled for autoclaving.

The inability to produce quantitative results by the initial disk susceptibility test was considered a distinct disadvantage. A semiquantitative test that used high- and low-concentration disks was developed. Bacteria were considered resistant if they grew up to the margins of both disks, whereas sensitive organisms showed zones of inhibition around both disks. Isolates were considered of intermediate susceptibility if they were inhibited only by the disk that contained the higher concentration of antibiotic.

DEVELOPMENT OF A STANDARDIZED DISK DIFFUSION PROCEDURE

By the end of the 1950s, the status of antimicrobial susceptibility testing in microbiology laboratories throughout the world was in chaos, primarily because

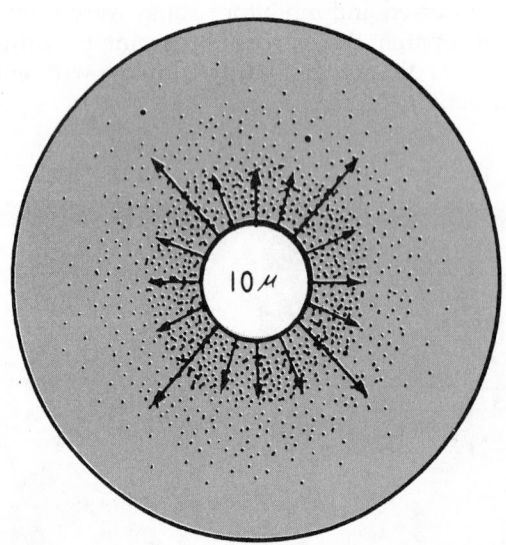

Figure 15-15
The principle of antibiotic diffusion in agar: The concentration of antibiotic decreases as the distance from the disk increases.

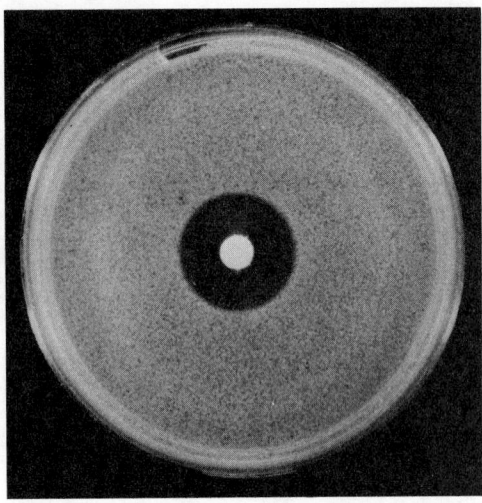

Figure 15-16
Disk antibiotic susceptibility plate showing the same principle as in Figure 15-15: At the area where the concentration of antibiotic is insufficient to prevent bacterial growth, a distinct margin can be seen.

of the lack of an acceptable standard procedure. The antibiotic concentrations in disks varied considerably, a wide variety of media was being employed, methods of inoculation differed from laboratory to laboratory, the length of incubation time was not uniform, and results were being interpreted by several criteria. A World Health Organization committee was formed to investigate this problem, and the deliberation of this committee provided the groundwork that led to the development of several standardized procedures.[294] The test that has become standard in the United States is based on the work of Bauer, Kirby, and coworkers.[14,15,182] The procedure for the disk diffusion test as recommended by the NCCLS is summarized in Chart 23.

If the test is properly performed, the edges of the inhibitory zones should be clear and easy to measure. Situations in which the technologist must learn to interpret unclear results correctly are listed in Box 15-3.

INTERPRETATION OF RESULTS

The zone size that is observed in a disk diffusion test has no meaning in and of itself. The interpretative standards provided by the NCCLS are derived from a correlation between zone sizes and MICs of those species that can be tested by the disk diffusion method. A prototype of a regression curve providing such a correlation is illustrated in Figure 15-21 (page 823). A large number of strains have been tested against a single antibiotic both by the disk diffusion technique and by a dilution method. Each triangle represents the results of both tests for a single strain. A regression line has been drawn through the many individual points. Once the regression line is established, an approximate MIC result can be inferred from any zone diameter. In this example, a zone size of 18 mm corresponds to an MIC of 6.25 μg/ml—the breakpoint of the broth dilution test illustrated in Figure 15-11.

BOX 15-3. CORRECTLY INTERPRETING ANTIBIOTICS: SPECIAL SITUATIONS

1. Motile organisms such as *Proteus mirabilis* or *P. vulgaris* may swarm when growing on agar surfaces, resulting in a thin veil that may penetrate into the zones of inhibition around antibiotic susceptibility disks (Fig. 15-17). This zone of swarming should be ignored; the outer margin, which is usually clearly outlined, should be measured. Similarly, with sulfonamide disks, growth may not be completely inhibited at the outer margin, resulting in a faint veil where 80% or more of the organisms are inhibited. Again, the outer margin of heavy growth inhibition should be used as the point of measurement.

2. The phenomenon shown in Figure 15-18 must be interpreted differently from that shown in Figure 15-17. Note that distinct colonies are present within the zone of inhibition. This does not represent swarming. Rather, these colonies are either mutants that are more resistant to the antibiotic than the major portion of the bacterial strain being tested or the culture is not pure and the separate colonies are of a different species. Isolation, identification, and susceptibility testing of the resistant colonies may be required to resolve this problem. If it is deter-

mined that the separate colonies represent a variant of a mutant strain, the bacterial species being tested must be considered resistant, even though a wide zone of inhibition may be present for the remainder of the growth.

3. Figure 15-19 demonstrates the difficulty in measuring one zone diameter when there is overlapping with adjacent antibiotic zones, or when the zone extends beyond the margin of the petri dish. Oval or elliptical zones may occur, and it is difficult to determine whether to measure the short or long diameters. Unless the zones are very wide and the organism being tested is obviously susceptible, the test must be repeated with more careful placement of the antibiotic disks so that overlapping will not occur.

4. Figure 15-20 illustrates a poorly prepared plate. The lines of streaking are irregular, leaving spaces between adjacent colonies. The margins of the zones are indistinct, making it difficult to pick the exact points at which to make the measurements. Readings should not be attempted on a poorly inoculated plate such as this, and the test should be repeated.

Thus, an antimicrobial agent that produces a zone diameter greater than 18 mm would theoretically have an MIC less than 6.25 µg/ml, and the organism would be considered susceptible; one producing a zone size less than 18 mm would, conversely, be considered resistant. In actual practice, regression curves are not that clearly defined, and a 2- to 4-mm zone may be established where it is not possible to determine whether the organism is susceptible or resistant (see Table 15-14). Isolates that produce an inhibitory zone in this range are characterized as intermediate in susceptibility. In studies conducted late in the 1950s, Bauer, Perry, and Kirby first demonstrated that bacterial strains tested against a given antibiotic tend to fall either into the resistant or the susceptible categories; only a small percentage (5% or less) fall into the intermediate range.[15] Thus, if a high percentage of intermediate re-

ports is issued by a certain laboratory, a re-examination of the procedure is indicated.

The interpretative guidelines for the disk diffusion test (see Table 15-14, page 817) permit the user to make approximations of the MIC for each of the antibiotics listed (last two columns) with zone diameters as determined by the disk diffusion technique. These correlates are not intended to match the breakpoints for susceptibility and resistance established for the dilution tests, but they do give the user an appreciation of the meaning of the report. For example, a microorganism showing an 11-mm zone of inhibition against ampicillin would be considered resistant at a level of greater than 32 µg/ml.

If the infection is in the lower urinary tract, however, very high concentrations of ampicillin are achieved, and the organism might be treatable even in the presence of an apparently resistant result. It may be

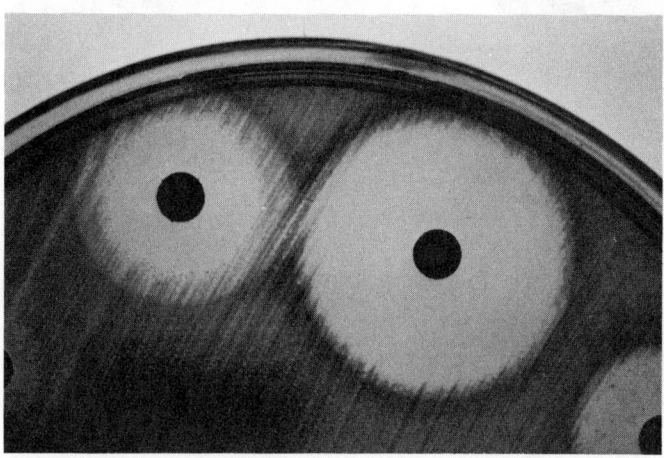

Figure 15-17
Photograph of an antibiotic susceptibility plate using a species of *Proteus* as the test organism: Note the swarming into the zone of inhibition at the peripheral margins. The second outer zone of growth inhibition should be used when measuring the width of the zone.

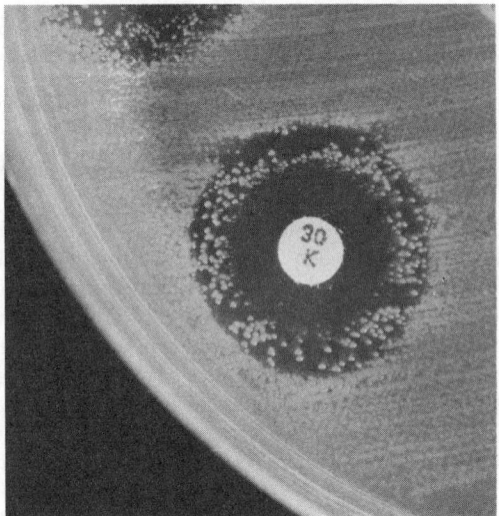

Figure 15-18
An antibiotic susceptibility plate in which colonies resistant to kanamycin are growing within the zone of inhibition: Biochemical tests must be performed to determine if the resistant strain is a mutant of the organisms being tested or represents a second species growing in mixed culture.

necessary to perform a dilution test to obtain a more precise result.

QUALITY CONTROL

Quality control should be performed each time a new lot of disks or agar is used. In the interim, controls should be tested each day the procedure is performed unless stringent criteria for weekly testing are met. The NCCLS has established limits on zone sizes that are acceptable for the quality control strains (Table 15-15, page 824); these limits provide a means by which to measure the accuracy of testing.

LIMITATIONS

The Bauer-Kirby test, as modified by the NCCLS, has been accepted as the standard technique for performing disk diffusion susceptibility tests, giving useful information in most instances. There are, however,

a few distinct limitations. The test should only be applied to bacterial species that have been thoroughly evaluated. Bacteria that grow slowly, need special nutrients, or require CO_2 or anaerobic conditions for growth should not be tested, unless the validity of the procedure has been documented.[120]

MICRODILUTION BROTH SUSCEPTIBILITY TEST

Concurrent with the development of a usable disk diffusion test, other investigators have attempted to simplify the broth dilution test. The microtube dilution procedure is similar in principle to the macrotube method, except that the susceptibility of microorganisms to antibiotics is determined in a series of microtube wells that are molded into a plastic plate. Each plate may contain 80, 96, or more wells, depending on the number and concentration of antibiotics that are to be included in the susceptibility test panel.

The advantages of the microtube method are that small volumes of reagents are used and that large numbers of bacteria can be tested simply and inexpensively against a panel of antibiotics. The intensive labor involved in preparing the multi-well plates has been a major impediment to their routine use.

A major advance in microbroth dilution testing was the development of instruments that dispensed replicate aliquots from tubes in which large volumes of antibiotic had been prepared. The precision of dilution in large volumes was combined with the ease of testing in microtiter plates. The Autospense (Sandy Springs Technologies, Inc, Gaithersburg, MD) (formerly Quickspense) instrument is commercially available and is employed in some hospital laboratories. If the resources are available, local production of plates allows the use of a tailored panel of antibiotics; users can change the panel at will. In Figure 15-22 (page 825), an early version of the Quickspense instrument is demonstrated. Dilutions are prepared in large volumes, after which the fluid is dispensed mechanically into the microtiter trays. After preparation of the dilutions is complete, antibiotic solutions can be dispensed into a large number of plates quickly. Such instruments combine the accuracy of preparing dilutions in large volumes with the convenience and economy of microtiter systems.

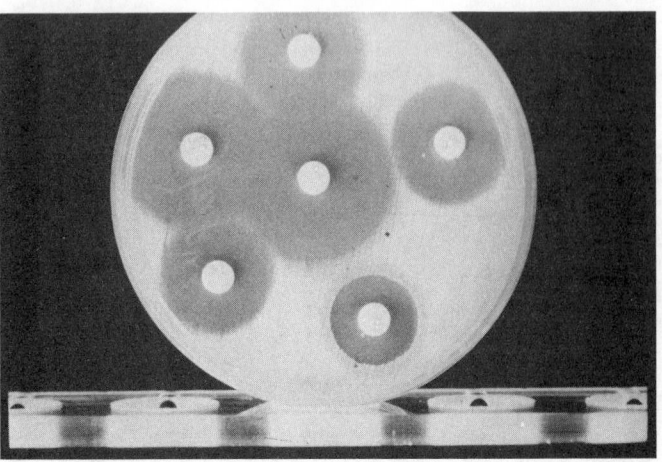

Figure 15-19
A poorly prepared antibiotic susceptibility plate showing objectionable overlapping of the zones of growth inhibition from adjacent disks.

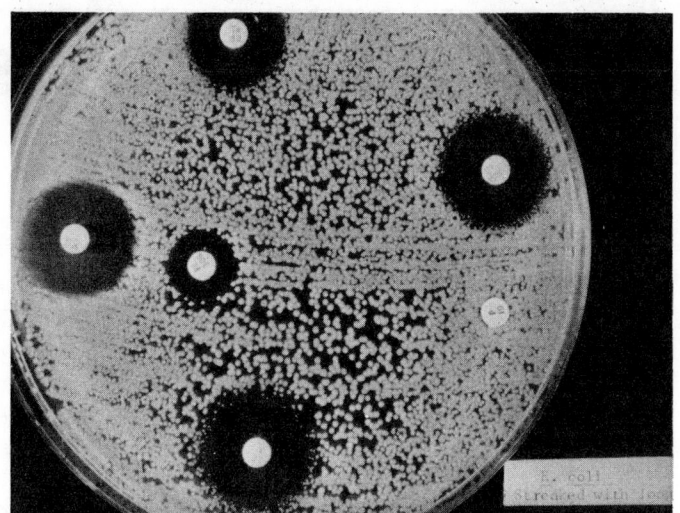

Figure 15-20
A poorly streaked antimicrobial susceptibility plate showing uneven growth: The zone margins are indistinct, compromising accurate measurement.

The antibiotic-containing plates must be frozen at −20°C or lower until used. Frozen prepared plates can be obtained from several commercial sources. Storage of large numbers of frozen microplates may be difficult in some laboratories. In this case, plates that contain lyophilized antibiotic solutions—the laboratory equivalent of instant coffee—may be purchased. Rehydration of the wells adds another step to the procedure, but the extended shelf-life of the freeze-dried plates is valuable, especially for laboratories in which small numbers of tests are performed. Both the frozen and lyophilized broth dilution systems have performed well in comparison to the reference methods.[41,82,84,210,235] As might be expected, the interlaboratory reproducibility of the commercial systems that use standardized batches of very large volume has been greater than that for homemade plates, even when the plates were prepared for investigational use.[82] Some of the commercial systems have not performed well in certain special situations, as discussed later.

The procedure for the microdilution broth test as recommended by the NCCLS is summarized in Chart 59. The interpretative guidelines suggested by the NCCLS, which should be reported along with or in place of the actual MIC values, are listed in Table 15-13. Separate guidelines for interpreting *Haemophilus* species, *Streptococcus pneumoniae*, and *Neisseria gonorrhoeae* have been published by the NCCLS. The guidelines for quality control are similar to those for the disk diffusion test (see Table 15-16, page 826).

End points are usually easily defined (Fig. 15-23). Examination of the microplates is facilitated by use of a viewing mirror (Fig. 15-24, page 827). Occasionally, growth may be inhibited in a well that is adjacent to wells with uninhibited growth (skipped well). If a single well is skipped and the interpretation of the result is not affected, the skipped well may be ignored. If multiple wells are skipped, if the skipped well occurs at a dilution that is critical for determining susceptibility of the isolate, or if multiple isolates demonstrate the

Figure 15-21
Prototype regression curve comparing MICs in micrograms per milliliter with zone size in millimeters: Each *triangle* represents the MIC (vertical axis) and inhibitory zone (horizontal axis) of a single isolate. A zone diameter of 18 mm corresponds with the MIC breakpoint of 6.25 μg/mL, a correlation that, theoretically, could be made for the test illustrated in Figures 15-11 and 15-12.

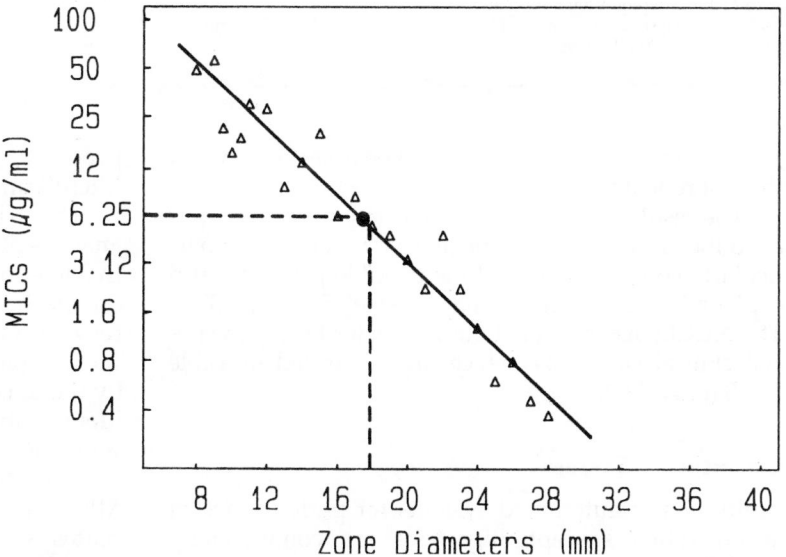

TABLE 15-15
CONTROL LIMITS FOR MONITORING ANTIMICROBIAL DISK SUSCEPTIBILITY TESTS; ZONE DIAMETER (mm) LIMITS FOR INDIVIDUAL TESTS ON MUELLER–HINTON MEDIUM WITHOUT BLOOD OR OTHER SUPPLEMENTS

ANTIMICROBIAL AGENT	DISK CONTENT	ESCHERICHIA COLI ATCC[b] 25922	STAPHYLOCOCCUS AUREUS ATCC 25923	PSEUDOMONAS AERUGINOSA ATCC 27853	ESCHERICHIA COLI ATCC 35218
Amikacin	30 µg	19–26	20–26	18–26	—
Amoxicillin/clavulanic acid	20/10 µg	19–25	28–36	—	18–22
Ampicillin	10 µg	16–22	27–35	—	—
Ampicillin/sulbactam	10/10 µg	20–24	29–37	—	13–19
Azithromycin	15 µg	—	21–26	—	—
Azilocillin	75 µg	—	—	24–30	—
Aztreonam	30 µg	28–36	—	23–29	—
Teicoplanin	30 µg		15–21	—	—
Tetracycline	30 µg	1–25	**24–30**	—	—
Ticarcillin	75 µg	24–30	—	22–28	—
Ticarcillin/clavulanic acid	75/10 µg	25–29	**29–37**	20–28	21–25
Tobramycin	10 µg	18–26	19–29	19–25	—
Trimethoprim	5 µg	21–28	19–26	—	—
Trimethoprim/sulfamethoxazole	1.25/23.75 µg	24–32	24–32	—	—
Trospectomycin	30 µg	10–16	15–20	—	—
Vancomycin	30 µg	—	**17–21**	—	—

NOTE 1: To determine whether the Mueller–Hinton medium has sufficiently low levels of thymidine and thymine, an *Enterococcus faecalis* (ATCC 29212 or 33186) may be tested with trimethoprim/sulfamethoxazole disks. An inhibition zone of ≥20 mm that is essentially free of fine colonies indicates a sufficiently low level of thymine and thymidine.
NOTE 2: Information in boldface type is considered tentative for 1 year.
[a] For control limits of gentamicin 120-µg and streptomycin 300-µg disks, use *E. faecalis* ATCC 29212 (gentamicin: 16 to 22 mm; streptomycin: 14 to 19 mm).
[b] ATCC is a registered trademark of the American Type Culture Collection.
NCCLS Vol. 15, No. 14, 1995.

phenomenon, the problem should be investigated and the test repeated.

The results of quality control testing may give clues as to the nature of the problem. Certain errors are particularly common. Some of the possible problems and explanations are summarized in Table 15-1 (page 828). The NCCLS has provided guidelines for testing in special clinical situations, which are illustrated in Table 15-18 (page 829).

COMMERCIAL SYSTEMS

Multiple semiautomated systems for performance of antimicrobial susceptibility tests are commercially available. The largest market share belongs to two products, Vitek (bioMérieux, Hazelwood, MO) and MicroScan (Dade International, West Sacramento, CA).

The Vitek instrument uses a computer-assisted analysis of growth in plastic cards to calculate an MIC. In some instances the calculation of the MIC depends on the bacterial identification. The additional accuracy provided by the computer-driven correlation of growth pattern and identification is counterbalanced by the uncertainty about the susceptibility result if the identification is not yet known or cannot be provided with adequate certainty by the system.

The MicroScan products are based on traditional MIC methodology. The line runs the gamut from plates—either frozen or lyophilized—that are interpreted manually to a semiautomated instrument, the

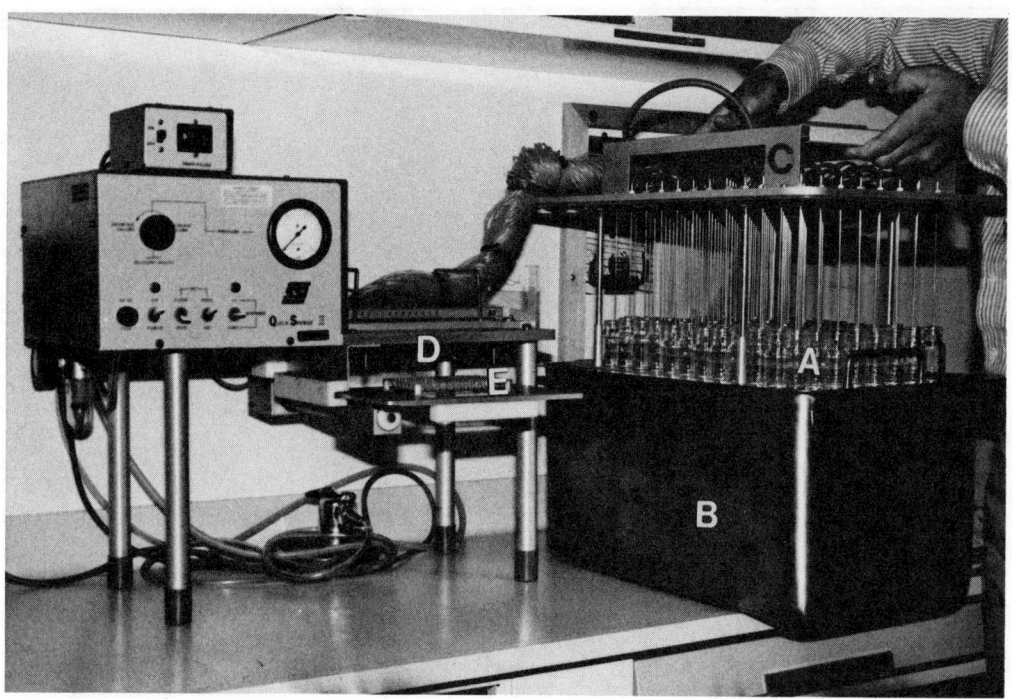

Figure 15-22
Quickspense instrument for dispensing fluid into microtiter plates: Dilutions of antibiotics are prepared in large volumes, using a set of 96 calibrated macrotubes (*A*). The tubes are placed in an air-tight dispensing chamber (*B*), the top of which contains a cannula for each macrotube (*C*). These cannulae are connected by plastic tubing to a set of 96 needles (*D*), through which antibiotic solutions are dropped into a microtiter plate (*E*). A measured volume is dispensed by introduction of pressure into the dispensing chamber.

"Walkaway." Biochemical reagents for bacterial identification are incorporated into the same microtiter plates. Traditional overnight incubation is used for most of the MicroScan products. The Walkaway system, however, incorporates a fluorescent detection system that will provide same-day identification and susceptibility testing for some organisms. A variety of other semi-automated systems is available, as well as several choices for purchase of commercially prepared microdilution plates, either frozen or lyophilized. In general the systems work well. In a recent evaluation of commonly isolated bacteria there were only 0.4% very major error rates with both MicroScan Walkaway and Vitek.[276] There were fewer than 5% minor errors with both systems. Current problems with both of these systems are discussed later.

Certain combinations of drug and bacterial species present difficulties for the instruments, and the laboratory must make other arrangements for testing these combinations. At one point difficulties in detecting resistance of *Staphylococcus aureus* to oxacillin were of great concern, but these methodologic problems seem to have been largely overcome by the major manufacturers. Discrepancies in results derived from automated instruments that are programmed to evaluate early phases of bacterial growth and those derived from the conventional 18-hour disk diffusion procedure may be encountered for *Escherichia coli* and *Klebsiella pneumoniae* against ampicillin and cephalothin. Presumably the longer incubation of the disk diffusion procedure is required to allow antibiotic action against these organisms and to avoid the falsely "sensitive" readings obtained from the rapid automated instruments. Problems in recognition of aminoglycoside-resistant enterococci have been encountered with several systems, but the companies have worked diligently to correct them. The current important "holes" in these systems are detection of pneumococcal resistance to β-lactam antibiotics, enterococcal resistance to vancomycin, and recognition of isolates that produce extended-spectrum β-lactamases, as discussed later. An optional software addition to the Vitek system provides useful assistance in recognition of potential producers of extended-spectrum β-lactamases. The major commercial suppliers of susceptibility testing equipment are constantly upgrading and improving procedures, reagents, and software. The analysis of advantages and problems is, therefore, very much a moving target. The reader who anticipates an equipment purchase is advised to consult with other users of the equipment who are respected in the local or national microbiology community.

Quality control of the automated results has been difficult and largely unsatisfactory. For most drug-organism combinations, the standard control strains

TABLE 15-16

ACCEPTABLE QUALITY CONTROL RANGES OF MINIMUM INHIBITORY CONCENTRATIONS (MICs; µg/mL) FOR REFERENCE STRAINS

ANTIMICROBIAL AGENT	STAPHYLOCOCCUS AUREUS ATCC[d] 29213	ENTEROCOCCUS FAECALIS ATCC 29212	ESCHERICHIA COLI ATCC 25922	PSEUDOMONAS AERUGINOSA ATCC 27853	ESCHERICHIA COLI ATCC 35218
Amikacin	1–4	64–256	0.5–4	1–4	—
Amoxicillin/clavulanic acid	0.12/0.06–0.5/0.25	0.25/0.12–1.0/0.5	2/1–8/4	—	4/2–16/8
Ampicillin	0.25–1	0.5–2	2–8	—	—
Ampicillin/sulbactam	—	—	1/0.5–4/2	—	4/2–16/8
Azithromycin	**0.5–2.0**	—	—	—	—
Azlocillin	2–8	1–4	8–32	2–8	—
Aztreonam	—	—	0.06–0.25	2–8	—
Sulfisoxazole[b]	32–128	32–128	8–32	—	—
Teicoplanin	0.25–1	0.06–0.5	—	—	—
Tetracycline	0.25–1	8–32	1–4	8–32	—
Ticarcillin	2–8	16–64	2–8	8–32	—
Ticarcillin/clavulanic acid	0.5/2–2/2	16/2–64/2	2/2–8/2	8/2–32/2	4/2–16/2
Tobramycin	0.12–1	8–32	0.25–1	0.25–1	—
Trimethoprim[b]	1–4	≤1	0.5–2	>64	—
Trimethoprim/ sulfimethoxazole (1/19)[b]	≤0.5/9.5	≤0.5/9.5	≤0.5/9.5	8/152–32/608	—
Trospectomycin	2–16	2–8	8–32	—	—
Vancomycin[c]	0.5–2	1–4	—	—	—

NOTE 1: These MICs were obtained in several reference laboratories by broth microdilution. If four or fewer concentrations are tested, quality control may be more difficult.
NOTE 2: Information in boldface type is considered tentative for 1 year.
[a] For control organisms for gentamicin and streptomycin high-level aminoglycoside screen tests for enterococci, see Table 7.
[b] Very medium-dependent, especially with enterococci.
[c] For control organisms for vancomycin screen test for enterococci, see Table 7.
[d] ATCC is a registered trademark of the American Type Culture Collection.
[e] A bimodal distribution of MICs; results at the extremes of the acceptable range should be suspect. Verify control validity with data from other control strains.
NCCLS Vol. 15, No. 14, 1995.

produce results that are at the extremes of the parameter measured and cannot be quantitated precisely.[130]

EPSILOMETER TEST (E-TEST, AB BIODISK, SWEDEN)

A recent addition to the diagnostic armamentarium is the E-test, which consists of antibiotic-impregnated strips that are placed on the surface of agar. The principle is an expansion of the disk diffusion method, and the protocol for preparing the inoculum is the same. The antibiotic content of the strips is graded, and the concentration is printed linearly along the strip (Fig. 15-25, page 830). After incubation the MIC is read from the point on the strip where the zone of growth inhibition passes. In contrast to the disk diffusion test, where the orientation of the disks does not matter, placing the E-test strips upside down on the agar will alter the results.[97] The same factors that influence the disk diffu-

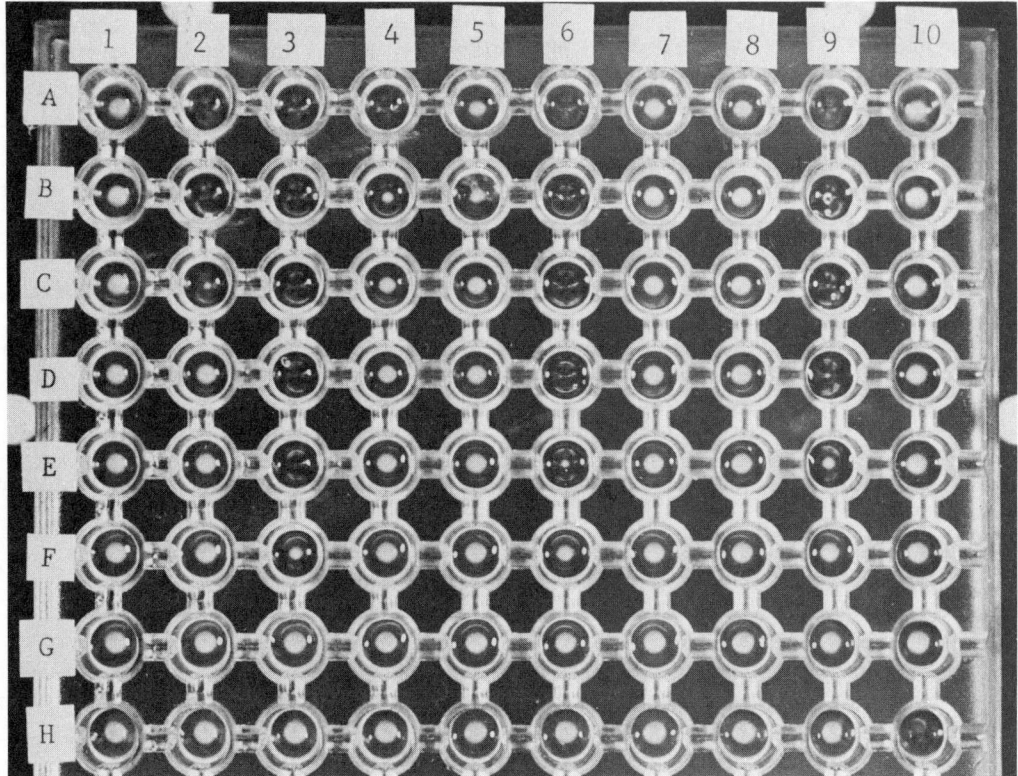

Figure 15-23
Microtube broth dilution antibiotic susceptibility plate: The *numbers* across the top indicate the different antibiotics being tested within each vertical column; the *letters* along the left border reflect the concentration of antibiotics contained within each well. The appearance of a button of bacterial growth in any well indicates resistance to that concentration of antibiotic.

sion susceptibility test apply to its stepchild, the E-test. Diffusion of antibiotics begins immediately after placement of the strip, which cannot, therefore, be moved once it has touched the agar. A poorly streaked plate may produce an irregular zone of inhibition at the MIC point. Swarming of *Proteus* spp. and mutant colonies within the zone of inhibition may be challenges with the E-test, as with disk diffusion.

The E-test has proven to be effective for general use,[9] and a variety of special situations: *Pseudomonas aeruginosa*,[128] *Pseudomonas aeruginosa* strains from cystic fibrosis patients,[157] *Stenotrophomonas maltophilia*,[110] *Campylobacter jejuni* (discrepancies with clindamycin, trimethoprim-sulfamethoxazole, and tetracycline),[110] *Helicobacter pylori*,[87] *Neisseria gonorrhoeae*,[274] coryneform bacteria,[158] nutritionally-deficient streptococci,[55] methicillin resistant staphylococci (with addition of 2% NaCl to agar)[110] and high-level aminoglycoside resistance in enterococci.[230] Tenover and colleagues found the E-test reliable for detection of vancomycin resistance in enterococci.[260] In contrast, the MICs of pneumococcus to vancomycin by E-test tend to be higher than microbroth dilution tests, producing results that are at the upper range of susceptible isolates, with quality control results above acceptable limits.[101]

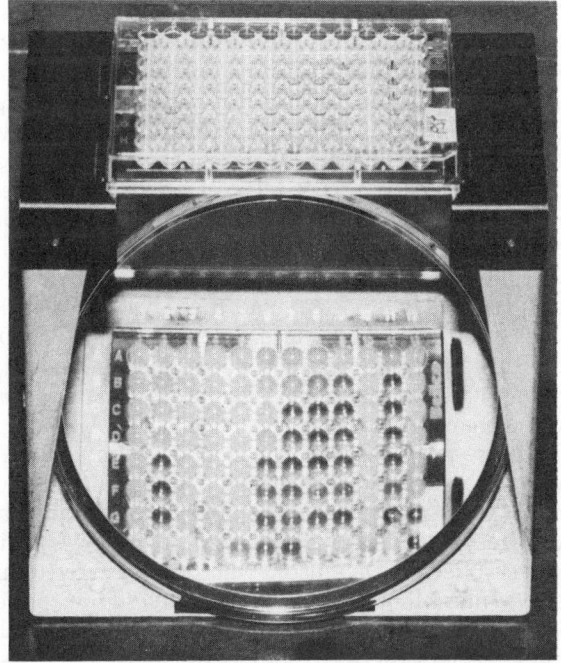

Figure 15-24
Viewing mirror for visualization of bacterial growth in broth microdilution test.

TABLE 15-17
TROUBLE-SHOOTING QUALITY CONTROL PROBLEMS IN SUSCEPTIBILITY TESTS

OBSERVATION	DIAGNOSIS	CORRECTIVE ACTION
MICs too large or zone sizes too small (isolates too resistant)	1. Inoculum too high 2. Deterioration of antibiotic 3. Change in QC* strain 4. Agar too deep 5. Incorrect reading of results	1. Check and adjust inoculum if necessary 2. Check potency of disks or powder; try new lot 3. Test new stock of QC strain 4. Check depth of agar 5. Repeat with multiple observers
MICs too small or zone sizes too large (isolates too susceptible)	1. Inoculum too low 2. Antibiotic too potent 3. Change in QC strain 4. Agar too thin 5. Incorrect reading of results	1. Check and adjust inoculum if necessary 2. Check potency of disks or powder; try new lot 3. Test new stock of QC strain 4. Check depth of agar 5. Repeat with multiple observers
Results for *Pseudomonas* and aminoglycosides out of control	1. Cation content incorrect	1. Use cation-supplemented broth or try different lot of agar
Results for *Pseudomonas* and carbenicillin out of control	1. Mutation of QC strain	1. Test new stock of QC strain
Aminoglycosides and macrolides too resistant; tetracycline too susceptible	1. Medium too acid	1. Check pH of media
Aminoglycosides and macrolides too susceptible; tetracycline too resistant	1. Medium too alkaline	1. Check pH of media
Trimethoprim MICs too large or zone sizes too small; results difficult to read	1. Excess thymidine in medium	1. Test medium with *Streptococcus faecalis* (ATCC 29212 or 33186); add thymidine phosphorylase or lysed horse blood

* QC, quality control.

SPECIAL ISSUES IN SUSCEPTIBILITY TESTING

β-LACTAMASES

β-Lactamases are heterogeneous bacterial enzymes that cleave the β-lactam ring of penicillins and cephalosporins to inactivate the antibiotic. β-Lactamases are found in a wide variety of gram-positive and gram-negative bacterial species. The enzymes produced by *Staphylococcus* species, *Haemophilus* species, *Moraxella (Branhamella) catarrhalis,* and *Neisseria gonorrhoeae* have been clinically most important. The significance of the conventional enzymes produced by many enteric bacteria is less clear, and these bacteria should not be tested for β-lactamase. The appearance of extended-spectrum β-lactamases in enteric bacteria, however, has focused increased attention on this resistance mechanism.

The presence of β-lactamases may be detected quickly, providing an early clue that an isolate will not respond to the β-lactam antibiotics in question. The chromogenic cephalosporin test, employing Nitrocefin (Cefinase, Becton-Dickinson Microbiology Systems, Cockeysville, MD), is the most sensitive. Filter-paper disks impregnated with Nitrocefin are commercially available. A loopful of a colony is smeared on the disk and placed in a closed Petri dish to prevent rapid desiccation. Organisms that contain β-lactamase will change the color of the disk from yellow to red. The re-

action usually occurs within 30 seconds, but tests are read finally after 15 minutes. A new chromogenic cephalosporin, S1 (International BioClinical, Inc., Portland, OR), performs in a very similar manner to Nitrocefin. In a multilaboratory study, the major difference between the two was greater sensitivity of S1 for the β-lactamase of *Bacteroides fragilis* in some of the participating laboratories.[49]

Acidometric tests are less expensive to perform but are less sensitive than the Nitrocefin assay. Opening of the β-lactam ring produces penicilloic acid, which is more acid than penicillin. The change in pH is detected by visual observation of an indicator dye, phenol red. A suspension of phenol red and penicillin G is adjusted with NaOH to pH 8.5 (the point at which the color changes to purple) and stored at −20°C for up to 1 week.[6] At the time of testing, a capillary tube is dipped into the phenol red solution until 1 cm of the tube is filled. The filled end of the tube is scraped across a bacterial colony to plug the tube, then incubated at room temperature for 60 minutes. A change in the phenol red indicator to yellow indicates the presence of β-lactamase.

In every case the Nitrocefin test has been the most sensitive and most specific method for measuring β-lactamases. It must be used when testing *Moraxella (Branhamella) catarrhalis.* There is little reason to use one of the other methods when the Nitrocefin test serves all purposes.

TABLE 15-18
MODIFICATIONS OF STANDARD METHODS FOR SPECIAL SITUATIONS

ORGANISM	METHOD	MEDIUM	INCUBATION	COMMENTS
Enterococcus spp.	Broth microdilution	Cation-supplemented Mueller–Hinton broth (CSMHB)	35°C; 16–24 h	Perform β-lactamase test; incubate plates 24 h for vancomycin
	Agar screen for high-level aminoglycoside resistance	Brain–heart infusion (BHI) agar + 500 μg/mL gentamicin or 2000 μg/mL streptomycin	35°C; 24–48 h	Incubate negative streptomycin screens for 48 h
	Broth screen for high-level aminoglycoside resistance	BHI broth + 500 μg gentamicin or 1000 μg streptomycin	35°C; 24–48 h	Incubate negative streptomycin screens for 48 h
	Agar screen for vancomycin resistance	BHI agar + 6 μg/mL vancomycin	35°C; 24 h	Growth of single colony indicates resistance
Penicillinase-resistant-penicillin (PRP) *Staphylococcus* spp.	Broth microdilution	CSMHB + 2% NaCl	30°–35°C; 24 h	Test only oxacillin; report result for all β-lactams
	Agar screen	Mueller–Hinton agar + 2% NaCl	30°–35°C; 24 h	Test only oxacillin; report result for all β-lactams; incubation may need to be extended to 48 h for coagulase-negative staphylococci
Haemophilus spp.	Broth microdilution	*Haemophilus* test medium or CSMHB with supplements	35°C; 20–24 h	Final volume of broth in wells should be 100 μL
	E-test	*Haemophilus* test medium or CSMHB with supplements	35°C; 20–24 h	
Streptococcus pneumoniae	Broth microdilution	CSMHB + 2–5% lysed horse blood	35°C; 20–24 h	Final volume of broth in wells should be 100 μL
	E-test	Mueller–Hinton agar with 5% sheep blood	35°C; 20–24 h; 5–7% CO_2 if necessary	Use horse blood when testing sulfonamides
Other streptococci	Broth microdilution	CSMHB + 2–5% lysed horse blood	35°C; 20–24 h	
	Agar dilution or E-test	Mueller–Hinton agar with 5% sheep blood	35°C; 20–24 h; 5–7% CO_2 if necessary	
Neisseria gonorrhoeae	Agar dilution	GC agar with supplements	35°C; 20–24 h; 5–7% CO_2	
Neisseria meningitidis	Broth microdilution	CSMHB	35°C; 24 h; 5–7% CO_2	
	Agar dilution	Mueller–Hinton agar	35°C; 24 h; 5–7% CO_2	

Adapted from Reference 183.

STAPHYLOCOCCUS SPECIES

The β-lactamases of staphylococci are induced by exposure to penicillins. They are responsible for most of the resistance to penicillin G and related compounds but are not active against the cephalosporins or the penicillinase-resistant penicillins, such as methicillin and nafcillin, unless produced in large amounts. De-tection of these enzymes is particularly difficult with the microbroth dilution test, because the bacteria in the relatively small inoculum used in this test may be killed before the enzyme is induced.

If the MIC of a staphylococcal strain to penicillin is greater than 0.25 μg/ml, the presence of a β-lactamase can be inferred. Isolates with penicillin MICs less than

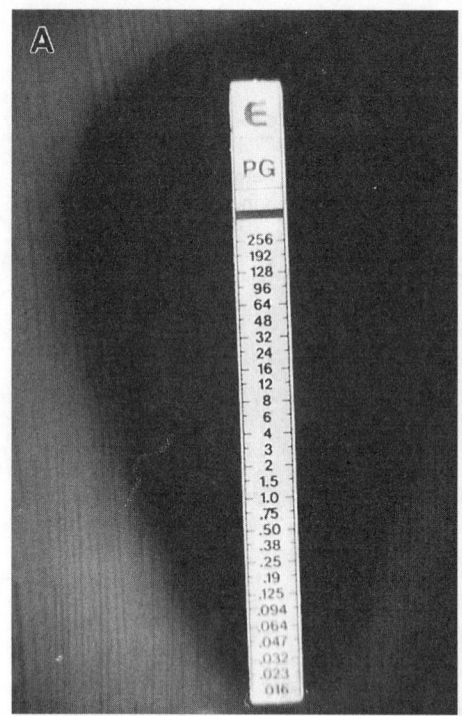
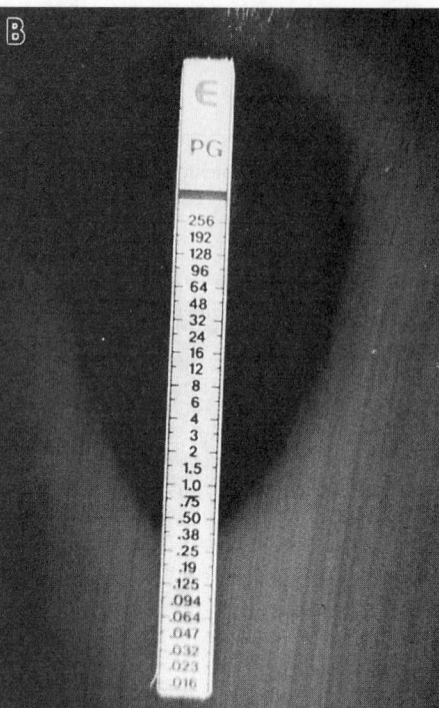

Figure 15-25
E-test for *Streptococcus pneumoniae* on Mueller–Hinton agar with blood: The plates have been prepared as for the disk diffusion test, after which the test strips have been applied. The MIC of the isolate is read where the line of growth inhibition crosses the strip. Panel **A** demonstrates a fully susceptible strain with an MIC of 0.016 µg/mL. Panel **B** demonstrates a strain with intermediate susceptibility and an MIC of 0.38 µg/mL.

0.03 µg/ml are considered non-producers and susceptible. Isolates for which the MIC falls between these limits (0.06 or 0.12 µg/ml) should be tested for the presence of β-lactamase before the results are reported. Use of bacterial growth from a well that contains a penicillin-class drug or from the edge of a zone of inhibition around a disk that contains a penicillin compound may induce activity and enhance detection of the enzyme. The results from the testing of penicillin can be extrapolated to ampicillin.

HAEMOPHILUS SPECIES

As many as 20% to 40% of type B *Haemophilus influenzae* isolates from serious infections produce β-lactamases.[50] Detection of the enzymes should be performed on any isolate that is considered a pathogen. A few strains have demonstrated resistance to ampicillin by other mechanisms, so a non-enzyme-producing strain should also be tested against ampicillin by a diffusion or dilution susceptibility test, at least for isolates from sterile sites.[17]

NEISSERIA GONORRHOEAE

Penicillinase-producing gonococci were detected initially in the Far East but are now widely distributed. All isolates should be tested for β-lactamase. As with *Haemophilus* species, some strains that are resistant to penicillin by nonenzymatic means have now been identified,[221] so that a susceptibility test should also be performed if the treatment fails.

MORAXELLA (BRANHAMELLA) CATARRHALIS

Moraxella (Branhamella) catarrhalis has been recognized in recent years as an important cause of upper respiratory tract infection and of nosocomial lower respiratory tract infection. Most strains produce β-lactamases, which are of two types. The most common enzyme (Ravasio type) is chromosomal, constitutive, tightly cell associated, and inhibited by β-lactamase inhibitors such as clavulanate and sulbactam.[46,66] A second, less common enzyme (1908 type) differs in several important respects. It is produced in 10- to 100-fold lower amounts than the Ravasio type. As a result, the quantitative susceptibility result may be in the susceptible range in the presence of a positive β-lactamase test. In the absence of good clinical data, these strains should probably be considered resistant. There is little reason to perform any test routinely other than β-lactamase on *Moraxella (Branhamella) catarrhalis* because the susceptibility of the organism to other antibiotics is predictable.[53] Doern and colleagues found that the Nitrocefin tube or disk test was the most effective means of detecting β-lactamase.[52] The subject has been reviewed by Doern and Jones.[48]

ENTEROCOCCUS SPECIES

Isolates of enterococci that produce β-lactamase have been identified.[179,201,203] This high-level resistance to penicillin can be detected by the Nitrocefin test. The β-lactamase, which resembles that of staphylococci, is carried on a plasmid,[180] but the enterococcal and staphylococcal plasmids themselves are not homologous.[277] Strains of *Enterococcus faecalis* that produce β-lactamase and also exhibit high-level resistance to aminoglycosides have become epidemic in some institutions.[288] If the Nitrocefin disk test is not performed on isolates, resistance to β-lactam antibiotics may not be recognized. In a survey of New Jersey laboratories by Tenover and colleagues a β-lactamase producing strain of *E. faecalis* was recognized as resistant to penicillin by only 66% of 76 participants and to ampicillin by a startling 8% of laboratories. Only three of the 76 laboratories recognized that the strain produced β-lactamase, emphasizing the importance of performing a β-lactamase test on enterococci, especially if they have been isolated from sterile sites.[261] A combination of piperacillin and tazobactam is effective against β-lactamase producing enterococci,[195] and it is possible that this combination will provide synergy with aminoglycosides for such strains.

EXTENDED-SPECTRUM β-LACTAMASES

During the early 1980s strains of *Klebsiella* spp. with reduced susceptibility to third-generation cephalosporins were noted in Europe. Resistance was mediated by new β-lactamases on plasmids that were soon passed on to *E. coli*. The new enzymes were derived from existing Class A plasmid β-lactamases in gram-negative bacteria, such as TEM-1 and SHV-1. There is now such a variety of enzymes with varying specificities that is impossible to make absolute statements about which antibiotics are affected and which are resistant. The most common enzymes in clinical isolates of *Klebsiella pneumoniae*, *Klebsiella oxytoca*, and *Escherichia coli* provide a high degree of resistance to ampicillin, piperacillin, ticarcillin, and cephalothin with reduced susceptibility to aztreonam and the third-generation cephalosporins, such as cefotaxime, ceftriaxone, and ceftazidime. For this reason they were named extended broad-spectrum (or extended-spectrum) β-lactamases.[118] The cephamycins, such as cefoxitin, cefotetan, and moxalactam, and the carbapenems, such as imipenem, are not affected. Synergy of β-lactams and clavulanate or sulbactam vary with the specific enzyme, but cannot be depended upon therapeutically for all strains. Extended-spectrum enzymes have derived from chromosomes as well as plasmids.[216] These resistant strains have become established in many hospitals, producing epidemic disease, especially in intensive care units. Risk factors for acquisition of strains in a French hospital were frequency of invasive procedures and length of stay in the hospital.[153] Colonization was a prerequisite for invasive infection. In other situations extensive use of third-generation cephalosporins, sometimes used appropriately for treatment of severe infections caused by bacteria resistant to other antibiotics, has led to the emergence of strains that produce the extended-spectrum enzymes.[173] The spread of infection can be reduced by implementation of standard infection control measures and restriction of the use of third-generation cephalosporins,[173] but the strains may later reappear.[223]

The producers of extended-spectrum β-lactamases demonstrate increasing resistance to third-generation cephalosporins with increasing bacterial inoculum (inoculum effect),[117] which is probably caused by the inability of the antibiotics to kill the bacteria as well as inhibit them.[173] The cephamycins, which often appear susceptible *in vitro*, also fail to exert bactericidal activity,[173] and the place of these antibiotics in therapy is unclear. Imipenem, which has bacteristatic and bactericidal activity, appears effective *in vitro* and is therapeutically active against strains that do not have other

mechanisms for resistance. When rats were infected experimentally with a strain of *Klebsiella pneumoniae* that produced a TEM-26 β-lactamase, the combinations of ampicillin-sulbactam and piperacillin-tazobactam were effective in reducing bacterial colony counts in intra-abdominal abscesses, but imipenem provided the most effective therapy.[222]

In addition to their broad spectrum of activity against antimicrobial agents, the extended-spectrum β-lactamase producers present an additional challenge, because current tests for antimicrobial susceptibility do not detect resistance to some antibiotics.[129] Ceftazidime is the best sentinel antibiotic for suspecting resistance, and this antibiotic may be the only one for which the decreased resistance actually reaches the breakpoint for interpretation of resistance in any of the commonly used testing systems.[129] Recognition of an epidemic of infection caused by extended-spectrum β-lactamases was delayed because disk diffusion susceptibility tests produced false reports of susceptibility.[173]

The presence of extended-spectrum β-lactamases can be suspected if an isolate of *Klebsiella pneumoniae* or *Escherichia coli* demonstrates resistance to ceftazidime, but susceptibility to other third-generation cephalosporins. Unfortunately some strains appear susceptible even to ceftazidime.[129] The enzymes are carried on plasmids that often mediate resistance to other antibiotics, such as aminoglycosides, tetracycline, and sulfonamides, so the appearance of unusual resistance patterns can also serve as a clue that the extended-spectrum enzymes are present.[68,129] Several methods have been suggested to augment the detection of this resistance mechanism. A double-disk synergy test with disks of cetotaxime and Augmentin placed 30 mm apart from center to center was effective at detecting resistance mediated by EBS-Bla type enzymes.[118] Thomson and Sanders evaluated two methods for detecting resistance.[263] A double disk test was performed with ampicillin-clavulanate disks surrounded by aztreonam and third-generation cephalosporin disks (separated by 30 mm center-to-center). Distortion of the zone sizes in a synergistic fashion (Fig. 15-26C) indicated production of enzyme. This method detected true resistance in 22 of 28 strains (79%). The second method was a three-dimensional test in which a circular hole in the agar was cut just inside the eventual position of antimicrobial disks. The hole was filled with bacterial inoculum. Otherwise the procedure followed the standard disk diffusion protocol. Distortion of the zone sizes at the point of the cut in the agar indicated the presence of enzyme. The three-dimensional test detected resistance in 26 of 28 isolates (93%), but the technique and interpretation are exacting.

OXACILLIN- AND VANCOMYCIN-RESISTANT STAPHYLOCOCCUS SPECIES

The resistance of *S. aureus* and *S. epidermidis* to penicillinase-resistant penicillins is particularly difficult to detect in the laboratory. These species are heteroresistant; that is, only a small fraction of the bacteria in a culture express resistance, a characteristic that is chromosomally mediated. Binding of methicillin to peni-

A AUTONOMY

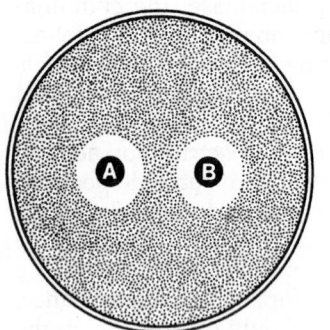

B ANTAGONISM

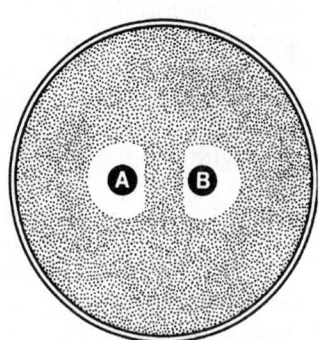

C SYNERGISM

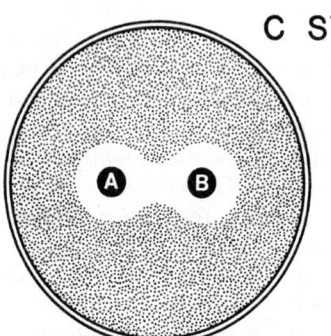
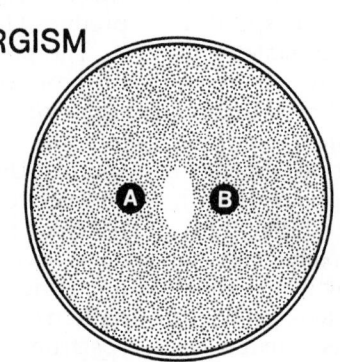

Figure 15-26
Diagram of potential interactions in disk diffusion test for bacterial synergy: Disks containing antibiotics *A* and *B* have been placed on Mueller–Hinton agar plates that have been inoculated with a bacterial isolate. Part **A** demonstrates additive or indifferent effects; each antibiotic produces a zone of inhibition that is not affected by the adjacent antibiotic. Part **B** demonstrates antagonistic effects, in which the inhibitory zones of each antibiotic are diminished in the presence of the other antibiotic. Part **C** demonstrates two possible manifestations of the synergistic interactions. On the *left*, an enlarged inhibitory zone occurs where the two antibiotics meet. On the *right*, neither antibiotic is inhibitory in its own right, but bacterial growth is inhibited where the two antibiotics diffuse together.

cillin binding protein 2a correlates with resistance to the antibiotic.[34] The resistant cells grow more slowly than the susceptible bacteria, unless incubated at reduced temperature. The relatively low inoculum used in the microdilution broth test may compromise detection of the small fraction of resistant cells. Variations in the ability of different lots of Mueller-Hinton agar to detect heteroresistance have been reported.[106]

In a study of 975 clinical isolates, Varaldo and colleagues found 122 strains of *S. aureus* (12.5%) that had borderline susceptibility to β-lactamase-resistant penicillins.[275] There are four potential mechanisms for this result. Initially, McDougal and Thornsberry reported that hyperproduction of β-lactamase is the mechanism by which some borderline-susceptible strains of *S. aureus* express resistance to oxacillin, and this appears to be the most common explanation.[166] The hyperproducing strains can be detected by performing an MIC test with a combination of β-lactamase inhibitor and a β-lactam antibiotic (Fig. 15-27). Chang and colleagues found that the MIC of *S. aureus* strains with an MIC of <64 µg/ml was reduced by four-fold to 32-fold if either 4 µg/ml of sulbactam or 8 µg/ml of tazobactam was added.[35] Addition of inhibitor to strains with an oxacillin MIC≥64 µg/ml did not alter the MIC, although these strains also produced β-lactamase. The mechanism for borderline susceptibility is not always

hyperproduction of conventional β-lactamase.[10] A β-lactamase that specifically hydrolyzes methicillin has been described.[162] A third mechanism is modification of the binding of antibiotic to normal penicillin binding proteins.[269] Finally, some strains with borderline susceptibility possess the mecA gene and produce penicillin binding protein 2a at a low level.[83] Some investigators have suggested that borderline strains can be discriminated by use of disks that contain ampicillin and a β-lactamase inhibitor,[147] but strains that are fully resistant may produce β-lactamase and appear susceptible to ampicillin-sulbactam.[275] Disks that contain both oxacillin and a β-lactamase inhibitor are not commercially available. Another approach is to perform a disk test for synergy between an oxacillin disk and a disk containing ampicillin-clavulanic acid or ampicillin-sulbactam. The two disks are placed adjacent to each other in an otherwise standardized disk diffusion test. If synergy is demonstrated (Fig. 15-26C) and the zone size around the oxacillin disk nearest the ampicillin-inhibitor disk would indicate susceptibility to oxacillin, hyperproduction of β-lactamase can be inferred as the mechanism for resistance.

The hyperproducing borderline strains usually have an MIC of 4 or 8 µg/ml. In contrast to the heteroresistant strains, which demonstrate multiple drug resistance, these strains are usually susceptible to other antibiotics.

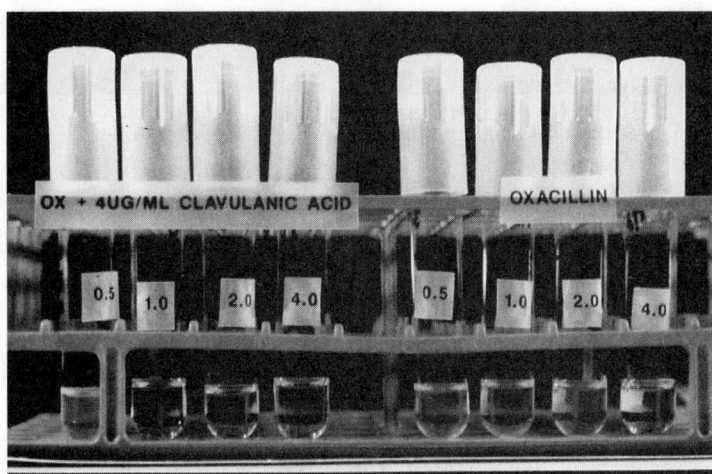

Figure 15-27
An isolate of *Staphylococcus aureus* with borderline susceptibility to oxacillin has been tested with and without the addition of clavulanic acid, an inhibitor of β-lactamase. In the absence of the inhibitor, the MIC of the strain is 4 µg/mL. After the addition of clavulanic acid the MIC is 1 µg/mL. The resistance of this strain is derived from the hyperproduction of β-lactamase.

Knapp and colleagues evaluated the Vitek GPS-SA card for borderline susceptible strains of *S. aureus* that lacked the mecA gene.[136] Vitek correctly characterized as susceptible 41 strains that grew in the Vitek card, but did not grow on agar screen plate and were susceptible by broth microdilution. Overall the accuracy of the card was 86%. The four isolates that were classified as resistant grew on the agar screen plate and were resistant also by broth microdilution, despite the fact that they lacked the mecA gene.

Experimental evidence from an animal model of endocarditis suggests that these borderline susceptible strains should respond to treatment with oxacillin just as do fully susceptible strains.[262] Limited clinical studies suggest the same conclusion.[99,161] If there is any question about clinical response, administration of vancomycin is the appropriate conservative treatment.

It is probable that no single procedure detects staphylococcal resistance to oxacillin with absolute reliability. It is also likely that false estimates of resistance can be generated by some manipulations, such as prolonged incubation of susceptibility tests.[38] The most reliable of the phenotypic methods is probably the agar dilution screen with 6 µg/ml of oxacillin. Although it is not yet generally available, molecular methods for detection of the mecA gene provide a modern approach that avoids all of the problems inherent in phenotypic variation.[196,299] Detection of oxacillin resistance is particularly troublesome in coagulase negative staphylococci. York and colleagues tested 44 strains of coagulase negative staphylococci that contained and expressed the mecA gene and an additional 97 strains that lacked the gene.[296] The sensitivities for detection of resistance by broth microdilution with 2% NaCl, the standardized disk diffusion test, and an agar screen with 4% NaCl and 6 µg/ml oxacillin were 50%, 84%, and 70% respectively at 24 hours and 77%, 82%, and 100% at 48 hours. The specificity of the tests for detecting strains without the gene were 100%, 89%, and 100% respectively at 24 hours. They recommend changing the breakpoint for susceptibility to oxacillin from 2 µg/ml to 1 µg/ml and performing an agar disk screen with incubation for 48 hours in suspect strains.

If there is a possibility of resistance to oxacillin in a clinically significant isolate of *Staphylococcus*, a variety of tests for detection of resistance should be performed. If resistance to oxacillin remains in question, other effective antibiotics, such as vancomycin alone or combined with rifampin, should be used.[7]

Guidelines to maximize detection of methicillin-resistant staphylococci are detailed in Box 15-4.

Resistance to cephalosporins among staphylococci is difficult to detect. There is clinical evidence that isolates of *S. aureus* that are resistant to oxacillin do not respond *in vivo* to cephalosporin therapy; the same phenomenon has also been suggested for *S. epidermidis*.[183] If resistance to nafcillin, oxacillin, or methicillin is demonstrated, the bacterial strain should be reported as resistant to other β-lactam antibiotics, including all cephalosporins, such as cefazolin or cephalothin, and the carbapenem antibiotic imipenem.

A strain of *S. haemolyticus* that developed resistance to vancomycin during treatment of a patient with recurrent episodes of peritonitis has been described.[238] Fortunately, no isolates of *S. aureus* have yet displayed resistance to vancomycin that has been confirmed *in vitro*, but that situation may change at any moment. Clinical isolates of methicillin-resistant *staphylococci* that are resistant to teicoplanin have been described, although they remained susceptible to vancomycin.[33,154] Even more ominous is the report that isolates of *S. aureus* with a fourfold decrease in susceptibility to vancomycin could be produced in the laboratory.[42] The change in susceptibility was correlated with the presence of a 39 kDa cytoplasmic protein. Furthermore, the enterococcal genes for resistance to vancomycin have been transferred in the laboratory to *S. aureus*.[193]

HAEMOPHILUS SPECIES

Haemophilus organisms require hemin (Factor X) and/or nicotinamide adenine dinucleotide (NAD) (Factor V) for growth. The validity of adding supplements both to dilution and also to diffusion susceptibility media has been established. A new supplement for *Haemophilus* has been suggested by Jorgensen and

BOX 15-4. MAXIMIZING DETECTION OF METHICILLIN-RESISTANT STAPHYLOCOCCI

1. For *S. aureus*, oxacillin is more likely to detect cross-resistance among penicillinase-resistant penicillins than other compounds. Cloxacillin and dicloxacillin should not be used. Nafcillin should not be used if the media contain blood.[183] Coudron and colleagues have suggested that methicillin may detect resistance in *S. epidermidis* better than oxacillin.

2. Addition of 2% NaCl to broth and 4% Na to agar that contains penicillinase-resistant penicillins enhances detection of resistance.[38,265] Baker and colleagues found, however, that use of 4% NaCl in agar media caused major error rates, and they recommend the use of 2% NaCl for agar dilution and E-test susceptibility methods.[8] They used the broth microdilution procedure and a DNA probe for the *mecA* gene as the reference standards.

3. The inoculum should be prepared by the alternative direct method, using colonies from fresh overnight plate (see Charts 23 and 59).

4. The cultures should be incubated at temperatures below 37°C to facilitate growth of resistant bacteria. A temperature of 35°C is a reasonable compromise for routine use. Incubation at 30°C may be used if resistance is highly suspected.

5. If the disk diffusion procedure is used, the edge of the apparent zone of inhibition should be examined closely. The border is sharp and clear when oxacillin-susceptible organisms are tested. Growth of oxacillin-resistant organisms "feathers" or "trails" as the disk is approached so that the inside edge of growth may be difficult to detect (Fig. 15-28).

6. Coudron and colleagues[38] found that two screening methods for detecting resistance to methicillin correlated with reference dilution tests on 91% or more of staphylococcal isolates; discrepancies were found primarily with strains that had borderline susceptibility. A bacterial inoculum adjusted to the density of a 0.5 McFarland turbidity standard is inoculated onto an agar plate that contains either 10 μg/mL of methicillin or 6 μg/mL of oxacillin. A 0.1-mL aliquot of the inoculum may be spread across the plate with a sterile glass rod. Alternatively, a swab may be dipped into the standardized suspension and then spotted onto the plate.

---

colleagues.[126] *Haemophilus* test medium consists of the following:

> Mueller-Hinton broth or agar
> Bovine hematin, 15 μg/ml
> Yeast extract, 5 mg/ml
> β-NAD, 15 μg/ml
> Thymidine phosphorylase, 0.2 IU/ml

The NCCLS has adopted the *Haemophilus* test medium, which may contain cation supplements if appropriate. The advantages of the medium include visual clarity and reliability of testing with trimethoprim-sulfamethoxazole.[126] Some investigators have experienced problems with the performance of both homemade and commercially prepared *Haemophilus* test medium.[172]

Proper preparation of the inoculum is very important for testing *Haemophilus* species. The alternate direct method of standardizing the bacterial suspension from an overnight culture should be used (see Charts 23 and 59).

Jorgensen and colleagues found a good correlation of the E-test and standardized microdilution tests for *Haemophilus influenzae*.[124] A recent study of susceptibility testing methods for *H. influenzae* documented a generally acceptable performance among commonly used methods.[86] The procedures and interpretations that have been developed for *H. influenzae* can be applied also to other *Haemophilus* spp.[123,124]

Antimicrobial susceptibility testing of *H. influenzae* has been reviewed by Doern and Jones.[48]

PENICILLIN ANTIBIOTICS

Doern and colleagues documented a prevalence of 15.2% for β-lactamase production in *Haemophilus influenzae*. The frequency of enzymatic degradation of ampicillin was 21% for encapsulated strains of *H. influenzae* type b and 12% for nonencapsulated strains of *H. influenzae*.[50] Isolates were more likely to produce β-lactamase if they were recovered from infants and young children rather than adults and if they were recovered from blood and cerebrospinal fluid rather than other fluids or tissues.

The incidence of β-lactamase production in a national collaborative survey was 20%, but once again there was a dichotomy between encapsulated and nonencapsulated strains.[51] The prevalence of the β-lactamase enzyme was 31.7% in type b strains and 15.6% in nonencapsulated strains of *H. influenzae*. Intrinsic resistance to ampicillin, not mediated by β-lactamase, was detected in only 0.1% of strains.

A repeat survey a few years later, limited to respiratory isolates, documented a prevalence of 16.5% for production of β-lactamase by *H. influenzae*. The frequency of resistance in encapsulated type b strains and in nonencapsulated strains was 29.5% and 15%, respectively.[121]

All isolates of *Haemophilus* species that are etiologic agents of serious infections should be tested for production of β-lactamase, preferably by the Nitrocefin procedure. Isolates from sterile body sites that do not produce the enzyme should be tested for intrinsic resistance if possible. In any event isolates should be re-

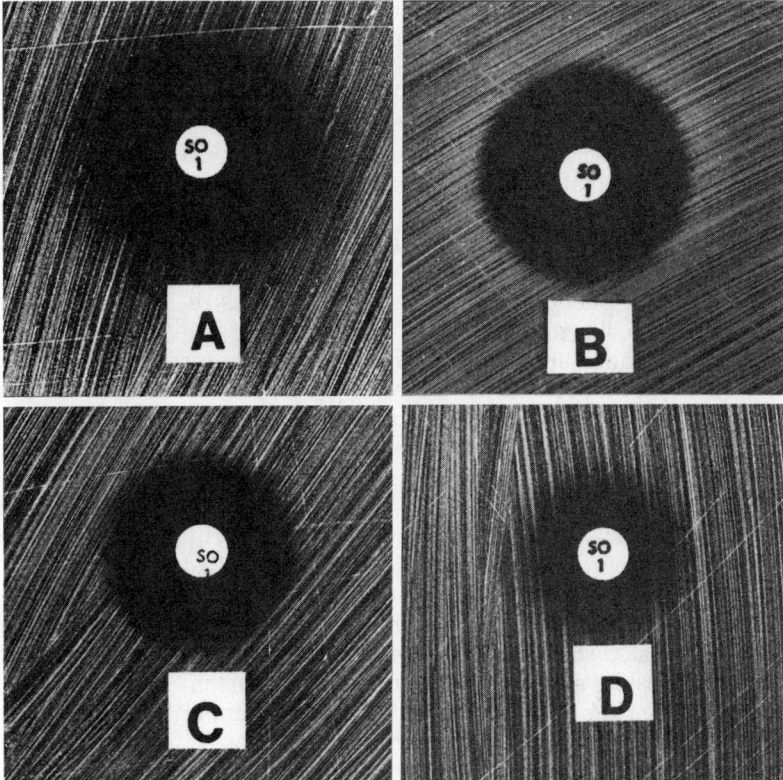

Figure 15-28
The effect of salt on the expression of methicillin resistance to staphylococci is shown: A susceptible strain was tested against a 1-µg oxacillin disk on Mueller–Hinton agar that had no supplemental salt (**A**) or that contained 4% NaCl (**B**). The zone of bacterial inhibition was unaffected by addition of the salt. A methicillin-resistant strain was also tested against oxacillin on Mueller–Hinton agar without (**C**), and with (**D**) the addition of 4% NaCl. Without salt, a clear zone of inhibition was produced (*C*), and the isolate would be considered susceptible. In the presence of salt there was a gradually decreasing growth or "feathering" right up to the disk; this organism should be considered resistant to oxacillin and other penicillinase-resistant penicillins.

ferred to a reference laboratory if there is any question about correlation of the laboratory and clinical results.

CHLORAMPHENICOL

For years the backup drug for serious *Haemophilus* infections was chloramphenicol. Although infrequent, resistance to this antibiotic has also developed. The frequency of resistance to chloramphenicol among isolates of *H. influenzae* was 0.5% in a national collaborative study.[51] In almost all instances resistance is mediated by enzymatic degradation.[81] Doern and colleagues have found the tube test significantly more accurate than a disk modification of the rapid assay for chloramphenicol acetyltransferase.[47]

CEPHALOSPORINS

The first-generation cephalosporins are poorly effective against *Haemophilus influenzae* and need not be tested. Second-generation cephalosporins, such as cefamandole and cefuroxime, are effective against *Haemophilus* species *in vitro*, but are least effective where they are needed most—for isolates that produce β-lactamase.[122] Therapeutic failures have been described with second-generation cephalosporin antibiotics. Third-generation cephalosporins, such as ceftriaxone, are uniformly effective against *H. influenzae*.

TRIMETHOPRIM-SULFAMETHOXAZOLE

Resistance of *Haemophilus influenzae* to trimethoprim-sulfamethoxazole can be detected in less than 1% of strains.[121] Although not the drug of choice for serious systemic disease, therapy with trimethoprim-sulfamethoxazole has been successful in treating pulmonary infections.

STREPTOCOCCUS PNEUMONIAE

For many years, penicillin was the standard treatment for pneumococcal infections and susceptibility testing was not indicated. The emergence of strains that are resistant to multiple antibiotics, including penicillin, has breached even this bastion of antimicrobial therapy. Strains that have MICs between 0.1 and 1.0 µg/ml are considered relatively resistant to penicillin; those with MICs greater than 1.0 µg/ml are designated as resistant. In one study, nearly 7% of patients in Denver who had pneumococcal bacteremia or meningitis were infected by relatively resistant strains.[113] What was once a small, local problem has become a large, world-wide concern. A total of 16.4% of the pneumococcal isolates submitted to the Centers for Disease Control and Prevention in 1991 and 1992 were resistant to one of the antimicrobial agents tested.[24] Intermediate resistance to penicillin was detected in 5.3% of isolates, and full resistance was present in 1.3%, compared to <0.02% in a previous survey performed in 1979 to 1987. In 1995 to 1996 at the University of Vermont, 15% of the pneumococcal isolates from serious infections demonstrated intermediate susceptibility and 5% of the strains were fully resistant to penicillin. Pneumococcal resistance to penicillin has been reviewed by Klugman[135], and a plan for dealing with the public health implications of this resistance has been developed by the Centers for Disease Control and Prevention.[32]

The mechanism of pneumococcal resistance to penicillin is the alteration of penicillin-binding proteins. *Streptococcus pneumoniae* does not produce β-lactamases. Multiple binding-proteins are involved in the acquisition of resistance, producing a step-wise decrease in susceptibility. It is interesting to note that 70% of clinical pneumococcal isolates that are resistant to penicillin also show defective lysis, a property that would also enhance their survival.[175] Two kinds of antibiotic pressure on pneumococci are hypothesized as explanations for the concordant phenomena. Pneumococcal strains resistant to penicillin may be clonal, but multiple pathways to resistance are possible, and resistant strains have emerged independently in diverse geographic locations. Penicillin resistance can be transferred horizontally from one pneumococcal strain to another, apparently by transformation.[56] Considerable variation in the genes for the altered proteins occurs from mismatch repair after the transfer. Penicillin resistance occurs with a variety of serogroups and among diverse strains that can be differentiated by molecular typing,[94,176] but this pattern could be produced by horizontal transfer among unrelated strains. Risk factors for serious infection with resistant strains include prior use of β-lactam antibiotics, age less than 15 years, infection in the upper respiratory tract, and nosocomial origin of infection.[16]

Pneumococci that are resistant to penicillin also have decreased susceptibility to other β-lactam antibiotics.[145] Imipenem, meropenem, cefotaxime, ceftriaxone, and cefpirome are more active than penicillin *in vitro*. Ampicillin, cefdinir, cefuroxime, cefoperazone, azlocillin, mezlocillin, piperacillin, cephalothin, and cefamandole demonstrate slightly less activity than penicillin. Oxacillin, cefixime, ceftizoxime, cefetamet, cefaclor, ceftazidime, cefoxitin, cefonicid, and latamoxef show very poor activity against resistant strains. The mechanism for resistance to these other β-lactam antibiotics is also an alteration in penicillin-binding proteins.[178]

Five percent sheep blood may be added to Mueller-Hinton agar and 2% to 5% lysed horse blood may be added to broth media for growth of *S. pneumoniae*. Quality control of these tests should include known resistant pneumococcal strains in addition to standard control organisms. Incubation in CO_2 is acceptable if necessary for growth of the strain. The *Haemophilus* test medium described earlier has been reported to work well for support of pneumococcal growth in broth microdilution tests,[125] although it has not worked well in all laboratories.

In most laboratories, the simplest screening test for resistance is a variation of the disk diffusion test. Although penicillin disks have been used in some studies, the procedure recommended by the NCCLS for detection of resistance to penicillin incorporates a 1-μg disk of oxacillin. Strains that have a zone diameter less than or equal to 19 mm should be reported as provisionally resistant to penicillin; confirmation by a dilution susceptibility test should be arranged (Fig 15-29). Swenson and colleagues found that oxacillin was a better predictor of penicillin susceptibility than was methicillin,[254] and nafcillin disks should not be used on agar-containing media.[182] The disk diffusion test does not differentiate strains that are relatively resistant (MIC of 0.1 to 1.0 μg/ml) from strains that are resistant (MIC >1.0 μg/ml). A strain of *S. pneumoniae* that is presumptively resistant to penicillin should be tested in a reliable broth dilution test.

Commercial susceptibility testing systems perform variably for detection of penicillin resistance in pneumococci.[259] The Pasco system (Difco, Wheatridge, CO) and the E-test were acceptable for all antibiotics, except for sulfamethoxazole with the E-test. The MicroMedia (Accumed, Westlake, OH) and MicroScan systems had an unacceptably high rate of minor errors, 16.4% and 63.6% respectively. Minor error rates for ceftriaxone and cefotaxime were lowest with the E-test and Sensitre (Accumed, Westlake, OH) methods (12.7%). Error rates were low when testing for erythromycin, tetracycline, and chloramphenicol, except for MicroScan, which produced an unacceptable frequency of very major errors with erythromycin (34.6%). The E-test has

Figure 15-29
Screening test for resistance of pneumococci to penicillin, using a 1-μg–oxacillin disk on Mueller–Hinton agar with sheep blood. A susceptible strain (*A*) shows a large zone of inhibition and can be reported as susceptible without further testing. The second strain (*B*) demonstrates a very small zone of inhibition. This strain could be susceptible, intermediate, or resistant (although the very small zone suggests that it will not be susceptible). In order to determine the correct interpretation an MIC test must be performed.

been evaluated independently in a collaborative study, which documented low minor error rates with penicillin (9.5%) and cefotaxime (5.4%) (see Fig. 15-25).[127] Vancomycin is the standard of therapy for resistant strains causing serious systemic infection. Hashemi and colleagues have noted that the E-test produces higher MIC results than does the microbroth dilution test, raising concern that reports of false resistance might result.[101]

Although some strains of relatively resistant pneumococci have responded to penicillin therapy,[197,278] meningitis may not be treated successfully because concentrations of antibiotic are lower in cerebrospinal fluid.[198] Strains that have an MIC greater than 1.0 μg/ml are unlikely to respond to penicillin therapy. Unfortunately, many of these overtly resistant strains are resistant to multiple antibiotics. The therapy of multiply-resistant pneumococci has been reviewed by Friedland and McCracken.[79]

NEISSERIA GONORRHOEAE

For many years the gonococcus was uniformly susceptible to penicillin and the therapeutic approach to gonococcal infection was relatively straightforward. In the mid 1970s strains of *Neisseria gonorrhoeae* that produced β-lactamase appeared[63] and spread rapidly.[242] This β-lactamase resembles the TEM enzyme found in enteric bacilli and *Haemophilus influenzae*. A second mechanism of resistance appeared a few years later when Dougherty and colleagues described resistant strains that lacked β-lactamase but contained altered penicillin-binding proteins.[54] These strains have produced epidemic as well as sporadic infection.[67]

A second weapon in the antigonococcal armamentarium was removed when a plasmid that mediated high-level resistance to tetracycline appeared in *N. gonorrhoeae*.[137] Resistance to quinolones has appeared in strains of *Neisseria gonorrhoeae* from Asia[255] and more recently in the United States.[31]

The tests recommended by the NCCLS for detection of chromosomally mediated resistance in *N. gonorrhoeae* are agar dilution and agar diffusion. The subject has been reviewed by Doern and Jones.[48] Either proteose peptone #3 agar with 1% hemoglobin and 1% Kellogg Supplement or DST agar with 5% lysed horse blood and 1% Kellogg Supplement may be used.[183] Agar diffusion tests are performed on GC agar base with X- and V-Factor supplement, but without hemoglobin.[182] Susceptibility plates for testing *N. gonorrhoeae* must be incubated at 35°C in CO_2. A zone of less than or equal to 26 mm in the disk diffusion test indicates resistance. A zone size of less than or equal to 19 mm usually indicates production of β-lactamase, but the β-lactamase test is preferred for assessing this mechanism of resistance. Criteria for interpretation of spectinomycin and tetracycline have been developed by the NCCLS. There have been no gonococcal strains resistant to ceftriaxone, so the resistant breakpoint has not been set.

Mueller-Hinton broth cannot be used for dilution tests because it lyses *N. gonorrhoeae*. Satisfactory results have been reported with trypticase soy broth supplemented with 1% hemoglobin and 1% X-Factor and V-Factor,[96,241] but the agar-based tests are preferred.

All isolates of *N. gonorrhoeae* should be tested for β-lactamase production, preferably using the Nitrocefin method. An agar dilution or disk diffusion test should be performed on β-lactamase negative isolates if the frequency of intrinsic resistance to penicillin or the prevalence of tetracycline resistance in the population is high. Any isolates from treatment failures should be tested locally or referred to a reference laboratory. The E-test has shown good correlation with agar dilution techniques for non-β-lactamase-producing strains,[274] but resistance may not be detected in strains that produce β-lactamase,[298] emphasizing the necessity for performing a test for β-lactamase production in all strains.

NEISSERIA MENINGITIDIS

Plasmid-mediated transfer of β-lactamase to *Neisseria meningitidis* has been documented.[45] In addition, strains have been described that are resistant on the basis of altered penicillin-binding proteins.[301] It appears that the altered membrane proteins were transferred to *Neisseria meningitidis* from commensal *Neisseria* spp.[22] The E-test has been evaluated for testing of *N. meningitidis* with mixed results. Pascual and colleagues have reported that this method overstates the degree of resistance and suggest that further evaluation of appropriate media is necessary.[200]

Susceptibility testing of meningococci to rifampin may occasionally be requested for epidemiologic purposes.[187] It is often difficult for the laboratory to generate a result in time to guide prophylaxis, which must start at the time the clinical diagnosis of meningococcal infection is made.

ENTEROCOCCUS SPECIES

The mainstay of antimicrobial therapy of serious enterococcal infections has been the use of combinations of β-lactam and aminoglycoside antibiotics.[111,272] The underpinnings of this approach have been seriously undermined in recent years. The subject has been reviewed by several authors.[105,144,229] The interactions among antibiotics and resistance mechanisms in enterococci are illustrated in Figure 15-10.

AMINOGLYCOSIDE ANTIBIOTICS

There are three mechanisms for enterococcal resistance to aminoglycosides. Aminoglycoside-modifying enzymes, which include phosphotransferases, nucleotidyltransferases, and an acetyltransferase, are produced constitutively on plasmids.[144] They resemble the enzymes found in staphylococci rather than those produced in gram-negative bacilli. Additional mechanisms include modification of the ribosomal target[61] and interference with transport of the antibiotic.

Detection of high-level resistance of enterococci to aminoglycosides is important because these strains are not inhibited synergistically by combination therapy with β-lactam antibiotics. Resistance of *E. faecium* to kanamycin, amikacin, netilmicin, and tobramycin can be assumed. Resistance of this species to gentamicin and streptomycin and of *E. faecalis* to all of the aminoglycosides can be predicted by *in vitro* testing with large concentrations of antibiotic in a dilution test or by disks with a high antibiotic content.[62,80,243] Concentrations of 1000 μg/ml of streptomycin by microdilution, 2000 μg/ml of streptomycin by agar dilution, and 500 μg/ml of gentamicin by either method are recommended as break points.[253] Growth of a single colony on agar dilution plates indicates resistance. Disks with 120 μg of gentamicin or 300 μg of streptomycin are recommended for the disk diffusion test. Resistance is indicated by ≤6 mm (no zone) and susceptibility by a zone of ≥10 mm. Strains with zones of 7 mm to 9 mm should be tested by dilution methods. Problems with detection of this resistance by commercial susceptibility systems have been addressed by the manufacturers.

β-LACTAM ANTIBIOTICS

Many strains of enterococci, particularly *Enterococcus faecium*, are intrinsically resistant to β-lactam antibiotics because they possess binding proteins with low affinity for these drugs. In particular, the cephalosporins are uniformly ineffective against enterococci and should not be tested. In general, ampicillin is more effective than penicillin *in vitro*. The recent emergence of enterococcal strains that produce β-lactamase has been discussed previously.

VANCOMYCIN

The last therapeutic resort for enterococci was vancomycin until Leclercq and colleagues described strains of *E. faecium* that contained a plasmid mediating resistance to the glycopeptide antibiotics vancomycin and teicoplanin.[143] Vancomycin-resistant isolates of *E. faecalis* have also been described.[188] Resistance to glycopeptides appears to be transferred by dissemination of a gene rather than a plasmid.[58] Three genetic mechanisms for resistance of enterococci to glycopeptides have been described.[229] The vanA gene complex is inducible and is carried on a family of plasmids in *E. faecium* and *E. faecalis*. It encodes high-level resistance to both vancomycin and teicoplanin. VanB is an inducible gene in *E. faecium* that mediates low-level resistance only to vancomycin by means of a carboxypeptidase. VanC is a constitutive chromosomal gene that mediates low-level resistance in *E. gallinarum*, an unusual clinical isolate.

Resistance to vancomycin, particularly that mediated by the vanB gene, is not reliably detected by all methods.

Unfortunately vancomycin resistant enterococci have taken a firm hold and have become epidemic in some hospitals and regions.[78,177] The characteristics of resistant strains vary over time and with geographic location. In a group of Connecticut hospitals the mean rate of high-level resistance to gentamicin was 29%; to ampicillin, 10% (all being isolates of *E. faecium*); and to vancomycin, 8%, but no isolates produced β-lacta-

mase.[202] Enterococci are pathogens-in-training in comparison to staphylococci and streptococci, but they can produce serious, life-threatening infections in hospitalized patients whose feces are colonized by resistant strains. Risk factors for colonization and invasive disease include serious illness and prior receipt of antibiotics, including vancomycin and drugs active against anaerobic bacteria.[60,177]

Detection of enterococcal resistance to vancomycin, particularly the vanB phenotype, in clinical laboratories is not optimal, primarily because commercially available testing systems, including the two most commonly used methods—Vitek AMS and various Microscan systems—do not pick up the moderate- and low-level resistance efficiently.[260] In a survey of New Jersey laboratories 96% of 76 clinical laboratories were able to recognize resistance in a strain of *E. faecium* with high-level resistance to vancomycin (MIC = 512 μg/ml), but only 27% of laboratories reported an *E. faecium* strain with moderate resistance (MIC = 64 μg/ ml) as resistant.[261] A strain of *E. faecalis* with low-level resistance (MIC = 32 μg/ml), a typical vanB phenotype, was recognized as resistant by only 16% of laboratories, and a strain of *E. gallinarum* with a typical vanC phenotype (MIC = 8 μg/ml) was correctly characterized by 74% of participants. In a comparative study from the Centers for Disease Control and Prevention, Tenover and colleagues evaluated ten commercial systems for detection of vancomycin resistance in enterococci.[260] A reference microdilution method was used as the standard for evaluation of 50 reference strains. An agar dilution screening test, the E-test, and some commercial microdilution systems (Sceptor [Becton-Dickinson Microbiology Systems, Cockeysville, MD], MicroMedia, Pasco, and Sensitre) performed well. Increased numbers of minor errors were seen with the disk diffusion test and other commercial microdilution systems (Alamar [Alamar Bioscience, West Sacramento, CA], Uniscept [bioMérieux], and conventional MicroScan panels). Very major error rates were produced by the Vitek system (10.3%) and the MicroScan Rapid system (20.7%), which was the only system to produce major errors (13.3%). On repeat testing with the Vitek very major errors were reduced to 3.4%, whereas the errors with the MicroScan Rapid system increased to 27.6%. A recent report confirms the ability of MicroScan conventional Positive Breakpoint Combo Type 6 panels to detect resistance among enterococci to ampicillin and vancomycin.[114] Fourteen of the fifteen incorrect results with vancomycin were in motile enterococci, which are less frequently isolated from serious infections than *E. faecium* and *E. faecalis*. There were no β-lactamase producing strains among the 132 isolates studied.

A commercial version of the agar screen test, the Remel Synergy Quad Plate, was not included in the study, but compares well to the reference test.[76] It incorporates 6 μg/ml of vancomycin into brain-heart infusion agar as recommended by Swenson and colleagues.[251]

The deficiency in the Vitek system appears to be related to the growth medium.[119] The manufacturers will undoubtedly work hard to resolve the problems with commercial systems as soon as possible, but it is important to query their representatives about the reliability of their systems for detection of this clinically important resistance. Vancomycin resistance in enterococci has been associated with more frequent episodes of recurrent bacteremia, persistent isolation of enterococci from primary sites of infection, increased frequency of endovascular infection, and increased mortality.[146]

Clinical microbiologists may be asked to screen feces for vancomycin-resistant enterococci to determine the prevalence of resistant organisms in an institution or to pinpoint patients at increased risk of invasive enterococcal infection. Several methods have been recommended. Barton and Doern found that bile esculin azide agar supplemented with 8 µg/ml of vancomycin was a useful screening medium.[13] Landman and colleagues compared five selective media, and found that Enterococcosel broth (Becton Dickinson, Cockeysville, MD), supplemented with 64 µg/ml of vancomycin and 60 µg/ml of aztreonam, was the most sensitive method.[140] Use of bile esculin azide agar with a 30 µg vancomycin disk was less sensitive, but would be easy to implement in most laboratories. Swabs collected from the rectum and the perirectal area provide equivalent results.[283]

LISTERIA MONOCYTOGENES

Microdilution broth tests may be performed in cation-supplemented Mueller-Hinton broth with 2% to 5% lysed horse blood. *Listeria monocytogenes* provides a good example of the care needed in extrapolating the zone size criteria in the disk diffusion test to bacteria that have not been evaluated. The diffusion test appears to be satisfactory for evaluation of *L. monocytogenes*, but susceptibilities to penicillin and ampicillin were not adequately determined by participants in proficiency test programs until the NCCLS clarified the zone sizes to be used for establishing breakpoints.[120]

STREPTOCOCCUS PYOGENES

Occasionally the laboratory may receive a request to perform a susceptibility test on an isolate of group A β-hemolytic *Streptococcus*. Such testing is appropriate for alternative drugs, such as erythromycin, if the patient is allergic to penicillin. To date there have been no strains of *Streptococcus pyogenes* resistant to penicillin *in vitro*. Therapeutic failures result from inadequate penetration of antibiotic into the crypts of the tonsils and adenoidal tissue where the bacteria may hide. In the absence of documented resistance and without a standardized, validated method for testing, acquiescence to such a test is more likely to cause problems than to solve them. If testing is believed to be indicated, any resistant results should be validated by a reference laboratory.

VIRIDANS STREPTOCOCCI

Although they are less frequent pathogens than pneumococci, viridans streptococci cause endocarditis and other serious infections (see Chap. 12). Alterations in penicillin-binding proteins have produced resistance to multiple β-lactam antibiotics among several of the species, including *S. mitis*[65] and *S. sanguis*.[302] It appears that the resistance in viridans streptococci originated in penicillin-resistant pneumococcal strains.[57] So far these resistant isolates have remained susceptible to vancomycin.

OTHER GRAM-POSITIVE BACTERIA

Vancomycin resistance is commonly found in strains of *Leuconostoc, Pediococcus,* and *Lactobacillus*.[252] These genera are infrequently pathogens, but on occasion they do produce bacteremia[163] and septicemia.[90] Resistance to vancomycin may be a useful clue to the correct identification, because streptococci, with which these genera may be confused, are uniformly susceptible to vancomycin.

RESISTANCE TO MACROLIDE-LINCOSAMIDE-STREPTOGRAMIN ANTIBIOTICS

Cross-resistance among macrolide antibiotics has been recognized for many years. It has become apparent that there are discrepancies between results with erythromcyin (a macrolide) and clindamycin (a lincosamide) when some strains of staphylococci and streptococci are tested. Sanchez and colleagues demonstrated that resistance to the whole group could be induced in a high proportion of isolates that were resistant to erythromycin.[231] They recommend that erythromycin only be tested and that induction tests be performed for coagulase-negative staphylococci from serious systemic infections before this group of antibiotics is used therapeutically.

DIRECT SUSCEPTIBILITY TESTING

Direct susceptibility testing of clinical specimens is not generally recommended because the inoculum is not standardized and mixed bacterial species are often present. Direct susceptibility testing of broth from positive blood culture bottles has correlated well with standard tests from isolated colonies. The tests have been performed both with unadjusted broth from the bottles[40] and after adjustment of the density of the culture by comparison to a 0.5 McFarland standard.[132] In addition, urine from patients with urinary tract infections may be tested directly if a single bacterial strain is present.[44] Some degree of mechanization has been achieved with the standard tests. Interpretation of the end points in microbroth dilution susceptibility tests by using commercially available microplate readers has compared well with visual inspection.[43] These instruments can be programmed to enter results directly into a computer and to provide interpretative correlates of susceptibility. An alternative system, which also performed well in comparison to traditional methods, incorporates a fluorescent dye into the microwells of bacterial inoculum; fluorescence that has been liberated by bacterial enzymatic alteration of the fluorescent substrates is measured.[248]

TESTS FOR DETERMINATION OF BACTERICIDAL ACTIVITY

INDICATIONS

The indications for determination of bactericidal activity are few.[187,267] The infection must either be a serious one in which antimicrobial activity that is lethal to the microbe is desired, because other host defense mechanisms are compromised, or be located in a site that is difficult to reach with antibiotics. Historically, streptococcal endocarditis has been the primary indication for determining bactericidal activity.

A large discrepancy exists between the concentrations of penicillins that are required to inhibit growth of enterococci and those concentrations that are lethal. Addition of an aminoglycoside to a penicillin antibiotic is often essential for successful treatment of the infection. This phenomenon is so prevalent among enterococci that documentation in the laboratory is no longer needed. Some nonenterococcal streptococci may also demonstrate this dichotomy. Recognition of these strains is important because addition of an aminoglycoside antibiotic to the therapeutic regimen should then be considered. It is not clear, however, that bactericidal testing must be done routinely.

Other situations in which bactericidal testing has been suggested include osteomyelitis, meningitis, and septicemia in patients who are neutropenic. Recently, an additional indication for bactericidal testing has been the possibility of "tolerance" in an isolate, especially in *Staphylococcus aureus*.[98,267] In light of the problems with methods, tests of bactericidal activity are clearly not routine, and the results should be interpreted with caution and some skepticism.[4]

Discrepancies between inhibitory and bactericidal values may also be found when staphylococci and enterococci are tested against vancomycin. The clinical significance of this phenomenon is not clear, and routine testing for bactericidal activity is not recommended.

DEFINITIONS

MINIMUM BACTERICIDAL CONCENTRATION

The minimum bactericidal concentration (MBC), in contrast to the MIC, is the lowest concentration in µg/ml of a drug that results in more than 99.9% killing of the bacteria being tested. Figure 15-30 illustrates a series of tubes from an MIC determination and agar plates on which subcultures have been made. Decreasing concentrations of antibiotic in tubes 2 through 9 (1 µg/ml to 128 µg/ml) were incubated with a bacterial isolate for 16 hours, vortexed, and reincubated for an additional 4 hours. After 20 hours, heavy growth is obvious in tubes 6 through 9 (1 µg/ml to 8 µg/ml), and light growth is apparent in tube 5 (16 µg/ml). Growth is also apparent in tube 10, which contains no antibiotic; no growth is present in tube 1, the sterility control. Subcultures were then made from tubes 2 through 5 to the surface of agar. Large numbers of bacteria are evident on plate 5, from a tube that contained barely visi-

ble growth, and on plate 4, from a tube that was visually clear after incubation for 20 hours. A small number of bacteria are present on plate 3, but the number is less than the calculated 99.9% reduction of the inoculum. Growth is entirely inhibited on plate 2. The MIC of this isolate is, therefore 64 µg/ml; the MBC is 128 µg/ml.

TOLERANCE

Tolerance is a term that has been used in several ways by different investigators to refer to combinations of drugs and microorganisms in which the bacteria are inhibited but not killed. The phenomenon occurs primarily, but not exclusively, with β-lactam antibiotics and gram-positive bacteria. Tolerance has little, if any meaning when discussing gram-negative bacteria.

Clinical concern has centered around tolerance of *Staphylococcus aureus* to β-lactam antibiotics. An operational definition of a tolerant strain is an isolate in which the MBC end points are five or more twofold dilutions greater than the MIC; that is, the MBC/MIC ratio is greater than 32 after incubation for 24 to 48 hours. The significance of tolerance has been clouded because the frequency with which the phenomenon is demonstrated varies greatly according to the method that is used (Table 15-19). For example, bacteria in the stationary phase are less susceptible to the lytic activity of β-lactam antibiotics than are bacteria that are growing rapidly. Bacteria that adhere to the wall of the tube above the meniscus may be shielded from the antibiotic and erroneously appear as resistant cells when the broth is subcultured.[258]

Tolerance may be demonstrated frequently in the laboratory, but failure to successfully treat an infection with a tolerant strain has been reported very infrequently.[228] It should be remembered that there are many reasons for failure of antimicrobial therapy in an individual patient. It is probably best to reserve assessment of tolerance for those strains that have not responded to appropriate antistaphylococcal chemotherapy.

The mechanism of bacterial tolerance is not completely understood.[98] Among the streptococci, it appears to be related to a deficiency in autolysins, which are enzymes that hydrolyze bonds in the bacterial cell wall.[267,268] Investigators have been able to produce tolerance in pneumococci by making the cell wall resistant to autolysins that are normally present; subsequently, they have returned the bacterial cells to the normal state by restoring the susceptibility of the cell wall to the autolytic enzymes.

Tolerance is presumably distinct from the "persister" phenomenon,[93] in which a very small fraction of resistant cells may remain even when bactericidal activity is present (one of the reasons for selecting 99.9% rather than 100% killing as the end point for most bactericidal tests). Tolerance may be related to the paradoxical or Eagle phenomenon,[59] in which increasing concentrations of antibiotic result in less killing, rather than an expected enhancement of bactericidal activity. Fontana and colleagues found that enterococcal strains expressed the paradoxical phenomenon, tolerance,

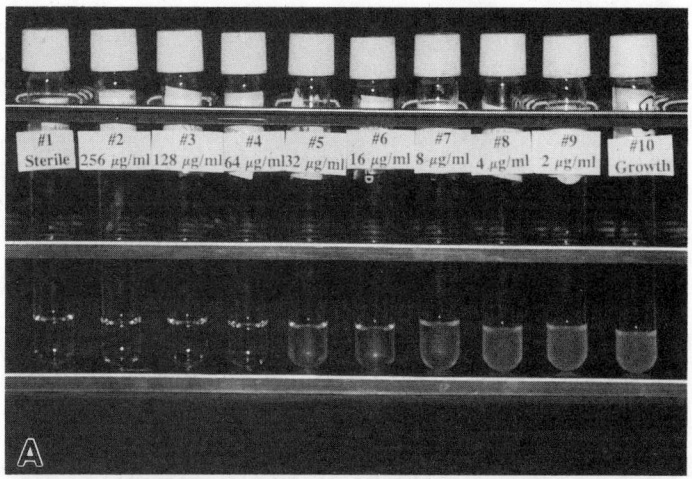

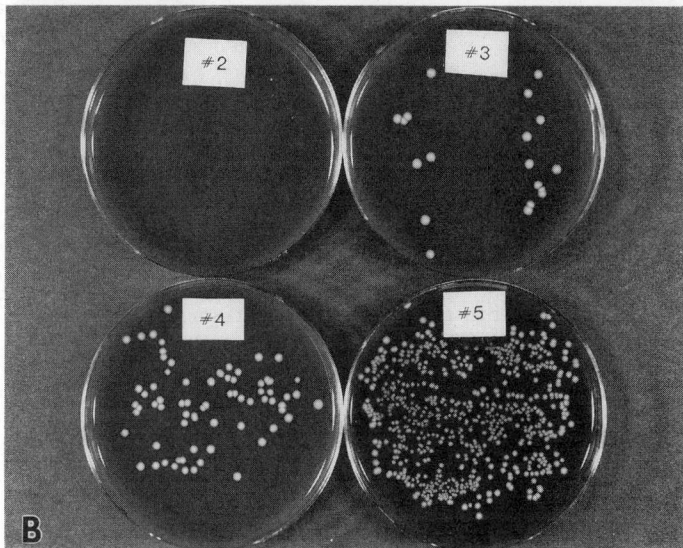

Figure 15-30

Test of minimum bactericidal concentration (MBC): (**A**) Visible growth was present in tubes 5 through 9, containing 2 to 32 µg/mL of antibiotic. The MIC of the isolate is, therefore, 64 µg/mL. (**B**) Subculture of tubes 3 through 5, containing 32 to 128 µg/mL, produced bacterial growth, but the number of colonies subcultured from tube 3 was less than the calculated 99.9% reduction of the inoculum. The MBC of the isolate is therefore 128 µg/mL.

both, or neither.[71] In this bacteriologic quagmire, the solid ground is the knowledge that combined aminoglycoside–β-lactam therapy must be used for serious enterococcal infection.

A satisfactory method for performing bactericidal tests has not been found. The method suggested by Schoenknecht and colleagues has corrected many of the methodologic difficulties.[237] That procedure is summarized in Chart 20. A proposed standard for macrotube and microdilution MBC tests has been published by NCCLS.[184]

Careful attention to detail is even more important in this test than in the determination of MICs. One author has stated that tolerant strains of *Staphylococcus aureus* have not been demonstrated in his laboratory since rigorous control of the MBC test has been instituted.[237] Pelletier and Baker were unable to demonstrate tolerance in 23 reputedly tolerant isolates of *S. aureus*.[207] For all these reasons bactericidal testing should not be done routinely.[187,207] If the tests are performed, it is important that all parties recognize the limitations. Reimer and colleagues have provided reference results for the bactericidal activity of the ATCC

quality control strains, both with and without serum in the broth.[218]

A disk diffusion method for demonstration of tolerance has been reported but has not been evaluated extensively.[211]

TESTING OF ANTIBIOTIC COMBINATIONS

A combination of two or more antibiotics may be needed for several reasons: 1) treatment of mixed infections when not all organisms are susceptible to the same antibiotic, 2) prevention or delay of development of bacterial resistance to an antibiotic, 3) ability to use nontoxic amounts of two antibiotics when toxic doses of a single antibiotic would be required, or 4) when combination therapy may be more effective against a single organism than the use of one antimicrobial agent alone.[139,160] King and colleagues have provided definitions of the types of interactions that may result.[133]

1. *Autonomous or indifferent:* the result with two drugs is equal to the result with the most effective drug by itself.

TABLE 15-19
Technical Factors That Influence Bactericidal Activity[237]

Variable	Effect of Variable on Results
Growth phase	Residual surviving bacteria in stationary phase; exaggerated paradoxic effect in late log phase
Type of tube or glassware	Adhesion varies with material and may produce erratic results or give impression of survivors
Inoculation	Adhesion above meniscus is minimized by a small-volume inoculum below the surface and avoidance of shaking
Mixing at 20 h	Vigorous vortexing is needed to resuspend the bacterial cells; care must be taken to avoid aerosols
Antibiotic carryover	Gives falsely low counts of survivors at >16 × MIC
Reincubation of MBC subculture plates	Up to 50% increase in colony counts after 72 h at >8 × MIC if paradoxic effect is present (increased survival of bacteria at higher concentration of drug after usual subculture incubation)

2. *Antagonistic:* the result with two drugs is significantly less than the best individual response.
3. *Additive:* the result with two drugs is equal to the combined action of each of the drugs used separately.
4. *Synergistic:* the result with two drugs is significantly better than the additive response.

Careful clinical and laboratory trials have established the value of combining antibiotics in many situations. Synergistic action occurs under several conditions: 1) when the antibiotics work sequentially or at different sites to inhibit synthesis of bacterial cell walls or block bacterial metabolism, 2) when the uptake of aminoglycosides into bacterial cells is enhanced by β-lactam antibiotics, and 3) when one member of the combination inhibits bacterial β-lactamase activity.[107]

The classic example of synergistic therapy is the use of a penicillin analogue and an aminoglycoside in the treatment of enterococcal endocarditis.[111] The molecular basis of this synergism has been clearly explained.[139] In brief, penicillin facilitates the entry of aminoglycosides into the bacterial cell but does not cause an irreversible defect by itself. Synergistic effects depend on the subsequent susceptibility of the bacterium to increased amounts of aminoglycoside. Many strains of *Enterococcus faecalis*, the most commonly isolated *Enterococcus* species, contain enzymes that inactivate aminoglycosides. Enzymes that inactivate streptomycin and kanamycin are more prevalent than those that inactivate gentamicin; for that reason, gentamicin is effective against more strains than are streptomycin and kanamycin.

There are many other mechanisms for bacterial synergism. Trimethoprim and the sulfonamides exert their individual antibacterial action at sequential points in the metabolism of folate to 1-carbon fragments, which are essential for the synthesis of amino acids. Sulfonamides compete with *p*-aminobenzoic acid and prevent the formation of 7,8-dihydropteroate, an early intermediary in the metabolic pathway. Trimethoprim inhibits a later metabolic stage, the conversion of dihydrofolic acid to tetrahydrofolic acid. Mammalian cells can bypass the metabolic blocks by importing preformed folates, but most bacterial cells are unable to do so; thus, the action of the antibiotics is directed selectively against the bacteria. Absence of the pyrimidine thymine is believed to be the mechanism of bacterial death, because addition of the nucleoside thymidine to media allows the bacteria to survive.

The results of *in vitro* tests for susceptibility of enterococci and trimethoprim-sulfamethoxazole must be viewed with caution because enterococci are able to bypass the action of the drugs by incorporating preformed exogenous folates. Several instances of discrepancies of *in vitro* results and clinical outcome have been reported.[91,300]

Trimethoprim and sulfamethoxazole represent one of the few examples in which routine combination therapy is rational. It is most important that antimicrobial combinations that might be used clinically are not antagonistic. Studies of synergism have a very important place, therefore, in the research laboratory.

Hospital microbiology laboratory personnel may occasionally be asked to assist the physician who wishes to employ combination therapy. Unfortunately, the tests for synergism, as currently performed, are cumbersome, labor intensive, and impractical for general use in most hospital laboratories. When both antibiotics in a combination exert independent activity, it may be difficult and rather arbitrary to decide when synergistic activity has been demonstrated. The polymicrobial nature of many infections in immunocompromised patients complicates the analysis even further.

COMMONLY USED TESTS

Krogstad and Moellering provide a detailed account of the theory and practice of synergy testing.[139] The following is a brief description of the most commonly used tests.

CHECKERBOARD ASSAY

If multiple antibiotics or multiple dilutions must be tested, a "checkerboard" assay may be useful.[109] The assay may be done in tubes or microtiter plates, in broth, or on agar. Broth is preferred if an assessment of bactericidal activity is also desired. Serial twofold dilutions of each drug are selected so that concentrations from one sixteenth to at least double the MIC are included (Fig. 15-31). Drug A is serially diluted along the ordinate, while drug B is diluted along the abscissa. The resulting checkerboard yields every combination of the two antibiotics, from a tube that contains the highest concentration of each at the opposite corner. The results of this test may be displayed graphically to

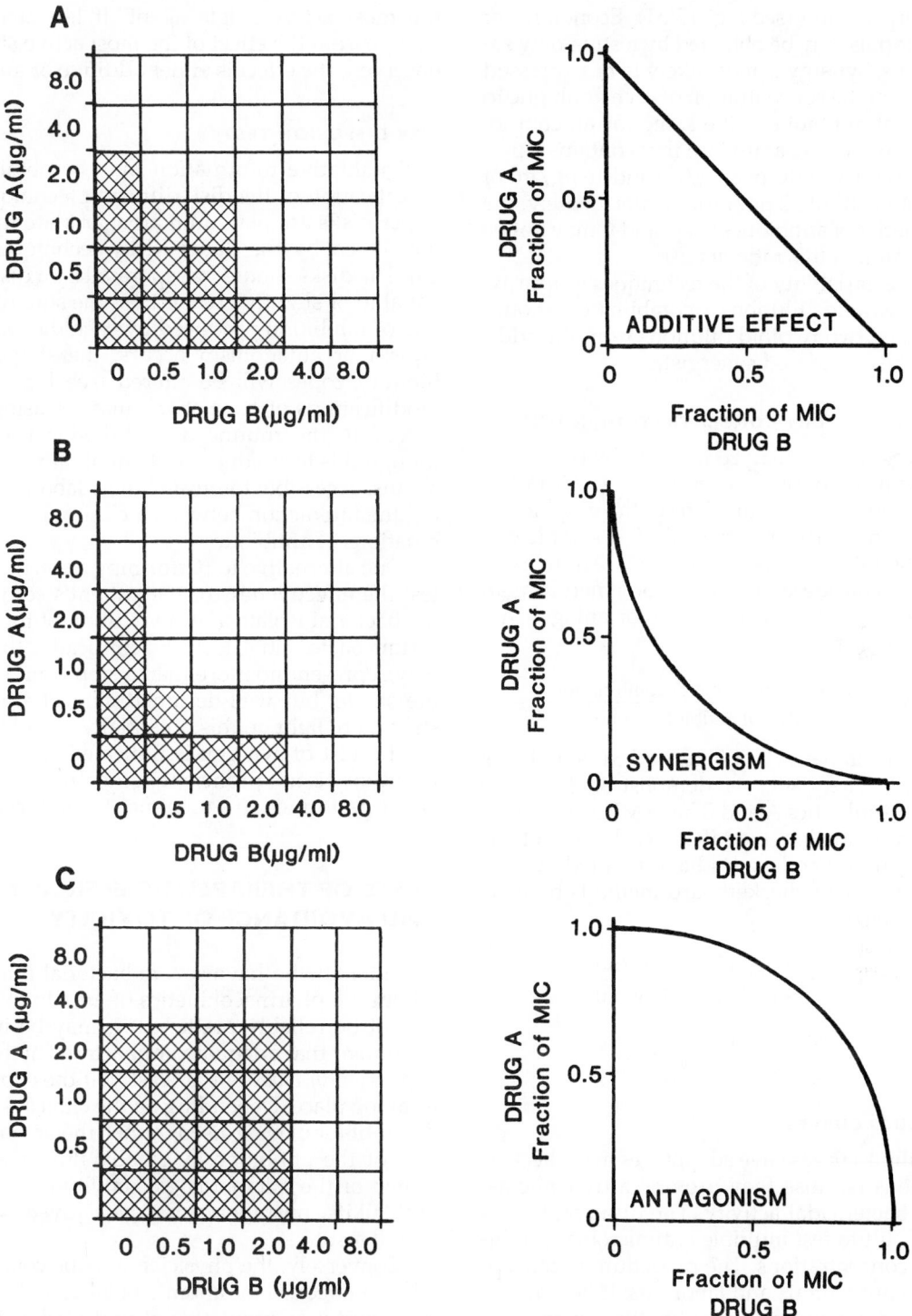

Figure 15-31

Checkerboard titration for antimicrobial synergy. Each square represents a tube or microtiter well. Increasing concentrations of antibiotic *A* are distributed along the vertical axis, and those of antibiotic *B* are distributed along the horizontal axis. The hatched squares indicate bacterial growth. In panel **A** the antibiotics demonstrate additive effect; the isobologram on the *right* is a straight line. Synergism is demonstrated in panel **B**, where the isobologram is concave. Antagonistic interactions in panel **C** result in a convex isobologram.

facilitate interpretation (see Fig. 15-31). Economies of time and materials may be obtained by testing only selected dilutions. Synergy is most likely to be expressed when the ratio of the concentration of each antibiotic to the MIC of that antibiotic is the same for all components of the mixture (eg, a mixture that contains 4 µg/ml of drug A with an MIC of 8 µg/ml and 16 µg/ml of drug B with an MIC of 32 µg/ml).[18] Unfortunately, the pharmacokinetics of antibiotics vary, and it may not be possible to maintain this ratio in vivo.

Because the variability of the techniques is approximately one twofold dilution, a combination should differ by at least two twofold dilutions from the additive result to be considered synergistic.

FRACTIONAL INHIBITORY CONCENTRATION INDEX

Many investigators analyze the data by constructing a fractional inhibitory concentration (FIC) index, which is mathematically equivalent to the graphic depiction of the checkerboard results.[18,139] A sample calculation of the FIC index is given below. An index of less than 0.5 is considered evidence for synergism; an index of greater than 2.0 is evidence for antagonism. For each antibiotic tested:

$$\text{FIC index} = \frac{\text{MIC of antibiotic in combination}}{\text{MIC of antibiotic alone}}$$

For example, in panel B of Figure 15-31, antibiotics A and B are synergistic, as demonstrated by the isobologram. Antibiotics A and B have MICs of 4.0 µg/ml alone; in combination, the MIC of each antibiotic is 1 µg/ml. Hsieh and colleagues have pointed out the inherent instability of checkerboard methods because of discontinuous dilutions.[109]

$$\text{FIC (A + B)} = \frac{1 \ \mu g/mL}{4 \ \mu g/mL} + \frac{1 \ \mu g/mL}{4 \ \mu g/mL}$$

$$= \frac{1}{4} + \frac{1}{4} = \frac{1}{2} = 0.5$$

KINETIC KILLING CURVES

Kinetic killing curves have advantages over checkerboard titrations because they provide a dynamic assessment of bactericidal activity. The disadvantage is that it is difficult to test multiple antimicrobial combinations and concentrations. The procedure is conceptually simple but tedious and laborious. If both drugs exert bactericidal activity, it may be difficult to separate additive from synergistic effects. An inoculum of 10^5 to 10^6 CFU/ml is added to a flask that contains a single concentration of both antibiotics and to flasks that contain the same concentration of each antibiotic separately. Quantitative cultures are performed immediately, the flasks are incubated at 35°C, and subsequent quantitative cultures are performed at several additional points over the succeeding 24 hours. The results are plotted on semilogarithmic paper (Fig. 15-32). Synergy is defined as a greater than 100-fold increase in killing at 24 hours, whereas antagonism results in at least a 100-fold decrease in killing as compared with

the most active single agent. If less than a tenfold change from the effect of the most active single drug is observed, the effect is either additive or autonomous.

DISK DIFFUSION TEST

Qualitative information may be obtained from a modification of the disk diffusion technique.[139] Filter-paper disks are placed on an agar plate that has been inoculated by the Bauer-Kirby technique (see Chart 23). The disks should be separated by a distance that is equal to or slightly greater than the sum of the diameters of inhibition produced by each disk alone. If synergism or antagonism occurs, the shape of the inhibitory zones will be altered (see Fig. 15-26). Such modifications of zone shape may occasionally be observed in the routine disk diffusion procedure. Although this technique is only qualitative, it is a simple means, accessible to most clinical laboratories, of testing the interaction between a clinical isolate and combinations of antibiotics.

One alternative to performing synergy studies is to test the effectiveness of the patient's serum in killing the bacterial isolate after institution of therapy (ie, the serum bactericidal test). Scientifically, this approach may represent no more than a step from the dark into the shade, but well-designed clinical studies should shed more light on this potentially useful test.

If a test of synergy is indicated clinically and the laboratory is not proficient in the procedure, the test is better performed in a reference laboratory.

TESTS OF THERAPEUTIC EFFICACY AND AVOIDANCE OF TOXICITY

In patients who have severe bacterial infections or in whom the pharmacokinetics of an administered drug cannot be reliably predicted, it may be important to document that adequate antibacterial activity is being expressed in vivo[5]—or at least that the expected action is taking place. Depending on the clinical situation and the antibiotic being used, either the actual concentration of the antibiotic in a body fluid may be determined or the microbiologic activity of the body fluid with all its constituents may be assayed (serum bactericidal test).

Conversely, the physician may be concerned about adverse effects, if the antimicrobial agent has toxic properties and if accumulation of undesirably high concentrations is a possibility. In this situation, a quantitative assay of the concentration of the drug is essential.

Serum is the body fluid that is assayed most frequently because it is most accessible, reflects best the overall interactions of antibiotic and patient, and has been studied most extensively. Before a laboratory measurement is performed, sufficient time should have elapsed after changes in antimicrobial therapy to allow equilibration of the antibiotic (usually two to three doses). In addition, any clinical manipulation that might alter the interpretation should be considered, such as the institution of hemodialysis that may

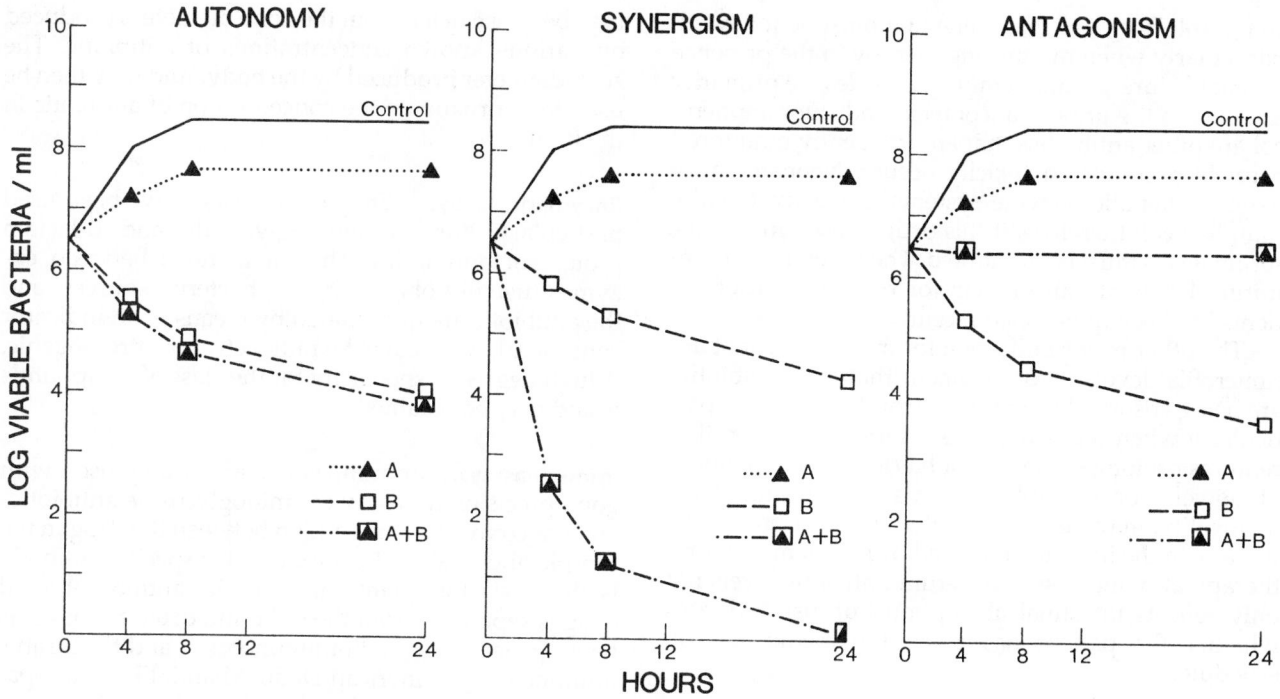

Figure 15-32
Time-kill curve for bactericidal effect and antimicrobial synergy: Tubes containing antibiotic *A*, antibiotic *B*, both antibiotics, or no antibiotic were inoculated with a bacterial isolate. The number of viable bacteria was quantitated by subculture to agar immediately after inoculation and after incubation for 4 and 18 hours. In each illustration, antibiotic *B* is bactericidal and antibiotic *A* is relatively ineffective; uninhibited growth occurs in the absence of any antibiotic. In the *first panel*, additive or autonomous effects are evident; bacterial killing is the same with the combination as with antibiotic *B* alone. Synergistic effects are demonstrated in the *middle panel*, in which the combination of antibiotics results in more rapid killing than does either antibiotic alone. Antagonism is illustrated in the *right panel*, in which the combination results in less bactericidal activity than does antibiotic *B* alone.

remove a drug from the serum more rapidly than the normal degradation process.

The most commonly selected times for obtaining specimens for drug assay are immediately before administration of a dose (trough level) or shortly thereafter (peak level, 30 minutes after completion of an intravenous infusion, 60 minutes after an intramuscular dose, or 60 to 120 minutes after an oral dose). The usefulness of determining both trough and peak levels has been documented only for the aminoglycosides. Antibiotic concentrations vary more at the peak than at the trough, especially after oral administration of the drug; if unexpectedly low levels are found after oral therapy, an assay at a later time, such as after 3 hours, may be considered. The time selected will depend on the clinical situation and whether the study is part of a pharmacokinetic analysis of the therapeutic regimen. Whatever the time or times selected for study, it is essential that both the time when the dose was given and the time when the specimen was collected be indicated accurately on the requisition. Labeling of the specimen as peak or trough is suboptimal. Similarly, it should not be assumed that the dose of antibiotic was given at the exact time specified on the order sheet. Coordination between physicians, nurses, phlebotomists, and

the laboratory is essential if interpretable data are to be generated and, even more importantly, if reporting of misleading data is to be avoided. In addition to information about the patient, the requisition should also contain a list of antibacterial compounds that the patient is receiving, particularly if a microbiologic assay of drug concentration is requested. The antimicrobial properties of some antineoplastic drugs should not be overlooked.

SERUM ANTIMICROBIAL LEVELS

INDICATIONS

The serum concentration of antibiotic (in micrograms per milliliter) should be determined if it is assumed that adequate levels cannot be achieved or if the toxic level is close to the optimum therapeutic level. The overwhelmingly prevalent indication for serum drug assays is the administration of aminoglycoside antibiotics. Many isolates of *Pseudomonas aeruginosa* have MICs to gentamicin of 4 to 8 µg/ml. These concentrations may not be achieved in all patients, even if recommended doses are administered. Gentamicin toxicity is a concern if concentrations exceed

10 μg/ml. It is clear that a fine line must be followed, particularly when monitoring therapy in the presence of renal failure, because aminoglycosides are primarily excreted in the urine. Vancomycin and chloramphenicol are other antibiotics that are frequently monitored because dose-related toxicity occurs. Neonates have deficient hepatic enzyme systems to inactivate chloramphenicol; therefore, if this drug is used in infants, serum levels must be monitored. The necessity of monitoring levels of vancomycin for management of patients has been questioned recently.[30]

The other major indication for measurement of antimicrobial levels is to document that oral antibiotics are being absorbed from the gastrointestinal tract, particularly when the patient has a serious infection that requires prolonged therapy or has lost a large segment of bowel. For example, patients with bacterial osteomyelitis may be treated initially with intravenous therapy in the hospital, followed by supplemental oral therapy at home. Assay of serum antibiotic levels not only reflects intestinal absorption but also indicates whether the patient has taken the medication on schedule.

METHODS FOR ASSAYING ANTIBIOTIC LEVELS

For many years, the standard means of quantitating antibiotics in biologic fluids was microbiologic assay, in which the antibacterial activity of fluids was tested against carefully selected indicator bacterial strains. Although this method is still useful, most modern clinical laboratories employ one of the chemical, physical, or immunologic procedures that have been developed in recent years. The techniques are often similar to those used for other drugs, referred to as therapeutic drug monitoring. These assays may be performed in clinical chemistry or microbiology laboratories; the volume of tests, local resources and interests, and efficiency of operation should determine the location. Much of the technology is more familiar to chemists than to microbiologists. On the other hand, microbiologists are often more conversant with the medical problems related to antimicrobial agents. At the very least, there should be close communication among those involved in the monitoring. The various procedures have been reviewed by Anhalt.[5]

Microbiologic Assay. It is difficult to match the precision and accuracy of the newer methods with microbiologic assays. If the patient is receiving multiple antibiotics, it may also be difficult to find an indicator bacterial strain that discriminates the drug of interest. The assay is usually performed by a modification of the disk diffusion test. Blank paper disks are impregnated with a series of concentrations of antibiotic and with the body fluid to be measured. A uniform suspension of the indicator bacterial strain is made in molten agar maintained at 50°C, after which the agar is poured into Petri dishes. After placement of the disks and overnight incubation of the Petri dishes at 35°C, the zone of bacterial inhibition will vary with the concentration of antibiotic in the disk. A standard curve

may be constructed from the zone diameters produced by various known concentrations of antibiotic. The zone diameter produced by the body fluid may then be used to approximate the concentration of antibiotic in the fluid.

Enzymatic Assays. Enzymatic assays have been used particularly for the aminoglycoside and β-lactam groups of antibiotics. The interactions between enzymes, usually obtained from bacterial sources, and the antibiotic are quantitated by means of an indicator compound, which may be radioactive or chromogenic. A high degree of specificity for the class of compounds tested may be obtained.

Immunoassays. Immunoassays are widely used with good precision for assay of aminoglycoside antibiotics and vancomycin. Competition between the drug in the sample and a labeled compound for specific antibody is the basis for quantitation. If the antibody-bound drug is separated from the unbound drug, the assay is heterogeneous (*eg*, radioimmunoassay and the Stratus immunoassay, American Dade, Miami, FL). If a separation is not performed and the bound drug is quantitated by changes that occur after binding to antibody, the assay is homogeneous (*eg*, EMITr, Syva Co, Palo Alto, CA; TDXr, Abbott Laboratories, North Chicago, IL; and TDAr, Miles Laboratories, Inc., Naperville, IL).

Chromatographic Drug Assays. Chromatographic drug assays are the most versatile assays because only minor modifications of equipment are necessary to test different drugs sequentially; however, these assays are less standardized than immunoassays and require greater preparation time. High-performance liquid chromatography accomplishes a physical separation of compounds on a chromatographic column, after which the separated peaks may be assayed by a variety of methods, most commonly by spectrophotometry.

SERUM ANTIMICROBIAL ACTIVITY (SCHLICHTER TEST)

In vitro measurements of the antibacterial activity of serum has been used for many years to assess the efficacy of antimicrobial therapy. The bactericidal test is also known as the serum killing power assay or the Schlichter test, although Schlichter and MacLean actually measured the inhibitory activity of serum in patients with bacterial endocarditis.[236] Inhibitory end points may be difficult to visualize in tubes that contain serum. Fisher modified Schlichter's test to include a subculture onto agar media for determination of bactericidal activity.[69] The subject has been thoroughly reviewed by Wolfson and Swartz,[292] Reller,[219] and Stratton.[249]

There is a logical rationale for the serum bactericidal test. Determination of the activity of drugs under conditions that more closely approximate the *in vivo* environment than do most other *in vitro* tests is an appealing concept. For example, some antibiotics are highly protein bound, so that only a fraction of the concentration that is measured in an antimicrobial assay is actually free in the serum. The serum bactericidal assay, in contrast, will measure only that fraction of antibiotic that is free for biologic activity.

Although the Schlichter test has been used for 40 years, Wolfson and Swartz noted that there had been only one prospective study in which a statistically significant correlation between the result of the test and clinical outcome was documented.[292] Serum bactericidal activity in nongranulocytopenic patients who had gram-negative sepsis was statistically predictive of outcome; the test may also be useful in granulocytopenic patients.[240]

Only recently has a multicenter prospective study of the original indication for the serum bactericidal test (to guide the therapy for bacterial endocarditis) been reported.[285] Using a standardized microdilution method, Weinstein and colleagues demonstrated that a peak titer of 1:64 and trough titer of 1:32 were 100% predictive of bacteriologic cure; failure to achieve these titers did not predict bacteriologic failure because many patients with streptococcal endocarditis were cured despite low serum bactericidal titers (see Chart 49 for further details).

There are other situations in which the serum bactericidal test may have clinical utility, but documentation is less extensive and less rigorous. Monitoring of therapy in patients with bacterial osteomyelitis, another infection in which bactericidal activity is desirable, is one instance. Statistical association of cure and failure with serum bactericidal levels in adults has been reported in a multicenter collaborative trial.[286] In patients who are receiving combinations of antibiotics, high serum bactericidal titers are associated with *in vitro* synergism against the infecting organism.[134] As mentioned previously, the serum bactericidal test may provide a useful alternative to synergy testing in the clinical laboratory. The test may also be useful as a substitute for or adjunct to measurement of antimicrobial concentrations when monitoring therapy for chronic infections after switching from parenteral to oral therapy.

Determination of the bactericidal activity of body fluids other than serum has been reported, but data are less extensive.[292]

For performance of the serum bactericidal test, the laboratory must have an isolate of the patient's organism and serum specimens (peak and/or trough) obtained as for antimicrobial assay. Weinstein and colleagues found that a peak serum sample was more useful than a trough specimen for predicting the outcome of therapy for endocarditis in adult patients.[285]

There are many variations of the serum bactericidal test, and the interpretation of significant titers has also varied. Woolfrey and colleagues demonstrated that the same methodologic variables that affected the measurement of MBCs of antibiotics were also important for the serum bactericidal assay.[293] They found that the microdilution procedure was less susceptible to methodologic variation than was the macrotube procedure. The inclusion of human serum in the diluent is important because some antibiotics are highly protein bound. The authors have chosen to provide details of a single microdilution protocol (see Chart 49) for which the interpretative criteria for patients with bacterial endocarditis[285] and for cancer patients with bacteremia[240] have been established. This microdilution method has the additional advantage that it can be applied to routine use in the clinical laboratory. A standard method for a macrotube and microdilution serum bactericidal test has been proposed by the NCCLS.[184]

More well-designed, prospective clinical studies are badly needed. Clinicians will undoubtedly continue to request the test because objective guidance of serious, refractory infections is greatly needed. Except in the few situations in which such data are available, the results should be interpreted with caution. Therapy should never be adjusted on the basis of this test alone.[292]

REFERENCES

1. ABRAHAM EP, CHAIN E: An enzyme from bacteria able to destroy penicillin. Nature 146:837, 1940
2. AHMAD MH, RECHENMACHER A, BOCH A: Interaction between aminoglycoside uptake and ribosomal resistance mechanisms. Antimicrob Agents Chemother 18:798–806, 1980
3. AMBLER RP: The structure of β-lactamases. Philos Trans R Soc London B 289:321–331, 1980
4. AMSTERDAM D: Assessing cidal activity of antimicrobial agents: Problems and pitfalls. Antimicrob Newsletter 7:49–56, 1990
5. ANHALT JP: Assays for antimicrobial agents in body fluids. In Balows A, Hausler WJ Jr, Herrmann KL et al (eds): *Manual of Clinical Microbiology*, pp 1192–1198. Washington, DC, American Society for Microbiology, 1991
6. ANHALT JP, WASHINGTON JA II (EDS): *Laboratory Procedures in Clinical Microbiology*, pp 281–313. New York, Springer-Verlag, 1985
7. ARCHER GL: *Staphylococcus epidermidis:* The organism, its disease, and treatment. Curr Clin Topics Infect Dis 5:25–48, 1984
8. BAKER CN, HUANG MB, TENOVER FC: Optimizing testing of methicillin-resistant *Staphlococcus* species. Diagn Microbiol Infect Dis 19:167–170, 1994
9. BAKER CN, STOCKER SA, CULVER DH, THORNSBERRY C: Comparison of the E test to agar dilution, broth microdilution, and agar diffusion susceptibility testing techniques by using a special challenge set of bacteria. J Clin Microbiol 29:533–538, 1991
10. BARG N, CHAMBERS H, KERNODLE D: Borderline susceptibility to antistaphylococcal penicillin is not conferred

exclusively by the hyperproduction of beta-lactamase. Antimicrob Agents Chemother 35:1975–1979, 1991

11. BARRY AL: Procedure for testing antimicrobial agents in agar medium: Theoretical considerations. In Lorian V (ed): *Antibiotics in Laboratory Medicine*, pp 1–26. Baltimore, Williams & Wilkins, 1986

12. BARRY AL, BADAL RE, HAWKINSON RW: Influence of inoculum growth phase on microdilution susceptibility tests. J Clin Microbiol 18:645–651, 1983

13. BARTON AL, DOERN GV: Selective media for detecting gastrointestinal carriage of vancomycin-resistant enterococci. Diagn Microbiol Infect Dis 23:119–122, 1995

14. BAUER AW, KIRBY WMM, SHERRIS JC ET AL: Antibiotic susceptibility testing by a standardized single disk method. Am J Clin Pathol 45:493–496, 1966

15. BAUER AW, PERRY DM, KIRBY WMM: Single-disk antibiotic-sensitivity testing of staphylococci. Arch Intern Med 104:208–216, 1959

16. BÉDOS J-P, CHEVRET C, CHASTANG C, GESLIN P, RÉGNIER, FRENCH COOPERATIVE PNEUMOCOCCUS STUDY GROUP: Epidemiological features of and risk factors for infection by *Streptococcus pneumoniae* strains with diminished susceptibility to penicillin: findings of a French survey. Clin Infect Dis 22:63–72, 1996

17. BELL SM, PLOWMAN D: Mechanisms of ampicillin resistance in *Haemophilus influenzae* from respiratory tract. Lancet 1:279–280, 1980

18. BERENBAUM MC: A method for testing for synergy with any number of agents. J Infect Dis 137:122–130, 1978

19. BISHOP RE, WEINER JH: Hypothesis: coordinate regulation of murein peptidase activity and AmpC β-lactamase synthesis in *Escherichia coli*. FEBS Letters 304:103–108, 1992

20. BLAZQUEZ J, BAQUERO MR, CANTON R, ALOS I, BAQUERO F: Characterization of a new TEM-type beta-lactamase resistant to clavulanate, sulbactam, and tazobactam in a clinical isolate of *Escherichia coli*. Antimicrob Agents Chemother 37:2059–2063, 1993

21. BLAZQUEZ J, MOROSINI M-I, NEGRI M-C, GONZALEZ-LEIZA M, BAQUERO F: Single amino acid replacements at positions altered in naturally occurring extended-spectrum TEM β-lactamases. Antimicrob Agents Chemother 39:145–149, 1995

22. BOWLER LD, ZHANG Q-Y, RIOU J-Y, SPRATT BG: Interspecies recombination between the *penA* genes of *Neisseria meningitidis* and commensal *Neisseria* species during the emergence of penicillin resistance in *N. meningitidis*: natural events and laboratory simulation. J Bacteriol 176:333–337, 1994

23. BOYCE JM, LONKS JR, MEDEIROS AA, PAPA EF, CAMPBELL S: Spurious oxacillin resistance in *Staphylococcus aureus* because of defective oxacillin disks. J Clin Microbiol 26:1425–1427, 1988

24. BREIMAN RF, BUTLER JC, TENOVER FC, ELLIOTT JA, FACKLAM RR: Emergence of drug-resistant pneumococcal infections in the United States. JAMA 271:1831–1835, 1994

25. BROOK I: Penicillin failure and copathogenicity in streptococcal pharyngotonsillitis. J Fam Pract 38:175–179, 1994

26. BRYAN LE, KEWAN S: Roles of ribosomal binding membrane potential and electron transport in bacterial uptake of streptomycin and gentamicin. Antimicrob Agents Chemother 23:835–845, 1983

27. BURNS JL, MENDELMAN PM, LEVY J, STULL TL, SMITH AL: A permeability barrier as a mechanism of chloramphenicol resistance in *Haemophilus influenzae*. Antimicrob Agents Chemother 27:46–54, 1985

28. BUSH K: β-lactamase inhibitors from laboratory to clinic. Clin Microbiol Rev 1:109–123, 1988

29. BUSH K, JACOBY GA, MEDEIROS AA: A functional classification scheme for β-lactamase and its correlation with molecular structure. Antimicrob Agents Chemother 39:1211–1233, 1995

30. CANTU TG, YAMANAKA-YUEN NA, LIETMAN PS: Serum vancomycin concentrations: reappraisal of their clinical value. Clin Infect Dis 18:533–543, 1994

31. CENTERS FOR DISEASE CONTROL AND PREVENTION: Fluoroquinolone resistance in *Neisseria gonorrhoeae*—Colorado and Washington, 1995. MMWR—Morbid Mortal Wkly Rep 44:761–764, 1995

32. CENTERS FOR DISEASE CONTROL AND PREVENTION: Defining the public health impact of drug-resistant *Streptococcus pneumoniae*: report of a working group. MMWR—Morbid Mortal Wkly Rep 45:Suppl RR-1, February 16, 1996

33. CERCENADO E, GARCIA-LEONI MF, DIAZ MD ET AL: Emergence of teicoplanin-resistant coagulase-negative staphylococci. J Clin Microbiol 34:1765–1768, 1996

34. CHAMBERS HF, SACHDEVA M: Binding of β-lactam antibiotics to penicillin-binding proteins in methicillin-resistant *Staphylococcus aureus*. J Infect Dis 161:1170–1176, 1990

35. CHANG S-C, HSIEH W-C, LUH K-T: Influence of β-lactamase inhibitors on the activity of oxacillin against methicillin-resistant *Staphylococcus aureus*. Diagn Microbiol Infect Dis 21:81–84, 1995

36. CHOW JW, SHLAES DM: Imipenem resistance associated with the loss of a 40 kDa outer membrane protein in *Enterobacter aerogenes*. J Antimicrob Chemother 28:499–504, 1991

37. COLLATZ E, LABIA R, GUTMANN L: Molecular evolution of ubiquitous β-lactamases towards extended-spectrum enzymes active against newer β-lactam antibiotics. Molec Microbiol 4:1615–1620, 1990

38. COUDRON PE, JONES DL, DALTON HP ET AL: Evaluation of laboratory tests for detection of methicillin-resistant *Staphylococcus aureus* and *Staphylococcus epidermidis*. J Clin Microbiol 24:764–769, 1986

39. COURVALIN P: Transfer of antibiotic resistance genes between gram-positive and gram-negative bacteria. Antimicrob Agents Chemother 38:1447–1451, 1994

40. COYLE MB, MCGONAGLE LA, PLORDE JJ ET AL: Rapid antimicrobial susceptibility testing of isolates from blood cultures by direct inoculation and early reading of disk diffusion tests. J Clin Microbiol 20:473–477, 1984

41. D'AMATO RF, ISENBERG HD, MCKINLEY GA ET AL: Collaborative evaluation of the UniScept qualitative antimicrobial susceptibility test. J Clin Microbiol 21:293–297, 1985

42. DAUM RS, GUPTA S, SABBAGH, MILEWSKI WM: Characterization of *Staphylococcus aureus* isolates with decreased susceptibility to vancomycin and teicoplanin: isolation and purification of a constitutively produced protein

associated with decreased susceptibility. J Infect Dis 166:1066–1072, 1992

43. DeGirolami PC, Eichelberger KA, Salfity LC et al: Evaluation of the AutoSCAN-3, a device for reading microdilution trays. J Clin Microbiol 18:1292–1295, 1983

44. Dennstedt FE, Stager CE, Davis JR: Rapid method for identification and susceptibility testing of *Escherichia coli* bacteriuria. J Clin Microbiol 18:150–153, 1983

45. Dillon JR, Tostowaryk W, Pauze M: Spread of penicillinase-producing and transfer plasmids from the gonococcus to *Neisseria meningitidis*. Lancet 1:779–781, 1983

46. Doern GV: Antimicrobial resistance among clinical isolates of *Haemophilus influenzae* and *Branhamella catarrhalis*. Clin Microbiol Newsletter 20:185–187, 1988

47. Doern GV, Daum GS, Tubert TA: *In vitro* chloramphenicol susceptibility testing of *Haemophilus influenzae*: Disk diffusion procedures and assays for chloramphenicol acetyltransferase. J Clin Microbiol 25: 1453–1455, 1987

48. Doern GV, Jones RN: Antimicrobial susceptibility testing of *Haemophilus influenzae, Branhamella catarrhalis*, and *Neisseria gonorrhoeae*. Antimicrob Agents Chemother 32: 1747–1753, 1988

49. Doern GV, Jones RN, Gerlach EH et al: Multicenter clinical laboratory evaluation of a β-lactamase disk assay employing a novel chromogenic cephalosporin, S1. J Clin Microbiol 33:1665–1667, 1995

50. Doern GV, Jorgensen JH, Thornsberry C et al: Prevalence of antimicrobial resistance among clinical isolates of *Haemophilus influenzae*: A collaborative study. Diagn Microbiol Infect Dis 4:95–107, 1986

51. Doern GV, Jorgensen JH, Thornsberry C et al: National collaborative study of the prevalence of antimicrobial resistance among clinical isolates of *Haemophilus influenzae*. Antimicrob Agents Chemother 32:180–185, 1988

52. Doern GV, Tubert TA: Detection of beta-lactamase activity among clinical isolates of *Branhamella catarrhalis* with six different beta-lactamase assays. J Clin Microbiol 25:1380–1383, 1987

53. Doern GV, Tubert TA: *In vitro* activities of 39 antimicrobial agents for *Branhamella catarrhalis* and comparison of results with different quantitative susceptibility test methods. Antimicrob Agents Chemother 32: 259–261, 1988

54. Dougherty TJ, Koller AE, Tomasz A: Penicillin-binding proteins of penicillin-susceptible and intrinsically resistant *Neisseria gonorrhoeae*. Antimicrob Agents Chemother 18:730–737, 1980

55. Douglas CP, Siarakas S, Gottlieb T: Evaluation of E-test as a rapid method for determining MICs for nutritionally variant streptococci. J Clin Microbiol 32: 2318–2320, 1994

56. Dowson CG, Hutchison A, Brannigan JA et al: Horizontal transfer of penicillin-binding protein genes in penicillin-resistant clinical isolates of *Streptococcus pneumoniae*. Proc Natl Acad Sci USA 86:8842–8846, 1989

57. Dowson CG, Hutchison A, Woodford N, Johnson AP, George RC, Spratt BG: Penicillin-resistant viridans streptococci have obtained altered penicillin-binding protein genes from penicillin-resistant strains of *Streptococcus pneumoniae*. Proc Natl Acad Sci USA 87: 5858–5862, 1990

58. Dutka-Malen S, Leclercq R, Coutant V et al: Phenotypic and genotypic heterogeneity of glycopeptide resistance determinants in gram-positive bacteria. Antimicrob Agents Chemother 34:1875–1879, 1990

59. Eagle H, Musselman AD: The rate of bacterial action of penicillin *in vitro* as a function of its concentration, and its paradoxically reduced activity at high concentrations against certain organisms. J Exp Med 88:99–131, 1948

60. Edmond MB, Ober JF, Weinbaum DL et al: Vancomycin-resistant *Enterococcus faecium* bacteremia: risk factors for infection. Clin Infect Dis 20:1126–1133, 1995

61. Eliopoulos GM, Farber BF, Murray BE et al: Ribosomal resistance of clinical enterococcal to streptomycin isolates. Antimicrob Agents Chemother 25:398–399, 1984

62. Eliopoulos GM, Wennersten C, Reiszner E et al: High-level resistance to gentamicin in clinical isolates of *Streptococcus (Enterococcus) faecium*. Antimicrob Agents Chemother 32:1528–1532, 1988

63. Elwell LP, Roberts M, Mayer LW et al: Plasmid-mediated beta-lactamase production in *Neisseria gonorrhoeae*. Antimicrob Agents Chemother 11:528–533, 1977

64. Eng RHK, Smith SM, Cherubin C: Inoculum effect of new beta-lactam antibiotics on *Pseudomonas aeruginosa*. Antimicrob Agents Chemother 26:42–47, 1984

65. Farber BF, Eliopoulos GM, Ward JI et al: Multiply resistant viridans streptococci: Susceptibility to β-lactam antibiotics and comparison of penicillin-binding protein patterns. Antimicrob Agents Chemother 24: 702–705, 1983

66. Farmer TA, Reading C: Beta-lactamases of *Branhamella catarrhalis* and their inhibition of clavulanic acid. Antimicrob Agents Chemother 21:506–508, 1982

67. Faruki H, Kohmescher RN, McKinney WP et al: A community-based outbreak of infection with penicillin-resistant *Neisseria gonorrhoeae* not producing penicillinase (chromosomally mediated resistance). N Engl J Med 313:607–611, 1985

68. Fernandez-Rodriguez A, Canton R, Perez-Diaz JC, Martinez-Beltran J, Picazo JJ, Baquero F: Aminoglycoside-modifying enzymes in clinical isolates harboring extended-spectrum β-lactamases. Antimicrob Agents Chemother 36:2536–2538, 1992

69. Fisher AM: A method for the determination of antibacterial potency of serum during therapy of acute infections: A preliminary report. Bull Johns Hopkins Hosp 90:313–320, 1952

70. Fleming A: On the antibacterial action of cultures of a penicillium with special reference to their use in isolation of *B. influenzae*. Br J Exp Pathol 110:226–236, 1929

71. Fontana R, Grossato A, Ligozzi M et al: *In vitro* response to bactericidal activity of cell wall-active antibiotics does not support the general opinion that enterococci are naturally tolerant to these antibiotics. Antimicrob Agents Chemother 34:1518–1522, 1990

72. Fontana R, Amalfitano G, Rossi L, Satta G: Mechanisms of resistance to growth inhibition and killing by beta-lactam antibiotics in enterococci. Clin Infect Dis 15:486–489, 1992

73. Fontana R, Grossato A, Rossi L, Cheng YR, Satta G: Transition from resistance to hypersusceptibility to

β-lactam antibiotics associated with loss of a low-affinity penicillin-binding protein in a *Streptococcus faecium* mutant highly resistant to penicillin. Antimicrob Agents Chemother 28:678–683, 1985

74. FOSTER JW, WOODRUFF HB: Microbiologic aspects of penicillin. J Bacteriol 46:187–202, 1943

75. FRAIMOW HS, JUNGKIND DL, LANDER DW, DELSO DR, DEAN JL: Urinary tract infection with an *Enterococcus faecalis* isolate that requires vancomycin for growth. Ann Intern Med 121:22–26, 1994

76. FREE L, SAHM DF: Investigation of the reformulated Remel Synergy Quad plate for detection of high-level aminoglycoside and vancomycin resistance. J Clin Microbiol 33:1643–1645, 1995

77. FRÉRE J-M, JORIS B: Penicillin-sensitive enzymes in peptidoglycan biosynthesis. CRC Crit Rev Microbiol 11:299–396, 1985

78. FRIEDEN TR, MUNSLIFF SS, LOW DE ET AL: Emergence of vancomycin-resistant enterococci in New York City. Lancet 342:76–79, 1993

79. FRIEDLAND IR, McCRACKEN GH JR: Management of infections caused by antibiotic-resistant *Streptococcus pneumoniae*. N Engl J Med 331:377–382, 1994

80. FULLER SA, LOW DE, SIMOR AE: Evaluation of a commercial microtiter system (MicroScan) using both frozen and freeze-dried panels for detection of high-level aminoglycoside resistance in *Enterococcus* spp. J Clin Microbiol 28:1051–1053, 1990

81. GAFFNEY DF, FOSTER TJ: Chloramphenicol acetyltransferases determined by R plasmids from gram-negative bacteria. J Gen Microbiol 109:351–358, 1978

82. GAVAN TL, JONES RN, BARRY AL: Evaluation of the Sensititre System for quantitative antimicrobial drug susceptibility testing: A collaborative study. Antimicrob Agents Chemother 17:464–469, 1980

83. GERBERDING JL, MIICK C, LIU HH, CHAMBERS HF: Comparison of conventional susceptibility tests with direct detection of penicillin-binding protein 2a in borderline oxacillin-resistant strains of *Staphylococcus aureus*. Antimicrob Agents Chemother 35:2574–2579, 1991

84. GERLACH EH, JONES RN, BARRY AL: Collaborative evaluation of the Microbial Profile System for quantitative antimicrobial susceptibility testing. J Clin Microbiol 17:436–444, 1983

85. GEHRLEIN M, LEYING H, CULLMANN W, WENDT S, OPFERKUCH W: Imipenem resistance in *Acinetobacter baumanii* is due to altered penicillin-binding proteins. Chemotherapy 37:405–412, 1991

86. GIGER O, MORTENSEN JE, CLARK RB, EVANGELISTA A: Comparison of five different susceptibility test methods for detecting antimicrobial agent resistance among *Haemophilus influenzae* isolates. Diagn Microbiol Infect Dis 24:143–153, 1996

87. GLUPCZYNSKI Y, LABBE M, HANSEN W, CROKAERT F, YOURASSOWSKY E: Evaluation of the E-test for quantitative antimicrobial susceptibility testing of *Helicobacter pylori*. J Clin Microbiol 29:2072–2075, 1991

88. GOLDMAN RC, CAPOBIANCO JO: Role of an energy-dependent efflux pump in plasmid pNE24-mediated resistance to 14- and 15-membered macrolides in *Staphylococcus epidermidis*. Antimicrob Agents Chemother 34:1973–1980, 1990

89. GOLDSTEIN FW, GUTMANN L, WILLIAMSON R ET AL: In vivo and in vitro emergence of simultaneous resistance to both beta lactam and aminoglycoside antibiotics in a strain of *Serratia marcescens*. Ann Microbiol (Inst Pasteur) 134A:329–337, 1983

90. GOLLEDGE CL, STINGEMORE N, ARAVENA M ET AL: Septicemia caused by vancomycin-resistant *Pediococcus acidilactici*. J Clin Microbiol 28:1678–1679, 1990

91. GOODHART GL: *In vivo* v. *in vitro* susceptibility of enterococcus to trimethoprim-sulfamethoxazole. JAMA 252:2748–2749, 1984

92. GUNKEL AG, HECHLER U, MARTIN HH: State of penicillin-binding proteins and requirements for their bactericidal interaction with beta-lactam antibiotics in *Serratia marcescens* highly resistant to extended-spectrum beta-lactams. J Gen Microbiol 137:243–252, 1991.

93. GUNNISON JB, FRAHER MA, JAWETZ E: Persistence of *Staphylococcus aureus* in penicillin in vitro. J Gen Microbiol 34:335–349, 1963

94. HACKENBECK R, BRIESE, CHALKLEY L ET AL: Antigenic variation of penicillin-binding proteins from penicillin-resistant clinical strains of *Streptococcus pneumoniae*. J Infect Dis 164:313–319, 1991

95. HACKENBECK R, ELLERBROOK H, BRIESE T, HANDWERGER S, TOMASZ A: Penicillin-binding proteins of penicillin-susceptible and -resistant pneumococci: immunological relatedness of altered proteins and changes in peptides carrying the β-lactam binding site. Antimicrob Agents Chemother 30:553–558, 1986

96. HALL WH, SCHIERL EA, MACCANI JE: Comparative susceptibility of penicillinase-positive and -negative *Neisseria gonorrhoeae* to 30 antibiotics. Antimicrob Agents Chemother 15:562–567, 1979

97. HAMILTON-MILLER JMT, SHAH S, YAN TS: Errors arising from incorrect orientation of E test strips. J Clin Microbiol 33:1966–1967, 1995

98. HANDWERGER S, TOMASZ A: Antibiotic tolerance among clinical isolates of bacteria. Rev Infect Dis 7:368–386, 1985

99. HANSEN SL, WALSH TJ: Detection of intrinsically resistant (heteroresistant) *Staphylococcus aureus* with the Sceptor and AutoMicrobic systems. J Clin Microbiol 25:412–415, 1987

100. HARTMAN BJ, TOMASZ A: Low-affinity penicillin-binding protein associated with β-lactam resistance in *Staphylococcus aureus*. J Bacteriol 158:513–516, 1984

101. HASHEMI FB, SCHUTZE GE, MASON EO JR: Discrepancies between results of E-test and standard microbroth dilution testing of *Streptococcus pneumoniae* for susceptibility to vancomycin. J Clin Microbiol 34:1546–1547, 1996

102. HAYS RC, MANDELL GL: pO₂, pH, and redox potential of experimental abscesses. Proc Soc Exp Biol Med 147:29–30, 1974

103. HECHLER U, VAN DEN WEGHE M, MARTIN HH, FRERE JM: Overproduced beta-lactamase and the outer-membrane barrier as resistance factors in *Serratia marcescens* highly resistant to beta-lactamase-stable beta-lactam antibiotics. J Gen Microbiol 135:1275–1290, 1989

104. HEDGE PJ, SPRATT BG: Amino acid substitutions that reduce the affinity of penicillin-binding protein 3 of *Escherichia coli* for cephalexin. Eur J Biochem 151:111–121, 1985

105. HERMAN DJ, GERDING DN: Antimicrobial resistance among enterococci. Antimicrob Agents Chemother 35: 1–4, 1991

106. HINDLER JA, INDERLIED CB: Effect of the source of Mueller-Hinton agar and resistance frequency on the detection of methicillin-resistant Staphylococcus aureus. J Clin Microbiol 21:205–210, 1985

107. HOLM SE: Interaction between β-lactam and other antibiotics. Rev Infect Dis 8:S305–S314, 1986

108. HORNE D, TOMASZ A: Hypersusceptibility of penicillin-treated group B streptococci to bactericidal activity of human polymorphonuclear leukocytes. Antimicrob Agents Chemother 19:745–753, 1981

109. HSIEH MH, YU CM, YU VL, CHOW JW: Synergy assessed by checkerboard. A critical analysis. Diagn Microbiol Infect Dis 16:343–349, 1993

110. HUANG MB, BAKER CN, BANERJEE S, TENOVER FC: Accuracy of the E-test for determining antimicrobial susceptibilities of staphylococci, enterococci, Campylobacter jejuni, and gram-negative bacteria resistant to antimicrobial agents. J Clin Microbiol 30:3243–3248, 1992

111. HUNTER TH: Use of streptomycin in treatment of bacterial endocarditis. Am J Med 2:436–442, 1947

112. HUOVINEN P: Trimethoprim resistance. Antimicrob Agents Chemother 31:1451–1456, 1987

113. ISTRE GR, HUMPHREYS JT, ALBRECHT KD ET AL: Chloramphenicol and penicillin resistance in pneumococci isolated from blood and cerebrospinal fluid: A prevalence study in metropolitan Denver. J Clin Microbiol 17: 472–475, 1983

114. IWEN PC, KELLY DM, LINDER J, HINRICHS SH: Revised approach for identification and detection of ampicillin and vancomycin resistance in Enterococcus species by using MicroScan panels. J Clin Microbiol 34:1779–1783, 1996

115. JABES D, NACHMAN S, TOMASZ A: Penicillin-binding protein families: evidence for the clonal nature of penicillin resistance in clinical isolates of pneumococci. J Infect Dis 159:16–25, 1989

116. JACOBY GA, ARCHER GL: New mechanisms of bacterial resistance to antimicrobial agents. N Engl J Med 324: 601–612, 1991

117. JACOBY GA, MEDEIROS AA: More extended-spectrum β-lactamases. Antimicrob Agents Chemother 35: 1697–1704, 1991

118. JARLIER V, NICOLAS M-H, FOURNIER G, PHILIPPON A: Extended broad-spectrum β-lactamases conferring transferable resistance to newer β-lactam agents in Enterobacteriaceae: hospital prevalence and susceptibility patterns. Rev Infect Dis 10:867–878, 1988

119. JETT B, FREE L, SAHM DF: Factors influencing the Vitek gram-positive susceptibility system's detection of vanB-encoded vancomycin resistance in enterococci. J Clin Microbiol 34:701–706, 1996

120. JONES RN, EDSON DC: Antibiotic susceptibility testing accuracy: Review of the College of American Pathologists Microbiology Survey, 1972–1983. Arch Pathol Lab Med 109:595–601, 1985

121. JORGENSEN JH, DOERN GV, MAHER LA ET AL: Antimicrobial resistance among respiratory isolates of Haemophilus influenzae, Moraxella catarrhalis, and Streptococcus pneumoniae in the United States. Antimicrob Agents Chemother 34:2075–2080, 1990

122. JORGENSEN JH, DOERN GV, THORNSBERRY C ET AL: Susceptibility of multiply resistant Haemophilus influenzae to newer antimicrobial agents. Diagn Microbiol Infect Dis 9:27–32, 1988

123. JORGENSEN JH, HOWELL AW, MAHER LA: Antimicrobial susceptibility testing of less commonly isolated Haemophilus species using Haemophilus test medium. J Clin Microbiol 28:985–988, 1990

124. JORGENSEN JH, HOWELL AW, MAHER LA: Quantitative antimicrobial susceptibility testing of Haemophilus influenzae and Streptococcus pneumoniae by using the E-test. J Clin Microbiol 29:109–114, 1991

125. JORGENSEN JH, MAHER LA, HOWELL AW: Use of Haemophilus test medium for broth microdilution antimicrobial susceptibility testing of Streptococcus pneumoniae. J Clin Microbiol 28:430–434, 1990

126. JORGENSEN JH, REDDING JS, MAHER LA ET AL: Improved medium for antimicrobial susceptibility testing of Haemophilus influenzae. J Clin Microbiol 25:2105–2113, 1987

127. JORGENSEN JH, FERRARO MJ, MCELMEEL ML, SPARGO J, SWENSON JM, TENOVER FC: Detection of penicillin and extended-spectrum cephalosporin resistance among Streptococcus pneumoniae clinical isolates by use of the E test. J Clin Microbiol 32:159–163, 1994

128. JOYCE LF, DOWNES J, STOCKMAN K, ANDREW JH: Comparison of five methods, including the PDM epsilometer test (E test), for antimicrobial susceptibility testing of Pseudomonas aeruginosa. J Clin Microbiol 30:2709–2713, 1992

129. KATSANIS GP, SPARGO J, FERRARO MJ, SUTTON L, JACOBY GA: Detection of Klebsiella pneumoniae and Escherichia coli strains producing extended-spectrum β-lactamases. J Clin Microbiol 32:691–696, 1994

130. KELLOGG JA: Inability to adequately control antimicrobial agents on AutoMicrobic System Gram-Positive and Gram-Negative Susceptibility Cards. J Clin Microbiol 21:454–456, 1985

131. KELLY JA, MOEWS PC, KNOX JR, ET AL: Penicillin target enzyme and the antibiotic binding site. Science 218:479–481, 1982

132. KIEHN TE, CAPITOLO C, ARMSTRONG D: Comparison of direct and standard microtiter broth dilution susceptibility testing of blood culture isolates. J Clin Microbiol 16:96–98, 1982

133. KING TC, SCHLESSINGER D, KROGSTAD DJ: The assessment of antimicrobial combinations. Rev Infect Dis 3:627–633, 1981

134. KLASTERSKY J, CAPPEL R, DANEAU D: Clinical significance of in vitro synergism between antibiotics in gram-negative infections. Antimicrob Agents Chemother 2: 470–475, 1972

135. KLUGMAN KP: Pneumococcal resistance to antibiotics. Clin Microbiol Rev 3:171–196, 1990

136. KNAPP CC, LUDWIG MD, WASHINGTON JA, CHAMBER HF: Evaluation of Vitek GPS-SA card for testing of oxacillin against borderline-susceptible staphylococci that lack mec. J Clin Microbiol 34:1603–1605, 1996

137. KNAPP JS, ZENILMAN JM, BIDDLE JW ET AL: Frequency and distribution in the United States of strains of Neisseria gonorrhoeae with plasmid-mediated, high-level resistance to tetracycline. J Infect Dis 155:819–822, 1987

138. KNOX JR, PRATT RF: Different modes of vancomycin and D-alanyl-D-alanine peptidase binding to cell wall peptide and a possible role for the vancomycin resistance protein. Antimicrob Agents Chemother 34: 1342–1347, 1990.

139. KROGSTAD DJ, MOELLERING RC: Antimicrobial combinations. In Lorian V (ed): *Antibiotics in Laboratory Medicine,* pp 537–595. Baltimore, Williams & Wilkins, 1986

140. LANDMAN D, QUALE JM, OYDNA E ET AL: Comparison of five selective media for identifying fecal carriage of vancomycin-resistant enterococci. J Clin Microbiol 34: 751–752, 1996

141. LAWRENCE RM, HOEPRICH PD: Totally synthetic medium for susceptibility testing. Antimicrob Agents Chemother 13:394–398, 1978

142. LECLERCQ R, CORUVALIN P: Bacterial resistance to macrolide, lincosamide, and streptogramin antibiotics by target modification. Antimicrob Agents Chemother 35:1267–1272, 1991

143. LECLERCQ R, DERLOT E, DUVAL J ET AL: Plasmid-mediated resistance to vancomycin and teicoplanin in *Enterococcus faecium*. N Engl J Med 319:157–161, 1988

144. LECLERCQ R, DUTKA-MALEN S, BRISSON-NOEL A, MOLINAS C, DERLOT E, ARTHUR M, DUVAL J, COURVALIN P: Resistance of enterococci to aminoglycosides and glycopeptides. Clin Infect Dis 15:495–501, 1992

145. LIÑARES J, ALONSO T, PÉREZ JL ET AL: Decreased susceptibility of penicillin-resistant pneumococci to twenty-four β-lactam antibiotics. J Antimicrob Chemother 30:279–288, 1992

146. LINDEN PK, PASCULLE AW, MANEZ R ET AL: Differences in outcomes for patients with bacteremia due to vancomycin-resistant *Enterococcus faecium* or vancomycin-susceptible *E. faecium*. Clin Infect Dis 22:663–670, 1995

147. LIU H, LEWIS N: Comparison of ampicillin/sulbactam and amoxicillin/clavulanic acid for detection of borderline oxacillin-resistant *Staphyloccus aureus.* Eur J Clin Microbiol Infect Dis 11:47–51, 1992

148. LIVERMORE DM: Permeation of β-lactam antibiotics into *Escherichia coli, Pseudomonas aeruginosa,* and other gram-negative bacteria. Rev Infect Dis 10:691–698, 1988

149. LIVERMORE DM: Interplay of impermeability and chromosomal β-lactamase activity in imipenem-resistant *Pseudomonas aeruginosa.* Antimicrob Agents Chemother 36:2046–2048, 1992

150. LIVERMORE DM: Determinants of the activity of β-lactamase inhibitor combinations. J Antimicrob Ther 31, Suppl A:9–21, 1993

151. LIVERMORE DM, DAVY KWM: Invalidity for *Pseudomonas aeruginosa* of an accepted model of bacterial permeability to β-lactam antibiotics. Antimicrob Agents Chemother 35:916–921, 1991

152. LORIAN V (ED): *Antibiotics in Clinical Medicine* (2nd ed). Baltimore, Williams & Wilkins, 1986

153. LUCET J-C, CHEVRET S, DECRÉ D ET AL: Outbreak of multiply resistant Enterobacteriaceae in an intensive care unit: epidemiology and risk factors for acquisition. Clin Infect Dis 22:430–436, 1996

154. MAINARDI J-L, SHLAES DM, GOERING RV, SHLAES JH, ACAR JF, GOLDSTEIN FW: Decreased teicoplanin susceptibility of methicillin-resistant strains of *Staphylococcus aureus.* J Infect Dis 171:1646–1650, 1995

155. MALQUIN F, BRYAN LE: Modification of penicillin-binding proteins as mechanisms of β-lactam resistance. Antimicrob Agents Chemother 30:1–5, 1986

156. MANDELL GL, PETRI WA JR: Antimicrobial agents: penicillins, cephalosporins, and other β-lactam antibiotics. In Hardman JG, Limbird LE (eds): Goodman & Gilman's The Pharmacological Basis of Therapeutics (9th ed), pp. 1073–1101. Mc-Graw-Hill, New York, 1996

157. MARLEY EF, MOHLA C, CAMPOS JM: Evaluation of E-test for determination of antimicrobial MICs for *Pseudomonas aeruginosa* isolates from cystic fibrosis patients. J Clin Microbiol 3191–3193, 1995

158. MARTINEZ-MARTINEZ L, ORTEGA MC, SUAREZ AI: Comparison of E-test with broth microdilution and disk diffusion for susceptibility testing of coryneform bacteria. J Clin Microbiol 33:1318–1321, 1995

159. MATES SM, ESENBERG ES, MANDEL LF ET AL: Membrane potential and gentamicin uptake in *Staphylococcus aureus.* Proc Natl Acad Sci USA 79:6693–6697, 1982

160. MARYMONT JHJ, MARYMONT J: Laboratory evaluation of antibiotic combinations: A review of methods and problems. Lab Med 12:47–55, 1980

161. MASSANARI RM, PFALLER MA, WAKEFIELD DS ET AL: Implications of acquired oxacillin resistance in the management and control of *Staphylococcus aureus* infections. J Infect Dis 158:702–709, 1988

162. MASSIDDA O, MONTANARI MP, VARALDO PE: Evidence for a methicillin-hydrolyzing β-lactamase in *Staphylococcus aureus* strains with borderline susceptibility to this drug. FEMS Microbiol Lett 92:223–227, 1992

163. MASTRO TD, SPIKA JS, LOZANO P ET AL: Vancomycin-resistant *Pediococcus acidilactici:* Nine cases of bacteremia. J Infect Dis 161:956–960, 1990

164. MAYER KH: Review of epidemic aminoglycoside resistance worldwide. Am J Med 80(suppl 6B):56–64, 1986

165. MAYER KH, OPAL SM, MEDEIROS AA: Mechanisms of antibiotic resistance. In Mandell GL, Bennett JE, Dolin R (eds): *Principles and Practice of Infectious Diseases,* (4th ed) Churchill Livingstone, New York, 1995, pp. 212–225

166. MCDOUGAL LK, THORNSBERRY C: The role of β-lactamase in staphylococcal resistance to penicillinase-resistant penicillins and cephalosporins. J Clin Microbiol 23: 832–839, 1986

167. MCMURRY L, PETRUCCI RE, LEVY SB: Active efflux of tetracycline encoded by four genetically different tetracycline resistance determinants in *Escherichia coli.* Proc Natl Acad Sci USA 71:3974–3977, 1980

168. MEDEIROS AA: β-Lactamases. Br Med Bull 40:18–27, 1984

169. MEDEIROS AA: Evolution and dissemination of β-lactamases accelerated by generation of β-lactam antibiotics. Clin. Infect. Dis. In Press.

170. MEDEIROS AA, O'BRIEN TF, ROSENBERG EY ET AL: Loss of OmpC Porin in a strain of *Salmonella typhimurium* causes increased resistance to cephalosporins during therapy. J Infect Dis 156:751–757, 1987

171. MENDELMAN PM, CHAFFIN DO, KRILOV LR ET AL: Cefuroxime treatment failure of nontypable *Haemophilus influenzae* meningitis associated with alteration of penicillin-binding proteins. J Infect Dis 162:1118–1123, 1990

172. MENDELMAN PM, WILEY EA, STULL TL ET AL: Problems with current recommendations for susceptibility testing

of *Haemophilus influenzae.* Antimicrob Agents Chemother 34:1480–1484, 1990

173. MEYER KS, URBAN C, EAGAN JA, BERGER BJ, RAHAL JJ: Nosocomial outbreak of *Klebsiella* infection resistant to late-generation cephalosporins. Ann Intern Med 119: 353–358, 1993

174. MEYER RD: *Legionella* infections: A review of five years of research. Rev Infect Dis 5:258–278, 1983

175. MOREILLON P, TOMASZ A: Penicillin resistance and defective lysis in clinical isolates of pneumococci: evidence for two kinds of antibiotic pressure operating in the clinical environment. J Infect Dis 157:1150–1157, 1988

176. MORENO F, CRISP C, JORGENSEN JH, PATTERSON JE: The clinical and molecular epidemiology of bacteremias at a university hospital caused by pneumococci not susceptible to penicillins. J Infect Dis 172:427–432, 1995

177. MORRIS JG JR, SHAY DK, HEBDEN JN ET AL: Enterococci resistant to multiple antimicrobial agents, including vancomycin. Establishment of endemicity in a university medical center. Ann Intern Med 123:250–259, 1995

178. MUÑOZ R, DOWSON CG, DANIELS M ET AL: Genetics of resistance to third-generation cephalosporins in clinical isolates of *Streptococcus pneumoniae.* Molec Microbiol 6:2461–2465, 1992

179. MURRAY BE, CHURCH DA, WANGER A ET AL: Comparison of two β-lactamase-producing strains of *Streptococcus faecalis.* Antimicrob Agents Chemother 30:861–864, 1986

180. MURRAY BE, MEDERSKI-SAMORAJ B, FOSTER SK ET AL: *In vitro* studies of plasmid-mediated penicillinase from *Streptococcus faecalis* suggest a staphylococcal origin. J Clin Invest 77:289–293, 1986

181. NAGARAJAN R: Antibacterial activities and modes of action of vancomycin and related glycopeptides. Antimicrob Agents Chemother 35:605–609, 1991

182. NATIONAL COMMITTEE FOR CLINICAL LABORATORY STANDARDS: Performance Standards for Antimicrobial Disk Susceptibility Tests (Approved Standard, M2-A5). Villanova, PA, National Committee for Clinical Laboratory Standards, 1993

183. NATIONAL COMMITTEE FOR CLINICAL LABORATORY STANDARDS: Methods for Dilution Antimicrobial Susceptibility Tests for Bacteria that Grow Aerobically (Approved Standard, M7-A3). Villanova, PA, National Committee for Clinical Laboratory Standards, 1993 Supplemental Tables Mico S5 1994

184. NATIONAL COMMITTEE FOR CLINICAL LABORATORY STANDARDS: Methods for Determining Bactericidal Activity of Antimicrobial Agents (Approved Standard, M26-P). Villanova, PA, National Committee for Clinical Laboratory Standards, 1987

185. NEU HC: The emergence of bacterial resistance and its influence on empiric therapy. Rev Infect Dis 5:S9–S20, 1983

186. NEYFAKH AA, BORSCH CM, KAATZ GW: Fluoroquinolone resistance protein NorA of *Staphylococcus aureus* is a multidrug efflux transporter. Antimicrob Agents Chemother 37:128–129, 1993

187. NEUMANN MA, SAHM DF, THORNSBERRY C ET AL: New developments in antimicrobial agent susceptibility testing: A practical guide. Cumitech 6A:1–26, 1991

188. NICAS TI, COLE CT, PRESTON DA ET AL: Activity of glycopeptides against vancomycin-resistant gram-positive bacteria. Antimicrob Agents Chemother 33:1477–1481, 1989

189. NICHOLAS RA, STROMINGER JL: Relations between beta-lactamases and penicillin-binding proteins: beta-lactamase activity of penicillin-binding protein 5 from *Escherichia coli.* Rev Infect Dis 10:733–738, 1988

190. NIKAIDO H: Outer membrane barrier as a mechanism of antimicrobial resistance. Antimicrob Agents Chemother 33:1831–1836, 1989

191. NIKAIDO H, ROSENBERG EY, FOULDS J: Porin channels in *Escherichia coli:* studies with β-lactams in intact cells. J Bacteriol 153:232–240, 1983

192. NIKAIDO H, VAARA M: Molecular basis of bacterial outer membrane permeability. Microbiol Rev 49:1–32, 1985

193. NOBLE WC, VIRANI Z, CREE RGA: Co-transfer of vancomycin and other resistance genes from *Enterococcus faecalis* NCTC 12201 to *Staphylococcus aureus.* FEMS Microbiol Lett 93:195–198, 1992

194. NORDMANN P, MARIOTTE S, NAAS T, LABIA R, NICOLAS MH: Biochemical properties of a carbapenem-hydrolyzing beta-lactamase from *Enterobacter cloacae* and cloning of the gene into *Escherichia coli.* Antimicrob Agents Chemother 37:939–946, 1993

195. OKHUYSEN PC, SINGH KV, MURRAY BE: Susceptibility of β-lactamase-producing enterococci to piperacillin with tazobactam. Diagn Microbiol Infect Dis 17:219–224, 1993

196. OLSSON-LILJEQUIST B, LARSSON P, RINGERTZ S, LÖFDAHL S: Use of a DNA hybridization method to verify results of screening for methicillin resistance in staphylococci. Eur J Clin Microbiol Infect Dis 12:527–533, 1993

197. PALLARES R, GUDIOL F, LINARES J ET AL: Risk factors and response to antibiotic therapy in adults with bacteremic pneumonia caused by penicillin-resistant pneumococci. N Engl J Med 317:18–22, 1987

198. PAREDES A, TABER LH, YOW MD ET AL: Prolonged pneumococcal meningitis due to an organism with increased resistance to penicillin. Pediatrics 58:378–381, 1976

199. PARR TR JR, BRYAN LE: Mechanism of resistance of an ampicillin-resistant, β-lactamase-negative clinical isolate of *Haemophilus influenzae* type b to β-lactam antibiotics. Antimicrob Agents Chemother 25:747–753, 1984

200. PASCUAL A, JOYANES P, MARTÍNEZ-MARTÍNEZ L, SUÁREZ AI, PEREA EJ: Comparison of broth microdilution and E-test for susceptibility of *Neisseria meningitidis.* J Clin Microbiol 34:588–591, 1996

201. PATTERSON JE, MASECAR BL, ZERVOS MJ: Characterization and comparison of two penicillinase-producing strains of *Streptococcus (Enterococcus) faecalis.* Antimicrob Agents Chemother 32:122–124, 1988

202. PATTERSON JE, SWEENEY AH, SIMMS M ET AL: An analysis of 110 serious enterococcal infections. Epidemiology, antibiotic susceptibility, and outcome. Medicine (Baltimore) 74:191–200, 1995

203. PATTERSON JE, ZERVOS MJ: Susceptibility and bactericidal activity studies of four β-lactamase-producing enterococci. Antimicrob Agents Chemother 33:251–253, 1989

204. PAYNE DJ, CRAMP R, WINSTANLEY DJ, KNOWLES DJ: Comparative activities of clavulanic acid, sulbactam, and

tazobactam against clinically important β-lactamases. Antimicrob Agents Chemother 38:767–772, 1994

205. PAYNE RH: Human infection with thymine-requiring bacteria. J Med Microbiol :33–42, 1978

206. PECHÈRE JC: Why are carbapenems active against *Enterobacter cloacae* resistant to third generation cephalosporins? Scand J Infect Dis, Suppl 78:17–21, 1991

207. PELLETIER LL JR, BAKER CB: Oxacillin, cephalothin, and vancomycin tube macrodilution MBC result reproducibility and equivalence to MIC results for methicillin-susceptible and reputedly tolerant *Staphylococcus aureus* isolates. Antimicrob Agents Chemother 324:374–377, 1988

208. PERL TM, PFALLER MA, HOUSTON A ET AL: Effect of serum on the *in vitro* activities of 11 broad-spectrum antibiotics. Antimicrob Agents Chemother 32:2234–2239, 1990

209. PETER K, KORFMANN G, WIEDEMANN B: Impact of the ampD gene and its product on beta-lactamase production in *Enterobacter cloacae*. Rev Infect Dis 10:800–805, 1988

210. PETERSON EM, EVANS KD, SHIGEI JT ET AL: Evaluation of four anti-microbic susceptibility testing systems for gram-negative bacilli. Am J Clin Pathol 86:619–623, 1986

211. PETERSON LR, DENNY AE, GERDING DN ET AL: Determination of tolerance to antibiotic bactericidal activity on Kirby-Bauer susceptibility plates. Am J Clin Pathol 74:645–650, 1980

212. PHILIPPON A, LABIA R, JACOBY GA: Extended-spectrum β-lactamases. Antimicrob Agents Chemother 33:1131–1136, 1989

213. PHILLIPS I, KING A, SHANNON K: Prevalence and mechanisms of aminoglycoside resistance. A ten-year study. Am J Med 80:48–55, 1986

214. POLLOCK HM, BARRY AL, GAVAN TL ET AL: Selection of a reference lot of Mueller-Hinton agar. J Clin Microbiol 24:1–6, 1986

215. POOLE K, KREBES K, MCNALLY C, NESHAT S: Multiple antibiotic resistance in *Pseudomonas aeruginosa*: evidence for involvement of an efflux operon. J Bacteriol 175:7363–7372, 1993

216. PÖRNULL KJ, GÖRANSSON E, RYTTING A-S, DORNBUSCH K: Extended-spectrum β-lactamases in *Eschericia coli* and *Klebsiella* spp. in European septicaemia isolates. J Antimicrob Chemother 32:559–570, 1993

217. QUINN JP, DUDEK EJ, DIVINCENZO CA ET AL: Emergence of resistance to imipenem during therapy for *Pseudomonas aeruginosa* infection. J Infect Dis 154:289–294, 1986

218. REIMER LG, STRATTON CW, RELLER LB: Minimum inhibitory and bactericidal concentrations of 44 antimicrobial agents against three standard control strains in broth with and without human serum. Antimicrob Agents Chemother 19:1050–1055, 1981

219. RELLER LB: The serum bactericidal test. Rev Infect Dis 8:803–808, 1986

220. RELLER LB, SCHOENKNECHT FD, KENNY MA ET AL: Antibiotic susceptibility testing of *Pseudomonas aeruginosa*: Selection of a control strain and criteria for magnesium and calcium content in media. J Infect Dis 130:454–462, 1974

221. RICE RJ, BIDDLE JW, JEANLOUIS YA ET AL: Chromosomally mediated resistance in *Neisseria gonorrhoeae* in the United States: Results of surveillance and reporting, 1983–1984. J Infect Dis 153:340–345, 1986

222. RICE LB, CARIAS LL, SHLAES DM: In vivo efficacies of β-lactam-β-lactamase inhibitor combinations against a TEM-26-producing strain of *Klebsiella pneumoniae*. Antimicrob Agents Chemother 38:2663–2664, 1994

223. RICE LB, WILLEY SH, PAPANICOLAOU GA ET AL: Outbreak of ceftazidime resistance caused by extended-spectrum β-lactamases at a Massachusetts chronic-care facility. Antimicrob Agents Chemother 34:2193–2199, 1990

224. RICHMOND MH, SYKES RB: The β-lactamases of gram-negative bacteria and their possible physiological role. Adv Microb Physiol 9:31–88, 1973

225. ROTSTEIN OD, PRUETT TL, SIMMONS RL: Mechanisms of microbial synergy in polymicrobial surgical infections. Rev Infect Dis 7:151–170, 1985

226. RUBENS CE, MCNEILL WF, FARRAR WE JR: Evolution of multiple-antibiotic-resistance plasmids mediated by transposable plasmid deoxyribonucleic acid sequences. J Bacteriol 140:713–719, 1979

227. RUSTHOVEN JJ, DAVIES A, LERNER SA: Clinical isolation and characterization of aminoglycoside-resistant small colony variants of *Enterobacter aerogenes*. Am J Med 67:702–706, 1979

228. SABATH LD, WHEELER N, LAVERDIERE M ET AL: A new type of penicillin resistance of *Staphylococcus aureus*. Lancet 1:443–447, 1977

229. SAHA V, GUPTA S, DAUM RS: Occurrence and mechanisms of glycopeptide resistance in gram-positive cocci. Infect Agents Dis 1:310–318, 1993

230. SANCHEZ ML, BARRETT MS, JONES RN: Use of the E-test to predict high-level resistance to aminoglycosides among enterococci. J Clin Microbiol 30:3030–3032, 1992

231. SANCHEZ ML, FLINT KK, JONES RN: Occurrence of macrolide-lincosamide-streptogramin resistances among staphylococcal clinical isolates at a university medical center. Diagn Microbiol Infect Dis 16:205–213, 1993

232. SANDERS CC, SANDERS WE JR, GOERING RV, WERNER V: Selection of multiple drug resistance to quinolones, beta-lactams, and aminoglycosides with special reference to cross-resistance between unrelated drug classes. Antimicrob Agents Chemother 26:797–801, 1984

233. SANDERS WE JR, SANDERS CC: Inducible beta-lactamases: clinical and epidemiologic implications for use of newer cephalosporins. Rev Infect Dis 10:830–838, 1988

234. SATTA G, CORNAGLIA G, MAZZARIOL A, GOLINI G, VALISENA S, FONTANA R: Target for bacteriostatic and bactericidal activities of β-lactam antibiotics against *Escherichia coli* resides in different penicillin binding proteins (dag). Antimicrob Agents Chemother 39:812–818, 1995

235. SCHIEVEN BC, HUSSAIN Z, LANNIGAN R: Comparison of American MicroScan dry and frozen microdilution trays. J Clin Microbiol 22:495–496, 1985

236. SCHLICHTER JG, MACLEAN H: A method of determining the effective therapeutic level in treatment of sub-acute bacterial endocarditis with penicillin. Am Heart J 34:209–211, 1947

237. SCHOENKNECHT FD: Bacterial tolerance to antimicrobial agents. Clin Microbiol Newsletter 8:72–74, 1986

238. SCHWALBE RS, STAPLETON JT, GILLIGAN PH: Emergence of vancomycin resistance in coagulase-negative staphylococci. N Engl J Med 316:927–931, 1987

239. SCOTT JR: Sex and the single circle: conjugative transposition. J Bacteriol 174:6005–6010, 1992

240. SCULIER JP, KLASTERSKY J: Significance of serum bactericidal activity in gram-negative bacillary bacteremia in patients with and without granulocytopenia. Am J Med 76:429–435, 1984

241. SHAPIRO MA, HEIFETZ CL, SESNIE JC: Comparison of microdilution and agar dilution procedures for testing antibiotic susceptibility of Neisseria gonorrhoeae. J Clin Microbiol 20:828–830, 1984

242. SIEGEL MS, THORNSBERRY C, BIDDLE JW ET AL: Penicillinase-producing Neisseria gonorrhoeae: Results of surveillance in the United States. J Infect Dis 137:170–175, 1978

243. SPIEGEL CA: Laboratory detection of high-level aminoglycoside-aminocyclitol resistance in Enterococcus spp. J Clin Microbiol 26:2270–2274, 1988

244. SPRATT BG: Resistance to antibiotics mediated by target alterations. Science 264:388–393, 1994

245. SPRATT BG: Distinct penicillin binding proteins involved in the division, elongation, and shape of Escherichia coli K12. Proc. Nat. Acad. Sci. USA 72:2999–3003, 1975

246. SPRATT BG, CROMIE KD: Penicillin-binding proteins of gram-negative bacteria. Rev. Infect. Dis. 10:699–711, 1988

247. SREEDHARAN S, ORAM M, JENSEN B, PETERSON LR, FISHER LM: DNA gyrase gyrA mutations in ciprofloxacin-resistant strains of Staphylococcus aureus: close similarity with quinolone resistance mutations in Escherichia coli. J Bacteriol 172:7260–7262, 1990

248. STANECK JL, ALLEN SD, HARRIS EE ET AL: Automated reading of MIC microdilution trays containing fluorogenic enzyme substrates with the Sensititre Autoreader. J Clin Microbiol 22:187–191, 1985

249. STRATTON CW: Serum bactericidal test. Clin Microbiol Rev 1:19–26, 1988

250. STRAUSBAUGH LJ, SANDE MA: Factors influencing the therapy of experimental Proteus mirabilis meningitis in rabbits. J Infect Dis 137:251–260, 1978

251. SWENSON JM, CLARK NC, FERRARO MJ ET AL: Development of a standardized screening method for selection of vancomycin-resistant enterococci. J Clin Microbiol 32:1700–1704, 1994

252. SWENSON JM, FACKLAM RR, THORNSBERRY C: Antimicrobial susceptibility of vancomycin-resistant Leuconostoc, Pediococcus, and Lactobacillus species. Antimicrob Agents Chemother 34:543–549, 1990

253. SWENSON JM, FERRARO MJ, SAHM DF ET AL: Multilaboratory evaluation of screening methods for detection of high-level aminoglycoside resistance in enterococci. J Clin Microbiol 33:3008–3018, 1995

254. SWENSON JM, HILL BC, THORNSBERRY C: Screening pneumococci for penicillin resistance. J Clin Microbiol 24:749–752, 1986

255. TANAKA M, MATSUMOTO T, KOBAYASHI I, UCHINO U, KUMAZAWA J: Emergence of in vitro resistance to fluoroquinolones in Neisseria gonorrhoeae isolated in Japan. Antimicrob Agents Chemother 39:2367–2370, 1995

256. TANZ RR, SHULMAN ST, SROKA PA, MARUBIO S, BROOK I, YOGEV R: Lack of influence of beta-lactamase-producing flora on recovery of group A streptococci after treatment of acute pharyngitis. J Pediatr 117:859–863, 1990

257. TAYLOR DE, CHAU A: Tetracycline resistance mediated by ribosomal protection. Antimicrob Agents Chemother 40:1–5, 1996

258. TAYLOR PC, SCHOENKNECHT FD, SHERRIS JC ET AL: Determination of minimum bactericidal concentrations of oxacillin for Staphylococcus aureus: Influence and significance of technical factors. Antimicrob Agents Chemother 23:142–150, 1983

259. TENOVER FC, BAKER CN, SWENSON JM: Evaluation of commercial methods for determining antimicrobial susceptibility of Streptococcus pneumoniae. J Clin Microbiol 34:10–14, 1996

260. TENOVER FC, SWENSON JM, OHARA CM, STOCKER SA: Ability of commercial and reference antimicrobial susceptibility testing methods to detect vancomycin resistance in enterococci. J Clin Microbiol 33:1524–1527, 1995

261. TENOVER FC, TOKARS J, SWENSON J ET AL: Ability of clinical laboratories to detect antimicrobial agent-resistant enterococci. J Clin Microbiol 31:1695–1699, 1993

262. THAUVIN-ELIOPOULOS C, RICE LB, ELIOPOULOS GM ET AL: Efficacy of oxacillin and ampicillin-sulbactam combination in experimental endocarditis caused by β-lactamase-hyperproducing Staphylococcus aureus. Antimicrob Agents Chemother 34:702–705, 1990

263. THOMSON KS, SANDERS CC: Detection of extended-spectrum β-lactamases in members of the family Enterobacteriaceae: comparison of the double-disk and three-dimensional tests. Antimicrob Agents Chemother 36:1877–1882, 1992

264. THOMSON KS, SANDERS CC, CHMEL H: Imipenem resistance in Enterobacter. Eur J Clin Microbiol Infect Dis 12:610–613, 1993

265. THORNSBERRY C, MCDOUGAL LK: Successful use of broth microdilution in susceptibility tests for methicillin-resistant (heteroresistant) staphylococci. J Clin Microbiol 18:1084–1091, 1983

266. TIPPER DJ, STROMINGER JI: Mechanism of action of penicillins: A proposal based on their structural similarity to acyl-d-alanine-d-alanine. Proc Natl Acad Sci USA 54:1133–1141, 1965

267. THRUPP LD: Susceptibility testing of antibiotics in liquid media. In Lorian V (ed): Antibiotics in Laboratory Medicine, pp 93–150. Baltimore, Williams & Wilkins, 1986

268. TOMASZ A: The mechanism of the irreversible antimicrobial effects of penicillin: How the beta-lactam antibiotics kill and lyse bacteria. Annu Rev Microbiol 33:113–137, 1979

269. TOMZSZ A, DRUGEON HB, DELENCASTRE HM, JABES D, MCDOUGALL L, BILLE J: New mechanism for methicillin resistance in Staphylococcus aureus: clinical isolates that lack the PBP2a gene and contain normal penicillin-binding proteins with modified penicillin-binding capacity. Antimicrob Agents Chemother 33:1869–1874, 1989

270. TORO CS, LOBOS SR, CALDERÓN I, RODRIGUEZ M, MORA GC: Clinical isolate of a porinless Salmonella typhi resistant to high levels of chloramphenicol. Antimicrob Agents Chemother 34:1715–1719, 1990

271. TUOMANEN E, LINDQUIST S, SANDE S, GALLENI M, LIGHT K, GAGE D, NORMARK S: Coordinate regulation of β-lacta-

mase induction and peptidoglycan composition by the *amp* operon. Science 251:201–204, 1991

272. TOMPSETT R, MCDERMOTT W: Recent advances in streptomycin therapy. Am J Med 7:371–381, 1949

273. UBUKATA K, NOBOGUCHI R, MATSUHASHI M ET AL: Expression and inducibility in *Staphylococcus aureus* of the Mec A gene, which encodes a methicillin-resistant *S. aureus*-specific penicillin-binding protein. J Bacteriol 171:2802–2885, 1989

274. VAN DYCK E, SMET H, PIOT P: Comparison of E-test with agar dilution for antimicrobial susceptibility testing of *Neisseria gonorrhoeae*. J Clin Microbiol 32:1586–1588, 1994

275. VARALDO PE, MONTANARI MP, BIAVASCO F, MANSO E, RIPA S, SANTACROCE F: Survey of clinical isolates of *Staphylococcus aureus* for borderline susceptibility to antistaphylococcal penicillins. Eur J Clin Microbiol Infect Dis 12:677–682, 1993

276. VISSER MR, BOGAARDS L, ROZENBERG-ARSKA M, VERHOEF J: Comparison of the autoSCAN-WA and Vitek Automicrobic systems for identification and susceptibility testing of bacteria. Eur J Clin Microbiol Infect Dis 11:979–984, 1992

277. WANGER AR, MURRAY BE: Comparison of enterococcal and staphylococcal beta-lactamase plasmids. J Infect Dis 161:54–58, 1990

278. WARD J: Antibiotic-resistant *Streptococcus pneumoniae*: Clinical and epidemiologic aspects. Rev Infect Dis 3:254–266, 1981

279. WASHINGTON JA II: Discrepancies between *in vitro* activity of and *in vivo* response to antimicrobial agents. Diagn Microbiol Infect Dis 1:25–31, 1983

280. WASHINGTON JA: Functions and activities of the area committee on microbiology of the National Committee for Clinical Laboratory Standards. Clin Microbiol Rev 4:150–155, 1991

281. WATANABE M, IYOBE S, INOUE M, MITSUHASHI S: Transferable imipenem resistance in *Pseudomonas aeruginosa*. Antimicrob Agents Chemother 35:147–151, 1991

282. WAXMAN DJ, STROMINGER JL: Penicillin-binding proteins and the mechanism of action of β-lactam antibiotics. Annu Rev Biochem 52:825–869, 1983

283. WEINSTEIN JW, TALLAPRAGADA S, FARREL P, DEMBRY L-M: Comparison of rectal and perirectal swabs for detection of colonization with vancomycin-resistant enterococci. J Clin Microbiol 34:210–212, 1996

284. WEINSTEIN MP, MURPHY JR, RELLER LB ET AL: The clinical significance of positive blood cultures: A comprehensive analysis of 500 episodes of bacteremia and fungemia in adults: II. Clinical observations, with special reference to factors influencing prognosis. Rev Infect Dis 5:54–70, 1983

285. WEINSTEIN MP, STRATTON CW, ACKLEY A ET AL: Multicenter collaborative evaluation of a standardized serum bactericidal test as a prognostic indicator in infective endocarditis. Am J Med 78:262–269, 1985

286. WEINSTEIN MP, STRATTON CW, HAWLEY HB ET AL: Multicenter collaborative evaluation of a standardized serum bactericidal test as a predictor of therapeutic efficacy in acute and chronic osteomyelitis. Am J Med 80:218–222, 1987

287. WEISBLUM B: Erythromycin resistance by ribosome modification. Antimicrob Agents Chemother 39: 577–585, 1995

288. WELLS VD, WONG ES, MURRAY BE, COUDRON PE, WILLIAMS DS, MARKOWITZ SM: Infections due to beta-lactamase-producing, high-level gentamicin-resistant *Enterococcus faecalis*. Ann Intern Med 116:285–292, 1992

289. WERTZ RK, SWARTZBERG JE: Computerized interpretation of minimum inhibitory concentration antimicrobic susceptibility testing. Am J Clin Pathol 75:312–319, 1981

290. WHITE RL, KAYS MB, FRIEDRICH LV, BROWN EW, KOONCE JR: Pseudoresistance of *Pseudomonas aeruginosa* resulting from degradation of imipenem in an automated susceptibility testing system with predried panels. J Clin Microbiol 29:398–400, 1991

291. WOOLFSON JS, HOOPER DC: Bacterial resistance to quinolones. Rev Infect Dis 11:S960–S968, 1989

292. WOLFSON JS, SWARTZ MN: Serum bactericidal activity as a monitor of antibiotic therapy. N Engl J Med 312: 968–975, 1985

293. WOOLFREY BF, LALLY RT, TAIT KR: Influence of technical factor variations on serum inhibition and bactericidal titers. J Clin Microbiol 23:997–1000, 1986

294. WORLD HEALTH ORGANIZATION: Standardization of methods for conducting microbic sensitivity tests. WHO Tech Rep Ser 210, 1961

295. YAO JDC, LOUIE M, LOUIE L, GOODFELLOW J, SIMOR AE: Comparison of E-test and agar dilution for antimicrobial susceptibility testing of *Stenotrophomonas (Xanthomonas) maltophilia*. J Clin Microbiol 33:1428–1430, 1995

296. YORK MK, GIBBS L, CHEHAB F, BROOKS GF: Comparison of PCR detection of mecA with standard susceptibility testing methods to determine methicillin resistance in coagulase-negative staphylococci. J Clin Microbiol 34:249–253, 1996

297. YOSHIMURA F, NIKAIDO H: Diffusion of β-lactam antibiotics through the porin channels of *Escherichia coli* K-12. Antimicrob Agents Chemother 27:84–92, 1985

298. YOUNG H, MOYES A, HOOD A: Penicillin susceptibility testing of penicillinase producing *Neisseria gonorrhoeae* by the E test: a need for caution. J Antimicrob Chemother 34:585–588, 1994

299. ZAMBARDI G, REVERDY ME, BLAND S, BES M, FRENEY J, FLEURETTE J: Laboratory diagnosis of oxacillin resistance in *Staphylococcus aureus* by a multiplex-polymerase chain reaction assay. Diagn Microbiol Infect Dis 19: 25–31, 1994

300. ZERVOS MJ, SCHABERG DR: Reversal of the *in vitro* susceptibility of enterococci to trimethoprim-sulfamethoxazole by folinic acid. Antimicrob Agents Chemother 28:446–448, 1985

301. ZHANG Q, JONES DM, SAEZ NIETO JA ET AL: Genetic diversity of penicillin-binding protein 2 genes of penicillin-resistant strains of *Neisseria meningitidis* revealed by fingerprinting of amplified DNA. Antimicrob Agents Chemother 34:1523–1528, 1990

302. ZITO ET, DANEO-MOORE L: Transformation of *Streptococcus sanguis* to intrinsic penicillin resistance. J Gen Microbiol 134:1237–1249, 1988

MYCOPLASMAS AND UREAPLASMAS

Mycoplasmas and ureaplasmas are organisms that differ from other bacteria in that they lack a rigid cell wall. Individual cells are bound only by a trilaminar unit membrane. In addition, the amount of genetic material comprising the genome of these organisms is quite small (molecular weight of 4.5×10^8 to 1×10^9 Da). Because of their lower genetic "IQ," these organisms have limited biosynthetic capabilities. Consequently, the cultivation of mycoplasmas and ureaplasmas requires an enriched medium containing precursors for nucleic acid, protein, and lipid biosynthesis. Precursors for nucleic acids and proteins are provided principally by the enriched basal peptone medium and yeast extract, and lipids are provided by the inclusion of serum. In fact, one of the principal criteria used in the taxonomic classification of these organisms is the requirement for the complex lipid cholesterol in the growth medium by certain mycoplasma and mycoplasma-like organisms.[301,307] All *Mycoplasma* species produce ATP by substrate-level phosphorylation effected by phosphoglyceric acid kinase and pyruvate kinase, two enzymes of the glycolytic pathway from glucose to pyruvate.[222] These two enzymes appear to be the major source of most of the

ATP synthesized by organisms in the class *Mollicutes*. These organisms are also much smaller than most bacteria, measuring 0.2 to 0.3 μm; hence, they are able to pass through bacteriologic filters. The lack of a typical bacterial cell wall containing peptidoglycans renders these organisms insensitive to cell wall–active antimicrobial agents, such as penicillins and cephalosporins.[19,239] Because of this, the recovery of these organisms from clinical specimens may have significant therapeutic implications.

Mycoplasmas and ureaplasmas have been recovered from humans, animals, birds, insects, and plants, although some species have a free-living existence in soil and water.[301] New species in both animals and plants are being continually identified and reported in the taxonomic literature. The human mycoplasmas belong to the genus *Mycoplasma* and to the genus *Ureaplasma*, which contains those mycoplasmas that are able to hydrolyze urea. Several species in the genus *Mycoplasma* and only one species in the genus *Ureaplasma*, *U. urealyticum*, are found in human clinical specimens.

With the exception of *M. pneumoniae*, the role of other mycoplasmas, specifically *M. hominis* and *U. urealyticum*, in human disease is controversial. *M. pneumoniae* is the well-recognized cause of atypical pneumonia, whereas *M. hominis* and *U. urealyticum* are

Color Plates for Chapter 16 are found between pages 784 and 785.

associated primarily with genital tract colonization and disease in adults and respiratory tract colonization and disease in newborns.[47,63,257] These two species are associated with and implicated as causative agents in a wide variety of pathologic conditions. However, these same species may also be isolated from asymptomatic individuals, suggesting that they may behave principally as opportunistic pathogens.[183,186,187] *M. genitalium*, a recently described fastidious human species, has been isolated from both the genital and respiratory tracts.[7,308] Its role in disease is also somewhat unclear. Other *Mycoplasma* species are found as part of the normal flora of the mouth, particularly in the gingival areas surrounding the teeth. In the late 1980s, another "new" mycoplasma, termed "*M. incognitus*" at that time, was detected in autopsy specimens from several patients who had AIDS and rapidly progressive disease, and it has been suggested that this organism may be either another opportunistic infection in these patients or may indeed behave as a sexually transmissible cofactor that hastens disease progression.[169,199] Several other newly described mycoplasmas have been isolated from human immunodeficiency virus (HIV)-infected patients, and these discoveries have spurred a renewed interest in the virulence factors of mycoplasmas and in methods for their detection and identification. In this chapter, emphasis will be placed on the clinical significance of *M. pneumoniae* and the genital mycoplasmas (*M. hominis* and *U. urealyticum*) and the methods used for the isolation of these bacteria in the clinical laboratory.

TAXONOMY OF MYCOPLASMAS AND UREAPLASMAS

Mycoplasmas and ureaplasmas are classified in the class *Mollicutes*. The name **mollicutes** means "soft skin," referring to the lack of a rigid bacterial cell wall.

Analysis of ribosomal RNA (rRNA) sequences have revealed that the mollicutes are most closely related to the bacillus–lactobacillus–streptococcus subdivision of the eubacteria, with the closest bacterial relatives being members of the clostridia, lactobacilli, and the genus *Erysipelothrix*.[216,242,331,332] In 1993, a proposal for revision of the taxonomy of the class *Mollicutes* was put forward by Tully and colleagues (Table 16-1).[303] According to this proposal, the class *Mollicutes* contains four orders: *Mycoplasmatales*, *Entomoplasmatales*, *Acholeplasmatales*, and *Anaeroplasmatales*. The order *Anaeroplasmatales* is composed of a single family (*Anaeroplasmataceae*) containing two species, *Anaeroplasma* and *Asteroleplasma*. These two species are strictly anaerobic in their metabolism. *Anaeroplasma* species require cholesterol for growth, whereas members of the genus *Asteroleplasma* do not. Both of these species are found in the rumens of cattle and sheep. Members of the order *Acholeplasmatales* do not require sterols for growth and are found preponderantly in plants, animals, and insects. The presence of these organisms in animal tissues is documented by the occurrence of acholeplasmas as contaminants in tissue culture media that are supplemented with animal serum. Two species, *Acholeplasma laidlawii* and *Acholeplasma ocula*, have been isolated from humans.[180,230,322] *A. laidlawii* is immunologically related to both *M. pneumoniae* and *M. genitalium*.[36] Because sterol compounds are not required for growth, acholeplasmas may be cultivated in medium lacking exogenous serum.

In the recent taxonomic proposal, a new order—*Entomoplasmatales*—was created to accommodate the families *Entomoplasmataceae* and *Spiroplasmataceae*. The *Entomoplasmataceae* contains two genera—*Entoplasma* and *Mesoplasma*—both of which are found in insects and plants.[303] The genus *Entoplasma* contains sterol-requiring species that grow optimally at 30°C, whereas the genus *Mesoplasma* contains species that do not require cholesterol but grow best at 30°C in cholesterol- or serum-free media supplemented with Tween 80

TABLE 16-1
TAXONOMY OF THE CLASS *MOLLICUTES*

ORDER	FAMILY	GENUS (NO. SPECIES)	STEROLS FOR GROWTH	HABITAT	COMMENTS
Mycoplasmatales	*Mycoplasmataceae*	*Mycoplasma* (>100)	Yes	Humans, animals	Optimal growth at 37°C; metabolize glucose or arginine, or both
		Ureaplasma (6)	Yes	Humans, animals	Optimal growth at 37°C; metabolizes urea
Entomoplasmatales	*Entomoplasmataceae*	*Entoplasma* (5)	Yes	Insects, plants	Optimal growth at 30°C
		Mesoplasma (4)	No	Insects, plants	Optimal growth at 30°C; grow in serum-free medium with 0.04% Tween 80
	Spiroplasmataceae	*Spiroplasma* (11)	Yes	Insects, plants	Optimal growth 30°–37°C
Acholeplasmatales	*Acholeplasmataceae*	*Acholeplasma* (9)	No	Animals, insects, plants	Optimal growth 30°–37°C
Anaeroplasmatales	*Anaeroplasmataceae*	*Anaeroplasma* (4)	Yes	Rumen of cattle, sheep	Anaerobic
		Asteroleplasma (1)	No	Rumen of cattle, sheep	Anaerobic

(0.04%). The family *Spiroplasmataceae* includes the single genus *Spiroplasma*. Members of the genus *Spiroplasma* are spiral-shaped mollicutes that require cholesterol for growth and are found in plants and insects. The genus *Spiroplasma* was formerly included in the order *Mycoplasmatales*.

Members of the order *Mycoplasmatales* require sterols, such as cholesterol, for cultivation in vitro. In the new taxonomic scheme, this order contains a single family—*Mycoplasmataceae*—containing the genus *Mycoplasma* and the genus *Ureaplasma*. The genus *Mycoplasma* contains over 100 species that inhabit a wide variety of plants and animals, including mammals, insects, birds, and reptiles, and may exist as commensels, parasites, and pathogens.[301,302] Thirteen *Mycoplasma* species have been isolated from humans (Table 16-2). *M. hominis*, *M. genitalium*, *M. fermentans*, *M. primatum*, *M. spermatophilum*, and *M. penetrans* are isolated primarily from the human genital tract, whereas *M. pneumoniae*, *M. salivarium*, *M. orale*, *M. buccale*, *M. faucium*, and *M. lipophilum* may be recovered from the human respiratory tract. The ecologic niche of *M. pirum* in humans is uncertain. *M. salivarium* is found in the gingival crevices and may play a role in certain types of periodontal disease. *M. orale*, *M. faucium*, *M. buccale*,

and *M. lipophilum* are considered part of the normal upper respiratory tract flora and are nonpathogenic. *M. fermentans* is a very infrequent isolate from the genital tract; however, this particular species is the same as "*M. incognitus*," the "virus-like infectious agent" recently recovered from AIDS patients (see later discussion).[245] *M. penetrans*, a relatively new addition to the genus, has been isolated from the urine of AIDS patients and along with *M. fermentans* may act as an opportunist or as a significant immunosuppressive agent itself (discussed later).

As with other bacteria, the human mycoplasmas recovered from clinical material differ in certain phenotypic characteristics that are exploited for their isolation and identification (Table 16-3). *M. pneumoniae* ferments glucose with the production of acidic end products, whereas *M. hominis* utilizes arginine, with the formation of basic end products. Cultivation of these organisms is dependent on the use of special agar and broth media that are enriched with factors required for mycoplasmal growth in addition to specific growth substrates, such as glucose and arginine. *M. pneumoniae* strains are antigenically homogeneous, with only one recognized serovar. The number of different *M. hominis* serovars is unknown. Genetic

TABLE 16-2
MYCOPLASMAS AND UREAPLASMAS ISOLATED FROM HUMANS

SPECIES	SITE(S) OF ISOLATION	ASSOCIATED DISEASES
Mycoplasma pneumoniae	Respiratory tract; genital tract (very rare); joint fluid aspirates (very rare)	Pneumonia, bronchitis, bronchiolitis, pharngitis, croup
M. orale	Oro- and nasopharynx	None
M. salivarium	Oro- and nasopharynx	None, questionable role in periodontal disease
M. buccale	Oro- and nasopharynx	None
M. faucium	Oro- and nasopharynx	None
M. lipophilum	Oro- and nasopharynx	None
M. primatum	Oro- and nasopharynx	None
M. hominis	Female genitourinary tract; tissues; blood	Vaginitis, cervicitis, postpartum sepsis, neonatal infections
M. genitalium	Genitourinary tract; respiratory tract; joint fluid aspirates (rare)	May be responsible for some cases of nongonococcal, nonchlamydial urethritis role in respiratory tract infections unknown; presence in joint fluid probably results from bacteremia and seeding of joint spaces
M. fermentans	Genitourinary tract; blood; internal tissues; urine	The "incognitus" strain has been isolated from AIDS and non-AIDS patients; postulated role as cofactor in the pathogenesis of HIV infection
M. penetrans	Genitourinary tract; urine	Possible role as cofactor in HIV pathogenesis; may be another opportunistic agent in AIDS
M. pirum	Isolated from peripheral blood of an AIDS patient (rare)	Recognized previously as a contaminant in tissue culture cells of human origin; role in pathogenesis of HIV infection is not known
Ureaplasma urealyticum	Genitourinary tract	Nongonococcal urethritis (NGU), upper genital tract infection, neonatal infections

TABLE 16-3
CHARACTERISTICS FOR THE IDENTIFICATION OF HUMAN *MYCOPLASMA* SPECIES

SITE OF ISOLATION AND SPECIES	UTILIZATION OF			OPTIMAL pH	TIME TO RECOVERY	GROWTH IN			SEROVARS
	GLUCOSE	ARGININE	UREA			AIR	CO_2	ANAEROBIC	
Respiratory tract									
M. pneumoniae	+	−	−	6.5–7.5	4–21 d	4+	4+	1+	1
M. salivarium	−	+	−	6.0–7.0	2–5 d	2+	NA	4+	1
M. orale	−	+	−	7.0	4–10 d	2+	NA	4+	1
Genital tract									
M. hominis	−	+	−	5.5–8.0	1–5 d	4+	4+	4+	Unknown
Ureaplasma urealyticum	−	−	+	5.5–6.5	1–4 d	4+	4+	4+	14
M. fermentans	+	+	−	7.0	4–21 d	2+	NA	4+	1
Respiratory/genital tracts									
M. genitalium	+	−	−	7.0	Slow	2+	3–4+	1+	Unknown
Acholeplasma laidlawii	+	−	−	6.0–8.0	1–5 d	4+	4+	4+	1

+, positive; − negative; NA, not available; 1+ to 4+, relative degree and rapidity of growth under optimal incubation conditions.

hybridization studies using rRNA probes have supported the serologic studies, with *M. pneumoniae* strains collected over many years displaying similar rRNA composition and *M. hominis* strains showing heterogeneous rRNA patterns.[17,35,337] In addition to certain ultrastructural similarities, both serologic cross-reactivities and genetic homologies have been described between *M. pneumoniae* and *M. genitalium*.[36,158,159]

The genus *Ureaplasma* comprises organisms within the family *Mycoplasmataceae* that are specifically able to hydrolyze urea. The genus currently contains six species: *U. urealyticum, U. diversum, U. gallorale, U. felinum, U. cati,* and *U. canigenitalium*.[4,92,93,108,144,260] *U. urealyticum* is recovered from the human respiratory and genital tracts.[260] As with the *Mycoplasma* species just described, the role of *U. urealyticum* as a primary pathogen in human disease is an area of debate and ongoing study. At the present time, 14 serotypes of *U. urealyticum* have been described in a variety of other animals and nonhuman primates.[4,240] These 14 serotypes are defined by reactivity of isolates with a panel of polyclonal antisera.[240] These serotypes have been subgrouped into two serotype clusters, or biovars, composed of types 1, 3, 6, and 14 (biovar 1) and types 2, 4, 5, 7, 8, 9, 10, 11, 12, and 13 (biovar 2).[91] Organisms belonging to biovar 1 have smaller genomes than the serotypes in biovar 2; biovar 1 has consequently been dubbed the "parvo" (small) biovar.[129] Monoclonal antibodies have been developed against serotypes 1, 3, and 6, and reaction of these defined antibodies on Western immunoblots with clinical isolates of *U. urealyticum* suggest that considerable antigenic diversity exists within the polyclonally defined serotypes.[32] However, this serologic grouping system has been supported by additional studies using cellular protein analysis and DNA restriction endonuclease patterns.[231] Analysis of rRNA with nucleic acid probes has demonstrated significant nucleotide sequence homology among serotypes of the same cluster, with less homology being noted between members of the different clusters. The degree of DNA–DNA hybridization among serotypes 1, 3, and 6 in biovar 1 is 91% to 92%, whereas that among serotypes 2, 4, 5, 7, and 8 in biovar 2 ranges from 69% to 97%. Immunoblot analyses of clinical isolates of *U. urealyticum* serotypes 1, 3, and 6 with monoclonal antibodies showed highly variable patterns compared with each other and with specific reference serotype strains, suggesting that a high degree of antigenic variation exists within and among the various serotypes.[32] Whether divergence in homology between the two biovars indicates separate species or subspecies status within the genus *Ureaplasma* has not yet been resolved. The members of these two biovars also demonstrate diffences in other properties, including restriction fragment length polymorphisms, whole-cell protein patterns on polyacrylamide gel electrophoresis, and sensitivity to manganese salts.[4,91,229,240,277] PCR techniques that detect biovar-specific 16S rRNA have also been developed; these techniques are currently being used to examine reference strains and clinical isolates to determine the relations between biovars and specific disease entities associated with *U. urealyticum*.[241,293]

The other *Ureaplasma* species are found exclusively in animals. *U. diversum* (three serovars) is found in the bovine and ovine respiratory and genital tracts; it is the etiologic agent of maternal and fetal infections, including amnionitis, abortion, low birth weight, infant pneumonia, and neonatal death. *U. gallorale* (one serovar) is a nonpathogenic species found in the respiratory tract of chickens and other fowl.[4,144] Two species—*U. felinum* and *U. cati*—have been recovered from the respiratory tracts of healthy domestic cats.[92] *U. canigenitalium*, the most recently described species, was isolated from oral, nasal, and prepuce cultures of dogs and comprises four serovars.[93] In addition to these six formally described species, genetically and antigenically distinctive avian, porcine, simian, bovine, and caprine–ovine ureaplasmas have also been described but have not been assigned definitive species status or epithets.[4,94,160]

VIRULENCE FACTORS
OF HUMAN MYCOPLASMAS

Potential virulence factors in human pathogenic mycoplasmas have not been extensively studied, but a few candidate factors have been described over the last few years. *M. pneumoniae* possesses a membrane-associated, 169-kDa protein called P1, which is known to mediate the adherence of *M. pneumoniae* to host cells.[115] Additional surface proteins have also been identified that interact along with P1 to promote adherence to target tissues.[6,48] Strains lacking P1 exhibit diminished capacities for binding to cells, and antibodies directed against P1 inhibit the adherence of *M. pneumoniae*.[6,109] Because adherence is a necessary first step for infection of susceptible mucosal surfaces, this protein represents a true virulence factor in this organism. In addition, individuals infected with *M. pneumoniae* produce a vigorous antibody response against this adhesin, suggesting that purified adhesin proteins may be useful in serologic tests for diagnosis of *M. pneumoniae* infections.[114,115] P50 and P100, two surface-localized polypeptides of *M. hominis*, function in adherence of this species to eucaryotic cells.[101] *M. hominis* also binds sulfated glycolipids in a time-, temperature-, and dose-dependent manner that can be inhibited by preincubation of the organisms with high molecular weight dextran sulfate.[208] Sulfated glycolipids and other glycoconjugates are present in high concentrations in the male and female urogenital tracts, and specific interaction of *M. hominis* with these molecules may help explain the urogenital tissue tropism of *M. hominis*. Isolates of *U. urealyticum* produce phospholipase enzymes in vitro.[58] These enzymes hydrolyze phospholipids, with the release of arachidonic acid. Because *U. urealyticum* is associated with amnionitis and perinatal morbidity and mortality (i.e., spontaneous abortions, prematurity, stillbirth), it has been postulated that female genital tract infection may initiate a sequence of pathologic events related to phospholipase production.[63] Release of arachidonic acids from amniotic membranes may lead to production of prostaglandins, which can trigger premature labor during pregnancy.[12] Phospholipases may also play a role in fetal lung disease related to respiratory tract infection with *U. urealyticum*.[249]

Over the last few years, several *Mycoplasma* species, including *M. fermentans*, *M. penetrans*, and *M. pirum*, have been isolated from patients with HIV infection. These organisms have been implicated as cofactors in the progression of HIV disease.[199] The mechanisms involved in their putative roles as cofactors include activation of the immune system, production of superantigens that stumulate the release of various immunomodulating cytokines, or production of free-radicals that contribute to oxidative stress observed in HIV infection. All three of these "AIDS-associated" mycoplasmas utilize glucose and hydrolyze arginine. Mycoplasmal arginine deaminase may cause depletion of arginine in infected macrophages. Arginine is a precursor for a molecule that is directly involved in macrophage-mediated cytotoxicity; therefore, depletion of arginine by mycoplasmal infection may result in diminished macrophage cytotoxicity. Mycoplasmas also release nucleases into the growth medium that degrade host cell nucleic acids to generate precursors for synthesis of their own nucleic acids. Lastly, the discovery of the AIDS-associated mycoplasmas provided evidence that, unlike other mycoplasmas causing infections in humans, these newly described species are able to invade cells and survive as intracellular pathogens. Invasion of cells has been documented for *M. fermentans*, *M. pirum*, and *M. penetrans*; in fact, the ability to "penetrate" into host cells provided the latter organism with its species name. The association of these organisms with intracellular locations in lymphocytes and macrophages helps explain the recovery of these organisms, especially, *M. fermentans* from the blood of AIDS patients.

CLINICAL SIGNIFICANCE
OF THE HUMAN *MYCOPLASMATACEAE*

MYCOPLASMA PNEUMONIAE

M. pneumoniae is one of many causes of a pneumonic process called atypical pneumonia, along with several viral (e.g., influenza, respiratory syncytial virus, adenoviruses), fungal (e.g., *Pneumocystis carinii*), and bacterial (e.g., *Chlamydia pneumoniae*, *Legionella pneumophila*) etiologies.[41] *M. pneumoniae* is one of the most common causes of respiratory tract illnesses, with over 2 million infections occurring annually in the United States alone. Similar to other organisms causing respiratory tract disease, *M. pneumoniae* is transmitted by airborne transfer of droplets containing the organisms. Although it is highly transmissible, only 3% to 10% of infected individuals develop symptoms consistent with bronchopneumonia, with the remainder being either asymptomatic or having a milder, bronchitis-like illness.[41] Infections may occur year-round, but the incidence of overt disease is highest in late fall and winter. Infection occurs in young children and in older adults, but most clinical disease is seen in children older than 5 years of age, in teenagers, and in young adults. Children younger than 3 years of age tend to develop upper respiratory tract infections, whereas older children and adults tend to develop pneumonia. Most infections caused by *M. pneumoniae* are relatively minor and include pharyngitis, tracheobronchitis, bronchiolitis, pharyngitis, and croup; up to one fifth of infections are actually asymptomatic and may represent reinfection.[70]

In susceptible hosts following exposure, the organism attaches to epithelial cells in the respiratory tract and multiplies. The organisms do not penetrate the epithelial cells of the respiratory tract but remain localized. Organisms may be recovered on culture during the incubation period and for several weeks during and after clinical illness, even in the presence of specific antibodies.[5] Following a 2- to 3-week incubation period, the clinical presentation of mycoplasmal pneumonia is usually insidious, rather than abrupt, with the gradual onset of constitutional and pneumonic symptoms that mimic influenza.[41] Most patients will develop fever (up to 39°C; 103°F) over a few days, with chills, malaise, sore throat, nasal congestion, and a dry, nonproductive cough appearing early in the course of disease. As lower respiratory tract symptoms develop, the sputum generally becomes more mucoid or mucopurulent; occasionally blood may be noted in the sputum.[41] Some patients may also complain of earaches, and on physical examination, an inflamed erythematous tympanic membrane may be observed. With the onset of pneumonic symptoms, patients may feel as if they have a "bad cold" or the "flu," yet will continue to function; hence, the application of the term "walking pneumonia" to this disease. On chest examination, localized rhonchi and scattered rales are usually detected, with no signs of consolidation. Findings on chest roentgenograms are consistent with a diffuse bronchopneumonia, generally involving multiple lobes of the lung, without consolidation. Radiographic patterns seen with *M. pneumoniae* pneumonia vary widely and may show peribronchial penumonia, atelectasis, nodular infiltrates, and hilar lymphadenopathy.[41] These radiologic findings usually appear more extensive than the physical examination of the patient would suggest. Pleural effusions are relatively rare in mycoplasmal pneumonia, occurring in up to 20% of patients.

M. pneumoniae pneumonia is generally self-limited, with resolution of most constitutional symptoms in 3 to 10 days without antimicrobial therapy.[41] Abnormalities on chest films generally resolve more slowly and may take anywhere from 10 days to 6 weeks for complete resolution. Although antimicrobial therapy with tetracycline or erythromycin significantly reduces the duration of signs and symptoms and hastens resolution of abnormalities seen on chest films, the organism is generally not eradicated from the respiratory tract by therapy.[41] In one study, throat cultures for *M. pneumoniae* were still positive 4 months after resolution of the infection.[70] Recurrences and relapses of pneumonia despite appropriate antimicrobial therapy have been reported, and the organism has been implicated in exacerbations of other pulmonary infections, including asthsma, chronic lung disease, and adult respiratory distress syndrome.[69]

Complications caused by *M. pneumoniae* infection are rare but protean in the numbers of organ systems that may be involved. These complications may be pulmonary (pleuritis, pneumothorax, respiratory distress syndrome, lung abscess), hematologic (hemolytic anemia secondary to the formation of cold agglutinins, intravascular coagulopathy, thrombocytopenia, paroxysmal cold hemoglobinuria), musculoskeletal (myalgias, arthralgias, arthritis), cardiovascular (pericarditis, myocarditis), dermatologic (maculopapular or urticarial rashes, erythema multiforme, erythema nodosum, and other rashes), or neurologic (meningoencephalitis, myelitis, neuropathies, motor deficits, Guillain-Barre syndrome).[33,41,70,134,145] Neurologic complications are apparently caused by direct invasion of the central nervous system by the organism, whereas the others are probably mediated by immunologic abnormalities in the host that may be induced by infection.[205] Ocular complications, including optic disk swelling, optic nerve atrophy, retinal exudation, and hemorrhage, have been reported in association with *M. pneumoniae* infection.[247]

Humoral and cellular immunodeficiency states also predispose individuals to more serious disease with *M. pneumoniae* as well as other mycoplasmas.[70,211,243] Individuals with hypogammaglobulinemia may suffer repeated bouts of *M. pneumoniae* pneumonia and have difficulty eliminating the organism from the repiratory tract despite adequate therapy. These patients often have severe upper and lower respiratory tract symptoms, with little or no infiltrates observed on chest radiography, and manifest significant complications, including rashes, joint pain, and frank arthritis.[123,243,288,291] *M. pneumoniae* may also cause severe disease in patients with conditions that abrogate cellular immunity, including HIV infection and sickle cell disease.[120,211]

Fulminant, disseminated *M. pneumoniae* infection is rare but has been reported. For example, Koletsky and Weinstein[142] reported a case of rapidly fatal, disseminated *M. pneumoniae* infection during which a 30-year-old female patient developed severe respiratory disease, pneumonia, cardiovascular collapse, and renal failure after a 9-day clinical course. The patient died within 24 hours of admission to the hospital. On autopsy, the organism was recovered from the lungs, kidneys, and brain. Tissue sections revealed bilateral consolidated pneumonia and disseminated intravascular coagulation.

M. pneumoniae may occasionally be isolated from extrapulmonary sites. These isolations have usually been from joint fluid aspirates or from systemic sites (e.g., CSF) of immunocompromised patients.[41] Goulet and coworkers[83] isolated *M. pneumoniae* from urogenital tract specimens of 22 female patients over a 2-year period. In addition, the organism was recovered from the urethra of one of three male sexual partners of a female patient who harbored the organism in her genital tract. *M. pneumoniae* has also been isolated from a tuboovarian abscess.[296] This organism has also been isolated from synovial fluid in mixed culture with *M. genitalium*, an organism that has also been recovered from both the genital and the respiratory tracts.[304]

MYCOPLASMA HOMINIS AND UREAPLASMA UREALYTICUM

Both *M. hominis* and *U. urealyticum* may be isolated from the genital tracts of asymptomatic men and women.[183,186,187] They are more frequently recovered from the lower genital tract of women, with vaginal isolation rates of 35% to 80% depending on the population studied. McCormack and colleagues demonstrated that rates of colonization with *M. hominis* and *U. urealyticum* in men varied from zero to 13% and 3% to 56%, respectively.[183,186] Similar data on women have shown that vaginal colonization rates for *M. hominis* and *U. urealyticum* range from zero to 31% and 8.5% to 77.5%, respectively, depending on age, race, sexual experience, and socioeconomic status.[183,185,187] Rates of genital tract colonization in both men and women are related to sexual activity, and individuals with multiple sexual partners are more likely to be colonized. Thus, the epidemiology of organism acquisition suggests that mycoplasmas are indeed sexually transmitted. Additional evidence for sexual acquisition is suggested by much lower isolation rates among women who use barrier contraceptives.[187] Given these data, it is clear that these organisms are exceedingly prevalent, particularly in the lower genital tracts of sexually active women.

Over the last several years, both *U. urealyticum* and *M. hominis* have been implicated in a variety of clinical conditions primarily related to lower genital tract colonization and infection, upper genital tract infections in women, and, rarely, upper genital tract infection and prostatitis in men.[63,65,95,117,215] Both organisms have been postulated to play roles in early and late endometritis, chorioamnionitis, and premature rupture of membranes.[60,61,63,87] The presence of these organisms in the upper female genital tract has also been associated statistically with prematurity, low birth weight infants, and infertility.[64,87,95,131] Controlled studies on the pathogenicity of the genital mycoplasmas are complicated because both organisms are highly prevalent in sexually active adults who usually are asymptomatic. To further confound issues of etiology, they are often recovered in culture along with other recognized genital tract pathogens, such as *Chlamydia trachomatis*, *Neisseria gonorrhoeae*, and group B streptococci.[2] These associations make it difficult to determine whether a pathologic condition is solely attributable to the presence of genital mycoplasmas per se. An excellant example of this dilemma is the condition now termed bacterial vaginosis. Both *M. hominis* and *U. urealyticum* are often isolated from women with this infection.[77,103,147] However, bacterial vaginosis is now believed to result from a complex interaction among aerobic and anaerobic bacterial organisms. The roles of genital mycoplasmas in this condition have not been elucidated or defined.

Studies on the pathogenicity of the genital mycoplasmas are further confounded by recovery of the organisms during or subsequent to the administration of antimicrobial agents for other genital tract pathogens.[45] Antimicrobial therapy for these other organisms may act to select for mycoplasmas that are resistant to the agents being used (e.g., penicillins and cephalosporins). After their recovery from a genital culture or a site of pathology, it becomes difficult to ascribe an etiologic role for the organisms in light of previous or ongoing antibiotic administration.

Both *U. urealyticum* and *M. hominis* have been isolated from blood cultures of women with postpartum fever.[55,63,65,148,188,204,221,323] About 10% of women with postpartum or postabortal fever will have either *M. hominis* or *U. urealyticum* isolated from blood cultures. In some cases, either or both mycoplasmas may be isolated from the blood along with other genital tract microorganisms, again confounding the etiologic role of the mycoplasmas. Postpartum bacteremia results from the ascension of the organisms from the site of colonization in the vagina into the endometrium, where the organism apparently causes an endometritis. Infection of the placental membranes and the amniotic fluid with mycoplasmas most frequently occurs in colonized women with premature rupture of the fetal membranes and preterm or prolonged labor.[18,74] From these sites, the organisms enter the bloodstream during and following labor and delivery or following a cesarean section.

The isolation of mycoplasmas from the lower genital tracts of pregnant women has been associated with adverse pregnancy outcomes, including the delivery of low birth weight infants.[47] In a study conducted by Kass and coworkers,[131] women who were colonized with *U. urealyticum* in the genital tract and who demonstrated a fourfold or greater antibody response to the organism showed an infant low birth weight rate of 30%, whereas colonized women who did not show this antibody response had an infant low birth weight rate of 7.3%. Furthermore, this antibody response was serotype-specific, suggesting that the additional low birth weight rate was related to recent infection with a new serotype of *U. urealyticum* that differed from the serotype or serotypes already present in the vagina. Treatment studies with either tetracycline or erythromycin have shown decreases in low birth weight rates, implying that eradication of mycoplasmas (or other organisms) from the genital tract may have a direct, beneficial effect on certain adverse outcomes of pregnancy.[131] Although it has been well established that healthy women who are colonized with *M. hominis* in the genital tract usually deliver healthy colonized infants, *M. hominis* has occasionally been associated, similar to *U. urealyticum*, with chorioamnionitis, abortion, stillbirth, and intrauterine fetal demise.[191]

Amniotic infections with *U. urealyticum* have also been demonstrated in asymptomatic women with intact fetal membranes; these infections were frequently associated with adverse pregnancy outcomes.[18,31,88,107] *U. urealyticum* can apparently initiate an intense inflammatory tissue response, with no associated symptomatology. Serologic evidence of an antibody response to these organisms and simultaneous recovery of ureaplasmas from the blood appear to confirm the possibility of silent amniotic infections.[31,61,78] Gray and associates[88] studied two groups of asymptomatic pregnant women, who were matched for maternal age, gestational age, and indications for amniocentesis. Transabdomenal amniocentesis specimens were cultured for mycoplasmas. Among the 86 women in the ureaplasma-negative group, there was a 1.2% incidence of spontaneous second trimester abortion and a prematurity rate of 9.3%, for an overall adverse outcome rate of 10.5%. However, the rate of adverse outcomes among the eight ureaplasma-positive women was 100%, representing an 8.6-fold greater risk of adverse outcome.[88] Adverse outcomes in these eight pregnancies included spontaneous abortion (75%), premature deliveries with a 50% mortality rate (25%), and hyaline membrane disease (seen in the single surviving infant). Introduction of the organisms into the amniotic fluid is also a crucial step in the development of chorioamnionitis and endometritis. In the study by Gray and coworkers,[88] histologic examination of placental tissues from the eight infected women revealed chorioamnionitis in all of them, and all seven lung tissue specimens from the infants showed pneumonia. Four of five placentas and three of five fetal lung tissue specimens that were cultured grew *U. urealyticum*. Horowitz and colleagues also showed that 50% of six women with positive midtrimester amniotic cultures for *U. urealyticum* had adverse pregnancy outcomes as compared with 12% of 123 women with negative amniotic fluid cultures.[107] Eschenbach[64] reviewed the lines of evidence relative to the contribution of *U. urea-*

lyticum to adverse outcomes of pregnancy and concluded that, although the presence of *U. urealyticum* in the lower genital tract was not associated with premature birth, the presence of the organism in the chorioamnion was strongly associated with histologic evidence of chorioamnionitis and weakly associated with premature birth as an outcome.

In some of these cases, ureaplasmas have been shown to contribute a priori to subsequent premature rupture of membranes and premature labor.[87] Colonization of the placenta permits infection of the endometrium, from which the organism can gain access to the blood. The recovery of *U. urealyticum* and *M. hominis* from endometrial tissue sometime after delivery has also established mycoplasmas and ureaplasmas, in particular, as probable causes of some cases of early- and late-onset endometritis.[65] Although it has been suggested by several workers and studies, a definite causal relation between genital mycoplasmas, salpingitis, and infertility has not been unequivocally demonstrated.[63,257,276]

U. urealyticum may play a role in spontaneous abortion that is related to its ability to cause chorioamnionitis. Joste and associates[127] examined 42 first trimester spontaneous abortions and 21 elective first trimester abortions and compared them histologically and culturally with 32 third trimester, preterm deliveries, 11 of which were culture-positive for *U. urealyticum*. Among specimens obtained from first trimester spontaneous abortions, 26% grew ureaplasmas compared with none of the 21 elective abortion specimens. Histologic evidence of chorioamnionitis did not correlate with culture positivity for the spontaneous abortion specimens. However, evidence of chorioamnionitis did correlate with positive ureaplasma cultures for the 11 third trimester, preterm deliveries. These workers postulated that early changes caused by *U. urealyticum* infection other than histologically evident chorioamnionitis may be responsible for the pathogenesis of spontaneous abortions related to ureaplasmal infection.[127]

Urinary tract infections caused by mycoplasmas have also been reported, and, again, most work in this area has been in pregnant women.[80] Determination of the significance of mycoplasmas in clean-catch urine specimens from women is difficult, owing to the likely contamination of the specimen from organisms colonizing the vagina and the distal urethra. Because of the recognized association between bacteriuria during pregnancy and the increased incidence of premature delivery and preeclampsia, Savige and coworkers[254] collected suprapubic bladder aspirates from 72 healthy pregnant women and 51 women with preeclampsia and cultured the urine specimens for mycoplasmas. *U. urealyticum* was isolated from the urine of 7% of the healthy women and from 20% of those with preeclampsia. In a subsequent study of bacteriuria in 340 pregnant women, the presence of *U. urealyticum* in the urine during the first trimester correlated with the development of preeclampsia during the third trimester of pregnancy.[80] Among the 21 women who developed preeclampsia, 29% had ureaplasmas present in urine during the first trimester compared with only 10% of the

patients who did not develop preeclampsia. Therefore, the development of preeclampsia was three times more likely in women who had ureaplasmas in the urine at the start of pregnancy than in those women who were culture-negative. Although the mechanisms involved in the pathogenesis of preeclampsia are unclear, it is suggested that ureaplasmas, similar to other bacteria involved in bacteriuria, may also contribute to adverse pregnancy outcome.

In men, *M. hominis* is relatively uncommon as a cause of clinical disease, and most research on mycoplasmas has concentrated on the association of *U. urealyticum* with nongonococcal, nonchlamydial urethritis. Although several studies have been done, the role of *U. urealyticum* in this clinical entity is still unclear.[2,183,186] Even though the data suggest that *U. urealyticum* is the cause of nongonococcal, nonchlamydial urethritis in some patients, it is not known what proportion of infections are due to the organism, and even if the organism is cultured from the urethra of a symptomatic man, its role as the causative agent may not be established. Studies of symptomatic men treated with antibiotics having differential activity between *Chlamydia trachomatis* and *U. urealyticum*, and cultures performed on men with persistent symptoms of urethritis following antigonococcal and antichlamydial therapies suggest that some cases of nongonococcal urethritis are caused by *U. urealyticum*.[45,281] The discovery of the fastidious species *M. genitalium* in men with nongonococcal urethritis has further clouded the issue of etiology and *U. urealyticum* in this clinical condition.[300,308] Although some studies have suggested a possible role for mycoplasmas in the etiology of prostatitis, the results have been inconclusive, partly because of the difficulty in collecting prostatic fluid specimens that are not contaminated by organisms present in the urethra.[215] *U. urealyticum* is rare as a cause of epididymitis; a single case has been reported from whom the organisms were isolated from an epididymal aspirate in association with a significant rise in antibodies to the organism.[117]

Infants born to mothers who are colonized with genital mycoplasmas are also frequently colonized themselves. In survey studies, 18% to 45% of neonates delivered to colonized mothers were also colonized with *M. hominis*, with positive cultures being obtained from the throat, the genital tract, or the urine.[60,63] The rate of vertical transmission of *U. urealyticum* ranges from 18% to 55% among full-term infants and from 29% to 55% among preterm infants.[248] Syrogiannopoulos and associates[278] cultured the throat, eyes, and vaginas of 193 full-term infants born to women colonized vaginally with *U. urealyticum*. Of these, 107 (55%) had *U. urealyticum* present in at least one culture site. Colonization may persist in these babies for prolonged periods with no ill effects to the child. In the latter study, 68%, 33%, and 37% of the infants who were colonized at birth in the throat, eyes, and vagina, respectively, were still colonized on follow-up at 3 months of age. Among the children who were colonized in the respiratory tract, there was no increased incidence of respiratory tract illnesses when compared with those children who were not colonized in this area. In a study performed in Israel, 24% of 99 preterm infants were colonized with mycoplasmas; *U. urealyticum* was isolated from 21 infants, and *M. hominis* was isolated from three infants.[112] In this study, the colonization rate was inversely correlated with gestational age, with 80% of infants younger than 28 weeks gestation colonized as opposed to 17.9% of infants at 28 to 36 weeks gestation.[112] Of the 27 infants requiring ventilatory assistance in this study, 22% had *U. urealyticum* isolated from lower respiratory tract secretions.

Several studies have indicated that *U. urealyticum* may indeed be associated with chronic lung disease, bronchopulmonary dysplasia, and systemic infection in premature infants.[214,271,313,317,324] Prospective studies have now shown a significant relation between *U. urealyticum* respiratory tract infection and the development of chronic lung disease of the newborn.[46,245,313,324,330] Cassell and others found that the recovery of *U. urealyticum* from the tracheas of infants weighing less than 1000 g, who also required ventilatory assistance, was associated with the development of bronchopulmonary dysplasia and associated conditions (e.g., hyaline membrane disease, patent ductus arteriosus, and pneumonia).[30] A subsequent study by Crouse and associates[46] showed that low birth weight infants with respiratory distress who had *U. urealyticum* recovered from tracheal cultures were more likely to show dysplasia and evidence of pneumonia on chest radiography than those without *U. urealyticum*. Nasopharyngeal or tracheal colonization of preterm infants with *U. urealyticum* is also associated with an elevated peripheral white blood cell count.[207] Sanchez and Regan[249] found that, among infants colonized with ureaplasmas in the respiratory tract, 30% developed chronic lung disease requiring mechanical ventilatory assistance, whereas only 8% of noncolonized neonates developed respiratory tract illness. Bloodstream infection with *U. urealyticum* has also been documented in newborn infants, and these infections have often been associated with coexisting respiratory tract infections.[23,30,317] These systemic infections are associated with urinary tract infection, preterm or prolonged membrane rupture, preterm labor, and chorioamnionitis in the mother, and with low birth weight, presence of congenital anomalies, and perinatal asphyxisa in the newborn.[317] The pathogenesis of this syndrome in the neonate has also been supported by animal models and reflects both the nature of these bacteria as opportunistic agents and the immunocompromised status of the premature infant. Studies with neonatal lung fibroblast cultures have demonstrated induction of cytokine release from these cells by infection with *U. urealyticum* in vitro, suggesting a possible role for cytokines in the pathogenesis of bronchopulmonary dysplasia in prematurity.[271] Serologic studies have shown that the neonate or fetus that is systemically infected with *U. urealyticum* mounts serovar-specific antiureaplasma IgM and IgG responses, providing additional evidence for the pathogenic potential of these organisms.[228] Unfortunately, full-term infants may also suffer adverse clinical outcomes with systemic *U. urealyticum* infection, and fatal congenital ureaplasma pneumonia in full-term infants has been described.[227]

Several reports and studies have also shown that both *U. urealyticum* and *M. hominis* may be infrequently recovered from the central nervous system as a cause of silent or clinically symptomatic meningitis in the newborn period.[313] Many cases of *M. hominis* central nervous system infections in the neonate have been described; most of these occurred in premature infants for whom prolonged rupture of membranes had been documented.[76,179,189,261] In a prospective study of 100 preterm infants, Waites and coworkers[320] isolated *U. urealyticum* from the cerebrospinal fluid (CSF) of eight babies and *M. hominis* from the CSF of five babies. Among the babies with *U. urealyticum* infection, six had intraventricular hemmorrhage, three developed hydrocephalus, and three died. None of the infants with *M. hominis* infections died, and only one had neurologic signs of meningitis. Gilbert and Drew,[79] however, reported a case of meningitis in a premature infant caused by *M. hominis* that ran a chronic course, with the development of intraventricular hemorrhage. In all of these infants, eradication of the organisms with antimicrobial therapy proved difficult.

In a study of 318 predominantly full-term infants with signs of suspected sepsis or meningitis born to primarily low-risk women, *M. hominis* was isolated from the CSF of nine infants and *U. urealyticum* was recovered from the CSF of five infants.[318] Of these 14 infected infants, 12 recovered without therapy and two died. Of these two, one infant with *M. hominis* died of *Haemophilus influenzae* sepsis, whereas the other, infected with *U. urealyticum*, developed intraventricular hemorrhage. This study suggested that mycoplasmas are more common in neonatal central nervous system infections than had been appreciated previously. Although central nervous system infections with *M. hominis* usually resolve spontaneously, ureaplasmas apparently can elicit an inflammatory response that is associated with intraventricular hemorrhage.[100]

In addition to central nervous system infections, mycoplasmas, particularly *M. hominis*, have also been isolated from other extragenital infections in both children and adults. Perinatally acquired *M. hominis* has been recovered from subcutaneous scalp abscesses at the site of forceps or monitor injuries, conjunctival infections, and submandibular lymph nodes in the newborn.[82,124,225] *M. hominis* was also isolated in multiple blood cultures from a 10-month-old child who had suffered severe burns.[51] In adults, *M. hominis* has been cultured from a wide variety of infections, including bacteremia, postoperative wounds, hematomas, septic arthritis, aspiration-associated empyema, septic thrombophlebitis, peritonitis, periorbital abscesses, and brain abscesses.[21,26,52,125,128,139,149,178,182,196,213,233,272] *M. hominis* bacteremia and postoperative sternal wound infection was documented in two patients following cardiothoracic surgery.[266] In a third case report of *M. hominis* sternal wound infection, *U. urealyticum* was also recovered.[220] Both *M. hominis* and *U. urealyticum* have been isolated from pericardial tissues or fluids of patients with pericardial effusions; these patients all had histories of recent cardiac surgery (coronary artery bypass surgery, aortic valve replacement, heart transplantation secondary to idiopathic dilated cardiomyopathy) or were immunocompromised (systemic lupus erythematosus, chronic obstructive pulmonary disease).[134] *M. hominis* was also isolated from a surgical wound infection following insertion of a silicone breast prosthesis.[250]

Mycoplasmas have been documented as opportunistic infectious agents in those with underlying diseases or conditions, such as hypogammaglobulinemia, Hodgkin's disease, systemic lupus erythematosus, transplantation, heart disease, leukemia, lymphoma, rheumatoid arthritis, and severe trauma.[38,75,81,130,176, 193,195,196,209,243,269,285,297] *M. hominis* and *U. urealyticum* septic arthritis has been reported in patients with hypogammaglobulinemia, hematologic malignancies, massive trauma, postpartum bacteremia, lupus erythematosus, and common variable immunodeficiency; this clinical entity likely occurs following hematologic seeding of the joint spaces.[25,38,126,140,190,283,297,316] In 1994, Kane and associates[130] reported the first case of respiratory tract infection with diffuse alveolar hemorrhage caused by *M. hominis* in a bone marrow tranplant recipient. *M. hominis* was isolated from postoperative perihepatic hematomas that developed in the abdomen of a liver transplant recipient a month after the transplant surgery.[116] Both *M. hominis* and *U. urealyticum* were isolated from a retroperitoneal hematoma 12 days after liver transplantation in a 45-year-old woman with fulminant hepatic failure.[89] Infections of prosthetic joints by *M. hominis* have also occurred, and *M. hominis* wound infections following open reduction of fractured mandibles and after cesarean sections have been reported as well.[218,266] Infections in the head, neck, and chest areas and in tissue contiguous with the genital tract may reflect the presence of these organisms in the adjacent respiratory and urogenital tracts, respectively.[194,233] For example, Kayser and Bhend[133] reported a case of paraspinal, intervertebral soft-tissue infection in a 45-year-old woman that developed 16 days after the patient underwent an abdominal hysterectomy.

M. hominis has also been isolated from the urine of patients with HIV infection. In a study by Chirgwin and colleagues[34] at the State University of New York in Brooklyn, *M. hominis* was isolated from 18% of the urine specimens obtained from 180 HIV-positive individuals and from 21% of urine specimens from 38 HIV-negative individuals. In this study, an additional 30 glucose-utilizing mycoplasmas were recovered only from the HIV-positive individuals.[34] Growth inhibition with species-specific antisera allowed identification of 18 of these isolates: 14 were identified as *M. fermentans* and four were identified as *M. pirum*. The remaining 12 isolates were nonviable on subculture.

MYCOPLASMA GENITALIUM

In 1980, Tully and coworkers isolated a previously undescribed and unusually fastidious mycoplasma from urethral specimens of two of 13 homosexual men with nongonococcal urethritis (NGU).[308] Ultrastructural analysis of these isolates indicated that the new organism shared several characteristics with *M. pneumoniae*. These characteristics included the tapering flasklike shape of the individual cells and the presence of a specialized apical structure that facilitated the adherence of the organism to tissue cells, erythrocytes, and inert material such as plastic and glass.[309] *M. genitalium* possesses a species-specific, 140-kDa protein called P140 that is a structural and functional counterpart of the 170-kDa P1 adhesin protein of *M. pneumoniae*.[200] Nonadherent variants of *M. genitalium* have an altered P140 adhesin or have lost the membrane-associated adhesin molecule.[192] *M. genitalium* and *M. pneumoniae* also contain a 43,000-Da cross-reactive protein that is also detectable on isolates of *Acholeplasma laidlawii*.[36] These shared antigenic epitopes are responsible for the cross-reactions observed with *M. genitalium* in most serologic tests for *M. pneumoniae* antibodies.[49,50] These tests have included complement fixation, indirect immunofluoresence assays, and metabolic inhibition and growth inhibition tests using heterologous antisera.[158,159] DNA hybridization studies have shown that the two organisms have 6.5% to 8.1% nucleotide sequence homology, the latter probably reflecting those genes that code for the antigenically cross-reactive proteins.[158,338] Other gene sequences are indeed unique for the two species, providing evidence that *M. pneumoniae* and *M. genitalium* are distinct species.[309]

M. genitalium has been isolated from both the genitourinary tract and the respiratory tract, but its role as a pathogen in these anatomic sites is unknown.[7,284,300] Although the organism can induce symptomatic genital tract infections in experimentally infected primates, evidence to indicate that *M. genitalium* may be associated with NGU in humans has largely awaited the development of molecular methods to detect the organism because culture is extremely difficult.[56,308] Failure to isolate the organisms in studies on urethritis may reflect inadequate specimens, media, or techniques. To circumvent the inherent problems related to culture of this fastidious organism, Hooten and coworkers[105] investigated the occurrence of *M. genitalium* in men using a species-specific nucleic acid probe. These workers detected the organism in 14% of 21 men with gonococcal urethritis, 10% of 30 men with chlamydial urethritis, 13% of 31 men with nongonococcal, nonchlamydial urethritis, and 27% of 37 men with recurrent or persistent urethritis. However, the organism was also detected in 12% of 84 men who had no genitourinary tract symptoms. These same workers also found that the organism was more commonly present in the urethras of homosexual men than heterosexual men. By using a PCR probe–based technique that detected the nucleotide sequence specific for the *M. genitalium* 140-kDa adhesin gene, Jensen and associates found *M. genitalium* DNA in 17% of urethral specimens from 99 men; 20% of specimens from symptomatic men were positive, whereas only 9% of specimens from asymptomatic men were positive.[121,122] In this study all attempts to culture the organism from PCR-positive specimens were unsuccessful. Horner and coworkers also used PCR probe technology for detection of *M. genitalium* and found that 23% of 103 men with signs or symptoms of acute NGU and 6% of 53 men without NGU were positive.[106] The presence of this organism in the male urogenital tract was independent of the presence of *Chlamydia trachomatis*. These workers concluded that *M. genitalium* was the etiologic agent in some cases of NGU; this was also supported by the clinical response of the infected men to treatment with doxycycline.[106] Blanchard and coworkers also used PCR to determine the prevalence of *M. genitalium* and *M. fermentans* in urethral and cervical sites of sexually active men and women.[15] *M. genitalium* was detected by PCR, but not by culture, in 11% of specimens from men and women with signs and symptoms of urethritis–cervicitis. *M. fermentans* was not detected by culture or by PCR in any of the urogenital specimens tested.

In 1988, Baseman and coworkers recovered *M. genitalium* along with *M. pneumoniae* from four of 16 frozen specimens collected from the upper respiratory tracts of military recruits during an *M. pneumoniae* vaccine trial in 1974 and 1975.[7] The role that the organism may play in respiratory tract disease is not clear, but it has been suggested that the association with *M. pneumoniae* may result in a synergistic infection that causes more severe pneumonic disease or may contribute to the pathogenesis of extrapulmonary complications of *M. pneumoniae* infection.[300] The presence of *M. genitalium* in the respiratory tract, with or without *M. pneumoniae*, and the immunologic cross-reactivity between the two organisms may not only complicate the infectious process in coinfected individuals but may also affect the immunologic response to infection. Such interactions, consequently, may interfere with the interpretation of serologic tests that are frequently used to diagnose *M. pneumoniae* infections. The use of PCR primers and nucleic acid probes that are specific for *M. pneumoniae* and *M. genitalium* may provide a solution to clinical and diagnostic problems by circumventing the need to cultivate these agents and clarifying the immune responses and consequent serologic cross-reactions that occur with these organisms.[110]

A few studies have addressed the detection and significance of *M. genitalium* in the female genital tract.[286] In a study performed in a sexually transmitted disease clinic in London, *M. genitalium* was detected by PCR in genital tract specimens from 20% of female patients.[210] Another study done in Copenhagen reported finding *M. genitalium* in endocervical specimens from five of 74 women.[122] Neither of these studies addressed the association of these isolates with the presence of disease or pathology. Although definitive data on the pathogenicity of this organism in the female genital tract are lacking, indirect evidence suggests that it may also be a player in both lower and upper genital tract infection. Serologic studies have documented elevated antibody titers to *M. genitalium* in some women with salpingitis that was not attributable to gonococci, chlamydia, or *M. hominis*, and chimpanzees experimentally inoculated with *M. genitalium* have developed upper and lower genital tract disease.[197,284] These issues await both confirmation and further clinical and laboratory study.

Besides the respiratory and genital tracts, *M. genitalium* has also been recovered from joint fluid aspirates of patients with arthritis. In a report on two such cases, *M. genitalium* was detected by PCR analysis in the knee joint of a 25-year-old man with Reiter's syndrome and in the knee joint of a 58-year-old man with seronegative rheumatoid arthritis.[287] Both *M. pneumoniae* and *M. genitalium* were detected in a knee joint fluid specimen from a patient with hypogammaglobulinemia, mycoplasma pneumonia, and polyarthritis following a bout of pneumonia.[304]

Similar to *M. fermentans*, *M. penetrans*, and *M. pirum*, *M. genitalium* has also been associated with HIV infection. Montagnier and colleagues detected *M. genitalium* by PCR in the blood of a patient with AIDS.[199] As with the other AIDS-associated mycoplasmas, the role of *M. genitalium* in the pathogenesis or progression of HIV disease is currently under intense investigation.

MYCOPLASMA FERMENTANS

In 1986, Lo and coworkers at the Armed Forces Institute of Pathology and the National Institutes of Health reported the isolation of a "novel virus" from Kaposi's sarcoma tissues of patients with AIDS.[161] This organism was isolated in tissue culture by transfection of the culture cells with material from Kaposi's sarcoma lesions. The putative agent was notable for its small size (140 to 280 nm), its membrane-bound morphology, and its location within the cytoplasm and nucleus of infected tissue culture cells. At this point, the organism was termed VLIA for "virus-like infectious agent."[170] Nucleic acid hybridization studies indicated a lack of significant relations between VLIA and several viruses but some nucleic acid sequence homologies with the rRNA of *Escherichia coli*, suggesting a relation between VLIA and bacterial organisms. It was eventually established that this novel organism was a mycoplasma, which was given the provisional name *Mycoplasma incognitus*.[169] Using immunohistochemical techniques employing monoclonal antibodies against this new agent, Lo and coworkers detected *M. incognitus* antigens in thymus, liver, spleen, lymph nodes, and brain tissue of patients with AIDS, and in placental tissues delivered by pregnant women with AIDS.[164] The histopathology of the infected tissues showed a range of responses; in some tissues no histologic changes were observed, whereas in others fulminant necrosis with inflammation was noted. Intraperitoneal inoculation of four silver leaf monkeys with this new agent resulted in a wasting syndrome that led to their deaths within 7 to 9 months.[172,174] These same workers also reported on six patients, from six different geographic areas, who presented with acute flulike illnesses that progressed to a syndrome of high, persistent fevers, lymphadenopathy, diarrhea, and heart, liver, and adrenal failure, resulting in death within 1 to 7 weeks. Examination of autopsy revealed fulminent necrosis of lymph node, lungs, liver, adrenal gland, heart, and brain tissues. Immunohistochemical techniques and electron microscopy revealed VLIA antigens in the areas of necrosis, and a labeled VLIA-specific DNA probe detected the genetic material of this agent in all of the infected tissues.[163] None of these patients was infected with HIV-1 or HIV-2. Nucleic acid hybridization and serologic studies were undertaken comparing this "new" mycoplasma with other *Mycoplasma* species. Hybridization profiles, restriction endonuclease mapping, and antigenic analyses with both polyclonal and monoclonal antibodies indicated that *M. incognitus* was not a new mycoplasma but a particular strain of *M. fermentans*, a fastidious, "nonpathogenic" mycoplasma found in the genital tract.[246,252]

The "incognitus" strain of *M. fermentans* was subsequently found to be associated with other pathology in AIDS patients. Bauer and colleagues[8] examined kidney tissues of 15 AIDS patients with light-microcopic evidence of AIDS-associated nephropathy. Tissues from all 15 patients showed positive immunofluorescent reactions with *M. fermentans* incognitus strain-specific monoclonal antibodies in glomerular endothelial and epithelial cells, glomerular basement membranes, tubular epithelial cells and casts, and mononuclear interstitial cells.[8] Mycoplasmal structures were observed with immunoelectron microcopy in the kidney tissues of all 15 patients as well. Renal tissues obtained from 15 AIDS patients without renal involvement and kidney tissue from non-AIDS patients with and without nephropathy did not reveal any mycoplasma organisms on histopathologic examination.[8] Ainsworth and associates[1] also reported a patient with HIV-associated nephropathy in whom *M. fermentans* was detected in renal tissues by PCR whom nephropathy first became clinically apparent; 18 months later, as the patient's disease progressed and renal function deteriorated, PCR detected *M. fermentans* in the patient's urine, throat, and peripheral blood. Lo and colleagues[173] reported an additional three non-AIDS patients who developed fulminant adult respiratory distress syndrome associated with *M. fermentans*; immunohistochemical and electron microscopic studies revealed the organisms in the patients' lungs and liver.

In addition to Lo and associates' report of an *M. fermentans* incognitus strain being associated with a fatal disease in non-AIDS patients, Macon and colleagues[177] reported on a 35-year-old homosexual man who developed Kaposi's sarcoma and T-cell lymphoma with a peripheral CD4 cell count of 43/mm³. He subsequently developed fatal pneumocystis pneumonia and disseminated cryptococcal infection. Multiple EIAs and Western immunoblots for HIV-1, HIV-2, HTLV-I, and HTLV-II antibodies were negative, as were retroviral cultures and PCR studies. Systemic *M. fermentans* infection was documented in this patient by immunohistochemical and PCR detection of the organism in both pre- and postmortem examination of tissue specimens. Beecham and coworkers[11] reported a similar case in a previously healthy 28-year-old nonimmunocompromised man who presented with a 7-day history of fever, abdomninal pain, diarrhea, rash, and shortness of breath. *M. fermentans* was detected in bone marrow biopsy specimens by both PCR and electron microscopy. In another report of a previously healthy HIV-seronegative man with AIDS-like symptoms of fever, malaise, weight loss, diarrhea, and extensive liver and spleen necrosis, treatment with doxycycline (300 mg/d, orally for 6 weeks) resulted in resolution of

the patient's symptoms and full recovery.[162] These studies suggest that *M. fermentans* organisms, or a specific strain of this species, are a potential systemic pathogen in patients who are not infected with HIV. This organism has also been investigated for its relation to chronic fatigue syndrome; none of 42 serum specimens from patients diagnosed with chronic fatigue syndrome reacted in an EIA test for detection of *M. fermentans* antibodies, suggesting that this *Mycoplasma* species is not involved in this chronic syndrome.[143]

Although it has been attempted in several studies, cultural isolation of *M. fermentans* is quite difficult. With PCR technology, Dawson and associates detected *M. fermentans* in 10 (43%) of 43 urine sediment specimens from patients with AIDS-associated nephropathy.[53] Of these PCR-positive samples, three specimens from two patients were culture-positive in modified SP-4, A-7, and Hayflick's media. Among these same patients, four cultures grew *U. urealyticum* and two grew *M. hominis*. None of 50 urine sediment specimens from 50 HIV-negative, healthy patients was culture- or PCR-positive for *M. fermentans*, although 23 specimens grew *U. urealyticum* and one specimen grew *M. hominis*. With the *M. fermentans* PCR assay, Katseni and coworkers[132] examined blood, throat, and urine specimens from 117 HIV-positive patients, 114 of whom were homosexual men, and from 73 HIV-seronegative patients attending an STD clinic in London. These workers detected *M. fermentans* in 10% of 117 peripheral blood mononuclear specimens, 23% of 65 throat specimens, and 8% of 55 urine specimens from the HIV-positive subjects. Among the 73 HIV-seronegative patients, *M. fermentans* was detected in peripheral blood mononuclear cells, throat, and urine specimens of 9%, 20%, and 6%, respectively. Hawkins and colleagues at the NIH detected *M. fermentans* DNA sequences in 11% of blood specimens from 55 HIV-seropositive patients but detected none in 26 HIV-seronegative, low-risk individuals.[96] Bebear and coworkers[9] in France cultured specimens and performed PCR analyses on throat, endocervical, urethral, urine, and peripheral blood mononuclear cell specimens from 105 HIV-positive individuals. Although PCR and cultures for *M. pneumoniae* and *M. genitalium* were uniformly negative, 26.7% of the 105 patients had *M. fermentans* detected by PCR in at least one site.[9] Detection of *M. fermentans* in these studies was not associated with the stage of HIV disease, the HIV-1 viral load, or the CD4 count.

M. fermentans, similar to the other AIDS-associated mycoplasmas, discussed later, is able to actively invade cultured cells, a property that was not previously associated with *Mycoplasma* species. Although an *M. fermentans* reference strains and the "incognitus" strain were able to invade HeLa cells, *M. fermentans* incognitus strains were more invasive when tested in tracheal explant cell cultures; incognitus strain organisms could be observed intracellularly, whereas the reference strain was observed only between and adherent to cells.[270,290] Intranasal infection of LEW rats with the incognitus strain and subsequent explant culture of the tracheal tissues of these animals also revealed intracellular localization of the organisms within the cultured cells.[270] The *M. fermentans* incognitus strain and other *M. fermentans* strains were able to cause ciliostasis and cytopathology in tracheal explant cultures, but the extent and severity of the cytopathology varied considerably from strain to strain. In vivo studies in animals also indicate that immunosuppression may allow *M. fermentans* to grow and flourish. Intravenous administration of *M. fermentans* incognitus strain killed BALB/c nude mice but did not kill immunocompetent BALB/c mice.[283]

Although some workers have noted differences between Lo's *M. fermentans* incognitus strain and other *M. fermentans* strains, others have noted no differences, Sasaki and coworkers[252] compared the characteristic of the original incognitus strain with three other reference and clinical isolates of *M. fermentans*. Restriction endonucleases treatment of the DNA from these strains showed similar patterns on polyacrylamide gel electrophorsis. Immunoblot profiles of cellular proteins were also similar, indicating a high degree of antigenic homogeneity among the four strains examined. Exposure of peripheral blood mononuclear cells (PBMCs) to these mycoplasmas resulted in significant increases in the production of interleukin-1β (IL-1β), IL-6, and tumor necrosis factor-α (TNF-α); these increases were observed after exposure to all four *M. fermentans* strains and were not restricted to the incognitus strain alone. Lastly, exposure of HIV-infected PBMCs to any of the *M. fermentans* strains resulted in a 1.8- to 4.3-fold enhancement of reverse transcriptase activity and a 3.3- to 7.0-fold increase in the production of p24 antigen in the culture. These workers concluded that the incognitus strain of *M. fermentans* was not unique when compared with other *M. fermentans* strains.[252]

Several investigators are currently examining the role of *M. fermentans* and other mycoplasmas as cofactors in the progression of HIV-associated disease. In vitro studies on HIV-infected CEM cells (a CD4-enriched T-lymphoblastoid tumor cell line) showed that treatment of the cells with tetracycline analogues or fluoroquinolones was able to inhibit the production of virus-induced cytopathic effects without inhibiting the replication and production of progeny virus.[154,206] Subsequent studies have indeed shown that *M. fermentans* acts synergistically with HIV-1 in lymphoblastoid and promonocytic cells to produce cell death; this ability has also been demonstrated to occur with other *Mycoplasma* species, including *M. penetrans*, *M. pirum*, and *M. arginini*.[155,171] Phillips and associates showed that mycoplasmal attachment to HIV-infected lymphocytes was associated with sites of viral budding, leading these investigators to surmise that attachment of mycoplasmas may trigger or enhance production of progeny virus by infected cells.[217]

Several mechanisms have been proposed whereby mycoplasmas such as *M. fermentans* may act as cofactors or immunomodulators in the production of HIV-associated disease.[199] Lymphocyte activation stimulates the replication of HIV, and *Mycoplasma* species,

including *M. fermentans*, have the capacity to behave as polyclonal activators of both B and T lymphocytes.[66,275] *M. fermentans* is able to induce the production of lymphokines (i.e., TNF, IL-1, and IL-6) in various cell types (i.e., monocytes, macrophages, astrocytes, and glial cells) in vitro.[73,202,203] Muhlradt and Frisch[201] isolated and partially purified a substance, which they termed MDHM (mycoplasma-derived high molecular weight material), that was membrane-associated, contained lipid, and existed in an aggregated form when purified. The presence of MDHM in nanogram-per-milliliter amounts activates macrophages to release nitric oxide, IL-6, and TNF. Another group identified a 48-kDa, hydrophobic, membrane-associated *M. fermentans* antigen, distinct from MDHM, that also stimulates the secretion of both TNF and IL-1 from cultured monocytes.[146] Second, some workers have proposed that *M. fermentans* may produce superantigens that bind to the major histocompatibility complex (MHC) proteins, thereby stimulating T-lymphocyte activation. A precedence for the production of superantigens by mycoplasmas already exists with the well-studied soluble T-cell mitogen produced by *M. arthriditis*.[43,223] Third, some have proposed that the production of peroxides and other reactive oxygen species (i.e., free radicals) by mycoplasmas or the production of enzymes that inactivate the normal intracellular catalase may induce HIV gene expression and activate viral replication. Peroxides and other reactive oxygen species induce HIV gene expression in vitro by *trans*-activation of viral promoter regions and contribute to programmed cell death.[28,151,255] Lastly, *M. fermentans* incognitus strain is able to fuse with both T cells and peripheral blood lymphocytes.[59] The delivery of mycoplasmal components into these cells may directly affect normal lymphocyte functions. In addition, the fusion of mycoplasmal and lymphocyte membranes may significantly change the structure or orientation of various receptors on the lymphocyte surface, thereby altering the binding, induction, or production of various lymphokines. These fundamental alterations in lymphocyte structure and function may influence attachment, integration, and gene expression of HIV.

In addition to its association with systemic infections and HIV disease, *M. fermentans*, similar to *M. genitalium*, may play a role in genital tract infection. Early in the recogition of *M. fermentans* and its role in HIV disease, this organism was detected in the placental tissues of two women with AIDS.[164] Blanchard and coworkers used culture and PCR methodology to examine the presence of both *M. genitalium* and *M. fermentans* in the genital tracts of sexually active adults and in the amniotic fluids of women with intact fetal membrane who were undergoing cesarean deliveries.[15] *M. genitalium* was detected by PCR, but not by culture, in 11% of of 94 men and 87 women with clinical symptoms of nongonococcal urethritis or cervicitis and was not detected by either method in any of 232 amniotic fluid specimens. On the other hand, *M. fermentans* was not detected by either method in any of the urogenital specimens but was detected by PCR in four of the 232 amniotic fluid specimens, suggesting that the organism may be transmitted transplacentally. Interestingly, two of the four patients with positive *M. fermentans* PCR results had histologic evidence of chorioamnionitis, implying that *M. fermentans* may also be a genital tract pathogen.[15]

MYCOPLASMA PENETRANS

In 1991, Lo and colleagues at the Armed Forces Institute of Pathology in Washington, D.C. reported the isolation of a unique *Mycoplasma* species from the urogenital tracts of homosexual men with HIV infection.[167] This organism exhibited unique morphologic characteristics, including a flask-shaped body composed of two compartments: one containing loosely packed, coarse granules consistent with ribosomal structures, and the other a tapered, smaller compartment containing densely packed fine granules.[166] This organism fermented glucose, hydrolyzed arginine but not urea, required cholesterol for growth, and could be cultivated in SP-4 medium. It was also able to adhere to and actively invade mammalian cells.[165] Intracellular organisms were observed to be inside of membrane-bound vesicles, with subsequent cell disruption and necrosis. This new species has been given the name *Mycoplasma penetrans*.[166]

Seroepidemiologic studies have documented a high frequency of antibodies against *M. penetrans* in HIV-infected individuals. Wang and associates found that 35.4% of serum samples from 444 HIV-1-infected patients were positive for antibodies against *M. penetrans*.[328] Among 234 men with AIDS, 41.5% were seropositive; 20.3% of 118 asymptomatic, HIV-1-infected individuals were also seropositive. Only one of 384 HIV-negative blood donors had antibodies against *M. penetrans*. Interestingly, 40% of 85 serum samples archived from patients with "GRID" (gay-related immunodeficiency), a term used in the early 1980s to describe AIDS, were also positive for anti-*M. penetrans* antibodies. Among 336 serum specimens from sexually transmitted diseases clinics in southern California, Brooklyn, and Milwaukee, only three were positive for *M. penetrans* antibodies. None of the 178 serum specimens obtained from HIV-1 seronegative individuals with other diseases or immunologic disorders (e.g., dialysis patients, systemic lupus erythematosus, rheumatoid arthritis, multiple sclerosis, leukemia, lymphoma, or other cancers) was positive for antibodies against *M. penetrans*.[328] Further seroepidemiologic studies by the same research group found similar high rates of mycoplasmal antibodies in both symptomatic and asymptomatic HIV-1-positive homosexual men but only 1% of 308 specimens from intravenous drug users and only 0.6% of 165 specimens from hemophiliacs with or without HIV-1 infection, suggesting that *M. penetrans* may be sexually transmitted.[329]

These workers also found an epidemiologic relation between the presence of antibodies to *M. penetrans* and the development of Kaposi's sarcoma (KS).[329] Grau and coauthors reported very similar findings on the presence of *M. penetrans* antibodies in a study conducted in France.[86] These workers found that positive *M. penetrans* serology was associated with both HIV-1 infection and with high-risk sexual practices among homosexual men and that the seroprevalence increased with progression of AIDS-related disease. However, the French research group reported no obvious association between *M. penetrans* infection and Kaposi's sarcoma.[86] Lo and colleagues examined *M. penetrans* seroprevalence and its association with the development of KS in a cohort of 33 HIV-seropositive and 31 HIV-seronegative homosexual men who were enrolled in an AIDS natural history study in New York City in 1984.[168] Testing of archived serum specimens from 1984 to 1985 revealed that 45.5% of the HIV-positive men and 22.5% of the HIV-negative men had antibodies against *M. penetrans*. These data suggest that *M. penetrans* was circulating as a probable sexually transmissible agent early in the AIDS epidemic and was not necessarily associated with HIV infection. Over the subsequent 8 years, nine men developed Kaposi's sarcoma; seven were *M. penetrans* antibody-positive and two were *M. penetrans* antibody-negative. Baseline seropositivity to *M. penetrans* was statistically associated with the subsequent development of KS, and, among the HIV-positive men, KS was more likely to occur among those men who had positive baseline serologies for *M. penetrans*. These workers concluded that *M. penetrans* infection may act as a cofactor with HIV in the subsequent development of KS.[168]

The exact role of *M. penetrans* in the pathogenesis of HIV infection is a subject of current investigations. Most of the work has centered on its putative role as a cofactor in HIV-associated disease progression. Sasaki and colleagues at the Institut Pasteur demonstrated that *M. penetrans* was able to activate human T lymphocytes to undergo blastogenesis followed by cell proliferation and expression of cell surface markers of activation.[251] These phenomena were observed with lymphocytes from healthy donors and from both symptomatic and asymptomatic HIV-infected patients. Characterization of the lymphocytes activated by exposure to *M. penetrans* showed that lymphocytes expressing either CD4 or CD8 underwent blastogenesis as a result. Activation activity was associated exclusively with cells of *M. penetrans* and not with culture supernatants.

MYCOPLASMA PIRUM

Although originally described in 1985, *M. pirum* has attracted some recent attention because it is another of the AIDS-associated mycoplasmas along with *M. fermentans* and *M. penetrans*. Before this association, *M. pirum* had been isolated only from cell cultures as a presumed contaminant, but the cell lines from which it was isolated were of human origin, and it is now thought that these mycoplasmas may have been in the cultured tissues naturally.[57] *M. pirum* has been isolated from peripheral blood mononuclear cells of a patient with HIV infection and has been detected by PCR in blood mononuclear cells of HIV-seropositive individuals.[84,85] Similar to *M. fermentans*, HIV-associated cytopathic effects in vitro are also enhanced by the presence of *M. pirum*, leading to the suggestion that, similar to *M. fermentans*, *M. pirum* may act as a cofactor in the pathogenesis of HIV-related conditions.[199]

M. pirum is closely related to *M. penetrans* and *M. pneumoniae* and, similar to these two other mycoplasmas, has a flask-shaped morphology and a "tip" by which the organism is able to attach to glass or plastic. The P1-like adhesin protein of *M. pirum* and the gene coding for it have been characterized.[295] Following attachment, *M. pirum*, as do *M. fermentans* and *M. penetrans*, is able to actively invade cells.[280] Research is actively underway to further define the interaction of *M. pirum* and other mycoplasmas with human cells and to investigate the role of these organisms, if any, in the pathogenesis of HIV-associated disease.

MYCOPLASMA SPERMATOPHILUM

M. spermatophilum is a newly described anaerobic *Mycoplasma* species that has been isolated from five sperm specimens and from a single female endocervical specimen; these six patients were attending an infertility clinic.[102] In culture, this obligately anaerobic species grew best at 35° to 37°C and produced a hemolysin that was able to lyse guinea pig, sheep, and human erythrocytes, although they did not hemadsorb or hemagglutinate these red cells. Colonies have the typical fried-egg appearance on agar media. This species requires sterols for growth and does not use glucose or hydrolyze either arginine or urea; it is not yet thought to be a pathogen.

HUMAN INFECTIONS DUE TO MYCOPLASMAS OF ANIMAL ORIGIN

M. arginini is one of the few mycoplasmas that is found in a number of animal hosts, including sheep and goats (respiratory and ocular tissues), cattle (respiratory tract, blood, udder, eyes, urogenital tract), and felines (respiratory tract). These animals may or may not exhibit pathologic symptoms, and the role of this organism in animal diseases is still unknown. Yechouran and colleagues reported a case of pneumonia complicated by fatal septicemia caused by *M. arginini* in a 64-year-old man with stage IVB non-Hodgkin's lymphoma, who was hypogammaglobulinemic and had been receiving prednisone.[336] Before his admission to the hospital, the patient had worked in a slaughterhouse, where he slaughtered sheep, cows, and chickens. *M. arginini* grew from three blood cultures: a bronchial brush specimen, a bronchoalveolar lavage specimen, and a Swan-Ganz catheter tip. Susceptibility testing of the isolate using a broth dilution procedure found that it was susceptible to tetracycline, doxycycline, and ciprofloxacin and resistant to erythromycin and streptomycin. This susceptibility pattern has also been found in *M. arginini* isolates recovered from animals. The authors of this case report suggested that the patient acquired his infection by inhalation of contaminated aerosols in the slaughterhouse setting.

Armstrong and colleagues reported a case of pulmonary infection caused by *M. canis* in a female patient who was receiving antineoplastic therapy for

metastatic carcinoma of the cervix.[3] The same organism was isolated from the respiratory tract of other family members and from the family dog, all of whom had upper respiratory tract infections at the same time.

CULTURE OF THE HUMAN MYCOPLASMAS FROM CLINICAL SPECIMENS

GENERAL CONSIDERATIONS

Human mycoplasmas can be divided into three groups on the basis of the utilization of three substrates: glucose, arginine, and urea (see Table 16-3). Depending on the species of mycoplasma that is being sought, an enriched peptone basal medium, containing yeast extract and serum, is supplemented with one of these three substrates and a pH indicator (usually phenol red) is added. *M. pneumoniae* metabolizes glucose to produce lactic acid, resulting in a shift to an acidic pH. *M. hominis* metabolizes arginine with the production of ammonia and a shift in pH from neutral to alkaline. Similarly, *U. urealyticum* produces urease enzymes that hydrolyze urea to ammonia, again resulting in an alkaline pH shift. *M. fermentans* produces acid from glucose and also metabolizes arginine.

Specimens for the isolation of mycoplasmas, particularly the more rapidly growing genital mycoplasmas, are routinely inoculated onto both solid agar media and into some type of selective–differential broth enrichment media. Most broth media formulations used for isolation of mycoplasmas are diphasic, with medium containing agar in the butt of a tube overlayed with broth of similar composition but without added agar. Media for isolation of mycoplasmas also contain antibiotics (e.g., ampicillin, penicillin, polymyxin B, and amphotericin) to inhibit contaminant bacteria and fungi. Thallium acetate was formerly commonly included as an antibacterial agent in media as well, but this compound is inhibitory for *U. urealyticum* and *M. genitalium* and is also highly poisonous for humans.[40]

Human mycoplasmas differ in their optimal pH for growth and in the atmospheric conditions that are required for successful recovery from clinical specimens (see Table 16-3). Media for the isolation of *M. pneumoniae* are buffered at an initial pH of about 7.8, whereas the growth medium for *M. hominis* is buffered at an initial neutral pH (7.0). *U. urealyticum* grows optimally in an environment with a slightly acid pH, so a primary isolation medium for this species is buffered at about pH 6.0. The optimal temperature for mycoplasmal growth is 35° to 37°C. *M. pneumoniae* and *M. hominis* grow well in air or in an atmosphere of 95% nitrogen and 5% carbon dioxide. *U. urealyticum* tends to be capnophilic, with optimal growth occurring in an atmosphere of 10% to 20% carbon dioxide and 80% to 90% nitrogen. An agar medium inoculated directly with specimens or subcultures from broths onto it should be incubated under the appropriate conditions described in the foregoing; a broth medium can always be incubated under aerobic conditions.

Broth media are generally inoculated with 0.1 to 0.2 mL of the specimen contained in a transport fluid. Agar plates are inoculated with a similar amount, and the inoculum is spread over the surface of the agar with a sterile bent glass rod. Agar plates are sealed with air-permeable cellophane tape to prevent the agar from drying out. Media for isolation of *M. pneumoniae* should be incubated for up to 4 weeks before a final culture report is made. Cultures for genital mycoplasmas should be incubated for 7 to 8 days; most positive broth cultures will be detected after 5 days incubation. Diphasic media are compared with coincubated tubes of the same media inoculated with sterile transport medium and with tubes inoculated with control mycoplasma strains to detect subtle differences in color or turbidity. Cultures should be inspected daily for subtle changes because the organisms die rapidly once growth occurs and the substrates are exhausted. If a potentially positive culture is detected visually in diphasic medium, the broth is subcultured onto a solid agar medium, such as SP-4 agar or A7 differential agar (see later discussion).

Identification of the mycoplasmas requires the recognition of typical colonies on solid media directly inoculated with the specimen or with a loopful of broth medium from a presumptively positive diphasic broth medium. Colonies on agar media can be directly examined under 30× to 100× magnification with peripherally incident light to ascertain morphology and growth characteristics. Supravital dyes, such as Dienes' stain, can be used to further characterize colonies and to differentiate them from artifacts. Various identification tests may be performed directly on solid medium, such as the hemadsorption test for presumptive identification of *M. pneumoniae*, or substrates such as arginine or urea, plus a phenol red indicator, may be incorporated in the agar to provide a direct assessment of substrate utilization and, therefore, a presumptive identification. Media for culture of respiratory and genital mycoplasmas and identification procedures for *M. pneumoniae* and *U. urealyticum* are detailed in Charts 21, 36, 45, 46, 47, and 68.

SPECIMEN COLLECTION

M. pneumoniae may be recovered from both upper and lower respiratory tract specimens, including throat swabs, nasopharyngeal swabs, throat washings, sputum, tracheal and transtracheal aspirate, bronchoscopy, bronchoalveolar lavage, and lung tissue specimens.[152] The organism may be recovered from these specimens throughout the course of the illness and for some time after symptomatic recovery. Because of the fastidious nature of these bacteria, culture media should be inoculated as soon after collection as possible. Culture media dispensed into small vials may be used for transport of swab specimens; other specimens (e.g., sputum, tissue, washings) may be transported to the laboratory in sterile screw-capped containers. Before inoculation of growth media, respiratory tract specimens should be homogenized by repeated drawing through a needle and syringe; sputolysin or other

chemical treatments for sputum liquefaction are toxic to mycoplasmas.

Genital mycoplasmas may be isolated from a variety of specimens. These include urethral, vaginal, and cervical swab specimens; prostatic secretions, semen, urine, blood, miscellaneous body fluids (cerebrospinal fluid, amniotic fluid, respiratory tract secretions, synovial fluid, pericardial fluid); and tissue (e.g., endometrial washings and biopsies, placental or amniotic tissues, fetal or abortus tissues, fallopian tube biopsies, uterine biopsies, wound biopsies, rectal tissues). Swab specimens should be obtained using rayon, calcium alginate, or cotton swabs, with either plastic or aluminum shafts. Swabs with wooden shafts should not be used because the wood itself may be toxic to ureaplasmas. If other genital tract pathogens are being sought simultaneously, rayon or Dacron swabs on plastic shafts are probably preferable because they are nontoxic to the other genital tract pathogens as well. Contact of the swab surfaces with antiseptic solutions, creams, jellies, or lubricants should be avoided. Swab specimens should not be allowed to dry and should be placed immediately into a transport or culture medium after collection. Other body fluids and tissue biopsy specimens should be submitted in sterile containers. Saline should not be used to moisten tissue specimens, for it may cause lysis of the organisms. In the laboratory, tissue specimens should be minced in sterile transport medium to produce a 10% (w/v) suspension and serially diluted 10- and 100-fold. This is necessary to prevent inhibition of mycoplasmal growth by organic materials such as hemoglobin, toxic phospholipids, antibodies, or complement that may be present in the tissue specimen. These dilutions are then used to inoculate growth media.

TRANSPORT MEDIA

A variety of transport media may be used for genital mycoplasma cultures. These include trypticase–soy broth with 0.5% bovine serum albumin, 2-sucrose-phosphate (2SP) broth with 10% heat-inactivated fetal calf serum (as is used for chlamydial cultures), or various types of mycoplasma growth media. Antibiotics are generally added to decrease contamination by other bacterial and fungal organisms. At the University of Illinois, we use a mycoplasma transport medium having the following formulation:

PPLO broth (Difco) 700 mL
Mycoplasma supplement (Difco) 300 mL
Phenol red (0.4% aqueous) 5.0 mL
Penicillin (100,000 U/mL) 5.0 mL
Polymyxin B (5,000 ug/mL) 10.0 mL
Amphotericin B (2 mg/mL) 2.5 mL
Final pH 6.0 ± 0.2, 25°C

PPLO broth contains beef heart infusion and peptones, and the mycoplasma supplement contains yeast extract and decomplemented horse serum. Penicillin, polymyxin B, and amphotericin B are added to inhibit gram-positive bacteria, gram-negative bacteria, and fungi, respectively. Specimens should be transported to the laboratory immediately and may be held up to 24 hours at 4°C before inoculation of growth media. If culture is delayed beyond this time, the specimen should be frozen at −70°C. Urine specimens for culture should be centrifuged and the sediment diluted 1:1 with transport medium before freezing. The protein stabilizers in the transport medium prevent loss of organism viability that may occur if urine specimens are frozen without this protective measure.

MEDIA FOR CULTURE OF MYCOPLASMAS

Several types of media have been described in the literature for the cultivation of *M. pneumoniae* and the genital mycoplasmas. As mentioned, most broth media are diphasic; that is, the tubes contain an agar phase that is overlayed with broth medium of similar composition. One medium recommended by the CDC for isolation of *M. pneumoniae* is called **methylene blue–glucose diphasic medium**.[215] This medium contains PPLO broth and agar, yeast extract, and serum supplements along with glucose, methylene blue, and phenol red. The methylene blue in the medium inhibits the growth of other human mycoplasmas that may be found in the respiratory tract, making the medium selective for *M. pneumoniae*. During growth of *M. pneumoniae*, the medium becomes more acidic and the phenol red turns color from salmon to yellow. At the same time, the organisms reduce the methylene blue and turn it from blue to colorless. Therefore, the color of the broth phase changes from purple to green or yellow-green, while the agar phase turns from a purple color to a yellow or yellow orange. This medium is used in conjunction with **mycoplasma glucose agar medium**. Colonies recovered either directly on this medium or from subcultures of positive broths are then subjected to inspection and identification procedures. The components and formulas for *M. pneumoniae* isolation medium are presented in Chart 46.

Another medium that is recommended for isolation of *M. pneumoniae* from clinical specimens is **SP-4 diphasic broth** and **SP-4 agar**.[305] These media were originally formulated for the cultivation of spiraplasmas, but they also provide superior recovery of *M. pneumoniae* and other human mycoplasmas (e.g., *M. genitalium*). In a comparative study conducted by Tully and coworkers, diphasic SP-4 medium recovered *M. pneumoniae* from 69 of 200 specimens that were negative when cultured by other "standard" methods.[305] As with the methylene blue–glucose diphasic medium, growth is detected by the change of the phenol red indicator from red to yellow indicating the production of acid from glucose.

Because *M. hominis* and *U. urealyticum* metabolize different substrates and differ in the pH for optimal growth, many laboratories use two types of agar media for their cultivation. In addition, diphasic broth and agar formulations of each medium type should be inoculated for optimal recovery of mycoplasmas. **H broth** and **H agar** are used to isolate *M. hominis* and are buffered at a neutral pH (7.0). Some formulations may also contain arginine as the growth substrate, with

both medium turbidity and a shift in the color of the phenol red indicator into the alkaline range being used to detect organism growth. **U broth** and **U agar**, used to isolate *U. urealyticum*, are buffered at a lower pH (5.5 to 6.0) and contain urea as the growth substrate. The latter media are also made more selective for *U. urealyticum* by the inclusion of lincomycin because ureaplasmas are resistant to this drug and *M. hominis* strains are susceptible. Medium formulations for isolation of genital mycoplasmas are found in Chart 47.

Several other media have been described in the literature for the isolation and identification of genital mycoplasmas. Broth media include the U-9 urease medium described by Shepard and Lunceford, bromthymol blue broth, S-2 Boston broth, and the SP-4 medium used for recovery of the respiratory tract mycoplasmas.[42,67,153,237,256,258,259,262,334] SP-4 medium should be supplemented with urea or arginine to specifically detect *U. urealyticum* and *M. hominis*, respectively. S-2 Boston broth is a single medium that contains enriched base medium, horse serum, yeast extract, phenol red indicator, L-cysteine, urea, and penicillin. Growth of *U. urealyticum* is detected by the appearance of a pink color in the medium, whereas growth of *M. hominis* is detected by a pale salmon-pink to orange color or by the appearance of slight turbidity. Shepard's **A7 differential agar medium** and various modifications of it (e.g., A7B and A8) are particularly useful because both *M. hominis* and *U. urealyticum* grow well on them and and can be easily differentiated from one another by colony morphology and by the direct detection of urease formation by the latter species (see later discussion).[256,258,259] As described in the following, presumptive identification of *M. hominis* and definitive identification of *U. urealyticum* can be obtained with this medium, without the need for additional tests or reagents.

ISOLATION AND IDENTIFICATION OF *MYCOPLASMA PNEUMONIAE*

In general, the growth of *M. pneumoniae* from clinical specimens is detected by the ability of these organisms to produce acid from glucose. Methylene blue–glucose diphasic medium is inoculated with 0.2 mL of the specimen in transport fluid. Tubes of media are simultaneouly inoculated with sterile tranport medium and with a positive control culture and are incubated along with the specimens. Broth cultures are incubated at 35°C with the caps tightened. Tubes are inspected daily for color changes in the medium and for turbidity for 4 weeks. The development of gross turbidity and an acid or alkaline shift of the indicator within 1 to 5 days is generally due to bacterial contamination. A slight, gradual shift in the pH indicator over an 8- to 15-day period without gross turbidity suggests a true positive culture. As soon as color changes in the medium are apparent, the broth must be subcultured to appropriate agar medium; as more acid accumulates in the medium, mycoplasmas rapidly become nonviable. At the earliest indication of growth, the broth is subcultured to agar medium (such as SP-4 agar) and incubated in air for 5 to 7 days. Inspection of the agar surface under the low power of the microscope will reveal small colonies of the organisms. In the absence of obvious color change in diphasic media, a blind subculture to agar media should be performed after 1 and 3 weeks incubation. A general scheme for the isolation of *M. pneumoniae* is shown in Figure 16-1.

M. pneumoniae may be identified by a variety of procedures, some of which are more involved than others. Tests that are easily adaptable to the clinical laboratory include the hemadsorption test (Chart 36) and the tetrazolium reduction test (Chart 68). In the hemadsorption procedure, colonies growing on the surface of the agar are flooded with a 0.2% to 0.4% suspension of washed guinea pig erythrocytes. After incubation, the surface of the plate is gently washed with sterile saline and examined under 50× to 100× magnification. Colonies of *M. pneumoniae* adsorb the erythrocytes to their surface and appear as round colonies studded with red blood cells (see Color Plate 16-1A). This procedure works best on colonies that are 5 to 7 days old; older colonies tend to lose their hemadsorbing properties. Other *Mycoplasma* species that inhabit the upper respiratory tract are negative in the hemadsorption test.

The tetrazolium reduction test exploits the unique ability of *M. pneumoniae* to reduce the colorless compound triphenyl tetrazolium to the red compound formozan. To perform the test, the agar surface bearing the suspected colonies is flooded with a solution of 2-(p-iodophenyl)-3-nitrophenyl-5-phenyl tetrazolium chloride (0.21%) and incubated at 35°C for an hour. Colonies of *M. pneumoniae* will appear reddish after 1 hour and may appear purple to black after 3 to 4 hours. Other mycoplasmas are negative with this test. The tetrazolium test can be performed even after the colonies are tested with the hemadsorption procedure.

Specific serologic methods may also be used for culture confirmation of *M. pneumoniae*.[39,42] The more rapid of these is the epifluorescence procedure. Agar medium containing colonies is flooded with *M. pneumoniae*-specific antibodies conjugated to fluorescein isothiocyanate, washed to remove unbound conjugate, and subsequently examined with a microscope equipped for epifluorescence procedures. Colonies of *M. pneumoniae* will fluoresce. Although considered to be the reference procedure, the growth inhibition test for identification of *M. pneumoniae* is also the most time-consuming procedure. In this test, an agar plate is inoculated as a lawn from a broth suspension of the isolate to be identified. A piece of filter paper impregnated with anti-*M. pneumoniae* antibodies is then placed on the agar surface. After incubation, inhibition of colonial growth will be observed surrounding the filter paper that is saturated with the species-specific antibodies.

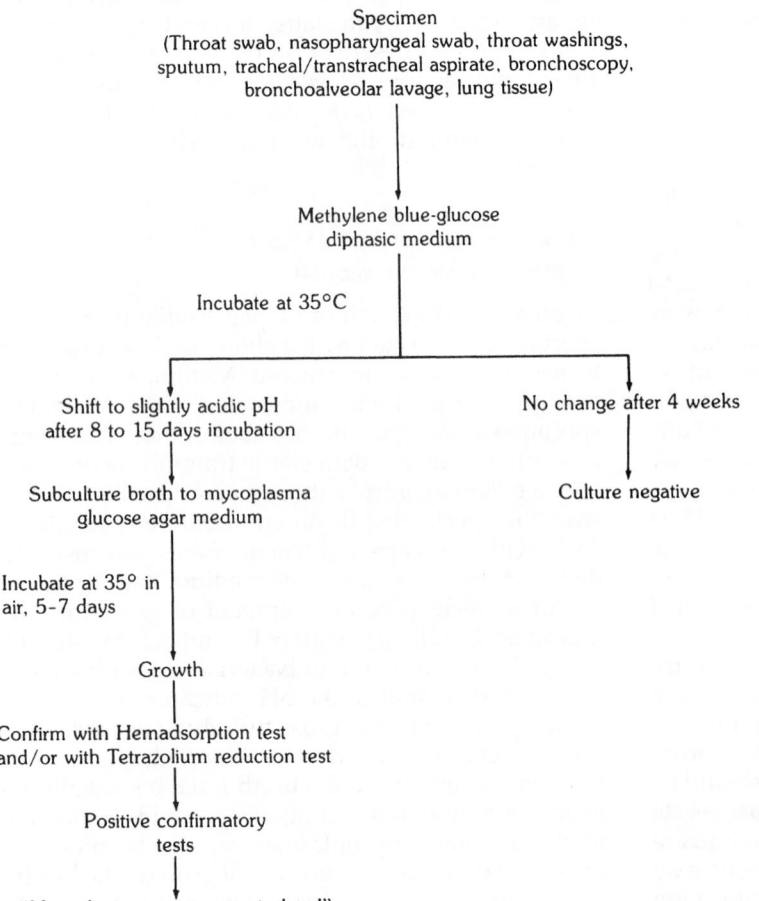

Figure 16-1.
Protocol for isolation of *Mycoplasma pneumoniae* from respiratory tract specimens.

Other technologies have also been applied to the diagnosis of *M. pneumoniae* respiratory tract infections. Cimolai and associates[37] described a rather novel culture-amplification technique similar to the shell vial methods currently used in virology. Conventional agar and broth cultures were set up in duplicate. During each day of incubation, aliquots from one set of broth specimens were tested by an immunoblot technique using a monoclonal antigen-capture antibody directed against the 43,000-Da membrane-associated adhesin of *M. pneumoniae*. The immunoblot method detected positive cultures in from 2 to 12 days (mean of 4.7 days), whereas conventional cultures were visibly positive in from 7 to 14 days (mean of 8.3 days). Marmion and colleagues described an antigen-capture enzyme immunoassay (EIA) using polyclonal antibodies directed against purified, P1 antigen as the capture antibody.[181] In a study of respiratory tract specimens from 234 patients, the antigen test detected four of four patients who were positive by culture and serology, and four of five patients who were positive by culture only. Interestingly, 43% of 23 patients who were culture-negative but seropositive and 71% of patients who had a diagnostic rise in antibody titer and had no culture done were positive in the antigen EIA. These findings indicated that the antigen test and probably other direct tests need to be confirmed by an assessment of the serologic antibody response to verify that the infection diagnosed by the direct test is a current infection and not the result of prolonged or continuing carriage of the organism from a previous infection.[181] Similar findings have been reported by others using a commercially available *M. pneumoniae* antigen EIA (Enzygnost-*Mycoplasma pneumoniae* Ag, Behringwerke, Germany).[141]

Because of the slow growth of *M. pneumoniae*, non–growth-dependent, direct specimen nucleic acid probe methods have been developed for the diagnosis of mycoplasmal respiratory tract infections. The *M. pneumoniae* DNA probe (Gen-Probe, Inc., San Diego CA) hybridizes with the 16S rRNA of the organism and uses a ^{125}I radioactive label to generate a detection signal. Tilton and coworkers compared the DNA probe with culture and found that the probe had a sensitivity of 100% and a specificity of 98% when compared with culture.[298] Another study by Dular and associates reported that the probe had both a sensitivity and a specificity of 89% compared with culture.[62] In both reports, the authors stressed the practical aspects of the probe as a rapid, sensitive, and timely approach to diagnosis because probe results are available in about 2 hours, whereas culture requires several weeks. In addition, the rapid diagnosis provided by the probe would eliminate the reliance on retrospective serologic testing (e.g., complement fixation) or nonspecific serologic markers (i.e., cold agglutinins) for diagnosis and would enable specific antimicrobial therapy to be initiated. The drawbacks of the probe include its relatively short 6-week shelf life, the need for additional equipment, the generation and disposal of radioactive wastes, and its expense. In addition, because the organisms may be harbored in the respiratory tract during convalescence, positive probe tests may be found in respiratory swab specimens collected from healthy individuals. Unfortunately, the Gen-Probe test was withdrawn from the market in 1992.

Molecular methods such as polymerase chain reaction (PCR) have also been used for detection of *M. pneumoniae* in a variety of specimen types.[24,29,54,175,181,253,263,299] Buck and coauthors described a PCR test in which the amplified DNA segment was a 375-base pair (bp) segment of the *M. pneumoniae* P1 adhesin protein.[24] For simulated clinical specimens, this test was able to detect a lower limit of between one and 10 organisms compared with a lower limit of 1000 organisms for cultural detection. Similar sensitivity has been reported by others using the same target DNA sequence.[29,54] Several investigators have designed species-specific probes for *M. pneumoniae* based on *M. pneumoniae*-specific 16S rRNA sequences and found that amplification and subsequent probe detection of these sequences in clinical specimens was more sensitive than culture.[253,299,314] By using PCR technology, Narita and coworkers detected *M. pneumoniae*-specific DNA in four of six cerebrospinal fluids specimens and in three of four serum specimens from patients with clinically and serologically confirmed *M. pneumoniae* central nervous system infection.[205] PCR "fingerprinting" technology has also been used to subtype isolates of *M. pneumoniae* based on nucleotide sequence divergence of the P1 cytoadhesin protein.[312]

ISOLATION AND IDENTIFICATION OF THE GENITAL MYCOPLASMAS

Mycoplasmas that may be recovered from the genital tract include *M. hominis*, *M. genitalium*, *M. fermentans*, and *U. urealyticum*. Whereas *M. hominis* and *U. urealyticum* are easily cultivated and usually grow within 1 to 5 days, *M. genitalium* and *M. fermentans* grow much more slowly and are more difficult to detect in culture. Furthermore, culture systems that are in current use for the recovery of genital mycoplasmas may not support optimal growth of these species. For example, the SP-4 medium described earlier for the isolation of *M. pneumoniae* is the optimal medium for *M. genitalium* because this organism is a glucose metabolizer, yet most laboratories do not employ glucose-containing culture media for culture of genital tract specimens. Furthermore, the slow growth of the organism on media precludes the clinical usefulness of such culture data. Nonculture methods (such as nucleic acid probes and PCR) show promise as techniques for detection of *M. genitalium*.[105,110] *M. fermentans* also utilizes glucose but is very slow growing. Because of these considerations, genital mycoplasmas other than *M. hominis* and *U. urealyticum* are generally not sought in genital tract specimens. Jensen and colleagues recently reported the successful isolation of *M. genitalium* from genital tract specimens.[119] From 11 PCR positive urethral specimens from patients with urethritis, nine were successfully propagated in Vero cell cultures. Growth in Vero cell culture was monitored by PCR. Of these nine isolates, six were adapted by serial passage to growth in Friis medium, a complex growth medium containing Hank's balanced salts solution, brain–heart infusion broth, "home-made" yeast extract, and up to 20% (v/v) horse serum. These six isolates required from one to 19 serial passages in Vero cell cultures before they could be adapted to growth in broth, and from two to six passages in broth before visible colonies were produced on an agar medium similar in formulation to the broth. In this report, the authors point out that, although the development of a medium able to support the growth of *M. genitalium* represented a major breakthrough, PCR methods were essential for initial detection and for monitoring the cultures for growth.

Appropriate specimens received in transport media are inoculated onto both broth and agar media. In general, about 0.2 mL of the specimen should be streaked onto agar media and placed in broth media. Broths may be incubated aerobically at 35°C, but plates should be incubated in a CO_2 incubator or a candle jar. Both organisms may also be recovered under anaerobic conditions. Plated media should be inspected daily under 40× magnification using oblique light to observe the "fried egg" colonies of *M. hominis* or the small, dense colonies of *U. urealyticum*. With broth cultures, any broths showing the slightest alkaline color change or turbidity should be subcultured to the appropriate plated media. In M broth, *M. hominis* produces a slight turbidity in addition to a change in color. In U broth, *U. urealyticum* will tend to produce a slight color change early in incubation with no distinct or obvious turbidity. In both cases, subcultures must be performed at these times to ensure recovery of viable bacteria because there is a rapid decrease in viability of the organisms once the pH has been elevated by substrate utilization and depletion. As with the primary culture plates, subcultures plates should be inspected daily. Most isolates of *M. hominis* and *U. urealyticum* will grow within 5 to 7 days. If growth is not detected on primary plates or broth subcultures after this time, the culture can be reported as negative for genital mycoplasmas. It is a good idea to freeze aliquots of positive broths at −70°C in case problems are encountered with viability on direct agar cultures or subcultures. The general scheme for isolation of genital mycoplasmas is presented in Figure 16-2.

Identification of genital mycoplasmas is generally quite easy and straightforward. *M. hominis* colonies grow in 1 to 5 days, have the typical fried egg colonial morphology, and are usually 50 to 300 μm in diameter. Colonies may be stained with the Dienes stain (Chart 21) to aid visualization (see Color Plate 16-1*B*). Further identification procedures are not necessary because rapidly growing, arginine-positive organisms exhibiting the typical colony morphology are invariably *M. hominis*. The small colonies of *U. urealyticum* may be difficult to distinguish from various artifacts, such as mammalian cells and cellular debris or materials present in serum. Because of these problems, suspect *U. urealyticum* colonies must be confirmed. This is done by exploiting the ability of *U. urealyticum* to hydrolyze urea. If the U agar medium contains urea and phenol red, the suspect ureaplasma colonies will be surrounded by a red halo.

Suspect *U. urealyticum* colonies may also be confirmed with the manganous chloride–urea test (Chart 45). In this test, an agar plate containing colonial growth is flooded with an aqueous solution of urea (1%) and 0.8% (w/v) manganous chloride. Hydrolysis of urea by urease liberates hydroxyl groups from water, and these hydroxyl moieties oxidize manganous chloride to insoluble manganese oxide, causing the deposition of a golden brown precipitate in the colonies themselves within a few minutes.

Shepard's A7 differential agar media and its modifications, A7B and A8 agars, have the urea and the ureahydrolysis detection reagent incorporated in the medium already, so flooding the plate with manganous chloride is not required.[256,258,259] A7 agar contains manganous sulfate as the precipitating agent along with penicillin (1000 U/mL) and amphotericin B (2.5 μg/mL). A7B differential agar is identical with A7 agar, except that the polyamine putrescine dihydrochloride (10 mM) is added to enhance the ureaplasma growth and development of the precipitate in the colonies. A8 differential agar incoporates calcium chloride (1 mM) as the divalent cation indicator for the detection of ammonia formation from urea, along with colistin (7.5 μg/mL), ampicillin (1 μg/mL), and amphotericin B (2.5 μg/mL). On all three media formulations, *M. hominis* appears with the characteristic fried egg morphology after 1 to 3 days on A7, A7B, and A8 differential agars. *U. urealyticum* colonies appear within 1 to 3 days and are 15 to 50 μm in diameter (depending on crowding). *U. urealyticum* colonies on A7 and A7B agars are dark brown owing to the accumulation of manganese oxide in the colony, whereas colonies on A8 differential agar are gold to light brown (see Color Plate 16-1*B*). Several comparative evaluations of A7, A7B, and A8 media indicate that they are probably the agar media of choice for culture of genital mycoplasmas and, when used with an appropriate broth medium (e.g., bromothymol blue broth, Boston broth), give the highest yield of positive cultures.[153,219,334] Because the growth charactertistics of *U. urealyticum* on these media are unique, further testing is not necessary. Both A7 and A8 differential agars are commercially available from Remel Laboratories (Lenexa, KA).

Definitive identification of *M. hominis* may be made by growth inhibition using specific antisera.[39] An indirect immunoperoxidase method has also been published for the identification of mycoplasmas.[111] This method employs filter paper strips that are impregnated with specific rabbit antisera to various mycoplasma species and are applied to mycoplasmal growth on an agar plate. After 1 hour, the papers are removed and the same spot is covered with another piece of filter paper impregnated with goat antirabbit antisera conjugated to horseradish peroxidase. After another hour incubation, the filter papers are removed and the plate is flooded with the enzyme substrate (1% 4-chloro-1-naphthol). The identity of the isolate is indicated by the appearance of a deep blue color where the initial species-specific antisera was placed on the plate.

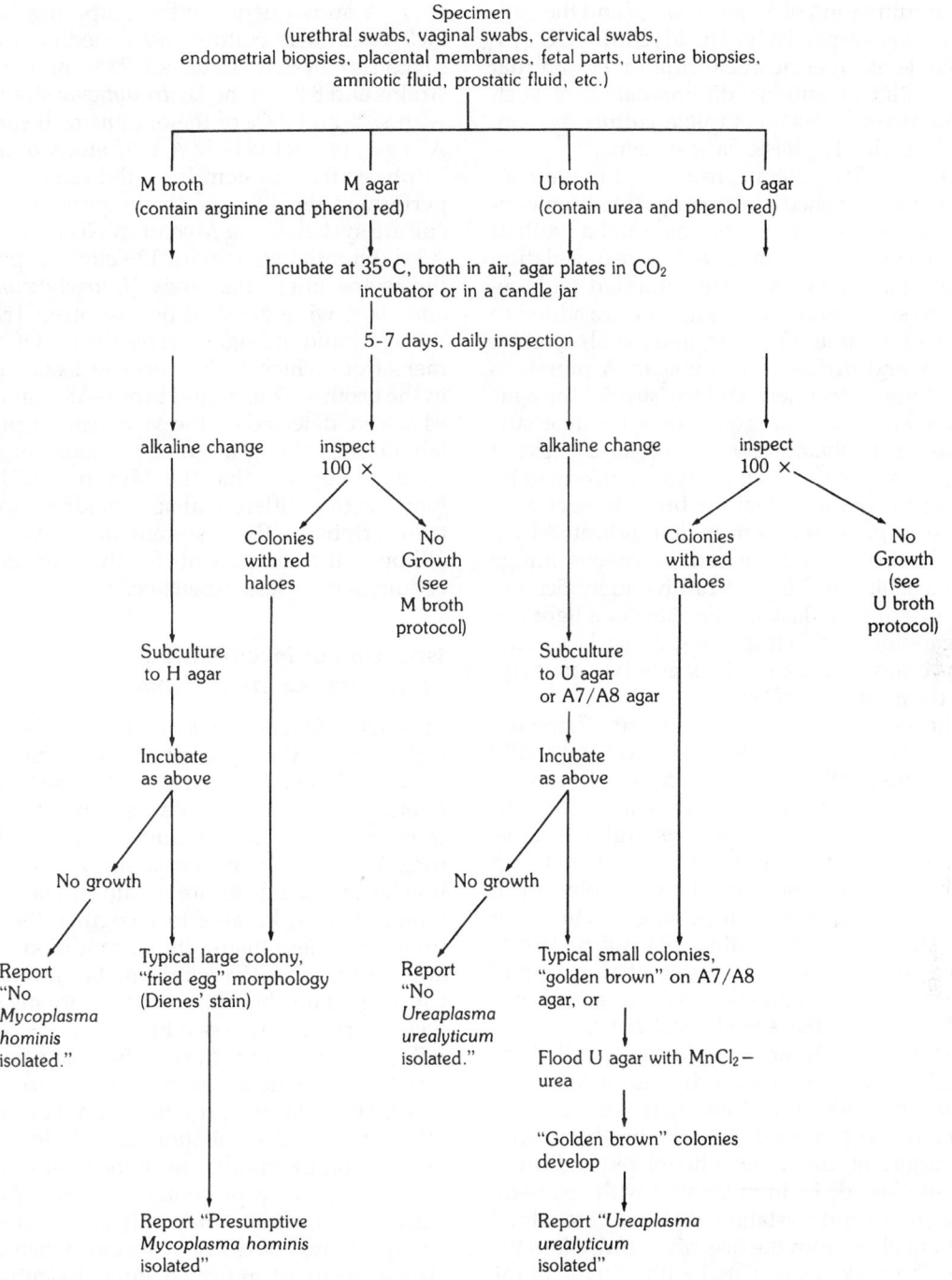

Figure 16-2.
Protocol for isolation of *Mycoplasma hominis* and *Ureaplasma urealyticum* from genital specimens.

This method produces results comparable with those of the antiserum growth inhibition procedure. Similar procedures, using both immunofluorescence and immunoperoxidase techniques, have been developed for use in mycoplasma studies in animals, where species having similar tissue tropisms may be present in mixed culture.[13]

PCR assays have also been developed using *M. hominis*-specific 16S rRNA sequences as the target for amplification and detection.[17] However, definitive species identification of large-colony mycoplasmas recovered from genital sites is generally not necessary.

COMMERCIAL MYCOPLASMA CULTURE SYSTEMS

The Mycotrim RS and Mycotrim Triphasic flask systems (Irvine Scientific, Irvine CA) are the only commercially available systems that have been used extensively for the cultivation of *M. pneumoniae* and the genital mycoplasmas, respectively. The Mycotrim GU system is available as an enrichment broth medium that can be used with conventional differential agars, such as A7 or A8 agars, or as a complete culture system, called the Mycotrim Triphasic flask system.

The Mycotrim RS system consists of a bottle containing a layer of enriched glucose agar medium containing phenol red indicator on one side and a broth of similar composition. Thirty minutes before inoculation with the specimen, disks that are saturated with cefaperazone, nystatin, and thallous acetate are added to the flasks to allow time for the antimicrobials to elute from the disk and diffuse into the agar. A pipette is used to add liquid specimens and to "streak" the agar surface. Swab specimens are rolled over the agar surface. The flask is incubated agar-side up for 2 weeks at 35° to 37°C. Reinoculation after 3 days is performed by manipulating the bottle so that the broth washes over part of the agar phase. Growth is first indicated by a change in the indicator from red to yellow-orange without noticeable turbidity. Definitive identification is made by placing the flask on the stage of a light microscope agar-side up and inspecting the surface of the agar for mycoplasma colonies. This may be done with or without the addition of Dienes stain.

Mycotrim GU broth and the Mycotrim Triphasic flask system are the only widely used, commercially available systems for the isolation and identification of the genital mycoplasmas *M. hominis* and *U. urealyticum*. Mycotrim GU broth contains arginine, urea, and phenol red indicator. This broth is inoculated with 0.1 mL of the specimen and is incubated aerobically at 35°C. The medium is observed for changes in the color of the indicator to a more alkaline pH; subculture to solid media, such as A7 or A8 differential agar; and subsequent incubation allows the recovery and identification of both *M. hominis* and *U. urealyticum*.

The Mycotrim Triphasic flask (formerly called the Mycotrim GU system) system is a diphasic system that contains modified A8 differential agar with calcium chloride in a tissue culture flask and a broth medium containing arginine, urea, and phenol red indicator. Before inoculation, disks impregnated with cefaperazone (100 µg/mL) and nystatin (50 U/mL) are added and allowed to elute from the disk and diffuse into the agar phase. The flask is inoculated with 0.10 mL of the specimen, and the broth–specimen mixture is washed over the agar phase. The flask is incubated at 35°C aerobically. Subculture is achieved by allowing the broth to wash over part of the agar phase after 24-hour incubation. With the appearance of a color change in the phenol red indicator from yellow to orange or orange-red, the agar phase is examined under the microscope for the typical fried egg colonies of *M. hominis* or the small, brown calcium oxide-stained colonies of *U. urealyticum*. Cultures are inspected daily and incubated for 7 days.

In a study published in 1985, Wood and associates[333] found that the Mycotrim GU system performed as well as the conventional method using arginine broth, urea broth, glucose agar, and A7B differential agar. A subsequent study comparing the Mycotrim GU system with culture on A7 medium found that the Mycotrim system detected 73% of the *M. hominis* strains and 84% of the *U. urealyticum* strains compared with 93% and 89% of the organisms being isolated on A7 agar, respectively.[219] A 1992 study of the Mycotrim Triphasic flask system from the same laboratory that performed the 1985 study compared the flask with a culture system using Mycotrim GU broth with A7 and A8 differential agars with 129 clinical specimens.[20] Of the 64 specimens that grew *U. urealyticum*, 25%, 98%, and 100% were detected on Mycotrim Triphasic agar, A7 agar, and A8 agar, respectively. Of the 18 specimens from which *M. hominis* was isolated, all 18 grew in the broth—A7 agar and broth–A8 agar cultures, and 94% were detected on the Mycotrim Triphasic agar. In laboratories doing a modest amount of mycoplasma work, it appears that the Mycotrim GU broth combined with a differential agar medium and the Mycotrim Triphasic flask system are fairly comparable, although the components for the "conventional" procedure may be less expensive.

ISOLATION OF MYCOPLASMAS ON ROUTINE CULTURE MEDIA

In general, *M. pneumoniae* and *U. urealyticum* are more fastidious in their growth requirements than *M. hominis*, and the latter species is the one that is most frequently recovered from sites other than the genital tract, such as blood, wounds, and joint fluids. Therefore, *M. hominis* may occasionally be isolated on routine bacteriologic culture medium. The clinical microbiologist must be able to recognize these organisms under these less-than-optimal conditions. *M. hominis* is able to grow on enriched media such as Columbia CNA agar and chocolate agar; the organism grows less well on tryptic soy-based blood agar.[212] The organisms will grow best under anaerobic conditions, with less rapid growth in an aerobic, CO_2-enriched environment. Mycoplasmal growth may not be apparent until after prolonged incubation (i.e., 72 to 96 hours), depending on the conditions of incubation and the numbers of organisms present. Colonies of *M. hominis* are extremely small and may only be detected as a "film" or "speckling" of the agar surface when examined by strong, incident, reflected light. Examination of this type of growth is facilitated by using a dissecting microscope. The colonies are difficult to pick up with a loop and will not stain with the Gram stain.

Suspected mycoplasma colonies from routine agar medium can be subcultured by cutting out a block of the blood agar and rubbing the side with the growth across the surface of a mycoplasma growth medium such as A7 differential agar. Another block should be aseptically removed and immersed in a broth medium such as H broth or Boston broth. Both broth and agar subcultures are then incubated and processed as described in the foregoing. Inspection of colony morphology, along with the growth rate and assessment of optimal incubation conditions for growth, will allow presumptive identfication of the species.

M. hominis may also be occasionally recovered from blood cultures, particularly in women with postpartum fever. Sodium polyanethol sulfonate (SPS), the anticomplementary and antiphagocytic additive that is present in most routine blood culture media, is toxic to mycoplasmas. In general, the higher the SPS content (0.025 versus 0.050%), the more inhibitory the media becomes for the recovery of mycoplasmas.[52] Mycoplasmas have been recovered from radiometric blood culture media (i.e., the BACTEC system), but the SPS will inhibit or delay organism recovery, depending on the SPS content of the broth. Smaron and coworkers isolated *M. hominis* from blood cultures using the radiometric BACTEC system with SPS-free media.[265] Organisms were detected in both aerobic and anaerobic blood culture vials after 3 to 7 days incubation. Blood bottles did not appear grossly positive, and growth indices on the instrument increased slowly over time. In addition, Gram stains from positive bottles failed to reveal any organisms, but they were visible when examined with the acridine orange stain. The addition of 10 mg/mL of gelatin to blood culture media has been demonstrated to partially overcome the inhibitory effects of SPS.[52] Also, the presence of sucrose in hypertonic blood culture media retards the growth of mycoplasmas.[52] In the BACTEC system, mycoplasmal growth may occur to some extent, but the growth index for the cultures may not exceed the threshold growth index value for positivity. Pratt explained this phenomenon by pointing out that CO_2 production by *M. hominis* results from arginine deaminase activity, which is produced by the organism late in the logarithmic growth phase. Limiting levels of [^{14}C] arginine may prevent mycoplasmal growth from reaching levels that "trip" the positive threshold of the BACTEC instrument.[226]

If *M. hominis* bacteremia is suspected, blood should optimally be inoculated at the patient's bedside into an SPS-free medium. Incubation of the cultures should be prolonged, and blind subcultures to appropriate agar and broth mycoplasma isolation medium, in addition to CNA agar, should be made at frequent intervals. Blood for recovery of mycoplasmas should be inoculated directly into the mycoplasma culture medium. The blood should be diluted 1:10 with growth medium, so culture of a substantial blood volume may require multiple vials of culture media.

NONCULTURE METHODS FOR MYCOPLASMA DETECTION AND IDENTIFICATION

Nonculture methods have also been examined for their ability to detect mycoplasmas. Hirai and colleagues developed an indirect fluorescent antibody (IFA) test for direct identification of *M. hominis* in vaginal specimens.[104] The staining of Vero cells that were infected with other *Mycoplasma* species, including *M. orale*, *M. salivarium*, and *M. fermentans*, demonstrated that the IFA procedure was specific for *M. hominis*. The IFA test was compared with culture on vaginal specimens collected from 193 healthy women. Among 22 culture-

positive specimens, 17 were positive with the IFA test. Interestingly, 48 of 171 specimens that were negative by culture were positive with the IFA test, suggesting that the IFA method was more sensitive than culture. These workers also demonstrated that the location of granular aggregates that were observed on vaginal epithelial cells stained with the Papanicolaou stain frequently corresponded to the areas of the smears that stained with the *M. hominis*-specific IFA reagents.[104]

Probe technology is also being exploited for detection of those mycoplasmas that are difficult to recover in culture, such as *M. genitalium*. Because of the recognized antigenic cross-reactivity between species and similarities in certain nucleotide sequences, nucleic acid probes for *M. genitalium* and *M. pneumoniae* must be constructed to specifically exclude homologous nucleotide sequences to prevent false-positive results.[338] Such carefully constructed DNA probes have been used along with gene amplification techniques and PCR to detect *M. pneumoniae*- and *M. genitalium*-specific nucleotide sequences directly in clinical specimens.[14,105,122] In one study, 10 of 150 genital specimens recovered from eight patients (three men and five women), were positive for *M. genitalium*.[122] These results were verified by Southern blot hybridization tests because cultures were not performed.

Because of the difficulty in cultural recovery of some *Mycoplasma* species, highly sensitive assays such as PCR have been developed. PCR methods have been developed for *U. urealyticum*, using the nucleotide sequence of the urease genes as the target for amplification and detection.[16,292] This test was able to detect as few as one colony-forming unit in specimens from the adult urogenital tract and amniotic fluids and endotracheal aspirates from newborn infants. Teng and coworkers[292] examined 50 clinical specimens (eight urethral swab specimens, eight urine specimens, 12 endocervical swab specimens, eight prostatic fluid specimens, and 14 semen specimens) by both culture and PCR. Cultures were positive for five specimens, and an additional four specimens produced appropriate pH changes in broth but did not grow on subculture to agar medium ("doubtful" positives). PCR was positive for all five culture-positive specimens, all four doubtful-positive specimens, plus three specimens (one prostatic fluid and two endocervical specimens) that were culture-negative. *M. fermentans* PCR methods detect a unique DNA sequence that appears repetitively in the genome of the organism, whereas those for detection of *M. hominis*, *M. penetrans* and *M. pirum* detect unique nucleotide sequences within the 16S rRNA of these species.[84,85,327]

SEROLOGIC TESTS FOR DIAGNOSIS OF *MYCOPLASMA PNEUMONIAE* INFECTION

Because of the limited availability of culture, the technical difficulties inherent in the culture techniques, and the amount of time required for culture results to become available, the diagnosis of *M. pneumoniae* infection is often made by a combination of clinical and serologic findings. Diagnosis on clinical grounds alone is difficult because many other pneumonic processes, particularly those caused by viruses, can present similarly.[5] The most widely used serologic test for diagnosis of *M. pneumoniae* infection is the complement fixation (CF) test. The antigen used in the test is a glycolipid from the organism that is extracted by chloroform–methanol (2:1 v/v).[138,315] The CF test measures predominantly early IgM antibodies to *M. pneumoniae* and detects IgG antibodies to a comparatively minor extent.[113] As with other serologic tests, a fourfold rise in CF titers between acute and convalescent serum specimens is diagnostic of recent or current infection with *M. pneumoniae*. The acute specimen should be collected as soon after disease onset as possible, with the convalescent specimen being collected 7 to 10 days later. Single CF titers of 32 or higher collected in the convalescent period are highly suggestive of recent infection.[138] CF titers begin to rise 7 to 10 days after infection with the organism and reach peak titers after 4 to 6 weeks.[5,113] Significant CF titers may persist beyond this time. Because the CF test measures primarily IgM antibodies, its usefulness for diagnosis of repeated infections caused by *M. pneumoniae* is less than those test methods that detect increases in other immunoglobulin classes (i.e., detection of changes in IgG along with IgM). The crude extract from *M. pneumoniae* that is used in the CF test is similar in structure to other bacterial and plant glycolipids, so cross-reactions of this antigen with other nonmycoplasmal antibodies may occur. CF titers for diagnosis of mycoplasmal pneumonia may be falsely positive in individuals with bacterial meningitis. In addition, some autoimmune conditions may also cause false-positive mycoplasmal CF serologic results.[113]

The sensitivity and the specificity of the CF test in retrospective diagnosis of *M. pneumoniae* infection varies depending on the time during the illness when specimens are collected, the availability of paired specimens, and the cutoff used for interpretation of titers from single serum specimens. In a study by Kenny and coworkers,[138] a fourfold rise in titer showed a sensitivity of only 53% in those patients who had pneumonia and were culture-positive. This sensitivity increased to 90% when single titers higher than 32 were included. Specificity of the CF test using either a fourfold titer increase or a titer of 32 or higher was 89%. A large 12-year study of the CF test and culture for diagnosis of *M. pneumoniae* found that the sensitivity and specificity of the CF test were 90% and 94%, respectively, whereas the sensitivity of culture was 64%.[113]

Enzyme immunoassays (EIAs) for the detection of *M. pneumoniae*-specific antibodies have also been developed. In general, these assays have proved to be more sensitive than the CF test; in one study, three of 65 sera that had CF titers of 16 had much higher titers in the EIA.[27] In this same study, EIA was less sensitive for antibody detection than the radioimmunoprecipitation assay. Fischer and associates[68] evaluated the MYCOPLASMELISA™ commercial EIA (Whittaker MA Bioproducts, Walkersville MD) in comparison with CF and found that the sensitivity and specificity of this assay for diagnosis of recent *M. pneumoniae* infection were 92.2% and 95%, respectively. Uldum and coworkers evaluated an EIA test for detection of both IgM and IgG anti-*M. pneumoniae* antibodies and compared their results with the CF test and the appearance of cold agglutinins.[311] These antibody EIA tests had a combined sensitivity of 97.8% and a specificity of 99.7%. No false-positive results were seen for patients with respiratory infection caused by other agents, and no false-positive IgM results because of rheumatoid factor were observed. These workers also noted that, in the EIA format, specimens from children and young adults were positive for IgM more frequently than specimens from adults, and specimens from older individuals tended to have fourfold or higher diagnostic IgG titer increases, probably because of previous infection and immunologic recall.

A microwell EIA procedure called the Sero *Mycoplasma pneumoniae* Test (Diatech Diagnostica, Israel) uses microtiter technology and an antibody-capture technique for detection of *M. pneumoniae*-specific IgM and total anti-*M. pneumoniae* antibodies. The microtiter wells are coated with anti-*M. pneumoniae* IgM and anti-*M. pneumoniae* IgM and IgG, respectively. The serum specimen is diluted 1:50 and and an aliquot is placed in each of the two microwells. After incubation and washing, alkaline phosphatase-labeled *M. pneumoniae* antigen is added. Following another incubation and wash step, the alkaline phosphatase substrate is added; the appearance of a yellow color in the well indicates that antibody present in the serum was captured and detected. Lieberman and coworkers evaluated this antibody-capture EIA and found it to be quite specific for *M. pneumoniae* antibodies (97.7%), but the sensitvity of the assay was only 61.2%.[156]

In recent years, several rapid serologic tests for *M. pneumoniae* have become commercially available. The Remel *M. pneumoniae* IgG–IgM antibody test system is a 5-minute EIA for simultaneous, qualitative detection of antibodies against *M. pneumoniae*. Patient serum is diluted and reacted with *M. pneumoniae* antigen that is immobilized on a permeable membrane. After rinsing, enzyme-labeled antihuman IgG–IgM is added and allowed to rinse through the membrane. After two washes, substrate–chromogen is added to the filter and allowed to react for 5 minutes. Thacker and Talkington evaluated this test with 50 paired serum samples and found that the Remel test detected antibodies in three specimens with CF titers of 32 and was positive for all but one specimen with CF titers of 64 or higher.[294] Microparticle agglutination assays have also been marketed for detection of *M. pneumoniae* antibodies. The Serodyne Color Vue IgG/IgM test (Serodyne, Indianapolis IN) uses latex particles coated with *M. pneumoniae* lipid antigen, whereas the Serodia-Myco II test (Fujire Bio, Japan) uses similarly sensitized gelatin particles. Both tests are performed by serially diluting heat-inactivated patient serum in a microtiter plate and adding a fixed aliquot of the latex or gelatin particles that are coated with *M. pneumoniae* lipid antigen to each of the dilution wells. After mixing on a microwell shaker and incubation, the endpoint is determined as the final dilution of serum causing agglutination of the antigen-sensitized particles. Thacker and Talkington evaluated the Serodyne 40-minute passive agglutination test and found it less sensitive than the Remel test described in the foregoing; only 68% of cases of mycoplasmal pneumonia could be serologically diagnosed with this kit, compared with 94% and 96% of cases being diagnosed by CF and Remel tests, respectively.[294] Lieberman and colleagues evaluated the Serodia-Myco II gelatin agglutination test and found the sensitivity, specificity, and predictive values of positive and negative tests to be 48.1%, 86.9%, 49.3%, and 86.3%, respectively.[156]

The purification and sequencing of the adhesin of *M. pneumoniae* and the recognition of specific immunodominant epitopes of this molecule may allow the manufacture of synthetic peptides that can be used as specific, chemically defined antigens in future serologic tests.[115] In addition, the use of species-specific epitopes will also eliminate possible false-positive serologic tests that may occur as a result of *M. genitalium* respiratory or urogenital tract infection and the host response to the cross-reacting antigens of the latter organism.[158,159]

A nonspecific serologic test that is often used to support the diagnosis of *M. pneumoniae* infection is the production of cold agglutinins. These agglutinins react in the cold with human erythrocyte I antigens. The I antigen is inactivated by α-glycosidase and the binding of cold agglutinins to these cells is inhibited by galactose.[335] Furthermore, when erythrocytes containing the I antigen are subjected to chloroform–methanol extraction, an antigen is extracted that will fix complement in the presence of anti-*M. pneumoniae* antibodies.[44] These data indicate that the I antigen of eythrocytes detected by cold agglutinins is similar in structure to certain antigenic determinants in the glycolipid membrane antigen of *M. pneumoniae*.[118] Similar to other IgM antibodies, cold hemagglutinins appear about 7 days after infection and peak after 4 to 5 weeks. Following this, titers decline rapidly, becoming undetectable after about 5 months. As with the CF and other serologic tests, a fourfold rise in cold agglutinin titers in the presence of a compatible clinical illness is suggestive of *M. pneumoniae* infection. The major drawback of using this test alone for presumptive diagnosis is that only about 50% of individuals with acute *M. pneumoniae* infection will have demonstrable cold agglutinin titers.[113] In addition, several other conditions can cause increases in cold agglutinins, including infectious mononucleosis, mumps, influenza, rubella, respiratory syncytial virus infections, adenovirus infections, peripheral vascular disease, and psittacosis.

EIA methods have also been described for the detection of serum antibodies against *M. hominis*, but these assays are not widely available.[22] By using Western immunoblot technology and a pool of sera from patients with *M. hominis* vaginal infections, Liepmann and colleagues identified antigens against which antibodies were consistently present.[157] These antigens were surface-exposed membrane antigens with molec-ular weights between 102 and 116 kDa. Sera containing antibodies reactive with these antigens were nonreactive against *M. pneumoniae* or *U. urealyticum*, indicating that these antibodies were specific for *M. hominis*. Easily performed methods for detecting antibody responses to genital mycoplasmas may be valuable in sorting out colonization versus infection with these bacteria, and may help target individuals, such as pregnant women, who may be at risk for more serious mycoplasma-associated disease.

ANTIMICROBIAL SUSCEPTIBILITY AND TREATMENT OF MYCOPLASMA INFECTIONS

Atypical pneumonia cause by *M. pneumoniae* is generally treated with tetracycline or erythromycin.[41] Although the organism may still be present in the upper respiratory tract during and after treatment, clinical manifestations of infection generally improve, and infiltrates on chest radiography usually disappear during therapy. Because of the difficulty in culturing the organism, its slow growth rate, and the lack of a readily available method, antimicrobial susceptibility testing of *M. pneumoniae* is neither necessary nor appropriate. Antimicrobial susceptibility testing of *M. pneumoniae* strains indicate that this organism is susceptible to a wide variety of antimicrobial agents, including the quinolones (ciprofloxacin, levofloxacin, ofloxacin, rufloxacin), clindamycin, lincomycin, tetracycline, doxycycline, minocycline, erthromycin, and aminoglycosides (gentamicin, streptomycin).[71] Some of the newer macrolide antibiotics, such as clarithromycin, azithromycin, and flurithromycin, are also highly active against *M. pneumoniae* and show a very narrow range of minimal inhibitor concentrations (MICs).[10,72]

Most isolates of both *M. hominis* and *U. urealyticum* are susceptible to tetracycline.[184] *M. hominis* strains are usually susceptible to clindamycin, but not erythromycin, whereas *Ureaplasma* strains are usually susceptible to erythromycin, but not to clindamycin.[19] In 1970, Braun and associates reported on the susceptibility of mycoplasmas and ureaplasmas using a metabolic inhibition technique.[19] In this study, *M. hominis* and *U. urealyticum* strains were inhibited by tetracycline, chloramphenicol, streptomycin, and gentamicin, and were resistant to the cell wall-active agents (i.e., cephalothin, ampicillin, and vancomycin). During the mid to late 1970s and early 1980s, strains of both species that were resistant to tetracyline were isolated and found to contain a genetic antimicrobial resistance determinant called *tetM*.[234,235] This determinant has also been found in other genital tract microorganisms, including group B streptococci, *Gardnerella vaginalis*, and *Neisseria gonorrhoeae*.[236] Strains of *U. urealyticum* that are resistant or intermediate in susceptibility to erythromycin and newer macrolides (e.g., flurithromycin) have also been described.[72,137,282] Most *M. hominis* strains are now resistant to erythromycin, and some are resistant to tetracycline and clindamycin. *M. hominis* strains are also resistant to flurithromycin, a newer macrolide antibiotic.[71] Tetracycline resistance has also been reported in strains of *U. urealyticum*; these strains also contain the *tetM* resistance determinant.[234,235,273] Erythromycin remains the drug of choice for the treatment of *U. urealyticum* non-CNS infections in neonates; CNS infections in this group of patients is best treated with tetracycline or chloramphenicol.[317] Strains of *U. urealyticum* are generally less susceptible to the quinolone antibiotics than either *M. pneumoniae* and or *M. hominis*.[71,135,136,150]

Renaudin and colleagues determined the susceptibilities of seven *M. genitalium* isolates using an agar dilution method and compared them with three *M. pneumoniae* strains.[232] Both species were susceptible to macrolides (erythromycin, spiramycin, roxithromycin, azithromycin, clarithromycin), clindamycin, tetracyline, doxycycline, minocycline, and the fluoroquinolones (ofloxacin, ciprofloxacin, lomefloxacin, sparfloxacin).

With use of a modified broth dilution procedure with SP-4 medium, Hayes and colleagues determined the antimicrobial susceptibilities of the *M. fermentans* incognitus strain along with reference strains of both *M. fermentans* (strain PG18 [ATCC 19989]) and *M. pneumoniae* (ATCC 15531).[97,99] As expected, all three mycoplasmas were resistant to cell wall-active agents (penicillin, ampicillin). Both the PG18 and the incognitus *M. fermentans* strains were resistant to erythromycin (mean MICs of erythromycin of 31.2 µg/mL and 43.0 µg/mL, respectively), whereas *M. pneumoniae* was susceptible to erythromycin (mean MIC of 0.0073 µg/mL). *M. fermentans* incognitus strain was susceptible to tetracycline, doxycycline, clindamycin, lincomycin, chloramphenicol, and ciprofloxacin. Both *M. fermentans* strains tested in this study were resistant to the aminoglycosides (gentamicin, kanamycin, streptomycin, and neomycin), whereas *M. pneumoniae* was susceptible. Aminoglycoside MICs for the incognitus strain of *M. fermentans* were higher than 1000 µg/mL for all four of these drugs, while the MICs for gentamicin, kanamycin, streptomycin, and neomycin for the PG18 strain were 15.6 µg/mL, 20.8 µg/mL, 18.2 µg/mL, and 52.1 µg/mL, respectively. Subsequent antimicrobial susceptibility testing of 24 additional *M. fermentans* isolates also indicated that this species is resistant to erythromycin and the aminoglycosides.[97] The subsequent study also documented that only ciprofloxacin and levofloxacin, both fluoroquinolone antimicrobial agents, had a significant bactericidal effect.[97] By using a modified broth dilution technique with Hayflick's broth, Hannon showed that azithromycin was more active against *M. fermentans* strains than either erythromycin or clarithromycin.[90]

Hayes and colleagues also examined the antimicrobial susceptibilities of *M. penetrans* isolates by a broth dilution procedure.[98] In their study of nine strains, all *M. penetrans* were susceptible to azithromycin, chloramphenicol, ciprofloxacin, clindamycin, doxycycline, erythromycin, levofloxacin, lincomycin, and tetracycline. All isolates were resistant to gentamicin and streptomycin. The fluoroquinolones were the only class of antimicrobial agents that demonstrated bactericidal, rather than bacteriostatic, activity against *M. penetrans*.[98]

With a macrodilution, metabolic inhibition assay, Poulin and colleagues examined the antimicrobial susceptibilties of several "AIDS-associated" mycoplasmas, including *M. fermentans* (a stock strain, two clinical isolates from AIDS patients, and the incognitus strain), *M. penetrans* (one strain), and *M. pirum* (one strain).[224] All isolates were susceptible to azithromycin, clarithromycin, clindamycin, doxycycline, ofloxacin, and tetracycline. *M. fermentans* strains and *M. pirum* were resistant to erythromycin, whereas *M. penetrans* was susceptible. These workers also found that dried Sensititre Gram-Positive MIC panels (BD Microbiology Systems) inoculated with a standardized suspension of the organisms in SP-4 broth produced results comparable with the metabolic inhibition method for all of the drugs tested by both methods. On the Sensititre panel, all strains tested were resistant to penicillin, ampicillin, cephalothin, imipenem, vancomycin, rifampin, and trimethoprim–sulfamethoxazole. *M. fermentans* strains and *M. penetrans* were resistant to gentamicin, whereas *M. pirum* was moderately susceptible.

Because of variability in antimicrobial susceptibility, methods for susceptibility testing on mycoplasmas have been devised, but are not widely available because they require special media and may incur considerable expense for routine clinical microbiology laboratories. Spaepen and Kundsin devised a relatively simple broth–disk elution procedure for susceptibility testing of ureaplasmas that is similar to those described in the past for testing anaerobic bacteria.[268] This procedure provided fairly reproducible results when inoculated with organisms grown in culture or with urine specimens containing organisms. Robertson and associates subsequently reported a standardized broth dilution method for determining MICs of antimicrobial agents for *U. urealyticum* strains.[239] In 1986, Kenny and associates published an agar dilution procedure for ureaplasma testing that appeared to yield more reproducible results that broth methods.[137]

In all of these procedures, problems that relate to the biological characteristics of the organisms and to the method itself may be encountered. Biological problems include the possibility of mixed cultures (e.g., both mycoplasmas and ureaplasmas) and the coexistence of susceptible and resistant populations in the same culture. The latter problem may be detected only in agar dilution-based systems, because colonies growing on antibiotic-containing media can be directly reidentified by urea hydrolysis or by serologic methods. Problems relating to the method include the lack of a standard medium for test performance, discrepancies related to the pH required for optimal mycoplasmal growth versus optimal antibiotic activity, the difficulty in standardization of inoculum size, the lack of standardized incubation times and conditions, and the lack of a standardized endpoint.[137] Because of these problems, susceptibility testing on mycoplasmas is usually performed only in larger institutions with special research interests in the therapy of genital mycoplasma infections.

REFERENCES

1. AINSWORTH JG, KATSENI V, HOURSHID S ET AL: *Mycoplasma fermentans* and HIV-associated nephropathy. J Infect 29:323–326, 1994

2. ALFA MJ, ROBERTSON JA: The co-existence of genital mycoplasmas and *Neisseria gonorrhoeae* isolated from the male urethra. Sex Transm Dis 11:131–136, 1984

3. ARMSTRONG D, YU BH, YAGODA A ET AL: Colonization of humans by *Mycoplasma canis*. J Infect Dis 124:607–609, 1971

4. BARILE MF: DNA homologies and serologic relationships among ureaplasmas from various hosts. Pediatr Infect Dis 5:S296–S299, 1986

5. BARTLETT JG, RYAN KJ, SMITH TF ET AL: Cumitech 7A: Laboratory Diagnosis of Lower Respiratory Tract Infections. Washington DC, American Society for Microbiology, 1987

6. BASEMAN JB, COLE RM, KRAUSE DC ET AL: Molecular basis for cytoadsorption of *M. pneumoniae*. J Bacteriol 151:1514–1522, 1982

7. BASEMAN JB, DALLO SF, TULLY JG ET AL: Isolation and characterization of *Mycoplasma genitalium* strains from the human respiratory tract. J Clin Microbiol 26:2266–2269, 1988

8. BAUER FA, WEAR DJ, ANGRITT P ET AL: *Mycoplasma fermentans* (incognitus strain) infection in the kidneys of patients with acquired immunodeficiency syndrome and associated nephropathy: a light microscopic, immunohistochemical, and ultrastructural study. Hum Pathol 22:63–69, 1991

9. BEBEAR C, DEBARBEYRAC B, CLERC M-T ET AL: Mycoplasmas in HIV-1 seropositive patients. Lancet 341:758–758, 1993

10. BEBEAR C, DUPON M, RENAUDIN H ET AL: Potential improvements in therapeutic options for mycoplasmal respiratory infections. Clin Infect Dis 17(suppl 1):S202–S207, 1993

11. BEECHAM HJ III, LO SC, LEWIS DE ET AL: Recovery from fulminant infection with *Mycoplasma fermentans* (incognitus strain) in non-immunocompromised host. Lancet 338:1014–1015, 1991

12. BEJAR R, CURBELO V, DAIRS C ET AL: Premature labor. Bacterial sources of phospholipase. Obstet Gynecol 57:479–482, 1981

13. BENCINA D, BRADBURY JM: Combination of immunofluorescence and immunoperoxidase techniques for serotyping mixtures of *Mycoplasma* species. J Clin Microbiol 30:407–410, 1992

14. BERNET C, GARRET M, DE BARBEYRAC B ET AL: Detection of *Mycoplasma pneumoniae* by using the polymerase chain reaction. J Clin Microbiol 27:2492–2496, 1989

15. BLANCHARD A, HAMRICK W, DUFFY L ET AL: Use of the polymerase chain reaction for detection of *Mycoplasma fermentans* and *Mycoplasma genitalium* in the urogenital tract and amniotic fluid. Clin Infect Dis 17(suppl 1):S272–S279, 1993

16. BLANCHARD A, HENTSCHEL J, DUFFY L ET AL: Detection of *Ureaplasma urealyticum* by polymerase chain reaction in the urogenital tracts of adults, in amniotic fluid, and in the respiratory tract of newborns. Clin Infect Dis 17(suppl 1):S148–S153, 1993

17. BLANCHARD A, YANEZ A, DYBVIG K, ET AL: Evaluation of intraspecies genetic variation within the 16S rRNA gene of *Mycoplasma hominis* and detection by polymerase chain reaction. J Clin Microbiol 31:1358–1361, 1993

18. BLANCO JD, GIBBS RS, MALHERBE H ET AL: A controlled study of genital mycoplasmas in amniotic fluid from patients with intra-amniotic infection. J Infect Dis 147:650–653, 1983

19. BRAUN P, KLEIN JO, KASS EH: Susceptibility of genital mycoplasmas to antimicrobial agents. Appl Microbiol 19:62–70, 1970

20. BROITMAN NL, FLOYD CM, JOHNSON CA ET AL: Comparison of commercially available media for detection and isolation of *Ureaplasma urealyticum* and *Mycoplasma hominis*. J Clin Microbiol 30:1335–1337, 1992

21. BROOKER RJ, EASON JD, SOLIMANO A: *Mycoplasma* surgical wound infection in a neonate. Pediatr Infect Dis J 13:751–752, 1994

22. BROWN MB ET AL: Measurement of antibody to *Mycoplasma hominis* by an enzyme-linked immunosorbent assay and detection of class-specific responses in women with postpartum fever. Am J Obstet Gynecol 156:701–708, 1987

23. BRUS F, VAN WAARDE WM, SCHOOTS C ET AL: Fatal ureaplasmal pneumonia and sepsis in a newborn infant. Eur J Pediatr 150:782–783, 1991

24. BUCK GE, O'HARA LC, SUMMERSGILL JT: Rapid, sensitive detection of *Mycoplasma pneumoniae* in simulated specimens by DNA amplification. J Clin Microbiol 30:3280–3283, 1992

25. BURDGE DR, REID GD, REEVE CF ET AL: Septic arthritis due to dual infection with *Mycoplasma hominis* and *Ureaplasma urealyticum*. J Rheumatol 15:366–368, 1988

26. BURKE DS, MADOFF S: Infection of a traumatic pelvic hematoma with *Mycoplasma hominis*. Sex Transm Dis 5:65–67, 1978

27. BUSOLO F, TONIN E, MELONI GA: Enzyme-linked immunosorbent assay for serodiagnosis of *Mycoplasma pneumoniae* infections. 18:432–435, 1983

28. BUTTKE TM, SANDSTROM PA: Oxidative stress as a mediator of apoptosis. Immunol Today 15:7–10, 1994

29. CADIEUX N, LEBEL P, BROUSSEAU R: Use of a triplex polymerase chain reaction for the detection and differentiation of *Mycoplasma pneumoniae* and *Mycoplasma genitalium* in the presence of human DNA. J Gen Microbiol 139:2431–2437, 1993

30. CASSELL GH, WAITES KB, CROUSE DT ET AL: Association of *Ureaplasma urealyticum* of the lower respiratory tract with chronic lung disease and death in very-low-birth-weight infants. Lancet 2:240–244, 1988

31. CASSELL GH, WAITES KB, GIBBS RS ET AL: Role of *Ureaplasma urealyticum* in amnionitis. Pediatr Infect Dis 5:S247–S252, 1986

32. CHENG X, NAESSENS A, LAUWERS S: Identification of serotype 1-, 3-, and 6-specific antigens of *Ureaplasma urealyticum* by using monoclonal antibodies. J Clin Microbiol 32:1060–1062, 1994

33. CHERRY JD: Anemia and mucocutaneous lesions due to *Mycoplasma pneumoniae* infections. Clin Infect Dis 17(suppl 1):S47–S51, 1993

34. CHIRGWIN KD, CUMMINGS MC, DeMEO LR ET AL: Identification of mycoplasmas in urine from persons infected with human immunodeficiency virus. Clin Infect Dis 17(suppl 1):S264–S266, 1993

35. CHRISTIANSEN G, ANDERSEN H: Heterogeneity among Mycoplasma hominis strains as detected by probes containing parts of ribosomal ribonucleic acid genes. Int J Syst Bacteriol 38:108–115, 1988

36. CIMOLAI N, BRYAN LE, TO M ET AL: Immunological cross-reactivity of a Mycoplasma pneumoniae membrane-associated protein antigen with Mycoplasma genitalium and Acholeplasma laidlawii. J Clin Microbiol 25:2136–2139, 1987

37. CIMOLAI N, SCHRYVERS A, BRYAN LE ET AL: Culture-amplified immunological detection of Mycoplasma pneumoniae in clinical specimens. Diagn Microbiol Infect Dis 9:207–212, 1988

38. CLOUGH W, CASSELL GH, DUFFY LB ET AL: Septic arthritis and bacteremia due to Mycoplasma resistant to antimicrobial therapy in a patient with systemic lupus erythematosus. Clin Infect Dis 15:402–407, 1992

39. CLYDE WA: Mycoplasma species identification based upon growth inhibition by specific antisera. J Immunol 92:958–965, 1964

40. CLYDE WA: Letter to the editors. Clin Microbiol Newslett 7:164–165, 1985

41. CLYDE WA: Clinical overview of typical Mycoplasma pneumoniae infections. Clin Infect Dis 17(suppl 1):S32–S36, 1993

42. CLYDE WA, KENNY GE, SCHACHTER J: Cumitech 19: Laboratory Diagnosis of Chlamydial and Mycoplasmal Infections. Washington DC, American Society for Microbiology, 1984

43. COLE BC, AHMED E, ARANEO BA ET AL: Immunomodulation in vivo by the Mycoplasma arthritidis superantigen, MAM. Clin Infect Dis 17(suppl 1):S163–S169, 1993

44. COSTEA N, YAKULIS VJ, HELLER P: The mechanism of induction of cold agglutinins by Mycoplasma pneumoniae. J Immunol 106:598–604, 1971

45. COUFALIK ED. TAYLOR-ROBINSON, CSONKA GW: Treatment of nongonococcal urethritis with rifampicin as a means of defining the role of Ureaplasma urealyticum. Br J Vener Dis 55:36, 1979

46. CROUSE DT, ODREZIN GT, CUTTER GR ET AL: Radiographic changes associated with tracheal isolation of Ureaplasma urealyticum from neonates. Clin Infect Dis 17(suppl 1):S122–S130, 1993

47. CUNNINGHAM CK: The role of genital mycoplasmas in neonatal disease. Clin Microbiol Newslett 12:147–149, 1990

48. DALLO SF, CHAVOYA A, BASEMAN JB: Characterization of the gene for a 30-kilodalton adhesin-related protein of Mycoplasma pneumoniae. Infect Immun 58:4163–4165, 1990

49. DALLO SF, CHAVOYA A, SU CJ ET AL: DNA and protein sequence homologies between the adhesins of Mycoplasma genitalium and Mycoplasma pneumoniae. Infect Immun 57:1059–1065, 1989

50. DALLO SF, HORTEN JR, SU CJ ET AL: Homologous regions shared by adhesin genes of Mycoplasma pneumoniae and Mycoplasma genitalium. Microb Pathog 6:69–73, 1989

51. DAN M, TYRRELL DLJ, STEMKE GW ET AL: Mycoplasma hominis septicemia in a burned infant. J Pediatr 99:743–745, 1981

52. DAVIES S, EGGINGTON R: Recovery of Mycoplasma hominis from blood culture media. Med Lab Sci 48:110–113, 1991

53. DAWSON MS, HAYES MM, WANG RY-H ET AL: Detection and isolation of Mycoplasma fermentans from urine of human immunodeficiency virus type 1-infected patients. Arch Pathol Lab Med 117:511–514, 1993

54. DeBARBEYRAC B, BERNET-POGGI C, FEBRER F ET AL: Detection of Mycoplasma pneumoniae and Mycoplasma genitalium in clinical samples by polymerase chain reaction. Clin Infect Dis 17(suppl 1):S83–S89, 1993

55. DE GIROLAMI PC, MADOFF S: Mycoplasma hominis septicemia. J Clin Microbiol 16:566–567, 1982

56. DEGUCHI T, GILROY CB, TAYLOR-ROBINSON D: Comparison of two PCR-based assays for detecting Mycoplasma genitalium in clinical specimens. Eur J Clin Microbiol Infect Dis 14:629–630, 1995

57. DEL GIUDICE RA, TULLY JG, ROSE DL, ET AL: Mycoplasma pirum sp. nov., a terminal structured mollicute from cell cultures. Int J Syst Bacteriol 35:285–291, 1985

58. DE SILVA NS, QUINN PA: Endogenous activity of phospholipases A and C in Ureaplasma urealyticum. J Clin Microbiol 23:354–359, 1986

59. DIMITROV DS, FRANZOSO G, SALMAN M ET AL: Mycoplasma fermentans (incognitus strain) cells are able to fuse with T lymphocytes. Clin Infect Dis 17(suppl 1):S305–S308, 1993

60. DINSMOOR MJ, RAMAMURTHY RS, GIBBS RS: Transmission of genital mycoplasmas from mother to neonate in women with prolonged membrane rupture. Pediatr Infect Dis J 8:843–847, 1989

61. DRISCOLL SG: Chorioamnionitis: perinatal morbidity and mortality. Pediatr Infect Dis 5:S273–S275, 1986

62. DULAR R, KAJIOKA R, KASATIYA S: Comparison of Gen-Probe commercial kit and culture technique for the diagnosis of Mycoplasma pneumoniae infection. J Clin Microbiol 26:1068–1069, 1988

63. EMBREE J: Mycoplasma hominis in maternal and fetal infections. Ann NY Acad Sci 549:56–64, 1988

64. ESCHENBACH DA: Ureaplasma urealyticum and premature birth. Clin Infect Dis 17(suppl 1):S100–S106, 1993

65. ESCHENBACH DA: Ureaplasma urealyticum as a cause of postpartum fever. Pediatr Infect Dis 5:S258–S261, 1986

66. FENG S-H, LO S-C: Induced mouse spleen B-cell proliferation and secretion of immunoglobulin by lipid-associated membrane proteins of Mycoplasma fermentans incognitus and Mycoplasma penetrans. Infect Immun 62:3916–3921, 1994

67. FIACCO V, MILLER MJ, CARNEY E ET AL: Comparison of media for isolation of Ureaplasma urealyticum and genital Mycoplasma species. J Clin Microbiol 20:862–865, 1984

68. FISCHER GS, SWEIMLER WI, KLEGER B: Comparison of MYCOPLASMELISA with complement fixation test for measurement of antibodies to Mycoplasma pneumoniae. Diagn Microbiol Infect Dis 4:139–145, 1986

69. FISCHMAN MARSCHALL KE, KISLAK W ET AL: Adult respiratory distress syndrome caused by Mycoplasma pneumoniae. Chest 74:471473, 1978

70. FOY HM: Infections caused by *Mycoplasma pneumoniae* and possible carrier state in different populations of patients. Clin Infect Dis 17(suppl 1):S37–S46, 1993

71. FURNERI PM, BISIGNANO G, CERNIGLIA G ET AL: In vitro antimycoplasmal activities of rufloxacin and its metabolite MF 922. Antimicrob Agents Chemother 38: 2651–2654, 1994

72. FURNERI PM, BISIGNANO G, CERNIGLIA G ET AL: In vitro antimycoplasmal activity of flurithromycin. J Antimicrob Chemother 35:161–165, 1995

73. GALLILY R, SALMAN M, TARSHIS M ET AL: *Mycoplasma fermentans* (incognitus strain) induces THF*alpha*, and IL-1 production by human monocytes and murine macrophages. Immunol Lett 34:27–30, 1992

74. GAUTHIER DW, MEYER WJ, BIENIARZ A: Expectant management of premature rupture of membranes with amniotic fluid cultures positive for *Ureaplasma urealyticum* alone. Am J Obstet Gynecol 170:587–590, 1994

75. GELFAND EW: Unique susceptibility of patients with antibody deficiency to mycoplasma infection. Clin Infect Dis 17(suppl 1):S250–S253, 1993

76. GEWITZ M, DINWIDDIE R, REES L ET AL: *Mycoplasma hominis*: a cause of neonatal meningitis. Arch Dis Child 54:231–239, 1979

77. GIBBS RS: Chorioamnionitis and bacterial vaginosis. Am J Obstet Gynecol 169:460–462, 1993

78. GIBBS RS, CASSELL GH, DAVIS JK ET AL: Further studies on genital mycoplasmas in intra-amniotic infection: blood cultures and serologic response. Am J Obstet Gynecol 154:717–726, 1986

79. GILBERT GL, DREW JH: Chronic *Mycoplasma hominis* infection complicating severe intraventricular hemorrhage in a premature neonate. Pediatr Infect Dis J 7: 817–818, 1988

80. GILBERT GL, GARLAND SM, FAIRLEY KF ET AL: Bacteriuria due to ureaplasmas and other fastidious organisms during pregnancy: prevalence and significance. Pediatr Infect Dis 5:S239–S243, 1986

81. GINSBURG KS, KUNDSIN RB, WALTER CW ET AL: *Ureaplasma urealyticum* and *Mycoplasma hominis* in women with systemic lupus erythematosus. Arthritis Rheum 35:429–433, 1992

82. GLASER JB, ENGELBERG M, HAMMERSCHLAG M: Scalp abscess associated with *Mycoplasma hominis* infection complicating intrapartum monitoring. Pediatr Infect Dis 2:468–470, 1983

83. GOULET M, DULAR R, TULLY JG ET AL: Isolation of *Mycoplasma pneumoniae* from the human urogenital tract. J Clin Microbiol 33:2823–2825, 1995

84. GRAU O, KOVACIC R, GRIFFAIS R ET AL: Development of a selective and sensitive polymerase chain reaction assay for the detection of *Mycoplasma pirum*. FEMS Microbiol Lett 106:327–334, 1993

85. GRAU O, KOVACIC R, GRIFFAIS ET AL: Development of PCR-based assays for the detection of two human molicute species: *Mycoplasma penetrans* and *Mycoplasma hominis*. Mol Cell Probes 8:139–148, 1994

86. GRAU O, SLIZEWICZ B, TUPPIN P ET AL: Association of *Mycoplasma penetrans* with human immunodeficiency virus infection. J Infect Dis 172:672–681, 1995

87. GRAVAT MG, ESCHENBACH DA: Possible role of *Ureaplasma urealyticum* in preterm premature rupture of the fetal membranes. Pediatr Infect Dis 5:S253–S257, 1986

88. GRAY DJ, ROBINSON HB, MALONE J ET AL: Adverse outcome in pregnancy following amniotic fluid isolation of *Ureaplasma urealyticum*. Prenat Diagn 12:111–117, 1992

89. HALLER M, FORST H, RUCKDESCHEL G ET AL: Peritonitis due to *Mycoplasma hominis* and *Ureaplasma urealyticum* in a liver transplant recipient. Eur J Clin Microbiol Infect Dis 10:172, 1993

90. HANNAN PCT: Antibiotic susceptibility of *Mycoplasma fermentans* strains from various sources and the development of resistance to aminoglycosides in vitro. J Med Microbiol 42:421–428, 1995

91. HARASAWA R, DYBVIG K, WATSON HL ET AL: Two genomic clusters among 14 serovars of *Ureaplasma urealyticum*. Syst Appl Microbiol 14:393–396, 1991

92. HARASAWA R, IMADA Y, ITO M ET AL: *Ureaplasma felinum* sp. nov. and *Ureaplasma cati* sp. nov. isolated from the oral cavities of cats. Int J Syst Bacteriol 40:45–51, 1990

93. HARASAWA R, IMADA Y, KOTANI H ET AL: *Ureaplasma canigenitalium* sp. nov., isolated from dogs. Int J Syst Bacteriol 43:640–644, 1993

94. HARASAWA R, STEPHENS EB, KOSHIMIZU K ET AL: DNA relatedness among established *Ureaplasma* species and unidentified feline and canine serogroups. Int J Syst Bacteriol 40:52–55, 1990

95. HARRISON HR: Cervical colonization with *Ureaplasma urealyticum* and pregnancy outcome: prospective studies. Pediatr Infect Dis 5:S266–S269, 1986

96. HAWKINS RE, RICKMAN LS, VERMUND SH ET AL: Association of mycoplasma and human immunodeficiency virus infection: detection of amplified *Mycoplasma fermentans* DNA in blood. J Infect Dis 165:581–585, 1992

97. HAYES MM, FOO H-H, KOTANI H ET AL: In vitro antibiotic susceptibility testing of different strains of *Mycoplasma fermentans* isolated from a variety of sources. Antimicrob Agents Chemother 37:2500–2503, 1993

98. HAYES MM, FOO H-H, TIMENETSKY J ET AL: In vitro antibiotic susceptibility testing of clinical isolates of *Mycoplasma penetrans* from patients with AIDS. Antimicrob Agents Chemother 39:1386–1387, 1995

99. HAYES MM, WEAR DJ, LO S-C: In vitro antimicrobial susceptibility testing for the newly identified AIDS-associated mycoplasma. Arch Pathol Lab Med 115:464–466, 1991

100. HEGGIE AD, JACOBS MR, BUTLER VT ET AL: Frequency and significance of isolation of *Ureaplasma urealyticum* and *Mycoplasma hominis* from cerebrospinal fluid and tracheal aspirate specimens from low birth weight infants. J Pediatr 124:956–961, 1994

101. HENRICH B, FELDMANN R-C, HADDING U: Cytoadhesins of *Mycoplasma hominis*. Infect Immun 61:2945–2951, 1993

102. HILL AC: *Mycoplasma spermatophilum*, a new species isolated from human spermatozoa and cervix. Int J Syst Bacteriol 41:229–233, 1991

103. HILL GB, LIVENGOOD CH: Bacterial vaginosis-associated microflora and effects of topical intravaginal clindamycin. Am J Obstet Gynecol 171:1198–1204, 1994

104. HIRAI Y, KANATANI T, ONO M ET AL: An indirect immunofluorescence method for detection of *Mycoplasma hominis* in vaginal smears. Microbiol Immunol 35:831–839, 1991

105. HOOTON TM, ROBERTS MC, STAMM W ET AL: Prevalence of *Mycoplasma genitalium* determined by DNA probe in men with urethritis. Lancet 1:266–268, 1988

106. HORNER PJ, GILROY CB, THOMAS BJ ET AL: Association of *Mycoplasma genitalium* with acute non-gonococcal urethritis. Lancet 342:582–585, 1993

107. HOROWITZ S, MAZOR M, ROMERO R ET AL: Infection of the amniotic cavity with *Ureaplasma urealyticum* in the midtrimester of pregnancy. J Reprod Med 40:375–379, 1995

108. HOWARD CJ, GOURLEY RN: Proposal for a second species within the genus *Ureaplasma*, *Ureaplasma diversum* sp. nov. Int J Syst Bacteriol 32:446–452, 1982

109. HU PC, COLE RM, HUANG YS ET AL: *Mycoplasma pneumoniae* infection: role of surface protein in the attachment organelle. Science 216:1126–1131, 1982

110. HYMAN HC, YOGEV D, RAZIN S: DNA probes for detection of *Mycoplasma pneumoniae* and *Mycoplasma genitalium*. J Clin Microbiol 25:726–728, 1987

111. IMADA Y, UCHIDA I, HASHIMOTO K: Rapid identification of mycoplasmas by indirect immunoperoxiase test using small square filter paper. J Clin Microbiol 25:17–21, 1987

112. IZRAELI S, SAMRA Z, SIROTA L ET AL: Genital mycoplasmas in preterm infants: prevalence and clinical significance. Eur J Pediatr 150:804–807, 1991

113. JACOBS E: Serological diagnosis of *Mycoplasma pneumoniae* infections: a critical review of current procedures. Clin Infect Dis 17(suppl 1):S79–S82, 1993

114. JACOBS E, BUCHHOLZ A, KLEINMAN B ET AL: Use of adherence protein of *Mycoplasma pneumoniae* as antigen for enzyme-linked immunosorbent assay (ELISA). Isr J Med Sci 23:709–712, 1987

115. JACOBS E, PILATSCHEK A, GERSTENECKER B ET AL: Immunodominant epitopes of the adhesin of *Mycoplasma pneumoniae*. J Clin Microbiol 28:1194–1197, 1990

116. JACOBS F, VAN DE STADT J, GELIN M ET AL: *Mycoplasma hominis* infection of perihepatic hematomas in a liver transplant recipient. Surgery 111:98–100, 1992

117. JALIL N ET AL: Infection of the epididymis by *Ureaplasma urealyticum*. Genitourin Med 62:342, 1988

118. JANNEY FA, LEE LT, HOWE C: Cold hemagglutinin cross-reactivity with *Mycoplasma pneumoniae*. Infect Immun 22:29–30, 1978

119. JENSEN JS, HANSEN HT, LIND K: Isolation of *Mycoplasma genitalium* strains from the male urethra. J Clin Microbiol 34:286–291, 1996

120. JENSEN JS, HEILMANN C, VALERIUS NH: *Mycoplasma pneumoniae* infection in a child with AIDS. Clin Infect Dis 19:207, 1994

121. JENSEN JS, ORSUM R, DOHN B ET AL: *Mycoplasma genitalium*: a cause of male urethritis? Genitourin Med 69:265–269, 1993

122. JENSEN JS, ULDUM SA, SONDERGARD-ANDERSEN J, VUUST J ET AL: Polymerase chain reaction for detection of *Mycoplasma genitalium* in clinical samples. J Clin Microbiol 29:46–50, 1991

123. JOHNSTON CLW, WEBSTER ADB, TAYLOR-ROBINSON D ET AL: Primary late-onset hypogammaglobulinemia associated with inflammatory polyarthritis and septic arthritis due to *Mycoplasma pneumoniae*. Ann Rheum Dis 42:108–110, 1983

124. JONES DM, TOBIN P: Neonatal eye infections due to *Mycoplasma hominis*. Br Med J 3:467–468, 1968

125. JONES K: Infection of a postpartum hematoma with *Mycoplasma hominis*. Clin Microbiol Newslett 10:63–64, 1988

126. JORUP-RONSTROM C, AHL T, HAMMARSTROM L ET AL: Septic osteomyelitis and polyarthritis with *Ureaplasma* in hypogammaglobulinemia. Infection 17:301–303, 1989

127. JOSTE NE, KUNDSIN RB, GENEST DR: Histology and *Ureaplasma urealyticum* culture in 63 cases of first trimester abortion. Am J Clin Pathol 102:729–732, 1994

128. KAILATH EJ, HARDY DB: Hematoma infected with *Mycoplasma hominis*. Sex Transm Dis 15:114–115, 1987

129. KAKULPHIMP J, FINCH LR, ROBERTSON JA: Genome sizes of mammalian and avian ureaplasmas. Int J Syst Bacteriol 41:326–327, 1991

130. KANE JR, SHENEP JL, KRANCE RA ET AL: Diffuse alveolar hemorrhage associated with *Mycoplasma hominis* respiratory tract infection in a bone marrow transplant recipient. Chest 105:1891–1892, 1994

131. KASS EH, LIN J-S, MCCORMACK WM: Low birth weight and maternal colonization with genital mycoplasmas. Pediatr Infect Dis 5:S279–S281, 1986

132. KATSENI VL, GILROY CB, RYAIT BK ET AL: *Mycoplasma fermentans* in individuals seropositive and seronegative for HIV-1. Lancet 341:271–273, 1993

133. KAYSER S, BHEND HJ: Lumbar pain caused by *Mycoplasma* infection. Infection 20:97–98, 1992

134. KENNEY RT, LI JS, CLYDE WA JR ET AL: Mycoplasma pericarditis: evidence of invasive disease. Clin Infect Dis 17(suppl 1):S58–S62, 1993

135. KENNY GE, CARTWRIGHT FD: Susceptibilities of *Mycoplasma hominis* and *Ureaplasma urealyticum* to two new quinolones, sparfloxacin and WIN 57273. Antimicrob Agents Chemother 35:1515–1516, 1991

136. KENNY GE, CARTWRIGHT FD: Susceptibilities of *Mycoplasma hominis*, *Mycoplasma pneumoniae*, and *Ureaplasma urealyticum* to a new quinolone, OPC 17116. Antimicrob Agents Chemother 37:1726–1727, 1993

137. KENNY GE, CARTWRIGHT FD, ROBERTS MC: Agar dilution method for determination of antibiotic susceptibility of *Ureaplasma urealyticum*. Pediatr Infect Dis 5:S332–S334, 1986

138. KENNY GE, KAISER GG, COONEY MK ET AL: Diagnosis of *Mycoplasma pneumoniae* pneumonia: sensitivities and specificities of serology with lipid antigen and isolation of the organism on soy peptone medium for identification of infections. J Clin Microbiol 28:2087–2093, 1990

139. KERSTEN RC, HAGLUND L, KULWIN DR ET AL: *Mycoplasma hominis* orbital abscess. Arch Ophthalmol 113:1096–1097, 1995

140. KIM SK: *Mycoplasma hominis* septic arthritis. Ann Plast Surg 20:163–166, 1988

141. KLEEMOLA M, RATY R, KARJALAINEN J ET AL: Evaluation of an antigen-capture enzyme immunoassay for rapid diagnosis of *Mycoplasma pneumoniae* infection. Eur J Clin Microbiol Infect Dis 12:872–975, 1993

142. KOLETSKY RJ, WEINSTEIN AJ: Fulminant *Mycoplasma pneumoniae* infection. Am Rev Respir Dis 122:491–469, 1980

143. KOMAROFF AL, BELL DS, CHENEY PR ET AL: Absence of antibody to *Mycoplasma fermentans* in patients with chronic fatigue syndrome. Clin Infect Dis 17:1074–1075, 1993

144. KOSHIMIZU K, HARASAWA R, PAN I-J ET AL: *Ureaplasma gallorale* sp. nov. from the oropharynx of chickens. Int J Syst Bacteriol 37:333–338, 1987

145. KOSKINIEMI M: CNS manifestations associated with *Mycoplasma pneumoniae* infections. Summary of cases at the University of Helsinki and review. Clin Infect Dis 17(suppl 1):S52–S57, 1993

146. KOSTYAL DA, BUTLER GH, BEEZHOLD DH: A 48-kilo-dalton *Mycoplasma fermentans* membrane protein induces cytokine secretion by human monocytes. Infect Immun 62:3793–3800, 1994

147. KROHN MA, HILLIER SL, NUGENT RP ET AL: The genital flora of women with intraamniotic infection. J Infect Dis 171:1475–1480, 1995

148. LAMEY JR, ESCHENBACH DA, MITCHELL SH ET AL: Isolation of mycoplasmas and bacteria from the blood of postpartum women. Amer J Obstet Gynecol 143:104–112, 1982

149. LEE Y-H, NERSASIAN RR, LAN NK ET AL: Wound infection with *Mycoplasma hominis*. JAMA 218:252–253, 1971

150. LEFEVRE JC, BAURIAUD R, GAUBERT E ET AL: In vitro activity of sparfloxacin and other antimicrobial agents against genital pathogens. Chemotherapy 38:303–307, 1992

151. LEGRAND-POELS S, VAIRA D, PINCEMAIL J ET AL: Activation of human immunodeficiency virus type 1 by oxydative stress. AIDS Res Human Retroviruses 6:1389–1397, 1990

152. LEHTOMAKI K, KLEEMOLA M, TUKIANEN P: Isolation of *Mycoplasma pneumoniae* from bronchoalveolar lavage fluid. J Infect Dis 155:1339-1341, 1987

153. LELAND DS, LAPWORTH MA, JONES RB ET AL: Comparative evaluation of media for isolation of *Ureaplasma urealyticum* and genital *Mycoplasma* species. J Clin Microbiol 16:709–714, 1982

154. LEMAITRE M, GUETARD D, HENIN Y ET AL: Protective activity of tetracycline analogs against the cytopathic effect of the human immunodeficiency viruses in CEM cells. Res Virol 141:5–16, 1990

155. LEMAITRE M, HENIN Y, DESTOUESSE F ET AL: Role of mycoplasma infection in the cytopathic effect induced by human immunodeficiency virus type 1 in infected cell lines. Infect Immun 60:742–748, 1992

156. LIEBERMAN D, LIEBERMAN D, HOROWITZ S ET AL: Microparticle agglutination versus antibody-capture enzyme immunoassay for diagnosis of community-acquired *Mycoplasma pneumoniae* pneumonia. Eur J Clin Microbiol Infect Dis 14:577–584, 1995

157. LIEPMANN MF, GIREAUDOT P, DELETREZ J ET AL: Use of the *Mycoplasma hominis* 102–116 kD proteins as antigen in an enzyme-linked immunosorbent assay. Microbios 65:7–13, 1991

158. LIND K: Serological cross-reactions between "*Mycoplasma genitalium*" and *Mycoplasma pneumoniae*. Lancet 2:1158–1159, 1982

159. LIND K, LINDHARDT BO, SCHUTTEN HJ ET AL: Serological cross-reactions between *Mycoplasma genitalium* and *Mycoplasma pneumoniae*. J Clin Microbiol 20:1036–1043, 1984

160. LIVINGSTON CW, GAUER BB: Isolation of T-strain mycoplasma from sheep and goats in Texas. Am J Vet Res 36:313–314, 1975

161. LO S-C: Isolation and identification of a novel virus from patients with AIDS. Am J Trop Med Hyg 35:675–676, 1986

162. LO S-C, BUCHHOLZ CL, WEAR DJ ET AL: Histopathology and doxycycline treatment in a previously healthy non-AIDS patient systemically infected with *Mycoplasma fermentans* (incognitus strain). Mod Pathol 6:750–754, 1991

163. LO S-C, DAWSON MS, NEWTON PB ET AL: Association of the virus-like infectious agent originally reported in patients with AIDS with acute fatal disease in previously healthy non-AIDS patients. Am J Trop Med Hyg 41:364–376, 1989

164. LO S-C, DAWSON MS, WONG DM ET AL: Identification of *Mycoplasma incognitus* infection in patients with AIDS: an immunohistochemical, in situ hybridization and ultrastructural study. Am J Trop Med Hyg 41:601–616, 1989

165. LO S-C, HAYES MM, KOTANI H ET AL: Adhesion onto and invasion into mammalian cells by *Mycoplasma penetrans*—a newly isolated mycoplasma from patients with AIDS. Mod Pathol 6:276–280, 1993

166. LO S-C, HAYES MM, TULLY JG ET AL: *Mycoplasma penetrans* sp. nov., from the urogenital tract of patients with AIDS. Int J Syst Bacteriol 42:357–364, 1992

167. LO S-C, HAYES MM, WANG RY-H ET AL: Newly discovered mycoplasma isolated from patients infected with HIV. Lancet 338:1415–1418, 1991

168. LO S-C, LANGE M, WANG R ET AL: Development of Kaposi's sarcoma is associated with serologic evidence of *Mycoplasma penetrans* infection: retrospective analysis of a prospective cohort study of homosexual men. First National Conference on Human Retroviruses and Related Infections, Program and Abstracts. 1993, abstr. 504, p 67.

169. LO S-C, SHIH JW-K, NEWTON PB ET AL: Virus-like infectious agent (VLIA) is a novel pathogenic mycoplasma: *Mycoplasma incognitus*. Am J Trop Med Hyg 51:586–600, 1989

170. LO S-C, SHIH JW-K, YANG N-Y ET AL: A novel virus-like infectious agent in patients with AIDS. Am J Trop Med Hyg 40:213–226, 1989

171. LO S-C, TSAI S, BENISH JR ET AL: Enhancement of HIV-1 cytocidal effects on CD4+ lymphocytes by the AIDS-associated mycoplasma. Science 251:1074–1076, 1991

172. LO S-C, WANG RY-H, NEWTON PB ET AL: Fatal infection of silver leaf monkeys with a virus-like infectious agent (VLIA) derived from a patient with AIDS. Am J Trop Med Hyg 40:399–409, 1989

173. LO S-C, WEAR DJ, GREEN SL ET AL: Adult respiratory distress syndrome with or without systemic disease associated with infections due to *Mycoplasma fermentans*. Clin Infect Dis 17(suppl 1):S259–S263, 1993

174. LO S-C, WEAR DJ, SHIH JW-K EL AL: Fatal systemic infections of nonhuman primates by *Mycoplasma fermentans* (incognitus strain). Clin Infect Dis 17(suppl):S283–S288, 1993

175. LUNEBERG E, JENSEN JK, FROSCH M: Detection of *Mycoplasma pneumoniae* by polymerase chain reaction and nonradiographic hybridization in microtiter plates. J Clin Microbiol 31:1088–1094, 1993

176. Luttrell LM, Kanj SS, Corey R et al: *Mycoplasma hominis* septic arthritis: two case reports and review. Clin Infect Dis 19:1067–1070, 1994

177. Macon WR, Lo S-C, Poiesz BJ et al: Acquired immunodeficiency syndrome-like illness associated with systemic *Mycoplasma fermentans* infection in a human immunodeficiency virus-negative homosexual man. Hum Pathol 24:554–558, 1993

178. Madoff S, Hooper DC: Nongenitourinary tract infections caused by *Mycoplasma hominis* in adults. Rev Infect Dis 10:602–613, 1988

179. Mardh P-A: *Mycoplasma hominis* infection of the central nervous system in newborn infants. Sex Transm Dis 10(suppl):331–334, 1983

180. Markham JG, Markham NP: *Mycoplasma laidlawii* in human burns. J Bacteriol 98:827–828, 1964

181. Marmion BP, Worswick JWDA, Kok T-W et al: Experience with newer techniques for the laboratory detection of *Mycoplasma pneumoniae* infection: Adelaide, 1978–1992. Clin Infect Dis 17(suppl 1):S90–S99, 1993

182. Martinez OV, Chan J, Cleary T et al: *Mycoplasma hominis* septic thrombophlebitis in a patient with multiple trauma: a case report and literature review. Diagn Microbiol Infect Dis 12:193–196, 1989

183. McCormack WM: *Ureaplasma urealyticum*: ecologic niche and epidemiologic considerations. Pediatr Infect Dis 5:S232–S233, 1986

184. McCormack WM: Susceptibility of mycoplasmas to antimicrobial agents: clinical implications. Clin Infect Dis 17(suppl 1):S200–S201, 1993

185. McCormack WM, Almeida PC, Bailey PE et al: Sexual activity and vaginal colonization with genital mycoplasmas. JAMA 221:1375–1377, 1972

186. McCormack WM, Lee Y-H, Zinner SH: Sexual experience and urethral colonization with genital mycoplasmas: a study in normal men. Ann Intern Med 78:696–698, 1973

187. McCormack WM, Rosner B, Alpert S et al: Vaginal colonization with *Mycoplasma hominis* and *Ureaplasma urealyticum*. Sex Transm Dis 13:67–70, 1986

188. McCormack WM, Rosner B, Lee Y-H et al: Isolation of genital mycoplasmas from blood obtained shortly after vaginal delivery. Lancet 1:596–599, 1975

189. McDonald JC, Moore DL: *Mycoplasma hominis* meningitis in a premature infant. Pediatr Infect Dis J 7:795–798, 1988

190. McDonald MI, Moore JO, Harrelson JM et al: Septic arthritis due to *Mycoplasma hominis*. Arthritis Rheum 26:1044–1047, 1983

191. Meis JF, van Kuppeveld FJ, Kreme JA et al: Fatal intrauterine infection associated with *Mycoplasma hominis*. Clin Infect Dis 15:753–754, 1992

192. Mernaugh GR, Dallo SF, Holt SC et al: Properties of adhering and nonadhering populations of *Mycoplasma genitalium*. Clin Infect Dis 17(suppl 1):S69–S78, 1993

193. Meyer RD, Clough W: Extragenital *Mycoplasma hominis* infections in adults: emphasis on immunosuppression. Clin Infect Dis 17(suppl 1):S243–S249, 1993

194. Miranda C, Alados JC, Molina JM et al: Posthysterectomy wound infection: a review. Diagn Microbiol Infection Dis 17:41–44, 1993

195. Miranda C, Carazo C, Banon R et al: *Mycoplasma hominis* infection in three renal transplant patients. Diagn Microbiol Infect Dis 13:329–331, 1990

196. Mokhbat JE, Peterson PK, Sabath LD et al: Peritonitis due to *Mycoplasma hominis* in a renal transplant recipient. J Infect Dis 146:713, 1982

197. Moller BR, Taylor-Robinson D, Furr PM: Serological evidence implicating *Mycoplasma genitalium* in pelvic inflammatory disease. Lancet 1:1102–1103, 1984

198. Montagnier L, Berneman D, Guetard D et al: Infectivity inhibition of HIV prototype strains by antibodies directed against a peptide sequence of mycoplasmas. CR Acad Sci III 311:425–430, 1990

199. Montagnier L, Blanchard A: Mycoplasmas as cofactors in infection due to human immunodeficiency virus. Clin Infect Dis 17(suppl 1):S309–S315, 1993

200. Morrison-Plummer J, Lazzell A, Baseman JB: Shared epitopes between *Mycoplasma pneumoniae* major adhesin protein P1 and a 140-kilodalton protein of *Mycoplasma genitalium*. Infect Immun 55:49–56, 1987

201. Muhlradt PF, Frisch M: Purification and partial biochemical characterization of a *Mycoplasma fermentans*-derived substance that activates macrophages to release nitric oxide, tumor necrosis factor, and interleukin-6. Infect Immun 62:3801–3807, 1994

202. Muhlradt PF, Quentmeier H, Schmitt E: Involvement of interleukin-1 (IL-1), IL-6, IL-2, and IL-4 in generation of cytolytic T cells from thymocytes stimulated by a *Mycoplasma fermentans*-derived product. Infect Immun 59:3962–3968, 1991

203. Muhlradt PF, Schade U: MDHM, a macrophage-stimulatory product of *Mycoplasma fermentans*, leads to in vitro interleukin-1 (IL-1), IL-6, tumor necrosis factor, and prostaglandin production and is pyrogenic in rabbits. Infect Immun 59:3969–3974, 1991

204. Naessens A, Foulen W, Breynaert J et al: Postpartum bacteremia and placental colonization with genital mycoplasmas and pregnancy outcome. Am J Obstet Gynecol 160:647–650, 1989

205. Narita M, Matsuzono Y, Togashi T et al: DNA diagnosis of central nervous system infection by *Mycoplasma penumoniae*. Pediatrics 90:250–253, 1992

206. Nozaki-Renard J, Iino T, Sato Y et al: A fluoroquinolone (DR-3355) protects human lymphocyte cell lines from HIV-1-induced cytotoxicity. AIDS 4:1283–1286, 1990

207. Ohlsson A, Wang E, Vearncombe M: Leukocytes counts and colonization with *Ureaplasma urealyticum* in preterm neonates. Clin Infect Dis 17(suppl 1):S144–S147, 1993

208. Olson LD, Gilbert AA: Characteristics of *Mycoplasma hominis* adhesion. J Bacteriol 175:3224–3227, 1993

209. Orange GV, Jones M, Henderson IS: Wound and perinephric haemotoma infection with *Mycoplasma hominis* in a renal transplant recipient. Nephrol Dial Transplant 8:1395–1396, 1993

210. Palmer HM, Gilroy CB, Claydon EJ et al: Detection of *Mycoplasma genitalium* in the genitourinary tract of women by the polymerase chain reaction. Int J STD AIDS 2:261–263, 1991

211. Parides GC, Bloom JW, Ampel NM et al: Mycoplasma and ureaplasma in bronchoalveolar lavage specimens from immunocompromised hosts. Diagn Microbiol Infect Dis 9:55–57, 1988

212. Pasculle AW: Recognition of *Mycoplasma hominis* in routine bacteriology specimens. Clin Microbiol Newslett 10:145148, 1988

213. PAYAN DG, SEIGAL N, MADOFF S: Infection of a brain abscess by *Mycoplasma hominis*. J Clin Microbiol 14:571–573, 1981

214. PAYNE NR, STEINBERG SS, ACKERMAN P ET AL: New prospective studies of the association of *Ureaplasma urealyticum* colonization and chronic lung disease. Clin Infect Dis 17(suppl 1):S117–S121, 1993

215. PEETERS MF ET AL: Role of mycoplasmas in chronic prostatitis. Yale J Med Biol 56:551, 1983

216. PETZEL JP, HARTMEN PA, ALLISON MJ: Pyrophosphate-dependent enzymes in walled bacteria phylogenetically related to the wall-less bacteria of the class *Mollicutes*. Int J Syst Bacteriol 39:413–419, 1989

217. PHILLIPS DM, PEARCE-PRATT R, TAN X ET AL: Association of human mycoplasmas with HIV-1 and HTLV-I in human lymphocytes. AIDS Res Hum Retroviruses 8:1863–1868, 1992

218. PHILLIPS LE, FARO S, POKORNY SF ET AL: Postcesarean wound infection by *Mycoplasma hominis* in a patient with persistent postpartum fever. Diagn Microbiol Infect Dis 7:193–197, 1987

219. PHILLIPS LE, GOODRICH KH, TURNER RM ET AL: Isolation of *Mycoplasma* species and *Ureaplasma urealyticum* from obstetrical and gynecological patients by using commercially available medium formulations. J Clin Microbiol 24:377–379, 1986

220. PIGRAU C, ALMIRANTE B, GASSER I ET AL: Sternotomy infection due to *Mycoplasma hominis* and *Ureaplasma urealyticum*. Eur J Clin Microbiol Infect Dis 14:597–598, 1995

221. PLATT R, LIN J-SL, WARREN JW: Infection with *Mycoplasma hominis* in postpartum fever. Lancet 22:1217–1221, 1980

222. POLLACK JD, JONES MA, WILLIAMS MV: The metabolism of AIDS-associated mycoplasmas. Clin Infect Dis 17(suppl 1):S267–S271, 1993

223. POSNETT DN, HODSTEV AS, KABAK S ET AL: Interaction of *Mycoplasma arthritidis* superantigen with human T cells. Clin Infect Dis 17(suppl 1):S170–S175

224. POULIN SA, PERKINS RE, KUNDSIN RB: Antibiotic susceptibilities of AIDS-associated mycoplasmas. J Clin Microbiol 32:1101–1103, 1994

225. POWELL DA, MILLER K, CLYDE WA: Submandibular adenitis in a newborn caused by *Mycoplasma hominis*. Pediatrics 63:798–799, 1979

226. PRATT BC: Recovery of *Mycoplasma hominis* from blood culture media. Med Lab Sci 48:350, 1991

227. QUINN PA, GILLAN JE, MARKESTAD T ET AL: Intrauterine infection with *Ureaplasma urealyticum* as a cause of fatal neonatal pneumonia. Pediatr Infect Dis 4:538–543, 1985

228. QUINN PA, LI HCS, TH'NG C ET AL: Serological response to *Ureaplasma urealyticum* in the neonate. Clin Infect Dis 17(suppl 1):S136–S143, 1993

229. RAZIN S, HARASAWA R, BARILE MF: Cleavage patterns of the mycoplasma chromosome, obtained by using restriction endonucleases, as indicators of genetic relatedness among strains. Int J Syst Bacteriol 33:201–206, 1983

230. RAZIN S, MICHMANN J, SHIMSHONI Z: The occurrence of mycoplasma (pleuropneumonia-like organisms, PPLO) in the oral cavity of dentulous and edentulous subjects. J Dent Res 43:402–405, 1964

231. RAZIN S, YOGEV D: Genetic relatedness among *Ureaplasma urealyticum* serotypes (serovars). Pediatr Infect Dis 5:S300–S304, 1986

232. RENAUDIN H, TULLY JG, BEBEAR C: In vitro susceptibilities of *Mycoplasma genitalium* to antibiotics. Antimicrob Agents Chemother 36:870–872, 1992

233. RIDGWAY EJ, ALLEN KD: *Mycoplasma hominis* abscess secondary to respiratory tract infection. J Infect 29:207–210, 1994

234. ROBERTS MC, KENNY GE: Dissemination of the *tetM* tetracycline resistance determinant to *Ureaplasma urealyticum*. Antimicrob Agents Chemother 29:350–352, 1986

235. ROBERTS MC, KENNY GE: *TetM* tetracycline-resistant determinants in *Ureaplasma urealyticum*. Pediatr Infect Dis 5:S338–S240, 1986

236. ROBERTS MC, KOUTSKY LA, HOLMES KK ET AL: Tetracycline-resistant *Mycoplasma hominis* strains contain streptococcal *tetM* sequences. Antimicrob Agents Chemother 28:141–143, 1985

237. ROBERTSON JA: Bromothymol blue broth: improved medium for detection of *Ureaplasma urealyticum* (T-strain mycoplasma). J Clin Microbiol 7:127–132, 1978

238. ROBERTSON JA, CHEN MC: Effects of manganese on the growth and morphology of *Ureaplasma urealyticum* (T-strain mycoplasmas). J Clin Microbiol 19:857–864, 1984

239. ROBERTSON JA, COPPOLA JE, HEISLER OR: Standardized method for determining antimicrobial susceptibility of strains of *Ureaplasma urealyticum* and their response to tetracycline, erythromycin, and rosaramicin. Antimicrob Agents Chemother 20:53–58, 1981

240. ROBERTSON JA, STEMKE GW: Expanded serotyping scheme for *Ureaplasma urealyticum* strains isolated from humans. J Clin Microbiol 9:673–678, 1982

241. ROBERTSON JA, VEKRIS A, BEBEAR C ET AL: Polymerase chain reaction using 16S rRNA gene sequences distinguishes the two biovars of *Ureaplasma urealyticum*. J Clin Microbiol 31:824–830, 1993

242. ROGERS MJ, SIMMONS J, WALKER RT ET AL: Construction of the mycoplasma evolutionary tree from 5S RNA sequence data. Proc Natl Acad Sci USA 82:1160–1164, 1995

243. ROIFMAN CM, RAO CP, LEDERMAN HM ET AL: Increased susceptibility to mycoplasma infections in patients with hypogammaglobulinemia. Am J Med 80:590–594, 1986

244. ROSE DL, KOCKA JP, SOMERSON NL ET AL: *Mycoplasma lactucae* sp. nov., a sterol-requiring mollicute from a plant surface. Int J Syst Bacteriol 40:138–142, 1990

245. RUDD PT, WAITES KB, DUFFY LB ET AL: *Ureaplasma urealyticum* and its possible role in pneumonia during the neonatal period and infancy. Pediatr Infect Dis 5:S288–S291, 1986

246. SAILLARD C, CARLE P, BOVE JM ET AL: Genetic and serologic relatedness between *Mycoplasma fermentans* strains and a mycoplasma recently identified in tissues of AIDS and non-AIDS patients. Res Virol 141:385–395, 1990

247. SALZMAN MB, SOOD SK, SLAVIN ML: Ocular manifestations of *Mycoplasma pneumoniae* infection. Clin Infect Dis 14:1137–1139, 1992

248. SANCHEZ PJ: Perinatal transmission of *Ureaplasma urealyticum*: current concepts based on review of the literature. Clin Infect Dis 16(suppl 1):S107–S111, 1993

249. SANCHEZ PJ, REGAN JA: *Ureaplasma urealyticum* colonization and chronic lung disease in low birth weight infants. Pediatr Infect Dis J 7:542–546, 1988

250. SANYAL D, THURSTON C: *Mycoplasma hominis* infection of a breast prosthesis. J Infect ??:210–211, 1991

251. SASAKI T, BLANCHARD A, WATSON HL ET AL: In vitro influence of *Mycoplasma penetrans* on activation of peripheral T lymphocytes from healthy donors or human immunodeficiency virus-infected individuals. Infect Immun 63:4277–4283, 1995

252. SASAKI T, SASAKI Y, KITA M ET AL: Evidence that Lo's mycoplasma (*Mycoplasma fermentans* incognitus) is not a unique strain among *Mycoplasma fermentans* strains. J Clin Microbiol 30:2435–2440, 1992

253. SASAKI Y, SHINTANI M, SHIMADA T ET AL: Detection and discrimination of *Mycoplasma pneumoniae* and *Mycoplasma genitalium* by the in vitro DNA amplification. Microbiol Immunol 36:21-27, 1992

254. SAVIGE JA, GILBERT GL, FAIRLEY KF ET AL: Bacteriuria due to *Ureaplasma urealyticum* and *Gardnerella vaginalis* in women with preeclampsia. J Infect Dis 148:605–607, 1983

255. SCHRECK R, RIEBER P, BAUERLE PA: Reactive oxygen intermediates as apparently widely used messengers in the activation of the NF-*kappa*B transcription factor and HIV-1. EMBO J 10:2247–2258, 1991

256. SHEPARD MC: Culture media for ureaplasmas. In Razin S, Tully JG, eds. *Methods in Mycoplasmatology*, vol 1, New York, Academic Press, 1983, pp 137–146.

257. SHEPARD MC: *Ureaplasma urealyticum*: overview with emphasis on fetal and maternal infections. Ann NY Acad Sci 549:48–55, 1988

258. SHEPARD MC, COMBS RS: Enhancement of *Ureaplasma urealyticum* growth on a differential agar medium (A7B) by a polyamine, putrescine. J Clin Microbiol 10:931–933, 1979

259. SHEPARD MC, LUNCEFORD CD: Differential agar medium (A7) for identification of *Ureaplasma urealyticum* (human T mycoplasmas) in primary cultures of clinical material. J Clin Microbiol 3:613–625, 1976

260. SHEPARD MC, LUNCEFORD CD, FORD DK ET AL: *Ureaplasma urealyticum* gen. nov., sp. nov.: proposed nomenclature for the human (T-strain) mycoplasmas. Int J Syst Bacteriol 24:160–171, 1974

261. SIBER GR, ALPERT S, SMITH AL ET AL: Neonatal central nervous system infection due to *Mycoplasma hominis*. J Pediatr 90:625–627, 1977

262. SILLIS M: Genital mycoplasmas revisited—an evaluation of a new culture medium. Br J Biomed Sci 50:89–91, 1993

263. SKAKNI L, SARDET A, JUST J ET AL: Detection of *Mycoplasma pneumoniae* in clinical samples from pediatric patients by polymerase chain reaction. J Clin Microbiol 30:2638–2643, 1992

264. SKOV JENSEN J, ULDUM SA, SONDERGARD-ANDERSEN J ET AL: Polymerase chain reaction for detection of *Mycoplasma genitalium* in clinical samples. J Clin Microbiol 29:46–50, 1991

265. SMARON MF, BOONLAYANGOOR S, ZIERDT CH: Detection of *Mycoplasma hominis* septicemia by radiometric blood culture. J Clin Microbiol 21:298–301, 1985

266. SMYTH EG, WEINBREN MJ: *Mycoplasma hominis* sternal wound infection and bacteremia. J Infect 26:315–319, 1993

267. SNELLER M, WELLBORNE F, BARILE MF ET AL: Prosthetic joint infection with *Mycoplasma hominis*. J Infect Dis 153: 174–175, 1986

268. SPAEPEN MS, KUNDSIN RB: Simple, direct broth–disk method for antibiotic susceptibility testing of *Ureaplasma urealyticum*. Antimicrob Agents Chemother 11: 267–270, 1977

269. SPENCER RC, BROWN CB: Septicemia in a renal transplant patient due to *Mycoplasma hominis*. J Infect 6:267–268, 1983

270. STADTLANDER CTK-H, WATSON HL, SIMECKA JW ET AL: Cytopathogenicity of *Mycoplasma fermentans* (including strain incognitus). Clin Infect Dis 17(suppl 1):S289–S301, 1993

271. STANCOMBE BB, WALSH WF, DERDAK S ET AL: Induction of human neonatal pulmonary fibroblast cytokines by hyperoxia and *Ureaplasma urealyticum*. Clin Infect Dis 17(suppl 1):S154–S157, 1993

272. STEFFENSON DO, DUMMER JS, GRANICK MS ET AL: Sternotomy infections with *Mycoplasma hominis*. Ann Intern Med 106:204–208, 1987

273. STIMSON JB, HALE J, BOWIE WR ET AL: Tetracycline-resistant *Ureaplasma urealyticum*: a cause of persistent nongonococcal urethritis. Ann Intern Med 94:192–194, 1981

274. STIPKOVITS L, RASHWAN A: Isolation of ureaplasmas from chickens. Proc Soc Gen Microbiol 3:158, 1976

275. STUART PM: Mycoplasmal induction of cytokine production and major histocompatibility complex expression. Clin Infect Dis 17(suppl 1):S187–S191, 1993

276. SWEET RL: Colonization of the endometrium and fallopian tubes with *Ureaplasma urealyticum*. Pediatr Infect Dis 5:S244–S246, 1986

277. SWENSON CE, VANHAMONT J, DUNBAR BS: Specific protein differences among strains of *Ureaplasma urealyticum* as determined by two-dimensional gel electrophoresis and a sensitive silver stain. Int J Syst Bacteriol 33: 417–421, 1983

278. SYROGIANNOPOULOS GA, KAPATAIS-ZOUMBOS K, DECAVALAS GO ET AL: *Ureaplasma urealyticum* colonization of full term infants: perinatal acquisition and persistence during early infancy. Pediatr Infect Dis J 9:236–240, 1990

279. TAYLOR-ROBINSON D: Evaluation of the role of *Ureaplasma urealyticum* in infertility. Pediatr Infect Dis 5: S262–S265, 1986

280. TAYLOR-ROBINSON D, DAVIES HA, SARATHCHANDRA P ET AL: Intracellular location of mycoplasmas in cultured cells demonstrated by immunocytochemistry and electron microscopy. Int J Exp Pathol 72:705–714, 1991

281. TAYLOR-ROBINSON D, EVANS RT, COUFALIK ED ET AL: Effect of short-term treatment of non-gonococcal urethritis with minocycline. Genitourin Med 62:19–21, 1986

282. TAYLOR-ROBINSON D, FURR PM: Clinical antibiotic resistance of *Ureaplasma urealyticum*. Pediatr Infect Dis 5: S335–S337, 1986

283. TAYLOR-ROBINSON D, FURR PM: Models of infection due to mycoplasmas, including *Mycoplasma fermentans*, in the genital tract and other sites in mice. Clin Infect Dis 17(suppl 1):S280–S282, 1993

284. TAYLOR-ROBINSON D, FURR PM, TULLY JG ET AL: Animal models of *Mycoplasma genitalium* urogenital infection. Isr J Med Sci 23:561–564, 1987

285. TAYLOR-ROBINSON D, FURR PM, WEBSTER ADB: *Ureaplasma urealyticum* in the immunocompromised host. Pediatr Infect Dis 5:S236–S238, 1986

286. TAYLOR-ROBINSON D, GILROY CB, HAY PE: Occurrence of *Mycoplasma genitalium* in different populations and its

clinical significance. Clin Infect Dis 17(suppl 1):S66–S68, 1993

287. TAYLOR-ROBINSON D, GILROY CB, HOROWITZ S ET AL: *Mycoplasma genitalium* in the joints of two patients with arthritis. Eur J Clin Microbiol Infect Dis 13:1066–1068, 1994

288. TAYLOR-ROBINSON D, GUMPEL JM,, HILL A ET AL: Isolation of *Mycoplasma pneumoniae* from the synovial fluid of a hypogammaglobulinaemic patient in a survey of patients with inflammatory polyarthritis. Ann Rheum Dis 37:180–182, 1978

289. TAYLOR-ROBINSON D, HAIG DA, WILLIAMS MH: Bovine T-strain mycoplasmas. Ann NY Acad Sci 143:517–518, 1967

290. TAYLOR-ROBINSON D, SARATHCHANDRA P, FURR PM: *Mycoplasma fermentans*—HeLa cell interactions. Clin Infect Dis 17(suppl 1):S302–S304, 1993

291. TAYLOR-ROBINSON D, WEBSTER ADB, FURR PM ET AL: Prolonged persistence of *Mycoplasma pneumoniae* in a patient with hypogammaglobulinemia. J Infect 2:171–175, 1980

292. TENG K, LI M, YU W ET AL: Comparison of PCR with culture for detection of *Ureaplasma urealyticum* in clinical samples from patients with urogenital infections. J Clin Microbiol 32:2232–2234, 1994

293. TENG L-J, ZHENG X, GLASS JI ET AL: *Ureaplasma urealyticum* biovar specificity and diversity are encoded in multiple-banded antigen gene. J Clin Microbiol 32: 1464–1469, 1994

294. THACKER WL, TALKINGTON DF: Comparison of two rapid commercial tests with complement fixation for serologic diagnosis of *Mycoplasma pneumoniae* infections. J Clin Microbiol 33:1212–1214, 1995

295. THAM TN, FERRIS S, BAHRAOUI E ET AL: Molecular characterization of the P1-like adhesin gene from *Mycoplasma pirum*. J Bacteriol 176:781–788, 1994

296. THOMAS M, JONES M, RAY S ET AL: *Mycoplasma pneumoniae* in a tubo-ovarian abscess. Lancet 2:774–775, 1975

297. TI TY, DAN M, STEMKE GW ET AL: Isolation of *Mycoplasma hominis* from the blood of men with multiple trauma and fever. JAMA 247:60–61, 1982

298. TILTON RC, DIAS F, KIDD H ET AL: DNA probe versus culture for detection of *Mycoplasma pneumoniae* in clinical specimens. Diagn Microbiol Infect Dis 10:109–112, 1988

299. TJHIE JH, VAN KUPPEVELD FJM, ROOSENDAAL R ET AL: Direct PCR enables detection of *Mycoplasma pneumoniae* in patients with respiratory tract infections. J Clin Microbiol 32:11–16, 1994

300. TULLY JG: The current enigma of *Mycoplasma genitalium*: new findings that affect mycoplasma identification in the clinical microbiology laboratory. Clin Microbiol Newslett 11:4–6, 1989

301. TULLY JG: Current status of the mollicute flora of humans. Clin Infect Dis 17(suppl 1):S2–S9, 1993

302. TULLY JG: Mollicute–host interrelationships: current concepts and diagnostic implications. In Tully JG, Razin S, eds. *Molecular and Diagnostic Procedures in Mycoplasmology*, vol 2, Academic Press, San Diego CA, 1996, pp 1–21.

303. TULLY JG, BOVE JM, LAIGRET F ET AL: Revised taxonomy of the Class *Mollicutes*: proposed elevation of a monophyletic cluster of arthropod-associated mollicutes to ordinal rank (*Entomoplasmatales* ord. nov.), with provision for familial rank to separate species with non-helical morphology (*Entomoplasmataceae* fam. nov.) from helical species (*Spiroplasmataceae*), and emended descriptions of the order *Mycoplasmatales*, Family *Mycoplasmataceae*. Int J Syst Bacteriol 43:378–385, 1993

304. TULLY JG, ROSE DL, BASEMAN JB ET AL: *Mycoplasma pneumoniae* and *Mycoplasma genitalium* mixture in synovial fluid isolate. J Clin Microbiol 33:1851–1855, 1995

305. TULLY JG, ROSE DL, WHITCOMB RF ET AL: Enhanced isolation of *Mycoplasma pneumoniae* from throat washings with a newly modified culture medium. J Infect Dis 139: 478–482, 1979

306. TULLY JG, SHIH JW-K, WANG RH-Y ET AL: Titers of antibody to *Mycoplasma* in sera of patients infected with human immunodeficiency virus. Clin Infect Dis 17(suppl 1):S254–S258, 1993

307. TULLY JG, TAYLOR-ROBINSON D: Taxonomy and host distribution of ureaplasmas. Pediatr Infect Dis 5:S292–S295, 1986

308. TULLY JG, TAYLOR-ROBINSON D, COLE RM ET AL: A newly discovered mycoplasma in the human genital tract. Lancet 1:1288–1291, 1981

309. TULLY JG, TAYLOR-ROBINSON D, ROSE DL ET AL: *Mycoplasma genitalium*, a new species from the human genital tract. Int J Syst Bacteriol 33:387–396, 1983

310. TULLY JG, TAYLOR-ROBINSON D, ROSE DL ET AL: Urogenital challenge of primate species with *Mycoplasma genitalium* and characteristics of infection induced in chimpanzees. J Infect Dis 23:2046–2054, 1986

311. ULDUM SA, JENSEN JS, SONDERGARD-ANDERSEN J ET AL: Enzyme immunoassay for detection of immunoglobulin M (IgM) and IgG antibodies to *Mycoplasma pneumoniae*. J Clin Microbiol 30:1198–1204, 1992

312. URSI D, IEVEN M, VANBEVER H ET AL: Typing of *Mycoplasma pneumoniae* by PCR-mediated DNA fingerprinting. J Clin Microbiol 32:2873–2875, 1994

313. VALENCIA GB, BANZON F, CUMMINGS M ET AL: *Mycoplasma hominis* and *Ureaplasma urealyticum* in neonates with suspected infection. Pediatr Infect Dis J 12:571–573, 1993

314. VAN KUPPEVELD FJ, JOHANSSON K-E, GALAMA JM ET AL: 16S rRNA based polymerase chain reaction compared with culture and serological methods for diagnosis of *Mycoplasma pneumoniae* infection. Eur J Clin Microbiol Infect Dis 13:401–405, 1994

315. VELLECA WM, BIRD BR, FORRESTER FT: Course 8228C: Laboratory diagnosis of mycoplasma infections. Atlanta, Centers for Disease Control, 1980

316. VERINDER DGR: Septic arthritis due to *Mycoplasma hominis*: a case report and review of the literature. J Bone Joint Surg (Br) 60B:224, 1978

317. WAITES KB, CROUSE DT, CASSELL GH: Systemic neonatal infection due to *Ureaplasma urealyticum*. Clin Infect Dis 17(suppl 1):S131–S135, 1993

318. WAITES KB, CROUSE DT, CASSELL GH: Therapeutic considerations for *Ureaplasma urealyticum* infections in neonates. Clin Infect Dis 17(suppl 1):S208–S214, 1993

319. WAITES KB, CROUSE DT, PHILIPS JB III ET AL: Ureaplasmal pneumonia and sepsis associated with persistent pulmonary hypertension of the newborn. Pediatrics 83: 79–85, 1989

320. WAITES KB, DUFFY LB, CROUSE DT ET AL: Mycoplasmal infections of cerebrospinal fluid in newborn infants from a community hospital population. Pediatr Infect Dis J 9:241–245, 1990

321. WAITES KB, RUDD PT, CROUSE DT ET AL: Chronic *Ureaplasma urealyticum* and *Mycoplasma hominis* infections of the central nervous system in preterm infants. Lancet 1:17–21, 1988

322. WAITES KB, TULLY JG, ROSE DL ET AL: Isolation of *Acholeplasma oculi* from human amniotic fluid in early pregnancy. Curr Microbiol 15:327–327, 1987

323. WALLACE RJ, ALPERT S, BROWNE K ET AL: Isolation of *Mycoplasma hominis* from blood cultures in patients with postpartum fever. Obstet Gynecol 51:181–185, 1978

324. WALSH WF, BUTLER J, COALSON J ET AL: A primate model of *Ureaplasma urealyticum* infection in the premature infant with hyaline membrane disease. Clin Infect Dis 17(suppl 1):S158–S162, 1993

325. WANG EEL, CASSELL GH, SANCHEZ PJ ET AL: *Ureaplasma urealyticum* and chronic lung disease of prematurity: critical appraisal of the literature on causation. Clin Infect Dis 17(suppl 1):S112–S116, 1993

326. WANG EEL, DRAYHA H, WATTS J ET AL: Role of *Ureaplasma urealyticum* and other pathogens in the development of chronic lung disease of prematurity. Pediatr Infect Dis J 7:547–551, 1988

327. WANG RY-H, HU WS, DAWSON MS ET AL: Selective detection of *Mycoplasma fermentans* by polymerase chain reaction and by using a nucleotide sequence within the insertion sequence-like element. J Clin Microbiol 30:245–248, 1992

328. WANG RY-H, SHIH JW-K, GRANDINETTI T ET AL: High frequency of antibodies to *Mycoplasma penetrans* in HIV-infected patients. Lancet 340:1312–1316, 1992

329. WANG RY-H, SHIH JW-K, WEISS SH ET AL: *Mycoplasma penetrans* infection in male homosexuals with AIDS: high seroprevalence and association with Kaposi's sarcoma. Clin Infect Dis 17:724–729, 1993

330. WIENTZEN RL: Genital mycoplasmas and the pediatrician. Pediatr Infect Dis J 9:232–235, 1990

331. WOESE CR: Bacterial evolution. Microbiol Rev 51:221–171, 1985

332. WOESE CR, MANILOFF J, ZABLEN LB: Phylogenetic analysis of the mycoplasmas. Proc Natl Acad Sci USA 77:494–498, 1980

333. WOOD JC, LU RM, PETERSON EM ET AL: Evaluation of Mycotrim-GU for isolation of *Mycoplasma* species and *Ureaplasma urealyticum*. J Clin Microbiol 22:789–792, 1985

334. YAJKO DM, BALSTON E, WOOD D ET AL: Evaluation of PPLO, A7B, E, and NYC agar media for the isolation of *Ureaplasma urealyticum* and *Mycoplasma* species from the genital tract. J Clin Microbiol 19:73–76, 1984

335. YAKULIS VJ, COSTEA N, HELLER P: *alpha*-Galactoside determinants of the I-antigen. Proc Soc Exp Biol Med 121:81N–N16, 1966

336. YECHOURON A, LEFEBVRE J, ROBSON HG ET AL: Fatal septicemia due to *Mycoplasma arginini*: a new human zoonosis. Clin Infect Dis 15:434–438, 1992

337. YOGEV D, HALACHMI D, KENNY GE ET AL: Distinction of species and strains of mycoplasmas (*Mollicutes*) by genomic DNA fingerprints with an rRNA probe. J Clin Microbiol 26:1198–1201, 1988

338. YOGEV D, RAZIN S: Common deoxyribonucleic acid sequences in *Mycoplasma genitalium* and *Mycoplasma pneumoniae* genomes. Int J Syst Bacteriol 36:426–430, 1986

MYCOBACTERIA

New techniques and revised algorithms for the recovery, identification, and susceptibility testing of mycobacteria are being implemented in many clinical laboratories in view of changes in the clinical manifestations and epidemiology of tuberculosis. In the short-term, conventional methods will continue to be used; however, rapid molecular-based techniques for the identification and susceptibility testing of *Mycobac-*

terium species recovered from clinical specimens are being introduced. At least two thirds of the basic and applied research papers relative to mycobacteriology and tuberculosis published in the current medical literature focus on potential laboratory applications of molecular techniques. Although the quest for pure research in molecular biology is an integral part of this evolution, the driving force for clinical laboratory personnel is to provide ever more rapid species identifications and antimycobacterial drug susceptibility profiles. As molecular-based procedures evolve from research laboratories into commercial products that receive Food and Drug Administration (FDA) approval, the ability to diagnose tuberculosis within days, rather than weeks, will theoretically be possible in most diagnostic laboratories.

TRENDS IN CLINICAL TUBERCULOSIS

The following are trends in the practice of mycobacteriology and tuberculosis control that must be addressed by laboratory personnel.

WORLDWIDE INCREASE IN THE INCIDENCE OF TUBERCULOSIS

The progressive decrease in the incidence of tuberculosis during the first eight decades of this century suddenly bottomed out early in the 1980s. As the incidence curve of tuberculosis approached zero baseline in many parts of the world by the late 1970s, many microbiologists had the supreme confidence that tuberculosis was about to be conquered. In fact, the opposite has happened. Currently, the rates of morbidity and mortality are rising as multidrug-resistant strains of several *Mycobacterium* species have emerged, primarily on the heels of the onset of the acquired immunodeficiency syndrome (AIDS) epidemic. An estimated 2 billion persons are currently infected with *M. tuberculosis* and other *Mycobacterium* species, and currently, an estimated 3 million people worldwide die annually from complications of this disease.[254] There are an estimated 8 million new cases each year, 95% of which occur in developing countries.[148] In industrialized countries, 80% of cases occur in persons older than 50 years of age; in developing countries 80% of cases occur between the ages of 15 and 50. An estimated 3 million persons with tuberculosis worldwide also have AIDS.[148] It has been estimated that 15 million persons in the United States are skin-test–positive or have clinical disease. The rates of increase are even greater in developing countries, primarily because of increased immigration of people from regions of high endemicity, declining socioeconomic conditions in densely populated cities, and the increasing number of human immunodeficiency virus (HIV)-infected individuals.

RAPIDLY PROGRESSIVE DISEASE

Recently acquired infections with *M. tuberculosis* often do not follow the classic, slowly progressive course of secondary disease; rather, a rapidly spreading miliary type of tuberculosis became the rule rather than the exception, particularly in patients with AIDS. Progression of disease is no longer measured in terms of months and years but in time frames of a few weeks.

Color Plates for Chapter 17 are found between pages 784 and 785.

The more rapid replication of mycobacteria at sites of infection, both of *M. tuberculosis* and particularly with strains belonging to the *M. avium–intracellular* complex, not only leads to high concentrations of organisms at these sites, septicemia, and miliary spread, but to treatment failures and the emergence of multidrug-resistant strains.

CHANGING PATTERNS OF PERSON-TO-PERSON TRANSMISSION

In a recent epidemiologic study of tuberculosis in New York City, Alland and associates[6] found that approximately 40% of the incident cases and two thirds of the drug-resistant cases resulted from recent human-to-human transmission rather than from reactivation of latent disease. Sullivan and coworkers[276] also have traced the emergence of *M. tuberculosis* strains resistant to the fluoroquinolones. Torrea and associates,[282] using chromosomal DNA fingerprinting analysis of *M. tuberculosis* recovered from 64 tubercular patients residing in French Polynesia, also found a pattern of common origin of strains among family members and nearby acquaintances, indicating considerable active transmission. Because many persons with active tuberculosis are heavily infected, the chances for transmission to an unsuspecting host are also increased. Health care workers, even in developed countries, are under increasing risk for contracting tuberculosis. Griffith and colleagues[87] report an outbreak of tuberculosis among 13 health care workers who either converted skin tests or developed active disease following exposures to undiagnosed index cases in as short as 2 hours time in the emergency room and 10 hours in a medical intensive care unit. Inherent in this increased risk of contracting tuberculosis is the greater chance for developing clinical disease and for acquiring multidrug-resistant strains, particularly against isoniazid, rifampin, and streptomycin.

IMPLEMENTATION OF MORE AGGRESSIVE INFECTION CONTROL AND EPIDEMIOLOGIC MEASURES

More aggressive measures are also being instituted to ensure that patients with a high index of suspicion for tuberculosis are promptly placed in isolation. Hospital personnel working in areas of high risk for acquiring tuberculosis, either those involved in direct patient care or in handling infected secretions, are required to follow isolation procedures and to don protective clothing and high-filtering masks. Ventilation systems in hospitals and in crowded settings, such as in prisons, nursing homes, and urban homeless shelters, where outbreaks of tuberculosis have been reported, are under intense scrutiny. Nardell and associates[198] found poor air quality in buildings fitted with air duct systems that deliver an inadequate mixture of outside air contributes to airborne infection. Problems will remain in unsuspected settings, however, such as the outbreak of tuberculosis among 41 patrons of a local bar reported by Kline and coauthors.[146] The index case was a homeless person who was a regular patron of the bar during a long asymptomatic interval before diagnosis. The possibility of heavy alcohol use among this population of patrons may have contributed to the high rate of infectivity.

TRENDS IN THE LABORATORY DIAGNOSIS OF TUBERCULOSIS

In response to these altered clinical and epidemiologic situations, several changes in laboratory practice have evolved over the past several years. Several new techniques have been introduced that are directed toward the more effective recovery of mycobacteria from clinical specimens, their rapid identification, and determination of their drug susceptibility profiles. The following is a brief summary of several of these new methods:

- **Use of automated and semi-automated instruments**—The period of recovery of mycobacteria from sputum and other specimens, including blood cultures, has been shortened by as much as 2 to 3 weeks.[192,234] The BACTEC 460 instrument can also be used for rapid drug susceptibility testing of frontline antituberculous drugs.[99] A rise in the growth index of an antibiotic-containing vial tested in the instrument within 3 to 5 days following inoculation with the test strain indicates drug resistance.
- **Use of broth culture media**—The rate of recovery and time to positivity of mycobacteria from clinical specimens have improved through the use of broth culture media. Two commercial systems are currently available for use in laboratories not having automated systems. The Septi-Chek AFB System (BBL) has proved useful in many laboratories. A new commercial product, the Mycobacteria Growth Indicator Tube (MGIT) System, has been introduced by Becton Dickinson (BBL Cat. No. 45111); it uses 7H9 broth and an O_2-sensitive fluorescent sensor to indicate microbial growth. Fluorescence usually occurs earlier in this system than does the visualization of turbidity in other broth systems or the detection of colonies on Löwenstein-Jensen (LJ) or synthetic agar.
- **Inoculation of clinical specimens to agar-based culture media** inoculation of a clear, agar-based culture medium, such as Middlebrook 7H10 or 7H11, permits the microscopic observation for microcolonies. Growth of colonies may be observed microscopically as early as 5 to 7 days after inoculation of smear-positive specimens. The morphology of the microcolonies can also be used for making early presumptive identifications of *M. tuberculosis* and *M. avium–intracellulare*. This information often provides a helpful guide to further workup of the isolate, particularly in selecting the appropriate nucleic acid probe assay.
- **Use of p-nitro-α-acetylamino-β-hydroxypropiophenone**—NAP is an antimycobacterial agent that selectively inhibits the growth of *M. tuberculosis* in broth culture media. After inoculation of a BACTEC culture vial containing NAP with the test organism, any rise in the growth index (which indicates resistance to NAP) after 3 days of incubation rules out *M. tuberculosis*.
- **Applications of gas–liquid chromatography, high-performance liquid chromatography, and mass spectrometry**—The composition of cell wall mycolic acids and fatty acid constituents, as determined by gas–liquid chromatography (GLC) and high-performance liquid chromatography (HPLC), provides profiles that are helpful in making a rapid species identification of mycobacteria recovered from clinical specimens.
- **Use of the lysis–centrifugation system blood culture tube**—The recovery of mycobacteria from peripheral blood and bone marrow samples may be improved by releasing intracellular mycobacterial cells into the blood culture broth, increasing the rate and reducing the time of recovery.
- **Recovery of mycobacteria from stool specimens**—Altered decontamination and concentration procedures are also being used to increase the recovery of mycobacteria from stool specimens, a useful diagnostic adjunct to the diagnosis of mycobacterial infections in patients with AIDS.
- **Introduction of nonisotopic nucleic acid probes**—Currently, several probes are commercially available for the culture confirmation of *M. tuberculosis* complex (*M. tuberculosis, M. bovis, M. africanum, M. microti*), *M. avium, M. intracellulare*, and *M. gordonae* (Accu-Probe; Roche Diagnostics, Nutley, NJ; Gen Probe, San Diego, CA). The library of probes will continue to grow as clinical syndromes related to mycobacteria other than *M. tuberculosis* (MOTT) become better defined.
- **Application of polymerase chain reaction technology**—By amplifying specific target sequences of DNA extracted from mycobacterial cells in clinical specimens, such as sputum, a rapid identification of *M. tuberculosis* infection may be possible. Although theoretically a specific DNA sequence from a single mycobacterial cell could be detected after polymerase chain reaction (PCR) amplification, Yajko and associates[325] determined that 42 colony-forming units (CFU) is the lower cutoff concentration in direct sputum specimens, which corresponds to eight CFU that can be recovered in culture from NALC–NaOH-processed specimens. The Amplified *Mycobacterium tuberculosis* Direct Test (Gen-Probe, San Diego CA), a PCR kit for the direct detection of mycobacteria in respiratory specimens, has recently been awarded FDA approval and is available for use in clinical laboratories.
- **Implementation of restriction endonuclease assays**—Following PCR amplification of target rRNA or DNA conserved sequences extracted from mycobacteria, the application of restriction endonuclease digestion procedures has been used, both to assist in making species identifications and in determining strain variance for epidemiologic studies.

896

Thus, the practical applications of molecular techniques, both as tools for rapid culture confirmation of culture isolates and in the direct detection of mycobacteria in clinical specimens, will permit earlier diagnosis of new cases and aggressive specific antitubercular therapy to help prevent the emergence of drug-resistant strains and human-to-human transmission.[215] The several new approaches outlined in the foregoing will be discussed in more detail later in this chapter.

THE CLINICAL LABORATORY

In reference to the overall organization of clinical laboratories and the necessity to provide more laboratory services, Salfinger[242,243] outlines what he refers to as a "fast-track" program. Three primary goals of the fast-track program are:

1. To use the most rapid and reliable technologies to achieve the shortest turnaround times possible for organism identification and susceptibility testing
2. To centralize such services to control costs
3. To have patients with non-*M. tuberculosis* infections confined to respiratory isolation rooms for as short a time as possible

The current practice of waiting for bacterial colonies to appear on solid agar, making species identifications without probe technology, and performing drug susceptibility tests only on solid media is too time-consuming. Which procedures and tests will be performed in the on-site, "point of care" laboratory and which will be sent to the specialty laboratory must be determined within each practice care community. In many practice settings, activities in the point of care laboratory may be limited to rapid turnaround procedures, such as screening acid-fast smears or setting up cultures. Other procedures, again to be determined by local health care personnel, will be performed in the regional specialty laboratory. Most of the techniques involved in direct identifications, such as high-performance liquid chromatography, nucleic acid probes, PCR, restriction endonuclease assays, and DNA sequencing, will be within the provence of the specialty laboratory. A team of health care workers, including clinicians, laboratory specialists, and support personnel must be established to determine how diagnostic approaches are to be coordinated within the fast-track program to ensure that the goals are being attained. Early diagnosis, prompt direct therapy, and respiratory isolation are the major ingredients to ensure not only cure of the infected patient but also to prevent the emergence of resistant strains and to interrupt person-to-person transmission of infections.

LABORATORY SAFETY

One additional trend in laboratory practice in response to the changing epidemiology of tuberculosis involves new guidelines for laboratory safety. With a growing national concern over biosafety relative to the handling of mycobacterial specimens and cultures in clinical microbiology laboratories, new stringent safety control standards conforming to the biosafety level 3 (BSL3) standard are now being recommended. Specifically, BSL3 practices are required for laboratories in which American Thoracic Society levels II and III activities (propagation and manipulation of cultures for *M. tuberculosis* or *M. bovis*) are being carried out. The following are the proposed biosafety requirements as specified by the U.S. Department of Health and Human Services (*Biosafety in Microbiological and Biomedical Laboratories*, 3rd ed, 1993):

> The BSL3 space, which houses the biologic safety cabinet (BSC) and centrifuge, should have nonpermeable walls and work surfaces, directional airflow (with the lowest air pressure in the laboratory), and a double-door air lock to prevent back flow of air. Air from the BSL space should be vented through HEPA (high efficiency particulate air) filters directly to the outside. Laboratories and hoods should be equipped with gauges to monitor air pressure, and a simple indicator can be constructed with light tissue paper to assess the flow of air through the suite.
>
> Because articles (including worker's arms) placed in a BSC may disrupt the laminar airflow and deflect contaminated air out the cabinet, anyone working in the cabinet and in the BSL3 space should wear protective clothing and respirators. Personnel must routinely be tested (annually) for respirator fit. Since splatter may occur, disposable gowns should be worn over scrub suit (street clothes should not be worn into the BSL3 space because they may become contaminated); gloves, caps, and shoe protection complete the protective personal accessories. Protective clothing should be removed and placed in a bag for autoclaving when work in the BSL3 is completed.

Each laboratory director must determine the extent to which renovations in current laboratory space may be required in their home laboratories. Renovations can run into many thousands of dollars and may not be cost-effective in certain environments. In such instances, a decision must be made if cultures for mycobacteria will be forwarded to a facility that can comply with the recommended standards.

PERSONS AT RISK

The following high-risk groups, designated by the CDC Advisory Council for the Elimination of Tuberculosis,[13] should be screened for tuberculosis:

1. Close contacts (those sharing the same household or other enclosed environments) of persons known or suspected to have tuberculosis
2. Persons infected with HIV
3. Persons who inject illicit drugs or other locally identified high-risk substance users (such as crack cocaine users)
4. Persons who have medical risk factors known to increase the chance for disease if infection occurs
5. Residents and employees of high-risk congregate settings (such as correctional institutions, nursing homes, mental institutions, other long-term residential facilities, and shelters for the homeless)

6. Health care workers who serve high-risk clients
7. Foreign-born persons, including children, recently arrived (within 5 years) from countries that have a high incidence or prevalence of tuberculosis
8. Some medically underserved low-income populations
9. High-risk racial or ethnic minority populations, as defined locally
10. Infants, children, and adolescents exposed to adults in high-risk categories.

It is recommended that local or state tuberculosis programs take the lead in determining the groups to be screened. In some locales, the local health departments should conduct the screening, or they should discuss the need for screening with other appropriate persons, such as the staff personnel of correctional facilities, hospital infection control officers, and operators of shelters. The reference cited provides several recommendations for conducting programs and handling specific high-risk groups.

SPECIMEN COLLECTION AND PROCESSING

Mycobacteria can potentially be recovered from a variety of clinical specimens, including upper respiratory collections (sputum, bronchial washes, bronchoalveolar lavage, bronchial biopsies, and such); urine, feces, blood, cerebrospinal fluid (CSF); tissue biopsies, and deep needle aspirations of virtually any tissue or organ.[149] Specimens that may contain mixed bacterial flora should be processed as soon after collection as possible to minimize the degree of overgrowth with contaminants.

RESPIRATORY SPECIMENS

Sputum samples collected by expectoration or by ultrasonic nebulization are best obtained shortly after the patient awakens in the morning, when mycobacteria are in the highest concentration. In the past, 24-hour sputum samples were required to have a sufficient concentration of mycobacteria present to maximize recovery; however, the extraction procedures currently being used are more efficient and require less sample to achieve the same degree of recovery. Twenty-four-hour collections are now discouraged because the sample containing the highest concentration of mycobacteria will be proportionately diluted by subsequent low-yield samples, and the chances for bacterial and fungal contamination during the prolonged collection process is significantly increased.[134]

The irregular and intermittent release of mycobacteria into the bronchial lumen from mucosal ulcers or loculated cavities often results in a variable pattern of recovery from respiratory secretions. Cultures obtained from patients with pulmonary or renal tuberculosis, in particular, may be positive on one day but negative on the next; thus, a minimum of three to five early-morning sputum or urine specimens, respectively, should be collected on successive 24-hour periods to maximize the chance of recovery of mycobacteria. All specimens should be transported promptly to the laboratory and refrigerated if processing is delayed.

BLOOD CULTURES

Several approaches may be used for the recovery of mycobacteria from blood cultures. Berlin and associates[16] report on the use of a biphasic system using modified 7H11 oleic acid albumin as the agar phase and brain–heart infusion as the broth phase—positive cultures for *M. avium–intracellulare* were obtained as early as 6 to 8 days. However, Agy and coworkers[3] report that only 43.8% of blood cultures from known blood culture-positive patients were recovered using a similar biphasic system. The use of the lysis–centrifugation blood culture system (Isolator; Wampole Laboratories, Cranberry NJ) has increased the yield and shortened the time of recovery of mycobacteria from blood cultures.[79,173] The lysis–centrifuge tube contains an anticoagulant and a lysing agent to effect rupture of both erythrocytes and neutrophils. Thus, intracellular mycobacteria are released into the broth milieu, further enriched by the lysis of the red blood cells. Each tube holds 5 mL of blood and cell lysis can be enhanced by gently inverting the tube several times immediately after adding the sample. Following centrifugation of the tube at 3000 g for 20 to 30 minutes, the eluate is discarded and 1.6 mL of sediment is divided into 0.2-mL aliquots for transfer to appropriate culture media.

In many laboratories, it is common practice to transfer one such aliquot to a BACTEC 12B blood culture vial. Wasilauskas and Morrell,[298,299] however, forewarn that the growth of *M. avium–intracellulare* (MAC) recovered from Isolator tubes may be inhibited when added to BACTEC 12B bottles compared with growth on solid media. The BACTEC (Becton Dickinson, Sparks, MD) is a semiautomated blood culture system that is based on the detection of radioactive $^{14}CO_2$ released in the blood culture vial from 1-[^{14}C]palmitic acid included in the broth medium (Middlebrook). They theorize that the lysis-anticoagulant reagent (LAR) contained within the Isolator tube may be toxic to MAC when the lysate is transferred to a closed liquid system, in contrast to subculture to solid media where the component is able to diffuse into the agar or evaporate into the overlying airspace. They cite an Isolator recovery study by Whittier and associates in which recovery of MAC from Septi-Check AFB biphasic media was superior to their recovery from the BACTEC 12B bottles inoculated in parallel.

However, Doern and Westerling[58,59] found that the inhibitory effect of LAR in BACTEC 12B bottles is minimized if a small inoculum (0.2 mL) of Isolator lysate is used. Wasilauskas and Morrell[299] provide the counterargument that using a smaller inoculum may compromise recovery in light infections. Perhaps, if a closed liquid system is to be used for transfer of lysis–centrifuged-processed blood specimens, inoculation of solid media in parallel may be in order, particularly in AIDS patients from whom the recovery of MAC organisms is highly likely.

The issue is avoided in many laboratories by using the BACTEC 13A bottle, which includes a lytic agent and can directly receive up to 5 mL of blood, thereby bypassing the potential problems associated with the Isolator system. In a study of 32 cases of mycobacterial sepsis,[3] growth was detected in 30 of the 13A vials (93.7%), on 27 Middlebrook 7H11 agar plates inoculated with sediment obtained from the Isolator tube (84.4%), and in 26 BACTEC 12B bottles inoculated with the Isolator sediment (81.2%). Growth was detected in the 13B vial and in the 12B vials at 14.2 and 13.7 days, respectively, compared with 20.8 days for the M7H11 plates. This study concluded that the BACTEC 13A vial is equal or better than the Isolator system, both in the rate and time of recovery of mycobacteria from blood cultures, a conclusion also reached by others.[316] Strand and associates[274] also found the BACTEC 13A vial comparable with the lysis–centrifugation/7H11 agar procedure in the rate of recovery (96.9% and 98.5%, respectively) and the time of detection of 64 blood cultures positive for *M. avium* and one for *M. tuberculosis*. Details of the BACTEC system and its applications in the mycobacteriology laboratory will be presented later in this chapter.

Whatever blood culture system is used, the policy of routinely obtaining at least two culture sets may not be cost-effective.[272] From a total of 1047 mycobacterial blood cultures obtained from 273 patients with disseminated *M. avium* complex infection, Stone and colleagues[272] found only one of the two bottles was positive in only four of 98 positive cultures (4%). In 85%, both bottles were negative, and in 11%, both bottles were positive. Thus, as a routine they recommend obtaining only a single blood culture for the diagnosis of mycobacterial septicemia and ordering a repeat culture only if there is strong clinical evidence of disseminated infection. The importance of obtaining blood cultures in patients with suspected tuberculosis has been stressed.[22] Fourteen percent of patients with disseminated tuberculosis had positive blood cultures (intravenous drug use and chronic alcoholism were risk factors); 26% to 42% of patients with AIDS in this study had mycobacterial infections at some time in the course of illness, and in 33%, positive blood cultures provided the initial recovery of the organism. Blood cultures positive for acid-fast bacilli, therefore, provide a noninvasive procedure for diagnosing disseminated disease.

STOOL SPECIMENS

In certain patients with AIDS, the concentration of mycobacteria, particularly *M. avium–intracellulare*, may be sufficiently high in the lower intestinal tract to be recovered in culture. Kiehn and associates[137] have outlined a procedure for processing stool specimens for mycobacterial culture:

- Stool specimens are collected in a clean (not necessarily sterile) container with a tightly fitting lid, as for routine bacterial cultures.
- A direct smear is first prepared from a small quantity of the specimen and stained for acid-fast bacilli,

using either the Ziehl-Neelsen or Kinyoun carbolfuchsin techniques or the rhodamine–auramine fluorescence method.

- If the smears are negative for acid-fast bacteria, the specimen is not further processed.
- If acid-fast bacilli are seen in the smear, 1 g of feces is suspended in 5 mL of Middlebrook 7H9 broth or equivalent and subjected to the same NaOH digestion–decontamination as used for sputum specimens, to be described later.
- Culture contamination with intestinal bacteria was not a problem following the digestion procedure.

One might raise the question of the significance of detecting mycobacteria in fecal samples. Conlon and coworkers,[42] in a study of 89 patients with AIDS-related enteropathy in Lusaka, Zambia, found that the symptom of chronic diarrhea did not correlate with the presence of mycobacteria in stool specimens. They conclude that mycobacteria play an insignificant role in the pathogenesis of enteropathy in AIDS patients. On the other hand, Chin and colleagues[33] found that the recovery of *M. avium–intracellulare* from stool specimens is predictive of disseminated disease. The technique described in the foregoing is workable; whether the procedure should be made available in a given laboratory must be an individual decision.

MISCELLANEOUS "STERILE" SPECIMENS

Specimens submitted for acid-fast culture that are normally sterile, such as cerebrospinal fluid, synovial fluid, and other body fluids, need not be decontaminated before culture. Processing can commence with centrifugation, as described in the following, and a small aliquot of the sediment transferred to an appropriate culture medium. Low-volume fluid samples can be added directly to approximately 10 mL of 7H9 or 7H11 broth and incubated directly. Urine samples can usually be processed without decontamination, centrifuged, and a portion of the sediment used for culture, as just described. The first morning sample rather than a 24-hour collection is preferred. It is the practice in some laboratories to set up bacterial cultures before culturing for mycobacteria to determine whether the specimens require decontamination. Also, 10 or 15 mL of 10% calcium chloride can be added to the urine sample until a precipitate forms to remove inhibitory factors. Following centrifugation, a portion of the sediment is cultured, as described earlier. Tissues and needle biopsy material should be placed in a small quantity of 7H9 or 7H11 broth as a holding medium. Depending on the size and nature of the material obtained, the specimen should be ground in a small amount of broth with a mortar and pestle and aliquots of the suspension transferred to appropriate culture media.

There is virtually no indication for obtaining material for mycobacterial culture with a swab because the hydrophobic nature of the lipid-containing cell wall of the bacteria inhibits transfer of the organisms from the swab to the aqueous culture medium. If a swab is received in the laboratory, the tip should be placed directly on the surface of the culture medium or into a tube containing approximately 5 mL of 7H9 broth and incubated for 4 to 8 weeks. Mycobacteria, if present, may be found forming colonies in the fibers of the swab at the junction with the culture media.

THE LABORATORY APPROACH TO THE RECOVERY AND IDENTIFICATION OF MYCOBACTERIA

The classic laboratory approach to the diagnosis of mycobacterial infections involving the phenotypic characterization of colonies growing on Löwenstein-Jensen medium using a battery of biochemical tests is too time-consuming for current applications. Figure 17-1 is

an algorithm that reflects the practice of processing sputum specimens in many clinical laboratories. Other specimens may require alternative treatment; however, in virtually all instances rapid procedures for the identification of *M. tuberculosis* and *M. avium–intracellulare* should be performed.

Smears should be prepared from the material submitted for acid-fast staining. Most laboratories use the auramine O stain for screening and follow up with a carbolfuchsin-based stain (Ziehl-Neelsen or Kinyoun) for confirmation of positive results. Most laboratories treat sputum specimens with the NALC–NaOH decontamination–digestion procedure for concentrating any mycobacterial cells that may be present. It is currently recommended that all sputum digests and other specimens be inoculated to broth culture media in addition to Löwenstein-Jensen media or Middlebrook agar. The

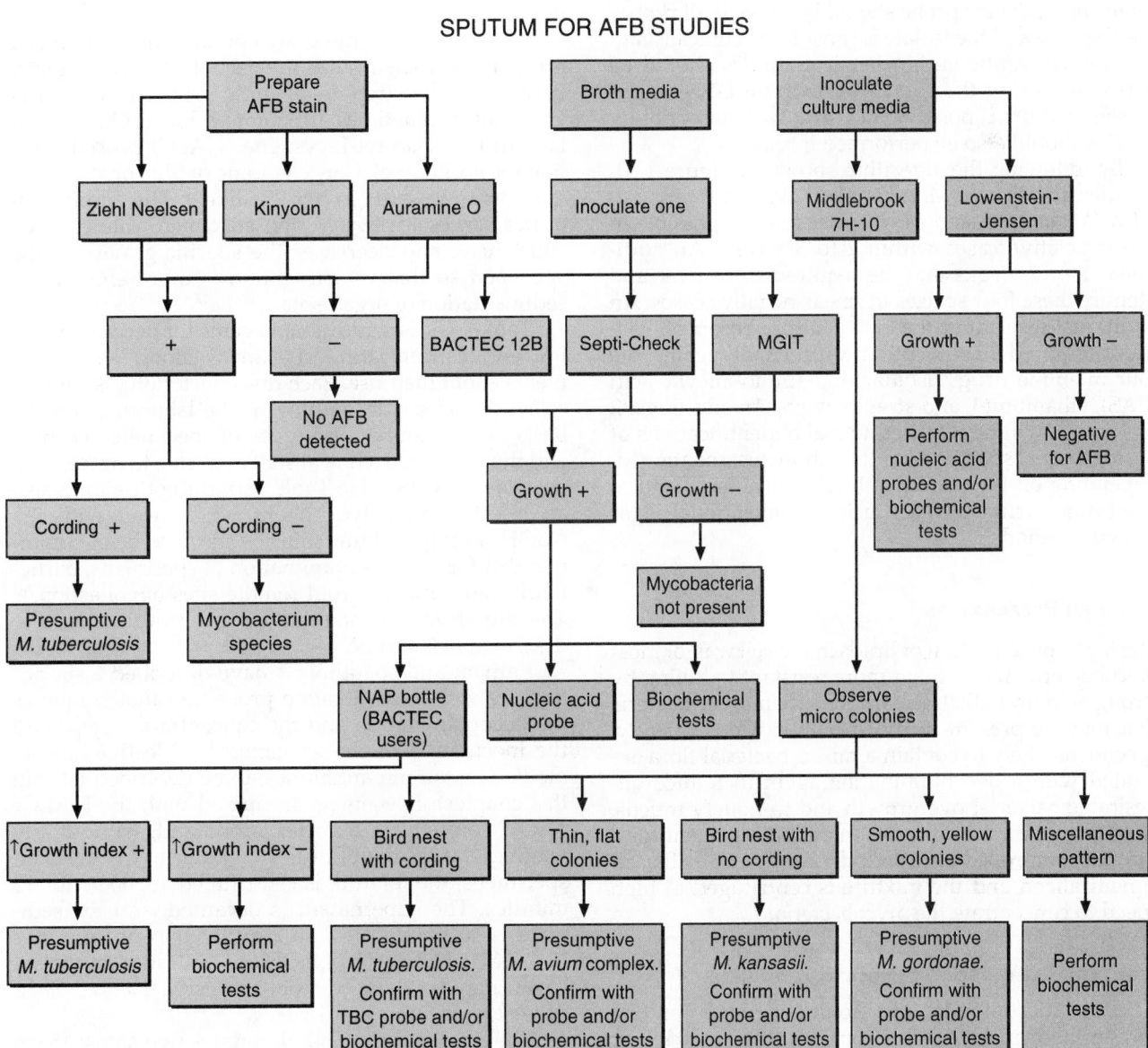

Figure 17-1.
An algorithm reflecting the practice of processing sputum specimens.

choices of broth cultures include the BACTEC 12A bottles in laboratories where a 460 BACTEC instrument is available or inoculation of the Septi-Chek or MGIT culture systems. If any of these cultures show evidence of growth, nucleic acid probe studies should be done as soon as the concentration of organisms exceeds the threshold of sensitivity for the assay. In laboratories using the BACTEC system, a NAP bottle should be inoculated to rule out *M. tuberculosis*.

Observation of microcolonies on Middlebrook agar may serve as a guide to which probe should be performed: if an interweaving pattern with cording is observed, a probe for *M. tuberculosis* should be performed; if the colonies are flat and transparent, the probe for *M. avium–intracellulare* is in order. Metchock and Diem[184] suggest that if smears are 3+ or 4+ positive and growth is detected within 5 days, a probe for *M. tuberculosis* should be done. For 1+ or 2+ positive smears that grow up in culture after 7 days, the *M. avium–intracellulare* probe should be done. If all probes are negative and the isolate is considered clinically significant, conventional biochemical studies should be performed using the colonies grown on Löwenstein-Jensen medium if positive. In vitro drug susceptibility studies should also be performed if required.

By following the algorithm shown in Figure 17-1, the identification of *M. tuberculosis*, *M. avium–intracellulare*, *M. kansasii*, and *M. gordonae* may be possible in smear-positive cases within 2 to 3 weeks. An additional 1 or 2 weeks may be required to recover and identify these four species in smear-negative cases. An additional week after the broth culture becomes positive is required for susceptibility test results against the four mainline drugs: isoniazid, *p*-aminosalicylic acid (PAS), ethambutol, and streptomycin. An additional 2 to 4 weeks will be required to make identifications of mycobacterial species other than those just mentioned, depending on the results of biochemical tests, and to determine drug profiles using conventional agar growth methods.

SPECIMEN PREPARATION

The high concentration of lipids in the cell wall of most mycobacteria makes them more resistant to killing by strong acid and alkaline solutions than other bacteria that may be present in the specimen. Consequently, specimens likely to contain a mixed bacterial flora are treated with a decontaminating agent to reduce undesirable bacterial overgrowth and to liquefy mucus. After treatment with the decontaminating agent for a carefully controlled time period, the acid or alkali used is neutralized and the mixture is centrifuged at high speed to concentrate the mycobacteria.

DIGESTION AND DECONTAMINATION AGENTS

Some decontaminating solutions, such as 6% sodium hydroxide, are so strong that they may kill or seriously injure mycobacteria to the point that they will grow only very slowly, if at all. Decreasing the strength of the acid or alkaline decontamination solution has resulted in an improved recovery of mycobacteria by culture but frequently at the price of overgrowth of the culture with contaminants. Exposure of specimens to strong sodium hydroxide, 5% oxalic acid, or other agents must be carefully timed to prevent excessive chemical injury to the mycobacterial cells.

The use of mild decontaminating agents, such as trisodium phosphate (TSP) alone or combined with benzalkonium chloride (Zephiran; Winthrop Laboratories, New York NY), is popular in some laboratories. Specimens containing large numbers of *M. tuberculosis* can withstand the action of these agents for as long as overnight, and careful timing of exposure is not required.[57] Specimens treated with TSP–Zephiran should be inoculated to an egg-based culture medium to neutralize the growth inhibition of the Zephiran. If agar-based media are used, neutralization of the Zephiran can be accomplished by adding lecithin. The standard digestion–decontamination procedure is shown in Box 17-1.

Usually, concentrated HCl or concentrated NaOH is employed to neutralize the decontaminating agents. Because of the strength of these solutions, a neutral endpoint is sometimes difficult to achieve. One advantage of the *N*-acetyl-L-cysteine (NALC) procedure is that the addition of a large volume of phosphate buffer makes strong shifts in pH less likely. The addition of buffer serves to "wash" the specimen, dilutes toxic substances, and decreases the specific gravity of the specimen so that centrifugation is more effective in sedimentation of organisms.

Table 17-1 lists additional agents for decontaminating and concentrating specimens along with comments about their use. Each mycobacteriologist should select the agents to employ in the laboratory on the basis of the number and types of specimens received and the time and technical staff available to process the specimens. As listed in Table 17-1, dithiothreitol is also an effective mucolytic agent when used with 2% NaOH. Cetylpyridium chloride has also been recommended for the decontamination of specimens, particularly those mailed from remote sites of collection.[262] The digestion–decontamination procedure is further described in Chart 22.

Ratnam and coauthors[229] have described a simplified acetylcysteine–alkaline procedure that combines the decontamination and the concentration steps and the inoculation of the specimen to selective culture media (containing antibiotics, to be described later in this chapter). Specimens are mixed with the NALC–NaOH solution on a vortex mixer and, without any waiting or addition of buffer or water to the digested specimens, the mixture is centrifuged at 3000 *g* for 15 minutes. The supernatant is decanted, and the sediment is suspended in 1 to 2 mL of phosphate buffer (0.067 M, pH 5.3). The NaOH concentration in the solution may be reduced from the usual 2% to 1.5% if necessary or feasible.

The modified method eliminates two steps: 15- to 20-minute decontamination time following digestion of specimens and the addition of phosphate buffer or water. According to these authors, the greatest killing

BOX 17-1. THE STANDARD DIGESTION–DECONTAMINATION PROCEDURE DEVELOPED BY KUBICA ET AL[155] AT THE CENTERS FOR DISEASE CONTROL

1. Prepare the acetylcysteine-alkali digestant as follows: Combine 50 mL of 2.94% trisodium citrate–3H$_2$O (0.1 M) with 50 mL of 4% NaOH. To this solution add 0.5 g of powdered N-acetyl-L-cysteine (NALC) just before use. The NaOH (which becomes a 2% solution after mixing equal parts with the specimen) serves as a decontaminating agent. Occasionally, the concentration of NaOH must be increased to 3% (6% original solution) during warm weather or in treating specimens from patients with large pulmonary cavities associated with persistent bacterial contamination. The NALC is a mucolytic agent without antibactericidal activity that liquifies mucus by splitting disulfide bonds. The mycobacteria are released when the mucus is liquefied, rendering them easy to concentrate by high-speed centrifugation.

2. Use 50 mL plastic centrifuge tubes with tightly fitting lids for the processing of all specimens. Add the NALC digestant mixture in a volume equal to that of the specimen. Typically, a volume of 10–15 mL of specimen is used. Tighten the screw cap.

3. Homogenize the mixture with a vortex mixer for 15–20 seconds or until well mixed and let stand at room temperature for 15–20 minutes, swirling the tubes periodically. Proper attention should be paid so that this digestion time does not exceed 20 minutes, because "overtreated" specimens result in fewer positive cultures.

4. After the digestion–decontamination step, add phosphate buffer, pH 6.8 (preferred over sterile water) up to the top ring in the tube. Mix well. The phosphate buffer makes strong shifts in pH less likely and also serves to "wash" the specimen, to dilute and neutralize toxic substances, and to reduce the specific gravity of the specimen so that centrifugation is more effective in the sedimentation of organisms.

5. Concentrate the specimen by centrifugation at 2000–3000 g for 15–20 minutes. A refrigerated centrifuge may be used at higher speeds to increase the yield of mycobacteria even more.

6. After centrifugation, decant all the supernatant carefully into a splash-proof can containing a phenolic disinfectant. Wipe the lip of the tube with a cotton ball soaked with 5% phenol. Add a small quantity of phosphate buffer, pH 6.8 (1–2 mL) and resuspend the sediment with a Pasteur pipette. Although addition of a small quantity of serum albumin has been advocated in the past, this is currently avoided as it increases the chances for contamination and a potential delay in the detection time.

7. Prepare smears on clean microscope slides for Ziehl-Neelsen (or Kinyoun) or fluorochrome staining, or both. Use either a sterile applicator stick or a flamed, 3-mm diameter bacteriologic loop and smear a portion of the sediment over an area 1 × 2 cm. If the quantity of sediment is very small, delay making smears until after the next step; i.e., the addition of albumin. Add 1 mL of sterile 0.2% bovine albumin.

8. Transfer a small quantity (0.2–0.4 mL) of the concentrate to an appropriate culture medium. Inoculation of a 1:10 dilution of the concentrate in sterile water to a second culture medium set is also done in some laboratories. Löwenstein-Jensen (LJ) slants and Middlebrook 7H10 or 7H11 agar plates are generally used.

---

of mycobacteria occurs during the first few minutes of exposure to the alkali digestion fluid, and as many as 10^4 mycobacteria may be lost depending on the species. The modified method eliminates the potential for specimens to drip from the cap or run down the outer surface of the tube when diluent is added after vortex mixing and reduces the chance for cross-contamination. Thus, the authors found the modified method to be simpler, faster, and safer than the original procedure, and the reduced manipulation is also likely to minimize the chance for cross-contamination in sequential specimen processing. Eliminating the initial digestion step had no adverse effects on the recovery of mycobacteria. In fact, at times, the addition of phosphate buffer or water actually resulted in poorer recovery, owing to a greater dissolution of the particulate matter in the specimens. Alkali tolerance was not a consistent feature among the mycobacterial species and strains tested, with the rapid growers being the most susceptible to a high pH. By reducing or eliminating the standard treatment time of 15 to 20 minutes or by decreasing the concentration of NaOH in the digestant solution from the usual 2% to either 1.5% or 1%, the adverse effects can be easily overcome.

Because of the emergence of drug-resistant strains of M. tuberculosis,[75] the performance of rapid laboratory tests to determine drug susceptibility profiles may be necessary to guide early therapy. Many of the new tests for identifying drug-resistance profiles are based on nucleic acid amplification procedures. Consequently, it may be necessary to store specimens or digested concentrates for future batch testing or for shipping to a distant reference laboratory. It may be advisable to render such samples noninfectious at early stages of processing to minimize the biohazard to laboratory workers. Williams and associates[314] found that ethanol fixation of sputum sediments containing M. tuberculosis served to render the bacteria nonviable, while still preserving the integrity of genomic DNA in a state suitable for testing by polymerase chain reaction techniques. In their studies, 0.25 mL of sputum sediments were diluted with 0.583 mL of 100% ethanol to bring the final ethanol concentration to 70%. They recommend storage of the ethanol-treated specimens

TABLE 17-1

COMMONLY USED AGENTS FOR DECONTAMINATION AND CONCENTRATION OF SPECIMENS

AGENT	COMMENTS
N-Acetyl-L-cysteine plus 2% NaOH	Mild decontamination solution with mucolytic agent NALC to free mycobacteria entrapped in mucus. Limit exposure to NaOH to 15 minutes.
Dithiothreitol plus 2% NaOH*	Very effective mucolytic agent used with 2% NaOH. Trade name of dithiothreitol is Sputolysin. Reagent is more expensive than NALC. Limit exposure to NaOH to 15 minutes.
Trisodium phosphate, 13% plus benzalkonium chloride (Zephiran)	Preferred by laboratories that cannot carefully control time of exposure to decontamination solution. Zephiran should be neutralized with lecithin and not inoculated to egg-based culture medium.
NaOH, 4%	Traditional decontamination and concentration solution. Time of exposure must be carefully controlled to no more than 15 minutes. NaOH, 4%, effects mucolytic action to promote concentration by centrifugation.
Trisodium phosphate, 13%	Can be used for decontamination of specimens when exposure time can be completely controlled. It is not as effective as TSP–Zephiran mixture.
Oxalic acid, 5%	Most useful in processing specimens that contain *Pseudomonas aeruginosa* as a contaminant.
Cetylpyridinium chloride, 1%, plus 2% NaCl†	Effective as a decontamination solution for sputum specimens mailed from outpatient clinics. Tubercle bacilli have survived 8-day transit without significant loss.

* See Shah and Dye.[253]
† See Smithwick et al.[262]

at 4°C if PCR testing is to be delayed. Zwadyk and coworkers[335] review several methods for rendering specimens safe for further testing. They discuss the killing effects and preservation of genomic DNA of mycobacteria in specimens after treatment with several disinfectants. They also introduced the technique of heating the samples at 100°C for 30 minutes in a boiling water bath or a forced-air oven, which both killed and lysed the mycobacteria, releasing short DNA fragments suitable for amplification.

CENTRIFUGATION

Rickman and Moyer[233] have called attention to the importance of carefully controlling centrifugal force in the recovery of mycobacteria from clinical specimens, particularly in the correlation of positive smears with positive cultures. The focus of this study is to understand the unique physical characteristics conferred on mycobacteria by the high lipid content of the cell wall (up to 30% dry weight). The lipid has the effect of making the specific gravity of the organism very low. If the organism is to be maximally sedimented during the centrifugation of the specimen, the specific gravity of the suspending fluid should be kept as low as possible, and the centrifugal force applied to the specimen should be as high as practical. Improved recovery of mycobacteria by culture occurred as the relative centrifugal force (RCF) was increased from 1260 to 3000 g (Table 17-2).[233] When the RCF was increased to 3800 g, a twofold increase in the correlation of positive smears to positive cultures from 40% to 82% was realized, or

more than a threefold increase from the correlation when the RCF was only 1260 g.

Subsequent evaluation for recovery of mycobacteria from sputum samples seeded with known concentrations of organisms following centrifugation has confirmed that the recovery rate increases with centrifugation time and speed.[228] However, the recovery rates in these experimental samples were not significantly lower when using an RCF of 2074 g for 20 minutes (67% to 71%) compared with the recovery at RCFs of 3005 g and 3895 g for 15 minutes (76% to 80%). Acid-fast smear sensitivity for 25,000 specimens processed with an RCF of 3800 g for 20 minutes was 71%. However, sensitivity was still 69% as determined for an additional 30,000 specimens processed in a similar manner but with an RCF of 2000 g. The authors conclude that the actual rates of recovery of viable mycobacteria from clinical specimens also depends on the method of treatment and individual species and strain differences of mycobacteria for alkali tolerance. Thus, although centrifugation at RCF of 3000 g for 15 minutes may be optimal for the recovery of mycobacteria from clinical specimens, the chances for recovery will not be substantially compromised in those laboratories where lower-cost centrifuges attaining only a maximum of 2074 g are available, if the time is increased to 20 minutes. As pointed out by Sommers and Good,[265] with the centrifugation forces produced at RCFs of 3000 g or higher, glass or plastic centrifuge tubes may collapse and must be placed in sealed cups. Also, considerable heat is generated at high speeds,

TABLE 17-2

EFFECT OF INCREASING CENTRIFUGAL FORCE ON POSITIVE SMEARS AND CULTURES FOR MYCOBACTERIA

	RELATIVE CENTRIFUGAL FORCE (g)		
	1260	*3000*	*3800*
Positive smears	1.8%	4.5%	9.6%
Positive cultures	7.1%	11.2%	11.6%
Correlation of positive smears/cultures	25%	40%	82%

(Adapted from Rickman TW, Moyer NP: Increased sensitivity of acid-fast smears. J Clin Microbiol II: 618–620, 1980).[233]

and refrigerated centrifuges may be required when RCFs exceed 3000 g.

BONE MARROW AND BIOPSY SPECIMENS

M. tuberculosis is a facultative intracellular parasite that may be present in macrophages of the bone marrow, liver, blood, and lymph nodes of patients with disseminated infections. Because tissue biopsies are usually not contaminated with other microorganisms, they can be homogenized and inoculated directly to culture media without the use of a decontaminating solution. Draining sinuses or other cutaneous lesions suspected of harboring mycobacteria are best cultured by obtaining a small portion of infected tissue or drainage. Fine-needle biopsies are also being used with increased frequency to obtain tissue material for culture from a variety of subcutaneous and deep visceral granulomas. In a study of 390 cases in which needle biopsies were obtained to diagnose suspected tuberculous lymphadenitis, the overall rate of smear positivity was 23.6%, and culture positivity was 35%.[225] Caseating lesions were more likely to produce positive cultures (40%) than noncaseating ones (9%).

MISCELLANEOUS LIQUID SPECIMENS

Liquid specimens (e.g., CSF, pleural fluid, or other) should be centrifuged, stained for acid-fast bacilli, and inoculated directly to liquid and solid culture media. Pleural fluid specimens are diluted with buffer in some laboratories to lower the specific gravity, thereby improving sedimentation of mycobacteria. Liquid specimens with a low protein content, such as CSF, can be filtered through a 0.22-μm cellulose nitrate membrane. The membrane can be cut into pieces, which can then be placed on or in different types of solid and liquid culture media.

Centrifuges used for the processing of specimens potentially containing acid-fast bacilli should be equipped with 50- or 250-mL centrifuge cups with aerosol-free tops that can be adapted to hold 50-mL centrifuge tubes. Such centrifuges need not be vented to the outdoor environment because of the danger of reverse airflow through the vent during windstorms. Precautions should be taken to prevent the sponta-

neous rupture of fluid surface tension membranes when inoculating broth cultures or liquid specimens. If such a membrane in an inoculation loop breaks, for example, droplet aerosols may be created that can persist in the air for long periods. Again, all such transfers must be performed in a biologic safety hood.

STAINING OF ACID-FAST BACILLI

The cell walls of mycobacteria, because of their high lipid content, have the unique capability of binding the fuchsin dye so that it is not destained by acid alcohol. This acid-fast–staining reaction of mycobacteria, along with their characteristic size and shape, is a valuable aid in the early detection of infection and in the monitoring of therapy for mycobacterial disease. The presence of acid-fast bacilli in the sputum, combined with a history of cough, weight loss, and chest radiographic evidence of a pulmonary infiltrate, is still presumptive evidence of active tuberculosis.

It has been estimated that when using standard concentrating techniques, approximately 10,000 (10^4) acid-fast bacilli per milliliter of sputum are required to detect microscopically. Patients with extensive disease shed large numbers of mycobacteria, with a good correlation between a positive smear and a positive culture. Many patients have minimal or less-advanced disease, and the correlation of positive smears to positive cultures in this group may be only 25% to 40%.

Acid-fast smears are also useful in following a patient's response to treatment. After antimycobacterial drugs are started, cultures become negative before the smears do, suggesting that the organisms are not capable of replicating but are capable of binding the stain. With continued treatment, more organisms are killed and fewer shed, so that assessing the number of organisms in the sputum during treatment can provide an early objective measure of response. Should the number of organisms fail to decrease after therapy is started, the possibility of drug resistance must be considered, and additional cultures and susceptibility studies should be obtained.

Two types of acid-fast stains are commonly used (Table 17-3):

1. Carbolfuchsin stains: a mixture of fuchsin with phenol (carbolic acid)
   a. Ziehl-Neelsen (hot stain)
   b. Kinyoun (cold stain)
2. Fluorochrome stain: auramine O, with or without a second fluorochrome, rhodamine

The carbolfuchsin and auramine O dyes used in the techniques of each of these stains bind to mycolic acid in the mycobacterial cell wall. Smears stained with the carbolfuchsin technique must be scanned with an oil-immersion objective. This limits the total area of a slide that can be viewed in a given unit of time. In contrast to the carbolfuchsin stains, smears stained by the auramine procedure can be scanned with a 25× objective, thereby increasing the field of view and reducing the time needed to scan a given area of the slide. Fluorochrome-stained smears require a strong light source—

TABLE 17-3
ACID-FAST–STAINING PROCEDURE

ZIEHL-NEELSEN PROCEDURE	KINYOUN COLD PROCEDURE	AURAMINE FLUROCHROME PROCEDURE
Carbolfuchsin: dissolve 3 g of basic fuchsin in 10 mL of 90%–95% ethanol. Add 90 mL of 5% aqueous solution of phenol.	**Carbolfuchsin:** dissolve 4 g of basic fuchsin in 20 mL of 90%–95% ethanol and then add 100 mL of a 9% aqueous solution of phenol (9 g of phenol dissolved in 100 mL of distilled water).	**Phenolic auramine:** dissolve 0.1 g of auramine O in 10 mL of 90%–95% ethanol and then add to a solution of 3 g of phenol in 87 mL of distilled water. Store the stain in a brown bottle.
Acid-alcohol: Add 3 mL of concentrated HCl *slowly* to 97 mL of 90%–95% ethanol, in this order. Solution may get hot!	**Acid-alcohol:** add 3 mL of concentrated HCl *slowly* to 97 mL of 90%–95% ethanol, in this order. Solution may get hot!	**Acid-alcohol:** add 0.5 mL of concentrated HCl to 100 mL of 70% alcohol.
Methylene blue counterstain: dissolve 0.3 g of methylene blue chloride in 100 mL of distilled water.	**Methylene blue counterstain:** dissolve 0.3 g of methylene blue chloride in 100 mL of distilled water.	**Potassium permanganate:** dissolve 0.5 g potassium permanganate in 100 mL of distilled water.
Procedure Cover a heat-fixed, dried smear with a small rectangle (2 × 3 cm) of filter paper. Apply 5–7 drops of carbolfuchsin stain to thoroughly moistened filter paper. Heat the stain-covered slide to steaming, but do not allow to dry. Heating may be done by gas burner or over an electric staining rack. Remove paper with forceps, rinse slide with water, and drain. Decolorize with acid-alcohol until no more stain appears in the washing (2 min). Counterstain with methylene blue (1–2 min). Rinse, drain, and air dry (1–2 min). Examine with 100× oil immersion objective. Mycobacteria are stained red and the background light blue.	**Procedure** Cover a heat-fixed, dried smear with a small rectangle (2 × 3 cm) of filter paper. Apply 5–7 drops of carbolfuchsin stain to thoroughly moisten filter paper. Allow to stand for 5 min. Add more stain if paper dries. Do not steam! Remove paper with forceps, rinse slide with water, and drain. Decolorize with acid-alcohol until no more stain appears in the washing (2 min). Counterstain with methylene blue (1–2 min). Rinse, drain, and air dry (1–2 min). Examine with 100× oil immersion objective. Mycobacteria are stained red and the background light blue.	**Procedure** Cover a heat-fixed, dried smear with carbol auramine and allow to stain for 15 min. Do not heat or cover with filter paper. Rinse with water and drain. Decolorize with acid-alcohol (2 min). Rinse with water and drain. Flood smear with potassium permanganate for 2 and not more than 4 min. Rinse with tap water. Drain. Examine with 25× objective using a mercury vapor burner and BG-12 filter or a strong blue light. Mycobacteria are stained yellowish-orange against a dark background.

either a 1200-W mercury vapor burner or a strong blue light with a fluorescein isothiocyanate (FITC) filter.

Fluorochrome-stained bacteria are bright yellow (rhodamine) or orange-red (rhodamine) against a dark background, allowing the slide to be scanned under lower magnification without losing sensitivity. The sharp contrast between the brightly colored mycobacteria and the dark background offers a distinct advantage in scanning the slide (see Color Plate 17-1A). Modifications of the auramine fluorochrome stain include the addition of rhodamine, giving a golden appearance to the cells, or the use of acridine orange as a counterstain, resulting in a red to orange background. False-positive reactions may be due to fluorescence of nonspecific tissue or cellular debris that can be mistaken for bacilli with the 25× objective. The 40× objective should be used to confirm any suspicious forms. Dead mycobacterial cells will also stain with rhodamine and auramine, leading to a smear-positive, culture-negative situation about 10% of the time. This feature is also important to remember when using acid-fast smears to

assess treatment efficacy—the presence of acid-fast bacilli in fluorochrome-stained smears does not necessarily indicate treatment failure and carbolfuchsin stains should also be performed. Fluorochrome-stained smears can be subsequently stained with carbolfuchsin; the opposite situation does not apply.

With carbolfuchsin, the acid-fast bacteria (AFB) stain bright red against either a blue or a green background, depending on the counterstain used (see Color Plate 17-1B). Although the Ziehl-Neelsen and the Kinyoun techniques are theoretically the same, it has been our experience that the former is more sensitive in detecting lightly staining organisms, particularly some strains of the rapidly growing *M. fortuitum–chelonei* complex. The property of acid-fastness is due to the thick, waxy capsule that surrounds the mycobacterial cells. For aqueous carbolfuchsin to penetrate through the wax, the capsule must be "softened." This is done with heat in the Ziehl-Neelsen procedure, much like the melting of a paraffin film in the hot rays of the sun. Dye that penetrates through the heat-softened capsule binds to the cell wall; then, when the bacterial cells cool after the heat is removed, the wax again hardens, protecting the bound dye from the action of the acid–alcohol decolorizer ("acid-fast"). In the Kinyoun, or "cold" technique, a surface-active agent is used to increase permeability of the dye through the waxy capsule; however, the re-formation of the waxy film may be incomplete, allowing most, if not all, of the bound dye to be extracted by the acid–alcohol decolorizer. Obviously, mycobacterial cells that are endowed with a thin waxy capsule will be more susceptible to decolorization, as may be the situation with many rapidly growing strains. In these circumstances, the use of a less stringent decolorizer, such as 1% HCl ("partial acid-fast" procedure), may disclose the innate acid-fast property. The carbolfuchsin-based procedure is described in Chart 9.

Although workers in various laboratories may be partial to either the carbolfuchsin- or the fluorescent-staining method, the specificity for detecting mycobacteria of the two methods seems about the same, with the possible exception of *M. fortuitum*. In a study of 15 strains of *M. fortuitum*,[131] five of the strains did not stain with auramine, but all 15 stained with carbolfuchsin. Uribe-Botero and associates,[286] who used Truant's auramine–rhodamine staining of routinely processed bone marrow aspirates and biopsies, describe considerable success in the detection of mycobacteria by fluorescent staining. In a study of 51 bone marrow specimens from 47 HIV-positive patients, mycobacteria were detected in 72%. If the fluorescent stain was positive, the positive predictive value for culturing mycobacteria was 87%. McCarter and Robinson,[179] in a study of 782 primary sputum smears evaluated blindly by the rhodamine–auramine method at both room temperature and at 37°C, found that the preparation stained at room temperature detected only 85.7% of the positive smears; 43.3% of the smears had more AFB in the 37°C stained smears compared with only 13.3% more AFB in the room temperature-stained smears. They conclude that staining at 37°C enhances the detection of AFB. Woods and coworkers[321] found no increase in the detection of acid-fast bacilli in 844 auramine O-stained cytocentrifuged sputum smears when compared with the traditional NALC–NaOH concentration method.

Because a significantly larger area of the smear can be scanned per unit of time with the auramine fluorochrome stain than with the carbolfuchsin method, the fluorochrome stain offers the advantage of greater sensitivity. Some workers use the fluorochrome method for scanning purposes and then confirm their findings by reexamining the preparation after destaining and restaining with carbolfuchsin method. After laboratory workers have become familiar with the auramine fluorochrome method, most prefer it over the carbolfuchsin procedure. The introduction of relatively low-cost blue-light illuminators has made fluorescence microscopy available to clinical laboratories where the detection and recovery of mycobacteria is offered as a service.[219] For use in laboratories where expensive illuminators may not be affordable, use of the UV ParaLens adaptor, a light-weight, portable, inexpensive epi-illuminator offers an alternative possibility. Patterson and associates[208] found a comparable sensitivity and specificity in the detection of fluorescing acid-fast bacilli using the UV ParaLens adapter when compared with Kinyoun-stained smears. Implementation of such an adapter offers applications in the examination of other fluorescing microorganisms such as *Giardia* and *Pneumocystis* species.

It should be emphasized that neither the auramine nor the auramine–rhodamine fluorochrome stain is a fluorescent antigen–antibody technique; rather, each is a direct physicochemical binding of the stain to the lipid-rich cell wall. The use of fluorescent-tagged antibodies to aid in the identification of various species of mycobacteria has been described, but they are not commonly used nor commercially available.

The recommendations of the American Lung Association for reporting mycobacteria seen on acid-fast–stained smears are given in Table 17-4. These recommendations are followed by many laboratories to provide consistency of observations between technologists in a given laboratory and uniformity of reporting from one laboratory to another. A summary of the fluorescent and carbolfuchsin-based techniques for the staining of mycobacteria can be found in Charts 9 and 31.

CULTURE OF SPECIMENS FOR RECOVERY OF MYCOBACTERIA

CULTURE MEDIA

The recovery of mycobacteria from agar culture media was poor when the first attempts were made late in the 19th century. Through experimentation it was found

---

TABLE 17-4

METHOD FOR REPORTING NUMBERS OF ACID-FAST BACILLI OBSERVED IN STAINED SMEARS*

NUMBER OF BACILLI OBSERVED	CDC METHOD REPORT	
0	Negative	(−)
1–2/300 fields	Number seen[†]	(±)
1–9/100 fields	Average no./100 fields	(1+)
1–9/10 fields	Average no./10 fields	(2+)
1–9 field	Average no./field	(3+)
More than 9/field	More than 9/field	(4+)

* Examination at ×800 to ×1000 is assumed. Magnifications less than ×800 should be clearly stated. If a microscopist uses consistent procedure for smear examination, relative comparisons of multiple specimens should be easy for the clinician, regardless of magnification used. To equate numbers of bacilli observed at less than ×800 with those seen under oil immersion , adjust counts as follows: for magnifications about ×650, divide count by 2; near ×450, divide by 4; near ×250, divide by 10; e.g., if 8 bacilli per 10 fields were seen at ×450, the count at ×1000 would be equivalent to about 2/10 fields (8 ÷ 4).

† Counts less than 3/3000 fields at ×800 to ×1000 are not considered positive; another specimen (or repeat smear of same specimen) should be processed if available.

(American Thoracic Society: Diagnostic standards and classification of tuberculosis and other mycobacterial diseases. Am Rev Respir Dis 123:343–358, 1981).

that a culture medium containing whole eggs, potato flour, glycerol, and salts solidified by heating to 85° to 90°C for 30 to 45 minutes was effective in isolating *M. tuberculosis*. The process of solidifying protein-containing medium by heat is known as inspissation. An inspissated culture medium is more subject to liquefaction from the effects of proteolytic enzymes produced by contaminating bacteria than a medium solidified by the addition of agar. However, it was soon discovered that the use of aniline dyes, such as malachite green or crystal violet, in the inspissated medium helped control contaminating bacteria. The concentration of dye must be carefully controlled; if too high, the growth of mycobacteria may also be inhibited along with the contaminating bacteria. Malachite green is the dye most commonly incorporated into nonselective culture media, in concentrations ranging between 0.0025 g/100 mL and 0.052 g/100 mL (Table 17-5).

NONSELECTIVE CULTURE MEDIA FOR RECOVERY OF MYCOBACTERIA

Several of the egg-based culture media for the recovery of mycobacteria are listed in Table 17-5. Löwenstein-Jensen medium is most commonly used in most clinical diagnostic laboratories; it is less inhibitory to the growth of mycobacteria than is Petragnani medium, which is used primarily to recover mycobacteria from specimens heavily contaminated with bacteria. Conversely, the American Thoracic Society (ATS) medium, which contains only 0.02 g/100 mL of malachite green, is less inhibitory to the growth of mycobacteria and is recommended for use in usually sterile specimens, such as CSF, pleural fluid, and tissue biopsies.

Because Löwenstein-Jensen medium is less sensitive in the recovery of mycobacteria from clinical specimens compared with broth culture media and Middlebrook 7H10 agar, and because detection of growth is delayed when positive, this medium is being dropped from routine use in many laboratories. The use of broth culture media followed by a DNA probe often establishes an organism identification before growth is visible on the LJ slant. Chromogenic studies and biochemical tests are most accurate when performed on subcultures from LJ medium. Thus, positive broth cultures are transferred to LJ medium in the event that the probe assays do not provide an identification when biochemical tests may be necessary.

MEDIA OF COHEN AND MIDDLEBROOK

During the 1950s, Cohen and Middlebrook developed a series of defined culture media for use in both research and clinical laboratories. These media were prepared from defined salts and organic chemicals; some contained agar, but all were found to require the addition of albumin for optimal growth of mycobacteria. The Middlebrook media that contain agar are transparent and allow early detection of growth after 10 to 12 days, instead of the 18 to 24 days of incubation required with other media. This is partly due to the inclusion of biotin and catalase to stimulate revival of damaged bacilli in clinical specimens. Albumin is also incorporated to bind toxic amounts of oleate and other compounds that might be released from spontaneous hydrolysis of Tween 80. The albumin does not appear to be metabolized by the bacilli.[301]

Not many of the earlier Cohen and Middlebrook culture media are used today. However, 7H9 is a popular liquid medium, and both 7H10 and 7H11 agar media are widely used for isolation and susceptibility testing. The antimycobacterial agents should be incorporated into the medium just before it solidifies to reduce the loss of activity known to occur with some drugs during the long heating period needed to prepare the inspissated egg-based media. This application will be discussed in more detail later in this chapter. 7H11 differs from 7H10 only in containing 0.1% casein hydrolysate, an additive that improves the rate and amount of growth of mycobacteria resistant to isoniazid (INH).[40] Both 7H10 and 7H11 contain malachite green but in 10 times smaller quantities than those usually used in egg-based media, explaining in part

TABLE 17-5
NONSELECTIVE MYCOBACTERIAL ISOLATION MEDIA

MEDIUM	COMPONENTS	INHIBITORY AGENT
Löwenstein-Jensen	Coagulated whole eggs, defined salts, glycerol, potato flour	Malachite green, 0.025 g/100 mL
Petragnani	Coagulated whole eggs, egg yolks, whole milk, potato, potato flour, glycerol	Malachite green, 0.052 g/100 mL
American Thoracic Society medium	Coagulated fresh egg yolks, potato flour, glycerol	Malachite green, 0.02 g/100 mL
Middlebrook 7H10	Defined salts, vitamins, cofactors, oleic acid, albumin, catalase, glycerol, dextrose	Malachite green, 0.0025 g/100 mL
Middlebrook 7H11	Defined salts, vitamins, cofactors, oleic acid, albumin, catalase, glycerol, 0.1% casein hydrolysate	Malachite green, 0.0025 g/100 mL

the higher incidence of contamination than on egg-based media.

One other advantage of the use of Middlebrook agar is that experienced mycobacteriologists can often make a presumptive identification of *M. tuberculosis* and other groups of mycobacteria within 10 days by examining early microcolonies on Middlebrook agar and observing certain well-defined morphologic features.[240] Photomicrographs of representative microcolonies are illustrated in Color Plate 17-1C (*M. tuberculosis*) and Color Plates 17-2A and 2B (*M. avium–intracellulare*).

Although essentially all culture media yield more growth and larger colonies of mycobacteria when incubated in 5% to 10% CO_2, the Middlebrook media absolutely require capneic incubation for proper performance. Exposure of 7H10 and 7H11 to strong light, or storage of the media at 4°C for more than 4 weeks may result in deterioration and release of formaldehyde, a chemical very inhibitory to mycobacteria.[187]

SELECTIVE MEDIA

Culture media containing antimicrobial agents are used to suppress bacterial and fungal contamination. Although certain antimicrobial agents are known to reduce contamination, they may also inhibit the growth of mycobacteria. Therefore, the times of exposure must be carefully controlled. The use of selective media can result in greatly improved recovery of mycobacteria. Table 17-6 lists the names and components of several selective media.

Currently, the selective medium described by Gruft,[90] which consists of Löwenstein-Jensen medium with penicillin, nalidixic acid, and RNA, is commonly used. Petran[213] subsequently described a selective medium containing cycloheximide, lincomycin, and nalidixic acid to control fungal and bacterial contaminants. By varying the concentrations of these agents, the medium can be prepared with either Löwenstein-Jensen or 7H10 base.

Selective 7H11 is a modification of an oleic acid agar medium first described by Mitchison.[188] The medium was originally designed for use with sputum specimens without the use of a decontaminating agent. Mitchison's medium contains carbenicillin, polymyxin, trimethoprim lactate, and amphotericin B. McClatchy[180] suggested reducing the concentration of carbenicillin from 100 μg/mL to 50 μg/mL and using 7H11 medium instead of oleic acid agar. He called this modification selective 7H11, or S7H11. With use of S7H11 medium with Löwenstein-Jensen and 7H11, recovery of mycobacteria is definitely improved, particularly when the S7H11 medium is used with the NALC–1% NaOH decontamination procedure.[180]

Subsequent to this report, a 3-year study comparing the use of S7H10 medium with undecontaminated specimens has shown significantly less contamination on S7H10 plates with homogenized specimens than on 7H10 medium with decontamination, using 2% NaOH with NALC. In addition, S7H10 medium recovered 18% more positive cultures, usually with more colonies per culture and with less contamination than did cultures inoculated onto 7H10 after 2% NaOH–NALC decontamination. In contrast to the recommendation in McClatchy's report, carbenicillin was left at 100 μg/mL instead of 50 μg/mL. Specimens inoculated directly to 7H10 plates were homogenized after the addition of equal quantities of NALC in 0.1 M sodium citrate at pH 8.1 and allowed to stand for 15 minutes before centrifugation. Inoculation of concentrated, but undecontaminated specimens, should pre-

TABLE 17-6
SELECTIVE MYCOBACTERIAL ISOLATION MEDIA

MEDIUM	COMPONENTS	INHIBITORY AGENTS
Gruft modification of Löwenstein-Jensen	Coagulated whole eggs, defined salts, glycerol, potato flour RNA—5 mg/100 mL	Malachite green, 0.025 g/100 mL Penicillin, 50 U/mL Nalidixic acid, 35 μg/mL
Löwenstein-Jensen	Coagulated whole eggs, defined salts, glycerol, potato flour	Malachite green, 0.025 g/100 mL Cycloheximide, 400 μg/mL Lincomycin, 2 μg/mL Nalidixic acid, 35 μg/mL
Middlebrook 7H10	Defined salts, vitamins, cofactors, oleic acid, albumin, catalase, glycerol, glucose	Malachite green, 0.0025 g/100 mL Cycloheximide, 360 μg/mL Lincomycin, 2 μg/mL Nalidixic acid, 20 μg/mL
Selective 7H11 (Mitchison's medium)	Defined salts, vitamins, cofactors, oleic acid, albumin, catalase, glycerol, glucose, casein hydrolysate	Carbenicillin, 50 μg/mL Amphotericin B, 10 μg/mL Polymyxin B, 200 U/mL Trimethoprim lactate, 20 μg/mL

dispose to recovery of fastidious or partially injured mycobacterial cells, sparing the additional injury of exposure to NaOH. Although the undecontaminated specimens on S7H10 recovered more mycobacterial species than the nonselective media, the antibiotics in the medium have a distinct inhibitory effect on the growth and colonial appearance of some species. During the development of 7H12 1-[^{14}C]palmitic acid broth medium, it was found that smaller amounts of the antibiotics were as effective as the higher concentrations used in S7H11. The antibiotics can be added to the broth culture before inoculation of the undecontaminated specimen.

INCUBATION

Different species of mycobacteria show striking dependence on the temperature of incubation for optimal growth. Species having a propensity for infecting skin, such as *M. marinum*, *M. ulcerans*, and *M. haemophilum*, grow best at the temperature of the skin (30° to 32°C) and very poorly or not at all at 37°C. *M. tuberculosis* grows best at 37°C and poorly or not at all at 30°C or 42° to 45°C (the body temperature of birds). *M. xenopi*, a species not commonly found as a cause of infection in humans, grows best at 42°C and has been implicated as an environmental contaminant in the hot water system of a large hospital.[89]

Optimal recovery of different mycobacterial species depends on the incubation of at least part of the concentrated specimen at a temperature most likely to promote growth of that species. An incubator set at 30°C should be used for all specimens from suspected skin or subcutaneous mycobacterial infections. If a 30°C incubator is not available, the specimens can be held in a temperature-monitored, closed box placed in a sheltered area away from warm or cool drafts. The temperature in the box should be between 24° and 25°C and recorded daily. An incubator maintained at 42°C can be helpful in recovering *M. xenopi*.

Mycobacteria grow best in an atmosphere of 3% to 11% CO_2 (Fig. 17-2). Use of CO_2 is mandatory if Middlebrook 7H11 medium is used. However, if lack of incubator space to maintain cultures is a problem, cultures can be removed from the CO_2 atmosphere after 7 to 10 days, for organisms will be in a log phase of growth and are less CO_2-dependent. For reasons that are not well understood, mycobacteria do not grow well in candle extinction jars. The CO_2 concentration in incubators should be monitored daily and a record kept of both the incubator temperature and the CO_2 level.

RAPID METHODS FOR ESTABLISHING A DIAGNOSIS

SENSITIVITY OF ACID-FAST SMEARS

One of the more practical and readily available methods to improve the rapid diagnosis of tuberculosis is to increase the RCF applied to clinical specimens to

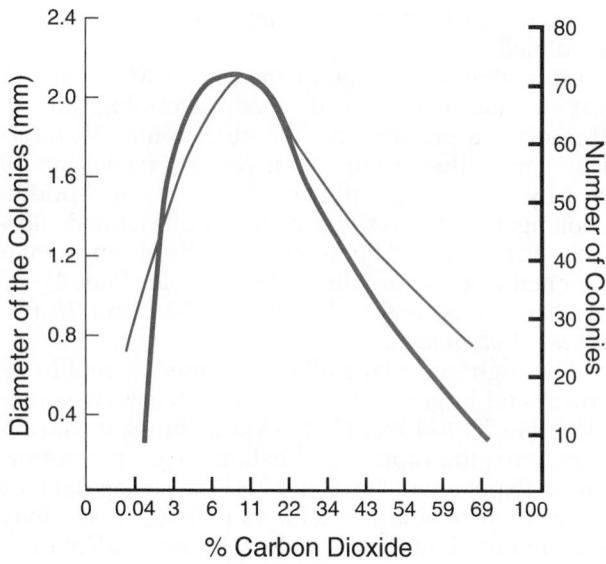

Figure 17-2.
Effect of CO_2 on the growth (colony size and number of colonies) of *M. tuberculosis* after primary isolation from sputum. (Redrawn from David HL: Bacteriology of the Mycobacterioses. DHEW Publication No. [CDC] 76-8316, Atlanta, USPHS Centers for Disease Control, Mycobacteriology Branch, 1976)

improve the sedimentation of the lipid-laden mycobacterial cells.[233] The improved correlation of positive smears to positive cultures has made the examination of an acid-fast–stained smear somewhat more reliable as an index of mycobacterial infection. Lipsky,[169] in a review of factors affecting the clinical value of microscopy for acid-fast bacilli, concludes that when the results of all specimens from each patient are considered in total, the acid-fast smear has a predictive value higher than 96% and remains one of the most rapidly performed tests in the detection of mycobacterial infections.

GAS–LIQUID AND HIGH-PERFORMANCE LIQUID CHROMATOGRAPHY

Analysis of cellular long-chain fatty acids by gas–liquid chromatography (GLC) has been used to aid in the characterization of mycobacteria. The pyrolysis gas–liquid method of Reiner,[230] in which long-chain mycolic acids are split into characteristic cleavage products, is largely restricted to research laboratories. Tisdale[280] has developed a GLC procedure for saponifying organisms in methanolic NaOH that permits the correct identification of most mycobacterial species based on chromatogram tracings and colonial characteristics. Guerrant and associates[91] have used acid methanolysis for isolating mycolic acid methyl esters from bacterial cells, a method that is not only less time-consuming than saponification techniques but is also more sensitive in detecting small numbers of cells. As little as a 1-mm loopful of organisms can be used, and the total time for analysis is less than 2 hours.[235]

A commercial system, the Microbial Identification System, (Microbial ID, Inc, Newark DE), consisting of a gas chromatograph (HP 5890A) and a computer (HP series 310, HP 98561A; Hewlett Packard Co, Palo Alto CA), is a rapid and reliable method for the culture confirmation of mycobacteria. The computer system includes a library of cell wall lipid patterns for 26 medically important *Mycobacterium* species, derived from isolates received from the American Type Culture Collection and including numerous clinical isolates. The use of negative-ion mass spectrometry to detect tuberculostearic acid in clinical specimens also holds promise for the rapid detection of mycobacteria in such specimens for those equipped with the necessary instruments.[159]

High-performance liquid chromatography (HPLC-FL) utilizing fluorescence detection of mycolic acid 6,7-dimethoxycoumarin esters has been used for the rapid identification of *M. tuberculosis* and *M. avium* directly from fluorochrome-stained, smear-positive sputum specimens and young BACTEC 12B cultures. In a study of 132 sputum specimens positive for *M. tuberculosis* and 48 positive for *M. avium–intracellulare*,[132] HPLC-FL made direct identifications with sensitivities of 56.8% and 33.3%, respectively. When performing HPLC-FL testing of cultures grown in BACTEC 12B bottles, sensitivities of 99.0% and 94.3% were achieved. The specificity was 100% in both evaluations. Cage[27] also successfully identified to the species level 117 of 126 (93%) mycobacteria grown in BACTEC 7H12B medium supplemented with oleic acid. Glickman and colleagues[81] describe a computer-based file containing patterns of mycolic acids characteristic of 45 species of *Mycobacterium*. By using their system in the evaluation of 1333 strains representing 24 *Mycobacterium* species, 97% were correctly identified (identification of *M. tuberculosis* was 99.85% accurate; of *M. avium* complex, 98% accurate). Thus, for those possessing the equipment and using computer-based pattern recognition files, mycobacteria can be identified accurately and rapidly using HPLC-generated chromatographic data.

USE OF BROTH CULTURE MEDIUM

For many years, those using the BACTEC 12B broth culture bottles have experienced a greater rate of recovery of *M. tuberculosis* and other *Mycobacterium* species 1 to 2 weeks earlier than cohorts who used only solid culture media. Therefore, the use of a broth culture medium for the early recovery of mycobacteria is now highly recommended; in fact, this has been added as a phase-deficiency item to the College of American Pathologists Inspection and Accreditation Checklist. Following are the semi-automated, automated and manual systems from which laboratory directors may choose.

AUTOMATED DETECTION SYSTEMS

Three semi-automated and automated mycobacteria detection systems are currently available: the time-honored and tested radiometric Bactec system, and the recently introduced non radiometric MB/BacT system (Organon Teknika Durham, NC) and the ESP Myco system (Difco Laboratories, Detroit, Michigan. Two viable alternates are the manual Septi-Chek System (BBL) the MGIT system (Becton Dickinson, Cockeysville, MD, for use in laboratories without automated systems.

BACTEC AFB SYSTEM

The components of the automated BACTEC 460 instrument (Becton Dickinson Diagnostic Instruments, Sparks, MD) include a scintillation counter, a needle aspiration assembly, and a movable track on which up to 60 culture bottles can be placed. The track is aligned so that each culture bottle passes, in turn, beneath the needle aspiration assembly at the rate of approximately one every 80 seconds. When the test bottle is immediately below the needle assembly, the needle is lowered through the rubber stopper into the headspace. A sample of the head gas is aspirated and delivered to the scintillation counter chamber. The head gas is replaced with a fresh bolus of 10% CO_2 immediately after the sample is aspirated. The instrument is fitted with a hood that provides HEPA-filtered air under negative pressure in the area of testing and a UV light source as an added safety feature. The needle is electrically heat sterilized during the interval before the next bottle is to be sampled.

The BACTEC 12B broth culture bottle is the key to operation. The bottle consists of a 20-mL glass vial with a short neck, the mouth of which is sealed with a thin rubber stopper. It contains 4 mL of broth culture medium consisting of Middlebrook 7H9 broth base, BSA, casein hydrolysate, catalase, and polyoxylene stearate as growth enhancers, small quantities of an antimicrobial mixture of polymyxin B, amphotericin B, nalidixic acid, trimethroprim, and azlocillin to suppress growth of contaminants, and ^{14}C-labeled palmitic acid as the growth detector. The vial is inoculated with 0.5 mL of the processed specimen and placed in a 35°C incubator. If mycobacteria are present in the inoculum, $^{14}CO_2$ is released into the headspace, the amount of which is a direct reflection of the amount of growth in the vial. The very sensitive radioactive detector system is used because the slowly metabolizing mycobacteria produce only trace quantities of CO_2. When a designated period of incubation has passed, usually about 3 days, the vials are placed on the track of the BACTEC 460 instrument in preparation for reading. The amount of radioactivity is measured in the aspirated head gas, which is translated into a numerical value called the growth index (GI). A GI higher than 10 is considered positive; however, acid-fast stains must be performed on a small aliquot of broth, for other bacteria may break through the antibiotic inhibition.

Both an increase in the yield of positive cultures from clinical specimens and lessening of the time to detection with use of the BACTEC system compared with conventional solid media have been reported.[205,249] The detection time for *M. tuberculosis* averages 9 to 14 days; it may be less than 7 days for some strains of mycobacteria other than *M. tuberculosis*. Disadvantages of the system include the cost of instrumentation, inability to observe colony morphology and detect mixed cultures, overgrowth by contaminants, need for disposal of radioactive materials, and extensive use of needles. Cases of pseudomycobacterial infections have been reported when the needle is incompletely sterilized following aspiration of a vial with a high concentration of organisms.[45,196] Specimens processed using reagents other than NALC–NaOH (such as benzalkonium chloride or Zephiran–trisodium phosphate) cannot be used with the BACTEC system because residual quantities in the broth potentially inhibit the growth of mycobacteria.

Initial studies of the sensitivity of this system in monitoring mycobacterial growth showed that an inoculum of 200 viable *M. tuberculosis* bacilli could be detected in 12 to 13 days, whereas if one waited for 14 to 17 days, as few as 20 viable bacilli could be detected.[185]

The value of the BACTEC in the detection of mycobacteria from sputum, blood, and other clinical specimens has been demonstrated in several field trial and clinical correlation studies.[14,25,85,104] In a multicenter collaborative study, the recovery of *M. tuberculosis* from clinical specimens known to be smear-positive can be accomplished by the BACTEC system in 14 days compared with 21 days by the standard culture method.[234] In this same study, the total time for isolation and drug susceptibility testing of *M. tuberculosis* was completed in an average of 18 days by the radiometric method in comparison with an average of 38 days using standard procedures. Similarly, smear-negative, culture-positive specimens were positive for growth of *M. tuberculosis* in an average of 14 days by the radiometric method compared with 25 days by the standard culture procedure.[50,192]

The capability of performing rapid mycobacterial drug susceptibility studies is an additional advantage of the BACTEC system.[99] The BACTEC instrument can also be used to differentiate *M. tuberculosis* and *M. bovis* from nontuberculous mycobacteria using blood culture vials containing *p*-nitro-acetylaminohydroxypropiophenone (NAP). *M. tuberculosis* and *M. bovis* cannot grow in NAP-containing culture media and, therefore, will not produce a positive GI after several days of incubation. The NAP test is presented in Chart 50. Detection of *M. tuberculosis* in contaminated clinical specimens can also be accomplished by using a 7H12A culture vial containing the same antimicrobial agents used in S7H11 agar, only in smaller concentrations (polymyxin, 50 µg/mL; amphotericin, 5 µg/mL; carbenicillin, 25 µg/mL; and trimethoprim, 2.5 µg/mL (PACT).

MB/BacT MYCOBACTERIA DETECTION SYSTEM

The MB/BacT is an automated system to detect mycobacteria, similar in design to the BacT/Alert blood culture system described in Chapter 3. The MB/BacT Process Bottles contains 10 mL of enhanced Middlebrook 7H9 broth in an atmosphere of CO_2, nitrogen and oxygen under vacuum. This bottle therefore provides suitable nutritional and environmental condi-

tions to recover the more commonly encountered *Mycobacterium* species for clinical specimens other than blood. One-half milliliter of reconstituted Mycobacteria antibiotic supplement (MAS), containing amphotericin B, azlocillin, nalidixic acid, polymyxin B, trimethroprim, and proprietary growth factors, is added to each bottle just before use to enhance the growth of *Mycobacterium* species and curtail the growth of contaminating bacteria that may survive the decontamination and concentration procedure. The bottom of each broth bottle is fitted with a gas-permeable sensor that changes from a dark green to a bright yellow when CO_2 is produced in the broth by metabolizing mycobacteria. Bottles are placed bottom down within individual wells in the incubation chamber, and reflected light is used to continuously monitor the production of microbial-generated CO_2.

Although multicenter field trials sponsored by the manufacturer indicate that the MB/BacT system recovered a higher percentage of mycobacteria with less time to detection when compared with conventional methods, and compared favorably in parallel cultures with the BACTEC 460 TB system, the overall performance when used in clinical settings remains to be determined. The colorimetric, nonradiometric detection of mycobacterial growth, eliminating the need for handling and disposing of radioisotopes, is a distinct advantage.

THE ESP MYCO SYSTEM

The ESP MYCO Culture System is an adaptation of the ESP Blood Culture System, described in Chapter 3. Each culture bottle, when placed in a special drawer in the incubation module, is attached to a sensor, consisting of a plastic housing, a recessed needle and a hydrophobic membrane. Thus each bottle is continuously monitored for any change in gas pressure due to the metabolic activity of microorganisms in the culture bottle. Significant pressure change may be signaled early from the consumption of oxygen; or, later with the production of gases by the metabolizing microorganisms.

Each bottle contains modified Middlebrook 7H9 medium, Casitone, glycerol and cellulose sponges. The sponges provide a growth platform for the mycobacteria, simulating the alveoli of the lungs. Immediately prior to specimen inoculation, each bottle is supplemented with an antibiotic mixture (PVNA) containing polymyxin B, vancomycin, nalidixic acid and amphotericin B.

Field trials sponsored by the manufacturer indicate that the total percentage of positive cultures detected by the ESP MYCO System compared favorably with the BACTEC 460 system. Of note, specimens from patients receiving antitubercular therapy were at times not positive in either broth system, indicating the need to inoculate solid culture media in parallel with the broth bottles. The results from this study further indicate that the ESP MYCO system detected positive cultures first about 3 times more frequently than the BACTEC 460 system and greater than 7 days sooner in about ½ of the cultures, presumably based on the early signal derived during the oxygen consumption phase of the growth cycle. Although the results of this field trial are impressive, the overall performance in clinical settings remains to be determined. The nonradiometric detection method used also precludes the need to handle and dipose of radioactive materials.

THE SEPTI-CHEK AFB SYSTEM

The Septi-Chek AFB System is a capped bottle containing 20.0 mL of modified Middlebrook 7H9 broth under 20% CO_2. A second component is a plastic tube, fitted on one end with a removable screw cap, within which is enclosed a two-faced paddle, on both surfaces of which are embedded solid culture media. One surface of the paddle is covered with nonselective Middlebrook 7H11 agar; the reverse side is divided into two sections, one containing modified LJ medium and the other containing chocolate agar to detect the growth of contaminating bacteria. The system is processed by removing the cap from the bottle containing the culture medium, to which is added 1.0 mL of a reconstituted supplement also provided by the manufacturer, composed of glucose, glycerin, oleic acid, pyridoxine, HCl, catalase, albumin, azlocillin, nalidixic acid, trimethoprim, polymyxin B, and amphotericin B. The supplemented broth is next inoculated with 0.5 mL of an NALC–NaOH-processed specimen. The screw cap is removed from the bottom of the paddle, and the assembly is secured to the broth culture bottle. The solid culture media on the paddle are inoculated by inverting the assembly, permitting the broth culture mixture to bathe all surfaces of the agar. The system is then placed into a 35°C incubator in an upright position. The agar surfaces and the culture media are examined every third day for the appearance of growth, after which, if negative, the assembly is again inverted to reinoculate the agar media. If growth is observed, acid-fast smears can be performed from isolated colonies growing on the agar surface, and subcultures of the broth to appropriate selective media can be made or can be prepared for DNA probe analysis.

In a four-center study in which over 3000 clinical specimens of various sources were studied, Isenberg and coworkers[119] found that the Septi-Chek system was more sensitive than LJ, 7H11, and BACTEC broth in the percentage of mycobacterial isolates recovered. The authors concluded that this better recovery rate could be attributed to the biphasic nature of the system and the advantage gained from repeated early exposure of the agar media to actively proliferating organisms in the broth phase. Compared with LJ and 7H11, the average number of days for recovery of mycobacteria was less for the Septi-Chek AFB system, averaging 3 days less for the detection of M. tuberculosis and 9 days less for M. avium–intracellulare. Although the time of recovery for the BACTEC system was less by an average of 3 days for M. tuberculosis and 12 days for M. avium–intracellulare compared with the Septi-Chek system, the former does not provide for isolated colonies; therefore, the time to final identification was

about equal between the two systems. Similar results were found in a follow-up study by D'Amato and associated[51] of the revised Septi-Chek AFB System, in which LJ agar was added to the paddle. A later study,[250] also confirmed that both the rate and time of recovery of M. tuberculosis, M. avium–intracellulare, and M. gordonae from smear-positive respiratory secretions were improved with the Septi-Chek AFB System compared with LJ medium. In this study, BACTEC 12A bottles detected growth of these Mycobacterium species earlier than Septi-Chek; however, as found in the previous study, the latter provided isolated colonies earlier and did not require special equipment for detection of growth.

MYCOBACTERIA GROWTH INDICATOR TUBE

The Mycobacteria Growth Indicator Tube (MGIT) system (BBL, Becton Dickinson Microbiology Systems, Hunt Valley, MD) consists of a 16× 100-mm round-bottomed glass tube containing 4 mL of modified 7H11 broth base, to which has been added 0.5 mL of OADC enrichment (oleic acid, bovine albumin, dextrose, and catalase) and 0.1 mL of PANTA antibiotic mixture (polymyxin B, amphotericin B, nalidixic acid, trimethoprim, azlocillin). The antibiotic mixture obviously inhibits the growth of contaminating bacteria; the OADC supplement provides oleic acid, an important metabolic stimulant for mycobacteria; albumin, to bind toxic free fatty acids; dextrose, as an energy source; and catalase, to destroy toxic peroxides that may be present in the medium. A fluorescent compound is embedded in silicone on the bottom of the tube. The fluorescent compound is sensitive to dissolved oxygen in the broth; that is, the presence of oxygen in the uninoculated medium serves to quench the emission of fluorescent light. As the actively growing bacteria consume the dissolved oxygen, the fluorescence is unmasked and can be detected by observing the tube under long-wave ultraviolet light (Wood's lamp). Growth may also be detected by observing a non-homogeneous turbidity or small grains or flakes in the culture medium.

In performing the test, the 0.1 mL of PANTA and 0.5 mL of OADC mixture are added aseptically to the tube, reconstituting the lyophilized medium. This is followed by 0.5 mL of specimen or specimen concentrate; adding more than 0.5 mL of specimen may adversely affect the performance of the tube. The cap is replaced, the ingredients mixed by inverting the tube several times, and the tube placed in a 37°C incubator. Tubes are read every other day starting on day 2. Tubes are read with a Wood's lamp, placing the tube with the test mixture between a positive (sodium sulfite solution) and a negative (uninoculated MGIT tube) control. Wear UV-protective goggles to observe for a bright orange color in the bottom of the positive tubes, with an orange reflection also seen on the meniscus. Positive tubes are stained for acid-fast bacilli, preferably using the Ziehl-Neelsen technique. Negative tubes are returned to the incubation rack and again observed at regular intervals for up to 6 weeks.

Hanna and coworkers[95] used the MGIT system to test 193 specimens (44 patients) from various body sites for the presence of *Mycobacterium* species. Of 32 patients, the sputum concentrates of which were positive for at least one acid-fast smear, MGIT cultures were positive in 31 (MTB, 25; MAI, 4; and *M. haemophilum*, 2). MGIT tubes were positive in an additional three smear-negative patients; the one false-negative MGIT test occurred in a patient with very few acid-fast bacilli seen on smear. The mean time to detection was 10.4 days (range 4 to 26 days). The two *M. haemophilum* isolates were recovered by adding an X (hemin) disk to the MGIT tube and incubating at 30°C. All positive reactions must be confirmed by an acid-fast stain because other oxygen-consuming bacteria may occasionally break through the PANTA antibiotic mixture. One major disadvantage is the high cost of each tube (about $8 per unit); however, this is offset to some degree as fluorescence is observed visually and does not require elaborate or costly equipment.

TECHNIQUES FOR THE IDENTIFICATION OF MYCOBACTERIA RECOVERED IN CULTURE

APPLICATIONS OF MOLECULAR BIOLOGY

As indicated by the algorithm presented earlier in this chapter, there is a movement in clinical laboratories away from the time-consuming and tedious task of performing biochemical tests to make a species identification of mycobacteria recovered in culture. More and more, nonculture methods based on molecular biology are being used in clinical laboratories for the culture confirmation of *Mycobacterium* species isolates recovered in culture. For example, the use of nucleic acid probe assays has virtually replaced conventional biochemical testing in the identification of *M. tuberculosis* and *M. avium–intracellulare*. Nucleic acid probes have also been produced for the direct identification of *M. kansasii* and *M. gordonae*, and it is only a matter of time before probes directed against other species will become available.

Three major applications for molecular techniques are available for use in clinical laboratories:

1. Culture confirmation of isolates recovered from clinical specimens using DNA probes
2. DNA fingerprinting and strain-typing of *Mycobacterium* species based on restriction fragment length polymorphism for use in epidemiologic studies
3. Direct detection of *M. tuberculosis* rRNA in sputum and other clinical specimens using nucleic acid amplification (PCR) and hybridization assays

The current medical literature relative to molecular diagnostics as applied to the direct and indirect identification of the mycobacteria is vast. It is difficult at this juncture to predict which of the several specific techniques will stand the test of time; therefore, it is equally difficult to determine what references and applications should be included in a general textbook. For those interested in brief descriptions of several scores of papers that have been published within the last decade relative to this topic, please see the supplementary section at the end of this chapter. Until we know the direction molecular diagnostics may be headed in reference to mycobacteriology, students should still focus on the more conventional techniques that are still used in most clinical laboratories. Study of these techniques also provides a fundamental understanding of the basic biology of mycobacteria and the role of the clinical laboratory in the diagnosis of tuberculosis.

IDENTIFICATION OF MYCOBACTERIUM SPECIES USING CONVENTIONAL METHODS

Although the applications of molecular techniques are being used with increasing frequency in establishing culture confirmation of mycobacteria recovered from clinical specimens, in epidemiologic studies and in direct testing of clinical specimens, conventional methods are still required to identify those *Mycobacterium* species for which molecular methods are not currently available.[104] Charts 1, 2, 9, 11, 22, 31, 34, 41, 42, 50, 52, 54, 62, 66, 71 and 73 provide a detailed presentation of the principles, reagents, procedures, and interpretation of various laboratory techniques, including digestion–decontamination methods, biochemical tests (that are included in identification Table 17-7), drug susceptibility testing, and DNA probe assays.

OPTIMAL TEMPERATURE FOR ISOLATION AND RATES OF GROWTH

As shown in Table 17-7, each *Mycobacterium* species has an optimum temperature for growth and a range of time of recovery in culture. The time of recovery will vary for the various types of media used—the average time of recovery of mycobacteria on egg-based media is about 21 days (as short as 3 to 5 days and as long as 60 days, depending on the species). Times of recovery are generally shorter by several days when using 7H10 or 7H11 agar if the technique of microscopic observation for microcolonies is employed (described later). The use of BACTEC vials, both for the inoculation of blood cultures and other body fluids, can shorten the times of detection considerably.[50,142,234]

For assessing the time of growth, any standard nonselective culture medium can be used, either in tubed slants or in petri plates. A well-isolated colony of the test organism is subcultured to a 7H9 broth containing Tween 80 and incubated for several days or until the medium is faintly turbid. The broth is diluted 1:100 and isolation streaks are made to the test medium, either in tubed slants or on petri plates, to obtain isolated colonies. To determine the growth rate accurately, it is necessary to use an inoculum sufficiently dilute to produce individual colonies. An inoculum of large numbers of slow-growing mycobacteria may form a visible colony within a few days and give an erroneous impression of the growth rate. *M. tuberculosis* stock cultures of known growth rates should be used as a control for slow-growing organisms; similarly, stock cultures of *M. fortuitum* can be used as a control comparison for rapidly growing organisms.

Petri plates of 7H10 agar or equivalent are preferred to the use of tubed media because the appearance of developing microcolonies can be studied with a dissecting or low-power microscopy. With experience, an assessment of the morphology of these microcolonies can be used in conjunction with the appearance of the cells in an acid-fast smear to make presumptive identifications of unknown isolates. Runyon[240] published guidelines by which the microcolonies of various species of mycobacteria can be distinguished by those who have gained experience in this approach.

In an unpublished 1988 study conducted in the clinical microbiology laboratory at the University of Illinois, Chicago, Parulekar and Koneman (personal communication) were able to detect the microcolonies of 29 smear-positive clinical sputum isolates of *Mycobacterium* species growing on 7H10 agar in an average of 6.1 days (range 3 to 12 days) compared with average recovery times of 32.4 days with Lowenstein-Jensen and 27.9 days with 7H11 agar using standard visual observations. The average detection time for these 29 isolates was 5.8 days by the BACTEC system, using radiometric 12B bottles. The results of this study indicate that mycobacteria can be detected by observing for microcolonies in the same shortened time period as that with the BACTEC system, providing all laboratories with a means for the early detection of mycobacteria when required. The microcolony method also allows an assessment of colony morphology, providing an additional piece of information not provided by the BACTEC system, which is helpful in making an early presumptive identification of an unknown *Mycobacterium* species.

PIGMENT PRODUCTION

The determination of whether an unknown *Mycobacterium* species isolate is capable of producing colony pigmentation in the dark (scotochromogen) or only after exposure to light (photochromogen) or not at all is helpful in making a final species identification (see Chart 2). *M. tuberculosis* fails to produce pigment, beyond a light buff color, even after exposure to light. The pigment-producing capabilities of other *Mycobacterium* species are listed in Table 17-7 (see Color Plates 17-2C through 2E).

NIACIN ACCUMULATION

All mycobacteria produce niacin; however, only *M. tuberculosis*, *M. simiae*, and occasional strains of *M. africanum*, *M. bovis*, *M. marinum*, and *M. chelonae* lack the enzyme necessary to further convert the niacin to niacin ribonucleotide. Thus, the determination of whether niacin has accumulated in the culture medium is a valuable differential test in identifying these species of mycobacteria, particularly *M. tuberculosis* (see Chart 52 for details). Reagent-impregnated filter paper strips have been developed that eliminate the necessity for using cyanogen bromide, a highly toxic substance, as required in the originally described method for performing this test. The development of a yellow color in the test medium incubated with a reagent strip is indicative of niacin accumulation and a positive test (see Color Plate 17-1D). It is essential to have sufficient growth on the primary egg-based medium, otherwise the risk of obtaining false-negative results is increased.

REDUCTION OF NITRATES TO NITRITES

Only a few species of mycobacteria, notably *M. tuberculosis*, produce nitroreductase, which catalyzes the reduction of nitrate to nitrite. The development of a red color on addition of sulfanilic acid and *N*-naphthylethylenediamine to an extract of the unknown culture is indicative of the presence of nitrite and a positive test (see Chart 54). The test must be carefully performed using three control cultures—one known to give a strong positive reaction, one giving a weak reaction, and the last a negative reaction. In addition to supporting the identification of *M. tuberculosis*, the nitrate reduction test is also a key test in the identification of *M. kansasii* and, in particular, *M. szulgai* (see Table 17-7 and Color Plates 17-1E and 2F).

TWEEN 80 HYDROLYSIS

Tween 80 is the trade name of a detergent that can be useful in identifying those mycobacteria that possess a lipase that splits the compound into oleic acid and polyoxyethylated sorbitol. This test is helpful in identifying *M. kansasii*, which can produce a positive result as quickly as 3 to 6 hours. Two scotochromogens with similar-appearing colonies, *M. gordonae* (positive) and *M. scrofulaceum* (negative), can be differentiated using the Tween-80 hydrolysis test. The Tween-80 hydrolysis reactions for other mycobacteria are listed in Table 17-8; the test procedure is described in detail in Chart 71, and a positive reaction is illustrated in Color Plate 17-2G.

CATALASE ACTIVITY

Most of the mycobacteria produce catalase; however, not all species are capable of producing a positive reaction after heating the culture at 68°C for 20 minutes (heat-stable catalase). Most strains of *M. tuberculosis* and other members of the *M. tuberculosis* complex do not produce heat-stable catalase, except for certain isoniazid (INH)-resistant strains, for which the results of this test are of particular value. Catalase activity can be semiquantitatively assessed by measuring the height achieved by the column of bubbles produced when hydrogen peroxide is added to a growing colony in a tube culture (see Chart 11). To perform this test, tubes of Lowenstein-Jensen medium must be poured in an upright position to produce a flat rather than a slanted surface. This surface is heavily inoculated with the test organism and incubated for 14 days before adding the hydrogen peroxide reagent. A column higher than 45 mm is considered a positive test (see Color Plate 17-2H). A quick assessment of catalase activity can be determined by placing a few drops of hydrogen perox-

(text continues on page 916)

TABLE 17-7
DIFFERENTIAL CHARACTERISTICS OF MYCOBACTERIA

| | OPTIMUM ISOLATION TEMPERATURE AND TIME FOR GROWTH | PIGMENTATION GROWTH IN | | NIACIN TEST | NITRATE REDUCTION | TWEEN 80 HYDROLYSIS— 10 DAYS |
		LIGHT	*DARK*			
M. tuberculosis	37°C 12–25 d	Buff	Buff	+	+	V
M. africanum	37°C 31–42 d	Buff	Buff	V	V	−
M. bovis	37°C 24–40 d	Buff	Buff	V	−	−
M. ulcerans	32°C 28–60 d	Buff	Buff	−	−	−
M. kansasii	37°C 10–20 d	Yellow	Buff	−	+	+
M. marinum	30°C 5–14 d	Yellow	Buff	V	−	+
M. simiae	37°C 7–14 d	Yellow	Buff	+	−	+/−
M. asiaticum	37°C 10–21 d	Yellow	Buff	−	−	+
M. szulgai	37°C 12–25 d	Yellow to orange	Yellow—37°C Buff—25°C	−	+	V
M. scrofulaceum	37°C 10 d	Yellow	Yellow	−	−	−
M. gordonae	37°C 10 d	Yellow to orange	Yellow	−	−	+
M. thermoresistible	45°C 7 d	Yellow	Yellow	−	+	+
M. flavescens	37°C 7–10 d	Yellow	Yellow	−	+	+
M. xenopi	42°C 14–28 d	Yellow	Yellow	−	−	−
M. avium complex	37°C 10–21 d	Buff to pale yellow	Buff to pale yellow	−	−	−
M. haemophilum	30°C 14–21 d	Gray	Gray	−	−	−
M. malmoense	37°C 21–28 d	Buff	Buff	−	−	+
M. shimoidei	37°C 14–28 d	Buff	Buff	−	−	+
M. genavense	37°C 14–28 d	Buff	Buff	−	−	+
M. celatum	37°C 14–28 d	Buff	Buff	−	−	−
M. gastri	37°C 10–21 d	Buff	Buff	−	−	+
M. terrae complex	37°C 10–21 d	Buff	Buff	−	V	+
M. triviale	37°C 10–21 d	Buff	Buff	−	+	+
M. fortuitum	37°C 3–5 d	Buff	Buff	−	+	V
M. chelonae						
spp. *chelonei*	28°C 3–5 d	Buff	Buff	V	−	V
spp. *abscessus*	35°C 3–5 d	Buff	Buff	−	−	V
M. smegmatis	37°C 3–5 d	Buff to yellow	Buff to yellow	−	+	+

(Continued)

	CATALASE		ARYLSUL-FATASE			IRON	GROWTH ON		
	SEMI-QUANTITATIVE	pH 7.0; 68°C	3 DAYS	UREASE	PYRAZIN-AMIDASE	UPTAKE	T_2H (1 µg/mL)	5% NaCl 28°C	MacCONKEY AGAR
M. tuberculosis	<45	−	−	+	+	−	+	−	−
M. africanum	>45	−	−	V	−	−	+	−	−
M. bovis	<45	−	−	+	−	−	−	−	−
M. ulcerans	>45	+	−	V	−	−	+	−	−
M. kansasii	>45	+	−	+	+	−	+	−	−
M. marinum	>45	−	V	+	+	−	+	−	−
M. simiae	>45	+	−	+	−	−	+	−	
M. asiaticum	>45	+	−	−	−	−	+	−	
M. szulgai	>45	+	−	+	−	−	+	−	−
M. scrofulaceum	>45	+	−	+	V	−	+	−	−
M. gordonae	>45	+	−	−	V	−	+	−	−
M. thermoresistible	>45	+	−	+		−		+	−
M. flavescens	>45	+	−	+	+	−	+	V	−
M. xenopi	<45	+	+	−	+	−	+	−	−
M. avium complex	<45	−	−	−	+	−	+	−	V
M. haemophilum	<45	−	−	−	+		+	−	
M. malmoense	<45	V	−	V	V	−	+	−	
M. shimoidei	<45	−	−	−	+	−	+	−	−
M. genavense	>45	+	−	+	+	−	+	−	−
M. celatum	<45	+	+	−	+	−	+	−	−
M. gastri	<45	−	−	+	−	−	+	−	−
M. terrae complex	>45	+	+	−	V	−	+	−	V
M. triviale	>45	+	V	−	V	−	+	+	
M. fortuitum	>45	+	+	+	+	+	+	+	+
M. chelonae									
spp. chelonei	>45	+	+	+	+	−	+	−	−
spp. abscessus	>45	+	+	+	+	−	+	+	+
M. smegmatis	>45	+	−			+	+	−	

+, positive; −, negative; V, variable; blank spaces, little or no data.

TABLE 17-8

NOMENCLATURE OF SELECT MYCOBACTERIA IN ORDER OF PRESENTATION

LEGITIMATE SPECIES NAME	RELATIVE PATHOGENICITY FOR HUMANS	EQUIVALENT RUNYON GROUP	ACCEPTABLE COMMON NAME	NAMES WITHOUT LEGITIMATE STANDING AND COMMENTS
M. tuberculosis	+++		Human tubercle bacillus	Causes human tuberculosis—highly contagious
M. bovis	+++		Bovine tubercle bacillus	Causes bovine and human tuberculosis; avirulent strains are used for BCG vaccines.
M. ulcerans	+++			Associated with skin infections in tropics—M. buruli
M. africanum	+++			Intermediate form between M. bovis and M. tuberculosis. It is found in northern and central Africa.
M. kansasii	+++	I photochromogen		Rare, nonpigmented, scotochromogenic, and niacin-positive strains
M. marinum	+++	I photochromogen		M. balnei, M. platypeocilus associated with skin infections
M. simiae	++	I photochromogen		M. habana—facultatively pathogenic; photoreactivity may be unstable; it is niacin positive
M. genavense	++			Grows only in broth culture. Propensity for causing pulmonary disseminated disease in patients with AIDS.
M. asiaticum	++	I photochromogen		Similar to M. simiae but differs antigenically
M. scrofulaceum	++	II scotochromogen		M. marinum—may cause cervical lymphadenitis
M. szulgai	+++	I photochromogen at 25°C II scotochromogen at 37°C		Associated with chronic pulmonary and extrapulmonary disease; distinctive lipid composition of cell walls
M. xenopi	++	III nonphotochromogen		M. littorale, M. xenopi grows slowly; best at 42°C; may contaminate hot-water systems.
M. celatum	+			Propensity for causing respiratory infections in patients with AIDS. Closely resembles M. xenopi.
M. gordonae	0/+	II scotochromogen	Tap water scoto-chromogens	M. aquae—occasionally pathogenic for humans.
M. thermo-resistible	+	II scotochromogen		Growth at 52°C. Potentially pathogenic. Slow-growing.
M. avium/intracellulare complex	+++	III nonphotochromogen*	Battey bacillus	M. batteyi, M. battey—frequently drug-resistant. Often cause of infection in patients with AIDS.
M. terrae	Rare	III nonphotochromogen	Radish bacillus	May be closely related to M. triviale
M. shimoidei	+			Resembles M. terrae complex. Rare cases of pulmonary infections.
M. triviale	0/+	III nonphotochromogen	V bacillus	Has been called atypical-atypical Mycobacterium
M. malmoense	+++	III nonphotochromogen		Slowly growing mycobacterium usually causing pulmonary disease.

(Continued)

TABLE 17-8 *(Continued)*				
NOMENCLATURE OF SELECT MYCOBACTERIA IN ORDER OF PRESENTATION				
LEGITIMATE SPECIES NAME	**RELATIVE PATHOGENICITY FOR HUMANS**	**EQUIVALENT RUNYON GROUP**	**ACCEPTABLE COMMON NAME**	**NAMES WITHOUT LEGITIMATE STANDING AND COMMENTS**
M. haemophilum	+++	III nonphotochromogen		Associated with skin lesions usually in immuno-suppressed patients.
M. fortuitum	+	IV rapid grower		*M. ranae; M. minetti*—skin and lung infections. It may cause disease in immunosuppressed host. May cause nosocomial infection.
M. cheloneae	+	IV rapid grower		May cause occasional skin disease. Includes two subspecies, *cheloneae* and *abscessus.* May cause nosocomial infection.

(After Sommers HM: The Clinically Significant Mycobacteria. Chicago, American Society of Clinical Pathologists, 1974)
* Strains recovered from patients with AIDS are often scotochromogenic.

ide on colonies growing on the surface of Middlebrook 7H10 agar and observing for rapid effervescence of bubbles (Color Plate 17-2*I*).

ARYLSULFATASE ACTIVITY

Determination of the activity of the enzyme arylsulfatase in mycobacteria is helpful in identifying certain species, notably in differentiating members of the rapidly growing *M. fortuitum–chelonei* complex (see Color Plate 17-2*J*) from group III nonphotochromogenic mycobacteria. Small quantities of this enzyme can also be produced by *M. marinum, M. kansasii, M. szulgai,* and *M. xenopi* (see Table 17-8). The development of a red color in the test medium, indicating a release of free phenolphthalein, is a positive test (see Chart 1). However, certain slower-growing species do not produce sufficient enzyme to give a consistently positive reaction.

UREASE ACTIVITY

Assessment of urease activity is an important test to differentiate *M. scrofulaceum* (positive) from *M. gordonae* (negative). It is also helpful in separating *M. gastri* (positive) from other members of the group III nonchromogenic mycobacteria (see Table 17-7). Determination of whether any given *Mycobacterium* species can produce urease can be performed either by inoculating the organism into distilled water containing a urea-base concentrate[317] or by use of filter paper disks containing urea that are added to distilled water.[208] Details of the urease test as applied to the identification of *Mycobacterium* species are presented in Chart 73 (see also Color Plate 17-2*K*).

PYRAZINAMIDASE

Another useful test in distinguishing *M. kansasii* and *M. marinum,* weakly niacin-positive *M. bovis* and *M. tuberculosis* and members of the *M. avium* complex from other species is the test for pyrazinamidase (all posi-

tive). Pyrazinamidase is an enzyme that deaminates pyrazinamide to form pyrazinoic acid, which produces a red band in the culture medium.[300] Details of this test are presented in Chart 62, and the end reaction is illustrated in Color Plate 17-2*L*.

IRON UPTAKE

Members of the *M. fortuitum–chelonei* complex have many similarities; however, it is occasionally necessary to distinguish between them. *M. fortuitum* has the ability to take up soluble iron salts from the culture medium, producing a rusty brown appearance on addition of an aqueous solution of 20% ferric ammonium citrate; *M. chelonei* lacks this property[301] (see Chart 42).

GROWTH INHIBITION BY THIOPHENE-2-CARBOXYLIC ACID HYDRAZIDE

Thiophene-2-carboxylic hydrazide (T_2H) selectively inhibits the growth of *M. tuberculosis,* whereas most other mycobacteria can grow in a medium containing this compound, which is helpful particularly in differentiating certain strains of *M. bovis* (see Chart 41 and Color Plate 17-1*F*). For example, 30% of *M. bovis* BCG strains may be weakly niacin positive, and others may be weak nitrate reducers, at times making differentiation of these strains from *M. tuberculosis* by these key tests somewhat difficult.

GROWTH IN 5% SODIUM CHLORIDE

The ability to grow on an egg-based culture medium containing 5% NaCl when incubated at 28°C is shared by *M. flavescens, M. triviale,* and the rapidly growing mycobacteria, with the exception of *M. chelonei* subspecies *chelonei* (see Table 17-8). Other mycobacteria do not tolerate this increased salt concentration. Slants of Lowenstein-Jensen medium containing 5% NaCl are commercially available. The test cannot be performed in an agar-based medium[154] (see Chart 66 for details).

GROWTH ON MACCONKEY AGAR

MacConkey agar, from which crystal violet has been removed, will support the growth of the *M. fortuitum–chelonaei* complex; most other *Mycobacterium* species cannot grow on this medium. The test procedure is detailed in Chart 34.

CLASSIFICATION OF MYCOBACTERIA

The features by which an unknown microorganism can be classified with the mycobacteria first of all requires that it is "acid-fast." **Acid-fast** is a term that is used to describe those bacteria that resist decolorization with acidified alcohol once they have been stained with carbolfuchsin. Certain bacterial species, notably *Nocardia* species and *Rhodococcus* species, retain carbolfuchsin only if a less stringent decolorizing agent is used (notably a low-concentration inorganic acid, such as 1% H_2SO_4 or 1% HCl). These species are referred to as being "partially acid-fast."

Wayne and Kubica[305] consider *Corynebacterium*, *Nocardia*, and *Rhodococcus* species to be clustered together in a supergenus based on many similarities. They have designated this cluster of organisms the CNM group. Details for the identification of these nonmycobacterial species have been presented in Chapter 13. Slow growth, the presence of faintly gram-positive, slightly curved or straight rods that rarely branch, resistance to lysozyme, and the patterns of reactions in the biochemical tests presented in the foregoing are the characteristics by which the mycobacteria can generally be recognized and by which species identifications can be made. However, the taxonomy and classification of *Mycobacterium* species has become somewhat complex and entailed.

In the late 1950s, as species of mycobacteria other than *M. tuberculosis* were being encountered with increasing frequency in medical practices, Runyon proposed the grouping of these "atypical" organisms based on growth rate and pigment production (see Box 17-2).

Advances in our knowledge of the genetics, cell structure, and aberrant phenotypic properties of old and newly discovered strains of the mycobacteria have advanced our knowledge beyond the neat packaging of species under the classic Runyon system of classification that has served clinical mycobacteriology laboratories for the past three decades. In addition, Sommers and Good[265] point out that certain strains of *M. kansasii*, for example, are either pigmented in the dark or are nonpigmented (qualifying for Runyon group II or group III, respectively). Pigmented strains of the *M. avium–intracellulare* complex are being encountered with increasing frequency. Therefore, a reliance on these phenotypic criteria may be misleading, and Sommers and Good advise that each isolate must be definitively identified and considered for its individual identity in light of the possible associated disease syndromes. In keeping with this new orientation, Woods and Washington[323] have suggested a clinically oriented classification of mycobacteria (Box 17-3), refined from an earlier published proposal by Wolinski.[319]

Nevertheless, for the traditionally trained mycobacteriologist, the splitting off of *M. tuberculosis* (and *M. bovis*) from mycobacteria other than *M. tuberculosis*

BOX 17-2. RUNYON'S CLASSIFICATION SCHEME*

Group I:	Photochromogens
Group II:	Scotochromogens
Group III:	Nonphotochromogens
Group IV:	Rapid Growers

* Does not include *M. tuberculosis* complex, including *M. bovis*.

BOX 17-3. WOODS AND WASHINGTON CLASSIFICATION SCHEME

Species Potentially Pathogenic in Humans

M. avium-intracellulare
M. kansasii
M. fortuitum–chelonae complex
M. scrofulaceum
M. xenopi
M. szulgai
M. malmoense
M. simiae
M. genavense
M. marinum
M. ulcerans
M. haemophilum
M. celatum

Saprophytic Mycobacteria Rarely Causing Disease in Humans

M. gordonae
M. asiaticum
M. terrae—triviale complex
M. shimoidei
M. gastri
M. nonchromogenicum
M. paratuberculosis

Species With an Intermediate Growth Rate

M. flavescens

Rapidly Growing Species

M. thermoresistible
M. smegmatis
M. vaccae
M. parafortuitum complex
M. phlei

(MOTT) and the preliminary separation of MOTT into the four Runyon groups will continue to provide a meaningful initial orientation. The fact that certain strains of the usually photochromogenic *M. kansasii* may be nonpigmented or even scotochromogenic, that some strains of *M. avium–intracellulare* may be lightly pigmented, and even that *M. szulgai* is scotochromogenic at 37°C but photochromogenic at 25°C (certainly disruptive to the Runyon scheme) does not mean that past orientations must be totally discarded, as will be discussed in the next section of this chapter.

LABORATORY IDENTIFICATION OF MYCOBACTERIA AND RELATED CLINICAL SYNDROMES

The identification of mycobacteria is not difficult but requires patience, familiarity with the endpoints of different identification characteristics, and a collection of control strains. Not every laboratory needs the ability to identify to the species level all mycobacterial isolates. The number of patients with tuberculosis in any given hospital is not large, and it may be prudent to use the services of a reference laboratory to provide definitive identifications and susceptibility testing of clinically important isolates recovered in the primary care laboratory. Each laboratory director or microbiology supervisor must determine the extent of services to be provided to meet the needs of the local clinical practice. Table 17-9 is a listing of the options for **extent** or **level** of services to be provided, in keeping with the inspection and accreditation guidelines provided by the College of American Pathologists.

Experience with the College of American Pathologists Special Mycobacterial Interlaboratory Survey over the past several years has shown that increasing numbers of laboratories are restricting their services for mycobacterial infections to the preparation and interpretation of acid-fast–stained smears, setting up primary cultures, and referring positive cultures to reference laboratories for identification and susceptibility testing.[264,322] Cost-containment measures imposed on most clinical laboratories and the commercial availability of nucleic acid probes that can provide more accurate and rapid results, are current forces that are prompting even more laboratories to provide services of no more than those required of level 1 or at the most level 2 laboratories. Results of the 1993 questionnaire[322] indicate that more laboratories are performing the

---

TABLE 17-9

LABORATORY SELF-DETERMINED EXTENTS OR LEVELS OF SERVICE AS PROPOSED BY THE COLLEGE OF AMERICAN PATHOLOGISTS AND THE AMERICAN THORACIC SOCIETY

COLLEGE OF AMERICAN PATHOLOGISTS EXTENTS OF SERVICE FOR PARTICIPATION IN MYCOBACTERIAL INTERLABORATORY COMPARISON SURVEYS	AMERICAN THORACIC SOCIETY LEVELS OF SERVICE FOR MYCOBACTERIAL LABORATORIES
1. No mycobacterial procedures performed	**Level I** 1a. Collect adequate clinical specimens, including aerosol-induced sputa 1b. Transport specimens to a higher level laboratory for isolation and identification. 1c. May prepare and examine smears for presumptive diagnosis or as a means of following the progress of diagnosed patients on chemotherapy
2. Acid-fast stain of exudates, effusions and body fluids, with inoculation and referral of cultures to reference laboratories for further identification	**Level II** 2a. May perform all functions of level I laboratories, and process specimens as necessary for culture on standard agar- or egg-based media 2b. Identify *M. tuberculosis* 2c. May perform drug susceptibility studies against *M. tuberculosis* with primary antituberculosis drugs 2d. Retain mycobacterial cultures for a reasonable time
3. Isolation of mycobacteria; identification of *M. tuberculosis* and preliminary identification of the atypical forms such as photochromogens, scotochromogens, nonphotochromogens, and rapid growers. Drug susceptibility testing may or may not be performed	**Level III** 3a. May perform all functions of laboratories at lower levels, and identify all *Mycobacterium* species from clinical specimens 3b. Perform drug susceptibility studies against mycobacteria 3c. Retain mycobacterial cultures for a reasonable time 3d. May conduct research and provide training
4. Definitive identification of mycobacteria isolated to the extent required to establish a correct clinical diagnosis and to aid in the selection of safe and effective therapy. Drug susceptibility testing performed	

fluorochrome-staining techniques (up to 61%), the BACTEC System (38%), susceptibility testing (61%), and nucleic acid probes for identification (51%). Identification of *M. tuberculosis* within 21 days of specimen receipt has increased to 41%, and this curve continues to rise.

Review of *Mycobacterium* Species: Laboratory Aspects and Clinical Correlations

Although a presumptive diagnosis of pulmonary tuberculosis can be made based on clinical history, presenting symptoms, physical examination, radiographic evidence of disease, and the presence of acid-fast bacilli in the sputum, the definitive diagnosis requires recovery of the causative organisms in culture. Several *Mycobacterium* species other than *M. tuberculosis* have emerged as important pathogens, each with differing potential for producing disease and often with unique antimycobacterial drug susceptibility profiles that must be determined by laboratory tests. The recent increase in the recovery of *Mycobacterium* species from a variety of extrapulmonary sites, including from such previously unlikely sources such as stool samples and blood cultures, requires that the clinician extend the differential diagnosis to include tuberculosis when evaluating an obscure case of infectious disease and that expanded test procedures be implemented in clinical microbiology laboratories. A presentation of the laboratory culture characteristics and the clinical manifestations of mycobacterial diseases for those species known to cause human infection and serving as strict or potential pathogens is listed in Box 17-4.

MYCOBACTERIUM TUBERCULOSIS COMPLEX

Mycobacterium tuberculosis. *M. tuberculosis,* as the most common cause of mycobacterial disease in humans, is often the major focus for making definitive identifications in many laboratories. As presented in the 1986 issue of *Bergey's Manual,*[305] the classic strains of *M. tuberculosis* can be phenotypically differentiated from *M. bovis* and the intermediate species, *M. microti* and *M. africanum.* However, several parameters, including analysis of antigenic extracts, target epitopes for monoclonal antibodies, and antigenic relatedness studies, suggest that *M. tuberculosis, M. bovis, M. microti,* and *M. africanum* represent a single species and currently are considered under the general term "*M. tuberculosis* complex."

A few relatively simple tests will identify most isolates, to some extent made easier in laboratories where the BACTEC system is used. The following are characteristics by which an identification of *M. tuberculosis* can be made:

1. Formation of nonpigmented, rough, buff colonies after 14 to 28 days' incubation at 37°C on Löwenstein-Jensen or Middlebrook media (see Color Plate 17-1*G* and 1*H*)

Box 17-4. *Mycobacterium* Species: Order of Presentation

***Mycobacterium tuberculosis* complex**

  M. tuberculosis
  M. bovis
  M. africanum
  M. ulcerans

Photochromogens

  M. kansasii
  M. marinum
  M. simiae
  M. genavense (genetically related to *M. simiae* but not chromogenic)
  M. asiaticum

Scotochromogens

  M. scrofulaceum
  M. szulgai (photochromogenic at 25°C)
  M. xenopi
  M. celatum (phenotypically related to *M. xenopi* but nonchromogenic)
  M. gordonae
  M. flavescens

Nonphoto Chromogens

  M. avium/intracellulare complex
  M. paratuberculosis
  M. terrae–triviale
  M. shimoidae

Rapid Growers

  M. fortuitum/chelonae complex
  M. thermoresistible

---

2. Appearance of microcolonies after 5 to 10 days incubation on Middlebrook 7H10 or 7H11 agars, with formation of serpentine cords owing to the production of "cording factor" (see Color Plate 17-1*C* and *I*)
3. Accumulation of niacin (*M. simiae,* certain strains of *M. bovis,* and occasional strains of *M. marinum* and *M. chelonae* may also be niacin-positive); therefore, this is not an absolute characteristic (see Color Plate 17-1*D*)
4. Reduction of nitrates to nitrites (see Color Plate 17-1*E*).
5. Ability to grow in the presence of thiophene-2-carboxylic acid hydrazide (T$_2$H; see Color Plate 17-1*F*)
6. Lack of catalase activity
7. Selective inhibition of growth in BACTEC 12A broth culture media containing *p*-nitro-acetyl-amino-hydroxypropiophenone (NAP; see Chart 50 for the details of this procedure).

The NAP inhibition of *M. tuberculosis* is used in many laboratories as a key test in making preliminary identifications, particularly for blood culture isolates. NAP selectively inhibits the ability of *M. tuberculosis* to release $^{14}CO_2$ from the radioactive 1-[^{14}C] palmitic acid contained in the medium.[160] The NAP BACTEC vial is also used for inoculation of other smear-positive specimens to enhance recovery and shorten the time for detection. Although the definitive identification of most NAP-negative mycobacteria strains still requires isolation and characterization by the spectrum of tests discussed before, those isolates that also produce microcolonies with serpentine cording on 7H10 agar can be presumptively identified and confirmed by the nucleic acid probe assay (see Color Plate 17-1C). The colonies visually appear "rough and buff" after 2 to 4 weeks incubation on Löwenstein-Jensen medium. These observations are sufficient criteria to warrant commencement of empiric therapy when clinically indicated.

Examination of the acid-fast–stained smear can also be helpful in supporting the presumptive identification. The typical cell morphology of *M. tuberculosis* as seen in acid-fast stains is a thin, slightly curved, bacillus measuring 0.3 to 0.6 by 1 to 4 µm, deeply red staining (strongly acid-fast), with a distinct beaded appearance (see Color Plate 17-1B). In the preparation of smears from cultures, the individual cells are often difficult to disperse, appearing as irregular aggregates, or lying in parallel strands. The presence of a *Mycobacterium* species can be suspected in Gram stains if poorly or nonstaining bacilli are observed surrounded by a clear halo (see Color Plate 17-1J). The crystal violet dye in the Gram stain reagent does not penetrate the thick, waxy lipid cell wall, and the organisms remain almost in negative relief against the background.

Mycobacterium bovis. *M. bovis* is now clustered in the *M. tuberculosis* complex. Phenotypic characteristics by which *M. bovis* can be differentiated from classic strains of *M. tuberculosis* include the following:

1. Most strains are niacin-negative.
2. Nitrates are not reduced to nitrites.
3. Pyrazinamidase is not produced.
4. Selective inhibition of growth by T₂H; *M. bovis* will not grow in medium containing T₂H.

The classic human strains have a very slow growth rate, producing "dysgonic"-appearing colonies on LJ medium. Thus, a problem in recognizing *M. bovis* may arise in laboratories where LJ cultures are discarded after 4 weeks, for often 6 to 8 weeks are required to observe visible growth. Growth of most strains is better on LJ medium than on Middlebrook 7H11 or equivalents. The medium most favorable for *M. bovis* contains 0.4% pyruvate without glycerol.[57] Typical colonies are buff, low, and small and may appear either smooth or rough on egg medium. On Middlebrook 7H11 agar, colonies are very thin and often show little or no stranding (referred to as "water droplet–like"). These colonies may also simulate dysgonic forms of *M. avium–intracellulare*. The latter are 68°C catalase-

positive, do not produce urease, and are pyrimizidase-positive. If pyruvate has been added to the medium, colonies may show serpentine cords similar to those of eugonic *M. tuberculosis*.

Certain laboratory strains of *M. bovis*, known as BCG (bacille Calmette-Geurin), which have been used as a vaccine in highly endemic areas of the world, simulate *M. tuberculosis* by being "eugonic," or more rapidly growing (3 to 4 weeks on LJ medium), having a rough, buff appearance and, in some cases, accumulating niacin. However, these strains remain T₂H-sensitive and can be differentiated on that basis.[88] The microscopic morphology of *M. bovis* cells in acid-fast–stained smears is not distinctive. They tend to be somewhat longer than *M. tuberculosis*, less curved, and less beaded.

Mycobacterium ulcerans. Most cases of *M. ulcerans* infections have been reported from Central and West Africa, Malaysia, New Guinea, Guyana, Mexico, and Australia. The name "Bairnsdale ulcer" has been used for the cutaneous lesions of *M. ulcerans* infections, named after the Australian town where the organism was first recognized by Alsop and Searls in the 1930s.[224] Most human infections occur in the tropical regions following rain forest disturbance.[102] It is postulated that the mycobacteria are carried from the soil into draining lacustrine systems, where they multiply over a period of months or years. Humans become infected by inhaling aerosolized organisms from these contaminated estuaries.

LABORATORY ASPECTS. *M. ulcerans* grows optimally at 33°C and not at all at 37°C. Rough, lightly buff or nonpigmented, convex to flat colonies, with irregular outline, often simulating those of *M. tuberculosis*, develop after 6 to 12 weeks. Microscopically the acid-fast cells are moderately long and rod-shaped, without banding or beading. *M. ulcerans* is biochemically inert, showing only heat-stable catalase activity among the several tests usually employed to identify mycobacteria.

PHOTOCHROMOGENS

Mycobacterium kansasii. Originally known as the "yellow bacillus" following the first description by Buhler and Pollak in 1953, *M. kansasii* is a photochromogen classified within the Runyon group I. Although infections occur throughout the United States, most cases have been reported from the southern states (Texas, Louisiana, Florida), Midwest (Illinois), and California. Kim and associates[140] report a decline in the overall incidence of disease in the United States over the past decade. Males are infected more frequently than females, with a ratio of 3:1. The disease is less common in children and individuals with higher incomes and better standards of living.[244]

LABORATORY ASPECTS. Typical strains of *M. kansasii* grow at approximately the same rate or slightly more rapidly than *M. tuberculosis* at 37°C. The distinctive feature is the dependence on light exposure for the pro-

CLINICAL CORRELATION BOX 17-1. *M. tuberculosis*

The recovery of *M. tuberculosis* from clinical specimens is almost always associated with infection, and tuberculosis is known to be a highly communicable disease. Most infections begin in the lungs where diffuse, finely nodular, or patchy infiltrates may be seen, primarily in the apical portions of the upper lobes, but also spreading to other foci in miliary or progressive exudative tuberculosis (see Color Plate 17-3A) as cavitary lesions, primarily in the apical portions of the upper lobes, or as a solitary tuberculoma or "coin lesion" that may be part of an old Ghon complex (see Color Plate 17-3B and 3C). Outbreaks in closed populations, such as in schools, ships, and crowded family groups are all too common. Disseminated or miliary spread of infection occurred in certain persons, usually those with malnutrition, immunosuppression, or other chronic debilitating diseases. Jereb and coworkers,[128] using restriction fragment length polymorphism (RFLP) by PCR, were able to pinpoint the source of an outbreak of *M. tuberculosis* among ten renal transplant patients in one hospital to a single patient who had posttransplant exposure in another hospital before transfer. The mean incubation time for the onset of tuberculosis in the newly infected renal transplant patients was 7.5 weeks. This situation illustrates how new molecular techniques can be helpful in detecting point sources of tuberculosis so that early isolation can be implemented to prevent nosocomial transmission of disease.

M. tuberculosis infections are most frequent among persons engaged in the following occupations:[32]

1. Persons with occupational tuberculosis exposure: funeral directors, health service personnel
2. Persons with occupational silica exposure: construction workers, brick and stone masons, carpenters, mining machine operators, and construction laborers
3. Low socioeconomic status occupations: food preparation and service workers
4. Unknown risk: farm operators, automobile racers and mechanics, butchers, entertainers

Reinfection or adult-type tuberculosis is a slowly progressive inflammatory process in the lungs, characterized by intense chronic granulomatous inflammation, usually with the formation of many Langhans-type giant cells, necrosis, and caseation, with the propensity of the process to break into bronchi (see Color Plate 17-3D). Large numbers of tubercle bacilli are spread to fresh foci within the lung when a cavity ruptures, and may be coughed up in profusion if the cavity breaks into a bronchus, potentially infecting others in close contact. Coughing, weight loss, low-grade fever, dyspnea, and chest pain are the usual clinical signs and symptoms of chronic progressive pulmonary tuberculosis. This is a description of the so-called secondary- or reinfection-type tuberculosis. In patients with AIDS, the disease takes on more of a primary type, characterized by more rapid progression, septicemia, and miliary dissemination, less focal fibrosis and caseation, and miliary dissemination to involve virtually any organ in the body.

Tuberculosis meningitis is a relatively rare disease in the United States, virtually always as a complication of primary pulmonary tuberculosis. Patients may be virtually asymptomatic, present with vague complaints of headaches, change in mentation, or, uncommonly, progress to manifestations of severe meningitis. In most instances, one of three laboratory measurements of cerebrospinal fluid will be altered: an increase in cell count, mostly lymphocytosis; a decrease in glucose levels; or an increase in protein concentrations, although any one of these parameters may be normal. In rare instances, all three parameters may be normal, providing little objective evidence for establishing the diagnosis. Acid-fast organisms may be observed in centrifuged specimens in about 37% of cases, a yield that increases with the number of spinal examinations performed. Pathologically, the meningeal involvement is most pronounced at the base of the brain, where visible changes range from a diffuse opacity to the presence of a thick gelatinous exudate, seen primarily in the area overlying the pons and adjacent to the optic chiasm (see Color Plate 17-3E).

Septicemia with *M. tuberculosis* is considered to be rare; however, Bouza and associates,[22] in a study of 285 patients with culture-proved tuberculosis in whom blood cultures were obtained, found that 50 (14%) had bacteremia. Of these, 81% were infected with the HIV virus. In 14 patients, blood was the first specimen from which organisms were recovered.

More than 93% of *M. tuberculosis* strains isolated from untreated patients are susceptible to antituberculosis drugs and respond promptly to treatment with two, or preferably three, drugs. The susceptibility testing of mycobacteria is presented later in this chapter.

duction of a visible yellow pigment (see Color Plates 17-2C and 2D) and the formation of reddish β-carotene crystals on prolonged incubation. The colonies are typically intermediate between fully rough and fully smooth (certain strains are totally one or the other). The microcolonies typically show elevated centers and curving strands of bacilli in the outer, thinner margins that may be confused with the serpentine cording of *M. tuberculosis*. The group of phenotypic properties, in addition to photochromogenicity, by which the identification of *M. kansasii* can be confirmed include:

1. Rapid hydrolysis of Tween within 3 days
2. Strong reduction of nitrate to nitrite

3. Rapid catalase reaction, including 68°C test
4. Strong pyrazinamidase activity

Less commonly, scotochromogenic or nonchromogenic strains may be encountered, including some strains with low catalase activity. The bacterial cells in acid-fast smear preparations are characteristically long and broad and distinctly cross-banded or barred (see Color Plate 17-2M), presumably from utilization of the fatty material of the medium. Although experienced mycobacteriologists may make a presumptive identification based on acid-fast stain, determination of phenotypic properties is usually required before a definitive identification can be made.

M. bovis produces tuberculosis typically in cattle but may also infect other animals, including dogs, cats, swine, rabbits, and possibly, certain birds of prey. Fanning and Edwards[67] traced 446 contacts of humans with domesticated elk in Alberta, Canada, 81 of whom were skin test-positive for *M. bovis*. Of these, 50 had been in contact with culture-positive animals, including one case of active *M. bovis* pulmonary infection diagnosed by a positive sputum specimen. With DNA fingerprinting assays with IS*6110* as the genetic marker, van Soolingen, et al.[290] were able to determine that the strains of *M. bovis* causing human infection in Argentina were transmitted from cattle, whereas the strains causing human disease among persons living in The Netherlands were contracted from animals other than cattle (various wild and zoo animals). In some areas in Scotland and in Czechoslovakia, where cattle and dairy farming is still the chief livelihood, *M. bovis* still may constitute as many as 39% of all cases of tuberculosis.[313] Human bovine pulmonary tuberculosis closely resembles that caused by *M.*

tuberculosis, in deference to Robert Koch, whose fame at the end dwindled among colleagues as he held firmly to the position that bovine tuberculosis caused only intestinal disease in humans. We now know that these two species are generally part of a complex, and *M. bovis* pulmonary tuberculosis is treated similarly to disease caused by *M. tuberculosis*.

During the time that humans physically milked cows much more frequently than today, cutaneous infections of the fingers were common, often with underlying osteomyelitis and osteoarthritis of the finger digits (see Color Plate 17-3F). A common site of recovery of *M. bovis* in clinical laboratories is from urine samples, as the bacille Calmette-Guérin (BCG) strain is used in bladder irrigations as an immunologic stimulant in the treatment of carcinoma in situ. This possibility should be considered when a slow-growing mycobacterium is recovered from urine samples, and any such isolate should not be passed off as a commensal. In some individuals, the BCG strain being used is not totally attenuated and may cause cystitis.

Mycobacterium marinum. In 1926, while investigating infectious diseases in saltwater fish, Aronson[9] discovered a new *Mycobacterium* species, later named *Mycobacterium marinum* ("of the sea").[305] The organism has also been called *M. platypoecilus* from infections observed in Mexican platyfish and also as *M. balnei* (a name referring to bath or spas). All are the same organism.

LABORATORY ASPECTS. *M. marinum*, when recovered from clinical specimens, grows optimally at 30° to 32°C. Growth is poor if it occurs at all at 37°C. Subcultures may grow at 37°C. Colonies appear in 8 to 14 days; those grown in the dark may appear nonpigmented. When exposed to light, a deep yellow pigment develops. Colonies vary between wrinkled and rough to smooth and hemispheric, particularly if grown on 7H10 or 7H11 agar (which contains oleic acid and albumin). Microscopically the cells are relatively long rods with frequent cross-barring.

Thus, photochromogenicity and preference for growth at 30°C are initial clues to the identification of *M. marinum*. The following are additional characteristics by which an identification can be made:

1. Some strains may accumulate niacin
2. Nitrates are not reduced to nitrites
3. Tween is hydrolyzed
4. Urease is positive
5. Pryazinamidase is produced
6. Heat-stable catalase is not produced

Mycobacterium simiae. Weiszfeiler and Karczag[308] named *M. simiae* in 1969, in recognition of the first recovery of the organism 4 years earlier by Karassova and colleagues, from *Macaca* rhesus monkeys imported into Hungary from India. This organism was subsequently found to be identical with a niacin-

positive strain of a group III mycobacterium recovered in Cuba by Valdivia and coworkers from patients with pulmonary tuberculosis. They named the organism *M. habana*, which subsequently has been shown to be the same organism as *M. simiae*.[305]

Infection presents as a painless "boil" or lump under the skin, which typically develops at the site of previous trauma, and proceeds into a shallow nonhealing ulcer, with a necrotic base within a few weeks. Some of the lesions studied by Igo and Murthy[116] were quite severe, with avascular coagulation necrosis extending deep into the subcutaneous fat. Satellite nodules that ulcerate may also develop. Successful therapy has been reported with application of local heat, excision, and grafting.[244] Igo and Murthy[116] provide the clinical, histologic, and microbiologic features of 46 cases of *M. ulcerans* infections studied in several villages along the Sepik River in New Guinea. Lesions are usually found on the lower extremities, and consist of shallow ulcers that develop in areas of subcutaneous induration at sites of previous trauma. Satellite nodules and superficial ulcers may develop. These are usually nonpainful unless secondarily infected. Delaporte et al.[55] report one of the first cases of *M. ulcerans* infections in a patient with AIDS. The patient was a 30-year-old pregnant Zairian woman, with a chronic, painful, ulcerating lesion of the knee. A superficial punch biopsy grew no organisms; a deeper biopsy of the fascia, however, revealed numerous acid-fast bacilli. The lesion healed with a 2-month regimen of isoniazid, rifampin, and ethambutol. Despite the association of *M. ulcerans* infection and AIDS in this patient, the association is too infrequent to serve as a marker.

CLINICAL CORRELATION BOX 17-4. *M. kansasii*

Chronic pulmonary disease simulating classic tuberculosis is the most common manifestation, classically involving the upper lobes. Cavitation with scarring is evident in most cases, and disease is slowly progressive.[244] Extrapulmonary or disseminated infections are less common, although cases of scrofula-like lymphadenitis, sporotrichosis-like cutaneous infections, osteomyelitis, soft-tissue infections, and tenosynovitis have been reported. Dillon et al.[56] in particular cite the progressive damage to the deep structures of the wrist and hand that can occur in cases of tenosynovitis. Disseminated disease may be seen in the presence of severe immunosuppression and has been reported in patients with AIDS. Jacobson and Isenberg,[123] in reporting an AIDS-related case of diffuse granulomatous interstitial pneumonitis caused by *M. kansasii*, indicate that only 0.2% of AIDS patients have superimposed *M. kansasii* infections. However, Valainis and coworkers,[289] reporting from Louisiana, a region endemic for *M. kansasii*, in a 60-month review of patients attending two major referral centers in New Orleans, found that 31.9% of HIV-1–infected patients were coinfected with *M. kansasii*. In a retrospective study of 35 patients, conducted in Kansas City,[13] the incidence of *M. kansasii* infections in patients with AIDS was three times higher than *M. tuberculosis* infections. Most patients responded to several different combinations of antituberculous drugs that included isoniazid, rifampin, ethambutol, and ciprofloxacin. Some patients tolerated therapy poorly; one developed isoniazid-induced hepatitis. The authors recommend that at least two active agents, such as ethambutol and rifampin, be used.

M. kansasii infections in patients with AIDS usually occurs during the late stages when CD4+ lymphocyte counts are fewer than 50, with serious and life-threatening complications in many cases. Levine and Chaisson[166] reviewed 19 patients with *M. kansasii* and HIV infection, 14 of whom had exclusive pulmonary infection, three had pulmonary and extrapulmonary disease, and two patients had extrapulmonary involvement exclusively. All patients with pulmonary infection presented with fever and cough of at least 2 weeks' duration. Focal upper lobe infiltrates, diffuse interstitial infiltrates, or thin-walled cavitary lesions, or a combination thereof, were seen on chest radiographs. Nine patients receiving antituberculosis therapy showed resolution of fever and respiratory symptoms, with clearing of the radiographic infiltrates. Other AIDS-related cases of *M. kansasii* infections have been reported.[108, 247] In the latter case, caseating granulomas were seen in the bowel wall and in the mesenteric lymph nodes, with accumulation of foamy histiocytes resembling Whipple's disease. Giladi and coauthors[77] report a case of catheter-associated *M. kansasii* peritonitis in a 62-year-old woman undergoing continuous ambulatory peritoneal dialysis, presumably the first such case report. Good response was achieved with combination therapy with isoniazid and rifampin and removal of the catheter. Tortoli and coworkers[283] found a cluster of *M. kansasii* strains that did not hybridize with the Accuprobe *M. kansasii* culture identification test (Gen Probe, San Diego, CA) that were distinctly associated with AIDS status. This suggests that *M. kansasii* may differ in virulence and that additional tests for identification may be required for Accuprobe-negative strains.

Strains of *M. kansasii* resistant to rifampin are being seen with increasing frequency. Wallace and coauthors[296] reported on 36 patients from whom rifampin-resistant *M. kansasii* had been isolated, 90% of whom had previously received therapy with this agent. The majority of patients, however, responded to a four-drug regimen, based on in vitro susceptibility studies, and sputum cultures converted to negative in 90% of those treated in a mean time of 11 weeks.

LABORATORY ASPECTS. Colonies develop within 2 to 3 weeks on egg-based media; they are typically smooth; and most strains are photochromogenic. Prolonged exposure to light may be required for those isolates that fail to produce pigment. The key identifying biochemical reactions are as follows:

1. Positive niacin accumulation
2. Hydrolysis of Tween (may be slow, requiring more than 10 days)
3. High thermostable catalase activity

Poor reproducibility of test reactions by some strains may make identification somewhat difficult. Some strains of *M. simiae* may be misidentified as members of the MAIS species.

Mycobacterium genavense. *M. genavense* is a newly described, slow-growing, nonpigmented, nontuberculous mycobacterium that causes infection in patients with AIDS. The organism was first recognized by Boettger and associates[21] by finding a unique pattern using DNA extracted from mycobacteria growing in BACTEC 13A blood culture media. Amplified gene fragments were sequenced directly, and electro-phoretic profiles were determined in 0.8% agarose gel stained with ethidium bromide. The authors studied 16 cases whose organisms had this unique DNA sequence profile and officially designated the organism *M. genavense* after the 28-year-old AIDS patient living in Geneva from whom the first isolate was recovered. Subsequently, Coyle and associates,[48] using assays for sequencing of the gene for 16S rRNA that had been extracted from unidentified mycobacterial isolates of 15 blood cultures obtained from seven patients with AIDS, also confirmed the identity of *M. genavense* as a separate species. The sequence pattern was most closely related to *M. simiae*; however, the clinical presentation, response to therapy, and autopsy manifestations more closely resemble infections with *M. avium* complex.[17] Histopathologically, *M. genavense* in HIV-positive patients produces lesions characterized by masses of foamy histiocytes and ill-defined granulomas, the development of which depends on the immunologic reactivity of the host.[177] In one autopsy series, small intestine, spleen, liver, and lymph nodes were most commonly involved; the lungs, myocardium, and kidney were spared, a distribution similar to that seen in subjects with *M. avium* complex diseases.

Typical infections involve the skin, usually resulting when traumatized skin comes in contact with inadequately chlorinated freshwater or saltwater (swimming pools, tropical fish aquariums, water-cooling towers). Fisher[70] recently reported three cases of cutaneous skin infection in lifeguards, citing this infection as a hazard of the trade. Included in the paper are good color photographs of the skin lesions. Several cases were seen in Denver, Colorado in the 1950s, secondary to massive contamination of the swimming pool spa in the mountain community of Glenwood Springs. Hoyt and associates[113] report several deep tissue infections and destructive tenosynovitis among fishermen in the Chesapeake Bay area. Several other citations of deep cutaneous infections, usually of the hands, and commonly associated with aquatic activity, such as cleaning of fish, include a case of tenosynovitis,[15] arthritis and bursitis,[37] and osteomyelitis.[114] Chemotherapy with some combination of drugs, such as rifampin and ethambutol, may be effective, but frequently, surgery may be required. Chemotherapy is least likely to be effective in patients previously treated with steroid injection, and avoidance of steroid injections is key to successful management.[37,130]

Some patients present with sporotrichosis-like lesions, with central spread along the lymphatics emanating from an ulcerated area at the primary site of inoculation.[205] More typically, the lesions present as tender, red or blue-red subcutaneous nodules, usually involving the elbow, knee, toe, or finger ("swimming pool granuloma"). Such lesions may be mistaken for rheumatoid nodules.[10] These authors cite other cases of deep subcutaneous infections, in some instances involving subcutaneous bursae, tendon sheaths, joints, and bone.

Treatment is usually directed to resecting the primary lesions if possible (curettage, electrodesiccation, excision). Antituberculous therapy may be required to cure chronic cases in which lymphatic spread is evident. Most strains are susceptible to rifampin and ethambutol but resistant to isoniazid and streptomycin.

The initial isolates were identified in samples obtained from AIDS patients in Switzerland[21] (thus the species name); however, as of February 1995, 54 patients with disseminated infections caused by *M. genavense* have been reported, the majority from Europe (37 cases), the remainder in North America (15) and Australia (2).[209] This geographic distribution may reflect more the awareness by health workers of this new species rather than select areas of endemicity. *M. genavense* may be underrecognized because it grows only in broth culture media (such as BACTEC 13A broth, in which it was first discovered) and requires prolonged incubation.[205] Fever, weight loss, diarrhea, hepatosplenomegaly, and anemia are the most common symptoms.

Mycobacterium asiaticum. *M. asiaticum* is phenotypically similar to *M. gordonae*; both have high catalase activity, hydrolyze Tween 80, and are negative for urease and nitrate reduction.[304] It is photochromogenic and is biochemically similar to *M. simiae*, except it is niacin negative. *M. asiaticum* has a distinct 16 rRNA profile, justifying a separate species status.[268]

Rare cases of human infection have appeared in the literature. The first indication that this disease could be pathogenic was in a report from Australia by Blacklock.[19] Of five cases reported, two had progressive cavitary pulmonary disease; three others had no evidence of progressive pulmonary disease, and the sputum isolates were thought to represent secondary colonization. The first case of pulmonary infection caused by *M. asiaticum* in the United States was isolated from a 62-year-old man living in Los Angeles.[277] Four isolates were reported from Florida.[82] Dawson and coworkers[53] recently report recovery of *M. asiaticum* from fluid aspirated from an olecranon bursa in a case of post-surgery infection. The infection cleared with drainage, regular dressing, and immobilization without the need for antimycobacterial therapy. *M. asiaticum* is photochromogenic and biochemically similar to *M. simiae* but is negative for niacin production.

SCOTOCHROMOGENS

Mycobacterium scrofulaceum. The species name *scrofulaceum*, derived from *scrofula* ("brood sow"), was named in 1956 by Prissick and Mason in reference to

Reports of human infection from *M. simiae* are relatively few. Isolated case reports of pulmonary infections occurring in France, Israel, Thailand, and the United States have been cited.[167] These authors report a case of a 43-year-old man with AIDS who developed disseminated mycobacterial infection. Organisms were recovered from blood, jejunal fluid, and duodenal and rectal biopsies. Although a few other cases of *M. simiae* infections have been reported in patients with AIDS, the association is infrequent and does not serve as a marker.[211] The Israeli experience with *M. simiae* is interesting, in that 399 strains were isolated from 287 persons during the period 1975 to 1981, primarily among inhabitants of the coastal plain of Tel Aviv.[163] Most of the isolates were commensal organisms related to environmental water sources. A few pulmonary infections occurred among patients from whom multiple isolates were recovered, usually complicating preexistent chronic pulmonary conditions.

Two cases of disseminated disease, with renal involvement following pulmonary infection, were reported.[239] Although most strains of *M. simiae* are resistant to antituberculous drugs by in vitro testing, a recent case of intra-abdominal disease was successfully treated with combination chemotherapy.[103]

the most common form of disease by this organism, cervical lymphadenitis in children.[221] *M. scrofulaceum*, however, is not the only mycobacterium causing cervical lymphadenitis. Gill and coauthors[78] reviewed the cases of 16 children with this disease; six were caused by *M. scrofulaceum*, four by *M. tuberculosis*, and four by *M. avium* complex. Therefore, culture and species identification of organisms isolated is required. *M. scrofulaceum* is uncommonly associated with AIDS. In 1985, 2% of mycobacterial infections in patients with AIDS in the United States were caused by *M. scrofulaceum*.[83] By 1989 the incidence of association was reported to be 15% in Sweden.[111]

Kirschner and associates[143] recovered large quantities of *M. scrofulaceum* from swamp water in several locations in Georgia, West Virginia, and Virginia, indicating environmental water sources are likely connected with the increased incidence of scrofula infections seen in these regions. High concentrations of organisms were found in warm water with low pH, low dissolved oxygen content, high soluble zinc levels, and high levels of humic and fulvic acids.

LABORATORY ASPECTS. Colonies of *M. scrofulaceum* grow slowly (4 to 6 weeks) at various temperatures (25°, 31°, and 37°C). They are typically smooth, buttery in consistency, and globoid, with pigmentation ranging from light yellow to deep orange (see Color Plate 17-2D). Pigment production is not dependent on light exposure; thus, the organism is included in the scotochromogen group II of Runyon.

Key biochemical test reactions include the following:

1. Failure to hydrolyze Tween
2. Nitrates are not reduced to nitrites
3. 68°C catalase test is positive
4. Urease is produced

Other-slow growing scotochromogens include certain strains of the *M. avium* complex, *M. gordonae*, and *M. szulgai*. Tween hydrolysis (the latter two are positive [*M. szulgai* may require 7 days or more], whereas *M. scrofulaceum* is negative) and urease activity (*M. scrofulaceum* hydrolyzes urea, whereas the other species, including pigmented strains of *M. avium* complex, are negative). Two groups of pigmented organisms within the *M. avium* complex, intermediate in biochemical reactivity with *M. scrofulaceum*, have been designated with the term MAIS complex.[98] One group of MAIS organisms produces a column of foam higher than 45 mm in the semiquantitative catalase test and is urease-negative; the other is catalase-negative but urease-positive.

Mycobacterium szulgai. *M. szulgai*, officially reported as a species in 1972 by Marks and coworkers,[176] is named after the Polish microbiologist T. Szulg.[305] The unique feature of this species is the temperature-dependent production of pigment—when grown at 37°C, the organism is scotochromogenic; it is photochromogenic when grown at room temperature (25°C). Therefore, to assess the photochromogenicity of an un-

known strain of *M. szulgai*, the light-exposed plates must be incubated at room temperature and not at 37°C. The scotogenic pigment produced at the higher temperature will mask any chance to visualize any photogenetic pigment that may be produced (see Chart 2).

LABORATORY ASPECTS. Growth is relatively rapid, with either smooth or rough colonies developing within 2 weeks at 37°C. Orange pigment may be observed, intensifying with exposure to continuous light. In acid-fast smear preparations, the bacterial cells appear as moderately long rods, with some cross-barring, reminiscent of *M. kansasii*. *M. szulgai* can be definitively identified by the following set of characteristics:

1. Slow hydrolysis of Tween
2. Nitrates reduced to nitrites
3. Positive catalase activity
4. Intolerance to 5% NaCl

Mycobacterium xenopi. *M. xenopi* (*Xenopus*, a genus of frog), was first isolated from an African toad.[305] Hot and cold water taps, including water storage tanks and hot water generators of hospitals, are potential sources for nosocomial infections. Previously considered to be nonpathogenic, *M. xenopi* has recently been incriminated in several infections. Wolinski[319] reported on 50

Maloney and associates[175] present three cases of human infections with *M. szulgai* and reviewed 24 previous cases reported in the literature before 1987. Lung infections were present in two thirds of the cases, and chest radiographs revealed unilateral or bilateral apical disease, with cavitation, simulating *M. tuberculosis*. A case of persistent lung infection caused by *M. szulgai* has also been reported.[41] Fever, cough, hemoptysis, and weight loss were common symptoms. Extrapulmonary infections with *M. szulgai* cited in the foregoing review include olecranon bursitis, tenosynovitis, and carpal tunnel syndrome, osteomyelitis, and localized cutaneous disease.

cases of human *M. xenopi* infections, primarily in England, France, Denmark, Australia, and the United States. Birds that frequent the costal regions in Great Britain constitute an important reservoir.

LABORATORY ASPECTS. *M. xenopi* colonies are slow-growing, small, erect, and produce characteristic yellow pigment (occasional strains are nonpigmented). Growth is more rapid at 42°C than 37°C; growth is absent at 25°C. Although previously included with the nonphotochromogenic mycobacteria, the brightly pigmented yellow colonies usually found on primary isolation suggest that the organism would be better considered with the scotochromogens. Colonies tend to be

rough, and an aerial mycelium may be evident. Examination of young microcolonies on 7H10 agar reveals a distinctive "bird's nest" appearance, with sticklike projections. Branching and filamentous extensions appear in older colonies, particularly those grown on cornmeal–glycerol agar.

Microscopically, acid-fast–stained smears reveal long, filamentous rods that are tapered at both ends, tending to arrange in palisades. The characteristics by which a species identification can be made are as follows:

1. Optimum growth at 42°C
2. Yellow scotochromogenic pigment
3. No niacin accumulation
4. Nitrate reduction-negative
5. Catalase produced at 68°C only
6. Arylsulfatase-positive
7. Pyrazinamidase-positive

Mycobacterium celatum. *M. celatum* is the proposed name for a new *Mycobacterium* species recently described by Butler and coauthors.[26] It most closely resembles *M. xenopi* phenotypically (in fact, it was not discovered until recently because it was hidden [*celatum*, "to conceal"] among strains of MAC and *M. xenopi*),[285] differing only in its poor growth at 45°C, growth of large colonies on 7H10 agar, and the production of only trace amounts of the fatty acid 2-docanosol.[205] This new species has been recovered from respiratory tract cultures, and less commonly from the blood, stool, and cerebrospinal fluid, in cultures ob-

Most human cases of *M. xenopi* infections have been pulmonary, resembling those seen in patients with *M. tuberculosis, M. kansasii,* or MAI infections. Multinodular densities, often showing cavitation and fibrosis, are often seen radiologically. Infections usually occur in patients with preexistent lung disease or predisposing conditions (alcoholism, malignancy, diabetes mellitus). Contreras and coauthors,[43] in reviewing 89 adult patients with pulmonary infections, report that *M. xenopi* was the second most frequent isolate (38% of cases). Similarly, in a review of cultures positive for nontuberculous mycobacteria, excluding *M. avium–intracellular* complex and *M. gordonae,* from 86 patients at the State University of New York–Health Sciences Center at Brooklyn, *M. xenopi* was the most common species isolated (33 cases).[250a] The majority of these isolates were recovered from respiratory specimens in patients with AIDS. The recovery of 28 isolates of *M. xenopi* from patients residing in the Ontario province of Canada has been reported.[257] In 19 patients, the isolate was considered insignificant; nine isolates were from middle-aged men with other chronic pulmonary diseases. In the province of Ontario, *M. xenopi* has been the second most common nontuberculous mycobacterial pathogen, second only to *M. avium–intracellulare.*

Intrapulmonary spread usually occurs in patients with AIDS[11]; in disseminated cases, organisms may also be re-

covered from bone marrow aspirates. *M. xenopi* infections are uncommonly found in HIV-positive patients. Two cases of HIV-infected men with symptomatic pulmonary infection—night sweats, cough, and pleuritic pain were reported.[124] *M. xenopi* grew in cultures of multiple respiratory specimens obtained from each patient. Both improved with multidrug therapy that included isoniazid and rifampin, which was unexpected in one case in whom in vitro resistance to isoniazid and rifampin was demonstrated. A case of pulmonary infection in a 39-year-old renal allograft recipient was reported.[306] Isolated cases of extrapulmonary infection involving bone, lymph node, epididymis, sinus tract, and a prosthetic temporomandibular joint have also been cited.[319] Infections of the lumbar spine have been reported,[222, 226] the latter in a 77-year-old immunocompetent woman presenting with a paravertebral abscess. An outbreak of 13 cases of pulmonary infection in residents of a housing project in Prague were reported.[259] The point source was thought to be the local water supply, as organisms were recovered from water faucets in five of the flats. Tortoli and coauthors,[285] reviewed the cases of 64 isolates of *M. xenopi* recovered from patients living in Florence, Italy during a 15-year period. The homogeneity of the biochemical, cultural, and antimicrobial sensitivity patterns of these isolates indicates there may be an endemic focus in the Florence area.

tained from patients residing in diverse geographic locations, including the United States, Finland, and Somalia. In the original report by Butler and co-authors,[26] approximately one third of the isolates were recovered from patients with AIDS. They also found cross-reactivity for eight of 20 strains with *M. tuberculosis* using the acridinium ester-labeled DNA probe, AccuProbe (Gen-Probe Inc., San Diego CA). This cross-reactivity with *M. tuberculosis* and the need for genomic sequencing or high-performance liquid chromatography of cell wall mycolic acids to make a correct identification will pose problems for those working in clinical laboratories. Tortoli and associates[285] report two cases in patients with AIDS. In the first patient, *M. celatum* was recovered from multiple blood cultures, first a cluster of four positive cultures, followed by a cluster of three additional positive cultures 9 months later. The second isolate was from a sputum culture, and the patient's pulmonary condition improved following combined drug treatment with clarithromycin, ciprofloxacin, and amikacin. Haase and coworkers[94] report a case of scrofula-like unilateral cervical lymphadenitis in an immunocompetent child.

Mycobacterium gordonae. Of the group of *Mycobacterium* species "rarely causing human infections," as designated in the outline presented in the foregoing, perhaps *M. gordonae* is recovered in clinical laboratories with greatest frequency. It is found particularly in aqueous environments, leading to the alternate designation of *M. aquae* or the "tap water bacillus."[305]

LABORATORY ASPECTS. *M. gordonae* is a scotochromogen, readily recognized by the smooth, deeply yellow-orange pigmented colonies that develop after 7 days of incubation at 37°C (see Color Plates 17-2E and 2M). The organism hydrolyzes Tween 80 and produces heat-stable catalase; it is urease-negative and does not reduce nitrates to nitrites. *M. gordonae* is resistant to isoniazid, streptomycin, and *p*-aminosalicylic acid (PAS) but is susceptible to rifampin and ethambutol.

M. flavescens is a scotochromogen that may phenotypically be confused with *M. gordonae*; however, *M. flavescens* possesses urease activity and reduces nitrates to nitrites, two characteristics not demonstrated by *M. gordonae*. *M. flavescens* is a commensal for humans and is not known to cause disease.[305]

NONPHOTOCHROMONGENS

Mycobacterium avium–intracellulare. *M. avium–intracellulare*, also known as the MAI complex (or MAC), is the same organism that caused an outbreak of pulmonary tuberculosis at the Battey State Hospital in Rome, Georgia in the 1950s and for some time carried the designation "Battey bacillus." MAI is widely distributed in water, soil, dust, animals, and poultry. For humans, the organism was considered of low pathogenicity and rarely caused disease. However, the AIDS epidemic has turned that around, so that currently only *M. tuberculosis* is being recovered with more frequency than MAC.[82]

Members of the *M. avium–intracellulare* complex of bacteria are ubiquitous, and they can be recovered from water estuaries, pools, soil, house dust, plants,

---

CLINICAL CORRELATION BOX 17-10. *M. gordonae*

Several isolated reports of infections in the literature are cited by Woods and Washington:[323] meningitis secondary to ventriculoatrial shunts, hepatoperitoneal disease, endocarditis in a prosthetic aortic valve, cutaneous lesions of the hand, and possible cases of pulmonary involvement. The case of peritonitis in a patient undergoing peritoneal dialysis,[170] suggests that infections with *M. gordonae*, being so prevalent in the environment, may emerge as a significant problem. It is believed that *M. gordonae* should not automatically be dismissed as a contaminant when isolated from clinical material.[307] The clinical characteristics were tabulated of 23 reported human cases of *M. gordonae* infection from the literature as of June 1992, that fit these criteria for inclusion.[307] The organ distribution of these previously reported cases was lungs in eight patients, soft tissue (7), peritoneal cavity (3), the cornea (1), and disseminated disease (5). They reported an additional case of disseminated disease in an 11-year-old girl. Multiple round granular lesions were seen scattered in both lung fields during an open lung biopsy. Necrotizing granulomatous inflammation was seen on histologic examination of biopsy material, including numerous acid-bast bacilli in acid-fast smears. Smooth, yellow colonies, later identified as *M. gordonae*, grew on solid media after 14 days incubation at 37°C in 8% CO_2. The patient recovered after 15 months

of antituberculous therapy, commencing with a combination of isoniazid, rifampin, amikacin, and ethambutol, followed by a 1-year course of rifampin and ethambutol.

Jarikre[125, 126] reported two cases of *M. gordonae* infections, each in 40-year-old housewives, one with a chronic urinary tract infection from whom *M. gordonae* was repeatedly recovered in urine specimens; the other, in a Pakistani patient with systemic infection, from whom the organism was recovered from sputum and urine. Liver biopsy revealed multiple granulomata from which *M. gordonae* was also recovered. The second patient responded dramatically on an antitubercular drug regimen of streptomycin, isoniazid, rifampin, and pyrazinamide. A case was reported[333] of chronic nodular cutaneous infection that presented histologically as classic tuberculoid granulomas teeming with acid-fast bacilli from which *M. gordonae* was recovered.

Wayne and Sramek,[304] however, after reviewing many of the previously reported alleged cases of *M. gordonae* infection, caution that organism descriptions and convincing clinical correlations often are lacking in many of the papers, and that its true pathogenicity remains in question. When recovered from specimens, each isolate must be accurately identified and a careful clinical correlation made to determine the clinical significance for what in most instances will be a contaminant.

and bedding materials. Natural sources of water, including potable water, pose considerable risk for acquiring human infections.[291] Waters that have moderate salinity (1 to 2 g% salt), relatively high acidity (pH 4.5 to 6.5), and are located at lower altitudes are ideal for supporting the propagation of *M. avium–intracellulare* organisms.[24] Human *M. avium–intracellulare* infections may occur from ingestion of contaminated water and food (the intestinal tract is thought to be the primary route of infection in AIDS patients) or by inhalation of organisms contained within aqueous aerosols. Wendt and coworkers[310] found *M. avium–intracellulare* organisms in droplet sizes of 0.7 to 3.3 mm above freshwater surfaces, sufficiently small to reach the alveolar spaces, and organisms may become highly concentrated in jet streams emanating from air–seawater interfaces. Although poultry, swine, and other species of birds and animals become infected and excrete organisms in the feces that can remain viable for long periods in soil, animal-to-human transmission is a rare event. Human-to-human transmission also is thought to be a minimal risk factor.[118]

M. avium–intracellulare is worldwide in distribution; however, endemic areas have been found in temperate geographic areas, including the United States, Canada, Great Britain, Europe, The Netherlands, and Japan.[118] From a 1979 survey in the United States, the overall prevalence of *M. avium–intracellulare* is 3.2 cases per 100,000 population, with highest incidences in Hawaii (10.8 cases), Connecticut (8.9 cases), Florida (8.4 cases), and Kansas (6.8 cases).[82] Although *M. gordonae* is the most frequent nontuberculous mycobacterium recovered from human sources, *M. avium–intracellulare* is most frequently associated with human disease. The rates of human infections with *M. avium–intracellulare* have remained stable or have slightly decreased in the non-AIDS population; in San Francisco, the overall increase in incidence of infections has paralleled the incidence of AIDS cases.[199] Of the 161,073 cases of AIDS reported to the CDC by December 1990, more than 12,000 cases of nontuberculous mycobacterial infections were also reported; in 96% of these *M. avium–intracellulare* was the agent.[112] HIV infection is the primary risk factor for disseminated infections with this organism.[203] In fact, it has been suggested that it may be an inevitable contributing cause of death in all HIV-infected patients who do not die of other causes.

LABORATORY ASPECTS. *M. avium–intracellulare* may appear as one of three colony variants: 1) smooth, opaque, and dome-shaped; 2) smooth, transparent, and flat; and 3) rough (see Color Plates 17-2*N* and 2*O*). The isolates recovered from AIDS patients most commonly produce the smooth, transparent, flat colony variant, as seen in microcolony observations (see Color Plates 17-2*A* and 2*B*). These flat, translucent colony types are more likely to be virulent[49,246] and to be multiply resistant to antimicrobial agents.[241] Although *M. avium* was originally classified in Runyon group III (nonchromogens), in the experience of many, most strains recovered from patients with AIDS have varying degrees of yellow pigmentation, intensifying as the colony ages. Doern and associates,[58] however, found that most of their strains were nonpigmented. Stormer and Falkingham[273] have determined that the strains recovered from HIV-positive patients are nonpigmented and tend to be more antibiotic-resistant than the pigmented strains.

Microscopic examination of acid-fast smears reveal cells that are typically short and coccobacillary. Early in culture and under certain conditions, long, thin bacilli may be seen. Staining is usually uniform without beading or banding. Although conventional carbolfuchsin-based stains, such as Ziehl-Neelsen and Kinyoun, are used in most laboratories, auramine–rhodamine staining with fluorescent microscopy may be helpful in some cases. Because mixed infections may occur, a predicted identification based on microscopic morphology alone is probably unwise.

Phenotypically, MAI complex strains are best characterized by a battery of negative reactions (see Table 17-7). The organism does produce heat-stable catalase and has the ability to grow on T_2H; otherwise, the biochemical reactions are inert. With the availability of a nucleic acid probe for the culture confirmation of *M. avium*, *M. intracellulare*, and *M. avium–intracellulare* complex, the delay in obtaining a species identification by conventional methods is no longer warranted. Although the applications of PCR for the direct identification of amplified nucleic acid targets of *M. avium–intracellulare* sputum and other clinical specimens, as discussed in another section of this chapter, is receiving much attention in research laboratories, a usable product for diagnostic laboratories is not available. With the recent commercial availability of a PCR system for the direct detection of *M. tuberculosis* DNA, a similar product for use with *M. avium–intracellulare* may also soon be available. Although it is common to perform the combination probe for *M. avium–intracellulare*, in some instances, it may be advisable to perform probes against each species because Yamori and Tsukamura[330] found that disease with *M. avium* appears to be worse than that caused by *M. intracellulare*.

Most strains of *M. avium–intracellulare* are resistant to the commonly used antituberculous drugs. The underlying mechanism of resistance is based on the impermeability of the molecularly complex cell wall.[227] The synthesis of aminoglycoside- and peptide-inactivating enzymes has not been demonstrated, although some strains do produce β-lactamases.[189] The surfactant effect on the cell wall of Tween 80 may potentiate the effect of certain antimicrobial agents; ethambutol also has an effect on cell wall permeability, reflecting how this agent may work synergistically to potentiate the effect of certain other antituberculous drugs.[110] Thus, ethambutol is usually included in the battery of drugs, such as INH, rifabutin, clofazimine, and others, used to treat patients with *M. avium–intracellulare* infection.[2] A U.S. Public Health Task Force has recommended that treatment of *M. avium–intracellulare* infection in patients with AIDS include a minimum of two agents, including one of the macrolides.[31] Individual decisions must be made on the basis of tolerance by the patient and the result of in vitro antimicrobial susceptibility studies.

Conditions predisposing individuals to pulmonary infections with *M. avium–intracellulare* include chronic obstructive pulmonary disease by whatever primary cause, bronchiectasis, chronic aspiration or recurrent pneumonia, inactive or active tuberculosis, pneumoconiosis, and bronchogenic carcinoma.[65] An association with cystic fibrosis has also been reported.[139] Pulmonary disease is also being seen in older women without predisposing conditions, termed Lady Windermere's syndrome, after Oscar Wilde's Victorian character who had the peculiar habit of suppressing a cough. In nonimmunosuppressed patients, pulmonary manifestations of MAI infections are similar to those of *M. tuberculosis*: cough, fatigue, weight loss, low-grade fever, and night sweats. Cavitary disease can usually be demonstrated radiologically, or solidary nodules or more diffuse infiltrates may be observed. Occasionally, patients may be asymptomatic.

The greatest upsurge in MAI infections during the past decade has been in patients with AIDS, to the point that, in some settings, MAI is more frequently recovered than *M. tuberculosis*. In a recent review of MAC infections in HIV-positive patients,[172] it was found that the MAC infections were usually disseminated and occurred late in the course of HIV infection. The risk of contracting *M. avium* infections in AIDS patients with CD4 counts are fewer than 50 is high (45% within 1 year after diagnosis).[33] When organisms were found in the sputum or gastrointestinal tract, 60% of patients had disseminated disease. Thus, these authors advise that AIDS patients with sputum or stool positive for *M. avium* should receive prophylactic therapy with rifabutin. Disseminated infections are characterized by intermittent fever, sweats, weakness, anorexia, and weight loss, that is relatively rapidly progressive. Abdominal pain or diarrhea with malabsorption was seen in some. Significant pulmonary involvement was not seen despite recovery of MAC organisms in sputum specimens. Bacteremia occurs in over 90% of patients with disseminated disease, with organisms found within the circulating monocytes. Colony counts as high as 10^6 CFU/mL have been reported, although counts in the range of 10^1 to 10^2 are more common.[324]

In a study of mycobacterial infections in 94 patients with AIDS,[190] significant pulmonary disease occurred in only about 25% of patients with MAC, in contrast to 83% of patients with *M. tuberculosis* infections who had pulmonary disease. Also, classic tuberculosis caused by *M.*

tuberculosis preceded the diagnosis of AIDS in two-thirds of the cases, in contrast with MAC infections, which were secondary complications of AIDS in all cases studied. Recently, disseminated disease caused by MAI has become more common. *M. avium–intracellulare* was recovered from 15 of 16 cases of tuberculosis meningitis.[121] The recovery of organisms from the spinal fluid always indicated disseminated disease, and prognosis in this group of patients was poor. The recovery of *M. avium–intracellulare* from sputum specimens is also an indicator of disseminated disease.[122]

From our experience, the following features of MAC infections in patients with AIDS seem evident. The organism load in biopsy or autopsy tissue sections is often extremely heavy, with intracellular bacterial aggregates often seen within large foamy macrophages, simulating the lepra cells seen in *M. leprae* infections (see Color Plates 17-2P and 17-3I and 3J). Involvement of the gastrointestinal tract also is often heavy. In some instances, large foamy macrophages, simulating the cells seen in Whipple's disease, seem to predominate the areas of inflammation. Patients with histologic evidence of gastrointestinal (and pulmonary) involvement invariably have disseminated disease.[33] Ingestion of contaminated water or food could well be the major mode of transmission. Lesions in other organs, notably the lungs, liver, spleen, and lymph nodes may also show a massive invasion with acid-fast bacilli. In some cases, little inflammation may be seen at the time of death. Necrotizing inflammation, rather than granuloma formation and caseation necrosis, is more characteristic of the histologic appearance of these lesions. Other investigators also have found heavy organism loads and atypical inflammatory reactions in AIDS patients with mycobacterial infections, and particularly cite the high incidence of mycobacterial septicemia and positive blood cultures in these patients.[97, 278, 332]

The MAC organisms have also been associated with scrofula-like cervical lymphadenitis in children.[141, 158] Woods and Washington[323] cite several other MAI infections, including granulomatous synovitis, genitourinary tract disease, cutaneous lesions, osteomyelitis, meningitis and colonic ulcers. In reference to the latter citation, that is, intestinal ulcer disease, evidence is growing that a causal relation exists between regional enteritis, or Crohn's disease, and mycobacteria, specifically a mycobacterium species closely related to *M. avium* and likely classified within the *M. avium–intracellulare* complex, *M. paratuberculosis*.

***Mycobacterium paratuberculosis* and Crohn's Disease.** Hermon-Taylor and coauthors[107] cite the work of a Glasgow surgeon, T. K. Dalziel, who in 1913 published a detailed description of chronic enteritis in humans. He proposed that the disease was caused by the same microorganisms as those responsible for Johne's disease, an ulcerative intestinal condition associated with chronic diarrhea in cattle. Johne's disease was known since 1895 and was thought to be associated with acid-fast bacilli, which could be seen in the tissues of infected animals but, in these early days, could not be cultured. Not long afterward, however, a slow-growing mycobacterium was finally recovered from the intestinal mucosa of infected animals, initially

known simply as Johne's bacillus but later identified as *M. paratuberculosis*.

In 1984, Chiodini and associates,[35] working with Hermon-Taylor and colleagues at St. George's Hospital in London, reported the recovery of an unclassified, extremely fastidious *Mycobacterium* species from three patients with Crohn's disease. After considerable effort, these workers identified the organism as belonging to the Runyon group III, closely related to the *M. avium–intracellulare* and *M. paratuberculosis* complex. Several additional cases linking *M. paratuberculosis* and Crohn's disease have been cited from the United States, The Netherlands, Australia, and France.[34] Further evidence that the Crohn's disease mycobacterium and *M. paratuberculosis* are the same was provided in yet another publication from the St. George's hospital group,[181] who recently demonstrated identical DNA restriction digests between these groups of organisms.

Gitnick and coauthors[80] report the recovery of fastidious mycobacteria, including *M. paratuberculosis*, from five of 82 surgically resected intestinal specimens from patients, 27 of whom had Crohn's disease. These isolates required between 4 and 8 months for cultivation—one reason why this organism has not been recovered in clinical laboratories. Prantera and coworkers[220] provide indirect evidence of the association of Crohn's disease with *M. paratuberculosis* by demonstrating high serum levels of antimycobacterial antibody that was demonstrated in patients following successful dapsone therapy, a phenomenon similar to that observed after treatment of classic cases of tuberculosis. With PCR and a portion of the *M. paratuberculosis* insertion sequence IS*900* as a probe, Sanderson and associates[245] were able to identify *M. paratuberculosis* DNA in 65% of rectal biopsy specimens in patients with Crohn's disease in comparison with only 4.3% and 12.5% of patients with ulcerative colitis and healthy persons, respectively. Similarly, Fidler and colleagues[69] found that the material obtained from granulomata of Crohn's disease tissues (31 biopsy samples in the study) were much more likely to amplify *M. paratuberculosis*-specific DNA on PCR than non-Crohn's disease tissues (10 biopsies of ulcerative colitis as negative controls). If indeed mycobacteria are the cause of intestinal diseases, new methods for prevention and treatment of these conditions, notably Crohn's disease, may be in order. The association has not been proved by Koch's postulates (See Cocito and coauthors[39] for a recent update on paratuberculosis).

***Mycobacterium terrae–triviale* Complex.** *M. triviale*, *M. gastri*, and *M. terrae* are other slow-growing nonphotochromogenic bacteria that, in the past, have not generally been known as pathogens but are encountered in the clinical laboratory. They can be differentiated by the characteristics listed in Table 17-7. *M. triviale* colonies may resemble those of MAI complex and in some instances may be so rough that they are confused with tubercle bacilli; however, these strains are niacin-negative and can grow in media containing 5% NaCl. *M. triviale* also hydrolyzes Tween 80 within 5 days; the MAI complex organisms are Tween-negative. *M. gastri* and *M. terrae* complex are other nonphotochromogenic species that may require biochemical differentiation (see Table 17-7). *M. terrae* is also known as the "radish bacillus," initially recovered from radish washings. Colonies of *M. terrae* tend to be smoother than the rough colonies of *M. triviale*.

Mycobacterium shimoidei. *M. shimoidei* has been proposed for an *M. terrae*-like organism recovered on multiple occasions over an 11-year period from a 56-year-old resident of Japan who had tuberculosis-like pulmonary disease.[305] In 1988, Imaeda and coworkers,[117] based on DNA homology studies, officially es-

---

CLINICAL CORRELATION BOX 17-12.
M. terrae–triviale COMPLEX

Members of the *M. terrae–triviale* complex have been incriminated in several cases of human infections, as cited by Woods and Washington:[323] septic arthritis caused by *M. triviale* in an infant, synovitis and osteomyelitis caused by *M. terrae* in a young man with Fanconi's pancytopenia, and possible disseminated *M. terrae* infection in a young woman with previous miliary tuberculosis. Several cases of pulmonary infection with *M. terrae* have been reported.[157, 281] Krishner and coauthors[152] report one case and cite six previous cases of respiratory infection. Peters and Morice[210] report a case of pulmonary *M. terrae* infection in a 64-year-old woman with ovarian carcinoma, presenting as caseating miliary infiltrates on chest radiographs and accompanied by a rash on the extremities. The lung and skin lesions cleared after 6 weeks of therapy with isoniazid, rifampin, and pyrazinamide, despite "resistance" of these drugs, as determined by in vitro susceptibility testing.

Petrini and coworkers[214] report a case of *M. terrae* tenosynovitis of the hand.[93] Both the tendon and tendon sheaths were swollen and chronic inflammation, granuloma formation, and necrosis were seen histologically. A case of tenosynovitis of the finger was reported[151] in a middle-aged fisherman who incurred puncture wounds while handling crappie fins.

---

tablished *M. shimoidei* as a distinct species. It differs phenotypically from members of the *M. terrae* complex by negative catalase and positive β-galactosidase reactions, and from *M. malmoense* by a positive acid phosphatase reaction. Because β-galactosidase and acid phosphatase reactions are rarely performed in clinical laboratories, species identification based on phenotypic properties may be difficult to establish.

Additional clinical cases have been reported since the index case just cited. *M. shimoidei* was the cause of pulmonary infections in patients living in Australia and in Germany,[100] the latter case complicating longstanding silicosis.[304] Initial therapy with isoniazid, propionamide, and rifampin failed because the organism was both isoniazid- and rifampin-resistant; a cure was effected with a 14-day course of streptomycin and isoniazid. Therefore, when a *Mycobacterium* species phenotypically similar to *M. terrae* complex or *M. malmoense* is recovered from respiratory specimens obtained from patients with pulmonary infections, *M. shimoidei* should be considered in the differential diagnosis, and a species identification should be attempted.

Mycobacterium malmoense. In 1977, Schroder and Juhlin[249] recovered a new *Mycobacterium* species from four patients with pulmonary disease. They called the organism *Mycobacterium malmoense*, after the Swedish city Malmo, in which these patients lived. The disease is also prevalent in Scotland.[73] The recovery of isolates has been reported from the United States: 12 strains by Good and associates,[82] in 1980, and more recently, from four patients with chronic lung disease by Albers and coworkers,[5] two of whom developed progressive disease.

LABORATORY ASPECTS. This organism typically grows slowly, some strains are seen as soon as 2 to 3 weeks of incubation at 37°C; however, some strains may require as long as 12 weeks before colonies become visible. This need for prolonged incubation beyond a period employed in most clinical laboratories may lead to underdiagnosis. Typical colonies of *M. malmoense* are grayish white, smooth, glistening, opaque, and domed. They are colorless, and exposure to light does not produce pigment. On acid-fast smears, the organisms appear coccoid or as short rods without cross-bands. The key biochemical tests by which *M. malmoense* can be identified are as follows:

1. No accumulation of niacin
2. Nitrate is not reduced to nitrite
3. Tween 80 is hydrolyzed
4. Catalase is produced at 68°C
5. Pryazinamidase is positive

Most strains are resistant to isoniazid, streptomycin, *p*-aminosalicylic acid, and rifampin but are susceptible to ethambutol (1 µg/mL) and cycloserine (16 µg/mL).

Mycobacterium haemophilum. Sompolinsky and associates[266] first recovered *M. haemophilum* in 1978 from a subcutaneous lesion of an Israeli patient with Hodgkin's disease. As the species name would indicate, *M. haemophilum* requires hemoglobin or hemin for growth. Chocolate agar, 5% sheep-blood Colombia agar, Mueller-Hinton agar with Fildes supplement, or LJ medium containing 2% ferric ammonium citrate are suitable for recovery of this organism.[323] McBride and associates[178] report success in the recovery of *M. haemophilum* using a medium containing Casman base, 5% heated sheep blood, and crystal violet. Because of the remote chance for recovery of this organism in most laboratories in the United States, use of an X factor strip in the area of inoculation on 7H10 agar, as suggested by Vadney and Hawkins,[288] offers a suitable solution in suspected cases.

As of February 1993, 22 human cases of *M. haemophilum* infection have been reported.[138] Most infections involve the skin and underlying tissue, possibly reflecting the propensity of the organism to grow at lower temperature.[153] Gupta and coworkers[93] report a case of osteomyelitis and skin infection in a patient with AIDS, successfully treated with minocycline. Kiehn and associates[138] reported four cases in immunocompromised patients, two with AIDS and two were allogeneic bone marrow transplant recipients. Because of the unique requirements for iron and lower temperature for optimum growth, these authors suggest that *M. haemophilum* should be considered when specimens from immunocompromised patients with unexplained illness fail to grow mycobacteria under routine culture conditions, or when acid-fast bacilli are seen on smear.

LABORATORY ASPECTS. Optimum growth occurs at 28° to 32°C; some strains grow at 20°C; little or no growth occurs at 37°C. Growth is stimulated by an incubation atmosphere of 10% CO_2. Typical colonies are rough or smooth after 2 to 4 weeks of incubation at 32°C on egg medium or 7H10 agar (supplemented with hemin or on the surface of which an "X-strip" has been placed, as discussed earlier). Pigment does not develop, even after exposure to light. Microscopically the cells are short, curved, and strongly acid-fast, without banding or beading. This organism is also biochemically inert, with the production of pyrazinamidase the only positive reaction among the commonly used tests to identify mycobacteria.

RAPID GROWERS

***Mycobacterium fortuitum–chelonae* Complex.** *M. fortuitum* was first described in 1938 by daCosta Cruz and was fully categorized in 1955 by Gordon and Smith.[305] *M. fortuitum* was unique among the mycobacteria by having a very rapid rate of growth (3 to 5 days). In the

---

CLINICAL CORRELATION BOX 17-13. *M. malmoense*

In the past decade, *M. malmoense* has been reported with increasing frequency as a pulmonary pathogen. More than 180 cases have been reported, most affecting patients with previous lung diseases, often middle-aged men with pneumoconioses.[334] Roentgenograms typically show a picture indistinguishable from *M. tuberculosis.* Jenkins and Tsukamura[127] describe two cases of cervical adenitis; Warren and associates[297] present a patient in the United States with chronic pulmonary disease. However, Albers and coworkers[5] believe that *M. malmoense* infections may be more common in the United States than suspected and is underreported, as some strains require 8 to 12 weeks or more of incubation before visible growth occurs, a period longer than cultures are held in most laboratories. Growth is significantly more rapid in specimens grown in BACTEC broth vials compared with delayed growth on Löwenstein-Jensen medium.[109] A broth culture medium should be employed in parallel to improve the yield of particularly slow-growing strains.[109] Recent case reports include a case of lymphadenitis in a 5-year-old girl;[217] septic cutaneous infection in a patient with hairy cell leukemia, cited by the authors as a distinct predisposing cause for mycobacterial infections;[28] and several cases of infection in HIV-positive patients.[38, 47, 315, 331] In one case,[28] the infection was successfully treated with ethambutol, cycloserine, and isoniazid, despite multiresistance in in vitro susceptibility tests. The lack of a clear correlation between in vitro susceptibility tests and clinical response was reported over a decade ago.[14] In their experience, omission of ethambutol from the therapeutic regimen, even if it showed resistance in in vitro studies, led to an unsatisfactory response.

Painful subcutaneous nodules, swellings, and ulcers that can progress into abscesses and draining fistulas are common clinical presentations. Rogers and coworkers[237] report cases of disseminated disease in patients with AIDS, in whom the skin lesions were multiple, involving the upper arm, hands, and feet (refer to this paper for excellent color photographs of these lesions). In a study of 13 patients with *M. haemophilum* infections culled from seven metropolitan hospitals in New York,[275] clinical manifestations included disseminated cutaneous lesions, bacteremia, diseases of the bones and joints, lymphatics, and lungs. The authors of this study stress that improper culture techniques may delay or even miss making a laboratory diagnosis, and that infections may be more common than realized.

Additional cases in patients with AIDS have been reported;[174] from the wrist and ankle at sites of severe tenosynovitis, and from a cutaneous lesion, lymph node, and eye of a male patient,[279] representing the first reported case of *M. haemophilum* infection in Canada (a second case of lymphadenitis in a 3-year-old Canadian girl was also included in this report). Lymphopenic patients are particularly at high risk for developing infections,[193] and renal dialysis and corticosteroid therapy were predisposing conditions of *M. haemophilum* infection,[86] raising the possibility of human-to-human transmission.

1923 edition of *Bergey's Manual*, another rapidly growing organism called *M. chelonae* was described, which had several metabolic characteristics in common with daCosta Cruz's organism. These two organisms have now been combined in the *M. fortuitum* complex. These mycobacteria are ubiquitous land and aquatic organisms that contaminate water supplies, including reagents and wash solutions used in hospitals.

LABORATORY ASPECTS. An unknown isolate can be suspected of belonging to the *M. fortuitum–chelonae* complex if growth of an acid-fast organisms is observed after 2 to 4 days of incubation. The young colonies of both species appear smooth and hemispherical, usually with a butyrous or waxy consistency. Colonies are typically nonchromogenic but may appear off-white or faintly cream-colored (see Color Plate 17-2Q). *M. fortuitum* produces branching, filamentous extensions from 1- to 2-day-old colonies on cornmeal–glycerol or Middlebrook 7H11 agar. Some strains produce rougher colonies with short aerial hyphae, best observed under a stereomicroscope. *M. chelonae* lacks these filamentous extensions.

Members of the *M. fortuitum–chelonae* complex also have the capability to grow on MacConkey agar without crystal violet. They also appear as smooth, dome-shaped colonies that may have a slight pink pigmentation (see Color Plate 17-2R). Growth may also be observed with some strains on routine 5% sheep blood agar, appearing as tiny pinpoint colonies (see Color Plate 17-2S). Microbiologists must be alert to this possibility and perform acid-fast stains in addi-

tion to Gram stains if the correct identification is to be made.

Microscopically, in acid-fast–stained preparations, the bacterial cells are generally pleomorphic, ranging from long filamentous forms to short, thick rods. Branching is absent or rudimentary at best; at times the cells may appear beaded or swollen, with nonstaining ovoid bodies present at one end. Some strains of *M. fortuitum* may grow within 48 hours on routine 5% sheep blood agar. The bacterial cells appear as short, slender, filamentous, faintly staining gram-positive bacilli (see Color Plate 17-2T). Silcox and associates[256] have identified the following characteristics for an isolate to belong to the *M. fortuitum–chelonae* complex:

1. Must be acid-fast
2. Lack of pigment production
3. Growth in less than 7 days at its optimum temperature
4. Evidence of arylsulfatase activity at 3 days
5. Grow at 28°C on special MacConkey agar (devoid of crystal violet)

Additional tests for characteristics can be performed to separate *M. fortuitum* from *M. chelonae*:

1. *M. chelonae* does not reduce nitrates (*M. fortuitum* is positive).
2. *M. chelonae* is incapable of assimilating iron from ferric ammonium citrate, a property uniquely possessed by *M. fortuitum* (see Chart 9).
3. *M. fortuitum* is susceptible to ciprofloxacin and pipemidic acid, but resistant to polymyxin B; *M. chelonae* has the opposite reactions.[270]

Subspecies identifications are possible with both organisms; however, this exercise has little clinical relevance but may be useful for certain epidemiologic applications. *M. fortuitum* exists in three biovariants: biovariant *fortuitum*, biovariant *peregrinum*, and an unnamed biovariant designated "third group"; *M. chelonae* has three subspecies, subsp. *chelonae*, subsp. *abscessus*, and an unnamed subspecies known as *M. chelonae*-like organisms.[305] The separation of these subspecies can be made biochemically (*M. fortuitum*, bv. *peregrinum* cannot assimilate mannitol; bv. *fortuitum* can, and *M. chelonei* subsp. *chelonei*; cannot grow on L-J medium containing 5% NaCl at 28°C, whereas subsp. *abscessus* can).

Mycobacterium smegmatis is another rapidly growing mycobacterium closely resembling *M. fortuitum*, differing only in its negative reaction in the 3-day arylsulfatase test, its ability to grow at 45°C, and delayed pigment production after 2 weeks incubation.[201]

Mycobacterium thermoresistible. As the species name would indicate, *M. thermoresistible* has the unique ability to grow at 52°C. This organism is potentially pathogenic; however, the infrequency of case reports indicates that exposure is either minimal or the organism is of very low virulence. Weitzman and coauthors[309] reported a case of *M. thermoresistible* human infection in an immunocompromised white female with fever, cough, and weight loss. Cavitary pulmonary disease

A wide variety of infections have been associated with *M. fortuitum* and *M. chelonae*, involving the lungs, skin, bone, central nervous system, prosthetic heart valves, and also in disseminated disease.[256, 323] Skin infections are particularly common, often evolving into draining subcutaneous abscesses.[96] Wallace and Brown[295] reviewed 100 skin, soft-tissue, or bone isolates of *M. chelonae* over a 10-year period. Cutaneous infection (53%), localized cellulitis or osteomyelitis (35%), and catheter infections (12%) were most commonly found. Underlying risk factors for disseminated infections included organ transplantation, rheumatoid arthritis, and autoimmune disorders; trauma and invasive medical procedures predisposed to localized infections. Previously, Wallace and coworkers[294] had reviewed 125 human infections caused by rapidly growing mycobacteria. *M. fortuitum* and *M. chelonae* were common isolates; 59% of these cases involved the skin (postsurgical wound infections, accidental trauma, needle injections).

A hospital ward outbreak of skin infections caused by *M. fortuitum* from exposure to a contaminated ice machine is reported;[162] contamination of an automated bronchoscope disinfection machine was another source of nosocomial infections.[74] A clinically distinctive cutaneous syndrome, associated with *M. chelonae* infections in renal transplant recipients, consisting of indolent, tender, nodular lesions on the extremities was reported.[46] Sporotrichoid spread of *M. chelonae* infections may occur in immunosuppressed patients;[194] rarely, cutaneous *M. chelonae* infections may represent the extension of disseminated disease.[60]

Several other clinical entities caused by *M. fortuitum–chelonae* complex have been recently reported. Several cases of *M. chelonae* keratitis have been reported both in soft[135] and hard[23] contact lens wearers. Most infections follow trauma, and response to topical antibiotic therapy is often not successful; therefore, keratoplasty is often required to effect a cure. It is recommended[232] that acid-fast smears of corneal scrapings be performed on any patient with chronic corneal ulcers. Patients receiving continuous ambulatory peritoneal dialysis are also at risk for acquiring *M. fortuitum/chelonae* peritonitis.[36, 63, 148, 183, 267] The collective recommendations are that mycobacterial cultures be performed on patients with peritonitis associated with continuous ambulatory peritoneal dialysis when routine cultures fail to reveal organisms and that *M. fortuitum–chelonae* be thought of when examining culture plates and Gram stains prepared from isolates recovered from peritoneal or dialysis fluids that have the appearance of poorly characterized diphtheroids. Removal of the catheter, drainage of fluid collections, and appropriate use of antimicrobial agents usually results in rapid cure.

Approximately 20 cases of pulmonary infection of varying degrees of severity caused by *M. fortuitum* have been reported.[165] *M. fortuitum*, being ubiquitous in many water sources, may colonize the respiratory tract of patients who have compromised local defense mechanisms or who are debilitated or immunocompromised, or who have long-standing chronic obstructive pulmonary disease. Invasive

respiratory tract procedures also serve as risk factors leading to infection. Burns and associates[25] studied an outbreak of positive *M. fortuitum* sputum cultures among 16 patients being treated on an alcoholism rehabilitation ward. Pulsed-field electrophoresis of large genomic DNA restriction enzyme fragments disclosed that the 16 isolates were identical. The point source was found to be a tap connected to the water line supplying the showers being used by these patients, and no further cases occurred after the showers were disconnected and decontaminated.

Several cases of *M. fortuitum–M. chelonae* catheter infections have been reported. Raad and coworkers[223] reviewed 15 infected cancer patients at M. D. Anderson Cancer Center, 9 caused by *M. fortuitum* and 6 by *M. chelonae*. Four bacteremic patients with associated catheter infections recovered after removal of the catheter and prompt institution of antibiotic therapy. Bacteremia recurred in seven patients in whom the catheter was left in place and who were treated with antibiotics alone. Patients with infections of the catheter tunnel required surgery for cure. Three cases of *M. chelonae* infections were reported[182] in febrile patients with neutropenia, which they consider a distinct risk factor for developing progressive and disseminated disease. Therefore, recovery of *M. chelonae* from respiratory specimens obtained from patients with fever and neutropenia should lead to empiric antibiotic therapy, with amikacin, cefoxitin, or erythromycin, antibiotics to which the organisms are usually susceptible.

Miscellaneous infections caused by the rapidly growing mycobacteria include an outbreak of *M. chelonae* otitis media in an office clinic setting when transfer occurred between patients from contaminated instruments,[171] aortitis following aortic valve replacement and sternal wound infection with *M. fortuitum*,[248] *M. fortuitum* endocarditis in a 54-year-old woman with chronic renal failure receiving hemodialysis,[258] a series of cardiac bypass-related infections,[309] rare cases of hepatitis and synovitis cited by Woods and Washington,[323] a retroperitoneal abscess infected with *M. chelonae* complicating a gunshot wound to the flank,[115] and a case of disseminated *M. fortuitum* infection in a patient with AIDS.[236] Two cases of *M. smegmatis* posttraumatic soft-tissue infections were reported[201] in a 21-year-old man and a 29-year-old woman who were involved in separate motor vehicle accidents. The former patient presented with a draining left leg lesion and inguinal adenopathy; the latter a chronically draining subcutaneous area of cellulitis of the posterolateral thigh. The authors also cite 12 cases of *M. smegmatis* infections reported in the literature, dispelling some doubt that this organism is nonpathogenic. Newton and Weiss[202] subsequently reported a case of aspiration pneumonia caused by *M. smegmatis*.

The rapidly growing mycobacteria vary in their in vitro susceptibilities.[114] Amikacin is predictably active; other aminoglycosides, cefoxitin, doxycycline, and erythromycin have also been selectively active. Newer agents that have shown in vitro activity against some strains include imipenem–cilastatin, amoxicillin–clavulanate and ciprofloxacin.[248]

was seen on radiographs. The organisms were recovered from sputum and a bronchoscopy specimen. Histologic examination of a lung biopsy revealed numerous microabscesses and granulomata with giant cells of the Langhans type, typical for tuberculosis. Wolfe

and Moore[318] reported a case of breast infection in a woman following augmentation mammaplasty.

The organism may grow slowly as a scotochromogen on primary isolation medium and may be mistaken for *M. gordonae*. Most strains of *M. gordonae* are urease-negative and do not grow in medium containing 6.5% sodium chloride.

SUSCEPTIBILITY TESTING

With the recent evolution of multidrug-resistant strains of *M. tuberculosis*, the need for prompt and accurate antimicrobial susceptibility testing has become a necessity. In a nationwide survey conducted by the CDC during the first quarter of 1991, *M. tuberculosis* isolates resistant to at least one antituberculous drug were found in 14.9% of cases; 3.3% of the isolates were resistant to both INH and rifampin.[31,62] In certain locales, notably New York City, isolates resistant to at least one drug, including emerging resistance to fluoroquinones[276] were recovered from 33% of cases, and the incidence of resistance to INH and rifampin was 19%. The random evolution of drug resistance of mycobacteria is independent of exposure to the agents.

The frequency of drug-resistant mutants in a culture of tubercle bacilli has been estimated to be about $1:10^5$ bacteria for INH and $1:10^6$ for streptomycin. If two drugs (i.e., INH and streptomycin) are taken together, the incidence of resistance will be the product of the two separately—$1:10^{11}$ organisms. Knowledge of the incidence of mutants becomes important because it has been determined that patients with an open pulmonary cavity may have a total bacillary population of 10^7 to 10^9 bacteria. Therefore, if these patients are treated with a single antituberculous agent, their cultures may soon show only resistant organisms to that agent, and thus treatment fails. Consequently, patients with tuberculosis must always be treated with two, or preferably three, drugs. Therefore, the failure of patients to take more than one of the drugs may lead to the rapid emergence of a specific drug-resistant tubercle bacillus (Fig. 17-3). After following a group of patients coinfected with *M. tuberculosis* and the AIDS virus, Nolan[204] has found that lack of compliance to antituberculous drug therapy is the primary reason for treatment failure. Lack of compliance may also contribute to the emergence of drug resistance.

A second principle of mycobacterial drug susceptibility testing is based on the in vitro correlation between the clinical response to an antimycobacterial agent and the result of in vitro susceptibility testing. If more than 1% of a patient's tubercle bacilli are resistant to a drug in vitro, therapy with that drug is not clinically useful. Therefore, most methods for drug susceptibility testing of mycobacteria must be capable of determining the proportion of bacilli susceptible and resistant to a given drug. When using agar dilution methods, the inoculum should be adjusted so that the number of spontaneously resistant mutants will not mislead the laboratory worker to interpret the culture as resistant. By the same token, there must be a sufficient number of colonies on the plate that the incidence of drug resistance in the range of 1% can be determined. This is best accomplished when 100 to 300 CFUs are present on each quadrant of a four-quadrant petri plate. To determine the incidence of resistance, it is usually necessary to inoculate two sets of susceptibility test

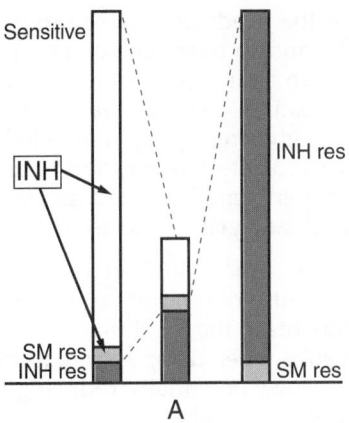

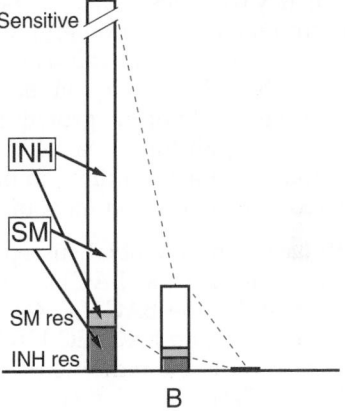

Figure 17-3.
Emergence of mycobacterial antimicrobial resistance with one- and two-drug therapy. (**A**) The patient is treated with only isoniazid (INH). Although the small number of streptomycin-resistant mutants are inhibited by the INH, the INH-resistant mutants are refractory and, in time, make up the majority of the population. This represents drug failure. (**B**) The patient is treated with both streptomycin and INH. The streptomycin-resistant mutants are inhibited by the INH, and the INH-resistant mutants are inhibited by streptomycin. Thus, neither of these mutant strains can overgrow and drug therapy is successful. (Redrawn from Crofton J: Some principles in the chemotherapy of bacterial infections. Br Med J 2:209–212, 1969)

plates, the second set with a 100-fold dilution of the inoculum used for the first set. This procedure is known as the **proportional susceptibility testing method**.

The test is performed in plastic petri dishes divided into four quadrants. Five milliliters of agar medium are placed into each quadrant, the first without any antimycobacterial agent to act as a growth control, the other three with varying concentrations of the drug to be tested. Although drugs have been incorporated in inspissated egg-based media in the past, the use of 7H10 agar as the base is currently preferred in most laboratories. The drugs to be tested are added after cooling the agar to 45°C, thereby decreasing the loss of activity that can occur during inspissation. An additional loss of drug activity may occur in egg-based media as the result of some agents binding to albumin and other proteins.

Because of the need for a more rapid turnaround time of results and to overcome certain problems inherent in in vitro agar dilution antituberculous drug susceptibility testing, use of a test based on broth medium culture is currently recommended because results are more accurate, precise, and obtained sooner than with tests performed on solid media.[118] Heifets[105] cites three disadvantages for the use of agar media:

1. The activity of some antituberculous drugs is compromised because of binding to the agar or to protein components in the medium.
2. The end results when using agar require prolonged incubation times, potentially reducing the potency of certain antimicrobials.
3. For unknown reasons, some *Mycobacterium* species lose their potency when tested in agar as opposed to growth in broth medium. For determining the endpoint of "susceptible" for *M. tuberculosis* tested in broth media, the 99% inhibition endpoint was equivalent to the failure of the growth index to increase in the test broth for at least 4 to 5 days following inoculation of a 1:100 dilution of the inoculum compared with an uninoculated broth control.

Most broth-based antimicrobial susceptibility testing for mycobacteria use the BACTEC radiometric, system, which includes the BACTEC 460 instrument fitted with a "TB hood" and BACTEC 12B bottles. The basis of this broth test is the radiometric detection of ^{14}C, released from 7H12 liquid medium containing 1-[^{14}C] palmitic acid by the metabolizing bacteria.[185] The BACTEC 460 instrument has been adapted in many laboratories to perform susceptibility tests. The principle of operation of the instrument involves aspiration of the headspace gas above the medium of an inoculated vial and quantitatively detecting the amount of radioactivity of the aspirate which, in turn, reflects the degree of growth in the vial. The headgas radioactivity counts are compared with a predetermined baseline level, and a growth index can be established. (See Chart 19 for details on the performance of this test.)

Several published studies confirm that the level of agreement between standard and radiometric susceptibility test methods exceeds 90%, at least for susceptible organisms.[161,234] Problems in the accuracy of the radiometric detection of resistant strains have been resolved by adjusting the concentration of antibiotic included in the culture vials.[101] For example, increasing the concentration of streptomycin from 4 to 6 µg/mL improved the correlation with 10 µg/mL in the 7H10 method; an adjustment of ethambutol to 2.5 µg/mL correlates with 5 µg/mL for resistant strains tested by the conventional method.[101,320] The sensitivity of the radiometric method in detecting isoniazid (INH) resistance also emerged as a problem. Hawkins and coworkers[101] determined that most discrepancies were caused by strains resistant to INH at 0.2 µg/mL but not at 0.1 µg/mL; therefore, reducing the concentration of drug in the INH vial to 0.1 µg/mL minimized the problem.

Currently, the drugs used in treating mycobacterial infections are those used primarily for classic tuberculosis, those for the mycobacteria other than *M. tubercu-*

losis (MOTT), and those used for treating leprosy.[330] The first-line drugs include isoniazid, rifampin, ethambutol, streptomycin, and pyrazinamide. The second-line drugs are *p*-aminosalicylic acid (PAS), cycloserine, ethionamide, kanamycin, amikacin, viomycin, and capreomycin.[263,269] The first-line drugs, excepting ethambutol, are considered bactericidal; the remaining included in the secondary list are to be used only when resistance to the primary drug develops. Table 17-10 lists the suggested concentrations of select drugs used for mycobacterial susceptibility testing.

Even if there is primary resistance to one drug, such as INH, treatment with the recommended triple-drug therapy provides adequate coverage. Susceptibility tests are necessary on mycobacterial isolates from patients who have shown relapses while receiving drug therapy. The probability of induced resistance in this group of patients is high. If susceptibility tests are not performed on isolates obtained from patients not previously seen by a laboratory, at least one culture should be saved for 6 months to 1 year in case the patient does not respond to therapy. Control strains for susceptibility studies should be run with each set of isolates tested. The controls should include a susceptible strain, an intermediate susceptible strain (e.g., *M. kansasii* resistant to 0.2 µg/mL INH, but susceptible to 1 µg/mL of INH), and a resistant strain. There are no standard methods for testing agents in combination. Although interpretive criteria of susceptibility and resistance are not established for testing multiple drugs in combination, the rate of killing as determined by time/kill curves may have more clinical relevance than the degree of killing.[200]

In vitro susceptibility testing of *M. avium–intracellulare* isolates using interpretative criteria applied to *M. tuberculosis* cannot be used as a guide for the treatment of patients with MAC disease.[118] MAC isolates are predictably resistant to isoniazid and pyrazinamide and are susceptible to rifampin and ethambutol only to varying degrees. All methods used for MAC organisms lack standardization, and prospective clinical tri-

---

TABLE 17-10
DRUG CONCENTRATION FOR PROPORTION METHOD OF SUSCEPTIBILITY TESTING USING VARIOUS CULTURE MEDIA

	DRUG CONCENTRATIONS (µg/mL)	
DRUG	*MIDDLEBROOK 7H10*	*LÖWENSTEIN-JENSEN*
Isoniazid	0.2, 1	0.2,1
Streptomycin	2	4
Rifampin	1	40
Ethambutol	2	2
Ethionamide	5	20
Kanamycin	5	20
Capreomycin	10	20
Cycloserine	20	30
Pyrazinamide	50	—

(McClatchy JK: In Lorian V (ed): Antibiotics in Laboratory Medicine. Baltimore, Williams & Wilkins, 1980)

als to determine the correlation between in vitro susceptibility results and clinical outcome have been lacking. Drug susceptibility profiles are more variable when testing *M. avium–intracellulare* than for *M. tuberculosis*, possibly because of a variation in colony morphology. The translucent colony variants are more resistant to antimicrobial agents than the rough strains. Also, the nonpigmented strains are more resistant than those producing pigment; however, the pigmented variants grow more rapidly and may mask the presence of slower-growing, nonpigmented strains.[273] Thus, testing of the more obvious pigmented strains may lead to a false-susceptible result.

For the susceptibility testing of rapidly growing species, the Etest (AB Biodisk North America Inc, Piscataway NJ) may be useful. Biehle and associates[18] performed Etests for 100 clinical strains of rapidly growing mycobacteria against six drugs: amikacin, cefoxitin, ciprofloxacin, clarithromycin, doxycycline, and imipenem. The Etest is an antibiotic-impregnated strip in which the test antibiotic is adsorbed to produce a concentration gradient from the top of the strip to the bottom, through at least 15-doubling dilutions. The diffusing antibiotic provides a continuous MIC gradient in the agar, which can be interpreted by reading the meniscus of growth inhibition against a calibration scale printed on the strip. These authors found an 85% agreement between the Etest results and agar dilution MICs within $\pm 1 \log^2$ and a 97% agreement at $\pm 2 \log^2$ dilutions. The rates of major and minor errors were 2.2% and 11.7%, respectively; there were no very major errors (disagreement of $\pm 3 \log^2$ dilutions or more). Interlaboratory agreement between Etest MICs determined in two separate laboratories was 81% within $\pm 1 \log^2$ dilution and 92% within $\pm 2 \log^2$ dilutions. They conclude that Etest may be an accurate and reproducible method for determining susceptibility of rapidly growing mycobacteria.

In conclusion, the radiometric susceptibility testing for *M. tuberculosis*, when performed according to well-controlled test conditions with the appropriate concentrations of drugs, is reliable for four of the front-line drugs: INH, streptomycin, ethambutol, and rifampin.[101] Susceptibility vials are commercially available for use in laboratories equipped with the BACTEC 460 instrument. Radiometric testing for secondary drugs has not yet been standardized. Readings can be made within 4 to 5 days, which is considerably shorter than the 3 to 7 weeks required using standard techniques. For a complete discussion of susceptibility tests for slow-growing nontuberculous mycobacteria and the rapidly growing *M. fortuitum–chelonae* complex of organisms, refer to Hawkins and Wallace.[101]

SHORT-COURSE THERAPY

Gosset[84] has provided a graphic illustration of the three most important types of tuberculous lesions harboring viable mycobacteria and the activity of the most important tuberculocidal agents in these lesions. It is postulated that, in a patient with pulmonary tu-

berculosis, three populations of mycobacteria are present:

1. Those located extracellularly in open cavities
2. Those located intracellularly in macrophages
3. Those in closed caseous lesions.

Organisms in each site have different metabolic activities and rates of replication.

The third characteristic listed is of considerable importance, because most mycobacteria are susceptible to the bactericidal effects of antibiotics only when they are preparing to divide. Because *M. tuberculosis* is an obligate aerobe, metabolic activity and the rate of replication will vary with the available oxygen supply. This rate may be high, as in a cavity where bacilli are undergoing rapid division, or low, with only infrequent replication of bacilli, as in closed caseous lesions. A tuberculous cavity may contain from 10^7 to 10^9 organisms actively multiplying in a neutral or slightly alkaline environment. Inasmuch as 1 of every 10^5 to 10^6 mycobacteria may be resistant to a single mycobacterial agent, the cavity may contain as many as 10^2 to 10^4 drug-resistant microorganisms. This potentially large population of drug-resistant bacilli underscores the need to use at least two bactericidal drugs for effective therapy of such lesions.

The second group of organisms found in a patient with tuberculosis is located in the phagosomes of macrophages. The intracellular environment in macrophages is acidic (pH 5.5), resulting in slow growth of mycobacteria. It has been estimated that macrophage phagosomes contain no more than a total of 10^4 to 10^5 organisms and, therefore, are not likely to contain many drug-resistant strains. Successful killing of mycobacteria in macrophages depends on the use of an antibiotic resistant to the acidic environment of macrophage phagolysosomes (e.g., pyrazinamide). This requirement excludes streptomycin and other aminoglycoside antibiotics that do not readily penetrate into macrophages and lose activity rapidly with a drop in pH.

The third population of mycobacteria present in patients with chronic tuberculosis is in the closed caseous lesion. These organisms are present in areas of necrosis where the blood supply is greatly diminished and the metabolic activity of any surviving organisms is presumably very low. There may be a total of 10^4 to 10^5 organisms in closed caseous lesions where, although the pH is neutral, multiplication is slow or intermittent.

Streptomycin, the first of the mycobactericidal agents, is most effective in killing actively multiplying extracellular organisms found in cavities. In contrast with INH and rifampin, streptomycin has little effect against organisms in closed caseous lesions or those in the acid phagosomes of macrophages. INH is active against all groups of rapidly dividing mycobacteria as well as against the slowly dividing mycobacteria found in the acid environment of macrophages. Although not as active as rifampin against organisms in the closed caseous lesions, INH does have some bactericidal effect on this group of mycobacteria. Rifampin is effective against all groups of organisms, particularly those in closed caseous lesions where the metabolic activity of the bacilli may be slow and episodic. Rifampin is the most universal antimycobacterial agent. Pyrazinamide is unique among the bactericidal agents effective against mycobacteria, in that it is active only at an acid pH and, hence, is effective only against those organisms in macrophage phagosomes.[64]

In contrast with the other agents just discussed, ethambutol is not considered to be a bactericidal drug and cannot be used with only one other drug in short-course therapy. It can, however, penetrate both the extracellular and intracellular environments of mycobacteria and can deter selection of resistant mutants. Recent studies have suggested that when ethambutol is used with three or four bactericidal drugs, it may play a role in shortening the duration of treatment.

In addition to the antituberculous drugs described in the foregoing, capreomycin, kanamycin, ethionamide, and cycloserine are also available in the United States. The first two agents are bactericidal to extracellular organisms in large cavities, whereas the second two are bacteriostatic to intracellular and extracellular organisms. However, when possible, therapy with streptomycin, isoniazid, and rifampin, pyrazinamide, or ethambutol, or a combination thereof, is preferred over the less commonly used agents.

The simplest regimen for the treatment of uncomplicated pulmonary tuberculosis is to administer INH and rifampin for a period of 9 months. Streptomycin or ethambutol may be added for the first 2 to 8 weeks. The 9-month period of therapy is in sharp contrast to the previously standard 18- to 24-month period necessary when using INH and ethambutol. The combination of INH and rifampin has introduced the concept of "short-course" therapy based on the ability of these two drugs to sterilize human tissue during a 9-month period.[73] One additional important aspect of short-course therapy is the finding that, following an initial month of therapy, both the INH and rifampin can be given twice weekly instead of daily. This schedule permits both a two thirds savings on the use of the expensive drug, rifampin, and a better compliance in patients taking the medication, particularly those considered to be unreliable. With this regimen, fewer than 3% of those who complete their course of therapy suffer a relapse. An important factor in the treatment of cavitary tuberculosis is the rapid elimination of organisms by the bactericidal action of INH and rifampin. This greatly reduces the emergence of drug-resistant organisms, resulting all too often when only a single bacterial agent is used.

AMERICAN THORACIC SOCIETY RECOMMENDATIONS

An ad hoc committee of the scientific assembly of the American Thoracic Society (ATS) on microbiology, tuberculosis, and pulmonary infections has published current recommendations for the treatment of tuberculosis in adults and children.[7] A summary of their recommendations can be found in Box 17-5.

SUMMARY

"The ultimate elimination of tuberculosis requires an organized and smoothly functioning network of primary and referral services based on cooperation between clinicians and public health officials, between health care facilities and community outreach programs, and between the private and public sectors of medical care."[7]

SUPPLEMENT: APPLICATIONS OF MOLECULAR BIOLOGY IN THE LABORATORY DIAGNOSIS OF MYCOBACTERIAL DISEASE: REVIEW OF THE CURRENT MEDICAL LITERATURE

USE OF NUCLEIC ACID PROBES IN CULTURE CONFIRMATION

Gen Probe, Inc, San Diego, California, has pioneered and brought to market single-stranded, ^{125}I-labeled DNA probes complementary to the rRNA of the following target organisms: M. tuberculosis complex, M. avium–intracellulare, M. avium, M. intracellulare (separate probes), M. kansasii, and M. gordonae. In brief, the principle of the test is that the rRNA released from the test bacterium through the action of a lysing agent, heat, and sonification, is hybridized with the single-stranded, ^{125}I-labeled DNA probe to form a stable DNA–RNA complex.[235] Following separation of the labeled complex from the unhybridized DNA, the radioactive DNA–RNA hybrids are counted. The test results are calculated as a percentage of input probe hybridization. The high levels of accuracy, specificity, and sensitivity of these probes in the culture confirmation of clinical Mycobacterium species have been authenticated in several studies.[61,136,197]

Recently, nonisotopic nucleic acid probes have become available, directed toward the identification of M. tuberculosis complex, M. avium, M. intracellulare, M. avium–intracellulare complex, and M. gordonae. These probes use an acridine ester-labeled, single-stranded DNA probe complementary to the rRNA of the target organism. The commercial kits have an extended shelf life of 6 months, extending the usefulness to a large number of laboratories. See Chart 24 for a detailed description of this procedure.

Separate studies[85,164] have confirmed that the nonisotopic acridinium–esther-labeled DNA probes, AccuProbes, commercially available from Gen-Probe (San Diego CA), for the culture confirmation of M. tuberculosis, M. avium–intracellulare, M. kansasii, and M. gordonae were equal in sensitivity and specificity to the isotopic ^{125}I-labeled probes previously on the market. The test requires 5 hours to perform; therefore, same-day reports are possible. These nonisotopic probes have a longer shelf life and are less hazardous to personnel, thus making them more available for use in clinical laboratories.

As recovery of mycobacteria in culture requires 2 to 3 weeks, several studies indicated that probe assays

BOX 17-5. ATS RECOMMENDATIONS FOR TREATMENT OF TUBERCULOSIS AND TUBERCULOSIS INFECTIONS

I. Preventive therapy for person with recent conversion of skin test.
  A. The criteria for interpretation of a positive skin test is:
    1. For adults and children with HIV infection, close contacts of infectious cases and those with fibrotic lesions on chest radiographs: a reaction of 5 mm or larger is considered positive
    2. For other at-risk adults and children, a reaction of 10 mm or larger is considered positive
    3. For persons without a defined risk factor for infection, a reaction of 15 mm or larger is considered positive. In general, persons not at risk for infection should not be skin tested
  B. For persons with a positive skin test, and any of the following risk factors, administer isoniazid for 6–12 months to decrease risk of future tuberculosis:
    1. Those with HIV infection (12-month regimen recommended)
    2. Those at risk for HIV infection with unknown HIV status
    3. Close contacts of sputum-positive persons with newly diagnosed infectious tuberculosis
    4. Persons with any of the following conditions known to increase the risk for tuberculosis:
      a. Diabetes mellitus
      b. Adrenocorticosteroid and immunosuppressive therapy
      c. Intravenous drug users
      d. Hematologic and reticuloendothelial malignancies
      e. End-stage renal disease
      f. Rapid weight loss or malnutrition
    5. In the absence of the foregoing risk factors, persons younger than 35 years with a positive skin test who belong to one or more of the following high-incidence groups should receive 6 months of prophylactic isoniazid therapy:
      a. Foreign born from a high-prevalence country
      b. Medically underserved, low-income persons from high-prevalence populations—blacks, Hispanics, Native Americans
      c. Residents of facilities for long-term care
    6. Persons older than 35 should have liver enzymes checked before commencement of therapy and monthly thereafter during the course of treatment
    7. Persons presumed to be infected with isoniazid-resistant organisms should be treated with rifampin

II. Therapy for persons with known tuberculosis by isoniazid-susceptible strains
  A. A 6-month regimen, beginning with isoniazid, rifampin, and pyrazinamide during the first 2 months, followed by isoniazid and rifampin for the following 4 months.
  B. Ethambutol should be included in the initial regimen until the results of drug susceptibility studies are available.
  C. The recommended regimen applies to both HIV-infected and noninfected persons. Therapy prolonged beyond the recommended period may be needed in HIV-infected persons, depending on the clinical and bacteriologic status.
  D. Alternatively, a 9-month regimen of isoniazid and rifampin is acceptable for persons who cannot, or should not, take pyrazinamide.
  E. Multiple drug-resistant tuberculosis poses difficult treatment problems. Treatment must be individualized based on in vitro susceptibility studies.
  F. Extrapulmonary tuberculosis should be managed according to the principles and with drug regimens outlined for pulmonary tuberculosis.
  G. A 4-month regimen of isoniazid and rifampin is acceptable therapy for adults who have active tuberculosis, but who are smear- and culture-negative, if there is little possibility of drug resistance.

III. Compliance with drug therapy is mandatory: any regimen is irrelevant if drugs do not enter the patient's body. Consider the following techniques:
  A. Ask patients routinely about compliance
  B. Periodic pill counts and urine tests may be used to monitor drug ingestion
  C. Carefully track persons who fail to return for follow-up visits
  D. Set hours of clinic visits to meet the needs of the patient
  E. Give observed treatment in the clinic, home, work place, or other location
  F. Offer incentives such as food, carfare, baby sitting services, or small gifts

could be performed on organisms recovered in broth culture, specifically in BACTEC bottles.[66,212] The technique involves aspirating 1.0 to 1.3 mL of fluid from a blood culture vial after a growth index of at least 100 is reached (GI = 999 achieves the highest level of sensitivity). The broth culture aliquot is placed into a 1.5-mL, screw-cap tube and placed into a microcentrifuge. Centrifugation at 9000 g for 5 to 7 minutes is used to concentrate the bacteria. After discarding the supernatant, the pellet is suspended in a sonication–lysate reagent, and the procedure is completed as described in the preceding paragraph. Kiehn and Edwards[136] combined the BACTEC TB system with the nucleic acid probe targeted to the rRNA of *M. avium* to rapidly identify this species when recovered from blood cultures of patients with AIDS. In a study conducted by Ellner and associates,[66] the combination of BACTEC recovery and DNA probe assay identified 89% of 176 isolates of *M. tuberculosis* and 89% of 110 isolates of *M. avium*. Most impressive was the reduction, by 5 to 7 weeks, of the time to final report compared with their conventional isolation and biochemical methods. Similarly, the rapid identification of *M. tuberculosis* was made[212] with the BACTEC TB–DNA probe combination in 83% of 64 cases, and in 92% of *M. avium* and 86% of *M. intracellulare* isolates.

In a study of 359 acid-fast–positive isolates in BACTEC 12 vials,[231] the following percentages of organisms were identified on initial direct screening of centrifuged pellets with species-specific nonisotopic, chemiluminescent AccuProbes (Gen-Probe, San Diego, CA): *M. tuberculosis* complex, 87.2%; *M. avium* complex, 78.6%; *M. kansasii*, 91.7%; and *M. gordonae*, 85.9%. The authors concluded that the lower percentage detection, when compared with previous studies, resulted in part from the centrifugal force used (3000 *g*, rather than 9,000 to 10,000 *g*). Where high-speed centrifuges are not available, extending the centrifugation time to 30 minutes may improve performance. To decrease the time of detection even more, Forbes and coworkers[71] applied PCR amplification to detect *M. tuberculosis* recovered in BACTEC 12B broth cultures. By using PCR, positive BACTEC 12B vials could be assayed when the growth index (GI) reached 10, shortening the time of incubation required for the GI to reach 100 or more. The use of PCR in this study resulted in a mean time to detection of *M. tuberculosis* of 9 days compared with 14 days by using nucleic acid probes from growth of BACTEC 12B subcultures on solid media. Kaminski and Hardy[133] suggest that the observation of cord formation in acid-fast stains performed on positive BACTEC 12B bottles can be used as a guide to immediately select the *M. tuberculosis* probe assay.

STRAIN TYPING AND DNA FINGERPRINTING SYSTEMS

The advent of molecular techniques permits strain-specific analysis of *M. tuberculosis* isolates for purposes of epidemiologic studies. The insertion sequence, IS*6110*, was specifically identified[30] as the target of a DNA probe to be used in fingerprint analysis. The IS*6110* was conserved in all of the *M. tuberculosis* strains studied, and was present in high copy numbers. The specific fingerprint technique described involved digestion of the genomic DNA with the restriction nuclease *Bam*HI, followed by separation of the fragments by agarose gel electrophoresis, transferring the DNA fragments to a nylon membrane, and hybridizing the membrane with cloned DNA segments representing two different portions of IS*6110*.

Several workers have used the insertion sequence IS*6110* as the target for conducting epidemiologic studies. Yang and associates[327] compared the fingerprinting patterns of 68 mycobacterial isolates obtained from HIV-seropositive patients with tuberculosis in the Dar es Salaam region of Tanzania, with 66 isolates recovered from HIV-negative patients living in the same region. They observed 101 different fingerprint patterns among this group of patients, with the level of diversity equal between the two. Of these isolates, 8.8% showed resistance to at least one drug; again, with no tendency to cluster within either of the groups. In a study of the IS*6110* fingerprint patterns of *M. tuberculosis* recovered from 64 patients living in French Polynesia,[282] 11 separate clusters were identified. Clustering of strains with identical patterns were identified among family groups, indicating that active transmission plays as significant a role as reactivation disease in French Polynesia. Similarly, in a subsequent study,[328] a high degree of likeness was found in IS*6110* fingerprint patterns among closely related individuals. One of the prevalent IS*6110*-defined clusters in Greenland accounted for 91% of 245 cases of tuberculosis in Denmark collected during the same period of time. These cases were traced to a group of immigrants from Greenland living in a small, defined geographic region in Denmark.

Van Soolingen and associates[290] detected 43 different IS*6110* fingerprint patterns of 153 *M. bovis* strains originating from cattle and humans in The Netherlands and Argentina, various animals in Dutch zoos, and in a wild park in Saudi Arabia, and from diseased seals and cats in Argentina. Strains presenting only a single band were characteristic for the strains recovered from cattle. Of the 20 human isolates from Argentina, 18 showed a single band, similar to that seen in the cattle strains, strongly suggesting bovine-to-human transmission. The fingerprint patterns of human *M. bovis* isolates from The Netherlands were diffuse, except for similar patterns in five patients, all living in Amsterdam and three of whom were from the same family. Cave and coworkers[29] found that the IS*6110* fragment length polymorphism patterns among six *M. bovis* isolates from one patient and 42 *M. tuberculosis* repeat isolates from 18 patients remained stable over a period of 8 months to 4.5 years and were not altered by changes in drug-resistance profiles. These cited studies illustrate the usefulness of restriction endonuclease analyses in epidemiologic studies of human and animal tuberculosis.

Several other DNA repetitive elements have been used as markers by a large number of researchers for the strain typing of *M. tuberculosis* and other *Mycobacterium* species. Space here permits only a few such applications from the plethora of research papers that have been published over the past 5 years. Hermans and coworkers[106] discovered a complex-specific mycobacterial DNA insert that hybridized specifically with DNA of *M. tuberculosis* complex strains. A nonrepetitive 158-base pair fragment of this sequence was amplified with PCR and used for the selective detection of mycobacteria from the *M. tuberculosis* complex directly in pleural fluid, bronchial washings, and biopsies, to a lower limit of sensitivity of 20 bacterial cells (about 103 cells in a sputum sample). Wiid and associates[312] used oligonucleotide GTG$_5$ as a marker for the identification of *M. tuberculosis* strains, which they found useful in cases where certain *M. tuberculosis* strains have few or no insertion elements such as IS*6110*. Friedman and colleagues[76] used PCR amplification of DNA segments located between two copies of repetitive elements IS*6110* and the polymorphic GC-rich repetitive sequence (PGRS). A PCR-amplified 439-bp segment of the 65-kDa heat-shock protein

(HSP) gene was used[271] to develop restriction fragment length polymorphism patterns of several rapidly growing *Mycobacterium* species including *M. fortuitum*, *M. chelonae*, *M. smegmatis*, and *M. mucogenicum*; the repetitive insertion sequence element IS1245 was used in a study[92] of human and animal isolates of *M. avium*; another study[238] used the repetitive insertion sequences IS1311 and IS900 as DNA probes in the restriction fragment length polymorphism of 75 clinical isolates of *M. avium*; and two markers, a newly identified 40-kDa protein (p40) and the insertion sequence IS901-IS902 were used[4] as molecular markers in the typing of 184 field strains of the *M. avium* complex.

Pulsed-field electrophoretic separation of restriction fragments generated by digestion of chromosomal DNA was used[326] in the typing of 16 strains of *M. haemophilum*, 12 of which showed similar patterns, including six from the same hospital; pulsed-field electrophoresis was also used[260] to identify several patients who were infected with more than one strain of *M. avium* complex. Random amplified polymorphic DNA, or RAPD (also referred to as arbitrary primer PCR) was used[168] in the study of several primers to determine which are most discriminatory in providing reproducible fingerprints in the strain typing of *M. tuberculosis*; RAPD was also used[1] in the typing of 15 strains of *M. tuberculosis*, with a PCR-amplified region separating the genes coding for 16S and 23S rRNA serving as the marker. These authors present molecular typing by RAPD as being more rapid and less technically demanding than most other molecular-typing methods. Also, smaller quantities of purified DNA are required than for other methods, allowing earlier analysis of young primary isolates of *M. tuberculosis*.

Kirschner and colleagues[144] have developed libraries of restriction fragment profiles of 16S rRNA subunits extracted from several *Mycobacterium* species that were previously characterized by biochemical tests or nucleic acid probes. The specific restriction endonuclease profile of an unknown *Mycobacterium* species can be easily compared with the library profile, providing a rapid nonculture means for making an accurate identification. Similarly, Avaniss-Aghajani and associates[12] developed a method for making identifications of mycobacterial isolates directly from water and clinical specimens. PCR was first used to amplify a portion of the small subunit rRNA (SSU) from 13 different species of mycobacteria, using a 5' PCR primer that carried a fluorescent label to allow detection of the amplified product. The PCR product was digested with restriction endonucleases and the sizes of the labeled restriction fragments were determined by an automated DNA sequencer. A library of 5' restriction fragment lengths produced by five different restriction endonucleases has been developed that can categorize 20 different *Mycobacterium* species. Each *Mycobacterium* species has a unique 5' restriction fragment length for each specific endonuclease, selections from which can be used to make identifications of unknown species. Advantages of this technique over rapid PCR methods include lower cost, the ability to characterize several

Mycobacterium species and to detect more than one *Mycobacterium* species in the same sample.

Strain-typing methods have also been used in the detection of drug-resistant strains of *M. tuberculosis*. In separate studies, Whelan and coworkers[311] and Felmlee and associates[68] used unique methods to detect mutations in the β-subunit of *M. tuberculosis* RNA polymerase (rpoB) to detect mutations most frequently associated with rifampin resistance. Plikaytis and coworkers,[218] in the study of an outbreak of multidrug resistant tuberculosis in New York City, used a multiplex PCR assay targeting a direct repeat of IS6110 with a 556-bp intervening sequence (NTF-1), to identify patients who were infected with what they designated the multidrug-resistant "W" strains of *M. tuberculosis*. Their assay correctly identified all 48 strain W isolates of *M. tuberculosis*, among a total of 193 strains studied. These studies indicate the degree of sophistication achieved by molecular techniques, yet the practical applications for which they are being used.

DIRECT DETECTION USING POLYMERASE CHAIN REACTION ASSAYS

Nolte and associates[206] independently developed a PCR assay for the rapid diagnosis of pulmonary tuberculosis. This paper is of interest to those who wish to learn background information relative to setting up a PCR assay. Recently, the FDA approval and commercial availability of the Amplified Mycobacterium Test (AMTD; Gen Probe, San Diego, CA), a PCR-based assay for the direct detection of mycobacterial DNA in sputum and other clinical specimens, represents a major advance in the diagnosis of tuberculosis in the United States. This is the culmination of several developmental studies and field trials over the past several years, leading to products that are standardized and designed in such a way that problems of contamination with extraneous DNA and inhibition of amplification reactions by endogenous inhibitors are minimized. These potential problems are underscored by the multilaboratory study reported by Noordhoek and coauthors.[207] They circulated among seven laboratories 200 sputum, saliva, and water samples containing known numbers of *M. bovis* BCG cells along with negative controls for PCR analysis, using the insertion sequence IS6110 as the target for DNA amplification. Each laboratory used its own protocol for pretreatment, DNA extraction, and detection of the amplification product. High levels of false-positive PCR results were found among the participating laboratories, ranging from 3% to 20% (with an extreme of 77% in one laboratory). This relatively poor performance resulted from lack of monitoring of each step of the procedure and underscores the necessity for careful quality control during all stages of the assay.

Even the availability of a commercial product does not preclude that users will encounter problems in implementation and use of the test. Laboratory directors and supervisors who elect to implement this test for the direct detection of mycobacteria in clinical specimens must ensure that the manufacturer's recommendations are closely followed and that quality control standards are rigidly enforced. Routine recovery methods must be run in parallel for each specimen received, and the clinical aspects of each case must be closely monitored, and open channels of communication between the laboratory and primary care physicians must be maintained throughout. With all of these provisions in place, the ability to diagnose new cases of tuberculosis early will have a major impact on therapy and prevention of human-to-human transfer of disease.

One of the early field trial studies of the Gen-Probe AMTD test was published by Jonas and coauthors[129] in 1993. In a study of 758 processed sputum sediments, 119 (16%) of which were positive for *M. tuberculosis*, the Gen-Probe assay performed with a sensitivity, specificity, positive and negative predictive value of 82%, 99%, 97%, and 96%, respectively, which were comparable with the results derived from culture and better than from smear analysis. It is beyond the scope of this text to review the dozen or so published works cited in that paper recognizing the contributions made by other researchers in the evolution of PCR applications to direct testing of specimens for mycobacteria. Subsequent studies determining the performance of AMTD have been published.[20,186,216] Vuorinen and associates[292] also conducted studies, comparing the performance of the Gen-Probe product with the Roche Amplicor *Mycobacterium tuberculosis* Test, a product that has been used extensively in Europe and still awaits FDA approval for use in the United States.

Miller and coworkers[186] performed a retrospective evaluation of three separate respiratory specimens from each of 250 patients using the AMTD, comparing the results with those of microscopy, culture, and patient chart review. Of these patients, 198 (from whom 594 specimens were collected), were negative for *M. tuberculosis* by culture and clinical criteria, and 52 were positive (156 specimens). The overall specificity of the AMTD was 98.5%. Of the 156 specimens obtained from the patients with tuberculosis, organisms were recovered from 142 (91%), acid-fast microscopy was positive for 105 (67.3%), and the AMTD was positive for 142 (91%). When all three specimens from each patient were tested, AMTD found all 52 patients positive for tuberculosis. In a study of 938 respiratory specimens, Pfyffer and associates[216] found that the AMTD test performed with a sensitivity of 93.9%, a specificity of 97.6%, a positive predictive value of 80.7%, and a negative predictive value of 99.3% after resolution of discrepant results by chart review. These authors conclude that the AMTD is highly sensitive and specific in detecting *M. tuberculosis* complex organisms within a few hours. The results of another study[20] were less encouraging. Of 617 respiratory tract specimens, 590 were culture- and AMTD-negative. Twenty-one cultures (3.4%) yielded *M. tuberculosis*; of these, 15 (71.4%) were detected by AMTD and six were missed. *M. tuberculosis* did not grow in culture from six AMTD-positive specimens (28.6%), obtained from three patients under treatment for tuberculosis. Thus, the sensitivity, specificity, negative and positive predictive values for AMTD were 71.4%, 99%, 99%, and 71.4%, respectively.

The test was judged to be easy to perform and highly specific by these authors, but wanting in sensitivity. They suggest that inclusion of an internal amplification control may be helpful.

Vuorinen and associates[292] tested 256 respiratory specimens obtained from 243 patients for the presence of *M. tuberculosis* complex with both the AMTD and PCR Roche Amplicor *Mycobacterium tuberculosis* Test (Amplicor PCR). When compared with the results of culture performed in parallel, the sensitivities of staining, AMTD and Amplicor PCR were 80.8%, 84.6%, and 84.6%, respectively. The specificities for these three tests were 99.1%, 98.7%, and 99.1%, respectively. The conclusions of these authors were that both nucleic acid amplification methods were rapid, sensitive, and specific for the detection of *M. tuberculosis* in respiratory specimens. Ichiyama and associates,[120] in a parallel study of 422 sputum samples obtained from 170 patients with mycobacterial infections, also found that the AMTD system and the AMPLICOR Mycobacterium system performed equally well, with agreement between the two of 98.7%.

D'Amato and colleagues[52] tested the Roche Amplicor test on 985 specimens from 372 patients. The sensitivity, specificity, and positive and negative predictive values compared with culture and clinical diagnosis were 66.7%, 99.6%, 91.7%, and 97.7%, respectively, comparable with culture results. The authors cite the great advantage of having test results available approximately 6.5 hours after the specimen arrived in the laboratory. Wobeser and coworkers[317] found that the Amplicor PCR assay performed with sensitivity, specificity, positive and negative predictive values of 79%, 99%, 93%, and 98%, respectively, in a study of 1480 clinical specimens obtained from 1155 patients. In smear-positive specimens, the sensitivity was 98% versus 59% for smear-negative specimens. The sensitivity and specificity of specimens demonstrating a positive growth index on the BACTEC 460 system were 98% and 100%, respectively. Delacourt and associates,[54] in a study of 68 children with various stages of tuberculosis, found that PCR was positive in 83.3% of 199 specimens obtained from children with active disease, but also in 38.9% of children without symptoms. The latter group may require renewed or continuation of therapy.

The Amplified Q-beta Replicase technique has also been used by several workers for the direct detection of *Mycobacterium* species. This method is based on reversible target capture (RTC) of *M. tuberculosis* 23S rRNA followed by Q-beta amplification of a replicable RNHA detector molecule. The details of this test can be found in the publications by Shah and coauthors.[251,252] They tested the digestion pellets obtained from 261 respiratory specimens, 34 of which were positive for *M. tuberculosis* (13%). The sensitivity, specificity, and positive and negative predictive values were 97.1%, 96.5%, 80.5%, and 99.5%, respectively, compared with culture. In a parallel study,[251] they tested spiked human sputum specimens and found that high levels of other mycobacterial rRNA organisms, including *M. avium* and *M. gordonae*, did not interfere with the sensitivity of the test. In a study of serial dilutions of *M. tuberculosis* cultures spiked into sputum and subjected to NALC–NaOH digestion and decontamination, An and associates[8] not only found that the Q-beta replicate assay was more sensitive than the PCR assay in the detection of mycobacteria (0.5 versus 5.0 CFU, respectively) but also that the assay was unaffected by inhibitors found in sputum that tend to compromise PCR amplification. Kulski and coworkers,[156] using multiplex PCR technique, were able to detect 38 *M. avium* and 2 *M. intracellulare* isolates from AIDS patients by direct testing of blood culture fluids, out of a total of 41 positive cultures.

These applications again highlight the potential for shortening to hours, rather than days and weeks, the detection and identification of Mycobacterium species directly in a variety of clinical specimens. Those working in molecular diagnostics have an interesting and bright future and the day may well come when the tedious and often marginally accurate species identifications described in some detail in this chapter will be relegated to the dust bins of antiquity.

REFERENCES

1. ABED Y, DAVIN-REGLI A, BOLLET C, DE MICCO P: Efficient discrimination of *Mycobacterium tuberculosis* strains by 16S–23S spacer region-based random amplified polymorphic DNA analysis. J Clin Microbiol 33:1418–1420, 1995
2. AGINS BD, BERMAN DS, SPICEHANDLER D, ET AL: Effect of combined therapy with ansamycin, clofazimine, ethambutol, and isoniazid for *Mycobacterium avium* infection in patients with AIDS. J Infect Dis 159:784–787, 1989
3. AGY MB, WALLIS CK, PLORDE JJ, ET AL: Evaluation of four mycobacterial blood culture media: BACTEC 13A, Isolator/BACTEC 12B, Isolator/Middlebrook agar and biphasic medium. Diagn Microbiol Infect Dis 12:303–308, 1989
4. AHRENS P, GIESE SB, KAUASEN J, INGLIS NF: Two markers, IS901-IS902 and p40, identified by PCR and by using monoclonal antibodies in *Mycobacterium avium* strains. J Clin Microbiol 33:1049–1053, 1995
5. ALBERS WM, CHANDLER KW, SOLOMON DA, GOLDMAN AL: Pulmonary disease caused by *Mycobacterium malmoense*. Am Rev Respir Dis 135:1375–1378, 1987
6. ALLAND D, KALKUT GE, MOSS AR, ET AL: Transmission of tuberculosis in New York City. An analysis by DNA fingerprinting and conventional epidemiologic methods. N Engl J Med 330:1710–1716, 1994
7. AMERICAN THORACIC SOCIETY: Ad Hoc Committee of the Scientific Assembly on Microbiology, Tuberculosis, and Pulmonary Infections: Treatment of tuberculosis and tuberculosis infection in adults and children. Clin Infect Dis 21:9–27, 1995
8. AN Q, BUXTON D, HENDRICKS A, ET AL: Comparison of amplified Q beta replicase and PCR assays for detection of *Mycobacterium tuberculosis*. J Clin Microbiol 33:860–867, 1995
9. ARONSON JD: Spontaneous tuberculosis in salt water fish. J Infect Dis 39:315–320, 1926
10. AUBREY M, FAM AG: A case of clinically unsuspected *Mycobacterium marinum* infection. Arthritis Rheum 30:1317–1318, 1987
11. AUSINA V, BARRIO J, LUGUIN M, ET AL: *Mycobacterium xenopi* infections in AIDS. Ann Intern Med 109:927–928, 1988
12. AVANISS-AGHAJANI E, JONES K, HOLTZMAN A, ET AL: Molecular technique for rapid identification of mycobacteria. J Clin Microbiol 34:98–102, 1996
13. BAMBERGER DM, DRIKS MR, GUPTA MR, ET AL: *Mycobacterium kansasii* among patients infected with human immunodeficiency virus in Kansas City. Clin Infect Dis 18:395–400, 1994
14. BANKS J, JENKINS PA, SMITH AP: Pulmonary infection with *Mycobacterium malmoense*—problems with treatment and diagnosis—a review of treatment and response. Tubercle 66:197–203, 1985
15. BECKMAN EN, PANKEY GA, MCFARLAND GB: The histopathology of *Mycobacterium marinum* synovitis. Am J Clin Pathol 83:457–462, 1985
16. BERLIN OG, ZAKOWSKI P, BRUCKNER DA, JOHNSON BL JR: New biphasic culture system for isolation of mycobacteria from blood cultures of patients with the acquired immunodeficiency syndrome. J Clin Microbiol 20:572–574, 1984
17. BERMAN SM, KIM RC, HAGHIGHAT D, ET AL: *Mycobacterium genavense* infection presenting as a solitary brain mass in a patient with AIDS: case report and review. Clin Infect Dis 19:1152–1154, 1994
18. BIEHLE JR, CAVALIERI SJ, SAUBOLLE MA, GETSINGER LJ: Evaluation of Etest for susceptibility testing of rapidly growing mycobacteria. J Clin Microbiol 33:1760–1764, 1995
19. BLACKLOCK ZM: *Mycobacterium asiaticum* as a potential pulmonary pathogen for humans: a clinical and bacteriological review of 5 cases. Am Rev Respir Dis 127:241–244, 1983
20. BODMER T, GURTNER A, SCHOPFER K, MATTER L: Screening of respiratory tract specimens for the presence of *Mycobacterium tuberculosis* by using the Gen-Probe Amplified *Mycobacterium tuberculosis* Direct Test. J Clin Microbiol 32:1483–1487, 1994
21. BOETTGER EC, TESKE A, KIRSCHNER P, ET AL: Disseminated "*Mycobacterium genavense*" infection in patients with AIDS. Lancet 340:76–80, 1992
22. BOUZA E, DIAZ-LOPEZ MD, MORENO S, ET AL: *Mycobacterium tuberculosis* bacteremia in patients with and without human immunodeficiency virus infection. Arch Intern Med 153:496–500, 1993
23. BROADWAY DC, KERR-MUIR MG, EYKYN SJ, PAMBAKIAN H: *Mycobacterium chelonei* keratitis: a case report and review of previously reported cases. Eye 8:134–142, 1994
24. BROOKS RW, PARKER BC, GRUFT H, FALKINGHAM JO 3RD: Epidemiology of infection by nontuberculous mycobacteria. V. Numbers of eastern United States soils and correlation with soil characteristics. Am Rev Respir Dis 130:630–633, 1983

25. BURNS DN, WALLACE RJ JR, SCHULTZ ME, ET AL: Nosocomial outbreak of respiratory tract colonization with *Mycobacterium fortuitum*: demonstration of the usefulness of pulsed-field gel electrophoresis in an epidemiologic investigation. Am Rev Resp Dis 144:1153–1159, 1991

26. BUTLER WR, O'CONNOR SP, YAKRUS MA, GROSS WM: Cross-reactivity of genetic probe for detection of *Mycobacterium tuberculosis* with newly described species *Mycobacterium celatum*. J Clin Microbiol 32:536–538, 1994

27. CAGE GD: Direct identification of *Mycobacterium* species in BACTEC 7H12B medium by high-performance liquid chromatography. J Clin Microbiol 32:521–524, 1994

28. CASTOR B, JUHLIN I, HENRIQUES B: Septic cutaneous lesions caused by *Mycobacterium malmoense* in a patient with hairy cell leukemia. Eur J Clin Microbiol Infect Dis 13:145–148, 1994

29. CAVE MD, EISENACH KD, MCDERMOTT PF, ET AL: IS*6110*: conservation of sequence in the *Mycobacterium tuberculosis* complex and its utilization in DNA fingerprinting. Mol Cell Probes 5:73–80, 1991

30. CAVE MD, EISENACH KD, TEMPLETON G: Stability of DNA fingerprint pattern produced with IS*6110* in strains of *Mycobacterium tuberculosis*. J Clin Microbiol 32:262–266, 1994

31. CENTERS FOR DISEASE CONTROL: National MDR-TB Task Force, national action plan to combat muiltidrug-resistant tuberculosis. MMWR 41:1–48, 1993

32. CENTERS FOR DISEASE CONTROL: Advisory Council for the Elimination of Tuberculosis: screening for tuberculosis and tuberculosis infection in high-risk populations. MMWR 44(RR-11), 1995

33. CHIN DP, HOPEWELL PC, YAJKO DM, ET AL: *Mycobacterium avium* complex in the respiratory or gastrointestinal tract and the risk of *M. avium* complex bacteremia in patients with human immunodeficiency virus infection. J Infect Dis 169:289–295, 1994

34. CHIODINI RJ: Crohn's disease and the mycobacterioses: a review and comparison of two disease entities. Clin Microbiol Rev 2:90–117, 1989

35. CHIODINI RJ, VAN KRUININGEN HJ, MERKAL RS, ET AL: Characteristics of an unclassified *Mycobacterium* species isolated from patients with Crohn's disease. J Clin Microbiol 20:966–971, 1984

36. CHOI CW, CHA DR, KWON YJ, ET AL: *Mycobacterium fortuitum* peritonitis associated with continuous ambulatory peritoneal dialysis. Korean J Intern Med 8:25–27, 1993

37. CHOW SP, IP FK, LAU JHK, ET AL: *Mycobacterium marinum* infection of the hand and wrists. J Bone Joint Surg 679A:1161–1168, 1987

38. CLAYDON EJ, COKER RJ, HARRIS JR: *Mycobacterium malmoense* infection in HIV positive patients. J Infec 23:191–194, 1991

39. COCITO C, GILOT P, COENE M, ET AL: Paratuberculosis. Clin Microbiol Rev 7:328–345, 1994

40. COHN ML, ET AL: The 7H11 medium for the culture of mycobacteria. Am Rev Respir Dis 98:295–296, 1976

41. COLLAZOS J, DIAZ F, RODRIQUEZ J, AYARZA R: Persistent lung infection due to *Mycobacterium szulgai*. Tubercle Lung Dis 74:412–413, 1993

42. CONLON CP, BRANDA HM, LUO NP, ET AL: Faecal mycobacteria and their relationship to HIV-related enteritis in Lusaka, Zambia. AIDS 3:539–541, 1989

43. CONTRERAS MA, CHEUNG OT, SANDERS DE, GOLDSTEIN RS: Pulmonary infections with nontuberculous mycobacteria. Am Rev Respir Dis 137:149–152, 1988

44. CONVILLE PS, KEISER JF, WITEBSKY FG: Comparison of three techniques for concentrating positive BACTEC 13A bottles of mycobacterial DNA probe analysis. Diagn Microbiol Infect Dis 12:309–313, 1989

45. CONVILLE PS, WITEBSKY FG: Inter-bottle transfer of mycobacteria by the BACTEC 460. Diagn Microbiol Infect Dis 12:401–405, 1989

46. COOPER JF, LICHTENSTEIN MJ, GRAHAM BS, SCHAFFNER W: *Mycobacterium chelonae*: a cause of nodular skin lesions with a proclivity for renal transplant recipients. Am J Med 86:173–177, 1989

47. COWLING P, GLOVER S, REEVES DS: *Mycobacterium malmoense* type II bacteremia contributing to death in a patient with AIDS. Int J SID AIDS 3:445–446, 1992

48. COYLE MB, CARLSON L, WALLIS C, ET AL: Laboratory aspects of *Mycobacterium genavense*, a proposed species isolated from AIDS patients. J Clin Microbiol 30:3206–3212, 1992

49. CROWLE AJ, TSANG AY, VATTER AE, MAY MH: Comparison of 15 laboratory and patient-derived strains of *Mycobacterium avium* for ability to infect and multiply in cultured human macrophages. J Clin Microbiol 24:812–821, 1986

50. D'AMATO JJ, COLLINS MT, ROTHLAUF MV, ET AL: Detection of mycobacteria by radiometric and standard plate procedures. J Clin Microbiol 17:1066–1073, 1983

51. D'AMATO RF, ISENBERG HD, HOCHSTEIN L, ET AL: Evaluation of the Roche Septi-Check AFB system for recovery of mycobacteria. J Clin Microbiol 29:2906–2908, 1991

52. D'AMATO RF, WALLMAN AA, HOCHSTEIN LH, ET AL: Rapid diagnosis of pulmonary tuberculosis by using Roche AMPLICOR *Mycobacterium tuberculosis* PCR test. J Clin Microbiol 33:1832–1834, 1995

53. DAWSON DJ, BLACKLOCK ZM, ASHDOWN LR, BOETTGER EC: *Mycobacterium asiaticum* as the probable causative agent in a case of olecranon bursitis. J Clin Microbiol 33:1042–1043, 1995

54. DELACOURT C, POVEDA JD, CHUREAU C, ET AL: Use of polymerase chain reaction for improved diagnosis of tuberculosis in children. J Pediatr 126(5 Pt 1):703–709, 1995

55. DELAPORTE E, ALFANDARI S, PIETTE F: *Mycobacterium ulcerans* associated with infection due to the human immunodeficiency virus. Clin Infect Dis 18:839, 1994

56. DILLON J, MILLSON C, MORRIS I: *Mycobacterium kansasii* infection of the wrists and hand. Br J Rheumatol 29:150–153, 1990

57. DIXON JMS, CITHBERT EH: Isolation of tubercle bacilli from uncentrifuged sputum on pyruvic acid medium. Am Rev Respir Dis 96:119–122, 1967

58. DOERN GV, WESTERLING JA: Optimum recovery of *Mycobacterium avium* complex from blood specimens of human immunodeficiency virus-positive patients by using small volumes of isolator concentrate inoculated into BACTEC 12B bottles. J Clin Microbiol 32:2576–2577, 1994

59. DOERN GV, WESTERLING JA: Optimum recovery of *Mycobacterium avium* complex from blood specimens of human immunodeficiency virus-positive patients by using small volumes of isolator concentrate inoculated

into BACTEC 12B bottles [letter response]. J Clin Microbiol 33:784–785, 1995

60. DRABICK JJ, DUFFY PE, SAMLASKA CP, SCHERBENSKE JM: Disseminated *Mycobacterium chelonei* subspecies *chelonei* infection with cutaneous and osseous manifestations. Arch Dermatol 126:1064–1067, 1990

61. DRAKE TA, HINDLER JA, BERLIN OGW, BRUCKNER DA: Rapid identification of *Mycobacterium avium* complex in culture using DNA probes. J Clin Microbiol 25:1442–1445, 1987

62. DRIVER CR, FRIEDEN TR, BLOCH AB, ET AL: Drug resistance among tuberculosis patients, New York City, 1991 and 1992. Public Health Rep 109:632–636, 1994

63. DUNMIRE RB 3D, BREYER JA: Nontuberculous mycobacterial peritonitis during continuous ambulatory peritoneal dialysis: case report and review of diagnostic and therapeutic strategies. Am J Kidney Dis 18:126–130, 1991

64. DUTT AK, SNEAD WW: Present chemotherapy for tuberculosis. J Infect Dis 146:698–705, 1982

65. EDZKORN ET, SIGFREDO A, MCALLISTER CK, ET AL: Medical therapy of *Mycobacterium avium–intracellulare* pulmonary disease. Am Rev Respir Dis 134:442–445, 1986

66. ELLNER PD, KIEHN TE, CAMMARATA R, HOSMER M: Rapid detection and identifiction of pathogenic mycobacteria by combining radiometric and nucleic acid probe methods. J Clin Microbiol 26:1349–1352, 1988

67. FANNING A, EDWARDS S: *Mycobacterium bovis* infection in human beings in contact with elk (*Cervus elaphus*) in Alberta, Canada. Lancet 338:1253–1255, 1991

68. FELMLEE TA, LIU Q, WHELEN AC, ET AL: Genotypic detection of *Mycobacterium tuberculosis* rifampin resistance: comparison of single-strand conformation polymorphism and dideoxy fingerprinting. J Clin Microbiol 33:1617–1623, 1995

69. FIDLER HM, THURRELL W, JOHNSON NM, ET AL: Specific detection of *Mycobacterium paratuberculosis* DNA associated with granulomatous tissue in Crohn's disease. Gut 35:506–510, 1994

70. FISHER AA: Swimming pool granulomas due to *Mycobacterium marinum*: an occupational hazard of lifeguards. Cutis 41:397–398, 1988

71. FORBES BA, HICKS KE: Ability of PCR assay to identify *Mycobacterium tuberculosis* in BACTEC 12B vials. J Clin Microbiol 32:1725–1728, 1994

72. FOX W, MITCHISON DA: Short course chemotherapy of pulmonary tuberculosis. Am Rev Respir Dis 111:315–353, 1975

73. FRANCE AJ, MCLEOD DT, CALDER MA, SEATON A: *Mycobacterium malmoense* infections in Scotland: an increasing problem. Thorax 42:593–595, 1987

74. FRASER VJ, JONES M, MURRAY PR, ET AL: Contamination of flexible fiberoptic bronchoscopes with *Mycobacterium chelonae* linked to an automated bronchoscope disinfection machine. Am Rev Respir Dis 145:853–85, 1992

75. FRIEDEN TR, STERLINE R, PABLOS-MENDEZ A, ET AL: The emergence of drug-resistant tuberculosis in New York City. N Engl J Med 328:521–526, 1993

76. FRIEDMAN CR, STOECKLE MY, JOHNSON WD JR, RILEY LW: Double-repetitive-element PCR method for subtyping *Mycobacterium tuberculosis* clinical isolates. J Clin Microbiol 33:1383–1384, 1995

77. GILADI M, LEE BE, BERLIN OG, PANOSIAN CB: Peritonitis caused by *Mycobacterium kansasii* in a patient undergoing continuous ambulatory peritoneal dialysis. Am J Kidney Dis 19:497–499, 1992

78. GILL MJ, FANNING EA, CHOMYC S: Childhood lymphadenitis in a harsh northern climate, due to atypical mycobacteria. Scand J Infect Dis 19:77–83, 1987

79. GILL VJ, PARK CH, STOCK F, ET AL: Use of lysis–centrifugation (Isolator) and radiometric (BACTEC) blood culture systems for the detection of mycobacteria. J Clin Microbiol 22:543–546, 1985

80. GITNICK G, COLLINS J, BEAMAN B, ET AL: Preliminary report on isolation of mycobacteria from patients with Crohn's disease. Dig Dis Sci 34:925–932, 1989

81. GLICKMAN SE, KILBURN JO, BUTLER WR, RAMOS LS: Rapid identification of mycolic acid patterns of mycobacteria by high-performance liquid chromatography using pattern recognition software and a mycobacterium library. J Clin Microbiol 32:740–745, 1994

82. GOOD RC, SNIDER DE: Isolation of non-tuberculous mycobacteria in the United States. J Infect Dis 146:829–833, 1980

83. GOOD RC: Opportunistic pathogens in the genus *Mycobacterium*. Annu Rev Microbiol 39:347–369, 1985

84. GOSSET J: Bacteriologic basis of short course chemotherapy for tuberculosis. Clin Chest Med 1:231, 1980

85. GOTTO M, OKA S, OKUZUMI K, ET AL: Evaluation of acridinium-ester-labeled DNA probes for identification of *Mycobacterium tuberculosis* and *Mycobacterium avium–intracellulare* complex in culture. J Clin Microbiol 219:2473–2476, 1991

86. GOUBY A, BRANGER B, OULES R, RAMUZ M: Two cases of *Mycobacterium haemophilum* infections in a renal dialysis unit. J Med Microbiol 25:299–300, 1988

87. GRIFFITH DE, HARDEMAN JL, ZHANG Y, ET AL: Tuberculosis outbreak among healthcare workers in a community hospital. Am J Respir Crit Care Med 152:808–811, 1995

88. GROSS WM, HAWKINS JE: Radiometric selective inhibition tests for differentiation of *Mycobacterium tuberculosis*, *Mycobacterium bovis* and other mycobacteria. J Clin Microbiol 21:565–568, 1985

89. GROSS W, HAWKINS J, MURPHY B: *Mycobacterium xenopi* in clinical specimens. I. Water as a source of contamination [abst]. Am Rev Respir Dis 113:78, 1976

90. GRUFT H: Isolation of acid-fast bacilli from contaminated specimens. Health Lab Sci 8:79–82, 1971

91. GUERRANT GO, LAMBERT MA, MOSS CW: Gas–chromatographic analysis of mycolic acid cleavage products in mycobacteria. J Clin Microbiol 13:899–907, 1981

92. GUERRERO C, BERNASCONI C, BURKI D, ET AL: A novel insertion element from *Mycobacterium avium*, IS1245, is a specific target for analysis of strain relatedness. J Clin Microbiol 33:304–307, 1995

93. GUPTA I, KOCHER J, MILLER AJ, ET AL: *Mycobacterium haemophilum* osteomyelitis in an AIDS patient. NJ Med 89:201–202, 1992

94. HAASE G, SKOPNIK H, BATGE S, BOETTGER EC: Cervical lymphadenitis caused by *Mycobacterium celatum*. Lancet 344:1021, 1994

95. HANNA BA, WALTERS SB, KODSI SE, ET AL: Detection of *Mycobacterium tuberculosis* directly from patient specimens with the mycobacteria growth indicator tube; a new rapid method. Presented at the American Society for Microbiology Annual meeting, Las Vegas, NV, May 23–27, 1994

946 MYCOBACTERIA

96. HANSON PJV, THOMAS JM, COLLINS JV: *Mycobacterium chelonei* and abscess formation in soft tissue. Tubercle 68:297–299, 1987

97. HAWKINS CC, GOLD JWM, WHIMBEY E, ET AL: *Mycobacterium avium* complex infections in patients with the acquired immune deficiency syndrome. Ann Intern Med 105:184–188, 1986

98. HAWKINS JE: Scotochromogenic mycobacteria which appear intermediate between *Mycobacterium avium–intracellulare* and *M. scrofulaceum*. Am Rev Respir Dis 116:963–964, 1977

99. HAWKINS JE: Rapid mycobacterial susceptibility tests. Clin Microbiol Newslett 8:101–104, 1986

100. HAWKINS JE, GROSS WM: Program Abst 23rd Intersci Conf Antimicrob Agents Chemother, abst 1045, 1983

101. HAWKINS JE, WALLACE RJ JR, BROWN BA: Antibacterial susceptibility tests: mycobacteria. Balows A (ed): *Manual of Clinical Microbiology*, 5th ed, Chap 108. Washington DC, American Society for Microbiology, 1991

102. HAYMAN J: Postulated epidemiology of *Mycobacterium ulcerans* infection. Int J Epidemiol 20:1093–1098, 1991

103. HEAP BJ: *Mycobacterium simiae* as a cause of intra-abdominal disease: a case report. Tubercle 70:217–221, 1989

104. HEIFETS LB: Gen-Probe test should not be considered final in *Mycobacterium tuberculosis* identification. J Clin Microbiol 27:229, 1989

105. HEIFETS LB: Qualitative and quantitative drug susceptibility tests in mycobacteriology. Am Rev Respir Dis 137:1217–1222, 1988

106. HERMANS PWM, SCHUTTEMA ARJ, VAN SOOLSINGEN D, ET AL: Specific detection of *Mycobacterium tuberculosis* complex strains by polymerase chain reaction. J Clin Microbiol 28:1204–1213, 1990

107. HERMON-TAYLOR J, MOSS M, TIZARD M, ET AL: Molecular biology of Crohn's disease mycobacteria. Baillieres Clin Gastroenterol 4:23–42, 1990

108. HIRASUNA JD: Disseminated *Mycobacterium kansasii* infection in the acquired immunodeficiency syndrome (AIDS). Ann Intern Med 107:784, 1987

109. HOFFNER SE, HENRIQUES B, PETRINI B, KALLENIUS G: *Mycobacterium malmoense*: an easily missed pathogen. J Clin Microbiol 29:2673–2674, 1991

110. HOFFNER SE, KRATZ M, OLSSON-LILJEQUIST B, ET AL: In-vitro synergistic activity between ethambutol and fluorinated quinolones against *Mycobacterium avium* complex. J Antimicrob Chemother 24:317–324, 1989

111. HOFFNER SE, PETRINI EB, PRENNAN PG, ET AL: AIDS and *Mycobacterium avium* serovars in Sweden. Lancet 2:336–337, 1989

112. HORSBURGH CR JR, CHIN DP, YAJKO DM, ET AL: Environmental risk factors for acquisition of *Mycobacterium avium* complex in persons with human immunodeficiency virus infection. J Infect Dis 170:362–367, 1994

113. HOYT RE, BRYANT JE, GLESSNER SF, ET AL: *Mycobacterium marinum* infections in a Chesapeake Bay community. Va Med 116:467–470, 1989

114. HURST LC, AMADIO PC, BADALAMENTE MA, ET AL: *Mycobacterium marinum* infections of the hand. J Hand Surg 12:428–435, 1987

115. IDEMYOR V, CHERUBIN CE: Retroperitoneal abscess caused by *Mycobacterium chelonae* and treatment. Ann Pharmacother 27:178–179, 1993

116. IGO JD, MURTHY DP: *Mycobacterium ulcerans* infection in Papua New Guinea: correlation of clinical, histological and microbiologic features. Am J Trop Med Hyg 38:391–392, 1988

117. IMAEDA T, BROSLAWSKI G, IMAEDA S: Genomic relatedness among mycobacterial species by nonisotopic blot hybridization. Int J Syst Bacteriol 38:151–156, 1988

118. INTERLIED CB, KLEMPER CA, BERMUDEZ LEM: The *Mycobacterium avium* complex. Clin Microbiol Rev 6:266–310, 1993

119. ISENBERG HD, D'AMATO RF, HEIFETS L, ET AL: Collaborative feasibility study of a biphasic system (Roche Septi-Check AFB) for rapid detection and isolation of mycobacteria. J Clin Microbiol 129:1719–1722, 1991

120. ICHIYAMA S, IINUMA Y, TAWADA Y, ET AL: Evaluation of the Gen-Probe amplified *Mycobacterium tuberculosis* direct test and Roche PCR-Microwell plate hybridization method (Amplicor *Mycobacterium*) for direct detection of mycobacteria. J Clin Microbiol 34:130–133, 1996

121. JACOB CN, HENEIN SS, HEURICH AE, KAMHOLZ S: Nontuberculous mycobacterial infection of the central nervous system in patients with AIDS. South Med J 86:638–640 Jun.

122. JACOBSON MA, HOPEWELL PC, YAJKO DM, ET AL: Natural history of disseminated *Mycobacterium avium* complex infection in AIDS. J Infect Dis 164:994–998, 1991

123. JACOBSON MA, ISENBERG WM: *M. kansasii* diffuse pulmonary infection in a patient with acquired immune deficiency syndrome. Am J Clin Pathol 91:236–238, 1989

124. JACOBY HM, JIVAS TM, KAMINSKI DA, ET AL: *Mycobacterium xenopi* infection masquerading as pulmonary tuberculosis in two patients infected with the human immunodeficiency virus. Clin Infect Dis 20:1299–1401, 1995

125. JARIKRE LN: Case report: disseminated *Mycobacterium gordonae* infection in an immunocompromised host. Am J Med Sci 302:382–384, 1991

126. JARIKRE LN: *Mycobacterium gordonae* genitourinary disease. Genitourin Med 68:45–46, 1992

127. JENKINS PA, TSUKAMURA M: Infections with *Mycobacterium malmoense* in England and Wales. Tubercle 60:71–76, 1979

128. JEREB JA, BURWEN DR, DOOLEY SW, ET AL: Nosocomial outbreak of tuberculosis in a renal transplant unit: application of a new technique for restriction fragment length polymorphism analysis of *Mycobacterium tuberculosis* isolates. J Infect Dis 168:1219–1224, 1993

129. JONAS V, ALDEN MJ, CURRY JI, ET AL: Detection and identification of *Mycobacterium tuberculosis* directly from sputum sediments by amplification of rRNA. J Clin Microbiol 31:2410–2416, 1993

130. JONES MW, WAHID IA: *Mycobacterium marinum* infections of the hand and wrist. Results of conservative treatment in twenty-four cases. J Bone Joint Surg 70:631–632, 1988

131. JOSEPH SW, VAICHULIS EMK, HOUK VN: Lack of auramine rhodamine fluorescene of Runyon group IV mycobacteria. Am Rev Resp Dis 95:114–115, 1967

132. JOST KC JR, DUNBAR DF, BARTH SS, ET AL: Identification of *Mycobacterium tuberculosis* and *M. avium* complex directly from smear-positive sputum specimens and BACTEC 12B cultures by high-performance liquid chromatography with fluorescence detection and computer-

driven pattern recognition models. J Clin Microbiol 33:1270–1277, 1995

133. KAMINSKI DA, HARDY DJ: Selective utilization of DNA probes for identification of *Mycobacterium* species on the basis of cord formation in primary BACTEC 12B cultures. J Clin Microbiol 33:1548–1550, 1995

134. KESTLE DG, KUBICA GP: Sputum collection for cultivation of mycobacteria: an early morning specimen or the 24 to 72 hour pool? Am J Clin Pathol 48:347–351, 1967

135. KHOOSHABEH R, GRANGE JM, YATES MD, ET AL: A case report of *Mycobacterium chelonae* keratitis and a review of mycobacterial infections of the eye and orbit. Tubercle Lung Dis 75:377–382, 1994

136. KIEHN TE, EDWARDS FF: Rapid identification using a specific DNA probe of *Mycobacterium avium* complex from patients with acquired immunodeficiency syndrome. J Clin Microbiol 25:1551–1552, 1987

137. KIEHN TE, EDWARDS FF, BRANNON P, ET AL: Infections caused by *Mycobacterium avium* complex in immuno-compromised patients: diagnosis by blood culture and fecal examination, antimicrobial susceptibility tests and morphological and seroagglutination characteristics. J Clin Microbiol 21:168–173, 1985

138. KIEHN TE, WHITE M, PURSELL KG, ET AL: A cluster of four cases of *Mycobacterium haemophilum* infection. Eur J Clin Microbiol 12:114–118, 1993

139. KILBY JM, GILLIGAN PH, YANKASKAS JR, ET AL: Nontuberculous mycobacteria in adult patients with cystic fibrosis. Chest 102:70–75, 1992

140. KIM TC, ARORA NS, ALDRICH TK, ROCHESTER DF: Atypical mycobacterial infections: a clinical study of 92 patients. South Med J 74:1304–1308, 1981

141. KINSELLA JP, CULVER K, JEFFRY RB, ET AL: Otomastoiditis caused by *Mycobacterium avium–intracellulare*. Pediatr Infect Dis J 6:289–291, 1986

142. KIRIHARA JM, HILLIER SL, COYLE MB: Improved detection times for *Mycobacterium avium* complex and *Mycobacterium tuberculosis* with the BACTEC radiometric system. J Clin Microbiol 22:841–845, 1985

143. KISCHNER RA JR, PARKER BC, FALKINHAM JO 3D: Epidemiology of infection by nontuberculous mycobacteria. *Mycobacterium avium, Mycobacterium intracellulare* and *Mycobacterium scrofulaceum* in acid, brown-water swamps of the southeastern United States and their association with environmental variables. Am Rev Respir Dis 145:271–275, 1992

144. KIRSCHNER P, SPRINGER B, VOGEL U, ET AL: Genotypic identification of mycobacteria by nucleic acid sequence determination: report of a 2-year experience in a clinical laboratory. J Clin Microbiol 31:1189–2282, 1993

145. KIRSCHNER P, VOGEL U, HEIN R, BOETTGER EC: Bias of culture techniques for diagnosing mixed *Mycobacterium genavense* and *Mycobacterium avium* infection in AIDS. J Clin Microbiol 32:828–831, 1994

146. KLINE SE, HEDEMARK LL, DAVIES SF: Outbreak of tuberculosis among regular patrons of a neighborhood bar. N Engl J Med 333:222–227, 1995

147. KOCHI A: The global tuberculosis situation and the new control strategy of the World Health Orginazation. Tubercle 71:1–6, 1991

148. KOLMOS HJ, BRAHM M, BRUUN B: Peritonitis with *Mycobacterium fortuitum* in a patient on continuous ambu-latory peritoneal dialysis. Scand J Infect Dis 24:801–803, 1992

149. KRASNOW I, WAYNE LG: Comparison of methods for tuberculosis laboratory. Appl Microbiol 28:915–917, 1969

150. KRASNOW I: Sputum digestion. I. The mortality rate of tubercle bacilli in various digestion systems. Am J Clin Pathol 45:352–355, 1969

151. KREMER LB, RHAME FS, HOUSE JH: *Mycobacterium terrae* tenosynovitis. Arthritis Rheum 32:132–134, 1988

152. KRISHNER KK, KALLAY MC, NOLTE FS: Primary pulmonary infection caused by *Mycobacterium terrae* complex. Diagn Microbiol Infect Dis 11:171–175, 1988

153. KRISTJANSSON M, BIELUCH VM, BYEFF PD: *Mycobacterium haemophilum* infection in immunocompromised patients: case report and review of the literature. Rev Infect Dis 13:906–910, 1991

154. KUBICA GP: Differential identification of mycobacteria. VII. Key features for identification of clinically significant mycobacteria. Am Rev Respir Dis 107:9–21, 11987

155. KUBICA GP, ET AL: Laboratory services for mycobacterial diseases. Am Rev Respir Dis 112:783–787, 1975

156. KULSKI JK, KHINSOE C, PRYCE T, CHRISTIANSEN K: Use of a multiplex PCR to detect and identify *Mycobacterium avium* and *M. intracellulare* in blood culture fluids of AIDS patients. J Clin Microbiol 33:668–674, 1995

157. KUZE F, MITSOUKA W, CHIBA W, ET AL: Chronic pulmonary infection caused by *M. terrae* complex: a resected case. Am Rev Respir Dis 128:561–565, 1983

158. LAI KK, STOTTMEIER KD, SHERMAN IH, MCCABE WR: Mycobacterial cervical lymphadenopathy. Relation of etiologic agents to age. JAMA 251:1286–1288, 1984

159. LARRSSONS L, ODHAM G, WESTERDAHL G, OLSSON B: Diagnosis of pulmonary tuberculosis by selected ion monitoring: improved analysis of tuberculostearate in sputum using negative-ion mass spectrometry. J Clin Microbiol 25:893–896, 1987

160. LASZLO A, GILL P, HANDZEL V, ET AL: Conventional and radiometric drug susceptibility testing of *Mycobacterium tuberculosis* complex. J Clin Microbiol 18:1225–1339, 1983

161. LASZLO AP, SIDDIQUI SH: Evaluation of a rapid radiometric differentiation test for the *Mycobacterium tuberculosis* complex by selective inhibition with *p*-nitro-acetylamino-hydroxy-propiophenone. J Clin Microbiol 19:694–698, 1984

162. LAUSSUCO S, BALTSCH AL, SMITH RW, ET AL: Nosocomial *Mycobacterial fortuitum* colonization from a contaminated ice machine. Am Rev Respir Dis 138:891–894, 1988

163. LAVY A, YOSHPE-PURER Y: Isolation of *Mycobacterium simiae* from clinical specimens in Israel. Tubercle 63:279–285, 1982

164. LEBRUN L, ESPINASSE F, POVEDA JD, ET AL: Evaluation of nonradioactive DNA probes for identification of mycobacteria. J Clin Microbiol 30:2476–2478, 1992

165. LESSING MP, WALKER MM: Fatal pulmonary infection due to *Mycobacterium fortuitum*. J Clin Pathol 46:271–272, 1993

166. LEVINE B, CHAISSON RE: *Mycobacterium kansasii*: a cause of treatable pulmonary disease associated with advanced human immunodeficiency virus (HIV) infection. Ann Intern Med 114:861–868, 1991

167. LEVY-FREBAULT V, PANGON B, BURE A, ET AL: *Mycobacterium simiae* and *Mycobacterium avium–intracellulare*

mixed infection in acquired immune deficiency syndrome. J Clin Microbiol 25:154–157, 1987

168. Linton CJ, Jalal H, Leeming JP, Millar MR: Rapid discrimination of *Mycobacterium tuberculosis* strains by random amplified polymorphic DNA analysis. J Clin Microbiol 32:2169–2174, 1994

169. Lipsky BA, Gates JA, Tenover FC, et al: Factors affecting the clinical value of microscopy for acid-fast bacilli. Rev Infect Dis 6:214–222, 1984

170. London RD, Damsker B, Neibert EP, et al: *Mycobacterium gordonae*: an unusual peritoneal pathogen in a patient undergoing continuous ambulatory peritoneal dialysis. Am J Med 85:703–704, 1988

171. Lowry PW, Jarvis WR, Oberle AD, et al: *Mycobacterium chelonei* causing otitis media in an ear nose and throat practice. N Engl J Med 319:978–982, 1988

172. MacDonnel KB, Glassroth J: *Mycobacterium avium* complex and other nontuberculous mycobacteria in patients with HIV infection. Semin Respir Infect 4:123–132, 1989

173. Macher AM, Kovacs JA, Gill V, et al: Bacteremia due to *Mycobacterium intracellulare* in the acquired immunodeficiency syndrome. Ann Intern Med 99:782–785, 1983

174. Males BM, West TE, Bartholomew WR: *Mycobacterium haemophilum* infection in a patient with acquired immune deficiency syndrome. J Clin Microbiol 25:186–190, 1987

175. Maloney JM, Clark RG, Stephans DS, et al: Infections caused by *Mycobacterium szulgai* in humans. Rev Infect Dis 9:1120–1126, 1987

176. Marks J, Jenkins PA, Tsukamura M: *Mycobacterium szulgai*—a new pathogen. Tubercle 53:210–214, 1972

177. Maschek H, Gerogii A, Schmidt RE, et al: *Mycobacterium genavense*. Autopsy findings in three patients. Am J Clin Pathol 101:95–99, 1994

178. McBride JA, McBride ME, Wolf JE Jr, et al: Evaluation of commercial blood-containing media for cultivation of *Mycobacterium haemophilum*. Am J Clin Pathol 98:282–286, 1992

179. McCarter YS, Robinson A: Detection of acid-fast bacilli in concentrated primary specimen smears stained with rhodamine–auramine at room temperature and at 37 degrees C. J Clin Microbiol 32:2487–2489, 1994

180. McClatchy JK, et al: Isolation of mycobacteria from clinical specimens by use of selective 7H11 medium. Am J Clin Pathol 65:412–415, 1976

181. McFadden JJ, Butcher PD, Chiodini R, Hermon-Taylor J: Crohn's disease-isolated mycobacteria are identical to *Mycobacterium paratuberculosis*, as determined by DNA probes that distinguish between mycobacterial species. J Clin Microbiol 25:796–801, 1987

182. McWhinney PH, Yates M, Prentice HG, et al: Infection caused by *Mycobacterium chelonae*: a diagnostic and therapeutic problem in the neutropenic patient. Clin Infect Dis 14:1208–1212, 1992

183. Merlin TL, Tzamaloukas AH: *Mycobacterium chelonae* peritonitis associated with continuous ambulatory peritoneal dialysis. Am J Clin Pathol 91:717–720, 1989

184. Metchock B, Diem L: Algorithm for use of nucleic acid probes for identifying *Mycobacterium tuberculosis* from BACTEC 12B bottles. J Clin Microbiol 33:1934–1937, 1995

185. Middlebrook G, Reggiardo Z, Tigertt WD: Automatable radiometric detection of growth of *Mycobacterium tuberculosis* in selective media. Am Rev Respir Dis 115:1066–1069, 1977

186. Miller N, Hernandez SG, Cleary TJ: Evaluation of Gen-Probe Amplified *Mycobacterium tuberculosis* Direct Test and PCR for direct detection of *Mycobacterium tuberculosis* in clinical specimens. J Clin Microbiol 32:393–397, 1994

187. Millner R, Stottmeir KD, Kubica GP: Formaldehyde: a photothermal activated toxic substance produced in Middlebrook 7H10 medium. Am Rev Respir Dis 99:603–607, 1969

188. Mitchison DA, et al: A selective oleic acid albumin agar medium for tubercle bacilli. J Med Microbiol 5:165–175, 1972

189. Mizuguchi Y, Ogawa M, Odou T: Morphological changes induced by β-lactam antibiotics in *Mycobacterium avium–intracellulare* complex. Antimicrob Agents Chemother 27:541–547, 1985

190. Modilevsky T, Sattler FR, Barnes PF: Mycobacterial disease in patients with human immunodeficiency virus infection. Arch Intern Med 149:2201–2205, 1989

191. Morbidity and Mortality Weekly Report: Proportionate mortality from pulmonary tuberculosis associated with occupations—28 states, 1979–1990. MMWR 44:14–19, 1995

192. Morgan MA, Horstmeier CD, DeYoung DR: Comparison of a radiometric method (BACTEC) and conventional culture media for recovery of mycobacteria from smear negative specimens. J Clin Microbiol 18:384–388, 1983

193. Moulsdale MT, Harper JM, Thatcher GN: Infection by *Mycobacterium haemophilum*, a metabolically fastidous acid-fast bacillus. Tubercle 64:29–36, 1983

194. Murdoch ME, Leigh IM: Sporotrichoid spread of cutaneous *M. chelonei* infection. Clin Exp Dermatol 14:309–312, 1989

195. Murphy DB, Hawkins JE: Use of urease test discs in the identification of mycobacteria. J Clin Microbiol 1:465–468, 1975

196. Murray P: Mycobacterial cross-contamination with the modified BACTEC 460 TB system. Diagn Microbiol Infect Dis 14:33–35, 1991

197. Musial CE, Tice LS, Stockman L, Roberts GD: Identification of mycobacteria from culture by using the Gen-Probe rapid diagnostic system for *Mycobacterium avium* complex and *Mycobacterium tuberculosis* complex. J Clin Microbiol 26:2120–2123, 1988

198. Nardell EA, Keegan J, Cheney SA, Etkind SC: Airborne infection. Theoretical limits of protection achievable by building ventilation. Am Rev Respir Dis 144:302–306, 1991

199. Nassos PS, Yajko DM, Sanders CA, Hadley WK: Prevalence of *Mycobacterium avium* complex in respiratory specimens from AIDS and non-AIDS patients in a San Francisco Hospital. Am Rev Respir Dis 143:66–68, 1991

200. National Committee for Clinical Laboratory Standards. Methods for determining bactericidal activity of antimicrobial agents (M26P). National Committee for Clinical Laboratory Standards, Villanova PA, 1987

201. NEWTON JA, WEISS PJ, BOWLER WA, OLDFIELD EC 3RD: Soft-tissue infection due to *Mycobacterium smegmatis*: report of two cases. Clin Infect Dis 16:531–533, 1993

202. NEWTON JA, WEISS PH: Aspiration pneumonia caused by *Mycobacterium smegmatis*. Mayo Clin Proc 69:296, 1994

203. NIGHTINGALE SD, BYRD LT, SOUTHERN PM, ET AL: Incidence of *Mycobacterium avium–intracellulare* complex bacteremia in human immunodeficiency virus-positive patients. J Infect Dis 165:1082–1085, 1992

204. NOLAN CM: Failure of therapy for tuberculosis in human immunodeficiency virus infection. Am J Med Sci 304:168–173, 1992

205. NOLTE FS, METCHOCK B: *Mycobacterium*. Murray PR (ed): *Manual of Clinical Microbiology*, 6th ed, Chap 31. Washington DC, ASM Press, 1995

206. NOLTE FS, METCHOCK B, MCGOWAN JE JR, ET AL: Direct detection of *Mycobacterium tuberculosis* in sputum by polymerase chain reaction and DNA hybridization. J Clin Microbiol 31:1777–1782, 1993

207. NOORDHOEK GT, KOLK AH, BJUNE G, ET AL: Sensitivity and specificity of PCR for detection of *Mycobacterium tuberculosis*: a blind comparison study among seven laboratories. J Clin Microbiol 32:277–284, 1994

208. PATTERSON KV, MCDONALD CL, MILLER BF, CHAPIN KC: Use of UV ParaLens adapter for detection of acid-fast organisms. J Clin Microbiol 33:239–241, 1995

209. PERCHERE M, OPRAVIL M, WALD A, ET AL: Clinical and epidemiologic features of infection with *Mycobacterium genavense*. Swiss HIV Cohort Study. Arch Intern Med 155:400–404, 1995

210. PETERS EJ, MORICE R: Miliary pulmonary infection caused by *Mycobacterium terrae* in an autologous bone marrow transplant patient. Chest 100:1449–1450, 1991

211. PETERS M, SCHURMANN D, MAYR AC, ET AL: Immunosuppression and mycobacteria other than *Mycobacterium tuberculosis*: results from patients with and without HIV infection. Epidemiol Infect 103:293–300, 1989

212. PETERSON EM, LU R, FLOYD C, ET AL: Direct identification of *Mycobacterium tuberculosis*, *Mycobacterum avium*, and *Mycobacterium intracellulare* from amplified primary cultures in BACTEC media using DNA probes. J Clin Microbiol 27:1543–1547, 1989

213. PETRAN EL, VERA HD: Media for selective isolation of mycobacteria. Health Lab Sci 8:2245, 1971

214. PETRINI B, SVARTENGREN G, HOFFNER SE, ET AL: Tenosynovitis of the hand caused by *Mycobacterium terrae*. Eur J Clin Microbiol 8:722–724, 1989

215. PFALLER MA: Application of new technology to the detection, identification, and antimicrobial susceptibility testing of mycobacteria. Am J Clin Pathol 101:329–337, 1994

216. PFYFFER GE, KISSLING P, WIRTH R, WEBER R: Direct detection of *Mycobacterium tuberculosis* complex in respiratory specimens by a target-amplified test system. J Clin Microbiol 32:918–923, 1994

217. PIERSIMONI C, FELICI L, PENATI V, LACCHINI C: *Mycobacterium malmoense* in Italy. Tubercle Lung Dis 76:171–172, 1995

218. PLIKAYTIS BB, MARDEN JL, CRAWFORD JT, ET AL: Multiplex PCR assay specific for multidrug-resistant strain W of *Mycobacterium tuberculosis*. J Clin Microbiol 32:1542–1546, 1994

219. POLLOCK HM, WIEMAN EJ: Smear results in the diagnosis of mycobacteriosis using blue light fluorescence microscopy. J Clin Microbiol 5:329–331, 1977

220. PRANTERA C, BOTHAMLEY G, LEVENSTEIN S, ET AL: Crohn's disease and mycobacteria: two cases of Crohn's disease with high anti-mycobacterial antibody levels cured by dapsone therapy. Biomed Pharmacother 43:295–299, 1989

221. PRISSICK FH, MASON AM: Cervical lymphadenitis in children caused by chromogenic mycobacteria. Can Med Assoc J 75:798–803, 1956

222. PROSSER AJ: Spinal infection with *Mycobacterium xenopi*. Tubercle 67:229–232, 1986

223. RAAD II, VARTIVARIAN S, KHAN A, BODEY GP: Catheter-related infections caused by the *Mycobacterium fortuitum* complex: 15 cases and review. Rev Infect Dis 13:1120–1125, 1991

224. RADFORD AJ: *Mycobacterium ulcerans* in Australia. Aust NZ J Med 5:162–169, 1975

225. RADHIKA S, GUPTA SK, CHAKRABARTI A, ET AL: Role of culture for mycobacteria in fine-needle aspiration diagnosis of tuberculous lymphadenitis. Diagn Cytopathol 5:260–262, 1989

226. RAHMAN MA, PHONGSATHORN V, HUGHES T, BIELAWSKA C: Spinal infection by *Mycobacterium xenopi* in a non-immunosuppressed patient. Tubercle Lung Dis 73:392–395, 1992

227. RASTOGI N, FREHEL C, RYTER A, ET AL: Multiple drug resistance in *Mycobacterium avium*: is the wall architecture responsible for the exclusion of antimicrobial agents? Antimicrob Agents Chemother 20:666–677, 1980

228. RATNAM SM, MARCH SB: Effect of relative centrifugal force and centrifugation time on sedimentation of mycobacteria in clinical specimens. J Clin Microbiol 23:582–585, 1986

229. RATNAM SM, STEAD FA, HOWES M: Simplified acetylcysteine–alkali digestion–decontamination procedure for isolation of mycobacteria from clinical specimens. J Clin Microbiol 25:1428–1432, 1987

230. REINER E: Identification of bacterial strains by pyrolysis–gas–liquid chromatography. Nature 206:1272–1274, 1965

231. REISNER BS, GATSON AM, WOODS GL: Use of Gen-Probe AccuProbes to identify *Mycobacterium avium* complex, *Mycobacterium tuberculosis* complex, *Mycobacterium kansasii*, and *Mycobacterium gordonae* directly from BACTEC TB broth cultures. J Clin Microbiol 32:2995–2998, 1994

232. RICHARDSON P, CRAWFORD GJ, SMITH DW, XANTHIS CP: *Mycobacterium chelonae* keratitis. Aust NZ J Ophthalmol 17:195–196, 1989

233. RICKMAN TW, MOYER NP: Increased sensitivity of acid fast smears. J Clin Microbiol 11:618–620, 1980

234. ROBERTS GD, GOODMAN NL, HEIFETS L, ET AL: Evaluation of the radiometric method for recovery of mycobacteria and drug susceptibility testing of *Mycobacterium tuberculosis* from acid-fast smear positive specimens. J Clin Microbiol 18:689–696, 1983

235. ROBERTS GD, KONEMAN EW, KIM YK: *Mycobacterium*. Balows A (ed): *Manual of Clinical Microbiology*, 5th ed, Chap 34. Washington DC, American Society for Microbiology, 1991

236. RODRIQUEZ-BARRADAS MC, CLARRIDGE J, DAROUICHE R: Disseminated *Mycobacterium fortuitum* disease in an AIDS patient. Am J Med 93:473-474, 1992

237. ROGERS PL, WALKER RE, LANE HC, ET AL: Disseminated *Mycobacterium haemophilum* infection in two patients with the acquired immunodeficiency syndrome. Am J Med 84:640-642, 1988

238. ROIS MP, PALENQUE E, GUERRERO C, GARCIA MJ: Use of restriction fragment length polymorphism as a genetic marker for typing *Mycobacterium avium* strains. J Clin Microbiol 33:1289-1391, 1995

239. ROSE HD, DORFF GJ, LAUWASSER M, ET AL: Pulmonary and disseminated *Mycobacterium simiae* infection in humans. Am Rev Respir Dis 126:1110-1113, 1982

240. RUNYON EH: Identification of mycobacterial pathogens utilizing colony characteristics. Am J Clin Pathol 54:578-586, 1970

241. SAITO H, TOMIOKA H: Susceptibilities of transparent, opaque, and rough colonial variants of *Mycobacterium avium* complex to various fatty acids. Antimicrob Agents Chemother 32:400-402, 1988

242. SALFINGER M, MORRIS AJ: The role of the microbiology laboratory in diagnosing mycobacterial diseases. Am J Clin Pathol 101(suppl 1):S6-13, 1994

243. SALFINGER M: Role of the laboratory in evaluating patients with mycobacterial disease. Clin Microbiol Newslett 17:108-111, 1995

244. SANDERS WE JR, HOROWITZ EA: Other mycobacteria species. Mandell GL, Douglas RG Jr, Bennett JE (eds): *Principles and Practice of Infectious Diseases*, 3rd ed, Chap 231. New York, Churchill Livingstone, 1990

245. SANDERSON JD, MOSS MT, TIOZARD ML, HERMON-TAYLOR: *Mycobacterium paratuberculosis* DNA in Crohn's disease tissue. Gut 33:890-896, 1992

246. SCHAEFER WB, DAVIS CL, COHN ML: Pathogenicity of transparent, opaque and rough variants of *Mycobacterium avium* in chickens and mice. Am Rev Respir Dis 102:499-506, 1970

247. SCHERER R, SABLE R, SONNENBERG M, ET AL: Disseminated infection with *Mycobacterium kansasii* in the acquired immunodeficiency syndrome. Ann Intern Med 105:710-712, 1986

248. SCHLOSSBERG D, AARON T: Aortitis caused by *Mycobacterium fortuitum*. Arch Intern Med 151:1010-1011, 1991

249. SCHRODER KH, JUHLIN I: *Mycobacterium malmoense* sp. nov. Int J Syst Bacteriol 27:241-246, 1977

250. SEWELL DL, RASHAD AL, ROURKE WJ, ET AL: Comparison of the Septi-Chek AFB and BACTEC systems and conventional culture for recovery of mycobacteria. J Clin Microbiol 31:2689-2691, 1993

250a. SHAFER RW, SIERRA MF: *Mycobacterium xenopi, Mycobacterium fortuitum, Mycobacterium kansasii*, and other nontuberculous mycobacteria in an area of endemicity for AIDS. Clin Infect Dis 15:161-162, 1992

251. SHAH JS, LIU J, BUXTON D, ET AL: Detection of *Mycobacterium tuberculosis* directly from spiked human sputum by Q-beta replicase-amplified assay. J Clin Microbiol 33:322-328, 1995

252. SHAH JS, LIU J, BUXTON D, ET AL: Q-beta replicase-amplified assay for detection of *Mycobacterium tuberculosis* directly from clinical specimens. J Clin Microbiol 33:1435-1441, 1995

253. SHAH RR, DYE WE: The use of dithiolthreitol to replace N-acetyl-L-cysteine for routine sputum digestion–decontamination for the culture of mycobacteria. Am Rev Respir Dis 94:454, 1966

254. SHINNICK TM, KING CH, QUINN FD: Molecular biology, virulence, and pathogenicity of mycobacteria. Am J Med Sci 309:92-98, 1995

255. SIDDIQUI SH, LIBONATI JP, MIDDLEBROOK G: Evaluation of a rapid radiometric method for drug susceptibility testing of *Mycobacterium tuberculosis*. J Clin Microbiol 13:908-912, 1981

256. SILCOX VA, GOOD RA, FLOYD MM: Identification of clinically significant *Mycobacterium fortuitum* complex isolates. J Clin Microbiol 14:686-691, 1981

257. SIMOR WE, SALIT IE, VELLEND H: Role of *Mycobacterium xenopi* in human disease. Am Rev Respir Dis 129:435-438, 1984

258. SINGH M, BOFINGER A, CAVE G, BOYLE P: *Mycobacterium fortuitum* endocarditis in a patient with chronic renal failure on hemodialysis. Pathology 24:197-200, 1992

259. SLOSAREK M, KUBIN M, JARESOVA M: Water-borne household infections due to *Mycobacterium xenopi*. Central Eur J Public Health 1:78-80, 1993

260. SLUTSKY AM, ARBEIT RD, BARBER TW, ET AL: Polyclonal infections due to *Mycobacterium avium* complex in patients with AIDS detected by pulsed-field gel electrophoresis of sequential clinical isolates. J Clin Microbiol 32:1773-1778, 1994

261. SMITH RL, YEW K, BERKOWITZ KA, ARANDA CP: Factors affecting the yield of acid-fast sputum smears in patients with HIV and tuberculosis. Chest 106:684-696, 1994

262. SMITHWICK RW, ET AL: Use of cetylpyridium chloride and sodium chloride for the decontamination of sputum specimens that are transported to the laboratory for the isolation of *Mycobacterium tuberculosis*. J Clin Microbiol 1:411-413, 1975

263. SNIDER DE JR, COHN DL, DAVIDSON PT, ET AL: Standard therapy for tuberculosis. Chest 87(suppl):S117-S124, 1985

264. SOMMERS HM: Special Mycobacterial Survey, Skokie, College of American Pathologists, 1976

265. SOMMERS HM, GOOD RC: *Mycobacterium*. Lennette EH (ed): *Manual of Clinical Microbiology*, 4th ed, Chap 22. Washington DC, American Society for Microbiology, 1985

266. SOMPOLINSKY D, LAGZIEL A, NAVEH D, YANKILEVITZ T: *Mycobacterium haemophilum* sp nov, a new pathogen of humans. Int J Syst Bacteriol 28:67-75, 1978

267. SORIANO F, RODRIQUEZ-TUDELA JL, GOMEZ-GARCES JL, VELO M: Two possibly related cases of *Mycobacterium fortuitum* peritonitis associated with continuous ambulatory peritoneal dialysis. Eur J Clin Microbiol Infect Dis 8:895-897, 1989

268. STAHL DA, URBANCE JW: The division between fast- and slow-growing species corresponds to natural relationships among the mycobacteria. J Bacteriol 172:116-124, 1990

269. STEAD WW, DUTT: Chemotherapy for tuberculosis today. Am Rev Respir Dis 125(suppl 3):94-101, 1982

270. STEELE LC, WALLACE RJ JR: Ability of ciprofloxacin but not pipemidic acid to differentiate all three biovariants

of *Mycabacterium fortuitum* from *Mycobacterium chelonae*. J Clin Microbiol 25:456–457, 1987

271. STEINGRUBE VA, GIBSON JL, BROWN BA, ET AL: PCR amplification and restriction endonuclease analysis of a 65-kilodalton heat shock protein gene sequence for taxonomic separation of rapidly growing mycobacteria. J Clin Microbiol 33:149–153, 1995

272. STONE BL, COHN DL, KANE MS, ET AL: Utility of paired blood cultures and smears in diagnosis of disseminated *Mycobacterium avium* complex infections in AIDS patients. J Clin Microbiol 32:842, 1994

273. STORMER RS, FALKINGHAM JO 3D: Differences in antimicrobial susceptibility of pigmented and unpigmented colonial variants of *Mycobacterium avium*. J Clin Microbiol 27:2459–2465, 1989

274. STRAND CL, EPSTEIN C, VERZOSA S, ET AL: Evaluation of a new blood culture medium for mycobacteria. Am J Clin Pathol 91:316–318, 1989

275. STRAUS WL, OSTROFF SM, JERNIGAN DB, ET AL: Clinical and epidemiologic characteristics of *Mycobacterium haemophilum*, an emerging pathogen in immunocompromised patients. Ann Intern Med 120:118–125, 1994

276. SULLIVAN EA, KREISWIRTH BN, PALUMBO L, KAPUR V, ET AL: Emergence of fluoroquinolone-resistant tuberculosis in New York City. Lancet 345:1148–1150, 1995

277. TAYLOR S: Pulmonary disease caused by *Mycobacterium asiaticum*. Tubercle 71:303–305, 1990

278. TENHOLDER MF, MOSER RJ, TELLIS CJ: Mycobacteria other than *M. tuberculosis*. Pulmonary involvement in patients with AIDS. Arch Intern Med 148:953–955, 1988

279. THIBERT L, LEBEL F, MARTINEAU B: Two cases of *Mycobacterium haemophilum* infection in Canada. J Clin Microbiol 28:621–623, 1990

280. TISDALL PA, ROBERTS GE, ANHALT JP: Identification of clinical isolates of mycobacteria with gas–liquid chromtography alone. J Clin Microbiol 10:506–514, 1979

281. TONNER JA, HAMMOND MD: Pulmonary disease caused by *Mycobacterium terrae* complex. South Med J 82:1279–1282, 1989

282. TORREA G, LEVEE G, GRIMONT P, ET AL: Chromosomal DNA fingerprinting analysis using the insertion sequence IS*6110* and the repetitive element DR as strain-specific markers for epidemiological study of tuberculosis in French Polynesia. J Clin Microbiol 33:1899–1904, 1995

283. TORTOLI E, SIMONETTI MT, LACCHINI C, ET AL: Tentative evidence of AIDS-associated biotype of *Mycobacterium kansasii*. J Clin Microbiol 32:1779–1782, 1994

284. TORTOLI E, PIERSIMONI C, BACOSI D, ET AL: Isolation of the newly described species *Mycobacterium celatum* from AIDS patients. J Clin Microbiol 33:137–140, 1995

285. TORTOLI E, SIMONETTI MT, LABARDI C, ET AL: *Mycobacterium xenopi* isolation from clinical specimens in the Florence area: review of 46 cases. Eur J Epidemiol 7:677–678, 1991

286. URIBE-BOTERO G, PRICHARD JG, KAPLOWITZ HJ: Bone marrow in HIV infections. A comparison of fluorescent staining and cultures in the detection of mycobacteria. Am J Clin Pathol 91:313–315, 1989

287. US PUBLIC HEALTH SERVICE TASK FORCE. Recommendations on prophyaxis and therapy for disseminated *Mycobacterium avium* complex for adults and adolescents infected with human immunodeficiency virus. Morbid Mortal Weekly Rep 42(RR-9):14–20, 1993

288. VADNEY FS, HAWKINS JE: Evaluation of a simple method for growing *Mycobacterium haemophilum*. J Clin Microbiol 22:884–885, 1985

289. VALAINIS GT, CARDONA LM, GREER DL: The spectrum of *Mycobacterium kansasii* disease associated with HIV-1 infected patients. J AIDS 4:516–520, 1991

290. VAN SOOLINGEN D, DE HAAS PE, HAAGSMA J, ET AL: Use of various genetic markers in differentiation of *Mycobacterium bovis* strains from animals and humans and for studying epidemiology of bovine tuberculosis. J Clin Microbiol 32:2425–2433, 1994

291. VON REYN CF, MASLOW JN, BARBER TW, ET AL: Persistent colonisation of potable water as a source of *Mycobacterium avium* infection in AIDS. Lancet 343:1137–1141, 1994

292. VUORINEN P, MIETTINEN A, VUENTO R, HALLSTROM O: Direct detection of *Mycobacterium tuberculosis* complex in respiratory specimens by Gen-Probe Amplified *Mycobacterium tuberculosis* Direct Test and Roche Amplicor *Mycobacterium tuberculosis* Test. J Clin Microbiol 33:1856–1859, 1995

293. WALLACE RJ JR, MUSSER JM, HULL SI: Diversity and sources of rapidly growing mycobacteria associated with infections following cardiac surgery. J Infect Dis 159:708–716, 1989

294. WALLACE RJ JR, SWENSON JM, SILCOX VA, ET AL: Spectrum of disease due to rapidly growing mycobacteria. Rev Infect Dis 5:657–679, 1983

295. WALLACE RJ JR, BROWN BA, ONYI GO: Skin, soft tissue, and bone infections due to *Mycobacterium chelonae chelonae*: importance of prior corticosteroid therapy, frequency of disseminated infections, and resistance to oral antimicrobials other than clarithromycin. J Infect Dis 166:405–412, 1992

296. WALLACE RJ JR, DUNBAR D, BROWN BA, ET AL: Rifampin-resistant *Mycobacterium kansasii*. Clin Infect Dis 18:736–743, 1994

297. WARREN NG, BODY BA, SILCOX VA, MATTHEWS JH: Pulmonary disease due to *Mycobacterium malmoense*. J Clin Microbiol 20:245–247, 1984

298. WASILAUSKAS B, MORRELL R JR: Inhibitory effect of the isolator blood culture system on growth of *Mycobacterium avium M. intracellulare* in BACTEC 12B bottles. J Clin Microbiol 32:654–657, 1994

299. WASILAUSKAS B, MORRELL R JR: Optimum recovery of *Mycobacterium avium* complex from blood specimens of human immunodeficiency virus-positive patients by using small volumes of isolator concentrate inoculated into BACTEC 12B bottles [letter]. J Clin Microbiol 33:784–785, 1995

300. WAYNE LG: Simple pyrazinamidase and urease tests for routine identification of mycobacteria. Am Rev Respir Dis 109:147–151, 1974

301. WAYNE LG: Microbiology of tubercle bacilli. Am Rev Respir Dis Suppl 125:31–41, 1982

302. WAYNE LG, DOUBEK JR: Diagnostic key to mycobacteria encountered in clinical laboratories. App Microbiol 16:925–931, 1968

303. WAYNE LG, KRASSNOW I: Preparation of tuberculosis testing medium by means of impregnated discs. Am J Clin Pathol 45:769–771, 1966

304. WAYNE LG, SRAMEK HA: Agents of newly recognized or infrequently encountered mycobacterial diseases. Clin Microbiol Rev 5:1–25, 1992

305. Wayne LG, Kubica GP: Genus *Mycobacterium*. Sneath PHA, Mair NS, Sharpe ME, Holt JG (eds): *Bergey's Manual of Systematic Bacteriology*, vol 2, pp 1436–1457. Baltimore, Williams & Wilkins, 1986

306. Weber J, Mettang T, Staerz E, et al: Pulmonary disease due to *Mycobacterium xenopi* in a renal allograft patient. Rev Infect Dis 11:964–969, 1989

307. Weinberger M, Berg SL, Feuerstein, et al: Disseminated infection with *Mycobacterium gordonae*: report of a case and critical review of the literature. Clin Infect Dis 14:1229–1239, 1992

308. Weiszfeiler JG, Karczag E: Synonymy of *Mycobacterium simiae* Karasseva et al, 1965 and *Mycobacterium habana* Valdiva et al. Int J Syst Bacteriol 26:474–477, 1971

309. Weitzman I, Osadczyi K, Corrado ML, Karp D: *Mycobacterium thermoresistible*: a new pathogen for humans. J Clin Microbiol 14:593–595, 1981

310. Wendt SL, George KL, Parker BC, et al: Epidemiology of infection by nontuberculous mycobacteria. III. Isolation of potentially pathogenic mycobacteria from aerosols. Am Rev Respir Dis 122:259–263, 1980

311. Whelen AC, Felmlee TA, Hunt JM, et al: Direct genotypic detection of *Mycobacterium tuberculosis* rifampin resistance in clinical specimens by using single-tube heminested PCR. J Clin Microbiol 33:556–561, 1995

312. Wiid IJ, Werely C, Beyers N, et al: Oligonucleotide (GTS)5 as a marker for *Mycobacterium tuberculosis* strain identification. J Clin Microbiol 32:1318–1321, 1994

313. Wilkins EGI, Griffiths RJ, Roberts C: Pulmonary tuberculosis due to *Mycobacterium bovis*. Thorax 41:685–687, 1986

314. Williams DL, Gillis TP, Dupree WG: Ethanol fixation of sputum sediments for DNA-based detection of *Mycobacterium tuberculosis*. J Clin Microbiol 33:1558–1561, 1995

315. Willocks L, Leen CL, Brettle RP, et al: Isolation of *Mycobacterium malmoense* from HIV–positive patients. J Infect 26:345–346, 1993

316. Witebsky FG, Keiser J, Conville P, et al: Comparison of BACTEC 13A medium and Du Pont Isolator for detection of mycobacteremia. J Clin Microbiol 26:1501–1505, 1988

317. Wobeser WL, Krajden M, Conly J, et al: Evaluation of Roche Amplicor PCR assay for *Mycobacterium tuberculosis*. J Clin Microbiol 34:134–139, 1996

318. Wolfe JM, Moore DF: Isolation of *Mycobacterium thermoresistible* following augmentation of mammaplasty. J Clin Microbiol 30:1036–1038, 1992

319. Wolinski E: Nontuberculous mycobacteria and associated diseases. Am Rev Respir Dis 119:107–159, 1979

320. Woodley CL: Evaluation of streptomycin and ethambutol concentrations for susceptibility testing of *Mycobacterium tuberculosis* by radiometric and conventional procedures. J Clin Microbiol 23:385–386, 1986

321. Woods GL, Pentony E, Boxley MJ, Gatson AM: Concentration of sputum by cytocentrifugation for preparation of smears for detection of acid-fast bacilli does not increase sensitivity of the fluorochrome stain. J Clin Microbiol 33:1915–1916, 1995

322. Woods GL, Witebsky FG: College of American Pathologists Mycobacteriology E Proficiency Testing Survey. Summary of participant performance, 1979–1992. Arch Pathol Lab Med 119:17–22, 1995

323. Woods GL, Washington JA II: Mycobacteria other than *Mycobacterium tuberculosis*: review of microbiologic and clinical aspects. Rev Infect Dis 9:275–294, 1987

324. Wong B, Edwards FF, Kiehn TE, et al: Continuous high-grade *Mycobacterium avium–intracellulare* bacteremia in patients with the acquired immune deficiency syndrome. Am J Med 78:35–40, 1985

325. Yajko DM, Wagner C, Tevere VJ, et al: Quantitative culture of *Mycobacterium tuberculosis* from clinical sputum specimens and dilution endpoint of its detection by the Amplicor PCR assay. J Clin Microbiol 33:1944–1947, 1995

326. Yakrus MA, Straus WL: DNA polymorphisms detected in *Mycobacterium haemophilum* by pulsed-field gel electrophoresis. J Clin Microbiol 32:1083–1084, 1994

327. Yang ZH, de Haas PE, van Soolingen D, et al: Restriction fragment length polymorphism *Mycobacterium tuberculosis* strains isolated from Greenland during 1992: evidence of tuberculosis transmission between Greenland and Denmark. J Clin Microbiol 32:3018–3025, 1994

328. Yang ZH, Mtoni I, Chonde M, et al: DNA fingerprinting and phenotyping of *Mycobacterium tuberculosis* isolates from human immunodeficiency virus (HIV)-seropositive and HIV-seronegative patients in Tanzania. J Clin Microbiol 33:1064–1069, 1995

329. Yao FDC, Moellering RC Jr: Antibacterial agents. Balows A (ed): *Manual of Clinical Microbiology*, 5th ed, Chap 108. Washington DC, American Society for Microbiology, 1991

330. Yamori S, Tsukamura M: Comparison of prognosis of pulmonary diseases caused by *Mycobacterium avium* and by *Mycobacterium intracellulare*. Chest 102:89–90, 1992

331. Yoganathan K, Elliot MW, Moxham J, et al: Pseudotumor of the lung caused by *Mycobacterium malmoense* infection in an HIV positive patient. Thorax 49:179–180, 1994

332. Young LS, Interlied CB, Berlin OG, Gottlieb MS: Mycobacterial infections in AIDS patients with emphasis on the *Mycobacterium avium* complex. Rev Infect Dis 8:1024–1033, 1986

333. Zala L, Nunzikere T, Braathen LR: Chronic cutaneous infection caused by *Mycobacterium gordonae*. Dermatology 187:301–302, 1993

334. Zaugg M, Salfinger, M, Opravil M, Luthy R: Extrapulmonary and disseminated infections due to *Mycobacterium malmoense*: case report and review. Clin Infect Dis 16:540–549, 1993

335. Zwadyk P Jr, Down JA, Myers N, Dey MS: Rendering of mycobacteria safe for molecular diagnostic studies and development of a lysis method for strand displacement amplification and PCR. J Clin Microbiol 32:2140–2146, 1994

SPIROCHETAL INFECTIONS

The 1980s was a good decade to buy stock in spirochetes. At one extreme, *Treponema pallidum*, a scourge of humans for centuries was almost eliminated by penicillin, but has staged a dramatic comeback that continues into the 1990s. At the other end of the spectrum *Borrelia burgdorferi*, recognized only 15 years ago, has become the most common spirochetal infection in the United States.[46]

This large and diverse group of bacteria includes pathogens and saprophytes. There are microaerophiles, strict anaerobes, species that have been cultured only in vivo, and some species that have never been cultured under any conditions. Some organisms have complex ecologic relations, and humans are only incidental victims. Other spirochetes infect only humans and must be transmitted directly from person to person.

TAXONOMY

The order *Spirochaetales* contains the major human pathogens. They are all helically shaped, motile bacteria that measure 0.1 to 3.0 μm in diameter by 5 to 120 μm in length.[43] The flagella of most spirochetes are encased within the multilayered outer membrane that is referred to as an outer sheath. The genus *Spirillum*,

Color Plates for Chapter 18 are found between pages 784 and 785.

however, has external flagella. In contrast with other bacteria, the spirochetes propel themselves by rotation through a liquid environment and are able to maintain their motility, even in high viscosity liquids.

The classification of the pathogenic spirochetes is detailed in Table 18-1. The pathogens are concentrated in three genera: *Treponema*, *Borrelia*, and *Leptospira*.

TREPONEMA

The four major pathogens in the genus *Treponema* are genetically related, infect only humans, and have not been cultivated for more than one passage in vitro. Despite these similarities they produce very different diseases.

TREPONEMA PALLIDUM SUBSPECIES PALLIDUM

T. pallidum subspecies *pallidum* (hereafter called *T. pallidum*) is the dominant pathogen among the spirochetes. *T. pallidum*, the cause of venereal syphilis, has been infamous for 500 years. It shares "100%" genetic homology with *T. pallidum* subspecies *pertenue*, which causes a nonvenereal cutaneous disease that differs in most aspects from syphilis.[168] One group of investigators, who tested a reference strain of each organism, reported a difference of only one nucleotide in the gene coding for a 19-kDa protein,[178] but the immunoreactivity of this protein was identical in the two subspecies.[177]

TABLE 18-1
CLASSIFICATION OF SPIROCHETES

ORGANISM	GEOGRAPHIC LOCATION	DISEASE
Order *Spirochaetales*		
Family *Spirochaetaceae*		
Genus III. *Treponema*		
T. pallidum	Worldwide	Venereal syphilis
subspecies *pallidum*		
T. pallidum	Tropical Asia, Africa, South and Central America	Yaws
subspecies *pertenue*		
T. pallidum	Africa, SE Asia, Middle East, Yugoslavia	Endemic, nonveneral syphilis
subspecies *endemicum*		
T. carateum	Central and South America	Pinta
"T. pallidum-like oral spirochetes"	Worldwide	Necrotizing gingivitis
Genus IV. *Borrelia*		
Borrelia spp.	Worldwide	Tick-borne relapsing fever
Borrelia recurrentis	South America, Europe, Africa, Asia	Louse-borne relapsing fever
Borrelia burgdorferi	North America, Europe	Lyme disease
Family *Leptospiraceae*		
Genus I. *Leptospira*		
Leptospira interrogans	Worldwide	Leptospirosis

Adapted from Krieg NR, Holt JR (eds): Bergey's Manual of Systematic Bacteriology, pp 38–64. Baltimore: Williams & Wilkins, 1984

The origin of *T. pallidum* is uncertain. The disease did not appear prominently in Europe until the 16th century. Fornaciari and colleagues studied a Renaissance mummy that contained structures identified by immunofluorescence and electron microscopy as *T. pallidum*.[84] Devotees of one school of thought believe that Columbus and his sailors brought the disease back from the New World.[26] These historians identify *T. pallidum* as the "Great Pox," whereas variola virus produced the "Small Pox." It is hypothesized that the Great Pox developed from a milder clinical disease in American Indians. There is abundant evidence of bone changes similar to those of syphilis in New World skeletons. Unfortunately, the question has not been answered definitively because the osseous lesions of venereal and nonvenereal syphilis are difficult to differentiate. Rothschild has suggested discriminators among treponemal species if adequate material is available.[211] Whatever the original source, each European country chose to associate the disease with its neighbor. To the English, syphilis was the "French disease." The French considered it the "Italian pox."

The clinical presentation of venereal syphilis is varied and complex. Sir William Osler, one of the founders of modern medicine, referred to the disease as "the great imitator" and admonished students that if they knew syphilis, they would know medicine. The clinical disease has been somewhat arbitrarily divided into a series of stages.[110,267,268]

INCUBATION PERIOD

The treponemes are introduced into the body through a mucous membrane or a cut or abrasion on the skin. It has been estimated epidemiologically that as many as 50% of sexual contacts of infectious persons escape infection. Experimental studies in human volunteers have documented, however, that the ID_{50} (the number of organisms needed to infect 50% of volunteers) for *T. pallidum* is as few as 57 organisms.[158] Shortly after inoculation the spirochetes are disseminated throughout the body, where they may eventually cause disease. The incubation period varies from 3 to 90 days, with a mean of 3 weeks.

PRIMARY SYPHILIS

This phase encompasses the development of the primary lesion at the site of inoculation. The inflammatory reaction creates an ulcerated lesion, called a chancre. The chancre has a clean, smooth base, and the edge is raised and firm. The ulcer is usually painless, although slightly tender. There is scant exudate unless the chancre is secondarily infected. There is usually a single primary chancre, but multiple primary ulcers may occur in patients with the acquired immunodeficiency syndrome (AIDS). The base contains spirochetes that can be visualized by darkfield microscopy or immunofluorescence after scraping of the lesion.

The chancre occurs at the inoculation site, most commonly on the genitalia. Occasionally, syphilis may occur without a visible ulcer.[241] The regional lymph nodes are enlarged, but painless and firm. The chancre heals in 3 to 6 weeks (range, 1 to 12 weeks).

The laboratory diagnosis of primary syphilis depends on demonstration of spirochetes in the lesions by darkfield microscopy or direct immunofluorescence in addition to serology.[111] Nontreponemal tests for syphilis are negative in 10% to 30% of patients with primary syphilis.[111,140]

SECONDARY SYPHILIS

The secondary phase of dissemination is the most florid part of the disease and is the period when organisms are most numerous. The secondary phase begins 2 to 8 weeks after the appearance of the chancre and lasts for a few days to months. The most dramatic presentation is a widespread rash, which may be macular, maculopapular, or pustular, but not vesicular. The rash in syphilis characteristically involves the palms of the hands and soles of the feet. In moist intertriginous areas broad, moist, gray-white plaques called condylomata lata are teeming with infectious spirochetes, which can be visualized by darkfield microscopy or immunofluorescence in scrapings of the lesions. Similarly, infectious lesions, called mucous patches, are found on mucous membranes. There may be loss of hair or thinning of the eyebrows.

Systemic symptoms include generalized lymphadenopathy, fever, and malaise. Virtually any organ may be involved in secondary syphilis. Keratitis, hepatitis, and osteitis can be found. Infection of the central nervous system occurs at any stage of syphilis, but is most common in the secondary phase.[219] Meningismus and headache are common. Aseptic meningitis may develop. Spirochetes can also be cultured from the cerebrospinal fluid (CSF), however, without any evidence of inflammation and without clinical disease.[151]

The borderline between the primary and secondary phases is not cleanly drawn. On occasion, the primary chancre may still be present when the secondary rash appears.

The laboratory diagnosis of secondary syphilis can usually be established easily by serologic techniques. The diagnosis of neurosyphilis is more difficult, as discussed later. Abnormalities of CSF in a patient with a serologic diagnosis of syphilis provide presumptive evidence that the nervous system has been involved.

LATENT SYPHILIS

Following the secondary phase, the disease becomes subclinical, although not necessarily dormant. The latent phase has been arbitrarily divided into an initial 4-year period, referred to as the early latent phase, and a subsequent late latent period.[45] During early latency relapses may occur, and the patient is infectious. Ninety percent of the relapses occur within the first year. The late latent period is of indefinite duration, and complications may never appear. During the latent stage of syphilis the presence of the disease can be detected only serologically.

LATE SYPHILIS

Late complications of syphilis include central nervous system disease, cardiovascular abnormalities, and tumors, called gummas, in any organ. Late neurovascular syphilis may be symptomatic or asymptomatic.[112] Asymptomatic disease is characterized by CSF abnormalities in the absence of symptoms.[219] Pleocytosis, elevated protein levels, or depressed glucose levels are usually found in the CSF. A positive serologic test, classically the VDRL assay, in the CSF defines the disease, although the spirochetes are rarely demonstrated by culture or more recently by molecular methods. Symptomatic infection is either meningovascular or parenchymatous, but there is considerable overlap in the categories. Meningovascular syphilis resembles the aseptic meningitis of the secondary stage. Any cranial nerve may be affected by the inflammation, and deafness or visual impairment may result. Parenchymatous disease may involve the neurons of either the cerebrum or the spinal cord. Cerebral involvement is manifested as a wide variety of neuropsychiatric disturbances, including physical changes, such as paralysis, and psychiatric problems, such as delusions of grandeur ("general paresis of the insane"). The posterior columns (sensory tracts) of the spinal cord are preferentially affected, causing severe pains and inability to perceive sensual impulses from the extremities. The disease, called tabes dorsalis, includes a peculiar "slapping" gait and deformed knees (Charcot's joints), which are caused by the lack of the feedback loop that tells the body to "go easy" on the joints.

The interval between primary disease and neurologic complication is 5 to 10 years for meningovascular syphilis, 15 to 20 years for general paresis, and 25 to 30 years for tabes dorsalis.

Cardiovascular Syphilis.   The cardiovascular lesion in tertiary (late) syphilis, syphilitic aortitis, occurs in approximately 10% of untreated cases. It is caused by inflammation in the small vessels that feed the aorta (syphilitic endarteritis) and affects primarily the ascending aorta. Two complications may result: an aortic aneurysm and dilatation of the aortic ring causing insufficiency and regurgitation of blood through the aortic valve. Aortic aneurysms may grow to such a size that they erode through the sternum and are visualized under the skin of the chest.

Late "Benign" Syphilis.   This phase is characterized by the formation of nonspecific granulomatous lesions called gummas. This lesion is the most common complication in late syphilis and occurs in approximately 15% of untreated patients. The formation of the granuloma indicates a fully active cellular immune response. The gumma, however, may destroy surrounding tissue as it enlarges.[206] Clinically, gummas are destructive mass lesions in virtually any organ and may be mistaken initially for carcinomas.

The laboratory diagnosis of late syphilis requires the demonstration of serologic reactivity with a treponemal or nontreponemal test. The only universally recognized test for the documentation of neurosyphilis is the nontreponemal VDRL test as adapted for spinal fluid. Unfortunately, this test is very insensitive, but other serologic tests are prone to nonspecificity. It has been suggested that the FTA-ABS test be used as a more sensitive screening test to eliminate patients with nonreactive spinal fluids from further consideration, but there is no currently approved test in the United States for this purpose.

Congenital Syphilis.   One of the greatest tragedies of syphilis is the intrauterine infection of the fetus.[275] Reflecting the increase in the general population, congenital syphilis has increased steadily since 1983.[68] Transplacental infection is most likely to occur during the primary or secondary stages of syphilis (see Color Plate 18-1A). The spirochetes may infect the fetus at any time during pregnancy, but the likelihood of clinical disease increases as the pregnancy progresses.

Many of the infected fetuses die. In some areas of the country congenital syphilis is the most common cause of nonimmune hydrops, a disease of the placenta that causes fetal death.[21] Of those who survive, half are asymptomatic and the remainder have the lesions of secondary syphilis without detectable primary lesions because they do not have a single primary portal of entry. Hepatosplenomegaly, meningitis, thrombocytopenia, anemia, and bone lesions characterize the infection.[148] Intrauterine infection of bone may result in visible abnormalities of bone and teeth, such as deformed tibias (saber shins) or teeth (mulberry molars). To prevent this tragedy, screening of women during pregnancy has been recommended. In high-risk populations it is additionally necessary to test maternal and neonatal sera for antibody at delivery. Cord blood is inferior to neonatal sera.[50]

The interpretation of serologic tests in congenital infection is difficult. Symptomatic infants born to untreated seropositive mothers require antimicrobial therapy. If the mother has received adequate penicillin therapy, congenital infection is unlikely, and the infant can be followed closely.[102] The VDRL test usually reverts to normal within 6 months and the FTA-ABS test within 1 year.[49] Traditional attempts to detect IgM antibody in the infant have floundered on the shoals of insensitivity and nonspecificity.[140] New approaches and variations of traditional approaches include modifications of methods for detection of IgM, use of immunoblots with defined antigens,[34] detection of spirochetes by direct immunofluorescence,[34] and detection of nucleic acid with amplification techniques.[215] In the absence of clear evidence that the mother has been adequately treated, empiric treatment of the infant is indicated until tests with sufficient sensitivity to eliminate the possibility of intrauterine infection are developed.

EPIDEMIOLOGY

Syphilis can be transmitted by only a few routes: sexual contact,[207] direct introduction into the vascular system by shared needles or transfusions,[48] direct cutaneous contact with infectious lesions, or transplacental transfer of spirochetes (Table 18-2).

Despite successful antitreponemal therapy and knowledge of the epidemiology for decades, the problem of syphilis remains and the incidence of infection is increasing. Between 1981 and 1989 the incidence of primary and secondary syphilis in the United States grew from 13.7 to 18.4 cases per 100,000 persons, an increase of 34%.[208] In 1987 congenital syphilis increased by 21%.[44] The only group in which syphilis decreased was white men, which was attributed to changes in sexual practice among homosexual men.[208] During this decade prostitution and cocaine abuse were recognized as risk factors for syphilis.[207] Cocaine use was as-

TABLE 18-2
TRANSMISSION OF SPIROCHETES

ORGANISM	TRANSMISSION
Treponema pallidum pallidum	Venereal
	Blood transfusion (human only)
T. pallidum pertenue	Direct skin contact (human only)
T. carateum	Direct skin contact (human only)
T. pallidum endemicum	Direct mucosal contact (human only)
	Contaminated eating or drinking vessels
Borrelia recurrentis	Human host, human louse vector (Pediculus humanus humanus)
Borrelia spp.	Rodents, primates, human host; tick vector (Ornithodoros, Rhipicephalus)
B. burgdorferi	Rodent, deer host; tick vector (Ixodes)
Leptospira interrogans	Rat hosts; contaminated water

sociated with both the development of syphilis and the failure to seek prenatal health care in an inner city population.[169]

A national epidemiologic study of syphilis seroreactivity indicated that race, age, education, income, and place of residence correlated with positivity.[97] An analysis of two recent outbreaks of primary and secondary syphilis has emphasized the problem. Transmission was heterosexual.[89,142] Men were usually diagnosed during the primary stage, whereas the primary lesion was often not detected in women, who were diagnosed during the early latent phase.[142] Reflecting major changes in American society in the last 50 years, a study of prenatal syphilis at Boston City Hospital documented a shift from married white women in 1951 to unmarried minority women in 1991. A positive serologic test was associated with substance abuse and the presence of other sexually transmitted diseases.[132]

Traditional epidemiologic techniques of partner notification are proving inadequate for changed socioeconomic circumstances of modern America.[10,89] Between 1983 and 1984 Alexander-Rodriguez and colleagues studied 285 girls and 2236 boys, aged 9 to 18 years, who were entering a detention facility.[5] The prevalence rate for gonorrhea was 3% in boys and 18.3% in girls. For syphilis the rate was 0.63% in boys and 2.5% in girls.

T. pallidum and human immunodeficiency virus (HIV) interact in several ways. It has been suggested that genital ulcers of a variety of etiologies facilitate the acquisition of HIV.[244] The immunosuppression that accompanies HIV infection may affect the serologic response to syphilis. As discussed later, in immunocompetent individuals serologic tests are uniformly reactive during the secondary phase of syphilis. Hicks and colleagues report a patient who was infected with HIV, had Kaposi's sarcoma, and developed secondary syphilis without a detectable serologic response.[106] Similarly, Haas and colleagues observed 109 homosexual men who had been treated for syphilis.[96] All of the men who had not been infected with HIV virus maintained their reactivity to treponemal antigen. In contrast, 7% of the men who had subclinical HIV infection and 38% of those with HIV disease had lost reactivity to the treponemal antigens. Conversely, biologic false-positive reactions in nontreponemal tests appear to be more common in HIV-infected patients than in those without HIV infection.[12,209] The mechanism for the association is unclear, and there are many potential confounding factors in these complicated patients. For instance, an association of biologic false-positive reactions has also been described in patients who are infected with hepatitis C virus.[265] Most positive nontreponemal tests in HIV-infected patients, however, do indicate syphilis.

Patients who are infected with HIV are more likely to present with secondary syphilis and with persistent chancres than non–HIV-infected patients.[116] Some investigators have suggested that the HIV epidemic has been accompanied by an increase in neurosyphilis,[173] but other investigators have not identified HIV as a risk factor for infection of the nervous system.[151] Unsuccessful treatment of syphilis in patients infected with HIV has been reported by several investigators.[30,151]

The standard of therapy for syphilis remains penicillin. Recent documentation of treatment failures, particularly in HIV-infected patients, has caused concern that the convenient regimen of long-lasting benzathine pencillin may be inadequate in some patients.[109,278] Alternative therapeutic choices for penicillin-allergic patients have limitations, but a third-generation cephalosporin, ceftriaxone, has been promising in clinical trials.[108] One of the uncommon complications of therapy is the Jarisch-Herxheimer reaction, which is both local and systemic. This reaction, which is associated with circulating endotoxin released from damaged organisms,[88] was classically noted in treated louse-borne relapsing fever.

IMMUNITY

Experimental studies using inbred strains of guinea pigs have documented the importance of the cellular immune system in resistance to *T. pallidum*.[188] Investigators were able to transfer delayed hypersensitivity reactions and partial resistance to infectious skin lesions by transfusing immune lymphoid cells.[188] In addition, the humoral response was partially protective because passive transfer of antibody ameliorated clinical symptoms.[189] There is firm evidence in humans that immunity to *T. pallidum* is partial or delayed in development. Congenitally infected infants have been reinfected as adolescents.[81] Similarly, human volunteers who previously had natural syphilis have been successfully reinfected.[158] The likelihood that reinfection will occur decreases with increasing time after primary infection.[82] A period of partial resistance develops, in which reinfection may occur without the presence of a chancre. By the late stage, the patient is completely immune to reinfection.

TREPONEMA PALLIDUM SUBSPECIES PERTENUE

T. pallidum subspecies *pertenue* (hereafter called *T. pertenue*) is the cause of yaws, a chronic, nonvenereal treponemal disease (see Table 18-1).[133] Yaws is endemic in central Africa and parts of the Indian subcontinent, South America, and Southeast Asia. There are primary, secondary, and tertiary stages of the disease. The skin and bones are primarily affected. Disease begins in childhood and is transmitted by contact with infectious skin lesions (see Table 18-2). In the tertiary phase the lesions may be gummatous. Benzathine penicillin is curative, although it may take months for the lesions to regress. Antibodies to *T. pertenue* are indistinguishable from antibodies to *T. pallidum*.[177]

TREPONEMA PALLIDUM SUBSPECIES ENDEMICUM

T. pallidum subspecies *endemicum* (hereafter called *T. endemicum*) is the cause of endemic, nonvenereal syphilis or bejel (see Table 18-1).[133] It is endemic in parts of Africa, the Middle East, India, and Asia. Infection occurs in childhood in rural areas with poor standards of hygiene. It is transmitted by contact with mucosal lesions or through contaminated drinking and eating utensils (see Table 18-2). The primary lesion of endemic syphilis is rarely seen, but the disease is otherwise similar to venereal syphilis. Benzathine penicillin is the therapy of choice. Correction of poor sanitation and hygiene may be preventive. Antibodies from patients with endemic syphilis cross-react with *T. pallidum*.

TREPONEMA CARATEUM

T. carateum, the etiologic agent of pinta, is probably the oldest of the human treponemes.[133] The disease is characterized by ulcerative or papulosquamous skin lesions that often depigment. Pinta is endemic in parts of South and Central America (see Table 18-1) and is spread by contact with infected skin lesions (see Table 18-2). There are no long-term systemic health effects, but the cosmetic disability is considerable. Antisera from patients with pinta cross-react with specific antigens of *T. pallidum*.[83]

LABORATORY DIAGNOSIS OF SPIROCHETAL DISEASES

The laboratory diagnosis of syphilis has been recently reviewed extensively by Larsen and colleagues,[140] and a cost-effective approach to diagnosis and therapy has been developed by Hart.[102]

The gold standard for diagnosis of syphilis is culture, which must be performed in vivo, usually by intratesticular inoculation of rabbits with clinical material (Table 18-3). The procedure is expensive and time-consuming, requiring several months for subculture of testicular material if the original animal does not seroconvert. For obvious reasons culture remains an investigative tool.[215]

In primary syphilis, before the appearance of antibody, direct detection of spirochetes in chancres is the

TABLE 18-3
CULTURE OF SPIROCHETES

ORGANISM	IN VIVO	IN VITRO
Treponema pallidum pallidum	Rabbit testis; hamster; guinea pig	None
T. pallidum pertenue	Rabbit testis; hamster; guinea pig	None
T. pallidum endemicum	Rabbit testis; hamster; guinea pig	None
T. carateum	None (chimpanzee ±)	None
Borrelia recurrentis	Various	Modified Kelly medium
Borrelia spp.	Various	Modified Kelly medium
B. burgdorferi	Various	Modified Kelly medium
Leptospira interrogans	Various	Fletcher medium; Khorthof medium; Tween 80–albumin medium

only means of diagnosis (Chart 17).[140] The traditional method has been darkfield microscopy of material scraped from the surface of a lesion (Fig. 18-1). Observation of spirochetal motility is integral to differentiation of *T. pallidum* from saprophytic spirochetes, so that the microscopy must be accomplished immediately after collection of the specimen, a feat that is very difficult for most clinical laboratories to accomplish.

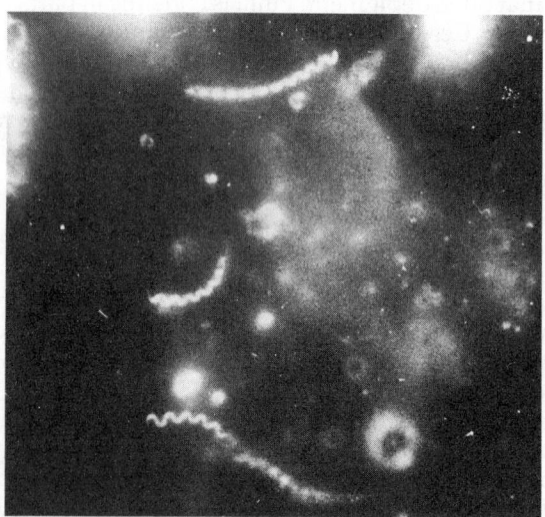

Figure 18-1.
Positive darkfield examination for *Treponema pallidum*. The tightly coiled spiral nature of the organisms is evident. The background consists of debris and occasional red blood cells, indicating an adequate specimen. × 1000. (Photomicrograph courtesy of Centers for Disease Control, Atlanta GA.)

Examination of oral lesions is not recommended because of the frequent presence of saprophytic treponemes in the mouth. Cutaneous and visceral lesions of secondary syphilis often contain large numbers of spirochetes, which can be demonstrated by darkfield microscopy of scrapings or imprints.

An alternative approach that is more satisfactory than darkfield microscopy is to demonstrate the presence of spirochetes in the lesions by immunofluorescence (see Color Plate 18-1B). Initially the diagnostic reagent was polyclonal rabbit antiserum to *T. pallidum* after absorption with the nonpathogenic Reiter strain of *T. phagadenis*. The immunofluorescence assay was equivalent to darkfield examination, but considerably more versatile.[56] More recently, monoclonal reagents with greater specificity have been developed.[111,119] Hook and colleagues demonstrated fluorescent treponemes in 30 of 30 patients with primary syphilis, 29 of whom also had positive darkfield examinations. An oral spirochete that is antigenically related to *T. pallidum* has been described in cases of necrotizing gingivitis,[205] so the possibility of falsely positive reactions exists when oral lesions are tested, even with a monoclonal antibody. Fluorescein-conjugated monoclonal antibody and control slides are available from the Centers for Disease Control and Prevention (CDC).

To perform the direct fluorescent antibody test for *T. pallidum* (DFA-TP), material from a lesion or tissue is collected as described for the darkfield examination, except that the material is allowed to dry on the slide (Chart 17). Alternatively the dried smears can be sent to a reference laboratory or the exudate may be collected in capillary tubes, which are then sealed and stored at 4°C for mailing. The direct immunofluorescence method has been effective for *T. pertenue* as well as *T. pallidum*.[192]

Spirochetes in formalin-fixed tissue can be demonstrated with one of several variations of a silver impregnation stain, such as the Steiner, Warthin-Starry, or Dieterle procedures (see Color Plate 18-1A).[270] Although finding spirochetes in the appropriate clinical situation is presumptive evidence of syphilis, the stain itself is nonspecific. Application of a fluoresceinated antibody provides specificity as well as sensitivity. Ito and colleagues found that *T. pallidum* in formalin-fixed tissues was stained well by polyclonal antisera after treatment of sections with either NH_4OH or trypsin, but absorption of the sera with the Reiter treponeme to increase specificity abrogated the reaction. Spirochetes were successfully demonstrated after absorption of a human serum with Reiter treponeme. Either NH_4OH or trypsin could be used to facilitate staining.[120] Subsequently, fluoresceinated monoclonal antibodies were successfully used on formalin-fixed tissue, again after treatment with NH_4OH or trypsin.[119]

SEROLOGIC TESTS

The serologic tests for syphilis can be divided into two groups: nontreponemal tests and treponemal tests. The two groups have distinctive characteristics that make them useful for different purposes. They are complementary, not mutually exclusive. The nontreponemal tests are most useful as screening tests. The treponemal tests should be reserved as confirmatory tests when a nontreponemal test is positive or when clinical suspicion of syphilis is high despite a nonreactive nontreponemal test. Hart has pointed out that the "greater" specificity of the treponemal tests is entirely an artifact of their current use as confirmatory tests after performance of a nontreponemal test.[102] When the tests are compared head to head as the initial serologic procedure, the VDRL nontreponemal test is actually as specific or more specific than the treponemal FTA-ABS test.[138] The general characteristics of these tests are summarized in Table 18-4.

The procedures for performance of these tests have been standardized and published in great detail by the U.S. Public Health Service.[139] Several of the procedures are summarized in the tables for pedagogic purposes. When these tests are performed in the laboratory, it is imperative that the manual or manufacturer's directions be consulted and followed exactly. The *Manual of Tests for Syphilis* even contains a classic typographic error: in Chapter 3 readers are instructed in the "Collection Procedure for Venus [*sic*] Blood."

Nontreponemal Tests. The nontreponemal tests take advantage of antibodies to a tissue lipid, called cardiolipin, that are produced as a byproduct of treponemal infection. The association was recognized early in this century when a variety of complement fixation tests were developed. The procedures in current use are predominantly flocculation tests. They use a form of cardiolipin that is complexed with cholesterol and lecithin. The most commonly used procedures are the Venereal Disease Research Laboratory (VDRL) and the rapid plasma reagin (RPR) tests. Other tests that have been used are the reagin screen test (RST), the unheated serum reagin (USR) test, and the toluidine red unheated serum test (TRUST).[140]

The nontreponemal tests have a sensitivity of 70% to 99%, depending on the stage of disease. The tests may not be positive in primary syphilis, so that they should be repeated after 1 week, 1 month, and 3 months if a negative result is obtained in a patient suspected of having syphilis. The sensitivity of these tests approaches 100% during the secondary phase of the disease. Plasma and cord blood should not be used because borderline reactions may be obtained.[137]

The nontreponemal tests are affected by antitreponemal therapy. As a result they are useful for following the progression of disease and response to therapy. The results of any positive test should be titered to an endpoint dilution. In addition, serum from patients with large amounts of antibody may produce a prozone phenomenon. When a prozone occurs, the relative concentrations of antibody and antigen are not in balance, and precipitation or flocculation does not occur. The false-positive results caused by the prozone phenomenon continue to be a clinical concern. The prozone results are often marked by a "rough" appearance to the flocculated antigen. Any serum that produces this rough appearance should be titered. In addition, serum should be diluted and retested if a patient with negative tests is strongly suspected of having syphilis on clinical grounds. In the general population the frequency of prozone reactions is sufficiently low that routine dilution of serum is not cost-effective.[71]

If the titer of the antibody does not fall progressively with treatment, the possibility of a treatment failure should be considered. There should be at least a fourfold decrease in antibody titer after 3 months of antitreponemal therapy. Patients who are treated in the late stages of syphilis or who are reinfected may develop titers that decline very slowly or remain stable. Some of these "chronic persisters" may maintain positive nontreponemal tests for life.[82]

The nontreponemal tests cannot be used to diagnose late syphilis, especially if treated, because the titer of antibody will eventually decline to undetectable levels.

The VDRL test has become the standard nontreponemal test. Preparation of the antigen must be done with great precision and attention to detail. It is the only serologic test that is universally accepted for the diagnosis of neurosyphilis. Examples of VDRL reactions are shown in Figure 18-2. The procedure is summarized in Chart 74.

The RPR test is an adaptation of the flocculation principle to a card format. The visibility of the flocculation is enhanced by incorporation of charcoal particles. The uses of the RPR test are similar to those of the VDRL test except that the RPR test cannot be used to test CSF. The simplicity of the RPR test has led most laboratories to adopt it as the primary screening test (Fig. 18-3). The procedure is described in Chart 64.

The specificity of the nontreponemal tests averages 98%, with a range from 93% to 99%. The lack of specificity is mostly a problem when the tests are used for screening populations with a low prevalence of syphilis, for whom positive reactions are likely to be false-positive. The false-positive reactions occur in patients who have other treponemal infections, but also in patients with diseases that elicit anticardiolipin antibodies. These "biologic false-positives" may be transient, usually from viral infections, or may be persistent, usually related to immunologically mediated diseases. Biologic false-positive reactions have been re-

TABLE 18-4
CHARACTERISTICS OF SEROLOGIC TESTS FOR SYPHILIS

TEST	TYPE	% POSITIVE AT INFECTIOUS STAGES		
		PRIMARY	*SECONDARY*	*LATE*
VDRL	Nontreponemal	70	99	1
RPR	Nontreponemal	80	99	0
FTA-ABS	Treponemal	85	100	98
TPHA	Treponemal	65	100	95
TPI	Treponemal	50	97	95

Adapted from Tramont EC. *Treponema pallidum* (syphilis). In Mandell GL, Douglas RG, Bennett JE (eds). Principles and Practice of Infectious Diseases, 3rd ed. Churchill Livingston, New York, 1990.

ported in drug addicts, a population at increased risk of developing syphilis.[128] As discussed earlier, patients with HIV infection also have an increased frequency of biologic false-positive reactions.[12,209] In one study, these positive reactions were associated with hepatitis C infection.[265] A positive reaction in a nontreponemal test should be confirmed, therefore, with a more specific treponemal test.

Pedersen and colleagues have evaluated an enzyme immunoassay that incorporates the VDRL antigen.[190] They found that the specificity of the nontreponemal test was improved when it was adapted to the enzyme immunoassay format. Harris and colleagues have developed an enzyme immunoassay that distinguishes between antibodies to syphilitic cardiolipin and cardiolipin antigens in patients with connective tissue diseases.[101] A commercial enzyme immunoassay that incorporates a treponemal antigen has proved specific and highly sensitive except in primary syphilis, for which the sensitivity was 82%.[144] These new approaches have not yet supplanted the traditional methods, but they may represent the tests of the future.

Treponemal Tests.   The treponemal tests incorporate specific treponemal antigens into the system. The traditional gold standard was the *T. pallidum* immobilization (TPI) test, in which the motility of live, virulent treponemes was inhibited by the presence of specific antibody. This expensive and cumbersome test has been replaced by the fluorescent treponemal antibody with absorption test (FTA-ABS). Subsequently, another test specific for treponemal antigens, the microhemagglutination test for *T. pallidum* (MHA-TP) was developed.

The FTA-ABS test is summarized in Chart 32. The specificity of the assay is increased by absorption of the test sera with a nonpathogenic spirochete, the Reiter strain of *T. phagadenis*. The FTA-ABS test has a higher rate of positivity in early syphilis than do the nontreponemal tests (see Table 18-4). The positivity rate approaches 100% in the secondary stage and remains so for life. It is not affected by antitreponemal therapy. The FTA-ABS test is, therefore, a good test for screening late syphilis, but it cannot be used to follow treatment. The degree of positivity in the FTA-ABS test has

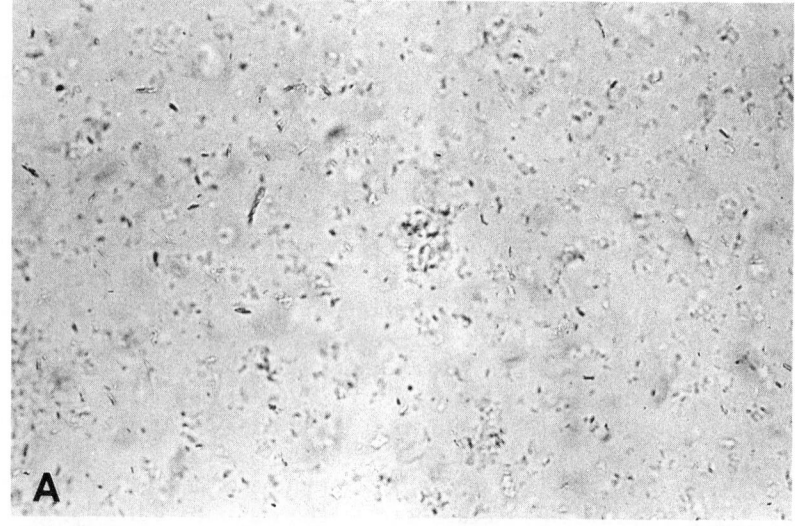
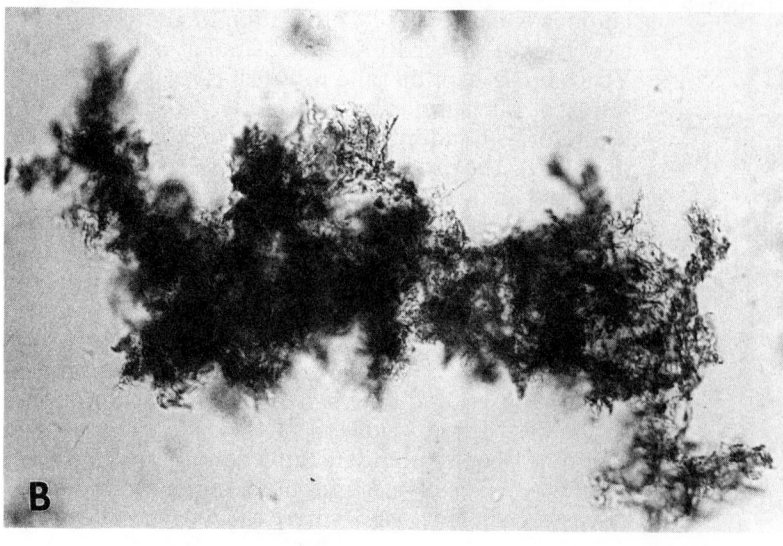

Figure 18-2.
VDRL test: The reactions in this test are evaluated microscopically. **(A)** Nonreactive serum. The particles of VDRL antigen are uniform and freely dispersed without clumping. **(B)** Reactive serum: The VDRL antigen particles are strongly agglutinated by this syphilitic serum. The individual particles have aggregated into sheaves and large clumps. × 100 (Courtesy of Burton Wilcke, PhD and Mary Celotti)

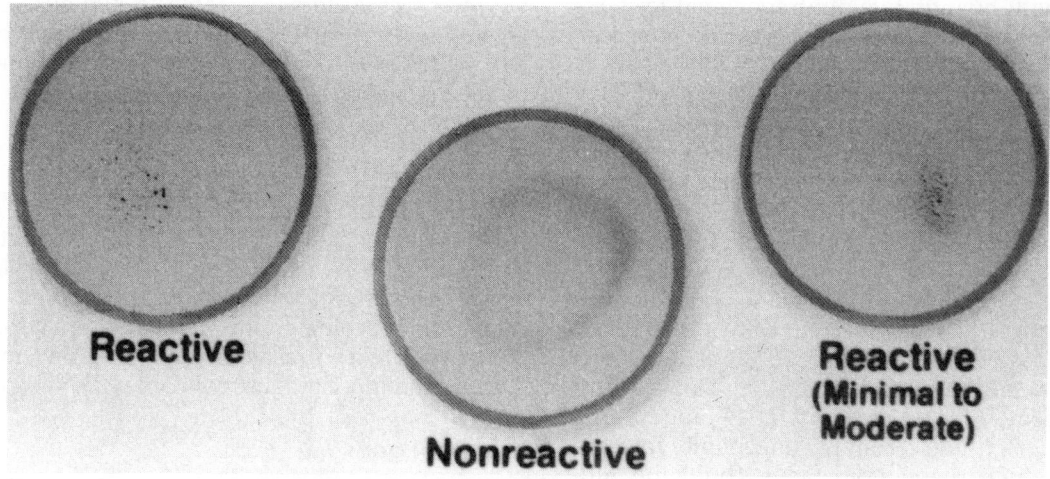

Figure 18-3.
RPR card test: The reactions in this test are read with the naked eye, using incandescent light illumination. This control card contains *Reactive* (R), *Weakly reactive* (W), and *Nonreactive* (N) sera. The modified VDRL antigen is made visible by complexing with charcoal particles. The charcoal–antigen particles are evenly dispersed and finely distributed in the nonreactive serum. The charcoal–antigen particles are grossly clumped. The serum with minimal to moderate activity produces small aggregates and clumps of charcoal–VDRL antigen particles.

no biologic meaning, so the intensity of fluorescence is not reported and positive sera are not titered. The specificity of the FTA-ABS test is very high. The biologic false-positive reactions of the nontreponemal tests do not occur with few exceptions. Sera from some patients, especially those with systemic lupus erythematosus or other connective tissue diseases, may produce an unusual beaded staining reaction.[135] It has been estimated that 1% of the normal population will have a positive FTA-ABS test.[139] Cross-reactions occur with other pathogenic treponemes. If the FTA-ABS test is used to screen populations with very low prevalences of syphilis, false-positive reactions may occur even with this very specific test.

A variation on the FTA-ABS test is the double-staining procedure. The test is very similar to the FTA-ABS, except that rhodamine-conjugated IgG antitreponemal antibody is used to locate the spirochetes. In the classic FTA-ABS test darkfield illumination is used to locate the spirochetes. The results of the traditional and double-staining procedures are comparable.[204]

The FTA-ABS test can be adapted to detect either IgG or IgM antibody. One advantage of detecting IgM antibody is to document infection in utero. Immunoglobulins of the G class cross the placenta and enter the fetal circulation, but IgM antibodies do not cross the placenta. IgM antibodies are made by the fetus in utero; therefore, the detection of specific antitreponemal IgM antibodies in a neonate indicates intrauterine infection.[6] There are potential problems with the IgM assays, however, and great care must be taken to validate a given assay before use. If antiglobulins, such as rheumatoid factors or anti-idiotype antibodies, are present in fetal sera, they will produce false-positive reactions. If present in excessive amounts, IgG anti-

body may block the antigenic sites, producing false-negative reactions. Rosen and colleagues demonstrated good performance with a research assay, but encountered problems when commercial reagents were used.[210]

The microhemagglutination test uses antigens specific to *T. pallidum*. The test is considerably less complicated than the FTA-ABS and does not require a fluorescence microscope. It is similar in performance to the fluorescent procedure, but it is less sensitive in early syphilis. The FTA-ABS test should be available to test sera that give equivocal reactions.[259]

RECENT INNOVATIONS: PROVISIONAL AND INVESTIGATIVE TESTS

Recently enzyme immunoassays for detection of specific treponemal antigens have appeared. An enzyme immunoassay to a recombinant membrane protein, TmpA, was similar to the microhemagglutination assay for diagnosis of syphilis at various stages.[118] A commercial enzyme immunoassay, the Bio-EnzaBead Assay (Organon Teknika Corp., Durham NC), performed well when tested against well-characterized antisera in two studies.[37,172] Another commercial assay for IgG and IgM, the Captia assay, also produced acceptable results, but gave positive reactions for IgM with some sera that contained rheumatoid factor.[144]

Disappointment in the performance of the IgM FTA-ABS test has prompted the investigation of other approaches. The 19S IgM FTA-ABS test includes fractionation of serum to obtain IgM specificity, rather than depending on antiglobulin reagents.[258] This test appears to avoid the problems of nonspecificity, so it can be used as a confirmatory procedure, but insensitivity prevents its use as a screening test. Sequential evaluation with quantitative nontreponemal tests remains the standard for laboratory evaluation of congenital syphilis.[140]

Modern molecular techniques may facilitate dissection of the issues. Sanchez and colleagues used Western blot analysis (immunoblots; see Chap. 1) to identify a 47-kDa antigen that was not seen in control patients and was correlated with intrauterine infection.[218] The sensitivity of immunoblotting for detection of IgM antibodies in 14 symptomatic neonates was 92%, whereas 83% of 12 asymptomatic neonates who were later proved to be infected were detected by Western blotting. Twenty-seven of 30 (90%) uninfected infants were correctly characterized.[167] Dobson and colleagues demonstrated reactivity to 47- and 37-kDa protein antigens in the serum of congenitally infected infants. Although rheumatoid factor could theoretically cause problems in the immunoblot assay, removing rheumatoid factor from the sera did not affect the results.[65] Immunoblots have also been used successfully as a confirmatory test for syphilis.[40] An advantage of this technology is that purified antigen can be used as the substrate, and the pattern of reactivity of sera can be used to determine positivity. If the criteria for determining positive immunoblot tests are not standardized, however, the variation in interpretation among laboratories can cause diagnostic problems. As understanding of the nature of the protein antigens of *T. pallidum* increases,[243] the number and quality of tests available in future years will undoubtedly expand.

Molecular techniques have also been applied to the direct detection of spirochetes in tissues and fluids. Investigators have concentrated their attention on intrauterine and central nervous system infection, because serologic techniques are not adequate for these important clinical problems.[94,179] DNA probes have not been sufficiently sensitive, so efforts have been focused on amplification techniques, such as polymerase chain reaction. Although the new technology is a valuable addition to the diagnostic armamentarium, the presence of inhibitors in clinical specimens yields false-negative tests that prevent use of amplification as a single tool for decision making, especially in CSF. False-positive reactions from contamination have been minimal in the research protocols, but it was necessary to address problems of nonspecificity in one study by using nested primers.[179] The close correlation of polymerase chain reaction and the impossibly impractical rabbit infectivity assays in other studies, however, suggests that this approach is the way of the future for difficult diagnostic problems.[215]

BORRELIA

Borrelia are helical bacteria that measure 0.2 to 0.5 μm in diameter and 3 to 20 μm in length with three to ten loose coils and 15 to 29 periplasmic flagella (see Color Plates 18-1C, D, and F). Those species that have been cultivated in vitro are microaerophilic (see Table 18-3). The bacteria are gram-negative and stain well with Giemsa's stain.[130] The human pathogens are transmit-

ted by insect vectors (see Table 18-2). Louse-borne relapsing fever is caused by *B. recurrentis*, tick-borne relapsing fever by a variety of species, and Lyme disease by *B. burgdorferi*.

RELAPSING FEVER

Relapsing fever is a distinctive clinical disease that was probably recognized by Herodotus in ancient Greece. There are two forms: 1) epidemic louse-borne disease and 2) endemic tick-borne relapsing fever. The epidemiologic, ecologic, and clinical characteristics are compared and contrasted in Table 18-5. Several old but still pertinent reviews are available.[36,77,239]

EPIDEMIOLOGY

Louse-borne relapsing fever is a disease that is fostered by poverty, crowding, and poor sanitation, as is louse-borne typhus fever. It has occurred in Africa, the Middle East, and Asia, but not in the New World. The human body louse inhabits humans only, and *B. recurrentis* is not transmitted vertically to succeeding generations of lice. The organism must be maintained by passage from louse to a human host and then back to another louse. The louse remains infected for its entire life. Epidemic disease thus occurs only under conditions of extreme deprivation. For the first half of this century epidemics occurred approximately every 20 years. In recent times, Ethiopia has been the only major geographic locus of infection.[36]

Tick-borne relapsing fever is distributed worldwide. Many soft-bodied ticks of the genus *Ornithodorus* carry distinctive borreliae. In the United States, the taxonomists have attempted to use the same name for tick and associated spirochete. Thus *O. hermsii* is the vector for *B. hermsii*. The epidemiologic characteristics of tick-

TABLE 18-5
CHARACTERISTICS OF RELAPSING FEVER

CHARACTERISTIC	LOUSE-BORNE	TICK-BORNE
Epidemiology	Epidemic	Usually endemic
Etiologic Agent	*B. recurrentis*	Various; *B. hermsii, B. turicatae, B. parkeri* in U.S.
Vector	*Pediculus humanus* ssp. *humanus*	Various; *Ornithidorus hermsii, O. turicatae, O. parkeri* in U.S.
Mean Duration of Primary Attack	5.5 d	3.1 d
Mean Duration (Range) of Asymptomatic Interval	9.25 d (3–27 d)	6.8 d (1–63 d)
Mean Number (Range) of Relapses	3 (0–13)	1 (0–3+)
Mean Duration of Relapse	1.9 d	2.5 d

Adapted from Southern PM Jr, Sanford JP. Relapsing fever. A Clinical and microbiological review. Medicine 48:129–149, 1969

borne relapsing fever depend on the habits of the local vector.[77] *O. hermsii* is the most common vector and *B. hermsii* the most common *Borrelia* in California, the Pacific Northwest, and Canada. *O. hermsii* lives in the remains of dead trees and parasitizes rodents, which often carry it into hunters' cabins. *O. parkeri* inhabits caves and burrows of ground squirrels and prairie dogs in the western United States. *B. parkeri* is a relatively infrequent pathogen of humans because of the inaccessibility of its vector. *O. turicata* inhabits caves and animal burrows in the western United States, Mexico, and South America, but it also has been found in closer association with humans under the foundations of houses in Texas. The tick-borne borreliae have a solid ecologic niche with virtually no possibility of eradication. The spirochete can be passed from generation to generation of ticks without intervention of a vertebrate host. *O. turicata* has been reported to survive in a starving state for 5 years,[77] and survival of borreliae in ticks without loss of infectivity has been reported for up to 12 years.[239]

Most tick-borne relapsing fever is endemic, afflicting the unfortunate person who becomes an incidental host. Under the right conditions, however, epidemic disease can occur. In 1968 there was an outbreak of tick-borne relapsing fever among 42 Boy Scouts and scoutmasters who were camping near Spokane, Washington.[266] Eleven of the 42 persons at risk developed clinical disease. In nine cases an exact incubation period could be calculated because they were only at risk for one night (mean 6.9 days; range, 3 to 9 days). The attack rate was higher in those who slept in abandoned cabins than in those who slept in tents, a fact that was also noted by Horton and Blaser in Colorado.[113] The authors noted poetic justice in the concentration of disease among scoutmasters and older scouts, who appropriated the cabins for themselves, leaving the younger scouts to "rough it."

In areas that have no indigenous relapsing fever spirochetes, importation of disease from endemic regions provides a diagnostic challenge.[51] Tick-borne infection is a more likely infection than louse-borne infection for tourists visiting Africa. Parasitologists should keep this diagnostic possibility in mind when examining smears collected for the detection of malaria parasites.

CLINICAL DISEASE

The clinical presentation of the two types of relapsing fever is similar. Differences in frequency and timing of relapses are noted in Table 18-5. *Ornithodorus* ticks feed on humans very inconspicuously and for short periods. Most patients, therefore, do not remember a tick bite. The onset of disease is typically abrupt with high fever, usually near 40°C (104°F), shaking chills, delirium, severe muscle aches, and pains in bones and joints. Hepatosplenomegaly and tenderness may be present, and the patient may be jaundiced. Characteristically there is a crisis after which the fever remits and the patient feels well. Fatalities are very uncommon. When relapses occur, each cycle tends to be less severe than the preceding one. Patients may develop a rash during the initial attack, but the rash does not usually appear in relapses. An outbreak of louse-borne relapsing fever in Ethiopian troops after the cessation of civil war provided an unfortunate recent opportunity to review the clinical features.[31] The case fatality rate was 3.6%, and 1.8% of patients had recrudescent disease.

Although penicillin is effective against borreliae, tetracycline or erythromycin are more effective at eliminating the spirochetes. Jarisch-Herxheimer (JH) reactions may occur during treatment. In the recent Ethiopian epidemic of louse-borne disease, 43% of patients experienced this complication.[31] Use of low-dose penicillin leads to more frequent relapses, but fewer JH reactions than tetracycline or larger doses of penicillin.[231] Administration of acetaminophen and hydrocortisone modified the changes in vital signs during the JH reaction, but did not prevent the dramatic rigor that occurs.[39] Transient increases in tumor necrosis factor and interleukins-6 and -8 correlate temporally with the reaction,[175] although not all investigators have been able to detect elevations of these cytokines. Control of the vector is also essential for the control of epidemic louse-borne infection.[260]

PATHOGENESIS

The borreliae enter the body through the bite of a tick or through contamination of abraded skin with infected hemolymph of crushed lice. Once in the body the spirochetes begin to undergo antigenic variation, which foils the ability of the immune system to produce an effective defense and facilitates recurrent episodes of disease. As many as 24 variants have been described, although some are more stable than others.[257] The variable antigens are spirochetal outer membrane proteins, which are produced by recombination between and within linear plasmids or by activation of silent genes.[131,202]

LABORATORY DIAGNOSIS

Relapsing fever borreliae can now be cultured in a modification[16] of Kelly's medium for borreliae,[129] but isolation is not a practical means of diagnosis in most situations. Similarly, although several serologic tests have been developed, they are not diagnostically useful. Approximately 5% of patients will have a positive VDRL test.[239]

The mainstay of diagnosis is demonstration of the spirochetes in body fluids, usually in peripheral blood smears (see Color Plate 18-1C). The diagnosis is often made in the hematology laboratory, because the clinical presentation can be enigmatic for physicians unaccustomed to the disease.[113] Horton and Blaser report a case in which the spirochetes were missed by an automated differential scanner, but were noted by an astute technologist who reviewed the smear.[113] In contrast to other spirochetes the relapsing fever borreliae are well stained by acid aniline dyes, such as Wright or Giemsa's stains. The borrelial spirochetes are thin, undulant, or overtly spiral organisms that are most visible when they are located between red blood cells (see Color Plate 18-1C). Felsenfeld advocates staining with Wright's stain followed by application of a 1% solution of crystal violet for 10 to 30 seconds.[77]

Borreliae are likely to be found in the blood during the febrile episodes. The sensitivity of staining peripheral smears is estimated at 70%.[239] Spirochetes are unlikely to be detected during the afebrile intervals between attacks, although they are still present in the body. Thick and thin films should be made as for malaria, because in some cases spirochetes will be detected only by examination of the thick film.[113]

Goldschmid and Mahomed used a microhematocrit centrifugation technique to concentrate the borreliae in and above the buffy coat,[92] but the procedure has not been widely used. Sciotto and colleagues used the fluorescent acridine orange technique to demonstrate borreliae in peripheral smears (see Color Plate 18-1D).[230] The fluorescence procedure greatly enhances the visibility of the spirochetes.

A monoclonal antibody for the identification of *B. hermsii* in peripheral blood smears and amplification techniques for identification of borrelial nucleic acid have been described but are not generally available.[196,228]

LYME DISEASE

In 1977, Steere and colleagues, at Yale University, reported that an epidemic of arthritis had been occurring in residents of several surrounding Connecticut communities since at least 1972.[253] The alarm had been sounded by two vigilant mothers. In 1975 a mother from Old Lyme, Connecticut informed the State Health Department of 12 cases of childhood arthritis in her small community of 5000 people. A second woman came to the Rheumatology Division at Yale University with a story of acute arthritis in herself, her husband, two children, and several neighbors. The disease in all the children had been diagnosed as juvenile rheumatoid arthritis, a clinical diagnosis that depends on exclusion of known causes of arthritis. The investigators at Yale believed that they were dealing with a new disease, which they named Lyme arthritis.

Steere and colleagues recognized that the arthritis was almost always preceded by a very distinctive skin rash, an erythematous papule that developed into a rapidly expanding annular lesion. Many of the physicians who examined the skin lesions believed that an insect bite had started the process, but an arthropod (in that case a tick) was recognized in only one patient. The nature of the primary lesion and the occurrence of cases in the summer and early fall suggested an arthropod vector. In that initial paper the authors noted the resemblance of the rash to a lesion called erythema chronicum migrans, which had been described in Europe, especially Scandinavia.

Little did the two mothers know what large waves would emanate from the rock they threw into their small Connecticut pool. Instead of discovering a new disease they had initiated an investigation that would unearth the cause of a century-old disease of worldwide proportions. The long history of European investigations is summarized in Box 18-1.[246]

In 1982, only 5 years after the original description of Lyme arthritis, Burgdorfer and colleagues determined the etiology by isolating a spirochete from the implicated tick vector, demonstrating that the spirochetes produced cutaneous lesions in rabbits and that the serum of patients with Lyme arthritis contained antibodies to the spirochete.[38] The next year Steere and associates clinched the issue by isolating a spirochete from blood, skin lesions, or CSF of infected patients as well as from ticks.[250] Shortly thereafter spirochetes were isolated from the lesions of erythema chronicum migrans and Bannwarth's syndrome in Europe.[1,199]

The newly isolated spirochete is related to other *Borrelia* species,[223] but shares almost no homology with species of *Treponema* and *Leptospira*.[117] It has been named *Borrelia burgdorferi*, in honor of Willy Burgdorfer, who first isolated the organism.[124] *B. burgdorferi* is the longest and narrowest of the borreliae. It contains numerous antigens that may be important for pathogenesis and diagnosis, including several outer surface proteins, OspA through OspF, that are located on plasmids, and a 41-kDa flagellar protein. Three genospecies are now recognized within the *B. burgdorferi* complex (*B. burgdorferi sensu lato*): *B. burgdorferi sensu stricto*, *B. garinii*, and *B. afzelii*. Strains found in the United States are relatively homogeneous and conform to the definition of *B. burgdorferi sensu stricto*. The immunologic homogeneity of almost all American strains was demonstrated by cross-protection studies in experimental animals.[149]

BOX 18-1. EUROPEAN INVESTIGATIONS OF LYME DISEASE

1921–1923:   Afzelius in Sweden and Lipschütz in Austria described erythema chronicum migrans. Later the chronic atrophic skin lesion described by Herxheimer in 1902 was recognized as part of the same process.

1944:   Bannwarth described a chronic radiculitis, sometimes preceded by erythema, accompanied by chronic lymphocytic meningitis, and cranial or peripheral neuritis. Later the disease was associated with ticks.

1948:   Lennhoff described the presence of spirochetes in the lesion of erythema chronicum migrans.

1951:   Hollström described the successful treatment of erythema chronicum migrans with penicillin.

The other two species are found in Europe[63] and Asia,[174] where they may produce mixed infections of humans and mice. *B. garinii* appears to be particularly associated with neuroborreliosis, whereas *B. afzelii* is associated with arthritis and skin lesions.[63,66] In the United States atypical strains of *B. burgdorferi* have been isolated from ticks along the eastern seaboard.[8,9] Some of the strains lacked the OspA protein that is often used in diagnostic reagents.

Isolates that do not fit into any of the recognized genospecies also occur. A new species, tentatively named *B. lonestari,* has been identified by molecular techniques in *Amblyomma americanum* ticks, but attempts at culture of the spirochete were unsuccessful.[19] These atypical strains have not yet been identified in humans, and understanding of their role in human disease awaits further studies.

Retrospective examination of *Ixodes ricinus* ticks that had been preserved in Hungarian and Austrian museums in 1884 and 1888, respectively, has documented the presence of DNA from a member of the *B. burgdorferi* complex.[162] Similarly, OspA sequences from

B. burgdorferi have been demonstrated by molecular techniques in white-footed mice that had been trapped in Massachusetts in 1894.[161] It appears, therefore, that the American and European foci have been independently present for at least a hundred years.

EPIDEMIOLOGY

Lyme disease is now the most common arthropod-borne infection in the United States. From 1982 to 1989 there was an 18-fold increase in cases reported to the Centers for Disease Control. From 1986 to 1989 the number of cases doubled each year, after which the incidence appeared to have reached a plateau. In 1994, however, 13,083 cases were reported from 44 states, a 58% increase over 1993 (Fig. 18-4).[46] Cases have been reported in almost every state, but they are concentrated in the Northeast, the North Central region, and the West Coast (Fig. 18-5). The infection is recognized around the entire northern hemisphere, including the Soviet republics.[62]

In the United States, the distribution of Lyme disease matches the distribution of ticks of the genus

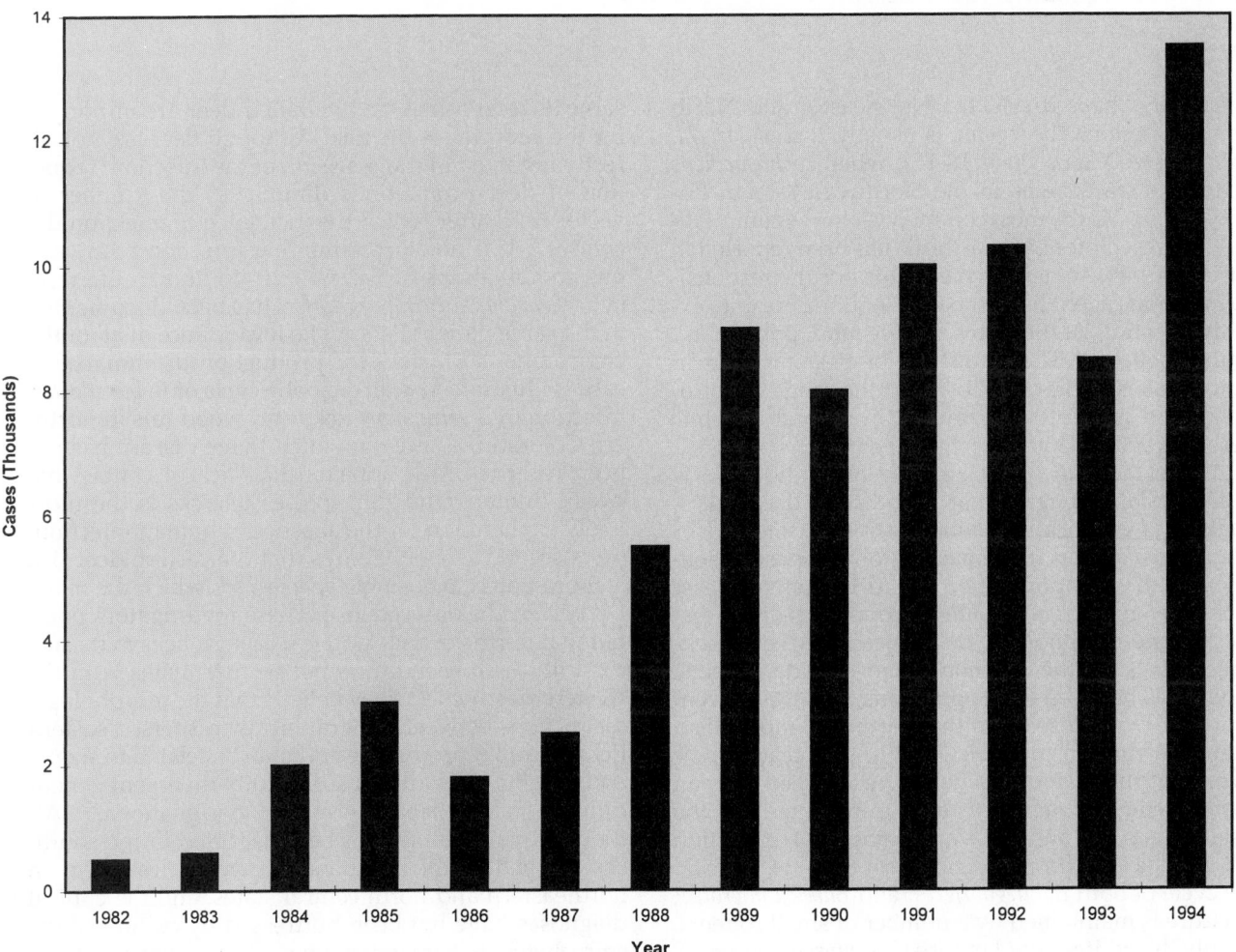

Figure 18-4.
Number of reported Lyme disease cases by year in the United States, 1982–1994. (Adapted from CDC: Lyme disease—United States, 1994. MMWR 44:459–462, 1995)

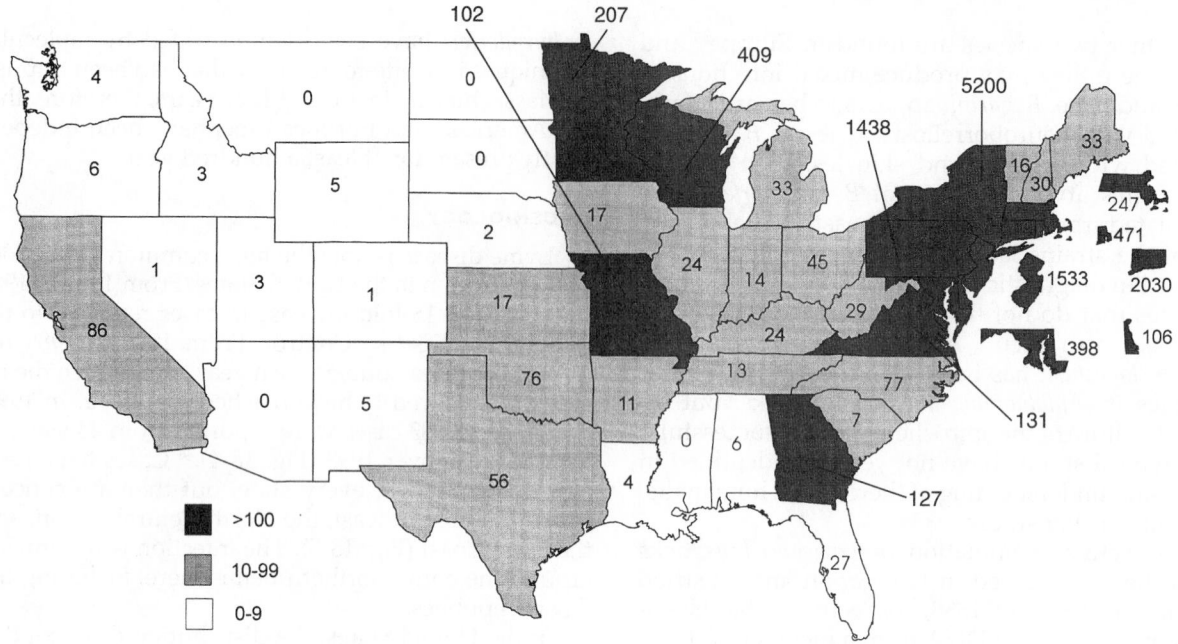

Figure 18-5.
Number of reported cases of Lyme disease by state in the continental United States, 1994.
There were no cases in Alaska or Hawaii. (Adapted from CDC: Lyme disease—United
States, 1994. MMWR 44:459–462, 1995)

Ixodes (see Chap. 20). In the Northeast[252] and North Central[91] regions the vector is usually *I. scapularis/I. dammini* (see Color Plate 18-1E), whereas *I. pacificus* carries the spirochetes in the Northwest.[221,252] In Europe, *I. ricinus* is the most common vector. A clinical illness that resembles Lyme arthritis has been reported in Australia,[85] where neither the vector nor the responsible infectious agent has yet been identified, despite extensive testing of ticks by culture and polymerase chain reaction.[213] The frequency of tick infection in some areas is as high as 75%,[7] and the range of spirochetal load in adult ticks caught in several endemic areas was 950 to 4350 spirochetes per tick.[35]

At the moment, the taxonomy of ixodid ticks is controversial. All agree that the western deer tick, *I. pacificus*, is genetically distinct from the eastern deer tick, *I. scapularis*. In 1979 investigators proposed separation of the tick population found in the Northeast into a new genus, *I. dammini*.[242] Proponents of the distinction cite morphologic differences between black-legged ticks in the far north and Florida, genetic differences between the populations, and the concentration of Lyme disease in the Northeast, rather than even distribution up and down the seaboard.[203] *Babesia microti*[242] and the newly recognized human granulocytic *Erlichia*[186] are also transmitted by the eastern deer tick and have a geographic distribution that matches the proposed northern clone of the tick. The cycle of both *B. burgdorferi*[146] and *Babesia microti*[242] in nature is maintained by a number of small rodents, notably the white-footed mouse (*Peromyscus leucopus*), which maintains an asymptomatic parasitemia or spirochetemia. Other small mammals, such as the Norway rat on Monhegan Island in Maine, may also

serve as reservoirs.[238] White-tailed deer are important for the survival of the tick. Although deer are not directly involved in transmission of the infection, reduction of deer populations diminishes the number of vector ticks after which the incidence of infection decreases.[61] It is not surprising that infection with various combinations of *Babesia microti*, human granulocytic *Erlichia*, and *B. burgdorferi* has been documented in the same patient.[24,160,171] The importance of all of the environmental factors for production of human disease is illustrated by an enzootic cycle of *B. burgdorferi* infection in *I. spinipalpis* ticks and wood rats in northern Colorado, an area in which Lyme disease has not been recorded.[164] It appears that lack of contact between humans and this species of ticks is the most likely explanation for the absence of human infection.

A second school believes that the eastern deer tick is represented by a single species, for which the name *I. scapularis* has precedence. These investigators point out that northern and southern eastern ticks mate successfully with each other, but neither mates with the western deer tick.[183] They believe that the morphologic distinctions between geographically dispersed eastern ticks are not reproducible and may be related to size,[115] and that the ticks are not sufficiently divergent genetically to justify separate species designations.[165] Although Lyme disease has been reported in the southeastern states, the frequency is much less than in northeastern and north central states, and the clinical diagnoses have not been buttressed by culture of the spirochetes. *B. burgdorferi*, however, has been isolated from southeastern ticks and has been transmitted by *I. scapularis* between experimental animals.[182] Opinion is now on the side of recognizing a single eastern tick species, *I. scapularis*,[240] but the argument has not been settled definitively.

The Lone Star tick, *Amblyomma americanum*, was named because of the star design on its body (see Chap. 20). *A. americanum* transmits *Rickettsia rickettsii* and *Franciscella tularensis*. *A. americanum* has been removed from patients with a lesion that resembles the erythema chronicum migrans lesion of Lyme disease,[42] spirochetes have been visualized in the ticks, and immunologic or genetic tests have suggested the presence of *B. burgdorferi* in the ticks.[226] Other investigators, however, have not been able to document infection with *B. burgdorferi* in those patients with skin lesions and exposure to *Amblyomma*.[42] Experimental transmission of *B. burgdorferi* has not been successful either with *A. americanum* or with *Dermacentor variabilis*, a vector of *R. rickettsii* and *F. tularensis*.[216] Recently genetic evidence has been presented that *A. americanum* in areas with "seronegative Lyme disease" is infected with a spirochete, tentatively named *B. lonestari*, that has not yet been cultivated.[19]

The life cycle of ixodid ticks involves three distinct stages and a life span of 2 years.[246] Ticks feed in late summer as larvae and the next year as nymphs (early spring) and adults (late summer). The larval and nymphal stages are so small that many patients do not recall having been bitten. The most effective tick stage for transmission appears to be the nymph, which is prevalent during the late spring and early summer when most cases of human disease occur. *B. burgdorferi* has been demonstrated in the saliva of infected *I. scapularis*, as well as in the hemolymph, suggesting that the infection is passed from tick to humans directly through the bite. From experimental data the ticks must remain attached for at least 24 hours to transmit the spirochetes effectively.[197] During the first 12 hours after attachment the body of the tick remains flat. After feeding for 24 hours, when approximately 5% of infected ticks transmit spirochetes, the posterior body of the nymph begins to extend. After 48 hours of feeding the posterior body is fully distended and appears opalescent; at this point approximately 50% of infected ticks transmit *Borrelia*. After 4 days of feeding, almost all infected ticks would have transmitted spirochetes, at which point the ticks are opaque and so bloated that the body is as thick as it is wide.[163] Attempts to culture spirochetes from skin immediately after removal of an infected tick in a hyperendemic area were successful in only 2 of 48 patients, on both of whom the tick had been attached for approximately 24 hours.[29]

Careful epidemiologic study of several endemic areas has documented the magnitude of the problem. On Fire Island, New York, 0.7% to 1.2% of summer residents developed symptomatic disease.[99] Four (3.1%) of 129 persons studied serologically at the beginning and end of the summer developed antibodies, but only 2 of the persons were symptomatic. In Great Island, Massachusetts, approximately 3% of the population developed Lyme disease each year, and 16% of the population developed the disease over the 4-year period of study.[256] In retrospect, the earliest case occurred in 1962. The clinical/subclinical ratio was estimated to be 1:1.

Cost-effectiveness analyses have been virtually unanimous in recommending that most patients who have been bitten by ticks not be treated prophylactically with antibiotics. Magid and colleagues, who attempted to quantify the analysis, recommended that patients not be treated if the risk of developing Lyme disease was less than 0.01.[153] Factors such as prolonged attachment of a feeding tick in an endemic region would increase the likelihood of transmission. If the tick is available for examination and is not an *Ixodes* species, or if Lyme disease is not endemic in the area, prophylaxis is clearly not indicated. Even in endemic areas it has not been proved in controlled trials that prophylactic therapy is justified routinely.[3,235]

CLINICAL DISEASE

The clinical manifestations of *B. burgdorferi* infection are protean.[246] This spirochete has been referred to as the "latest great imitator,"[245] following in the tracks of its relative *T. pallidum*. As in syphilis the manifestations of Lyme disease may be catalogued into three stages.

Stage one is the stage in which the tick bite elicits the classic lesion, erythema (chronicum) migrans. The expanding erythematous skin lesion presents in multiple locations and in varying extents.[28] In New Jersey, 93% of the patients developed erythema migrans and approximately half had systemic symptoms including lymphadenopathy.[33] At this stage the spirochete is most easily cultivated, and it may be visualized in as many as 40% of biopsy specimens by silver impregnation staining.[28]

The second stage of Lyme disease results from previous dissemination of the spirochete throughout the body.[247] The polymerase chain reaction was approximately three times more sensitive for detecting spirochetemia than was culture of the organisms. Borrelial DNA was documented in the serum of 14 of 76 patients (18.4%) with erythema migrans. The number of clinical symptoms was the strongest independent predictor of spirochetemia.[93] It appears that the spirochetemia is both low level and intermittent.[271] Examination of CSF fluid of patients with erythema chronicum migrans documented borrelial DNA in eight of 12 patients, four of whom had no neurologic abnormalities or symptoms. Spirochetal DNA was documented in the CSF taken from four of nine patients with neurologic symptoms.[150] The most common lesions are acute arthritis[254] and meningitis.[185] Bowen and colleagues documented arthritis in 26% of their patients, meningitis in 10%, and cranial nerve palsies in 8%.[33] The meningitis may appear purulent.[32] Secondary cutaneous lesions, infection of the eye, hepatitis, and myocardial damage may occur.

The third and chronic phase of the disease is characterized by chronic skin lesions, chronic neurologic symptoms, and chronic arthritis.[254] The recurrent episodes of arthritis diminish in frequency and severity each year, but some patients develop chronic synovitis and permanent disability.

As in syphilis, *B. burgdorferi* may be transmitted from mother to infant,[220,274] but the full effects of congenital infection are not yet known. Survival of the spirochete has been demonstrated experimentally for as long as 45 days in stored red blood cells, so that transmission in blood transfusions is possible.[13] To date, however, the risk remains theoretical. No instances of transfusion-associated Lyme disease were encountered among 149 patients who received more than 600 units of blood in an area that is endemic for Lyme disease. One patient contracted babesiosis for a risk of 0.17%.[90]

The manifestations of Lyme disease in Europe are similar to those in the United States, but arthritis may be relatively underrepresented and chronic meningitis relatively overrepresented,[246] perhaps because of the presence of the neurotropic species, *B. garinii*, in Europe.[63] Conversely, widespread disseminated infection appears to be more common in the United States than in Europe.[246]

The initial therapy of Lyme disease was penicillin or tetracycline, which are effective in many cases.[248,251] Treatment failures with both antibiotics have been described.[57,64] Recently, a clinical trial of ceftriaxone in late Lyme disease documented a greater efficacy of that antibiotic than penicillin.[58] Ceftriaxone and erythromycin were most effective against *B. burgdorferi* in vitro, but ceftriaxone and tetracycline were most effective in an animal model.[123] Despite therapy the long-term prognosis for patients with Lyme disease includes an increased likelihood of impaired musculoskeletal function and verbal memory.[234] Although the symptoms of chronic Lyme disease may be nonspecific, there is no evidence that the chronic fatigue syndrome is caused by *B. burgdorferi*.[53]

Symptomatic infection appears not to occur in wildlife, but domestic animals may develop disease. Kornblatt and colleagues have described Lyme arthritis in dogs.[134] Duray has described the surgical pathology of Lyme disease.[69]

PATHOGENESIS

B. burgdorferi is antigenically complex.[18,20] Subculture of the organisms in vitro is associated with loss of virulence, but the mechanisms are unknown.[246] A lipopolysaccharide has been demonstrated,[22] but other investigators have not demonstrated classic enteric lipopolysaccharide.[262] Endotoxin has not been detected in patients.[224] Antigenic variation, as observed in other *Borrelia* spp., occurs only to a limited extent.[17] The terminal portion of the OspB surface protein appears to be important for protection in experimental models, and a mutant with a truncated protein was able to escape immunologic surveillance.[80]

The manifestations of disease are possibly caused both by direct invasion of the organism and by immunopathologic mechanisms, perhaps at different stages of the disease. Spirochetes have been demonstrated in the original skin lesions,[28] heart,[60] and joints.[125] As in syphilis, spirochetes may be detected in CSF in the absence of inflammation.[195] Evidence for an immunologic component includes hyperactivity of B lymphocytes during the course of the disease[237] and the presence of

immune complexes in arthritic joints.[100] Borrelial DNA may be detected in the joint fluid of 85% of patients with Lyme arthritis, even though culture of the spirochete from this site is very uncommon, suggesting that the relation between pathogen and host is not straightforward.[176] Patients with persistent joint disease after treatment are also more likely to have T-cell clones that are reactive with OspA protein than are patients whose disease has responded to treatment.[145] One potential clue to neurologic disease is the observation that antibodies directed against the 41-kDa flagellin antigen of *B. burgdorferi* cross-react with a neuroblastoma cell line.[78]

Entry of *B. burgdorferi* into cultured endothelial cells is enhanced by binding to plasminogen,[52] at least partly, mediated, by interaction of plasminogen with OspA.[86] A strain with a mutant OspB protein that showed diminished invasiveness of human umbilical vein endothelial cells also showed decreased virulence for experimental animals.[214] The frequency of intracellular invasion by spirochetes in human infection is unknown.

Both neutrophils and monocytes phagocytize and subsequently kill *B. burgdorferi* effectively,[194] even in the absence of specific antibody. The receptor for the Fc fragment of antibody may be important for adherence of spirochetes before phagocytosis.[25]

LABORATORY DIAGNOSIS

Lyme disease may be diagnosed by culture of the spirochete, by demonstration of the spirochetes in tissue using immunologic or molecular techniques, or by documentation of a serologic response. The erythema migrans lesion is specific, and Lyme disease may be most confidently diagnosed if this lesion is present.

B. burgdorferi has been isolated in cell-free medium (see Table 18-3). The process is relatively easy when infected ticks are triturated and cultured (see Color Plate 18-1*E*). Unfortunately, the yield from human specimens is too low to be diagnostically useful.[23,201,249,250] Subculture from broth to agar results in the formation of spirochetal colonies with varying morphology.[136] The medium of choice is a modification of Kelly's medium for spirochetes[129] that was developed by Barbour (Box 18-2).[16] Additional modifications to that medium have been suggested.[198]

Citrated blood should be cultured. Tubes are incubated at 34° to 37°C in the dark. They are examined by darkfield microscopy after incubation for 2 to 3 weeks. The identity of any spiral organisms detected must be confirmed by specific immunofluorescence reagents.

Detection of spirochetes in tissues by morphologic means is also insensitive for most specimens and stages of the disease. Any of the silver impregnation methods for demonstration of spirochetes in tissue (Warthin-Starry, Steiner, Dieterle) may be used to stain the organisms, but specific identification must be confirmed with antisera, because the silver stains detect any type of bacterium.

Molecular amplification techniques have demonstrated greater sensitivity than culture or morphologic detection in peripheral blood[93] and joint fluid.[193] In contrast, culture was more sensitive than an amplification assay when various organs of experimentally infected animals were tested[184] and when skin lesions from humans with erythema migrans were examined.[229] The sensitivity of polymerase chain reaction is less in CSF than in urine in patients with symptomatic neurologic disease.[141] After treatment borrelial DNA could no longer be detected in urine. Borrelial antigen was also detected in urine by the polymerase chain reaction using nested primers in 26 patients with erythema migrans.[225] DNA was initially detected in 92% of the patients, but in only 2 of 16 patients (13%) after 8 weeks of therapy. A role exists for molecular techniques in documenting acute infection or sorting out difficult cases, but the tests still remain experimental.

The diagnostic method of choice by default is serologic analysis. Immunofluorescence and enzyme immunoassays have been used most commonly. Indirect immunofluorescence,[157] quantitative fluorescence immunoassay,[191] and a fluoroimmunoassay[105] have been recommended, but many investigators have found the enzyme immunoassay to be more satisfactory.[54,212] Antibody may be absent early, but is usually present after several weeks.[246] A response to OspA tends to occur late, but may be detected in low titer or complexed to spirochetes early in the course of infection if special techniques are used.[227] A response to the OspC protein or the less specific flagellin antigen occurs more commonly in early sera.[156] For maximum sensitivity in early Lyme disease use of an IgM assay has been recommended, either by immunofluorescence[170] or immunoblot[4] techniques. Specific IgM titers may remain elevated throughout the course of illness and even years after treatment, so the presence of IgM cannot be used to establish acute infection.[98] Collection of a second specimen 8 to 14 days after the baseline sample has been recommended for documentation of seroconversion in early Lyme disease.[227]

Examination of spinal fluid for intrathecally produced antibodies has been performed for the diagnosis of neuroborreliosis. The presence of higher titers of antibody in cerebrospinal fluid than in peripheral blood documents infection of the nervous system.[277] Given the many difficulties with serologic analysis of peripheral blood, these approaches should be reserved for experienced reference laboratories, which have documented the efficacy of their tests.

Most currently available assays use sonicated whole spirochetes, and the reagents are not standardized. As a result there have been serious problems with reproducibility and with accuracy, compounding the difficulties of clinical diagnosis. In a proficiency testing program as many as 21% of participants failed to recognize the presence of antibody at a titer of 512 or higher.[14] With lower concentrations of antibody as many as 55% of participants failed to recognize the serum as positive. Conversely, the false-positive rate was up to 7% with a polyvalent conjugate and as high as 27% with an IgG conjugate. Reproducibility of results when the same serum was submitted as a challenge at different times was also suboptimal. The fact that these proficiency testing problems are present in the real world is emphasized by the report from a Lyme referral center, where 45% of patients who had been referred with an incorrect diagnosis of Lyme disease had had positive serologic tests for *B. burgdorferi* that could not be confirmed in the reference laboratory.[255] Furthermore, in a single laboratory only 16.3% of positive results using an enzyme immunoassay could be confirmed with an immunoblot.[55] The authors argue that insensitivity of the immunoblot does not explain the results, because more cases of erythema migrans were detected with the immunoblot than with the enzyme immunoassay.

Our clinical colleagues have not been successful in dealing with this enigmatic disease either. At one university Lyme disease clinic, 38% of children were overdiagnosed and 8% were underdiagnosed.[74] One quarter of the patients who had been diagnosed correctly were subsequently treated incorrectly. In a study of diagnostic tests at a prepaid health care plan in California, only 19% of laboratory tests were ordered because the physician suspected Lyme disease.[147] Fully 60% of the tests were ordered as a part of a battery of tests for patients with vague complaints. In an area where Lyme disease is uncommon, such indiscriminant test ordering stacks the deck against serologic tests that already have more than enough problems of their own!

Cross-reactions with a variety of infectious agents have been found in sera from patients suspected of having Lyme disease. Sera of patients with other borrelial infections,[155] treponemal infections,[27,114,200] HIV,[200] Epstein-Barr virus,[27] and rickettsial infections[27] may react in assays for *B. burgdorferi*. Reports on cross-reaction with leptospira antisera are conflicting.[155,200] Although cross-reactions develop with specific treponemal antigens, the VDRL test is not positive in patients with Lyme disease.[246] The nonspecific reactions have been reported to be concentrated in the IgG2 class of antibodies in several instances.[233]

As often happens, interpretation of serologic results is most straightforward when it is least needed, that is, when the classic erythema chronicum migrans rash occurs. When the presentation is atypical, the diagnosis is usually serologic and the possibility of misleading results with serious consequences is magnified. Steere has pointed out that serologic evidence of infection may be correct but that the Lyme disease may be subclinical and the patient's problems caused by another agent.[246]

Kaell and colleagues described four patients from an area endemic for Lyme disease who had confusing multisystemic disease that was initially attributed to *B. burgdorferi*.[127] All four patients had antibodies to the spirochete, and three of the four had positive Western blot tests; however, continued study revealed that the cause of the illness in all four cases was subacute bacterial endocarditis. Subsequently, these investigators demonstrated increased antibodies to *B. burgdorferi* in 13 of 30 patients (43%) with nonspirochetal endocarditis.[126] The specificity of Lyme serology in this population was only 60%. When immunoblots were performed, only 1 patient had a pattern of reactivity that suggested prior exposure to the spirochete. The authors hypothesize that cross-reactions with the infecting bacterium might be responsible for the high frequency of nonspecific results.

Two major types of approach to the serologic problems have been taken: development of immunoblots (Western blots) and a search for defined—and, therefore, reproducible—antigens that react with the sera of most infected patients.

Immunoblots have served as reference tests for HIV and might serve the same function in Lyme disease.[95] Immunoblots are clearly not, however, an absolute gold standard for *B. burgdorferi*. Dattwyler and colleagues have reported patients who had vigorous T-cell proliferative responses when exposed to *B. burgdorferi* antigen, but lacked antibody by immunofluorescence and by Western blot analysis.[59] They concluded that the patients had Lyme disease without a serologic response, but normal persons may have a similar blastogenic response to borrelial antigens.[246,261]

The presence of positive Western blots in patients with bacterial endocarditis indicates that immunoblotting is not per se a guarantee of specificity.[127] As in HIV infection the immunoblot can be used to improve the specificity of other immunoassays.[55] Dressler and colleagues developed criteria for positive immunoblots in a retrospective study.[67] The best discrimination was obtained if detection of two of the eight most common IgM bands (18, 21, 28, 37, 41, 45, 58, and 93 kDa) was required for positivity in early disease and detection of at least five of the ten most common IgG bands (18, 21, 28, 30, 39, 41, 45, 58, 66, and 93 kDa) was required for diagnosis after the first weeks of infection. Application of these criteria to more than 300 patients in a prospective study yielded a sensitivity of 32% and a specificity of 100% for the IgM test. The sensitivity and specificity of the IgG test were 83% and 95%, respectively. Slightly different criteria have been suggested by Engstrom and colleagues.[73] Their criteria for positivity of IgM immunoblots include recognition of at least two of the following proteins: 24 (OspC), 39, and 41 (flagellin) kDa. The sensitivities of the IgG and IgM immunoblots in 55 patients with documented erythema migrans were 58.5% and 54.6% respectively, at the time of diagnosis and 100% after an additional 8 to 12 days. Ma and associates have emphasized the importance of antibody to the 39-kDa antigen for specific diagnosis.[152]

The Centers for Disease Control and Prevention and Association of State and Territorial Public Health Laboratory Directors currently recommend the IgM criteria of Engstrom and the IgG criteria of Dressler.[47] By using these criteria Aguero-Rosenfeld and associates observed positive IgM immunoblots at the time of initial study in 43% of a group of 46 patients with culture-positive erythema migrans and in 84% of the patients 8 to 14 days later.[4] Although 89% of patients developed antibodies to *B. burgdorferi*, IgG immunoblots were positive by the recommended criteria in only 22% of convalescent sera. After 1 year 38% of the IgM immunoblots were still positive. IgM antibodies reactive with 39-, 58-, 60-, 66-, and 93-kDa antigens were most often seen in the first month after diagnosis, and these investigators suggest that the presence of these bands may be helpful in suggesting recent infection in patients from endemic areas.[4]

Hilton and colleagues suggest that two additional antigens be added to the criteria for IgG positivity: 31-kDa (OspA) and 34-kDa (OspB) antigens.[107] Of 136 patients evaluated for Lyme disease, 4 (8%) would have been considered positive only if these two antigens were included in the criteria. These 4 patients had erythema migrans or arthritis and lived in endemic zones. It is obvious that the criteria for interpretation of immunoblots are still evolving.

Fine-tuning of the criteria for positive serologic tests will undoubtedly continue, but confirmation of an indeterminate or questionable result with an enzyme immunoassay should be sought by performing an immunoblot in an experienced laboratory.

Attempts to improve the specificity of serologic diagnosis also include development of recombinant antigens for enzyme immunoassays, predominantly

OspA,[79,156] OspB,[79,156] and OspC.[87,156] Recognition of antigenic diversity among strains may be important for greater sensitivity in certain regions.[264]

The current status of laboratory diagnosis of Lyme disease has been reviewed recently.[154] The CDC recommends a two-step approach to diagnosis. An enzyme immunoassay or immunofluorescence assay with high sensitivity should be used as the initial test. Negative sera need not be studied further, but convalescent sera should be collected if clinically indicated. Positive results should be confirmed with both IgM and IgG immunoblots.[47]

LEPTOSPIRA

Leptospira are motile, obligately aerobic helical rods that measure 0.1 μm in diameter and 6 to 12 μm in length. They are gram-negative and are only faintly stained by aniline dyes. Darkfield microscopy must be used to visualize unstained leptospira (Fig. 18-6). Two species of *Leptospira* are currently recognized: *L. interrogans*, which contains all of the human pathogens, and the saprophytic species, *L. biflexa*. *L. interrogans* contains many individual serotypes that cause human disease. Antigenically related serovars are collected into serogroups for classification purposes. The type strain is *L. interrogans* serovar *icterohaemorrhagiae*,[122] and the clinical disease is leptospirosis. Several thorough reviews, although old, still reflect the state of knowledge in many areas.[70,75,103,104]

Yasuda and colleagues studied the DNA relatedness between serogroups and serovars of *Leptospira*.[276] On genetic grounds they proposed at least five new species among the human pathogens. The nucleic acid analysis

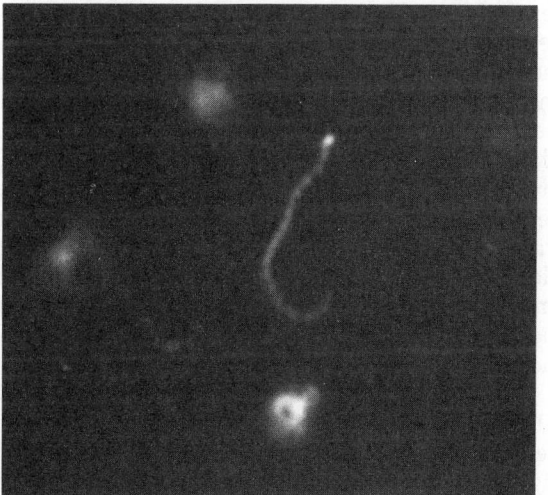

Figure 18-6.
Darkfield examination of *Leptospira interrogans* culture. The spiral coils, which are not clearly demonstrated, appear as alternating bright and dark areas. The very bright upper end of the organism may represent the hooked end that many leptospira possess. It is easy for inexperienced observers to confuse cell debris and artifacts with leptospira in clinical specimens. ×1000. (Photomicrograph courtesy of David Miller, DVM, MS)

did not correlate well with the serologic classification. A single serovar might be found in several species.

LEPTOSPIROSIS

EPIDEMIOLOGY

Leptospira are distributed worldwide and infect many types of domestic and wild animals. Humans become incidental, "dead-end" hosts because transmission from humans to animals or to other humans does not occur. Rats have been classically associated with this disease, but sheep, cattle, dogs, and other domestic animals may be infected. In the wild, foxes, raccoons, skunks, shrews, and hedgehogs carry the leptospires. Associations between serovars and animal species exist, such as *L. interrogans* sv. *icterohaemorrhagiae* and rats or *L. interrogans* sv. *canicola* and dogs. Several different serovars of *Leptospira* may be carried by a single animal genus, however, and a single serovar may be associated with more than one animal host. In general, the animal hosts are not symptomatic and do not develop antibody despite overwhelming infection.[75]

Leptospirosis has been traditionally considered an occupational disease, concentrated among workers in sewers, rice fields, sugar cane fields, and abattoirs. In the 1970s in the United States, however, only 30% of the persons for whom an occupation was reported to the CDC were exposed at work. There were children, homemakers, and retired or unemployed persons among the infected. It has been suggested that increasing leisure time and more frequent forays into the countryside have increased the likelihood of casual exposure. Leptospirosis has been reported in association with kayaking.[236] Epidemiologic factors that were associated with leptospirosis in Hawaii included catchment of rainwater for household use, contact with cattle and cattle urine, or handling of animal tissues.[217] Feigin and colleagues documented a small epidemic in University City, Missouri, an upper–middle-class suburb of St. Louis.[76] They were able to isolate *Leptospira interrogans* sv. *icterohaemorrhagiae* from rats and house pets and from soil in the yards of homes. Some of the dogs from whom they isolated leptospires had been immunized with commercially available anti-*Leptospira* vaccines. Epidemic disease may occur from a common source, as was recently found in a waterborne outbreak in Italy.[41] In that epidemic it was suggested that an outbreak associated with a town fountain was caused by a hedgehog trapped in a water reservoir. A recent outbreak in Illinois was traced to a contaminated pond; a drought was hypothesized to have increased the risk of exposure to infected animal excreta.[121] Leptospira are distributed worldwide, so that imported disease must be considered in travelers.[269]

CLINICAL DISEASE

Classic leptospirosis is a biphasic disease, which consists of an initial septicemic phase and a secondary immune phase. The severity ranges from subclinical infection to fatal systemic disease, known as Weil's disease after the man who first described icterohemorrhagic fever in 1886. In severe cases the two phases merge together and an asymptomatic interval may not be recognized.

Surveys of workers at occupational risk have demonstrated antibodies without a recognized episode of leptospirosis in 5% to 16% of those tested. In patients who are recognized to have leptospiral infection, Weil's disease occurs in 5% to 10%.[75]

The initial septicemic phase of the disease is abrupt in onset, ushered in by high fever, severe headache, malaise, and muscle aches. Eye pain, photophobia, and conjunctival suffusion or even hemorrhage are characteristically present. It should be emphasized that inflammation or true conjunctivitis is conspicuously absent. Pulmonary infiltrates are relatively common, but disease is usually mild. Leptospirosis presenting as adult respiratory distress syndrome has been described.[72,180] Patients may present with rashes that are macular, maculopapular, urticarial, or hemorrhagic. A distinctive pretibial rash accompanied an epidemic of *L. interrogans* sv. *autumnalis* infection and was named Fort Bragg fever. This pretibial rash has accompanied infections with other serovars.

After an asymptomatic interval of 1 to 3 days, the immune phase of the infection develops. The Jarisch-Herxheimer reaction has been reported after early treatment.[72] Leptospires are rapidly cleared from the blood and CSF, and an inflammatory process develops. A CSF pleocytosis will develop in 90% of patients during the second week of illness, but only half of these patients have symptoms of aseptic mengingitis. *L. interrogans* was responsible for 5% to 13% of cases of aseptic meningitis in one series.[75]

The hallmarks of Weil's disease are jaundice and acute renal failure. The jaundice and other signs of liver dysfunction appear as early as the third week and as late as the ninth week after infection.

The diagnosis of classic infection is relatively straightforward, but the diagnosis is considerably more difficult in the average case without an occupational exposure. Schmid and associates reported a very unusual case of leptospirosis, in which the clinical symptoms mimicked Lyme disease. The etiologic agent was a previously unrecognized leptospira, which they named "*L. inadai*" sv. *lyme*.[222]

PATHOLOGY AND PATHOGENESIS

The pathogenesis of leptospirosis, for the most part, is unknown. It is clear that there is a vasculitis in severe cases. It has been suggested that the ability of the spirochetes to bore through tissue allows them to penetrate privileged sites, such as the aqueous humor of the eye. The spirochetes produce a hemolysin, which may contribute to hyperbilirubinemia, but hepatic damage is probably more important. Abnormalities in the liver range from distorted liver cords to multiple foci of necrosis.[11] Renal damage is concentrated in the convoluted tubules, which undergo focal necrosis.

LABORATORY DIAGNOSIS

Laboratory diagnosis of leptospirosis may be by culture of the spirochete, by demonstration of the organisms in specimens, or by serology.

Direct demonstration of *Leptospira* may be attempted by darkfield examination of blood, CSF, or urine. Centrifugation at low speed of oxalated or heparinized blood to remove cellular elements and then at high speed to concentrate leptospira has been recommended. Unfortunately, the direct examination results in rapid but erroneous diagnoses, because fibrils or extrusions from red blood cells are misinterpreted as spirochetes. Although examination of CSF and urine are somewhat less treacherous, similar caveats apply.[75] Direct identification of leptospira with labeled antisera has been described but reagents are not available commercially. Recently *L. interrogans* has been detected in clinical specimens with DNA probes.[143,263]

L. interrogans is by far the easiest of the pathogenic serotypes to culture. The most commonly used media are Fletcher's semisolid medium, Khorthof's liquid medium, or bovine serum albumin–Tween 80 medium, which may be either liquid or solid. The media may be stored at room temperature for long periods. Antibiotics are usually added when the specimen, such as urine, is likely to be contaminated with bacteria, but some of the antibiotics also inhibit leptospira at the required concentration. A combination of fosfomycin and 5-fluorouracil has been found effective when used with Korthof's medium, but the authors caution that the results cannot automatically be transferred to other *Leptospira* media.[181]

L. interrogans can be isolated freely from blood and CSF during the first week of illness. During the immune stage the organisms disappear from the blood and CSF. The kidney, however, is a privileged site and *Leptospira* are excreted in the urine for up to 1 month (see Color Plate 18-1*G*).

It is recommended that at least four 5-mL tubes of culture media from two different lots be inoculated with the clinical specimen. For recovery of fastidious serotypes, 0.4% to 1.0% sterile rabbit serum may be added to the bovine serum albumin–Tween 80 medium. Only small volumes of blood or urine should be inoculated, because larger volumes will introduce interfering substances. Media should be inoculated with 1 to 2 drops of specimen per tube. If the procedure cannot be done at the bedside, oxalated or heparinized blood may be sent to the laboratory. A triturated clot may also be inoculated, but citrated blood may be inhibitory. When urine is tested, an undiluted specimen and a tenfold dilution should be inoculated. When CSF is used, 0.5 to 5.0 mL should be inoculated.

The cultures are incubated in the dark at 28° to 30°C for up to 6 weeks and examined weekly by darkfield microscopy for the presence of leptospira (see Fig. 18-6). Growth is often delayed for several weeks but occurs considerably earlier in Tween 80–albumin medium. Leptospira typically grow as a band 0.5 to 1.0 cm below the surface of semisolid media (see Color Plate 18-1*H*).

Manca and colleagues reported recovery of *L. interrogans* from simulated specimens and from human blood using a commercial radiometric blood culture system. They used Stuart's medium and Middlebrook TB (12A) medium that had been supplemented with bovine serum albumin, catalase, and casein hydrolysate and labeled with ^{14}C-fatty acids. The time to recovery in human blood was 2 to 5 days.[159]

Diagnosis of leptospirosis by culture is definitive, but the techniques are specialized and difficult for most laboratories to maintain when the disease is of low prevalence. The mainstay of diagnosis in most hospitals is, therefore, serologic analysis; and the gold standard is the microagglutination test, using live leptospira. Formalin-killed leptospira are also used, but may result in somewhat lower sensitivity. This reference test is serovar-specific, so that a large number of antigens must be tested against the sera. Commercially available serogroup-specific leptospiral antigens are used in a macroscopic agglutination test that may be used to screen sera. Positive reactions should be confirmed in a reference laboratory with the use of the microagglutination test.

Several versions of hemagglutination tests have been less commonly used. Seki and colleagues described a rapid microcapsule agglutination test,[232] but this test has not been evaluated by other investigators. Several groups have reported enzyme immunoassays that appear promising.[2,187,273] IgM antibody is most specific for current infection. The assays appear to function well and may eventually replace the cumbersome microagglutination test, but cross-reactions do occur.[187] More work is necessary before these procedures can be accepted as new gold standards.

Recently molecular amplification techniques have been employed successfully for the diagnosis of leptospirosis.[15,166] Leptospiral DNA was present in urine even in the early stages of infection, when spirochetemia predominates. These assays are not widely available, but may find a place in reference laboratories.

SPIRILLUM MINOR (RAT-BITE FEVER)

Spirillum minor is a short, thick, tightly coiled spiral rod that measures 0.2 to 0.5 μm in diameter by 3 to 5 μm in length. It produces a large proportion of rat-bite fever in Asia, but rarely occurs in the United States. Transmission is, as the name implies, by rat bite. Human-to-human transmission has not been documented. One to four weeks after the bite a systemic illness, characterized by chills, headache, and fever, occurs. The site of the bite, which had healed, reactivates and is accompanied by regional lymphadenitis and a blotchy rash. Relapsing fever may occur for weeks, months, or years. The most serious complication is infectious endocarditis.[272]

Spirillum minor cannot be cultured in vivo, and no specific serologic tests are available. As many as 50% of infected patients have false-positive serologic tests for syphilis. The spirochetes may be visualized in blood, exudates, or tissue using Giemsa's or Wright's stain or darkfield microscopy.

REFERENCES

1. ACKERMAN R, KABATZKI J, BOISTEN HP, ET AL: Spirochäten-Ätiologie der Erythema-chronicum-migrans-Krankheit. Dtsch Med Wochenschr 109:92–97, 1984
2. ADLER B, MURPHY AM, LOCARNINI SA, ET AL: Detection of specific and antileptospiral immunoglobulins M and G in human serum by solid-phase enzyme-linked immunosorbent assay. J Clin Microbiol 11:452, 1980
3. AGRE F, SCHWARTZ R: The value of early treatment of deer tick bites for the prevention of Lyme disease. Am J Dis Child 147:945–947, 1993
4. AGUERO-ROSENFELD ME, NOWAKOWSKI J, BITTKER S, COOPER D, NADELMAN RB, WORMSER GP: Evolution of the serologic response to Borrelia burgdorferi in treated patients with culture-confirmed erythema migrans. J Clin Microbiol 34:1–9, 1996
5. ALEXANDER-RODRIGUEZ T, VERMUND SH: Gonorrhea and syphilis in incarcerated urban adolescents: prevalence and physical signs. Pediatrics 80:561–564, 1987
6. ALFORD CA, POLT SS, CASSADY GE, STRAUMFJORD JV, REMINGTON JS: Gamma-M-fluorescent treponemal antibody in the diagnosis of syphilis. N Engl J Med 280:1086–1091, 1969
7. ANDERSON JF: Epizootiology of Borrelia in Ixodes tick vectors and reservoir hosts. Rev Infect Dis 11(suppl 6):S1451–S1459, 1989
8. ANDERSON JF, FLAVELL RA, MAGNARELLI LA, ET AL: Novel Borrelia burgdorferi isolates from Ixodes scapularis and Ixodes dentatus ticks feeding on humans. J Clin Microbiol 34:524–529, 1996
9. ANDERSON JF, MAGNARELLI LA, MCANINCH JB: New Borrelia burgdorferi antigenic variant isolated from Ixodes dammini from upstate New York. J Clin Microbiol 26:2209–2212, 1988
10. ANDRUS JK, FLEMING DW, HARGER DR, ET AL: Partner notification: can it control epidemic syphilis? Ann Intern Med 112:539–543, 1990
11. AREAN VM: The pathologic anatomy and pathogenesis of fatal human leptospirosis (Weil's disease). Am J Pathol 40:393–423, 1962
12. AUGENBRAUN MH, DEHOVITZ JA, FELDMAN J, CLARKE L, LANDESMAN S, MINKOFF HM: Biological false-positive syphilis test results for women infected with human immunodeficiency virus. Clin Infect Dis 19:1040–1044, 1994
13. BADON SJ, FISTER RD, CABLE RG: Survival of Borrelia burgdorferi in blood products. Transfusion 29:581–583, 1989
14. BAKKEN LL, CASE KL, CALLISTER SM, BOURDEAU NJ, SCHELL RF: Performance of 45 laboratories participating in a proficiency testing program for Lyme disease serology. JAMA 268:891–895, 1992
15. BAL AE, GRAVEKAMP C, HARTSKEERL RA, DE MEZA-BREWSTER J, KORVER H, TERPSTRA WJ: Detection of leptospires in urine by PCR for early diagnosis of leptospirosis. J Clin Microbiol 32:1894–1898, 1994
16. BARBOUR AG: Isolation and cultivation of Lyme disease spirochetes. Yale J Biol Med 57:521–525, 1984

17. BARBOUR AG: Molecular biology of antigenic variation in Lyme borreliosis and relapsing fever: a comparative analysis. Scand J Infect Dis Suppl 77:88–93, 1991

18. BARBOUR AG, HEILAND RA, HOWE TR: Heterogeneity of major proteins in Lyme disease borreliae: a molecular analysis of North American and European isolates. J Infect Dis 152:478–484, 1985

19. BARBOUR AG, MAUPIN GO, TELTOW GJ, CARTER CJ, PIESMAN J: Identification of an uncultivable *Borrelia* species in the hard tick *Amblyomma americanum*: possible agent of a Lyme disease-like illness. J Infect Dis 173:403–409, 1996

20. BARBOUR AG, TESSIER SL, HAYES SF: Variation in a major surface protein of Lyme disease spirochetes. Infect Immun 45:94–100, 1984

21. BARTON JR, THORPE EM JR, SHAVER DC, HAGER WD, SIBAI BM: Nonimmune hydrops fetalis associated with maternal infection with syphilis. Am J Obstet Gynecol 167:56–58, 1992

22. BECK G, HABICHT GS, BENACH JL, COLEMAN JL: Chemical and biologic characterization of a lipopolysaccharide extracted from the Lyme disease spirochete (*Borrelia burgdorferi*). J Infect Dis 152:108–117, 1985

23. BENACH JL, BOSLER EM, HANRAHAN JP, ET AL: Spirochetes isolated from the blood of two patients with Lyme disease. N Engl J Med 308:740–742, 1983

24. BENACH JL, COLEMAN JL, HABICHT GS, MacDONALD A, GRUNWALDT E, GIRON JA: Serological evidence for simultaneous occurrences of Lyme disease and babesiosis. J Infect Dis 152:473–477, 1985

25. BENACH JL, FLEIT HB, HABICHT GS, COLEMAN JL, BOSLER EM, LANE BP: Interactions of phagocytes with the Lyme disease spirochete: role of the Fc receptor. J Infect Dis 150:497–507, 1984

26. BENDITT J: The syphilized world. Sci Am 260:30, 1989

27. BERARDI VP, WEEKS KE, STEERE AC: Serodiagnosis of early Lyme disease: analysis of IgM and IgG antibody responses by using an antibody-capture enzyme immunoassay. J Infect Dis 158:754–760, 1988

28. BERGER B: Erythema chronicum migrans of Lyme disease. Arch Dermatol 120:1017–1021, 1984

29. BERGER BW, JOHNSON RC, KODNER C, COLEMAN L: Cultivation of *Borrelia burgdorferi* from human tick bite sites: a guide to the risk of infection. J Am Acad Dermatol 32:Pt 1):184–187, 1995

30. BERRY CD, HOOTON TM, COLLIER AC, LUKEHART SA: Neurologic relapse after benzathine penicillin therapy for secondary syphilis in a patient with HIV infection. N Engl J Med 316:1587–1589, 1987

31. BORGNOLO G, HAILU B, CIANCARELLI A, ALMAVIVA M, WOLDEMARIAM T: Louse-borne relapsing fever. A clinical and an epidemiological study of 389 patients in Asella Hospital, Ethiopia. Trop Geogr Med 45:66–69, 1993

32. BOURKE SJ, BAIRD AG, BONE FJ, BAIRD DR, STEVENSON RD: Lyme disease with acute purulent meningitis. Br Med J 297:460, 1988

33. BOWEN GS, GRIFFIN M, HAYNE C, SLADE J, SCHULZE TL, PARKIN W: Clinical manifestations and descriptive epidemiology of Lyme disease in New Jersey, 1978 to 1982. JAMA 251:2236–2240, 1984

34. BROMBERG K, RAWSTRON S, TANNIS G: Diagnosis of congenital syphilis by combining *Treponema pallidum*-specific IgM detection with immunofluorescent antigen detection for *T. pallidum*. J Infect Dis 168:238–242, 1993

35. BRUNET LR, SPIELMAN A, TELFORD SR 3RD: Short report: density of Lyme disease spirochetes within deer ticks collected from zoonotic sites. Am J Trop Med Hyg 53:300–302, 1995

36. BRYCESON ADM, PARRY EHO, PERINE PL, WARRELL DA, VUKOTICH D, LEITHEAD CS: Louse-borne relapsing fever—a clinical and laboratory study of 62 cases in Ethiopia and reconsideration of the literature. Q J Med 39:129–170, 1970

37. BURDASH NM, HINDS KK, FINNERTY JA, MANOS JP: Evaluation of the syphilis Bio-EnzaBead assay for detection of treponemal antibody. J Clin Microbiol 25:808–811, 1987

38. BURGDORFER W, BARBOUR AG, HAYES SF, BENACH JL, GRUNWALDT E, DAVIS JP: Lyme disease—a tick-borne spirochetosis. Science 216:1317–1319, 1982

39. BUTLER T, JONES PK, WALLACE CK: *Borrelia recurrentis* infection: single-dose antibiotic regimens and management of the Jarisch-Herxheimer reaction. J Infect Dis 137:573–577, 1978

40. BYRNE RE, LASKA S, BELL M, LARSON D, PHILLIPS J, TODD J: Evaluation of a *Treponema pallidum* Western immunoblot assay as a confirmatory test for syphilis. J Clin Microbiol 30:115–122, 1992

41. CACCIAPUOTI B, CICERONI L, MAFFEI C, ET AL: A waterborne outbreak of leptospirosis. Am J Epidemiol 126:535–545, 1987

42. CAMPBELL GL, PAUL WS, SCHRIEFER ME, CRAVEN RB, ROBBINS KE, DENNIS DT: Epidemiologic and diagnostic studies of patients with suspected early Lyme disease, Missouri, 1990–1993. J Infect Dis 172:470–480, 1995

43. CANALE-PAROLA E: Spirochetales. In Krieg NR, Holt JR (eds): Bergey's Manual of Systematic Microbiology. Baltimore, Williams & Wilkins, 1984

44. CENTERS FOR DISEASE CONTROL: Syphilis and congenital syphilis—United States, 1985–1988. MMWR 37:486–489, 1988

45. CENTERS FOR DISEASE CONTROL AND PREVENTION: Comparison of early and late latent syphilis—Colorado, 1991. MMWR 42:155–157, 1993

46. CENTERS FOR DISEASE CONTROL AND PREVENTION: Lyme disease—United States, 1994. MMWR 44:459–462, 1995

47. CENTERS FOR DISEASE CONTROL AND PREVENTION: Recommendations for test performance and interpretation from the Second National Conference on Serologic Diagnosis of Lyme Disease. MMWR 44:590–591, 1995

48. CHAMBERS RW, FOLEY HT, SCHMIDT PJ: Transmission of syphilis by fresh blood components. Transfusion 9:32–34, 1969

49. CHANG SN, CHUNG KY, LEE MG, LEE JB: Seroreversion of the serological tests for syphilis in the newborns born to treated syphilitic mothers. Genitourin Med 71:68–70, 1995

50. CHABRA RS, BRION LP, CASTRO M, FREUNDLICH L, GLASER JH: Comparison of maternal sera, cord blood, and neonatal sera for detecting presumptive congenital syphilis: relationship with maternal treatment. Pediatrics 91:88–91, 1993

51. COLEBUNDERS R, DE SERRANO P, VAN GOMPEL A, ET AL: Imported relapsing fever in European tourists. Scand J Infect Dis 25:533–536, 1993

52. COLEMAN JL, SELLATI TJ, TESTA JE, KEW RR, FURIE MB, BENACH JL: *Borrelia burgdorferi* binds plasminogen, resulting in enhanced penetration of endothelial monolayers. Infect Immun 63:2478–2484, 1995

53. COYLE PK, KRUPP LB, DOSCHER C, AMIN K: *Borrelia burgdorferi* reactivity in patients with severe persistent fatigue who are from a region in which Lyme disease is endemic. Clin Infect Dis 18(Suppl 1):S24-27, 1994

54. CRAFT JE, GRODZICKI RL, STEERE AC: Antibody response in Lyme disease: evaluation of diagnostic tests. J Infect Dis 149:789–795, 1984

55. CUTLER SJ, WRIGHT DJ: Predictive value of serology in diagnosing Lyme borreliosis. J Clin Pathol 47:344–349, 1994

56. DANIELS KC, FERNEYHOUGH HS: Specific direct fluorescent antibody detection of *Treponema pallidum*. Health Lab Sci 14:164–171, 1977

57. DATTWYLER RJ, HALPERIN JJ: Failure of tetracycline therapy in early Lyme disease. Arthritis Rheum 30:448–450, 1987

58. DATTWYLER RJ, HALPERIN JJ, VOLKMAN DJ, LUFT BJ: Treatment of late Lyme borreliosis—randomised comparison of ceftriaxone and penicillin. Lancet 1:1191–1194, 1988

59. DATTWYLER RJ, VOLKMAN DJ, LUFT BJ, HALPERIN JJ, THOMAS J, GOLIGHTLY MG: Seronegative Lyme disease. Dissociation of specific T- and B-lymphocyte responses to *Borrelia burgdorferi*. N Engl J Med 319:1441–1446, 1988

60. DE KONING J, HOOGKAMP-KORSTANJE JA, VAN DER LINDE MR, CRIJNS HJ: Demonstration of spirochetes in cardiac biopsies of patients with Lyme disease. J Infect Dis 160:150–153, 1989

61. DEBLINGER RD, WILSON ML, RIMMER DW, SPIELMAN A: Reduced abundance of immature *Ixodes dammini* (Acari: Ixodidae) following incremental removal of deer. J Med Entomol 30:144–150, 1993

62. DEKONENKO EJ, STEERE AC, BERARDI VP, KRAVCHUK LN: Lyme borreliosis in the Soviet Union: a cooperative US–USSR report. J Infect Dis 158:748–753, 1988

63. DEMAERSCHALCK I, BEN MESSAOUD A, DE KESEL M, ET AL: Simultaneous presence of different *Borrelia burgdorferi* genospecies in biological fluids of Lyme disease patients. J Clin Microbiol 33:602–608, 1995

64. DIRINGER MN, HALPERIN JJ, DATTWYLER RJ: Lyme meningoencephalitis: report of a severe, penicillin-resistant case. Arthritis Rheum 30:705–708, 1987

65. DOBSON SR, TABER LH, BAUGHN RE: Recognition of *Treponema pallidum* antigens by IgM and IgG antibodies in congenitally infected newborns and their mothers. J Infect Dis 157:903–910, 1988

66. DRESSLER F, ACKERMANN R, STEERE AC: Antibody responses to the three genomic groups of *Borrelia burgdorferi* in European Lyme borreliosis. J Infect Dis 169:313–318, 1994

67. DRESSLER F, WHALEN JA, REINHARDT BB, STEERE AC: Western blotting in the serodiagnosis of Lyme disease. J Infect Dis 167:392–400, 1993

68. DUNN RA, WEBSTER LA, NAKASHIMA AK, SYLVESTER GC: Surveillance for geographic and secular trends in congenital syphilis—United States, 1983–1991. MMWR CDC Surveill Summ 42:59–71, 1993

69. DURAY PH: The surgical pathology of human Lyme disease. An enlarging picture. Am J Surg Pathol 11(suppl 1):47–60, 1987

70. EDWARDS GA, DOMM BM: Human leptospirosis. Medicine 39:117, 1960

71. EL-ZAATARI MM, MARTENS MG, ANDERSON GD: Incidence of the prozone phenomenon in syphilis serology. Obstet Gynecol 84:609–612, 1994

72. EMMANOUILIDES CE, KOHN OF, GARIBALDI R: Leptospirosis complicated by a Jarisch-Herxheimer reaction and adult respiratory distress syndrome: case report. Clin Infect Dis 18:1004–1006, 1994

73. ENGSTROM SM, SHOOP E, JOHNSON RC: Immunoblot interpretation criteria for serodiagnosis of early Lyme disease. J Clin Microbiol 33:419–427, 1995

74. FEDER HM JR, HUNT MS: Pitfalls in the diagnosis and treatment of Lyme disease in children. JAMA 274:66–68, 1995

75. FEIGIN RD, ANDERSON DC, HEATH CW: Human leptospirosis. Crit Rev Clin Lab Sci 5:413–467, 1975

76. FEIGIN RD, LOBES LA JR, ANDERSON D, ET AL: Human leptospirosis from immunized dogs. Ann Intern Med 79:777, 1973

77. FELSENFELD O: Borreliae, human relapsing fever, and parasite–vector–host relationships. Bacteriol Rev 29:46, 1965

78. FIKRIG E, BERLAND R, CHEN M, WILLIAMS S, SIGAL LH, FLAVELL RA: Serologic response to the *Borrelia burgdorferi* flagellin demonstrates an epitope common to a neuroblastoma cell line. Proc Natl Acad Sci USA 90:183–187, 1993

79. FIKRIG E, HUGUENEL ED, BERLAND R, RAHN DW, HARDIN JA, FLAVELL RA: Serologic diagnosis of Lyme disease using recombinant outer surface proteins A and B and flagellin. J Infect Dis 165:1127–1132, 1992

80. FIKRIG E, TAO H, KANTOR FS, BARTHOLD SW, FLAVELL RA: Evasion of protective immunity by *Borrelia burgdorferi* by truncation of outer surface protein B. Proc Natl Acad Sci USA 90:4092–4096, 1993

81. FIUMARA NJ: Acquired syphilis in three patients with congenital syphilis. N Engl J Med 290:1119–1120, 1974

82. FIUMARA NJ: Reinfection primary, secondary, and latent syphilis: the serologic response after treatment. Sex Transm Dis 7:111–115, 1980

83. FOHN MJ, WIGNALL S, BAKER-ZANDER SA, LUKEHART SA: Specificity of antibodies from patients with pinta for antigens of *Treponema pallidum* subspecies *pallidum*. J Infect Dis 157:32–37, 1988

84. FORNACIARI G, CASTAGNA M, TOGNETTI A, TORNABONI D, BRUNO J: Syphilis in a Renaissance Italian mummy. Lancet 2:614, 1989

85. FRASER JR: Lyme disease challenges Australian clinicians: the implications of Australia's first reported case of Lyme arthritis. Med J Aust 1:101–102, 1982

86. FUCHS H, WALLICH R, SIMON MM, KRAMER MD: The outer surface protein A of the spirochete *Borrelia burgdorferi* is a plasmin(ogen) receptor. Proc Natl Acad Sci USA 91:12594–12598, 1994

87. FUNG BP, MCHUGH GL, LEONG JM, STEERE AC: Humoral immune response to outer surface protein C of *Borrelia burgdorferi* in Lyme disease: role of the immunoglobulin M response in the serodiagnosis of early infection. Infect Immun 62:3213–3221, 1994

88. GELFAND JA, ELIN RJ, BERRY FW JR, FRANK MM: Endotoxemia associated with the Jarisch-Herxheimer reaction. N Engl J Med 295:211–213, 1976

89. GERBER AR, KING LC, DUNLEAVY GJ, NOVICK LF: An outbreak of syphilis on an Indian reservation: descriptive epidemiology and disease-control measures. Am J Publ Health 79:83–85, 1989

90. GERBER MA, SHAPIRO ED, KRAUSE PJ, CABLE RG, BADON SJ, RYAN RW: The risk of acquiring Lyme disease or babesiosis from a blood transfusion. J Infect Dis 170: 231–234, 1994

91. GODSEY MS JR, AMUNDSON TE, BURGESS EC, ET AL: Lyme disease ecology in Wisconsin: distribution and host preferences of *Ixodes dammini*, and prevalence of antibody to *Borrelia burgdorferi* in small mammals. Am J Trop Med Hyg 37:180–187, 1987

92. GOLDSCHMID JM, MAHOMED K: The use of the microhematocrit technic for the recovery of *Borrelia duttonii* from the blood. Am J Clin Pathol 58:165–169, 1972

93. GOODMAN JL, BRADLEY JF, ROSS AE, ET AL: Bloodstream invasion in early Lyme disease: results from a prospective, controlled, blinded study using the polymerase chain reaction. Am J Med 99:6–12, 1995

94. GRIMPREL E, SANCHEZ PJ, WENDEL GD, ET AL: Use of polymerase chain reaction and rabbit infectivity testing to detect *Treponema pallidum* in amniotic fluid, fetal and neonatal sera, and cerebrospinal fluid. J Clin Microbiol 29:1711–1718, 1991

95. GRODZICKI RL, STEERE AC: Comparison of immunoblotting with indirect enzyme-linked immunosorbent assay using different antigen preparations for diagnosing early Lyme disease. J Infect Dis 157:790–797, 1988

96. HAAS JS, BOLAN G, LARSEN SA, CLEMENT MJ, BACCHETTI P, MOSS AR: Sensitivity of treponemal tests for detecting prior treated syphilis during human immunodeficiency virus infection. J Infect Dis 162:862–866, 1990

97. HAHN RA, MAGDER LS, ARAL SO, JOHNSON RE, LARSEN SA: Race and the prevalence of syphilis seroreactivity in the United States population: a national sero-epidemiologic study. Am J Publ Health 79:467–470, 1989

98. HAMMERS-BERGGREN S, LEBECH AM, KARLSSON M, SVENUNGSSON B, HANSEN K, STIERNSTEDT G: Serological follow-up after treatment of patients with erythema migrans and neuroborreliosis. J Clin Microbiol 32: 1519–1525, 1994

99. HANRAHAN JP, BENACH JL, COLEMAN JL, ET AL: Incidence and cumulative frequency of endemic Lyme disease in a community. J Infect Dis 150:489–496, 1984

100. HARDIN JA, STEERE AC, MALAWISTA SE: The pathogenesis of arthritis in Lyme disease: humoral immune responses and the role of intra-articular immune complexes. Yale J Biol Med 57:589–593, 1984

101. HARRIS EN, GHARAVI AE, WASLEY GD, HUGHES GR: Use of an enzyme-linked immunosorbent assay and of inhibition studies to distinguish between antibodies to cardiolipin from patients with syphilis or autoimmune disorders. J Infect Dis 157:23–31, 1988

102. HART G: Syphilis tests in diagnostic and therapeutic decision making. Ann Intern Med 104:368–376, 1986

103. HEATH CW JR, ALEXANDER AD, GALTON MM: Leptospirosis in the United States (concluded). Analysis of 483 cases in man, 1949–1961. N Engl J Med 273:915–922, 1965

104. HEATH CW JR, ALEXANDER AD, GALTON MM: Leptospirosis in the United States. Analysis of 483 cases in man. N Engl J Med 273:857–864, 1965

105. HECHEMY KE, HARRIS HL, WETHERS JA, ET AL: Fluoroimmunoassay studies with solubilized antigens from *Borrelia burgdorferi*. J Clin Microbiol 27:1854–1858, 1989

106. HICKS CB, BENSON PM, LUPTON GP, TRAMONT EC: Seronegative secondary syphilis in a patient infected with the human immunodeficiency virus (HIV) with Kaposi sarcoma. A diagnostic dilemma. Ann Intern Med 107:492–495, 1987

107. HILTON E, DEVOTI J, SOOD S: Recommendation to include OspA and OspB in the new immunoblotting criteria for serodiagnosis of Lyme disease. J Clin Microbiol 34: 1353–1354, 1996

108. HOOK EW, RODDY RE, HANDSFIELD HH: Ceftriaxone therapy for incubating and early syphilis. J Infect Dis 158:881–884, 1988

109. HOOK EW III: Treatment of syphilis: current recommendations, alternatives, and continuing problems. Rev Infect Dis 11:S1511–S1517, 1989

110. HOOK EW III, MARRA CM: Acquired syphilis in adults. N Engl J Med 326:1060–1069, 1992

111. HOOK EW III, RODDY RE, LUKEHART SA, HOM J, HOMES KK, TAM MR: Detection of *Treponema pallidum* in lesion exudate with a pathogen-specific monoclonal antibody. J Clin Microbiol 22:241–244, 1985

112. HOOSHMAND H, ESCOBAR MR, KOPF SW: Neurosyphilis. A study of 241 patients. JAMA 219:726–729, 1972

113. HORTON JM, BLASER MJ: The spectrum of relapsing fever in the Rocky Mountains. Arch Intern Med 145.871–875, 1985

114. HUNTER EF, RUSSELL H, FARSHY CE, SAMPSON JS, LARSEN SA: Evaluation of sera from patients with Lyme disease in the fluorescent treponemal antibody-absorption test for syphilis. Sex Transm Dis 13:232–236, 1986

115. HUTCHESON HJ, OLIVER JH JR, HOUCK MA, STRAUSS RE: Multivariate morphometric discrimination of nymphal and adult forms of the blacklegged tick (Acari: Ixodidae), a principal vector of the agent of Lyme disease in eastern North America. J Med Entomol 32:827–842, 1995

116. HUTCHINSON CM, HOOK EW 3RD, SHEPHERD M, VERLEY J, ROMPALO AM: Altered clinical presentation of early syphilis in patients with human immunodeficiency virus infection. Ann Intern Med 121:94–100, 1994

117. HYDE FW, JOHNSON RC: Genetic relationship of Lyme disease spirochetes to *Borrelia*, *Treponema*, and *Leptospira* spp. J Clin Microbiol 20:151–154, 1984

118. IJSSELMUIDEN OE, SCHOULS LM, STOLZ E, ET AL: Sensitivity and specificity of an enzyme-linked immunosorbent assay using the recombinant DNA-derived *Treponema pallidum* protein TmpA for serodiagnosis of syphilis and the potential use of TmpA for assessing the effect of antibiotic therapy. J Clin Microbiol 27:152–157, 1989

119. ITO F, HUNTER EF, GEORGE RW, POPE V, LARSEN SA: Specific immunofluorescent staining of pathogenic treponemes with a monoclonal antibody. J Clin Microbiol 30:831–838, 1992

120. ITO F, HUNTER EF, GEORGE RW, SWISHER BL, LARSEN SA: Specific immunofluorescence staining of *Treponema pallidum* in smears and tissues. J Clin Microbiol 29:444–448, 1991

121. JACKSON LA, KAUFMANN AF, ADAMS WG, ET AL: Outbreak of leptospirosis associated with swimming. Pediatr Infect Dis J 12:48–54, 1993

122. JOHNSON RC, FAINE S: *Leptospira* Noguchi 1917. In Bergey's Manual of Systematic Bacteriology, pp 62–67. Baltimore, Williams & Wilkins, 1984

123. JOHNSON RC, KODNER C, RUSSELL M: In vitro and in vivo susceptibility of the Lyme disease spirochete, *Borrelia burgdorferi*, to four antimicrobial agents. Antimicrob Agents Chemother 31:164–167, 1987

124. JOHNSON RC, SCHMID GP, HYDE FW, STEIGERWALT AG, BRENNER DJ: *Borrelia burgdorferi* sp. nov.: Etiologic agent of Lyme disease. Int J Syst Bacteriol 34:496–497, 1984

125. JOHNSTON YE, DURAY PH, STEERE AC, ET AL: Lyme arthritis. Spirochetes found in synovial microangiopathic lesions. Am J Pathol 118:26–34, 1985

126. KAELL AT, REDECHA PR, ELKON KB, ET AL: Occurrence of antibodies to *Borrelia burgdorferi* in patients with nonspirochetal subacute bacterial endocarditis. Ann Intern Med 119:1079–1083, 1993

127. KAELL AT, VOLKMAN DJ, GOREVIC PD, ET AL: Positive Lyme serology in subacute bacterial endocarditis: a study of four patients. JAMA 264:2916–2918, 1990

128. KAUFMAN RE, WEISS S, MOORE JD, FALCONE V, WIESNER PJ: Biological false positive serological tests for syphilis among drug addicts. Br J Vener Dis 50:350–353, 1974

129. KELLY R: Cultivation of *Borrelia hermsii*. Science 173:443–444, 1971

130. KELLY RT: *Borrelia* Swellengrebel 1907. In Bergey's Manual of Systematic Bacteriology, pp 57–62. Baltimore, Williams & Wilkins, 1984

131. KITTEN T, BARRERA AV, BARBOUR AG: Intragenic recombination and a chimeric outer membrane protein in the relapsing fever agent *Borrelia hermsii*. J Bacteriol 175:2516–2522, 1993

132. KLASS PE, BROWN ER, PELTON SI: The incidence of prenatal syphilis at the Boston City Hospital: a comparison across four decades. Pediatrics 94:24–28, 1994

133. KOFF AB, ROSEN T: Nonvenereal treponematoses: yaws, endemic syphilis, and pinta. J Am Acad Dermatol 29:519–535, 1993

134. KORNBLATT AN, URBAND PH, STEERE AC: Arthritis caused by *Borrelia burgdorferi* in dogs. J Am Vet Med Assoc 186:960–964, 1985

135. KRAUS SJ, HASERICK JR, LANTZ MA: Fluorescent treponemal antibody-absorption test reactions in lupus erythematosus. Atypical beading pattern and probable false-positive reactions. N Engl J Med 282:1287–1290, 1970

136. KURTTI TJ, MUNDERLOH UG, JOHNSON RC, AHLSTRAND GG: Colony formation and morphology in *Borrelia burgdorferi*. J Clin Microbiol 25:2054–2058, 1987

137. LARSEN SA: Syphilis. Clin Lab Med 9:545–557, 1989

138. LARSEN SA, HAMBIE EA, PETTIT DE, PERRYMAN MW, KRAUS SJ: Specificity, sensitivity, and reproducibility among the fluorescent treponemal antibody-absorption test, the microhemagglutination assay for *Treponema pallidum* antibodies, and the hemagglutination treponemal test for syphilis. J Clin Microbiol 14:441–445, 1981

139. LARSEN SA, HUNTER EF, KRAUS SJ: Manual of Tests for Syphilis, 8th ed. Washington DC. American Public Health Association, 1990

140. LARSEN SA, STEINER BM, RUDOLPH AH: Laboratory diagnosis and interpretation of tests for syphilis. Clin Microbiol Rev 8:1–21, 1995

141. LEBECH AM, HANSEN K: Detection of *Borrelia burgdorferi* DNA in urine samples and cerebrospinal fluid samples from patients with early and late Lyme neuroborreliosis by polymerase chain reaction. J Clin Microbiol 30:1646–1653, 1992

142. LEE CB, BRUNHAM RC, SHERMAN E, HARDING GK: Epidemiology of an outbreak of infectious syphilis in Manitoba. Am J Epidemiol 125:277–283, 1987

143. LEFEBVRE R: DNA probe for detection of the *Leptospira interrogans* serovar *hardjo* genotype *hardjo-bovis*. J Clin Microbiol 25:2236–2238, 1987

144. LEFEVRE JC, BERTRAND MA, BAURIAUD R: Evaluation of the Captia enzyme immunoassays for detection of immunoglobulins G and M to *Treponema pallidum* in syphilis. J Clin Microbiol 28:1704–1707, 1990

145. LENGL-JANSSEN B, STRAUSS AF, STEERE AC, KAMRADT T: The T helper cell response in Lyme arthritis: differential recognition of *Borrelia burgdorferi* outer surface protein A in patients with treatment-resistant or treatment-responsive Lyme arthritis. J Exp Med 180:2069–2078, 1994

146. LEVINE JF, WILSON ML, SPIELMAN A: Mice as reservoirs of the Lyme disease spirochete. Am J Trop Med Hyg 34:355–360, 1985

147. LEY C, LE C, OLSHEN EM, REINGOLD AL: The use of serologic tests for Lyme disease in a prepaid health plan in California. JAMA 271:460–463, 1994

148. LIU CC, SO WC, LIN CH, YEH TF: Congenital syphilis: clinical manifestations in premature infants. Scand J Infect Dis 25:741–745, 1993

149. LOVRICH SD, CALLISTER SM, LIM LC, DUCHATEAU BK, SCHELL RF: Seroprotective groups of Lyme borreliosis spirochetes from North America and Europe. J Infect Dis 170:115–121, 1994

150. LUFT BJ, STEINMAN CR, NEIMARK HC, ET AL: Invasion of the central nervous system by *Borrelia burgdorferi* in acute disseminated infection. JAMA 267:1364–1367, 1992

151. LUKEHART SA, HOOK EW, BAKER-ZANDER SA, COLLIER AC, CRITCHLOW CW, HANDSFIELD HH: Invasion of the central nervous system by *Treponema pallidum*: implications for diagnosis and treatment. Ann Intern Med 109:855–862, 1988

152. MA B, CHRISTEN B, LEUNG D, VIGO-PELFREY C: Serodiagnosis of Lyme borreliosis by Western immunoblot: reactivity of various significant antibodies against *Borrelia burgdorferi*. J Clin Microbiol 30:370–376, 1992

153. MAGID D, SCHWARTZ B, CRAFT J, SCHWARTZ JS: Prevention of Lyme disease after tick bites—a cost-effectiveness analysis. N Engl J Med 327:534–541, 1992

154. MAGNARELLI LA: Current status of laboratory diagnosis for Lyme disease. Am J Med 98:10S–12S, 1995

155. MAGNARELLI LA, ANDERSON JF, JOHNSON RC: Cross-reactivity in serological tests for Lyme disease and other spirochetal infections. J Infect Dis 156:183–188, 1987

156. MAGNARELLI LA, FIKRIG E, PADULA SJ, ANDERSON JF, FLAVELL RA: Use of recombinant antigens of *Borrelia burgdorferi* in serologic tests for diagnosis of Lyme borreliosis. J Clin Microbiol 34:237–240, 1996

157. MAGNARELLI LA, MEEGAN JM, ANDERSON JF, CHAPPELL WA: Comparison of an indirect fluorescent-antibody test with an enzyme-linked immunosorbent assay for serological studies of Lyme disease. J Clin Microbiol 20:181–184, 1984

158. MAGNUSON HJ, THOMAS EW, OLANSKY S, KAPLAN BI, DE MELLO L, CUTLER JC: Inoculation syphilis in human volunteers. Medicine 35:33–82, 1956

159. MANCA N, VERARDI R, COLOMBRITA D, RAVIZZOLA G, SAVOLDI E, TURANO A: Radiometric method for the rapid detection of *Leptospira* organisms. J Clin Microbiol 23:401–493, 1986

160. MARCUS LC, STEERE AC, DURAY PH, ANDERSON AE, MAHONEY EB: Fatal pancarditis in a patient with coexistent Lyme disease and babesiosis. Demonstration of spirochetes in the myocardium. Ann Intern Med 103:374–376, 1985

161. MARSHALL WF 3RD, TELFORD SR, 3RD, RYS PN, ET AL: Detection of *Borrelia burgdorferi* DNA in museum specimens of *Peromyscus leucopus*. J Infect Dis 170:1027–1032, 1994

162. MATUSCHKA FR, OHLENBUSCH A, EIFFERT H, RICHTER D, SPIELMAN A: Antiquity of the Lyme-disease spirochaete in Europe. Lancet 346:1367, 1995

163. MATUSCHKA FR, SPIELMAN A: Risk of infection from and treatment of tick bite. Lancet 342:529–530, 1993

164. MAUPIN GO, GAGE KL, PIESMAN J, ET AL: Discovery of an enzootic cycle of *Borrelia burgdorferi* in *Neotoma mexicana* and *Ixodes spinipalpis* from northern Colorado, an area where Lyme disease is nonendemic. J Infect Dis 170:636–643, 1994

165. MCLAIN DK, WESSON DM, OLIVER JH JR, COLLINS FH: Variation in ribosomal DNA internal transcribed spacers 1 among eastern populations of *Ixodes scapularis* (Acari: Ixodidae). J Med Entomol 32:353–360, 1995

166. MERIEN F, BARANTON G, PEROLAT P: Comparison of polymerase chain reaction with microagglutination test and culture for diagnosis of leptospirosis. J Infect Dis 172:281–285, 1995

167. MEYER MP, EDDY T, BAUGHN RE: Analysis of Western blotting (immunoblotting) technique in diagnosis of congenital syphilis. J Clin Microbiol 32:629–633, 1994

168. MIAO RM, FIELDSTEEL AH: Genetic relationship between *Treponema pallidum* and *Treponema pertenue* two noncultivable human pathogens. J Bacteriol 141:427–429, 1980

169. MINKOFF HL, MCCALLA S, DELKE I, STEVENS R, SALWEN M, FELDMAN J: The relationship of cocaine use to syphilis and human immunodeficiency virus infections among inner city parturient women. Am J Obstet Gynecol 163:521–526, 1990

170. MITCHELL PD, REED KD, ASPESLET TL, VANDERMAUSE MF, MELSKI JW: Comparison of four immunoserologic assays for detection of antibodies to *Borrelia burgdorferi* in patients with culture-positive erythema migrans. J Clin Microbiol 32:1958–1962, 1994

171. MITCHELL PD, REED KD, HOFKES JM: Immunoserologic evidence of coinfection with *Borrelia burgdorferi*, *Babesia microti*, and human granulocytic *Erlichia* species in residents of Wisconsin and Minnesota. J Clin Microbiol 34:724–727, 1996

172. MOYER NP, HUDSON JD, HAUSLER WJ JR: Evaluation of the Bio-EnzaBead test for syphilis. J Clin Microbiol 25:619–623, 1987

173. MUSHER DM, HAMILL RJ, BAUGHN RE: Effect of human immunodeficiency virus (HIV) infection on the course of syphilis and on the response to treatment. Ann Intern Med 113:872–881, 1990

174. NAKAO M, MIYAMOTO K: Mixed infection of different *Borrelia* species among *Apodemus speciosus* mice in Hokkaido, Japan. J Clin Microbiol 33:490–492, 1995

175. NEGUSSIE Y, REMICK DG, DEFORGE LE, KUNKEL SL, EYNON A, GRIFFIN GE: Detection of plasma tumor necrosis factor, interleukins 6, and 8 during the Jarisch-Herxheimer Reaction of relapsing fever. J Exp Med 175:1207–1212, 1992

176. NOCTON JJ, DRESSLER F, RUTLEDGE BJ, RYS PN, PERSING DH, STEERE AC: Detection of *Borrelia burgdorferi* DNA by polymerase chain reaction in synovial fluid from patients with Lyme arthritis. N Engl J Med 330:229–234, 1994

177. NOORDHOEK GT, COCKAYNE A, SCHOULS LM, MELOEN RH, STOLZ E, VAN EMBDEN JD: A new attempt to distinguish serologically the subspecies of *Treponema pallidum* causing syphilis and yaws. J Clin Microbiol 28:1600–1607, 1990

178. NOORDHOEK GT, HERMANS PWM, PAUL AN, ET AL: *Treponema pallidum* subspecies *pallidum* (Nichols) and *Treponema pallidum* subspecies *pertenue* (CDC 2575) differ in at least one nucleotide: comparison of two homologous antigens. Microb Pathog 6:29–42, 1989

179. NOORDHOEK GT, WOLTERS EC, DE JONGE EJ, VAN EMBDEN JDA: Detection by polymerase chain reaction of *Treponema pallidum* DNA in cerebrospinal fluid from neurosyphilis patients before and after antibiotic treatment. J Clin Microbiol 29:1976–1984, 1991

180. O'NEIL KM, RICKMAN LS, LAZARUS AA: Pulmonary manifestations of leptospirosis. Rev Infect Dis 13:705–709, 1991

181. OIE S, KOSHIRO A, KONISHI H, YOSHII Z: In vitro evaluation of combined usage of fosfomycin and 5-fluorouracil for selective isolation of *Leptospira* species. J Clin Microbiol 23:1084–1087, 1986

182. OLIVER JH JR, CHANDLER FW JR, LUTTRELL MP, ET AL: Isolation and transmission of the Lyme disease spirochete from the southeastern United States. Proc Natl Acad Sci USA 90:7371–7375, 1993

183. OLIVER JH JR, OWSLEY MR, HUTCHESON HJ, ET AL: Conspecificity of the ticks *Ixodes scapularis* and *I. dammini* (Acari: Ixodidae). J Med Entomol 30:54–63, 1993

184. PACHNER AR, RICALTON N, DELANEY E: Comparison of polymerase chain reaction with culture and serology for diagnosis of murine experimental Lyme borreliosis. J Clin Microbiol 31:208–214, 1993

185. PACHNER AR, STEERE AC: The triad of neurologic manifestations of Lyme disease: meningitis, cranial neuritis, and radiculoneuritis. Neurology 35:47–53, 1985

186. PANCHOLI P, KOLBERT CP, MITCHELL PD, ET AL: *Ixodes dammini* as a potential vector of human granulocytic ehrlichiosis. J Infect Dis 172:1007–1012, 1995

187. PAPPAS MG, BALLOU WR, GRAY MR, ET AL: Rapid serodiagnosis of leptospirosis using the IGM-specific dot-ELISA: comparison with the microscopic agglutination test. Am J Trop Med Hyg 34:346–354, 1985

188. PAVIA CS, NIEDERBUHL CJ: Adoptive transfer of anti-syphilis immunity with lymphocytes from *Treponema pallidum*-infected guinea pigs. J Immunol 135:2829–2834, 1985

189. PAVIA CS, NIEDERBUHL CJ: Acquired resistance and expression of a protective humoral immune response in guinea pigs infected with *Treponema pallidum* Nichols. Infect Immun 50:66–72, 1985

190. PEDERSEN NS, ORUM O, MOURITSEN S: Enzyme-linked immunosorbent assay for detection of antibodies to the

venereal disease research laboratory (VDRL) antigen in syphilis. J Clin Microbiol 25:1711–1716, 1987

191. PENNELL DR, WAND PJ, SCHELL RF: Evaluation of a quantitative fluorescence immunoassay (FIAX) for detection of serum antibody to *Borrelia burgdorferi*. J Clin Microbiol 25:2218–2220, 1987

192. PERINE PL, NELSON JW, LEWIS JO, ET AL: New technologies for use in the surveillance and control of yaws. Rev Infect Dis 7:295, 1985

193. PERSING DH, RUTLEDGE BJ, RYS PN, ET AL: Target imbalance: disparity of *Borrelia burgdorferi* genetic material in synovial fluid from Lyme arthritis patients. J Infect Dis 169:668–672, 1994

194. PETERSON PK, CLAWSON CC, LEE DA, GARLICH DJ, QUIE PG, JOHNSON RC: Human phagocyte interactions with the Lyme disease spirochete. Infect Immun 46:608–611, 1984

195. PFISTER HW, PREAC-MURSIC V, WILSKE B, EINH:AUPL KM, WEINBERGER K: Latent Lyme neuroborreliosis: presence of *Borrelia burgdorferi* in the cerebrospinal fluid without concurrent inflammatory signs. Neurology 39:1118–1120, 1989

196. PICKEN RN: Polymerase chain reaction primers and probes derived from flagellin gene sequences for specific detection of the agents of Lyme disease and North American relapsing fever. J Clin Microbiol 30:99–114, 1992

197. PIESMAN J, MATHER TN, SINSKY RJ, SPIELMAN A: Duration of tick attachment and *Borrelia burgdorferi* transmission. J Clin Microbiol 25:557–558, 1987

198. POLLACK RJ, TELFORD SR 3RD, SPIELMAN A: Standardization of medium for culturing Lyme disease spirochetes. J Clin Microbiol 31:1251–1255, 1993

199. PREAC-MURSIC V, WILSKE B, SCHIERZ G, PFISTER HW, EINHAUPL K: Repeated isolation of spirochetes from the cerebrospinal fluid of a patient with meningoradiculitis Bannwarth. Eur J Clin Microbiol 3:564–565, 1984

200. RAOULT D, HECHEMY KE, BARANTON G: Cross-reaction with *Borrelia burgdorferi* antigen of sera from patients with human immunodeficiency virus infection, syphilis, and leptospirosis. J Clin Microbiol 27:2152–2155, 1989

201. RAWLINGS JA, FOURNIER PV, TELTOW GJ: Isolation of *Borrelia* spirochetes from patients in Texas. J Clin Microbiol 25:1148–1150, 1987

202. RESTREPO BI, BARBOUR AG: Antigen diversity in the bacterium *B. hermsii* through "somatic" mutations in rearranged *vmp* genes. Cell 78:867–876, 1994

203. RICH SM, CAPORALE DA, TELFORD SR 3RD, KOCHER TD, HARTL DL, SPIELMAN A: Distribution of the *Ixodes ricinus*-like ticks of eastern North America. Proc Natl Acad Sci USA 92:6284–6288, 1995

204. RIGGSBEE JH, LAMKE CL: An evaluation of the double-staining procedure for the fluorescent treponemal antibody-absorption (FTA-ABS) test. Lab Med 12:232–234, 1981

205. RIVIERÉ GR, WAGONER MA, BAKER-ZANDER SA, ET AL: Identification of spirochetes related to *Treponema pallidum* in necrotizing ulcerative gingivitis and chronic periodontitis. N Engl J Med 325:539–543, 1991

206. RODRIGUEZ S, TEICH DL, WEINMAN MD, GREENE JM, KEROACK MA, APSTEIN MD: Gummatous syphilis: a reminder. J Infect Dis 157:606–607, 1988

207. ROLFS RT, GOLDBERG M, SHARRAR RG: Risk factors for syphilis: cocaine use and prostitution. Am J Public Health 80:853–857, 1990

208. ROLFS RT, NAKASHIMA AK: Epidemiology of primary and secondary syphilis in the United States, 1981 through 1989. JAMA 264:1432–1437, 1990

209. ROMPALO AM, CANNON RO, QUINN TC, HOOK EW 3RD: Association of biologic false-positive reactions for syphilis with human immunodeficiency virus infection. J Infect Dis 165:1124–1126, 1992

210. ROSEN EU, RICHARDSON NJ: A reappraisal of the value of the IgM fluorescent treponemal antibody absorption test in the diagnosis of congenital syphilis. Pediatrics 87:38–42, 1975

211. ROTHSCHILD BM, ROTHSCHILD C: Treponemal disease revisited: skeletal discriminators for yaws, bejel, and venereal syphilis. Clin Infect Dis 20:1402–1408, 1995

212. RUSSELL H, SAMPSON JS, SCHMID GP, WILKINSON HW, PLIKAYTIS B: Enzyme-linked immunosorbent assay and indirect immunofluorescence assay for Lyme disease. J Infect Dis 149:465–470, 1984

213. RUSSELL RC, DOGGETT SL, MUNRO R, ET AL: Lyme disease: a search for a causative agent in ticks in south-eastern Australia. Epidemiol Infect 112:375–384, 1994

214. SADZIENE A, BARBOUR AG, ROSA PA, THOMAS DD: An OspB mutant of *Borrelia burgdorferi* has reduced invasiveness in vitro and reduced infectivity in vivo. Infect Immun 61:3590–3596, 1993

215. SANCHEZ PJ, WENDEL GD JR, GRIMPREL E, ET AL: Evaluation of molecular methodologies and rabbit infectivity testing for the diagnosis of congenital syphilis and neonatal central nervous system invasion by *Treponema pallidum*. J Infect Dis 167:148–157, 1993

216. SANDERS FH JR, OLIVER JH JR: Evaluation of *Ixodes scapularis*, *Amblyomma americanum*, and *Dermacentor variabilis* (Acari: Ixodidae) from Georgia as vectors of a Florida strain of the Lyme disease spirochete, *Borrelia burgdorferi*. J Med Entomol 32:402–406, 1995

217. SASAKI DM, PANG L, MINETTE HP, ET AL: Active surveillance and risk factors for leptospirosis in Hawaii. Am J Trop Med Hyg 48:35–43, 1993

218. SANCHEZ PJ, MCCRACKEN GH JR, WENDEL GD, OLSEN K, THRELKELD N, NORGARD MV: Molecular analysis of the fetal IgM response to *Treponema pallidum* antigens: implications for improved serodiagnosis of congenital syphilis. J Infect Dis 159:508–517, 1989

219. SCHECK DN, HOOK EW 3RD: Neurosyphilis. Infect Dis Clin North Am 8:769–795, 1994

220. SCHLESINGER PA, DURAY PH, BURKE BA, STEERE AC, STILLMAN MT: Maternal–fetal transmission of the Lyme disease spirochete, *Borrelia burgdorferi*. Ann Intern Med 103:67–68, 1985

221. SCHMID GP, HORSLEY R, STEERE AC, ET AL: Surveillance of Lyme disease in the United States, 1982. J Infect Dis 151:1144–1149, 1985

222. SCHMID GP, STEERE AC, KORNBLATT AN, ET AL: Newly recognized *Leptospira* species ("*Leptospira inadai*" serovar *lyme*) isolated from human skin. J Clin Microbiol 24:484–486, 1986

223. SCHMID GP, STEIGERWALT AG, JOHNSON SE, ET AL: DNA characterization of the spirochete that causes Lyme disease. J Clin Microbiol 20:155–158, 1984

224. Schmid GP, Verardo L, Highsmith AK, Weisfeld JS: Failure to detect endotoxin in sera from patients with Lyme disease. J Infect Dis 150:616, 1984

225. Schmidt B, Muellegger RR, Stockenhuber C, et al: Detection of *Borrelia burgdorferi*-specific DNA in urine specimens from patients with erythema migrans before and after antibiotic therapy. J Clin Microbiol 34:1359–1363, 1996

226. Schulze TL, Bowen GS, Bosler EM, et al: *Amblyomma americanum*: a potential vector of Lyme disease in New Jersey. Science 224:601–603, 1984

227. Schutzer SE, Coyle PK, Dunn JJ, Luft BJ, Brunner M: Early and specific antibody response to OspA in Lyme disease. J Clin Invest 94:454–457, 1994

228. Schwan TG, Gage KL, Karstens RH, Schrumpf ME, Hayes SF, Barbour AG: Identification of the tick-borne relapsing fever spirochete *Borrelia hermsii* by using a species-specific monoclonal antibody. J Clin Microbiol 30:790–795, 1992

229. Schwartz I, Wormser GP, Schwartz JJ, et al: Diagnosis of early Lyme disease by polymerase chain reaction amplification and culture of skin biopsies from erythema migrans lesions. J Clin Microbiol 30:3082–3088, 1992

230. Sciotto CG, Lauer BA, White WL, et al: Detection of *Borrelia* in acridine orange-stained blood smears by fluorescence microscopy. Arch Pathol Lab Med 107:384–386, 1983

231. Seboxa T, Rahlenbeck SI: Treatment of louse-borne relapsing fever with low dose penicillin or tetracycline: a clinical trial. Scand J Infect Dis 27:29–31, 1995

232. Seki M, Sato T, Arimitsu Y, et al: One point method for serological diagnosis of leptospirosis: a microcapsule agglutination test. Epidemiol Infect 99:399–405, 1987

233. Seppala IJ, Kroneld R, Schauman K, Forsen KO, Lassenius R: Diagnosis of Lyme borreliosis: non-specific serological reactions with *Borrelia burgdorferi* sonicate antigen caused by IgG2 antibodies. J Med Microbiol 40:293–302, 1994

234. Shadick NA, Phillips CB, Logigian EL, et al: The long-term clinical outcomes of Lyme disease. A population-based retrospective cohort study. Ann Intern Med 121:560–567, 1994

235. Shapiro ED, Gerber MA, Holabird NB, et al: A controlled trial of antimicrobial prophylaxis for Lyme disease after deer-tick bites. N Engl J Med 327:1769–1773, 1992

236. Shaw RD: Kayaking as a risk factor for leptospirosis. Mo Med 89:354–357, 1992

237. Sigal LH, Steere AC, Dwyer JM: In vivo and in vitro evidence of B cell hyperactivity during Lyme disease. J Rheumatol 15:648–654, 1988

238. Smith RP Jr, Rand PW, Lacombe EH, et al: Norway rats as reservoir hosts for Lyme disease spirochetes on Monhegan Island, Maine. J Infect Dis 168:687–691, 1993

239. Southern P, Sanford JP: Relapsing fever. A clinical and microbiological review. Medicine 48:129–149, 1969

240. Spach DH, Liles WC, Campbell GL, Quick RE, Anderson DE Jr, Fritsche TR: Tick-borne diseases in the United States. N Engl J Med 329:936–947, 1993

241. Sperling LC, Hicks K, James WD: Occult primary syphilis: the nonerosive chancre. J Am Acad Dermatol 23:514–515, 1990

242. Spielman A, Clifford CM, Piesman J, Corwin RM: Human babesiosis on Nantucket Island, USA: description of the vector, *Ixodes (Ixodes) dammini*, n. sp. (Acarina: Ixodidae). J Med Entomol 15:218–234, 1979

243. Stamm LV, Dallas WS, Ray PH, Bassford PJ Jr: Identification, cloning, and purification of protein antigens of *Treponema pallidum*. Rev Infect Dis 10(suppl 2):S403–S407, 1988

244. Stamm WE, Handsfield HH, Rompalo AM, Ashley RL, Roberts PL, Corey L: The association between genital ulcer disease and acquisition of HIV infection in homosexual men. JAMA 260:1429–1433, 1988

245. Stechenberg BW: Lyme disease: the latest great imitator. Pediatr Infect Dis J 7:402–409, 1988

246. Steere AC: Lyme disease. N Engl J Med 321:586–596, 1989

247. Steere AC, Bartenhagen NH, Craft JE, et al: The early clinical manifestations of Lyme disease. Ann Intern Med 99:76–82, 1983

248. Steere AC, Green J, Schoen RT, et al: Successful parenteral penicillin therapy of established Lyme arthritis. N Engl J Med 312:869–874, 1985

249. Steere AC, Grodzicki RL, Craft JE, Shrestha M, Kornblatt AN, Malawista SE: Recovery of Lyme disease spirochetes from patients. Yale J Biol Med 57:557–560, 1984

250. Steere AC, Grodzicki RL, Kornblatt AN, et al: The spirochetal etiology of Lyme disease. N Engl J Med 308:733–740, 1983

251. Steere AC, Hutchinson GJ, Rahn DW, et al: Treatment of the early manifestations of Lyme disease. Ann Intern Med 99:22–26, 1983

252. Steere AC, Malawista SE: Cases of Lyme disease in the United States: locations correlated with distribution of *Ixodes dammini*. Ann Intern Med 91:730, 1979

253. Steere AC, Malawista SE, Snydman DR, et al: Lyme arthritis. An epidemic of oligoarticular arthritis in children and adults in three Connecticut communities. Arthritis Rheum 20:7–17, 1977

254. Steere AC, Schoen RT, Taylor E: The clinical evolution of Lyme arthritis. Ann Intern Med 107:725–731, 1987

255. Steere AC, Taylor E, McHugh GL, Logigian EL: The overdiagnosis of Lyme disease. JAMA 269:1812–1816, 1993

256. Steere AC, Taylor E, Wilson ML, Levine JF, Spielman A: Longitudinal assessment of the clinical and epidemiological features of Lyme disease in a defined population. J Infect Dis 154:295–300, 1986

257. Stoenner HG, Dodd T, Larsen C: Antigenic variation of *Borrelia hermsii*. J Exp Med 156:1297–1311, 1982

258. Stoll BJ, Lee FK, Larsen S, et al: Clinical and serologic evaluation of neonates for congenital syphilis: a continuing diagnostic dilemma. J Infect Dis 167:1093–1099, 1993

259. Su SJ, Huang S, Chung CY, Yang HM, Chow YO: Evaluation of the equivocal test results of *Treponema pallidum* haemagglutination assay. J Clin Pathol 43:166–167, 1990

260. Sundnes KO, Haimanot AT: Epidemic of louse-borne relapsing fever in Ethiopia. Lancet 342:1213–1215, 1993

261. Tai KF, Ma Y, Weis JJ: Normal human B lymphocytes and mononuclear cells respond to the mitogenic and cytokine-stimulatory activities of *Borrelia burgdorferi* and its lipoprotein OspA. Infect Immun 62:520–528, 1994

262. TAKAYAMA K, ROTHENBERG RJ, BARBOUR AG: Absence of lipopolysaccharide in the Lyme disease spirochete, *Borrelia burgdorferi*. Infect Immun 55:2311, 1987

263. TERPSTRA WJ, SCHOONE GJ, LIGTHART GS, TER SCHEGGET J: Detection of *Leptospira interrogans* in clinical specimens by in situ hybridization using biotin-labelled DNA probes. J Gen Microbiol 133:911–914, 1987

264. THEISEN M, FREDERIKSEN B, LEBECH AM, VUUST J, HANSEN K: Polymorphism in ospC gene of *Borrelia burgdorferi* and immunoreactivity of OspC protein: implications for taxonomy and for use of OspC protein as a diagnostic antigen. J Clin Microbiol 31:2570–2576, 1993

265. THOMAS DL, ROMPALO AM, ZENILMAN J, HOOVER D, HOOK EW 3RD, QUINN TC: Association of hepatitis C virus infection with false-positive tests for syphilis. J Infect Dis 170:1579–1581, 1994

266. THOMPSON RS, BURGDORFER W, RUSSELL R, FRANCIS BJ: Outbreak of tick-borne relapsing fever in Spokane County, Washington. JAMA 210:1045–1050, 1969

267. TRAMONT EC: *Treponema pallidum* (syphilis). In Mandell GL, Bennett JE, Dolin R (eds): Principles and Practice of Infectious Diseases, 4th ed. New York, Churchill Livingstone, 1995

268. TRAMONT E: Syphilis in adults: from Christopher Columbus to Sir Alexander Fleming to AIDS. Clin Infect Dis 21:1361–1371, 1995

269. VAN CREVEL R, SPEELMAN P, GRAVEKAMP C, TERPSTRA WJ: Leptospirosis in travelers. Clin Infect Dis 19:132–134, 1994

270. VAN ORDEN AE, GREER PW: Modification of the Dieterle spirochete stain. Histotechnology 1:51–53, 1977

271. WALLACH FR, FORNI AL, HARIPRASHAD J, ET AL: Circulating *Borrelia burgdorferi* in patients with acute Lyme disease: results of blood cultures and serum DNA analysis. J Infect Dis 168:1541–1543, 1993

272. WASHBURN RG: *Spirillum minor* (Rat-bite fever). In Mandell GL, Bennett JE, Dolin R (eds): Principles and Practice of Infectious Diseases, 4th ed, pp. 2155–2156. New York, Churchill Livingstone, 1995

273. WATT G, ALQUIZA LM, PADRE LP, ET AL: The rapid diagnosis of leptospirosis: a prospective comparison of the dot enzyme-linked immunosorbent assay and the genus-specific microscopic agglutination test at different stages. J Infect Dis 157:840–842, 1988

274. WEBER K, BRATZKE HJ, NEUBERT U, WILSKE B, DURAY PH: *Borrelia burgdorferi* in a newborn despite oral penicillin for Lyme borreliosis during pregnancy. Pediatr Infect Dis J 7:286–289, 1988

275. WENDEL GD: Gestational and congenital syphilis. Clin Perinatol 15:287–303, 1988

276. YASUDA PH, STEIGERWALT AG, SULZER KR, KAUFMANN AF, ROGERS F, BRENNER DJ: Deoxyribonucleic acid relatedness between serogroups and serovars in the family *Leptospiraceae* with proposals for seven new *Leptospira* species. Int J Syst Bacteriol 37:407–415, 1987

277. ZBINDEN R, GOLDENBERGER D, LUCCHINI GM, ALTWEGG M: Comparison of two methods for detecting intrathecal synthesis of *Borrelia burgdorferi*-specific antibodies and PCR for diagnosis of Lyme neuroborreliosis. J Clin Microbiol 32:1795–1798, 1994

278. ZENKER PN, ROLFS RT: Treatment of syphilis, 1989. Rev Infect Dis 12(suppl 6):S590–S609, 1990

MYCOLOGY

The primary care physician, the surgical pathologist, and the microbiologist must work in consort to establish the diagnosis of a fungal infection.[183] The primary care physician is responsible for recognizing the signs and symptoms of fungal infections and for seeing that appropriate specimens are properly collected and transported to the laboratory in optimal condition without delay.[218] At particular risk for acquiring fungal infections are individuals who are immunosuppressed or who have reduced numbers or compromised function of the circulating polymorphonuclear leukocytes. Recipients of organ transplants, particularly during the posttransplant period of immunosuppression; pa-

tients with malignant neoplasms, particularly those with leukemia and lymphoma; and patients with a variety of debilitating immunologic and metabolic disorders, including systemic lupus erythematosus and other collagen vascular diseases, diabetes mellitus, dysgammaglobulinemia, and alcohol or IV drug abuse can in particular be singled out.[296]

The presenting symptoms in this group of patients may be atypical, vague, and nonspecific, reducing the chance for making a clinical diagnosis. Low-grade fever, night sweats, weight loss, lassitude, easy fatigability, cough, and chest pain are common presenting symptoms. Deep-seated or disseminated fungal diseases may mimic other infections such as tuberculosis, brucellosis, syphilis, sarcoidosis, or disseminated carcinomatosis. Careful examination of the skin and mucous membranes should always be performed because

Color Plates for Chapter 19 are found between pages 784 and 785.

systemic fungal infections may often present with mucocutaneous lesions. Rippon[296] describes ulcerating lesions in the intestine, larynx, pharynx, genitals, and tongue as complications of chronic disseminated histoplasmosis; up to 50% of patients with blastomycosis have verrucous or pustular lesions of the skin, which may be the presenting symptom, or ulcerating granulomas of mucous membranes, reported in such sites as the larynx,[94] the esophagus,[214] tongue,[221] and the mouth[253]; Prichard and coworkers[279] describe the cutaneous manifestations of disseminated coccidioidomycosis in patients with AIDS, and Yoswiak and coauthors[379] describe "red lumps on shins" as being a cardinal sign of that disease.

Signs and symptoms related to pulmonary infection are listed in Table 19-1; those for infections in extrapulmonary sites are listed in Table 19-2.

Prior treatment with corticosteroids or cytotoxic agents is also a risk factor. A history of recent travel to, or previous habitation in, a region of the world endemic for fungal infections; participation in activities or occupations that bring one in direct skin contact with infected animals or with contaminated materials; or the possibility of ingestion or inhalation of fungal spores should also be taken into consideration.

Laboratory tests may reveal nonspecific inflammatory responses. The erythrocyte sedimentation rate (ESR) may be increased, the levels of serum enzymes or gamma globulin may be high, and low-grade neutrophilia or monocytosis may be present. Radiologic findings may be helpful; however, often the presence of pulmonary infiltrates or inflammatory processes in other organs are nonspecific. In some patients with severely compromised resistance, general symptoms or laboratory and radiographic abnormalities may be totally lacking. Fine-needle biopsies play an important role in the rapid diagnosis of fungal infections, particularly those involving subcutaneous tissues.[203] The flip side, however, is the case reported by Carter and associates[56] of cutaneous blastomycosis resulting from inoculation of the skin with yeast forms following a fine-needle aspiration of an active lesion in the left upper lobe of the lung.

The primary role of the surgical pathologist is to establish the diagnosis of fungal infections based on the observation of characteristic forms in stained tissue sections. Of equal importance is their role in establishing protocols, in conjunction with the surgical service, to ensure that specimens likely to contain fungal elements are not prematurely placed in fixatives. The as-

---

TABLE 19-1
SIGNS AND SYMPTOMS OF PULMONARY MYCOSES

TYPE OF INFECTION	SIGNS AND SYMPTOMS
General	A transient influenza-like syndrome or pneumonia that localizes in one lobe or spreads to other lobes seen in early infection.
	Cough, minimal sputum production, dyspnea, tachypnea, hemoptysis.
	Chest pain, frequently pleuritic in nature.
	Rales or rhonchi and a pleural friction rub may be detected on auscultation.
	Roentgenogram of the chest may reveal small pulmonary infiltrates and hilar adenopathy or more diffuse and confluent opacities.
Allergic broncho-pulmonary	Symptoms characteristic of asthma: nonproductive cough, wheezing, tightness in the chest.
	Episodic bronchospasm.
	Segmental atelectasis caused by mucous plugging of bronchioles.
	Charcot-Leyden crystals and eosinophils in sputum; peripheral blood eosinophilia.
	Cutaneous hypersensitivity reaction to antigens of *Aspergillus* spp.
	Elevated serum IgE concentration and IgG anti-aspergillus antibodies.
Fungus ball	Growth of fungus colony within a preexistent cavity.
	Hemoptysis, despite little or no invasion of cavity wall.
	Dissemination is rare, even in patients receiving corticosteroids.
Invasive	Symptoms of acute pneumonia.
	Low-grade, undulant fever.
	Cough may be productive or nonproductive; chest pain usually present.
	Progressive dyspnea and shortness of breath.
	Hemoptysis may indicate infarction and parenchymal necrosis.
	Chest radiographs may reveal a diffuse infiltrate emanating from the hilum, finely nodular fibrosis, multifocal abscesses, or cavitation, depending on the fungus species. Clues to specific agents:
	"Millet seed" fibrosis: histoplasmosis
	Peripheral coin lesion: coccidioidomycosis
	Cavitary lesions: histoplasmosis or coccidioidomycosis
	Fungus ball: aspergillosis, pseudallescheriosis, zygomycosis
	Allergic bronchopulmonary disease: *Aspergillus fumigatus, A. flavus*

TABLE 19-2
SIGNS, SYMPTOMS AND PROBABLE AGENTS OF EXTRAPULMONARY MYCOSES

TYPE OF INFECTION	SIGNS AND SYMPTOMS
Cutaneous	Superficial scaling lesions, varying in size, shape, and color, of the thorax or back: tinea versicolor secondary to *Malassezia furfur* infection. Itching, scaling lesions known as tinea or ringworm: dermatophytosis Thickened, crusting, hyperkeratotic, exophytic fungoid affliction known as favus: *Trichophyton tonsurans, T. violaceum,* and *T. schoenleinii).* Scaling or crusting lesions confined to the moist intertriginous areas of skin suggest yeast infections: *Candida albicans.* Primary subcutaneous pustular infection at the site of inoculation with proximal spread and evolution of secondary skin ulcers along the course of the lymphatics: *Sporothrix schenckii.* Nonhealing pustules, ulcers, or draining sinuses: disseminated dimorphic fungal diseases and mycetomas secondary to a variety of fungal agents. Purpuric lesions and subcutaneous cysts: phaeohyphomycosis. Fungating, discolored, hemorrhagic lesions: chromomycosis.
CNS	Insidious onset of headaches that increase in frequency and severity, accompanied by nausea, irritability, and clumsiness; cryptococcosis. Meningitis and meningoencephalitis: Zygomycosis, particularly in diabetics. Brain abscesses: *Xylophyla bantiana,* other dematiaceous fungi; *Aspergillus* species.
Urinary tract	Pyelitis and pyelonephritis associated with administration of long-term antibiotics, cortisteroids, immunosuppressants, antineoplastic drugs, and prolonged insertion of indwelling catheters for urinary drainage, particularly in elderly women: Candidiasis. Limited pyuria, lower abdominal pain, frequency of urination: nonbacterial cystitis in middle-aged women: *Torulopsis glabrata.*
Ocular infections	Conjunctivitis, corneal infections, and keratoconjunctivitis: *Fusarium* spp., *Aspergillus* spp., *Cladosporium* spp., *Acremonium* spp., and others. Intraocular infections, usually following trauma or eye surgery: *Candida albicans, Aspergillus* spp., or *Zygomyces* spp.
Endocarditis	Low-grade fever, cardiac murmurs, positive echogram: *Candida* spp., *Aspergillus* spp., *Paecilomyces* spp.[171]
Sinusitis	Facial pain and cutaneous hyperemia, headache, low-grade fever, radiographic evidence of filling of a sinus or fluid levels: *Aspergillus fumigatus, Sporothrix schenckii, Alternaria* spp., and *Pseudallescheria boydii.*[149]

tute surgical pathologist will also be alert to preparing touch preparations or obtaining samples for cultures of suspicious lesions observed while cutting in tissue specimens or performing autopsies. In all too many cases, a definitive diagnosis of a fungal infection cannot be made on the study of tissue sections alone, and the lack of a corroborative positive culture leaves too many cases unsolved.

The microbiologist and supporting staff play a major role in establishing a definitive diagnosis of fungal infections. Laboratory protocols must be firmly established for the prompt, direct examination and processing of cultures soon after receipt in the laboratory, for the preparation of wet mounts and stained smears and slides for microscopic examination, for the selection and appropriate inoculation and incubation of culture media, and for the examination, biochemical characterization, and final identification of any yeast or mold that is recovered. Issuing a timely, succinct, and clearly written final report and the availability for direct consultation on any complicated cases complete the obligations of those working in the microbiology laboratory. These several items are discussed in more detail in the following.

CLASSIFICATION AND TAXONOMY OF HUMAN MYCOSES

The opening paragraphs of this chapter describe the practical and functional elements of the practice of clinical mycology. The classification of the mycotic diseases seen from the vantage point of the clinician must be reconciled with the taxonomy of the several genera and species of fungi that are encountered in the clinical laboratory. As indicated in the foregoing, the better the understanding and communication between these two spheres of activity, the more likely that the correct diagnosis for the patient with a fungus infection will be established. The task becomes more difficult because neither the clinical nor the laboratory orientations to mycotic diseases and their etiologic agents remain static, and an ongoing dialogue is necessary.

For example, the clinical classification of human fungal infections, as outlined in Table 19-3, can only serve clinicians as a broad guideline. Approaching the grouping of mycotic diseases based on the site of involvement can no longer be separated into the classic and, at one time neatly defined, categories of "deep-seated" or "systemic," "subcutaneous," and "superfi-

TABLE 19-3

CLASSIFICATION OF THE MORE COMMONLY ENCOUNTERED HUMAN MYCOSES
AND THEIR ETIOLOGIC AGENTS

DEEP-SEATED MYCOSES	OPPORTUNISTIC MYCOSES	SUBCUTANEOUS MYCOSES	SUPERFICIAL MYCOSES
Blastomycosis *Blastomyces dermatitidis*	Aspergillosis *Aspergillus fumigatus* *A. flavus* *A. niger* *A. terreus*	Maduromycosis (Mycetoma) *Acremonium* spp. *Exophiala jeanselmei* *Pseudallescheria boydii* *Nocardia* spp.	Black piedra *Piedraia hortae*
Coccidioidomycosis *Coccidioides immitis*			Tinea nigra *Phaeoannelomyces wernickii*
Cryptococcosis *Cryptococcus neoformans*	Candidosis *Candida albicans* *Candida* spp.	Chromoblastomycosis *Cladosporium carionii* *Fonsecaea* spp. *Phialophora* spp.	Tinea versicolor *Malassezia furfur*
Histoplasmosis *Histoplasma capsulatum*	Geotrichosis *Geotrichum candidum*		Dermatomycoses *Microsporum* spp. *Trichophyton* spp. *Epidermophyton floccosum*
Paracoccidioidomycosis (South American blastomycosis) *Paracoccidioides brasiliensis*	Phaeohyphomycosis *Alternaria* spp. *Curvularia* spp. *Drechslera/Bipolaris* spp. *Exophiala* spp. *Wangiella* spp.	Phaeohyphomycosis (cutaneous) *Alternaria* spp. *Cladosporium* spp. *Xylohypha emmonsii* *Exophiala* spp. *Phialophora* spp. *Wangiella dermatitidis*	Mycotic keratitis *Fusarium* spp. *Aspergillus* spp. *Candida* spp.
Sporotrichosis (unusual) *Sporothrix schenckii*	Hyalohyphomycosis (rare) *Acremonium* spp. *Fusarium* spp. *Paecilomyces* spp. *Penicillium* spp. *Scedosporium* spp. (*Pseudallescheria* spp.)	Sporotrichosis *Sporothrix schenckii*	Onychomycosis *Candida* spp. *Aspergillus* spp. *Trichosporon beigelii* *Geotrichum candidum*
	Zygomycosis *Rhizopus* spp. *Mucor* spp. *Cunninghamella* spp.		Tinea unguium *Trichophyton* spp. *Epidermophyton floccosum*

cial," as outlined in Table 19-3. For example, the fungal agent *Malassezia furfur*, which historically caused only the superficial dermatomycosis tinea versicolor now is an agent of disseminated infections in patients receiving parenteral nutrition through indwelling catheters.[124, 205]

The term **deep-seated** or **systemic** has referred to a group of fungal infections caused by agents that inherently can be highly virulent, that can invade deeply into tissues and organs, and that have the capability of spreading widely throughout the body. From a classic perspective, most of these infections have been caused by the dimorphic fungi; that is, those species that exist in mold form in the environment ("room temperature incubation") but as yeasts when incubated at 35° to 37°C (body temperature). Currently, because of the increased number of individuals who are immunosuppressed or who have severely compromised cellular immunity, other fungal agents, formerly considered only as "contaminants," are causing systemic disease. One prime example is the hyaline mold *Penicillium marnettei*, which causes a disseminated reticuloen-

dothelial infection clinically that is pathologically indistinguishable from histoplasmosis. Although uncommon, certain agents of deep-seated mycoses, notably *Blastomyces dermatitidis* and *Histoplasma capsulatum*, can cause primary cutaneous and subcutaneous infection without evidence of dissemination.

Sporothrix schenckii, classically classified in the subcutaneous group of mycoses as the agent of lymphocutaneous infection, may also cause invasive and systemic disease. Other agents within the subcutaneous group, notably certain species of *Cladosporium* and *Xylohypha*, can cause brain abscesses. Case reports of virtually every fungus listed in Table 19-3 causing endocarditis can be found in the literature, particularly among intravenous (IV) drug users.

The term **opportunistic** is used for any nonpathogenic fungus that can cause subcutaneous and disseminated infections. These are fungi, usually of inherent low or limited virulence, that nevertheless can cause local or disseminated disease in individuals who are debilitated, who are immunosuppressed, or who carry intravascular or prosthetic devices. *Aspergillus* species,

Candida species, and the *Zygomycetes* (mucormycosis) are the three groups of fungi that were classically considered opportunistic. Recently, localized and deep-seated infections have been ascribed to several other species of light (hyaline) and dark (dematiaceous) rapidly growing molds that formerly were considered contaminants.

Therefore, current mycologists must accept that a variety of fungal species can cause virtually all clinical forms of mycoses and that recovery of the etiologic agent is necessary to establish a diagnosis. The onus now shifts to the laboratory mycologists who must work with a classification of fungal agents that provides meaningful information to the clinician who is faced with making a diagnosis of clinical disease. To cause less confusion, the generic and all-inclusive terms **phaeohyphomycosis** and **hyalohyphomycosis** have been suggested to designate those mycoses (both systemic and subcutaneous) caused by fungi that appear dark or black from the production of a yellow or brown-pigmented mycelium or by those species that produce colorless, transparent (hyaline) hyphae respectively.[123] This has been done to relieve the clinician of trying to remember which of several fungal agents are either commonly associated with a given infection or can be considered as contaminants.

The approach used in this chapter is to focus on that select number of mycotic agents that most commonly cause human mycoses. By working within this limited list, clinicians will become familiar with the more important agents of disease. It is our suggestion that the specific agents recovered be named to genus or species levels along with comments in the report that indicate the potential clinical significance of those fungi that are either uncommon or for which a recent name change has occurred. The director and supervisor of each mycology laboratory must assume this responsibility so that situations such as those cited by McGinnis and Salkin[212] do not occur. They report the case of *Cunninghamella* infection that was overlooked because the physician did not recognize this fungus as an agent of zygomycosis. Other genera within the class *Zygomycetes*, such as *Saksenaea*, *Mortierella*, *Conidiobolus*, and *Basidiobolus* are being incriminated as agents of zygomycosis.[31,172] When any of these fungi are encountered in clinical specimens, they can be reported with the genus level as long as a comment indicates that they belong to the "zygomycetes," a term that may be more familiar to most clinicians.

CLASSIC TAXONOMY AND DEFINITION OF RELATED TERMS

Clinical mycologists must develop a functional classification of those select fungal species that cause the majority of human infections. This classification must take into account the phylogenetic taxonomy of fungi that has evolved from academic mycologists. Table 19-4 is a revised taxonomy of medically important fungi (abridged to the class division) derived from the simplified taxonomic scheme presented by Dixon and

TABLE 19-4

THE MAJOR GROUPS OF MEDICALLY IMPORTANT FUNGI— A SIMPLIFIED TAXONOMIC SCHEME

Class: *Zygomycetes*
　Order: *Mucorales*
　　Genera:
　　　Rhizopus, Mucor, Rhizomucor, Absidia, Cunninghamella, Saksenaea
　Order: *Endomophthorales*
　　Genera:
　　　Basidiobolus, Conidiobolus
Class: *Ascomycetes*
　Order: *Endomycetales*
　　Genera:
　　　Saccharomyces, Pichia
　　Telomorphs of some *Candida* spp.
　Order: *Onygenales*
　　Genera:
　　　Arthroderma (telemorphs of *Trichophyton* and *Microsporum* spp.)
　　　Ajellomyces (telemorphs of *Histoplasma* spp. and *Blastomyces* spp.)
　　Telomorphs of some *Aspergillus* and *Penicillium* spp.
Class: *Deuteromycetes*
　Order: *Cryptococcales*
　　Genera:
　　　Candida, Cryptococcus, Trichosporon, Pityrosporum
　Order: *Moniliales*
　　Family: *Moniliaceae*
　　Genera:
　　　Epidermophyton, Coccidioides, Paracoccidioides, Sporothrix, Aspergillus
　　Family: *Dematiaceae*
　　Genera:
　　　Phialophora, Fonsecaea, Exophiala, Wangiella, Xylohypha, Bipolaris, Alternaria
　Order: *Sphaeropsidales*
　　Genera:
　　　Phoma
Class: *Oomycetes*
　Genera:
　　Pythium

Fromtling.[88] (For the derivation of the most common mycologic terms, see Box 19-1). The simplified taxonomy as presented can be better understood if the derivation and meaning of each of the terms used in the nomenclature of class, order, and genera are explained. The term **mycology** itself is derived from the Greek word *mykes*, a direct counterpart of the Latin word *fungus*, in turn thought to be a modification of the Greek word *sponges*, from which our word "sponge" is derived.

In a broad context, fungi are members of the plant kingdom that are devoid of leaves, stems, or roots. They are further characterized by lacking chlorophyll; therefore, they require an external carbon source, which they derive either as saprophytes by adhering to and decomposing nonliving organic matter or as parasites by invading living plants and animals (including humans), in which they may or may not be associated with disease. Fungi are eukaryotic; that is, each cell

BOX 19-1. DERIVATION OF COMMONLY USED MYCOLOGIC TERMS

The first class of fungi listed in Table 19-4 is the class *Zygomycetes*. The term **zygo** is derived from the Greek *zygon*, meaning a fusion or joining in the manner of a yoke. This derivation refers to the sexual phase of reproduction in which there is a joining or fusion of the two independent sex cells to form a zygospore. The previous designation, "phycomycete" (from the Greek *phykos*, seaweed), for this group of fungi has been more correctly replaced by the term "zygomycete." The term for the order *Mucorales* is derived from the Latin, *mucere*, to be moldy or musty. The order *Mucorales* includes those zygomycetes that can reproduce both asexually, by forming spores within saclike sporangia, and sexually, by the formation of zygospores. Thus, the frequently used term, **mucormycosis**, refers to a mycosis that can be caused by any of the fungal species included in the *Mucorales*, not just infections caused by the species *Mucor*. Most human zygomycoses are caused by fungi belonging to this order.

The order *Endomycetales* (*endo*, within; *myces*, fungus) includes those zygomycetes that produce only sexually, with the production of ascospores. The only medically significant member of this order is *Saccharomyces* species. The word **telomorph**, as used in Table 19-4, refers to the sexual form of a fungus. Most mycologists feel that every fungus has a sexual phase that may manifest if the correct environmental conditions and nutritional requirements are provided. Thus, as seen in Table 19-4, *Arthroderma* refers to the sexual forms, or telomorphs of the dermatophyte genera *Trichophyton* and *Microsporum*; *Ajellomyces* to the telomorphs of *Blastomyces* and *Histoplasma* spp. (not seen in cultures or specimens in clinical laboratories). The term **onygenales** is from the Greek, *onych*, referring to claw or nail (thus, onychomycosis is an infection of the nail). Accordingly, the order *Onygenales* includes those fungi that infect nails. The term for the order *Eurotiales* is derived from Greek, *euros*, mold, and by definition, includes those fungi in which sexually derived spores are contained within a closed ascocarp (cleistothecium). Experienced mycologists have seen the cleistothecia produced by certain *Aspergillus* spp., notably strains of *A. nidulans* and *A. glaucus*.

The class *Basidiomycetes* includes the mushrooms, which are only indirectly of medical importance because of the mycotoxins they produce. The term **basidio** is directly from the Latin, referring to a clublike organ in which spores are formed by both mitosis and meiosis, resulting in four spores called basidiospores.

The class *Deuteromyces* (Latin *deutero*, second), refers to the "fungi imperfecti"; that is, those fungi in which only an asexual phase of reproduction has been observed. Included are most species of fungi of medical importance. The subclass *Blastomycetes* (Greek *blasto*, budding) includes the order *Cryptococcales* (Greek *kryptos*, hidden or covered), or those fungi that are yeastlike throughout most of their life cycle. In contrast, the subclass *Hyphomycetes* (Greek *hyphe*; web), includes those fungi in which a mycelium is produced. The order *Moniliales* (Latin *monile*; necklace) includes those fungi imperfecti in which spores are borne directly off the hyphae (conidia) and not aggregated within fruiting bodies. This includes most of the important hyaline and dematiaceous molds. In older usage, the term "monilia" or "monoliasis" referred specifically to infections with *Candida* species, probably because early workers recognized the formation of pseudohyphae giving rise to blastoconidia. The archaic term **torula** (Latin *torus*; protuberance or bulge), in contrast, referred to infections with cryptococci, which formed only buds ("bulges") and not pseudohyphae.

The order *Sphaeropsidales* (Greek *sphairo*; sphere) includes the single medically important genus *Phoma* (there are hundreds of species of *Sphaeropsidales* that inhabit and cause disease in plants). This order of fungi has the characteristic of forming large, spherical spore-bearing structures called pycnidia (Greek *pycno*; skin). Pycnidia are asexually derived fruiting bodies and contain conidia, in contrast with the sexually derived cleistothecia and perithecia, which contain asci and ascospores. In practice, one can distinguish these in microscopic mounts by pressing down on the coverslip with the tip of a pencil to "pop open" the spherical fruiting body and looking to see if conidia or ascospores are released.

---

possesses a nucleus, nuclear membrane, endoplasmic reticulum, Golgi apparatus, and mitochondria. They also possess a rigid cell wall composed of chitin (*N*-acetyl-D-glucosamine) linked by β1-4 glycoside bonds, mannans (polymers of glucose in α- or β-glycoside bonds), and sometimes cellulose. These cell wall constituents adsorb several dyes, which, after the application of special stains, permits their identification in laboratory mounts and in tissue sections.

Single-cell fungal forms are known as yeasts; those with multiple cells forming a filamentous mycelium are known as molds. Fungi reproduce by spores, either sexually or asexually, that may be derived directly from the vegetative mycelium or from the surface of special aerial fruiting bodies. The morphology,

arrangement, and mode of derivation of spores serve as important criteria by which genus and species identifications can be made.

FUNCTIONAL TAXONOMY FOR USE IN CLINICAL MYCOLOGY LABORATORIES

Although the simplified taxonomy suggested by Dixon and Fromtling[88] is phylogenetically correct and has meaning to academic mycologists, it is of less relevance to the clinical mycologist in the day-to-day task of making accurate genus–species identifications. The system map found in Box 19-2 includes those fungi that are most commonly encountered in clinical laboratories and that are involved in the vast majority of mycoses.

BOX 19-2. SYSTEM MAP OF COMMONLY ENCOUNTERED FUNGI IN CLINICAL LABORATORIES

Zygomycetes

Rhizopus spp.

Absidia spp.

Syncephalastrum spp.

Circinella spp.

Cunninghamella spp.

Aspergillus

Aspergillus fumigatus

A. flavus

A. niger

A. terreus

Halinohyphomyces

Penicillium spp.

Paecilomyces spp.

Scopulariopsis spp.

Acremonium spp.

Fusarium spp.

Trichoderma spp.

Gliocladium spp.

Scedosporium spp.

Chrysosporium

Sepedonium spp.

Beauveria spp.

Phaeohyphomyces

Alternaria spp.

Ulocladium spp.

Stemphilium spp.

Epicoccum spp.

Curvularia spp.

Bipolaris spp.

Phoma spp.

Chaetophoma spp.

Aureobasidium spp.

Phaeoannellomyces spp.

Xylohypha (Cladophialophora) gartiana

Chromomycosis

Cladosporium carionii

Phialophora verrucosum

Fonsecaea pedrosi

Exophiala spp.

Wangiella spp.

Dermatophytes

Microsporium canis

M. gypseum

Trichophyton rubrum

T. mentagrophytes

T. tonsurans

E. floccosum

Dimorphic

Blastomyces dermatitidis

Coccidioides immitis

Histoplasma capsulatum

Sporothrix schenckii

Paracoccidioides brasiliensis

Yeasts

Candida spp.

C. albicans

Cryptococcus spp.

C. neoformans

Torulopsis glabrata

Trichosporon spp.

Geotrichum spp.

Malassezia furfur

LABORATORY APPROACH TO THE DIAGNOSIS OF FUNGAL INFECTIONS

SPECIMEN COLLECTION AND TRANSPORT

General guidelines for the collection and transport of specimens for culture have been given in Chapter 2. Physicians, nurses, ward personnel, and laboratory technologists must work in developing joint protocols that ensure the proper collection and prompt transport of specimens for fungus cultures. The selection of appropriate collection devices and transport containers, affixing labels that include pertinent patient information, and establishing a means of communication for special requests are possibly the most important considerations in ensuring the accurate diagnosis of mycotic infections.

Although prompt delivery of specimens to the laboratory is to be encouraged, several fungal species, including *Histoplasma capsulatum*, *Blastomyces dermatitidis*, *Cryptococcus neoformans*, and *Aspergillus* species, can be recovered from samples that have been in transit for as long as 16 days.[306] Sealed, sterile transport containers, however, should be used for all liquid or moist specimens. However, skin scrapings, nail fragments, and hairs can be transported in an envelope, petri dish, or other convenient conveyance. Because many specimens contain contaminating bacteria that may compromise their quality, 50,000 U of penicillin, 100,000 μg of streptomycin, or 0.2 mg of chloramphenicol can be added per milliliter of specimen if it is anticipated that transit will be prolonged (such as transport through the mail).[184] Directions for the proper packaging and labeling of specimens for shipping and mailing are discussed in Chapter 2.

Recommendations for the collection of several common specimen types for fungal cultures as formulated by the American Thoracic Society are listed in Table 19-5.[306]

SPECIMEN PROCESSING

Once received in the laboratory, a specimen should be examined as soon as possible. Swab specimens are generally inadequate for the recovery of fungi; attempts should be made to receive aspirated material or tissue biopsies. Direct wet mounts or smears should be prepared if appropriate, and a portion of the specimen transferred to appropriate fungal culture media. This last step is also important in the ultimate recovery of fungi and cannot be slighted or delegated to marginally trained personnel.

DIRECT EXAMINATION

It is highly recommended that a direct microscopic examination be made on most specimens submitted for fungal culture. Not only may this provide an immediate presumptive diagnosis for the physician, but it may also aid in the selection of an appropriate culture medium. Table 19-6 lists the observations one might make in stained smears and the presumptive identifications that may be possible. Following are a few additional comments relative to the initial examination and processing of specimens.

A phase-contrast microscope is a valuable adjunct in the direct examination of specimens. The advantages include the following: 1) mounts can be made and examined quickly; 2) there is no need for direct staining; and 3) the objects can be clearly visualized. Presumptive identification of fungi on the basis of direct microscopic examination of material from clinical

TABLE 19-5

RECOMMENDATIONS FOR COLLECTION OF SPECIMENS FOR FUNGUS CULTURE: AMERICAN THORACIC SOCIETY[306]

SPECIMEN	RECOMMENDED PROCEDURE
Sputum	The first early-morning sample should be collected after rising, but before breakfast. Patients are instructed to rinse their mouths with water vigorously immediately before coughing ½ to 1 ounce of sputum into a sterile-screw-capped container. Sputum induction with a heated aerosol saline suspension may be required if an adequate specimen cannot be obtained.
Bronchoscopy	Bronchial brushings, biopsy, or bronchoalveolar lavage fluid should be transported promptly to the laboratory in sterile, sealed containers. Middlebrook 7H11 broth is used in some laboratories as a transport medium because mycobacteria will also be preserved. A postbronchoscopy sputum sample should be collected when possible.
Cerebrospinal fluid	As much cerebrospinal fluid (CSF) as possible should be used for the culture of fungi. If processing is to be delayed, samples should be left at room temperature and not be refrigerated as CSF is an adequate fluid culture medium in which fungal elements can survive until subcultured.
Urine	The first early-morning urine sample is preferred; random samples are acceptable. Specimens should be collected aseptically in sterile, screw-capped containers and sent immediately for processing. If a delay in processing beyond 2 h is anticipated, the urine sample should be placed in a 4°C refrigerator to inhibit the overgrowth of rapidly growing bacteria.
Prostatic secretions	Some deep-seated mycoses, notably blastomycosis and, less commonly, histoplasmosis or coccidioidomycosis, may be diagnosed by collecting prostatic secretions. The bladder is first emptied, followed by prostatic massage. Secretions should be inoculated directly into appropriate fungal culture media; also, 5–10 mL of urine should be collected in a separate container.
Exudates	The skin over pustular lesions should be disinfected and exudates aspirated using a sterile needle and syringe. The syringe also serves as a transport container if the needle is capped. Biopsy of the lesion may be necessary if the aspirate fails to yield fungi.
Skin, nails, hair	First swab the area of skin to be sampled with 70% alcohol to remove surface bacterial contaminants. Sample the peripheral, erythematous, growing margin of typical "ringworm" lesions, scraping with the side of a glass micro-scope slide or the edge of a scalpel blade. Infected nails should be sampled from beneath the nail plate to obtain softened material from the nail bed. If this is not possible, scrape away the surface of the nail before collecting shavings from the deeper portions. Hairs should be collected from areas of scaling or alopecia, or those that fluoresce when viewed under a Wood's (long wavelength) ultraviolet lamp.
Tissue biopsies	Tissue biopsies of suspected sites of infection should be transported in a sterile gauze moistened with physiologic, nonbacteriostatic, sterile saline solution in a screw-capped container. The specimen should not be frozen or allowed to dehydrate prior to culture.
Blood	Biphasic agar–broth bottles designed specifically for fungal cultures are superior to routine bottles used for the recovery of bacterial pathogens. Lysis–centrifugation systems, such as the Isolator (Wampole Laboratories, Cranbury NJ) are also highly recommended, particularly for the recovery of *H. capsulatum* and other yeasts.

specimens is shown in Table 19-6. A series of excellent photomicrographs illustrating several fungal forms that commonly may be observed microscopically in direct examination of various body fluids have been published by Merz and Roberts.[218]

SELECTION AND INOCULATION OF CULTURE MEDIA

The battery of culture media for the recovery of fungi from clinical specimens need not be elaborate.[124] Although the recovery rate may be somewhat enhanced by using a variety of isolation media, considerations of cost, storage and incubator space, and technologist time generally dictate a more conservative approach in most laboratories. Table 19-7 lists various culture sites,

techniques for processing and inoculating specimens, and recommended culture media.

Two general types of culture media are essential to ensure the primary recovery of all clinically significant fungi from clinical specimens. One medium should be nonselective; that is, one that will permit the growth of virtually all fungal species. The use of Sabouraud's dextrose agar as a primary recovery medium is discouraged, except for the recovery of dermatophytes from cutaneous samples or yeasts from vaginal cultures.[184] Rather, either inhibitory mold agar or Sabhi agar is recommended to improve the recovery of certain of the more fastidious or slow-growing fungi. Sabouraud's dextrose agar (2%) can be used to subculture fungi recovered on enriched medium to enhance

TABLE 19-6
PRESUMPTIVE IDENTIFICATION OF FUNGI BASED ON DIRECT MICROSCOPIC EXAMINATION
OF MATERIAL FROM CLINICAL SPECIMENS

DIRECT MICROSCOPIC OBSERVATIONS	PRESUMPTIVE IDENTIFICATION
Hyphae relatively small (3–6 μm) and regular in size, dichotomously branching at 45° angles with distinct cross-septa	*Aspergillus* spp.
Hyphae irregular in size, ranging from 6 to 50 μm ribbonlike, and devoid of septa	Zygomycetes (Phycomycetes) *Rhizopus–Mucor–Absidia*
Hyphae small (2–3 μm) and regular, some branching, with rectangular arthrospores sometimes seen; found only in skin, nail scrapings, and hair	Dermatophyte group *Microsporum* spp. *Trichophyton* spp. *Epidermophyton* spp.
Hyphae regular in diameter, 3–6 μm, parallel walls, irregular branching, septate, dark yellow, brown, or hyaline.	*Phaeohyphomyces* spp. *Hyalohyphomyces* spp.
Hyphae, distinct points of constriction simulating link sausages (pseudohyphae), with budding yeast forms (blastospores) often seen	*Candida* spp.
Yeast forms, cells spherical and irregular in size (5–20 μm), classically with a thick polysaccharide capsule (not all cells are encapsulated), with one or more buds attached by a narrow constriction	*Cryptococcus neoformans* *Cryptococcus* spp. nonencapsulated
Small budding yeast, relatively uniform in size (3–5 μm), with a single bud attached by a narrow base, extracellular or within macrophages	*Histoplasma capsulatum*
Yeast forms, large (8–20 μm), with cells appearing to have a thick, double-contoured wall, with a single bud attached by a broad base	*Blastomyces dermatitidis*
Large, irregularly sized (10–50 μm), thick-walled spherules, many of which contain small (2–4 μm), round endospores	*Coccidioides immitis*

sporulation and provide the more characteristic colonial morphology. Czepak's agar should be used for the subculture of *Aspergillus* species if colonial morphology is an important identifying criterion for any given unknown isolate.

A second medium, more selective for the recovery of fungi, should also be used. Combinations of antibiotics, including penicillin (20 U/mL) and streptomycin (40 U/mL), gentamicin (5 μg/mL), and chloramphenicol (16 μg/mL), can be used to inhibit the growth of bacteria. Cycloheximide (Actidione) in a concentration of 0.5 mg/mL, may be added to prevent the overgrowth of certain rapidly growing environmental molds that may contaminate the culture plates. However, opportunistic pathogenic fungi, including *C. neoformans* and *A. fumigatus* may be partially or totally inhibited by cycloheximide.

For the recovery of the more fastidious dimorphic fungi, such as *B. dermatitidis* and *H. capsulatum*, an enriched agar base, such as brain–heart infusion, must be used. Antibiotic combinations may be added because the incubation of the plates or tubes may require 1 month or more. For optimal recovery of these organisms, the addition of 5% to 10% sheep blood is also recommended; however, if blood is used, it may be necessary to subculture to a less-enriched medium, such as Sabouraud's dextrose agar or potato dextrose

agar, so that the more characteristic sporulation can be observed.

It is currently recommended that all fungal cultures be incubated at a controlled 30°C. Incubation of a second set of plates at 35°C for the recovery of the yeast forms of dimorphic fungi is not cost-effective. Any mold recovered in primary culture that is suggestive of a dimorphic species can be subcultured to brain–heart infusion agar containing 10% sheep blood or to cottonseed conversion medium (Traders Protein Division, Fort Worth TX) (if *B. dermatitidis* is suspected) and incubated for 7 to 10 days at 35°C to accomplish in vitro yeast conversion. The exoantigen extraction test or species-specific nucleic acid probe assays are currently recommended in lieu of the in vitro conversion procedure for confirming the identification of *B. dermatitidis*, *H. capsulatum*, *C. immitis*, and *P. brasiliensis*.[113,114] These procedures are described in Charts 24 and 27.

The commercial availability of reagents (Nolan Biologicals, Tucker GA) provides clinical laboratories with the capability to easily and accurately identify these species of dimorphic fungi without the need for the more time-consuming mold conversion studies.[114] Exoantigen test reagents are also available for the identification of a variety of fungi, including *Aspergillus* species, *Penicillium marneffei*, *Pseudallescheria boydii*, *Sporothrix schenckii*, and dematiaceous fungi belonging

TABLE 19-7
GUIDELINES FOR DIRECT EXAMINATION AND PROCESSING OF SPECIMENS SUBMITTED FOR FUNGAL CULTURES

Respiratory	The sputum quality-grading system described in Chapter 2 is not applicable to specimens submitted for fungal cultures. Select the most purulent or blood-flecked parts of the sample. If the sample is highly viscid, it should be homogenized by adding a small pinch of crystalline N-acetyl-L-cystine to the specimen. NaOH or other digesting agents, used for the processing of specimens for the recovery of mycobacteria, should not be used. Prepare a wet mount of the homogenized sample for direct microscopic examination and inoculate about 0.5 mL to each of the culture media to be used. Because respiratory secretions are often contaminated with bacteria, media containing antibiotics should be used. A combination of a nonselective agar, such as inhibitory mold agar or Sabhi agar, and an inhibitory agar such as brain–heart infusion with chloramphenicol and cycloheximide are recommended.
Cerebrospinal fluid	CSF samples may be centrifuged at 1500–2000 g for 20 min and the sediment inoculated onto the surface of noninhibitory culture media, such as inhibitory mold agar or SabHi agar. Preferably, if more than 2 mL of fluid is available, pass fluid through a 0.45-μm membrane filter, using a Swinnex syringe attachment. Place the filtrate side of the filter paper face down on the surface of appropriate culture medium. The paper should be repositioned to other sites on the medium using sterile forceps on an every-other-day schedule. If only a scant amount of fluid is provided, spot inoculate the surface of the agar medium directly in 3- or 4-drop aliquots. The India ink (nigrosin is an acceptable substitute) mounts may be prepared when *Cryptococcus neoformans* is suspected. To prepare the mount, either a drop of the centrifuged sediment or a small amount of material from the surface of the membrane is mixed with a drop of India ink on a microscope slide. A coverslip is applied and the mount microscopically examined for the presence of encapsulated, budding yeast forms.
Urine	Centrifuge about 10 mL of urine sample, then inoculate 0.5 mL of sediment to both a noninhibitory agar, such as inhibitory mold agar or Sabhi agar, and to an inhibitory medium, such as brain–heart infusion agar, containing chloramphenicol and cycloheximide. Direct mounts can be prepared and examined microscopically for yeast or hyphal forms.
Skin, nails, hair	Skin scales, nail scrapings, and hairs should be examined after potassium hydroxide treatment. The KOH preparation is made by emulsifying the specimen in a drop of 10% KOH on a microscope slide. The purpose of the KOH is to clear out any background scales or cell membranes that may be confused with hyphal elements. Clearing can be accelerated by gently heating the mixture over the flame of a Bunsen burner. A coverslip is applied, and the specimen is examined for the presence of narrow, regular hyphae that characteristically break up into arthroconidia. The visualization of hyphae is improved by adding calcofluor white to the potassium hydroxide reagent and examining with a fluorescent microscope fitted with filters of appropriate wavelengths.[85] With hairs, mosaic arrangement of spores may be seen on the surface of the shaft (ectothrix infection) or hyphal fragments and arthroconidia may be seen internally (endothrix infection). Skin scales, nail scrapings, or hairs should be placed directly on the surface of the culture medium, such as brain–heart infusion agar with chloramphenicol and cycloheximide (commercially available as Mycosel or Mycobiotic agars). With a straight inoculating wire, submerge a few of the fragments beneath the agar surface. Examine in the areas of inoculation at frequent intervals for the appearance of surface colonies. Hold cultures for a minimum of 30 days before discarding as negative.
Tissue	When processing tissues for the recovery of fungi, the use of a mortar and pestle or a tissue grinder should be avoided. The hyphal forms can easily be destroyed by grinding, making it difficult to recover viable organisms in culture (particularly if the aseptate hyphae of one of the *Zygomycetes* are present). Rather, mince the tissue into 1-mm cubes with sterile scissors or a sharp scalpel blade, and place the tiny fragments directly onto the agar, submerging them slightly beneath the surface with an inoculating needle. A 5-to 10-mL sample of tissue homogenate, bone marrow, or fluid specimen sediment should be placed onto the surface of appropriate culture media. Nonselective culture media, without antibiotics, such as inhibitory mold agar or Sabhi, are probably adequate, as these specimens are usually sterile and antibiotic inhibition is not necessary.
Blood	Commercial blood culture bottles, designed for the recovery of bacteria from blood are not suitable for the recovery of many fungal species. The Isolator System (Wampole Laboratories, Cranbury NJ) has shown much promise in the more direct recovery of fungi from blood samples obtained from patients with mycotic sepsis. If this system is used, carefully follow the instructions of the manufacturer. In particular, care must be taken during the subculture stage to avoid contamination with environmental organisms. Working in a laminar airflow hood during this procedure has been advocated.

to the *Cladosporium*, *Exophiala*, and *Wangiella* genera. Nucleic acid probes for the culture confirmation of *B. dermatitidis*, *H. capsulatum*, and *C. immitis* are commercially available (Accuprobes, GenProbe Inc., La Jolla CA) and are discussed later in this chapter.

All fungal cultures should be incubated for a minimum of 30 days before discarding as negative, even if plates appear contaminated with bacteria or other fungi. We have seen colonies of *H. capsulatum*, for example, growing on the surface of colonies of *C. albicans* or contaminating molds.

The use of culture tubes or plates is optional. For low-volume laboratories staffed with personnel who may not be as familiar with the handling of fungi or where incubator and storage space may be at a premium the use of tubes is recommended. Large culture tubes (150 × 25 mm) with tightly fitted, screw-cap lids are recommended. The media should be poured in thick slants to prevent dehydration during the prolonged incubation period. After the medium is inoculated, be sure not to screw down the cap too tightly because it is necessary for the fungi to "breathe" if they are to survive.

Petri dishes have the advantage of providing a larger surface of growth, making the cultures easier to examine and subculture. Fungal colonies in mixed culture are easier to separate and work with individually. Plate cultures will become dehydrated during the prolonged incubation period if provisions are not made to keep them humidified. Pour the agar to a depth of 6 to 8 mm in the dishes, tape down the lids (use a type of tape through which air can diffuse), place the plates into loosely closed plastic bags or wrappers. Also use an incubator with a humidity of at least 50% to minimize loss of moisture from the culture during incubation. A flat pan of water can be placed on the bottom shelf of the incubator to raise the ambient humidity.

IDENTIFICATION OF FUNGAL CULTURE ISOLATES

PRELIMINARY OBSERVATIONS

The identification of an unknown fungal isolate recovered from a clinical specimen need not be difficult if a few preliminary observations are made. In most instances, it is not difficult to distinguish the smooth, pasty to mucoid colony of a yeast growing on the surface of the primary isolation medium from the cottony or wooly presentation of a mold. Exceptions include the young yeastlike colonies of the dimorphic fungus, *Sporothrix schenckii*, and the dematiaceous species, *Exophiala jeanselmei* and *Wangiella dermatitidis*, which will assume the more characteristic mold form as the colonies mature. Conversely, colonies of *Geotrichum* species and *Trichosporon* species may at times appear yeastlike, and at other times, a distinct low aerial mycelium may be observed.

The immediate task for the clinical microbiologist or mycologist when an unknown fungus is encountered is to determine the potential pathogenicity of the isolate. Every isolate must be considered potentially pathogenic; however, certain groups, including the dimorphic fungi, the dermatophytes, and certain of the slow-growing black molds, are almost always associated with disease when recovered from clinical specimens. Therefore, these fungi must be identified without fail, and answers must be forthcoming as soon as possible so that antifungal therapy can be instituted. The following are observations that may be helpful in making this initial decision.

INITIAL OBSERVATIONS IN THE STUDY OF FUNGUS ISOLATES

APPEARANCE OF THE GROWTH

The dimorphic fungi and the dermatophytes, in particular, produce delicate hyphae, no more than 1 to 2 mm in diameter, which give the mold form of the colonies a cobweb or hairlike appearance (see Color Plate 19-5A). Therefore, whenever delicate hyphae are observed, either visually or microscopically, the possibility of an obligate pathogen should be considered. The jet black reverse surface of a colony can be used to distinguish the dematiaceous group of fungi from their hyaline counterparts. This can be an important first step in making an identification.

RATE OF GROWTH

The rate of growth on primary recovery may be of some help in making a preliminary identification. The saprobic molds generally produce mature colonies within 3 to 5 days. However, in cases of heavy infections, for which the concentration of organisms in tissues and secretions may be high, the usual recovery times of 10 days or more for dimorphic fungi may be considerably shortened. Therefore, a rapid rate of growth is merely a guide, not an absolute criterion.

COLONY PIGMENTATION

Many strains of the hyaline group of saprobic molds produce pigmented conidia that impart a brightly colored surface to the colony, ranging from pastel to dark green, blue, yellow, orange, and red. The greater the sporulation, the more granular or sugary the colony surface appears (see Color Plates 19-2 and 19-4 for representative colonies). Although the vegetative hyphae of certain strains of the dimorphic molds, particularly *Coccidioides immitis*, may appear lightly pigmented, the deeper, granular pigmentation of the colony surface rarely develops. Certain fungi produce water-soluble pigments that diffuse into the agar and color the underside of the colony. The wine-red diffusible pigment produced by *Trichophyton rubrum* is a helpful clue in making an identification (see Color Plate 19-4E).

GROWTH ON MEDIA CONTAINING ANTIFUNGAL AGENTS

Most strains of the dimorphic fungi can grow in the presence of antifungal agents, specifically on culture media containing cycloheximide. Most strains of the rapidly growing saprobes are inhibited.

BOX 19-3. HELPFUL CLUES IN THE GENUS–SPECIES IDENTIFICATION OF FUNGI

1. A white or gray-brown, wooly or cottony mold, that grows from border to border in the petri dish without producing a colony margin, is characteristic of one of the *Zygomycetes* (see Color Plate 19-1*A* and 1*B*).

2. A mold that grows from border to border in the petri dish in the form of a green or green-yellow lawn is characteristic of *Trichoderma* or *Gliocladium* spp. (see Color Plate 19-2*H*).

3. A hyaline mold that produces a distinctive rose-red, lavender, or red-purple pigment is highly suggestive of *Fusarium* spp. (see Color Plate 19-2*F*).

4. A hyaline mold that produces a cottony colony, with a house mouse gray surface, is highly suggestive of *Pseudallescheria boydii* (specifically, the anamorph named *Scedosporium monosporium*; see Color Plate 19-2*G*).

5. A hyaline mold producing a marginated colony with a green, granular surface surrounded by a white apron is suggestive of *Penicillium* spp. or *Aspergillus fumigatus* (see Color Plate 1*C* and 2*A*).

6. A dematiaceous mold that grows very slowly, producing a small buttonlike colony with a delicate hairlike surface, is suggestive of *Cladosporium carionii, Phialophora* spp. or *Fonsecaea* spp. (see color Plate 19-3*D* and 3*E*).

7. A black yeast is most suggestive of *Aureobasidium pullulans*. However, young colonies of *Exophiala* spp., *Wangiella* spp., and *Sporothrix schenckii* may also present as black yeasts (see Color Plates 3*H* and 5*H*).

8. A yeast colony that is distinctly mucoid indicates the presence of capsular material and is suggestive of *Cryptococcus* spp. (see Color Plate 19-6*C*). An orange-pigmented yeast (that may also appear mucoid) is suggestive of *Rhodotorula* spp. (see Color Plate 19–6*F*).

9. A slower-growing colony that appears to have both mold and yeast components (see Color Plate 19-5*A*) or has a prickly appearance (see Color Plate 19-5*D*) suggests one of the dimorphic molds.

DIMORPHIC GROWTH

The dimorphic fungi grow in one of two forms: 1) a mold form (the environmental and infective form) when incubated at ambient or room temperature (22°C to 30°C); and 2) a yeast form (invasive form) when incubated nearer body temperature 30°C to 35°C. The presumptive identification of a dimorphic mold that has been recovered at ambient temperature must be confirmed by demonstrating conversion to the yeast form when incubated at 35°C on an appropriate culture medium, or, more quickly and easily, by detecting specific antigen through exoantigen assays or through the use of a nucleic acid probe assays when available.[252,328] Representative mold and yeast colonies are shown in Color Plate 19-5. Box 19-3 lists several other colony characteristics that may provide an early clue to making a presumptive identification.

With experience, each microbiologist and mycologist begins to learn the colonial presentations of the various yeasts and molds that are endemic in any given locale. Because colonial characteristics may vary depending on the environmental conditions, the culture media used, and strain differences, microscopic confirmation is obviously necessary before a final report can be issued.

PREPARATION OF MOUNTS FOR STUDY

The tease mount (Fig. 19-1), the transparency tape preparation (Fig. 19-2), and the microslide technique (Fig. 19-3) are three commonly used methods for the microscopic examination of filamentous molds.[184] In each instance, a portion of the mold colony is mounted in a drop of lactophenol aniline (cotton) blue stain on a microscope slide. A coverslip is positioned over the drop and gently pressed to disperse the sample more evenly throughout the mounting fluid to facilitate microscopic examination.

THE TEASE MOUNT

With a pair of dissecting needles or pointed applicator sticks, dig out a small portion of the colony to be examined, including some of the subsurface agar.

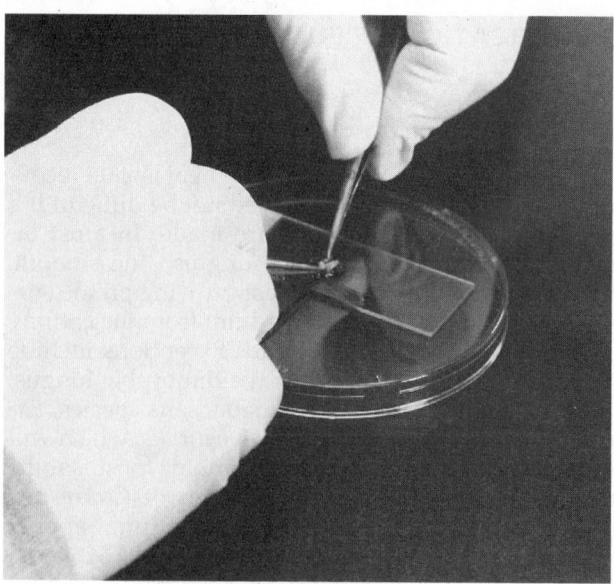

Figure 19-1
Tease mount preparation illustrating dissection of the colony fragment with needles in a drop of lactophenol aniline blue prior to placement of the cover slip.

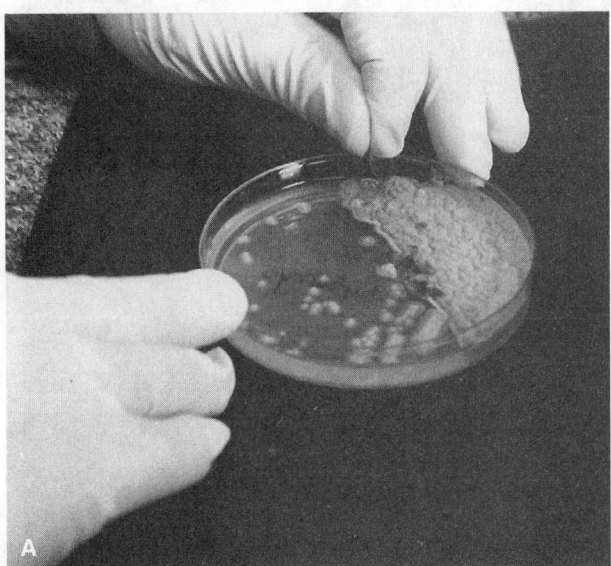

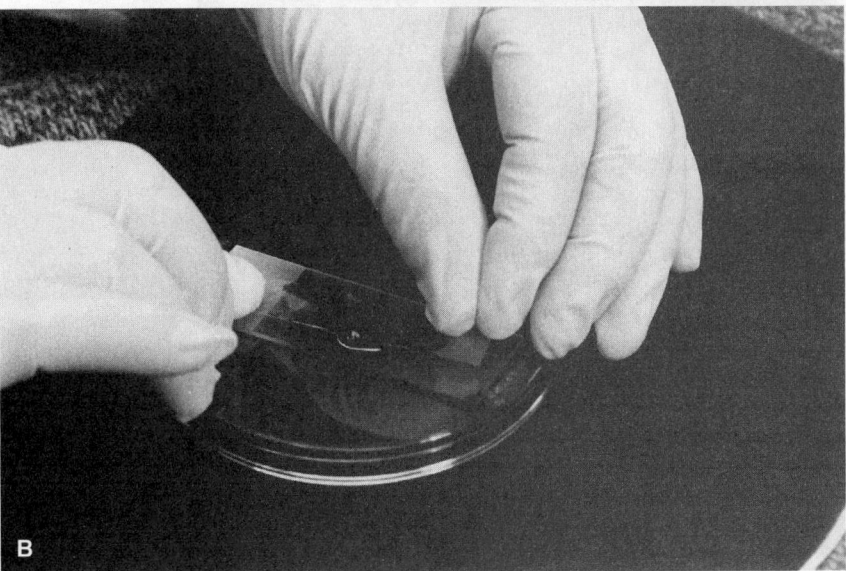

Figure 19-2
(**A**) Scotch tape preparation: sticky side of tape being pressed to the surface of a fungus colony. (**B**) Scotch tape preparation: stretching the inoculated scotch tape preparation over a drop of lactophenol aniline blue on a microscope slide.

Place the colony fragment on a microscope slide in a drop of lactophenol aniline blue, tease the colony apart with the dissecting needles, and overlay with a coverslip (see Fig. 19-1). Gentle pressure on the surface of the coverslip with the eraser end of a pencil may help disperse the mount, particularly if small chunks of agar are present. Examine the preparation microscopically, first under the low-power (10×) objective and then under high-power (40×), or under oil immersion (100×) if suspicious fungal structures are seen. Teasing the colony often disrupts the delicate fruiting structures of the filamentous molds, making it difficult in some instances to observe the characteristic spore arrangements necessary for a definitive identification.

SCOTCH TAPE PREPARATION

The Scotch tape method of preparing cultures for microscopic examination is often helpful because the spore arrangements of the more delicate filamentous molds are better preserved. With the unfrosted, clear cellophane tape, press the sticky side gently but firmly to the surface of the colony, picking up a portion of the aerial mycelium (see Fig. 19-2A). This operation should always be performed under a biologic safety hood. Care must also be taken that the exposed fingers do not come in contact with the mold surface. For maximum safety, gloves should be worn. The preparation is made by placing a drop of lactophenol aniline blue stain on a microscope slide. Stick one end of the tape to the surface of the slide adjacent to the drop of stain. Then stretch the tape over the stain, gently lowering it so that the mycelium becomes permeated with stain (see Fig. 19-2B). Pull the tape taut and then stick the opposite end to the glass, avoiding as much as possible the trapping of air bubbles. Some practice may be needed in removing the sticky surface of the tape if gloves are worn.

The preparation can now be examined microscopically in the same manner described for the tease mount preparation, with the exception that the use of oil

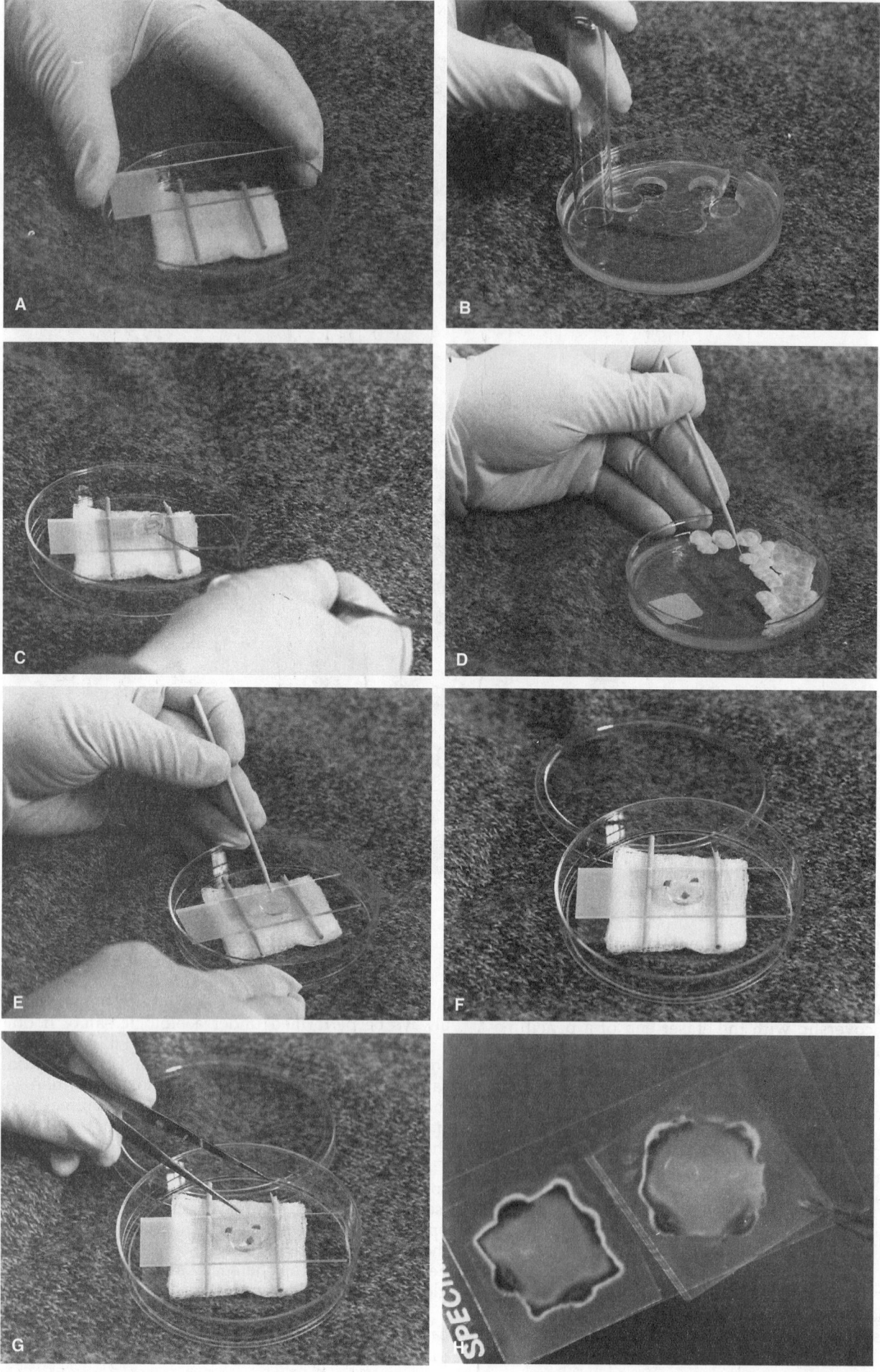

immersion is generally less than satisfactory because of interference from the substance of the tape. This method is inexpensive, rapid, simple to perform, and with few exceptions allows one to make an accurate identification.

THE MICROSLIDE CULTURE TECHNIQUE

In instances for which neither the tease mount nor the Scotch tape preparations establish an accurate identification, or when permanent slide mounts are desired for further study or for use of student study, the microslide culture technique is recommended. Although somewhat tedious to perform, high-quality preparations in which the spore structures and arrangements are beautifully preserved can be made. The technique is as follows:

1. Place a round piece of filter paper or gauze flat into the bottom of a sterile petri dish. Place a pair of thin glass rods or applicator sticks cut to length to fit on top of the filter paper to serve as supports for a 3 by 1-in. glass microscope slide (Fig. 19-3A).
2. Place a block or plug of cornmeal or potato dextrose agar on the surface of the microscope slide (Figs. 19-3B and C). Two blocks, separated by about 1 in. (2.5 cm), can be placed on the same microscope slide if more than one mount is desired (see Fig. 19-3A).
3. Inoculate the margins of the agar plug in three or four places with a small portion of the colony to be studied, using a straight inoculating wire or the tip of a dissecting needle (see Fig. 19-3D, E and F).
4. Gently heat a coverslip by passing it quickly through the flame of a Bunsen burner and immediately place it directly on the surface of the inoculated agar block. Heating the coverslip produces a tight seal between the bottom of the coverslip and the surface of the agar, which is briefly melted by the warm glass.
5. Pipette a small amount of water into the bottom of the petri dish to saturate the filter paper or the gauze. Place the lid on the petri dish and incubate the assembly at room temperature (or 30°C) for 3 to 5 days (see Fig. 19-3E).
6. When growth visually appears to be mature, the coverslip can be gently lifted from the surface of the agar with a pair of forceps, taking care not to disrupt the mycelium adhering to the bottom of the coverslip any more than necessary (see Fig. 19-3G).
7. Place the coverslip on a small drop of lactophenol aniline blue applied to the surface of a second 3 by 1-in. glass slide. The mount can be preserved for future study by rimming the outside margins of the coverslip with mounting fluid or clear fingernail polish. This activity should be performed under a biologic safety hood (see Fig 19-3H).
8. After the coverslip has been removed from the agar block (or blocks), the agar block itself can be removed by prying it away from the glass slide with

Figure 19-3
Microculture preparation sequence. See text for details.

an applicator stick. This operation is performed over a beaker or pan containing 5% phenol decontamination fluid, into which the agar blocks are allowed to fall. The mycelium adhering to the surface of the original glass slide after the block is removed can also be stained with lactophenol aniline blue and a coverslip overlaid, serving as a second stained mount. Again, the mount can be preserved for future study by rimming the coverslip with mounting fluid or fingernail polish, as previously described.

One should not be concerned if the agar blocks completely dry out before harvesting the coverslip. Even if the coverslip is firmly adherent to the surface of the glass, a drop of lactophenol aniline blue can be placed adjacent to one margin of the slide. By capillary action the stain will diffuse between the undersurface of the coverslip and the glass slide. In fact, there is often less disruption of the mycelial elements and superior preparations are the result.

Each of these preparations permits the microscopic study of filamentous molds.

TERMS USEFUL IN THE EXAMINATION OF FUNGI

In the examination of fungal colonies and microscopic mounts, the following are terms useful in describing various observations:

1. The fundamental microscopic unit of a fungus is the threadlike structure called a **hypha**. Several hyphae combine to form the matt of growth known as the **mycelium**. Hyphae that are subdivided into individual cells by transverse walls or septat are called **septate**; those without walls are **aseptate**. Pseudohyphae form from elongation of budding yeast cells (blastoconidia), and show sausage-like constructions between segments. (Fig. 19-4).
2. The portion of the mycelium that extends into the substratum of the culture medium and is responsible for absorbing water and nutrients, is the **vegetative mycelium**; the portion that projects above the substrate is the **aerial mycelium**, also called the **reproductive mycelium** because special spore or conidia-bearing fruiting bodies derive from this portion.
3. The identification and classification of fungi are primarily based on the morphologic differences in reproductive structures and the manner in which spores or conidia are formed from specialized cells called **conidiogenous cells**.

Three general types of reproduction are commonly observed in the fungal species of medical importance: vegetative sporulation, aerial sporulation, and sexual sporulation.

VEGETATIVE REPRODUCTION

Three types of spores or conidia may form directly from the vegetative mycelium: **blastoconidia**, **chlamydospores**, and **arthroconidia** (the old term for vegetative spores was **thallospore**). The term **spore** should be

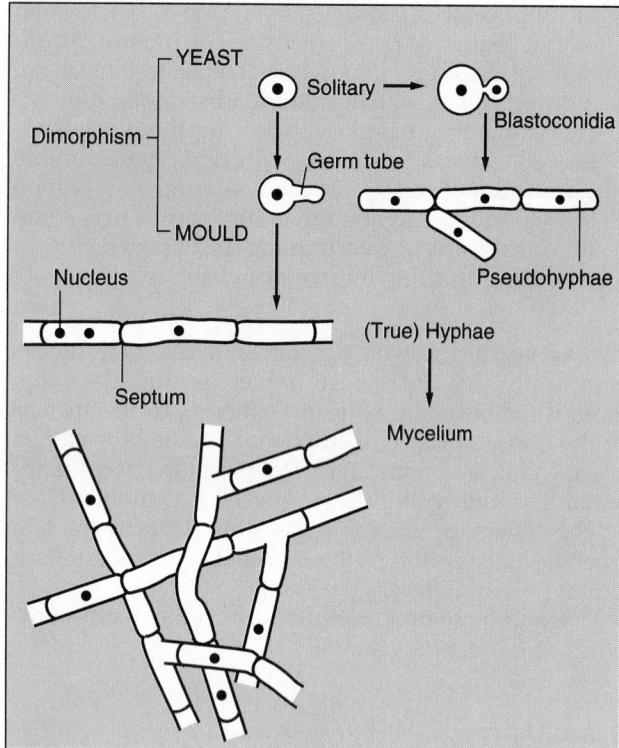

Figure 19-4
Simplified sketches of basic fungal morphology.

reserved for only those reproductive elements that arise from meiosis (sexual reproduction), such as ascospores, oospores, or zygospores) or from mitosis (asexual reproduction) within a sporangium (as with the *Zygomycetes*). The term **endospore** is also used for spores produced within a confined space (the tissue form of *Coccidioides immitis*, for example). All other asexual "spores" are conidia. Therefore, the terms blastoconidia and arthroconidia are correct; the designations blastospores and arthrospores are incorrect. Although chlamydoconidia is the correct terminology, the term chlamydospores is retained in most circles.

Blastoconidia are the familiar budding forms characteristically produced by yeasts. A bud scar (dysjuncter) often remains at the point where the conidium becomes detached. **Chlamydoconidia** (chlamydospores) are formed from preexistent cells in the hyphae, which become thickened and often enlarged. Chlamydoconidia may be found within (intercalary), along the side (sessile), or at the tip (terminal) of the hyphae. This type of conidiation is characteristic of *Candida albicans*. **Arthroconidia** also are formed from preexistent cells in the hyphae, which become enlarged and thickened. On reaching maturity, these conidia are released by lysis of adjacent hyphal cells. This type of sporulation is characteristic of the mold form of *Coccidioides immitis* and *Geotrichum* species, among others.

AERIAL REPRODUCTION

Emanating from the hyphae and extending from the mycelial surface are specialized fruiting bodies that give rise to a variety of spores or conidia. Fruiting bod-

ies may form closed sacs called **sporangia**, within which spores called **sporangiospores** are produced (Fig. 19-5). The specialized hyphal segment that holds up or supports the sporangium is called the **sporangiophore** (the suffix "phore" [Greek *phoros*] means "bearing"). This type of sporulation is characteristic of the *Zygomycetes*. Many other fungi produce elaborate fruiting bodies that give rise to spores produced from the surface, to which the term **conidia** (dust) is applied. The specialized hyphal segment that supports a conidia-bearing fruiting head is called a **conidiophore**.

The conidiophore may branch into secondary spore-producing segments, called **phialides**. A **phialide**, by definition, is a conidiogenous cell that produces conidia from a locus inside its apex, which does not increase in width or length during conidiogenesis (in contrast with the processes of annelide formation, in which the tip of the phialide cyclically extends and retracts when conidia are formed, leaving a succession of scars or rings). This property of branching into phialides is characteristic of the fingerlike fruiting body of *Penicillium* species. Conidia may be borne singly, in long chains, or in tightly bound clusters. Tiny one-celled conidia, usually borne either directly from the sides of the hyphae or supported by a hairlike conidiophore, are called **microconidia**, in contrast with the much larger, multicelled **macroconidia** that assume a variety of sizes and shapes. A multicelled macroconidia that is divided by both transverse and longitudinal septations giving a mosaic appearance is a **dictyospore**, more commonly referred to as **muriform** (resembling a stone wall). The term **aleureospore** refers to a conidium, usually a macroconidium, that by definition is attached to the hyphae by a supporting cell that fractures when the conidium is released (e.g., *Microsporium canis*).

When conidia form in chains, the process whereby those that are produced from a conidium at the apex, such that the oldest cell is at the base, is known as

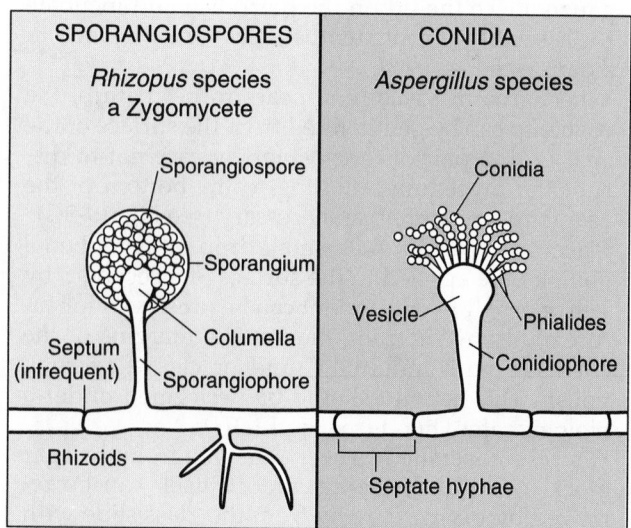

Figure 19-5
Simplified sketches of aerial mycelium.

acropetal (e.g., *Penicillium* species); **basipetal sporulation** refers to that process by which a new conidium forms at the base of the chain, pushing all other conidia in the chain ahead such that the oldest conidium is at the tip (e.g., *Paecilomyces* species).

SEXUAL SPORULATION

Sexual sporulation requires the merging and nuclear recombination of two specialized fertile cells (each having undergone meiosis) arising on the aerial hyphae (Fig. 19-6).

If the reproductive cells formed by fusion of morphologically identical cells, often from the same hyphae (homothallic), the spore is called a **zygospore**, characteristic of the *Zygomycetes*. If the fusing reproductive cells are derived from two different cells, often derived from separate hyphal segments, the resulting spore is called an **oospore**.

The sexual spores of several members of the class **Ascomycetes**, previously mentioned, which are of medical importance, are called **ascospores**. For example, certain strains of *Aspergillus* species, notably of the *A. nidulans* and *A. glaucus* groups, produce large, closed, baglike structures called cleistothecia, which in turn contain smaller baglike structures called asci (see Figs. 19-6 and 19-18). Within each ascus are four ascospores, the product of meiotic division. Medically important fungi other than *Aspergillus* species in which sexual sporulation may be observed include *Saccharomyces* species and *Pseudallescheria boydii*.

The sexual form of a fungus is known as a **teleomorph**, in contrast to the term **anamorph**, which refers to the various asexual reproductive forms or structures produced by an imperfect fungus (such as phialides, annellides, branching chains, and such). Thus, for example, *P. boydii* is the telomorph of this species, and various "perfect" forms, such as cleistothecia, asci, and ascospores may be observed. *Scedosporium monospo-*

rium is the imperfect form of this species, producing primarily single-celled conidia as the chief anamorphic form. This brief orientation to the filamentous molds will serve as points of reference for the several groups of fungi to be discussed in the next sections.

LABORATORY AND CLINICAL CHARACTERISTICS OF SPECIFIC GROUPS OF FILAMENTOUS MOLDS

THE ZYGOMYCETES AND ZYGOMYCOSIS

The *Zygomycetes* are a group of fungi that are widely distributed in nature as environmental inhabitants of soil, dung, and vegetable matter. Humans usually become infected through inhalation of airborne spores (sinus and pulmonary disease) or through ingestion of contaminated foodstuffs (gastrointestinal disease). A proclivity to invade blood vessels may result in disseminated disease and the formation of metastatic foci in many organs.

LABORATORY PRESENTATION

A fungal isolate can be suspected of belonging to the *Zygomycetes* if it grows rapidly over the entire surface of the agar plate as a gray-white, brown, or gray-brown, cottony or wooly colony, without a distinct margin (see Color Plates 19-1*A* and 1*B*). The term "lid lifter" has been used to describe the rapid and prolific growth of this fungus. As the colony matures, the mycelium may darken and show a black pepper effect as myriads of sporangia are formed.

Microscopically, the characteristic features are the presence of broad, ribbonlike, aseptate hyphae (occasionally, septa may be seen in older cultures, particularly at the terminal portions of the sporangiophores) and the production of sporangiospores within sporan-

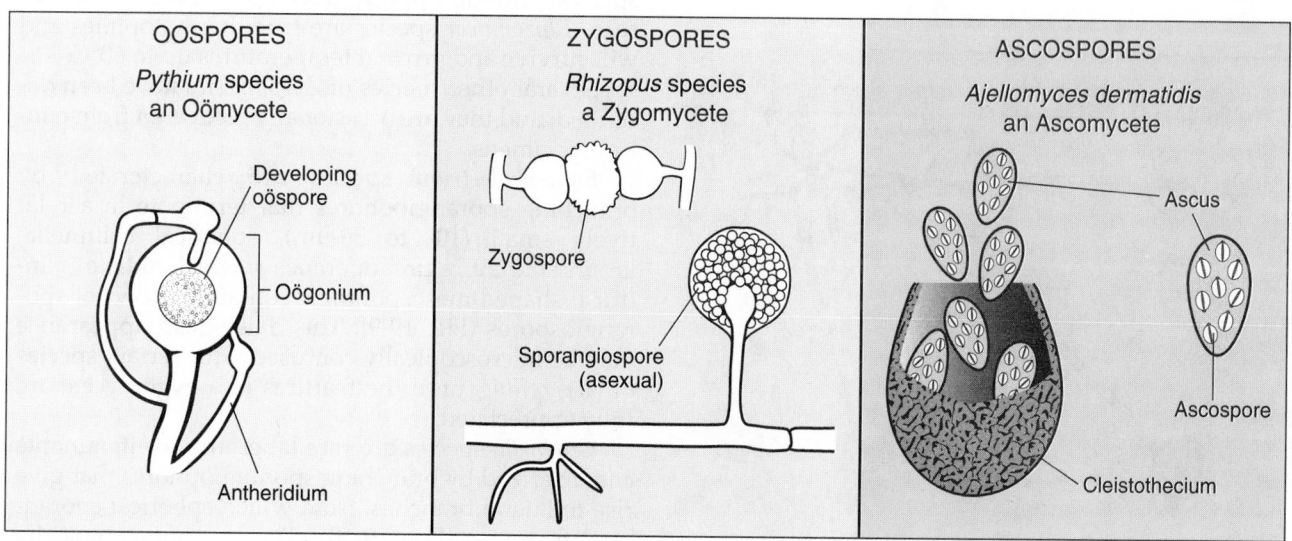

Figure 19-6
Simplified sketches of sexual reproduction.

gia. The sporangia are borne at the tips of unbranched or branched sporangiophores that terminate in a bulbous swelling called the **columella**. The presence of rootlike structures, called **rhizoids**, is a helpful feature in making genus identifications (Fig. 19-7).

The genera of fungi of medical importance that are included within the class *Zygomycetes* include the two more common isolates, *Rhizopus* and *Mucor*, and less commonly encountered, *Absidia, Rhizomucor, Syncephalastrum, Circinella, Cokeromyces, Basidiobolus, Saksenaea,* and *Apophysomyces. Rhizopus* species is distinguished by the production of rootlike structures called rhizoids that lie on the stolon immediately adjacent to the points of derivation of the sporangiophores (see Fig.19-7). This "nodal" derivation of the sporangiophores is contrary to the "internodal" derivation of the rhizoids by *Absidia* species, which lie on the stolon between the sporangiophores.

The rhizoids of *Absidia* species are typically delicate, in contrast with the coarser and more-spiked rhizoids of *Rhizopus* species. The sporangiophores of *Rhizopus* species are generally simple but occasionally may branch; the sporangiophores of *Absidia* species usually branch freely (Fig. 19-8). The columella of *Rhizopus* species often collapses at maturity, taking on a drooping umbrella shape. The columella of *Absidia* are semicircular, have a knob at the top, and rest within a widened flange at the tip of the conidiophore, called an apophysis.

R. rhizopodoformis and *R. arrhizus* are the species most commonly associated with human infections[296]; however, because there is rarely a clinical indication, species identifications are not made in most laboratories. Chlamydoconidia may occasionally be seen; zygospores are not seen in either of these species (but may be seen in *R. stolonifer,* a rare species encountered as a laboratory contaminant).

Mucor species do not produce rhizoids. The sporangiophores may be simple but tend to branch; the sporangium is large (up to 100 μm), spherical, and disintegrates on maturity, with release of many sporan-

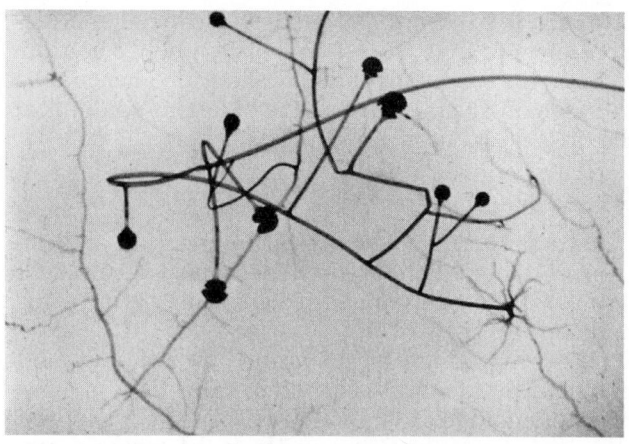

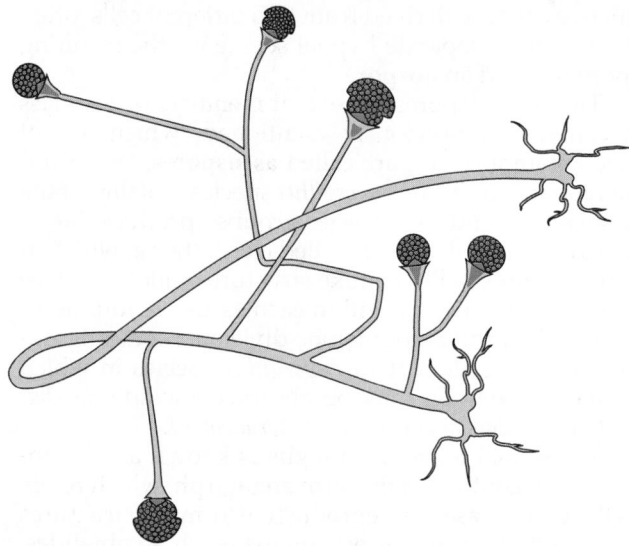

Figure 19-8
Sketch and photomicrograph of *Absidia* species.

giospores. *Rhizomucor* species are similar to *Mucor* species, although poorly developed rhizoids may be seen. *Rhizomucor* species are true thermatophiles and will survive and grow at temperatures up to 60°C.

Several other species of *Zygomycetes* have been described, and they are occasionally recovered from clinical specimens.

Syncephalastrum species are characterized by branching sporangiophores that terminate in a relatively small (10- to 50-μm), spherical columella, around the entire circumference of which radiate cylindrical-shaped mesosporangia containing rows of sporangiospores (Fig. 19-9). This daisy-head appearance may be microscopically confused with certain species of *Aspergillus,* until the features of a zygomycete are fully appreciated.

Circinella species are rare laboratory contaminants characterized by branching sporangiophores that give rise to lateral branches, from which spherical sporangia are borne (Fig. 19-10). The sporangia typically curve inward and may be encrusted with calcium oxalate crystals.

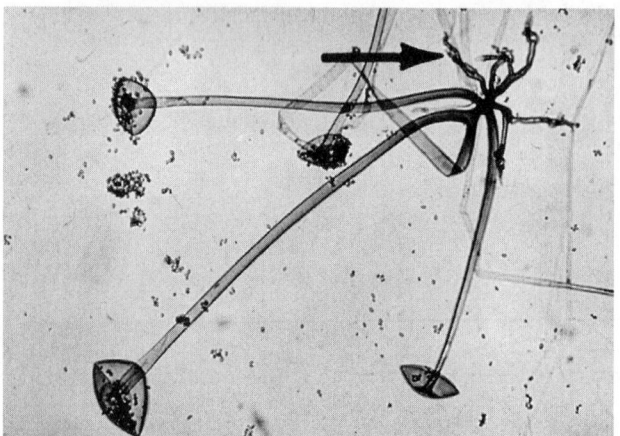

Figure 19-7
Photomicrograph of *Rhizopus* species. Note the root-like rhizoids (*arrow*) at the base of the conidiophores.

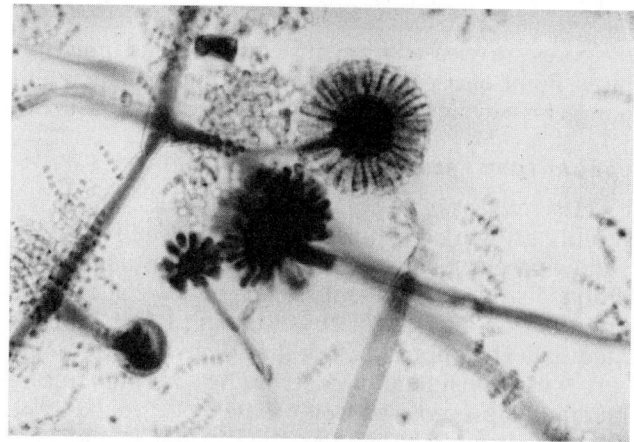

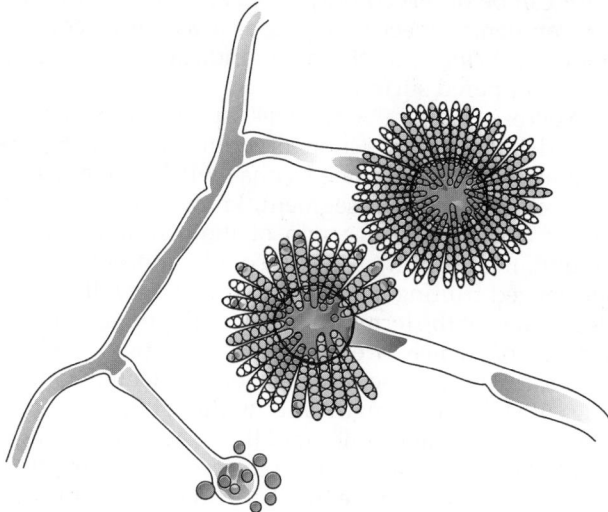

Figure 19-9
Sketch and photomicrograph of *Syncephalastrum* species.

Cunninghamella species (*C. bertholletiae* is most commonly recovered from clinical specimens) are characterized by branched sporangiophores that terminate in a spherical vesicle from which secondary spherical sporangiolas (tiny sporangia without columella) are derived from the surface, each attached to the vesicle by a delicate pedicle (Fig. 19-11).

HISTOPATHOLOGY

The ribbonlike, broad, aseptate hyphae of the *Zygomycetes* as described in the foregoing are generally distinct from other hyphal-producing fungi in tissue sections. The hyphae range from 3 to 25 µm in width, have nonparallel walls, and often tend to break up into small fragments (Fig. 19-12, page 1004). The hyphae often do not stain well, even with periodic acid-Schiff (PAS) or Gomori's methenamine silver (GMS) fungal stains. The background tissue reaction is typically purulent, and both intact and fragmented hyphae are usually seen amid a sea of segmented neutrophils. Occasional septa may be observed. Hyphae cut in cross-section can also mimic spores or small immature spherules of *Coccidioides immitis*, potentially leading to

an incorrect conclusion. Members of the *Zygomycetes* also have a propensity to invade blood vessels, causing hemorrhagic infarction (one reason why the gross tissue often appears charred). They can also present as a fungus ball in body cavities and, occasionally, the typical fruiting heads, complete with sporangia and sporangiospores may be observed.

ASPERGILLUS SPECIES AND ASPERGILLOSIS

The aspergilli compose a group of rapidly growing, hyaline molds that commonly cause opportunistic infections in humans. Of the some 700 *Aspergillus* species described by Raper and Fennell in their classic text,[286] only 19 species have been cited by Rinaldi[293] as causing human infections; of these, only four species are recovered with any frequency from hospitalized patients: *A. fumigatus* (the species causing most allergic pulmonary and invasive diseases), *A. flavus*, *A. niger*, and *A. terreus*. Thus, with this focus, the task of identifying *Aspergillus* species in clinical laboratories is manageable.

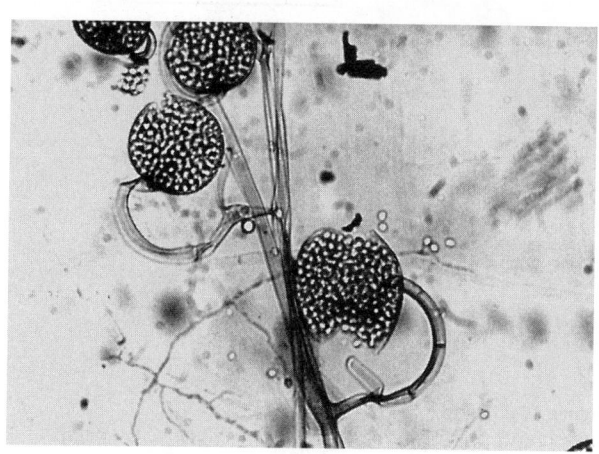

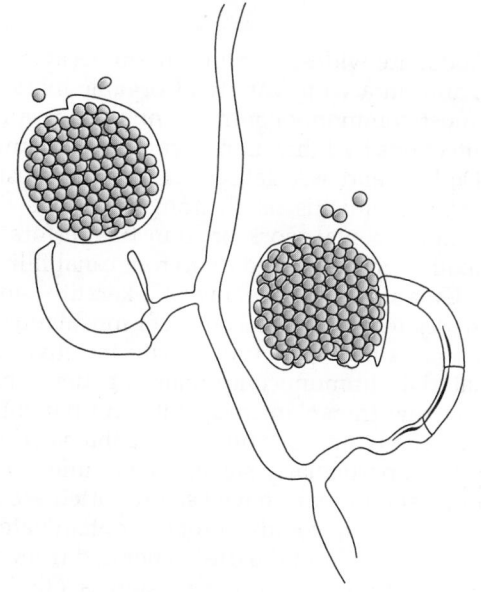

Figure 19-10
Sketch and photomicrograph of *Circinella* species.

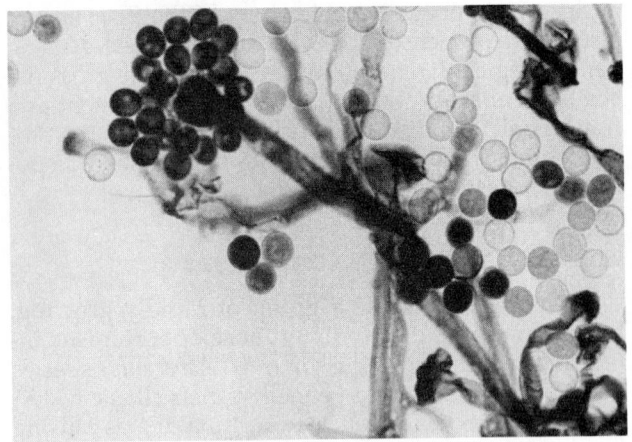

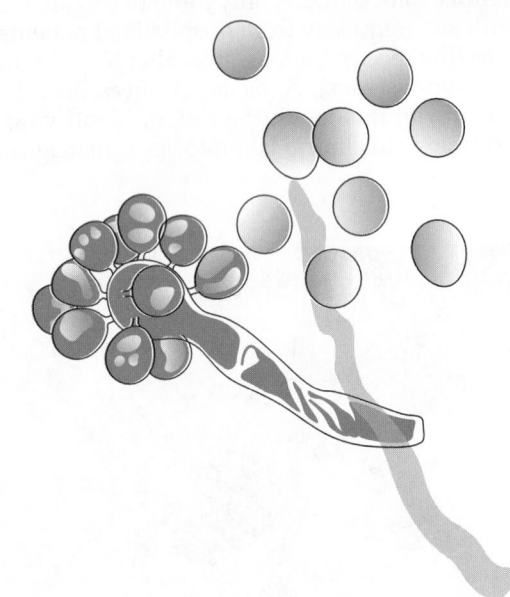

Figure 19-11
Sketch and photomicrograph of *Cunninghamella* species.

Conidia are widespread in soil, on decaying vegetation, and on a wide variety of organic matter. Humans most commonly contract sinus and respiratory tract infections by inhalation of conidia-contaminated dust. De Foer and associates[82] suggest that most cases of aspergilla sinusitis result from oral–sinus fistulae complicating dental work or from the perforation of the maxillary sinus secondary to root canal filling materials. Cutaneous disease, mycotic keratitis, and otomycosis result from direct contact or inoculation of the affected parts from penetration with infective vegetative materials. Immunocompromised patients, notably bone marrow transplant recipients and patients with leukemia and lymphoma undergoing intensive chemotherapy, are particularly susceptible to infection. Several hospital outbreaks have been reported secondary to dissemination of conidia through contaminated ventilation ducts[2] or from the dust generated from nearby construction projects.[246] Rhame[290] suggests that the incidence of nosocomial aspergillosis in any given institution occurs in direct proportion to the mean ambient airborne spore count and is highest when minibursts of spores are released from dust, clothing, and other surfaces. Point-of-use filters, high filtration efficiency, and a high air exchange are effective protective measures.

LABORATORY PRESENTATION

Aspergillus species can be suspected in culture if a rapidly growing (within 3 to 5 days), usually yellow, yellow-green, yellow-brown or green, granular colony, with a distinct margin and a white peripheral apron is observed on an agar plate containing fungal culture medium. The appearance of the colonial morphology can vary considerably, depending on the culture media being used (see Color Plate 19-1C to 1H). The classic morphology, as described in Raper and Fennel[286] can be observed only on Czapek's agar. Certain environmental species may appear as white, cottony colonies; *A. niger*, as the name indicates, produces a black, peppered surface.

Microscopically, *Aspergillus* species are characterized by the production of uniform, 4- to 6-μm–diameter, hyaline, septate hyphae with parallel walls. A specialized hyphal segment, known as a foot cell, serves as the base of origin of the conidiophore. In mounts made from cultures, conidiation occurs in a specialized fruiting body composed of a swollen vesicle situated at the terminus of a conidiophore, from the surface of which are borne one or two rows of phialides, giving rise to chains of pigmented conidia (Fig. 19-13). The length and width of the conidiophores, the size and contour of the vesicle, the arrangement of the phialides, and the color, size, and length of chains of the conidia are the structures used in making species identifications.[286]

The following outlines the colonial morphology and microscopic appearance of the four clinically significant *Aspergillus* species listed earlier.

Aspergillus fumigatus.   The colonies of *A. fumigatus* are granular to cottony and usually have some shade of green, green-gray, or green-brown pigmentation (see Color Plate 19-1C). A white apron is seen at the periphery at the growing margin.

Microscopically, the conidiophores are relatively long (300 to 500 μm), the vesicles are 30 to 50 μm in diameter, club-shaped and covered on the top half with only a single row of phialides, giving rise to long chains of spherical to slightly ovoid conidia that tend to sweep toward the central axis (Fig. 19-14, page 1005).

Aspergillus flavus.   The colonies of *A. flavus* are granular to wooly and have some shade of yellow or yellow-brown; see Color Plate 19-1D). Microscopically, the conidiophores are long (400 to 800 μm) and tend to be roughened just beneath a globose vesicle measuring 25 to 45 μm in diameter (Fig. 19-15, page 1005). Phialides arise from the entire circumference of the vesicle surface and may have one row (uniseriate), or more characteristically, two rows (biseriate) of phialides. Conidia are spherical, smooth, or slightly roughened with maturity and form relatively long chains.

CLINICAL CORRELATION BOX 19-1. DISEASES ASSOCIATED WITH *ZYGOMYCETES*

Rhinocerebral, pulmonary, cutaneous, and disseminated forms of disease are most commonly encountered with the *Zygomycetes*:

1. *Rhinocerebral disease:* Headache, unilateral retroorbital pain, and fever may begin insidiously or be rapidly progressive. Sinusitis is a common presenting symptom. Patients with diabetic acidosis are most likely to develop a rapidly invasive disease characterized by edema of the eyelids, proptosis, malar anesthesia, and internal and external ophthalmoplegia. A thick, dark, blood-tinged nasal discharge may be observed, the nasal turbinates may appear blackened or a necrotic ulcer of the palate may be present. Cerebral involvement usually occurs by direct extension of nasal, sinus, or orbital disease, manifest by headache, drowsiness, semistupor, and nuchal rigidity. Localized cerebral disease is uncommon, occurring most frequently among intravenous drug abusers.[221] Confusion and mood disturbances may be the presenting signs. Space-occupying lesions and brain abscesses are seen in drug addicts. Once cerebral symptoms set in, the process is often rapidly fatal.

2. *Pulmonary:* The onset of disease may be insidious or sudden—chest pain, hemoptysis, sputum production, and cough are seen in varying degrees of severity. Patients with hematologic malignancies are particularly at high risk; however, disease may be seen in patients without underlying disease.[188] Infiltrates, ill-defined or diffuse, localized (lesions may cavitate or fungus ball involvement may be seen), or diffuse fine nodules (miliary pattern) may be seen radiologically. Subacute pulmonary disease is usually intrabronchial, with the formation of mucin plugs. The pleura may occasionally be involved.[122]

3. *Cutaneous:* Cutaneous disease usually occurs secondary to trauma and soil contamination,[250, 344] in patients with burns,[74] and episodically, from direct implantation with Elastoplast bandages.[258] Occasionally, subcutaneous involvement by hematogenous spread may complicate disseminated disease. Lesions ranging from small violaceous plaques, to cellulitis, ulceration, and gangrene may be seen.

4. *Disseminated:* Disseminated disease may involve virtually any organ, occurring from secondary spread from the lung, the sinuses, or rarely, from the gastrointestinal tract.[296] Most commonly affected are persons who are immunosuppressed because of their age (the very young and the very old), drug users, or those with underlying diseases, such as hematologic malignancies (particularly during periods of leukopenia), diabetes mellitus, and lupus erythematosus.[41, 314] The use of deferoxamine in dialysis patients has also been cited as a predisposing cause.[43] Symptoms most commonly reflect local organ thrombosis and infarction.

CLINICAL CORRELATION BOX 19-2. INFECTIONS WITH UNCOMMON *ZYGOMYCETES* SPECIES

Similar to *Cunninghamella* spp., *Cokeromyces* spp. also form sporangiolas, the pedicles of which, however, twist and curve back on themselves. Kemma and coauthors[172] report a case of *C. recurvatus* endocervicitis in a 37-year-old insulin-dependent person with diabetes and cite reports of three instances of recovery of this fungus as probably commensals or contaminants from genitourinary specimens. They cite the ability to grow at 42°C, the ability to assimilate nitrate as the sole nitrogen source, the inability to utilize sucrose or ferment glucose, and the susceptibility to cycloheximide, as characteristics helpful in separating *Cokeromyces* spp. from other zygomycetes. *Basidiobolus* and *Conidiobolus* spp., belonging to the order *Endophthalmorales* and reported in rare cases of rhinofacial[337] and disseminated diseases,[294] also form sporangiola. *Basidiobolus* spp. can be suspected if masses of zygospores, measuring from 20 to 50 μm in diameter with a prominent beak, and chlamydoconidia in addition to the sporangiola, are observed. The sporangiola of *Conidiobolus* spp. are single-celled and appear as large conidia (25 to 45 μm). Spores, often covered by short, hairlike appendages called villae, may be ejected from the sporangiola, and can travel a distance of 30 mm. *Mortierella* spp. is characterized by the formation of sporangia that lack a columella and produce small, spiny, or echinulate sporangiospores, called sytlospores.

Apophysomyces elegans, the cause of several recently reported infections,[69, 198, 215, 268] forms long sporangiophores that terminate in large sporangia, with prominent funnel-shaped apophyses. Meis and associates[215] report on a recent case of *A. elegans* osteomyelitis of the humerus of a healthy 69-year-old man, unusual in that the patient was neither immunosuppressed nor a diabetic. The infection was rapidly progressive, despite amphotericin B therapy, indicating that zygomycosis can progress in patients without underlying disease. They tabulate nine additional cases of *A. elegans* infections from the literature, most in patients without underlying disease, involving the skin or subcutaneous tissue following trauma or surgery. *Saksenaea vasiformis* is characterized by the formation of flask-shaped sporangia supported by very short sporangiophores that may arise adjacent to rhizoids. Bearer and coworkers[31] report a case of posttraumatic zygomycosis of a right arm wound caused by *S. vasiformis* in a 49-year-old patient with diabetes and cite three previous cases caused by this agent from the recent literature. For those interested in studying these rare isolates in more detail, refer to Richardson and Shankland.[289]

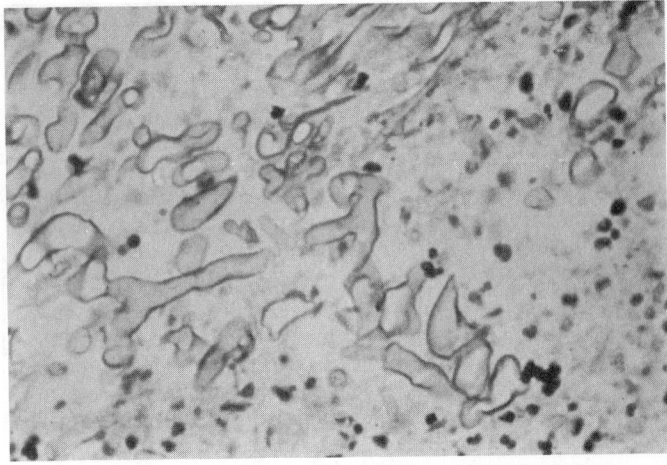

Figure 19-12
Tissue section showing irregular-sized, broad, aseptate hyphal forms of one of the *Zygomycetes* species (H&E, oil immersion).

Aspergillus niger. The colonies of *A. niger* are instantly recognized—the surface is covered by a dense aggregate of jet-black conidia, giving a characteristic peppered effect (see Color Plate 19-1*E*). The underside of the colony is buff or yellow-gray, distinguishing *A. niger* from the dematiaceous fungi, to be described later.

Microscopically, conidiation is extremely profuse, to the extent that the vesicles are obscured by dense aggregates of 3- to 5-μm diameter, spherical, black conidia that become roughened with maturity (Fig. 19-16). The vesicles, when visible, are globose and measure up to 75 μm in diameter.

Aspergillus terreus. The colonies of *A. terreus* are cinnamon buff, brown, or orange-brown (see Color Plate 19-1*F*). Radial folds emanating from the center of the colony are often observed.

Microscopically the vesicles are relatively small (10 to 16 μm in diameter) and dome-shaped. The phialides are biseriate; uniquely the proximal, primary phialides are shorter (5 to 8 μm) than the secondary phialides (8 to 12 μm), producing an upward sweeping appearance, simulating a long net of hair pulled into a hair dryer (Fig. 19-17, *right*, page 1007). Smooth, elliptical conidia measure 2 to 2.5 μm in diameter and are formed in long chains. Also unique to *A. terreus*, 6- to 7-μm–diameter microconidia, supported by a single, short conidiophore, are borne laterally from the hyphal cells (Fig. 19-17, *left*).

Because any of the aforementioned four species can be an environmental contaminant when recovered in culture, it is usually necessary to recover the same strain from repeated specimens before its clinical significance can be established. When *Aspergillus* species other than the four discussed in the foregoing are recovered, they are usually considered environmental contaminants, and a report "*Aspergillus* species, no further identification" can be issued. However, if they also are recovered from repeated samples and appear to be clinically significant, a definitive identification may be necessary. If local resources are not available to make species identification, the services of a reference laboratory should be considered.

Certain species, such as *A. nidulans* and *A. glaucus* (colonies are shown in Color Plates 19-1*G* and 1*H*), which may rarely be recovered from cases of human infections, may form sexually derived ascospores contained within saclike structures called cleistothecia (Fig. 19-18). These species are rarely encountered from clinical specimens, and these telomorphic structures are

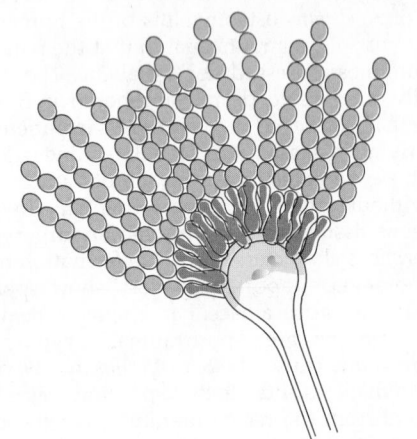

Figure 19-13
Sketch and photomicrograph of *Aspergillus* species (generic).

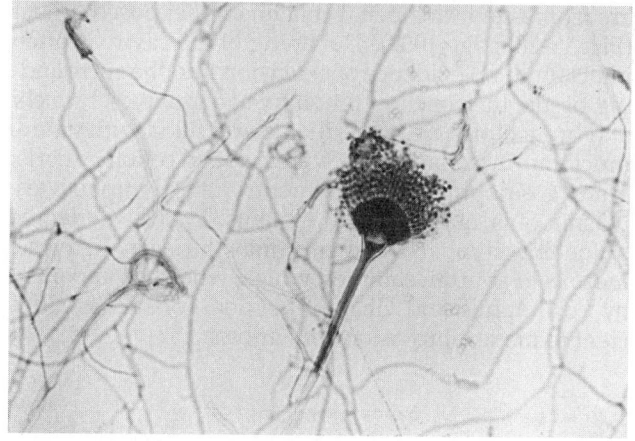

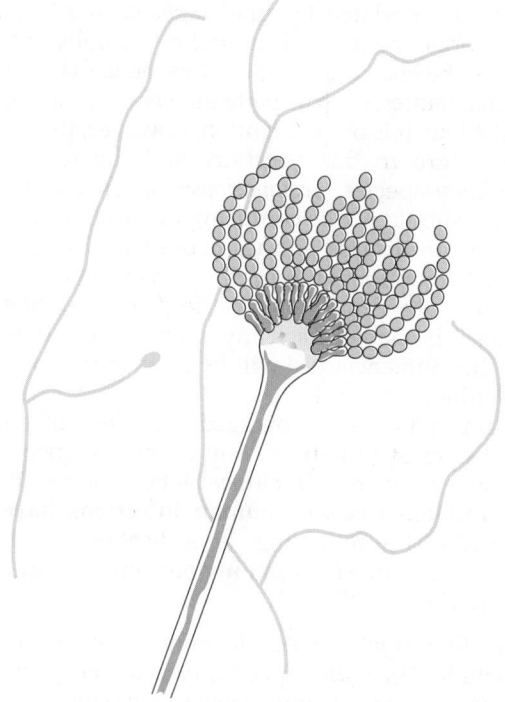

Figure 19-14
Sketch and photomicrograph of *Aspergillus fumigatus*.

uncommonly seen. Tong and coauthors[341] report a fatal case of cerebral aspergillosis caused by *A. nidulans*, presenting as abscesses deep within the right temporal lobe.

Serodiagnosis has been of little help in the diagnosis of invasive aspergillosis. The presence or absence of anti-aspergillus antibodies reflects more a preexisting humoral condition than pathology.[28] Progress has been limited by the lack of dependable and standardized antigens.[185] Several studies to detect various aspergillus antigens in serum and urine have been developed in research laboratories; however, a commercially available usable product is still wanting. Stynen and coworkers,[332] using a sandwich enzyme-linked immunosorbent assay, were able to detect *A. fumigatus* galactomannan in the sera of nine patients with invasive aspergillosis, with a sensitivity of detection as low as 1 ng/mL of antigen. Detection of serum antigen was superior to testing of urine.

Melchers and associates[216] report progress in the application of polymerase chain reaction (PCR) in identifying genus-specific sequences in the 18S rRNA extracted from several *Aspergillus* species. *Aspergillus* species were detected in bronchoalveolar lavage (BAL) fluid of four neutropenic patients with proved aspergillosis, even though organisms were recovered in only one case. However, the results of Bretagne and colleagues[50] are far more pessimistic. When using a competitive PCR assay, they found false-positive detection of *Aspergillus* species in BAL specimens of 12 patients (25% of those tested) who did not develop invasive aspergillosis. In this assay, a 1-kb mitochondrial DNA fragment of *A. fumigatus* was sequenced, with the primers used allowing amplification of the DNAs from several *Aspergillus* species but not that of other fungi or yeasts. Several reasons for the low positive predictive value in their study were discussed by the authors; however, their conclusion is that PCR currently is not a viable tool in the diagnosis of invasive aspergillosis. The early diagnosis of invasive aspergillosis thus remains elusive.

HISTOPATHOLOGY

The hyphae of *Aspergillus* species as observed in stained tissue sections are characteristically hyaline, septate, and regular in outline and have parallel walls. They average 3 to 6 μm in diameter (Fig. 19-19, page 1009). The regular dichotomous branching at 45-degree

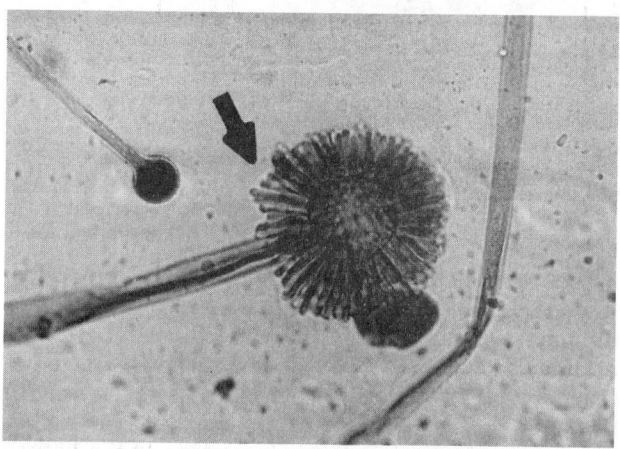

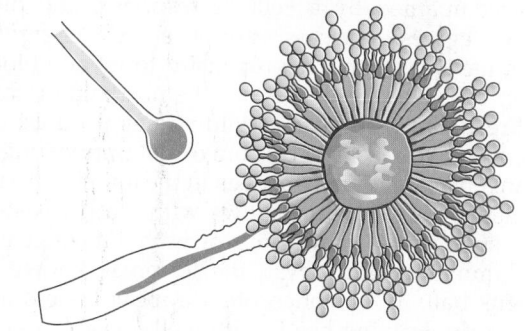

Figure 19-15
Sketch and photomicrograph of *Aspergillus flavus*.

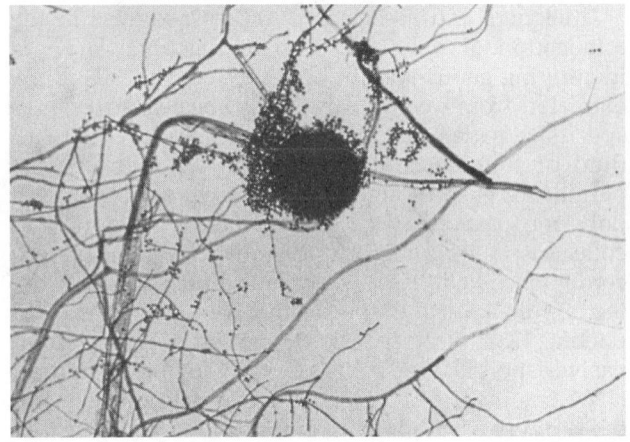

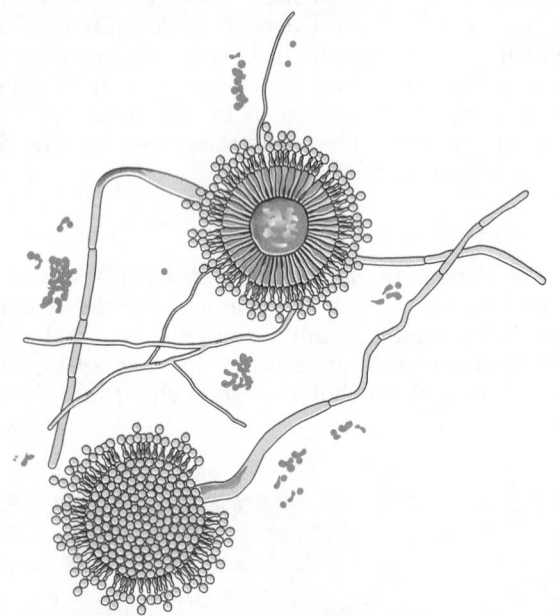

Figure 19-16
Sketch and photomicrograph of *Aspergillus niger.*

angles is a helpful differential feature from other hyphae-producing fungi. The hyphae do not stain well in hematoxylin and eosin (H&E) sections but are well outlined in PAS- and GMS-stained sections. The tissue reaction in immunocompetent hosts infected with these fungi may first be purulent and then granulomatous; more commonly, hyphal invasion of the tissues is unaccompanied by a cellular response, and only varying degrees of necrosis are observed. *Aspergillus* species have a particular propensity to invade blood vessels, causing thrombosis and hemorrhagic infarction. Presumably because certain strains produce oxalic acid, local deposits of calcium oxalate, appearing as birefringent crystals, may be seen in the invaded tissue.

When a fungal colony grows within a preexistent cavity, such as in a nasal sinus or within a congenital or inflammatory lung cyst, the lesion is known as a fungus ball. The hyphae often appear lifeless and stain poorly. Fruiting heads with well-formed vesicles and chains of conidia may be seen within cavities that are connected to open bronchi and exposed to air (Fig. 19-20, page 1009). The lining of the cavity is often intact, with no evidence of extension into the surrounding tissue. In bronchopulmonary aspergillosis, bronchi and bronchioles are often dilated and filled with viscid, mucinous material in which are trapped cellular debris, many eosinophils, scattered neutrophils, lymphocytes, plasma cells, and hyphal fragments. Typical 45-degree branching hyphal fragments may be seen in direct mounts of sputum samples, which, when accompanied by eosinophils and Charcot-Leyden crystals, is sufficient to make a provisional diagnosis.

AGENTS OF HYALOHYPHOMYCOSIS

The suggestion by Ajello[4,5] that infections caused by a variety of unrelated hyaline *Hyphomycetes* be categorized under the general umbrella "hyalohyphomycosis" may be less confusing to physicians than using individual names, such as penicilliosis, scopulariopsosis, and the like. It is our contention, however, that we may have outgrown this necessity and the reporting of *Penicillium* species, *Scopulariopsis* species, as the case may be, should not be confusing to the clinician. When referring to disease entities caused by this group of fungi, the option of reporting "hyalohyphomycosis secondary to *Penicillium* species," or "*Scopulariopsis* species," is viable. Each mycologist must determine how this nomenclature will be used in the local practice setting.

Hundreds of recognized species of hyaline saprobes exist in nature; only a few are encountered with any frequency in clinical laboratories. Of these, only isolated cases of human infections have been reported. The following is a list of the hyaline *Hyphomycetes* most commonly encountered in clinical laboratories.

1. Hyaline *Hyphomycetes* forming conidia in chains include *Aspergillus* species, *Penicillium* species, *Paecilomyces* species, and *Scopulariopsis* species.
2. Those forming conidia in clusters include *Acremonium* species, *Fusarium* species, *Gliocladium* species, and *Trichoderma* species.
3. Those forming conidia borne singly include *Beauvaria* species and *Pseudallescheria boydii* (*Scedosporium apiospermum*).

LABORATORY PRESENTATION

Colonies of the hyaline hyphomycetes typically mature within 3 to 5 days on culture media free of antifungal agents. As the colonies mature and sporulation takes place, the surface of the colonies become sugary, powdery, or granular. Photographs of the colonies of the more frequently encountered species are illustrated in Color Plate 19-2. The colonies of *Penicillium* species generally are various shades of green, although yellow and yellow-brown variants are encountered (see Color Plate 19-2A). A narrow white apron is generally seen at the outer growing margin of the colony. The colonies of *P. marneffei* are unique by

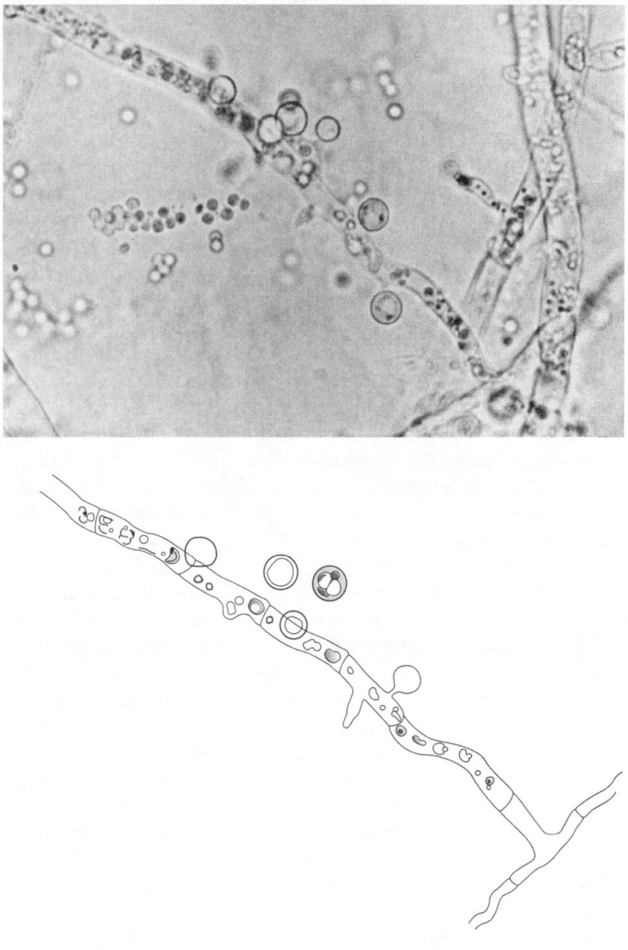

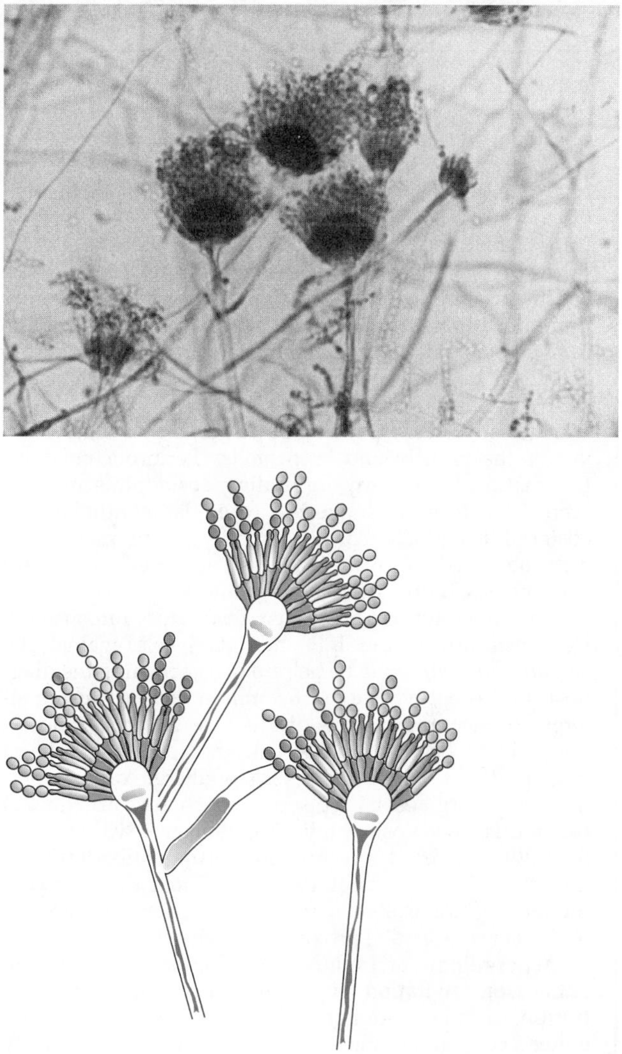

Figure 19-17
Sketch and photomicrograph of *Aspergillus terreus*.

producing abundant water-soluble red pigment that diffuses into the culture medium (see Color Plate 19-2*B*). However, as other *Penicillium* species may also produce red pigment, it may be advisable to forward suspicious strains to a reference laboratory where "yeast" conversion studies, exoantigen extraction tests, or nucleic acid probes may be performed to confirm the identification. The colonies of *Paecilomyces* species may also have various shades of light green, similiar to those of *Penicillium* species; however, colonies often are tan or yellow-brown (see Color Plate 19-2*C*). *Scopulariopsis* species have a distinctive colony, characterized by a yellow brown, granular colony with radial rugae emanating from the center to the periphery (see Color Plate 19-2*D*). A dematiaceous variant, producing a dark gray colony with a black underside, called *S. brumptii*, may occasionally be encountered. The colonies of *Acremonium* species are generally less wooly and granular but are glabrous in appearance,

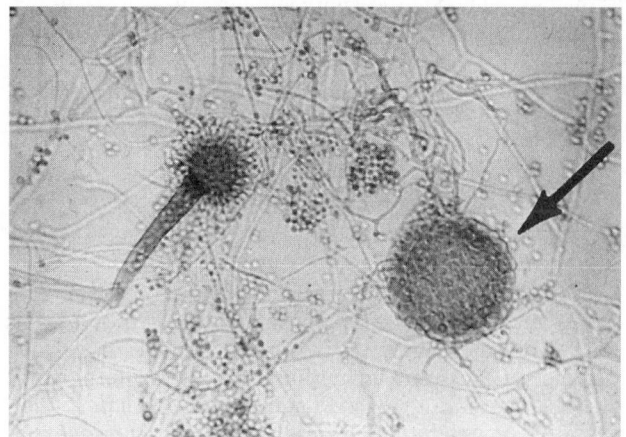

Figure 19-18
Photomicrograph of *Aspergillus glaucus* (to show cleistothecium).

CLINICAL CORRELATION BOX 19-3. ASPERGILLOSIS

Aspergillosis may present as well-defined clinical syndromes involving a variety of sites and organ systems: pulmonary,[85] disseminated,[293, 296] central nervous system,[46, 341, 354] cutaneous,[44] endocardial,[75] and nasoorbital.[82, 156, 222, 350] Pulmonary aspergillosis can be further divided into allergic bronchopulmonary,[192, 316] colonizing (fungus ball),[241, 293, 296] and invasive forms.[85, 380] These clinical forms of pulmonary disease constitute a continuous spectrum, ranging from invasive disease in the severely immunosuppressed patient, to hypersensitivity reactions in hyperactive patients, to noninvasive colonization of the bronchial tree in otherwise normal persons with previously diseased areas of the lung.[114]

Allergic bronchopulmonary aspergillosis chiefly involves the bronchi and bronchioles. Peribronchiolar inflammation with many infiltrating eosinophils may be seen. This form is suggested when large numbers of eosinophils and Charcot-Leyden crystals are microscopically observed in mucin plugs expectorated in sputum specimens. Chronic disease may, after several years, lead to bronchiolar fibrosis and severe respiratory impairment. Demonstrating serum IgE and IgG levels against *Aspergillus fumigatus* may be helpful in establishing the diagnosis of this entity. The most common species causing allergic bronchopulmonary disease are *A. flavus* and *A. fumigatus*.[380] Lee[192] suggests that the following criteria must pertain to make a diagnosis of allergic bronchopulmonary aspergillosis: 1) episodic bronchial obstruction, 2) peripheral blood eosinophilia, 3) cutaneous reactivity to *A. fumigatus* antigen, 4) precipitating serum antibodies to *A. fumigatus*, 5) elevated total serum IgE, 6) history of pulmonary infiltrates, 7) elevated serum IgE and serum IgG to *A. fumigatus*, and 8) proximal bronchiectasis.

Aspergilloma or fungus ball infections may develop either from cavitation within an area of pulmonary infiltration, or, more commonly, within a preexistent cavity, either a congenital lung cyst or in an inflammatory cavity (commonly secondary to old tuberculosis). The fungus ball consists of a tangled mass of hyphae, often dead. Aspergillomas involving the paranasal sinuses have been reported.[222] In cases of pulmonary aspergillomas, cavities in which air is supplied through an open bronchus may contain viable fruiting heads, the detection of which can lead to a definitive diagnosis. In most cases, the fungus ball remains confined to the cavity without invasion of the surrounding parenchyma. However, Nolan and Long[241] warn that aspergillomas should not be considered an indolent condition, as cases of intermittent or exsanguinating hemoptysis have been reported; and, on occasion, erosion into adjacent structures may result in morbidity or death.

Invasive pulmonary aspergillosis occurs almost exclusively in patients who are immunosuppressed or neutropenic, particularly in transplant recipients and those with leukemias and lymphomas.[280, 353] Although *A. fumigatus* and *A. flavus* are the two species most commonly involved, *A. terreus* has also recently been incriminated.[377] Woods and associates[377] reported on four cases of disseminated disease caused by *A. terreus*, and reviewed five additional cases reported in the medical literature. In immunocompetent individuals with only structural lung damage, saprophytic growth of *Aspergillus* spp. is the rule.[110] Of 2315 consecutive autopsies, Boon and coworkers[46] found 32 cases of invasive aspergillosis (1.4% of all cases, but 10.7% of a subpopulation considered at "high risk"). Liver transplant recipients were at higher risk than renal transplant recipients, presumably because these patients receive more immunosuppressive therapy.[139] Denning and Stevens,[85] in a review of over 2000 cases of aspergillosis culled from the literature, found that aspergillosis in bone marrow transplant patients is particularly devastating, with a mortality rate of 94% in reported cases despite therapy. The overall rate of response to amphotericin B therapy of all cases reviewed in this series was 55%.

Invasive pulmonary aspergillosis often presents first as pneumonia, often necrotizing,[280] with symptoms of cough, fever, and signs of respiratory distress. Pleural invasion may result in chest pain and a pleural friction rub. Because of the propensity for advancing hyphae to invade blood vessels, disseminated disease with metastatic spread to the CNS and other organs is possible. The brain was the most common site of extrapulmonary spread in the series of Boon and coworkers.[46]

The acquired immunodeficiency syndrome (AIDS) per se is not considered a risk factor for invasive pulmonary aspergillosis. In a series of AIDS patients with aspergillosis reviewed by Singh and associates,[321] 79% had known predisposing risk factors, including neutropenia, corticosteroid use, and intravenous drug abuse. Although aspergillosis was initially included as an AIDS-defining infection, the CDC later reversed its position and deleted it as a case definition of AIDS.[321] Aspergillosis occurs in the later stages of AIDS, and when diagnosed, has a dismal prognosis, which can only be improved by early diagnosis.[176] Meyer and colleagues[219] report three cases of aspergillus sinusitis in patients with AIDS, a condition that occurs in the later stages of disease when the CD4+ lymphocyte counts are fewer than 50/mm³.

---

owing to the production of a very delicate mycelium. Colonies may be white or various shades of light pastel green and yellow (see Color Plate 19-2E). Colonies that have a distinct lavender, rose-red, or magenta surface pigmentation point immediately to *Fusarium* species (see Color Plate 19-2F). *Pseudallescheria boydii* (*Scedosporium apiospermum* is the name of the asexual anamorph) also has a distinct colony characterized by a house mouse gray, silky surface on which tiny water droplets tend to aggregate (see Color Plate 19-2G). In contrast with the other hyaline fungi, the colonies of which have a distinct margin, those of *Gliocladium* species and *Trichoderma* species grow from rim to rim in the petri dish as a dense green or yellow lawn (see Color Plate 19-2H). *Beauveria* species usually produce nondescript, delicate cottony, white colonies.

Microscopically the hyphae are clear (hyaline), relatively broad (4 to 8 μm in diameter) and have uniform, parallel walls with distinct septations. Genus and species identifications are made by observing for the fruiting heads characteristic for each. Conidia may form in long chains, in dense clusters, or singly, borne

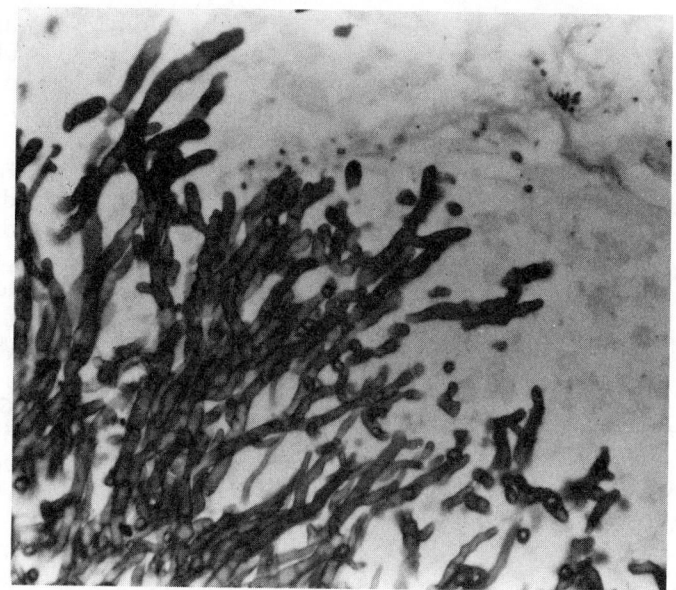

Figure 19-19
Tissue section of lung illustrating invasion with hyphal forms of *Aspergillus* species. The individual hyphae are uniform (measure 3 to 4 µm in diameter), have parallel walls, and show dichotomous 45°-angle branching and septations (oil immersion, GMS stain).

from individual conidiophores. These arrangements are helpful in the initial categorization of these molds, as indicated by the foregoing listing, particularly in certain direct microscopic preparations when the conidia often become dislodged from the parent fruiting structures.

The distinctive microscopic features of *Aspergillus* species are conidiophores, terminating in a swollen vesicle that supports one or two rows of phialides from which chains of conidia are produced. In contrast, the conidiophores of *Penicillium*, *Paecilomyces*, and *Scopulariopsis* species have primary branches called metulae that, in turn, branch into phialides, giving the appearance of a brush or broom (*penicillus* and *scopula* are Latin and Greek derivatives respectively for "broom" or "brush").

The following are illustrations depicting the key microscopic features of the hyaline group of fungi:

***Penicillium* Species.**   In *Penicillium* species, small spherical conidia are borne in long chains from the tips of phialides, the tips of which are blunt and appear

chopped off (Fig. 19-21). The branching metulae and phialides give the characteristic "penicillus" fruiting head.

***Paecilomyces* Species.**   A branching, "penicillus-like" fruiting head is also formed in *Paecilomyces* species; however, in contrast with the *Penicillium* species, the terminal ends of the phialides are long and tapered. Because the conidia of paecilomyces are formed basipetally, the older, terminal conidia tend to be larger and darker staining than the more proximal ones (Fig. 19-22).

***Scopulariopsis* Species.**   The conidia of *Scopulariopsis* species are two to three times larger than those of *Penicillium* species, are lemon-shaped, rough-walled, and formed in chains. The conidia of *Scopulariopsis* species are anneloconidia, produced from the protruded tip of the previous conidium that then retracts, forming scars that appear as rings or annelides at the base of the newly formed cell (Fig. 19-23). Remnants of these pro-

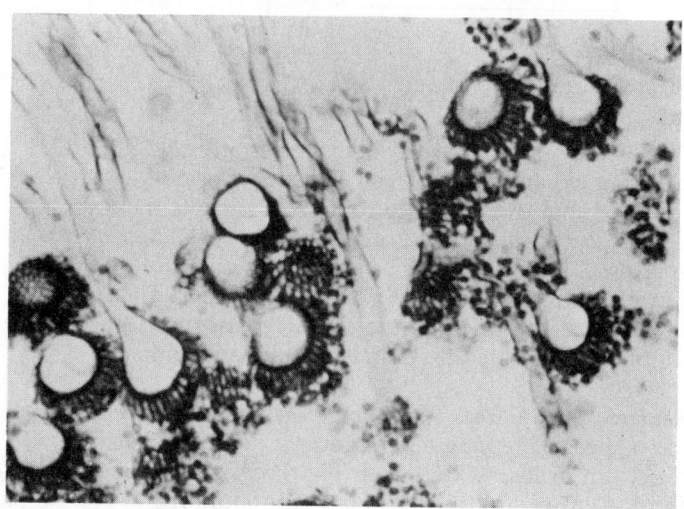

Figure 19-20
Photomicrograph of material from an aspergillus fungus ball infection, showing club-shaped vesicles with sporulation only from the top half of the vesicles, characteristic of *A. fumigatus* (H&E, high power).

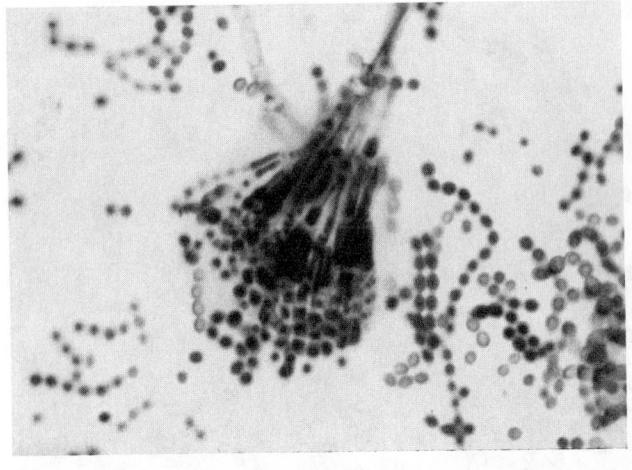

liptical, and arrange in a "diphtheroidal pattern," simulating the topography of the cerebral cortex, thus probably giving rise to the old designation, *Cephalosporium* species.

Fusarium Species. *Fusarium* species are unique in producing both micro- and macroconidia. The microconidia, similar in size, shape, and arrangement, are identical with those of *Acremonium* species; however, the telltale large, pointed, sickle-form, multicellular macroconidia are distinctive for *Fusarium* species (Fig. 19-25).

Gliocladium Species. Branching phialides are tapered at the tips, supporting a tight cluster of small, spherical conidia, much as approximated fingertips of the hand might hold a ball (Fig. 19-26).

Trichoderma Species. The phialides of *Trichoderma* species are similar in appearance to those of *Paecilomyces* species, broadened at the base and pointed at the tip (Fig. 19-27, page 1013). In contrast, here the spherical conidia are aggregated into tight clusters instead of into long chains. The phialides extend in pairs opposite one another from the sides of the hyphae at approximately 45-degree angles.

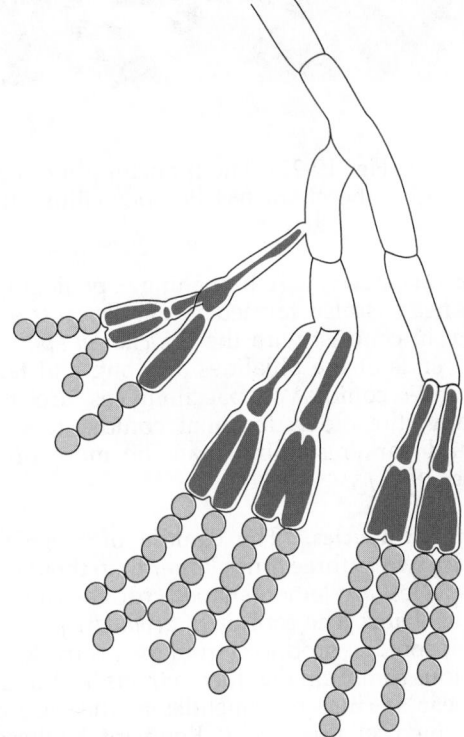

Figure 19-21
Sketch and photomicrograph of *Penicillium* species.

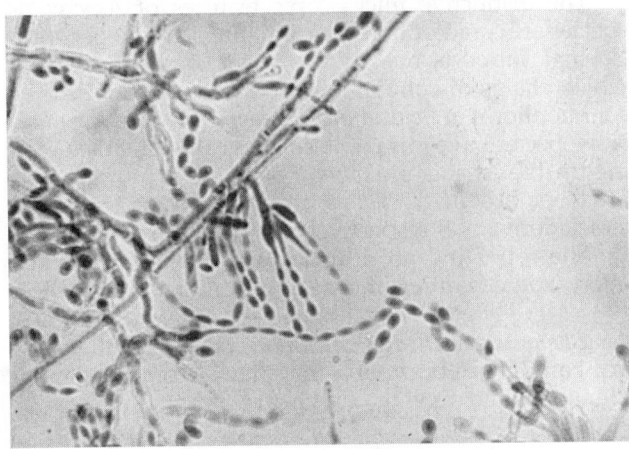

trusions appear as stubby rodlike connectors between the two cells.

Microascus and *Chaetomium* species are thought to be teleomorphic states of *Scopulariopsis* species.

The fungi that produce conidia in clusters include *Gliocladium*, *Trichoderma*, *Acremonium*, and *Fusarium* species. Color photographs of typical colonies for these fungi are shown in Color Plate 19-2*E*, *F* and *H*. The following are the microscopic characteristics by which these fungi can be differentiated from one another.

Acremonium Species. The conidiophores of *Acremonium* species are long and extremely delicate, measuring 1 µm or less in diameter (Fig. 19-24). The conidia form in clusters at the tips of the conidiophores, are el-

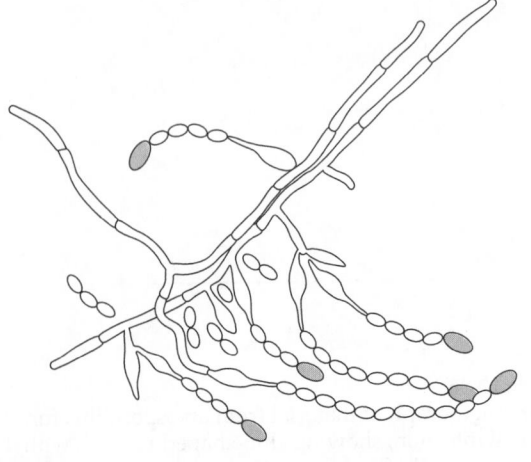

Figure 19-22
Sketch and photomicrograph of *Paecilomyces* species.

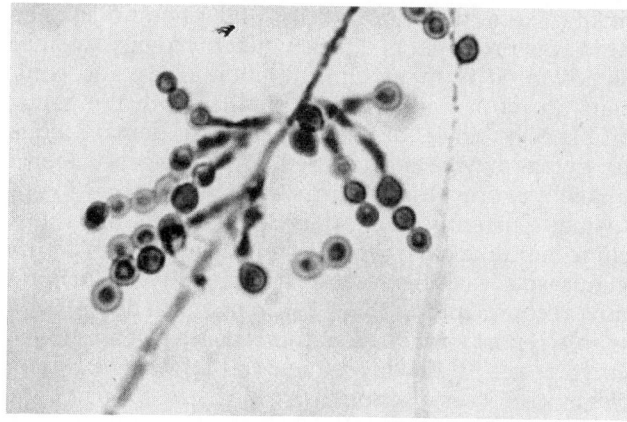

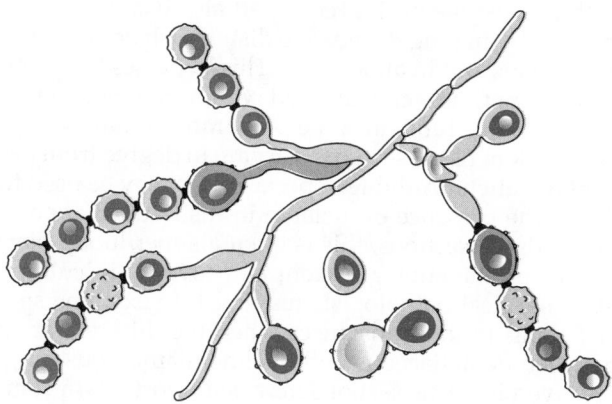

Figure 19-23
Sketch and photomicrograph of *Scopulariopsis* species.

Several hyaline fungi produce conidia singly from separate conidiophores. Those more commonly encountered in clinical laboratories include *Scedosporium, Chrysosporium, Sepedonium,* and *Beauveria* species.

Scedosporium apiospermum (**anamorphic form**), also known as *Pseudallescheria boydii* (sexual or **telomorphic** form) is the species most commonly encountered in clinical practices. *Scedosporium inflatum*, a newly designated species, also causes human infections. Both produce a characteristic house mouse gray, silky surface on which tiny water droplets tend to aggregate (Color Plate 19-2G). Dark pigment may extend to the reverse surface, suggesting a dark fungus.

The colonies of *Chrysosporium* species are not distinctive. A white to gray, cottony or wooly mycelium develops after 2 to 4 days of incubation.

In *Beauveria* species, the colonies are similar to those of *Chrysosporium* species, also producing a white, cottony or wooly surface. The underside of the colony is a light buff.

MICROSCOPIC FEATURES

The following summarizes the key microscopic features for the identification of this group of hyaline fungi.

Scedosporium **Species.** In *Scedosporium* species, single, relatively large (4- to 9-μm) lemon-shaped or pyriform

conidia, are borne, usually singly (or in small clusters), from a simple or branched conidiophore (Fig. 19-28). Baglike structures, called **cleistothecia**, which contain sexually derived (telomorphic) spores called **ascospores**, may be rarely observed (*Pseudallescheria boydii*). The phialides of *S. proliferans* (*inflatum*) are broad at the base and narrow at the tip, simulating an urn.

Chrysosporium **Species.** In *Chrysosporium* species, subglobose to pyriform conidia are borne singly at the tips of long lateral conidiophores. Conidia often have a broad basal scar. The microscopic appearance of *Chrysosporium* species closely resembles that of *Blastomyces dermatitidis*, and either exoantigen extraction or nucleic acid probe testing may be required to make the differentiation.

Sepedonium **Species.** Large, spherical, bluntly spiked macroconidia, simulating those of *Histoplasma capsulatum*, are characteristic of *Sepedonium* species (Fig. 19-29). Smaller, ovate conidia, borne singly from short conidiophores, may also be observed.

Beuveria **Species.** In *Beuveria* species, tiny, globose microconidia are densely aggregated around delicate, short, branching conidiophores that uniquely bend to form zig-zag turns (a bent-knee appearance that is called **geniculate**; Fig. 19-30). A conidium is borne in one plane, the conidiophore turns before bearing an-

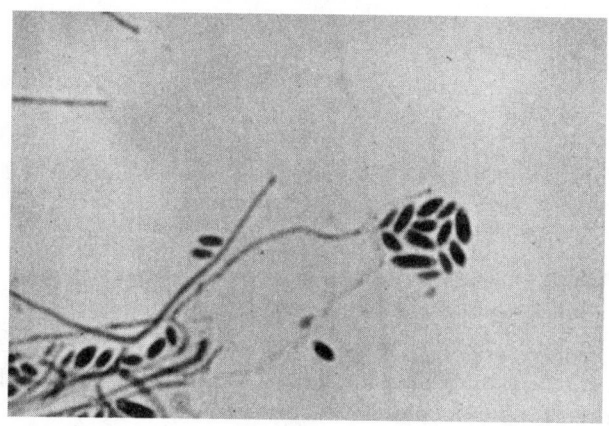

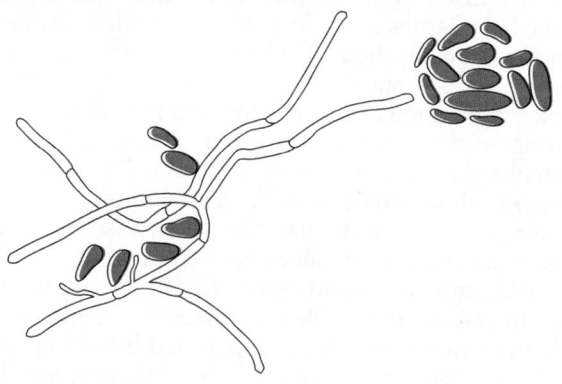

Figure 19-24
Sketch and photomicrograph of *Acremonium* species.

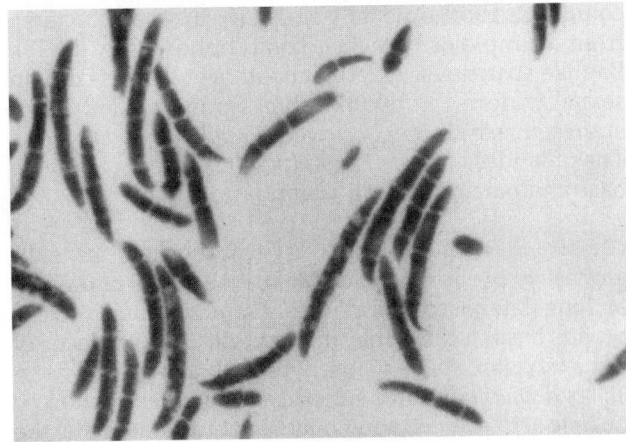

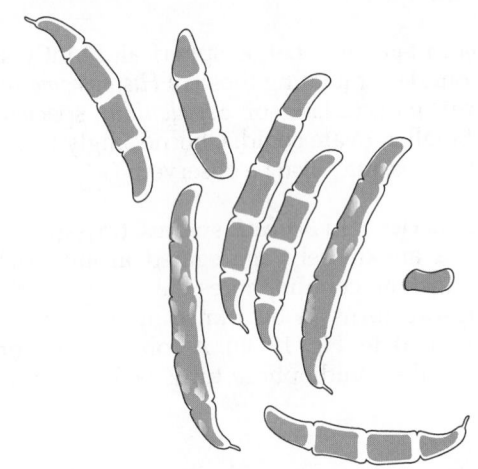

Figure 19-25
Sketch and photomicrograph of *Fusarium* species.

other conidium in another plane, and so forth. This type of conidiation is called **sympodial**.

AGENTS OF CHROMOBLASTOMYCOSIS, EUMYCOTIC MYCETOMAS, AND PHAEOHYPHOMYCOSIS

The concept of "phaeohyphomycosis" was first proposed by Ajello and coworkers[4,5] in 1974 to "cover all infections of a cutaneous, subcutaneous and systemic nature caused by hyphomycetous fungi that develop in the host tissues in the form of dark-walled, dematiaceous septate mycelial elements." A tissue section of a necrotic subcutaneous abscess illustrating irregular dark, fragmented hyphae, 4- to 6-μm in width, is characteristic of the fungal elements seen in a lesion of phaeohyphomycosis. Thus, as originally described, **phaeohyphomycosis** was a histopathologic entity rather than any particular clinical disease or fungal species as identified in laboratory culture.

Although Ajello and associates[4] originally limited the clinical entities related to phaeohyphomycosis to subcutaneous lesions and deep-seated infections, particularly brain abscesses, phaeohyphomycosis has been used since to describe a variety of additional lesions caused by dematiaceous fungi, including si-

nusitis, keratitis, endocarditis, and pneumonia. The term was proposed at a time when mycology was not as advanced in many clinical laboratories, and clinicians in particular were not familiar with the genus and species names of the large array of dematiaceous fungi that may be encountered. Thus, the general term phaeohyphomycosis was proposed to obviate any confusion. Currently, clinical microbiologists and most clinicians alike have become familiar with many of the genus–species designations, and many mycologists are now recommending that the generic term be replaced with a report such as "keratomycosis caused by *Bipolaris* species"[153] or "mycetoma caused by *Phialophora richardsiae*,"[266] as examples.

Linking the clinical disease or source of the isolate with the genus–species recovered also has the advantage of eliminating the need to distinguish between dematiaceous and hyaline fungi. This bypasses the problems sometimes encountered when the hyphae of dematiaceous fungi in some preparations may not appear dark in tissue sections, varying in degree from patient to patient. Although special stains may be used to detect the presence of melanin in the hyphae appearing in tissue sections, this is often a superfluous exercise when the etiologic agent is recovered in culture. Only surgical pathologists may wish to examine special stains in those instances when the differentiation between dematiaceous and hyaline filamentous fungi observed in tissue sections may be important. In communicating with clinicians, it is probably best to avoid

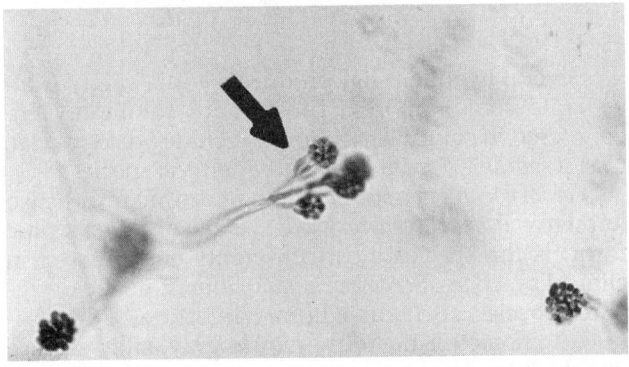

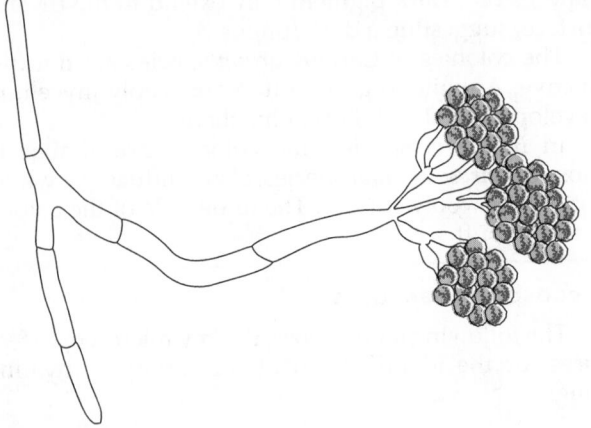

Figure 19-26
Sketch and photomicrograph of *Gliocladium* species.

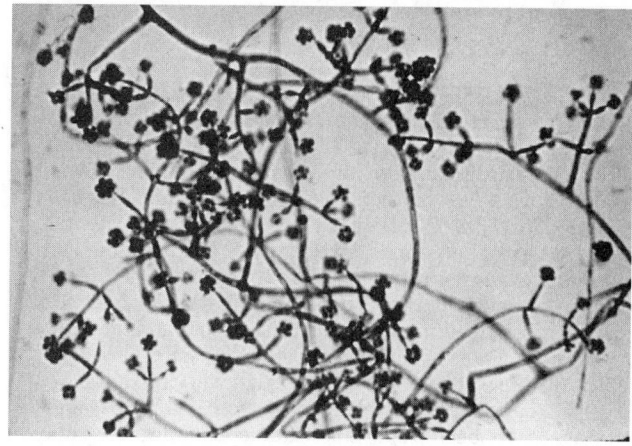

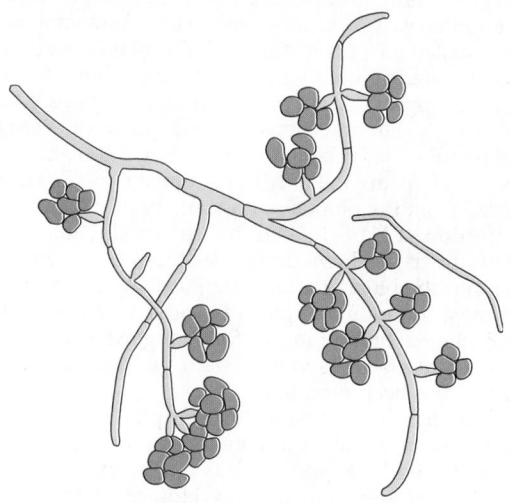

Figure 19-27
Sketch and photomicrograph of *Trichoderma* species.

the terms phaeohyphomycosis and hyalohyphomycosis and instead report out the genus–species names for each isolate.

A list of the genus and species of the more commonly encountered agents for these diseases includes the agents of chromomycosis and mycetoma, including *Phialophora verrucosum*, *Cladosporium carrionii* (*Cladophialophora carrionii*), *Fonsecaea pedrosoi*, *F. compacta*, *Exophiala jeanselmei*, and *Wangiella dermatitidis*, and the agents of phaeohyphomycosis, including *Alternaria* species, *Aureobasidium pullulans*, *Bipolaris* species, *Drechslera* species, *Cladosporium* species, *Curvularia* species, *Exophiala jeanselmei*, *Excerohilum* species, *Phaeoannellomyces* species, *Phoma* species, and *Xylohypha emmonsii*.

LABORATORY IDENTIFICATION

The dematiaceous fungi can be suspected in culture by observing the dark gray, brown, or black, wooly, hairy, or velvety surface colonies that have a black pigmentation on the reverse (see Color Plate 19-3*A* and 3*B*). Although it may no longer be appropriate to subdivide the dematiaceous fungi into "pathogenic" and

"saprobic" groups, the agents causing classic cases of chromoblastomycosis, namely *Cladosporium carrionii* (this name will be retained here, although McGinnis and Rinaldi[211] indicate that the currently accepted name is *Cladophialophora carrionii*), *Phialophora verrucosum*, and *Fonsecaea pedrosoi* grow more slowly than several molds that are commonly recovered as environmental contaminants in clinical laboratories but that can on occasion cause phaeohyphomycosis. In addition, *Cladosporium carrionii* does not grow at temperatures higher than 37°C, which separates it from the saprobic *Cladosporium* species that can grow at 42°C. Therefore, the recovery of a dematiaceous fungus in the laboratory must be considered potentially significant, and a clinical correlation is in order. The colony morphology of select dematiaceous molds is illustrated in Color Plate 19-3.

Microscopically, the dematiaceous molds are characterized by a dark yellow-brown mycelium composed of uniform hyphae with parallel walls and distinct septations. The various genera and species are identified based on morphologic differences in fruiting bodies and conidiation. The dematiaceous molds can be broadly divided into three groups: 1) those produc-

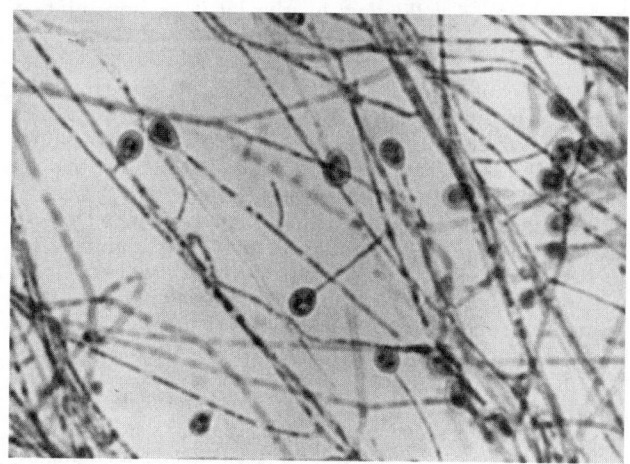

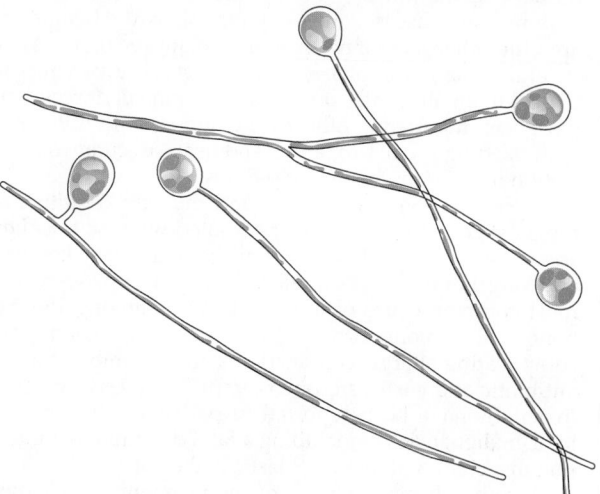

Figure 19-28
Sketch and photomicrograph of *Scedosporium* species.

CLINICAL CORRELATION BOX 19-4.
AGENTS OF HYALOPHOMYCOSIS

Several literature reports of infections with the *Hyphomycetes* group of fungi have been cited by Rippon.[296] Five cases of penicilliosis caused by *Penicillium marneffei* were reported from Thailand in patients with a variety of underlying disorders, including tuberculosis, lupus erythematosus, and lymphoreticular neoplasms.[154] *P. marneffei* infections have also been reported in patients with AIDS[8] and in a patient with osteomyelitis.[59] Small intracellular bodies resembling the yeast forms of *Histoplasma capsulatum* have been observed in histologic sections obtained from these lesions. Kaufman and associates at the CDC[165] developed monoclonal antibodies against the yeastlike culture filtrate antigens of *P. marneffei* from which, after absorption with yeast forms of *H. capsulatum*, they developed a sensitive indirect fluorescent antibody reagent. They were able to detect *P. marneffei* yeastlike forms in 43 isolates and in tissue section from six humans with penicilliosis marneffei. No false-positive results were found in the study of tissue sections containing *H. capsulatum* yeast forms. LoBuglio and Taylor[194] report the development of primers for the amplification of *P. marneffei* that may have future application in a PCR-based identification system that may be useful in detecting this agent in clinical materials.

Rippon[296] reports several cases of infections secondary to *Paecilomyces* spp.: mycotic keratitis, an outbreak of endophthalmitis following intraocular lens implantation from contamination of the disinfectant used for surgical instruments, endocarditis, and cutaneous cellulitis. Cases of cutaneous cellulitis caused by *P. lilacinus* were reported in an immunocompromised patient.[152, 233] The species causing the latter infection was *P. variotii*, which is pathogenic in normal and cortisone-treated mice. A case of deep subcutaneous infection of the left forearm with *P. lilacinus* was reported[57] in a renal transplant patient, which responded to oral griseofulvin therapy. These authors reviewed 42 cases of human mycoses caused by *Paecilomyces* spp., usually in conjunction with prosthesis implants or immunosuppression. Most strains of *P. lilacinus* are resistant to amphotericin B; most strains of *P. variotii* are susceptible. A case of cutaneous hyalohyphomycosis caused by an unidentified species that simulated squamous cell carcinoma has been reported.[123] *Scopulariopsis* spp. have been reported to cause infections of nails, subcutaneous tissue, and the lungs.[173] Two patients were described[234] with invasive disease, one receiving intensive chemotherapy, the other a bone marrow transplant recipient. Also, several human cases of *S. brevicaulis* mycosis involving the toenail in an allogeneic bone marrow transplant recipient have been reported[273]; others were hypersensitivity pneumonitis, fungus ball formation, and deep subcutaneous infection in an immunosuppressed host.

Mycetoma, onychomycosis, and mycotic keratitis are the most common infections associated with *Acremonium* spp.; *Fusarium* spp. also commonly cause mycotic keratitis and onychomycosis.[296] In fact, *Fusarium* spp. were the most common cause of mycotic keratitis among 156 patients with mycotic corneal ulcer disease, most commonly complicating allergic conjunctivitis and a combination of antibiotic and corticosterone therapy.[346] Invasive fusarial infections have been reported in patients with hematologic malignancies,[173] including a fatal disseminated infection in a child with lymphoblastic leukemia.[187]

A comprehensive review of the taxonomy, mycology, laboratory features, and clinical syndromes related to *Fusarium* spp. has been published.[235, 236] These authors also cite *Fusarium* spp. as the most common cause of mycotic keratitis in the United States, usually following corneal trauma from ocular implantation of vegetable fragments or soil matter during outdoor activities. Fungal keratitis has been reported in 4% to 27% of contact lens wearers, with *Fusarium* spp. being recovered most frequently.[369] Predisposing conditions include improper lens care; the presence of an underlying corneal infection, such as herpes simplex infection, and the prolonged use of local corticosteroid and antibiotic medication. Cases of onychomycosis, manifesting as a milky white disintegration of the toenails, with varying degrees of swelling and tenderness at the base of the nails, following trauma have been reported. Cutaneous infections may occur, either from direct penetration of the skin by contaminated vegetative material, or from the bloodstream in cases of disseminated infections. Accumulation of excessive moisture within intertriginous parts of the skin, or burn, trauma, or immunosuppression are predisposing conditions.[14] Various forms of skin infections include pustules, vesicles, painful nodules, necrotizing ulcers, and mycetoma.

Fusarium spp. are the only opportunistic molds readily recovered from the bloodstream, usually in patients with skin infection. It is postulated that the production of toxins leads to tissue breakdown, facilitating the entry of fusaria into the bloodstream.[15] Multiorgan dissemination occurs most commonly in patients with chronic leukemia, aplastic anemia, lymphoma, or following extensive burns. Disseminated infections in bone marrow transplant recipients have also been reported.

Scedosporium apiospermum (telomorph *Pseudallescheria boydii*) has been involved in a variety of infections, as recently reviewed by Rippon.[296] It is one of the more common causes of subcutaneous mycetomas in the United States. Pulmonary infections with *S. apiospermum* often resemble infections with *Aspergillus* spp., and the hyphae have a similar appearance in stained tissue sections. The presence of soft to firm white to yellow, spherical grains points to infection with *Scedosporium* spp. Sinusitis, including fungus ball infections, meningitis, osteomyelitis, endocarditis, mycotic keratitis, endophthalmitis, and otomycosis are other scedosporium infections extensively reviewed by Rippon. Perez and coauthors[262] report a case of *Pseudallescheria boydii* brain abscess in association with an infected central venous catheter.

Scedosporium prolificans (*inflatum*) is cited as an emerging pathogen,[304] with 15 human cases of infection reported. Also, another 11 cases of *S. inflatum* infection, almost always in patients who had penetrating trauma or surgery, have been reported.[371] *Scedosporium* spp. are resistant to amphotericin B, miconazole and ketoconazole, and other antimycotic agents, one important reason for differentiating them from *Aspergillus* spp. A nosocomial outbreak of four fatal cases of *S. prolificans* (*inflatum*) was reported[9] in patients with severe neutropenia, secondary to leukemia therapy. The infections occurred sequentially within a 1-month period in two rooms during a phase of hospital reconstruction when the patients were housed in a provisional hematology unit. The authors conclude that, despite the inability to recover *S. proliferans* from the patients' rooms or adjacent corridors, circumstantial evidence indicated a nosocomial outbreak. Antifungal susceptibility tests performed on the isolates revealed resistance to amphotericin B, ketoconazole, and miconazole, confirming the resistance profile previously observed by others.

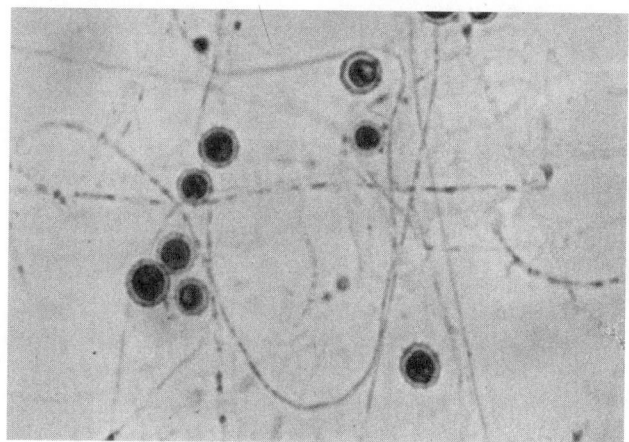

Figure 19-29
Photomicrograph of *Sepedonium* species.

ing multicelled macroconidia divided by both longitudinal and transverse septa (muriform macroconidia); 2) those in which the macroconidia are divided only by transverse septa; and 3) those that produce one celled conidia.

Macroconidia With Transverse and Longitudinal Septa

ALTERNARIA SPECIES. Characteristic in *Alternaria* species are the formation of chains of multicelled, macroconidia that are separated by both cross and longitudinal septa (**muriform**; Fig. 19-31). The macroconidia are shaped like drumsticks, with the elongated beak of one conidium butting against the rounded, blunt end of the next.

ULOCLADIUM SPECIES. The conidia in *Ulocladium* species are more spherical than those of *Alternaria* species, do not chain, and are borne from short, twisted bent-knee, or **geniculate**, conidiophores (Fig. 19-32; see Color Plate 19-3C).

STEMPHILIUM SPECIES. The muriform macroconidia in *Stemphilium* species appear as bales of cotton at the swollen tips of a straight, nongeniculate conidiophore (Fig. 19-33).

EPICOCCUM SPECIES. The hyphae in *Epicoccum* species typically form focal repeated branching and re-branching of certain threads, forming masses known as **sporodochia** (Fig. 19-34). Short conidiophores arise from these masses, bearing multicelled, muriform, spherical to slightly club-shaped macroconidia, that may be roughened on the surface giving a blackish wartlike appearance.

Macroconidia With Transverse Septa

CURVULARIA SPECIES. The macroconidia of *Curvularia* species are easy to recognize, having four to five cells separated by transverse septa, borne sympodially from twisted conidiophores (Fig. 19-35). The center cells grow more rapidly than those at the ends, producing a curved or "boomerang" appearance.

BIPOLARIS SPECIES. The designation *Bipolaris* is derived from the property of this mold to produce germ tubes (when a water mount of conidia is examined after incubation at 25°C for 8 to 24 hours) that arise from both ends of the base of the conidium in parallel with the long axis of the cell. The distinguishing feature of the mold is the production of cylindrical, smooth-walled, multi-celled macroconidia from conidiophores that have kneelike bends (**geniculate**) in a **sympodial** arrangement (Fig. 19-36).

DRECHSLERA SPECIES. *Drechslera* species also produce cylindrical, multicelled conidia from geniculate conidiophores similar to *Bipolaris* species. The conidia have nonprotruding, rounded contours at the base. In saline mounts, a single germ tube, derived midway between the base of the conidium and the septum and extending at right angles to the long axis, is a key identifying feature. There is current sentiment that the separate designation of *Drechslera* may not be necessary, and in practice most clinical isolates showing the morphologic features described will be *Bipolaris* species.

EXSEROHILUM SPECIES. The conidia of *Exserohilum* species are similar to those of *Bipolaris* species, except they are longer and more pencil-shaped, have more cells and an extended, prominent protruding hilum (Fig. 19-37).

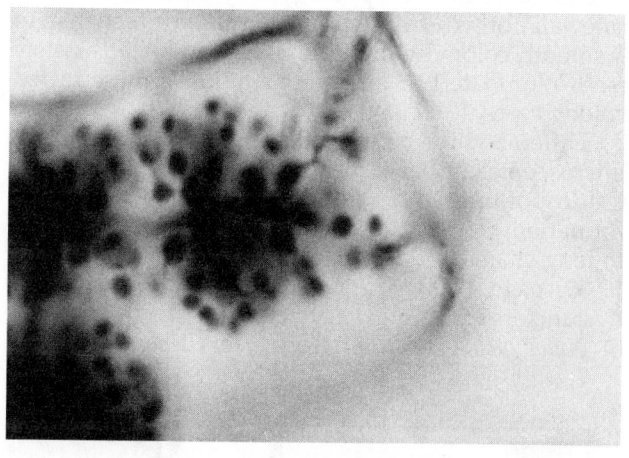

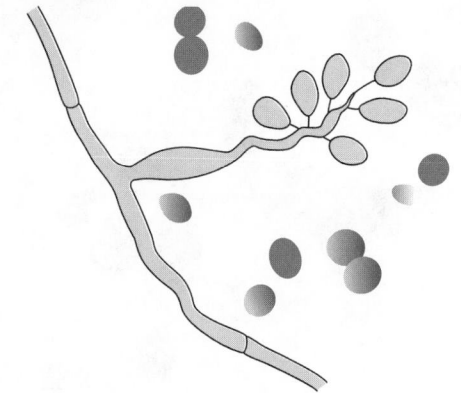

Figure 19-30
Sketch and photomicrograph of *Beauveria* species.

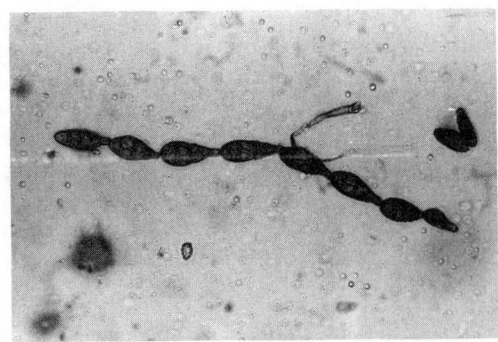

Figure 19-31
Photomicrograph of *Alternaria* species.

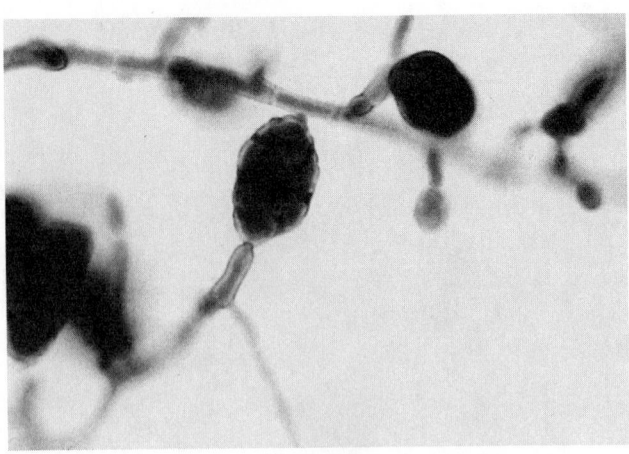

HELMINTHOSPORIUM SPECIES. *Helminthosporium* species is a rare isolate in most clinical laboratories. This fungus produces simple, straight (nongeniculate) conidiophores that give rise to multicelled macroconidia that are attached laterally by prominent pores (Fig. 19-38). This mode of conidiation is called **rhinocladiella**.

Chromoblastomycosis. The agents causing most cases of classic chromoblastomycosis and mycetoma, namely, *Cladosporium carrionii*, *Phialophora verrucosum*, and *Fonsecaea pedrosoi*, can be suspected in the laboratory when a slow-growing black mold is encountered. The gross colony morphology may vary from a delicate hairy brown-black surface, a velvety green mat, to a smooth colony, with almost a leathery consistency (see Color Plate 19-3 for demonstration of these varied colony types).

Differentiation between these three genera is made microscopically based on differences in sporulation. Cladosporium-type sporulation is characterized by the formation of freely branching hyphae that give rise to long chains of dark-staining, elliptical conidia (Fig. 19-39, page 1018). The conidia often show scars or dysjunctors at the sites of attachment. The sporulation of *Xylohypha bantianum* (formerly *Cladosporium tri-*

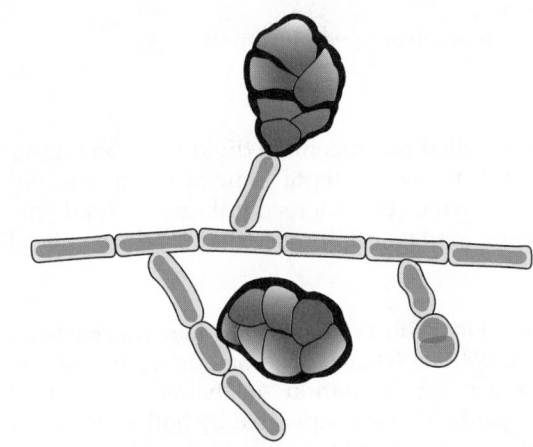

Figure 19-33
Sketch and photomicrograph of *Stemphilium* species.

choides) is also of the cladosporium type; however, it can be differentiated from *C. carrionii* by only sparsely branching, forming long chains of conidia with as many as 30 cells each and producing nonpigmented conidia without dysjunctors.[210] *X. bantianum* grows at 43°C and does not liquify gelatin, two features that also help separate this fungus from *Cladosporium* spe-

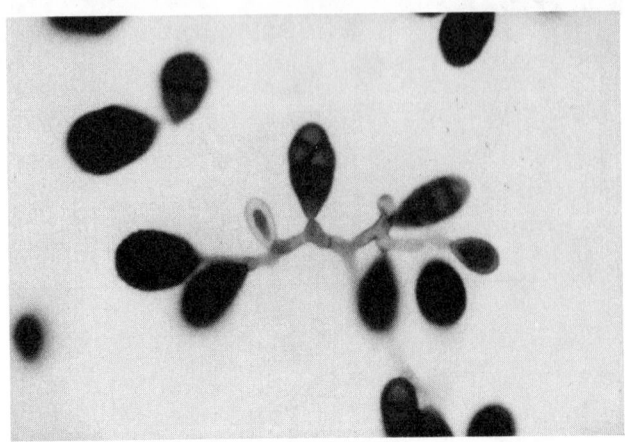

Figure 19-32
Photomicrograph of *Ulocladium* species.

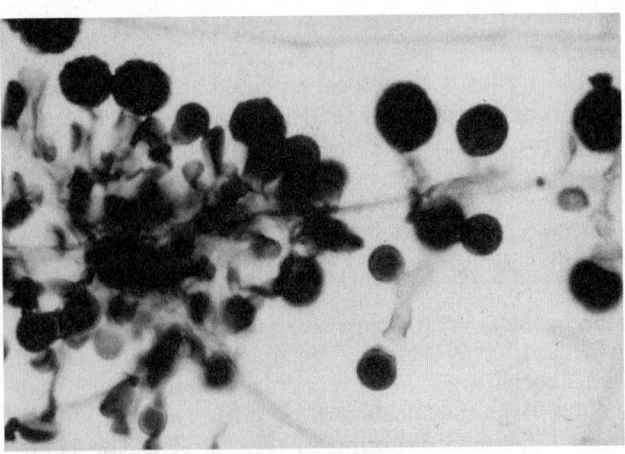

Figure 19-34
Photomicrograph of *Epicoccum* species.

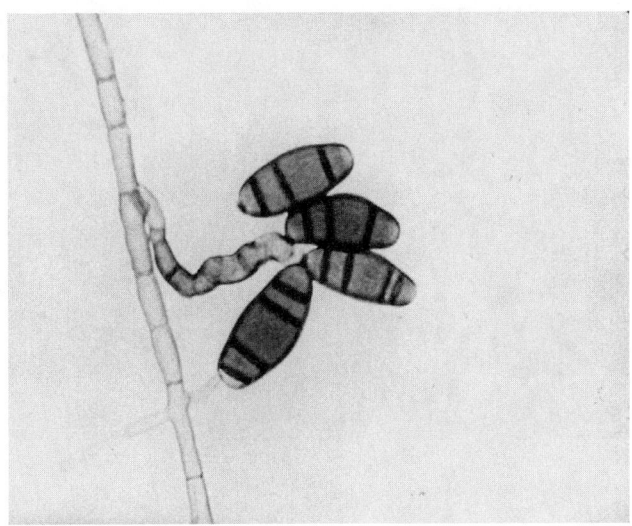

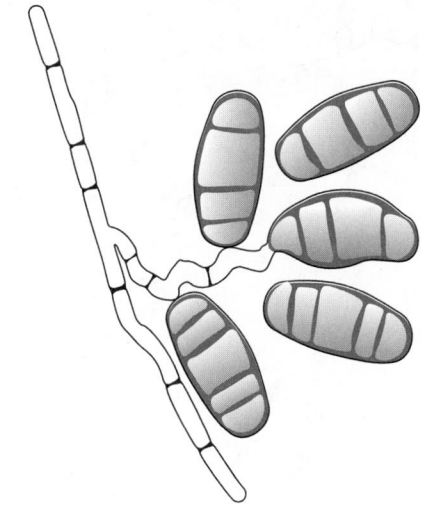

Figure 19-35
Sketch and photomicrograph of *Curvularia* species.

cies. McGinnis and Rinaldi[211] are proposing further name changes, namely that certain members of the genus *Cladosporium* be renamed *Cladophialophora*; that is, *Cladophialophora carrionii* and *Cladophialophora bantianum*. This proposed name change has not yet gained universal acceptance.

The phialophora-type sporulation is characterized by the production of flask-shaped or urn-shaped phialides ranging from 4 to 7 μm in length, terminating in a collarette from the neck of which are borne tight clusters of spherical to elliptical, hyaline conidia (Fig. 19-40). The collarettes for *P. verrucosum* are typically urn-shaped. The phialides of *P. richardsiae*, a common agent recovered from phaeohyphomycotic cysts, tend to be narrower and longer than those of *P. verrucosum*. The collarettes are distinctly more flattened and saucer-shaped. The elliptical to cylindrical conidia also tend to cluster in balls at the tips of the phialides; however, they may also be seen aligned singly in Indian file fashion along the walls of the phialides and adjacent hyphae.

Acrotheca sporulation is characteristic of *Fonsecaea* species. In this type of sporulation, conidia arise from

short denticles attached laterally to the sides of conidiogenous cells, which periodically swell, turn sympodially, and produce additional conidia that appear in circumferential clusters at points of septation. Some strains may also show the rhinocladiella type sporulation in which rows of elliptical conidia are borne directly from either side of the conidiophore (Fig. 19-41). Commonly cladosporium-type sporulation and rarely phialophora-type sporulation may be admixed in certain strains of *Fonsecaea* species. *F. pedrosoi* and much less commonly *F. compacta* are the species most commonly involved as agents of chromoblastomycosis. The latter is morphologically similar to *F. pedrosoi* except the conidial heads are arranged more compactly.

Exophiala jeanselmei (formerly *Phialophora jeanselmei*) and *Wangiella dermatitidis* have similar gross colony and microscopic characteristics. Immature colonies may appear initially as black yeasts, with only budding yeast-like cells seen microscopically. However, as the colony matures, a delicate, hairlike or velvety, gray-brown to black mycelium covers the surface. The genus *Exophiala* was created by Carmichael in 1966 to include those dematiaceous fungi that produce conidiogenous cells with annellides. According to Kwon-Chung,[187] this genus currently now includes several clinically important species formerly classified as *Phialophora* or *Cladosporium*: *E. jeanselmei* (formerly *Phialophora jeanselmei*), *E. spinifera* (*P. spinifera*), *E. wernickii* (*Cladosporium wernickii*), and *E. dermatitidis* (*P. dermatitidis*, *Wangiella der-*

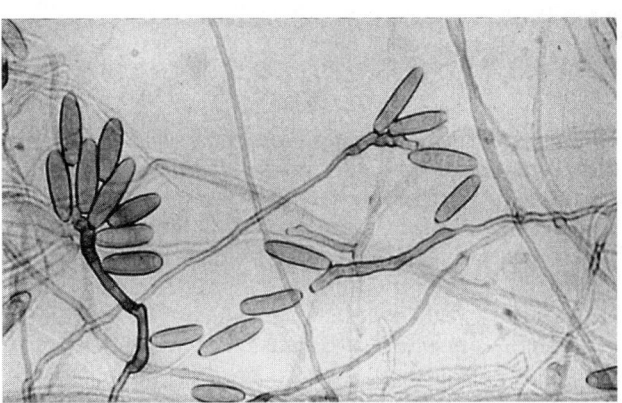

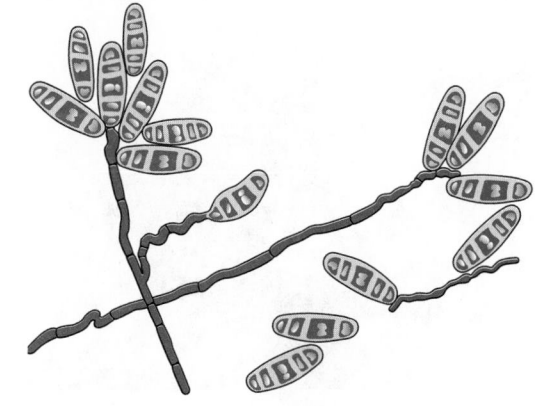

Figure 19-36
Sketch and photomicrograph of *Bipolaris* species.

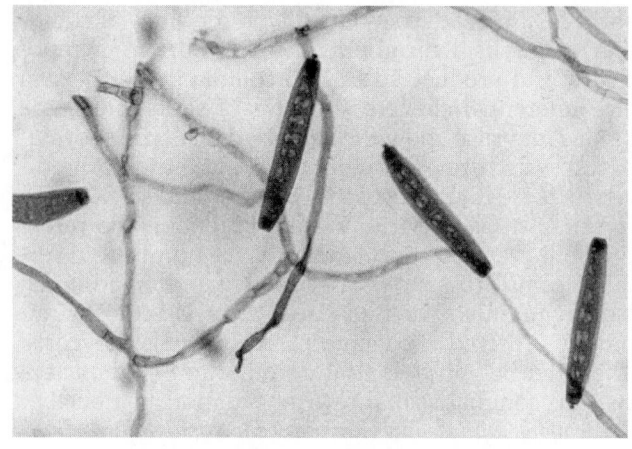

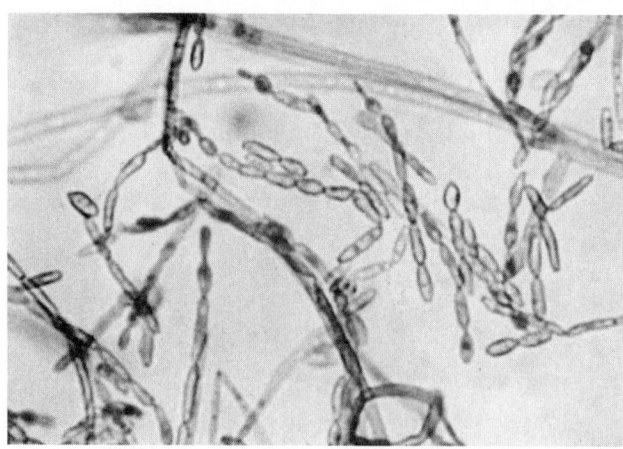

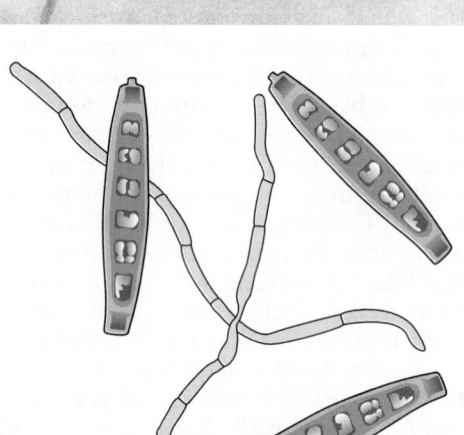

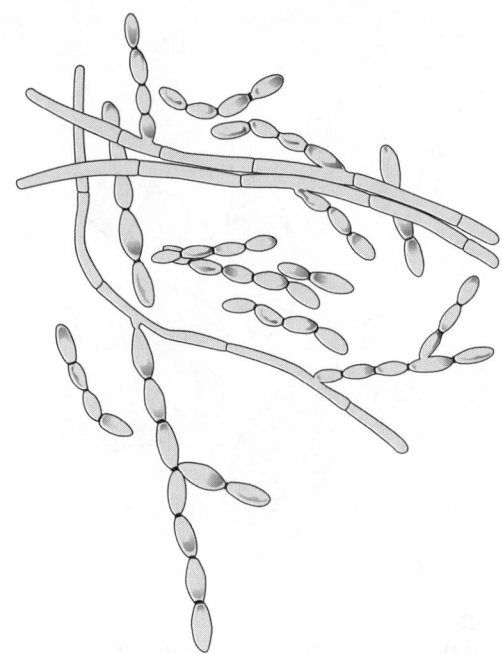

Figure 19-37
Sketch and photomicrograph of *Exserohilum* species.

matitidis). The genus designation *Wangiella* has also re-sulted in confusion. McGinnis considered that the phialides produced by what was formerly called *Phialophora dermatitidis* did not contain collarettes, and he proposed that a new genus, which he designated *Wangiella*, was required to accommodate these strains. Kwon-Chung, on the other hand, feels that the genus *Wangiella* is unnecessary because the "phialides with-out collarettes, although short, produce annellides as determined by scanning electron microscopic observa-

Figure 19-39
Sketch and photomicrograph of *Cladosporium* species.

tions." Thus, the old *Phialophora dermatitidis* has cur-rently been transferred to the genus *Exophiala*, and the genus *Wangiella* is considered a synonym.

Microscopically, the background mycelium of *Ex-ophiala* species is yellow-brown and distinctly septate hyphae. The conidiophores (in this case called a annel-lophores because conidiation occurs from annelids rather than from phialides) are of varying length but tend to be long (up to 12 µm), have tapered to pointed tips, and are borne at obtuse or right angles from the hyphae (Fig. 19-42). The tapered tip is reflective of the elongation and narrowing that occurs as successive conidia are formed; with exacting lighting and focus-ing, ringlike terminal annellations may be observed. *E. jeanselmei* is an agent of chromoblastomycosis which has also been incriminated in disseminated disease in immunocompromised patients.[296]

Other species of black yeasts include *Aureobasidium pullulans* and *Phaeoannelomyces wernickii* (formerly *Ex-*

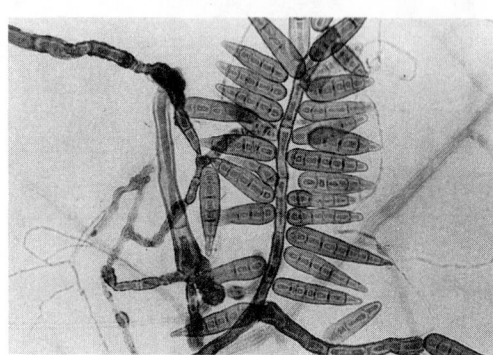

Figure 19-38
Photomicrograph of *Helminthosporium* species.

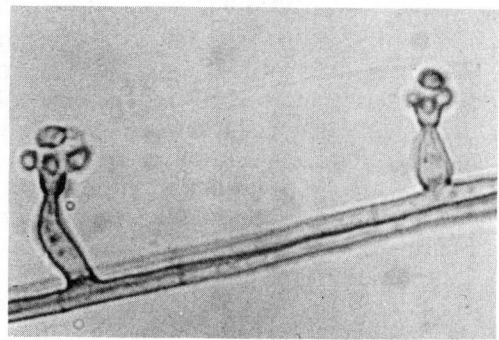

Figure 19-40
Photomicrograph of *Phialophora* species.

ophiala wernickii). Both of these species have been cited as agents of phaeohyphomycosis.[213,305,309] *A. pullulans* grows as a smooth, pasty black yeast (see Color Plate 19-3*H*). The genus *"Phaeoannellomyces"* was created in 1985, by McGinnis, Schell and Carson[213] "to accommodate those black yeasts that are characterized by the development of yeast cells that function as annellides" (*phaeo*, dark; *annello*, annellides; *myces*, fungus). According to the McGinnis scheme, *Phaeoannellomyces wernickii* forms yeasts with two cells, differentiating it from *Phaeoannellomyces elegans* that forms single-celled yeasts.

Microscopic features include two anamorphs: a segmentation of the hyphae into deep-staining, thick-walled arthroconidia-like structures, and small, hyaline, elliptical blastoconidia formed from roughened denticles along the walls of these hyphae. *P. wernickii* (*Exophiala wernickii*) microscopically produces two-celled yeast cells. According to McGinnis and associates,[213,309] these yeast cells form annellides from their distal segments, therefore warranting their inclusion in the new genus *Phaeoannellomyces* (Fig. 19-43). Rippon,[296] on the other hand, prefers to retain the genus designation *Exophiala* for those strains causing tinea nigra, in which the annellide-producing anamorph has not been observed. Engleberg and coworkers[99] have reported a case of phaeohyphomycotic cyst caused by *P. elegans*. The yeast cells with this species are unicellular and may develop thick dark walls and pseudohyphae upon maturity.

Controversy still exists whether the genus *"Phaeoannellomyces"* has taxonomic legitimacy. Kwon-Chung[187] has found that "the yeast-like colonial characteristics are invariably unstable, and the colony becomes mycelial as the cultures are maintained in the laboratory." She goes on to describe a culture of *P. elegans* referred to her laboratory that on arrival had already taken on the morphologic characteristics indistinguishable from those of *Exophiala jeanselmei*. Thus, based on these observations, Kwon-Chung argues against creating a separate genus designation for the yeast form because she feels they are both synonymous. Perhaps in response to this finding, the McGinnis school cited earlier has suggested the term **synanamorph** to designate one of several anamorphic forms with which a fungus may present.

***Aureobasidium* Species.** *Aureobasidium pullulans* grows as a smooth, pasty, black yeast (see Color Plate 19-3*H*). Microscopically, two anamorphs may be recognized: segmented hyphae that are deep-staining, thick-walled, and arthroconidia-like and small, hyaline, elliptical blastoconidia formed from roughened denticles along the walls of these hyphae (Fig. 19-44).

THE DERMATOPHYTES

The dermatophytes are a distinct group of fungi that infect the skin, hair, and nails of humans and animals, producing a variety of cutaneous infections, colloquially known as "ringworm." With the advent of griseofulvin and topical antifungal compounds, the laboratory identification of the dermatophytes is now less frequently required. In most clinical practices, physicians prepare a KOH mount of skin scales, nail scrapings, or hairs and microscopically observe for typical

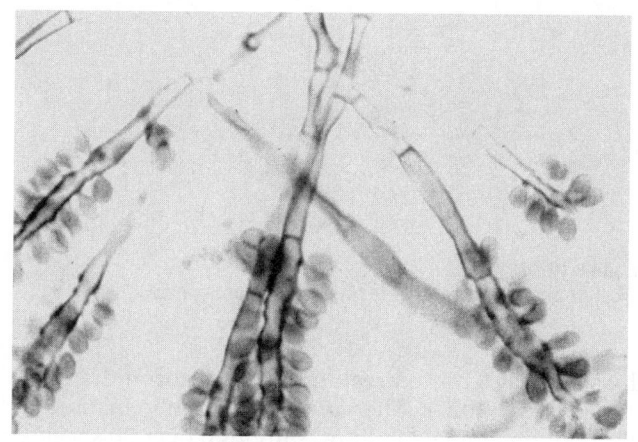

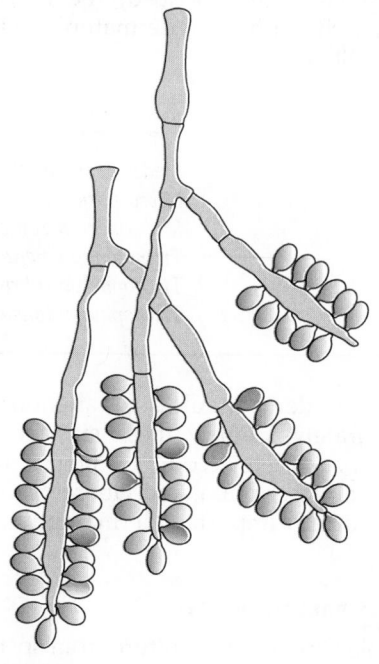

Figure 19-41
Sketch and photomicrograph of *Fonsecaea* species (Rhinocladiella type sporulation).

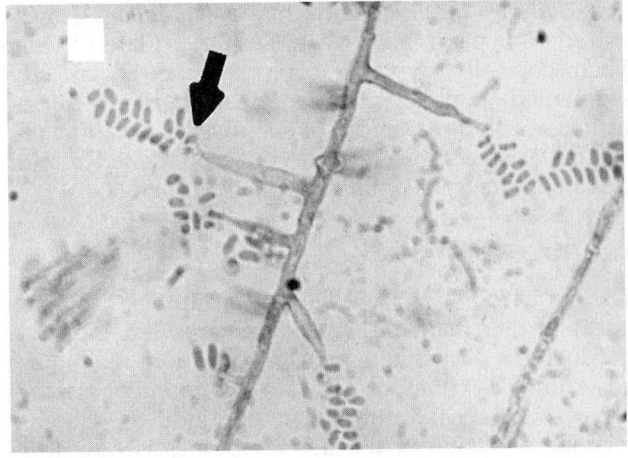

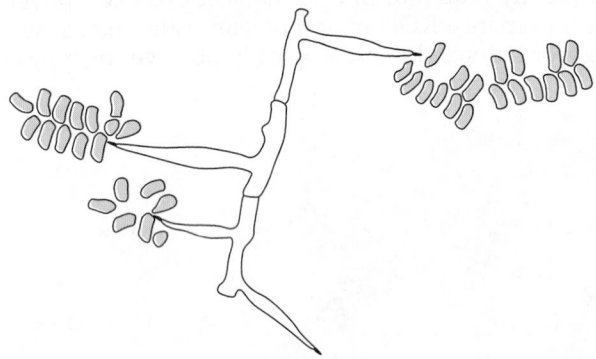

Figure 19-42
Sketch and photomicrograph of *Exophiala* species.

hyphae that tend to break up into arthroconidia (Fig. 19-46, page 1023). Therapy is commonly instituted without obtaining a culture. Although over 30 species of dermatophytes are described, the following six cause the majority of human dermatophyte infections in the United States:

GENUS	SPECIES
Epidermophyton	Epidermophyton floccosum
Microsporum	Microsporum canis
	Microsporum gypseum
Trichophyton	Trichophyton mentagrophytes
	Trichophyton rubrum
	Trichophyton tonsurans

Beginning students should focus attention on being able to accurately identify these six dermatophyte species. For a complete account of the ecology, distribution, clinical description, and laboratory identification of all medically important dermatophytes, refer to Rippon.[296]

LABORATORY PRESENTATION

Any mold recovered in culture from specimens labeled skin, nail, or hair should be suspected of being one of the dermatophyte species. One must be alert, however, that other pathogenic fungi, including the di-

morphic molds, can also involve the skin and may have microscopic features similar to the dermatophytes. Making a misidentification could have grave consequences. Observing typical hyphal segments in direct KOH mounts of skin scales (see Fig. 19-46, page 1023) or either ectothrix or endothrix invasion of infected hairs are helpful preliminary findings (Fig. 19-47, page 1023). Because the colonies of the various strains of dermatophytes vary considerably in rates of growth, morphology, and pigment production, even within the same species, the genus and species designations depend on observing microscopic features. However, a few colony characteristics, when present, may be helpful in identifying a given species. Representative dermatophyte colonies are illustrated in Color Plate 19-4.

Microsporum canis produces colonies that are cottony or wooly and may be suspected when a lemon-yellow pigmentation around the growing periphery or the underside of the colony is observed (see Color Plate 19-4A). *M. gypseum* typically sporulates heavily, imparting a sugary, granular surface that is cinnamon brown to buff in color (see Color Plate 19-4B). *T. mentagrophytes* produces a variety of colonial variants; however, only two basic patterns are generally recognized: fluffy (see Color Plate 19-4C) and granular (see Color Plate 19-4D). The latter colony type is generally from animal reservoirs (zoophilic) and has a greater ten-

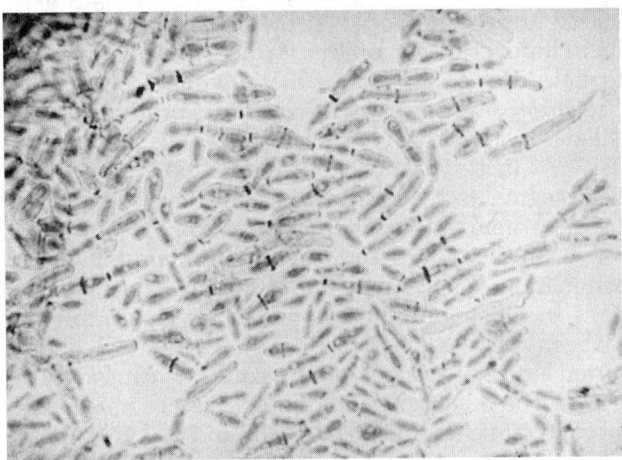

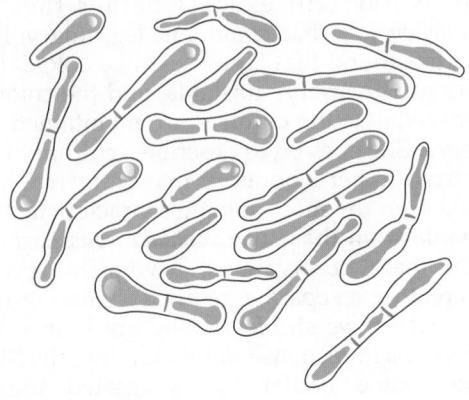

Figure 19-43
Sketch and photomicrograph of *Phaeoannelomyces* species.

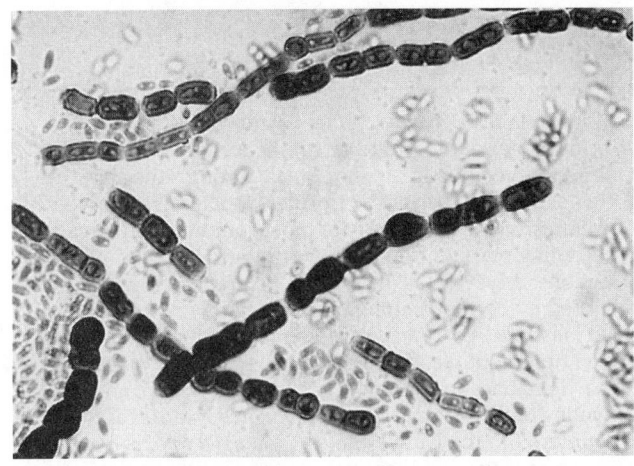

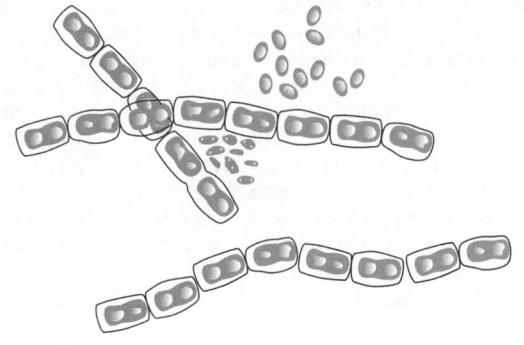

Figure 19-44
Sketch and photomicrograph of *Aureobasidium* species.

dency to be associated with inflammatory dermatoses in humans.

T. rubrum generally produces a deep, water-soluble, burgundy-red pigment that diffuses into the agar, particularly when grown on potato dextrose or corn-meal agars (see Color Plate 19-4*E* and 4*F*). *T. mentagrophytes* can also form a similar pigment; however, it is usually less intense than *T. rubrum* and is usually minimally evident on potato dextrose and cornmeal agars (see Color Plate 19-4*F*). The colonies of *T. tonsurans* are typically flat, granular, buff to tan-brown in color, and rugose, with folds radiating outward from the center (see Color Plate 19-4*G*). The colonies of *E. floccosum* growing on Sabouraud's dextrose or Mycosel agars are typically khaki or green-yellow and have a low aerial mycelium, giving a "suede" appearance to the surface (see Color Plate 19-4*H*). Gentle folds are usually seen.

Microscopically, the dermatophytes produce delicate, narrow, hyaline, septate hyphae. A variety of vegetative structures, including chlamydoconidia, favic chandeliers, pectinate bodies and nodular organs may be seen. Spiral hyphae are particularly abundant in many cultures of *T. mentagrophytes*. These vegetative structures are nonspecific and cannot be used to suggest species identifications.

SPECIES IDENTIFICATION BASED ON MICROSCOPIC FEATURES

The Genus *Microsporum*.   The chief distinguishing microscopic feature of the genus *Microsporum* is the presence of multicelled macroconidia that have thick, rough walls (Fig. 19-48). At times, it may be necessary to observe a given macroconidium under oil immersion magnification to determine if the surface echinulations are present. Usually, microconidia are present only in small numbers, unevenly dispersed, generally oval to elliptical, and have no distinguishing morphologic features. *M. canis* produces barrel-shaped, multicelled macroconidia that are pointed and slightly turned to one side at the tip (Fig. 19-48).

The macroconidia of *M. gypseum* generally are more numerous than found with *M. canis*, are less barrel-shaped, and have rounded tips (Fig. 19-49). These fea-

---

CLINICAL CORRELATION BOX 19-5.
CHROMOBLASTOMYCOSIS

Chromoblastomycosis was the term originally used to describe a cutaneous and subcutaneous infection characterized by the formation of elevated, roughened verrucous vegetations, most commonly spreading over the dorsal surfaces of the feet and lower leg, caused by a group of slow-growing, dematiaceous fungi belonging to the genera *Phialophora*, *Cladosporium*, and *Fonseceae*. These agents gain entrance to the skin through traumatic wounds and penetrating injuries. Dematiaceous hyphal elements may be seen in the tissues; however, more diagnostic is the presence of muriform, light yellow-staining yeast bodies grouped in clusters or in short chains, known as "Medlar bodies" or "copper pennies" (Figure 19-45). Microabscesses, granulomatous nodules, extreme acanthosis, and pseudoepitheliomatous hyperplasia, with varying degrees of fibrosis and scarring, are the common histologic changes. Local spread of the infection is common, and prognosis for complete cure is poor; although combina-

tions of heat treatment (pocket warmers) and regimen of 5-flucytosine have been efficacious.[334]

Wortman[378] reports a case of chromoblastomycosis caused concurrently by *F. pedrosoi* and *Nocardia brasiliensis*, complicating a traumatic penetrating injury. Four indigenous cases of chromoblastomycosis caused by *F. pedrosoi* were reported from New Zealand. The report of chromomycosis caused by *Exophiala spinifera*[25] illustrates the extended spectrum of dematiaceous organisms that can cause various clinical diseases. Clinical and biologic cure of chromoblastomycosis caused by *F. pedrosoi* is reported[283] in 8 of 19 (42%) Brazilian patients, who were treated with itraconazole, 4 of whom had severe lesions that were cured in a mean time after 17.6 months of therapy. This study indicates that even severe cases of chromomycosis may not be hopeless, and that newer antifungal agents are worth a trial.

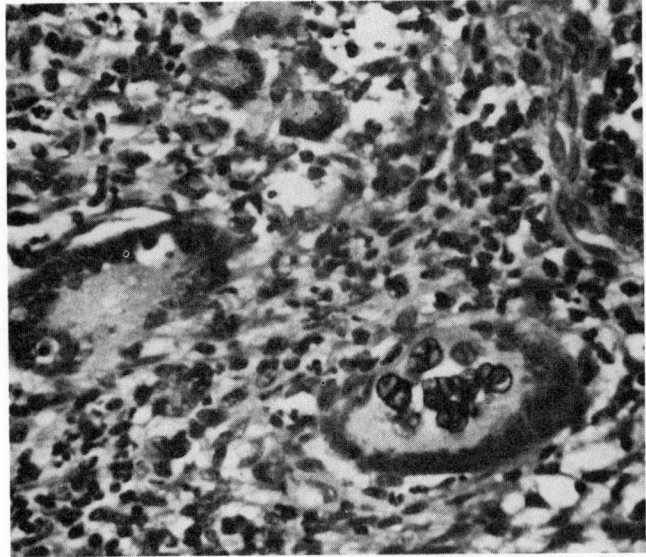

Figure 19-45
Photomicrograph of the tissue section from a case of subcutaneous chromoblastomycosis. Note the inclusion of several sclerotic bodies within the giant cell shown in the *lower right* quadrant of the field (oil immersion, H&E).

CLINICAL CORRELATION BOX 19-6. MYCETOMA

Mycetoma refers to subcutaneous infections in which the tissue is markedly swollen with the formation of deeply penetrating sinus tracts that break through the superficial skin and discharge purulent material. The feet (Madura foot) and hands are most commonly involved, becoming markedly swollen and deformed in serious infections. Mycetomas have two primary causes: those caused by bacteria belonging to the family *Actinomycetes* (*Actinomyces*, *Nocardia*, and *Streptomyces* spp.); and the true fungi (eumycotic mycetomas), primarily caused by the dematiaceous fungus *Exophiala jeanselmei* and the hyaline mold, *Pseudallescheria boydii* in sporadic cases encountered in the United States. *Madurella* spp. is a more common cause in other parts of the world, particularly western and eastern Africa. Suppurating abscesses, purulent draining sinus tracts, and varying degrees of granulomatous inflammation are seen histologically. Often white, grey, brown, or yellow "grains" or granules ("sulfur" granules), including necrotic debris admixed with either branching filamentous bacteria (actinomycotic mycetomas) or true hyphal elements, usually club or swollen, are the telltale signs of mycetomatous infections. Turiansky and associates[342] report an unusual case of mycetoma by *Phialophora verrucosa*, an unusual agent of subcutaneous phaeohyphomycosis.

CLINICAL CORRELATION BOX 19-7. PHAEOHYPHOMYCOSIS

The term phaeohyphomycosis has been used for a variety of superficial, cutaneous, subcutaneous, and systemic fungal infections caused by several species of dematiaceous saprobic fungi.[208, 309] Rippon[296] has divided the clinical spectrum of phaeohyphomycosis into superficial, cutaneous, mycotic keratitis, subcutaneous, and invasive or systemic forms of infection. The superficial infections include black piedra, caused by *Piedraia hortae*, and tinea nigra, caused by *Exophiala* (*Phaeoannellomyces*) *wernickii*. Onychomycosis is the most common form of cutaneous phaeohyphomycosis. Rinaldi and associates[295] recently report a case of onychomycosis caused by *Curvularia* spp. Subcutaneous phaeohyphomycotic cysts are also increasing in frequency. A case of a phaeohyphomycotic cyst of the foot caused by *Phialophora richardsiae* was reported[266] in a 60-year-old woman, who incurred a penetrating injury to the site some 40 years before. Eight other cases caused by this agent were culled from the past literature, including *Phoma minutella*[24] and *Phaeoannellomyces elegans*.[213]

The paranasal sinuses are also a common site of infection with dematiaceous fungi. Adam and colleagues[1] report nine cases of sinusitis presenting as allergic rhinitis or nasal polyposis, caused by *Bipolaris* and *Excerohilum* spp. A case of *Exserohilum rostratum* sinusitis and parasinusitis was reported[22] that progressed to the formation of multiple intracranial mucoceles. Also, cases of maxilloethmoid sinusitis caused by *Drechslera* spicifera[324]—the same organism, renamed *Bipolaris spicifera*—was more recently recovered from three cases of sinusitis.[119] These authors advise that one of the phaeohyphomyctic fungi should be considered in patients with nasal polyps or sinusitis that is refractory to conventional medical therapy.

Most cases of human central nervous system phaeohyphomycosis have been caused by *Xylohypha bantiana* (*Cladophialophora bantiana*[211]; formerly *Cladosporium bantianum* or *C. trichoides*).[211, 309] Infections are most frequently found in young men with chronic headache for approximately 8 weeks' duration. Resectable lesions consist of discrete demarcated masses surrounded by a gliotic capsule; poorly resectable lesions are poorly delineated, often accompanied by multiple satellite abscesses. Patients with the latter disease generally have a poor prognosis, with fatal outcomes reported in 45% of neurosurgically treated patients.[89]

Several cases of mycotic keratitis caused by various species of dematiaceous fungi, including *Curvularia*, *Excerohilum*, *Phialophora*, and *Phoma* spp. have been listed by Rippon.[296] A recent case of mycotic keratitis caused by *Curvularia lunata* has been reported.[295]

Systemic disease occurs most commonly in immunocompromised hosts. Such infections commonly begin in the lungs, after inhalation of conidia, which leads to invasive infections that may disseminate to distal organs. A case of disseminated *Curvularia* sp. infection has recently been reported[274]; *Xylohypha bantiana* (*Cladophialophora bantiana*)[211] was the cause of a cerebral abscess.[137] Several cases of invasive, systemic, and disseminated infections caused by many species of phaeohyphomycotic fungi listed by Rippon,[296] usually occurring in immunosuppressed patients, have occurred, with the primary sites of infection being the lungs, sinuses, or traumatic sites in the skin. Included are cases of endocarditis, resulting from implantation during surgery, or intravenous injection of contaminated materials by drug users.

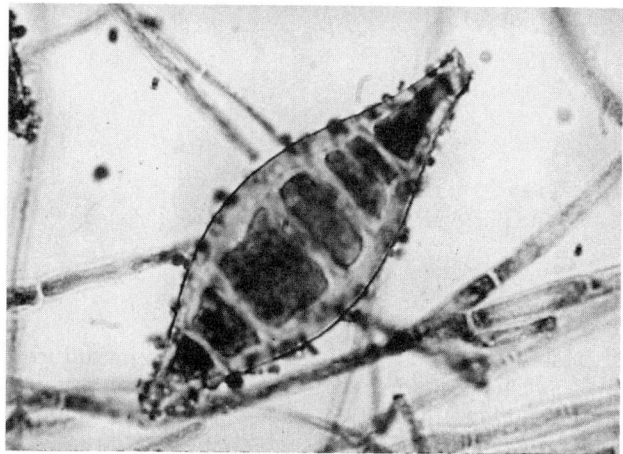

Figure 19-46
Photomicrograph of a KOH preparation of skin scales illustrating a hyphal segment of one of the dermatophytic fungi. Note that the hyphal fragment is breaking up into tiny arthroconidia (oil immersion).

tures are not always clearcut, and other criteria, such as the site and nature of the infection, a history of exposure to animals, and the colonial morphology, may be helpful in making the differential identification.

The Genus *Trichophyton*. In the genus *Trichophyton*, macroconidia are typically absent or present only in small numbers (Fig. 19-50). They are elongated, pencil-shaped, and multicelled and have thin, smooth walls. Small, 1- to 2-μm, regular-sized microconidia are usually abundant, particularly in cultures of *M. mentagrophytes*, where they tend to cluster in grapelike masses (en grappe). Spiral hyphae may also be seen (Fig. 19-50).

The microconidia of *T. rubrum* tend to be tear-shaped, regular in size, and are usually distributed on either side of the hyphal strands, producing a "bird-on-the-fence" appearance. Macroconidia are uncommon, but when seen are pencil-shaped and have thin, smooth walls. (Fig. 19-51).

If the microscopic morphology is not distinctive, urease and hair-baiting tests can be performed. The hair-baiting test is performed by placing a lock of hair into a petri dish containing water. The water is next inoculated with a portion of the unknown colony. *T. men-*

tagrophytes will invade the hair shaft within 7 to 10 days, producing conical-shaped holes; *T. rubrum* is non-invasive.[3,302] *T. mentagrophytes* can also be distinguished because most strains will convert Christensen's urea agar to a red color within 1 to 2 days; *T. rubrum* is typically negative in that time frame (a faint red color in the slant may be seen after 5 days' incubation).

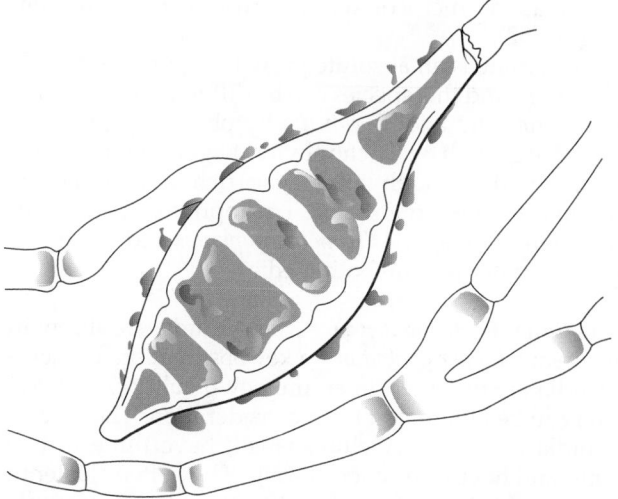

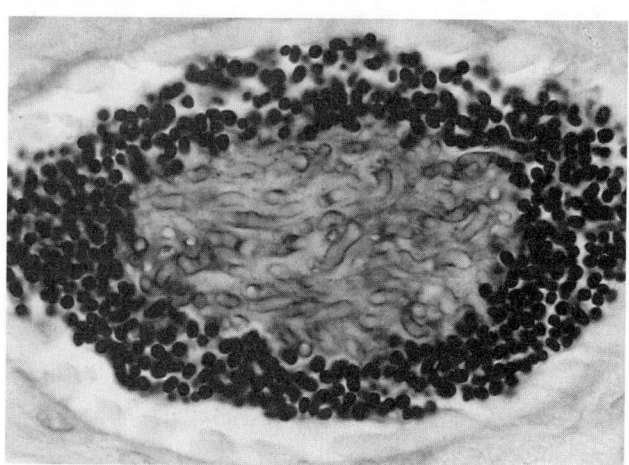

Figure 19-47
Photomicrograph of skin section in cross-section through a hair follicle filled with hyphae and conidia.

Figure 19-48
Sketch and photomicrograph of *Microsporum canis*.

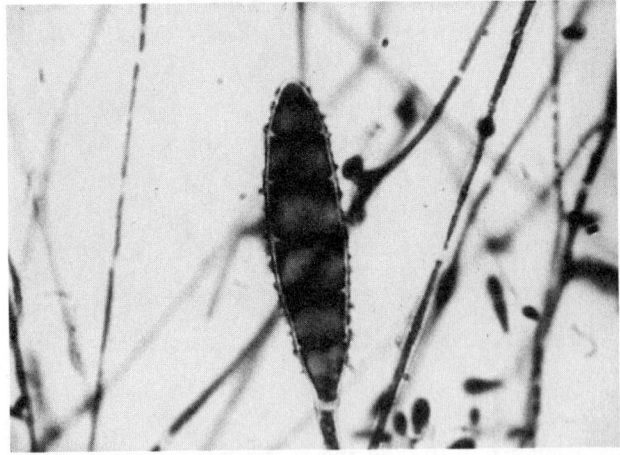

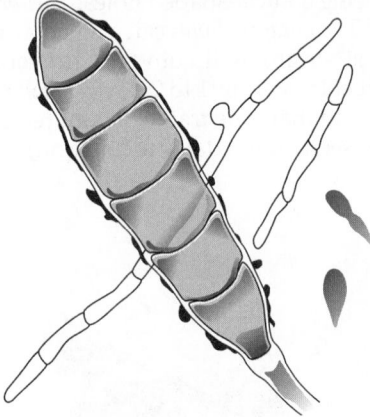

Figure 19-49
Sketch and photomicrograph of *Microsporum gypseum*.

Macroconidia are virtually never seen in cultures of *T. tonsurans*. However, microconidia are usually present and are distinctive. They vary considerably in size, and many elongated, club-shaped or large balloon-shaped forms admixed with the smaller oval or tear-shaped microconidia are also usually present (Fig. 19-52).

Thiamine is an absolute growth requirement for *T. tonsurans*, and this species can be differentiated from *T. mentagrophytes* and *T. rubrum* by observing the comparative growth on Trichophyton 1 agar (devoid of thiamine) and Trichophyton 4 agar (rich in thiamine). *T. tonsurans* grows poorly on Trichophyton 1 agar but luxuriently on agar 4; *T. mentagrophytes* and *T. rubrum* grow equally well on both media.

The Genus *Epidermophyton*.   Microconidia are absent in the genus *Epidermophyton*—a key observation. If microconidia are observed in an unknown culture, *E. floccosum* can be eliminated from consideration. The macroconidia are typically club-shaped, have three to five cells, and have thin, smooth walls. They often cluster in groups of three or four (Fig. 19-53). Chlamydoconidia are also typically present, particularly in older cultures.

DIMORPHIC MOLDS

Dimorphism refers to the ability of certain species of fungi to grow in two forms depending on the environmental conditions: 1) as a mold when growing or incubated at 25°C to 30°C; and 2) as a yeast when incubated at 35°C to 37°C. The mold form is the infective form, and humans contract disease by inhaling dust or having direct penetration of skin or mucous membranes with soil contaminated with environmental conidia. Infection in organs and tissues is produced by the yeast form. The dimorphic fungi responsible for specific mycotic diseases are *Blastomyces dermatitidis*, *Histoplasma capsulatum*, *Coccidioides immitis*, *Sporothrix schenckii*, and *Paracoccidioides brasiliensis*.

Because 30°C incubation is recommended for the recovery of dimorphic fungi from clinical specimens, it is the mold form that is most commonly isolated. For confirmation of an unknown mold as a dimorphic fungus, conversion to the yeast form must be demonstrated. This can be accomplished by transferring a small portion of the mold colony to a slant of brain–heart infusion agar containing 10% sheep blood. Cotton seed agar is effective for the conversion of *B.*

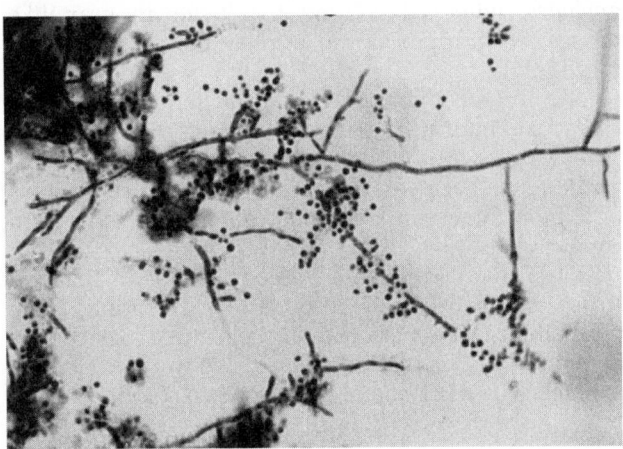

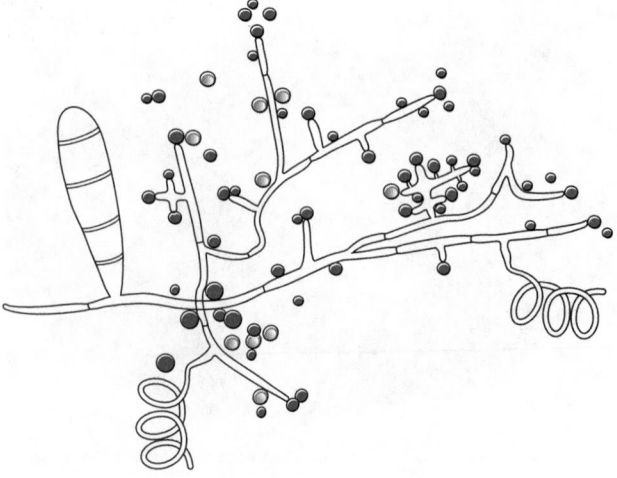

Figure 19-50
Sketch and photomicrograph of *Trichophyton mentagrophytes*.

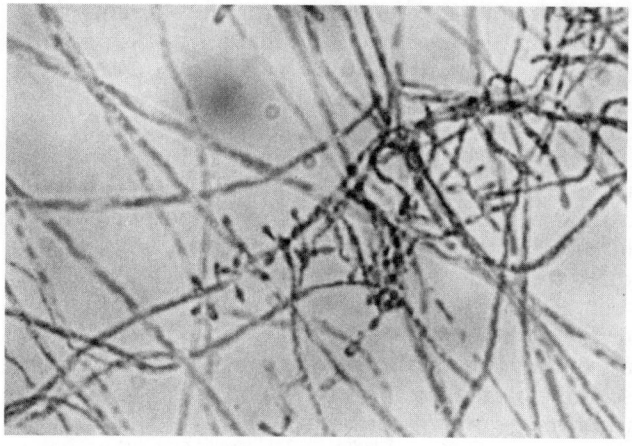

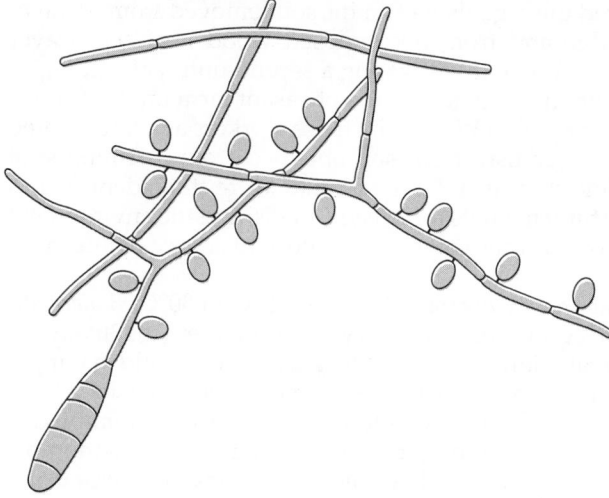

Figure 19-51
Sketch and photomicrograph of *Trichophyton rubrum*.

able for the performance of exoantigen tests, as reviewed by Sekhon and associates.[313] Nucleic acid probes are now commercially available for the culture confirmation of *H. capsulatum* and other dimorphic molds, to be presented in more detail later.

One of the dimorphic fungi may be suspected in culture if 1) it is slow growing (although in heavy infections, growth of *C. immitis* may be as soon as 3 to 5 days); 2) growth is not inhibited by culture media containing cycloheximide; 3) the colonies have cobweb or hairlike texture; 4) the hyphae appear very thin and arrange in parallel, ropelike masses when examined microscopically; 5) conversion from the mold form to the yeast form can be demonstrated, or the exoantigen extraction test reveals a specific precipitin, or positive results from the DNA probe for *B. dermatitidis*, *H. capsulatum*, or *C. immitis* are forthcoming. The colonial characteristics of the dimorphic fungi are shown in Color Plate 19-5.

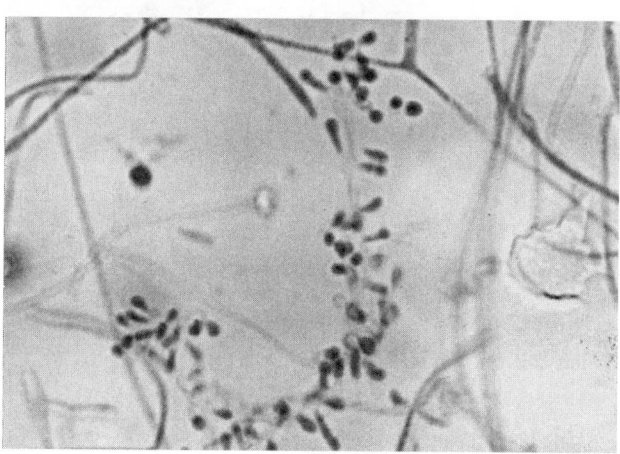

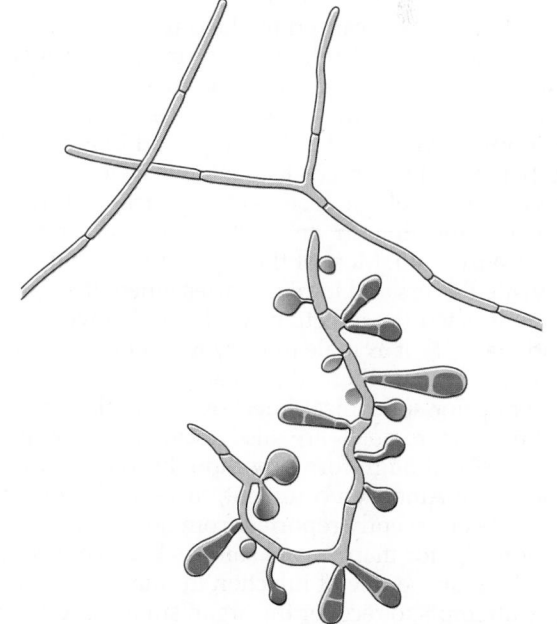

Figure 19-52
Sketch and photomicrograph of *Trichophyton tonsurans*.

dermatitidis, which usually can be accomplished within 3 days. A few drops of brain–heart infusion broth may be added to provide moisture during incubation. The screw cap must be left loose to allow the culture to breathe. More than one transfer may be required before complete conversion takes place. See Color Plate 19-5*A* for a representative dimorphic colony showing a yeastlike central portion, surrounded concentrically by a delicate, cobweb mycelial growth.

Because the conversion of *H. capsulatum* may be difficult, even after multiple subcultures, and *C. immitis* cannot be converted to the spherule form with the techniques commonly used in microbiology laboratories, exoantigen extraction of the mycelium or nucleic acid probe assays may be used to establish a rapid and accurate identification.[170,251,328] The exoantigen procedure is detailed in Chart 27. In brief, the mycelial matt of a mature subculture of the unknown mold is overlaid with aqueous merthiolate solution, 1:5000. After 24 hours of extraction, the aqueous extract is filtered and concentrated, before reacting with specific antiserum in an agar, double-diffusion test system. The appearance of species-specific precipitin bands confirms the identification. Commercial reagents are avail-

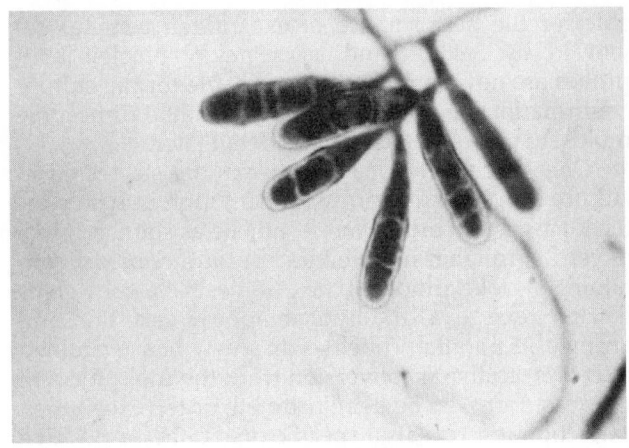

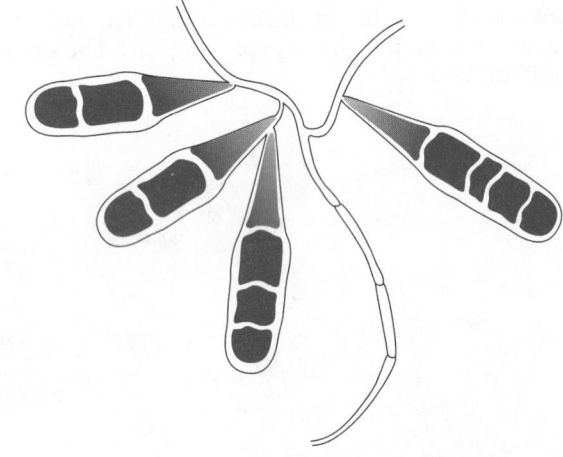

Figure 19-53
Sketch and photomicrograph of *Epidermophyton floccosum.*

BLASTOMYCES DERMATITIDIS AND BLASTOMYCOSIS

Blastomycosis is caused by the dimorphic mold, *B. dermatitidis*, a natural inhabitant of moist, warm soil. Most cases in the United States occur sporadically in regions around the Great Lakes, adjacent to the upper Mississippi River and its tributaries, and in the southeast. Baumgardner and colleagues[30] reviewed the clinical and epidemiologic aspects of 73 patients with blastomycosis residing in an endemic region of north central Wisconsin. Most of these patients lived near or had visited rivers and local estuaries where they probably contracted the infection. Vaaler and coworkers[343] found that 30% of 39 male forestry workers in northern Minnesota and northern Wisconsin had serologic evidence of prior subclinical infections with blastomycosis. Endemic regions are also located in southern Canada.[162] Although formerly thought to be confined to the North American continent, cases of blastomycosis have been recently reported from South Africa.[34,138]

Although for many years soil has been considered to be the main source of infection in humans, until recently attempts to recover the organism from soil samples have generally been unsuccessful. In the soil, this fungus is in the mycelial form. A soil of high organic or humus content (60% to 70%), an alkaline pH, and critical concentrations of moisture from recent rains, dew, or mist are the conditions optimal for recovery of the organism from dirt, wood, or other environmental sources. Only within very short periods when these conditions are exacting, conidiation will occur.[80] Conidia may become airborne if the soil is dug, plowed, or if buried stumps or logs are dislodged. The airborne conidia are sufficiently small to reach the alveoli when inhaled, causing primary pulmonary disease. Dogs that root around in infected soil or serve as hunting animals are particularly susceptible to acquiring infections.[19] Klein and associates,[180] while investigating an outbreak of blastomycosis among 89 elementary school children and 10 adults who attended an environmental camp in northern Wisconsin (48 contracted disease, one-half of whom were symptomatic), recovered the organism from the soil removed from a beaver lodge and from decomposed wood near the beaver dam. While investigating a second outbreak among 12 residents and guests of a pheasant farm on the Tomorrow River in Wisconsin, these workers again recovered the organism from soil obtained from a fishing spot along the river.[181] River banks were thus identified as natural habitats for *B. dermatitidis*, and the environment around waterways is an important source of infection.

Laboratory Presentation. At 25°C to 30°C, *B. dermatitidis* grows on laboratory medium after 7 to 30 days of incubation as a white to gray-brown mold having a delicate, silky or hairlike appearance (see Color Plate 19-5*B*). If conversion to the yeast form is attempted, a prickly stage may be seen during transformation before typical yeastlike colonies are observed (see Color Plate 19-5*C*). When conversion is complete, the colony has the typical appearance of a yeast.

Microscopically, the mold form is characterized by regular delicate, hyaline septate hyphae ranging from 1 to 2 μm in width. The most important diagnostic feature is the oval or pyriform, 2- to 4-μm–diameter, single-celled conidia borne singly at the tips of long or short conidiophores, simulating lollipops (Fig. 19-54, page 1029).

The 35°C form consists of round, thick-walled yeast cells (6 to 15 μm in diameter) that have single buds attached by a broad base (Fig. 19-55, page 1029). During the prickly or incomplete conversion phase, a combination of swollen hyphae and poorly defined budding forms may be seen.

Although it is not difficult to convert mycelial cultures of *B. dermatitidis* to the yeast forms in the laboratory, exoantigen extraction tests[170] and nucleic acid probe assays[355] are available for a more rapid culture confirmation. Results for the exoantigen test are available within 48 to 72 hours; from probe assays, within 2 hours after the assay is set up. Padhye and associates[252] correctly identified all 74 *B. dermatitidis* isolates within 2 hours using Accuprobe, a chemiluminescent DNA probe assay commercially available (Gen-Probe, Inc, San Diego CA). Similarly, Stockman and coworkers,[328] using the AccuProbe reagent kit (GenProbe, Inc, San Diego CA), demonstrated 87.8% sensitivity and 100% specificity in testing 65 target strains of *B. dermatitidis*

CLINICAL CORRELATION BOX 19-8. TINEA INFECTIONS

The term **tinea**, dating back to the Middle Ages, refers to the circular holes in garments produced by the clothes moth, an appearance similar to the ringlike lesions of the skin produced by dermatophytic fungi. The term is now used to describe the various clinical syndromes caused by the dermatophytes. Tinea infections are also common in dogs, cats, horses, cattle, and other animals, providing a source for human zoophilic infections. The following is a brief summary of the several clinical types of tinea infections.

1. *Tinea capitis* (ringworm of the scalp): Several types of infection may be observed: 1) gray-patch ringworm, a communicable ectothrix infection of children caused by *Microsporum audouini* (formerly quite prevalent in the United States but currently encountered infrequently) or *M. canis*; 2) inflammatory ectothrix infection with *T. mentagrophytes*, of animal origin; 3) black-dot ringworm, an endothrix infection, in which infected, degenerate hairs break off at the skin surface producing what appears to be a black dot, caused by *T. tonsurans*; and 4) fungating exophytic masses (kerions) produced by *T. tonsurans*, or favus infections caused by *T. schoenleini* (in Scandinavia and northern Europe) and by *T. violaceum* (in southern Mediterranean Europe). Tinea capitis is most frequently incurred either from direct contact with an infected child, or from a variety of fomites; an asymptomatic adult carrier state may contribute to persistence of infection in a given setting.[23] In a recent study of dermatophyte infection in 202 children residing in Kuwait, tinea capitis was the most common infection site and *M. canis* was the most prevalent species (96% of cases in this series).[6] Contact with infected domestic pets was found in 52% of cases, and a familial occurrence of similar infections was seen in 56% of cases.

2. *Tinea corporis* (ringworm of the body): Typical annular lesions on the skin of the smooth parts of the body, which have a spreading, hemorrhagic border, are caused most commonly by *T. rubrum*, *T. mentagrophytes*, and *T. tonsurans*. *T. tonsurans* is now recovered with increasing frequency as the cause of tinea corporis in the United States. Recently, three health care workers in a suburban Chicago hospital contracted *T. tonsurans* infections while caring for a disabled child who had the disease. This experience indicates that person-to-person spread can occur, and that appropriate preventive measures may be required in these situations. *T. rubrum*, in particular, is well suited to survive on the surface of the skin, leading to chronic infection, often for a lifetime.[77] The mannans of *T. rubrum* appear to be better able to suppress cell-mediated immune reactions than are mannans from other fungi, thereby evading host response and permitting survival. *T. rubrum* can also survive off the human body as spores in desquamated skin scales, promoting person-to-person transmission in various human habitats. Zoophilic *T. canis* and geophilic *T. gypseum* infections are also occasionally encountered in clinical practice.

3. *Tinea barbae* (ringworm of the bearded area): This zoophilic infection has most commonly been found among farm workers. *T. mentagrophytes* is the most common agent, and the lesions tend to be inflammatory.

4. *Tinea cruris* (ringworm of the groin): The lesions tend to be circinate and serpiginous with inflammatory, vesicular, enlarging margins, most commonly caused by *Epidermophyton floccosum*. This infection may reach epidemic proportions in athletes, soldiers, and ship crews among whom towels, linen, and clothing may be shared.

5. *Tinea pedis* (ringworm of the feet; athlete's foot): This is the most common fungal infection in humans, typically manifesting as itching, scaling, or seeping skin lesions on the soles of the feet or in the clefts between the toes, or both. Infections are most common during the warm, humid months. *T. mentagrophytes*, *T. rubrum*, and *T. floccosum* are the dermatophyte species most commonly recovered. Nielsen,[239] in a study of dermatophytosis in northern Sweden, found that *T. mentagrophytes* occurred with greatest frequency. The increased amount of keratin on the soles of the feet and the palms of the hands makes these two sites selectively vulnerable to infection with *T. mentagrophytes* and other dermatophytes. The capability of *T. rubrum* to survive as spores in desquamated skin scales makes these hyperkeratotic areas particularly vulnerable to contracting infections from contaminated bath towels, locker room floors, and other human habitats.

6. *Tinea unguium* (ringworm of the nails): **Tinea unguium** is the term used to describe involvement of the nails by dermatophyte fungi, to be differentiated from **onychomycosis**, which refers to nail infections caused by a wide variety of nondermatophytic fungi, including *Aspergillus* spp., *C. albicans*, *Geotrichum* spp., and several species of hyaline and dematiaceous hyphomycetes. Tinea unguium infections begin at the lateral or distal edge of the nail plate and result in paronychial inflammation. As the lesion progresses, the nail becomes thickened and brittle, with accumulation of subungual keratinized debris. The dermatophytes most commonly involved are *T. rubrum*, *T. mentagrophytes*, and *E. flocossum*. Other commonly encountered forms of tinea are discussed by Rippon.[296]

In a study[200] of 100 consecutive diabetic patients, no higher incidence of dermatophyte infections was found, compared with a control population. Dermatophyte infections of one type or another were found in 31% of the diabetics, and in 33% of the control group. Thus, contrary to popular notion, diabetes mellitus apparently does not predispose to dermatophytosis. In a study of 84 cases of dermatophytosis among German children birth to 17 years of age,[380] interesting epidemiologic perspectives are provided. Tinea capitis was at peak incidence in the early school years, caused primarily by *M. canis*; *T. rubrum* tinea pedis was the most common infection among adolescents, with peak months of infection in this series being January and September.

CLINICAL CORRELATION BOX 19-9. MISCELLANEOUS SUPERFICIAL FUNGAL INFECTIONS

One of the more commonly encountered superficial infections of the skin is tinea (pityriasis) versicolor, caused by *Malassezia furfur*, a lyophilic yeast that is a commensal of normal skin. Because of the accumulation of sebum and skin oils, the organism proliferates during times of poor hygiene, when washing and bathing are not possible for prolonged periods. *M. furfur* is a common commensal of the skin. It was recovered from skin scrapings in 8 of 25 (32%) premature infants[277]; the incidence of colonization reaches as high as 84% in older infants.[20] The infection is manifest early on by irregular patches of hypopigmentation or hyperpigmentation, particularly noticeable on exposure to sunlight. Intermittent areas of scaling, with variegated hues varying between light yellow and dark brown, may be observed as the infection progresses, accounting for the term **versicolor**. Folliculitis may be seen in more severe cases in which the infection extends into the hair shafts and sebaceous glands. The skin of the chest, back, and upper arms is most commonly involved. The condition is chronic; irritation and inflammation are usually absent, although mild pruritus may be experienced in some patients.

The diagnosis usually can be readily established by directly observing the skin for a characteristic yellow fluorescence when viewed with a Wood's lamp, or by microscopically observing for tight clusters of spherical yeast cells admixed with hyphal fragments (a picture colloquially known as "spaghetti and meat balls") in KOH-, lactophenol aniline-, or methylene blue-stained preparations made from superficial skin scrapings taken from areas of involvement.[202] The organism can be recovered in culture on Sabouraud's dextrose agar that has been overlaid with long-chain fatty acids, such as those contained in virgin olive oil. Yeastlike colonies, creamy in consistency, develop slowly after 2 to 4 days incubation at 35°C (growth at 25° does not occur). Microscopically, 1 by 2- to 2 by 4-µm, broadly budding yeast cells are observed, which are described as being "bottle shaped," with a collarettelike thickening seen at the junction of the mother and daughter cells. *M. pachydermatis*, a second species of *Malassezia*, is a cause of otitis externa of dogs. It may be found as a commensal on human skin and does not require oil for recovery in culture.

Recently, several cases of *M. furfur* and *M. pachydermatis* systemic infections and septicemia have been reported, most commonly associated with deep-line vascular catheters in patients receiving parenteral therapy.[124, 205, 317] Many of the emulsions used for parenteral therapy are rich in long-chain fatty acids. An ideal microenvironment is established at the catheter site at which a small amount of the oily emulsion can pool, supporting growth of the endogenous lipophilic organisms present on the skin surface. The catheter provides a barrier break in the skin through which the proliferating organisms can enter the blood stream. The lungs, in which there is vascular lipid deposition of the parenteral emulsions, provide an ideal site for dissemination of the organism.[202] Three cases of severe bronchopneumonia and respiratory failure in three premature infants in whom Broviac catheters were in place, are reported.[292] Two of these patients died. Some of these cases were in premature infants.[317] All three had fatal outcomes, characterized by massive involvement of the lungs, and endocardial vegetations were present in two. Risk factors included young gestational age (younger than 26 weeks), hyaline membrane disease, duration of ventilation, and duration of antimicrobial therapy. Thirty-two cases of *M. furfur* and *M. pachydermatis* systemic infections were referred to the Centers for Disease Control in Atlanta.[124] The patients had similar febrile syndromes with both species, including infections of the lungs and other organs. The diagnosis of catheter-related septicemia can best be made by recovering organisms in blood cultures drawn from infected catheters.[205] Blood culture bottles, however, do not appear visually cloudy, and they often do not give an "alert" in continuous reading systems; therefore, subculture to blood agar overlaid with virgin olive oil may be necessary to recover the organism.

Superficial cutaneous infections also include the tropical disease tinea nigra palmaris, manifesting as spreading, sharply marginated, flat, nonscaling areas of pigmentation, primarily involving the palms of the hands. The causative agent is *Exophiala wernickii*.[296] Black piedra, manifest as hard, brown to black encrustations on the shafts of hairs is caused by the black fungus, *Piedraia hortae*. White piedra, in which encrusted granules of the hair shafts are lighter and generally softer than those of black piedra, is caused by *Trichosporon beigelii*.

---

and 219 nontarget other fungi, respectively. Cross-reactivity of the probe assay has been demonstrated against *P. brasiliensis*; however, in a practical sense, this is of little concern in evaluating patients residing in the United States.

Differential Considerations. The mold form of *P. brasiliensis* is also characterized by the presence of single conidia, morphologically similar to those of *B. dermatitidis*. Certain strains of *Histoplasma capsulatum* also produce microconidia in early culture that can be confused with those of *B. dermatitidis*; however, after additional incubation, the larger, characteristic, rough-walled macroconidia usually form, and the correct identification can be made. The anamorphic form (*Scedosporium apiospermum*) of *Pseudallescheria boydii* and

the saprobe *Chrysosporium* species also produce "lollipops"; however, these two organisms are inhibited by cycloheximide-containing media and cannot be converted to yeast forms. They also are negative in the exoantigen and probe assays. *P. brasiliensis* yeast forms also range from 6 to 15 µm; however, in contrast with *B. dermatitidis*, they produce multiple buds, simulating a mariner's wheel (Fig. 19-56). In tissue sections, occasional strains of *B. dermatitidis* produce giant yeastlike cells, overlapping the size range of immature spherules of *Coccidioides immitis*, with which they may be confused (Fig. 19-57).[359] Usually, occasional broad-based budding forms or more mature spherules containing endospores may be observed, depending on whether *B. dermatitidis* or *C. immitis*, respectively, is the true cause of the infection (Fig. 19-58).

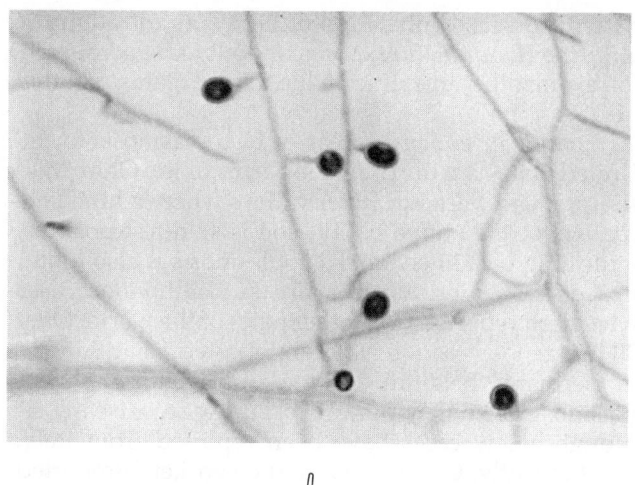

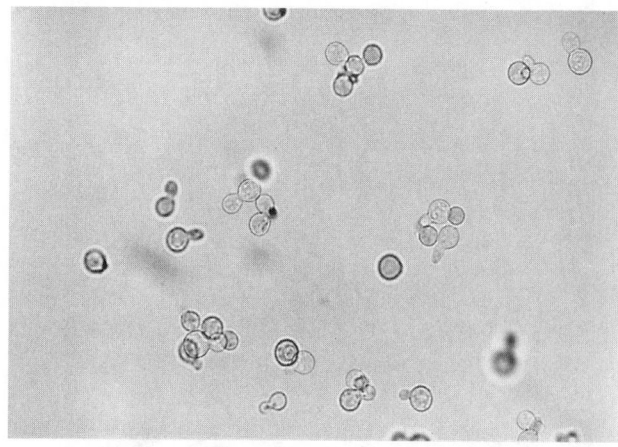

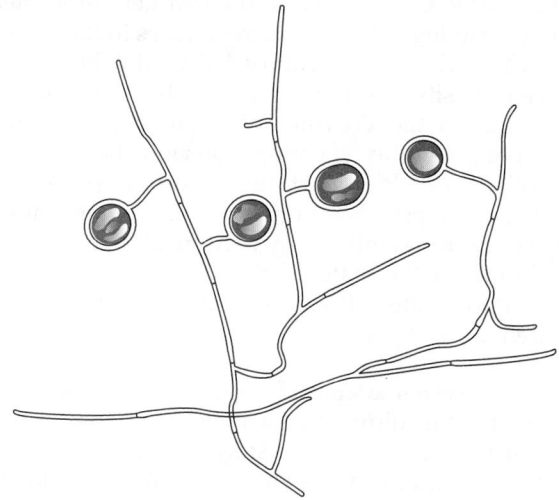

Figure 19-54
Sketch and photomicrograph of *Blastomyces dermatitidis* (mold).

Figure 19-55
Sketch and photomicrograph of *Blastomyces dermatitidis* (yeast).

HISTOPLASMOSIS

Histoplasmosis, caused by the dimorphic fungus *Histoplasma capsulatum* is the most common systemic fungal disease in the United States. The mycelial form is present in warm, moist soil rich in organic content, particularly where there are heavy accumulations of bird or bat excreta. Bird roosts, chicken houses, caves, or old buildings frequented by bats are potentially highly infective areas. Disruption of these areas by bulldozing or clean-up efforts may expose humans to large numbers of airborne spores. Titelli and coauthors[340] report the case of recurrent pulmonary histoplasmosis in a bulldozer operator who worked in Africa for a long period in extremely dusty conditions without any protection. In this patient, three episodes of *H. capsulatum* pneumonia recurred during an 18-month period. Amphotericin B failed to elimi-

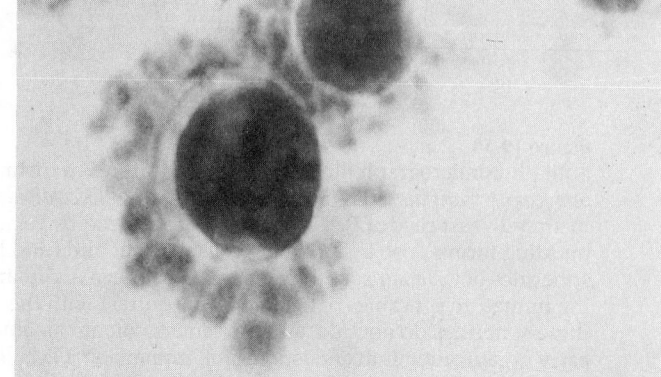

Figure 19-56
Photomicrograph of a yeast form of *Paracoccidioides brasiliensis,* showing a large central yeast cell and multiple peripheral buds, simulating a mariner's wheel (oil immersion).

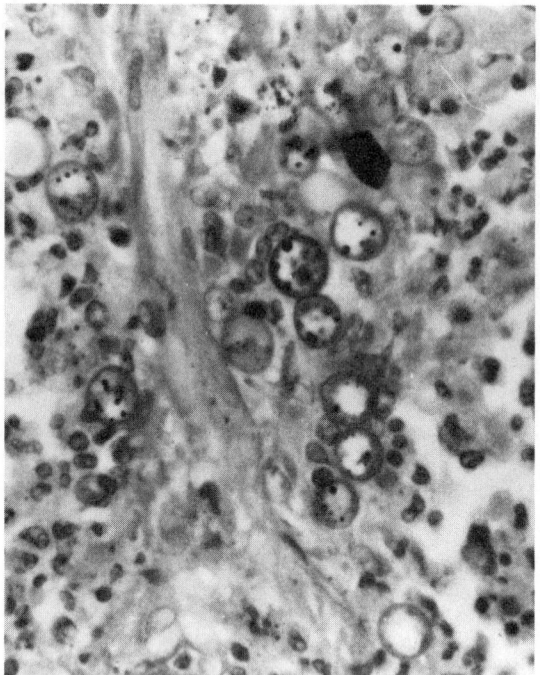

Figure 19-57
Photomicrograph of purulent tissue reaction, including multiple large yeast forms (12 to 15 μm in diameter) of *Blastomyces dermatitidis,* simulating immature spherules of *Coccidioides immitis.* The size of the yeast forms can be estimated by comparing with the nuclei of the background inflammatory cells (averaging 3 to 6 μm in diameter). Note the budding form with the broad-based bud in the *center* of the field; occasional other yeast cells have single rudimentary buds.

nate the disease. Inhalation of high concentrations of airborne *H. capsulatum* spores undoubtedly accounted for the inability to eradicate the microorganism in this case.

The major endemic areas of histoplasmosis in the United States are the drainage basins of the Ohio, Mississippi, and Missouri River valleys where a high percentage of the native population is skin-test-positive, indicating past infection. Histoplasmosis is also found in Central America; only rare autochthonous cases have been reported from other parts of the world. Only 30 indigenous cases have been reported from Europe; in Germany, Belgium, Holland and Denmark, histoplasmosis is known as an "exo-European" disease, although a few cases have been reported from Italy. Most recently, Confalonieri and coworkers[72] reported two new histologically documented cases in Italian patients who had never been abroad. A relatively high incidence of positive histoplasmin skin tests in a survey carried out in the Province of Cremona, Italy confirmed the possibility of endogenous infections. Lopes and colleagues[196,197] report two cases in successive studies of *H. capsulatum* peritonitis in women undergoing continuous ambulatory peritoneal dialysis, who were living in the state of Rio Grande do Sul, the southernmost state in Brazil, a region not considered to be endemic.

Laboratory Presentation. *H. capsulatum* develops on enriched fungal culture media after 10 to 30 days of incubation at 25°C to 30°C, as a silky or hairlike, white to gray-tan mold, appearing similar to the mold forms

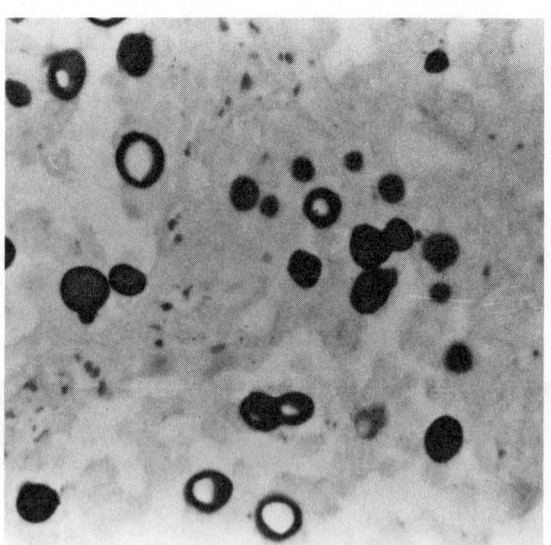
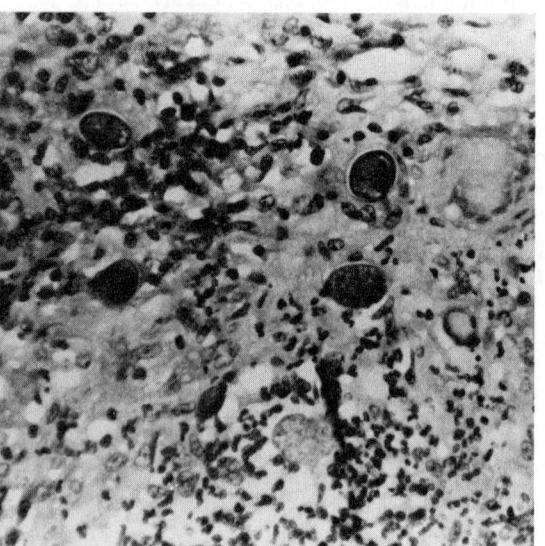

Figure 19-58
Split photomicrograph illustrating useful features in distinguishing the yeast forms of *Blastomyces dermatitidis* from immature spherules of *Coccidioides immitis.* In the *left frame* are illustrated yeast cells of *B. dermatitidis* characterized by relatively large size and broad-based budding forms. Also included are cells without buds and hollow centers, simulating spherules of *C. immitis.* In the *right frame* is shown an inflammatory tissue reaction, including immature spherules of *C. immitis.* In contrast with the yeast forms of *B. dermatitidis,* these spherules do not bud, and the centers contain an amorphous material that suggests early organization into endospores (oil immersion, GMS [*left*] and H&E [*right* frame]).

CLINICAL CORRELATION BOX 19-10. BLASTOMYCOSIS

Blastomycosis has been divided into five categories by Rippon[296]: 1) primary pulmonary, that may present either as an inapparent, self-limiting illness, or with severe symptoms; 2) chronic cutaneous disease, either with or without occult osseous lesions; 3) single-organ system involvement that may be occult for many years; 4) generalized systemic, multiorgan disease, running a rapid course; and 5) self-limited inoculation blastomycosis.

In most clinical settings, blastomycosis almost always begins in the lungs as the primary pulmonary form of the disease, which occasionally may be progressive and severe, but most commonly resolves spontaneously after a brief flulike syndrome.[49] Dry cough, low-grade fever, weight loss, night sweats, pleuritic chest pain, and myalgias may be presenting symptoms early in acute infections.[30] Persistent, localized chest pain, weight loss, night sweats, and malaise may indicate progression into a chronic form of the disease. Meyer and associates[220] describe ten patients with overwhelming pulmonary infection, manifest as the adult respiratory distress syndrome (ARDS), with marked reduction in alveolar oxygenation. Numerous, broad-based, budding yeast forms were seen microscopically in bronchial secretions. In establishing the diagnosis, even in disseminated cases, recovery of B. dermatitidis yeast forms from blood cultures is extremely rare.[231] Hebert and coauthors[134] warn that late, rapidly progressing relapses may occur several months following apparent cure after a full course of therapy (ketoconazole). Physicians are advised to follow patients for a sufficiently long period after therapy to be sure that a cure has been effected.

Several cases of extrapulmonary infections have been reported in the recent medical literature. Lopez and associates[198] report a case of intraocular infection in a 45-year-old man with disseminated disease. They review an additional ten cases from the literature, ranging from keratitis to panophthalmitis. A case of temporal bone osteomyelitis, secondary to B. dermatitidis, manifesting as serous otitis media was reported.[104] Orthopedic manifestations of blastomycosis are common. The metaphyses of long bones and small bones are most frequently involved; metaphyseal lesions tended to be eccentric, well-circumscribed, and lytic in 17 patients.[201] A rare case of primary blastomycosis of the soft tissues of the hand, progressing to loss of function, was reported.[33] The genitourinary tract, particularly the prostate gland, epididymis, and kidney; the brain, with local abscess formation; lymph nodes; and the adrenal gland are other extrapulmonary sites of involvement culled from the earlier literature.[187] These reports indicate the array of clinical syndromes that may complicate infections with B. dermatitidis.

Skin or mucous membrane involvement usually indicates systemic disease and, frequently, may be the initial lesions. In review of a large series of blastomycosis diagnosed at the Mayo Clinic between 1960 and 1990,[287] involvement of the skin and mucous membranes (including the larynx) were quite common, often with clinical and histologic features resembling well-differentiated squamous cell carcinoma. Blastomycosis should be considered in the differential diagnosis of any patient with nonhealing skin lesions associated with risk factors such as living in an endemic area and having an occupation or vocation involving frequent contact with soil.[361] Single or multiple ulcerating papules or pustules of the skin, usually involving the face, hands, or lower legs, may slowly progress into an ulcerated verrucous granuloma, with an advancing serpiginous border. Primary cutaneous lesions may occur at the site of penetrating injuries of the skin; systemic spread from primary cutaneous lesions does not occur.

Blastomycosis has not been considered as one of the AIDS-defining infections; nevertheless, in some practice settings, a marked increase in incidence occurring in immunocompromised hosts, from 3% before 1977 to 24% in the period 1978 to 1991, was noted.[256] The disease also appeared to be more aggressive in immunocompromised patients.[363] For example, two friends were studied in parallel—one with AIDS—who were infected with the same strain of B. dermatitidis (proved by restriction endonuclease analysis). The patient with AIDS developed severe, progressive, fatal pulmonary blastomycosis, despite aggressive treatment with fluconazole and amphotericin B; his HIV-negative friend responded completely to the same course of therapy. The authors concluded that cellular immunity plays a critical role in the progression of disease in patients with blastomycosis. This conclusion appears to be supported[131] by autopsy findings of two AIDS patients with blastomycosis. Both had a rapidly progressive course, with massive pulmonary involvement seen at autopsy and extensive extrapulmonary disease also noted in several organs, including the leptomeninges. Patients with AIDS, when coinfected with B. dermatitidis, particularly late in the course when the CD4 count has dropped below 200 cells/mm³, are prone to rapidly progressive pulmonary infection with overwhelming dissemination to other organs, including the central nervous system.[257] Six of 15 patients included in this study had fatal outcomes within 21 days after blastomycosis was diagnosed.

of B. dermatitidis. If conversion can be successfully accomplished, the colonies appear as typical yeasts (see Color Plate 19-5E).

Microscopically, the hyphae are delicate, averaging 1 to 2 μm in diameter. Early in culture, microconidia that resemble those of B. dermatitidis and Trichophyton rubrum begin to develop along the hyphae in a sleeve-like pattern. The diagnostic form that often develops only after the colony becomes mature or after prolonged incubation is the large, rough-walled macroconidia, ranging between 5 and 15 μm in diameter (Fig. 19-59). Early on, these macroconidia may have smooth walls; however, after additional incubation the rough, spiked appearance usually is recognizable.

The mold form of H. capsulatum is often difficult to convert to the yeast form in culture. Consequently, the exoantigen test or the nucleic acid probe test is recommended to rapidly confirm the final identification. The cultures need not be mature for probe testing. Huffnagle and Gander[149] demonstrated 100% specificity and sensitivity in probing 95 mold-phase fungi, including 41 isolates of H. capsulatum and a variety of other molds. By using a chemiluminescent, acridinium ester-labeled, single-stranded DNA probe complementary

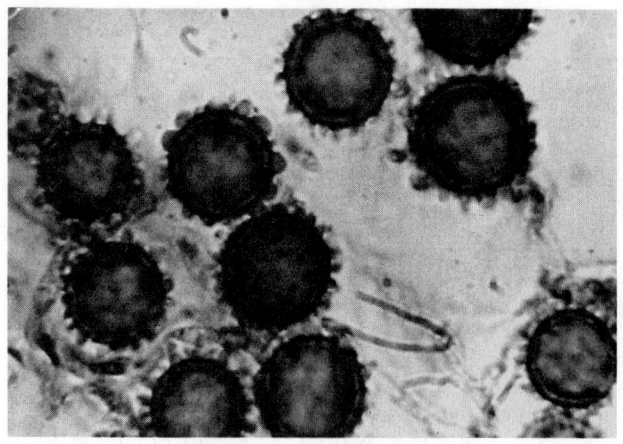

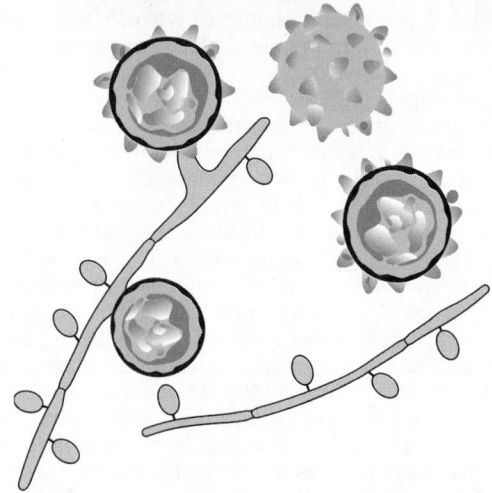

Figure 19-59
Sketch and photomicrograph of *Histoplasma capsulatum* (mold).

to the rRNA of *H. capsulatum* mold forms, Padhye and associates[251] correctly identified 103 of 105 *H. capsulatum* cultures within 2 hours. Similarly, Hall and coworkers[129] correctly identified 53 of 54 isolates of *H. capsulatum* with an acridinium ester-labeled probe, and Stockman and colleagues,[328] using the AccuProbe (GenProbe Inc San Diego CA) reagent kit, demonstrated 100% sensitivity and specificity in the study of 86 strains of *H. capsulatum* and 154 other nontarget fungi, respectively. The age of the culture, medium for isolation, and morphologic state did not affect the results, which indicates that an identification can be made before characteristic spores are produced.

The yeast forms appear microscopically as 2- to 3-μm–diameter, spherical to oval blastoconidia, often with single buds attached by narrow necks. When seen in tissue sections, these yeast forms are clustered within reticuloendothelial cells and are surrounded by a halo giving the false impression of a capsule (Fig. 19-60).

Differential Considerations. In cultures where only the sleevelike arrangement of microconidia are seen, *H. capsulatum* mold forms may closely simulate the microscopic presentation of *Trichophyton rubrum* or *Sporothrix schenckii*. Confusing *H. capsulatum* with *T. rubrum* may occur if the specimen is from a cutaneous lesion that is submitted to the laboratory labeled "skin scraping"; however, *T. rubrum* grows more rapidly and usually produces a colony with a wine-red pigment that diffuses into the agar. It is not dimorphic and is exoantigen- and probe-negative when tested against *H. capsulatum*. *S. schenckii*, which also clinically produces focal, ulcerating, cutaneous lesions, may be more difficult to differentiate from *H. capsulatum* in early culture, and an exoantigen test or probe assay may be necessary. In the mold form, most strains of *S. schenckii* produce microconidia that arrange in the typical daisylike arrangement at the tip of a delicate conidiophore (Fig. 19-64). By sharply focusing the field of view the hairlike attachments of each individual conidium to the conidiophore can be observed. *S. schenckii* is usually easy to convert to the yeast form, and the elongated, cigar-shaped cells are easy to distinguish from the spherical yeast forms of *H. capsulatum* (Fig. 19-65). The lollipop-appearing microconidia of *H. capsulatum* can closely resemble those of *B. dermatitidis*.

Diagnosis by Direct Methods. As the diagnosis of histoplasmosis may be made by identifying the small, intracellular budding yeast cells in tissue sections or stained smears, or by detecting antigen in body fluids. Blumenfeld and associates[42] were able to identify intracytoplasmic organisms in both Diff-Quick and Papanicolaou-stained smears of bronchoalveolar lavage fluid. Follow-up stains with methenamine silver revealed budding yeasts in an intracellular location, confirming that they were *H. capsulatum*. *H. capsulatum* antigen was detected in bronchoalveolar lavage fluid in 19 of 27 cases (70.3%) of pulmonary histoplasmosis studied by Wheat and coworkers,[365] making it a useful test in diagnosis of pulmonary histoplasmosis in patients with AIDS. The diagnosis of histoplasmosis may be difficult to confirm by culture or histologic examination of tissue in some cases. Wheat and colleagues have found that the detection of *H. capsulatum* polysaccharide antigen, using radioimmunoassay techniques, in bronchoalveolar fluid, urine, and blood may be useful both as a diagnostic test and in assessing the efficacy of therapy in cases of progressive disease. In a study of 226 patients, 18 years old or younger in whom *H. capsulatum* antigen was detected in urine specimens by radioimmunoassay and who had at least one other corroborating standard test, Fojtasek and colleagues[108] found that 85% had disseminated disease and 15% had self-limited pulmonary disease.

In an outbreak of histoplasmosis in Indianapolis, Williams and coworkers,[370] in a study of 195 patients, detected antigen in 92%, 21%, and 39% of patients with the disseminated, chronic pulmonary, and self-limited forms, respectively. Tests for antigen are most useful in patients with clinical findings of disseminated infection, or during the first month of illness in cases of severe pulmonary involvement when serologic tests for antibodies may be negative.

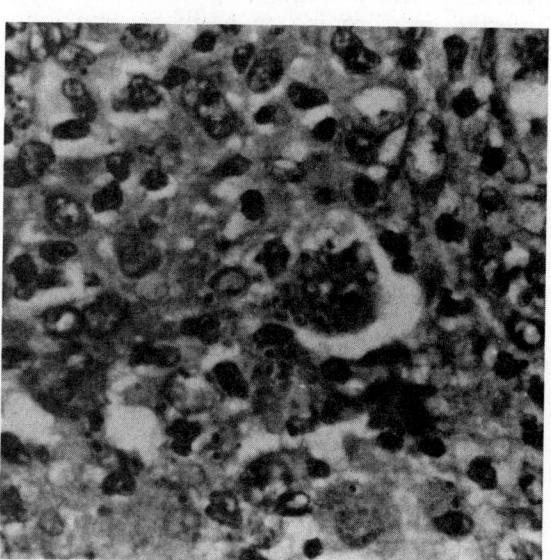 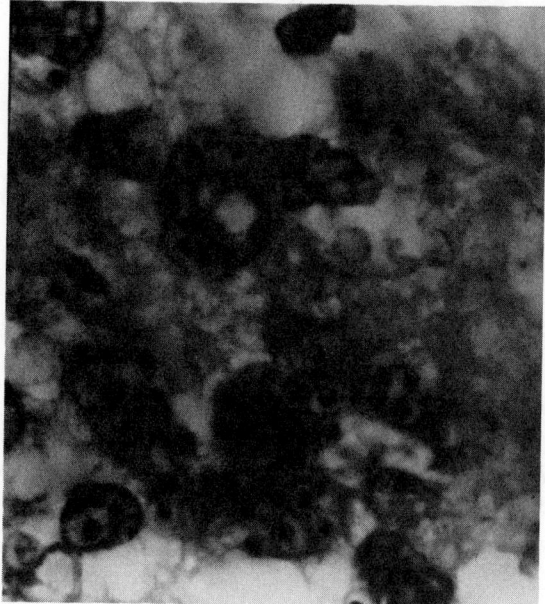

Figure 19-60

Split frame of a tissue section revealing large macrophages containing intracytoplasmic, 2- to 3-μm–diameter, pseudoencapsulated yeast forms of *Histoplasma capsulatum*. The *left frame,* taken at low-power magnification, illustrates the granulomatous nature of the inflammatory reaction and yeast-containing macrophages centrally; the *right frame,* taken under oil immersion, better illustrates the morphology of the individual yeast cells. The clear halos around the yeast bodies do not represent true capsules, but rather, a shrinking fixation artifact. (Courtesy G. D. Roberts)

COCCIDIOIDES IMMITIS AND COCCIDIOIDOMYCOSIS

The dimorphic fungus *C. immitis*, the causative agent of coccidioidomycosis, is endemic in hot, dry, alkaline soil in the lower Sonoran, Western, and Southwestern desert regions of the United States and semiarid regions in northern Mexico and Central America.[363] The arthroconidia that develop from the mycelial form of the fungus mature under the intense heat of the subsurface desert sand and easily become wind borne. These conidia, being small and light, are highly infectious for humans, resulting in primary pulmonary disease when they are inhaled. Cutaneous manifestations usually occur as a complication of disseminated disease; primary cutaneous disease may result from inoculation of open skin lesions with contaminated sand or dust, but reported cases are quite rare. The high prevalence of an acute self-limited pulmonary disease in Kern County, California, historically known as San Joaquin Valley fever, is now known to be caused by *C. immitis*; thus, coccidioidomycosis has been called "valley fever."

In a 1992 survey, the reported cases of coccidioidomycosis in California had increased threefold compared with a similar survey conducted in 1986.[226] Striking increases were particularly reported to the California State Department of Health from the San Joaquin Valley counties of Kern and Tulare, where new cases tripled up to 1200 in 1991 and to 4541 in 1992.[255] A five-year drought ended in March of 1991 when there was abundant rain. This drought rain cycle

was again repeated in the spring of 1992. Construction of new buildings and the arrival of susceptible immigrants into the endemic areas also contributed to this striking increase in incidence. Also, with the increase in mass travel throughout the world, infections are being seen increasingly in locales outside the endemic areas, which poses a diagnostic challenge for clinicians practicing in virtually every corner of the globe.[376] Sporadic exotic infections in nonendemic regions of the world have resulted from contact with contaminated fomites such as Indian pottery and packing material shipped from Arizona, clothing and various agricultural products imported from endemic areas, and conidia-bearing California-grown cotton.[254,299]

Laboratory Presentation. If the concentration of organisms is high in the primary specimen, colonies may grow on fungal culture media as soon as 3 to 5 days after inoculation. More commonly 1 or 2 weeks are required to recover the organism. At 25°C to 35°C incubation, the colonies typically have a delicate cobweb appearance and are white to gray-tan (see Color Plate 19-5F), although some strains with a light pastel orange to yellow pigmentation may be encountered. With age, the colonies may take on a more powdery appearance as arthroconidia are formed. On blood-containing media, the colonies may show a greenish discoloration from the accumulation of oxidized hemoglobin by-products leached from the degenerating red cells. Laboratory personnel must be particularly

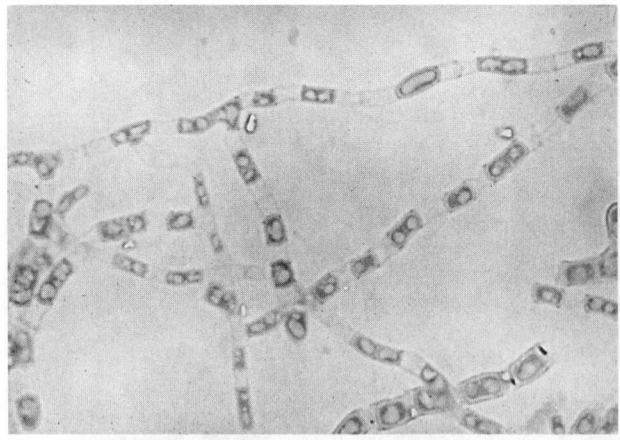

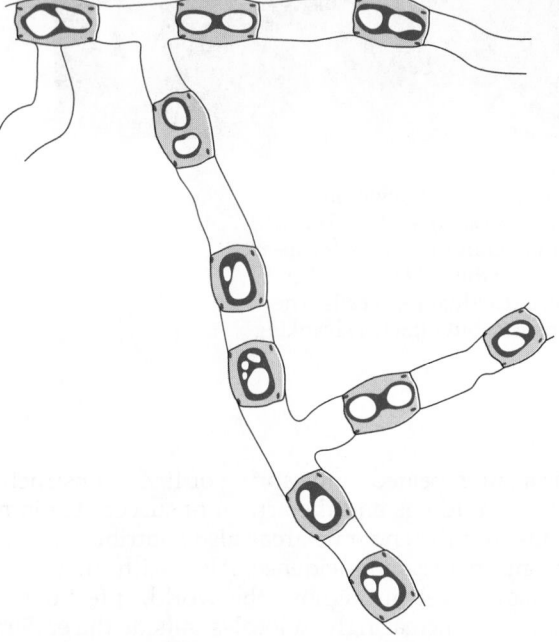

Figure 19-61
Sketch and photomicrograph of *Coccidioides immitis* (mold).

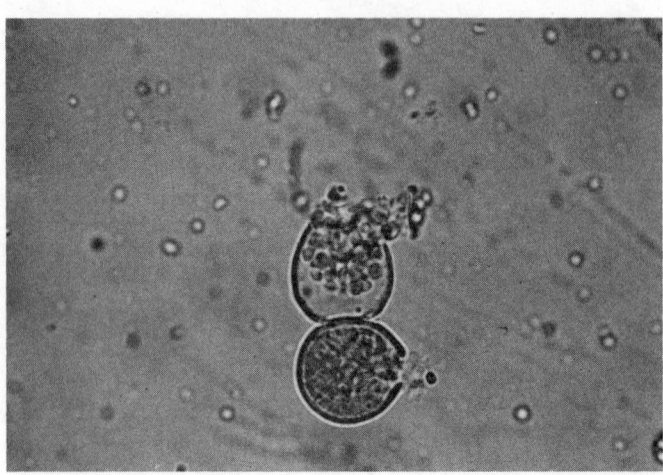

careful not to work in the open air with any fungal culture suspected of being *C. immitis* because the highly infective arthroconida can easily become airborne and are easily inhaled (Fig. 19-61).

The microscopic observation of delicate hyphae that break up into alternately staining arthroconidia is sufficient to suspect *C. immitis* (see Fig. 19-61). Typically, mature arthroconidia are thick-walled and barrel-shaped.

Conversion of the mold form to the spherule form is possible under special cultural conditions; however, this technique is beyond the capabilities of most clinical laboratories. A typical spherule containing and extruding endospores is shown in Figures 19-62 and 19-63. In the tissues and organs of the body, *C. immitis* produces thick-walled spherules measuring 10 to 60 μm in diameter. When mature endospores (2 to 4 μm in diameter) form within the spherules, a presumptive diagnosis can be made, as previously discussed.

When present in pulmonary cavities exposed to the air through an open bronchus, *C. immitis* may produce hyphal forms with or without the presence of spherules. Wages and coauthors[352] report a case of coccidioides meningitis in a 31-year-old man in fluid obtained from a ventriculoperitoneal shunt in which only hyphal forms were seen. The diagnosis was confirmed by recovering the fungus in cultures, the identification of which was confirmed by a DNA probe assay.

Differential Considerations.   *Malbranchia* and *Gymnoascus* species also produce alternate staining arthroconidia that tend to be more rectangular than barrel-shaped but can be difficult to distinguish from *C. immitis*. Growth of these species are inhibited in cycloheximide-containing culture media and they are negative in the exoantigen and probe assays. *Trichosporon* and *Geotrichum* species also produce arthroconidia, but these arthroconidia are typically rectangular and regularly staining, without the alternate skip areas characteristic of *C. immitis*. *Oospora* species, which also produce regularly staining arthroconidia from hyphae that branch freely, are rarely encountered in clinical laboratories. The differential considerations in observ-

Figure 19-62
Two spherules of *Coccidioides immitis* lying adjacent to one another, simulating the broad-based budding yeast cells of *Blastomyces dermatitidis*. Note the formation of endospores, particularly well illustrated in the *upper spherule,* with fracture of the capsules and extrusion of endospores (oil immersion, phase contrast). (Courtesy G. D. Roberts)

Most cases of histoplasmosis resolve after an acute pulmonary illness of varying degrees of severity, characterized by fever, headache, chills, cough, and chest pain. Underlying pneumonia and enlargement of the mediastinal lymph nodes are often seen. In fewer than 1% of patients, a chronic pulmonary form may develop, characterized by persistent cough, low-grade fever, and occasional episodes of hemoptysis. Cavitary lesions may develop in adults, or one or more thick, laminated, calcified "histoplasmomas" may be seen radiographically. Mediastinal granuloma formation, followed by fibrosing mediastinitis and esophagitis, is a rare complication, but cases have been reported.[207] Dyspnea, hemoptysis, postobstructive pneumonia, and superior vena cava obstruction are associated complications. The intense fibrosis found in these patients renders surgery difficult. A rare complication of pleural effusion and pericardial fibrosis has been reported.[177] This patient later developed constrictive pericarditis, confirmed at autopsy. Because H. capsulatum is an obligate intracellular organism residing in macrophages of the reticuloendothelial system, varying degrees of hepatomegaly, splenomegaly, and lymphadenopathy may be seen in cases of acute and chronic disseminated disease, which usually occurs in immunosuppressed hosts.

Progressive disseminated histoplasmosis is often an AIDS-defining illness, being the first manifestation in 50% to 75% of AIDS patients with histoplasmosis.[158, 315, 363] The clinical manifestations are fever, fatigue, and weight loss, the latter often presenting as a wasting disease. Forty-eight AIDS patients with progressive disseminated histoplasmosis were culled from 66 cases of histoplasmosis among 1300 cases of AIDS diagnosed in the Houston, Texas, metropolitan area between 1983 and 1987 (5% prevalence rate).[155] Fever, weight loss, and splenomegaly were the most common presenting signs. One-third of the patients had hematologic abnormalities; the diagnosis was made by biopsy or culture of the bone marrow in 69% of the cases. A 4% prevalence of histoplasmosis was similarly found[240] among 980 AIDS patients seen in Dallas, Texas; examination of the peripheral smear and bone marrow established the diagnosis in 88% of these patients. In addition, five cases of disseminated histoplasmosis were found[148] in patients with AIDS; all had fungemia and three died within 4 weeks after the diagnosis was established.

The presence of AIDS typically renders histoplasmosis refractory to therapy. Bone marrow and peripheral blood specimens in 13 patients with AIDS and disseminated histoplasmosis were reviewed.[186] Anemia, leukopenia, or thrombocytopenia was found in 12, 10, and 7 patients, respectively. Circulating organisms in blood smears or buffy coat preparations in five patients were associated with normoblasts circulating in the peripheral blood and severe absolute monocytopenia. The marrow specimens revealed one of four morphologic patterns: 1) no morphologic evidence of infection (two patients, one with positive bone marrow culture); 2) discrete granulomas (two patients); 3) lymphohistiocytic aggregates (six patients); and 4) diffuse macrophage infiltrates (three patients). Lysis–centrifugation for recovery of organism from blood cultures and examination of the bone marrow, peripheral blood smear, and respiratory secretions may make the diagnosis.

Other organ systems involved with histoplasmosis in patients with AIDS, as recorded in the recent medical literature, include the CNS, which may take the form of chronic meningitis, cerebral or spinal cord mass lesions, simulating neoplasms or encephalitis.[13, 364] CNS manifestations were present in 10% to 20% of patients with disseminated histoplasmosis,[364] and this organism may be the cause of chronic meningitis with no other evidence for dissemination in some patients. Cerebral or spinal cord mass lesions, resembling neoplasms or abscesses, and encephalitis were the most common forms of presentation in this series.

Histoplasmosis of the gastrointestinal tract may also occur, in which ulcers or a mass, often mimicking inflammatory bowel disease or carcinoma,[62] usually of the small bowel may be seen. Rare cases of constrictive colonic histoplasmosis have been reported.[120] Two cases of histoplasmosis presenting as annular constricting lesions of the right colon are reported,[67] and also a case of colonic histoplasmosis in a young HIV antibody-positive homosexual man who presented with acute diarrhea.[70] Diagnosis was made by flexible sigmoidoscopic biopsy. At colonoscopy, skip areas with plaques, ulcers, and pseudopolyps were observed.

Cases of histoplasmosis of the oropharynx have also been reported, in which lesions can be mistaken for carcinoma on initial presentation,[142] particularly when the vocal cords are involved.[322] A review of the literature[308] showed fewer than 100 cases of laryngeal carcinoma reported since the first case described in 1952. These authors report an additional case presenting as laryngitis, with papillomatosis of the vocal cords, in a 44-year-old woman. Pulido and associates[281] report a case of histoplasma endophthalmitis following cataract extraction, further showing the range of infections caused by this organism.

Cutaneous lesions may be the initial presentation for histoplasmosis in about 10% of cases and may serve as a marker for AIDS. Erythematous or hyperpigmented papules, pustules, folliculitis, eczematous changes, erythema multiforme, and rosacealike rashes are the more common skin manifestations.[363] In four patients with AIDS, a disseminated histoplasmosis with multiple small (up to 3 mm in diameter) erythematous maculopapules on the extremities, face and trunk, often centered around hair follicles were observed.[58] Histologically, perivascular infiltrates, with conspicuous leukocytoclasis, the lack of a macrophage response, and absence of granulomas, and organisms lying free in the dermis, intraneurally and in skin appendages were distinct differences seen in non-AIDS patients. Cutaneous lesions of histoplasmosis were described[96] in three patients with AIDS as multiple discrete papules on the extremities, trunk, and face, some of which were follicular. A sparse perivascular infiltrate, with segmented neutrophils, lymphocytes, and occasional histiocytes were seen, without granuloma formation. Perivascular leukocytoclasis in the dermis and the extracellular distribution of organisms was also found in these patients.

Although genitourinary tract fungal infections are more commonly seen in blastomycosis, histoplasmosis cases have been reported, particularly in patients with AIDS. A case of prostatic abscess occurred after therapy for pulmonary histoplasmosis,[381] and a case of massive granulomatous orchitis and epididymitis with caseous necrosis have been reported.[160]

The use of the lysis–centrifuge blood culture tubes is the optimal technique for recovering H. capsulatum yeast forms from the blood in suspected cases of disseminated disease,[259] significantly increasing the yield of positive cultures and shortening the time of recovery. The superiority of this system is also supported by the observations, from a study[230] of 182 fungal isolates of all types, that H. capsulatum was recovered only in the lysis–centrifugation system.[230] Early diagnosis is important, because dissemination can be rapidly progressive and fatal in patients with AIDS.

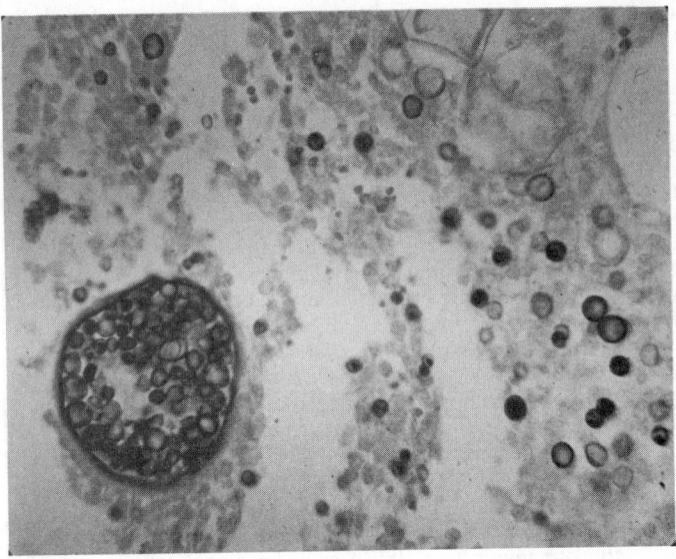

Figure 19-63
Large mature *Coccidioides immitis* spherule (*lower left*) packed with endospores. Note the presence of the free endospores in the surrounding tissue, simulating the yeast forms of *Histoplasma capsulatum* or *Cryptococcus neoformans* (oil immersion, GMS stain). (Courtesy G. D. Roberts)

ing for the presence of spherules in tissue sections have been discussed previously.

Culture confirmation of *C. immitis* can most rapidly and accurately be accomplished by using the chemiluminescent DNA probe (Accuprobe; Gen-Probe, Inc, San Diego CA). Padhye and associates,[252] in a study of 72 mycelial cultures of *C. immitis* referred to the CDC for review, report that all were accurately identified within 48 hours, in contrast to negative results for several other heterologous arthroconidia-forming fungi (several strains of *Malbranchea* and *Geotrichum* species). Stockman and colleagues[328] found that the AccuProbe reagent kit performed with 99.2% sensitivity in the culture confirmation of 121 target strains of *C. immitis* and with 100% specificity against 164 strains of other fungi.

The serologic diagnosis of coccidioidomycosis is conventionally made by detecting antibodies by one of three techniques: tube precipitin, latex agglutination (primarily detecting immunoglobulin IgM), and complement fixation (primarily detecting IgG). Currently, the enzyme immunoassay (EIA) is rapid, easy to interpret, and bypasses the anticomplement interference often encountered with traditional assays. In a study of 47 serum and cerebrospinal fluid specimens from human cases with confirmed coccidioidomycosis,[168] the Premier EIA assay (Meridian Diagnostics, Inc, Cincinnati OH) detected both IgG and IgM antibodies in all cases, a 100% sensitivity when compared with the results of tube precipitin and complement fixation tests run in parallel. The EIA, however, was not absolutely specific, as cross-reacting antibodies from a few patients with blastomycosis and from patients with noncoccidioidal disease led to false-positive readings.

SPOROTRICHOSIS

Sporotrichosis, caused by the dimorphic fungus *Sporothrix schenckii*, is primarily a subcutaneous mycosis found worldwide. In the United States, the disease is most prevalent in the Midwest, particularly in the states bordering the Missouri and Mississippi River Valleys. From 1978 to 1992, only 55 cases of cutaneous sporotrichosis had been reported in European countries other than Italy; in Italy alone, 58 cases were reported in this time period.[27] The mycelial form of the fungus, from which the infective conidia are produced, resides in the soil and lives on plants and plant debris. Recently, Sigler and coauthors[318] reported on several cases of blood and human skin isolates of *S. cyanescens*, a recently described species thought to be primarily a commensal of the skin. Blood invasion may occur by extension of skin organisms through breaks in the skin associated with indwelling intravenous catheters.

Sporotrichosis has also been known as the rose gardener's disease because the primary lesion often presents as a nonhealing ulcer of the skin of the fingers, hands, forearm, or feet, which develops 1 or 2 weeks after skin puncture by an infected rose thorn or other contaminated vegetation. Cases have been reported in greenhouse workers and orchid growers who handle sphagnum moss. Coles and colleagues[71] reviewed 84 cases involving persons living in 25 states who became infected after handling Wisconsin evergreen seedlings packed in sphagnum moss. The use of gloves when handling any packaged plants and the use of alternative packing material, such as cedar wood chips or shredded paper, are suggested measures to minimize transmission of infection. Masonry workers who handle old bricks and miners and others who come in close contact with soil and vegetative material are also highly susceptible. Infection occurs as organisms gain access to the deeper portions of the skin by trauma or through cracks or fissures of the skin or through the bites of insects or animals that act as carriers of the conidia.

Cooper and associates[73] report a case of laboratory-acquired infection in a New York researcher studying isolates from the 1980 epidemic in the United States. There had been no evidence of trauma or a penetrating injury to the skin, suggesting that *S. schenckii* may be capable of invading healthy skin. Distant inoculation of secondary sites is also possible, as indicated by an-

CLINICAL CORRELATION BOX 19-12. COCCIDIOIDOMYCOSIS

The clinical manifestations of coccidioidomycosis and progression of disease differ in patients who are immunocompetent and those with AIDS. Most primary infections of the classic disease are confined to the lungs and are self-limited. Sixty percent of infected individuals are asymptomatic; many skin test-positive patients do not remember having symptoms. Those who are symptomatic experience an acute, short-term flulike, lower respiratory tract infection with varying degrees of cough, sputum production, chest pain, fever, and arthralgia. Manifestations of bacterial pneumonia are unusual, although two such cases are reported[199] that were complicated by extrapulmonary dissemination and sepsis. Only 2% of infected individuals ultimately develop chronic pulmonary disease with sequelae. Solitary "coin lesions" or granulomas that may cavitate, usually located peripherally within the lung parenchyma, are common residual findings in previously infected individuals, particularly those not living in endemic areas. Erythema nodosum (particularly in women) and erythema multiforme of the trunk and extremities may develop. In only about 0.5% of cases does the disease disseminate, most commonly in persons of Filipino, native African, Mexican, and Asian ancestry. Muscles, tendons, bones, joints, and skin are common sites of dissemination; the CNS and genital organs are less commonly involved. Ampel and associates[10] report that of 15 patients with *C. immitis* fungemia, 11 had a diffuse miliary pneumonia on chest radiographs. All patients died within 1 month of the positive blood culture.

In a retrospective review of 77 patients having coccidioidomycosis during AIDS infection, Fish and coworkers[105] defined six categories of disease, based on primary clinical presentation: group 1, focal pulmonary disease (20 patients); group 2, diffuse pulmonary disease (31); group 3, cutaneous coccidioidomycosis (4); group 4, coccidioidal meningitis established by a positive coccidioidal complement texation serology of 1:16 or greater in the CSF; group 5, extrathoracic lymph node or liver involvement (7); and group 6, positive coccidioidal serology, without a clinical focus of infection (6). Coccidioidal serologies were positive in 83% of these patients (39% for TP antibodies, 74% for CF antibodies); 11 of the 12 seronegative patients had diffuse pulmonary disease. At the time of follow-up, 32 of the 77 patients had died, most commonly those with diffuse pulmonary disease (group 2). Antoniskis and associates[17] found that two of eight patients with coccidioidomycosis and HIV infection were repeatedly seronegative, concluding that histopathology and culture remain the most reliable methods for establishing the diagnosis in patients with AIDS.

Several other conditions coexistent with coccidioidomycosis have also been reported in the recent literature: a case of disseminated coccidioidomycosis in a liver transplant recipient detected by a percutaneous liver biopsy[90]; three cases of coccidioidal peritonitis in patients undergoing continuous ambulatory peritoneal dialysis[11]; a rare case of genital tract infection associated with peritonitis in a woman undergoing therapy for Hodgkin's disease[53]; and a case of coccidioidomycosis of the knee,[189] presenting 11 years after treatment and presumed cure of the primary infection. A case of coccidioidomycosis was diagnosed in an axillary lymph node biopsy obtained from a 76-year-old woman with a mammogram suggestive of malignancy.[323] A case of disseminated coccidioidomycosis was reported[141] in a black man that was diagnosed by observing spherules in a needle biopsy of a subcutaneous neck mass. Moorthy and colleagues[228] draw attention to the increase in coccidioidomycotic iridocyclitis in conjunction with the recent epidemic in the Southwest region of the United States, forewarning that the diagnosis should be suspected in any person who has granulomatous iridocyclitis associated with an iris mass that does not respond to corticosteroid therapy. These case reports indicate the diversity of clinical presentations of coccidioidomycosis.

Whether pregnancy predisposes to infection with *C. immitis* is still questionable. Wack and coworkers,[351] recognizing many previous studies in which coccidioidomycosis during pregnancy was considered a devastating disease with high mortality, nevertheless found only 10 cases of coccidioidomycosis in 47,120 pregnancies among women living in Tucson, Arizona. The infection resolved in 7 of the women in whom coccidioidomycosis was diagnosed during the first or second trimester; whereas the disease became disseminated in 2 of 3 women who were diagnosed in the third trimester. Improvement in medical care and the introduction of antifungal therapy relatively early in the course of coccidioidomycosis may account for the lower current mortality rate among pregnant women, in comparison with the several fatalities reported in the older literature.[348] Nevertheless, it is recommended[267] that pregnant women, wherever they reside, who develop persistent respiratory symptoms of pleuritic pain and productive cough, should be questioned about recent travel or residency in an endemic area and examined carefully for toxic erythema, erythema nodosum, or erythema multiforme. If complement fixation titers are high, aggressive treatment with amphotericin B should be begun, both to prevent dissemination in the mother, but also to minimize the possibility of placental transfer to the fetus.

Infection with HIV is also a risk factor for coccidioidomycosis in endemic areas,[12] which represents the third most frequently reported opportunistic infection in this condition.[363] In a study of 602 AIDS patients in the United States with disseminated coccidioidomycosis,[157] approximately 60% resided in endemic locales; the remaining 40% were inhabitants of 35 nonendemic states. Those living in endemic counties were more likely to be injecting drug users or past recipients of blood products. Of AIDS patients with coccidioidomycosis, 63% in this series died within 1 year, indicating the high likelihood of devastating progression of infection in this population. In contrast with immunocompetent individuals, in whom the detection of circulating plasma anticoccidioidal complement-fixing antibodies without evidence of active disease is extremely unusual, this is not true in the AIDS population.[18] In endemic areas, serum serology studies should be performed on all patients with a diagnosis of AIDS, even in the absence of symptoms. In the study by Arguinchona and associates,[18] asymptomatic individuals with positive serologies went on to develop active coccidioidomycosis, and a trend toward reduction in active disease was found in those who received antifungal therapy. In a study of 54 patients with coccidioidomycosis, 19 of whom also had AIDS,[87] transbronchial biopsy was 100% sensitive in yielding a rapid diagnosis, in contrast with cytologic examination of bronchial fluid or bronchoalveolar lavage, which provided a diagnosis in only 34% of cases.

other case.[169] A 56-year-old woman with sporotrichosis on the cheek also developed a second lesion on the knee, presumably from distant autoinoculation. Although rare, cases of zoonotic transmission of infection have also been reported: a veterinarian acquired infection from a cat[288] and an 84-day-old girl had fixed cutaneous sporotrichosis also transmitted by a cat.[284] Use of gloves by veterinarians when handling animals with cutaneous ulcers and protection of infants from infected animals are obvious preventive measures.

Laboratory Presentation. After incubation at 25°C to 30°C for 2 to 7 days, *S. schenckii* may appear as a white to yellow mold (see Color Plate 19-5G); however, yeastlike colonies may also appear at this temperature. The authors recently encountered both white and darkly pigmented yeasts that grew overnight on routine blood agar isolation plates. Typically with maturation, the colony develops a wrinkled or folded membranous surface that tends to turn dark brown or black (see Color Plate 19-5H). Conversion of the mold to the yeast form usually occurs within 2 or 3 days when a subculture is incubated at 35°C to 37°C. *S. cyanescens* differs from *S. schenckii* by producing lavender pigmentation of the colonies, susceptibility to cycloheximide (inhibition of growth on Mycosel agar), a strong urease reaction, and the inability to convert to a yeast form.[318]

Microscopically, the hyphae are very delicate, ranging between 1 and 2 μm in diameter. Small, one-celled, round or oval microconidia (3 to 6 μm in diameter) develop laterally along the hyphae in a sleevelike pattern. The arrangement of the conidia in flowerettes atop a long, slender conidiophore simulating daisy petals may be seen in the mature colony (Fig. 19-64).

By focusing up and down with the microscope and using an oil immersion objective, the characteristic hairlike attachments between the conidia and the conidiophore (from which the species name is derived) can be observed. *S. cyanescens* has an appearance similar to *S. schenckii*, except that secondary conidia are formed, appearing as budding yeast cells borne from the tips of the primary conidia (see the paper by Sigler[318] for excellent photomicrographs).

The yeast forms are 2 to 4 μm in dimension and tend to be oval or elliptical, often with a single bud (Fig. 19-65). Most helpful in making the microscopic identification of *S. schenckii* yeast forms is the observation of cigar-shaped forms measuring 3 by 10 μm. These yeast forms may be difficult to seen in stained human tissue sections, and animal inoculation may be required to demonstrate them. Fig. 19-66 is a methenamine silver-stained section of a subcutaneous granuloma that is packed with elliptical yeast cells. Note the cigar-shaped daughter buds from a few of the mother cells.

PARACOCCIDIOIDOMYCOSIS (SOUTH AMERICAN BLASTOMYCOSIS)

Paracoccidioidomycosis is a progressive subacute to chronic systemic granulomatous fungal infection caused by the thermally dimorphic fungus *Paracoccid-*

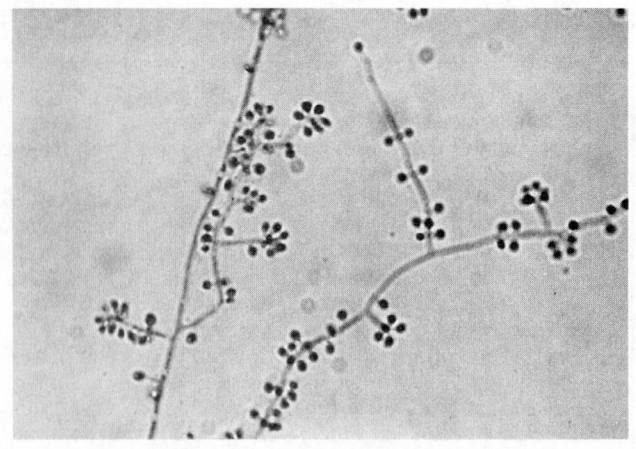

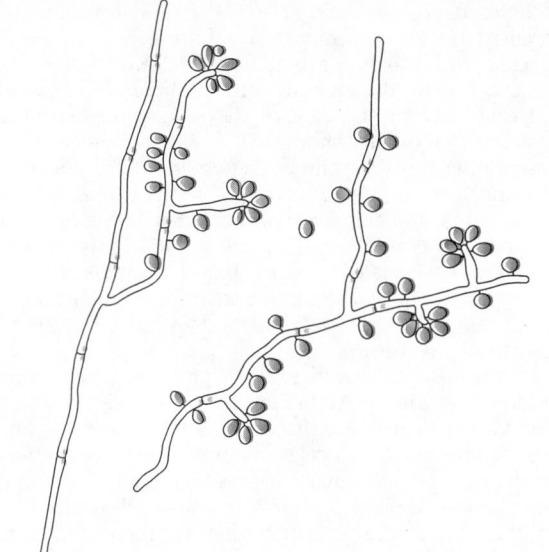

Figure 19-64
Sketch and photomicrograph of *Sporothrix schenckii* (mold).

ioidomyces brasiliensis. It is the most common systemic mycosis in Latin America, with an estimated 10 million people in the entire area of endemicity infected as of 1977.[118] In South America, most cases have been reported from Brazil, Colombia, and Venezuela; endemic areas also exist in southern Mexico and in all countries in Central America except Belize and Nicaragua.[51] Countries in the Caribbean Islands, the Guyanas, and Chile have been free of reported disease. In endemic areas, most cases occur in and around humid forested regions. The disease most frequently involves adults older than 30 years of age, is rare in children, and occurs in men over women with an overall ratio of 15:1. Although most patients are agriculturists, cases have been reported in individuals with rare direct exposure to soil and vegetation. Whites are more prone to develop infections than native Indians; immigrants coming to endemic areas tend to develop more severe infection.[51] Individuals carrying human leukocyte antigens HLA-B40, A9, and B13 may have a higher risk of infection.[116]

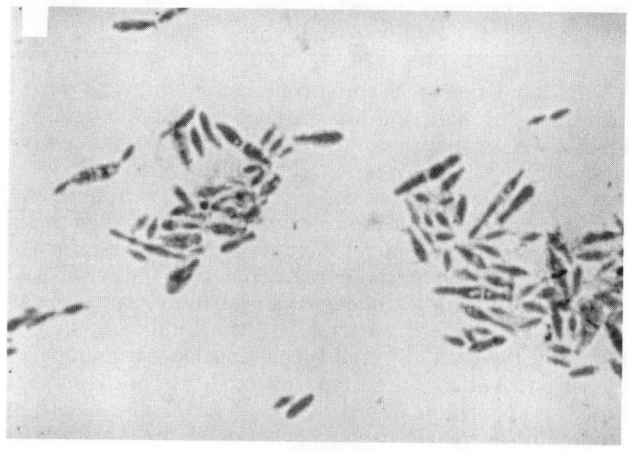

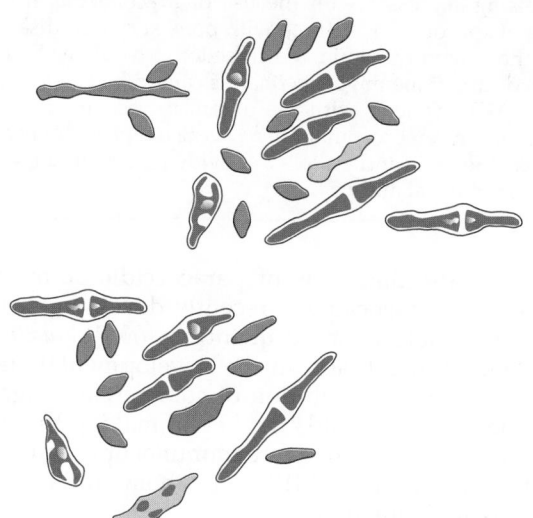

Figure 19-65
Sketch and photomicrograph of *Sporothrix schenckii* (yeast).

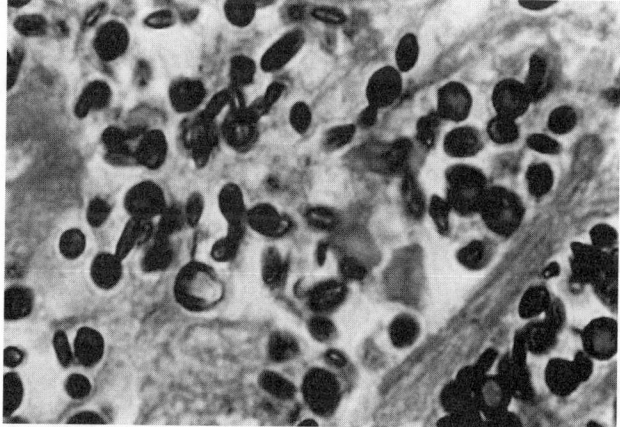

Figure 19-66
Photomicrograph of a cutaneous biopsy from a case of sporotrichosis revealing numerous spherical to oval yeast cells, some of which show elongated, cigar-shaped buds (high-power, methenamine silver stain).

Laboratory Diagnosis. The diagnosis of paracoccidioidomycosis can be most quickly established by directly demonstrating in clinical materials the 10- to 30-μm spherical, thick-walled yeast cells with multiple daughter buds, each attached by a narrow-necked bud (Fig. 19-67). These yeast forms may be best observed in KOH mounts, either directly or using calcofluor white or immunofluorescence reagents. Occasionallly, the budding daughter cells may form short chains. In tissue sections the background inflammation is usually granulomatous admixed with varying concentrations of polymorphonuclear leukocytes. The diagnosis is established by finding the multibudding yeast forms described in the foregoing, best seen in PAS- or GMS-stained sections.

When incubated at 25°C to 30°C, *P. brasiliensis* grows very slowly over 10 to 30 days as a silky, white to gray-tan mold. Microscopically, delicate, hyaline, septate hyphae make up the background mycelium. Characteristic oval, nonpigmented, 2- to 4-μm conidia are borne singly from short, slender conidiophores directly from the hyphae, in a lollipop fashion, similar in appearance to those produced by *B. dermatitidis*.

Conversion to the yeast form is slow. The mother yeast cells of *P. brasiliensis* observed in culture are 6 to 15 μm in diameter and appear similar to those of *B. dermatitidis*, except that multiple narrow-necked buds of the former are easy to distinguish from the single, broad-based budding forms seen for the latter.

Brummer and coauthors[51] have reviewed the several immunodiagnostic approaches for the diagnosis of paracoccidioidomycosis. Following diagnosis and for the first year thereafter, elevated serum levels of specific IgG antibodies can be detected; elevated IgM antibody levels are usually not seen, except in cases of extensive lymph node involvement. Mendes-Giannini and colleagues[217] demonstrated IgG-, IgA-, and IgM-specific antibodies to a 43-kDa antigen of *P. brasiliensis* in patients with paracoccidioidomycosis and further demonstrated that a lowering of the titers during a course of treatment was correlated with an improvement in symptoms. Monoclonal antibodies against this 43-kDa glycoprotein have been prepared in research laboratories; however, commercial reagents are not currently available.

P. brasiliensis antigens derived from culture filtrates or whole yeast cells that have been used to assist in making diagnoses fall into three general categories: cell wall-derived, cytoplasmic (intracellular), and culture filtrate (exocellular).[54] Cell wall antigens prepared for use in precipitation and immunodiffusion tests have cross-reactivity with other fungi; therefore, their usefulness in skin testing and serologic testing is limited. Several citations are given by Brummer and coauthors[51] to the work of Fava-Netto, who developed cytoplasmic yeast-form polysaccharide antigens that have been successfully used for the diagnosis of paracoccidioidomycosis in complement fixation assays. Several antigens have been electrophoretically identified in yeast-phase filtrates of *P. brasiliensis* cultures suitable for use in exoantigen tests.

CLINICAL CORRELATION BOX 19-13. SPOROTRICHOSIS

The appearance of a small, red, painless pustule on an extremity, together with the appearance of multiple, linearly placed secondary pustular or ulcerating lesions along the proximal lymphatics is sufficient to suggest sporotrichosis. The primary pustule may slowly enlarge, ulcerate, and discharge a small amount of serosanguineous exudate. Varying degrees of cellulitis, with swelling and redness of the surrounding subcutaneous tissue, may be observed. The secondary satellite lesions present initially as verrucous, erythematoid plaques or scaly patches, often developing into ulcers that also exude purulent material. Bacterial superinfections may confuse the gross appearance.

Extracutaneous sporotrichosis occasionally occurs with spread to joints, tendon sheaths, bursae, bone, and muscle.[373] Chowdhary and coauthors[63] report a case of polyarticular sporotrichal arthritis; an additional case of bilateral polyarticular arthritis of the wrists and elbows has also been reported.[282] Although arthritis is an uncommon manifestation of sporotrichosis, these two cases indicate the broadened spectrum of disease that may be caused by this fungus. England and Hochholzer[98] report on eight cases of primary pulmonary sporotrichosis in patients fol-lowing inhalation of airborne conidia, an otherwise rare occurrence. Cough, sputum production, and low-grade fever are the usual presenting symptoms. Disseminated sporotrichosis has been reported in patients with AIDS.[193]

Disseminated sporotrichosis is uncommon in individuals infected with HIV. Four cases, three of whom died despite aggressive antifungal therapy, are reported.[260] Progressive infection was most common in those individuals with CD4 cell counts of fewer than $100/mm^3$. In the one patient who survived, a decline in serum antibodies were traced to the 6-month regimen of itraconazole therapy. Heller and Fuhrer[136] also report a fatal case of disseminated sporotrichosis in a patient with AIDS, also associated with severe CD4 lymphocyte depletion. There was promising success[374] with the use of itraconazole in six cases of sporotrichosis, three with bone and joint disease and three with disseminated infection. The alleged first proved case of meningoencephalitis caused by *S. schenckii* in an AIDS patient, with the organism recovered from postmortem cerebrospinal fluid was also reported.[91] Invasions of the brain and vessels was evident in the tissue sections obtained at autopsy.

The exoantigen test, using reagents recently refined by Camargo and colleagues,[54] has been cited as reliable in the culture confirmation of *P. brasiliensis*. Indirect immunofluorescent techniques, immunoenzymatic assays, and most recently, PCR amplification tests were cited as having been used by many investi-gators in the diagnosis of paracoccidioidomycosis. Goldani and associates[117] recently developed a PCR assay that detects small quantities of *P. brasiliensis* antigen. Although still in the developmental stages and awaiting the evolution of commercial reagents, PCR nevertheless holds the key to making the diagnosis in patients with severe immunosuppression, including those with AIDS, in whom antibody responses are inadequate.

YEASTS: CLINICAL DISEASES AND LABORATORY IDENTIFICATION

Each laboratory director and supervisor must decide to what extent yeast isolates are to be identified. Because yeasts are considered normal flora in the oropharynx and gastrointestinal tract, their recovery from throat swabs, sputum, bronchial washings, gastric washings, and stool specimens is of questionable clinical significance. Yeasts may also be recovered from urine cultures, nail scrapings, and vaginal specimens, the significance of which must be determined by the clinical history. The repeated isolation of yeasts from a series of clinical specimens from the same patient usually indicates infection with the organism recovered, and identification of the isolates is necessary. Another clinical situation in which species identification is justified is when a yeast is recovered from normally sterile body fluids, such as blood, CSF, or fluids aspirated from the joints, pleural cavity, or pericardial sac.

One approach to the identification of yeast isolates is shown in Figure 19-68. Most yeasts grow well on routine blood agar isolation plates, and special fungal media are not required. The colonies generally are entire, slightly domed or flat, smooth and buttery in consistency, or roughened and pasty as the colony

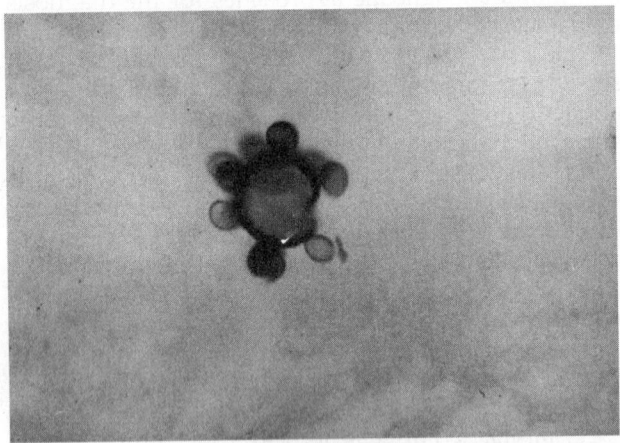

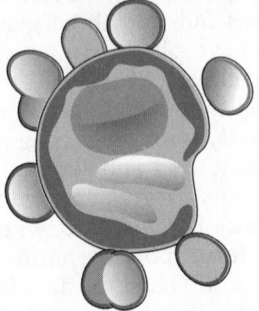

Figure 19-67
Sketch and photomicrograph of *Paracoccidioides brasiliensis* (yeast).

matures. An aerial mycelium does not develop, although spiderlike extensions may occasionally radiate from the periphery of the colony. If a distinct aerial mycelium is observed, the possibility of a dimorphic fungus must be considered, or one of the yeastlike fungi that can form true mycelia, such as *Geotrichum* or *Trichosporon* species, must be considered. A colony with a mucoid appearance and consistency suggests capsule formation and may provide an initial clue to the identification of *Cryptococcus neoformans*.

LABORATORY APPROACH TO YEAST IDENTIFICATION

The Germ Tube Test. The first step in the identification of an unknown yeast isolate is to perform a germ tube test (Box 19-4). A **germ tube** is defined as a filamentous extension from a yeast cell that is about half the width and three to four times the length of the cell (Fig. 19-69). The true germ tube of *Candida albicans* has no constriction at the point of origin; early pseudohyphae of *C. tropicalis* may be confused but characteristically show a point of constriction adjacent to the mother cell. The new cellular material that composes a germ tube, according to Odds,[243] represents **true hyphae** that, by definition, do not show

points of constriction. A constricted germ tube represents a pseudohyphae formation derived from a budding process of the blastoconidia. In the authors' experience, both constricted and nonconstricted "germ tubes" may be seen in the germ tube test for *C. albicans*; however, if the preparation appears to contain only constricted germ tubes, one should seriously consider the possibility of *C. tropicalis* or other *Candida* species. When the differentiation may be clinically significant, carbohydrate assimilation studies should be performed.

An alternative germ tube test, combining the assessment of chlamydospores in one agar, has been modified in the microbiology laboratory at the University of Vermont.[107] The surface of a 2% Tween oxgall caffeic acid (TOC) agar plate is streaked with a small portion of an isolated colony suspected of being *C. albicans*. A sterile coverslip is lightly overlaid on the agar surface in an inoculate area. To avoid accumulation of moisture, do not press the coverslip to the agar. Incubate the plate at 35°C in 10% CO_2 for 2 hours. Leave the lid of the petri dish slightly ajar during this incubation period so that the medium will be fully permeated with CO_2. Examine the area of inoculation under the microscope for the formation of germ tubes. If germ tubes are present, the test is posi-

CLINICAL CORRELATION BOX 19-14.
PARACOCCIDIOIDOMYCOSIS

The mycelial form of *P. brasiliensis* resides in the soil, and humans develop pulmonary infection by inhalation of the small 4-µm–diameter conidia. On reaching the distal portion of the pulmonary parenchyma, the conidia develop into yeast cells that may be confined locally or propagate and disseminate to distal organs in progressive disseminated disease. In a competent host, local growth is retarded, and the infection may end without development of a lesion. A rapidly progressive and widely disseminated juvenile form of the disease (about 5% of total cases) occurs in children and young adults with severely depressed cell-mediated immunity. Involvement of the organs of the reticuloendothelial system and dysfunction of the bone marrow may be so severe as to simulate a lymphoproliferative disorder.[195] The prognosis is poor.

In the chronic, adult form, the disease is slowly progressive and remains primarily confined to the lungs. The pulmonary lesions as seen by radiography are nodular, infiltrative, fibrotic, or cavitary, preferentially localized to the lower lobes of the lungs.[195] Cough, expectoration of sputum, and shortness of breath are the more common pulmonary symptoms, often accompanied by low-grade intermittent fever, weight loss, and anorexia. The chronic disease may be mild, moderate, or severe, depending on the patient's general condition and immune status; severe fibrosis, leading to chronic obstructive pulmonary disease and cor pulmonale, is the fatal sequela. Lesions of the skin and oral and nasal mucosa are commonly found in patients with the chronic multifocal form of the disease.

The incidence of paracoccidioidomycosis has not increased in recent years to the extent of other mycoses in

patients with AIDS. One reason for the scarcity of coinfection in patients with AIDS may be the widespread use of trimethoprim–sulfamethoxazole as prophylaxis for *Pneumocystis carinii* pneumonia, an agent also very effective against *P. brasiliensis*.[118] Because of the difficulty in establishing a diagnosis in AIDS patients, paracoccidioidomycosis may be more prevalent than believed. Reactivation of latent disease most likely serves as the pathogenesis of paracoccidioidomycosis in patients with AIDS. The clinical manifestation encountered among the 27 AIDS patients reported by Goldani and Sugar[118] ran the spectrum from indolent infection to a rapidly progressive course, the latter being found in the majority, with dissemination to extrapulmonary organs found in 19 of the 27 (70.4%). Disseminated disease was the most common form, with lung, skin, and lymph nodes being the most common sites of infection. Prolonged fever, lymphadenopathy, hepatosplenomegaly, and cutaneous lesions were most commonly encountered; in fact, these represent a cadre of symptoms that may serve as a marker for AIDS. The diagnosis is best made by direct examination and culture of sputum specimens, skin biopsies, and lymph node aspirates. PCR assay of these specimens promises to greatly enhance the chances for making a diagnosis.

Trimethoprim–sulfamethoxazole, amphotericin B, and ketoconazole, either administered singly or in combination therapy, have been the agents most commonly used for the treatment of AIDS patients with paracoccidioidomycosis; however, about half of the patients treated in the Goldani and Sugar[118] series died, despite aggressive therapy.

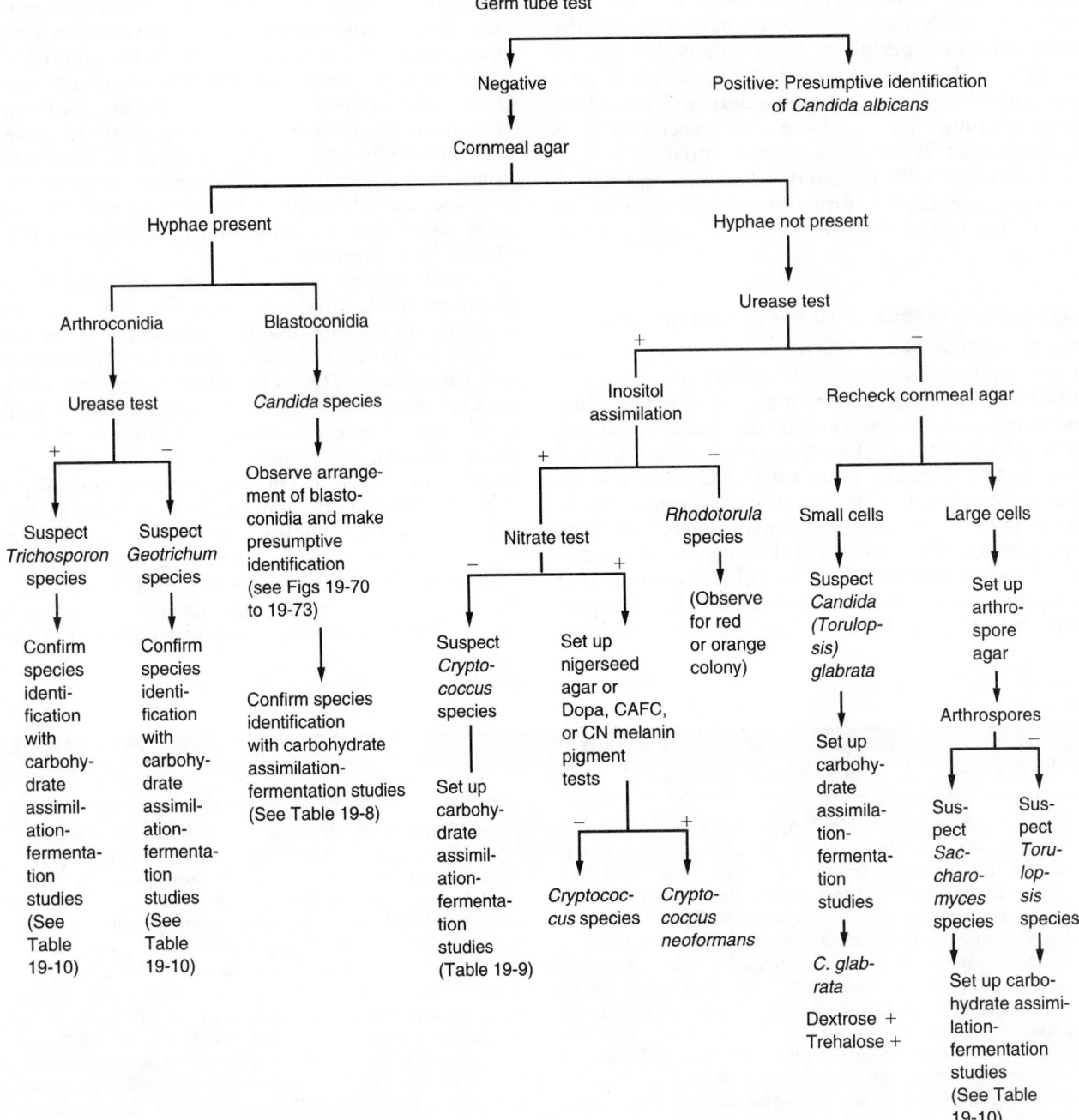

Figure 19-68
Identification schema for the workup of commonly encountered yeasts.

tive, a presumptive identification of *C. albicans* can be reported, and further testing is not necessary. If germ tubes are not observed, the plate can be incubated for an additional 24-48 hours and the presence of chlamydospores observed. *C. stellatoidea*—considered a phenotypic variant of *C. albicans*—and *C. tropicalis* can rarely produce germ tubes.[339] If a definitive identification of a given isolate is clinically necessary, on occasion, biochemical confirmation may be required. Berardinelli and Opheim[32] have also described a germ tube induction medium, consisting of three parts of

rabbit coagulase plasma with EDTA (BBL Microbiology Systems) and with two parts of Tryp-Soy broth (Scott Laboratories, Inc), which in their hands is more accurate and less expensive than other commercial germ tube media.

If germ tubes are not observed, a report "*Candida* not *C. albicans*" may be issued; however, about 5% of *C. albicans* are germ tube–negative.[303] False-negative results may also occur if too heavy an inoculum of yeast cells is used. If a definitive identification is clinically indicated, further testing must be carried out. A portion of the unknown colony should be inoculated onto a cornmeal agar plate and to the surface of a Christensen's urea agar slant (or the rapid urease test [see Box 19-6] should be performed). *C. albicans* does not produce urease; *C. neoformans* quickly converts urea agar to a pink color. Tween 80 (polysorbate) in a final concentration of 0.02% should be added to the cornmeal agar to reduce surface tension and enhance the formation of hyphae and blastoconidia (Box 19-5).

Cornmeal Agar Preparations. The cornmeal agar preparations should be examined for the presence of hyphae, blastoconidia, chlamydoconidia, or arthroconidia. The cornmeal morphology of several select species of yeasts is shown in Figures 19-70 through 19-73. If hyphae are present, first determine whether they are pseudohyphae, resulting from the pinching off process of blastoconidiation (and, therefore, have regular points of constriction), or whether they are true hyphae breaking up into arthroconidia. If the cornmeal growth reveals pseudohyphae and blastoconidia, the unknown yeast belongs to the genus *Candida*. Many times it may be possible to make a species identification based on the morphology and specific arrangement of the blastoconidia.

The production of chlamydospores is diagnostic of *C. albicans* (Fig. 19-70, *left*). *C. albicans* may also be tentatively identified if compact clusters of blastoconidia are formed at regular intervals along the pseudohyphae (Fig. 19-70, *right*). Smaller numbers of blastoconidia, widely spaced, singly or in small clusters, along the hyphae are more consistent with *C. tropicalis* (Fig. 19-71).

The formation of spider or "match-stick" colonies that satellite along the streak lines is suggestive of *C. parapsilosis* (Fig. 19-72); certain strains may also produce giant hyphae. A "long-in-stream" arrangement of the blastoconidia is the characteristic leading to a presumptive identification of *C. kefyr (pseudotropicalis)* (Fig. 19-73). This pattern may also be seen with *C. kruzei*.

If there is difficulty in deriving a presumptive identification from these growth patterns on cornmeal agar, carbohydrate fermentation or assimilation tests may be required for final species identification. The carbohydrate fermentation test assesses the ability of various species of yeast to form gas from different carbohydrates. Because endogenous carbohydrates adsorbed in the cell wall often produce false-positive reactions, fermentation studies are rarely performed in most clinical laboratories. Rather, they have been replaced by carbohydrate assimilation tests, in which the ability of different species of yeasts to grow in various single carbohydrate substrates is determined (see Chart 8). The specific fermentation and assimilation reactions of several species of *Candida* when tested with a number of carbohydrates are listed in Table 19-8.

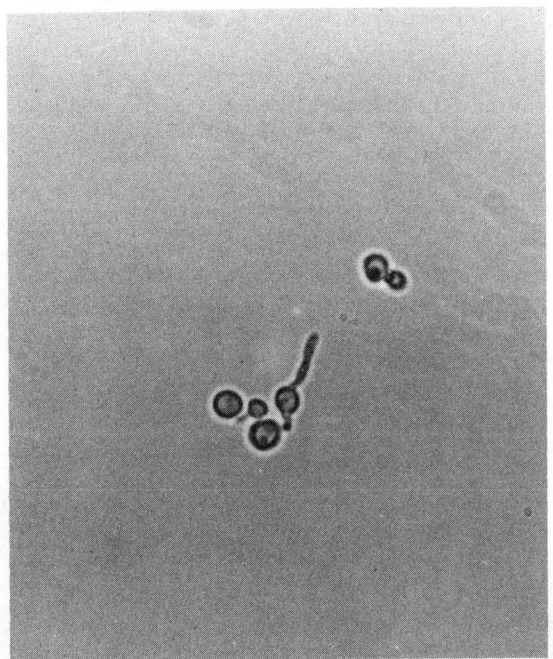

Figure 19-69
Photomicrograph of a germ tube, characteristic of *Candida albicans* (oil immersion).

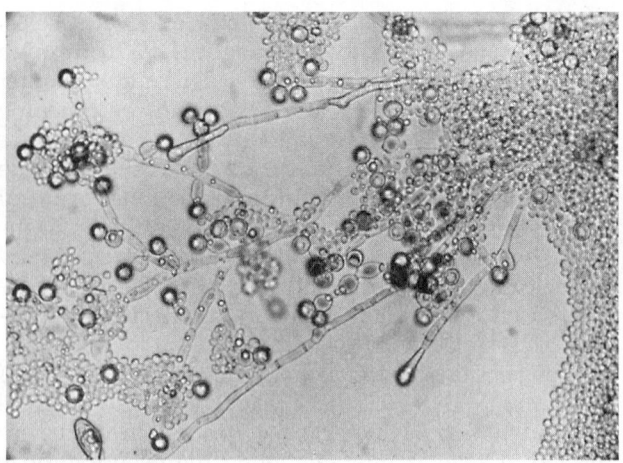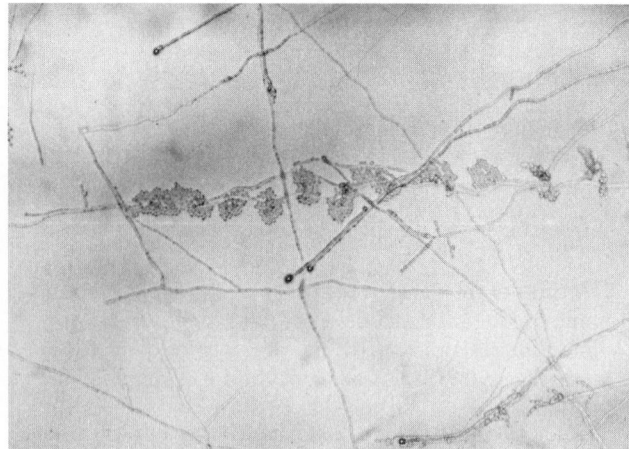

Figure 19-70
Photomicrographs of cornmeal agar preparation of *Candida albicans*.

The availability of packaged systems for the biochemical characterization of yeasts, described in more detail later in this chapter, has brought definitive species identification within the capability of virtually all laboratories. Yet, because of the relatively high cost of these products and the questionable clinical significance of many yeast isolates, it would seem prudent for microbiologists to make preliminary observations leading to, at least, a presumptive identification before subjecting every yeast recovered in the laboratory to a kit analysis. Each laboratory supervisor must also assess the accuracy of the system selected in keeping with the yeasts commonly recovered.

CANDIDA ALBICANS

Because *C. albicans* is the species of yeast most frequently cultured from clinical specimens, initial laboratory studies should be directed to its identification before additional costly tests are performed. (The mor-

phology of a typical colony is shown in Color Plate 19-6*A*.) Demonstration of the spiderlike colonies on eosin methylene blue (EMB) agar (see Color Plate 19-6*B*); or observation of the production of chlamydospores on cornmeal agar (Fig. 19-71, *left*) is an acceptable method for identifying *C. albicans*. The rapid germ tube test is used in most laboratories. Except for strains of *C. stellatoidea*, generally considered a phenotypic variant of *C. albicans*,[187] and rare strains of *C. tropicalis*, only *C. albicans* forms germ tubes under the test conditions (Fig. 19-69).[339] *C. albicans* is a common colonizer of human skin and mucous membranes. An average of 25% to 30% of individuals harbor *C. albicans* in their oral cavity, with higher incidence in infants, young children, and persons with AIDS.[187] Figure 19-74 is a photomicrograph of a gram stained smear obtained from oral secretions of a patient with "thrush." Note the distinct pseudohyphae and budding blastoconidia. Poor oral hygiene and dentures increases the oral carriage rate. Approximately 50% of persons har-

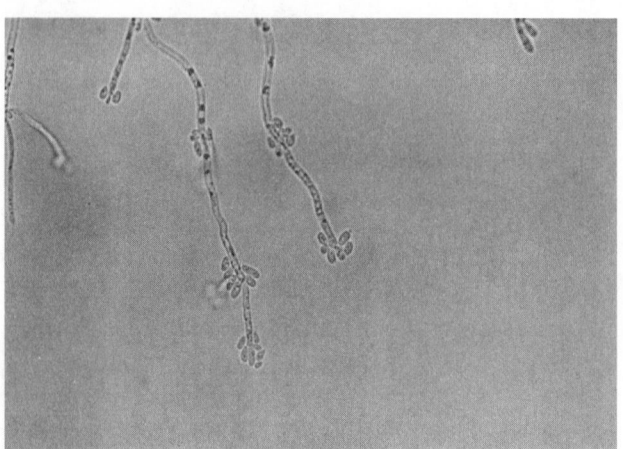

Figure 19-71
Photomicrograph of cornmeal agar preparation of *Candida tropicalis*.

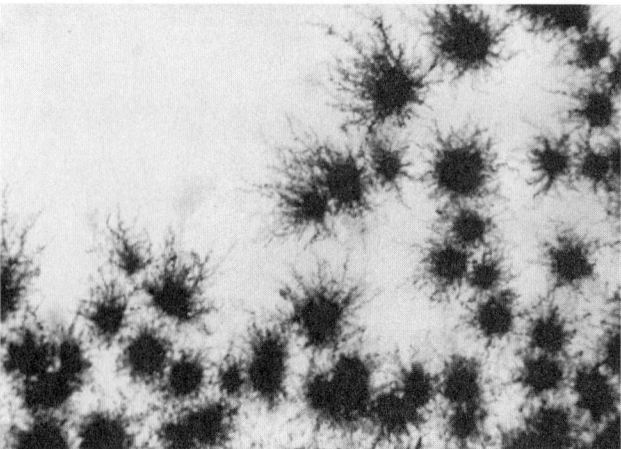

Figure 19-72
Photomicrograph of cornmeal agar preparation of *Candida parapsilosis*.

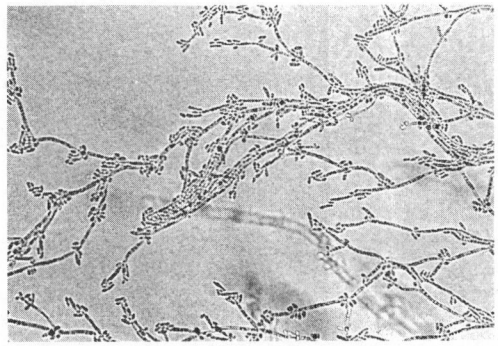

Figure 19-73
Photomicrograph of cornmeal agar preparation of *Candida kefyr*.

bor *C. albicans* in their gastrointestinal tract, and about 30% of females have vaginal colonization at one time or another. Vaginal carriage is particularly prevalent during pregnancy.

The ability of certain strains of *C. albicans* to undergo phenotypic "switching"—that is, the formation of different-appearing colony types, particularly those showing discontinuous fringe formation, when cultured on specific synthetic culture media—has a strong association with virulence and tissue invasion.[325] Jones and associates[159] investigated 59 strains of *C. albicans* divided into three groups: 1) isolates from feces; 2) iso-

lates from vaginal secretions; and 3) isolates causing clinically invasive disease. The rate of phenotypic switching demonstrated by the latter group was significantly in excess of that seen with the commensal isolates. The authors conclude from their work, and that obtained from other studies, that phenotypic switching between various forms allows a strain to select the phenotype optimal for invasion. *C. albicans* also expresses at least three types of surface adhesion molecules to facilitate attachment to epithelial surfaces, followed by deeper penetration of keratinized epithelia through the production of aspartyl proteinase and hyphal formation.[146,244]

CANDIDA SPECIES OTHER THAN CANDIDA ALBICANS

Species of *Candida*, other than *C. albicans*, are normal flora of cutaneous and mucocutaneous surfaces and are only rarely incriminated as agents of clinical disease. Nevertheless, several *Candida* species have been incriminated as agents of virtually every form of candidiasis, as reflected in numerous reports in the recent medical literature. Wingard,[372] in a review of 1591 cases of candidal infections published in 37 reports between 1952 and 1992, found that non–*Candida albicans* species were the causative agents in 46% of systemic infections: *C. tropicalis* accounted for 25% of the infections, *C. glabrata* for 8%, *C. parapsilosis* for 7%,

TABLE 19-8
BIOCHEMICAL CHARACTERISTICS OF MEDICALLY IMPORTANT *CANDIDA* SPECIES

	ASSIMILATION OF											
	MALTOSE	SUCROSE	TREHALOSE	GALACTOSE	CELLOBIOSE	XYLOSE	RAFFINOSE	LACTOSE	DULCITOL	MELIBIOSE	UREASE	NO₃–NO₂
Candida albicans	+	+	+	+	−	+	−	−	−	−	−	−
C. catenulata	+	−	+	+	−	+	−	−	−	−	−	−
C. guilliermondii	+	+	+	+	+	+	+	−	+	+	−	−
C. kefyr	−	+	−	+	+	+	+	−	−	−	−	−
C. krusei	−	−	−	−	−	−	−	+	−	−	+	−
C. lambica	−	−	−	−	−	+	−	−	−	−	−	−
C. lipolytica	−	−	−	−	−	−	−	−	−	−	+	−
C. lusitaniae	+	+	+	+	+	+	−	−	−	−	−	−
C. parapsilosis	+	+	+	+	−	+	−	−	−	−	−	−
C. rugosa	−	−	−	+	−	+	−	−	−	−	−	−
C. tropicalis	+	+	+	+	+	+	−	−	−	−	−	−
C. zeylanoides	−	−	+	−	−	+	−	−	−	−	−	−

Simplified grid and algorithm for the identification of *Candida* species. Glucose assimilation does not appear on this chart because all *Candida* species assimilate glucose; therefore, this characteristic has a separatory value of zero and does not discriminate between any species pair. Carbohydrate fermentation reactions also are omitted in this chart because these tests are rarely performed in most laboratories because of the variability in reactivity caused by contaminant carbohydrate adsorbed to the cell wall. The sequence of carbohydrates is arranged by descending order of the separatory values. *C. albicans* is usually identified either by observing germ tube formation or the production of chlamydospores on cornmeal agar. Notice that the grid does not allow the differentiation between *C. lusitaniae* and *C. tropicalis*; assimilation of arabinose is necessary to make the separation biochemically. *C. albicans* and *C. parapsilosis* also cannot be biochemically separated in this grid; however, this is not an issue even for germ tube-negative strains of *C. albicans* because the cornmeal morphology is distinctly different.

and *C. krusei* for 4%. From these reports, patients with leukemia were more likely to be infected with *C. albicans* or *C. tropicalis*; bone marrow transplant recipients were more likely to be infected with *C. krusei* or *C. lusitaniae*. An extensive review of new and emerging yeast pathogens has been published by Hazen.[133] In this review, 30 emerging yeast pathogens are cross-linked with 168 references for those interested in pursuing this subject in greater detail. Although of the non–*C. albicans* species *C. parapsilosis* and *C. glabrata* (particularly isolates in blood cultures), *C. krusei*, *C. guilliermondii*, *C. lipolytica*, and

---

CLINICAL CORRELATION BOX 19-15. *CANDIDA ALBICANS*

The infectious disease manifestations of *C. albicans* are primarily of three types, mucocutaneous, cutaneous, and systemic. Candidiasis of the mucous membranes may involve the oral cavity, the vaginal canal, the trachea and bronchi, and the alimentary canal, including esophagitis, gastritis, enteric, and perianal disease. Infections of the skin commonly involve the moist, intertriginous areas, such as in the webs of the fingers and toes, beneath the female breasts, in the armpits, and in the folds of the groin. Infection of the nails proper is known as onychomycosis; or paronychia if the folds of skin encasing the nails are involved. Diaper rash infection of neonates is also a common manifestation. Chronic mucocutaneous candidiasis is an opportunistic infection of skin and mucous membranes associated with several genetic defects involving compromised leukocyte function or the endocrine system. Chronic granulomatous disease, thymic dysplasia with and without hypogammaglobulinemia, hypoparathyroidism, and chronic granulomatous disease, the latter involving a myeloperoxidase defect of phagocytes precluding post-phagocytic killing of yeast forms, are among the predisposing conditions discussed by Rippon.[296] Systemic candidiasis is a relatively rare condition, occurring primarily as a terminal event in patients with debilitating, neoplastic (blast crisis of leukemias and lymphoma, for example), immunosuppressive diseases and following organ transplant, particularly during an acute rejection syndrome.

Oral candidiasis, a condition known as thrush (a term derived from the Scandinavian word *trosk*), is the most common clinical manifestation of candidiasis in humans. The infection is manifest as white patches or plaques on the buccal mucosa and tongue,[29] which may coalesce into a membrane in more serious infections. These adhere firmly to the epithelium, revealing a reddened, edematous base when removed. The diagnosis can be made by observing microscopically the characteristic pseudohyphae and blastoconidia in gram-stained preparations of smears prepared from some of the exudate (see Fig. 19-74).

Alteration of the normal flora secondary to prolonged antibiotic therapy, low pH of the salivary secretions in newborns, hypertrophy of the papillae of the tongue ("black hairy tongue"), and chronic glossitis are predisposing causes.[29] Oral candidiasis is seen in virtually 100% of patients with AIDS and often may be the initial sign.[182] Candidiasis is also the most common cause of opportunistic mucosal infections in HIV-positive women.[150a] These workers demonstrated that candidal vaginitis was not associated with significant reduction in CD4 lymphocyte counts, in contrast with those with oropharyngeal candidiasis in whom counts were reduced, and in those with esophageal involvement in whom CD4 counts were always below 0.1×10^9/L. Vaginal candidiasis in non-AIDS females, characterized by the production of a thick yellow, milky discharge, is often associated with diabetes, pregnancy, and the use of oral contraceptives.

Candidiasis of the urinary tract is relatively rare, manifesting as cystitis (more commonly caused by *Torulopsis* (*Candida*) *glabrata* and pyelonephritis, either ascending from a bladder infection or from hematogenous spread from a distant primary site of infection.[106] Aggregates of pseudohyphae and blastoconidia may be seen histologically in glomeruli, presumably in a microenvironment conducive to growth because of the lowered pH from Na^+ and H^+ ion exchanges.

A low pH environment may also explain the relatively high incidence of candidiasis at the gastroesophageal junction, particularly in patients with hematologic malignancy. Dysphagia, retrosternal pain, upper gastrointestinal bleeding, and nausea are associated symptoms. Esophageal candidiasis may also occur as an extension of oropharyngeal thrush, particularly in newborns. The diagnosis of candida enteritis is difficult to establish, because of the known colonization in the colon. Gupta and Ehrinpreis[125] report on ten elderly, malnourished, and critically ill patients with candida-associated diarrhea, based primarily on recovery of predominantly *C. albicans* from stool specimens, with decreased normal flora and the absence of other identifiable causes of the diarrhea. The diarrhea in these cases was secretory, without evidence of blood, pus, or mucus in stool specimens.

Endocarditis is most often seen in persons with pre-existing valvular disease, particularly following episodes of septicemia associated with the use of indwelling catheters, prolonged intravenous infusions, and intravenous drug abuse. Candidal septicemia may also be seen in patients receiving long-term antibiotics and corticosteroids. Although most strains of *C. albicans* can be recovered from blood cultures in most commercially available blood culture bottles, Marcelis and associates[204] report that culture media containing resin (specifically BACTEC PLUS high blood volume resin was used in their study) may enhance recovery, particularly in patients receiving antibiotics.

Candidal meningitis is a rare condition, secondary to dissemination from sites of infection in the gastrointestinal or respiratory tracts, or from septic emboli released from infected heart valves: Cases of CNS candidiasis are reported[103] in infants in intensive care nurseries secondary to intravenous therapy; cases of superinfection following acute bacterial meningitis were reported[115] in adults who have incurred CNS trauma or surgical intervention. They counsel that any patient with bacterial meningitis who do not improve with antimicrobial chemotherapy should be investigated for a *Candida* superinfection.

Rippon[296] cites five conditions that predispose to *C. albicans* infection: 1) extreme youth, during the period before normal flora is established; 2) physiologic conditions, such as pregnancy, endocrine dysfunctions, and diabetes mellitus; 3) prolonged administration of antibiotics that alter bacterial flora; 4) general debility, including immunosuppression, in particular AIDS, and defects in leukocyte function; and 5) barrier breaks secondary to a variety of surgical procedures and insertion of indwelling catheters.

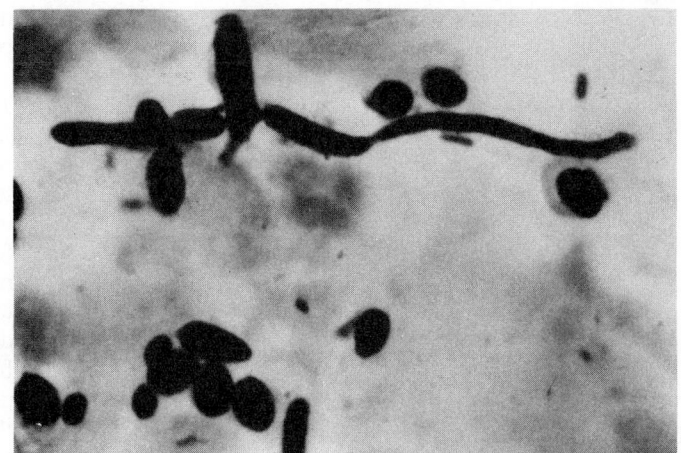

Figure 19-74
Photomicrograph of gram-stained sputum showing pseudohyphae and budding blastoconidia characteristic of *Candida albicans* (oil immersion).

C. kefyr (C. pseudotropicalis) were on the increase, Hazen[133] also mentions the emergence and significant increase in incidence of *Malassezia, Rhodotorula, Hansenula,* and *Trichosporon* species as non–*Candida* species isolates from clinical materials, with several citations to specific case reports of infections caused by these agents.

Several causes have been proposed for the sudden emergence of so many new species of yeasts as agents of infections. Included are the use of broad-spectrum antibiotics and antineoplastic agents, the administration of vancomycin, intravenous catheterization, and the increased number of patients with neutropenia and immunosuppression.[133] The possibility that widespread use of fluconazole accounts for the relative decrease in recovery of *C. albicans* from blood cultures, relative to other *Candida* species, has been proposed.[178] Cross-contamination by hospital personnel may also account for increases in yeast infections in certain environments. For example, a recent survey of hospital personnel[331] revealed that 70% of nurses and nonnursing hospital personnel carried yeasts on their hands, with *Rhodotorula* species and *C. parapsilosis* being those most frequently recovered.

Additional cases of infections with unusual *Candida* species culled from the literature include *C. utilis* fungemia in a 5-year-old AIDS victim associated with catheter implantation[7]; *C. norvegensis* peritonitis and invasive disease in a patient receiving peritoneal dialysis[238]; nail and skin infections from *C. ciferrii*[83]; a case of endophthalmitis secondary to *C. famata*[285]; and report of several cases of *C. lusitaniae* infections in patients with underlying predisposing conditions—leukemia, multiple myeloma, alcoholic hepatitis, bone marrow transplant, and traumatic accident.[40,126] Rippon[296] has linked several of these species with distinct clinical syndromes:

1. *C. parapsilosis*: paronychia, endocarditis, otitis externa, endophthalmitis, septic arthritis, and peritonitis[360]
2. *C. tropicalis*: vaginitis, intestinal infections, bronchopulmonary and systemic infections

3. *C. guilliermondii*: endocarditis, cutaneous candidiasis, and onychomycosis
4. *C. krusei*: rarely, endocarditis and vaginitis
5. *C. zeylanoides*: onychomycosis

The laboratory identification of the medically important *Candida* species is summarized in Table 19-8. Conventional biochemical tests or the use of one of several commercial systems described in more detail later are helpful in identifying these species. Cornmeal agar preparations should be set up as a quality control check. The morphology of more commonly encountered *Candida* species are shown in Figs. 19-70 and 19-73. Again, careful clinical correlations are necessary before accepting a *Candida* species isolate as being clinically significant and in need of a definitive identification.

YEASTS FORMING ARTHROCONIDIA

If the cornmeal agar growth reveals true hyphae and arthroconidia, *Trichosporon* and *Geotrichum* species are the most likely possibilities. Both produce arthroconidia on cornmeal agar and occasionally may be difficult to distinguish from one another. *Trichosporon* species, in addition to producing arthroconidia, also produce blastoconidia, rabbit-ear–like buds extending from both corners of the arthroconidia (Fig. 19-75). This feature is not commonly seen in cornmeal mounts but may be better observed in malt extract broth incubated at room temperature.

The arthroconidia of *Geotrichum* species may produce a hyphal extension from one corner, producing a structure colloquially known as "hockey sticks" (Fig. 19-76). Most species of *Trichosporon* produce urease; species of *Geotrichum* do not. Carbohydrate fermentation and assimilation studies, discussed later, may be required to differentiate species within these two genera if the results of the urease test are equivocal.

Trichosporon beigelii, classically the cause of white piedra, is the species most commonly encountered in clinical laboratories. Hoy and coauthors[147] review 19

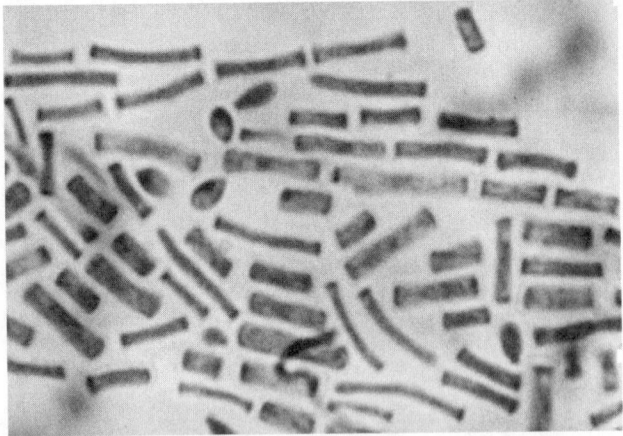

Figure 19-75
Photomicrograph of *Trichosporon beigelii* illustrating arthroconidia, one of which is showing the characteristic budding yeasts from two corners, simulating a "rabbit ears."

cases of disseminated *T. beigelii* infections in patients with a variety of neoplastic diseases being treated at M. D. Anderson Hospital in Houston over a 10-year period. Nonspecific febrile illness or pneumonia were the most common clinical manifestations among this group of patients. Three-fourths of these patients died, and the diagnosis was not suspected before their death in 25% of the autopsied cases. At autopsy, the findings were similar to those seen in patients with disseminated candidal infections. Histologically, the blastoconidia of *T. beigelii* also appeared similar to those of *Candida* species, although pseudohyphal formation was much less evident in the *T. beigelii* lesions. The authors also present the findings of disseminated *T. beigilii* infections in 24 patients with

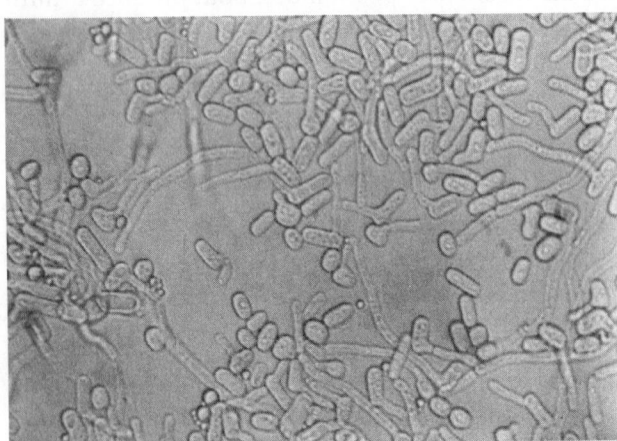

Figure 19-76
Photomicrograph of *Geotrichum candidum* illustrating arthroconidia, a few of which show the characteristic germ tube-like extension from one corner, simulating a "hockey stick."

neoplastic and nonneoplastic diseases culled from the past literature.

Disseminated infections have also been seen with *Trichosporon capitatum*, recently renamed *Blastoschizomyces capitatus*.[301] Martino and associates[206] have reviewed the clinical, pathologic, and microbiologic features of 12 patients with disseminated *B. capitatus* infections. Most of these patients were being treated for leukemia, lymphoma, or other hematologic malignancies that lead to neutropenia. The clinical presentation in patients with *B. capitatus* infections did not differ among these patients from those with other fungal infections, with evidence of hepatosplenic and pulmonary involvement evident in most cases. *B. capitatus* assimilates only glucose and galactose, in contrast to *T. beigelii*, which assimilates most carbohydrates, providing a ready means for identifying the two species. D'Antonio and coworkers[78] report a case of osteomyelitis and intervertebral diskitis secondary to *B. capitatus*, also in a leukemic patient. The source of infection was an infected central venous catheter. The formation of annelloconidia that undergo schizogonic division to form abundant arthroconidium-like structures, the capability of growing at 45°C, resistance to cycloheximide, and the incapability to produce urease were additional characteristics used in making the species identification of the isolate recovered from the laminectomy fragments removed in this case.[78]

Disseminated infections with *Geotrichum* species are less commonly encountered. The autopsy case of disseminated *G. candidum* infection in a patient with acute leukemia[163] is an unusual occurrence but does illustrate the potential virulence of this yeast. *G. candidum* assimilates only glucose, galactose, and xylose, which, except for the xylose utilization, is a pattern similar to that of *T. capitatus*.

YEASTS THAT DO NOT FORM HYPHAE IN CORNMEAL AGAR

Several yeasts do not produce pseudohyphae in cornmeal preparations. In these instances, the appropriate portion of the scheme outlined in Figure 19-68 must be followed. The yeast cells that are present (blastoconidia) should be examined carefully for the presence of a capsule, and if seen, it is highly suggestive for the presence of *Cryptococcus neoformans*.

CRYPTOCOCCOSIS AND *CRYPTOCOCCUS NEOFORMANS*

C. neoformans is a yeast with natural habitat in the soil, particularly in dirt with an alkaline pH and rich in nitrogen. These latter conditions are optimally achieved in soil mixed with the excreta of turkeys, pigeons, starlings, and other birds. *C. neoformans* yeast cells may become highly concentrated in the feces of birds that have the habit of picking for food in contaminated soil. Thus, humans who are exposed to dirt and dust containing bird droppings, such as poultry farm workers and groundskeepers of city parks in endemic areas, are particularly at risk for contracting cryptococcosis. Because bats also serve as mechanical carriers of *C. neoformans*, archaeologists and explorers who frequent bat-infested caves are also at increased risk.

Before the onset of the AIDS epidemic, the annual incidence of cryptococcal infections in the United States was estimated at one to two new cases per million population.[311] Specifically, 1264 cases in the United States were reported between 1965 and 1977. The frequency has increased until cryptococcosis now constitutes the fourth most common opportunistic infection in patients with AIDS.[272] Currie and Casadavall[76] calculate the prevalence rate of cryptococcosis among HIV-infected individuals in New York City to be 6.1% to 8.5% (1994), representing 1277 cases in 1991 alone, more than the 12-year incidence in the entire United States as cited in the foregoing. Of all cases of cryptococcosis in New York City in 1991, 96% were HIV-related. Incidence rates are even higher in other parts of the world; for example, cryptococcosis in AIDS patients living in sub-Saharan, equatorial Africa approaches 30%.[275] During initial therapy, up to 15% of these patients die; 60% succumb within 1 year. An excellent comprehensive review of cryptococcosis in the era of AIDS has been published by Mitchell and Perfect.[224]

Laboratory Identification of *Cryptococcus neoformans.*
A yeast isolate can be suspected as a *Cryptococcus* species when a mucoid colony is observed on primary recovery medium (see Color Plate 19-6C). The formation of a long string when one retracts an inoculating needle from the surface of the colony is one clue that abundant capsular material may be present. An India ink or nigrosin preparation can be made from a small inoculum of such a colony, and the presence of irregularly sized yeast cells, 4 to 10 μm in diameter and surrounded by capsular material, is also supporting evidence (Fig. 19-77). The capsule, however, may be lost in cells obtained from cultures, particularly after one or more passes in subculture. The spherical shape, irregular size and separation by capsular material are also helpful clues to the identification of Cryptococcus neoformans in tissue sections (see Figs. 19-78).

If a species of *Cryptococcus* is suspected in the identification of an unknown yeast, *C. neoformans* must be specifically ruled in or out by biochemical or serologic testing because of its potential pathogenicity for humans. Table 19-9 lists the differential features by which *C. neoformans* can be differentiated from other *Cryptococcus* species.

A positive urease test result also suggests *Cryptococcus* species (Box 19-6). The test also can be performed by using Christensen's urea agar. Strong urease-producing strains of *C. neoformans* often begin to produce a color change within 2 hours at 35°C.[162] Alternatively, one can use the rapid selective urease test described by Zimmer and Roberts,[382] for which positive test readings can be made within 10 to 30 minutes.

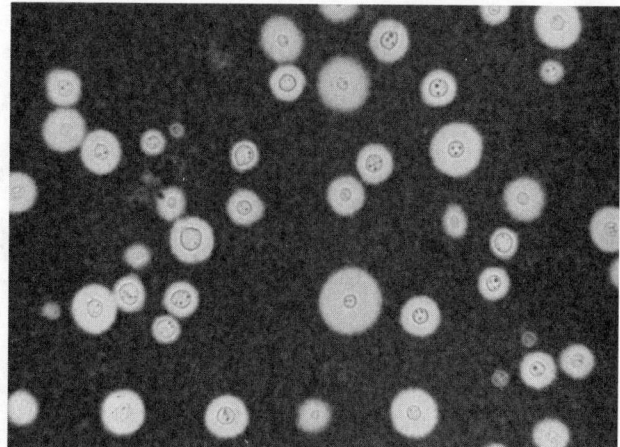

Figure 19-77
Photomicrograph of an India ink preparation illustrating the irregular-sized, encapsulated, spherical yeast cells of *Cryptococcus neoformans.*

Species of *Rhodotorula*, *Candida krusei*, and *Trichosporon* species also produce urease. *C. krusei* and *Trichosporon* species produce hyphae on cornmeal, the former with blastoconidia, the latter with arthroconidia. *Rhodotorula* species, as the name indicates (*rhodo*, "red"), produce orange or orange-red colonies (Color Plate 19-6,F) and inositol is not assimilated, two characteristics that are usually sufficient to exclude them from *Cryptococcus* species.

The inability of *C. neoformans* to reduce nitrates to nitrites is another helpful presumptive test in screening suspected colonies. Rhodes and Roberts[291] have described an easy and rapid modification of the nitrate reduction test, using semisolid indole nitrate medium and a heavy inoculum of the organism. The production of a red color after adding sulfanilic acid and α-naphthylamine to a 48- to 72-hour culture indicates a positive test result.

A rapid nitrate reduction test has also been described by Hopkins and Land,[145] which uses a cotton-tipped applicator that has been impregnated with an inorganic nitrate substrate (Box 19-7).

The niger seed agar test of Staib and Senskau[326] is quite useful for detecting and identifying *C. neoformans*. The plate is heavily inoculated with the test organism and is incubated at 37°C for at least 1 week. The production of a red-brown or maroon pigment is characteristic of *C. neoformans* (see Color Plate 19-6D).

The same agar can also be used to confirm the identification of *C. neoformans*. Ferric ammonium sulfate, 0.015%, is substituted for the caffeic acid in the TOC formula. A dehydrated caffeic acid paper disk is then placed in the area of inoculation. If the unknown colony is *C. neoformans*, a deep maroon-black pigment develops adjacent to the disk.

C. neoformans produces phenoloxidase, an enzyme that is necessary for the metabolism of 3,4-dihydroxy-

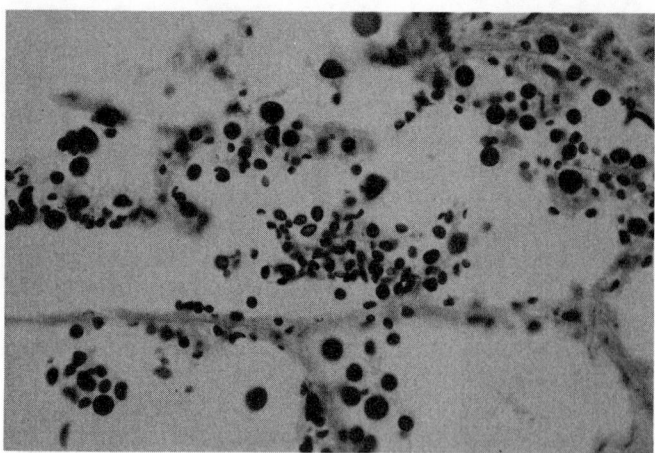

Figure 19-78
Photomicrograph of a GMS-stained section of lung illustrating yeast forms of *Cryptococcus neoformans*. Note that the yeast cells are widely separated by spaces previously filled with capsular polysaccharide and vary considerably in size. Occasional budding forms attached by a narrow base are observed (oil immersion). (Courtesy G. D. Roberts)

phenylalanine (DOPA) and other phenolic compounds in the pathway of melanin synthesis.[242] It was determined that the compound 3,4-dihydrocinnamic acid (caffeic acid) is the melanin-producing substrate in niger seed agar (see Color Plate 19-6D). Hopfer and Groschel have described a caffeic acid test for the rapid identification of *C. neoformans*.[144] Subsequently, Wang and coauthors[356] described a more convenient modification of the caffeic acid test that uses filter paper disks impregnated with a caffeic acid–ferric citrate reagent.

The media or test systems containing DOPA, an immediate precursor in the metabolic synthesis of melanin, should be used for the detection of pigment production.[164,356] The niger seed agar and caffeic acid tests just described lack the necessary de-

gree of sensitivity and specificity in demonstrating pigment production by some strains of *C. neoformans*, a problem that is virtually eliminated by using test media containing DOPA as the phenoloxidase substrate. *C. neoformans* (CN) medium contains DOPA as the substrate for phenoloxidase, glucose, glycine, glutamine, asparagine, and the pH indicator phenol red. The medium is available from Flow Laboratories (Roslyn NY) and is 92% sensitive and 99% specific for the rapid identification of *C. neoformans*.

Kaufmann and Merz[164] have described two rapid pigmentation tests that are highly sensitive for the detection of melanin pigment production by *C. neoformans*, a cornmeal–Tween-80 agar containing caffeic acid, and a new phenoloxidase test using a

TABLE 19-9
BIOCHEMICAL CHARACTERISTICS OF MEDICALLY IMPORTANT *CRYPTOCOCCUS* SPECIES

	ASSIMILATION OF											
	MALTOSE	SUCROSE	TREHALOSE	GALACTOSE	CELLOBIOSE	XYLOSE	RAFFINOSE	LACTOSE	DULCITOL	MELIBIOSE	UREASE	NO₃-NO₂
Cryptococcus neoformans	+	+	+	+	+	+	+	−	+	−	+	−
Cryptococcus albidus	+	+	+	+	+	+	+	+	+	+	+	+
Cryptococcus laurentii	+	+	+	+	+	+	+	+	+	+	+	−
Cryptococcus luteolus	+	+	+	+	+	+	+	−	+	+	+	−
Cryptococcus terreus	+	−	+	+	+	+	−	+	−	−	+	+
Cryptococcus uniguttulatus	+	+	−	−	−	+	+	−	−	−	+	−

Simplified grid and algorithm for the identification of *Cryptococcus* spp. Glucose assimilation does not appear on this chart because all *Cryptococcus* spp. assimilate glucose; therefore, this characteristic has a separatory value of zero and does not discriminate between any species pair. Carbohydrate fermentation reactions also are omitted in this chart, for these tests are rarely performed in most laboratories because of the variability in reactivity caused by contaminant carbohydrate adsorbed to the cell wall. This scheme would rarely be used to identify *C. neoformans*, because it is the only *Cryptococcus* spp. that produces phenol oxidase, which is detected by using niger seed (birdseed) agar or the caffeic acid test. All other species have at least one characteristic by which it can be separated from a closely related mate.

BOX 19-6. PROCEDURE FOR A RAPID UREASE TEST

1. The tip of a cotton applicator, impregnated with Christensen's urease agar base, is swept across the surface of two or three isolated colonies of the organism to be studied.

2. The inoculated applicator is placed into a test tube containing 3 drops of 1% benzalkonium chloride (an exact pH of 4.86 ± 0.01 is critical for accurate test results).

3. The tip of the swab is swirled firmly against the bottom of the tube to embed the organism into the cotton fibers.

4. The tube is plugged with cotton and incubated at 45°C.

5. The tube is examined at 10, 15, 20 and 30 minutes—a positive test result is indicated by the development of a red-purple color.

DOPA–ferric citrate-impregnated blotting paper strip. Clinical isolates of *C. neoformans* produce a dark brown to black pigment in these test systems within 60 to 90 minutes. When used in conjunction with the rapid urease test of Zimmer and Roberts[382] and the rapid nitrate reduction test of Hopkins and Land,[145] rapid definitive identification of *C. neoformans* is possible. If the results of these two tests are equivocal, carbohydrate assimilation tests may be necessary to identify members of the *Cryptococcus* genus. Carbohydrate fermentation tests produce less reliable results and are no longer commonly performed in clinical laboratories. The carbohydrate fermentation and assimilation reactions for several species of *Cryptococcus* are listed in Table 19-9.

BOX 19-7. PROCEDURE FOR A RAPID NITRATE REDUCTION TEST

1. The tip of the applicator is swept across two or three colonies of the yeast to be tested. The inoculate swab is then swirled against the bottom of an empty test tube to embed the yeast cells within the fibers of the swab.

2. The tube and swab are incubated for 10 minutes at 45°C. The swab is incubated for 10 minutes at 45°C.

3. The swab is removed and 2 drops each of α-naphthylamine and sulfanilic acid reagents are added to the tube.

4. The swab is replaced in the tube to allow it to absorb the reagents and the immediate development of a red color indicates a positive reaction.

Nucleic acid probe technology offers the possibility of making a rapid culture confirmation of *C. neoformans*.[345] Huffnagle and Gander,[149] using the *Cryptococcus neoformans* AccuProbes (Gen-Probe, La Jolla, Ca), demonstrated 100% sensitivity and specificity in the identification of 42 *C. neoformans* isolates.

OTHER NONHYPHAL-FORMING YEASTS OF MEDICAL IMPORTANCE

Several other species of yeasts recovered from clinical specimens may be of clinical significance. Of these, *Torulopsis glabrata* is most frequently recovered, primarily from the urinary tract of females with cystitis. Table 19-10 lists the biochemical characteristics by which these species of yeasts can be differentiated.

TORULOPSIS (CANDIDA) GLABRATA

If a yeast is recovered on blood agar from a clinical specimen, particularly the urine, that grows as small, glossy, smooth colonies (see Color Plate 19-6E) and that produces tiny, regular-sized yeast cells in compact clusters in cornmeal agar preparations, without the formation of pseudohyphae, *T. glabrata* should be considered. *T. glabrata* is the accepted name for this organism, according to McGinnis and Rinaldi.[211] Kwon-Chung and Bennett,[187] on the other hand, indicating that "the name *Torulopsis* has not been settled to everyone's satisfaction," prefer the genus designation *Candida*, arguing that failure to produce pseudohyphae is an arbitrary separation between the genera *Candida* and *Torulopsis* because rare pseudohyphal-producing strains of the latter have been identified, and that the genus *Candida* "is known to include yeasts with diverse physiologic and morphologic characteristics." We elect not to enter this taxonomic quagmire, but from a purely practical standpoint, prefer to use *Torulopsis* as the genus designation. Strains that we encounter in the clinical laboratory do not produce pseudohyphae. The observation of small, regular-sized, compact clusters of yeast cells in cornmeal agar preparations and in tissue sections is a characteristic of *T. glabrata*, which is strikingly different from the pseudohyphae produced by other *Candida* species.

T. glabrata is an agent of urinary tract infections, constituting about 20% of all yeast isolates from urine specimens.[112] Cases of endocarditis,[55] meningitis,[16] and disseminated infection[140] caused by *T. glabrata* have been reported in the recent literature. *T. glabrata* assimilates both glucose and trehalose, an assimilation pattern that is helpful in making the laboratory identification.

RHODOTORULA SPECIES

The observation of a red or orange-red yeast is diagnostic of *Rhodotorula* species (see Color Plate 19-6F).

The recovery of *C. neoformans* from clinical specimens must always be considered significant unless proved otherwise. This is not true for other *Cryptococcus* species, when contamination or recovery of a commensal is more likely. Although the incidence of cryptococcosis has been relatively low in the past (about 300 cases per year in the United States), the current observation that *C. neoformans* is one of a select group of microorganisms causing infection in patients with AIDS will elicit renewed efforts to obtain cultures for laboratory identification. Human cryptococcosis generally manifests clinically as pulmonary, CNS, and disseminated or visceral forms of disease. Cutaneous and osseous forms of disease are less common occurrences. It should be remembered that CNS disease may occur without evidence of disease elsewhere; likewise, lungs and other organs can be involved in the absence of CNS disease. Primary cryptococcal infection of the skin is rare; usually cutaneous disease is a manifestation of systemic infection.[128]

Central nervous system cryptococcosis may be insidious in onset, with mild headaches, memory lapses, or personality changes being the only clues. Low-grade fever may also be present. As the disease progresses, signs and symptoms suggestive of meningitis include nuchal rigidity, tenderness of the neck, and positive knee and leg flexion tests (Brudzinki's and Kernig's signs). In cases of localized cryptococcomas, localizing signs, such as paralysis, hemiparesis, and jacksonian seizures, may be evident. Depending on the location of the cryptococcoma, blurring of vision, diplopia, ophthalmoplegia, slurred speech, double vision, and unsteadiness of gait may occur. Papilledema is generally a sign of increased intracranial pressure. Weight loss, malaise, persistence of fever, nausea, vomiting, and dizziness may be experienced as the disease progresses. In progressive fulminant or fatal cases, mental changes may be marked (agitation, irritability, confusion, hallucinations, psychosis) developing into delirium, coma, and finally death. In disseminated cases, all viscera and organ systems may be involved. Ulcerative or nodular cutaneous manifestations occur in 5% of patients; osseous lesions occur in 10%.

The diagnosis of CSF cryptococcosis can be made by observing typical encapsulated, singly budding yeast cells in the cerebrospinal fluid in an India ink preparation (Fig. 19-77), or recovering the organism in culture. The time-honored India ink preparation, rapid and easy to perform, is nevertheless positive in only about 50% of non–HIV-infected patients, and in 74% to 88% of HIV-positive patients.[39] More commonly, the diagnosis is made by detecting cryptococcal antigen in CSF, using either commercially available anticryptococcal globulin-sensitized latex particles; or, with an enzyme immunoassay using polyclonal antibody capture and monoclonal detection methods.[109] The latex tests provide quantitative results, making prognostication and assessment of efficacy of therapy theoretically possible. However, prognostic information gained from antigen quantitation after the course of therapy is of limited value and the trauma of repeated spinal taps is unwarranted.[276] However, during therapy of acute disease, an unchanged or increased titer of antigen was correlated with clinical and microbiologic failure to respond to therapy.

Tanner and associates[335] evaluated the performance of five commercial kit systems (Calas [Meridian Diagnostics], Crypto-LA [International Biological Labs], MycoImmune [MicroScan], Immy [Immunomycologies], and Premier [Meridian Diagnostics]) compared with culture. These systems performed equally well, with 93% to 100% sensitivity and 93% to 98% specificity in detecting cryptococcal antigen in CSF. Kiska and coworkers[179] found the performance of CRYPO-LEX (Trinity Laboratories, Raleigh, NC), a new latex agglutination test, to be 97% to 100% sensitive and specific in detecting cryptococcal antigen in either blood or serum of 67 patients with cryptococcosis. False-positive latex agglutination reactions for cryptococcal antigen in serum may be found in the presence of rheumatoid factor and other macroglobulins in patients with systemic lupus erythematosus and sarcoidosis. These false-positive reactions can be neutralized by pretreatment of the serum with pronase,[329] or by treatment with 2-β-mercaptoethanol (2-ME).[367] Boom and associates[45] caution that inoculating loops that have been used to sample colonies from chocolate agar surfaces should not be placed back in the sample in making a second subculture. Syneresis fluid, obtained from the surface of chocolate agar plates, even in trace amounts, can result in false-positive latex agglutinations. Certain disinfectants and soaps[39] may also produce false-positive test results, and those performing assays must guard against these contaminants. Heelan and coworkers[135] also suggest that the latex test be performed before subcultures are made, as the platinum wire inoculating loop may contain interfering substances.

These interference factors do not present a problem with EIA-based assays. Engler and Shea[100] demonstrated that the Premier EIA assay (Meridian Diagnostics, Cincinnati OH) did not produce false-positive reactions with serum specimens containing syneresis fluid, rheumatoid factor, or the interference factors in 23 sera obtained from patients with systemic lupus erythematosus. This increase in specificity is to be expected when species-specific monoclonal antibodies are used in the assay. Chapin-Robertson and colleagues[61] also found that urine serves as an alternative fluid for the detection of cryptococcal antigen. In a study of 21 cases of cryptococcosis in AIDS patients, cryptococcal antigen was found in the urine in all cases in whom antigen was also present in the CSF or serum specimens.

The natural history, clinical presentation, diagnosis, and therapy of primary pulmonary cryptococcosis has been elucidated in a review of 41 patients.[174] The authors were able to establish the diagnosis when an abnormal chest roentgenogram was associated with the isolation of *C. neoformans* from respiratory secretions or the observation of mucicarmine-positive, typically appearing organisms in sections of lung tissue (see Fig. 19-78). Most patients in their series had underlying conditions predisposing to cryptococcal infection: immunosuppressive therapy (28/41), diabetes mellitus (20/41), hematologic or lymphoreticular malignancies (12/41), recent renal transplant (10/41), and connective tissue diseases or chronic active hepatitis (5/41). Seven of the patients had no detectable underlying abnormalities. Constitutional symptoms predominated—fever and malaise occurred in over one-half of the patients. Chest pain, dyspnea, weight loss, and night sweats, in varying combinations, were observed in

(continued)

from one quarter to one third of the patients. Only 7 of the patients complained of cough. Seven patients were asymptomatic and studied only because of abnormal roentgenograms. The abnormalities observed on chest x-ray films included circumscribed mass lesions, alveolar or interstitial infiltrates, abscesses with air–fluid levels or cavitary lesions (7/41), solitary coin lesions, and multiple small rounded opacities. In contrast with what previous reports lead one to believe, the lung lesions as disclosed radiographically in this series were not confined to the lower lobes. Pleural effusion was seen in 7 of their patients. In 4 patients, the pulmonary lesions were observed 4 to 5 weeks before onset of CNS disease, leading the authors to conclude that the primary focus of cryptococcosis occurs in the lung, which may resolve spontaneously even in the face of dissemination.

Cryptococcosis is commonly associated with AIDS. In the study of a series of 106 patients with AIDS,[64] cryptococcosis was the initial manifestation in 45%. Witt and associates[375] also report a case of a previously healthy man in whom bone marrow and mediastinal cryptococcosis were the first manifestations of AIDS. In a study of 68 HIV-positive patients,[69] *C. neoformans* was the initial AIDS-defining illness in 51 (75%). Most of these patients presented with CNS symptoms, most commonly fever, headache, and altered mental status. These findings were consistent with the symptoms reported in non-AIDS patients with CNS cryptococcosis; in contrast to non–HIV-infected patients, those in the study here cited rarely had signs of meningeal inflammation, such as meningismus, photophobia, and cranial nerve palsies. Many of these patients had normal CSF profiles, with positive India ink capsule stains, indicating an increased fungal load with diminished host response.

Primary pulmonary cryptococcosis may also herald the diagnosis of AIDS; however, in studies independently reported,[191, 358] the diagnosis may not be made because of the lack of primary signs, symptoms, or radiographic findings. They suggest that the Riu stain (commonly used to demonstrate bacterial flagellae) as an excellent way to demonstrate organisms in smears prepared from bronchoscopic brushings or needle aspirates. In an autopsy study of 11 patients with AIDS and cryptococcosis,[113] several patterns of infection were found: diffuse interstitial infiltration involving all lobes, mixed interstitial and intra-alveolar infiltrates, and nodular infiltrates diffusely dispersed. Cellular inflammation and granuloma formations were uncommon. In a study of 18 AIDS patients with advanced cryptococcal meningitis,[93] pulmonary symptoms were experienced up to 4 months before the development of CNS symptoms. They advocate more aggressive attempts to diagnose pulmonary cryptococcosis in AIDS patients with low CD4 counts who develop pneumonia symptoms, particularly the full identification of any yeast species recovered from sputum and bronchoalveolar lavage fluid specimens.

In cornmeal agar preparations, pseudohyphae are not formed; rather, regular-sized yeast cells, averaging 5 μm in diameter, often with single buds, are observed. *Rhodotorula* species are urease-positive. Recovery of these organisms in clinical specimens is generally of academic interest only because only rare infections caused by this yeast have been reported.

MALASSEZIA FURFUR

As discussed before in the dermatophyte section, *M. furfur* is the cause of superficial infections of the skin known as tinea (pityriasis) versicolor. Systemic infections and septicemia have also been reported, most commonly associated with deep-line vascular catheters in patients receiving parenteral therapy. Many of the emulsions used for parenteral therapy are rich in long-chain fatty acids. An ideal microenvironment is established at the catheter site where a small amount of the oily emulsion can pool, supporting growth of the endogenous lipophilic organisms present on the skin surface. The catheter provides a barrier break in the skin through which the proliferating organisms can enter the blood stream.

The organism can be recovered in culture on Sabouraud's dextrose agar or 5% sheep blood agar that has been overlaid with long-chain fatty acid, such as contained in olive oil. Yeastlike colonies, creamy in consistency, develop slowly after 2 to 4 days' incubation at 35°C (growth at 25°C does not occur; see Color Plate 19-6G).

SACCHAROMYCES SPECIES

Saccharomyces species are not considered pathogenic for humans, although isolated cases of septicemia have been reported.[66,101,237] Tawfik and associates[336] report a case of polymicrobic pneumonia including *S. cerevisiae* in a patient with AIDS. This yeast was also recovered from cultures of lungs, spleen, oral mucosa, and small intestine at autopsy, indicating disseminated disease. They also review eight previously reported cases of saccharomyces infections in patients with a variety of underlying conditions, including two receiving hemodialysis in treatment of chronic renal failure, another receiving long-term steroids in treatment of chronic obstructive pulmonary disease, a cardiac prosthetic valve recipient, and a burn victim. Infections in two patients were associated with ingestion of Brewer's yeast, one of whom was cured after discontinuation of the ingestion.

Saccharomyces species produce large yeast cells in cornmeal preparations and also produce ascospores when grown on ascospore agar medium (see Color Plate 19-6H). This medium contains potassium acetate (10 g), yeast extract (2.5 g), glucose (1 g), agar (30 g), and distilled water (1 L). The unknown colony is inoc-

TABLE 19-10

Biochemical Characteristics of Medically Important Miscellaneous yeasts

	ASSIMILATION OF											
	MALTOSE	*SUCROSE*	*TREHALOSE*	*GALACTOSE*	*CELLOBIOSE*	*XYLOSE*	*RAFFINOSE*	*LACTOSE*	*DULCITOL*	*MELIBIOSE*	*UREASE*	*NO₃-NO₂*
Torulopsis glabrata	−	−	+	−	−	−	−	−	−	−	−	−
Rhodotorula rubra	+	+	+	+	+	+	+	−	−	−	−	−
Saccharomyces cerevisiae	+	+	+	+	−	−	+	−	−	−	−	−
Hansonella anomala	+	+	+	+	+	+	−	−	−	−	−	+
Trichosporon beigelii	+	+	+	+	+	+	+	+	+	+	+	−
Geotrichum candidum	−	−	−	+	−	+	−	−	−	−	−	−
Blastoschizomyces capitatus	−	−	−	+	−	−	−	−	−	−	−	−
Protetheca wickerhamii	−	−	+	+	−	−	−	−	−	−	−	−

Simplified grid and algorithm for the identification of the yeasts included. Glucose assimilation does not appear on this chart because all yeast species included here assimilate glucose; therefore, this characteristic has a separatory value of zero and does not discriminate between any species pair. Carbohydrate fermentation reactions are also omitted in this chart, for these tests are rarely performed in most laboratories because of the variability in reactivity caused by contaminant carbohydrate adsorbed to the cell wall. Most of the species included here are identified by alternative methods. *T. glabrata* is usually identified by its colonial morphology both on blood agar or Sabouraud's dextrose agar, together with selective assimilation of glucose and trehalose; *R. rubra* usually produce distinctive orange-red colonies that, coupled with a rapid positive urease reaction, are distinctive; *T. beigelii* and *G. candidum* are initially suspected because both produce arthroconidia in cornmeal agar preparations. Most strains of *T. beigelii* are urease-positive and produce blastoconidia that bud from two corners of the arthroconidia; *G. candidum* is urease-negative and produces germ tubelike extensions from one corner of the arthroconidia, simulating hockey sticks; *B. capitatus* is morphologically difficult to distinguish from *T. beigelii*, but is asaccharolytic; both *H. anomala* and *S. cerevisiae* produce ascospores when grown on ascospore agar, but their caplike, rather than spherical, morphology and the ability to assimilate cellobiose are features identifying *H. anomala*; and *P. wickerhamii* is generally recognized by identifying sporangia in direct preparations, although the selective assimilation of trehalose and galactose as shown here is distinctive.

ulated onto the surface of an ascospore agar plate and incubated at 30°C for up to 10 days. Ascospores are acid-fast and appear as large, thick-walled structures when stained with the Kinyoun stain.

PACKAGED YEAST IDENTIFICATION KITS

Several packaged kits for identifying yeasts have been introduced by commercial companies. Bowman and Ahearn,[48] in a study conducted not long after three of the kits had been introduced, found that the API 20C system (Analytab Products, Plainview NY) gave 95% agreement with conventional methods, the Micro Drop system (Clinical Sciences, Whippany NJ) 84% agreement, and the Uni-Yeast-Tek system (Remel Laboratories, Lenexa KS) 99% agreement. The three systems currently used in the majority of clinical microbiology laboratories are the 20C yeast identification system, the Uni-Yeast-Tek system and the VITEK yeast identification card. Two additional systems have also been recently introduced.

The current API 20C yeast identification system has an improvement over the first-generation strip. The carbohydrate fermentation tests included in the initial system have been eliminated, and the 20 cupules in the present version contain freeze-dried carbohydrate substrates that do not degrade after prolonged storage. The cupules are easy to inoculate with the yeast sus-

pension to be tested, and the oil or wax overlay used in the first-generation strip to maintain an anaerobic environment is no longer required.

The individual cupules in the strip are inoculated with a yeast suspension in molten agar, and the unit is incubated for 72 hours at 30°C. The organisms grow only in cupules in which the specific carbohydrate has been assimilated, producing a cloudiness in the agar medium that is easy to visualize against bold lines printed on the plastic surface behind the cupules. Nineteen assimilation tests can be determined (one cupule is used as a growth control), and the manufacturer provides a profile index by which the pattern of assimilation reactions can be used to establish the identity of the yeast. Thus, it may be necessary to obtain cultures from multiple sites, particularly in urine samples, to make the diagnosis in suspected cases.

Beushing and colleagues[37] found a 97% agreement between the API 20C system and conventional methods in a study of 505 yeast strains. Of the 17 strains incorrectly identified, one or more assimilation results were incorrect or the numerical code numbers derived for the assimilation pattern were not listed in the profile index. However, these deficiencies have been corrected. The density of the inoculum must be carefully regulated—if the suspension is too heavy, false-positive results can occur; if too light, false-negative results tend to occur.

The Uni-Yeast-Tek system (Remel Laboratories, Lenexa KS) consists of a multicompartmented plastic dish, with each compartment containing a different carbon assimilation agar medium. Also incorporated is a central well containing cornmeal–Tween 80 agar for determining mycelial growth and chlamydospore production. Urea agar, nitrate assimilation agar, and additionally, a 0.05% glucose–2.6% beef extract broth for performing the germ tube test are provided. The carbohydrate concentrations vary from 1% to 4% and include sucrose, lactose, maltose, cellobiose, soluble starch, trehalose and raffinose.

Each of the compartments is inoculated through a small portal on the side of the well with 1 drop of distilled water suspension of the yeast to be tested, equal in turbidity to a McFarland 4 standard. The cornmeal agar is inoculated by making two or three parallel slashes into the agar with an inoculating needle containing a small portion of the yeast colony to be tested. A number 1 flame-sterilized coverslip is placed over the area of inoculation. The plastic dish is incubated for 2 to 7 days at 30°C or 35°C. The carbohydrate assimilation compartments are observed for a blue to yellow (positive test) color change, the nitrate medium for a blue to blue-green (nitrate reduction) color change, and the cornmeal agar is examined microscopically for the presence of hyphae and blastoconidia.

In a current study of this system, for which the database has been recently expanded to include biotype numbers for additional yeast species, Salkin and coworkers[303] found only a 40% agreement with the API 20C system, using the manufacturer's criteria of reliable identification without additional tests. The problems cited by the authors include the need to incorporate the results of the germ tube test in making a final identification; however, about 5% of C. albicans strains are germ tube-negative, potentially leading to a false identification. However, the authors did not include the germ tube test in their evaluation of this system; therefore, all C. albicans isolates were considered unidentifiable (however, in defense of the system, an agar medium is included to detect chlamydospores, which will still identify those strains of C. albicans that are germ tube-negative).

VITEK YEAST BIOCHEMICAL CARD

The VITEK yeast identification system (YBC) uses a disposable plastic card containing tiny wells for the testing of 26 conventional biochemical tests and 4 negative controls. The card is inoculated with a standardized suspension of the yeast to be identified, using the negative pressure filling module provided by the manufacturer. The inoculated card is then placed into a reader incubator unit, designed to read the turbidity in each well once each hour. The readings are electronically transferred into a computer file. Once a pattern of turbidity reactions match an established profile stored in the computer database, an organism identification is printed. An acceptable identification is set at ≥85% confidence; readings less than the 85% break point

must be further evaluated with morphologic studies and supplemental tests in order to make an acceptable identification.

In a study of 409 germ tube-negative isolates, including Geotrichum species, Penn and associates[261a] found that the VITEK YBC system correctly identified 89.7% of the isolates, compared to 99.3% for the API 20E system run in parallel. The YBC compared unfavorably in the identification of Candida tropicalis, C. krusei, Trichosporon species, and non–C. neoformans cryptococci. The results for the YBC system were improved by incubating the card for an additional 24 hours, because the misidentificaiton of several strains of Candida tropicalis as Candida parapsilosis were based on a false negative reaction for a single determinant, N-acetylglucosamine. The reaction turned posititve after an additional 24 hours incubation, providing a correct identification. The authors stress the need to observe the colonial morphology of any yeast isolate on cornmeal agar before blindly accepting the identification provided by any of the yeast identification systems.

Dooley and associates[92] also found that the Vitek Yeast Biochemical card identified commonly encountered yeasts, C. albicans, C. tropicalis, C. parapsilosis, C. neoformans, and T. glabrata with acceptable accuracy (93% of strains tested); however, it performed poorly in the identification of many uncommonly isolated species, with "no identification" constituting 79% of the identification failures. Assessment of colonial morphology on cornmeal agar or equivalent is recommended for a quality assurance check on all isolates identified by commercial systems. These are presented in more detail later in this chapter.

THE RAPID YEAST PLUS SYSTEM

The RapID Yeast Plus System (Innovative Diagnostic Systems, Norcross, GA) has recently been introduced for the identificaiton of unknown yeast isolates. The system is comprised of a panel of 18 reaction cavities molded into the periphery of a plastic disposable tray. Each cavity contains a dehydrated conventional or chromogenic substrate. A suspension of the unknown yeast to be tested, using a fluid provided by the manufacturer, is placed into the inoculation tray and delivered to each of the cavities by gently tilting and rocking the device to achieve an even distribution of the inoculum. After incubating the panel at 30°C for 48 hours, the first six cavities containing carbohydrate substrates are read directly for a color change; cavities 7–14 are read after adding a reagent "A," and the remaining cavities read after adding a reagent "B." The reactions are recorded on a special report form. An octal code number is derived by interpreting the positive and negative results, which is compared to a series of profile numbers recorded in a code compendium book. In a study of 500 field trial clinical and reference isolates tested in the research laboratories of the manufacturer, a correlation of 95.2% in correct identifications between the RapID and the API 20C systems was found. This system is easy to use and offers a rapid and accurate system for identifying most clinically significant yeasts. Again, cornmeal agar morphology studies should always be performed as a quality control check. The system is designed for the identification of isolates in pure culture, and cannot be used for the direct testing of clinical specimens. The manufacturer's specifications are to be strictly followed for optimum results.

THE BACTCARD CANDIDA TEST

Two commercial products are available for the presumptive identificaiton of *Candida albicans*, serving as a substitute for the more labor intensive germ tube test. The BactCard Candida test (Remel Laboratories, Lenexa, KS) consists of a card on which are placed two sparate reagent impregnated test circles, one for the detection of proline aminopeptidase (PRO), the other for β-galactosaminidase (MUGAL) activities. The test is simply performed by rehydrating each reagent test circle with a reagent supplied by the manufacturer. Using an applicator stick, each test circle is then inoculated with the top portion of a well-isolated colony of the yeast to be identified and incubated for 5 minutes at room temperature. L-proline-β-naphthylamide is impregnated in the PRO circle; a red color develops within 30 seconds after addition of a color developer supplied by the manufacturer if the yeast possesses proline aminopeptidase activity. The MUGAL circle is impregnated with 4-methylumbelliferyl-N-acetyl-b-D-galactosamine; a bright blue florescence develops within 30 seconds in the area of inoculation upon release of 4-methylumbelliferone by yeasts possessing β-galactosaminidase activity. Although many species of yeasts may demonstrate rectivity for one or the other of these substrates, only *Candida albicans* will produce a positive reaction for both. The test must be performed only on well-isolated colonies of a pure culture. Testing of isolates less than 18 hours old may result in false-negative reactions; false-positive reactions may occur if the reagent circles are read more than 30 seconds after adding the color developing reagents.

The Murex *C. albicans* test (Murex Diagnostics, Norcross, GA) utilizes a combination of p-nitrophenyl-N-acetyl-beta-D-galactosaminide (NGL) and L-proline-beta-naphthylamide (PRO) for the presumptive identification of *Candida albicans* from culture media. Both of these reagents are impregnated on a dried filter paper disk. The test is performed by placing a disk in a small tube provided by the manufacturer. The disk is rehydrated with a drop of demineralized water following which a visible "paste" of a well-isolated yeast colony to be tested is rubbed into the disk. The cap is placed on the tube and incubated for 30 minutes at 35°C. After incubation, one drop of 0.3% sodium hydroxide is added to the disk. If the yeast possesses NGL, a yellow color will develop almost immediately. One drop of color developer supplied by the manufactuerer is then added to the disk. The presence of PRO activity is indicated by the development of a red color within 1 minute. If both tests are positive, a pre-sumptive identification of *C. albicans* can be made; if one or both of the tests is negative, additional tests must be performed to identify the unknown yeast. Just as with the traditional germ tube procedure, each of these reagent substrate tests provides presumptive results, and serves only as part of an overall scheme for making a definitive yeast identification.

Odds and Bernaerts[245] describe the use of a new medium, CHROMagar Candida (CHROMagar Company, Paris, France), for the identification of important *Candida* species. CHROMagar is a proprietary product that allows the differentiation of *C. albicans*, *C. krusei*, and *C. tropicalis* by observing for different colors of isolated colonies growing on the agar surface. Colonies of *C. albicans* appeared smooth and green; *C. tropicalis* produced dark blue-gray colonies with a halo of dark brown-purple in the surrounding agar; and *C. krusei* produced rough, spreading colonies with pink centers and a white edge. Color photographs are included in the paper to illustrate these colonies. In a study of 285 isolates of *C. albicans* isolates, 54 of *C. tropicalis*, and 43 of *C. krusei*, the authors found that presumptive identifications based on these distinctive morphologic colony types was possible with 99% sensitivity and specificity. Rousselle and coauthors[300] describe two commercially available media, Albicans ID and Fluoro agar, for the rapid presumptive identification of *C. albicans*. On Albicans ID agar, *C. albicans* grows as distinctive blue colonies. On the Fluoroplate agar, *C. albicans* is the only *Candida* species (with the exception of rare strains of *C. tropicalis*) that appear as smooth fluorescent colonies. The authors report 93.8% sensitivity and 98.6% specificity of these two media in the selective identification of 352 strains of *C. albicans* among a total of 723 yeast isolates of various species.

Molecular methods for direct detection of *C. albicans* in clinical specimens, for epidemiologic studies and for the diagnosis of invasive disease are being developed in research laboratories. Holmes and coauthors[143] describe a PCR amplification technique for the detection of *C. albicans* in clinical specimens using primers complementary to extracted 5S rDNA and the adjacent non-transcribed spacer region in yeast chromosomal DNA. Miyakawa and associates[225] were able to detect *C. albicans* cells in human blood by a PCR reaction that amplifies a species-specific 125-bp region of target DNA. The sensitivity in their experiments was about three *C. albicans* cells per 0.1 mL of blood. Robert and coworkers,[297] who used random amplified polymorphic DNA, were able to type 32 strains of *C. albicans* obtained from various anatomic sites (wound swabs, mouth swabs, urine, and blood) in patients confined to a burn unit. In this particular study, 22 different strains were identified. In follow-up studies over a 9-month period, seven patterns were identified among 84 isolates from 18 patients, with one pattern identifying isolates from seven of 18 patients. Room-to-room transfer of this common isolate was determined. De Bernardis and colleagues,[81] used a dot immunobinding assay and a monoclonal antibody against mannoprotein antigen of *C. albicans* and were able to detect, with high sensitivity and specificity, circulating mannoprotein (MP) antigen of *Can-*

dida species in the sera of neutropenic patients with proved invasive candidiasis compared with a control group without disease. Although these techniques are still limited to individual studies in research settings, the availability of commercial reagents may provide for broader applications in the near future.

The use of these systems requires technical skills and sufficient familiarity with each test performed to enable accurate interpretations. Before deciding to use one of these systems in a laboratory, such factors as cost, stability, and adaptability to individual needs must be taken into account.

ANTIFUNGAL SUSCEPTIBILITY TESTING

Considerable advances in the standardization of techniques for antifungal susceptibility tests have been made over the past 5 years, primarily through the efforts of several individuals serving on the National Committee for Clinical Laboratory Standards (NCCLS) Subcommittee on Antifungal Susceptibility tests.[271] After extensive testing in seven reference laboratories of 10 candidate yeast strains for potential use in the quality control of antifungal susceptibility tests, excellent performance within established quality control (QC) limits was consistently found for *Candida parapsilosis* ATCC 22019 and *C. krusei* ATCC 6258 when tested by broth dilution against amphotericin B, flucytosine (5FC), and fluconazole.[271] These two catalogued strains, therefore, have been established as the quality control standards for anyone performing antifungal susceptibility tests against these three drugs. From results of a previous multicenter study,[269] *C. albicans* ATCC 90028, *C. parapsilosis* ATCC 22018, *C. tropicalis* ATCC 750, and *Saccharomyces cerevisiae* ATCC 9763 also performed well within the desired 3-log dilution range for each of the foregoing three antifungal agents and can be used for method development and training. Pfaller and Barry[268] developed a colorimetric broth microdilution method, that uses an oxidation–reduction indicator (Alamar Biosciences, Inc, Sacramento CA) that provided a more clearcut endpoint reaction. This colorimetric test was in 98% agreement with the standard noncolorimetric microdilution test for amphotericin B and 5FC, but only 84% for fluconazole, in a study of 600 clinical yeast isolates. In a parallel study of 100 coded yeast isolates,[270] tested in six reference laboratories, agreement between the colorimetric and standard microdilution antifungal susceptibility tests were 96.2% for fluconazole and 92.7% for amphotericin B. Thus, both methods can be recommended. In a comparative study of 273 yeast isolates, including several commonly encountered species, tested Barchiesi and coworkers[26] also validated the NCCLS-recommended microdilution test against amphotericin B, fluconazole, itraconazole, and flucytosine when tested against the standard macrodilution technique. Although these studies demonstrate excellent laboratory quality control, the degree to which in vitro antifungal susceptibility test results of the several drugs tested can be used to predict in vivo clinical response remains an open question. However, now that the techniques have been standardized, valid clinical studies are now possible.

SEROLOGIC DIAGNOSIS OF FUNGAL DISEASE

The details of serologic diagnosis of fungal infections have been reviewed by Kaufman and Riess[167] and are summarized in Table 19-5. The general principles of serologic diagnosis and interpretations of the more common pathogenic fungi have also been prepared in an official statement by the American Thoracic Society.[315] Selections of this data are included in Table 19-11. A recent review of the role of serodiagnostic tests in the diagnosis of fungal disease by Davies and Sarosi[79] is now somewhat dated but is still worthy of attention. Fungal serology is currently performed only in select reference laboratories. The time-honored procedures, including tube precipitin, immunodiffusion, latex agglutination, and complement fixation tests have given way in many laboratories to newer, more sensitive technologies, including immunoassay (EIA) techniques that utilize species-specific monoclonal antibodies, nucleic acid probe assays, and polymerase chain reaction (PCR).

As a general rule, single species-specific serologic reactions in titers of 1:32 or higher generally indicate disease; however, demonstrating a rising titer of fourfold or more in samples drawn 3 weeks apart generally has greater significance. Titers lower than 1:32, or less than a fourfold increase between the paired samples, usually indicate the presence of either early infection or nonspecific cross-reactivity with other antigens. Antibodies of the IgM class (using tube precipitin, latex agglutination, or immunodiffusion methods) are commonly detectable about 2 weeks after the disease is acquired and indicate recent infection. Usually IgM antibodies are no longer detectable after 6 months. The presence of IgG antibodies (detected by complement fixation tests or by immunodiffusion) appear shortly after the rise in IgM titer, do not peak until about 6 to 12 weeks, and may remain elevated for many months after infection. Thus, a single elevated IgG antibody titer cannot be used to distinguish between recent and remote infections.

The serodiagnosis for opportunistic infections, in particular in an attempt to diagnose disseminated and invasive candidiasis and aspergillosis, remains disappointing.[86] Immunosuppressed patients may have a poor immune response or defects in cell-mediated immune functions that compromise antibody production. Many of the opportunistic organisms, particularly *Candida* species, are ubiquitous in the environment and commonly colonize the mucous membranes of humans. Establishing antibody threshold levels to distinguish invasive disease from mucous membrane colonization have been difficult.

More promising is the current focus on identifying fungal antigens in blood and body fluids using the new EIA and nucleic acid probe assays.

TABLE 19-11
SEROLOGIC TESTS USEFUL IN THE DIAGNOSIS OF MYCOTIC DISEASE

Aspergillosis

Immunodiffusion: One or more precipitin bands suggest active disease. IgG antibodies are present in most patients with aspergillomas; IgG and IgE antibodies are present in most patients with allergic bronchopulmonary aspergillosis. Serologic tests are less useful for diagnosis of invasive disease. False-positive results are common in patients with pulmonary infections caused by other fungi and in tuberculosis. Positive cultures are required before the presence of precipitin bands can be considered clinically diagnostic. Tests for direct detection of *Aspergillus* antigen are being developed but are not yet commercially available.

Blastomycosis

Complement Fixation: CF tests using the crude antigen blastomycin prepared from culture filtrates were neither sensitive nor specific, with cross-reactions with histoplasmin being common. Because antibody was detected in only about one-third of patients with active disease, this antigen is no longer used. Using a more purified antigen called Antigen A or AWSE, which consists of alkali and water-soluble extract derived from yeast phase cultures, gave positive results in only 10% of patients with acute pulmonary blastomycosis, in 40% with chronic pulmonary blastomycosis, and in only 50% with disseminated disease.

Immunodiffusion: More specific than the CF test. Test is positive in 60% of patients with chronic pulmonary disease and in 80% of patients with disseminated blastomycosis.

EIA: With the AWSE antigen, EIA detects about 75% of patients with acute blastomycosis and is quite specific when titers of 1:32 or higher are detected. Detection rates exceeding 90% are found in chronic pulmonary and in disseminated disease.

Candidiasis

Tests measuring antibody to *Candida* antigens are not currently useful. Up to 50% of patients with invasive *Candida* infections have had negative tests. Tests such as RIA and EIA do not distinguish patients with invasive infection from patients who are merely colonized. Tests for direct detection of circulating *Candida* antigens are not yet standardized or available outside research circles.

Coccidioidomycosis

Complement Fixation: This is the most important test to perform. Sixty percent of patients with symptomatic primary infection have a positive CF test (titer of 1:2 or greater) by 4 weeks and 80%–90% by 8 weeks. A rising titer or a titer of 1:16 usually indicates active disease. Many asymptomatic or minimally symptomatic patients never develop a positive CF test. In symptomatic, but self-limited disease, the CF test is positive in about 75% of cases; in disseminated disease it is positive in more than 95% with titers of 1:32 or higher in the majority (not as sensitive in immunosuppressed patients). CF of the CSF is positive in about 60% of patients with coccidioidal meningitis. Because the complex antigen coccidioidin shares determinants with antigens of *H. capsulatum* and *B. dermatitides,* low CF titers (1:2 to 1:4) in patients without current coccidioidomycosis may represent cross-reactivity. Low CF titers also may reflect a remote *Coccidioides* infection, because low-level titers can remain elevated for years following acute infection.

Cryptococcosis

Tests for cryptococcal antibodies are not useful. Tests give false-negative results in more than half of patients with known cryptococcal infection. Cross-reactions are frequent in patients with other fungal disease.

Latex Agglutination: LA assay for cryptococcal polysaccharide antigen is positive in the CSF of more than 90% of patients with cryptococcal meningitis (sensitivity of India ink preparation is only 50%; culture only 70%). Most negative tests occur early in infection when symptoms are mild. Titers of 1:32 or higher occur in 90% of patients with fatal infections. Persistent titers of 1:8 or greater at the completion of therapy portend relapse. Serum antigen tests are positive in about 50% of patients with cryptococcal meningitis and in about 10% of patients with serious nonmeningeal disease. False-positive tests are usually of low titer (1:4 or less), often associated with rheumatoid-like substances. Treatment of the specimen with pronase reduces false-positive results.

Histoplasmosis

Complement Fixation: CF against yeast antigen is more sensitive than ID, but is less specific. Background positivity with titers 1:16 or less may be found in 10% of persons living in endemic areas. A single titer of 1:32 or higher or a fourfold increase is diagnostic of current histoplasmosis in the appropriate clinical setting. CF has poor sensitivity during the acute pulmonary phase of disease, but is positive in 80% of patients after 4 or more weeks of illness, and in those with chronic cavitary or disseminated disease. False-positive results occur in patients with tuberculosis, aspergillosis, blastomycosis, and coccidioidomycosis. Increased titers may be seen following recent histoplasmin skin tests.

Immunodiffusion: ID is the least sensitive and of little value as a screening test. It may have value when the serum is anticomplementary in the CF test, when the CF titer is low, or in detecting early infection when the ID M band is more specific than CF. The presence of both an H and an M band indicates active infection, but occurs in only about 20% of persons with a positive M band. An isolated H band almost never occurs. Disappearance of an H band following therapy may indicate regression of disease.

Sporotrichosis

Latex Agglutination: Titers of 1:80 or higher usually indicate active infection. Most positive tests are seen in extracutaneous infections; titers are negative in most cases of primary skin infections.

(Adapted from Davies SF, Sarosi GA: Role of serodiagnostic tests and skin tests in the diagnosis of fungal disease.
Clin Chest Med 8:135–146, 1987)

REFERENCES

1. ADAM RD, PAQUIN ML, PETERSEN EA, ET AL: Phaeohyphomycosis caused by the fungal genera *Bipolaris* and *Excerohilum*. A report of 9 cases and review of the literature. Medicine 65:203–217, 1986

2. AISNER JA, SCHIMPFF SC, ET AL. *Aspergillus* infection in cancer patients: association with fire-proofing materials in a new hospital. JAMA 235:411–412, 1976

3. AJELLO L, GEORG IK: In vitro hair cultures for differentiation between atypical isolates of *Trichophyton mentagrophytes* and *Trichophyton rubrum*. Mycopathol Mycol Appl 8:3–11, 1957

4. AJELLO L: Hyalohyphomycosis: a disease entity whose time has come. Newsl Med Mycol Soc NY 10:305, 1982

5. AJELLO L: Hyalohyphomycosis and phaeohyphomycosis: two global disease entities of public health importance. Eur J Epidemiol 2:243–251, 1986

6. AL-FOUZAN AS, NANDA A, KUBEC K: Dermatophytosis of children in Kuwait: a prospective survey. Int J Dermatol 32:798–801, 1993

7. ALSINA A, MASON M, UPHOFF RA: Catheter-associated *Candida utilis* fungemia in a patient with acquired immunodeficiency syndrome: species verification with molecular probe. J Clin Microbiol 26:621–624, 1988

8. ALVAREZ S: Systemic infection by *Penicillium decumbens* in a patient with acquired immunodeficiency syndrome. J Infect Dis 162:283, 1990

9. ALVAREZ M, PONGA BL, RAYON C, ET AL: Nosocomial outbreak caused by *Scedosporium prolificans (inflatum)*: four fatal cases in leukemic patients. J Clin Microbiol 33:3290–3295, 1995

10. AMPEL NM, RYAN KJ, CARRY PJ, ET AL: Fungemia due to *Coccidioides immitis*. An analysis of 16 episodes in 15 patients and a review of the literature. Medicine 65:312–321, 1986

11. AMPEL NM, WHITE JD, ET AL: Coccidioidal peritonitis associated with continuous ambulatory peritoneal dialysis. Am J Kidney Dis 11:512–514, 1988

12. AMPEL NM, DOLS CL, GALGIANI JN: Coccidioidomycosis during human immunodeficiency virus infection: results of a prospective study in a coccidioidal endemic area. Am J Med 94:235–240, 1993

13. ANAISSIE E, FAINSTEIN V, SAMO T, ET AL. Central nervous system histoplasmosis. An unappreciated complication of the acquired immunodeficiency syndrome. Am J Med 84:215–217, 1988

14. ANAISSIE E, KANTARJIAN H, JONES P: *Fusarium*. A newly recognized fungal pathogen in immunosuppressed patients. Cancer 57:2141–2145, 1986

15. ANAISSIE E, LEGRAND C, HACHEM R, ET AL: Recovery of *Fusarium* sp from the bloodstream using a rabbit model of systemic fusariosis. Abstr Annu Meet Am Soc Microbiol 90:413, 1990 (abstr F-28)

16. ANHALT E, ALVAREZ J, BERT R: *Torulopsis glabrata* meningitis. South Med J 79:916, 1986

17. ANTONISKIS D, LARSEN RA, AKIL B, ET AL: Seronegative disseminated coccidioidomycosis in patients with HIV infection. AIDS 4:691–693, 1990

18. ARGUINCHONA HL, AMPEL NM, DOLS CL, ET AL: Positive coccidioidal serologies in HIV-infected patients without evidence of active coccidioidomycosis. Int Conf AIDS Aug 7–12 10:160, 1994 (abstr PB0654)

19. ARMSTRONG CW, JENKINS SR, KAUFMAN L, ET AL: Common-source outbreak of blastomycosis in hunters and their dogs. J Infect Dis 155:568–570, 1987

20. ASCHNER JL, PUNSALANG A JR, MANISCALCO WM, MENEGUS MA: Percutaneous central venous catheter colonization with *Malassezia furfur*: incidence and clinical significance. Pediatrics 80:535–539, 1987

21. ATKINSON JB, CONNOR DH, ROBINOWITZ M: Fungal infections: a review of autopsy findings in 60 patients. Hum Pathol 15:935–942, 1984

22. AVIV JE, LAWSON W, BOTTONE EJ, ET AL: Multiple intracranial mucoceles associated with phaeohyphomycosis of the paransal sinus. Arch Otolaryng Head Neck Surg 116:1210–1213, 1990

23. BABEL DE, ROGERS AL, BENEKE ES: Dermatophytosis of the scalp: incidence, immune response, and epidemiology. Mycopathologia 109:69–73, 1990

24. BAKER JG, SALKIN IF, FORGACS P, ET AL: First report of subcutaneous phaeohyphomycosis of the foot caused by *Phoma minutella*. J Clin Microbiol 25:2395–2397, 1987

25. BARBA-GOMEZ JF, MAYORGA J, MCGINNIS MR, ET AL: Chromoblastomycosis caused by *Exophiala spinifera*. J Am Acad Dermatol 26:367–370, 1992

26. BARCHIESI F, COLOMBO AL, MCGOUGH DA, RINALDI MG: Comparative study of broth macrodilution and microdilution techniques for in vitro antifungal susceptibility testing of yeasts by using the National Committee for Clinical Laboratory Standards' proposed standard. J Clin Microbiol 32:2494–2500, 1994

27. BARILE F, MASTROLONARDO M, LOCONSOLE F, RANTUCCIO F: Cutaneous sporotrichosis in the period 1978–1992 in the province of Bari, Apulia, southern Italy. Mycoses 36:181–185, 1993

28. BARNES RA: *Aspergillus* infection: does serodiagnosis work? Serodiagn Immunother Infect Dis 5:135–138, 1993

29. BASSIOUNY A, EL-REFAI HA, ET AL: *Candida* infection of the tongue and pharynx. J Laryngol Otol 98:609–611, 1984

30. BAUMGARDNER DJ, BUGGY BP, MATTSON RJ, ET AL: Epidemiology of blastomycosis in a region of high endemicity in north central Wisconsin. Clin Infect Dis 15:629–635, 1992

31. BEARER EA, NELSON PR, CHOWERS MY, DAVIS CE: Cutaneous zygomycosis cuased by *Saksenaea vasiformis* in a diabetic patient. J Clin Microbiol 32:1823–1824, 1994

32. BERARDINELLI C, OPHEIM DJ: New germ tube induction medium for the identification of *Candida albicans*. J Clin Microbiol 22:861–862

33. BERGMAN BA, BROWN RE, KHARDORI N: Blastomycosis infection of the hand. Ann Plast Surg 33:330–332, 1994

34. BERKOWITZ I, DIAMOND TH: Disseminated *Blastomyces dermatitidis* infection in a non-endemic area. A case report. S Afr Med J 71:717–719, 1987

35. BERLINGER NT, FREEMAN TJ: Acute airway obstruction due to necrotizing tracheobronchial aspergillosis in immunocompromised patients: a new clinical entity. Ann Otol Rhinol Laryngol 29:718–720, 1989

36. Bethlem NM, Lemle A, Bethlem E, Wanke B. Paracoccidioidomycosis. Semin Respir Med 12:81–86, 1991

37. Beushing WJ, Kurek K, Roberts GK: Evaluation of the modified API 20C system for identification of clinically important yeasts. J Clin Microbiol 9:565–569, 1979

38. Blazar BR, Hurd DD, Snover DC, et al: Invasive *Fusarium* infections in bone marrow transplant recipients. Am J Med 77:645–651, 1984

39. Blevens LB, Fenn J, Segal H, et al: False-positive cryptococcal antigen latex agglutination caused by disinfectants and soaps. J Clin Microbiol 33:1674–1675, 1995

40. Blinkhorn RJ, Adelstein D, Spagnuolo PJ: Emergence of a new opportunistic pathogen, *Candida lusitaniae*. J Clin Microbiol 27:236–240, 1989

41. Bloxham CA, Carr S, Ryan DW, et al. Disseminated zygomycosis and systemic lupus erythematosus. Intensive Care Med 16:201–207, 1990

42. Blumenfeld W, Gan GL: Diagnosis of histoplasmosis in bronchoalveolar lavage fluid by intracytoplasmic localization of silver-positive yeast. Acta Cytol 35:710–712, 1991

43. Boelaert JR, vanRoost GF, Vergauwe PL, et al: The role of desferrioxamine in dialysis-associated mucormycosis: report of three cases and review of the literature. Clin Nephrol 29:261–266, 1988

44. Bohler K, Metze D, Poitschek C, Jurecka W: Cutaneous aspergillosis. Clin Exp Dermatol 15:446–450, 1990

45. Boom WH, Piper DJ, Rouff KL, et al: New cause for false-positive results with the cryptococcal antigen test by latex agglutination. J Clin Microbiol 22:856–857, 1985

46. Boon AP, Adams DH, Buckels J, McMaster P: Cerebral aspergillosis in liver transplantation. J Clin Pathol 43:114–118, 1990

47. Boon AP, O'Brien D, Adams DHJ: 10 year review of invasive aspergillosis detected at necropsy. J Clin Pathol 44:452–454, 1991

48. Bowman PL, Ahearn DG: Evaluation of commercial systems for the identification of clinical yeast isolates. J Clin Microbiol 4:49–53, 1976

49. Bradsher RW: Blastomycosis. Clin Infect Dis 14(suppl 1):S82–S90, 1992

50. Bretagne S, Costa J, Marmorat-Khoung A, et al: Detection of *Aspergillus* species DNA in bronchoalveolar lavage samples by competitive PCR. J Clin Microbiol 33:1164–1168, 1995

51. Brummer E, Castaneda E, Restrepo A: Paracoccidioidomycosis: an update. Clin Microbiol Rev 6:89–117, 1993

52. Brummund W, Resnick A, Fink FN, Kurup VP: *Aspergillus fumigatus*-specific antibodies in allergic bronchopulmonary aspergillosis and aspergilloma: evidence for a polyclonal antibody response. J Clin Microbiol 25:5–9, 1987

53. Bylund DJ, Nanfro JJ, Marsh WL Jr: Coccidioidomycosis of the female genital tract. Arch Pathol Lab Med 110:232–235, 1986

54. Camargo ZP, Taborda CP, Rodreiquez EG, Travassos LR: The use of cell-free antigens of *Paracoccidioides brasiliensis* in serological tests. J Med Vet Mycol 29:31–38, 1991

55. Carmody TJ, Kane KK: *Torulopsis* (*Candida*) *glabrata* endocarditis involving a bovine pericardial xenograft heart valve. Heart Lung 15:40–42, 1986

56. Carter RR 3d, Eilson JP, Turner HR, Chapman SW: Cutaneous blastomycosis as a complication of transthoracic needle aspiration. Chest 91:917–918, 1987

57. Castro LG, Salebian A, Sotto MN: Hyalohyphomycosis by *Paecilomyces lilacinus* in a renal transplant patient and a review of human *Paecilomyces* species infections. J Med Vet Mycol 28:15–26, 1990

58. Chalub E, Sambuelli R, Armando R, Bistoni A: Histologic response of disseminated histoplasmosis in AIDS patients with skin lesions. Int Conf AIDS, Aug 7–12, 10(2):148, 1994 (abstr PB0605)

59. Chan YF, Woo KC: *Penicillium marneffei* osteomyelitis. J Bone Joint Surg 72:500–503, 1990

60. Chandler FW, Kaplan W, Ajello L: Histopathology of Mycotic Diseases. Chicago, Year Book Medical Publishers, 1980

61. Chapin-Robertson K, Bechtel C, Waycott S, et al: Cryptococcal antigen detection from the urine of AIDS patients. Diag Microbiol Infect Dis 17:197–201, 1993

62. Chappell MS, Mandell W, Grimes MM, Neu HC: Gastrointestinal histoplasmosis. Dig Dis Sci 33:353–360, 1988

63. Chowdhary G, Weinstein A, Klein R, Mascarenhas BR: Sporotrichal arthritis. Ann Rheum Dis 50:112–114, 1991

64. Chuck SL, Sande MA: Infections with *Cryptococcus neoformans* in the acquired immunodeficiency syndrome. N Engl J Med 21:794–799, 1989

65. Chutrasakul C, Chantarakul N: Mucormycosis in the severely burned patient. Report of two cases with extensive destructive lesions. J Med Assoc Thail 66:132–138, 1983

66. Cimolai N, Gill MJ, Church D: *Saccharomyces cerevisiae* fungemia: a case report and review of the literature. Diagn Microbiol Infect Dis 8:113–117, 1987

67. Cimponeriu D, LoPresti P, Lavelanet M, et al: Gastrointestinal histoplasmosis in HIV infection: two cases of colonic pseudocancer and review of the literature. Am J Gastroenterol 89:129–131, 1994

68. Clarke A, Skelton J, Fraser RS: Fungal tracheobronchitis. Report of 9 cases and review of the literature. Medicine 70:1–14, 1991

69. Clarke RA, Greer D, Atkinson W, et al: Spectrum of *Cryptococcus neoformans* infection in 68 patients infected with human immunodeficiency virus. Rev Infect Dis 12:768–777, 1990

70. Clarkston WK, Bonacini M, Peterson I: Colitis due to *Histoplasma capsulatum* in the acquired immune deficiency syndrome. Am J Gastroenterol 86:913–916, 1991

71. Coles FB, Schuchat A, Hibbs JR, et al: A multistate outbreak of sporotrichosis associated with sphagnum moss. Am J Epidemiol 36:475–487, 1992

72. Confalonieri M, Nanetti A, Gandola L, et al: Histoplasmosis capsulati in Italy: autochthonous or imported? Eur J Epidemiol 110:435–439, 1994

73. Cooper CR, Dixon DM, Salkin IF: Laboratory-acquired sporotrichosis. J Med Vet Mycol 30:169–171, 1992

74. Cooter RD, Lim IS, Ellis DH, Leitch IO: Burn wound zygomycosis caused by *Apophysomyces elegans*. J Clin Microbiol 28:2151–2153, 1990

75. Cox JN, diDio F, Pizzolato GP, et al: Aspergillus endocarditis and myocarditis in a patient with the im-

munodeficiency syndrome. A review. Virchows Arch 417:255–259, 1990

76. CURRIE BP, CASADEVALL A: Estimation of the prevalence of cryptococcal infection among patients infected with the human immunodeficiency virus in New York City. Clin Infect Dis 19:1029–1033, 1994

77. DAHL MV, GRANDO SA: Chronic dermatophytosis: what is special about *Trichophyton rubrum*? Adv Dermatol 9:97–109, 1994

78. D'ANTONIO D, PICCOLOMINI R, FIORITONI G, ET AL: Osteomyelitis and intervertebral discitis caused by *Blastoschizomyces capitatus* in a patient with acute leukemia. J Clin Microbiol 32:224–227, 1994

79. DAVIES SF, SAROSI GA: Role of serodiagnostic tests and skin tests in the diagnosis of fungal disease. Clin Chest Med 8:135–146, 1987

80. DAVIES SF, SAROSI GA: Blastomycosis. Eur J Clin Microbiol Infect Dis: 8:474–479, 1989

81. DE BERNARDIS F, GIRMENIA C, BOCCANERA M, ET AL: Use of a monoclonal antibody in a dot immunobinding assay for detection of circulating mannoprotein of *Candida* spp. in neutropenic patients with invasive candidiasis. J Clin Microbiol 31:3146–3242, 1993

82. DEFOIER C, FOSSION E, VAILLANT JM: Sinus aspergillosis. J Craniomaxillofac Surg 18:33–40, 1990

83. DEGENTILE L, BOUCHARA JP, CIMON B, CHABASSE D: *Candida cifferrii*: clinical and microbiological features of an emerging pathogen. Mycosis 34:125–128, 1991

84. DENNING DW, WILLIAMS AH: Invasive pulmonary aspergillosis diagnosed by blood culture and successfully treated. Br J Dis Chest 81:300–304, 1987

85. DENNING DW, STEVENS DA: Antifungal and surgical treatment of invasive aspergillosis: review of 2121 published cases. Rev Infect Dis 12:1147–1201, 1990

86. DE REPINTIGNY L, REIS E: Current trends in immunodiagnosis of candidiasis and aspergillosis. Rev Infect Dis 6:301–312, 1984

87. DITOMASSO JP, AMPEL NM, SOBONYA RE, BLOOM JW: Bronchoscopic diagnosis of pulmonary coccidioidomycosis. Comparison of cytology, culture, and transbronchial biopsy. Diagn Microbiol Infect Dis 18:83–87, 1994

88. DIXON DM, FROMTLING RA: Morphology, taxonomy and classification of the fungi. In Murray PR, ed. Manual of Clinical Microbiology, 6th ed. Washington DC, American Society for Microbiology, 1995, Chap 59

89. DIXON DM, WALSH TJ, MERZ WG, McGINNIS MR: Infections due to *Xylohypha bantiana* (*Cladosporium trichoides*). Rev Infect Dis 11:515–525, 1990

90. DODD LG, NELSON SD: Disseminated coccidioidomycosis detected by percutaneous liver biopsy in a liver transplant recipient. Am J Clin Pathol 93:141–144, 1990

91. DONABEDIAN H, O'DONNELL E, OLSZEWSKI C, ET AL: Disseminated cutaneous and meningeal sporotrichosis in an AIDS patient. Diagn Microbiol Infect Dis 18:111–115, 1994

92. DOOLEY DP, BECKIUS ML, JEFFREY BS: Misidentification of clinical yeast isolates by using the updated Vitek yeast biochemical card. J Clin Microbiol 32:2889–2892, 1994

93. DRIVER JA, SAUNDERS CA, HEINZE-LACEY B, SUGAR AM: Cryptococcal pneumonia in AIDS: is cryptococcal

meningitis preceded by clinically recognizable pneumonia? J AIDS Hum Retrovirol 9:168–171, 1995

94. DUMICH PS, NEEL HB: Blastomycosis of the larynx. Laryngoscope 93:1266–1270, 1983

95. EDWARDS JE: *Candida* species. In Mandell GL, Douglas RG Jr, Bennett JE, eds. Principles and Practice of Infectious Diseases, 3rd ed. New York, Churchill Livingstone, 1990, Chap 235, pp 1943–1958

96. EIDBO J, SANCTHEZ RL, TSCHEN JA, ELLNER KM: Cutaneous manifesations of histoplasmosis in the acquired immune deficiency syndrome. Am J Surg Pathol 17:110–116, 1993

97. ENG RHK, PERSON A: Serum cryptococcal antigen determination in the presence of rheumatoid factor. J Clin Microbiol 14:700–702, 1981

98. ENGLAND DM, HOCHHOLZER I: Primary pulmonary sporotrichosis: report of eight cases with clinicopathologic review. Am J Surg Pathol 9:193–204, 1985

99. ENGLEBERG NC, JOHNSON J IV, BLEUSTEIN J, ET AL: Phaeohyphomycotic cyst caused by a recently described species, *Phaeoannellomyces elegans*. J Clin Microbiol 25:605–608, 1987

100. ENGLER HD, SHEA YR: Effect of potential interference factors on performance of enzyme immunoassay and latex agglutination assay for cryptococcal antigen. J Clin Microbiol 32:2307–2308, 1994

101. ESCHETE ML, WEST BC: *Saccharomyces cerevisiae* septicemia. Arch Intern Med 140:1539, 1980

102. ESCURO RS, JACOBS M, GERSON SL, ET AL: Prospective evaluation of a candida antigen detection test for invasive candidiasis in immunocompromised adult patients with cancer. Am J Med 87:621–627, 1989

103. FAIX RG: Systemic *Candida* infections in infants in intensive care nurseries: high incidence of central nervous system involvement. J Pediatr 105:616–622, 1984

104. FARR RC, GARDNER G, ACKER JD, ET AL: Blastomycotic cranial osteomyelitis. Am J Otol 13:582–586, 1992

105. FISH DG, AMPEL NM, GALGIANI JN, ET AL: Coccidioidomycosis during human immunodeficiency virus infection. A review of 77 patients. Medicine 69:384–391, 1990

106. FISHER JF: Urinary tract infections due to *Candida albicans*. Rev Infect Dis 4:1107–1118, 1982

107. FLEMING WH III, HOPKINS JM, LORD GA: New culture medium for presumptive identification of *Candida albicans* and *Cryptococcus neoformans*. J Clin Microbiol 5:236–243, 1977

108. FOJTASEK MF, KLEIMAN MB, CONNOLLY-STRINGFIELD P, ET AL: The *Histoplasma capsulatum* antigen assay in disseminated histoplasmosis in children. Pediatr Infect Dis J 13:801–805, 1994

109. FRANK UK, NISHIMURA SL, LI NC, ET AL: Evaluation of an enzyme immunoassay for detection of cryptococcal capsular polysaccharide antigen in serum and cerebrospinal fluid. J Clin Microbiol 31:94–101, 1993

110. FRASER RS: Pulmonary aspergillosis: pathologic and pathogenic features. Pathol Annu 28:231–277, 1993

111. FRASER VJ, KEATH EJ, POWDERLY WG: Two cases of blastomycosis from a common source: use of DNA restriction analysis to identify strains. J Infect Dis 163:1278–1381, 1991

112. FRYE KR, DONOVAN JM, DRACH GW: *Torulopsis glabrata* urinary tract infections. J Urol 139:1245–1249, 1988
113. GAL AA, KOSS MN, HAWKINS J, ET AL: The pathology of pulmonary cryptococcal infections in the acquired immunodeficiency syndrome. Arch Pathol Lab Med 110:502–507, 1986
114. GEFTER WB: The spectrum of pulmonary aspergillosis. J Thorac Imaging 7:56–74, 1992
115. GELFAND MS, MCGEE ZA, KAISER AB, ET AL: Candidal meningitis following bacterial meningitis. South Med J 83:567–570, 1990
116. GOLANDI LZ, MONTEIRO CMC, DONALDI EA, ET AL: HLA antigens in Brazilian patients with paracoccidioidomycosis. Mycopathologia 114:89–91, 1991
117. GOLDANI LZ, MAIN AI, SUGAR AM: Cloning and nucleotide sequence of a specific DNA fragment from *Paracoccidioides brasiliensis*. J Clin Microbiol 33:369–372, 1995
118. GOLDANI LZ, SUGAR AM: Paracoccidioidomycosis and AIDS: an overview. Clin Infect Dis 21:1275–1281, 1995
119. GOURLEY DS, WHISMAN BA, JORGENSEN NL, ET AL: Allergic *Bipolaris* sinusitis: clinical and immunopathologic characteristics. J Allergy Clin Immunol 85:583–591, 1990
120. GRAHAM BD, MCKINSEY DS, DRIKS MR, SMITH DL: Colonic histoplasmosis in acquired immunodeficiency syndrome. Report of two cases. Dis Colon Rectum 34:185–190, 1991
121. GRAY LD, ROBERTS GK: Experience with the use of pronase to eliminate interference factors in the latex agglutination test for cryptococcal antigen. J Clin Microbiol 26:2450–2451, 1988
122. GREEN WR, BOUCHETTE D: Pleural mucormycosis (zygomycosis). Arch Pathol Lab Med 110:441–442, 1986
123. GRIFFIN TD, MCFARLAND JP, JOHNSON WC: Hyalohyphomycosis masquerading as squamous cell carcinoma. J Cutan Pathol 18:116–119, 1991
124. GUEHO E, SIMMONS RB, PRUITT WR, ET AL: Association of *Malassezia pachydermatis* with systemic infections of humans. J Clin Microbiol 25:1789–1790, 1987
125. GUPTA TP, EHRINPREIS MN: Candida-associated diarrhea in hospitalized patients. Gastroenterology 98:780–785, 1990
126. HADFIELD TL, SMITH MB, WINN RE, ET AL: Mycoses caused by *Candida lusitaniae*. Rev Infect Dis 9:1006–1012, 1987
127. HAGEAGE GJ JR, HARRINGTON BH: Use of calcofluor white in clinical mycology. Lab Med 15:109–111, 1984
128. HAIGHT DO, ESPERANZA LE, GREENE JN: Case report: cutaneous manifestations of cryptococcosis. Am J Med Sci 308:192–195, 1994
129. HALL GS, PRATT-RIPPIN K, WASHINGTON JA: Evaluation of a chemiluminescent probe assay for identification of *Histoplasma capsulatum* isolates. J Infect 22:179–182, 1991.
130. HALL J, HEIMANN P, COSTAS C: Airway obstruction caused by *Aspergillus* tracheobronchitis in an immunocompromised patient. Crit Care Med 18:575–576, 1990
131. HARDING CV: Blastomycosis and opportunistic infections in patients with acquired immunodeficiency syndrome. An autopsy study. Arch Pathol Lab Med 115:1133–1136, 1991
132. HAYNES KA, LATGE JP, ROGERS TR: Detection of *Aspergillus* antigens associated with invasive infection. J Clin Microbiol 28:2040–2044, 1990
133. HAZEN KC: New and emerging yeast pathogens. Clin Microbiol Rev 8:462–478, 1995
134. HEBERT CA, KING JW, GEORGE RB: Late dissemination of pulmonary blastomycosis during ketoconazole therapy. Chest 95:240–242, 1989
135. HEELAN JS, CORPUS L, KISSIMIAN N: False-positive reactions in the latex agglutination test for *Cryptococcus neoformans* antigen. J Clin Microbiol 29:1260–1261, 1991
136. HELLER HM, FUHRER J: Disseminated sporotrichosis in patients with AIDS: case report and review of the literature. AIDS 5:1243–1246, 1991
137. HENEY C, SONG E, KELLEN A, ET AL: Cerebral phaeohyphomycosis caused by *Xylohypha bantiana*. Eur J Clin Microbiol Infect Dis 8:984–988, 1989
138. HERWITZ MD, KALLENBACH JM, ROHR A, ET AL: Blastomycosis. A case report. S Afr Med J 70:622–624, 1986
139. HIBBERD PL, RUBIN RH: Clinical aspects of fungal infection in organ transplant recipients. Clin Infect Dis 1:S33–40, 1994
140. HICKEY WF, SOMMERVILLE LH, SCHOEN FJ: Disseminated *Candida glabrata*: report of a uniquely severe infection and a literature review. Am J Clin Pathol 80:724–727, 1983
141. HICKS MJ, GREEN LK, CLARRIDGE J: Primary diagnosis of disseminated coccidioidomycosis by fine needle aspiration of a neck mass. A case report. Acta Cytol 38:422–426, 1994
142. HILTBRAND JB, MCGUIRT WF: Oropharyngeal histoplasmosis. South Med J 83:227, 1990
143. HOLMES AR, CANNON RD, SHEPHERD MG, JENKINSON HF: Detection of *Candida albicans* and other yeasts in blood by PCR. J Clin Microbiol 32:228–231, 1994
144. HOPFER RL, GROSCHEL D: Six hour pigmentation test for the identification of *C. neoformans*. J Clin Microbiol 2:96–98, 1975
145. HOPKINS JM, LAND GA: Rapid method for determining nitrate utilization by yeasts. J Clin Microbiol 5:497–500, 1977
146. HOSTETTER MK: Adhesins and ligands involved in the interaction of *Candida* spp. with epithelial and endothelial surfaces. Clin Microbiol Rev 7:29–42, 1994
147. HOY J, HSU KC, ROLSTON K, ET AL: *Trichosporon beigelii* infection: a review. Rev Infect Dis 8:959–967, 1986
148. HUANG CT, MCGARRY T, COOPER S, ET AL: Disseminated histoplasmosis in the acquired immunodeficiency syndrome. Report of five cases from a nonendemic area. Arch Intern Med 147:1181–1184, 1987
149. HUFFNAGLE KE, GANDER RM: Evaluation of Gen-Probe's *Histoplasma capsulatum* and *Cryptococcus neoformans* AccuProbes. J Clin Microbiol 31:419–421, 1993
150. HULSHOF CM, VANZANTEN RA, SLUITERS JF, ET AL: *Penicillium marneffei* infection in an AIDS patient. Eur J Clin Microbiol Infect Dis 9:370, 1990
151. ISENBERG HD, TUCCI V, CINTRON F, ET AL: Single-source outbreak of *Candida tropicalis* complicating coronary bypass surgery. J Clin Microbiol 27:2426–2428, 1989
152. JADE KB, LYONS MF, GNANN JR: *Paecilomyces lilacinus* cellulitis in an immunocompromised patient. Arch Dermatol 122:1169–1170, 1986
153. JAY WM: Ocular involvement in mycotic sinusitis caused by *Bipolaris*. Am J Ophthalmal 105:366–370, 1988

154. JAYANETRA P, NITIYANANT P, AJELLO A, ET AL: *Penicillium marneffei* in Thailand: report of five human cases. Am J Trop Med Hyg 33:637–644, 1984

155. JOHNSTON PC, KHARDORI N, NAJJAR AF, ET AL: Progressive disseminated histoplasmosis in patients with acquired immunodeficiency syndrome. Am J Med 85: 152–158, 1988

156. JONATHAN D, LUND V, MILROY C: Allergic aspergillus sinusitis. J Laryngol Otol 103:1181–1183, 1989

157. JONES JL, FLEMING PL, CIESIELSKI CA, ET AL: Coccidioidomycosis among persons with AIDS in the United States. J Infect Dis 171:961–966, 1995

158. JONES PG, COHEN RL, BATES DH, ET AL: Disseminated histoplasmosis, invasive pulmonary aspergillosis and other opportunistic infections in a homosexual patient with acquired immune deficiency syndrome. Sex Transm Dis 10:202–204, 1983

159. JONES S, WHITE G, HUNTER PR: Increased phenotypic switching in strains of *Candida albicans* associated with invasive infections. J Clin Microbiol 32:2869–2870, 1994

160. KAHN DG, THOMMES J: Granulomatous orchitis and epididymitis secondary to *Histoplasma capsulatum* and CMV in AIDS. Int Conf AIDS, July 19–24, 8(3):93, 1992 (abstr PuB 7267)

161. KANE J, FISHER JB: The differentiation of *Trichophyton rubrum* and *Trichophyton mentagrophytes* by use of Christensens' urea broth. Can J Microbiol 17:911–913, 1971

162. KANE J, RICHTER J, KRAJDEN S, ET AL: Blastomycosis—a new endemic focus in Canada. J Can Med Assoc 129: 728–731, 1983

163. KASSAMALI H, ANAISSIE E, RO J, ET AL: Disseminated *Geotrichum candidum* infection. J Clin Microbiol 25: 1782–1783, 1987

164. KAUFMANN CS, MERZ WG: Two rapid pigmentation tests for identification of *Cryptococcus neoformans*. J Clin Microbiol 15:339–341, 1982

165. KAUFMAN L, STANDARD PG, ANDERSON SA, ET AL: Development of specific fluorescent-antibody test for tissue form of *Penicillium marneffei*. J Clin Microbiol 33:2136–2138, 1995

166. KAUFMAN L, BLUMER S: Cryptococcosis: the awakening giant [abstr]. In Proceedings of the Fourth International Conference on the Mycoses. PAHO scientific publication 356:176–182, 1977

167. KAUFMAN L, REECE E: Serodiagnosis of fungal diseases. In Lennette EH, ed. Manual of Clinical Microbiology, 4th ed. Washington DC, American Society for Microbiology, l985, pp 924–944

168. KAUFMAN L, SEKHON AS, MOLEDINA N, ET AL: Comparative evaluation of commercial premier EIA and microimmunodiffusion and complement fixation tests for *Coccidioides immitis* antibodies. J Clin Microbiol 33:618–619, 1995

169. KAUFMAN L, STANDARD PG, WEEKS RJ, ET AL: Detection of two *Blastomyces dermatitidis* serotypes by exoantigen analysis. J Clin Microbiol 18:110–114, 1983

170. KAUFMAN L, STANDARD PG: Specific and rapid identification of medically important fungi by exoantigen detection. Annu Rev Microbiol 41:209–221, 1987

171. KAUFMAN SM: *Curvularia* endocarditis following cardiac surgery. Am J Clin Pathol 56:466–470, 1971

172. KEMMA ME, NERI RC, ALI R, SALKIN IF: *Cokeromyces recurvatus*, a mucoraceous zygomycete rarely isolated in clinical laboratories. J Clin Microbiol 32:843–845, 1994

173. KENNEDY MJ, SIGLER L: *Aspergillus, Fusarium*, and other opportunistic moniliaceous fungi. In Murray PR, ed. Manual of Clinical Microbiology, 6th ed. Washington DC, American Society for Microbiology, 1995, Chap 64

174. KERKERING TM, DUMA RJ, SHADOMY S: The evolution of pulmonary cryptococcosis: clinical implications from a study of 41 patients with and without compromising host factors. Ann Intern Med 94:611–616, 1981

175. KHARDORI N, HAYAT S, ROLSTON K, BODEY GP: Cutaneous *Rhizopus* and *Aspergillus* infections in five patients with cancer. Arch Dermatol 125:952–956, 1989

176. KHOO SH, DENNING DW. Invasive aspergillosis in patients with AIDS. Clin Infect Dis 19(suppl 1):S41–S48, 1994

177. KILBURN CD, McKINSEY DS: Recurrent massive pleural effusion due to pleural, pericardial and epicardial fibrosis in histoplasmosis. Chest 100:1715–1717, 1991

178. KIM JH, YUN SK, IHM CW: Cutaneous sporotrichosis and distant autoinoculation. J Dermatol 22:72–73, 1995

179. KISKA DL, ORKISZEWSKI DR, HOWELL D, GILLIGAN PH: Evaluation of new monoclonal antibody-based latex agglutination test for detection of cryptococcal polysaccharide antigen in serum and cerebrospinal fluid. J Clin Microbiol 32:2309–2311, 1994

180. KLEIN BS, VERGERONT JM, ROBERTS RJ, ET AL: Isolation of *Blastomyces dermatitidis* in soil associated with a large outbreak of blastomycosis in Wisconsin. N Engl J Med 314:529–534, 1986

181. KLEIN BS, VERGERONT JM, DISALVO, ET AL: Two outbreaks of blastomycosis along rivers in Wisconsin. Isolation of *Blastomyces dermatitidis* from riverbank soil and evidence of transmission along waterways. Am Rev Respir Dis 136:1333–1338, 1987

182. KLEIN RS, HARRIS CA, ET AL: Oral candidiasis in high risk patients as the initial manifestation of acquired immunodeficiency syndrome. N Engl J Med 31:354–358, 1984

183. KONEMAN EW, ROBERTS GD: Mycotic disease. In Henry JB, ed. Clinical Diagnosis and Management by Laboratory Methods, 18th ed. Philadelphia, WB Saunders, 1991, Chap 45

184. KONEMAN EW, ROBERTS GD: Practical Laboratory Mycology, 3rd ed. Baltimore, Williams & Wilkins, 1985

185. KURUP VP, KUMAR A: Immunodiagnosis of aspergillosis. Clin Microbiol Rev 4:439–456, 1991

186. KURTIN PJ, McKINSEY DS, GUPTA MR, DRIKS M: Histoplasmosis in patients with acquired immunodeficiency syndrome: hematologic and bone marrow manifestations. Am J Clin Pathol 93:367–372, 1990

187. KWON-CHUNG KJ, BENNETT JE: Medical Mycology. Philadelphia, Lea & Febiger, 1992

188. LAKE FR, McALEER R, TRIBE AD: Pulmonary mucormycosis without underlying systemic disease. Med J Aust 149:323–325, 1988

189. LANZ B, SELAKOVICH WG, COLLINS DH, GARVIN KL: Coccidioidomycosis of the knee with a 26-year follow-up evaluation. A case report. Clin Orthop 234:183–187, 1988

190. LAWRENCE RM, SNODGRASS WT, REICHEL GW, ET AL: Systemic zygomycosis caused by *Apophysomyces elegans.* J Med Mycol 24:57–65, 1986

191. LEE CH, LAN RS, TSAI YH, ET AL: Riu's stain in the diagnosis of pulmonary cryptococcosis. Introduction of a new diagnostic method. Chest 93:467–470, 1988

192. LEE TM, GREENBERGER PA, PATTERSON R, ET AL: Stage V (fibrotic) allergic bronchopulmonary aspergillosis. A review of 17 cases followed from diagnosis. Arch Intern Med 147:319–323, 1987

193. LIPSTEIN-KRESH E, ISENBERG HD, SINGER C, ET AL: Disseminated *Sporothrix schenckii* infection with arthritis in a patient with acquired immunodefiency syndrome. J Rheumatol 12:805–808, 1985

194. LOBUGLIO IF, TAYLOR JW. Phylogeny and PCR identification of the human pathogenic fungus *Penicillium marneffei.* J Clin Microbiol 33:85–89, 1995

195. LONDERO AT, MELO IS: Paracoccidioidomysosis in childhood. A critical review. Mycopathologia 82:49–55, 1983

196. LOPES JO, ALVES SH, BENEVENGA JP, ET AL: *Histoplasma capsulatum* peritonitis associated with continuous ambulatory peritoneal dialysis. Mycopathologia 122:101–102, 1993

197. LOPES JO, ALVES SH, BENEVENGA JP, ROSA AC: The second case of peritonitis due to *Histoplasma capsulatum* during continuous ambulatory peritoneal dialysis in Brazil. Mycoses 37:161–163, 1994

198. LOPEZ R, MASON JO, PARKER JS, PAPPAS PG: Intraocular blastomycosis: case report and review. Clin Infect Dis 18:805–807, 1994

199. LOPEZ AM, WILLIAMS PL, AMPEL NM: Acute pulmonary coccidioidomycosis mimicking bacterial pneumonia and septic shock: a report of two cases. Am J Med 95:236–239, 1993

200. LUGO-SOMOLINOS A, SANCHEZ JL: Prevalence of dermatophytosis in patients with diabetes. J Am Acad Dermatol 26:908–910, 1992

201. MACDONALD PB, BLACK GB, MACKENZIE R: Orthopaedic manifestations of blastomycosis. J Bone Joint Surg 72:860–864, 1990

202. MARCON MJ, POWELL DA: Human infections due to *Malassezia* spp. Clin Microbiol Rev 5:101–119, 1992

203. MAMIKUNIAN C, GATTI WM, REYES CV: Subcutaneous blastomycosis: diagnosis by fine-needle aspiration cytology. Otolaryngol Head Neck Surg 101:607–610, 1989

204. MARCELIS L, VERHAEGEN J, VANDEVEN J, ET AL: Evaluation of Bactec high blood volume resin media. Diagn Microbiol Infect Dis 15:385–391, 1992

205. MARCON MJ, POWELL DA: Epidemiology, diagnosis and management of *Malassezia furfur* systemic infection. Diagn Microbiol Infect Dis 7:161–175, 1987

206. MARTINO P, VENDITTI M, MICOZZI A, ET AL: *Blastoschizomyces capitatus*: an emerging cause of invasive fungal disease in leukemia patients. Rev Infect Dis 12:570–581, 1990

207. MATHISEN DJ, GRILLO HC: Clinical manifestation of mediastinal fibrosis and histoplasmosis. Ann Thorac Surg 54:1053–1057, 1992

208. MCGINNIS MR: Chromoblastomycosis and phaeohyphomycosis: new concepts, diagnosis and mycology. J Am Acad Dermatol 8:1–15, 1983

209. MCGINNIS MR, AJELLO L, SCHELL WA: Mycotic diseases: a proposed nomenclature. Int J Dermatol 24:9–15, 1986

210. MCGINNIS MR, BORELLI D, PADHYE AA, AJELLO L: Reclassification of *Cladosporium bantianum* in the genus *Xylohypha.* J Clin Microbiol 23:1148–1151, 1986

211. MCGINNIS MR, RINALDI MG: Selected medically important fungi and some common synonyms and obsolete names. Clin Infect Dis 21:777–778, 1995

212. MCGINNIS MR, SALKIN IF: Identification of molds commonly used in proficiency tests. Lab Med 17:138–142, 1986

213. MCGINNIS MR, SCHELL WA, CARSON J: *Phaeoannellomyces* and the *Phaeococcomycetaceae*. New dematiaceous blastomycete taxa. J Med Vet Mycol 232:179–188, 1985

214. MCKENSIE R, KHAKOO R: Blastomycosis of the esophagus presenting with gastrointestinal bleeding. Gastroenterology 88:1271–1273, 1984

215. MEIS JFGM, JAN KULLBERG B, PRUSZCZYNSKI M, VETH RPH: Severe osteomyelitis due to the zygomycete *Apophysomyces elegans.* J Clin Microbiol 32:3078–3081, 1994

216. MELCHERS WJG, VERWEIJ PE, VAN DEN HURK P, ET AL: General primer-mediated PCR for detection of *Aspergillus* species. J Clin Microbiol 32:1710–1717, 1994

217. MENDES-GIANNINI MJ, BUENO JP, SHIKANAI-YASUDA MA, ET AL: Antibody response to the 43 kDa glycoprotein of *Paracoccidioides brasiliensis* as a marker for the evaluation of patients under treatment. Am J Trop Med Hyg 43:200–206, 1990

218. MERZ WG, ROBERTS GD: Detection and recovery of fungi from clinical specimens. In Murray PR, ed. Manual of Clinical Microbiology, 6th ed. Washington DC, American Society for Microbiology, 1995, Chap 60

219. MEYER RD, BAULTIER CR, YAMASHITA JT, ET AL: Fungal sinusitis in patients with AIDS: report of 4 cases and review of the literature. Medicine 73:69–78, 1994

220. MEYER KC, MCMANUS EJ, MAKI DG: Overwhelming pulmonary blastomycosis associated with the adult respiratory distress syndrome. N Engl J Med 329:1231–1236, 1993

221. MILLER HS, NANCE MA, BRUMMITT CF, ET AL: Fungal infections associated with intravenous drug abuse: a case of localized cerebral phycomycosis. J Clin Psychiatry 49:320–322, 1988

222. MILROY CM, BLANSHARD JD, LUCAS S, MICHAELS L: Aspergillosis of the nose and paranasal sinuses. J Clin Pathol 42:123–127, 1989

223. MINAMOTO G, ARMSTRONG D: Fungal infections in AIDS. Histoplasmosis and coccidioidomycosis. Infect Dis Clin North Am 2:447–456, 1988

224. MITCHELL TG, PERFECT JR: Cryptococcosis in the era of AIDS—100 years after the discovery of *Cryptococcus neoformans.* Clin Microbiol Rev 8:515–548, 1995

225. MIYAKAWA U, MABUCHI T, FUKAZAWA Y: New method for detection of *Candida albicans* in human blood by polymerase chain reaction. J Clin Microbiol 31:3344–3347, 1993

226. MMWR MORB MORTAL WKLY REP: Coccidioidomycosis—United States, 1991–1992.22:21–24, 1993

227. MONHEIT JE, COWAN DF, MOORE DG: Rapid detection of fungi in tissues using calcofluor white and fluorescence microscopy. Am J Clin Pathol 82:597–601, 1984

228. MOORTHY RS, RAO NA, SIDIKARO Y, FOOS RY: Coccidioidomycocis iridocyclitis. Ophthalmology 101:1923–1928, 1994

229. MORDUCHOWICZ G, SHMUELI D, SHAPIRA Z, ET AL: Rhinocerebral mucormycosis in renal transplant recipients: report of three cases and review of the literature. Rev Infect Dis 8:441–446, 1986.

230. MURRAY PR: Comparison of the lysis–centrifugation and agitated biphasic blood culture system for detection of fungemia. J Clin Microbiol 29:96–98, 1991.

231. MUSIAL CE, COCKERILL FR 3D, ROBERTS GD: Fungal infections of the immunocompromised host: clinical and laboratory aspects. Clin Microbiol Rev 1:349–364, 1988.

232. MYSKOWSKI PL, BROWN AD, ET AL: Mucormycosis following bone marrow transplantation. J Am Acad Dermatol 9:111–115, 1983

233. NAIDU J, SINGH SM: Hyalohyphomycosis caused by *Paecilomyces variotii*: a case report, animal pathogenicity and "in vitro" sensitivity. Antonie Leeuwenhoek 62:225–230, 1992

234. NEGLIA JP, HURD DD, FERRIERI P, SNOVER DC: Invasive scopulariopsis in the immunocompromised host. Am J Med 83:1163–1166, 1987

235. NELSON PE, TOUSSOUN TA, MARASAS WFO: *Fusarium* species: An illustrated manual for identification. State College, PA, Pennsylvania State University Press, 1983

236. NELSON PE, DIGNANI MC, ANAISSIE EJ: Taxomony, biology, and clinical aspects of *Fusarium* species. Clin Microbiol Rev 7:479–504, 1994

237. NIELSEN H, STENDERUP J, BRUUN B: Fungemia with *Saccharomycetaceae*. Report of four cases. Scand J Infect Dis 22:581–584, 1990

238. NIELSEN H, STENDERUP J, BRUUN B, LADEFOGED J: *Candida norvegensis* peritonitis and invasive disease in a patient on continuous ambulatory peritoneal dialysis. J Clin Microbiol 28:1664–1665, 1990

239. NIELSEN PG: Hereditary palmoplantar keratoderma and dermatophytosis in the northernmost county of Sweden (Norrbotten). Acta Derm Venereol Suppl (Stockh) 188:1–60, 1994

240. NIGHTINGALE SD, PARKS JM, POU DK, ET AL: Disseminated histoplasmosis in patients with AIDS. South Med J 83:624–630, 1990

241. NOLAN MT, LONG JP, MACREAN DP, FITZGERALD MX: Aspergillosis and lung fibrosis. Ir J Med Sci 154:336–342, 1985

242. NURUDEEN TA, AHEARN DG: Regulation of melanin production by *Cryptococcus neoformans*. J Clin Microbiol 10:724–729, 1979

243. ODDS FC: *Candida* and Candidosis. Baltimore, University Park Press, 1979

244. ODDS FC: Pathogenesis of *Candida* infections. J Am Acad Dermatol 32:52–55, 1994

245. ODDS FC, BERNAERTS R: CHROMagar Candida, a new differential isolation medium for presumptive identification of clinically important *Candida* species. J Clin Microbiol 32:1923–1929, 1994

246. OPAL SM, ASP AA, ET AL: Efficacy of infection control measures during a nosocomial outbreak of disseminated aspergillosis associated with hospital construction. J Infect Dis 153:634–637, 1986

247. PADGE AA, KAPLAN W, NEUMAN MA, ET AL: Subcutaneous phaeohyphomycosis caused by *Exophiala spinifera*. Sabouraudia 22:498–500, 1984

248. PADHYE AA: Fungi causing eumycotic mycetoma. In Murray PR, ed. Manual of Clinical Microbiology, 6th ed. Washington DC, American Society for Microbiology, 1995, Chap 68

249. PADHYE AA, HELWIG WB, WARREN NG, ET AL: Subcutaneous phaeohyphomycosis caused by *Xylohypha emmonsii*. J Clin Microbiol 26:709–712, 1988

250. PADHYE AA, KOSHI G, ANANDI V, ET AL: First case of subcutaneous zygomycosis caused by *Saksenaea vasiformis*. Diagn Microbiol Infect Dis 9:69–77, 1988

251. PADHYE AA, SMITH G, MCLAUGHLIN D, STANDARD PG, KAUFMAN L: Comparative evaluation of a chemiluminescent DNA probe and an exoantigen test for rapid identification of *Histoplasma capsulatum*. J Clin Microbiol 30:3108–3111, 1992

252. PADHYE AA, SMITH G, STANDARD PG, ET AL: Comparative evaluation of chemiluminescent DNA probe assays and exoantigen tests for rapid identification of *Blastomyces dermatitidis* and *Coccidioides immitis*. J Clin Microbiol 32:867–870, 1994

253. PAGE LR, DRUMMOND JF, ET AL: Blastomycosis with oral lesions. Report of two cases. Oral Surg 47:157–160, 1979

254. PAPPAGIANIS D: Epidemiology of coccidioidomycosis. In McGinnis MR, ed. Current Topics of Medical Mycology. New York, Springer-Verlag, 1988, pp 199–238.

255. PAPPAGIANIS D: Marked increase in cases of coccidioidomycosis in California, 1991, 1992 and 1993. Clin Infect Dis 19(suppl 1):S14–S18, 1994

256. PAPPAS PG, POTTAGE JC, POWDERLY WG, ET AL: Blastomycosis in patients with the acquired immunodeficiency syndrome. Ann Intern Med 116:845–853, 1992

257. PAPPAS PG, THRELKELD MG, BEDSOLE GD, ET AL: Blastomycosis in patients with the acquired immunodeficiency syndrome. Medicine 72:311–325, 1993

258. PATTERSON JE, BARDEN GE, BIA FJ: Hospital-acquired gangrenous mucormycosis. Yale J Biol Med 59:453–459, 1986

259. PAYA CV, ROBERTS GD, COCKERILL FR III: Laboratory methods for the diagnosis of disseminated histoplasmosis: clinical importance of the lysis–centrifugation blood culture technique. Mayo Clin Proc 62:480–485, 1987

260. PENN C, HINTHORN D, O'CONNOR M, GOLDSTEIN E: Sporotrichosis in AIDS. Int Conf AIDS Jun 6–11, 9:371, 1993 (abstr PO-BO9-1413)

261. PENN RL, LAMBERT RS, GEORGE RB: Invasive fungal infections: the use of serologic tests in diagnosis and management. Arch Intern Med 143:1215–1220, 1983

261a. PENN JP, SEGAL H, BARLAND B, ET AL: Comparison of updated Vitek yeast biochemical card and API 20C yeast identification systems. J Clin Microbiol 32:1184–1187,1994

262. PEREZ RE, SMITH M, MCCLENNDON J, ET AL: *Pseudallescheria boydii* brain abscess. Complication of an intravenous catheter. Am J Med 84:359–362, 1988

263. PERFECT JR: Cryptococcosis. Infect Dis Clin North Am 3:77–102, 1989

264. PERSELL KJ, TELZAK EE, ARMSTRONG D: *Aspergillus* species colonization and invasive disease in patients with AIDS. Clin Infect Dis 14:141–148, 1992

265. PERTHAM ES, SEAL RME: *Aspergillus* prosthetic valve endocarditis. Thorax 31:380–390, 1976

266. PETRAK DL, KONEMAN EW, ESTUPINAN RC, JACKSON JC: *Phialophora richardsiae* infection in humans. Rev Infect Dis 10:1195–1203, 1988

267. PETERSON CM, SCHUPPERT K, KELLY PC, ET AL: Coccidioidomycosis in pregnancy. Obstet Gynecol Surv 48: 149–156, 1993

268. PFALLER MA, BARRY AL: Evaluation of a novel colorimetric broth microdilution method for antifungal susceptibility testing of yeast isolates. J Clin Microbiol 32:1992–1996, 1994

269. PFALLER MA, BALE M, BUSCHELMAN B, ET AL: Selection of candidate quality control isolates and tentative quality control ranges for in vitro susceptibility testing of yeast isolates by National Committee for Clinical Laboratory Standards proposed standard methods. J Clin Microbiol 32:1650–1653, 1994

270. PFALLER MA, VU Q, LANCASTER M, ET AL: Multisite reproducibility of colorimetric broth microdilution method for antifungal susceptibility testing of yeast isolates. J Clin Microbiol 32:1625–1628, 1994

271. PFALLER MA, BALE M, BUSCHELMAN B, ET AL: Quality control guidelines for National Committee for Clinical Laboratory Standards recommended broth macrodilution testing of amphotericin B, fluconazole, and flucytosine. J Clin Microbiol 33:1104–1107, 1995

272. PHILLIPS P, DOWD A, JEWESSON P, ET AL: Nonvalue of antigen detection immunoassays for diagnosis of candidemia. J Clin Microbiol 28:2320–2326, 1990

273. PHILLIPS P, WOOD WS, PHILLIPS G, RINALDI MG: Invasive hyalohyphomycosis caused by *Scopulariopsis brevicaulis* in a patient undergoing allogeneic bone marrow transplant. Diagn Microbiol Infect Dis 12:429–432, 1989

274. PIERCE NF, MILLAN JC, BENDER BS, CURTIS JL: Disseminated *Curvularia* infection. Additional therapeutic and clinical considerations with evidence of medical cure. Arch Pathol Lab Med 110:959–961, 1986

275. POWDERLY WG: Cryptococcal meningitis and AIDS. Clin Infect Dis 17:837–842, 1993

276. POWDERLY WG, CLOUD GA, DISMUKES WE, SAAG MS: Measurement of cryptococcal antigen in serum and cerebrospinal fluid: value in the management of AIDS-associated cryptococcal meningitis. Clin Infect Dis 18: 789–792, 1994

277. POWELL DA, HAYES J, DURRELL DE, ET AL: *Malassezia furfur* skin colonization of infants hospitalized in intensive care units. J Pediatr 111:217–220, 1987

278. PRICE MF, LAROCCO MT, GENTRY LO: Fluconazole susceptibilities of *Candida* species and distribution of species recovered from blood cultures over a 5-year period. Antimicrob Agents Chemother 38:1422–1424, 1994

279. PRICHARD JB, SOROTZKIN RA, JAMES RE 3D: Cutaneous manifestations of disseminated coccidioidomycosis in the acquired immunodefiency syndrome. Cutis 39: 203–205, 1987

280. PURSELL KJ: Invasive pulmonary aspergillosis complicating neoplastic disease. Semin Respir Infect 7:96–103, 1992

281. PULIDO JS, ET AL: *Histoplasma* endophthalmitis after cataract extraction. Ophthalmology 97:217–220, 1990

282. PURVIS RS, DIVEN DG, DRECHSEL RD, ET AL: Sporotrichosis presenting as arthritis and subcutaneous nodules. J Am Acad Dermatol 28:879–884, 1993

283. QUEIROZ-TELLES F, PURIM KS, FILLUS NH, ET AL: Itraconazole in the treatment of chromoblastomycosis due to *Fonsecaea pedrosoi*. Int J Dermatol 31:805–812, 1992

284. RAFAAL ES, RASMUSSEN JE: An unusual presentation of fixed cutaneous sporotrichosis: a case report and review of the literature. J Am Acad Dermatol 25:928–932, 1991

285. RAO NA, NERENBERG AV, FORSTER DJ: *Torulopsis candida* (*Candida famata*) endophthalmitis simulating *Propionibacterium acnes* syndrome. Arch Ophthalmol 109: 1718–1721, 1991

286. RAPER KB, FENNELL DL: The Genus *Aspergillus*. Baltimore, Williams & Wilkins, 1965

287. REDER PA, NEEL HB 3D, NEEL HB: Blastomycosis in otolaryngology: review of a large series. Laryngoscope 103:53–58, 1993

288. REED KD, MOORE FM, GEIGER GE, STEMPER ME: Zoonotic transmission of sporotrichosis: case report and review. Clin Infect Dis 16:384–387, 1993

289. RICHARDSON MD, SHANKLAND GS: *Rhizopus, Rhizomucor, Absidia*, and other agents of systemic and subcutaneous zygomycosis. In Murray PR, ed. Manual of Clinical Microbiology, 6th ed. Washington DC, American Society for Microbiology, 1995, Chap 66

290. RHAME FS: Prevention of nosocomial aspergillosis. J Hosp Infect 18:466–467, 1991

291. RHODES JC, ROBERTS GD: Comparison of four methods for determining nitrate utilization by cryptococci. J Clin Microbiol 1:9–10, 1975

292. RICHET HM, MCNEIL MM, EDWARDS MC, JARVIS WR: Cluster of *Malassezia furfur* pulmonary infection in infants in a neonatal intensive-care unit. J Clin Microbiol 27:1197–1200, 1989

293. RINALDI MG: Invasive aspergillosis. Rev Infect Dis 5:1061–1077, 1983

294. RINALDI MG: Zygomycosis. Infect Dis Clin North Am 3:19–41, 1989

295. RINALDI MG, PHILLIPS P, SCHWARTZ JG, ET AL: Human *Curvularia* infections. Report of five cases and review of the literature. Diag Microbiol Infect Dis 6:27–39, 1987

296. RIPPON JW: Medical Mycology: The Pathogenic Fungi and the Pathogenic Actinomycetes, 3rd ed. Philadelphia, WB Saunders, 1988, p 482

297. ROBERT F, LEBRETON F, BOUGNOUX ME, ET AL: Use of random amplified polymorphic DNA as a typing method for *Candida albicans* in epidemiological surveillance of a burn unit. J Clin Microbiol 33:2366–2371, 1995

298. ROGERS AL, KENNEDY MJ: Opportunistic hyaline hyphomycetes. In Balows A, ed. Manual of Clinical Microbiology, 5th ed. Washington DC, American Society for Microbiology, 1991, pp 659–673

299. ROTHMAN PE, ET AL: Coccidioidomycosis: possible fomite transmission. Am J Dis Child 118:792–801, 1969

300. ROUSSELLE P, FREYDIERE AM, COUILLEROT PJ, ET AL: Rapid identification of *Candida albicans* by using Albicans ID and Fluoroplate agar plates. J Clin Microbiol 32: 3034–3036, 1994

301. SALKIN IF, GORDON MA, SAMSONOFF WM, RIEDER CL: *Blastoschizomyces capitatus*, a new combination. Mycotaxon 22:373–380, 1985

302. SALKIN IF, HOLLICK GE, HURD NJ, ET AL: Evaluation of human hair sources for the in-vitro hair perforation test. Am Rev Respir Dis 132:1373–1379, 1985

303. SALKIN IF, LAND GA, HURD NJ, ET AL: Evaluation of YeastIdent and Uni-Yeast-Tek yeast identification systems. J Clin Microbiol 25:624–627, 1987

304. SALKIN IF, McGINNIS MR, DYKSTRA MJ, RENALDI MG: *Scedosporium inflatum*, an emerging pathogen. J Clin Microbiol 26:498–503, 1988

305. SALKIN IF, MARTINEZ JA, KEMMA ME: Opportunistic infection of the spleen caused by *Aureobasidium pullulans*. J Clin Microbiol 23:828–831, 1986

306. SAROSI GA, ET AL: Laboratory diagnosis of mycotic and specific fungal infections. Am Rev Respir Dis 132: 1373–1379, 1985

307. SAROSI GA, JOHNSON PC: Disseminated histoplasmosis in patients infected with human immunodeficiency virus. Clin Infect Dis 14(suppl 1):S60–67, 1992

308. SATALOFF RT, WILBORN A, PRESTIPINO A, ET AL: Histoplasmosis of the larynx. Am J Otolaryngol 14:199–205, 1993

309. SCHELL WA, PASARELL L, SALKIN IF, McGINNIS MR: *Bipolaris, Exophiala, Scedosporium, Sporothrix*, and other dematiaceous fungi. In Murray PR, ed. Manual of Clinical Microbiology, 6th ed. Washington DC, American Society for Microbiology, 1995, Chap 67

310. SCHNELLER FR, GULATI SC, CUNNINGHAM TB, ET AL: Fusarium infections in patients with hematologic malignancies. Leuk Res 14:961–966, 1990

311. SCHOLER H: Diagnosis of cryptococcosis and monitoring of chemotherapy. Mykosen 28:5–16, 1995

312. SEAWORTH BJ, KWON-CHUNG KJ, HAMILTON JD, ET AL: Brain abscess caused by a variety of *Cladosporium trichoides*. Am J Clin Pathol 79:747–752, 1983

313. SEKHON AS, DiSALVO AF, STANDARD PG, ET AL: Evaluation of commercial reagents to identify the exoantigens of *Blastomyces dermatitidis, Coccidioides immitis* and *Histoplasma* species cultures. Am J Clin Pathol 82: 206–209, 1984

314. SENNESH J, COOPER JN, PERFECT JR: Disseminated zygomycosis: report of four cases and review. Rev Infect Dis 11:741–754, 1989

315. SEROSI GA, ET AL: Laboratory diagnosis of mycotic and specific fungal infections. Am Rev Resp Dis 132: 1373–1379, 1985

316. SHAH A, KHAN ZU, CHATURVEDI S, ET AL: Allergic bronchopulmonary aspergillosis with coexistent aspergilloma: a long-term follow up. J Asthma 26: 109–115, 1989

317. SHEK YH, TUCKER MC, VICIANA AL, ET AL: *Malassezia furfur*–disseminated infection in premature infants. Am J Clin Pathol 92:595–603, 1989

318. SIGLER L, HARRIS JL, DIXON DM, ET AL: Microbiology and potential virulence of *Sporothrix cyanescens*, a fungus rarely isolated from blood and skin. J Clin Microbiol 28:1009–1015, 1990

319. SIMON GB, BERSONET SD, ET AL: Blastomycosis of the tongue. S Afr Med J 52:82–83, 1977

320. SINGH N, YU VL, RIHS JD: Invasive aspergillosis in AIDS. South Med J 84:822–827, 1991

321. SINGH G, WIJESURENDRA CS, GREEN JT: Disseminated aspergillosis in the acquired immunodeficiency syndrome. Int J STD AIDS 5:63–66, 1994

322. SMALL JM, LARSEN RA, PERIC-GOLIA L: The frequency of fungal involvement in abnormal vocal cord biopsy specimens. Arch Pathol Lab Med: 110:141–143, 1986

323. SMITH MA, ANDERSON AE, KOSTROFF K: An unusual case of coccidioidomycosis. J Clin Microbiol 32:1063–1064, 1994

324. SOBOL SM, LOVE RG, STUTMAN HR ET AL: Phaeohyphomycosis of the maxillary ethmoid sinus caused by *Drechslera spicefera*—a new fungal pathogen. Laryngoscope 94:620–627, 1984

325. SOLL DR: High frequency switching in *Candida albicans*. Clin Microbiol Rev 5:183–203, 1992

326. STAIB F, SENSKAU M: Der Bruanfarbeffkt (BFEP) bei *Cryptococcus neoformans* auf *Guizzotia abyssinica*-keratininagar in abhangigkeit voms ausgans pH-wert. Zentralbl Bakteriol (Orig A) 225:113–124, 1973

327. STECK WD: Blastomycosis. Dermatol Clin 7:241–250, 1989

328. STOCKMAN L, CLARK KA, HUNG JM, ROBERTS GD: Evaluation of commercially available acridinium ester-labeled chemiluminescent DNA probes for culture identification of *Blastomyces dermatitidis, Coccidioides immitis, Cryptococcus neoformans*, and *Histoplasma capsulatum*. J Clin Microbiol 31:845–850, 1993

329. STOCKMAN L, ROBERTS GD: Specificity of the latex test for cryptococcal antigen: a rapid, simple method for eliminating interference factors. J Clin Microbiol 17:945–947, 1983

330. STRAND CL: Role of the microbiology laboratory in the diagnosis of opportunistic infections in persons infected with human immunodeficiency virus. Arch Pathol Lab Med 114:277–283, 1990

331. STRAUSBAUGH LJ, SEWELL DL, WARD T, ET AL: High frequency of yeast carriage on hands of hospital personnel. J Clin Microbiol 32:2299–2300, 1994

332. STYNEN D, GORIS A, SARFATI J, LATGE JP: New sensitive sandwich enzyme-linked immunosorbent assay to detect galactofuran in patients with invasive aspergillosis. J Clin Microbiol 33:497–500, 1995

333. SUMMERFELL RC, RICHARDSON SE, KANE J: *Fusarium proliferatum* as an agent of disseminated infection in an immunosuppressed patient. J Clin Microbiol 26:82–87, 1988

334. TAGAMI H, GINOZA M, IMAIZUMI S, URANO-SUEHISA S: Successful treatment of chromoblastomycosis with topical heat therapy. J Am Acad Dermatol 10:615–619, 1984

335. TANNER DC, WEINSTEIN MP, FEDORCIW B, ET AL: Comparison of commercial kits for detection of cryptococcal antigen. J Clin Microbiol 1680–1684, 1994

336. TAWFIK OW, PAPASIAN CJ, DIXON AY, POTTER LM: *Saccharomyces cerevisiae* pneumonia in a patient with acquired immune deficiency syndrome. J Clin Microbiol 27:1689–1691, 1989

337. TAYLOR GD, SEKHON AS, TYRRELL DL, GOLDSAND G: Rhinofacial zygomycosis caused by *Conidiobolus coronatus*: a case report including in-vitro sensitivity to antimycotic agents. Am J Trop Med Hyg 36:398–401, 1987

338. THOMSON RB JR, ROBERTS GD: A practical approach to the diagnosis of fungal infections of the respiratory tract. Clin Lab Med 2:242–321, 1982

339. TIERNO PM JR, MILSTOC M: Germ tube-positive *Candida tropicalis*. Am J Clin Pathol 68:284–295, 1977

340. TITELLI M, MICHELONE G, CAVANNA C: Recurrent *Histoplasma capsulatum* pneumonia: a case report. Microbiologica 15:89–93, 1992

341. TONG QJ, CHAI WX, WANG ZF, ET AL: A case of cerebral aspergillosis caused by *Aspergillus nidulans*. Chin Med J (Engl) 103:518–522, 1990

342. Turiansky GW, Benson PM, Sperling LC, et al: *Phialophora verrucosa*: a new cause of mycetoma. J Am Acad Dermatol 32:311–315, 1995

343. Vaaler AK, Bradsher RW, Davies SF: Evidence of subclinical blastomycosis in forestry workers in northern Minnesota and northern Wisconsin. Am J Med 89: 470–476, 1990

344. Vainrub B, Macareno A, Mandel S, Musher DM: Wound zygomycosis (mucormycosis) in otherwise healthy adults. Am J Med 84:546–548, 1988

345. Varma A, Kwon-Chung KS: Restriction fragment polymorphism in mitochondrial DNA of *Cryptococcus neoformans*. J Gen Microbiol 135:3353–3362, 1989

346. Vajpayee RB, Gupta SK, Bareja U, Kishore K: Ocular atopy and mycotic keratitis. Ann Ophthalmol 22: 369–372, 1990

347. Valenstein P, Schell WA: Primary intranasal *Fusarium* infection. Arch Pathol Lab Med 110:751–754, 1986

348. Vanbergen WS, Fleury FJ, Cheatle EL: Fatal maternal disseminated coccidioidomycosis in a nonendemic area. Am J Obstet Gynecol 124:661–663, 1976

349. Vartian CU, Shales DM, Padhye AA, et al: *Wangiella dermatitidis* in an IV drug user. Am J Med 78:703–707, 1985

350. Vollier AF, Peterson DE, DeJongh CA, et al: *Aspergillus* sinusitis in cancer patients. Cancer 58:366–371, 1986

351. Wack EE, Ampel NM, Galgiani NJ, Bronnimann DA: Coccidioidomycosis during pregnancies. Chest 94: 376–379, 1988

352. Wages DS, Helfend L, Finkle H: *Coccidioides immitis* presenting as a hyphal form in a ventriculoperitoneal shunt. Arch Pathol Lab Med 119:91–93, 1995

353. Walsh TJ: Invasive pulmonary aspergillosis in patients with neoplastic diseases. Semin Respir Infect 5:111–122, 1990

354. Walsh TJ, Hier DB, Caplan LR: Aspergillosis of the central nervous system: clinicopathological analysis of 17 patients. Ann Neurol 18:574–582, 1985

355. Walsh TJ, Mitchell TG, Larone DH: *Histoplasma, Blastomyces, Coccidioides*, and other dimorphic fungi causing systemic mycoses. In Murray PR, ed. Manual of Clinical Microbiology, 6th ed. Washington DC, American Society for Microbiology, 1995, Chap 63

356. Wang HS, Zeimis RT, Roberts GD: Evaluation of caffeic acid-ferric citrate test for rapid identification of *Cryptococcus neoformans*. J Clin Microbiol 6:445–449, 1977

357. Warren NG, Hazen KC: *Candida, Cryptococcus*, and other yeasts of medical importance. In Murray PR, ed. Manual of Clinical Microbiology, 6th ed. Washington DC, American Society for Microbiology, 1995, Chap 61

358. Wasser L, Talavera W: Pulmonary cryptococcosis in AIDS. Chest 92:692–695, 1987

359. Watts JC, Chandler FW, Mihalov ML, et al: Giant forms of *Blastomyces dermatitidis* in the pulmonary lesions of blastomycosis. Potential confusion with *Coccidioides immitis*. Am J Clin Pathol 93:575–578, 1990

360. Weems JJ Jr: *Candida parapsilosis*: epidemiology, pathogenicity, clinical manifestations, and antimicrobial susceptibility. Clin Infect Dis 14:756–766, 1992

361. Weingardt J, Li YP: North American blastomycosis. Am Fam Physician 43:1245–1248, 1991

362. Weitzman I, Kane J, Summerbell RC: *Trichophyton, Microsporum, Epidermophyton*, and agents of superficial mycoses. In Murray PR, ed. Manual of Clinical Microbiology, 6th ed. Washington DC, American Society for Microbiology, 1995, Chap 65

363. Wheat J: Endemic mycoses in AIDS. A clinical review. Clin Microbiol Rev 8:146–159, 1995

364. Wheat LJ, Batteiger DE, Sathapatayavongs B: *Histoplasma capsulatum* in the central nervous system. A clinical review. Medicine 69:244–260, 1990

365. Wheat LJ, Connolly-Stringfield P, Williams B, et al: Diagnosis of histoplasmosis in patients with the acquired immunodeficiency syndrome by detection of *Histoplasma capsulatum* polysaccharide antigen in bronchoalveolar lavage fluid. Am Rev Respir Dis 145: 1421–1424, 1992.

366. Wheat LJ, Kohler RB, Tewari RP: Diagnosis of disseminated histoplasmosis by detection of *Histoplasma capsulatum* antigen in serum and urine specimens. N Engl J Med 314:83–88, 1986

367. Whittier S, Hopper RI, Gilligan P: Elimination of false-positive serum reactivity in latex agglutination test for cryptococcal antigen in human immunodeficiency virus-infected population. J Clin Microbiol 32: 2158–2161, 1994

368. Wieden MA, Steinbronn KK, Padhye AA, et al: Zygomycosis caused by *Apophysomyces elegans*. J Clin Microbiol 22:522–526, 1985

369. Wilhelmus DR, Robinson NM, Font RA, et al: Fungal keratitis in contact lens wearers. Am J Ophthalmol 106:708–714, 1988

370. Williams B, Fojtasek M, Connolly-Stringfield P, Wheat J: Diagnosis of histoplasmosis by antigen detection during an outbreak in Indianapolis, Ind. Arch Pathol Lab Med 118:1205–1208, 1994

371. Wilson CM, O'Rourke EJ, McGinnis MR, Salkin IF: *Scedosporium inflatum*: clinical spectrum of a newly recognized pathogen. J Infect Dis 161:102–107, 1990

372. Wingard JR: Importance of *Candida* species other than *C. albicans* as pathogens in oncology patients. Clin Infect Dis 20:115–125, 1995

373. Winn RE: Systemic fungal infections: Diagnosis and treatment: I. Sporotrichosis. Infect Dis Clin North Am 2:899–911, 1988

374. Winn RE, Anderson J, Piper J, et al: Systemic sporotrichosis treated with itraconazole. Clin Infect Dis 17:210–217, 1993

375. Witt D, McKay D, Schwam L: Acquired immune deficiency syndrome presenting as bone marrow and mediastinal cryptococcosis. Am J Med 82:149–150, 1987

376. Wong JS, Herman SJ, de Hoyos A, Weisbrod GL: Pulmonary manifestations of coccidioidomycosis. Can Assoc Radiol J 45:87–92, 1994

377. Woods GL, Goldsmith JC: *Aspergillus* infection of the central nervous system in patients with acquired immunodeficiency syndrome. Arch Neurol 47:181–184, 1990

378. Wortman PD: Concurrent chromoblastomycosis caused by *Fonsecaea pedrosoi* and actinomycetoma caused by *Nocardia brasiliensis*. J Am Acad Dermatol 32:390–392, 1995

379. YU VL, MUDER RR, POORSATTAR A: Significance of isolation of *Aspergillus* from the respiratory tract in diagnosis of invasive pulmonary aspergillosis. Result from a three-year prospective study. Am J Med 81:249–254, 1986

380. ZIENICKE HC, KOPRTING HC, LUKACS A, BRAUN-FALCO O: Dermatophytosis in children and adolescents: epidemiological, clinical, and microbiological aspects changing with age. J Dermatol 18:438–446, 1991

381. ZIGHELBOIM J, GOLDFARB RA, MODY D, ET AL: Prostatic abscess due to *Histoplasma capsulatum* in a patient with the acquired immunodeficiency syndrome. J Urol 147:166–168, 1992

382. ZIMMER BL, ROBERTS GD: Rapid selective urease test for presumptive identification of *Cryptococcus neoformans*. J Clin Microbiol 10:380–381, 1979

PARASITOLOGY

The basic tenets of parasitology were well established at the turn of the 20th century.[107] The life cycles of virtually all parasites afflicting humans have now been well studied, and preventive measures are in effect in most of the developed and many of the developing countries in the world to minimize the incidence and prevalence of parasitic diseases. Yet, human parasites still account for inestimable loss of life, widespread morbidity, and the retardation of economic development in many countries. To quote a recent report,[357] "prevalence rates (of parasitic diseases) are of such staggering magnitude that the mind has difficulty in conceiving the descriptive statistics." To continue from this report, "the total number of protozoan and helminthic infections currently existing worldwide far outnumbers the total world population since multiple infections is the rule rather than the exception."

Color Plates for Chapter 20 are found between pages 784 and 785.

Box 20-1 is a list of the estimated worldwide prevalence rates of select individual parasitic diseases, based on data from the World Health Organization (WHO) and other sources, in the order of presentation in this chapter.

In the United States, certain parasite species are encountered more frequently than others, and expertise in their identification must remain foremost. From a Centers for Disease Control and Prevention (CDC) intestinal parasite surveillance program, parasitic forms were found in 64,901 (15.6%) of the over 400,000 stool samples examined.[45] *Giardia lamblia* was found in 3.8% of all stool specimens, *Trichuris trichiura* ova in 2.7%, *Ascaris lumbricoides* ova in 2.3%, *Enterobius vermicularis* ova in 1.6% (not a true reflection of the incidence of this disease, for stool specimen examination is not the most sensitive method for establishing a diagnosis), and *Entamoeba histolytica* in 0.6% of all stool specimens. Diphyllobothriasis, including sparganosis and anisakiasis, is also seen with increased frequency as ingestion

PARASITIC DISEASE	GLOBAL PREVALENCE (MILLIONS OF PEOPLE)
Amebiases	500
Giardiasis	200
Ascariasis	800
Trichuriasis (whipworm)	800
Hookworm	900
Strongyloidiasis	50–100
Enterobius (pinworm)	42 (developed countries)
Taenia (cysticercosis)	1% of population in endemic countries)
Diphyllobothriasis	5–10
Schistosomiasis	200
Fascioliasis	1–2
Clonorchiasis	20 (China)
Paragonimiasis	4–5
Malaria	100–270
Leishmaniasis	12
Trypanosomiasis (African)	20,000 new cases/year
Trypanosomiasis (Chagas')	15
Onchocerciasis	20
Filariasis	90
Echinococcus disease	1/100,000–150/100,000

* The incidence figures recorded here are rough estimates only and intended only to illustrate the huge magnitude of infections. There are variations in numbers published in different sources which probably reflect incomplete access to information or to differences in extrapolation of known data to the population at large.

of fresh fish becomes more in vogue. Private practitioners and public health officials must be on the alert for a possible increase in taenia infections, including neurocysticercosis and other parasitic diseases, with the advent of the North American Free Trade Agreement and a more free exchange of foodstuff between North American countries.[291]

Box 20-2 is a summary of the parasites found by Bruckner and associates in a 6-month survey of stool specimen examinations on outpatients treated at Olive View Medical Center and Harbor General Hospital in Los Angeles.[35]

Other protozoa were identified in about 3% of all stool specimens in this study; other nematodes in 3%, and cestodes in 0.5%.

In a study of 274 homosexual men in Chicago with symptomatic diarrhea, 39% of the stool specimens contained E. nana, 26% E. histolytica, 14% E. coli, 9% E. hartmanni, and 8% G. lamblia.[258] The high rates of protozoal infections in this select population are consistent with similar high prevalence rates in New York City[346] and San Francisco.[215] Vermund and coworkers[329] found that the AIDS epidemic has had a definite influence on the relative prevalence of parasitic diseases. For example, Cryptosporidium species, rarely recognized in humans

before 1983, constituted 13.8% of all pathogenic protozoa in 1984. By 1986, Strongyloides stercoralis was approaching the incidence of Trichuris trichiura as the most frequent nematode at the New York Columbia–Presbyterian Medical Center, in a survey of 41,958 stool specimens submitted for examination during the period 1971 through 1984.

Blood and tissue parasitic infections are relatively rare in the United States. About 2000 to 3000 cases of malaria were reported annually during the Vietnam War, an incidence that dropped to 471 cases in 1976. Three years later, the incidence dropped even further—only 165 cases were reported during the first 6 months of 1979. However, owing to the recent influx of refugees from Vietnam, Laos, Cambodia, Africa, and other regions of the world, 566 cases were reported during the first 6 months of 1980, a 243% increase in incidence over the same period in 1979. This incidence of new cases has held, with minor annual variations, through 1988, when 1099 cases were reported to the CDC.[47]

Although the vast majority of patients with newly diagnosed malaria in the United States have been foreign-born or recent returnees from endemic regions, anopheline vectors are found in many locales. For example, cryptic cases of malaria have been reported from San Diego County in California and from Bay County in Florida.[125] None of the affected individuals gave a history of recent foreign travel, recent blood transfusions, or use of intravenous drugs. Each, however, had frequented or camped in mosquito-infested areas adjacent to encampments of migrant workers. Epidemiologic studies revealed that none of the migrant workers had a clinical history suggestive of malaria; however, the competent mosquito vector, Anopheles hermsi, was found along the San Luis Rey River in California. The conclusion from study of these isolated cases is that malaria must be included in the differential diagnosis of any patient with acute onset of cyclic fever, even if the history of recent foreign travel is lacking. More recently, Newton and associates[244] report that as of December 20, 1993, 112 cases of im-

ORGANISM	OLIVE VIEW (1350 SAMPLES)	HARBOUR GENERAL (493 SAMPLES)
Giardia lamblia	14.5%	8.7%
Endolimax nana	13.0%	8.5%
Entamoeba coli	10.5%	7.7%
Entamoeba histolytica	4.5%	5.3%
Ascaris lumbricoides	3.9%	2.0%
Hymenolepis nana	3.3%	1.4%
Dientamoeba fragilis	2.1%	2.8%

* Other protozoa were identified in about 3% of all stool specimens in this study; other nematodes in 3% and cestodes in 0.5%.

ported malaria were diagnosed in U.S. Marine Corps personnel returning from Somalia. *Plasmodium vivax* was detected in the great majority (87%), with *Plasmodium falciparum* found in eight (7%) cases and *P. malariae* in only a single case. Mixed *P. vivax* and *P. falciparum* infections were noted in six patients (5%).

The incidence of disease is not the only criterion that microbiologists must consider when determining where to concentrate their efforts in diagnostic parasitology. For example, the parasitic forms of *E. histolytica* must be identified without fail, although clinical correlation is needed to determine the clinical significance of any given isolate because most of those infected may be harboring commensal strains of *Entamoeba dispar* (to be discussed in detail later in this chapter). In a study of several institutions reporting an overly high incidence of amebiasis, Krogstad and associates[188] discovered that segmented neutrophils, when observed in saline mounts of stool specimens, were often misidentified as amebic cysts by inexperienced laboratory personnel. This misidentification not only deprives patients with nonparasitic diarrheal diseases from receiving appropriate therapy but may lead to unnecessary treatment with potentially toxic antiamebic drugs. Stained smears of feces and concentrated stool preparations should always be examined to differentiate suspicious amebic forms from inflammatory cells.

Because of expanded international travel, students and technologists working in diagnostic laboratories must maintain a broad acquaintance with all parasitic diseases. Trade agreements between countries, some endemic for parasitic diseases, also open up borders to the influx of goods that potentially are contaminated with animal parasites. Travelers from the United States to foreign lands must also remember that a variety of parasitic diseases are endemic in most developing countries. For example, over 20% of Muslim pilgrims for Jaj or Omra were infected with parasites.[289] Specific risk factors and preventive measures to be taken by travelers are presented in some detail later in this chapter.

Several factors serve to maintain a relatively high prevalence of food-borne parasitic diseases in many parts of the world.[66] Even in better-developed countries, political and social changes with influx of refugees from areas of high endemicity serve to make eradication among certain enclaves difficult to accomplish. Behavioral patterns of living, dietary habits, and ancient practices of animal husbandry continue to provide animal parasites with opportunities for survival and proliferation. For example, even in well-developed countries, such as West Germany, toxoplasmosis remains highly prevalent, with about 4% of the German population becoming infected per year.[148] The prevalence of sarcocystis and *Taenia saginata* infections also remains high in Germany, with the latter affecting about 900,000 people, giving an average annual prevalence of 1.5%. *Taenia solium* and *Trichinella spiralis* infections are rare because of improved methods of breeding and keeping pigs. However, infections with *Diphyllobothrium latum* and *Opisthorchis felineus* are on the increase, particularly in the north coastal regions where ingestion of uncooked freshwater fish has become a delicacy.

The almost universal eating of raw fish and water plants among most people living in Eastern Asia also leads to a high prevalence of parasitic diseases in which lake and sea life serve as intermediate or secondary hosts. *Clonorchis sinensis*, the Chinese liver fluke and closely related *Opisthorchis viverrini*; *Fasciolopsis buski*, the giant intestinal fluke; and *Angiostrongylus cantonensis*, the rat lung fluke that cause eosinophilic meningitis in humans, are found with great frequency in many southeast Asian countries. Anisikiasis, gnathostomiasis, paragonimiasis, and sparganosis, parasitic diseases acquired by humans by the ingestion of raw seafood, are on the rise in Japan.[170] However, infections with *T. spiralis*, *T. saginata*, and *T. solium* are also on the rise in Korea, Laos, Japan, Thailand, and other southeast Asian countries, as changes in eating habits now include ingestion of raw pork, beef, and wild game.[170,307]

A recent nationwide survey of the distribution of human parasites in China[367] revealed an overall infection rate of 63.2%, ranging from a low of 17.5% in Heilong-Jiang province to 94.7% in Hainan. Polyparasitism was found among 43.3% of those infected, with 56 different species being detected. The highest incidence of infections are among those living in rural areas, particularly among peasants and farmers. Preventive measures, such as adequate inspection of food products, changes in dietary habits and farming practices, improvement in sanitation and general education of the public, remain long-term goals with short-term failures. The advent of free-market commerce also is good news for the survival and dissemination of food-borne parasites.

Of the "blood and tissue" parasites, malaria has an estimated worldwide prevalence of at least 100 million, with 1 million deaths per year occurring in Africa alone.[362] An estimated 905 million people are at risk for contracting lymphatic filariasis, 81.6 million of whom are infected with *Wuchereria bancrofti*, with most cases occurring in China, India, and Indonesia. Species of sandflies causing visceral leishmaniasis have been found in 70 countries; 110,000 cases per year occur in India alone. The tsetse fly has been found in 36 countries; prevalence figures for African trypanosomiasis have been impossible to derive. In many locales, however, sleeping sickness is a major problem. Approximately 65 million people in South America have potential exposure to reduviid bugs; the prevalence of Chagas' disease is approximately 15 million.

Also, the frequent occurrence of certain parasitic infections in patients with AIDS has spurred a new interest in clinical parasitology among laboratory workers in nonendemic areas.[219] *Pneumocystis carinii*, *Toxoplasma gondii*, *Cryptosporidium* species, and *Isospora* species are the most common parasitic infections in patients with AIDS.[174] *Entamoeba histolytica* and *Giardia lamblia* are also found with increasing frequency in male homosexuals; however, these are often avirulent strains, and symptoms are minimal or absent.

RISK AND PREVENTION OF PARASITIC INFECTIONS

The risk factors in acquiring parasitic infections during travel to infested areas of the world and prophylactic measures have been reviewed by Warren and Mahmoud.[338] At lowest risk is the business person who stays in first-class hotels in large cities for short periods. At the opposite end of the spectrum are volunteers and missionaries who live in tents or native dwellings in rural settings.

Most parasitic diseases are contracted either through ingestion of contaminated food or water or through the sting or bite of an arthropod vector. Drinking untreated water or brushing teeth with contaminated water can be particularly hazardous. Because most intestinal parasites withstand freezing, contaminated ice water is equally unsafe. Hot tap water is relatively safe because the infective forms of most intestinal parasites are heat-sensitive; however, tap water may not consistently exceed the critical temperature of 43°C (110°F), and safety cannot be guaranteed. The ingestion of fresh, unpasteurized milk should also be avoided in endemic areas. Bottled milk and carbonated beverages are usually safe.

Undercooked meats or raw freshwater fish can transmit flukes, tapeworm, nematodes, such as *Trichinella spiralis*, and the bradyzoites of *Toxoplasma gondii*. Raw vegetables are relatively safe if peeled before eating; however, lettuce and other leafy vegetables are particularly difficult to rid of infective parasitic eggs and cysts.

Precautions should be taken to avoid insect bites in tropical regions. The use of screens, bug bombs, insect repellents, and long-sleeved protective clothing is highly recommended. Travelers to foreign countries, particularly to underdeveloped regions in the tropical or subtropical climates, should consult local health authorities about appropriate immunization programs. Travelers to areas where malaria is endemic should receive chemoprophylactic drugs. Local state health authorities should be consulted by individuals planning to visit certain countries to determine the magnitude and geographic distribution of the different malarial parasites and which prophylactic regimen should be initiated.

Travelers to tropical regions should also be warned against swimming in natural freshwater estuaries. The infective cercariae of *Schistosoma* species abound in many freshwater rivers, lakes, and canals and can easily penetrate the unbroken skin of an unsuspecting wader. Chlorine in the concentration used in swimming pools may not make the water safe. Schistosomal cercariae that infest humans are not found in seawater; however, swimmer's itch may occur after wading in brackish water following penetration of the skin by cercariae of species that infect animals. Examining physicians should make an effort to obtain any history of recent travel into regions where parasitic diseases are endemic and question patients carefully about the conditions under which they lived. The laboratory should be informed if a physician suspects a parasitic disease so that relevant specimens can be collected and the proper procedures carried out for optimal recovery of the diagnostic forms.

Immunosuppressed patients, particularly AIDS patients, are especially susceptible to opportunistic infections with *P. carinii*, *T. gondii*, *Cryptosporidium* species, *Isospora belli*, and *Strongyloides stercoralis*.[165,195] Isolation of patients with pneumocystis pneumonia from other immunocompromised or debilitated patients should be considered because there is recent evidence that the disease is communicable.[113] Patients with Hodgkin's disease and AIDS have a particular predisposition to develop meningoencephalitis caused by *T. gondii*. Latent strongyloidiasis in patients with a variety of immunocompromised conditions, including AIDS,[142,186] lymphoma,[123] renal transplantation with impaired T-lymphocyte function,[82] and corticosteroid therapy,[56] among others, may develop into severe or even fatal disseminated disease. Therefore, stool examinations to screen for *S. stercoralis* larvae have been recommended on all patients before they receive immunosuppressive drugs.[124,179]

CLINICAL MANIFESTATIONS OF PARASITIC DISEASE

The most common symptom of intestinal parasitic infection is diarrhea, which may be bloody or purulent. Cramping abdominal pain may be a prominent feature in those diseases in which the bowel mucosa or wall is invaded by the parasite, such as in infections with hookworms, Manson's or oriental schistosomes, or intestinal flukes. Heavy infection with *Ascaris lumbricoides* can result in small-bowel obstruction. Patients with tapeworms may be asymptomatic except for weight loss despite increased appetite and food intake. Bloating, belching, and steatorrhea may be seen in patients with giardiasis.

Peripheral blood eosinophilia (15% to 50%) is one of the more important markers for parasitic infestation. Eosinophilia may also be seen in various body secretions, such as sputum, diarrheal stools, suppurative exudates, or fluids from pseudocysts or various body cavities. However, the lack of eosinophils in either the blood or body fluids does not preclude the diagnosis of those parasitic diseases in which eosinophilia is not a common manifestation or the load of parasites may be light. A generalized urticarial skin rash, thought to be a hypersensitivity reaction secondary to metabolic or lytic products of dead organisms that are absorbed into the circulation, may also suggest parasitic infection.

Hepatosplenomegaly is a common manifestation of leishmaniasis (kala azar) and liver fluke infection. Portal hypertension, in particular, can be caused by *Schistosoma japonicum*, and jaundice is a common presenting sign. Space-occupying cystic lesions of the liver, brain, and other organs can be found in amebiasis, echinococcosis, and cysticercus (larval stage of *T. solium*) infections.

Suprapubic pain, frequency of urination, and hematuria are highly suggestive of *S. haematobium* infection. Transient pneumonitis may be experienced during the larval migratory phases of ascaris or hookworm infections. Cough, chest pain, and hemoptysis, together with the formation of parabronchial cysts, are common manifestations of the lung fluke, *Paragonimus westermani.* Low-grade fever, weight loss, facial edema, and skeletal muscle pain indicate possible infection with *Trichinella spiralis.* Focal itching of the skin may occur at the sites of penetration of hookworm larvae or schistosome cercariae.

Generalized constitutional symptoms are more commonly experienced after infections with the blood parasites. Fever, chills, night sweats, lassitude, myalgias, and weight loss are common manifestations of malaria, leishmaniasis, and trypanosomiasis. Varying degrees of hepatosplenomegaly and lymphadenopathy are also seen with these diseases. Neurologic signs and symptoms secondary to encephalitis, meningitis, or localizing neuropathies may be seen in a variety of parasitic diseases. Central nervous system (CNS) involvement is commonly diffuse in African trypanosomiasis (sleeping sickness), falciparum malaria, and toxoplasmosis, whereas space-occupying abscesses or cysts are more commonly seen with *Entamoeba histolytica,* *T. solium* (cysticercosis), and *Echinococcus granulosus* infections. Cardiac myopathy is one of the most serious complications of South American trypanosomiasis (*Trypanosoma cruzi*). Huge swellings of the legs, arms, and scrotum (elephantiasis) are common symptoms of filariases because the adult worms block the lymphatic vessels, resulting in extensive chronic inflammation and fibrosis. Localized subcutaneous nodules or serpiginous inflammatory areas in the skin may be seen in diseases such as onchocerciasis, dracunculiasis, or cutaneous larval migrans from hookworms of dogs and other animals.

A succinct overview of the clinical and laboratory aspects of several common and uncommon parasitic diseases has been published.[316]

COLLECTION, TRANSPORT, AND PROCESSING OF SPECIMENS

Appropriate specimens must be collected from the patient and transported to the laboratory sufficiently preserved to permit the detection and identification of any parasitic forms. The diagnosis of parasitic infections relies largely on macroscopic or microscopic examination of feces, urine, blood, sputum, and tissues. The implementation of reliable laboratory processing techniques is an integral step. It is not possible to review more than a few of the commonly used laboratory procedures that can aid in the recovery and identification of parasitic forms in clinical specimens. For a succinct and practical overview of these procedures, the reader is referred to Garcia and Bruckner[120] and to Melvin and Smith.[231]

FECAL SPECIMENS

Stool specimens should be collected in a clean, wide-mouthed container with a tightly fitted lid. Specimens that are admixed with water (e.g., contamination from the toilet bowl or bed pan) or urine are unsuitable because trophozoites may lose their motility or undergo lysis. Medications containing mineral oil, bismuth, antibiotics, antimalarials, or other chemical substances may compromise the detection of intestinal protozoa. Thus, examination of specimens must be delayed for 1 week or more after diagnostic procedures (barium enema) or therapy is stopped. Patients who have received a barium enema may not excrete organisms in their stools for at least 1 week following the enema.[120,231] The lid should be tightly fitted to the container immediately after collection of the sample to maintain adequate moisture. Every specimen container must be properly labeled, as outlined in Chapter 2.

The collection of three fecal specimens usually suffices to make the diagnosis of intestinal parasitic diseases—two obtained on successive days during normal bowel movement and a third after a Fleet's phosphosoda or magnesium sulfate purge. Cathartics with an oil base should be avoided because oils retard motility of trophozoites and distort the morphology of the parasites. A total of six specimens, collected on successive days, may be required if intestinal amebiasis or giardiasis is suspected. Examination of more than six samples in a 10-day period rarely yields additional information. Post-therapy specimens should be examined 3 to 4 weeks after treatment of patients with protozoan infections and 5 to 6 weeks after therapy for taenia infections.

PRESERVATION OF CLINICAL SPECIMENS

Many stool specimens for examination of ova and parasites are collected either at home, in a physician's office, or in a clinic some distance from the laboratory that performs the examination. Because trophozoites disintegrate rapidly after defecation and do not encyst, liquid stool specimens should be examined within 30 minutes after collection (not 30 minutes after receipt in the laboratory), or semiformed stools within 60 minutes, to detect motile trophozoites, particularly in suspected infections with *E. histolytica.* Formed stools, in which trophozoites are not expected, may be examined up to 24 hours after passage. Stool specimens should never be frozen and thawed or placed in an incubator because parasitic forms may deteriorate rapidly.

Several preservatives are available for permanent fixation of stool specimens that must be sent to reference laboratories for analysis. Ten percent formalin-saline (100 mL formaldehyde in 900 mL 0.85% sodium chloride) is a time-honored fixative. Some parasitologists prefer a formula containing 5% formalin, which is purported to be less damaging to protozoa and emits less formalin vapor into the laboratory environment. One disadvantage of formalin-fixed stool specimens is the unsuitability for the preparation of permanent-stained smears. Polyvinyl alcohol (PVA) is widely used because the performance of concentration procedures and the preparation of permanent-stained smears are both possible. The details of stool preparation and preservation methods are found in Chart 28.

Garcia and Ash[117] have proposed the assembly of a fecal collection kit for clinical use, along with specific instructions for the collection and preservation of fecal specimens. The kit includes all containers, vials containing appropriate fixative solutions, applicator sticks, preservatives, labels, and instructions necessary for proper collection. Para-paks (Meridian Diagnostics Inc., Cincinnati OH) and Fekal-kits (Trend Scientific Inc., Minneapolis MN) are commercially available stool collection and preservation kits.

VISUAL EXAMINATION

Freshly passed stool specimens submitted for parasitologic study should be visually examined for the presence of barium, oils, or other materials that may render them unacceptable for further processing. Patches of blood or mucin should be specifically selected for microscopic study because they may be derived directly from ulcers or purulent abscesses where the concentration of amebae may be highest.

Visual examination can also be used to determine the appropriate procedures to perform, as outlined by Melvin and Smith.[231] Formed stools are unlikely to contain trophozoites; thus, wet mounts are usually unnecessary and only concentrates need to be prepared. Helminth eggs and larvae and protozoan cysts can be seen in the sediment of concentrates. The preparation of stained smears is helpful in identifying cysts found in wet mounts.

PROCESSING FRESH STOOL SPECIMENS FOR OVA AND PARASITE EXAMINATION

Three preparations should be made for liquid and soft stool specimens submitted for parasitic examinations: 1) direct wet mounts, 2) concentrates, and 3) permanent-stained smears.

Direct saline mounts are valuable for the detection of motile trophozoites (a relatively uncommon event in most clinical laboratories). Helminth eggs and larvae and protozoan cysts may also be observed in direct saline mounts; the addition of a drop of iodine may aid visualization of these forms. For fecal specimens that are watery or liquid, centrifugation of the specimen alone may suffice because trophozoites do not concentrate well from liquid stools, and cysts that may be present can be seen in the sediment. The direct examination may be omitted for the processing of semiformed stools because any parasitic forms present will still be detected in the concentrated preparation.

Final identifications of parasites should not be made from examination of direct mounts alone; rather, permanent-stained smears should be prepared and examined to confirm the characteristic morphologic features. Permanent stains should be prepared on any specimens for which a delay in transport is anticipated. Mix 1 to 2 drops of the specimen with 3 to 4 drops of polyvinyl-alcohol, spread over the surface of

a glass slide, and allow to air-dry. Or, a small amount can be added to an equal volume of Schaudinn's fixative in a capped tube.

Preparation of Direct Wet Mounts. The saline mount is made by emulsifying a small portion of fecal material in a drop of physiologic saline on a microscope slide and overlaying the mixture with a coverslip. Mounts should be just thick enough that newspaper print can be read through the slide. If the mounts are too thick, particularly iodine preparations, parasitic forms often stain poorly and may be difficult to differentiate from background debris. If the smear is too thin, parasitic forms in low numbers may be diluted out and missed during routine microscopic examination. Saline mounts are prepared to observe the motility of trophozoites. Protozoan cysts also appear more refractile on saline preparations than on iodine preparations. Definitive identification of either trophozoites or protozoan cysts is difficult in saline mounts because the internal structures are often poorly delineated and permanent-stained smears should always be prepared.

Iodine is used as a stain to highlight the internal structures of internal parasites. One percent solutions of iodine (for example, D'Antoni's iodine, prepared by adding 1.0 g potassium iodide and 1.5 g powdered iodine crystals to 100 mL of distilled water) should be used. Lugol's iodine, used for Gram stains, in full strength is too strong to stain protozoan forms but can be used if a freshly prepared solution is diluted 1:5 with distilled water (having the appearance of strong tea). Examination of iodine mounts alone, however, may not be satisfactory because trophozoites are no longer motile. Both saline and iodine mounts can be prepared on a single microscope slide making it easy to compare any suspicious forms.

Concentration Methods. Eggs, cysts, and trophozoites are often in such low numbers in fecal material that they are difficult to detect in direct smears or mounts; therefore, concentration procedures should always be performed. The two most commonly used are 1) flotation and 2) sedimentation (see Chart 22 for details). Both are designed to separate intestinal protozoa and helminth eggs from excess fecal debris.

When fecal material is concentrated by the flotation technique, eggs and cysts float to the top of the zinc sulfate solution with its high specific gravity of 1.18. In contrast, the specific gravity of protozoa and many of the helminth eggs is lower; for example, a hookworm egg is 1.055; an ascaris egg, 1.110; a trichiura egg, 1.150; and *G. lamblia* cysts, 1.060. Cysts and eggs that float to the top of the heavier zinc sulfate suspension are collected by placing a coverslip on the surface of the meniscus at the top of the tube. The oocysts of *Cryptosporidium* species can be better concentrated using Schaeffer's flotation technique.[7]

Operculated trematode and cestode eggs may not be detected because the high concentration of the zinc sulfate suspension causes the opercula to pop open, fill with fluid, and sink to the bottom of the tube. Bartlett and associates[20] have described a modified zinc sulfate flotation technique that may be adapted for use with specimens that have been formalin-fixed. The formalin fixation not only prevents operculated eggs from popping so that they can be detected in flotation eluates but also prevents the distortion of parasitic forms caused by salt solutions of high specific gravity. All flotation techniques have the advantage that most of the interfering background debris is eliminated.

Concentration of intestinal parasites by sedimentation techniques, using either gravity or centrifugation, leads to a good recovery of protozoa, eggs, and larvae, although they may be more difficult to detect in microscopic mounts and in stained smears because of the comparatively large amount of background debris. In keeping with OSHA requirements, ethyl acetate has been substituted for diethyl ether in the formalin concentration procedure. Young and associates[365] have demonstrated that ethyl acetate is less flammable and less hazardous to use than diethyl ether, and the capability to concentrate cysts and eggs is not compromised. Care must be taken during the washing steps in the procedure to decant the supernatant carefully; otherwise, a significant number of parasitic forms can be lost. Neimeister and coworkers[242] have demonstrated that Hemo-De (PMP Medical Industries, Inc, Irving TX and distributed by Fisher Scientific Co, Pittsburgh, PA) is an effective replacement for ethyl acetate. Hemo-De is a solvent with a specific gravity and solubility similar to that of ethyl acetate, is nonflammable, nontoxic, and is biodegradable (classified as GRAS [generally regarded as safe]) by the U.S. Food and Drug Administration).

Permanent-Stained Smears. Although temporary wet mounts of fecal material for direct microscopic examination facilitate the rapid detection of intestinal parasites in fecal specimens, the identification of *E. histolytica* or other protozoan infections can be greatly enhanced by preparing permanent-stained smears. The morphology of cysts and trophozoites is better visualized in stained smears that can be used as permanent mounts for future study, for use in teaching collections, and for consultation with experts when unusual forms are observed. Because smaller protozoan organisms may be missed if only direct smear and concentration methods are employed, it is recommended[120] that permanent stains be prepared as part of the examination of every stool specimen submitted for parasitologic examination. Shetty and Brabhu,[301] in a review of 1285 stool specimens from patients with diarrhea and dysentery, also demonstrated that fecal preservation and subsequent staining was superior to wet mount examination for detection of amebic and giardial trophozoites.

Two permanent stains commonly used to visualize intestinal protozoa in fecal smears are 1) the iron hematoxylin stain and 2) the modified (Wheatley's) Gomori's trichrome stains. The iron hematoxylin stain is the time-honored technique used for the most exacting definition of the morphology of intestinal parasites. The staining procedure is somewhat difficult to control and is best performed by an experienced person to achieve optimum results. The trichrome stain is widely used in diagnostic laboratories because it is easy to perform and good results are obtained with both fresh and PVA-preserved fecal material. However, Shetty and Brabhu[301] have demonstrated that, although the trichrome and the iron hematoxylin stains were comparable for the detection of cysts and trophozoites of the entamoebas, the trophozoites of *G. lamblia* stained better with iron hematoxylin. These staining procedures are reviewed in detail in Chart 70.

Permanent-stained smears are prepared by spreading a thin film of fecal material on the surface of a glass slide. Smears should be prepared from fresh specimens if possible and immediately placed in fixative. An old, thick smear that has been inadequately fixed may result in failure of the organisms to stain. The fixatives recommended are either PVA or Schaudinn's solution. Markell and Quinn[216] have demonstrated that more specimens are positive for cysts and trophozoites and more organisms are seen per slide with PVA than with Schaudinn's fixative.

PVA is recommended for use on fecal specimens that will be delayed more than 1 hour in transport to the laboratory. The staining time required for PVA-fixed smears is generally longer than the standard time indicated in Chart 70 and must be adjusted by the person performing the procedure. The most effective PVA is prepared with Schaudinn's fixative that has a mercuric chloride base; substitutes, such as copper sulfate, are inferior. When properly stained, the organisms have a blue-green to purple cytoplasm and red to purple-red chromatin against a green-staining background. Helminth eggs and larvae have a red or purple appearance. Remember that *T. trichiura* eggs and *G. lamblia* cysts do not concentrate as well from PVA as from formalin-fixed material, that the morphology of larval forms of *Strongyloides stercoralis* is poor in PVA-fixed stools, and that *Isospora belli* may be missed completely.

Garcia and Bruckner[120] have described other techniques for the examination of fecal specimens, particularly useful for detecting infections with hookworms *Strongyloides* and *Trichostrongylus*. These include the Harade-Mori filter-paper strip culture technique, the filter paper–slant culture method, the charcoal culture technique, the Baermann procedure for culture of strongyloides larvae, methods for performing egg counts, and techniques for hatching schistosome eggs. These techniques are beyond the needs of most clinical laboratories, but on occasion, may be useful.

With the advent of diarrheal syndromes, particularly in patients with AIDS associated with sporozoan organisms, namely, *Cryptosporidium* species, *Cyclospora* species, and *Microsporum* species, additional stains may be required in the examination of liquid and soft stools. The oocysts of *Cryptosporidium* species and *Cyclospora* species stain well with the modified acid-fast stain, in which 1% sulfuric acid is used as the decolorizer. A fluorescent antibody method is also available for the detection of *Cryptosporidium* species, often in combination with a monoclonal antibody directed against *G. lamblia* cysts (discussed in detail later in this chapter). Remember that fresh or formalin-fixed material must be used to perform the acid-fast or the monoclonal antibody techniques; PVA-preserved specimens cannot be used.

The tiny organisms of *Microsporum* species do not stain well with most stains. Two modified trichrome-staining methods, the Weber stain and the Ryan stain, can be recommended. These are described in detail later in this chapter.

INTESTINAL SPECIMENS OTHER THAN STOOL

Parasites such as *G. lamblia* and *S. stercoralis* commonly inhabit the duodenum and jejunum. Samples of duodenal contents may be required to demonstrate these organisms. A saline wet mount can be prepared from the aspirated material and examined microscopically. If motile organisms are seen, examination of a second iodine preparation may be helpful to highlight the internal structures so that a definitive identification can be made.

Duodenal contents can be examined by the string test.[167] The implement used is a weighted gelatin capsule containing a coiled length of nylon string (commercially available as Enterotest from HEDECO, Palo Alto CA). One end of the string, which is taped to the face of the patient, protrudes from the capsule. The capsule is swallowed and peristalsis carries the weighted string into the duodenum. After 4 to 6 hours, the string is removed and any bile-stained mucus adhering to the distal end is used to prepare direct mounts and stained smears for microscopic study. The examination of duodenal contents should be performed only on patients with signs and symptoms suggestive of giardiasis. McHenry and associates[227] obtained duodenal aspirates from 144 patients who were undergoing endoscopy for other reasons. In only one patient (0.7%) was *G. lamblia* recovered.

Enterobius vermicularis infection of the rectal canal is best detected using cellulose tape. To perform the examination, the adhesive surface of a 3- or 4-inch strip of clear cellulose tape is applied to the perianal folds of a patient suspected of having pinworm infection. Specimens collected in the early morning, soon after the patient arises and before bathing, are optimal for detecting ova. A tongue blade can be used to provide a firm backing for the tape. The tape is then placed adhesive side down on a glass microscope slide and examined for the characteristic ova of *E. vermicularis*. A commercially available "paddle" with a flat, sticky surface ("Swube"-Falcon 2012 disposable applicator, Falcon, Oxnard CA) can be used to obtain the specimen.

Histologic examination of a sigmoid biopsy may be necessary in some cases of *Entamoeba histolytica* infection, when repeated stool examinations fail to reveal organisms. The processing of these specimens is described later in this chapter.

EXTRAINTESTINAL SPECIMENS

SPUTUM

On rare occasions, the larval stages of hookworm, *A. lumbricoides* or *S. stercoralis*, or the eggs of *P. westermani* may be seen in sputum samples. The preparation

of a direct saline mount is usually sufficient. If the sputum is unusually thick or mucoid, an equal quantity of 3% N-acetyl-L-cysteine or 3% sodium hydroxide (or undiluted chlorine bleach) can be added to liquefy the specimen, mixed for 2 or 3 minutes, and the specimen centrifuged. After centrifugation, a wet mount of the sediment is prepared for microscopic examination. If for any reason examination of the sputum specimen is delayed, 10% formalin should be added to preserve helminth eggs or larvae.

URINE AND BODY FLUIDS

Samples of large volume should be allowed to settle for 1 or 2 hours. About 50 mL can then be taken from the bottom sediment for centrifugation. The highly concentrated sediment can then be examined by preparing a direct wet mount. If objects suggestive of parasites are seen, examination of an iodine preparation may be helpful in highlighting the diagnostic internal structures.

TISSUE BIOPSIES AND ASPIRATES

Cutaneous ulcers (as seen in leishmaniasis), skin nodules (seen in onchocerciasis and in *Mansonella streptocerca* infections), and lymph nodes may be either aspirated with a fine needle or biopsies taken. In suspected cases of cutaneous leishmaniasis, material should be aspirated with a needle and syringe from beneath the ulcer bed. A "skin snip" can be obtained to diagnose subcutaneous leishmanial disease by grasping with a forceps or elevating with the tip of a needle a small portion of skin. The tip of the small "cone" of skin is then sliced with a sharp surgical or razor blade. The snip should be sufficiently deep to include the dermal papillae but not so deep as to produce bleeding. Biopsies of rectal and bladder mucosa may be indicated to identify the characteristic ova in cases of suspected intestinal or urinary schistosomiasis.

All biopsy tissue must be submitted to the laboratory without the addition of formalin fixative. If a delay in processing cannot be prevented, the specimens should be placed in PVA fixative. If the specimen is soft, a small portion should be scraped free and placed in a drop of saline for wet mount examination. Impression smears should also be prepared by pressing a freshly cut surface of the tissue against the surface of a glass slide and placing the slide immediately into a fixative, such as Schaudinn's solution. Trichrome and other stains can be applied. The remaining portion of the biopsy material should then be submitted for histologic examination.

CORNEAL SCRAPINGS OR BIOPSY

Corneal scrapings are helpful in making the diagnosis in suspected cases of suspected acanthamoeba keratitis. The corneal scrapings obtained by a physician are placed on a slide and fixed in methyl alcohol for 3 to 5 minutes. Garcia and Bruckner[120] suggest that staining should be done using calcofluor white, a textile whitener that is commercially available. A solution of 0.1% calcafluor white and 0.1% Evans blue is dissolved in distilled water. A few drops of this solution are placed on the methanol-fixed smear for 5 minutes. The slide is then tipped and the fluid drained into an absorbent paper towel, a cover slip added, and the slide examined for apple-green amebic cysts (trophozoites do not stain), which will have an apple-green or blue-white fluorescence, depending on the exciter light–filter combination used.

MUSCLE

The characteristic spiral larval forms of *T. spiralis* are best demonstrated in a tease mount made from a skeletal muscle biopsy. Garcia and Bruckner[120] suggest that the biopsy material be treated with a digestion fluid before examination. The digestion fluid is prepared by adding 5 g of pepsin to a mixture of 1000 mL of distilled water and 7 mL of concentrated HCl. The tissue is placed in a wide-mouth Erlenmeyer flask and digestion fluid is added in a ratio of one part tissue to 20 parts fluid. The digestion mixture is held at 37°C for 12 to 24 hours. After digestion, examine a few drops of the eluate under the microscope for the presence of larvae. If none are seen, centrifuge a 15-mL aliquot of the mixture and examine the sediment.

BLOOD

A drop of anticoagulated blood can be placed on a microscope slide, a coverslip put in place, and the specimen microscopically examined for large, often motile, extraerythrocytic forms, such as trypanosomas and microfilaria. When first examining a stained blood film, screen the smear under low-power magnification (250× or less) in search of these larger parasitic forms, which may be missed if only oil immersion is used. The morphology of intraerythrocytic plasmodia (malaria, babesia, theileria) is best observed in Wright's- or Giemsa-stained peripheral blood films.

Blood smears prepared for the detection of malaria should be collected specifically for that purpose and not allowed to remain on a blood collection tray during collection rounds. Smears should be prepared on anticoagulated blood samples as soon after collection as possible because the long exposure to the anticoagulant may compromise staining. The morphology of mature schizonts and gametocytes in particular may be altered. Also, sexual stages continue to develop during storage of the blood sample in a warm laboratory environment, or following exposure of the blood sample to air, gametocytes may exflagellate, releasing gametes into the plasma that can be confused microscopically with *Borrelia* species. Merozoites, particularly those of *Plasmodium vivax*, may be released from mature schizonts and reinvade erythrocytes in which they may appear similar to the small "accolade" ring forms of *P. falciparum*.

Both thin and thick blood films should be prepared. The thin blood smear, used primarily for the definitive species identification of plasmodia and other intraerythrocytic parasites, is prepared exactly as for a differential blood count. The thin feathered end should be at least 12 mm long, show no overlapping of erythrocytes, and be centrally placed, with free margins on either side. Care must be taken in preparing the thin film to see that the feathered edge is evenly spread and free of holes, streaks, or other artifacts.

Thick blood smears, which allow examination of a large quantity of blood, are especially useful in detecting malarial parasites in light infections. Place 2 or 3 drops to cover an area the size of a dime. Blood should be obtained from a finger stick and allowed to flow freely; "milking" of the finger should be avoided. Continue stirring the drop for about 30 seconds to prevent formation of fibrin clots. Allow the film to air-dry in a dust-free area. Once the film is dry, the blood should be laked by placing the slide in water or a buffer solution immediately before staining.

If anticoagulated blood is used (which currently is almost the universal practice), stirring is not necessary because fibrin strands do not form. Potassium EDTA is the anticoagulant of choice. Garcia (personal communication) has described a technique by which both a thick and thin smear can be accomplished on the same slide. Place 2 or 3 drops of anticoagulated blood at one end of a glass slide, then, with an applicator stick pressed flat, smear the drop over the surface of the remainder of the slide using a continuous circular motion. Both thick and thin areas will develop where the concentric circles intersect. At least three specimens should be taken on successive days if initial samples are negative for parasites.

Both thin and thick smears should be stained as soon as possible after preparation (always within 48 hours) with Giemsa or Wright's stain. Remember that the pH of both the stain and the buffer must be carefully controlled between 7.0 and 7.2; the stains used in the routine hematology laboratory are closer to pH 6.8, eliminating any possibility of observing Schuffner's dots. The use of automated-staining instruments is to be avoided. Thick smears may require a slightly longer exposure to the stain than the time used for the thin smear preparations.

It is recommended that at least 300 oil fields be microscopically examined at 1000× magnification on the thin film and approximately 100 fields on the thick film. The number of organisms may be very few in patients in relapse, in those who have an early infection, or in those who have received inadequate treatment or partial prophylaxis. In these instances, the number of fields examined should be doubled. Proper interpretation of the thick smear requires considerable experience, and positive controls for comparison should be made available.

IDENTIFICATION AND DIFFERENTIATION OF PARASITES

Although certain clinical signs and symptoms may suggest the possibility of a parasitic disease, the final diagnosis is made by demonstrating the causative organism in properly collected specimens. Because many artifacts resemble parasitic forms, the final identification must always rest on well-established morphologic criteria. Microscopic interpretations, in particular, cannot be left to guesswork, and a laboratory diagnosis of a parasitic disease should not be rendered until adequate identifying features can be clearly and objectively demonstrated.

One problem faced by both the new student and the instructor of clinical parasitology is the lack of a unified approach to the taxonomy of the parasites. The traditional approach of separating the parasites into various morphologic groups (protozoa, nematodes, cestodes, trematodes, and so forth) is followed in this text with the full realization that a certain degree of clinical and laboratory correlation may be lost. For example, even though hookworms and pinworms are taxonomically included with the nematodes, there are considerable differences in their life cycles, modes of infection, and the seriousness of the diseases they cause. In fact, each species of parasite is unique unto itself, and attempts to group them by whatever criteria will meet with some degree of failure.

The microscope to be used for the examination of parasites must have an eyepiece fitted with an accurately calibrated ocular micrometer. The procedure for calibrating an ocular micrometer is presented in Chart 6. The ability to measure exactly the size of parasitic forms encountered in clinical specimens is often vital to the correct identification of the parasites. In the discussions that follow, emphasis is placed on the size ranges of various diagnostic parasite forms that are reviewed.

LIFE CYCLES OF HUMAN PARASITES

Many of the life cycles of human parasites are included in the sections on the laboratory identification that follow. This is not done to imply that students must memorize every phase of every life cycle; rather, the life cycles are helpful in pinpointing the infective, invasive, and diagnostic forms of each parasite, an awareness of which is necessary to make a diagnosis.

Figure 20-1 has been designed to provide an overall orientation to the life cycles of parasites of importance to humans. Parasites can be divided into three major groups on the basis of their life cycles: 1) those having no intermediate hosts, 2) those using one intermediate host, and 3) those for which two intermediate hosts are necessary.

Most parasites that have no intermediate host are transmitted directly between humans (or animal to animal) through fecally contaminated food or water. This is true for most of the protozoa and for nematodes such as *Enterobius vermicularis* and *Trichuris trichiura*. Human-to-human transmission occurs through the transfer of cysts or ova that can survive external environmental conditions and contaminate food and water supplies. The eggs of *Ascaris lumbricoides*, *T. trichiura*, and the hookworms require a period of maturation after the stool is passed into the environment before they become infective. The life cycle of *A. lumbricoides*, although following the fecal to oral route without the need for a secondary host, is more entailed as the hatching larvae after ingestion enter the circulation and pass

through the lungs before being swallowed from oral secretions. The mode of infection for the hookworms and *Strongyloides stercoralis* is not fecal–oral; rather, it is through the direct penetration of bare skin by filariform larvae lying in contaminated dung or soil.

Parasites requiring one intermediate host commonly select either a large mammal, rodent, crustacean, or insect vector within which they complete their life cycle, a process that can be either simple or complex. For example, the human intestine serves as the primary site for the adult worms of *T. solium* and *T. saginata*. The pig and cow, respectively, are secondary hosts for these tapeworms in which larvae reside in skeletal muscle. However, the larval form of the disease (cysticercosis) may develop in humans if ova of *T. solium*, specifically, are ingested, leading to the formation of cysts in the liver, brain, and other organs. Echinococcosis is another cystic larval disease in humans in which the dog is the primary host harboring the adult echinococcal tapeworm in the intestine. Sheep normally serve as the secondary host in which the cystic lesions develop in many organs following ingestion of infective eggs. The life cycle is completed when dogs and other carnivores ingest the larval-infected offal of dead sheep.

Parasites involving crustaceans and insects usually go through a complex series of developmental stages before the infective form is released. In malaria, for example, the plasmodia undergo sexual gametogenesis within the mosquito before infective sporozoites are injected back into a human host. A similar life cycle is characteristic of other blood parasitic infections, such as trypanosomiasis, leishmaniasis, and filariasis.

Parasites that require two intermediate hosts (*Diphyllobothrium latum* and most trematodes) follow similar life cycles. Eggs that are passed from the primary host hatch in a suitable aqueous environment and release free-swimming, ciliated miracidia. These are usually ingested by a snail (a crustacean cyclops with *D. latum*), within which multiplication division takes place in cystlike spaces known as rediae. Thus, a single miracidium is multiplied into numerous free-swimming, infective cercariae. The cercariae, in turn, invade the flesh of crustaceans or fish, in which they become encysted as metacercaria. A second host becomes infected by ingesting the metacercaria in raw or inadequately cooked crab or fish meat. In the life cycle of *Fasciola* species and *Fasciolopsis* species, the cercariae become attached as encapsulated metacercaria to water plants. Human infections occur by ingesting poorly cooked infected plants.

INTESTINAL PROTOZOA

Four broad groups of intestinal protozoa are currently recognized: 1) the amebae, 2) the flagellates, 3) the ciliates, and 4) the coccidia.[196] The task of learning the differential features of these protozoa is somewhat lessened when one recognizes that only a few species are of medical importance within each of these major groups. The species that will be discussed in this chapter are listed in Box 20-3.

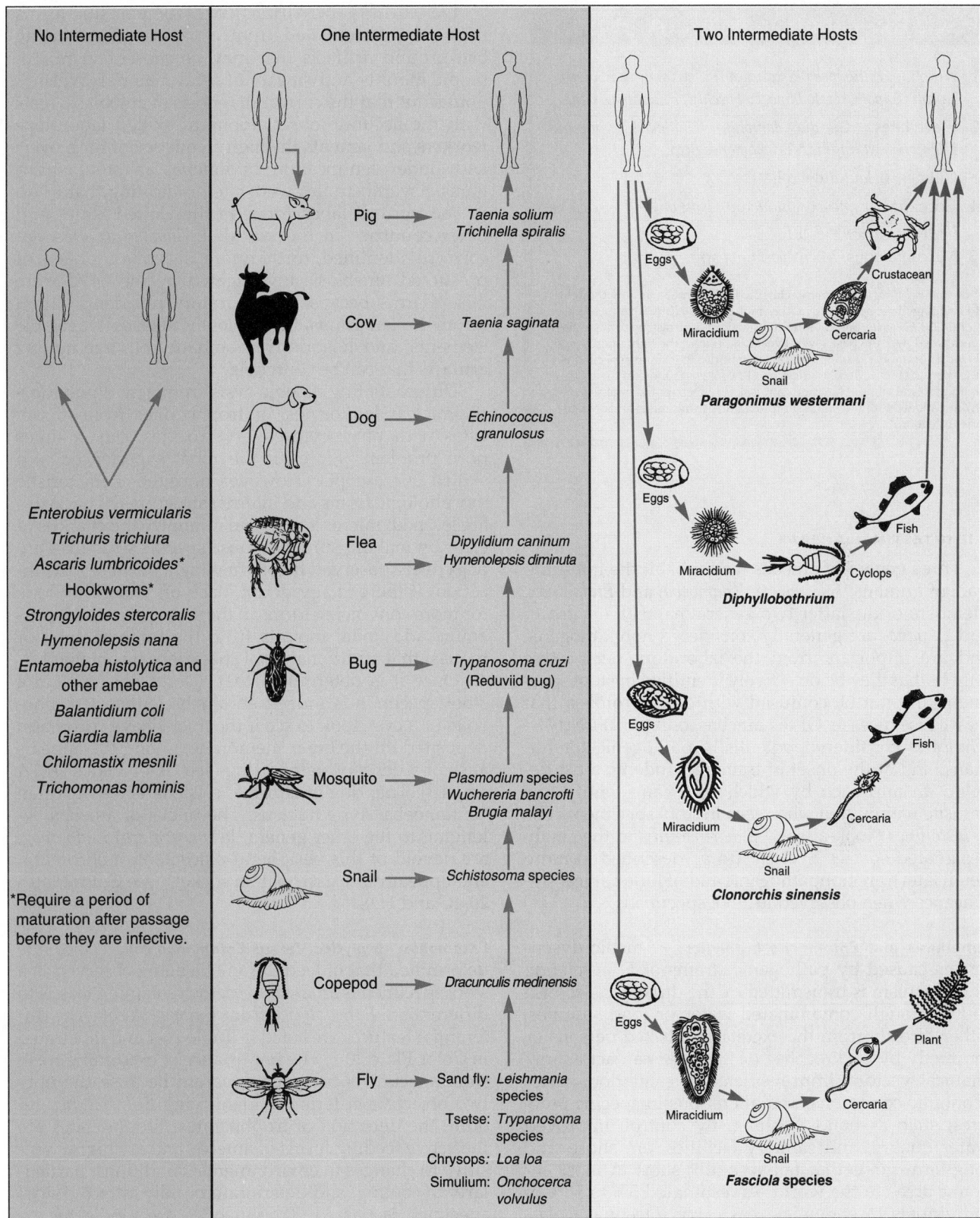

Figure 20-1
An overview of the life cycles of parasites of importance to humans.

THE INTESTINAL AMEBAE

Three genera of amebas may inhabit the intestinal tract of humans: *Entamoeba*, *Iodamoeba*, and *Endolimax*. Members of the latter two genera, namely, *I. butschlii* and *E. nana*, are generally considered nonpathogenic and are important from the laboratory perspective only in that they be objectively identified in stool specimens and not be confused with other protozoa that may cause disease. Of the amebas, only *Entamoeba histolytica* is considered potentially pathogenic for humans, and at the onset of training, students must develop an approach by which they can identify this parasite without fail when seen in stool specimens. The *E. histolytica* "look-alikes," *E. hartmanni* and the newly designated species *E. dispar* (to be described in more detail later), are nonpathogenic and of little clinical significance when observed in stool specimens.

Amebiasis and *Entamoeba histolytica*. Amebic dysentery is caused by pathogenic strains of *E. histolytica*. The organism is transmitted by the direct fecal-to-oral route through contaminated water or food supplies, either directly from the excreta of infected persons or indirectly by cockroaches or flies that can act as mechanical vectors. Improvements in sanitation, socioeconomic conditions, and alterations in specific practices, such as hand washing, fly control, improved water quality, and sanitary facilities, are short- and long-term goals that fall woefully short in most endemic areas in the world. An estimated 5% to 50% of individuals in endemic areas carry intestinal *E. histolytica*. Of these, 10% develop invasive, dysenteric bowel disease and 0.5% develop extraintestinal disease, most commonly liver abscesses. Of those with liver abscesses, 2% to 10% die. The death rate can reach as high as 70% in persons with fulminant colitis. The life cycle of *E. histolytica*, as prototype for all intestinal amebas, is shown in Figure 20-2.

LABORATORY IDENTIFICATION. True parasitic forms must be differentiated from a variety of confusing background artifacts that may be present in microscopic mounts and smears of fecal material. Welsh[332] points out that the correct diagnosis of amebiasis rests with the accurate observations of skilled laboratory workers and laments the high frequency of both over- and underidentification of amebas in stool specimens. Several studies were cited indicating that in up to one third of laboratories in the United States and other countries in the world, *E. histolytica* was not correctly identified; furthermore, several outbreaks of presumed amebiasis investigated by the CDC were false alarms because of laboratory misidentification errors. Pollen grains, incompletely digested vegetable elements, and host-derived somatic cells are among artifacts that can be confusing.

Differentiating amebic cysts from active polymorphonuclear leukocytes, or trophozoites from monocytes with phagocytosed erythrocytes, can at times pose problems for even the most experienced and skilled microscopist. However, once the characteristic morphologic forms and internal structures of parasites are learned, microscopists can minimize the chances of error by making sure that those specific structures are objectively observed before making a positive identification. If there is any doubt, back off and either look for more convincing forms in the same preparation, examine additional mounts from the same sample, or request that additional stool specimens be obtained.

Once it is determined that a form observed in a stool specimen is indeed an ameba, either a trophozoite or a cyst, look to see if the nuclei have chromatin deposited on the outer membrane, giving the appearance of a densely stained ring (see Color Plates 20-1*A* and 1*B*). This ring of chromatin is characteristic of an "entamoeba"-type nucleus. The nuclei of amebas belonging to the other genera, *Iodamoeba* and *Endolimax*, are devoid of this peripheral placement of chromatin and appear more as a "ball in socket" (see Color Plates 20-1*C* and 1*D*).

***Entamoeba histolytica* Versus *Entamoeba coli*.** Once it is determined that indeed the ameba being observed in a stool specimen is an *Entamoeba*, the remaining task is to differentiate *E. histolytica* from *Entamoeba coli*. The differential features are listed in Table 20-1 and illustrated in Color Plate 20-1. The importance of examining fresh stool specimens becomes apparent because the only two objective criteria for identifying *E. histolytica* require the detection of trophozoites. Trophozoites are the active feeding forms of amebas and are highly sensitive to changes in environmental conditions, particularly to cooling, and deteriorate rapidly after the stool specimen is passed. Trophozoites are motile by extruding one or more pseudopods.

The trophozoites of *E. histolytica* have a unidirectional motility (i.e., they extend pseudopods only along one plane and actually will "walk" off the edge of the field of focus when observed in a microscopic mount). The trophozoites of *E. coli*, on the other hand, extend pseudopods in multiple planes and "wander" aim-

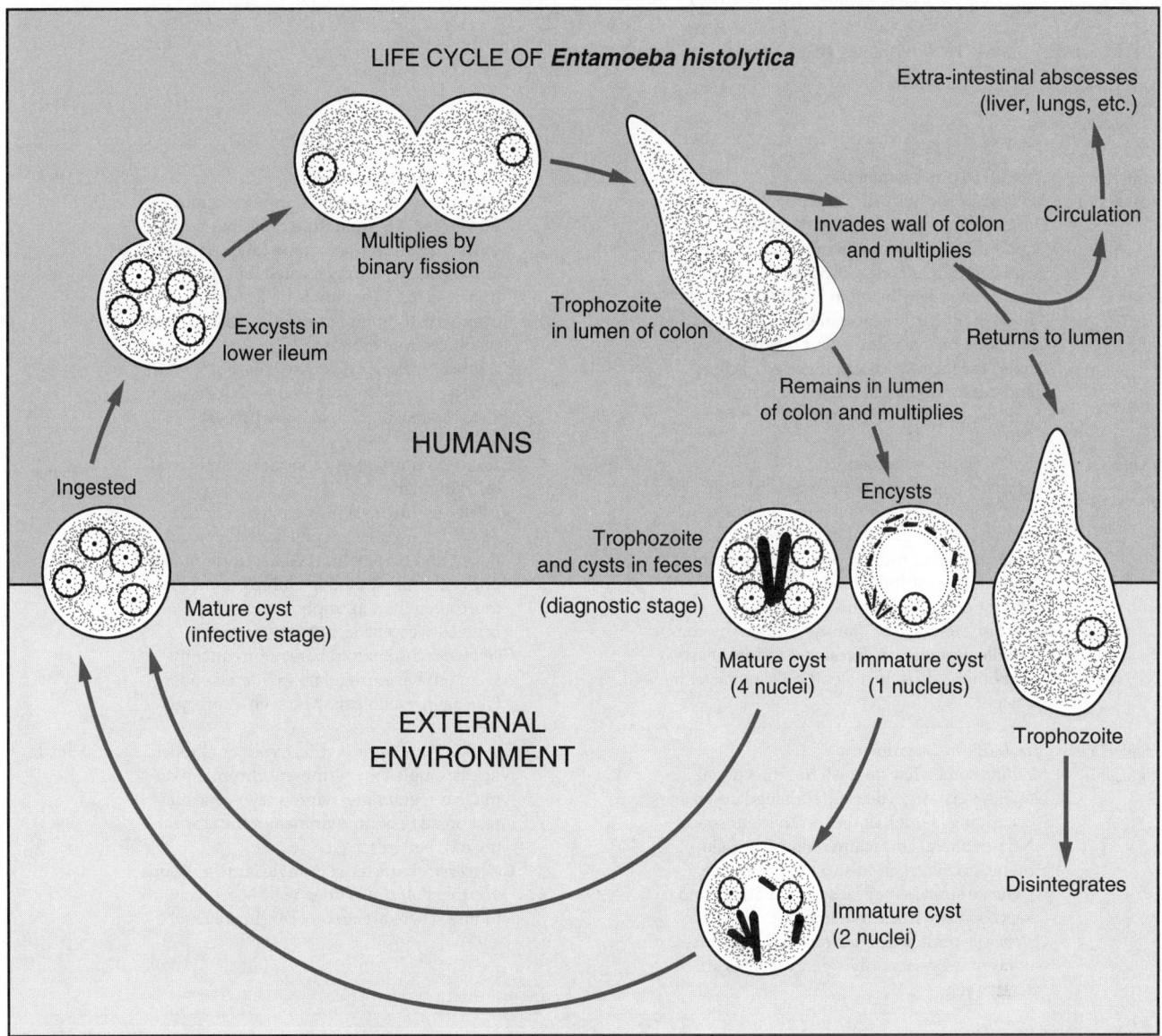

Figure 20-2
Life cycle of *Entamoeba histolytica*.

lessly in one direction then the other. The trophozoites of *E. histolytica* also have the unique capability of ingesting erythrocytes; it is extremely rare that ingested red cells will be seen in *E. coli* trophozoites. Gonzalez-Ruiz and coworkers[128] found that erythrophagocytic strains of *E. histolytica* always demonstrate a pathogenic zymodeme pattern, confirming that erythrocyte phagocytosis is virtually 100% specific and predictive of infection with invasive strains.

All other identifying characteristics between these two amebas, as listed in Table 20-1, are secondary, may be inconsistent, and can lead to only a presumptive identification when observed. However, if more than four nuclei are observed in any amebic cyst, *E. histolytica* can be ruled out. The intranuclear karyosomes of *E. histolytica*, whether observed in trophozoites or cysts, tend to be tiny and centrally placed in contrast to

the relatively larger and eccentric karyosomes of *E. coli*. The ring of nuclear chromatin of *E. histolytica* is evenly dispersed and beadlike in contrast with the blotchy distribution seen in *E. coli* (see Color Plate 20-1E).

The cytoplasm of *E. histolytica* trophozoites tends to be smooth or finely granular (because powerful proteolytic enzymes completely digest phagocytosed particles) in contrast with the "junky" cytoplasm seen in *E. coli* trophozoites. Although chromatoidal bars are seen in only about 10% to 15% of cysts, when present, those of *E. histolytica* have smooth, rounded ends in contrast with the fragmented and frayed appearance of those seen in *E. coli* (see Color Plates 20-1F and 1G). By combining two or more of these features when observing several amebic forms in a given microscopic mount, a highly presumptive, if not definitive, diagnosis can usually be rendered.

TABLE 20-1

INTESTINAL AMEBAE: KEY FEATURES FOR LABORATORY IDENTIFICATION

SPECIES	TROPHOZOITES	PLATE REFERENCE	CYSTS	PLATE REFERENCE
Entamoeba histolytica	*Size:* 12–60 µm, asymmetric *Motility:* purposeful, directional *Nucleus:* single and spherical. Karyosome tiny, spherical, with a smooth border, compact, and centrally placed. Chromatin is delicate and evenly distributed in beadlike arrangement on nuclear membrane. *Cytoplasm:* finely granular and contractile vacuoles are inconspicuous. Ingested bacteria and yeasts are absent. Presence of ingested red blood cells is diagnostic.	20-1*A, B, I*	*Size:* 10–20 µm, spherical *Nucleus:* 4 are present in mature cyst; may be fewer than 4 in immature cysts, but never more than four. Karyosome tiny, compact, and usually centrally located, but may vary in position. Chromatin is delicate and evenly distributed in beadlike fashion along the nuclear membrane. *Cytoplasm:* 10% of cysts may have chromatoid bars with smooth, rounded ends. Glycogen vacuole may be seen in early precyst.	20-1*F, K*
Entamoeba coli	*Size:* 15–50 µm, asymmetric *Motility:* sluggish and nonpurposeful. Short pseudopodia extend in many directions. *Nucleus:* single, spherical. Karyosome relatively large and eccentrically located. Chromatin is irregularly distributed in uneven clumps along nuclear membrane. *Cytoplasm:* tends to be "junky" with many contractile vacuoles, undigested bacteria, yeasts, and other debris. Red blood cells are never ingested.	20-1*E*	*Size:* 10–35 µm, usually spherical, rarely oval or triangular *Nucleus:* mature cyst may contain 8 or rarely 16 nuclei. Immature cysts have 1–8 nuclei. Peripheral chromatin is coarse and granular, unevenly distributed in clumps; somewhat more even than in trophozoites. Karyosome is usually eccentric, but may be central. *Cytoplasm:* chromatoid bars not frequently seen, but have irregular, splintered ends. Glycogen vacuole may be seen in precyst.	20-1*G, L*
Iodamoeba bütschlii	*Size:* 6–25 µm, asymmetric *Motility:* somewhat sluggish but directional *Nucleus:* very large, densely staining karyosome occupying about half the intranuclear space. No peripheral chromatin on nuclear membrane, giving a ball-in-socket appearance. Delicate strands may be seen radiating from karyosome to nuclear membrane. *Cytoplasm:* undigested bacteria and food vacuoles may be seen. Glycogen vacuoles are rarely seen.		*Size:* 6–15 µm, asymmetric, ovoid or elliptical *Nucleus:* single. No peripheral chromatin on nuclear membrane. Large karyosome may rest on edge of nuclear membrane, appearing as a ball in socket. *Cytoplasm:* characteristic single large glycogen vacuole that stains deep yellow-brown with iodine. There are no other inclusions.	20-1*C, D*
Endolimax nana	*Size:* 6–15 µm, asymmetric *Motility:* sluggish, forming many short, blunt pseudopodia *Nucleus:* single, with no peripheral chromatin on nuclear membrane. There is a large central karyosome giving a ball-in-socket appearance. *Cytoplasm:* finely vacuolated and may contain undigested bacteria	20-1*H*	*Size:* 5–14 µm, oval *Nucleus:* 1–4 may be present, but immature cysts with fewer than four are rarely seen. There is no peripheral chromatin on nuclear membrane. There are large, deeply staining central karyosomes, giving distinct ball-in-socket effect. *Cytoplasm:* not distinctive. It is fairly uniform with small granules or oval masses rarely seen.	20-1*H*

The critical observation of an "endamoeba"-type nucleus when observing an amebic form in a microscopic mount also can be extremely helpful in two other situations. Often the precysts of both *E. histolytica* and *E. coli* (intermediate forms at that phase in the life cycle when a trophozoite begins to encyst) can form prominent intracytoplasmic vacuoles, closely simulating the glycogen mass characteristic of *Iodamoeba bütschlii* (see Color Plate 20-1C). *E. hartmanni* develops

both trophozoites and cysts that are in the size range of *Endolimax nana*. Again, differentiating endamoeba-type nuclei characteristic of the former from the ball-in-socket presentation of the latter will minimize confusion between these two species.

Dientamoeba fragilis is now classified as a flagellate,[363] even though it does not possess flagella when observed with the light microscope. In practice, this organism may appear more as an amebic trophozoite than a flagellate in microscopic mounts. Nevertheless, following this suggested taxonomic change, *D. fragilis* is discussed later in the section on flagellates.

E. polecki is another member of the *Entamoeba* genus that may rarely be found in human stool specimens, particularly in individuals who may have close association with pigs. Considerable experience is necessary before the microscopic forms of this organism can be objectively identified in stool specimens. The trophozoite resembles *E. coli* in size, the sluggish pattern of motility, eccentricity of the nuclear karyosome, and junky appearance of the cytoplasm. The cysts typically have only one nucleus (never more than two), with a small, eccentric karyosome and fine, even distribution of chromatin along the nuclear membrane. Small, multiple, iodine-positive glycogen masses may be seen in the cytoplasm. A case of human infection has been reported in a Japanese refugee.[189]

I. butschlii can be identified by demonstrating the large, iodine-positive–staining glycogen vacuole in the cyst (the structure from which the genus name is derived; see Color Plates 20-1C). Early precysts of *E. coli* and, less frequently of *E. histolytica*, may also have a cytoplasmic inclusion that appears similar (see Color Plate 20-1D). The cysts of *I. butschlii* have only a single nucleus, with a large karyosome, giving a ball-in-socket appearance, in contrast to the cysts of *Entamoeba* species, which have multiple nuclei, with small karyosomes and margination of chromatin along the inner nuclear membrane. Other details for identifying this ameba are listed in Table 20-1.

Endolimax nana can be suspected on initial examination by its small size, ranging from 5 to 8 μm. The cysts have up to four nuclei, each with a relatively large, blotlike karyosome (see Color Plate 20-1H). *Entamoeba hartmanni*, although in the same size range as *E. nana*, can be distinguished primarily because it possesses an entamoeba-type nucleus in contrast with the ball-in-socket nucleus of *E. nana*. Details for identifying this ameba can be found in Table 20-1.

NONPATHOGENIC *ENTAMOEBA HISTOLYTICA*: UPDATE. For some time it has been known that the presence of *E. histolytica* cysts in stool specimens does not necessarily indicate active infection.[302] Only certain strains are capable of tissue invasion and cytolysis. Isoenzyme electrophoresis in starch gel has been used to study cell extracts obtained from amebae grown in axenic cultures. From the reactivity of four enzymes—glucose phosphate isomerase, phosphoglucomutase, L-malate: NADP, oxidoreductase, and hexokinase—18 so-called zymodeme patterns have been identified by Sargeaunt and colleagues.[287,288] Only those *E. histolytica* strains demonstrating certain zymodeme patterns are associated with human infections. Although 20% or more of homosexual men attending sexually transmitted disease clinics may harbor intestinal *E. histolytica*, only nonpathogenic zymodeme patterns have been demonstrated.[6] Weinke and associates[343] demonstrated practical applications of zymodeme determinations by identifying five travelers in whom pathogenic zymodemes for *E. histolytica* were correlated with invasive disease and positive serology, in contrast with a group of 320

CLINICAL CORRELATION BOX 20-1. *ENTAMOEBA HISTOLYTICA*

The disease syndromes resulting from infection with *E. histolytica* have been outlined by Guerrant.[138] Most humans infected with *E. histolytica* (80% to 99%) are asymptomatic, as determined by observing for excreted cysts in fecal-screening examinations or from the data of serologic surveys. A majority of those infected have disease limited to the gastrointestinal tract, following an incubation period on the average of 1 to 4 weeks. The typical lesions are "button-hole" ulcers, so-called because the trophozoites that penetrate through the mucosa are unable to digest the musculature of the bowel wall and, therefore, extend laterally along the submucosa. (Color Plate 20-1I illustrates several trophozoites in the submucosa.) Lower abdominal pain, low-grade fever, and bloody diarrhea, with or without tenesmus, are the usual presenting symptoms. Pregnancy, malnutrition, underlying metabolic diseases, and corticosteroid therapy predispose to more serious disease. Complications are relatively uncommon, developing in 1% to 4% of patients, and include bowel perforation and peritonitis. Cases of paracecal amebomas, at times forming an annular inflammatory mass simulating colonic carcinoma, have been reported. Davidson and coworkers[73] report a recent case of paracecal ameboma with fistulae extending into the appendix and into the urinary bladder.

Extraintestinal amebiasis occurs with varying frequency in different geographic areas. In Mexico, about one in every five infected individuals develop invasive disease, compared with only 1:100 to 1:1000 in the United States. The onset of symptoms may be within days after the acute bout of dysentery, or delayed by months or even years. The liver is the most common organ of extraintestinal involvement. Adams and McLeod[3] report that in up to 50% of cases of amebic liver abscesses, a history of intestinal amebiasis is lacking and trophozoites or cysts cannot be detected in stool specimens. Symptoms include weight loss, low-grade fever, weakness and vague right upper quadrant discomfort and point between the ribs on palpation. Anemia, leukocytosis and an elevated alkaline phosphatase are other supporting findings. The diagnosis is usually made by observing the characteristic single, large defect in the right lobe with a liver scan. Direct extension into the pleura or pericardium or metastatic foci in the brain, lung and kidney are uncommon events. Recent unusual cases of extraintestinal amebiasis have been reported—the pericardium,[30] endometritis in association with actinomycosis in a patient wearing an intrauterine contraceptive device,[12] and the skin of the face in a 17-month-old child.[16]

male homosexuals who had neither pathogenic zy- modemes nor symptoms of amebiasis. The rates of cyst excretion by asymptomatic and symptomatic individ- uals among a group of homosexuals studied by Key- stone and coworkers[174] were similar.

Sufficient biochemical, immunologic, and genetic data have now been gathered to support Sargeaunt's premise that what appears microscopically as a single morphotype, E. histolytica, in fact represents two distinct organisms, one pathogenic, the other nonpathogenic. Interestingly, the first indication of this dichotomy came from Emile Brumpt in 1925.[260] Diamond and Clark[83] have officially retained the name of the classic patho- genic strain as Entamoeba histolytica (Schaudinn, 1903) and given the nonpathogenic strain the designation En- tamoeba dispar (Brumpt, 1925). These two workers had previously described the nonpathogenic Laredo strain of E. histolytica, which has the unique property of grow- ing at room temperature (25° to 30°C).[58] These workers have officially assigned the Laredo strain within the species, Entamoeba moshkovskii.

Although commercial reagents are not yet available for the differentiation of E. histolytica from E. dispar, it is only a matter of time before one or more approaches currently being developed in research laboratories will reach diagnostic clinical parasitology laboratories. Wonsit and associates[355] developed a murine mono- clonal antibody against a crude lysate of a pathogenic strain of E. histolytica that showed a 97.6% specificity for detection of antigen in stool specimens of 40 pa- tients in whom E. histolytica trophozoites were ob- served microscopically. Tannich and Burchard[319] were able to differentiate pathogenic from nonpathogenic laboratory strains of E. histolytica by a sensitive assay that combined extraction of a 482 DNA segment, oligonucleotide primers, polymerase chain reaction amplification, and endonuclease digestion of the am- plified DNA. Similarly, Katzwinkel-Wladarsch and coworkers,[171] using a simple DNA extraction method and PCR amplification, were able to detect E. histolyt- ica-specific antigen directly in stool specimens contain- ing as few as one trophozoite per milligram of feces. Acuna-Soto and associates[2] also used PCR to detect E. histolytica antigen in formalin-fixed stool specimens from nine patients with intestinal amebiasis. Gonzalez- Ruiz and colleagues[127] developed an invasive strain- specific monoclonal antibody against E. histolytica used in a capture enzyme-linked immunosorbent assay (ELISA) test that could detect antigen in clinical speci- mens to an equivalent of as few as 72 trophozoites per well. The sensitivity of this test was 87% and the speci- ficity 100% in a field study of amebic dysentery in pa- tients from Bangladesh.

From the observations that nonpathogenic strains of E. histolytica exist, the controversial notion that asymptomatic homosexual patients who are excreting only cysts do not require treatment has evolved. Alla- son-Jones and coauthors[6] also make the comment that in no instance have pathogenic and nonpathogenic zy- modeme patterns coexisted in the amebas recovered from the same individual, and there is no indication that nonpathogen-to-pathogen mutations occur. How-

ever, Richman and Kerdel[273] have recently reported ex- perimental studies in which a change in zymodeme patterns was accompanied by a change in virulence of E. histolytica isolates that acquired the ability to pro- duce liver abscesses in hamsters and to destroy mono- layers of tissue cell cultures. They conclude that a zy- modeme pattern is not a stable inherent property of amebas, and that they may change and cannot neces- sarily be used as the basis for arbitrating the issue of therapy. Thus, the final decision of whether to treat asymptomatic patients who are excreting cysts re- mains with the attending physicians. If therapy is not prescribed, the patients should at least be informed that they are carrying potentially virulent organisms and to practice preventive measures accordingly. Metronidazole (Flagyl) is the treatment of choice when indicated.

Geurrant[138] and Ravdin[271] also discuss other viru- lence mechanisms characteristic of E. histolytica that produce disease: 1) chemically defined adherence factors (galactose-specific adhesin) that determine whether the organism can attach to the bowel mucosa and act as an important virulence mechanism; 2) the secretion of cytotoxins, including hyaluronidase, trypsin, pepsin, gelatinase, and hydrolytic enzymes for casein, fibrin, and hemoglobin, and 3) the production of proteolytic enzymes. The host uses several defenses to protect against invasion by parasites.[260] Pancreatic proteases, bile salts, and bacterial glycosidases may destroy the galactose-specific adhesin on the amoeba surface and block adherence. Colonic mucins, produced in re- sponse to contact of the epithelial cells by ameba, can also effectively block adherence by binding the carbo- hydrate-recognition domain of the galactose adhesin. Humans who have debilitating disease, are malnour- ished, or have defective immune responses are partic- ularly prone to both intestinal and extraintestinal dis- ease. The aforementioned papers should be consulted for in-depth presentations of research findings that may have practical implications beyond the scope of discussion here.

Identification of the galactose adherence protein as a virulence factor for pathogenic strains of E. histolytica has led to additional applications. Abd-Alla and asso- ciataes[1] have developed an epitope-specific mono- clonal antibody for use in ELISA to detect this antigen in serum and feces. In a study of 15 stool samples ob- tained from patients with intestinal amebiasis, all had a positive ELISA GIAP result; of these, the epitope- specific monoclonal antibody identified eight subjects with pathogenic strains. Overall they demonstrated 94% specificity for the detection of E. histolytica infec- tion. The GIAP antigen also serves as a candidate for developing a colonization-blocking vaccine, as this epitope is antigenically conserved and has a high- affinity interaction with the galactose-terminal colonic mucin glycoproteins.

Healy and Smith[145] reviewed several serologic tests that can be used in the diagnosis of amebiasis. Such studies are indicated when the etiologic agent is diffi- cult to detect, such as in cases of liver abscesses, when interfering substances prevent the detection of organisms in conventional studies of stool specimens, and as an epidemiologic tool in determining prevalence of disease in a given population. Sensitivities of serologic testing for liver abscesses have been 95% to 100% and 85% to 95% for the detection of invasive intestinal disease. The presence of antiamebic antibodies may not correlate with the clinical status or the intensity of infection.[340] Antibodies may persist for years following initial exposure, and thus their presence does not necessarily differentiate between past and present infection. Methods for the detection of antigen are also emerging. Newer techniques evolving in research laboratories are showing promise. Sensitive and specific serodiagnosis of invasive amebiasis has been demonstrated[206] by immunoblotting and ELISA techniques to detect a specific recombinant surface protein of pathogenic E. histolytica, and results[68] from an in-house rapid latex agglutination test to detect E. histolytica antigen in sera of patients with extraluminal amoebiasis were comparable with other standard serologic techniques used in parallel. Although commercial reagents are not currently available, it is only a matter of time before serologic techniques will be within reach of clinical laboratories, in addition to the few reference laboratories that currently provide services.

Protozoa of Uncertain Classification

BLASTOCYSTIS HOMINIS. B. hominis, once thought to be a yeast, has recently been classified as a protozoan, specifically an ameba, based on the following characteristics outlined by Zierdt:[369] 1) the organism has no cell wall; 2) it grows only in the presence of bacteria and not on fungal media; 3) it has a preference for alkaline pH and a mildly hypotonic environment; 4) it reproduces by binary fission and not by budding; 5) it extends and retracts pseudopods and ingests bacteria; and 6) it is optimally active at 37°C, does not grow at 25°C, and is killed at 4°C.

Morphologically, B. hominis appear as irregularly sized spherical cells ranging from 5 to 15 μm in diameter, although smaller forms may occasionally be found (see Color Plate 20-1J). A homogeneous-staining (green in trichrome stains) central body occupying 70% or more of the cell is characteristic, with nuclear material either scattered in undefined fragments between the central body and the outer membrane, or as one or two elongated masses in a bipolar distribution. MacPherson and MacQueen[208] point out the morphologic variability in size, shape, nuclear detail, and central body characteristics between cells, which may account to some extent for the differences in the incidence of detection of B. hominis in various reported case studies.

Several reports[114,193,327,369] provide evidence that B. hominis may be a cause of gastrointestinal disease. Recurrent diarrhea without fever, episodes of vomiting, and cramping abdominal pain have been the chief symptoms. Garcia and associates,[118] in a review of more than 6000 stool specimens, found that 289 were positive for B. hominis (in two thirds of the cases, it was the only parasite found). Within this group, gastrointestinal symptoms were noted in 24 patients, the majority of whom had underlying debilitating disease or were im-

munosuppressed. These workers conclude that B. hominis may be a pathogen when no other agent is found and when the parasite burden is high. This conclusion is supported by the cases of recurrent diarrhea reported by Vannatta[327] and Lebar,[193] in which numerous B. hominis (5/HPF) sere seen in stool samples, and cultures for bacterial pathogens and tests for rotovirus particles were negative. The symptoms subsided when these patients received antiprotozoal therapy.

Although these case reports seem to indicate that B. hominis may be an intestinal pathogen in humans, the pathogenesis is still unclear, and further studies are required before proof will be conclusive. Markell and Udkow,[217] in a study of 32 persons with B. hominis infection in whom at least six stool examinations were performed, found that 27 had other recognized pathogens—E. histolytica, G. lamblia, or Dientamoeba fragilis. In all of these cases, symptoms subsided with therapy. In the five remaining cases in whom only B. hominis was found, treatment with iodoquinol eradicated the organisms, but symptoms more consistent with irritable bowel syndrome persisted. Thus, as also counselled by Wolf and coworkers,[350] other pathogenic organisms must be eliminated from consideration before common commensal parasites are incriminated. Nagler and associates,[235] in a study of 12 patients with exacerbated inflammatory bowel disease in whom stool specimens were also positive for B. hominis, also conclude that this organism is not a significant pathogen for this entity. All of their patients improved on medical therapy, three to treatment with corticosteroids alone and one with bowel rest without medication. Five patients failed to improve with metronidazole therapy, but four responded to subsequent courses of corticosteroids.

Until the issue of pathogenicity is settled, clinical laboratory parasitologists should still indicate the detection of B. hominis in stool specimens in the final report. Some form of quantitation should be made (rare, few, moderate, many); specifically, the presence of five or more B. hominis forms per high power field (HPF) is considered to be in the moderate to many category and is reported by most laboratories. The clinician must evaluate whether such reports have clinical significance and decide whether to treat based on the clinical presentation.

INTESTINAL FLAGELLATES

As the name implies, all flagellates possess an organelle of motility, the flagellum, which serves as a means for locomotion. Other structures also serve as an integral part of the locomotor organelle (namely, the kinetoplast, to which the flagella are attached, and the axostyle and parabasal bodies). Therefore, when any of these structures is identified in a parasitic form, the parasite can be tentatively grouped with the flagellates. Unlike the ameba, which assume variable shapes, the flagellates are more rigid and tend to retain distinctive shapes, a feature often helpful in their identification.

Giardia lamblia, Chilomastix mesnili, Trichomonas hominis, and Dientamoeba fragilis are the species of flagellates commonly seen in human stool specimens. The differential features by which these four flagellates can be identified are listed in Table 20-2 and are illustrated in Color Plate 20-2.

Giardia lamblia. *G. lamblia* is the number 1 parasite-caused gastrointestinal disease in the United States[200,227,262] and has become a major worldwide public health problem.[298] It was found in 3.8% of 414,820 stool specimens submitted to state health laboratories in the United States as part of a 1976 CDC intestinal parasitic surveillance study.[45] Over 50 waterborne outbreaks were reported to the WHO involving some 20,000 people.

The life cycle is also simply completed by a fecal–oral route of transmission, with the cysts providing for a long-term survival under adverse environmental conditions. Cysts commonly find their way into streams and wells from inadequately controlled sewer systems, and mountain streams down river from residential areas are commonly contaminated. Multiplication occurs in the trophozoite form within the human, dividing by binary fission. An illustration of the life cycle representative of the intestinal flagellates is found in Figure 20-3.

The organism is not difficult to identify in microscopic mounts of fecal specimens. The trophozoite is bilaterally symmetrical and has two nuclei, one on either side of a central axostyle (giving the appearance of a "monkey face"; see Color Plate 20-2*B*). The trophozoites remain motile in the bowel lumen, and the organisms attach to the surface of epithelial cells (see Color Plate 20-2*A*). In wet preparations, a graceful "falling-leaf" motility can be a helpful identifying feature, distinguishing it from *C. mesnili*, which has a slower, stiff motion, and from *T. hominis*, which is quick, jerky, and darting.

G. lamblia cysts are distinctly oval in outline, measuring 8 to 12 µm, have a thin smooth membrane, and contain four nuclei clustered at one end, a longitudinal parabasal body near the center of the cell, and fibrils (see Color Plate 20-2*C*). Light bile staining is often seen, and there is a tendency for the cytoplasm to retract slightly from the cell wall. Once recognized, both the trophozoites and cysts are easily recognized, even under lower magnifications, making screening of specimens somewhat less tedious.

Because of irregular shedding of organisms in the feces, several samples obtained on nonsuccessive days may be required to establish a diagnosis in suspected cases, particularly in chronic disease. In one study,[147] 53% of the patients had complaints referable to giardiasis that existed for 6 months or more. The yield can be improved by preparing stained smears from concentrated fecal specimens because organisms may often be missed if only saline mount procedures are performed.[120,301] However, Heymans and associates[147] found that the "triple fecal test," that is, the examination of three stool specimens on nonconsecutive days, had a sensitivity of 95.7% in detecting organisms in known cases of giardiasis. Organisms were found in only three of 109 patients on whom duodenal biopsies

were performed after negative stool examinations (false-negative rate of 2.8%). Similarly, McHenry and coworkers[227] found only one positive aspirate in 144 duodenal aspirates in patients with nonspecific gastrointestinal symptoms. The conclusion can be drawn, therefore, that extraordinary procedures need not be performed to establish the diagnosis in the great majority of cases.

In highly suspected cases where a diagnosis has not been established, the string test is an alternative to duodenal aspiration or biopsy procedures.[167] The device used consists of a weighted capsule containing gelatin and a tightly wound string (available as Enterotest; Hedeco Corp., Mountain View CA). The capsule is swallowed and the end of the string is taped to the side of the cheek. After approximately 5 hours, the string is removed and the adherent material is stripped onto the surface of one or more glass slides. A small amount of material can be mixed with 1 or 2 drops of saline, a coverslip applied, and examined directly for the presence of diagnostic forms. A permanent-stained slide can be prepared if the wet mount results are equivocal.

Garcia and coauthors[119] reported 100% sensitivity and specificity in the detection of *G. lamblia* cysts and *Cryptosporidium* species oocysts in fecal specimens using the Merifluor (Meridian Diagnostics, Inc., Cincinnati OH) direct immunofluorescence detection system. The cysts of *Giardia* species appeared as oval, apple-green fluorescing forms measuring 11 to 14 µm in diameter; the cryptosporidial oocysts measured 4 to 6 µm in diameter and also displayed a bright apple-green fluorescence. The investigators cite the ability to screen smears under low power magnification and the ability to detect forms in low concentration as major advantages of the direct fluorescent system. It is not uncommon to find organisms by the fluorescent procedure that are not observed by routine ova and parasite examination.

Currently, success has been reported in the use of several immunologic methods to directly detect *G. lamblia* antigen in fecal specimens.[163,350] ELISA, using antibodies prepared against a variety of giardia antigens, has been the technology most often used. Knisley and colleagues,[181] who used rabbit and goat antisera following immunization with giardia trophozoites, report sensitivities of 92% and 87% and specificities of 87% and 91%, respectively; Carlson and coworkers[43] report a 97% correlation between enzyme immunoassay and direct microscopic examination on 353 specimens from human subjects in the United States. Stibbs,[312] using a monoclonal antibody-based antigen-capture enzyme immunoassay for the detection of *G. lamblia* antigen in human stool specimens, also found a 97% correlation with microscopic examinations, including formalin-fixed specimens (the absorbance was actually increased in 20 of 26 *G. lamblia*-positive specimens tested, both formalinized and unfixed).

Rosoff and associates[277] have evaluated a commercially available enzyme immunoassay (EIA; ProSpecT/ Giardia, Alexon Inc., Mountain View CA) that detects giardia-specific antigen 65 (GAS 65). All of 93 specimens

SPECIES	TROPHOZOITES	PLATE REFERENCE	CYSTS	PLATE REFERENCE
Giardia lamblia	*Size:* 9–21 μm long, 5–15 μm wide; pear-shaped with tapering end *Motility:* active, "falling leaf" *Nucleus:* 2, laterally placed. No peripheral chromatin and difficult to see in unstained mounts. There are small, central karyosomes. *Cytoplasm:* uniform and finely granular. Two median bodies appear as a mustache on the axostyle. Sucking disks occupy half of ventral surface. *Flagella:* 4 lateral, 2 ventral. They are often difficult to see.	20-2A, B	*Size:* 8–12 μm long, 7–10 μm wide; oval *Nucleus:* 4. Karyosomes are smaller than in trophozoites and tend to be eccentrically placed. There is no peripheral chromatin on nuclear membrane. *Cytoplasm:* clear space between cyst wall and cytoplasm gives an easy-to-recognize halo effect. Ill-defined longitudinal fibrils may be seen. Four median bodies are present.	20-2C
Chilomastix mesnili	*Size:* 6–20 μm long, 5–7 μm wide, round on one end, tapering to other *Motility:* stiff, rotary *Nucleus:* single and large, placed anteriorly at rounded end. Small central or eccentric karyosome with radiating filaments, difficult to see in unstained mounts. *Cytoplasm:* may be vacuolated. Prominent cytostome extending over half of body length. Spiral groove across ventral surface may be difficult to see. *Flagella:* 3 anterior and 1 in cytostome	20-2D	*Size:* 6–10 μm long, 4–6 μm wide; lemon-shaped with anterior knob *Nuclei:* 1, difficult to see in unstained mounts. There is an indistinct central karyosome. *Cytoplasm:* curved cytostome with fibrils, appearing as a "shepherd's crook," often difficult to see	20-2E
Trichomonas hominis	*Size:* 7–15 μm long, 4–7 μm wide; teardrop shaped *Motility:* active, nervous, jerky *Nucleus:* single, anterior. Small central karyosome. There is uneven distribution of chromatin on nuclear membrane. *Cytoplasm:* central, longitudinal axostyle. There is a longitudinal impression (costa) at attachment of undulating membrane that runs the full length of the body (*T. vaginalis* extends only half the body distance). *Flagella:* 3 to 5 anterior, 1 posterior. They are usually difficult to see.	20-2F	No cyst form known	
Dientamoeba fragilis	*Size:* 5–12 μm, asymmetric. There may be considerable variation in size and shape in same specimen. *Motility:* active and purposeful *Nucleus:* 1 or 2. Very delicate nuclear membrane and may be difficult to see. Karyosome is composed of 4–8 chromatin granules that tend to become separated, giving a shattered appearance. *Cytoplasm:* very vacuolated and may contain numerous undigested bacteria. *Note:* permanent stain is necessary for identification.	20-2G	No cyst stage known	
Balantidium coli	*Size:* 50–100 μm long, 40–70 μm wide; oval *Motility:* rotary, boring *Nucleus:* 1 kidney-bean–shaped macronucleus; 1 tiny round micronucleus immediately adjacent to the macronucleus *Cytoplasm:* many food vacuoles and contractile vacuoles; distinct anterior cytostome *Cilia:* body surface is covered with spiral, longitudinal rows of cilia.	20-2H, I	*Size:* 50–75 μm in diameter, spherical to ellipsoid *Nucleus:* 1 kidney-shaped macronucleus; 1 tiny spherical micronucleus lying within "hoff" of macronucleus (may be difficult to see) *Cytoplasm:* small vacuoles persist. Cilia retracted within. There is a thick, tough cyst wall.	

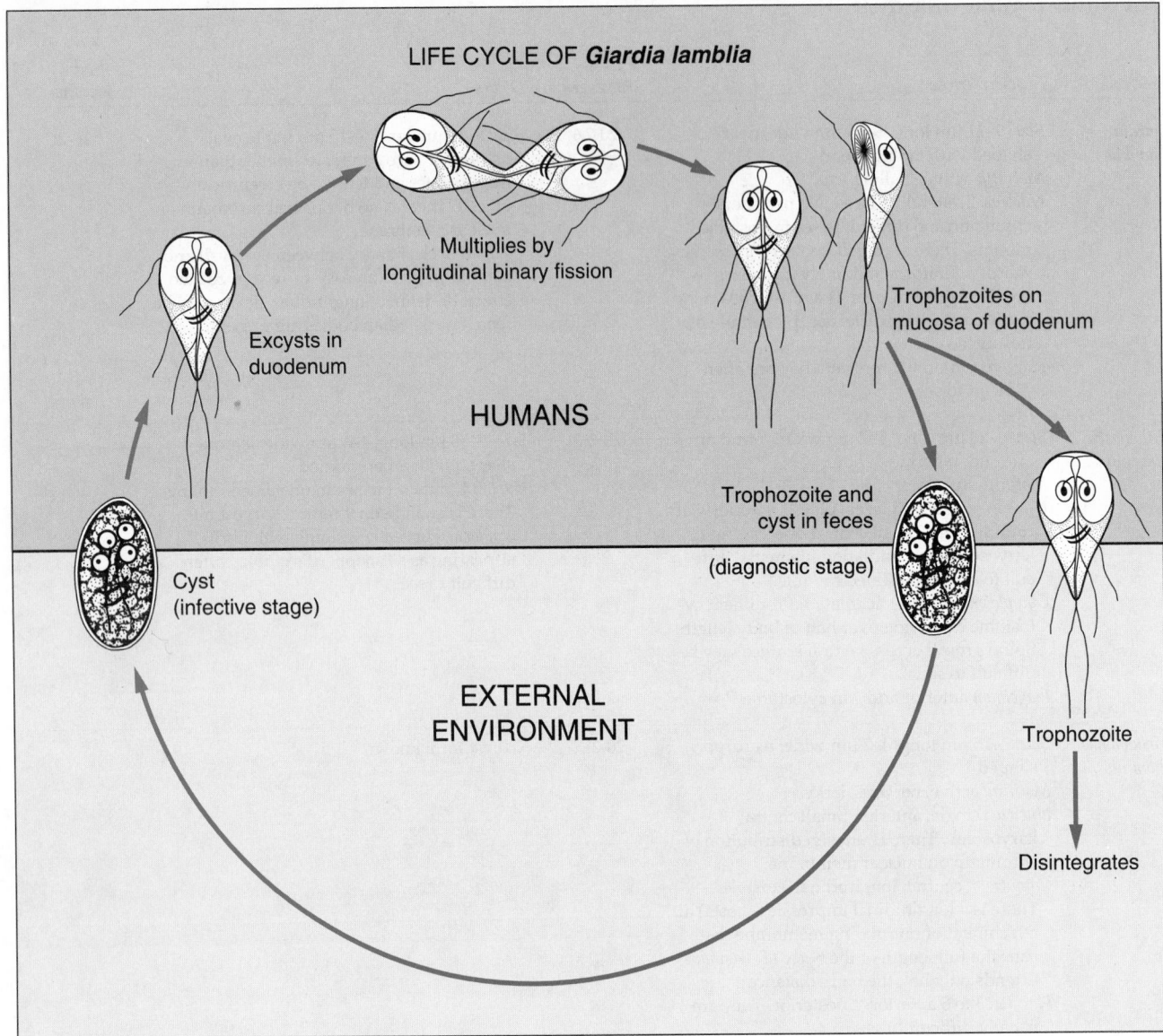

Figure 20-3
Life cycle of *Giardia lamblia*.

obtained from symptomatic and giardia O- and P-positive stool specimens gave strongly positive visual and spectrophotometric results. Of 232 randomly collected specimens, six O + P-negative specimens gave positive EIA results. Clinical evidence was strong that these six patients in fact had giardiasis. With these results taken into account, the EIA test performed with a sensitivity of 96% and a specificity of 100%. Scheffler and Van Etta[292] also evaluated the ProSpecT/Giardia kit and found a sensitivity of 95%, specificity of 100%, positive predictive value of 99.5%, and a negative predictive value of 100%, relative to conventional microscopy, in the study of 223 formalin-preserved stool specimens.

Other Intestinal Flagellates
CHILOMASTIX MESNILI. The most helpful feature in identifying *C. mesnili* is the large anterior nucleus placed immediately beneath the outer membrane and

the presence of a prominent cytosome (see Color Plate 20-2*D*). Three anterior flagella can often be seen by reducing the amount of condenser light and sharpening the focus. The cysts may be difficult to identify because the internal structures are not always well-defined; the lemon-shape and presence of a hyaline knob are helpful features (see Color Plate 20-2*E*). This flagellate is not pathogenic to humans and does not require treatment.

TRICHOMONAS HOMINIS. T. hominis may be somewhat more difficult to definitively identify because it is fragile and does not stain well. The trophozoite has a tear-drop shape and possesses a single anterior-placed nucleus, which is still remote from the outer membrane, helping to distingish it from *C. mesnili* (see Color Plate 20-2*F*). An undulating membrane extends the full length of the organism, theoretically serving as a helpful feature in distinguishing *Trichomonas vaginalis*, the undulating membrane of which extends only

CLINICAL CORRELATION BOX 20-2. *GIARDIA LAMBLIA*

G. lamblia is a known cause of acute diarrhea, abdominal pain and, in some cases, constitutional symptoms, such as weight loss and lassitude.[350,351] In chronic cases, malabsorption and steatorrhea simulating sprue may be experienced. The exact mechanism by which *G. lamblia* causes disease is not completely known. Physical occlusion of the mucosa, bile salt deconjugation, enterotoxin excretion, prostaglandin release, and injury to the mucosal epithelial cell brush border are several hypotheses reviewed by Smith and Wolfe.[305]

Most infections are sporadic, contracted after exposure to contaminated food or water under a variety of circumstances. Waterborne outbreaks have been cited[305] in locales as diverse as Colorado, Russia, New York, and among campers in the western United States. In a follow-up on the Aspen–Snowmass outbreak, only two cases of giardiasis were found among 225 visitors,[191] a rate far lower than that reported during the previously cited outbreak. Other waterborne outbreaks have more recently been reported[109] among individuals drinking water from an unfiltered municipal water supply in Dunedin, New Zealand; in a chlorinated community water supply in Penticton, British Columbia;[234] among preschool children drinking from school water supplies in Lesothro;[103] and, from use of a new hotel water slide, which was cleansed by both bromidization and sand filtration.[133]

The risk to campers has been reviewed,[155,304] the latter reported an outbreak caused by leakage of a sewage-effluent irrigation system into a potable water system adjacent to a state park campground in Arizona. Hopkins and Juranek[156] report a waterborne outbreak in 31 of 93 university students and faculty participating in a geology field trip in Colorado, related to ingestion of untreated stream water. Buret and associates[41] also warn of the zoonotic potential of giardiasis in domestic animals, indicating that ruminants, such as calves and lambs, may serve as reservoirs.

Children attending day care centers are perhaps at greatest risk for contracting giardiasis. Novotny and coworkers[245] found a 16% prevalence among children attending day care facilities in Denver, Colorado. Risk factors included increasing duration of attendance, time per week attending, low family income, large family size, and frequency of travel to the Colorado mountains. Eight of 97 children, 2 to 5 years old, were found to harbor *G. lamblia* cysts in a day care center in southern Ontario, Canada.[356] Three recurrent outbreaks were reported in a large day care facility in Wisconsin, with attack rates of 47%, 17%, and 37%, respectively.[311] Attack rates were highest for ambulatory diapered children and in those attending the center more than 40 hours per week. Teaching personnel appropriate diapering practices and hand-washing techniques were countermeasures taken.

The high prevalence of giardiasis is a worldwide problem, with endemic areas reported in England, Russia, several countries in Eastern Europe, and many coastal areas of the Mediterranean.[359] Recent reports reveal that *G. lamblia* was found in 10% of children residing in the Ain-Shams and El-Mowassa orphanages in Cairo;[289] giardiasis was the most common parasitic disease (11.63%) found among Muslims coming for the annual "Haj and Omra" pilgrimages to Mecca.

The drugs of choice in the treatment of giardiasis, when clinically indicated, are quinacrine (Atabrine) or metronidazole (Flagyl).

---

one half the distance of the body. In practice this is a moot point, as the undulating membranes are not seen in regular trichrome-stained smears; rather, they require mounts of anexic cultures. Trichomonads in stool specimens will most likely be *T. hominis*, although in females, *T. vaginalis* may contaminate the specimen. *T. hominis* is not pathogenic in humans.

DIENTAMOEBA FRAGILIS. The trophozoite typically has two nuclei with karyosomes fragmented into four to eight granules (about 20% have a single nucleus). Single-nucleated forms of *D. fragilis* may be difficult to differentiate from the trophozoites of *E. nana*. Relatively broad-lobed, clear pseudopods provide purposeful motility. A cyst stage has not been identified. Further identifying features are listed in Table 20-2, and a two-nucleated trophozoite is illustrated in Color Plate 20-2G.

D. fragilis produces a syndrome characterized by diarrhea, abdominal pain, and anal pruritus. Microbiologists in clinical laboratories must be aware that *D. fragilis* is being recovered from stool specimens with increasing frequency. It has been reported in 1.4% to 19% of specimens submitted for routine examination and in up to 47% of defined populations, such as inmates in mental institutions.[363] A high prevalence has also been reported among certain groups of Arizona Native Americans. In some settings, identification of *D. fragilis* in stool specimens is as frequent as *G. lamblia*. In fact, in laboratories where *G. lamblia* is being identified to the exclusion of *D. fragilis*, a review of collection and diagnostic methods may be in order. Because the cytoplasm is so delicate, *D. fragilis* may be difficult to identify in wet mounts, and study of a permanently stained preparation is virtually mandatory if morphologic details are to be studied.

Grendon and associates[134] warn that failure to use recommended stool fixation and permanent-staining techniques virtually precludes identification of *D. fragilis*. To increase probability, they strongly recommend that all stools submitted for examination be fixed in polyvinyl alcohol, sodium acetate–acetic acid–formalin or Schaudinn's fixatives, and that all specimens, regardless of consistency, be permanently stained before microscopic examination. Sawangjaroen and associates,[290] in a study of 260 consecutive patients with diarrhea in Brisbane, conclude that culture for *D. fragilis* is more sensitive than microscopy. Chan and colleagues[51] successfully used an indirect fluorescent antibody assay to improve screening of preserved fecal specimens for *D. fragilis* and further suggest that the development of ELISAs to detect *D. fragilis* antigens in fecal specimens would improve detection.

Because *D. fragilis* does not have an identified cyst state, direct food- or waterborne transfer from host to host is less likely. The nine times higher incidence of *D. fragilis* in patients with pinworm infection suggests that the *Enterobius vermicularis* eggs may be infected with the flagellate and serve as the chief vector for transfer to humans. This possibility may also explain why almost 50% of reported cases of dientamebiasis occurs in patients younger than 20 years of age. The drugs of choice in include tetracycline or metronidazole.

INTESTINAL CILIATES: *BALANTIDIUM COLI*

B. coli is the only member of the ciliates known to infect humans. The mode of transmission from humans to humans is by a simple fecal–oral route, and an intermediate host is not required for completion of the life cycle. The life cycle of *B. coli* is illustrated in Figure 20-4.

Laboratory Identification. It is generally easy to recognize *B. coli* in stool specimens because of its large size (100 μm or more in diameter), an outer membrane covered with short cilia, and its large kidney-shaped macronucleus (see Color Plate 20-2*H*). When observed in wet mounts, the trophozoite has a rotary, boring motility. In iodine mounts, the trophozoite stains yellow-brown, and the macronucleus is quite visible. The cyst measures 50 to 65 μm and can be recognized by the single large macronucleus.

B. coli is found primarily in swine and less commonly in other animals. Human balantidiosis is most prevalent where pigs are raised and slaughtered. Reports of infection are uncommon, with most coming from Latin America, the Far East, and New Guinea. In-

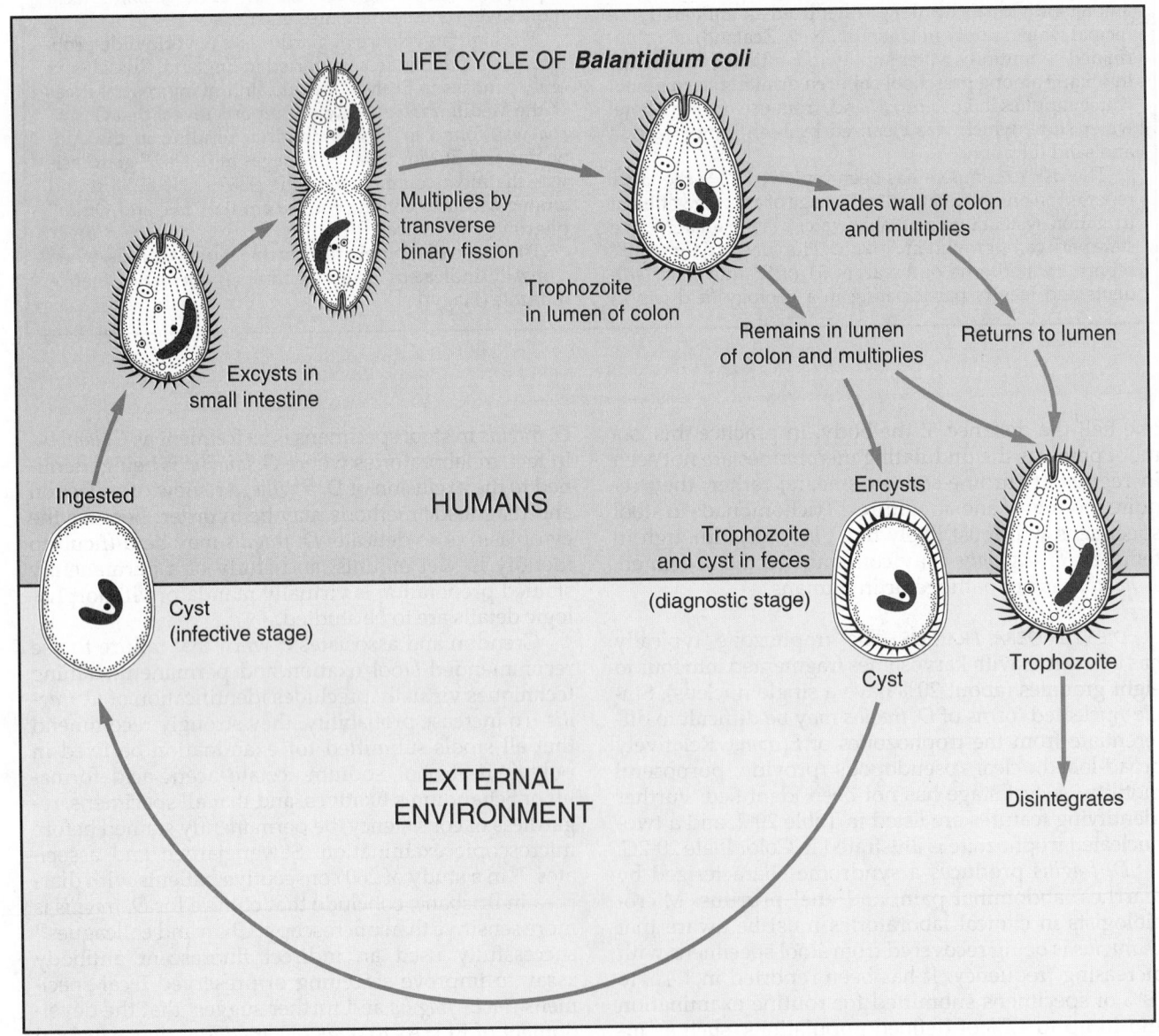

Figure 20-4
Life cycle of *Balantidium coli*.

festation in humans is generally noninvasive, asymptomatic, and self-limited. In debilitated patents carrying a heavy load of trophozoite, bloody dysentery, severe dehydration, or, in rare instances, death may result. Color Plate 20-2I illustrates several *B. coli* trophozoites invading the submucosa of the bowel in a rare fatal case of balantidium infection. Intestinal ulcers, mesenteric lymphadenitis, and rare extraintestinal extension to liver, lung, and other organs have been reported in isolated autopsy cases.[180]

The drugs of choice are tetracycline or, alternatively, diiodohydroxyquine or metronidazole.

COCCIDIA SPECIES

The *Coccidia*, a subgroup of protozoa within the subphylum Sporozoa, are obligate tissue parasites with sexual and asexual stages in their life cycles. Included in this group are the malarial parasites in the blood, *Plasmodium* species, the tissue protozoan *Toxoplasma gondii*, and the intestinal coccidia—*Cryptosporidium* species, *Isospora belli*, *Sarcocystis* species, and *Cyclospora* species (see Table 20-3 for key morphologic features).

The life cycle of most coccidia requires an external intermediate host, such as a cat, calf, or other animal, in which sporogenesis and oocyst formation take place. After ingestion of infective oocysts by a human host, the released sporocysts invade the mucosal epithelial cells for completion of all or part of their life cycle. The *Coccidia* species have six stages in their life cycle: 1) excystation (release of infective sporozoites from the oocysts); 2) asexual reproduction of the sporozoites (mesozoites); 3) formation of male and female gametocytes from mature sporozoites; 4) fertilization of the female gametocyte; 5) formation of the oocyst wall; and 6) formation of sporozoites in the oocyst. The life cycle of *I. belli*, as representative of the coccidia, is shown in Figure 20-5.

Humans become infected either by 1) ingesting food or water contaminated with highly infective oocysts (the sexual form) that were passed in the feces of certain herbivorous and carnivorous animals or by humans, or 2) by ingesting tissues infected with sporozoites (the asexual form). After ingestion of contaminated food or water, the oocysts are digested in the stomach, and infective sporozoites are released. The sporozoites, in turn, may invade the intestinal epithelial cells and can enter the circulation and invade mammalian cells throughout the body. Animal tissues containing sporozoites (e.g., undercooked meats) serve as the second mode of infection for humans. When ingested, these sporozoites directly invade intestinal epithelial cells and can enter the circulation in a manner similar to those released from oocysts.

Some of the sporozoites remain in the intestinal epithelial cells and form male (micro) and female (macro) gametocytes. Fertilization occurs, and oocysts are formed to complete the life cycle. These sexual and asexual phases in the life cycles of the various intestinal coccidia can occur in the definitive animal host, in humans, or in both, depending on the species. The following is a brief review of the three types of human coccidian infections of the intestine.

Cryptosporidium. Cryptosporidia are minute coccidian protozoa that have been known to be associated with enterocolitis in a variety of domestic animals, including calves, pigs, and chickens.[9] This microorganism cannot be added to the list of agents of human diarrheal disease, except in individuals with immunodeficiency, especially patients with AIDS.[69,70,239] In fact, the detection of *Cryptosporidium* parvum or of *I. belli* in patients not suspected of having AIDS should lead to testing for HIV infection.[259] Humans become infected either from direct contact with infected animals or from ingestion of fecally contaminated food or water. Water-borne transmission is particularly troublesome for *Cryptosporidium*

TABLE 20-3

INTESTINAL COCCIDIA: KEY FEATURES FOR LABORATORY IDENTIFICATION OF FECAL FORMS

SPECIES	IDENTIFYING FEATURES	PLATE REFERENCE
Isospora belli	Mature oocysts measure 25–30 μm, are ellipsoid, and have a thin, smooth wall and 2 internal spherical sporocysts (4 sporozoites may also be seen inside). Immature oocysts enclose only a single granular mass (zygote).	
Sarcocystis spp.	Mature oocysts have a thin, smooth wall that appears collapsed around two internal spherical sporocysts. In fully mature oocysts, a total of 4 sporozoites may be seen inside.	
Cryptosporidium spp.	Oocysts average 4–5 μm in diameter, are spherical or oval, and have smooth outer walls. Four naked sporozoites may be seen within mature oocyst (sporocysts not present). Oocysts appear bright red when stained with conventional acid-fast techniques.	20-2J
Cyclospora spp.	Mature organisms measure 8–9 μm in diameter and appear as wrinkled spheres with well-defined nonrefractile external walls and internal granular material. Organisms fluoresce under ultraviolet illumination and are variably staining with carbolfuchsin stains, appearing deep red when stain is taken up optimally.	20-2K

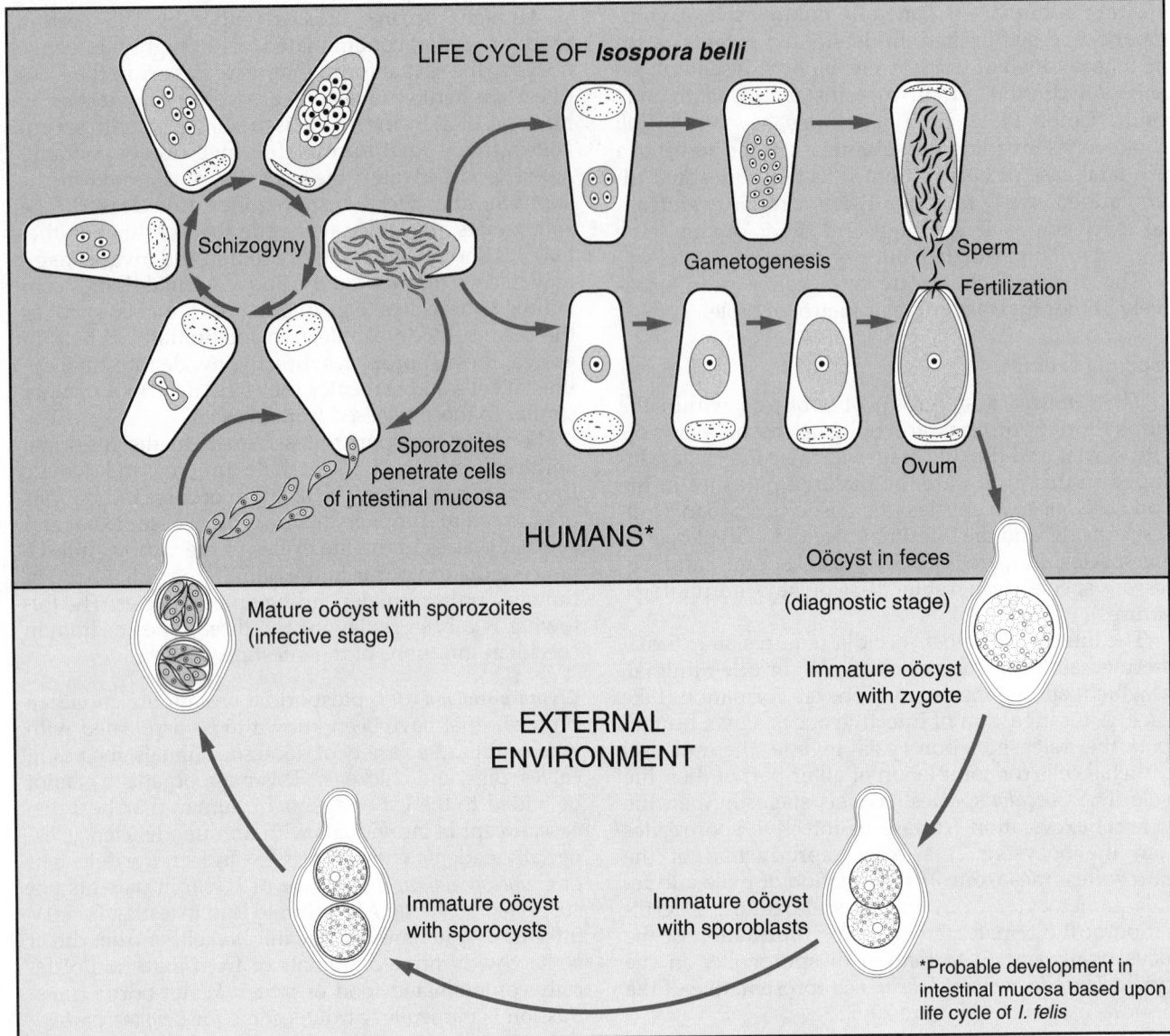

LIFE CYCLE OF *Isospora belli*

Schizogyny

Sporozoites penetrate cells of intestinal mucosa

Gametogenesis

Sperm

Fertilization

Ovum

HUMANS*

Oöcyst in feces

(diagnostic stage)

Mature oöcyst with sporozoites (infective stage)

Immature oöcyst with zygote

EXTERNAL ENVIRONMENT

Immature oöcyst with sporocysts

Immature oöcyst with sporoblasts

*Probable development in intestinal mucosa based upon life cycle of *I. felis*

Figure 20-5
Life cycle of *Isospora belli*.

parvum because the oocysts are not eliminated by chlorination and may persist in posttreatment water supplies.[304] The clinical syndrome includes a cholera-like, watery or mucous diarrhea, persistent gastroenteritis with varying degrees of vomiting, and abdominal cramping, malabsorption, and low-grade fever.

The organism during all stages of development is confined to the microvilli of intestinal epithelial cells. Thus, the diagnosis can be made in hematoxylin and eosin (H & E)-stained sections of small bowel by observing the tiny oocysts, often in huge numbers, attached to the surface of the epithelial cells lining the villi (see Color Plate 20-2J, *left* and Fig. 20-6). Oocysts have a propensity to adhere to the brush border of the epithelial cells, with loss or degeneration of the microvilli at the attachment zone.[239] The loss of microvilli may result in the impaired digestion, malabsorption, and diarrhea that make up the clinical syndrome.

Oocysts are ovoid to spherical, measure 5 to 6 μm in diameter, and appear highly refractile when observed in flotation preparations (Fig. 20-7). Small granules may be observed internally or, with phase contrast microscopy, up to four slender, bow-shaped sporozoites may be seen in each oocyst.[69,70,239] The identification is most commonly made by identifying the red-staining, 4 to 6 μm in diameter spherical oocysts in acid-fast–stained stool preparations (see Color Plate 20-2J, *right*). The infective oocysts are immediately passed in the feces. Calves and other animals serve as a major source for human infections, and human-to-human transmission can occur.[183]

Oocyst-positive stools occur between 7 and 28 days after infection, with a mean incubation period of 7.2 days. In a study of 84 children with cryptosporidium-related diarrhea, Stehr-Green and colleagues[310] found that shedding of oocysts ranged from 8 to more than 50

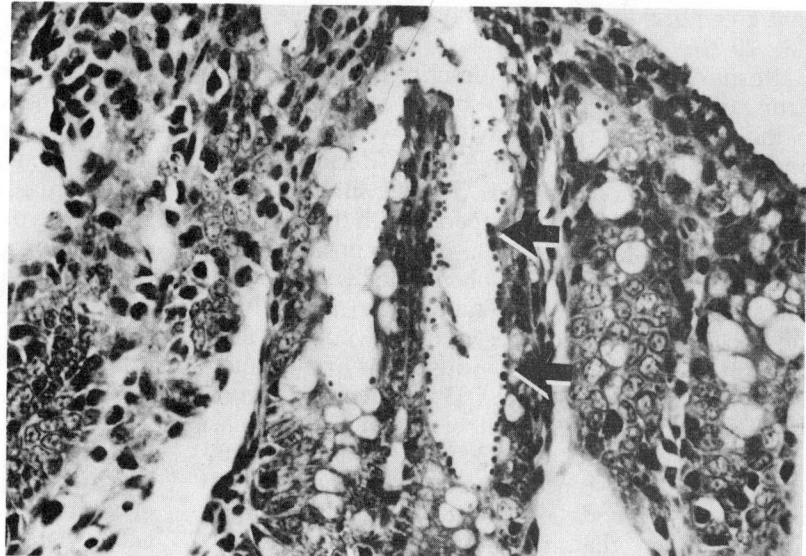

Figure 20-6
Section of mouse intestinal mucosa infected with *Cryptosporidium parvum*, illustrating the tiny oocysts on the surface epithelium (*arrows*; original magnification ×320). (Courtesy of Bruce C. Andersen)

days, with no relation between duration of shedding and severity of diarrhea. Shepherd and coworkers,[299] on the other hand, in a study of 49 patients, found that most stopped shedding by 20 days, with symptoms related to shedding in 25 of the 49. Thus, duration of diarrhea and the onset and length of time of oocyst shedding are patient dependent.[166]

The diagnosis can also be made by identifying oocysts in fecal specimens. With heavy infections, the concentration techniques routinely used for the recovery of eggs and parasites in most laboratories are adequate for the recovery of cryptosporidial oocysts. With light infections, Sheather's sugar flotation method is recommended and can be performed, as described by Garza[122] (Box 20-4).

Weber and coworkers[340] have successfully used a modified formalin–ethyl acetate (FEA) stool concentration technique to detect cryptosporidial oocysts in stool specimens. Following the usual FEA procedure, the sediment was layered and floated over a hypertonic saline solution to separate parasites from stool debris. This technique showed the most significant improvement in the recovery of oocysts from stool specimens that were formed and not fatty.

A modified acid-fast stain can also be used to detect cryptosporidial oocysts in air-dried, methanol-fixed smears prepared directly from a fecal sample.[122] The carbolfuchsin stain is applied to the smear in the same manner as the routine acid-fast stain; however, 1% H_2SO_4 is used as the decolorizer instead of acid alcohol. The oocysts appear bright pink-red against the

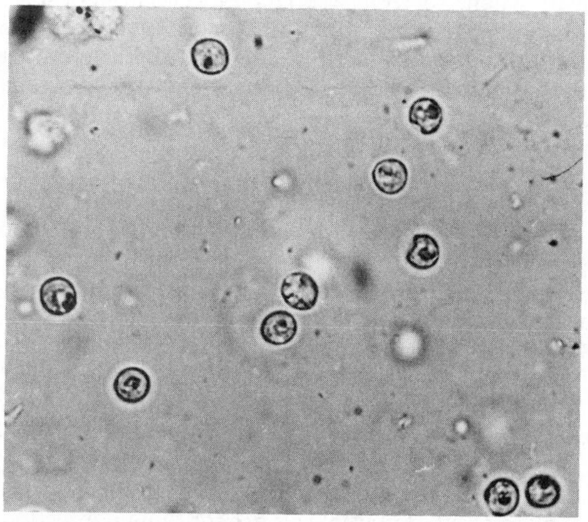

Figure 20-7
Oocysts of *Cryptosporidium parvum* as observed in a fecal floatation preparation (original magnification ×1280). (Courtesy of Bruce C. Andersen)

BOX 20-4. SHEATHER'S FLOTATION TECHNIQUE FOR RECOVERY OF CRYPTOSPORIDIUM OOCYSTS IN FECAL SPECIMENS

1. A heavy suspension of feces is made in physiologic saline solution and strained through gauze into a centrifuge tube to one-half full.

2. Add an equal volume of Sheather's sugar solution (500 g of sucrose, 320 mL of distilled water and 6.5 g of melted phenol) to bring the surface of the liquid slightly above the top of the tube. Gently mix the suspension with an applicator stick.

3. Place an 18 mm² or 22 mm² coverslip on the surface of the suspension and let stand undisturbed for 45 minutes.

4. Gently remove the coverslip and mount it on a glass slide. Observe under phase contrast microscopy for the spherical, highly refractile 5-µm–diameter oocysts.

light green background of the counterstain (see Color Plate 20-2*J*).

Rusnak and coworkers[281] describe a method of detecting cryptosporidium oocysts in fecal smears using an indirect fluorescence assay (IFA) with monoclonal antibodies (reagents available from Meridian Diagnostics, Inc., Cincinnati OH). The sensitivity of this IFA test was 100% when compared with the modified Ziehl-Neelsen acid-fast stain on 56 positive fecal smears (specificity was 97% when tested with 63 negative stool specimens). Acridine orange (AR) staining can also be used to detect oocysts. Arrowood and Sterling,[11] in study comparing various stains for the detection of oocysts, found that of 32 positive smears prepared from formalin-fixed stool specimens, acid-fast stains detected 40.6%, AR 93.8%, a monoclonal antibody direct fluorescence technique 93.8%, an indirect monoclonal antibody method 81.3%, and a biotinylated indirect diaminobenzidine method 71.9%. Oocysts can also be identified with the IFA technique applied to tissue sections; intracellular trophozoites do not react with the antibody.[204]

An indirect, double-antibody ELISA for the detection of cryptosporidium antigens in fecal specimens has been described by Ungar.[323] In a study of 62 frozen stool specimens from patients with cryptosporidiosis, 51 were positive by ELISA (sensitivity 82.3%). The specificity was 96.7% in the testing of 182 negative stool specimens. When reagents become commercially available, ELISA may provide a direct rapid method for diagnosing intestinal cryptosporidium infections.

Kehl and associates[176] found that two enzyme immunoassays, The ProSpect *Cryptosporidium* microtiter assay (Alexon, Inc., Mountain View CA) and Color Vue *Cryptosporidium* assay (Seardyn Inc., Indianapolis IN) and a direct immunofluorescent assay, Merifluor *Cryptosporidium* kit (Meridian Diagnostic, Cincinnati OH) were equally sensitive and specific for the detection of cryptosporidium oospores, although the immunofluorescent procedure was considered easiest to read and required the least hands-on technologist time. An antigen capture ELISA (LMD Laboratories, Carlsbad CA) was sensitive and specific in the detection of cryptosporidium oocysts in human diarrheal stool specimens.[243]

Isospora belli. Isosporiasis, an illness characterized by diarrhea and malabsorption, was formerly only rarely encountered and was considered to be of limited clinical significance. Currently, *I. belli* is being seen in increasing frequency as one of the causes of the diarrheal syndrome in AIDS patients.[79,306] Fever, headache, steatorrhea, and weight loss may occur in protracted cases; deaths due to water loss and electrolyte imbalance have been reported in overwhelming infections.[180] The drug of choice is trimethoprim–sulfamethoxazole.

Human *I. belli* infections differ from those of other coccidia in that both the sexual and the asexual forms inhabit the human intestine, and a second host is not required to complete the life cycle. Human-to-human transmission can occur after ingesting infective oocysts in fecally contaminated food and water; thus, the dis-

---

CLINICAL CORRELATION BOX 20-3. *CRYPTOSPORIDIOSIS*

Cryptosporidiosis in AIDS patients often is particularly troublesome because of the prolonged diarrhea that worsens progressively. Therapeutic regimens have been largely unsuccessful to date, and complications in severe infections may lead to death. One exception has been reported[286] in a 22-year-old, HIV-positive homosexual man. A small-bowel biopsy revealed typical villous atrophy and infiltration of the lamina propria with neutrophils, simulating celiac disease. Treatment with metronidazole effected a remission, and the patient was disease-free for 3 years. An excellent review of the clinical, epidemiologic, and parasitic aspects of cryptosporidiosis has been published.[239]

Hart and Baxby[144] also draw attention to the importance of cryptosporidiosis as a potential cause of diarrhea in immunocompetent humans, particularly in children. Children attending day care centers particularly are at high risk.[146] Alpert and associate[7] tested stool specimens over a 2-month period from 53 children attending a day care center, 23 were positive (43%). In an August 1989 study at a day care center in Georgia,[318] 39 of 79 children (49%) and three of 23 staff members (13%) were shedding oocysts in their stools. Thirty of 39 (77%) of the infected children had mild to moderate diarrhea, the remainder were asymptomatic. Those at highest risk were younger than 36 months of age, in diapers, and not toilet trained.

Other studies reveal similarly high prevalence among this population of children: 80 of 186 (43%) children attending a day care center in Tulsa[146] and 9 of 30 5-year-olds from day care centers in west-central Colorado.[86]

The prevalence of *Cryptosporidium* species in stool specimens varies with different population groups around the world. Two reports from Israel reveal widely divergent prevalences: 13.5% of 221 Israeli children with diarrhea hospitalized at the Hebrew University Hadassah Medical School[285] compared with 3.25% at the Edith Wolfson Hospital in Holon.[71] The infection rate was greatest in late summer and autumn. Those with cryptosporidium-positive stools were significantly more malnourished than those free of infection. The incidence of recovery was 0.5% of 2197 patients admitted to the Royal Victoria Infirmary in Newcastle upon Tyne, United Kingdom;[218] 1.4% recovery at the Childrens Hospital in London;[21] 2.5% at the Fairfield Infectious Diseases Hospital in Victoria, Australia;[29] 4.1% in Pretoria, South Africa;[309] and 4.2% in New Zealand.[35] El Ahraf and coworkers[100] found that 2% of stray dogs (vs. 3% of humans) in San Bernardino County, California, were passing *Cryptosporidium* species oocysts, representing another possible source for human infection.

Most infections are self-limited, and therapy has been disappointing. Spiramycin has been tried, but results are still inconclusive.

ease is not a zoonosis. The oocysts are the diagnostic forms seen in human fecal specimens. They measure 25 to 30 μm in diameter, have thin, smooth walls, and are nonmotile. Immature oocysts contain only one sporocyst; more typically, mature oocysts contain two sporocysts and are the characteristic forms seen in stool specimens (Fig. 20-8). Four sporozoites may be seen within each sporocyst.

***Sarcocystis* species.**   *Sarcocystis* species use two mammals for the sexual and asexual phases of their life cycles. Humans may serve as either the intermediate or the definitive host. As intermediate host, encysted sporozoites from various *Sarcocystis* species have been identified in skeletal and cardiac muscle at autopsy.[24] This form is usually asymptomatic, although a history of polymyositis and eosinophilia have been reported in rare cases. As the definitive host, the sexual cycle of the organism develops in the subepithelial portion of the small-bowel mucosa. Humans acquire the intestinal form of the disease by ingesting poorly cooked infected beef or pork. Intestinal infections are associated with *S. hominis* or *S. suishiominis* (formerly *Isospora hominis*) and are often asymptomatic but may on occasion result in a diarrheal syndrome similar to that produced by *I. belli*. The diagnostic forms in stool specimens are mature, 25- by 33-μm oocysts containing two sporocysts, appearing similar to those of *I. belli*. Single sporocysts measuring 13 to 17 μm may also be seen.

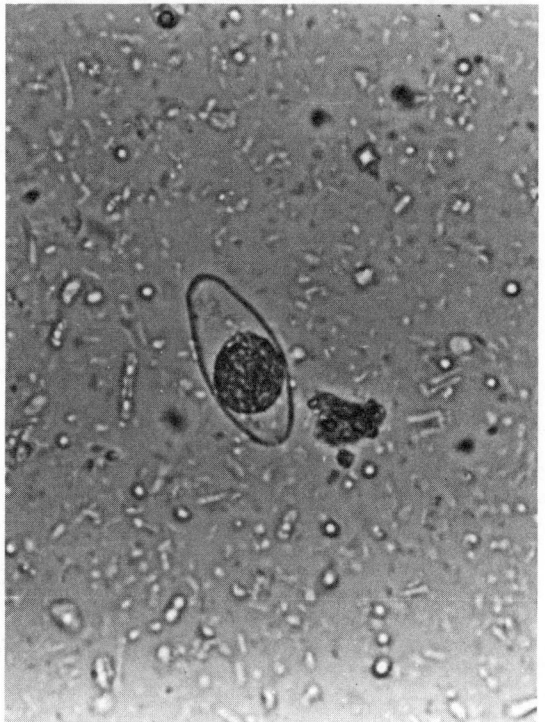

Figure 20-8
Immature cyst of *Isospora belli* containing a single sporozoite. These oocysts average 25 to 30 μm by 15 to 20 μm, are typically ellipsoidal and nonmotile, and have a smooth, thin wall and a single granular zygote within. Mature oocysts contain two sporozoites.

***Cyclospora* species.**   The organisms now included in the genus *Cyclospora* were originally thought to be cyanobacteria or blue-green algae-like organisms.[201,250] *Cyclospora* species have morphologic characteristics similar to *Isospora* species and *Cryptospsoridium parvum*, except that they have two sporocysts per oocyte and two sporozoites per sporocyst. *Isospora* species have two sporocysts per oocyst and four sporozoites per sporocyst; *Cryptosporidium* parvum has four "naked," or nonencysted, sporozoites per oocyst. The species name, *Cyclospora cayatenensis*, honors the Unversidad Peruana Cayetano Heredia in Lima, Peru, the institution where much of the original epidemiologic and taxonomic research was done.

In unstained, unconcentrated stools, the oocysts of *Cyclospsora* species appear as nonrefractile, spherical to oval, slightly wrinkled bodies measuring 8 to 10 μm in diameter (almost twice the size of the oocysts of *Cryptosporidium parvum*), with an internal cluster of membrane-bound globules.[26] They are acid-fast and stain with a faint pink or pink-red color; older cells may fail to stain[26,202] (see Color Plate 20-2*K*). The oocysts stain orange red with safranin; they do not stain with iron hematoxylin, Grocott-Gomori methenamine silver, iodine, or periodic acid–Schiff.[202]

The life cycle, although not completely understood, is thought to be similar to that of *Cryptosporidium* species. Sporozoites excyst from oocysts in the digestive tract soon after ingestion in contaminated food or water. The sporozoites enter the epithelial cells in the small intestine. The mechanism by which diarrhea is produced is not known; endoscopy reveals moderate to marked erythema of the distal duodenum. Duodenal and jejunal biopsies reveal blunting of jejunal villi, villous atrophy, and crypt hyperplasia of varying degrees. The absence of fecal leukocytes and erythrocytes indicates that the process is not invasive; impaired D-xylose absorption implies a malabsorption type syndrome.

Illness usually follows ingestion of water and occurs primarily in the warm summer months. Powdered milk diluted with water before consumption has also been implicated.[361] In a Chicago outbreak at Cook County Hospital, house staff and employees in a dormitory developed diarrhea following failure of the dormitory's water pump.[360] Cyclospora-linked disease often occurs as "traveler's diarrhea," with several literature citations of diarrhea occurring in travelers returning from Haiti, Mexico, Guatemala, Puerto Rico, Morocco, Cambodia, Pakistan, India, the Solomon Islands, and particularly Nepal.[152,265] However, Ooi and coauthors[249] report three residents of New England who developed diarrheal syndromes but had no history of recent foreign travel. Infections with *Cyclospora* species should be considered in the differential diagnosis of community-acquired diarrhea, even in the absence of foreign travel.

The incubation period is 2 to 7 days. Onset of diarrhea may be abrupt (68% of cases) or gradual (32%).[293] Watery diarrhea, which is self-limited in immunocompetent patients (rarely lasting more than 12 days), may be accompanied by mild nausea, abdominal cramping, fatigue, and malaise.[360,361] In immunoincompetent patients, the diarrhea may be prolonged, lasting 4 to 6 weeks, simulating tropical sprue. Cyclospora infections are common in patients with AIDS. Of 450 patients with AIDS, Pappe and associates[252] found *Cryptosporidium* species in the stool specimens of 135 (30%), *I. belli* in 12%, *Cyclospora* in 11%, *G. lamblia* in 3%, and *E. histolytica* in 1%. No specific pharmacotherapy has proved effective.[252] Oral trimethorpim–sulfamethoxazole has been effective in the treatment of some cases;[360] metronidazole, norfloxacin, quinacrine, nalidixic acid, and diloxanide furoate have been used with varying success in other cases. In patients with AIDS, treatment is often limited to supportive care with hydration and nutritional supplements, although Pappe and coworkers[252] found trimethoprim–sulfamethoxazole effective in some cases.

Directors and supervisors of microbiology laboratories must decide whether stool specimens are to be routinely examined for the presence of *Cryptosporidium* and *Cyclospora* organisms. In practice settings where stool specimens are received from many AIDS patients, the preparation of routine acid-fast stains of fecal smears can be recommended.

Microsporidia

MICROSPORIDIUM SPECIES. The microsporidia are obligate intracellular parasites that are sufficiently unique to be classified into a separate phylum, *Microspora*.[196] The unique feature of the *Microspora* is the production of spores that contain a complex tubular extrusion mechanism by which the infective material, "sporoplasm," is injected into host cells. This occurs after ingestion by the host, stimulated by changes in pH and in ionic concentration of the intestinal contents. The coiled tubule is everted and penetrates the host cell.

Approximately 80 genera and over 700 species are included in this collective "catch all" group called *Microsporidium*, which primarily cause disease in a variety of nonhuman hosts of commercial import, including insects, fish, laboratory rodents, rabbits, fur-bearing animals, and primates.[38] They are true eukaryotes (perhaps arising as a very early branch of the eukaryotes), having a nucleus, a nuclear envelope, and an array of intracytoplasmic membranes. Within the phylum are several genera, only four of which cause disease in humans: *Encephalitozoon, Nosema, Pleistophora*, and *Enterocytozoon*. A fifth recently named genus, *Septata*, has been found to be closely linked to *Enterocytozoon* and is no longer given separate genus status. Species differentiation is virtually impossible by light microscopy.

By electron microscopy, the identification of spores with a polar tube is characteristic of all genera. Members of the genus *Encephalitozoon* are enclosed in a host-produced, phagosomelike, limiting vesicle. Both *Enterocytozoon* species and *Nosema* species develop in direct contact with host cell cytoplasm without a limiting vesicle; *Nosemia* species are distinguished by having paired, abutted nuclei.[37,38]

The diagnostic microsporidia spores are small, ranging from 1.5 × 2.5 μm to 2.5 × 4.0 μm.[297] They are oval to cylindrical and possess thick walls that render them environmentally resistant and difficult to stain. A transverse pink-staining band midway in the cells is a helpful identifying feature (see Color Plate 20-2L). The spores stain poorly with hematoxylin and eosin (H & E) but can be better visualized with Gram, acid-fast, periodic acid–Schiff (PAS), Giemsa, or modified trichrome stains, the latter to be described in Box 20-5. They are gram-positive and acid-fast; in PAS stain an anterior PAS-positive granule is observed.[121] The stain devised by Weber and associates[341] can be highly recommended for the detection of microsporidia spores in duodenal aspirates and in fecal material.

DeGirolami et al[78] found that both Weber's modified trichome stain and the fluorochrome Uvitex 2B stains were equally and highly sensitive, compared with duodenal biopsies, in detecting microsporidia spores in smears of duodenal aspirates biopsy material from 43 patients. Ryan and coworker[282] describe a modified stain in which the phosphotungstic acid is decreased in concentration to 0.25 g/100 mL, and aniline blue instead of fast green was used as the counterstain. Each staining procedure requires 90 minutes, and selection between the Weber and the Ryan stain is one of personal preference. Kokoskin and coworkers[184] found that performing the stain at a temperature of 50°C and decreasing the time of staining to 10 minutes produced a deeper, easier to interpret stain. Because

---

BOX 20-5. WEBER STAIN FOR THE DETECTION OF MICROSPORIDIA SPORES IN STOOL AND DUODENAL ASPIRATES[351]

1. Prepare slides for light microscopic examination of stool by taking a 10-μL aliquot of unconcentrated liquid stool concentrate in 10% formalin (12:3 ratio), spread thinly over an area 45 × 25 mm.

2. Fix smears in methanol for 5 minutes.

3. Stain for 90 minutes in the Weber chromotrope-based stain. To prepare the stain, mix Chromotrope 2R (Harleco, Gibbstown NJ) 6.0 g; fast green (Allied Chemical & Dye, New York) 0.15 g; and phosphotungstic acid, 0.70 g. Allow these ingredients to stand ("ripen") for 30 minutes in 3 mL glacial acetic acid. Then mix with 100 mL of distilled water.

4. After staining, rinse slides in acid alcohol (4.5 mL of acetic acid and 995.5 mL of 90% ethyl alcohol) for 10 seconds and then rinse briefly in 95% alcohol.

5. Successively dehydrate smears in 95% alcohol for 5 minutes, 100% alcohol for 10 minutes, and Hemo-De (xylene substitute; Fisher Scientific, Pittsburgh PA) for 10 minutes.

6. Examine 100 oil immersion fields per slide, a reading time of approximately 10 minutes. Look for the small 1- to 4-μm cylindrical spores that stain bright pink-red. The demonstration of a pink-red, beltlike stripe that girds the spores diagonally or equatorial is virtually diagnostic (see Color Plate 20-2L).

the microsporidia spores are very small and may resemble bacteria or tiny yeast cells, staining of positive control material is always necessary when performing either of these stains.

Although all species of microsporidia may cause disseminated infections and organisms may be found in several organs, including liver, kidney, and brain, *Enterocytozoon bieneusi* is the species that tends to preferentially infect enterocytes in the small-bowel mucosa, particularly in patients with AIDS.[108] However, several case reports[264] indicate that *E. bieneusi* may colonize the bile duct epithelium, leading to cholangitis. The estimated prevalence of microsporidia intestinal infection in AIDS patients may be as high as 12%[184] or even higher if special techniques, including cytocentrifugation, fluorescent antibody detection, and serology, are used.

Encephalitozoon cuniculi is most commonly associated with disseminated infection, with a propensity for infecting the brain and kidneys. *Nosema corneum* has been found in several cases of keratoconjunctivitis;[46] however, *E. cuniculi* and *E. hellem* have also been recovered from the cornea and conjunctiva in AIDS patients with keratoconjunctivitis.[85] Conjunctivitis, scleritis, sensation of foreign body, and blurred vision are common presenting symptoms.

Those with experience may be able to identify the characteristic, tiny 2-μm–diameter intracytoplasmic spores in stained tissue sections of intestinal biopsies. Spores are best demonstrated using Brown-Brenn or Brown-Hopps tissue Gram stains, or Giemsa-stained touch preparations. Organisms may also be seen in semithin plastic sections stained with methylene blue–azure II with basic fuchsin or toluidine blue counterstains.[37,38] Positive control slides should always be performed in parallel when using any of these stains. Spores have also been demonstrated in CSF and urine by the use of immunofluorescence light microscopy.[297] As laboratory workers begin to use the various techniques described in the foregoing and become more familiar with the morphology of *Microsporidium* species by light microscopy, the prevalence of infections will undoubtedly increase, and the chances for underdiagnosis will be reduced.

Aldras and coworkers[5] demonstrated the superiority of detecting microsporidia spores in the stools of AIDS patients in indirect immunofluorescence antibody stains using polyclonal antisera to *E. cuniculi* and *E. hellum* and monoclonal antibodies raised against *E. hellem*.

Several techniques for the nonmicroscopic detection of microsporidial spores are in the research laboratories, waiting for a future time when the laboratory diagnosis may be simplified. Zierdt and associates[370] used a variety of polyclonal mouse and rabbit antisera raised against *E. cuniculi* and *E. hellum* spores in an indirect fluorescent antibody assay to successfully identify microsporidial spores in 11 of 12 fecal samples, in addition to detection of antigen in colon and duodenal fluids and in duodenal biopsy touch preparations. Abd-Alla and colleagues[1] also successfully used monoclonal antibodies raised against *E. hellem* in an indirect

immunofluorescence to detect microsporidial spores in formalin-fixed stool and urine specimens. Franzen and coworkers[108] successfully used microsporidian DNA amplification by PCR on six known positive duodenal biopsy specimens to detect a 353-bp DNA fragment specific for *E. bieneusi*. They suggest that PCR may be a useful approach to diagnosing microsporidiosis in HIV-infected patients.

There is no known effective therapy for microsporidiosis. Limited experience in treating intestinal infections caused by *E. bieneusi* with pyrimethamine, metronidazole, or trimethoprim–sulfamethoxazole (SXT) may be effective. One of three patients reported by Rijpstra and coauthors[274] may have responded to 50 mg/day of pyrimethamine received as prophylaxis for recurrent cerebral toxoplasmosis. Diarrhea improved in another patient reported by Current and Owen[70] after treatment with (SXT), but the infection in this case was not eliminated.

For a comprehensive review of human microsporidial infections, including over 250 references, see Weber and coauthors,[340,341] who introduce several new diagnostic techniques that will "facilitate future studies on the incidence, risk factors, origins of infection, modes of transmission, clinical manifestations, pathogenesis and treatment of this emerging pathogen."

NEMATODES

The nematodes are helminth roundworms, the adults of which are characterized by a tapered, cylindrical body, with longitudinally oriented muscles and a triradiate esophagus. The species of intestinal nematodes (roundworms) that most commonly infect humans include *Ascaris lumbricoides*; *Trichuris trichiura*; hookworms: *Necator americanus*, *Ancylostoma duodenale*; *Strongyloides stercoralis*; *Enterobius vermicularis*; *Capillaria philippinensis*; and *Trichostrongylus* species.

Worldwide, an estimated 1 billion persons are infected with intestinal nematodes.[32,40] The morbidity from these infections is generally underestimated, and even infections of moderate intensity may result in developmental consequences for school-aged children.[52] The worldwide prevalence of several individual nematode infections has been reported in publications by the WHO.[316] Ascariasis is the most common nematode infection worldwide, involving some 800 million persons. Between 700 and 900 million persons are infected with hookworm (mostly *Ancylostoma duodenale*), 0.2% of whom suffer from severe anemia. The magnitude of strongyloidiasis is similar to that of hookworm, with up to 10% of certain populations being infected. The overall incidence of *Trichuris trichiura* infections is not known, although a 90% prevalence has been cited in certain populations in Cameroon, Malaysia, and in Caribbean countries. Vermund and colleagues[329] found that *T. trichiura* was the most common nematode recovered from 41,958 stool specimens submitted to the Columbia-Presbyterian Medical Center in New York during the period 1971 to 1984. Of the cestodes, *Taenia solium* is particularly prevalent in Latin America, where an estimated 1% of the population is infested.

Neurocysticercosis is also highly prevalent there, involving some 350,000 persons.

The key features for laboratory identification of the more commonly encountered nematodes are listed in Table 20-4 and are illustrated in Color Plate 20-3. *Trichostrongylus* species, endemic in the Orient, the Middle East, and Africa, and *Capillaria philippinensis*, prevalent in the Philippines, Thailand, and the region of the South China Sea, are rarely seen in the United States.

The life cycles of this group of helminths vary in complexity and modes of infection. These nematodes do not have an intermediate host in their life cycle (see Fig. 20-1); however, most require a stage outside of the human host for the ova to develop into an infective form. The egg or ovum is a mature gamete produced by adult females residing in the intestine and passed with the feces. This form is the resting stage, serving as the diagnostic or infective form. The ova of most nematode species require an intermediate time of development in the external environment to develop into a larval and often infective stage, depending on the temperature, moisture, and nature of the soil into which they are passed. Life cycle drawings may be found in the section devoted to each of the nematode species discussed in this chapter. A collection of life cycles can be found in the CDC publications by Melvin and coauthors.[229,230]

ASCARIASIS AND *ASCARIS LUMBRICOIDES*

It is estimated that *A. lumbricoides* affects about 25%, or 1 billion, of the world's population.[40] The highest prevalence is in malnourished people residing in developing countries. Areas with modern water and waste treatment have a low incidence of disease. The life cycle does not involve an external intermediate host; however, it is somewhat complex, requiring a period for ova maturation in the external environment and a transpulmonary larval migratory phase in humans that may result in transient asthma-like symptoms in heavy infections. The life cycle of *A. lumbriciodes* is illustrated in Figure 20-9, page 1102.

Laboratory Identification. The laboratory diagnosis of ascariasis is made either by observing the adult worms as they protrude from body orifices or in situ in the intestine or contiguous duct systems (as seen at surgery or at autopsy), or more commonly by detecting the characteristic ova in stool specimens. The adult worms measure between 15 and 35 cm in length, with the males being smaller and identified by their curved tail. The cuticle is smooth and lacks the annular muscular striations characteristic of earthworms (see Color Plate 20-3A). The key features of the adults and ova are listed in Table 20-4.

The eggs measure about 60 × 45 μm, are yellow-brown (bile stained), oval or spherical, and characteristically have a thick, transparent, hyaline shell, covered by an albuminous coat (see Color Plate 20-3B). Eggs that have had prolonged exposure to pancreatic secretions may be devoid of the albuminous coat (decorticoid). Fertilized eggs can be recognized by the cleav-

age of the internal yolk; internal organization is lacking in unfertilized ova. Color Plate 20-3C illustrates embryonated eggs in the late stages of larval formation. Unfertilized, decorticate ova may resemble vegetable cells and can be extremely difficult to recognize in stool specimens; however, in most instances, examination of additional fields will usually reveal the characteristic thick, outer mammillated, albuminoid eggs.

Unfertilized *A. lumbricoides* ova are too heavy to float in the zinc sulfate flotation procedure and may be missed if the sediment is not also examined. The presence of only unfertilized ova in stool specimens may indicate infection with a single female worm. One adult female *A. lumbricoides* can produce about 200,000 ova per day; therefore, the enumeration of ova in fecal specimens using egg counts, a valuable procedure in evaluating the magnitude of hookworm infections, does not necessarily reflect the worm load. (See page 1103 for Clinical Correlation.)

TRICHURIASIS AND *TRICHURIS TRICHIURA* (WHIPWORM)

The overall incidence of *T. trichiura* infections is not known, although a 90% prevalence has been cited in certain populations in Cameroon, Malaysia, and in Caribbean countries. Vermund and coworkers[329] found that *T. trichiura* was the most common nematode recovered from 41,958 stool specimens submitted to the Columbia-Presbyterian Medical Center in New York during 1971 to 1984.

The life cycle of *T. trichiura* follows a simple fecal–oral route of transmission without an intermediate phase in an external host. The ova, however, must mature in the external environment, requiring a period of about 21 days under favorable conditions before they become infective. The life cycle is illustrated in Figure 20-10, page 1104.

Adult trichuris worms measure between 30 and 50 mm in length, with males being slightly smaller than females. The worm derives its colloquial name, "whipworm," from the thin, anterior, whiplike head (see Color Plate 20-3D). In fact, because the head, rather than the tail, is at the tip of the whip, the genus name should be *Trichocephalus*, replacing the incorrect designation *Trichuris* ("thread-tail"). In intestinal infections, the head is buried in the mucosa of the large bowel; therefore, adults are rarely seen in stool specimens. Males have a 360-degree caudal coil.

The ova measure in the range of 54 × 22 μm and are among the more easy to recognize in microscopic preparations by their distinct barrel shape and refractile hyaline polar plugs at either end (see Color Plate 20-3E). Only the eggs of *Capillaria philippinensis* may be confused; however, their polar plugs are less prominent and the shell is thicker and striated (see Fig. 20-13).

PINWORM INFECTIONS AND *ENTEROBIUS VERMICULARIS*

The life cycle of *E. vermicularis* is quite simple, requiring no external host, with the fecal to oral route being the main means of human-to-human transmission similar to that of the amebas. In most cases, eggs

SPECIES	HABITAT OF ADULT	INFECTIVE FORM	DIAGNOSTIC FORMS	PLATE REFERENCE
Ascaris lumbricoides	Small and large intestine of humans; may migrate into bile duct or pancreatic duct.	Fertile eggs	*Fertile eggs:* 60 × 45 µm, round or ovoid, with thick shell covered by a thick albuminous coat; inner cell in various stages of cleavage. They have a brown color. *Decorticate eggs:* Digestive enzymes may dissolve the albuminous coat, leaving the ovum with a smooth decorticate surface. *Infertile eggs:* 90 × 40 µm, elongated. Shell is often thin with loss of mamillated albuminous covering. Internal material is a mass of nondescript globules. *Adult worms:* 25–35 cm in length. Males are smaller than females and have a curved tail. White longitudinal streaks on either side of body and lack of muscular segments are helpful identifying features.	20-3B, C 20-3A
Trichuris trichiura	Large intestine	Fertile eggs	*Egg:* 54 × 22 µm, elongate, barrel-shaped with polar hyaline "plug" at either end. Shell is yellow to brown; plugs are colorless. *Adult worms:* 35–45 mm, long, attenuated whiplike anterior portion; short, thick, handlelike posterior.	20-3E 20-3D
Enterobius vermicularis	Large intestine, appendix, perianal area	Eggs	*Eggs:* 55 × 26 µm, elongate, asymmetric with one side flattened, the other convex. Shell is thin and smooth, and fully developed larvae are usually observed in cellulose tape preparations. *Adult worms:* 3 × 5 mm to 1 cm, white with a pointed tail. Paraoral alae (wings) are diagnostic.	20-3G 20-3F, H
Ancylostoma duodenale	Small intestine. Scolex of adult is firmly attached to mucosa by two pairs of chitinous teeth.	Filariform larvae that penetrate skin	*Rhabditiform larvae:* occasionally seen in stool specimens that have sat at room temperature for many days before being examined. They can be distinguished from rhabditiform larvae of *Strongyloides stercoralis* by the hookworm's long buccal cavity. *Eggs:* 60 × 40 µm, oval ellipsoid. Shells are thin-walled, smooth, and colorless. Internal cleavage is usually well developed at 4- to 8-cell stage, which characteristically pulls away from the shell leaving an empty space. *Head of adult:* presence of two pairs of chitinous teeth.	20-3K, right 20-3I 20-3J (left)
Necator americanus	Small intestine. Scolex of adult is firmly attached to mucosa by cutting plates.	Filariform larvae that penetrate skin	*Eggs:* 65 × 40 µm. They are morphologically similar to *A. duodenale.* *Rhabditiform larvae:* similar to *A. duodenale.* *Head of adult:* mouth part filled with sharp cutting plates.	20-3I 20-3J (right)
Strongyloides stercoralis	Small intestine	Filariform larvae Self-infections may occur if passage of stool is delayed and filariform larvae develop.	*Eggs:* usually not seen in stool specimens, but similar to those of hookworm. *Rhabditiform larvae:* this is the form most commonly seen in stool specimens. By the time the ova reach the large intestine, most have hatched. The larvae measure 0.75–1 mm in length and 75 µm in diameter. *Strongyloides* rhabditiform larvae can be distinguished from those of hookworm by their short buccal cavity and by the presence of a prominent genital primordium. *Filariform larvae:* rarely found. Long, slender form with a notched tail. They are highly infectious.	20-3I 20-3K, left

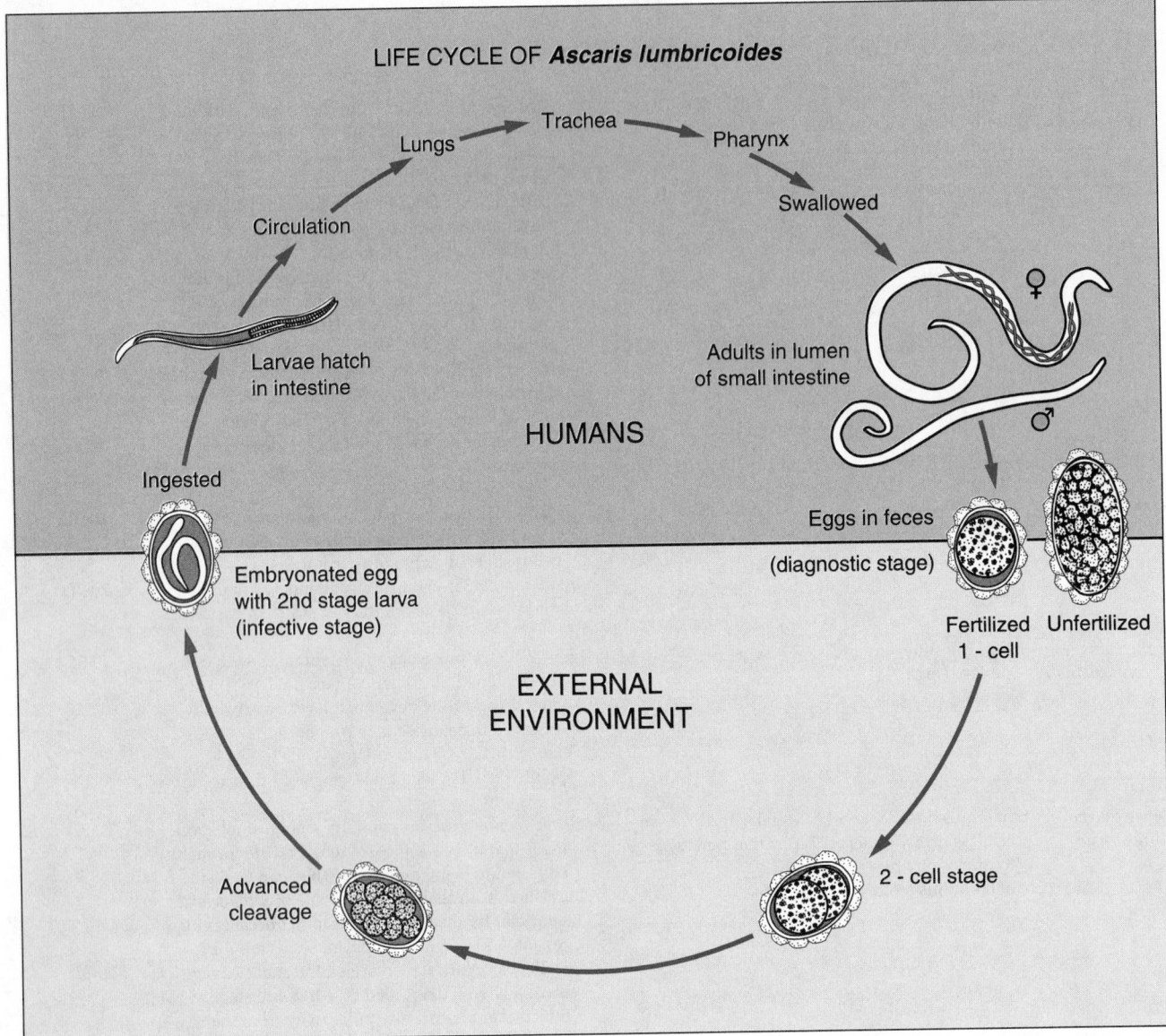

LIFE CYCLE OF *Ascaris lumbricoides*

Lungs → Trachea → Pharynx

Circulation

Swallowed

Larvae hatch in intestine

Adults in lumen of small intestine

HUMANS

Ingested

Eggs in feces

(diagnostic stage)

Embryonated egg with 2nd stage larva (infective stage)

Fertilized 1 - cell   Unfertilized

EXTERNAL ENVIRONMENT

2 - cell stage

Advanced cleavage

Figure 20-9
Life cycle of *Ascaris lumbricoides.*

have matured at the time they are detected in stool specimens or on mounts prepared from the perianal skin. Well-developed larvae are often observed in these specimens.

The adult female worm measures approximately 8 to 13 mm long by 0.4 mm in diameter. It can be recognized by the cuticular, winglike alar expansion at the anterior end (see Color Plate 20-3F) and the long pointed tail ("pin"). The diagnosis of *E. vermicularis* (pinworm) infection is most commonly made through the use of the cellulose acetate ("Scotch tape") test technique by which the sticky side of a piece of transparent tape is pressed on the perianal skin. Yield is best in children if the test is performed early in the morning when worm migration is maximal, immediately on waking before bowel movement.

The ova measure approximately 30 × 50 µm in size, have a thin, smooth, transparent shell, are oval in outline, asymmetric, with one side flattened. A well-developed larva is usually contained (see Color Plate 20-3G). See page 1105 for Clinical Correlation.

HOOKWORMS

Ancylostoma duodenale is the old-world hookworm, and *Necator americanus* is the new-world species, as defined by the areas of endemic disease. Because their life histories are essentially the same and the two species cannot be differentiated by the appearance of their eggs, the general term "hookworm" is commonly used for both species. An estimated 700 to 900 million people worldwide are infected with hookworm (mostly *A. duodenale*), 0.2% of whom suffer from severe anemia.

Although a second host is not required for the completion of the life cycle, there are significant differences that set hookworms apart from other nematodes.

CLINICAL CORRELATION BOX 20-4. *ASCARIS LUMBRICOIDES*

Patients with light infections may be asymptomatic. In heavy intestinal infections, abdominal pain, discomfort, and diarrhea are common findings. In contrast with hookworms, for which a heavy worm load is prerequisite to the presence of disease, a human intestinal infestation with only one *A. lumbricoides* worm may be important. Ascarid adults have the propensity to migrate and wander into the bile ducts, pancreatic duct, or lumen of the appendix, or may rarely penetrate the bowel. A fatal case of pancreatitis in which a single *A. lumbricoides* worm was found impacted within the ampulla of Vater has been reported.[209] Appendicitis, pancreatitis, biliary obstruction, and hepatic abscess formation, all are potential complications that can occur, even in light infections.[141] Recurrent pancreatitis secondary to an impacted calcified ascaris remnant within the duct of Wirsung in a 20-year-old woman has been reported,[187] and a case of granulomatous peritonitis in response to ascaris ova[335] are examples of these complications.

This propensity for ascarids to wander from the bowel lumens is particularly notable during drug therapy—one reason why inadequate or incomplete courses of treatment can be particularly dangerous. Adult worms may protrude from the rectum or be coughed up in heavy infections. Intestinal obstruction, intussusception, volvulus, or bowel perforation are other potential complications of heavy infection. Intestinal obstruction occurs in approximately 2 of every 1000 persons infected; this condition is fatal in 6:100,000 children.[321] Baird and associates[19] report a fatal case of ascariasis in a 2-year-old black South African girl, from whom 796 *A. lumbricoides* worms, weighing an aggregate of 550 g, were removed at autopsy. Torsion and gangrene of the heavily worm-infested ileum was the cause of death. Worms were also recovered from the stomach, esophagus, intrahepatic and extrahepatic bile ducts, and the gallbladder. An estimated 20,000 persons worldwide die of ascariasis annually.[321]

Treatment is with mebendazole (Vermox), given orally at a dose of 100 mg twice daily for 3 days, which comes in 100-mg chewable tablets. Side effects include abdominal pain and diarrhea, particularly if infection is heavy and many worms are expelled. Use of the drug is contraindicated during pregnancy.

Hookworm eggs are usually passed in early cleavage and, in about 24 hours, hatch into the first larval stage, the free-feeding rhabditiform larva. About 5 to 7 days later, the rhabditiform larva transforms into the third-stage filariform larva, which is the infective form for humans. Depending on the temperature and moisture content of the soil, filariform larva can remain infective for up to 6 weeks. Humans become infected by penetration of the filariform larva on skin contact. An illustration of the life cycle is shown in Figure 20-11.

The laboratory diagnosis is usually made by observing the characteristic ova in stool specimens. It is important that the eggs of the hookworms be identified because of the potentially severe disease associated with infections with this nematode. The ova of both *A. duodenale* and *N. americanus* are identical, and also cannot be distinguished from those of *Strongyloides stercoralis*. They measure approximately 60 × 40 μm and are distinctly oval. The shells are thin, smooth, transparent, and unpigmented. The yolk cells retract, leaving a clear space beneath the shell (see Color Plate 20-3I).

The adult worms, which measure up to 1.5 cm in length, reside in the upper intestine where they are firmly attached to the mucosa by the biting action of cutting mouth parts. The male worms are distinguished by their frayed posterior bursa. Observation of the mouth parts can be used to distinguish between the two species. *A. duodenale* has two pairs of chitinous teeth (see Color Plate 20-3J); the mouthpart of *N. americanus* is fitted with a pair of cutting plates.

Nutrition for the adult hookworms is derived by leaching blood from the host. Each adult worm can ingest up to 0.05 mL/day of blood; thus, in heavy infections, a substantial amount of blood can be lost, and severe iron deficiency anemia may develop in a short time. Consequently, fecal egg counts may be indicated in assessing the severity (worm burden) in certain cases. Adult female hookworms produce only about 2500 to 5000 eggs per day; thus, the fecal egg counts may reflect the number of adult hookworms and, in turn, indicate the severity of infection. A concentration of more than 2000 hookworm ova per milliliter of feces in women and children and more than 5000 per milliliter in males is usually associated with anemia. Egg-counting techniques are described by Garcia and Bruckner.[120]

After eggs are passed in the feces and reach warm, moist soil, they hatch into filariform larvae. These can be distinguished by observing for the long buccal cavity (see Color Plate 20-3K, *right*) as compared with the short buccal cavity of the filariform larvae of *S. stercoralis* (see Color Plate 20-3K, *left*).

STRONGYLOIDIASIS AND *STRONGYLOIDES STERCORALIS*

Peculiarities in the life cycle set infections with *S. stercoralis* apart from those of other nematodes. For example, the laboratory diagnosis of strongyloidiasis is usually made by observing motile rhabditiform larvae rather than ova in stool specimens (see Color Plate 20-3K). Strongyloides ova cannot be distinguished from those of the hookworms; however, this is of little practical concern as larval development is so quick that only rhabditiform larvae (or rarely filariform larvae) and no ova are microscopically seen in fecal specimens. Theoretically, the rhabditiform larvae of *Strongyloides* species must be distinguished from those of hookworms. However, again, it is not of practical concern because hookworm rhabditiform larvae are rarely seen in stool specimens. Only in cases of fecal impaction, or when stool specimens have been delayed in transit to the laboratory or examined only after some delay, will the ova have

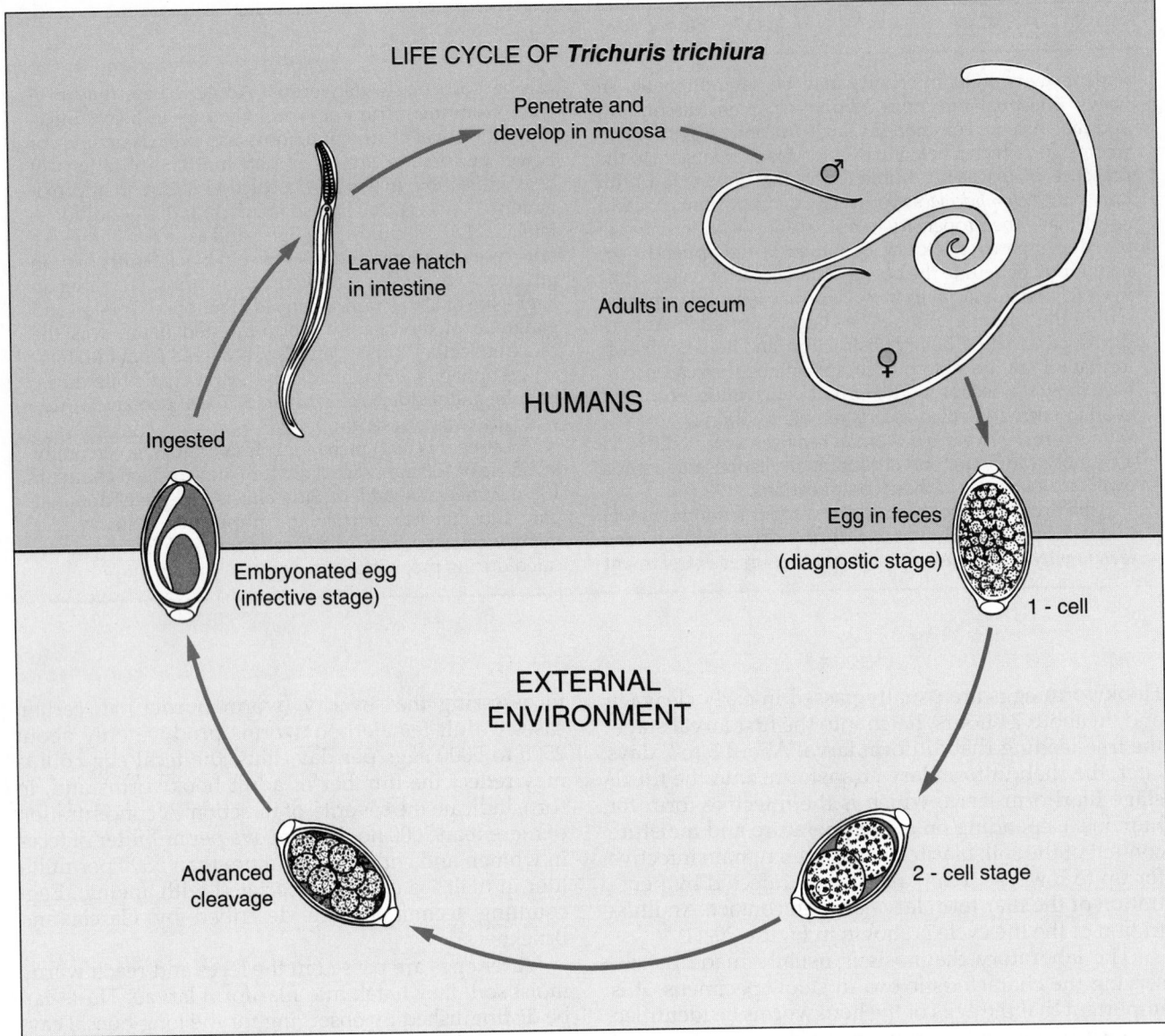

Figure 20-10
Life cycle of *Trichuris trichiura*.

time to hatch the rhabditiform larvae. Second, in the absence of host immunity, rhabditiform larvae may transform into filariform larva while still in the intestine, leading potentially into a disseminated hyperinfection syndrome, described in more detail in Clinical Correlation Box 20-8. A life cycle is illustrated in Figure 20-12.

The rhabditiform larvae of *S. stercoralis* have a short buccal cavity (see Color Plate 20-3K), in contrast with a long buccal cavity for the rhabditiform larvae of the hookworms (see Color Plate 20-3K). *S. stercoralis* rhabditiform larvae also have a prominent genital primordium about one third the distance from the tail. These differences are listed in Table 20-4.

In light infections, the Baermann technique or the agar plate culture method may be helpful in establishing a diagnosis.[120] de Kaminsky[80], in a study of 427 stool samples, found that an additional 33 cases were

diagnosed using a modified Baerman technique and 28 additional cases were diagnosed using the agar plate culture method.

TRICHOSTRONGYLUS SPECIES

Uncommonly detected in the United States, *Trichostrongylus* species are small adult nematodes, similar to the hookworms, that reside with heads buried in small intestinal epithelium. Adult worms typically inhabit the gastrointestinal tracts of sheep, cattle, goats, and other herbivores. Although third-stage larvae lie on grass and vegetation, infection is by oral ingestion because these larva lack the ability to invade skin. Also, in human infections, because they do not possess the special mouth parts characteristic of hookworms, leaching of blood does not occur. Heavy infections may produce abdominal pain, diarrhea, and mild eosinophilia, but for the most part symptoms are minimal. The ova resemble those of the hookworm but are longer (78 to 98 μm by 40 to 50 μm) with pointed ends. It is important to recognize these subtle differences in egg morphology so that an incorrect diagnosis of hookworm infection is not made. Thiabendazole, 25 mg/kg every 12 hours for 2 days is the recommended treatment.

CAPILLARIA PHILIPPINENSIS

C. philippinensis is an extremely small nematode, the adults measuring from 1.5 to 3.9 mm in length and in width from 5 μm at the filamentous head to 30 μm in midbody. After considerable research to find the reservoir hosts, it is now believed that fish-eating birds are natural hosts within a fish–bird life cycle.[67] Humans become infected when they eat poorly cooked fish commonly consumed by birds.

The gradual onset of abdominal pain, gurgling stomach, and intermittent diarrhea over a 4- to 8-week period is the common presenting clinical picture. Severe protein-losing enteropathy, malabsorption of fats and sugars, and a low xylose excretion rate are commonly seen. Fluid loss and electrolyte imbalances, characterized by low plasma levels of potassium, sodium, and calcium, are seen. Immunoglobulin E (IgE) is at high levels, with IgG, IgM, and IgA being at low levels. In fatal cases, heavy infection in the jejunum, fatty metamorphosis of the liver, vacuolization of the cytoplasm of renal proximal convoluted tubular cells and of myocardial cells, with heavy cytoplasmic deposition of lipochrome pigment were seen. Focal mucosal atrophy at sites of the organism's invasion was seen in histologic sections of the small intestine.[67]

The disease is endemic in the Philippines, Thailand, and regions adjacent to the South China Sea. Local eating habits include ingestion of raw animal organs and the use of intestinal juices from animals to season rice and other foodstuffs. Uncooked crabs and small freshwater fish are also considered a food delicacy in many indigenous populations. Infection with *C. philippinensis* always causes illness and may lead to death if untreated. From 1967 to 1990, 1884 confirmed cases of intestinal capillariasis were documented, of which 110 people died.[67] Cases of intestinal capillariasis have also been reported from Japan, Egypt,[366] and Iran.[14] From a stool examination, the condition may be confused with *T. trichiura* because the ova have a similar appearance. However, the ova of *C. philippinensis* have less conspicuous polar plugs and a thick, striated shell (Fig. 20-13, page 1109). A misidentification could lead to unnecessary morbidity or even death as cases of *T. trichiura* often go untreated.

INTESTINAL CESTODES

The cestodes are a subclass of helminths comprising true tapeworms, which have a scolex and a series of hermaphroditic body segments. The cestodes of human importance are *Taenia saginata*, *T. solium*, *Diphyllobothrium latum*, *Hymenolepis nana*, *H. diminuta*, and *Dipylidium caninum*.

The body of an adult cestode or tapeworm, called the strobila, consists of two parts, a scolex and the proglottides (see Color Plate 20-4*A*). The scolex is the

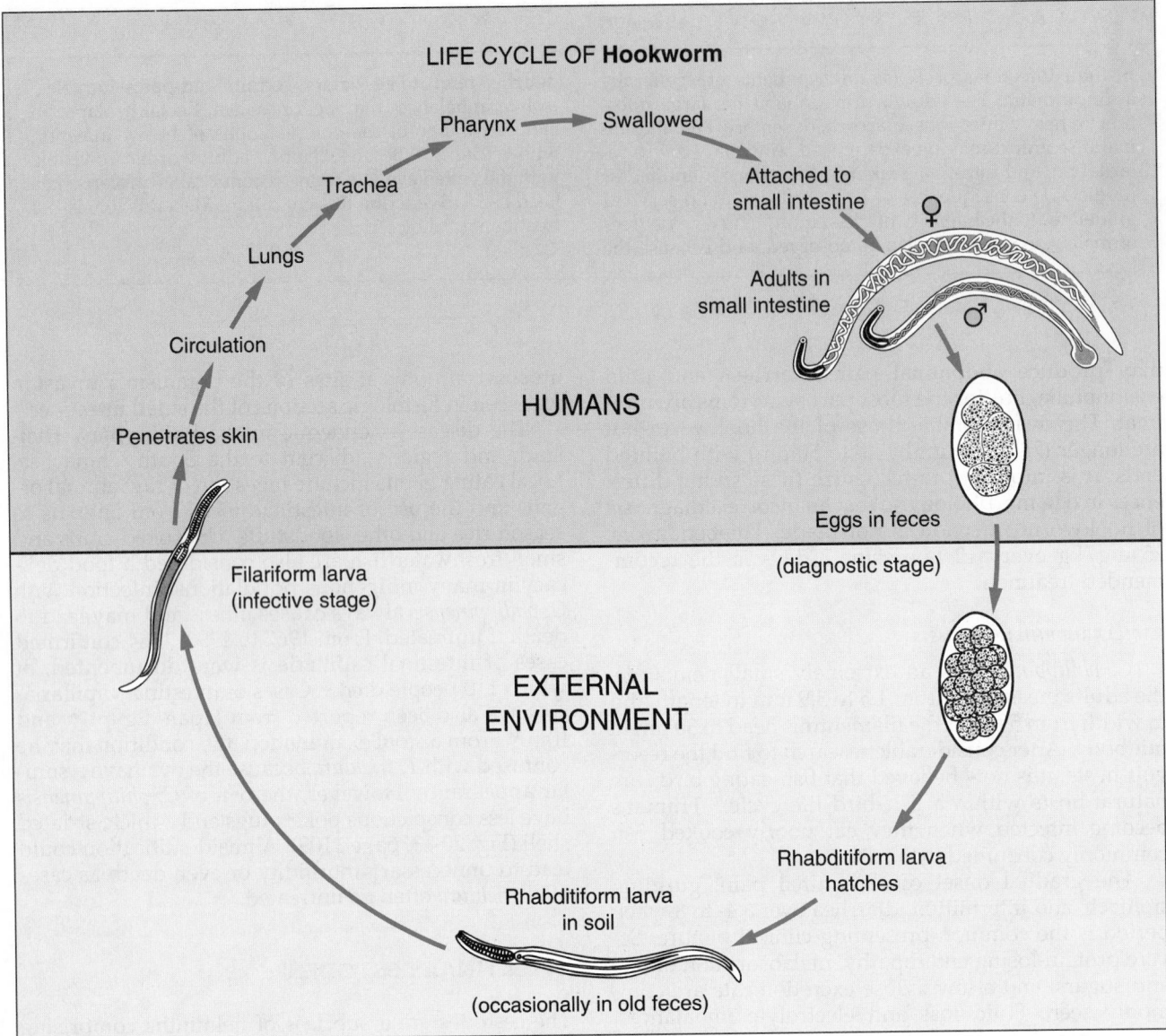

Figure 20-11
Life cycle of a hookworm.

anterior portion, with hooklets or suckers by which the worm can attach and anchor to the intestinal mucosa. The crown of the scolex, called the rostellum, may be fitted with hooklets (armed; see Color Plate 20-4*B*), or may be devoid of hooklets and smooth (unarmed). These morphologic differences are helpful in establishing a species identification.

The major portion of the body of a tapeworm is composed of a long series of segments called proglottides. Each proglottid possesses male and female reproductive structures, the uterine branches of which are packed with ova when mature (see Color Plate 20-4*C*). The ova are passed in the feces, in which they are observed in microscopic mounts to establish a laboratory diagnosis. Subtle differences in the size, shape,

and internal structures of proglottides serve as aids in establishing a species identification.

With the exception of *H. nana*, with which human-to-human transmission of infections may occur through ingestion of fecally contaminated food or water that contains infective eggs, the life cycles of the cestodes require one or more intermediate hosts to support stages of larval development. For example, humans with an intestinal tapeworm infection pass feces containing mature ova that can contaminate vegetative matter, soil, or fresh water. Tapeworm eggs ingested by cows, pigs, and fish, for example, hatch in the intestines of these intermediate hosts, liberating larvae that penetrate the bowel mucosa and migrate

(text continues on page 1109)

CLINICAL CORRELATION BOX 20-7. *HOOKWORMS*

Symptoms may occur relative to various stages of the life cycle. Skin infections may be experienced at the sites of filariform larval invasion, particularly when humans are infected with nonhuman hookworm species commonly involving other animals ("ground itch").[333] Loeffler's syndrome in lungs and eosinophilia may be seen during the pulmonary larval migratory stage. In a heavy infection of 500 or more worms, the host could be bled the equivalent of ½ to 1 pint of blood per week, producing severe hypochromic, iron deficiency anemia and marked erythroid hyperplasia of the bone marrow. Weakness, fatigue, growth retardation, peripheral edema, and congestive heart failure may be complications in severe infections. Of major concern worldwide is the lack of mental development in millions of children infected with hookworms.[158] Diarrhea, abdominal pain, and nausea are manifestations of the intestinal phase of infection. Thirty-five of 684 soldiers who took part in the Grenada military operations developed hookworm infections,[117] most commonly associated with ground exposure near homes with compromised sanitation. Mebendazole, 100 mg orally every 12 hours for 3 days is the recommended treatment.

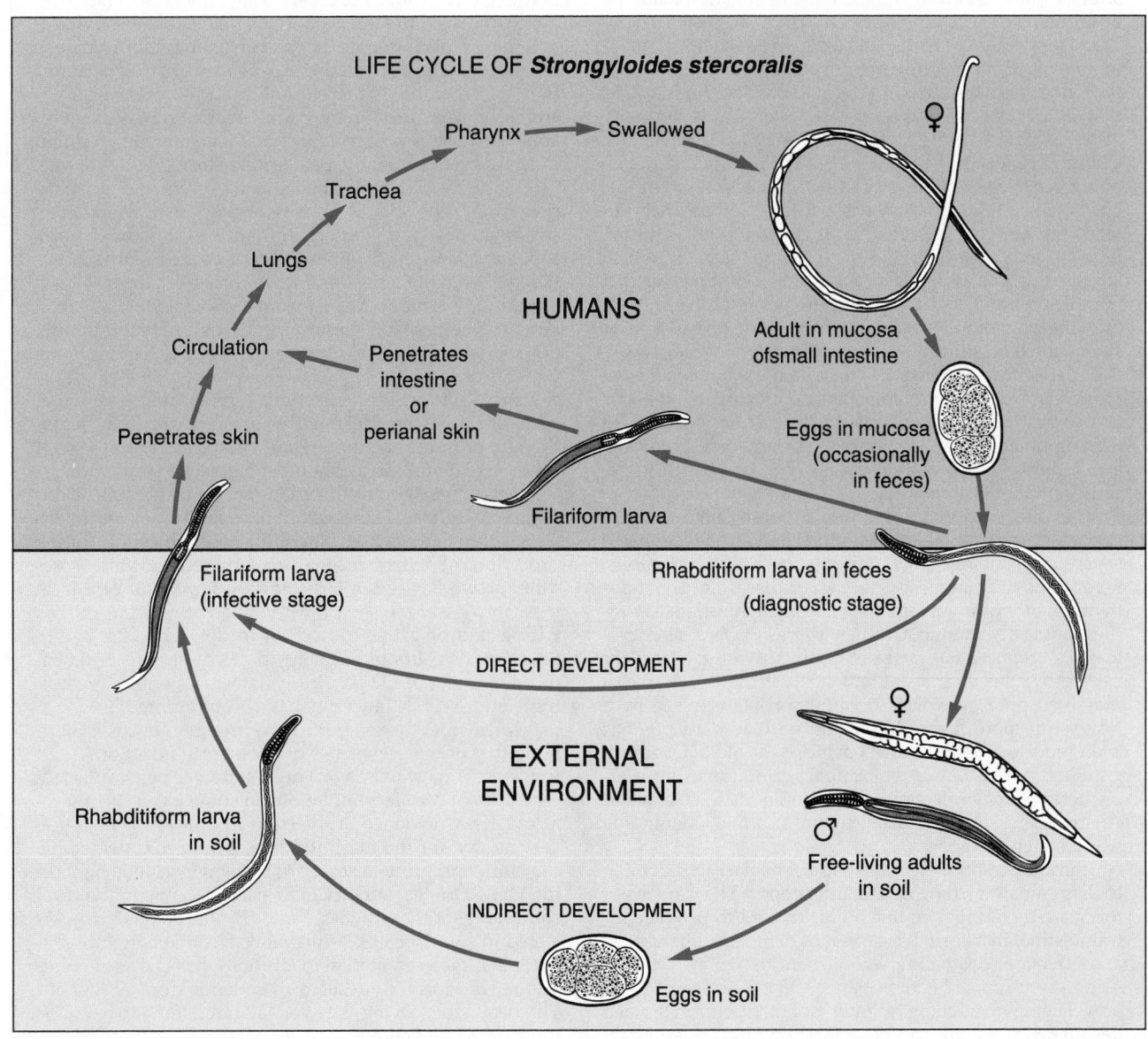

Figure 20-12
Life cycle of *Strongyloides stercoralis*.

CLINICAL CORRELATION BOX 20-8. *STRONGYLOIDIASIS*

Skin irritation and pruritus in the form of low-grade chronic dermatitis may be seen at the portal of entry.[55] The full-blown ground itch, characteristic of hookworm cutaneous infections, usually does not occur. Leighton and MacSween,[194] however, report a case of a 74-year-old woman with a 65-year history of urticarial-like eruptions since childhood, which were finally correlated with long-term persistence of hyperinfection strongyloidiasis. The case for making a diagnosis of disseminated strongyloidiasis through recognition of filariform larvae in skin biopsies has also been made.[131]

With a heavy infective dose, pulmonary disease suggestive of Loeffler's pneumonia, with wheezing and eosinophilia, may occur; or in cases of hyperinfection syndrome, to be described in the following, full-blown pneumonia, with cough and shortness of breath, may develop. Harris and associates[143] report two cases of disseminated strongyloidiasis in which the diagnosis was first made by observing larvae in the sputum. They suggest that immunosuppressed patients who develop nonbacterial pneumonia, particularly in the presence of eosinophilia, should have both stool and sputum samples checked for infection with *S. stercoralis.* Long-term corticosteroid therapy may also predispose to disseminated strongyloides infections. Chu and coauthors[56] describe a case of pneumonia developing in a 65-year-old man with steroid-dependent chronic obstructive pulmonary disease. Strongyloides rhabditiform larvae were detected in an expectorated sputum. Dunlap and associates[94] also report a case in which strongyloidiasis manifested as asthma, pointing out that not all hyperinfected patients show eosinophilia. In general, the pneumonitis caused by nematode larvae is transient and characterized by cough and fever; in more severe cases, it is characterized by chest pain, dyspnea, and hemoptysis. Delarocque Astagneau and coworkers[81] report a case of obstructive jaundice caused by papillary necrosis of the ampulla of Vater secondary to strongyloides infection, and indicate that strongyloidiasis should be added to the causes of papillary stenosis.

The intestinal manifestations of strongyloides infections vary from few if any symptoms in light infections, to severe necrotizing bowel disease in heavy infections. Symptoms may suggest peptic ulcer disease in some patients; in others, involvement of the small intestine may radiographically mimic Crohn's disease. Dees and colleagues[76] report a rare case of bleeding from a gastric ulcer caused by a heavy infestation with *S. stercoralis.* A case of massive upper gastrointestinal hemorrhage caused by a heavy infection of the duodenum with *S. stercoralis* has been reported[27] that occurred in a 29-year-old black immigrant from Africa. A case of jejunal perforation complicating *S. stercoralis* infection of the bowel in a 65-year-old Australian ex-prisoner-of-war who also had pneumonia was also reported.[173]

Immunosuppressed hosts are particularly vulnerable to disseminated strongyloides infections.[31] The propensity for *S. stercoralis* eggs to hatch quickly and to produce intraintestinal filariform larvae makes patients vulnerable to autoinfection, producing a condition known as hyperinfection syndrome.[162] (Color Plate 20-3L is a section of small bowel being invaded by recently molted filariform larvae.) Because *S. stercoralis* can be carried by humans as a sub-clinical infestation for many years following initial contact, patients who develop disseminated strongyloidiasis need not have had a recent exposure. Purtilo and associates,[268] after observing the absence of granulomatous tissue response to larvae in several autopsy cases of fatal strongyloidiasis, conclude that an intact cell-mediated immune system is necessary to keep the organism in check. Once immunity is compromised or abrogated, hyperinfection, with dissemination of larvae to many organs and tissues, is likely to occur in patients harboring the parasite. Genta[123] offers the alternative argument that corticosteroids, rather than working through suppression of immunity, may in fact act directly on the worm as "molting hormones" that directly promote organism proliferation, making disseminated disease a more likely possibility.

Mortality rates as high as 50% have been reported in naturally or iatrogenically compromised patients with hyperinfection strongyloidiasis.[153] Klein and associates[179] reiterate the need to screen stool specimens for strongyloidiasis in patients living in endemic areas for whom a course of immunosuppressive therapy is planned. Hyperinfection syndrome is further complicated because of the increased risk of developing gram-negative sepsis, presumably because intestinal bacteria can invade through mucosal breaks from the penetrating strongyloides larvae.

Recipients of organ transplants represent another high-risk group who should have stool examinations to detect strongyloides larvae before immunosuppressive therapy is begun.[74] Recipients of renal allografts are highly susceptible to hyperinfection strongyloidiasis because of their impaired T-lymphocyte function.[82] Strongyloidiasis can remain quiescent for many years, becoming manifest only at the onset of immunosuppressive therapy.[82] Lymphoma patients are another high-risk group susceptible to opportunistic strongyloides infection,[123] reiterating again that such infections are treatable, and candidates for chemotherapy or immunosuppression who reside or have spent time in endemic areas should be screened for strongyloidiasis. Often chronic infections are light and may be difficult to diagnose. Examination of several stool specimens on successive days may be required; or the concentration procedure of Baermann may be indicated. In this procedure, active larvae are induced to migrate out of a fecal mass into a water reservoir through a wire screen covered with a pad of gauze (described in detail by Garcia and Bruckner).[120] Although strongyloides hyperinfection syndrome has not been specifically associated with HIV positivity and AIDS, a few cases have been reported.[142, 165]

Worldwide, the magnitude of strongyloidiasis is similar to that of the prevalence of hookworm infections, with upward of an estimated 800 million people being infected, with 10% of certain populations in some locales being infected. The incidence of infection in any given region is very spotty, for the filariform larvae require considerable moisture and grow best where the water table is high. In the United States, strongyloidiasis is endemic in the rural south and southeast, with 3% to 5% of persons being infected in some locales.[333] Infections also have high prevalence in inmates in mental institutions, prisons, and immigrants who formerly resided in endemic tropical regions. Thiabendazole, 25 mg/kg every 12 hours for 2 to 5 days is the treatment of choice.

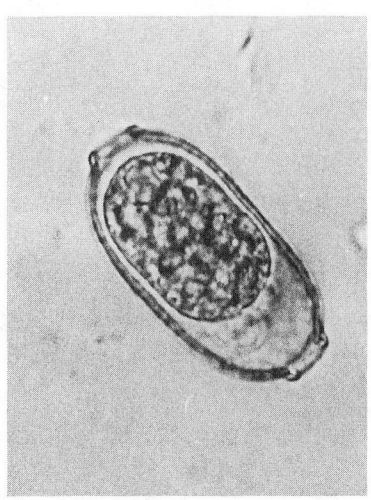

Figure 20-13
Photomicrograph of an ovum of *Capillaria philippinensis*, measuring about 50 by 35 μm. Note their resemblance to the eggs of *Trichuris trichiura*; they differ in that the bipolar hyaline plugs are less prominent and more flattened, and have a shell that is somewhat thickened with distinct striations.

into the skeletal muscle or flesh. The larvae become encysted in a form called cysticercus, or "bladder worm." Humans become infected by eating raw or poorly cooked beef, pork, or fish infested with the cysticerci. The life cycle of *T. solium* is illustrated in Figure 20-14. The key laboratory features for the identification of intestinal cestodes are found in Table 20-5.

TAENIA SOLIUM AND TAENIA SAGINATA

Differentiation of *T. saginata* from *T. solium* is more than an academic exercise. Humans acquire the intestinal infections with an adult *Taenia* tapeworm through ingestion of larval infected, poorly cooked pork (*T. solium*) or beef (*T. saginata*). Intestinal infections with the adult tapeworms of these two species produce similar symptoms in humans, as discussed in Clinical Correlation Box 20-9. However, humans may also serve as the intermediate host if the ova of *T. solium* are ingested. In this case, the larvae circulate widely in the circulation, with a propensity to lodge in the brain, producing a disease called cysticercosis. Laboratory workers must be careful when handling the ova-packed proglottides of *T. solium* to avoid inadvertent hand-to-mouth transmission. Human cysticercosis does not occur with *T. saginata*; however, as the true identity may not be immediately known, care must be taken when handling any proglottides.

The laboratory diagnosis of taenia tapeworm infections is usually made by observing the characteristic eggs in microscopic mounts of fecal material. The eggs for the two species are morphologically identical. They are spherical, measure approximately 30 by 45 μm in diameter, and have a thick shell with radial striations (see Color Plate 20-4*D*). Three pairs of hooklets may be observed internally, in a structure called an onchosphere. Comparative features by which *T. saginata* and *T. solium* can be differentiated are shown in Box 20-6 (also see Table 20-5, page 1112).

Chapman and associates[54] have developed a species-specific DNA probe that differentiates *T. solium* ova from those of *T. saginata*. Without going into details, the authors describe the isolation and characterization of recombinant clones that contain repetitive DNA sequences (a 158-bp sequence for *T. solium* and an unrelated *T. saginata* sequence that encodes a portion of the mitochondrial cytochrome *c* oxidase I gene, each specifically hybridizing with genomic DNA from either species). When such a probe becomes commercially available, a rapid, sensitive, and noninvasive diagnostic test for the detection of *T. solium* ova may become possible.

DIPHYLLOBOTHRIUM LATUM

D. latum, the human giant fish tapeworm, uses two intermediate hosts in the development of its larval forms. Endemic areas include the cold clear lake regions of Scandinavia, northern Europe, northern Japan, the upper Midwest of the United States, Canada, and Alaska. The cycle can be traced as follows: eggs are passed with fecal material into fresh water; after several days coracidia hatch and release miracidia; these, in turn, are ingested by invertebrate copepoda (cyclops), which serve as the first intermediate host; copepoda serve as one of the major food sources for a variety of freshwater fish in North America. These fish serve as the second intermediate host. After further maturation in the fish, plerocercoid larvae of the parasite (spargana) develop within the flesh of the fish. Humans become infected by ingesting these plerocercoid larvae in raw or poorly cooked fish. In the human intestine, the larvae develop into the adult worm. The life cycle is illustrated in Figure 20-15, page 1114.

The laboratory diagnosis of *D. latum* infection in humans is commonly made by identifying the characteristic operculated eggs in stool specimens (see Color Plate 20-4*G*). They measure approximately 55 to 75 μm by 40 to 55 μm in size, are elongated, have a smooth shell, with an inconspicuous unshouldered operculum at one end and a knoblike thickening at the other. The differentiation of *D. latum* eggs from those of *Paragonimus westermani* (discussed later) may be difficult, and a careful clinical history may be required. *P. westermani* ova have a distinct shouldered operculum (see Color Plate 20-5*L*) that is usually sufficiently visible to differentiate it from *D. latum* ova, which have no operculum.

The strobila measures from 3 to 10 m in length and has over 3000 proglottides. Although the proglottides are rarely passed in the stool, they are distinctive because the individual segments are broader than they are long (*latum*, Latin for broad). A nondescript coiled uterus in the form of a compact rosette is seen centrally within each segment (see Color Plate 20-4*H*).

The scolex, rarely recovered from stool specimens, is almond-shaped and measures 2 to 3 mm by 1 mm. Two deep dorsoventral suctorial grooves (*bothria*: pit), demarcated by lateral liplike folds (*phyllon*: leaves) is also distinctive (see Color Plate 20-4*I*).

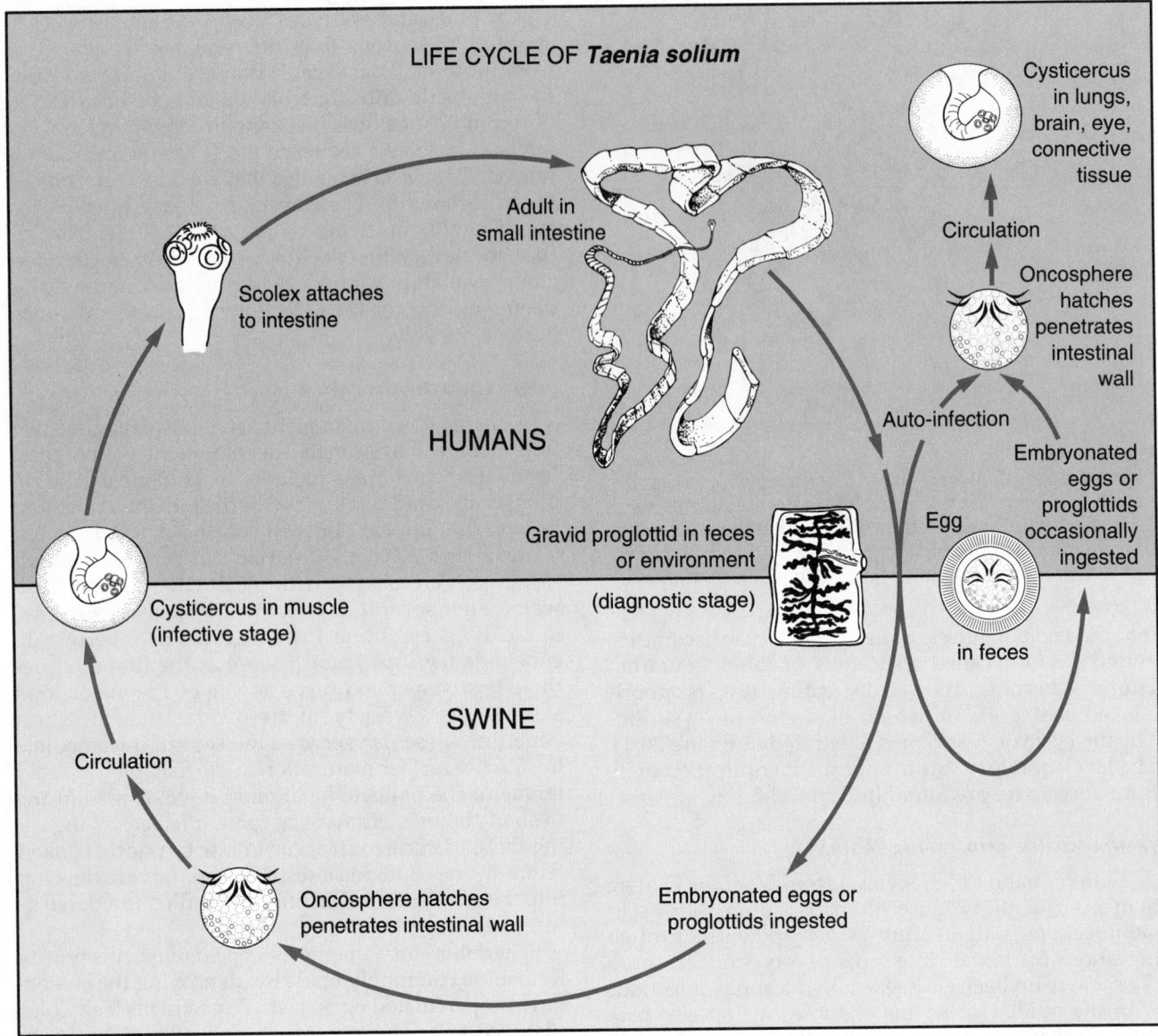

Figure 20-14
Life cycle of *Tinea solium.*

HYMENOLEPIS NANA AND HYMENOLEPIS DIMINUTA

An intermediate host is not necessary in the life cycle of *H. nana.* Human-to-human transmission of ova is by the fecal to oral route; humans serve as both intermediate and definitive host. Larval development occurs in the villi of the upper part of the small intestine following ingestion of an infective ovum. Upon hatching, larvae penetrate the villi, develop into a cysticercoid state in the proximal wall before migrating back into the lumen where, as adult worms, they attach to the mucosal lining. Humans serve as the accidental host for *H. diminuta,* the rat tapeworm, through the ingestion of infected *Tribolium* or *Tenebrio* "meal beetles." The life cycle of *H. diminuta* is illustrated in Figure 20-16, page 1115.

H. nana, perhaps the most frequently encountered tapeworm worldwide, is most commonly seen in children.[25] The adult worms of *H. nana* are small, measuring no longer than 4.6 cm when mature, and often simulate mucous threads; thus, they are not commonly seen in stool specimens. The tiny scolex has a protruding, armed scolex with a row of 20 to 30 hooklets (see Color Plate 20-4J, *left*).

The laboratory diagnosis is usually made by microscopically detecting the characteristic ova in mounts or stained smears of fecal specimens. The ova are morphologically distinctive, having a smooth outer shell and an inner membrane, containing a hexacanth (six hooklets) embryo (see Color Plate 20-4J, *right*). The ova of *H. nana* are smaller (47×57 μm) than those of *H.*

diminuta (58 × 86 µm). Look for the presence of slender polar filaments arising from thickenings on either side of the membrane of the hexacanth embryo and extending into the space beneath the shell. If they are present, *H. nana* can be identified, for *H. diminuta* is devoid of polar filaments.

DIPYLIDIUM CANINUM

The life cycle of *D. caninum* is similar to that of *H. diminuta*. Humans serve as an accidental host and become infected following ingestion of dog or cat fleas that are infected with the cysticercoid form of *D. caninum*. The adult tapeworm resides in the intestine of dogs or cats. The eggs, discharged in the feces, are ingested by several species of dog fleas or lice, within the body cavity of which develops the infective cysticercoids. Upon ingestion of a dog flea by a human, the cysticercoid larva penetrates the small intestinal mucosa and develops in situ into an adult worm. Human infections particularly occur in children who have more intimate contact with household pets.

The strobila ranges from 15 to 70 cm in length and possesses 60 to 175 proglottides. The scolex is rhomboidal and possesses a retractile conical armed rostellum. The proglottides measure 12 × 2.7 mm and are distinctive for possessing a double genital pore (dipylidium; see Color Plate 20-4K). Proglottides may detach from the strobila and migrate singly or as short chains from the anus of cats and dogs, appearing as tiny grains of rice when deposited on the carpet or floor.

The laboratory diagnosis in human infections is usually made by microscopically observing the characteristic egg packets (see Color Plate 20-4L). Each packet contains 15 to 25 globular eggs, each measuring 35 to 60 µm in diameter, containing an oncosphere with six hooklets.

Infected individuals usually have minimal or no symptoms. In heavy infections, symptoms are usually limited to indigestion, appetite loss, and vague abdominal discomfort. Praziquantel is the treatment of choice; niclosamide is also effective.[241] Human infection is preventable by keeping pet dogs and cats free of tapeworms and fleas.

TREMATODES

The trematodes are a class of helminths including all the flukes that are parasites for humans. Flukes are leaflike and flat, hermaphroditic except for the schistosomes, and possess two suckers—one oral, through which the digestive tract opens; the other ventral, for attachment. The trematodes of human importance are the liver flukes *Fasciola hepatica* and *Clonorchis sinensis*; the giant intestinal fluke *Fasciolopsis buskii*; the schistosomes *Schistosoma mansoni*, *S. haematobium*, *S. japonicum*; and the lung fluke *Paragonimus westermani*.

The key features for laboratory identification of these flukes are listed in Table 20-6, page 1117.

The life cycles of the flukes are similar, requiring two intermediate hosts before the stages that are infective for humans develop (*Schistosoma* species are an exception). The initial stages of the life cycles are virtually identical; that is, eggs passed into water (fecal contamination from open privies on bridges over canals or lakes) hatch either immediately or following a short period of embryonation. Free-swimming miracidia are released, which are either ingested or penetrate into the flesh of the first intermediate host—a snail. Within the snail, the miracidia transform into a second larval stage known as a sporocyst (schistosomes) or a redia (the trematodes). This developmental period may be as short as 3 weeks for *C. sinensis* and as long as 12 weeks for *F. hepatica*. The purpose of this larval stage in the snail is to provide an environment for replication of hundreds of cercaria. As a prototype for the flukes, except the schistosomes, an illustration of the life cycle of *F. hepatica* is shown in Figure 20-17.

The mode of infection for various cercariae varies with the species. For example, mature schistosome cercariae, with characteristic forked tails (see Color Plate 20-5A), after release from the snail, infect humans who wade or swim in infested waters. Cercariae directly penetrate the water-softened skin without requiring a second intermediate host. A mild inflammatory response may occur at the sites of cercarial penetration. *C. sinensis* cercariae infect freshwater fish; those of *P. westermani* use various species of crustaceans (crabs or crayfish); and those with *F. hepatica* and *F. buski* attach to a variety of water plants (water chestnut or watercress), on which they form encysted structures known as metacercariae. These metacercariae are more resistant to environmental stresses than free-swimming cercariae and can survive for several weeks or months. Humans become infected by ingesting the metacercariae contained in the raw or undercooked flesh of fish or crustaceans that are attached to the leaves or stems of water plants.

SCHISTOSOMES

The name **schistosome** is derived from the appearance of the adult male, the body of which has a longitudinal genital groove, or canal, that serves as a receptacle for the female during copulation (see Color Plate 20-5B). Three *Schistosoma* species, *S. mansoni*, *S. haematobium*, and *S. japonicum*, cause the majority of human

(text continues on page 1114)

TABLE 20-5

INTESTINAL CESTODES: KEY FEATURES FOR LABORATORY IDENTIFICATION

SPECIES	HABITAT OF ADULT	INFECTIVE FORM	DIAGNOSTIC FORMS	PLATE REFERENCE
Taenia saginata	Small intestine	Cysticercus larvae in beef muscle	*Eggs:* 31 × 43 μm, spherical or subspherical, with thick shell with prominent radial striations. Embryonated oncosphere possessing three pairs of hooklets within the shell is diagnostic of the genus (*Taenia* species identification cannot be made on the basis of egg morphology). *Proglottids:* longer than wide. Gravid segments have a central uterine stem with 15–20 lateral branches on each side. They are motile when first passed. *Scolex:* 4 suckers characteristic of the genus with a bare crown devoid of a hooked rostellum. Scolex is 2 mm in diameter.	20-4D
Taenia solium	Small intestine (Extraintestinal cysticercosis may develop in humans with this species, with encysted larvae infecting the heart, eye, central nervous system, and other viscera.)	Cysticercus larvae in pork muscle (Plate 20-4E and F) Eggs or gravid proglottids leading to cysticercus infection	*Eggs:* identical to those of *T. saginata.* Species identification is not possible from ova morphology. *Proglottids:* longer than wide. Gravid segments have a central uterine stem with 8–13 lateral stems, in contrast with those of *T. saginata,* which have more. *Scolex:* 4 suckers characteristic of the genus, with a rostellum armed with a double row of 25–30 large and small, brown chitinous hooks.	20-4D 20-4C 20-4B
Hymenolepis nana	Small intestine	Eggs	*Eggs:* 40 × 60 μm, oval or subspherical. Shell consists of 2 distinct membranes: the outer membrane is relatively thin and has a smooth surface; the inner membrane has 2 opposite poles from which 4–8 filaments arise and spread between the 2 membranes (differential feature from *H. diminuta,* which is devoid of filaments). Inside the inner membrane is an oncosphere with 3 pairs of hooklets (hexacanth ovum). *Adult worm:* may rarely be found in stool specimens, where it can be confused with thin strands of mucin. It measures less than 40 mm (1.5 in.) long and has indistinct, broader-than-long proglottids, a tiny scolex with 4 suckers, and a protruding rostellum with a ring of 20–30 spines.	20-4J, right 20-4J, left
Hymenolepis diminuta	Small intestine	Cysticercoid larvae in various species of fleas, cockroaches, moths, and "meal beetles," which are inadvertently ingested by humans	*Eggs:* 70–85 μm long, 60 × 80 μm wide, round to oval. They have appearance similar to the eggs of *H. nana,* except the more spherical inner membrane has no protruding filaments. *Adult worm:* Rarely found in stool specimens. Proglottid segments are not distinctive. The scolex is tiny and spherical and has 4 deep, spherical suckers and a rounded rostellum devoid of hooklets.	
Diphyllobothrium latum	Small intestine	Plerocercoid larvae in flesh of freshwater fish	*Eggs:* 60 × 75 μm long, 40 × 50 μm wide. The eggs are oval or elliptical. An inconspicuous nonshouldered operculum is seen at one of the lateral ends with a small terminal knob at the other. Shell is thin and smooth. Internal cleavage is not organized and extends to the shell, completely filling the inner area. *Proglottids:* wider than long, containing a nondescript uterine structure in the center of the proglottid with the appearance of a rosette *Scolex:* shaped like a rounded spatula, with a shallow longitudinal groove bordered on either side by liplike folds	20-4G 20-4H 20-4I

(Continued)

TABLE 20-5   *(Continued)*

INTESTINAL CESTODES: KEY FEATURES FOR LABORATORY IDENTIFICATION

SPECIES	HABITAT OF ADULT	INFECTIVE FORM	DIAGNOSTIC FORMS	PLATE REFERENCE
Dipylidium caninum	Small intestine	Cysticercoid larvae that develop in the body cavity of cat or dog fleas and lice, which are inadvertently ingested by humans	*Eggs:* egg packet usually seen, which is a sac enclosing 5 to 15 spherical eggs. Each egg measures 35 × 40 μm, is spherical, and encloses an inner oncosphere with six delicate hooklets.	20-4L
			Proglottids: longer than wide, barrel shaped, and have a double set of reproductive structures with two genital pores for each segment, one on each side (other *Taenia* species have only one genital pore).	20-4K
			Scolex: conical or ovoid rostellum with 30 to 150 small thornlike hooks arranged in several rows. Rostellum may retract into a depression in upper portion of scolex.	

CLINICAL CORRELATION BOX 20-9. *TAENIA SOLIUM AND TAENIA SAGINATA*

Intestinal symptoms are usually insignificant. Passage of proglottides in stool may be the first indication of disease. Epigastric pain, vague abdominal discomfort, nervousness, and increase in appetite may be experienced. Weight loss is minimal. Eosinophilia is usually moderate.

Cysticercosis refers to the development of extraintestinal, encysted larval forms of *T. solium* in various organs following ingestion of gravid ova in fecally contaminated food or water. Although most human cases are caused by *T. solium,* other species of animal tapeworms can, on rare occasions, also produce morphologically similar cysticerci. The CNS is involved in 60% to 96% of patients, a condition known as neurocysticercosis[226, 266] (see Color Plates 20-4E and 3F). Most patients with neurocysticercosis have more than one cyst, with as many as 200 cysts found in one autopsy case.[226] Symptoms vary considerably from patient to patient. Lesions in the cerebral cortex may result in seizures or localizing neurologic deficits. Cranial nerve palsies, in particular involving the fifth and seventh nerves, and abnormal reflexes are commonly found. Cysticercosis is the most frequently identified cause of epilepsy in young adults living in endemic areas, and it is the sole manifestation in up to one-third of cases.[226] Focal seizures occur in up to three-quarters of those infected. Intraventricular brain cysts may obstruct the flow of CSF, leading to symptoms of acute intracranial hypertension (headache, vertigo, nausea, vomiting, papilledema, and visual disturbances may occur); sudden death resulting from occlusion of the fourth ventricle has been reported.[34] Changes in personality and mental status are present in 40% of patients.[226] Symptoms may occur up to 30 years after exposure.[88]

Cysticercosis is prevalent in many parts of the world. A recent field survey of 1502 infected aborigines in ten mountainous districts/towns in Taiwan, Korea, North Sumatra, and Indonesia revealed the common habit of eating raw meat and viscera of wild or domestic animals.[104]

Among the aborigines, 73% ate wild boar, 66% flying squirrel, 65% wild goat, 49% wild rats, 46% monkey, and the others habitually ingested raw flesh and viscera of several other small animals.

Cysticercosis is highly prevalent in Mexico and Latin America, where an estimated 350,000 persons are infected. The disease has been found in 2% to 3% of autopsy cases in Mexico City, accounting for 25% of all intracranial masses found by computed tomography scans.[266] Until the last decade, neurocysticercosis has been uncommon in the United States (only a few hundred cases recorded since surveillance began in 1857);[266] however, a marked increase has been recently noted, parallel with the increased immigration of peoples from Mexico, Central and South America, and Asia.[63] In 1989, cysticercosis became a reportable disease in California.[99] During the first year, 134 cases were reported, nearly all (117) of Hispanic background and most of whom had immigrated from *T. solium* endemic countries. In addition to the higher incidence of disease in California, several individual cases have also been reported from various diverse areas in the United States, including Texas, Colorado, Pennsylvania, and Missouri.[226] Indirect hemagglutination serologic assays for confirming the diagnosis of cysticercosis in suspected cases are available through the CDC in Atlanta. A titer of 1:64 or higher is usually indicative of active infection.[136]

The invasive larvae (onchospheres) are susceptible to antibody and complement, but develop only after the larvae have transformed into the antibody-resistant metacestodes.[345] In fact, antibody may bind by Fc receptors to the worm, which may use it as a source of protein. Taeniaestatin and other parasite molecules may interfere with lymphocyte proliferation and macrophage function, thereby paralyzing the cellular immune response. Praziquantel and albendazole have been extensively tested and successfully used for treatment of neurocysticercosis, usually in combination with cortisteroids.[339]

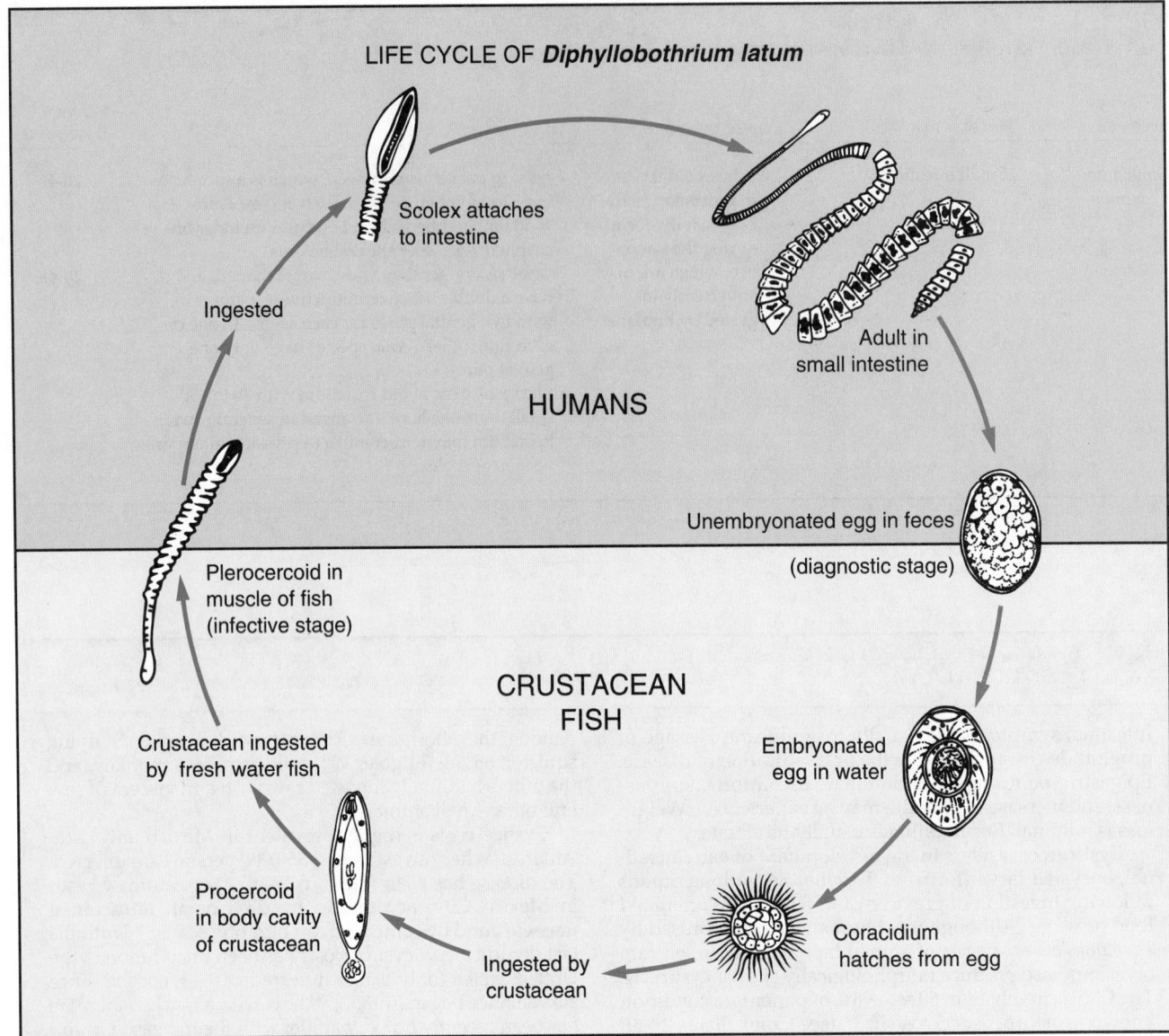

LIFE CYCLE OF *Diphyllobothrium latum*

Scolex attaches to intestine

Ingested

Adult in small intestine

HUMANS

Unembryonated egg in feces

(diagnostic stage)

Plerocercoid in muscle of fish (infective stage)

CRUSTACEAN FISH

Embryonated egg in water

Crustacean ingested by fresh water fish

Procercoid in body cavity of crustacean

Ingested by crustacean

Coracidium hatches from egg

Figure 20-15
Life cycle of *Diphyllobothrium latum*.

infections. *S. mekongi*, which resembles *S. japonicum*, and *S. intercalatum*, whose ova resemble those of *S. haematobium* but whose clinical illness mimicks *S. mansoni* infection, are two other species with limited geographic distributions in the Mekong basin and in Central and West Africa, respectively.[314]

The life cycle is similar to that of other flukes except that a second intermediate host is not required to transmit disease. Eggs that are passed in the feces into freshwater lakes, canals, and the like, hatch under suitable conditions, releasing a free-swimming miracidium. The miracidium penetrates the tissues of an appropriate snail, within which it undergoes maturation division to form hundreds of cercariae. The free-swimming cercariae released from infected snails have the capability of directly penetrating the water-

softened skin of unsuspecting swimmers and waders in freshwater estuaries. Once in the subcutaneous tissues, the heads of the cercariae enter the circulation. They migrate to the portal venous system where they develop into adult flukes. The life cycle is illustrated in Figure 20-18.

Depending on the species, the schistosome adults may be located in various areas in the portal vein system: 1) in the portal veins of the large intestine for *S. mansoni* and *S. intercalatum*; 2) in the small intestine for *S. japonicum* and *S. mekongi*; and 3) in the veins of the urinary bladder for *S. haematobium*. Although the adult worms, which measure about 2.5 to 3 cm in length and 0.5 mm in diameter when mature, may cause portal vein obstruction at the sites where they reside, disease is more commonly caused by the extensive tissue dam-

CLINICAL CORRELATION BOX 20-10. *DIPHYLLOBOTHRIUM LATUM*

Patients may harbor an adult worm for up to 20 years. Intestinal symptoms are minimal. Large adult worms may cause mechanical bowel obstruction, accompanied by abdominal pain and diarrhea. In a minority of patients infected with *D. latum*, particularly in northern Europe and specifically in Finland, megaloblastic anemia is not uncommon, secondary to the selective competition of the parasite for intraintestinal vitamin B_{12}.

Humans may also become infected with the larval plerocercoids of diphyllobothrioid tapeworms closely related to *D. latum*, causing an infection known as sparganosis.

Adult worms are found in dogs and cats; the larval form develops in humans following ingestion of larval-infected copepoda or the raw flesh of amphibians and reptiles. The plerocercoid larvae (sparganum) develop into pruritic nodules in the subcutaneous tissues over a period of months. Peripheral blood eosinophilia is a nonspecific clue to the possibility of sparganosis; however, the characteristic larvae must be demonstrated in subcutaneous nodules before a definitive diagnosis can be made. A single 2-g dose of niclosamide in the form of 0.5-gram chewable tablets is the treatment of choice.

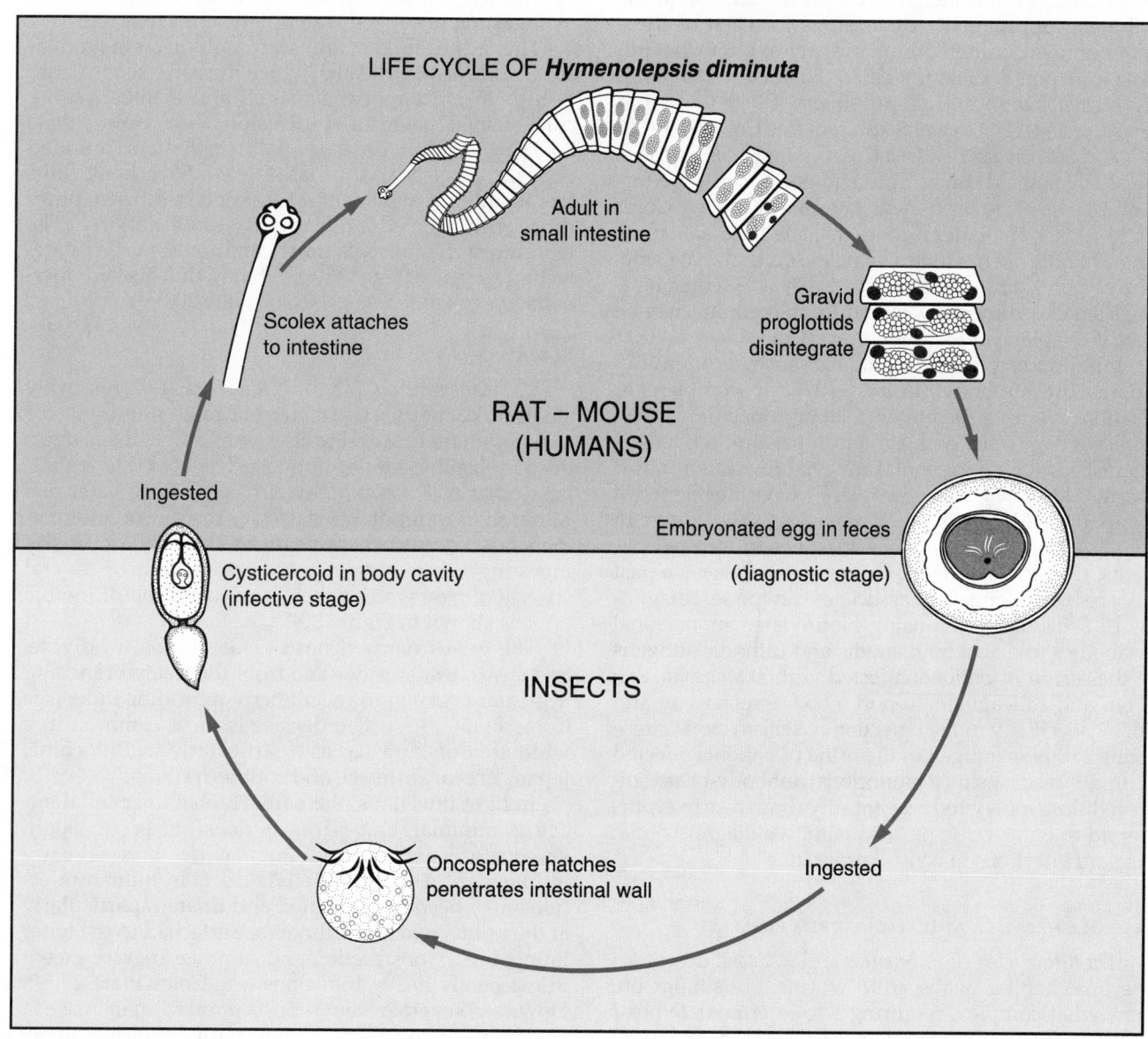

Figure 20-16
Life cycle of *Hymenolepsis diminuta*.

In contrast with infections with *Taenia* and *Diphyllobothrium* species, in which only one worm inhabits the intestine, up to 1000 *H. nana* worms may be present in heavy infections. Symptoms in light infections may be absent; anorexia, abdominal pain, diarrhea, headache, and nervousness may be seen in heavy infections. Peripheral eosinophilia is mild to moderate (4% to 16%). Autoinfection, in which ova hatch in the intestine and reinfect by the normal life cycle, described in the foregoing, may result in a high worm burden that can cause severe complications in immunosuppressed patients. The treatment is niclosamide, 2 g/day for 5 days in adults; 1 g initial dose followed by 500 mg/day for 6 days in children. This prolonged therapy is needed because onchospheres develop in the jejunal villi, and cysticercoids emerge in the lumen of the intestine about 4 days after the initial treatment.

age that results from the deposition of the myriad of eggs that are produced daily by the female.[314]

The laboratory diagnosis is made by detecting the characteristic ova in stool or, in cases of *S. haematobium* infections, in the urine. The ova are very large, in the following approximate dimensions for each of three commonly encountered human species: 116 to 180 μm × 45 to 58 μm (*S. mansoni*); 112 to 180 μm by 40 to 70 μm (*S. haematobium*); and 75 to 90 μm × 60 to 68 μm (*S. japonicum*). The ova of *S. mansoni* (see Color Plate 20-5*C*) and *S. haematobium* (see Color Plate 20-5*D*) are distinctly oval; these can be differentiated because the former possesses a prominent lateral spine (see Color Plate 20-5*C*), the latter a more delicate terminal spine. The ova of *S. intercalatum* also possess a terminal spine. The ova of *S. japonicum* are broadly oval to semispherical; a small rudimentary, lateral, knoblike spine may be seen if the plane of focus is correct (Color Plate 20-5*E*).

Immunodiagnostic techniques, such as immunofluorescent antibody, ELISA, RIA, or complement fixation, are used in reference laboratories to help establish a diagnosis. With a monoclonal antibody raised against a 15-kDa tegumental antigen of *S. mansoni* adult worms, Da Silva and coworkers[72] have developed a competitive ELISA that they report as 94% sensitive in the detection of *S. mansoni* antibodies in infected patients. Considerable work has been done over the past decade by De Jonge and associates[77] in the serodiagnosis of schistosomiasis using biotinylated monoclonal antibodies to detect both anodic and cathodic antigens in the serum of patients infected with *S. mansoni*. Van Etten and colleagues[325] report a 95.5% sensitivity and 96.7% specificity in the detection of schistosomal circulating cathodic antigen in the urine of patients infected with *S. mansoni* using a monoclonal antibody-coated nitrocellulose–polyvinyl reagent strip. Such a strip is purported to be of value in the qualitative diagnosis of *S. mansoni* infections in control programs.

FASCIOLA HEPATICA AND FASCIOLOPSIS BUSKI

The life cycles of *F. hepatica* and *F. buski*, except for the final habitat of the adult worms, are similar but somewhat complex, requiring two intermediate hosts (see life cycle drawings, Fig. 20-17 and 20-18, pages 1118 and 1119). After discharge of mature ova into canals, lakes, streams, and the like, a free-swimming miracidium emerges, which burrows into the flesh of an appropriate snail. Within the snail, maturation and multiplication take place, ultimately leading to the release of hundreds of free-swimming, straight-tailed cercariae. The cercariae attach to water plants and encyst as infective metacercariae. Humans become infected by ingesting uncooked water plants thus infected.

The adult flukes are seen only if removed at surgery. *F. hepatica* adults, which measure 20 to 30 mm × 8 to 13 mm, appear flattened and leaflike, with a cone-shaped anterior protrusion (see Color Plate 20-5*F*); the adult flukes of *F. buski* have a rounded cephalic end (see Color Plate 20-5*G*). Each adult fluke has an anterior and a ventral sucker and is hermaphroditic, with a convoluted uterus seen anteriorly. The laboratory diagnosis is most commonly made by detecting the very large (150 × 80 μm), thin-walled operculated eggs in feces (see Color Plate 20-5*H*).

CLONORCHIS SINENSIS

C. sinensis, the Chinese liver fluke, is a relatively small fluke that varies in size (12 to 20 mm by 3 to 5 mm) when mature and resides within the biliary ducts or in the gallbladder of humans. The life cycle is similar to that of *F. hepatica*, except that a freshwater fish rather than water plants is used as the second intermediate host. Humans become infected with *C. sinensis* by ingesting the raw or poorly cooked flesh of several species of freshwater fishes. An illustration of the life cycle is shown in Figure 20-19, page 1121.

The genus name (from the Greek *clon*, to divide, and *orchis*, testis) is derived from the freely branching testicular organ in the adult hermaphroditic fluke (see Color Plate 20-5*I*). The disease is most common in a wide area of the Far East, particularly in Indochina, Japan, Korea, Formosa, and southern China.

In light infections, the parenchymal liver cell damage is minimal, and cirrhosis does not occur. Slight leukocytosis and eosinophilia may be observed early in infection. Although the bile ducts in human infections may become thickened and dilated, particularly at the points where the flukes are attached to the inner lining, biliary obstruction and jaundice are rare except in extremely heavy infections (see Color Plate 20-5*J*). However, several recent reports point to an increase in cholangiocarcinoma associated with *C. sinensis* infections.[295,300] In Hong Kong and other areas of the Far East, *C. sinensis* and *Opisthorchis viverrini* are the most common causes of cholangiocarcinoma.[300] In most

TABLE 20-6
TREMATODES: KEY FEATURES FOR LABORATORY IDENTIFICATION

SPECIES	HABITAT OF ADULT	INFECTIVE FORM	DIAGNOSTIC FORMS	PLATE REFERENCE
Schistosoma mansoni	Male and female flukes reside together in the portal system venules, primarily those of the large intestine.	Forked tailed cercariae that penetrate skin of humans wading in freshwater canals	*Adult flukes:* The female is 1.6 cm long and resides in the gynecophoral canal of the male, which is 1 cm long. Rarely seen as a diagnostic form.	20-5B
			Cercaria: The infective cercaria of the schistosomes has a forked tail. Not used as a diagnostic form.	20-5A
			Eggs: 115–180 μm long, 45–70 μm wide. Elongated with a prominent lateral spine near the more-rounded posterior end; anterior end tends to be somewhat pointed and slightly curved. When embryonated, the ovum may contain a mature miracidium.	20-5C
Schistosoma haematobium	Male and female flukes reside together in the portal system venules, primarily those of the urinary bladder.	Forked tailed cercariae that penetrate skin of humans wading in freshwater canals	*Eggs:* 110–170 μm long, 40 to 70 μm wide. Elongated with a rounded anterior end and a prominent spine from the terminus of the more tapered posterior end. Embryonated ovum may contain a mature miracidium.	20-5D
Schistosoma japonicum	Male and female flukes reside together in the portal system venules, primarily those of the small intestine.	Forked tailed cercariae that penetrate skin of humans wading in freshwater canals	*Eggs:* 70–100 μm long, 55–65 μm wide. Oval or sub-spherical. A small rudimentary knob or delicate spine may be seen on the lateral wall. Because it is often located in a depression in the shell, this small spine is often difficult to see.	20-5E
Fasciola hepatica	Bile ducts	Metacercariae encysted on water plants that are ingested by humans	*Eggs:* 150 × 80 μm. Elliptical to oval. The shell is thin, with a smooth surface, and an indistinct operculum is located at one end. The internal cleavage material is poorly organized and extends to the shell margins without leaving a clear space. Ova cannot be distinguished from those of *F. buski.*	20-5H
			Adult fluke: It measures 3 × 1.2 cm and can be distinguished from that of *F. buski* because of the elongated cone-shaped anterior end.	20-5F
Fasciolopsis buski	Small intestine	Metacercariae encysted on water plants that are ingested by humans	*Eggs:* indistinguishable from *F. hepatica*	20-5H
			Adult fluke: It measures 2.0–7.5 cm long by 0.8–2 cm wide and in addition to its generally larger size, it can be distinguished from *F. hepatica* by its broadly rounded anterior end.	20-5G
Clonorchis sinensis	Bile ducts	Metacercariae encysted in flesh of freshwater fish	*Eggs:* 27–35 μm long, 14–17 μm wide. Broad, round posterior end and concave constriction at anterior end give this relatively small egg an urnlike appearance. A convex operculum is seen resting on shoulders. A small knob often is present at the posterior end.	20-5K
			Adult fluke: measures 1.5 × 0.5 cm. Bottle-shaped head, anterior uterus, and posterior branched testes.	20-5I, J
Paragonimus westermani	Cystic cavities in the lung	Metacercariae encysted in flesh of various crustaceans (crayfish, crabs)	*Eggs:* 65–120 μm long, 40–70 μm wide. Ovoid or elongated, somewhat asymmetric, with one edge flattened. A flattened operculum rests on shouldered area, a distinguishing feature from *D. latum.* Shell is thick, but smooth, and internal cleavage fills entire area.	20-5L
			Adult fluke: It measures about 12 × 7 mm and up to 5 mm in thickness, making it rounder than other flukes. Rarely seen as a diagnostic form.	

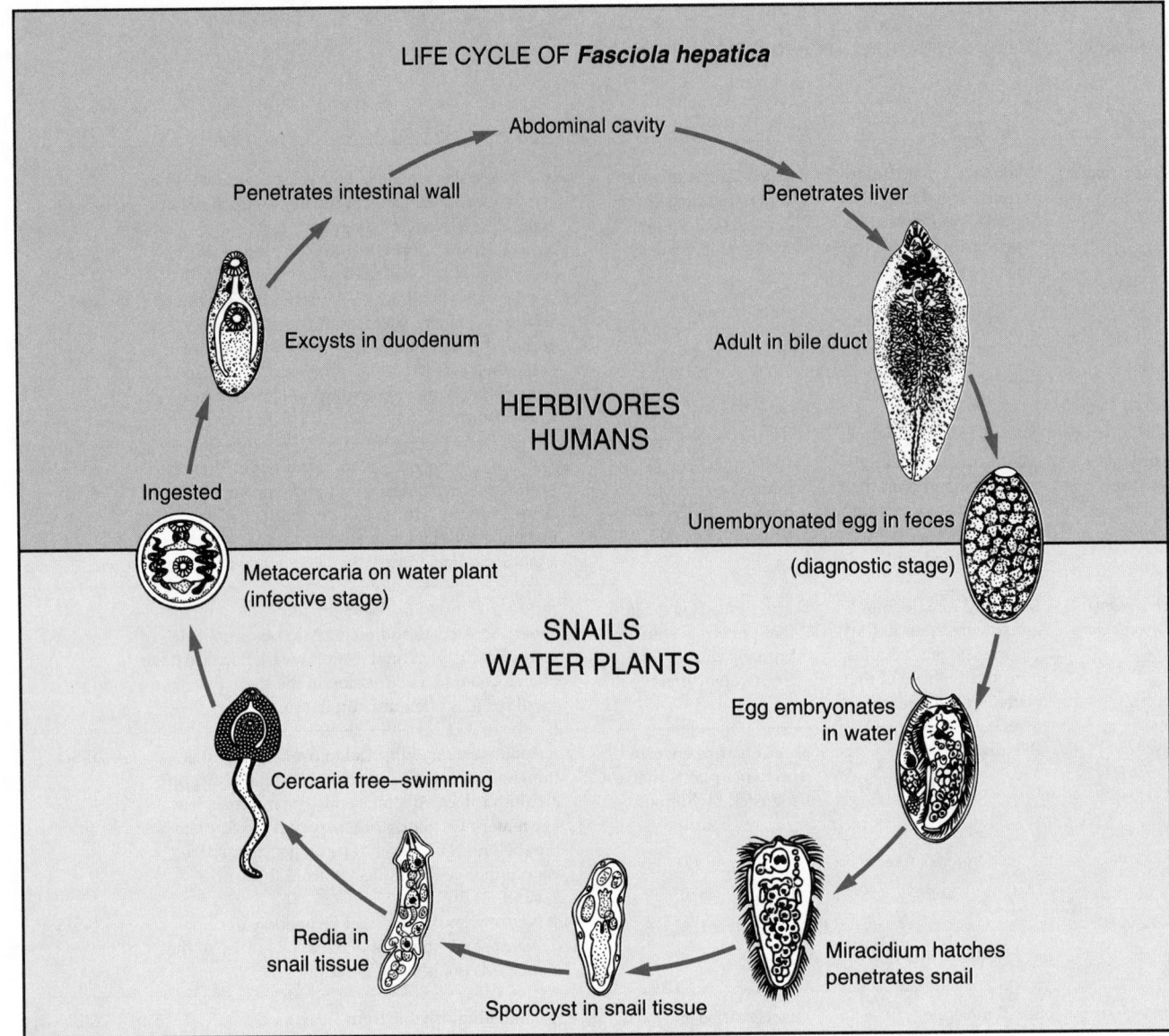

LIFE CYCLE OF *Fasciola hepatica*

Abdominal cavity

Penetrates intestinal wall

Penetrates liver

Excysts in duodenum

Adult in bile duct

HERBIVORES
HUMANS

Ingested

Unembryonated egg in feces

Metacercaria on water plant
(infective stage)

(diagnostic stage)

SNAILS
WATER PLANTS

Egg embryonates
in water

Cercaria free–swimming

Redia in
snail tissue

Miracidium hatches
penetrates snail

Sporocyst in snail tissue

Figure 20-17
Life cycle of *Fasciola hepatica.*

cases, the disease tends to remain low grade and chronic, with organisms persisting for four or five decades, producing only minor symptoms of abdominal distress, intermittent diarrhea, and liver pain or tenderness. In isolated instances, however, severe hepatobiliary disease, with biliary obstruction and hepatic fibrosis, has been reported.[338]

The laboratory diagnosis is made by identifying the characteristic, small, urn-shaped eggs in stool specimens. The typical ovum measures about 29 × 16 µm, generally has a light yellow-brown pigmentation from bile staining, and possesses a prominent convex operculum that rests on "shoulders" (see Color Plate 20-5K). A small median protuberance may be microscopically observed posteriorly when in the correct plane of focus. This egg is morphologically similar to those of *Heterophyes heterophyes* and *Metagonimus yokogawai*, two small

intestinal flukes that are also prevalent in the Far East and infect humans who ingest raw or pickled fish.

Because parasite eggs may be shed only after 8 or more weeks following infection, or intermittently thereafter, serologic tests have been used in reference laboratories for the diagnosis of fascioliasis. Espino and associates[101] developed a sandwich ELISA using antibodies against *F. hepatica* excretory-secretory (ES) antigens to detect circulating parasite antigen in humans with fascioliasis. The authors indicated that the antigen detection test had the advantage over several antibody detection methods because serum titers may remain elevated even after cure. In a later follow-up study, Espino and Finlay[102] report on the development of a mouse monoclonal antibody raised against *F. hepatica* ES antigens and a rabbit polyclonal antibody–peroxidase conjugate detector to identify fasciola ES

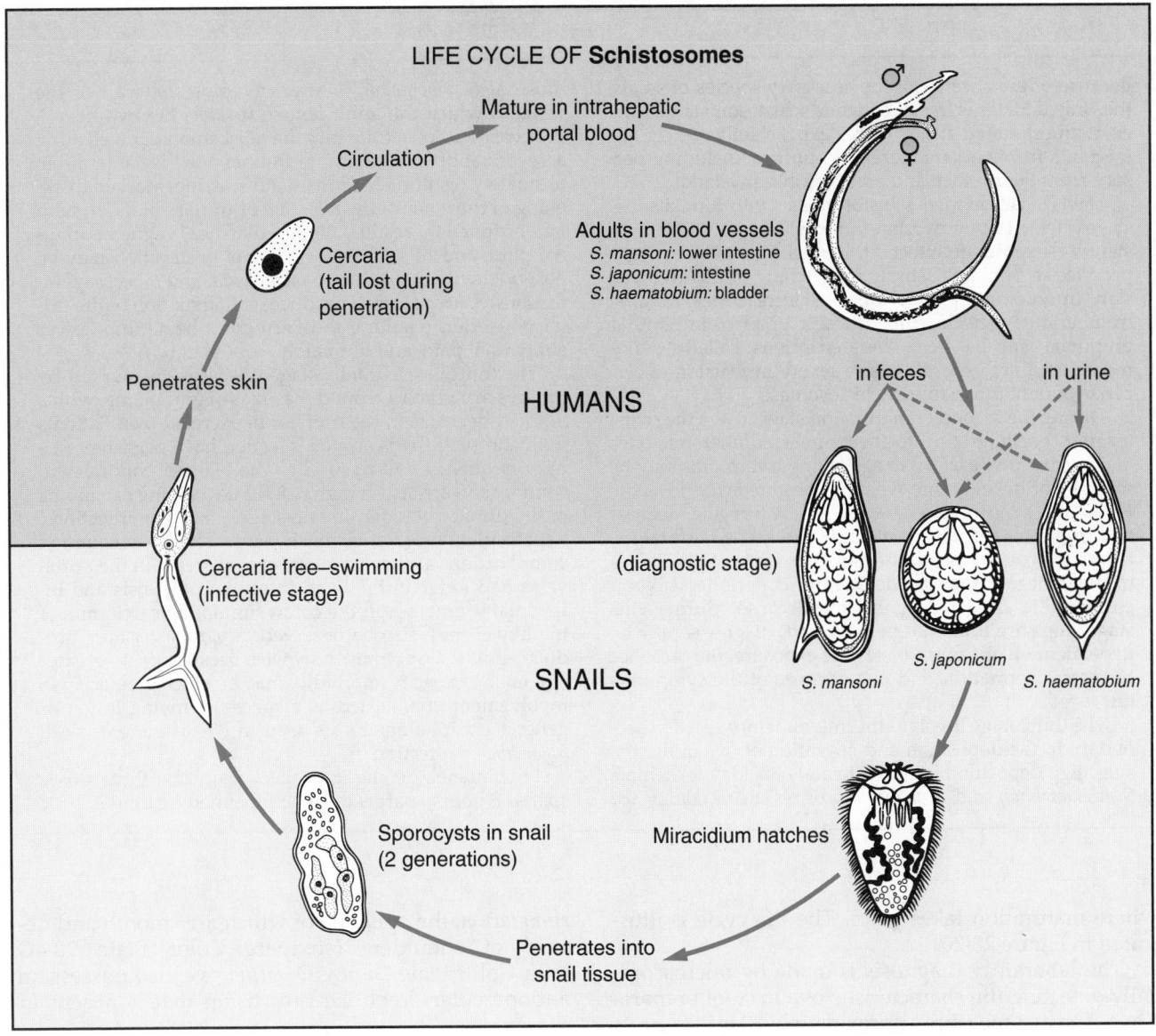

Figure 20-18
Life cycle of *Schistosoma* species.

antigen in stool specimens. The investigators cite the advantages of detecting antigen in stool specimens over serum as 1) avoiding the problem of immune complex formation that decreases the potential rate of detection and 2) circumventing venipuncture in many regions of the world where the procedure is objectionable. The authors also used the stool antigen detection test to advantage as a test for cure.

Praziquantel 25 mg/kg orally for three doses spaced 8 hours apart is the recommended treatment.

PARAGONIMUS WESTERMANI

P. westermani and other *Paragonimus* species are lung flukes causing disease endemic in West Africa, the Orient, and certain regions of Central and South America. The adult worms measure approximately 8 to 16 mm × 4 to 8 mm in size, are spoon-shaped with one end contracted, the other elongated. Anterior and ventral suckers are of equal size.

The life cycle of these flukes represents a classic example of **organotropism**; that is, the special affinity a parasite has to seek out and reside within a given organ. Humans become infected following ingestion of raw or poorly cooked crab meat or crayfish, the flesh of which contains encysted metacercariae. Following ingestion, the metacercariae hatch in the duodenum, releasing larvae that attach to the duodenal mucosa. The larvae then penetrate the full thickness of the bowel wall and enter the abdominal cavity. They transmigrate to the diaphragm and enter the pleural space. The larvae then bore into the peripheral lung tissue,

Because of the absence of the necessary species of snails, the United States is free of endemic schistosomiasis. However, an estimated 400,000 cases exist, chiefly among immigrants from endemic foreign countries, including persons from Puerto Rico and other Caribbean islands.[213]

Davis[75] has divided schistosomiasis into four distinct stages, which often overlap in individuals who are constantly reexposed to infection. Cercarial invasion early on produces a prickling sensation or itching of the involved skin. In nonimmune individuals, skin reactions, ranging from minute petechiae to urticaria or pruritic papular eruptions may be seen. These eruptions, called "swimmer's itch," are generally more severe in reaction to cercariae of nonhuman (bird) schistosomes.

During the second or maturation stage, when the schistosomes are migrating to their preferred anatomic sites and pairing preparatory to egg laying, symptoms may be minimal or develop into what has been referred to as the Katayama syndrome, characterized by varying degrees and mixtures of fever, malaise, backache, arthralgia, anorexia, cough, headache, and toxemia. Mild hepatosplenomegaly may be detected and peripheral blood eosinophilia may be significant. Because, during this stage, eggs are often not yet excreted, diagnosis may be dependent on eliciting a history of exposure, the presence of typical dermatitis, and one or more of the symptoms just listed.

The third stage involves the inflammatory reaction secondary to the deposition and migration of ova in the tissues. Egg deposition is approximately 300/day for female *S. haematobium* and *S. mansoni* worms and 3000/day for those of *S. japonicum*.[212] After invading the wall of the veins in which the adult female resides, the ova have a propensity to penetrate into the adjacent viscera, eliciting a severe suppurative and granulomatous inflammation, ultimately resulting in fibrosis and scarring. Marked thickening of the walls of the intestine or urinary bladder, with loss of function, results. Bloody diarrhea, vague abdominal pain, and in severe cases, bowel obstruction may be observed with *S. mansoni*, *S. japonicum*, and *S. mekongi* infections. *S. haematobium* produces inflammation of the urinary bladder, resulting in intermittent hematuria, lower abdominal pain, and ultimately, contraction.

The fourth, or chronic, stage of disease is marked by progressive fibrosis around the areas of granuloma, with a marked decrease in the number of excreted ova. Patients with chronic *S. haematobium* infection have persistent urinary frequency and dysuria as the bladder continues to contract and are also at high risk for developing carcinoma of the urinary bladder. In late-stage *S. mansoni* infections, hepatosplenomegaly, cirrhosis, and ascites are common complications as the ova are swept upstream in the portal veins and lodge in the liver. Intestinal polyposis and inflammatory masses in the colon simulating carcinoma of the bowel may also be observed. *S. japonicum* may produce similar symptoms; however, because of its greater egg-laying capacity, morbidity may be much greater. CNS involvement, manifested as a space-occupying lesion or general encephalopathy, is seen in 3% of patients with *S. japonicum* infection.[248]

Praziquanel, 20 mg/kg taken orally for three doses spaced 8 hours apart is the recommended treatment.

where maturation takes place. The life cycle is illustrated in Figure 20-20.

The laboratory diagnosis is made by microscopically detecting the characteristic ova in stool preparations. The ova measure approximately 80 to 120 μm × 48 to 60 μm, are dark yellow-brown, and have a thick, smooth shell with a prominent shouldered operculum. The presence of this shoulder serves to distinguish the *Paragonimus* ova from those of *Diphyllobothrium latum*, the opercula of which are smooth and devoid of shoulders (compare Color Plate 20-4G with Color Plate 20-5L). *D. latum* ova also possess an antiopercular, knoblike protrusion that is absent in *P. westermani*.

Chills, fever, and marked eosinophilia may be seen during this migratory phase. In time, the adult fluke comes to reside within a small pseudocyst in the lung tissue. The cyst enlarges as the adult fluke grows

The flukes can attach to the pharyngeal mucosa and cause local laryngopharyngitis, called **halzoun**, if raw sheep or goat liver infected with adolescent worms are ingested. Human fascioliasis is manifested by headache, chills, fever, and right upper quadrant pain. Hepatomegaly, jaundice, diarrhea, and anemia may occur in severe infections; hepatic biliary cirrhosis is a late complication. Praziquantel 25 mg/kg three times a day for 6 days is the recommended treatment regimen.

F. buski, a fluke similar to *F. hepatica* except that it is somewhat larger (20 to 75 mm by 8 to 20 mm) and has a rounded, instead of a conical, anterior portion (see Color Plate 20-5F). These flukes reside in the small intestine and, by means of a small oral sucker, attach to the intestinal mucosa. Local mucosal ulcers produce varying degrees of epigastric pain, nausea, and diarrhea, especially in the morning. Ascites and intestinal obstruction may be seen in heavy infections. Laboratory diagnosis is made by identifying the large eggs in the feces, which are identical in appearance to those of *F. hepatica*. Praziquanel in a single 25 mg/kg dose is the recommended treatment.

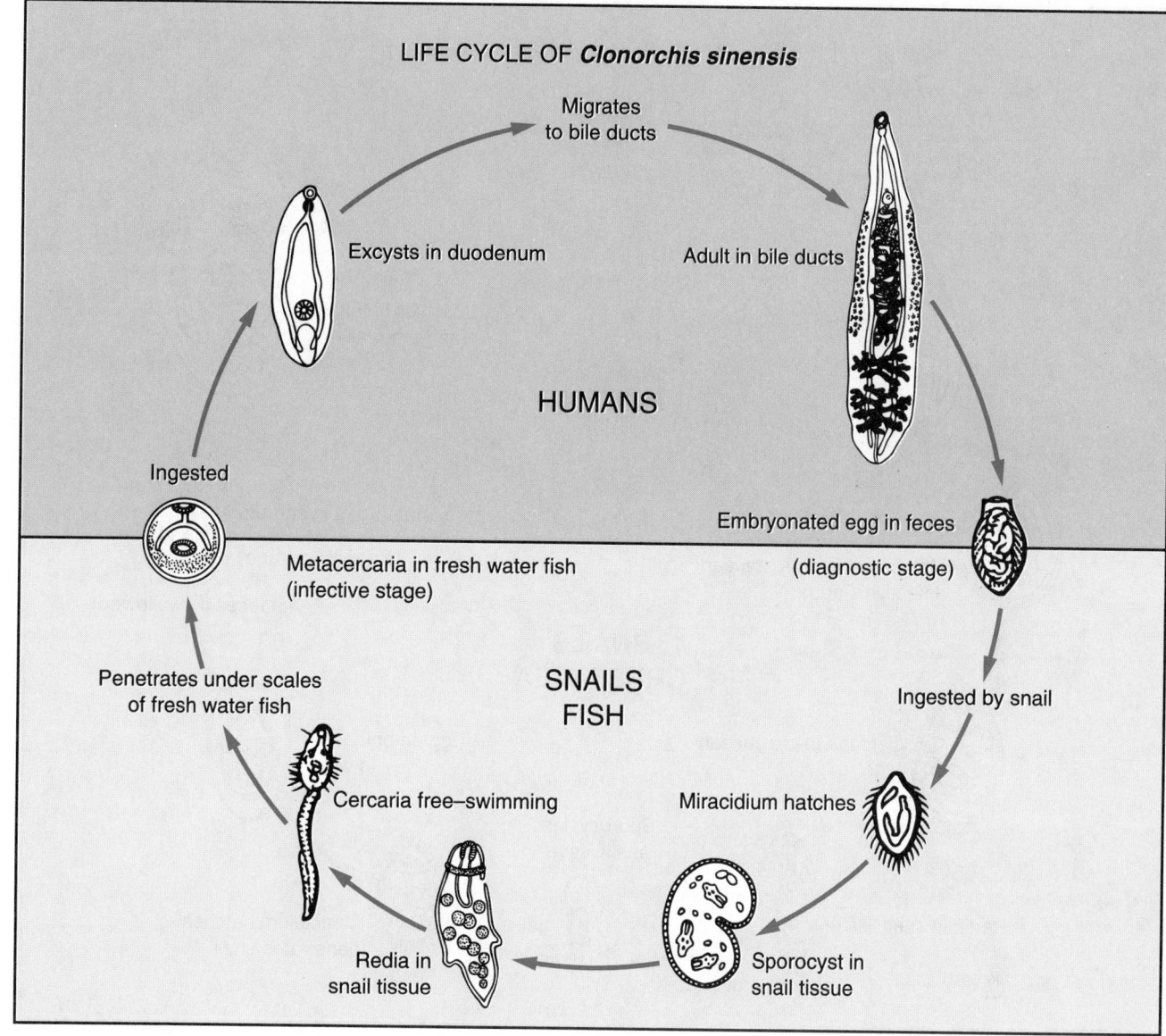

LIFE CYCLE OF *Clonorchis sinensis*

Migrates to bile ducts

Excysts in duodenum

Adult in bile ducts

HUMANS

Ingested

Embryonated egg in feces
(diagnostic stage)

Metacercaria in fresh water fish
(infective stage)

SNAILS
FISH

Penetrates under scales
of fresh water fish

Ingested by snail

Cercaria free–swimming

Miracidium hatches

Redia in
snail tissue

Sporocyst in
snail tissue

Figure 20-19
Life cycle of *Clonorchis sinensis*.

and may break into an adjacent bronchiole. When a pseudocyst ruptures into a bronchus, coughing and hemoptysis are common symptoms. Eggs produced by mature flukes are discharged into the bronchi and are ultimately swallowed by the patient from secretions coughed into the oropharynx.

The disease tends to become chronic, leading to varying degrees of pulmonary fibrosis and scarring. Intermittent chest pain, fever, and chills may be late manifestations. Abdominal paragonimiasis may occur if the fluke remains localized to the abdomen. Dull abdominal tenderness and bloody diarrhea are the chief complaints. Rare cases of cerebral disease have been reported, which must be differentiated from echinococcosis. Praziquantel, 25 mg/kg tid for 2 days, followed by 30 to 50 mg/kg every other day for 10 to 15 days is recommended.

BLOOD AND TISSUE PARASITES

Parasites found in the blood or in other organs are usually discussed separately from those inhabiting the gastrointestinal tract. However, it should be understood that blood and tissue parasites include protozoa, nematodes, and cestodes, with various forms of their life cycles that are morphologically similar to their intestinal counterparts. For example, *Toxoplasma gondii* is a tissue coccidian, the trypanosomas are hemoflagellates, visceral and cutaneous larval migrans are caused by the larval forms of dog or cat ascarid nematodes, and echinococcosis is the larval form of a dog cestode. The plasmodia responsible for malaria are sporozoa that also have an intestinal counterpart, *Isospora hominis*, that may be found in feces.

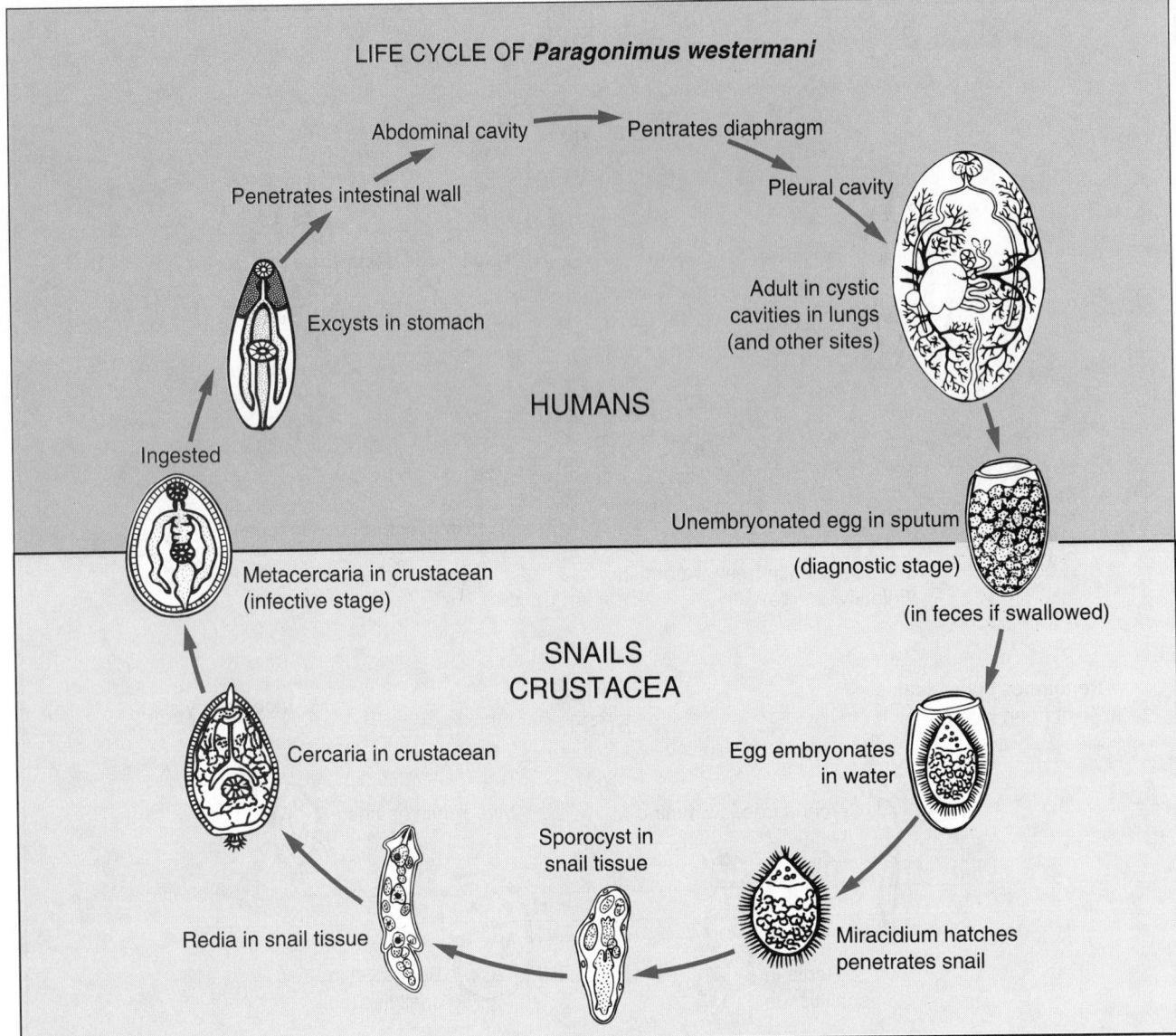

LIFE CYCLE OF *Paragonimus westermani*

Abdominal cavity → Pentrates diaphragm

Penetrates intestinal wall

Pleural cavity

Excysts in stomach

Adult in cystic
cavities in lungs
(and other sites)

HUMANS

Ingested

Unembryonated egg in sputum

(diagnostic stage)

Metacercaria in crustacean
(infective stage)

(in feces if swallowed)

SNAILS
CRUSTACEA

Cercaria in crustacean

Egg embryonates
in water

Sporocyst in
snail tissue

Redia in snail tissue

Miracidium hatches
penetrates snail

Figure 20-20
Life cycle of *Paragonimus westermani*.

In general, the life cycles of the blood and tissue parasites are more complex than those of their intestinal counterparts. Most of the blood parasites are transmitted to humans by an arthropod vector within which the sexual phase of the life cycle develops. Many parasites causing tissue infections use various insects for the development of intermediate stages in their life cycles.

Tissue parasites may be either intracellular or extracellular, depending on the species and the phase of the parasitic cycle. An outline of human blood and tissue parasites, which will also serve as a guide to the discussion for the remainder of this chapter, is listed in Box 20-7.

MALARIA AND *PLASMODIUM* SPECIES

In the United States, most cases of malaria are found in travelers, foreign-born students, or refugees who have been exposed to mosquitos in endemic areas.[362] Newton and coauthors[244] report that as of December 20, 1993, 112 imported cases of malaria were detected in U.S. Marines returning from Somalia. *P. vivax* was identified in 97 (85%) cases and *P. falciparum* in eight (7%) cases. Mixed *P. vivax* and *P. falciparum* infections were noted in six soldiers. Only one case of *P. malariae* was found. Occasionally, plasmodia have been transmitted by blood transfusions or blood-contaminated syringes and needles shared by drug addicts. The diagnosis of malaria is often clinically overlooked in the United States because of the rarity of the disease in most locales. In 1980, 566 cases were reported to the CDC, a 243% increase in incidence over the 165 cases reported in 1988.[47] The worldwide prevalence is in the neighborhood of 100 million; 1 million deaths a year occur in Africa alone. Most cases occurred in refugees, principally from Southeast Asia.

Clinicians must, therefore, remain alert to the possibility of malaria in certain populations. Another reason for misdiagnosis is that the cardinal symptoms, chills and fever, are associated with so many other diseases that malaria tends to be overlooked as a possible diagnosis in nonendemic areas. The higher mortality rate in American civilian hospitals (8.5%) for falciparum malaria as compared with that in military hospitals (0.7%) has been attributed to delays in establishing a diagnosis.[362]

The life cycle of the plasmodium parasite has two phases: a sexual cycle, known as sporogony, which takes place within the intestinal tract of the mosquito; and an asexual cycle, known as schizogony, which occurs in the human host. Sporozoites, the infective form for humans, are found in the salivary glands of female anopheline mosquitos. Saliva containing infective sporozoites is injected into the blood stream of humans through the mosquito proboscis. After circulating in the peripheral blood for about 20 to 30 minutes, the sporozoites enter the parenchymal cells of the liver, where they begin to multiply (the exoerythrocytic states). In about 10 days, multiple small forms, called merozoites, break out of the liver cells and are released into the circulation, where they seek out and penetrate erythrocytes.

Within the erythrocytes (intraerythrocytic cycle), a series of developmental stages takes place (see Color Plates 20-6A through 6F). These organisms develop into a "ring form," known as the trophozoite, which, depending on the species, enlarges and divides into a segmented state known as the schizont. The individual segments of the schizonts are merozoites. When mature, the schizonts rupture the erythrocytes, and merozoites are released into the circulation. These merozoites then seek out uninfected erythrocytes, and the cycle continues. An illustration of the life cycle is shown in Figure 20-21.

After several erythrocyte cycles have taken place, certain of the merozoites transform into sexual macrogametocytes (female) and microgametocytes (male). When a plasmodium-free mosquito bites a human infected with malaria, these gametocytes are ingested along with the trophozoite-infected erythrocytes as part of the blood meal. In the stomach of the mosquito, the male microgametocytes develop six to eight flagella. The microgametocytes break free to penetrate the female macrogametocytes and produce fertilized zygotes. These zygotes then enter the stomach wall of the mosquito, where sporozoites eventually break out into the body cavity and migrate to the salivary glands. When the mosquito bites a new host, sporozoites are squeezed from the salivary glands and injected through the proboscis.

Laboratory Identification. Laboratory identification of the malarial parasites in humans is made by studying stained thin and thick peripheral blood smears, as previously described. Smears should be obtained at different times of the day from patients with suspected infections because parasitemia may be intermittent, and the number of circulating parasites may vary.

Three species of *Plasmodium* most commonly cause human malaria: *P. vivax, P. falciparum,* and *P. malariae*. A fourth species, *P. ovale*, is rare in much of the world but relatively common in western Africa. The differential features of the three common species are reviewed in Table 20-7. The microscopic morphology of the intraerythrocytic forms is illustrated in Color Plate 20-6A through 6F.

The laboratory identification of the various *Plasmodium* species is not difficult if an orderly approach based on the observation of a few key morphologic structures is followed. It is quite important that infections with *P. falciparum* be recognized as early as possible because the disease can be particularly severe, rapidly progressing to a fatal outcome. A suggested laboratory approach to the identification of *Plasmodium* species is presented in Box 20-8 (see Table 20-7).

The identification of *Plasmodium* species is usually not difficult if the principles described above are applied. Problems arise, however, in the interpretation of peripheral smears in patients who have been partially or inadequately treated and in whom normal maturation of the parasites may be blocked and only atypical forms are observed. The peripheral blood picture may also be confusing if a given individual is doubly infected with more than one *Plasmodium* species.

BABESIA SPECIES

The status of infections with *B. microti* in the United States has recently been updated by Persing and coauthors.[256] *B. microti* causes most human infections in nonsplenectomized individuals; *B. bovis* and *B. divergens* are other species causing infections in splenectomized persons. *B. microti* shadows *Borrelia burgdorferi*, the spiro-

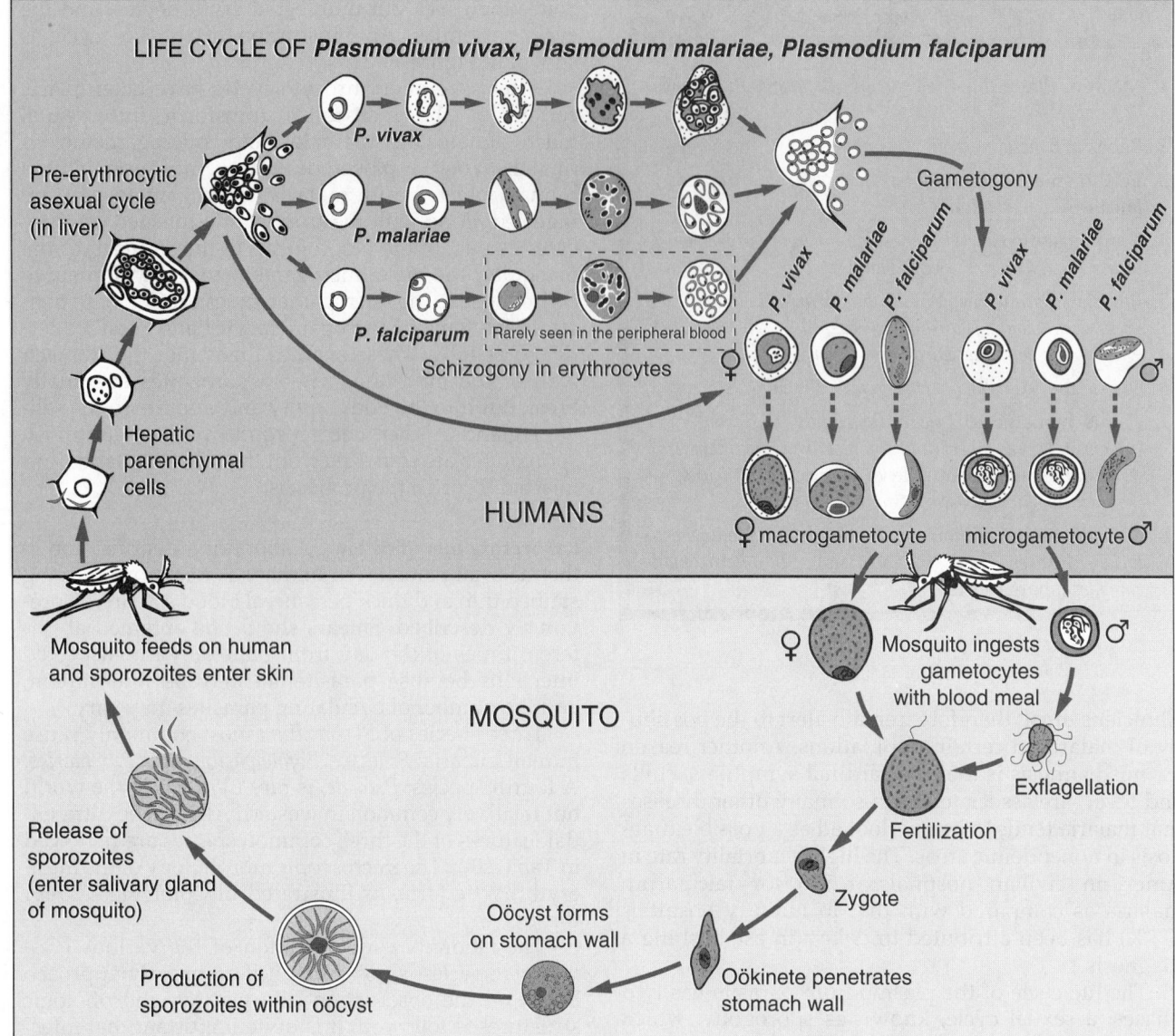

Figure 20-21
Life cycle of *Plasmodium malariae*.

chete causing Lyme disease, as both agents have the white-footed mouse, *Peromyscus leucopus*, as the main reservoir host. Most outbreaks have occurred in the northeastern regions of the United States, particularly in Connecticut, Nantucket Island, Long Island, and Cape Cod. The predominant vector for both agents is the *Ixodes dammini* tick, 40% of which are coinfected. The much lower incidence of babesiosis relative to Lyme disease in humans living in endemic areas may reflect the tendency of *B. microti* to produce subclinical infections. Serologic studies indicate that 10% of *B. burgdorferi*-seropositive Connecticut natives also have antibodies against *B. microti*, indicating that infections are far more frequent than previously suspected.

The laboratory diagnosis is most commonly made by detecting the intraerythrocytic parasitic inclusions, which appear as tiny rings, ranging between 1.0 and 3.0

μm, resembling the early trophozoites of *P. falciparum*. The nuclei are very small, and one or two chromatin dots may be seen. Mature forms may appear as doublets, simulating rabbit ears; or in tetrads, resembling a Maltese cross. The erythrocytes are not enlarged, are normochromic, and do not develop stippling.

As pointed out by Persing and coauthors,[256] the symptoms in early babesiosis may be minimal: malaise, anorexia, and fatigue—nonspecific symptoms that are easily confused with other infectious diseases. The diagnostic intraerythrocytic forms described in the foregoing are scarce during the early stages of infection and may be missed, even by experienced microscopists. Mattia and coworkers[224] used a buffy coat technique to improve the detection of parasitemia in cases of babesiosis. Persing and colleagues, to aid in making the diagnosis in early infection, generated *B. microti*-

TABLE 20-7

PLASMODIA: KEY FEATURES FOR LABORATORY IDENTIFICATION

SPECIES	APPEARANCE OF ERYTHROCYTES	TROPHOZOITES	SCHIZONTS	GAMETOCYTES	SPECIAL FEATURES
Plasmodium vivax	Enlarged and pale; Schüffner's dots usually prominent.	*Early:* ring relatively large (one third the size of red blood cell). Rings with 2 nuclei or cells with 2 or 3 rings may be seen (Plate 20-6C) *Mature:* Ameboid, with delicate pseudopodia that flow to fill the entire red blood cell.	12–24 segments (merozoites); pigment fine grained and inconspicuous. (Plate 20-6D)	Round to oval and almost completely fill red blood cell. Large chromatin mass. Pigment is coarse and evenly distributed. (Plate 20-6E)	Length of asexual cycle (fever cycle) is 48 h (benign tertian). Be alert for possibility of mixed species infection when *P. vivax* forms are identified.
Plasmodium falciparum	Normal size; Maurer's dots or clefts are rarely seen.	Ring forms extremely small, occupying no more than one-fifth of red blood cell. Double nuclei are common, and multiple rings per red blood cell are usual. Appliqué forms plastered on the red blood cell membrane are virtually diagnostic (Plate 20-6A)	Not normally seen except in fulminant disease; 24 or more segments are characteristic.	Characteristic crescent- or banana-shaped forms are virtually diagnostic. Microgametocytes stain lighter blue than macrogametocytes. (Plate 20-6B)	The ratio of infected to normal red blood cells is high. Intermediate ring forms or schizonts are not commonly seen in the peripheral blood. Length of asexual cycle is 48 h (malignant tertian).
Plasmodium malariae	Normal size; no dots or clefts form.	*Early:* similar to *P. vivax*, except staining is deeper blue and the cytoplasm of the ring is broader. Double rings are rare. *Mature:* less tendency to become ameboid; rather, it forms a ribbon or band (Plate 20-6F, *left*)	More than 12 segments are rarely seen. Merozoites arrange in rosettes. Pigment is abundant and coarse, often in aggregates within "hoff" of rosettes (Plate 20-6F, *right*).	Not distinctive and resemble those of *P. vivax*. Red blood cells are not enlarged. Pigment usually more abundant in *P. vivax* and tends to be coarse and unevenly distributed.	Asexual cycle lasts 72 h (quartan). Identification of *P. malariae* is often made after either *P. vivax* or *P. falciparum* has been excluded by their more distinctive morphologic features.

specific DNA sequence information by universal primer amplification of a portion of a nuclear 16S-like gene. The sequence information was then used to synthesize specific primers for use in PCR for DNA amplification. Although still in the research stages, future developments may lead to the availability of commercial reagents that can enhance the diagnosis of babesiosis.

HEMOFLAGELLATES: *LEISHMANIA* SPECIES AND *TRYPANOSOMA* SPECIES

The protozoan family Trypanosomatidae includes members from the genera *Leishmania* and *Trypanosoma*, which are flagellates that inhabit the blood and tissues of humans. Four stages of development of the parasites may be observed. The adult or trypanosomal forms have an elongated body, with a whiplike posterior flagellum that is attached by a delicate undulating membrane that runs the length of the body. Three species are associated with human disease: *T. gambiense* and *T. rhodesiense* cause African sleeping sickness, whereas *T. cruzi* is responsible for South American trypanosomiasis. The least developed forms of these protozoa, called the amastigote or leishmanial forms, are devoid of a flagella and are found as intracellular parasites in reticuloendothelial cells. *L. donovani*, the cause of visceral kala-azar in humans, and *L. tropica* complex, the agents of cutaneous tropical sores, are the leishmanial species most commonly associated with human diseases. *T. cruzi* also exists as a leishmanial form, infecting heart muscle fibers or the cells of other visceral organs. The leptomonas ancrithidial stages of develop-

BOX 20-8. LABORATORY APPROACH TO IDENTIFICATION OF *PLASMODIUM* SPECIES

1. First rule out *P. falciparum*. This species is potentially the most dangerous, and infections should be diagnosed as early as possible. In the peripheral smear look for:

   Tiny ring forms that occupy less than one third the diameter of the erythrocyte. Often multiple forms are seen within one erythrocyte; with two nuclei in the same ring. Infections may be heavy, involving 20% or more of the erythrocytes in fulminant infections. The tiny rings often are plastered on the erythrocyte cell membrane, known as an "aplique" effect (see Color Plate 20-6*A*).

   Developing ring forms, or schizonts, are not observed. The only forms usually seen except in terminal, fulminant situations, are early ring forms and gametocytes.

   The presence of banana- or crescent-shaped gametocytes (see Color Plate 20-6*B*). These may be absent in early stages of infection and usually begin to appear only 7 to 10 days after onset of fever.

2. If the foregoing picture is not seen, next make an objective identification of *P. vivax*. Look for:

   Infected erythrocytes that are somewhat irregular in shape, enlarged, pale, and contain prominent pink–red-staining granules, called Schüffner's dots (see Color Plate 20-6*C*).

   All stages of ring forms may be present. Young rings measure larger than one third the diameter of the infected erythrocyte. As the trophozoites mature, they begin to fill the erythrocyte with "flowing" or "ameboid" cytoplasm. More than one nucleus is evident in preparation for the formation of seg-

mented forms, known as a schizont. The schizonts of *P. vivax* comprise 12 to 14 or more individual segments, known as merozoites (see Color Plate 20-6*D*).

   Gametocytes are large and circular (note—any single-celled nucleus occupying more than one-half the cell diameter is a gametocyte). Any trophozoite that grows this large will always divide, forming early schizonts, with two or more segments. Malarial pigment in the form of finely granular, brownish pigment may be abundant (see Color Plate 20-6*E*).

3. Although the identification of *P. malariae* is often by exclusion, if the characteristics of *P. falciparum* and *P. vivax*, as described in the foregoing, have not been observed, look for the following features by which an objective identification can be made:

   Developing trophozites that extend to the borders of the erythrocyte membrane in bridging "bands" (see Color Plate 20-6*F, left*).

   Infected erythrocytes that are not enlarged nor pale. Schüffner's dots are absent.

   Schizonts that comprise no more than 6 to 12 segments, with the nuclear segments arranging to form a "rosette" (see Color Plate 20-6*F, right*).

   Malarial pigment that is abundant and more coarse (or even "chunky") than seen with *P. vivax*.

   Gametocytes are contained within normal-sized erythrocytes free of Schüffner's dots. Aggregates of coarse, dark brown-staining malarial pigment may be present.

ment are harbored within the insect vector, the latter representing the infective form for humans. Key features for laboratory identification of the hemoflagellates are listed in Table 20-8, page 1128.

Leishmaniasis and *Leishmania* species. Human leishmaniasis may take two forms, a disseminated disease (kala-azar) involving the liver, spleen, and other parts of the reticuloendothelial system, and a primary cutaneous form, clinically manifesting as ulcers or "sores" of the skin and mucous membranes (see Color Plate 20-6*G*). Humans become infected through the regurgitation of the promastigotic infective forms of the parasite into the subcutanaeous tissue at the time several species of *Phlebotomus* sandflies take a blood meal.

A small skin papule develops at the site of the sandfly bite but rarely progresses to an ulcer. The promastigotes transform into amastigotes, which proliferate locally in the subcutaneous tissue into amastigotic forms that disseminate throughout the reticuloendothelial system to involve the spleen, liver, bone marrow, and lymph nodes in which the organisms are found as obligate intracellular parasites (see Color Plate

20-6*H*). The simple life cycle is then completed when amistigotes are again taken up by a sandfly during a subsequent blood meal. The amastigotes transform into infective promastigotes in the midgut of the fly.

Visceral leishmaniasis is caused by several species belonging to the *Leishmania donovani* complex: *L. donovani donovani*, *L. donovani infantum*, and *L. donovani chagasi*. The incubation period is in the range of 3 to 8 months. Whether the disease progresses depends on the capability of the host's T lymphocytes to activate macrophages to kill the parasites.

Symptoms may be mild and self-limited in light, contained infections, or there may be the sudden onset of symptoms, including spiking fevers (a pattern of two or three peaks per day), anorexia, malaise, and a feeling of ill health, simulating typhoid fever or malaria. If the disease progresses and becomes chronic, persistence of low-grade fever, vague abdominal pain, enlargement of the abdomen from hepatomegaly, and splenomegaly (which can become enormous), generalized lymphadenopathy, anemia and leukopenia may become pronounced. Secondary infections, jaundice, cachexia, bleeding disorders with frequent epistaxis

Fever is the constant presenting symptom of infections with all *Plasmodium* species. Temperature spikes commence 7 to 10 days following the bite of an infected anopheles mosquito during a period when the organisms are undergoing preerythrocyte multiplication in the cells of the liver. Prodromal symptoms of headache, myalgia, malaise, and fatigue suggestive of a flulike syndrome may be experienced during this period. However, once a brood of merozoites leave the hepatic cells and invade the erythrocytes, the regularly spaced fever cycles begin. The periodicity of each episode of high fever is related to the rupture of erythrocytes as merozoites are released into the circulation. The designations of this fever cycle, "tertian" malaria, for *P. vivax* and *P. falciparum* malaria, and "quartan" malaria for *P. malariae* malaria is somewhat confusing. The fever spikes for tertian malaria occur on an every-other-day schedule; however, because any given fever episode is counted as day 1, the next spike will not occur until the third day (thus, tertian). Similarly, the fever spikes of quartan malaria occur on an every-3-day cycle; however, counting the first episode as day 1, the next spike will occur on the fourth day. Such classic fever patterns, however, may often be irregular and cannot be relied on exclusively to make a presumptive diagnosis.

Each fever episode is characterized by a short "cold" period lasting for approximately 1 hour when the skin is cold and the lips and nailbeds appear cyanotic owing to peripheral vasoconstriction. This short period is followed by the sudden onset of the "hot period" when the skin feels warm and dry and fever spikes up to 105° to 106°F (40.5° to 41.1°C) are experienced, lasting 3 to 6 hours. Headaches, chest and back pain, tachycardia, cough, vomiting, and delirium of varying degrees of severity accompany the fever spikes. Fatigue and sleep follow each febrile episode. Patients are essentially asymptomatic between febrile episodes.

Hemolytic anemia, splenomegaly, and tender hepatomegaly are found to varying degrees. Patients are highly susceptible to rupture of the spleen and deep palpation of the left upper abdomen and flank should be avoided during physical examination. Lymphadenopathy is absent and always points to some other condition if lymph nodes are enlarged. Of greatest concern are the CNS complications that may occur secondary to *P. falciparum* infections. The erythrocytes infected with *P. falciparum* trophozoites undergo membrane changes that cause them to become "sticky" and adhere to specific receptors on the endothelial cell lining of capillaries.[57] The microcirculation of the brain is particularly vulnerable to blockage with *P. falciparum*-infected erythrocytes, resulting in small areas of cerebral infarction and hemorrhage.[4] Disturbances in consciousness, ranging from somnolence to coma, behavioral changes, hallucinations, motor seizures, and occasionally tremors, focal muscle paralysis, and other localizing signs, may be present. A rapidly progressive downhill course, leading to death may occur in fulminant cases.

Individuals planning travel to parts of the world endemic for malaria should consult with local public health authorities for advice on protection and prophylaxis. Recommendations to travelers for prophylaxis while in endemic regions is published periodically by the CDC.[49] The type of prophylaxis to recommend will be based on whether the places of anticipated travel have a high risk of acquiring chloroquine-resistant malaria, whether the person had previous reactions to antimalarial drugs, and whether or not medical care will be readily available. Chloroquine prophylaxis should begin 1 to 2 weeks before anticipated travel and extend for 4 weeks after return. Chloroquine-resistant strains of *P. falciparum* have been found in all regions endemic for malaria, except the Dominican Republic, Haiti, Central America west of the Panama Canal, and the Middle East, including Egypt.[49] Travel doses of Fansidar (combination of sulfadoxine and pyrimethamine) should be readily available, and taken promptly if sudden onset of a febrile illness is experienced. In such cases, obtaining prompt medical attention is mandatory because of the potential life-threatening nature of *P. falciparum* infections and the potential of experiencing complications of drug therapy. The use of a new prophylactic drug effective against chloroquine-resistant strains of *P. falciparum*, mefloquine (Lariam), has been recommended by the CDC.[49] It has fewer side effects than Fansidar.

and petechiae and ecchymoses of the extremities, and dysentery are complications that can lead to considerable morbidity or even death in fulminant cases. Sodium stibogluconate (Pentostam) 20 mg/kg per day given IM or IV for 20 days is the recommended treatment regimen.

The laboratory diagnosis of disseminated leishmaniasis (kala-azar) is made by demonstrating amastigotes in stained smears, imprints, or biopsies of infected tissues. The organisms are oval, intracellular, and very small, averaging 2 to 4 μm, simulating the yeast cells of *Histoplasma capsulatum* (see Color Plate 20-6H). The leishmania amastigotes possess a barlike kinetoplast adjacent to the nucleus, a structure that is helpful in distinguishing these organisms from the yeast forms of *H. capsulatum*.

Primary cutaneous leishmaniasis includes both Old World and New World diseases. The Old World disease, or Oriental sore, is most commonly caused by members of the *L. tropica* complex (including *L. major*, *L. tropica minor*, and *L. aethiopica*). This form of disease is endemic in the tropical and subtropical regions of Asia Minor, China, the southern Mediterranean, India, and Africa. At the site of insect bites on exposed parts of the body, the promastigotes injected into the skin are taken up by the reticuloendothelial cells in which they develop into the amastigotes. The species causing cutaneous leishmaniasis do not circulate except in very rare instances. An intensely pruritic papule develops that, in the course of several weeks or months, progresses to a chronic well-circumscribed ulcer with a raised, erythematous margin and a shallow bed. The ulcers caused by *L. major* tend to be moist and multiple; those of *L. tropica minor* are drier and tend to crust over. Most lesions are benign and self-healing, and

TABLE 20-8
HEMOFLAGELLATES: KEY FEATURES FOR LABORATORY IDENTIFICATION

SPECIES	ARTHROPOD VECTOR	SITES OF INFECTION	DIAGNOSTIC FORMS	PLATE REFERENCE
Leishmania donovani	Phlebotomus fly Leptomonad forms in fly proboscis are infective forms for humans.	Intracellular parasites of reticuloendothelial cells: bone marrow, liver, spleen, and lymph nodes. Organisms do not circulate in peripheral blood. Species in the *L. tropica*, *L. braziliensis*, and *L. mexicana* complexes cause mucocutaneous ulcers.	Ovoid 2- to 4-μm forms seen intracellularly in tissue sections. Morphology best seen in Giemsa-stained touch preparations. Presence of rod-shaped kinetoplast adjacent to nucleus helps to distinguish *Leishmania* from the fungus *Histoplasma capsulatum* or the parasite *Toxoplasma gondii*	20-6G, H
Trypanosoma gambiense *T. rhodesiense*	Tsetse fly Metacyclic trypanosomal form in salivary gland of fly is infective form for humans.	In early infection, the parasites may be found in lymph nodes and circulating in the bloodstream. In later infections, the organism may invade the central nervous system, producing sleeping sickness.	The organisms are long, slender, spindle-shaped forms, measuring 15–30 μm in length and 1.5–4 μm in width. A single flagellum takes its origin from a dotlike kinetoplast located posterior to the central nucleus. The flagellum runs along an undulating membrane that projects beyond the anterior point of the organism.	20-6I
T. cruzi	Triatomid bug (known also as reduviid or kissing bug; 20-6K) Metacyclic trypanosome in bug feces is infective form for humans.	Early in infection, the trypanosome form is found circulating in the blood. A chronic disease form is characterized by leishmanial forms in reticuloendothelial cells or in heart muscle. The leishmanial forms do not circulate in the blood but can be seen only in stained tissue sections.	The circulating trypanosomal organisms are similar to those of *T. gambiense* and *T. rhodesiense*. Characteristic C-forms are characteristic when seen, but are rarely diagnostic. Leishmanial forms in tissues are morphologically similar to those of *L. donovani*.	20-6J 20-6L

permanent immunity develops. The cutaneous lesions of *L. aethiopica* may not ulcerate but often result in deep, spreading subcutaneous infections, and this species also has the propensity to cause disseminated disease indistinguishable from *L. donovani* infections.[255]

New World cutaneous leishmaniasis is caused by the *L. braziliensis* complex (also including *L. braziliensis gyanensis* and *L. braziliensis panamensis*), which is endemic in almost all states in South America and in several regions in Latin America, and by the *L. mexicana* complex, including several separate species endemic in various regions in Mexico, Guatemala, Venezuela, and in the Amazon Basin of Brazil. The *L. braziliensis* complex of organisms causes aggressive, chronic cutaneous ulcers, with mucous membrane (oral, nasal, pharyngeal) spread, a clinical picture called espundia. Organisms of the *L. mexicana* complex are more likely to produce self-limiting cutaneous ulcers (60% of lesions occur on the ear lobes, producing what are known as "Chiclero ulcers"). The mucous membranes are less commonly involved, although *L. peruviana* is likely to produce a more diffuse cutaneous disease, known as "uta" in Peru. Stibogluconate sodium is the treatment of choice.

The laboratory diagnosis is made by demonstrating the intracellular leishmanial organism in impression smears or tissue sections prepared from active lesions

(see Color Plate 20-6H). Biopsies should be obtained from the elevated, inflamed margin of the lesion; aspirates should be obtained by extending the tip of the needle deep beneath the ulcer bed. Culture methods, used primarily in laboratories serving practices in endemic areas, are described in detail by Garcia and Bruckner.[120] Lopez-Velez and coauthors[205] also describe a culture method using buffy coat samples from peripheral blood that was successful in diagnosing leishmaniasis in AIDS patients presenting with atypical clinical pictures. Animal inoculation techniques are also used in these laboratories for diagnosing infections when parasite concentrations are low.

ELISA techniques, using species-specific monoclonal antibodies[168] and DNA probes,[348] have been successful in the direct detection of leishmania antigen in extracts of tissue samples in laboratories where reagents are available. Piarroux and associates,[261] who used a PCR assay amplifying a repeated sequence from the *L. infantum* genome, in a study of 73 patients with a working clinical diagnosis of visceral leishmaniasis, demonstrated superior sensitivity of the method (82%) in making the diagnosis compared with examination of bone marrow aspirates (55%) and myeloculture (55%). They conclude that PCR may serve as an aid in diagnosing visceral leishmaniasis in immunocompromised patients. Rodriquez and coworkers,[275] who used a PCR-hybridization technique that employed oligonucleotides directed against conserved regions of kinetoplast DNA, were able to detect the presence of leishmania cells in 98% of patients clinically diagnosed as having cutaneous leishmaniasis by the Montenegro skin test. They further believe the technique is epidemiologically valuable in making the taxonomic discrimination between species.

Trypanosomiasis. Human trypanosomiasis is caused by a flagellate protozoan that inhabits the blood and tissues. The adult form, which measures 1.5 to 30 μm long and 1.5 to 3.5 μm wide, has an elongated body, with a whip-like posterior flagellum that is attached by a delicate undulating membrane that runs the length of the body. Wild game serve as the reservoir host. A central nucleus

and a posterior kinetoplast are usually easily seen. These diagnostic forms can be readily seen in stained smears of peripheral blood (see Color Plate 20-6*I*) and in the CSF in cases of active infection. However, in chronic or light infections, Bailey and Smith,[17] in a study of blood samples obtained from 134 patients with *Trypanosoma gambiense* infection, found the quantitative buffy coat test, developed for malaria diagnosis, the most sensitive diagnostic test for the detection of trypanosomal forms.

The life cycle involves animals and humans as the definitive host, in which the mature trypanosomas circulate and divide in the peripheral blood and ultimately invade into the CNS; and an intermediate host, the tsetse fly, in which the immature forms develop in the salivary gland, ultimately forming infective metacyclic trypanomastigotes. The life cycle is illustrated in Figure 20-22.

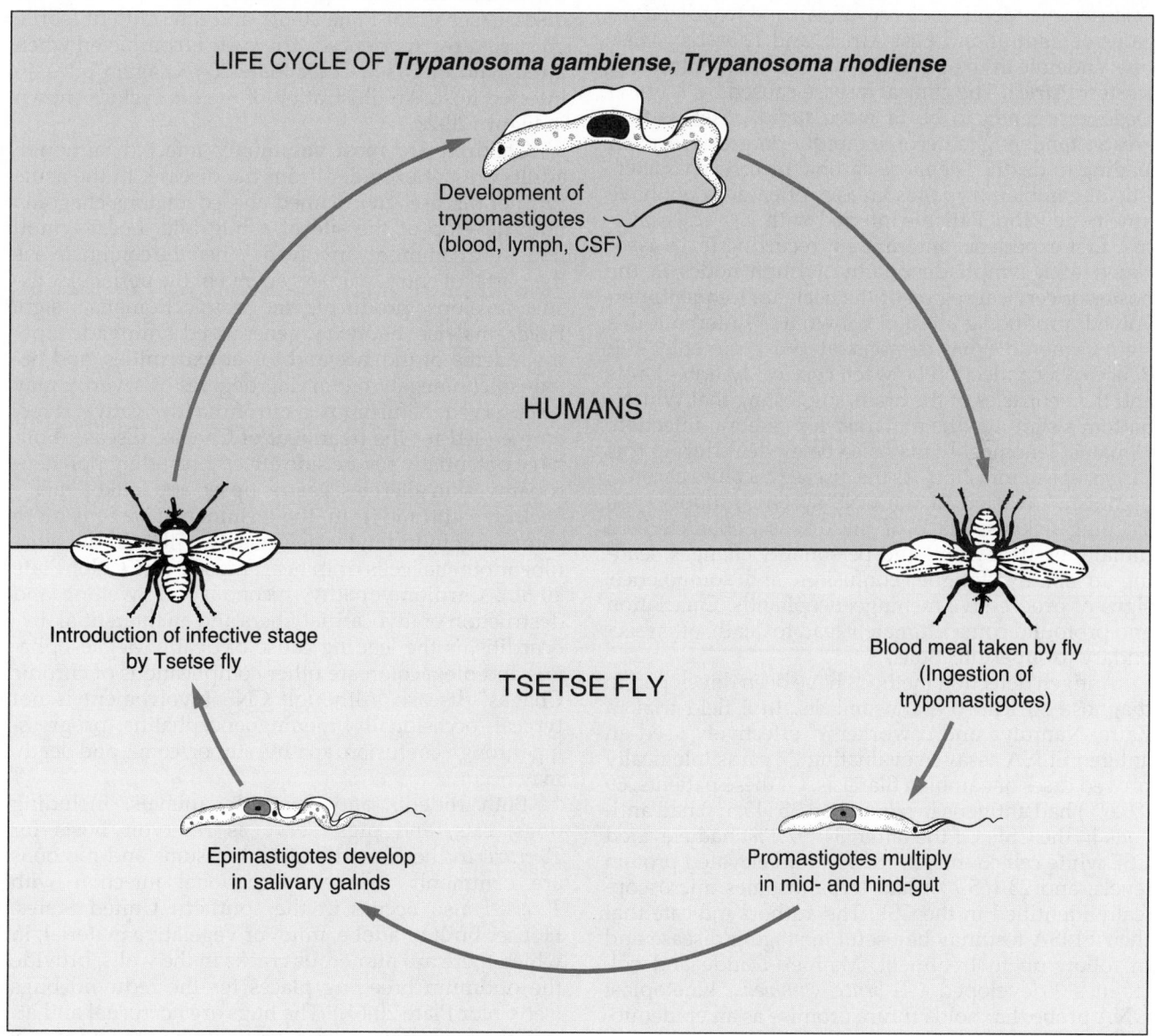

Figure 20-22
Life cycle of *Trypanosoma gambiense* and *T. rhodesiense*.

Approximately 50 million persons are at risk for African trypanosomiasis; 20,000 new cases are diagnosed each year.[358] In the African form of the disease, humans become infected through the bites of infected *Glossina* tsetse flies that harbor the infective procyclic trypanomastigotes in their salivary glands. Tsetse flies are found only in Africa. A chancre develops at the site of the insect bite, within which, over a period of several weeks, the trypanosomes undergo multiplication and maturation. Ultimately, they invade the lymphatics and blood stream, widely disseminating to lymph nodes and ultimately to the CNS. Organism multiplication continues to take place in the blood stream despite humoral immunity of the infected host, a fundamental difference from *T. cruzi*. This capacity is due to the unique property of these organisms to periodically change the antigenic structure of the glycoproteins within their surface membranes.[91]

African trypanosomiasis, also known as sleeping sickness, is caused by one of two species, *T. brucei rhodesiense*, endemic in the savannah and woodland regions of Central and East Africa, and *T. brucei gambiense*, endemic in the tropical rain forests of central and western Africa. The clinical disease caused by *T. brucei rhodesiense* tends to be of more rapid onset, with a greater tendency to become rapidly progressive, even leading to death. The more chronic picture, characteristic of gambian trypanosomiasis, often does not have time to develop. Patients infected with *T. brucei gambiense* first experience intermittent recurring fever associated with lymphadenopathy. Lymph nodes in the posterior cervical region of the neck are frequently involved, producing a lesion known as Winterbottom's sign. Ormerod[251] has demonstrated experimental evidence of a connection between cervical lymph glands and the ventricles of the brain, suggesting that Winterbottom's sign may be a marker for cerebral infection. Hepatosplenomegaly may also be evident during this early stage of infection. As the disease becomes chronic, organism invasion of the CNS system produces the sleeping-sickness stage of the disease, characterized initially by behavioral and personality changes, leading to apathy, fatigue, confusion, and somnolence, signs of progressive meningoencephalitis. Emaciation and profound coma ultimately lead to death, often secondary to superinfections.

Antigen detection methods have been developed to diagnose African trypanosomiasis. In a field trial in Zaire, Nantulya and coworkers[237] effectively used an antigen ELISA assay in evaluating 77 parasitologically proved cases of gambian filariasis. Of these patients, 69 (89.6%) had antigens in serum and 35 (45.5%) had antigens in the CSF. Of the latter, 34 (97.1%) had elevated CSF white cell counts, 29 (82.9%) had elevated protein levels, and 23 (65.7%) had trypanosomes microscopically identified in the CSF. The authors indicate that their ELISA test may be useful in staging disease and in follow-up to treatment. Mathieu-Daude and colleagues[221] developed a *T. brucei gambiense* kinetoplast DNA probe that holds future promise as an epidemiologic and survey tool.

Suramin or pentamidine are the drugs of choice. Malarsoprol may be used in later stages with CNS disease.

SOUTH AMERICAN TRYPANOSOMIASIS: CHAGAS' DISEASE. South American trypanosomiasis (also known as Chagas' disease) caused by *T. cruzi*, is found from the southern United States through Latin and South America to Argentina. An estimated 10 to 12 million people are infected, approximately half of whom live in Brazil.[84] Although *T. cruzi* has been found in dogs, wild mammals, and insect vectors in the southern part of the United States, autochthonous human cases have been reported only very rarely.[140,320]

The life cycle of *T. cruzi* differs from the African species in that the triatomid or reduviid bug serves as the arthropod vector, and that visceral organs may be infected with the leishmanial form of the parasite. Humans become infected when the trypanosomal-infected fecal matter is discharged into the wound when the bug feeds. The bite is quite painful, and the infected feces are rubbed into the wound. In the human host, the C-shaped trypanosomes circulate in the bloodstream during the early acute phase of the disease (see Color Plate 20-6*J*), and intermittent febrile episodes are experienced. The cycle is completed when a reduviid bug (see Color Plate 20-6*K*) again bites an infected host. An illustration of the life cycle is shown in Figure 20-23.

Children are most commonly infected, although adults are not excluded from the disease. In the acute form of disease, an inflamed and edematous chagoma may develop at the site of a bug bite. Local lymph nodes are commonly involved. When the conjunctiva is the portal of entry, painless edema of the periocular tissue develops, producing the classic Romana's sign. Fever, malaise, anorexia, generalized lymphadenopathy, edema of the face and lower extremities, and hepatosplenomegaly of varying degrees of severity may be observed. Nifurtimox, a nitrofuran derivative, is recommended for the treatment of Chagas' disease. Both have potentially severe side effects, including polyneuropathy, skin allergies, gastric upset, and leukopenia.

In the chronic form, the leishmanial stage is more commonly found in tissues, usually either in the reticuloendothelial cells or in heart muscle (see Color Plate 20-6*L*). Cardiomyopathy, secondary to swelling and destruction of myocardial fibers and an interstitial myocarditis, is the leading cause of death. Megaesophagus and megacolon are other complications of chronic Chagas' disease. Although CNS involvement is not typical, occasionally, meningoencephalitis, progressing through confusion, apathy, stupor, coma, and death, may occur.

Both rodents and domestic animals, including dogs, cats, and pigs, serve as reservoir hosts for *T. cruzi*. In the United States, opossums and raccoons are commonly infected. Occasional infection with *T. cruzi* also occurs in the southern United States. Houses built of adobe, mud, or vegetative material, in which there are numerous cracks in the walls, provide the optimum breeding places for the reduviid bugs (see Color Plate 20-6*K*). The bugs are nocturnal and attack their sleeping victims. Prevention of the disease is therefore aimed at improving housing conditions.

T. rangeli is another trypanosomal organism transmitted to humans by reduviid bugs. Human infections

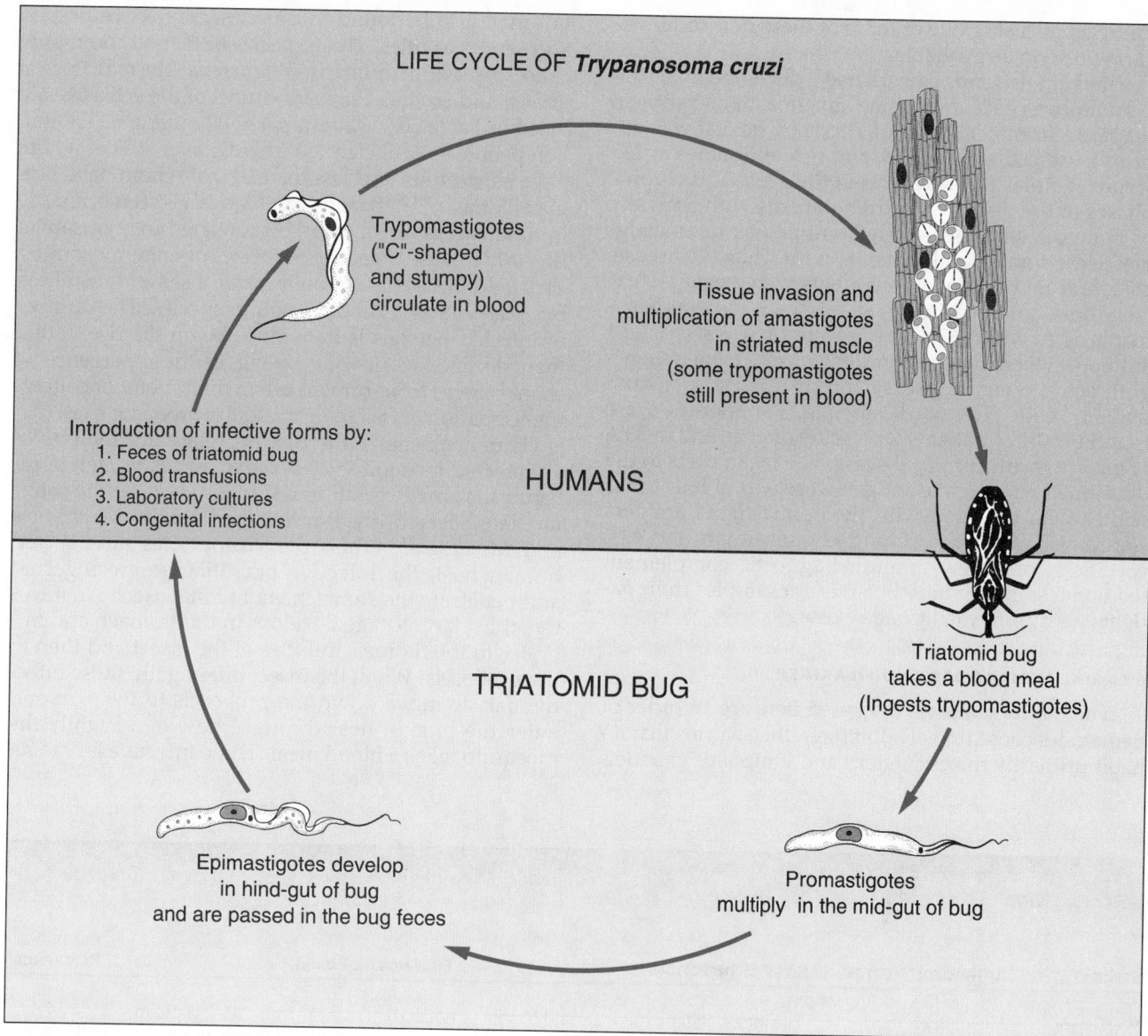

LIFE CYCLE OF *Trypanosoma cruzi*

Trypomastigotes
("C"-shaped
and stumpy)
circulate in blood

Tissue invasion and
multiplication of amastigotes
in striated muscle
(some trypomastigotes
still present in blood)

Introduction of infective forms by:
1. Feces of triatomid bug
2. Blood transfusions
3. Laboratory cultures
4. Congenital infections

HUMANS

TRIATOMID BUG

Triatomid bug
takes a blood meal
(Ingests trypomastigotes)

Epimastigotes develop
in hind-gut of bug
and are passed in the bug feces

Promastigotes
multiply in the mid-gut of bug

Figure 20-23
Life cycle of *Trypanosoma cruzi*.

are usually asymptomatic. The trypanomastigotes can be identified in thick and thin smears of peripheral blood and morphologically resemble those seen in African trypanosomiasis. However, unless a careful clinical history is obtained, a misdiagnosis of *T. cruzi* infection may be made. Serologic testing may be of value in differentiating *T. rangeli* infections from Chagas' disease; however, double infections may occur, producing confusing results. Hudson and coworkers,[159] in an immunologic study of a group of Colombian patients in the area of Tibu, hope to elucidate what effect infections with *T. rangeli* may have on the course of Chagas' disease in patients with coinfections.

Serodiagnostic methods are being developed to detect *T. cruzi* serum antibodies to aid in the diagnosis of Chagas' disease. Godsel and associates[126] identified in the serum of patients with Chagas' disease a new recombinant antigen called FCaBP, a 24-kDa flagellar calcium-binding protein. This protein may be used as a component of a multiple recombinant antigen preparation effective in screening for *T. cruzi* in donor blood supplies. Tanowitz and coauthors,[320] in a comprehensive review of Chagas' disease, discuss the importance of screening donor blood for this disease. The issue affects not only individuals living in countries with endemic disease, but also is of concern in the United States where upward of 50,000 immigrants from endemic countries may be infected. Avila and associates[14,15] also suggest a sensitive screening test for diagnosing chronic Chagas' disease in blood bank donors. They demonstrated a 100% sensitivity compared with serologic tests in the detection of PCR-amplified products of *T. cruzi* kinetoplast minicircle DNA in 114 blood samples obtained from chronic chagasic and nonchagasic patients, using a specific digoxigenin-labeled oligonucleotide probe. One hopes that commercial reagents using one or more of these new technologies will soon be available.

Matsumoto and coworkers[223] developed an immunofluorescence test using an amastigote antigen prepared from a Y strain of *T. cruzi*. The test was applied to detecting IgG, IgM, and IgA antibodies in 238 serum samples from patients in the acute and chronic phases of the disease and from patients with a variety of nonchagastic diseases. IgG antibodies to amastigotes were found in all patients with Chagas' disease; all sera from nonchagastic patients were negative (except those obtained from patients with visceral leishmaniasis, in which 63% cross-reactivity was seen). IgM antibodies were detected in 100% of sera from patients with acute Chagas' disease and in 7.5% of sera from patients with chronic disease; IgA antibodies were found in 60% of patients with acute disease and in 33% of patients with chronic disease. The mean titers to the developed amastigotic antigen were two to four times higher than obtained with the epimastigote antigen. Garcia and associates[116] found 92% sensitivity and 99% specificity of a new immunodiagnostic complement fixation test in the study of 66 serum samples from patients with confirmed Chagas' disease.

FILARIAL NEMATODES AND FILARIASIS

The filarial parasites discussed here are an order of nematodes consisting of adult threadlike worms that inhabit primarily the circulatory and lymphatic channels but may also be found in muscles, connective tissues, and serous cavities. Three species of filariae commonly cause disease in humans: *Wuchereria bancrofti, Brugia malayi,* and *Loa loa.* The key features of these filariae are listed in Table 20-9. An estimated 90 million to 150 million people are afflicted worldwide, over 90% of whom have bancroftian and less than 10% of whom have brugian filariasis.[214,236] Bancroftian filariasis is seen primarily in urban areas in Southeast Asia related to poor sanitation and intense breeding of species of *Culex* mosquitos. Brugian filariasis is mainly a rural disease transmitted by *Anopheles* and *Aedes* mosquito species. The number of infected persons is thought to be on the rise, rather than decline, worldwide owing to the emergence of shanty towns from rural to urban migrations, encouraging formation of favorable mosquito breeding sites.[337]

Humans acquire the disease following the bite of an infected mosquito (*W. bancrofti* and *B. malayi*) or tabanid flies for *L. loa.* Biting midges serve as the intermediate hosts for the nonsheathed species *M. perstans* and *M. ozzardi.* When the vector bites an infected human host, the infective microfilariae are ingested and penetrate the stomach wall of the insect. An infective third larval stage develops in the stomach and migrates to the thoracic muscles of the insect and then to the proboscis. When the insect bites again, these infective larvae move down the proboscis to the skin and enter the human host through the wound while the mosquito takes a blood meal. These infective larvae re-

TABLE 20-9
FILARIA: KEY FEATURES TO LABORATORY IDENTIFICATION

SPECIES	ARTHROPOD VECTOR	SITES OF INFECTION	DIAGNOSTIC FORMS	PLATE REFERENCE
Wuchereria bancrofti	Mosquitoes: third-stage larvae in mosquito proboscis is infective form for humans.	The long slender adult male and female nematodes reside in the lymphatic channels throughout the body, primarily in the legs and pelvis. The lymphatics become blocked, leading, in the chronic form of the disease, to marked swelling and edema of the legs, arms, and scrotum, a condition known as elephantiasis.	*Microfilariae:* measuring 245–295 µm in length × 7.5–10 µm width, these forms can be easily seen in direct microscopic examinations of blood, especially when collected at night. *W. bancrofti* microfilariae have a sheath, and the column of nuclei terminate 15–20 µm proximal to the tail, leaving a clear space.	20-7*A*
Brugia malayi	Mosquitoes: the infective form, is the same as *W. bancrofti.*	Similar disease as with *W. bancrofti*	*Microfilariae:* appear similar to those of *W. bancrofti* and are also released into the bloodstream with nocturnal periodicity. They differ from *W. bancrofti* in that 2 nuclei, spaced about 10 µm apart from the main column, extend into the tip of the tail.	20-7*B*
Loa loa	Tabanid flies (*Chrysops dimidiata*): the infective form is the same as for *W. bancrofti.*	The adult worms migrate through the subcutaneous tissue and may be visualized particularly beneath the thin conjunctival epithelium of the eye (for this reason, *L. loa* is known as the eye worm). Calabar swellings may occur in other parts of the skin, a helpful diagnostic clue.	*Microfilariae:* appear similar to those of *W. bancrofti* and *B. malayi,* except that the column of nuclei extends completely to the tip of the tail section. A sheath is present. Microfilariae are released by the adult worms on a diurnal schedule.	20-7*C*

produce locally in the subcutaneous tissue and ultimately enter the peripheral lymphatics where they find their way to lymph nodes and lymphatic channels in various parts of the body. Over a period of several weeks, the larvae develop into white, threadlike adult worms. The lymphatics of the lower extremities and the epitrochlear and femoral lymph nodes are the sites most commonly involved. An illustration of the life cycle of *W. bancrofti* as a prototype for the filarial worms is shown in Figure 20-24.

The laboratory diagnosis is made by observing circulating microfilariae in stained peripheral blood smears.[135] Microfilariae circulate in the peripheral blood with a regular periodicity; those of *W. bancrofti* and *B. malayi* are nocturnal, and those of *L. loa* are diurnal. Therefore, to diagnose bancroftian filariasis, blood should be optimally obtained between midnight and 2:00 A.M. In cases of light infections or when samples

are collected at suboptimal times, membrane filtration, centrifugation, sedimentation (Knott's concentration), and preparation of thick smears are techniques that may help detect circulating microfilariae.[272] Long and coauthors[203] describe an interesting approach to the laboratory diagnosis of filariasis using an acridine orange–microhematocrit tube technique. A microhematocrit tube incorporating heparin, EDTA, and acridine orange serves as the basis for this test. After centrifugation, parasites become concentrated in the buffy coat and can be visualized through the clear glass wall of the tube. The acridine orange stains the DNA of the parasites, and the morphologic characteristics, including the nuclear patterns in the tail sections, can be examined by fluorescence microscopy in making a species identification.

Mature female worms produce myriads of prelarvae, known as microfilariae, that circulate in the blood

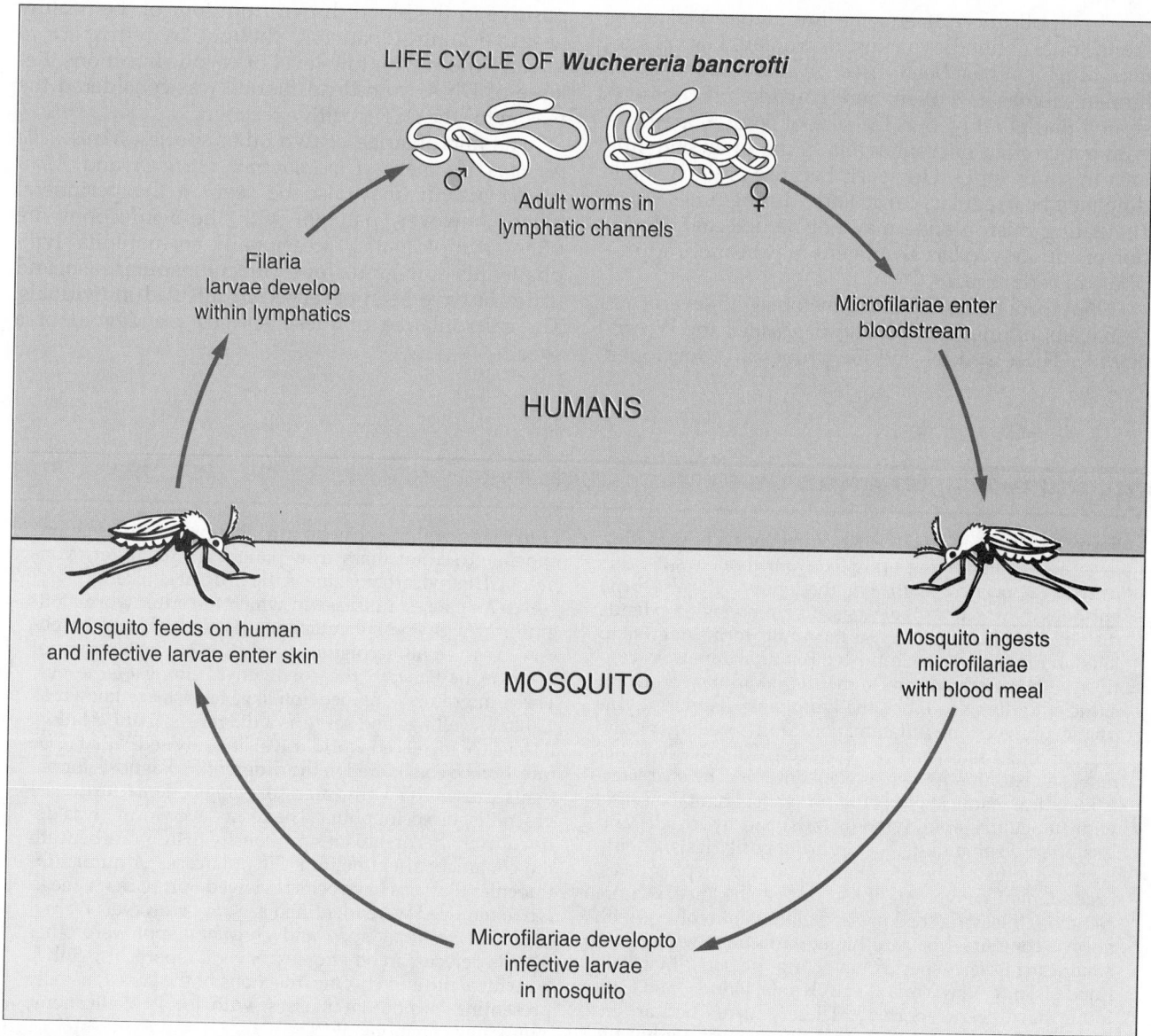

Figure 20-24
Life cycle of *Wuchereria bancrofti*.

and serve as the mode of transmission when the mosquito vector takes a blood meal. Microfilaria measure between 240 and 300 μm in length and about 7 μm in width. They are ribbonlike and can be seen in microscopic mounts of anticoagulated blood by their undulating motion, displacing the red blood cells from side to side as they move. In stained peripheral blood smears, a prominent sheath that extends beyond the tail section may be observed. The sheath is a close-fitting membrane that envelops the microfilariae of pathogenic filarial worms, representing the remnants of the ovum membrane from which it was derived. Identification of the three pathogenic species can be made by observing the size and the pattern of extension of nuclei into the tail sections, as described in Table 20-9 and illustrated in Color Plates 20-7A to 7C. The microfilariae of W. bancrofti do not extend into the tail section; those of B. malayi have two nuclei extending into the tail, spaced about 10 μm apart, and an uninterrupted column of nuclei extends into the tail with Loa loa.

The application of enzyme immunoassays using monoclonal antibodies against microfilarial larval surface antigens has been used in the diagnosis of human filariasis.[198] Weil and coworkers[342] demonstrated filarial antigen in the sera of 56 of 57 patients with bancroftian microfilaremia living in an endemic area in south India. However, because antigen shedding may be irregular, particularly during times when circulating microfilariae may not be detected, detection of antibody to larval antigens may be more appropriate in certain cases.[87]

DNA probes have been developed in several research laboratories for B. malayi, B. pahangi, and W. bancrofti.[228] These species-specific probes are developed based on identifying repeated DNA sequences in each species. In a double-blind study of patients with suspected filariasis in Indonesia, McReynolds and co-workers[228] found a 98.5% agreement between a DNA probe they developed against B. malayi microfilariae and conventional microscopic techniques in 642 specimens tested. According to these workers, the ability to detect either filarial antigen or antibody would preclude the necessity for obtaining night blood and would not require the presence of circulating microfilariae, helpful in diagnosing occult infections. Field studies are currently underway in China and other endemic regions. See Grimaldi and Tesh[135] for a review of various clinical laboratory procedures for diagnosing leishmaniasis, including the use of nuclear probes and various serologic techniques.

Lizotte and associates[199] demonstrated a 100% correct identification of 66 microfilaria-positive samples collected in a field trial in Indonesia, with a PCR-based assay using the Hha I family of highly repeated DNA sequences from Brugia species. The PCR assay was also positive in the blood drawn from four of the healthy negative control patients, thought in retrospect to identify those with low-level or cryptic infections. Release of DNA from dead filariae was considered the reason for the PCR-positive reaction.

The microfilariae of two other species, Mansonella perstans (formerly Dipetalonema perstans) and Mansonella ozzardi, may also be seen in the peripheral blood; however, patients with these infections are often asymptomatic. Occasionally eosinophilia, lymphadenitis, low-grade fever, maculopapular rash, and urticaria have been observed in infected individuals. The microfilariae of these species are devoid of a sheath.

CLINICAL CORRELATION BOX 20-15. FILARIASIS

Early in W. bancrofti and B. malayi infections, a bout of high fever and chills, lasting up to 5 days before subsiding, is usually associated with lymphadenitis. These febrile episodes may recur as the persistent lymphangitis extends distally from lymph nodes, as the adult worms migrate to take up final residence in the lymphatic channels. In contrast with the schistosomes, the filarial adult worms are sufficiently large to block the lymphatic channels. Lymphatic obstruction, inflammation, and swelling of the surrounding tissues evolve, producing extensive lymphadema, a condition known as elephantiasis. The characteristic clinical manifestation of W. bancrofti is genital disease, with funiculitis, epididymo-orchitis, and hydrocele, and less often elephantiasis.[75, 254] In brugian filariasis, adenolymphadenitis of the inguinal region and elephantiasis, predominantly involving the leg below the knee, is more common,[254] leaving the knee and elbow uninvolved, with normal contours.[75] Several human infections with North American Brugia species involving persons living in Rhode Island, New York, Pennsylvania, Florida, and California have been reported.[18] These patients had an enlarged lymph node containing a single worm within the lymphatic channels. Clark and Lieber[59] also report a case of filariasis of the spermatic cord that presented as an unexplained scrotal mass in a patient in Rochester, Minnesota. Diethylcarbamazine is the drug of choice.

Loa loa causes a disease in which the adult worms migrate through the subcutaneous tissue and may be observed as a small, serpiginous elevation of the thin parts of the skin or beneath the conjunctival lining of the eye. These migratory, angioedema skin lesions are known as Calibar swellings and serve as a diagnostic manifestation. Because of increased world travel, it is advised[269] that L. loa infection be considered in the differential diagnosis for patients presenting with migratory angioedema, urticarial vasculitis, or eosinophilia. The term "eye worm" was derived from this organism's propensity to infiltrate beneath the conjunctival epithelium. Fifty-six cases of human intraocular filariasis have been reviewed.[23] In 10 cases, the filariae removed were identified as L. loa. However, W. bancrofti, Dipetalonema spp., and Dirofilaria spp. were other filariae detected in other cases. Several reports also link L. loa with acute and chronic infections of the breast, usually presenting as nodular masses, with focal calcifications, simulating carcinoma.[42, 190]

Onchocerciasis and *Onchocerca volvulus*. Onchocerciasis is a filarial worm disease that primarily involves the subcutaneous skin in the form of dense fibrous nodules ranging in diameter from 5 to 25 mm, at the sites of bites of the vector, the *Simulian*, black or buffalo fly. The fly has its main habitat in the underbrush lining the banks of fast-moving streams. African onchocerciasis occurs mainly in the Congo Basin, Zaire, Angola, and the Sudan; in the Americas, it is found in the highlands of Guatemala, the states of Oaxaca and Chiapas in Mexico, in Columbia, and in northeastern Venezuela. The nodules are more likely to be distributed in the trunk, thighs, and arms in African subjects, but more likely in the neck and shoulders in inhabitants of Central America.

In the life cycle, humans become infected by bites from the simulian fly, which possess in their mouth parts the infective third-stage larval forms. The adult worms develop in tangled masses within nodules beneath the skin (Fig. 20-25), and the females produce microfilaria (see Color Plate 20-7D). The microfilariae remain localized to the infected sites and do not circulate in the peripheral blood except in rare instances (Fig. 20-26). The life cycle is completed when a black fly again bites a diseased human at one of the infected sites, picking up the microfilariae in the mouth parts. The microfilariae then develop in the fly until they mature into the third-stage, infective larval forms. An illustration of the life cycle is shown in Figure 20-27.

The diagnosis is clinically suspected when a patient from an endemic area presents with pruritic, subcutaneous nodules with associated dermatitis, loss of elasticity, and hyperpigmentation. The laboratory diagnosis is established by demonstrating microfilariae in teased snips of skin. Ogunrinade and associates[246] evaluated an enzyme immunoassay using recombinant *O. volvulus* antigens OC 3.6 and OC 9.3 as an aid in diagnosing patients with suspected onchocerciasis. Forty of the 42 (95%) serum samples they tested from patients with known onchocerciasis were reactive with the OC 3.6 antigen, whereas 81% were positive for the OC 9.3 antigen. Further studies revealed that the OC 3.6 antigen was most helpful in detecting prepatent infections in humans; the OC 9.3 antigen was more sensitive in patients with mature, patent infections.

Although the microfilariae may remain localized to the site of infection, they may wander through the adjacent skin and reach other tissues, including the eye. Ocular involvement is the most serious complication, often leading to varying degrees of loss of sight, known as "river blindness." The eye serves as a trap for wandering microfilariae which may be found either dead or alive in the anterior chamber, the cornea, choroid, and vitreous humor. The mechanical action or effects from secretory toxins released by the adult worm in a hypersensitive patient accounts for the development of blindness. The enzyme immunoassay described in the foregoing may be helpful in establishing the diagnosis in patients presenting primarily with river blindness.

Treatment consists of the surgical removal of detectable nodules when efficacious. Diethylcarbamazine, beginning with small doses plus suramin are the drugs of choice if surgical excisions are not feasible. Cutaneous and systemic side effects from death of the microfilariae may require coverage with anti-inflammatory drugs. Mebendazole and benzimidazole derivatives are alternatives with fewer side effects.

Dracunculiasis. *Dracunculus medinensis* is a tissue roundworm often grouped with the filariae. *D. medinensis* is the guinea worm that probably represents the "fiery serpent" of biblical lore.[151] Hopkins and Ruiz-Tiben[157] report that much progress has been made in complying with the 1986 WHO mandate to have dracunculiasis be the next disease to be eradicated (by 1995). Although much progress has been made in reducing the incidence of disease, of the 100 million people in India, Pakistan, and 17 African countries who are at risk, an estimated 3 million are still infected as of 1992. A program of intensive case detection and containment, with rewards for reporting of cases, promises to dramatically reduce disease by the end of the century. Humans acquire the infection through ingestion of infected copepoda. The larvae develop into adult worms in the serous cavities and the gravid females migrate to the subcutaneous tissue. These female worms can measure as long as 100 cm and cause a burning sensation and ulceration of the skin at the sites of infection. They can be removed surgically from

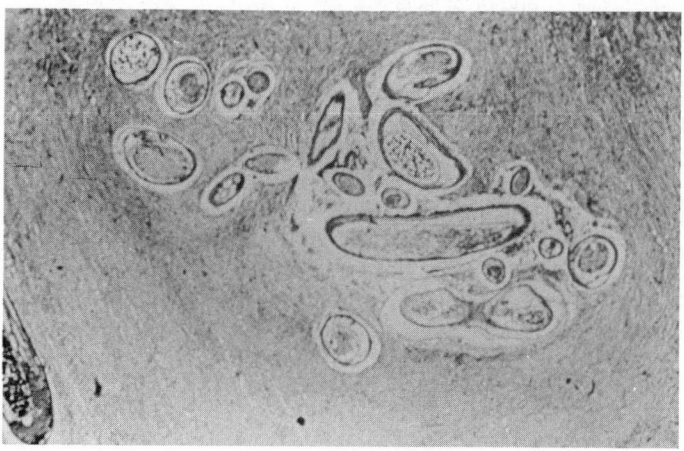

Figure 20-25
High-power view of histologic section of subcutaneous nodule of *Onchocerca volvulus* infestation. The irregular circular structures in the *center* of the photograph are many nematode adults cut in cross-section.

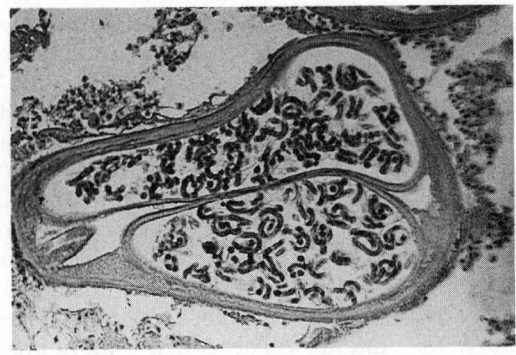

Figure 20-26
Section through the ovary of a female *O. volvulus* female worm illustrating the production of myriads of microfiliaria (H & E section, ×400).

the subcutaneous tissue by winding them slowly on a stick. The life cycle of the parasite is complete when the larvae produced by the female escape from the skin blister and are discharged into water in which the copepoda live.

Dirofilariasis. *Dirofilaria* species, transmitted by mosquitos, are filarial parasites commonly infecting animals. In the definitive host, most commonly the dog, the infective larval forms injected into the subcutaneous tissue from the proboscis of the mosquito enter into the circulation and ultimately find their way to the heart, where they develop into adults (dog heart worms; see Color Plate 20-7E). The diagnosis in dogs may be made by observing circulating microfilariae in the peripheral blood. When humans, as accidental

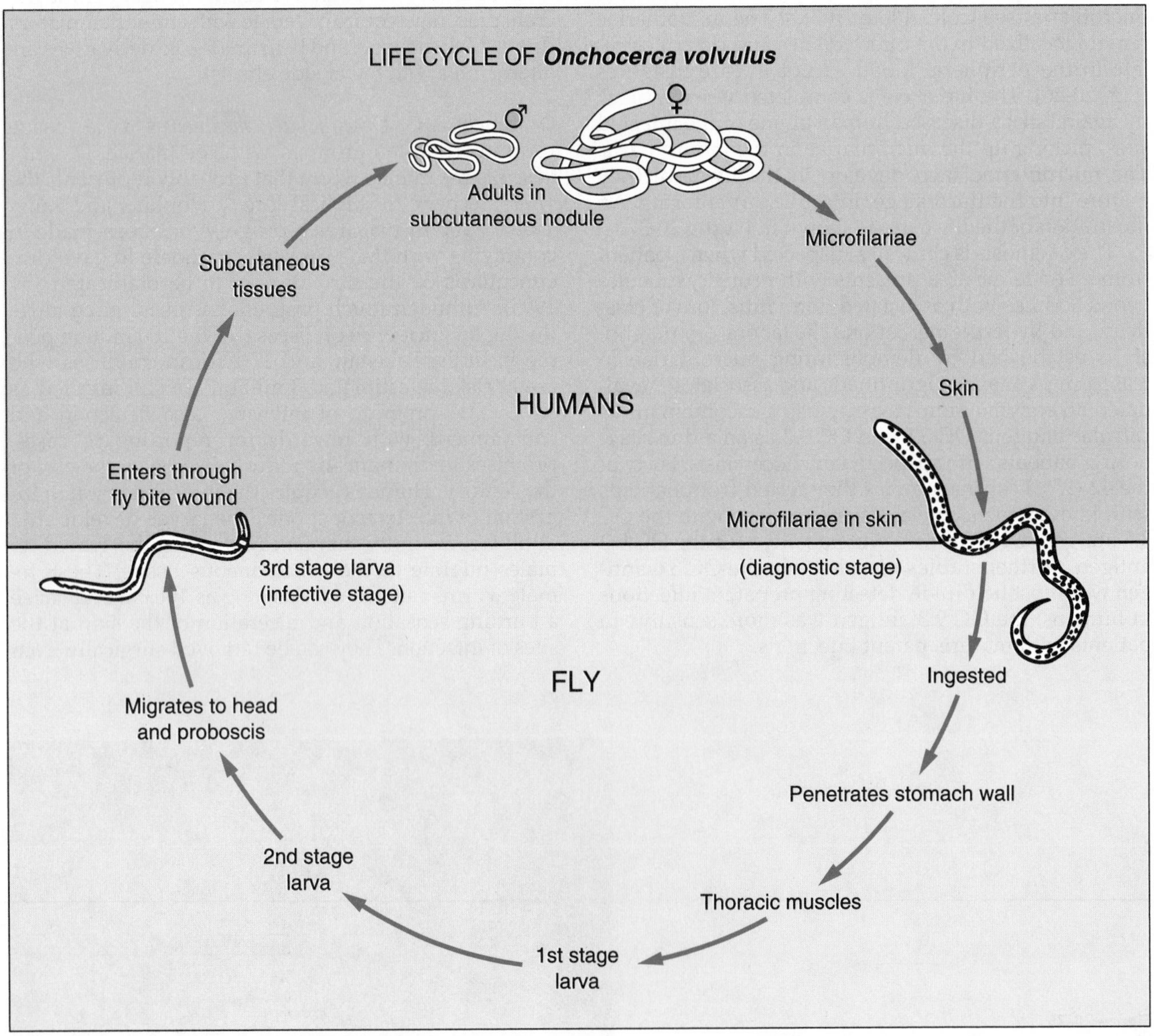

LIFE CYCLE OF *Onchocerca volvulus*

♂   ♀
Adults in
subcutaneous nodule

Microfilariae

Subcutaneous
tissues

Skin

HUMANS

Enters through
fly bite wound

Microfilariae in skin

3rd stage larva
(infective stage)

(diagnostic stage)

FLY

Ingested

Migrates to head
and proboscis

Penetrates stomach wall

2nd stage
larva

Thoracic muscles

1st stage
larva

Figure 20-27
Life cycle of *Onchocerca volvulus*.

hosts, are bitten by infected mosquitos, the larvae are incapable of completing their life cycle because they are in the wrong host, rather they lodge in and obstruct pulmonary arterioles, where they develop into local granulomatous nodules that may, on occasion, reach sufficient size to be diagnosed as "coin lesions" radiologically. Microfilariae never circulate in human blood. The diagnosis is made by histologic observation of immature filarial larvae within the pulmonary granulomatous nodules.

TISSUE PROTOZOAN INFECTIONS

Toxoplasma gondii. *T. gondii* is a protozoan parasite that has a particular propensity to infect the CNS in humans. As is characteristic of other coccidia, the life cycle of *T. gondii* has both sexual and asexual stages.

The sexual stage occurs in the intestine of cats, where infective oocysts 10 to 12 μm in diameter are excreted in the feces. The asexual stage commonly occurs in a variety of herbivorous and carnivorous animals and also in humans. Cockroaches, earthworms, snails, and slugs may serve as transport hosts for oocysts. The life cycle is illustrated in Figure 20-28.

Three modes of transmission lead to most human infections: 1) directly from ingestion of infective oocysts in food (e.g., unwashed leafy vegetables) or water contaminated with cat feces; 2) indirectly, from ingestion of the raw or undercooked meat of animals that had ingested oocysts (it is estimated that 25% of lamb and pork meat sold at supermarkets contains viable tissue cysts); and 3) transplacental transfer to the fetus from a mother infected during pregnancy. Maternal infection rates during the reproductive years is es-

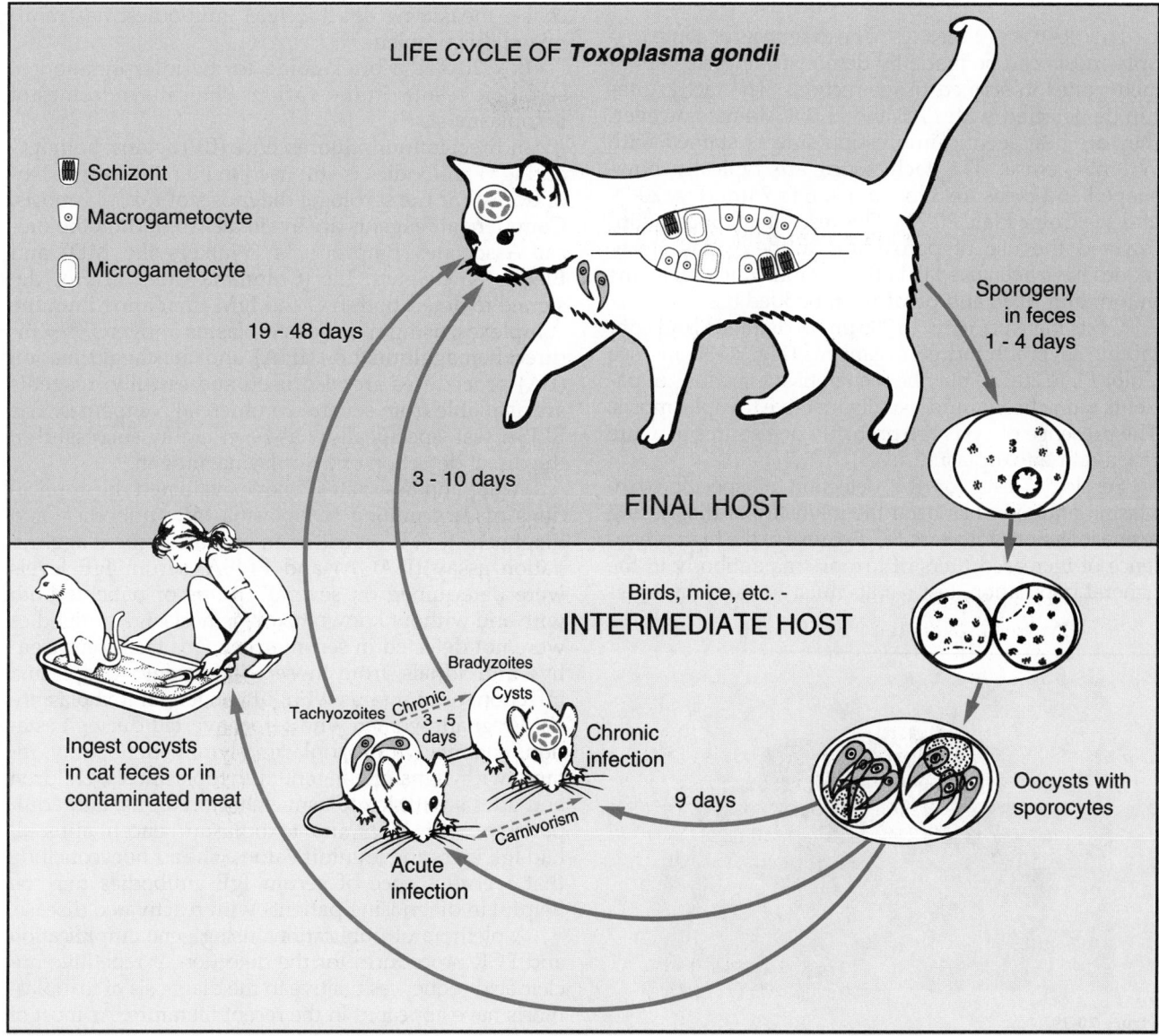

Figure 20-28
Life cycle of *Toxoplasma gondii*.

timated at between 3% and 5%.[111] Pregnant women should be strongly advised to avoid the handling of cats and the ingestion of undercooked meat.[110]

Two parasitic stages may be involved in human infections. After ingestion of oocysts or the encysted infective forms in uncooked meat, tachyzoites are released in the small intestine and first invade the mucosal epithelial cells, from which they enter the circulation, and then are widely distributed throughout the body. Considerable tissue damage may occur as the tachyzoites destroy the cells they parasitize; however, as the immune response develops, the tachyzoites become less active and ultimately aggregate within membrane-enclosed cysts. Although inactive, the tachyzoites within these cysts may remain viable for weeks or for years. Most commonly, they ultimately disintegrate and become enmeshed in a hyaline scar or undergo calcification. The detection of intracerebral calcification in skull roentgenograms is one method for establishing previous infection.

LABORATORY DIAGNOSIS. The diagnosis of acute toxoplasmosis can be made by demonstrating clusters of tachyzoites in stained tissue sections. The tachyzoites can be detected with PAS and H & E stains; however, they are best seen in impression smears stained with Wright-Giemsa. The tachyzoites are typically bow-shaped and measure 3 to 4 μm × 6 to 7 μm (Fig. 20-29 and see Color Plate 20-7F). Fluorescent antibody staining and the use of peroxidase–antiperoxidase techniques have been used to better demonstrate organisms in formalin-fixed and paraffin-embedded tissues.

Cysts measuring up to 200 μm in diameter and containing several hundred organisms (Fig. 20-30 and see Color Plate 20-7G) may be seen in tissue sections of patients with chronic and usually inactive toxoplasmosis. The presence of cysts are probably one source of acute reactivation toxoplasmosis.

Serologic tests for the detection of specific toxoplasma antibody has been the mainstay of diagnosing active infections for years.[22,225] Because of the high prevalence of increased titers of toxoplasma antibody in the general population, test results must be carefully interpreted before a definitive diagnosis can be established. The time honored Sabin-Feldman dye test, based on the principle that live T. gondii tachyzoites lose their affinity for methylene blue dye in the presence of immune serum, being both sensitive and specific, still serves as the reference method. Nonetheless, it has been replaced by newer techniques in most reference laboratories to bypass the necessity of having to work with live organisms. Also, this test measures IgG antibodies, which appear in the serum within 1 to 2 weeks following infection; peak in 6 to 8 weeks; and decline over the next few months but never completely disappear in postinfection patients. Because serum titers as high as 1:512 can persist for many years in normal persons, interpretations of single samples must be made with care.

The presence of IgM antibodies is highly suggestive of recent or active infection.[93] False-positive IgM antibody results may be caused by the presence of rheumatoid factor or competing IgG antibodies. The use of ELISA techniques or indirect immunofluorescence, measuring specific IgM antibodies, has minimized this problem.[169,198]

Box 20-9 is a brief guide to the interpretation of serologic results in the various clinical syndromes of toxoplasmosis.[225]

Indirect immunofluorescence (IIF) against both IgG and IgM antibodies is still used in many reference laboratories for the serologic diagnosis of toxoplasmosis. Commercial reagents are available from Microbiological Associates Bioproducts (Walkersville MD) and Electro-Nucleonics, Inc (Columbia MD). ELISA, designed to detect both IgG and IgM circulating immune complexes, using specific toxoplasma antigens,[238,326] indirect hemagglutination (IHA), and latex agglutination (LA) procedures are also used successfully; reagents are available from several commercial companies. The ELISA test, specifically, has been highly successful in the direct detection of toxoplasma antigen.[198]

Wong and associates[354] have evaluated the applications of determining toxoplasma IgE antibodies as a diagnostic test. With use of an immunosorbent agglutination assay (ISAGA) and ELISA, serum IgE levels were determined on several groups of patients both with and without known toxoplasmosis. IgE antibodies were not detected in serum specimens from seronegative individuals, from those with chronic toxoplasma infection, or in infants without congenital toxoplasmosis. Pregnant women who seroconverted during gestation, patients with toxoplasmic lymphadenopathy, infants with signs of congenital toxoplasmosis, children and adults with toxoplasmic chorioretinitis, and adult patients with AIDS and toxoplasmic encephalitis all had IgE titers above cutoff values. The authors conclude that recrudescence of serum IgE antibodies may be helpful in diagnosing patients with reactivated disease.

A plethora of publications using gene amplification and PCR procedures for the detection of repetitive nucleic acid sequences relative to the diagnosis of toxoplasmosis have appeared in the recent literature. As most of these newer techniques are works-in-progress in various research laboratories, it is only a matter of time before commercial reagents become available for use in diag-

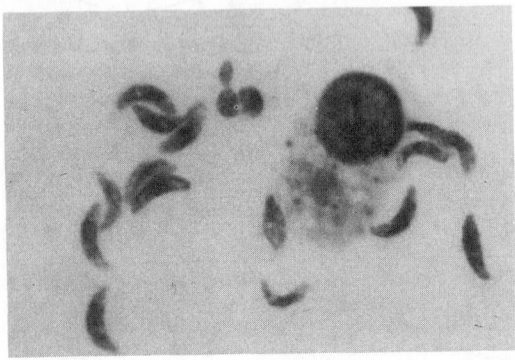

Figure 20-29
High-power view of Giemsa-stained impression smear demonstrating toxoplasma trophozoites. Note characteristic bow shape and central dark-staining nucleus (×1000).

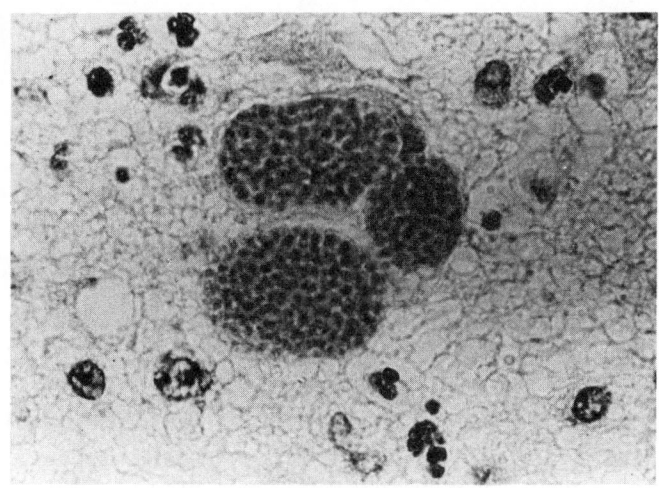

Figure 20-30
High-power view of the toxoplasmal pseudocysts illustrated in Figure 20-28. Each pseudocyst contains several scores of trophozoites. These pseudocysts are most commonly seen in patients with latent disease. Note the absence of an inflammatory reaction adjacent to these pseudocysts (H & E × 1000).

nostic microbiology laboratories. It is beyond the scope of this text to discuss these new advances in any detail. The references cited in the following may be of interest to those who are on the cutting edge of this new technology.

Several reports describe the *T. gondii B1* gene as the marker to be detected by gene amplification by PCR.[106,150,175,253] Several conclusions emerge from review of these studies. The *B1* gene amplification procedure is sufficiently sensitive to detect a single isolated parasite and as few as 10 parasites in a background of 100,000 leukocytes.[253] Gene amplification techniques are more sensitive and may replace cell culture as the method of choice in detecting toxoplasma para-

sitemia.[150] The use of gene amplification assays is particularly promising in the diagnosis of toxoplasma parasitemia in AIDS patients who have unexplained fever and/or central nervous system abnormalities.[106] Examination of blood by PCR may also be useful in diagnosing extracerebral toxoplasmosis from the local reactivation of latent brain cysts.[96] Dupon and coworkers,[95] also found the PCR examination of CSF or blood to be a valuable adjunct in detecting reactivation of latent cerebral toxoplasmosis. In addition to detecting the *T. gondii B1* nucleic acid sequences, they cite other studies successfully using p30, TGR1 genes, and the 18S rDNA as targets.

BOX 20-9. INTERPRETATIONS OF SEROLOGIC RESULTS IN CLINICAL SYNDROMES OF TOXOPLASMOSIS

I. *Acute acquired toxoplasmosis in an immunocompetent patient:* The diagnosis can be highly suspected if
  A. Seroconversion from negative to positive is demonstrated.
  B. A twofold increase in titer between a baseline sample and a repeat test 3 weeks later.
  C. A high IgM titer with a single high IgG titer (greater than 1:1000).
  D. A low titer in the DS-IgM-ELISA test indicates that the infection was acquired 4 months or more before. *Note:* A negative dye or IFA test result in an immunocompetent person virtually precludes the diagnosis of acute toxoplasmosis.

II. *Acute acquired toxoplasmosis in an immunoincompetent patient:* The criteria cited for immunocompetent patients apply to immunoincompetent individuals as well. However, IgM antibody or twofold rises in IgG antibody often is not detected; therefore, a negative test does not rule out acute toxoplasmosis. Organisms must be demonstrated in tissue biopsies or impression

smears of aspirates before a secure diagnosis can be made in this group of patients.

III. *Ocular toxoplasmosis:* The diagnosis can be suspected if
  A. Low titers of IgG antibody are found in the presence of a typical retinal lesion.
  B. If *C* is equal to or greater than 8 using the following formula when testing aqueous humor fluid:

$$C = \frac{\text{Antibody titer in fluid} \times \text{concentration of gamma globulin in serum}}{\text{Antibody titer in serum} \times \text{concentration of gamma globulin in body fluid}}$$

IV. *Congenital toxoplasmosis:* The diagnosis of toxoplasma infection in the neonate can be established if
  A. There is a persistent or rising titer in the dye or IFA test
  B. A positive IgM test at any titer after birth in the absence of a placental leak (DS-IgM-ELISA test preferred)

Adapted from McCabe and Remington.[225]

A broad spectrum of signs and symptoms may be encountered in cases of human toxoplasmosis. Given the high prevalence of seropositivity in certain populations, reported as high as 90% in some regions of El Salvador, Tahiti, and France (an average of 20% in the United States),[225] millions of healthy people are or have been infected with *T. gondii*. Yet, symptoms are absent or overlooked in all but about 10% of cases, and the incidence of progressive disease is very low.

Symptomatic acute toxoplasmosis in immunocompetent humans presents as generalized lymphadenopathy, particularly of the cervical area of the neck. If accompanied by sore throat, fever, and myalgias, the disease complex may simulate infectious mononucleosis. The disease is usually self-limited; however, overt disseminated disease may rarely develop. Myocarditis, pneumonitis, and encephalitis may occur in varying degrees of severity, and may mimic other disseminated diseases, such as tuberculosis, sarcoidosis, tularemia, lymphoma, or leukemia. The outcome may be fatal in severe cases. Pyrimethamine, 75 mg/d for 3 days and 25 mg for 3 to 4 weeks thereafter in combination with sulfadiazine, 500 mg four times daily, is the recommended adult therapy. Children should receive pyrimethamine 2 mg/kg for 3 days followed by 1 mg/kg for 3 weeks in combination with sulfadiazine 25 mg/kg four times per day.

Immunosuppressed persons are highly susceptible to infection with *T. gondii*, either acquired from new exposures or from reactivation of old disease. A marked increase in incidence of symptomatic disease has been found among homosexual men and parenteral drug abusers.[353] In fact, AIDS or drug abuse should be suspected for any patient with a diagnosis of toxoplasmosis.

The disease often localizes in the CNS with symptoms of encephalitis (Fig. 20-31) or meningoencephalitis, or manifests as a space-occupying lesion.[207,279] The disease can progress rapidly and usually terminates in death if the compromised immune status remains unchanged. Pulmonary, cardiac, and lymphoreticular disease may also be present. The CSF typically shows high protein levels and an increase in mononuclear inflammatory cells.

Tachyzoites circulating in the blood of an infected pregnant woman transmigrate the placenta and are widely distributed in the fetal tissues. Term infants with a full component of maternal IgG antibody often withstand the infections; premature or antibody-deficient infants are more susceptible to developing progressive disease. General symptoms, such as splenomegaly, jaundice, fever, and lymphadenopathy, may be seen. The CNS is particularly susceptible and symptoms may vary. Impaired vision, convulsions, mental retardation, spasticity, hydrocephalus, microcephalus, and deafness are among the more common symptoms. Newborns who are asymptomatic at birth may develop late-onset disease; spinal or subarachnoid punctures should be performed in suspected cases to make the diagnosis. Grover and associates[137] recently report the application of PCR in the early diagnosis of congenital toxoplasma infection. This technique is based on direct lysis of pelleted amniotic fluid cells followed by PCR amplification of a gene sequence specific for *T. gondii*. The PCR correctly identified the presence of *T. gondii* in five amniotic fluid samples obtained from four patients with proved congenital infection in the study cited.

Vitreous exudate and bilateral retinochoroiditis of the macula are common ocular signs of congenital toxoplasmosis. Symptoms may not manifest until the second or third decade of life. Chorioretinitis with blurred vision, photophobia, and ocular pain may be seen in acquired cases; however, it is usually unilateral.

Pneumocystis carinii.   *P. carinii* is a microorganism the exact classification of which is still uncertain. Morphologically *P. carinii* appears to be a protozoan and has been considered by many as a sporozoan with a reproductive life cycle including schizogony and the periodic release of trophozoites. However, others favor the possibility of it being a fungus, namely an ascosporogenous yeast that, in keeping with other fungi, takes up the methenamine silver stain. Edman and coworkers[98] and later Stranger and associates,[313] using techniques that classify organisms based on an analysis of DNA sequences, also have demonstrated that *P. carinii* genetically is more closely aligned with the fungi. Hadley and Ng,[139a] in the 1995 edition of the *ASM Manual*, include the separate chapter on *P. carinii* in the mycology section of the text, citing the following features suggesting phylogenetic relatedness to fungi:

1. Cyst wall ultrastructure similar to that of fungal cell wall
2. Lamellar cristae in the mitochondria (protozoans have tubular cristae)
3. Formation of intracystic bodies resembling the formation of ascospores by the ascomycetes
4. Highest homology of the more conserved domains of the 16S rRNA subunit with that of ascomycetes
5. Homology of the protein synthesis elongation factor EF-3 with that of the ascomycete *Saccharomyces cerevisiae*
6. Separate proteins for thymidylate synthase and dihydrofolate reductase (protozoa produce a single bifunctional protein)
7. Homology of the sequence encoding pneumocystis thymidylate synthase with that of an ascomycete

The foregoing features notwithstanding, the practical laboratory consideration remains that *P. carinii* cannot be cultured on common laboratory or cell-free culture systems. Therefore, it is unlikely that the laboratory diagnosis of *P. carinii* will be relegated to the mycology section of most clinical laboratories in the near future. The considerations raised by Frenkel and associates[112] have not been completely addressed. Thus, for the current edition of this text, and until the taxonomists officially reclassify *P. carinii* as an ascomycete, we elect not to make the shift to the chapter on mycology and leave it here for the present. Laboratory workers will continue to approach the detection and identification of this organism as before and will

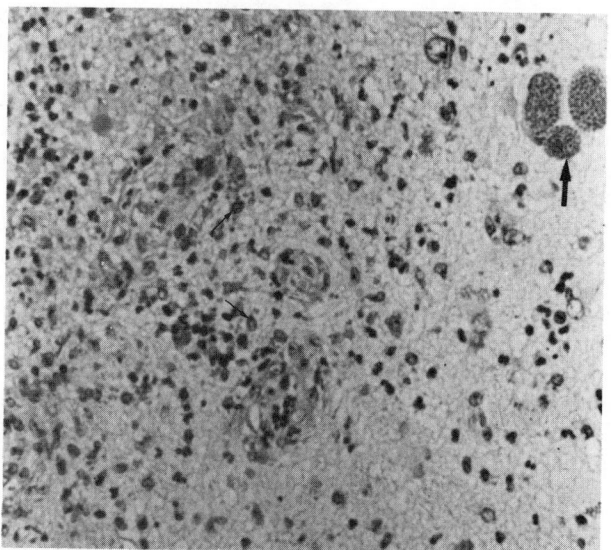

Figure 20-31
Tissue section of brain of a patient dying with AIDS illustrating a central area of necrosis characterized by capillary endothelial proliferation, vascular thrombosis, and a perivascular infiltration with mononuclear inflammatory cells. Tiny spherical forms (*small arrows*), suspicious for intracellular trophozoites, can be seen in the areas of necrosis; diagnostic toxoplasma pseudocysts are seen in the *upper right corner* (*large arrows*). This most likely represents a case of latent toxoplasmosis with immunosuppression-induced exacerbation of disease (H & E × 450).

be able to find the description here, albeit perhaps with the use of the index.

P. carinii is the etiologic agent of two distinct clinical forms of pneumocystosis: 1) epidemic plasma cell pneumonia, occurring in debilitated or premature infants between 3 and 6 months of age who have severe IgG and IgA deficiency; and 2) hypoergic, hypoimmune pneumocystosis, occurring sporadically in both adults and children who are receiving immunosuppressive drugs or prolonged antibiotic therapy.[113,336]

Beginning in the 1920s and extending into the 1950s, several epidemics of fatal plasma cell pneumonia were reported in nurseries, foundling homes, or hospitals with large populations of immunosuppressed children in Germany, France, Switzerland, Sweden, Finland, Italy, Hungary, and other European countries.[113] The etiology of the plasma cell pneumonia was not known until 1951 when Vanek[324] demonstrated the causative microorganisms in the alveolar exudates of infected patients.

The sporadic form occurs clinically only in relatively few patients who are receiving immunosuppressive therapy, usually in treatment of leukemia, lymphocytic neoplasms and immunodeficiency disease, and in transplant recipients.[336] Whereas epidemic plasma cell pneumonia probably involves human-to-human transmission, the sporadic form more likely represents activation of an inapparent chronic infection or carrier state, a situation similar to the delayed

clinical manifestations of slow virus infection. The possibility of a carrier state for *P. carinii* may also explain the relatively common coexistence of pneumocystosis with cytomegalovirus and herpes infections.

Pneumocystosis is among the more common causes of nonbacterial pneumonia in immunocompromised hosts in the United States[10] and is a leading cause of death in patients with AIDS.[185,220,232] Pifer and associates[263] also found *P. carinii* to be a common agent of pneumonia in pediatric patients with AIDS, many of whom acquired the disease through blood transfusions. Several reports in the recent medical literature cite an increasing incidence of extrapulmonary pneumocystosis, primarily in patients with AIDS. Cohen and Stroeckle[61] reviewed 37 such cases, 19 of which occurred in the absence of recognized pneumonia. The possible modes of infection among these patients included blood and lymphatic dissemination, unmasking of latent infections in extrapulmonary sites, or primary infections at these sites.

Following are select extrapulmonary sites of involvement as cited in these papers: bone marrow in a patient with coexistent malignant lymphoma and AIDS;[278] liver in a patient with concurrent pneumonia;[283] a plaquelike tumor of the small intestine in a patient without pneumonia;[44] skin of the right ear;[64] the temporal bone in two patients;[33] and the thyroid in two independently reported cases, one in a 38-year-old African-American with diffuse enlargement of the left lobe[115] and the other in a 38-year-old man with thyroiditis.[92]

Dyspnea, fever, nonproductive cough, cyanosis, rales, and hepatosplenomegaly are the most common clinical signs and symptoms of pulmonary pneumocystosis. The disease may be fulminant and rapidly fatal, particularly in the sporadic form.[336] Although the fatality rate is high among untreated patients, pneumocystosis is curable in most cases by instituting prompt antimicrobial therapy. Trimethoprim–sulfamethoxazole or pentamidine are the drugs usually chosen.

Histologically, pulmonary pneumocystosis is characterized by an alveolar exudation having a foamy or honeycomb matrix. A heavy interstitial infiltrate with chronic inflammatory cells, notably plasma cells, is seen in infants with the epidemic form of the disease, a component not present in sporadic pneumocystosis.[10] The honeycomb effect, as seen in H & E-stained tissue sections, is due to the presence of cysts measuring 5 to 8 μm in diameter, best demonstrated by Gomori methenamine silver (GMS) stain, or the rapid toluidine blue stain described by Chalvardjian and Grawe.[50] The cyst walls absorb the GMS stain, and the organisms appear deep blue-black (see Color Plate 20-7H, *left*). Schwartz and coauthors[296] currently report that plastic embedding of bronchial or lung biopsies, staining with silver methenamine borate with a toluidine blue counterstain, and high-resolution light microscopy permits simultaneous observation of both the cyst wall and the intracystic sporozoites. Schumann and Swensen[294] report that the Papanicolaou stain is equally as sensitive as the GMS stain in detecting pneumocystis organisms in bronchoalveolar lavage specimens, precluding the need for using more complicated staining techniques.

Because yeast cells, particularly those of *Torulopsis glabrata* and *Histoplasma capsulatum*, may morphologically simulate *P. carinii* cysts in GMS-stained tissue sections, further studies, including cultures, may be required to confirm the diagnosis. The morphology of *P. carinii* cysts can best be demonstrated in GMS-stained touch preparations made from a fresh cut of lung surface or in smears of respiratory secretions. The cysts stain pale blue-gray, and most appear collapsed and empty. The diagnostic forms are those that contain internal structures appearing as opposing parentheses.

Bronchoalveolar lavage (BAL) has proved to be a superior method for the recovery and demonstration of *P. carinii* organisms.[129] The procedure is performed using a flexible fiberoptic bronchoscope with an outer diameter of 6 mm. The tip of the bronchoscope is wedged in a segmental bronchus in a lobe of lung judged by chest radiograph to be affected. Aliquots of 35 mL of sterile 0.9% saline solution are injected through the biopsy channel of the bronchoscope. The injected saline solution is aspirated into a sterile sputum trap. The total amount of saline solution used is 70 to 250 mL, of which 40% to 70% is removed. Smears are prepared from the centrifuged sediment and are processed as previously described.

Recent studies indicate that induced sputum specimens, when properly collected, are also valuable in establishing a diagnosis of pneumocystis pneumonia in a significant proportion of patients.[28,178,368] Although the sensitivity of detection is in the range of only 56% to 78% in cases ultimately proved to be positive, this technique is rapid, low-cost, and innocuous. Thus, even with this relatively low sensitivity, the need for more invasive procedures can be eliminated in from over one-half to three-fourths of cases.

The use of Gram-Weigert and Giemsa stains on fresh lung specimens can be recommended. Gram-Weigert stains, which take 20 minutes to perform, may be used to detect cysts, but not trophozoites of *P. carinii* in frozen sections and impression smears. Cysts are 5 to 7 μm in diameter and stain blue to purple. Traditional Giemsa stains, which take 45 to 60 minutes, have been useful in demonstrating trophozoites, which measure 1.5 to 4 μm in diameter and stain with red nuclei and light blue cytoplasm. An even more rapid, modified Giemsa stain, commercially marketed as Diff-Quick, reduces the time for staining to 10 minutes. The cell walls do not stain; rather, one observes small bluish-staining spheres within which several reddish-staining trophozoites may be observed (see Color Plate 20-7H, *right*).

Cregan and coworkers[65] found this stain to be inexpensive, easy to prepare, and suitable for identification of sporozoites and also of cysts (which appear negatively stained). However, because of the heavy staining of background material, particularly when examining induced sputum, bronchoscopy, or bronchoalveolar lavage specimens, interpretation of smears requires a high level of technical expertise. Although the staining time is "quick," the extra time required to search for pneumocystis organisms makes the overall procedure not so rapid. This time for search can be reduced if the microscopist screens bits of cyst-containing foamy appearing debris, which represent aggregates of alveolar secretions where the pneumocystis organisms reside.

A rapid and easily prepared modified toluidine blue O stain for *P. carinii* has been described by Gosey and associates.[129] The stain employs a sulfonation reagent that removes background material, leaving the *P. carinii* cysts easy to visualize. They found that adding the coverslip to the slide while it was still moist with xylene resulted in a brighter, easier to read slide. The major advantage of the stain is that reports can be issued within 1 hour after receipt of specimens.

Organisms can also be demonstrated by immunofluorescent techniques, using fluorescein-tagged antibodies prepared from immune rats or immunized rabbits, or from serum pooled from humans with active disease. In a study of 100 mixed induced sputum and bronchoalveolar lavage specimens,[65] both the direct and indirect immunofluorescence assays were 92% sensitive in detecting *P. carinii* organisms. A new direct immunofluorescence method using a monoclonal antibody is commercially available from Genetic Systems, Inc., Seattle, Washington. Wolfson and coworkers[352] found a specificity of greater than 99% and a false-positive rate of less than 1% in detecting *P. carinii* in bronchoalveolar lavage specimens obtained from 67 patients with AIDS. Although the staining procedure takes approximately 1 hour to complete, screening is very rapid, making the overall time of detection comparable with the Diff-Quick procedure.

A presumptive serodiagnosis can be made in suspected cases of pneumocystis infections.[334] Complement fixation (CF) titers of 1:4 or higher usually indicate active disease. Latex agglutination tests for *P. carinii* have proved positive in only about one third of patients with known disease. However, serodiagnosis is somewhat complicated because *P. carinii* is a ubiquitous organism, and many individuals have background titers from previous exposure. In one study,[317] 90% of patients with *P. carinii* pneumonia had anti-*P. carinii* antibody titers of 1:40 or higher, as assayed by indirect immunofluorescence. Antibody titers occurred in early stages of pneumonia and reached peak levels during the febrile stage. However, these authors found that high titers did not necessarily reflect acute active infections; rather, they were also seen in patients with old subclinical infections. Thus, serial monitoring of patients is necessary to demonstrate a fourfold or greater increase in antibody titer before a diagnosis could be confirmed.

The applications of PCR-based assays in the detection of *P. carinii* DNA offer new laboratory possibilities in the rapid and accurate diagnosis of pneumocystis infections. Olsson and associates,[247] using a primer pair selected from a published sequence of the thymidylate synthase gene of *P. carinii*, were able to amplify and demonstrate *P. carinii* DNA in 30 of 42 sputum samples obtained from immunosuppressed patients (in contrast to only 21 of 42 samples positive by indirect immunofluorescence). The PCR in particular was more sensitive than IFL in detecting *P. carinii* in a subgroup of patients receiving prophylactic chemotherapy.

Other recent PCR-based studies were by Tamburrini and coworkers,[315] who describe a rapid two-step procedure for the diagnosis of *P. carinii* infections, and Roux and associates,[280] who also compared PCR detection of parasitic forms in BAL, induced sputum, and blood samples relative to that of standard-staining techniques. In a study of 67 BAL specimens, their PCR technique detected *P. carinii* in 100% of an untreated HIV-seropositive subgroup of patients, although the authors admit that this technique had no diagnostic advantage over direct-staining methods. The advantage of PCR was in a subgroup of seven PCR-negative patients undergoing treatment, in whom the parasite burden was low in respiratory secretions, yet in whom rare cysts were identified in BAL specimens by IFI. They conclude that PCR may be able to discriminate false-positive specimens that are without genetic material and, therefore, presumably indicate drug efficacy in treated cases.

MISCELLANEOUS LARVAL TISSUE PARASITE INFECTIONS

Humans may be inadvertent intermediate or accidental hosts for several nematodes and cestodes that have life cycles in other animals. The adults of these species normally reside in the intestinal tract or select tissues of the definitive hosts; humans become infected by ingesting either the larvae in poorly cooked meat, or by the fertile ova. Of particular concern in the United States is the potential increased exposure to a variety of helminthic parasites through the ingestion of uncooked seafood in the form of dishes such as sushi, sashimi, lomi lomi salmon, pickled herring, and the like. Because humans are not the natural definitive host for certain of these parasites, the larvae often aimlessly wander among tissues and organs, either forming cysticercoid lesions or areas of granulomatous inflammation. The following larval parasitic diseases will be discussed: nematodes, including *Trichinella spiralis* (pig, bear, walrus intestinal nematode), *Toxocara canis* or *Toxocara cati* (dog and cat ascarids), *Ancylostoma braziliense* or *A. caninum* (dog and cat hookworms), *Anisakis* species (fish or sea mammal nematodes), *Gnathostoma spinigerum* (dog and cat gastric nematode), *Angiostrongylus* species; and cestodes, including *Echinococcus granulosus* (dog tapeworm), *Echinococcus multilocularis* (dog, fox, wolf, cat tapeworm), *Multiceps* species (coenurosis), *Spirometra mansonoides* (sparganum; dog or cat *Diphyllobothrium* tapeworm).

Trichinosis. Trichinosis is a disease of carnivores caused by infection with the nematode *Trichinella spiralis*, resulting from ingestion of raw or poorly cooked meat. The life cycle is illustrated in Figure 20-32. Humans are accidental hosts and are most commonly infected through ingestion of pork or pork products that contain encysted larvae.[132] Infections have also been reported after ingestion of poorly cooked bear meat.[60] Smoking, salting, or drying the meat does not destroy the infective larval forms; however, prolonged freezing (20 days in the average home freezer) decontaminates the meat. The disease has a worldwide distribution; in the United States, 4% of human cadavers were found to be infected in 1968.[132] Fewer than 50 new cases are currently reported each year in the United States,[48] a tribute to the meat inspection program and the stringent laws against feeding uncooked garbage to pigs.

The larvae are released in the intestine, where they burrow into the villi. After molting, the trichinellae develop into adult male and female worms, measuring from 2 to 4 mm in length. The average life span of the adults in the intestine is about 4 months; however, during that time each female releases as many as 3000 larval offspring. These larvae enter the circulation and are deposited throughout the tissues of the body, where most are killed. However, many of those that reach the skeletal muscle become encysted and survive. These larval forms coil 2½ times on themselves and are associated with granulomatous foci of infection within muscle fibers (Fig. 20-33 and see Color Plate 20-7I). The adjacent muscle fibers undergo degeneration so that a cyst measuring about 0.25 to 0.50 mm develops. In time, these inflammatory cystic lesions may undergo calcification. Wakelin[331] poses the interesting possibility that host immunity acts to limit parasite survival; however, it also helps to ensure transmission by allowing the host to survive, providing time for the infective stages of the parasite to mature.

Most infections are subclinical. The minimal number of ingested larvae required to produce symptoms is about 100, and a fatal dose is estimated to be 300,000.[132] Fever, muscle pain and aching, periorbital edema, and peripheral blood eosinophilia are the cardinal features by which a clinical diagnosis can be made. Mebendazole 100 mg three times a day for 3 days is the recommended therapy.

LABORATORY DIAGNOSIS. The laboratory diagnosis of trichinosis is most commonly made by detecting the spiral larvae in muscle tissue (see Fig. 20-33 on page 1145 and Color Plate 20-7I). The deltoid muscle of the upper arm or the gastrocnemius muscle of the calf are usually selected for biopsy. The specimen may be examined by first digesting the muscle fibers with trypsin and then mounting some of the digested tissue on a microscope slide, or by preparing a tease preparation of the muscle tissue in a drop of saline solution and squeezing it between two microscope slides. Linear or spiral larval forms may also be observed in stained tissue sections, although their morphology is not as well delineated.

Mahannop and coworkers,[211] using crude antigens obtained from the infective stage larvae of *T. spiralis* in an ELISA system for detecting serum IgG antibodies to *T. spiralis*, reported a 100% sensitivity in a group of patients with confirmed trichinelliasis. They found cross-reactions in sera collected from patients with capillariasis, gnathostomiasis, opisthorchiasis, and strongyloidiasis. Similarly, Raungkunaporon and associates[270] reported 81% and 92% sensitivities for the

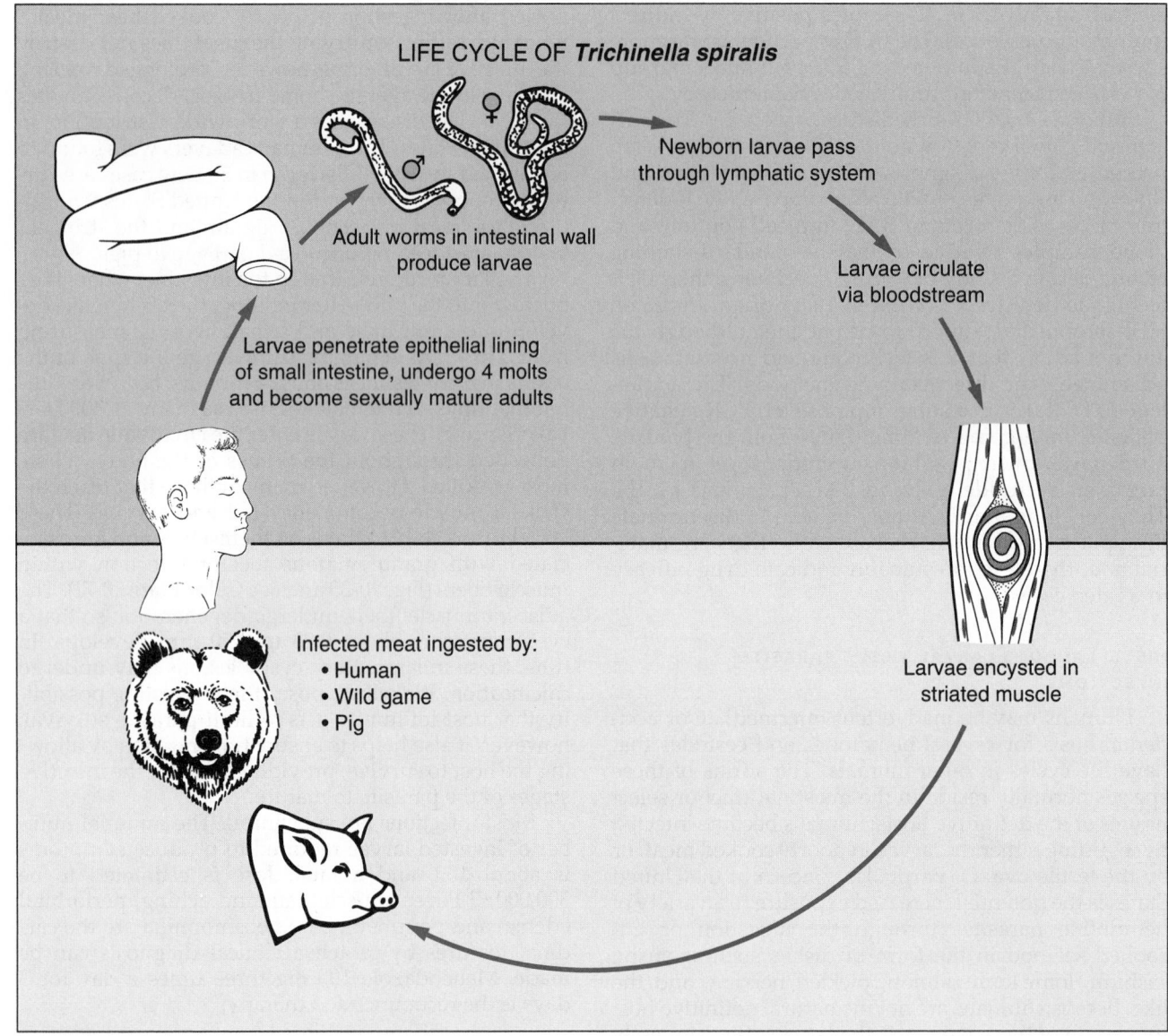

Figure 20-32
Life cycle of *Trichinella spiralis*.

detection of trichinosis antigens by indirect ELISA and Western blotting assays, respectively.

Visceral Larval Migrans. *Toxocara canis*, the dog intestinal roundworm with a life cycle similar to that of human *Ascaris lumbricoides*, is the most common cause of larva migrans. Larva migrans is a condition in which the larvae of nematode parasites of lower animals migrate into the tissues of humans without further development. Larva migrans may be caused by many different species of parasites and may affect either cutaneous or visceral tissues, depending on the body areas affected and the parasites involved.

In *T. canis* infection, humans become an accidental host through ingestion of embryonated eggs in the soil. The disease is most common in children because of their close association with dogs and their inadvertent ingestion of soil. The embryonated eggs hatch in the in-

testine of the human host, liberating the larvae which, in turn, penetrate the bowel wall and enter the circulation. However, because humans are abnormal hosts, the lung cycle is not completed; rather, the larvae are filtered out in various organs, chiefly the liver. They may cause local tissue reactions or granulomas, but the larvae eventually die out with no sequelae. The infection can be suspected in a child with hepatomegaly, nonspecific pulmonary disease, and a high peripheral blood eosinophilia.

Buijs and coauthors[39] report that the seroprevalence of toxocara in the Netherlands is 11% in The Hague and 6% in Rotterdam. They found a significant correlation of recurrent asthma and bronchitis in toxocara-seropositive children. They speculate that elevated allergen-specific IgE in these patients may account for the asthma. Jacquier and associates[164] evaluated a commercial ELISA kit marketed by Biokema-Affinity Prod-

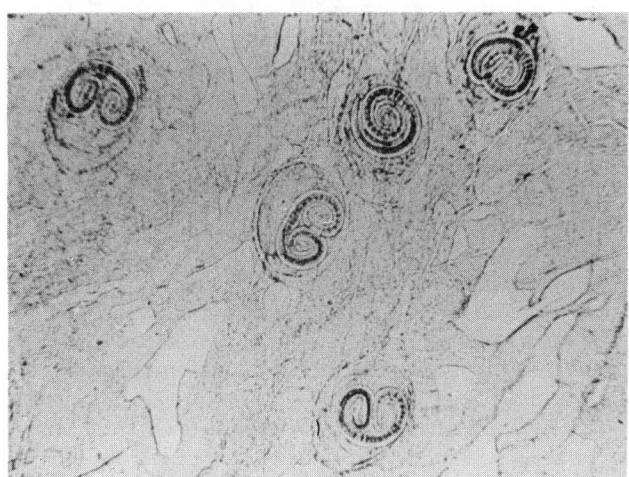

Figure 20-33
High-power view of tease preparation of skeletal muscle showing infestation with *T. spiralis* larvae.

ucts, Crissier-Lausanne, Switzerland, which is based on excretory–secretory antigen derived from second-stage *T. canis* larvae. In a survey of 1000 serum samples randomly collected from healthy blood donors and children in Switzerland, the seroprevalence of toxocariasis was 2.7%. Of the positive samples, the Biokema kit had an overall diagnostic sensitivity of 91% and a specificity of 86%. The lower specificity was due to cross-reactivity with some other helminth infections.

Cutaneous Larval Migrans. The filariform larvae of dog or cat hookworms, commonly of the species *Ancylostoma braziliense* and *A. caninum*, are capable of penetrating the exposed skin of humans, producing a pruritic, papular condition known as "creeping eruption." The larvae penetrate deeply into the subcutaneous tissue and produce linear tracts that extend for several millimeters each day. This deep tissue migration may lead to lung infections. *Ancylostoma* species infections must be included in the differential diagnosis when peripheral blood eosinophilia and Charcot-Leyden crystals are microscopically detected in sputum samples. The diagnosis is made by a history of exposure and the presence of subcutaneous linear tracts. Biopsies of suspicious lesions are of little help in establishing a diagnosis, showing only an eosinophilic cellular infiltrate.

Anisakiasis. Anisakiasis is a zoonotic disease in which humans, through the ingestion of raw, pickled, smoked, or poorly cooked seafood such as sushi, sashimi, pickled herrings, and the like, become an accidental host for the larval nematodes belonging to the genera *Anisakias*, *Phocanema*, and *Contracaecum*. The number of infections in the United States has increased as raw fish dishes, such as lomi lomi salmon, sushi, and sashimi have become popular. Doardorff and Kent[89] report that only wild-caught salmon were infected; those pen-reared were free of infection. Thus, knowing the origin of the fresh fish may help in avoiding infections.

After entering the stomach with the raw fish meal, the larvae penetrate into the wall, forming small tunnels and burrows amid a dense granulomatous inflammatory reaction.[284] In some cases, mucosal ulcers can be identified. Nausea and vomiting may be experienced within 24 hours after ingesting contaminated fish. Later manifestations include sharp, periodic, upper abdominal pain and diarrhea, at times simulating gastritis, duodenal ulcer, or on occasion, acute appendicitis. Larvae may on occasion migrate beyond the stomach producing metastatic infections in the omentum, liver, pancreas, and lungs.[284] Minamoto and coauthors[233] report two cases of anisakiasis of the colon. Matsumoto and associates[222] report the endoscopic and radiologic findings in six patients with colon infections. Luminal narrowing and thumbprinting, with demonstration of the worm in four cases were the radiologic features of these cases. Treatment consists of surgically excising the areas of granulomatous inflammation including the worm.

Ikeda and associates[161] report on the successful treatment of nine patients with gastric anisakiasis by removing the causative larval worms through an endoscope, which immediately alleviated the acute abdominal pain. Yaquihashi and associates[364] report on the successful diagnosis of anisakiasis using a microenzyme-linked immunosorbent assay, with a monoclonal antibody directed against a specific *A. simplex* antigen. However, this approach is limited to a few research or reference laboratories because commercial reagents are not currently available. Surgical removal of the worm granuloma or thiabendazole, 25 mg/kg three times a day for 3 days is the recommended therapy.

Gnathostomiasis. *Gnathostoma spinigerum* is a nematode that normally infects the intestinal tract of cats and dogs. However, humans may become accidental hosts by ingesting poorly cooked or pickled seafoods. The disease is endemic in the Far East. In the cat or dog, ingested larvae develop in the stomach or intestinal wall into adults that produce granulomatous lesions. In humans, however, the larvae do not mature, rather they penetrate the gastric wall and migrate throughout the tissues. Deep cutaneous or subcutaneous tunnels may develop, simulating cutaneous larva migrans, or hard nonpitting painful swellings may occur. A recent case of intestinal gnathostomiasis was reported by Hira and associates[149] in a Thai resident living in Kuwait, who presented with acute pain in the right iliac fossa. A mass of the terminal ileum and cecum was removed, revealing an immature male *G. spinigerum* worm. Nawa[240] reports that, in addition to *G. spinigerum*, three other *Gnathostoma* species cause disease in humans living in Japan: *G. hispidum*, *G. nipponicum*, and *G. doloresi*. Cases of infections with *G. hispidum* and *G. nipponicum* occurred in patients eating raw loaches imported from Taiwan, Korea, and mainland China; *G. doloresi* infections were secondary to eating raw slices of freshwater fishes.

These helminth infections, although rare, must be included in the differential diagnosis of various obscure visceral and cutaneous diseases, particularly in persons native to the Orient or in individuals with the habit of ingesting raw seafood. Surgical removal of the worm granuloma or drug treatment with mebendazole, or both, are recommended.

Angiostrongyliasis.   Human angiostrongyliasis is caused by the larvae of nematodes, the adults of which live in rats as the definitive host. The disease presents in humans in two clinical forms depending on the species: *A. cantonensis*, endemic in Thailand, Tahiti, and Taiwan, among other South Pacific locales, causes a syndrome of meningitis, eosinophilic pleocytosis in the CSF, and peripheral blood eosinophilia (known as eosinophilic meningitis). *A. costaricensis*, the rat lungworm, endemic primarily in Costa Rica, with reported cases also in Mexico and in Central and South America, causes abdominal disease primarily of the distal small intestine and ascending colon, the sites of penetration by the developing larvae.

The adult female produces eggs at the site of infection in the rat lung, which are then swallowed and passed in the feces. Slugs, land snails, and other mollusks (less commonly also freshwater prawns, land crabs, and frogs) ingest these eggs and serve as an intermediate host within which the infective third-stage larvae develop. Humans acquire the infection by ingesting foods, usually leafy vegetables, contaminated with infected snails and slugs. After ingestion by humans, the larvae migrate to the brain causing eosinophilic meningitis. Symptoms vary from mild headache, stiff neck, and weakness, to more full-blown symptoms including nausea, vomiting, pruritic skin rash, and a variety of neurologic symptoms, including paresthesias, fourth and sixth cranial nerve palsies, and in heavy infections, coma and death.

Witoonpanich and coauthors[349] report two fatal cases out of three infected in one family. Two days after ingestion of pila snails, all three patients developed a generalized itchy maculopapular rash followed by myalgia, marked paresthesia, fever, and headache. Weakness of the extremities, urine retention, and cloudiness of consciousness, progressing to coma were experienced by the two patients with a fatal outcome. Autopsy revealed multiple tracks and cavities with the presence of *A. cantonensis* in the brain and various levels of the spinal cord.

In the normal host, the rat, *A. costaricensis* adults occupy arteries and arterioles of in the ileocecal part of the intestine. Eggs deposited in the rat tissue hatch and escape in the feces. Slugs also serve as intermediate hosts, and humans become infected by ingesting slug-contaminated foods. The larvae penetrate the tissues in the ileocecal portion of the human intestine, including the appendix, where a combination of the adult worms and the deposited eggs causes a severe granulomatous inflammatory reaction, resulting in the formation of a tumorlike mass. Hulbert and associates[160] report two cases of *A. costaricensis* infections in children acquired within the United States. One patient presented with symptoms suggestive of acute appendicitis, the other with a possible Meckel's diverticulum.

The diagnosis is usually made in patients in endemic areas on the basis of the symptoms described, together with increased eosinophils seen in the spinal fluid and in the peripheral blood. An ELISA serologic test has been described;[182] however, this test is not readily available.

Echinococcosis (Hydatid Disease).   Echinococcosis, or hydatid disease, is possibly one of the more difficult parasitic diseases to understand because of the peculiar cystic lesions that form when the larval stages of the parasite invade the viscera. Two species with somewhat different morphology and patterns of behavior may be encountered, *Echinococcus granulosus* and *E. multicellularis*. Humans serve as accidental hosts for both species. The normal life cycle of *E. granulosa* involves dogs or foxes as the definitive hosts, within the intestines of which the adult tapeworms reside. They measure about 3 to 6 mm in length and possess three proglottides and a scolex armed with a double row of hooklets (Fig. 20-34). Sheep, cattle, or swine serve as the intermediate hosts and develop cystic larval disease to be described in the following. *E. multilocularis* differs slightly in this regard because the definitive hosts are dogs, foxes, wolves, and cats, whereas the intermediate hosts are small rodents, including squirrels, field mice, and voles. If humans are infected, they are also intermediate hosts in whom the larval form of the parasite is harbored. The life cycle is illustrated in Figure 20-35.

Hexacanth eggs, closely resembling those of *Taenia* species, are passed in dog feces and become embryonated in the soil. Under normal circumstances, these eggs are ingested by the natural intermediate hosts— sheep, cattle, or swine, or by the small rodents mentioned for *E. multilocularis*. The larvae are released from the eggs in the intestines of the intermediate hosts and, by means of their hooklets, bore through the bowel wall and enter the circulation.

The circulating embryos are filtered out in the capillaries of various organs, usually the liver because it is

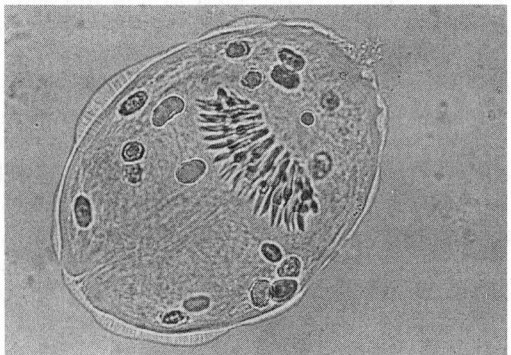

Figure 20-34
Photomicrograph of a single grain of "hydatid sand" illustrating a protoscolex with a prominent row of hooklets, representing the anlage of the armed rostellum of the adult worm (×1000).

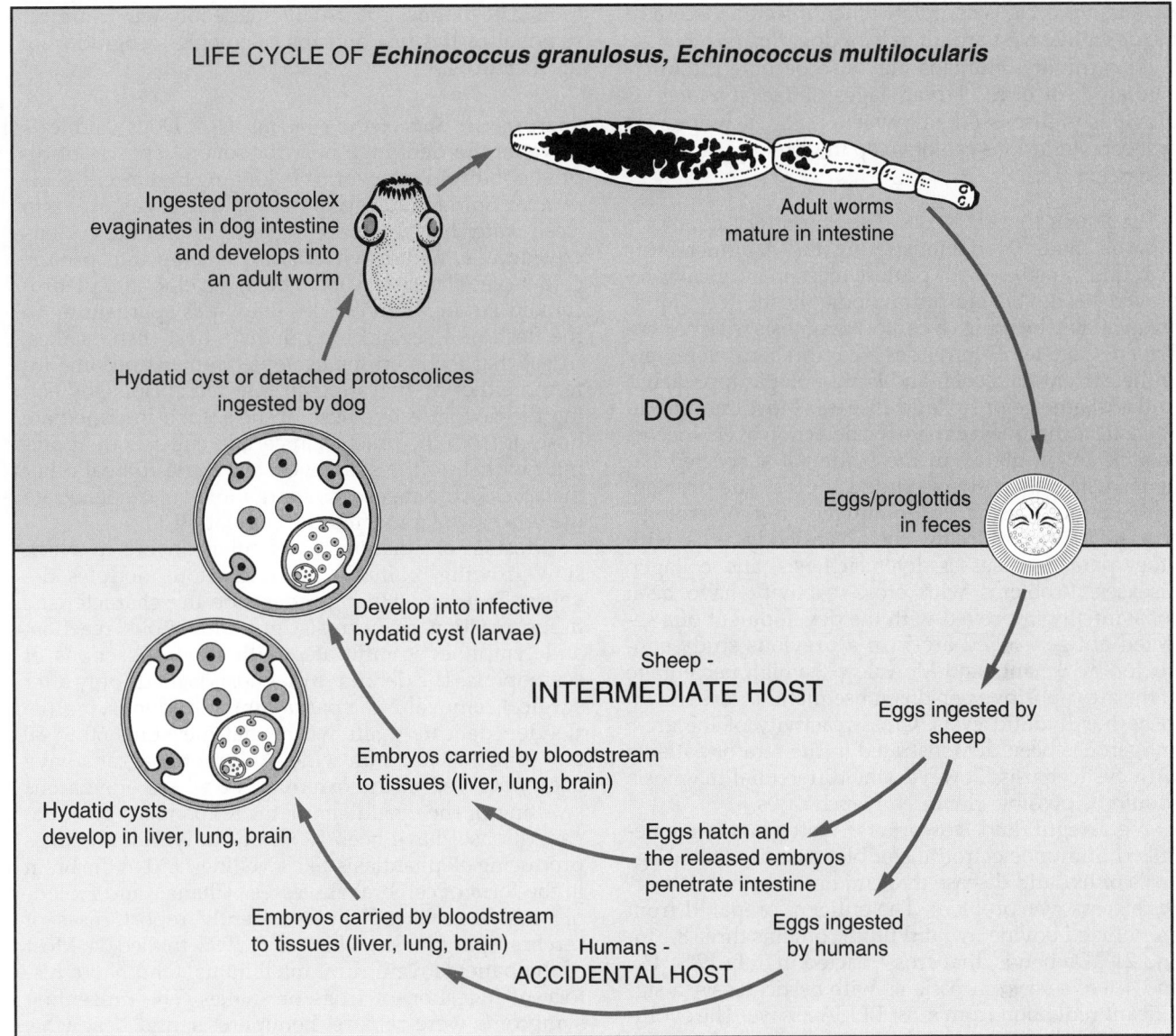

LIFE CYCLE OF *Echinococcus granulosus, Echinococcus multilocularis*

Ingested protoscolex evaginates in dog intestine and develops into an adult worm

Adult worms mature in intestine

Hydatid cyst or detached protoscolices ingested by dog

DOG

Eggs/proglottids in feces

Develop into infective hydatid cyst (larvae)

Sheep - INTERMEDIATE HOST

Eggs ingested by sheep

Embryos carried by bloodstream to tissues (liver, lung, brain)

Hydatid cysts develop in liver, lung, brain

Eggs hatch and the released embryos penetrate intestine

Embryos carried by bloodstream to tissues (liver, lung, brain)

Humans - ACCIDENTAL HOST

Eggs ingested by humans

Figure 20-35
Life cycle of *Echinococcus granulosus.*

the first organ to drain the mesenteric blood. Within the organ, *E. granulosus* produces a single multilayered cyst (see Color Plate 20-7J), or small cysts called *bladder worms* may form. The cysts of *E. multilocularis*, as the species name would imply, have multiple locules. Multiple cysts up to 5 cm in diameter, resembling what Aristotle called hailstones, may be seen in some cases.

The inner lining of the cyst is a germinal membrane from which numerous protoscoleces develop. These form as tiny polypoid structures (brood capsules) that line the inner reproductive membrane from which large numbers of daughter cysts (hydatid sand) are produced (see Color Plate 20-7J, *left*). When the embryos break free from the membrane and float in the fluid within the cyst, they are known as hydatid sand or individually as protoscolices (see Color Plate 20-7J, *right*). If examined under the microscope, each grain of

sand is, in fact, a tiny embryonic beginning of a new tapeworm, complete with an inverted scolex, with a rostellum armed with hooklets (see Fig. 20-35). The cysts of *E. granulosis* slowly grow and usually remain quiescent for many years. Only rarely do cysts rupture, at times into the biliary tract, and at other times through the liver capsule into the peritoneal cavity. If the cyst should rupture, either spontaneously in the body or during surgery, the danger of death from anaphylactic shock is high. Metastatic cystic lesions can also develop in virtually any of the visceral organs if the primary cyst ruptures. If cyst material seeds the peritoneal lining, massive proliferation can occur with vascular invasion and spread to other organs. Brain cysts may also occasionally be found. The cysts of *E. multilocularis* grow more rapidly, with invasion of hepatic parenchyma simulating a carcinoma.

The life cycle is complete when infected viscera of the definitive host are eaten by a dog, fox, or other related carnivore. Humans may also become the intermediate host of the larval stages of *Taenia solium*, as previously discussed, in which bladder worms or cysticercoid lesions can develop in virtually any of the visceral organs.

LABORATORY DIAGNOSIS. The laboratory diagnosis may be made by demonstrating the daughter cysts or brood capsules with protoscolices in surgically removed tissue. Several immunodiagnostic techniques are available by which a clinical diagnosis may be confirmed. Gottstein[130] provides a comprehensive review of the current molecular and immunologic approaches to the diagnosis of hydatid disease. Most immunodiagnostic techniques involve the detection of echinococcus-specific antibody in the serum of suspected patients, using a variety of crude antigens. The problem with methods using crude antigens is the serologic cross-reactivity of echinococcal antibody tests with other parasite diseases, liver cirrhosis, and collagen diseases. Problems with cross-reactivity have been substantially improved with the development of a selected antigen called arc-5. In a previous study conducted by Schantz and McAuley,[291] a high percentage of the arc-5-positive persons subsequently were shown to harbor hydatid cysts. Cross-reactivity of the arc-5 antigen has been demonstrated in the sera of patients with cysticercosis; however, the differential diagnosis should be possible clinically in such cases.

Verastegui and coworkers[328] offer an enzyme-linked immunoelectrotransfer blot assay for the diagnosis of hydatid disease that circumvents the cysticercosis crossover problem. The antigen, prepared from lyophilized bovine hydatid fluid, contains three 8-, 16- and 21-kDa bands, that cross-reacted in only 12%, 4%, and 4% of sera from patients with cysticercosis, a significant reduction from most ELISA assays. The evolution of PCR coupled with the production of specific DNA probes has great promise in the diagnosis of echinococcal disease, particularly in the detection of target antigen in fine-needle biopsy material obtained from suspicious lesions.[130]

Multiceps Species: Coenurosis. Coenurosis is another human disease related to a dog tapeworm, a taenia-like cestode of the genus *Multiceps*, in which the normal intermediate hosts are sheep, cattle, horses, and other herbivorous animals. Humans become infected by ingesting food or water contaminated with dog feces containing multiceps eggs. The disease in humans involves primarily the CNS, where the migrating larvae develop into echinococcal-type cysts, individually known as a coenurus. These cysts differ from echinococcal cysts by having multiple scolices, but no brood capsules or daughter cysts. Symptoms are often those of a space-occupying lesion, including headache, vomiting, and localizing neurologic symptoms, such as hemiplegia, paraplegia, aphasia, and seizures. Basal arachnoiditis leading to the posterior fossa syndrome and internal hydrocephalus are also presenting symptoms. The diagnosis is usually made following surgical removal of the cyst and the histologic recognition of the coenurus.

Sparganosis: *Spirometra mansonoides*. Dogs and cats serve as the definitive host for several species of diphyllobothroid tapeworms belonging to the genus *Spirametra*. Spirametra eggs passed in dog or cat feces into fresh water hatch and are ingested by minute cyclops crustaceans, within which they develop into procercoid larvae. These larvae, in turn, develop into pleurocercoid larvae, individually known as sparganum, in the flesh of a second intermediate host (fish, snakes, frogs) that feeds on the cyclops. Humans become infected either by ingesting an infected cyclops, by eating the raw, infective flesh of the second intermediate host, or from the practice in certain cultures of applying raw fish to the skin, eyes, or vagina to heal other maladies. After ingestion, sparganum larvae penetrate the bowel wall and enter the circulation.

Most lesions in humans are subcutaneous in which slow-growing, painful, red, edematous nodules develop. Tsou and Huang[322] describe the characteristic tissue reaction as necrosis, granulomatous reaction, and lymphocytic infiltrates with focal collections of eosinophils. The definitive diagnosis is made only after surgical removal of a sparganum and identifying the slender, delicate white worm that measures 60 to 80 mm long × 1 to 2 mm wide. Aberrant spargana have been observed in the external eye where edematous swelling of the eyelid simulates Romana's sign (Chagas' disease) have been reported, in lymph channels producing elephantiasis-like swellings and in the brain in the form of cerebral abscesses.[8] Chang[53] and Holodniy and associates[154] independently report cases of cerebral sparganosis, which as of 1992, totaled 34. Most of the patients were rural inhabitants, who had a history of ingestion of frogs or snakes. The presenting symptoms were seizure, hemiparesis, and headache. The cerebral hemispheres, particularly the frontoparietal lobes, were most commonly involved. The basal ganglia and cerebellum were generally spared.

SEROLOGIC DIAGNOSIS OF PARASITIC INFECTIONS

The serologic approach to the evaluation of parasitic diseases is most applicable when invasive techniques other than the routine examination of blood, feces, or other body fluids are required to establish a diagnosis.[169] For example, the infective parasitic forms in toxoplasmosis, extraintestinal amebiasis, trichinosis, and cysticercosis are often lodged deep within tissues and organs, and either deep-needle or open surgical biopsies are needed to confirm the diagnosis. In such cases, serologic diagnosis may be possible if several potential problems, as outlined by Garcia and Bruckner are considered:[120]

1. Certain parasites that pass through several developmental phases may not provide sufficiently con-

stant or continuous antigenic stimuli to elicit antibody formation.

2. Antibody responses in specific cases may be lacking, either because of a limited antigenic stimulus or because a relevant antigen is not present in the test system.

3. The antigens employed in assays are often poorly defined heterogeneous mixtures or extracts of parasitic forms. Such antigen preparations may show cross-reactivity or inadequate sensitivity, making interpretation difficult.

4. Patients living in endemic areas may have higher baseline antibody titers than those in nonendemic areas; thus, if possible, changes in titer must be ascertained.

5. Reliable test kits for general diagnostic use are often not available from commercial sources. Even when available, the incidence of parasitic disease is usually so low in most laboratories that the reagents become outdated. In addition, these tests may be performed too infrequently for laboratory personnel to feel comfortable in making interpretations.

The status of serologic testing for a number of parasitic diseases has been well summarized by Wilson and coauthors.[347] Several of the applications of antibody and antigen detection provided in that review are reflected in short sections included within the discussion of each animal parasite in this text. We have elected to include such discussions within each section, rather than having a stand-alone presentation here. Much of the details of the various methods currently being used in research laboratories is beyond the scope of this text. In a practical sense, the volume of parasitic diseases encountered in most practice settings in the United States is low to nonexistent, making serologic testing impractical in most diagnostic microbiology laboratories. In most instances, cases and specimens are referred to local and regional reference laboratories, including the various state public health laboratories. Each reference laboratory will have in operation a mixture of time-honored and newer technologies that is unique to that laboratory, and consultation is necessary to learn which application and the types of specimens required may be most applicable.

The various serodiagnostic tests for parasitic diseases as reviewed by Walls[344] still serve as the standards in most reference laboratories. Box 20-10 is the list of serologic tests performed at the CDC for various parasitic diseases, along with the titers considered to be diagnostically significant, as originally published by Walls[344].

The IHA test has the advantage that a variety of antigens can be absorbed to tanned erythrocytes, providing a single method for detection of many diseases. The test is easy to perform and does not require special equipment. A tendency toward nonspecific activity can be minimized by using nonsensitized cell controls. According to Walls,[344] IHA is the method of choice for the serodiagnosis of amebiasis, cysticercosis, echinococcosis, filariasis, and strongyloidiasis.

The IIF uses particulate antigens and is, therefore, more specific than the IHA test. The test is more diffi-

---

BOX 20-10. SEROLOGIC TESTS PERFORMED AT THE CDC

DISEASE	TEST	DIAGNOSTIC TITERS
African trypanosomiasis	IFA	≥1:16
Amebiasis	IHA	≥1:256
Ascariasis	ELISA	≥1:32
Chagas' disease	CF, IHA	≥1:8; 1:64
Cysticercosis	IHA	≥1:64
Echinococcosis	IHA	≥1:256
Fascioliasis	IHA	≥1:128
Filariasis	IHA	≥1:128
Leishmaniasis	IIF	≥1:16
Malaria	IIF	≥1:64
Paragonimiasis	CF	≥1:8
Pneumocystosis	IIF	≥1:16
Schistosomiasis	IIF	≥1:16
Strongyloidiasis	IHA	≥1:64
Toxocariasis	ELISA	≥1:32
Toxoplasmosis	IIF, IgM-IIF	≥1:256, 1:16
Trichinosis	Bentonite floc	≥1:16

---

cult to perform and interpret, and special immunofluorescence microscopy and technical expertise are required. However, the ability to use specific fluorescent-tagged G, M, and A antiglobulins gives IIF the distinct advantage of potentially identifying the stage of parasitic disease. Walls recommends IIF or the serodiagnosis of leishmaniasis, malaria, schistosomiasis, and toxoplasmosis.[344]

ELISA is based on the same principle as IIF, except that an enzyme label and color readout is used instead of fluorescence. ELISA is highly sensitive and specific and can be used with almost any antigen; however, strict quality control is required because technical variations and nonspecific reagent binding are likely. The ELISA procedure has wider use in the serodiagnosis of parasitic diseases; it is currently the primary test for toxocariasis and for the detection of IgM antibody in toxoplasmosis.

The complement fixation test is used only infrequently for the serodiagnosis of Chagas' disease, paragonimiasis, and leishmaniasis. Immunoelectrophoresis and double-diffusion precipitin tests are rarely employed and have ancillary roles in the diagnosis of amebiasis, cysticercosis, and trichinelliasis. Agglutination procedures, using carrier particles such as latex, bentonite, and cholesterol are available only at reference centers such as the CDC. Bentonite flocculation is still recommended for the serodiagnosis of trichinelliasis and is performed in a few reference laboratories. Other newer methods including possible applications of nucleic acid probes and polymerase chain reactions are presented within the sections devoted to a discussion of each major parasite group.

Most of the advances in diagnostic clinical parasitology over the past 5 years involve the introduction of new serologic techniques for the detection of antibodies and antigens in blood and other fluids and secretions. Enzyme immunoassays (EIA), indirect hemagglutination inhibition (IHA) assays, indirect and direct fluorescent assays, and complement fixation constitute the spectrum of procedures used in larger clinical and reference parasitology laboratories. Application of molecular biology into diagnostic parasitology, or to use Persing's sound bite,[257] "from trenches to benches," is an exciting evolution coming from within research laboratories.

Enthusiasm, however, must be tempered by certain realities as pointed out by Weiss.[344] A number of new molecular assays for the diagnosis of parasitic diseases have been included in this text as short segments in the sections on laboratory diagnosis of the various parasites. These citations focus on the work currently being performed in research laboratories; however, as pointed out by Weiss,[354] very few of the new techniques have been subjected to field trials or large-scale clinical evaluations. The practical applications of PCR can be cited as an example. PCR provides a great increase in the sensitivity and specificity of DNA probe assays, resulting from the enhanced signals produced by the thousand times replication of targeted repetitive species-specific DNA sequences. This offers the possibility of quickly and directly identifying target antigens in very low concentrations or in trace amounts in clinical specimens. However, PCR is currently available only in a few diagnostic laboratories because of the high expense and technical demands of the method. A separate laboratory facility must be provided and great care must be taken in the handling of specimens to prevent contamination with extraneous DNA. All of this costs money and requires special training of personnel. These high expenses, along with the limited availability of equipment and reagents, will preclude widespread use of PCR in developing countries, at least in the short term. However, the day when

amplification methods become standard in many clinical laboratories is sooner rather than later. These direct diagnostic techniques will not only aid in the early diagnosis of parasitic diseases in humans, but will also provide the opportunity to study parasite-harboring vectors, leading to the prevention of parasitic diseases through more effective vector control. Automation, market forces, technical expertise and the need for shortening the turn-around time to establish a diagnosis of parasitic disease are all working to bring molecular biology "to the benches."

DRUGS COMMONLY USED IN THE TREATMENT OF PARASITIC DISEASES

Drug therapy of parasitic diseases is directed to interrupting the invasive capabilities of the parasites. Infections that occur primarily within the gastrointestinal tract are best treated with compounds that are poorly absorbed, resulting in high concentrations of active drug within the intestinal lumen. Agents that are well absorbed and achieve high serum and tissue levels are required for the treatment of invasive parasitic diseases, particularly the larval forms. In some cases of extraintestinal amebiasis, a combination of a nonabsorbable drug to treat any residual organisms in the intestine and an adsorbable agent to treat the visceral forms may be required. Many parasites exist in a cyst form, which may be poorly penetrated by many of the drugs, leading to potential reactivation of infection at a later date. A prime example is the inactive, encysted forms of *Toxoplasma gondii*, which are drug resistant and prone to reactivate when immunity is lost, particularly in patients with AIDS, who are rarely cured.

Table 20-10 summarizes the mode of action and other attributes of the more commonly used antiparasitic drugs.

TABLE 20-10
DRUGS COMMONLY USED IN THE TREATMENT OF PARASITIC INFECTIONS

DRUG	TYPE OF AGENT	MODE OF ACTION	COMMENTS
Amphotericin B	Polyene macrolide	Increases cell membrane permeability leading to a loss by leakage, first of ions and then of other cellular contents. Binding is effected by sterols in membrane.	Mammalian cells may also be affected with severe side effects. Used in treatment of infections with *Acanthamoeba* species and in advanced cases of mucocutaneous leishmaniasis.
Chloroquine	4 amino quinoline (quinine)	The concentration of drug achieved in malarial parasitized erythrocytes is several hundred times greater than in normal erythrocytes. The drug binds to ferriprotoporphyrin IX (FP), a degradation product of the hemoglobin present in the parasite food vacuole. The complex of chloroquine with FP is lytic for the parasite.	Mainstay of malarial therapy for over two decades. *P. falciparum* drug resistance occurs in strains that can somehow sequester FP so that it does not bind to chloroquine. Chloroquine is not curative for *P. vivax*.

(Continued)

TABLE 20-10   *(Continued)*
DRUGS COMMONLY USED IN THE TREATMENT OF PARASITIC INFECTIONS

DRUG	TYPE OF AGENT	MODE OF ACTION	COMMENTS
Emetine	Alkaloid (cycloheximide)	Directly lethal to trophozoites of *E. histolytica* by causing degenerative changes in the trophozoites. The drug causes interruption of cell division by irreversibly inhibiting protein synthesis by preventing movement of mRNA along the 60s ribosomal subunit.	Used in the therapy for severe intestinal amebiasis or amebic liver abscess as an alternative to metronidazole. Mammalian cells are also affected, resulting in severe side effects and limiting its therapeutic use.
Diethylcarbamazine citrate (Hetrazan)	Piperazine derivative (two nitrogens in benzene ring)	The drug is thought to alter surface properties and mobilization of microfilariae, causing them to leave the circulation through a specific neuromuscular effect. The microfilariae become trapped in the liver and are subject to phagocytosis.	Used primarily in the treatment of filarial infections. The drug is well absorbed, reaching peak serum concentrations within 3 hours, and is widely distributed throughout the body.
Ivermectin	A 22,23 dihydro derivative of avermectin B, a complex macrocyclic lactone produced by *Streptomyces avermitilis*	The drug acts on gamma-aminobutyric acid (GABA) receptors on the parasite musculature. Inhibitory neurons that cause release of GABA from presynaptic terminals are stimulated, in essence blocking signal transmission from interneurons to excitatory neurons. The effect is the loss of locomotor activity by the parasite, making normally motile parasites highly susceptible to various host defenses.	The drug has a broad spectrum of antinematodal activity but has no effects on flukes and tapeworms. It has been effectively used in onchocerciasis, cutaneous visceral larval migrans, *Angiostrongylus meningitis,* and various gastrointestinal nematode infections.
Mebendazole	Benzimidazole—benzine + five ring structure, including three carbon and two nitrogen molecules	Selective inhibition of glucose uptake in nematodes and cestodes, leading to increased utilization of parasite glycogen; parasites are thereby deprived of their main energy sources. Under action of the drug, the parasite is immobilized and in vitro larval development is interrupted.	Mebendazole is active against nematodes and used primarily in the treatment of trichuriasis, ascariasis, hookworm, and strongyloides infections. The drug is minimally absorbed from the gastrointestinal tract, thus being most effective in the treatment of intraintestinal worms.
Melarsoprol	Arsenical (a dimercaprol derivative of melarsen oxide)	Arsenoxides attach to trypanosomes by covalent bonding—sulfur groups in arsenoxide exert lethal effect by blocking essential biologically active glycolytic enzymatic groups. Arsenicals react with sulfhydryl groups, leading to inactivation of various enzymes synthesized by the parasite for glycolysis.	Used in the treatment of trypanosomiasis. The drug enters parasite cells more rapidly than human cells, and thus is more toxic to the parasite. The drug crosses the blood-brain barrier and enters the cerebrospinal fluid, making it highly effective in the treatment of CNS infection.
Metronidazole (Flagyl)	5-nitroimidazole	Metronidazole is metabolized into derivatives, including superoxide radicals, that interfere with DNA metabolism in parasites, causing extensive breaks in the DNA strands and interrupting the helical structure. Protein synthesis in the parasite is thus disrupted.	Used in the treatment of invasive amebiasis and also for infections with *Trichomonas vaginalis* and *Giardia lamblia.* Because only 10% of the drug is bound to serum proteins, it reaches high concentrations in the tissues, including lung, bile, bone, liver, and brain, exceeding levels required to inhibit the organisms against which it is active.

(Continued)

TABLE 20-10   *(Continued)*
DRUGS COMMONLY USED IN THE TREATMENT OF PARASITIC INFECTIONS

DRUG	TYPE OF AGENT	MODE OF ACTION	COMMENTS
Niclosamide	Heterocyclic pyrazinoisoquino-line derivative	The oxidative phosphorylation of mitochondria of cestodes is interrupted. The effect on mature adult worms is lethal, inducing complete muscular paralysis in certain species. The drug induces the scoleces to detach and the worms to disintegrate before they are eliminated in the feces.	Niclosamide is an alternative drug for the treatment of tapeworms. Treatment for *Hymenolepis* worms is increased to 5 days because onchospheres develop in the jejunal villi, and cysticercoids emerge into the intestinal lumen about 4 days later.
Praziquantel: (Pyrazinoquinoline)	8-amino-quinoline derivative	The drug acts by increasing the membrane permeability to calcium, causing contractions and paralysis of the musculature of worms. Neuromuscular effects lead to increased motility and spastic paralysis, causing the worms to detach and disintegrate in the intestine.	Used for the treatment of schistosomiasis, cysticercosis, tapeworm infections, and liver, lung, and intestinal flukes. The drug achieves excellent therapeutic levels in the liver, bile, and muscle tissue, and crosses the blood-brain barrier to reach the brain and spinal fluid as well.
Primaquine	Tetrahydral pyrimidine	The drug is gametocidal and sporonticidal for all species of human malaria. Its mechanism of action is unknown, although inhibition of DNA synthesis is most likely.	Primaquine is a poor blood schizonticide but is effective against exoerythrocytic hypnozoites. Therefore, it is effective in preventing relapses due to *P. vivax* and *P. ovale*. Radical cure of malaria can be effected by a combination of chloroquine and primaquine therapy.
Pyrantel pamoate	Naphthylamine sulfonic acid, a polyanion dye	Pyrantel (and its analogues) acts as a cholinergic antagonist, causing the depolarization of muscle cells within the parasite, leading to irreversible contractures.	Used primarily in the treatment of infections with ascaris, hookworms, pinworms, and *Trichostrongylus*. The drug is insoluble in water and poorly absorbed from the gastrointestinal tract, leading to little toxicity.
Suramin		The drug inhibits glycerol 3-phosphate oxidase and glycerol 3-phosphate dehydrogenase, preventing reoxidation of nicotinamide-adenine dinucleotide and decreasing adenosine triphosphate synthesis. This interruption in metabolism is lethal to the parasite.	The drug is widely distributed in the body but, because of avid protein binding in the serum, does not pass the blood-brain barrier. The drug is used in the treatment of early trypanosomiasis; however, as it does not penetrate into the central nervous system, it is not effective in the treatment of progressive CNS disease.
Thiabendazole	Benzimidazole	Mechanism of action unknown.	The drug is well suited for the treatment of disseminated strongyloides infection and any larval forms causing visceral and cutaneous larval migrans. The bulk of absorbed drug is metabolized in the liver and excreted as metabolites in the urine.

(Continued)

TABLE 20-10 *(Continued)*
DRUGS COMMONLY USED IN THE TREATMENT OF PARASITIC INFECTIONS

DRUG	TYPE OF AGENT	MODE OF ACTION	COMMENTS
Stibogluconate sodium	An antimony-containing compound	The drug is thought to act on sulfhydryl-containing enzymes within the parasite, decreasing the flow of glucose into the tricarboxylic acid cycle, resulting in the accumulation of glycolytic byproducts that are toxic to the developing amastigotes.	Used primarily in the treatment of leishmaniasis. After intramuscular or intravenous administration, a serum peak is achieved in 2 hours, and over 90% of the drug is excreted within 8 hours. However, the drug does gradually accumulate in the tissues, explaining why long courses of therapy are necessary.

REFERENCES

1. ABD-ALLA MD, JACKSON TF, GATHIRAM V, et al: Differentiation of pathogenic *Entamoeba histolytica* infections from nonpathogenic infections by detection of galactose-inhibitable adherence protein (GIAP) antigen in sera and feces. J Clin Microbiol 28:2845–2850, 1993

2. ACUNA-SOTO R, SAMUELSON J, DE GIROLAMI P, et al: Application of the polymerase chain reaction to the epidemiology of pathogenic and nonpathogenic *Entamoeba histolytica*. Am J Trop Med Hyg 48:48–70, 1993

3. ADAMS EB, MACLAUD IN: Invasive amebiasis. II. Amebic liver abscess and its complications. Medicine 56:325–334, 1977

4. AIKAWA M, TSEKI M, BARNWELL JW, et al: The pathology of human cerebral malaria. Am J Trop Med Hyg 43:30–37, 1990

5. ALDRAS AM, ORENSTEIN JM, KOTLER DP, et al: Detection of microsporidia by indirect immunofluorescence antibody test using polyclonal and monoclonal antibodies. J Clin Microbiol 32:608–612, 1994

6. ALLASON-JONES E, MINDEL A, SARGEAUNT P, WILLIAMS P: *Entamoeba histolytica* as a commensal intestinal parasite in homosexual men. N Engl J Med 315:353–356, 1986

7. ALPERT G, BELL LM, KIRKPATRICK CE, et al: Outbreak of cryptosporidiosis in a day-care center. Pediatrics 77:152–157, 1986

8. ANDERS K, FOLEY K, STERN WE, BROWN WJ: Intracranial sparganosis: an uncommon infection. J Neurosurg 60:1282–1286, 1984

9. ANDERSON BX: Cryptosporidiosis. Lab Med 14:55–56, 1983

10. ARMSTRONG D, ROSEN PP, et al: *Pneumocystis carinii* pneumonia: a cluster of eleven cases. Ann Intern Med 82:772–777, 1975

11. ARROWOOD MJ, STERLING CR: Comparison of conventional staining methods and monoclonal antibody-based methods for *Cryptosporidium* oocyst detection. J Clin Microbiol 27:1490–1495, 1989

12. ARROYO G, QUINN JA Jr: Association of amoeba and actinomyces in an intrauterine contraceptive device user. Acta Cytol 33:298–300, 1989

13. ASH LR, ORIHEL TC: Tissue helminths. Balows A (ed), *Manual of Clinical Microbiology*, 5th ed, Chap 70. Washington DC, American Society for Microbiology, 1991

14. AVILA HA, SIGMAN DS, COHEN LM, et al: Polymerase chain reaction amplification of *Trypanosoma cruzi* kinetoplast minicircle DNA isolated from whole blood lysates: diagnosis of chronic Chagas' disease. Mol Biochem Parasitol 48:211–222, 1991

15. AVILA HA, PEREIRA JB, THIEMANN O, et al: Detection of *Trypanosoma cruzi* in blood specimens of chronic chagasic patients by polymerase chain reaction amplification of kinetoplast minicircle DNA: comparison with serology and xenodiagnosis. J Clin Microbiol 31:2421–2426, 1993

16. BAEZ MJ, RAMIREZ BARBA EJ: Cutaneous amebiasis of the face: a case report. Am J Trop Med Hyg 35:69–71, 1986

17. BAILEY JW, SMITH DH: The quantitative buffy coat for the diagnosis of trypanosomes. Trop Doc 24:54–56, 1994

18. BAIRD JK, ALPERT LI, FRIEDMAN R, et al: North American brugian filariasis: report of nine infections of humans. Am J Trop Med Hyg 35:1205–1209, 1986

19. BAIRD JK, MISTREY M, PIMSLER M, CONNOR DH: Fatal human ascariasis following secondary massive infection. Am J Trop Med Hyg 35:314–318, 1986

20. BARTLETT MS, HARPER K, SMITH N, et al: Comparative evaluation of a modified zinc sulfate flotation technique. J Clin Microbiol 7:524–528, 1977

21. BAXBY D, HART CA: The incidence of cryptosporidiosis: a two-year prospective survey in a children's hospital. J Hyg (Lond) 96:107–111, 1986

22. BEAMAN M, McCABE RE, WONG SY, REMINGTON JS: *Toxoplasma gondii*. Mandell GL, Bennett JE, Dolin R (eds), *Principles and Practices of Infectious Diseases*, Chap 257. New York, Churchill Livingstone, 1995

23. BEAVER PC: Intraocular filariasis: a brief review. Am J Trop Med Hyg 40:40–45, 1989

24. BEAVER PC, GADGEL PK, MORERA P: Sarcocystis in man: a review and report of five cases. Am J Trop Med Hyg 28:819–844, 1979

25. BEAVER PC, JUNG RC, CUPP EW: *Clinical Parasitology*, 9th ed. Philadelphia, Lea & Febiger, 1984

26. BERLIN OGW, NOVAK SM, PORCHEN RK: Recovery of *Cyclospora* organisms from patients with prolonged diarrhea. Clin Infect Dis 18:606–609, 1994

27. BHATT RD, CHAPPELL MS, SMILOW PC, DAS KM: Recurrent massive upper gastrointestinal hemorrhage due to *Strongyloides stercoralis* infection. Am J Gastroenterol 85:1034–1036, 1990

28. BIGBY TD, MARGOLSKEE D, CURTIS JL, et al: The usefulness of induced sputum in the diagnosis of *Pneumocystis carinii* pneumonia in patients with the acquired immunodeficiency syndrome. Am Rev Respir Dis 133:515–518, 1986

29. BIGGS BA, MEGNA R, WICKREMESINGHE S, DWYER B: Human infection with *Cryptosporidium* spp: results of a 24-month survey. Med J Aust 147:175–177, 1987

30. BLACKETT K: Amoebic pericarditis. Int J Cardiol 21:183–187, 1988

31. BRADLEY SL, DINES DE, BREWER NS: Disseminated *Strongyloides stercoralis* in an immunosuppressed host. Mayo Clin Proc 53:332–335, 1978

32. BRATTON RL, NESSE RE: Ascariasis. An infection to watch for in immigrants. Postgrad Med 93:171–173, 1993

33. BREDA SD, HAMMERSCHLAG PE, GIOLIOTTI F, SCHINELLA R: *Pneumocystis carinii* in the temporal bone as a primary manifestation of the acquired immunodeficiency syndrome. Ann Otol Rhinol Laryngol 95:427–431, 1988

34. BROWN WJ, VOGE M: Cysticercosis: a modern day plague. Seidel JS (ed), *Parasitic Infections.* Pediatr Clin North Am 32:953–969, 1985

35. BRUCKNER DA, GARCIA LS, VOGE M: Intestinal parasites in Los Angeles, California. Am J Med Technol 45:1020–1024, 1979

36. BRUCKNER DA: Amebiasis. Clin Microbiol Rev 5:356–369, 1992

37. BRYAN RT: "Microsporidia." Mandell GL, Bennett JE, Dolin R (eds), *Principles and Practices of Infectious Diseases*, Chap 264. New York, Churchill Livingstone, 1995

38. BRYAN RT, CALI A, OWEN RL, SPENCER HC: *Microsporidia*: opportunistic pathogens in patients with AIDS. Sun T (ed), *Progress in Clinical Parasitology*, 2. Philadelphia, Field and Wood, 1991

39. BUIJS J, BARSBOOM G, VAN GEMUND J, et al: Toxocara seroprevalence in 5-year-old elementary schoolchildren: relation with allergic asthma. Am J Epidemiol 140:839–847, 1994

40. BUNDY DA: Immunoepidemiology of intestinal helminthic infections. 1. The global burden of intestinal nematode disease. Trans R Soc Trop Med Hyg 88:259–261, 1994

41. BURET A, DEN HOLLANDER N, WALLIS PM, et al: Zoonotic potential of giardiasis in domestic ruminants. J Infect Dis 162:231–237, 1990

42. CAREME B, PARAISO D, GOMBE-MBALAWA C: Calcifications of the breast probably due to *Loa loa*. Am J Trop Med Hyg 42:65–66, 1990

43. CARLSON JR, SULLIVAN PS, HARRY DJ, et al: Enzyme immunoassay for the detection of *Giardia lamblia*. Eur J Clin Microbiol Infect Dis 7:538–540, 1988

44. CARTER TR, COOPER PH, PETRI WA JR, et al: *Pneumocystis carinii* infection of the small intestine in a patient with acquired immune deficiency syndrome. Am J Clin Pathol 89:683–697, 1988

45. CENTERS FOR DISEASE CONTROL: Intestinal parasite surveillance: United States 1976. MMWR 27:167, 1978

46. CENTERS FOR DISEASE CONTROL: Microsporidian keratoconjunctivitis in patients with AIDS. MMWR 39:188–189, 1990

47. CENTERS FOR DISEASE CONTROL: Summary of malarial diseases 1988. MMWR 37:3, Oct 6, 1988

48. CENTERS FOR DISEASE CONTROL: Trichinosis, 36:2, Nov 1987

49. CENTERS FOR DISEASE CONTROL: Recommendations for the prevention of malaria among travelers. MMWR 39:3, Mar 9, 1990

50. CHALVARDJAN AM, GRAWE LA: A new procedure for the identification of *Pneumocystis carinii* cysts in tissue sections and smears. J Clin Pathol 16:383–384, 1963

51. CHAN FT, GUAN MX, MACKENZIE AM: Application of indirect immunofluorescence to detection of *Dientamoeba fragilis* trophozites in fecal specimens. J Clin Microbiol 31:1710–1714, 1993

52. CHAN MS, MEDLEY GF, JAMISON D, BUNDY DA: The evaluation of potential global morbidity attributable to intestinal nematode infections. Parasitology 109:373–387, 1994

53. CHANG KH, CHI JG, CHO SY, et al: Cerebral sparganosis: analysis of 34 cases with emphasis on CT features. Neuroradiology 34:1–8, 1992

54. CHAPMAN A, VALLEJO V, MOSSIE KG, et al: Isolation and characterization of species-specific DNA probes from *Taenia solium* and *Taenia saginata* and their use in an egg detection assay. J Clin Microbiol 33:1283–1288, 1995

55. CHAUDHRY AZ, LONGWORTH DL: Cutaneous manifestations of intestinal helminthic infections. Dermatol Clin 7:275–290, 1989

56. CHU E, WHITLOCK WL, DIETRICH RA: Pulmonary hyperinfection syndrome with *Strongyloides stercoralis*. Chest 97:1475–1477, 1990

57. CHULEY JD, OCKENHOUSE CF: Host receptors for malaria-infected erythrocytes. Am J Trop Med Hyg 43:6–14, 1990

58. CLARK CG, DIAMOND LS: The Laredo strain and other "*Entamoeba histolytica*-like" amoeba are *Entamoeba moshkovskii*. Mol Biochem Parasitol 46:11–18, 1991

59. CLARK MR, LIEBER MM: Genital filariasis in Minnesota. Urology 28:518–520, 1986

60. CLARK PS, BROWNSBERGER KM, SASLOW AR, et al: Bear meat trichinosis: epidemiologic, serologic, and clinical observations from two Alaskan outbreaks. Ann Intern Med 76:951–956, 1972

61. COHEN OJ, STROECKLE MY: Extrapulmonary *Pneumocystis carinii* infections in the acquired immunodeficiency syndrome. Arch Intern Med 151:1205–1214, 1991

62. COOPER ES, THYTE-ALLENG CA, FINZI-SMITH JS, MACDONALD TT: Intestinal nematode infections in children: the pathophysiological price paid. Parasitology 104 (suppl):S91–103, 1992

63. COULDWELL WT, APUZZO ML: Cysticercosis cerebri. Neurosurg Clin North Am 3:471–481, 1992.

64. COULMAN CU, GREENE I, ARCHIBALD RM: Cutaneous pneumocystosis. Ann Intern Med 106:396–398, 1987

65. CREGAN P, YAMAMOTO A, LUM A, et al: Comparison of four methods for rapid detection of *Pneumocystis carinii* in respiratory specimens. J Clin Microbiol 28:2432–2436, 1990

66. CROMPTON DWT, SAVIOLL L: Intestinal parasitic infections and urbanization. Bull WHO 71:1–9, 1993

67. CROSS JH: Intestinal capillariasis. Clin Microbiol Rev 5:120–129, 1992

68. CUMMINS AJ, MOODY AH, LALLOO K, CHIODINI PL: Rapid latex agglutination test for extraluminal amoebiasis. J Clin Pathol 47:647–648, 1994.

69. CURRENT WL: The biology of *Cryptosporidium*. ASM News 54:605–611, 1988

70. CURRENT WL, OWENS RL: Cryptosporidiosis and microsporidiosis. Farthing MJG, Keusch FT (eds), *Enteric Infection: Mechanisms, Manifestations and Management*. London, Chapman & Hall Medical, 1989

71. DAN M, GUTMAN R: Prevalence of cryptosporidiosis in Israeli children with diarrhoeae. J Infect 21:139–141, 1990

72. DA SILVA AJ, PIUVERZAM MR, DE MOURA H, et al: Rapid competitive enzyme-linked immunosorbent assay using a monoclonal antibody reacting with a 15-kilodalton tegumental antigen of *Schistosoma mansoni* for serodiagnosis of schistosomiasis. J Clin Microbiol 31:2315–2319, 1993

73. DAVIDSON BR, NEOPTOLEMOS JP, WATKIN D, TALBOT IC: Invasive amoebiasis: an unusual presentation. Gut 29:682–685, 1988

74. DAVIDSON RA, FLETCHER RH, CHAPMAN EE: Risk factors for strongyloidiasis—a controlled study. Arch Intern Med 144:321–325, 1984

75. DAVIS A: Recent advances in schistosomiasis. Q J Med 226:95–110, 1986

76. DEES A, BATENBURG PL, UMAR HM, et al: *Strongyloides stercoralis* associated with a bleeding gastric ulcer. Gut 31:1414–1415, 1990

77. DE JONGE N, RABELLO ALT, KRUGER FW, et al: Levels of the schistosome circulating anodic and cathodic antigens in the serum diagnosis of schistosomiasis patients from Brazil. Trans R Soc Trop Med Hyg 85:756–759, 1991

78. DEGIROLAMI PC, EZRATTY CR, DESAI G, et al: Diagnosis of intestinal microsporidiosis by examination of stool and duodenal aspirate with Weber's modified trichrome and Uvitex 2B stains. J Clin Microbiol 33:805–810, 1995

79. DE HOVITZ JA, PAPE JW, BONCY J, JOHNSON WD Jr: Isosporiasis in AIDS. N Engl J Med 315:87, 1986

80. DEKAMINSKY RG: Evaluation of three methods for laboratory diagnosis of *Strongyloides stercoralis* infection. J Parasitol 79:277–280, 1993

81. DELAROCQUE ASTAGNEAU E, HADENGUE A, DEGOTT C, et al: Biliary obstruction resulting from *Strongyloides stercoralis* infection. Report of a case. Gut 35:705–706, 1994

82. DEVAULT GA JR, KING JW, ROHR MS, ET AL: Opportunistic infections with *Strongyloides stercoralis* in renal transplantation. Rev Infect Dis 12:653–671, 1990

83. DIAMOND LS, CLARK CG: A redescription of *Entamoeba histolytica* Schaudinn, 1903 (Emended Walker, 1911) separating it from *Entamoeba dispar* Brumpt, 1925. J Eukaryotic Microbiol 40:340–344, 1994

84. DIAZ JCP: Control of Chagas' disease in Brazil. Parasitol Today 3:336–341, 1987

85. DIDIER ES, DIDIER PJ, FRIEDBERG DN, et al: Isolation and characterization of a new human microsporidian, *Encephalitozoon hellum* (n. sp.), from three AIDS patients with keratoconjunctivitis. J Infect Dis 163:617–621, 1991

86. DIERS J, MCCALLISTER GL: Occurrence of *Cryptosporidium* in home day care centers in west-central Colorado. J Parasitol 75:637–638, 1989

87. DISSANAYAKE S, ISMAIL MN: Immunodiagnosis of bancroftian filariasis. Ciba Found Symp 127:203–224, 1987

88. DIXON HBF, LIPSCOMB FM: Cysticercosis: an analysis and follow-up of 450 cases. Med Res Council Spec Rep 299:1–58, 1961

89. DOARDORFF TL, KENT MLP: Prevalence of larval *Anisakis simplex* in pen-reared and wild-caught salmon (*Salmonidae*) from Puget Sound, Washington. J Wildlife Dis 25:416–419, 1989

90. DOARDORFF TL, KAYES SG, FUDUMURA T: Human anisakiasis transmitted by marine food products. Hawaii Med J 50:9–16, 1991

91. DONELSON JE: Antigenic variation in African trypanosomes. Contrib Microbiol Immunol 8:138–175, 1987

92. DRUCKER DJ, BAILEY D: Thyroiditis as the presenting manifestation of disseminated extrapulmonary *Pneumocystis carinii* infection. J Clin Endocrinol Metab 71:1663–1665, 1990

93. DUERMEYER W, VANDERVEEN J: Specific detection of IgM-antibodies by ELISA, applied in hepatitis-A. Lancet 2:684–685, 1978

94. DUNLAP NE, SHIN MS, POLT SS, et al: Strongyloidiasis manifested as asthma. South Med J 77:77–78, 1984

95. DUPON M, CAZENAVE J, PELLEGRIN JL, et al: Detection of *Toxoplasma gondii* by PCR and tissue culture in cerebrospinal fluid and blood of human immunodeficiency virus-seropositive patients. J Clin Microbiol 33:2421–2426, 1995

96. DUPOUY-CAMET J, DE SOUZA SL, MASLO C, et al: Detection of *Toxoplasma gondii* in venous blood from AIDS patients by polymerase chain reaction. J Clin Microbiol 31:1866–1869, 1993

97. EBERHARD ML, LAMMIE PJ: Laboratory diagnosis of filariasis. Clin Lab Med 11:997–1010, 1991

98. EDMAN JC, KOVACS JA, MASUR H, et al: Ribosomal RNA sequence shows *Pneumocystis carinii* to be a member of the fungi. Nature 334:519–522, 1988

99. EHNERT KL, ROBERTO RR, BARRETT L, et al: Cysticercosis: first 12 months of reporting in California. Bull Pan Am Health Organ 26:165–172, 1992

100. EL-AHRAF A, TACAL JV JR, SOBIH M, et al: Prevalence of cryptosporidiosis in dogs and human beings in San Bernardino County, California. J Am Vet Med Assoc 198:631–634, 1991

101. ESPINO AM, MARCET R, FINLAY CM: Detection of circulating excretory secretory antigens in human fascioliasis by sandwich enzyme-linked immunosorbent assay. J Clin Microbiol 28:2637–2640, 1990

102. ESPINO AM, FINLAY CM: Sandwich enzyme-linked immunosorbent assay for detection of excretory secretory antigens in human fascioliasis. J Clin Microbiol 32:190–193, 1994

103. ESREY SA, COLLETT J, MIKIOTIS MD, et al: The risk of infection from *Giardia lamblia* due to drinking water supply, use of water and latrines among preschool children in rural Lesotho. Int J Epidemiol 18:248–253, 1989

104. FAN PC, CHUNG WC, SOH CT, KOSMAN ML: Eating habits of East Asian people and transmission of taeniasis. Acta Trop 50:305–315, 1992

105. FARRINGTON M, WINTERS S, WALKER C, et al: Cryptosporidium antigen detection in human feces by reverse passive hemagglutination assay. J Clin Microbiol 32:2755–2759, 1994

106. FILICE GA, HITT JA, MITCHELL CD, et al: Diagnosis of toxoplasma parasitemia in patients with AIDS by gene detection after amplification with polymerase chain reaction. J Clin Microbiol 31:2327–2331, 1993

107. FOSTER WE: *A History of Parasitology.* Edinburgh, E & S Livingstone, 1965

108. FRANZEN C, MULLER A, HEGENER P, et al: Detection of microsporidia (*Enterocytozoon bieneuzi*) in intestinal biopsy specimens from human immunodeficiency virus-infected patients by PCR. J Clin Microbiol 33:2294–2296, 1995

109. FRASER GG, COOKE KR: Endemic giardiasis and municipal water supply. Am J Public Health 81:760–762, 1991

110. FRENKEL JK, DUBEY JP: Toxoplasmosis and its prevention in cats and man. J Infect Dis 126:664–673, 1972

111. FRENKEL JK: Toxoplasmosis. Pediatr Clin N Am 32:917–932, 1985

112. FRENKEL JK, BARTLETT MS, SMITH JW: RNA homology and the classification of *Pneumocystis carinii.* Diag Microbiol Infect Dis 13:1, 1990

113. GAJDUSEK EC: *Pneumocystis carinii* as the cause of human disease: historical perspectives and magnitude of the problem. Introductory remarks. Natl Cancer Inst Monogr 43:1–10, 1976

114. GALLAGHER PG, VENGLARCIK JS III: *Blastocystis hominis* enteritis. Pediatr Infect Dis 4:556–557, 1985

115. GALLANT JE, ENRIQUEZ RE, COHEN KI, ET AL: *Pneumocystis carinii* thyroiditis. Am J Med 84:303–306, 1988

116. GARCIA E, RAMIREZ LE, MENTEON V, SOTELO J: Diagnosis of American trypanosomiasis (Chagas' disease) by the new complement fixation test. J Clin Microbiol 33:1034–1035, 1995

117. GARCIA LS, ASH LR: *Diagnostic Parasitology: Clinical Laboratory Manual.* 2nd ed. St Louis, CV Mosby, 1979

118. GARCIA LS, BRUCKNER DA, CLANCY MN: Clinical relevance of *Blastocystis hominis.* Lancet 1:1233–1234, 1984

119. GARCIA LS, SCHUM AC, BRUCKNER DA: Evaluation of a new monoclonal antibody combination reagent for direct fluorescence detection of *Giardia* cysts and *Cryptosporidium* oocysts in human fecal specimens. J Clin Microbiol 30:3255–3257, 1992

120. GARCIA LS, BRUCKNER DA: *Diagnostic Medical Parasitology.* 2nd ed. Washington DC, American Society for Microbiology, 1994

121. GARCIA LS, SHIMIZU RY, BRUCKNER DA: Detection of microsporidial spores in fecal specimens from patients diagnosed with cryptosporidiosis. J Clin Microbiol 32:1739–1741, 1994

122. GARZA D: Diarrhea caused by a universal coccidian parasite. Lab Med 14:283–286, 1983

123. GENTA RM, MILES P, FIELDS K: Opportunistic *Strongyloides stercoralis* infection in lymphoma patients. Report of a case and review of the literature. Cancer 63:1407–1411, 1989

124. GENTA RM: Dysregulation of strongyloidiasis: a new hypothesis. Clin Microbiol Rev 5:345–355, 1992

125. GINSBERG M, HUNT S, BARTZEN M, et al: Mosquito-transmitted malaria—California and Florida. MMWR 40:106–108, 1991

126. GODSEL LM, TIBBETTS RS, OLSON CL, et al: Utility of recombinant flagellar calcium-binding protein for serodiagnosis of *Trypanosoma cruzi* infection. J Clin Microbiol 33:2082–2085, 1995

127. GONZALEZ-RUIZ A, HAQUE R, REHMAN T, et al: Diagnosis of amebic dysentery by detection of *Entamoeba histolytica* fecal antigen by an invasive stain-specific monoclonal antibody-based enzyme-linked immunosorbent assay. J Clin Microbiol 32:964–1970, 1994

128. GONZALEZ-RUIZ A, HAQUE R, AGUIRRE A, et al: Value of microscopy in the diagnosis of dysentery associated with invasive *Entamoeba histolytica.* J Clin Pathol 47:236–239, 1994

129. GOSEY LL, HOWARD RM, WITEBSKY FG, et al: Advantages of a modified toluidine blue-O stain and bronchoalveolar lavage for the diagnosis of *Pneumocystis carinii* pneumonia. J Clin Microbiol 22:803–807, 1985

130. GOTTSTEIN B: Molecular and immunological diagnosis of echinococcosis. Clin Microbiol Rev 5:248–261, 1992

131. GORDON SM, GAL AA, SOLOMON AR, BRYAN JA: Disseminated strongyloidiasis with cutaneous manifestations in an immunocompromised host. J Am Acad Dermatol 32:255–259, 1994

132. GOULD SE: The story of trichinosis. Am J Clin Pathol 55:2–11, 1970

133. GREENSMITH CT, STANWICK RS, ELLIOT BE, FAST MV: Giardiasis associated with the use of a water slide. Pediatr Infect Dis J 7:91–94, 1988

134. GRENDON JH, DIGIACOMO RF, FROST FJ: *Dientamoeba fragilis* detection methods and prevalence: a survey of state public health laboratories. Public Health Rep 106:322–325, 1991

135. GRIMALDI G JR, TESH RB: Leishmaniases of the New World: current concepts and implications for the future. Clin Microbiol Rev 6:230–250, 1993

136. GRISOLIA JS, WIDERHOLD WC: CNS cysticercosis. Arch Neurol 39:540–544, 1982

137. GROVER CM, THULLIEZ P, REMINGTON JS, BOOTHROYD JC: Rapid prenatal diagnosis of congenital toxoplasma infection by using polymerase chain reaction and amniotic fluid. J Clin Microbiol 28:2295–2301, 1990

138. GUERRANT RL: The global problem of amebiasis: current status, research needs, and opportunities for progress. Rev Infect Dis 8:218–227, 1986

139. GUHL F, HUDSON L, MARINKELLE CJ, et al: Clinical *Trypanosoma rangeli* infection as a complication of Chagas' disease. Parasitology 94:475–484, 1987

140. HAGAR JM, RAHIMTOOLA SH: Chagas' disease in the United States. N Engl J Med 763–768, 1991

141. HAMALOGLU E: Biliary ascariasis in fifteen patients. Int Surg 77:77–79, 1992

142. HARCOURT-WEBSTER JN, SCARAVILLI F, DARWISH AH: *Strongyloides stercoralis* hyperinfection in an HIV positive patient. J Clin Pathol 44:346–348, 1991

143. HARRIS RA JR, MUSHER DM, FAINSTEIN V, et al: Disseminated strongyloidiasis: diagnosis made by sputum examination. JAMA 244:65–68, 1980

144. HART CA, BAXBY D: Cryptosporidiosis in immunocompetent patients. N Engl J Med 313:1018–1019, 1985

145. HEALY GR, SMITH JW: Intestinal and urogenital protozoa. Murray PR (ed), *Manual of Clinical Microbiology*, 6th ed, Chap 106. Washington DC, American Society for Microbiology, 1995

146. HEIJBEL H, SLAINE K, SEIGEL B, et al: Outbreak of diarrhea in a day care center with spread to household members: the role of *Cryptosporidium*. Pediatr Infect Dis 6:532–535, 1987

147. HEYMANS HS, ARONSON DC, VAN HOOFT MA: Giardiasis in childhood: an unnecessarily expensive diagnosis. Eur J Pediatr 146:401–403, 1987

148. HINZ E: Current status of food-borne parasitic zoonoses in West Germany. Southeast Asian J Trop Med Public Health 22 (suppl):78–84, 1991

149. HIRA PR, NEAFIE R, PRAKASH B, et al: Human gnathostomiasis: infection with an immature male *Gnathostoma spinigerum*. Am J Trop Med Hyg 41:91–94, 1989

150. HITT JA, FILICE GA: Detection of *Toxoplasma gondii* parasitemia by gene amplification, cell culture, and mouse inoculation. J Clin Microbiol 30:3181–3184, 1992

151. HOEPLI R: *Parasites and Parasitic Infection in Early Medicine and Science*. Singapore, University of Malaya Press, 1959

152. HOGE CW, SCHLIM DR, RAJAH R, et al: Epidemiology of diarrhoeal illness associated with coccidian-like organisms among travelers and foreign residents in Neap. Lancet 349:1175–1179, 1993

153. HOLCOMBE DJ: A case of *Strongyloides stercoralis* in central Louisiana. J La State Med Soc 141:22–24, 1989

154. HOLODNIY M, ALMENOFF J, LOUTIT J, STEINBERG GK: Cerebral sparganosis: case report and review. Rev Infect Dis 13:155–159, 1991

155. HOLTAN NR: Giardiasis. A crimp in the life-style of campers, travelers and others. Postgrad Med 83:54–57, 59–61, 1988

156. HOPKINS RS, JURANEK DD: Acute giardiasis: an improved clinical case definition for epidemiologic studies. Am J Epidemiol 15:402–407, 1991

157. HOPKINS DR, RUIZ-TIBEN E: Surveillance for dracunculiasis, 1981–1991. CDC Surveillance Summaries. MMWR 42:1–13, 1992

158. HOTEZ PJ, PRITCHARD DI: Hookworm infection. Sci Am 272:68–74, 1995

159. HUDSON L, GUHL F, DESANCHEZ N, et al: Longitudinal studies of the immune response of Colombian patients infected with *Trypanosoma cruzi* and *T. rangeli*. Parasitology 96:449–460, 1988

160. HULBERT TV, LARSEN RA, CHANDRASOMA PT: Abdominal angiostrongyliasis mimicking acute appendicitis and Meckel's diverticulum: report of a case in the United States and review. Clin Infect Dis 14:836–840, 1992

161. IKEDA K, KUMASHIRO R, KIFUNE T: Nine cases of acute gastric anisakiasis. Gastrointest Endosc 35:304–308, 1989

162. INGRA-SIEGMAN Y, KAPILA R, SEN P, et al: Syndrome of hyperinfection with *Strongyloides stercoralis*. Rev Infect Dis 3:397–407, 1981

163. ISAAC-RENTON, JL: Immunological methods of diagnosis in giardiasis: an overview. Ann Clin Lab Sci 21:116–122, 1991

164. JACQUIER P, GOTTSTEIN B, STINGELIN Y, ECKERT J: Immunodiagnosis of toxocarosis in humans: evaluation of a new enzyme-linked immunosorbent assay kit. J Clin Microbiol 29:1831–1835, 1991

165. JANDA WM: The acquired immunodeficiency syndrome. Clin Microbiol Newslett 4:169–171, 1982

166. JOKIPII I, JOKIPII AM: Timing of symptoms and oocyts excretion in human cryptosporidiosis. N Engl J Med 315:1643–1647, 1986

167. JONES JE: String test for diagnosing giardiasis. Am Fam Physician 34:123–126, 1986

168. JONES TC, JOHNSON WD JR, BARRETTO AC, et al: Epidemiology of American cutaneous leishmaniasis due to *Leishmania braziliensis braziliensis*. J Infect Dis 156:73–83, 1987

169. KAGAN IG, NORMAL L: Serodiagnosis of parasitic diseases. Rose NR, Freidman HG: *Manual of Clinical Immunology*, pp 382–409, 1976

170. KAMIYA M, OOI HK: Current status of food-borne parasitic zoonoses in Japan. Southeast Asian J Trop Med Public Health 22:48–53, 1991

171. KATZWINKEL-WLADARSCH S, LOSCHER T, RINDER H: Direct amplification and differentiation of pathogenic and nonpathogenic *Entamoeba histolytica* DNA from stool specimens. Am J Trop Med Hyg 51:115–118, 1994

172. KELLEY PW, TAKAFUJI ET, WIENER H, et al: An outbreak of hookworm infection associated with military operations in Grenada. Milit Med 154:55–59, 1989

173. KENNEDY S, CAMPBELL RM, LAWRENCE JE, et al: A case of severe *Strongyloides stercoralis* infection with jejunal perforation in an Australian ex-prisoner-of-war. Med J Aust 150:92–93, 1989

174. KEYSTONE JS, KEYSTONE DL, PROCTOR EM: Intestinal parasitic infections in homosexual men: prevalence, symptoms and factors in transmission. Can Med Assoc J 123:512–514, 1980

175. KHALIFA KES, ROTH A, ROTH B, et al: Value of PCR for evaluating occurrence of parasitemia in immunocompromised patients with cerebral and extracerebral toxoplasmosis. J Clin Microbiol 32:2813–2819, 1994

176. KEHL KSC, CICIRELLO H, HAVENS PL: Comparison of four different methods for detection of *Cryptosporidium* species. J Clin Microbiol 33:416–418, 1995

177. KIM CW: The significance of changing trends in trichinellosis. Southeast Asian J Trop Med Public Health 22(suppl):316–320, 1991

178. KIRSCH CM, AZZI RL, YENOLIDA GG, JENSEN MA: Analysis of induced sputum in the diagnosis of *Pneumocystis carinii* pneumonia. Am J Med Sci 61:386–391, 1990

179. KLEIN RA, CLERI DJ, DOSHI V, et al: Disseminated *Strongyloides stercoralis*: a fatal case eluding diagnosis. South Med J 76:1438–1440, 1983

180. KNIGHT R: Giardiasis, isosporiasis and balantidiasis. Clin Gastroenterol 7:31–47, 1978

181. KNISLEY CV, ENGLEKIRK PG, PICKERING LK, et al: Rapid detection of *Giardia* antigen in stool with the use of enzyme immunoassays. Am J Clin Pathol 91:704–708, 1989

182. KO RC, et al: First report of human angiostrongyliasis in Hong Kong diagnosed by computerized axial tomography (CAT) and enzyme-linked immunosorbent assay. Trans R Soc Trop Med Hyg 78:354–355, 1984

183. KOCH KL, PHILLIPS DJ, AGER RC, et al: Cryptosporidiosis in hospital personnel—evidence of person to person transmission. Ann Intern Med 102:593–596, 1985

184. KOKOSKIN E, GYORKOS TW, CAMUS A, et al: Modified technique for efficient detection of microsporidia. J Clin Microbiol 32:1974–1975, 1994

185. KOVACS JA, HIEMENZ JW, MACHER AM, et al: *Pneumocystis carinii* pneumonia: a comparison between patients with acquired immunodeficiency syndrome and patients with other immunodeficiencies. Ann Intern Med 100:663–671, 1984

186. KRAMER MR, GREGG PA, GOLDSTEIN M, et al: Disseminated strongyloidiasis in AIDS and non-AIDS immunocompromised hosts: diagnosis by sputum and bronchoalveolar lavage. South Med J 83:1226–1229, 1990

187. KRIGE JE, LEWIS G, BORNMAN PC: Recurrent pancreatitis caused by a calcified ascaris in the duct of Wirsung. Am J Gastroenterol 82:256–257, 1987

188. KROGSTAD KF, SPENCER JD JR, HEALY GR, et al: Amebiasis: epidemiologic studies in the United States 1971–1974. Ann Intern Med 88:89–97, 1978

189. KUROKI T, YAMAI S, KOYAMA T: *Entamoeba polecki* infection in a Southeast Asian refugee in Japan. Jpn J Med Sci Biol 42:25–29, 1989

190. LANG AP, LUCHSINGER IS, RAWLING EG: Filariasis of the breast. Arch Pathol Lab Med 111:757–759, 1987

191. LAPHAM SC, HOPKINS RS, WHITE MC, et al: A prospective study of giardiasis and water supplies in Colorado. Am J Public Health 77:354–355, 1987

192. LAWANDE RV, DUGGAN MBG, CONSTANTINIDOU M, et al: Primary amoebic meningoencephalitis in Nigeria. Report of two cases in children. J Trop Med Hyg 82:84–88, 1979

193. LEBAR WD, LARSEN EC, PATEL K: Afebrile diarrhea and *Blastocystis hominis*. Ann Intern Med 103:806, 1985

194. LEIGHTON PM, MACSWEEN HM: *Strongyloides stercoralis*. The cause of an urticarial-like eruption of 65 years' duration. Arch Intern Med 150:1747–1748, 1990

195. LEVINE GI: Parasitic diseases. Diseases associated with acquired immunodeficiency syndrome. Primary Care 18:129–152, 1991

196. LEVINE ND, CORLISS JO, COX FEG, et al: A newly revised classification of the protozoa. J Protozool 27:37–58, 1980

197. LIM PK: Recent advances in diagnostic techniques in filariasis. Southeast Asian J Trop Med Public Health 24(suppl 2):45–50, 1993

198. LIN T, CHIN-SEE MW, HALBERT SP, et al: An enzyme immunoassay for immunoglobulin-M antibodies to *Toxoplasma gondii* which is not affected by rheumatoid factors or immunoglobulin-G antibodies. J Clin Microbiol 23:77–82, 1986

199. LIZOTTE MR, SUPALI T, PARTONO F, WILLIAMS SA: A polymerase chain reaction assay for the detection of *Brugia malayi* in blood. Am J Trop Med Hyg 51:314–321, 1994

200. LOKEN S: Giardiasis: diagnosis and treatment. Nurse Pract 11:20–22, 26–32, 1986

201. LONG EG, EBRAHIMZADEH A, WHITE EH, et al: Alga associated with diarrhea in patients with acquired immunodeficiency syndrome and in travelers. J Clin Microbiol 28:1101–1104, 1990

202. LONG EG, WHITE EH, CARMICHAEL WW, et al: Morphologic and staining characteristics of a cyanobacterium-like organism associated with diarrhea. J Infect Dis 164:199–202, 1991

203. LONG GW, RICKMAN LS, CROSS JH: Rapid diagnosis of *Brugia malayi* and *Wuchereria bancrofti* filariasis by an acridine orange/microhematocrit tube technique. J Parasitol 76:278–281, 1990

204. LOOSE JH, SEDERARAN DJ, COOPER HS: Identification of *Cryptosporidium* in paraffin-embedded tissue sections with the use of a monoclonal antibody. Am J Clin Pathol 91:206–209, 1989

205. LOPEZ-VALEZ R, LAGUNA F, ALVAR J, et al: Parasitic culture of buffy coat for diagnosis of visceral leishmaniasis in human immunodeficiency virus-infected patients. J Clin Microbiol 33:937–939, 1995

206. LOTTER H, MANNWEILER E, SCHREIER M, TANNICH E: Sensitive and specific serodiagnosis of invasive amebiasis by using a recombinant surface protein of pathogenic *Entamoeba histolytica*. J Clin Microbiol 30:3163–3167, 1992

207. LUFT BJ, BROOKS RG, CONLEY FK, et al: Toxoplasmic encephalitis in patients with acquired immune deficiency syndrome. JAMA 252:913–917, 1984

208. MACPHERSON EW, MACQUEEN WM: Morphological diversity of *Blastocystis hominis* in sodium acetate–acetic acid–formalin-preserved stool samples stained with iron hematoxylin. J Clin Microbiol 32:267–268, 1994

209. MADDERN GJ, DENNISON AR, BLUMGART LH: Fatal ascaris pancreatitis: an uncommon problem in the west. Gut 33:402–403, 1992

210. MAHANNOP P, SETASUBAN P, MORAKOTE N: Immunodiagnosis of human trichinellosis and identification of specific antigen for *Trichinella spiralis*. Int J Parasitol 25:87–94, 1995

211. MAHANNOP P, CHAICUMPA W, SETASUBAN P, et al: Immunodiagnosis of human trichinellosis using excretory–secretory (ES) antigen. J Helminthol 66:297–304, 1992

212. MAHMOUD AAF: Trematodes (schistosomiasis) and other flukes. Mandell GL, Bennett JE, Dolin R (eds), *Principles and Practices of Infectious Diseases*, Chap 268. New York, Churchill Livingston, 1995

213. MADWAR MA, EL TAHAWY M, STRICKLAND GT: The relationship between uncomplicated schistosomiasis and hepatitis B infection. Trans R Soc Trop Med Hyg 83:233–236, 1989

214. MAK JW: Epidemiology of lymphatic filariasis. Ciba Found Symp 127:5–14, 1987

215. MARKELL EK, HAVENS RF, KURITSBURO RA, et al: Intestinal protozoa in homosexual men in the San Francisco Bay area; prevalence and correlates of infection. Am J Trop Med Hyg 32:239–245, 1984

216. MARKELL EK, QUINN PM: Comparison of immediate polyvinyl alcohol (PVA) fixation with Schaudinn's fixation for the demonstration of protozoa in stool specimens. Am J Trop Med Hyg 26:1139–1142, 1977

217. MARKELL EK, UDKOW MP: *Blastocystis hominis*: pathogen or fellow traveler? Am J Trop Med Hyg 35:1023–1026, 1986

218. MARSHALL AR, AL-JUMAILI IJ, FENWICK GA, et al: Cryptosporidiosis in patients at a large teach-in hospital. J Clin Microbiol 25:172–173, 1987

219. MARX JL: Spread of AIDS sparks new health concern. Science 219:42–43, 1983

220. MASUR H, LANE HC, KOVACS, et al: NIH Conference. *Pneumocystis* pneumonia: from bench to clinic. Ann Intern Med 111:813–826, 1989

221. MATHIEU-DAUDE F, BICART-SEE A, BOSSENO MF, et al: Identification of *Trypanosoma brucei gambiense* group I

by a specific kinetoplast DNA probe. Am J Trop Med Hyg 50:13–19, 1994

222. MATSUMOTO T, IIDA M, KIMURA Y, et al: Anisakiasis of the colon: radiologic and endoscopic features in six patients. Radiology 183:97–99, 1992

223. MATSUMOTO TK, HOSHINO-SHIMIZU S, NAKAMURA PM, et al: High resolution of *Trypanosoma cruzi* amastigote antigen in serodiagnosis of different clinical forms of Chagas' disease. J Clin Microbiol 31:1486–1492, 1993

224. MATTIA AR, WALDRON MA, SIERRA LS: Use of the quantitative buffy coat system for detection of parasitemia in patients with babesiosis. J Clin Microbiol 31:2816–2818, 1993

225. MCCABE RE, REMINGTON JS: *Toxoplasma gondii*. Mandell GI, Douglas RG Jr, Bennett JE (eds), *Principles and Practices of Infectious Diseases*, Chap. 255. New York, Churchill Livingstone, 1989

226. MCCORMICK GF, CHI-SHING ZEE, HEIDEN J: Cysticercosis cerebri: review of 127 cases. Arch Neurol 39:534–539, 1982

227. MCHENRY R, BARTLETT MS, LEHMAN GA, O'CONNER KW: The yield of routine duodenal aspiration for *Giardia lamblia* during esophagogastroduodenoscopy. Gastrointest Endosc 33:425–426, 1987

228. MCREYNOLDS LA, POOLE C, HONG Y, et al: Recent advances in the application of molecular biology in filariasis. Southeast Asian J Trop Med Public Health 24(suppl 2):55–63, 1993

229. MELVIN M, BROOKE MM, HEALY GR: Common blood and tissue parasites of man: life cycle charts. DHEW Publication 1234. Washington DC, US Government Printing Office, 1969

230. MELVIN DM, BROOKE MM, SUDAN EH: Common intestinal helminths of man: life cycle charts. DHEW Publication 1234. Washington DC, US Government Printing Office, 1974

231. MELVIN DM, SMITH JW: Intestinal parasitic infections. Problems in laboratory diagnosis. Lab Med 10:207–210, 1979

232. MILLS J: *Pneumocystis carinii* and *Toxoplasma gondii* infections in patients with AIDS. Rev Infect Dis 8:1001–1011, 1986

233. MINAMOTO T, SAWAQUICHI K, OAINO T, MAI M: Anisakiasis of the colon: report of two cases with emphasis on the diagnostic and therapeutic value of colonoscopy. Endoscopy 23:50–52, 1991

234. MOORHEAD WP, GUASPARINI R, DONOVAN CA, et al: Giardiasis outbreak from a chlorinated community water supply. Can J Public Health 81:358–362, 1990

235. NAGLER J, BROWN M, SOAVE R: *Blastocystis hominis* in inflammatory bowel disease. J Clin Gastroenterol 16:109–112, 1993

236. NANDURI J, KAZURA JW: Clinical and laboratory aspects of filariasis. Clin Microbiol Rev 2:39–50, 1989

237. NANTULYA VM, DOUA F, MOLISHO S: Diagnosis of *Trypanosoma brucei gambiense* sleeping sickness using an antigen detection enzyme-linked immunosorbent assay. Trans R Soc Trop Med Hyg 86:42–45, 1992

238. NAOT Y, DESMONTS G, REMINGTON JS: IgM enzyme-linked immunosorbent assay test for diagnosis of congenital toxoplasma infection. J Pediatr 92:232–236, 1984

239. NAVIN TR, JURANEK DD: Cryptosporidiosis: clinical, epidemiological and parasitic review. Rev Infect Dis 6:313–317, 1984

240. NAWA Y: Historical review and current status of gnathostomiasis in Asia. Southeast Asian J Trop Med Public Health 22 (suppl):217–219, 1991

241. NEAFIE RC, MARTY AM: Unusual infections in humans. Clin Microbiol Rev 6:34–56, 1993

242. NEIMEISTER R, LOGAN AL, EGLETON JH: Modified trichrome staining technique with xylene substitution. J Clin Microbiol 22:306–307, 1985

243. NEWMAN RD, JAEGER KL, WUHIB T, et al: Evaluation of an antigen capture enzyme-linked immunosorbent assay for detection of *Cryptosporidium* oocysts. J Clin Microbiol 31:2080–2084, 1993

244. NEWTON JA Jr, SCHNEPF GA, WALLACE MR, et al: Malaria in US Marines returning from Somalia. JAMA 272:397–399, 1994

245. NOVOTNY TE, HOPKINS RS, SHILLAM P, JANOFF EN: Prevalence of *Giardia lamblia* and risk factors for infection among children attending day-care facilities in Denver. Public Health Rep 105:72–75, 1990

246. OGUNRINADE AF, CHANDRASHEKAR R, EBBERHARD ML, WEIL GJ: Preliminary evaluation of recombinant *Onchocerca volvulus* antigens for serodiagnosis of onchocerciasis. J Clin Microbiol 31:1741–1745, 1993

247. OLSSON M, ELVIN K, LOFDAHL S, LINGER E: Detection of *Pneumocystis carinii* DNA in sputum and bronchoalveolar lavage samples by polymerase chain reaction. J Clin Microbiol 31:221–226, 1993

248. OLVEDA RM, DOMINGO EO: *Schistosoma japonicum*. Mahmoud AAF (ed), *Clinical Tropical Medicine and Communicable Diseases*, pp 397–418. London, Bailliere-Tindall, 1987

249. OOI WW, ZIMMERMAN SK, NEEDHAM CA: *Cyclospora* species as a gastrointestinal pathogen in immunocompetent hosts. J Clin Microbiol 33:1267–1269, 1995

250. ORGETA YR, STERLING CR, GILMAN RH, et al: *Cyclospora* species—a new protozoan pathogen of humans. N Engl J Med 328:1308–1312, 1993

251. ORMEROD WE: Hypothesis: the significance of Winterbottom's sign. J Trop Med Hyg 94:338–340, 1991

252. PAPPE JW, VERDIER RI, BONEY M, et al: *Cyclospora* infection in adults infected with HIV. Clinical manifestations, treatment and prophylaxis. Ann Intern Med 121:654–657, 1994

253. PARMLEY SF, GOEBEL FD, REMINGTON JS: Detection of *Toxoplasma gondii* in cerebrospinal fluid from AIDS patients by polymerase chain reaction. J Clin Microbiol 30:3000–3002, 1992

254. PARTONA F: The spectrum of disease in lymphatic filariasis. Ciba Found Symp 127:15–31, 1987

255. PEARSON RD, DE QUEIROZ SOUSA A: *Leishmania* species: visceral (kala-azar), cutaneous and mucosal leishmaniasis. Mandell GL, Bennett JE, Dolin R (eds), *Principles and Practices of Infectious Diseases*, Chap 254. New York, Churchill Livingston, 1995

256. PERSING DH, MATHIESEN D, MARSHALL WF, et al: Detection of *Babesia microti* by polymerase chain reaction. J Clin Microbiol 30:2097–2103, 1992

257. PERSING DH: Polymerase chain reaction: trenches to the benches. J Clin Microbiol 29:1281–1285, 1991

258. PETERS LS, SABLE R, JANDA WM, et al: Prevalence of enteric parasites in patients attending a homosexual outpatient clinic. J Clin Microbiol 24:684–685, 1986

259. PETERS CS, KATHPALIA SB, CHITTOM-SWIALTO AL, et al: *Isospora belli* and *Cryptosporidium* sp from a patient not suspected of having acquired immunodeficiency syndrome. Diagn Microbiol Infect Dis 8:197–199, 1987

260. PETRI WA JR, CLARK CG, DIAMOND LS: Host-parasite relationships in amebiasis: conference report. J Infect Dis 169:483–484, 1994

261. PIARROUX R, GAMBARELLI F, DUMON H, et al: Comparison of PCR with direct examination of bone marrow aspiration, myeloculture, and serology for diagnosis of visceral leishmaniasis in immunocompromised patients. J Clin Microbiol 32:746–749, 1994

262. PICKERING LK, ENGELKIRK PG: *Giardia lamblia*. Pediatr Clin North Am 35:565–577, 1988

263. PIFER LL, WOODS DR, EDWARDS CC, et al: *Pneumocystis carinii* serologic study in pediatric acquired immunodeficiency syndrome. Am J Dis Child 142:36–39, 1988

264. POL S, ROMANA CA, RICHARD S, et al: *Microsporidia* infection in patients with the human immunodeficiency virus and unexplained cholangitis. N Engl J Med 328:95–99, 1993

265. POLLOK RCG, BENDALL RP, MOODY A, et al: Traveler's diarrhoea associated with cyanobacterium-like bodies [letter]. Lancet 340:556–557, 1992

266. POLLY SM: Neurocysticercosis. Infect Dis Newslett 5:89–91, Dec 1986

267. PORTER JD, GAFFNEY, C, HEYMANN D, PARKIN W: Foodborne outbreak of *Giardia lamblia*. Am J Public Health 80:1259–1260, 1990

268. PURTILLO DT, MYERS WM, CONNOR DH: Fatal strongyloidiasis in immunocompromised patients. Am J Med 56:488–493, 1974

269. RAKITA RM, WHITE AC JR, KIELHOFNER MA: *Loa loa* infection as a cause of migratory angioedema: report of three cases from the Texas Medical Center. Clin Infect Dis 17:691–694, 1993

270. RAUNGKUNAPORN Y, WATT G, KARNASUTA C, et al: Immunodiagnosis of trichinellosis: efficacy of somatic antigen in early detection of human trichinellosis. Asian Pacific J Allergy Immunol 12:39–42, 1994

271. RAVDIN JI: Pathogenesis of disease caused by *Entamoeba histolytica*: studies of adherence, secreted toxins and contact-dependent cytolysis. Rev Infect Dis 8:247–260, 1986

272. RAWLINS SC, CHAILETT P, RAGOONANANSINGH RN, et al: Microscopical and serological diagnosis of *Wuchereria bancrofti*. West Indian Med J 43:75–79, 1994

273. RICHMAN TB, KURDEL FA: Amebiasis and trypanosomiasis. Exp Parasitol 62:142–148, 1986

274. RIJPSTRA AC, CANNING EU, VAN KETEL RJ, et al: Use of light microscopy to diagnose small-intestinal microsporidiosis in patients with AIDS. J Infect Dis 157:827–831, 1988

275. RODRIQUEZ N, GUZMAN B, RODAS A, et al: Diagnosis of cutaneous leishmaniasis and species discrimination of parasites by PCR and hybridization. J Clin Microbiol 32:2246–2252, 1994

276. ROMBO L, EDWARDS G, WARD SA, et al: Seven patients with relapses of *Plasmodium vivax* or *P. ovale* despite primaquine treatment. Trop Med Parasitol 38:49–50, 1987

277. ROSOFF JD, SANDERS CA, SONNAD SS, et al: Stool diagnosis of giardiasis using a commercially available enzyme immunoassay to detect giardia-specific antigen 65 (GAS 65). J Clin Microbiol 27:1997–2002, 1989

278. ROSSI JF, ELEDJAN JJ, DELAGE A, et al: *Pneumocystis carinii* infection of bone marrow in patients with malignant lymphoma and acquired immunodeficiency syndrome. Original report of three cases. Arch Intern Med 150:450–452, 1990

279. ROSSITCH E JR, CARRAZANA EJ, SAMUELS MA: Cerebral toxoplasmosis in patients with AIDS. Am Fam Physician 41:867–873, 1990

280. ROUX P, LAVRARD I, POIROT JL, et al: Usefulness of PCR for detection of *Pneumocystis carinii* DNA. J Clin Microbiol 32:2324–2326, 1994

281. RUSNAK J, HADFIELD TL, RHODES MM, GAINES JK: Detection of *Cryptosporidium* oocysts in human fecal specimens by an indirect immunofluorescence assay with monoclonal antibodies. J Clin Microbiol 27:1135–1136, 1989

282. RYAN NJ, SUTHERLAND G, COUGHLAN K, et al: A net trichrome-blue stain for detection of microsporidial species in urine, stool and nasopharyngeal specimens. J Clin Microbiol 31:3264–3269, 1993

283. SACHS JR, GREENFIELD SM, SOHN II, TURNER JL: Disseminated *Pneumocystis carinii* infection with hepatic involvement in a patient with the acquired immune deficiency syndrome. Am J Gastroenterol 86:82–85, 1991

284. SAKANARI JA, MCKERROW JH: Anasakiasis. Clin Microbiol Rev 2:278–284, 1989

285. SALLON S, DECKELBAUM RJ, SCHMID II, et al: *Cryptosporidium*, malnutrition and chronic diarrhea in children. Am J Dis Child 142:312–315, 1988

286. SALTZBERG DM, KOTLOFF KL, NEWMAN JL, FASTIGGI R: *Cryptosporidium* infection in acquired immunodeficiency syndrome: not always a poor prognosis. J Clin Gastroenterol 13:94–97, 1991

287. SARGEAUNT PG, WILLIAMS JE: Electrophoretic isoenzyme patterns of *Entamoeba histolytica* and *Entamoeba coli*. Trans R Soc Trop Med Hyg 72:164–166, 1978

288. SARGEAUNT PG, BAVEJA UK, NANDA R, ANAND BS: Influence of geographical factors in the distribution of pathogenic zymodemes of *Entamoeba histolytica*: identification of zymodeme XIV in India. Trans R Soc Trop Med Hyg 78:96–101, 1984

289. SARWAUT MA, AL SHAIBY AL: Parasitic infections among patients of Al Nour specialized hospital. J Egypt Soc Parasitol 23:321–827, 1993

290. SAWANGJAROEN N, LUKE R, PROVIC P: Diagnosis by faecal culture of *Dientamoeba fragilis* infections in Australian patients with diarrhoea. Trans R Soc Trop Med Hyg 87:163–165, 1993

291. SCHANTZ PM, MCAULEY J: Current status of food-borne parasitic zoonoses in the United States. Southeast Asian J Trop Med Public Health 22(suppl):65–71,1991

292. SCHEFFLER EH, VAN ETTA LL: Evaluation of rapid commercial enzyme immunoassay for detection of *Giardia lamblia* in formalin-preserved stool specimens. J Clin Microbiol 32:1807–1808, 1994

293. SCHLIM DR, COHEN MT, EATON M, et al: An alga-like organism associated with an outbreak of prolonged diarrhea among foreigners in Nepal. Am J Trop Med Hyg 45:383–389, 1991

294. SCHUMANN GB, SWENSEN JJ: Comparison of Papanicolaou's stain with the Gomori methenamine silver (GMS) stain for the cytodiagnosis of *Pneumocystis carinii* in bronchoalveolar lavage (BAL) fluid. Am J Clin Pathol 95:583–586, 1991

295. SCHWARTZ DA: Cholangiocarcinoma with liver fluke infection: a preventable source for morbidity in Asian immigrants. Am J Gastroenterol 81:76–79,1986

296. SCHWARTZ DA, MUNNER RG, KATZ SM: Plastic embedding evaluation of *Pneumocystis carinii* pneumonia in AIDS. Simultaneous demonstration of cyst and sporozoite forms. Am J Surg Pathol 11:304–309, 1987

297. SHADDUCK JA, GREELEY E: Microsporidia and human infections. Clin Microbiol Rev 2:158–165, 1989

298. SHANDERA WX: From Leningrad to the day-care center. The ubiquitous *Giardia lamblia*. West J Med 153:154–159, 1990

299. SHEPHERD RC, REED CL, SINHA GP: Shedding of oocysts of *Cryptosporidium* in immunocompetent patients. J Clin Pathol 41:1104–1106, 1988

300. SHER L, SHUNZABURO I, LEBEAU G, ZAJKO AB: Hilar cholangiocarcinoma associated with *Clonorchis*. Dig Dis Sci 34:1121–1123, 1989

301. SHETTY N, BRABHU T: Evaluation of faecal preservation and staining methods in the diagnosis of acute amoebiasis and giardiasis. J Clin Pathol 41:694–699, 1988

302. SINGH BN: *Pathogenic and Non-pathogenic Amoebae*. New York, John Wiley & Sons, 1975

303. SMITH JW, GUTIERREZ Y: Medical parasitology. Henry JB (ed), *Clinical Diagnosis and Management by Laboratory Methods*, Chap 46. Philadelphia, WB Saunders, 1991

304. SMITH HV, PATTERSON WJ, HARDIE R, et al: An outbreak of waterborne cryptosporidiosis caused by post-treatment contamination. Epidemiol Infect 103:703–715, 1989

305. SMITH JW, WOLFE MS: Giardiasis. Annu Rev Med 31:373, 1980

306. SOAVE R: Cryptosporidiosis and isosporiasis in patients with AIDS. Infect Dis Clin North Am 2:485, 1988

307. SOH CT: Current status of food-borne parasitic zoonoses in Korea. Southeast Asian J Trop Med Public Health 22:54–55, 1991

308. STARKO KM, LIPPY EC, DOMINQUEZ LB, et al: Campers' diarrhea outbreak traced to water-sewage link. Public Health Rep 101:527–531, 1986

309. STEELE AD, GOVE E, MOEWE PJ: Cryptosporidiosis in white patients in South Africa. J Infect 19:281–285, 1989

310. STEHR-GREEN JK, MCCAIG L, REMSEN HM, et al: Shedding of oocysts in immunocompetent individuals infected with *Cryptosporidium*. Am J Trop Med Hyg 36:338–342, 1987

311. STEKETEE RW, REID S, CHENG T, et al: Recurrent outbreaks of giardiasis in a child day care center, Wisconsin. Am J Public Health 79:485–490, 1989

312. STIBBS HH: Monoclonal antibody-based enzyme immunoassay for *Giardia lamblia* antigen in human stool. J Clin Microbiol 2k7:2582–2588, 1989

313. STRANGER SL, STRINGER JR, BLASE MA, et al: *Pneumocystis carinii*: sequence from ribosomal RNA implies a close relationship with fungi. Exp Parasitol 68:450–461, 1989

314. STRICKLAND GT, ABDEL-WAHAB M: Schistosomiasis. Strickland GT (ed), *Hunters Tropical Medicine*, 7th ed. Philadelphia, WB Saunders, 1991

315. TAMBURRINI E, MENCARINI P, DE LUCA A, et al: Simple and rapid two-step polymerase chain reaction for diagnosis of *Pneumocystis carinii* infection. J Clin Microbiol 31:2788–2789, 1993

316. TAN JS: Common and uncommon parasitic infections in the United States. Med Clin North Am 62:1059–1081, 1978

317. TANABE L, FIRITA T, KATSUMOTO U, et al: Serologic observations of *Pneumocystis carinii* infection in humans. J Clin Microbiol 22:1058–1060, 1985

318. TANGERMANN RH, GORDON S, WIESNER P, KRECKMAN L: An outbreak of cryptosporidiosis in a day-care center in Georgia. Am J Epidemiol 133:471–476, 1991

319. TANNICH E, BURCHARD GD: Differentiation of pathogenic from nonpathogenic *Entamoeba histolytica* by restriction fragment analysis of a single gene amplified in vitro. J Clin Microbiol 29:250–255, 1991

320. TANTOWITZ HB, KORCHHOFF LV, SIMON D, et al: Chagas' disease. Clin Microbiol Rev 5:400–419, 1992

321. TIETZE PE, TIETZE PH: The roundworms. *Ascaris lumbricoides*. Primary Care 18:23–41, 1991

322. TSOU MH, HUANG TW: Pathology of subcutaneous sparganosis: report of two cases. J Formosan Med Assoc 92:649–653, 1993

323. UNGAR BL: Enzyme-linked immunoassay for detection of *Cryptosporidium* antigens in fecal specimens. J Clin Microbiol 28:2491–2495, 1990

324. VANEK J, JIROVEC O, LUKES J: Interstitial plasma cell pneumonia in infants. Ann Pediatr 180:1, 1953

325. VAN ETTEN L, FOLMAN CC, EGGELTE TA: Rapid diagnosis of schistosomiasis by antigen detection in urine with a reagent strip. J Clin Microbiol 2404–2406, 1994

326. VAN KNAPEN F, PANGGPBEN SO, VAN LEUDSEN J: Demonstration of toxoplasma antigen containing complexes in active toxoplasmosis. J Clin Microbiol 22:645–650, 1985

327. VANNATA JB, ADAMSON D, MUJLLICAN K: *Blastocystis hominis* infection presenting as recurrent diarrhea. Ann Intern Med 102:495–496, 1985

328. VERASTEGUI M, MORO P, GUEVEREA A, et al: Enzyme-linked immunoelectrotransfer blot test for diagnosis of human hydatid disease. 30:1557–1561, 1992

329. VERMUND SH, LALLEUR F, MACLEOD S: Parasitic infections in a New York City hospital: trends from 1971 to 1984. Am J Pub Health 76:1024–1026, 1986

330. VINAYAK VK, et al: Specific circulating immune complexes in amoebic liver abscess. J Clin Microbiol 23:1088–1090, 1986

331. WAKELIN D: *Trichinella spiralis*: immunity, ecology and evolution. J Parasitol 79:488–94, 1993

332. WELSH JA: Problems in recognition and diagnosis of amebiasis: estimation of the global magnitude of morbidity and mortality. Rev Infect Dis 8:118–238, 1986

333. WALDEN J: Parasitic diseases. Other roundworms. Trichiuris, hookworm and strongyloides. Primary Care 18:53–74, 1991

334. WALLS KW, SMITH JW: Serology of parasitic infections. Lab Med 10:329–336, 1979

335. WALTER H, KRISHNASWAMI H: Granulomatous peritonitis caused by *Ascaris* eggs: a report of three cases. J Trop Med Hyg 92:17–19, 1989

336. WALZER PD: *Pneumocystis carinii*. Mandell GL, Bennett JE, Dolin R (eds), *Principles and Practices of Infectious Dis-*

eases, 4th ed, Chap 258. New York, Churchill Livingston, 1995

337. WAMAE CN: Advances in the diagnosis of human lymphatic filariases: a review. E Afr Med J 74:171–182, 1994

338. WARREN KS, MAHMOUD AAF: Algorithms in the diagnosis and management of exotic diseases. XII. Prevention of exotic diseases: advice to travelers. J Infect Dis 133:596–601, 1976

339. WEBBE G: Human cysticercosis: parasitology, pathology, clinical manifestations and available treatment. Pharmacol Ther 64:175–200, 1994

340. WEBER R, BRYAN RT, JURANEK DD: Improved stool concentration procedure for detection of *Cryptosporidum* oocysts in fecal specimens. J Clin Microbiol 30:2869–2873, 1992

341. WEBER R, BRYAN RT, SCHWARTS DA, OWEN RL: Human microsporidial infections. Clin Microbiol Rev 7:426–461, 1994

342. WEIL GJ, JAIN DC, SANTHANASA S, et al: A monoclonal antibody-based enzyme immunoassay for detecting parasite antigenemia in bancroftian filariasis. J Infect Dis 156:350–355, 1987

343. WEINKE T, FRIEDRICH-JANICKE B, HOPP P, JANITSCHKE K: Prevalence and clinical importance of *Entamoeba histolytica* in two high-risk groups: travelers returning from the tropics and male homosexuals. J Infect Dis 161:1029–1031, 1990

344. WEISS JB: DNA probes and PCR for diagnosis of parasitic infections. Clin Microbiol Rev 8:113–130, 1995

345. WHITE AC JR, TATO P, MOLINARI JL: Host-parasite interactions in *Taenia solium* cysticercosis. Infect Agents Dis 1:185–193, 1992

346. WILLIAMS DC, SHOOKHOFF HB, FELMAN YM, et al: High rates of protozoal infections in selected homosexual men attending a venereal disease clinic. Sex Transm Dis 5:155–157, 1978

347. WILSON M, SCHANTZ P, PIENIAZEK N: Diagnosis of parasitic infections: immunologic and molecular methods. Murray PR (ed), *Manual of Clinical Microbiology*, 6th ed, Washington DC, ASM Press, 1995

348. WIRTH DF, ROGERS WO, BARKER R JR, et al: Leishmaniasis and malaria: new tool for epidemiologic analysis. Science 234:975–979, 1986

349. WITOONPANICH R, et al: Eosinophilic myelomeningoencephalitis caused by *Angiostrongylus cantonensis*: a report of three cases. Southwest Asian J Trop Med Public Health 22:262–267, 1991

350. WOLF MS: Symptomatology, diagnosis and treatment. Erlandsen SL, Meyer EA (eds), *Giardia and Giardiasis*. New York, Plenum, 1984.

351. WOLF MS: Giardiasis. Clin Microbiol Rev 5:93–100, 1992

352. WOLFSON JS, WALDRON MA, SIERRA LS: Blinded comparison of a direct immunofluorescent monoclonal antibody staining method and a Giemsa staining method for identification of *Pneumocystis carinii* in induced sputum and bronchoalveolar lavage specimens of patients infected with human immunodeficiency virus. J Clin Microbiol 28:2136–2138, 1990

353. WONG B, GOLD JWM, BROWN AE, et al: Central nervous system toxoplasmosis in homosexual men and parenteral drug abusers. Ann Intern Med 100:36–42, 1984

354. WONG SY, JAJDU MP, RAMIREZ R, et al: Role of specific immunoglobulin E in diagnosis of acute toxoplasma infection and toxoplasmosis. J Clin Microbiol 31:2952–2959, 1993

355. WONSIT R, THAMMAPALERD N, THARAVANIJ S, et al: Enzyme-linked immunosorbent assay based on monclonal and polyclonal antibodies for the detection of *Entamoeba histolytica* antigens in fecal specimens. Trans R Soc Trop Med Hyg 86:166–169, 1992

356. WOO PT, PATERSON WB: *Giardia lamblia* in children in day-care centers in southern Ontario, Canada, and susceptibility of animals to *G. lamblia*. Trans R Soc Trop Med Hyg 80:56–59, 1986

357. WORLD HEALTH ORGANIZATION: Parasitic Diseases Programme. Major parasitic infections: a global view. World Health Stat Q 39:145–160, 1986

358. WORLD HEALTH ORGANIZATION: Epidemiology and control of African trypanosomiasis: report of a WHO expert committee. WHO Tech Rep Ser 739:36–58, 1986

359. WRIGHT RA AND VERNON TM: Epidemic giardiasis at a resort lodge. Rocky Mt Med J 73:208–211, 1976

360. WURTZ R, KOCKA FE, PETERS CS, et al: Clinical characteristics of seven cases of diarrhea associated with a novel acid-fast organism in the stool. Clin Infect Dis 16:136–138, 1991

361. WURTZ R: *Cyclospora*: A newly identified intestinal pathogen of humans. Clin Infect Dis 18:620–626, 1994

362. WYLER DJ: *Plasmodium* species (malaria). Mandell G, Bennett JE, Dolin R (eds), *Principles and Practice of Infectious Diseases*, 4th ed, Chap 253. New York, Churchill Livingstone, 1995

363. YANG J, SCHOLTON T: *Dientamoeba fragilis*: A review with notes on epidemiology, pathogenicity, mode of transmission and diagnosis. Am J Trop Med Hyg 26:16–22, 1979

364. YAQUIHASHI A, SATO N, TAKAHASHI S, et al: A serodiagnostic assay by microenzyme-linked immunosorbent assay for human anisakiasis using a monoclonal antibody specific for *Anisikiasis* larvae antigen. J Infect Dis 161:995–998, 1990

365. YOUNG DK, BULLOCK SL, MILVIN DM, et al: Ethyl acetate as a substitute for diethyl ether in the formalin– ether sedimentation technique. J Clin Microbiol 10: 852–853, 1979

366. YOUSSEF FG, MIKHAIL EM, MANSOUR HS: Intestinal capillariasis in Egypt: a case report. Am J Trop Med Hyg 40:195–196, 1989

367. YU S, XU L, JIANG Z, et al: Report on the first nationwide survey of the distribution of human parasites in China. Chin J Parasit Dis 12:241–247, 1994

368. ZAMAN MK, WOOTEN OJ, SUPRAHMANYA B, et al: Rapid noninvasive diagnosis of *Pneumocystis carinii* from induced liquefied sputum. Ann Intern Med 109:7–10, 1988

369. ZIERDT, CH: *Blastocystis hominis*: an intestinal protozoan parasite of man. Public Health Lab 36:147–160, 1978

370. ZIERDT CH, GILL VJ, ZIERDT WS: Detection of microsporidian spores in clinical samples by indirect fluorescent-antibody using whole-cell antisera to *Encephalitozoon cuniculi* and *Encephalitozoon heelem*. J Clin Microbiol 31:3071–3074, 1993

APPENDIX I

ECTOPARASITES AND OTHER INVERTEBRATES IN THE CLINICAL LABORATORY: A BRIEF GUIDE*

Ectoparasites are organisms that live in or on the skin of a host, from which they receive nourishment. The relation is, therefore, parasitic or possibly symbiotic. Intimacy of contact varies from the time required for a blood meal to days, weeks, or even months of association. Organisms that contact a host casually (e.g., house flies) or without deriving benefit (e.g., scorpions, bees, and spiders) are not, strictly speaking, ectoparasites.[42]

Arthropods are invertebrates with jointed appendages (hence, the name) and a chitinous exoskeleton. They have long been recognized as direct or indirect causes of human disease and may produce damage to the human host in their own right. Alternatively, they may serve as the vectors for transmission of infectious agents and entry of the agent into the human host. In some instances, the arthropod serves as a mere carrier, depositing the infectious agent in the proximate environment where it can contact the potential victim. An example of such a scenario is the transmission of bacterial pathogens from one site to another on the bodies of flies or cockroaches.[4,30] A much more intimate relation occurs when the arthropod is the direct mediator of cellular damage or when a biting insect transmits an infectious agent into the tissue of the victim. Such biting insects ingest the infectious agent when they take a blood meal from an infected human or from an infected nonhuman mammal, which is referred to as a **reservoir of infection**. When an insect bites an animal or human, it often injects salivary secretions that contain enzymes and anticoagulants designed to permit the ingestion of a blood meal. If the infectious agent has moved from the gut of the insect into the hemolymph and subsequently made its way to the salivary glands, the infection is transmitted in the salivary secretions at the time of the bite.[29] If the infectious agent is present in the gut—with or without infectious material in the saliva—the microbial agent may be excreted in the feces when the arthropod defecates after ingestion of the blood meal. Entry of the agent from the feces into the injection site is facilitated when the host scratches the site of irritation.

The list of medically significant arthropods continues to expand, as does the list of diseases they can produce. At the same time, clinical laboratories are receiving increasing numbers of specimens for identification. Many arthropods that are very important in human infectious disease are rarely, if ever, seen in clinical microbiology laboratories because the insects were not seen, were exterminated, or were not collected for examination. Other important insects, such as scorpions, are seen in localized geographic distributions. On the other hand, clinical microbiologists may be called on to identify insects that caused alarm at their presence even though they have done no harm.

This section is designed to assist the reader in understanding the medical significance and laboratory identification of arthropods that may be encountered commonly in the clinical laboratory. An abbreviated classification schema is detailed in Table 20-11 and select definitions and related taxonomy of the ectoparasites of importance to humans are listed in Box 20-11. The reader is referred to several excellent reference texts for more detailed information.[14–17,26,33,37]

SUBMISSION OF SPECIMENS TO THE LABORATORY

Because of the diversity of specimens dealt with in medical entomology, it is difficult to recommend a single method for submission of specimens. In general, 70% ethanol will work well for most specimens as a preservative, also preventing escape or autoinfection. It should be added to the specimen in a clean container so that the arthropod is completely submersed.

Formalin and sterile saline may be satisfactory but generally have more disadvantages when compared with ethanol. Flying insects should be killed using gases, such as chloroform, and then preserved as a dry mount.[16] Garcia and coworkers list a recipe for Berelese's medium, which they suggest is a good solution to use for most specimens.[16] Killing in hot water has been suggested for examination of fly larvae.[15] If in doubt, check with the facility that will be handling the specimen for specific recommendations.

The materials and techniques required for examination of arthropods are simple. Low magnification can be obtained with a hand lens or optimally with a stereomicroscope. Low to moderate power magnification can also be obtained with a low power objective (e.g., 2× or 4×) and a compound microscope. A good light source is essential for observation. Fiberoptic lights provide excellent illumination without heating and excessive drying of the specimen. Lights with flexible arms allow maximal control of the illumination angle. The specimen can be manipulated best with a pair of dissecting needles.

In the exceptional circumstance that culture of the potential pathogen from the vector is under consideration, the insect must be unfixed. If the specimen was fixed before submission to the laboratory, modern molecular methods allow specific identification of infectious agents by immunofluorescence or DNA hybridization–amplification.

---

*With a contribution by Fred W. Westenfeld.

TABLE 20-11
CLASSIFICATION OF ARTHROPODS OF MEDICAL IMPORTANCE

CLASS	ORDER OR SUBCLASS	EXAMPLES	DIRECT INJURY OR INFECTIONS TRANSMITTED
Diplopoda		Millipedes	Direct
Chilopoda		Centipedes	Direct
Hexapoda (Insecta)	Hemiptera	Bedbugs Kissing bugs	Direct
Hexapoda (Insecta)	Siphonaptera	Fleas	Direct
Hexapoda (Insecta)	Anopleura	Sucking lice	Direct; typhus; trench fever; relapsing fever
Hexapoda (Insecta)	Dictyoptera	Cockroaches	Sanitation problems; allergic reactions
Hexapoda (Insecta)	Hymenoptera	Ants, wasps, bees	Direct
Hexapoda (Insecta)	Coleoptera	Beetles	Direct
Hexapoda (Insecta)	Diptera	Flies, mosquitoes, midges	Direct; arboviruses; parasitic infection; *Bartonella*; *Francisella*
Hexapoda (Insecta)	Lepidoptera	Moths, butterflies, caterpillars	Direct
Pentastomida		Tongue worms	Direct
Arachnida	Subclass: Scorpiones	Scorpions	Direct
Arachnida	Subclass: Araneae	Spiders	Direct
Arachnida	Subclass: Acari	Ticks, mites, chiggers	Direct; *Borrelia*; arboviruses; *Ehrlichia*; *Rickettsia*; *Francisella*

ARACHNIDA: TICKS, MITES, AND SPIDERS

TICKS

Ticks are either "hard" or "soft." Hard ticks have mouthparts that extend outward and, therefore, are easily visible when looking straight down at the specimen. In addition, they have a dorsal hard plate or shield, known as a scutum. Soft ticks do not possess a scutum, and their mouthparts are positioned toward the middle of the ventral side, so that they are not observable when viewed from above.

There are major differences in the biology of soft and hard ticks.[17] Soft ticks are relatively resistant to desiccation and are often found in hot, dry climates. They inhabit animal burrows and dens or abandoned huts and cabins. Soft ticks may go through several nymphal molts, and adults may take more than one blood meal and lay more than one batch of eggs. They are adapted to obtaining a rapid blood meal, so they need not remain attached to a mammalian host for long periods.

Conversely, hard ticks are susceptible to desiccation, and they are found in areas with woods or brush, where there is ready access to mammalian hosts. Most hard ticks that parasitize humans proceed through three developmental stages—larval, nymphal, and adult—each of which takes a single blood meal. Complete feeding may require several days.[17]

Identification of common ticks to the level of the genus can be accomplished with reasonable accuracy if clinical microbiologists are willing to familiarize themselves with the major taxonomic characters. It is important to recognize several general principles for observation of ticks. Male and females of the same species have different appearances. An unfed (flat) and engorged (round) tick of the same sex and species can appear dramatically different. Finally, an engorged hard tick may be so swollen that its distinguishing scutum is obscured, leading the inexperienced observer to identify it as a soft tick.[17]

It is extremely difficult to identify ticks to the species level, a task that should be left to expert entomologists, who are usually available for consultation through local health departments or universities. Fortunately, the situation is somewhat simplified by the limited number of species that commonly feed on humans and the geographically defined (if often extensive) distribution of these species. Therefore, the possibilities are relatively defined and limited if a submitted tick has been feeding on a person. In contrast, the possibilities for a tick that has been found on vegetation or free in the environment are poorly defined, and the choices are much greater. Goddard relates a personal experience in which 30% of the ticks collected and identified in a study of Mississippi ticks were assigned to species that do not occur in the United States.[17]

BOX 20-11. ECTOPARASITES: DEFINITIONS AND TAXONOMY

Arthropoda: Phylum of organisms having a hard, jointed exoskeleton and symmetrical paired, jointed legs. Of the five classes of arthropods, only the *Arachnida* and the *Insecta* serve as vectors of human disease.

Class *Arachnida* (ticks, mites, and spiders): a class of arthropods characterized by the absence of wings, presence of four pairs of legs, and fusion of the head and thorax into a cephalothorax.

Ticks are larger than mites, have a leathery body that is either hairless or covered with short hairs, an exposed hypostome and a pair of spiracles near the cosze of the fourth pair of legs. They are divided into the argasid, or soft ticks (*Ornithodoros* species being of human importance), and the ixodid, or hard ticks, including the genera *Dermacentor*, *Amblyomma* and *Ixodes*, which are responsible for transmitting the agents of several rickettsial, viral, bacterial, and spirochetal diseases.

Mites are smaller than ticks, do not have a leathery covering, and have a hypostome that may be unarmed. Of importance to humans are the trombiculid mites, causing chiggers, and the mange mites of the family *Sarcoptidae*, which include *S. scabiei*, the agent of scabies, and *Demodex folliculorum*, which infest the hair follicles and sebaceous glands.

Spiders are unsegmented, have a hairy abdomen to which are attached four pairs of legs through a slender constriction. They also possess a pair of poisonous jaws through which venom flows from a pair of glands in the cephalothorax. The brown recluse, black widow, and the hobo spiders most commonly cause painful and toxic bites in humans.

Class *Insecta* (flies, mosquitoes, bugs, fleas and lice): a class of arthropods, including organisms with a body divided into three parts, head, thorax and abdomen, and possessing three pairs of legs. The order *Hemiptera* includes winged or wingless bugs and lice that have mouth parts adapted for piercing and sucking; the order *Diptera* (two winged) include flies, gnats and mosquitos, and the order *Siphonaptera* includes the fleas, which are wingless and have mouth parts adapted for blood sucking.

Flies are two winged insects that serve as vectors for the transmission of several agents of human disease. Included are the *Phlebotomus* sandflies (leishmaniasis), *Simulium* black fly (onchocerciasis), Chrysops deer fly (*Loa loa*), and the *Glossina* or tsetse fly (trypanosomiasis). Mosquitos transmit a variety of viral, protozoan, and helminth diseases, most notably malaria and fliariasis. Humans may also be infested with the larval forms of flies, a condition known as myiasis.

The biting and blood sucking "bugs" of importance in human disease include *Cimex lectularius*, the common bedbug, and the "kissing bugs" of the family *Reduviidae*, which transmit the causative agent of South American trypanosomiasis (Chagas disease).

Fleas are small, brown, wingless, laterally compressed, bloodsucking insects most notably cited as vectors for transmission of the agents of bubonic plague and typhus. Fleas are also involved in the transmission of parasitic diseases, including the dog tapeworm, *Dipylidium caninum*, and the rat tapeworm, *Hymenolepis diminuta*.

Lice are dorsoventrally flattened, wingless insects that include three species of importance to humans: *Pediculus humanus* var. *capitis* (head louse), *Pediculus humanus* var. *corporis* (body louse) and *Phthirus pubis* (crab louse). The order includes both biting and sucking lice; however, only the latter, in the suborder *Anoplura*, are ectoparasitic for humans.

IXODES SPP.

Relation to Disease

Ixodes ticks are also known as black-legged ticks, deer ticks, or bear ticks. They transmit the causative bacterial agent of Lyme disease, *Borrelia burgdorferi*[8,12]; *Babesia microti*, a protozoan parasite that causes babesiosis[36]; and the newly described agent of human granulocytic ehrlichiosis.[24] The vector for a newly described babesia-like organism in the western United States has not been defined.[25a]

Identification

Ticks belonging to the genus *Ixodes* are hard ticks and easily identified by a characteristic "U"-shaped groove anterior to the anus (see Color Plate 20-8*A*). They have no colored markings on the scutum (see Color Plate 20-8*B*).

Geographic Distribution

A small number of *Ixodes* spp. both seek human hosts frequently[13] and are competent at maintaining and transmitting the pathogens mentioned before.[27] The

primary human-seeking vectors within the genus are *I. scapularis* (*dammini*) in the eastern and north central United States (Lyme disease, babesiosis, and granulocytic ehrlichiosis), *I. pacificus* in the western United States (Lyme disease), *I. ricinus* in Europe, and possibly *I. persulcatus* in Japan.[7,19] Other ixodid ticks may harbor and transmit *Borrelia burgdorferi*, but do not encounter humans frequently enough to cause disease commonly.[23] Nymphs of the northern form of *I. scapularis* (*dammini*) feed on small mammals, especially rodents, deer, and birds; also on humans, and other large mammals. Adult ticks prefer deer and occasionally feed on humans. The southern form of *I. scapularis* and *I. pacificus* have similar preferences, but lizards figure more prominently in their preferences.[17]

DERMACENTOR SPP.

Relation to Disease

Dermacentor spp. transmit *Rickettsia rickettsii*, which causes Rocky Mountain spotted fever.[35] This genus has also been associated with tularemia,[35] tick paralysis,[35]

Colorado tick fever,[35] and possibly *Salmonella* infection.[14]

Identification

Dermacentor spp. are "hard" ticks. They possess small mouth parts, which are as long as the basis capituli. White markings on the scutum are characteristic of this genus and also of *Amblyomma* spp. (see Color Plate 20-8C). Eleven festoons are present.[15]

Geographic Distribution

The Rocky Mountain wood tick, *D. andersoni*, is the primary vector of human pathogens in the western United States and Canada. Nymphs prefer small mammals, whereas adults seek out cattle, sheep, deer, and other large mammals, including humans. In the eastern United States the primary species of concern is the American dog tick, *D. variabilis*. This species occurs throughout the country except in parts of the Rocky Mountain region.[17] Nymphs feed on rodents or other small animals, whereas adults take their blood meal preferentially from dogs, but will happily bite humans if available.

AMBLYOMMA SPP.

Relation to Disease

Amblyomma spp. may transmit *Francisella tularensis* and also cause tick paralysis. This genus may also transmit Rocky Mountain spotted fever and human monocytic ehrlichiosis (*Ehrlichia chaffeensis*), although it does not appear to be as important as *Dermacentor* spp. in the life cycle of these pathogens.[35] It has been suggested that *A. americanum* transmits *Borrelia burgdorferi*, but recent evidence indicates that the infectious agent is actually an as yet uncultivated spirochete, tentatively named *Borrelia lonestari*.[3]

Identification

Amblyomma americanum females have a characteristic white marking (the "lone star") on the scutum, which usually contains two "eyes." Mouthparts are quite long, three to four times as long as the basis capituli (see Color Plate 20-8D).

Geographic Distribution

Amblyomma americanum occurs in the East and Midwest from central Texas north to Iowa and New Jersey or New York. This tick is voracious and catholic in its preferences, willing to feed on birds and on virtually any available mammal, including humans.

ORNITHODOROS SPP.

Relation to Disease

Ornithodoros spp. transmit the *Borrelia* spp. that cause endemic relapsing fever.

Identification

Ornithodoros spp. are soft ticks. By definition their mouthparts are not visible from above, and they do not have a scutum. They have a prominent hypostome covered with teeth (see Color Plate 20-8E).

Geographic Distribution

It is difficult to differentiate among the several species that may transmit relapsing fever. In the northwestern United States and western Canada *O. hermsi* is the primary vector. This species feeds on small rodents as well as humans and typically inhabits cracks and crevices in shacks and cabins. A famous outbreak in a Boy Scout troop was concentrated in senior scouts and scoutmasters, who commandeered an abandoned cabin, leaving the younger scouts to spend their night unbitten under the stars.[39]

In the Southwest and southern Midwest the common vector is *O. turicata*, which is found on a variety of small and large mammals, rodents, birds, and reptiles. This species is often found in animal burrows.

MITES

Numerous species of mites exist in nature. Species of the family Trombiculiae (chigger mites) produce intense itching or dermatitis as they feed transiently. Members of the genus *Leptotrombidium* transmit scrub typhus in Southeast Asia and Australia.[43] House dust mites in the genus *Dermatophagoides* serve as allergens for certain individuals. The mouse mite, *Liponyssoides* (*Allodermanyssus*) *sanguineus*, transmits *Rickettsia akari*, the agent of rickettsialpox.[18] The itch mite, *Sarcoptes scabei*, and the follicle mite, *Demodex folliculorum*, are the two mites that have an intimate and prolonged parasitic association with humans.

SARCOPTES SCABEI (SCABIES)

Relation to Disease

Sarcoptes scabei is known as the "itch mite." The mite causes mange by burrowing into the skin and laying eggs in the burrows. Resulting larval and nymphal stages of the mite live in the burrows and adjacent hair follicles. Fecal deposits left by the mites provoke intense itching, leading to significant irritation and hair loss.

Identification

Microscopic examination of skin scrapings reveals the characteristic mite (see Color Plate 20-8F), which measures 0.2 to 0.4 mm in length.

Geographic Distribution

Itch mites are distributed worldwide.

DEMODEX FOLLICULORUM (HAIR FOLLICLES); DEMODEX BREVIS (SEBACEOUS GLANDS)

Relation to Disease

Infections are usually found on the face. Organisms can cause pruritus and local tissue reaction as they burrow in the skin. They are also found, however, in asymptomatic individuals.

Identification

Microscopic examination of specimens from skin reveals the characteristic mite, which measures 0.1 to 0.4 mm in length.

Geographic Distribution
Follicle mites are distributed worldwide.

SPIDERS

Thousands of species of spiders exist in nature. Most possess potent toxins, but only a small number are capable of penetrating human skin when biting.[15]

LOXOSCELES RECLUSA

Relation to Disease
Loxosceles reclusa, known commonly as the brown recluse spider, prefers to exist in stored clothes and sleeping bags, basements, closets, and other sites with reduced human activity.[15,16] Their venom is injected through biting, and can cause serious desquamation and necrosis of skin. Large doses of venom are associated with dissemination and significant mortality.

Identification
The brown recluse spider is characterized by its yellow to brown coloration, 1- to 2-cm size, and a violin- or fiddle-shaped marking on its head (see Color Plate 20-9G).[15,16] There are several related species, which may require expert help for correct identification.

Geographic Distribution
The brown recluse spider is found in most of the continental United States except for the extreme western sections.

LACTRODECTUS MACTANS

Relation to Disease
Several species of widow spiders exist. *Lactrodectus mactans*, the most common black widow spider, may cause a serious systemic reaction, even death, after injection of its venom. Fortunately, most patients are not gravely ill and recover quickly.[15,16] Most bites occur on the hands.[37] Male spiders produce mild or no symptoms after their bite.[17]

Identification
The black widow female is 3 cm long (including legs), glossy black, and displays a characteristic red hourglass marking on her abdomen (see Color Plate 20-9H).[15,16,37] Differentiation among related species is difficult and best left to experts.

Geographic Distribution
Different species of widow spiders exist throughout the entire continental United States. *Latrodectus mactans* occurs from southern New England south to Florida and west to California and Oregon; it is more common in the southern part of the range. The northern black widow spider, *L. variolus* is present in New England and southern Canada south to Florida and west to eastern Texas, Oklahoma, and Kansas; it is more common in the northern part of its range.

TEGENARIA AGRESTIS

Relation to Disease
In recent years, there have been increasing reports of toxic reactions to the bite of the hobo spider, *T. agrestis*. Many bites are not followed by serious reactions, but some bites may produce a lesion that closely resembles that of the brown recluse spider. Erythema is followed by blistering and then ulceration. An eschar forms and subsequently sloughs, with or without formation of a scar. Systemic effects are usually mild but may be severe. The male spider is more venomous than the female.[11]

Identification
Hobo spiders are brown with gray markings. They are moderately large, measuring 7 to 14 mm in body length and 27 to 45 mm in leg span.

Geographic Distribution
Tegenaria agrestis is distributed throughout the Pacific Northwest, southwestern Canada, and the Alaskan panhandle. The distribution of this spider does not overlap that of *Loxosceles reclusa*. The hobo spider builds funnel-shaped webs in damp, moist places, such as wood piles and crawl spaces. It is rarely found above foundation or ground level.

INSECTA: FLIES, BUGS, FLEAS, AND LICE

MYIASIS-PRODUCING FLY LARVAE

Myiasis occurs when fly larvae infect humans either accidentally or by penetrating skin directly to form subcutaneous skin lesions, for the purpose of feeding on tissue. Imported cases of myiasis are increasing owing to more frequent travel to endemic areas.[6,40] The two most common genera that parasitize humans are *Dermatobia* and *Cordylobia*. Flies in the genera *Wohlfarhtia*, *Cochliomyia*, *Hypoderma*, and *Oestrus* affect humans much less commonly and will not be discussed here.[14,15,17,33]

DERMATOBIA HOMINIS (HUMAN BOT FLY)
Relation to Disease
The fascinating life cycle of this organism requires some discussion to understand infection. The female attaches her eggs to another insect vector, often a mosquito. While the insect is biting a host, the eggs release larvae which immediately penetrate the skin. Larvae mature in the skin for approximately 6 to 12 weeks, after which they leave the subcutaneous tissue for the soil, where they require another 3 weeks of maturation before an adult fly emerges.[6,33,40]

While in the skin, the larvae produce a lesion that resembles a "boil," which is often quite pruritic and occasionally painful. Complete excision of the larvae eliminates the disease and allows confirmation of the diagnosis. Secondary bacterial infections of the lesions occur occasionally.

Identification
Larvae range in size from several millimeters to 18 to 25 mm, depending on maturity at the time of excision. Rows of spines that are easily visible with a dissecting microscope encircle them (see Color Plate 20-8G). Larval stages may have a distinct "flask" shape, with a long tapered neck. Microscopic examination of the spiracles (stigmal plates) are useful when making an identification.[15,16]

Geographic Distribution
Dermatobia hominis is common in Central and South America.[6,15,31]

CORDYLOBIA ANTHROPOPHAGA (TUMBU FLY)

Relation to Disease
Larvae emerge from eggs that have contaminated bed linen, clothing or other materials and penetrate the host's skin shortly after contact.[6,20] Development in the subdermal layer occurs much faster than with *Dermatobia hominis*, usually within 2 weeks,[6] reducing the relative number of imported cases.[20] Patients are generally exposed to a larger number of eggs, so numerous lesions are more likely with *Cordylobia* infection than with *Dermatobia*.[6]

Identification
Larvae reach 7 to 12 mm at maturation. Their more conical shape readily distinguishes them from *Dermatobia*.[20] Spiracles appear at the widest end.

Geographic Distribution
Cordylobia is primarily found in sub-Saharan Africa.

OTHER FLIES

Several other medically important flies warrant brief discussion, although specimens are rarely submitted to clinical laboratories.

Sandflies belonging to the genera *Lutzomyia* and *Phlebotomus* are responsible for transmission of leishmaniasis. These flies are hairy, small, and tend to have wings held in an erect "V" shape. *Chrysops* sp., commonly known as deer flies, are involved in transmission of *Loa loa*, the African eye worm. Black flies (*Simulium* sp.) are the vectors for the microfilariae causing onchocerciasis. Different *Simulium* species exist in distinct geographic regions, but all reproduce in fast-flowing waterways near which the largest number of bites occur. Tsetse flies (*Glossina* sp.) exist only in tropical Africa and transmit African trypanosomiasis (sleeping sickness). These elongated flies possess a powerful proboscis capable of inflicting painful bites.[37]

MOSQUITOES

Mosquitoes are responsible for transmitting diseases causing greater morbidity and mortality than any other arthropod.[15,16,37]

Relation to Disease
Mosquitoes produce pruritic skin lesions that appear shortly after taking a blood meal. They are also capable of transmitting serious infections. *Anopheles* spp. are the arthropod vectors responsible for transmitting malaria. Filariasis is spread by some *Aedes* spp., *Mansonia* spp., and *Anopheles* spp. A variety of arthropod-borne viruses (arboviruses) use *Aedes* spp., *Culex* spp., *Culiseta* spp., *Haemagogus* spp., and *Sabethes* spp. as vectors of serious infections, such as equine encephalitis, yellow fever, and dengue.[9,28,37] Both male and female mosquitoes feed on nectar and pollinate flowers. The female mosquito must take a blood meal to complete development of eggs.[17]

Identification
Mosquitoes are dainty-appearing, flying insects easily recognized by most. Identification to genus and species level requires significant experience and should be left to the experts. Mosquito bites are sufficiently common that patients rarely bring specimens to the clinical laboratory for identification.

Geographic Distribution
Mosquitoes are found worldwide, but individual species have well-defined environmental niches. For instance, classic yellow fever was an urban disease, because the primary vector, *Aedes aegypti*, was limited to standing water in the vicinity of human dwellings. It was hoped that the disease could be completely eliminated by controlling the mosquito vector. Unfortunately, control of urban yellow fever revealed a sylvatic cycle among monkeys and several forest mosquito species, and it soon became clear that the virus could be controlled, but never eliminated (unless we are successful at destroying all of the rain forests).[37]

"BUGS"

Bedbugs (*Cimex* spp.) and reduviid (Family Reduviidae) bugs suck the blood of vertebrates, including humans, and may act as important vectors in transmission of disease.[15,37] They are nocturnal, feeding at night, hiding and resting during the day. The common bedbug (*C. lectularius*) is occasionally submitted to microbiology laboratories for identification.

CIMEX LECTULARIUS

Relation to Disease
The common bedbug can cause numerous small lesions on the skin wherever a blood meal was taken. The severity of the lesions is related to the sensitivity of the individual. Bedbugs feed primarily at night, otherwise hiding in the bed linen, loose wallpaper, and mattresses.[15] They do not act as vectors of infectious agents.

Identification
Bedbugs are light to orangish-brown, 5 mm long × 3 mm wide.[15,16] Adults have small, nonworking wing appendages (see Color Plate 20-8H).

Geographic Distribution
Cimex lectularius is distributed worldwide, although more common in temperate zones, whereas *C. hemipterus* is more common in tropical climates.[37]

KISSING BUGS: *PANSTRONGYLUS* SPP., *RHODNIUS* SPP., AND *TRIATOMA* SPP.

Relation to Disease
The family Reduviidae has several popular names. These bugs are sometimes known as "cone-nose bugs" from the elongated shape of their head. The majority of the group are known as assassin bugs from their lethal aggression against other insects. Assassin bugs may also bite humans and cause painful lesions.[17]

Medically, the most important group are the "kissing bugs," so-named because they may take their blood meals from the skin around the lips. Kissing bugs transmit the causative agent of Chagas disease, *Trypanosoma cruzi*. They are unable to bite through clothing, so lesions are most common on exposed parts of the body.[17] Feces containing *T. cruzi* are deposited on the host while feeding. Subsequent scratching of pruritic skin at the bite site introduces organisms into the wound. Transmission also occurs when fecally contaminated fingers are rubbed in the eyes, nose, or mouth.[37]

Identification
Unlike bedbugs, reduviid (triatomid) bugs possess functioning wings. They range in size from 1 to 4 cm, are more elongate than bedbugs, and have relatively long, thin heads (see Color Plate 20-9A).[15,16,37]

Geographic Distribution
Kissing bugs occur in southern portions of the United States and in Central and South America.

FLEAS

Relation to Disease
Fleas may cause irritating, itchy bites after sucking blood from a host. Those species that transmit the most serious human infections most commonly are considered here. The Oriental rat flea, *Xenopsylla cheopis*, is the classic vector of plague[22] and murine typhus.[17] *Tunga penetrans*, the "jigger" flea found in Africa and in Central and South America, penetrates the skin and lays eggs inside the host (see Color Plate 20-9B).

The cat flea, *Ctenocephalides felis*, and the dog flea, *Ctenocephalides canis*, can infect either species of domestic animal (see Color Plate 20-9C). In North America the dog flea is uncommon and most human disease is caused by the cat flea.[17] Either species can bite humans. The dog tapeworm, *Dipylidium caninum*, may occasionally infect humans when a flea containing the cysticercoid stage of the tapeworm is accidentally ingested.[15,16] Several species of fleas, in addition to other insects, may transmit the larvae of the rat tapeworm, *Hymenolepis diminuta* to humans. Recently it has been recognized that endemic plague may be associated with exposure to cats, and endemic typhus, caused by *Rickettsia typhi*, may be transmitted by the cat flea.[34,41] A newly described rickettsia, known as the ELB agent,[32] also infects the cat flea.[41] This new rickettsial organism can be maintained by transovarial transmission in cat fleas.[2] In developed countries cats may be more important than rats in transmission of these infections.

Identification
Recognition of fleas is relatively easy. They are wingless, and have long, muscular legs[15,16,37] hanging down from a body that looks "hunched over" (see Color Plates 20-9B and 20-9C). Speciation of fleas is very difficult, usually requiring considerable expertise.

Geographic Distribution
Fleas are found worldwide, following the distribution of the mammalian host. *Xenophylla cheopis* is associated primarily with brown rats (*Rattus norvegicus*, also known as Norwegian sewer rats) and black rats (*Rattus rattus*, also known as house or roof rats). *Ctendocephalides* spp. are found on cats and dogs.

LICE

Lice are a considerable public health concern, producing diseases that range from relatively benign to life-threatening. As agents of direct injury they cause minor, yet irritating skin and hair infestations. As arthropod vectors they are capable of transmitting important bacterial pathogens. Although individual species are associated with different parts of the body, some overlap does occur.

PEDICULUS HUMANUS

Relation to Disease
Pediculus humanus (the human body louse) parasitizes most parts of the human body other than the head. Body lice are primarily found in the hairier regions, where they migrate back and forth from clothing to skin to take blood meals.[15] Feeding causes irritating, pruritic bite wounds, a general characteristic of infestations with lice. Most eggs, called nits, are laid on clothing.

Body lice transmit *Borrelia recurrentis*, the causative agent of relapsing fever,[5,38] and *Rickettsia prowazekii* and *Bartonella* (*Rochalimaea*) *quintana*,[21] which cause epidemic typhus and trench fever, respectively.[15,37] In relapsing fever, crushed lice release organisms onto the skin that then enter through abrasions. Typhus and trench fever agents, which are present in louse feces, enter when scratched into the skin by the host.[37] The mortality rate in untreated epidemic typhus may be as high as 60%,[37] perhaps because of the presence of other complicating factors, but antimicrobial therapy effectively controls the infection.[25]

Body lice are spread by fairly close contact with infected individuals. Shared clothing, bedding, and close communal habitation are associated with transmission.[15] Not surprisingly, louse-borne infections occur under conditions of extreme privation, such as war and famine.

Identification
Body lice reach 2 to 4 mm in length, with a relatively long, slender abdomen. They have three pairs of legs, with clawlike hooks on the ends that aid in securing the louse to its host (see Color Plate 20-9D).

Geographic Distribution
Body lice occur worldwide.

PEDICULUS CAPITIS

Relation to Disease

Head lice produce irritating infections of the head, hair, and neck regions. They infect only humans; pets and other animals are not susceptible. Unlike the body louse, head lice do not serve as vectors for transmission of bacteria, although secondary bacterial infection of the bite wound may occur.[10] The 1-mm–sized nits (eggs) are most often glued to a hair shaft near the scalp (see Color Plate 20-9E).

Infestations are most common in children.[10] They occur through close contact and sharing of fomites such as combs, hats, and scarves.[15]

Identification

Head lice closely resemble body lice. Although size overlap does occur, they may be slightly shorter than body lice, averaging 1 to 3 mm.[1] The elongated abdomen and the three pairs of legs with hooks are virtually identical with those found on the body louse. Nits are easily confused with dandruff, seborrheic scales, hair spray, or fungal infection (see Color Plate 20-9E).[10] Specimens should be submitted to experts for confirmation.

Geographic Distribution

The head louse is found throughout the world.

PHTHIRUS PUBIS

Relation to Disease

Phthirus pubis, also known as the crab or pubic louse, causes an irritating infection of the pubic area. It may be found less frequently in the armpits, chest, thighs, and short facial hairs of mustaches, eyebrows, and eyelashes.[1,15] The lice leave a pruritic bite wound on the skin after taking a blood meal. Secondary infection of the bite wound may occur, but is uncommon. Nits are laid on the lower portion of hair shafts as with head lice. Pubic lice do not transmit infectious agents. Transmission occurs primarily through intimate contact.

Identification

Pubic lice are 1 to 2 mm long and have a short, round abdomen. Their shape has been described as "turtle-like."[1] Pubic lice possess three pairs of legs, with claws that appear larger and thicker than those of the body or head louse (see Color Plate 20-9F).

Geographic Distribution

Pubic lice can be found worldwide.

REFERENCES

1. ANONYMOUS: Lice and Scabies: *From Infestation to Disinfestation*. Kenilworth NJ, Reed & Carnrick, 1976
2. AZAD AF, SACCI JB JR, NELSON WM, DASCH GA, SCHMIDTMANN ET, CARL M: Genetic characterization and transovarial transmission of a typhus-like rickettsia found in cat fleas. Proc Natl Acad Sci USA 89:43–46, 1992
3. BARBOUR AG, MAUPIN GO, TELTOW GJ, CARTER CJ, PIESMAN J: Identification of an uncultivable *Borrelia* species in the hard tick *Amblyomma americanum*: possible agent of a Lyme disease-like illness. J Infect Dis 173:403–409, 1996
4. BENNETT G: Cockroaches as carriers of bacteria. Lancet 341:732, 1993
5. BORGNOLO G, HAILU B, CIANCARELLI A, ALMAVIVA M, WOLDEMARIAM T: Louse-borne relapsing fever. A clinical and an epidemiological study of 389 patients in Asella Hospital, Ethiopia. Trop Geogr Med 45:66–69, 1993
6. BREWER TF, WILSON ME, GONZALEZ E, FELSENSTEIN D: Bacon therapy and furuncular myiasis. JAMA 270:2087–2088, 1993
7. BURGDORFER W: Discovery of the Lyme disease spirochete and its relation to tick vectors. Yale J Biol Med 57:515–520, 1984
8. BURGDORFER W, BARBOUR AG, HAYES SF, BENACH JL, GRUNWALDT E, DAVIS JP: Lyme disease—a tick-borne spirochetosis. Science 216:1317–1319, 1982
9. CALISHER CH: Medically important arboviruses of the United States and Canada. Clin Microbiol Rev 7:89–116, 1994
10. CARSON DS: Detection and treatment of pediculosis capitis. Internal Medicine for The Specialist 11:74–86, 1990
11. CENTERS FOR DISEASE CONTROL AND PREVENTION: Necrotic arachnidism—Pacific Northwest, 1988–1996. MMWR 45:433–436, 1996
12. EWING C, SCORPIO A, NELSON DR, MATHER TN: Isolation of *Borrelia burgdorferi* from saliva of the tick vector, *Ixodes scapularis*. J Clin Microbiol 32:755–758, 1994
13. FALCO RC, FISH D: Ticks parasitizing humans in a Lyme disease endemic area of southern New York State. Am J Epidemiol 128:1146–1152, 1988
14. FAUST EC, RUSSELL PF, JUNG RC: *Craig and Faust's Clinical Parasitology*, 8th ed. Philadelphia, Lea & Febiger, 1970
15. FRITSCHE TR, PFALLER MA: Arthropods of medical importance. In Murray PR, Baron EJ, Pfaller MA, Tenover FC, Yolken RH(eds): Manual of Clinical Microbiology, 6th ed. Washington, ASM Press, 1995
16. GARCIA L, BRUCKNER DA: Diagnostic Medical Parasitology, 2nd ed. Washington, ASM Press, 1993
17. GODDARD J: *Physician's Guide to Arthropods of Medical Importance*. Boca Raton, CRC Press, 1993
18. KASS EM, SZANIAWSKI WK, LEVY H, LEACH J, SRINIVASAN K, RIVES C: Rickettsialpox in a New York City hospital, 1980 to 1989. N Engl J Med 331:1612–1617, 1994
19. KAWABATA M, BABA S, IGUCHI K, YAMAGUTI N, RUSSELL H: Lyme disease in Japan and its possible incriminated tick vector, *Ixodes persulcatus*. J Infect Dis 156:854, 1987
20. LANE RP, LOVELL CR, GRIFFITHS WAD, SONNEX TS: Human cutaneous myiasis—a review and report of three cases due to *Dermatobia hominis*. Clin Exp Dermatol 12:40–45, 1987
21. LOGAN JS: Trench fever in Belfast, and the nature of the "relapsing fevers" in the United Kingdom in the nineteenth century. Ulster Med J 58:83–88, 1989
22. MANN JM, MARTONE WJ, BOYCE JM, KAUFMANN AF, BARNES AM, WEBER NS: Endemic human plague in New Mexico—risk factors associated with infection. J Infect Dis 140:397–401, 1979

23. MAUPIN GO, GAGE KL, PIESMAN J, et al: Discovery of an enzootic cycle of *Borrelia burgdorferi* in *Neotoma mexicana* and *Ixodes spinipalpis* from northern Colorado, an area where Lyme disease is nonendemic. J Infect Dis 170: 636–643, 1994

24. PANCHOLI P, KOLBERT CP, MITCHELL PD, et al: *Ixodes dammini* as a potential vector of human granulocytic ehrlichiosis. J Infect Dis 172:1007–1012, 1995

25. PERINE PL, CHANDLER BP, KRAUSE DK, et al: A clinico-epidemiological study of epidemic typhus in Africa. Clin Infect Dis 14:1149–1158, 1992

25a. Persing DH, Herwaldt BL, Glaser C, et al: Infection with a babesia-like organism in Northern California. N Engl J Med 332:298–303, 1995.

26. PETERS W: A Colour Atlas of Arthropods in Clinical Medicine. London, Wolfe Publishing, 1992

27. PIESMAN J, SINSKY RJ: Ability of *Ixodes scapularis*, *Dermacentor variabilis*, and *Amblyomma americanum* (Acari: Ixodidae) to acquire, maintain, and transmit Lyme disease spirochetes (*Borrelia burgdorferi*). J Med Entomol 25: 336–339, 1988

28. RAMIREZ-RONDA CH, GARCIA CD: Dengue in the Western Hemisphere. Infect Dis Clin North Am 8:107–128, 1994

29. RIBEIRO JM, MATHER TN, PIESMAN J, SPIELMAN A: Dissemination and salivary delivery of Lyme disease spirochetes in vector ticks (Acari: Ixodidae). J Med Entomol 24:201–205, 1987

30. ROSEF O, KAPPERUD G: House flies (*Musca domestica*) as possible vectors of *Campylobacter fetus* subsp. *jejuni*. Appl Environ Microbiol 45:381–383, 1983

31. SCHEMBRE DB, SPILLERT CR, KHAN MY, LAZARO EJ: *Dermatobia hominis* myiasis masquerading as an infected sebaceous cyst. Can J Surg 33:145–146, 1990

32. SCHRIEFER ME, SACCI JB JR, DUMLER JS, BULLEN MG, AZAD AF: Identification of a novel rickettsial infection in a patient diagnosed with murine typhus. J Clin Microbiol 32: 949–954, 1994

33. SERVICE MW: Guide to Medical Entomology. London, MacMillan Press, 1980

34. SORVILLO FJ, GONDO B, EMMONS R, et al: A suburban focus of endemic typhus in Los Angeles County: association with seropositive domestic cats and opossums. Am J Trop Med Hyg 48:269–273, 1993

35. SPACH DH, LILES WC, CAMPBELL GL, QUICK RE, ANDERSON DE JR, FRITSCHE TR: Tick-borne diseases in the United States. N Engl J Med 329:936–947, 1993

36. SPIELMAN A, CLIFFORD CM, PIESMAN J, CORWIN RM: Human babesiosis on Nantucket Island, USA: description of the vector, *Ixodes* (*Ixodes*) *dammini*, nov. sp. (Acarina: Ixodidae). J Med Entomol 15:218–234, 1979

37. STRICKLAND GT: *Hunter's Tropical Medicine*, 7th ed. Philadelphia, WB Saunders, 1991

38. SUNDNES KO, HAIMANOT AT: Epidemic of louse-borne relapsing fever in Ethiopia. Lancet 342:1213–1215, 1993

39. THOMPSON RS, BURGDORFER W, RUSSELL R, FRANCIS BJ: Outbreak of tick-borne relapsing fever in Spokane County, Washington. JAMA 210:1045–1050, 1969

40. WESTENFELD F: Cutaneous myiasis caused by *Dermatobia hominis*. Clin Microbiol Newslett 15:3, 1993

41. WILLIAMS SG, SACCI JB JR, SCHRIEFER ME, et al: Typhus and typhuslike rickettsiae associated with opossums and their fleas in Los Angeles County, California. J Clin Microbiol 30:1758–1762, 1992

42. WILSON BB: Ectoparasites: introduction. In Mandell GL, Bennett JE, Dolin R (eds): *Principles and Practice of Infectious Diseases*, 4th ed. p. 2258, New York, Churchill Livingstone, 1995

43. YAMASHITA T, KASUYA S, NODA N, NAGANO I, KANG JS: Transmission of *Rickettsia tsutsugamushi* strains among humans, wild rodents, and trombiculid mites in an area of Japan in which tsutsugamushi disease is newly endemic. J Clin Microbiol 32:2780–2785, 1994

APPENDIX II

FREE-LIVING AMEBAE

Small, free-living water and soil amebae of the genera *Naegleria* and *Acanthamoeba* are capable of producing opportunistic infections in humans. The major diseases produced by this group are forms of devastating, usually fatal meningoencephalitis and *Acanthamoeba* keratitis, an ulcerative, vision-threatening infection involving the cornea of the eye, caused by certain species of *Acanthamoeba* but not *Naegleria*.[28] The free-living amebae are not related to the intestinal amebae discussed previously and do not inhabit the intestines of humans or other mammals.

ECOLOGY, EPIDEMIOLOGY, PATHOGENESIS, AND DISEASE

Naegleria and *Acanthamoeba*, along with many other genera of free-living amebae, have a worldwide distribution in various freshwater habitats, including rivers, lakes, ponds, hot springs and spas, domestic water systems, air-conditioning systems, humidifiers, and cooling towers.[18,19] They are believed to play a role in a hypersensitivity pneumonitis known as humidifier fever.[39] They are ubiquitous in soils, dust, air, and composts; have been found on the surfaces of vegetables; and have been isolated from sewage sludge and fresh water polluted by domestic or industrial waste. *Acanthamoeba* species have been isolated from sea water, especially associated with discharges of inadequately treated sewage from hotels and municipal sewage effluents (D. A. Munson: personal communication, 1991 and reference 19). *Naegleria* and *Acanthamoeba* have also been found associated with thermally polluted discharges in ponds and lakes connected with electric power plants, nuclear power plants, or thermal polluting factories.[18,19]

In nature, free-living amebae feed on bacteria, including *Legionella* species,[3,35,39,42] and the amebae form cysts that tend to be more resistant to adverse environmental conditions (such as drying in soil) than the vegetative ameboid forms. De Jonckheere and Van de Voorde reported that the cysts of some strains of *Acanthamoeba* are highly resistant to chlorine and not killed by the usual concentrations of chlorine maintained in municipal or domestic water supplies or in chlorinated swimming pools.[20] On the other hand the cysts of *Naegleria fowleri* were more sensitive to chlorine; these authors concluded that viable *N. fowleri* are not likely to be found in clean water where low concentrations of chlorine (eg, 0.5 µg free available chlorine per milliliter) are maintained.[20] Rowbotham was the first to point out that *L. pneumophila* can grow within *Acanthamoeba* species, thus providing an explanation of how nutritionally fastidious legionnellae can maintain viability in pristine, low-nutrient waters.[39] *Legionella* species also proliferate within various other free-living amebae.[42] It has been speculated that legionellae could be aerosolized through the air to humans in droplets of water while residing within amebae.[39] This makes sense, especially if amebic cysts could protect legionellae from chlorine in domestic water supplies (see Chapter 8).

In addition, free-living amebae, including *Naegleria fowleri*, *Hartmanella* species, and various *Acanthamoeba* species, have been isolated from the throats and nasal passages of humans[1,6,26,38,42,43]—probably as cysts that were inhaled with dust in the air, in aerosols, or were present in ingested food or water.[16] Trophozoites of *Naegleria* or *Acanthamoeba* have not been demonstrated in the human nasopharynx in absence of CNS disease.[16]

Primary Amebic Meningoencephalitis

Prior to 1958, none of the free-living water and soil amebae were recognized as pathogenic. Then Culbertson and associates observed an ameba contaminant in tissue culture cells.[17] This strain, now call *Acanthamoeba culbertsoni* strain A-1, when instilled intranasally into young mice or various other animals, produced infection within the nasal mucosa and submucosa that spread from there along the olfactory nerve through the cribriform plate of the skull to produce invasion of the brain and a rapidly fatal meningoencephalitis.[12,13,17] Based on his experimental work with animals, Culbertson predicted that similar disease could occur in humans.[12,15,17] In 1965, the first human case was reported in a child from Australia by Fowler and Carter.[22] The following year, three additional cases were reported by Butt from Florida, who called the disease "primary amebic meningoencephalitis."[9] Thus, conceptually, primary amebic meningoencephalitis differed from amebic disease of the CNS involving *Entamoeba histolytica* because primary amebic meningoencephalitis was *not* "secondary" to amebic disease of the colon.

It is now known that the portal of entry for *Naegleria* is the nose and the true "primary" site of the infection is the upper respiratory tract.[10,13,16] Most patients with *Naegleria* CNS infections have been children or young adults who were swimming in lakes or rivers or otherwise had an opportunity for water (containing *Naegleria*) to enter the nose.[3,4,29,31] After infecting the nasal mucosa, *N. fowleri* then spread along the olfactory nerve, through the cribriform plate into the brain via the route originally observed in animals by Culbertson and colleagues.[12,17] Pathologic findings in humans with acute meningoencephalitis caused by *N. fowleri* have been remarkably similar to those seen originally in the experimental animal models by Culberston and associates with *Acanthamoeba culbertsoni* strain A-1 (the most virulent of the *Acanthamoeba* species).[9,10,13–16,23,28,30] Other *Acanthamoeba* species are not so virulent and tend to produce subacute or chronic brain abscesses, with or without granulomas.

In humans, CNS disease associated with *Acanthamoeba* species have not been as common as that produced by *N. fowleri*. More than 140 cases of primary amebic meningoencephalitis have been estimated to have occurred worldwide, whereas only 40 or more cases of *Acanthamoeba* CNS infections have been reported.[28] Most patients with *Acanthamoeba* CNS disease have been immunocompromised and have not had a history of exposure to water.[16,28,30,31] However, since *Acanthamoeba* cysts may be present in soil or dust, it is possible that the organisms could have been inhaled into the nasal cavity or even the lower respiratory tract.[16] It is conceivable that in humans *Acanthamoeba* species might spread either from the nasal cavity to the brain by way of the olfactory nerve or intravascularly from the lungs or possibly from skin lesions (reported rarely) to the brain.[16,31]

N. fowleri produces a diffuse and fulminant meningoencephalitis characterized by large areas of hemorrhagic necrosis, especially involving the olfactory bulbs, frontal lobes, base of the brain, proximal spinal cord, and/or temporal lobes of the brain. The parietal lobes and occipital cortex may also be involved. Acute purulent exudate is found in the leptomeninges and within the cortex. Amebic trophozoites are scattered or may be seen focally in clusters within necrotic cortex. They especially show a predilection for blood vessels; small arteries, arterioles, veins, venules, and capillaries may be surrounded by 10- to 15-µm *Naegleria* trophozoites containing large prominent nucleoli.[13,15,31]

Within the brain, *Acanthamoeba* species produce acute inflammation in early stages of the disease in animals. However, species less virulent than *A. culbertsoni* strain A-1 tend to produce focal or multifocal chronic abscesses, with or without granulomas (including presence of foreign body giant cells). Trophozoites and cysts may be focal or scattered in small numbers throughout involved areas but may be located in perivascular spaces and can be seen within the walls of small vessels in association with perivascular hemorrhage and intravascular thrombosis. Amebic cysts are seen within tissue in *Acanthamoeba* infections but have not been observed in tissues infected with *Naegleria*.[13,15,31]

Acanthamoeba Keratitis

Acanthamoeba keratitis is a serious, often devastating infection of the cornea involving certain species of *Acanthamoeba* (eg, *A. polyphaga*, *A. castellanii*, *A. rhysodes*, *A. culbertsoni*, and *A. hatchetti*).[5,28,33] Since the first case was described in 1975,[24] more than 200 cases have been reported worldwide.[28] Until about 1984, the majority of infections were associated with trauma to the cornea and exposure to contaminated water; more recently, many cases have been associated with the use of contact lenses, especially daily-wear or extended-wear soft contact lenses.[5,11,33,41] Other factors involved in *Acanthamoeba* keratitis include trauma to the cornea and the use of contaminated homemade saline or tap water rinses to clean lenses, the failure to disinfect lenses properly or as often as recommended by manufacturers, and wearing lenses while swimming.[8,28,41] Acanthamoebae may be present in contact lens cases and contact lens wash solutions, and they are capable of adhering to contact lens surfaces.[8,27,33,41,44] *Acanthamoeba* keratitis presents as an ophthalmologic emergency. It occurs commonly in children, mostly in persons 12 years of age and older, but also is common in young adults and less common in older persons.[41] The infection progresses relentlessly with corneal ulceration and may result in blindness. It is difficult to diagnose and treat. The disease has often been misdiagnosed as herpes simplex keratitis, fungal keratitis, or bacterial (or mycobacterial) infection, sometimes resulting in delays of weeks or months before a diagnosis has been made and proper treatment is begun. Detailed clinical findings have been published elsewhere in several excellent reviews.[27,33,37,41,44]

LABORATORY INVESTIGATION

Collection and Transport of Specimens

When amebic disease is suspected, fresh cerebrospinal fluid or tissue (*eg*, corneal biopsy, corneal scrapings, CNS tissue) should be collected aseptically and examined immediately. Specimens intended for culture must never be frozen or refrigerated and should be maintained at 20°C to 30°C during transport to the laboratory or prior to processing within the laboratory.[3,14] If immediate examination is not possible or not practical, amebae have survived in sterile fluid or otherwise sterile tissue for several days at room temperature prior to processing in the laboratory. If a transport medium is needed for transport of tissue biopsy samples or corneal scrapings, the minimal essential medium used in virology laboratories is preferred (see Chapter 21) over Page's ameba saline (D. Place, F. Curtis, E. Powell, and A. Newsome: personal communication, 1991).

Direct Microscopic Examination

Small drops of cerebrospinal fluid, other body fluids, or tissue suspensions should be examined in wet mounts (on slides under coverslips) by light microscopy, under reduced light, or by phase microscopy for motile trophozoites (using a 40 × objective). Keeping the microscope stage warmed to 30°C to 37°C may enhance motility, especially of *Acanthamoeba* species.[14] *Naegleria* may be actively motile at 22°C to 25°C, but the motility of *Acanthamoeba* species at room temperature is very sluggish. These amebae tend to be more actively motile than leukocytes, and the nuclei and nucleoli of *Naegleria* and *Acanthamoeba* species differ from those of granulocytes or macrophages.

Material to be stained on slides should first be fixed in 10% neutral buffered formalin. After the slide is air dried it can then be stained with trichrome, the Papanicolaou stain, or hematoxylin and eosin.[3,14] Tissue sections should be stained with hematoxylin and eosin. Other stains preferred for direct examination preparations by some include lactophenol cotton blue, Giemsa's, acridine orange, and calcofluor white.[28] Certain reference and research laboratories, such as those of the CDC and of the Department of Pathology at the Indiana University Medical Center have developed specific indirect fluorescent antibody procedures or indirect immune coagglutination procedures that provide rapid direct immunologic identification of amebae in specimens.[3,28]

Culture of Free-Living Amebae

Culbertson's method for culturing amebae with *Escherichia coli* on salt-free, water agar,[14] a slight modification of Singh's original procedure, has proven to be useful for culturing body fluids, suspensions of eye tissue, and other specimens. Agar plates are prepared with 20 to 25 ml of 1.5% agar in distilled water (without nutrients and no salt added). A loopful or one drop of a heavy suspension of *E. coli*, from a 24- to 48-hour blood agar plate culture, is spread in the center of the plate in an area 1 cm in diameter.

Alternatively, the *E. coli* can be spread as an X-streak (with 2 streaks of *E. coli* suspension that intersect in the middle of the plate, C. G. Culbertson: personal communication, 1989). The inoculum (a drop of cell suspension, sediment, or tissue fragments) is placed on top of the center of the bacterial spot and the plate is sealed with tape. Duplicate plates are incubated at 30°C and 37°C, or a single plate is incubated at 34°C to 35°C. After 18 to 24 hours of incubation, the plate is kept sealed and examined agar side up with a 10× objective. Alternatively, an inverted microscope can be used. If no amebae are seen, the plate is reincubated and examined daily for 10 days. The amebae may be in clusters of cells or will appear as small refractile bodies that migrate from the inoculum, often leaving irregular trails or tortuous tracks behind them where they have moved through the bacteria.[14] Individual amebae can be transferred from the agar to a slide to view as a wet mount or stained preparation. Subculture can be made by cutting out a plug of agar at the "front" containing amebae (using a sterile scalpel) from outside the zone of bacteria, where the amebae are more likely to be free of bacteria, and then transferring the amebae to another water agar plate containing *E. coli* (the addition of amphotericin B in final concentration of 2.5 mg/ml in the agar aids in minimizing fungal contaminants) (E. Powell: personal communication, 1991). From there, the amebae are transferred to a broth medium (*eg*, trypticase-soy broth) containing antibiotics (*eg*, penicillin 1000 µ/ml and streptomycin 0.1 mg/ml final concentration).

After the amebae are free of bacteria (axenic), they can be transferred to trypticase-soy broth without antibiotics to be used as a growth medium.[3,14] *Naegleria* will not grow in trypticase-soy broth unless it contains 10% sterile fetal calf serum. The growth of amebae in trypticase-soy broth is optimized by using plastic tissue culture tubes so that the amebae will attach to the tubes.[3,14] The cultures are incubated at 35°C almost horizontally at a 15° to 20° angle, analogous to what is often done with cell cultures in virology laboratories. Not all amebae grow in trypticase-soy broth. Alternative media include Plate Count Broth (Difco Laboratories, Detroit, MI) and broth media recommended in the American Type Culture Collection Catalogue (12301 Parklawn Drive, Rockville, MD 20852-1776) including ATCC Medium #354 (*Acanthamoeba* Medium), ATCC Medium #1034 (PYNFH medium), and ATCC medium #997 (Fresh Water Amoeba Medium) (E. Powell: personal communication, 1991). Neroad and co-workers[34] have also described a chemically defined medium for cultivating pathogenic and high temperature tolerant species of *Naegleria*.

Tissue Culture

The more virulent free-living amebae (*eg, A. culbertsoni* strain A-1) grow in mammalian cell cultures including monkey kidney, McCoy cells, and others, and may produce cytopathogenic effects (CPE) resembling those seen with viruses.[17,43] Less virulent amebae may grow poorly in tissue (cell) culture without producing CPE. Amebae can be extremely difficult to see when growing with tissue culture cells; fluid should be removed from a tissue culture tube or flask, centrifuged at 500–800 g (×5 min), or can be prepared using a Cytospin™, then the sediment is used to prepare a wet mount that is examined by phase or light microscopy using low illumination. Alternatively the slide preparation can be dried, fixed in formalin, and stained with H&E to aid in observing amebic features.[3] Once isolated in tissue culture, isolates can be transferred to a broth medium and/or to water agar with *E. coli* (as described in the preceding section).

Morphologic Features

When rounded up, the trophozoites of *Naegleria* are 8 to 15 μm and usually smaller than those of *Acanthamoeba* species, which are usually 10 to 25 μm in diameter.[2,4] The nuclei of both genera are similar and contain large, prominent nucleoli. *Naegleria* have one or more smooth, lobate pseudopodia and are actively motile at room temperature or 35°C to 37°C. *Acanthamoeba* species are very sluggish at 22°C to 25°C but may become more actively motile at 35°C and 37°C. Acanthamoebae have numerous, spiny pseudopodia on their surface called acanthopodia. *Naegleria* species are characterized by a temporary ameboflagellate stage; when *Naegleria* trophozoites are put in distilled water, they may develop pear-shaped, actively motile forms containing two or more flagella (within 1 to 3 hours). The cysts of acanthamoebae are more thick-walled than those of *Naegleria* and have distinctive appearances that aid in identification of the species level.[36] In addition, *Naegleria* species produce a distinctive form of mitosis (promitosis) in which the nuclear membrane remains intact.[36] In contrast, acanthamoebae produce a more classic type of mitosis (metamito-

sis) in which the nucleolus and nuclear membrane disappear and the mitotic spindle appears with the chromosomes in metaphase.[14,36,59,194] For more detailed descriptive information, readers are referred to references[3,14,16,25,28,36].

Identification of *Naegleria* and *Acanthamoeba* beyond the genus level requires not only a detailed morphologic study but also the use of other procedures, including tests with species-specific immunologic reagents (eg, immunofluorescent antibody tests, coagglutination tests) and tests for pathogenicity (in mice). Identification of *Naegleria* or *Acanthamoeba* to species level may be useful in an epidemiologic investigation or research projects, but its practical value for the clinical laboratory to assist clinicians in the management of patients has not been demonstrated. Looking to the future, Flores and associates[21] have described the use of specific monoclonal antibodies and applications of flow cytometry as an aid in the separation of *Naegleria fowleri* and *Acanthamoeba* species; experimental nucleic acid probes are also available to make this separation (see Chapter 1).

INTERPRETATION OF THE SIGNIFICANCE OF FREE-LIVING AMEBAE ISOLATED IN CULTURE

Because free-living amebae are ubiquitous in water, soil, dust, and the air, it is possible that cysts, carried about in the air, could contaminate the surface of a corneal scraping, tissue biopsy, or fluid specimen during the time of specimen collection, processing, inspection of primary plates for growth, or following prolonged incubation. Amebae could also be on the skin, lid margin, or in the conjunctival sac of an eye without causing keratitis, although this has not been demonstrated. Thus, as emphasized by Allen and Culbertson, personnel should not accept positive cultures of amebae, by themselves, as being clinically significant with respect to causing disease, unless trophozoites can be demonstrated on direct microscopic examination of the specimen, or can be seen microscopically within the tissue by histopathologic examination.[3]

TREATMENT

At least two patients with *Naegleria* meningoencephalitis have survived. Each received amphotericin B. One of the patients, in addition to receiving amphotericin B, also received miconazole, rifampin, and sulfasoxazole.[3,7,37,40] The treatment of choice for *Acanthamoeba* CNS disease has not been established, since most cases have been diagnosed at autopsy. However, Culbertson and associates found that sulfadiazine was highly active against some strains of *Acanthamoeba* in animal models *in vivo*.[3,16] The treatment of *Acanthamoeba* keratitis has been successful in several patients using an intensive treatment protocol involving topical propamidine isethionate (Brolene drops) and neomycin sulfate–polymyxin B sulfate–gramicidin drops (Neosporin Ophthalmic Solution).[32,33,37,45]

REFERENCES

1. ABRAHAM SN, LAWANDE RV: Incidence of free-living amoebae in the nasal passages of local population of Zaria, Nigeria. J Trop Med Hyg 85:217–222, 1982
2. ADAMS EB, MACLAUD IN: Invasive amebiasis: II. Amebic liver abscess and its complications. Medicine 56:325–334, 1977
3. ALLEN SD, CULBERTSON CG: *Naegleria* and *Acanthamoeba*. In Feigin R, Cherry J (eds): *Textbook of Pediatric Infectious Diseases*, 3rd ed, chap 182. Philadelphia, WB Saunders, 1992 (in press)
4. ARROWOOD MJ, STERLING CR: Comparison of conventional staining methods and monoclonal antibody-based methods for *Cryptosporidium* oocyst detection. J Clin Microbiol 27:1490–1495, 1989
5. AURAN JD, STARR MB, JAKOBIEC FA: *Acanthamoeba* keratitis: A review of the literature. Cornea 6:2–26, 1987
6. BADENOCH PR, GRIMMOND TR, CADWGAN J et al: Nasal carriage of free-living amoebae. Microb Ecol Health Dis 1:209–211, 1988
7. BLACKETT K: Amoebic pericarditis. Int J Cardiol 21: 183–187, 1988
8. BRANDT FH, WARE DA, VISVESVARA GS: Viability of *Acanthamoeba* cysts in ophthalmic solutions. Appl Environ Microbiol 55:1144–1146, 1989
9. BUTT CG: Primary amebic meningoencephalitis. N Engl J Med 274:1473–1476, 1966
10. CARTER RF: Description of a *Naegleria* sp. isolated from two cases of primary amoebic meningoencephalitis, and of the experimental pathological changes induced by it. J Pathol 100:217–244, 1970
11. Centers for Disease Control: *Acanthamoeba* keratitis associated with contact lenses—United States. MMWR 35: 405–408, 1986
12. CULBERTSON CG: Pathogenic *Acanthamoeba* (*Hartmanella*). Am J Clin Pathol 35:195–202, 1961
13. CULBERTSON CG: The pathogenicity of soil amebas. Ann Rev Microbiol 25:231–254, 1971
14. CULBERTSON CG: Soil amoeba infection. In Lennette EH, Spaulding EH, Truant JP (eds): *Manual of Clinical Microbiology*. 2nd ed, pp 602–604. Washington, DC, American Society for Microbiology, 1974
15. CULBERTSON CG: Amebic meningoencephalitides. In Binford CH, Connoe DH (eds): *Pathology of Tropical and Extraordinary Diseases, An Atlas*, vol 1, pp 317–324. Washington, DC, Armed Forces Institute of Pathology, 1976
16. CULBERTSON CG: Amebic meningoencephalitis. Antibiot Chemother 30:28–53, 1981
17. CULBERTSON CG, SMITH JW, MINNER JR: *Acanthamoeba*: Observations on animal pathogenicity. Science 127:1506, 1958
18. DEJONCKHEERE JF: Epidemiology. In Rondanelli EG (ed): *Amphizoic Amoebae Human Pathology*, pp 127–147. Padua, Italy, Piccin Nuova Libraria, 1987
19. DE JONCKHEERE JF: Ecology of *Acanthamoeba*. Rev Infect Dis 13 (suppl 5):S385–S387, 1991
20. DE JONCKHEERE JF, VAN DE VORDE H: Differences in destruction of cysts of pathogenic and nonpathogenic *Naegleria* and *Acanthamoeba* by chlorine. Appl Environ Microbiol 31:294–297, 1976
21. FLORES BM, GARCIA CA, STAMM WE, TORIAN BE: Differentiation of *Naegleria fowleri* from *Acanthamoeba* species by using monoclonal antibodies and flow cytometry. J Clin Microbiol 28:1999–2005, 1990
22. FOWLER M, CARTER RF: Acute pyogenic meningitis probably due to *Acanthamoeba* sp: A preliminary report. Br Med J 2:740–742, 1965
23. JOHN DT: Primary amoebic meningoencephalitis and the biology of *Naegleria fowleri*. Ann Rev Microbiol 36: 101–123, 1982
24. JONES DB, VISVESVARA GS, ROBINSON NM: *Acanthamoeba polyphaga* keratitis and *Acanthamoeba* uveitis associated with fatal meningoencephalitis. Trans Ophthalmol Soc UK 95:221–232, 1975
25. KILVINGTON S, LARKIN DFP, WHITE DG, BEECHING JR: Laboratory investigation of *Acanthamoeba* keratitis. J Clin Microbiol 28:2722–2725, 1990
26. LAWANDE RV, ABRAHAM SN, JOHN I, EGLER LJ: Recovery of soil amebas from the nasal passages of children during the dusty harmattan period in Zaria. Am J Clin Pathol 71:201–203, 1979
27. LINDQUIST TD, SHER NA, DOUGHMAN DJ: Clinical signs and medical therapy of early *Acanthamoeba* keratitis. Arch Ophthalmol 106:73–77, 1988
28. MA P, VISVESVARA GS, MARTINEZ AJ et al: *Naegleria* and *Acanthamoeba* infection: Review. Rev Infect Dis 12:490–513, 1990
29. MARCIANO-CABRAL F: Biology of *Naegleria* spp. Microbiol Rev 52:114–133, 1988
30. MARTINEZ AJ: Is *Acanthamoeba* encephalitis an opportunistic infection? Neurology 30:567–574, 1980.
31. MARTINEZ AJ: Free-Living Amebas: *Natural History, Prevention, Diagnosis, Pathology, and Treatment of Disease*. Boca Raton, FL, CRC Press, 1985
32. MOORE MB: Parasitic infections. In Kaufman HE, Barron BA, McDonald MB et al (eds): *The Cornea*, pp 271–297. New York, Churchill Livingstone, 1988
33. MOORE MB, MCCULLEY JP: *Acanthamoeba* keratitis associated with contact lenses: Six consecutive cases of successful management. Br J Ophthalmol 73:271–275, 1989
34. NEROAD TA, VISVESVARA GS, DAGGETT PM: Chemically defined media for the cultivation of *Naegleria*: Pathogenic and high temperature tolerant species. J Protozool 30:383–387, 1983
35. NEWSOME AL, BAKER RL, MILLER RD et al: Interactions between *Naegleria fowleri* and *Legionella pneumophila*. Infect Immun 50:449–452, 1985
36. PAGE FC: A *New Key to Freshwater and Soil Gymnamoebae*, pp 1–122. Ambleside, Cumbria, Freshwater Biological Association, The Ferry House, 1988
37. PETRI WA JR, RARDIN JI: Free-living amebae, in Mandell GL, Douglas RG Jr, Bennett JE (eds): *Principles and Practices of Infectious Diseases*, chap 250. New York, Churchill Livingstone, 1990
38. RIVERA F, ROSAS I, CASTILLO M et al: Pathogenic and free-living protozoa cultured from the nasopharyngeal and oral regions of dental patients: II. Environmental Research 39:364–371, 1986

39. ROWBOTHAM TJ: Preliminary report on the pathogenicity of *Legionella pneumophila* for freshwater and soil amoebae, J Clin Pathol 33:1179–1183, 1980

40. SEIDEL JS, HARMATZ P, VISVESVARA GS et al: Successful treatment of primary amebic meningoencephalitis. N Engl J Med 306:346–348, 1982

41. STEHR-GREEN JK, BAILEY TM, VISVESVARA GS: The epidemiology of *Acanthamoeba* keratitis in the United States. Am J Ophthalmol 107:221–336, 1989

42. WADOWSKY RM, BUTLER LJ, COOK MK et al: Growth-supporting activity for *Legionella pneumophila* in tap water cultures and impliction of Hartmanellid amoebae as growth factors. Appl Environ Microbiol 54:2677–2682, 1988

43. WANG SS, FELDMAN HA: Isolation of *Hartmannella* species from human throats. N Engl J Med 277:1174–1179, 1967

44. WILHELMUS KR, JONES DB (guest eds): International symposium on *Acanthamoeba* and the eye. Rev Infect Dis 13 (suppl 5):S450, 1991

45. WRIGHT P, WARHURST D, JONES BR: *Acanthamoeba* keratitis successfully treated medically. Br J Ophthalmol 69:778–782, 1985

DIAGNOSIS OF INFECTIONS CAUSED BY VIRUSES, *CHLAMYDIA*, *RICKETTSIA*, AND RELATED ORGANISMS

INTRODUCTION

Diagnostic virology is a recent addition to the services offered by clinical microbiology laboratories. Three distinct stages have evolved as laboratory workers have provided clinicians with objective data to evaluate patients with viral infections.

HISTORICAL REVIEW

The first stage, of historical interest, spanned the years during which the existence of infection by submicroscopic particles was established. For many decades after Carlos Finlay hypothesized that yellow fever was transmitted by the bite of a mosquito, the only means available for isolation of viral agents was the inoculation of animals or embryonated eggs. Embryonated chicken eggs are still inoculated today for surveillance of infections caused by influenza A virus if cell culture is not available. Furthermore, the inoculation of rodents remains essential for the recovery of certain viruses, such as coxsackievirus A and the togaviruses. New agents continue to be uncovered only by the use of subhuman primates (kuru and Creutzfeldt-Jakob viruses)[289] and even human volunteers (Norwalk agent of infectious gastroenteritis).[436]

EVOLUTION OF CELL CULTURE TECHNIQUES

The next major breakthrough in diagnostic virology was provided by Enders and colleagues, who demonstrated that the virus that caused poliomyelitis could be isolated in nonneural cells in vitro.[239] In the 1950s and 1960s there was a rapid expansion of knowledge about clinical features, epidemiology, and diagnosis of common viral infections, largely provided by the expanding use of cell culture. Diagnostic efforts, which were an integral part of the clinical studies, were incorporated into university and government research laboratories. The high cost of definitive identification of isolates, the absence of effective antiviral chemotherapy, and the paucity of cell culture facilities all combined to limit the importation of these tests into the diagnostic microbiology laboratory.

EVOLUTION OF DIAGNOSTIC VIROLOGY SERVICES

In the past 15 years, several events have promoted and facilitated the provision of diagnostic virology services by laboratories of different sizes and backgrounds:

1. Situations have arisen in which important clinical decisions depend on prompt and accurate viral diagnosis. The risk for the newborn of maternal herpes simplex infection was recognized in the early 1970s.[601] Investigators, who recognized the association of neonatal herpes with active herpetic infection of the maternal genital tract, developed protocols to screen mothers for herpesvirus shedding.[62] Careful study, however, documented serious problems with the screening protocols.[27] The American College of Obstetrics and Gynecology no longer advocates routine genital cultures for herpes simplex virus in pregnant women[11] (see page 1211). This impetus to the development of diagnostic virology services in many hospitals has, nevertheless, left an enduring legacy.

   The enormous publicity given to genital herpes infections in nonpregnant patients has undoubtedly stimulated even more requests for diagnostic laboratory support. Many patients and physicians would like to know with certainty whether a lesion is herpetic. Although the disease is not life-threatening in a healthy patient, there may be considerable morbidity and there is enormous social concern. Genital infections may be caused by either type 1 or type 2 herpes simplex virus, which is discussed later in this chapter. The ready availability of reliable typing sera allows laboratories to differentiate the two viruses after they are isolated in culture.

2. The availability of effective antiviral chemotherapy for herpes simplex encephalitis[877] and for respiratory syncytial virus infection[775] has further emphasized the importance of reliable laboratory diagnostic support. Antiviral chemotherapy is also useful for influenza A virus infection in selected patients.[219,790] Although ganciclovir therapy for cytomegalovirus (CMV) infections is not curative, it has provided a first tool for combatting potentially lethal or blinding infections in immunosuppressed patients.[241] Resistance to antiviral agents has fortunately been rare to date, but such resistance can be induced in the laboratory and has been reported in patients.[186,470] When immunosuppressed patients, such as those infected with the human immunodeficiency virus (HIV), fail to respond to antiviral therapy or relapse promptly after cessation of therapy, development of drug resistance must be considered.[708] As chemotherapeutic agents against other viruses are introduced, these resilient infectious agents will undoubtedly respond by developing resistance. In the future it may even become necessary to determine routinely the susceptibility of certain viral isolates to potential therapeutic agents, as we have done for many years with bacterial pathogens.

3. A ready commercial supply of diverse mammalian cell cultures has made isolation of viruses feasible for many laboratories.

4. An expanding list of reliable immunologic reagents and molecular techniques has also enhanced the ability of laboratories to identify many viruses rapidly and definitively. Increasingly, kits for direct identification of specific agents in clinical specimens or for isolation and identification of the agent in culture are being marketed commercially.

Color Plates for Chapter 21 are found between pages 784 and 785.

1178

Economic pressures are making it imperative to provide clinically useful and cost-effective results. The time is right for virology to enter the diagnostic laboratory.

DIAGNOSTIC VIROLOGY MYTHS

Several traditional reservations about the appropriateness of diagnostic virology services are no longer relevant.[223]

1. Myth #1. *The isolation of a viral pathogen is of academic interest only.* The impact of viral diagnosis on clinical decisions has already been mentioned. The expense and potential toxicity of some of the therapeutic regimens, such as ribavirin for respiratory syncytial virus infection, must be considered. The adverse consequences of ignoring treatable viral infections provide even more compelling arguments for efficient diagnosis. Recognition of enteroviral meningoencephalitis facilitates cessation of antibacterial therapy and the early discharge of some patients from the hospital.[155] Similarly, viral infection in the neonatal period may be difficult to distinguish clinically from bacterial infection.[190] Although effective therapy for most viral infections does not yet exist, identification of the virus directly affects management of the patient by permitting the clinician to design rational therapy and to assess the child's prognosis.[440,753,881]

2. Myth #2. *Viral diagnosis is of epidemiologic interest only in the community.* Several instances of hospital-acquired viral infections have been reported. Nosocomial outbreaks of respiratory[203,242,325,345,348,434,863] and gastrointestinal viral disease[791] are well documented. Many viruses may, on occasion, cause serious nosocomial infection. Nosocomial transmission may occur from patient to patient or from hospital staff to patient.[714,869] It is important, therefore, to maintain high levels of immunization in health care workers when possible and to monitor the etiology of nosocomial respiratory disease.

3. Myth #3. *Viral diagnosis is too slow to be clinically useful.* As many as 25% to 50% of the isolates of herpes simplex virus may be recovered within the first day, a rate comparable to the isolation of bacteria from blood culture; by 72 hours, as many as 85% to 95% of the cultures become positive.[93] More than 90% of isolates may be detected within 24 hours if the inoculum is centrifuged onto cell monolayers and the cells stained with fluorescent antiserum to the virus.[311,735] Even isolation of the recalcitrant CMV, which usually requires 2 weeks or more for isolation by traditional techniques, may be facilitated by centrifugation of some specimens onto susceptible tissue culture cells.[309]

4. Myth #4. *The diagnosis of viral infections is prohibitively expensive.* Definitive identification of all viral isolates to the level of serotype requires large stocks of specific antisera and the use of cumbersome neutralization tests. For several reasons, guidance can be provided both expeditiously and relatively inexpensively for management of patients without such complex procedures:

- *Clinical clues to viral disease diagnosis*: In some instances, the suspect virus (eg, herpes simplex or CMV) can be defined clearly from clinical data and the diagnostic evaluation tailored accordingly, much as the bacteriologist does for group A β-hemolytic streptococci in throat cultures.

- *Cytopathic effects in cell culture*: Often a presumptive identification, entirely sufficient for clinical management, can be established by demonstrating the pattern of cytopathic effect in various types of cell culture. For example, management of aseptic meningitis is facilitated by the identification of an enterovirus,[155] which can be accomplished presumptively when a skilled technologist observes the characteristic viral cytopathic effect. Further identification to the level of serotype is expensive and usually does not provide essential clinical information.

- *Direct viral detection*: The increasing availability of dependable immunofluorescent and immunoenzymatic reagents now makes identification of certain important groups of viruses economical, even including the serotype in some cases. Reagents are available, often from multiple commercial sources, for detecting herpesviruses,[39,311,318] adenoviruses,[505,571] and myxoviruses.[145,245,496,571,573,889] Commercial reagents for direct detection of enteroviruses in clinical specimens are not available, although monoclonal antibodies that are specific for individual serotypes or react widely with the group are commercially available and can be used for detection or identification of enteroviruses after amplification in culture.[459]

In the molecular age nucleic acid hybridization or amplification assays have been developed for virtually every infectious agent that has been cultured and, most usefully, for some that have not yet been cultured. A few have already made the transition to routine use, and more will undoubtedly follow.

- *Single agent infections*: Most viral infections are caused by a single agent. Only rarely is it necessary, therefore, to incur the expense of working up multiple isolates from a single specimen, as happens often with specimens that have been submitted to a bacteriology laboratory. Dual infections do occur,[831] however, and the laboratory worker should be alert to this possibility when faced with confusing results. Mixed infections have been reported in transplant recipients.[4]

5. Myth #5. *We do not need viral culture because we can do serologic tests.* Serologic tests are valuable accessory tools in the diagnosis of viral diseases.[87] Serum antibody is a useful marker for prior exposure to a virus that induces solid, long-lasting immunity; for example, one can determine whether a young woman is at risk of developing rubella infection by measuring her serum antibody levels. Demonstration of an immunologic response to an infectious agent is a valuable adjunct to virologic diagnosis, particularly if the virus has been recovered from a mucosal sur-

face. The likelihood that an isolate of adenovirus from the throat of an infant has caused an infection is greater if the infant develops antibody to adenovirus. Infections by some viruses, such as the togaviruses (arthropod-borne or arboviruses), hepatitis viruses, and Epstein-Barr virus (the primary cause of infectious mononucleosis), are diagnosed primarily by serologic techniques.

Serologic tests should never divert attention away from virologic diagnosis, which is more rapid and more definitive. In almost every instance, the time required for identification of viruses that commonly produce infection in the United States is less if a specimen is cultured than if acute and convalescent sera are analyzed for development of specific antibody.[543,648] On the one hand, immunologic specificity makes serologic screening difficult; on the other hand, immunologic cross-reactivity can complicate the interpretation of a positive result. For example, antibodies that cross react among all the herpesviruses do not exist, so that multiple reagents must be used for serologic examination; but differentiation between serotypes of herpes simplex virus on serologic grounds is also difficult because of extensive cross-reactions.[32,338] As is discussed below, even the diagnostic requirement for IgM antibody or a fourfold increase in antibody may be flawed, especially in evaluation of infections produced by the herpesvirus group.

LEVELS OF SERVICE

Each laboratory director or supervisor must decide the level of service that is appropriate for local clinical needs. It is far better to limit the scope of effort to those tests that can be performed with high proficiency than to attempt broad coverage when resources are insufficient. Several likely levels of service can be imagined and are listed in Box 21-1.

Most small hospital laboratories will probably fit into levels 1 or 2,[778] whereas larger community hospital and university laboratories may offer services at levels 3 or 4. These hospitals are most likely to serve the patients who need comprehensive virology services. It is feasible to use such laboratories as regional diagnostic resources.

TAXONOMY

Many viral infections, such as influenza, chickenpox, measles, and hepatitis, were well characterized clinically long before the etiologic agent was recognized. Once isolated, the virus was given the name of the corresponding clinical condition. In an attempt to bring order to the scheme of classification, taxonomists have used modern knowledge of viral structure and antigenic composition when naming viruses.[593] Names have a Latin stem, but the conventions of bacterial nomenclature have not been followed completely. Families and genera have been delineated, but the designation of viruses at the species level has not yet been

---

BOX 21-1. LEVELS OF DIAGNOSTIC SERVICE

Level 1. No virology services performed. Specimens are collected for transfer to a reference laboratory.

Level 2. Limited virology procedures performed. Such laboratories may or may not also have the capability to detect viral or chlamydial antigens in body secretions and fluids. These laboratories also may or may not have the capability to inoculate specimens to tissue culture for transfer to reference laboratories.

Level 3. These laboratories are able to recover selected viral groups that grow in commonly used cell cultures. They may also perform limited identification of selected agents, for which transportation, cell isolation, and simple immunologic confirmation systems are commercially available, with referral of other isolates to reference laboratories.

Level 4. These laboratories are expected to have personnel with a high degree of expertise in virology who are able to isolate all of the common viral groups and to perform *clinically relevant* identifications.

---

accomplished. Rather, the vernacular names are used most commonly as species designations. In the absence of formal binomial nomenclature, the vernacular names should not be capitalized or italicized. For instance, the name herpes simplex virus should be used, not *Herpes simplex*. In some instances, the traditional names, derived from clinical usage, have been incorporated into the official nomenclature. For example, the smallpox and cowpox viruses have been assigned to the family Poxviridae.

Much of viral taxonomy derives from detailed knowledge of viral structure. Viruses are among the smallest of infectious agents (Fig. 21-1). The poxviruses, which are the largest members of the virus family and similar in size to the smallest bacteria, are close to the resolution of the light microscope; an electron microscope is necessary to visualize all other viruses.

Almost without exception, viruses contain either DNA or RNA, but not both. The center of any viral particle, the ribonucleoprotein core, contains coiled nucleic acid and protein.[363] Around the core is a protective shell composed of repeating protein units called capsomeres, which, in the aggregate, make up the capsid shell. With the nucleoprotein core, the nucleocapsid unit is complete. The architecture of most viruses has a symmetry that is either helical, similar to nucleic acid, or icosahedral, the architecture of a geodesic dome. These two symmetries, illustrated in Figure 21-2, provide the most efficient means for assembling the structural shells, an economy that is essential for these very small particles with limited genetic resources.

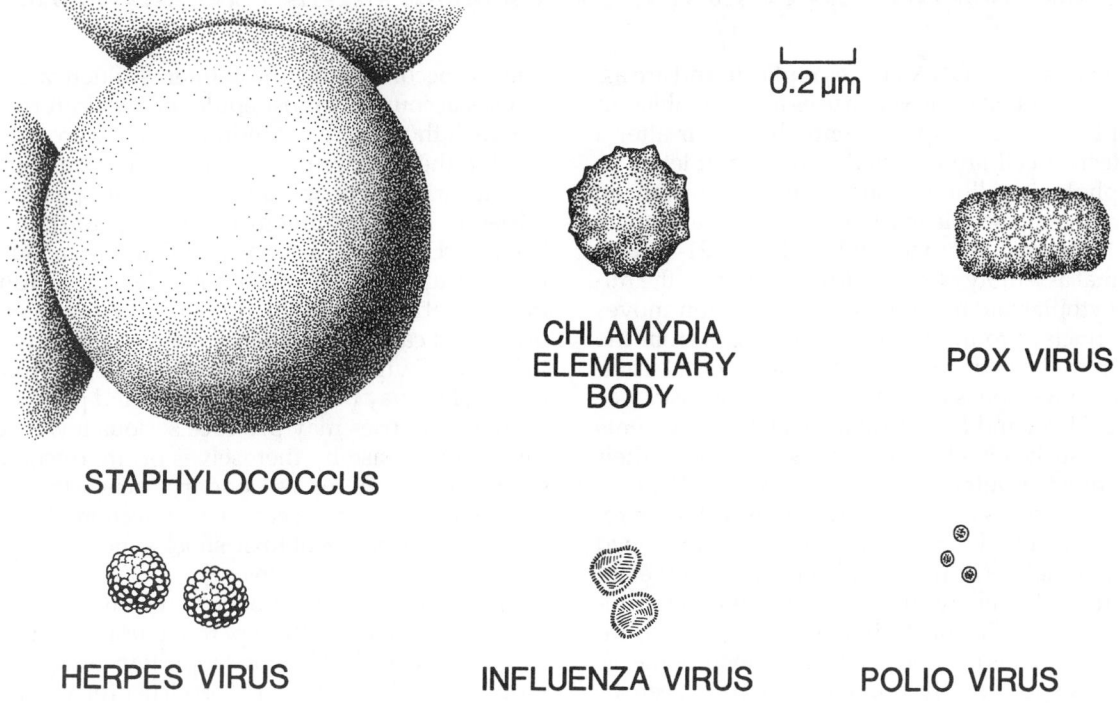

Figure 21-1
Viruses are the smallest of infectious agents. The relative size of a bacterium, *Staphylococ- cus,* is compared with *Chlamydia,* with the largest virus group (poxvirus), and with one of the smallest viruses (poliovirus, a member of the enterovirus group).

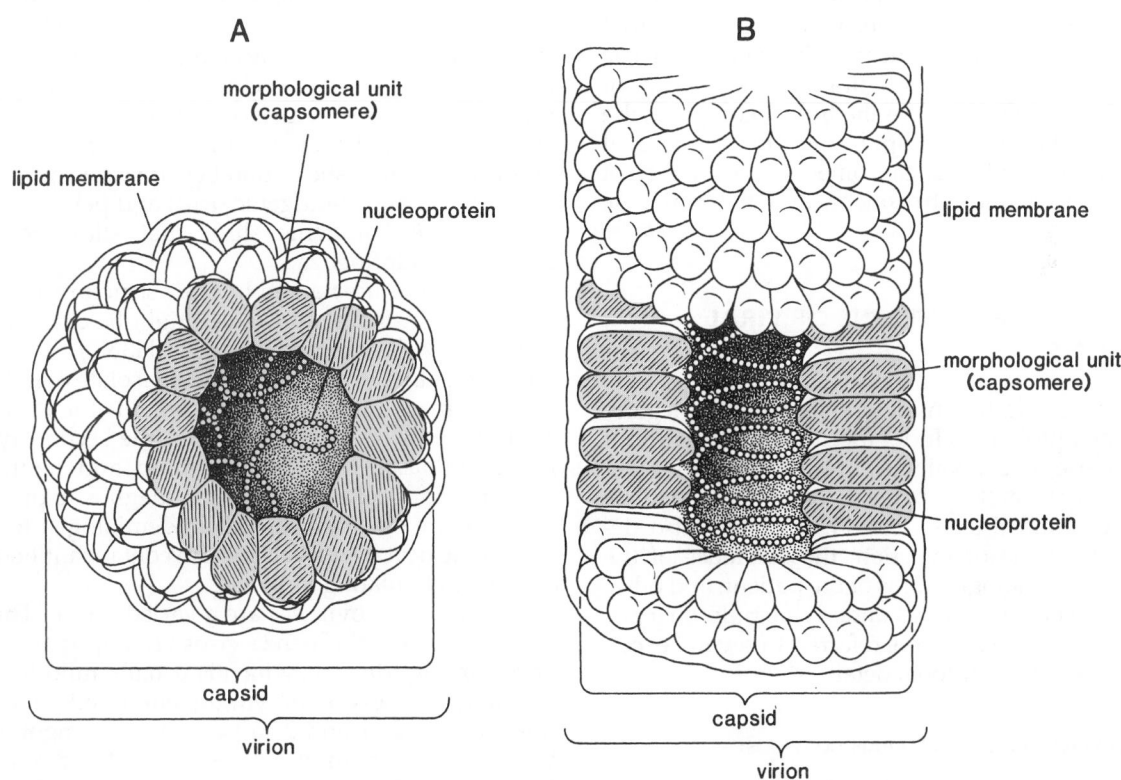

Figure 21-2
Viruses are constructed with great economy. A central nucleoprotein core is surrounded by a protein capsid, which is made up of individual capsomeres. Some viruses also have a lipoprotein membrane around the nucleocapsid. The two most common organizational patterns of symmetry are icosahedral (**A**) and helical (**B**). Ultra-structurally, the icosahedral viruses appear round, although the facets may occasionally be visualized (see the illustration of adenovirus in Table 21-2).

As a general rule, DNA viruses replicate and are assembled in the nucleus; RNA viruses are assembled in the cytoplasm. The complex events that occur after a virus infects a cell are reflected only incompletely in the morphologic cellular changes. In some instances, however, one can see clearly how the virus has appropriated the genetic resources of the cell (Fig. 21-3A and B). The final assembly of some viruses occurs at the nuclear or cytoplasmic membrane. As the virion moves from the nucleus to the cytoplasm or passes from the cytoplasm to the extracellular space, an external lipid-containing envelope is added to the nucleocapsid (see Figs. 21-2, 21-3A and F, and Table 21-2). Lipid solvents inactivate such enveloped viruses, whereas their nonenveloped counterparts are not affected. Replication of some viruses results in death of the cell with release of the assembled nucleocapsids. The enveloped viruses that mature at the cytoplasmic membrane are released from the cell by "budding" through the membrane (see Figs. 21-3F and 21-16). In this process the envelope accumulates portions of the lipid membrane, as well as virus-specified glycoproteins that have been inserted into that membrane.

The major groups of viruses are summarized in Tables 21-1 and 21-2. Illustrative electron micrographs of negatively stained viral particles (kindly provided by Frederick A. Murphy) are juxtaposed to a brief description of the families and genera. The list is not exhaustive, but includes the most important human pathogens. Structural and biochemical features that are used for classification include the type of nucleic acid (DNA or RNA), the configuration or symmetry of the nucleocapsid (helical, icosahedral, or complex), the presence or absence of a lipid envelope, the size of the virion, the number of capsomeres, the stability of the virion to chemical treatment, and the antigenic composition.

CLINICAL MANIFESTATIONS OF VIRAL INFECTIONS

The clinical manifestations of viral infection are legion. General symptoms include fever with or without chills, malaise, and myalgias. Specific symptoms derive primarily from the propensity of the virus to infect various cells and tissues (tropism) but may also depend on the route of infection, the virulence of the strain, the immunologic status of the patient, and other predisposing factors, such as underlying pulmonary or cardiac disease. The reader is referred to several excellent textbooks for additional details.[248,261]

ORTHOMYXOVIRUSES AND PARAMYXOVIRUSES

The orthomyxoviruses, which include influenza A, B, and C viruses, produce a wide variety of respiratory infections.[14,222] The influenza or "flu" syndrome begins with the abrupt onset of headache, fever, chills, and dry cough; later, high fever, myalgias, malaise, and anorexia appear. In young children gastrointestinal symptoms may be prominent. Almost all cases of influenza occur during the winter. Influenza A and B viruses account for most epidemic respiratory disease in which there is excess mortality. They are rarely isolated in the absence of infection. Influenza A virus infects a variety of mammalian and avian species. Transmission of swine influenza from pigs to humans has been described occasionally.[868] Concern about infection of humans with swine virus led to a nationwide immunization campaign in 1976, with unexpected and unwanted cases of Guillain-Barré syndrome resulting. Influenza C virus is an uncommon cause of human infection, but may produce bronchitis and pneumonia.[581] Influenza viruses may produce serious lower respiratory tract disease by themselves or, more commonly, set up the patient for a secondary bacterial infection.[863] A recent twist on the secondary infection scenario has been the production of toxic shock syndrome by the invading *Staphylococcus aureus*.[527]

The structure and function of influenza virus are intimately related both to pathogenesis and to laboratory diagnosis.[484] The nucleoprotein antigen in the viral core defines the type of virus; for example, influenza A or B. This antigen is stable and is recognized by many of the diagnostic antisera, which are able to detect all circulating strains of a particular type. Two glycoprotein antigens on the surface of the influenza virion are important for pathogenesis, epidemiology, and immunotherapy. The dominant antigen is the hemagglutinin, which is responsible for attachment to respiratory epithelial cells and therefore an important target for influenza vaccines. The surface neuraminidase enzyme participates in entry of the virus into the cell. These surface antigens are constantly changing, so that they are a moving target for therapeutic and diagnostic antibodies. It is the constant, incremental change (antigenic drift) and periodic, quantum change (antigenic shift) that allow recurring epidemics of influenza.

The viruses are named by their structure and geography. For instance, an isolate might be characterized influenza A/Leningrad/360/86 (H3N2). The name means that this strain was the 360th isolate of influenza A in Leningrad in 1986 and it contains the third antigenic type of hemagglutinin and the second type of neuraminidase. The hemagglutinin and neuraminidase are not useful antigens for diagnostic purposes, but they are essential for the epidemiologist to study so that the next year's vaccine can contain antibodies to currently circulating antigens.

The paramyxoviruses are a varied group. The four serotypes of parainfluenza virus are important causes of respiratory disease, which is usually mild in adults but may be severe in young children.[14,838] Parainfluenza viruses 1 and 2 cause croup (laryngotracheobronchitis) in children between ages 2 and 6. Parainfluenza virus 3 is an important cause of bronchiolitis in children younger than age 2 years; infections occur all year long, with peaks in the fall and spring.

Mumps virus produces infectious parotitis. It frequently causes aseptic meningitis, which is usually mild, and may also affect the pancreas and gonads.

(text continues on page 1192)

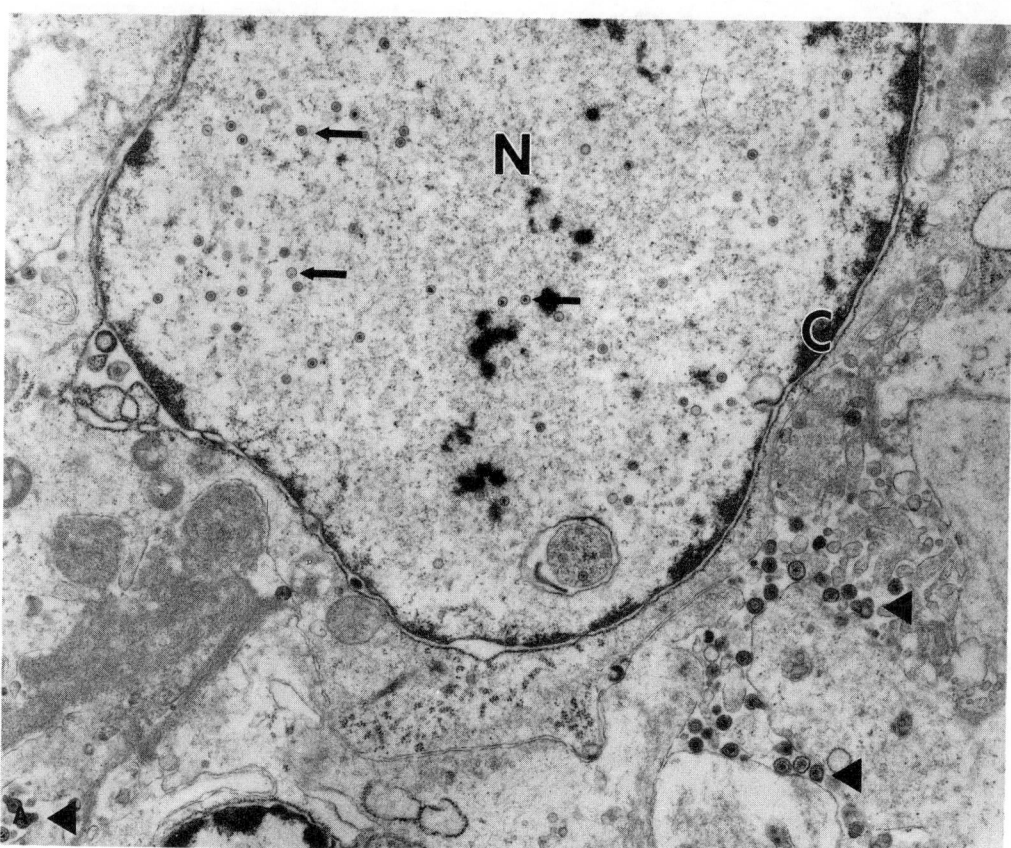

Figure 21-3

(**A**) Ultrastructure of viruses. Herpes simplex virus. The herpesviruses are assembled in the nucleus of the cell (**N**). The cellular chromatin (**C**) is pushed to the edge of the nucleus by the viral deoxyribonucleoprotein, which stains lightly in the micrograph. This material corresponds to the eosinophilic intranuclear inclusion seen with the light microscope (see Color Plate 21-1). Naked (nonenveloped) virions (**arrows**) are assembled in the nucleus. Outside the cell, some mature virions that have acquired a lipid envelope from the cell (**arrowheads**) are visible (MRC-5 cells, infected with herpes simplex virus, type 1, ×22,400). (**B**) Adenovirus. Adenoviruses are assembled in the nucleus (**N**). They have icosohedral symmetry and are not enveloped. They are often closely packed in paracrystalline arrays (**arrows**). As the viruses accumulate, the whole nucleus may become filled with virions, producing the inclusions seen with the light microscope (see Color Plate 21-1*E*) (Infected HEp-2 cells ×22,400). (**C**) Respiratory syncytial virus is assembled in the cytoplasm and matures at the cell membrane. Inclusions may be seen in the cytoplasm of infected cells, both in vivo and in vitro (see Color Plate 21-1*G*). The inclusions (**arrows**) are intracytoplasmic and are composed of fibrillar ribonucleoprotein. Contrast the density of the nucleolus (**arrowhead**) with that of the inclusions (infected HEp-2 cells, ×3,150). (**D**) Coxsackievirus B. The enteroviruses are small RNA-containing viruses that have icosohedral symmetry and are often packed in a paracrystalline array (**arrows**). They are assembled in the cytoplasm. Inclusions are not seen with the light microscope (infected rhesus monkey kidney cells, ×56,000). (**E**) Rabies virus. This bullet-shaped rhabdovirus is assembled in the cytoplasm. The fibrillar nucleoprotein (**P**) and the elongated viruses (**arrows**) are found together. The mass of viral material corresponds to the Negri body, which is seen with the light microscope (see Color Plate 21-1*H*). The internal structure that may be seen in classic Negri bodies comes from the incorporation of cytoplasmic material into the body of the inclusion (Infected human brain, ×25,000). (**F**) Eastern equine encephalitis virus. This togavirus illustrates the maturation of virus particles at the surface of the cell. Mature virions (**arrows**) are present in the extracellular space. A maturing (**budding**) virion is denoted by the dense nucleoprotein core and a condensation of the cellular membrane where the envelope is forming (**arrowhead**). Some viruses, such as the myxoviruses, insert their hemagglutinins into the membrane at this stage; they can be detected by the adherence of red blood cells to the viral hemagglutinin in the cell membrane (hemadsorption) (Infected mouse brain, ×60,000). (**E**, courtesy of Daniel Perl; **F**, courtesy of Frederick Murphy). *(Figure continues on pages 1184–1186)*

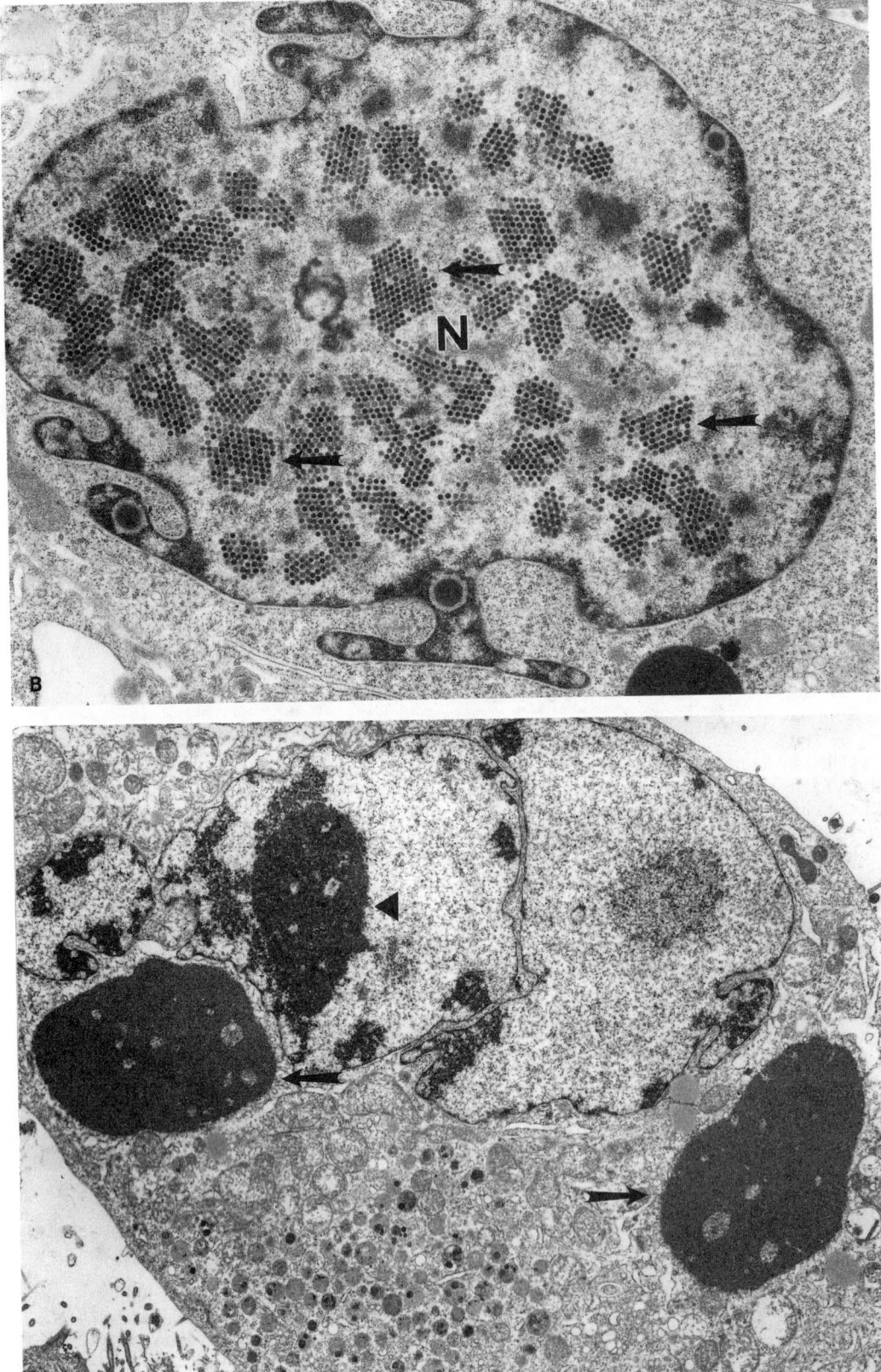

Figure 21-3 *(Continued)*

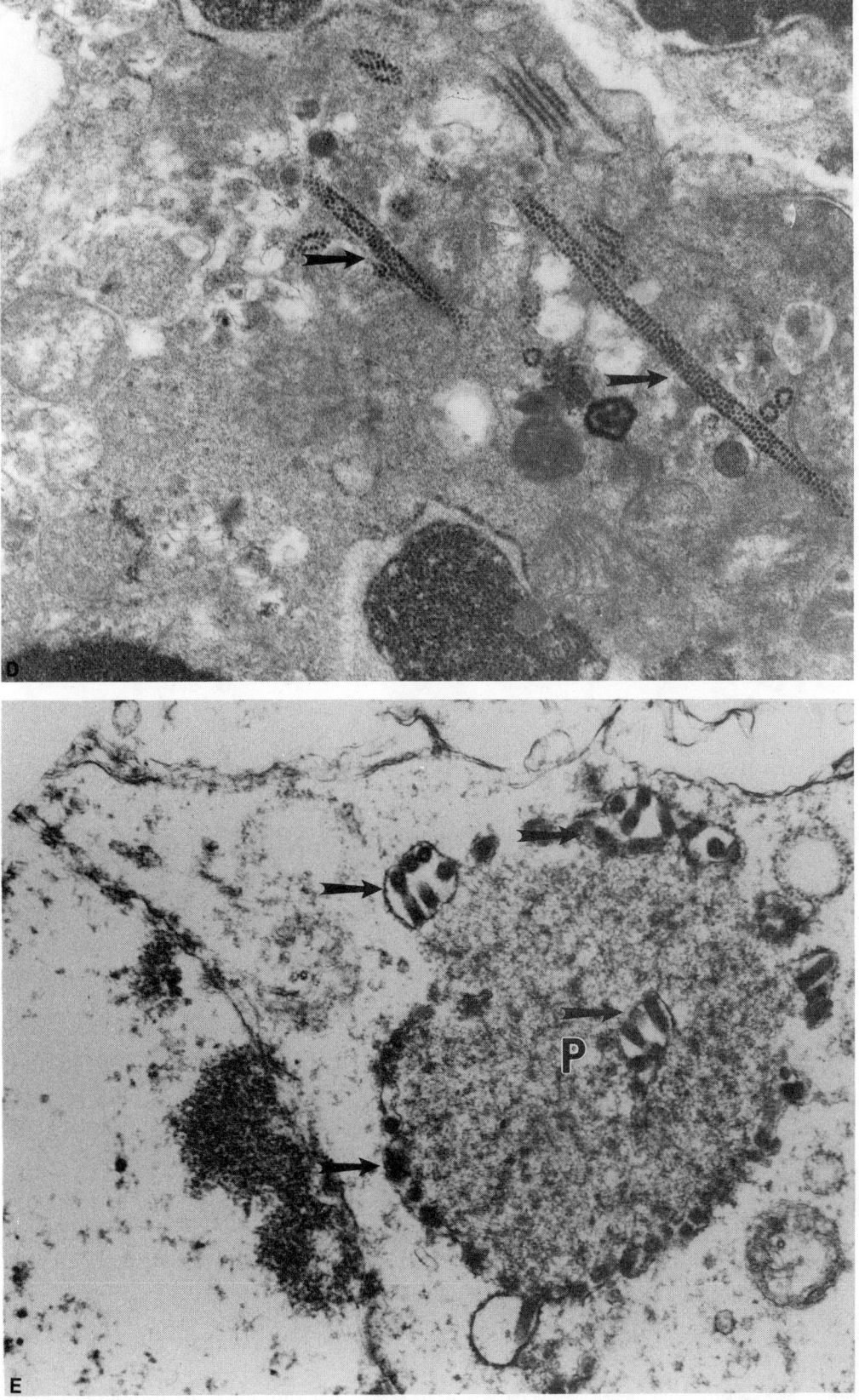

Figure 21-3 *(Continued)*

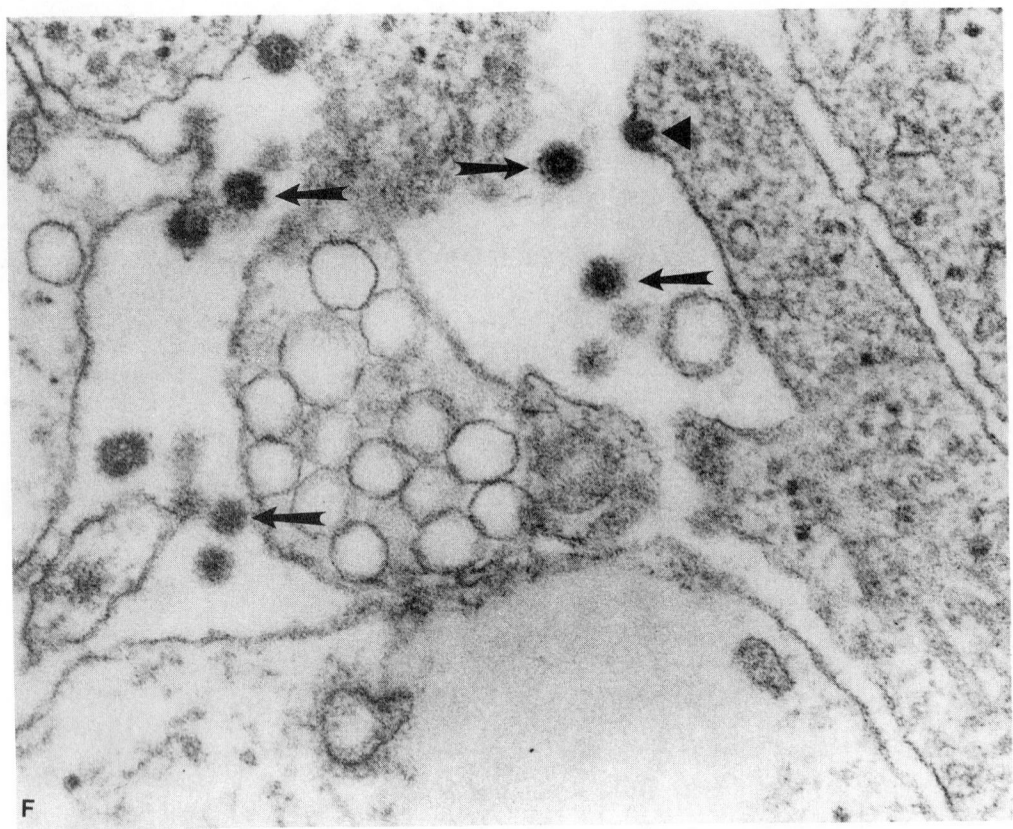

Figure 21-3 *(Continued)*

TABLE 21-1		
CLASSIFICATION OF RNA VIRUSES		

Family: *Orthomyxoviridae*
  Size: 100 nm, spherical or pleomorphic
  Symmetry: Helical
  Lipid envelope: Present
  Antigens: Hemagglutinin and neu-
    raminidase
  Genus: *Influenzavirus*
    Types: Influenza A
          Influenza B

  Genus: Unnamed
    Type: Influenza C
  Natural habitat: Humans and animals
  Distribution: Worldwide
  Mode of transmission: Aerosol droplet
    spread from person to person; rarely
    animal to person
  Route of infection: Respiratory

Diseases: Respiratory infections including coryza (common cold), tracheobronchitis, and pneumonia. Extrapulmonary
symptoms are prominent in the influenza syndrome; rarely, extrapulmonary disease such as myocarditis
may be present.

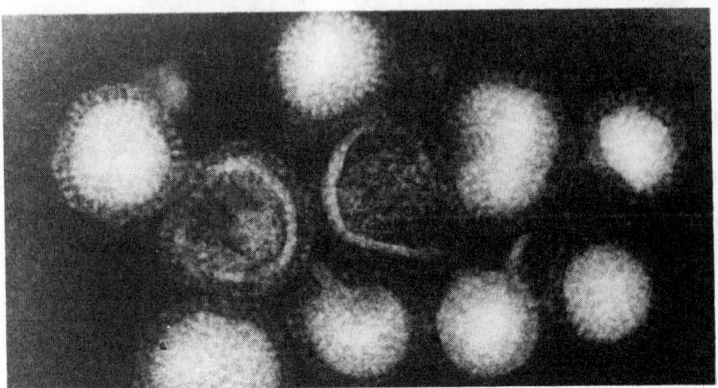

Influenzavirus A. The particles are roughly spherical but
irregular. The internal helical structure is difficult to appreciate, but the fringelike projections of hemagglutinin
and neuraminidase are shown well. ×135,000.

(Continued)

TABLE 21-1 *(Continued)*
CLASSIFICATION OF RNA VIRUSES

Family: *Paramyxoviridae*
Size: 150–300 nm, spherical or pleomorphic
Symmetry: Helical
Lipid envelope: Present
Genus: *Paramyxovirus*
    Types: Parainfluenza viruses 1
            through 4
            Mumps virus
Antigens: Hemagglutinin and neuraminidase
Genus: *Morbillivirus*
    Type: Measles virus

Antigens: Nucleocapsid; envelope
  hemagglutinin; no strain variation
Genus: *Pneumovirus*
    Type: Respiratory syncytial virus
    (RSV)
Antigens: No hemagglutinin or neuraminidase
Natural habitat: Humans
Distribution: Worldwide
Mode of transmission: Droplet aerosol or
  direct inoculation

Route of infection: Respiratory
Diseases: Common cold, tracheobronchitis, rarely pneumonia (parainfluenza); tracheobronchitis and pneumonia especially in young children (RSV); parotitis, pancreatitis, orchitis, meningitis (mumps); rash, pneumonia, encephalitis, subacute sclerosing panencephalitis (measles).

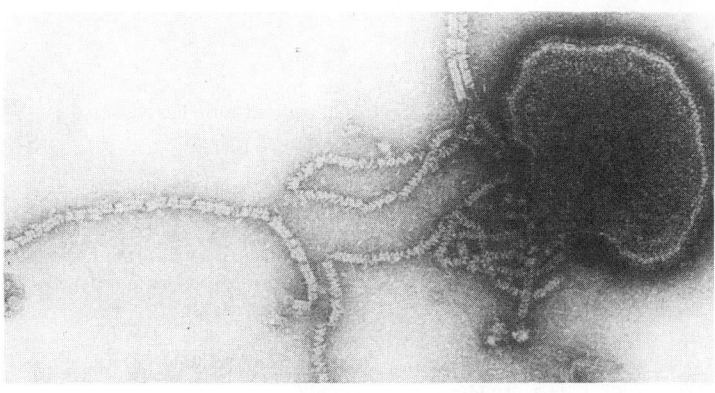

Parainfluenzavirus 1. The irregular virion has been disrupted, releasing a long strand of uncoiled RNA. The hemagglutinin fringes on the virion are evident. ×72,000.

Family: *Rhabdoviridae*
Size: 50–95 nm by 130–389 nm, bullet-shaped
Symmetry: Helical
Lipid envelope: Present
Genus: *Vesiculovirus*
    Type: vesicular stomatitis virus (VSV)

Genus: *Lyssavirus*
    Type: Rabies virus
Natural habitat: Wild and domestic
  animals
Distribution: Worldwide

Mode of transmission: Infected secretions, rabies usually transmitted by bite
Route: Cutaneous or respiratory
Diseases: Encephalitis (rabies); veterinary diseases (VSV)

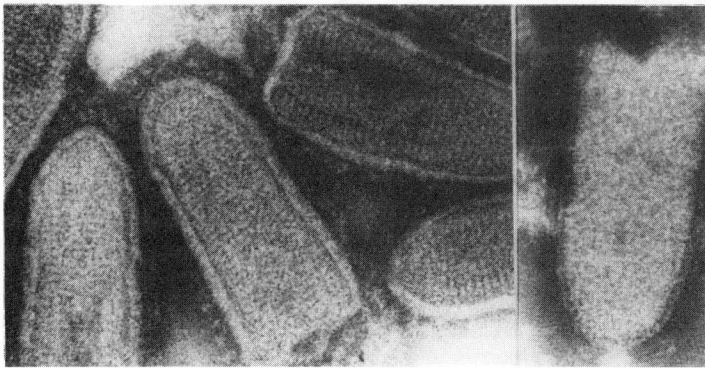

Vesicular stomatitis virus. The bullet shape of the virion is evident. The coiled helical nature of the internal ribonucleoprotein is reflected in the striations. ×216,000.

(Continued)

TABLE 21-1 *(Continued)*
CLASSIFICATION OF RNA VIRUSES

Family: Proposed family: *Filoviridae*
Size: 80 nm by 800–1000 nm, filamentous
Symmetry: Helical
Lipid envelope: Present

Genus: None established
Types: Marburg virus
        Ebola virus
Natural habit: Nonhuman primates

Distribution: Africa, Philippines
Mode of transmission: Unknown, but
    close contact required
Diseases: Hemorrhagic fever with fatality
    rates as high as 90%

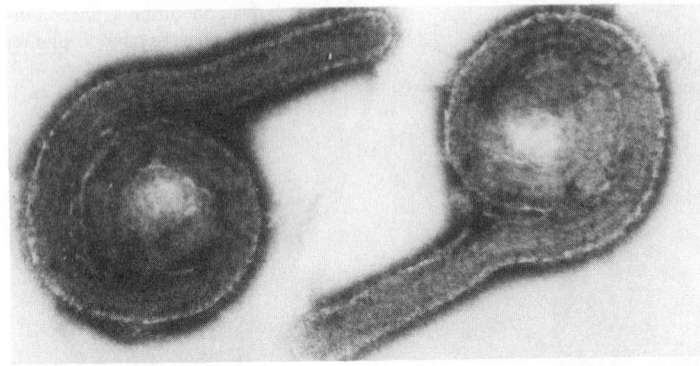

Ebola virus. Long, filamentous form has assumed a "crook" shape. ×59,000.

Family: *Bunyaviridae*
Size: 90–120 nm
Symmetry: Helical
Lipid envelope: Present
Antigens: Surface hemagglutinin

Genus: *Bunyavirus*
    Types: California encephalitis virus
           LaCrosse virus
           Hantavirus
Natural habitat: Small mammals
Distribution: Worldwide; in U.S. primarily in Midwest and north central regions

Mode of transmission: Bite of infected
    mosquitoes or exposure to rodent
    excreta (hantavirus)
Diseases: Febrile illness; aseptic
    meningitis; respiratory failure
    (hantavirus)

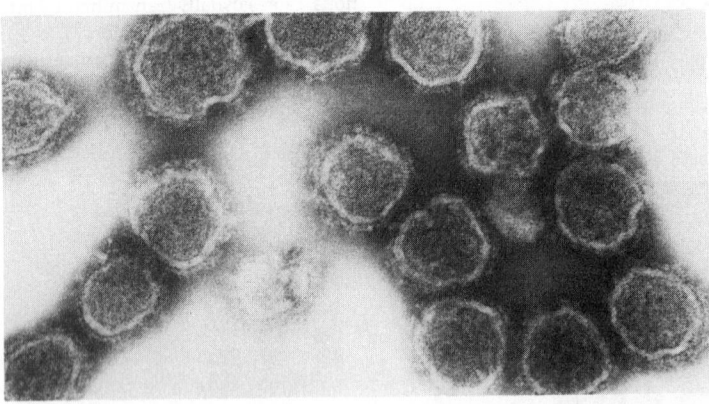

LaCrosse virus. Irregular virus particles; the lipid envelope and surface projections are evident. × 117,000.

(Continued)

TABLE 21-1   *(Continued)*
CLASSIFICATION OF RNA VIRUSES

Family: *Coronaviridae*
Size: 80–130 nm, pleomorphic with large, clubbed projections
Symmetry: Helical
Lipid envelope: Present

Genus: *Coronavirus*
Natural habitat: Humans and animals
Distribution: Worldwide
Transmission: Person-to-person, presumably by aerosol

Route of infection: Respiratory
Diseases: Common cold; rarely lower respiratory disease

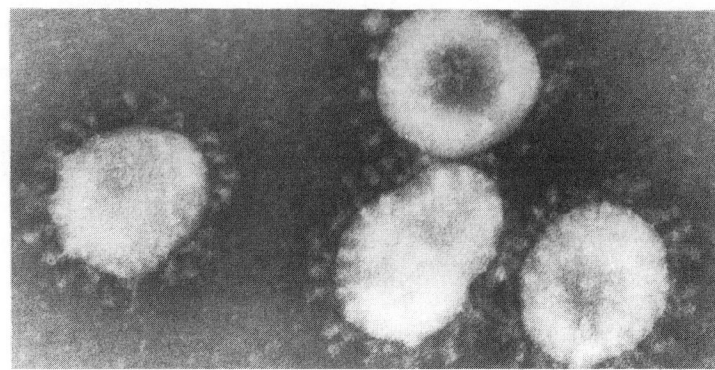

Human coronavirus OC43. The club-shaped projections are the most distinctive features of these pleomorphic particles. ×180,000.

Family: *Picornaviridae*
Size: 22–30 nm, 60 subunits
Symmetry: Icosahedral
Lipid envelope: Absent
Genus: *Enterovirus*
    Types: Poliovirus 1, 2, 3
        Coxsackievirus A, 23 types
        Coxsackievirus B, types 1–6
        Echovirus, 31 types
        Enterovirus 68–71

Genus: *Rhinovirus*
    Types: Rhinovirus, 100 types
Natural habitat: Human gastrointestinal tract; survives in environment (enterovirus); human upper respiratory tract (rhinovirus)
Distribution: Worldwide

Transmission: Fecal–oral from human-to-human or contaminated water (enterovirus); human respiratory tract by aerosol or on hands (rhinovirus)
Route of infection: Gastrointestinal (enterovirus); respiratory (rhinovirus)
Diseases: Febrile illness, meningitis, encephalitis, myocarditis (enteroviruses); common cold (rhinoviruses)

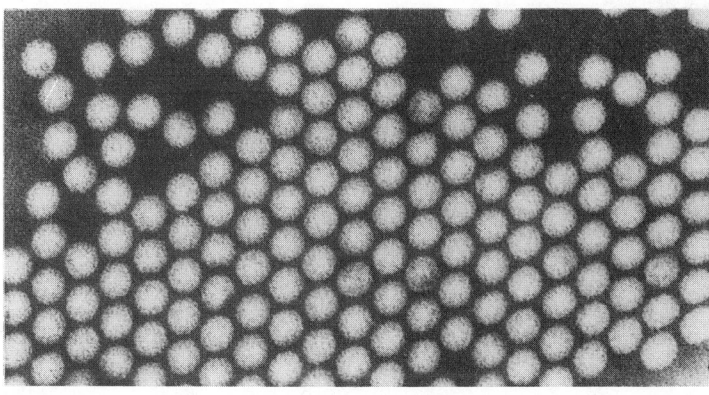

Poliovirus 1. The particles are small, regular, and nonenveloped. ×180,000.

(Continued)

TABLE 21-1 *(Continued)*
CLASSIFICATION OF RNA VIRUSES

Family: *Caliciviridae*
Size: 35–39 nm
Symmetry: Icosahedral
Lipid envelope: Absent
Genus: *Calcivirus*
    Types: Possibly Norwalk agent
        Other gastroenteritis agents

Natural habitat: Human gastrointestinal
    tract; other agents infect animals
Distribution: Worldwide

Transmission: Fecal–oral; contaminated
    water
Portal of entry: Gastrointestinal
Diseases: Gastroenteritis

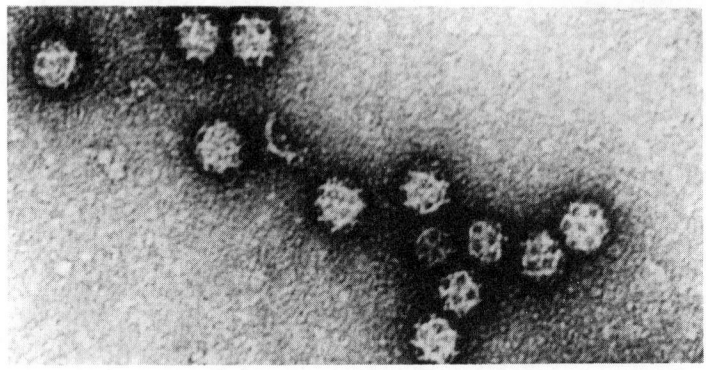

Swine exanthemata virus. Very small, regular particles with prominent cuplike depressions. The surface depressions of the human Norwalk-like viruses are not as pronounced.

Family: *Reoviridae*
Size: 60–80 nm, variable morphology
Symmetry: Icosahedral
Lipid envelope: Absent
Genus: *Reovirus*

Genus: *Rotavirus*
Natural habitat: Gastrointestinal tract of
    humans (reovirus and rotavirus) and
    animal (rotavirus)
Distribution: Worldwide

Transmission: Fecal–oral by direct con-
    tact; animal to human
Portal of entry: Gastrointestinal tract
Diseases: Gastroenteritis (rotavirus); none
    (reovirus)

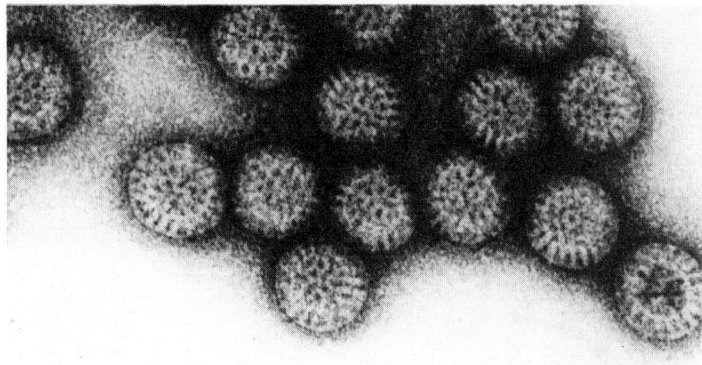

Human rotavirus. The distinctive feature of the *Reoviridae* is the presence of a double shell, each with icosahedral symmetry. ×135,000.

(Continued)

TABLE 21-1 *(Continued)*
CLASSIFICATION OF RNA VIRUSES

Family: *Togaviridae*
  Size: 40–70 nm
  Symmetry: Icosahedral
  Lipid envelope: Present
  Genus: *Alphavirus*
    Type: Group A arboviruses
  Genus: *Flavivirus*
    Type: Group B arboviruses
      Hepatitis E virus

Genus: *Rubivirus*
    Type: Rubella virus
  Natural habitat: Small mammals and insects (arboviruses); humans (rubella)
  Transmission: By mosquito or tick vectors (arboviruses); aerosols or transplacental (rubella)

Portal of entry: Cutaneous (arboviruses); respiratory or vascular (rubella)
  Diseases: Hepatitis, meningitis, encephalitis, arthritis, febrile illness (arboviruses); rash illness, congenital infection (rubella)

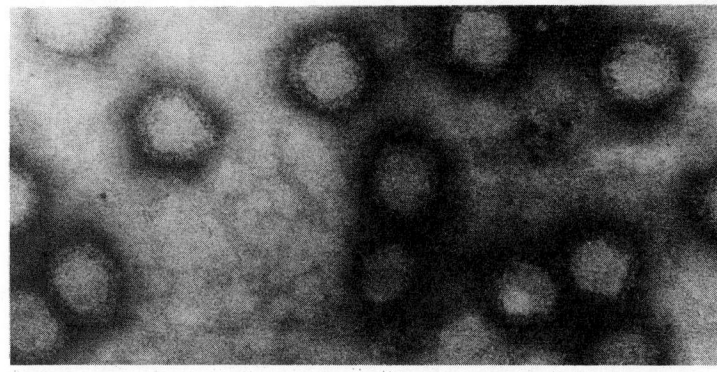

Rubella virus. The spherical virions have a lipid membrane and surface hemagglutinin projections. ×135,000.

Family: *Retroviridae*
  Size: 80–100 nm
  Symmetry: Unknown
  Lipid envelope: Present
  Subfamily: *Oncovirinae*
    Types: Human T-cell leukemia/lymphoma virus (HTLV), types 1–2

Human immunodeficiency virus (HIV), types 1 and 2
  Natural habitat: Humans
  Distribution: Worldwide
  Transmission: Unknown (HTLV); transfusions or contaminated needles, sex acts (HIV)

Portal of entry: Unknown (HTLV); intravenous or venereal (HIV)
  Diseases: T-cell leukemia and lymphoma (HTLV); acquired immunodeficiency syndrome (AIDS) (HIV)

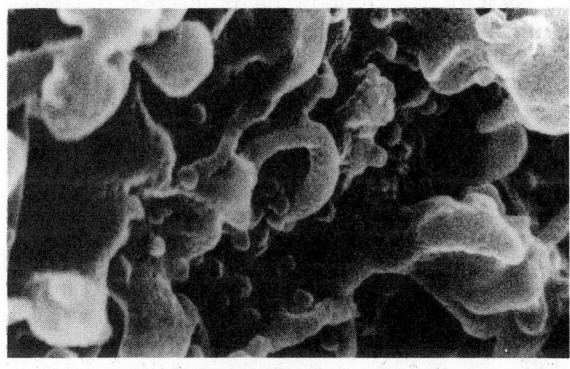

Human immunodeficiency virus. Scanning electron micrograph of human T lymphocyte with virus particles budding from surface.

(Continued)

TABLE 21-1 *(Continued)*
Classification of RNA Viruses

Family: *Arenaviridae*
  Size: 50–300 nm
  Symmetry: Unknown
  Lipid envelope: Present
  Genus: *Arenavirus*
    Types: Lassa virus
    Lymphocytic choriomeningitis virus

Machupo virus (Bolivian hemorrhagic fever)
Junin virus (Argentinian hemorrhagic fever)
Guanarito virus (Venezuelan hemorrhagic fever)
Sabiá (Brazilian hemorrhagic fever)
Natural habitat: Small mammals

Distribution: Worldwide (LCM); South America (Machupo, Junin, Guanarito and Sabiá); Africa (Lassa)
Transmission: Secretions from infected rodents or patients
Portal of entry: Respiratory
Diseases: Febrile illness, meningitis (LCM); hemorrhagic fever (others)

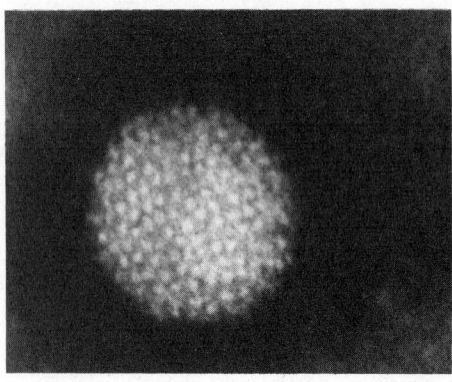 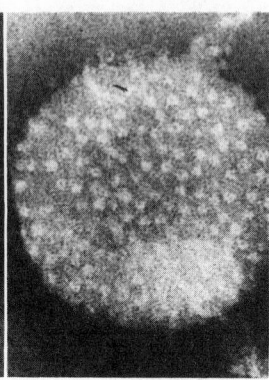

Lymphocytic choriomeningitis virus. The spherical virus has large surface projections. The name is derived from the Latin word *arena* (sand), which was suggested by the internal ribosomelike particles that are seen by transmission electron microscopy. ×225,000.

The introduction of effective vaccines has greatly reduced the incidence of mumps virus infection. At the Mayo Clinic mumps virus was isolated 185 times in the 1960s but only 3 times in the 1970s.[777]

Measles virus (rubeola virus) is unlikely to be encountered in the clinical laboratory,[777] but unfortunately the virus has made a clinical comeback. Laxity in monitoring and enforcing immunization practices has led to explosive outbreaks both in young adults, who may have waning immunity, and in children, especially in inner city areas where levels of immunization are low.[107] The affliction of varsity sports teams and cancellation of highly visible sports contests are guaranteed to get the attention of the media and the public. The public health implications of exposure in our mobile society was illustrated by an epidemic of 247 cases that began in a ski area in Breckenridge, Colorado.[120] After dispersal of infected individuals, cases of measles were detected in 10 states. The need for primary and booster immunization campaigns is suggested by infection of preschool- and school-age children.[537]

Two factors minimize the likelihood of isolating measles virus: the diagnosis is usually made on clinical grounds, and specimens are often not submitted to the laboratory. Additionally, virus is isolated from respiratory secretions and urine only early in the course of the infection. The diagnostic rash is produced by complexes of viral antigen and antibody. Thus, at the time the diagnosis is made by a physician the virus is being neutralized and cultures are likely to be negative. Atypical clinical symptoms were seen formerly in patients who had received early inactivated measles vaccines,[19] but this phenomenon is no longer prevalent. Pneumonia and encephalitis are the most serious complications of measles.[238,426] In addition, measles virus (or a variant thereof) rarely produces a chronic encephalitis known as subacute sclerosing panencephalitis.[650]

The diagnosis of most myxovirus and paramyxovirus infections is by clinical observation or by culture, with serology playing an adjunctive role. Methods for detection of viral antigen have been developed but not yet widely accepted. The importance of laboratory confirmation of measles cases is illustrated by examining sites where multiple viruses that produce skin rashes circulate concurrently. Dengue virus, an arbovirus in the flavivirus group, produces a rash that resembles measles. Dengue virus serotypes are endemic in Puerto Rico, where 28% of all laboratory confirmed cases of dengue infection met the official clinical criteria for a diagnosis of measles.[213] Of 94 patients with rashes that met the clinical criteria for measles, 22 (23%) patients were confirmed to have measles, but 32 (34%) of the patients had laboratory evidence of recent dengue infection. It is easy to see how both patients and clinicians could be confused about the correct diagnosis without adequate laboratory support. More importantly, public health officials cannot take appropriate control measures without the correct diagnosis. Transmission of dengue is controlled by interrupting mosquito transmission, whereas spread of measles virus is eliminated by isolation of infected patients and immunization of susceptible individuals.

PICORNAVIRUSES

The picornaviruses, which include the rhinoviruses and the enteroviruses, constitute the other large and important group of RNA viruses. The rhinoviruses are frequent causes of the common cold. They are acid labile and do not infect the gastrointestinal tract. Trans-

(text continues on page 1196)

TABLE 21-2
CLASSIFICATION OF DNA VIRUSES

Family: *Herpesviridae*
Size: 100–200 nm
Symmetry: Icosahedral
Lipid envelope: Present
Subfamily: *Alphaherpesvirinae*
    Types: Herpes simplex virus 1 and 2
    Varicella-zoster virus (VZV)
Subfamily: *Betaherpesvirinae*
    Type: Cytomegalovirus (CMV)

Subfamily: *Gammaherpesvirinae*
Type: Epstein-Barr virus (EBV)
Unclassified: Human herpesvirus-6 (HHV6)
                Human herpesvirus-7 (HHV7)
                Human herpesvirus-8 (HHV8)
Natural habitat: Humans; related viruses are
    found in animals
Distribution: Worldwide
Transmission: By infected oral or genital se-
    cretions, by blood, or transplacentally

Portal of entry: Respiratory, cutaneous, in-
    travascular, transplacental
Diseases: Neonatal sepsis, pharyngitis, cervi-
    citis, local skin lesions, pneumonia, esoph-
    agitis (herpes simplex), congenital infec-
    tion, hepatitis, mononucleosis, pneumonia
    (CMV); chickenpox (VZV); pharyngitis,
    mononucleosis, hepatitis (EBV); exanthem
    subitum (HHV6 and HHV7); Kaposi's
    sarcoma and lymphoma (HHV8)

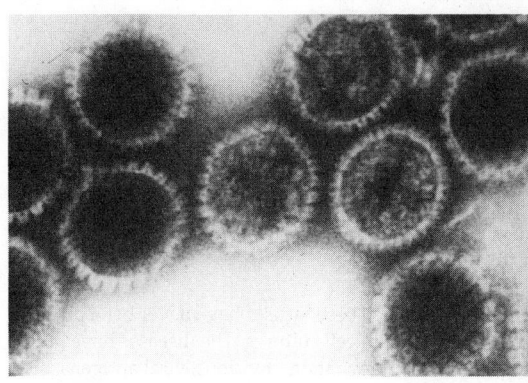 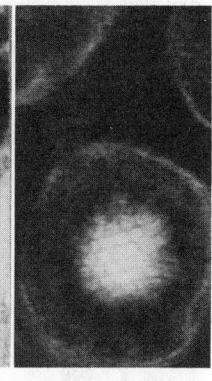

Herpes simplex virus. (*Left*) Naked nucleocapsids demonstrate the regular structure of the virion. Clearly defined structural units appear to have a central depression. (*Right*) Enveloped particle has, in addition, a lipid membrane derived from the infected cell. ×189,000.

Family: *Adenoviridae*
Size: 70–90 nm; 252 capsomeres
Symmetry: Icosahedral
Lipid envelope: Absent
Genus: *Mastadenovirus*
    Types: Adenovirus, types 1–37
    Enteric adenovirus, types 40–41

Natural habitat: Humans (other genera of
    adenoviridae infect animals)
Distribution: Worldwide
Transmission: Fecal–oral, ? aerosol droplet
Portal of entry: Gastrointestinal, res-
    piratory.

Diseases: Conjunctivitis, keratitis, pharyn-
    gitis, tracheobronchitis, pneumonia, cys-
    titis; gastroenteritis (types 40–41)

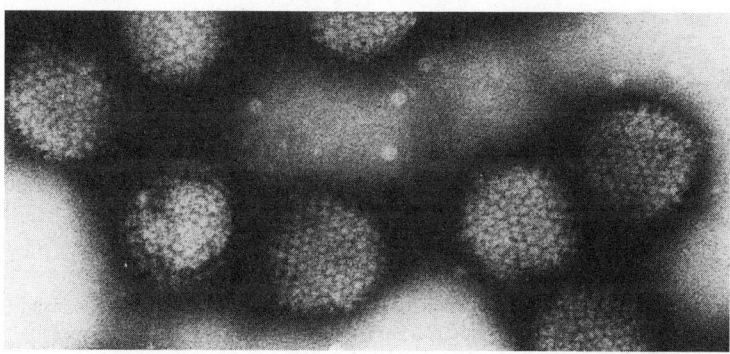

Adenovirus, type 5. The regular arrangement of the structural units of the virion is clearly evident. ×234,000.

(Continued)

TABLE 21-2 *(Continued)*
CLASSIFICATION OF DNA VIRUSES

Family: *Papovaviridae*
Size: 45–55 nm
Symmetry: Icosahedral
Lipid envelope: Absent
Genus: *Papillomavirus*
    Types: Human wart viruses
Genus: *Polyomavirus*
Types: BK virus
      JC virus
      SV40 virus

Natural habitat: Humans and animals; the viruses are largely species-specific
Distribution: Worldwide
Transmission: By contact with infected secretions; viruses remain dormant in tissue

Portal of entry: Cutaneous, genital, or respiratory (papilloma); ? respiratory (polyoma)
Diseases: Cutaneous, genital and laryngeal warts (papilloma); progressive multifocal leukoencephalopathy (polyoma)

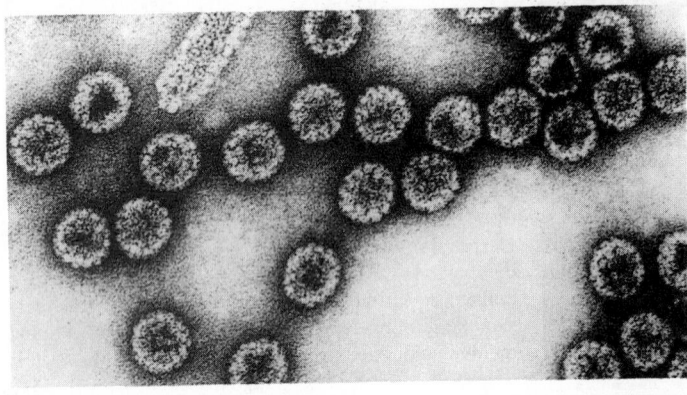

Human wart virus. These viruses have never been propagated successfully in cell cultures. The diseases have been associated by demonstration of virions, viral antigens, or nucleic acid in lesions. ×135,000.

Family: *Parvoviridae*
Size: 18–26 nm
Symmetry: Icosahedral
Lipid envelope: Absent
Genus: *Parvovirus*
    Types: Possibly Norwalk agent; human parvovirus-like agent (HPLA)

Natural habitat: Humans, animals, and insects; viruses are species-specific
Distribution: Worldwide
Transmission: Unknown

Portal of entry: Unknown
Diseases: Gastroenteritis, erythema infectiosum (fifth disease) of childhood; hemolytic disease

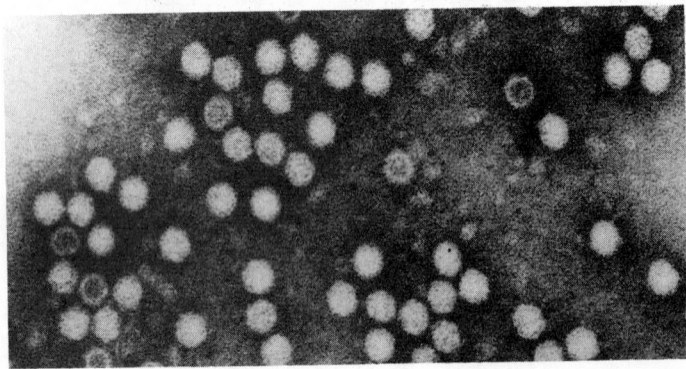

H-1 virus. The virions are very small and regular in size and shape. Parvoviruses are unusual in that they contain single-stranded DNA.

(Continued)

TABLE 21-2 *(Continued)*
CLASSIFICATION OF DNA VIRUSES

Family: Proposed family:
Hepadnaviridae
  Size: 42 nm
  Symmetry: Unknown
  Lipid envelope: Present
  Genus: None established
    Types: Hepatitis B-like viruses

Antigens: Surface antigen (HBsAg)
  Core antigen (HBcAg)
  Early antigen (HBeAg)
Natural habitat: Humans
Distribution: Worldwide
Transmission: Infected secretions and
  blood

Portal of entry: Transfusions, cutaneous
  by shared implements, close contact
  (mechanisms probably various)
Diseases: Hepatitis, cirrhosis, hepatocellular carcinoma

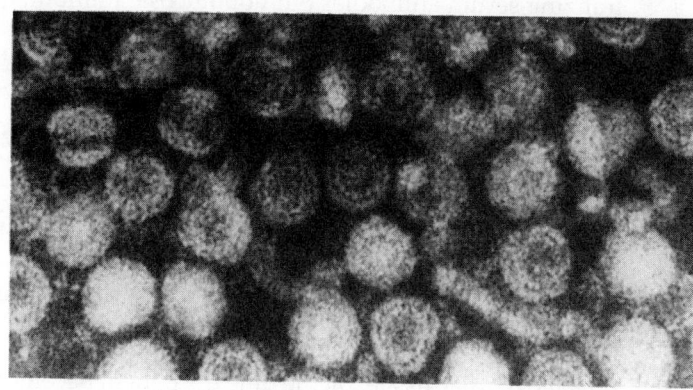

Hepatitis B virus. These 42-nm particles, which are the infectious agent, were originally known as Dane particles.
×225,000.

Family: *Poxviridae*
  Size: 300–450 nm by 170–260 nm; brick
    shaped
  Symmetry: Unknown
  Lipid envelope: Absent
  Subfamily: *Chordopoxvirinae*
    Genus: *Orthopoxvirus*
      Types: Variola (smallpox)
        Vaccinia virus
        Cowpox virus
        Monkeypox virus

Genus: *Parapoxvirus*
  Type: Orf virus
Natural habitat: Humans and animals
Distribution: Worldwide, variola exists
  now only in two research laboratories

Transmission: From infected humans or
  animals
Portal of entry: Respiratory
Diseases: Cutaneous ulcerative lesions;
  smallpox (eradicated)

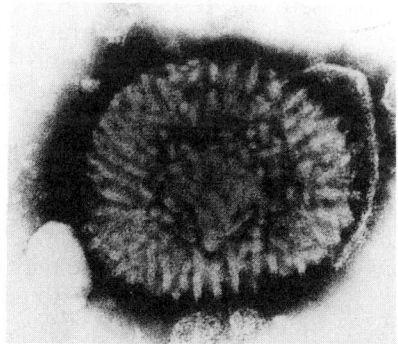

Vaccinia virus. The convoluted outer coat of these large,
brick-shaped particles is evident. When smallpox existed,
negative-stain electron microscopy was a useful tool for
differentiation of the pocks from those of varicella. ×49,500.

mission of rhinoviruses probably occurs by generation of respiratory aerosols,[568] as has been suggested for other respiratory viruses. This hardy virus may also be transmitted through contact with contaminated inanimate surfaces.[20,340]

There are so many rhinovirus serotypes (100 at present) that immunologic diagnosis is impractical. Culture is infrequently requested because rhinovirus infections are uncomfortable, but almost never life-threatening.

The classic enteroviruses are polioviruses 1 through 3, coxsackieviruses A and B, and echoviruses. The coxsackie group received its name from a small town in upstate New York where the first isolates were recovered. "Echo" stands for *e*nteric *c*ytopathic *h*uman *o*rphan, a name applied before the pathogenic potential of the viruses was appreciated. Subsequently, other members of the genus have been recognized and designated enteroviruses 68 through 71. Enteroviruses can be isolated from 40% to 80% of patients with aseptic meningitis.[154] Many more cases of sporadic and epidemic aseptic meningitis are probably caused by enteroviruses, based on the finding that the epidemic curve for all cases of aseptic meningitis parallels exactly the curve for those cases from which enteroviruses have been isolated. The peak incidence is in the summer and early fall.

The enteroviruses, especially coxsackievirus B, also produce myocarditis, pericarditis, and epidemic pleurodynia. An association of these viruses with cardiomyopathy, a noninflammatory disorder of cardiac muscle, has also been suggested but is controversial.[829] Coxsackievirus A causes herpangina and hand-foot-and-mouth disease. The enteroviruses also produce febrile disease with rash, which is usually maculopapular but can rarely be vesicular.[201] Two recently recognized pathogenic enteroviruses are enterovirus 70, which causes epidemic hemorrhagic conjunctivitis,[556,634] and enterovirus 71, which produces central nervous system (CNS) infection including polio-like paralysis.[156,562]

Enteroviral infection is most common in infants and young children. Paradoxically, paralytic poliovirus disease is most prevalent in young adults. Spread of enteroviruses is facilitated by poor hygiene and sanitation and by crowding. In populations among which virus spreads actively (low socioeconomic groups), infection occurs at an early age and paralytic disease is infrequent. Persons in high socioeconomic groups escape infection as infants and are more likely to develop paralysis after infection as a teenager. A similar phenomenon has been documented with varicella-zoster virus, Epstein-Barr virus, and rubella virus. Fortunately, paralytic disease was almost entirely caused by virulent poliovirus serotypes and has been virtually eradicated by immunization in most countries. Wild-type poliovirus has now been eradicated from the Western Hemisphere.[116] The last case of paralytic disease occurred in a 2-year-old boy in Peru. Paralytic disease may be caused by traditional coxsackieviruses and enteroviruses, but only very rarely. The production of paralytic disease

by enterovirus 71 has been noted.[156] Most cases of paralytic poliomyelitis are now caused by the attenuated (Sabin) vaccine strains.[563] There is consequently periodic discussion of the value of returning to an inactivated vaccine.[564]

The pathogenesis of most enterovirus infections includes primary infection of the respiratory or gastrointestinal tracts followed by viremia and infection of a distant target organ, such as skin, heart, or meninges. The inactivated (Salk) poliovirus vaccine elicits neutralizing serum antibodies but not mucosal immunity. The vaccine works because the serum antibodies block the viremic spread to the meninges.[563] The inability of the Salk vaccine to prevent mild gastrointestinal infection is not a serious problem for the individual patient, although it does allow continued circulation of the virulent strain.

The symptoms of most enterovirus infections are produced by direct viral cytopathic effect on the target organ. Meningoencephalitis is accompanied by productive infection of the CNS by actively replicating virus. The clinical syndrome of myocarditis, however, is caused by an immunologic reaction to enterovirus-infected cardiac tissue. By the time the patient becomes symptomatic the virus has usually been eliminated from the heart.

It is clear from the pathogenesis of enteroviral infection that culture of patients with aseptic meningitis (productive infection) makes sense, but culture of patients with myocarditis (immunopathologic disease) is unlikely to yield a viral isolate.

Extensive cross-reactions among the enteroviruses make serologic diagnosis of these infections impractical. The diagnosis can be made only if a virus has been isolated from the patient or if the clinical syndrome defines the serotypes of interest. Clinicians often request serologic testing for the six coxsackievirus B serotypes in cases of myocarditis. The rationale for the request is statistical, based on the predominance of these serotypes in myocarditis, and practical, in that the number of serotypes is limited.

Isolation of an enterovirus from a sterile body fluid is proof that the virus is the cause of the disease. Cerebrospinal fluid (CSF) should be cultured, even in the absence of a cellular response if meningitis is evident clinically.[154] Blood culture may be useful,[673] and virus may be recovered from both serum and white blood cell fractions.[672] Enteroviruses may be isolated more frequently from the upper respiratory tract and, especially, from feces than from internal organs. It is more difficult to associate isolates from the respiratory and gastrointestinal tracts with disease because these viruses may be excreted in the feces for long periods in the absence of clinical symptoms.[424] Asymptomatic fecal passage of enteroviruses is most prevalent in infants and young children,[730] the age groups in which symptomatic disease is also most common. The echoviruses and coxsackievirus B serotypes can be reliably isolated in cell culture, but inoculation of suckling mice must be performed for isolation of all coxsackievirus A serotypes. A prototype commercial system has been developed for direct detection of enteroviral RNA in

CSF.[900] There is a clear role for direct detection of enteroviruses in a timely fashion that could affect the management of the patient, including use of antibacterial agents. Viral cultures play such a role in a small subset of patients, as discussed previously.[155] A result that was available more rapidly than viral culture would expand the subset of patients, but would probably not be necessary for all patients with aseptic meningitis.

RESPIRATORY SYNCYTIAL VIRUS

Respiratory syncytial virus causes recurrent respiratory infections from infancy through adult life. Epidemics are common and may be hospital associated.[242,348] There are two distinct serologic groups of respiratory syncytial virus (A and B). A single group predominates in most epidemics.[589] Waris reported that the two groups produced epidemics in Finland in an alternating cycle.[855] Epidemics in nurseries have been recognized for many years. Recently, outbreaks of respiratory syncytial virus disease have been described in nursing homes.[251] Infection is concentrated in the winter months, although summertime infection may occur in warm climates.[856]

Infection is spread by large particle droplets and by fomites (contaminated environmental particles, such as dust), rather than by small particle aerosols.[347,349] Almost all seronegative infants who are exposed to their first epidemic become infected, but immunity is incomplete. As a result, the rate of nosocomial infection may be almost 50% unless active measures to control transmission are undertaken.[348] Wearing gowns and masks does not prevent transmission.[592] A combination of techniques is required to prevent transmission: (1) active monitoring of respiratory infection in new admissions, (2) limitation of visitors, (3) cohorting of infants such that infected patients are separated from susceptible infants, and (4) various control measures.[347] Successful control measures have included use of gowns and gloves (as opposed to gowns and masks).[501] The explanation for this dichotomy is probably the predominance of direct transfer over aerosol dissemination as a means of infection by this virus. Good laboratory diagnostic support is needed not only for managing the individual patient, but also for limiting nosocomial spread of the infection. Jacobsen and colleagues noted that reliance on direct immunofluorescence tests, the reference procedure for direct detection of viral antigen, would have resulted in correct placement of children in a cohorting scheme in 92% of cases.[416] They considered the direct fluorescence test a reliable method, except for patients with a very high risk of serious disease, such as infants with bronchopulmonary dysplasia.

Respiratory syncytial virus may produce croup, bronchitis, bronchiolitis, or interstitial pneumonia. It is the most common cause of respiratory disease in hospitalized infants who are younger than 1 year of age.[415] Respiratory syncytial virus infections are often severe in young children. If congenital heart disease[528] or immunologic deficiency is present,[351] the disease may be lethal; in one study, 8 (73%) of 11 infants with congenital heart disease and pulmonary hypertension died.[528] Many previously normal children, especially infants, are sufficiently ill that ventilatory support is required. Apnea is a prominent part of the syndrome.[165] Although debate continues about the efficacy of ribavirin therapy,[558] reports of its efficacy have fueled the demand for efficient and speedy laboratory diagnostic support.[775] Recently, administration of respiratory syncytial virus immune globulin to high-risk infants has successfully prevented respiratory syncytial virus infection.[334,335]

Immunity to respiratory syncytial virus is short lived and incomplete.[352] Antibody to surface glycoproteins is partially protective, but reinfections occurred in 25% of volunteers, no matter what the level of antibody or number of previous infections. Recurrent infections in older children and adults are less severe than those in neonates. It was once believed that respiratory syncytial virus infections in adults were very mild. Hall and associates[354] demonstrated lower respiratory tract infection in 10 adult patients during a prospective study; the illness was sufficiently severe to result in an average of 6 days lost from work. The serious nature of respiratory syncytial virus infection in immunocompromised adults has been recognized.[379] In one study, 4 of 11 immunocompromised adults died of respiratory syncytial virus pneumonia.[240] Serious respiratory syncytial virus infection occurs also in the elderly and in adults with chronic diseases, such as diabetes, cirrhosis, and chronic obstructive pulmonary disease.[337,817]

The diagnosis of respiratory syncytial virus infection is best accomplished by direct detection of antigen in clinical specimens. Culture of this labile virus is definitive but difficult to accomplish in a timely fashion. Serology is used primarily for epidemiology studies.

RHABDOVIRUSES

Many other important RNA viruses have been described, some of which cause highly lethal infections. These viruses are primarily tropical and are therefore less likely to be encountered by clinical laboratories than are the picornaviruses and the myxoviruses. Among these are the rhabdoviruses, including the agent of rabies, which is important worldwide.

The diagnosis of rabies is made by detection of viral antigen in clinical specimens from animals or humans. Culture of rabies virus is infrequently performed because of the simplicity, accuracy, and speed of direct immunofluorescence. This historical scourge is endemic in wild animals in the United States but is extremely uncommon in humans.[114] Human exposure continues, however, from hunting dogs exposed to infected wild animals, from infected bats, and from domestic animals. Great anxiety is caused by possible exposures because of the lethality of the infection. The cost of preventing human disease can be enormous, as was shown in New Hampshire when a large number of individuals were potentially exposed to a rabid kitten in a pet store.[128] The estimated cost for epidemiologic investigation and prophylaxis was $1.5 million. Ongoing epizootic disease in raccoons in the eastern United States is of particular concern because of the frequency with which these aggressive animals invade human habitations. It is sometimes impossible to identify any source for human rabies.[776] The molecular structure of rabies strains reflects their animal host. It is now possible to identify the likely source of a viral isolate from its nucleic acid composition. A case of inadvertent surgical transmission of rabies in a corneal transplant has been reported.[401] Interested readers should consult a recently revised treatise on the subject.[36]

ARENAVIRUSES

The arenaviruses are a family of RNA viruses that share fascinating biologic characteristics.[661] Their natural host is a variety of rodents, which are persistently infected without an effective host response or symptomatic disease. Infectious virus is excreted in the urine, which is the source of human infection. Those at risk of infection are, therefore, individuals who come in contact with infected rodent excreta, either in their homes or at work in the fields. Person-to-person transmission occurs regularly only with Lassa virus, usually in health care workers who have been exposed to infected body fluids, especially at autopsy. Several of the hemorrhagic fever viruses appear to have been transmitted to sexual partners by convalescent men. The infected patient does not pose a significant risk to individuals with casual contact. Laboratory infections have been an uncommon, but regular risk of these agents. Most recently a laboratory worker was infected with Sabiá virus.[121] The sources of infection have been aerosolization of culture fluids and probably rodent urine. Epidemics of lymphocytic choriomeningitis virus have occurred among laboratory workers who worked with hamsters and among individuals who owned hamsters as pets.[329]

The major human pathogens, the geographic distribution, rodent reservoir, clinical disease, and date of discovery are summarized in Table 21-3. Lymphocytic choriomeningitis (LCM) virus was discovered during investigation of the St. Louis encephalitis virus epidemic in 1933.[22] It was soon recognized that the virus caused aseptic meningitis in humans.[715] The frequency of infection is probably underestimated, because clinicians do not suspect the infection and diagnostic tools are not readily available. Investigators found antibody to LCM virus in 5.1% of healthy women in Birmingham, Alabama.[800] Junin virus was the first recognized arenavirus cause of hemorrhagic fever, Argentinian hemorrhagic fever in the pampas region.[640] The mysteries of the epidemiology were unraveled a few years later by Karl Johnson et al. during investigation of an outbreak of Bolivian hemorrhagic fever in the Beni province, caused by Machupo virus.[425] Further notoriety for the viruses followed the recognition of severe hemorrhagic disease in several West African countries, caused by Lassa virus.[275] The most recent additions also come from South America: Guanarito virus in Venezuela[733] and Sabiá virus in Brazil.[173] The old viruses are still with us, an outbreak of Bolivian hemorrhagic fever having occurred in 1994 in the provinces of El Beni and Santa Cruz.[122]

The arenaviruses have a distinctive morphology (see Table 21-1) that led to the recognition of the group.[594] They are roughly spherical, enveloped particles with prominent ribosome-like structures in the center. The name of the group derives from the Latin arenosus (sandy), which was suggested by the internal particles. The original proposal, arenoviruses, was subsequently modified to arenaviruses to avoid confusion with adenoviruses. Laboratory diagnosis is usually made by one of several serologic techniques. Virus can be isolated from blood by inoculation of animals or cell cultures, most commonly Vero cells. These tests should be reserved for reference laboratories with Biosafety level 4 containment facilities.

FILOVIRUSES

For many years the only known member of this group was Marburg virus, which caused a mysterious, fatal illness among monkey handlers in a laboratory in Marburg, Germany in 1967.[454] The source of the virus was African green monkeys, but attempts to identify the agent in freshly caught monkeys in Africa were unsuccessful. Over the next decade there were few isolations

TABLE 21-3
CHARACTERISTICS OF ARENAVIRUSES PATHOGENIC FOR HUMANS

VIRUS	GEOGRAPHIC DISTRIBUTION	RODENT HOST	HUMAN DISEASE	FATALITY RATE	DATE OF DISCOVERY
Lymphocytic choriomeningitis (LCM) virus	Europe, North and South America	*Mus domesticus; Mus musculus*	Aseptic meningitis	<1%	1933 (St. Louis)
Junin virus	Argentina	*Calomys musculinus*	Hemorrhagic fever	15–30%	1958
Machupo virus	Bolivia	*Calomys callosus*	Hemorrhagic fever	25%	1963
Lassa virus	West Africa	*Mastomys* species	Hemorrhagic fever	15%	1969
Guanarito virus	Venezuela	*Zygodontomys brevicauda; Sigmodon alsoni*	Hemorrhagic fever	25%	1990
Sabiá virus	Brazil	Unknown	Hemorrhagic fever	? 30%	1990

of the virus, which remained a curiosity, albeit a lethal one. In 1977 a new virus, designated Ebola virus, was isolated from simultaneous outbreaks of disease in Zaire and the Sudan. The outbreaks shared epidemiologic and clinical characteristics, and the viruses were closely related, although antigenically distinct.[709] The disease was characterized by high fever, shock, involvement of multiple organ systems, and diffuse hemorrhage. The mortality rate for Marburg virus was 25%; for Ebola-Sudan, 50%, and for Ebola-Zaire, 90%. As with Marburg, the source of the infection was unknown, but transmission was clearly associated with exposure to body fluids of infected patients.[44] The medical staff of some of the small mission hospitals were decimated by the mysterious disease.

The two epidemics in remote areas of Sudan and Zaire caused alarm in public health and infectious disease circles, but did not make an impact on the general public. That situation changed dramatically when a large outbreak occurred in 1995 in Kikwit, Nigeria. More than 300 cases occurred over a short period of time, approximately one-third of the cases were in health care workers, and the fatality rate was approximately 80%.[126] The epidemic was eventually controlled by introducing strict barrier precautions to prevent families and health care workers from having contact with secretions of infected patients. The source of this extensive epidemic was not clear.

A third strain of Ebola virus was identified in the Ivory Coast in 1994. Conjecture about the source in nature of Ebola virus had focused on monkeys because of the simian origins of Marburg virus, but no hard evidence had been found to support the hypothesis. In the Ivory Coast, however, a laboratory worker who had autopsied a sick chimpanzee in the field developed a febrile, dengue-like illness that did not respond to antimalarial therapy. Subsequently diarrhea and a pruritic rash developed, but the worker recovered from the infection. She had been participating in an investigation of the second of two outbreaks of fatal hemorrhagic disease that was decimating a large chimpanzee colony. A strain of Ebola virus most closely related to the Zaire type was isolated from the patient's blood.[504]

Additional evidence for a simian source of Ebola virus comes from an epidemic of lethal infection among cynomolgus monkeys in two animal holding facilities—the first in Reston, Virginia,[417] the second in Texas.[134] In both cases the animals had been imported from the Philippines, and the virus was antigenically distinct from the strains isolated in Zaire, Sudan, and the Ivory Coast. Only five cases of human infection with the Reston strain of Ebola virus have been documented, all of which were asymptomatic.[108] There was evidence of transmission of infection from animal to animal by aerosols, a terrifying epidemiologic characteristic that has fortunately been missing from the human epidemics. Data indicating epidemic disease among captive cynomolgus monkeys in the Philippines before export have also been reported. The fatality rate among infected monkeys was 82%, and monkeys held in a group cage were more likely to develop infection than those held in individual cages.[368]

The filoviruses are RNA viruses with a characteristic ultrastructure (see Table 21-1) and a distinctive filamentous morphology that gives the family its name.[448] The two viruses, Marburg and Ebola, can be distinguished by ultrastructural morphology, and the types of Ebola virus are antigenically distinct.[256]

Laboratory diagnosis is accomplished in reference laboratories by direct detection of antigens, by cell culture or inoculation of animals, or by serologic techniques. The Vero cell line supports the growth of virus in vitro and is used in some clinical laboratories. Most of these viruses require Biosafety level 4 isolation procedures for containment of biohazard and are restricted to high security government laboratories. Guidelines for management of patients with suspected viral hemorrhagic fever have been promulgated.[127]

TOGAVIRUSES

The Togaviridae and Bunyaviridae now include most of the viruses that were previously known as arboviruses (arthropod-borne viruses). Both groups are single-stranded RNA viruses with a lipid envelope.[94] The togaviruses were named for their lipid "toga" that surrounds the virus (see pages 1186 and 1191). These biologically diverse agents have a complex ecology; they usually infect small mammals or birds (reservoir) and are transmitted from animal to animal by ticks or mosquitoes (vector). Many of these viruses are also maintained by transovarial passage from insect to larva. Humans are accidental hosts when they are inadvertently infected instead of the usual animal reservoirs.

There are two divisions within the Togaviridae. The alphaviruses (formerly group A arboviruses) contain the agents of eastern equine encephalitis, western equine encephalitis, and Venezuelan encephalitis. The flaviviruses (formerly group B arboviruses) include the agents of St. Louis encephalitis, dengue (breakbone fever), and yellow fever.

Small numbers of cases of eastern equine encephalitis and western equine encephalitis infections occur each year. Human disease may be presaged by increased incidence of illness in horses. Epidemics of St. Louis encephalitis occur approximately every 10 years in the southern part of the United States, especially in Texas, in the Gulf Coast states, and in Florida. The reservoir for St. Louis encephalitis virus is birds, and the mosquito vectors vary with the geographic location. Disease is most severe in the elderly, and cases are concentrated in heavily wooded neighborhoods with poor screening of homes.

Dengue fever is prevalent in the Caribbean[688] and in Southeast Asia.[298] Imported cases are seen in the United States with increasing frequency, and indigenous transmission of the virus in the United States has been reported occasionally, most commonly in Texas.[123] A most unusual route of entry into the United States was uncovered when infected mosquitoes were found in stagnant water that had accumulated in tires imported from Southeast Asia. Uncomplicated dengue infection is an undifferentiated febrile disease, sometimes accompanied by a rash and arthralgias or arthritis. The differential diagnosis includes other viral infections, such as rubella. There are four distinct serotypes of dengue virus. Halstead has hypothesized that serial infection with different serotypes triggers immunopathologic mechanisms that produce the dengue hemorrhagic fever syndrome.[355] Formerly limited to Southeast Asia, the lethal hemorrhagic form of the disease has occurred in the Caribbean with increasing frequency.[124]

Although some arboviruses can be isolated in cell culture, inoculation of infant mice is necessary for reliable isolation of most agents. The encephalitis viruses are infrequently isolated from specimens other than brain tissue. Potential biohazards mandate the high security that is available only in a few reference laboratories. For all of these reasons, serology is the mainstay of diagnosis of arbovirus infections.

The other major virus in the Togaviridae, rubella virus, has an entirely different biology from that of the arboviruses. Rubella virus produces an acute febrile illness with a maculopapular rash (German measles) and may cause arthritis. If a pregnant woman is infected, especially in the first trimester, infection of the fetus may occur; the resultant infection in the infant may be asymptomatic but may result in severe congenital abnormalities or death of the fetus. Diagnosis of rubella infections is almost always serologic.

BUNYAVIRUSES

The Bunyaviridae are a large and diverse group of viruses, which are transmitted to humans by arthropod vectors, principally ticks and mosquitoes, and from the excreta of rodents. There are four medically important genera: 1) Bunyavirus, including the Cali-

fornia encephalitis virus group; 2) Nairovirus, including Congo-Crimean hemorrhagic fever virus; 3) Phlebovirus, including Rift Valley fever virus and sandfly fever virus; and 4) Hantavirus, including the agents of Korean hemorrhagic fever, nephropathic epidemica, and hantavirus pulmonary syndrome.[94]

CALIFORNIA ENCEPHALITIS VIRUSES

The most important of the bunyaviruses in the United States is the California encephalitis group of viruses. Despite the name "California," these viruses produce disease most commonly in midwestern and north central states. The California encephalitis viruses commonly produce aseptic meningitis, a disease that occurs in the summer and is clinically indistinguishable from enteroviral disease.[26,94] Most patients recover uneventfully from their infection.

HANTAVIRUSES

The hantaviruses are a steadily expanding group of viruses that have moved from exotic infectious agents to endemic threats in the United States. The uniform characteristics of the group include asymptomatic, persistent infection of a rodent host, probable transmission to humans through infected rodent excreta, and infection of the vascular endothelium. The current status of the viruses, their rodent host, and associated clinical diseases are summarized in Table 21-4.

During the Korean War a severe hemorrhagic fever was recognized among American soldiers. Shock and renal failure, which were prominent symptoms, provided the descriptive name hemorrhagic fever with renal symptoms (HFRS).[85,773] Fever, thrombocytopenia,

---

TABLE 21-4
HANTAVIRUSES: THEIR HOSTS AND CLINICAL DISEASES

VIRUS	GEOGRAPHIC DISTRIBUTION	RODENT HOST	CLINICAL DISEASE
Hantaan	Far East; ? Balkans and Central Europe	*Apodemus* species	Hemorrhagic fever with renal symptoms (HFRS)
Seoul	Far East; ? worldwide	*Rattus rattus* *Rattus norvegicus* (Urban rats)	Mild HFRS
Belgrade	Yugoslavia	Unknown	HFRS
Puumala	Scandinavia; Europe	Voles	Nephropathia epidemica
Prospect Hill	United States	Microtine rodents	Rare asymptomatic infection
Sin Nombre Convict Creek	Western United States	*Peromyscus maniculatus* (deer mouse)	Hantavirus pulmonary syndrome (HPS)
Bayou	Louisiana	Unknown	HPS
Black Creek Canal	Florida	*Sigmodon hispidus* (cotton rats)	Unknown
Not Yet Named	Northeastern United States	Unknown	HPS

and renal failure comprise the classic clinical picture. The return of platelets presages restoration of normal renal function. Shock and multiorgan failure, simulating bacterial sepsis, characterize the most severe cases. Less common manifestations include retroperitoneal hemorrhage and pulmonary edema. Some patients experience undifferentiated febrile illness with normal renal function. A clinical syndrome of severe hepatic disease has been described in Greece, where the prevalent strains resemble the virus associated with infections in Korea.[234]

Subsequent to the documentation of disease in Korea, it was recognized that this severe clinical syndrome occurred in the eastern Soviet Union and Manchuria.[97] The etiologic agent was not isolated until 1982, when Hantaan virus (named after a Korean river where epidemic disease had occurred) was isolated.[502] This virus produces asymptomatic, persistent infection in its rodent host, *Apodemus agrarius*. Subsequently, a second, related agent, Seoul virus, which produces less severe infection, was isolated. The rodent hosts of Seoul virus are urban rats, *Rattus norvegicus* and *Rattus rattus*. Seoul virus has been found in laboratory rats and produced infection in laboratory workers.[211] There are no documented cases of Hantaan virus infection in the United States, but cases of Seoul virus–induced HFRS have been documented serologically in Baltimore.[305] The rat-associated hantaviruses in the United States have been frequently associated with hypertensive renal disease but not with other chronic renal diseases.[306] Although hypertensive renal disease is not usually associated with infectious agents, the lesson of *Helicobacter pylori* and gastritis should caution us against dismissing the association out of hand. A Balkan version of HFRS is caused by Belgrade virus, and a virus indistinguishable from Hantaan virus has also been documented in that region.[313]

A milder version of this infection, known as nephropathia epidemica, is produced by Puumala virus and occurs in Scandinavia.[83] The virus produces asymptomatic infections in voles; in humans it is an acute febrile disease with lower back pain and polyuria but with mild or no hemorrhagic manifestations and without shock. Patients recover without sequelae.[483] The symptoms are frequently nonspecific, and the clinical diagnosis was correct in only 28% of cases in one Finnish study.[599] Severe HFRS caused by Puumala-like virus has been reported in Germany[912] and Yugoslavia.[214] Puumala virus is associated with voles in Scandinavia, but the Yugoslavian strain was isolated from mice, *Mus musculus*.

Prospect Hill virus, which was the first indigenous hantavirus recognized in the United States,[503] is most closely related to Puumala virus. It was first recognized by D. Carleton Gajdusek, who won a Nobel Prize for his study of kuru (see page 1223), on his farm in rural Maryland. The virus is widely distributed throughout the United States, but appears to have infected few humans and has not caused clinical disease.

The spotlight focused on hantaviruses in 1993 when an outbreak of severe respiratory disease occurred in the Four Corners area of the southwestern United States.[226] The patients had a prodromal syndrome of fever, myalgia, cough or dyspnea, gastrointestinal symptoms, and headache, which progressed rapidly to irreversible pulmonary edema. With amazing rapidity the causative agent was recognized as a new member of the hantavirus genus, named Sin Nombre virus (initially named Four Corners virus).[477,611] A closely related virus, termed Convict Creek virus, was isolated concurrently from the California-Nevada border region. The rodent host of Sin Nombre virus is the deer mouse, *Peromyscus maniculatus*.[153] It is hypothesized that heavy rains increased food sources, causing a great increase in the number of rodents, increasing the frequency of contact between humans and mice, and altering the epidemiology from sporadic, endemic disease to epidemic infection.[409] There is no evidence of human-to-human transmission of hantavirus pulmonary syndrome. Retrospective diagnosis of cases of infection with Sin Nombre or a related virus dating back as far as 1978 has been made by immunoperoxidase staining of stored paraffin-embedded tissue.[911] All of the 12 infections identified retrospectively had occurred west of the Mississippi River, most in the Far West.

Subsequent to the discovery of Sin Nombre virus other related hantaviruses have been identified in the United States, including Louisiana,[585] Florida,[718] and the northeastern United States.[119] The frequency of hantavirus infection outside of the endemic areas is unknown. A serologic survey of patients hospitalized with community-acquired pneumonia in Baltimore, where Seoul virus infections have been documented and near the home of Prospect Hill virus, did not yield any cases of hantavirus pulmonary syndrome.[34]

The lung is the target organ pathologically as well as clinically.[618,910] Edema and fibrin deposition with focal hyaline membranes in the airspaces are accompanied by an interstitial mononuclear exudate. Large immunoblastic cells infiltrate many organs. The hematologic findings include left-shifted neutrophilic leukocytosis, thrombocytopenia, circulating immunoblasts, and (in severe cases) hemoconcentration. Viral antigen is concentrated in endothelial cells, particularly in the pulmonary vasculature, and virus-like particles may be seen in those cells.[910] Hantaviral antigens are also found in follicular dendritic cells, macrophages, and lymphocytes. It is of interest that Hantaan virus infects human endothelial cells in vitro.[654]

HUMAN GASTROENTERITIS VIRUSES

Viral gastroenteritis is second only to viral respiratory disease as a cause of morbidity in the United States. The incidence of viral gastroenteritis has been estimated at approximately 11% per year.[216] Mortality is rare. In the past decade much has been learned about the etiologic agents, but only about 50% of infectious gastroenteritis can be assigned an etiology. Most of these agents have been identified by immunoelectron microscopy. In this technique immune serum is mixed with a virus suspension or a stool specimen. Clumping of the submicroscopic viral particles can be observed when negatively stained preparations are examined with the electron microscope. Most of these agents cannot be cultivated easily. Therefore, details of their composition are not known; for convenience they will be discussed with the most common pathogen, the rotaviruses.

The agents of viral gastroenteritis can be divided into six groups. The classification is embryonic because of limited knowledge about some of the agents:

> Rotaviruses
> Norwalk-like agents
> Caliciviruses
> Astroviruses
> Other small round viruses
> Enteric adenoviruses

The frequency of these viruses in the United States is summarized in Table 21-5. The data come from a multicenter study, using electron microscopy.[511] The identification of agents in this study was entirely morphologic.

Many aspects of these viral gastrointestinal infections are similar. They produce acute vomiting or diarrhea, which is usually mild, self-limited, and noninflammatory. Bloody diarrhea does not occur. Microscopic analysis of biopsies from human volunteers who have been fed these infectious agents show blunting of intestinal villi and mild inflammatory changes in the submucosa, changes that are indicative of small bowel malabsorption. Damaged cells at the tips of the villi are replaced by cells from the bases of the crypts over 5 to 10 days. Diarrhea that lasts more than 7 to 10 days is unlikely to be viral. Treatment is by replacement of lost fluid and electrolytes, usually caused by vomiting. Unfortunately immunity appears to be only partial.[216]

Of note is the absence of conventional intestinal viruses from the list of pathogens. There is little evidence that enteroviruses or respiratory adenoviruses cause gastrointestinal disease.

Laboratory diagnosis of viral gastroenteritis can be accomplished by a variety of means, some of which are

commercially available. This subject has been reviewed by Christensen.[162] The first question clinicians and microbiologists must ask is whether diagnosis of individual patients is necessary. It is important to remember that the necessity for having diagnostic tests with which to understand the biology of the disease does not mean that those tests must be used on individual patients. The similarity in pathophysiology and clinical features of the infections, the lack of specific antiviral therapy, the commonality of supportive therapy, the infrequency of serious complications, and the need for similar infection control mechanisms regardless of etiology make it hard to justify routine use of the necessary battery of expensive diagnostic tests. At least one-half of the infections will remain undiagnosed, and most of the patients will be well before the results are obtained. Diagnostic support for severe infections and for large epidemics is important, but best accomplished in reference laboratories where the gamut of possibilities can be tested.

ROTAVIRUSES

Rotaviruses are the most important human pathogens in the Reoviridae. The reoviruses themselves are not associated with human disease, but they have been useful in the study of molecular mechanisms of viral pathogenesis.[760] "Reo" stands for *r*espiratory-*e*nteric *o*rphan, from the source of virus isolates and the lack of association with clinical disease. Rotavirus got its name from the wheel-like appearance of the virion in electron micrographs (see Table 21-1).

The rotaviruses contain both human and animal pathogens, but animal rotaviruses do not infect humans. Human rotaviruses have been classified serologically, with most pathogenic human strains in the United States and Europe falling into group A. Human rotavirus is a common cause of gastroenteritis in infants and young children.[436] The clinical presentation is varied, but vomiting and dehydration are prominent features in comparison to gastroenteritis produced by other viruses. The combination of vomiting and a seasonal occurrence in the winter months has led investigators to name the condition "winter vomiting disease." The frequency and specificity of respiratory symptoms in rotavirus infection is controversial.[162,435] It is possible that the prevalence of vomiting in rotavirus infection reflects the age of the patient rather than a property of the virus, because Norwalk virus produces significantly more vomiting in infants than in adults.[437] Uhnoo and Svensson studied the comparative features of group A, subgroups 1 and 2 in Swedish infants.[836] Patients with subgroup 1 strains developed fever up to 39°C significantly more often than those with subgroup 2, but infants who had subgroup 2 infections were sicker, hospitalized more frequently, and more likely to have respiratory symptoms. The frequency of diarrhea and vomiting in the two groups was similar.

Chronic rotavirus infection may occur in immunosuppressed children. In adults, rotavirus infection is usually asymptomatic. These viruses are notorious

---

TABLE 21-5

PREVALENCE OF VIRAL AGENTS OF GASTROENTERITIS IN THE UNITED STATES AND CANADA

Number positive	8262
Rotavirus	48%
Astrovirus	2.4%
Calicivirus	1.3%
SRV/SRSV	10.0/0.4%*
Adenovirus	17.2%†
Coronavirus	6.6%†
Other	14.6%

* Small round virus/small round structured virus, including Norwalk-like agents
† Includes both respiratory and intestinal strains
Adapted from Lew, J.F., et al: Six-year retrospective surveillance of gastroenteritis viruses identified at ten electron microscopy centers in the United States and Canada. Pediatr Infect Dis J 9:709–714, 1990

causes of nosocomial infection, including epidemics, in children.[271]

Rotaviruses were discovered, using electron microscopy, and were associated with human disease using immunoelectron microscopy.[436] The most common diagnostic methods used in clinical laboratories have been the identification of viral antigen with a variety of enzyme immunoassays and latex agglutination tests. False-positive test results have been the primary problem with these assays. The reliability of enzyme immunoassays in diagnosing neonatal infections has been questioned in particular, especially with early versions of the tests. Commercial products that include confirmatory assays, such as a blocking enzyme immunoassay, are preferred.[435] Many other diagnostic approaches, including molecular probes, have been developed. The reader is referred to the thorough review by Christensen for details of individual tests.[162]

Although human rotavirus has been difficult to culture, new approaches have allowed recovery of the agent in as many as three-fourths of specimens that were positive by other means. Hasegawa and colleagues isolated human rotaviruses from 17 of 21 clinical specimens that contained rotavirus by electron microscopy or immune adherence hemagglutination.[364] Cytopathic effect developed in cynomolgus monkey kidney cells that were fed with trypsin-containing media. The viruses are fastidious, however, and cell culture has not become a standard diagnostic tool.

NORWALK-LIKE VIRUSES

The Norwalk agent of gastroenteritis was recognized as a 27-nm particle in stool specimens from an outbreak of community gastroenteritis in Norwalk, Ohio.[436] Subsequently, similar RNA viruses have been isolated from other epidemics.[215,826] These viruses are often called small, round, structured viruses. Their taxonomic place is not entirely clear.

Norwalk-like viruses have produced epidemics of disease frequently and also cause sporadic infection.[437] These viruses produce infection and active disease in persons of all ages, in contrast to most of the other viral agents, which produce symptomatic disease predominantly in infants and young children. The Norwalk-like agents have been associated with contaminated food and water and are one of the possibilities to consider when a patient has recently ingested shellfish.[583]

Laboratory diagnosis is still a research tool because the Norwalk-like viruses cannot be grown in cell culture. Immunoelectron microscopy is the reference method. Research immunoassays have been developed for some strains but cannot detect unrecognized serotypes.

CALICIVIRUSES

The caliciviruses are small RNA viruses that resemble the Norwalk agents but are morphologically distinct. They derive their name from the cuplike depressions (chalice or calyx) visible in the particles (see Table 21-1). The human caliciviruses have been reported primarily in epidemic and sporadic gastroenteritis of young children.[216] The human strains have not been cultivated successfully in cell cultures. Diagnosis is by electron microscopy.

ASTROVIRUSES

The astroviruses also contain RNA and have been difficult to cultivate in vitro, although a few strains have been successfully grown.[162] They derive their name from their star-shaped ultrastructural appearance. Astroviruses are shed in large numbers in the stool but appear to be less pathogenic than the Norwalk-like agents. They have produced epidemic disease in young children, on pediatric wards, in day care centers,[512] and in nursing homes.[216] In one recent study they were the second most common virus (after rotavirus) identified in children with diarrhea.[376] Concurrent infection with astroviruses and caliciviruses has been described.[327] Diagnosis is primarily by electron microscopy because these viruses do not grow in cell cultures.

ENTERIC CORONAVIRUSES

The role of coronaviruses in gastroenteritis is uncertain. Both morphologically typical and atypical virions (coronavirus-like particles) are found.

ENTERIC ADENOVIRUSES

A causative association of the classic adenovirus serotypes with diarrheal disease could not be established, but "noncultivable" serotypes were demonstrated by immunoelectron microscopy. Adenovirus types 40 and 41, which do not grow well in the usual tissue culture cells, are intestinal pathogens.[198] These enteric adenoviruses are the second most common cause of viral gastroenteritis in infants. They produce sporadic infection, although epidemics have been described.[152] Most patients are younger than 2 years of age.

Although these enteric adenovirus serotypes have been designated as noncultivable, they will grow in cell line 293, which was originally derived from transformed human embryonic kidney cells,[81,816] and in HEp-2 cells.[660] Molecular methods for detecting the antigens or genome of these viruses have been developed and made commercially available.[162]

CORONAVIRUSES

The coronaviruses are causes of the common cold.[870] Most require use of organ culture for reliable isolation and are unlikely to be encountered in the clinical laboratory.

ORBIVIRUSES

Orbiviruses are primarily animal pathogens. The group includes, however, the virus of Colorado tick fever, an undifferentiated febrile illness that is usually mild and self-limited.

RETROVIRUSES

The retroviruses are RNA viruses; they were so named because they contain an enzyme that transcribes RNA into DNA, a reversal of the normal sequence in which DNA is transcribed into RNA. For many years, these viruses were known to cause tumors in animals. In the 1970s, two viruses that caused T-cell lymphocytic lymphomas in humans were recognized and named human T-cell lymphoma virus (HTLV-I and HTLV-II). This discovery was extremely important biologically, but the tumors are uncommon.

The retrovirus group assumed sudden prominence and increased notoriety in 1983 when a third human retrovirus was identified as the cause of the acquired immunodeficiency syndrome (AIDS).[314] AIDS had been recognized clinically several years earlier when opportunistic infections were detected in young men who were homosexual, bisexual, or drug addicts but did not have conventional risk factors for *Pneumocystis* pneumonia or candidiasis.[323,550]

Similar viruses were isolated in several laboratories and named variously HTLV-III, lymphadenopathy-associated virus (LAV), and AIDS-related virus (ARV). An expert panel settled on the name, human immunodeficiency virus (HIV).[171] Although HIV was first isolated in 1983, retrospective analysis of frozen serum and tissue suggested that a similar virus had infected a sexually active teenage boy in St. Louis in 1968.[294] Subsequently, a serologically related virus was isolated and named HIV-2. The distribution of HIV-1 is worldwide. HIV-2, found predominantly in West Africa, also produces an acquired immunodeficiency syndrome.[167] Cases of HIV-2 infection have been reported in the United States, but most patients have had some connection with West Africa.[106] There are immunologic cross-reactions between HIV-1 and HIV-2.[820] Specific immunoassays must be performed both to distinguish between the two infections and also to detect the type-specific antigens with maximum sensitivity.[315] To complicate matters further, at least one patient has been identified who was infected with both viruses.[695] HIV is a member of the lentivirus (*lenti* = slow) subfamily of the Retroviridae. Other viruses in this group produce chronic infections with long periods of clinical latency. Some of these animal retroviruses also produce immunodeficiency, such as simian immunodeficiency virus and feline leukemia virus. Infection across species has not been demonstrated.

The ability of HIV to vary its antigenic makeup within an individual patient under pressure from the immune system or antiviral chemotherapy has been recognized.[344,727] In addition, more systematic variation is now becoming apparent.[408] Within the group of isolates characterized as HIV-1 there are two groups. The group M strains are composed of 8 subtypes (A–H), of which subtype B accounted for 48% of isolates in one database. Subtype B strains make up the overwhelming majority of the isolates in the United States. The group O strains show greater genetic divergence from the prototype strains. These variant strains were first recognized in West Africa and are still concentrated in that part of the world.[206] Although there was no evidence of the group O strains in 1072 stored serum samples from the United States,[644] a case of imported group O infection has recently been recognized in Los Angeles.[137] The current assays for antibody to HIV-1 are quite variable in their ability to detect antibody to the group O stains.[137,521]

There is no question that HIV is the plague of the latter half of the 20th century. It has changed the face of our society and will continue to wreak havoc for many years to come, especially in the third world.[320] By 1990, AIDS had become the second most common cause of death in men aged 25 to 44. It is expected to be among the top five killers of women in this age group by the early 1990s.[111] As of mid-1996 the United Nations estimated that 21.8 million people worldwide were infected with HIV.[18] Of these a staggering 63% live in subsaharan Africa, 23% live in South and Southeast Asia, and 6% live in Latin America. Western Europe and the United States are home to 2.2% and 3.7% of infected individuals, respectively. By 1995, the World Health Organization estimated that there were 4.5 million cases of AIDS worldwide.[131] As of October 31, 1995, there were 501,310 individuals with AIDS in the United States.[131] HIV-2 remains a rare infection in the United States. As of 1995, only three transfusion-related cases of HIV-2 infection had been reported to the Centers for Disease Control and Prevention (CDC).[130]

The discussion below is a brief attempt to capture some of the most salient features of this multifaceted virus and the diseases it produces. It is a tribute to modern science that an infectious agent was reported only 3 years after the first reports of the clinical syndrome. Without the modern armamentarium of molecular biology and virology, we would still be defenseless against this scourge.

The HIV-1 virion is icosahedral and contains 72 external spikes.[330] It is considerably more complex than HTLV-1 and HTLV-2, consonant with its more complicated natural history. The gene products can be divided into three groups (Box 21-2). The viral proteins

---

BOX 21-2. GENE PRODUCTS OF HIV-1 VIRION

1. The gag proteins (group-specific antigen/core) are a part of the viral nucleocapsid, providing stability for the shell and binding directly to the genomic RNA.

2. The pol proteins (polymerase) are enzymatic proteins that are crucial to the life cycle of the virus. The most famous of the pol proteins is the RNA-dependent DNA polymerase or reverse transcriptase.

3. The env proteins (envelope) are envelope glycoproteins that are critical for interactions with the outside world. These proteins are responsible for adhering to target cells (gp120) and for production of cytopathic cell fusion (gp41). The envelope also includes host cell components that are picked up as the virus buds through the cell membrane.

TABLE 21-6

MAJOR ANTIGENS OF HUMAN IMMUNODEFICIENCY VIRUS,
TYPE I

GENE	GENE PRODUCTS
Group-specific antigen/ core (*GAG*)	p(rotein)18, p24, p55
Polymerase (*POL*)	p31, p51, p66
Envelope (*ENV*)	gp(glycoprotein)41, gp120, gp160

Adapted from Centers for Disease Control: Interpretation and use of the Western blot assay for serodiagnosis of human immunodeficiency virus type 1 infections. MMWR 38 (S7):1–7, 1989.

that represent the most important diagnostic antigens are summarized in Table 21-6.

The gp120 envelope protein holds the initial key for entry of HIV-1 virus into the patient. This protein has a remarkable affinity for a receptor on the surface of cells throughout the body, known as the CD4 receptor. The CD4 receptor, which invites the entry of the HIV-1 virus into its cell, is found on T-helper lymphocytes, macrophages, and Langerhans cells in the skin. It has been hypothesized that uncircumcised men are more likely to develop HIV infection because the prepuce is a rich source of Langerhans cells as well as macrophages and lymphocytes.[2] The enhanced susceptibility to HIV infection in patients with genital ulcers may result from the accessibility of CD4+ macrophages and lymphocytes in the inflamed bases of the ulcers.[794] Macrophages provide the vehicle for transport to distant organs, such as the brain.[464] The most important viral targets, however, are the CD4+ T lymphocytes.[490] These "helper" lymphocytes are the "Times Square" of the cellular immune system. Without them the body is at increased risk for many opportunistic infections. In addition to the T-cell abnormality, defective response of B cells to T cell-independent antigens has also been documented.[491]

The initial encounter with HIV-1 virus produces a transient febrile disease, which may be accompanied by lymphadenopathy, pharyngitis, or a diffuse rash.[447] During the acute illness high levels of circulating virus are present in the absence of specific antibody.[166,189] In the natural course of the infection antibody develops within several weeks to several months. The duration of the antibody-negative, virus-positive window has been estimated to be a median of 2.1 months, with 95% of seroconversions occurring within 5.8 months.[394] The window is important because there are to date few practical means for detecting infectivity until antibody develops.

The ensuing subclinical phase of the disease is accompanied by antibody, circulating p24 antigen,[250] low levels of circulating virus, and infectious immune complexes.[264] Testing of blood products for p24 antigen before transfusion has been recently introduced in an attempt to narrow the window of seronegativity, although weeks to months still remain between infection and appearance of antigenemia. During the chronic

viremia, repetitive mutations in the viral genome thwart the attempts of the host immune system to eliminate the infection.[344,727] The onset of clinical illness is associated with an increase in the quantity of virus, both within peripheral blood mononuclear cells and in plasma.[385]

A wide spectrum of clinical conditions may result after HIV-1 infection. The CDC classification of HIV disease is summarized in Tables 21-7, 21-8, and 21-9.[98] The 1987 surveillance definition of AIDS was amended in 1993 by the addition of pulmonary tuberculosis, recurrent pneumonia, invasive cervical cancer, or severe immunosuppression in an HIV-infected individual (<200 CD4+ T lymphocytes/μL or a CD4+ T-lymphocyte percentage of total lymphocytes <14%).[115] The correlation between absolute counts of CD4+ T lymphocytes and percentage of total lymphocytes is shown in Table 21-10. The change in definition had a significant effect on the number of cases classified as AIDS in national statistics. In 1993, there were 103,500 cases of AIDS in individuals more than 13 years old, an increase of 111% over 1992. In 1993, however, 54% of the cases were a result of the expanded case definition. Following the earlier definition there would have been 48,068 cases in 1993, a 2% decrease from 1992.[118] Separate guidelines have been issued for classification of infections in children less than 13 years of age.[92]

Longitudinal follow-up of HIV-1 infected men with lymphadenopathy has indicated increasing risk of developing AIDS after the third year of lymphadenopathy.[439] By far the most serious stage is the period of severe lymphocytopenia and opportunistic infection (AIDS) resulting from HIV destruction of helper T lymphocytes, followed by a profound immunosuppression. The patient is then rendered defenseless against many infectious agents, especially those normally contained by the cellular immune system.

The infectious complications of HIV infection include viral, fungal, mycobacterial, bacterial, and parasitic infections. The practice of infectious disease and clinical microbiology has been irrevocably altered by HIV. Numerous previously uncommon or exotic infections have become commonplace in centers that have large numbers of HIV-infected patients. Old rules must be thrown out when the patient is so severely immunosuppressed as are patients with AIDS or patients with major organ transplants. Anything is possible, and the host inflammatory response that has been associated with a particular infectious agent may or may not be present. What would be "shotgun" microbiology in a normal patient becomes good practice in this group of patients. Integration of clinical, epidemiologic, and laboratory data is needed to decide which laboratory resources must be tapped for an individual patient.

Strand has discussed the role of the microbiology laboratory in support of patients with HIV disease.[804] The most common opportunistic infections that afflict patients with AIDS are listed in Tables 21-8 and 21-9. Some of the infections are characteristic of a particular phase of the disease. For instance, oral candidiasis is often a presenting feature of the disease.[458] *Pneumocys-*

TABLE 21-7
Demographic Characteristics of Patients with AIDS in the United States by Date of Report, 1981–1995

Characteristic	No. Cases 1981–1987 (%)	No. Cases 1988–1992 (%)	No. Cases 1993–1995 (%)
Sex			
Male	46,317 (92)	177,807 (87.5)	204,356 (82.5)
Female	4,035 (8)	25,410 (12.5)	43,383 (17.5)
Race/Ethnicity			
White non-Hispanic	30,104 (59.8)	102,551 (50.5)	105,516 (42.6)
Black non-Hispanic	12,794 (25.4)	63,319 (31.2)	94,158 (38)
Hispanic, any race	7,039 (14)	35,213 (17.3)	45,135 (18.2)
Asian/Pacific Islander	309 (0.6)	1339 (0.7)	1,809 (0.7)
American Indian/Alaskan Native	67 (0.1)	433 (0.2)	783 (0.3)
Exposure Category			
Men who have sex with men	32,246 (64)	110,934 (54.6)	111,257 (44.9)
Injecting-drug users	8,639 (17.2)	49,093 (24.2)	67,708 (27.3)
Men who have sex with men and inject drugs	4,193 (8.3)	14,252 (7)	13,984 (5.6)
Hemophilia	505 (1)	1744 (0.9)	2009 (0.8)
Heterosexual contact	1,248 (2.5)	12,335 (6.1)	24,958 (10.1)
Transfusion recipients	1,285 (2.6)	3,894 (1.9)	2,521 (1)
Perinatal transmission	608 (1.2)	3,084 (1.5)	2,432 (1)
No risk reported	1,628 (3.2)	7,881 (3.9)	7,566 (3.1)
Region			
Northeast	19,544 (38.8)	62,282 (30.6)	74,769 (30.2)
Midwest	3,770 (7.5)	20,352 (10)	24,914 (10.1)
South	12,960 (25.7)	65,926 (32.4)	86,462 (34.9)
West	13,550 (26.9)	46,675 (23)	53,729 (21.7)
U.S. Territories	516 (1)	7,889 (3.9)	7,566 (3.1)
TOTAL	**50,352**	**203,217**	**247,741**

Adapted from Centers for Disease Control and Prevention: First 500,000 AIDS cases—United States, 1995. MMWR 44:849–853, 1995.

TABLE 21-8
1993 Revised Classification System Among Adolescents and Adults Positive for HIV

	Clinical Categories		
CD4+ T-Lymphocyte Categories	*(A)* ASYMPTOMATIC, ACUTE (PRIMARY) HIV, OR PERSISTENT GENERALIZED LYMPHADENOPATHY	*(B)* SYMPTOMATIC, NOT (A) OR (C) CONDITIONS (SEE TABLE 21-9)	*(C)* AIDS-INDICATOR CONDITIONS (SEE TABLE 21-9)
(1) ≥500/μL	A1	B1	C1*
(2) 200–499/μL	A2	B2	C2*
(3) <200/μL	A3*	B3*	C3*

* Categories added to previous definition in 1993 classification.
The lowest accurate, but not necessarily the most recent CD4+ T-lymphocyte count should be used for classification.
Castro KG, Ward JW, Slutsker L et al: 1993 revised classification system for HIV infection and expanded surveillance case definition for AIDS among adolescents and adults. MMWR 41:No. RR-17, 1992.

TABLE 21-9

ANCILLARY CONDITIONS (CATEGORY B) AND CONDITIONS INCLUDED IN THE 1993 AIDS
SURVEILLANCE CASE DEFINITION (CATEGORY C)

Category B
Bacillary angiomatosis
Candidiasis, oropharyngeal (thrush)
Candidiasis, vulvovaginal; persistent, frequent, or poorly responsive to therapy
Cervical dysplasia (moderate or severe)/carcinoma in situ
Constitutional symptoms, such as fever (38.5°C) or diarrhea lasting >1 month
Hairy leukoplakia, oral
Herpes zoster (shingles), involving at least two distinct episodes or more than one dermatome
Idiopathic thrombocytopenic purpura
Listeriosis
Pelvic inflammatory disease, particularly if complicated by tubo-ovarian abscess
Peripheral neuropathy
Other unspecified conditions

Category C
Candidiasis of bronchi, trachea, or lungs
Candidiasis, esophageal
Cervical cancer, invasive*
Coccidioidomycosis, disseminated or extrapulmonary
Cryptococcosis, extrapulmonary
Cryptosporidiosis, chronic intestinal (>1 month's duration)
Cytomegalovirus disease (except liver, spleen, lymph nodes)
Cytomegalovirus retinitis with loss of vision
Encephalopathy, HIV related
Herpes simplex: chronic ulcers (>1 month's duration); or bronchitis, pneumonitis, or esophagitis
Histoplasmosis, disseminated or extrapulmonary
Isosporiasis, chronic intestinal (>1 month's duration)
Kaposi's sarcoma
Lymphoma, Burkitt's (or equivalent term)
Lymphoma, immunoblastic (or equivalent term)
Lymphoma, primary, of brain
Mycobacterium avium complex or *Mycobacterium kansasii*, disseminated or extrapulmonary
Mycobacterium tuberculosis, any site (pulmonary* or extrapulmonary)
Mycobacterium, other species or unidentified species, disseminated or extrapulmonary
Pneumocystis carinii pneumonia
Pneumonia, recurrent*
Progressive multifocal leukoencephalopathy
Salmonella septicemia, recurrent
Toxoplasmosis of brain
Wasting syndrome due to HIV

* Added to previous definition in the 1993 classification.
Castro KG, Ward JW, Slutsker L et al: 1993 revised classification system for HIV infection and expanded surveillance case definition for AIDS among adolescents and adults. MMWR 41:No. RR-17, 1992.

tis carinii pneumonia first occurs when lymphocyte counts are relatively high early in the disease process. *Mycobacterium avium* complex infections tend to occur late in the disease, when the CD4+ lymphocyte count is low.[393] Although infections with cell-associated pathogens (facultative intracellular organisms) are most closely associated with defects in cellular immunity, bacterial infections for which humoral immunity is an important host defense are also more common in HIV-infected patients.[612] The risk of bacterial pneumonia is increased in patients infected with HIV. It is greatest in abusers of intravenous drugs and in patients whose CD4+ T-lymphocyte count is <200/mm³.[384] The search for the etiology of an oppor-

TABLE 21-10

EQUIVALENCES BETWEEN ABSOLUTE NUMBERS OF CD4+
T LYMPHOCYTES AND PERCENTAGE OF TOTAL LYMPHOCYTES

CD4+ T LYMPHOCYTE CATEGORY	CD4+ T LYMPHOCYTES/μL	CD4+ PERCENTAGE OF TOTAL LYMPHOCYTES
(1)	≥500	≥29
(2)	200–499	14–28
(3)	<200	<14

Castro KG, Ward JW, Slutsker L et al: 1993 revised classification system for HIV infection and expanded surveillance case definition for AIDS among adolescents and adults. MMWR 41:No. RR-17, 1992.

tunistic infection should not stop when the first agent is identified because many of the infections in AIDS patients are polymicrobial.[682] As therapy for HIV infection and for infectious complications of the immunodeficiency has improved, the pattern of infections encountered has changed. An analysis of autopsies from Los Angeles in 1982–1993 documented a decrease in the number of fatal infections caused by *Pneumocystis carinii*, bacterial sepsis, CMV, *Mycobacterium avium* complex, and *Toxoplasma gondii* in 1989–1993 compared to 1982–1988.[457]

Not all disease is caused by opportunistic infection. The HIV virus itself is cytopathic and produces clinical disease such as encephalitis[89] and AIDS-related dementia.[518] Collapse of the cellular immune system and its surveillance mechanisms leads to neoplastic complications, some of which may be virus induced.[356] A previously unusual neoplasm, Kaposi's sarcoma, has occurred frequently in patients with AIDS, often as an early manifestation of the disease (see page 1215). Other manifestations of disease may have an immunopathologic mechanism or the mechanisms are unknown.[57] Some infections that might have been predicted to afflict AIDS patients, such as legionellosis and aspergillosis, are relatively uncommon. The cellular immune system undoubtedly contributes to the control of invasive aspergillosis and legionellosis, but other mechanisms, not destroyed by HIV-1, are presumably also important.

HIV-1 is excreted in the saliva,[333] milk,[633] semen,[908] and other body fluids,[284] but transmission of infection has been documented to occur only after exposure to blood or genital secretions. The importance of maternal milk in the transfer of virus from mother to child is unclear.

The most important groups at risk of HIV infection are those who have received blood products (recipients of blood transfusions, hemophiliacs), those who have shared contaminated needles (drug addicts), those who have had sexual intercourse with an infected individual, and children of an infected mother.[284] At the outset of the epidemic most of the sexually transmitted infections in the United States and Europe were between homosexual men, but heterosexual transmission was soon documented.[362] Heterosexual transmission of HIV-1 virus has been dominant in Africa from the beginning of the epidemic.[320] The risk of transmission of HIV infection from mother to infant and the severity of disease in the infant are directly related to the severity of infection in the mother at the time of delivery.[67] A correlate of this observation is the direct relationship of the level of p24 antigen in the bloodstream of infants with the severity of clinical disease, regardless of the age at which the HIV infection is recognized.[639] Rupture of membranes more than 4 hours before delivery also increases the risk of transfer of HIV-1 from mother to infant.[486]

The effects of changes in sexual practice of white male homosexuals, increasing transmission of HIV among abusers of intravenous drugs and crack cocaine, and increasing heterosexual transmission are listed in Table 21-7. An increasing proportion of infections occurred in women, in abusers of intravenous

drugs, and in nonwhite non-Hispanic individuals between 1981 and 1995. Longitudinal studies have demonstrated that consistent use of condoms is a highly effective means of preventing heterosexual transmission of HIV.[199] Between 1989 and 1994 the incidence of AIDS among white, non-Hispanic men who have sex with men was relatively stable, whereas the rates among Hispanic and especially black non-Hispanic men who have sex with men rose dramatically.[125]

The risk of transmitting HIV in blood transfusions has been dramatically reduced by screening all units of blood for antibody and asking members of high-risk groups not to donate blood. The result has been a steadily decreasing incidence of transfusion-related HIV infection as the sensitivity of the tests used for screening blood products before transfusion has increased. A review of more than 4.1 million blood donations in the United States has produced the following statistics:[480]

- One donation in every 360,000 was made during the seronegative window.
- One donation in every 2,600,000 was from an HIV-positive donor but missed because of a falsely negative laboratory test.
- 15% to 42% of donations during the seronegative window were discarded because of seropositivity for agents other than HIV.
- One case of HIV transmission occurred for every 450,000 to 660,000 donations.
- 18 to 27 infectious donations are available for transfusion every year.

Therapy of HIV infection has represented a constant battle between the virus and the pharmaceutical industry, resulting in alternating exhilaration and despair among patients and health care workers. The first line of treatment is the use of inhibitors of viral reverse transcriptase, most prominently zidovudine (AZT). These drugs interfere with viral replication, but the virus has shown a disturbing propensity for mutation to altered forms of reverse transcriptase that do not interact with the drugs.[383] Combination chemotherapy with other nucleoside analogs, such as didanosine, zalcitabine, or lamivudine (3TC) has improved antiviral effect without increasing toxicity significantly. The latest addition to the therapeutic armamentarium is an expanding group of drugs that inhibit viral protease, such as ritonavir.[191,538] The protease inhibitors have a potent antiviral effect in their own right. The combination of zidovudine, zalcitabine, and saquinavir (another protease inhibitor) had a greater antiviral effect than zidovudine and either of the other two drugs alone.[174]

The therapeutic end point of greatest clinical interest is the prevention or reversal of HIV-related disease. Unfortunately, the time required to assess therapeutic interventions with this endpoint is too great for practical advances in therapy. Investigators have used a series of surrogate measures of antiviral effect: measurement of quantitative CD4+ T-lymphocyte counts, quantitative viral culture, quantitative determination of p24 antigen in peripheral blood, and quantitative measurement of cell-associated viral RNA using molecular amplification techniques. The quantitative assessment of viremia, especially by molecular amplification methods, is sometimes referred to as **viral load testing**. The efficacy of certain surrogate markers for predicting the subsequent course of HIV infection has been assessed by the Veterans Affairs Study Group on AIDS.[624] They found that progression of HIV infection to AIDS was strongly correlated with baseline CD4+ T-lymphocyte counts and plasma levels of HIV-1 RNA, but not with baseline levels of β_2-microglobulin. A decrease of at least 75% in the level of plasma HIV-1 RNA in the 6 months after therapy with zidovudine accounted for 59% of the treatment effect (defined as absence of progression to AIDS). If an increase of 10% in CD4+ T-lymphocytes was added to the decrease in viral load, 79% of the treatment effect could be accounted for. Mellors and colleagues found that the frequency with which HIV-1 RNA could be detected in plasma samples was an independent predictor of progression to AIDS and the future status of CD4+ T-lymphocyte cell counts.[561] The level of p24 antigen has received less attention than detection of viral RNA in recent clinical investigations because the amplification techniques for quantitation of viral RNA are more sensitive indicators.[700]

The particularly thorny question of determining whether infants born to HIV-infected mothers are themselves infected has also been addressed by use of molecular amplification techniques. Paul and colleagues found that the most useful algorithm for congenital infection was a baseline polymerase chain reaction (PCR) test followed by PCR on a second sample.[645] Two consecutive positive results confirmed infection in the infant. Two negative results reconfirmed at 6 months of age established that the infant was not infected.

The measurement of CD4+ T lymphocytes has become a routine procedure for many clinical immunology laboratories. Guidelines for the performance of CD4+ T-lymphocyte determinations in HIV-infected individuals have been issued by CDC.[613] Viral culture is time consuming and difficult. Quantitation of viral RNA has been a research procedure but is rapidly becoming a standard of clinical care. The recent availability of a quantitative commercial PCR test for HIV-1 RNA (Amplicor-HIV, Roche Diagnostics) will undoubtedly accelerate the trend toward use of this surrogate marker. The laboratory diagnosis by determination of antibody to HIV is discussed on page 1258, and the direct detection of viral RNA by molecular methods is briefly reviewed on page 1254.

Special concern has been expressed about transfer of HIV to and from health care workers. This virus is transmitted by the same mechanisms as hepatitis B virus. Fortunately, HIV is much less contagious than hepatitis B virus and continuing surveillance has discovered very few cases of nosocomial transmission.[536] High rates of infection in African hospitals appear to reflect community infection rather than nosocomial transmission.[600] Only one instance of transmission from a health care worker to a patient is on record. The mechanisms of a highly publicized transmission from an HIV-1 infected dentist to multiple patients have not been elucidated,[110] but enormous public concern has

resulted. A case-control study of HIV infection in health care workers after exposure to infectious material documented an association with the following factors:[132]

Deep injury
Device visibly contaminated with the source patient's blood
Procedures involving placement of a needle directly in the source patient's vein or artery
Terminal illness in the source patient
Failure of health care worker to receive zidovudine

Provisional recommendations for chemoprophylaxis of health care workers who have been exposed to HIV-contaminated fluids are related to the extent of the risk.[136] Prophylaxis with multiple antiviral agents should be recommended for those at highest risk of infection. For those with lesser risk antiviral therapy should be offered to workers. If the exposure involves minimal risk, such as exposure to urine, chemotherapy is not recommended.

The most recalcitrant problem in AIDS control is the population of drug addicts who share needles. Infected addicts may pass their infections on both with additional contaminated needles and by sexual contact.

HERPESVIRUSES

Viruses of the human herpesvirus group are the most frequent isolates in general laboratories. The group consists of the following:

Herpes simplex virus, type 1
Herpes simplex virus, type 2
Human cytomegalovirus
Epstein-Barr virus
Varicella-zoster virus
Human herpesvirus-6
Human herpesvirus-7
Human herpesvirus-8

Most members of the herpesvirus group can integrate their DNA with that of the host cell, produce a latent infection in lymphoid cells or ganglia of the CNS, and subsequently reactivate to cause recurrent disease. In general, the primary infections are more severe than are recurrences. The primary infections produced by several viruses of this group are more severe when they occur in adolescence or adulthood, rather than childhood. The viruses circulate more freely and earlier in life among low socioeconomic groups and not until adolescence in more affluent society. The infections in high socioeconomic groups therefore tend to be more severe.

HERPES SIMPLEX VIRUS

Herpes simplex virus causes a wide variety of infections.[178,806] Two serotypes of the virus infect humans. Shared antigens between types 1 and 2 make serologic differentiation difficult,[226,338] but reliable monoclonal antibodies for typing isolated viruses have been developed.[656] In healthy persons, infections of the oral cavity and genital tract predominate. Type 1 infections are most common in the upper body, whereas type 2 infections produce genital lesions; but there are exceptions to the rule. As many as one-third of isolates from the genital tract represent type 1 strains. In contrast, very few isolates from the oral cavity are type 2 strains. Typing of herpes isolates from genital sites provides valuable prognostic information because genital infections caused by type 1 herpes simplex virus are less likely to recur than are those caused by type 2 virus.[481,698] In a group of 457 women who had a primary genital infection (defined by absence of antibody to type 2 virus and a positive culture of genital lesions), 89% had a recurrence after a median time of 391 days.[55] There were at least six recurrences during the first year in 38% of patients, and 20% of individuals had more than 10 recurrences. A sequential study of patients with recurrent infection demonstrated that the patient was asymptomatic and lacked visible lesions during one-third of the period that the patient shed virus.[843] Genital infections with either viral type are more likely to recur than oral infections with the same type.[481] In addition, the mechanism of infection may be different for the two serotypes. Exposure to type 1 virus begins in childhood, with 25% to 50% of college students having developed antibody. Acquisition of antibody to type 2 virus does not begin until the teens and continues throughout the period of sexual activity.[338] Immunoblots have been developed for reliable characterization of type-specific antibody, but they are not marketed currently. The commercially available enzyme immunoassays do not distinguish between antibodies to the two serotypes reliably.[32] Isolation of type 2 virus from a genital site implies sexual transmission, whereas the route of transmission for type 1 virus may be by autoinoculation with oral secretions.

Herpesvirus is passed from person to person by infected secretions or lesions. Infection is usually sporadic, but an epidemic of cutaneous infection at a wrestling camp (herpes gladiatorum) has been described.[54]

The most serious herpes simplex virus infections are encephalitis, which most commonly affects the temporal lobe and the orbital aspect of the frontal lobe in adults, and disseminated infection in newborn infants, which may be acquired either during or after birth. Herpes simplex virus causes sporadic encephalitis. In the neonatal period the infecting strains are type 2, reflecting their origin in the maternal genital tract. Type 1 strains are overwhelmingly predominant in older children and adults. The diagnosis can be made most definitively by brain biopsy and culture,[879] but the availability of nontoxic antiviral chemotherapy[877] has prompted clinicians to treat patients empirically, thus avoiding an invasive procedure. Unfortunately, other potentially treatable diseases may be missed as a result. Whitley and colleagues studied 432 patients who underwent brain biopsy for suspected herpes encephalitis as a part of a national collaborative chemotherapy trial.[878] Herpes simplex encephalitis was identified in 45% of the patients. Another 18% had other identifiable infectious diseases, half of which were

treatable. Thus, 10% of the total population had a treatable infection that would have been missed without the brain biopsy. Until recently the only noninvasive diagnostic test was the electroencephalogram, in which abnormal temporal lobe discharges are characteristic if present. The advent of sophisticated imaging techniques has revolutionized the clinical approach.[827] Magnetic resonance imaging (MRI) is more sensitive than computed tomography. Herpesvirus encephalitis occurs very rarely, if ever, in the presence of a normal MRI study. Lesions are not limited, however, to unilateral temporal lobe lesions. The abnormalities by MRI may be multifocal or diffuse.[744] At the beginning of the illness the only abnormalities may be in the electroencephalogram.[719]

Herpes simplex virus is infrequently isolated from CSF. In the national collaborative study, an isolate was recovered from CSF in only 2 of 45 (4%) of biopsy-proven cases of herpes encephalitis.[602] Serologic diagnosis is too insensitive, nonspecific, and slow to be of use in therapeutic decisions.[602] Use of molecular techniques to detect antibodies in CSF has not been successful in correcting specificity problems and does not speed the process.[432] A major diagnostic advance has been the use of molecular amplification techniques for detection of herpesvirus genome in the CSF of patients with encephalitis or meningoencephalitis (see page 1254).

Herpesvirus remains latent in spinal ganglia after the initial infection. Type 1 virus is recovered from thoracic ganglia and type 2 virus is recovered from sacral ganglia.[41] Herpetic aseptic meningitis does occur uncommonly, usually caused by type 2 virus.[822] Viral meningitis is characteristically associated with a normal level of glucose in the CSF in contrast to the markedly diminished levels of glucose in bacterial meningitis. The cerebrospinal glucose level in herpes meningitis, however, may be very low, and the cell count may be in the thousands.[582] Early in the course of any viral meningitis, neutrophils may predominate and suggest the possibility of a bacterial process. Herpes simplex virus, usually type 2, also causes recurrent lymphocytic meningitis (Mollaret's meningitis); the culture is almost uniformly negative, but viral genome can be demonstrated in the CSF by PCR.[819]

Neonatal herpes infection is estimated to occur in 1:2000 to 1:5000 deliveries.[876] It is almost always symptomatic and frequently fatal.[809] In a collaborative study the mortality rate was 50% to 60% in infants with disseminated infection who were treated with acyclovir or vidarabine.[875] In contrast, no fatalities occurred among infants with disease limited to the nose, eyes, or mouth. The diagnosis is suggested by the development of vesicular skin lesions, but these may be absent in 20% of patients.[809] Poor prognostic factors include disseminated disease, comatose state at admission to the hospital, disseminated intravascular coagulation, or prematurity.[875]

The high morbidity and mortality of infant disease has prompted great efforts to diagnose maternal infection. Most cases of neonatal herpes simplex virus infection are contracted during vaginal delivery and can be prevented by cesarean section. Complex protocols for screening pregnant women have been developed but unfortunately have not worked well. Asymptomatic maternal infection at the time of delivery occurs regularly,[677] although the risk of infants appears to be low if the infection is recrudescent and maternal antibody to type 2 virus is present.[82] Many women do not recognize their primary genital infection. In one study specific antibody to type 2 herpes simplex virus was detected in 439 of 1355 pregnant women without a clinical history of genital herpes (32%).[280] Asymptomatic shedding of virus in late pregnancy and at delivery was detected in 5 of 1160 cultures (0.43%). During the pregnancy 43 of the women who had antibody to type 2 virus recognized their first symptomatic genital infection.

Cultures of the mother taken in the days or weeks before delivery do not predict well the results at the time of delivery.[27] The American College of Obstetrics and Gynecology recommends that if the patient is symptomatic, the lesions should be cultured for herpesvirus and the infant delivered by cesarean section. If the patient is asymptomatic and lesions are not visible, vaginal delivery is permissible.[11] The authors of a position paper from the Infectious Diseases Society of America recognize the difficulty of constructing detailed guidelines.[676] Their general recommendations are based on virologic, serologic, and clinical features. Viral culture is suggested for documentation of the etiology of symptomatic lesions. In the asymptomatic woman who is known to be infected with herpesvirus, they recommend viral culture only at the time of delivery. Swabs from maternal cervix, vulva (at the sites of usual recurrence), vaginal secretions, and from the infant's oropharynx can be combined. They emphasize that their recommendations do not constitute a standard of care.

Persons with compromised defense mechanisms are predisposed to herpes simplex esophagitis,[3] tracheobronchitis,[762] or pneumonia[324,689] and disseminated infection, including hepatitis.[687] Herpes simplex infections may be necrotizing and may suggest a bacterial etiology if the characteristic inclusions (see page 1251) are not recognized or viral cultures are not done.[606,857,886] Immunosuppression is not a prerequisite for lower respiratory tract infection or esophagitis.[210] The risk factors for lower respiratory tract infection include intubation, suggesting that the pathogenesis may be similar to that of bacterial pneumonia—aspiration of contaminated oropharyngeal secretions.[324,689] Patients with extensive burns are at risk for infection both of the denuded skin and of the lower respiratory tract.[268] Disseminated herpes simplex virus infection can rarely produce severe, even lethal disease in the mother as well as the infant.[906] There are three patterns of infection, which usually occurs in the second or third trimester: 1) encephalitis without hepatic involvement 2) hepatitis with or without abnormalities of the CNS, and 3) disseminated skin lesions.

Infection of the eye includes conjunctivitis, which may be accompanied by fever, photophobia, and re-

gional lymphadenopathy. Herpetic keratitis, which has a branching or dendritic appearance, is the second most common cause of corneal blindness (after trauma) in the United States.[876]

Herpes simplex virus is one of the viral causes of pharyngitis and tonsillitis, usually as a primary infection. The mucosa may be ulcerated, and lesions may be limited to the posterior pharynx.[312] Necrotizing tonsillitis may mimic bacterial peritonsillar abscess.[857] Hemorrhagic cystitis has been reported as a part of disseminated infection[204] and herpetic proctitis may occur in homosexual men.[319]

The diagnosis of herpes simplex infection is usually made by isolation of virus from an infected lesion. Herpes simplex viremia is uncommonly detected, but has been reported recently in pediatric patients with neonatal infection or immunosuppression, some of whom did not have cutaneous lesions.[797] Direct detection of virus in the lesions by histologic or cytologic examination (presumptive) or by immunologic techniques (definitive) can be accomplished in some lesions and sites. Serologic diagnosis is at present only useful for establishing immune status in donors or recipients of transplants.

Isolates of herpes simplex virus resistant to acyclovir, which were initially a laboratory phenomenon, have now become a clinical reality, especially in immunosuppressed patients, some of whom do not respond to chemotherapy.[186,619] Resistant isolates have been recovered, although less frequently in immunocompetent patients with recurrent genital herpes.[470]

CYTOMEGALOVIRUS

Cytomegalovirus (CMV) is one of a family of related viruses that are specific for a particular species.[76] Mouse CMV does not infect humans and vice versa. CMV was first isolated from mice by Margaret Smith, who subsequently isolated the human virus from the salivary gland tissues of an infected infant. She recognized the species specificity of the virus, although the reviewers of her initially rejected paper did not![866] Isolation of the human virus was reported concurrently by Smith, Weller, and Rowe. With the generosity of a gentleman, who also happens to be a Nobel Prize winner, Dr. Weller gives Dr. Smith the credit for the primacy of her discovery. CMV is an opportunistic pathogen that may produce persistent, even lifelong infections.[59] It was recognized many decades ago as a human pathogen by the peculiar cytopathology it produces (see Color Plate 21-1D). Initially, investigators considered CMV as a protozoan invader of human tissue.[420]

This virus is associated with leukocytes and may be transmitted with a blood transfusion[273,507] or transplanted organ.[386] When detected by monoclonal antibodies or genetic probes, CMV is concentrated in the neutrophil fraction of the buffy coat,[736] rather than in the mononuclear fraction. Replicating virus is found in both fractions, so that material for culture should include all leukocytes. Virus is also excreted in saliva and in semen.[492] Venereal transmission has been strongly suggested by epidemiologically related clusters of cases.[161,492] CMV may be passed from mother to offspring through the placenta,[792] in cervical secretions during delivery,[702] or in breast milk.[366]

The variety of infectious diseases produced by this pathogen is great and includes congenital infection, neonatal infection, heterophil-negative infectious mononucleosis, hepatitis, pneumonia in immunosuppressed patients, and disseminated infection in immunosuppressed patients. At the same time it may be extremely difficult to decide whether an individual patient has CMV-induced disease or is only persistently infected, because replicating virus is found in normally sterile organs and body fluids in the absence of clinical disease.[726] Multiple genetic variants of CMV have been found in a single infected patient.[159] It is relatively easy to document infection by culturing the virus or demonstrating the presence of specific antibody. Detection of CMV antigenemia is more sensitive than viral culture, is commercially available, and has replaced culture in many laboratories (see page 1253).[283,551,659,840] Positive staining of leukocytes with a commercial kit for detection of antigenemia has been reported in patients in whom CMV infection could not be substantiated,[658] but the assay is generally considered acceptably specific. Detection of CMV DNA by PCR is even more sensitive but is not yet commercially available.[70,915] Diagnosis of congenital infection by PCR of peripheral blood from symptomatic infants has been reported to be 100% sensitive, but identical sensitivity was achieved with the readily available culture of urine for CMV.[607]

In contrast to documentation of CMV *infection*, proof that a particular *disease process* is caused by CMV often requires biopsy and histologic examination. Even then the assessment is not always easy. For instance, some patients excrete CMV in their urine for years without ill effect, especially those who were congenitally infected.[703] Recovery of CMV from bronchoalveolar lavage correlates poorly with CMV pneumonia,[726] which ultimately must be diagnosed by putting all facts together, often including the results of lung biopsy. Detection of serum antibody is the most sensitive method for determining if the patient has ever been infected by CMV. The presence of serum antibody is of little use, however, in determining if the patient is currently infected or if CMV disease is present, although there is a presumption that virus may persist in some host cells or tissue.[500,543,648] Viruria is the most sensitive method for detection of active infection, but it is a poor indicator of active CMV clinical disease. Likewise recent studies indicate that viremia is not a good predictor of clinically significant CMV disease in patients with HIV infection[500] or in recipients of liver transplants, with the possible exception of seronegative patients who have received a transplant from a seropositive donor (a situation that is avoided if possible).[35] The antigenemia assay provides the greatest promise of useful information for managing immunosuppressed patients who are infected with CMV. The mean number of CMV-positive cells in HIV-infected agents without clinically evident disease was 2.1,

whereas the mean number of infected cells in patients with clinically evident disease was 76.[551] In a study of patients who were infected with HIV or had received organ transplants, there were 23 patients who had not received ganciclovir for more than 24 hours and developed clinically apparent CMV disease within 2 weeks.[487] Of these 23 patients, 4 individuals had low-level antigenemia (maximum number of CMV-positive cells = 0–2), 3 patients had intermediate-level antigenemia (maximum number of cells = 22–44), and 16 patients had high-level antigenemia (maximum number of cells = >50). Careful prospective studies of quantitative antigenemia will be required to establish the true value of this technique for managing patients. Surprisingly, quantitative antigenemia assays may be more useful than culture in assessing the clinical efficacy (as opposed to the virologic efficacy) of ganciclovir. In a study of 10 renal transplant patients who were treated with ganciclovir for CMV disease, CMV blood cultures rapidly became negative regardless of the clinical response.[839] In eight of nine cases with clinical improvement the level of antigenemia decreased within a week, whereas the number of positive cells actually increased initially in three patients who did not respond to therapy. The best cutoff point for determining CMV disease has yet to be determined. One group of investigators, who used commercial monoclonal antibodies (Biotest Diagnostics Corp., Denville, NJ), found that a cutoff of five antigen positive cells per slide was necessary to achieve a specificity of 81% to 87%.[51] In the process the sensitivity was reduced from 91% to 67%. Patients with CMV retinitis, in particular, often had very few antigen-positive cells in their peripheral blood. For such studies to be useful clinically, it will be essential that they be performed with readily available commercial reagents. It is not safe to assume that reports of investigations with research reagents will be uniformly applicable.

Recently, circulating endothelial cells identified as infected with CMV by immunofluorescence have been described in a research setting.[655] The number of circulating endothelial cells correlated with the level of antigenemia and with the clinical status.

Paradoxically, quantitative molecular amplification may actually be less useful for assessing disease status because of its greater sensitivity. CMV DNA can be detected in serum far longer than either antigen or viable virus after resolution of a clinical episode or initiation of therapy, sometimes in the absence of CMV RNA, suggesting that the DNA represents latent, nonreplicating virus.[693] In heart transplants, detection of CMV only by PCR was never associated with overt clinical symptoms.[301]

A latent virus or one that is clinically silent may reactivate to produce disease. An individual patient may experience CMV disease after reactivation of a latent infection or after a primary exposure to the virus. The distinction is prognostically important because primary infections are clinically more severe[60] and more likely to cause symptomatic disease in a neonate.[793]

Some situations can be manipulated to increase the odds against primary infections. For example, transplant recipients can be screened so that seronegative patients do not receive blood or an organ from a seropositive donor.[71] In some studies administration of CMV immune globulin to seronegative recipients of potentially infected kidneys had a protective effect.[784]

Virus infection of previously healthy persons usually manifests as a self-limited mononucleosis syndrome.[172,398] As in Epstein-Barr virus infection there is evidence for CMV mononucleosis that the symptoms are produced by cytotoxic lymphocytes, which attempt to eliminate the CMV-infected cells.[683]

The spectrum of disease is considerably broader in patients who are immunosuppressed, depending on the extent of immunocompromise. In patients who are moderately immunocompromised, such as renal transplant patients, CMV pneumonia is a common manifestation.[181] When immunosuppression is more extreme, extensive, overwhelming infection may result. Recipients of heart, liver, or bone marrow transplants or HIV-infected patients may experience hepatitis,[79] destructive retinitis,[285] or previously unheard of complications such as perforation through an infected intestinal wall.[278]

An additional complication in organ recipients is the association of CMV infection with rejection of the renal[520] or cardiac[326] transplant. The pathogenesis of the process is unclear. Although a glomerulopathy has been described in transplanted kidneys of CMV-infected patients,[706] the pathology of the rejected kidneys usually suggests an immunologic rather than an infectious process. To complicate matters even further evidence suggests that patients who receive a transplanted heart and are infected with CMV develop more superinfections with bacteria and fungi than do transplant recipients who are free of CMV.[690]

Most congenitally and neonatally acquired infection is asymptomatic, but some infants who appear normal at birth may develop subtle symptoms.[703] At the other extreme is disseminated infection with multiorgan disease and severe congenital abnormalities, such as microcephaly. The frequency of intrauterine transmission of CMV has been estimated at 30% to 40%, and the risk of an adverse outcome is increased during the first half of the gestation.[792]

Treatment of CMV infections is unsatisfactory because the available drugs are toxic and do not eradicate the virus. When therapy is stopped, relapse is common. The urgency of overwhelming disease and impending blindness requires the use of available therapy regardless of limitations.[493] New drugs are being developed and tested because of the pressing need for effective therapy.[529]

Drew has reviewed the laboratory diagnosis of CMV infections,[224] and Klevjer-Anderson has discussed the diagnostic significance of CMV serology.[460]

EPSTEIN-BARR VIRUS

Epstein-Barr virus (EBV) is the primary cause of infectious mononucleosis. This versatile virus produces disease that ranges from acute self-limited infection to malignant neoplasms. The mononucleosis syndrome consists of fever, malaise, exudative pharyngitis, lymphadenopathy, and atypical lymphocytes circulating in the peripheral blood. Splenomegaly is common, and rupture of the spleen is a serious complication.[642] Acute hepatitis may also be a part of the syndrome.[179,874]

The virus was originally recognized during studies of Burkitt's lymphoma in Africa[711] and only later associated with mononucleosis.[614] The virus gains entry to the body by infecting the pharyngeal epithelium.[770] Its primary target, however, is the circulating B lymphocyte, which it infects and then immortalizes.[713] The result of this interaction is a polyclonal stimulation of the humoral immune system, which produces an array of antibodies to many antigens. At the same time, the cellular immune system is triggered to fight the EBV infection. It is the activated T lymphocytes that are seen in the peripheral blood smear as atypical lymphocytes.[643,723] The circle is completed when virus is excreted through the oral mucosa into the saliva.[299,615] Young children usually have an asymptomatic or minimally symptomatic infection, and the diagnostic heterophil antibody test is often negative.[396]

If integration of the EBV genome into certain types of cells occurs, a neoplasm may result instead of an acute infection. The unregulated growth of EBV in patients with HIV infection, who have lost the regulatory control of cellular immunity, may lead to increased EBV-related tumors.[64] Most of these tumors are of B-lymphocyte lineage, such as Burkitt's lymphoma and primary lymphoma of the brain,[387] but nasopharyngeal carcinoma has also been associated strongly with EBV.[711] A subset of gastric[10] and colonic[907] carcinomas has also been ascribed to infection with EBV. A variety of other processes include lymphocytic interstitial pneumonia[40] and hemophagocytic syndrome.[288] Establishing association of a latent or persistent virus such as EBV is not enough do prove a causal relationship, which can only come from repetitive association and careful molecular analysis.

In the mid 1980s it was suggested that a poorly defined syndrome of chronic fatigue might represent chronic EBV infection.[103] Chronic EBV infection does exist and may be troublesome,[751,828] but the nonspecific syndrome of chronic fatigue does not appear to be EBV related.[194]

The laboratory diagnosis of acute EBV infection is serologic (see page 1256). The mainstay of diagnosis, the heterophil antibody test, was described decades before the viral etiology was elucidated.[195] The major viral antigens that are useful diagnostically are listed in Table 21-11.

The cells that best support viral replication with shedding of infectious particles are epithelial cells of the oropharynx. Saliva from acutely ill or chronically infected patients contains viable virus, which can be demonstrated by co-cultivation with normal peripheral blood lymphocytes.[299,615] Alternatively, peripheral blood lymphocytes of infected individuals can be cultured in the presence of an agent that depletes T lymphocytes, such as cyclosporin A.[898] The diagnosis of neoplastic manifestations must be by molecular demonstration that the virus has been integrated into

TABLE 21-11

DIAGNOSTIC ANTIGENS OF EPSTEIN-BARR VIRUS

PHASE OF REPLICATION	ANTIGEN	COMMENTS
Latent Phase	EBNA (EB-nuclear antigen)	Group of neoantigens in infected cells; responsible for immortalization
	LDMA (lymphocyte detected membrane antigen)	Target for the T-cell immune response to the EBV-infected cell
Early Replication Phase	EA (early antigen); "D" (diffuse); "R" (restricted; ie, localized)	Indicates onset of viral replication
Late Replication Stage	VCA (viral capsid antigen)	Indicates complete viral particles are being assembled; IgG and IgM responses detected
	MA (membrane antigen)	Responsible for viral neutralization

Miller G: Epstein-Barr virus. In Fields BN, Knipe DM (eds): Virology, 2nd ed. New York, Raven Press, 1990.

the genome of the malignant cells. Cells from EBV-induced tumors can often be cultured as immortalized cell lines in vitro. The detection of EBV in tissue specimens has been reviewed recently.[10]

VARICELLA-ZOSTER VIRUS

Varicella-zoster virus (VZV) causes chickenpox as a primary infection.[29] The virus may remain latent in the sensory ganglia of the spinal cord for many years before reactivating and producing disease for a second time.[535] The reactivated disease resembles chickenpox but is limited to the dermatome that is innervated by the infected nerve. The reactivation disease is known as shingles.[391] The dermatome of most concern is the ophthalmic branch of the trigeminal nerve because destructive corneal infection may occur as part of the reactivation disease. Before the identity of the processes was recognized, the virus of chickenpox was called varicella virus and that of shingles was called herpes zoster. The virus and its clinical manifestations has been reviewed recently.[28]

Varicella-zoster virus produces considerable discomfort in healthy persons and may produce pneumonia, but in immunosuppressed individuals the disease can become a life-threatening disseminated infection.[570] Pregnant women are at increased risk of developing severe varicella,[236] and neonates who are born within 4 days of their mother's infection are at great risk because maternal antibodies have not yet developed.[302] The risk of embryopathy in the fetus after maternal VZV infection in the first 20 weeks of pregnancy is approximately 2%.[641]

Conventional wisdom states that immunity to varicella is lifelong and that all subsequent disease is recrudescent. Reinfection has been suggested, however, by careful serologic study of immune persons in a house with a fresh case of chickenpox.[30] Housemates

who had preexisting antibody remained well but developed increased antibody titers, indicating subclinical infection.

Sensitive serologic tests such as indirect immunofluorescence to membrane antigen are good markers for immunity to VZV (see page 1258).[883] Insensitive tests such as complement fixation are not adequate markers of susceptibility. There is great concern in hospitals for the safety of immunosuppressed patients who come in contact with an infected person. Exposure may occur unwittingly because patients with VZV are infectious shortly before the onset of the characteristic rash.[29] Measures to reduce risk include use of immune health care personnel for immunosuppressed patients and limitation of visitors. Prompt administration of zoster immune globulin after inadvertent exposure has a protective effect.[84]

HUMAN HERPESVIRUS-6

A new addition to the list of pathogens in the herpes group is human herpesvirus-6 (HHV-6). This virus was first isolated from patients with lymphoproliferative disorders and named human B-lymphotropic virus.[732] The virus has the morphologic structure of a herpesvirus but is genetically unrelated to the five previously identified herpesviruses. Thus it was named human herpesvirus-6. There are two currently recognized subtypes, designated A and B. This virus shares with EBV the ability to grow in human lymphocytes. In contrast to EBV, which infects lymphocytes in a latent stage and does not actively grow in the cells, HHV-6 appears to produce only productive infection in human lymphocytes (ie, mature infectious viral particles are produced in the infected cells).[652]

HHV-6 can be isolated by the same techniques used for HTLV, HIV, and EBV, so it is not surprising that early isolates were made serendipitously from patients with neoplastic disease or who were at risk for HIV infection. The relationship of HHV-6 to the lymphoproliferative disorders originally described is unclear. Rather it produces a common childhood disease called exanthem subitum (also known as roseola infantum, roseola subitum, Duke disease, or fourth disease).[468,897] Exanthem subitum occurs in children between 6 months and 3 years of age. In one study of sera from 25 healthy infants, all children who were at least 44 months old had antibody to HHV-6.[896] Exanthem subitum begins with an abrupt fever, which is followed by a rash as the fever subsides on the third or fourth day. Febrile convulsions occur in approximately 8% of acutely infected patients.[31] Hall and colleagues have described the spectrum of HHV-6 disease in children presenting to the emergency room with acute illnesses.[350] Cases were identified by culture of peripheral blood mononuclear cells, by serology, and by PCR testing of peripheral blood. There were no cases of HHV-6 among 582 infants and young children with acute nonfebrile illnesses or among 352 controls without acute illness. Among children with acute febrile illnesses 160 of 1653 patients (9.7%), ranging in age from 2 weeks to 25 months, had HHV-6 infection. The most common clinical presentations were fever with otitis media (30%), fever of undetermined cause or possible sepsis (29%), and exanthem subitum (27%). A typical rash was only noted at the initial visit, however, in 6% of the children. HHV-6 infections accounted for 20% of 365 visits to the emergency department for febrile illnesses in children between the ages of 6 and 12 months. Twenty-one of the acutely ill children (13%) were hospitalized. The most common complication of the infection was seizures, which occurred in 29% of children between the ages of 12 and 18 months and in 36% of children who were older than 18 months. HHV-6 accounted for one-third of febrile seizures in children less than 2 years of age. The etiology of the seizures may be high fever, but HHV-6 has been detected in the CSF of a patient with seizures and CSF pleocytosis. The virus was detected at a time when the child was no longer viremic.[905] Evidence of possible reactivation was found by serology (16%) or by PCR (6%), but not by viral culture. Other investigators have reported the reactivation of HHV-6, but not EBV, another lymphotropic herpesvirus, in children who were experiencing an acute measles infection, an illness that has been associated with temporary immunosuppression.[808] A variety of other serious complications has been reported, including fatal disseminated infection in an apparently immunocompetent 13-month-old girl.[674] In this case intranuclear inclusions suggestive of herpesvirus were identified as HHV-6 by in situ hybridization. The understanding of the full spectrum of HHV-6 infection awaits further experience.

Most individuals are infected with this virus during childhood. Sera from 25 of 26 healthy adults (96%) had antibodies to HHV-6.[896] Shedding of HHV-6 in the saliva of healthy adults has been reported by some investigators,[509] but not by others.[895] In immunosuppressed adults HHV-6 has produced interstitial pneumonitis after bone marrow transplantation[96] and disseminated infection in a patient with HIV infection,[463] documented in both cases by culture of the virus. Infected cells were identified in tissue by immunohistochemistry. These cases presumably represent reactivation of latent virus in mononuclear cells. Active infection with HHV-6 has also been documented by serology and culture in a group of adults with fatigue and neurologic disease (chronic fatigue syndrome).[88] It is clear that viable virus was present in these individuals, presumably representing reactivation, but it was not established that the virus was causally related to the clinical symptoms.

Viral culture, molecular techniques, and serologic diagnosis of HHV-6 infection are available in reference laboratories.

HUMAN HERPESVIRUS-7

In 1990 a new herpesvirus was isolated from CD4+ T-lymphocytes of a healthy individual, using techniques that cause activation of T cells.[281] The virus, which was named human herpesvirus-7 (HHV-7), is distinct from but closely related to HHV-6.[896] The two viruses do not produce cross-immunity. Children are infected with HHV-7 at a slightly later age than with HHV-6.[896] In a group of 25 healthy infants none had antibody to HHV-7 at 25 months of age, whereas most had encountered HHV-6. By 75 months of age all of the children tested had antibodies to HHV-7 and 25 of 26 healthy adults (96%) had antibodies.[896] The spectrum of clinical disease appears similar to that of HHV-6. In a study of 22 cases of HHV-7 infection, 47.1% of the children had exanthem subitum as the clinical presentation. More serious disease has also been reported with HHV-7, although the difficulties of establishing causality with the latent herpesviruses makes certainty difficult without extensive experience. A patient who was initially thought to have chronic EBV infection with hepatosplenomegaly and pancytopenia was found to be actively infected with HHV-7.[443]

The chronicity of HHV-7 infections is also indicated by the frequency with which the virus can be isolated from approximately 75% of saliva specimens taken from healthy adults.[895] The receptor for HHV-7 is the CD4 epitope on lymphocytes, the same receptor that HIV uses as a primary point of contact with its target cell.[523] In the laboratory the two viruses compete with each other for the receptor, and HHV-7 produces interference with the growth of HIV.

HUMAN HERPESVIRUS-8

The latest addition to the group of lymphotropic herpesviruses is the Kaposi's-sarcoma-associated herpesvirus, which has been named human herpesvirus-8 (HHV-8). As implied by the name, the virus was first detected in tissue from Kaposi's sarcoma in patients with HIV infection, using molecular techniques.[142] Subsequent investigation demonstrated that the viral gene sequences were present in several clinical types of Kaposi's sarcoma: that occurring in patients with AIDS, classic Kaposi's sarcoma unrelated to HIV infection, and Kaposi's sarcoma in homosexual men who are not infected with HIV.[579] The sequences have been identified in AIDS-related body cavity-based lymphomas, which also contained genetic sequences from EBV.[139] Finally (perhaps), HHV-8 sequences have been found in tissue from multicentric Castleman's disease, an atypical lymphoid hyperplasia, which may progress to lymphoma or Kaposi's sarcoma.[786] The sequences are also found in nonneoplastic tissue of HIV-infected patients with Kaposi's sarcoma.[142] Using sensitive amplification techniques, HHV-8 gene sequences have been demonstrated in peripheral blood mononuclear cells from 5 of 56 HIV-negative healthy individuals (9%).[61] Viral gene sequences have also been demonstrated in prostate tissue and semen of healthy individuals, but it has not been definitively established that sexual transmission occurs.[577]

Human herpesvirus-8 has not yet been cultured in vitro. At present, molecular techniques are required to detect the presence of virus, and the results of infection are neoplasia, rather than an inflammatory process. These infections will be faced more frequently by the surgical pathologist than the clinical microbiologist.

B VIRUS

In the 1930s a virus of the herpes group was isolated from a patient who developed a fatal neurologic disease after being bitten by a monkey. About the same time, Sabin isolated a virus from another patient who developed transverse myelitis after a monkey bite.[729] He named the isolate B virus after the afflicted patient. It has also been called herpesvirus simiae, which is something of a misnomer because a variety of herpesviruses are found in monkeys. The recommended taxonomic name is cercopithecine herpesvirus 1. At least 25 cases of herpes B virus infection have been documented in humans, of which 16 were fatal.[860]

The B virus is unusual because it crosses species lines. It is indigenous to Old World monkeys, such as rhesus and cynomolgus, in which it produces a latent infection. Localized human infections have been reported,[56] but most are severe and systemic. An animal bite is the usual means of infection, but infection after a needle-stick injury has been reported.[23] A vesicular eruption often develops around the bite and is followed by regional lymphadenopathy and fever. Encephalitis, transverse myelitis, or visceral necrosis accompanies systemic spread. Fierer and colleagues have reported a remarkable case in which B virus was isolated from a patient who presented with the syndrome of ophthalmic zoster infection.[262]

Two recent events have called attention to B virus. The first documented episode of human-to-human transmission occurred as a part of a cluster of cases at a research facility.[104] The second event was the discovery that monkey kidney cells that had been commercially supplied for diagnostic laboratories were contaminated with B virus. No human infections resulted, but the cells were recalled.[867] The ability of B virus to replicate in monkey kidney monolayers has been known for years.[890] In fact, the stress of processing the kidneys may stimulate activation of latent B virus. The cytopathic effect of the virus consists of cell enlargement and fusion, which may spread through the monolayer. Cowdry type A inclusions identical to those of herpes simplex virus or VZV will be seen in stained cell preparations. Subculture to other monkey kidney cells or to rabbit kidney cells (commonly used for isolation of herpes simplex virus) will transmit the virus.

Antiviral chemotherapy with acyclovir or ganciclovir has been used in a few patients, most of whom survived.[23,193] The single fatality among three infected workers at an animal facility in Michigan was not treated until late in the course of a serious infection.[193]

ADENOVIRUSES

Adenoviruses were originally recognized when spontaneous degeneration occurred in adenoidal tissue cultures. They were called adenoid degeneration (AD), adenoid-pharyngeal-conjunctival (APC), or acute respiratory disease (ARD) agents.[759] These viruses can be present in the pharynx and in the feces without causing disease. Designation of an infectious agent as the etiologic agent must be done carefully so that one is not misled by a fortuitous association. For instance, at one time adenoviruses were considered causes of the pertussis syndrome because they were isolated in the absence of the common bacterial cause, *Bordetella pertussis*. The role of adenovirus in a pertussis syndrome is controversial. It has been suggested that being fastidious, *B. pertussis* may not have been recovered in many cases of whooping cough while the adenoviruses represented incidental isolates or copathogens.[399]

Adenoviruses produce approximately 5% of the acute respiratory disease in children younger than the age of 5 years and may be responsible for 10% of childhood pneumonia.[73] They produce an exudative pharyngitis that can mimic group A β-hemolytic streptococcal disease.[725] In one pediatric hospital, adenoviruses were responsible for otitis, pharyngitis, and gastroenteritis.[724] Certain serotypes are associated with acute conjunctivitis, with or without pharyngitis. Adenovirus disease may be sporadic or may occur in epidemics, such as an outbreak of pharyngitis associated with a swimming pool.[651,834] Lower respiratory tract disease, such as bronchiolitis obliterans[49] or pneumonia,[227,750] occurs uncommonly. Severe pneumonia can also be part of disseminated infection in immunosuppressed patients.[380,469,764]

Adenovirus types 11 and 21 cause acute hemorrhagic cystitis in children.[765] Encephalitis has been reported rarely.[872]

Adenovirus infections of the gastrointestinal tract were discussed earlier with the other viral causes of gastroenteritis. The major adenoviral infections and their associated serotypes are summarized in Table 21-12.

The diagnosis of adenovirus infections is best accomplished by isolation of the virus. Serotyping of isolates is not necessary for clinical purposes in most situations. Direct detection of antigen or genome has been

TABLE 21-12
ADENOVIRUS INFECTIONS

SYNDROME	AGE GROUPS	SEROTYPES
Acute febrile pharyngitis	Young children	1, 2, 3, 5, 6, 7
Pharyngoconjunctival fever	School-age children	3, 7, 14
Acute respiratory disease	Military recruits	3, 4, 7, 14, 21
Pneumonia	Young children	1, 2, 3, 7
Pneumonia	Military recruits	4, 7
Epidemic keratoconjunctivitis	All	8, 11, 19, 37
Pertussis-like syndrome	Young children	5
Acute hemorrhagic cystitis	Young children	11, 21
Gastroenteritis	Young children	40, 41

Horwitz MS: Adenoviruses. In Fields BN, Knipe DM (eds): Virology, 2nd ed. New York, Raven Press, 1990.

attempted but not entirely successfully in the respiratory tract. Serology plays a secondary role in diagnosis.

POXVIRUSES

The king of the poxvirus group was the variola virus, the etiologic agent of smallpox, which has now passed from endangered species status into extinction.[257] Known stocks of virus remain only in the United States and Russia, and the genome has been sequenced. Destruction of all existing virus has been discussed and planned, but not yet accomplished.[220] Orthopoxviruses of animals, such as cowpox and monkeypox viruses, can occasionally infect humans. The origin of vaccinia virus is unclear; it has many characteristics of a distinct species but may have been derived by recombination between other viruses.

The parapoxviruses include agents causing diseases in sheep (orf or contagious pustular dermatitis virus) and in cows (milker's node or pseudocowpox virus). They may also produce localized infections in humans who are occupationally exposed to the viruses. Molluscum contagiosum virus, which has never been cultured, causes a localized hypertrophic skin lesion that has a diagnostic histologic appearance. The poxviruses are unlikely to be isolated in the clinical laboratory.

PAPOVAVIRUSES

The papovaviruses, a diverse group of DNA viruses, are made up of the papilloma (Pa), polyoma (PO), and vacuolating (VA) viruses. The subgroups differ greatly in their biology. The vacuolating viruses are indigenous to animals and will be encountered by microbiologists only as contaminating agents in monkey kidney cell cultures.

POLYOMAVIRUSES

The most important of the human polyomaviruses is the JC virus, which produces a destructive encephalitis (progressive multifocal leukoencephalopathy) in immunocompromised patients.[704,705] SV40 (simian virus 40) also produces the disease, another example of a monkey virus crossing species barriers. The histologic appearance, including intranuclear viral inclusions, of progressive multifocal leukoencephalopathy is diagnostic.

Polyomaviruses are frequently reactivated in recipients of transplants, often longer after transplantation than other latent human viruses.[25] JC virus and BK virus are most frequently found. Both have been associated with a severe hemorrhagic cystitis in recipients of bone marrow transplants.[24,25]

The polyomaviruses are cultured in vitro only with great difficulty. BK virus will grow in common cell lines, such as human diploid fibroblasts, but several days to weeks are required before cytopathic effect is evident.[815] JC virus is difficult to culture. The most sensitive cell type is primary human fetal glial cells, which is not an easy reagent to acquire.

PAPILLOMAVIRUSES

The human papillomaviruses (HPV) cause common warts, sexually transmitted venereal warts, and tumors of the respiratory and genital tracts. The viral nature of warts was known early in the 20th century when they were transferred with cell-free filtrates, and Shope defined the rabbit papillomavirus as the cause of papillomas in 1933.[406] Study of HPV was impeded until molecular techniques sufficient for the task were developed in the 1970s.

More than 60 genetic types of HPV have been described. There are strong associations between certain genotypes and clinical lesions (Table 21-13). The common wart is the most common lesion, but most attention has been focused on the genital infections, including the association with neoplasia. Crum and colleagues have lucidly analyzed the problems and challenges.[184] Sexual partners of patients who are infected with HPV are also frequently infected and the disease processes are concordant. Male partners of women with condylomata (usually infected with HPV-6 or HPV-11) have condylomata, macules, or papules, whereas male sexual partners of women with cervical intraepithelial neoplasia (usually infected with HPV-16,18 or 33) have penile intraepithelial neoplasia.[45]

The association of HPV with cervical neoplasia has been constructed from many studies, but the evidence is not yet conclusive that HPV is the sole factor.[184] Brescia and associates have reviewed current concepts of cervical neoplasia and its relationship to HPV infection.[74] Rather than a dramatic shift from normal to neoplastic epithelium in the cervix, there is a continuous spectrum, recognized as increasingly severe grades of cervical intraepithelial neoplasia. The final stage in the process is the development of overt malignancy, invasive carcinoma, which may be either glandular or

TABLE 21-13

ASSOCIATION OF SELECTED HUMAN PAPILLOMAVIRUSES (HPV) WITH CLINICAL DISEASE

VIRAL TYPE	CLINICAL DISEASE	NEOPLASTIC POTENTIAL
HPV-1	Deep plantar wart	Not described
HPV-2	Common wart	Not described
	Mosaic wart	
HPV-3	Flat wart	Not described
HPV-4	Common wart	Not described
HPV-5	Plaques in epidermodysplasia verruciformis	Squamous carcinoma May develop in sun-exposed areas
HPV-6	Genital: Exophytic condyloma Flat condyloma Giant condyloma Respiratory papillomas Conjunctival papillomas	Weak association, especially vulva
HPV-7	Common Butcher's warts	Not described
HPV-11	See HPV-6	See HPV-6
HPV-16	Genital: Bowenoid papulosis Flat condyloma	Strong association in cervix and vulva
HPV-18	Genital: Flat condyloma	Strong association in cervix; infrequently found in precursor lesions
HPV-31, 33, 35	Genital: Cervix	Moderate association in flat condyloma

Adapted from Shah KV, Howley PM: Papillomaviruses. In Fields BN, Knipe DM (eds): Virology, 2nd ed. New York, Raven Press, 1990.

squamous. Likewise there is a continuum in the expression of HPV genes and antigens.[699] In the normal epithelium the cells of the basal layer progressively differentiate to form keratinized squamous epithelium at the surface. As the cervical epithelial changes progress from mildly dysplastic to severely dysplastic, the following changes occur: 1) the cells become less differentiated throughout the epithelium, 2) the chromosomal content of the nuclei becomes increasingly abnormal, 3) the expression of HPV gene products (antigens) becomes less intense, and 4) the expression of HPV genes is increasingly difficult to demonstrate. The diagnostic cellular characteristic of the HPV infected cell is koilocytosis, a perinuclear clearing in the squamous epithelium accompanied by nuclear atypia.[884] The appearance of koilocytic atypia in exfoliated cervical cells is shown in Figure 21-4. Nuovo and colleagues were able to detect HPV DNA in 65% of lesions that had koilocytic atypia but in only 11.7% of lesions that lacked this abnormality.[621] As the lesions dedifferentiate, however, it becomes increasingly difficult to demonstrate HPV DNA.

Although a variety of HPV types may be found in flat warts, there is a preponderance of certain types, especially HPV-16, in neoplastic lesions and precancers that have a high risk of progression to neoplasia.[185] It is not possible to determine the viral type from the histologic abnormalities,[431] but associations between particular viral types and neoplasms have been suggested. For instance, in one study HPV-16 was associated with keratinizing squamous carcinomas, while HPV-18 was relatively concentrated in adenocarcinomas.[880] It is of interest that the HPV genome is integrated into several tumor cell lines that were derived from genital tumors.

The famous HeLa cell line, originally derived from a cervical adenocarcinoma, contains HPV-18 DNA.[899] The association of certain HPV types with neoplastic or benign conditions is not absolute. Cases of cervical[304] and vulvar[691,811] carcinoma have been linked to HPV-6 or HPV-11. HPV DNA has been found in extragenital neoplasms, such as anal squamous cell carcinoma[290] or anaplastic carcinoma of the lung,[807] but the associations are more preliminary than those with cervical neoplasia.

The cellular biology of HPV supports a role in the development of neoplasia. The viral types most closely associated with cervical cancer, particularly HPV-16, are capable of transforming cells in culture so that they lose their normal growth control mechanisms. The DNA from these types integrates into host DNA,[669] in one case near cellular oncogenes.[232] The viral integration may cause chromosomal rearrangement[499] and lead to abnormal cellular differentiation in vitro.[552] Zur Hausen has put forth the hypothesis that cervical neoplasia is the result of failure of a primal cellular surveillance mechanism that was designed to control persisting viral genomes.[916]

Epidemiologic evidence of association between HPV and cervical neoplasia is provided by the histopathologic studies discussed earlier and from analyses of exfoliated cervical cells. De Villiers and colleagues studied 9295 endocervical smears stained by the Papanicolaou technique and examined for HPV DNA.[200] They found that HPV infection was identified in approximately 10% of normal endocervical smears but in 35% to 40% of malignant and premalignant abnormalities. Reeves and colleagues also found a statistically significant association of HPV, particularly

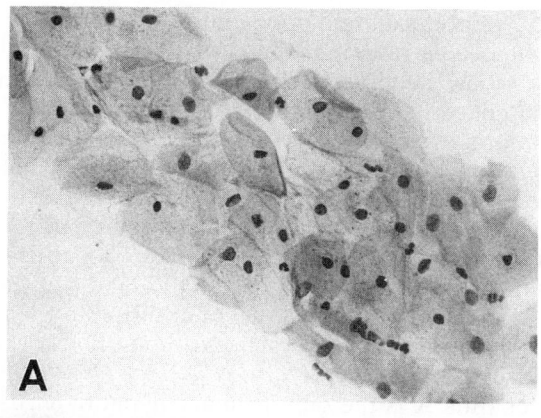

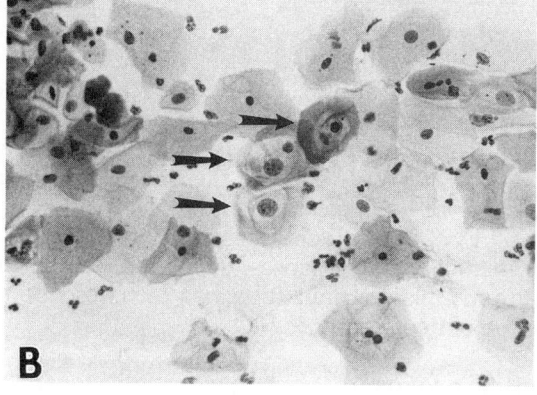

Figure 21-4
Papanicolaou stain. (**A**) Normal exfoliated cervical squamous epithelial cells. The nucleus is small and compact, and the cytoplasm is abundant in these mature, keratinized epithelial cells. (**B**) Koilocytic atypia. The nuclei in some of these superficial cells are enlarged with coarse, clumped chromatin, and there is a pallor or clearing in the cytoplasm (**arrow**) (×250).

HPV-16 or HPV-18, with cervical cancer in Latin America.[697] The rates of infection in women without carcinoma were also extraordinarily high in this study. The theory that HPV causes cervical cancer was not supported by a large epidemiologic study of women in Denmark and Greenland.[456] Contrary to expectations, there was an inverse relationship between HPV infection and cervical neoplasia in the two countries.

Papillomavirus DNA has been demonstrated in normal cervical epithelium adjacent to genital warts[258] and cancer.[531] Failure to remove all the infected tissue may lead to recurrences. HPV DNA can also be demonstrated in 5%[620] to 10%[200] of women with normal cervical smears or biopsies.

With the information currently available, routine detection of HPV DNA in clinical specimens cannot be recommended. There is a place for judicious use of the technology in selected patients who are clinical problems.

PARVOVIRUSES

As the name implies, the parvoviruses are very small; they are unusual in that they contain single-stranded DNA.[180] The only human parvovirus, known as B19,

has been demonstrated to cause a common childhood febrile illness with rash. Erythema infectiosum is also known as fifth disease (the fifth childhood disease after rubeola, rubella, varicella, and roseola). It is characterized by fever and a characteristic "slapped cheek" rash in young children.[667] Most persons are immune by the time they reach adulthood, but susceptible persons may experience arthritis or arthralgias.[754] This pattern of mild rash illness in childhood and severe arthritis in adults resembles that of rubella virus. The rash in erythema infectiosum is maculopapular, but a vesiculopustular lesion has been reported in an adult.[604]

Parvovirus B19 has an affinity for immature red blood cell precursors. The receptor on human erythrocytes for parvovirus B19 is the P antigen, and individuals who lack that antigen are naturally resistant to infection.[80] Unfortunately, very few individuals lack the P erythrocyte antigen. Parvovirus B19 can produce transient anemia in normal persons[885] and severe chronic anemia[478,479] or aplastic crisis[158] in patients with malignancies or hemoglobinopathies. If pregnant women undergo a primary parvovirus infection, fatal erythroblastosis fetalis with hydrops may result.[12] In this case the virus produces severe chronic anemia, whereas in immunologic erythroblastosis (Rh disease) antibodies to the fetal red blood cells do the damage. A viral hemophagocytic syndrome in children and adults has been associated with human parvovirus.[590,766] Transmission of parvovirus infection from heavily infected patients to susceptible health care workers has been documented.[52]

The clinical manifestations of human parvovirus infection during an epidemic in Cadiz, Spain included hematologic manifestations in 13.9% of 43 patients, dermatologic lesions in 53.4%, arthralgias or arthritis in 20.9%, and infection in pregnancy in 7.0% patients (two of these women suffered abortions). Fever and lymphadenopathy were presenting complaints in 37% of the patients.[293]

Parvovirus DNA can be detected in the sera of acutely infected individuals for less than 1 month by DNA hybridization techniques, but DNA was detectable in most patients by a sensitive nested PCR assay for 3 months and in some patients for longer than 1 year.[597]

Parvovirus B19 has not been cultured in vitro. Virus has been detected in blood morphologically, immunologically, or genetically.[580] The basophilic, intranuclear inclusions of parvovirus can be seen in bone marrow aspirates after staining with hemtoxylin-eosin or the Wright-Giemsa technique if the smears are first fixed with formalin. The inclusions can also be seen in formalin-fixed paraffin-embedded tissue.[472] Antibodies may be measured by enzyme immunoassay.[15] It has been suggested that saliva can be used instead of serum for detection of antibodies.[187] Serologic and molecular virologic methods are complementary techniques for assessing maternal infection.[913] In situ detection of viral DNA has been recommended for detection of virus in fetal cord blood.

HEPATITIS VIRUSES

Many viruses can produce infectious damage to the liver. EBV and CMV occasionally cause symptomatic hepatitis as a part of the mononucleosis syndrome. The primary hepatitis viruses are a diverse group. The "alphabet soup" of hepatitis is summarized in Table 21-14.

HEPATITIS A VIRUS

Hepatitis A virus produces sporadic and epidemic infectious hepatitis. The disease has been known since antiquity, but the virus was not identified until the 1970s. Hepatitis A virus was first classified as enterovirus 72 based on biochemical and physical features.[339] Subsequently, it was recognized that there were considerable differences from classical enteroviruses. It has now been transferred into a new genus, *Hepatovirus*, within the family *Picornaviridae*.[574]

Hepatitis A virus produces acute self-limited hepatitis. The incubation period between exposure and clinical disease is short (< 1 month). For 7 to 10 days before clinical illness there is noncytopathic viral replication in hepatocytes, viremia, and fecal shedding of infectious virus.[212] A period of viral replication with hepatocyte damage, including classic "ballooning" degeneration of liver cells, follows. At this point the communicable period is almost complete. Hepatitis A virus infection is rarely transmitted by blood transfusions because little virus is present in the blood and the duration of viremia is limited. Transmission of infection to patients with hemophilia in clotting factor concentrate, which contains samples from many donors, has been described in Europe and the United States.[135] Massive hepatic necrosis and postinfectious cirrhosis are rare.[548] Chronic hepatitis and neoplasia are not complications.

Hepatitis A is transmitted by contaminated food and water.[783] Bivalve shellfish from contaminated waters have produced numerous outbreaks because they are often eaten raw or steamed to a temperature that does not kill the virus.[465] The transmission of hepatitis A virus, like EBV and poliovirus, is determined by sanitation and socioeconomic condition. Virus circulates freely under conditions of poor sanitation and infects humans at an early age, when the infection is usually asymptomatic. More affluent citizens escape infection until adulthood, when symptomatic hepatitis results.[388] (See "Poliovirus," page 1196, and "Epstein-Barr Virus," page 1213.) A recent addition to the risk factors is certain sexual practices among homosexual and bisexual men.[374]

Hepatitis A is the only primary hepatitis virus to have been cultured in vitro. The virus will grow in a variety of simian cells, most notably early passages of African green monkey kidney cells.[63] Culture is not a viable diagnostic option, however, because recovery from primary specimens is not reliable. Hepatitis A is diagnosed serologically by detection of specific IgM antibody.[686,783,810] Very early in the infection IgM antibody may not be detectable, so the test should be repeated 2 weeks later if clinical suspicion is high.[382] An experimental two-step process, using monoclonal antibodies and DNA hybridization, has been described for detection of hepatitis A.[418]

HEPATITIS B VIRUS

Hepatitis B virus is a DNA hepadnavirus. It produces acute and chronic hepatitis and is an etiologic agent of hepatocellular carcinoma. Hepatitis B virus has a long incubation period (45–120 days) and is transmitted primarily by parenteral means. Until routine screening of blood products for this virus was begun, hepatitis B was the most common cause of transfusion-associated hepatitis. Other parenteral routes have included acupuncture[101] and tattooing.[588] Hepatitis B antigen has been demonstrated in mosquitoes, but

TABLE 21-14
PRIMARY VIRAL CAUSES OF HEPATITIS

VIRUS	TAXONOMY	TRANSMISSION	CHRONICITY	NEOPLASIA
Hepatitis A	Hepatovirus RNA	Enteric: Water Food Shellfish	No	No
Hepatitis B	Hepadnavirus DNA	Parenteral: Blood Sexual Needles Enteric	Yes	Yes
Hepatitis C	? Togavirus 27-nm virions RNA	Parenteral: Blood	Yes	?
Hepatitis D	42- to 47-nm virion RNA	Parenteral	Yes	No
Hepatitis E	27- to 34-nm virion	Enteric	? No	? No

transmission of infection by arthropods has not been authenticated.[675] This virus can be transmitted by sexual contact[378] and has produced epidemic disease in male homosexuals, prostitutes, and abusers of intravenous drugs.[721] Perinatal infection occurs,[628] but breast milk does not appear to play a role in transmission.[48] In contrast to hepatitis A virus, hepatitis B virus may produce fulminant fatal acute hepatitis, called massive hepatic necrosis. It has been suggested that a mutation in the virus may cause this severe manifestation.[513,630]

The array of mechanisms for transmission of hepatitis B virus infection recalls HIV. The concentration of hepatitis B virus in blood and body fluids is much greater than HIV, however, and nosocomial infection is consequently a greater problem. This virus is the most common viral laboratory-acquired infection.[666] A nosocomial outbreak traced to contaminated spring-loaded devices for collecting capillary blood has been reported.[668] The prevalence of hepatitis B virus infection is greater in dentists, a high-risk group, than in the general population,[586] and an outbreak of infection has been traced to an oral surgeon.[714] Transmission of infection from surgeons to patients is uncommon, but it has occurred in the absence of any identified breeches of infection control protocols.[361]

Hepatitis B virus is a 47-nm spherical virus that possesses several antigens of importance for diagnosis and pathogenesis. There are three envelope polypeptides that come under the designation HBsAg (hepatitis B surface antigen), HBcAg (hepatitis B core antigen), and HBeAg (hepatitis B e antigen). This virus has not been cultured in vitro, but the variety of antigens and corresponding antibodies provide ample tools for documenting clinical disease. DNA and DNA polymerase are not commonly measured. Although not absolute, the presence of e antigen correlates well with the presence of DNA and DNA polymerase and with viral infectivity.[7] The fascinating story of the discovery of Australia antigen (now known as HBsAg) and its relationship to hepatitis has been reviewed by Blumberg.[68] It serves as a reminder that no one can predict where basic research will have its impact. Who would have predicted that a research group interested in genetic polymorphisms of blood proteins would discover the key to the most important cause of human hepatitis?

For reasons that are unclear, some persons who are infected with hepatitis B virus develop antibody and clear the virus from their system, whereas others continue to circulate viral antigens. A subset of these chronic carriers develops chronic liver disease. Another serious complication of this infection is the integration of viral DNA into the genome of the liver cells and the development of hepatocellular carcinoma.[757] The serologic diagnosis of hepatitis B infections is discussed on page 1256.

Along with the knowledge of hepatitis B biology has come an effective vaccine, which can provide financial savings as well as prevent disease if used wisely.[591] Unfortunately some populations most in need of protection respond poorly to the vaccine and are incompletely protected.[343]

HEPATITIS C VIRUS

After diagnostic reagents for hepatitis A and B viruses became available it became obvious that there were other causes of transfusion-associated hepatitis.[255] The unknown virus or viruses were dubbed non-A, non-B hepatitis. Thanks to the sophisticated technology of molecular biology we now recognize hepatitis C as the cause of most cases of transfusion-associated non-A, non-B hepatitis. Aach and colleagues have estimated that 91% of non-A, non-B transfusion hepatitis is caused by hepatitis C virus.[1] Choo and colleagues used the blood of a chronically infected chimpanzee to create a genomic library of DNA strands that were complementary to the DNA and RNA in the serum (cDNA).[157] They used the serum of a patient with documented non-A, non-B hepatitis as a source of antibody. After screening 1 million clones they found one that reacted with the serum, providing them with the first portion of the single-stranded RNA genome. The genetic sequence of hepatitis C virus is most closely related to the flaviviruses (group B arboviruses) and pestiviruses (animal viruses), and it has been placed taxonomically in the family *Flaviviridae*.[276] Hepatitis C virus consists of a group of heterogeneous genotypes, currently 6 types and 11 subtypes, which have defined geographic distributions.[767] Types 1, 2, and 3 are distributed worldwide, with types 1a and 1b accounting for approximately 60% of infections. Type 4 is found predominantly in the Middle East; type 5, in South Africa; and type 6, in Hong Kong.

The epidemiology of hepatitis C infections has many similarities to hepatitis B, but some significant differences are apparent. The most common route of spread is through blood products, including immune globulin,[65] surgery, and intravenous drug abuse.[567] Screening of blood products for hepatitis C virus has substantially reduced the risk of transmission by this route.[218] Sexual transmission occurs, but the frequency is much less than in hepatitis B infection.[631,864] Likewise, transmission of the virus occurs vertically from mother to infant, the risk increasing with increasing maternal viral titers, but the frequency appears to be less than in hepatitis B.[627] The frequency of antibody to hepatitis C among health care workers in Baltimore was similar to that in the general population, suggesting that workers are exposed to low levels of virus or that the transmissibility is not great.[824] Transmission of infection from a cardiac surgeon to a patient has been documented.[247] The level of viremia is similar in infections caused by various genotypes,[774] but it has been suggested that some genotypes, such as type 2, are more frequently associated with cirrhosis than are other types.[671]

Acute hepatitis C virus infection is often less severe than that of hepatitis B, but the frequency of chronic hepatitis C disease is high.[476] Fulminant hepatic failure may rarely result from the initial infection.[322] The subject has been reviewed by Iwarson and colleagues.[414] Cirrhosis is a significant complication of chronic infection. In one study 37% of patients had cirrhosis at the time of diagnosis, an additional 5% developed cirrhosis within the next 4 years, and 20% of patients had progression of histologic damage at the time of a second biopsy.[567] Hepatitis C infection is an independent risk factor for hepatocellular carcinoma after the development of cirrhosis.[768] Extrahepatic immunologic manifestations, such as cryoglobulinemia and rheumatoid factors, are a prominent part of hepatitis C infection, as they are for hepatitis B.[647] Some patients with hepatitis C infection respond to therapy with interferon-α, especially those with a low level of viremia.[497] Reinfection is common with hepatitis C, indicating that neutralizing antibodies are not produced, and raising the specter that an effective vaccine will not be possible.[252]

The laboratory diagnosis of hepatitis C infections is primarily serologic, but molecular amplification techniques are beginning to find a place in routine testing. The first generation of enzyme immunoassays lacked sensitivity and specificity, but the second and third generations have improved substantially on the early tests.[1,144,498] Low-level or absence of reactivity reliably predicts the absence of hepatitis C RNA in serum of all patients, although false-negative tests have been noted in a small number of cases by some investigators.[259] False-positive tests have been noted in patients who had been recently immunized with influenza virus antigens.[530] IgM antibody is detectable in serum of patients with acute disease, disappears during resolution of the acute infection, and may reappear before a biochemical relapse, even in the absence of detectable RNA in serum.[684]

Although greatly improved, the third-generation immunoassays are not perfect.[259] Analogous to serologic evaluation of human immunodeficiency virus infections, immunoblots using recombinant antigens are used to confirm the results of second- and third-generation enzyme immunoassays.[259] There have been three generations of these immunoblot tests (RIBA). Approximately 10% of the immunoblots produce indeterminate results.[646] Approximately half the patients with indeterminate RIBA results have detectable viral RNA in the serum. The explanation for the other indeterminate results is unclear but is not related to the infecting genotype.

The most recent addition to the therapeutic armamentarium is the use of amplification methods for detection of viral RNA in serum, which has been extensively reviewed.[471] The selection of the primers for amplification is important for maximum sensitivity. Bukh and colleagues reported that use of primers from the 5' noncoding (NC) region of the genome was the most sensitive method and resulted in a threefold greater frequency of positivity than use of primers from the nonstructural (NS) 3-like region of the gene.[90] An evaluation of a commercial polymerase chain reaction for hepatitis C RNA noted good correlation when the viral load was low, but the commercial test yielded less virus when high copy numbers were present.[722] The discrepancy would not be significant for detection of infection, but potentially could affect decisions that depend on accurate assessment of viral load. Detection of hepatitis C viral load is in its infancy. A cautionary note was sounded by the report that only 5 of 31 (16%) laboratories performed faultlessly in assessing 12 plasma samples for virus.[909]

HEPATITIS D VIRUS

Hepatitis D virus, also known as the delta agent, is a 35-nm double-shelled RNA virus that is incapable of multiplication without the surface antigen of hepatitis B.[390] The maturing delta virus covers itself in the HBsAg coat before infecting other cells. Thus the biology of hepatitis D is inextricably tied to that of hepatitis B. Hepatitis D can produce infection and disease only in patients who are concurrently infected with hepatitis B or who are producing HBsAg from a previous infection. Not surprisingly, hepatitis D virus infection is concentrated in pockets of populations with hepatitis B virus infection, such as drug addicts and homosexual men.[202]

When co-infection occurs, the clinical disease is similar to that of hepatitis B and is usually self-limited.[390] When hepatitis D infects a patient who is a chronic carrier of hepatitis B, the clinical disease is much more severe, disease becomes chronic in as many as 80% of cases, and fatality rates may be dramatically increased to as high as 12%.[102]

Diagnosis of acute delta hepatitis is difficult because the antibody response is transient. Chronic hepatitis D virus infection can be documented by a serologic assay.[680]

HEPATITIS E VIRUS

The newest addition to the alphabet soup of hepatitis viruses is a 27-nm labile RNA virus.[701] Hepatitis E virus produces an enterically transmitted acute hepatitis that most closely resembles that of hepatitis A. The viral genome has been cloned by techniques similar to those used to identify hepatitis C. The taxonomic status of this virus is not yet clear. It has similarities to the caliciviruses, but its closest genetic relative is rubella virus, currently classified as a togavirus.[681] Large waterborne epidemics of disease are produced under conditions of poor sanitation,[605] but the infection has not yet been recognized as a cause of indigenous disease in the United States. Travelers to endemic areas, however, have returned to the United States with the infection.[117] The diagnosis is made serologically, with an enzyme-linked immunosorbent assay (ELISA),[316] which remains an experimental procedure.

OTHER HEPATITIS VIRUSES

The transmission of a hepatitis virus from a surgeon to marmosets was reported in 1967.[205] The virus was named hepatitis virus GB after the source patient. It has been determined that there are two viruses, designated GB-A and GB-B, which are members of the flavivirus group.[769] Recently, a third related virus, hepatitis virus GB-C, has been described as a cause of persistent infection in patients on maintenance hemodialysis.[549] None of the 16 infected patients had evidence of active liver disease, raising the question about whether it is premature to call the agent a hepatitis virus. Other investigators have reported an agent designated hepatitis G virus that appears to be the same as the hepatitis GB-C virus.[515] (Hepatitis F virus has been described, but not substantiated.) These new viruses were detected and characterized by molecular cloning, following the examples of hepatitis C and E viruses. We can expect new hepatitis viruses to surface in the future. In a study of waterborne hepatitis in India, most cases were caused by agents that were closely related to hepatitis E virus, but some outbreaks appear to have been caused by as yet undescribed agents.[21] In addition, a variety of other viruses, such as EBV, CMV, herpes simplex virus, and adenovirus can cause hepatitis. The taxonomists may eventually run out of letters of the alphabet!

TRANSMISSIBLE SPONGIFORM ENCEPHALOPATHIES

The transmissible spongiform encephalopathies are a fascinating group of CNS infections that are defined by a distinctive cellular pathology, which produces a vacuolated appearance to the cerebral white matter. The infections and their natural host are:

Scrapie—sheep
Bovine spongiform encephalopathy (BSE)—cattle
Transmissible mink encephalopathy—mink
Kuru—humans
Creutzfeldt-Jakob disease (CJD)—humans
Gerstmann-Sträussler-Scheinker syndrome (GSS)—humans

The etiologic agents of these infections have not been completely characterized. Their small size and transmissible nature suggest that they are viruses, but no nucleic acids have been identified definitively. The agents are more resistant to inactivation by x-rays, ultraviolet light, and harsh chemical treatment, including immersion in 10% formalin, than any other known infectious agent. Griffith has proposed the heretical notion that the agents may be replicating proteins without any nucleic acid.[332] A protease-resistant protein that is rod shaped by electron microscopy has been identified in these infections.[678] These abnormal proteins have been named prions. They aggregate into fibrillary tangles that resemble amyloid protein, and the agents have also been called transmissible amyloids. The prion protein is a modified version of a normal cellular protein.[626] The nature of the transmissible agent remains controversial. Two theories have been proposed: 1) that the prion protein is itself the infectious agent and 2) that the prion protein participates in the pathologic process, but the actual agent is as yet unidentified, probably a small virus.[150]

The first human disease to be recognized was kuru, which occurred among a remote, isolated tribe of aborigines in the New Guinea highlands.[289] Gajdusek won a Nobel Prize for unraveling the mysterious disease that began with cerebellar ataxia and a shivering-like tremor, progressed to complete loss of motor and speech function, and resulted in death within a year. The agent was transmitted through the practice of rit-ual cannibalism as part of the mourning ritual for the dead. Transmission of the infection was stopped when the tribe was convinced to alter their practices. Subsequently, it was recognized that two rare human dementias—CJD and a variant, GSS—were caused by a similar agent. The infections produce the rapid onset of dementia with memory loss and behavioral problems at some point in most patients. Death occurs within months to a year after onset.

Bovine spongiform encephalopathy (BSE) appeared in southern England in 1986, and approximately 100,000 cases had been documented by the end of 1993.[72] Scrapie has been passed from sheep to cattle experimentally,[303] and it has been conjectured that the disease was transmitted to cattle through sheep brains included in feed as a protein supplement.[72] What was an economic disaster turned into a political and scientific nightmare in 1996 when it was announced that some cases of "atypical Creutzfeld-Jakob disease" in England may have been contracted by eating meat from cows with BSE.[133] The British government underreacted, the European governments overreacted, and a crisis with more politics than science ensued. At this writing there are no scientific evaluations of the problem, but it is reported that many experts question whether a problem even exists. BSE has not been documented in cattle in the United States, but the potential exists.

There are no readily available diagnostic tests for the spongiform encephalopathies. The diagnosis is usually made clinically and confirmed by pathologic analysis of brain tissue. Elaborate precautions must be taken in the autopsy room and histology laboratory because the agents of these infections survive formalin fixation and even survive embedding in paraffin blocks.

CLINICAL CLASSIFICATION OF VIRAL INFECTIONS

Although the virologic taxonomy is important scientifically, clinical schemes of classification have practical validity when considering an individual patient. The clinical syndromes and associated viruses that are most commonly encountered are summarized in Table 21-15. Note that viruses from varying taxonomic groups may produce the same symptoms.

Among the many viruses that are pathogens for humans, only a small number produce the majority of infections in western countries. The frequency of recovery of viruses from clinical specimens at the University of Vermont and at the Mayo Clinic is summarized in Table 21-16. In both laboratories, herpes simplex was by far the most common virus recovered. Differences in populations of patients, orientation of the laboratory (for instance, hospital laboratory versus reference laboratory), and availability of other diagnostic laboratories (such as those in state health departments) will all influence the types of viruses recovered.

TABLE 21-15
CLINICAL SYNDROMES ASSOCIATED WITH VIRAL INFECTIONS

ORGAN SYSTEM	SYNDROME	MORE LIKELY AGENTS	LESS LIKELY AGENTS
Respiratory	Coryza: "Cold"	Rhinovirus Coronavirus Adenovirus Parainfluenza 3	Influenza A or B Parainfluenza 1 or 2 RSV Enterovirus
	Pharyngitis	Adenovirus Herpes simplex Enterovirus Epstein-Barr virus	Influenza A or B RSV Parainfluenza 1 or 2 Rhinovirus Coronavirus
	Croup	Parainfluenza 1–3	Influenza A RSV Measles Coronavirus
	Bronchiolitis	Parainfluenza 3 RSV	Adenovirus Parainfluenza 1–2 Influenza A or B Rhinovirus
	Pneumonia	Influenza A RSV Parainfluenza 3 Adenovirus Cytomegalovirus (immunosuppressed patients)	Parainfluenza 1–2 Rhinovirus Epstein-Barr virus Influenza B
	Pleurodynia	Coxsackievirus B	Coxsackievirus A Echovirus
Central nervous system	Aseptic meningitis	Echovirus Coxsackievirus A Coxsackievirus B Mumps virus	LCM Herpes simplex 2 Varicella-zoster Adenovirus Bunyaviruses
	Encephalitis	None frequent	Herpes simplex 1 Togaviruses Bunyaviruses Epstein-Barr virus Enteroviruses Rabies virus Cytomegalovirus
Gastrointestinal	Diarrhea (infants)	Rotavirus Adenovirus 40–41	Adenovirus Enterovirus Norwalk-like virus Coronavirus
	Diarrhea (adults)	Norwalk-like virus	Rotavirus Adenovirus Enterovirus
	Hepatitis	Hepatitis A Hepatitis B Hepatitis C	Epstein-Barr virus Cytomegalovirus Hepatitis D Hepatitis E
	Parotitis	Mumps virus	Parainfluenza viruses

(Continued)

TABLE 21-15 *(Continued)*
CLINICAL SYNDROMES ASSOCIATED WITH VIRAL INFECTIONS

ORGAN SYSTEM	SYNDROME	MORE LIKELY AGENTS	LESS LIKELY AGENTS
Cutaneous	Vesicular rash	Herpes simplex Varicella-zoster	Echovirus Coxsackievirus A Vaccinia
	Maculopapular rash	Echovirus Coxsackievirus Human herpesvirus-6 Human herpesvirus-7	Adenovirus Epstein-Barr virus Dengue virus Measles virus Rubella virus
	Petechial rash	None frequent	Adenovirus Echovirus Coxsackievirus Hemorrhagic fever viruses
Urogenital	Hemorrhagic cystitis	None frequent	Adenovirus Herpes Simplex 1 virus

Cardiac	Myocarditis/
	  pericarditis
		Coxsackievirus A, B
		Echovirus
			Adenovirus
			  Herpes Simplex 1 virus
			Influenza A
			Mumps virus

Ocular	Keratitis/ conjunctivitis	Herpes simplex Varicella-zoster Adenovirus	Vaccinia Measles virus

RSV, respiratory syncytial virus; LCM, lymphocytic choriomeningitis virus
Adapted from McIntosh K: Diagnostic virology. In Fields BN, Knipe DM, Melnick JL, et al (eds): Virology, 2nd ed, chap 16, pp 411–440. New York, Raven Press, 1990

DIAGNOSIS OF VIRAL INFECTIONS

The primary diagnostic technique for most viral infections is the isolation of the virus in cell culture. Serologic techniques may also be useful, especially if the virus was isolated from a nonsterile site. In some instances, serologic diagnosis is the only practical approach in a clinical laboratory. Direct detection of antigen in body fluids or tissues has also been effective for some viruses. The list of agents for which direct detection of antigen is useful will undoubtedly continue to expand. In Table 21-17, the methods most commonly used in hospital laboratories to diagnose viral infections are summarized. The advantages and disadvantages of each of these approaches are compared in Table 21-18. There are several excellent reference texts on diagnostic virology that should be consulted for additional information.[407,506,595,720,787]

COLLECTION OF SPECIMENS FOR DIAGNOSIS

In general, an attempt should be made to obtain material from the organ or organs that are infected. For the most common viral infections of the skin, the cutaneous lesions are the best specimens for culture. For diagnosis of infections of the respiratory and gastrointestinal tracts, secretions from those regions should be cultured. Recommended specimens for viral culture are listed in Table 21-19.

Most viruses enter the body through the respiratory or gastrointestinal tracts. Although the most obvious clinical manifestations of disease may occur in a distant organ, it is often appropriate to collect a specimen from the point of entry. Sampling of multiple sites is particularly useful if it is difficult to obtain a specimen from an internal organ or if the virus is difficult to isolate from the target organ. For example, the skin is most dramatically involved in measles infection, but measles virus may be isolated from the respiratory tract or from the urine. Similarly, the cardiac and central nervous systems are commonly affected in serious enteroviral infection, but the virus may be isolated from the upper airways or from the gastrointestinal tract.

If the virus is rarely isolated from these nonsterile sites (as is the case with measles), recovery of a virus establishes an etiologic diagnosis. If the virus is recovered from sites where it may be found in the absence of disease (eg, the enteroviruses in throat or stool specimens), the recovery of a potentially pathogenic virus provides a presumptive diagnosis.

Viruses colonize mucosal surfaces less frequently than do bacteria[341] but may be present more commonly during the months when increased circulation of viruses occurs—the winter for respiratory viruses and the summer for enteroviruses. The frequency with which enteroviruses colonize the gastrointestinal tract is greatest in infants and least in adults. In Cincinnati, the carrier rate for echoviruses was 5.2% among 1- to

TABLE 21-16
FREQUENCY OF ISOLATION OF VIRUSES

	MAYO CLINIC, 1974–1982		UNIV. OF VERMONT, 1980–1990
	INTERNAL	EXTERNAL	
Total isolates	4181	581	3014
% of total isolates			
Herpes simplex virus	43.8	82.2	84.0
Enterovirus	16.2	8.1	4.2
Influenza virus	10.0	0.3	0.4
Adenovirus	7.8	2.2	0.9
Cytomegalovirus	6.6	5.8	3.3
Varicella-zoster	6.6	0.7	1.5
Parainfluenza virus	5.6	0.7	0.9
Rhinovirus	2.2	0.0	0.1
Respiratory syncytial virus	0.9	0.0	4.4
Mumps virus	0.1	0.0	0.0
Unidentified	0.2	0.0	0.3
Total	100.0	100.0	100.0

* Adapted from Smith TF: Clinical uses of the diagnostic virology laboratory. Med Clin North Am 67:935–951, 1983

4-year-old children, 2.6% in 5- to 9-year-old children, and only 0.2% in 10- to 14-year-old children.[730] Herpes simplex virus[514] and CMV[386] may produce chronic infections and be shed intermittently into secretions and fluids.

The association of a clinical illness with a virus that has been recovered from a nonsterile site may be strengthened by demonstration of a serologic response to the isolated virus.

The optimal specimens for viral culture are aspirates of fluids, exudates, or secretions; tissues; washings of the upper airways; or stool specimens. Swab specimens, which are convenient, may also be obtained from these sites. Smith and associates isolated respiratory viruses from 12.5% of throat swabs that had already been processed for bacterial culture.[781] Calcium alginate swabs are toxic to herpes simplex virus,[182] and there is suggestive evidence that calcium alginate is toxic to respiratory syncytial virus also.[279] If the specimen is processed immediately or if the swab is removed from the transport medium, the toxicity of calcium alginate can be minimized, but it is best to avoid this material if possible.[58] Some investigators prefer not to use swabs with wooden shafts.

There are well-documented situations in which swabs are inferior to aspirates.[346] Aspirates or washings are probably optimal for recovery of all respiratory viruses,[849] although it is difficult to separate specimen type from swab characteristics and other variables in published reports.[279] Toxicity of swab material for certain viruses has already been mentioned. In addition, irreversible adsorption of viruses and infected cells to the swabs reduces the inoculum available for cell cultures. Levin and colleagues examined in a quantitative fashion the effect of swabs on recovery of VZV.[508]

Cotton and alginate swabs were immersed in stock suspensions of VZV; after only 5 minutes at 4°C, 80% to 90% of the viral particles had been lost.

McIntosh and colleagues detected more respiratory syncytial virus antigen in nasopharyngeal aspirates than in nasopharyngeal swabs.[373] Treuhaft and colleagues were able to isolate respiratory syncytial virus from 84% of infants in a mean of 4.2 days,[830] when nasopharyngeal aspirates were cultured. Concurrently, nasopharyngeal and throat swabs were collected from the same patients; respiratory syncytial virus was isolated from only 45% of the nasopharyngeal swabs in a mean of 5.5 days and from 39% of the throat swabs in a mean of 5.7 days. These investigators used alginate swabs in their study.

Rectal swabs are less valuable specimens than stool for the isolation of enterovirus but may be used if stool cannot be obtained.[565]

Viremia occurs frequently during viral infections but is not often detected. CMV viremia occurs regularly and can be detected by several methods (see pages 1212 and 1253).

Recently, respiratory syncytial virus antigen has been demonstrated in circulating peripheral blood monocytes.[217] Prather and colleagues have suggested that blood may be a useful specimen for diagnosis of enteroviral infection because they were able to isolate virus from 14 of 31 frozen serum specimens that had been collected from patients with enteroviral disease.[672,673]

To culture vesicular skin lesions, the skin should be cleansed with an alcohol swab and allowed to dry for at least 1 minute.[785] The vesicle should then be unroofed with a sterile scalpel and a sterile swab touched several times to the base. The swab should be placed in a viral transport medium, as described below. Alternatively, the contents of the vesicle may be aspirated with a tuberculin syringe and 26-gauge needle, if the vesicle is sufficiently large. Material for a Tzanck preparation can be collected by vigorously scraping the base of the lesion with the edge of a scalpel blade; the material on the blade is then touched to a glass slide and allowed to air dry.[785]

As a general rule, the frequency with which viruses are recovered decreases as the duration of illness increases so that every effort should be made to obtain specimens as early in the infection as possible.

TRANSPORTATION AND STORAGE OF SPECIMENS

Aspirates, fluids, and tissues should be transported to the laboratory in a sterile, leakproof container. Every effort should be made to minimize the interval between collection of the specimen and its inoculation into cell culture. Inoculation of cell cultures at the bedside has been recommended for some fragile viruses.[346] Ray and Minnich, however, found no significant effect on the rate of viral isolation when delays in transport were as great as 24 hours.[694] Bromberg and colleagues found that delays of up to 3 hours did not compromise the isolation of respiratory syncytial virus.[77] At the University of Vermont we have found the recovery of respiratory

TABLE 21-17

METHODS FOR DIAGNOSIS OF VIRAL INFECTIONS

VIRUS GROUP	ANTIGEN DETECTION	VIRUS ISOLATION	SEROLOGY
Adenoviruses	Described, but not generally available	Primary method	Paired sera required
Enteroviruses	Not available	Primary method	Not generally available; viral isolate required
Epstein-Barr virus	Not available	Not generally available	Primary method
Herpesviruses	Useful for VZV; CMV antigen; adequacy for herpes simplex varies	Primary method	Not useful except for immune status
Orthomyxoviruses	Influenza A enzyme immunoassay	Primary method	Paired sera required
Paramyxoviruses	Described, but not generally available	Primary method	Paired sera required
Rotaviruses	Primary method	Not generally available	Not practical for single cases
Rhabdoviruses	Primary method in reference laboratories	Primary method in reference laboratories	Useful for assessment of immunity
RSV	Useful for rapid diagnosis	Primary method	Paired sera required
Togaviruses (arboviruses and rubella)	Not available	Not generally available	Primary method

CMV, cytomegalovirus; VZV, varicella-zoster virus; RSV, respiratory syncytial virus

syncytial virus to be significantly greater in specimens that are inoculated into cell cultures within 1 hour than in specimens that are inoculated after a delay of up to 6 hours. When specimens that contain a labile virus must be transported to a reference laboratory, direct detection of antigen should be considered as an alternative.

Swabs should be placed into a transport medium that includes antibiotics; dry swabs are not acceptable. The type of transport medium is probably not critical. Huntoon and colleagues compared Stuart's (as used for bacterial cultures), Hanks', and Leibovitz-Emory media that had been incorporated into Culturette swabs by

the manufacturer (Marion Scientific, Kansas City, MO). Although the greatest number of isolates was recovered in Hanks' medium, the differences among the three media were not statistically significant.[411] Traditionally, a nutrient medium has been supplemented with a source of protein in an attempt to stabilize fragile viruses and with antibiotics to minimize bacterial contamination. The formula for such a medium, veal infusion broth (VIB), is given in Table 21-20. The sucrose–phosphate–glutamate (SPG) medium that was designed for *Chlamydia* is also an effective transport medium for viral specimens;[854] the formula for SPG

TABLE 21-18

COMPARISON OF DIAGNOSTIC METHODS

METHOD	TIME	ADVANTAGES	DISADVANTAGES
Culture	Days to weeks	Specificity and sensitivity maximum; isolate available for characterization	Cell culture facilities needed; time for diagnosis may be long
Direct detection	Hours to 1 day	Speed of diagnosis; used for viruses difficult to culture	False-positives and -negatives; hard to batch tests
Serology	Weeks	Assessment of immunity or response to virus isolated from nonsterile site; used for viruses difficult to culture	Potential cross-reaction; need for acute and convalescent specimens

TABLE 21-19
RECOMMENDED SPECIMENS FOR VIRAL CULTURE

SYNDROME	OPTIMAL SPECIMENS	PERMISSIBLE ALTERNATES AND ADDITIONAL SPECIMENS
Coryza Croup	Nasopharyngeal aspirate	Nasopharyngeal swab
Pharyngitis	Throat washing or swab	
Bronchiolitis Pneumonia	Nasopharyngeal aspirate Tracheal aspirate Lung aspirate or biopsy	Nasopharyngeal swab
Pleurodynia	Nasopharyngeal aspirate *plus* feces	Nasopharyngeal swab Rectal swab

Aseptic meningitis
Encephalitis
Transverse myelitis
	Spinal fluid
	(Use of feces, rectal swabs, and nasopharyngeal
	   specimens controversial)
		(Rectal swab)
		(Nasopharyngeal swab)
		Brain biopsy for herpes simplex; urine for measles
		   or mumps

Gastroenteritis	Feces	Rectal swab
Parotitis	Nasopharyngeal aspirate *plus* urine	Nasopharyngeal swab
Vesicular rash	Aspirate or swab of vesicle	
Maculopapular rash	Nasopharyngeal aspirate *plus* feces	Nasopharyngeal swab Rectal swab
Hemorrhagic cystitis	Urine	
Myocarditis Pericarditis	Nasopharyngeal aspirate *plus* feces	Urine for mumps virus Nasopharyngeal swab Rectal swab
Keratitis Conjunctivitis	Conjunctival or corneal scraping *plus* nasopharyngeal aspirate	Conjunctival or corneal swab Nasopharyngeal swab

Adapted from McIntosh K: Diagnostic virology. In Fields BN, Knipe DM, Melnick JL, et al (eds): Virology, 2nd ed.,
chap 16, pp 411–440. New York, Raven Press, 1990

medium is shown in Table 21-21. Commercial viral[423] and chlamydial[42] transport systems have also been reported to be suitable for herpes simplex virus.

Specimens should be refrigerated until they are inoculated into cell cultures. To select the best temperature for storage, one must balance the decrease in viral titer that occurs progressively at 4°C against the sudden decrease that occurs when specimens are frozen and thawed. It is clear that 1) the specimens should be maintained at −70°C if they are to be stored for a very long time (weeks or months) and 2) the best temperature is 4°C if the delay will be short (less than 24 hours). A reasonable recommendation is that specimens be refrigerated for up to 96 hours and frozen at −70°C if the delay will be longer.[555] The very worst temperature is −20°C, especially in a frost-free freezer, where repeated cycles of defrosting and freezing are extremely traumatic to all forms of life. Specimens should never be frozen in the freezing compartment of a standard refrigerator. Johnson has thoroughly reviewed the transport of specimens for viral diagnosis.[422]

ISOLATION OF VIRUSES IN CULTURE

Although a few of the largest hospital laboratories may have facilities for inoculation of animals, most diagnostic facilities are restricted to the use of in vitro analogs. For laboratories that cannot perform cell cultures, inoculation of embryonated eggs is a useful means for surveillance of influenza A virus infections.[381] Eggs are less convenient to manipulate than cell cultures and pose a greater potential biohazard.

PREPARATION AND MAINTENANCE OF CELL CULTURES

Cell culture is the cultivation in vitro of dissociated single cells. Tissue and organ culture is the maintenance in vitro of a portion of an organ, usually for short, delimited periods of time. The use of organ culture has been restricted almost completely to the research laboratory. For example, cultures of trachea have been used to isolate human coronaviruses, most of which do not grow in cell culture. Occasionally,

TABLE 21-20
VEAL INFUSION BROTH TRANSPORT MEDIUM

Veal infusion broth powder (BBL)	15 g
Distilled water	600 mL
Gelatin	3.0 g
Mix and autoclave 15 min, 15 lb, 121°C	
Cool and add antibiotics:	
Gentamicin (50 mg/mL)	0.6 mL
Amphotericin B (250 μg/mL) [Fungizone]	6.0 mL
Penicillin (100,000 U/mL)	2.0 mL
Aliquot 3 mL in sterile vials; store frozen, preferably at −70°C	

TABLE 21-21
SUCROSE–PHOSPHATE–GLUTAMATE TRANSPORT MEDIUM

Sucrose	75.00 g
KH_2PO_4	0.52 g
Na_2HPO_4	1.22 g
Glutamic acid	0.72 g
Distilled water, to	1000 mL
Adjust pH to 7.4–7.6 and autoclave	
Cool and add the following:	
Bovine serum, to	5%
Gentamicin	50 μg/mL
Vancomycin	100 μg/mL
Nystatin	25 U/mL

Nash P, Krenz MM: Culture media. In Balows A, Hausler WJ Jr, Herrmann KL, et al (eds): Manual of Clinical Microbiology, 5th ed, pp 1238–1239. Washington DC, American Society for Microbiology.

organ and cell cultures must be combined. For example, an explant of infected brain and an indicator monolayer of susceptible cells was used for the isolation of measles virus from patients with subacute sclerosing panencephalitis.[650] Other references are available for readers who desire more detailed information than can be provided in this chapter.[282,745]

Cell cultures are of three types (Table 21-22). Primary cell cultures consist of a mixture of cells, usually kidney or lung, obtained by dissociation of cells from the minced organ. These cells can be maintained in culture for a limited time only. Once subcultured in vitro a primary cell culture becomes a cell line. The most commonly used cell lines are composed of fibroblasts, obtained from skin or embryonic lung. A cell line is diploid if at least 75% of the cells have a normal complement of chromosomes. A cell line is heteroploid if more than 25% of the cells have an abnormal complement of chromosomes.

The life expectancy of normal diploid cells is approximately 50 serial doublings in vitro;[367] those cell lines that have been transferred at least 70 times are considered to be established cell lines. These established or continuous lines may be derived from normal tissue, as was the Vero cell line from African green monkey renal cells. Alternatively, they may originate from neoplastic epithelium, such as the HeLa cells that came from a cervical adenocarcinoma and the HEp-2 cells that were derived from a carcinoma of the larynx. The appearance of uninoculated cell cultures is illustrated in Figure 21-5. The fibroblastic cells are usually long, spindly, and oriented in parallel, whereas the established cell lines consist of polygonal epithelial cells. The primary cultures naturally contain a mixture of cell types.

Conditions for growth and maintenance of cell cultures vary considerably, and only a few generalizations are possible. The temperature of incubation is optimal at 36°C to 37°C but may be lowered to 35°C after confluence of cells is achieved. This maneuver may facilitate isolation of viruses, such as myxoviruses and rhinoviruses, that grow optimally at 33°C. A physiologic pH must be maintained. Usually a CO_2-bicarbonate buffering system is used, CO_2 being supplied by the metabolizing cells in a closed tube or flask. In an open system a CO_2-air mixture must be provided. Buffering compounds that do not depend on CO_2-bicarbonate, such as HEPES buffer (N-2-hydroxyethylpiperazine-N'-2-ethanesulfonic-acid), may be used in open systems if an incubator with CO_2 is not available. A pH indicator is often included in the media to monitor closely shifts in pH during incubation. Phenol red, which is red at physiologic pH, turning yellow at acidic pH and purple at alkaline pH, is frequently used.

Essential vitamins and amino acids must be supplied in viral culture media. These compounds are stable when stored at 4°C, except for L-glutamine, which must be replenished periodically.[584] Eagle's Minimum

TABLE 21-22
TYPES OF CELL CULTURES

TYPE OF CULTURE	CHARACTERISTICS	EXAMPLES	PRIMARY USE
Primary	Diploid; mixed cell types; 1 or 2 passages	Primary monkey kidney	Influenza; parainfluenza; some enteroviruses
Cell lines	Diploid; fibroblasts; limited passage (<50–70)	Human diploid fibroblast (WI-38, MRC-5, or HEL)	Herpes simplex; cytomegalovirus; varicella-zoster; rhinovirus
Established cell lines	Heteroploid; continuous passage in vitro	HeLa; HEp-2	Adenovirus; respiratory syncytial virus

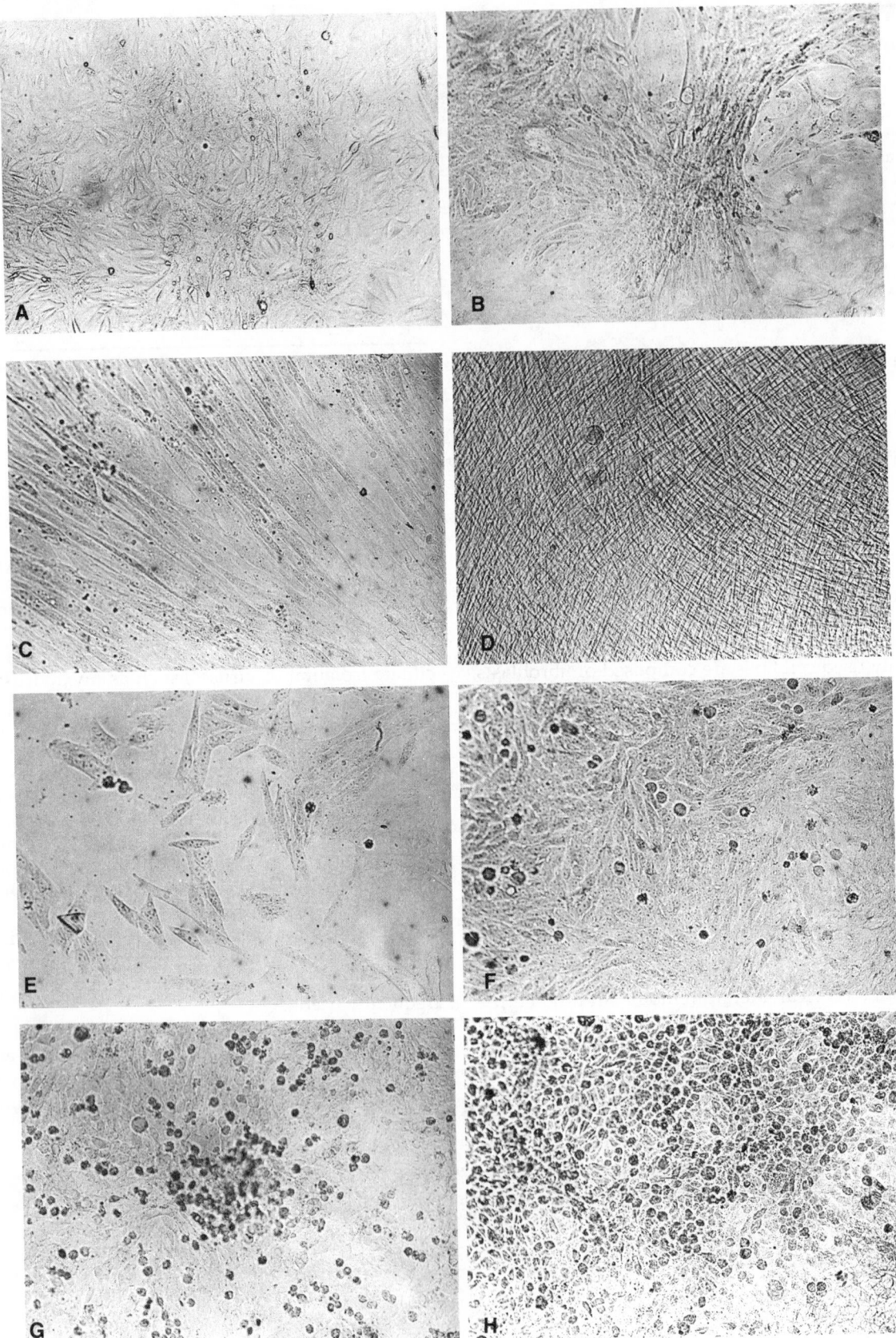

Figure 21-5

Essential Medium (MEM) is the most commonly used, both for growth and for maintenance of cells (Table 21-23). It is usually supplemented with small amounts of serum (up to 5%) for maintenance of a monolayer after cells have reached confluent growth. To enhance initial growth, larger amounts of serum (usually 10%) are used. It is important that the serum be free of infectious agents, including the mycoplasmas, and not contain antibodies to any viruses that might be present in clinical specimens. For this reason, either fetal, newborn, or agammaglobulinemic calf serum is most commonly used. Other formulations, such as Medium 199 or RPMI 1640, contain a richer mixture of nutrients and may be optimal for maintenance of some cell lines. Two forms of balanced salt solution are most frequently used, both for washing of cells and for incorporation into complete media (Table 21-24). The formulations of Hanks' and Earle's solutions differ in several respects, notably the amount of buffering capacity. The two solutions are used virtually interchangeably, but Earle's balanced salt solution with its greater buffering power may be desirable for prolonged maintenance of monolayers.

CONTAMINATION OF CELL CULTURES

Contamination of media is reduced by inclusion of antibiotics. Penicillin (200 µg/mL) and streptomycin (200 µg/mL) or gentamicin (50 µg/mL) are commonly used for suppression of bacterial growth; amphotericin B (1.25 µg/mL) is used for inhibition of fungal growth.[407] The use of antibiotics does not substitute, however, for careful aseptic technique.

Contamination of culture media by *Mycoplasma* species is a common and troublesome problem.[554] *Mycoplasma* species usually are introduced in the serum additives or from contaminated stock viruses; once in the culture, they are very difficult to eradicate. The effects on the cells include suboptimal growth and disturbances in the interactions of cells and viruses. The presence of contaminating *Mycoplasma* species may be monitored by recovering them in culture, by staining for *Mycoplasma* DNA, by biochemical measurement of uracil incorporation, or by nucleoside phosphorylase activity techniques. Commercial suppliers of cells should document their efforts at surveillance and quality control.

In addition, cell cultures may be contaminated with viruses (usually ones that were present in the original tissue)[407] or even with other cells.[608] The most frequent type of viral contamination is the presence of indigenous simian viruses in primary monkey cell cultures, such as the vacuolating agent (SV40), foamy viruses, or the monkey parainfluenza virus (SV5). Simian viruses that have hemagglutinins (eg, SV5 virus) may produce misleading results if hemadsorption tests are performed to detect human respiratory viruses. When myxoviruses are sought, it is important to perform control hemadsorption tests on uninoculated tubes from the same lot of cells that was used for the clinical specimens (see Chart 35; Fig. 21-12E). The frequency with which tubes in a shipment of monkey kidney cells are contaminated may vary from 5% to 100%. Reserving a few uninoculated tubes for hemadsorption controls is not foolproof. If an unusual number of patients have hemadsorbing viruses on a given day, the possibility of simian virus contamination should be considered. Contamination of a commercial lot of A-549 cells with infectious bovine rhinotracheitis virus caused diagnostic problems in several laboratories.[269] The cytopathic effect in the contaminated monolayers resembled herpes simplex virus, but the agent could not be typed with

◀ **Figure 21-5**

Normal cell cultures. (**A**) Normal rhesus monkey kidney monolayer. This primary culture is just at confluence—there are no spaces between the cells, but cells have not begun to pile on each other. The variability of the cells in the monolayer is a reflection of their origin from diverse cell types (×180). (**B**) Normal rhesus monkey kidney monolayer. After continued incubation, areas of more luxuriant growth have become evident. The variability of the cells in the monolayer can still be appreciated (×180). (**C**) Normal MRC-5 fibroblast monolayer. These diploid fibroblastic cells have the elongated, spindly character of their type. They are just reaching confluence; a few spaces remain between some of the cells (×180). (**D**) Normal MRC fibroblast monolayer. After continued incubation, the criss-cross pattern of fibroblasts piled one on top of the other is apparent. The detail of the individual cells is less apparent. Such senescent monolayers should not be inoculated (×180). (**E**) Normal HEp-2 cells. An established cell line has been subcultured, and new cells have begun to grow. There are large spaces between individual cells, which have a spindle shape as they spread over the new glass surface (×180). (**F**) Normal HEp-2 cells. The subcultured cells have now multiplied to the point of confluence but are still easily visible as distinct polygonal cells. The ideal point for inoculation of most viruses is at this stage or slightly earlier (×180). (**G**) Normal HEp-2 cells. After continued incubation, the cell line has multiplied so that cells are piled one on top of the other. Cells that are dividing or detaching from the glass appear rounded. As the monolayers age, they become less susceptible to the cytopathic effect of viruses, and it becomes increasingly difficult to detect the cytopathic effect visually. (**H**) Normal McCoy cells. This established cell line, the origin of which is unknown, is pictured at a point where confluent growth has been obtained. The cells are compact and polygonal. Specimens should be inoculated at this stage or when the cells are slightly less confluent (×180).

TABLE 21-23
EAGLE'S MINIMUM ESSENTIAL MEDIUM (MEM)

COMPONENT	CONSTITUENTS	STORAGE
Base	Hanks' or Earle's balanced salt solutions (BSS)	4°C 4°C
L-Amino acids	Arginine, histidine, lysine, tryptophane, phenylalanine, threonine, leucine, valine, isoleucine, methionine, tyrosine, cysteine	4°C
Vitamins	Nicotinamide, pyridoxal, thiamine, pantothenic acid, choline, *i*-inositol, riboflavin, biotin, folic acid	−20°C −20°C
Labile amino acids	L-glutamine (added at time of use)	−20°C
Antibiotics	Gentamicin (50 µg/mL) or penicillin (200 U/mL) and streptomycin (200 µg/mL) added at time of use	−20°C
Growth medium	10% fetal, newborn, or agammaglobulinemic calf serum	4°C
Maintenance medium	0–2% calf serum	4°C

Adapted from Hsiung GD: Diagnostic Virology Illustrated by Light and Electron Microscopy, 3rd ed. New Haven, Yale University Press, 1982; Schmidt NJ: Cell culture techniques for diagnostic virology. In Lennette EH, Schmidt NJ (eds): Diagnostic Procedures for Viral, Rickettsial and Chlamydial Infections, 5th ed, pp 65–139. Washington DC, American Public Health Association, 1979

available antisera. An additional problem was the inhibition by the contaminant virus of adenovirus that was in two of the specimens. The adenovirus isolates were subsequently recovered by inoculation of a new lot of A-549 cells with residual specimen.

An extremely rare but potentially serious problem can be caused by the presence of pathogenic viruses in the tissues of monkeys. Although fortunately very rare, the simian herpes virus and Marburg virus, which produces a hemorrhagic fever, have caused lethal laboratory infections. These agents provide justification for working with primary cell cultures of simian origin in a biologic safety cabinet.

Contamination of cell cultures with other cells has resulted in the erroneous supposition that a new cell line has been established in more than one research laboratory. In fact, a hardy HeLa cell may have found its way into the flask and taken over.[608] In the diagnostic laboratory, cross-contamination of an established cell line onto a diploid cell line or primary cell culture may give the appearance of cytopathic effects in the victimized cell culture (Fig. 21-6*D*).

TECHNICAL ASPECTS OF CELL CULTURE

A variety of containers is used for the support of cell monolayers. The most common cell cultures in use are commercially available in tubes or vials that are ready for inoculation of specimens. Many laboratories may prefer, for reasons of economy, to maintain cell lines in their own laboratories. T-shaped plastic flasks have generally replaced glass bottles for the propagation of cell lines (Fig. 21-7).

Cell lines may be maintained in the laboratory by dissociation of cells, which are then distributed into new vessels (Box 21-3).

Established monolayers are dissociated by brief incubation in a solution of trypsin or a mixture of ethylenediaminetetraacetic acid (EDTA), which is also known as versene, and trypsin. Damage to cells may occur if the suspension of trypsin is too concentrated or if the contact is too prolonged. Neutralization of the trypsin is provided by serum in the growth medium that is added after cells have been dissociated. Detachment of the cells from the surface may be enhanced physically by agitation or by scraping with a rubber-

TABLE 21-24
BALANCED SALT SOLUTIONS

	PER LITER OF 10 × SOLUTION	
	EARLE'S	*HANKS'*
NaCl	68.0 g	80.0 g
KCl	4.0 g	4.0 g
CaCl$_2$	2.0 g	1.4 g
MgSO$_4$ · 7H$_2$O	2.0 g	2.0 g
NaH$_2$PO$_4$ · 12H$_2$O		1.2 g
NaH$_2$PO$_4$ · H$_2$O	1.4 g	
KH$_2$PO$_4$		0.6 g
Glucose	10.0 g	10.0 g
Phenol red, 1%	20.0 mL	16.0 mL
2.8% NaHCO$_3$ (added to 1 × solution)		1.25%
8.8% NaHCO$_3$ (added to 1 × solution)	2.5%	

Adapted from Schmidt NJ: Cell culture techniques for diagnostic virology. In Lennette EH, Schmidt NJ (eds): Diagnostic Procedures for Viral, Rickettsial and Chlamydial Infections, 5th ed, pp 65–139. Washington DC, American Public Health Association, 1979

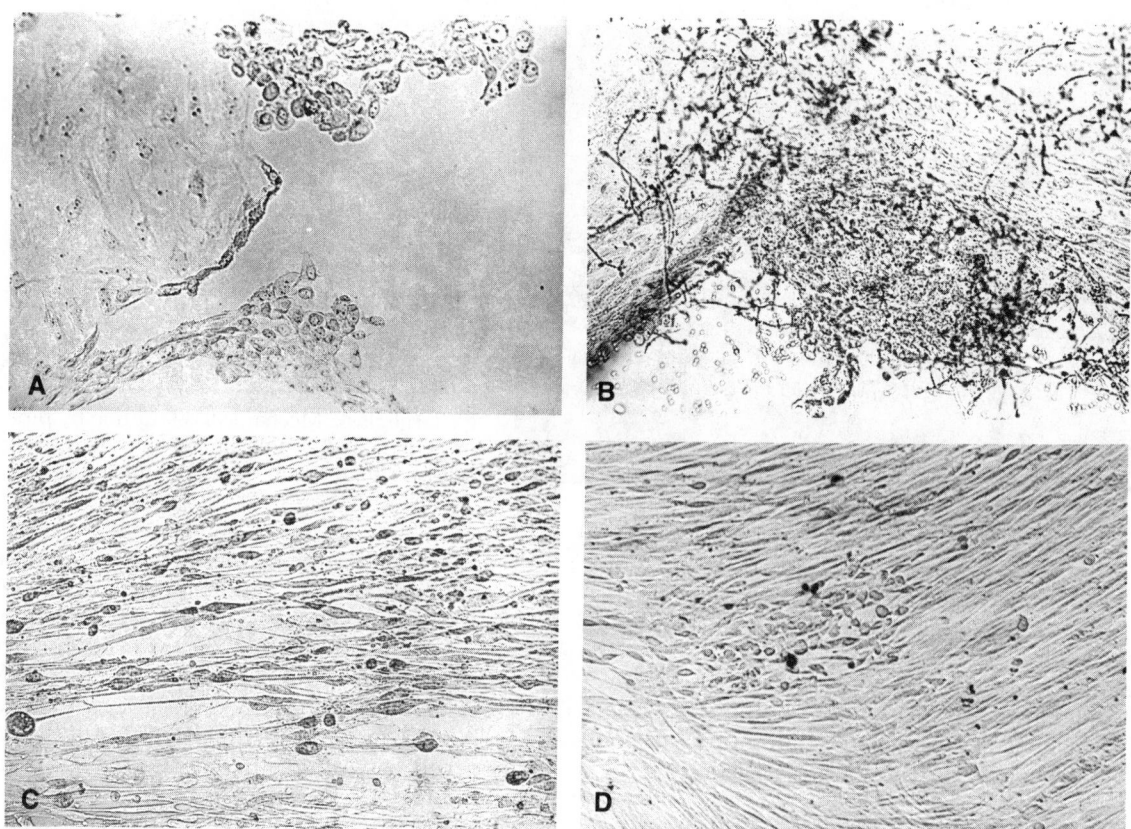

Figure 21-6

Artifacts in cell culture. (**A**) Rhesus monkey kidney cells. The tube has been inoculated with a specimen that contained nonspecific toxic material. Cells in the monolayer have rounded up focally, and many cells have detached from the glass. The nonviral effect can be distinguished from viral cytopathic effect by the overall pattern, by the rapidity of occurrence, and by the inability to reproduce the nonspecific effect after subculture into fresh monolayers (×180). (**B**) Rhesus monkey kidney cell culture. A stool specimen was inadequately decontaminated before inoculation. Bacteria and fungal hyphae are evident on the monolayer, which is granular and will soon degenerate. The media may become acidic and cloudy. Retreatment of the specimen with additional antibiotics is necessary. The specimen may also be filtered, but cell-associated viruses may be lost (×180). (**C**) MRC-5 fibroblasts. A filtrate of stool that contained *Clostridium difficile* was inoculated onto the monolayer 24 hours earlier. The generalized disorganization of the monolayer with rounding and sloughing of cells is typical of this toxin. Specific identification of the cause of toxicity is provided by neutralization of the effect with specific antiserum. *C. difficile* toxin may give an initial impression of viral cytopathic effect, but the effect will not be reproduced when material from the suspect tube is subcultured onto additional monolayers (×180). (**D**) MRC-5 fibroblasts. Focal cell rounding and enlargement appeared on these fibroblasts that had been inoculated with cerebrospinal fluid, suggesting viral cytopathic effect. The atypical progression of the cytopathic effect and observation that some of the foci were superimposed on the fibroblasts suggested cellular contamination. HEp-2 cells were subsequently recovered from the tube and demonstrated to have a karyotype that was identical to that of the HEp-2 cells used in the laboratory. The mechanism by which the contamination occurred was never elucidated (×180).

tipped glass rod, a device known as a "rubber police-man" (see Fig. 21-7). The dissociated cells are then dispensed into tubes for inoculation of specimens or into additional flasks for continued propagation of stock cells. The density of the suspension can be adjusted to provide confluent monolayers after 1 or more days of incubation. After inoculation of clinical specimens, the same protocol may be used to prepare infected cells for subculture to additional monolayers.

Round-bottomed glass tubes (16 × 125 mm) are the most commonly used containers for viral isolation (Fig. 21-8). These tubes are incubated at a 5° fixed angle, so that the monolayer forms on one side of the tube. The heaviest aggregation occurs near the center and at the butt of the tubes; the thinnest layer is at the edges and toward the mouth. Round Petri dishes or glass slides, onto which are affixed plastic chambers, are less frequently used for diagnostic purposes. The slide-cham-

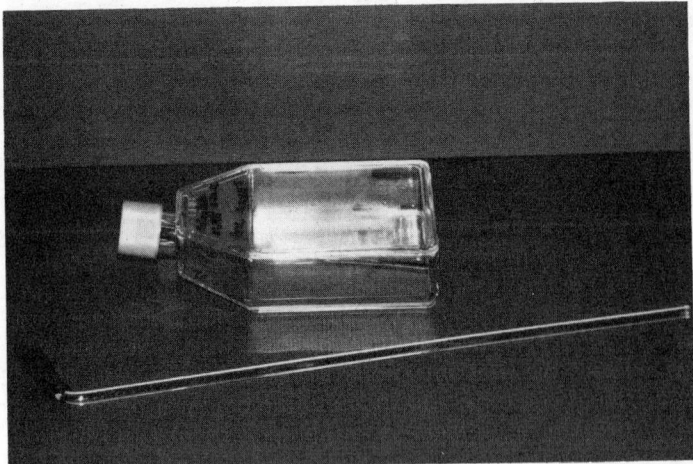

Figure 21-7

T-shaped plastic flask and rubber-tipped glass rod, known as a "rubber policeman." Monolayers of cell lines may be grown in large flasks. Many individual tubes for virus culture may be prepared from a single large flask. Mechanical disruption by pipetting or by the "rubber policeman" helps to dislodge the cells during trypsinization for subculture.

ber system is expensive but useful if morphologic study of an undisrupted monolayer is planned.

Recently, shell vials, originally used for isolation of *Chlamydia trachomatis*, have been used to increase the frequency and speed with which viruses are isolated. A cell monolayer is prepared on a round glass coverslip that has been placed on the bottom of a flat-bottomed vial (Fig. 21-9). If the inoculum is centrifuged onto the monolayer, as is essential for the recovery of *C. trachomatis*, and the monolayer stained with fluorescein-conjugated antiserum or tested with a molecular probe, almost all isolates of herpes simplex virus can be detected within 24 hours.[244,311,735] The recovery of herpes simplex virus in conventional culture is sufficiently rapid that addition of an expensive procedure can be questioned. A far more dramatic improvement in the speed of isolation has been reported for CMV.[270,309] The technique is more sensitive than conventional culture for most specimens other than blood, but use of both approaches maximizes results.[685] The shell vial technique is still useful but less productive with blood specimens, only partly because of toxicity of the specimen. Heparin is usually recommended as the best anticoagulant. Kimpton and colleagues found that none of the anticoagulants they studied damaged cell-associated CMV, but heparin and EDTA killed cell-free virus.[451] They reported that sodium citrate was the preferred choice, but clinical studies have not been performed. In a clinical study, recovery of CMV was equivalent when the blood sample was collected in EDTA-lithium or heparin vacutainer tubes.[802] White blood cell separators that provide both neutrophils and monocytes are superior to physical separation of the buffy coat.[405] The results are influenced significantly by the number of leukocytes in the sample, many of which come from leukopenic patients.[517]

The gain from shell vial culture comes both from centrifugation and from the use of a fluoresceinated monoclonal of high quality.[421] Even supposedly uniform reagents, such as monoclonal antibodies, may vary from lot to lot. Nonspecific staining of cell nuclei may occur with some lots of antisera. The appearance of a shell vial culture containing CMV is shown in Color Plate 21-2*F*. Paya and colleagues have studied the number of shell vials required for each specimen.[649] They found that three vials were required for maximal yield from blood specimens, whereas two vials were needed for urine, bronchoalveolar lavage, and tissue. Fedorko and colleagues found that the age of fibroblasts in the shell vials was important for recovery of cytomegalovirus. Old monolayers (8–15 days) were less sensitive for virus recovery but more sensitive to toxic components in the specimens.[253] Most laboratories depend on commercial suppliers for shell vials, and it is difficult for manufacturers to provide young monolayers. Pretreatment of monolayers with dexamethasone and dimethyl sulfoxide enhanced detection of CMV in confluent monolayers,[871] but this finding was unfortunately not confirmed in a clinical study.[254]

Gleaves and colleagues have reported success with still a third cell-associated herpesvirus, VZV.[307] They examined 68 specimens from 60 patients. VZV was identified by some method in 57% of patients. The sensitivity of diagnostic techniques in decreasing order was direct immunofluorescence of skin scrapings, shell vial culture, and conventional culture. Schirm and colleagues have confirmed the utility of

---

BOX 21-3. PROCEDURE FOR MAINTAINING CELL LINES

1. The monolayer is washed with phosphate-buffered saline, pH 7.5.

2. A suspension of 0.25% trypsin or equal parts of 0.25% trypsin and 1:2000 versene is added for 15 to 30 seconds, then removed.

3. The monolayer is incubated at 35°C until the cells have dissociated. Gentle shaking of the flask may enhance dissociation.

4. Growth medium is added and the cells resuspended at the concentration desired for subculture. Alternatively, the cells may be divided arbitrarily (1:2 or 1:3) as dictated by past experience.

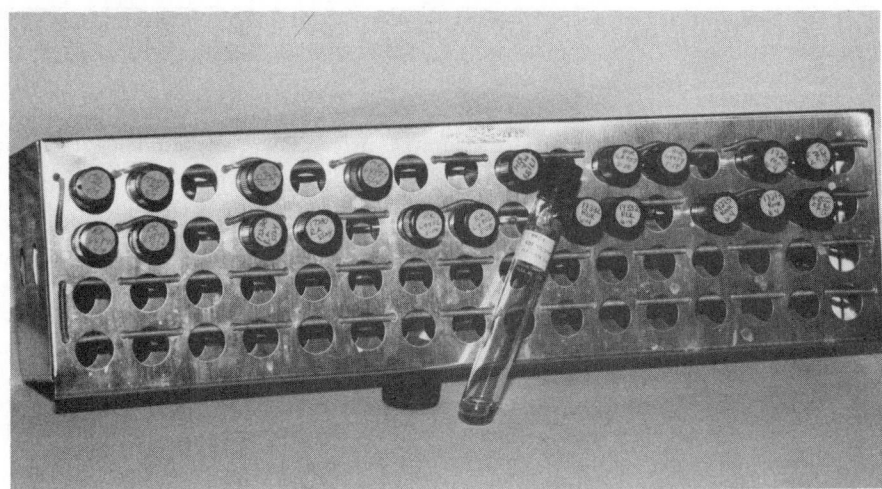

Figure 21-8
Viral culture tubes are slanted at a fixed angle of 5° in a stationary rack. Metal springs hold the tubes in place. Round labels for the tops of the tubes facilitate identification of cultures without removing the tubes from the racks.

shell vial culture for VZV.[743] They were able to detect half of the positive patients within 3 days using shell vials and a monoclonal antibody, whereas the conventional tube method detected a third of the patients after a mean of 7.5 days. Pérez and colleagues detected an equivalent number of isolates in shell vials and conventional tubes.[657] One factor in the yield of cell cultures is the choice of cell lines. Human diploid fibroblasts have been used most commonly, but the addition of rhesus monkey kidney cells[873] or A-549 cells[75] substantially improves the recovery rate in conventional tube cultures. The enhanced recovery is less evident with shell vial cultures.[75] Presumably the shell vial centrifugation technique increases contact of inoculum with monolayer, but the exact mechanisms are unknown.

The shell vial technique has been applied also to viruses other than the herpes group, including influenza virus,[46,245,755,801] adenovirus,[243,848] and BK virus.[544]

Several investigators have had luck with variations on the shell vial theme. Hughes and colleagues enhanced detection of herpes simplex virus by using continuous high-speed rolling of conventional cell culture tubes.[410] Oefinger and colleagues obtained enhanced

recovery of CMV by centrifuging both shell vials and conventional tubes.[625]

SELECTION OF CELL CULTURES FOR ISOLATION OF VIRUSES

The minimum requirements for isolation of viruses in culture are a primary culture of simian kidney cells (for isolation of myxoviruses and enteroviruses) and a diploid cell line of human origin (essential for isolation of CMV, rhinovirus, and VZV; useful for isolation of herpes simplex virus). The addition of an established cell line of human origin (eg, HEp-2) is also useful for isolation of adenovirus and respiratory syncytial virus.

Other cell lines may provide satisfactory substitutes for these three basic cell types if isolation of a specific virus is desired. The additional cell lines may be used as substitutes for simian cells if they are not available; alternatively, they may be used selectively to enhance the isolation rate of specific viruses during seasons when infections would be expected. There are no substitutes for human diploid fibroblasts. Some diagnostic alternatives for specific viral groups are summarized in Box 21-4.

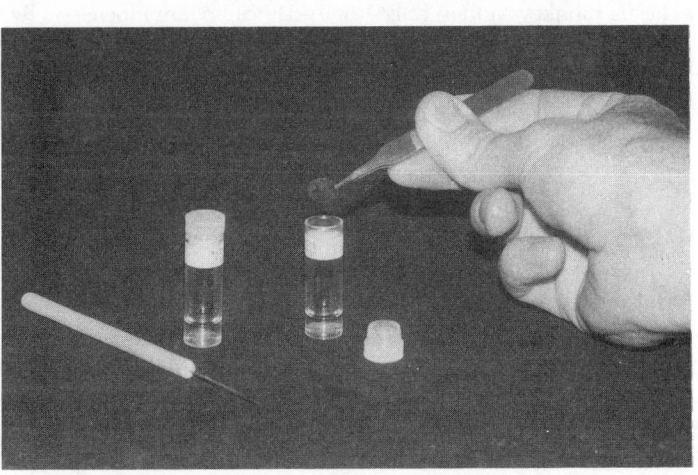

Figure 21-9
Shell vials for isolation of *Chlamydia trachomatis* and viruses. The vials are round with a flat bottom and contain a round coverslip on which the cells are grown. The top may be rubber or plastic as shown here. The coverslip is removed with forceps or with a needle.

BOX 21-4. ALTERNATIVE CELL CULTURES FOR SPECIFIC VIRAL GROUPS

Myxoviruses

Myxoviruses may be isolated in the Madin-Darby canine kidney (MDCK) continuous cell line.[277,559] Meguro and colleagues isolated influenza virus more frequently in MDCK cells than in either embryonated eggs or monkey kidney cells. Addition of trypsin (2 µg/mL) and EDTA (0.9 µg/mL) to the medium did not increase the number of isolates, but shortened the time required for detection of viral growth.[559] Parainfluenza viruses were also isolated, but less frequently than in monkey kidney cells. Frank and colleagues found that LLC-MK2 cells were an acceptable substitute for monkey kidney cells as an isolation system for parainfluenza viruses.[277] Influenza A virus may be isolated efficiently in embryonated eggs.[381]

Herpes Simplex Virus

Herpes simplex virus may be isolated more quickly and more reliably in primary cultures of guinea pig embryo or rabbit kidney than in human embryonic lung fibroblasts.[489] In our laboratory, the relative performance of fibroblasts and rabbit kidney cells has varied considerably with different lots or sources of cells. The primary cultures support the growth of fewer viruses so that a presumptive identification of herpes simplex viruses can be made with somewhat greater certainty if growth occurs in these cells. Conversely, use of these cells has the disadvantage that they must be used in addition to fibroblasts. Local preparation of the primary cultures is not an option for most laboratories.

Herpes simplex virus can also be isolated in established cell lines, which are less expensive than primary cell cultures. Vero cells (derived from African green monkey kidneys) are more sensitive than are HeLa or HEp-2 cells. Salmon and colleagues found that a continuous line of mink lung cells was equivalent to primary rabbit kidney cells and more sensitive than either human lung fibroblasts or Vero cells for isolation of herpes simplex virus.[734] Chang and colleagues, however, found that the mink cells did not support the growth of herpes simplex as well as rabbit kidney cells or a variety of human fibroblasts.[141]

Varicella-Zoster Virus

Varicella-zoster virus can be recovered more reliably if rhesus monkey kidney cells[873] or A-549 cells[75] are inoculated in addition to human diploid fibroblasts, as discussed previously.

Enteroviruses

Isolation of enteroviruses may be enhanced by use of additional cell lines. Serotypes of coxsackievirus A that normally require inoculation of suckling mice can be isolated in RD cells, which were derived from a human rhabdomyosarcoma.[749] Both the rate and speed of isolation of coxsackievirus B is enhanced in BGM cells, a continuous African green monkey kidney cell line.[566] Inoculation of primary monkey kidney cultures is still necessary for isolation of echoviruses. The extra expense incurred must be balanced against the earlier provision of results that may influence clinical decisions.[155]

Adenoviruses

Some virologists consider primary human embryonic kidney cells to be the optimal system for recovery of adenoviruses.[73, 286] These cells may be difficult and expensive to obtain; furthermore, not all laboratories have found them essential.[779] Adenoviruses, particularly fastidious adenoviruses (serotypes 40 and 41), may be isolated with greater frequency in cell line 293, which is a continuous line of human embryonic kidney cells that have been transformed with type 5 adenovirus.[81, 816] The cells contain approximately 12% of the adenovirus 5 genome. Although other viruses, such as enteroviruses and herpes simplex virus, may be isolated in these cells, they are not sufficiently sensitive to substitute for fibroblasts or primary monkey kidney cultures. Some virologists have assumed that an adenovirus isolated in conventional cell lines, such as HEp-2, is not a "noncultivable" enteric adenovirus. Perron-Henry and colleagues isolated 40% of enteric adenoviruses in HEp-2 cells, so such an assumption is not warranted.[660]

Miscellaneous

Recently A-549 cells, derived from a human carcinoma, have been shown to be effective at isolating herpes simplex virus, adenovirus, and enteroviruses but not respiratory syncytial virus, rhinovirus, or influenza A virus.[893] This cell line can be locally maintained in laboratories that have adequate cell culture facilities. Minnich and colleagues have isolated measles virus in approximately 65% of nasopharyngeal-throat swabs from patients with clinical measles.[572] By using A-549 cells in shell vials and a fluoresceinated monoclonal antibody they were able to recover most isolates in 24 to 48 hours.

The quality and provenance of the cells used for isolation are important. Careful studies of cloned fibroblasts from a single fetus demonstrated a large variation in the degree to which the clones supported the growth of respiratory viruses.[835] Variants of established cell lines, such as HeLa and HEp-2, differ also in the sensitivity with which they support some viruses. It is important to ensure that the selected cell variant is of adequate sensitivity.

Once a cell line has been found acceptable, multiple aliquots should be frozen in liquid nitrogen. Cells for daily use may be maintained in continuous culture. The original stock should be used periodically to replenish the working stock, so that the cells do not mutate to a state that is less susceptible to viral growth.

Rhesus and cynomolgus monkey kidney cells are comparable for isolation of myxoviruses. MRC-5 fibroblasts, on the other hand, have been reported to be more sensitive than WI-38 fibroblasts for the isolation of CMV.[331] The sensitivity of all diploid cell lines decreases as the number of passages increases. Some commercial suppliers are now using cells that have been subcultured as many as 30 times. The lowest passage level from a reliable supplier should be sought. If cell sheets, particularly those of established cell lines, are too thick, recovery of viruses may be reduced and evaluation of cytopathic effects is difficult. For some viruses, islands of cells or a barely confluent monolayer are preferable to a fully confluent cell sheet.[830]

Additionally, the cells must be in sufficiently good condition to last the several weeks necessary for isolation of slowly growing viruses. Contamination with *Mycoplasma* species should be avoided if maximal isolation rates are to be ensured. Viruses, such as VZV, that spread directly from cell to cell rather than through the culture medium, require a healthy monolayer. Use of growth medium with 10% serum may enhance development and progression of cytopathic effects caused by these viruses,[865] although we have not been impressed that this manipulation is necessary. In contrast, serum contains inhibitors of myxoviruses and paramyxoviruses. The maintenance medium in the cells used for these viruses (usually primary monkey kidney) should be free of serum.

INOCULATION AND INCUBATION OF CELL CULTURES

Transport vials that contain swabs should be vortexed and material from the swab expressed into the medium, which contains antibiotics. Tissues are minced and homogenized in a small volume of transport broth. It may be necessary to suspend fecal specimens in 10 volumes of transport medium. Feces, tissues, and respiratory aspirates that contain excessive debris or mucus may be clarified by low-speed centrifugation. Antibiotics are present in most transport and tissue culture media. If bacterial or fungal contamination of the specimen is expected, additional antibiotics should be added to the specimen before inoculation (penicillin and streptomycin or gentamicin plus amphotericin at twice the concentration used in cell culture media).[407] After processing, the specimen may be inoculated into the culture media. Alternatively, the inoculum may be placed directly onto the monolayer after most of the culture media has been removed. The more direct contact of viral particles with cells enhances infectivity and may increase both the number of isolates and the speed with which they are recovered. After adsorption of the inoculum onto the monolayer for 30 to 60 minutes at 36°C to 37°C, the medium is replaced and incubation of the culture is continued. Toxic substances in the specimen may also be more evident after adsorption of the inoculum. If two tubes of each cell type are used, one may be inoculated by introducing a specimen into the medium and the other by adsorption. Any remaining specimen should be retained at 4°C or frozen at −70°C in case toxicity or bacterial contamination occurs. If bacterial or fungal

growth results, additional antibiotics may be added to the specimen. The specimen may be passed through a 0.45-μm micropore filter before additional cultures are inoculated, but viruses that are cell associated, such as CMV and VZV, may be lost when infected cells are trapped in the filter.[508] Nonspecific toxicity to the monolayer is usually evident within 24 hours; the specimen may then be reinoculated after making a 1:10 dilution in balanced salt solution. The pH of the specimen should also be checked and adjusted to neutrality if the specimen is very acid or alkaline. If nonspecific degeneration of the monolayer occurs after incubation for several days, the cells and fluid may be subcultured onto fresh monolayer.

Monolayers should be incubated at 36°C to 37°C for recovery of most viruses. The optimal temperature of incubation for respiratory viruses, especially rhinovirus, is 33°C, but recovery of other viruses may be reduced at this temperature. Use of a roller drum (Fig. 21-10) facilitates isolation of pathogens in primary monkey kidney and diploid fibroblast cells, especially from respiratory specimens.

Two weeks of incubation is adequate for the recovery of most other viruses. Less than 10% of isolates that are not CMV were recovered after 14 days at the Mayo Clinic.[375] CMV may require longer incubation, but Gregory and Menegus found that 92% of CMV isolates were recovered within 14 days when MRC-5 fibroblasts were used.[331] If the recovery of only herpes simplex virus is sought, the period of incubation may be further abbreviated to 7 days. Centrifugation of the inoculum and detection of antigen will dramatically shorten the detection time for several viruses, includ-

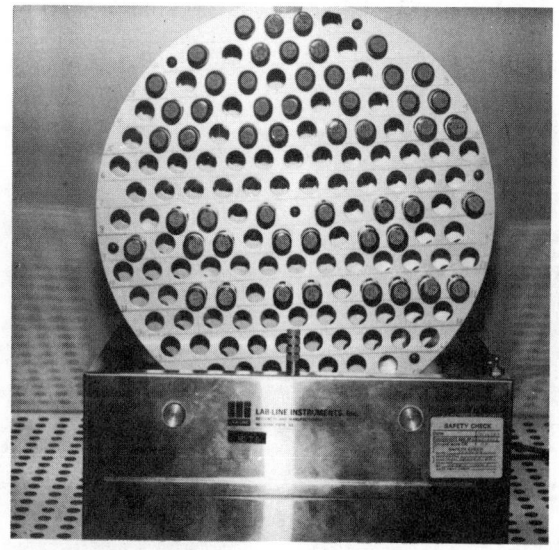

Figure 21-10
Roller drum for viral cultures. The cytopathic effect of many viruses, especially those that cause respiratory infection, is enhanced by slow rotation of the tubes, so that one revolution occurs every 3 minutes.

ing CMV and VZV. Hemadsorption tests should be performed after incubation of primary monkey kidney cells for 5 and 10 days.

DETECTION OF VIRUS AND PROVISIONAL IDENTIFICATION

CYTOPATHIC EFFECT

The most common method for detecting a virus is examination of cultures for virus-induced damage to the monolayers or cytopathic effect. Monolayers should be examined daily if herpes simplex virus is sought and at least three times a week if more slowly growing viruses are suspected. Glass tubes can be examined with a conventional light microscope, using simple holders to prevent the round tubes from rolling on the microscope stage (Fig. 21-11). If the monolayer is to be examined in shell vials, an inverted microscope must be used.

Provisional identification of the specific virus (or at least the virus group) can often be provided on the basis of the type of cytopathic effect and the type of cell that is affected. Typical patterns of cytopathic effect and the rate of isolation for viruses most commonly isolated in hospital laboratories are summarized in Table 21-25.

When one examines a culture in the laboratory, the pattern of cytopathic effect is known but the name of the virus is not. A flow chart for analyzing cytopathic effect in a clinical specimen is presented in Table 21-26. This table represents the most common patterns of cytopathic effect. The inclusion of all possible combinations for all strains would make the table unwieldy and probably useless.

The effects of the virus on the cells may be subtle initially. Although quantitation of the viral inoculum based on the extent of cytopathic effect is not precise, it is useful to make a laboratory record of the semiquan-

titative estimate for comparative purposes (1+ = less than 25% of the monolayer affected; 2+ = 25% to 50%; 3+ = 51% to 75%; 4+ = more than 75%). These estimates make it easier to document progression of cytopathic effect and establish the presence of a cytopathic agent. It may be necessary to subculture the cells from a tube with possible cytopathic effect onto fresh monolayers. If possible, such a subculture should be performed after cytopathic effect has reached 2+, using trypsinization, physical disruption of the monolayer with a "rubber policeman," or several cycles of quick freeze/thawing. Then, an aliquot is inoculated onto the type of cell in which cytopathic effect was originally observed and any other cell type that might aid in making a provisional diagnosis.

Viral cytopathic effects for three commonly used cell cultures are demonstrated sequentially in Figures 21-12 through 21-15. In most cases early and late changes have been depicted.

There are relatively few ways in which cells can express cytotoxicity. Rounding is a common expression of damage, but cells may appear either swollen or shrunken and granular or glassy. Some viruses produce factors that cause cell fusion, leading to the formation of multinucleated giant cells, which are also called syncytial cells; respiratory syncytial virus, parainfluenza viruses 2 and 3, measles virus, and mumps virus can produce syncytial giant cells. In addition, herpes simplex virus and VZV produce smaller multinucleated giant cells.

Not all isolates of respiratory syncytial virus produce syncytial cells. Production of the F(usion) glycoprotein by the virus is required for cell fusion. Shahrabadi and Lee demonstrated that calcium must be present in the culture medium for respiratory syncytial virus-induced fusion of HEp-2 cells to occur.[758] The formation of syncytial giant cells also appears re-

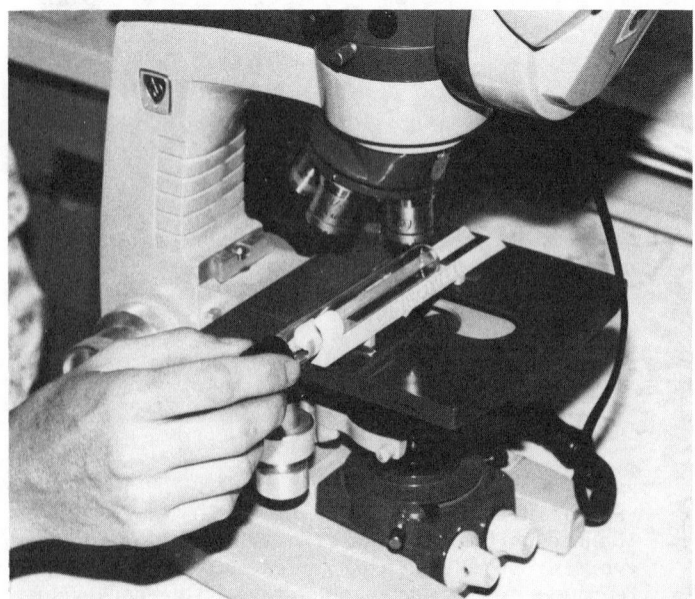

Figure 21-11
Examinaton of cultures for cytopathic effect can be performed with an inverted or a traditional microscope. A rack, which fits in the specimen holder of the microscope stage, prevents the round tubes from rolling. High magnification is not possible but is not needed for recognition and characterization of cytopathic effect.

TABLE 21-25
DIFFERENTIAL DIAGNOSIS OF VIRAL CYTOPATHIC EFFECT

VIRUS	CELL CULTURE			DAYS TO ISOLATION		DESCRIPTION
	PMK	HDF	HEP-2	MAYO MEAN*	MT. ZION MEAN†	
Influenza virus	+++	−	−	4	3.8	None or focal enlarged granular cells followed by sloughing; rapid progression
Parainfluenza virus	+++	+	+	11	6.4	None or focal rounding and multi-nucleated giant cells (types 2 and 3)
Respiratory syncytial virus	++	+	+++	8.3	6.1	Enlarged, glassy syncytial giant cells; or granular, rounded cells
Mumps virus	+++	+	−	6.9		Enlarged, syncytial giant cells
Measles virus	+	−	+			Vacuolated, syncytial giant cells; rarely isolated
Poliovirus	+++	+++	+++	4.6		Random, swollen, glassy cells; rapid progression and detachment of cells from glass
Coxsackievirus B	+++	+	+++	3.5	4.2	Focal, swollen, glassy cells; detachment from glass
Echoviruses	+++	+++	+	3.9	4.2	Focal, swollen, glassy cells; detachment from glass
Rhinovirus	+	+++	−	6.6		Focal, swollen, or granular cells
Adenovirus	++	+	+++	6.2	6.4	Enlarged, clustered cells (bunches of grapes or lattice)
Herpes simplex virus	++	+++	++	3.5	2.7	Enlarged or shrunken granular cells starting at edge; rapid progression and sloughing; may have giant cells
Varicella-zoster virus	++	++	−	7.6	6.1	Discrete, elongated foci of enlarged or shrunken cells; slow contiguous progression enhanced by use of growth medium
Cytomegalovirus	−	+++	−	10	5.8	Compact foci of enlarged cells; slow, contiguous progression

+++, Optimal cells for detection of cytopathic effect (CPE); ++, CPE frequent, may be best available system for detection of CPE; +, CPE may occasionally be observed; −, CPE does not usually occur; PMK, primary monkey kidney cells; HDF, human diploid fibroblast cells; HEp-2, human continuous cell line
* From the Mayo Clinic, abstracted from Herrmann EC Jr: Experience in providing a viral diagnostic laboratory compatible with medical practice. Mayo Clin Proc 42:112–123, 1967; and Herrmann EC Jr: Efforts toward a more useful viral diagnostic laboratory. Am J Clin Pathol 56:681–686, 1971
† From Mount Zion Hospital and Medical Center, San Francisco, abstracted from Drew WL: Controversies in viral diagnosis. Rev Infect Dis 8:814–824, 1986
Adapted from McIntosh K: Diagnostic virology. In Fields BN, Knipe DM, Melnick JL, et al (eds): Virology, 2nd ed., chap 16, pp 411–440. New York, Raven Press, 1990

lated, at least in part, to the concentration of glutamine in the culture medium.[539]

Cytopathic effect usually starts focally and often is most readily seen at the edges of the monolayer, where the density of cells is low. For viruses that spread from cell to cell through the culture media, the cytopathic effect progresses from focality to totality, sometimes with great rapidity. If the number of virions in the specimen is very large, most of the monolayer may be infected simultaneously; in this case, widespread degeneration must be differentiated from nonspecific cytotoxicity by subculture of fluid to fresh

TABLE 21-26
Differential Diagnosis of Viral Cytopathic Effect

PRIMARY ISOLATION IN:			RBC HAd	CPE Type	VIRUS SUSPECTED	COMMENTS AND ANCILLARY TESTS	CONFIRMATION
PMK	HDF	HEP-2					
+	+	+	−	Swelling/ shrinking/ hyaline	Poliovirus		NT, FA
				Syncytium in HEp-2 and PMK	Respiratory syncytial virus		FA, NT, EIA
				Rounded, swollen cells, especially in fibroblasts	Herpes simplex	Growth in rabbit kidney	FA, EIA
				Swollen clusters/ lattice	Adenovirus		NT, FA, CF
+	+	−	−	Swelling/ shrinking/ hyaline	Echovirus Coxsackievirus A		NT, FA
				Focal, linear swelling/giant cells	Varicella-zoster	Cell association on passage	NT, FA
				Swelling/ shrinking	Rhinovirus	pH 3 stability	NT
			+ (Guinea pig)	Large, granular syncytium	Mumps	Rarely isolated	HAI, NT
+	−	+	−	Swelling/ shrinking/ hyaline	Coxsackievirus B		NT, FA
				Swollen clusters/lattice	Adenovirus		NT, FA, CF
			+ (Monkey)	Vacuolated syncytium	Measles	Rarely isolated; clinical history; HAd	NT, FA
			+ (Guinea pig)	Rounding, syncytium	Parainfluenza 2 and 3	HAd	FA, HAI
+	−	−	+ (Guinea pig)	None/ rounding	Influenza Parainfluenza 1–3	HAd 4C = 20C HAd 4C < 20C	HAI, FA, CF HAI, FA, CF
				Syncytium	Parainfluenza 2, 3	HAd	HAI, FA, CF
				Large, granular syncytium	Mumps	Rarely isolated	HAI, NT
			+ (Monkey)	Vacuolated syncytium	Measles	Rarely isolated; clinical history; HAd	NT, FA
−	+	−	−	Focal/enlarged cells	Cytomegalovirus	Cell association	FA, H&E
				Focal, linear plaques	Varicella-zoster	Cell association; H&E	FA, CF
				Focal/swelling	Rhinovirus	pH 3 stability	NT

PMK, primary monkey kidney cells; HDF, human diploid fibroblast cells; HEp-2, human continuous cell line; CPE, cytopathic effect HAd, hemadsorption; FA, immunofluorescence; NT, neutralization test; CF, complement fixation; EIA, enzyme-linked immunosorbent assay; H&E, stain for inclusions

cell cultures. For viruses that spread directly from cell to cell (CMV and VZV) the cytopathic effect progresses more slowly and by local extension of the initial foci.

It is, of course, somewhat artificial to try to capture the considerable variability of a biologic process in a single photographic frame. In a clinical laboratory, it will be possible to examine other parts of the monolayer, view other cell cultures, and even reexamine a suspicious culture after incubation for a few more hours. It will often be possible, therefore, to detect cytologic changes that are even earlier than those that make convincing photographs.

HEMAGGLUTINATION AND HEMADSORPTION

Many viruses contain surface components that agglutinate red blood cells from various species of animals. Some viruses, primarily those of the myxovirus and paramyxovirus groups, also insert the hemagglutinins into the membrane of the infected cell as the virus matures at the cytoplasmic membrane. Some isolates of influenza A virus and the parainfluenza viruses may be detected only by hemagglutination or hemadsorption (see Fig. 21-12A and B).

The hemagglutination test is performed less frequently than the hemadsorption test for detection of isolates in cell culture but is required if eggs have been inoculated. Hemagglutination of red blood cells is observed in tubes or microtiter plates after addition of fluid from infected cultures or eggs. If characterization of the strain is necessary, inhibition of viral hemagglutination by specific antiviral serum is the most economical procedure (see Chart 37). New strains of influenza viruses are typed by this method in reference laboratories; cross-reacting inhibition by antisera against previous strains allows an assessment of how closely related the new strain is to previous isolates.[221]

The hemadsorption test for myxoviruses (see Fig. 21-12A through E) is performed by adding fresh guinea pig red blood cells to an infected monolayer (see Chart 35).[842] The test can be performed without damage to the monolayer, after which incubation of the cell culture can be continued. Agglutination of the red blood cells in the fluid phase may be observed in addition to hemadsorption. The processes of hemadsorption and hemagglutination are shown in Figure 21-16. The temperature at which hemadsorption is optimal has some differential diagnostic value.[779] Most isolates of influenza A virus adsorb red blood cells as efficiently at 20°C as at 4°C. In contrast, 60% to 80% of parainfluenza virus 1 through 3 isolates produce better hemadsorption at 4°C; if absorbed tubes are warmed to room temperature, the red blood cells will elute from the monolayer. Slightly more than one-half of the isolates of parainfluenza virus 4 and mumps virus, both uncommon isolates in most clinical laboratories, adsorb red blood cells better at 20°C.

Hemadsorption is more convenient than hemagglutination for testing the presence of virus in most clinical laboratories. Hemadsorption inhibition can also be used to identify isolates, but it is much more wasteful of antisera than is hemagglutination inhibition.

LIGHT MICROSCOPY

As they replicate, some viruses produce masses of nucleoprotein and virions in various stages of assembly. The anatomic pathologist or cytologist uses these viral inclusions to detect the presence of a viral infection and identify the agent presumptively.[151,427,805] Although the characteristics of cytopathic effect in unstained monolayers are usually sufficient to render a provisional diagnosis, the virologist may gain additional information simply by staining the cells with hematoxylin and eosin, with the Papanicolaou stain, or with acridine orange (see Color Plate 21-1).

ELECTRON MICROSCOPY

For laboratories with access to an electron microscope, the ultrastructural morphology of an isolate may identify the group to which it belongs.[6,593] Negative-staining electron microscopy is simple and may be accomplished rapidly on supernatant fluid or lysed cells. This technique may be particularly useful for differentiation of nonspecific toxicity from a large viral inoculum.

BIOCHEMICAL DIFFERENTIATION

The cytolytic changes produced by rhinoviruses may resemble those of enteroviruses, although rhinoviruses replicate less rapidly and demonstrate the lability of the rhinovirus group to an acid environment. To make this assessment, aliquots of infected cell culture are adjusted to pH 3.0 or 7.4 for 3 hours. Then an estimate of the infectivity is obtained by inoculating serial 10-fold dilutions of the aliquots into cell cultures. A reduction in infectivity of 2 to 4 $\log_{10}$ should be observed if the virus is a rhinovirus.[407]

CELL ASSOCIATION

The demonstration of the association of virions with infected cells is useful to differentiate members of the herpesvirus group. Herpes simplex virus is released freely into the culture medium, whereas CMV and VZV remain cell associated. Herpes simplex virus rapidly infects the whole monolayer (see Fig. 21-14B). The cytopathic effect of CMV and VZV is usually focal (see Fig. 21-14E through H), because virions do not spread through the medium. Occasionally, however, large numbers of viral particles in the inoculum may produce widespread cytopathic effect resembling that of herpes simplex. Subculture of the culture medium and disrupted cells separately documents the cell association of the isolate.

Other presumptive tests that have been used include characterization of the type of nucleic acid in the virion and the sensitivity of enveloped viruses to ether.

DETECTION OF VIRAL ANTIGENS

In addition to confirmation of the identity of a cytopathic agent, demonstration of specific antigens in culture has been used as a method for detecting the presence of a virus, even in the absence of cytopathic effect.[245,309,311,572,735] Tests for antigen may be performed after a brief incubation if rapid diagnosis is desired. Alternatively, antigen tests may be performed after a specified incubation before reporting the absence of virus. This technique should work well if the virus can be targeted precisely on clinical grounds. The most dramatic improvements in the rapidity with which isolates are detected will occur with those viruses that have the slowest growth in conventional systems, such as respiratory syncytial virus, cytomegalovirus, and varicella-zoster virus (see page 1252 and Color Plate 21-2D and F).

(text continues on page 1245)

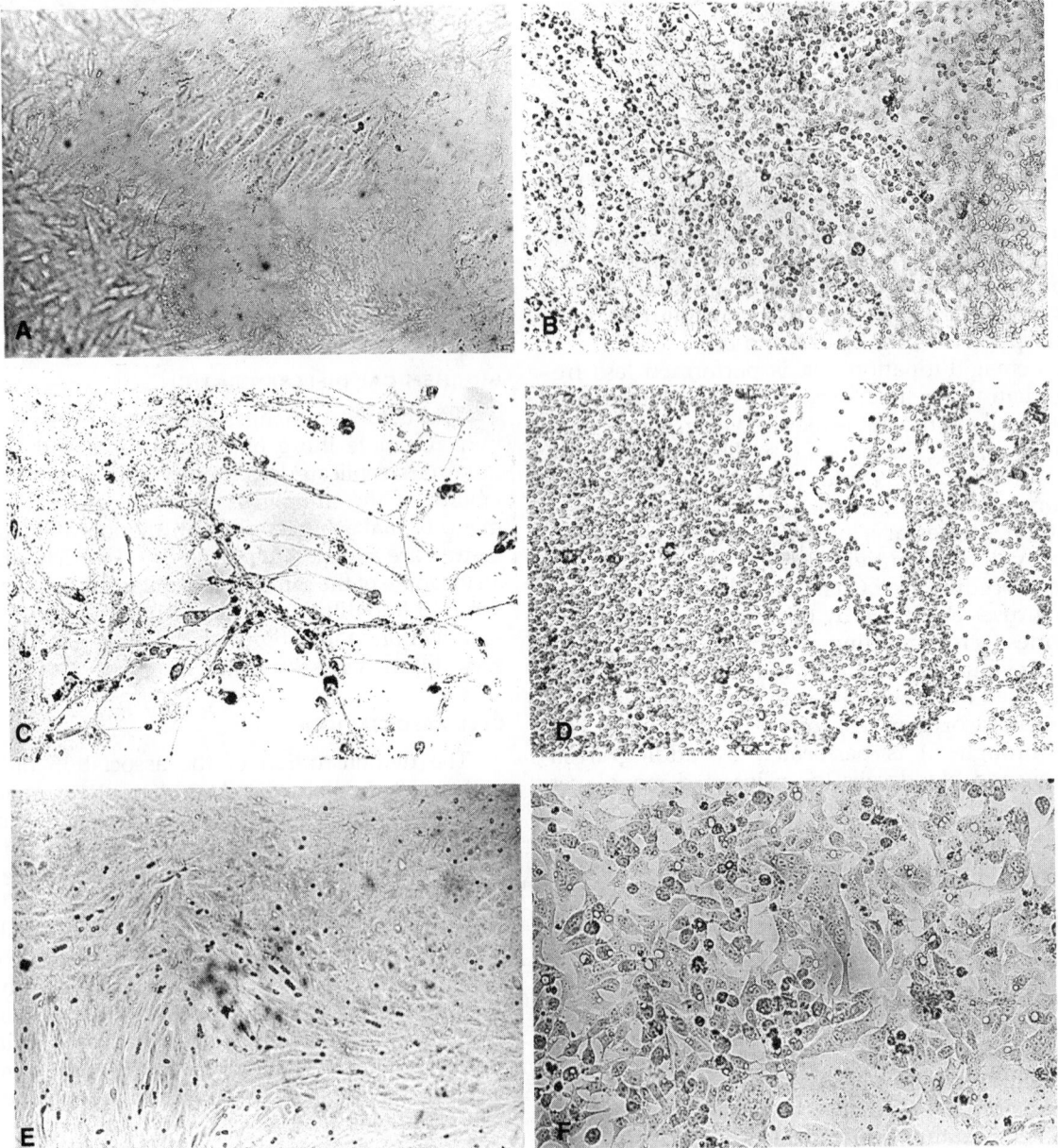

Figure 21-12

Cytopathic effect of myxoviruses. (**A**) Rhesus monkey kidney cells infected with influenza A virus. This isolate produces no cytopathic effect in the monolayer. A hemadsorption test identified the presence of a virus. Many of the current strains of influenza A virus and most strains of influenza B virus produce cytopathic effect, which often develops more rapidly than that produced by the parainfluenza viruses (×180). (**B**) Rhesus monkey kidney cells infected with influenza A virus. The monolayer is intact but is covered with numerous guinea pig red blood cells. The red cells have adhered to the viral hemagglutinins on the surface of the infected cells. Hemagglutination of red blood cells in the fluid phase by free virus can often be detected but is not shown in the photograph (×180). (**C**) Rhesus monkey kidney cells infected with parainfluenza virus 3. The monolayer has degenerated, and cells have fallen off the glass. Many of the remaining cells are enlarged or granular. Often, isolates of parainfluenza viruses do not produce obvious cytopathic effect and must be detected by hemadsorption (×180). (**D**) Rhesus monkey kidney cells infected with parainfluenza virus 3. A hemadsorption test has been performed. The remaining cells are covered with guinea pig red blood cells that have attached to the viral hemagglutinin on the cell membranes (×180). (**E**) Rhesus monkey kidney cells that are uninfected demonstrate a negative hemadsorption test. A few guinea pig red blood cells have stuck to the monolayer, but the massive adherence of red blood cells that characterizes a positive test is not present. The settled cells are also dislodged more easily from an uninfected monolayer than from a myxovirus-infected monolayer by shaking the tube. (**F**) HEp-2 cells infected with parainfluenza virus 3. Large multinucleated giant cells (known as *syncytial cells*) have formed in the monolayer by fusion of adjacent cells. This type of cytopathic effect is characteristic of parainfluenza viruses 2 and 3 in monkey kidney cells and parainfluenza virus 3 in HEp-2 cells. Syncytial cells are also formed by other viruses, notably respiratory syncytial virus. The parainfluenza viruses can be differentiated from respiratory syncytial virus easily by performance of a hemadsorption test (×180).

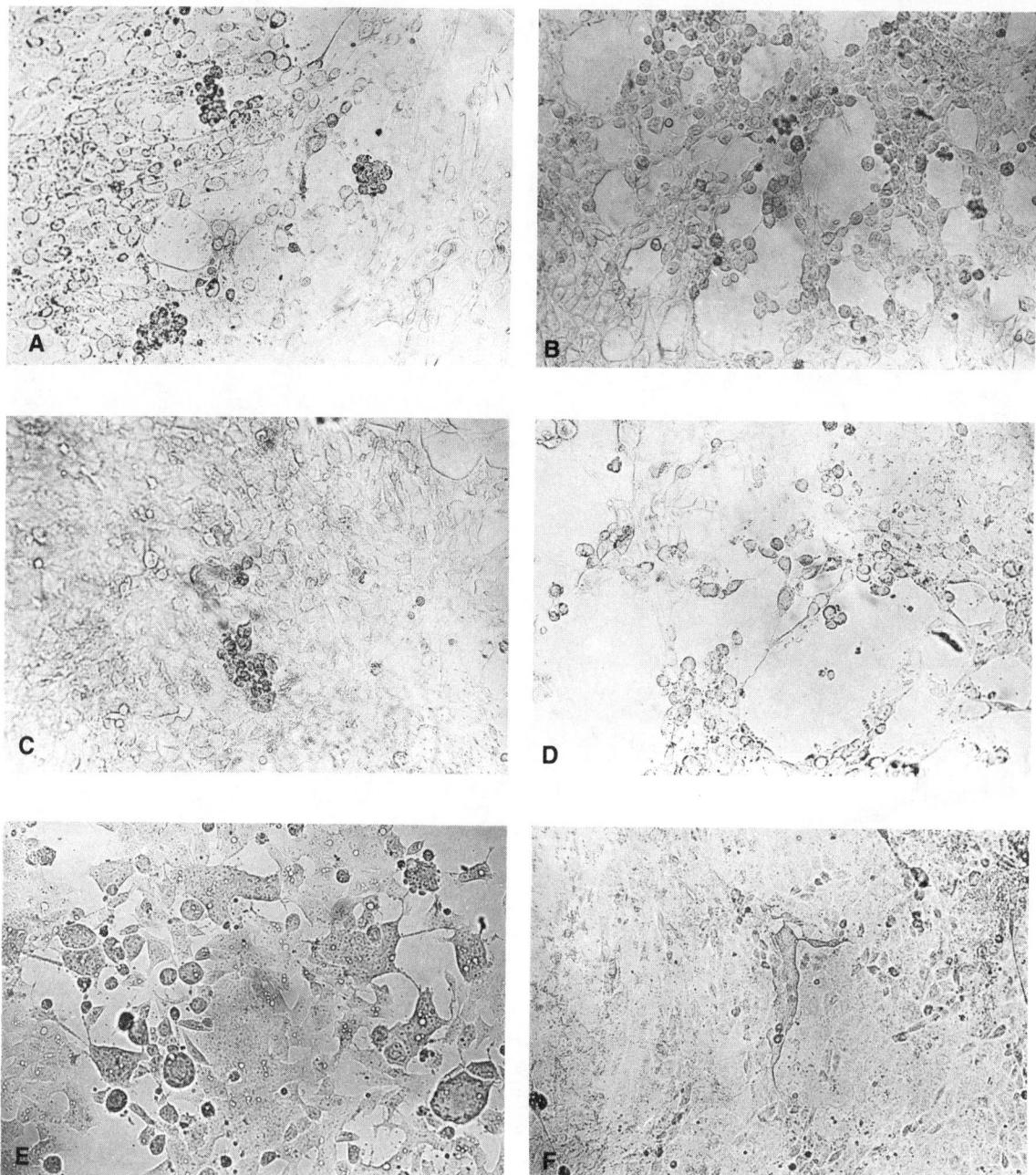

Figure 21-13
Cytopathic effect of other respiratory viruses. (**A**) HEp-2 cells infected with adenovirus. Several foci of enlarged, granular cells are evident. Adenovirus cells are often clustered like bunches of grapes, much as are staphylococci in a Gram stain (×180). (**B**) HEp-2 cells infected with adenovirus. Most of the cells in the monolayer are now rounded; many cells have detached from the glass, leaving multiple holes. In several places, clustering of cells can be seen. Strands of cytoplasm connect some of the residual infected cells, producing the beginning of a lattice effect. (× 180). (**C**) Rhesus monkey kidney cells infected with adenovirus. One cluster of granular, enlarged cells is evident. A preliminary report could be issued if multiple foci were present in the culture. If only a few are present, it would be best to observe the monolayer for progression of cytopathic effect. (× 180). (**D**) Rhesus monkey kidney cells infected with adenovirus. The extent of cytopathic effect has increased considerably. Clustered, swollen cells with intercellular cytoplasmic bridges are evident. Many cells have detached from the glass. Eventually, there will be only scattered cells left on the glass tube as evidence that a monolayer was once present. (× 180). (**E**) HEp-2 cells infected with respiratory syncytial virus. Many of the cells in the monolayer have been fused by the virus to form syncytial giant cells, much like those formed by parainfluenza viruses. Other cells are enlarged or have detached from the glass. A hemadsorption test on this monolayer would be negative. (× 180). (**F**) Rhesus monkey kidney cells infected with respiratory syncytial virus. One large syncytium has formed in the monolayer. One could differentiate this isolate from parainfluenza virus by hemadsorption or by identification of specific antigen.

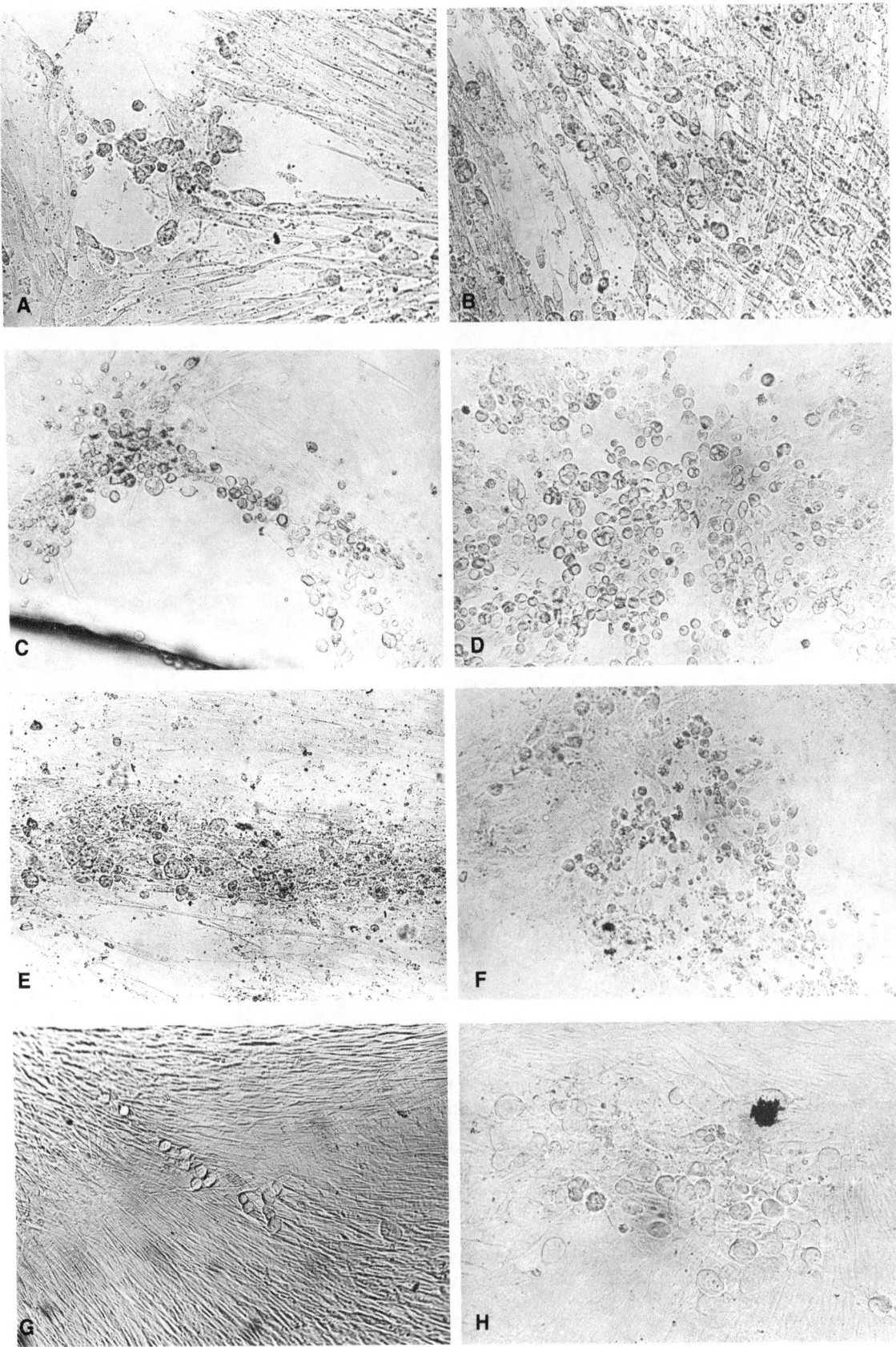

Figure 21-14

Although most laboratories will not encounter rubella virus, Schmidt and colleagues have reported that immunoperoxidase staining of RK-13 or BSC-1 cells facilitated the detection of this fastidious virus.[747]

Amplification detection systems designed to produce rapid diagnosis have not always worked sufficiently well to replace conventional culture techniques. For example, only 25 of 45 isolates (56%) of influenza viruses were detected by immunofluorescence staining of shell vial cultures that had been incubated for 24 hours.[245]

ARTIFACTS AND NONVIRUS-INDUCED CHANGES

As cells age in culture, morphologic changes unrelated to viral infection may occur (see Fig. 21-5). The density of cells in diploid cell lines and, in particular, established cell lines may become very high; dying or dividing cells may appear rounded or granular. Scattered atypical cells occur in any culture and are especially noticeable in less dense areas, such as the edge of the monolayer, where viral cytopathic effect may also become apparent first. It is important, therefore, to maintain uninoculated controls of cells from the same batch as those used for specimens.

Primary monkey kidney cells may be infected with simian viruses that produce a variety of degenerative changes,[407] including a foamy or vacuolated appearance in the monolayer.

The presence of extraneous cells that settle on the monolayer may also cause confusion (see Fig. 21-6D). Cytopathic effect may be mimicked because the contaminating cells differ in appearance from the original monolayer. Usually a virus that produces focal abnormalities in the monolayer, such as CMV, is simulated. The artifact may be suspected because the cells are on top of the monolayer, rather than becoming an integral part. Contaminating cells may be of human origin, such as epithelial or mesothelial cells present in the specimen, or may have originated in other cell cultures, particularly if a subculture from one cell line to another has been performed.

A variety of nonviral agents or substances in clinical specimens may be toxic to cell monolayers (see Fig. 21-6A). If bacterial or fungal growth occurs (see Fig. 21-6B), the nature of the problem is obvious; the specimen must then be treated again with antibiotics or filtered and inoculated into additional cell cultures.

Usually the nature of the cytotoxicity is unknown. The ordinary remedy is to dilute the specimen and inoculate additional monolayers. Howell and associates found that the toxicity of semen from patients with AIDS could be avoided by inoculating the monolayer with a cell pellet, obtained by high-speed centrifugation.[404] CMV, which is a frequent pathogen in patients with AIDS, is associated with leukocytes. On the other hand, toxic substances were concentrated in the supernatant fraction.

◀ **Figure 21-14**

Cytopathic effect of herpesviruses. (**A**) MRC-5 fibroblasts infected with herpes simplex virus. There is a focus of enlarged, rounded cells in the monolayer. Many cells have detached from the glass. Such foci will enlarge rapidly, and the entire monolayer is usually involved within a few days ($\times 180$). (**B**) MRC-5 fibroblasts infected with herpes simplex virus. Cytopathic effect has progressed so that virtually every cell in the monolayer is affected. Again, the cells are enlarged, even ballooned, and granular. This type of generalized cytopathic effect can occasionally be seen with cytomegalovirus if very large quantities of virus are present, as in patients with AIDS. Cytomegalovirus can be distinguished from herpes simplex by identification of specific antigens and by demonstration that transfer of cells is necessary to transfer the cytopathic effect to new cultures efficiently. ($\times 180$) (**C**) Rhesus monkey kidney cells infected with herpes simplex. As often happens at the outset, this focus of cytopathic effect is at the edge of the monolayer. Enlarged, ballooned cells surround the center of the focus, where the cells have already detached from the glass. ($\times 180$). (**D**) HEp-2 cells infected with herpes simplex virus. There is a large focus of swollen cells in the monolayer. Some of the cells have the appearance of multinucleated giant cells, although it is difficult to delineate the cellular structure in an unstained preparation at low magnification. ($\times 180$). (**E**) MRC-5 fibroblasts infected with varicella-zoster virus. A cytopathic focus consists of large swollen cells and granular degenerated cells. The focus is elongating in the direction of the underlying fibroblasts. The slow appearance and slow progression of the foci are characteristic. Transfer of cytopathic effect requires the inclusion of infected cells. The cytopathic effect has some similarities to that of cytomegalovirus; the foci of cytomegalovirus tend to be more compact and spread centrifugally without such a pronounced linear orientation. ($\times 180$) (**F**) Rhesus monkey kidney cells infected with varicella-zoster virus. A focus of enlarged, swollen cells is less distinctive than the cytopathic effect in MRC-5 cells. It can be differentiated from that produced by herpes simplex virus by the speed with which it appears and progresses. Cytomegalovirus does not produce cytopathic effect in monkey cells. ($\times 180$) (**G**) WI-38 fibroblasts infected with cytomegalovirus. There is a small focus of enlarged, granular cells in the monolayer. ($\times 180$) (**H**) MRC-5 fibroblasts infected with cytomegalovirus. A developing focus of cytopathic effect is evident. The cells are swollen, and the focus is quite compact. Cytopathic effect of cytomegalovirus appears late and progresses slowly. It tends to be more compact and less linear than that of varicella-zoster virus. Differentiation from varicella is by clinical history, by demonstration of multinucleated giant cells in varicella monolayers, and by the demonstration of specific antigen ($\times 180$).

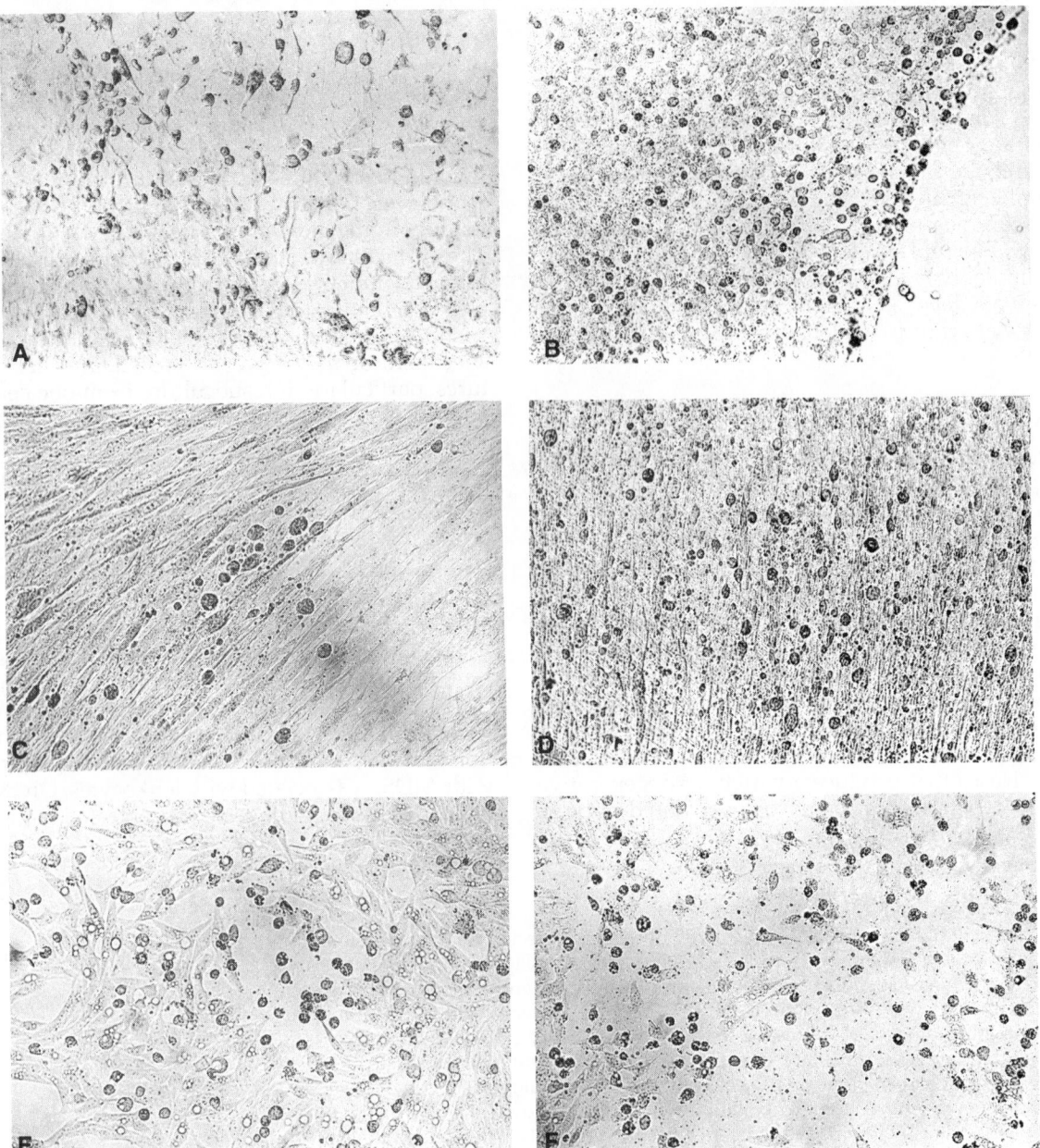

Figure 21-15

Cytopathic effect of enteroviruses. **(A)** Rhesus monkey kidney cells infected with coxsackievirus B. There is a focus of cytopathic effect in which cells are either small and shrunken or enlarged. Some of the cells have a refractile or glassy appearance that is typical of enteroviral cytopathic effect. Elongated "tadpole" cells are also typical of the cytopathology produced by this group of viruses (×180). **(B)** Rhesus monkey kidney cells infected with coxsackievirus B. Cytopathic effect progresses relatively rapidly with the enteroviruses; poliovirus may cause complete destruction of the monolayer overnight. In this photomicrograph virtually every cell in the monolayer has been damaged, and large segments of the cell sheet (*lower right*) have peeled off entirely (×180). **(C)** MRC-5 fibroblasts infected with echovirus 11. An early focus of enteroviral cytopathic effect is evident. The cells appear enlarged and granular. It would be very difficult at this stage to guess the identity of the virus. Most isolates of echovirus grow well in human diploid fibroblasts, whereas isolates of coxsackievirus do not (×180). **(D)** MRC-5 fibroblasts infected with echovirus 11. Cytopathic effect has extended to involve almost the entire monolayer. Virus is spread extracellularly through the medium so that cytopathic effect tends to change from focal to generalized in nature relatively rapidly (×180). **(E)** HEp-2 cells infected with coxsackievirus B. A small focus of cytopathic effect in the HEp-2 cells is manifested by rounded, shrunken granular cells and detachment of cells from the glass. Early cytopathic effect is much more difficult to recognize if the cell sheet is too heavy and the cells are piled one on top of the other (×180). **(F)** HEp-2 cells infected with coxsackievirus B. Almost all of the cells in the monolayer have detached from the glass. Those that remain are abnormal. Most coxsackievirus B isolates grow well in HEp-2 cells, whereas coxsackievirus A and echovirus do not (×180).

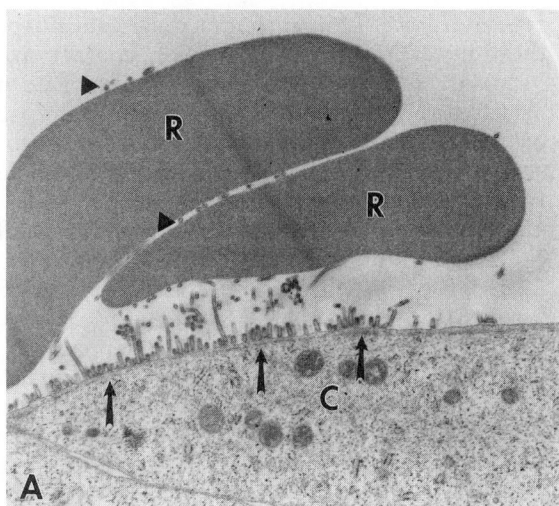 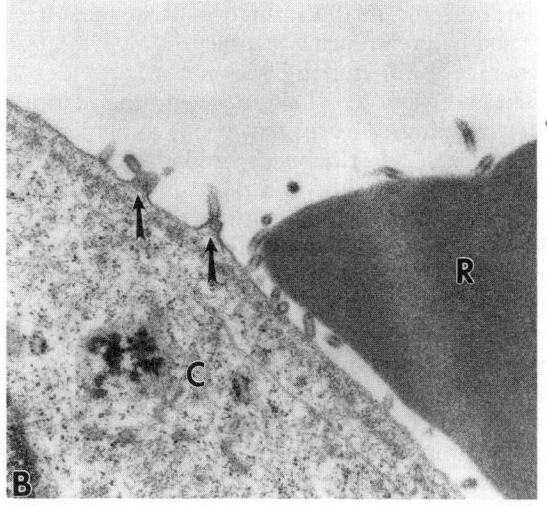

Figure 21-16
Electron microscopy of hemadsorption and hemagglutination of influenza A virus.
(**A**) Two red blood cells (**R**) have adhered to a monolayer of rhesus monkey kidney cells
(**C**). The glue that holds them together is the large number of influenza virions that are
"budding" from the surface of the kidney cells (**arrows**) or adhering to the red blood cells
(**arrowheads**) (×35,000). (**B**) At higher magnification, the bulges in the cell membrane at
the point of budding can be seen clearly (**arrows**). The hemagglutinin and neuraminidase
spikes on the virus particles appear as a "fringe" (×80,000).

On occasion the cytopathic effect may be "specific," although the cause is unexpected and perhaps unwanted. *Clostridium difficile* toxin in fecal specimens (see Fig. 21-6C) may produce cytopathic effect resembling enteroviral damage.[748]

Gentry and associates reported the isolation of *Trichomonas vaginalis* in BHK cell cultures.[297] The flagellates produced a cytopathic effect that mimicked that of herpes simplex virus; the cytopathic effect was reproduced when viable *Trichomonas* or lysates from axenic cultures were added to cell cultures. Motile trichomonads could be seen when the cultures were inspected closely.

Isolation of *Pneumocystis carinii* from patients with AIDS has been reported. It is difficult to propagate this protozoan parasite serially in the laboratory, but organisms have been grown in cell cultures, including MRC-5 human diploid fibroblasts.[494] The *P. carinii* isolates produced a cytopathic effect that resembled viral effects. *Toxoplasma gondii* may be recovered in cell culture lines, such as human diploid fibroblasts, although the sensitivity of culture has not been evaluated.

DEFINITIVE IDENTIFICATION OF ISOLATES

In a diagnostic laboratory the combination of clinical history and cytopathic effect provides sufficient information to identify some viruses, including herpes simplex, CMV, VZV, adenovirus, and respiratory syncytial virus. Enteroviruses can usually be identified to the genus level. Complete identification of isolates, including serotyping, requires immunologic characterization of the viral antigens.

The traditional method for preparing antisera has been to inject the antigen into a laboratory animal, usually a rabbit. The animal then makes polyclonal antibody to a variety of determinants (epitopes) on the antigen. Little more than a decade ago the immunologic world was revolutionized by the fusion of antibody-producing plasma cells with a malignant plasma cell tumor. The hybrid cells maintain the antibody-producing capability of one parent and the neoplastic capability for indefinite multiplication of the other parent.[466]

This new monoclonal antibody technology has been aggressively applied to many areas of research, including virology.[903] The reagents have the great advantage that a continuous, unchanging source of antibody is ensured. No longer is it necessary to worry that the "new rabbit is not as good as the old rabbit was." The monoclonal reagents also have the capability of recognizing very small segments (epitopes) of the antigen, so that more sophisticated schemes for typing isolates are possible. The monoclonal reagents are not infallible, however, and there are even some potential disadvantages. Although the epitopes with which the monoclonal reagents react are narrowly defined, cross-reactions may still occur if that epitope is shared by other antigens.[516] If the monoclonal reagents are too narrowly defined, they may not detect all isolates.[670,814] (See Chapter 1 for further information.)

Immunologic tests can be adapted either for identification of antigens or antibodies against those antigens. The most specific immunologic test for the majority of viral infections is the neutralization assay (Chart 51). The identification of an unknown viral isolate is made by analyzing the degree to which antisera of known reactivity prevent the virus from infecting tissue culture cells, eggs, or animals.[745] The disadvantages of the neutralization test are the time and expense required for its performance. It is most frequently used in a reference laboratory.

The hemagglutination inhibition test provides a convenient and economical alternative to the neutralization test for those viruses that produce hemagglutinins (Chart 37). The principle is similar to that of the neutralization test, but the end point is inhibition of the virus-mediated agglutination reaction rather than inhibition of infectivity.[221] Reference sera of known reactivity are used to characterize a viral isolate.

The complement-fixation test has been a mainstay of viral diagnosis for many years (Chart 14). That complement fixation can be adapted for use with a large number of antigens and that large numbers of specimens can be tested are major advantages. On the other hand, the complement-fixation test is cumbersome to perform and is relatively insensitive, and sera that have anticomplementary activity cannot be tested. Although other assays, especially enzymatic assays, have replaced the complement-fixation test for detecting many viruses, it is still used in some laboratories.[635]

Many viral tests are important for epidemiologic analysis, but, with the exception of the myxoviruses,

are rarely necessary for routine diagnostic purposes. In those instances in which complete characterization is necessary (eg, paralytic disease), the isolate may be sent to a reference laboratory. A thorough discussion of antigenic characterization, which is beyond the scope of this chapter, may be found in textbooks of virology and viral diagnosis.[261,407,506,787]

For many hospital laboratories immunofluorescence and immunoenzyme assays provide a viable alternative by which definitive identification of many viruses to the genus level can be made. Fortunately, the expanding catalogue of commercially available reagents, which are of increasingly high quality, simplifies the task. The enteroviruses and rhinoviruses are notable exceptions because their complicated antigenic composition makes definitive identification difficult without neutralization tests.

Immunofluorescence and immunoenzyme assays are similar in principle, differing mainly in the detection system. The immunofluorescence test (Chart 39) has been used for many years and in many variations. Several variations of the procedure are illustrated graphically in Figure 21-17. The direct fluorescent

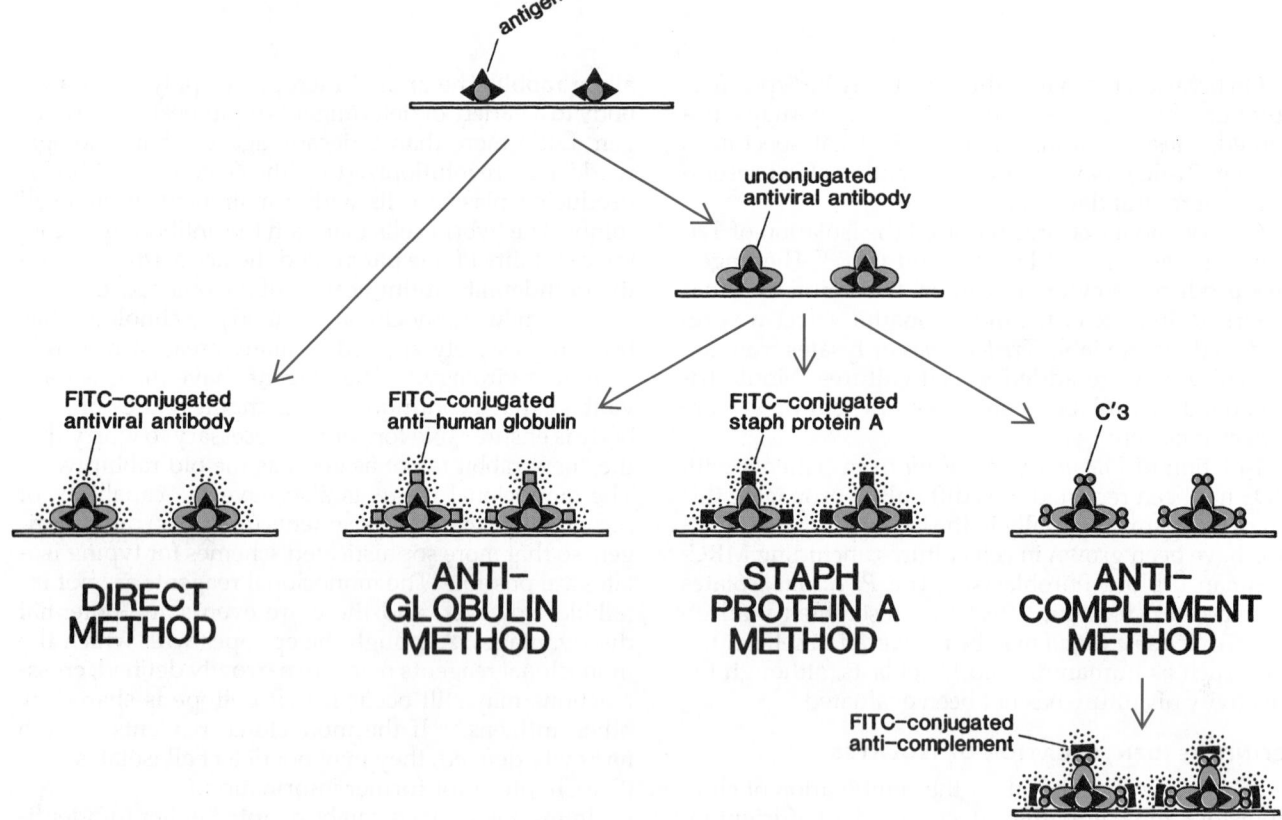

Figure 21-17
Fluorescence assays are performed in a variety of ways. Antigen is first fixed to a microscope slide by treatment with acetone, alcohol, or heat, depending on the nature of the antigen. For direct diagnosis of infections this antigen is, in fact, the clinical specimen. For serologic diagnosis, a known antigen is attached to the solid-phase. The simplest method for identifying antigen in clinical specimens is the direct method. The indirect methods are usually more sensitive because they involve several amplification steps; the anticomplement method is probably the most sensitive of these techniques. Along with increased sensitivity, however, goes increased risk of nonspecific reactions. If antibody is to be detected, one of the indirect methods must be used.

assay test is the simplest to perform, but specific conjugated antisera are required. Indirect immunofluorescent tests—using antiglobulin, staphylococcal protein A, or complement—are more sensitive but often suffer from lower specificity. In contrast to the direct test, multiple conjugated reagents are not needed to perform the indirect test, but the procedure is more time consuming because of the multiple steps required.

The solid phase of immunoenzymatic tests can be the specimen itself, placed on a glass slide. In this case, the reaction is detected visually with a microscope. Solid phase immunoassays can also be performed in tubes or microtiter trays (Chart 25). Several of the variations of the serologic enzyme immunoassay are depicted in Figure 21-18. For detection or identification of antigen, the wells are usually coated with an antiserum, which can be IgM, as illustrated, or can be whole immunoglobulin.

Enzyme and fluorescence immunoassays can be considered equivalent for most applications, although the fluorescence tests have been slightly more sensitive in some situations.[392,780] Nonspecificity has been a problem in enzyme immunoassays, and controls for specificity should be available. On the other hand, visual as-

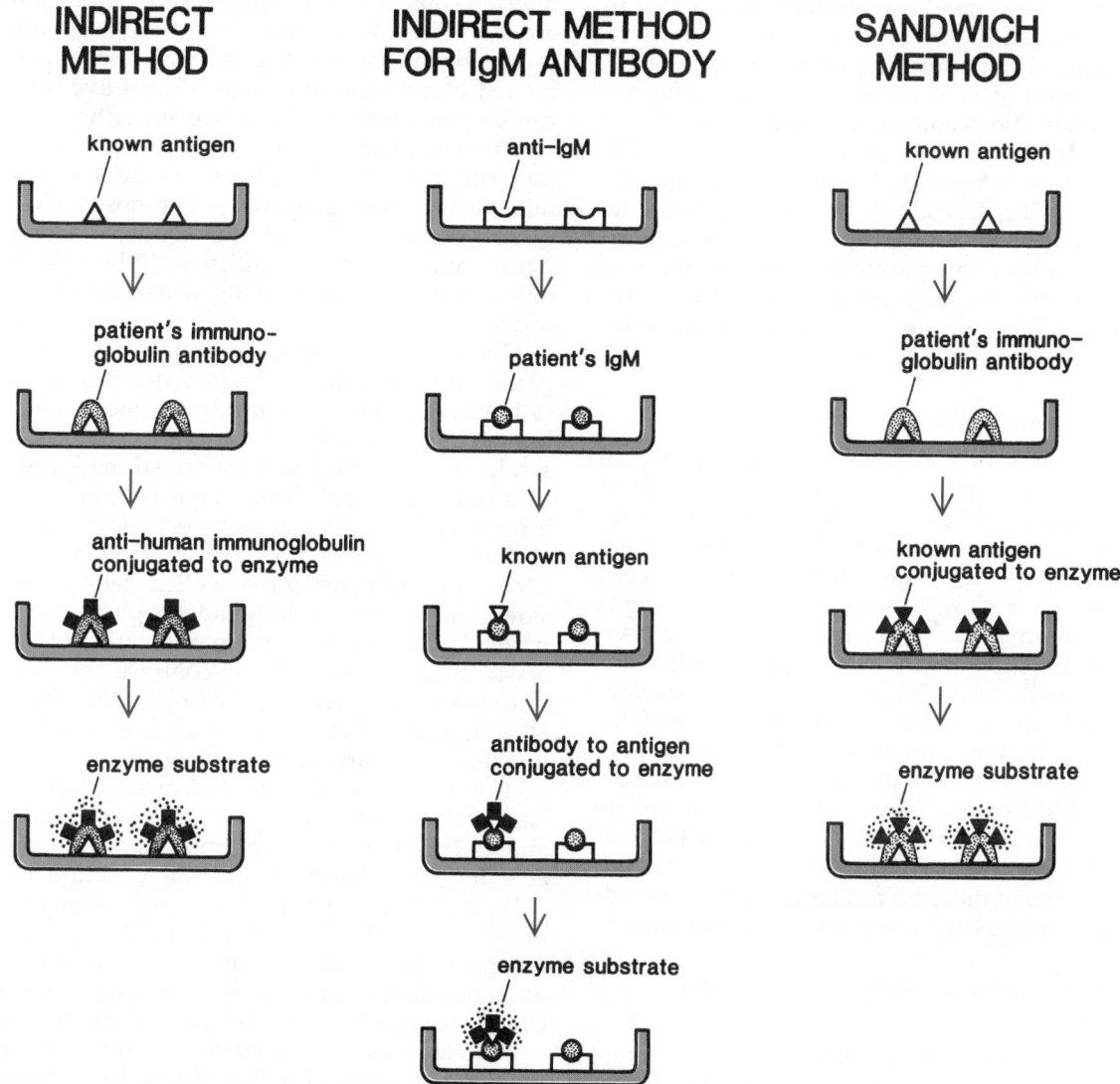

Figure 21-18

Enzyme immunoassays may be performed by a great variety of methods. If antibody is to be measured, antigen is placed on the solid phase as capture layer. After reaction of the antigen with the patient's serum, the detection layer may be either an antiglobulin reagent or enzyme-labeled antigen. Although immunoglobulin class-specific (usually IgM or IgG) antiglobulins may be used to detect class-specific antibody responses, the preferred method for detection of IgM responses is to coat the solid phase with anti-IgM to capture any IgM in the patient's serum. Subsequently, the specificity of that captured IgM is tested with specific antigen. If direct detection of the agent in clinical specimens is desired, the first step is usually to coat the solid phase with specific antibody against the antigen to capture the antigen from the specimen. Subsequently, the presence of a reaction is detected by addition of enzyme-conjugated antibody to the antigen of interest.

says, such as direct immunofluorescence, are subject to considerable viewer-to-viewer variation. Assays in which a positive reaction is determined microscopically have two advantages: 1) the cellularity (and the quality) of the specimen can be judged and 2) the relationship of the antigen to the cells can be assessed.[223]

The decision as to which assay to use will depend on local resources, experience, and the volume of tests. Immunofluorescence is simpler than most immunoassays if a small number of specimens is to be tested. When the number of specimens increases and the tests can be performed in batches, immunoenzyme assays or newer molecular probes become more attractive because automated systems can be used.

Positive and negative controls must be included in these tests. The specificity of the immunoenzyme assay can be enhanced by performing a blocking test.[78]

Identification of viral isolates by nucleic acid hybridization has also been accomplished.[143,160,263,616,696,841] The new technique of DNA amplification by the PCR technique has also been applied to many diagnostic problems (see Chapter 1).[176,208,763] We are well into the molecular age but only at the beginning of the application of these tools to diagnostic problems. In the next few years as commercial reagents and kits become increasingly available, the appropriate uses of these sophisticated tools will be clearer.

STORAGE OF VIRAL ISOLATES

If the necessity for additional characterization of an isolate seems probable, infected cell culture fluid should be frozen at −70°C. If the laboratory has the resources, it is good practice to retain all isolates for a period of time. A general rule is that mammalian cells should be frozen slowly, whereas infectious agents should be frozen quickly. The dramatic decrease in viability that accompanies the freezing process is minimized if the cultures are snap frozen and if a stabilizing agent is included in the medium. A mixture of dry ice and alcohol is a convenient means for snap freezing viral isolates. Many stabilizing agents have been used. Howell and Miller found that the sucrose phosphate broth that is used for transport of swabs for isolation of *Chlamydia* functioned as well as 70% sorbitol for maintenance of some of the most fastidious viruses, including cytomegalovirus and respiratory syncytial virus.[403]

SUMMARY OF DETECTION AND IDENTIFICATION OF VIRUSES

The orthomyxoviruses, paramyxoviruses, and respiratory syncytial virus (see Figs. 21-12 and 21-13) produce a variety of cytopathic effects in cell culture. Many isolates of influenza and parainfluenza viruses produce no visible changes in the monolayer and must be detected by other means. Cytopathic strains may be differentiated from other viruses with similar effects by noting the restriction of cytopathic effect to monkey kidney cells and by demonstration of hemadsorption, as described earlier. Multinucleated giant cells occur in monolayers that have been infected with measles, respiratory syncytial (see Fig. 21-13E and F), parain-

fluenza (see Fig. 21-12F), and mumps viruses; they are produced by virus-directed fusion of adjacent cells (syncytium formation). Such cells may also be seen in infected patients (see Color Plate 21-1F and G).[151,805]

Isolates are definitively identified by immunologic means. Antisera of good quality are available for most of the common myxoviruses. The genus or type of virus (eg, influenza A virus or respiratory syncytial virus) may be identified by immunofluorescence of infected cells. Characterization of strains of influenza viruses must be performed by hemagglutination inhibition.

Adenoviruses (see Fig. 21-13A through D) can be identified presumptively by observing the characteristic cytopathology in cell cultures. Clusters of swollen infected cells or a lattice appearance to the monolayer are typical. Adenoviruses can be placed into subgroups by the pattern of agglutination with rhesus and rat red blood cells, after which definitive serotyping can be performed.[441] Group-specific antigens that are common to all adenovirus serotypes have been identified, and monoclonal antibodies to the common determinants have been prepared.[138] For most clinical applications, confirmation of the genus adenovirus by immunofluorescence is sufficient. If the type of adenovirus must be determined, neutralization tests are necessary.

The herpesvirus group produces a variety of cytopathic effects in cell culture. EBV does not grow in the cell cultures commonly used in clinical laboratories; human infections with this virus are usually diagnosed serologically. CMV and VZV are strongly cell associated (see Fig. 21-14E through H). They are difficult to grow in cell culture, and they grow slowly. Successful subculture requires transfer of infected cells. Both CMV and VZV produce swollen cells in foci that slowly enlarge by direct spread; the plaques of VZV, in particular, tend to follow the orientation of the fibroblastic tissue culture cells. In contrast, herpes simplex virus is spread extracellularly (see Fig. 21-14A through D); cytopathic effect starts focally but rapidly spreads to affect other parts of the monolayer.

Centrifugation of the inoculum onto the monolayer has accelerated the recovery of herpes simplex, VZV, and CMV. Monoclonal antibodies have proved valuable for both detection and identification of CMV, VZV, and herpes simplex virus. Separation of isolates of herpes simplex into types 1 and 2 was not entirely reliable with polyclonal antisera. Monoclonal antisera are more discriminatory,[39,274,317] although some monoclonal reagents have not detected all strains.[814] A fluoresceinated monoclonal antibody that reacts with both types of herpes simplex virus has been developed,[308] so that virologists who do not wish to type isolates may operate with one reagent. Enteroviruses grow relatively rapidly in cell cultures, producing a widespread cytopathic effect (see Fig. 21-15). Affected cells may be shrunken and granular or may have a refractile, glassy appearance. Most serotypes of coxsackievirus A do not grow well in commonly used cell cultures. Isolates of coxsackievirus B usually do not grow well in human diploid fibroblast lines; echovirus strains do not grow well in HEp-2 cells. Definitive identification of an enterovirus requires immunologic identification, usually with a neutralization test.

DIRECT DETECTION OF VIRUSES IN CLINICAL SPECIMENS

The desire for greater rapidity in diagnosis of viral infections has been stimulated by the availability of rapid diagnostic methods in other areas of the laboratory and by the development of effective antiviral chemotherapy. A variety of methods is available, ranging from the traditional to the experimental.[707,710]

LIGHT MICROSCOPIC DETECTION OF INCLUSIONS

The detection of viral inclusions in smears or tissues by light microscopy has been the traditional means of directly demonstrating viral infections.[151,805] In general, those viruses that are assembled in the nucleus (usually DNA viruses) produce intranuclear inclusions, whereas cytoplasmic assembly (predominantly RNA containing viruses) yields cytoplasmic inclusions.

Intranuclear inclusions are produced in cells that have been infected by herpes simplex virus, VZV, CMV, adenovirus, and papovaviruses. The inclusions of herpes simplex (see Color Plate 21-1A and B) and VZV are indistinguishable. Nuclei have a homogeneous, eosinophilic or slightly basophilic appearance, and granular, basophilic nuclear chromatin is pushed against the edge of the nuclear membrane. Other infected cells may have a more eosinophilic inclusion that is accentuated by a halo between the inclusion and the nuclear membrane. This halo is an artifact of fixation but is useful diagnostically. Ultrastructurally, the inclusions are composed of a mixture of deoxyribonucleoprotein and assembled virions (see Fig. 21-3A); as the virions pass through the nuclear membrane, they pick up a lipid-containing membrane. The infected cells may be mononuclear or multinuclear.

Cytomegalovirus produces basophilic inclusions in an enlarged cell (see Color Plate 21-1D). These distinctive cells, which are pathognomonic of CMV infection, were originally believed to be protozoa that were invading tissue.[420] A halo is often present around the inclusion. Granular, basophilic inclusions may be found in the cytoplasm of some infected cells.

A variety of inclusions may be found in adenovirus infections. Early inclusions are eosinophilic and may closely resemble herpesvirus-infected cells. Inclusions become more basophilic as they mature and increasingly fill the nucleus (see Color Plate 21-1E). Eventually, they become extremely basophilic and may completely distort the cell; these diagnostic cells are referred to as "smudge cells" and must be distinguished from uninfected cells with hyperchromatic nuclei. The adenovirus inclusions are composed of nucleoprotein and numerous virions, which often demonstrate a paracrystalline array because their icosahedral shape permits tight packing of the particles (see Fig. 21-3B).

The intranuclear inclusions of the papovavirus group will not be encountered frequently by clinical virologists because these viruses are difficult or impossible to grow in culture. The inclusions in human warts begin as granular eosinophilic matter, later condensing into rounded, basophilic masses; cytoplasmic inclusions in the epidermal cells of warts are condensed keratin and are not virus specific. The inclusions in progressive multifocal leukoencephalopathy occur in astrocytes and oligodendroglia (nonnerve cells that perform a supportive function); the inclusions vary from small granular material to large basophilic masses that fill the nucleus.

Intracytoplasmic inclusions may be found in cells that have been infected by respiratory syncytial virus, rabies virus, and viruses of the pox group. The intracytoplasmic inclusions of respiratory syncytial virus are brightly eosinophilic (see Color Plate 21-1G); they are present regularly in cell culture but less frequently in clinical specimens. Ultrastructurally, the inclusions of respiratory syncytial virus consist of fibrillar ribonucleoprotein (see Fig. 21-3C). The intracytoplasmic inclusions of rabies virus are known as Negri bodies (see Color Plate 21-1H). They may be single or multiple and occur in neurons that look otherwise healthy. The edges of the inclusions are sharply defined as if bounded by a membrane. Clear spaces or basophilic stippling, which may be seen within the inclusion, result from the incorporation of some cytoplasmic material into the mass of viral ribonucleoprotein (see Fig. 21-3E). Fortunately, the intracytoplasmic inclusions of the poxviruses, known as Guarneri bodies, are unlikely to be encountered today.

Intranuclear and intracytoplasmic inclusions are found in measles infection. During the prodromal stage of measles, giant cells appear in lymphoid tissue throughout the body. These so-called Warthin-Finkeldey giant cells contain as many as 100 nuclei and rarely may contain inclusion bodies. A second type of giant cell may arise later from epithelial tissue, such as that lining the lower respiratory tract. There are fewer nuclei in these giant cells, but inclusions are almost constant. The intranuclear inclusions resemble those produced by the herpesviruses, may be single or multiple, and vary in their degree of eosinophilia (see Color Plate 21-1F).

Detection of inclusions provides valuable information in selected clinical situations. The Tzanck test, performed by preparing a Giemsa-stained smear of vesicular scrapings, can be used to document the presence of a herpesvirus by demonstrating multinucleated giant cells (see Color Plate 21-1C). Hematoxylin-eosin or the Papanicolaou stain may also be used. The nuclei should have a ground-glass and molded or multifaceted appearance.[785] Intranuclear inclusions, which are accentuated in histologic sections by the artifactual halo produced by the fixation of tissues in formalin, may not always be visualized in the smears. A presumptive diagnosis of herpes infection can be made, although differentiation between herpes simplex virus and VZV is not possible by morphology alone.

Solomon and colleagues found positive Tzanck tests in 11 patients with clinical chickenpox (varicella virus) and in 12 of 15 patients (80%) with shingles (herpes zoster virus). However, varicella virus was recovered in only 7 of the 11 patients with chickenpox.[785] Multinucleated giant cells or inclusions or both were demonstrated in skin lesions from 18 of 21 patients (86%) from whom herpes simplex virus was isolated.[587] An analysis of the proficiency with which dermatologists correctly interpreted a study set of 10 smears demonstrated a "reverse learning curve" (or loss of neuronal synapses with increasing age!).[336] Second- and third-year residents correctly interpreted a mean of 91% of the slides; dermatologists in practice for less than 10 years scored a mean of 84% correct answers; dermatologists in practive for more than 10 years got 67% of the samples correct on average.

Although the direct smears have worked well in the study of skin lesions, the sensitivity has unfortunately been low for other applications. Only a minority of culture-positive specimens from the genital tract[823] or the respiratory tract[603] contained inclusion-bearing cells. Similarly, Nahmias and colleagues found intranuclear inclusions in only 56% of 113 cases of herpes simplex encephalitis.[602] The specificity was considerably higher (86%) than the sensitivity in this collaborative study of antiviral chemotherapy, but false-positive results are potentially dangerous if therapy for another condition, such as bacterial brain abscess, is omitted. Intranuclear inclusions were reported in 10 patients from whom herpes simplex virus was not isolated; in 7 of these patients, an alternative diagnosis not associated with inclusions was established. These results emphasize the importance of careful and informed use of "simple" morphologic tests.

The sensitivity of histologic or cytologic detection of CMV in lung tissue has varied from 38% to 70%.[310,342,603]

ELECTRON MICROSCOPIC DETECTION OF VIRAL PARTICLES

Electron microscopy can be applied to the study of both clinical specimens and cell cultures, either in thin sections of tissue or by negative stain microscopy. The inaccessibility of electron microscopes to most clinical laboratories and the sampling errors inherent in examination of small samples of tissue have deterred routine application of this technique in making viral disease diagnoses. The use of electron microscopy was specific for the diagnosis of herpes simplex encephalitis in one study (98%), but herpes virions were detected in only 45% of the cases.[602] The technique has been used effectively in the detection of viral agents of gastroenteritis,[436] especially those that are not recovered by conventional cell culture (rotavirus, Norwalk-like agents, and enteric adenoviruses). Ultrastructural diagnosis remains, however, a research technique in most laboratories.

IMMUNOLOGIC DETECTION OF VIRAL ANTIGEN

Immunologic and, more recently, molecular techniques have been used effectively to expedite diagnoses of certain viral infections. Immunofluorescence or immunoenzyme stains of clinical specimens or tissues and enzyme-linked immunosorbent assays on specimens are frequently used techniques (see Charts 25 and 39; Figs. 21-17 and 21-18).

These techniques have many advantages and have functioned well when applied by trained persons. The risks of erroneous results are great in the absence of proper equipment and training.[223] For almost all procedures, culture of the infectious agent remains the standard. Whenever possible, cultures should be done in parallel with rapid immunologic tests, until proficiency at the technique is demonstrated.

Respiratory Viruses. The diagnosis of infections caused by respiratory syncytial virus has been evaluated most extensively in clinical studies. The sensitivity of either immunofluorescence[392,433,495] or ELISA[5,373,392,813] has been 80% to 95%, with immunofluorescence being perhaps slightly more sensitive. Procedures using monoclonal antibodies have performed well,[433,449] although it is important to obtain monoclones that react broadly with wild respiratory syncytial virus strains.[670] Stout and colleagues have reported the successful use of a monoclonal antibody pool against a panel of respiratory viruses in an indirect immunofluorescence test.[803] The specificity of this test has been greater than 90%, and many of the apparent false-positive results probably reflect the difficulty of recovering this labile virus in cell culture. Collection of an adequate specimen is essential for reliable detection of antigen. Nasal aspirates have been superior to nasal and throat swabs in most studies.[346,373] The results of testing bronchoalveolar lavage fluid by culture and direct immunofluorescence have been concordant with nasal specimens in a very limited number of cases.[209] Immunofluorescence is best performed on sedimented cells after washing of the cells to remove mucus (see Color Plate 21-2E). The multiple washes are laborious and time consuming. Anestad and colleagues were able to detect respiratory syncytial virus antigen in 17 of 18 positive smears after the specimens were spread on a slide without washing.[16,17] The experience of each laboratory with the fluorescence reagents available should determine whether the serial washes are necessary. Smears of cells should be fixed in cold acetone, stained as described for cell cultures, and examined with a high-quality fluorescent microscope.

In contrast to the fluorescence procedure, results of the ELISA test for respiratory syncytial virus are improved if the fluid rather than the cells is tested.[496] Membrane enzyme immunoassays for respiratory syncytial virus have been introduced. They have slightly less sensitivity and specificity than immunofluorescence tests performed by experienced observers, but they can be performed by less experienced personnel and more quickly than immunofluorescence.[444,475] Influenza A virus, influenza B virus, and parainfluenza viruses 1 through 3 have also been detected in clinical specimens.[557,571] The increasing availability of commercial reagents, including monoclonal antibodies, for detection of these viruses will make testing easier.

Herpes Group Viruses. Direct antigenic detection of herpes simplex virus in vesicular lesions of the skin has been reliable. Virus was detected in all 15 vesicular lesions of the buttocks[852] and 23 of 24 penile lesions[853] in two studies in which the investigators used a commercial enzyme immunoassay. Lafferty and colleagues found that a combination of culture and direct immunofluorescence provided the maximal yield from lesions on the external genitalia.[482]

Unfortunately, as is the case with light microscopy, results from direct antigen detection procedures have not been entirely satisfactory in the two clinical situations of most concern—diagnosis of herpes encephalitis and evaluation of pregnant women near term. For example, the sensitivity of immunofluorescence for the diagnosis of herpes simplex encephalitis was 70% and the specificity was 91% in a large collaborative study.[602]

Although the commercial enzyme immunoassays performed well on skin lesions, reports indicate that only 40% to 70% of cervical specimens that contained virus were positive.[756,852,853] To date, these methods have not been evaluated completely. Immunofluorescence may be better suited to evaluate vesicular cervical lesions but cannot be used for detection of asymptomatic viral shedding.

Direct detection of VZV has also been reported. Several investigators have found that immunofluorescence and enzyme immunoassay both detected more cases than did viral culture.[225,746,914] In these cases, the cultures appear to represent false-negative results. Although laboratory confirmation of VZV infection is usually not necessary, the results of direct examination may be useful in problem cases.

Monoclonal antibodies have facilitated the rapid immunologic diagnosis of CMV infections in patients' specimens as well as in cell culture. Hackman and colleagues were able to detect CMV by immunofluorescence in 25 of 27 lung biopy specimens from which the virus was subsequently cultured;[342] light microscopic inclusions were demonstrated in only 20 of the specimens. Preliminary studies with bronchoalveolar lavage specimens from immunosuppressed patients[177,235,545] have yielded greatly differing estimates of sensitivity, varying from 31.6% to 100%. The numbers of patients in these studies were small, the antibodies were different, and the composition of the patient groups may have been different. The correlation of immunologic detection of viral antigen in tissue (without inclusions or histopathologic abnormalities) and clinical disease is not clear.

The efficacy of the CMV antigenemia test has been discussed on page 1212. Several viral antigens have been evaluated, of which the most common is the pp65 cytoplasmic antigen. Commercial sources of monoclonal antibodies to this antigen are available.[659] It cannot be assumed that commercial reagents will perform in the same manner as research reagents on which published reports have been based.[300]

Methodologic variables in the antigenemia assay have been assayed. Immunofluorescence is more sensitive than immunoperoxidase or other immunoenzymatic methods, and formalin fixation of smears is preferable to methanol-acetone fixation.[300] Blood for detection of CMV antigenemia may be collected either in EDTA or in lithium-heparinized tubes.[802] White blood cell separators that provide both neutrophils and monocytes are superior to physical separation of the buffy coat.[405] Preparation of the leukocyte fraction by 6% dextran sedimentation (Macrodex; Parmacia, Uppsala, Sweden) and the Polymorphprep separation procedure (Nycomed Pharma AS, Majorstua, Norway) provided equivalent results.[292] The effects of delay in processing have also been studied. In one study 49 positive samples were tested within 2 to 4 hours of receipt, then stored at 4°C for 24 hours before retesting by the same protocol. On first testing there were 41 positive samples, while 40 positive tests were recorded the next day, a statistically insignificant difference.[617] Nine specimens were positive only on initial testing, but eight specimens were positive only on the second day. In a separate study 19 of 20 specimens (95%) remained positive after storage at room temperature for 24 hours, although the average quantitative result decreased by 44%.[69] A correlation between the concentration of leukocytes in the specimen, many of which come from leukopenic patients, and CMV blood culture has been documented.[517] It is reasonable to expect a similar influence of leukocyte concentration on the results of the antigenemia assay. An advantage of morphologic assays, such as the antigenemia test, is that the adequacy of the specimen can be determined individually and directly.

Other Viruses. Human rotavirus is difficult to recover in cell culture.[851] Infections by these viruses can be diagnosed effectively either by an enzyme immunoassay or by latex agglutination. The sensitivity for both methods has ranged from 80% to 90%; the specificity has been 90% to 100%.[163,164,825] Krause and colleagues have questioned the reliability of the Rotazyme immunoassay in neonates.[473]

MOLECULAR TECHNIQUES

Nucleic acid hybridization holds great promise in the diagnosis of viral infections because of its molecular specificity. Cloned fragments of DNA or RNA that are complementary to the viral nucleic acid of interest (molecular probe) carrying either an enzyme or a radioactive marker can be reacted directly with a clinical specimen.[233,488,636] The reaction may either be performed in situ on a tissue section or in a test tube. After separating the unreacted nucleic acid from the mixture, the hybridized nucleic acid is quantitated either by measuring radioactivity or the quantity of color generated from the enzyme-labeled substrate. More recently, amplification techniques such as the polymerase chain reaction and ligase chain reaction have been introduced into clinical settings (see Chapter 1).

This technique is now emerging from research laboratories into the clinical laboratory. It has been applied successfully to the diagnosis of adenovirus,[263,616,841] CMV,[160,788,837] and herpes simplex virus[272,287] infections. Undoubtedly the initial blush of enthusiasm will be tempered by clinical experience. Probes that are both sensitive and practical will have to be developed. Many of the research probes have used gamma-particle emitting radioisotopes, which are potentially hazardous, require expensive equipment for detection of emissions, and have short half-lives. Enzymatic alternatives have been developed,[616,837] but sensitivity in comparison to the "gold standard" of culture remains a problem.

Although the molecular probes should provide the ultimate in specificity, pitfalls do exist. For instance, if probes against obligate intracellular parasites, such as viruses, include part of the cellular DNA (or if the cell and virus have DNA in common), unwanted reactions with normal tissue can occur. Cross-reactions may occur if the gene sequence that has been selected is shared with other agents.[522]

Commercially available kits have already received limited testing. Forghani and colleagues detected herpes simplex virus DNA in 16 of 17 stored human brain specimens from which the virus had been cultured previously.[272] Another probe was less successful in detecting herpesvirus in cervical specimens;[287] the sensitivity of indirect immunofluorescence and nucleic acid hybridization was 77.1% and 71.4%, respectively, in comparison with cell culture.

Molecular diagnosis has been applied commercially to HPV because the virus cannot be cultured and immunologic reagents do not detect latent virus. Several methods have been used successfully, but the requirement for radiolabeled probes has limited its application. The standard method has been Southern blot analysis. In this technique DNA in the specimen is digested and electrophoresed through an agarose gel, which separates the DNA species by size. The nucleic acids are then transferred to nitrocellulose paper, after which the "blot" is treated with a specific nucleotide probe to the virus of interest. The appropriate reactions are detected by radioautography. The Southern blot procedure is complex, expensive, and time consuming, but it is the most specific and sensitive nonamplification method. A radioautograph of papillomavirus DNA is demonstrated in Figure 21-19, where the separate bands of DNA can be seen. Other methods involve concentrating the DNA directly on a solid surface. If the digested DNA is filtered through nitrocellulose, a dot or slot blot (depending on shape) is produced (Fig. 21-20). If the DNA is captured by filtration, the test is described as a filter in situ hybridization test. The sensitivity of the in situ and dot blot methods has ranged from 60% to 90% of the reference Southern blot, depending on procedure and detection method.[99,560,638] In one study cervical swabs and cytobrush scrapings were equivalent for detecting papillomavirus infection.[653] Questionable reactions should be confirmed by the Southern blot procedure, by which the pattern of separated DNA species can be visualized.

DNA survives fixation and embedding in paraffin, so that "archaeological" analysis can be done of stored surgical specimens. Fortunately the fixative of choice is buffered formalin,[622] commonly used in surgical laboratories, but degradation of DNA does occur.

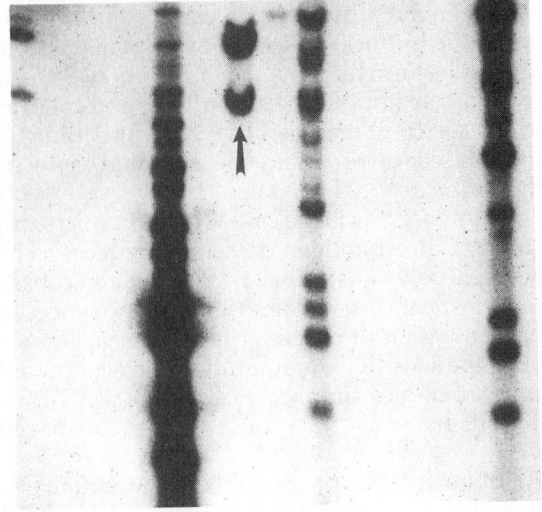

Figure 21-19
Southern blot of human papillomavirus DNA. Multiple specimens have been treated to release DNA from cells, after which the DNA was electrophoresed in agarose. Subsequently the electrophoresed DNA was transferred (blotted) onto nitrocellulose paper, reacted with ^{32}P-labeled probes for human papillomaviruses 6, 11, 16, 18, 31, 33, and 35. A radioautograph of the blot is shown here. Where the probes recognized papillomavirus genes, the radiolabel has darkened the x-ray film. Some lanes have no papillomavirus DNA, and others have multiple bands. To determine what papillomavirus is present, individual probes must be reacted when mixed infections are present. One lane contains HeLa cells which are infected with human papillomavirus, type 18 (**arrow**). (Courtesy K. DeGrove)

Amplification techniques have been applied to virtually every human viral pathogen in the research setting. Already a clinically relevant role has been established for these procedures in certain clinical situations, as described below.

Herpes Simplex Virus. Molecular amplification techniques are finding a secure place in the diagnosis of herpes simplex virus encephalitis, which has previously been exceedingly difficult to diagnose without a brain biopsy. The sensitivity of PCR assays has been reported as 75% to almost 100%, depending on the details of the assay.[33,832,679] The assays are not yet commercially available, so the detailed performance of any "home-brew" test should be investigated.

Hepatitis C Virus. Molecular techniques for detection of hepatitis C virus in blood specimens are beginning to make a place for themselves in the clinical laboratory (see page 1221).

Human Immunodeficiency Virus. Various amplification assays have been used by investigators in clinical trials of anti-HIV chemotherapy. Three assays for quantitative determination of HIV-1 levels in plasma are now commercially available.[700] Revets and colleagues evaluated commercial versions of quantitative PCR, the

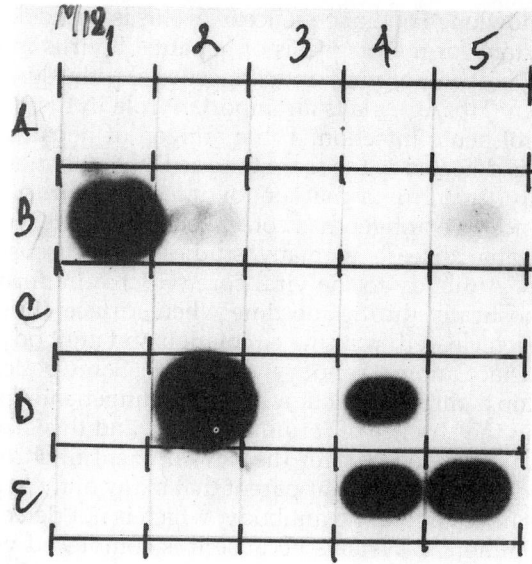

Figure 21-20

Dot blot of human papillomavirus DNA. Digested DNA from multiple specimens has been filtered directly onto nitrocellulose paper without prior electrophoresis in agar. The blots have been reacted with ^{32}P-labeled probes against human papillomavirus types 16 and 18. Specimens B1, D2, D4, E4, and E5 were positive, causing exposure of the x-ray film in these locations. Specimens B2 and B5 contained reactivity that was greater than background activity, which could be nonspecific or could represent shared nucleic acid sequences with another papillomavirus type.

nucleic acid sequence-based amplification (NASBA), and the branched DNA (bDNA) signal amplification techniques. There was no significant difference among the assays in quantitation of baseline levels of RNA or in quantitating changes in RNA after institution of antiviral chemotherapy. All of the assays were more sensitive than measurement of p24 antigenemia.

SELECTION OF TESTS FOR RAPID DIAGNOSIS

The choice of a technique for direct detection of virus must depend on the availability of equipment, on the experience of personnel, and on the number of specimens to be tested. Microscopic detection of inclusions is simple and inexpensive but relatively insensitive; it works well for documentation of herpetic skin lesions. Electron microscopy has restricted indications. Microscopic solid phase immunoassays (immunofluorescence and enzyme assays) have advantages over assays for soluble antigens: 1) the location and type of staining can be assessed morphologically and 2) small numbers of specimens may be processed quickly. These attributes may be outweighed by the disadvantages of subjectivity in interpretation and the need to acquire an expensive microscope for fluorescence.

Enzyme immunoassay is most useful when a large number of specimens are to be tested or when the specimens can be collected and tested in a batch. The end point can be read with a spectrophotometer, eliminating subjective decisions.

To study tissue sections for viral elements, immunoperoxidase has the advantage over other markers in that viral antigens are generally available for reaction without additional treatment. Endogenous peroxidases in the sections must be blocked completely. Before immunofluorescence for detection of some antigens can be performed, fixed, embedded tissue must be treated with a proteolytic agent, such as trypsin.[140,389]

Trained personnel who are familiar with these techniques are essential. It is important also to have available a "gold standard," such as viral culture, at least until experience with the technique has been obtained.

SEROLOGIC DIAGNOSIS OF VIRAL INFECTIONS

Serologic tests are the mainstay of diagnosis for certain viral infections, such as those caused by hepatitis viruses, EBV, and rubella virus. Wherever recovery of the virus in culture is difficult or impossible, documentation of an immunologic response to the agent will continue to be important. In certain cases, such as the evaluation of rubella infections, serologic diagnosis may be as rapid a culturing the virus, even if one has to wait 2 or 3 weeks for collection of a convalescent serum specimen. In those situations in which culture of the virus is reliable and readily available, serologic diagnosis has a supportive or adjunctive role.

General immunologic principles also apply when establishing a diagnosis of viral disease using serologic methods. Antibodies to many viral antigens remain for months or years after an acute infection. Demonstration of a significant increase (generally considered a fourfold rise) in titer of antibody is considered diagnostic of recent infection with the agent.

If antibodies are not present in the initial specimen, this diagnostic increase in antibody titer is referred to as a seroconversion. In this case, the infection probably represents a primary encounter with the virus. The infection may be either primary or reactivation of a latent infection if antibodies are present, even in low titer, at the time of initial testing.[602] The serologic diagnosis of herpetic infections is frequently complicated by recrudescent disease. For example, in a patient with CNS disease, oral herpetic lesions may be reactivated by the stress of the acute illness. A serologic response that may result from the reactivated oral lesions could be misinterpreted as evidence that the CNS disease was caused by herpesvirus.

Serologic cross-reactions within many virus groups and even across groups do exist, notably, among enteroviruses, paramyxoviruses, and togaviruses. All serologic diagnoses must be considered, therefore, to some degree presumptive.

A fourfold or greater decrease in antibody titer suggests an infection at some time in the past. Most antibodies disappear slowly, however, so that it is usually difficult to be sure how recent the infection was.

The clinical setting must be kept in mind when assigning a diagnosis. Even a seroconversion documents only a recent infection with the agent; association with the clinical illness is by inference.

HEPATITIS B VIRUS AND EPSTEIN-BARR VIRUS

There are a few exceptions to the general rule that a seroconversion must be documented to establish a diagnosis. In a few viral infections, antibodies to a variety of antigens appear at different times after infection and persist for varying lengths of time. It may be possible to establish a definitive diagnosis with a single serum when an antibody is detected that appears only acutely. The two prime examples are infectious mononucleosis caused by EBV (Fig. 21-21) and hepatitis B (Fig. 21-22) infections. In both cases, certain antibodies, such as IgG antibody to EBV persist for long periods; a seroconversion to these antigens must be detected. Other antibodies, such as those against the early antigen (EA) of EBV, appear transiently and may serve as markers of acute infection.

If the infectious agent is not eliminated by the immune response, the presence of antibody means that the patient may still harbor the microbe. For instance, patients who have antibody to CMV, which often produces a latent infection, are more likely to transmit the virus if blood or an organ is transplanted.[386]

Knowledge of the sequence of events is particularly important for the diagnosis of hepatitis B virus infection. Detection of viral antigen, especially the surface antigen (HbsAg), plays an important role in the diagnosis of acute infection. The e antigen of hepatitis B virus is detected at the same time as DNA polymerase activity, which is a marker for infectious virus; the presence of e antigen has correlated with acute, communicable disease in many studies,[596] as discussed above. Antibody to the viral core (HBc) is important diagnostically during the time when surface antigen has been cleared from the circulation and antibody to the surface antigen is not yet detectable. Some patients develop a chronic infection in which antigenemia persists in the absence of serum antibody, and this group has an increased risk for the development of chronic liver disease. It is now apparent that many of these patients have circulating antibody, which is not detected by commercial systems because it is complexed with antigen.[547] In addition, it has been demonstrated that some patients who have circulating antibody and no detectable surface antigen have circulating viral DNA

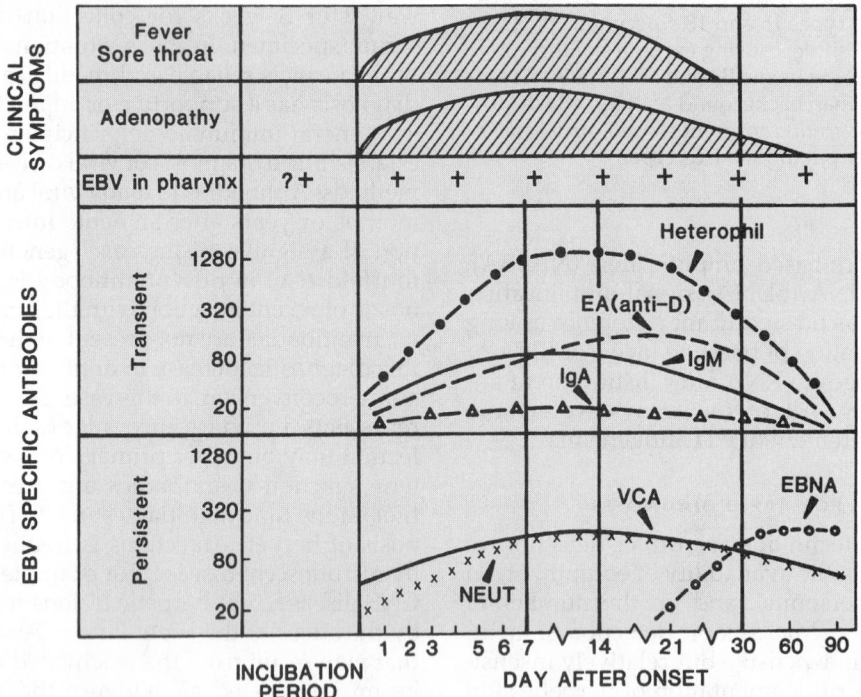

Figure 21-21

The time course of Epstein-Barr virus (EBV) infections and the serologic response. Although virus may be identified in oral secretions, the techniques for culture are difficult and are available only in research laboratories. The heterophil antibody response is the classic means of documenting infectious mononucleosis and is still the most useful test. The transient appearance of heterophil antibody, IgM antibody to viral capsid antigen, and antibody to early antigen (EA) allows one to associate the presence of antibody with the present illness. Neutralizing antibody and IgG antibody to viral capsid antigen (VCA) persist for months or years. These tests are useful to determine that the patient has been infected previously and is therefore immune; they may also be useful diagnostically if the first specimen is collected sufficiently early and a seroconversion is documented. If the patient is seen late in the course of the illness, diagnosis may be made by detection of a seroconversion to viral nuclear antigen (EBNA). (Modified with permission from James C. Niederman, Yale University School of Medicine.)

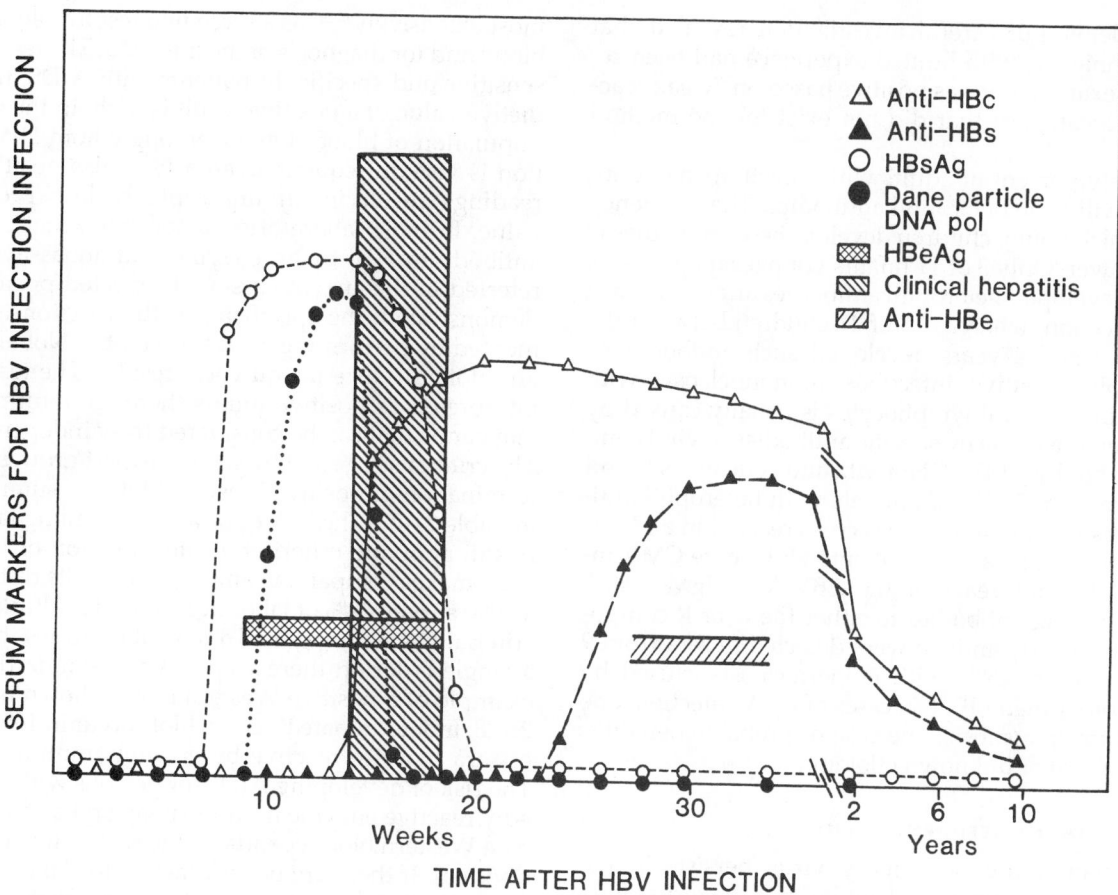

Figure 21-22
The appearance of antigens and antibodies after self-limited infection with hepatitis B virus is an example of how knowledge of the biology of infection led to very effective diagnostic strategies, although the virus itself was difficult or impossible to culture. One must look for both antigen and antibody to detect cases efficiently. Hepatitis B surface antigen (HBs) appears first; after it is cleared from the blood, antibody to that antigen can be detected (antiHBs). There may be a time, however, when antigen has been cleared but antibody is not detectable; measurement of antibody to the core antigen (anti-HBc) will cover that possibility. The presence of HBs does not equal acute, self-limited infection because some persons become carriers. (Modified with permission from William S. Robinson, MD, Stanford University Medical Center)

detectable by amplification techniques for as long as 5 years.[569]

Likewise the diagnosis of infectious mononucleosis can be made on a single serum if antibody to early antigen *and* IgM antibody to viral capsid antigen (VCA) are present. A high titer of IgG antibody to VCA in the absence of both antibody to EA and IgM antibody to VCA suggests a past infection.

The most common test for detecting infections by EBV is the heterophil antibody test. Heterophil antibodies are immunoglobulins that react with substances from another species. In the course of an EBV infection antibodies are produced to a variety of extraneous antigens. Agglutinins for sheep and horse red blood cells, hemolysins for beef red blood cells, and antibodies to the *Proteus* OX19 antigen of the Weil-Felix test are all produced. The heterophil antibodies that are very specific for infectious mononucleosis are

absorbed by beef red blood cells but not by guinea pig kidney. The Paul-Bunnell-Davidsohn differential test for infectious mononucleosis is designed to characterize these heterophil antibodies; it is highly specific for EBV and confirmatory for making the laboratory diagnosis of infectious mononucleosis.[195] A variety of simplified tests for detecting the heterophil response in infectious mononucleosis are now available commercially; most test agglutination of horse red blood cells after appropriate absorption of the sera.[267,397] Results that do not conform to clinical or hematologic data should be evaluated by performing the differential tube test or testing for EBV specific antibodies. The agglutination tests for heterophil antibody are "simple" tests, which can be performed by "anyone" with no difficulty. In 1990 a pseudoepidemic of infectious mononucleosis was recognized in Puerto Rico.[112] Quality control and proficiency testing results gave no hint of problems, but careful investigation revealed that two technicians with limited experience had been reporting examinations as positive based on "weak reactivity," a category that did not exist for the method used.

Ninety percent of adults with infectious mononucleosis will have heterophil antibodies. The frequency with which young children develop these antibodies is much lower. Only 3 of 11 infants younger than 2 years of age developed heterophil antibodies after a primary EBV infection, whereas 16 of 21 children between the ages of 2 and 4 years developed such antibodies.[396] Heterophil-negative infectious mononucleosis with circulating atypical lymphocytes is usually caused by EBV (demonstrable by specific antibodies to viral components) or by CMV.[395] Horwitz and colleagues found that sera from 38.1% of patients with heterophil antibody-positive mononucleosis cross reacted in an IgM-CMV test, but sera from patients with acute CMV infection did not react in the EBV VCA-IgM test.[395] Cross-reacting antibodies to either the D or R component of the early antigen were detected in sera from 9 of 36 patients (25%) with mononucleosis caused by agents other than EBV (six cases of CMV infection, one case of toxoplasmosis, one case of probable hepatitis, and one case of unknown etiology).

HUMAN IMMUNODEFICIENCY VIRUS

Human immunodeficiency virus persists in patients who have developed antibody to the virus. Serologic tests for HIV have been used as a screening tool because isolation of the virus in cell culture is difficult and not readily available. The reference serologic method is a Western blot procedure, in which sera are reacted with viral proteins that have been separated by polyacrylamide gel electrophoresis and transferred onto nitrocellulose paper. This test requires considerable expertise and care in performance. Several other, more easily performed assay systems have been developed. An enzyme immunoassay has been evaluated

most extensively[95,291] as a screening test for blood-bank blood and for diagnosis of the infection. The test is both sensitive and specific. In patients with AIDS, the predictive value of a positive result is high. In the general population of blood donors, among whom HIV infection is very infrequent, even a few false-positive test readings result in an unacceptably low predictive value. In most laboratories, a specimen that contains antibody to HIV by an enzyme immunoassay is first retested in the enzyme assay; if repeated positivity is demonstrated, the specificity of the reaction is documented by performing a Western blot.[175] Not all Western blots produce unequivocal results. The test is not interpreted as positive unless there are multiple protein bands that can be considered truly independent.[105] The criteria suggested by several expert groups for determination of positive Western blots are summarized in Table 21-27. The lack of uniformity among laboratories in applying criteria for interpretation of Western blots makes comparison among test results difficult. In a 1990 survey 22% of laboratories used multiple sets of criteria. Even among the 78% of laboratories that used a single criterion there were several standards.[113] An example of a positive Western blot is shown in Figure 21-23. Indeterminate Western blots occur in 10% to 20% of sera that are reactive by enzyme immunoassay.[100] The risk of developing AIDS for persons with a repeatedly reactive enzyme immunoassay and an indeterminate Western blot depends on the risk factors of the individual. If there are no risk factors for HIV infection, the patient or donor does not require further followup. As noted earlier there is a finite period of time shortly after infection with HIV when infectious virus may be present in the absence of detectable antibody.

VARICELLA-ZOSTER VIRUS

The reference serologic method for detection of antibody to VZV has been fluorescent antibody to membrane antigen assay, which requires considerable experience. Commercial versions of this assay and some

---

TABLE 21-27
Criteria for Positive Western Blot for Antibody to Human Immunodeficiency Virus

Organization	Criteria
Association of State and Territorial Public Health Laboratory Directors/CDC	Any two of: p24 gp41 gp120/gp160
FDA Licensed DuPont Test	p24 and p31 and gp41 or gp120/gp160
American Red Cross	≥3 bands: 1 from each gene product group: GAG and POL and ENV
Consortium for Retrovirus Serology Standardization	≥2 bands: p24 or p31 plus gp41 or gp120/gp160

Adapted from Centers for Disease Control: Interpretation and use of the Western blot assay for serodiagnosis of human immunodeficiency virus type 1 infections. MMWR 38 (S7):1–7, 1989

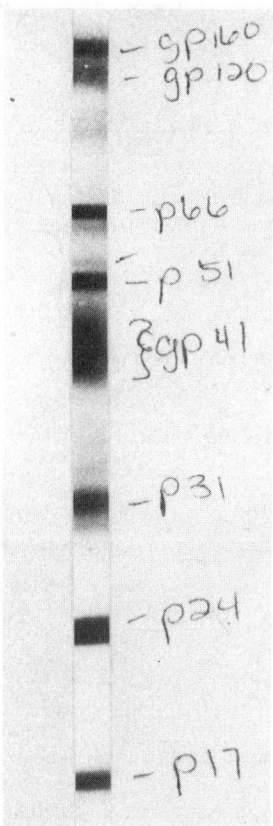

Figure 21-23
Western blot for HIV-1 antibody. Disrupted virus was electrophoresed through polyacrylamide gel, after which it was transferred (blotted) onto nitrocellulose paper. Patient's serum was then reacted with the nitrocellulose strips, after which enzyme-labeled anti-human immunoglobulin was added to the strips. Development of the enzyme reaction revealed multiple bands with this serum from an HIV-1 infected patient. The electrophoresis separated the various proteins and glycoproteins by molecular weight. The bands are labeled here according to the viral protein they have detected.

enzyme immunoassays have not functioned optimally.[38] A latex agglutination assay compared favorably to the fluorescent test,[461,799] and was more sensitive than an enzyme immunoassay.[799] When measured against cell-mediated immune responses to VZV (blastogenesis after exposure of peripheral blood mononuclear cells to viral antigen), the latex test was slightly more sensitive than an enzyme immunoassay and correlated well with cell-mediated immunity at titers ≥1:8.[862]

ANTI-IGM ANTIBODIES

In general, IgM antibody appears earlier than IgG after an acute infection and is more transient. Additionally, IgM does not readily cross the placenta, so that demonstration of this antibody in a neonate indicates a congenital or perinatal infection, rather than passive transfer of antibody from the mother.

Demonstration of IgM antibody to any antigen suggests, therefore, a recent infection. The test should be used only in laboratories in which the results have been carefully evaluated, because several theoretical and practical pitfalls may produce an erroneous interpretation. Most importantly, critical clinical decisions are often dependent on accurate results.

It is extremely important that the procedure for detection of the IgM class be demonstrably specific. The presence of IgM antibody is usually tested by demonstration of a decrease in titer after removal of IgM, by documenting residual activity after removal of IgG, by using specific antiglobulins directed against IgM, or by a combination of these approaches.

If an anti-IgM antibody is used to determine the acuteness of an infection, the specificity of the antiglobulin must be documented. False-negative results may be generated if there are very high levels of IgG, which may block the sites that would have reacted with IgM. False-positive results may be encountered if antiglobulins, such as rheumatoid factor, are present in the patient's serum. If a serum reacts with multiple antigens (ie, rubella, CMV, herpes simplex virus, and *Toxoplasma gondii*), an antiglobulin should be suspected.

Finally, although IgM antibody in serum is usually transient, there are documented instances in which IgM antibody has persisted for months or even years. Furthermore, it is now recognized that IgM can be detected when a latent infection is reactivated.[223]

MISCELLANEOUS SEROLOGIC PROCEDURES

A wide variety of procedures can be used for serologic diagnosis of viral infections (Table 21-28). The indirect immunofluorescence, enzyme immunoassay, hemagglutination inhibition, complement-fixation, and neutralization tests are outlined in Charts 14, 25, 37, 39, and 51. The reader is referred to manuals of immunologic tests for additional details.[720] Enzyme immunoassay and immunofluorescence tests are gaining increasing popularity in clinical laboratories; many of these tests are available commercially in kit form.

The complement-fixation test, which has been a mainstay of viral diagnosis, is complex and cumbersome to perform. It is still a useful test, but it has been supplanted by newer procedures, such as enzyme immunoassay, for the detection of many viral antigens and antibodies. Likewise the neutralization test may be necessary for certain purposes but is too time consuming and expensive for routine use.

The hemagglutination inhibition test is essential for testing strain-specific immunity to myxoviruses and remains the reference test for rubella infections. A variety of methods is preferred to the hemagglutination inhibition test for the diagnosis of rubella in many hospital laboratories.[237] Most tests work well in a reference laboratory, but the need for better standardization of results in the field has been emphasized.[377] A simple card agglutination test, which can be used as a screening test for rubella antibodies, has performed well with negative and strongly positive sera but less well with sera that are near the interpretative cutoff for positivity.[771] Cremer and colleagues found that a commercial enzyme immunoassay was more sensitive for detection

TABLE 21-28
SEROLOGIC DIAGNOSIS OF VIRAL INFECTIONS

VIRUS	TESTS PERFORMED	COMMENTS
Respiratory Infections		
Influenza A and B	CF; HAI	CF used for stable type-specific antigen; HAI used for strain-specific antigen
Parainfluenza virus	HAI; CF; EIA	Cross-reactions common with other paramyxoviruses
Respiratory syncytial	CF; EIA	EIA most sensitive method
Adenovirus	CF; EIA	Group-specific antigen
Central Nervous System Infections		
Enteroviruses	CF; NT; EIA	Not generally available; used in conjunction with isolation of virus
Mumps virus	HAI; IFA; EIA	Cross-reactions with other paramyxoviruses
Herpes simplex virus	CF; IHA; EIA; IFA	Not useful for diagnosis
Rabies virus	RFFIT; IFA	For diagnosis or confirmation of immune status
Hepatitis		
Hepatitis A	RIA; EIA	IgM antibody for diagnosis
Hepatitis B	RIA; EIA	IgM anti-HBc (core antigen) diagnostic; antigen detection preferred
Cutaneous Infections		
Measles virus	HI; IFA; EIA; CF	For immune status or diagnosis
Varicella-zoster virus	CF	For diagnosis only
	IFA; FAMA	For immune status
Other Infections		
Cytomegalovirus	CF; IHA; EIA; IFA	Limited value except screening of blood or organ donors
Rubella	HI; EIA; IFA; LA	Preferred method of diagnosis
Epstein-Barr virus	Heterophil test	Preferred method; may be negative, especially in children
	IFA for various antigens	For diagnosis of problem cases

CF, complement fixation; HAI, hemagglutination inhibition; EIA, enzyme immunoassay; NT, viral neutralization; IFA, immunofluorescence; RFFIT, rabies fluorescent focus test; RIA, radioimmunoassay; IHA, indirect hemagglutination; FAMA, fluorescent antibody to membrane antigen assay
Adapted from Herrmann KL: Viral serology. In Lennette EH, Balows A, Hausler WJ Jr, et al (eds): Manual of Clinical Microbiology, 4th ed, pp 921–923. Washington DC, American Society for Microbiology, 1985

of acute rubella infection than either the hemagglutination inhibition assay or a complement-fixation test.[183] In many immunology or microbiology laboratories the availability of equipment for detection of antibodies, such as spectrophotometers for enzyme immunoassays, or experience with a particular methodology will influence the choice of methods.

DIAGNOSIS OF OTHER VIRAL INFECTIONS

Diagnosis of some viral infections is beyond the scope of most hospital laboratories because the infections are rare or exotic, the etiologic agents are hazardous, or special diagnostic facilities are necessary. Tests for rabies, arboviral infections, and viral hemorrhagic fevers are usually performed in a reference laboratory, such as those in state departments of health or at the CDC.

INFECTIONS WITH *CHLAMYDIA* SPECIES

Chlamydiae are obligately intracellular bacterial pathogens. Three species of *Chlamydia* produce human disease. *Chlamydia psittaci* causes acute respiratory infections, usually transmitted from infected birds.[742] Infections by *Chlamydia trachomatis*, which includes 15

serologic variants (serovars), are much more common.[738] Serovars L1, L2, and L3 produce a sexually transmitted disease, lymphogranuloma venereum. Trachoma, a chronic conjunctivitis often complicated by blindness, is associated with serovars A, B1, B2, and C. The newest member of the genus, *Chlamydia pneumoniae*, was originally referred to as the TWAR bacillus, using the initials of two patients from whom the bacterium was isolated. Genetic studies demonstrate that the three species are closely related.[296]

All of the chlamydia may be isolated in embryonated eggs and cell culture. Recovery of *C. psittaci* in cell culture should not be attempted unless stringent isolation facilities are available for protection of laboratory personnel. Care to prevent laboratory-acquired infections should also be exercised if the serovars that cause lymphogranuloma venereum are suspected.

CHLAMYDIA TRACHOMATIS

CLINICAL FEATURES AND EPIDEMIOLOGY

Inclusion conjunctivitis (an infection distinguished from trachoma by the absence of corneal scarring), pneumonia in neonates,[50] and sexually transmitted infections in adults, all of which are caused by serovars D through K, are the chlamydial diseases of most importance for diagnostic laboratories. It has been suggested on serologic grounds that community-acquired pneumonia in adults may also be caused by *C. trachomatis*.[467] The antibodies detected in this study, however, may have been directed against the newly recognized species, *C. pneumoniae*, the apparent reactivity with *C. trachomatis* representing an unsuspected cross-reaction. The sexually transmitted infections include urethritis,[553] mucopurulent cervicitis,[86] and salpingitis.[812] The sexually transmitted and neonatal infections are, in fact, directly connected. Schachter and colleagues followed 131 infants born to mothers from whose cervix *C. trachomatis* was cultured.[739] Eighteen percent of the infants developed culture-confirmed inclusion conjunctivitis, and 16% had neonatal chlamydial pneumonia. Lan and colleagues used PCR technology to investigate the distribution of *C. trachomatis* serovars in a group of asymptomatic young women who were invited to participate in a screening program (serovars E, I, and D in decreasing order) and in a group of randomly selected patients at an inner city gynecology clinic (serovars F, E, and G in decreasing order).[485] The effects of geography on the distribution of serovars is not known.

Nettleman and colleagues suggested that empiric treatment of three groups of patients was the most cost-effective approach: (1) all patients who attended a sexually transmitted disease clinic, (2) men with either high or low risk of infection, and (3) women at high risk.[609] Cultures were indicated for women at low risk of infection. Others consider confirmation of the etiology worth the relatively modest cost of the tests, especially if disease of the upper genital tracts is a possibility.

COLLECTION OF SPECIMENS

Cervical and ocular specimens are best collected by scraping the mucosa. Swabs are readily available and minimally traumatic. Wooden-tipped swabs and swabs made of calcium alginate should be avoided; some cotton swabs have been toxic to *Chlamydia*; Dacron or rayon material is preferred.[170] Despite the use of acceptable types of swabs, some lots may be toxic to *Chlamydia*, so that pretesting of lots is recommended.[664] Urethral and nasopharyngeal specimens may be collected with a fine swab on a flexible wire. The swab should be inserted 3 to 5 cm into the urethra. Semen and purulent urethral discharge are not considered adequate specimens for culture.[170] *C. trachomatis* can be detected in first morning urine specimens with some enzyme immunoassays and with amplification techniques, as discussed later.

Cervical specimens are collected from the endocervix after carefully removing mucus. The isolation rate is increased if a urethral and cervical swab are placed in the same transport vial. The cytobrush, used for collection of Papanicolaou smears, has been reported to be superior to swabs by some investigators[430] but not others.[861] The cytobrush cannot be used in pregnant women. Lesions in the rectum and fallopian tube should be sampled under direct visualization by anoscopy or laparoscopy.

Direct detection of *C. trachomatis* by immunofluorescence is done after application of the specimen to a clean glass slide. The type and manner of collection of specimens is the same as for diagnosis by culture. The slide should be fixed according to the manufacturer's instructions as quickly as possible. For the commonly used Microtrak reagent (Syva Co., Palo Alto, CA), fixation in methanol enhanced detection of organisms in comparison to fixation in acetone.[430]

ISOLATION OF *CHLAMYDIA TRACHOMATIS* IN CELL CULTURE

Although chlamydiae are bacteria, they are obligate intracellular pathogens. Methods for isolation in culture are similar to those employed in the virology laboratory. It is essential, however, that the infective elementary bodies of chlamydiae be centrifuged onto the monolayer in a shell vial (see Fig. 21-9). Isolation of the bacteria is optimized if a force of 3000 $\times g$ for 60 minutes can be achieved.[780] Cells that have been irradiated or treated with a metabolic inhibitor are used for culture of *C. trachomatis*. Cycloheximide-treated McCoy cells are the most commonly used cell line;[902] cycloheximide (1 µg/mL) is included in the tissue culture media that are used after infection of the monolayer. Polybrene, a polycation that has been used to enhance the infectivity of retroviruses, also enhances the number of chlamydial inclusions and the rate of isolation from clinical specimens.[737] Sabet and colleagues successfully used HeLa 229 cells that had been treated with DEAE-dextran and cycloheximide for isolation of *C. trachomatis*.[728] Buffalo green monkey cells are reportedly superior to McCoy cells.[474]

Inclusion bodies of *C. trachomatis* contain glycogen, which may be stained with iodine. After incubation for 48 to 72 hours, the coverslips are removed and stained with iodine or, for somewhat greater sensitivity, with a fluoresceinated monoclonal antibody[796] (see Color Plate 21-2C). Species-specific monoclonal antibodies directed against outer membrane proteins and genus-specific antibodies directed against lipopolysaccharide are available. Chlamydial inclusions are well demarcated, cytoplasmic structures. Additional sensitivity may be achieved by subculturing growth in a vial if the culture is negative after a single passage, but the expense of the procedure is increased considerably.

Micromethods for culture have been described in which 96-well microplates are seeded with McCoy cells either before or at the time of inoculation with the clinical specimen.[818,902,904] The wells are examined microscopically after staining with iodine or fluorescein-conjugated antiserum. The microplates are considerably more economical than the individual shell vials and have been found to be of equivalent sensitivity by several investigators.[902,904] Other investigators, however, consider the micromethod less sensitive than conventional culture.[429,516] Much of the argument over whether blind subculture increases the recovery of *Chlamydia* probably derives from varying protocols for primary culture.[429] In general, there is little yield from blind subculture if vessels with a large surface are inoculated and a monoclonal antibody is used to detect inclusions. Micromethods benefit from routine subculture.

DIRECT DETECTION OF *CHLAMYDIA TRACHOMATIS* IN CLINICAL SPECIMENS

If large numbers of chlamydial inclusion bodies are present, a diagnosis may be established easily by staining smears by the Giemsa or Gimenez methods.[372] The Gimenez stain, which contains carbolfuchsin, is preferred because the inclusions are colored well, but the Giemsa stain is more generally available. The inclusions, which are located in the cytoplasm of epithelial cells, often have a perinuclear location and must be distinguished from artifacts, such as fragmented nuclei (see Color Plate 21-2A). The frequency with which inclusions are detected in smears is highest in neonatal conjunctivitis, lower in inclusion conjunctivitis of adults and in trachoma, and lowest in urethritis and cervicitis, where inclusions are rarely found. The advent of commercially available monoclonal antibodies to species-specific antigens of *C. trachomatis* has revolutionized the rapid diagnosis of this infection. The monoclonal antibodies detect the elementary particle and inclusions of all serovars with considerably greater sensitivity than histochemical stains.

Immunofluorescence. A direct immunofluorescence test (Microtrak; Syva Co., Palo Alto, CA) has been evaluated most extensively. The sensitivity of the test for detection of genital infections has ranged from 60% to 100%, and the specificity has been very high.[795,818] The large variation in sensitivity may reflect, in part, differences in the prevalence of chlamydial infection in various populations.[43] The direct test may be particularly valuable when long delays are inevitable between the collection of a specimen and the initiation of culture.[882] Interpretation of the test requires trained personnel and high-quality (ie, expensive) equipment. Although the antibody is of monoclonal origin, at least one of the antigens of *C. trachomatis* resembles the lipopolysaccharide of enteric bacteria[623] and probable cross-reactions with other bacteria have been reported.[516] Many different immunofluorescence reagents are now on the market. In general, the fluorescence of reagents that are directed against the major outer membrane proteins is brighter and the bacterial morphology is more consistent.[168] Antibodies to *C. trachomatis* lipopolysaccharide cross react with other *Chlamydia* species, which may be an advantage or disadvantage, depending on the objective of the user.

Elementary bodies are the infectious form that is seen in clinical specimens. They are small (0.25–0.35 μm) and round with sharp, well-defined margins (see Color Plate 21-2B). Smears should be examined with a 40× or 63× objective, and the identity of fluorescing particles should be confirmed with a 100× objective. At the higher magnification, a central, more darkly staining region can often be discerned in the structures. Although the elementary bodies are very small, they often occur in small clusters, even when only few in number. When the infection is heavy, there is greater variation in the size and shape of elementary bodies and inclusion bodies may be seen occasionally.

Distinguishing the morphology of the tiny, fluorescing particles from debris is of prime importance. Particulate debris often has a yellowish color and can be visualized as refractile structures with incident white light. In contrast, specific fluorescence has an apple-green color and the elementary bodies cannot be seen with white light. The color of the specific fluorescence, however, may appear yellow-green if there is abundant background material that fluoresces red in the presence of a counterstain. A minimum number (defined by the manufacturer) of well-defined elementary bodies should be observed before the smear is reported as positive. The smear should be examined completely for at least 3 minutes before a negative interpretation is reported. Genital specimens that are acellular or contain only mature squamous cells are suboptimal. Brunham and colleagues studied the correlation of inflammatory exudate and recovery of *C. trachomatis* in 100 randomly selected women.[86] More than 10 polymorphonuclear neutrophils per oil immersion field were observed in 17 (89%) of 19 women from whom *C. trachomatis* was isolated. The presence of at least five columnar epithelial cells on a slide increased the sensitivity of the test from 70% to 92% in one study.[665] Unfortunately, the scanty cellular content of the specimen will not be known until after the test has been performed, but the information should be conveyed to the clinician.

The direct immunofluorescence procedure is even more sensitive for detection of inclusion conjunctivitis than for genital infection, as might be expected from the experience with Giemsa-stained smears. Two groups of investigators identified all infants with neonatal chlamydial conjunctivitis using the direct procedure.[53,692] In contrast, the sensitivity of Giemsa-stained smears was only 42%.

In a small number of patients, the direct immunofluorescence test has been used to diagnose neonatal chlamydial pneumonia.

The direct immunofluorescence test has almost achieved the status of another diagnostic "gold standard" when performed by highly trained personnel who use high-quality fluorescence microscopes. The influence of inadequate skill and training on the results of this reliable but subjective test can be devastating.[519]

Howard and colleagues studied the effect of specimen quality on detection of elementary bodies.[402] If the slide contained no columnar or transitional epithelial cells, only 0.78% of slides were positive for *C. trachomatis*. If fewer than 25 columnar/transitional cells were present, 2.8% of slides were positive. 8.8% of slides were positive when more than 25 columnar/transitional cells were present.

Enzyme Immunoassay. Enzyme immunoassays for *C. trachomatis* are also available. The original commercial assay has been evaluated most thoroughly (Chlamydiazyme; Abbott Laboratories, North Chicago, IL). The sensitivity of the enzyme assay has varied from 70% to 100%, partially depending on the source of the specimen.[149,428,510] The specificity of a modified test appears to have been improved,[149,428] although one recent collaborative study documented a sensitivity of only 57% in comparison to culture.[534] The correlation of culture and enzyme immunoassay decreased in subgroups at low risk of disease. A disturbingly low specificity was observed with the original assay and with a modified assay also.[510,534] Most of the positive results that were not supported by culture occurred with cervical specimens from asymptomatic women.

In most comparative studies the sensitivity of direct immunofluorescence and enzyme immunoassay has been similar. The nonspecificity of enzyme assays[445,534] has been recognized by the commercial suppliers, some of whom now provide confirmatory blocking assays with their kits. Another approach to increasing specificity has been to centrifuge specimens that were positive by enzyme immunoassay and examine the sediment by direct immunofluorescence.[576] In the process, of course, the test becomes more expensive and less timely. The problem of nonspecificity in a population with low prevalence requires that confirmatory steps be taken.

Some investigators have recommended that urine sediments from male patients with urethritis be examined for *C. trachomatis* by the enzyme immunoassay.[752] The advantage of this noninvasive procedure to the patient is obvious. Unfortunately, not all investigators have had success with urine specimens[782] and problems with nonspecificity of the enzyme immunoassay may be magnified.[207] Molecular amplification methods provide another, superior approach to this problem, as discussed later.[148]

The choice of tests for diagnosis of chlamydial infection will depend on local needs. If the population of patients to be tested is expected to have a low prevalence of chlamydial infection (eg, patients from private obstetric practices), culture will probably be the most sensitive and specific diagnostic modality. Immediacy of diagnosis is not usually an issue. If facilities for culture are not readily available and transportation of specimens is difficult, one of the methods for detection of antigen may be preferable.

SEROLOGIC DIAGNOSIS

Antibodies to *C. psittaci* and the lymphogranuloma venereum serovars of *C. trachomatis* can be detected by the complement-fixation test. A microimmunofluorescence test for antibodies to *C. trachomatis* is more sensitive for diagnosis of lymphogranuloma venereum infections and can also be used to document infections by other serovars. This test is less widely available and multiple antigens must be tested. It is most useful for seroepidemiologic studies of populations at high risk of chlamydial infection.

MOLECULAR TECHNIQUES

The first commercial molecular test applied to *C. trachomatis* was a DNA probe against rRNA (Gen-Probe, Inc., San Diego, CA). The sensitivity of the test has ranged from approximately 80% to 95%, depending on the population of patients tested, the source of the specimen, the version of the test evaluated, and the "gold standard" applied. The importance of patient population is illustrated by a study that used the relatively insensitive first generation of the test.[894] The sensitivity of the Gen-Probe PACE assay overall was 80%, but the sensitivity was 94% in emergency room patients and 74% in outpatient clinic patients. Improvements in the assay (PACE2) and in methods for collection of specimens have improved the performance of the test, with most recent reports yielding sensitivities at the upper end of the range.[400,462]

Falsely positive probe tests may occur if swabs other than those supplied by the manufacturer are used. Additionally, samples that produce results near the positive cutoff may be erroneously characterized as positive. An indeterminate zone has been introduced in many laboratories, and tests that fall in that range are repeated. A confirmatory competitive assay for these specimens is now available. Woods and Garza have reported that they were able to confirm the results of presumptively positive direct probe test with a competitive assay in 100% of specimens that gave a reading of more than 1500 relative light units (RLU), in 79% of specimens that gave a RLU reading between 1000 and 1500, and in 59% of specimens that gave a RLU of less than 1000.[892]

When head-to-head comparisons with enzyme immunoassays and the DNA probe have been performed, the sensitivity and specificity of the probe has been equivalent or superior to the immunoassay. In contrast to some enzyme immunoassays the probe test is not approved for testing urine specimens, but as discussed above, the enzyme immunoassay is not the optimal test for this purpose.

The probe test has been approved for use with genital and ocular specimens. In a study of ocular specimens from an area endemic for trachoma, the Gen-Probe test had a sensitivity and specificity of 87% and 91%, respectively, in comparison to culture.[197] The sensitivity and specificity of direct immunofluorescence on the same patients were 48% and 97%, respectively. The poor results of immunofluorescence may relate to the low numbers of inclusions in patients with trachoma in comparison to individuals with acute conjunctivitis.

A new dimension has been introduced to chlamydial diagnosis by application of amplification tests, the PCR (Roche Molecular Systems, Branchburg, NJ), and ligase chain reaction (LCR) (Abbott Laboratories, North Chicago, IL). The adjusted sensitivity of the Roche Amplicor assay for endocervical specimens has been 89% to 97%.[47,772] The reference standard was a positive culture or confirmation of the molecular reaction with a second set of primers. The adjusted sensitivity of culture was 86% and 72% in the two studies, whereas the enzyme immunoassay tested had an adjusted sensitivity of 61%. The specificity of the PCR was 99.7% to 100%. Culture was absolutely specific. When applied to voided urine specimens the sensitivity of the PCR was 91.7% to 95% and the specificity was 99.5% to 99.8%.[47,419]

The target of the LCR is plasmid DNA. A confirmatory assay uses primers directed against a portion of the gene that encodes outer membrane protein. In a comparative study of LCR and culture for detection of *C. trachomatis* from endocervical specimens, the sensitivity of culture and LCR was 65% and 94%, respectively. The specificity of LCR was more than 99%. Discrepant tests were resolved by direct immunofluorescence and use of the second set of primers. Investigators have focused attention on the first voided urine specimen of the day in men and women. The sensitivity of LCR on first voided urine specimens from women ranges from 86% to 96%, and the specificity approaches 100%.[148,740] In a study where the adjusted sensitivity of the LCR was 96% on urine specimens, the sensitivity of the Chlamydiazyme (Abbott Laboratories, North Chicago, IL) was only 37% in women and 68% in men. The sensitivity of culture of the male urethra was 38%, perhaps reflecting the difficulty of getting adequate urethral samples.[148]

The role of the amplification techniques is most clearly established for diagnosis of urethritis in men or urethritis without cervicitis in women with the added bonus that the test can be performed on a specimen obtained by noninvasive means. The sensitivity of the amplification procedures for cervical specimens is also increased over nonamplified methods, but the advantages are not so great as with urethral/urine specimens.

OTHER METHODS FOR DIAGNOSIS

Cytologic detection of *Chlamydia* has not generally been considered reliable. Kiviat and colleagues, however, have reported a cytologic inflammatory pattern that suggested strongly the presence of chlamydial infection.[455] If "transparent" lymphocytes and increased numbers of histiocytes were present, *C. trachomatis* was isolated in 53% of patients; in the absence of those findings *C. trachomatis* was isolated only from 4% of patients. If these cytologic features are noted in a cervical smear, specific tests for chlamydia should be considered.

A bewildering array of diagnostic products is now available for diagnosing *Chlamydia* infections, including tests designed to be performed in a physician's office. The careful microbiologist will scrutinize the claims closely and wait for multiple, careful, objective evaluations to be published.

DIAGNOSIS OF SEXUAL ABUSE

Among the less attractive aspects of *Chlamydia* infections is the occurrence of the organism in sexually abused children.[192] The test of choice for investigation of suspected sexual abuse is the culture. Tests for chlamydial antigen or even genes are potentially nonspecific[358,446] and will probably not stand up in court.

CHLAMYDIA PSITTACI

Chlamydia psittaci is the causative agent of psittacosis or ornithosis. The source of infection is a variety of birds, especially psittacine species such as parakeets.[360]

An outbreak of psittacosis occurred at a turkey processing plant in North Carolina.[109] Many organ systems may be affected in the natural host. In humans the primary infectious target is the lung.[741] The resulting pneumonia is usually subacute or chronic, but acute, fulminating infection can result.[91] *C. psittaci* is a cause of endocarditis.[850]

The diagnosis of psittacosis is usually accomplished by serology, the traditional test being complement fixation. The microimmunofluorescence test has become the reference serologic test for this infection. Complement-fixing antibodies to *C. psittaci* were detected in 36 of 78 sera (46%) submitted for chlamydial serology.[888] An additional 12 sera (15%) were positive by microimmunofluorescence, and a further 9 sera had antibodies to *C. pneumoniae* by microimmunofluorescence.

The organism can be isolated in cell culture using methods designed for *C. trachomatis*, but this agent has great potential for producing laboratory infections, so great care should be taken with the specimen. Species-specific antisera are necessary for definitive identification of the isolate. If the monolayer reacts with antibodies to the lipopolysaccharide, but not the outer membrane protein of *C. trachomatis*, it suggests that another *Chlamydia* species is present. Presumptive identification of *C. psittaci* directly in respiratory secretions has been reported by using antisera to chlamydial lipopolysaccharide.[629] The PCR has been used to identify isolated *C. psittaci* in culture.[246]

CHLAMYDIA PNEUMONIAE

Chlamydia pneumoniae was originally isolated from patients with respiratory infections and was first called TWAR after the source patients. It produces sporadic and epidemic lower respiratory disease that is characterized as atypical pneumonia.[328,662] It has been estimated that 10% of pneumonias worldwide are caused by *C. pneumoniae*,[442] but most infections do not require admission to the hospital. Asymptomatic infection occurs in 2% to 5% of individuals. *C. pneumoniae* was detected by culture or PCR in the nasopharynx of 2 of 104 (1.9%) asymptomatic adults.[413] The prevalence of antibody to *C. pneumoniae* in this population was 82%.

Primary infection occurs in children and young adults, but immunity is not solid and reinfections are common in adults.[442] The onset of pneumonia is often insidious without purulent sputum or leukocytosis. The chest radiograph varies from normal to extensive involvement, and there are no diagnostic features. In primary infection the most common pattern is unilateral alveolar infiltrates.[533] Chronic pulmonary infections occur, and patients may be symptomatic for weeks or months.[357]

Chlamydia pneumoniae is a cause of pharyngitis alone and in combination with other agents[412] and may be a cause of culture-negative endocarditis.[542] It has been linked epidemiologically to coronary heart disease.[731]

Chlamydia pneumoniae can be cultured in the laboratory using HeLa 229 cells with dextran, HL cells,[169] HEp-2 cells,[716,526] or NCI-H 292 cells.[526,887] If HL cells or 292 cells are used, it may not be necessary to treat the monolayers or to perform blind passage.[887] Eagle's minimal essential medium or sucrose–phosphate–glutamate with an added protein source, such as fetal calf serum, as used for viruses and *C. trachomatis*, are useful transport media.[524] Laboratory-adapted strains of *C. pneumoniae* are relatively stable, but wild-type strains are more labile and do not survive well for more than a few hours even at 4°C. Samples should be frozen, preferably at −70°C if they cannot be processed on the day of collection. Fluorescein-conjugated monoclonal antisera are available for detection and identification of isolates in culture.[578] Cultures are incubated for 72 hours. Incubation in serum-free medium has been reported to increase the infectivity of laboratory-adapted strains for HL cells 10- to 50-fold and to increase the number of inclusions produced by a wild-type strain.[525]

Most infections are diagnosed serologically. The serology may be more complicated than presently realized. Antigenic variation among isolates was sufficiently great in one study that some patients only produced measurable antibody against their own isolate.[66] The proposed serologic diagnostic criteria for acute infection are an IgM titer of ≥1:16 or an IgG titer of ≥512 by microimmunofluorescence. Hyman and colleagues found that 19 of 101 asymptomatic adults (19%) fulfilled these criteria,[413] so demonstration of seroconversion in acute and convalescent specimens is the most reliable serologic approach. Molecular amplification methods for direct detection of *C. pneumoniae* in respiratory specimens have been developed because of the difficulties inherent in cultural and serologic approaches.[295]

INFECTIONS WITH *RICKETTSIA* AND RELATED ORGANISMS

The order Rickettsiales includes the genera *Rickettsia*, *Coxiella*, *Rochalimaea*, *Ehrlichia*, *Bartonella*, and several newly identified pathogens. Infections caused by *Rochalimaea* and *Bartonella*, including cat-scratch fever, are discussed in Chapter 8.[858,859] The most numerous and important genus is *Rickettsia*.

RICKETTSIA AND COXIELLA

CLINICAL FEATURES AND EPIDEMIOLOGY

Rickettsia species infect vascular endothelial cells. The clinical manifestations of infection are consequently protean and may reflect damage to any organ system. The skin and brain are most frequently involved symptomatically. *Rickettsia* can be divided into the typhus, scrub typhus, and spotted fever groups (Table 21-29). The agent of Q fever, *Coxiella burnetii*, is also an obligate intracellular pathogen. The primary means of transmission of rickettsial infections is by the bite of an infected arthropod. Q fever may also be transmitted through infected milk or by aerosol.

Epidemic typhus has been one of the great scourges of mankind, appearing during periods of crowding and starvation. *R. prowazekii* has been demonstrated in

TABLE 21-29
RICKETTSIAL INFECTIONS

DISEASE	SPECIES	INSECT VECTOR
Typhus Group		
Epidemic typhus	*R. prowazekii*	Human louse
Murine typhus	*R. typhi*	Flea
Relapsing typhus (Brill-Zinsser)	*R. prowazekii*	
Spotted Fever Group		
Rocky Mountain spotted fever	*R. rickettsii*	Ixodid ticks
Boutonneuse fever (Mediterranean spotted fever)	*R. conorii*	Ixodid ticks
Rickettsialpox	*R. akari*	Mites
Scrub Typhus Group		
Scrub typhus	*R. tsutsugamushi*	Mites
Q Fever Group		
Q fever	*C. burnettii*	Tick (animals)

flying squirrels in the eastern United States,[891] and a small number of associated human infections have occurred.

In the United States, the most important rickettsial infection is Rocky Mountain spotted fever.[844] This multisystemic febrile disease is usually accompanied by a skin rash that begins on the extremities.[369,452,845] The infection is widely distributed throughout the country, wherever the tick vectors exist (see Chapter 20; appendix I). Paradoxically, the infection is more common in the midwestern and south central states than in the western and mountain states.[188,365] The therapy for Rocky Mountain spotted fever is doxycycline or chloramphenicol in patients who are allergic to tetracyclines.[845] Patients who are treated appropriately within the first 5 days of illness are less likely to die than those who are not treated or who are treated later.[453]

Q fever, which is highly contagious, usually causes asymptomatic infection, undifferentiated febrile disease, granulomatous hepatitis, or atypical pneumonia.[541,789,833] It may be transmitted through milk, products of conception, or excreta of infected cattle, sheep, and goats. Epidemics have occurred in laboratories where sheep were used for research purposes.[353] A chronic form of the infection may result in subacute bacterial endocarditis.[450] Rash is rare in Q fever.

COLLECTION OF SPECIMENS

Culture of *Rickettsia* is performed only in reference laboratories. Blood or biopsy tissue from a lesion should be frozen at −70°C. Direct immunofluorescence may be performed on a frozen or formalin-fixed biopsy or autopsy specimen. Rickettsial infections are usually diagnosed serologically, using acute and convalescent sera.

ISOLATION OF *RICKETTSIA* AND *COXIELLA* IN CULTURE

Rickettsia and *Coxiella* may be isolated in small laboratory animals or in embryonated eggs.[846] *Coxiella burnetii* has been isolated in shell vial cultures of human embryonic lung fibroblasts from blood of 17% of untreated patients with acute Q fever and 53% of untreated patients with chronic disease.[598] All of these bacteria are highly infectious when they are aerosolized. They have been responsible for many laboratory-acquired infections, some of which were fatal.[632] Isolation of the agents should be attempted only in laboratories where adequate containment of infection is possible. Whole blood or biopsied tissues may be cultured.

DIRECT DETECTION OF ANTIGEN IN CLINICAL SPECIMENS

Antigens of *Rickettsia rickettsii*, the cause of Rocky Mountain spotted fever, can be detected directly by staining sections of infected skin lesions using the direct or indirect immunofluorescence technique.[846] The sensitivity of the procedure is approximately 70%, and the specificity approaches 100%. Usually, petechial skin lesions are biopsied. The rickettsiae are most likely to be in the blood vessel at the center of the lesion, so it is important to ensure that such vessels are included in the tissue section. Antigens can also be demonstrated in paraffin-embedded, formalin-fixed specimens if the section is treated first with trypsin to unmask antigens.[847] Although the immunofluorescence test is valuable for making an early diagnosis of Rocky Mountain spotted fever, it is available in very few laboratories.

SEROLOGIC DIAGNOSIS

Most diagnoses of rickettsial infections are made by serology. In recent years, the microimmunofluorescence assay has become the reference test.[663] This procedure appears to be the most sensitive and specific method for the diagnosis of rickettsial infections.[438] The degree of cross-reaction among rickettsial species varies from patient to patient.[663] Cross-reactions are strongest within the rickettsial subgroups. It may be difficult to distinguish between epidemic and endemic typhus or between Rocky Mountain spotted fever and rickettsialpox.[846] Antibodies first appear 7 to 10 days after infection. A fourfold rise in serum antibody is desired for diagnosis, but a single titer of more than 1:64 is highly suggestive.

The microimmunofluorescence test requires highly trained personnel and a fluorescence microscope. Latex agglutination tests, which are now commercially available for Rocky Mountain spotted fever, are in more general use. The latex tests appear to produce positive reactions only during an acute infection, so a single positive test is diagnostic.[370] The sensitivity has ranged from 70% to 95%.[370,438] The complement-fixation test was once the diagnostic standard,[761] and it remains a valid very specific serologic tool. As the newer tests have been developed, however, it has become apparent that the complement-fixation test is insensitive for rickettsial diagnosis.[438,610] After infection by *Coxiella burnetti*, antibodies may be produced to two biologic phases of the organism. Antibodies to phase II are produced first. Antibodies to phase I, which appear weeks or months later, may reach high levels in patients with Q fever endocarditis. If complement-fixation antibodies to both phases of *Coxiella* are high in a patient with culture-negative endocarditis, a diagnosis of Q fever is likely.[450,789] Interested readers should consult the recent comprehensive review of Q fever by Marrie and colleagues.[540]

Historically, the most common diagnostic test for rickettsial disease has been the Weil-Felix test, in which anti-rickettsial antibodies that cross react with strains of *Proteus* species are detected. The test originated from the chance observation that sera from patients with typhus agglutinated strains of *Proteus vulgaris*. As experience with immunologically specific serologic tests has been accumulated, it has become apparent that the Weil-Felix test is both insensitive and nonspecific.[371,438,846] In some populations, a positive Weil-Felix test result has been more common in those who did not have Rocky Mountain spotted fever than in those who were infected.[846] All of these facts argue strongly for the relegation of this test to the archives.

EHRLICHIA SPECIES

The tribe Ehrlichieae are *Rickettsia*-like bacteria that infect a variety of animal species, producing diseases such as tropical canine pancytopenia and Potomac horse fever.[712] They are obligate intracellular parasites and, like rickettsia, grow in the cytosol of infected cells.

Human ehrlichial infection, which is a recently recognized phenomenon, is caused by two distinct species: *Ehrlichia chaffeensis*, which infects human monocytic cells,[13,196] and an as yet unnamed species that infects granulocytic cells (currently designated the human granulocytic *Ehrlichia*).[146] Both species are transmitted to humans by ticks and produce febrile illness with leukopenia, thrombocytopenia, and elevated serum aminotransferase.[229]

Human monocytic ehrlichiosis, caused by *Ehrlichia chaffeensis*, was recognized first. It is distributed widely through the southeast, midwest, and far west of the United States. The most common vector is the lonestar tick, *Amblyomma americanum* (see Chapter 18 and Chapter 20, appendix I).[8] In areas where tick vectors are prevalent seroconversions to *Rickettsia rickettsii* occurred in 2.5% and to *E. chaffeensis* in 1.3% of military personnel.[901] In southern Georgia human monocytic ehrlichiosis was seven to eight times more prevalent than Rocky Mountain spotted fever.[266] Contact with ticks is a risk factor for both ehrlichiosis and Rocky Mountain spotted fever.[8] An outbreak of monocytic ehrlichiosis occurred in a golf-oriented retirement community (community A) that abutted a natural wildlife area.[798] Cases were not recognized at a nearby community and golf course (community B) that were not surrounded by a natural area. The prevalence of antibody to *E. chaffeensis* in community A was 12.5%, whereas in community B the prevalence was 3.3%. Thousands of *A. americanum* ticks were found in community A, but only three ticks were detected in community B. The risk factors for developing ehrlichiosis included tick bites, contact with wildlife, failure to use insect repellent, and golfing. Among golfers those at greatest risk were the hookers and slicers, who were constantly retrieving their balls from the rough. The moral is that if you golf in a rural area, you should wear insect repellent and hit the ball straight.

The clinical symptoms of monocytic ehrlichiosis range from nonspecific febrile disease to severe systemic infection with multiorgan failure.[229,265] Prolonged fever may be the only clinical symptom.[717] In one study of 237 infected patients, 60.8% were hospitalized.[265] Severe monocytic ehrlichiosis with failure of multiorgan systems has been mistaken for thrombotic thrombocytopenic purpura[546] and toxic shock syndrome.[260]

The most effective chemotherapy for monocytic ehrlichiosis is tetracycline or chloramphenicol.[265] The median time for recovery of hospitalized patients was 16 days for patients treated with tetracycline, 12 days for those treated with chloramphenicol, and 27 days for patients who received other antibiotics. Patients who did not receive tetracycline or chloramphenicol until 8 or more days after the onset of illness were more likely to suffer severe illness or die. Three of 49 outpatients (6.1%) who were treated with one of these two antibiotics were subsequently hospitalized in contrast to 35 of 38 outpatients (92%) who received other antibiotics. Persistent infection resulting in death has been reported in a patient who had been treated with both tetracycline and chloramphenicol.[231]

Masses of ehrlichieae (morula) may be seen within the cytoplasm of infected monocytes (Color Plate 21-2G), but these diagnostic structures are infrequently seen with *E. chaffeensis* infection.[229] The diagnosis is made serologically, by culture of the agent,[147] or by molecular methods.[9,249] A variant strain of *E. chaffeensis* has been described, and the full antigenic diversity of the species is probably not yet appreciated.[230]

The most recent addition to the list of pathogenic *Ehrlichia* is the human granulocytic agent, which was first recognized in Minnesota and Wisconsin by an alert infectious disease physician, who recognized the similarity of the intracellular granulocytic inclusions to those described in *E. chaffeensis* infection.[37,146] The agent of human granulocytic ehrlichiosis has not yet been named. It is closely related to *Ehrlichia phagocytophila* and *Ehrlichia equi*, the agent of Potomac fever in horses.[228,532] The vector for the human granulocytic *Ehrlichia* is *Ixodes scapularis (dammini)* (See Chapter 18 and Chapter 20, Appendix I), the same vector that transmits Lyme disease and babesiosis.[637] Patients in the north central United States appear from serologic studies to have been infected with all three pathogens.[575] Not surprisingly, the distribution of human granulocytic ehrlichiosis is expanding to cover the range of the host tick. Infections have now been reported from New York,[129] Connecticut,[359] and Massachusetts.[821]

The clinical disease appears to be similar to that produced by *E. chaffeensis*. Laboratory diagnosis is still in its infancy. Intracellular inclusions (morula) in granulocytes (Color Plate 21-2H) appear to be more common than are inclusions in monocytic ehrlichiosis,[37] but there may be an ascertainment bias without readily available laboratory diagnostic support. Culture of the organism in vitro has been reported,[321] but confirmation of most cases is by serologic techniques, which are not yet widely available.

Ehrlichia sennetsu produces a self-limited febrile disease with neutropenia in humans. The differential diagnosis includes infectious mononucleosis and scrub typhus. The organism is isolated by inoculation of mice.

REFERENCES

1. AACH, RD, STEVENS CE, HOLLINGS FB ET AL: Hepatitis C virus infection in post-transfusion hepatitis. An analysis with first- and second-generation assays. N Engl J Med 325:1325–1329, 1991

2. ACKERMAN SJ: HIV-1 link prompts circumspection on circumcision. J NIH Res 3:44–46, 1991

3. AGHA FP, LEE HH, NOSTRANT TT: Herpetic esophagitis: A diagnostic challenge in immunocompromised patients. Am J Gastroenterol 81:246–253, 1986

4. AGUADO S, ONA M, MARTINEZ A ET AL: Concomitant infection with three types of virus in a renal transplant recipient. Nephron 48:161–163, 1988

5. AHLUWALIA GS, HAMMOND GW: Comparison of cell culture and three enzyme-linked immunosorbent assays for the rapid diagnosis of respiratory syncytial virus from nasopharyngeal aspirate and tracheal secretion specimens. Diagn Microbiol Infect Dis 9:187–192, 1988

6. ALMEIDA JD: Uses and abuses of diagnostic electron microscopy. Curr Top Microbiol Immunol 104:147–158, 1983

7. ALTER HJ, SEEFF LB, KAPLAN PM ET AL: Type B hepatitis: The infectivity of blood positive for e antigen and DNA polymerase after accidental needlestick exposure. N Engl J Med 295:909–913, 1976

8. ANDERSON BE, SIMS KG, OLSON JG ET AL: *Amblyomma americanum:* A potential vector of human ehrlichiosis. Am J Trop Med Hyg 49:239–244, 1993

9. ANDERSON BE, SUMNER JW, DAWSON JE, TZIANABOS T ET AL: Detection of the etiologic agent of human ehrlichiosis by polymerase chain reaction. J Clin Microbiol 30:775–780, 1992

10. AMBINDER RF, MANN RB: Detection and characterization of Epstein-Barr virus in clinical specimens. Am J Pathol 145:239–252, 1994

11. AMERICAN COLLEGE OF OBSTETRICS AND GYNECOLOGY: Perinatal herpes simplex virus infections. ACOG Tech Bull 122:1–5, 1988

12. ANAND A, GRAY ES, BROWN T ET AL: Human parvovirus infection in pregnancy and hydrops fetalis. N Engl J Med 316:183–186, 1987

13. ANDERSON BE, DAWSON JE, JONES DC, ET AL: *Ehrlichia chaffeensis*, a new species associated with human ehrlichiosis. J Clin Microbiol 29:2838–2842, 1991

14. ANDERSON LJ, PATRIARCA PA, HIERHOLZER JC ET AL: Viral respiratory illnesses. Med Clin North Am 67:1009–1030, 1983

15. ANDERSON LJ, TSOU C, PARKER RA ET AL: Detection of antibodies and antigens of human parvovirus B19 by enzyme-linked immunosorbent assay. J Clin Microbiol 24:522–526, 1986

16. ANESTAD G, BREIVIK N, THORESEN T: Rapid diagnosis of respiratory syncytial virus and influenza A virus infections by immunofluorescence: Experience with a simplified procedure for the preparation of cell smears from nasopharyngeal secretions. Acta Path Microbiol Immunol Scand 91:267–271, 1983

17. ANESTAD G, MAEHLE OR: Rapid diagnosis of respiratory syncytial (RS) virus infection by immunofluorescence: A simplified procedure for the preparation of nasopharyngeal suction specimens. Acta Pathol Microbiol Scand 89:285–287, 1981

18. ANONYMOUS: New AIDS drugs spawn a global pill chase. Patients head to U.S., turn to mail order, black markets. *Wall Street Journal* July 8, 1996, p. A6

19. ANNUNZIATO D, KAPLAN MH, HALL WW ET AL: Atypical measles syndrome: Pathologic and serologic findings. Pediatrics 70:203–209, 1982

20. ANSARI SA, SPRINGTHORPE VS, SATTAR SA ET AL: Potential role of hands in the spread of respiratory viral infections: Studies with human parainfluenza virus 3 and rhinovirus 14. J Clin Microbiol 29:2115–2119, 1991

21. ARANKALLE VA, CHADHA MS, TSAREV SA ET AL: Seroepidemiology of water-borne hepatitis in India and evidence for a third enterically-transmitted hepatitis agent. Proc Natl Acad Sci USA 91:3428–3432, 1994

22. ARMSTRONG C, LILLIE RD: Experimental lymphocytic choriomeningitis of monkeys and mice produced by a virus encountered in studies of the 1933 St. Louis encephalitis virus epidemic. Public Health Rep 49:1019–1027, 1934

23. ARTENSTEIN AW, HICKS CB, GOODWIN BS JR, HILLIARD JK: Human infection with B virus following a needlestick injury. Rev Infect Dis 13:288–291, 1991

24. ARTHUR RR, SHAH KV, BAUST SJ ET AL: Association of BK viruria with hemorrhagic cystitis in recipients of bone marrow transplants. N Engl J Med 315:230–234, 1986

25. ARTHUR RR, SHAH KV, CHARACHE P ET AL: BK and JC virus infections in recipients of bone marrow transplants. J Infect Dis 158:563–569, 1988

26. ARTSOB H: Distribution of California serogroup viruses and virus infections in Canada. Prog Clin Biol Res 123:277–290, 1983

27. ARVIN AM, HENSLEIGH PA, PROBER CG ET AL: Failure of antepartum maternal cultures to predict the infant's risk of exposure to herpes simplex virus at delivery. N Engl J Med 315:796–800, 1986

28. ARVIN AM: Varicella-zoster virus. Clin Microbiol Rev 9:361–381, 1996

29. VARICELLA-ZOSTER VIRUS. IN FIELDS BN, KNIPE DM, HOWLEY PM ET AL (EDS): Fields Virology (3rd ed), pp 2547–2585. Philadelphia, Lippincott-Raven, 1996

30. ARVIN AM, KOROPCHAK CM, WITTEK AE: Immunologic evidence of reinfection with varicella-zoster virus. J Infect Dis 148:200–205, 1983

31. ASANO Y, YOSHIKAWA T, SUGA S ET AL: Clinical features of infants with primary human herpesvirus 6 infection (exanthem subitum, roseola infantum). Pediatrics 93:104–108, 1994

32. ASHLEY R, CENT A, MAGGS V, NAHMIAS A, COREY L: Inability of enzyme immunoassays to discriminate between infections with herpes simplex virus types 1 and 2. Ann Intern Med 115:520–526, 1991

33. AURELIUM E, JOHANSSON B, SKÖLDENBERG B, STALAND Å, FORSGREN M: Rapid diagnosis of herpes simplex encephalitis by nested polymerase chain reaction assay of cerebrospinal fluid. Lancet 337:189–192, 1991

34. AUWAERTER PG, OLDACH D, MUNDY LM ET AL: Hantavirus serologies in patients hospitalized with community-acquired pneumonia. J Infect Dis 173:237–239, 1996

35. BADLEY AD, PATEL R, PORTELA DF ET AL: Prognostic significance and risk factors of untreated cytomegalovirus viremia in liver transplant recipients. J Infect Dis 173:446–449, 1996

36. BAER GM: The Natural History of Rabies (2nd ed). Boca Raton, FL, CRC Press, 1991

37. BAKKEN JS, DUMLER JS, CHEN SM, ECKMAN MR, VAN ETTA LL, WALKER DH: Human granulocytic ehrlichiosis in the upper Midwest United States. A new species emerging? JAMA 272:212–218, 1994

38. BALFOUR HH JR, EDELMAN CK, DIRKSEN CL ET AL: Laboratory studies of acute varicella and varicella immune status. Diagn Microbiol Infect Dis 10:149–158, 1988

39. BALKOVIC ES, HSIUNG GD: Comparison of immunofluorescence with commercial monoclonal antibodies to biochemical and biological techniques for typing clinical herpes simplex virus isolates. J Clin Microbiol 22:870–872, 1985

40. BARBERA JA, HAYASHI S, HEGELE RG, HOGG JC: Detection of Epstein-Barr virus in lymphocytic interstitial pneumonia by in situ hybridization. Am Rev Respir Dis 145:940–946, 1992

41. BARINGER JR: Recovery of herpes simplex virus from human sacral ganglions. N Engl J Med 291:828–830, 1974

42. BARNARD DL, FARNES K, RICHARDS DF ET AL: Suitability of new *Chlamydia* transport medium for transport of herpes simplex virus. J Clin Microbiol 24:692–695, 1986

43. BARNES RC, KATZ BP, ROLFS RT ET AL: Quantitative culture of endocervical *Chlamydia trachomatis*. J Clin Microbiol 28:774–780, 1990

44. BARON RC, McCORMICK JB, ZUBEIR OA: Ebola hemorrhagic fever in southern Sudan: Hospital dissemination and intrafamilial spread. Bull World Health Organ 61:997–1003, 1983

45. BARRASSO R, DEBRUX J, CROISSANT O ET AL: High prevalence of papillomavirus-associated penile intraepithelial neoplasia in sexual partners of women with cervical intraepithelial neoplasia. N Engl J Med 317:916–923, 1987

46. BARTHOLOMA NY, FORBES BA: Successful use of shell vial centrifugation and 16- to 18-hour immunofluorescent staining for the detection of influenza A and B in clinical specimens. Am J Clin Pathol 92:487–490, 1989

47. BASS CA, JUNGKIND DL, SILVERMAN NS, BONDI JM: Clinical evaluation of a new polymerase chain reaction assay for detection of *Chlamydia trachomatis* in endocervical specimens. J Clin Microbiol 31:2648–2653, 1993

48. BEASLEY RP, STEVENS CE, SHIAO I ET AL: Evidence against breast-feeding as a mechanism for vertical transmission of hepatitis B. Lancet 2:740–741, 1975

49. BECROFT DM: Bronchiolitis obliterans, bronchiectasis, and other sequelae of adenovirus type 21 infection in young children. J Clin Pathol 24:72–82, 1971

50. BEEM MO, SAXON EM: Respiratory-tract colonization and a distinctive pneumonia syndrome in infants infected with *Chlamydia trachomatis*. N Engl J Med 296:306–310, 1977

51. BEK B, BOECKH M, LEPENIES J ET AL: High-level sensitivity of quantitative pp65 cytomegalovirus (CMV) antigenemia assay for diagnosis of CMV disease in AIDS patients and follow-up. J Clin Microbiol 34:457–459, 1996

52. BELL LM, NAIDES SJ, STOFFMAN P ET AL: Human parvovirus B19 infection among hospital staff members after contact with infected patients. N Engl J Med 321:485–491, 1989

53. BELL TA, KUO CC, STAMM WE ET AL: Direct fluorescent monoclonal antibody stain for rapid detection of infant *Chlamydia trachomatis* infections. Pediatrics 74:224–228, 1984

54. BELONGIA EA, GOODMAN JL, HOLLAND EJ ET AL: An outbreak of herpes gladiatorum at a high-school wrestling camp. N Engl J Med 325:906–910, 1991

55. BENEDETTI J, COREY L, ASHLEY R: Recurrence rates in genital herpes after symptomatic first-episode infection. Ann Intern Med 121:847–854, 1994

56. BENSON PM, MALANE SL, BANKS R ET AL: B virus (Herpesvirus simiae) and human infection. Arch Dermatol 125:1247–1248, 1989

57. BESCHORNER WE, BAUGHMAN K, TURNICKY RP ET AL: HIV-associated myocarditis: Pathology and immunopathology. Am J Pathol 137:1365–1371, 1990

58. BETTOLI EJ, BREWER PM, OXTOBY MJ ET AL: The role of temperature and swab materials in the recovery of herpes simplex virus from lesions. J Infect Dis 145:399, 1982

59. BETTS RF: Syndromes of cytomegalovirus infection. Adv Intern Med 26:447–466, 1980

60. BETTS RF, FREEMAN RB, DOUGLAS RG JR ET AL: Clinical manifestations of renal allograft derived primary cytomegalovirus infection. Am J Dis Child 131:759–763, 1977

61. BIGONI B, DOLCETTI R, DE LELLIS L ET AL: Human herpesvirus 8 is present in the lymphoid system of healthy persons and can reactivate in the course of AIDS. J Infect Dis 173:542–549, 1996

62. BINKIN NJ, KOPLAN JP, CATES WJ: Preventing neonatal herpes: The value of weekly viral cultures in pregnant women with recurrent genital herpes. JAMA 251: 2816–2821, 1984

63. BINN LN, LEMON SM, MARCHWICKI RH ET AL: Primary isolation and serial passage of hepatitis A virus strains in primate cell cultures. J Clin Microbiol 20:28–33, 1984

64. BIRX DL, REDFIELD RR, TOSATO G: Defective regulation of Epstein-Barr virus infection in patients with acquired immunodeficiency syndrome (AIDS) or AIDS-related disorders. N Engl J Med 314:874–879, 1986

65. BJØRO K, FRØLAND SS, YUN Z, SAMDAL HH, HAALAND T: Hepatitis C infection in patients with primary hypogammaglobulinemia after treatment with contaminated immune globulin. N Engl J Med 331:1607–1611, 1994

66. BLACK CM, JOHNSON JE, FARSHY CE ET AL: Antigenic variation among strains of *Chlamydia pneumoniae*. J Clin Microbiol 29:1312–1316, 1991

67. BLANCHE S, MAYAUX M-J, ROUZIOUX C ET AL: Relation of the course of HIV infection in children to the severity of the disease in their mothers at delivery. N Engl J Med 330:308–312, 1994

68. BLUMBERG BS: Australia antigen and the biology of hepatitis B. Science 197:17–25, 1977

69. BOECKH M, WOOGERD PM, STEVENS-AYERS T, RAY CG, BOWDEN RA: Factors influencing detection of quantitative cytomegalovirus antigenemia. J Clin Microbiol 32:832–834, 1994

70. BOLAND GJ, DE WEGER RA, TILANUS MG, VERVERS C, BOSBOOM-KALSBEEK K, DE GAST GC: Detection of cytomegalovirus (CMV) in granulocytes by polymerase chain reaction compared with the CMV antigen test. J Clin Microbiol 30:1763–1767, 1992

71. BOWDEN RA, SAYERS M, FLOURNOY N ET AL: Cytomegalovirus immune globulin and seronegative blood products to prevent primary cytomegalovirus infection after marrow transplantation. N Engl J Med 314:1006–1010, 1986

72. BRADLEY R, WILESMITH JW: Epidemiology and control of bovine spongiform encephalopathy (BSE). Br Med Bull 49:932–959, 1993

73. BRANDT CD, KIM HW, VARGOSKO AJ ET AL: Infections in 18,000 infants and children in a controlled study of respiratory tract disease: I. Adenovirus pathogenicity in relation to serologic type and illness syndrome. Am J Epidemiol 90:484–500, 1969

74. BRESCIA RJ, JENSON AB, LANCASTER WD ET AL: The role of human papillomaviruses in the pathogenesis and histologic classification of precancerous lesions of the cervix. Hum Pathol 17:552–559, 1986

75. BRINKER JP, DOERN GV: Comparison of MRC-5 and A-549 cells in conventional culture tubes and shell vial assays for the detection of varicella-zoster virus. Diagn Microbiol Infect Dis 17:75–77, 1993

76. BRITT WJ, ALFORD CA: Cytomegalovirus. In Fields BN, Knipe DM, Howley PM et al (eds): Fields Virology (3rd ed), pp 2493–2523. Philadelphia, Lippincott-Raven, 1996

77. BROMBERG K, DAIDONE B, CLARKE L ET AL: Comparison of immediate and delayed inoculation of HEp-2 cells for isolation of respiratory syncytial virus. J Clin Microbiol 20:123–124, 1984

78. BROMBERG K, TANNIS G, DAIDONE B ET AL: Comparison of Ortho respiratory syncytial virus enzyme-linked immunosorbent assay and HEp-2 cell culture. J Clin Microbiol 22:1071–1072, 1985

79. BRONSTHER O, MAKOWKA L, JAFFE R ET AL: Occurrence of cytomegalovirus hepatitis in liver transplant patients. J Med Virol 24:423–434, 1988

80. Brown KE, Hibbs JR, Gallinella G et al: Resistance to parvovirus B19 infection due to lack of virus receptor (erythrocyte P antigen). N Engl J Med 330:1192–1196, 1994

81. Brown M, Petric M: Evaluation of cell line 293 for virus isolation in routine viral diagnosis. J Clin Microbiol 23:704–708, 1986

82. Brown ZA, Benedetti J, Ashley R et al: Neonatal herpes simplex infection in relation to asymptomatic maternal infection at the time of labor. N Engl J Med 324:1247–1252, 1991

83. Brummer-Korvenkontion M, Vaheri A, Hovi T et al: Nephropathia endemica: Detection of antigen in bank voles and serologic diagnosis of human infection. J Infect Dis 141:131–134, 1980

84. Brunell PA, Gershon AA, Hughes WT et al: Prevention of varicella in high risk children: A collaborative study. Pediatrics 50:718–722, 1972

85. Bruno P, Hassell LH, Brown J, Tanner W, Lau A: The protean manifestations of hemorrhagic fever with renal syndrome. A retrospective review of 26 cases from Korea. Ann Intern Med 113:385–391, 1990

86. Brunham RC, Paavonen J, Stevens CE et al: Mucopurulent cervicitis: The ignored counterpart in women of urethritis in men. N Engl J Med 311:1–6, 1984

87. Bryan JA: The serologic diagnosis of viral infection: An update. Arch Pathol Lab Med 111:1015–1023, 1987

88. Buchwald D, Cheney PR, Peterson DL et al: A chronic illness characterized by fatigue, neurologic and immunologic disorders, and active human herpesvirus type 6 infection. Ann Intern Med 116:103–113, 1992

89. Budka H, Costanzi G, Cristina S et al: Brain pathology induced by infection with the human immunodeficiency virus (HIV): A histological, immunocytochemical, and electron microscopical study of 100 autopsy cases. Acta Neuropathol 75:185–198, 1987

90. Bukh J, Purcell RH, Miller RH: Importance of primer selection for the detection of hepatitis C virus RNA with the polymerase chain reaction assay. Proc Natl Acad Sci USA 89:187–191, 1992

91. Byrom NP, Walls J, Mair HJ: Fulminant psittacosis. Lancet 1:353–356, 1979

92. Caldwell MB, Oxtoby MJ, Simonds RJ, Lindegren ML, Rogers MF: 1994 revised classification system for human immunodeficiency virus infection in children less than 13 years of age. MMWR 42:RR-12, 1994

93. Callihan DR, Menegus MA: Rapid detection of herpes simplex virus in clinical specimens with human embryonic lung fibroblast and primary rabbit kidney cell cultures. J Clin Microbiol 19:563–565, 1984

94. Calisher CH: Medically important arboviruses of the United States and Canada. Clin Microbiol Rev 7:89–116, 1994

95. Carlson JR, Bryant ML, Hinrichs SH et al: AIDS serology testing in low- and high-risk groups. JAMA 253:3405–3408, 1985

96. Carrigan DR, Drobyski WR, Russler SK et al: Interstitial pneumonitis associated with human herpesvirus-6 infection after bone marrow transplantation. Lancet 338:147–149, 1991

97. Casals J, Henderson B, Hoogstraal H, Johnson KM, Shelokov A: A review of Soviet viral hemorrhagic fevers. J Infect Dis 122:437–453, 1970

98. Castro KG, Ward JW, Slutsker L et al: 1993 revised classification system for HIV infection and expanded surveillance case definition for AIDS among adolescents and adults. MMWR Morb Mortal Wkly Rep 41:No. RR-17, 1992

99. Caussy D, Orr W, Daya AD et al: Evaluation of methods for detecting human papillomavirus deoxyribonucleotide sequences in clinical specimens. J Clin Microbiol 26:236–243, 1988

100. Celun CL, Coombs RW, Lafferty W, et al: Indeterminate human immunodeficiency virus type 1 Western blots: seroconversion risk, specificity of supplemental tests, and an algorithm for evaluation. J Infect Dis 164:656–664, 1991

101. Centers for Disease Control: Hepatitis B associated with acupuncture—Florida. MMWR Morb Mortal Wkly Rep 30:1–3, 1981

102. Centers for Disease Control: Delta hepatitis—Massachusetts. MMWR Morb Mortal Wkly Rep 33:493–494, 1984

103. Centers for Disease Control: Chronic fatigue possibly related to Epstein-Barr virus—Nevada. MMWR Morb Mortal Wkly Rep 35:350–352, 1986

104. Centers for Disease Control: B-virus infection in humans—Pensacola, Florida. MMWR Morb Mortal Wkly Rep 36:289–296, 1987

105. Centers for Disease Control: Interpretation and use of the Western blot assay for serodiagnosis of human immunodeficiency virus type 1 infections. MMWR Morb Mortal Wkly Rep 38(S-7):1–7, 1989

106. Centers for Disease Control: Update: HIV-2 infection—United States. MMWR Morb Mortal Wkly Rep38:572–580, 1989

107. Centers for Disease Control: Update: Measles outbreak. MMWR Morb Mortal Wkly Rep 39:317–326, 1990

108. Centers for Disease Control: Update: Filovirus infection in animal handlers. MMWR Morb Mortal Wkly Rep 39:221, 1990

109. Centers for Disease Control: Psittacosis at a turkey processing plant—North Carolina, 1989. MMWR Morb Mortal Wkly Rep 39:460–469, 1990

110. Centers for Disease Control: Update: Transmission of HIV infection during an invasive dental procedure—Florida. MMWR Morb Mortal Wkly Rep 40:21–33, 1991

111. Centers for Disease Control: Mortality attributable to HIV infection/AIDS—United States, 1981–1990. MMWR Morb Mortal Wkly Rep 40:41–44, 1991

112. Centers for Disease Control: Pseudo-outbreak of infectious mononucleosis—Puerto Rico, 1990. MMWR Morb Mortal Wkly Rep 40:552–555, 1991

113. Centers for Disease Control: Interpretive criteria used to report Western blot results for HIV-1 antibody testing—United States. MMWR Morb Mortal Wkly Rep 40:692–695, 1991

114. Centers for Disease Control: Human rabies—Texas, Arkansas, and Georgia, 1991. MMWR Morb Mortal Wkly Rep 40:765–769, 1991

115. Centers for Disease Control and Prevention: 1993 Revised classification system for HIV infection and expanded surveillance case definition for AIDS among adolescents and adults. MMWR Morb Mortal Wkly Rep 41:No. RR-17, 1992

116. CENTERS FOR DISEASE CONTROL AND PREVENTION: Update: Eradication of paralytic poliomyelitis in the Americas. MMWR Morb Mortal Wkly Rep 41:681–683, 1992

117. CENTERS FOR DISEASE CONTROL AND PREVENTION: Hepatitis E among U.S. travelers, 1989–1992. MMWR Morb Mortal Wkly Rep 42:1–4, 1993

118. CENTERS FOR DISEASE CONTROL AND PREVENTION: Update: Impact of the expanded AIDS surveillance case definition for adolescents and adults on case reporting—United States, 1993. MMWR Morb Mortal Wkly Rep 43:160–170, 1994

119. CENTERS FOR DISEASE CONTROL AND PREVENTION: Hantavirus pulmonary syndrome—northeastern United States. MMWR Morb Mortal Wkly Rep 43:548–556, 1994

120. CENTERS FOR DISEASE CONTROL AND PREVENTION: Interstate measles transmission from a ski resort—Colorado, 1994. MMWR Morb Mortal Wkly Rep 43:627–629, 1994

121. CENTERS FOR DISEASE CONTROL AND PREVENTION: Arenavirus infection: Connecticut. MMWR Morb Mortal Wkly Rep 43:635–636, 1994

122. CENTERS FOR DISEASE CONTROL AND PREVENTION: Bolivian hemorrhagic fever—El Beni department, Bolivia, 1994, MMWR Morb Mortal Wkly Rep 43:943–946, 1994

123. CENTERS FOR DISEASE CONTROL AND PREVENTION: Dengue surveillance—United States, 1986–1992. MMWR Morb Mortal Wkly Rep 43:No. SS-2, 1994

124. CENTERS FOR DISEASE CONTROL AND PREVENTION: Imported dengue—United States, 1993–1994. 44:353–356, 1995

125. CENTERS FOR DISEASE CONTROL AND PREVENTION: Update: Trends in AIDS among men who have sex with men—United States, 1989–1994. MMWR Morb Mortal Wkly Rep 44:401–404, 1995

126. CENTERS FOR DISEASE CONTROL AND PREVENTION: Update: Outbreak of Ebola viral hemorrhagic fever—Zaire, 1995. MMWR Morb Mortal Wkly Rep 44:468–475, 1995

127. CENTERS FOR DISEASE CONTROL AND PREVENTION: Update: Management of patients with suspected viral hemorrhagic fever—United States. MMWR Morb Mortal Wkly Rep 44:475–479, 1995

128. CENTERS FOR DISEASE CONTROL AND PREVENTION: Mass treatment of humans exposed to rabies—New Hampshire, 1994. MMWR Morb Mortal Wkly Rep 44:484–486, 1995

129. CENTERS FOR DISEASE CONTROL AND PREVENTION: Human granulocytic ehrlichiosis—New York, 1995. MMWR Morb Mortal Wkly Rep 44:593–595, 1995

130. CENTERS FOR DISEASE CONTROL AND PREVENTION: Update: HIV-2 infection among blood and plasma donors—United States, June 1992–June 1995. MMWR Morb Mortal Wkly Rep 44:603–606, 1995

131. CENTERS FOR DISEASE CONTROL AND PREVENTION: First 500,000 AIDS cases—United States, 1995. MMWR Morb Mortal Wkly Rep 44:849–853, 1995

132. CENTERS FOR DISEASE CONTROL AND PREVENTION: Case-control study of HIV seroconversion in health-care workers after percutaneous exposure to HIV-infected blood—France, United Kingdom, and United States, January 1988–August 1994. MMWR Morb Mortal Wkly Rep 44:929–933, 1995

133. CENTERS FOR DISEASE CONTROL AND PREVENTION: World Health Organization consultation on public health issues related to bovine spongiform encephalopathy and the emergence of a new variant of Creutzfeldt-Jakob disease. MMWR Morb Mortal Wkly Rep 45:295–303, 1996

134. CENTERS FOR DISEASE CONTROL AND PREVENTION: Ebola-Reston virus infection among quarantined nonhuman primates—Texas, 1996. MMWR Morb Mortal Wkly Rep 45:314–316, 1996

135. CENTERS FOR DISEASE CONTROL AND PREVENTION: Hepatitis A among persons with hemophilia who received clotting factor concentrate—United States, September–December 1995. MMWR Morb Mortal Wkly Rep 45:29–32, 1996

136. CENTERS FOR DISEASE CONTROL AND PREVENTION: Update: Provisional public health service recommendations for chemoprophylaxis after occupational exposure to HIV. MMWR Morb Mortal Wkly Rep 45:468–472, 1996

137. CENTERS FOR DISEASE CONTROL AND PREVENTION: Identification of HIV-1 group O infection—Los Angeles County, California, 1996. MMWR Morb Mortal Wkly Rep 45:561–565, 1996

138. CEPKO CL, WHETSTONE CA, SHARP PA: Adenovirus hexon monoclonal antibody that is group specific and potentially useful as a diagnostic reagent. J Clin Microbiol 17:360–364, 1983

139. CESARMAN E, CHANG Y, MOORE PS, SAID JW, KNOWLES DM: Kaposi's sarcoma-associated herpesvirus-like DNA sequences in AIDS-related body-cavity-based lymphomas. N Engl J Med 332:1186–1191, 1995

140. CHANDLER FW, GORELKIN L: Immunofluorescence staining of adenovirus in fixed tissues pretreated with trypsin. J Clin Microbiol 17:371–373, 1983

141. CHANG RS, ARNOLD D, CHANG YY ET AL: Relative sensitivity of cell culture systems in the detection of herpes simplex viruses. Diagn Microbiol Infect Dis 5:135–141, 1986

142. CHANG Y, CESARMAN E, PESSIN MS ET AL: Identification of herpesvirus-like DNA sequences in AIDS-associated Kaposi's sarcoma. Science 266:1865–1869, 1994

143. CHAPMAN NM, TRACY S, GAUNTT CJ ET AL: Molecular detection and identification of enteroviruses using enzymatic amplification and nucleic acid hybridization. J Clin Microbiol 28:843–850, 1990

144. CHAUDHARY RK, MACLEAN C: Detection of antibody to hepatitis C virus by second-generation enzyme immunoassay. Am J Clin Pathol 99:702–704, 1993

145. CHEESEMAN SH, PIERIK LT, LEOMBRUNO D ET AL: Evaluation of a commercially available direct immunofluorescent staining reagent for the detection of respiratory syncytial virus in respiratory secretions. J Clin Microbiol 24:155–156, 1986

146. CHEN SM, DUMLER JS, BAKKEN JS, WALKER DH: Identification of a granulocytotropic *Ehrlichia* species as the etiologic agent of human disease. J Clin Microbiol 32:589–595, 1994

147. CHEN SM, POPOV VL, FENG HM, WEN J, WALKER DH: Cultivation of *Ehrlichia chaffeensis* in mouse embryo, Vero, BGM, and L929 cells and study of *Ehrlichia*-induced cytopathic effect and plaque formation. Infect Immun 63:647–655, 1995

148. CHERNESKY MA, JANG D, LEE H ET AL: Diagnosis of *Chlamydia trachomatis* infections in men and women by

testing first-void urine by ligase chain reaction. J Clin Microbiol 32:2682–2685, 1994

149. CHERNESKY MA, MAHONY JB, CASTRICIANO S ET AL: Detection of *Chlamydia trachomatis* antigens by enzyme immunoassay and immunofluorescence in genital specimens from symptomatic and asymptomatic men and women. J Infect Dis 154:141–148, 1986

150. CHESEBRO B, FIELDS BN: Transmissible spongiform encephalopathies: A brief introduction. In Fields BN, Knipe DM, Howley PM et al (eds): Fields Virology (3rd ed), pp 2845–2849. Philadelphia, Lippincott-Raven, 1996

151. CHEVILLE NF: Cytopathology in Viral Diseases. Basel, *S. Karger, 1975*

152. CHIBA S, NAKATA S, NAKAMURA I ET AL: Outbreak of infantile gastroenteritis due to type 40 adenovirus. Lancet 2:954–957, 1983

153. CHILDS JE, KSIAZEK TG, SPIROPOULOU CF ET AL: Serologic and genetic identification of *Peromyscus maniculatus* as the primary rodent reservoir for a new hantavirus in the southwestern United States. J Infect Dis 169:1271–1280, 1994

154. CHONMAITREE T, BALDWIN CD, LUCIA HL: Role of the virology laboratory in diagnosis and management of patients with central nervous system disease. Clin Microbiol Rev 2:1–14, 1989

155. CHONMAITREE T, MENEGUS MA, POWELL KR: The clinical relevance of "CSF viral culture": A two-year experience with aseptic meningitis in Rochester, NY. JAMA 247:1843–1847, 1982

156. CHONMAITREE T, MENEGUS MA, SCHERVISH SEM ET AL: Enterovirus 71 infection: Report of an outbreak with two cases of paralysis and a review of the literature. Pediatrics 67:489–493, 1981

157. CHOO Q, KUO G, WEINER AJ ET AL: Isolation of a cDNA clone derived from a blood-borne non-A, non-B viral hepatitis genome. Science 244:359–362, 1989

158. CHORBA T, COCCIA P, HOLMAN RC ET AL: The role of parvovirus B19 in aplastic crisis and erythema infectiosum (fifth disease). J Infect Dis 154:383–393, 1986

159. CHOU S: Reactivation and recombination of multiple cytomegalovirus strains from individual organ donors. J Infect Dis 160:11–15, 1989

160. CHOU S, MERIGAN TC: Rapid detection and quantitation of human cytomegalovirus in urine through DNA hybridization. N Engl J Med 308:921–925, 1983

161. CHRETIEN JH, McGINNISS CG, MULLER A: Venereal causes of cytomegalovirus mononucleosis. JAMA 238:1644–1645, 1977

162. CHRISTENSEN ML: Human viral gastroenteritis. Clin Microbiol Rev 2:51–89, 1989

163. CHRISTY C, VOSEFSKI D, MADORE HP: Comparison of three enzyme immunoassays to tissue culture for the diagnosis of rotavirus gastroenteritis in infants and young children. J Clin Microbiol 28:1428–1430, 1990

164. CHUDZIO T, KASATIYA S, IRVINE N ET AL: Rapid screening test for the diagnosis of rotavirus infection. J Clin Microbiol 27:2394–2396, 1989

165. CHURCH NR, ANAS NG, HALL CB ET AL: Respiratory syncytial virus-related apnea in infants: Demographics and outcome. Am J Dis Child 138:247–250, 1984

166. CLARK SJ, SAAG MS, DECKER WD ET AL: High titers of cytopathic virus in plasma of patients with symptomatic primary HIV-1 infection. N Engl J Med 324:954–960, 1991

167. CLAVEL F, MANSINHO K, CHAMARET S ET AL: Human immunodeficiency virus type 2 infection associated with AIDS in West Africa. N Engl J Med 316:1180–1185, 1987

168. CLES LD, BRUCH K, STAMM WE: Staining characteristics of six commercially available monoclonal immunofluorescence reagents for direct diagnosis of *Chlamydia trachomatis* infections. J Clin Microbiol 26:1735–1737, 1988

169. CLES LD, STAMM WE: Use of HL cells for improved isolation and passage of *Chlamydia pneumoniae.* J Clin Microbiol 28:938–940, 1990

170. CLYDE WA, KENNY GE, SCHACHTER J: Diagnosis of *Chlamydia* infection. In Cumitech, pp 1–19. Washington, DC, American Society for Microbiology, 1984

171. COFFIN J, HAASE A, LEVY JA ET AL: Human immunodeficiency viruses. Science 232:697, 1986

172. COHEN JI, COREY GR: Cytomegalovirus infection in the normal host. Medicine 64:100–114, 1985

173. COIMBRA TLM, NASSAR ES, BURATTINI MN ET AL: New arenavirus in Brazil. Lancet 343:391–392, 1994

174. COLLIER AC, COOMBS RW, SCHOENFELD DA ET AL: Treatment of human immunodeficiency virus infection with saquinavir, zidovudine, and zalcitabine. N Engl J Med 334:1011–1017, 1996

175. CONCENSUS CONFERENCE. The Impact of Routine HTLV-III Antibody Testing of Blood and Plasma Donors on Public Health. JAMA 256:1778–1783, 1986

176. CONE RW, HOBSON AC, PALMER J ET AL: Extended duration of herpes simplex virus DNA in genital lesions detected by the polymerase chain reaction. J Infect Dis 164:757–760, 1991

177. CORDONNIER C, ESCUDIER E, NICHOLAS JC, ET AL: Evaluation of three assays on alveolar lavage fluid in the diagnosis of cytomegalovirus pneumonitis after bone marrow transplantation. J Infect Dis 155:495–500, 1987

178. COREY L, SPEAR PG: Infections with herpes simplex viruses (2). N Engl J Med 314:749–757, 1986

179. COREY L, STAMM WE, FEORINO PM ET AL: HBsAg-negative hepatitis in a hemodialysis unit: Relation to Epstein-Barr virus. N Engl J Med 293:1273–1278, 1975

180. COTMORE S, TATTERSALL P: Characterization and molecular cloning of a human parvovirus genome. Science 226:1161–1165, 1984

181. CRAIGHEAD JE: Pulmonary cytomegalovirus infection in the adult. Am J Pathol 63:487–504, 1971

182. CRANE LR, GUTTERMAN PA, CHAPEL T ET AL: Incubation of swab materials with herpes simplex virus. J Infect Dis 141:531, 1980

183. CREMER NE, HAGENS SJ, FUKUCHI R: Improved serological diagnosis of rubella. J Clin Microbiol 18:743–744, 1983

184. CRUM CP, BARBER S, ROCHE JK: Pathobiology of papillomavirus-related cervical diseases: Prospects for immunodiagnosis. Clin Microbiol Rev 4:270–285, 1991

185. CRUM CP, MITAO M, LEVINE RU ET AL: Cervical papillomaviruses segregate within morphologically distinct precancerous lesions. J Virol 54:675–681, 1985

186. CRUMPACKER CS, SCHNIPPER LE, MARLOWE SI ET AL: Resistance to antiviral drugs of herpes simplex virus iso-

lated from a patient treated with acyclovir. N Engl J Med 306:343–346, 1982

187. CUBEL RCN, OLIVEIRA SA, BROWN DWG, COHEN BJ, NASCIMENTO JP: Diagnosis of parvovirus B19 infection by detection of specific immunoglobulin M antibody in saliva. J Clin Microbiol 34:205–207, 1996

188. D'ANGELO LJ, BREGMAN DJ, WINKLER WG: Rocky Mountain spotted fever in the United States: Use of age-specific incidence to determine public health policy for a vector-borne disease. South Med J 75:3–5, 1982

189. DAAR ES, MOUDGIL T, MEYER RD ET AL: Transient high levels of viremia in patients with primary human immunodeficiency virus type 1 infection. N Engl J Med 324:961–964, 1991

190. DAGAN R, POWELL KR, HALL CB ET AL: Identification of infants unlikely to have serious bacterial infection although hospitalized for suspected sepsis. J Pediatr 107: 855–860, 1985

191. DANNER SA, CARR A, LEONARD JM ET AL: A short-term study of the safety, pharmacokinetics, and efficacy of ritonavir, an inhibitor of HIV-1 protease. N Engl J Med 333:1528–1533, 1995

192. DATTEL BJ, LANDERS DV, COULTER K ET AL: Isolation of *Chlamydia trachomatis* from sexually abused female adolescents. Obstet Gynecol 72:240–242, 1988

193. DAVENPORT DS, JOHNSON DR, HOLMES GP, JEWETT DA, ROSS SC, HILLIARD JK: Diagnosis and management of human B virus (herpesvirus simiae) infections in Michigan. Clin Infect Dis 19:33–41, 1994

194. DAVID AS, WESSELY S, PELOSI AJ: Postviral fatigue syndrome: Time for a new approach. Br Med J [Clin Res] 296:696–699, 1988

195. DAVIDSOHN I, LEE CL: The laboratory in the diagnosis of infectious mononucleosis with additional notes on epidemiology, etiology and pathogenesis. Med Clin North Am 46:225–244, 1962

196. DAWSON JE, ANDERSON BE, FISHBEIN DB, ET AL: Isolation and characterization of an *Ehrlichia* sp. from a patient diagnosed with human ehrlichiosis. J Clin Microbiol 29:2741–2745, 1991

197. DEAN D, PALMER L, PANT CR, COURTRIGHT P, FALKOW S, OHANLEY P: Use of a *Chlamydia trachomatis* DNA probe for detection of ocular chlamydiae. J Clin Microbiol 27:1062–1067, 1989

198. DE JONG JC, WIGAND R, KIDD AH ET AL: Candidate adenoviruses 40 and 41: Fastidious adenoviruses from human infant stool. J Med Virol 11:215–231, 1983

199. DE VINCENZI I, THE EUROPEAN STUDY GROUP ON HETEROSEXUAL TRANSMISSION OF HIV: A longitudinal study of human immunodeficiency virus transmission by heterosexual partners. N Engl J Med 331:341–346, 1994

200. DE VILLIERS E, WAGNER D, SCHNEIDER A ET AL: Human papillomavirus infections in women with and without abnormal cervical cytology. Lancet 2:703–706, 1987

201. DECHAMPS C, PEIGUE-LAFEUILLE HH, LAVERAN H ET AL: Four cases of vesicular lesions in adults caused by enterovirus infections. J Clin Microbiol 26:2182–2183, 1988

202. DECOCK KM, GOVINDARAJAN S, CHIN KP ET AL: Delta hepatitis in the Los Angeles area: A report of 126 cases. Ann Intern Med 105:108–114, 1986

203. DEFABRITUS AM, RIGGIO RR, DAVID DS ET AL: Parainfluenza type 3 in a transplant unit. JAMA 241:384–386, 1979

204. DEHERTOGH DA, BRETTMAN LR: Hemorrhagic cystitis due to herpes simplex virus as a marker of disseminated herpes infection. Am J Med 84:632–635, 1988

205. DEINHARDT F, HOLMES AW, CAPPS RB, POPPER H: Studies on the transmission of human viral hepatitis to Marmoset monkeys. I. Transmission of disease, serial passages, and description of liver lesions. J Exp Med 125:673–688, 1967

206. DE LEYS R, VANDERBORGHT B, VANDEN HAESEVELDE M ET AL: Isolation and partial characterization of an unusual human immunodeficiency retrovirus from two persons of west-central African origin. J Virol 64:1207–1216, 1990

207. DEMAIO J, BOYD RS, RENSI R ET AL: False-positive Chlamydiazyme results during urine sediment analysis due to bacterial urinary tract infections. J Clin Microbiol 29:1436–1438, 1991

208. DEMMLER GJ, BUFFONE GJ, SCHIMBOR CM ET AL: Detection of cytomegalovirus in urine from newborns by using polymerase chain reaction DNA amplification. J Infect Dis 158:1177–1184, 1988

209. DERISH MT, KULHANJIAN JA, FRANKEL LR, SMITH DW: Value of bronchoalveolar lavage in diagnosing severe respiratory syncytial virus infections in infants. J Pediatr 119:761–763, 1991

210. DESIGAN G, SCHNEIDER RP: Herpes simplex esophagitis in healthy adults. South Med J 78:1135–1137, 1985

211. DESMYTER J, JOHNSON KM, DECKERS C ET AL: Laboratory rat associated outbreak of haemorrhagic fever with renal syndrome due to Hantaan-like virus in Belgium. Lancet 1:1445–1448, 1983

212. DIENSTAG JL, FEINSTONE SM, KAPIKIAN AZ ET AL: Faecal shedding of hepatitis-A antigen. Lancet 1:765–767, 1975

213. DIETZ VJ, NIEBURG P, GUBLER DJ, GOMEZ I: Diagnosis of measles by clinical case definition in dengue-endemic areas: Implications for measles surveillance and control. Bull World Health Organ 70:745–750, 1992

214. DIGLISIC G, XIAO SY, GLIGIC A ET AL: Isolation of a Puumala-like virus from *Mus musculus* captured in Yugoslavia and its association with severe hemorrhagic fever with renal syndrome. J Infect Dis 169:204–207, 1994

215. DOLIN R, REICHMAN RC, ROESSNER KD ET AL: Detection by immune electron microscopy of the Snow Mountain agent of acute viral gastroenteritis. J Infect Dis 146:184–189, 1982

216. DOLIN R, TREANOR JJ, MADORE HP: Novel agents of viral enteritis in humans. J Infect Dis 155:365–376, 1987

217. DOMURAT F, ROBERTS NJ JR, WALSH EE ET AL: Respiratory syncytial virus infection of human mononuclear leukocytes in vitro and in vivo. J Infect Dis 152:895–902, 1985

218. DONAHUE JG, MUÑOZ A, NESS PM ET AL: The declining risk of post-transfusion hepatitis C virus infection. N Engl J Med 327:369–373, 1992

219. DOUGLAS RG JR: Prophylaxis and treatment of influenza. N Engl J Med 322:443–450, 1990

220. DOWDLE WR: Destruction of the smallpox virus: Why the debate? Clin Microbiol Newsletter 17:101–102, 1995

221. DOWDLE WA, KENDAL AP, NOBLE GR: Influenza viruses. In Lennette EH, Schmidt NJ (eds): Diagnostic Procedures for Viral, Rickettsial and Chlamydial Infections (5th ed), pp 585–609. Washington, DC, American Public Health Association, 1979

222. DOWDLE WR, COLEMAN MT, GREGG MB: Natural history of influenza type A in the United States, 1957–1972. Prog Med Virol 17:91–135, 1974

223. DREW WL: Controversies in viral diagnosis. Rev Infect Dis 8:814–824, 1986

224. DREW WL: Diagnosis of cytomegalovirus infection. Rev Infect Dis 101:S468–S476, 1988

225. DREW WL, MINTZ L: Rapid diagnosis of varicella-zoster virus infection by direct immunofluorescence. Am J Clin Pathol 73:699–701, 1980

226. DUCHIN JS, KOSTER FT, PETERS CJ ET AL: Hantavirus pulmonary syndrome: A clinical description of 17 patients with a newly recognized disease. N Engl J Med 330:949–955, 1994

227. DUDDING BA, WAGNER SC, ZELLER JA ET AL: Fatal pneumonia associated with adenovirus type 7 in three military trainees. N Engl J Med 286:1289–1292, 1972

228. DUMLER JS, ASANOVICH KM, BAKKEN JS, RICHTER P, KIMSEY R, MADIGAN JE: Serologic cross-reactions among *Ehrlichia equi, Ehrlichia phagocytophila,* and human granulocytic *Ehrlichia.* J Clin Microbiol 33:1098–1103, 1995

229. DUMMLER JS, BAKKEN JS: Ehrlichial diseases of humans: Emerging tick-borne infections. Clin Infect Dis 20:1102–1110, 1995

230. DUMLER JS, CHEN SM, ASANOVICH K, TRIGIANI E, POPOV VL, WALKER DH: Isolation and characterization of a new strain of *Ehrlichia chaffeensis* from a patient with nearly fatal monocytic ehrlichiosis. J Clin Microbiol 33:1704–1711, 1995

231. DUMLER JS, SUTKER WL, WALKER DH: Persistent infection with *Ehrlichia chaffeensis.* Clin Infect Dis 17:903–905, 1993

232. DURST M, CROCE CM, GISSMANN L ET AL: Papillomavirus sequences integrate near cellular oncogenes in some cervical carcinomas. Proc Natl Acad Sci USA 84:1070–1074, 1987

233. EDBERG SC: Principles of nucleic acid hybridization and comparison with monoclonal antibody technology for the diagnosis of infectious diseases. Yale J Biol Med 58:425–442, 1985

234. ELISAF M, STEFANAKI S, REPANTI M ET AL: Liver involvement in hemorrhagic fever with renal syndrome. J Clin Gastroenterol 17:33–37, 1993

235. EMANUEL D, PEPPARD J, STOVER D ET AL: Rapid immunodiagnosis of cytomegalovirus pneumonia by bronchoalveolar lavage using human and murine monoclonal antibodies. Ann Intern Med 104:476–481, 1986

236. ENDERS G: Varicella-zoster virus infection in pregnancy. Prog Med Virol 29:166–196, 1984

237. ENDERS G: Serologic test combinations for safe detection of rubella infections. Rev Infect Dis 71:S113–S122, 1985

238. ENDERS JF, McCARTHY K, MITUS A ET AL: Isolation of measles virus at autopsy in cases of giant-cell pneumonia without rash. N Engl J Med 261:875–881, 1959

239. ENDERS JF, WELLER TH, ROBBINS FC: Cultivation of the Lansing strain of poliomyelitis virus in cultures of various human embryonic tissues. Science 109:85–87, 1949

240. ENGLUND JA, SULLIVAN CJ, JORDAN MC ET AL: Respiratory syncytial virus infection in immunocompromised adults. Ann Intern Med 109:203–208, 1988

241. ERICE A, JORDAN MC, CHACE BA ET AL: Ganciclovir treatment of cytomegalovirus disease in transplant recipients and other immunocompromised hosts. JAMA 257:3082–3087, 1987

242. ERIKSSON M, FORSGREN M, SJOBERG S ET AL: Respiratory syncytial virus infection in young hospitalized children: Identification of risk patients and prevention of nosocomial spread by rapid diagnosis. Acta Paediatr Scand 72:47–51, 1983

243. ESPY MJ, HIERHOLZER JC, SMITH TF: The effect of centrifugation on the rapid detection of adenovirus in shell vials. Am J Clin Pathol 88:358–360, 1987

244. ESPY MJ, SMITH TF: Detection of herpes simplex virus in conventional tube cell cultures and in shell vials with a DNA probe kit and monoclonal antibodies. J Clin Microbiol 26:22–24, 1988

245. ESPY MJ, SMITH TF, HARMON MW ET AL: Rapid detection of influenza virus by shell vial assay with monoclonal antibodies. J Clin Microbiol 24:677–679, 1986

246. ESSIG A, ZUCS P, SUSA M ET AL: Diagnosis of ornithosis by cell culture and polymerase chain reaction in a patient with chronic pneumonia. Clin Infect Dis 21:1495–1497, 1995

247. ESTEBAN JI, GÓMEZ J, MARTELL M ET AL: Transmission of hepatitis C virus by a cardiac surgeon. N Engl J Med 334:555–560, 1996

248. EVANS AS (ED): Viral Infections of Humans: Epidemiology and Control. New York, Plenum, 1982

249. EVERETT ED, EVANS KA, HENRY RB, McDONALD G: Human ehrlichiosis in adults after tick exposure. Diagnosis using polymerase chain reaction. Ann Intern Med 120:730–735, 1994

250. EYSTER ME, BALLARD JO, GAIL MH ET AL: Predictive markers for the acquired immunodeficiency syndrome (AIDS) in hemophiliacs: Persistence of p24 antigen and low T4 cell count. Ann Intern Med 110:963–969, 1989

251. FALSEY AR, WALSH EE, BETTS RF: Serologic evidence of respiratory syncytial virus infection in nursing home patients. J Infect Dis 162:568–569, 1990

252. FARCI P, ALTER HJ, GOVINDARAJAN S ET AL: Lack of protective immunity against reinfection with hepatitis C virus. Science 258:135–140, 1992

253. FEDORKO DP, ILSTRUP DM, SMITH TF: Effect of age of shell vial monolayers on detection of cytomegalovirus from urine specimens. J Clin Microbiol 27:2107–2109, 1989

254. FEDORKO DP, ILSTRUP DM, SMITH TF: Effect of treatment of shell vial cell cultures with dimethyl sulfoxide and dexamethasone and age of MRC-5 monolayers for detection of cytomegalovirus. Diagn Microbiol Infect Dis 13:41–44, 1990

255. FEINSTONE SM, KAPIKIAN AZ, PURCELL RH ET AL: Transfusion-associated hepatitis not due to viral hepatitis type A or B. N Engl J Med 292:767–770, 1975

256. FELDMANN H, NICHOL ST, KLENK H-D, PETERS CJ, SANCHEZ A: Characterization of filoviruses based on differences in structure and antigenicity of the virion glycoprotein. Virology 199:469–473, 1994

257. FENNER F: Poxviruses. In Fields BN, Knipe DM, Howley PM et al (eds): Fields Virology (3rd ed), pp 2673–2702. Philadelphia, Lippincott-Raven, 1996

258. FERENCZY A, MITAO M, NAGAI N ET AL: Latent papillomavirus and recurring genital warts. N Engl J Med 313:784–788, 1985

259. FEUCHT HH, ZOLLNER B, POLYWKA S, LAUFS R: Study on reliability of commercially available hepatitis C virus antibody tests. J Clin Microbiol 33:620–624, 1995

260. FICHTENBAUM CJ, PETERSON LR, WEIL GJ: Ehrlichiosis presenting as a life-threatening illness with features of the toxic shock syndrome. Am J Med 95:351–357, 1993

261. FIELDS BN, KNIPE DM, HOWLEY PM ET AL (EDS): Fields Virology (3rd ed). Philadelphia, Lippincott-Raven, 1996

262. FIERER J, BAZELEY P, BRAUDE AI: Herpes B virus encephalomyelitis presenting as ophthalmic zoster. Ann Intern Med 79:225–228, 1973

263. FIFE KH, ASHLEY R, SHIELDS AF ET AL: Comparison of neutralization and DNA restriction enzyme methods for typing clinical isolates of human adenovirus. J Clin Microbiol 22:95–100, 1985

264. FISCUS SA, WALLMARK EB, FOLDS JD ET AL: Detection of infectious immune complexes in human immunodeficiency virus type 1 (HIV-1) infections: Correlation with plasma viremia and CD4 cell counts. J Infect Dis 164:765–769, 1991

265. FISHBEIN DB, DAWSON JE, ROBINSON LE: Human ehrlichiosis in the United States, 1985 to 1990. Ann Intern Med 120:736–743, 1994

266. FISHBEIN DB, KEMP A, DAWSON JE, GREENE NR, REDUS MA, FIELDS DH: Human ehrlichiosis: Prospective active surveillance in febrile hospitalized patients. J Infect Dis 160:803–809, 1989

267. FLEISHER GR, COLLINS M, FAGER S: Limitations of available tests for diagnosis of infectious mononucleosis. J Clin Microbiol 17:619–624, 1983

268. FOLEY FD, GREENAWALD KA, NASH G ET AL: Herpesvirus infection in burned patients. N Engl J Med 282:652–656, 1970

269. FONG CKY, LANDRY ML: An adventitious viral contaminant in commercially supplied A-549 cells. Identification of infectious bovine rhinotracheitis virus and its impact on diagnosis of infection in clinical specimens. J Clin Microbiol 30:1611–1613, 1992

270. FORBES BA, BARTHOLOMA NY: Detection of cytomegalovirus in clinical specimens using shell vial centrifugation and conventional cell culture. Diagn Microbiol Infect Dis 10:121–124, 1988

271. FORD-JONES EL, MINDORFF CM, GOLD R ET AL: The incidence of viral-associated diarrhea after admission to a pediatric hospital. Am J Epidemiol 131:711–718, 1990

272. FORGHANI B, DUPUIS KW, SCHMIDT NJ: Rapid detection of herpes simplex virus DNA in human brain tissue by in situ hybridization. J Clin Microbiol 22:656–658, 1985

273. FOSTER KM, JACK I: A prospective study of the role of cytomegalovirus in post-transfusion mononucleosis. N Engl J Med 280:1311–1316, 1969

274. FRAME B, MAHONY JB, BALACHANDRAN N ET AL: Identification and typing of herpes simplex virus by enzyme immunoassay with monoclonal antibodies. J Clin Microbiol 20:162–166, 1984

275. FRAME JD, BALDWIN JM, GOCKE DJ, TROUP JM: Lassa fever, a new virus disease of man in West Africa. I. Clinical description and pathological findings. Am J Trop Med Hyg 19:670–676, 1970

276. FRANCKI RI, FAUQUET CM, KNUDSON DL, BROWN F: Classification and nomenclature of viruses. Arch Virol S2:223–233, 1991

277. FRANK AL, COUCH RB, GRIFFIS CA ET AL: Comparison of different tissue cultures for isolation and quantitation of influenza and parainfluenza viruses. J Clin Microbiol 10:32–36, 1979

278. FRANK D, RAICHT RF: Intestinal perforation associated with cytomegalovirus infection in patients with acquired immune deficiency syndrome. Am J Gastroenterol 79:201–205, 1984

279. FRAYHA H, CASTRICIANO S, MAHONY J ET AL: Nasopharyngeal swabs and nasopharyngeal aspirates equally effective for the diagnosis of viral respiratory disease in hospitalized children. J Clin Microbiol 27:1387–1389, 1989

280. FRENKEL LM, GARRATY EM, SHEN JP, WHEELER N, CLARK O, BRYSON YJ: Clinical reactivation of herpes simplex virus type 2 infection in seropositive pregnant women with no history of genital herpes. Ann Intern Med 118:414–418, 1993

281. FRENKEL N, SCHIRMER EC, WYATT LS ET AL: Isolation of a new herpesvirus from human CD4+ T cells. Proc Natl Acad Sci USA 87:748–752, 1990

282. FRESHNEY RI: Culture of Animal Cells: A Manual of Basic Technique. New York, Alan R. Liss, 1983

283. FREYMUTH F, GENNETAY E, PETITJEAN J ET AL: Comparison of nested PCR for detection of DNA in plasma with pp65 leukocytic antigenemia procedure for diagnosis of human cytomegalovirus infection. J Clin Microbiol 32:1614–1618, 1994

284. FRIEDLAND GH, KLEIN RS: Transmission of the human immunodeficiency virus. N Engl J Med 317:1125–1135, 1987

285. FRIEDMAN AH, ORELLANA J, FREEMAN WR ET AL: Cytomegalovirus retinitis: A manifestation of the acquired immune deficiency syndrome (AIDS). Br J Ophthalmol 67:372–380, 1983

286. FRIEDMAN HM, FORRER CB: Diagnosis of viral respiratory infections in the 1980s. Clin Lab Med 2:383–391, 1982

287. FUNG JC, SHANLEY J, TILTON RC: Comparison of the detection of herpes simplex virus in direct clinical specimens with herpes simplex virus-specific DNA probes and monoclonal antibodies. J Clin Microbiol 22:748–753, 1985

288. GAFFEY MJ, FRIERSON HF JR, MEDEIROS LJ, WEISS LM: The relationship of Epstein-Barr virus to infection-related (sporadic) and familial hemophagocytic syndrome and secondary (lymphoma-related) hemophagocytosis: An in situ hybridization study. Hum Pathol 24:657–667, 1993

289. GAJDUSEK DC: Unconventional viruses and the origin and disappearance of Kuru. Science 197:943–960, 1977

290. GAL AA, SAUL SH, STOLER MH: In situ hybridization analysis of human papillomavirus in anal squamous cell carcinoma. Mod Pathol 2:439–442, 1989

291. GALLO D, DIGGS JL, SHELL GR ET AL: Comparison of detection of antibody to the acquired immune deficiency syndrome virus by enzyme immunoassay, immunofluorescence, and Western blot methods. J Clin Microbiol 23:1049–1051, 1986

292. GARCÍA A, NIUBÒ J, BENÍTEZ MA, VIQUEIRA M, PÉREZ JL: Comparison of two leukocyte extraction methods for cytomegalovirus antigenemia assay. J Clin Microbiol 34:182–184, 1996

293. GARCIA-TAPIA AM, FERNANDEZ-GUTIÉRREZ DEL ALAMO C, GIRÓN JA ET AL: Spectrum of parvovirus B19 infection: analysis of an outbreak of 43 cases in Cadiz, Spain. Clin Infect Dis 21:1424–1430

294. GARRY RF, WITTE MH, GOTTLIEB AA ET AL: Documentation of an AIDS virus infection in the United States in 1968. JAMA 260:2085–2087, 1988

295. GAYDOS CA, FOWLER CL, GILL VJ, EIDEN JJ, QUINN TC: Detection of Chlamydia pneumoniae by polymerase chain reaction-enzyme immunoassay in an immunocompromised population. Clin Infect Dis 17:718–723, 1993

296. GAYDOS CA, PALMER L, QUINN TC, FALKOW S, EIDEN JJ: Phylogenetic relationship of Chlamydia pneumoniae to Chlamydia psittaci and Chlamydia trachomatis as determined by analysis of 16S ribosomal DNA sequences. Int J Syst Bacteriol 43:610–612, 1993

297. GENTRY GA, LAWRENCE N, LUSHBAUGH W: Isolation and differentiation of herpes simplex virus and Trichomonas vaginalis in cell culture. J Clin Microbiol 22:199–204, 1985

298. GEORGE R: Dengue haemorrhagic fever in Malaysia: A review. Southeast Asian J Trop Med Public Health 18:278–283, 1987

299. GERBER P, NONOYAMA M, LUCAS S, PERLIN E, GOLDSTEIN LI: Oral excretion of Epstein-Barr virus by healthy subjects and patients with infectious mononucleosis. Lancet 2:988–989, 1972

300. GERNA G, REVELLO MG, PERCIVALLE E, MORINI F: Comparison of different immunostaining techniques and monoclonal antibodies to the lower matrix phosphoprotein (pp65) for optimal quantitation of human cytomegalovirus antigenemia. J Clin Microbiol 30:1232–1237, 1992

301. GERNA G, ZIPETO D, PAREA M ET AL: Monitoring of human cytomegalovirus infections and ganciclovir treatment in heart transplant recipients by determination of viremia, antigenemia, and DNAemia. J Infect Dis 164:488–498, 1991

302. GERSHON AA, RAKER R, STEINBERG S ET AL: Antibody to varicella-zoster virus in parturient women and their offspring during the first year of life. Pediatrics 58:692–696, 1976

303. GIBBS CJ JR, SAFAR J, CERONI M, DIMARTINO A, CLARK WW, HOURIGAN JL: Experimental transmission of scrapie to cattle. Lancet 335:1275, 1990

304. GISSMANN L, WOLNIK L, IKENBERG H ET AL: Human papillomavirus types 6 and 11 DNA sequences in genital and laryngeal papillomas and in some cervical cancers. Proc Natl Acad Sci USA 80:560–563, 1983

305. GLASS GE, WATSON AJ, LEDUC JW, CHILDS JE: Domestic cases of hemorrhagic fever with renal syndrome in the United States. Nephron 68:48–51, 1994

306. GLASS GE, WATSON AJ, LEDUC JW, KELEN GD, QUINN TC, CHILDS JE: Infection with a ratborne hantavirus in US residents is consistently associated with hypertensive renal disease. J Infect Dis 167:614–620, 1993

307. GLEAVES CA, LEE CF, BUSTAMANTE CI ET AL: Use of murine monoclonal antibodies for laboratory diagnosis of varicella-zoster virus infection. J Clin Microbiol 26:1623–1625, 1988

308. GLEAVES CA, RICE DH, BINDRA R ET AL: Evaluation of a HSV specific monoclonal antibody reagent for laboratory diagnosis of herpes simplex virus infection. Diagn Microbiol Infect Dis 12:315–318, 1989

309. GLEAVES CA, SMITH TF, SHUSTER EA ET AL: Comparison of standard tube and shell vial cell culture techniques for the detection of cytomegalovirus in clinical specimens. J Clin Microbiol 21:217–221, 1985

310. GLEAVES CA, SMITH TF, WOLD AD ET AL: Detection of viral and chlamydial antigens in open-lung biopsy specimens. Am J Clin Pathol 83:371–374, 1985

311. GLEAVES CA, WILSON DJ, WOLD AD ET AL: Detection and serotyping of herpes simplex virus in MRC-5 cells by use of centrifugation and monoclonal antibodies 16 h post inoculation. J Clin Microbiol 21:29–32, 1985

312. GLEZEN WP, FERNALD GW, LOHR JA: Acute respiratory disease of university students with special reference to the etiologic role of herpesvirus hominis. Am J Epidemiol 101:111–121, 1975

313. GLIGIC A, DIMKOVIC N, XIAO SY ET AL: Belgrade virus: A new hantavirus causing severe hemorrhagic fever with renal syndrome in Yugoslavia. J Infect Dis 166:113–120, 1992

314. GLUCKMAN JC, KLATZMANN D, MONTAGNIER L: Lymphadenopathy-associated-virus infection and acquired immunodeficiency syndrome. Annu Rev Immunol 4:97–117, 1986

315. GNANN JW JR, MCCORMICK JB, MITCHELL S ET AL: Synthetic peptide immunoassay distinguishes HIV type 1 and HIV type 2 infections. Science 237:1346–1349, 1987

316. GOLDSMITH R, YARBOROUGH PO, REYES GR ET AL: Enzyme-linked immunosorbent assay for diagnosis of acute sporadic hepatitis E in Egyptian children. Lancet 339:328–331, 1992

317. GOLDSTEIN LC, COREY L, MCDOUGALL JK ET AL: Monoclonal antibodies to herpes simplex viruses: Use in antigenic typing and rapid diagnosis. J Infect Dis 147:829–837, 1983

318. GOLDSTEIN LC, MCDOUGALL J, HACKMAN R ET AL: Monoclonal antibodies to cytomegalovirus: Rapid identification of clinical isolates and preliminary use in diagnosis of cytomegalovirus pneumonia. Infect Immun 38:273–281, 1982

319. GOODELL SE, QUINN TC, MKRTICHIAN E ET AL: Herpes simplex virus proctitis in homosexual men: Clinical, sigmoidoscopic, and histopathological features. N Engl J Med 308:868–871, 1983

320. GOODGAME RW: AIDS in Uganda: Clinical and social features. N Engl J Med 323:383–389, 1990

321. GOODMAN JL, NELSON C, VITALE B ET AL: Direct cultivation of the causative agent of human granulocytic ehrlichiosis. N Engl J Med 334:209–215, 1996

322. GORDON FD, ANASTOPOULOS H, KHETTRY U: Hepatitis C infection: A rare cause of fulminant hepatic failure. Am J Gastroenterol 90:117–120, 1995

323. GOTTLIEB MS, SCHROFF R, SCHANKER HM ET AL: Pneumocystis carinii pneumonia and mucosal candidiasis in previously healthy homosexual men: Evidence for a new acquired cellular immunodeficiency. N Engl J Med 305:1425–1431, 1981

324. GRAHAM BS, SNELL JDJ: Herpes simplex virus infection of the adult lower respiratory tract. Medicine 62:384–393, 1983

325. GRAMAN PS, HALL CB: Epidemiology and control of nosocomial viral infections. Infect Dis Clin North Am 3:815–841, 1989

326. GRATTAN MT, MORENO-CABRAL CE, STARNES VA ET AL: Cytomegalovirus infection is associated with cardiac allograft rejection and atherosclerosis. JAMA 261:3561–3566, 1989

327. GRAY JJ, WREGHITT TG, CUBITT WD ET AL: An outbreak of gastroenteritis in a home for the elderly associated with astrovirus type 1 and human calicivirus. J Med Virol 23:377–381, 1987

328. GRAYSTON JT, DIWAN VK, COONEY M ET AL: Community- and hospital-acquired pneumonia associated with *Chlamydia* TWAR infection demonstrated serologically. Arch Intern Med 149:169–173, 1989

329. GREGG MB: Recent outbreaks of lymphocytic choriomeningitis in the United States of America. Bull World Health Organ 52:549–554, 1975

330. GREENE WC: The molecular biology of human immunodeficiency virus type 1 infection. N Engl J Med 324:308–317, 1991

331. GREGORY WW, MENEGUS MA: Practical protocol for cytomegalovirus isolation: Use of MRC-5 cell monolayers incubated for 2 weeks. J Clin Microbiol 17:605–609, 1983

332. GRIFFITH JS: Self-replication and scrapie. Nature 215:1043–1044, 1967

333. GROOPMAN JE, SALAHUDDIN SZ, SARNGADHARAN MG ET AL: HTLV-III in saliva of people with AIDS-related complex and healthy homosexual men at risk for AIDS. Science 226:447–449, 1984

334. GROOTHUIS JR, SIMOES EAF, HEMMING VG, THE RESPIRATORY SYNCYTIAL VIRUS IMMUNE GLOBULIN STUDY GROUP: Respiratory syncytial virus (RSV) infection in preterm infants and the protective effects of RSV immune globulin (RSVIG). Pediatrics 95:463–467, 1995

335. GROOTHUIS JR, SIMOES EAF, LEVIN MJ ET AL: Prophylactic administration of respiratory syncytial virus immune globulin to high-risk infants and young children. N Engl J Med 329:1524–1530, 1993

336. GROSSMAN MC, SILVERS DN: The Tzanck smear: Can dermatologists accurately interpret it? J Am Acad Dermatol 27:403–405, 1992

337. GUIDRY GG, BLACK-PAYNE CA, PAYNE DK, JAMISON RM, GEORGE RB, BOCCHINI JA JR: Respiratory syncytial virus infection among intubated adults in a university medical intensive care unit. Chest 100:1377–1384, 1991

338. GUINAN ME, WOLINKSY SM, REICHMAN RC: Epidemiology of genital herpes simplex virus infection. Epidemiol Rev 7:127–146, 1985

339. GUST ID, COULEPIS AG, FEINSTONE SM ET AL: Taxonomic classification of hepatitis A virus. Intervirology 20:1–7, 1983

340. GWALTNEY JM JR: Transmission of experimental rhinovirus infection by contaminated surfaces. Am J Epidemiol 116:828–833, 1982

341. HABLE KA, WASHINGTON JA II, HERRMANN EC JR: Bacterial and viral throat flora: Comparison of findings in children with acute upper respiratory tract disease and in healthy controls during winter. Clin Pediatr 10:199–203, 1971

342. HACKMAN RC, MYERSON D, MEYERS JD ET AL: Rapid diagnosis of cytomegaloviral pneumonia by tissue immunofluorescence with a murine monoclonal antibody. J Infect Dis 151:325–329, 1985

343. HADLER SC, FRANCIS DP, MAYNARD JE ET AL: Long-term immunogenicity and efficacy of hepatitis B vaccine in homosexual men. N Engl J Med 315:209–214, 1986

344. HAHN BH, SHAW GM, TAYLOR ME ET AL: Genetic variation in HTLV-III/LAV over time in patients with AIDS or at risk for AIDS. Science 232:1548–1553, 1986

345. HALL CB, DOUGLAS RG JR: Nosocomial influenza infection as a cause of intercurrent fevers in infants. Pediatrics 55:673–677, 1975

346. HALL CB, DOUGLAS RG JR: Clinically useful method for the isolation of respiratory syncytial virus. J Infect Dis 131:1–5, 1975

347. HALL CB, DOUGLAS RG JR, GEIMAN JM: Possible transmission by fomites of respiratory syncytial virus. J Infect Dis 141:98–102, 1980

348. HALL CB, DOUGLAS RG JR, GEIMAN JM ET AL: Nosocomial respiratory syncytial virus infections. N Engl J Med 293:1343–1346, 1975

349. HALL CB, GEIMAN JM, DOUGLAS RG: Modes of transmission of respiratory syncytial virus. J Pediatr 99:100–103, 1981

350. HALL CB, LONG CE, SCHNABEL KC ET AL: Human herpesvirus-6 infection in children. A prospective study of complications and reactivation. N Engl J Med 331:432–438, 1994

351. HALL CB, POWELL KR, MACDONALD NE ET AL: Respiratory syncytial viral infection in children with compromised immune function. N Engl J Med 315:77–81, 1986

352. HALL CB, WALSH EE, LONG CE ET AL: Immunity to and frequency of reinfection with respiratory syncytial virus. J Infect Dis 163:693–698, 1991

353. HALL CJ, RICHMOND SJ, CAUL EO ET AL: Laboratory outbreak of Q fever acquired from sheep. Lancet 1:1004–1006, 1982

354. HALL WJ, HALL CB, SPEERS DM: Respiratory syncytial virus infection in adults: Clinical, virologic, and serial pulmonary function studies. Ann Intern Med 88:203–205, 1978

355. HALSTEAD SB, NIMMANNITYA S, COHEN SN: Observations related to pathogenesis of dengue hemorrhagic fever: IV. Relation of disease severity to antibody response and virus recovered. Yale J Biol Med 42:311–328, 1970

356. HAMILTON-DUTOIT SJ, PALLESEN G, FRANZMANN MB ET AL: AIDS-related lymphoma: Histopathology, immunophenotype, and association with Epstein-Barr virus as demonstrated by in situ nucleic acid hybridization. Am J Pathol 138:149–163, 1991

357. HAMMERSCHLAG MR, CHIRGWIN K, ROBLIN PM ET AL: Persistent infection with *Chlamydia pneumoniae* following acute respiratory illness. Clin Infect Dis 14:178–182, 1992

358. HAMMERSCHLAG MR, RETTIG PJ, SHIELDS ME: False positive results with the use of chlamydial antigen detection tests in the evaluation of suspected sexual abuse in children. Pediatr Infect Dis J 7:11–14, 1988

359. HARDALO CJ, QUAGLIARELLO V, DUMLER JS: Human granulocytic ehrlichiosis in Connecticut: Report of a fatal case. Clin Infect Dis 21:910–914, 1995

360. HARDING HB: The epidemiology of sporadic urban ornithosis. Am J Clin Pathol 38:230–243, 1962

361. HARPAZ R, VON SEDILEIN L, AVERHOFF FM ET AL: Transmission of hepatitis B virus to multiple patients from a surgeon without evidence of inadequate infection control. N Engl J Med 334:549–554, 1996

362. HARRIS C, SMALL CB, KLEIN RS ET AL: Immunodeficiency in female sexual partners of men with the acquired immunodeficiency syndrome. N Engl J Med 308:1 181–1184, 1983

363. HARRISON SC, WILEY DC, SKEHEL JJ: Virus structure. In Fields BN, Knipe DM, Howley PM et al: Fields Virology (3rd ed), pp 59–99. Philadelphia, Lippincott-Raven, 1996

364. HASEGAWA AK, MATSUNO S, INOUYE S ET AL: Isolation of human rotaviruses in primary cultures of monkey kidney cells. J Clin Microbiol 16:387–390, 1982

365. HATTWICK MAW, O'BRIEN RJ, HANSON BF: Rocky Mountain spotted fever: Epidemiology of an increasing problem. Ann Intern Med 84:732–739, 1976

366. HAYES K, DANKS DM, GIBAS H ET AL: Cytomegalovirus in human milk. N Engl J Med 287:177–178, 1972

367. HAYFLICK L: The limited in vitro lifetime of human diploid cell strains. Exp Cell Res 37:614–636, 1965

368. HAYES CG, BURANS JP, KSIAZEK TG ET AL: Outbreak of fatal illness among captive macaques in the Philippines caused by an Ebola-related filovirus. Am J Trop Med Hyg 46:664–671, 1992

369. HAZARD GW, GANZ RN, NEVIN RW ET AL: Rocky Mountain spotted fever in the eastern United States: Thirteen cases from the Cape Cod area of Massachusetts. N Engl J Med 280:57–62, 1969

370. HECHEMY KE, ANACKER RL, PHILIP RN ET AL: Detection of Rocky Mountain spotted fever antibodies by a latex agglutination test. J Clin Microbiol 12:144–150, 1980

371. HECHEMY KE, STEVENS RW, SASOWSKI S ET AL: Discrepancies in Weil-Felix and microimmunofluorescence test results for Rocky Mountain spotted fever. J Clin Microbiol 9:292–293, 1979

372. HENDRICKSON DA, KRENZ MM: Reagents and stains. In Lennette EH, Balows A, Hausler WJ Jr (eds): Manual of Clinical Microbiology, pp 1289–1314. Washington, DC, American Society for Microbiology, 1991

373. HENDRY RM, MCINTOSH K: Enzyme-linked immunosorbent assay for detection of respiratory syncytial virus infection: Development and description. J Clin Microbiol 16:324–328, 1982

374. HENNING KJ, BELL E, BRAUN J, BARKER ND: A community-wide outbreak of hepatitis A: Risk factors for infection among homosexual and bisexual men. Am J Med 99:132–136, 1995

375. HERRMANN EC JR: Experience in providing a viral diagnostic laboratory compatible with medical practice. Mayo Clin Proc 42:112–123, 1967

376. HERRMANN JE, TAYLOR DN, ECHEVERRIA P ET AL: Astroviruses as a cause of gastroenteritis in children. N Engl J Med 324:1757–1760, 1991

377. HERRMANN KL: Available rubella serologic tests. Rev Infect Dis 7:S108–S112, 1985

378. HERSH T, MELNICK JL, GOYAL RK ET AL: Nonparenteral transmission of viral hepatitis type B (Australia antigen-associated serum hepatitis). N Engl J Med 285:1363–1364, 1971

379. HERTZ MI, ENGLUND JA, SNOVER D ET AL: Respiratory syncytial virus-induced acute lung injury in adult patients with bone marrow transplants: A clinical approach and review of the literature. Medicine 68:269–281, 1989

380. HIERHOLZER JC: Adenoviruses in the immunocompromised host. Clin Microbiol Rev 5:262–274, 1992

381. HIGGINS PG, ELLIS EM: The isolation of influenza viruses. J Clin Pathol 25:521–524, 1972

382. HIRATA R, HOSHINO Y, SAKAI H, MARUMO F, SATO C: Patients with hepatitis A with negative IGM-HA antibody at early stages. Am J Gastroenterol 90:1168–1169, 1995

383. HIRSCH MS, KAPLAN JC, D'AQUILA RT: Antiviral agents. In Fields BN, Knipe DM, Howley PM et al (Eds.) Fields Virology (3rd ed), pp 431–466. Philadelphia, Lippincott-Raven, 1996

384. HIRSCHTICK RE, GLASSROTH J, JORDAN MC ET AL: Bacterial pneumonia in persons infected with the human immunodeficiency virus. N Engl J Med 333:845–851, 1995

385. HO DD, MOUDGIL T, ALAM M: Quantitation of human immunodeficiency virus type 1 in the blood of infected persons. N Engl J Med 321:1621–1625, 1989

386. HO M, SUWANSIRIKUL S, DOWLING JN ET AL: The transplanted kidney as a source of cytomegalovirus infection. N Engl J Med 293:1109–1112, 1975

387. HOCHBERG FH, MILLER G, SCHOOLEY RT ET AL: Central-nervous-system lymphoma related to Epstein-Barr virus. N Engl J Med 309:745–748, 1983

388. HOLLINGER FB, TICEHURST J: Hepatitis A virus. In Fields BN, Knipe DM, Howley PM et al (eds): Fields Virology (3rd ed), pp 735–782. Philadelphia, Lippincott-Raven, 1996

389. HONDO R, KURATA T, SATO S ET AL: Enzymatic treatment of formalin-fixed and paraffin-embedded specimens for detection of antigens of herpes simplex, varicella-zoster and human cytomegaloviruses. Jpn J Exp Med 52:17–25, 1982

390. HOOFNAGLE JH: Type D (Delta) hepatitis. JAMA 261:1321–1325, 1989

391. HOPE-SIMPSON RE: The nature of herpes zoster: A long-term study and a new hypothesis. Proc R Soc Med 58:9–20, 1965

392. HORNSLETH A, FRIIS B, ANDERSEN P ET AL: Detection of respiratory syncytial virus in nasopharyngeal secretions by ELISA: Comparison with fluorescent antibody technique. J Med Virol 10:273–281, 1982

393. HORSBURGH CR JR: Mycobacterium avium complex infection in the acquired immunodeficiency syndrome. N Engl J Med 324:1332–1338, 1991

394. HORSBURGH CR JR, OU CY, JASON J ET AL: Duration of human immunodeficiency virus infection before detection of antibody. Lancet 2:637–639, 1989

395. HORWITZ CA, HENLE W, HENLE G ET AL: Heterophil-negative infectious mononucleosis and mononucleosis-like illness. Laboratory confirmation of 43 cases. Am J Med 63:947–957, 1977

396. HORWITZ CA, HENLE W, HENLE G ET AL: Clinical and laboratory evaluation of infants and children with Epstein-Barr virus-induced infectious mononucleosis: Report of 32 patients (aged 10–48 months). Blood 57:933–938, 1981

397. HORWITZ CA, HENLE W, HENLE G ET AL: Spurious rapid infectious mononucleosis test results in noninfectious

mononucleosis sera: The role of high-titer horse agglutinins. Am J Clin Pathol 78:48–53, 1982

398. HORWITZ CA, HENLE W, HENLE G ET AL: Clinical and laboratory evaluation of cytomegalovirus-induced mononucleosis in previously healthy individuals: Report of 82 cases. Medicine 65:124–134, 1986

399. HORWITZ MS: Adenoviruses. In Fields BN, Knipe DM, Howley PM et al (eds): Fields Virology (3rd ed.), pp 2149–2171. Philadelphia, Lippincott-Raven, 1996

400. HOSEIN IK, KAUNITZ AM, CRAFT SJ: Detection of cervical *Chlamydia trachomatis* and *Neisseria gonorrhoeae* with deoxyribonucleic acid probe assays in obstetric patients. Am J Obstet Gynecol 167:588–591, 1992

401. HOUFF SA, BURTON RC, WILSON RW ET AL: Human-to-human transmission of rabies virus by corneal transplant. N Engl J Med 300:603–604, 1979

402. HOWARD C, FRIEDMAN DL, LEETE JK, ET AL: Correlation of the percent of positive *Chlamydia trachomatis* direct fluorescent antibody detection tests with the adequacy of specimen collection. Diagn Microbiol Infect Dis 14:233–237, 1991

403. HOWELL CL, MILLER MJ: Effect of sucrose phosphate and sorbitol on infectivity of enveloped viruses during storage. J Clin Microbiol 18:658–662, 1983

404. HOWELL CL, MILLER MJ, BRUCKNER DA: Elimination of toxicity and enhanced cytomegalovirus detection in cell cultures inoculated with semen from patients with acquired immunodeficiency syndrome. J Clin Microbiol 24:657–660, 1986

405. HOWELL CL, MILLER MJ, MARTIN WJ: Comparison of rates of virus isolation from leukocyte populations separated from blood by conventional and Ficoll-Paque/Macrodex methods. J Clin Microbiol 10:533–537, 1979

406. HOWLEY PM: Papillomavirinae and their replication. In Fields BN, Knipe DM, Howley PM et al (eds): Fields Virology (3rd ed), pp 2045–2076. Philadelphia, Lippincott-Raven, 1996

407. HSIUNG GD: Diagnostic Virology Illustrated by Light and Electron Microscopy. New Haven, CT, Yale University Press, 1982

408. HU DJ, DONDERO TJ, RAYFIELD MA ET AL: The emerging genetic diversity of HIV. The importance of global surveillance for diagnostics, research, and prevention. JAMA 275:210–216, 1996

409. HUGHES J, PETERS CJ, COHEN ML, MAHY BWJ: Hantavirus pulmonary sundrome: An emerging infectious disease. Science 262:850–851, 1993

410. HUGHES JH, HAMPARIAN VV, MAVROMOUSTAKIS CT: Continuous high-speed rolling versus centrifugation for detection of herpes simplex virus. J Clin Microbiol 27:2884–2886, 1989

411. HUNTOON CJ, HOUSE RF JR, SMITH TF: Recovery of viruses from three transport media incorporated into culturettes. Arch Pathol Lab Med 105:436–437, 1981

412. HUOVINEN P, LAHTONEN R, ZIEGLER T ET AL: Pharyngitis in adults: The presence and coexistence of viruses and bacterial organisms. Ann Intern Med 110:612–616, 1989

413. HYMAN CL, ROBLIN PM, GAYDOS CA, QUINN TC, SCHACHTER J, HAMMERSCHLAG MR: Prevalence of asymptomatic nasopharyngeal carriage of *Chlamydia pneumoniae* in subjectively healthy adults: Assessment by polymerase chain reaction-enzyme immunoassay and culture. Clin Infect Dis 20:1174–1178, 1995

414. IWARSON S, NORKRANS G, WEJSTÅLR: Hepatitis C: Natural history of a unique infection. Clin Infect Dis 20:1361–1370, 1995

415. JACOBS JW, PEACOCK DB, CORNER BD ET AL: Respiratory syncytial and other viruses associated with respiratory disease in infants. Lancet 1:871–876, 1971

416. JACOBSEN D, ACKERMAN P, PAYNE NR: Rapid identification of respiratory syncytial virus infections by direct fluorescent antibody testing: Reliability as a guide to patient cohorting. Am J Infect Control 19:73–78, 1991

417. JAHRLING PB, GEISBRT TW, DALGARD DW ET AL: Preliminary report: Isolation of Ebola virus from monkeys imported to the USA. Lancet 335:502–505, 1990

418. JANSEN RW, NEWBOLD JE, LEMON SM: Combined immunoaffinity cDNA-RNA hybridization assay for detection of hepatitis A virus in clinical specimens. J Clin Microbiol 22:984–989, 1985

419. JASCHEK G, GAYDOS CA, WELSH LE, QUINN TC: Direct detection of *Chlamydia trachomatis* in urine specimens from symptomatic and asymptomatic men by using a rapid polymerase chain reaction assay. J Clin Microbiol 31:1209–1212, 1993

420. JESIONEK K: Ueber unen Befund von Protozoen-artigen gebilden in den Organen eines hereditarluetischen Foetus. Munchen Med Wochenschr 51:1905–1907, 1904

421. JESPERSEN DJ, DREW WL, GLEAVES CA ET AL: Multisite evaluation of a monoclonal antibody reagent (Syva) for rapid diagnosis of cytomegalovirus in the shell vial assay. J Clin Microbiol 27:1502–1505, 1989

422. JOHNSON FB: Transport of viral specimens. Clin Microbiol Rev 3:120–131, 1990

423. JOHNSON FB, LEAVITT RW, RICHARDS DF: Evaluation of the virocult transport tube for isolation of herpes simplex virus from clinical specimens. J Clin Microbiol 20:120–122, 1984

424. JOHNSON GM, MCABEE GA, SEATON ED, LIPSON SM: Suspect value of non-CSF viral cultures in the diagnosis of enteroviral CNS infection in young infants. Dev Med Child Neurol 34:876–884, 1992

425. JOHNSON KM, WIEBENGA NH, MACKENZIE RB ET AL: Virus isolations from human cases of hemorrhagic fever in Bolivia. Proc Soc Exp Biol Med 118:113–118, 1965

426. JOHNSON RT, GRIFFIN DE, HIRSCH RL ET AL: Measles encephalomyelitis—clinical and immunologic studies. N Engl J Med 310:137–141, 1984

427. JOHNSTON WW, FRABLE WJ: The cytopathology of the respiratory tract: A review. Am J Pathol 84:372–424, 1976

428. JONES MF, SMITH TF, HOUGLUM AJ ET AL: Detection of *Chlamydia trachomatis* in genital specimens by the Chlamydiazyme test. J Clin Microbiol 20:465–467, 1984

429. JONES RB, VAN DER POL B, KATZ BP: Effect of differences in specimen processing and passage technique on recovery of *Chlamydia trachomatis*. J Clin Microbiol 27:894–898, 1989

430. JUDSON BA, LAMBERT PP: Improved Syva MicroTrak *Chlamydia trachomatis* direct test method. J Clin Microbiol 26:2657–2658, 1988

431. KADISH AS, BURK RD, KRESS Y ET AL: Human papillomaviruses of different types in precancerous lesions of the uterine cervix: Histologic, immunocytochemical and ultrastructural studies. Hum Pathol 17:384–392, 1986

432. KAHLON J, CHATTERJEE S, LAKEMAN FD ET AL: Detection of antibodies to herpes simplex virus in the cerebrospinal fluid of patients with herpes simplex encephalitis. J Infect Dis 155:38–44, 1987

433. KAO CL, MCINTOSH K, FERNIE B ET AL: Monoclonal antibodies for the rapid diagnosis of respiratory syncytial virus infection by immunofluorescence. Diagn Microbiol Infect Dis 2:199–206, 1984

434. KAPIKIAN AZ, BELL JA, MASTROTA FM ET AL: An outbreak of parainfluenza 2 (croup-associated) virus infection: Association with acute undifferentiated febrile illness in children. JAMA 183:112–118, 1963

435. KAPIKIAN AZ, CHANOCK RM: Rotaviruses. In Fields BN, Knipe DM, Howley PM et al (eds): Fields Virology (3rd ed), pp 1657–1708. Philadelphia, Lippincott-Raven, 1996

436. KAPIKIAN AZ, WYATT RG, DOLIN R ET AL: Visualization by immune electron microscopy of a 27-nm particle associated with acute infectious nonbacterial gastroenteritis. J Virol 10:1075–1081, 1972

437. KAPLAN JE, GARY GW, BARON RC ET AL: Epidemiology of Norwalk gastroenteritis and the role of Norwalk virus in outbreaks of acute nonbacterial gastroenteritis. Ann Intern Med 96:756–761, 1982

438. KAPLAN JE, SCHONBERGER LB: The sensitivity of various serologic tests in the diagnosis of Rocky Mountain spotted fever. Am J Trop Med Hyg 35:840–844, 1986

439. KAPLAN JE, SPIRA TJ, FISHBEIN DB ET AL: A six-year follow-up of HIV-infected homosexual men with lymphadenopathy: Evidence for an increased risk for developing AIDS after the third year of lymphadenopathy. JAMA 260:2694–2697, 1988

440. KAPLAN MH, KLEIN SW, MCPHEE J ET AL: Group B coxsackievirus infections in infants younger than three months of age: A serious childhood illness. Rev Infect Dis 5:1019–1032, 1983

441. KASEL JA: Adenoviruses. In Lennette EH, Schmidt NJ (eds): Diagnostic Procedures for Viral, Rickettsial and Chlamydial Infections (5th ed), pp 229–255. Washington, DC, American Public Health Association, 1979

442. KAUPPINEN M, SAIKKU P: Pneumonia due to *Chlamydia pneumoniae*: Prevalence, clinical features, diagnosis, and treatment. Clin Infect Dis 21:S244–S252, 1995

443. KAWA-HA K, TANAKA K, INOUE M ET AL: Isolation of human herpesvirus 7 from a child with symptoms mimicking chronic Epstein-Barr virus infection. Br J Haematol 84:545–548, 1993

444. KELLOGG JA: Culture vs direct antigen assays for detection of microbial pathogens from lower respiratory tract specimens suspected of containing the respiratory syncytial virus. Arch Pathol Lab Med 115:451–458, 1991

445. KELLOGG JA, SEIPLE JW, MURRAY CL ET AL: Effect of endocervical specimen quality on detection of *Chlamydia trachomatis* and on the incidence of false-positive results with the Chlamydiazyme method. J Clin Microbiol 28:1108–1113, 1990

446. KELLOGG ND, HUSTON RL, FOULDS M: *Chlamydia trachomatis* infections in children evaluated for sexual abuse. Fam Med 23:59–61, 1991

447. KESSLER HA, BLAAUW B, SPEAR J ET AL: Diagnosis of human immunodeficiency virus infection in seronegative homosexuals presenting with an acute viral syndrome. JAMA 258:1196–1199, 1987

448. KILEY MP, BOWEN ETW, EDDY GA ET AL: Filoviridae: A taxonomic home for Marburg and Ebola viruses? Intervirology 18:24–32, 1982

449. KIM HW, WYATT RG, FERNIE BF ET AL: Respiratory syncytial virus detection by immunofluorescence in nasal secretions with monoclonal antibodies against selected surface and internal proteins. J Clin Microbiol 18:1399–1404, 1983

450. KIMBROUGH RC, ORMSBEE RA, PEACOCK M ET AL: Q fever endocarditis in the United States. Ann Intern Med 91:400–402, 1979

451. KIMPTON CP, MORRIS DJ, CORBITT G: Inhibitory effects of various anticoagulants on the infectivity of human cytomegalovirus. J Virol Methods 24:301–306, 1989

452. KIRK JL, FINE DP, SEXTON DJ, MUCHMORE HG: Rocky Mountain spotted fever. A clinical review based on 48 confirmed cases, 1943–1986. Medicine (Baltimore) 69:35–45, 1990

453. KIRKLAND KB, WILKINSON WE, SEXTON DJ: Therapeutic delay and mortality in cases of Rocky Mountain spotted fever. Clin Infect Dis 20:1118–1121, 1995

454. KISSLING RE, ROBINSON RQ, MURPHY FA, WHITFIELD SG: Agent of disease contracted from green monkeys. Science 160:888–890, 1968

455. KIVIAT NB, PETERSON M, KINNEY-THOMAS E ET AL: Cytologic manifestations of cervical and vaginal infections: II. Confirmation of *Chlamydia trachomatis* infection by direct immunofluorescence using monoclonal antibodies. JAMA 253:997–1000, 1985

456. KJAER SK, TEISEN C, HAUGAARD BJ ET AL: Risk factors for cervical cancer in Greenland and Denmark: a population based cross-sectional study. Int J Cancer 44:40–47, 1989

457. KLATT EC, NICHOLS L, NOGUCHI TT: Evolving trends revealed by autopsies of patients with the acquired immunodeficiency syndrome. 565 autopsies in adults with the acquired immunodeficiency syndrome, Los Angeles, Calif, 1992–1993. Arch Pathol Lab Med 118:884–890, 1994

458. KLEIN RS, HARRIS CA, SMALL CB ET AL: Oral candidiasis in high-risk patients as the initial manifestation of the acquired immunodeficiency syndrome. N Engl J Med 311:354–358, 1984

459. KLESPIES SL, CEBULA DE, KELLEY CL, GALEHOUSE D, MAURER CC: Detection of enteroviruses from clinical specimens by spin amplification shell vial culture and monoclonal antibody assay. J Clin Microbiol 34:1465–1467, 1996

460. KLEVJER-ANDERSON P: Diagnostic significance of cytomegalovirus serology. Clin Microbiol Newsletter 9:36–38, 1987

461. KLEVJER-ANDERSON P, ANDERSON LW: Comparison of a new latex agglutination assay with indirect immunofluorescence to detect varicella-zoster antibodies. Diagn Microbiol Infect Dis 17:247–249, 1993

462. KLUYTMANS JA, GOESSENS WH, VAN RIJSOORT-VOS JH, NIESTERS HG, STOLZ E: Improved performance of PACE 2 with modified collection system in combination with probe competition assay for detection of *Chlamydia trachomatis* in urethral specimens from males. J Clin Microbiol 32:568–570, 1994

463. KNOX KK, CARRIGAN DR: Disseminated active HHV-6 infections in patients with AIDS. Lancet 343:577–578, 1994

464. KOENIG S, GENDELMAN HE, ORENSTEIN JM ET AL: Detection of AIDS virus in macrophages in brain tissue from AIDS patients with encephalopathy. Science 233:1089–1093, 1986

465. KOFF RS, GRADY GF, CHALMERS TC ET AL: Viral hepatitis in a group of Boston hospitals: III. Importance of exposure to shellfish in a nonepidemic period. N Engl J Med 276:703–710, 1967

466. KOHLER G, MILSTEIN C: Continuous cultures of fused cells secreting antibody of predefined specificity. Nature 256:495–497, 1975

467. KOMAROFF AL, ARONSON MD, SCHACHTER J: *Chlamydia trachomatis* infection in adults with community-acquired pneumonia. JAMA 245:1319–1322, 1981

468. KONDO K, HAYAKAWA Y, MORI H ET AL: Detection by polymerase chain reaction amplification of human herpesvirus 6 DNA in peripheral blood of patients with exanthem subitum. J Clin Microbiol 28:970–974, 1990

469. KONERU B, JAFFE R, ESQUIVEL CO ET AL: Adenoviral infections in pediatric liver transplant recipients. JAMA 258:489–492, 1987

470. KOST RG, HILL EL, TIGGES M, STRAUS SE: Brief report: Recurrent acyclovir-resistant genital herpes in an immunocompetent patient. N Engl J Med 329:1777–1782, 1993

471. KRAJDEN M: Molecular detection of hepatitis C virus: Impact of detection methodology on clinical and laboratory correlations. Crit Rev Clin Lab Sci 32:41–66, 1995

472. KRAUSE JR, PENCHANSKY L, KNISELY AS: Morphological diagnosis of parvovirus B19 infection: A cytopathic effect easily recognized in air-dried, formalin-fixed bone marrow smears stained with hematoxylin-eosin or Wright-Giemsa. Arch Pathol Lab Med 116:178–180, 1992

473. KRAUSE PJ, HYAMS JS, MIDDLETON PJ ET AL: Unreliability of Rotazyme ELISA test in neonates. J Pediatr 103:259–262, 1983

474. KRECH T, BLECKMANN M, PAATZ R: Comparison of buffalo green monkey cells and McCoy cells for isolation of *Chlamydia trachomatis* in a microtiter system. J Clin Microbiol 27:2364–2365, 1989

475. KRILOV LR, LIPSON SM, BARONE SR, KAPLAN MK, CIAMICIAN Z, HARKNESS SH: Evaluation of a rapid diagnostic test for respiratory syncytial virus (RSV): Potential for bedside diagnosis. Pediatrics 93:903–906, 1994

476. KROGSGAARD K, WANTZIN P, MATHIESEN LR ET AL: Early appearance of antibodies to hepatitis C virus in community acquired acute non-A, non-B hepatitis is associated with progression to chronic liver disease: The Copenhagen Hepatitis Acuta Programme. Scand J Infect Dis 22:399–402, 1990

477. KSIAZEK TG, PETERS CJ, ROLLIN PE ET AL: Identification of a new North American hantavirus that causes acute pulmonary insufficiency. Am J Trop Med Hyg 52:117–123, 1995

478. KURTZMAN G, FRICKHOFEN N, KIMBALL J ET AL: Pure red-cell aplasia of 10 years' duration due to persistent parvovirus B19 infection and its cure with immunoglobulin therapy. N Engl J Med 321:519–523, 1989

479. KURTZMAN GJ, COHEN B, MEYERS P ET AL: Persistent B19 parvovirus infection as a cause of severe chronic anaemia in children with acute lymphocytic leukaemia. Lancet 2:1159–1162, 1988

480. LACKRITZ EM, SATTEN GA, ABERLE-GRASSE J ET AL: Estimated risk of transmission of the human immunodeficiency virus by screened blood in the United States. N Engl J Med 333:1721–1725, 1995

481. LAFFERTY WE, COOMBS RW, BENEDETTI J ET AL: Recurrences after oral and genital herpes simplex virus infection: Influence of site of infection and viral type. N Engl J Med 316:1444–1449, 1987

482. LAFFERTY WE, KROFFT S, REMINGTON M ET AL: Diagnosis of herpes simplex virus by direct immunofluorescence and viral isolation from samples of external genital lesions in a high-prevalence population. J Clin Microbiol 25:323–326, 1987

483. LAHDEVIRTA J: Clinical features of HFRS in Scandinavia as compared with East Asia. Scnd J Infect Dis 36:93–95, 1982

484. LAMB RA, KRUG RM: Orthomyxoviridae: The viruses and their replication. In Fields BN, Knipe DN, Howley PM et al (eds): Fields Virology (3rd ed), pp 1353–1395. Philadelphia, Lippincott-Raven, 1996

485. LAN J, MELGERS I, MEIJER CJLM ET AL: Prevalence and serovar distribution of asymptomatic cervical *Chlamydia trachomatis* infections as determined by highly sensitive PCR. J Clin Microbiol 33:3194–3197, 1995

486. LANDESMAN SH, KALISH LA, BURNS DN ET AL: Obstetrical factors and the transmission of human immunodeficiency virus type 1 from mother to child. N Engl J Med 334:1617–1623, 1996

487. LANDRY ML, FERGUSON D. Comparison of quantitative cytomegalovirus antigenemia assay with culture methods and correlation with clinical disease. J Clin Microbiol 31:2851–2856, 1993

488. LANDRY ML, FONG CK: Nucleic acid hybridization in the diagnosis of viral infections. Clin Lab Med 5:513–529, 1985

489. LANDRY ML, MAYO DR, HSIUNG GD: Comparison of guinea pig embryo cells, rabbit kidney cells, and human embryonic lung fibroblast cell strains for isolation of herpes simplex virus. J Clin Microbiol 15:842–847, 1982

490. LANE HC, DEPPER JM, GREENE WC ET AL: Qualitative analysis of immune function in patients with the acquired immunodeficiency syndrome. N Engl J Med 313:79–84, 1985

491. LANE HC, MASUR H, EDGAR LC ET AL: Abnormalities of B-cell activation and immunoregulation in patients with the acquired immunodeficiency syndrome. N Engl J Med 309:453–458, 1983

492. LANG DJ, KUMMER JF, HARTLEY DP: Cytomegalovirus in semen: Persistence and demonstration in extracellular fluids. N Engl J Med 291:121–123, 1984

493. LASKIN OL, CEDERBERG DM, MILLS J ET AL: Ganciclovir for the treatment and suppression of serious infections caused by cytomegalovirus. Am J Med 83:201–207, 1987

494. LATORRE CR, SULZER AJ, NORMAN LG: Serial propagation of *Pneumocystis carinii* in cell line cultures. Appl Environ Microbiol 33:1204–1206, 1977

495. LAUER BA: Comparison of virus culturing and immunofluorescence for rapid detection of respiratory syncytial

virus in nasopharyngeal secretions: Sensitivity and specificity. J Clin Microbiol 16:411–412, 1982

496. LAUER BA, MASTERS HA, WREN CG ET AL: Rapid detection of respiratory syncytial virus in nasopharyngeal secretions by enzyme-linked immunosorbent assay. J Clin Microbiol 22:782–785, 1985

497. LAU JYN, DAVIS GL, KNIFFEN J ET AL: Significance of serum hepatitis C virus RNA levels in chronic hepatitis C. Lancet 341:1501–1504, 1993

498. LAVANCHY D, MAYERAT C, MOREL B ET AL: Evaluation of third-generation assays for detection of anti-hepatitis C virus (HCV) antibodies and comparison with presence of HCV RNA in blood donors reactive to c100-3 antigen. J Clin Microbiol 32:2272–2275, 1994

499. LAZO PA: Rearrangement of both alleles of human chromosome 8 in HeLa cells, one of them as a result of papillomavirus DNA integration. J Biol Chem 263:360–367, 1988

500. LAZZAROTTO T, DAL MONTE P, BOCCUNI MC, RIPALTI A, LANDINI MP: Lack of correlation between virus detection and serologic tests for diagnosis of active cytomegalovirus infection in patients with AIDS. J Clin Microbiol 30:1027–1029, 1992

501. LECLAIR MM, FREEMAN J, SULLIVAN BF ET AL: Prevention of nosocomial respiratory syncytial virus infections through compliance with glove and gown isolation precautions. N Engl J Med 317:329–334, 1987

502. LEE H, BAEK LJ, JOHNSON KM: Isolation of Hantaan virus, the etiologic agent of Korean hemorrhagic fever, from wild urban rats. J Infect Dis 146:638–644, 1982

503. LEE P, AMYX HL, GAJDUSEK DC ET AL: New hemorrhagic fever with renal syndrome-related virus in indigenous wild rodents in United States. Lancet 2:1405, 1982

504. LE GUENNO, B, FORMENTRY P, WYERS M, GOUNON P, WALKER F, BOESCH C: Isolation and partial characterization of a new strain of Ebola virus. Lancet 345:1271–1274, 1995

505. LEHTOMAKI K, JULKUNEN I, SANDELIN K ET AL: Rapid diagnosis of respiratory adenovirus infections in young adult men. J Clin Microbiol 24:108–111, 1986

506. LENNETTE EH, SCHMIDT NJ (EDS): Diagnostic Procedures for Viral, Rickettsial and Chlamydial Infections (5th ed). Washington, DC, American Public Health Association, 1979

507. LERNER PI, SAMPLINER JE: Transfusion-associated cytomegalovirus mononucleosis. Ann Surg 185:406–410, 1977

508. LEVIN MJ, LEVENTHAL S, MASTERS HA: Factors influencing quantitative isolation of varicella-zoster virus. J Clin Microbiol 19:880–883, 1984

509. LEVY JA, FERRO F, GREENSPAN D, LENNETTE ET: Frequent isolation of HHV-6 from saliva and high seroprevalence of the virus in the population. Lancet 335:1047–1050, 1990

510. LEVY RA, WARFORD AL: Evaluation of the modified Chlamydiazyme immunoassay for the detection of chlamydial antigen. Am J Clin Pathol 86:330–335, 1986

511. LEW JF, GLASS RI, PETRIC M ET AL: Six-year retrospective surveillance of gastroenteritis viruses identified at ten electron microscopy centers in the United States and Canada. Pediatr Infect Dis J 9:709–714, 1990

512. LEW JF, MOE CL, MONROE SS ET AL: Astrovirus and adenovirus associated diarrhea in children in day care settings. J Infect Dis 164:673–678, 1991

513. LIANG TJ, HASEGAWA K, RIMON N ET AL: A hepatitis B virus mutant associated with an epidemic of fulminant hepatitis. N Engl J Med 324:1705–1709, 1991

514. LINDGREN KM, DOUGLAS RG JR, COUCH RB: Significance of herpesvirus hominis in respiratory secretions of man. N Engl J Med 278:517–523, 1968

515. LINNEN J, WAGES J JR, ZHANG-KECK ZY ET AL: Molecular cloning and disease association of hepatitis G virus: A transfusion-transmissible agent. Science 271:505–508, 1996

516. LIPKIN ES, MONCADA JV, SHAFER MA ET AL: Comparison of monoclonal antibody staining and culture in diagnosing cervical chlamydial infection. J Clin Microbiol 23:114–117, 1986

517. LIPSON SM, FALK LH, LEE S-H: Effect of leukocyte concentration and inoculum volume on the laboratory identification of cytomegalovirus in peripheral blood by the centrifugation culture—antigen detection methodology. Arch Pathol Lab Med 120:53–56, 1996

518. LIPTON SA, GENDELMAN HE: Dementia associated with the acquired immunodeficiency syndrome. N Engl J Med 332:934–940, 1995

519. LIVENGOOD CH III, SCHMITT JW, ADDISON WA ET AL: Direct fluorescent antibody testing for endocervical *Chlamydia trachomatis*: Factors affecting accuracy. Obstet Gynecol 72:803–809, 1988

520. LOPEZ C, SIMMONS RL, MAUER SM ET AL: Association of renal allograft rejection with virus infections. Am J Med 56:280–289, 1974

521. LOUSSERT-AJAKA I, LY TD, CHAIX ML ET AL: HIV-1/Hiv-2 seronegativity in HIV-1 subtype O infected patients. Lancet 343:1393–1394, 1994

522. LURAIN NS, THOMPSON KD, FARRAND SK: Rapid detection of cytomegalovirus in clinical specimens by using biotinylated DNA probes and analysis of cross-reactivity with herpes simplex virus. J Clin Microbiol 24:724–730, 1986

523. LUSSO P, SECCHIERO P, CROWLEY RW, GARZINO-DEMO A, BERNEMAN ZN, GALLO RC: CD4 is a critical component of the receptor for human herpesvirus 7: Interference with human immunodeficiency virus. Proc Natl Acad Sci USA 91:3872–3876, 1994

524. MAASS M, DALHOFF K: Transport and storage conditions for cultural recovery of *Chlamydia pneumoniae*. J Clin Microbiol 33:1793–1796, 1995

525. MAASS M, ESSIG A, MARRE R, HENKEL W: Growth in serum-free medium improves isolation of *Chlamydia pneumoniae*. J Clin Microbiol 31:3050–3052, 1993

526. MAASS M, HARIG U: Evaluation of culture conditions used for isolation of *Chlamydia pneumoniae*. Am J Clin Pathol 103:141–148, 1995

527. MACDONALD KL, OSTERHOLM MT, HEDBERG CW ET AL: Toxic shock syndrome: A newly recognized complication of influenza and influenzalike illness. JAMA 257:1053–1058, 1987

528. MACDONALD NE, HALL CB, SUFFIN SC ET AL: Respiratory syncytial viral infection in infants with congenital heart disease. N Eng J Med 307:397–400, 1982

529. MacGregor RR, Graziani AL, Weiss R et al: Successful foscarnet therapy for cytomegalovirus retinitis in an AIDS patient undergoing hemodialysis: Rationale for empiric dosing and plasma level monitoring. J Infect Dis 164:785–787, 1991

530. MacKenzie WR, Davis JP, Peterson DE, Hibbard AJ, Becker G, Zarvan BS: Multiple false-positive serologic tests for HIV, HTLV-1, and hepatitis C following influenza vaccination, 1991. JAMA 268:1015–1017, 1992

531. MacNab JCM, Walkinshaw SA, Cordiner JW et al: Human papillomavirus in clinically and histologically normal tissue of patients with genital cancer. N Engl J Med 315:1052–1058, 1986

532. Madigan JE, Richter PJ Jr, Kimsey RB, Barlough JE, Bakken JS, Dumler JS: Transmission and passage in horses of the agent of human granulocytic ehrlichiosis. J Infect Dis 172:1141–1144, 1995

533. McConnell CT Jr, Plouffe JF, File TM et al: Radiographic appearance of Chlamydia pneumoniae (TWAR strain) respiratory infections. CBPIS Study Group. Community-based Pneumonia Incidence Study. Radiology 192:819–824, 1994

534. Magder LS, Klontz KC, Bush LH et al: Effect of patient characteristics on performance of an enzyme immunoassay for detecting cervical Chlamydia trachomatis infection. J Clin Microbiol 28:781–784, 1990

535. Mahalingham R, Wellish M, Wolf W et al: Latent varicella-zoster viral DNA in human trigeminal and thoracic ganglia. N Engl J Med 323:627–631, 1991

536. Marcus R, CDC Cooperative Needlestick Surveillance Group: Surveillance of health care workers exposed to blood from patients infected with the human immunodeficiency virus. N Engl J Med 319:1118–1123, 1988

537. Markowitz LE, Preblud SR, Orenstein WA et al: Patterns of transmission in measles outbreaks in the United States, 1985–1986. N Engl J Med 320:75–81, 1989

538. Markowitz M, Saag M, Powderly WG et al: A preliminary study of ritonavir, an inhibitor of HIV-1 protease, to treat HIV-1 infection. N Engl J Med 333:1534–1539, 1995

539. Marquez A, Hsiung GD: Influence of glutamine on multiplication and cytopathic effect of respiratory syncytial virus. Proc Soc Exp Biol Med 124:95–99, 1967

540. Marrie TJ: Q Fever: The Disease. Boca Raton, FL, CRC Press, 1990

541. Marrie TJ: Coxiella burnetti (Q fever) pneumonia. Clin Infect Dis 21:S253–S264, 1995

542. Marrie TJ, Harczy M, Mann OE et al: Culture-negative endocarditis probably due to Chlamydia pneumoniae. J Infect Dis 161:127–129, 1990

543. Marsano L, Perrillo RP, Flye MW et al: Comparison of culture and serology for the diagnosis of cytomegalovirus infection in kidney and liver transplant recipients. J Infect Dis 161:454–461, 1990

544. Marshall WF, Telenti A, Proper J et al: Rapid detection of polyomavirus BK by a shell vial cell culture assay. J Clin Microbiol 28:1613–1615, 1990

545. Martin WJ, Smith TF: Rapid detection of cytomegalovirus in bronchoalveolar lavage specimens by a monoclonal antibody method. J Clin Microbiol 23:1006–1008, 1986

546. Marty AM, Dumler JS, Imes G, Brusman HP, Smrkovski LL, Frisman DM: Ehrlichiosis mimicking thrombotic thrombocytopenic purpura. Case report and pathological correlation. Hum Pathol 26:920–925, 1995

547. Maruyama T, McLachlan A, Lino S, Koike K, Kurokawa K, Milich DR: The serology of chronic hepatitis B infection revisited. J Clin Invest 91:2586–2595, 1993

548. Masada CT, Shaw BW Jr, Zetterman RK, Kaufman SS, Markin RS: Fulminant hepatic failure with massive necrosis as a result of hepatitis A infection. J Clin Gastroenterol 17:158–162, 1993

549. Masuko K, Mitsui T, Iwano K et al: Infection with hepatitis GB virus C in patients on maintenance hemodialysis. N Engl J Med 334:1485–1490, 1996

550. Masur H, Michelis MA, Greene JB et al: An out-break of community-acquired Pneumocystis carinii pneumonia: Initial manifestation of cellular immune dysfunction. N Engl J Med 305:1431–1438, 1981

551. Mazzulli T, Rubin RH, Ferraro MJ et al: Cytomegalovirus antigenemia: Clinical correlations in transplant recipients and in persons with AIDS. J Clin Microbiol 31:2824–2827, 1993

552. McCance DJ, Kopan R, Fuchs E et al: Human papillomavirus type 16 alters human epithelial cell differentiation in vitro. Proc Natl Acad Sci USA 85:7169–7173, 1988

553. McCutchan JA: Epidemiology of venereal urethritis: Comparison of gonorrhea and nongonococcal urethritis. Rev Infect Dis 6:669–688, 1984

554. McGarrity GJ, Sarama J, Vanaman V: Cell culture techniques. ASM News 51:170–183, 1985

555. McIntosh K: Diagnostic virology. In Fields BN, Knipe DM, Howley PM et al (eds): Fields Virology (3rd ed), pp 401–430. Philadelphia, Lippincott-Raven, 1996

556. McMoli TE, Bordoh AN, Munube GM et al: Epidemic acute haemorrhagic conjunctivitis in Lagos, Nigeria. Br J Ophthalmol 68:401–404, 1984

557. McQuillin J, Madeley CR, Kendal AP: Monoclonal antibodies for the rapid diagnosis of influenza A and B virus infections by immunofluorescence. Lancet 2:911–914, 1985

558. Meert KL, Sarnaik AP, Gelmini MJ, Lieh-Lai MW: Aerosolized ribavirin in mechanically ventilated children with respiratory syncytial virus lower respiratory tract disease: A prospective, double-blind, randomized trial. Crit Care Med 22:566–572, 1994

559. Meguro H, Bryant JD, Torrence AE et al: Canine kidney cell line for isolation of respiratory viruses. J Clin Microbiol 9:175–179, 1979

560. Melchers WJG, Herbrink P, Walboomers JMM et al: Optimization of human papillomavirus genotype detection in cervical scrapes by a modified filter in situ hybridization test. J Clin Microbiol 27:106–110, 1989

561. Mellors JW, Kingsley LA, Rinaldo CR Jr et al: Quantitation of HIV-1 RNA in plasma predicts outcome after seroconversion. Ann Intern Med 122:573–579, 1995

562. Melnick JL: Enterovirus type 71 infections: A varied clinical pattern sometimes mimicking paralytic poliomyelitis. Rev Infect Dis 62:S387–S390, 1984

563. Melnick JL: Enteroviruses: Polioviruses, coxsackieviruses, echoviruses, and newer enteroviruses. In Fields BN, Knipe DM, Howley PM et al (eds): Virology

(3rd ed), pp 655–712. Philadelphia, Lippincott-Raven, 1996

564. MELNICK JL: Current status of poliovirus infections. Clin Microbiol Rev 9:293–300, 1996

565. MELNICK JL, WENNER HA, PHILLIPS CA: Enteroviruses. In Lennette EH, Schmidt NJ (eds): Diagnostic Procedures for Viral, Rickettsial and Chlamydia Infections (5th ed), pp 471–534. Washington, DC, American Public Health Association, 1979

566. MENEGUS MA, HOLLICK GE: Increased efficiency of group B coxsackievirus isolation from clinical specimens by use of BGM cells. J Clin Microbiol 15:945–948, 1982

567. MERICAN I, SHERLOCK S, MCINTYRE N, DUSHEIKO GM: Clinical, biochemical and histological features in 102 patients with chronic hepatitis C virus infection. Q J Med 86:119–125, 1993

568. MESCHIEVITZ CK, SCHULTZ SB, DICK EC: A model for obtaining predictable transmission of rhinoviruses in human volunteers. J Infect Dis 150:195–201, 1984

569. MICHALAK TI, PASQUINELLI C, GUILHOT S, CHISARI FV: Hepatitis B virus persistence after recovery from acute viral hepatitis. J Clin Invest 93:230–239, 1994

570. MILIAUSKAS JR, WEBBER BL: Disseminated varicella at autopsy in children with cancer. Cancer 53:1518–1525, 1984

571. MINNICH L, RAY CG: Comparison of direct immunofluorescent staining of clinical specimens for respiratory virus antigens with conventional isolation techniques. J Clin Microbiol 12:391–394, 1980

572. MINNICH LL, GOODENOUGH F, RAY CG: Use of immunofluorescence to identify measles virus infections. J Clin Microbiol 29:1148–1150, 1991

573. MINNICH LL, RAY CG: Comparison of direct and indirect immunofluorescence staining of clinical specimens for detection of respiratory syncytial virus antigen. J Clin Microbiol 15:969–970, 1982

574. MINOR P: Picornaviridae. Arch Virol S2:320–326, 1991

575. MITCHELL PD, REED KD, HOFKES JM: Immunoserologic evidence of coinfection with *Borrelia burgdorferi, Babesia microti,* and human granulocytic *Erlichia* species in residents of Wisconsin and Minnesota. J Clin Microbiol 34:724–727, 1996

576. MONCADA J, SCHACHTER J, BOLAN G ET AL: Confirmatory assay increases specificity of the Chlamydiazyme test for *Chlamydia trachomatis* infection of the cervix. J Clin Microbiol 28:1770–1773, 1990

577. MONINI P, DE LELLIS L, FABRIS M, RIGOLIN F, CASSAI E: Kaposi's sarcoma-associated herpesvirus DNA sequences in prostate tissue and human semen. N Engl J Med 334:1168–1172, 1996

578. MONTALBAN GS, ROBLIN PM, HAMMERSCHLAG MR: Performance of three commercially available monoclonal reagents for confirmation of *Chlamydia pneumoniae* in cell culture. J Clin Microbiol 32:1406–1407, 1994

579. MOORE PS, CHANG Y: Detection of herpesvirus-like DNA sequences in Kaposi's sarcoma in patients with and those without HIV infection. N Engl J Med 332:1181–1185, 1995

580. MORI J, FIELD AM, CLEWLEY JP ET AL: Dot blot hybridization assay of B19 virus DNA in clinical specimens. J Clin Microbiol 27:459–464, 1989

581. MORIUCHI H, KATSUSHIMA N, NISHIMURA H, NAKAMURA K, NUMAZAKI Y: Community-acquired influenza C virus infection in children. J Pediatr 118:235–238, 1991

582. MORRISON RE, MILLER MH, LYON LW ET AL: Adult meningoencephalitis caused by herpesvirus hominis type 2. Am J Med 56:540–544, 1974

583. MORSE DL, GUZEWICH JJ, HANRAHAN JP ET AL: Widespread outbreaks of clam- and oyster-associated gastroenteritis: Role of Norwalk virus. N Engl J Med 314:678–681, 1986

584. MORTON HJ: A survey of commercially available tissue culture media. In Vitro 6:89–108, 1970

585. MORZUNOV SP, FELDMANN H, SPIROPOULOU CF ET AL: A newly recognized virus associated with fatal case of hantavirus pulmonary syndrome in Louisana. J Virol 69:1980–1983, 1995

586. MOSLEY JW, EDWARDS VM, CASEY G ET AL: Hepatitis B virus infection in dentists. N Engl J Med 293:729–734, 1975

587. MOTYL MR, BOTTONE EJ, JANDA JM: Diagnosis of herpesvirus infections: Correlation of Tzanck preparation with viral isolation. Diagn Microbiol Infect Dis 2: 157–160, 1984

588. MOWAT NAG, ALBERT-RECHT F, BRUNT PW ET AL: Outbreak of serum hepatitis associated with tatooing. Lancet 1:33–34, 1973

589. MUFSON MA, BELSHE RB, ORVELL C ET AL: Respiratory syncytial virus epidemics: Variable dominance of subgroups A and B strains among children, 1981–1986. J Infect Dis 157:143–148, 1988

590. MUIR K, TODD WTA, WATSON WH, FITZSIMONS E: Viral-associated haemophagocytosis with parvovirus-B19-related pancytopenia. Lancet 339:1139–1140, 1992

591. MULLEY AG, SILVERSTEIN MD, DIENSTAG JL: Indications for use of hepatitis B vaccine, based on cost-effectiveness analysis. N Engl J Med 307:644–652, 1982

592. MURPHY D, TODD JK, CHAO RK ET AL: The use of gowns and masks to control respiratory illness in pediatric hospital personnel. J Pediatr 99:746–750, 1981

593. MURPHY FA: Virus taxonomy. In Fields BN, Knipe DM, Howley PM et al (eds): Fields Virology (3rd ed), pp 15–57. Philadelphia, Lippincott-Raven, 1996

594. MURPHY FA, WEBB PA, JOHNSON KM, WHITFIELD SG: Morphologic comparison of Machupo with lymphocytic choriomeningitis virus: Basis for a new taxonomic group. J Virol 4:535–541, 1969

595. MURRAY PR, BARON EJ, PFALLER MA, TENOVER FC, YOLKER RH (EDS): Manual of Clinical Microbiology (8th ed). Washington, ASM Press, 1995

596. MUSHAHWAR IK, MCGRATH LC, DRNEC J ET AL: Radioimmunoassay for detection of hepatitis B e antigen and its antibody: Results of clinical evaluation. Am J Clin Pathol 76:692–697, 1981

597. MUSIANI M, ZERBINI M, GENTILOMI G, PIAZZI M, GALLINELLA G, VENTUROLI S: Parvovirus B19 clearance from peripheral blood after acute infection. J Infect Dis 172:1360–1363, 1995

598. MUSSO D, RAOULT D: *Coxiella burnetii* blood cultures from acute and chronic Q-fever patients. J Clin Microbiol 33:3129–3132, 1995

599. MUSTONEN J, BRUMMER-KORVENKONTIO M, HEDMAN K, PASTERNACK A, PIETILA K, VAHERI A: Nephropathia epi-

demica in Finland: A retrospective study of 126 cases. Scand J Infect Dis 26:7–13, 1994

600. N'GALY B, RYDER RW, BILA K ET AL: Human immunodeficiency virus infection among employees in an African hospital. N Engl J Med 319:1123–1127, 1988

601. NAHMIAS AJ, JOSEY WE, NAIB ZM ET AL: Perinatal risk associated with maternal genital herpes simplex virus infection. Am J Obstet Gynecol 110:825–837, 1971

602. NAHMIAS AJ, WHITLEY RJ, VISINTINE AN ET AL: Herpes simplex virus encephalitis: Laboratory evaluations and their diagnostic significance. J Infect Dis 145:829–836, 1982

603. NAIB ZM, STEWART JA, DOWDLE WR ET AL: Cytological features of viral respiratory tract infections. Acta Cytol 12:162–171, 1968

604. NAIDES SJ, PIETTE W, VEACH LA ET AL: Human parvovirus B19-induced vesiculopustular skin eruption. Am J Med 84:968–972, 1988

605. NAIK SR, AGGARWAL R, SALUNKE PN, MEHROTRA NN: A large, waterborne viral hepatitis E epidemic in Kanpur, India. Bull World Health Organ 70:597–604, 1992

606. NASH G: Necrotizing tracheobronchitis and bronchopneumonia consistent with herpetic infection. Hum Pathol 3:283–291, 1972

607. NELSON CT, ISTAS AS, WILKERSON MK, DEMMLER GJ: PCR detection of cytomegalovirus DNA in serum as a diagnostic test for congenital cytomegalovirus infection. J Clin Microbiol 33:3317–3318, 1995

608. NELSON-REES WA, FLANDERMEYER R, HAWTHORNE PK: Banded marker chromosomes as indicators of intraspecies cellular contamination. Science 184: 1093–1096, 1974

609. NETTLEMAN MD, JONES RB, ROBERTS SD ET AL: Cost-effectiveness of culturing for Chlamydia trachomatis: A study in a clinic for sexually transmitted diseases. Ann Intern Med 105:189–196, 1986

610. NEWHOUSE VF, SHEPARD CC, REDUS MD ET AL: A comparison of the complement fixation, indirect fluorescent antibody, and microagglutination tests for the serological diagnosis of rickettsial diseases. Am J Trop Med Hyg 28:387–395, 1979

611. NICHOL ST, SPIROPOULOU CF, MORZUNOV S ET AL: Genetic identification of a hantavirus associated with an outbreak of acute respiratory illness. Science 262:914–917, 1993

612. NICHOLS L, BALOGH K, SILVERMAN M: Bacterial infections in the acquired immunodeficiency syndrome. Clinicopathologic correlations in a series of autopsy cases. Am J Clin Pathol 92:787–790, 1989

613. NICHOLSON JKA, McDOUGAL JS, HEARN TL ET AL: 1994 revised guidelines for the performance of CD4+ T-cell determinations in persons with human immunodeficiency virus (HIV) infections. MMWR—Morb Mortal Wkly Rep 43:No. RR-3, 1994

614. NIEDERMAN JC, EVANS AS, SUBRAHMANYAN L ET AL: Prevalence, incidence and persistence of EB virus antibody in young adults. N Engl J Med 282:361–365, 1970

615. NIEDERMAN JC, MILLER G, PEARSON HA ET AL: Infectious mononucleosis: Epstein-Barr-virus shedding in saliva and oropharynx. N Engl J Med 294:1356–1359, 1976

616. NIEL C, GOMES SA, LEITE JPG ET AL: Direct detection and differentiation of fastidious and nonfastidious aden-

oviruses in stools by using a specific nonradioactive probe. J Clin Microbiol 24:785–789, 1986

617. NIUBÓ J, PÉREZ JL, CARVAJAL A, ARDANUY C, MARTIN R: Effect of delayed processing of blood samples on performance of cytomegalovirus antigenemia assay. J Clin Microbiol 32:1119–1120, 1994

618. NOLTE KB, FEDDERSEN RM, FOUCAR K ET AL: Hantavirus pulmonary syndrome in the United States: A pathological description of a disease caused by a new agent. Hum Pathol 26:110–120, 1995

619. NUGIER F, COLIN JN, AYMARD M, LANGLOIS M: Occurrence and characterization of acyclovir-resistant herpes simplex virus isolates: Report on a two-year sensitivity screening survey. J Med Virol 36:1–12, 1992

620. NUOVO GJ: Correlation of histology with human papillomavirus DNA detection in the genital tract. Gynecol Oncol 31:176–183, 1988

621. NUOVO GJ, BLANCO JS, SILVERSTEIN SJ ET AL: Histologic correlates of papillomavirus infection of the vagina. Obstet Gynecol 72:770–774, 1988

622. NUOVO GJ, SILVERSTEIN SJ: Comparison of formalin, buffered formalin, and Bouin's fixation on the detection of human papillomavirus deoxyribonucleic acid from genital lesions. Lab Invest 59:720–724, 1988

623. NURMINEN M, LEINONEN M, SAIKKU P ET AL: The genus-specific antigen of Chlamydia: Resemblance to the lipopolysaccharide of enteric bacteria. Science 220: 1279–1281, 1983

624. O'BRIEN WA, HARTIGAN PM, MARTIN D ET AL: Changes in plasma HIV-1 RNA and CD4+ lymphocyte counts and the risk of progression to AIDS. N Engl J Med 334:426–431, 1996

625. OEFINGER PE, SHAWAR RM, LOO SH ET AL: Enhanced recovery of cytomegalovirus in conventional tube cultures with a spin-amplified adsorption. J Clin Microbiol 28:965–969, 1990

626. OESCH B, WESTAWAY D, WLCHLI M ET AL: A cellular gene encodes scrapie PrP 27–30 protein. Cell 40:735–746, 1985

627. OHTO H, TERAZAWA S, SASAKI N ET AL: Transmission of hepatitis C virus from mothers to infants. N Engl J Med 330:744–750, 1994

628. OKADA K, KAMIYAMA I, INOMATA M ET AL: e Antigen and anti-e in the serum of asymptomatic carrier mothers as indicators of positive and negative transmission of hepatitis B virus to their infants. N Engl J Med 294: 746–749, 1976

629. OLDACH DW, GAYDOS CA, MUNDY LM, QUINN TC: Rapid diagnosis of Chlamydia psittaci pneumonia. Clin Infect Dis 17:338–343, 1993

630. OMATA M, EHATA T, YOKOSUKA O ET AL: Mutations in the precore region of hepatitis B virus DNA in patients with fulminant and severe hepatitis. N Engl J Med 324: 1699–1704, 1991

631. OSMOND DH, PADIAN NS, SHEPPARD HW, GLASS S, SHIBOSKI SC, REINGOLD A: Risk factors for hepatitis C virus seropositivity in heterosexual couples. JAMA 269: 361–365, 1993

632. OSTER CN, BURKE DS, KENYON RH ET AL: Laboratory-acquired Rocky Mountain spotted fever: The hazard of aerosol transmission. N Engl J Med 297:859–863, 1977

633. OXTOBY MJ: Human immunodeficiency virus and other viruses in human milk: Placing the issues in broader perspective. Pediatr Infect Dis J 7:825–835, 1988

634. PAL SR, SZUCS G, MELNICK JL: Rapid immunofluorescence diagnosis of acute hemorrhagic conjunctivitis caused by enterovirus 70. Intervirology 20:19–22, 1983

635. PALMER DF, WHALEY SD: Complement fixation test. In Rose NR, Friedman H, Fahey JL (eds): Manual of Clinical Immunology, pp 57–66. Washington, DC, American Society for Microbiology, 1986

636. PALVA A, RANKI M: Microbial diagnosis by nucleic acid sandwich hybridization. Clin Lab Med 5:475–490, 1985

637. PANCHOLI P, KOLBERT CP, MITCHELL PD ET AL: *Ixodes dammini* as a potential vector of human granulocytic ehrlichiosis. J Infect Dis 172:1007–1012, 1995

638. PAO CC, LAI C, WU S ET AL: Detection of human papillomaviruses in exfoliated cervicovaginal cells by in situ DNA hybridization analysis. J Clin Microbiol 27:169–173, 1989

639. PAPAEVANGELOU V, POLLACK H, RIGAUD M ET AL: The amount of p24 antigenemia and not the time of first detection of virus predicts the clinical outcome of infants vertically infected with human immunodeficiency virus. J Infect Dis 173:574–578, 1996

640. PARODI AS, GREENWAY DJ, RUGGIERO HR ET AL: Sobre la etiologia del brote epidémico de Junin (nota previa). Dia Méd 30:62, 1958

641. PASTUSZAK AL, LEVY M, SCHICK B ET AL: Outcome after maternal varicella infection in the first 20 weeks of pregnancy. N Engl J Med 330:901–905, 1994

642. PATEL JM, RIZZOLO E, HINSHAW JR: Spontaneous subcapsular splenic hematoma as the only clinical manifestation of infectious mononucleosis. JAMA 247:3243–3244, 1982

643. PATTENGALE PK, SMITH RW, PERLIN E: Atypical lymphocytes in acute infectious mononucleosis: Identification by multiple T and B lymphocyte markers. N Engl J Med 291:1145–1148, 1974

644. PAU CP, HU DJ, SPRUILL C ET AL: Surveillance for human immunodeficiency virus type 1 group O infections in the United States. Transfusion 36:398–400, 1996

645. PAUL MO, TETALI S, LESSER ML ET AL: Laboratory diagnosis of infection status in infants perinatally exposed to human immunodeficiency virus type 1. J Infect Dis 173:68–76, 1996

646. PAWLOTSKY J-M, BASTIE A, PELLET C ET AL: Significance of indeterminate third-generation hepatitis C virus recombinant immunoblot assay. J Clin Microbiol 34:80–83, 1996

647. PAWLOTSKY J-M, ROUDOT-THORAVAL F, SIMMONDS P ET AL: Extrahepatic immunologic manifestations in chronic hepatitis C and hepatitis C serotypes. Ann Intern Med 122:169–173, 1995

648. PAYA CV, SMITH TF, LUDWIG J ET AL: Rapid shell vial culture and tissue histology compared with serology for the rapid diagnosis of cytomegalovirus infection in liver transplantation. Mayo Clin Proc 64:670–675, 1989

649. PAYA CV, WOLD AD, ILSTRUP DM ET AL: Evaluation of number of shell vial cell cultures per clinical specimen for rapid diagnosis of cytomegalovirus infection. J Clin Microbiol 26:198–200, 1988

650. PAYNE FE, BAUBLIS JV, ITABASHI HH: Isolation of measles virus from cell cultures of brain from a patient with subacute sclerosing panencephalitis. N Engl J Med 281:585–589, 1969

651. PAYNE SB, GRILLI EA, SMITH AJ ET AL: Investigation of an outbreak of adenovirus type 3 infection in a boys boarding school. J Hyg 93:277–283, 1984

652. PELLETT PE, BLACK JB: Human herpesvirus-6. In Fields BN, Knipe DM, Howley PM et al (eds): Fields Virology (3rd ed), pp 2587–2608. Philadelphia, Lippincott-Raven, 1996

653. PENG H, ROTH P, CAUSSY D ET AL: Comparison of the cytobrush and cotton swabs in sampling cervical cells for filter in situ hybridization detection of human papillomavirus types 16 and 18 DNA. Acta Cytol 32:311–313, 1988

654. PENSIERO MN, SHAREFIKIN JB, DIEFFENBACK CW, HAY J: Hantaan virus infection of human endothelial cells. J Virol 66:5929–5936, 1992

655. PERCIVALLE E, REVELLO MG, VAGO L, MORINI F, GERNA G: Circulating endothelial giant cells permissive for human cytomegalovirus (HCMV) are detected in disseminated HCMV infections with organ involvement. J Clin Invest 92:663–670, 1993

656. PEREIRA L, DONDERO DV, GALLO D ET AL: Serological analysis of herpes simplex virus types 1 and 2 with monoclonal antibodies. Infect Immun 35:363–367, 1982

657. PÉREZ JL, NIUBÒ J, MARISCAL D, TUBAU F, SALVÁ J, MARTÍ R: Evaluation of a monoclonal antibody for detection of varicella-zoster virus infections using a shell vial technique. Eur J Clin Microbiol Infect Dis 12:875–879, 1993

658. PÉREZ JL, MARISCAL D, TUBAU F, NIUBÒ J, MARTIN R: Evaluation of the CMV-vue antigenemia assay for rapid detection of cytomegalovirus in peripheral blood leukocytes. Diagn Microbiol Infect Dis 19:15–18, 1994

659. PÉREZ JL, NIUBÒ J, ARDNUY C ET AL: Comparison of three commercially available monoclonal antibodies directed against pp65 antigen for cytomegalovirus antigenemia assay. Diagn Microbiol Infect Dis 21:21–25, 1995

660. PERRON-HENRY DM, HERRMANN JE, BLACKLOW NR: Isolation and propagation of enteric adenoviruses in HEp-2 cells. J Clin Microbiol 26:1445–1447, 1988

661. PETERS CJ, BUCHMIER M, ROLLIN PE, KSIAZEK TG: Arenaviruses In Fields BN, Knipe DM, Holey PM et al (eds): Fields Virology (3rd ed), pp 1521–1551, Philadelphia, Lippincott-Raven, 1996

662. PETHER JVS, SAN-PIN W, GRAYSTON JT: *Chlamydia pneumoniae*, strain TWAR, as the cause of an outbreak in a boy's school previously called psittacosis. Epidemiol Infect 103:395–400, 1989

663. PHILIP RN, CASPER EA, ORMSBEE RA ET AL: Microimmunofluorescence test for the serological study of Rocky Mountain spotted fever and typhus. J Clin Microbiol 3:51–61, 1976

664. Philips RS, Hanff PA, Holmes MD et al: *Chlamydia trachomatis* cervical infection in women seeking routine gynecologic care: Criteria for selective testing. Am J Med 86:515–520, 1989

665. PHILLIPS RS, HANIFF PA, KAUFFMAN RS ET AL: Use of a direct fluorescent antibody test for detecting *Chlamydia trachomatis* cervical infection in women seeking routine gynecological care. J Infect Dis 156:575–581, 1987

666. PIKE RM: Past and present hazards of working with infectious agents. Arch Pathol Lab Med 102:333–336, 1978

667. PLUMMER FA, HAMMOND GW, FOWARD K ET AL: An erythema infectiosum-like illness caused by human parvovirus infection. N Engl J Med 313:74–79, 1985

668. POLISH LB, SHAPIRO CN, BAUER F ET AL: Nosocomial transmission of hepatitis B virus associated with the use of a spring-loaded finger-stick device. N Engl J Med 326:721–725, 1992

669. POPESCU NC, AMSBAUGH SC, DIPAOLO JA: Human papillomavirus type 18 DNA is integrated at a single chromosome site in cervical carcinoma cell line SW756. J Virol 51:1682–1985, 1987

670. POTHIER P, NICOLAS JC, DE SAINT MAUR GP ET AL: Monoclonal antibodies against respiratory syncytial virus and their use for rapid detection of virus in nasopharyngeal secretions. J Clin Microbiol 21;286–287, 1985

671. POZZATO G, KANEKO S, MORETTI M ET AL: Different genotypes of hepatitis C virus are associated with different severity of chronic liver disease. J Med Virol 43:291–296, 1994

672. PRATHER SL, DAGAN R, JENISTA JA ET AL: The isolation of enteroviruses from blood: A comparison of four processing methods. J Med Virol 14:221–227, 1984

673. PRATHER SL, JENISTA JA, MENEGUS MA: The isolation of nonpolio enteroviruses from serum. Diagn Microbiol Infect Dis 2:353–357, 1984

674. PREZIOSO PJ, CANGIARELLA J, LEE M ET AL: Fatal disseminated infection with human herpes-virus-6. J Pediatr 120:921–923, 1992

675. PRINCE AM, METESELAAR D, KAFUKO GW ET AL: Hepatitis B antigen in wild-caught mosquitoes in Africa. Lancet 2:247–250, 1972

676. PROBER GG, COREY L, BROWN ZA ET AL: The management of pregnancies complicated by genital infections with herpes simplex virus. Clin infect Dis 15:1031–1038, 1992

677. PROBER CG, HENSLEIGH PA, BOUCHER FD ET AL: Use of routine viral cultures at delivery to identify neonates exposed to herpes simplex virus. N Engl J med 318:887–891, 1988

678. PRUSINER SB, MCKINLEY MP, BOWMAN KA ET AL: Scrapaie prions aggregate to form amyloid-like birefringent rods. Cell 35:349–358, 1983

679. PUCHHAMMER-STÖCKL E, POPOW-KRAUPP T, HEINZ FX ET AL: Establishment of PCR for the early diagnosis of herpes simplex encephalitis. J Med Virol 32:77–82, 1990

680. PUIG J, FIELDS HA: Development of an enzyme immunoassay using recombinant expressed antigen to detect hepatitis delta virus antibodies. J Clin Microbiol 27:2222–2225, 1989

681. PURCELL RH: Hepatitis E virus. In Fields BN, Knipe DM, Howley PM et al (eds): Fields Virology (3rd ed), pp 2831–2843. Philadelphia, Lippincott-Raven, 1996

682. QUINN TC, STAMM WE, GOODELL SE ET AL: The polymicrobial origin of intestinal infections in homosexual men. N Engl J Med 309:576–582, 1983

683. QUINNAN GVJ, BURNS WH, KIRMANI N ET AL: HLA-restricted cytotoxic T lymphocytes are an early immune response and important defense mechanism in cytomegalovirus infections. Rev Infect Dis 6:156–163, 1984

684. QUIROGA JA, HERRERO M, CASTILLO I, NAVAS S, PARDO M, CARRENO V: Long-term follow-up study of serum IgM antibody to hepatitis C virus (HCV), HCV replication, and liver disease outcome in chronic hepatitis C. J Infect Dis 170:669–673, 1994

685. RABELLA N, DREW WL: Comparison of conventional and shell vial cultures for detecting cytomegalovirus infection. J Clin Microbiol 28:807, 1990

686. RABINOWITZ M, HALLAK A, GRUNBERG J ET AL: A modified, solid phase radioimmunoassay for the differential diagnosis of acute and convalescent phases of hepatitis A infection. Am J Clin Pathol 88:738–742, 1987

687. RAGA J, CHRYSTAL V, COOVADIA HM: Usefulness of clinical features and liver biopsy in diagnosis of disseminated herpes simplex infection. Arch Dis Child 59:820–824, 1984

688. RAMIREZ-RONDA CH: Dengue in Puerto Rico: Clinical manifestations and management from 1960s to 1987. Puerto Rico Health Sci J 6:113–118, 1987

689. RAMSEY PG, FIFE KH, HACKMAN RC ET AL: Herpes simplex virus pneumonia: Clinical, virologic, and pathologic features in 20 patients. Ann Intern Med 97:813–820, 1982

690. RAND KH, POLLARD RB, MERIGAN TC: Increased pulmonary superinfections in cardiac-transplant patients undergoing primary cytomegalovirus infection. N Engl J Med 298:951–953, 1978

691. RANDO RF, SEDLACEK TV, HUNT J ET AL: Verrucous carcinoma of the vulva associated with an unusual type 6 human papillomavirus. Obstet Gynecol 67:70S–74S, 1986

692. RAPOZA PA, QUINN TC, KIESSLING LA ET AL: Assessment of neonatal conjunctivitis with a direct immunofluorescent monoclonal antibody stain for Chlamydia. JAMA 255:3369–3373, 1986

693. RATNAMOHAN VM, MATHYS JM, MCKENZIE A, CUNNINGHAM AL: HCMV-DNA is detected more frequently than infectious virus in blood leucocytes of immunocompromised patients: A direct comparison of culture-immunofluorescence and PCR for detection of HCMV in clinical specimens. J Med Virol 38:252–259, 1992

694. RAY CG, MINNICH LL: Regional diagnostic virology services: Are satellite laboratories necessary? JAMA 247:1309–1310, 1982

695. RAYFIELD M, DE COCK K, HEYWARD W ET AL: Mixed human immunodeficiency virus (HIV) infection in an individual: Demonstration of both HIV type 1 and type 2 proviral sequences by using polymerase chain reaction. J Infect Dis 158:1170–1175, 1988

696. REDFIELD DC, RICHMAN DD, ALBANIL S ET AL: Detection of herpes simplex virus in clinical specimens by DNA hybridization. Diagn Microbiol Infect Dis 1:117–128, 1983

697. REEVES WC, CAUSSY D, BRINTON LA ET AL: Case-control study of human papillomaviruses and cervical cancer in Latin America. Int J Cancer 40:450–454, 1987

698. REEVES WC, COREY L, ADAMS HG ET AL: Risk of recurrence after first episodes of genital herpes: Relation to HSV type and antibody response. N Engl J Med 305:315–319, 1981

699. REID R, CRUM CP, HERSCHMAN BR ET AL: Genital warts and cervical cancer: III. Subclinical papillomaviral infection and cervical neoplasia are linked by a spectrum of continuous morphologic and biologic change. Cancer 53:943–953, 1984

700. REVETS H, MARISSENS D, DE WIT S ET AL: Comparative evaluation of NASBA HIV-1 RNA QT, AMPLICOR-HIV Monitor, and QUANTIPLEX HIV RNA immunod-

eficiency virus type 1 RNA in plasma. J Clin Microbiol 34:1058–1064, 1996

701. Reyes GR, Purdy MA, Kim JP et al: Isolation of a cDNA from the virus responsible for enterically transmitted non-A, non-B hepatitis. Science 247:1335–1338, 1990

702. Reynolds DW, Stagno S, Hosty TS et al: Maternal cytomegalovirus excretion and perinatal infection. N Engl J Med 289:1–5, 1973

703. Reynolds DW, Stagno S, Stubbs G et al: Inapparent congenital cytomegalovirus infection with elevated cord IgM levels. N Engl J Med 290:291–296, 1974

704. Richardson E: Progressive multifocal leukoencephalopathy. N Engl J Med 265:815–823, 1961

705. Richardson EP: Progressive multifocal leukoencephalopathy 30 years later. N Engl J Med 318:315–316, 1988

706. Richardson WP, Colvin RB, Cheeseman SH et al: Glomerulopathy associated with cytomegalovirus viremia in renal allografts. N Engl J Med 305:57–63, 1981

707. Richman D, Schmidt N, Plotkin S et al: Summary of a workshop on new and useful methods in rapid viral diagnosis. J Infect Dis 150:941–951, 1984

708. Richman DD: Selection of AZT-resistant variants of HIV by therapy. J NIH Res 3:83–87, 1991

709. Richman DD, Cleveland PH, McCormick JB, Johnson KM: Antigenic analysis of Ebola virus: Identification of two Ebola virus serotypes. J Infect Dis 147:268–271, 1983

710. Richman DD, Cleveland PH, Redfield DC et al: Rapid viral diagnosis. J Infect Dis 149:298–310, 1984

711. Richtsmeier WJ, Wittels EG, Mazur EM: Epstein-Barr virus-associated malignancies. Crit Rev Clin Lab Sci 25:105–136, 1987

712. Rikihisa Y: The tribe Ehrlichieae and ehrlichial diseases. Clin Microbiol Rev 4:286–308, 1991

713. Rickinson AB, Kieff E: Epstein-Barr virus. In Fields BN, Knipe DM, Howley PM et al (eds): Fields Virology (3rd ed), pp 2397–2446. Philadelphia, Lippincott-Raven, 1996

714. Rimland D, Parkin WE, Miller GB Jr et al: Hepatitis B outbreak traced to an oral surgeon. N Engl J Med 296:953–958, 1977

715. Rivers TM, Scott TFM: Meningitis in man caused by a filterable virus. Science 81:439–440, 1935

716. Roblin PM, Dumornay W, Hammerschlag MR: Use of HEp-2 cells for improved isolation and passage of Chlamydia pneumoniae. J Clin Microbiol 30:1968–1971, 1992

717. Roland WE, McDonald G, Caldwell CW, Everett ED: Ehrlichiosis—a cause of prolonged fever. Clin Infect Dis 20:821–825, 1995

718. Rollin PE, Ksiazek TG, Elliott LH et al: Isolation of Black Creek Canal virus, a new hantavirus from Sigmodon hispidus in Florida. J Med Virol 46:35–39, 1995

719. Rose JW, Stroop WG, Matsuo F, Henkel J: Atypical herpes simplex encephalitis: Clinical, virologic, and neuropathologic evaluation. Neurology 42:1809–1812, 1992

720. Rose NR, Friedman H, Fahey JL (eds): Manual of Clinical Laboratory Immunology (3rd ed). Washington, DC, American Society for Microbiology, 1986

721. Rosenblum L, Darrow W, Witte J et al: Sexual practices in the transmission of hepatitis B virus and preva-

lence of hepatitis delta virus infection in female prostitutes in the United States. JAMA 267:2477–2481, 1992

722. Roth WK, Lee J-H, Rüster B, Zeuzem S: Comparison of two quantitative hepatitis C virus reverse transcriptase PCR assays. J Clin Microbiol 34:261–264, 1996

723. Royston I, Sullivan JL, Periman PO et al: Cell-mediated immunity to Epstein-Barr virus-transformed lymphoblastoid cells in acute infectious mononucleosis. N Engl J Med 293:1159–1163, 1975

724. Ruuskanen O, Meurman O, Sarkkinen H: Adenoviral diseases in children: A study of 105 hospital cases. Pediatrics 76:79–83, 1985

725. Ruuskanen O, Sarkkinen H, Meurman O et al: Rapid diagnosis of adenoviral tonsillitis: A prospective clinical study. J Pediatr 104:725–728, 1984

726. Ruutu P, Ruutu T, Volin L et al: Cytomegalovirus is frequently isolated in bronchoalveolar lavage fluid of bone marrow transplant recipients without pneumonia. Ann Intern Med 112:913–916, 1990

727. Saag MS, Hahn BH, Gibbons J et al: Extensive variation of human immunodeficiency virus type-1 in vivo. Nature 334:440–444, 1988

728. Sabet SF, Simmons J, Caldwell HD: Enhancement of Chlamydia trachomatis infectious progeny by cultivation in HeLa 229 cells treated with DEAE-Dextran and cycloheximide. J Clin Microbiol 20:217–222, 1984

729. Sabin AB: Studies of B virus: I. The immunological identity of a virus isolated from a human case of ascending myelitis associated with visceral necrosis. Br J Exp Pathol 15:248–268, 1934

730. Sabin AB: The significance of viruses recovered from the intestinal tracts of healthy infants and children. Ann NY Acad Sci 66:226–230, 1956

731. Saikku P, Leinonen M, Tenkanen L et al: Chronic Chlamydia pneumoniae infection as a risk factor for coronary heart disease in the Helsinki Heart Study. Ann Intern Med 116:273–278, 1992

732. Salahuddin SZ, Ablashi DV, Markham PD et al: Isolation of a new virus, HBLV, in patients with lymphoproliferative disorders. Science 234:596–601, 1986

733. Salas R, De Manzione N, Tesh RB et al: Venezuelan haemorrhagic fever. Lancet 338:1033–1036, 1991

734. Salmon VC, Stanberry LR, Overall JC Jr: More rapid isolation of herpes simplex virus in a continuous line of mink lung cells than in Vero or human fibroblast cells. Diagn Microbiol Infect Dis 2:317–324, 1984

735. Salmon VC, Turner RB, Speranza MJ et al: Rapid detection of herpes simplex virus in clinical specimens by centrifugation and immunoperoxidase staining. J Clin Microbiol 23:683–686, 1986

736. Saltzman RL, Quirk MR, Jordan MC: Disseminated cytomegalovirus infection: Molecular analysis of virus and leukocyte interactions in viremia. J Clin Invest 81:75–81, 1988

737. Sankar-Mistry P, Albota V, Knelsen B: Effect of polybrene on isolation of Chlamydia trachomatis from clinical specimens. J Clin Microbiol 22:671–673, 1985

738. Schachter J: Chlamydial infections. N Engl J Med 298:428–434, 1978

739. Schachter J, Grossman M, Sweet RL et al: Prospective study of perinatal transmission of Chlamydia trachomatis. JAMA 255:3374–3377, 1986

740. SCHACHTER J, MONCADA J, WHIDDEN R ET AL: Noninvasive tests for diagnosis of *Chlamydia trachomatis* infection: Application of ligase chain reaction to first-catch urine specimens of women. J Infect Dis 172:1411–1414, 1995

741. SCHAFFNER W, DRUTZ DJ, DUNCAN GW, KOENIG MG: The clinical spectrum of endemic psittacosis. Arch Intern Med 119:433–443, 1967

742. SCHAFFNER W, DRUTZ DJ, DUNCAN GW ET AL: The clinical spectrum of endemic psittacosis. Arch Intern Med 119:433–443, 1967

743. SCHIRM J, MEULENBERG JJ, PASTOOR GW ET AL: Rapid detection of varicella-zoster virus in clinical specimens using monoclonal antibodies on shell vials and smears. J Med Virol 28:1–6, 1989

744. SCHLESINGER Y, BUTLER RS, BRUNSTROM JE, MORAN CJ, STORCH GA: Expanded spectrum of herpes simplex encephalitis in childhood. J Pediatr 126:234–241, 1995

745. SCHMIDT NJ: Cell culture techniques for diagnostic virology. In Lennette EH, Schmidt NJ (eds): Diagnostic Procedures for Viral, Rickettsial and Chlamydial Infections (5th ed), pp 65–139. Washington, DC, American Public Health Association, 1979

746. SCHMIDT NJ, GALLO D, DEVLIN V ET AL: Direct immunofluorescence staining for detection of herpes simplex and varicella-zoster virus antigens in vesicular lesions and certain tissue specimens. J Clin Microbiol 12:651–655, 1980

747. SCHMIDT NJ, HO HH, CHIN J: Application of immunoperoxidase staining to more rapid detection and identification of rubella virus isolates. J Clin Microbiol 13:627–630, 1981

748. SCHMIDT NJ, HO HH, DONDERO ME: *Clostridium difficile* toxin as a confounding factor in enterovirus isolation. J Clin Microbiol 12:796–798, 1980

749. SCHMIDT NJ, HO HH, LENNETTE EH: Propagation and isolation of group A coxsackieviruses in RD cells. J Clin Microbiol 2:183–185, 1975

750. SCHONLAND M, STRONG ML, WESLEY A: Fatal adenovirus pneumonia: Clinical and pathological features. S Afr Med J 50:1748–1751, 1976

751. SCHOOLEY RT, CAREY RW, MILLER G ET AL: Chronic Epstein-Barr virus infection associated with fever and interstitial pneumonitis: Clinical and serologic features and response to antiviral chemotherapy. Ann Intern Med 104:636–643, 1986

752. SELLORS J, MAHONY J, JANG D ET AL: Rapid, on-site diagnosis of chlamydial urethritis in men by detection of antigens in urethral swabs and urine. J Clin Microbiol 29:407–409, 1991

753. SELLS CJ, CARPENTER RL, RAY CG: Sequelae of central-nervous-system enterovirus infections. N Engl J Med 293:1–4, 1975

754. SEMBLE EL, AGUDELO CA, PEGRAM PS: Human parvovirus B19 arthropathy in two adults after contact with childhood erythema infectiosum. Am J Med 83:560–562, 1987

755. SENO M, KANAMOTO Y, TAKAO S ET AL: Enhancing effect of centrifugation on isolation of influenza virus from clinical specimens. J Clin Microbiol 28:1669–1670, 1990

756. SEWELL DL, HORN SA: Evaluation of a commercial enzyme-linked immunosorbent assay for the detection of herpes simplex virus. J Clin Microbiol 21:457–458, 1985

757. SHAFRITZ DA, SHOUVAL D, SHERMAN HI ET AL: Integration of hepatitis B virus DNA into the genome of liver cells in chronic liver disease and hepatocellular carcinoma: Studies in percutaneous liver biopsies and postmortem tissue specimens. N Engl J Med 305:1067–1073, 1981

758. SHAHRABADI MS, LEE PW: Calcium requirement for syncytium formation in HEp-2 cells by respiratory syncytial virus. J Clin Microbiol 26:139–141, 1988

759. SHENK T: Adenoviridae: The viruses and their replication. In Fields BN, Knipe DM, Howley PM et al (eds): Fields Virology (3rd ed), pp 2111–2148. Philadelphia, Lippincott-Raven, 1996

760. SHARPE AH, FIELDS BN: Pathogenesis of viral infections: Basic concepts derived from the reovirus model. N Engl J Med 312:486–497, 1985

761. SHEPARD CC, REDUS MA, TZIANABOS T ET AL: Recent experience with the complement fixation test in the laboratory diagnosis of rickettsial diseases in the United States. J Clin Microbiol 4:277–283, 1976

762. SHERRY MK, KLAINER AS, WOLFF M ET AL: Herpetic tracheobronchitis. Ann Intern Med 109:229–233, 1988

763. SHIBATA D, MARTIN WJ, APPLEMAN MD ET AL: Detection of cytomegalovirus DNA in peripheral blood of patients infected with human immunodeficiency virus. J Infect Dis 158:1185–1192, 1988

764. SHIELDS AF, HACKMAN RC, FIFE KH ET AL: Adenovirus infections in patients undergoing bone-marrow transplantation. N Engl J Med 312:529–533, 1985

765. SHINDO K, KITAYAMA T, URA T ET AL: Acute hemorrhagic cystitis caused by adenovirus type 11 after renal transplantation. Urol Int 41:152–155, 1986

766. SHIRONO K, TSUDA H: Parvovirus B19-associated haemophagocytic syndrome in healthy adults. Br J Haematol 89:923–926, 1995

767. SIMMONDS P, HOLMES EC, CHA T-A ET AL: Classification of hepatitis C virus into six major genotypes and a series of subtypes by phylogenetic analysis of the NS-5 region. J Gen Virol 74:2391–2399, 1993

768. SIMONETTI RG, CAMMÀ C, FIORELLO F ET AL: Hepatitis C virus infection as a risk factor for hepatocellular carcinoma in patients with cirrhosis. A case-control study. Ann Intern Med 116:97–102, 1992

769. SIMONS JN, PILOT-MATIAS TJ, LEARY TP ET AL: Identification of two flavivirus-like genomes in the GB hepatitis agent. Proc Natl Acad Sci USA 92:3401–3405, 1995

770. SIXBEY JW, NEDRUD JG, RAAB-TRAUB N ET AL: Epstein-Barr virus replication in oropharyngeal epithelial cells. N Engl J Med 310:1225–1230, 1984

771. SKENDZEL LP, WILCOX KR, EDSON DC: Evaluation of assays for the detection of antibodies to rubella: A report based on data from the College of American Pathologists Surveys of 1982. Am J Clin Pathol 80:594–598, 1983

772. SKULNICK M, CHUA R, SIMOR AE ET AL: Use of the polymerase chain reaction for the detection of *Chlamydia trachomatis* from endocervical and urine specimens in an asymptomatic low-prevalence population of women. Diag Microbiol Infect Dis 20:195–201, 1994

773. SMADEL J: Epidemic hemorrhagic fever. Am J Public Health 43:1327–1330, 1951

774. SMITH DB, DAVIDSON F, YAP P-L ET AL: Levels of hepatitis C virus in blood donors infected with different viral genotypes. J Infect Dis 173:727–730, 1996

775. SMITH DW, FRANKEL LR, MATHERS LH ET AL: A controlled trial of aerosolized ribavirin in infants receiving mechanical ventilation for severe respiratory syncytial virus infection. N Engl J Med 325:24–29, 1991

776. SMITH JS, FISHBEIN DB, RUPPRECHT CE ET AL: Unexplained rabies in three immigrants in the United States: A virologic investigation. N Engl J Med 324:205–211, 1991

777. SMITH TF: Clinical uses of the diagnostic virology laboratory. Med Clin North Am 67:935–951, 1983

778. SMITH TF: Diagnostic virology in the community hospital: Extent and options. Postgrad Med 75:215–223, 1984

779. SMITH TF (ED): Laboratory Procedures in Clinical Microbiology, pp 537–624. New York, Springer-Verlag, 1985

780. SMITH TF, BROWN SD, WEED LA: Diagnosis of *Chlamydia trachomatis* infections by cell cultures and serology. Lab Med 13:92–100, 1982

781. SMITH TF, MARTIN WJ, WASHINGTON JA II: Isolation of viruses from single throat swabs processed for diagnosis of group A beta-hemolytic streptococci by fluorescent antibody technic. Am J Clin Pathol 60:707–710, 1973

782. SMITH TF, WEED LA: Comparison of urethral swabs, urine, and urinary sediment for the isolation of chlamydia. J Clin Microbiol 2:134–135, 1975

783. SNYDMAN DR, DIENSTAG JL, STEDT B ET AL: Use of IgM-hepatitis A antibody testing: Investigating a common-source, food borne outbreak. JAMA 245:827–830, 1981

784. SNYDMAN DR, WERNER BG, HEINZE-LACEY B ET AL: Use of cytomegalovirus immune globulin to prevent cytomegalovirus disease in renal-transplant recipients. N Engl J Med 317:1049–1054, 1987

785. SOLOMON AR, RASMUSSEN JE, WEISS JS: A comparison of the Tzanck smear and viral isolation in varicella and herpes zoster. Arch Dermatol 122:282–285, 1986

786. SOULIER J, GROLLET L, OKSENHENDLER E ET AL: Kaposi's sarcoma-associated herpesvirus-like DNA sequences in multicentric Castleman's disease. Blood 86:1276–1280, 1995.

787. SPECTER S, LANCZ GJ: Clinical Virology Manual. New York, Elsevier, 1986

788. SPECTOR SA, RUA JA, SPECTOR DH ET AL: Detection of human cytomegalovirus in clinical specimens by DNA-DNA hybridization. J Infect Dis 150:121–126, 1984

789. SPELMAN DW: Q fever: A study of 111 consecutive cases. Med J Aust 1:547–553, 1982

790. SPERBER SJ, HAYDEN FG: Antiviral chemotherapy and prophylaxis of viral respiratory disease. Clin Lab Med 7:869–896, 1987

791. SRINIVASAN G, AZARCON E, MULDOON MR ET AL: Rotavirus infection in normal nursery: Epidemic and surveillance. Infect Control 5:478–481, 1984

792. STAGNO S, PASS RF, CLOUD G ET AL: Primary cytomegalovirus infection in pregnancy: Incidence, transmission to fetus, and clinical outcome. JAMA 256:1904–1908, 1986

793. STAGNO S, PASS RF, DWORSKY ME ET AL: Congenital cytomegalovirus infection: The relative importance of primary and recurrent maternal infection. N Engl J Med 306:945–949, 1982

794. STAMM WE, HANDSFIELD HH, ROMPALO AM ET AL: The association between genital ulcer disease and acquisition of HIV infection in homosexual men. JAMA 260:1429–1433, 1988

795. STAMM WE, HARRISON HR, ALEXANDER ER ET AL: Diagnosis of *Chlamydia trachomatis* infections by direct immunofluorescence staining of genital secretions: A multicenter trial. Ann Intern Med 101:638–641, 1984

796. STAMM WE, TAM M, KOESTER M ET AL: Detection of *Chlamydia trachomatis* inclusions in McCoy cell cultures with fluorescein-conjugated monoclonal antibodies. J Clin Microbiol 17:666–668, 1983

797. STANBERRY LR, FLOYD-REISING SA, CONNELLY BL ET AL: Herpes simplex viremia: Report of eight pediatric cases and review of the literature. Clin Infect Dis 18:401–407, 1994

798. STANDAERT SM, DAWSON JE, SCHAFFNER W ET AL: Ehrlichiosis in a golf-oriented retirement community. N Engl J Med 333:420–425, 1995

799. STEINBERG SP, GERSHON AA: Measurement of antibodies to varicella-zoster virus by using a latex agglutination test. J Clin Microbiol 29:1527–1529, 1991

800. STEPHENSEN CB, BLOUNT SR, LANFORD RE ET AL: Prevalence of serum antibodies against lymphocytic choriomeningitis virus in selected populations from two U.S. cities. J Med Virol 38:27–31, 1992

801. STOKES CE, BERNSTEIN JM, KYGER SA ET AL: Rapid diagnosis of influenza A and B by 24-h fluorescent focus assays. J Clin Microbiol 26:1263–1266, 1988

802. STORCH GA, GAUDREAULT-KEENER M, WELBY PC: Comparison of heparin and EDTA transport tubes for detection of cytomegalovirus in leukocytes by shell vial assay, pp65 antigenemia assay, and PCR. J Clin Microbiol 32:2581–2583, 1994

803. STOUT C, MURPHY MD, LAWRENCE S ET AL: Evaluation of a monoclonal antibody pool for rapid diagnosis of respiratory viral infections. J Clin Microbiol 27:448–452, 1989

804. STRAND CL: Role of the microbiology laboratory in the diagnosis of opportunistic infections in persons infected with human immunodeficiency virus. Arch Pathol Lab Med 114:277–283, 1990

805. STRANO AJ: Light microscopy of selected viral diseases (morphology of viral inclusion bodies). Pathol Ann 11:53–75, 1976

806. STRAUS SE, ROONEY JF, SEVER JL ET AL: NIH Conference: Herpes simplex virus infection: Biology, treatment, and prevention. Ann Intern Med 103:404–419, 1985

807. STREMLAU A, GISSMAN L, IKENBERG H ET AL: Human papillomavirus type 16 related DNA in an anaplastic carcinoma of the lung. Cancer 55:1737–1740, 1985

808. SUGA S, YOSHIKAWA T, ASANO Y, NAKASHIMA T, KOBAYASHI I, YAZAKI T: Activation of human herpesvirus-6 in children with acute measles. J Med Virol 38:278–282, 1992

809. SULLIVAN BJZ, HULL HF, WILSON C ET AL: Presentation of neonatal herpes simplex virus infections: Implications for a change in therapeutic strategy. Pediatr Infect Dis 5:309–314, 1986

810. SUPRAN EM, CRASKE J, HART RJ ET AL: Report of a joint DMRQC/Organon field trial to detect hepatitis A IgM by ELISA. J Clin Pathol 36:1111–1115, 1983

811. SUTTON GP, STEHMAN FB, EHRLICH CE ET AL: Human papillomavirus deoxyribonucleic acid in lesions of the female genital tract: Evidence for type 6/11 in squamous

carcinoma of the vulva. Obstet Gynecol 70:564–568, 1987

812. SWEET RL, BLANKFORT-DOYLE M, ROBBIE MO ET AL: The occurrence of chlamydial and gonococcal salpingitis during the menstrual cycle. JAMA 255:2062–2064, 1986

813. SWENSON PD, KAPLAN MH: Rapid detection of respiratory syncytial virus in nasopharyngeal aspirates by a commercial enzyme immunoassay. J Clin Microbiol 23:485–488, 1986

814. SWIERKOSZ EM, ARENS MQ, SCHMIDT RR ET AL: Evaluation of two immunofluorescence assays with monoclonal antibodies for typing of herpes simplex virus. J Clin Microbiol 21:643–644, 1985

815. TAKEMOTO K, MULLARKEY M: Human papovaviruses, BK strain: Biological studies including antigenic relationship to simian virus 40. J Virol 12:625–631, 1973

816. TAKIFF HE, STRAUS SE, GARON CF: Propagation and in vitro studies of previously noncultivable enteral adenoviruses in 293 cells. Lancet 2:832–834, 1981

817. TAKIMOTO CH, CRAM DL, ROOT RK: Respiratory syncytial virus infections on an adult medical ward. Arch Intern Med 151:706–708, 1991

818. TAM MR, STAMM WE, HANDSFIELD HH ET AL: Culture-independent diagnosis of Chlamydia trachomatis using monoclonal antibodies. N Engl J Med 310:1146–1150, 1984

819. TEDDER DG, ASHLEY R, TYLER KL, LEVIN MJ: Herpes simplex virus infection as a cause of benign recurrent lymphocytic meningitis. Ann Intern Med 121:334–338, 1994

820. TEDDER RS, O'CONNOR T, HUGHES A ET AL: Envelope cross-reactivity in Western blot for HIV-1 and HIV-2 may not indicate dual infection. Lancet 2:927–930, 1988

821. TELFORD SR, LEPORE TJ, SNOW P, WARNER CK, DAWSON JE: Human granulocytic ehrlichiosis in Massachusetts. Ann Intern Med 123:277–279, 1995

822. TERNI M, CACCIALANZA P, CASSAI E ET AL: Aseptic meningitis in association with herpes progenitalis. N Engl J Med 285:503–504, 1971

823. THIN RNT, ATIA W, PARKER JDJ ET AL: Value of Papanicolaou-stained smears in the diagnosis of trichomoniasis, candidiasis, and cervical herpes simplex virus infection in women. Br J Vener Dis 51:116–118, 1975

824. Thomas DL, Factor SH, Kelen GD, Washington AS, Taylor E Jr, Quinn TC: Viral hepatitis in health care personnel at The Johns Hopkins Hospital. The seroprevalence of and risk factors for hepatitis B and hepatitis C infection. Arch Intern Med 153:1705–1712, 1993

825. THOMAS EE, PUTERMAN ML, KAWANO E ET AL: Evaluation of seven immunoassays for detection of rotavirus in pediatric stool samples. J Clin Microbiol 26:1189–1193, 1988

826. THORNHILL TS, WYATT RG, KALICA AR ET AL: Detection by immune electron microscopy of 26- to 27-nm viruslike particles associated with two family outbreaks of gastroenteritis. J Infect Dis 135:20–27, 1977

827. TIEN RD, FELSBERG GJ, OSUMI AK: Herpesvirus infections of the CNS: MR findings. AJR Am J Radiol 161:167–176, 1993

828. TOBI M, STRAUS SE: Chronic Epstein-Barr virus disease: A workshop held by the National Institute of Allergy and Infectious Diseases. Ann Intern Med 103:951–953, 1985

829. TRACY S, WIEGAND V, MCMANUS B ET AL: Molecular approaches to enteroviral diagnosis in idiopathic cardiomyopathy and myocarditis. J Am Coll Cardiol 15:1688–1694, 1990

830. TREUHAFT MW, SOUKUP JM, SULLIVAN BJ: Practical recommendations for the detection of pediatric respiratory syncytial virus infections. J Clin Microbiol 22:270–273, 1985

831. TRISTRAM DA, MILLER RW, MCMILLAN JA ET AL: Simultaneous infection with respiratory syncytial virus and other respiratory pathogens. Am J Dis Child 142:834–836, 1988

832. TROENDLE-ATKINS J, DEMMLER GJ, BUFFONE GJ: Rapid diagnosis of herpes simplex virus encephalitis by using the polymerase chain reaction. J Pediatr 123:376–380, 1993

833. TSELENTIS Y, GIKAS A, KOFTERIDIS D ET AL: Q fever in the Greek island of Crete: Epidemiologic, clinical, and therapeutic data from 98 cases. Clin Infect Dis 20:1311–1316, 1995

834. TURNER M, ISTRE GR, BEAUCHAMP H ET AL: Community outbreak of adenovirus type 7a infections associated with a swimming pool. South Med J 80:712–715, 1987

835. TYRRELL DAJ, MIKA-JOHNSON M, CHAPPLE PJ: Clones of cells from a human embryonic lung: Their growth and susceptibility to respiratory viruses. Arch Virol 61:69–85, 1979

836. UHNOO I, SVENSSON L: Clinical and epidemiological features of acute infantile gastroenteritis associated with human rotavirus subgroups 1 and 2. J Clin Microbiol 23:551–555, 1986

837. UNGER ER, BUDGEON LR, MYERSON D ET AL: Viral diagnosis by in situ hybridization: Description of a rapid simplified colorimetric method. Am J Surg Pathol 10:1–8, 1986

838. VAININONP R, HYYPI T: Biology of parainfluenza viruses. Clin Microbiol Rev 7:265–275, 1994

839. VAN DEN BERG AP, TEGZESS AM, SCHOLTEN-SAMPSON A ET AL: Monitoring antigenemia is useful in guiding treatment of severe cytomegalovirus disease after organ transplantation. Transpl Int 5:101–106, 1992

840. VAN DER BIJ W, SCHIRM J, TORENSMA R ET AL: Comparison between viremia and antigenemia for detection of cytomegalovirus in blood. J Clin Microbiol 26:2531–2535, 1988

841. VIRTANEN M, PALVA A, LAAKSONEN M ET AL: Novel test for rapid viral diagnosis: Detection of adenovirus in nasopharyngeal mucus aspirates by means of nucleic-acid sandwich hybridisation. Lancet 1:381–383, 1983

842. VOGEL J, SHELOKOV A: Adsorption-hemagglutination test for influenza virus in monkey kidney tissue culture. Science 126:358–359, 1957

843. WALD A, ZEH J, SELKE S, ASHLEY RL, COREY L: Virologic characteristics of subclinical and symptomatic genital herpes infections. N Engl J Med 333:770–775, 1995

844. WALKER DH: Rocky Mountain spotted fever: A disease in need of microbiological concern. Clin Microbiol Rev 2:227–240, 1989

845. WALKER DH: Rocky Mountain spotted fever: A seasonal alert. Clin Infect Dis 20:1111–1117, 1995

846. WALKER DH, BURDAY MS, FOLDS JD: Laboratory diagnosis of Rocky Mountain spotted fever. South Med J 73:1443–1449, 1980

847. WALKER DH, CAIN BG: A method for specific diagnosis of Rocky Mountain spotted fever on fixed, paraffin-embedded tissue by immunofluorescence. J Infect Dis 137:206–209, 1978

848. WALPITA P, DAROUGAR S: Double-label immunofluorescence method for simultaneous detection of adenovirus and herpes simplex virus from the eye. J Clin Microbiol 27:1623–1625, 1989

849. WANER JL: Isolation and identification of viruses from respiratory specimens. Newsletter Pan Am Group Rapid Viral Diagn 12:1–4, 1986

850. WARD C: Acquired valvular heart-disease in patients who keep pet birds. Lancet 2:734–736, 1974

851. WARD RL, KNOWLTON DR, PIERCE MJ: Efficiency of human rotavirus propagation in cell culture. J Clin Microbiol 19:748–753, 1984

852. WARFORD AL, LEVY RA, REKRUT KA: Evaluation of a commercial enzyme-linked immunosorbent assay for detection of herpes simplex virus antigen. J Clin Microbiol 20:490–493, 1984

853. WARFORD AL, LEVY RA, STRONG CA ET AL: Comparison of two commercial enzyme-linked immunosorbent assays for detection of herpes simplex virus antigen. Am J Clin Pathol 85:229–232, 1986

854. WARFORD AL, REKRUT KA, LEVY RA ET AL: Sucrose phosphate glutamate for combined transport of chlamydial and viral specimens. Am J Clin Pathol 81:762–764, 1984

855. WARIS M: Pattern of respiratory syncytial virus epidemics in Finland: Two-year cycles with alternating prevalence of groups A and B. J Infect Dis 163:464–469, 1991

856. WASHBURNE JF, BOCCHINI JA JR, JAMISON RM: Summertime respiratory syncytial virus infection: Epidemiology and clinical manifestations. South Med J 85:579–583, 1992

857. WAT PJ, STRICKLER JG, MYERS JL, NORDSTROM MR: Herpes simplex infection causing acute necrotizing tonsillitis. Mayo Clin Proc 69:269–271, 1994

858. WEAR DJ, MALATY RH, ZIMMERMAN LE ET AL: Cat-scratch disease bacilli in the conjunctiva of patients with Parinaud's oculoglandular syndrome. Ophthalmology 92:1282–1287, 1985

859. WEAR DJ, MARGILETH AM, HADFIELD TL ET AL: Cat-scratch disease: A bacterial infection. Science 221:1403–1405, 1983

860. WEIGLER BJ: Biology of B virus in macaque and human hosts: A review. Clin Infect Dis 14:555–567, 1992

861. WEILAND TL, NOLLER KL, SMITH TF ET AL: Comparison of Dacron-tipped applicator and cytobrush for detection of chlamydial infections. J Clin Microbiol 26:2437–2438, 1988

862. WEINBERG A, HAYWARD AR, MASTERS HB, OGU IA, LEVIN MJ: Comparison of two methods for detecting varicella-zoster virus antibody with varicella-zoster virus cell-mediated immunity. J Clin Microbiol 34:445–446, 1996

863. WEINGARTEN S, FRIEDLANDER M, RASCON D ET AL: Influenza surveillance in an acute-care hospital. Arch Intern Med 148:113–116, 1988

864. WEINSTOCK HS, BOLAN G, REINGOLD L, POLISH LB: Hepatitis B virus infection among patients attending a clinic for sexually transmitted diseases. JAMA 269:392–394, 1993

865. WELLER TH: Varicella and herpes zoster. In Lennette EH, Schmidt NJ (eds): Diagnostic Procedures for Viral, Rickettsial and Chlamydial Infections (5th ed), pp 375–398. Washington, DC, American Public Health Association, 1979

866. WELLER TH: Cytomegalovirus: The difficult years. J Infect Dis 122:532–539, 1970

867. WELLS DL, LIPPER SL, HILLIARD JK ET AL: Herpesvirus simiae contamination of primary rhesus monkey kidney cell cultures: CDC recommendations to minimize risks to laboratory personnel. Diagn Microbiol Infect Dis 12:333–336, 1989

868. WELLS DL, HOPFENSPERGER DJ, ARDEN NH ET AL: Swine influenza virus infections. Transmission from ill pigs to humans at a Wisconsin agricultural fair and subsequent probable person-to-person transmission. JAMA 265:478–481, 1991

869. WENZEL RP, DEAL EC, HENDLEY JO: Hospital-acquired viral respiratory illness on a pediatric ward. Pediatrics 60:367–371, 1977

870. WENZEL RP, HENDLEY JO, DAVIES JA ET AL: Coronavirus-infections in military recruits: Three-year study with coronavirus strains OC43 and 229E. Am Rev Respir Dis 109:621–624, 1974

871. WEST PG, ALDRICH B, HARTWIG R ET AL: Enhanced detection of cytomegalovirus in confluent MRC-5 cells treated with dexamethasone and dimethyl sulfoxide. J Clin Microbiol 26, 12:2510–2514, 1988

872. WEST TE, PAPASIAN CJ, PARK BH ET AL: Adenovirus type 2 encephalitis and concurrent Epstein-Barr virus infection in an adult man. Arch Neurol 42:815–817, 1985

873. WESTENFELD FW, WINN WC JR: Recovery of varicella-zoster virus in diploid fibroblast and monkey kidney cell cultures. Am J Clin Pathol 102:733–735, 1994

874. WHITE NJ, JUEL JBE: Infectious mononucleosis hepatitis. Semin Liver Dis 4:301–306, 1984

875. WHITLEY R, ARVIN A, PROBER C ET AL: Predictors of morbidity and mortality in neonates with herpes simplex virus infections. N Engl J Med 324:450–454, 1991

876. WHITLEY RJ: Herpes simplex viruses. In Fields BN, Knipe DM, Howley PM et al (eds): Fields Virology (3rd ed), pp 2297–2342. Philadelphia, Lippincott-Raven, 1996

877. WHITLEY RJ, ALFORD CA, HIRSCH MS ET AL: Vidarabine versus acyclovir therapy in herpes simplex encephalitis. N Engl J Med 314:144–149, 1986

878. WHITLEY RJ, COBBS CG, ALFORD CA JR ET AL: Diseases that mimic herpes simplex encephalitis: Diagnosis, presentation, and outcome. NIAID Collaborative Antiviral Study Group. JAMA 262:234–239, 1989

879. WHITLEY RJ, SOONG S, LINNEMAN C ET AL: Herpes simplex encephalitis: Clinical assessment. JAMA 247:317–320, 1982

880. WILCZYNSKI SP, BERGEN S, WALKER J ET AL: Human papillomaviruses and cervical cancer: Analysis of histopathologic features associated with different viral types. Hum Pathol 19:697–704, 1988

881. WILFERT CM, THOMPSON RJJ, SUNDER TR ET AL: Longitudinal assessment of children with enteroviral meningitis during the first three months of life. Pediatrics 67:811–815, 1981

882. WILLIAMS T, MANIAR AC, BRUNHAM RC ET AL: Identification of Chlamydia trachomatis by direct immuno-fluores-

cence applied in specimens originating in remote areas. J Clin Microbiol 22:1053–1054, 1985

883. WILLIAMS V, GERSHON AA, BRUNELL PA: Serologic response to varicella-zoster membrane antigens measured by direct immunofluorescence. J Infect Dis 130:669–672, 1974

884. WINKLER B, CRUM CP, FUJII T ET AL: Koilocytic lesions of the cervix: The relationship of mitotic abnormalities to the presence of papillomavirus antigens and nuclear DNA content. Cancer 53:1081–1087, 1984

885. WODZINSKI MA, LILLEYMAN JS: Transient erythroblastopenia of childhood due to human parvovirus B19 infection. Br J Haematol 73:127–131, 1989

886. WOLFSEN HC, BOLEN JW, BOWEN JL, FENSTER LF: Fulminant herpes hepatitis mimicking hepatic abscesses. J Clin Gastroenterol 16:61–64, 1993

887. WONG KH, SKELTON SK, CHAN YK: Efficient culture of Chlamydia pneumoniae with cell lines derived from the human respiratory tract. J Clin Microbiol 30:1625–1630, 1992

888. WONG KH, SKELTON SK, DAUGHARTY H: Utility of complement fixation and microimmunofluorescence assays for detecting serologic responses in patients with clinically diagnosed psittacosis. J Clin Microbiol 32: 2417–2421, 1994

889. WONG DT, WELLIVER RC, RIDDLESBERGER KR ET AL: Rapid diagnosis of parainfluenza virus infection in children. J Clin Microbiol 16:164–167, 1982

890. WOOD W, SHIMADA FT: Isolation of strains of virus B from tissue cultures of cynomolgus and rhesus monkey. Can J Public Health 45:509–518, 1954

891. WOODMAN DR, WEISS E, DASCH GA ET AL: Biological properties of Rickettsia prowazekii strains isolated from flying squirrels. Infect Immun 16:853–860, 1977

892. WOODS GL, GARZA DM: Use of Gen-Probe probe competition assay as a supplement to probes for direct detection of Chlamydia trachomatis and Neisseria gonorrhoeae in urogenital specimens. J Clin Microbiol 34: 177–178, 1996

893. WOODS GL, YOUNG A: Use of A-549 cells in a clinical virology laboratory. J Clin Microbiol 26:1026–1028, 1988

894. WOODS GL, YOUNG A, SCOTT JC JR, BLAIR TM, JOHNSON AM: Evaluation of a nonisotopic probe for detection of Chlamydia trachomatis in endocervical specimens. J Clin Microbiol 28:370–372, 1990

895. WYATT LS, FRENKEL N: Human herpesvirus 7 is a constitutive inhabitant of adult human saliva. J Virol 66: 3206–3209, 1992

896. WYATT LS, RODRIGUEZ WJ, BALACHANDRAN N, FRENKEL N: Human herpesvirus 7: Antigenic properties and prevalence in children and adults. J Virol 65:6260–6265, 1991

897. YAMINISHI K, OKUNO T, SHIRAKI K ET AL: Identification of human herpesvirus-6 as a causal agent for exanthem subitum. Lancet 1:1065–1067, 1988

898. YAO QY, RICKINSON AB, EPSTEIN MA. A re-examination of the Epstein-Barr virus carrier state in healthy seropositive indviduals. Int J Cancer 35:35–42, 1985

899. YEE C, KRISHNAN-HEWLETT I, BAKER CC ET AL: Presence and expression of human papillomavirus sequences in human cervical carcinoma cell lines. Am J Pathol 119:361–366, 1985

900. YERLY S, GERVAIX A, SIMONET V, CAFLISCH M, PERRIN L, WUNDERLI W: Rapid and sensitive detection of enteroviruses in specimens from patients with aseptic meningitis. J Clin Microbiol 34:199–201, 1996

901. YEVICH SJ, SANCHEZ JL, DEFRAITES RF ET AL: Seroepidemiology of infections due to spotted fever group rickettsiae and Ehrlichia species in military personnel exposed in areas of the United States where such infections are endemic. J Infect Dis 171:1266–1273, 1995

902. YODER BL, STAMM WE, KOESTER CM ET AL: Microtest procedure for isolation of Chlamydia trachomatis. J Clin Microbiol 13:1036–1039, 1981

903. YOLKEN RH: Use of monoclonal antibodies for viral diagnosis. Curr Top Microbiol Immunol 104:177–195, 1983

904. YONG DCT, PAUL NR: Micro direct inoculation method for the isolation and identification of Chlamydia trachomatis. J Clin Microbiol 23:536–538, 1986

905. YOSHIKAWA T, NAKASHIMA T, SUGA S ET AL: Human herpesvirus-6 DNA in cerebrospinal fluid of a child with exanthem subitum and meningoencephalitis. Pediatrics 89:888–890, 1992

906. YOUNG EJ, CHAFTIZADEH E, OLIVEIRA VL, GENTA RM: Disseminated herpesvirus infection during pregnancy. Clin Infect Dis 22:51–58, 1996

907. YUEN ST, CHUNG LP, LEUNG SY, LUK IS, CHAN SY, HO J: In situ detection of Epstein-Barr virus in gastric and colorectal adenocarcinomas. Am J Surg Pathol 18: 1158–1163, 1994

908. ZAGURY D, BERNARD J, LEIBOWITCH J ET AL: HTLV-III in cells cultured from semen of two patients with AIDS. Science 226:449–451, 1984

909. ZAAIJER HL, CUYPERS HT, REESINK HW, WINKEL IN, GERKEN G, LELIE PN: Reliability of polymerase chain reaction for detection of hepatitis C virus. Lancet 341: 722–724, 1993

910. ZAKI SR, GREER PW, COFFIELD LM ET AL: Hantavirus pulmonary syndrome: Pathogenesis of an emerging infectious disease. Am J Pathol 146:552–579, 1995

911. ZAKI SR, KHAN AS, GOODMAN RA ET AL: Retrospective diagnosis of hantavirus pulmonary syndrome, 1978–1993. Arch Pathol Lab Med 120:134–139, 1996

912. ZEIER M, ZOLLER L, WEINREICH T, PADBERG-WOLF E, ANDRASSY K, RITZ E: Severe hemorrhagic complications from infection with nephropathia epidemica strain of Hantavirus. Clin Nephrol 38:190–192, 1992

913. ZERBINI M, MUSIANI, M, GENTILOMI G, VENTUROLI S, GALLINELLA G, MORANDI R: Comparative evaluation of virological and serological methods in prenatal diagnosis of parvovirus B19 fetal hydrops. J Clin Microbiol 34:603–608, 1996

914. ZIEGLER T: Detection of varicella-zoster viral antigens in clinical specimens by solid-phase enzyme immunoassay. J Infect Dis 150:149–154, 1984

915. ZIPETO D, REVELLO MG, SILINI E ET AL: Development and clinical significance of a diagnostic assay based on the polymerase chain reaction for detection of human cytomegalovirus DNA in blood samples from immunocompromised patients. J Clin Microbiol 30:527–530, 1992

916. ZUR HAUSEN H: Intracellular surveillance of persisting viral infections: Human genital cancer results from deficient cellular control of papillomavirus gene expression. Lancet 2:489–491, 1986

CHARTS

CHARTS

CHART 1   ARYLSULFATASE

I. Principle

Arylsulfatase is an enzyme that splits free phenolphthalein from the tripotassium salt of phenolphthalein disulfite. The test for the identification of *Mycobacterium* species is performed in a tube containing a substrate of phenolphthalein in oleic acid agar (Wayne). After 3 (or 14) days of incubation of a subculture of the unknown species, the appearance of a pink color after addition of sodium carbonate indicates a positive reaction.

II. Specimen

Mature colony of the unknown *Mycobacterium* species recovered from clinical material, grown on an LJ slant or on Middlebrook 7H-10 agar. Prepare a suspension of the organism in sterile water and incubate for 3 days (14 days)

III. Materials

A. Equipment
   1. Biologic safety cabinet

B. Media
   1. Arylsulfatase stock substrate
      a. Dissolve 2.6 g of phenolphthalein disulfate tripotassium salt in 50 mL of sterile deionized water.
      b. Sterilize by membrane filtration (0.22-μm–pore size filter)
      c. Store in the refrigerator at 2°–8°C
      d. Shelf life is indefinite if stored properly. Discard if solution becomes cloudy
   2. Arylsulfatase broth: 3-day test
      a. Aseptically add 2.5 mL of stock substrate to 200 mL of sterile Dubos Tween broth.
      b. Aseptically dispense 2.0 mL amounts into screw-cap test tubes (16 × 125 mm)
      c. Store at 2°–8°C. Discard if the solution becomes cloudy
   3. Arylsulfatase broth: 2-week test
      a. Aseptically add 7.5 mL of stock substrate to 200 mL of sterile Dubos Tween broth
      b. Aseptically dispense 2.0 mL amounts into screw-cap test tubes (16 × 125 mm)
      c. Store at 2°–8°C.

   Wayne's arylsulfatase agar is commercially available from several sources.

C. Reagents
   1. 2 N sodium carbonate (Na_2CO_3): Dissolve 10.6 g of anhydrous sodium carbonate in 100 mL of distilled water.

IV. Quality Control

A. Three-Day Test
   1. Positive Control: *Mycobacterium fortuitum* ATCC 6841 (if positive control is negative, repeat tests with a fresh subculture of the positive organism. If the negative controls are positive, repeat the tests with a new lot of media)
   2. Negative Control: *Mycobacterium intracellulare* ATCC 13950
   3. Uninoculated medium and reagent only: No color

B. Fourteen-Day Test
   1. Positive control: *Mycobacterium fortuitum* ATCC 23292
   2. Negative control: *Mycobacterium intracellulare* ATCC 13950
   3. Uninoculated medium and reagent only: No color

V. Procedure
   1. Inoculate each tube of substrate with a lightly turbid suspension of the test organism in sterile water. Thoroughly emulsify the culture in the broth.

2. Incubate tube for 3 days or 14 days (2-week test) at 35°C in the non-CO_2 incubator
3. Following incubation, add 1 mL of the 2 N sodium carbonate reagent, mix and observe for color change.

VI. Results

A. Interpretation (Readout or Calculations)

Visually observe for a color change from pale pink to deep red. The lack of color change indicates a negative reaction.

VII. Procedure Notes

Include an actively growing control organism with each batch of test. For slow growers, use a 3- to 5-week subculture; for rapid growers, a 1- to 3-week subculture. If the positive control is negative, repeat the tests with a fresh subculture of the positive organism. If the negative controls are positive, repeat the tests with a new lot of media.

VIII. Limitation of Procedure

A. False-negative results can be due to control cultures that are too old.

B. False-positive results may occur if medium contains free phenolphthalein.

IX. Bibliography

Kubica GP, Ridgon AL: The arylsulfatase activity of mycobacteria. III. Preliminary investigation of rapidly growing mycobacteria. Am Rev Respir Dis 83:737–740, 1961

Kubica GP, Vestal AL: The aryl sulfatase activity of acid-fast bacilli: I. Investigation of stock cultures of mycobacteria. Am Rev Respir Dis 83: 728–732, 1961

Lutz B: Arylsulfatase test. In Isenberg HD: Mycobacteriology Section, Clinical Microbiology Procedure Handbook. Washington DC, American Society for Microbiology, 1992

Wayne LG: Recognition of *Mycobacterium fortuitum* by means of a three-day phenolphthalein sulfatase test. Am J Clin Pathol 36:185–187, 1961

CHART 2   ASSESSMENT OF PHOTOREACTIVITY OF MYCOBACTERIA

I. Principle

The appearance of yellow pigment in the colonies of photochromogenic mycobacteria is the result of yellowish-orange carotene crystals that are produced by actively metabolizing microorganisms after exposure to bright light. Scotochromogenic species have the capability of producing yellow pigment without exposure to light; however, the type of pigment is unknown. The pigmentation of young colonies of mycobacteria after growth in the dark or following exposure to light can be an important aid in the identification of certain *Mycobacterium* species.

II. Specimen

A primary broth culture of the test organism, diluted sufficiently to produce isolated colonies when inoculated to agar culture.

III. Materials

A. Equipment
   1. Biologic safety cabinet
   2. 37°C incubator

B. Supplies
   1. Sterile screw-cap test tubes, 20 × 110 or 20 × 125 mm
   2. Sterile Pasteur pipettes
   3. Inoculating wires and loops

C. Medium
   1. Three slants of Lowenstein-Jensen medium
   2. Three Middlebrook 7H10 agar plates

IV. Standards and Controls (include controls with each batch of tests)

  A. Positive photochromogen: *M. kansasii* ATCC 12478

  B. Positive scotochromogen: Stock strains of *M. scrofulaceum* or *M. gordonae*

  C. Negative chromogen: *M. tuberculosis* ATCC 25177

V. Procedure

   1. Inoculate the surfaces of three Lowenstein-Jensen slant media or three Middlebrook 7H11 agar plates with fluid from a dilute broth culture of the organism to be tested. Wrap two of the tubes or plates with aluminum foil; leave the third exposed to the ambient light in the incubator.

   2. Incubate one of the wrapped tubes or plates at 25°–30°C; the other wrapped tubes or plates at 37°C.

   3. Several days after growth is noted in the light-exposed control tube or plate, examine the wrapped tubes or plates for growth.

   4. If early growth is detected in the wrapped tubes or plates, expose one of each pair to a strong light for approximately 5 hours. A 100-W tungsten bulb or fluorescent equivalent is adequate. Loosen the cap of the culture tube during this period of light exposure.

   5. Following exposure to light, the tube or plate is returned to the incubator and inspected after 24 to 48 hours for the appearance of yellow pigment.

VI. Results

  A. Interpretation

   Mycobacteria that are scotochromogenic produce an equal amount of pigment whether light exposed or left in the dark. *M. scrofulaceum, M. gordonae, M. flavescens, M. xenopi,* and *M. szulgai* (the latter is scotochromogenic only when incubated at 37°C) compose the scotochromogenic group.

   Mycobacteria that are photochromogenic produce yellow pigment only after exposure to light. The more commonly encountered photochromogens include *M. kansasii, M. marinum, M. simiae,* and *M. asiaticum.*

   Nonchromogenic mycobacteria are incapable of producing pigment either in the dark or after exposure to light. *M. tuberculosis, M. bovis, M. ulcerans, M. fortuitum, M. chelonae,* and classic strains of *M. avium* are the more commonly encountered nonchromogens.

VII. Procedure Notes

  When *M. szulgai* is suspected, the light-exposed tubes or plates should be incubated at 25°C for 3–5 days. If incubated at 37°C, the photochromogenic potential will be masked by the development of the scotochromogenic pigment at that temperature.

VIII. Limitation of Procedure

  Currently, a high proportion of strains of *M. avium–intracellulare* recovered from patients with AIDS show pigment production. Thus, certain strains previously classified as nonchromogens may indeed be chromogenic. This departure, along with the temperature-dependent chromogenicity of *M. szulgai,* are reasons currently brought forth against the validity of the classic Runyoun classification of the mycobacteria.

IX. Bibliography

Wayne LG, Doubek SR: The role of air in the photochromogenic behavior of *M. kansasii.* Am J Clin Pathol 42:431–435, 1964

CHART 3   BACITRACIN AND SXT SUSCEPTIBILITY TESTS

I. Principle

Susceptibility to low concentrations of the polypeptide antibiotic bacitracin and to the combination sulfonamide trimethoprim–sulfamethoxazole (SXT) provides an easy and inexpensive method for the presumptive identification of both group A and group B β-hemolytic streptococci. Although still used in many laboratories, this test has largely been supplanted by reliable and relatively inexpensive serologic procedures.

Group A streptococci are susceptible to relatively low concentrations of bacitracin and are resistant to SXT. Group B streptococci are resistant to both antibiotics. Other β-hemolytic streptococci show varying susceptibility to bacitracin, but these organisms are usually susceptible to SXT. Therefore, the performance of the SXT test along with the bacitracin test increases the sensitivity and predictive value of the bacitracin test.

II. Reagents

A. Sheep blood agar plate

B. Taxo "A" bacitracin differential disks (0.04 units/disk)

C. SXT disks (trimethoprim–sulfamethoxazole, 1.25 µg/23.75 µg)

III. Quality Control

A. Bacitracin S, SXT R: Group A streptococcus

B. Bacitracin R, SXT R: Group B streptococcus

C. Bacitracin S or R, SXT S: β-Hemolytic streptococcus, groups C, F, or G

IV. Procedure

1. Pick three to four isolated colonies of the β-hemolytic streptococcus and streak the inoculum down the center of half of a blood agar plate.
2. Using a sterile swab or a bacteriologic loop spread the inoculum as a lawn over the entire half of the plate.
3. Aseptically place a Taxo "A" bacitracin disk and an SXT disk on the inoculated area. Make sure that the disks are spaced evenly. Using flamed forceps, gently tamp down the disks so that they adhere to the agar surface.
4. Incubate the plate in ambient air at 35°C.

V. Results

A. Interpretation
1. Susceptible (S): Any zone around either of the disks
2. Resistant (R): Growth up to the edge of the disk

Bacitracin	SXT	Identification
S	R	Presumptive Group A
R	R	Presumptive Group B
S/R	S	Not groups A or B

3. Results should be reported as "β-hemolytic streptococci, presumptive group A, by bacitracin/SXT", or "β-hemolytic streptococci, presumptively not group A by bacitracin/SXT".
4. Because these tests are generally performed on throat isolates, for which group A streptococci are being sought, the presumptive group B is generally not reported.

VI. Limitations of Test

Only β-hemolytic streptococci should be tested, because many α-hemolytic streptococci (including pneumococci) are susceptible to low concentrations of bacitracin.

No data are available to indicate that zones of inhibition should be measured. Interpretation of SXT susceptibility may be difficult, because the organisms may grow slightly before total inhibition of growth occurs.

The lawn of bacterial inoculum should be confluent. Too light of an inoculum will cause non–group A streptococci to appear susceptible to bacitracin.

CHART 4   BILE–ESCULIN TEST

I. Principle

The bile–esculin test is based on the ability of certain bacteria, notably the group D streptococci and *Enterococcus* species, to hydrolyze esculin in the presence of bile (4% bile salts or 40% bile). Esculin is a glycosidic coumarin derivative (6-β-glucoside-7-hydroxycoumarin). The two moieties of the molecule (glucose and 7-hydroxycoumarin) are linked together by an ester bond through oxygen. For this test, esculin is incorporated into a medium containing 4% bile salts.

Bacteria that are bile–esculin-positive are, first of all, able to grow in the presence of bile salts. Hydrolysis of the esculin in the medium results in the formation of glucose and a compound called esculetin. Esculetin, in turn, reacts with ferric ions (supplied by the inorganic medium component ferric citrate) to form a black diffusable complex.

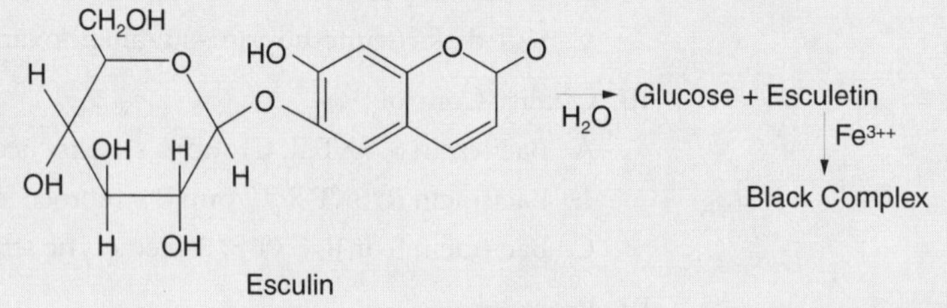

Esculin

II. Materials

A. Medium

Bile–esculin agar medium is prepared as agar slants or plates. The medium has the following formula:

Peptone	5 g
Beef extract	3 g
Oxgall (bile)	40 g
Esculin	1 g
Ferric citrate	0.5 g
Agar	15 g
Distilled water	1 L
pH = 7.0	

III. Quality Controls

A. Positive control: *Enterococcus* species (e.g., *E. faecalis*)

B. Negative control: Viridans streptococcus, not group D

IV. Procedure

1. With an inoculating wire or loop, touch two or three morphologically similar streptococcal colonies and inoculate the slant of the bile esculin medium with an S-shaped motion, or streak the surface of a bile esculin plate for isolation.

2. Incubate the tube or plate at 35°C for 24–48 hours in an ambient air incubator.

V. Results

A. Interpretation

Diffuse blackening of more than half of the slant within 24–48 hours indicates esculin hydrolysis. On plates, black haloes will be observed around isolated colonies and any blackening is considered positive. All group D streptococci will be bile–esculin-positive within 48 hours.

VI. Limitations of Test

Some viridans streptococci (approx. 3%) may also hydrolyze esculin in the presence of bile.

CHART 5 BILE SOLUBILITY TEST

I. Principle

Bile salts, specifically sodium deoxycholate and sodium taurocholate, have the capability to selectively lyse *Streptococcus pneumoniae* when added to actively growing bacteria in agar or broth media. *S. pneumoniae* produces autolytic enzymes (autolysins) that account for the central depression or umbilication characteristic of older pneumococcal colonies on agar media. The addition of bile salts activates the autolysins and accelerates the natural lytic reaction observed with cultures or pneumococci.

The bile solubility test can be performed either with a broth culture of the organism or with colonies growing on agar media. The turbidity of a broth suspension visibly clears on addition of bile salts if the organism is soluble. On agar medium, bile-soluble colonies "disappear" when drops of the reagent are placed on them. Because sodium deoxycholate may precipitate at a pH of 6.5 or less, the broth culture medium used must be adjusted to pH of 7.0 to prevent false-negative reactions.

II. Media and Reagents
   1. A pure culture of the test organism grown at 35°C for 18 to 24 hours in Todd-Hewitt broth (or equivalent)
   2. Sheep blood agar plate
   3. Sodium deoxycholate (10% for tube test, 2% for plate test)
   4. Phenol red solution (1% aqueous)
   5. Sodium hydroxide (NaOH) solution, 0.10 N

III. Quality Control

   A. Positive (bile-soluble) control: *Streptococcus pneumoniae*
   B. Negative (bile-insoluble) control: Viridans streptococci

IV. Procedure

   A. *Broth Test*
   1. Transfer approximately 0.5 mL of an 18- to 24-hour broth culture to two clean test tubes. Alternatively, a suspension of the organism may be prepared from growth on agar media in phosphate-buffered saline, pH 7.0. If the latter is done, the pH need not be readjusted.
   2. Add 1 drop of the phenol red indicator to each tube.
   3. Add 0.10 N NaOH to adjust the pH to 7.0 (indicator a light pink color)
   4. Add 0.5 mL of 10% sodium deoxycholate to one of the tubes (labeled "test")
   5. Add 0.5 mL sterile normal saline to the other tube (labeled "control")
   6. Gently agitate both test tubes and place them in an incubator or a water bath at 35°C for 3 hours, checking hourly.

   B. *Plate Test*
   1. To a few well-isolated colonies on the test organism growing on sheep blood agar, place a drop of 2% sodium deoxycholate.
   2. Without inverting the plate, place it in a 35°C incubator for 30 minutes.

V. Results

   A. Interpretation
   1. *Broth Test*
      Bile-soluble (positive reaction): there is visible clearing of the suspension in the tube containing the sodium deoxycholate, with no change in the saline control suspension.
      Bile-insoluble (negative reaction): there is no change in the turbidity of the sodium deoxycholate-containing tube relative to the control saline suspension.

2. *Plate Test*

Bile-soluble (positive reaction): colonies on which the reagent was placed disappear, leaving a partially hemolyzed area where the colony had been.

Bile-insoluble (negative reaction): colonies where the reagent was placed remain intact and visible.

VI. Limitations of Test

Only 86% of pneumococcal strains will lyse completely and additional testing (e.g., quelling tests) may be required for the remaining, incompletely lysed strains.

CHART 6   CALIBRATION OF THE OCULAR MICROMETER

I. Principle

Ability to measure accurately the size of trophozoites, eggs, or other parasitic forms is often necessary in making a species identification. This measurement can be made with a calibrated scale called a micrometer. The ocular micrometer, a small, round glass disk etched with a fixed scale, is inexpensive and easy to use, and is recommended for routine laboratory use.

Ocular micrometers are etched with a fixed scale, usually consisting of 50 parallel lines. Depending on the magnifying power of the set of objectives used in a compound microscope, each division in the ocular micrometer represents different measurements. Therefore, for each set of oculars and objectives used, the ocular scale must be calibrated using a stage micrometer etched with a scale (0.1-mm and 0.01-mm divisions are commonly used). It is important to remember that a calibration for a given set of oculars and objectives cannot be interchanged with corresponding components from another microscope.

II. Materials

1. Ocular micrometer with fixed scale (American Optical Co., Buffalo NY)
2. Stage micrometer scaled with 0.1-mm and 0.01-mm divisions (American Optical Co.)
3. Standard compound microscope

III. Procedure

1. Remove the ocular from the microscope to be used. If a binocular microscope is used, it is customary to remove the right × 10 ocular.
2. Unscrew the eye lens (top lens) of the ocular and insert the micrometer wafer so that it rests on the diaphragm ring inside the ocular. Place the micrometer with the engraved side down. The micrometer should be handled with lens paper and every effort made to prevent lint from adhering to the surface.
3. Replace the ocular in the housing. When viewed through the ocular, the micrometer scale appears as a series of lined divisions, illustrated in *A*.
4. Place the stage micrometer under the objective of the microscope that is to be calibrated. Bring into view the stage micrometer scale, which appears as a series of lines divided into 0.1-mm and 0.01-mm divisions, as shown in the simulated view through the microscope in *B*.
5. Adjust the stage micrometer so that the 0 line on the ocular micrometer is exactly superimposed with the 0.0 line on the stage micrometer scale. When viewed under high magnification (×450), the superimposition of the two scales appears as in the simulated view through the microscope shown in *C*.
6. Without further manipulation, look across the two scales and find the next pair of lines that exactly coincide. In *D* (a simulated high-power × 450 view), the coinciding lines are the 40 mark on the ocular scale and 0.09-mm mark on the stage micrometer scale (*arrow*).

IV. Calculation

The object of the calibration is to determine the width in micrometers of each ocular scale division, when calibrated against the stage micrometer scale. Thus, as illustrated in

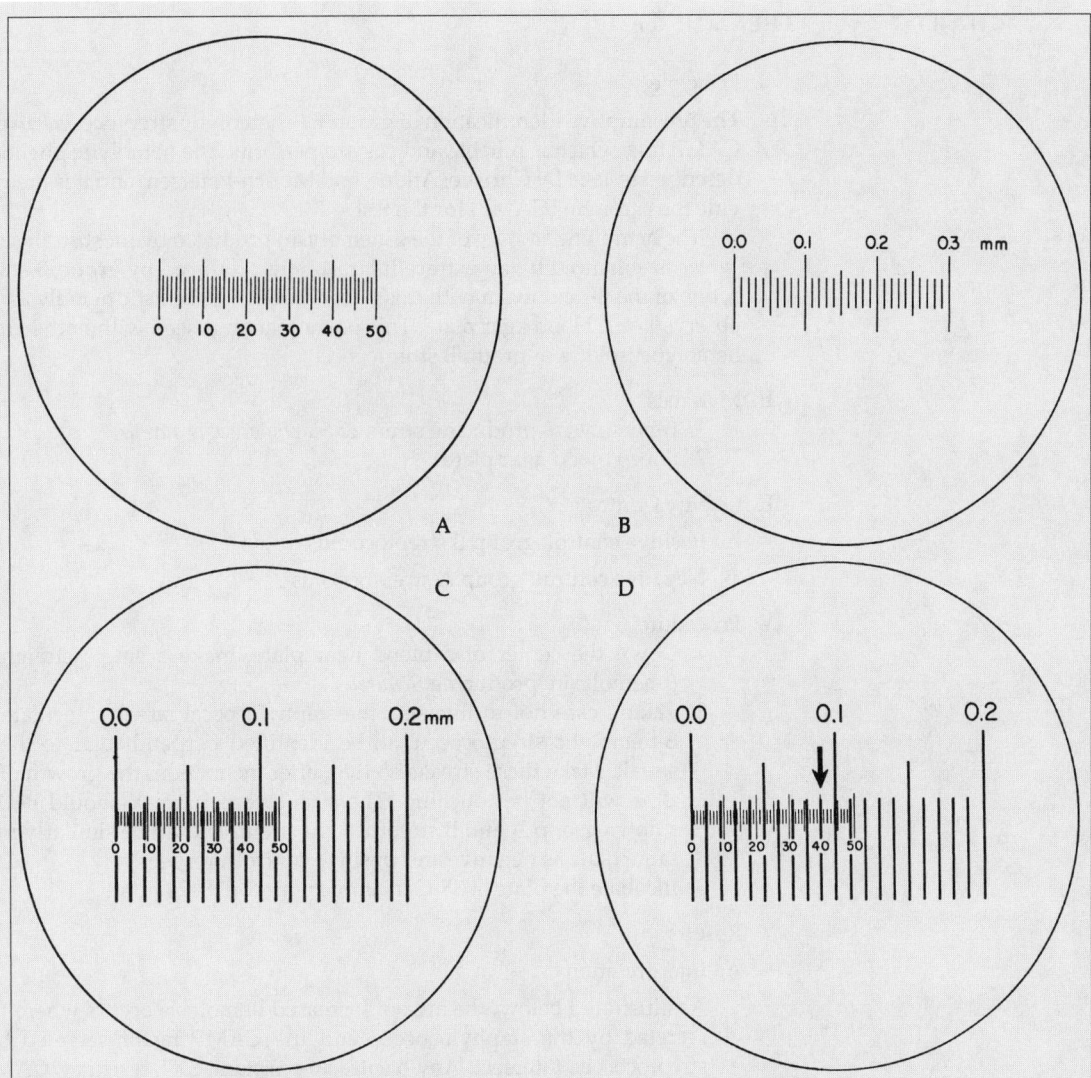

the drawing, 40 units on the ocular scale are equal to 0.09 mm on the stage micrometer scale.

Therefore, each ocular division is equal to 0.09 mm/40, or 0.00225 mm. Because there are 1000 μm in each millimeter, each ocular micrometer division in the calibration illustrated here is equal to 0.00225 × 1000, or 2.25 μm.

Thus, if an object that is viewed under the microscope occupies 10 ocular scale divisions, it would measure 2.25 × 10, or 22.5 μm.

This same calculation can be used for the calibration of any set of oculars and objectives, substituting the appropriate numbers.

V. Bibliography

Garcia GS, Ash LR: Diagnostic Parasitology: Clinical Laboratory Manual, pp 42, 43. St Louis, CV Mosby, 1975

Koneman EW, Richie LE, Tiemann C: Practical Laboratory Parasitology, pp 12–14. New York, Medcom Press, 1974

CHART 7   THE CAMP TEST

I. Principle

The presumptive identification of group B β-hemolytic streptococci can be done with the CAMP test, which is reliable and easy to perform. The hemolytic phenomenon was first described in 1944 by Christie, Atkins, and Munch-Petersen, and it is their names that provide the acronym (CAMP) for the test.

The hemolytic activity of the β-hemolysin produced by most strains of *Staphylococcus aureus* is enhanced by an extracellular protein produced by group B streptococci. Interaction of the β-hemolysin with this factor causes "synergistic hemolysis," which is easily observed on a blood agar plate. This phenomenon is seen with both hemolytic and non-hemolytic isolates of group B streptococci.

II. Materials

    1. β-hemolysin–producing strain of *Staphylococcus aureus*
    2. Sheep blood agar plate

III. Quality Control

  A. Positive control: group B streptococcus

  B. Negative control: group A streptococcus

IV. Procedure

    1. Down the center of a blood agar plate, make a single straight line streak of β-hemolysin–producing *S. aureus.*
    2. Taking care not to intersect the staphylococcal streak, inoculate a streak of the β-hemolytic streptococcus to be identified perpendicular to the staphylococcal streak. Make these streaks so that, after incubation, the growth of the two organisms will not be touching. The streptococcal streak should be 3 to 4 cm long. Known group A and B streptococcal strains should be similarly inoculated on the same plate as negative and positive controls, respectively.
    3. Incubate the plate at 35°C in ambient air for 18–24 hours.

V. Results

  A. Interpretation

As illustrated below, the area of increased hemolysis occurs where the β-hemolysin secreted by the staphylococcus and the CAMP factor secreted by the group B streptococcus intersect. Any bacitracin-resistant, SXT-resistant, CAMP test-positive, β-hemolytic streptococcus can be reported as "β-hemolytic streptococcus, presumptive group B by CAMP test."

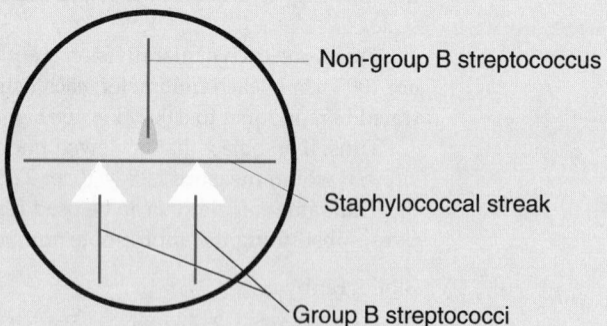

VI. Limitations

Some group A streptococci will be CAMP test-positive if the test plate is incubated in a candle jar, in a CO_2 atmosphere, or under anaerobic conditions. Therefore, ambient air incubation should be used.

CHART 8   CARBOHYDRATE ASSIMILATION TEST FOR YEAST IDENTIFICATION

I. Principle

The assessment of the ability of yeasts to utilize carbohydrates is based on the use of carbohydrate-free yeast nitrogen-base agar and observing for the presence of growth around
carbohydrate-impregnated filter paper disks after an appropriate period of incubation.

II. Specimen

Isolated colonies on an appropriate recovery culture medium of the yeast to be identified.

III. Materials
   A. Supplies
      1. Inoculation wires or loops
      2. Sterile transfer pipettes
      3. Sterile plastic, 100 mL petri dishes
      4. 10-mm–diameter blank filter paper disks
      5. Millipore or Nucleopore filter
   C. Reagents
      1. Yeast nitrogen-base agar
         a. Prepare a 2% agar solution (20 g of agar per liter of distilled water). Autoclave
            for 15 minutes at 121°C at 15 psi.
         b. Dissolve 6.7 g of yeast nitrogen-base in 100 mL distilled water. Adjust pH to 6.2
            to 6.4 by adding 1 N NaOH.
         c. Sterilize by filtration.
         d. Add 88 mL of yeast nitrogen base and 100 mL of the filter-sterilized bromcresol
            purple indicator, as prepared for the carbohydrate fermentation test, to 1 L of
            the 2% agar solution. Pour into sterile, plastic petri dishes, approximately
            20 mL/plate.
      2. Carbohydrate-impregnated filter paper disks
         These are commercially available. They can be prepared in-house by soaking filter
         paper disks, 10 mm in diameter, in 1% solutions of the carbohydrates to be tested
         and allowed to dry before use.

IV. Quality Control

Each newly prepared batch of yeast nitrogen base agar and new carbohydrate disks must
be tested with positive- and negative-reacting yeasts for each carbohydrate to be tested.

V. Procedure
   1. With a sterile transfer pipette, flood the surface of a yeast nitrogen-base plate with
      a suspension of yeast in saline equivalent to a McFarland standard 4.
   2. Aspirate the excess suspension using the same pipette. Let the surface of the agar
      dry for about 5 minutes.
   3. Place carbohydrate disks on the agar and press down firmly with the tip of a
      flamed forceps.
   4. Incubate plate at 30°C for 24 hours and record results.

VI. Results

A positive test is the observation of visible growth around a carbohydrate disk, which indicates that the sugar contained has been assimilated by the yeast species under study.

VII. Procedure Notes
   1. The carbohydrate disks should be placed sufficiently far apart so that the zone of
      diffusion from one carbohydrate disk does not overrun the diffusion zone of an-
      other. Placing one disk in each outer quadrant of the plate and one in the center is
      recommended.
   2. If growth on the plate is not sufficiently concentrated to enable a reading, reincu-
      bate for 24 hours and read again.
   3. The test is best read by removing the top of the petri dish and tilting the bottom of
      the plate while viewing against bright indirect light.
   4. Read only for the presence or absence of growth; the size of the zone or the density
      of growth around a disk is unimportant.

VIII. Bibliography

Warren NG, Shadomy HJ: Yeasts of Medical Importance. In Balows A (ed): Manual of Clinical Microbiology, 5th ed, Chap 80. Washington DC, American Society for Microbiology, 1991

CHART 9   CARBOL FUCHSIN STAINS

I. Principle

The carbolic acids within the lipid-rich, waxy cell wall of mycobacteria have the unique capability of binding fuchsin dye so that it is not destained by acid alcohol. The Ziehl–Neelsen stain is known as the "hot stain" as heat is used for the dye to penetrate through the cell wall. The Kinyoun stain is known as a "cold stain" because the high concentration of phenol in the reagent serves to "dissolve" the lipid material in the cell wall, allowing penetration of the carbol fuchsin dye without the use of heat. Once stained, the cell wall holds the die "fast," giving the characteristic red color.

II. Specimen

A smear is prepared either directly from the specimen or from a suspension of organisms obtained from colonies grown on primarily culture media.

III. Materials

A. Equipment: 3″ × 1″ glass slides and reagents

B. Media: Not applicable

C. Reagents
1. Carbolfuchsin (commercially available)
2. Acid–alcohol (commercially available)
3. Methylene blue counterstain (commercially available)

IV. Quality Control

A. Unstained positive control smears (*M. tuberculosis*) and negative control smears (*Nocardia asteroides*) have been prepared.

B. Control smears are reviewed before the patient smears are read to confirm that the mycobacteria stain acid-fast:
1. Positive: *Mycobacterium* spp.: magenta red against blue background
2. *N. asteroides:* no acid-fast cells; background blue

C. If control slide is unacceptable, review procedures and reagent preparation. Unacceptable control slides include the following:
1. Bacilli in positive control do not fluoresce or do not stain red
2. Negative control remains red after destaining or fluoresces
3. Background is not properly decolorized or gives nonspecific fluorescence

V. Procedure

A. Ziehl–Neelsen
1. Place a 2 × 3-cm filter paper strip on the slide to help hold the stain on the slide and filter undissolved crystals.
2. Flood the paper strip with Ziehl–Neelsen carbolfuchsin.
3. Using a Bunsen burner or electric staining rack, heat the slide slowly until steaming, but short of boiling.
4. Stain for 5 minutes. If the stain dries, add more stain without heating.
5. Carefully remove the paper slip from the slide using forceps.
6. Rinse the slide thoroughly with water.
7. Flood the smear with 3% acid–alcohol decolorizer for 2 minutes.
8. Rinse with water and drain excess water.
9. Flood the slide with methylene blue counterstain for 1 minute. Do not blot.
10. Examine the smear with a × 100 oil immersion objective.

B. Kinyoun
1. Heat fix smears on slide warmer at 72°–75°C.

2. Cover the smear with the Kinyoun's carbolfuchsin reagent. A small 2″ × 3″ rectangular piece of filter paper can be placed over the smear and the stain applied to the filter paper to avoid spilling over the sides of the smear. Do not steam.
3. Stain for 5 minutes.
4. Remove the filter paper with forceps, rinse the stain off the slide with distilled water.
5. Decolorize for 3 minutes with acid–alcohol or until no red stain appears.
6. Flood smear for 3–4 minutes with methylene blue counterstain.
7. Rinse dry and examine under a × 100 oil immersion objective.

VI. Results

Examine smears with a × 100 oil immersion objective and report as follows:

Smear Observation	Report
1 or 2 per 300 fields (3 sweeps)	Doubtful, repeat
1–9 per 100 fields	Rare, 1+
1–9 per 10 fields	Few, 2+
1–9 per immersion field	Numerous, 3+
9 per field	4+

VII. Procedure Notes
1. Avoid under decolorization with acid-alcohol. Organisms that are truly acid-fast are difficult to overdecolorize.
2. Avoid making thick smears, which may interfere with proper decolorization.
3. If an inordinate number of smear-positive, culture-negative results are encountered, check water reservoirs for contaminating acid-fast organisms. Transfer of material from slide to slide and from immersion oil are other possible sources of false-positive smear results.
4. Strong counterstains may mask the presence of acid-fast bacilli. Brilliant green may have a slight advantage over methylene blue as a counterstain.

VIII. Limitation of Procedure
1. Acid-fast smears do not stand alone, and final interpretation must always be correlated with culture results.
2. Organisms other than mycobacteria may demonstrate various degrees of acid-fastness: *Rhodococcus* spp., *Nocardia* spp, *Legionella micdadei*, and the cysts of *Cryptosporidium* spp. Use differences in smear morphology and correlation with culture appearance and other biochemical tests.
3. Rapidly growing mycobacteria may stain poorly or not at all. The Ziehl–Neelsen stain may provide better staining than the Kinyoun method for weak acid–fast organisms.

IX. Bibliography

Berlin OGW. Mycobacteria. In Baron EJ, Finegold SM (eds). Bailey and Scott's Diagnostic Microbiology, 8th ed, pp 597–640. St. Louis, CV Mosby, 1990

Ebersole LL: Acid-fast stain procedures, in Isenberg HD. Mycobacteriology Section, Clinical Microbiology Procedure Handbook, Washington DC. American Society for Microbiology, 1992

Kent PT, Kubica GP. Public Health Mycobacteriology: A Guide for the Level III Laboratory. US Department of Health and Human Services Publication (CDC) 86-21654, 1985

CHART 10   CATALASE

I. Principle

Catalase is an enzyme that decomposes hydrogen peroxide (H_2O_2) into water and oxygen. Chemically, catalase is a hemoprotein, similar in structure to hemoglobin, except that the four iron atoms in the molecule are in the oxidized (Fe^{3+}), rather than the reduced (Fe^{2+}), state. Excluding the streptococci, most aerobic and facultative bacteria possess catalase activity.

Hydrogen peroxide forms as one of the oxidative end products of aerobic carbohydrate metabolism. If allowed to accumulate, it is lethal to bacterial cells. Catalase converts hydrogen peroxide into oxygen and water as shown by the following reaction:

$$2H_2O_2 \rightarrow 2H_2O + O_2 \text{ (gas bubbles)}$$

The catalase test is most commonly used to differentiate members of the *Micrococcaceae* from members of the *Streptococcaceae*.

II. Reagents

The hydrogen peroxide reagant must be tested with positive and negative control organisms each day or immediately before unknown bacteria are tested.

A. Hydrogen peroxide 3% stored in a brown bottle under refrigeration.

B. An 18- to 24-hour culture of the organism to be tested

III. Quality Control

The hydrogen peroxide reagent must be tested with positive and negative control organisms each day or immediately before unknown bacteria are tested.

A. Positive control: *Staphylococcus aureus*

B. Negative control: *Streptococcus* species

IV. Procedure
  1. With an inoculating needle or a wooden applicator stick, transfer growth from the center of a colony to the surface of a glass slide.
  2. Add 1 drop of 3% hydrogen peroxide and observe for bubble formation.

V. Results

A. Interpretation

The rapid and sustained appearance of bubbles or effervescence constitutes a positive test. Because some bacteria possess enzymes other than catalase that can decompose hydrogen peroxide, a few tiny bubbles forming after 20 to 30 seconds is not considered a positive test. In addition, catalase is present in red blood cells, so care must be taken to avoid carryover of red blood cells with the colony material.

CHART 11   **CATALASE 68°C**

I. Principle

Catalase splits hydrogen peroxide into water and oxygen. The evolution of oxygen appears as bubbles. Some forms of catalase are inactivated by heating at 68°C for 20 minutes, a valuable identifying feature for certain *Mycobacterium* species. The hydrogen peroxide used for the identification of *Mycobacterium* species differs from that used to detect catalase in other types of bacteria, by using a 30% concentration (Superoxal) in a strong detergent solution (10% Tween-80). The detergent helps disperse the hydrophobic tightly clumped mycobacteria from large aggregates to individual bacilli, maximizing the detection of catalase.

II. Specimen

Mature colony of the unknown *Mycobacterium* species recovered from clinical material, grown on an LJ slant or on Middlebrook 7H-10 agar.

III. Materials

A. Equipment
  1. 68°C water bath or heat block

B. Media
  1. Middlebrook 7H9 broth
  2. Lowenstein-Jensen deeps in 25- × 150-mm screw-cap test tubes

C. Reagents
  1. 30% hydrogen peroxide (commercially available as Superoxol)
  2. 10% Tween-80
  3. M/15 phosphate buffer (0.067 M)

IV. Quality Control

 A. Negative control: *M. tuberculosis* ATCC 15177, bubbles at 22–25°C, but not at 68°C.

 B. Positive control: *M. fortuitum* ATCC 6841, bubbles at 22–25°C and at 68°C.

 C. Controls are included with each batch of tests.

V. Procedure

 A. Heat-stable catalase test
  1. Set up one screw-cap tube per organism specimen to be tested in sterile water.
  2. Label each tube with the number of the specimen.
  3. Add 0.5 mL of sterile 0.067 M phosphate buffer to each tube.
  4. Inoculate the buffer with a spadeful of growth from an actively growing subculture of the organism to be tested (2–4 weeks old).
  5. Thoroughly emulsify the culture in the buffer.
  6. Incubate the tubes in a 68°C water bath for exactly 20 min.
  7. Remove the tubes from the water bath. Cool to room temperature.
  8. Add 0.5 mL of freshly prepared Tween-80–hydrogen peroxide reagent.
  9. Allow the tubes to sit at room temperature for 20 minutes. Do not shake the tubes.
  10. Visually observe for the evolution of bubbles.

 B. Semiquantitative catalase test
  1. Inoculate a liquid medium, such as Dubos Tween broth or Middlebrook 7H9 broth with a spadeful or loopful of the culture to be tested. Include controls.
  2. Incubate for 7 days at 37°C.
  3. Mix for 5–10 seconds on a vortex mixer.
  4. Transfer 6 drops to a Lowenstein-Jensen deep (prepared in 25- × 150-mm tubes).
  5. Incubate the deeps for 14 days at 37°C. Be sure caps are loose.
  6. Add 1 mL of freshly prepared Tween-80–hydrogen peroxide reagent. Avoid contact of reagent with skin.
  7. Allow tests to sit at room temperature for 5 minutes.
  8. Measure the column of bubbles.

VI. Results

 A. Interpretation (Readout or Calculations)
  1. Heat-stable catalase test: The appearance of bubbles indicates a positive test; lack of bubbles is a negative reaction. *M. tuberculosis* and other mycobacteria lose their catalase activity when heated to 68°C.
  2. Semiquantitative catalase test:

   High catalase reaction: >45 mm of foam
   Low catalase reaction: <45 mm of foam

VII. Procedure Notes

 Failure of control cultures to give expected results is usually due to the use of cultures that are too old—use only actively growing cultures.

VIII. Limitation of Procedure

 False-negative results can be due to use of cultures with inadequate growth, the use of cultures that are too old, or reagents that are outdated. Inadequate growth may result from an inadequate inoculum or from screwing screw-cap lids too tightly.

 False-positive results may occur if the culture contains catalase-positive, contaminating bacterial species.

IX. Bibliography

Kubica GP, et al: Differential identification of mycobacteria: I. Tests on catalase activity. Am Rev Respir Dis 95:400–405, 1966

Lutz B: Catalase tests. In Isenberg HD (ed). Clinical Microbiology Procedure Handbook, Mycobacteriology Section. Washington DC, American Society for Microbiology, 1992

CHART 12   CITRATE UTILIZATION

I. Principle

Sodium citrate is a salt of citric acid, a simple organic compound found as one of the metabolites in the tricarboxylic acid cycle (Krebs cycle). Some bacteria can obtain energy in a manner other than by the fermentation of carbohydrates by using citrate as the sole source of carbon. The measurement of this characteristic is important in the identification of many members of the *Enterobacteriaceae*. Any medium used to detect citrate utilization by test bacteria must be devoid of protein and carbohydrates as sources of carbon.

The utilization of citrate by a test bacterium is detected in citrate medium by the production of alkaline by-products. The medium includes sodium citrate, an anion, as the sole source of carbon, and ammonium phosphate as the sole source of nitrogen. Bacteria that can use citrate can also extract nitrogen from the ammonium salt, with the production of ammonia (NH^+), leading to alkalinization of the medium from conversion of the NH_3^{2+} to ammonium hydroxide (NH_4OH). Bromthymol blue—yellow below pH 6.0 and blue above pH 7.6—is the indicator.

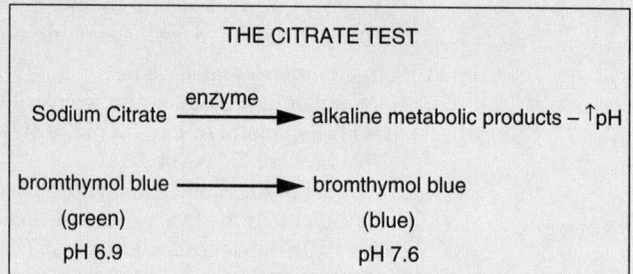

THE CITRATE TEST

Sodium Citrate —enzyme→ alkaline metabolic products – ↑pH

bromthymol blue ———→ bromthymol blue
(green)   (blue)
pH 6.9   pH 7.6

II. Media and Reagents

The citrate medium most commonly used is the formula of Simmons. The medium is poured into a tube on a slant. The formula of Simmons citrate medium is shown below:

Ammonium dihydrogen phosphate	1 g
Dipotassium phosphate	1 g
Sodium chloride	5 g
Sodium citrate	2 g
Magnesium sulfate	0.20 g
Agar	15 g
Bromthymol blue	0.08 g
Distilled water to	1 L

Final pH = 6.9

III. Quality Control

Each new batch of medium should be tested with a positive- and a negative-reacting organism. The following species are suggested controls:

A. Positive control—*Enterobacter aerogenes*

B. Negative control—*Escherichia coli*

IV. Procedure

1. A well-isolated colony is picked from the surface of a primarily isolation medium and inoculated as a single streak on the slant surface of the citrate agar tube. The tube is incubated at 35°C for 24 to 48 hours.

V. Results

A. Interpretation

A positive test is represented by the development of a deep blue color within 24 to 48 hours, indicating that the test organism has been able to utilize the citrate contained in the medium, with the production of alkaline products (see Color Plate 4–4D). A positive test may also be read without a blue color if there is visible colonial growth along the inoculation streak line. This is possible because, for growth to be visible, the organism must enter the log phase of growth, possible only if carbon and nitrogen have been assimilated. A positive interpretation from reading the streak line can be confirmed by incubating the tube for an additional 24 hours, when a blue color usually develops.

VI. Bibliography

BBL Manual of Products and Laboratory Procedures, 5th ed, pp 115 and 138. Cockeysville MD, BioQuest, 1968

Blazevic DJ, Ederer GM: Principles of Biochemical Tests in Diagnostic Microbiology, pp 15–18. New York, John Wiley & Sons, 1975

Koser SA: Utilization of the salts of organic acids by the colon–aerogenes groups. J Bacteriol 8:493–520, 1923

MacFaddin JF: Biochemical Tests for Identification of Medical Bacteria, 2nd ed, pp 59–63. Baltimore, Williams & Wilkins, 1980

Simmons JS: A culture medium for differentiating organisms of typhoid–colon aerogenes groups and for isolation of certain fungi. J Infect Dis 39:209–214, 1926

CHART 13 COAGULASE TEST

I. Principle

Coagulase is a protein of unknown chemical composition having a prothrombinlike activity capable of converting fibrinogen into fibrin, which results in the formation of a visible clot in a suitable test system. Coagulase is believed to function in vivo by producing a fibrin barrier at the site of staphylococcal infection. This probably plays a role in localizing the abscesses (e.g., carbuncles and furuncles). In the laboratory, the coagulase test is used to identify *Staphylococcus aureus* and differentiate it from the other species of staphylococci.

Coagulase is present in two forms, bound and free, each having different properties that require the use of separate testing procedures.

Bound coagulase (slide test): Bound coagulase, also known as clumping factor, is attached to the bacterial cell wall and is not present in culture filtrates. Fibrin strands are formed between the bacterial cells when suspended in plasma (fibrinogen), causing them to clump into visible aggregates.

Free coagulase (tube test): Free coagulase is a thrombin-like substance present in culture filtrates. When a suspension of coagulase-producing organisms is prepared in plasma in a test tube, a visible clot forms as the result of coagulase reacting with a serum substance (coagulase-reacting factor) to form a complex which, in turn, reacts with fibrinogen to produce the fibrin clot.

II. Media and Reagents

Rabbit plasma with EDTA (commercially available in lyophilized form). Reconstituted plasma should be refrigerated.

III. Quality Control

Coagulability of plasma may be tested by adding one drop of 5% calcium chloride to 0.5 mL of the reconstituted plasma. A clot should form within 10 to 15 seconds. A known *Staphylococcus aureus* strain and a *Staphylococcus epidermidis* strain serve as positive and negative control strains, respectively. Each reconstituted vial of rabbit plasma with EDTA should be tested with 18- to 24-hour cultures of the control strains.

IV. Procedure
1. *Slide test* (bound coagulase): Place two drops of sterile water or saline in two circles drawn on a glass slide with a wax pencil. Gently emulsify colony material from the organism to be identified in liquid in each of the circles. Place a drop of coagulase plasma in the suspension in one of the circles and mix with a wooden applicator stick. Place another drop of water or saline in the other circle as a control. Rock the slide back and forth, observing for agglutination of the test suspension.
2. *Tube test* (free coagulase): Emulsify a small amount of the colony growth of the organism in a tube containing 0.5 mL of coagulase plasma. Incubate the tube at 35°C for 4 hours and observe for clot formation by gently tilting the tube. If no clot is observed at that time, reincubate the tube at room temperature and read again after 18 hours.

V. Results
    A. Interpretation
        1. *Slide test:* A positive reaction will be detected within 10 to 15 seconds of mixing the plasma with the suspension by the formation of a white precipitate and agglutination of the organisms in the suspension. The test is considered negative if no agglutination is observed after 2 minutes. The saline control should remain smooth and milky. If the control suspension agglutinates as well, the test is noninterpretable. All strains that are coagulase positive can be reported as *Staphylococcus aureus.* All strains producing negative slide tests must be tested with the tube coagulase test.
        2. *Tube test:* The tube coagulase test is considered positive if any degree of clotting is noted. The tube should be gently tilted and not agitated, since this may disrupt partially formed clotted material. Fibrinolysins produced by the organism may also dissolve the clot soon after formation. Tube tests that are negative after 4 hours should be incubated at room temperature overnight and read after 18 hours.

CHART 14	COMPLEMENT FIXATION (CF) TEST

I. Principle

The complement fixation test is one of the major traditional tests for demonstration of infectious antigens and antibodies. It requires a veritable zoo of reagents and numerous preparatory steps. There are almost as many versions as there have been users; the microtiter version developed at the Centers for Disease Control (LBCF test) includes rigorous controls and is commonly employed. The CF test does not depend on hemagglutinating activity of the virus, but the antibodies must fix complement, and the sera must be free of anticomplementary activity. The test has been superseded, in many instances, by newer tests, such as enzyme immunoassay (EIA).

The terminal components of the complement cascade, C789 (the attack complex), can damage cell membranes in the presence of specific antibody, which fixes complement to the cell surface. In the CF test, erythrocytes are used as the target cell, because complement-induced leakiness of the membrane can be visualized or measured colorimetrically as an increase in free hemoglobin. In the presence of specific antibodies to an infectious agent, any complement in the system is bound, leaving no residual complement for reaction with antibodies to the indicator erythrocytes. Thus, the presence of specific antibody is indicated by the absence of hemolysis.

II. Materials and Reagents

Sheep erythrocyte suspension
Hemolysin (rabbit anti-sheep red cell antibody)
Guinea pig complement, free of antibodies to the agent of interest
Barbital-buffered diluent
Plastic microtiter plate
Centrifuge adapter for microtiter plates
Water bath for incubation of plates
Color standards for judging hemolysis (prepared by lysing various concentrations of red cells)

III. Quality Control

Known positive antibody or antigen
Known negative antibody or antigen
Serum control without antigen (to detect anticomplementary activity)
Antigen controls without serum (to detect anticomplementary activity)
Tissue control (the cells or tissue in which the antigen was prepared)
Buffer control without antigen or antibody
Back titration of complement to document the use of 5 CH_{50} units
Cell control to demonstrate absence of hemolysis
Reference hemolysis standards

IV. Procedure

1. *Sensitization of Erythrocytes*

Serial dilutions of hemolysin are incubated with a 2.8% solution of sheep red cells in barbital buffer. As the concentration of hemolysin increases, the percentage hemolysis will increase to a plateau level. The concentration of hemolysin that represents the second point on the plateau is used for the test.

2. *Quantitation of Complement*

Varying amounts of a 1:400 dilution of cold, reconstituted guinea pig complement are incubated with sensitized cells. The volume of complement that produces 50% lysis of the red cells (CH_{50} unit) is calculated from the graphed results of the hemolysis. The complement stock may be aliquoted and frozen at $-70°C$, but adequate reactivity must be demonstrated before use in the test.

3. *The Complement Fixation Test*

A block titration of serial dilutions of both antigen and antibody is performed in the presence of 5 CH_{50} units of complement at 4°C for 18 hours. Serum is heated at 56°C for 30 minutes to inactivate any endogenous complement. The characteristics of either the antigen or antibody will be known; the serial dilutions of the known reagent may be abbreviated to include the dilution on each side of the expected optimum. Subsequently, sheep red cells that have been sensitized with the optimal dilution of hemolysin are incubated at 37°C for 30 minutes. Plates are centrifuged at low speed to sediment the unlysed erythrocytes.

V. Results

A. Interpretation

The highest dilution of antigen or antibody that provides 3+ to 4+ fixation of complement (<30% hemolysis) is the endpoint. All reagents must be free of anticomplementary activity, the correct quantity of complement must have been added, and the control specimens must react as expected.

VI. Bibliography

Hsiung GD: Diagnostic Virology, 3rd ed. New Haven, Yale University Press, 1982
Standardized diagnostic complement fixation method and adaptation to microtest. US Public Health Service Publ. 1228 (Public Health Monogr. 74), Atlanta, 1965

CHART 15   CYSTINE–TELLURITE BLOOD AGAR

I. Principle

Cystine–tellurite blood agar is a medium used for the primary isolation of *Corynebacterium diphtheriae*. It has advantages over Tinsdale medium in being easier to prepare and having a longer shelf life.

The potassium tellurite in this medium serves to inhibit growth of most normal bacterial inhabitants of the upper respiratory tract, including most species of *Streptococcus* and *Staphylococcus*. *C. diphtheria* grows well, producing grayish or black colonies after 24 to 48 hours of incubation.

II. Media and Reagents

A. *Formula*

Heart infusion agar, 2% solution	100 mL
Potassium tellurite, 0.3% solution	15 mL
L-Cystine	5 mg
Sheep blood	5 mL

B. *Preparation*

Melt the sterile heart infusion agar solution and cool to 45°C or 50°C. Carefully maintain this temperature while performing subsequent steps. Aseptically add the sterile potassium tellurite solution (previously sterilized by autoclaving) and the sheep blood. Mix thoroughly. Add the cystine powder, mix well, and pour the medium into sterile petri dishes. Rotate the flask frequently while pouring into plates because the cystine does not go entirely into solution.

III. Procedure

Streak the plate with the clinical material to be cultured to obtain well-isolated colonies.

IV. Results

A. Interpretation

C. diphtheriae develops gray or black colonies after 24 to 48 hours of incubation. On occasion, colonies of staphylococci not inhibited by the medium also appear black; however, these can be distinguished by their characteristic Gram stain reaction.

Three biotypes of *C. diphtheriae* can be distinguished on cystine–tellurite blood agar: 1) biotype *gravis* colonies are flat, dark gray with radial striations, and dry and have an irregular edge; 2) biotype *mitis* colonies are small, black, shiny, and convex with an entire edge and have a moist appearance; 3) biotype *intermedius* colonies are small and flat and have a raised, black center.

V. Bibliography

Frobisher M Jr: Cystine–tellurite agar for *C. diphtheriae*. J Infect Dis 60:99–105, 1937

CHART 16   CYTOCHROME OXIDASE

I. Principle

The cytochromes are iron-containing hemoproteins that act as the last link in the chain of aerobic respiration by transferring electrons (hydrogen) to oxygen, with the formation of water. The cytochrome system is found in aerobic, or microaerophilic, and facultatively anaerobic organisms, so the oxidase test is important in identifying organisms that either lack the enzyme or are obligate anaerobes. The test is most helpful in screening colonies suspected of being one of the *Enterobacteriaceae* (all negative) and in identifying colonies suspected of belonging to other genera such as *Aeromonas, Pseudomonas, Neisseria, Campylobacter*, and *Pasteurella* (positive).

The cytochrome oxidase test uses certain reagent dyes, such as *p*-phenylenediamine dihydrochloride, that substitute for oxygen as artificial electron acceptors. In the reduced state, the dye is colorless; however, in the presence of cytochrome oxidase and atmospheric oxygen, *p*-phenylenediamine is oxidized, forming indophenol blue.

MECHANISM OF THE CYTOCHROME OXIDASE REACTION

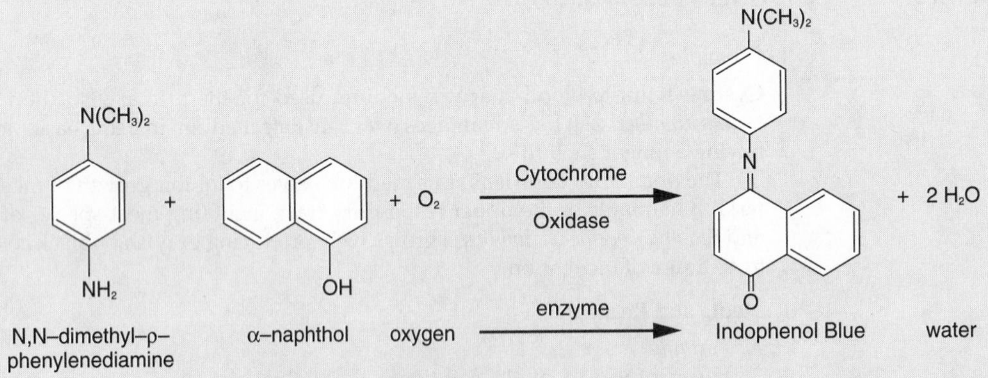

II. Media and Reagents

A. Tetramethyl-*p*-phenylenediamine dihydrochloride, 1% (Kovac's reagent)

B. Dimethyl-*p*-phenylenediamine dihydrochloride, 1% (Gordon and McLeod's reagent)

C. Commercial disks and reagents

1. Difco Laboratories (Detroit, MI):

Bacto differentiation disks, oxidase
Spot test oxidase reagent
Dryslide™ Oxidase

2. Remel (Lenexa, KS)

Bactidrop oxidase

III. Quality Control

Bacterial species showing positive and negative reactions should be run as controls at frequent intervals. The following can be suggested:

A. Positive control—*Pseudomonas aeruginosa*

B. Negative control—*Escherichia coli*

IV. Procedure

The test is commonly performed by one of two methods: 1) the direct plate technique, in which 2 to 3 drops of reagent are directly added to isolated bacterial colonies growing on plate medium; and 2) the indirect paper strip procedure, in which either a few drops of the reagent are added to a filter paper strip or commercial disks or strips impregnated with dried reagent are used. The tetramethyl derivative of *p*-phenylenediamine is recommended because the reagent is more stable in storage and is more sensitive to the detection of cytochrome oxidase and is less toxic than the dimethyl derivative. In either method, a loopful of suspected colony is smeared into the reagent zone of the filter paper.

V. Results

A. Interpretation

Bacterial colonies having cytochrome oxidase activity develop a deep blue color at the inoculation site within 10 seconds (Color Plate 4–1G). Any organism producing a blue color in the 10- to 60-second period must be further tested because it probably does not belong to the *Enterobacteriaceae*. Stainless steel or Nichrome inoculating loops or wires should not be used for this test because surface oxidation products formed when flame sterilizing may result in false-positive reactions.

VI. Bibliography

Gordon J, McLeod JW: The practical application of the direct oxidase reaction in bacteriology. J Pathol Bacteriol 31:185–190, 1928

MacFaddin JF: Biochemical Tests for Identification of Medical Bacteria, 2nd ed, pp 249–260. Baltimore, Williams & Wilkins, 1980

Steel KJ: The oxidase reaction as a taxonomic tool. J Gen Microbiol 25:297–306, 1961

Weaver DK, Lee EKH, Leahy MS: Comparison of reagent impregnated paper strips and conventional methods for identification of *Enterobacteriaceae*. Am J Clin Pathol 49:494–499, 1968

CHART 17   DARKFIELD MICROSCOPY OF GENITAL LESIONS

I. Principle

Darkfield detection of spirochetes allows presumptive diagnosis of syphilis during the primary phase before antibody has developed. There are few contaminating spirochetes in genital sites, so detection of spirochetes with a morphology compatible with *Treponema pallidum* subspecies *pallidum* provides a solid diagnosis. The prevalence of spirochetes in the oral cavity necessitates caution. The test is best not performed in the oral cavity; if spirochetes are seen there, their identity must be established by specific immunologic means.

II. Equipment and Reagents

Microscope with transmitted light and a darkfield consenser. Use a 10× objective to focus the specimen and center the darkfield condenser. Use a 40× to 63× objective to search the specimen. Final identification is made with a 100× objective.

Microscope slides, 1″ × 3″. Thickness should match that recommended in microscope manual

Coverglass #1, 22 mm × 22 mm

Immersion oil, nondrying, Cargille type A or equivalent

Lens paper and lens cleaner

Applicator sticks
Sterile saline
Disinfectant, such as iodine or 70% alcohol

III. Quality Control

A scraping of gingival mucosa may be used as a control with which to set up the dark-field condenser.

IV. Procedure

A. *Collection of Specimen*
   1. General
      a. Remove any scab or crust covering the lesion.
      b. Remove any exudate with a gauze sponge.
      c. If necessary, compress the base of the lesion or apply a suction cup to promote accumulation of tissue fluid on ulcer surface.
      d. Apply a glass slide with a sterile bacteriologic loop.
      e. Place a glass coverslip on the specimen and press it down to remove bubbles.
      f. Examine immediately.
   2. Dry papulosquamous lesions of the skin
      a. Gently remove the superficial layer of skin, trying not to cause bleeding.
      b. Compress the lesion if very little fluid appears
      c. Touch a microscope slide to the lesion or transfer a small amount of fluid to a slide with a bacteriologic loop.
      d. Alternatively, a small amount of sterile saline can be injected into the lesion, aspirated back, and placed on a slide.
      e. Cover slip and examine immediately.
   3. Cervical/vaginal lesions
      a. Under visualization with a bivalve speculum, remove any cervical or vaginal discharge.
      b. Obtain serous exudate with a bacteriologic loop.
      c. If necessary, serous exudate can be produced by compressing the lesion with a Kelly clamp.
      d. Prepare slides as above.
   4. Mucous patches
      a. Using a sterile bacteriologic loop, collect some of the mucus and place it on a glass slide.
      b. Place a cover slip on the slide and examine immediately.

V. Examination of the Specimen

Prepare the darkfield microscope before collection of the specimen.
Using a 40× to 63× objective search the slide systematically.
When a suspicious structure is found, examine under 100× magnification.
When observation is completed, discard the slide in disinfectant.
Characteristics of *T. pallidum* and saprophytic genital species, *T. refringens*.

Characteristic	*T. pallidum*	*T. refringens*
Morphology		
Shape	Delicate corkscrew shape	Loose coiled, coarse
Length	6–14 μm	8–20 μm
Width	0.25–0.3 μm	0.4–0.75 μm
Spiral wave length	Approx. 1.0–1.5 μm	
Motility		
Translation	Slow, deliberate back and forth movement	Rapid, writhing motion
Rotation	Slow to rapid rotation (corkscrew); may rotate in place	Active serpentine rotation
Flexion	Rotation accompanied by soft bending and twisting Bending occurs stiffly in middle of organism	Marked flexion
Distortion	May occur as a ring or attached to cells	None noted

VI. Results

A. Interpretation

False-positive results may occur if oral spirochetes are not confirmed or if characteristic motility of genital spirochetes is misinterpreted.

A few red blood cells in the preparation are a sign that exudate was obtained, but the specimen should not be bloody. Bubbles should be carefully removed.

False-negative results may be obtained if insufficient exudate was obtained, if there was too long an interval between collection and examination, if the lesion is late, or if the patient has been treated with antitreponemal drugs.

VII. Bibliography

Larson SA, Hunter EF, Kraus SJ (eds): Manual of Tests for Syphilis, 8th ed., Washington DC, American Public Health Association, 1990

CHART 18   DECARBOXYLASES

I. Principle

Decarboxylases are a group of substrate-specific enzymes that are capable of reacting with the carboxyl (COOH) portion of amino acids, forming alkaline-reacting amines. This reaction, known as decarboxylation, forms carbon dioxide as a second product. Each decarboxylase enzyme is specific for an amino acid. Lysine, ornithine, and arginine are the three amino acids routinely tested in the identification of the *Enterobacteriaceae*. The specific amine products are as follows:

Lysine   → Cadaverine
Ornithine   → Putrescine
Arginine   → Citrulline

The conversion of arginine to citrulline is a dihydrolase, rather than a decarboxylase reaction, in which an NH_2 group is removed from arginine as a first step. Citrulline is next converted to ornithine, which then undergoes decarboxylation to form putrescine.

Moeller decarboxylase medium is the base most commonly used for determining the decarboxylase capabilities of the *Enterobacteriaceae*. The amino acid to be tested is added to the decarboxylase base before inoculation with the test organism. A control tube, consisting of only the base without the amino acid, must also be set up in parallel. Both tubes are anaerobically incubated by overlaying with mineral oil. During the initial stages of incubation, both tubes turn yellow, owing to the fermentation of the small amount of glucose in the medium. If the amino acid is decarboxylated, alkaline amines are formed and the medium reverts to its original purple color.

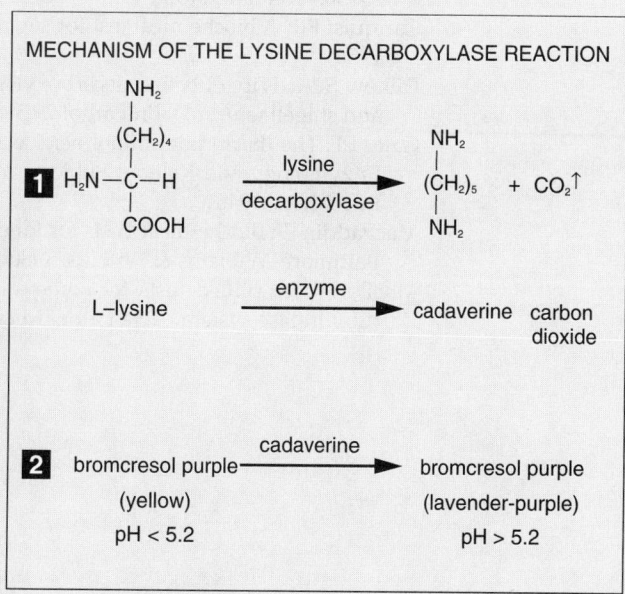

II. Media and Reagents

A. *Moeller Decarboxylase Broth Base*

Peptone	5 g
Beef extract	5 g
Bromcresol purple	0.01 g
Cresol red	0.005 g
Glucose	0.5 g
Pyridoxal	0.005 g
Distilled water to	1 L

Final pH = 6.0

B. Amino Acid

Add 10 g (final concentration = 1%) of the L (*levo*)-form of the amino acid (lysine, ornithine, or arginine). Double this amount if the D (*dextro*)-L-form is to be used, because only the L-form is active.

III. Quality Control

The following organisms are suggested for positive and negative controls:

AMINO ACID	POSITIVE CONTROL	NEGATIVE CONTROL
Lysine	*Enterobacter aerogenes*	*Enterobacter cloacae*
Ornithine	*Enterobacter cloacae*	*Klebsiella pneumoniae*
Arginine	*Enterobacter cloacae*	*Enterobacter aerogenes*

IV. Procedure

From a well-isolated colony of the test organism previously recovered on primary isolation agar, inoculate two tubes of Moeller decarboxylase medium, one containing the amino acid to be tested, the other to be used as a control tube devoid of amino acid. Overlay both tubes with sterile mineral oil to cover about 1 cm of the surface and incubate at 35°C for 18 to 24 hours.

V. Results

A. Interpretation

Conversion of the control tube to a yellow color indicates that the organism is viable and that the pH of the medium has been lowered sufficiently to activate the decarboxylase enzymes. Reversion of the tube containing the amino acid to a blue-purple color indicates a positive test owing to the formation of amines from the decarboxylation reaction (see Color Plate 4–4F).

VI. Bibliography

Blazevic DJ, Ederer GM: Principles of Biochemical Tests in Diagnostic Microbiology, pp 29–36. New York, John Wiley & Sons, 1975

Carlquist PR: A biochemical test for separating paracolon groups. J Bacteriol 71:339–341, 1956

Falkow S: Activity of lysine decarboxylase as an aid in the identification of salmonellae and shigellae. Am J Clin Pathol 29:598–600, 1958

Gale EF: The bacterial amino acid decarboxylases. In Nord FF (ed): Advances in Enzymology and Related Subjects of Biochemistry, vol. 6. New York, Interscience Publishers, 1946

MacFaddin JF: Biochemical Tests for Identification of Medical Bacteria, 2nd ed, pp 78–93. Baltimore, Williams & Wilkins, 1980

Moeller V: Simplified tests for some amino acid decarboxylases and for the arginine dihydrolase system. Acta Pathol Microbiol Scand 36:158–172, 1955

CHART 19   DETECTION, IDENTIFICATION, AND DRUG SUSCEPTIBILITY TESTING
OF *M. TUBERCULOSIS* BY RADIOMETRIC INSTRUMENTATION

I. Principle

The metabolism of [^{14}C]palmitic acid to $^{14}CO_2$ by members of the genus *Mycobacterium* is a sensitive and specific method to recover, identify, and test mycobacteria for drug susceptibility. $^{14}CO_2$ is detected in the ion chamber of the BACTEC 460 (Becton Dickinson Instruments Systems, Sparks MD). Because of the sensitivity of the instrument to detect $^{14}CO_2$, the ability to assess growth in the presence of one of several antituberculous drugs incorporated into the media provides a rapid method to determine drug resistance. Clinical specimens can be scanned for activity every day. Growth is determined by finding increasing readings for $^{14}CO_2$ in the ion chamber.

II. Specimen

A positive culture for suspected *M. tuberculosis* (as determined by growth inhibition in a NAP bottle run in parallel, or by observing cord formation in acid-fast stain or on examination of microcolonies on a clear Middlebrook 7H10 plate) from a BACTEC 12A blood culture vial that has reached a growth index of 500 or more is used.

III. Materials

A. Equipment: BACTEC 460 instrument

B. Media

1. BACTEC 12A broth culture vials (two per unknown)
2. BACTEC NAP vial
3. BACTEC 12A broth culture vials, one each including the following antituberculous drugs:
   a. Isoniazid
   b. Streptomycin
   c. Rifampin
   d. Ethambutol

IV. Quality Control

Quality control of the antibiotic-containing vials is performed by the manufacturer before shipment. Local practice must dictate whether it is necessary to perform a quality control check on each new lot of antibiotic-containing vials with a strain of *M. tuberculosis* that has a known resistance profile.

V. Procedure

1. The procedure starts by detecting a BACTEC-positive 12A vial that has reached a growth index of 100 and determining that acid-fast bacilli are present.
2. Inoculate 1 mL of the culture into a vial containing 12A medium plus *p*-nitroacetyl-aminohydroxypropiophenone (NAP; see Chart 50). Also inoculate 1 mL of the positive culture into a third vial containing 12A medium only.
3. If growth is inhibited after 3 to 5 days incubation, the isolate is either *M. tuberculosis* or *M. bovis;* no inhibition of growth indicates that the organism is a *Mycobacterium* species other than *M. tuberculosis*, in which case a BACTEC susceptibility test cannot be performed.
4. If growth is inhibited in the NAP bottle, observe the growth index in the 12A vial without NAP that had been inoculated in parallel. When the growth index reaches 500, the concentration is sufficient to perform antimycobacterial susceptibility studies against the unknown strain of *M. tuberculosis.*
5. Inoculate 0.1 mL of the positive culture into each of the drug-containing vials provided by the manufacturer (currently isoniazid, streptomycin, rifampin, and ethambutol) and with representative control strains.
6. At the same time, inoculate another vial of 12A medium without drugs with 0.1 mL of a 1:100 dilution of the positive culture used to inoculate the drug-containing vials. This will be equivalent to 1% growth in the proportion method for drug susceptibility testing.
7. Incubate the vials and read daily until the growth index of the control vial reaches 30. Then record the growth index of the drug-containing vials.

VI. Results

   A. Interpretation

   If the increase in growth index in drug-containing medium is more than the change in growth index in the control (30 or greater), the *M. tuberculosis* strain is growing in the presence of that drug and is considered resistant.

VII. Procedure Notes

The final drug concentrations in each of the drug-containing vials is 90% of the stated concentration because of the dilution factor (2.0 mL of medium plus 0.1 mL of drug solution plus 0.1 mL of inoculum = 2.2 mL).

VIII. Bibliography

Damato JJ, Collins MT, Rothlauf MV, et al: Detection of mycobacteria by radiometric and standard plate procedures. J Clin Microbiol 17:1066–1073, 1983

Gross WM, Hawkins JE: Radiometric selective inhibition tests for differentiation of *Mycobacterium tuberculosis, Mycobacterium bovis* and other mycobacteria. J Clin Microbiol 21:565–568, 1985

Morgan MA, Horstmeier CD, DeYoung DR: Comparison of a radiometric method (BACTEC) and conventional culture media for recovery of mycobacteria from smear-negative specimens. J Clin Microbiol 18:384–388, 1983

Roberts GD, Goodman NL, Heifets L, et al: Evaluation of the radiometric method for recovery of mycobacteria and drug susceptibility testing of *Mycobacterium tuberculosis* from acid-fast smear positive specimens. J Clin Pathol 18:689–696, 1983

CHART 20   DETERMINATION OF MINIMUM BACTERICIDAL CONCENTRATION

I. Principle

The minimum bactericidal concentration (MBC) of an antibiotic is the concentration of antibiotic that kills at least 99.9% of a standardized bacterial inoculum. The indications for the test are few, primarily nonenterococcal streptococcal endocarditis and the possibility of tolerance in a staphylococcal infection that has not responded to usual therapy. Great care is needed in the interpretation of the results.

A few antibiotics inhibit bacterial growth without actually killing the microorganisms, but most modern antibiotics exert lethal activity. The concentration of drug that inhibits growth is very close to the concentration that produces death of the bacteria (within one to two, twofold dilutions). In some situations there is a larger difference between the inhibitory and lethal concentrations. Tolerance has been operationally defined as a difference that is at least 32-fold (see text for a more complete discussion).

II. Materials and Reagents

   1. Mueller-Hinton broth for performance of MIC test
   2. 1.0 and 0.5 McFarland turbidity standards
   3. Scrupulously clean, acid-washed borosilicate glass tubes
   4. Vortex mixer
   5. Eppendorf or similar micropipette
   6. Nutrient agar plates, such as blood agar, for subculture from broth

III. Procedure

   A. *Preparation of the Inoculum*
   1. Subculture the test organism and quality control organisms onto appropriate medium (usually a blood agar plate) and incubate overnight at 35°C.
   2. Inoculate a tube that contains 2 mL of saline or Mueller-Hinton broth with five or more colonies from the agar plate and adjust turbidity to match a McFarland 1 standard (approximately 10^8 CFU/mL).
   3. Transfer 0.1 mL of the turbid broth into 10 mL of Mueller-Hinton broth; incubate in shaking water bath or equivalent at 35°C until turbid (5 to 6 hours for rapid growers). The relevant control organism should be inoculated into 3 mL of broth and incubated without shaking until turbid. This represents a midexponential phase of growth.

4. Prepare twofold serial dilutions of the antibiotic in 2 mL of Mueller-Hinton broth. Use acid-washed borosilicated glass tubes.
5. Standardize the inoculum of the patient's organism and the control strain by adjusting to a McFarland 0.5 standard in 3 mL of saline or broth.
6. Dilute the adjusted inocula 1:10 (approximately 5×10^6 CFU/mL).
7. Using an Eppendorf or equivalent pipette, dispense 0.1 mL of the diluted inoculum into the tubes that contain serial dilutions of antibiotic. Insert the tip well under the surface of the broth; avoid any contact between the tip and the walls of the tube. Rinse the tip five times. The same tip may be used if the tubes are inoculated from the lowest to the highest concentration of antibiotic. The final inoculum size is approximately 2.5×10^5 CFU/mL.
8. Incubate the tubes for 20 hours at 35°C.

B. *Quantitation of the Inoculum*
1. From the final dilution of the inoculum (approximately 5×10^6 CFU/mL), perform four serial tenfold dilutions in Mueller-Hinton broth (final concentration of 5×10^2 CFU/mL).
2. In duplicate, dispense 0.1 mL onto the surface of a blood agar plate. Spread the inoculum evenly with a sterile bent glass rod.
3. Incubate the plates at 35°C overnight.

C. *Determination of MIC*
1. After overnight incubation, determine the MIC of the quality control strain by visual inspection of the tubes.
2. For the patient's sample only, vortex the tubes without growth vigorously for 15 seconds to resuspend any bacteria that might have adhered to the walls of the tube. *Caution:* Avoid aerosols.
3. Reincubate the tubes for an additional 4 hours.
4. Determine the MIC of the patient's strain by visual inspection of the tubes.

D. *Subculture for Determination of MBC*
1. After the 4-hour additional incubation, again vortex the visually clear tubes containing the patient's isolate. Spread 0.1 mL from each tube across the surface of dried blood agar plates with sterile bent glass rods.
2. Incubate the plates overnight (or longer for a slow-growing organisms) at 35°C.

IV. Results

A. Interpretation
1. *Determination of the MBC*
   a. Count the bacterial colonies on each MBC subculture plate.
   b. Determine the number of colonies in the original inoculum by counting a dilution of the quantitative subculture that yields between 20 and 200 colonies after incubation for the same length of time that the MBC subcultures were incubated. With practice at preparing the inoculum, only the estimated endpoint dilution need be subcultured in duplicate onto agar.

The MBC is the lowest concentration of antibiotic that produced a 99.9% kill. For example, if the fourth plate in the inoculum quantitation contained 45 colonies, the actual inoculum was 4.5×10^5 CFU/mL (45 colonies/0.1 mL $\times$ 3 serial tenfold dilutions = $45 \times 10 \times 10^3 = 45 \times 10^4 = 4.5 \times 10^5$). A three $\log_{10}$ reduction (99.9% kill) should result in a concentration of 4.5×10^2 CFU/mL. Subculture of 0.1 mL from such a tube should result in 45 colonies on the subculture plate. Therefore, any concentration of antibiotic that produces fewer than 45 colonies after subculture is considered bactericidal. If growth of bacteria reappears at concentrations of antibiotic higher than the apparent MBC endpoint, the presence of a paradoxic effect may be noted. The clinical interpretation of such a test is problematic.

A discrepancy of at least five twofold dilutions between MIC and the MBC is the most common definition of *tolerance*. Care must be taken to minimize the chance of laboratory artifacts producing the appearance of tolerance. Clinically, an additional antibiotic should be considered in the therapy for such an infection.

V. Bibliography

Reimer LG, Stratton CW, Reller LB: Minimum inhibitory and bactericidal concentrations of 44 antimicrobial agents against three standard control strains in broth with and without human serum. Antimicrob Agents Chemother 19:1050–1055, 1981

Stratton CW, Cooksey RC: Susceptibility tests: Special tests. In Balows A, Hasler WJ Jr, Herrmann KL, et al (eds). Manual of Clinical Microbiology, 5th ed., pp 1153–1165. Washington DC, American Society for Microbiology, 1990

Taylor PC, Schoenknecht FD, Sherris JC et al: Determination of minimum bactericidal concentrations of oxacillin for *Staphylococcus aureus:* Influence and significance of technical factors. Antimicrob Agents Chemother 23:142–150, 1983

CHART 21   DIENE'S STAIN PROCEDURE FOR IDENTIFICATION OF MYCOPLASMAS

I. Principle

Mycoplasma colonies from genital cultures are easily identified by observing typical colonies on agar medium. Visualization of colonial morphology is facilitated by application of Dienes' stain directly to the agar surface.

Dienes' stain is a nonspecific stain that imparts a contrasting appearance to *Mycoplasma* colonies on agar, allowing easier visualization of colony morphology and characteristics.

II. Reagents

A. Modified Dienes' Stain (stock solution)

Methylene blue	2.5 g
Azure II	1.25 g
Maltose	10.0 g
Na$_2$CO$_3$	0.25 g
Distilled water	100 mL

Dienes' stain working solution is prepared by diluting an aliquot of the stock solution 1:3 with distilled water.

III. Procedure

1. Flood an agar plate containing mycoplasmal growth with 1 mL of Dienes' stain working solution
2. *Immediately rinse the agar surface with distilled water to remove the stain.*
3. Decolorize the medium by adding 1 mL of 95% ethanol. Leave in contact with the agar for 1 minute, then remove. Repeat the wash step a second time.
4. Rinse the plate with distilled water and allow to dry
5. Observe for colonies under the low power of a microscope (50 to 100×).

IV. Results

A. Interpretation

Mycoplasmas with the "fried-egg" colony morphology will stain with a dark blue center and a light blue periphery and will appear highly granular. The agar background will be clear or slightly violet.

Mycoplasmas other than *M. pneumoniae* will remain stained; *M. pneumoniae* reduces the methylene blue after a time and will become colorless. If the isolate is from the genital tract and produces typical colonies and staining, the isolate can be reported as *M. hominis.*

V. Bibliography

Velleca WM, Bird BR, Forrester FT: Laboratory Diagnosis of Mycoplasma Infections. Atlanta, U.S. Department of Health and Human Services, 1980

CHART 22   DIGESTION AND DECONTAMINATION: *N*-ACETYL-L-CYSTEINE–SODIUM HYDROXIDE (NALC)

I. Principle

Mycobacteria are optimally recovered from clinical specimens when they are released from mucin, body fluids, and cells (digestion.) *N*-Acetyl-L-cysteine (NALC) is a mucolytic agent that in concentrations of 0.5% to 2% can rapidly digest tenacious sputum and other mucoid specimens within 2 minutes. Growth of mycobacteria in culture media is also enhanced when the concentration of competing organisms is minimal (decontamination). The addition of 4% sodium hydroxide to the digestion mixture to reach a final concentration of 2% is the most commonly used decontaminating agent.

II. Specimen

A. Type of Specimen

Any specimen that is mucoid in consistency or is known to be contaminated with bacteria should undergo digestion and decontamination. Included are all respiratory specimens, gastric lavage fluid, stools, urine (when Gram stain shows the presence of bacteria), postmortem tissue, and biopsy samples.

B. Patient Preparation

When collecting specimens through a contaminated area, such as collection of expectorated sputum, every effort should be made to cleanse or decontaminate the area. For example, before patients are asked to produce an expectorated sputum, they should rinse out their mouth two or three times with water or a proprietary mouth wash. The skin adjacent to a biopsy site should be carefully cleaned with iodine followed by an alcohol swab.

C. Special Collection Procedures

In patients suspected of having pulmonary tuberculosis who cannot produce adequate sputum, an induced sputum should be collected. In instances where diagnosis has been difficult to establish, invasive procedures, such as bronchial brush biopsies, bronchial washings, or bronchoalveolar lavage may be required.

D. Special Handling Conditions

All specimens submitted for the culture of mycobacteria must be handled in a properly functioning biohazard hood. Care must also be taken in the preparation, examination, and storage of stained smears, as all acid-fast bacilli may not be killed in the fixation and staining procedure. Care must be taken not to produce aerosols when subcultures are made, when specimens are centrifuged, and when various biochemical tests are performed.

III. Materials

A. Equipment
1. Centrifuge with aerosol-free centrifuge cups
2. Vortex mixer

B. Supplies
1. Discard container containing disinfectant solution
2. Sterile 50-mL conical polypropylene screw-cap tubes (aerosol-free and graduated)
3. 10 mL sterile transfer pipette
4. Clean, unscratched, 1″ × 3″ microscope slides

C. Reagents
1. N-Acetyl-L-cysteine (NALC) digestant–decontaminant: TB base digestant, 50 mL (available commercially)
2. TB phosphate buffer: 0.067 M, pH 6.8, 250 mL (commercially available)
3. N-Acetyl-L-cysteine (NALC): Mucomyst, 20% solution (commercially available from Bristol Laboratories, Evansville IN)

IV. Quality Control

The percentage of clinical specimens that grow bacterial contaminants in TB cultures following the digestion and decontamination procedure should average about 3%. A contamination rate significantly less than 3% may indicate overly harsh decontamination and the concentration of NaOH should be reduced. A contamination rate significantly greater than 5% suggests either too weak a decontamination or incomplete digestion. Increasing the concentration of NaOH or the time of exposure, or both, may correct this problem.

V. Procedure
1. Add 1.5 mL NALC to 50 mL TB base digestant to make a working solution.
2. Add a volume of working NALC–NaOH solution (no more than 24 hours old) equal to the volume of specimen in a sterile 50-mL conical polypropylene screw-cap centrifuge tube. If more than 20 mL of specimen is submitted, use a sterile transfer pipette to select 10 mL of the most purulent, blood, or mucoid portion. Secure the cap tightly.

3. Agitate the tube on a vortex mixer for not more than 30 seconds. Be sure to move the tube so that the NALC–NaOH comes in contact with the entire inner surface of the tube.
4. Let the tube stand for 15 minutes at room temperature to decontaminate the specimen.
5. Dilute the mixture to the 50-mL mark with either sterile distilled water or sterile 0.067 phosphate buffer (pH 6.8). This will reduce the continued action of the NaOH and lower the viscosity of the mixture.
6. Recap the tube tightly and invert several times to mix the contents.
7. Centrifuge the tube at 3000 3 g for 15 to 20 minutes. Use aerosol-free sealed centrifuge cups.
8. Pour the supernatant into a splash-proof discard container filled with disinfectant.
9. Use a sterile 3-mm–diameter bacteriologic loop or the end of two sterile wooden applicator sticks to remove a portion of the sediment, and prepare a smear over an area 1×2 cm on a new, clean, unscratched glass slide.
10. Suspend the remaining sediment in 1 to 2 mL of TB buffer or sterile distilled water if media are to be inoculated immediately. Otherwise, suspend the sediment in 1 to 2 mL of sterile 0.2% bovine albumin fraction V. If the amount of the sediment is very small, reconstitute the sediment in 1 mL only.
11. Add 3 drops to each side of a 7H11 agar slant
12. Inoculate 0.5 mL into BACTEC vial

VI. Results

Not applicable

VII. Procedure Notes
1. Excessive agitation of the NALC–NaOH solution should be avoided because NALC is unstable in the presence of oxygen.
2. Bovine albumin serves to buffer the inoculum and enhance adhesion of the sample to solid media
3. Sterile water only should be used: Tap water may contain environmental mycobacteria that can confuse observations of stained smears and contaminate culture media.

VIII. Limitation of Procedure

The concentration of NaOH and the time of exposure of specimen to reagent during the decontamination procedure must be carefully controlled to avoid undue loss of mycobacterial cells during this procedure.

IX. Bibliography

Good RC, Silcox V, Kilburn JO: Tuberculosis and other mycobacterioses. In Balows A, Hausler WJ (eds). Diagnostic Procedures for Bacterial, Mycotic and Parasitic Infections, 6th ed, pp. 675–703. Washington DC, American Public Health Association, 1985

Kubica GP, Dye WE, Cohn ML, Middlebrook G: Sputum digestion and decontamination with N-Acetyl-L-cysteine–sodium hydroxide for culture of mycobacteria. Am Rev Respir Dis 87:775–779, 1963

Strong BE, Kubica GP: Isolation and Identification of *Mycobacterium tuberculosis:* A Guide for the Level II Laboratory. US Public Health Service publication 81-8390. Atlanta, Centers for Disease Control, 1976

CHART 23   DISK DIFFUSION (BAUER-KIRBY) SUSCEPTIBILITY TEST

I. Principle

Continued evaluation and revision of the disk diffusion procedure has been performed by a committee of the NCCLS. Designating a national standard test for disk diffusion has not only permitted more exacting quality control, but has also allowed valid comparison of results among different laboratories using the procedure. The committee publishes periodic updates that incorporate new information and changes that have been suggested by users. It is important to maintain currency of the procedure.

The principle of the disk diffusion procedure has been discussed in the text. The zone diameters that are generated by the test are meaningless without reference to the minimum inhibitory concentration (MIC) correlates and interpretative guidelines published by the NCCLS.

II. Media and Reagents
   1. Bacterial isolate from an infectious process
   2. Nutrient broth (soybean–casein digest broth is recommended) for growth of the inoculum
   3. McFarland 0.5 standard for adjusting the turbidity of the inoculum
   4. Vortex mixer for suspension of the inoculum
   5. Viewbox for comparison of broth with standard. A photometer may be used if satisfactory results are documented.
   6. Mueller-Hinton 150-mm agar plates from a lot that produces satisfactory quality control results. The pH must be 7.2 to 7.4, and the depth must be approximately 4 mm.
   7. Calipers, ruler, or template for measuring the diameters of inhibitory zones

III. Quality Control

Reference strains of *Staphylococcus aureus*, *Escherichia coli*, and *Pseudomonas aeruginosa* should be tested each time a new batch of disks or agar is used. Additional controls should be performed each day the test is done, unless the laboratory can justify weekly quality control by conformance to published criteria (see Tables 15-15 and 15-17).

IV. Procedure
   A. *Preparation of Inoculum*
      1. With a wire loop or Dacron-tipped swab, touch the tops of four or five similar-appearing, well-isolated colonies on an agar plate culture. Transfer the growth to a tube that contains 4 to 5 mL of a suitable broth medium.
      2. Allow the culture to incubate at 35°C until it matches the turbidity of the standard prepared in the foregoing. Vigorously agitate the standard on a mechanical vortex mixer immediately before use. Use adequate light to read the tube against a white background with a contrasting black line. Add sterile saline or broth if necessary to obtain a turbidity visually comparable with that of the standard. Alternatively, a direct broth or saline suspension of colonies from an 18- to 24-hour agar plate may be adjusted to the standard. In this case, the bacteria must have been grown on a nutrient, nonselective medium, such as blood agar. Commercially available devices to standardize the inocula without adjustment of turbidity and without preincubation in broth media have also performed acceptably.
      3. Within 15 minutes after adjusting the turbidity of the inoculum suspension to that of the standard, dip a sterile nontoxic cotton swab into the inoculum suspension and rotate the swab several times with firm pressure on the inside wall of the tube to remove excess fluid.
      4. Inoculate the dried surface of a Mueller-Hinton agar plate that has been brought to room temperature by streaking the swab three times over the entire agar surface, rotating the plate approximately 60° to ensure an even distribution of the inoculum. Replace the lid of the dish. Allow 3 to 5 minutes, but no longer than 15 minutes, for the surface of the agar to dry before adding the antibiotic disks.
   B. *Alternative Inoculum Preparation*
      1. Make a direct saline or broth suspension of colonies from a nutrient nonselective agar plate that has been incubated for 18 to 24 hours.
      2. Immediately adjust the inoculum to the standard density, as before.
      3. This method is recommended for *Haemophilus* species, *Neisseria gonorrhoeae*, *Streptococcus pneumoniae*, and *Staphylococcus* species.
   C. *Testing of Antibiotics*
      1. Place the appropriate antimicrobial-impregnated disks on the surface of the agar, using either forceps or a multidisk dispenser.
      2. Gently tamp each disk down onto the agar to provide uniform contact. Do not move a disk once it has contacted the agar, because some of the drug diffuses almost immediately. Disks must be evenly distributed on the agar so that they are no closer than 24 mm from center to center.
      3. Invert the plates and place them in a 35°C air incubator for 16 to 18 hours.

V. Results

A. Interpretation

Measurement of zone diameters: Although zones of inhibition of growth may be set as early as 4 hours after inoculation with some of the more rapidly growing bacteria and become visible shortly thereafter, 16 to 18 hours is the standard time at which the zone diameters are measured. With the use of sliding calipers, a ruler, or a template, the zones of complete growth inhibition around each of the disks are carefully measured to within the nearest millimeters; the diameter of the disk is included in this measurement.

All measurements are made with the unaided eye while viewing the back of the petri dish with reflected light against a black, nonreflecting background. The plates should be viewed from a directly vertical line of sight to avoid any parallax that may result in misreadings. Susceptibility plates prepared with blood must be viewed from the agar surface and measurements made with the cover of the petri dish removed, again using reflected light to illuminate the plate. Common problems in delineation of zone sizes are discussed in the text.

An interpretative correlate (susceptible, moderately susceptible, intermediate, or resistant) is provided by reference to published guidelines (see Table 15-14). Zones that fall into the intermediate range should be considered equivocal; if therapy with the drug is desired, a dilution susceptibility test should be performed to clarify the issue.

VI. Bibliography

National Committee for Clinical Laboratory Standards: Performance Standards for Antimicrobial Disk Susceptibility Tests, (approved Standard M2-A4). Villanova, PA, National Committee for Clinical Laboratory Standards, 1984

CHART 24   DNA PROBES FOR THE IDENTIFICATION OF MYCOBACTERIA (ADAPTED FROM STOCKMAN)

I. Principle

A commercially manufactured system, AcuProbe Culture Confirmation Tests is available for identification of isolates of several species of mycobacteria (*M. tuberculosis* complex, *M. avium, M. intracellulare, M. gordonae, M. avium* complex, and *M. kansasii*). The system is based on the use of DNA probes that are complementary to species-specific rRNA. The mycobacterial cells are lysed by sonication, heat killed, and exposed to DNA that has been labeled with a chemiluminiscent tag. The labeled DNA probe combines with the organism's rRNA to form a stable DNA–RNA hybrid. A selection reagent "kills" the signal on all unbound DNA. Chemiluminescence produced by DNA–RNA hybrids is measured in a luminometer.

II. Specimen

Any actively growing culture less than 1 month old recovered on solid or broth medium (Middlebrook 7H9, 7H10, 7H11, 7H11 Selective or Lowenstein-Jensen) may be used.

III. Materials

A. Reagents

Reagent	Description	Storage Temperature (°C)
Lysing tubes	Lyophilized glass beads and buffer	23–25
Probe reagent	Tubed lyophilized species-specific DNA	4
Reagent 1	Specimen diluent	23–25
Reagent 2	Probe diluent	23–25
Reagent 3	Selection reagent	23–25
Detection I	H_2O_2 in nitric acid solution containing 1 N NaOH	23–25
Detection II	H_2O_2 in nitric acid solution containing 1 N NaOH	23–25
Ultrasonic enhancer	Detergent-like solution to increase sonication	23–25

B. Supplies
1. Micropipettes (100 μl)
2. Micropipettor (300 μL)
3. Repipettor (300 μL)
4. Repipettor syringes
5. Plastic sterile inoculating loops (1 μg)

C. Equipment
1. Luminometer (Leader 1, Leader 250, or PAL)
2. Vortex mixer
3. Water or dry bath, 90° ± 5°C
4. Water or dry bath, 60° ± 5°C

IV. Quality Control

A. Frequency and tolerance of controls
1. Run a positive and negative control with each batch of organisms to be tested.
2. If controls are not set within limits, check age of culture (should be less than 2 months old), level of water in sonicator, quality of sonicator (by observing waving water patterns while sonicator is on; water should "dance"), and temperature of hybridization; if necessary, run a tritium standard.

B. Control Organisms

Probe to be Tested	Control	
	Positive	*Negative*
M. avium	*M. avium* ATCC 25291	*M. intracellular* ATCC 13950
M. intracellulare	*M. intracellulare* ATCC 13950	*M. avium* ATCC 25291
M. tuberculosis complex	*M. tuberculosis* ATCC 14470	*M. avium* ATCC 25291
M. gordonae	*M. gordonae* ATCC 14470	*M. scrofulaceum* ATCC 19073
M. avium complex	*M. intracellulare* ATCC 13950	*M. gordonae* ATCC 14470
M. kansasii	*M. kansasii* ATCC 12478	*M. tuberculosis* ATCC 25177

V. Procedure
1. Add 1 cupful of ultrasonic enhancer to the water in the sonicator. Degas the water for 15 minutes. Turn on 95°C water bath (or heat block) and 60°C water bath (or heat block).
2. Add 100 mL of reagent 1 (specimen diluent) and 100 mL of reagent 2 (probe diluent) to each lysing tube.
3. Working in a biologic safety cabinet, transfer a loopful (1 mL) of test organism into the lysing tube. Twirl the loop against the side of the tube to remove the entire inoculum.
4. Place the lysing tubes in the sonicator. Ensure that the water level is high enough to cover the contents of the tube. Do not allow the tubes to touch the sides of the sonicator. Sonicate at room temperature for 15 minutes.
5. Place the lysing tubes in the 95°C water bath (or heat block) for 15 minutes.
6. Allow the tubes to cool at room temperature for 5 minutes.
7. Pipette 100 mL of the killed lysate into the probe reaction tube.
8. Incubate the tubes for 15 minutes at 60°C in the water bath (or heat block).
9. Pipette 300 mL of reagent 3 (selection reagent) into each tube. Recap and vortex the tubes, and immediately place them back into the 60°C water bath (or heat block). Incubate for 5 minutes.
10. Prepare the luminometer for operation by completing a wash cycle. To prevent static buildup and to ensure that no residue is present on the outside of the tube, wipe each tube with a damp tissue before inserting it into the luminometer. Read each tube and controls. The luminometer records relative light units (RLU).

VI. Results

A. A positive result is >30,000 RLU.

B. Signals lower than 30,000 RLU are considered negative.

C. Repeat any test with a result between 20,000 and 29,999 RLU.

VII. Procedure Notes

    A. It is important to maintain the $60° \pm 1°C$ dry bath, because annealing of the DNA–RNA hybrid is temperature-sensitive.

    B. The water level of the sonicator should be sufficiently high to cover the hybridization buffer, beads, and organism.

    C. Other sources of error include failure to vortex after addition of the organism–buffer mixture to the probe tube and after addition of reagent 3, which inactivates the acridinium ester not bound to rRNA.

    D. This method is currently being evaluated for use with BACTEC bottles.

VIII. Limitations of the Procedure

    A. This method cannot be used directly on fresh clinical specimens; it is for culture confirmation only.

    B. A small number of biochemically determined *M. avium* complex isolated will not produce a positive result with the *M. avium* complex probe. The taxonomic status of these strains is currently uncertain.

    C. The *M. tuberculosis* complex culture confirmation test does not differentiate between *M. tuberculosis, M. bovis, M. bovis* BCG, *M. africanum,* and *M. microti*

    D. The *M. avium* complex culture confirmation does not differentiate between *M. avium* and *M. intracellulare.*

IX. Bibliography

Gen-Probe, Inc.: Product Information: AcuProbe Mycobacterium Culture Confirmation Tests. Gen-Probe, Inc., San Diego CA, 1990

Stockman L: Identification of Mycobacteria in DNA probes. In Isenberg HD (ed): Clinical Microbiology Procedure Handbook. Washington DC, American Society for Microbiology, 1992

CHART 25   ENZYME-LINKED IMMUNOSORBENT ASSAY (EIA)

I. Principle

EIA provides a useful alternative to immunofluorescence for identification of a viral isolate or documentation of a serologic response. The advantages of the method are that large numbers of specimens can be processed, and the subjectivity of immunofluorescence tests can be obviated. The disadvantages are that the procedure is time-consuming if employed for small numbers of specimens and morphologic assessment of the reaction cannot be performed.

The principle of EIA is similar to that of immunofluorescence. Antigen and antibody, one of which must be known, are reacted. Color is generated by the interaction of a chromogenic substrate and an enzyme that has been coupled to the detector antibody. As for radioimmunoassay, a variety of approaches to this assay have been developed. The most commonly employed is the direct solid-phase system, in which specific antibody coats the solid-phase to serve as a capture layer, and enzyme-conjugated specific antibody is the detector. An indirect method, which requires only a single labeled reagent, may also be used.

If antibody is to be tested, the solid-phase is reacted with a known antigen, after which the patient's serum is incubated as the first layer in an indirect test (see Fig. 21–18). IgM-specific antibody can be detected by coating the solid phase with specific anti-IgM, followed sequentially by test serum, known antigen, and enzyme-conjugated antibody to that antigen (see Fig. 21–18).

II. Materials and Reagents

    A. Plastic microtiter plates or beads as a substrate.

    B. Antibody to coat the solid-phase. F(ab)2 fragments may be utilized to minimize nonspecific interactions.

    C. Antigen to coat the solid-phase or to react with coating antibody.

    D. Carbonate-bicarbonate buffer (pH 9.6) for coating.

    E. PBS–Tween 20 for dilution of serum

F. Detecting antibody—may be conjugated to enzyme

G. Detection reagent for indirect test—enzyme-conjugated antibody to globulin of species used for detecting antibody (or staphylococcal protein A if F(ab)2 or antigen has been used to coat the plastic)

H. Chromogenic substrate—defined by enzyme system.

I. Colorimeter or spectrophotometer.

III. Quality Control

A. Known positive serum or antigen

B. Known negative serum or antigen

C. Buffer control (no serum or antigen)

IV. Procedure

1. The coating layer is incubated with the solid-phase in carbonate buffer and a moist chamber at 4°C for 18 to 24 hours.

2. The coating solution is removed, and the solid-phase is washed five times with PBS–Tween. Each succeeding layer is added, after washing with PBS–Tween. The time and temperature of incubation varies with the assay.

V. Results

A. Interpretation

1. After incubation of enzyme conjugate and chromogenic substrate, the reaction is stopped chemically.

2. Color may be assessed visually or with a spectrophotometer.

3. Positive results are defined by comparison with the negative control. Values higher than a group of negative spectrums or two to three times higher than the mean of a group of negative controls are considered positive. Endpoint dilution may also be employed.

VI. Bibliography

Yolken RH: Prospects for solid-phase immunoassays in the diagnosis of respiratory infections. In Coonrod JD, Kunz LJ, Ferraro MJ (eds.): The Direct Detection of Microorganisms in Clinical Samples, Orlando FL, Academic Press, 1983

CHART 26   ESCULIN HYDROLYSIS TEST

I. Principle

Esculin medium without bile is useful in differentiating several species on nonfermenting bacilli. Esculin is a substituted glucoside that can be hydrolyzed by certain bacteria to yield glucose and esculetin. Esculin is a fluorescent compound that fluoresces under long-wave UV light at 360 nm. When esculin is hydrolyzed, fluorescence is lost, and the medium turns black due to the reaction of esculetin with the ferric ions in the medium. Several species of *Chryseobacterium*, *Sphingobacterium*, as well as *C. luteola*, *B. vesicularis*, *S. paucimobilis*, *S. maltophilia*, *A. radiobacter*, and some species of *B. cepacia*, *B. pseudomallei*, and *O. anthropi* are esculin positive.

II. Media and Reagents

The formula for Esculin medium is as follows:

Esculin Agar Modified:

esculin	1 g
ferric citrate	0.5 g
heart infusion agar	40 g
distilled water to	1 L

Esculin Broth:

heart muscle, infusion	10 g
peptic digest of animal tissue	10 g
sodium chloride	5 g
esculin	1 g
distilled water to	1 L

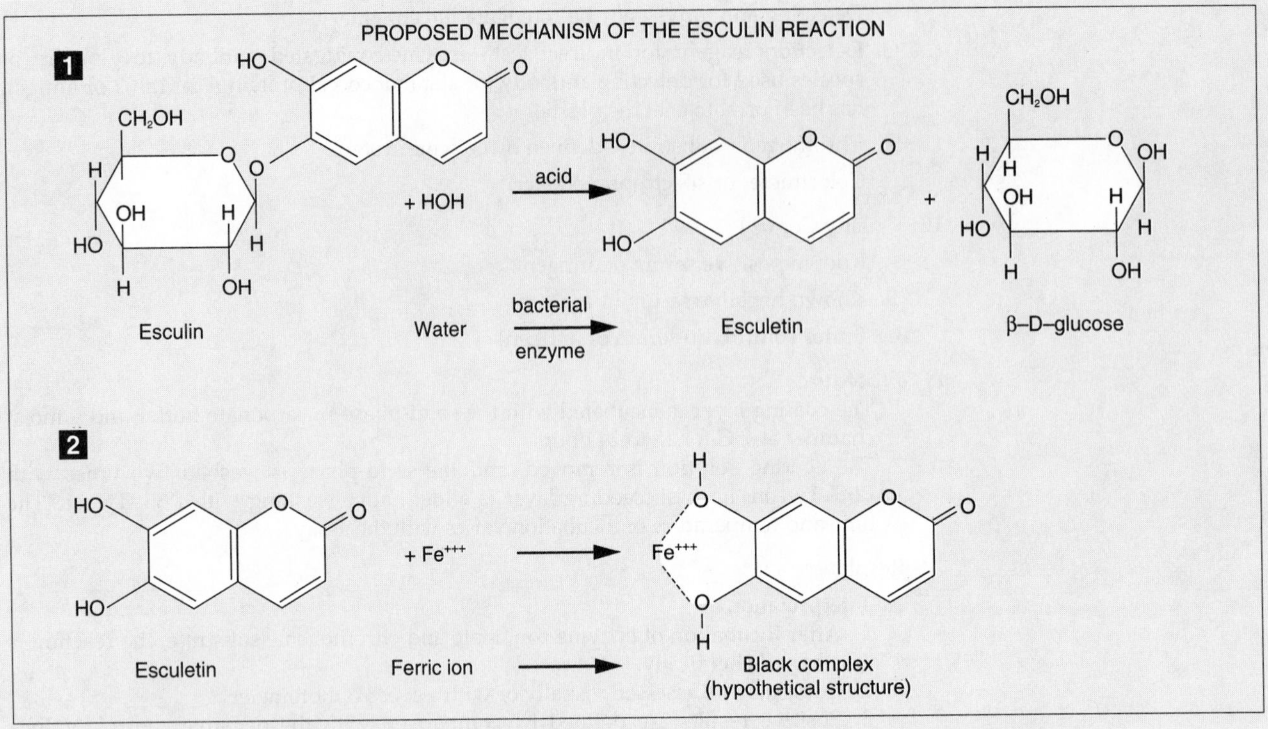

PROPOSED MECHANISM OF THE ESCULIN REACTION

III. Quality Control

    A. Positive control: *Aeromonas hydrophila* ATCC 7965

    B. Negative control: *P. aeruginosa* ATCC 27853

IV. Procedure

After touching the center of one well-isolated colony with a sterile inoculation loop or wooden stick, inoculate the organism onto the surface of the agar slant or into the broth. Incubate for 18 to 24 h at 35°C.

V. Results

    A. Interpretation

The development of a black color or the loss of fluorescence under UV light (360 nm) is interpreted as a positive test. Fluorescence or lack of a black color is interpreted as a negative test

VI. Bibliography

MacFaddin JF: *Biochemical Tests for Identification of Medical Bacteria*, 2nd ed., pp 4–12, Williams & Wilkins, Baltimore, 1980

Shigei J: Test methods used in the identification of commonly isolated aerobic gram-negative bacteria, p. 1.19.38-1.19.40. In H.H. Isenberg (ed.), *Clinical Microbiology Procedures Handbook*, vol. 1. American Society for Microbiology, Washington DC, 1992

CHART 27   EXOANTIGEN EXTRACTION

I. Principle of Test

Isolates of the dimorphic fungi *Blastomyces dermatitidis*, *Coccidioides immitis*, *Histoplasma capsulatum*, and *Paracoccidioides brasiliensis* may, on occasion, not sporulate or produce atypical colony and microscopic features, making identification on morphologic criteria difficult. The mycelial elements of these dimorphic fungi produce water-soluble, cell-free antigens that can be extracted in aqueous solutions and reacted with their homologous antibodies to produce visible precipitin reactions when placed in an appropriate double-diffusion agar test system. Exoantigens homologous to *B. dermatitidis* precipitin A; to *C. immitis* precipitin HS, HL, or F; to *H. capsulatum* precipitins H or M; or to *P. brasiliensis* precipitins 1 (E) and 2 can be detected, thus providing a relatively rapid method for making a definitive species identification.

II. Specimen

    A. Type of Specimen

    A mold form isolate suspected of being one of the dimorphic fungi recovered on an appropriate fungus isolation medium. The isolate need not show typical colony or morphologic features, but must be sufficiently mature to produce the exoantigen to be tested.

    B. Special Handling Conditions

    All work with open cultures should be performed in a properly functioning biohazard hood. Gloves should be worn when making direct manipulations with the culture plates, and precautions should be taken to see that the mycelial elements do not become aerosolized or come in direct contact with skin.

III. Materials

    A. Equipment
      1. Filter apparatus fitted with a 0.45-μm Nalgene filter.
      2. Amicon Minicon Macrosulate B-15 Concentrator or equivalent.

    B. Supplies
      1. Glass or plastic transfer pipettes
      2. Micropipettes suitable to deliver solution to diffusion plates.

    C. Reagents
      1. Aqueous merthiolate solution, 1:5,000
      2. Noble agar (or equivalent) immunodiffusion slide and template for cutting 6- to 8-mm diameter wells in a configuration of six in a circle at a distance of 10 mm apart. Specially prepared immunodiffusion slides are commercially available from Immuno Mycologics, Norman OK, or from Nolan Scott Biological Laboratories, Tucker GA.

IV. Quality Control

Set up control reagents in parallel with the test samples, either as prepared in-house from known strains of the fungal species to be tested, or as supplied by the manufacturer. Precipitin bands should be observed for each of the control samples against which readings of the unknown samples can be compared.

V. Procedure

    1. Overlay the surface of mycelial growth, as recovered either on a plate or a tube slant, with aqueous merthiolate (be sure the entire surface of the mycelium is covered to render the culture safe to handle during this phase of the procedure).
    2. Allow the solution to remain in contact with the culture for 24 hours.
    3. After the extraction is complete, filter the aqueous extract through a 0.45 filter.
    4. Concentrate 5 mL of the filtered extract 50 times for cultures in which *H. capsulatum* or *B. dermatitidis* are suspected; or 25 times if *C. immitis* or *P. brasiliensis* are suspected.
    5. With a micropipette, transfer a small quantity of the concentrated extract to be tested into appropriate wells in the microdiffusion plate in such a way that control sera are placed adjacent to each of the unknown specimens to be tested.
    6. Allow microdiffusion to take place for 24 hours at 25°C.

VI. Procedure Notes

    1. Be sure that the cultures during the extraction phase and the agar diffusion plates during the incubation phase are covered and not allowed to dehydrate.
    2. When transferring the concentrated extract to the agar diffusion wells, make sure each well is completely filled so that a slightly convex meniscus is visible.
    3. To increase the sensitivity for *B. dermatitidis*, incubate the immunodiffusion plates at 37°C for 48 hours. As the precipitin bands are visually sharper when plates are incubated at 25°C, it may be wise to set up *B. dermatitidis* extracts under both conditions.

VII. Results

After the incubation period, tilt the slides to catch strong transmitted light in such a way that precipitin bands can be visualized clearly. Compare the reactions of the unknown concentrates with those of the positive controls. *C. immitis* can be identified by the presence of IDCF, IDTP, or IDHL antigens; *H. capsulatum* by the presence of H or M bands; *B. dermatitidis* by the presence of A or B antigens and *P. brasiliensis* by one (E) or two or three antigens.

VIII. Limitation of Procedure

A. Cultures must be sufficiently mature for adequate exoantigen to be extracted. If insufficient exoantigen is available, it may be difficult to interpret the presence or absence of very thin or obscure precipitin bands.

B. False-positive results can arise if an excess of aqueous merthiolate solution is used during the extraction phase.

C. *B. dermatitidis* produces the weakest antigen and may be associated with false-negative results. Prolonged incubation at 37°C as indicated before may help to resolve this problem.

IX. Bibliography

Huppert M, Sun SH, Rice EH: Specificity of exoantigens for identifying cultures of *Coccidioides immitis*. J Clin Microbiol 8:346–348, 1978

Kaufman L, Standard P, Padhye AA: Exoantigen tests for the immunoidentification of fungal cultures. Mycopathologia 82:3–12, 1983

Kaufman L, Standard PG: Specific and rapid identification of medically important fungi by exoantigen detection. Annu Rev Microbiol 41:209–215, 1987

Sekhon AS, et al: Evaluation of commercial reagents to identify the exoantigens of *Blastomyces dermatitidis, Coccidioides immitis,* and *Histoplasma* species cultures. Am J Clin Pathol 82:206–209, 1984

CHART 28   FECAL CONCENTRATION TECHNIQUES FOR THE RECOVERY OF INTESTINAL PARASITES

I. Principle

The number of parasitic forms in fecal specimens is often too low to be observed microscopically in direct wet mounts or stained smear preparations. Therefore, concentration procedures must be employed to detect them. The two most commonly used techniques are *sedimentation* and *flotation*.

A. Sedimentation

The specific gravity of protozoan cysts and helminth ova is greater than water or saline–fecal suspensions and they tend to settle out. This process can be accelerated by light centrifugation. A formalin–ethyl acetate mixture is often added to the fecal suspension to clear out the fecal debris and fix the parasitic forms that may be present.

B. Flotation (Method of Bartlett and Co-workers[17])

Protozoan cysts and helminth ova of low specific gravity can be made to float on the surface of a solution with a high specific gravity. Zinc sulfate solution, with a specific gravity of 1.180, is most commonly used. The parasites that float to the surface can be collected by skimming the top of the solution with a wire loop.

II. Media and Reagents

A. Sedimentation

Formalin, 10% solution
Ethyl acetate

B. Flotation

10% formalin
Zinc sulfate (ZnSO$_4$, specific gravity 1.195) Add 400 g of ZnSO$_4$ into 1 L of warm tap water. Mix thoroughly. Check with a good hygrometer and adjust the specific gravity to 1.195 to 1.200. Store in a tightly stoppered container. Check the specific gravity weekly.

III. Procedure

A. Sedimentation

1. Thoroughly mix a portion of stool specimen about the size of a walnut into 10 mL of saline solution. This suspension should yield about 1 or 2 mL of sediment.
2. Filter the emulsion through fine mesh gauze into a conical centrifuge tube.
3. Centrifuge at RCF = 600 × g (about 2000 rpm) for 1 minute. The quantity of sediment following this first centrifugation step should be between 0.75 mL for fresh specimens and 0.5 mL for formalinized feces.

4. Decant the supernatant and wash the sediment with 10 mL of saline solution. Centrifuge again and repeat washing until supernatant is clear.

5. After the last wash, decant the supernatant and add 10 mL of 10% formalin to the sediment. Mix and let stand for 5 minutes.

6. Add 1 or 2 mL of ethyl acetate. Stopper the tube and shake vigorously.

7. Centrifuge at RCF = 450 × g (about 1500 rpm) for 1 minute. Four layers should result as follows: (1) top layer of ethyl acetate; (2) plug of debris; (3) layer of formalin; and (4) sediment.

8. Free the plug of debris from the sides of the tube by ringing with an applicator stick. Carefully decant the top three layers.

9. With a pipette, mix the remaining sediment with the small amount of remaining fluid and transfer 1 drop each to a drop of saline and iodine on a glass slide, cover with a coverslip, and examine microscopically for the presence of parasitic forms.

B. Flotation

1. Add 1 part feces (a quantity sufficient to yield about 0.75 mL of sediment) to 3 to 5 parts of 10% formalin. Mix thoroughly and allow to fix for at least 30 minutes.

2. Strain the well-mixed fecal–formalin suspension through one layer of gauze into a round-bottom tube (100 × 26 mm) to within ¾ in. (19.05 mm) of the rim.

3. Centrifuge the suspension at RCF = 600 × g (about 2000 rpm) for 3 to 5 minutes. Let centrifuge come to rest without mechanical breaking.

4. Decant the supernatant and drain the last drop onto a clean section of paper towel.

5. Add ZnSO₄ solution to within 1 in. (25 mm) of the rim of the tube.

6. With two applicator sticks, resuspend the packed sediment until no coarse particles remain.

7. Immediately centrifuge the suspension for 1.5 minutes at RFC 5 450 × g (about 1500 rpm). Again, allow the centrifuge to stop without mechanical breaking.

8. Carefully transfer the tube to a rack that will hold it in an upright position. Allow the tube to stand for 1 minute.

9. With a wire loop 7 mm in diameter and bent at a right-angle at the stem, transfer 2 loops of surface film to a drop of 0.85% saline and to a drop of Dobell & O'Connor iodine on a 3 × 2 in. glass side. Mix each suspension.

10. Place a clean, 22 × 30-mm No. 1 coverslip on each fluid mount. Examine microscopically within 1 hour. Hold mounts in a moisturized petri dish if they are not to be examined immediately.

IV. Procedure Notes

A. Sedimentation

The sedimentation procedure can also be used to process polyvinyl alcohol (PVA)-fixed specimens. The flotation mount should be prepared within 1 hour after preparation because cysts and ova begin to resettle after that time. If the sediment cannot be immediately examined when first prepared in the sedimentation technique, a small amount of 10% formalin can be added and the tube tightly capped to prevent drying for examination at a future time. Errors may occur if too little or too much feces are used in the sedimentation procedure (see third step in the foregoing).

B. Flotation

Zinc sulfate flotation techniques have the general advantage that the background fecal debris is eliminated, exposing any cysts or eggs that may be present. This modification using a formalin-fixed fecal sample clears the internal structures of the protozoan cysts, prevents distortion caused by the high salt concentration, and prevents popping and sinking of operculated eggs. The method is not suitable for recovery of *Schistosoma* eggs.

V. Bibliography

A. Sedimentation

Garcia LS, Ash LR: Diagnostic Parasitology: Clinical Laboratory Manual, 2nd ed. St. Louis, CV Mosby, 1979

Koneman EW, Richie IE, Tiemann C: Practical Laboratory Parasitology. Baltimore, Williams & Wilkins, 1974

Smith JW, Gutierrez Y: Medical parasitology. In Henry JB (ed): Todd, Sanford, and Davidsohn's Clinical Diagnosis and Management by Laboratory Methods, 16th ed, chap 51. Philadelphia, WB Saunders, 1979

Young KH, Bullock SL, Melvin DM et al: Ethyl acetate as a substitute for diethyl ether in the formalin–ether sedimentation technique. J Clin Microbiol 10:852–853, 1979

B. Flotation
Bartlett MS, Harper K, Smith N et al: Comparative evaluation of a modified zinc sulfate flotation technique. J Clin Microbiol 7:524–528, 1977

Smith JW, Gutierrez Y: Medical parasitology. In Henry JB (ed): Todd, Sanford, and Davidsohn's Clinical Diagnosis and Management by Laboratory Methods, 16th ed, chap 51. Philadelphia, WB Saunders, 1979

CHART 29   FLAGELLAR STAIN

I. Principle

Most motile bacteria possess flagella, the shape, number, and position of which are important characteristics in the differentiation of genera and species identification, particularly when biochemical reactions are weak or equivocal. The Leifson staining technique (or modification) is most commonly employed in clinical laboratories and is not difficult to perform, providing exact details are followed in each step of the procedure.

Bacterial flagella can be stained by alcoholic solutions of rosaniline dyes that form a precipitate as the alcohol evaporates in the staining procedure. Basic fuchsin (pararosaniline acetate) serves as the primary stain with tannic acid added to the solution as a mordant. A counterstain, such as methylene blue, may be used to better visualize the bacteria in instances in which the primary stain is weak or does not react at all with the bacterial cell wall.

II. Media and Reagents

A. Leifson method
1. Basic fuchsin, 1.2% in 95% alcohol
   a. Commercial product must be certified for flagellar stain.
   b. Pararosaniline acetate is preferred. If the dye solution is a mixture of pararosaniline acetate and pararosaniline hydrochloride, the hydrochloride compound must not compose more than two thirds of the solution.
   c. The stain must have the odor of acetic acid to be satisfactory.
   d. When new stain is prepared, at least 1 day must be allowed for the dye to enter completely into solution.
2. Tannic acid, 3% in water
   a. The suspension must have a light yellow color to be satisfactory.
   b. Add phenol in a 1:200 concentration to discourage emergence of molds during storage.
3. Sodium chloride, 1.5% in water
4. Final stain
   a. Combine the three stock solutions in equal volumes. The stain is ready for use immediately after preparation and should be stored in a tightly stoppered bottle.
   b. A precipitate will form during storage. This should not be disturbed; rather, remove the staining solution from the top with a pipette.
   c. Shelf life of the staining solution is 1 week at room temperature, 1 month in the refrigerator, and indefinite if frozen.

B. Ryu method
1. Solution
   a. 5% phenol, 10.0 mL
   b. Powdered tannic acid, 2.0 g
   c. Saturated aluminum potassium sulfate 12-hydrate (crystals) (prepare 14 g potassium alum in 100 mL distilled H_2O), 10.0 mL
2. Solution II
   a. Saturated solution of crystal violet in alcohol (prepare 12 g in 100 mL of 95% ethanol)
3. Final stain
   a. Ten parts of solution I (mordant) are mixed with one part of solution II and stored in a plastic bottle at room temperature

III. Quality Control

The following bacterial species may serve as controls:

A. Positive: peritrichous, *Escherichia coli;* polar, monotrichous, *Pseudomonas aeruginosa;* multitrichous, *Burkholderia cepacia*

B. Negative: *Acinetobacter baumannii*

IV. Procedure

A. Leifson method

1. Using a young culture on an appropriate agar medium, prepare a light suspension of the bacteria in water.

2. Place 2 drops of the bacterial suspension toward one end of an acid-cleaned microscope slide. Allow to air dry. With a wax pencil, draw a perpendicular line on the glass surface toward the opposite end from the dried suspension.

3. Place the slide on a tilted rack and overlay the dried bacterial suspension with a thin film of stain. The wax pencil mark prevents the stain from running off the end of the slide.

4. Stain for 5 to 15 minutes, allowing a precipitate to form as the alcohol evaporates. The staining time is decreased if the stain is fresh, if the room temperature is high, if there are air currents in the laboratory, or if the layer of stain is thin. The opposite effects increase the staining time.

5. When a precipitate forms, rinse the slide gently with distilled water, drain off excess water, and allow to air dry.

B. Ryu method

1. Prepare the smear by picking up some young growth from carbohydrate-free culture medium on an inoculating needle and lightly touching the center of each of 2 drops of distilled water on a new, precleaned slide. Let the drops air dry at room temperature.

2. Flood the air-dried smears with the staining solution for 1 to 5 minutes (some trial and error may be needed to determine the time that best produces satisfactory staining of the flagella, but avoids excessive debris in the background). Wash the staining solution off in tap water.

3. After the smears have dried, examine them under the oil immersion objective of the microscope. Cell bodies and flagella stain violet.

V. Results

A. Interpretation

Observe the stained slide under the oil immersion (100 ×) objective of the microscope. Dark-staining red to blue-black flagella should be observed. Compare morphology with the photomicrographs provided in Leifson's *Atlas of Bacterial Flagellation*, cited in the bibliography, and see also, Fig. 5-3.

VI. Bibliography

Clark WA: A simplified Leifson flagella stain. J Clin Microbiol 3:632–634, 1976
Leifson E: Atlas of Bacterial Flagellation. New York, Academic Press, 1960
Ryu E: A simple method of staining bacterial flagella. Kitasato Arch Exp Med 14:218–219, 1937

CHART 30   FLUORESCENCE–DENITRIFICATION

I. Principle

The ability to produce fluorescein pigment and to reduce nitrate or nitrite completely to nitrogen gas are two important characteristics in the identification of the pseudomonads and other nonfermentative bacilli. Fluorescence denitrification (FN) medium is formulated to detect these two characteristics. Fluorescence–lactose nitrate (FLN) medium is a modification in which lactose and phenol red indicator are added to permit detection of acid formed from utilization of lactose, which is helpful in identifying the strongly lactose-positive group of nonfermenters.

A. Fluorescence test

Fluorescein is an organic luminescent pigment that on excitation with ultraviolet light emits a green-yellow fluorescence. A few of the nonfermentative bacilli, notably *Pseudomonas aeruginosa*, are capable of producing fluorescein, detection of which is helpful in their identification. Fluorescence of colonies may not be detected on an ordinary isolation medium, such as blood agar or MacConkey agar; rather, media containing cationic salts, such as magnesium sulfate (included in FN medium), which act as activators or coactivators to intensify luminescence, often must be used.

B. Denitrification test

The reduction of nitrate to nitrogen gas (N_2) or nitrous oxide (N_2O) is called denitrification and is shown by the following chemical equation:

$$2\,NO_3^- + 10\,e^- + 12\,H^- \rightarrow N_2 \uparrow + 6\,H_2O$$

In this reduction process, five electrons are accepted by the nitrate radical, resulting in formation of nitrogen gas and six molecules of water. The denitrification test is helpful in the separation of *Pseudomonas stutzeri* group (most strains are positive) from other nonfermentative bacilli (see Table 5–6).

II. Media and Reagents

A. The formula for FN medium is as follows:

Proteose peptone 3 (Difco Laboratories, Detroit MI)	1 g
Magnesium sulfate $\cdot 7H_2O$	0.15 g
Dipotassium hydrogen phosphate	0.15 g
Potassium nitrate	0.2 g
Sodium nitrite	0.05 g
Agar	1.5 g
Distilled water to	100 mL

pH = 7.2

1. Suspend all the ingredients except the magnesium sulfate in distilled water. The magnesium sulfate is dissolved separately in a small amount of water before adding to the agar medium to avoid the formation of an insoluble precipitate.
2. If FLN medium is to be prepared, add 2 g of lactose and 0.002 g of phenol red indicator. Dispense 4 mL of medium into 13-mm screw-cap tubes and let solidify to give a deep and a slant of approximately equal length.
3. Sellers medium, available commercially, is also suitable for determination of fluorescence and denitrification by nonfermentative bacteria.

B. The formula for nitrate/nitrite reduction medium is as follows:

Heart infusion broth (Difco Laboratories, Detroit MI),*	25 g
Potassium nitrate C.P.	2 g
Distilled water to	1 L

pH = 7.0

III. Quality Control

The following organisms are appropriate controls:

Positive fluorescence/positive denitrification: *Pseudomonas aeruginosa*
Negative fluorescence/positive denitrification: *Pseudomonas stutzeri*
Negative fluorescence/negative denitrification: *Escherichia coli*

IV. Procedure

Inoculate the medium by stabbing the deep with a heavy suspension of the culture and then streaking the slant. Incubate at 35°C for 24 to 48 hours.

V. Results

A. Interpretation

Examine the tube for fluorescence with an ultraviolet light source (Wood's lamp). A bright yellow-green glow constitutes a positive test. The presence of gas bubbles in the deep of the medium indicates that nitrogen gas has been produced from denitrification, and a yellow slant with FLN medium indicates acid has been produced from the utilization of lactose by the microorganism. In broth medium, nitrogen gas formation is detected by noting the presence of a gas bubble in the upper portion of the inverted Durham tube, Color Plate 5-2B.

VI. Bibliography

Pickett MJ, Pedersen MM: Screening procedure for partial identification of nonfermentative bacilli associated with man. Appl Microbiol 16:1631–1632, 1968

*Agar is omitted from broth medium and inverted Durham tubes added to detect gas.

CHART 31 FLUORESCENT STAIN: AURAMINE O; AURAMINE–RHODAMINE

I. Principle

Acid-fast organisms emit a bright yellow fluorescence when activated with a short-wave ultraviolet light. The potassium permanganate counterstain causes the nonspecific background debris to fluoresce a pale yellow, in contrast with the bright yellow appearance of acid-fast bacilli.

II. Specimen

Smear prepared either directly from the specimen or from a suspension of organisms obtained from colonies grown on primary culture media.

III. Materials

A. Equipment
   1. 3″ × 1″ glass slides

B. Reagents
   1. Auramine O
      a. Solution 1: Dissolve 1.5 g of Auramine O in 10 mL of 95% ethanol.
      b. Solution 2: Dissolve 3.0 g of phenol crystals in 87 mL of distilled water
      c. Working solution: Combine solutions 1 and 2. Label with name of reagent and dates of preparation and expiration. Shelf life is 3 months if stored in a brown bottle.
   2. Auramine–rhodamine
      a. Solution 1: Dissolve 1.5 g of Auramine O and 0.75 g of rhodamine B in 75 mL of glycerol
      b. Solution 2: Mix 10 mL of phenol with 50 mL distilled water
      c. Working solution: Combine solutions 1 and 2 and mix for 24 hours with a magnetic stirrer. Filter stain through glass wool and store in a glass bottle. Affix a label with the name of the reagent and dates of preparation and expiration. Shelf life is 3 months if stored in a brown bottle.
   3. Permanganate counterstain: 0.5%
      a. Dissolve 0.5 g of potassium permanganate in 100 mL distilled water.
      b. Affix a label with the name of the reagent and dates of preparation and expiration.
   4. 0.5% acid alcohol decolorizer
      a. Add 0.5 mL of concentrated hydrochloric acid to 100 mL of 70% ethanol.
      b. Affix label with name of reagent and dates of preparation and expiration.
      c. Shelf life is 3 months when stored at room temperature.

C. Special Supplies
   1. Fluorescent microscope fitted with a BG-12 or 52112 primary filter and an OG-1 barrier filter.

D. Biosafety Instructions
   1. Handle all slides carefully. Heat fixing may not kill all of the mycobacteria. Dispose all slides into a biohazard container.
   2. Heat-sterilize bacteriologic loops in the electric incinerator contained in the biologic safety hood.
   3. Perform all operations in a biosafety hood. Place a paper towel soaked with disinfectant under the field of operation. Thoroughly clean all work surfaces with a disinfectant solution before and after use:
   4. Carcinogenic—AB
   5. Work under the hood in the special chemistry laboratory

IV. Quality Control

A. Control Materials To Be Used

A positive and negative control smear for mycobacteria is included with each run of stains. Control slides are reviewed before the patient smears are read to confirm that the positive control contains mycobacteria that fluoresce and that the negative smear has no fluorescing cells.
   1. Positive control: *Mycobacterium* spp; bacilli with yellow to orange fluorescence

2. Negative control: *Nocardia asteroides*; no fluorescing cells

If either control smears are unacceptable, reagent preparations and procedure are checked

V. Procedure
1. Heat fix smears on slide warmer at 72° to 75°C.
2. Flood surface of the smear with Auramine O stain. Let stand at room temperature for 15 minutes.
3. Rinse with tap water. Drain.
4. Decolorize with 0.5% acid alcohol for 2 minutes.
5. Rinse with tap water. Drain.
6. Flood smear for 2 minutes with 0.5% potassium permanganate counterstain.
7. Rinse with tap water. Drain.
8. Air dry. *Do not blot.*
9. Observe the smear as soon as possible using the fluorescent microscope. If there is a delay, refrigerate the smears at 4°C in the dark.

VI. Results

A. Interpretation (Readout or Calculations)

Acid-fast bacilli (AFB) are 1 to 10 μm long, and appear as slender, rod-shaped bacilli emitting a bright yellow fluorescence, against the pale yellow background. First scan the smears briefly with the 25× objective; move to the 63× objective to confirm the bacterial morphology of any suspicious fluorescing forms. Thoroughly examine each slide for the presence of acid-fast bacilli. Mycobacteriologists recommend that a minimum of 100 fields be examined before a smear is reported as negative. Three passes along the long axis of the slide or nine passes along the short axis usually provides ample area for reading, and minimizes the possibility of reading the same area more than once.

B. Reporting Format

The American Lung Association recommends the following method for fuchsin stains, also applicable to fluorescent stains:

Number of Bacilli	Report
0	No AFB seen
1–2 on entire smear	Report number seen and ask for repeat
1–9 per 10 fields	Rare or 1+
1–9 per field	Few or 2+
10–90 per field	Numerous or 3+
>90 per field	4+

VII. Procedure Notes

Fluorochrome-stained smears may be directly restained with any of the carbolfuchsin staining procedures. This is done to confirm positive slides and to study the morphology of the organisms present.

VIII. Limitation of Procedure

Organisms other than mycobacteria, including *Rhodococcus* spp., *Nocardia* spp., *Legionella micdadei*, and the cysts of *Cryptosporidium* and *Isospora* spp. may demonstrate varying degrees of acid-fastness. These can often be suggested by differences in morphology; recovery of contaminating bacteria in subcultures may be necessary in equivocal cases.

Rapidly growing mycobacteria may vary in their abilities to retain acid-fast dyes. Most species will not fluoresce in fluorochrome-stained smears and a carbolfuchsin procedure is recommended.

Dead acid-fast bacilli may still stain positive in fluorescent stains, a feature that must be considered when using smears to assess efficacy of treatment.

IX. Bibliography

Joseph SW, Vaichulis EMK, Houk VN: Lack of Auramine Rhodamine fluorescence of Runyon Group IV mycobacteria. Am Rev Respir Dis 95:114–115, 1967

Koneman EW, Allen SD, Janda WM, Schreckenberger PC, Winn WC Jr: Color Atlas and Textbook of Diagnostic Microbiology, 4th ed, pp 713–715, Philadelphia, JB Lippincott, 1992

Pollock HM, Wieman EJ: Smear results in the diagnosis of mycobacteriosis using blue light fluorescence microscopy. J Clin Microbiol 5:329–331, 1977

Uribe-Botero G, Prichard JG, Kaplowitz HJ: Bone marrow in HIV infections: A comparison of fluorescent staining and culture in the detection of mycobacteria. Am J Clin Pathol 91:313–315, 1989

CHART 32 FLUORESCENT TREPONEMAL ANTIBODY ABSORBTION TEST (FTA-ABS)

I. Principle

The fluorescent treponemal antibody-absorption test (FTA-ABS) is an indirect fluorescent antibody technique (see Chap. 21). The patient's serum, which has been diluted 1:5 in sorbent (an extract from cultures of *Treponema phagadenis*, the Reiter treponeme), is layered on a microscope slide to which *T. pallidum* subsp. *pallidum* has been fixed. If the patient's serum contains antibody to *T. pallidum*, it will coat the treponeme. When fluorescein isothiocyanate (FITC)-labeled antihuman globulin is added, it will fix to any patient's antibodies that have become affixed to the spirochete. The fluorescent reaction is visible when viewed by fluorescence microscopy.

II. Materials

A. Equipment

Incubator, 35° to 37°C
Water bath, adjustable to 56°C
Safety pipetting devices
Micropipettors delivering 10 to 200 µL
Loop, bacteriologic standard, 2 mm, 26 gauge, platinum
Bibulous paper
Slide board with moist chamber and paper towels
Staining dishes, glass or plastic, with removable slide carriers
Microscope slides, 1 × 3 in., with frosted end, 1-mm thick, with two etched circles, 1 cm inside diameter
Coverslips, No. 1, 2-mm square
Test tubes (12 × 75 mm) and holders
Discard containers and disinfectants
Disposable latex gloves, safety glasses and protective clothing
Fluorescence microscope set up for fluorescein microscopy
Mixer; Vortex Jr. or equivalent

B. Reagents

1. Purchased

a. *T. pallidum* antigen: A suspension of *T. pallidum* (Nichols strain) extracted from rabbit testicular tissue and washed in phosphate-buffered saline to remove rabbit globulin.

b. Fluorescein isothiocyanate (FITC)-labeled antihuman IgG.

c. Sorbent: Prepared from cultures of nonpathogenic Reiter treponemes, usually with no preservative added. Frequently dispensed in 5 mL amounts and freeze-dried, but also sold in liquid state.

d. Reactive control serum: A pool of human serum samples obtained from syphilitic donors that are 4+ reactive. Used to prepare 4+ serum controls and minimally reactive 1+ control. The 1+ control demonstrates the minimal degree of fluorescence reported as reactive and is used as a reading standard.

e. Nonspecific control serum: A serum pool obtained from nonsyphilitic individuals. No preservative is added. This control demonstrates a ≥2+ nonspecific reactivity at a 1:5 dilution in PBS and essentially no staining when diluted 1:5 in sorbent.

f. Oil: Low fluorescence, nondrying, immersion oil, type A, Cargille No. 1248.

g. Acetone: ACS reagent grade.

2. Prepared
    a. Phosphate-buffered saline, pH 7.2.
    b. 2% Tween-80 (polysorbate 80) in PBS. Heat the reagents in a 56°C water bath. To 49 mL of sterile PBS, add 1 mL of Tween-80, by measuring from the bottom of a pipette and rinsing the pipette in the mixture. Check pH and adjust to pH 7.2 with 1 N NaOH. Discard if a precipitate develops or the pH changes.
    c. Mounting medium: Add 1 part PBS to 9 parts glycerin (reagent grade).
    d. Distilled water.

III. Preparing Test Reagents

A. *T. pallidum Antigen*
    1. Rehydrate antigen according to manufacturer's instructions. Opened vials, stored at 2° to 8°C, are stable for 1 week.
    2. To prepare slides, mix antigen suspension thoroughly on a mixer for 10 seconds. Determine by darkfield examination that treponemes are adequately dispersed before making slides for the FTA-ABS test.
    3. Wipe slides with clean gauze to remove dust particles. Clean slides by sonic vibration or alcohol wiping if treponemes are not clearly observed after staining.
    4. Prepare very thin *T. pallidum* antigen smears within each circle by using a 2-mm wire loop. Place one loop of antigen within the two 1-mm circles. Allow to air dry at least 15 minutes.
    5. Fix slides in acetone for 10 minutes and air dry. Fix no more than 60 slides with 200 mL of acetone. Store acetone-fixed smears at −20°C. Do not thaw and refreeze smears.
    6. Store unopened vials of antigen at 2° to 8°C. The unopened antigen is stable until the expiration date.

B. *Titration of Antihuman IgG Globulin*
    1. Rehydrate conjugate according to directions. If the conjugate is cloudy, centrifuge it at 500 × g for 10 minutes. Aliquot in small volumes and store at −20°C. Do not refreeze thawed conjugate, but store at 2° to 8°C.
    2. Prepare 4+ and 1+ dilutions of the reactive control serum to determine conjugate working dilution.
    3. Run the control pattern with a reference or a known conjugate. An example is shown:

Conjugate Dilutions	Nonspecific Staining Control (PBS)	Reactive (4+) Control Serum (1:5 in PBS)	Reaction (1+) Control Serum
Reference Conjugate			
Dilution 1:400	−	4+	1+
New Conjugate			
1:12.5	<1+	4+	3+
1:25	−	4+	3+
1:50	−	4+	3+
1:100	−	4+	2+
1:200*	−	4+	1+
1:400	−	4+	<1+
1:800	−	3+	±

*The dilution selected for the working titer is 1:200, one doubling dilution below the 4+ endpoint (1:400), 1 + staining with the 1 + control dilution (1:200), and no nonspecific staining for three doubling dilutions below the working dilution (1:25).

C. *Sorbent*
    1. Rehydrate freeze-dried material with sterile distilled water or according to manufacturer's instructions. The rehydrated sorbent may be stored at 2° to 8°C or at −20°C. It can be used as long as acceptable reactivity is obtained and the product is not contaminated.

D. *Test Serum*
    1. Observe recommended safety precautions for handling human serum.
    2. Heat the test and control sera at 56°C for 30 minutes before testing.
    3. Reheat previously heated test sera for 10 minutes at 56°C on the day of testing.

E. *Control Test*
1. Rehydrate serum according to manufacturer's instructions.
2. Aliquot in 0.25 mL amounts and store at −20° for as long as acceptable reactivity is obtained.
3. Prepare the following controls for each test run:
   a. Reactive (R) 4+ control serum: a syphilitic serum showing 4+ fluorescence in the unabsorbed test and only slightly reduced fluorescence in the absorbed test. To produce unabsorbed serum, add 50 μL of reactive control serum into a tube containing 200 μL PBS and mix well. To produce absorbed serum, transfer 50 μL of Reactive control serum into a tube containing 200 μL of sorbent and mix well.
   b. Minimally reactive (MR) control serum: This is a dilution in PBS of the reactive control serum, which will give the minimal degree of fluorescence (1+) considered reactive.
   c. Nonspecific (NS) control serum: a nonsyphilitic serum showing ≥2+ fluorescence in the unabsorbed test. To produce the unabsorbed serum, transfer 50 μL of nonspecific control serum into a tube containing 200 μL of PBS and mix well. To produce the absorbed serum, transfer 50 μL of nonspecific control serum into a tube containing 200 μL of nonspecific control serum into a tube containing 200 μL of sorbent and mix well.
   d. Controls for nonspecific staining by conjugate consist of an antigen smear overlaid with 30 μL of PBS in place of serum and an antigen smear overlaid with 30 μL of sorbent in place of serum.

F. *The FTA-ABS Test*

1. Identify previously prepared antigen slides by numbering the frosted end.
2. Number each tube and slide to correspond to the test serum and the control serum to be used.
3. Prepare reactive (4+), minimally reactive (1+), and nonspecific control serum dilutions in sorbent or PBS according to the directions.
4. Pipette 200 μL of sorbent into a test tube for each test serum.
5. Add 50 μL of the heated test serum to the appropriate tube and mix eight times.
6. Cover the appropriate antigen smears with 30 μL of the reactive (4+), minimally reactive (1+), and nonspecific control serum dilutions.
7. Cover the appropriate antigen smears with 30 μL of the PBS and 30 μL of the sorbent for nonspecific-staining controls a and b. The controls should give the following pattern:

CONTROL PATTERN FOR THE FTA-ABS TEST

Reactive control	a. 1:5 PBS dilution	R4+
	b. 1:5 Sorbent dilution	R(4+−3+)
Minimally reactive control	1+ Control dilution	R1+
Nonspecific serum	a: 1:5 PBS dilution	R(2+−4+)
controls	b. 1:5 Sorbent dilution	N−±
Nonspecific-staining	a. Antigen, PBS, conjugate	N
controls	b. Antigen, sorbent, conjugate	N

8. Cover the appropriate antigen smears with 30 μL of the test serum dilutions.
9. Prevent evaporation by placing slides in a moist chamber and incubate at 35° to 37°C for 30 minutes.
10. At the completion of the incubation perform the following rinses:
    a. Place slides in slide carriers and rinse 5 seconds with running PBS.
    b. Place slides in staining dish containing PBS for 5 minutes.
    c. Agitate slides by dipping them in and out of the PBS at least 30 times.
    d. Using fresh PBS, repeat the above two steps.
    e. Rinse slides for 5 seconds in running distilled water and gently blot with bibulous paper.
11. Dilute FITC-labeled antihuman IgG to its working titer in PBS containing 2% Tween-80 and place approximately 30 μL of the diluted conjugate on each smear.
12. Repeat incubation and rinsing of slides.
13. Mount slides immediately by placing a small drop of mounting medium on each smear and applying a cover glass.

14. Place slides in a darkened room and read within 4 hours.
15. Check smear by darkfield microscopy using the tungsten lamp first, to verify the presence of treponemes on the smear, then read FITC (test) fluorescence.
16. Using the minimally reactive (1+) control slide as the reading standard, record the intensity of fluorescence of the treponemes:

RECORDING INTENSITY OF FLUORESCENCE

Reading	Intensity of Fluorescence
2+ to 4+	Moderate to strong
1+*	Equivalent to minimally reactive (1+) control
± to <1+	Visible staining but less than 1+
−	None or vaguely visible but without distinct fluorescence
Atypical**	Varied: treponemes appear to be "moth eaten" or to have "beads" of fluorescence throughout their length

*Retest all specimens that initially give a 1+ intensity of fluorescence.
**Atypical or beaded pattern of fluorescence has been described in patients with lupus and other autoimmune diseases.

17. Report the result as follows:

REPORTING SYSTEM FOR FTB-ABS TEST

Initial Test Reading	Repeat Test Reading	Report
4+		Reactive
3+		Reactive
2+		Reactive
1+	>1+	Reactive
1+	1+	Reactive Minimal*
1+	<1+	Nonreactive
<1+		Nonreactive
N		Nonreactive
Beaded fluorescence		Atypical Fluorescence Observed**

*In the absence of evidence of treponemal infection, this test result should be considered equivocal. A second specimen should be obtained 1–2 weeks after the initial specimen and submitted to the laboratory for serologic testing.
**Beaded fluorescence has been observed in serum from patients with active systemic lupus erythematosus and from patients with other autoimmune diseases. The DNA absorption procedure can be requested from the Treponemal Pathogenesis and Immunobiology Branch, Division of Sexually Transmitted Diseases, CDC, Atlanta, GA 30333. The request must be routed through the appropriate State Health Department.

IV. Acceptable Variations

1. Reading of slides may be delayed beyond 4 hours if slides are protected from light and stored at 2° to 8°C. For the test to be valid with a delayed reading, *the complete control pattern must be clearly satisfactory when the slides are read.*

2. Conjugate that has been filter-sterilized and contains a preservative, such as sodium azide, to prevent bacterial contamination may be stored at 2° to 8°C. Any precipitate or cloudiness must be removed by centrifugation.

3. Slides may be held from 30 minutes to 1 hour in PBS if the test is interrupted. For the results to be valid, control slides must react appropriately when the test is read.

4. Multicircle slides may be used rather than the two-circle slide. Add only 10 μL volumes to the antigen smears. Exercise care in handling and washing slides to prevent serum runover.

5. With accurate micropipettors, the 1:5 test dilution may be prepared by pipetting 25 μL of serum into 100 μL of diluent.

V. Sources of Error

1. If reagent evaluation procedures are not strictly followed, results will be unreliable.

2. If multicircle slides are used and serum from one well is allowed to run onto another well, serum from a person without syphilis may appear reactive.

3. If microscope slides are not clean, the test may be difficult to read and the results unreliable.

4. If the FTA-ABS test is used as a screening procedure, rather than to confirm the reactive results of a nontreponemal test, or as a specific diagnostic test in patients with signs or symptoms of late syphilis, the positive predictive value of the FTA-ABS test is decreased.

5. If the microscope is not properly aligned and the control pattern is not obtained, the test results are invalid.

6. If reagents become bacterially contaminated, the antibody may be reduced and the results may be invalid.

7. If reagent storage instructions are not followed, the reagents will not produce satisfactory control results.

8. If frozen antigen slides are thawed and refrozen, the treponemes will be difficult to see and the test results will be unsatisfactory.

9. If a serum is bacterially contaminated or is excessively hemolyzed, the test results may be invalid.

10. If antigen slides are not dried and stored according to the procedure or if too much volume is placed on the slide, the antigen may wash off. One loop of antigen is sufficient for two 1-cm circles.

11. If too many smears are fixed in a given volume of acetone, the background staining may be increased.

12. If rehydrated antigen does not adhere to the slide, too few treponemes may be observed.

13. If a precipitate is observed in conjugate preparation, nonspecific staining may be observed.

14. If the atypical staining pattern of beaded fluorescence is not recognized, these specimens may be incorrectly reported as reactive.

15. If FTA-ABS slides are read on a microscope equipped with incident illumination, the nonreactive slides must be examined by darkfield examination for the presence of treponemes.

VI. Test Limitations

1. The FTA-ABS test is not intended for routine use or as a screening procedure. Its greatest value is in distinguishing true-positive nontreponemal results from false-positive results and to establish the diagnosis of late latent or late syphilis.

2. Problems arise when the FTA-ABS test is used as a screening procedure, because approximately 1% of the general population will be falsely positive.

3. Although false-positive results in the FTA-ABS test are often transient and the cause is unknown, a definite association has been made between false-positive FTS-ABS results and the diagnosis of discoid, systemic, and drug-induced varieties of lupus erythematosus.

4. Unexplained FTA-ABS reactive results may occur in elderly patients.

VII. Bibliography

Larson SA, Hunter EF, Kraus SJ (eds). Manual of Tests for Syphilis (8th ed). Washington DC, American Public Health Association, 1990

CHART 33 FURAZOLIDONE DISK TEST

I. Principle

There are several methods available for differentiation of staphylococci from micrococci (Table 11–3). One of these is susceptibility to the compound furoxone (also called furazolidone). This test is performed as a disk susceptibility procedure: staphylococci are susceptible to this compound, whereas micrococci are resistant.

II. Reagents
1. Furazolidone disks, 100 µg (FX 100, BD Microbiology Systems)
2. Sheep blood agar plate

III. Quality Control

Known strains of *Staphylococcus* (either *S. aureus* or a coagulase-negative strain) and *Micrococcus* species should be tested with each new lot of disks, or on a weekly basis.

IV. Procedure
1. Prepare a suspension of the organism to be tested in sterile distilled water or broth. The suspension should be equivalent to a 0.5 MacFarland turbidity standard.
2. With a swab, spread the organism suspension onto one-half of a blood agar plate.
3. Aseptically place an FX disk in the center of the inoculated area, and gently tamp the disk so it adheres to the agar surface.
4. Incubate the plate at 35°C in an ambient air incubator for 18 to 24 hours.

V. Results

A. Interpretation
1. *Micrococcus* species are FX-resistant and will have zones of 6 mm (no zone) to 9 mm.
2. *Staphylococcus* species are FX-susceptible and will have zones of inhibition of 15 mm or larger.

CHART 34 GROWTH ON MACCONKEY AGAR

I. Principle

The ability to grow on special MacConkey agar, formulated without crystal violet, differentiates *M. fortuitum* and *M. cheloniae*, which can grow within 5 days, from other rapidly growing mycobacteria that show only slight growth after 11 days.

II. Specimen

A mature colony of the unknown *Mycobacterium* species recovered from clinical material, grown on an LJ slant or on Middlebrook 7H-10 agar is tested.

III. Materials

A. Equipment: None

B. Media: MacConkey agar without crystal violet. Purchased from Remel Laboratories. Stored in the walk-in refrigerator at 4°C.

C. Reagents: None

D. Supplies: None

IV. Quality Control

A. Positive control: *M. fortuitum* ATCC 6841

B. Negative control: *M. phlei* ATCC 11758; uninoculated medium and reagent only

V. Procedure
1. Inoculate a fresh MacConkey plate with 3 drops of the organism grown for 7 to 10 days in 7H9 broth and streak for isolation.
2. Incubate at 28° to 30°C for 11 days without CO_2.
3. At 5 and 11 days, visually observe the surface of the agar plate for the presence of colony growth.

VI. Results

A. Interpretation (Readout or Calculations)

A positive test for *M. fortuitum* will show growth along the entire streak area and possibly a color change in the medium in 5 days. The absence of growth indicates a negative test.

VII. Procedure Notes

Include controls with each batch of tests. If results are not as expected, repeat tests with fresh control organisms and a new lot of media.

VIII. Limitation of Procedure

About 25% of *M. smegmatus* strains grow on MacConkey agar without crystal violet. To obviate any diagnostic difficulties, the 3-day arylsulfatase test may be used to separate *M. smegmatus* (negative) from mycobacteria belonging to the *M. fortuitum–chelonae* complex (positive).

IX. Bibliography

Jones WD, Kubica GP: The use of MacConkey agar for differential typing of *M. fortuitum.* Am J Med Technol 30:182–195, 1946

Lutz B: Nitrate reduction. In Isenberg HD (ed): Clinical Microbiology Procedure Handbook, Mycobacteriology Section. Washington DC, American Society for Microbiology, 1992

CHART 35   HEMADSORPTION (HAD) TEST

I. Principle

The hemadsorption test is the simplest method of identifying the presence of an orthomyxovirus or paramyxovirus. Identification of the isolate may also be accomplished by testing inhibition of hemadsorption, but the hemagglutination inhibition (HAI) test is less cumbersome and is cheaper to perform.

Among the viruses that produce agglutination of red cells, the orthomyxoviruses and paramyxoviruses mature at the plasma membrane of infected cells. As they "bud" at the plasma membrane, they insert virally specified hemagglutinins into the membrane. The presence of infected cells in a monolayer can be detected by adherence of the red cells to the monolayer. Because some simian viruses that may be present in monkey tissue also produce hemagglutinins, it is important to include uninfected monolayers as controls.

II. Materials and Reagents

A. Infected and control primary monkey kidney cells

B. 0.4% solution of fresh, washed guinea pig erythrocytes in serum-free medium

III. Quality Control

A. Positive control (hemagglutinating virus)

B. Negative control (uninfected monolayer)

IV. Procedure

1. Add 0.2 mL of guinea pig erythrocytes for each 1 mL of medium.
2. Incubate in a slanted rack for 1 hour at 4°C.
3. Observe microscopically for agglutination in the fluid phase and adherence of erythrocytes to the monolayer.
4. Incubate the cultures for an additional 1 hour at 20°C.
5. Observe again for agglutination and adherence.

V. Results

A. Interpretation

Agglutination of erythrocytes in the fluid phase or adherence of red cells to the monolayer. If HAD occurs in the negative control, the test is invalid. Elution of erythrocytes at 20°C suggests the presence of parainfluenza virus 1–3.

VI Bibliography

Smith TF: Viruses. In Washington JA (ed): Laboratory Procedures in Clinical Microbiology, 2nd ed. New York, Springer-Verlag, 1985

CHART 36   HEMADSORPTION TEST FOR IDENTIFICATION OF *MYCOPLASMA PNEUMONIAE*

I. Principle

Among the respiratory mycoplasmas, *M. pneumoniae* is the only species that will specifically absorb red blood cells. This property, therefore, provides a method for the presumptive identification of *M. pneumoniae*.

When colonial growth is noted on mycoplasma isolation media inoculated with respiratory tract specimens, a suspension of guinea pig erythrocytes is placed on the agar surface for a given time, and then washed off. *M. pneumoniae* colonies will adsorb some of the red cells to the colony surface.

II. Reagents

A. Mycoplasma glucose agar with suspicious colonies present.

B. Washed guinea pig erythrocytes (0.2% to 0.4%) suspended in mycoplasma broth medium.

III. Quality Control

A. Positive control: *M. pneumoniae*

B. Negative control: *Mycoplasma* species

IV. Procedure

1. Flood the surface of the agar plate with 2 mL of the red cell suspension.
2. Incubate the plate at 35°C for 30 minutes and rotate the plate occasionally to prevent the red cells from settling out.
3. Wash the surface of the plate three times with 3 mL of mycoplasma broth by gently rotating the plate. Remove wash fluid by aspiration with a pipet.
4. Examine the colonies at 50 to 100× magnification under a dissecting microscope.

V. Results

A. Interpretation
1. Positive test: Colonies with RBCs adsorbed onto the surface = *M. pneumoniae*.
2. Negative: Colonies with no RBCs adsorbed = *Mycoplasma* species, not *M. pneumoniae*

VI. Bibliography

Manchee RJ, Taylor-Robinson D: Hemadsorption and hemagglutination by mycoplasmas. J Gen Microbiol 50:465, 1968

CHART 37   HEMAGGLUTINATION INHIBITION (HAI) TEST

I. Principle

The nucleic acids of many viruses encode surface proteins that agglutinate the red cells of a variety of species. The phenomenon is most commonly employed for diagnosis of infections produced by orthomyxoviruses, paramyxoviruses, and the arboviruses–togaviruses (including rubella), flaviviruses, and bunyaviruses. The presence of virus in infected cell cultures can be detected by hemagglutination; the identity of the virus or of antibodies in a patient's serum can be determined by specific inhibition of that hemagglutination. Although influenza viruses can be detected by hemadsorption (see Chart 35), typing of the isolate is done most efficiently by hemagglutination inhibition. Reagents and conditions for the test vary by virus.

Reaction of viral hemagglutinins with red cells results in a lattice of agglutinated cells which settle irregularly in a tube or microtiter well. Unagglutinated cells settle in a compact button.

II. Materials and Reagents

1. Red cells from an appropriate species (chicken, goose, guinea pig, trypsinized human O) collected in Alsever's solution or heparin
2. Diluent at appropriate pH
3. Solutions to remove nonspecific hemagglutinins from serum
4. Infected culture fluid or standard antigen for serology

III. Quality Control

A. Known positive serum

B. Known negative serum

C. Serum and cells without antigen (to detect nonspecific agglutination)

D. Back titration of hemagglutination activity of the antigen (to ensure that 4 HAU were tested)

IV. Procedure

A. Determination of Hemagglutinating Titer

1. A diluted suspension of red cells is incubated at 4°C or room temperature with serial dilutions of antigen until red cells in tubes without virus settle in a compact button (1 to 4 hours). The highest dilution that produces partial or complete agglutination represents 1 hemagglutinating unit (HAU).

B. Treatment of Sera

1. Removal of nonspecific inhibitors in sera is necessary for most viruses. Removal may be accomplished by physical means, such as kaolin; by enzymes, such as neuraminidase or the receptor-destroying enzyme (RDE) of *Vibrio cholerae;* or by a combination. The choice varies with the virus to be tested.

C. Inhibition Test

1. A dilution of antigen that contains 4 HAU is mixed with appropriate red cells and serial twofold dilutions of treated serum. The suspension is incubated as for the hemagglutination test.

V. Results

A. Interpretation

The end point is the last well at which partial or complete agglutination of the red cells occurs. A smooth or jagged shield of cells or an irregular button indicates agglutination. Observation of the movement of the button of red cells when the plate is tilted may help to clarify the end point.

VI. Bibliography

Hsiung GD: Diagnostic Virology, 3rd ed. New Haven, Yale University Press, 1982

Lennette EH, Schmidt NJ (eds): Diagnostic Procedures for Viral, Rickettsial, and Chlamydial Infections, 5th ed. Washington DC, American Public Health Association, 1979

Smith TF: Viruses. In Washington JA (ed): Laboratory Procedures in Clinical Microbiology, 2nd ed. New York, Springer-Verlag, 1985

CHART 38   HYDROLYSIS OF XANTHINE, HYPOXANTHINE, TYROSINE, AND CASEIN

I. Principle

Aerobic actinomycetes may be characterized by their ability to hydrolyze xanthine, hypoxanthine, tyrosine, and casein. These compounds are incorporated into nutrient agar, and the organisms are seeded heavily on the agar surface. Results are interpreted by observing for clearing of the medium under and around the bacterial growth, indicating hydrolysis.

II. Media and Reagents

A. Xanthine, hypoxanthine, and tyrosine suspensions

1. Basal Medium

Beef extract	3.0 g
Peptone	5.0 g
Agar	15.0 g
Distilled water	1 L

2. Suspensions

Tyrosine	0.5 g
Xanthine	0.4 g
Hypoxanthine	0.4 g
Distilled water	100 mL

Heat the basal medium to bring the ingredients into solution and place 100-mL aliquots into 250-mL flasks. Sterilize by autoclaving at 15 psi for 15 minutes. Allow medium to cool almost to solidification. To each aliquot, add 10 mL of xanthine, hypoxanthine, or tyrosine suspensions. The suspensions are autoclaved before adding to the basal media. It is essential that the granules of xanthine, tyrosine, and hypoxanthine be kept in suspension until the medium solidifies; hence, the addition of the biochemical granules and the pouring of the medium into petri dishes should be done when the basal medium has cooled just short of solidification. The media are poured into sterile 15 × 100-mm petri dishes.

   3. Casein Medium
      a. Solution A
         (1) Skim milk (powdered)   10.0 g
         (2) Distilled water   100 mL
      b. Solution B
         (1) Agar   2.0 g
         (2) Distilled water   100 mL

Autoclave solutions A and B separately, allow each to cool to about 50°C, and combine A with B and pour into 15 × 100-mm petri dishes.

III. Quality Control

   A. Negative controls: *Nocardia asteroides*

   B. Positive controls: *Streptomyces* species

IV. Procedure

Each xanthine, hypoxanthine, tyrosine, and casein plate is commonly divided into wedge-shaped thirds, providing an area to inoculate positive and negative controls along with the organism to be identified. The plates are incubated at 30°C and read at the following times:

   1. Casein hydrolysis   Read after 2 weeks
   2. Xanthine hydrolysis   Read after 3 weeks
   3. Hypoxanthine hydrolysis Read after 3 weeks
   4. Tyrosine hydrolysis   Read after 3 weeks

V. Results

   A. Interpretation

Casein hydrolysis is read by observing for a complete clearing to transparency of the white, milky medium. The other three hydrolysis tests are read by observing the dissolution of the crystalline compounds around the colonies growing on the media.

VI. Bibliography

Gordon RE, Mihm JM: Identification of *Nocardia caviae* (Erickson) nov. comb. Ann NY Acad Sci 98:628–636, 1962

CHART 39   **IMMUNOFLUORESCENCE TESTS**

I. Principle

Immunofluorescence tests provide a useful means of identifying viral antigen directly in clinical specimens and of providing specific immunologic identification of isolates in the laboratory. If the antigen is known, the presence of specific antibodies in a test serum may also be documented.

Antiserum is conjugated to fluorescein isothiocyanate. After incubation of antiserum and antigen, the presence of a reaction is detected by observation of fluorescence in a microscope that is equipped with a source of ultraviolet light. A sequence of filters is used to generate exciting light of optimal wavelength and to block light of harmful wavelengths before viewing.

II. Materials and Reagents
   1. Direct test: fluoresceinated specific globulin
   2. Indirect test: unconjugated specific globulin and fluoresceinated anti-immunoglobulin. Reagents are diluted to the optimal dilution (two- to fourfold below the last dilution that shows 3 to 4+ fluorescence with a known positive specimen)

3. Phosphate-buffered saline solution
4. Alkaline-buffered glycerol
5. High-quality fluorescence microscope. Epifluorescence with interference filters is preferred. A tungsten light source is adequate for fluorescein.

III. Quality Control

A positive and negative control should be included in each run or on each day of testing. The optimal controls are a specific antiserum that has been absorbed with the antigen of interest or blocked by an unlabeled specific serum.

IV. Procedure
1. The specimen is fixed to a scrupulously clean glass slide, usually by cold acetone, which increases accessibility of the immunoglobulin to intracellular structures. Testing of cell cultures for viruses is performed when CPE is 2+ to 3+; for *Chlamydia,* after incubation for 48 to 72 hours.
2. If antibody is to be tested, a known antigen is fixed to the slide, after which the indirect test is performed with the patient's serum as the first reagent.
3. In the direct test for antigen, the specific antiserum is conjugated to the fluorescent compound and reacted in a single step.
4. A two-step procedure is employed in the indirect test for antigen:
   a. A nonconjugated specific antibody is reacted.
   b. After washing to remove unreacted globulin, a fluorescent antibody to immunoglobulin of the species used for step 1 is reacted.
5. The incubation is performed in a moist chamber for 30 to 60 minutes at either room temperature or 37°C.
6. Slides are rinsed three times in PBS and mounted in alkaline-buffered glycerol.

V. Results

A. Interpretation

Specific fluorescence (usually >1+, preferably 3+ to 4+) that has the pattern expected of the antigen sought and is not present in the negative controls is a positive result (see Fig. 21–17).

VI. Bibliography

McIntosh K, Pierik L: Immunofluorescence in viral diagnosis. In Coonrod JD, Kunz LP, Ferraro MJ (eds): The Direct Detection of Microorganisms in Clinical Samples. Orlando FL, Academic Press, 1983

Riggs JL: Immunofluorescent staining. In Lennette EH, Schmidt NJ (eds): Diagnostic Procedures for Viral, Rickettsia, and Chlamydial Infections, 5th ed. Washington DC, American Public Health Association, 1979

CHART 40   INDOLE

I. Principle

Indole, a benzyl pyrrole, is one of the metabolic degradation products of the amino acid tryptophan. Bacteria that possess the enzyme tryptophanase are capable of hydrolyzing and deaminating tryptophan with the production of indole, pyruvic acid, and ammonia. Indole production is an important characteristic in the identification of many species of microorganisms, being particularly useful in separating *Escherichia coli* (positive) from members of the *Klebsiella–Enterobacter–Hafnia–Serratia* group (mostly negative).

The indole test is based on the formation of a red complex when indole reacts with the aldehyde group of *p*-dimethylaminobenzaldehyde. This is the active chemical in Kovac and Ehrlich reagents, shown in the Media and Reagents section. A medium rich in tryptophan must be used. In practice, combination media such as sulfide indole motility (SIM), motility indole ornithine (MIO), or indole nitrate are used. Rapid spot tests, using filter paper strips impregnated with *p*-dimethylaminocinnamaldehyde reagent, are useful in screening for bacteria that are prompt indole producers.

MECHANISM OF THE INDOLE REACTION

1 tryptophan → (tryptophanase) → indole + $H_3C-C(=O)-COOH$ + NH_3

tryptophan   (enzyme) →   indole   pyruvic acid   ammonia

2 indole + p-N,N-dimethylamino-benzaldehyde → (acid condensation) → Quinoidal red-violet compound + H_2O

indole   ρ-N,N-dimethylamino-benzaldehyde   →   Quinoidal red-violet compound di [4-(indole-3-yl-methylene)-2,5-cyclohexadien-1-ylidene]-dimethyl-ammonium salt (pink- red)   water

II. Media and Reagents

A. Tryptophan broth (1% tryptophan)

Peptone or pancreatic digest of casein (trypticase)	2 g
Sodium chloride	0.5 g
Distilled water	100 mL

B. Kovac reagent

Pure amyl or isoamyl alcohol	150 mL
p-Dimethylaminobenzaldehyde	10 g
Concentrated HCl	50 mL

C. Ehrlich's reagent

p-Dimethylaminobenzaldehyde	2 g
Absolute ethyl alcohol	190 mL
Concentrated HCl	40 mL

III. Quality Control

Each new batch of medium or reagent should be tested for positive and negative indole reactions. The following organisms serve well as controls:

A. Positive control: *Escherichia coli*

B. Negative control: *Klebsiella pneumoniae*

IV. Procedure

Inoculate tryptophan broth (or other suitable indole media) with the test organism and incubate at 35°C for 18 to 24 hours. At the end of this time, add 15 drops of reagent down the inner wall of the tube. If Ehrlich reagent is used, this step should be preceded by the addition of 1 mL xylene. This is not necessary with Kovac reagent.

V. Results

A. Interpretation

The development of a bright fuchsia red color at the interface of the reagent and the broth (or the xylene layer) within seconds after adding the reagent is indicative of the presence of indole and is a positive test (see Color Plates 4–4C and 5-2C).

VI. Bibliography

Blazevic DJ, Ederer GM: Principles of Biochemical Tests in Diagnostic Microbiology, pp 63–67, New York, John Wiley & Sons, 1975

Isenberg HD, Sundheim LH: Indole reactions in bacteria. J Bacteriol 75:682–690, 1958

MacFaddin JF: Biochemical Tests for Identification of Medical Bacteria, 2nd ed, pp 173–183. Baltimore, Williams & Wilkins, 1980

Miller JM, Wright JW: Spot indole test: Evaluation of four reagents. J Clin Microbiol 15:589–592, 1982

Vracko R, Sherris JC: Indole-spot test in bacteriology. Am J Clin Pathol 39:429–432, 1963

CHART 41   INHIBITION BY THIOPHENE-2-CARBOXYLIC ACID HYDRAZIDE (T$_2$H, 1 μg/mL)

I. Principle

Thiophene-2-carboxylic acid hydrazide has the property of inhibiting *M. bovis*, but not other species of mycobacteria, a helpful feature differentiating *M. bovis* from *M. tuberculosis*.

II. Specimen

A 3- to 4-week-old culture of the test organism growing on Lowenstein-Jensen medium or Middlebrook 7H10 agar.

III. Materials

A. Equipment
1. Biologic safety cabinet
2. 10% CO$_2$ incubator at 37°C

B. Supplies
1. Sterile applicator sticks
2. Sterile 9.0 mL water blanks
3. Sterile deionized water
4. Quadrant petri dishes

C. Media
1. TCH susceptibility medium (10 μg/mL)
   a. Make two 200-mL batches of Middlebrook 7H10 medium in separate flasks.
   b. Sterilize by autoclaving. Cool to 50°C in a water bath.
   c. Pipette 5.0 mL of cooled medium from one of the flasks into quadrants I and III of a quadrant petri dish.
   d. Add 2.0 mL of a 1000 μg/mL TCH stock solution into the remaining flask (final concentration of 10 μg/mL). Swirl well to mix.
   e. Dispense 5.0 mL of this medium into quadrants II and IV of each plate.
   f. Protect the plates from light by covering with brown paper. Store plates at 2° to 8°C; shelf life is approximately 1 month.

IV. Quality Control

A. Positive control: *M. bovis* ATCC 35734 (susceptible to TCH at 10 μg/mL)

B. Negative control: *M. tuberculosis* ATCC 25177 (resistant)

V. Procedure

1. Prepare a suspension of the unknown mycobacterium in sterile water equivalent to a McFarland 1 standard.
2. Dilute to make a suspension of 10^{-3} to 10^{-4} in sterile deionized water.
3. Inoculate 3 drops of each dilution onto a control quadrant and a TCH quadrant on the quadrant plates.
4. Cover the plates with brown paper to prevent exposure to light, letting the plates sit at room temperature to allow adsorption of the inoculum.
5. Place each plate into a CO$_2$-permeable zipper bag, invert the plates, and incubate at 37°C in 8% to 10% CO$_2$ for 3 weeks.
6. After incubation, count the colonies on the control quadrant and on the quadrant that contains the TCH at 10 μg/mL.

VI. Results

A. Calculate the percentage of resistance as follows:

Number of colonies on quadrant containing TCH × 100 =
percentage of colonies resistant on control quadrant

B. Record the test culture as resistant to TCH if the derived number is higher than 1%.

VII. Bibliography

Harrington R, Karlson AG: Differentiation between *M. tuberculosis* and *M. bovis* by in vitro procedures. Am J Vet Res 27:1193–1196, 1967

Lutz B: Identification tests for mycobacteria: Inhibition by thiophene-2-carboxylic acid hydrazide. In Isenberg HD (ed): Clinical Microbiology Procedure Handbook. Washington DC, American Society for Microbiology, 1992

Wayne LG, et al: Highly reproducible techniques for use in systematic bacteriology in the genus *Mycobacterium:* Tests for niacin and catalase and for resistance to isoniazid, thiophene 2-carboxylic acid hydrazide, hydroxylamine and *p*-nitrobenzoate. Int J Syst Bacteriol 26:311–318, 1976

CHART 42   IRON UPTAKE

I. Principle

The ability to take up iron from an inorganic iron-containing reagent helps to differentiate *Mycobacterium fortuitum* and *M. phlei* (positive) from *M. chelonae*, which does not take up iron.

II. Specimen

Mature colony of the unknown *Mycobacterium* species recovered from clinical material, grown on an LJ slant.

III. Materials

A. Equipment
   1. Biologic safety hood
   2. 28° to 30°C incubator
   3. Sterile Pasteur pipettes

B. Media
   1. Lowenstein-Jensen slants (purchased from Remel Laboratories)

C. Reagents
   20% ferric ammonium citrate
   1. Add 20 g of ferric ammonium citrate to 100 mL of deionized water
   2. Swirl to dissolve
   3. Autoclave for 15 minutes at 121°C
   4. Store in the refrigerator at 2° to 8°C

IV. Quality Control

A. Positive control: *M. fortuitum,* ATCC 6841

B. Negative control: *M. chelonae,* ATCC 35751; uninoculated medium and reagent only

V. Procedure
   1. Use an actively growing (1- to 2-week-old) subculture of a rapidly growing mycobacterium on a Lowenstein-Jensen slant.
   2. Add as many drops of sterile 20% ferric ammonium citrate as there are millileters of medium in the slant. For example, for 8 mL of medium, add 8 drops of ferric ammonium citrate.
   3. Reincubate the slant at 28° to 30°C for up to 3 weeks.
   4. Visually examine the surface of the slants for the presence of a dark, rust brown color.

VI. Results

The color of a truly positive iron uptake test will be very dark rust. A positive reaction seen in a rapidly growing strain of mycobacteria is indicative of *M. fortuitum.*

VII. Procedure Notes

If the results are not as expected, check the ages and purity of the control and test cultures. Repeat the tests with new ferric ammonium citrate reagent and new control cultures.

VIII. Limitation of Procedure

Some isolates of *M. chelonae* will turn tannish brown, a color sometimes referred to as "turtlelike," giving a false-positive reaction. Look for a very dark rust color.

IX. Bibliography

Lutz B: Iron uptake. In Isenberg HD (ed) Clinical Microbiology Procedure Handbook, Mycobacteriology Section. Washington DC, American Society for Microbiology, 1992
Silcox VA, Good RA, Floyd MM: Identification of clinically significant *Mycobacterium fortuitum* complex. J Clin Microbiol 14:686–691, 1981

CHART 43   LOEFFLERS' METHYLENE BLUE STAIN

I. Principle

Methylene blue is a simple stain that is particularly useful in the identification of *Corynebacterium* species.

The metachromatic granules of *C. diphtheriae* readily take up methylene blue dye and appear deep blue. Although some authors have stated that the cytoplasmic granule formation characteristic of *C. diphtheriae* is rarely seen with saprophytic species of *Corynebacterium*, this criterion is unreliable and cannot be used for definitive identification of *C. diphtheriae* without further studies.

II. Media and Reagents

Methylene blue (80% dye content)	0.3 g
Ethyl alcohol (95%)	30 mL
Distilled water	100 mL

III. Procedure
1. Heat-fix the smear. Flood the surface of the smear with the methylene blue-staining solution for 1 minute. Wash the slide with water and blot dry.
2. In the past it was necessary to add alkali to the above solution before use. However, methylene blue dyes prepared in recent years do not require this additional step because acid impurities found in older stains have been removed.

IV. Results

A. Interpretation

The corynebacteria are pleomorphic bacilli that range in size from 0.5 to 1.0 μm in width and from 2 to 6 μm in length and appear as straight, curved, or club-shaped rods. Characteristic for the microorganisms are the metachromatic granules that take up the methylene blue stain and appear dark blue. Although this finding is characteristic of the corynebacteria, species of *Propionibacterium*, some of the actinomycetes, pleomorphic strains of streptococci, and other bacteria may also morphologically resemble the corynebacteria and must be differentiated by other cultural and biochemical characteristics.

CHART 44   LOEFFLERS' SERUM MEDIUM

I. Principle

Loeffler's serum medium is used primarily for the recovery of *C. diphtheriae* from clinical specimens. Because of this serum content, the medium may also be used more generally to determine the proteolytic activity of various microorganisms.

C. diphtheriae produces cells with characteristic morphologic features on Loeffler medium. The medium is also helpful in the determination of pigment production by some bacteria.

II. Media and Reagents

A. Formula

Beef serum	70 g/L
Infusion dextrose broth (dry powder)	2.5 g/L
Egg (whole, dried)	7.5 g/L

Final pH = 7.6

B. Preparation

1. To rehydrate the medium, dissolve 80 g of Loeffler medium (BBL) in 1 L of distilled water and warm to 42° to 45°C. The powder should be gradually added while the flask is gently rotated to minimize mixing air into the suspension.

2. The medium should be dispensed in tubes and coagulated-sterilized in the autoclave as follows:

    a. When the suspension is uniform, dispense in tubes.

    b. Arrange the tubes in a slant position not more than four deep with several layers of newspaper or paper towels below and above the tubes to prevent rapid coagulation.

    c. Tightly close the autoclave, turn on the steam, and allow pressure to remain at 10 psi for 20 minutes.

    d. During this time allow no air or steam to escape.

    e. Adjust the steam inlet valve and open the air escape valve such as to maintain a pressure of 10 psi. Abrupt changes in pressure may cause the medium to bubble.

    f. Close the outlet valve when all air has been replaced by steam and allow the pressure to reach 15 psi and hold there for 15 minutes.

    g. Allow the autoclave to cool slowly. When properly prepared the slants are smooth and grayish white. The slants should be incubated before inoculation for 24 hours at 35°C as a sterility check.

III. Procedure

1. When *C. diphtheriae* is suspected, inoculate the Loeffler medium as soon as possible after collection of the specimen.

2. Examine the slants for growth after 8 to 24 hours of incubation.

3. Prepare smears and stain with methylene blue.

IV. Results

A. Interpretation

See Chart 43 for interpretation of these stained smears.

V. Comment

Because Loeffler medium is difficult to prepare, purchase of commercially prepared medium in sealed tubes is recommended.

VI. Bibliography

BBL Manual of Products and Laboratory Procedures, 5th ed, pp 118–119. Cockeysville MD, BBL, Division of Becton, Dickinson, and Co, 1973

Buck T: A modified Loeffler's medium for cultivating *Corynebacterium diphtheriae*. J Lab Clin Med 34:582–583, 1949

CHART 45   MANGANOUS CHLORIDE–UREA TEST FOR IDENTIFICATION OF *UREAPLASMA UREALYTICUM*

I. Principle

Of the human mycoplasmas, *U. urealyticum* is the only species that is able to hydrolyze urea to ammonia. This property not only facilitates isolation of the organism, but also provides a rapid and convenient way to identify the species in culture. The manganous chloride ($MnCl_2$)–urea test provides a visual method for detecting ammonia formation by *U. urealyticum*.

Urease activity of *U. urealyticum* is detected by exposing the colonies to a solution of $MnCl_2$ in the presence of urea. The urease of the organism hydrolyzes urea to ammonia, and then the following reaction occurs:

$$2NH_3 + 2 H_2O \rightarrow 2NH_4OH \rightarrow 2NH_4^+ + 2OH^-$$
$$MnCl_2 + 2OH^- \rightarrow MnO_2 + 2 HCl$$

The manganese oxide formed in the reaction is insoluble and forms a dark brown precipitate around the colonies. This reaction is then detected under a dissecting microscope.

II. Reagents

    A. $MnCl_2$–urea Reagent

Urea (Sigma, St Louis MO)	1.0 g
$MnCl_2$ (Fisher Scientific)	0.8 g
Distilled water	100 mL

    B. Sterilize by filtration, dispense in 3-mL aliquots, and freeze at $-20°C$

    C. Growth of suspect colonies on agar medium

III. Quality Control

    A. Positive control: *U. urealyticum*

    B. Negative control: *M. hominis*

IV. Procedure

    1. Flood the plate with 2 to 3 mL of the $MnCl_2$–urea reagent.

    2. After 5 minutes at room temperature, examine the colonies under 50 to 100× magnification with a dissecting microscope.

V. Results

    A. Interpretation

    Colonies of *U. urealyticum* will stain a dark brown. Other mycoplasmas (e.g., *M. hominis*) will remain unstained.

VI. Comments

This test works optimally on colonies that are not too crowded together on agar medium. Colonies should not be older than 48 hours when the test is performed.

VII. Bibliography

Shepard MC, Howard DR: Identification of "T" mycoplasmas in primary agar cultures by means of a direct test for urease. Ann NY Acad Sci 174:809, 1970

CHART 46   MEDIUM FOR ISOLATION OF *MYCOPLASMA PNEUMONIAE*

I. Base reagents for preparation of complete media

    A. Mycoplasma base agar: This medium may be prepared using commercial PPLO agar as directed according to the package insert, or may be prepared from raw materials using the following formula:

Beef heart infusion	50 g
Peptone	10 g
NaCl	5 g
Purified agar	14 g
Distilled water	1 L

    Mix together and melt the agar in a boiling water bath. Dispense in 70-mL aliquots and autoclave at 15 psi for 15 minutes. Store at 4°C.

    B. Yeast Extract

    1. Purchase commercial 25% yeast extract or prepare as follows: Weigh out 250 g of active bakers' yeast and place in 1 L of distilled water. Heat to boiling, cool, and filter to remove particulate matter. Adjust the pH to 8.0, and filter-sterilize.

    2. Yeast extract (20 mL) is then mixed with uninactivated horse serum (10 mL) in a 2:1 ratio and frozen in 30-mL aliquots at $-20°C$.

C. Phenol red solution (0.4%): Phenol red (1 g) is dissolved in 3 mL of 1 N NaOH and then 247 mL of distilled water is added. Solution is filter-sterilized and stored at 4° to 8°C.

D. Methylene blue solution (1%): Methylene blue (1 g) is dissolved in 100 mL distilled water and autoclaved for 15 minutes.

E. Thallium acetate solution (10%): Thallium acetate (10 g) is dissolved in 100 mL of distilled water and filter-sterilized.

F. Glucose solution: Glucose (50 g) is dissolved in 100 mL distilled water and filter-sterilized.

G. Penicillin solution: Penicillin powder is dissolved in distilled water to achieve a concentration of 100,000 units/mL.

II. Methylene Blue–Glucose Diphasic Medium
1. Melt 70 mL of mycoplasma agar in a boiling water bath. Cool to 50°C and add 30 mL prewarmed yeast extract–serum.
2. Add the following:

Methylene blue solution (1%)	0.1 mL
Phenol red solution (0.4%)	0.5 mL
Glucose solution	2.0 mL
Thallium acetate solution (10%)	0.25 mL
Penicillin solution	3.0 mL

3. Adjust the pH to 7.8 with sterile 1N NaOH.
4. Dispense agar in 1-mL aliquots into sterile 13 × 100-mm screw-capped tubes.
5. Mix 140 mL of mycoplasma broth (A, above, without agar) with 60 mL of the yeast extract–serum. Add the following to this mixture:

Methylene blue solution (1%)	0.2 mL
Phenol red solution	1.0 mL
Glucose solution	4.0 mL
Thallium acetate solution (10%)	6.0 mL
Penicillin solution	0.5 mL

Adjust the pH to 7.8 with sterile 1N NaOH. Dispense 2.0 mL into each of the tubes containing the solidified agar medium.

III. Mycoplasma Glucose Agar Medium
1. Melt 70 mL of mycoplasma agar in a boiling water bath. Cool to 50°C.
2. Prewarm 30 mL of yeast extract–serum and mix with the agar medium.
3. Aseptically add the following reagents:

Glucose solution	2.0 mL
Thallium acetate solution (10%)	0.25 mL
Penicillin solution	3.0 mL

4. Adjust the pH to 7.8 with sterile 1N NaOH.
5. Dispense 6 mL of medium into 60 × 15-mm petri dishes. Allow to cool. Store media at 4°C.

IV. SP-4 Medium (also used for culture of *M. pneumoniae*, but mostly for culture of highly fastidious species)
A. Basal medium

Mycoplasma Broth Base (BBL)	3.5 g/L
Bacto Tryptone (Difco)	10.0 g/L
Bacto Peptone (Difco)	5 g/L
Glucose	5.0 g/L
Deionized water	615 mL

Adjust to pH 7.5 to 7.6
Autoclave at 121°C, 15 minutes

B. Sterile supplements

CMRL 1066 Tissue Culture Supplement with glutamine (Gibco)	50.0 mL
Fresh yeast extract (25% solution)	35.0 mL
Yeastolate (2% solution)	100.0 mL
Fetal bovine serum (heated to 56°C for 1 hour)	170.0 mL
Penicillin (100,000 U/mL stock)	10 mL
Phenol red solution (0.1%, aqueous)	20 mL

C. Final formulation

Combine basal medium (615 mL) with supplements (385 mL) and dispense aseptically in 3-mL volumes into 4-mL, screw-capped vials.

V. Bibliography

Velleca WB, Bird BR, Forrester FT: Laboratory Diagnosis of *Mycoplasma* Infections. Atlanta, U.S. Department of Health and Human Services, 1980.

CHART 47   MEDIUM FOR ISOLATION OF THE GENITAL MYCOPLASMAS

I. U Broth and U agar for isolation of *Ureaplasma urealyticum*

A. U broth

1. Add the following to 70 mL of Mycoplasma broth base (BBL) (see Chart 46):

Yeast extract–horse serum	30 mL
Urea solution (50%)	0.1 mL
Phenol red solution (0.4%)	0.5 mL
Penicillin solution	0.5 mL
Polymyxin B solution (5000 µg/mL)	0.5 mL
Lincomycin solution (1500 µg/mL)	1.0 mL
Amphotericin B solution (5000 µg/mL)	0.1 mL

2. Adjust the pH to 6.0 with 1N HCl.
3. Dispense in 2-mL aliquots into sterile 12 × 75-mm screw-capped tubes or sterile 1-dram vials. Store at 4° to 8°C.

B. U agar

1. Add 30 g of trypticase–soy broth to 1 L distilled water. Add 11.3 g of purified agar (e.g., Noble agar, Ion agar 2) and heat to boiling to dissolve. Dispense into 80-mL aliquots and store refrigerated.
2. Melt 80 mL of the agar base in a boiling water bath and cool to 50°C. Adjust the pH to 6.0 with 1N HCl.
3. In a separate sterile flask, combine the following:

Horse serum	2.0 mL
Phenol red solution (0.4%)	0.5 mL
Urea solution (50%)	0.1 mL
Penicillin solution	0.5 mL
Lincomycin solution (1500 µg/mL)	1.0 mL

4. Add the agar to the contents of the flask, mix, and dispense 3-mL aliquots into 60 × 15-mm petri plates. Place in plastic bags and store at 4° to 8°C.

II. H broth and H agar for isolation of *Mycoplasma hominis*

A. H broth

1. Add the following to 70 mL of Mycoplasma broth base (BBL) (see Chart 46).

Yeast extract/horse serum	30 mL
L-Arginine hydrochloride (30%)	0.66 mL
Phenol red solution (0.4%)	0.5 mL
Penicillin solution	0.5 mL
Polymyxin B (5000 µg/mL)	1.0 mL
Amphotericin B (5000 µg/mL)	0.1 mL

2. Adjust the pH to 7.0 with 1N HCl.
3. Dispense in 2-mL aliquots into sterile 12 × 75-mm screw-capped tubes or 1-dram vials. Store at 4° to 8°C.

B. H agar

1. Melt 70 mL of mycoplasma agar base in a boiling water bath and let cool to 50°C.
2. Adjust the pH of the agar to 7.0 with 1N HCl.
3. Prewarm 30 mL of yeast extract–serum and add the following:

L-Arginine hydrochloride (30%)	0.66 mL
Phenol red solution (0.4%)	0.5 mL
Penicillin solution	0.5 mL

4. Mix the agar base with the yeast extract–serum and additives and dispense 3-mL aliquots into 60 × 15-mm agar plates. Store in plastic bags at 4° to 8°C.

III. Bibliography

Velleca WM, Bird BR, Forrester FT: Laboratory Diagnosis of Mycoplasma Infections. Atlanta, U.S. Department of Health and Human Services, 1980

CHART 48   **METHYL RED**

I. Principle

Methyl red is a pH indicator with a range between 6.0 (yellow) and 4.4 (red). The pH at which methyl red detects acid is considerably lower than the pH for other indicators used in bacteriologic culture media. Thus, to produce a color change, the test organism must produce large quantities of acid from the carbohydrate substrate being used.

The methyl red test is a quantitative test for acid production, requiring positive organisms to produce strong acids (lactic, acetic, formic) from glucose through the mixed acid fermentation pathway (see Fig. 4–2). Because many species of the *Enterobacteriaceae* may produce sufficient quantities of strong acids that can be detected by methyl red indicator during the initial phases of incubation, only organisms that can maintain this low pH after prolonged incubation (48 to 72 hours), overcoming the pH-buffering system of the medium, can be called methyl red positive.

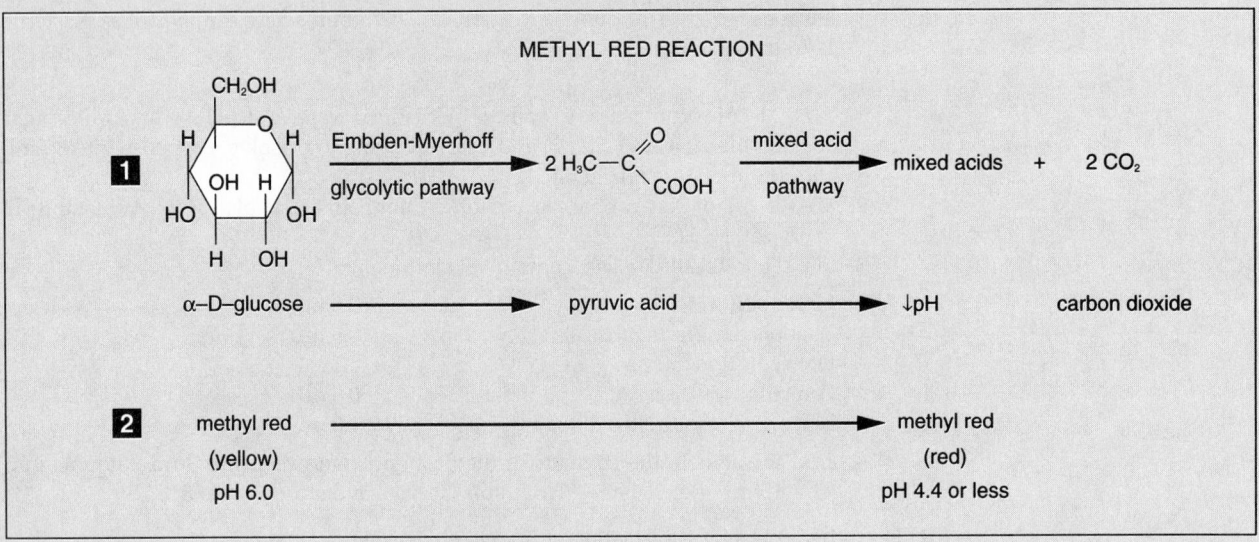

METHYL RED REACTION

II. Media and Reagents

The medium most commonly used is methyl red–Voges–Proskauer (MR/VP) broth, as formulated by Clark and Lubs. This medium also serves for the performance of the Voges–Proskauer test.

A. MR/VP broth

Polypeptone	7 g
Glucose	5 g
Dipotassium phosphate	5 g
Distilled water to	1 L
Final pH = 6.9	

B. Methyl red pH indicator

Methyl red, 0.1 g, in 300 mL of 95% ethyl alcohol
Distilled water, 200 mL

III. Quality Control

Positive and negative controls should be run after preparation of each lot of medium and after making each batch of reagent. Suggested controls include the following:

A. Positive control: *Escherichia coli*

B. Negative control: *Enterobacter aerogenes*

IV. Procedure

1. Inoculate the MR/VP broth with a pure culture of the test organism. Incubate the broth at 35°C for 48 to 72 hours (no fewer than 48 hours).
2. At the end of this time, add 5 drops of the methyl red reagent directly to the broth.

V. Results

A. Interpretation

The development of a stable red color in the surface of the medium indicates sufficient acid production to lower the pH to 4.4 and constitutes a positive test (see Color Plate 4–4C). Because other organisms may produce smaller quantities of acid from the test substrate, an intermediate orange color between yellow and red may develop. This does not indicate a positive test.

VI. Bibliography

Barry AL et al: Improved 18-hour methyl red test. Appl Microbiol 20:866–870, 1970

Blazevic DJ, Ederer GM: Principles of Biochemical Tests in Diagnostic Microbiology, pp 75–77. New York, John Wiley & Sons, 1975

Clark WM, Lubs HA: The differentiation of bacteria of the colon–aerogenes family by the use of indicators. J Infect Dis 17:160, 1915

MacFaddin JF: Biochemical Tests for Identification of Medical Bacteria, 2nd ed, pp 209–214. Baltimore, Williams & Wilkins, 1980

CHART 49

MICRODILUTION SERUM BACTERICIDAL TEST FOR MONITORING THERAPY OF BACTERIAL ENDOCARDITIS, OSTEOMYELITIS, AND GRAM-NEGATIVE BACTEREMIA

I. Principle

The serum bactericidal test has been used for many years, but with little evidence from well-designed prospective studies that the results correlated with clinical outcome. Results obtained with the following standardized test were statistically significantly correlated with bacteriologic cure in patients with bacterial endocarditis. The outcome of the infection, a more complex endpoint, was not predicted by the test. An association with a favorable clinical response has also been documented in patients with gram-negative bacteremia and with osteomyelitis.

The rationale of the serum bactericidal test is logical and intuitively appealing. The serum of a patient who is being treated for an infection is tested for in vitro activity against the very bacterial strain that produced the infection. The antibacterial activity comes principally from antibiotics in the serum. Antibody, complement, and other serum factors may also exert antibacterial effects, especially against gram-negative bacteria.

II. Materials and Reagents

1. Peak or trough serum specimen from patient. The serum should be tested fresh. If a delay of more than 2 hours is anticipated, the specimen should be frozen.
2. Isolate of infecting bacterium from patient
3. Mueller-Hinton broth supplemented with a 50 mg CA^{2+} and 20 mg Mg^{2+} per liter (MHB-S)
4. Pooled normal human serum. The serum should be screened for hepatitis B virus antigen and antibodies to human immunodeficiency virus (HIV). The pH of the serum should be adjusted to 7.3 to 7.4 with 0.1N NaOH or 0.1 N HCl, clarified by filtration through a 0.8-μm filter, and sterilized by filtration through a 0.45-μm filter. It should then be tested for antibacterial activity. A microbiologic assay may be done, or an MBC test, using the serum in the diluent, may be done with ATCC reference strains, using published guidelines for expected results in the presence of serum. β-Lactamase testing may be done by the acidometric method.
5. Nutrient broth, such as Mueller-Hinton broth or trypticase–soy broth, for preparation of inoculum
6. Microtiter plate
7. Micropipettes or droppers for delivering inoculum in 50 μL volume

8. Antibiotic-free agar, such as Mueller-Hinton agar, for subculture of broth–serum mixture
9. Multipoint inoculator with which to transfer the broth–serum mixture to agar for determination of bactericidal activity

III. Methods

A. Preparation of Serum Dilutions
1. Heat pooled normal serum at 56°C for 30 minutes to inactivate complement.
2. Prepare a 1:1 mixture of MHB-S and heat-inactivated human serum (MHB-S/HS).
3. In triplicate rows, add 50 μL of MHB-S/HS to wells 2 through 10.
4. Add 100 μL of patient's serum to well 1.
5. Remove 50 μL from well 1 and transfer to well 2. Mix by pipetting and transfer 50 μL to well 3. Continue through well 9. Discard the 50 μL of serum–broth mix from well 9. Note that the patient's serum is not transferred into well 10, which is a normal serum control. After the bacterial inoculum is added, serial dilutions of the test serum will range from 1:2 to 1:512.

B. Preparation of Inoculum
1. The inoculum is prepared as for the MIC test (see Chart 59). Inoculate a portion of five similar-appearing colonies into nutrient broth and incubate at 35°C until turbid (3 to 5 hours). Adjust the turbidity to that of a 0.5 McFarland standard.
2. Dilute the adjusted broth with MHB-S/HS so that each well will contain 5×10^5 CFU/mL (5×10^4 CFU per well). The adjustment will depend on the volume of inoculum introduced. A 0.05-mL pipette dropper may be used to deliver 50 μL to each well (to obtain 5×10^4 CFU in 50 μL, the inoculum should have a concentration of 1×10^6 CFU/mL; therefore, a 1:200 dilution of the 0.5 McFarland standard would be required).
3. Perform serial tenfold dilutions of the inoculum (10^2 to 10^4) in nutrient broth, and spread an aliquot of each inoculum over the surface of the agar with a sterile, bent-glass rod.

C. Incubation
1. Seal the plate in a plastic bag, with plastic tape, or with a tight-fitting plastic cover.
2. Incubate the tray and inoculum plates at 35°C in an air incubator for 20 hours.
3. Shake the tray by hand to mix the contents of the wells and continue incubation of tray and plates for 4 hours (total incubation, 24 hours).

D. Determination of Bactericidal Activity
1. Subculture the contents of each well onto a nutrient agar plate, using a replicate inoculator that removes 10 μL from each well. The subcultures should be done in duplicate. Incubate the plate for 24 hours in air at 35°C.
2. Confirm that the expected inoculum has been delivered (5×10^5 CFU/mL; range 5×10^4 to 5×10^6 CFU/mL) by enumerating colonies on the dilution plate that contains 20 to 200 colonies.

IV. Results

A. Interpretation

The first well that produces no growth after subculture of the wells onto the agar is the lethal endpoint. For example, if no growth is observed after subculture of the third well, the serum bactericidal activity is 1:8.

Bacteriologic cure was demonstrated in all patients with endocarditis who had a peak titer higher than or equal to 64 or a trough titer higher than or equal to 32. Statistical correlation of response was best with a peak serum titer higher than or equal to 1:32 (predictive value for cure = 98.9%; predictive value for failure = 28.6%) or a trough serum titer higher than or equal to 1:8 (predictive value for cure = 97.6%; predictive value for failure = 21.2%) in patients with endocarditis. Bacteriologic failure was predicted less successfully, because many patients with lower titers responded well to therapy.

A favorable clinical outcome (98% of patients) in severely granulocytopenic patients with gram-negative bacillary bacteremia was correlated with a peak titer higher than or equal to 1:16. A favorable response (87% of patients) was correlated with a peak titer higher than or equal to 1:8 in nongranulocytopenic patients.

In acute osteomyelitis trough titers higher than or equal to 1:2 predicted cure of the infection, whereas trough titers of less than 1:2 predicted failure. In chronic infection of bone, trough titers higher than or equal to 1:4 predicted cure; titers of less than 1:4 predicted an unfavorable clinical outcome. Peak titers were too widely dispersed to be useful in either acute or chronic osteomyelitis.

V. Bibliography

Reller LB, Stratton CW: Serum dilution test for bactericidal activity: II. Standardization and correlation with antimicrobial assays and susceptibility tests. J Infect Dis 136:196–204, 1977

Sculier JP, Klastersky J: Significance of serum bactericidal activity in gram-negative bacillary bacteremia in patients with and without granulocytopenia. Am J Med 76:429–435, 1984

Stratton CW, Reller LB: Serum dilution test for bactericidal activity: I. Selection of a physiologic diluent. J Infect Dis 136:187–195, 1977

Weinstein MP, Stratton CW, Ackley A et al: Multicenter collaborative evaluation of a standardized serum bactericidal test as a prognostic indicator in infective endocarditis. Am J Med 78:162–269, 1985

Weinstein MP, Stratton CW, Hawley HB et al: Multicenter collaborative evaluation of a standardized serum bactericidal test as a predictor of therapeutic efficacy in acute and chronic osteomyelitis. Am J Med 80:218–222, 1987

CHART 50   NAP Test (p-Nitro-α-acetylamino-β-hydroxypropiophenone); (BACTEC)

I. Principle

Members of the *Mycobacterium tuberculosis* complex do not grow in the presence of p-nitro-α-acetylamino-β-hydroxypropiophenone (NAP). Each BACTEC vial contains 5 μg of NAP. When 1 mL of an actively growing culture in 12B medium is added to this vial, the growth of mycobacteria belonging to the *M. tuberculosis* complex is inhibited. MOTT do not demonstrate significant inhibition. The presence of growth is detected by monitoring $^{14}CO_2$ production by the radioactive detector of the instrument, the absence of which (no increase in the growth index) is consistent with the *M. tuberculosis* complex.

II. Specimen

BACTEC 12B medium with a growth index > 50

III. Materials

A. Equipment
   1. BACTEC 560 instrument (Becton Dickinson)
   2. Carbon dioxide tank containing 5% to 10% CO_2 and 90% to 95% air attached to the instrument
   3. BACTEC TB hood (Becton Dickinson)
   4. Biologic safety cabinet
   5. Incubator, well calibrated at 37° ± 1°C
   6. Vortex mixer

B. Supplies
   1. Disposable tuberculin syringes with permanently attached needles
   2. Amphyl disinfectant
   3. Gloves, masks, gowns
   4. Cotton or gauze pads
   5. Alcohol swabs

C. Media and Reagents
   1. Middlebrook 7H12 (BACTEC 12B) medium (contains 7H9 broth base, bovine serum albumin, casein hydrolysate, catalase, and ^{14}C-labeled substrate)
   2. BACTEC NAP vials

IV. Quality Control

A. Medium: Quality control of the 12B medium is done by the manufacturer.

B. Include *M. tuberculosis* ATCC 27294 and *M. kansasii* ATCC 35775 as controls.

C. Test the control organisms along with test cultures at least once a month and each time a new lot of NAP is used. The growth index of *M. tuberculosis* should be flat; that of *M. kansasii* should show an ascending curve with time of incubation.

V. Procedure
1. Read vials positive for AFB daily until the growth index (GI) reaches approximately 50 to 100.
2. Mix medium well and aseptically transfer 1 mL of the culture medium from this vial into a NAP vial.
3. Clean the vial tops with Amphyl then with 70% ethyl alcohol.
4. Shake vial to mix.
5. Read both the original and inoculated NAP vials daily for 2 to 5 days and record the GI reading.
6. For cultures where the GI has passed 100, dilution is necessary before performing the NAP test. The following table should be used to determine the dilution:

GI Reading	Dilution
50–100	No dilution
101–200	0.8 mL into 4 mL 7H12/12B
201–400	0.6 mL into 4 mL 7H12/12B
401–600	0.4 mL into 4 mL 7H12/12B
601–800	0.3 mL into 4 mL 7H12/12B
801–999	0.2 mL into 4 mL 7H12/12B

Mix the dilution thoroughly and transfer 1.0 mL of the contents to a NAP test vial. Incubate the remaining dilution and test as a control for the assay.

VI. Results

A. Reporting
1. Reporting is done within 2 to 7 days, with an average of 4 days.
Report as: NAP test indicates *M. tuberculosis* complex, if growth index is flat; NAP test indicates MOTT, if growth index increases.
2. The *M. tuberculosis* complex should not be reported in fewer than 4 days.
3. Among mycobacteria other than the *M. tuberculosis* complex, certain strains of *M. kansasii*, *M. gastri*, *M. szulgai*, *M. terrae*, and *M. triviale* are partially inhibited by NAP. In such instances, there is a longer lag phase in the presence of NAP, and results interpreted in the first 2 to 4 days may be misleading. Incubate further, and test for an additional 2 to 3 days before reporting.
4. Optimum incubation temperature is critical for the NAP test. Some mycobacteria (*M. marinum*, *M. chelonae*) grow at 30°C. There will be inhibition by NAP at 37°C in such cases. The test results will be clear and can be reported within 4 days if the cultures are incubated at 30°C. The NAP test for specimens originating from wounds or skin should be incubated at 37° and 30°C.

B. Interpretation
1. Interpretation of NAP results: The daily GI of the control vial (original culture vial) will continue to increase or decrease. In the NAP vial, increase or decrease depends on the species of mycobacteria:
a. TB complex: Two consecutive significant decreases in GI after the inoculation = TB complex; slight but not significant increase in the first 2 days and then no increase, or as a decrease in GI = TB complex
b. MOTT: Daily GI reading increase to over 400 within 4 days = MOTT; no increase of slight decrease in the first 1 or 2 days after inoculation and then two consecutive daily significant increases following day 2 = MOTT

VII. Limitations of the Procedure

The NAP test is successful in differentiating the *M. tuberculosis* complex from MOTT only if pure isolated cultures are used. A mixed culture of TB and MOTT will result in an increase of GI indicating MOTT only. Contamination with bacteria can also result in false increases in GI; therefore, acid-fast and in some cases a Gram stain should be performed to confirm a mixed culture or bacterial contamination.

VIII. Bibliography

Siddiqi SH: BACTEC NAP test. In Isenberg HD (ed): Clinical Microbiology Procedure Handbook, Mycobacteriology Section. Washington DC, American Society for Microbiology, 1992

CHART 51   NEUTRALIZATION TEST

I. Principle

The neutralization of viral infectivity is the most sensitive and specific method for determining the identity of an isolate and for determining the presence of specific antibodies in a patient's serum. For some viruses (e.g., enteroviruses), it is the only practical means of identification, because extensive cross-reactions plague other immunologic tests. Unfortunately, the procedure is expensive and time-consuming. For viral groups that contain multiple serotypes, preliminary identification of an isolate may be made by pooling sera. Specific identification may be accomplished by testing the individual components of a positive pool. For enteroviruses, a group of eight "intersecting pools" have been constructed; each serotype is included in multiple pools, so the identification may be pinpointed by examination of the composition of those pools that produce neutralization.

If neutralizing antibody is present, virus cannot attach to cells, and infectivity is blocked. A fraction of infective virus may remain even in the presence of specific antiserum, so that infection may be delayed, rather than blocked completely. To identify viral isolates, antisera of known reactivity are employed. For serologic testing, suspensions of reference viruses are tested against test sera.

Any endpoint of viral infectivity may be employed:

Cytopathic effect: used most commonly and described in the following
Hemadsorption or hemagglutination: for myxoviruses and paramyxoviruses
Metabolic inhibition (colorimetric): acidification of phenol red-containing medium by growing cells if virus replication has been neutralized
Plaque reduction: cells infected by many viruses can be detected by overlaying the monolayer with a nutrient agar solution that contains a vital dye, such as neutral red. Infected cells appear as colorless "plaques" against the red background of viable cells. Reduction in the number of plaques indicates neutralization.

II. Materials and Methods
1. Monolayers of cells that will support viral growth
2. Viral isolate or reference virus
3. Patient's serum or reference serum
4. 37°C water bath for preliminary incubation of virus and antibody
5. Incubator for incubation of monolayers
6. Microscope for observation of CPE

III. Quality Control

Tubes are inoculated with serum only to document toxicity of the serum for the cell cultures. A back titration of the viral inoculum is performed to document that an appropriate challenge has been used; an abbreviated scheme, which includes the dilutions just above and below the expected $TCID_{50}$, is used.

IV. Procedure

A. Preparation of Challenge Inoculum (100 $TCID_{50}$)

The viral inoculum is usually held constant, and the concentration of serum is varied. Alternatively, a single dilution of serum may be interacted with varying dilutions of virus. The classic scheme detailed below is expensive and requires the use of many tubes. For some viruses, the procedure may be performed in microtiter trays, into which the cells and inoculum are introduced simultaneously. Alternatively, an approximation of the standard inoculum may be achieved by employing an arbitrary dilution of virus, usually 10^{-1} or 10^{-2}, depending on the extent and rapidity with which CPE develops.

Serial tenfold dilutions of virus are inoculated in duplicate onto appropriate monolayers; CPE is determined at each dilution. The dilution at which 50% of the cultures are infected ($TCID_{50}$) is determined statistically, most often by the method of Reed and Muench. Ideally, the whole range of infectivity from 0 to 100% should be encompassed by the selected dilutions, but the method can be used if there is a logical progression and the results are not erratic.

$$\text{Proportionate distance} = \frac{(\% \text{ infection at dilution next above } 50\%) - 50\%}{(\% \text{ infection next above } 50\%) - (\% \text{ infection next below } 50\%)}$$

$$\text{Negative log TCID}_{50} = \text{Negative log of dilution next above 50\% infection} +$$
$$\text{proportionate distance} \times \text{dilution factor (log}_{10})$$

$$\text{TCID}_{50} = \text{antilog of log TCID}_{50}$$

B. Example

Virus Dilution	CPE+	CPE−	Cumulative Infected	Cumulative Uninfected	Ratio	%
10^{-1}	6	0	24	0	24/24	100
10^{-2}	6	0	18	0	18/18	100
10^{-3}	6	0	12	0	12/12	100
10^{-4}	2	2	6	2	6/8	75
10^{-5}	4	4	4	6	4/10	40
10^{-6}	0	6	0	12	0/12	0
10^{-7}	0	6	0	18	0/18	0

By simple inspection, one can see that the TCID_{50} lies between 10^{-4} and 10^{-5}; 100 TCID_{50} is between 10^{-2} and 10^{-3}.

$$\text{Proportionate distance} = \frac{75 - 50}{75 - 40} = 25/35 = 0.7$$

$$\text{Negative log TCID}_{50} = -4.0 + (0.7 \times -1) = -4.0 - 0.7 = -4.7$$
(Dilution factor is -1 because tenfold serial dilutions were used in this example)

$$\text{Log dilution containing 100 TCID}_{50} = -2.7$$

$$\text{Dilution containing 100 TCID}_{50} = \text{antilog } -2.7 = 1{:}500$$

1. Standardization of antibody for identification of an isolate is performed by determination of the dilution that neutralizes 100 TCID_{50} of virus (1 antibody unit): 50 to 100 antibody units are used in the test.
2. Mixtures of serum and virus are prepared. Preincubation of the mixture may be performed for 30 to 60 minutes at 37°C, room temperature, or 4°C. Prolonged incubation at 37°C may result in loss of labile viruses.
3. For each mixture 0.2 ml is added to fresh monolayers in duplicate or triplicate.
4. The monolayers are incubated at 37°C and examined for the development of CPE.

V. Results

A. Interpretation

The dilution of serum that neutralizes the challenge inoculum represents the reciprocal of the titer. The reference serum that neutralizes the infectivity of an unidentified isolate establishes the identification of that isolate.

VI. Bibliography

Hsiung GD: Diagnostic Virology, 3rd ed. New Haven, Yale University Press, 1982

Schmidt NJ: Cell culture techniques for diagnostic virology. In Lennette EH, Schmidt NJ (eds): Diagnostic Procedures for Viral, Rickettsia, and Chlamydial Infections, 5th ed. Washington DC, American Public Health Association, 1979

Smith TF: Viruses. In Washington JA (ed): Laboratory Procedures in Clinical Microbiology, 2nd ed. New York, Springer-Verlag, 1985

CHART 52   NIACIN ACCUMULATION

I. Principle

All *mycobacteria* species produce niacin ribonucleotide; however, virtually all strains of *M. tuberculosis, M. simiae* and some strains of *M. chelonae* lack the enzymes to further convert niacin to nicotinamide adenine dinucleotide (NAD). Niacin accumulates in the culture medium from which it can be extracted with sterile water or physiologic saline. The extract is placed in a small test tube to which is added a reagent-impregnated niacin filter strip (Difco Laboratories, Detroit MI)

II. Specimen

A longer than 3-week-old heavy growth on Lowenstein-Jensen of the organism to be tested. Growth on other culture media do not produce sufficient niacin to produce a positive test reaction by this method.

III. Materials

A. Equipment
   1. Biologic safety cabinet
   2. 37°C incubator

B. Supplies
   1. Sterile screw-cap test tubes, 20 × 110 or 20 × 125 mm
   2. Sterile Pasteur pipettes
   3. Sterile 5 mL pipettes

C. Reagents
   1. Niacin filter paper strips (Difco)
   2. Sterile H_2O

IV. Standards and Controls (include controls with each batch of tests):

A. Positive control: *M. tuberculosis* ATCC 25177

B. Negative control: *M. intracellulare* ATCC 13950

V. Procedure

   1. Flood the surface of the Lowenstein-Jensen slant over the heavy growth of the test organism with 1 mL sterile H_2O. Stab the medium with the tip of the pipette to allow access of the water to the underlying medium.
   2. Tilt the tube so the water covers the surface of the slant. Let stand for 20 to 30 minutes.
   3. Rotate the tube so that the slant faces downward. Carefully remove 0.6 mL of extract without touching the slant and transfer to the screw-cap test tube.
   4. Using a pair of forceps, drop a niacin test strip with the arrow pointing downward into the tube. Stopper the tube immediately.
   5. Gently shake the tube and repeat shaking after 5 and 10 minutes.
   6. After 12 to 15 minutes, and not longer than 30 minutes, read the test for the presence of a yellow color.

VI. Results

A. Interpretation

The development of a yellow color indicates a positive test. If a culture resembles *M. tuberculosis*, but the niacin test is negative, reincubate the slant for an additional 2 to 4 weeks and repeat the test.

VII. Limitation of Procedure

False-negative reactions may occur. Reasons include 1) an insufficient amount of growth on the slant, 2) failure to stab the agar if the growth is confluent, and 3) the presence of contaminating bacteria that may have metabolized any niacin that may have accumulated.

M. simiae and occasional strains of *M. bovis*, *M. marinum*, and *M. chelonae* may accumulate niacin in the test medium. These species can be readily differentiated from *M. tuberculosis* by several key characteristics described in the interpretation section of this manual.

VIII. Bibliography

Gangadharam PR, Droubi DSA: A comparison of four different methods for testing the production of niacin by mycobacteria. Am Rev Respir Dis 104:434–437, 1971

Kilburn JO, Kubica GP: Reagent impregnated paper for detection of niacin. Am J Clin Pathol 50:530–531, 1968

Konno K, et al: Niacin metabolism in mycobacteria. Am Rev Respir Dis 93:41–46, 1966

Lutz B: Nitrate reduction. In Isenberg HD (ed): Clinical Microbiology Procedure Handbook, Mycobacteriology Section. Washington DC, American Society for Microbiology, 1992

Runyon EH, Selin MJ, Hawes HW: Distinguishing mycobacteria by the niacin test. Am Rev Tubercu 79:663–665, 1959

Young WE Jr et al: Development of paper strip test for the detection of niacin produced by mycobacteria. Appl Microbiol 20:949–945, 1970

CHART 53 NITRATE REDUCTION: GENERAL APPLICATIONS

I. Principle

The capability of an organism to reduce nitrates to nitrites is an important characteristic used in the identification and species differentiation of many groups of microorganisms. All *Enterobacteriaceae* except certain biotypes of *Pantoa agglomerans* and certain species of *Serratia* and *Yersinia* demonstrate nitrate reduction. The test is also helpful in identifying members of the *Haemophilus, Neisseria,* and *Moraxella* genera.

Organisms demonstrating nitrate reduction have the capability of extracting oxygen from nitrates to form nitrites and other reduction products. The chemical equation is

$$NO_3^- + 2e^- + 2H \rightarrow NO_2 + H_2O$$
$$\text{Nitrate} \qquad\qquad \text{Nitrite}$$

The presence of nitrites in the test medium is detected by the addition of α-naphthylamine and sulfanilic acid, with the formation of a red diazonium dye, *p*-sulfobenzene-azo-α-naphthylamine. See Figure in Chart 54.

II. Media and Reagents

A. Nitrate Broth or Nitrate Agar (Slant)

Beef extract	3 g
Peptone	5 g
Potassium nitrate (KNO$_3$)	1 g
Agar (nitrite-free)	12 g
Distilled water to	1 L

B. Reagent A

α-Naphthylamine	5 g
Acetic acid (5 N), 30%	1 L

C. Reagent B

Sulfanilic acid	8 g
Acetic acid (5 N), 30%	1 L

III. Quality Control

It is important to test each new batch of medium and each new formulation of test reagents for positive and negative reactions. The following organisms are suggested:

A. Positive control: *Escherichia coli*

B. Negative control: *Acinetobacter baumannii*

IV. Procedure

1. Inoculate the nitrate medium with a loopful of the test organism isolated in pure culture on agar medium and incubate at 35°C for 18 to 24 hours.
2. At the end of incubation, add 1 mL each of reagents A and B to the test medium, in that order.

V. Results

A. Interpretation

The development of a red color within 30 seconds after adding the test reagents indicates the presence of nitrites and represents a positive reaction for nitrate reduction (see Color Plate 4–1*H*). If no color develops after adding the test reagents, this may indicate either that nitrates have not been reduced (a true negative reaction) or that they have been reduced to products other than nitrites, such as ammonia, molecular nitrogen (denitrification), nitric oxide (NO) or nitrous oxide (N$_2$O), and hydroxylamine. Because the test reagents detect only nitrites, the latter process would lead to a false-negative reading. Thus, it is necessary to add a small quantity of zinc dust to all negative reactions. Zinc ions reduce nitrates to nitrites, and the development of a red color after adding zinc dust indicates the presence of residual nitrates and confirms a true negative reaction.

VI. Bibliography

Finegold SM, Martin WJ, Scott EG: Bailey and Scott's Diagnostic Microbiology, 5th ed, p 490. St Louis, CV Mosby, 1978

MacFaddin JF: Biochemical Tests for Identification of Medical Bacteria, 2nd ed, pp 236–245. Baltimore, Williams & Wilkins, 1980

Wallace GI, Neave SL: The nitrite test as applied to bacterial cultures. J Bacteriol 14:377–384, 1927

CHART 54   NITRATE REDUCTION: MYCOBACTERIA

I. Principle

Mycobacteria producing nitroreductase are capable of catalyzing the reduction of nitrate to nitrite. In the reaction, oxygen is extracted from nitrate according to the following formula:

$$NO_3 + 2e^- + 2H \rightarrow NO_2 + H_2O$$

The nitrate produced is detected by the addition of α-naphthalamine and sulfanilic acid, forming the red diazonium dye, p-sulfobenzene-azo-α-naphthalamine.

II. Specimen

A 3- to 4-week-old culture of the test organism growing on Lowenstein-Jensen medium or other coagulated egg medium.

III. Materials

A. Equipment
1. Biologic safety hood
2. 37°C water bath or heating block

B. Supplies
1. Sterile Pasteur pipettes
2. Sterile forceps

C. Reagents
1. Nitrate test substrate (0.01 M) in M/45 phosphate buffer (0.02 M, pH 7.0)

NaNo₃	0.8 g
KH2PO₄	1.17 g
Na₂HPO₄	1.93 g
H₂O	999 mL (final volume)

PROPOSED MECHANISM OF THE NITRATE REDUCTION REACTION

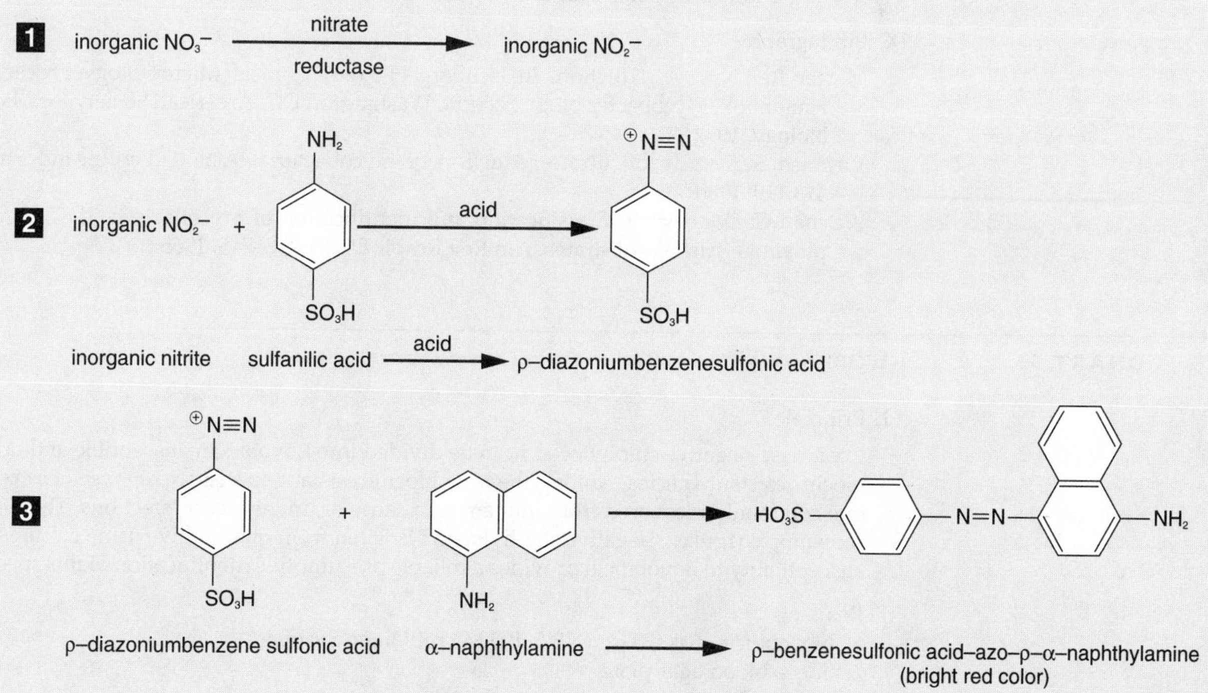

Dissolve and mix the chemicals. Adjust pH to 7.0. Autoclave and store and dispense in 2.0-mL aliquots in sterile tubes. When stored at 2° to 8°C, the shelf life is 1 to 2 months.

2. 0.2% sulfanilimide: Completely dissolve 0.1 g of sulfanilamide in 50 mL of deionized water. It may be necessary to warm the water to 47° to 50°C for complete solubility. If stored in brown-glass bottles at 2° to 8°C, the shelf life is about 1 month.

3. 0.1% N-(1-naphthyl)ethylenediamine dihydrochloride: Dissolve 0.05 g of N-(1-naphthyl)ethylenediamine dihydrochloride in 50 mL of deionized water. The shelf life is 1 month if stored in a brown-glass bottle at 2° to 8°C.

IV. Quality Control

A. Positive control: *M. tuberculosis* ATCC

B. Negative control: *M. avium* complex ATCC

C. Negative reagent control: Uninoculated tube containing appropriate substrate

V. Procedure

1. Emulsify one loopful or spadeful of colonies from solid medium into 2 mL of nitrate substrate.

2. Shake by hand to mix and incubate at 35° to 37°C for 2 hours.

3. Add reagents to mixture in the following order:

   1 drop concentrated HCl
   2 drops of 0.2% sulfanilamide
   2 drops of 0.1% N-(1-naphthyl)ethylenediamine dihydrochloride

4. Allow mixture to sit at room temperature for 5 minutes.

5. Read for the development of a pink to red color.

VI. Results

The appearance of a red or pink color is indicative of a positive test. A quantitative reading can be made by comparing with nitrate reduction standards. Quantitation is not performed in most laboratories.

VII. Procedure Notes

If no color change occurs, confirm negative results by adding a small amount of zinc dust. A deep red to pink color after the addition of zinc dust indicates that nitrate was reduced. Reagents are stored at 2° to 8°C in the refrigerator, away from direct light.

VIII. Limitation of Procedure

The color may fade rapidly in some instances and can lead to a false-negative test if a reading is not made soon after the reagents are added.

IX. Bibliography

Master RN: Nitrate reduction. In Isenberg HD (ed): Clinical Microbiology Procedure Handbook, Mycobacteriology Section. Washington DC, American Society for Microbiology, 1992

Virtanen S: A study of nitrate reduction of mycobacteria. Acta Tuberc Scand Suppl 418:119, 1960

Wayne LC, Doubek SR: Classification and identification of mycobacteria: II. Tests employing nitrite as substrates. Am Rev Respir Dis 91:478–745, 1965

CHART 55   NOVOBIOCIN DISK TEST

I. Principle

Coagulase-negative staphylococci can be divided into novobiocin-susceptible and novobiocin-resistant species. Among the novobiocin-resistant species, *S. saprophyticus* is the one commonly recovered from humans as a cause of urinary tract infections. Therefore, screening coagulase-negative staphylococci isolated from quantitative urine cultures for susceptibility to novobiocin provides a reliable presumptive identification of this species.

II. Reagents

1. Novobiocin disks, 5 μg (NB 5, BD Microbiology Systems)

2. Sheep blood agar plate

III. Quality Control

A known *S. saprophyticus* strain and a *S. epidermidis* strain should be tested with each new lot of novobiocin disks or on a weekly basis.

IV. Procedure
1. Prepare a suspension of the organism to be identified in sterile distilled water or broth.
2. The suspension should be equivalent in turbidity to a 0.5 McFarland standard.
3. With a sterile swab, spread some of the suspension over half of a blood agar plate.
4. Aseptically place a novobiocin disk on the inoculated area. Susceptibility to furazolidone (see Chart 33) may be assessed on the same plate by placing the disks about 4 cm apart on the inoculated area. Gently tamp the disk(s) with sterile forceps to assure contact with the agar surface.
5. Incubate the plate aerobically for 18 to 24 hours at 35°C.

V. Results

A. Interpretation
1. *S. saprophyticus* are novobiocin-resistant and will show zones of inhibition of 6 mm (no zone) to 12 mm.
2. Other coagulase-negative staphylococci and *S. aureus* are novobiocin-susceptible and will show zones of 16 mm or larger.

CHART 56   OPTOCHIN SUSCEPTIBILITY TEST

I. Principle

Ethylhydrocupreine hydrochloride (optochin), a quinine derivative, selectively inhibits the growth of *Streptococcus pneumoniae* at very low concentrations (5 μg/mL or less). Optochin may also inhibit other viridans streptococci, but only at much higher concentrations. The test has a sensitivity of more than 95%, is simple to perform, and is inexpensive.

Optochin is water-soluble and diffuses readily into agar medium. Therefore, filter paper disks impregnated with optochin can be used in a disk diffusion test format to determine susceptibility of suspected pneumococci and, thereby, confirm their identity as such. *S. pneumoniae* cells surrounding the disk are lysed owing to changes in the surface tension, and a zone of inhibition is produced.

II. Media and Reagents
1. Well-isolated colonies of the organism to be tested on sheep blood agar
2. Sheep blood agar plate
3. Optochin disks (5 μg): Bacto Differentiation Disks, Optochin (Difco)
           Taxo "P" disks (BBL)
4. Disks should be stored at 4°C when not in use.

III. Quality Control

A. Positive control: *Streptococcus pneumoniae*

B. Negative control: Viridans streptococcus or *Enterococcus faecalis*

IV. Procedure
1. Using an inoculating loop or wire, select three to four well-isolated colonies of the organism to be tested and streak onto one-half to a one-third of a blood agar plate. The inoculated area should be about 3 cm².
2. Place an optochin disk in the upper third of the streaked area. Tamp down the disk with flamed forceps so that the disk adheres firmly to the agar surface.
3. Incubate the plate at 35°C for 18 to 24 hours in a candle jar or in 5% to 7% CO_2.

V. Results

A. Interpretation

A viridans streptococcus can be presumptively identified as *S. pneumoniae* if it shows a zone of inhibition of 14 mm or more around a 6-mm (Taxo A) disk, or a zone of 16 mm or more around a 10-mm disk (Bacto). Organisms showing zones smaller than these should be tested for bile solubility.

VI. Limitations of Procedure

Occasionally, viridans streptococci will show small zones of inhibition around the optochin disk. These organisms, however, will not be bile-soluble.

CHART 57   O-NITROPHENYL-β-D-GALACTOPYRANOSIDE

I. Principle

o-Nitrophenyl-β-D-galactopyranoside (ONPG) is structurally similar to lactose, except that orthonitrophenyl has been substituted for glucose, as shown in the following chemical reaction:

ORTHONITROPHENYL–β–D–GALACTOPYRANOSIDE

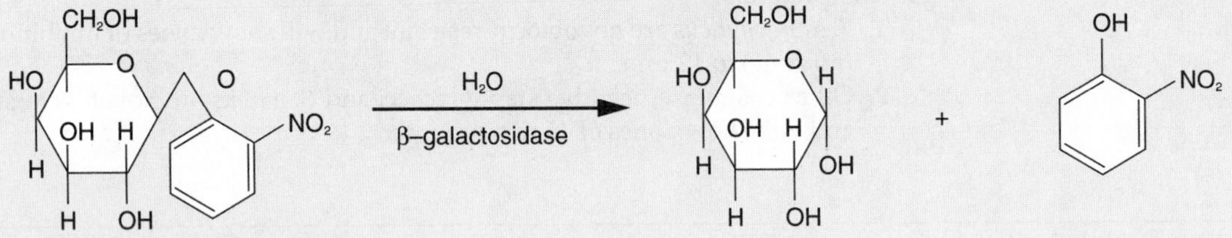

Orthonitrophenyl–β–D–Galactopyranoside (ONPG) (colorless)   →   Galactose   +   Orthonitrophenol (yellow)

H₂O / β–galactosidase

On hydrolysis, through the action of the enzyme β-galactosidase, ONPG cleaves into two residues, galactose and *o*-nitrophenol. ONPG is a colorless compound; *o*-nitrophenol is yellow, providing visual evidence of hydrolysis.

Lactose-fermenting bacteria possess both lactose permease and β-galactosidase, two enzymes required for the production of acid in the lactose fermentation test. The permease is required for the lactose molecule to penetrate the bacterial cell where the β-galactosidase can cleave the galactoside bond, producing glucose and galactose. Non–lactose-fermenting bacteria are devoid of both enzymes and are incapable of producing acid from lactose. Some bacterial species appear to be non–lactose-fermenters because they lack permease, but do possess β-galactosidase and give a positive ONPG test. So-called late lactose fermenters may be delayed in their production of acid from lactose because of sluggish permease activity. In these instances, a positive ONPG test may provide a rapid identification of delayed lactose fermentation.

II. Media and Reagents
  1. Sodium phosphate buffer, 1 M, pH 7.0
  2. *o*-Nitrophenyl-β-D-galactopyranoside (ONPG), 0.75 M (Buffered ONPG tablets are commercially available.)
  3. Physiologic saline
  4. Toluene

III. Quality Control

  A. Positive control: *Escherichia coli*

  B. Negative control: *Proteus* species

IV. Procedure

Bacteria grown in medium containing lactose, such as Kligler iron agar (KIA) or triple-sugar iron (TSI) agar, produce optimal results in the ONPG test. A loopful of bacterial growth is emulsified in 0.5 mL of physiologic saline to produce a heavy suspension. One drop of toluene is added to the suspension and vigorously mixed for a few seconds to release the enzyme for the bacterial cells. An equal quantity of buffered ONPG solution is added to the suspension, and the mixture is placed in a 37°C water bath.

When using ONPG tablets, a loopful of bacterial suspension is added directly to the ONPG substrate resulting from adding 1 mL of distilled water to a tablet in a test tube. This suspension is also placed in a 37°C water bath.

V. Results

A. Interpretation

The rate of hydrolysis of ONPG to o-nitrophenol may be rapid for some organisms, producing a visible yellow color reaction within 5 to 10 minutes (see Color Plate 4–4A). Most tests are positive within 1 hour; however, reactions should not be interpreted as negative before 24 hours of incubation. The yellow color is usually distinct and indicates that the organism has produced o-nitrophenol from the ONPG substrate through the action of β-galactosidase.

VI. Bibliography

Belliveau RR, Grayson JW Jr, Butler TJ: A rapid, simple method of identifying *Enterobacteriaceae.* Am J Clin Pathol 50:126–128, 1968

Blazevic DJ, Ederer GM: Principles of Biochemical Tests in Diagnostic Microbiology, pp 83–85. New York, John Wiley & Sons, 1975

Lederberg J: The beta-d-galactosidase of *Escherichia coli,* strain K-12. J Bacteriol 60:381–392, 1950

Lowe GH: The rapid detection of lactose fermentation in paracolon organisms by the demonstration of β-galactosidase. J Med Lab Technol 19:21–25, 1962

MacFaddin JF: Biochemical Tests for Identification of Medical Bacteria, 2nd ed, pp 120–128. Baltimore, Williams & Wilkins, 1980

CHART 58 OXIDATIVE–FERMENTATIVE TEST (HUGH AND LEIFSON)

I. Principle

Saccharolytic microorganisms degrade glucose either fermentatively or oxidatively, as shown in Figure 5–1. The end products of fermentation are relatively strong mixed acids that can be detected in a conventional fermentation test medium. However, the acids formed in oxidative degradation of glucose are extremely weak, and the more sensitive oxidation–fermentation medium of Hugh and Leifson (OF medium) is required for their detection.

The OF medium of Hugh and Leifson differs from carbohydrate fermentation media as follows:

The concentration of peptone is decreased from 1% to 0.2%
The concentration of carbohydrate is increased from 0.5% to 1.0%.
The concentration of agar is decreased from 1.5% to 0.3%, making it semisolid.

The lower protein/carbohydrate ratio reduces the formation of alkaline amines that can neutralize the small quantities of weak acids that may form from oxidative metabolism. The relatively larger amount of carbohydrate serves to increase the amount of acid that can potentially be formed. The semisolid consistency of the agar permits acids that form on the surface of the agar to permeate throughout the medium, making interpretation of the pH shift of the indicator easier to visualize. Motility can also be observed in this medium.

II. Media and Reagents

For comparison, the formulas for a conventional carbohydrate fermentation medium and OF medium are as follows:

CARBOHYDRATE FERMENTATION MEDIUM		OF MEDIUM OF HUGH AND LEIFSON	
Peptone	10 g	Peptone	2 g
Sodium chloride	5 g	Sodium chloride	5 g
D-glucose	5 g	D-glucose	10 g
Bromcresol purple	0.02 g	Bromthymol blue	0.03 g
Agar*	15 g	Agar	3.0 g
Distilled water to	1 L	Dipotassium phosphate	0.30 g
pH = 7.0		Distilled water to	1 L
		pH =7.1	

The OF sugar reactions listed in the Weaver CDC tables, described in Chapter 5, are based on tests using a "special" base with phenol red as the indicator:

Bacto casitone, 2 g
Bacto agar, 3 g
Phenol red, 1.5% aqueous, 2 mL
Distilled water to equal 1 L

The basal medium is adjusted to a pH of 7.3 and autoclaved. Carbohydrate solutions are passed through a Seitz filter and added to the basal medium to a final concentration of 1.0%. Studies at the CDC revealed that the correlation of test results between the Difco and the special CDC OF basal media are excellent and that either can be used when making interpretations from the Weaver tables.

OF medium should be poured without a slant into tubes with an inner diameter of 15 to 20 mm to increase surface area.

III. Quality Control

   A. Glucose fermenter: *Escherichia coli*

   B. Glucose oxidizer: *Pseudomonas aeruginosa*

   C. Nonsaccharolytic: *Moraxella* species

IV. Procedure

Two tubes are required for the OF test, each inoculated with the unknown organism, using a straight needle, stabbing the medium three to four times halfway to the bottom of the tube. One tube of each pair is covered with a 1-cm layer of sterile mineral oil or melted paraffin, leaving the other tube open to the air. Incubate both tubes at 35°C and examine daily for several days.

V. Results

   A. Interpretation

   Acid production is detected in the medium by the appearance of a yellow color. In the case of oxidative organisms, color production may be first noted near the surface of the medium. Following are the reaction patterns:

OPEN TUBE	COVERED TUBES	METABOLISM
Acid (Yellow)	Alkaline (Green)	Oxidative
Acid (Yellow)	Acid (Yellow)	Fermentative
Alkaline (Green)	Alkaline (Green)	Nonsaccharolytic

   These color reactions are shown in Color Plate 5–1D. For slower growing species, incubation for 3 days or longer may be required to detect positive reactions.

VI. Bibliography

BBL Manual of Products and Laboratory Procedures, 5th ed, pp 129–130. Cockeysville MD, BioQuest, 1973

Hugh R, Leifson E: The taxonomic significance of fermentative versus oxidative metabolism of carbohydrates by various gram-negative bacilli. J Bacteriol 66:24–26, 1953

MacFaddin JF: Biochemical Tests for Identification of Medical Bacteria, 2nd ed, pp 260–268. Baltimore, Williams & Wilkins, 1980

CHART 59   PERFORMANCE OF MICRODILUTION BROTH SUSCEPTIBILITY TESTS

I. Principle

The microdilution test is an adaptation of the reference macroscopic test. Large numbers of isolates can be tested against multiple drugs easily, so the procedure is well adapted to routine use. This test generates more quantitative information, which may be useful in certain circumstances, than does the disk diffusion test.

The principle of the microdilution test is the same as that of the macroscopic test. Bacterial isolates are exposed to serial dilutions of each antimicrobial agent, after which the concentration of drug that inhibits growth is determined by visual inspection.

II. Media and Reagents

   1. Nutrient broth (soybean-casein digest broth is recommended)
   2. 0.5 McFarland standard for adjusting inoculum

3. White background with black lines for comparison of turbidity of inoculum with 0.5 McFarland standard

4. Frozen or lyophilized microtiter plates containing antibiotics in cation-supplemented Mueller-Hinton broth

5. Multiprong inoculators—either wire loops or disposable plastic pins

6. Viewing mirror and template for visualization of endpoints. A photometric or fluorometric analysis of endpoints may be done if demonstrated to be equivalent to visual inspection.

III. Quality Control

Quality control should be performed with each new lot of plates. During use controls may be performed daily or at weekly intervals if strict criteria have been fulfilled.

The organisms used for the dilution test are *Staphylococcus aureus* (ATCC 29213), *Enterococcus faecalis* (ATCC 29212), *Escherichia coli* (ATCC 25922), *Pseudomonas aeruginosa* (ATCC 27583), *Neisseria gonorrhoeae* (ATCC 49226), and *Haemophilus influenzae* (ATCC 49247). Note that the *S. aureus* strain differs from that used in the disk diffusion test. *E. coli* (ATCC 35218) may be used to control combinations that include clavulanic acid, a β-lactamase inhibitor.

IV. Procedure

A. Preparation of Inoculum

At least five similar-appearing colonies are selected, as described in the disk diffusion test. The turbidity of an actively growing broth culture is adjusted to the density of a 0.5 McFarland standard. A direct method, in which bacteria from a plate that has been incubated overnight are adjusted directly, has also produced satisfactory results. The extent to which the inoculum must be diluted further will depend on the system, because replicate inoculating devices deliver various volumes of fluid. Each well should contain approximately 5×10^5 CFU/mL.

B. Inoculation of Plates

Inoculate the bacterial suspension into each well of the microplate within 15 minutes of adjusting the density of the inoculum. One well should contain bacteria without antibiotic (growth control), and one well should contain broth only (sterility control). If the volume of the inoculum exceeds 10% of the volume of the well, the dilution effect on the antimicrobial agent must be calculated. To prevent drying, seal the plates in a plastic bag, with plastic tape, or with a tight-fitting plastic cover. A portion of a nutrient agar plate, such as blood agar, should be inoculated to detect contamination.

C. Incubation

Incubate the plates at 35°C for 16 to 20 hours in a forced air incubator. Do not place more than four plates in a stack, so that a uniform temperature of incubation is maintained.

V. Results

A. Interpretation

The MIC is the lowest concentration of antibiotic that inhibits growth of the isolate. It may be determined by viewing the wells with the unaided eye, comparing the growth in the wells that contain antibiotics with that in the growth control well. A viewing mirror, with which the bottom of the microtubes may be visualized, facilitates observation. A template on which the contents of each well are detailed is useful. The endpoints may also be determined in a semiautomated fashion.

Refer to the guidelines for interpretation of MIC results as susceptible, moderately susceptible, intermediate, or resistant (see Table 15–13).

Examine the purity plate and repeat the test if contamination is present.

VI. Bibliography

National Committee for Clinical Laboratory Standards: Methods for Dilution Antimicrobial Susceptibility Tests for Bacteria That Grow Aerobically (approved Standard M7-A2). Villanova PA, National Committee for Clinical Laboratory Standards, 1985

CHART 60   PHENYLALANINE DEAMINASE

I. Principle

Phenylalanine is an amino acid that on deamination forms a keto acid, phenylpyruvic acid. Of the *Enterobacteriaceae*, only members of the *Proteus, Morganella,* and *Providencia* genera possess the deaminase enzyme necessary for this conversion.

The phenylalanine test depends on the detection of phenylpyruvic acid in the test medium after growth of the test organism. The test is positive if a visible green color develops on addition of a solution of 10% ferric chloride.

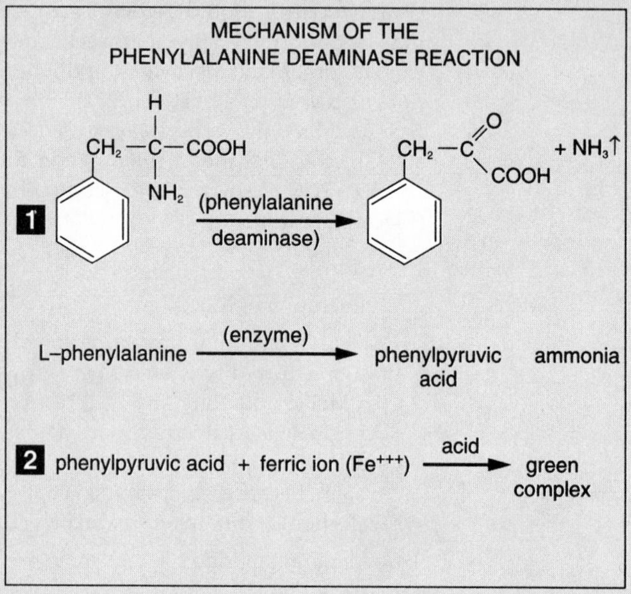

MECHANISM OF THE
PHENYLALANINE DEAMINASE REACTION

1 L-phenylalanine $\xrightarrow{\text{(enzyme)}}$ phenylpyruvic acid   ammonia

2 phenylpyruvic acid + ferric ion (Fe^{+++}) $\xrightarrow{\text{acid}}$ green complex

II. Media and Reagents

Phenylalanine agar is poured as a slant into a tube. Meat extracts or protein hydrolysates cannot be used because of their varying natural content of phenylalanine. Yeast extract serves as the carbon and nitrogen source. The formula is shown below:

Medium:

DL-Phenylalanine	2 g
Yeast extract	3 g
Sodium chloride	5 g
Disodium phosphate	1 g
Agar	12 g
Distilled water to	1 L
pH = 7.3	

Reagent:

Ferric chloride	12 g
Concentrated HCl	2.5 mL
Distilled water to	100 mL

III. Quality Control

Each new batch of medium or reagent must be tested with positive- and negative-reacting organisms. The following are suggested:

A. Positive control: *Proteus* species

B. Negative control: *Escherichia coli*

IV. Procedure

The agar slant of the medium is inoculated with a single colony of the test organism isolated in pure culture of primary plating agar. After incubation at 35°C for 18 to 24 hours, 4 or 5 drops of the ferric chloride reagent are added directly to the surface of the agar. As the reagent is added, the tube is rotated to dislodge the surface colonies.

V. Results

A. Interpretation

The immediate appearance of an intense green color indicates the presence of phenylpyruvic acid and a positive test (see Color Plate 14–4*E*).

VI. Bibliography

Blazevic DJ, Ederer GM: Principles of Biochemical Tests in Diagnostic Microbiology, pp 23–28. New York, John Wiley & Sons, 1975

Hendriksen SD: A comparison of the phenylpyruvic acid reaction and urease test in the differentiation of *Proteus* from other enteric organisms. J Bacteriol 60:225–231, 1950

Hendriksen SD, Closs K: The production of phenylpyruvic acid by bacteria. Acta Pathol Microbiol Scand 15:101–113, 1938

MacFaddin JF: Biochemical Tests for Identification of Medical Bacteria, 2nd ed, pp 269–274. Baltimore, Williams & Wilkins, 1980

Shaw C, Clarke PH: Biochemical classification of *Proteus* and *Providencia* cultures. J Gen Microbiol 13:155–161, 1955

CHART 61   PYR TEST

I. Principle

The PYR test was first described by Facklam and coauthors in 1982 and, since that time, has gained acceptance as a rapid test for the presumptive identification of both group A β-hemolytic streptococci and enterococci. Whereas the original test was described as a 16- to 20-hour agar test, subsequent PYR test formats include a 4-hour broth assay and several rapid (10 to 15 minutes) tests where the PYR reagent is impregnated in filter paper disks or strips that are inoculated with the organism to be tested. The PYR test also appears on several of the kits systems for identification of streptococci and streptococcus-like bacteria. This chart describes the 4-hour broth PYR test.

The substrate used for the PYR test is L-pyrrolindonyl-β-naphthylamide. This compound is hydrolyzed by a specific bacterial aminopeptidase enzyme. Hydrolysis of the substrate by this enzyme releases free β-naphthylamide, which is detected by the addition of *N,N*-dimethylaminocinnamaldehyde. This detection reagent couples with the naphthylamide to form a red Shiff base.

II. Media and Reagents
1. PYR broth (Todd-Hewitt broth with 0.01% L-pyrrolidonyl-β-naphthylamide) dispensed into sterile tubes in 0.20-mL volumes
2. PYR reagent (0.01% *p*-dimethylaminocinnamaldehyde)

III. Quality Control

A. Positive: *Enterococcus faecalis* or group A streptococcus

B. Negative: Group B streptococcus

IV. Procedure
1. With a sterile bacteriologic loop, pick up the growth of two to three morphologically similar colonies and emulsify them in the small volume of PYR broth.
2. Incubate the tube at 35°C for 4 hours.
3. Add 1 drop of the PYR reagent and observe for color change. The reaction should be read and recorded 1 minute after reagent addition.

V. Results

A. Interpretation
1. Positive: the development of a deep cherry red color within a minute of reagent addition
2. Negative: a yellow or orange color

VI. Procedure Notes

It is essential that testing be performed before the PYR test to determine that the organism is a streptococcus (i.e., gram-positive cocci, catalase-negative). Other organisms (e.g., some aerococci, staphylococci, nutritionally variant streptococci, *Arcanobacterium haemolyticum*) may also be PYR positive.

CHART 62   PYRAZINAMIDASE

I. Principle

The deamidation of pyrazinamide to pyrazinoic acid in 4 days is a useful phenotypic characteristic by which *M. marinum* (positive) can be differentiated from *M. kansasii* (negative) and by which weakly niacin-positive strains of *M. bovis* (negative) can be distinguished from *M. tuberculosis* complex (positive).

II. Specimen

Mature colonies of the unknown *Mycobacterium* species recovered from clinical material, grown on an LJ slant or on Middlebrook 7H-10 agar.

III. Materials

A. Equipment: None

B. Medium

1. Pyrazinamidase substate medium

a. Dissolve 6.5 g of Dubos broth base in 1 L distilled water.

b. Add

Pyrazinamide	0.1 g
Sodium pyruvate	2.0 g
Agar	15 g

c. Heat to dissolve. Dispense in 50.0-mL amounts into screw-cap tubes.

d. Autoclave for 15 minutes at 121°C.

e. Allow agar to harden with tubes in upright position.

f. Shelf life is 6 months when stored at 2° to 8°C. Discard if agar appears dehydrated or contaminated.

C. Reagents

1% ferrous ammonium sulfate (prepare immediately before use): Place 0.1 g of ferrous ammonium sulfate in sterile screw-cap test tubes. Add 10 mL of sterile deionized water immediately before use, and allow the crystals to dissolve.

D. Supplies

1. Sterile applicator sticks

2. Sterile 1.0- or 5.0-mL pipettes

IV. Quality Control

A. Positive control: *M. intracellulare* ATCC 13950

B. Negative control: *M. kansasii* ATCC 12478

V. Procedure

1. Inoculate a large loopful of growth from an actively growing subculture to the surface of two pyrazinamidase agar deeps.

2. Incubate the tubes with caps loose at 37°C.

3. Remove one of the tubes from the incubator after 4 days. Remove one of the control tubes also.

4. Add 1.0 mL of freshly prepared 1% ferrous ammonium sulfate to each tube.

5. Examine the tubes for a pink band in the agar after 30 minutes at room temperature.

6. Refrigerate any negative tubes for 4 hours more and reexamine for the presence of a pink band.

VI. Results

A. Interpretation

After 4 hours, examine the tubes for a pink band in the reagent layer on the surface of the agar (positive reaction), using incident room light against a white background. Repeat the procedure with the remaining tube after 7 days incubation.

VII. Procedure Notes

Perform all tests under a biologic safety hood.

VIII. Bibliography

Wayne LG: Simple pyrazinamidase and urease tests for routine identification of mycobacteria. Am Rev Respir Dis 109:147–151, 1974

Lutz B: Identification tests for mycobacteria: Pyrazinamidase. In Isenberg HD (ed): Clinical Microbiology Procedure Handbook. Washington DC, American Society for Microbiology, 1992

CHART 63   RAPID CARBOHYDRATE UTILIZATION TEST FOR IDENTIFICATION OF *NEISSERIA* SPECIES

I. Principle

The rapid carbohydrate utilization test procedures have largely supplanted the use of cystine–tryptic digest semisolid agar with carbohydrates for the identification of *Neisseria* species. The procedure described is a modification of the procedure described in *Cumitech 4* from the American Society for Microbiology.

The rapid carbohydrate utilization test employs a balanced phosphate-buffered saline solution containing phenol red indicator. Small (0.10-mL) aliquots of the buffer are distributed in a series of tubes, one for each carbohydrate tested. Single drops of the individual carbohydrates (20% w/v) are added to individual tubes. A heavy suspension of the organism to be tested is prepared in the buffer without carbohydrates, and 1 drop of this suspension is added to each of the carbohydrate tubes. After 4 hours of incubation, the reactions are interpreted. Production of acid from carbohydrates is indicated by a change in the color of the phenol red indicator from red to yellow.

II. Media and Reagents

A. Phosphate balanced salts solution (BBS): a 10 × stock solution having the following formula:

K$_2$HPO$_4$	0.40 g
KH$_2$PO$_4$	0.10 g
KCl	8.0 g
Distilled water	100 mL

Filter sterilize and store at 4° to 8°C

B. Working Solution

Add 10 mL of the 10 × BSS to 90 mL of distilled water. After this, 0.5 to 0.8 mL of a 1% aqueous solution of phenol red is added to the solution, so that the final product is "cherry red." This working solution is then filter-sterilized. To ensure that the distilled water is the proper pH, the use of pharmacy-grade sterile distilled water is recommended.

C. Stock Carbohydrate Solutions

Weigh out 10 g each of glucose, maltose, sucrose, and lactose (and, if desired, fructose) individually. Each is dissolved in 50 mL of distilled water. The solutions are filter-sterilized, dispensed into sterile vials, and frozen at 20°C. It is important that "reagent-grade" carbohydrates be used, because the maltose from some bacteriologic media vendors may be contaminated with glucose. Carbohydrates may be obtained from Sigma Chemical Company (St. Louis MO), Fisher Scientific Company (Fairlawn NJ), or Mallinckrodt Chemical Works (St Louis MO).

III. Quality Control

A. Positive glucose: *N. gonorrhoeae*

B. Positive maltose: *N. meningitidis*

C. Positive lactose: *N. lactamica*

D. Positive sucrose and fructose: *N. mucosa*

IV. Procedure

1. A series of nonsterile 12 × 75-mm tubes are labeled with the carbohydrate to be tested. Generally, glucose, maltose, sucrose, and lactose are tested. Some laborato-

ries will also include fructose in the test battery. An additional tube, labeled with the isolate or specimen number, is also included for preparation of the inoculum.

2. For each of the carbohydrate tubes, 0.10 mL of working BSS is added to each of the tubes. For the inoculum tube, 0.30 to 0.40 mL of BSS is placed in the tube.

3. A single drop of each of the carbohydrates is added to the appropriately labeled tube with a Pasteur pipette.

4. A heavy suspension of the organism to be tested is prepared in the inoculum tube using a sterile bacteriologic loop. The inoculum is prepared from an 18- to 24-hour, pure chocolate agar subculture of the organism. The inoculum suspension is carefully vortexed to obtain a uniform, heavy suspension.

5. Single drops of the inoculum suspension are added to each of the carbohydrate-containing tubes. The tubes are briefly agitated to ensure thorough mixing and are placed in an incubator or water bath at 35°C for 4 hours.

V. Results

A. Interpretation

The development of a yellow color in any of the carbohydrate-containing tubes indicates utilization of that carbohydrate by the organism. Negative carbohydrate utilization tests remain red or red-orange.

VI. Bibliography

Janda WM: Identification of *Neisseria* species and *Branhamella catarrhalis.* In: Identification of Aerobic Gram-Positive and Gram-Negative Cocci, pp 115–131. Washington DC, American Society for Microbiology, 1986

Kellogg DS, Holmes KK, Hill GA: Cumitech 4, Marcus S, Sherris JC (eds): Laboratory Diagnosis of Gonorrhea. Washington DC, American Society for Microbiology, 1976

CHART 64	RAPID PLASMA REAGIN (RPR) CARD TEST

I. Principle

The RPR (circle) Card Test was instituted as the routine screening test in the Maryland State Department of Health Laboratories on January 13, 1964. The main advantages of the RPR over the VDRL test are that the serum does not have to be heat-treated, interpretations are made macroscopically instead of microscopically, the antigen is stable, and components are disposable. Tests can be performed rapidly and inexpensively, thereby making the technique suitable for large-volume operations. The sensitivity and specificity of the RPR test are equal to those of the VDRL and other nontreponemal serologic tests.

The RPR antigen suspension is a carbon-containing cardiolipin antigen that detects "reagin," an antibody-like substance present in the plasma and sera of persons with syphilis or previous exposure to the treponema spirochete. When a specimen contains specific antibody, flocculation occurs with coagglutination of the carbon particles of the RPR card antigen, appearing as black clumps against a white background of the plastic-coated card. This coagglutination can be read macroscopically; nonreactive specimens have a smooth, milky light-gray color.

II. Equipment, Supplies, and Reagents

1. Disposable, calibrated 20-gauge needle without bevel, silicone treated
2. Plastic antigen dispensing bottle, 1 dram
3. Plastic-coated RPR cards with ten circles, each approximately 18 mm in diameter
4. Dispenstirs, a disposable (plastic) dispensing-stirring device that delivers 50 μL
5. Mechanical rotator, fixed speed or adjustable to 100 ± 2 rpm, circumscribing a circle 3⁄4 in. in diameter on a horizontal plane
6. Humidifying cover for rotator
7. High-intensity incandescent lamp
8. Safety pipetting device with disposable tip that delivers 50 μL
9. Discard containers and disinfectants
10. Disposable latex gloves, safety glasses, and protective clothing
11. RPR antigen suspension (a variation of the VDRL antigen): a stabilized combination of 0.003% cardiolipin, 0.020–0.022% lecithin, 0.09% cholesterol, 10% choline

chloride, 0.0125 M EDTA, 0.1875% charcoal, 0.1 M Na$_2$HPO4, 0.01 M KH$_2$PO$_4$, 0.1% thimerosal, and distilled water

12. Control serum samples: lyophilized reactive (R), minimally reactive (MR), and nonreactive (N) control serum specimens on a card

13. 0.9% saline as a diluent

III. Procedures

A. Testing Accuracy of Antigen Needle
1. Check the calibrated needle periodically to be sure that it delivers 60±2 drops/mL (17 μL). The accuracy of the test depends on the amount of antigen used.
2. Consult the procedure for calibrating needles in the VDRL test (see Chart 74).

B. Testing and Storing the Antigen Suspension
1. Store ampules of antigen at 2° to 8°C. Do not store in the bright sunlight. Do not store above 29°C and do not freeze. Antigen in an opened ampule is stable for up to 12 months.
2. Attach the needle hub to the fitting on the plastic dispensing bottle. Open the ampule after shaking it to resuspend the particles. Squeeze the dispensing bottle to collapse it, insert the needle into the ampule, and withdraw all the antigen suspension into the dispensing bottle. Shake the dispensing bottle gently before each series of antigen drops is delivered.
3. Test each lot of antigen suspension in parallel with an antigen of known standard reactivity before putting it into use.
4. At each routine test run, test the reactivity of the antigen with control cards or sera of known reactivity. Use only suspensions that produce appropriate activity.
5. After completion of the days work, remove the needle from the antigen-dispensing bottle, rinse in distilled water, and air dry. Do not wipe the needle (an action that will remove the silicone coating).

C. Preparing and Storing Specimens
1. Either serum or plasma may be tested. Plasma is obtained by collecting blood into a tube that contains EDTA as an anticoagulant.
2. Do not test specimens that are grossly contaminated, excessively hemolyzed, or chylous.

D. Performing the Qualitative Test
1. All reagents should be at room temperature (23° to 29°C) before tests are performed.
2. Place 50 μL of serum or plasma into an 18-mm circle of the RPR test card, using a disposable Dispenstir or a safety pipetting device.
3. With the inverted Dispenstir (closed end) or flat toothpicks, spread the serum or plasma to fill the entire circle, but not to extend beyond the bounds of the circle.
4. Gently shake the antigen-dispensing bottle to resuspend the particles.
5. While holding the dispensing bottle and needle in a vertical position, dispense several drops to clear the needle of air. Then add exactly 1 free-falling drop (17 μL) of antigen suspension to each circle containing serum or plasma. Do not mix the antigen and serum or plasma.
6. Place the card on the mechanical rotator under a humidifying cover. Rotate the card for 8 minutes at 100 ± 2 rpm.
7. Immediately remove the card from the rotator. Briefly rotate and tilt the card by hand to aid in differentiating nonreactive from minimally reactive results. Read the test reactions in the "wet" state, using a high-intensity incandescent light, without magnification.
8. Report the results as follows:

Reading	Report
Characteristic clumping ranging from marked and intense (reactive) to slight but definite (minimally reactive)	Reactive (R)
Slight roughness or no clumping	Nonreactive (N)

9. Perform the quantitative test on serum specimens showing any degree of reactivity or "roughness."

IV. Performing the Quantitative Test
1. Quantitate to an endpoint all serum specimens with reactive or rough nonreactive results in the qualitative test. Test each specimen undiluted (1:1) and in 1:2, 1:4, 1:8, and 1:16 dilutions.

2. Place 50 μL of 0.9% saline in circles numbered 2 through 5. Do not spread the saline.
3. Using a safety pipette device, place 50 μL of serum in circle 1 and 50 μL of serum in circle 2.

   Mix the saline and the serum in the circle by drawing the mixture up and down in the safety pipette eight times. Avoid forming bubbles.
4. Transfer 50 μL from circle 2 (1:2) to circle 3 and mix.
5. Transfer 50 μL from circle 3 (1:4) to circle 4 and mix.
6. Transfer 50 μL from circle 4 (1:8) to circle 5 (1:16) and mix. Discard the last 50 μL.
7. With the broad end of a clean Dispenstir, spread the serum dilution to fill the entire surface of circle 5, the highest dilution (1:16). With the same Dispenstir, do the same for circles 4 (1:8), 3 (1:4), 2 (1:2), and 1 (undiluted).
8. Gently shake the dispensing bottle to resuspend the antigen particles.
9. Holding the antigen-dispensing bottle in a vertical position, dispense 1 or 2 drops to clear the needle of air. Then add exactly 1 free-falling drop (17 μL) of antigen suspension in each circle. Do not mix.
10. Place the card on the rotator under the humidifying cover and rotate the card for 8 minutes at 100 ± 2 rpm.
11. Immediately remove the card from the rotator; briefly, rotate and tilt the card by hand (three or four to-and-fro motions) to aid in differentiating nonreactive from minimally reactive results. Read the results in the wet state with the unaided eye, using a bright incandescent light.
12. Report the results in terms of the highest dilution that has given a reactive result, including a minimally reactive result, as follows:

Serum Dilutions					Report
Undiluted	1:2	1:4	1:8	1:16	
RM	N	N	N	N	Reactive, undiluted
R	R	R	N	N	Reactive, 1:4 dilution
R	R	R	RM	N	Reactive, 1:8 dilution

R, Reactive; RM, Reactive, minimally; N, nonreactive
Note: Report the result as either reactive or nonreactive; there is no minimally reactive report in the RPR card test

V. Results

A. Interpretation
   1. Clinicians must combine the results of this test with the clinical and epidemiologic information. The predictive value of a positive RPR test is increased if the specimen is also reactive in a specific treponemal test, such as the FTA-ABS.
   2. A reactive test indicates present or past inadequately treated infection or a false-positive reaction. Technical false-positive reactions may be detected by a negative RPR test when repeated. Biologic false-positive reactions are detected by a negative specific treponemal test, such as the FTA-ABS test.
   3. A negative test in the absence of clinical symptoms may indicate no infection or adequately treated infection in the past. A negative test may also occur during the incubation period before the first symptoms have manifested. A negative test in the presence of clinical symptoms may occur during early primary syphilis, as a prozone during secondary syphilis, or occasionally in tertiary syphilis.
   4. When the quantitative RPR test is performed on patients with syphilis, a fourfold rise in titer may indicate an active infection, a reinfection, or failure of therapy. A fourfold fall in titer usually means adequate syphilis therapy.
   5. All reactive qualitative RPR tests should be titered to an endpoint and the endpoint titer reported. Very high RPR card titers may occur in patients with HIV infection. Very high false-positive titers may occur in patients with lymphomas.

B. Acceptable Variations
   1. Prepare a 1:16 dilution for further quantitation, using 50 μL of specimen to 750 μL of 0.9% saline.
   2. If, after screening, the serum to be quantitated seems likely to exceed 1:16, prepare all dilutions directly on the card, using a 1:50 nonreactive serum as the diluent beginning with circle 6 (1:32) and continuing for the remainder of the card.

VI. Sources of Error

1. If the temperatures of the sera, reagents or testing area are lower than 23°C, test reactivity decreases; if temperatures are higher than 29°C, test reactivity increases.
2. If the speed of the mechanical rotator is too fast or too slow, improper mixing of antigen and antibody will yield unpredictable results.
3. If the card is excessively rotated and tilted by hand after removal from the rotator, a false-positive reaction may occur.
4. If lighting produces a glare on the card, results may be obscured.
5. If the antigen is outdated or not tested for standard reactivity, results may be unpredictable.
6. If the serum is unevenly spread in the circle, the antigen and antibody may not mix properly.
7. If hemolyzed, contaminated, or improperly collected serum or plasma samples are tested, the reaction may be masked.
8. If plasma specimens are stored at −20°C for longer than 1 week, the specimens become unsuitable for testing.
9. If the moistened humidifying cover is not used to cover tests as they are being rotated, proper humidity will not be maintained, and test components may dry on the card, causing false-positive reactions to occur.

VII. Test Limitations

1. The RPR card tests cannot be used to test spinal fluids.
2. A prozone reaction may be encountered occasionally. In a prozone reaction, complete or partial inhibition of reactivity occurs with undiluted serum. The prozone phenomenon may be so pronounced that only a rough reaction is produced in the qualitative test by a serum that will be strongly positive in the quantitative test. Any specimen that produces any degree of roughness or reactivity in the qualitative test should be retested in the quantitative test.
3. The RPR test may be reactive in persons from areas where yaws, pinta, or nonvenereal syphilis is endemic. As a general rule, residual titers from these infections will be less than 1:8.
4. Biologic false-positive reactions occur occasionally, particularly in persons who abuse drugs; who have diseases such as lupus erythematosus, mononucleosis, malaria, leprosy, or viral pneumonia; or who have been recently vaccinated.
5. Nontreponemal test titers of persons who have been treated in latent or late stages of syphilis or who have been reinfected do not decrease as rapidly as those who are treated in early primary infection. Some of these individuals may become "serofast," retaining their reactivity for life.

VIII. Bibliography

Fiumara NJ. Serologic responses to treatment of 128 patients with late latent syphilis. Sex Transm Dis 6:243–246, 1979

Larson SA, Hunter EF, Karus SJ (eds): Manual of Tests for Syphilis, 8th ed. Washington DC, American Public Health Association, 1990

CHART 65   SALT TOLERANCE TEST

I. Principle

Ability to grow in the presence of variable amounts of sodium chloride (NaCl) is a test that has been used to characterize several bacteria, including the viridans streptococci. It is particularly useful, however, for presumptive identification of the enterococcal group D organisms, which have the specific ability to grow in the presence of 6.5% NaCl incorporated into either a broth or an agar medium. This test, along with the bile esculin test, is used in many laboratories to distinguish *Enterococcus* species from the group D streptococci, *S. bovis* and *S. equinus*.

Heart infusion broth is a general-purpose nutritional broth that is used for the cultivation of many bacteria. It normally contains 0.5% NaCl. By increasing the salt concentration to 6.5%, the medium becomes semiselective for the growth of enterococci.

II. Medium

1. 6.5% NaCl broth has the following formula:

Heart infusion broth	25 g
Sodium chloride	60 g
Indicator (1.6 g of bromcresol purple in 100 mL of 95% ethanol)	1 mL
Glucose	1 g
Distilled water	1 L

2. The indicator may be omitted.

3. Dispense into tubes in 3- to 5-mL volumes and autoclave at 121°C for 15 minutes.

III. Quality Control

A. Positive growth: *Enterococcus faecalis*

B. Negative growth: *Streptococcus bovis*

IV. Procedure

1. Inoculate two or three colonies into broth.
2. Incubate overnight at 35°C in ambient air incubator.

V. Results

A. Interpretation

A positive test is the presence of obvious bacterial growth in the medium, with or without a color change in the indicator. If the organism is bile esculin-positive and grows in the 6.5% NaCl broth, the organism is an *Enterococcus* species. If the organism is bile esculin-positive and fails to grow in the 6.5% NaCl broth, the organism is a group D streptococcus.

VI. Limitations of Procedure

1. If the medium is inoculated too heavily, inoculum may be interpreted as growth, resulting in a false-positive reaction.
2. To prevent interpretation of the test as falsely negative, agitate the tube gently before reading, as the growth may settle out during incubation.
3. Up to 80% of group B streptococci may be salt-tolerant, as will occasional isolates of group A streptococci. Aerococci may also be bile esculin-positive and may grow in 6.5% NaCl.

CHART 66   SODIUM CHLORIDE TOLERANCE: MYCOBACTERIA

I. Principle

Of the slowly growing mycobacteria, only *M. triviale* grows in media containing 5% NaCl; of the medically significant rapidly growing mycobacteria, only *M. chelonae* subsp *chelonae* fail to grow in such media.

II. Specimen

A 3- to 4-week-old culture of the test organism growing on Lowenstein-Jensen medium or other coagulated egg medium.

III. Materials

A. Equipment
1. Biologic safety hood
2. Slant racks

B. Supplies
1. Sterile applicator sticks
2. Sterile 1.0-mL pipettes
3. McFarland 1 standard

C. Media
1. Lowenstein-Jensen without 5% NaCl in slants
2. Lowenstein-Jensen with 5% NaCl in slants
3. Dubos Tween or Middlebrook 7H9 broth

IV. Quality Control

A. Positive control: *M. fortuitum* ATCC 6841

B. Negative control: *M. gordonae* ATCC 14470

Set up controls for each new lot number of medium received. Reject medium if results on control organisms are not as expected. Purchase Lowenstein-Jensen with and without NaCl in the same size tubes for consistency in interpretation.

V. Procedure

1. Use an actively growing culture (2 to 4 weeks for slow growers; 1 to 2 weeks for rapid growers). Make a suspension of organisms in Middlebrook 7H9 broth equal to a McFarland 1 standard.
2. Take one Lowenstein-Jensen slant with 5% NaCl and one slant without 5% NaCl and inoculate into each tube, 0.1 mL of the described suspension.
3. Incubate the slants with the caps loose in a 5 to 10% CO$_2$ incubator. Lie slants flat in a rack during incubation. Incubate for 1 week at 29° to 30°C for rapid growers and 37°C for slow growers. Stand negative tubes up straight; incubate 3 more weeks. Visually examine slants weekly for growth.

VI. Results

1. When numerous colonies are seen on the control slant and more than 50 colonies on the medium containing 5% NaCl, record the test as positive.
2. When there are colonies on the control slant and no visible growth on the slant containing NaCl, continue incubation for up to 4 weeks.

VII. Procedure Notes

Use the slant without 5% NaCl to check for viability of the organism. It is not necessary to have equal growth in both tubes. If the organism does not grow on the slant without 5% NaCl, repeat the test.

VIII. Limitation of Procedure

Some strains of *M. fortuitum* and *M. chelonae* grow on a NaCl-containing media only at temperatures lower than 35°C. For this reason all test specimens should be incubated at 29° to 30°C.

IX. Bibliography

Lutz B: Sodium chloride tolerance. In Isenberg HD (ed): Clinical Microbiology Procedure Handbook, Mycobacteriology Section. Washington DC, American Society for Microbiology, 1992

Silcox VA, Good RA, Floyd MM: Identification of clinically significant *Mycobacterium fortuitum* complex. J Clin Microbiol 14:686–691, 1981

CHART 67   TEST FOR X AND V FACTOR REQUIREMENTS

I. Principle

X factor (hemin, hematin) and V factor (NAD) are required either singly or in combination to support the growth of various species of *Haemophilus* on agar media. Filter paper strips or disks impregnated with X and V factors are commercially available.

X and V factors, each being water-soluble, readily diffuse in agar culture media. Filter paper disks or strips impregnated with these factors are placed on the surface of a medium deficient in these factors, such as trypticase–soy or brain–heart infusion agar, which has been inoculated as a lawn with the test organism. Factor requirements of the organism are then determined, after overnight incubation, by observing the patterns of growth around the paper strips or disks (see following illustration).

II. Media and Reagents

1. Paper strips or disks impregnated with X and V factors
2. An agar medium deficient in X and V factors. Trypticase-soy or brain-heart infusion agars are suitable
3. Brain-heart infusion broth

III. Quality Control

    A. *Haemophilus parainfluenzae:* requires V factor only

    B. *Haemophilus influenzae:* requires both X and V factors

IV. Procedure

    1. From a pure culture of the organism to be identified, prepare a light suspension of the growth in the brain–heart infusion broth. Be careful when transferring the growth not to pick up any of the hemin-containing medium from the culture plate. From this suspension, inoculate the surface of the factor-deficient agar medium.

    2. Place an X and a V factor strip on the surface of the agar in the area of inoculation.

    3. Position the strips about 1 cm apart.

    4. Incubate the plate in 3% to 5% CO_2 at 35°C for 18 to 24 hours.

V. Results

    A. Interpretation

    Visually inspect the agar surface, observing closely for visible growth between or around one or more of the strips or disks. The following patterns indicate the need for X factor only (*left*), V factor only (*center*), or both X and V factors (*right*):

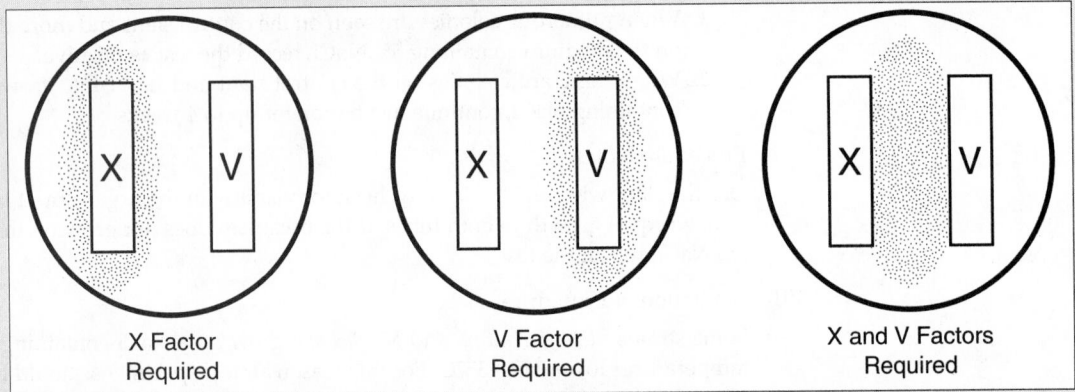

X Factor Required   V Factor Required   X and V Factors Required

VI. Bibliography

    Parker RH, Hoeprich PD: Disk method for rapid identification of *Haemophilus* sp. Am J Clin Pathol 37:319–327, 1963

CHART 68   TETRAZOLIUM REDUCTION TEST FOR THE PRESUMPTIVE IDENTIFICATION OF *MYCOPLASMA PNEUMONIAE*

I. Principle

    M. pneumoniae is able to reduce the colorless compound tetrazolium to the red-colored compound formozan. Among the large-colony mycoplasmas, this is a unique feature of *M. pneumoniae* and provides the laboratory with a rapid and easy method for identification of *M. pneumoniae* colonies directly on isolation medium.

    By using enzymes that are associated with the cell membrane of the organism, *M. pneumoniae* can reduce the compound 2-(*p*-iodophenyl)-3-nitrophenyl-5-phenyl tetrazolium chloride to formozan, a red-insoluble compound that precipitates in the cells and renders the colony red to purple-black on prolonged exposure to the substrate.

II. Reagents

    1. Isolated colonies on mycoplasma glucose agar

    2. 2-(*p*-iodophenyl)-3-nitrophenyl-5-phenyl tetrazolium chloride (Aldrich Chemical Co.)–0.21 g/100 mL distilled water. Sterilize by filtration and store in brown-glass bottle at room temperature.

III. Quality Control

    A. Positive control: *M. pneumoniae*

    B. Negative control: *Mycoplasma* species

IV. Procedure
1. Flood the surface of the agar plate containing the colonies of the organism with 2 mL of the tetrazolium reagent.
2. Incubate the plate at 35°C for 30 to 60 minutes (incubation for 60 minutes intensifies reactions that are already apparent at 30 minutes).
3. Examine the colonies under 50 to 100× magnification with a dissecting microscope.

V. Results
A. Interpretation
1. Positive test: Colonies of *M. pneumoniae* will visibly darken, becoming red to purple after 60 minutes. On prolonged incubation (3 to 4 hours), the colonies will become black.
2. Negative test: No color change will be noted after 60 minutes.

VI. Comments

Although equivalent to the hemadsorption test, tetrazolium reduction can be performed on the same plate after doing the hemadsorption procedure.

VII. Bibliography

Johnson JE, Smith TF: A simplified tetrazolium reduction test for *Mycoplasma pneumoniae.* Med Lab Sci 33:235, 1976

CHART 69 TINSDALES' AGAR (AS MODIFIED BY MOORE AND PARSONS)

I. Principle

Tinsdale medium supports the growth of all species of *Corynebacterium* while inhibiting the growth of normal inhabitants of the upper respiratory tract. Moore and Parsons modified the original Tinsdale formula, simplifying the composition, but retaining the specificity for the recovery of *C. diphtheriae* and *C. ulcerans.*

The potassium tellurite is deposited within the colonies of *Corynebacterium,* turning them black, Tinsdale medium is cystine–sodium thiosulfate tellurite, which is specifically helpful in the identification of *C. diphtheriae,* colonies of which are surrounded by a brown halo (see Plate 13–2F).

II. Media and Reagents
A. Formula (modified Tinsdale base)

Thiotone peptone	20 g
Sodium chloride	5 g
Agar	14 g
L-Cystine	0.24 g
Sodium thiosulfate	0.24 g
Distilled water	1 L

B. Preparation
1. Suspend 39 g of powder in 1 L of distilled water and heat with agitation. Boil for 1 minute. Autoclave for 15 minutes at 121°C.
2. Cool the modified base to 50°C and add:

Sterile bovine serum	100 mL
Tellurite solution, 1%	30 mL

3. Pour 15 to 20 mL of this medium into petri dishes and allow to harden.
4. The Tinsdale agar base medium without serum and tellurite is stable indefinitely if stored in closed screw-capped tubes or bottles. However, the medium is ordinarily stable for only 2 or 3 days when stored in the refrigerator following the addition of serum and tellurite.

III. Procedure

Streak the plate so as to obtain well-isolated colonies. It is recommended that the agar be stabbed at intervals, because browning of the medium can be detected early in the stab areas.

IV. Results

A. Interpretation

A brown halo around the colony is considered presumptive evidence of *C. diphtheriae*. This can sometimes be seen after 10 to 12 hours of incubation, although 48 hours may be required for the appearance of typical dark-brown halos. The only related species other than *C. diphtheriae* that produces this halo is *C. ulcerans*. Other bacteria, such as coagulase-positive staphylococci, grow well on this medium, but do not have a brown halo. Bacteria, such as species of *Proteus* that produce a heavy, diffuse blackening of the medium, can be distinguished by their Gram stain reaction and biochemical characteristics.

V. Bibliography

Moore MS, Parsons EI: A study of modified Tinsdale's medium for the primary isolation of *Corynebacterium diphtheriae*. J Infect Dis 102:88–93, 1958

Tinsdale GFW: A new medium for the isolation and identification of *C. diphtheriae* based on production of hydrogen sulfide. J Pathol Bacteriol 59:61–66, 1947

CHART 70   TRICHROME-STAINING TECHNIQUE FOR FECAL SMEARS

I. Principle

Because the refractive index of protozoan cysts and some helminth ova is near that of water, staining techniques are required to study the details of their internal structures. Permanent stains also enhance the detection of *Entamoeba histolytica*, the most important disease-producing amoeba for humans. The trichrome staining technique is a rapid procedure that gives results for routine purposes.

The trichrome stain is a modification of the Gomori stain, which contains chromotrope 2R and light green SF as the primary-staining agents. Smears made from fresh fecal material must be fixed; PVA samples are already fixed and need no additional treatment.

II. Media and Reagents

A. Schaudinn's Fixative Solution

1. Saturated mercuric chloride ($HgCl_2$)

$HgCl_2$	100 g
Distilled water	1 L

2. In a fume hood, boil until the $HgCl_2$ is dissolved and let stand to cool until crystals form.

B. Stock Solution

$HgCl_2$	600 mL
Ethyl alcohol, 95%	300 mL

1. Immediately prior to use add 6 mL of glacial acetic acid per 100 mL of stock solution.

C. Gomori Trichrome Stain

Chromotrope 2R	0.6g
Light green SF	0.3 g
Phosphotungstic acid	0.7 g
Acetic acid (glacial)	1 mL
Distilled water	100 mL

1. Add 1 mL of glacial acetic acid to the dry components. Allow mixture to stand for 15 to 30 minutes and then add the 100 mL of distilled water. A good stain is purple.

D. Iodine–Alcohol Solution

1. Add sufficient iodine crystals to 70% alcohol to make a dark, concentrated stock solution. At the time of use, dilute the desired amount of stock solution with 70% alcohol until a port wine working solution is obtained. The exact concentration is not critical.

III. Quality Control

It is recommended that several smears of material containing parasitic organisms of known staining properties be stained in parallel with each unknown smear. If staining is of poor quality, the smears may have been too thick or poorly fixed, or residual $HgCl_2$ may not have been removed owing to use of an alcohol–iodine mixture that was too weak. Cloudy preparations may result if dehydration is incomplete owing to failure to change alcohol solutions that may have become contaminated with water. Staining quality can be improved by draining slides between transfers from one reagent to another.

IV. Procedure

A. Preparation of Material
 1. With a small portion of the fresh stool specimen, prepare two smears on the microscope slides using sticks or a brush. The material should be spread thin enough that newsprint can be read through the smear.
 2. Immerse the smears immediately in Schaudinn's fixative solution and allow to fix for a minimum of 30 minutes. Overnight fixation is preferred.
 3. If the specimen is liquid, mix several drops of fecal material with 3 or 4 drops of PVA on a slide and let dry for several hours in a 37°C incubator.
 4. If the specimen is in PVA, pour some of the mixture onto a paper towel to absorb out the PVA. Prepare slides of the material from the paper towels as described. Let dry for several hours in a 37°C incubator.

B. Staining Technique
 1. After smears have properly fixed and dried, place the slides in 70% ethyl alcohol and leave for 5 minutes.
 2. Place in alcohol–iodine working solution for 2 to 5 minutes.
 3. Wash with two changes of 70% alcohol, one for 5 minutes and one for 2 to 5 minutes.
 4. Place in trichrome stain solution for 10 minutes.
 5. Place in 90% ethyl alcohol, acidified (1% acetic acid) for up to 5 seconds.
 6. Dip once in 100% ethyl alcohol.
 7. Place in two changes of 100% ethyl alcohol for 2 to 5 minutes each.
 8. Remove alcohol with two changes of xylene or tuoluene, 2 to 5 minutes each.
 9. Add mounting medium and overlay with a No. 1 coverslip.
 10. Examine under oil immersion for parasitic forms.

V. Results

A. Interpretation

The cytoplasm of thoroughly fixed and well-stained cysts and trophozoites is blue green, tinged with purple. The nuclear chromatin, chromatoid bodies, and ingested red blood cells appear red or red-purple. Background material is green.

VI. Bibliography

Garcia LS, Ash LR: Diagnostic Parasitology: Clinical Laboratory Manual, 2nd ed. St Louis, CV Mosby, 1979

Pruneda RC, Cartwright GW, Melvin DM: Laboratory diagnosis of parasitic diseases. In Koneman EW, Britt MS (eds): Clinical Microbiology, Lecture 15. Bethesda MD, Health and Education Resources, 1977

CHART 71   TWEEN-80 HYDROLYSIS

I. Principle

Tween-80 is the trade name of the polyethylene derivative of sorbitan monooleate. Some *Mycobacterium* species possess an enzyme that releases oleic acid from the Tween-80. The color change from orange to pink is due to hydrolysis of Tween-80, which modifies the optical rotation of light passing through the substrate.

II. Specimen

Mature colony of the unknown *Mycobacterium* species recovered from clinical material, growth on an LJ slant.

III. Materials
  A. Supplies
     1. Sterile applicator sticks
     2. Screw cap tubes (12 × 100 mm) containing 2.0 mL of deionized water per tube
  B. Media
     1. Lowenstein-Jensen slants (purchased from Remel Laboratories)
  C. Reagents
     1. Tween-80 hydrolysis reagent (purchased from Remel Laboratories)
     2. 2 drops of Difco reagent added to distilled water in screw-capped tubes.
  D. Equipment
     1. Biohazard hood

IV. Quality Control
  A. Positive control: *M. kansasii*, ATCC 12478 incubated for 12 days
  B. Negative control: Stock culture of *M. intracellulare* ATCC 13950
  C. Negative reagent: Uninoculated tube of substrate, incubated for 12 days

V. Procedure
  1. Add 2 drops of Tween reagent to 1 mL of sterile distilled water in screw-cap tubes.
  2. Inoculate a loopful of the organism to be tested.
  3. Incubate at 35°C in the dark with caps tight.
  4. Visually read tubes at 24 hours. If negative, read again at 5 and 10 days. Compare the color of the liquid with that in the control tubes.

VI. Results

A positive result is recorded when the liquid, not the cells, turns from light orange to pink or red. *M. kansasii* usually turns positive within 24 hours. Read again at 3, 5, and 10 to 12 days. Record results and discard positives. Discard all tubes at 12 days.

VII. Procedure Notes

Keep Tween hydrolysis reagent in the dark. Do not store or incubate tubes in the light. The red color of a positive reaction is not due to a pH change, rather to release of neutral red.

VIII. Bibliography

Lutz B: Tween-80 hydrolysis. In Isenberg HD (ed): Clinical Microbiology Procedure Handbook, Mycobacteriology Section. Washington DC, American Society for Microbiology, 1992

Kilburn JO, et al: Preparation of a stable mycobacterial Tween hydrolysis test substrate. App. Microbiol 26:826, 1973

Wayne LG, Doubek JR, Russell RL: Classification and identification of mycobacteria: I Tests employing Tween-80 as substrate. Am Rev Respir Dis 90:588–597, 1964

CHART 72　　Urease: Conventional

I. Principle

Urea is a diamide of carbonic acid with the formula

$$NH_2 - \overset{\displaystyle O}{\overset{\|}{C}} - NH_2.$$

All amides are easily hydrolyzed with the release of ammonia and carbon dioxide.

Urease is an enzyme possessed by many species of microorganisms that can hydrolyze urea following the chemical reaction

$$NH_2 - \overset{\displaystyle O}{\overset{\|}{C}} - NH_2 + 2HOH \xrightarrow{\text{Urease}} CO_2 + H_2O + 2NH_3 \rightleftharpoons (NH_4)_2CO_3$$

The ammonia reacts in solution to form ammonium carbonate, resulting in alkalinization and an increase in the pH of the medium.

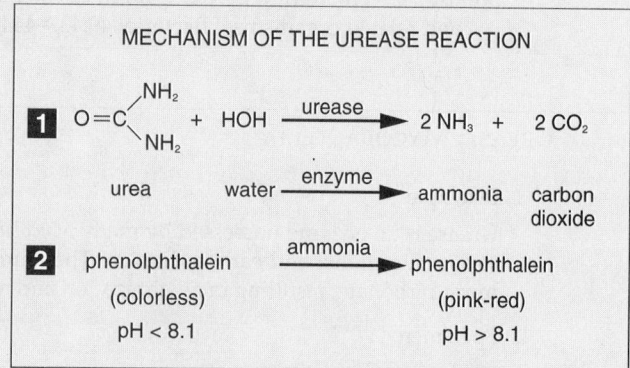

II. Media and Reagents

Stuart's urea broth and Christensen's urea agar are the two media most commonly used in clinical laboratories for the detection of urease activity.

STUART'S UREA BROTH	
Yeast extract	0.1 g
Monopotassium phosphate	9.1 g
Disodium phosphate	9.5 g
Urea	20 g
Phenol red	0.01 g
Distilled water to	1 L

Final pH = 6.8

CHRISTENSEN'S UREA AGAR	
Peptone	1 g
Glucose	1 g
Sodium chloride	5 g
Monopotassium phosphate	2 g
Urea	20 g
Phenol red	0.012 g
Agar	15 g
Distilled water to	1 L

Final pH = 6.8

III. Quality Control

Positively and negatively reacting control organisms should be run with each new batch of medium. The following organisms are suggested:

A. Positive control: *Proteus* species

B. Positive control (weak): *Klebsiella* species

C. Negative control: *Escherichia coli*

IV. Procedure

The broth medium is inoculated with a loopful of a pure culture of the test organism; the surface of the agar slant is streaked with the test organism. Both media are incubated at 35°C for 18 to 24 hours.

V. Results

A. Interpretation

Organisms that hydrolyze urea rapidly may produce positive reactions within 1 or 2 hours; less active species may require 3 or more days. The reactions are as follows:
1. Stuart's broth
   Red color throughout the medium indicates alkalinization and urea hydrolysis
2. Christensen's agar
   Rapid urea splitters (*Proteus* species): red color throughout medium
   Slow urea splitters (*Klebsiella* species): red color initially in slant only, gradually converting the entire tube
3. No urea hydrolysis: medium remains original yellow color (see Color Plate 4–4E).

VI. Bibliography

BBL Manual of Products and Laboratory Procedures, 5th ed, p 154. Cockeysville MD, BioQuest, 1968

Christensen WB: Urea decomposition as a means of differentiating *Proteus* and paracolon cultures from each other and from *Salmonella* and *Shigella* types. J Bacteriol 52: 461–466, 1946

MacFaddin JF: Biochemical Tests for Identification of Medical Bacteria, 2nd ed, pp 298–308. Baltimore, Williams & Wilkins, 1980

Stuart CA, Van Stratum E, Rustigian R: Further studies on urease production by *Proteus* and related organisms. J Bacteriol 49:437–444, 1945

CHART 73   UREASE: MYCOBACTERIA

I. Principle

Urease is an enzyme possessed by many *Mycobacterium* species that can hydrolyze urea to form ammonia and carbon dioxide. The ammonia reacts in solution to form ammonium carbonate, resulting in alkalinization and an increase in the pH of the medium.

II. Specimen

A. Type of Specimen

Mature colony of the unknown *Mycobacterium* species recovered from clinical material, grown on an LJ slant.

III. Materials

A. Equipment
1. Biologic safety hood
2. 37°C incubator

B. Medium
1. Urea broth
   a. Add 10 g of Difco Bacto urea agar base concentrate to 90 mL of sterile deionized water. Mix well to dissolve.
   b. Aseptically aliquot 3.0 mL portions into sterile screw-cap test tubes.
   c. Store at 2° to 8°C; shelf life is 1 month.

IV. Quality Control

A. Positive control: *M. kansasii* ATCC 12478

B. Negative control: *M. avium/intracellulare* ATCC 13950

V. Procedure
1. Inoculate each substrate tube with a spadeful of growth from an actively growing culture. Thoroughly emulsify the culture in the broth.
2. Incubate at 35°C for 5 days.
3. Visually read the tubes at 1, 3, and 7 days.

VI. Results

Color change from yellow to dark pink or red indicates a positive reaction. No color change is a negative reaction.

VII. Procedure Notes

Repeat tests that appear slightly pink; if the repeat test result is still ±, report as negative.

VIII. Limitation of Procedure
1. False-positive tests are usually due to incorrect interpretation of results, incubation beyond 5 days, or contaminated test or control cultures.
2. False-negative results are due to the use of an incorrect medium (i.e., one used for testing bacteria other than acid-fast bacilli), insufficient inoculum, or cultures that are too old.

IX. Bibliography

Kent PT, Kubica GP: Public Health Mycobacteriology: A Guide for the Level III Laboratory. US Department of Health and Human Services, publication (CDC) 86-21654-6, Atlanta, Centers for Disease Control, 1985

Lutz B: Identification tests for mycobacteria: Urease. In Isenberg HD (ed): Clinical Microbiology Procedure Handbook. Washington DC, American Society for Microbiology, 1992

Murphy DB, Hawkins JE: Use of urease disks in the identification of mycobacteria. J Clin Microbiol 1:465–468, 1975

CHART 74   VENEREAL DISEASE RESEARCH LABORATORY (VDRL) SLIDE TEST ON SERUM

I. Principle

The VDRL slide test is the reference nontreponemal antibody test for syphilis. It is the only generally recognized test for diagnosing neurosyphilis.

The VDRL is a nontreponemal microflocculation test. It uses an antigen that contains cardiolipin, lecithin, and cholesterol. The antigen forms microscopic clumps when mixed with antibodies to cardiolipin complex.

II. Equipment and Reagents

A. Equipment
1. Nondisposable needles without a bevel
   a. Serum test: 18 gauge
2. Bottles: 30-mL, round, narrow-mouthed, 35 mm in diameter, with glass stoppers and *flat inner-bottom surface* (Corning Glass Works, Corning NY, cat. no. LG-1 MW-90530).
3. Safety pipetting device with disposable tip to deliver 50 μL.
4. Pipettes, serologic, graduated to tip:
   a. 1.0 mL, graduated in 1/100 mL
   b. 5.0 mL, graduated in 1/10 mL
   c. 10.0 mL, graduated in 1/10 mL
5. Slides
   a. Serum test: 2 $\times$ 3 in., with 12 paraffin or ceramic rings approximately 14 mm in diameter (rings must be high enough to prevent spillage during rotation).
   b. 12 concavities measuring 16 mm in diameter and 1.75 mm in depth.
6. Slide holder for 2 $\times$ 3-in. slides.
7. Ringmaker to make paraffin rings if ceramic rings not used.
8. Mechanical rotator adjustable to 180$\pm$2 rpm, circumscribing a circle 19 mm in diameter on a horizontal plane.
9. Discard containers or disinfectants, disposable latex gloves.
10. Humidifying covers (in dry climates).

B. Reagents
1. VDRL antigen: Store in the dark at room temperature or in refrigerator. Discard vials that contain a precipitate.
2. VDRL-buffered saline, pH 6.0 $\pm$ 0.1 (1.0% NaCl) (purchased or prepared).
3. Control serum samples: Reactive (R), weakly reactive (W), nonreactive (N).
4. 0.9% saline.
5. 10.0% saline.

III. Procedures for Serum Tests

A. Preparing the Antigen Suspension
1. Prepare a fresh VDRL antigen suspension each day. The temperature of all reagents should be at 23° to 29°C.
2. Pipette 0.4 mL of VDRL-buffered saline to the bottom of a round, 30-mL, glass-stoppered bottle with a flat inner surface.
3. Add 0.5 mL VDRL antigen directly into the saline while continuously but gently rotating the bottle on a flat surface. Add antigen drop by drop at a rate allowing approximately 6 seconds for each 0.5 mL of antigen. Keep the pipette tip in the upper third of the bottle and do not splash saline onto the pipette tip. The proper speed of rotation is obtained when the center of the bottle circumscribes a 2-in. in diameter circle approximately three times per second.
4. Expel the last drop of antigen from the pipette without touching the pipette to the saline. Continue rotation of the bottle for 10 seconds.
5. Add 4.1 mL buffered saline from a 5-mL pipette.
6. Cap the bottle and shake it from bottom to top and back approximately 30 times in 10 seconds. The antigen suspension must be used within 8 hours.
7. Mix the suspension by gently swirling it each time it is used. Do not mix it by forcing it back and forth through the syringe and needle.

B. Testing Accuracy of Antigen Suspension Needle
1. The accuracy of the test depends on the amount of antigen dispensed. Check the calibrated needle periodically for accuracy.

2. For the qualitative and quantitative tests on serum, dispense the antigen suspension from a syringe fitted with an 18-gauge needle without a bevel, which will deliver 60±2 drops of antigen suspension per millileter (17 μL/drop) when held vertically.

3. Place the needle on a 2-mL syringe or on a 1-mL pipette and fill the syringe or pipette with VDRL antigen suspension. Holding the syringe or pipette vertically, count the number of drops delivered in 0.5 mL. The needle is correctly calibrated if 30 drops ± 1 drop are delivered in 0.5 mL.

   Adjust or replace the needle if it does not meet the specifications.

C. Testing and Storing the VDRL Antigen Suspension

1. Prepare a fresh antigen suspension each day. Store the suspension at room temperature, 23° to 29°C.

2. Test the antigen suspension with control sera that are reactive, weakly reactive, and nonreactive.

3. Use only suspensions that reproduce the established reactivity pattern of the controls.

4. After completing the day's tests, discard the antigen suspension and clean the dispensing needle and syringe by rinsing with water, alcohol, and acetone, in that order. Remove the needle from the syringe after cleaning.

D. Preparing and Storing Specimens

1. Observe recommended safety precautions for handling human sera.

2. Centrifuge clotted blood at room temperature at 1500 to 2000 rpm for 5 minutes to sediment the cellular elements.

3. Transfer the serum to a clean, dry test tube and heat it in a 56°C water bath for 30 minutes.

4. Recentrifuge any specimen that contains debris after heat inactivation.

5. Reheat the serum at 56°C for 10 minutes if testing is delayed more than 4 hours.

6. Specimens must be at room temperature (23° to 29°C) at the time of testing.

E. Performing the Qualitative Test on Serum

1. With all reagents at room temperature, place 50 μL of serum into one ring of a paraffin- or ceramic-ringed slide, using a safety pipetting device. Do not use glass slides with concavities, wells, or glass rings.

2. Gently resuspend the VDRL antigen suspension.

3. Holding the VDRL antigen suspension dispensing needle and syringe in a vertical position, dispense several drops to clear the needle of air. Then add exactly 1 free-falling drop (17 μL) of antigen suspension to each circle that contains serum.

4. Place the slide on a mechanical rotator. Rotate for 4 minutes at 180 ± 2 rpm. In a dry climate, cover the slide with a moist humidifying cover during rotation.

5. Immediately after the completion of rotation, remove the slide from the rotator and read the test results microscopically, using a 10× ocular and a 10× objective.

6. Report the results as follows:

Reading	Report
Medium or large clumps	Reactive (R)
Small clumps	Weakly Reactive (W)
No clumping or slight roughness	Nonreactive (N)

7. Test quantitatively to an endpoint all serum specimens that produce reactive, weakly reactive, or "rough" nonreactive results in the qualitative test.

F. Performing the Quantitative Test in Serum

1. Quantitate the serum samples to an endpoint titer. Quantitative tests through the 1:8 dilution for three serum specimens may be performed on one slide.

2. Place 50 μL of 0.9% saline in circles numbered 2 through 4, but do not spread the saline.

3. Using a safety pipetting device, place 50 μL of serum in both circle 1 and circle 2.

4. Mix the saline and the serum in circle 2 by drawing the mixture up and down in the safety pipette eight times. Avoid formation of bubbles.

5. Transfer 50 μL from circle 2 (1:2) to circle 3 and mix.

6. Transfer 50 μL from circle 3 to circle 4 and mix. Discard the last 50 μL.

7. Gently resuspend the VDRL antigen suspension.

8. Holding the VDRL antigen suspension-dispensing needle and syringe in a vertical position, dispense several drops to clear the needle of air. Then add exactly 1 free-falling drop (17 μL) of antigen suspension to each circle.

9. Place the slide on the mechanical rotator. Rotate the slide for 4 minutes at 180 ± 2 rpm. Add a humidifying cover in dry environments.

10. Immediately after rotation, read the test microscopically using a 10× ocular and a 10× objective.

11. If the highest dilution tested (1:8) is reactive proceed as follows:

    a. Prepare a 1:8 dilution of the test specimen. Add 0.1 mL serum to 0.7 mL of 0.9% saline and mix thoroughly.

    b. Place 50 μL of 0.9% saline into the second, third, and fourth paraffin rings in a row on the slide. Prepare additional serial dilutions for strongly reactive specimens.

    c. Add 50 μL of the 1:8 dilution of the test specimen to paraffin rings 1 and 2.

12. Report titers in terms of the highest dilution that produces a reactive (not a weakly reactive) result:

Serum Dilutions						Report
Undiluted	1:2	1:4	1:8	1:16	1:32	
R	W	N	N	N	N	Reactive, undiluted, 1 dil.
R	R	W	N	N	N	Reactive, 1:2 dilution, 2 dils
R	R	R	W	N	N	Reactive, 1:4 dilution, 4 dils
W	W	R	R	W	N	Reactive, 1:8 dilution, 8 dils
N (Rough)	W	R	R	R	N	Reactive, 1:16 dilution, 16 dils
W	N	N	N	N	N	Weakly Reactive, undiluted, 0 dil

IV. Results

A. Interpretation

1. The VDRL test is an aid in the diagnosis of syphilis. A positive test may indicate a past or present infection. False-positive results occur because of laboratory error, infection with other treponemes, or the presence of antibodies unrelated to treponemal infection. The predictive value of a positive VDRL result is increased when combined with a reactive treponemal test, such as the fluorescent treponemal antibody absorption test (see Chart 32) or the microhemagglutination test.

2. A nonreactive result may indicate no infection, adequately treated infection, or infection in the remote past. A nonreactive result may be obtained in incubating or early primary syphilis. Prozone phenomena occur, especially with high titers in secondary syphilis. Sera should be diluted if a rough result is obtained or if clinical information indicates the likelihood of syphilis.

3. A fourfold increase in titer may indicate a reinfection or treatment failure. A fourfold decrease in titer in early syphilis usually indicates adequate therapy.

4. All sera should be titered to the endpoint. Unusually high titers may be seen in some patients who are concurrently infected with human immunodeficiency virus, type 1. Unusually high false-positive titers may be seen in some patients with lymphomas.

V. Sources of Error

1. Reactivity is decreased if the specimen, testing area, or reagents are at temperatures lower than 23°C. Reactivity is increased if any of these are at temperatures higher than 29°C.

2. Test results are unpredictable if hemolyzed, contaminated, or extremely turbid sera are tested.

3. Reactivity will be unpredictable if reagents are outdated, inadequately tested, or if procedures are not followed strictly. Forcing the VDRL antigen through the needle and syringe repetitively will cause the suspension to lose reactivity.

VI. Test Limitations

1. The prozone phenomenon described in the foregoing may produce false-negative results on high-titered sera.

2. The VDRL antigen suspension must be prepared daily.

3. The VDRL-CSF test should be performed only if the serum test is reactive.

4. Plasma cannot be used for the VDRL test.

5. Biologic false-positive results occur with cardiolipin antigens, especially in specimens from persons who abuse drugs; who have diseases such as lupus erythematosus, mononucleosis, malaria, leprosy, or viral pneumonia; or who have recently been immunized.

6. Note: The VDRL slide test on CSF is similar to the serum test, but there are important methodologic differences (see bibliography). Only reactive and nonreactive results are reported on CSF.

VII. Bibliography

Larson SA, Hunter EF, Karus SJ (eds): Manual of Tests for Syphilis, 8th ed. Washington DC, American Public Health Association, 1990

CHART 75   VOGES–PROSKAUER TEST

I. Principle

Voges–Proskauer is a double eponym, named after two microbiologists working at the beginning of the 20th century. They first observed the red color reaction produced by appropriate culture media after treatment with potassium hydroxide. It was later discovered that the active product in the medium formed by bacterial metabolism is acetyl methyl carbinol, a product of the butylene glycol pathway.

Pyruvic acid, the pivotal compound formed in the fermentative degradation of glucose, is further metabolized through various metabolic pathways, depending on the enzyme systems possessed by different bacteria. One such pathway results in the production of acetoin (acetyl methyl carbinol), a neutral-reacting end product. Organisms such as members of the *Klebsiella–Enterobacter–Hafnia–Serratia* group produce acetoin as the chief end product of glucose metabolism and form smaller quantities of mixed acids. In the presence of atmospheric oxygen and 40% potassium hydroxide, acetoin is converted to diacetyl, and α-naphthol serves as a catalyst to bring out a red complex.

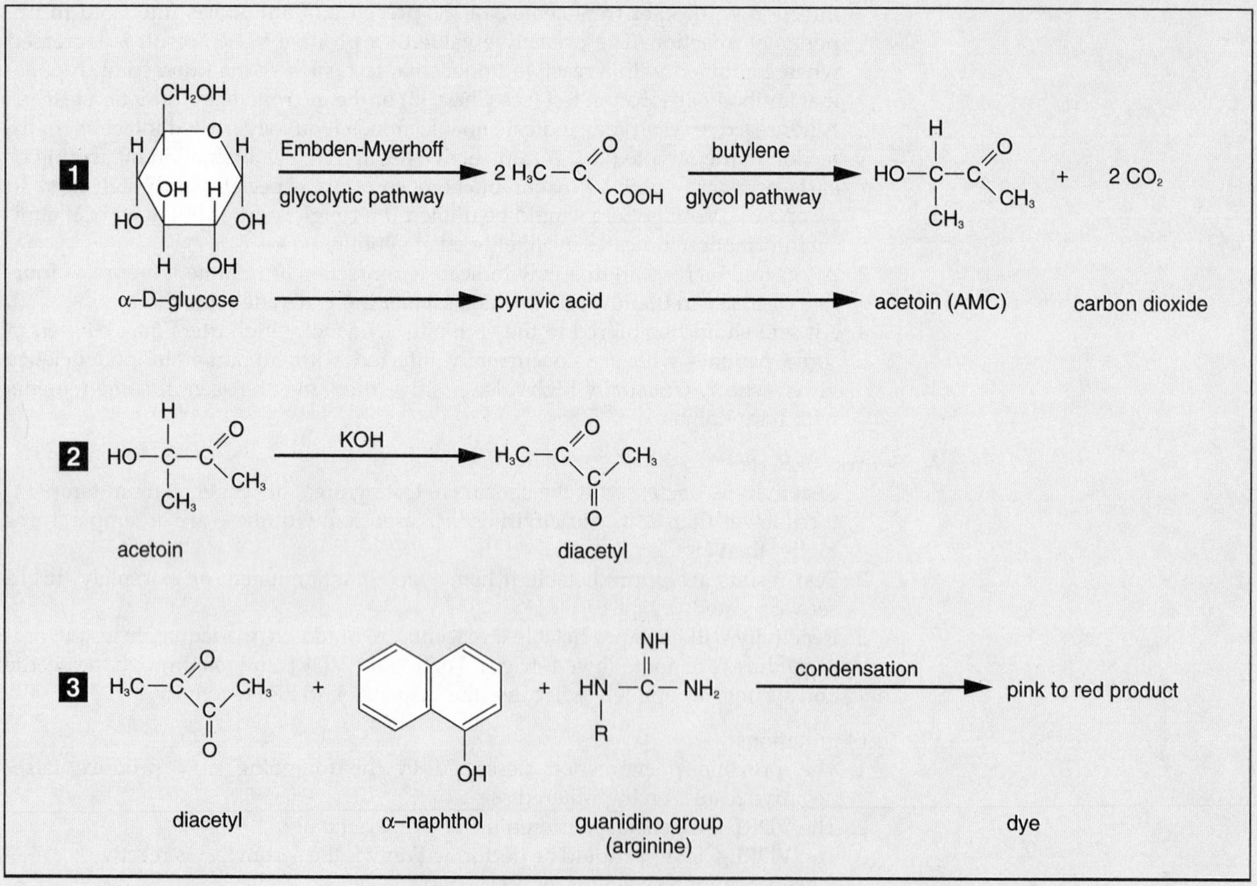

II. Media and Reagents

A. Media

1. The medium is the MR/VP broth described in Chart 48.

B. Reagents
   1. α-Naphthol, 5% color intensifier

α-Naphthol	5 g
Absolute ethyl alcohol	100 mL

   2. Potassium hydroxide, 40%, oxidizing agent

Potassium hydroxide	40 g
Distilled water to	100 mL

III Quality Control

Positive and negative controls should be run after preparation of each lot of medium and after making each batch of reagent. Suggested controls include the following:

A. Positive Control: *Enterobacter aerogenes*

B. Negative Control: *Escherichia coli*

IV. Procedure

Inoculate a tube of MR/VP broth with a pure culture of the test organism. Incubate for 24 hours at 35°C. At the end of this time, aliquot 1 mL of broth to a clean test tube. Add 0.6 mL of 5% α-naphthol, followed by 0.2 mL of 40% KOH. It is essential that the reagents be added in this order. Shake the tube gently to expose the medium to atmospheric oxygen and allow the tube to remain undisturbed for 10 to 15 minutes.

V. Results

A. Interpretation

A positive test is represented by the development of a red color 15 minutes or more after addition of the reagents, indicating the presence of diacetyl, the oxidation product of acetoin (see Color Plate 4–4D). The test should not be read after standing for over 1 hour because negative Voges-Proskauer cultures may produce a copper-like color, potentially resulting in a false-positive interpretation.

VI. Bibliography

Barritt MM: The intensification of the Voges–Proskauer reaction by the addition of α-naphthol. J Pathol Bacteriol 42:441–454, 1936

Barry AL, Feeney KL: Two quick methods for Voges–Proskauer test. Appl Microbiol 15:1138–1141, 1967

Blazevic DJ, Ederer GM: Principles of Biochemical Tests in Diagnostic Microbiology, pp 105–107. New York, John Wiley & Sons, 1975

MacFaddin JF: Biochemical Tests for Identification of Medical Bacteria, 2nd ed, pp 308–320. Baltimore, Williams & Wilkins, 1980

Voges O, Proskauer B: Beitrag zue Ernährungsphysiologie und zur Differential-diagnose der Bakterien der hämorrhagischen Septicamia. Z. Hyg 28:20–32, 1898

INDEX